Alvarez

OBSTETRICS
Normal and Problem Pregnancies

OBSTETRICS
Normal and Problem Pregnancies

Steven G. Gabbe, MD
Emeritus Chief Executive Officer
The Ohio State University Wexner Medical Center
Professor of Obstetrics and Gynecology
The Ohio State University College of Medicine
Columbus, Ohio

Jennifer R. Niebyl, MD
Professor
Department of Obstetrics and Gynecology
University of Iowa Hospitals and Clinics
Iowa City, Iowa

Joe Leigh Simpson, MD
Senior Vice President for Research and Global Programs
March of Dimes Foundation
White Plains, New York;
Professor of Obstetrics and Gynecology
Professor of Human and Molecular Genetics
Herbert Wertheim College of Medicine
Florida International University
Miami, Florida

Mark B. Landon, MD
Richard L. Meiling Professor and Chair
Department of Obstetrics and Gynecology
The Ohio State University College of Medicine
Columbus, Ohio

Henry L. Galan, MD
Professor
Department of Obstetrics and Gynecology
University of Colorado School of Medicine;
Co-Director
Colorado Fetal Care Center
Colorado Institute for Maternal and Fetal Health
Aurora, Colorado

Eric R.M. Jauniaux, MD, PhD
Professor of Obstetrics and Fetal Medicine
Institute for Women's Health
University College London
London, United Kingdom

Deborah A. Driscoll, MD
Luigi Mastroianni Professor and Chair
Department of Obstetrics and Gynecology
Perelman School of Medicine at the University
 of Pennsylvania
Philadelphia, Pennsylvania

Vincenzo Berghella, MD
Professor
Department of Obstetrics and Gynecology
Director
Maternal-Fetal Medicine
Jefferson Medical College of Thomas Jefferson
 University
Philadelphia, Pennsylvania

William A. Grobman, MD, MBA
Arthur Hale Curtis Professor
Department of Obstetrics and Gynecology
The Center for Healthcare Studies
Feinberg School of Medicine
Northwestern University
Chicago, Illinois

SEVENTH 7 EDITION

ELSEVIER

ELSEVIER

1600 John F. Kennedy Blvd.
Ste 1800
Philadelphia, PA 19103-2899

OBSTETRICS: NORMAL AND PROBLEM PREGNANCIES,
SEVENTH EDITION

ISBN: 978-0-323-32108-2

Previous editions copyrighted © 2012 by Saunders, an imprint of Elsevier, Inc. and © 2007, 2002, 1996, 1991, and 1986 by Churchill Livingstone, an imprint of Elsevier, Inc.

Library of Congress Cataloging-in-Publication Data

Names: Gabbe, Steven G., editor.
Title: Obstetrics : normal and problem pregnancies / [edited by] Steven G. Gabbe [and 8 others].
Other titles: Obstetrics (Gabbe)
Description: Seventh edition. | Philadelphia, PA : Elsevier, [2017] | Includes bibliographical references and index.
Identifiers: LCCN 2016006912 | ISBN 9780323321082 (hardcover)
Subjects: | MESH: Pregnancy | Obstetrics–methods | Pregnancy Complications
Classification: LCC RG524 | NLM WQ 200.1 | DDC 618.2–dc23 LC record available at
    http://lccn.loc.gov/2016006912

Executive Content Strategist: Kate Dimock
Content Development Manager: Lucia Gunzel
Publishing Services Manager: Patricia Tannian
Senior Project Manager: Carrie Stetz
Design Direction: Renee Duenow

Printed in China

Last digit is the print number: 9 8 7 6 5 4 3 2 1

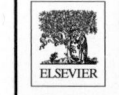

Three of us met on the obstetrics service at The New York Hospital and Cornell University Medical College in 1968. Two of us (J.R.N. and J.L.S.) were residents, and one (S.G.G.) was a medical student. We became friends, and, as our careers moved ahead, we continued to see each other at national meetings. About 35 years ago, at one of these conferences, we were approached by Lynne Herndon, then with Churchill Livingstone, and asked if we would like to collaborate on a new obstetrics book. We were honored to be asked.

We believed a new book was needed and thought that our different areas of interest would complement each other. We decided to prepare a multiple-author textbook, inviting our friends and colleagues to join us. The book was targeted to residents and fellows in training. Of course, we were all in different cities, and this was before the internet, word processors, or fax, so preparing a book like this was a challenge. Yes, it was much more work than we imagined, but it was exciting to read each new chapter and watch the book come together. We were then, and we remain today, extremely thankful to our authors for their outstanding state-of-the-art contributions. Although it has been challenging to keep up with the rapid advances in our field, our authors, including many who have written chapters in every edition, made sure we did.

The first edition of the book was very well received. We were honored by this response and so pleased that the publisher encouraged us to do a second edition, and we accepted. Then a third, a fourth, a fifth, and a sixth followed in the next three decades. Over the years, we invited an outstanding group of editors to join us, and we have had great support from our publishers, now Elsevier.

This seventh edition is the last we will edit. Although we all continue to see patients and teach, we believe the time has come to pass the baton to our colleagues, Dr. Landon, Dr. Galan, Dr. Jauniaux, Dr. Driscoll, Dr. Berghella, and Dr. Grobman. Because *Obstetrics: Normal and Problem Pregnancies* has been the single most important contribution of our professional careers, we are honored they have decided to dedicate this edition to us. We thank them very much, and we thank you, our readers, for your loyalty and support over the years.

Steven G. Gabbe, MD
Jennifer R. Niebyl, MD
Joe Leigh Simpson, MD

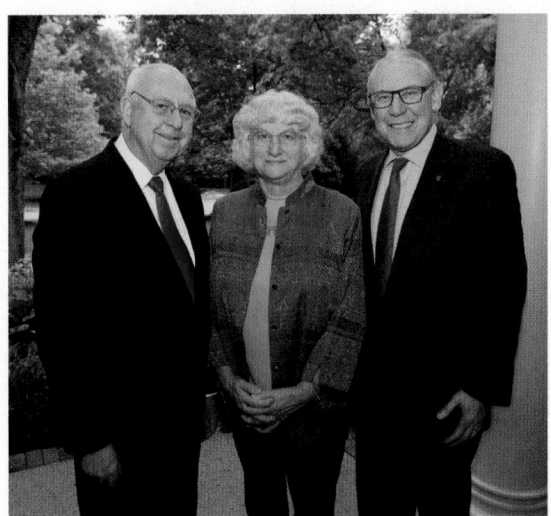

Joe Leigh Simpson, Jennifer R. Niebyl, and Steven G. Gabbe
(photograph courtesy Kevin Fitzsimons)

Contributors

Kjersti Aagaard, MD, PhD, MSCI
Associate Professor
Department of Obstetrics and Gynecology
Baylor College of Medicine
Houston, Texas

Kristina M. Adams Waldorf, MD
Associate Professor
Department of Obstetrics and Gynecology
University of Washington
Seattle, Washington

Margaret Altemus, MD
Associate Professor
Department of Psychiatry
Yale University School of Medicine
New Haven, Connecticut

George J. Annas, JD, MPH
Professor and Chair
Department of Health Law, Bioethics & Human Rights
Boston University School of Public Health
Boston, Massachusetts

Kathleen M. Antony, MD, MSCI
Department of Obstetrics and Gynecology
University of Wisconsin School of Medicine and Public
  Health
Madison, Wisconsin

Jennifer L. Bailit, MD, MPH
Clinical Director
Family Care Service Line
Metrohealth Medical Center
Cleveland, Ohio

Ahmet Alexander Baschat, MD
Director
Johns Hopkins Center for Fetal Therapy
Department of Gynecology and Obstetrics
Johns Hopkins Hospital
Baltimore, Maryland

Vincenzo Berghella, MD
Professor
Department of Obstetrics and Gynecology
Director
Maternal-Fetal Medicine
Jefferson Medical College of Thomas Jefferson University
Philadelphia, Pennsylvania

Helene B. Bernstein, MD, PhD
Director, Division of Maternal-Fetal Medicine
Departments of Obstetrics and Gynecology, Microbiology, and
  Immunology
SUNY Upstate Medical University
Syracuse, New York

Amar Bhide, MD
Consultant in Fetal Medicine
Fetal Medicine Unit
St. George's Hospital
London, United Kingdom

Meredith Birsner, MD
Assistant Professor
Department of Maternal-Fetal Medicine
Thomas Jefferson University
Philadelphia, Pennsylvania

Debra L. Bogen, MD
Associate Professor of Pediatrics
Department of Psychiatry and Clinical and Translational
  Sciences
University of Pittsburgh School of Medicine
Division of General Academic Pediatrics
Children's Hospital of Pittsburgh of UPMC
Pittsburgh, Pennsylvania

D. Ware Branch, MD
Professor
Department of Obstetrics and Gynecology
University of Utah School of Medicine
Salt Lake City, Utah

Gerald G. Briggs, AB, BPharm
Clinical Professor of Pharmacy
University of California–San Francisco
San Francisco, California;
Adjunct Professor of Pharmacy Practice
University of Southern California–Los Angeles
Los Angeles, California;
Adjunct Professor
Department of Pharmacotherapy
Washington State University
Spokane, Washington

Haywood L. Brown, MD
Professor and Chair
Department of Obstetrics and Gynecology
Duke University
Durham, North Carolina

Brenda A. Bucklin, MD
Professor of Anesthesiology and Assistant Dean
Clinical Core Curriculum
Department of Anesthesiology
University of Colorado School of Medicine
Denver, Colorado

Graham J. Burton, MD, DSc
Centre for Trophoblast Research
Physiology, Development and Neuroscience
University of Cambridge
Cambridge, United Kingdom

Mitchell S. Cappell, MD, PhD
Chief
Division of Gastroenterology and Hepatology
William Beaumont Hospital;
Professor of Medicine
Oakland University William Beaumont School of Medicine
Royal Oak, Michigan

Jeanette R. Carpenter, MD
Department of Maternal-Fetal Medicine
Obstetric Medical Group of the Mountain States
Salt Lake City, Utah

Patrick M. Catalano, MD
Dierker-Biscotti Women's Health and Wellness Professor
Director, Center for Reproductive Health at MetroHealth
Director, Clinical Research Unit of the Case Western Reserve
    University CTSC at MetroHealth
Professor of Reproductive Biology
MetroHealth Medical Center/Case Western Reserve University
Cleveland, Ohio

Suchitra Chandrasekaran, MD, MSCE
Assistant Professor
Department of Obstetrics and Gynecology
University of Washington
Seattle, Washington

David F. Colombo, MD
Department of Obstetrics, Gynecology, and Reproductive
    Biology
Spectrum Health
College of Human Medicine
Michigan State University
Grand Rapids, Michigan

Larry J. Copeland, MD
Professor
Department of Obstetrics and Gynecology
The Ohio State University
Columbus, Ohio

Jason Deen, MD
Assistant Professor of Pediatrics
Adjunct Assistant Professor of Medicine
Division of Cardiology
Seattle Children's Hospital
University of Washington Medical Center
Seattle, Washington

COL Shad H. Deering, MD
Chair, Department of Obstetrics and Gynecology
Assistant Dean for Simulation Education
F. Edward Hebert School of Medicine
Uniformed Services University of the Health Sciences
Chair, Army Central Simulation Committee
Bethesda, Maryland

Mina Desai, MSc, PhD
Associate Professor
Department of Obstetrics and Gynecology
David Geffen School of Medicine at Harbor-UCLA Medical
    Center
Los Angeles, California

Gary A. Dildy III, MD
Professor and Vice Chair of Quality and Patient Safety
Director, Division of Maternal-Fetal Medicine
Department of Obstetrics and Gynecology
Baylor College of Medicine;
Chief Quality Officer, Obstetrics and Gynecology
Service Chief, Maternal-Fetal Medicine
Texas Children's Hospital
Houston, Texas

Mitchell P. Dombrowski, MD
Professor and Chief
Department of Obstetrics and Gynecology
St. John Hospital
Detroit, Michigan

Deborah A. Driscoll, MD
Luigi Mastroianni Professor and Chair
Department of Obstetrics and Gynecology
Perelman School of Medicine at the University of Pennsylvania
Philadelphia, Pennsylvania

Maurice L. Druzin, MD
Professor and Vice Chair
Department of Obstetrics and Gynecology
Stanford University School of Medicine
Stanford, California

Patrick Duff, MD
Professor
Associate Dean for Student Affairs
Department of Obstetrics and Gynecology
University of Florida
Gainesville, Florida

Thomas Easterling, MD
Professor
Department of Obstetrics and Gynecology
University of Washington
Seattle, Washington

Sherman Elias, MD[†]
John J. Sciarra Professor and Chair
Department of Obstetrics and Gynecology
Feinberg School of Medicine
Northwestern University
Chicago, Illinois

M. Gore Ervin, PhD
Professor of Biology
Middle Tennessee State University
Murfreesboro, Tennessee

Michael R. Foley, MD
Chairman
Department of Obstetrics and Gynecology
Banner University Medical Center
Professor
University of Arizona College of Medicine
Phoenix, Arizona

Karrie E. Francois, MD
Perinatal Medical Director
Obstetrics and Gynecology
HonorHealth
Scottsdale, Arizona

Steven G. Gabbe, MD
Emeritus Chief Executive Officer
The Ohio State University Wexner Medical Center
Professor of Obstetrics and Gynecology
The Ohio State University College of Medicine
Columbus, Ohio

Henry L. Galan, MD
Professor
Department of Obstetrics and Gynecology
University of Colorado School of Medicine;
Co-Director
Colorado Fetal Care Center
Colorado Institute for Maternal and Fetal Health
Aurora, Colorado

Etoi Garrison, MD, PhD
Associate Professor, Division of Maternal-Fetal Medicine
Department of Obstetrics and Gynecology
Vanderbilt Medical Center
Nashville, Tennessee

Elizabeth E. Gerard, MD
Associate Professor
Department of Neurology
Northwestern University
Chicago, Illinois

Robert Gherman, MD
Associate Director
Prenatal Diagnostic Center and Antepartum Testing Unit
Division of Maternal-Fetal Medicine
Franklin Square Medical Center
Baltimore, Maryland

William M. Gilbert, MD
Regional Medical Director
Women's Services
Department of Obstetrics and Gynecology
Sutter Medical Center Sacramento;
Clinical Professor
Department of Obstetrics and Gynecology
University of California–Davis
Sacramento, California

Laura Goetzl, MD, MPH
Professor and Vice Chair
Department of Obstetrics and Gynecology
Temple University
Philadelphia, Pennsylvania

Bernard Gonik, MD
Professor and Fann Srere Endowed Chair of Perinatal Medicine
Department of Obstetrics and Gynecology
Division of Maternal-Fetal Medicine
Wayne State University School of Medicine
Detroit, Michigan

Mara B. Greenberg, MD
Director of Inpatient Perinatology
Obstetrics and Gynecology
Kaiser Permanente Northern California
Oakland Medical Center
Oakland, California

Kimberly D. Gregory, MD, MPH
Vice Chair
Women's Healthcare Quality & Performance Improvement
Department of Obstetrics and Gynecology
Cedars Sinai Medical Center
Los Angeles, California

William A. Grobman, MD, MBA
Arthur Hale Curtis Professor
Department of Obstetrics and Gynecology
The Center for Healthcare Studies
Feinberg School of Medicine
Northwestern University
Chicago, Illinois

Lisa Hark, PhD, RD
Director
Department of Research
Wills Eye Hospital
Philadelphia, Pennsylvania

Joy L. Hawkins, MD
Professor
Department of Anesthesiology
University of Colorado School of Medicine
Aurora, Colorado

†Deceased.

Wolfgang Holzgreve, MD, MBA
Professor of Obstetrics and Gynaecology
Medical Director and CEO
University Hospital Bonn
Bonn, Germany

Jay D. Iams, MD
OB Lead
Ohio Perinatal Quality Collaborative
Emeritus Professor of Obstetrics and Gynecology
The Ohio State University
Columbus, Ohio

Michelle M. Isley, MD, MPH
Assistant Professor
Department of Obstetrics and Gynecology
The Ohio State University
Columbus, Ohio

Eric R.M. Jauniaux, MD, PhD
Professor of Obstetrics and Fetal Medicine
Institute for Women's Health
University College London
London, United Kingdom

Vern L. Katz, MD
Clinical Professor
Department of Obstetrics and Gynecology
Oregon Health Science University
Eugene, Oregon

Sarah Kilpatrick, MD, PhD
Head and Vice Dean
Department of Obstetrics and Gynecology
Director
Division of Maternal-Fetal Medicine
University of Minnesota
Minneapolis, Minnesota

George Kroumpouzos, MD, PhD
Clinical Associate Professor
Department of Dermatology
Alpert Medical School of Brown University
Providence, Rhode Island

Daniel V. Landers, MD
Professor and Vice Chair
Department of Obstetrics, Gynecology, and Women's Health
University of Minnesota
Minneapolis, Minnesota

Mark B. Landon, MD
Richard L. Meiling Professor and Chair
Department of Obstetrics and Gynecology
The Ohio State University College of Medicine
Columbus, Ohio

Susan M. Lanni, MD
Associate Professor of OBGYN and Maternal-Fetal Medicine
Director, Labor and Delivery
Virginia Commonwealth University
Richmond, Virginia

Gwyneth Lewis, OBE, MBBS, DSc, MPH
Leader
International Women's Health Research
Institute for Women's Health
University College London
London, United Kingdom

Charles J. Lockwood, MD, MHCM
Dean, Morsani College of Medicine
Senior Vice President
USF Health
Professor of Obstetrics & Gynecology and Public Health
University of South Florida
Tampa, Florida

Jack Ludmir, MD
Professor
Department of Obstetrics and Gynecology
Perelman School of Medicine at the University of Pennsylvania
Philadelphia, Pennsylvania

A. Dhanya Mackeen, MD, MPH
Clinical Assistant Professor
Temple University School of Medicine
Department of Obstetrics, Gynecology, and Reproductive
  Services
Director of Research
Division of Maternal-Fetal Medicine
Geisinger Health System
Danville, Pennsylvania

George A. Macones, MD, MSCE
Professor and Chair
Department of Obstetrics and Gynecology
Washington University in St. Louis School of Medicine
St. Louis, Missouri

Brian M. Mercer, MD
Professor and Chairman
Department of Reproductive Biology
Case Western Reserve University–MetroHealth Campus
Chairman, Department of Obstetrics and Gynecology
Director, Women's Center
MetroHealth Medical Center
Cleveland, Ohio

Jorge H. Mestman, MD
Professor
Departments of Medicine and Obstetrics & Gynecology
Keck School of Medicine of the University of Southern
  California
Los Angeles, California

David Arthur Miller, MD
Professor of Obstetrics, Gynecology, and Pediatrics
Keck School of Medicine of the University of Southern
  California
Children's Hospital of Los Angeles
Los Angeles, California

Emily S. Miller, MD, MPH
Assistant Professor
Department of Obstetrics and Gynecology
Division of Maternal-Fetal Medicine
Feinberg School of Medicine
Northwestern University
Chicago, Illinois

Dawn Misra, MHS, PhD
Professor and Associate Chair for Research
Department of Family Medicine & Public Health Sciences
Wayne State University School of Medicine
Detroit, Michigan

Kenneth J. Moise Jr, MD
Professor of Obstetrics, Gynecology, and Reproductive
   Sciences and Pediatric Surgery
Director
Fetal Intervention Fellowship
UTHealth School of Medicine at Houston;
Co-Director
The Fetal Center
Children's Memorial Hermann Hospital
Houston, Texas

Mark E. Molitch, MD
Martha Leland Sherwin Professor of Endocrinology
Division of Endocrinology, Metabolism, and Molecular
   Medicine
Northwestern University Feinberg School of Medicine
Chicago, Illinois

Chelsea Morroni, MBChB, DTM&H, DFSRH, Mphil, MPH, PhD
Clinical Lecturer
EGA Institute for Women's Health and Institute for Global
   Health
University College London
London, United Kingdom;
Senior Researcher
Wits Reproductive Health and HIV Institute (Wits RHI)
University of the Witwatersrand
Johannesburg, South Africa

Roger B. Newman, MD
Professor and Maas Chair for Reproductive Sciences
Department of Obstetrics and Gynecology
Medical University of South Carolina
Charleston, South Carolina

Edward R. Newton, MD
Professor
Department of Obstetrics and Gynecology
Brody School of Medicine
Greenville, North Carolina

Jennifer R. Niebyl, MD
Professor
Department of Obstetrics and Gynecology
University of Iowa Hospitals and Clinics
Iowa City, Iowa

COL Peter E. Nielsen, MD
Commander
General Leonard Wood Army Community Hospital
MFM Division Director
Obstetrics and Gynecology
Fort Leonard Wood, Missouri

Jessica L. Nyholm, MD
Assistant Professor
Department of Obstetrics, Gynecology and Women's Health
University of Minnesota
Minneapolis, Minnesota

Lucas Otaño, MD, PhD
Head, Division of Obstetrics and Fetal Medicine Unit
Department of Obstetrics and Gynecology
Hospital Italiano de Buenos Aires
Buenos Aires, Argentina

John Owen, MD, MSPH
Professor
Department of Obstetrics and Gynecology
Division of Maternal-Fetal Medicine
University of Alabama at Birmingham
Birmingham, Alabama

Teri B. Pearlstein, MD
Associate Professor of Psychiatry and Human Behavior and
   Medicine
Alpert Medical School of Brown University;
Director
Women's Behavioral Medicine
Women's Medicine Collaborative, a Lifespan Partner
Providence, Rhode Island

Christian M. Pettker, MD
Associate Professor
Department of Obstetrics, Gynecology, and Reproductive
   Sciences
Yale University School of Medicine
New Haven, Connecticut

Diana A. Racusin, MD
Maternal Fetal Medicine Fellow
Department of Obstetrics and Gynecology
Baylor College of Medicine
Houston, Texas

Kirk D. Ramin, MD
Professor
Department of Obstetrics, Gynecology, and Women's Health
University of Minnesota
Minneapolis, Minnesota

Diana E. Ramos, MD, MPH
Director
Reproductive Health
Los Angeles County Public Health;
Adjunct Assistant Clinical Professor
Keck University of Southern California School of Medicine
Los Angeles, California

Roxane Rampersad, MD
Associate Professor
Department of Obstetrics and Gynecology
Washington University in St. Louis School of Medicine
St. Louis, Missouri

Leslie Regan, MD, DSc
Chair and Head
Department of Obstetrics and Gynaecology at St. Mary's
    Campus
Imperial College;
Vice President, Royal College of Obstetricians &
    Gynaecologists
Chair, FIGO Women's Sexual & Reproductive Rights
    Committee
Chair, National Confidential Enquiry into Patient Outcome
    and Death
London, United Kingdom

Douglas S. Richards, MD
Clinical Professor
Division of Maternal-Fetal Medicine
Intermountain Medical Center
Murray, Utah;
Clinical Professor
Division of Maternal-Fetal Medicine
University of Utah School of Medicine
Salt Lake City, Utah

Roberto Romero, MD, DMedSci
Chief, Program for Perinatal Research and Obstetrics
Division of Intramural Research
Eunice Kennedy Shriver National Institute of Child Health
    and Human Development
Perinatology Research Branch
National Institutes of Health
Bethesda, Maryland;
Professor, Department of Obstetrics and Gynecology
University of Michigan
Ann Arbor, Michigan;
Professor, Department of Epidemiology and Biostatistics
Michigan State University
East Lansing, Michigan

Adam A. Rosenberg, MD
Professor
Department of Pediatrics
Children's Hospital of Colorado
University of Colorado School of Medicine
Aurora, Colorado

Michael G. Ross, MD, MPH
Distinguished Professor
Department of Obstetrics and Gynecology
David Geffen School of Medicine at Harbor-UCLA Medical
    Center;
Distinguished Professor
Community Health Sciences
Fielding School of Public Health at UCLA
Los Angeles, California

Paul J. Rozance, MD
Associate Professor
Department of Pediatrics
University of Colorado School of Medicine
Aurora, Colorado

Ritu Salani, MD, MBA
Associate Professor
Department of Obstetrics and Gynecology
The Ohio State University
Columbus, Ohio

Philip Samuels, MD
Professor
Residency Program Director
Department of Obstetrics and Gynecology, Maternal-Fetal
    Medicine
The Ohio State University Wexner Medical Center
Columbus, Ohio

Nadav Schwartz, MD
Assistant Professor
Department of Obstetrics and Gynecology
Perelman School of Medicine at the University of Pennsylvania
Philadelphia, Pennsylvania

Lili Sheibani, MD
Peter E. Nielsen, MD, Clinical Instructor
Obstetrics and Gynecology
University of California–Irvine
Orange, California

Baha M. Sibai, MD
Director
Maternal-Fetal Medicine Fellowship Program
Department of Obstetrics, Gynecology and Reproductive
    Sciences
University of Texas Medical School at Houston
Houston, Texas

Colin P. Sibley, PhD, DSc
Professor of Child Health and Physiology
Maternal and Fetal Health Research Centre
University of Manchester
Manchester, United Kingdom

Hyagriv N. Simhan, MD
Professor and Chief
Division of Maternal-Fetal Medicine
Executive Vice Chair
Obstetrical Services Department
University of Pittsburgh School of Medicine;
Medical Director of Obstetric Services
Magee-Women's Hospital of UPMC
Pittsburgh, Pennsylvania

Joe Leigh Simpson, MD
Senior Vice President for Research and Global Programs
March of Dimes Foundation
White Plains, New York;
Professor of Obstetrics and Gynecology
Professor of Human and Molecular Genetics
Herbert Wertheim College of Medicine
Florida International University
Miami, Florida

Dorothy K.Y. Sit, MD
Department of Psychiatry
University of Pittsburgh Medical Center
Pittsburgh, Pennsylvania

Karen Stout, MD
Director
Adult Congenital Heart Disease Program
Department of Internal Medicine
Division of Cardiology
University of Washington;
Professor of Internal Medicine/Pediatrics
Department of Pediatrics
Division of Cardiology
Seattle Children's Hospital
Seattle, Washington

Dace S. Svikis, PhD
Professor
Department of Psychology
Institute for Women's Health
Virginia Commonwealth University
Richmond, Virginia

Elizabeth Ramsey Unal, MD, MSCR
Assistant Professor
Department of Obstetrics and Gynecology
Division of Maternal-Fetal Medicine
Southern Illinois University School of Medicine
Springfield, Illinois

Annie R. Wang, MD
Department of Dermatology
Alpert Medical School of Brown University
Providence, Rhode Island

Robert J. Weber, MS, PharmD
Administrator
Pharmacy Services
Assistant Dean
College of Pharmacy
The Ohio State University Wexner Medical Center
Columbus, Ohio

Elizabeth Horvitz West, MD
Resident Physician
Department of Obstetrics and Gynecology
University of California–Irvine
Irvine, California

Janice E. Whitty, MD
Professor and Director of Maternal-Fetal Medicine
Department of Obstetrics and Gynecology
Meharry Medical College
Nashville, Tennessee

Deborah A. Wing, MD, MBA
Professor
Department of Obstetrics and Gynecology
University of California–Irvine
Orange, California

Katherine L. Wisner, MD
Asher Professor of Psychiatry and Obstetrics and Gynecology
Director
Asher Center for Research and Treatment of Depressive
   Disorders
Department of Psychiatry
Feinberg School of Medicine
Northwestern University
Chicago, Illinois

Jason D. Wright, MD
Sol Goldman Associate Professor
Chief, Division of Gynecologic Oncology
Department of Obstetrics and Gynecology
Columbia University College of Physicians and Surgeons
New York, New York

Preface

The seventh edition of *Obstetrics: Normal and Problem Pregnancies* is being delivered to you prematurely! Do we have your attention? Good. We don't mean the book is incomplete. In fact, this edition may have more new information than any we've done before, which is why it is being published just 4 years since the sixth edition, rather than on our usual 5-year cycle. We want to be sure our readers have access to the best, most advanced resource to guide them as they learn and practice obstetrics today. We were able to accomplish this accelerated process thanks to the hard work of our editors, our contributing authors, and our publisher, Elsevier.

As we have done in the past, we surveyed our readers and leaders in the field to assess content that needed to be added and revised. You will find four new chapters in the seventh edition: "Vaginal Birth After Cesarean Delivery," "Placenta Accreta," "Obesity in Pregnancy," and "Improving Global Maternal Health: Challenges and Opportunities." The first three topics have become more important in our day-to-day obstetric practice, and the chapter on global maternal health is a "must read" for anyone providing obstetric care abroad. In addition to the two appendices on normal values in pregnancy and the anatomy of the pelvis, we have added a third—a glossary of the most frequently used key abbreviations—for easy reference.

We also welcome two new editors to the seventh edition: Drs. Vincenzo Berghella and William Grobman, both recognized leaders in our field who have authored chapters in past editions. We again thank our chapter authors for their outstanding contributions. We welcome nearly 30 new authors, and we recognize six who have written chapters in every edition: Drs. George J. Annas, D. Ware Branch, Mark B. Landon, Adam A. Rosenberg, Philip Samuels, and Baha Sibai. During this past year, we lost a beloved friend and colleague, Sherman Elias, who had coauthored the chapter on legal and ethical issues in obstetric practice with Dr. Annas for the first six editions. Sherman is and will continue to be missed by so many of us.

Readers will find that we have expanded the use of bolded statements and key points to enhance mastery of each chapter. Our chapter on obstetric ultrasound now contains more than 100 images (in print and online), providing an important resource for normal and abnormal fetal anatomy. Our seventh edition's online features include an exciting new resource: videos to accompany several chapters to enhance learning in areas such as cesarean delivery and operative vaginal delivery.

The seventh edition would not have been possible without outstanding support from our publisher, Elsevier, and its expert and dedicated team, Lucia Gunzel, Kate Dimock, and Carrie Stetz, as well as members of our own staff who have provided invaluable editorial and secretarial assistance, including Kenzie Palsgrove and Susan DuPont (Columbus, Ohio), Nancy Schaapveld (Iowa City), and Lisa Prevel (New York).

As noted on the dedication page, this will be the last edition three of us (S.G.G., J.R.N., J.L.S.) will edit. It has been a privilege for us to contribute to this book over the last four decades. We are confident our coeditors will make the book even better, and we wish them great success.

Whether our readers are beginning their careers or have had many years of clinical experience, we hope they will find the seventh edition of this textbook to be a valuable and supportive resource in today's challenging health care climate. And, we hope they appreciate its earlier arrival!

Steven G. Gabbe, MD
Jennifer R. Niebyl, MD
Joe Leigh Simpson, MD
Mark B. Landon, MD
Henry L. Galan, MD
Eric R.M. Jauniaux, MD, PhD
Deborah A. Driscoll, MD
Vincenzo Berghella, MD
William A. Grobman, MD, MBA

Contents

[†]Deceased.

Video Contents

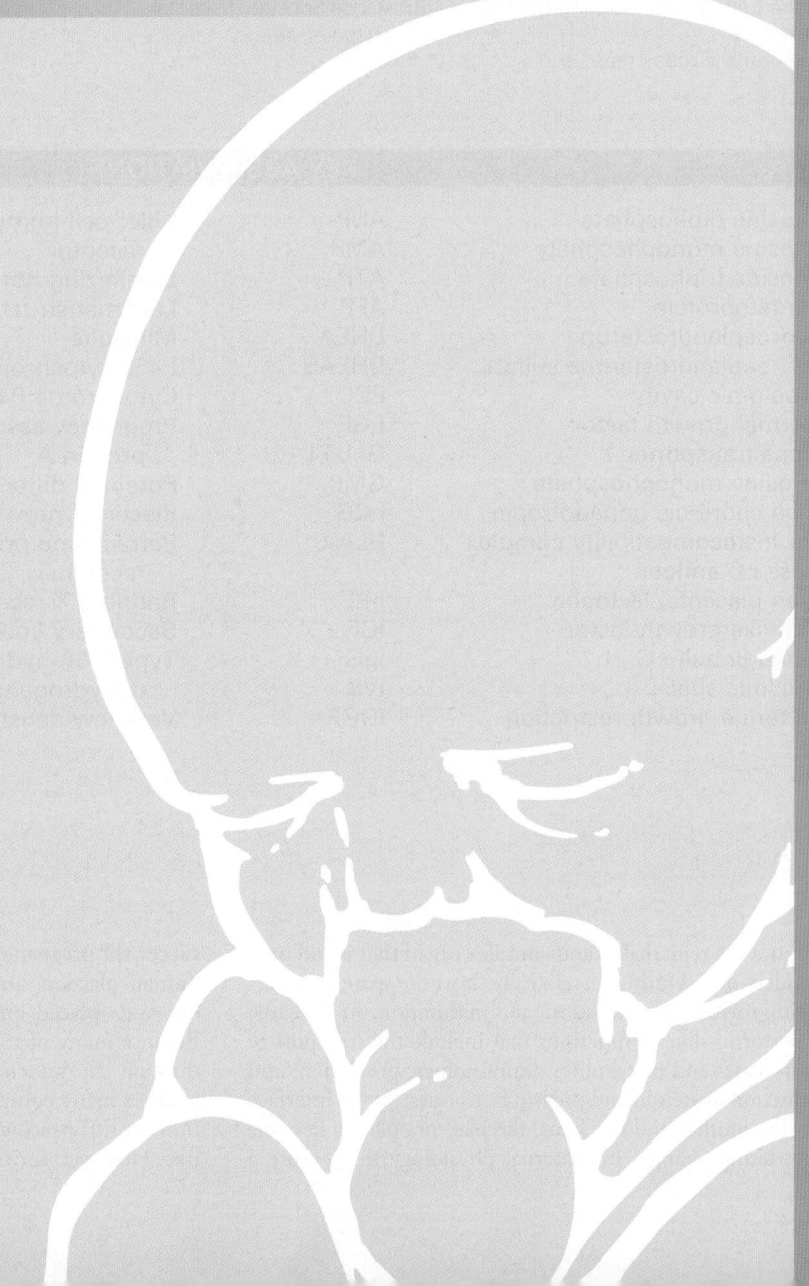

Physiology

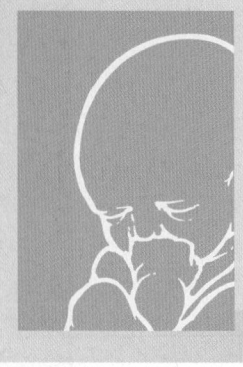

CHAPTER 1

Placental Anatomy and Physiology

GRAHAM J. BURTON, COLIN P. SIBLEY, and ERIC R.M. JAUNIAUX

KEY ABBREVIATIONS

Adenosine diphosphate	ADP	Killer-cell immunoglobulin-like receptor	KIR
Adenosine monophosphate	AMP	Luteinizing hormone	LH
Adenosine triphosphate	ATP	Last menstrual period	LMP
Alpha-fetoprotein	AFP	Millivolts	mV
Dehydroepiandrosterone	DHEA	P450 cytochrome aromatase	P450arom
Dehydroepiandrosterone sulfate	DHEAS	Cytochrome P450scc	P450scc
Exocoelomic cavity	ECC	Pregnancy-associated plasma protein A	PAPP-A
Epidermal growth factor	EGF		
Glucose transporter 1	GLUT1	Potential difference	PD
Guanosine monophosphate	GMP	Placental growth hormone	PGH
Human chorionic gonadotropin	hCG	Peroxisome proliferator–activated receptor	PPAR
Major histocompatibility complex class I C antigen	HLA-C		
Human placental lactogen	hPL	Retinoid X receptor	RXR
Insulin-like growth factor	IGF	Secondary yolk sac	SYS
Immunoglobulin G	IgG	Type 1 3ß-hydroxysteroid dehydrogenase	3ß-HSD
Intervillous space	IVS		
Intrauterine growth restriction	IUGR	Very-low-density lipoprotein	VLDL

The placenta is a remarkable and complex organ that is still only partly understood. During its relatively short life span, it undergoes rapid growth, differentiation, and maturation. At the same time it performs diverse functions that include the transport of respiratory gases and metabolites, immunologic protection, and the production of steroid and protein hormones. As the interface between the mother and her fetus, the placenta plays a key role in orchestrating changes in maternal physiology that ensure a successful pregnancy. This chapter reviews the structure of the human placenta and relates this to the contrasting functional demands placed on the organ at different stages of gestation. Because many of the morphologic features are best understood through an understanding of the organ's development, and because many complications of pregnancy arise through aberrations in this process, we approach the subject from this perspective. However, for the purposes of orientation and to introduce some basic terminology, we first provide a brief description of the macroscopic appearance of the delivered organ, with which readers are most likely to be familiar.

PLACENTAL ANATOMY
Overview of the Delivered Placenta
At term, the human placenta is usually a discoid organ, 15 to 20 cm in diameter, approximately 3 cm thick at the center, and weighing on average 450 g. Data show considerable individual variation, and placentae are also influenced strongly by the mode of delivery. **Macroscopically, the organ consists of two surfaces or plates: the *chorionic plate*, to which the umbilical cord is attached, and the *basal plate* that abuts the maternal endometrium.** Between the two plates is a cavity that is filled with maternal blood, delivered from the endometrial spiral arteries through openings in the basal plate (Fig. 1-1). This cavity is bounded at the margins of the disc by the fusion of the chorionic and basal plates, and the smooth chorion, or *chorion laeve,* extends from the rim to complete the chorionic sac. The placenta is incompletely divided into between 10 and 40 lobes by the presence of septa created by invaginations of the basal plate. The septa are thought to arise from differential resistance of the maternal tissues to trophoblast invasion and may help to compartmentalize, and hence direct, maternal blood flow through the organ. **The fetal component of the placenta comprises a series of elaborately branched villous trees that arise from the inner surface of the chorionic plate and project into the cavity of the placenta.** This arrangement is reminiscent of the fronds of a sea anemone wafting in the seawater of a rock pool. Most commonly, each villous tree originates from a single-stem villus that undergoes several generations of branching until the functional units of the placenta, the **terminal villi**, are created. These consist of an epithelial covering of trophoblast and a mesodermal core that contains branches of the umbilical arteries and tributaries of the umbilical vein. Because of this repeated

branching, the tree takes on the topology of an inverted wine glass, often referred to as a *lobule*, and two to three of these may "sprout" within a single placental lobe (see Fig. 1-1). As will be seen later, **each lobule represents an individual maternal-fetal exchange unit.** Near term, the continual elaboration of the villous trees almost fills the cavity of the placenta, which is reduced to a network of narrow spaces collectively referred to as the *intervillous space* **(IVS)**. The maternal blood percolates through this network of channels and exchanges gases and nutrients with the fetal blood that circulates within the villi before draining through the basal plate into openings of the uterine veins. **The human placenta is therefore classified in comparative mammalian terms as being of the villous hemochorial type, although as we shall see, this arrangement only pertains to the second and third trimesters of pregnancy.**[1] **Prior to that, the maternal-fetal relationship is best described as deciduochorial.**

Placental Development
Development of the placenta is initiated morphologically at the time of implantation, when the embryonic pole of the blastocyst establishes contact with the uterine epithelium. At this stage, the wall of the blastocyst comprises an outer layer of unicellular epithelial cells, the trophoblast, and an inner layer of extraembryonic mesodermal cells derived from the inner cell mass; together these layers constitute the chorion. The earliest events have never been observed in vivo for obvious ethical reasons, but they are thought to be equivalent to those that take place in the rhesus monkey.

Attempts have also been made to replicate the situation in vitro by culturing in vitro fertilized human blastocysts on monolayers of endometrial cells. Although such reductionist systems cannot take into account the possibility of paracrine signals that emanate from the underlying endometrial stroma, the profound differences in trophoblast invasiveness displayed by various species are maintained. In the case of the human, the trophoblast

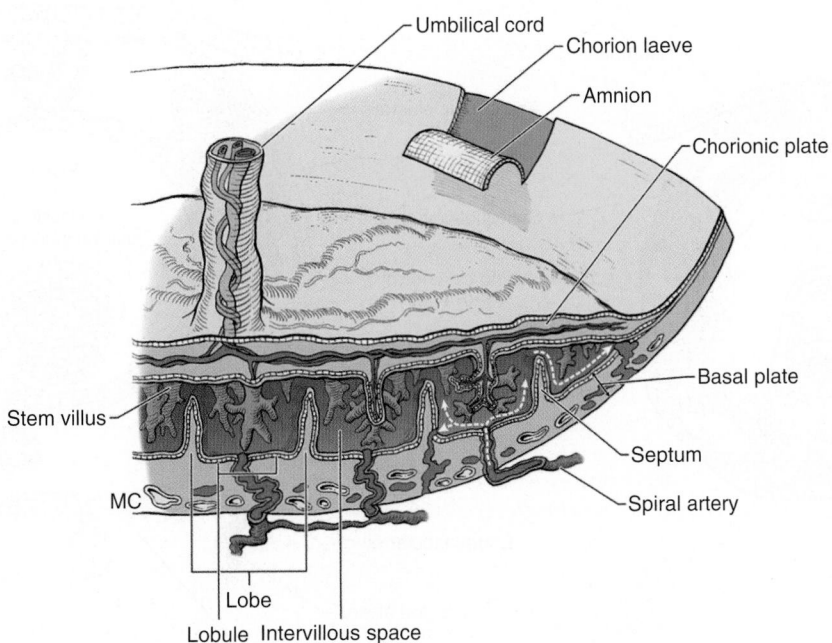

FIG 1-1 Diagrammatic cross section through a mature placenta shows the chorionic and basal plates that bound the intervillous space. The villous trees arise from stem villi attached to the chorionic plate and are arranged as lobules centered over the openings of the maternal spiral arteries. MC, maternal circulation.

in contact with the endometrium undergoes a syncytial transformation, and tongues of syncytiotrophoblast begin to penetrate between the endometrial cells. No evidence suggests cell death is induced as part of this process, but gradually the conceptus embeds into the stratum compactum of the endometrium.

Recent ultrasound and comparative data indicate that upgrowth and encapsulation by the endometrium may be just as important as trophoblast invasion in this process.[2] The earliest ex vivo specimens available for study are estimated to be around 7 days postfertilization, and in these, the conceptus is almost entirely embedded. A plug of fibrin initially seals the defect in the uterine surface, but by days 10 to 12, the epithelium is restored.

By the time implantation is complete, the conceptus is surrounded entirely by a mantle of syncytiotrophoblast (Fig. 1-2, *A*). This multinucleated mantle tends to be thicker beneath the conceptus, in association with the embryonic pole, and it rests on a layer of uninucleate cytotrophoblast cells derived from the original wall of the blastocyst. **Vacuolar spaces begin to appear within the mantle and gradually coalesce to form larger lacunae, the forerunners of the IVS.** As the lacunae enlarge, the intervening syncytiotrophoblast is reduced in thickness and forms a complex lattice of trabeculae (see Fig. 1-2, *B*). Soon after, starting around day 12 after fertilization, the cytotrophoblast cells proliferate and penetrate into the trabeculae. On reaching their tips approximately 2 days later, the cells spread laterally and establish contact with those from other trabeculae to form a new layer interposed between the mantle and the endometrium, the *cytotrophoblastic shell* (see Fig. 1-2, *C*). Finally, at the start of the third week of development, mesodermal cells derived from the extraembryonic mesoderm invade the trabeculae, bringing with them the hemangioblasts from which the fetal vascular circulation differentiates. The mesoderm

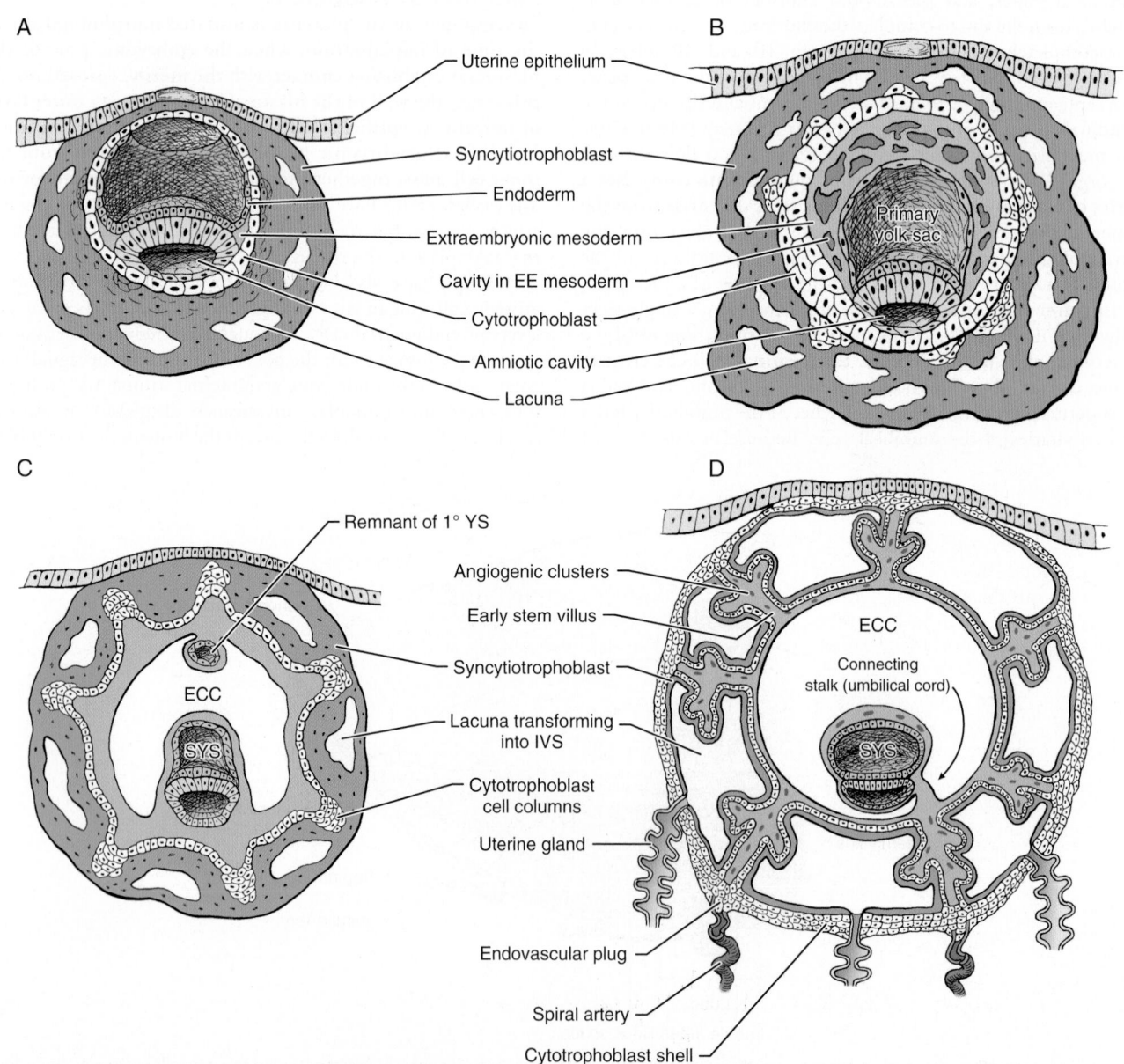

FIG 1-2 Schematic representation of early placental development between days 9 and 16 postfertilization. *ECC,* extracoelomic cavity; *EE,* extraembryonic; *IVS,* intervillous space; *SYS,* secondary yolk sac; *YS,* yolk sac.

cells do not penetrate right to the tips of the trabeculae, and these remain as an aggregation of cytotrophoblast cells—the *cytotrophoblast cell columns,* which may or may not have a covering of syncytiotrophoblast (see Fig. 1-2, *C*). Proliferation of the cells at the proximal ends of the columns and their subsequent differentiation contribute to expansion of the cytotrophoblastic shell. Toward the end of the third week, the rudiments of the placenta are therefore in place. **The original wall of the blastocyst becomes the chorionic plate, the cytotrophoblastic shell is the precursor of the basal plate, and the lacunae form the IVS** (Fig. 1-2, *D*). The trabeculae are the forerunners of the villous trees, and repeated lateral branching gradually increases their complexity.

Initially, villi form over the entire chorionic sac, but toward the end of the first trimester, they regress from all except the deep pole, where they remain as the definitive discoid placenta. Abnormalities in this process may account for the persistence of villi at abnormal sites on the chorionic sac and, hence, the presence of accessory or succenturiate lobes. Also, excessive asymmetric regression may result in the umbilical cord being attached eccentrically to the placental disc.

Amnion and Yolk Sac

While these early stages of placental development are taking place, the inner cell mass differentiates and gives rise to the amnion, the yolk sac, and the bilaminar germ disc. The amnion, the yolk sac, and the fluid compartment in which they lie play an important role in the physiology of early pregnancy; their development will be described. The initial formation of these sacs has been controversial over the years, due mainly to the small number of specimens available for study. However, there now appears to be consensus that the amnion extends from the margins of the epiblast layer over the future dorsal surface of the germ disc, whereas the primary yolk sac extends from the hypoblast layer around the inner surface of the trophoblast, separated from it by a loose reticulum thought to be derived from the endoderm. Over the next few days, considerable remodeling of the yolk sac occurs that involves three closely interrelated processes. First, formation of the primitive streak in the germ disc and the subsequent differentiation of definitive endoderm lead to displacement of the original hypoblast cells into the more peripheral regions of the primary yolk sac. Second, the sac greatly reduces in size, either because the more peripheral portion is nipped off, or because it breaks up into a number of vesicles. Third, the reticulum splits into two layers of mesoderm except at the future caudal end of the germ disc, where it persists as a mass; this is the connecting stalk that links the disc to the trophoblast. One layer lines the inner surface of the trophoblast, contributing to formation of the chorion, and the other covers the outer surfaces of the amnion and yolk sac. In between these layers is a large fluid-filled space, the *exocoelomic cavity* (ECC). **The net result of this remodeling is the formation of a smaller secondary yolk sac (SYS); connected to the embryo by the vitelline duct, it floats within the ECC** (see Fig. 1-2, *D*).

The ECC is a conspicuous feature ultrasonographically that can be clearly visualized using a transvaginal probe toward the end of the third week after fertilization (fifth week of gestational age). Between 5 and 9 weeks of pregnancy, it represents the largest anatomic space within the chorionic sac. **The SYS is the first structure that can be detected ultrasonographically within that space, and its diameter increases slightly between 6 and 10 weeks of gestation to reach a maximum of 6 to 7 mm, and then it decreases slightly.** Histologically, the SYS consists of an inner layer of endodermal cells linked by tight junctions at their apical surface and bearing a few short microvilli. Their cytoplasm contains numerous mitochondria, whorls of rough endoplasmic reticulum, Golgi bodies, and secretory droplets; this gives them the appearance of being highly active synthetic cells. With further development, the epithelium becomes folded to form a series of cyst-like structures or tubules, only some of which communicate with the central cavity. The function of these spaces is not known, although it has been proposed that they serve as a primitive circulatory network in the earliest stages of development because they may contain nonnucleated erythrocytes. On its outer surface, the yolk sac is lined by a layer of mesothelium derived from the extraembryonic mesoderm. This epithelium bears a dense covering of microvilli, and the presence of numerous coated pits and pinocytotic vesicles gives it the appearance of an absorptive epithelium. Although no direct evidence has yet been obtained of this function in the human, transport proteins for glucose and folate have been immunolocalized to this layer.[3] Experiments in the rhesus monkey have revealed that the mesothelial layer readily engulfs horseradish peroxidase, and the proposed transport function is reinforced by the presence of a well-developed capillary plexus immediately beneath the epithelium that drains through the vitelline veins to the developing liver.

However, by week 9 of pregnancy, the SYS begins to exhibit morphologic evidence of a decline in function. This appears to be independent of the expansion of the amnion, which is gradually drawn around the ventral surface of the developing embryo. As it does this, it presses the yolk sac remnant against the connecting stalk, thus forming the umbilical cord. By the end of the third month, the amnion abuts the inner surface of the chorion, and the ECC is obliterated. The fusion of the amnion and chorion and elimination of the ECC can be seen by ultrasound at around 15 weeks of gestation.

Maternal-Fetal Relationship During the First Trimester

For the placenta to function efficiently as an organ of exchange, it requires adequate and dependable access to the maternal circulation. Establishing that access is arguably one of the most critical aspects of placental development, and over recent years, it has certainly been one of the most controversial. As the syncytiotrophoblastic mantle enlarges, it soon comes in close proximity to superficial veins within the endometrium. These undergo dilation to form sinusoids, which are subsequently tapped into by the syncytium. As a result, maternal erythrocytes come to lie within the lacunae, and their presence has in the past been taken by embryologists as indicating the onset of the maternal circulation to the placenta. If this is a circulation, however, it is entirely one of venous ebb and flow, possibly influenced by uterine contractions and other forces. Numerous traditional histologic studies have demonstrated that arterial connections are not established with the lacunae until much later in pregnancy,[4,5] although the exact timing was not known for many years. The advent of high-resolution ultrasound and Doppler imaging has appeared to answer this question, for in normal pregnancies most observers agree that moving echoes indicative of significant fluid flow cannot be detected within the IVS until 10 to 12 weeks of gestation.

It is now well accepted on the basis of evidence from a variety of techniques that a major change in the maternal circulation to the placenta takes place at the end of the first trimester. First, direct vision into the IVS during the first trimester with a hysteroscope reveals the cavity to be filled with a clear fluid rather than with maternal blood.[6] Second, perfusion of pregnant hysterectomy specimens with radiopaque and other media demonstrates little flow into the IVS during the first trimester, except perhaps at the margins of the placental disc.[4] Third, the oxygen concentration within the IVS is low (<20 mm Hg) prior to 10 weeks of pregnancy, and it rises threefold between weeks 10 and 12.[7] This rise is matched by increases in the mRNA concentrations encoding and in activities of the principal antioxidant enzymes in the placental tissues that confirm a change in oxygenation at the cellular level.[7] The mechanism that underlies this change in placental perfusion relates to the phenomenon of extravillous trophoblast invasion.

Extravillous Trophoblast Invasion and Physiologic Conversion of the Spiral Arteries

During the early weeks of pregnancy, a subpopulation of trophoblast cells migrates from the deep surface of the cytotrophoblastic shell into the endometrium. Because these cells do not take part in the development of the definitive placenta, they are referred to as *extravillous trophoblast*. Their activities are, however, fundamental to the successful functioning of the placenta, for their presence in the endometrium is associated with the physiologic conversion of the maternal spiral arteries. The cytologic basis of this phenomenon is still not understood, but the net effect is the loss of the smooth muscle cells and elastic fibers from the media of the endometrial segments of the arteries and their subsequent replacement by fibrinoid.[8,9] Some evidence suggests that this is a two-stage process. Very early in pregnancy, the arteries display endothelial basophilia and vacuolation, disorganization of the smooth muscle cells, and dilation. Because these changes are observed equally in both the decidua basalis and parietalis, and because they are also seen within the uterus in cases of ectopic pregnancies, they must be independent of local trophoblast invasion. Instead, it has been proposed that these changes result from activation of decidual renin-angiotensin signaling. Slightly later, during the first few weeks of pregnancy, the invading extravillous trophoblasts become closely associated with the arteries and infiltrate their walls. **Further dilation ensues, and as a result, the arteries are converted from small-caliber vasoreactive vessels into funnel-shaped flaccid conduits.**

The extravillous trophoblast population can be separated into two subgroups: the *endovascular trophoblast* migrates in a retrograde fashion down the lumens of the spiral arteries, replacing the endothelium; and the *interstitial trophoblast* migrates through the endometrial stroma. **In early pregnancy, the volume of the migrating endovascular cells is sufficient to occlude, or plug, the terminal portions of the spiral arteries as they approach the basal plate (Fig. 1-3).[4,5] It is the dissipation of these plugs toward the end of the first trimester that establishes the maternal circulation to the placenta.** The mechanism of unplugging of the arteries is unknown at present but could potentially reflect changes in endovascular trophoblast motility or alterations in maternal hemodynamics. Trophoblast invasion is not equal across the implantation site; rather it is greatest in the central region, where it has presumably been established the

longest. It is to be expected, therefore, that the plugging of the spiral arteries will be most extensive in this region, and this may account for the fact that maternal arterial blood flow is most often first detectable ultrasonographically in the peripheral regions of the placental disc.[10] **Associated with this blood flow is a high local level of oxidative stress, which can be considered physiologic because it occurs in all normal pregnancies. It has recently been proposed that this stress induces regression of the villi over the superficial pole of the chorionic sac, so forming the chorion laeve (Fig. 1-4).[10]**

Under normal conditions, the interstitial trophoblast cells invade as far as the inner third of the myometrium, where they fuse and form multinucleated giant cells. **It is essential that the process is correctly regulated; excessive invasion can result in complete erosion of the endometrium and the condition known as *placenta accreta* (see Chapter 21).** As they migrate, the trophoblast cells interact with cells of the maternal immune system present within the decidua, in particular macrophages and uterine natural killer (NK) cells. These interactions may play a physiologic role in regulation of the depth of invasion and in the conversion of the spiral arteries. Uterine NK cells accumulate in the endometrium during the secretory phase of the nonpregnant cycle and are particularly numerous surrounding the spiral arteries at the implantation site. Despite their name, no evidence suggests that they destroy trophoblast cells. On the contrary, their cytoplasm contains numerous granules with a diverse array of cytokines and growth factors. **Extravillous trophoblast cells express the polymorphic human leukocyte C-antigen (HLA-C) that binds to killer cell immunoglobulin-like receptors (KIRs) on the NK cells. Recent evidence indicates that a degree of activation of the NK cells is necessary for successful pregnancy, most likely because of the release of factors that mediate spiral artery remodeling. Hence, combinations of HLA-C antigen and KIR subtypes that are generally inhibitory are associated with a high risk of pregnancy complications,[11] which emphasizes the importance of immunologic interactions to reproductive success.**

Physiologic conversion of the spiral arteries is often attributed with ensuring an adequate maternal blood flow to the placenta, but such comments generally oversimplify the phenomenon. By itself, the process cannot increase the volume of blood flow to the placenta because it only affects the most distal portion of the spiral arteries. **The most proximal part of the arteries, where they arise from the uterine arcuate arteries, always remains unconverted, and will act as the rate-limiting segment. These segments gradually dilate in conjunction with the rest of the uterine vasculature during early pregnancy, most probably under the effects of estrogen; as a result, the resistance of the uterine circulation falls, and uterine blood flow increases from approximately 45 mL/min during the menstrual cycle to around 750 mL/min at term or 10% to 15% of maternal cardiac output.**

By contrast, the terminal dilation of the arteries will substantially reduce both the rate and pressure with which that maternal blood flows into the IVS. Mathematic modeling has demonstrated that physiologic conversion is associated with a reduction in velocity from 2 to 3 m/sec in the nondilated section of a spiral artery to approximately 10 cm/sec at its mouth.[12] **This reduction in the velocity will ensure that the delicate villous trees are not damaged by the momentum of the inflowing blood. Slowing the rate of maternal blood flow across the villous trees will also facilitate exchange, whereas lowering the**

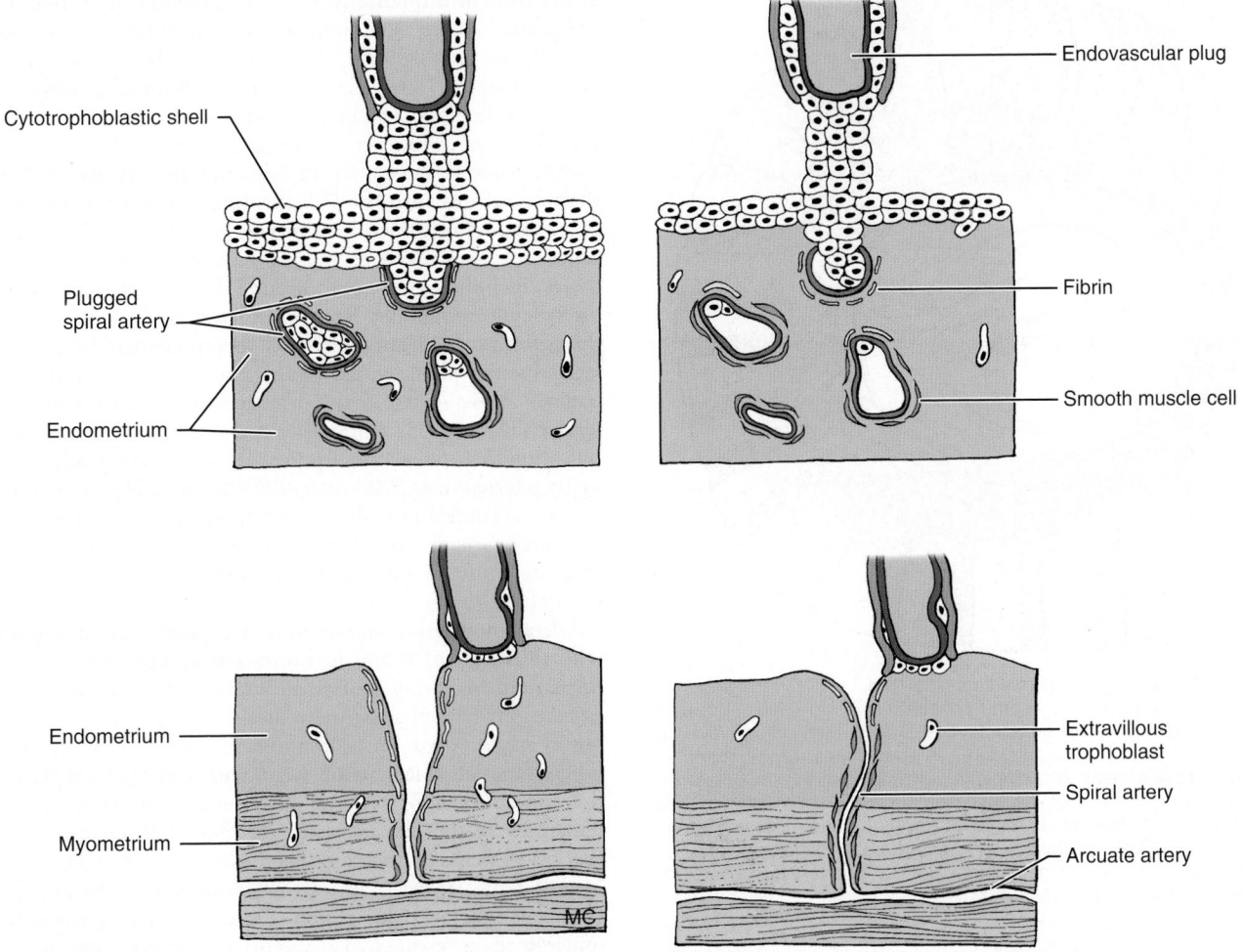

FIG 1-3 During early pregnancy, the tips of the maternal spiral arteries are occluded by invading endovascular trophoblast cells, which impedes flow into the intervillous space. The combination of endovascular and interstitial trophoblast invasion is associated with physiologic conversion of the spiral arteries. Both processes are deficient in preeclampsia, and the retention of vascular smooth muscle may increase the risk of spontaneous vasoconstriction and hence may result in an ischemia-reperfusion type injury to the placenta. MC, maternal circulation.

pressure in the IVS is important to prevent compression and collapse of the fetal capillary network within the villi. Measurements taken in the rhesus monkey indicate that the pressure at the mouth of a spiral artery is only 15 mm Hg and within the IVS is on average 10 mm Hg. The pressure within the fetal villous capillaries is estimated to be approximately 20 mm Hg, providing a pressure differential that favors their distension of 5 mm Hg.

Many complications of pregnancy are associated with defects in extravillous trophoblast invasion and failure to establish the maternal placental circulation correctly. In the most severe cases, the cytotrophoblastic shell is thin and fragmented; this is observed in approximately two thirds of spontaneous miscarriages.[13] Reduced invasion may reflect defects inherent in the conceptus, such as chromosomal aberrations, or it may be due to thrombophilia, endometrial dysfunction, or other problems in the mother. The net result is that onset of the maternal circulation is both precocious and widespread throughout the developing placenta, consequent upon absent or incomplete plugging of the maternal arteries.[10] Hemodynamic forces coupled with excessive oxidative stress within the

placental tissues[14] are likely to be major factors that contribute to loss of these pregnancies.

In milder cases, the pregnancy may continue, but it is complicated later by preeclampsia, intrauterine growth restriction (IUGR), or a combination of the two. The physiologic changes are either restricted to only the superficial endometrial parts of the spiral arteries or are absent all together (see Fig. 1-3). In the most severe cases of preeclampsia associated with major fetal growth restriction, only 10% of the arteries may be fully converted, compared with 96% in normal pregnancies.[15] There is still debate as to whether this is due to an inability of the interstitial trophoblast to invade the endometrium successfully, or whether having invaded sufficiently deeply, the trophoblast cells fail to penetrate the walls of the arteries. These two possibilities are not mutually exclusive and may reflect different etiologies.

Whatever the causation, there are several potential consequences to incomplete conversion of the arteries. First, because of the absence of the distal dilation, maternal blood will enter the IVS with greater velocity than normal, forming jetlike spurts that can be detected ultrasonographically. The villous trees are

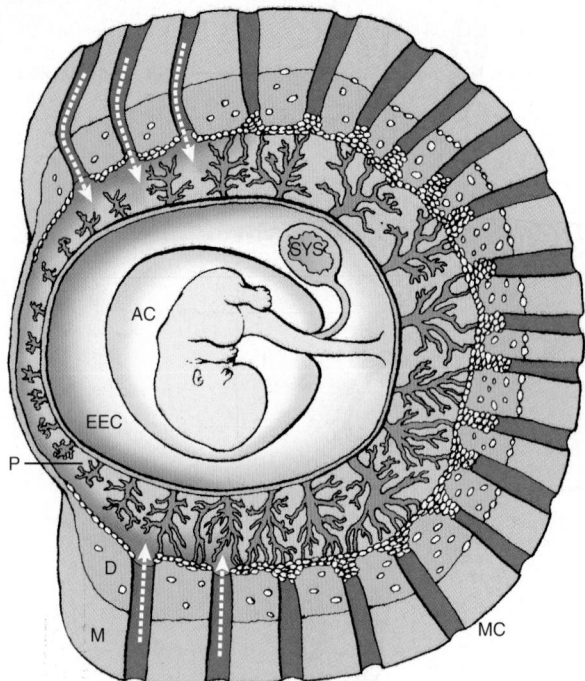

FIG 1-4 Onset of the maternal circulation (MC) starts in the periphery of the placenta (*arrows*), where trophoblast invasion—and hence plugging of the spiral arteries—is least developed. The high local levels of oxidative stress are thought to induce villous regression and formation of the chorion laeve. AC, amniotic cavity; D, decidua; ECC, exocoelomic cavity; P, placenta; M, myometrium; SYS, secondary yolk sac. (Modified from Jauniaux E, Cindrova-Davies T, Johns J, et al. Distribution and transfer pathways of antioxidant molecules inside the first trimester human gestational sac. *J Clin Endocrinol Metab.* 2004;89:1452-1459.)

often disrupted opposite these spurts, which leads to the formation of intervillous blood lakes, and the altered hemodynamics within the IVS result in thrombosis and excessive fibrin deposition. Second, incomplete conversion will allow the spiral arteries to maintain greater vasoreactivity than normal. Evidence from rhesus monkeys and humans shows that spiral arteries are not continuously patent but that they undergo periodic constriction independent of uterine contractions.[10,16] It has recently been proposed that exaggeration of this phenomenon due to the retention of smooth muscle in the arterial walls may lead to a hypoxia-reoxygenation–type injury in the placenta, which culminates in the development of oxidative stress. **Placental oxidative stress is a key factor in the pathogenesis of preeclampsia, and clinical evidence suggests that hypoxia-reoxygenation is a more physiologic stimulus for its generation than simply reduced uterine perfusion.**[17] The third consequence of incomplete conversion is that the distal segments of the arteries are frequently the site of acute atherotic changes.[18] These are likely to be secondary changes, possibly induced by the involvement of these segments in the hypoxia-reoxygenation process or their abnormal hemodynamics; however, if the lesions become occlusive, they will further impair blood flow within the IVS, which contributes to the growth restriction.

Role of the Endometrium During the First Trimester

Signals from the uterine epithelium and secretions from the endometrial glands play a major role in regulating receptivity

at the time of implantation, but the potential contribution of the glands to fetal development once implantation is complete has largely been ignored. This has been due to the general assumption that once the conceptus is embedded within the uterine wall, it no longer has access to the secretions in the uterine lumen. However, a review of archival placenta in situ hysterectomy specimens has revealed that **the glands discharge their secretions into the IVS through openings in the basal plate throughout the first trimester** (see Fig. 1-2).[19] The secretions are a heterogenous mix of maternal proteins; carbohydrates, including glycogen; and lipid droplets phagocytosed by the syncytiotrophoblast. Recently, it has been demonstrated that the pattern of sialylation of the secretions changes between the late secretory phase of the nonpregnant cycle and early pregnancy.[20] A loss of terminal sialylic acid caps occurs, which will render the secretions more easily degradable by the trophoblast following their phagocytic uptake. The fact that glycodelin, formerly referred to as *PP14* or α_2-*PEG,* is derived from the glands and yet accumulates within the amniotic fluid with concentrations that peak at around 10 weeks' gestation indicates that the placenta must be exposed to glandular secretions extensively throughout the first trimester.

Ultrasonographic measurements suggest that an endometrial thickness of 8 mm or more is necessary for successful implantation, although not all studies have found such an association. Nonetheless, these measurements are in line with observations based on placenta-in-situ specimens, in which an endometrial thickness of over 5 mm was reported beneath the conceptus at 6 weeks of gestation.[21] Gradually, over the remainder of the first trimester, the endometrium regresses so that by 14 weeks of gestation, the thickness is reduced to 1 mm. Histologically, there is also a transformation in the glandular epithelial cells over this period. During early pregnancy, they undergo characteristic hypersecretory morphologic changes, the so-called Arias-Stella reaction,[22] and their cytoplasm contains abundant organelles and large accumulations of glycogen.[19,21] These changes are likely a response to placental lactogens and prolactin from the decidua, which represents a servomechanism by which the placenta induces upregulation of its own nutrient supply. However, by the end of the first trimester, the cells are more cuboidal, and secretory organelles are much less prominent, although the lumens of the glands are still filled with secretions.

The overall picture is that the glands are most prolific and active during the early weeks of pregnancy, and that their contribution gradually wanes during the first trimester. This would be consistent with a progressive switch from histotrophic to hemotrophic nutrition as the maternal arterial circulation to the placenta is established. The glands should not be considered solely as a source of nutrients; their secretions are also rich in growth factors such as leukemia inhibitory factor, vascular endothelial growth factor (VEGF), epidermal growth factor, and transforming growth factor beta (TGF-β).[21] Receptors for these factors are present on the villous tissues, so the glands may play an important role in modulating placental proliferation and differentiation during early pregnancy, as in other species. The change in sialylation in early pregnancy will ensure that any of the secretions that gain access to the maternal circulation via the uterine veins will be rapidly cleared in the maternal liver. Hence, a unique proliferative microenvironment can be created within the IVS of the early placenta without placing the mother's tissues at risk of excessive stimulation. Attempts to correlate the functional activity of the glands with pregnancy outcome have met with mixed success. Thus reduced concentrations of mucin 1, glycodelin, and leukemia inhibitory factor have been reported in uterine flushings from women who have suffered repeated miscarriages.[23] However, a recent study has shown no significant association between the expression of these markers within the endometrium and outcome.[24] This difference may reflect impairment in the secretory, rather than the synthetic, machinery of the gland cells, although further work is required to confirm this point.

From the evidence available, it would appear that the functional importance of the endometrial glands to a successful pregnancy extends well beyond the time of implantation.

Topology of the Villous Trees

One of the principal functions of the placenta is diffusional exchange, and the physical requirements for this impose the greatest influence on the structure of the organ. The rate of diffusion of an inert molecule is governed by Fick's law, so it is proportional to the surface area for exchange divided by the thickness of the tissue barrier. A large surface area will therefore facilitate exchange, and this is achieved by repeated branching of the villous trees.

The villous trees arise from the trabeculae interposed between the lacunae (see Fig. 1-2) through a gradual process of remodeling and lateral branching. Initially, the different branches have an almost uniform composition, and the villi can be separated only by their relative size and position in the hierarchical branching pattern. At this stage, the mesodermal core is loosely packed, and at the proximal end of the trees, it blends with the extraembryonic mesoderm that lines the ECC. The stromal cells possess sail-like processes that often link together to form fluid-filled channels orientated parallel to the long axis of the villi. Macrophages are often seen within these channels, so it is possible they function as a primitive circulatory system prior to vasculogenesis. In this way proteins derived from the uterine glands could freely pass into the coelomic fluid, and it is notable that the macrophages within the channels are strongly immunoreactive for maternal glycodelin[19] secreted from the glands.

Toward the end of the first trimester, the villi begin to differentiate into their principal types. **The connections to the chorionic plate become remodeled to form stem villi, which represent the supporting framework of each villous tree.**[25] These progressively develop a compact fibrous stroma and contain branches of the chorionic arteries and accompanying veins. The arteries are centrally located and are surrounded by a cuff of smooth muscle cells. **Although these have the appearance of resistance vessels, physiologic studies indicate that under normal conditions, the fetal placental circulation operates under conditions of full vasodilation.** Stem villi contain only a few small caliber capillaries, and so they play little role in placental exchange.

After several generations of branching, stem villi give rise to intermediate villi. These are longer and more slender in form and can be of two types: immature and mature. The former are seen predominantly in early pregnancy and represent a persistence of the nondifferentiated form as indicated by the presence of fluid-filled stromal channels. Mature intermediate villi provide a distributing framework, and terminal villi arise at intervals from their surface. Within the core are arterioles and venules

but also a significant number of nondilated capillaries, which suggest a limited capacity for exchange.

The main functional units of the villous tree are, however, the terminal villi. There is no strict definition as to where a terminal villus starts, but they are most often short, stubby branches up to 100 μm in length and approximately 80 μm in diameter that arise from the intermediate villi (Fig. 1-5).[25] They are highly vascularized, but by capillaries alone, and they are highly adapted for diffusional exchange, as will be seen later.

This differentiation of the villi coincides temporally with the development of the lobular architecture, and the two processes are most likely interlinked. Lobules can be first identified during the early second trimester, following onset of the maternal circulation, when it is thought hemodynamic forces may shape the villous tree. Convincing radiographic and morphologic evidence shows that maternal blood is delivered into the center of the lobule and that it then disperses peripherally, as in the rhesus monkey placenta.[26] Consequently, it is to be expected that an oxygen gradient will exist across the lobule, and differences in the activities and expression of antioxidant enzymes within the villous tissues suggest strongly that this is the case. Other metabolic gradients (e.g., glucose concentration) may also exist, and together these may exert powerful influences on villous differentiation. Villi in the center of the lobule, where the oxygen concentration will be highest, display morphologic and enzymatic evidence of relative immaturity, and so this is considered to be the germinative zone. By contrast, villi in the periphery of the lobule are better adapted for diffusional exchange.

Elaboration of the villous tree is a progressive event that continues at a steady pace throughout pregnancy, and by term, the villi present a surface area of 10 to 14 m². This may be significantly reduced in cases of IUGR, although this principally reflects an overall reduction in placental volume rather than maldevelopment of the villous tree.[27] In cases of preeclampsia alone, villous surface area is normal and is only compromised with associated growth restriction.[27] Attempts have recently been made to monitor placental growth longitudinally during pregnancy using ultrasound. Although the data show considerable individual variability, they indicate that in cases of growth restriction or macrosomia, placental volume is significantly reduced or increased, respectively, at 12 to 14 weeks. **These findings suggest that ultimate placental size has its origins firmly in the first trimester.**

PLACENTAL HISTOLOGY

The epithelial covering of the villous trees is formed by the syncytiotrophoblast. As its name indicates, this is a true multinucleated syncytium that extends without lateral intercellular clefts over the entire villous surface. In essence, the syncytiotrophoblast acts as the endothelium of the IVS, and everything that passes across the placenta must pass through this layer, either actively or passively. This tissue also performs all hormone synthesis in the placenta, and so a number of potentially conflicting demands are placed upon it.

The syncytiotrophoblast is highly polarized, and one of its most conspicuous features is the presence of a dense covering of **microvilli** on the apical surface. In the first trimester, the microvilli are relatively long (approximately 0.75 to 1.25 μm in length and 0.12 to 0.17 μm in diameter), but as pregnancy advances, they become shorter and more slender, being approximately 0.5 to 0.7 μm in length and 0.08 to 0.14 μm in diameter at term.

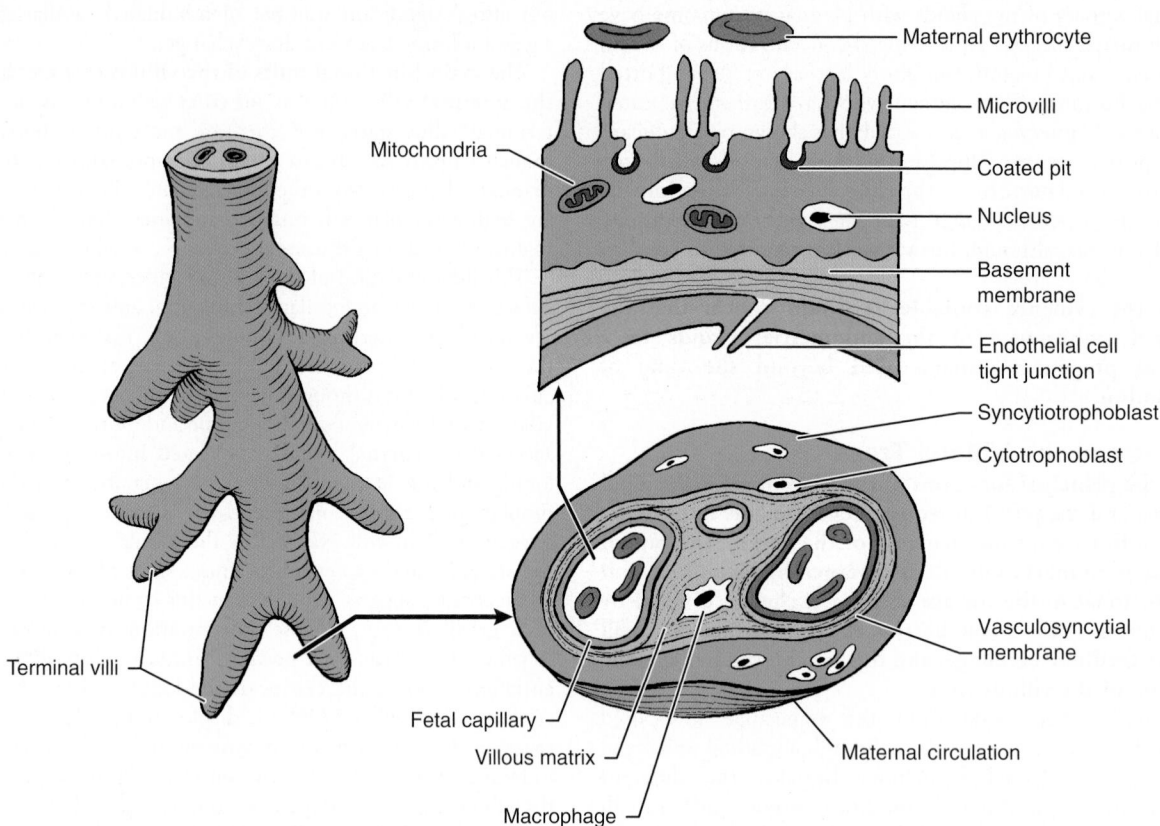

FIG 1-5 Diagrammatic representation of an intermediate villus with terminal villi arising from the lateral surface.

The microvillous covering is even over the villous surface, and measurements of the amplification factor provided vary from 5.2 to 7.7. Many receptors and transport proteins have been localized to the microvillous surface by molecular biologic and immunohistochemical techniques, as will be discussed later. The receptors are thought to reside in lipid rafts, and once bound to their ligand, they migrate to the base of the microvilli, where clathrin-coated pits are present (see Fig. 1-5).[28] Receptor-ligand complexes are concentrated in the pits, which are then internalized. Disassociation of ligands such as cholesterol may occur in the syncytioplasm, whereas other ligands, such as immunoglobulin G, are exocytosed at the basal surface.

Support for the microvillous architecture is provided by a substantial network of actin filaments and microtubules that lie just beneath the apical surface. Also present within the syncytioplasm are numerous pinocytotic vesicles, phagosomes, lysosomes, mitochondria, secretory droplets, strands of endoplasmic reticulum, Golgi bodies, and lipid droplets.[28] **The overall impression is of a highly active epithelium engaged in absorptive, secretory, and synthetic functions. Therefore it is not surprising that the syncytiotrophoblast has a high metabolic rate, consuming approximately 40% of the oxygen taken up by the fetoplacental unit.**[29]

The syncytiotrophoblast is a terminally differentiated tissue; consequently, mitotic figures are never observed within its nuclei. It has been suggested that this condition, which is frequently observed in the fetal cells at the maternal-fetal interface in other species, reduces the risk of malignant transformation in the trophoblast and so protects the mother. Whatever the reason, **the syncytiotrophoblast is generated by the recruitment of progenitor cytotrophoblast cells,** which are uninucleate and lie on a well-developed basement membrane immediately beneath the syncytium. A proportion represents progenitor cells that undergo proliferation, with daughter cells that undergo progressive differentiation.[30] Consequently, a range of morphologic appearances are seen, from cuboidal resting cells with a general paucity of organelles to fully differentiated cells that closely resemble the overlying syncytium.[28] Ultimately, membrane fusion takes place between the two, and the nucleus and cytoplasm are incorporated into the syncytiotrophoblast. Early in pregnancy, the cytotrophoblast cells form a complete layer beneath the syncytium, but as pregnancy advances, the cells become separated and are seen less frequently in histologic sections. In the past this observation was interpreted as being indicative of a reduction in the number of cytotrophoblast cells and therefore a reduction in the proliferative potential of the trophoblast layers. More recent stereologic estimates have revealed a different picture, however, because the total number of these cells increases until term.[31] The apparent decline results from the fact that villous surface area increases at a greater rate, and so cytotrophoblast cell profiles are seen less often in any individual histologic section.

The stimuli that regulate cytotrophoblast cell proliferation are not fully understood. In early pregnancy, prior to 6 weeks, epidermal growth factor (EGF) may play an important role; expression of both the factor and its receptor are localized principally to these cells. EGF is also strongly expressed in the epithelium of the uterine glands,[21] and in the horse, a tight spatial and temporal correlation exists between glandular expression and proliferation in the overlying trophoblast. Later during the first trimester, insulin-like growth factor II (IGF-II) can be immunolocalized to the cytotrophoblast cells, as can the receptor for hepatocyte growth factor—a powerful mitogen expressed by the mesenchymal cells, which provides the possibility of paracrine control. Environmental stimuli may also be important, and hypoxia has long been known to stimulate cytotrophoblast proliferation in vitro. A greater number of cell profiles are also observed in placentae from high altitudes, where they are exposed to hypobaric hypoxia, and in conditions associated with poor placental perfusion. However, whether this represents increased proliferation or decreased fusion with the syncytiotrophoblast is uncertain.

The factors that regulate and mediate fusion are equally uncertain. Growth factors such as EGF, granulocyte-macrophage colony-stimulating factor (GM-CSF), and VEGF are able to stimulate fusion in vitro, as are the hormones estradiol and human chorionic gonadotropin (hCG). By contrast, TGF-β, leukemia inhibitory factor, and endothelin inhibit the process, which suggests that the outcome in vivo depends on a balance between these opposing influences. One of the actions of hCG at the molecular level is to promote the formation of gap junctions between cells, and strong experimental evidence suggests that communication via gap junctions is an essential prerequisite in the fusion process.[32] Whether membrane fusion is initiated at the sites of gap junctions is not known at present, but much interest has been paid recently to other potential mechanisms of fusion. One such is the externalization of phosphatidylserine on the outer leaflet of the cell membrane, although whether this represents part of an apoptotic cascade that is only completed in the syncytiotrophoblast or is inherent to cytotrophoblastic differentiation remains controversial. Another is the expression of human endogenous retroviral envelope proteins HERV-W env and HERV-FRD env, commonly referred to as *syncytin 1* and *syncytin 2,* respectively. The first protein entered the primate genome approximately 25 million years ago, the second over 40 million years ago, and these are considered to have fusigenic and immunomodulatory roles.[33] Expression of syncytin appears to be necessary for syncytial transformation of trophoblast cells in vitro, and ectopic expression in other cell types renders them fusigenic. **Syncytin interacts with the amino acid transporter protein ASCT2, and the expression of both is influenced by hypoxia in trophoblast cell lines in vitro. This could provide an explanation for the increased number of cytotrophoblast cells observed in placentae from hypoxic pregnancies.**

Although it is clear that the cascade of events that control cytotrophoblastic proliferation and fusion has yet to be fully elucidated, it appears to be tightly regulated in vivo. Thus the ratio of cytotrophoblastic to syncytial nuclei remains at approximately 1:9 throughout pregnancy,[31] although it may be perturbed in pathologic cases. Recent evidence from immunohistochemistry and the incorporation of fluorouridine suggests that a constant proportion of the nuclei (approximately 80%) are transcriptionally active across gestation,[34] which enables the tissue to respond more rapidly and independently to challenges. **Nuclei that are transcriptionally inactive are sequestered together into aggregates known as *syncytial knots*. These nuclei display dense heterochromatin and also show evidence of oxidative changes, which suggests they are aged or damaged in some way.[35] Syncytial knots become more common in later pregnancy and are taken by pathologists as a marker of syncytial well-being, the so-called Tenney-Parker change.**

Integrity of the Villous Membrane

One situation that may alter the balance of the two populations of nuclei is damage to the trophoblast layers and the requirement for repair. Isolated areas of syncytial damage, often referred to as sites of *focal syncytial necrosis,* are a feature of all placentae, although they are more common in those from pathologic pregnancies. Their origin remains obscure but they could potentially arise from altered hemodynamics within the IVS or from physical interactions between villi. One striking example of the latter is the rupture of syncytial bridges that form between adjacent villi and lead to circular defects on the surface 20 to 40 μm in diameter. Disruption of the microvillous surface leads to the activation of platelets and to the deposition of a fibrin plaque on the trophoblastic basement membrane. Apoptosis of syncytial nuclei has been reported in the immediate vicinity of such plaques, but whether this reflects cause or effect has yet to be determined. With time, cytotrophoblast cells migrate over the plaque, differentiate, and fuse to form a new syncytiotrophoblastic layer. As a result, the plaque is internalized, and the integrity of the villous surface is restored. In the interim, however, these sites are nonselectively permeable to creatinine and may represent a paracellular route for placental transfer.[36]

In the past, more widespread apoptosis in the syncytiotrophoblast has been reported, with the interpretation that this reflects increased turnover of the trophoblast in pathologic conditions. However, recent research has clarified that although rates of apoptosis are increased in preeclampsia and IUGR, the cell death is confined to the cytotrophoblast cells.[37]

Extensive damage to the syncytiotrophoblast is seen in cases of missed miscarriage, in which complete degeneration and sloughing of the layer can occur.[10,14] Although apoptosis and necrosis are increased among the cytotrophoblast cells, the remaining cells differentiate and fuse to form a new and functional syncytial layer. A similar effect is observed when villi from either first trimester or term placentae are maintained under ambient conditions in vitro.

Thus it is likely that considerable turnover of the syncytiotrophoblast takes place over the course of a pregnancy, although in the absence of longitudinal studies, it is impossible to determine the extent of this phenomenon. Nonetheless, it is clear that the villous membrane cannot be considered an intact physical barrier and that other elements of the villous trees may play important roles in regulating maternal-fetal transfer.

Placental Vasculature

The development of the fetal vasculature begins during the third week after conception (the fifth week of pregnancy) with the de novo formation of capillaries within the villous stromal core. Hemangioblastic cell cords differentiate under the influence of growth factors such as basic fibroblast growth factor and VEGF.[38] By the beginning of the fourth week, the cords have developed lumens, and the endothelial cells become flattened. Surrounding mesenchymal cells become closely apposed to the tubes and differentiate to form pericytes. During the next few days, connections form between neighboring tubes to form a plexus, and this ultimately unites with the allantoic vessels developing in the connecting stalk to establish the fetal circulation to the placenta.

Exactly when an effective circulation is established through these vessels is difficult to determine. First, the connection between the corporeal and extracorporeal fetal circulations is initially particularly narrow, which suggests there can be little flow. Second, the narrow caliber of the villous capillaries, coupled with the fact that the fetal erythrocytes are nucleated during the first trimester and hence are not readily deformable, will ensure that the circulation presents a high resistance to flow. This is reflected in the Doppler waveform obtained during the first trimester, and the resistance gradually falls as the vessels enlarge over the ensuing weeks.

Early in pregnancy, there are relatively few pericytes, and the capillary network is labile and undergoes considerable remodeling. **Angiogenesis continues until term and results in the formation of capillary sprouts and loops. Both of these processes contribute to the elaboration of terminal villi.**[39] **The caliber of the fetal capillaries is not constant within intermediate and terminal villi, and frequently on the apex of a tight bend, the capillaries become greatly dilated and form sinusoids. These regions may help to reduce vascular resistance and facilitate distribution of fetal blood flow through the villous trees.**[39] **Equally important is the fact that the dilations bring the outer wall of the capillaries into close juxtaposition with the overlying trophoblast. The trophoblast is locally thinned, and as a result, the diffusion distance between the maternal and fetal circulations is reduced to a minimum** (see Fig. 1-5). **Because of their morphologic configuration, these specializations are referred to as** *vasculosyncytial membranes,* **and they are considered the principal sites of gaseous and other diffusional exchanges.** The arrangement can be considered analogous to that in the alveoli of the lung, where the pulmonary capillaries indent into the alveolar epithelium in order to reduce the thickness of the air-blood diffusion barrier. Thinning of the syncytial layer will not only increase the rate of diffusion into the fetal capillaries, it will also reduce the amount of oxygen extracted by the trophoblast en route. The syncytiotrophoblast is highly active metabolically because of the increased rates of protein synthesis and ionic pumping, but by having an uneven distribution of the tissue around the villous surface, the oxygen demands of the fetus and the placenta can be separated to a large extent.

It is notable that development of vasculosyncytial membranes is seen to its greatest extent in the peripheral regions of a placental lobule, where the oxygen concentration is lowest, and also in placentae from high altitudes. In both instances, it is associated with enlargement of the capillary sinusoids and may be viewed as an adaptive response aimed at increasing the diffusing capacity of the placental tissues. Conversely, an increase in the thickness of the villous membrane is often seen in cases of IUGR and in placentae from cigarette smokers. As mentioned earlier, the hydrostatic pressure differential across the villous membrane is an important determinant of the diameter of the capillary dilations and hence of the villous membrane thickness. Raising the pressure in the IVS not only compresses the capillaries, it also increases the resistance within the umbilical circulation. Both effects will impair diffusional exchange, which highlights the importance of full conversion of the spiral arteries.

Vascular changes are observed in many complications of pregnancy,[40] **where they may underpin changes in the topology of the villous tree. Increased branching of the vascular network is observed in placentae from high altitudes, which causes the terminal villi to be shorter and more clustered than normal. At present, no experimental data indicate that this has any impact on placental exchange; but in theory, this shortening of the arteriovenous pathway may lead to increased efficiency.**

PLACENTAL PHYSIOLOGY

The placenta provides the fetus with all its essential nutrients, including water and oxygen, and it gives a route for clearance of fetal excretory products in addition to producing a vast array of protein and steroid hormones and factors necessary for the maintenance of pregnancy. In the first trimester, the SYS and the extraembryonic coelom play an important role in protein synthesis and as an additional transport pathway inside the gestational sac. In the last two trimesters, the majority (95%) of maternofetal exchange takes place across the chorioallantoic placenta.

Physiology of the Secondary Yolk Sac and Exocoelomic Cavity

Now that development of the placenta and the extraembryonic membranes has been covered, we turn to their physiologic roles during pregnancy. Phylogenetically, the oldest membrane is the yolk sac, and the SYS plays a major role in the embryonic development of all mammals. **The function of the yolk sac has been most extensively studied in laboratory rodents. It has been demonstrated that it is one of the initial sites of hematopoiesis, it synthesizes a variety of proteins, and it is involved in maternal-fetal transport.**

The endodermal layer of the human SYS is known to synthesize several serum proteins in common with the fetal liver, such as alpha-fetoprotein (AFP), alpha$_1$-antitrypsin, albumin, prealbumin, and transferrin. With rare exceptions, the secretion of most of these proteins is confined to the embryonic compartments, and the contribution of the SYS to the maternal protein pool is limited.[41] This can explain why their concentrations are always higher in the ECC than in maternal serum. AFP is also produced by the embryonic liver from 6 weeks until delivery; it has a high molecular weight (±70 kDa) and, conversely to hCG, is found in similar amounts on both sides of the amniotic membrane. **Analysis of molecular variants of AFP that have an affinity for concanavalin A have demonstrated that AFP molecules within both the coelomic and amniotic fluids are mainly of yolk sac origin, whereas maternal serum AFP molecules are principally derived from the fetal liver.**[42] **These results suggest that the SYS also has an excretory function and secretes AFP toward the embryonic and extraembryonic compartments. By contrast, AFP molecules of fetal liver origin are probably transferred from the fetal circulation to the maternal circulation, mainly across the placental villous membrane.**

The potential absorptive role of the yolk sac membrane has been evaluated by examining the distribution of proteins and enzymes between the ECC and SYS fluids and by comparing the synthesizing capacity of SYS, fetal liver, and placenta for hCG and AFP.[43] The distribution of the trophoblast-specific hCG in yolk sac and coelomic fluids, together with the absence of hCG mRNA expression in yolk sac tissues, provided the first biologic evidence of its absorptive function. Similarities in the composition of the SYS and coelomic fluids suggest that a free transfer for most molecules occurs between the two corresponding compartments. Conversely, an important concentration gradient exists for most proteins between the ECC and amniotic cavity, indicating that transfer of molecules is limited at the level of the amniotic membrane.

These findings suggest that the yolk sac membrane is an important zone of transfer between the extraembryonic and

embryonic compartments, and that the main flux of molecules occurs from outside the yolk sac—that is, from the ECC—in a direction toward its lumen and subsequently to the embryonic gut and circulation. The recent identification of specific transfer proteins on the mesothelial covering,[3] and of the multifunctional endocytic receptors megalin and cubilin,[44] lends further support to this concept. When after 10 weeks of gestation, the cellular components of the wall of the SYS start to degenerate, this route of transfer is no longer functional, and most exchanges between the ECC and the fetal circulation must then take place at the level of the chorionic plate.

The development and physiologic roles of the ECC are intimately linked with that of the SYS, for which it provides a stable environment. The concentrations of hCG, estriol, and progesterone are higher in the coelomic fluid than in maternal serum[41] and strongly suggest the presence of a direct pathway between the trophoblast and the ECC. Morphologically, this may be via the villous stromal channels and the loose mesenchymal tissue of the chorionic plate. Protein electrophoresis has also shown that the coelomic fluid results from an ultrafiltrate of maternal serum with the addition of specific placental and SYS bioproducts. For the duration of the first trimester, the coelomic fluid remains straw colored and more viscous than the amniotic fluid, which is always clear. This is mainly due to the higher protein concentration in the coelomic fluid than in the amniotic cavity. The concentration of almost every protein is higher in coelomic fluid than in amniotic fluid, ranging from 2 to 50 times higher depending on the molecular weight of the protein investigated.[41] The coelomic fluid has a very slow turnover, so the ECC may act as a reservoir for nutrients needed by the developing embryo. These findings suggest that the ECC is a physiologic liquid extension of the early placenta and an important interface in fetal nutritional pathways. Molecules such as vitamin B$_{12}$, prolactin, and glycodelin (placental protein 14, PP14) are known to be mainly produced by the uterine decidua.[41] This pathway may be pivotal in providing the developing embryo with sufficient nutrients before the intervillous circulation becomes established.[19]

Some analogies can be drawn between the ECC and the antrum within a developing graafian follicle. It has been suggested that the evolution of the latter was necessary to overcome the problem of oxygen delivery to an increasing large mass of avascular cells. Because the contained fluid has no oxygen consumption, it will permit diffusion more freely than an equivalent thickness of cells. However, because neither follicular nor coelomic fluids contain an oxygen carrier, the total oxygen content must be low. An oxygen gradient will inevitably exist between the source and the target, whether it be an oocyte or an embryo. Measurements in human patients undergoing in vitro fertilization (IVF) have demonstrated that the oxygen tension in follicular fluid falls as follicle diameter, assessed by ultrasound, increases. Thus diffusion across the ECC may be an important route of oxygen supply to the embryo before the development of a functional placental circulation, but it will maintain the early fetus in a low-oxygen environment. This may serve to protect the fetal tissues from damage by O$_2$ free radicals and may prevent disruption of signaling pathways during the crucial stages of embryogenesis and organogenesis. The presence in the ECC of molecules with a well-established antioxidant role—such as taurine, transferrin, vitamins A and E, and selenium—supports this hypothesis. Associated with this, the low-oxygen environment may also favor the maintenance of "stemness" in embryonic and placental stem cells. It is notable that the proliferative capacity of the placenta rapidly reduces at the end of the first trimester,[30] which may reflect loss of growth factor stimulation from the endometrial glands or the rise in intraplacental oxygen concentration.

Placental Metabolism and Growth

The critical function of the placenta is illustrated by its high metabolic demands. For example, placental oxygen consumption equals that of the fetus, and it exceeds the fetal rate when expressed on a weight basis (10 mL/min/kg).[45] Glucose is the principal substrate for oxidative metabolism by placental tissues. Of the total glucose leaving the maternal compartment to nourish the uterus and its contents, placental consumption may represent up to 70%. In addition, a significant fraction of placental glucose uptake derives from the fetal circulation. Although one third of placental glucose may be converted to the three-carbon sugar lactate, placental metabolism is not heavily anaerobic. Instead, because the placental tissues are not capable of metabolizing lactate, this may represent a mechanism by which energy resources can be protected for use by the fetal kidneys and liver. During the first trimester, activity is high in the polyol pathways.[46]

These phylogenetically old carbohydrate pathways enable nicotinamide adenine dinucleotide (NAD$^+$) and nicotinamide adenine dinucleotide phosphate (NADP$^+$) to be regenerated independent of lactate production and thereby permit glycolysis to be maintained under the low-oxygen conditions. Metabolomic profiling confirms that first-trimester tissues are not compromised energetically, and the ratio of adenosine triphosphate (ATP) to adenosine diphosphate (ADP) is the same at 8 weeks of gestation as it is at term. The factors that regulate short-term changes in placental oxygen and glucose consumption are uncertain at present, although in pregnancies at high altitudes, the placenta appears to spare oxygen for fetal use at the cost of increased placental utilization of glucose.

The regulation of placental growth is incompletely understood, although dramatic advances have recently been made in the study of imprinted genes. Such genes are expressed in a parent-of-origin manner: paternally expressed genes generally promote placental growth, whereas maternally expressed genes provide restraint. Approximately 100 imprinted genes have been identified at present; these are expressed in the placenta and also in the brain, where they regulate reproductive behaviors such as nest building. Imprinting is achieved through epigenetic mechanisms that are particularly sensitive to environmental factors such as hypoxia, maternal diet, and stress. Perturbations of imprinting therefore represent a possible mechanism linking extrinsic changes to alterations in placental differentiation and function.

Normal term placental weight averages 450 g, which represents approximately one seventh (one sixth with cord and membranes) of the fetal weight. Large placentae, either ultrasonographically or at delivery, may prompt investigation into possible etiologies: increased placental size has been associated with maternal anemia, fetal anemia associated with erythrocyte isoimmunization, and hydrops fetalis secondary to fetal α-thalassemia with hemoglobin Bart's. The association of a large placenta with maternal diabetes mellitus is also recognized, possibly a result of insulin-stimulated mitogenic activity or enhanced angiogenesis. Enlarged placentae are also found in cloned animals, presumably because of defects in the expression of imprinted genes, and in animals in which specific gene products have been deleted. **In humans, an increased ratio of placental size to fetal weight is associated with increased morbidity for the offspring, both in the neonatal period and subsequently.**

An array of growth-promoting peptide hormones (factors) have been characterized in placental tissue at the protein and/or receptor levels. These include the insulin receptor, IGF-I and IGF-II, EGF, leptin, placental growth factor, placental growth hormone, placental lactogen, and a variety of cytokines and chemokines, each of which has been shown to play an important role in fetal/placental development. **IGF-I and IGF-II are polypeptides with a high degree of homology to human proinsulin; both are produced within the placenta and in the fetus and mother, both circulate bound to carrier proteins, and they are 50 times more potent than insulin in stimulating cell growth.** EGF increases RNA and DNA synthesis and cell multiplication in a wide variety of cell types. The integrated physiologic role of these and other potential placental growth factors in regulating placental growth remains to be fully defined; however, the development of null-mutation mouse models for IGF-I, IGF-II, IGF-Ir, and IGF-IIr—as well as for the EGF receptor—have provided evidence in this regard.[47] Specifically, the EGF receptor appears important in placental development, as does IGF-II. Knockout of IGF-II results in diminished placental size, whereas deletion of the *H19* gene that regulates imprinting of the IGF-II clearance receptor results in an increase in placental size.

Conversely, **exposure to chronic hypoxia at high altitudes, nutrient deprivation, infection, and malperfusion due to deficient remodeling of the spiral arteries all lead to a small placenta and fetal IUGR.** Inhibition of protein synthesis through activation of the integrated stress response pathways, formerly referred to as *endoplasmic reticulum stress* or the *unfolded protein response*, and deactivation of the mTOR/AKT pathway appears to be a common feature in many cases.[48] Translational arrest also appears to reduce complexes of the mitochondrial electron transport chain at the protein, but not mRNA, level at high altitudes, which renders ATP levels lower in these placentae compared with sea level controls.[49] Modeling these changes in placental cell lines in vitro leads to a reduction in the rate of cell proliferation. Exposure to exogenous corticosteroid may also result in diminished placental size and represents another pathway through which stress and undernutrition may act.

Placental Transport

For the bulk of pregnancy, the chorioallantoic placenta is the major site of exchange of nutrients (including oxygen) and of waste products of fetal metabolism (including carbon dioxide) between mother and fetus. As described above, histotrophic nutrition occurs in early pregnancy, and the yolk sac probably contributes to the uptake of nutrients and their transport to the embryo. However, once blood flow to the IVS begins at around 10 weeks of gestation, exchange across the barrier between maternal and fetal circulations within the villi will be predominant, although there may be some limited transfer between maternal blood in the endometrium and the fluid of the amniotic sac. As discussed below, many of the transport mechanisms required to effect exchange are present in the placenta by 10 weeks, and these may be upregulated or downregulated throughout the rest of pregnancy to meet the requirements of fetal growth and homeostasis. The impact of perturbations of nutrient transport on fetal growth has recently been reviewed.[50]

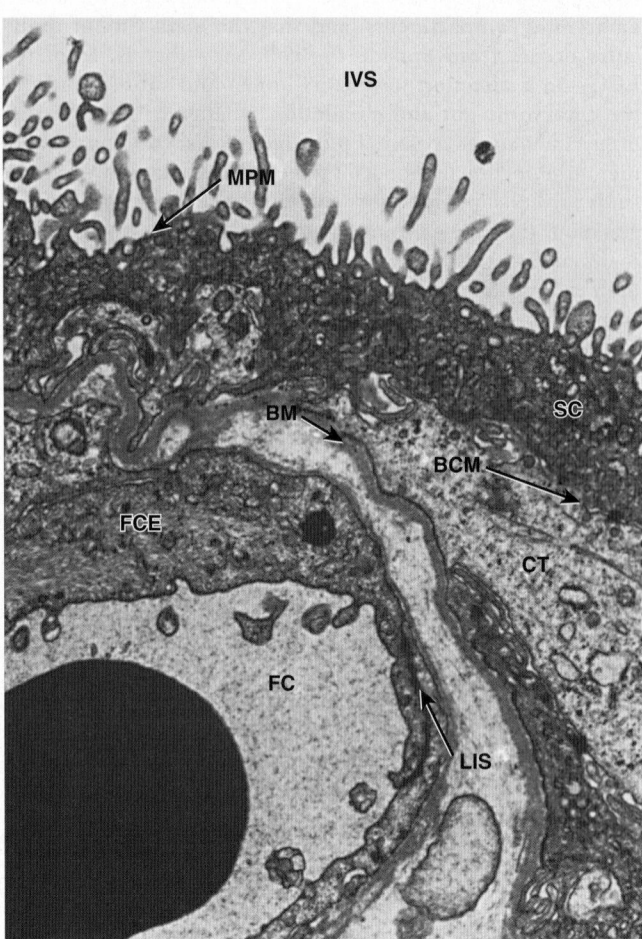

FIG 1-6 Electron micrograph of human placenta demonstrates the cellular and extracellular components with which solutes must interact in moving from the maternal intervillous space (IVS) to the lumen of the fetal capillary (FC). BCM, basal cell membrane of the syncytiotrophoblast cell; CT, cytotrophoblast; FCE, fetal capillary endothelial cell; LIS, lateral intercellular space of fetal endothelial cell; MPM, microvillous plasma membrane of the syncytiotrophoblast; SC, syncytiotrophoblast. (Courtesy Kent L. Thornburg, PhD, Center for Developmental Health, Oregon Health Science University, Portland.)

For a molecule to reach fetal plasma from maternal plasma and vice versa, it must cross the syncytiotrophoblast, the matrix of the villous core, and the endothelium of the fetal capillary (Fig. 1-6). **The syncytiotrophoblast is the transporting epithelium and is considered to be the major locus of exchange selectivity and regulation. However, both the matrix and endothelium will contribute to the properties of the placenta as an organ of exchange because both contribute to the thickness of the barrier; they may also act as a size filter in that the finite width of the space between the endothelial cells is likely to restrict the diffusion of larger molecules.**

The fact that the syncytiotrophoblast is a true syncytium, with no obvious intercellular or extracellular water-filled spaces, suggests that it forms a tight barrier. However, physiologic data suggest that this is not the case (see below). Nevertheless, regulated exchange most likely occurs predominantly across the two opposing plasma membranes, the *microvillous* (maternal facing) and *basal* (fetal facing) membranes.

Maternal-fetal exchange across the placenta may occur, broadly, by one of four mechanisms: (1) bulk flow/solvent

drag, (2) diffusion, (3) transporter-mediated mechanisms, and (4) endocytosis/exocytosis.

Bulk Flow/Solvent Drag

Differences in hydrostatic and osmotic pressures between the maternal and fetal circulations within the exchange barrier drive water transfer by bulk flow, which drags along dissolved solutes. These solutes are filtered as they move through the components of the barrier. Water movement may be via paracellular channels (see below) or across the plasma membranes. The latter may be enhanced by the presence of aquaporins, integral membrane proteins that form water pores in the plasma membrane.

Hydrostatic pressure gradients will be created by differences in maternal and fetal blood pressure and vascular resistances on the maternal and fetal sides of the placenta. Although the actual pressures are impossible to measure in vivo at this time, evidence suggests that they are lower in the IVS than in the fetal capillaries. Because this would drive water from the fetus to the mother, which is incompatible with fetal growth, clearly a deficit exists in our knowledge and understanding; the assumptions involved in assessing the hydrostatic pressures could simply be wrong. On the other hand, fetal-maternal water transfer driven by hydrostatic pressures may be opposed, and exceeded by, maternal-fetal water transfer driven by osmotic pressure gradients created by the active transport of solute to the fetus across the syncytiotrophoblast. These forces may well be altered as gestation proceeds. Altogether, this is an important area in which further research is required.

Diffusion

Diffusion of any molecule occurs in both directions across any barrier. When a concentration gradient exists—and/or for charged species, an electrical gradient—one of these unidirectional fluxes (rates of transfer) is greater in one direction than it is in the other so that there is a net flux in one direction. Net flux (*Jnet*) of solute across the placenta for an uncharged molecule may be described by an adaptation of Fick's law of diffusion:

$$Jnet = (AD/l)(Cm - Cf) \text{ moles/unit time}$$

where *A* is the surface area of the barrier available for exchange, *D* is the diffusion coefficient in water of the molecule (smaller molecules will have a larger D), *l* is the thickness of the exchange barrier across which diffusion is occurring, *Cm* is the mean concentration of the molecule in maternal plasma, and *Cf* is the mean concentration of solute in the fetal circulation.

Small, relatively hydrophobic molecules such as O_2 and CO_2 will diffuse rapidly across the plasma membranes of the barrier, so their flux is dependent much more on the concentration gradients than on the surface area of the barrier available for exchange or the thickness of the exchange barrier across which diffusion is occurring. Because this concentration gradient is affected predominantly by the blood flows in both circulations, the diffusion of such molecules is said to be *flow limited*. This explains why reductions in uterine or umbilical flow may result in fetal asphyxia and, consequently, growth restriction.

By contrast, **hydrophilic molecules such as glucose and amino acids will not diffuse across plasma membranes easily; rather their concentration gradients are maintained, and flux**

will be determined predominantly by barrier surface area and thickness. Flux of such "membrane-limited" molecules is not affected by blood flow unless blood flow is dramatically reduced, but it will be altered if abnormal placental development results in reduced surface area of the barrier available for exchange or increased thickness of the barrier; evidence suggests that this occurs in idiopathic IUGR.[27]

In Fick's equation, the term *AD/l* is equivalent to what is described as the permeability of a membrane. Measurements of the passive permeability of the placenta have been made in vivo[51] and in vitro[52] utilizing hydrophilic molecules that would be unlikely to be affected by blood flow and which are not substrates for transporter proteins. These measurements show that **an indirect relationship exists between permeability and the molecular size of the hydrophilic tracer.** Such a relationship is explained, most simply, by the presence of extracellular water-filled channels, or pores, across the exchange barrier through which the molecules can diffuse. The existence of this "paracellular permeability pathway" has been controversial because of the syncytiotrophoblast being syncytial, with no obvious paracellular channels. However, transtrophoblastic channels may be present that are not normally visible by electron microscopy. Furthermore, the areas of syncytial denudation that occur in every placenta may provide a route through which molecules may diffuse.[52]

Rates of transfer of hydrophobic molecules by flow-limited diffusion may change over gestation because, as described in previous sections, both uteroplacental and fetoplacental blood flows change. Changes in concentration—and for charged molecules, changes in electrical gradients—between maternal and fetal plasma will also affect rates of transfer. Gestational changes do occur in the maternal and fetal plasma concentrations of solutes, and this affects driving forces. For example, **glucose and amino acid concentrations in maternal plasma increase over gestation, which is due at least in part to the effects of insulin resistance in pregnancy, and of hormones such as human placental lactogen (hPL).** If expressed across the placental exchange barrier, a maternal-fetal electrical potential difference (PD_{mf}) will have an effect on the exchange of ions. In the human, the PD_{mf} is small but significant between maternal and fetal circulations (-2.7 ± 0.4 mV fetus negative) in mid gestation[53] and zero or close to it at term.[54] A PD between the mother and the coelomic cavity has been measured in first-trimester pregnancies.[55] No change was apparent in this PD value (8.7 ± 1 mV fetus negative) between 9 and 13 weeks' gestation, which was somewhat higher than the PD across the syncytiotrophoblast (3 mV) measured using microelectrodes in term placental villi in vitro. The in vitro PD across the microvillous membrane of human syncytiotrophoblast decreases between the early (median, -32 mV) and late first trimester (median, -24 mV), with a small subsequent fall at term (-21 mV). This suggests that as pregnancy progresses, the driving force for cation flux into the syncytiotrophoblast decreases, and for anions it increases.

Transporter Protein–Mediated Processes

Transporter proteins are integral membrane proteins that catalyze transfer of solutes across plasma membranes at faster rates than would occur by diffusion. Transporter proteins are a large and diverse group of molecules generally characterized by showing substrate specificity. That is, one transporter or class of transporters will predominantly

transfer one substrate or class of substrates (e.g., amino acids) by having appropriate saturation kinetics (i.e., raising the concentration of a substrate solute will not infinitely increase the rate at which it is transferred on transporters) and by being competitively inhibitable (two structurally similar molecules will compete for transfer by a particular transporter protein). Transporter proteins are found most abundantly in the placenta in the microvillous and basal plasma membranes of the syncytiotrophoblast. A detailed description of all these is beyond the scope of this chapter but may be found in work by Atkinson and colleagues.[56] In overview, channel proteins form pores in the plasma membrane and allow diffusion of ions such as K^+ and Ca^{2+}, and transporters allow facilitated diffusion down concentration gradients, such as the GLUT1 glucose transporter. *Exchange transporters,* such as the Na^+/H^+ exchanger involved in pH homeostasis of the syncytiotrophoblast and fetus, and *cotransporters,* such as the system-A amino acid transporter—which cotransports small hydrophilic amino acids such as alanine, glycine, and serine with Na^+—require the maintenance of an ion gradient through secondary input of energy, often via Na^+/K^+ATPase. Finally, *active transporters* directly utilize ATP to transfer against concentration gradients; these include the Na^+/K^+ATPase and the Ca^{2+}ATPase, which pumps Ca^{2+} across the basal plasma membrane from syncytiotrophoblast cytosol toward the fetal circulation.

Gestational changes in the flux of solutes through transporter proteins could result from changes in the number of transporters in each plasma membrane, their turnover (i.e., the rate of binding to and release from the transporter), or their affinity for solute as well as from changes in the driving forces acting on them, such as electrochemical gradients and ATP availability. A variety of evidence shows that such developmental changes do occur. Using the technique of isolating and purifying microvillous plasma membrane and radioisotopic tracers to measure transport rates in vesicles formed from these membranes, it has been shown that the V_{max} of the Na^+-dependent system-A amino acid transporter increases by about fourfold per milligram of membrane protein between the first trimester and term. The activity of the system-y^+ cationic amino acid (e.g., arginine, lysine) transporter increases over gestation, whereas the activity of the system-y^+L transporter decreases.[57] This decrease in system-y^+L activity is due to a decrease in the affinity of the transporter for substrate and is accompanied by an increased expression of 4F2hc monomer of the dimer protein.[57] The reason for this decline is not known but could well be associated with a specific fetal need. **Glucose transporter 1 (GLUT1) expression in microvillous membrane increases between the first trimester and term.**[58] Na^+/H^+ exchanger activity is lower in first-trimester microvillous membrane vesicles compared with that at term,[59] a result borne out by studies on the intrasyncytiotrophoblast pH of isolated placental villi from these two stages in gestation. Interestingly, the expression of the NHE1 isoform of this exchanger in the microvillous membrane does not change across gestation, but the expression of both of its NHE2 and NHE3 isoforms increases between weeks 14 and 18 and term.[59] In contrast, no difference is apparent in Cl^-/HCO_3^- exchanger activity or, by Western blotting, expression of its AE1 isoform between first trimester and term. Our understanding of how these gestational changes are regulated is currently sparse; studies in knockout mice suggest that hormones from the fetus such as IGF-II, which signals demand for the nutrients required

for growth, are important, but much further work is needed in this area.

Endocytosis/Exocytosis
Endocytosis is the process by which molecules become entrapped in invaginations of the microvillous plasma membrane of the syncytiotrophoblast, which eventually pinch off and form vesicles within the cytosol. Such vesicles may diffuse through the intracellular compartment, and if they avoid fusion with lysosomes, they eventually fuse with the basal plasma membrane and undergo exocytosis, releasing their contents into the fetal milieu. **Evidence suggests that immunoglobulin G (IgG) and other large proteins may cross the placenta by this mechanism.**[56,60] Specificity and the ability to avoid lysosomal degradation during the endocytosis phase may be provided by the presence of receptors for IgG in the microvillous membrane invaginations and vesicles. However, this mechanism of transfer and its gestational regulation, if any, is still not well understood.

A Selective Barrier
In addition to facilitating maternal-fetal transfer, the placenta also acts as a selective barrier that prevents certain substances and maternal hormones from either crossing to the fetus or crossing in an active form. Members of the multidrug-resistance protein (MRP) family, the breast-cancer–resistant protein (BCRP), and P-glycoprotein are present on the apical surface of the syncytiotrophoblast and in the endothelium of the villous capillaries at term. These transporters mediate the efflux of a wide range of anionic and cationic organic compounds in an ATP-dependent manner, and their expression at the mRNA level shows a general increase toward term. **Within the syncytioplasm are a range of cytochrome P450 (CYP) enzymes. Although more restricted than in the liver, placental CYP-mediated metabolism is capable of detoxifying several drugs and foreign chemicals.** Alcohol dehydrogenase is also present, along with glutathione transferase and N-acetyltransferase. This combination of efflux transporters and defensive enzymes provides a degree of protection to the fetus against exposure to potentially noxious xenobiotics, although many drugs and chemicals can still cross and act as teratogens.

The syncytiotrophoblast also expresses the enzyme 11-β-hydroxysteroid dehydrogenase 2 (11β-HSD2), which oxidizes maternal cortisol into the inactive metabolite, cortisone. This process allows the fetal hypothalamic-pituitary-adrenal (HPA) axis to develop in isolation from maternal cortisol and also protects the fetal tissues against the growth-inhibitory effects of corticosteroids. However, the activity of placental 11β-HSD2 can be perturbed in pathologic pregnancies associated with growth restriction, and raised fetal levels of cortisol may contribute to the developmental programming of organ systems.

Substance-Specific Placental Transport
Respiratory Gases
The transfer of the primary respiratory gases, oxygen and carbon dioxide, is likely to be flow limited. Thus, the driving force for placental gas exchange is the partial pressure gradient between the maternal and fetal circulations. Early in gestation, the human embryo develops in a low-oxygen environment. Such an environment appears to be necessary for the avoidance of teratogenesis and the maintenance of stem

cell populations. After about week 10 of gestation, the placenta becomes important as a respiratory organ. Indeed, estimates of human placental diffusing capacities predict that the placenta's efficiency as an organ of respiratory gas exchange allows equilibrium of oxygen and carbon dioxide between the maternal IVS and the fetal capillaries. However, this prediction varies from the observed 10 mm Hg difference in oxygen tension between the umbilical and uterine veins and between the umbilical vein and IVS. By contrast, the PCO_2 difference from the umbilical to the uterine vein is small (3 mm Hg). PO_2 differences could be explained by areas of uneven distribution of maternal-to-fetal blood flows or shunting; this limits fetal and maternal blood exchange, a process that may be an active one, as in the lung. The most important contribution, however, is likely the high metabolic rate of the placental tissues. Thus trophoblast cell O_2 consumption and CO_2 production lower umbilical vein O_2 tension and increase uterine vein CO_2 tension to a greater degree than could be explained by an inert barrier for respiratory gas transfer.

The arteriovenous difference in the uterine circulation and the venoarterial difference in the umbilical circulation widen during periods of reduced blood flow. **Proportionate O_2 uptake increases and O_2 consumption remains unchanged over a fairly wide range of blood flows. Thus both uterine and umbilical blood flows can fall significantly without decreasing fetal O_2 consumption.**[61] **Conversely, unilateral umbilical artery occlusion is associated with significant fetal effects.**

Carbon dioxide is carried in the fetal blood both as dissolved carbon dioxide and as bicarbonate. Because of its charged nature, fetal to maternal bicarbonate transfer is limited. However, CO_2 likely diffuses from fetus to mother in its molecular form, and $[HCO_3^-]$ does not contribute significantly to fetal CO_2 elimination.

Glucose

Placental permeability for D-glucose is at least 50 times greater than the value predicted on the basis of size and lipid solubility. Specific transporter proteins of the GLUT family are present on both the microvillous and basal membranes of the syncytiotrophoblast, although they are at greater density in the former.[58] This distribution may provide additional uptake capacity to meet the metabolic demands of the syncytium. **The primary human placental glucose transporter is GLUT1, a sodium-independent facilitated transporter, unlike the sodium-dependent transporters found in the adult kidney and intestine.** This transporter is not insulin sensitive. Placental GLUT1 can be saturated at high substrate concentrations; 50% saturation is observed at glucose levels of approximately 5 mM (90 mg/dL). Thus glucose transfer from mother to fetus is not linear, and transfer rates decrease as maternal glucose concentrations increase. This effect is reflected in fetal blood glucose levels following maternal sugar loading. **Modification of transporter expression within the placenta also occurs in response to maternal diabetes.** In this setting, GLUT1 expression is thought to increase on the rate-limiting basal membrane, while it remains constant on the maternal-facing microvillous membrane.[62] Alterations in transporter expression may also depend on gestational stage (e.g., early in pregnancy, GLUT4 may be present within the placenta) and maternal nutrition/placental blood flow. A third transporter, GLUT3, has also been noted in the fetal-facing placental endothelium. Its presence within the syncytiotrophoblast remains controversial.

Amino Acids

Amino acid concentrations are generally higher in fetal umbilical cord plasma than in maternal plasma. Like monosaccharides, amino acids enter and exit the syncytiotrophoblast via specific membrane transporter proteins. These proteins allow amino acids to be transported against a concentration gradient into the syncytiotrophoblast, and subsequently—if not directly—into the fetal circulation.

Multiple class-specific transporter proteins mediate neutral, anionic, and cationic amino acid transport into the syncytiotrophoblast. These include both sodium-dependent and sodium-independent transporters.[63] In many cases, amino acid entry is coupled to sodium in cotransport systems located at the microvillous membrane facing the maternal IVS; the system-A amino acid transporter—for which glycine, alanine, and serine are substrates—is a good example of such a cotransport system. As long as an inwardly directed sodium gradient is maintained, trophoblast cell amino acid concentrations will exceed maternal blood levels. **The sodium gradient is maintained by Na^+/K^+ATPase located on the basal or fetal side of the syncytiotrophoblast. In addition, high trophoblast levels of amino acids transported by sodium-dependent transporters can "drive" uptake of other amino acids via transporters that function as "exchangers"** (Fig. 1-7).[63] Examples of these include ASCT1 and y^+LAT/4F2HC. Still other transporters function in a sodium-independent fashion. Individual amino acids may be transported by single or multiple transport proteins, and transport systems have been defined in human placenta. A list of the transporters and their changes in IUGR is found in Table 1-1).

SNAT1 and SNAT2, sodium-dependent transporters with activity localized on both the microvillous and basal membranes of the syncytiotrophoblast, are responsible for the system-A transporter activity of the neutral amino acids described above. SNAT4, with similar substrate specificity, is present early in gestation. Other sodium-dependent transport activities localized

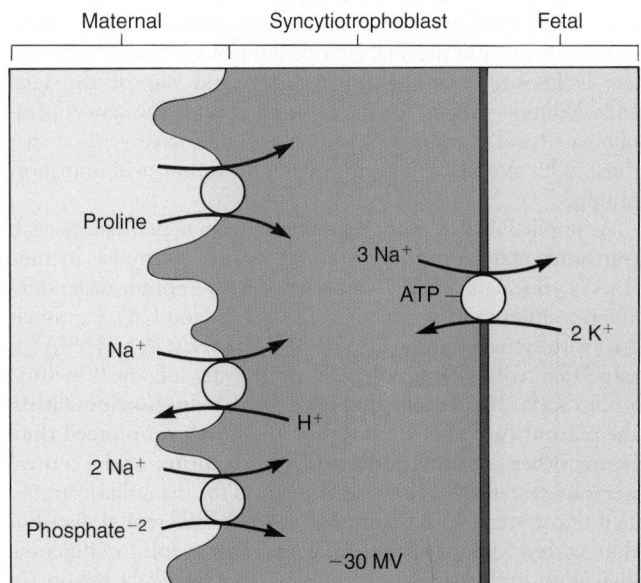

FIG 1-7 Pathways for sodium entry into the syncytiotrophoblast and exit to the fetal circulation. ATP, adenosine triphosphate. (Data from references 101-104.)

TABLE 1-1   CHANGES IN ACTIVITY OF TRANSPORTER PROTEINS IN THE MICROVILLOUS AND BASAL PLASMA MEMBRANES OF PLACENTAE FROM PREGNANCIES COMPLICATED BY INTRAUTERINE GROWTH RESTRICTION*

TRANSPORTER	MVM	BM	REFERENCE
System A	Decreased	No change	91
System L (leucine)	Decreased	Decreased	92
System y⁺/y⁺L (arginine/lysine)	No change	Decreased	57, 92
System β	Decreased	No change	93
Na⁺-independent taurine	No change	Decreased	93, 94
GLUT1	No change	No change	91, 95
Na⁺/K⁺ATPase	Decreased	No change	96
Ca²⁺ATPase	Not present	Increased	97
Na⁺/H⁺ exchanger	Decreased	Activity not present	98
H⁺/lactate	No change	Decreased	99

*Compared with normal pregnancies.
ATPase, adenosine triphosphatase; *BM*, basal membrane; *MVM*, microvillous membrane.

to the microvillous membrane include that for β-amino acids such as taurine (TauT) and perhaps glycine transport via system GLY. Sodium-independent transporters that mediate neutral amino acid transfer on the microvillous membrane include system L (LAT-1, 2/4F2HC), which exhibits a high affinity for amino acids with bulky side chains such as leucine, and y⁺LAT/4F2HC, which is capable of transporting both neutral and cationic amino acids such as lysine and arginine. The aforementioned transporters are heterodimeric and require the combination of two distinct proteins with the cell membrane for transport to occur. Cationic amino acids may also be transported by the sodium-independent transport protein CAT1, whereas anionic amino acids (glutamate, aspartate) are transported by the sodium-dependent transport proteins EAAT1 through EAAT4. Basal membrane transport activities are similar; however, a predominance of sodium-independent transport and exchange (e.g., ASCT1) allows flow of amino acids down their concentration gradients into the fetal endothelium/blood space. Although less is known regarding transfer into and out of the fetal endothelium—which, for the most part, abuts the syncytiotrophoblast basal membrane—available studies have verified that these cells also have a complement of amino acid transport proteins.

As implied earlier, **more than one protein may mediate each transport activity within a single tissue.** Examples include EAAT1 through EAAT5, associated with sodium-dependent anionic amino acid transfer; CAT1, CAT2, and CAT2a, associated with system-y+ activity; and SNAT1, SNAT2, and SNAT4, associated with sodium-dependent transfer of small neutral amino acids. **The reasons that underlie this duplication within the placenta are unclear, but they are more pronounced than in any other organ with the possible exception of the central nervous system.** Certainly, as is the case for the anionic amino acid transporters EAAT1 through EAAT5, differential distribution within various tissue elements plays a role. Differential regulation within single cell types is another likely reason. In isolated trophoblast cells, system-A activity (sodium-dependent transfer of small neutral amino acids) is upregulated by the absence of amino acids partially because of an increase in carrier

affinity. Conversely, increases in trophoblast amino acid concentrations may suppress uptake (transinhibition). These mechanisms serve to maintain constant trophoblast cell amino acid levels during fluctuations in maternal plasma concentrations. **Insulin has also been shown to upregulate this transport activity, as has IGF-I.**

The coordination between placental/fetal metabolism and amino acid transfer is illustrated by the anionic amino acids glutamate and aspartate, which are poorly transported from mother to fetus. **Glutamate, however, is produced by the fetal liver from glutamine and is then taken up across the basal membrane of the placenta. Within the placenta, the majority of glutamate is metabolized and utilized as an energy source.** As a result, sodium-dependent anionic amino acid transfer activity is of particular importance on the basal membrane, as is system-ASC (ASCT1) activity, which is responsible for the uptake of serine—also produced by the fetal liver—into the placenta.

Lipids

Esterified fatty acids (triglycerides) are present in maternal serum as components of chylomicrons and very-low-density lipoproteins (VLDLs). Before transfer across the placenta, lipoprotein lipase interacts with these particles and releases free fatty acids, which are relatively insoluble in plasma and circulate bound to albumin owing to their hydrophobic nature. As a result, fatty acid transfer involves dissociation from maternal protein and subsequent association with placental proteins, first at the plasma membrane (FABPpm) and then after transfer into the cell (thought to be via FAT/CD36 and FATP) with intracytoplasmic binding proteins. Transfer out of the syncytiotrophoblast is less well understood but is thought to occur via interaction with FAT/CD36 and FATP, which are present at both the microvillous and basal membrane surfaces. Subsequently, interaction with fetal plasma proteins occurs. Placental fatty acid uptake is in part regulated by peroxisome proliferator–activated receptor γ (PPARγ) and retinoid X receptor (RXR). In turn, long-chain polyunsaturated fatty acids (PUFAs) taken up by the placenta can be metabolized into PPAR ligands, thus affecting the expression of an array of placental genes, including those that influence fatty acid metabolism and transfer. **Fatty acids may also be oxidized within the placenta as a source of energy.** Although precise interactions and mechanisms remain uncertain, it is clear that lipid uptake is of profound importance to fetal development. Targeted deletion of the gene encoding FATP4 (*Slc27a4*), found within the placenta, results in fetal lethality.[64]

Early studies documented that placental fatty acid transfer increases logarithmically with decreasing chain length (C16 to C8) and then declines somewhat for C6 and C4. However, more recent work has clarified the fact **that essential fatty acids are, in general, transferred more efficiently than are nonessential fatty acids.**[65] Of these, docosahexaenoic acid seems to be transferred more efficiently than arachidonic acid; oleic acid is transferred least efficiently. As in the case of amino acids discussed earlier, **the fetus is significantly enriched in long-chain PUFAs compared with the mother.** Such selectivity may also relate to the composition of triglycerides in maternal serum because lipoprotein lipase preferentially cleaves fatty acids in the two positions. In general, **fatty acids transferred to the fetus reflect maternal serum lipids and diet.** Placental fatty transfer has been recently reviewed.[65] **Evidence also suggests that the placental secretion of leptin, a hormone generally secreted by**

adipocytes, may promote maternal lipolysis, thus providing both placenta and fetus the means by which to ensure an adequate lipid supply. Another possible mechanism by which lipids may be excreted from the placenta involves the synthesis and secretion of apolipoprotein (apo) B–containing lipoproteins. The relative importance of this pathway in the human placenta is unclear. Placental uptake and excretion of cholesterol is discussed in the section on receptor-mediated endocytosis.

Water and Ions

Water transfer from mother to fetus is determined by a balance of osmotic, hydrostatic, and colloid osmotic forces at the placental interface. Calculation of osmotic pressure from individual solute concentrations is unreliable because osmotic pressure forces depend on the membrane permeability to each solute. Thus sodium and chloride, the principal plasma solutes, are relatively permeable across the placenta and would not be expected to contribute important osmotic effects. As a result, although human fetal plasma osmolality is equal to or greater than maternal plasma osmolality, these measured values do not reflect the actual osmotic force on either side of the membranes.[66] Coupled with findings that hydrostatic pressure may be greater in the umbilical vein than in the IVS, these data do not explain mechanisms for fetal water accumulation. Alternatively, **colloid osmotic pressure differences and active solute transport probably represent the main determinants of net water fluxes—approximately 20 mL/day. It is likely, however, given the large (3.6 L/hr) flux of water between mother and fetus that more active mechanisms, including perhaps controlled changes in end-vessel resistance, play a significant role.** In fact, water flux occurs through both transcellular and paracellular pathways. Water channels (aquaporins 1, 3, 8, and 9) have been identified within the placenta, but their roles relative to water flux within the fetal placental unit have not been discerned.

In comparison to other epithelia, the specialized placental mechanisms for ion transport are incompletely understood. Multiple mechanisms of sodium transport exist in syncytiotrophoblast membranes (see Fig. 1-7). The maternal-facing microvillous membrane contains, at a minimum, 1) multiple amino acid cotransporters; 2) a sodium phosphate cotransporter, in which two sodium ions are transported with each phosphate radical; 3) a sodium-hydrogen ion antiport that exchanges one proton for each sodium ion that enters the cell; and 4) other nutrient transporters. In addition, both sodium and potassium channels have been described. A membrane potential with the inside negative (-30 mV) would promote sodium entry from the IVS, and this probably exists.[67] The fetally directed basal side of the cell contains the Na^+/K^+ATPase. The microvillous or maternal-facing trophoblast membrane has an anion exchanger (AE1) that mediates chloride transit across this membrane in association with Cl^- conductance pathways (channels) present in both the microvillous and basal membranes.[68] Paracellular pathways also play an important role. The integration and regulation of these various mechanisms for sodium and chloride transport from mother to fetus is not completely understood; however, accumulating evidence suggests that mineralocorticoids may regulate placental sodium transfer. Further, sodium-hydrogen exchange, mediated by multiple members of the NHE family (NHE1, NHE2, and NHE3), is regulated both over gestation and in response to IUGR, as is expression of Na^+/K^+ATPase.

Calcium

Calcium is an essential nutrient for the developing fetus, and ionized calcium levels are higher in fetal than in maternal blood. Higher fetal calcium levels are due to a syncytiotrophoblast basal membrane ATP-dependent Ca^{2+} transport system that exhibits high affinity (nanomolar range) for calcium. Indeed, analogous to amino acid and sodium-hydrogen exchange proteins, multiple isoforms of the plasma membrane calcium ATPase (PMCAs 1 through 4) are expressed within the placenta[69]; the placental expression of PMCA3 has been linked to intrauterine bone accrual. Sodium-calcium exchange (NCX) proteins may also play a role in the extrusion of calcium from the trophoblast—again, multiple isoforms are expressed within the placenta. A variety of calcium channels have been identified in both the apical and basal membranes; TRPV6 plays a significant role in calcium uptake into the syncytiotrophoblast.[69] Intracellular calcium is bound by multiple calcium-binding proteins, which have been identified within the placenta; these include CaBP9k, CaBP28k, CaBP57k, oncomodulin, S-100P, S-100α, and S-100β. **CaBP9k** in particular is thought to have a regulatory and perhaps rate-limiting role. Calcium transport across the placenta is increased by the calcium-dependent regulatory protein **calmodulin,** regulated by 1,25 dihydroxycholecalciferol, calcitonin, parathyroid hormone–related protein, and parathyroid hormone.

Placental Nutrient Supply and Intrauterine Growth Restriction

The term *placental insufficiency* has been used as a cause of IUGR but has been poorly understood until recently. It is often taken as being synonymous with *reduced uteroplacental blood flow* or *reduced umbilical blood flow.* Doppler measurements of such blood flows have been of assistance in diagnosing and assessing the severity of IUGR but are limited in value.[70] It is now clear that other variables that determine the capacity of the placenta to supply nutrients may also contribute to IUGR. For example, **in IUGR, the surface area of the exchange barrier is decreased and its thickness decreased,**[27] and such changes are likely to markedly decrease the passive permeability of the placenta. Furthermore, **considerable evidence now shows that the activity and expression of transporter proteins in the syncytiotrophoblast is altered in IUGR.**[71,72] The reported data are summarized in Table 1-1. As can be seen, activity of several transporters decrease, at least one increases, and others show no change at all. This variation in response could reflect whether a change in the placenta is *causative* in IUGR (e.g., the decrease in system-A amino acid transporter activity) or *compensatory* (e.g., the increase in Ca^{2+} ATPase activity) and could also reflect differential regulation of the transporters. Understanding these placental phenotypes of IUGR may well give clues to novel means of diagnosing and even treating the condition.

Vasomotor Control of the Umbilicoplacental Circulation

The placenta represents an extensive extracorporeal vascular bed that must be perfused by the fetal heart. In addition, for efficient exchange, flow in the maternal and placental circulations must be matched as closely as possible. Hence, **there must be local control of vascular resistance within the fetal placental vascular bed.** The principal resistance vessels in the placental circulation are the muscular arteries contained within the stem villi. In the absence of any nerves within the placenta, vasomotor control must be performed by local paracrine factors. Nitric oxide, carbon monoxide, and hydrogen sulfide have been identified as having powerful vasodilatory effects.[73] It is thought that under normal conditions, the villous vascular bed is fully dilated, and it might constrict under hypoxic conditions to redistribute flow to better perfused areas of the placenta, analogous to the situation in the lung. It is notable that expression of the enzyme cystathionine γ-lyase, which synthesizes hydrogen sulfide, is reduced in the smooth muscle that surrounds the resistance arteries in growth-restricted placentae that display abnormal umbilical artery Doppler waveforms,[73] which suggests it plays an important physiologic role.

Placental Endocrinology

The human placenta is an important endocrine organ. It signals the presence of the conceptus to the mother in early pregnancy and optimizes the intrauterine environment and maternal physiology for the benefit of fetal growth. **Two major groups of hormones are produced: the** *steroid hormones,* **progesterone and the estrogens, and** *peptide hormones,* **such as human chorionic gonadotropin (hCG) and hPL.** All are predominantly synthesized in the syncytiotrophoblast, and although the synthetic pathways have been generally elucidated, the factors that regulate secretion are still largely unknown. During early pregnancy, the hormones increase maternal food intake and energy storage, whereas later they mobilize these resources for use by the fetus.

Progesterone

During the first few weeks of pregnancy, progesterone is mainly derived from the corpus luteum; gradually, as the placental mass increases, this organ's contribution becomes dominant with the production of around 250 mg/day of progesterone. The corpus luteum regresses at around 9 weeks, and at that stage, it is no longer essential for the maintenance of a pregnancy.

Placental synthesis of progesterone begins with the conversion of cholesterol to pregnenolone, as in other steroid-secreting tissues. Placental tissues are poor at synthesizing cholesterol, and so they utilize maternal cholesterol derived from low-density lipoproteins (LDLs) taken up in coated pits on the surface of the syncytiotrophoblast. Conversion of cholesterol to pregnenolone occurs on the inner aspect of the inner mitochondrial membrane, catalyzed by cytochrome P450scc (CYP11A1), and in other steroidogenic tissues, the delivery of cholesterol to this site is the principal rate-limiting step in progesterone synthesis. There, delivery is facilitated by the steroidogenic acute regulatory (StAR) protein, which binds and transports cholesterol, but this protein is not present in the human placenta.[74] Instead, a homologue, MLN64, may carry out a similar function; freshly isolated cytotrophoblast cells appear to contain concentrations of cholesterol that are near saturating for progesterone synthesis, which indicates that supply of the precursor is not rate limiting.[75] Side-chain cleavage requires molecular oxygen, but it is unclear whether the conditions that prevail during the first trimester are rate limiting. The rate of production of pregnenolone from radiolabeled cholesterol by placental homogenates in vitro increases throughout the first trimester, and both the concentration and activity of P450scc increase in placental mitochondria from the first trimester to term. These changes, coupled with the expansion of the syncytiotrophoblast, most likely account for the increase in progesterone synthesis observed.

Side-chain cleavage also requires a supply of electrons, and this is provided by nicotinamide adenine dinucleotide phosphate (NADPH) through a short electron transport chain in the mitochondrial matrix that involves adrenodoxin reductase and its redox partner adrenodoxin. Preliminary studies in Tuckey's[74] laboratory suggest that the transport of electrons to P450scc is rate limiting for the enzyme's activity at mid pregnancy, and so further research on the factors that regulate expression and activity of adrenodoxin reductase during gestation is clearly needed.

The resultant pregnenolone is then converted to progesterone by the enzyme type 1 3β-hydroxysteroid dehydrogenase (3β-HSD), principally in the mitochondria. The activity of 3β-HSD in placental tissues is significantly higher than that of cytochrome P450scc, and so this step is unlikely to ever be rate limiting for the production of progesterone. **Once secreted, the principal actions of the hormone are to maintain quiescence of the myometrium, although it may have immunomodulatory and appetite stimulatory roles as well.** In addition, our new data on the importance of histotrophic nutrition during the first few weeks of pregnancy suggest that **progesterone may be essential to maintain the secretory activity of the endometrial glands.**

Estrogens

The human placenta lacks the enzymes required to synthesize estrogens directly from acetate or cholesterol, and so it uses the precursor dehydroepiandrosterone sulfate (DHEAS) supplied by the maternal and fetal adrenal glands in approximately equal proportions near term. Following uptake by the syncytiotrophoblast, DHEAS is hydrolyzed by placental sulfatase to dehydroepiandrosterone (DHEA), which is further converted to androstenedione by 3β-HSD. Final conversion to estradiol and estrone is achieved by the action of P450 cytochrome aromatase (P450arom; CYP19), which has been immunolocalized to the endoplasmic reticulum. The syncytiotrophoblast can also utilize 16-OH DHEAS produced by the fetal liver, converting this to 16α-OH androstenedione through the action of 3β-HSD and then to estriol through the action of P450arom. Because approximately 90% of placental estriol production is reliant on fetal synthesis of the precursor 16-OH DHEAS, maternal estriol concentrations have, in the past, been taken clinically as an index of fetal well-being.

Although the synthesis of estrogens can be detected in placental tissues during the early weeks of gestation, secretion significantly increases toward the end of the first trimester. By 7 weeks' gestation, more than 50% of maternal circulating estrogens are of placental origin. Recent analysis of the transcriptional regulation of the *CYP19A1* gene has shown it to be oxygen responsive through a novel pathway that involves the basic helix-loop-helix transcription factor MASH-2.[76] Production of MASH-2 is increased under physiologically low-oxygen conditions and leads to repression of *CYP19A1* gene expression. Hence the change in oxygenation that occurs at the end of the first trimester[7] may stimulate placental production of estrogens.

Human Chorionic Gonadotropin

Human chorionic gonadotropin (hCG) is secreted by the trophoblast at the blastocyst stage and can be detected in the maternal blood and urine approximately 8 to 10 days after fertilization. Its principal function is to maintain the corpus luteum until the placenta is sufficiently developed to take over production of progesterone. It is a heterodimeric glycoprotein (approximately 38,000 Da) that consists of α and β subunits and is principally derived from the syncytiotrophoblast. **The α subunit is common to that of thyroid-stimulating hormone (TSH), luteinizing hormone (LH), and follicle-stimulating hormone (FSH) and is encoded by a single gene located at chromosome 6q12-21. It is the β subunit that determines the biologic specificity of hCG, and this evolved by a duplication event at the *LHB* gene locus.** Mapping has revealed that in the human, six copies of the CGB gene are located together with a single copy of the *LHB* gene at chromosome 19p13.3. Polymerase chain reaction (PCR)–based techniques have revealed that at least five of the genes, and possibly all six, are transcribed in vivo during normal pregnancy. Most of the steady-state hCGβ mRNAs are transcribed from *CGB* genes 5, 3, and 8 but with the levels of expression being β5 > β3 = β8 > β7, β1/2.[77] The β subunits of LH and hCG share 85% amino acid sequence homology and are functionally interchangeable. One of the principal differences between the two is the presence of a 31–amino acid carboxyl-terminal extension in hCGβ compared with a shorter 7–amino acid stretch in LHβ. This extension is hydrophilic, contains four *O*-glycosylated serine residues, and is thought to act as a secretory routing signal that targets release of hCG from the apical membrane of the syncytiotrophoblast.

Assembly of hCG involves a complex process of folding, in which a strand of 20 residues of the β subunit is wrapped around the α subunit, and the two are secured by a disulfide bond. Combination of the subunits occurs in the syncytiotrophoblast prior to the release of intact hCG, and because only limited storage exists in cytoplasmic granules, secretion is largely thought to reflect de novo synthesis. Oxidizing conditions promote combination of the subunits in vitro, most likely through their effects on the disulfide bond, and so the wave of physiologic oxidative stress observed in placental tissues at the transition from the first to second trimesters[7] may influence the pattern of secretion in vivo.

Concentrations of the hCG dimer in maternal blood rise rapidly during early pregnancy, peak at 9 to 10 weeks, and subsequently decline to a nadir at approximately 20 weeks. The physiologic role of the hCG peak is unknown, and the serum concentration far exceeds that required to stimulate LH receptors in the corpus luteum. In any case, the corpus luteum is coming to the end of its extended life, and so the peak may therefore merely reflect other physiologic events. Production of the β subunit follows the same pattern, whereas the maternal serum concentration of the α subunit continues to rise during the first and second trimesters. **Synthesis of the β subunit is therefore considered to be the rate-limiting step.** Early experiments that used primary placental cultures revealed that cyclic adenosine monophosphate (cAMP) plays a key role in the biosynthesis of both subunits, and subsequent work showed it to increase both the transcription and the stability of the α- and β-mRNAs. The kinetics were different for the two subunits, however, which suggests that the effect occurs through separate pathways or transcription factors. Possible regulatory elements within the α and β genes were extensively reviewed by Jameson and Hollenberg.[78]

Another theory that has been proposed is that intact hCG may modulate its own secretion in an autocrine/paracrine fashion through the LH/hCG receptor.[79] This G protein–coupled receptor has been identified on the syncytiotrophoblast of the mature placenta and contains a large extracellular domain that binds intact hCG with high affinity and specificity. However, during early pregnancy, the receptors in the placenta are truncated and probably functionless until 9 weeks. Hence, in the absence of self-regulation, maternal serum concentrations of hCG may rise steeply, until the expression of functional LH/hCG receptors on the syncytiotrophoblast toward the end of the first trimester brings it under control. Reduced synthesis of the functional receptor may underlie the raised serum concentrations of hCG that characterize cases of Down syndrome (trisomy 21).[80]

In addition to changes in the rate of secretion, hCG also exhibits molecular heterogeneity in both its protein and carbohydrate moieties; also, the ratio of the different isoforms secreted changes with gestational age. For the first 5 to 6 weeks of gestation, hyperglycosylated isoforms of the β subunit predominate (hCG-H), resembling the pattern seen in choriocarcinoma.[81] These isoforms are particularly released by extravillous trophoblast, and they stimulate invasion through autocrine/paracrine pathways rather than having traditional endocrine activity. **Reduced levels of hCG-H in the maternal serum have been linked with miscarriage and poor obstetric outcome,[81] and they may reflect impaired development of the extravillous trophoblast. This in turn would lead to deficient spiral artery remodeling.** In normal pregnancies, these hyperglycosylated isoforms decline after the first trimester and are replaced by those that predominate for the remainder of the pregnancy. Midtrimester maternal concentrations of hCG were also found to be raised in a retrospective study of early-onset preeclampsia,[82] and recently a link between the serum concentration and the severity of maternal oxidative stress has been reported.[83] These data reinforce the putative link between the secretion of hCG and the redox status of the trophoblast.

Placental Lactogen
Human placental lactogen (hPL), also known as *chorionic somatotropin,* is a single-chain glycoprotein (22,300 Da) that has a high degree of amino acid sequence homology with both human growth hormone (96%) and prolactin (67%). Therefore it has been suggested that the genes that encode all three hormones arose from a common ancestral gene through repeated gene duplication. Thus **hPL has both growth-promoting and lactogenic effects, although the former are of rather low activity. The hormone is synthesized exclusively in the syncytiotrophoblast and is secreted predominantly into the maternal circulation, where it can be detected from the third week of gestation onward.** Concentrations rise steadily until they plateau at around 36 weeks of gestation, at which time the daily production rate is approximately 1 g. The magnitude of this effort is reflected by the fact that at term, production of hPL accounts for 5% to 10% of total protein synthesis by placental ribosomes, and the encoding mRNA represents 20% of the total placental mRNA.

Little is known regarding the control of hPL secretion in vivo, and maternal concentrations correlate most closely with placental mass. Evidence suggests that calcium influx into the syncytiotrophoblast or an increase in the external concentration in albumin can cause the release of hPL from placental explants in vitro, and this does not appear to be mediated by activation of the inositol phosphate, cAMP, or cyclic guanosine monophosphate (cGMP) pathways.

The actions of hPL are well defined, both as an appetite stimulant and for its effects on maternal metabolism. It

promotes lipolysis, which increases circulating free fatty acid levels, and in the past it was also thought to act as an insulin antagonist, thereby raising maternal blood glucose concentrations. However, it is now thought that placental growth hormone is more important in this respect. Placental lactogen also promotes growth and differentiation of the mammary glandular tissue in anticipation of lactation.

Placental Growth Hormone

Placental growth hormone (PGH) is expressed from the hGH-V gene *GH2*, which is in the same cluster as *CSH1*, and it differs from pituitary growth hormone by only 13 amino acids.[84] PGH is secreted predominantly by the syncytiotrophoblast into the maternal circulation in a nonpulsatile manner and cannot be detected in the fetal circulation. Between 10 and 20 weeks of gestation, PGH gradually replaces pituitary growth hormone, which then becomes undetectable until term. In contrast to hPL, PGH has high growth-promoting but low lactogenic activities.

Secretion of PGH is not modulated by growth-hormone releasing hormone but rather appears to be rapidly suppressed by raised glucose concentrations both in vivo and in vitro.[84] Through its actions on maternal metabolism, PGH increases nutrient availability for the fetoplacental unit and promotes lipolysis and also gluconeogenesis. It is also one of the key regulators of maternal insulin sensitivity and IGF-I concentrations. Although IGF-I does not cross into the fetal circulation, it does have a powerful influence on fetal growth through its effects on maternal metabolism, maternal-fetal nutrient portioning, placental transporter expression, and placental growth and blood flow. Circulating levels of PGH correlate with birthweight and are reduced in cases of IUGR.[84]

Leptin

Leptin is secreted by adipose tissue and normally feeds back on the hypothalamus to suppress appetite and food intake. However, pregnancy is a state of central leptin resistance that allows the mother to lay down adipose reserves. During pregnancy, leptin is secreted in large quantities by the syncytiotrophoblast, regulated in part through hCG and 17β-estradiol.[85] Expression correlates closely with maternal serum concentrations and peaks at the end of the second and during the early third trimesters. The hormone has local stimulatory effects on placental transporter expression and has central effects on appetite.

Pregnancy-Associated Plasma Protein A

Pregnancy-associated plasma protein A (PAPP-A) is a macromolecular glycoprotein that is increased in the serum of pregnant women from 5 weeks' gestation, and it continuously rises until the end of pregnancy. It is mainly produced by the villous trophoblast and, during pregnancy, its synthesis is upregulated by progesterone. It is a key regulator of IGF bioavailability, which is essential for normal fetal development, and low maternal serum levels of PAPP-A have been associated with a higher risk of preeclampsia and poor fetal growth during the second half of pregnancy.[86] Ultrasound measurements of the basal surface area indirectly reflect development of the definitive placenta. The finding of a relationship between basal surface area and PAPP-A levels in maternal serum, and also between basal surface area and birthweight centile, suggests that a combination of these parameters could be useful in identifying placenta-related disorders from the end of the first trimester of pregnancy.[87]

Sex Differences in Placental Function

Increasing evidence suggests sex differences in placental development and function, and in particular to its responses to various stressors.[72,88] Differences are found in growth factor pathways—with concentrations of IGF-I being higher in the cord blood of female fetuses, whereas the reverse is true for growth hormone—and placental cytokine production. Males grow faster in utero than females but have a smaller placenta in relation to fetal weight, which suggests that the organ is more efficient. However, this may mean that the functional reserve is less and that, as a result, male fetuses are more vulnerable to developmental programming under adverse conditions.[89] Dimorphic patterns of placental gene expression may underlie the greater risk of preeclampsia, growth restriction, and prematurity associated with male babies. For example, in preeclamptic pregnancies, the placentae of boys show significantly higher levels of proinflammatory cytokines and activation of apoptosis, which is associated with more pronounced nuclear factor κB (NFκB) signaling.[90] This is an area of active research, and greater consideration needs to be paid to the sex of the fetus in future placenta studies.

SUMMARY

The placenta must be one of the most complex human organs. While growing and differentiating, it performs the functions of many organ systems in the fetus—such as the lungs, kidneys, and liver—that are still immature. Although principally considered an organ of exchange, the placenta also has a major endocrine role. It orchestrates a variety of physiologic responses in the mother that sustain the pregnancy and ensure appropriate allocation of nutrient resources to both parties. Imprinted genes are key players in regulating placental differentiation and function, and their epigenetic status is sensitive to environmental factors. These genes provide a mechanism by which the placenta is able to adapt to meet changing fetal demands and maternal supply. Impaired placental development is frequently associated with fetal growth restriction, and developmental programming of the major organ systems may influence the life-long health of the offspring. Placentation therefore has clinical impact that extends far beyond the 9 months of pregnancy.

KEY POINTS

- The mature human placenta is a discoid organ that consists of an elaborately branched fetal villous tree bathed directly by maternal blood of the villous hemochorial type. Normal term placental weight averages 450 g and represents approximately one seventh (one sixth with cord and membranes) of the fetal weight.

- Continual development throughout pregnancy leads to progressive enlargement of the surface area for exchange (12 to 14 m² at term) and reduction in the mean diffusion distance between the maternal and fetal circulations (approximately 5 to 6 μm at term).

- The maternal circulation to the placenta is not fully established until the end of the first trimester; hence organogenesis takes place in a low-oxygen environment of approximately 20 mm Hg, which may protect against free radical–mediated teratogenesis. Uterine blood flow at term averages 750 mL/min, or 10% to 15% of maternal cardiac output.
- During the first trimester, the uterine glands discharge their secretions into the placental intervillous space and represent an important supply of nutrients, cytokines, and growth factors prior to the onset of the maternal-fetal circulation.
- The exocoelomic cavity acts as an important reservoir of nutrients during early pregnancy, and the secondary yolk sac is important in the uptake of nutrients and their transfer to the fetus.
- Oxygen is a powerful mediator of trophoblast proliferation and invasion, villous remodeling, and placental angiogenesis.
- Ensuring an adequate maternal blood supply to the placenta during the second and third trimesters is an essential aspect of placentation and is dependent upon physiologic conversion of the spiral arteries induced by invasion of the endometrium by extravillous trophoblast during early pregnancy. Many complications of pregnancy, such as preeclampsia, appear to be secondary to deficient invasion.
- All transport across the placenta must take place across the syncytial covering of the villous tree, the syncytiotrophoblast, the villous matrix, and the fetal endothelium, each of which may impose its own restriction and selectivity. Exchange will occur via one of four basic processes: (1) bulk flow/solvent drag, (2) diffusion, (3) transporter-mediated mechanisms, and (4) endocytosis/exocytosis.
- The rate of transplacental exchange will depend on many factors, such as the surface area available, the concentration gradient, the rates of maternal and fetal blood flows, and the density of transporter proteins. Changes in villous surface area, diffusion distance, and transporter expression have been linked with IUGR.
- The placenta is an important endocrine gland that produces both steroid and peptide hormones, principally from the syncytiotrophoblast. Concentrations of some hormones are altered in pathologic conditions—for example, human chorionic gonadotropin in trisomy 21—but in general, little is known regarding control of endocrine activity.

Acknowledgment

The section on placental metabolism and growth is based on material prepared by Dr. Donald Novak from Chapter 2 of the previous edition of this text.

REFERENCES

1. Jauniaux E, Gulbis B, Burton GJ. The human first trimester gestational sac limits rather than facilitates oxygen transfer to the fetus-a review. *Placenta.* 2003;24(suppl A):S86-S93.
2. Gellersen B, Reimann K, Samalecos A, et al. Invasiveness of human endometrial stromal cells is promoted by decidualization and by trophoblast-derived signals. *Hum Reprod.* 2010;25:862-873.
3. Jauniaux E, Johns J, Gulbis B, et al. Transfer of folic acid inside the first-trimester gestational sac and the effect of maternal smoking. *Am J Obstet Gynecol.* 2007;197(58):e1-e6.
4. Hustin J, Schaaps JP. Echographic and anatomic studies of the materno-trophoblastic border during the first trimester of pregnancy. *Am J Obstet Gynecol.* 1987;157:162-168.
5. Burton GJ, Jauniaux E, Watson AL. Maternal arterial connections to the placental intervillous space during the first trimester of human pregnancy: the Boyd Collection revisited. *Am J Obstet Gynecol.* 1999;181:718-724.
6. Schaaps JP, Hustin J. In vivo aspect of the maternal-trophoblastic border during the first trimester of gestation. *Trophoblast Res.* 1988;3:39-48.
7. Jauniaux E, Watson AL, Hempstock J, et al. Onset of maternal arterial bloodflow and placental oxidative stress: a possible factor in human early pregnancy failure. *Am J Pathol.* 2000;157:2111-2122.
8. Pijnenborg R, Vercruysse L, Hanssens M. The uterine spiral arteries in human pregnancy: facts and controversies. *Placenta.* 2006;27:939-958.
9. Harris LK. Review: Trophoblast-vascular cell interactions in early pregnancy: how to remodel a vessel. *Placenta.* 2010;31(suppl):S93-S98.
10. Jauniaux E, Hempstock J, Greenwold N, et al. Trophoblastic oxidative stress in relation to temporal and regional differences in maternal placental blood flow in normal and abnormal early pregnancies. *Am J Pathol.* 2003;162:115-125.
11. Hiby SE, Apps R, Sharkey AM, et al. Maternal activating KIRs protect against human reproductive failure mediated by fetal HLA-C2. *J Clin Invest.* 2010;120:4102-4110.
12. Burton GJ, Woods AW, Jauniaux E, et al. Rheological and physiological consequences of conversion of the maternal spiral arteries for uteroplacental blood flow during human pregnancy. *Placenta.* 2009;30:473-482.
13. Hustin J, Jauniaux E, Schaaps JP. Histological study of the materno-embryonic interface in spontaneous abortion. *Placenta.* 1990;11:477-486.
14. Hempstock J, Jauniaux E, Greenwold N, et al. The contribution of placental oxidative stress to early pregnancy failure. *Hum Pathol.* 2003;34:1265-1275.
15. Brosens IA. The utero-placental vessels at term - the distribution and extent of physiological changes. *Trophoblast Res.* 1988;3:61-67.
16. Martin CB, McGaughey HS, Kaiser IH, et al. Intermittent functioning of the uteroplacental arteries. *Am J Obstet Gynecol.* 1964;90:819-823.
17. Burton GJ, Yung HW, Cindrova-Davies T, et al. Placental endoplasmic reticulum stress and oxidative stress in the pathophysiology of unexplained intrauterine growth restriction and early onset preeclampsia. *Placenta.* 2009;30(suppl A):S43-S48.
18. Meekins JW, Pijnenborg R, Hanssens M, et al. A study of placental bed spiral arteries and trophoblast invasion in normal and severe pre-eclamptic pregnancies. *Br J Obstet Gynaecol.* 1994;101:669-674.
19. Burton GJ, Watson AL, Hempstock J, et al. Uterine glands provide histiotrophic nutrition for the human fetus during the first trimester of pregnancy. *J Clin Endocrinol Metab.* 2002;87:2954-2959.
20. Jones CJ, Aplin JD, Burton GJ. First trimester histiotrophe shows altered sialylation compared with secretory phase glycoconjugates in human endometrium. *Placenta.* 2010;31:576-580.
21. Hempstock J, Cindrova-Davies T, Jauniaux E, et al. Endometrial glands as a source of nutrients, growth factors and cytokines during the first trimester of human pregnancy: a morphological and immunohistochemical study. *Reprod Biol Endocrinol.* 2004;2:58.
22. Arias-Stella J. The Arias-Stella reaction: facts and fancies four decades after. *Adv Anat Pathol.* 2002;9:12-23.
23. Mikolajczyk M, Skrzypczak J, Szymanowski K, et al. The assessment of LIF in uterine flushing - a possible new diagnostic tool in states of impaired infertility. *Reprod Biol.* 2003;3:259-270.
24. Tuckerman E, Laird SM, Stewart R, et al. Markers of endometrial function in women with unexplained recurrent pregnancy loss: a comparison between morphologically normal and retarded endometrium. *Hum Reprod.* 2004;19:196-205.
25. Kaufmann P, Sen DK, Schweikert G. Classification of human placental villi. 1. Histology. *Cell Tissue Res.* 1979;200:409-423.
26. Ramsey EM, Donner MW. *Placental Vasculature and Circulation. Anatomy, Physiology, Radiology, Clinical Aspects, Atlas and Textbook.* Stuttgart: Georg Thieme; 1980:101.
27. Mayhew TM, Ohadike C, Baker PN, et al. Stereological investigation of placental morphology in pregnancies complicated by pre-eclampsia with and without intrauterine growth restriction. *Placenta.* 2003;24:219-226.

28. Jones CJ, Fox H. Ultrastructure of the normal human placenta. *Electron Microsc Rev*. 1991;4:129-178.

29. Carter AM. Placental oxygen consumption. Part I: in vivo studies-a review. *Placenta*. 2000;21(suppl A):S31-S37.

30. Hemberger M, Udayashankar R, Tesar P, et al. ELF5-enforced transcriptional networks define an epigentically regulated trophoblast stem cell compartment in the human placenta. *Hum Mol Genet*. 2010;19: 2456-2467.

31. Mayhew TM, Leach L, McGee R, et al. Proliferation, differentiation and apoptosis in villous trophoblast at 13-41 weeks of gestation (including observations on annulate lamellae and nuclear pore complexes. *Placenta*. 1999;20:407-422.

32. Frendo JL, Cronier L, Bertin G, et al. Involvement of connexin 43 in human trophoblast cell fusion and differentiation. *J Cell Sci*. 2003;116:3413-3421.

33. Mangeney M, Renard M, Schlecht-Louf G, et al. Placental syncytins: Genetic disjunction between the fusogenic and immunosuppressive activity of retroviral envelope proteins. *Proc Natl Acad Sci U S A*. 2007; 104:20534-20539.

34. Fogarty NM, Mayhew TM, Ferguson-Smith AC, et al. A quantitative analysis of transcriptionally active syncytiotrophoblastic nuclei across human gestation. *J Anat*. 2011;219:601-610.

35. Fogarty NM, Ferguson-Smith AC, Burton GJ. Syncytial knots (Tenney-Parker changes) in the human placenta: evidence of loss of transcriptional activity and oxidative damage. *Am J Pathol*. 2013;183: 144-152.

36. Brownbill P, Mahendran D, Owen D, et al. Denudations as paracellular routes for alphafetoprotein and creatinine across the human syncytiotrophoblast. *Am J Physiol Regul Integr Comp Physiol*. 2000;278: R677-R683.

37. Longtine MS, Chen B, Odibo AO, Zhong Y, Nelson DM. Villous trophoblast apoptosis is elevated and restricted to cytotrophoblasts in pregnancies complicated by preeclampsia, IUGR, or preeclampsia with IUGR. *Placenta*. 2012;33(5):352-359.

38. Burton GJ, Charnock-Jones DS, Jauniaux E. Regulation of vascular growth and function in human placenta. *Reproduction*. 2009;138: 895-902.

39. Kaufmann P, Bruns U, Leiser R, et al. The fetal vascularisation of term placental villi. II. Intermediate and terminal villi. *Anat Embryol (Berl)*. 1985;173:203-214.

40. Mayhew TM, Charnock Jones DS, Kaufmann P. Aspects of human fetoplacental vasculogenesis and angiogenesis. III. Changes in complicated pregnancies. *Placenta*. 2004;25:127-139.

41. Jauniaux E, Gulbis B. Fluid compartments of the embryonic environment. *Hum Reprod Update*. 2000;6:268-278.

42. Jauniaux E, Gulbis B, Jurkovic D, et al. Protein and steroid levels in embryonic cavities in early human pregnancy. *Hum Reprod*. 1993;8: 782-787.

43. Gulbis B, Jauniaux E, Cotton F, et al. Protein and enzyme patterns in the fluid cavities of the first trimester gestational sac: relevance to the absorptive role of the secondary yolk sac. *Mol Hum Reprod*. 1998;4:857-862.

44. Burke KA, Jauniaux E, Burton GJ, et al. Expression and immunolocalisation of the endocytic receptors megalin and cubilin in the human yolk sac and placenta across gestation. *Placenta*. 2013;34:1105-1109.

45. Hauguel S, Challier JC, Cedard L, et al. Metabolism of the human placenta perfused in vitro: glucose transfer and utilization, O2 consumption, lactate and ammonia production. *Pediatr Res*. 1983;17:729-732.

46. Jauniaux E, Hempstock J, Teng C, et al. Polyol concentrations in the fluid compartments of the human conceptus during the first trimester of pregnancy; maintenance of redox potential in a low oxygen environment. *J Clin Endocrinol Metab*. 2005;90:1171-1175.

47. Fowden AL, Sibley C, Reik W, et al. Imprinted genes, placental development and fetal growth. *Horm Res*. 2006;65(suppl 3):50-58.

48. Yung HW, Calabrese S, Hynx D, et al. Evidence of placental translation inhibition and endoplasmic reticulum stress in the etiology of human intrauterine growth restriction. *Am J Pathol*. 2008;173:451-462.

49. Colleoni F, Padmanabhan N, Yung HW, et al. Suppression of mitochondrial electron trnasport chain function in the hypoxic human placenta: a role for miR-210 and protein synthesis inhibition. *PLoS ONE*. 2013;8: e55194.

50. Desforges M, Sibley CP. Placental nutrient supply and fetal growth. *Int J Dev Biol*. 2010;54:377-390.

51. Bain MD, Copas DK, Taylor A, et al. Permeability of the human placenta in vivo to four non-metabolized hydrophilic molecules. *J Physiol*. 1990;431:505-513.

52. Brownbill P, Edwards D, Jones C, et al. Mechanisms of alphafetoprotein transfer in the perfused human placental cotyledon from uncomplicated pregnancy. *J Clin Invest*. 1995;96:2220-2226.

53. Stulc J, Svihovec J, Drabkova J, et al. Electrical potential difference across the mid-term human placenta. *Acta Obstet Gynecol Scand*. 1978;57: 125-126.

54. Mellor DJ, Cockburn F, Lees MM, et al. Distribution of ions and electrical potential differences between mother and fetus in the human at term. *J Obstet Gynaecol Br Commonw*. 1969;76:993-998.

55. Ward S, Jauniaux E, Shannon C, et al. Electrical potential difference between exocelomic fluid and maternal blood in early pregnancy. *Am J Physiol*. 1998;274:R1492-R1495.

56. Atkinson DE, Boyd RDH, Sibley CP. Placental transfer. In: Neill JD, ed. *Placental Transfer*. Amsterdam: Elsevier; 2006:2787-2846.

57. Ayuk PT, Theophanous D, D'Souza SW, et al. L-arginine transport by the microvillous plasma membrane of the syncytiotrophoblast from human placenta in relation to nitric oxide production: effects of gestation, preeclampsia, and intrauterine growth restriction. *J Clin Endocrinol Metab*. 2002;87:747-751.

58. Illsley NP. Glucose transporters in the human placenta. *Placenta*. 2000;21:14-22.

59. Hughes JL, Doughty IM, Glazier JD, et al. Activity and expression of the Na(+)/H(+) exchanger in the microvillous plasma membrane of the syncytiotrophoblast in relation to gestation and small for gestational age birth. *Pediatr Res*. 2000;48:652-659.

60. Sibley CP, Boyd RDH. Mechanisms of transfer across the human placenta. In: Polin PA, Fox WW, Abman SH, eds. *Fetal and Neonatal Physiology*. Philadelphia: Saunders; 2004:111-122.

61. Wilkening RB, Meschia G. Fetal oxygen uptake, oxygenation, and acid-base balance as a function of uterine blood flow. *Am J Physiol*. 1983;244:H749-H755.

62. Baumann MU, Deborde S, Illsley NP. Placental glucose transfer and fetal growth. *Endocrine*. 2002;19:13-22.

63. Lewis RM, Brooks S, Crocker IP, et al. Review: Modelling placental amino acid transfer–from transporters to placental function. *Placenta*. 2013; 34(suppl):S46-S51.

64. Gimeno RE, Hirsch DJ, Punreddy S, et al. Targeted deletion of fatty acid transport protein-4 results in early embryonic lethality. *J Biol Chem*. 2003;278:49512-49516.

65. Duttaroy AK. Transport of fatty acids across the human placenta: a review. *Prog Lipid Res*. 2009;48:52-61.

66. Dancis J, Kammerman S, Jansen V, et al. Transfer of urea, sodium, and chloride across the perfused human placenta. *Am J Obstet Gynecol*. 1981; 141:677-681.

67. Birdsey TJ, Boyd RD, Sibley CP, et al. Microvillous membrane potential (Em) in villi from first trimester human placenta: comparison to Em at term. *Am J Physiol*. 1997;273:R1519-R1528.

68. Riquelme G. Placental chloride channels: a review. *Placenta*. 2009;30: 659-669.

69. Belkacemi L, Bedard I, Simoneau L, et al. Calcium channels, transporters and exchangers in placenta: a review. *Cell Calcium*. 2005;37:1-8.

70. Sibley CP, Turner MA, Cetin I, et al. Placental phenotypes of intrauterine growth. *Pediatr Res*. 2005;58:827-832.

71. Sibley CP. Understanding placental nutrient transfer–why bother? New biomarkers of fetal growth. *J Physiol*. 2009;587:3431-3440.

72. Brett KE, Ferraro ZM, Yockell-Lelievre J, et al. Maternal-fetal nutrient transport in pregnancy pathologies: the role of the placenta. *Int J Mol Sci*. 2014;15:16153-16185.

73. Cindrova-Davies T, Herrera EA, Niu Y, et al. Reduced cystathionine gamma-lyase and increased miR-21 expression are associated with increased vascular resistance in growth-restricted pregnancies: hydrogen sulfide as a placental vasodilator. *Am J Pathol*. 2013;182:1448-1458.

74. Tuckey RC. Progesterone synthesis by the human placenta. *Placenta*. 2005;26:273-281.

75. Tuckey RC, Kostadinovic Z, Cameron KJ. Cytochrome P-450scc activity and substrate supply in human placental trophoblasts. *Mol Cell Endocrinol*. 1994;105:103-109.

76. Mendelson CR, Jiang B, Shelton JM, et al. Transcriptional regulation of aromatase in placenta and ovary. *J Steroid Biochem Mol Biol*. 2005; 95:25-33.

77. Bo M, Boime I. Identification of the transcriptionally active genes of the chorionic gonadotropin beta gene cluster in vivo. *J Biol Chem*. 1992; 267:3179-3184.

78. Jameson JL, Hollenberg AN. Regulation of chorionic gonadotropin gene expression. *Endocr Rev*. 1993;14:203-221.

79. Licht P, Losch A, Dittrich R, et al. Novel insights into human endometrial paracrinology and embryo-maternal communication by intrauterine microdialysis. *Hum Reprod Update.* 1998;4:532-538.

80. Banerjee S, Smallwood A, Chambers AE, et al. A link between high serum levels of human chorionic gonadotrophin and chorionic expression of its mature functional receptor (LHCGR) in Down's syndrome pregnancies. *Reprod Biol Endocrinol.* 2005;3:25.

81. Cole LA. Hyperglycosylated hCG, a review. *Placenta.* 2010;31:653-664.

82. Shenhav S, Gemer O, Sassoon E, et al. Mid-trimester triple test levels in early and late onset severe pre-eclampsia. *Prenat Diagn.* 2002;22: 579-582.

83. Kharfi A, Giguere Y, De Grandpre P, et al. Human chorionic gonadotropin (hCG) may be a marker of systemic oxidative stress in normotensive and preeclamptic term pregnancies. *Clin Biochem.* 2005;38:717-721.

84. Lacroix MC, Guibourdenche J, Frendo JL, et al. Human placental growth hormone–a review. *Placenta.* 2002;23(suppl A):S87-S94.

85. Tessier DR, Ferraro ZM, Gruslin A. Role of leptin in pregnancy: consequences of maternal obesity. *Placenta.* 2013;34:205-211.

86. Kalousova M, Muravska A, Zima T. Pregnancy-associated plasma protein A (PAPP-A) and preeclampsia. *Adv Clin Chem.* 2014;63:169-209.

87. Suri S, Muttukrishna S, Jauniaux E. 2D-Ultrasound and endocrinologic evaluation of placentation in early pregnancy and its relationship to fetal birthweight in normal pregnancies and pre-eclampsia. *Placenta.* 2013;34: 745-750.

88. Clifton VL. Review: Sex and the human placenta: mediating differential strategies of fetal growth and survival. *Placenta.* 2010;31(suppl): S33-S39.

89. Eriksson JG, Kajantie E, Osmond C, et al. Boys live dangerously in the womb. *Am J Hum Biol.* 2010;22:330-335.

90. Muralimanoharan S, Maloyan A, Myatt L. Evidence of sexual dimorphism in the placental function with severe preeclampsia. *Placenta.* 2013;34(12): 1183-1189.

91. Jansson T, Ylven K, Wennergren M, et al. Glucose transport and system A activity in syncytiotrophoblast microvillous and basal plasma membranes in intrauterine growth restriction. *Placenta.* 2002;23:392-399.

92. Jansson T, Scholtbach V, Powell TL. Placental transport of leucine and lysine is reduced in intrauterine growth restriction. *Pediatr Res.* 1998;44:532-537.

93. Norberg S, Powell TL, Jansson T. Intrauterine growth restriction is associated with a reduced activity of placental taurine transporters. *Pediatr Res.* 1998;44:233-238.

94. Roos S, Powell TL, Jansson T. Human placental taurine transporter in uncomplicated and IUGR pregnancies: cellular localization, protein expression and regulation. *Am J Physiol Regul Integr Comp Physiol.* 2004;287:R886-R893.

95. Jansson T, Wennergren M, Illsley NP. Glucose transporter protein expression in human placenta throughout gestation and in intrauterine growth retardation. *J Clin Endocrinol Metab.* 1993;77:1554-1562.

96. Johansson M, Karlsson L, Wennergren M, et al. Activity and protein expression of Na+/K+ ATPase are reduced in microvillous syncytiotrophoblast plasma membranes isolated from pregnancies complicated by intrauterine growth restriction. *J Clin Endocrinol Metab.* 2003;88:2831-2837.

97. Strid H, Bucht E, Jansson T, et al. ATP dependent Ca2+ transport across basal membrane of human syncytiotrophoblast in pregnancies complicated by intrauterine growth restriction or diabetes. *Placenta.* 2003;24: 445-452.

98. Johansson M, Glazier JD, Sibley CP, et al. Activity and protein expression of the Na+/H+ exchanger is reduced in syncytiotrophoblast microvillous plasma membranes isolated from preterm intrauterine growth restriction pregnancies. *J Clin Endocrinol Metab.* 2002;87:5686-5694.

99. Settle P, Mynett K, Speake P, et al. Polarized lactate transporter activity and expression in the syncytiotrophoblast of the term human placenta. *Placenta.* 2004;25:496-504.

100. Boyd CA, Lund EK. L-proline transport by brush border membrane vesicles prepared from human placenta. *J Physiol.* 1981;315:9-19.

101. Whitsett JA, Wallick ET. [3H]ouabain binding and Na+-K+-ATPase activity in human placenta. *Am J Physiol.* 1980;238:E38-E45.

102. Lajeunesse D, Brunette MG. Sodium gradient-dependent phosphate transport in placental brush border membrane vesicles. *Placenta.* 1988;9:117-128.

103. Balkovetz DF, Leibach FH, Mahesh VB, et al. Na+-H+ exchanger of human placental brush-border membrane: identification and characterization. *Am J Physiol.* 1986;251:C852-C860.

104. Bara M, Challier JC, Guiet-Bara A. Membrane potential and input resistance in syncytiotrophoblast of human term placenta in vitro. *Placenta.* 1988;9:139-146.

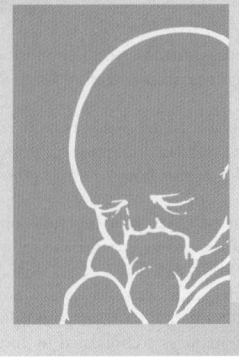

CHAPTER 2

Fetal Development and Physiology

MICHAEL G. ROSS and M. GORE ERVIN

KEY ABBREVIATIONS

2,3-Diphosphoglycerate	2,3-DPG
α-Melanocyte–stimulating hormone	α-MSH
Adrenocorticotropic hormone	ACTH
Angiotensin-converting enzyme	ACE
Angiotensin II	AII
Arginine vasopressin	AVP
Atrial natriuretic factor	ANF
Carbon dioxide	CO_2
Corticotropin-like intermediate lobe peptide	CLIP
Corticotrophin-releasing factor	CRF
Cyclic adenosine monophosphate	cAMP
Epidermal growth factor	EGF
Epidermal growth factor receptor	EGF-R
Glomerular filtration rate	GFR
Insulin-like growth factor	IGF
Oxygen	O_2
Thyrotropin-releasing hormone	TRH
Thyroid-stimulating hormone	TSH
Thyroxine	T_4
Triiodothyronine	T_3
Vascular endothelial growth factor	VEGF

In obstetric practice, recognition of normal fetal growth, development, and behavior often suggests an expectant management plan. However, abnormalities may require clinical strategies for fetal assessment and intervention. The basic concepts of placental and fetal physiology provide the building blocks necessary for understanding pathophysiology and thus mechanisms of disease. Throughout this chapter, we have reviewed the essential tenets of fetal physiology and have related this information to normal and abnormal clinical conditions.

Much of our knowledge of fetal physiology derives from observations made in mammals other than humans. We have attempted to include only those observations reasonably applicable to the human fetus and in most instances have not detailed the species from which the data were obtained. Should questions arise regarding the species studied, the reader is referred to the extensive bibliography.

UMBILICAL BLOOD FLOW

Fetal blood flow to the umbilical circulation represents approximately 40% of the combined output of both fetal ventricles.[1] Over the last third of gestation, increases in umbilical blood flow are proportional to fetal growth so that umbilical blood flow remains constant when normalized to fetal weight. Human umbilical venous flow can be estimated through the use of triplex ultrasonography. Although increases in villous capillary number represent the primary contributor to gestation-dependent increases in umbilical blood flow, the factors that regulate this change are unknown; however, a number of important angiogenic peptides and factors, including vascular endothelial growth factor (VEGF), have been identified.[2] Short-term changes in umbilical blood flow are primarily regulated by perfusion pressure. **The relationship between flow and perfusion pressure is linear in the umbilical circulation.** As a result, small (2 to 3 mm Hg) increases in umbilical vein pressure evoke proportional decreases in umbilical blood flow. Because both the umbilical artery and vein are enclosed in the amniotic cavity, pressure changes caused by increases in uterine tone are transmitted equally to these vessels without changes in umbilical blood flow. **Relative to the uteroplacental bed, the fetoplacental circulation is resistant to vasoconstrictive effects of infused pressor agents, and umbilical blood flow is preserved unless cardiac output decreases. Thus despite catecholamine-induced changes in blood flow distribution and increases in blood pressure during acute hypoxia, umbilical blood flow is maintained over a relatively wide range of oxygen tensions.** Endogenous vasoactive autacoids have been identified; nitric oxide may also be important. Endothelin-1, in particular, is associated with diminished fetoplacental blood flow.[3]

AMNIOTIC FLUID VOLUME

Mean amniotic fluid volume (AFV) increases from 250 to 800 mL between 16 and 32 weeks of gestation. Despite considerable variability, the average volume remains stable up to 39 weeks and then declines to about 500 mL at 42 weeks (Fig. 2-1). Amniotic fluid index (AFI) values across gestation are found in Chapter 35. The origin of amniotic fluid during the first trimester of pregnancy is uncertain. Possible sources include a transudate of maternal plasma through the chorioamnion or a transudate of fetal plasma through the highly permeable fetal skin before keratinization. The origin and dynamics of amniotic fluid are better understood beginning in the second trimester, when the fetus becomes the primary determinant. **AFV is maintained by a balance of fetal *fluid production* (lung liquid and urine) and *fluid resorption* (fetal swallowing and flow across the amniotic and/or chorionic membranes to the fetus or maternal uterus; Fig. 2-2).**[4]

The fetal lung secretes fluid at a rate of 300 to 400 mL/day near term. Chloride is actively transferred from alveolar capillaries to the lung lumen, and water follows the chloride gradient. Thus lung fluid represents a nearly protein-free transudate with an osmolarity similar to that of fetal plasma. Fetal lung fluid does not appear to regulate fetal body fluid homeostasis, just as fetal intravenous volume loading does not increase lung fluid secretion. Rather, **lung fluid likely serves to maintain lung expansion and facilitate pulmonary growth. Lung fluid must decrease at parturition to provide for the transition to respiratory ventilation.** Notably, several hormones that increase in fetal plasma during labor (i.e., catecholamines, arginine vasopressin [AVP]) also decrease lung fluid production. With the reduction of fluid secretion, the colloid osmotic gradient between fetal plasma and lung fluid results in lung fluid resorption across the pulmonary epithelium and clearance via lymphatics. **The absence of this process explains the increased incidence of transient tachypnea of the newborn, or "wet lung," in infants delivered by cesarean section in the absence of labor.**

Fetal urine is the primary source of amniotic fluid, and outputs at term vary from 400 to 1200 mL/day. Between 20 and 40 weeks' gestation, fetal urine production increases about tenfold in the presence of marked renal maturation. The urine is normally hypotonic, and the low osmolarity of fetal urine accounts for the hypotonicity of amniotic fluid in late gestation relative to maternal and fetal plasma. Numerous fetal endocrine factors that include AVP, atrial natriuretic factor (ANF), angiotensin II (AII), aldosterone, and prostaglandins can alter fetal renal blood flow, glomerular filtration rate, and urine flow rates.[5] In response to fetal stress, endocrine-mediated reductions in fetal urine flow may explain the association between fetal hypoxia and oligohydramnios. The regulation of fetal urine production is discussed further under "Fetal Kidney" later in this chapter.

Fetal swallowing is believed to be a major route of amniotic fluid resorption, although swallowed fluid contains a mixture of amniotic and tracheal fluids. Human fetal swallowing has been demonstrated by 18 weeks' gestation,[6] with daily swallowed volumes of 200 to 500 mL near term. Similar to fetal urine flow, daily fetal swallowed volumes (per body weight) are markedly greater than adult values. With the development of fetal neurobehavioral states, fetal swallowing occurs primarily during active sleep states associated with respiratory and eye movements.[7] Moderate elevations in fetal plasma osmolality increase the number of swallowing episodes and volume swallowed, indicating the presence of an intact thirst mechanism in the near-term fetus.

Because amniotic fluid is hypotonic with respect to maternal plasma, there is a potential for bulk water removal at the amniotic-chorionic interface with maternal or fetal plasma. Although fluid resorption to the maternal plasma is likely minimal, intramembranous flow from amniotic fluid to fetal placental vessels may contribute importantly to amniotic fluid resorption. Thus **intramembranous flow may balance fetal**

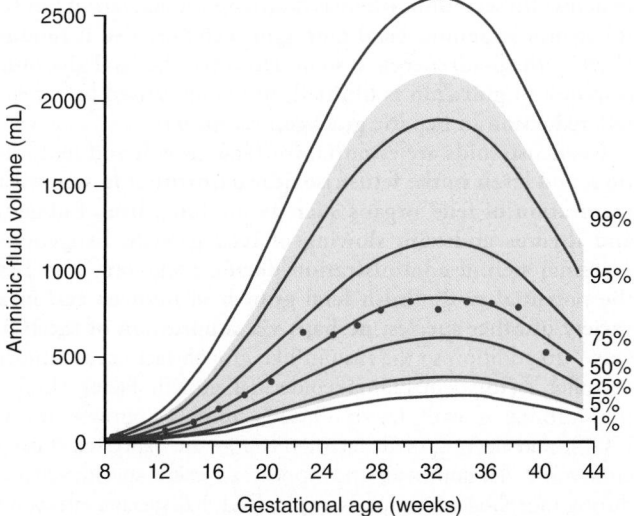

FIG 2-1 Normal range of amniotic fluid volume in human gestation. (From Beall MH, van den Wijngaard JP, van Gemert MJ, Ross MG. Amniotic fluid water dynamics. *Placenta.* 2007;28:816-823.)

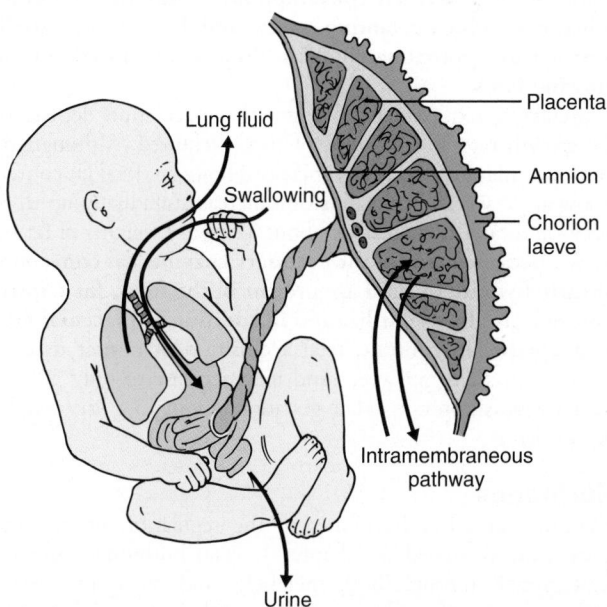

FIG 2-2 Water circulation between the fetus and amniotic fluid. The major sources of amniotic fluid water are fetal urine and lung liquid, and the routes of absorption are through fetal swallowing and intramembranous flow. (From Beall MH, van den Wijngaard JP, van Gemert MJ, Ross MG. Amniotic fluid water dynamics. *Placenta.* 2007;28:816-823.)

urine and lung-liquid production with fetal swallowing to maintain normal AFVs.

The mechanisms by which water is transferred across the amnion into fetal vessels remains uncertain, but evidence implicates the presence of water channels within the amnion and, as discussed previously, the placental trophoblast and fetal endothelium. Aquaporins 1, 3, 8, and 9 are found within the placenta and fetal membranes. Mice deficient in aquaporin 1 develop polyhydramnios, which suggests an important role for this protein in intramembranous water transfer.[8] Aquaporins 1 and 3, important in transplacental water flow, are regulated by AVP and by cyclic adenosine monophosphate (cAMP), and they show changes in expression throughout gestation.[9]

FETAL GROWTH AND METABOLISM
Substrates

Nutrients are utilized by the fetus for two primary purposes: oxidation for energy and tissue accretion. Under normal conditions, glucose is an important substrate for fetal oxidative metabolism. The glucose utilized by the fetus derives from the placenta rather than from endogenous glucose production. However, based on umbilical vein–umbilical artery glucose and oxygen (O_2) concentration differences, glucose alone cannot account for fetal oxidative metabolism. In fact, glucose oxidation accounts for only two thirds of fetal carbon dioxide (CO_2) production.[10] Thus **fetal oxidative metabolism depends on substrates in addition to glucose.** A large portion of the amino acids taken up by the umbilical circulation are used by the fetus for aerobic metabolism instead of protein synthesis. Fetal uptake for a number of amino acids actually exceeds their accretion into fetal tissues. In addition, other amino acids—notably glutamate—are taken up by the placenta from the fetal circulation and are metabolized within the placenta.[11] **In fetal sheep, and likely in the human fetus as well, lactate also is a substrate for fetal oxygen consumption.**[10] **Thus the combined substrates—glucose, amino acids, and lactate—essentially provide the approximately 87 kcal/kg required daily by the growing fetus.**

Metabolic requirements for new tissue accretion depend on the growth rate and the type of tissue acquired. Although the newborn infant has relatively increased body fat, fetal fat content is low at 26 weeks. Fat acquisition increases gradually up to 32 weeks and rapidly thereafter (about 82 g [dry weight] of fat per week). **Because many of the necessary enzymes for conversion of carbohydrate to lipid are present in the fetus, fat acquisition reflects glucose utilization in addition to placental fatty acid uptake.** In contrast, fetal acquisition of nonfat tissue is linear from 32 to 39 weeks and may decrease to only 30% of the fat-acquisition rate in late gestation (about 43 g [dry weight] per week).

Hormones

The roles of select hormones in the regulation of placental growth are discussed in Chapter 1. Fetal hormones influence fetal growth through both metabolic and mitogenic effects. **Although growth hormone and growth hormone receptors are present early in fetal life, and growth hormone is essential to postnatal growth, growth hormone appears to have little role in regulating fetal growth.** Instead, changes in insulin-like growth factor (IGF), IGF-binding proteins, or IGF receptors explain the apparent reduced role of growth hormone on fetal growth. Most if not all tissues of the body produce IGF-I and IGF-II, and both are present in human fetal tissue extracts after 12 weeks' gestation. Fetal plasma IGF-I and -II levels begin to increase by 32 to 34 weeks' gestation. **The increase in IGF-I levels directly correlates with increase in fetal size, and a reduction in IGF-I levels is associated with growth restriction.**[12] **In contrast, no correlation has been found between serum IGF-II levels and fetal growth.** However, a correlation has been noted between small offspring and genetic manipulations that result in decreased IGF-II messenger RNA production. IGF-II knockout mice are small, and knockout of the IGF-II receptor results in fetal overgrowth.[13] Thus tissue IGF-II concentrations and localized IGF-II release may be more important than circulating levels in supporting fetal growth.

IGF binding proteins (IGFBPs) modulate IGF-I and II concentrations in serum, with IGFBP1 having an inhibitory and IGFBP3 a comparatively stimulatory effect. As such, diminished fetal concentrations of IGFBP3 and enhanced concentrations of IGFBP1 have been associated with smaller fetal size.[14]

A role for insulin in fetal growth is suggested from the increases in body weight and in heart and liver weights in infants of diabetic mothers. Insulin levels within the high physiologic range increase fetal body weight, and increases in endogenous fetal insulin significantly increase fetal glucose uptake. In addition, fetal insulin secretion increases in response to elevations in blood glucose, although the normal rapid insulin response phase is absent.[15] Plasma insulin levels sufficient to increase fetal growth also may exert mitogenic effects, perhaps through insulin-induced IGF-II receptor binding. Separate receptors for insulin and IGF-II are expressed in fetal liver cells by the end of the first trimester. Hepatic insulin receptor numbers (per gram tissue) triple by 28 weeks, whereas IGF-II receptor numbers remain constant. Thus, although infants of diabetic mothers are at increased risk of cardiac defects, the growth patterns of these infants indicate that insulin levels may be most important in late gestation (see Chapter 40). Although less common, equally dramatically low birthweights are associated with the absence of fetal insulin. Experimentally induced hypoinsulinemia causes a 30% decrease in fetal glucose utilization and decreases fetal growth.

As in the adult, β-adrenergic receptor activation increases fetal insulin secretion, whereas β-adrenergic activation inhibits insulin secretion. Fetal glucagon secretion also is modulated by the β-adrenergic system. However, the fetal glycemic response to glucagon is blunted, probably caused by a relative reduction in hepatic glucagon receptors.

Corticosteroids are essential for fetal growth and maturation, and levels in the fetus rise near parturition in step with maturation of fetal organs such as the lung, liver, kidneys, and thymus and with slowing of fetal growth. Exogenous maternal steroid administration during pregnancy also has the potential to diminish fetal growth in humans and in a variety of other species, perhaps via suppression of the IGF axis.[14] In addition to the insulin-like growth factors, a number of other factors—including epidermal growth factor (EGF), transforming growth factor (TGF), fibroblast growth factor (FGF), and nerve growth factor (NGF)—are expressed during embryonic development and appear to exert specific effects during morphogenesis; for example, EGF has specific effects on lung growth and on differentiation of the secondary palate, and normal sympathetic adrenergic system development is dependent on NGF. However, the specific role of these factors in regulating fetal growth remains to be defined. **Similarly, the fetal thyroid also is not important for overall fetal growth but is important for central nervous system development.**

Substantial evidence now exists to support the view that several cell-specific growth factors and their cognate receptors play an essential role in placental growth and function in a number of species. Growth factors identified to date include family members of EGF, TGF-β, NGF, IGF, hematopoietic growth factors, VEGF, and FGF. The expression, ontogeny, and regulation of most but not all of these growth factors have been explored; in addition, a number of cytokines also play a role in normal placental development. In vitro placental cell culture studies support the concept that **growth factors and cytokines exert their functions locally, promoting proliferation and differentiation through their autocrine and/or paracrine mode of actions.** For example, EGF promotes cell proliferation, invasion, or differentiation depending on the gestational age. Hepatocyte growth factor and VEGF stimulate trophoblast DNA replication, whereas TGF-β suppresses cytoplast invasion and endocrine differentiation. In support of local actions, functional receptors for various growth factors have been demonstrated on trophoblast and other cells. Various intracellular signal proteins and transcription factors that respond to growth factors are also expressed in the placenta. A number of elegant studies have identified alterations in growth factors and growth factor receptors in association with placental and fetal growth restriction. Placental defects in growth factor and receptor pathways, explored through the use of transgenic and mutant mice, have provided potential mechanisms for explaining complications of human placental development.[16] **An illustrative example is EGF, a potent mitogen for epidermal and mesodermal cells that is expressed in human placenta. EGF is involved in embryonal implantation, it stimulates syncytiotrophoblast differentiation in vitro, and it modulates production and secretion of human chorionic gonadotropin (hCG) and human placental lactogen (hPL).** The effects of EGF are mediated by EGF-receptor (EGF-R), a transmembrane glycoprotein with intrinsic tyrosine kinase activity. EGF-R is expressed on the apical microvillus plasma membrane fractions from early, middle, and term whole placentae. Placental EGF-R expression is regulated by locally expressed parathyroid hormone–related protein, which is important in placental differentiation and maternal-fetal calcium flux.[17,18] Decreased EGF-R expression has been demonstrated in association with intrauterine growth restriction (IUGR). **Targeted disruption of EGF-R has been shown to result in fetal death as a result of placental defects.[19] Overexpression of EGF-R activity results in placental enlargement.[20]**

The EGF family now consists of at least 15 members, many of which have been identified in human placenta. Future studies should reveal whether EGF family members play distinct or overlapping functions in mediating placental growth.

Control of fetal growth may occur via the impact of growth factors/hormones on the placenta or may occur as a direct result of action in and on the fetus. It is clear that nutrition may play a role in these processes. However, the number of genes and gene products known to control or affect fetal growth continues to increase. **Imprinted genes, expressed primarily from maternally or paternally acquired alleles, play a particularly important role in controlling fetal growth.[21] Abnormalities in the expression of these genes often result in fetal overgrowth or undergrowth.** Environmental influences, such as alterations in gene methylation or in modification of histones associated with genes, may further alter gene expression and thus fetal growth, making this a rich area for further exploration.

FETAL CARDIOVASCULAR SYSTEM
Development

The heart and the vascular system develop from splanchnic mesoderm during the third week after fertilization. The two primordial heart tubes fuse to form a simple contractile tube early in the fourth week, and the cardiovascular system becomes the first functional organ system. **During weeks 5 to 8, this single-lumen tube is converted into the definitive four-chambered heart through a process of cardiac looping (folding), remodeling, and partitioning.** However, an opening in the interatrial septum, the foramen ovale, is present and serves as an important right-to-left shunt during fetal life.

During the fourth embryonic week, three primary circulations characterize the vascular system. The *aortic/cardinal circulation* serves the embryo proper and is the basis for much of the fetal circulatory system. Of note the left sixth aortic (pulmonary) arch forms a connection between the left pulmonary artery and the aorta as the ductus arteriosus. **The ductus arteriosus also functions as a right-to-left shunt by redistributing right ventricular (RV) output from the lungs to the aorta and fetal and placental circulations.** The *vitelline circulation* develops in association with the yolk sac, and although it plays a minor role in providing nutrients to the embryo, its rearrangement ultimately provides the circulatory system for the gastrointestinal (GI) tract, spleen, pancreas, and liver. The *allantoic circulation* develops in association with the chorion and the developing chorionic villi and forms the placental circulation, comprised of two umbilical arteries and two umbilical veins. **In humans, the venous pathways are rearranged during embryonic weeks 4 to 8, and only the left umbilical vein is retained. Subsequent rearrangement of the vascular plexus associated with the developing liver forms the ductus venosus, a venous shunt that allows at least half of the estimated umbilical blood flow (70 to 130 mL/min/kg fetal weight after 30 weeks' gestation) to bypass the liver and enter the inferior vena cava.[22]**

Placental gas exchange provides well-oxygenated blood that leaves the placenta (Fig. 2-3) via the umbilical vein. In addition to the ductus venosus, small branches into the left lobe of the liver and a major branch to the right lobe account for the remainder of the umbilical venous flow. Left hepatic vein blood combines with the well-oxygenated ductus venosus flow as it enters the inferior vena cava. Because right hepatic vein blood combines with the portal vein (only a small fraction of portal vein blood passes through the ductus venosus), right hepatic vein blood is less oxygenated than its counterpart on the left,[22] and a combination of right hepatic/portal drainage with blood returning from the lower trunk and limbs further decreases the oxygen content. Although both ductus venosus blood and hepatic portal/fetal trunk bloods enter the inferior vena cava and the right atrium, little mixing occurs. **This stream of well-oxygenated ductus venosus blood is preferentially directed into the foramen ovale by the valve of the inferior vena cava and the crista dividens on the wall of the right atrium. This shunts a portion of the most highly oxygenated ductus venosus blood through the foramen ovale with little opportunity for mixing with superior vena cava/coronary sinus**

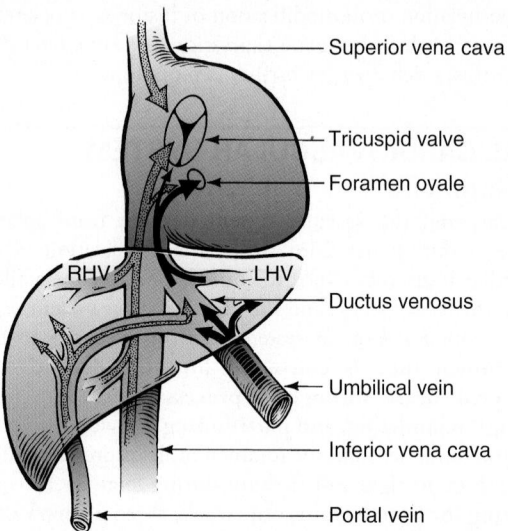

FIG 2-3 Anatomy of the umbilical and hepatic circulation. *Black arrows* represent nutrient-rich and oxygen-rich blood. LHV, left hepatic vein; RHV, right hepatic vein. (From Rudolph AM. Hepatic and ductus venosus blood flows during fetal life. *Hepatology.* 1983;3:254-258.)

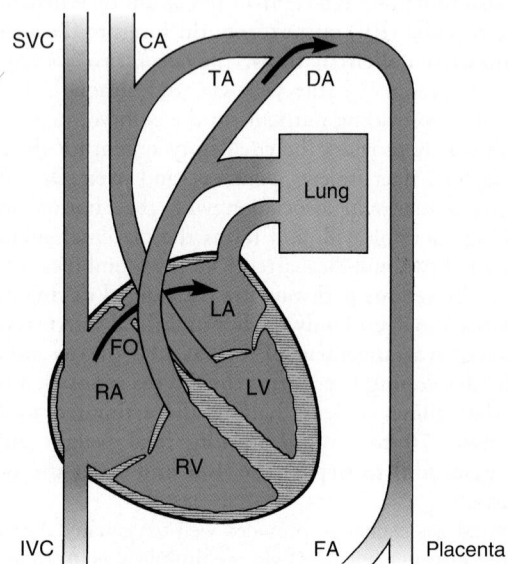

FIG 2-4 Anatomy of the fetal heart and central shunts. CA, carotid artery; DA, ductus arteriosus; FA, femoral artery; FO, foramen ovale; IVC, inferior vena cava; LA, left atrium; LV, left ventricle; RA, right atrium; RV, right ventricle; SVC, superior vena cava; TA, thoracic aorta. (From Anderson DF, Bissonnette JM, Faber JJ, Thornburg KL. Central shunt flows and pressures in the mature fetal lamb. *Am J Physiol.* 1981;241:H60-H66.)

venous return (Fig. 2-4; see also Fig. 2-3). **As a result, left atrial filling results primarily from umbilical vein–ductus venosus blood, with a small contribution from pulmonary venous flow. Thus blood with the highest oxygen content is delivered to the left atrium and left ventricle and ultimately supplies blood to the upper body and limbs, carotid and vertebral circulations, and the brain.** Inferior vena cava flow is greater than the volume that can cross the foramen ovale. The remainder of the oxygenated inferior vena cava blood is directed through the tricuspid valve (see Fig. 2-3) into the right ventricle (see Fig. 2-4) and is accompanied by venous return from the superior

vena cava and coronary sinus. However, the very high vascular resistance in the pulmonary circulation maintains mean pulmonary artery pressure 2 to 3 mm Hg above aortic pressure and directs most of the RV output through the ductus arteriosus and into the aorta and the fetal and placental circulations.[22]

Fetal Heart

The adult cardiovascular system includes a high-pressure (95 mm Hg) system and a low-pressure pulmonary circuit (15 mm Hg) driven by the left and right ventricles working in series. Although the ejection velocity is greater in the left ventricle than in the right, equal volumes of blood are delivered into the systemic and pulmonary circulations with contraction of each ventricle. The stroke volume is the volume of blood ejected by the left ventricle with each contraction, and cardiac output is a function of the stroke volume and heart rate (70 mL/beat × 72 beats/min = 5040 mL/min). For a 70-kg adult man, cardiac output averages 72 mL/min/kg. In addition to heart rate, cardiac output varies with changes in stroke volume, which in turn is determined by venous return (preload), pulmonary artery and aortic pressures (afterload), and contractility.

In contrast to the adult heart, where the two ventricles pump blood in a series circuit, the unique fetal shunts provide an unequal distribution of venous return to the respective atria, and ventricular output represents a mixture of oxygenated and deoxygenated blood. **Thus the fetal right and left ventricles function as two pumps that operate in parallel, rather than in series, and cardiac output is described as the combined ventricular output. RV output exceeds 60% of biventricular output[23] and is primarily directed through the ductus arteriosus to the descending aorta** (see Fig. 2-4). **As a result, placental blood flow, which represents approximately 40% of the combined ventricular output, primarily reflects RV output. Because of the high pulmonary vascular resistance,[23] the pulmonary circulation receives only 5% to 10% of the combined ventricular output.** Instead, left ventricular (LV) output is primarily directed through the aortic semilunar valve and aortic arch to the upper body and head. Estimates of fetal LV output average 120 mL/min/kg body weight. If LV output is less than 40% of the combined biventricular output,[23] total fetal cardiac output would be above 300 mL/min/kg. The distribution of the cardiac output to fetal organs is summarized in Table 2-1,[1] with fetal hepatic distribution reflecting only the portion supplied by the hepatic artery. In fact, hepatic blood flow derives principally from the umbilical vein and to a lesser extent the portal vein,[24] and represents about 25% of the total venous return to the heart.

The placenta receives approximately 40% of the combined ventricular output, which means the single umbilical vein also conducts this volume of the combined ventricular output toward the fetus. At least half of the umbilical venous blood bypasses the liver via the ductus venosus, and the remainder traverses the hepatic circulation. The combination of umbilical vein blood, hepatic portal blood, and blood returning from the lower body contributes approximately 69% of the cardiac output that enters the right atrium from the inferior vena cava. Flow across the foramen ovale accounts for approximately one third (27%) of the combined cardiac output.[23] Pulmonary venous return to the left atrium is low and represents approximately 7% of combined ventricular output. Thus the left atrium accounts for only about 34% (27% + 7%) of the combined ventricular output. Because a volume of inferior vena cava venous return

TABLE 2-1	DISTRIBUTION OF CARDIAC OUTPUT TO FETAL ORGANS
ORGAN	**BIVENTRICULAR CARDIAC OUTPUT (%)**
Placenta	40
Brain	13
Heart	3.5
Lung	7
Liver	2.5 (hepatic artery)
Gastrointestinal tract	5
Adrenal glands	0.5
Kidney	2.5
Spleen	1
Body	25

Data from Rudolph AM, Heymann MA. Circulatory changes during growth in the fetal lamb. *Circ Res.* 1970;26(3):289.

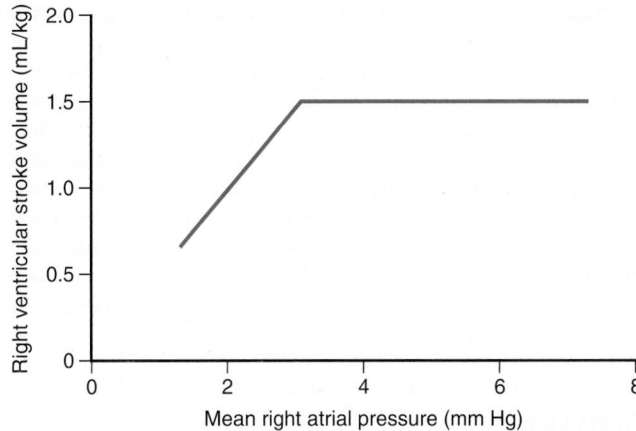

FIG 2-5 Stroke volume of the fetal right ventricle as a function of mean right atrial pressure. (From Thornburg KL, Morton MJ. Filling and arterial pressures as determinants of RV stroke volume in the sheep fetus. *Am J Physiol.* 1983;244:H656-H663.)

equivalent to 27% of the combined ventricular output is shunted across the foramen ovale, 42% remains in the right atrium and contributes to RV output. With another 21% from the superior vena cava and 3% from the coronary circulation, RV output accounts for 66% of the combined ventricular output. However, only 7% of RV output enters the pulmonary circulation, leaving 59% entering the aorta via the ductus arteriosus. Similarly, 24% of the combined ventricular output derived from the left ventricle is distributed to the upper body and brain, with approximately 10% combining with RV output in the aorta. Thus 69% of the combined ventricular output reaches the descending aorta, and 40% of this accounts for placental flow, with the remainder distributed to the fetal abdominal organs and lower body.

Consistent with the greater contribution of the right ventricle to combined ventricular output, coronary blood flow to the myocardium reflects the greater stroke volume of the right side, and RV free wall and septal blood flows are higher than in the left ventricle.[25] **It is not surprising then that fetal ventricular wall thickness is greater on the right side relative to the left.** As in the adult, fetal ventricular output depends on heart rate, pulmonary artery and aortic pressures, and contractility. The relationship between mean right atrial pressure (the index often used for ventricular volume at the end of diastole) and stroke volume is depicted in Figure 2-5. The steep ascending limb represents the length–active tension relationship for cardiac muscle in the right ventricle.[26] Under normal conditions, fetal right atrial pressure resides at the break point in this ascending limb, and increases in pressure do not increase stroke volume. Thus **the contribution of Starling mechanisms to increasing right heart output in the fetus is limited. In contrast, decreases in venous return and right atrial pressure decrease stroke volume.** Compared with the left ventricle, the fetal right ventricle has a greater anteroposterior dimension, which increases both volume and circumferential radius of curvature. This anatomic difference increases the radius/wall thickness ratio for the right ventricle and produces increased wall stress in systole and a decrease in stroke volume when afterload increases.[25] Because the right ventricle is sensitive to afterload, a linear inverse relationship exists between stroke volume and pulmonary artery pressure.[26]

The relationship between atrial pressure and stroke volume in the left ventricle is similar to that shown in Figure 2-5 for the right ventricle. Although the break point occurs near the normal

value for left atrial pressure, a small amount of preload reserve remains.[25] In distinction to the fetal right ventricle, the left side is not sensitive to aortic pressure increases. Thus postnatal increases in systemic blood pressure do not decrease LV stroke volume, and LV output increases to meet the needs of the postnatal systemic circulation. Although Starling mechanism–related increases in stroke volume are limited, especially in the right side of the heart, late-gestation fetal heart β-adrenergic receptor numbers are similar to those in the adult, and circulating catecholamine–induced increases in contractility may increase stroke volume by 50%.

Although the fetal heart rate (FHR) decreases during the last half of gestation, particularly between 20 and 30 weeks, the FHR averages more than twofold above resting adult heart rates. If analysis is confined to episodes of low heart rate variability, mean heart rate decreases from 30 weeks to term. However, if all heart rate data are analyzed, mean heart rate is stable at 142 beats/min over the last 10 weeks of gestation. Variability in mean heart rate over 24 hours includes a nadir between 2 AM and 6 AM and a peak between 8 AM and 10 AM. Most FHR accelerations occur simultaneously with limb movement, which primarily reflects central neuronal brainstem output. Also, movement-related decreases in venous return and a reflex tachycardia may contribute to heart rate accelerations.[27] **Because ventricular stroke volumes decrease with increasing heart rate, fetal cardiac output remains constant over a heart rate range of 120 to 180 beats/min.** The major effect of this inverse relationship between heart rate and stroke volume is an alteration in end-diastolic dimension. If end-diastolic dimension is kept constant, no fall in stroke volume occurs, and cardiac output increases.

At birth, major changes in vascular distribution occur with the first breath. Alveolar expansion and the associated increase in alveolar capillary oxygen tension induce a marked decrease in pulmonary microvascular resistance. This decrease in pulmonary vascular resistance has two effects. First, an accompanying decrease occurs in right atrial afterload and right atrial pressure. Second, the increase in pulmonary flow increases venous return into the left atrium and therefore increases left atrial pressure. The combined effect of these two events is to increase left atrial pressure above right atrial pressure, which leads to a physiologic closure of the foramen ovale. The return of the highly oxygenated blood from the lungs to the left atrium, left ventricle, and aorta and the decrease in pulmonary vascular resistance, and hence pulmonary trunk pressure, allows backflow of oxygen-rich blood into the ductus arteriosus. **This local increase in ductus arteriosus oxygen tension alters the ductus response to prostaglandins and causes a marked localized vasoconstriction. Concurrent spontaneous constriction (or clamping) of the umbilical cord stops placental blood flow, reduces venous return, and perhaps augments the decrease in right atrial pressure.**

Regulation of Cardiovascular Function

Autonomic Regulation

Through reflex stimulation of peripheral baroreceptors, chemoreceptors, and central mechanisms, the sympathetic and parasympathetic systems have important roles in the regulation of FHR, cardiac contractility, and vascular tone. The fetal sympathetic system develops early, whereas the parasympathetic system develops somewhat later.[28] Nevertheless, in the third trimester, increasing parasympathetic tone accounts for the characteristic decrease in FHR with periods of reduced FHR reactivity. As evidence, FHR increases in the presence of parasympathetic blockade with atropine. **Opposing sympathetic and parasympathetic inputs to the fetal heart contribute to R-R interval variability from one heart cycle to the next and to basal heart rate variability over periods of a few minutes. However, even when sympathetic and parasympathetic inputs are removed, a level of variability remains.**

Fetal sympathetic innervation is not essential for blood pressure maintenance when circulating catecholamines are present. Nevertheless, fine control of blood pressure and FHR requires an intact sympathetic system. In the absence of functional adrenergic innervation, hypoxia-induced increases in peripheral, renal, and splanchnic bed vascular resistances and blood pressure are not seen.[29] However, hypoxia-related changes in pulmonary, myocardial, adrenal, and brain blood flows occur in the absence of sympathetic innervation, which indicates that both local and endocrine effects contribute to regulation of blood flow in these organs.

Receptors in the carotid body and arch of the aorta respond to pressor or respiratory gas stimulation with afferent modulation of heart rate and vascular tone. Fetal baroreflex sensitivity, in terms of the magnitude of decreases in heart rate per millimeter of mercury increase in blood pressure, is blunted relative to the adult.[30] However, **fetal baroreflex sensitivity more than doubles in late gestation.** Although the set point for FHR is not believed to depend on intact baroreceptors, FHR variability increases when functional arterial baroreceptors are absent.[31] The same observation has been made for fetal blood pressure. Thus fetal arterial baroreceptors buffer variations in fetal blood pressure during body or breathing movements.[31] Changes in baroreceptor tone likely account for the increase in mean fetal blood pressure normally observed in late gestation. In the absence of functional chemoreceptors, mean arterial pressure is maintained[31] while peripheral blood flow increases. Thus peripheral arterial chemoreceptors may be important to maintenance of resting peripheral vascular tone. **Peripheral arterial chemoreceptors also are important components in fetal reflex responses to hypoxia; the initial bradycardia is not seen without functional chemoreceptors.**

Hormonal Regulation

Adrenocorticotropic hormone (ACTH) and catecholamines are discussed in the sections that describe the fetal adrenal and thyroid glands later in this chapter.

ARGININE VASOPRESSIN

Significant quantities of arginine vasopressin (AVP) are present in the human fetal neurohypophysis by completion of the first trimester. Ovine fetal plasma AVP levels increase appropriately in response to changes in fetal plasma osmolality induced directly in the fetus[32] **or via changes in maternal osmolality.**[33] Because of functional high- and low-pressure baroreceptors and chemoreceptor afferents, decreases in fetal intravascular volume or systemic blood pressure[34,35] also increase fetal AVP secretion. Thus in the late-gestation fetus as in the adult, AVP secretion is regulated by both osmoreceptor and volume/baroreceptor pathways. Hypoxia-induced AVP secretion has been demonstrated beyond mid pregnancy of ovine gestation, and reductions in fetal PO_2 of 10 mm Hg (50%) evoke profound increases in fetal plasma AVP levels (about 2 pg/mL to 200 to 400 pg/mL or more). Thus, because fetal AVP responsiveness to hypoxia is augmented relative to the adult (as much as fortyfold), and fetal responsiveness appears to increase during the last half of gestation, **hypoxemia is the most potent stimulus known for fetal AVP secretion.**

The cardiovascular response pattern to AVP infusion includes dose-dependent increases in fetal mean blood pressure and decreases in heart rate at plasma levels well below those required for similar effects in the adult. Receptors (V1) distinct from those that mediate AVP antidiuretic effects in the kidney (V2) account for AVP contributions to fetal circulatory adjustments during hemorrhage, hypotension, and hypoxia.[36] Corticotropin-releasing factor (CRF) effects of AVP may contribute to hypoxia-induced increases in plasma ACTH and cortisol levels. In addition to effects on FHR, cardiac output, and arterial blood pressure, AVP-induced changes in peripheral, placental, myocardial, and cerebral blood flows directly parallel the cardiovascular changes associated with acute hypoxia. Because many of these responses are attenuated during AVP receptor blockade, AVP effects on cardiac output distribution may serve to facilitate oxygen availability to the fetus during hypoxic challenges. However, other hypoxia-related responses, including decreases in renal and pulmonary blood flows and increased adrenal blood flow, are not seen in response to AVP infusions.

RENIN–ANGIOTENSIN II

Fetal plasma renin levels are typically elevated during late gestation.[37] A variety of stimuli that include changes in tubular sodium concentration; reductions in blood volume, vascular pressure, or renal perfusion pressure; and hypoxemia all increase fetal plasma renin activity. The relationship between fetal renal perfusion pressure and plasma renin activity is similar to that of adults. Consistent with the effects of renal nerve activity on renin release in adults, fetal renin gene expression is directly modulated by renal sympathetic nerve activity. **Although fetal plasma AII levels increase in response to small changes in blood volume and hypoxemia, fetal AII and aldosterone levels do not increase in proportion to changes in plasma renin activity. This apparent uncoupling of the fetal renin-angiotensin-aldosterone system and the increase in newborn AII levels may relate to the significant contribution of the placenta to plasma AII clearance in the**

fetus relative to the adult. Also, limited angiotensin-converting enzyme (ACE) availability due to reduced pulmonary blood flow and direct inhibition of aldosterone secretion by the normally high circulating ANF levels may contribute. Thus, reductions in AII production and aldosterone responses to AII, augmented AII and aldosterone clearances, and the resulting reductions in AII and aldosterone levels and feedback inhibition of renin may account for the elevated renin and reduced AII and aldosterone levels typically observed during fetal life.

AII infusion increases fetal mean arterial blood pressure. In contrast to AVP-induced bradycardia, fetal AII infusion increases heat rate (after an initial reflex bradycardia) through both a direct effect on the heart and decreased baroreflex responsiveness. Both hormones increase fetal blood pressure similar to the levels seen with hypoxemia. However, AII does not reduce peripheral blood flow, perhaps because circulation to muscle, skin, and bone is always under maximum response to AII, which thereby limits increases in resting tone. AII infusions also decrease renal blood flow and increase umbilical vascular resistance, although absolute placental blood flow does not change. Whereas the adult kidney contains both AII-receptor subtypes (AT_1 and AT_2), the AT_2 subtype is the only form present in the human fetal kidney. Maturational differences in the AII receptor subtype expressed would be consistent with earlier studies that demonstrated differing AII effects on fetal renal and peripheral vascular beds. Thus, the receptors that mediate AII responses in the renal and peripheral vascular beds differ during fetal life.

Fetal Hemoglobin

The fetus exists in a state of aerobic metabolism, with arterial blood PO_2 values in the 20 to 35 mm Hg range but with no evidence of metabolic acidosis. Adequate fetal tissue oxygenation is achieved by several mechanisms. Of major importance are the higher fetal cardiac output and organ blood flows. A higher hemoglobin concentration (relative to the adult) and an increase in oxygen-carrying capacity of fetal hemoglobin also contribute. The resulting leftward shift in the fetal oxygen dissociation curve relative to the adult (Fig. 2-6) increases fetal blood oxygen saturation for any given oxygen tension. For example, at a partial pressure of 26.5 mm Hg, adult blood oxygen saturation is 50%, whereas fetal oxygen saturation is 70%. Thus at a normal fetal PO_2 of 20 mm Hg, fetal whole-blood oxygen saturation may be 50%.

The basis for increased oxygen affinity of fetal whole blood resides in the interaction of fetal hemoglobin with intracellular organic phosphate 2,3-diphosphoglycerate (2,3-DPG). The fetal hemoglobin (HgbF) tetramer is composed of two α-chains (identical to adult) and two γ-chains. The latter differ from the γ-chain of adult hemoglobin (HgbA) in 39 of 146 amino acid residues. Among these differences is the substitution of serine in the γ-chain of HgbF for histidine at the β-143 position of HgbA, which is located at the entrance to the central cavity of the hemoglobin tetramer. Due to a positively charged imidazole group, histidine can bind with the negatively charged 2,3-DPG. Binding of 2,3-DPG to deoxyhemoglobin stabilizes the tetramer in the reduced form. Because serine is nonionized and does not interact with 2,3-DPG to the same extent as histidine, the oxygen affinity of HgbF is increased, and the dissociation curve is shifted to the left. If HgbA or HgbF is removed from the erythrocyte and stripped of organic phosphates, the oxygen affinity for both hemoglobins is similar. However, addition of equal amounts of 2,3-DPG to the hemoglobins decreases

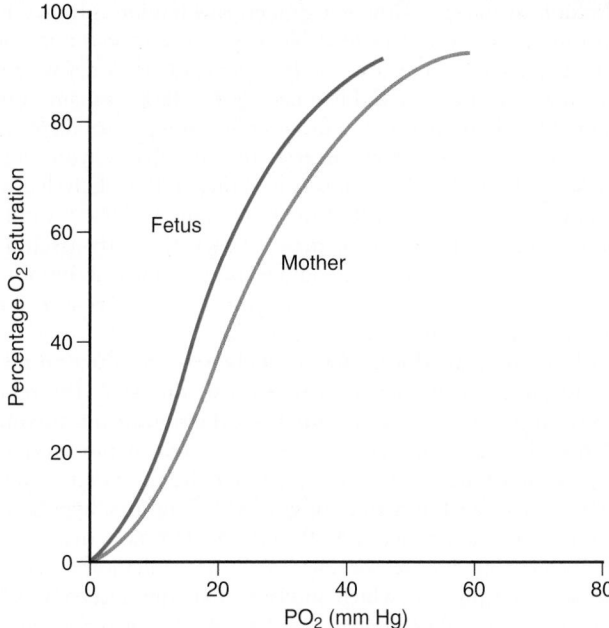

FIG 2-6 Oxyhemoglobin dissociation curves of maternal and fetal human blood at pH 7.4 and 37° C. (Modified from Hellegers AE, Schruefer JJ. Normograms and empirical equations relating oxygen tension, percentage saturation, and pH in maternal and fetal blood. *Am J Obstet Gynecol.* 1961;81:377-384.)

HgbA oxygen affinity (dissociation curve shifts to the right) to a greater extent than for HgbF. Thus, even though overall oxygen affinities are similar, differences in 2,3-DPG interaction result in a higher oxygen affinity for HgbF.

The proportion of HgbF to HgbA changes between 26 and 40 weeks' gestation. HgbF decreases linearly from 100% to about 70% so that HgbA accounts for 30% of fetal hemoglobin at term. This change in expression from γ- to β-globulin synthesis takes place in erythroid progenitor cells. Although the basis for this switching is not yet known, our understanding of human globin gene regulation has provided important insights into several fetal hemoglobin disorders, such as the thalassemias and sickle cell anemia. Duplication of the α-genes on chromosome 16 provides the normal fetus with four gene loci. The genes for the remaining globins are located on chromosome 11 and consist of $^{G}\gamma$, $^{A}\gamma$, δ, and β. The two γ-genes differ in the amino acid in position 36, glycine versus alanine. HgbA synthesis is dictated by the γ- and β-genes, HgbF by α and γ, and $HgbA_2$ by α and δ. Sequences in the δ region may be responsible for the relative expression of the γ-gene such that fetal hemoglobin persists when these are absent.

FETAL KIDNEY

Overall fetal water and electrolyte homeostasis is primarily mediated by fetal–maternal exchange across the placenta. However, urine production by the fetal kidney is essential to maintenance of AFV and composition. Although absolute glomerular filtration rate (GFR) increases during the third trimester, GFR per gram of kidney weight does not change because GFR and fetal kidney weight increase in parallel. The genesis of new glomeruli is complete by about 36 weeks. Subsequent increases in GFR reflect increases in glomerular surface area for filtration, effective filtration pressure, and capillary filtration coefficient. Although glomerular filtration is related to hydrostatic pressure, and fetal blood pressure increases in the third trimester, both renal blood flow per gram of kidney weight and filtration fraction (GFR/renal plasma flow) remain constant.[38] Newborn increases in filtration fraction parallel increases in arterial pressure, which suggests that the lower hydrostatic pressure within the glomerulus contributes to the relatively low filtration fraction and GFR of the intrauterine kidney.[38] A mild glomerulotubular imbalance may describe the early-gestation fetus. However, renal tubular sodium and chloride reabsorptions increase in late gestation such that glomerulotubular balance is maintained in the third-trimester fetus.[38]

Although fetal GFR is low, the daily urine production rate is substantial, equaling 60% to 80% of the AFV. The relatively large urine output results from the significant portion of the filtered water (20%) that is excreted in the form of hypotonic urine. The positive free-water clearance that characterizes fetal renal function originally led to the hypothesis that the fetal kidney lacked AVP receptors. However, ovine fetal renal collecting duct responses to AVP can be demonstrated in the second trimester, which indicates that diminished urine-concentrating ability is not caused by AVP receptor absence. Fetal renal V_2 receptors mediate AVP-induced tubular water reabsorption, and functional V_2 receptors are present in the fetal kidney by the beginning of the last third of gestation.[36] In addition, AVP-induced cAMP production is not different from that of the adult, and AVP-induced apical tubular water channels (aquaporin 2) are expressed in the fetal kidney. In fact, the selective AVP V_2 receptor agonist dDAVP appropriately increases fetal renal water reabsorption without affecting blood pressure or heart rate.[36] Thus V_2 receptors mediate AVP effects on fetal urine production and AFV.[36] Instead, **the reduced concentrating ability of the fetal kidney primarily reflects reductions in proximal tubular sodium reabsorption, short juxtamedullary nephron loops of Henle, and limited medullary interstitial urea concentrations.**

Although fetal plasma renin activity levels are high, effective uncoupling of AII production from plasma renin activity and a high placental clearance rate for AII serve to minimize increases in fetal plasma AII levels. Limiting fluctuations in fetal plasma AII levels may be advantageous for fetal renal function regulation. For example, fetal AII infusion increases fetal mean arterial pressure and renal and placental vascular resistances. In contrast, fetal treatment with the ACE inhibitor captopril increases plasma renin activity and decreases arterial blood pressure, renal vascular resistance, and filtration fraction, and urine flow effectively ceases. Given the potential for AII to decrease placental blood flow, uncoupling of renin-induced angiotensin I production, limited ACE activity, and augmented placental AII clearance may protect the fetal cardiovascular system from large increases in plasma AII levels. Collectively, plasma AII levels appear to be regulated within a very narrow range, and this regulation may be important to overall fetal homeostasis.

Atrial natriuretic factor (ANF) granules are present in the fetal heart, and fetal plasma ANF levels are elevated relative to the adult. Fetal plasma ANF levels increase in response to volume expansion, and ANF infusion evokes limited increases in ovine fetal renal sodium excretion. Fetal ANF infusion also decreases fetal plasma volume with minimal effect on blood pressure. These observations suggest that ANF actions in the fetus are primarily directed at volume homeostasis and have minimal cardiovascular effects.

The ability of the fetal kidney to excrete titratable acid and ammonia is limited relative to the adult. In addition, the threshold for fetal renal bicarbonate excretion—defined as the excretion of a determined amount of bicarbonate per unit GFR—is much lower than in the adult. That is, fetal urine tends to be alkaline at relatively low plasma bicarbonate levels, despite the high fetal arterial PCO_2. Because fetal renal tubular mechanisms for glucose reabsorption are qualitatively similar to those in the adult, fetal renal glucose excretion is limited. In fact, the maximum ability of the fetal kidney to reabsorb glucose exceeds that of the adult when expressed as a function of GFR.

FETAL GASTROINTESTINAL SYSTEM
Gastrointestinal Tract

Amniotic fluid contains measurable glucose, lactate, and amino acid concentrations, which raises the possibility that fetal swallowing could serve as a source of nutrient uptake. Fetal swallowing contributes importantly to somatic growth and GI development as a result of the large volume of ingested fluid. **About 10% to 15% of fetal nitrogen requirements may result from swallowing of amniotic fluid protein.[39] Amino acids and glucose are absorbed and utilized by the fetus if they are administered into the fetal GI tract.[40] Furthermore, intragastric ovine fetal nutrient administration partially ameliorates fetal growth restriction induced by maternal malnutrition.[41]**

Further evidence for the role of swallowing in fetal growth results from studies that have demonstrated that impairment of fetal rabbit swallowing at 24 days' gestation (term = 31 days) induces an 8% weight decrease (compared with controls) by 28 days.[42] The fetal GI tract is directly affected, and esophageal ligation of fetal rabbit pups results in marked reductions in gastric and intestinal tissue weight and gastric acidity.[42] Reductions in GI and somatic growth were reversed by fetal intragastric infusion of amniotic fluid.[42] Similarly, esophageal ligation of 90-day ovine fetuses (term = 145 to 150 days) induces a 30% decrease of small intestine villus height[43] and a reduction in liver, pancreas, and intestinal weight.[44]

Although ingestion of amniotic fluid nutrients may be necessary for optimal fetal growth, trophic growth factors within the amniotic fluid also importantly contribute. Thus the reduction in fetal rabbit weight induced by esophageal ligation is reversed by gastric infusion of EGF. Studies in human infants support the association of fetal swallowing and GI growth because upper GI tract obstructions are associated with a significantly greater rate of human fetal growth restriction as compared with fetuses with lower GI obstructions.[45]

Blood flow to the fetal intestine does not increase during moderate levels of hypoxemia. The artery–mesenteric vein difference in oxygen content is also unchanged so that at a constant blood flow, intestinal oxygen consumption can remain the same during moderate hypoxemia. **However, with more pronounced hypoxemia, fetal intestinal oxygen consumption falls as blood flow decreases, and the oxygen content difference across the intestine fails to widen. The result is a metabolic acidosis in the blood that drains the mesenteric system.**

Liver

Near term, the placenta is the major route for bilirubin elimination. Less than 10% of an administered bilirubin load is excreted in the fetal biliary tree over a 10-hour period; about

20% remains in plasma. Thus the fetal metabolic pathways for bilirubin and bile salts remain underdeveloped at term. The cholate pool size (normalized to body surface area) is one third and the synthetic rate is one half the adult levels. In premature infants, cholate pool size and synthesis rates represent less than half and one third, respectively, of term infant values. In fact, premature infant intraluminal duodenal bile acid concentrations are near or below the level required to form lipid micelles.[46]

The unique attributes of the fetal hepatic circulation were detailed during the earlier discussion of fetal circulatory anatomy. Notably, the fetal hepatic blood supply primarily derives from the umbilical vein. The left lobe receives its blood supply almost exclusively from the umbilical vein (with a small contribution from the hepatic artery), whereas the right lobe receives blood from the portal vein as well. **The fetal liver under normal conditions accounts for about 20% of total fetal oxygen consumption.** Because hepatic glucose uptake and release are balanced, net glucose removal by the liver under normal conditions is minimal. During episodes of hypoxemia, β-adrenergic receptor–mediated increases in hepatic glucose release account for the hyperglycemia characteristic of short-term fetal hypoxemia.[47] **Hypoxia severe enough to decrease fetal oxygen consumption selectively reduces right hepatic lobe oxygen uptake, which exceeds that of the fetus as a whole. In contrast, oxygen uptake by the left lobe of the liver is unchanged.**

FETAL ADRENAL AND THYROID GLANDS
Adrenal Glands
The fetal anterior pituitary secretes ACTH in response to stress, which includes hypoxemia. The associated increase in cortisol exerts feedback inhibition of the continued ACTH response.[48] In the fetus and adult, proopiomelanocortin posttranslational processing gives rise to ACTH, corticotropin-like intermediate lobe peptide (CLIP), and α-melanocyte–stimulating hormone (α-MSH). The precursor peptide preproenkephalin is a distinct gene product that gives rise to the enkephalins. Fetal proopiomelanocortin processing differs from the adult. For example, although ACTH is present in appreciable amounts, the fetal pituitary contains large amounts of CLIP and α-MSH. The fetal ratio of CLIP plus α-MSH to ACTH decreases from the end of the first trimester to term. Because pituitary corticotropin-releasing hormone (CRH) expression is relatively low until late gestation, AVP serves as the major CRF in early gestation. With increasing gestational age, fetal cortisol levels progressively increase secondary to hypothalamic-pituitary axis maturation. Cortisol is important to pituitary maturation because it shifts corticotrophs from the fetal to the adult type, and it impacts adrenal maturation through regulation of ACTH receptor numbers.[49]

On a body-weight basis, the fetal adrenal gland is an order of magnitude larger than in the adult. This increase in size is due to the presence of an adrenal cortical definitive zone and a so-called fetal zone that constitutes 85% of the adrenal at birth. Cortisol and mineralocorticoids are the major products of the fetal definitive zone, and fetal cortisol secretion is regulated by ACTH but not human chorionic gonadotropin (hCG). Low-density lipoprotein (LDL)–bound cholesterol (see "Receptor-Mediated Endocytosis and Exocytosis" in Chapter 1) is the major source of steroid precursor in the fetal adrenal. Because the enzyme 3α-hydroxysteroid dehydrogenase is lacking

in the fetal adrenal, dehydroepiandrosterone sulfate (DHEAS) is the major product of the fetal zone. At mid gestation, DHEAS secretion is determined by both ACTH and hCG. Both fetal ACTH and cortisol levels are relatively low during most of gestation, and no clear correlation has been found between plasma ACTH levels and cortisol production. This apparent dissociation between fetal ACTH levels and cortisol secretion may be explained by 1) differences in ACTH processing, and the presence of the large-molecular-weight proopiomelanocortin processing products CLIP and α-MSH may suppress ACTH action on the adrenal until late gestation, when ACTH becomes the primary product; 2) fetal adrenal definitive zone ACTH responsiveness may increase; or 3) placental ACTH and/or posttranslational processing intermediates may affect the adrenal response to ACTH.

Resting fetal plasma norepinephrine levels exceed epinephrine levels approximately tenfold. The fetal plasma levels of both catecholamines increase in response to hypoxemia, and norepinephrine levels are invariably higher than epinephrine levels. Under basal conditions, norepinephrine is secreted at a higher rate than epinephrine, and this relationship persists during a hypoxemic stimulus. Plasma norepinephrine levels increase in response to acute hypoxemia but decline to remain above basal levels with persistent (>5 min) hypoxemia. In contrast, adrenal epinephrine secretion begins gradually but persists during 30 minutes of hypoxemia. These observations are consistent with independent sites of synthesis and regulation of the two catecholamines.[50] Although the initial fetal blood pressure elevation during hypoxemia correlates with increases in norepinephrine, afterward the correlation between plasma norepinephrine and hypertension is lost.

Thyroid Gland
The normal placenta is impermeable to thyroid-stimulating hormone (TSH), and triiodothyronine (T$_3$) transfer is minimal.[51] However, appreciable levels of maternal thyroxine (T$_4$) are seen in infants with congenital hypothyroidism (see Chapter 42). **By week 12 of gestation, thyrotropin-releasing hormone (TRH) is present in the fetal hypothalamus, and TRH secretion and/ or pituitary sensitivity to TRH increases progressively during gestation. Extrahypothalamic sites, including the pancreas, also may contribute to the high TRH levels observed in the fetus. Measurable TSH is present in the fetal pituitary and serum, and T$_4$ is measurable in fetal blood by week 12 of gestation.** Thyroid function is low until about 20 weeks, when T$_4$ levels increase gradually to term. TSH levels rise markedly between 20 and 24 weeks then slowly decrease until delivery. **Fetal liver T$_4$ metabolism is immature, characterized by low T$_3$ levels until week 30. In contrast, reverse T$_3$ levels are high until 30 weeks and decline steadily thereafter until term.**

FETAL CENTRAL NERVOUS SYSTEM
Clinically relevant indicators of fetal central nervous system function are body movements and breathing movements. Fetal activity periods in late gestation are often termed *active* or *reactive* and *quiet* or *nonreactive*. The *active cycle* is characterized by clustering of gross fetal body movements, a high heart rate variability, heart rate accelerations (often followed by decelerations), and fetal breathing movements. The *quiet cycle* is noted by absence of fetal body movements and a low variability in the fetal heart period. In this context, *fetal heart*

period variability refers to deviations in the model heart rate period averaged over short periods (seconds)[52] and is distinct from beat-to-beat variability. In the last 6 weeks of gestation, the fetus is in an active state 60% to 70% of the time. The average duration of quiet periods ranges from 15 to 23 minutes (see Table 4 in Visser and colleagues[52] for a review).

The fetal electrocorticogram shows two predominant patterns: low-voltage, high-frequency and high-voltage, low-frequency electrocortical patterns. *Low-voltage, high-frequency* activity is associated with bursts of rapid eye movement (REM) and fetal breathing movements. Similar to REM sleep in the adult, inhibition of skeletal muscle movement is most pronounced in muscle groups that have a high percentage of spindles. Thus the diaphragm, which is relatively spindle free, is not affected. Fetal body movements during low-voltage electrocortical activity are reduced relative to the activity seen during *high-voltage, low-frequency* electrocortical activity.[53] Polysynaptic reflexes elicited by stimulation of afferents from limb muscles are relatively suppressed when the fetus is in the low-voltage state.[54] Short-term hypoxia[53] or hypoxemia inhibits reflex limb movements, and the inhibitory neural activity arises in the midbrain area.[54] Fetal cardiovascular and behavioral responses to maternal cocaine use previously have been attributed to reductions in uteroplacental blood flow and resulting fetal hypoxia. However, fetal sheep studies indicate that acute fetal cocaine exposure evokes catecholamine, cardiovascular, and neurobehavioral effects in the absence of fetal oxygenation changes.[55] It is not yet clear whether cocaine-induced reductions in fetal low-voltage electrocortical activity reflect changes in cerebral blood flow or a direct cocaine effect on norepinephrine stimulation of central regulatory centers. However, these observations are consistent with the significant neurologic consequences of cocaine use during pregnancy (see Chapter 55).

Fetal breathing patterns are rapid and irregular in nature and are not associated with significant fluid movement into the lung.[56] **The central medullary respiratory chemoreceptors are stimulated by CO_2,**[57] **and fetal breathing is maintained only if central hydrogen ion concentrations remain in the physiologic range. That is, central (medullary cerebrospinal fluid) acidosis stimulates respiratory incidence and depth, and alkalosis results in apnea. Paradoxically, hypoxemia markedly decreases breathing activity, possibly as a result of inhibitory input from centers above the medulla.**[58]

Glucose is the principal substrate for oxidative metabolism in the fetal brain under normal conditions. During low-voltage electrocortical activity, cerebral blood flow and oxygen consumption are increased relative to high-voltage values, with an efflux of lactate. During high voltage, the fetal brain shows a net uptake of lactate.[59] The fetal cerebral circulation is sensitive to changes in arterial oxygen content, and despite marked hypoxia-induced increases in cerebral blood flow, cerebral oxygen consumption is maintained without widening of the arterial-venous oxygen content difference across the brain.[60] Increases in CO_2 also cause cerebral vasodilation. However, the response to hypercarbia is reduced relative to that of the adult.

SUMMARY

The fetus and placenta depend on unique physiologic systems to provide an environment that supports fetal growth and development in preparation for transition to extrauterine life. Because specific functions of the various physiologic systems are often gestation specific, differences between the fetus and adult of one species are often greater than the differences between systems. Thus the clinician or investigator concerned with fetal life or neonatal transition must fully appreciate these aspects of fetal physiology and their application to their area of study or treatment.

KEY POINTS

- Mean amniotic fluid volume increases from 250 to 800 mL between 16 and 32 weeks and decreases to 500 mL at term.
- Fetal urine production ranges from 400 to 1200 mL/day and is the primary source of amniotic fluid.
- The fetal umbilical circulation receives approximately 40% of fetal combined ventricular output (300 mL/mg/min).
- Umbilical blood flow is 70 to 130 mL/min after 30 weeks' gestation.
- Fetal cardiac output is constant over a heart rate range of 120 to 180 beats/min.
- The fetus exists in a state of aerobic metabolism, with arterial PO_2 values in the 20 to 25 mm Hg range.
- Glucose, amino acids, and lactate are the major substrates for fetal oxidative metabolism.
- Approximately 20% of the fetal oxygen consumption of 8 mL/kg/min is required in the acquisition of new tissue.
- By week 12 of gestation, thyrotropin-releasing hormone is present in the fetal hypothalamus.
- Fetal activity periods in late gestation are often termed *active* or *reactive* and *quiet* or *nonreactive*.

REFERENCES

1. Rudolph AM, Heymann MA. Circulatory changes during growth in the fetal lamb. *Circ Res.* 1970;26:289-299.
2. Cheung CY, Brace RA. Developmental expression of vascular endothelial growth factor and its receptors in ovine placenta and fetal membranes. *J Soc Gynecol Investig.* 1999;6:179-185.
3. Thaete LG, Dewey ER. Neerhof MG. Endothelin and the regulation of uterine and placental perfusion in hypoxia-induced fetal growth restriction. *J Soc Gynecol Investig.* 2004;11:16-21.
4. Beall MH, van den Wijngaard JP, van Gemert MJ, Ross MG. Amniotic fluid water dynamics. *Placenta.* 2007;28:816-823.
5. Robillard JE, Ramberg E, Sessions C, et al. Role of aldosterone on renal sodium and potassium excretion during fetal life and newborn period. *Dev Pharmacol Ther.* 1980;1:201-216.
6. Abramovich DR. Fetal factors influencing the volume and composition of liquor amnii. *J Obstet Gynaecol Br Commonw.* 1970;77:865-877.
7. Harding R, Sigger JN, Poore ER, Johnson P. Ingestion in fetal sheep and its relation to sleep states and breathing movements. *Q J Exp Physiol.* 1984;69:477-486.
8. Mann SE, Ricke EA, Torres EA, Taylor RN. A novel model of polyhydramnios: amniotic fluid volume is increased in aquaporin 1 knockout mice. *Am J Obstet Gynecol.* 2005;192:2041-2044.
9. Beall MH, Wang S, Yang B, et al. Placental and membrane aquaporin water channels: correlation with amniotic fluid volume and composition. *Placenta.* 2007;28:421-428.
10. Hay WW Jr, Myers SA, Sparks JW, et al. Glucose and lactate oxidation rates in the fetal lamb. *Proc Soc Exp Biol Med.* 1983;173:553-563.

11. Battaglia FC. Glutamine and glutamate exchange between the fetal liver and the placenta. *J Nutr.* 2000;130:974S-977S.
12. Forbes K, Westwood M. The IGF axis and placental function: a mini review. *Horm Res.* 2008;69:129-137.
13. Constancia M, Hemberger M, Hughes J, et al. Placental-specific IGF-II is a major modulator of placental and fetal growth. *Nature.* 2002;417: 945-948.
14. Murphy VE, Smith R, Giles WB, Clifton VL. Endocrine regulation of human fetal growth: the role of the mother, placenta, and fetus. *Endocr Rev.* 2006;27:141-169.
15. Hay WW, Meznarich HK, Sparks JW, et al. Effect of insulin on glucose uptake in near-term fetal lambs. *Proc Soc Exp Biol Med.* 1985;178: 557-564.
16. Fowden AL. The insulin-like growth factors and feto-placental growth. *Placenta.* 2003;24:803-812.
17. El-Hashash AH, Esbrit P, Kimber SJ. PTHrP promotes murine secondary trophoblast giant cell differentiation through induction of endocycle, upregulation of giant-cell-promoting transcription factors and suppression of other trophoblast cell types. *Differentiation.* 2005;73:154-174.
18. Bond H, Dilworth MR, Baker B, et al. Increased maternofetal calcium flux in parathyroid hormone-related protein-null mice. *J Physiol.* 2008;586: 2015-2025.
19. Threadgill DW, Dlugosz AA, Hansen LA, et al. Targeted disruption of mouse EGF receptor: effect of genetic background on mutant phenotype. *Science.* 1995;269:230-234.
20. Dackor J, Li M, Threadgill DW. Placental overgrowth and fertility defects in mice with a hypermorphic allele of epidermal growth factor receptor. *Mamm Genome.* 2009;20:339-349.
21. Frost JM, Moore GE. The importance of imprinting in the human placenta. *PLoS Genet.* 2010;6:e1001015-1-9.
22. Rudolph AM. Hepatic and ductus venosus blood flows during fetal life. *Hepatology.* 1983;3:254-258.
23. Anderson DF, Bissonnette JM, Faber JJ, Thornburg KL. Central shunt flows and pressures in the mature fetal lamb. *Am J Physiol.* 1981;241: H60-H66.
24. Edelstone DI, Rudolph AM, Heymann MA. Liver and ductus venosus blood flows in fetal lambs in utero. *Circ Res.* 1978;42:426-433.
25. Thornburg KL, Morton MG. Filling and arterial pressures as determinants of left ventricular stroke volume in fetal lambs. *Am J Physiol.* 1986;251: H961-H968.
26. Thornburg KL, Morton MJ. Filling and arterial pressures as determinants of RV stroke volume in the sheep fetus. *Am J Physiol.* 1983;244: H656-H663.
27. Bocking AD, Harding R, Wickham PJ. Relationship between accelerations and decelerations in heart rate and skeletal muscle activity in fetal sheep. *J Dev Physiol.* 1985;7:47-54.
28. Assali NS, Brinkman CR III, Woods JR Jr, et al. Development of neurohumoral control of fetal, neonatal, and adult cardiovascular functions. *Am J Obstet Gynecol.* 1977;129:748-759.
29. Iwamoto HS, Rudolph AM, Miskin BL, Keil LC. Circulatory and humoral responses of sympathectomized fetal sheep to hypoxemia. *Am J Physiol.* 1983;245:H767-H772.
30. Dawes GS, Johnston BM, Walker DW. Relationship of arterial pressure and heart rate in fetal, newborn and adult sheep. *J Physiol.* 1980;309: 405-417.
31. Itskovitz J, LaGamma EF, Rudolph AM. Baroreflex control of the circulation in chronically instrumented fetal lambs. *Circ Res.* 1983;52:589-596.
32. Weitzman RE, Fisher DA, Robillard J, et al. Arginine vasopressin response to an osmotic stimulus in the fetal sheep. *Pediatr Res.* 1978;12:35-38.
33. Ervin MG, Ross MG, Youssef A, et al. Renal effects of ovine fetal arginine vasopressin secretion in response to maternal hyperosmolality. *Am J Obstet Gynecol.* 1986;155:1341-1347.
34. Rose JC, Meis PJ, Morris M. Ontogeny of endocrine (ACTH, vasopressin, cortisol) responses to hypotension in lamb fetuses. *Am J Physiol.* 1981; 240:E656-E661.
35. Ross MG, Ervin MG, Leake RD, et al. Isovolemic hypotension in ovine fetus: plasma arginine vasopressin response and urinary effects. *Am J Physiol.* 1986;250:E564-E569.
36. Ervin MG, Ross MG, Leake RD, Fisher DA. V1- and V2-receptor contributions to ovine fetal renal and cardiovascular responses to vasopressin. *Am J Physiol.* 1992;262:R636-R643.
37. Robillard JR, Nakamura KT. Neurohormonal regulation of renal function during development. *Am J Physiol.* 1988;254:F771-F779.
38. Lumbers ER. A brief review of fetal renal function. *J Dev Physiol.* 1984;6:1-10.
39. Pitkin RM, Reynolds WA. Fetal ingestion and metabolism of amniotic fluid protein. *Am J Obstet Gynecol.* 1975;123:356-363.
40. Charlton VE, Reis BL. Effects of gastric nutritional supplementation on fetal umbilical uptake of nutrients. *Am J Physiol.* 1981;241:E178-E185.
41. Charlton V. Johengen M: Effects of intrauterine nutritional supplementation on fetal growth retardation. *Biol Neonate.* 1985;48:125-142.
42. Wesson DE, Muraji T, Kent G, et al. The effect of intrauterine esophageal ligation on growth of fetal rabbits. *J Pediatr Surg.* 1984;19:398-399.
43. Trahair JF, Harding R, Bocking AD, et al. The role of ingestion in the development of the small intestine in fetal sheep. *Q J Exp Physiol.* 1986;71:99-104.
44. Avila C, Harding R, Robinson P. The effects of preventing ingestion on the development of the digestive system in the sheep fetus. *Q J Exp Physiol.* 1986;71:99-104.
45. Pierro A, Cozzi F, Colarossi G, et al. Does fetal gut obstruction cause hydramnios and growth retardation? *J Pediatr Surg.* 1987;22:454-457.
46. Lester R, Jackson BT, Smallwood RA, et al. Fetal and neonatal hepatic function. II. *Birth defects.* 1976;12:307-315.
47. Jones CT, Ritchie JW, Walker D. The effects of hypoxia on glucose turnover in the fetal sheep. *J Dev Physiol.* 1983;5:223-235.
48. Wood CE, Rudolph AM. Negative feedback regulation of adrenocorticotropin secretion by cortisol in ovine fetuses. *Endocrinology.* 1983;112: 1930-1936.
49. Challis JR, Brooks AN. Maturation and activation of hypothalamic-pituitary adrenal function in fetal sheep. *Endocrinol Rev.* 1989;10: 182-204.
50. Padbury J, Agata Y, Ludlow J, et al. Effect of fetal adrenalectomy on catecholamine release and physiological adaptation at birth in sheep. *J Clin Invest.* 1987;80:1096-1103.
51. Fisher DA. Maternal-fetal thyroid function in pregnancy. *Clin Perinatol.* 1983;10:615-626.
52. Visser GH, Goodman JD, Levine DH, Dawes GS. Diurnal and other cyclic variations in human fetal heart rate near term. *Am J Obstet Gynecol.* 1982;142:535-544.
53. Natale R, Clewlow F, Dawes GS. Measurement of fetal forelimb movements in the lamb in utero. *Am J Obstet Gynecol.* 1981;140:545-551.
54. Blanco CE, Dawes GS, Walker DW. Effect of hypoxia on polysynaptic hindlimb reflexes of unanesthetized foetal and newborn lambs. *J Physiol.* 1983;339:453-466.
55. Chan K, Dodd PA, Day L, et al. Fetal catecholamine, cardiovascular, and neurobehavioral responses to cocaine. *Am J Obstet Gynecol.* 1992;167: 1616-1623.
56. Dawes GS, Fox HE, Leduc BM, et al. Respiratory movements and rapid eye movement sleep in the foetal lamb. *J Physiol.* 1972;220:119-143.
57. Connors G, Hunse C, Carmichal L, et al. Control of fetal breathing in human fetus between 24 and 34 weeks gestation. *Am J Obstet Gynecol.* 1989;160:932-938.
58. Dawes GS, Gardner WN, Johnson BM, Walker DW. Breathing activity in fetal lambs: the effect of brain stem section. *J Physiol.* 1983;335:535-553.
59. Chao CR, Hohimer AR, Bissonnette JM. The effect of electrocortical state on cerebral carbohydrate metabolism in fetal sheep. *Brain Res Dev Brain Res.* 1989;49:1-5.
60. Jones MD, Sheldon RE, Peeters LL, et al. Fetal cerebral oxygen consumption at different levels of oxygenation. *J Appl Physiol Respir Envorion Exerc Physiol.* 1977;43:1080-1084.

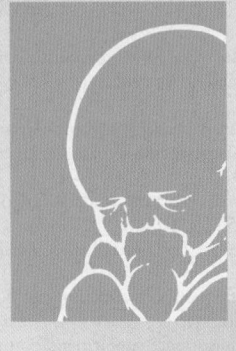

CHAPTER 3

Maternal Physiology

KATHLEEN M. ANTONY, DIANA A. RACUSIN, KJERSTI AAGAARD, and GARY A. DILDY III

KEY ABBREVIATIONS

Activated protein C	APC	Glomerular filtration rate	GFR
Adrenocorticotropic hormone	ACTH	Human chorionic gonadotropin	hCG
Alanine aminotransferase	ALT	Mean arterial pressure	MAP
Arginine vasopressin	AVP	Nitric oxide	NO
Aspartate aminotransferase	AST	Parathyroid hormone	PTH
Atrial natriuretic peptide	ANP	Peak expiratory flow	PEF
Blood pressure	BP	Plasminogen activator inhibitor	PAI
Blood urea nitrogen	BUN	Premature ventricular contraction	PVC
Body mass index	BMI	Pulmonary capillary wedge pressure	PCWP
Brain natriuretic peptide	BNP	Rapid eye movement	REM
Cardiac output	CO	Red blood cell	RBC
Colloidal oncotic pressure	COP	Renin-angiotensin-aldosterone system	RAAS
Corticosteroid-binding globulin	CBG	Restless legs syndrome	RLS
Corticotropin-releasing hormone	CRH	Stroke volume	SV
Deoxycorticosterone	DOC	Systemic vascular resistance	SVR
Forced expiratory volume in 1 second	FEV_1	Thyroid-stimulating hormone	TSH
Forced vital capacity	FVC	Thyroxine-binding globulin	TBG
Free thyroxine index	FTI	Total lung capacity	TLC
Functional residual capacity	FRC	Total thyroxine	TT4
Gastroesophageal	GE	Total triiodothyronine	TT3
Gestational weight gain	GWG	White blood cell	WBC

OVERVIEW

Pregnancy is characterized by major adaptations in the maternal anatomy, physiology, and metabolism that are necessary to achieve a successful pregnancy. Hormonal changes significantly alter the maternal physiology and persist throughout both pregnancy and the postpartum period. These adaptations are profound and affect nearly every organ system, and complete understanding of these changes is necessary to differentiate between physiologic alterations and pathology. This chapter describes maternal adaptations in pregnancy and gives specific clinical correlations to describe how these changes may affect care. A complete understanding of these adaptations will also facilitate adequate counseling of patients regarding the physiology that underlies various "normal" symptoms that they may experience.

Many changes in routine laboratory values caused by pregnancy are described in the following text. For a comprehensive review of normal reference ranges for common laboratory tests by trimester, please refer to Appendix A.

GESTATIONAL WEIGHT GAIN

Pregnancy is generally characterized as a period of weight gain. **Studies on the mean gestational weight gain (GWG) of normal-weight women giving birth to term infants ranged from 22.0 to 36.8 lb during pregnancy.**[1] The recommendations for weight gain during pregnancy have also evolved over time. In the early twentieth century, doctors frequently recommended that women gain between 15 and 20 pounds.[1] However, since that era, our understanding of the contributors to GWG have become more sophisticated, and simultaneously, the body composition of the reproductive-aged population has significantly changed. Thus **we now have more tailored recommendations for GWG that are body mass index (BMI) specific.**[1]

GWG consists of the maternal contribution and the weight of the products of conception. The maternal contribution includes increases in the circulating blood volume, increased mass of the uterus and breasts, increased extracellular fluid, and fat mass accretion.[1] The majority of the accumulated fat mass is subcutaneous, but visceral fat also increases.[2] **The products of conception—the placenta, fetus, and amniotic fluid—comprise approximately 35% to 59% of the total GWG.**[3] The pattern of GWG is most commonly described as sigmoidal with mean weight gains being highest in the second trimester,[4] but the pattern depends on BMI. The Institute of Medicine (IOM) has issued BMI-specific GWG guidelines based upon these BMI differences (Table 3-1). However, since the publication of these guidelines, emerging evidence suggests that among women who are obese, **adverse pregnancy outcomes may be minimized by limiting GWG even further**; future guidelines may even endorse weight loss.[5,6]

CARDIOVASCULAR SYSTEM

Heart

Some of the most profound physiologic changes of pregnancy take place in the cardiovascular system in order to maximize oxygen delivery to both the mother and fetus. The combination of displacement of the diaphragm and the effect of pregnancy on the shape of the rib cage displaces the heart upward and to the left. The heart also rotates along its long axis, thereby resulting in an increased cardiac silhouette on imaging studies. No change is evident in the cardiothoracic ratio. Other radiographic findings include an apparent straightening of the left-sided heart border and increased prominence of the pulmonary conus. **It is therefore important to confirm the diagnosis of cardiomegaly with an echocardiogram and not simply to rely on radiographic imaging.**

Eccentric cardiac hypertrophy is commonly noted in pregnancy. It is thought to result from expanded blood volume in the first half of pregnancy and progressively increasing afterload in later gestation. These changes, similar to those found in response to exercise, enable the pregnant woman's heart to work more efficiently. Unlike the heart of an athlete that regresses rapidly with inactivity, the pregnant woman's heart decreases in size less rapidly and takes up to 6 months to return to normal.[7]

Cardiac Output

One of the most remarkable changes in pregnancy is the tremendous increase in cardiac output (CO). A review of 33 cross-sectional and 19 longitudinal studies revealed that CO increased significantly beginning in early pregnancy and peaked at an average of 30% to 50% above preconceptional values.[8] In a longitudinal study using Doppler echocardiography, CO increased by 50% at 34 weeks from a prepregnancy value of 4.88 to 7.34 L/min (Fig. 3-1).[8,9] In twin gestations, CO incrementally increases an additional 20% above that of singleton pregnancies. By 5 weeks' gestation, CO has already risen by more than 10%. By 12 weeks, the rise in output is 34% to 39% above nongravid levels, which accounts for about 75% of the total increase in CO during pregnancy. **Although the literature is not clear regarding the exact point in gestation at which CO peaks, most studies point to a range between 25 and 30 weeks.**[9] The data on whether the CO continues to increase in the third trimester are very divergent, with equal numbers of good longitudinal studies showing a mild decrease, a slight increase, or no change.[8] Thus little to no change is likely during this period. This apparent discrepancy appears to be explained by the small number of individuals in each study and the probability that the course of CO during the third trimester is determined by factors specific to the individual.[8] For example, maternal CO in the third trimester is significantly correlated with fetal birthweight and maternal height and weight.[10]

TABLE 3-1	GESTATIONAL WEIGHT GAIN RECOMMENDATIONS	
	TOTAL WEIGHT GAIN	MEAN (RANGE) IN LB/WK AFTER FIRST TRIMESTER
Underweight prepregnancy BMI (<18.5 kg/m²)	28-40 lb	1 (1-1.3)
Normal prepregnancy BMI (18.5-24.9 kg/m²)	25-35 lb	1 (0.8-1)
Overweight prepregnancy BMI (25.0-29.9 kg/m²)	15-25 lb	0.6 (0.5-0.7)
Obese prepregnancy BMI (≥30 kg/m²)	11-20 lb	0.5 (0.4-0.6)

From Rasmussen KM, Yaktine AL, eds. Committee to Reexamine IOM Pregnancy Weight Guidelines, Institute of Medicine, National Research Council. *Weight Gain During Pregnancy: Reexamining the Guidelines.* Washington DC: The National Academies Press; 2009.
BMI, body mass index.

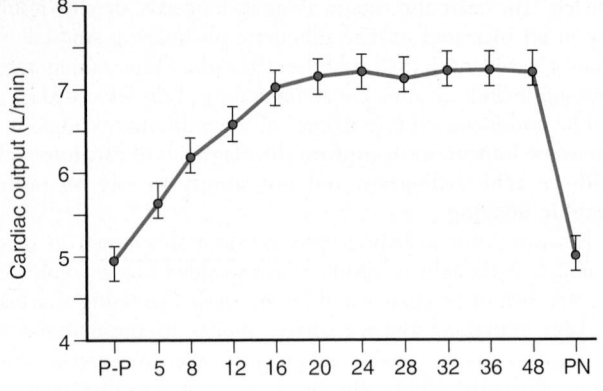

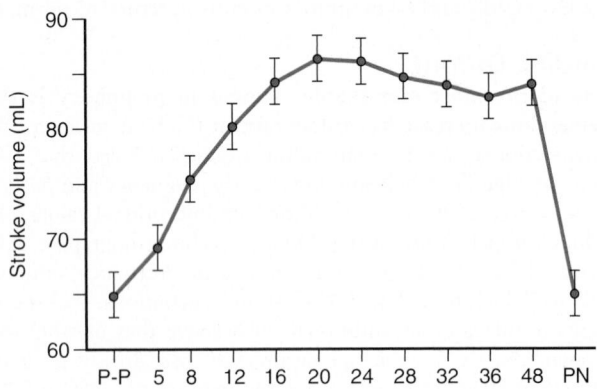

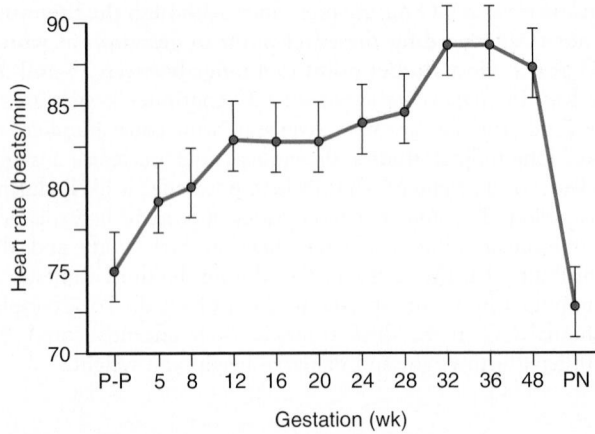

FIG 3-1 Increase in cardiac output, stroke volume, and heart rate from the nonpregnant state throughout pregnancy. PN, postnatal; P-P, pre-pregnancy. (From Hunter S, Robson S. Adaptation of the maternal heart in pregnancy. *Br Heart J.* 1992;68:540.)

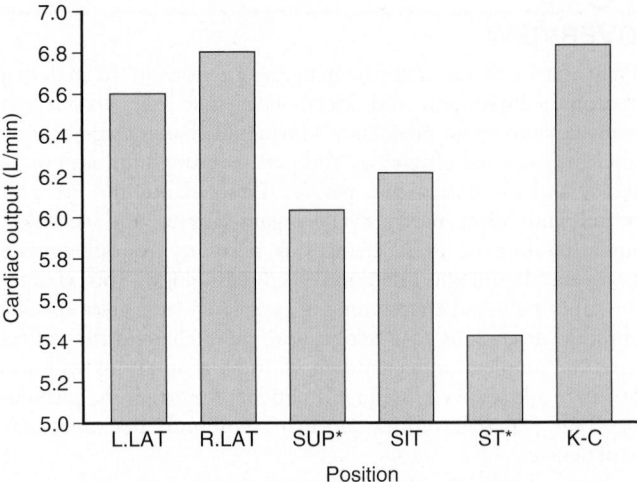

FIG 3-2 Effect of position change on cardiac output during pregnancy. *$P < .05$. K-C, knee-chest; *L.LAT,* left lateral; *R.LAT,* right lateral; *SIT,* sitting; *ST,* standing; *SUP,* supine. (From Clark S, Cotton D, Pivarnik J, et al. Position change and central hemodynamic profile during normal third-trimester pregnancy and postpartum. *Am J Obstet Gynecol.* 1991;164:883.)

Most of the increase in cardiac output is directed to the uterus, placenta, and breasts. In the first trimester, as in the nongravid state, the uterus receives 2% to 3% of CO and the breasts 1%. The percentage of CO that goes to the kidneys (20%), skin (10%), brain (10%), and coronary arteries (5%) remains at similar nonpregnant percentages, but because of the overall increase in CO, this results in an increase in absolute blood flow of about 50%. By term, the uterus receives 17% (450 to 650 mL/min) and the breasts 2%, mostly at the expense of a reduction of the fraction of the CO going to the splanchnic bed and skeletal muscle. The absolute blood flow to the liver is not changed, but the overall percentage of CO is significantly decreased.

Cardiac output (CO) is the product of stroke volume (SV) and heart rate (HR; CO = SV × HR), both of which increase during pregnancy and contribute to the overall rise in CO. An initial rise in the HR occurs by 5 weeks' gestation and continues until it peaks at 32 weeks' gestation at 15 to 20 beats above the nongravid rate, an increase of 17%. The SV begins to rise by 8 weeks of gestation and reaches its maximum at about 20 weeks at 20% to 30% above nonpregnant values.

Cardiac output in pregnancy depends on maternal position. In a study in 10 normal gravid women in the third trimester, using pulmonary artery catheterization, **CO was noted to be highest in the knee-chest and lateral recumbent positions at 6.9 and 6.6 L/min, respectively.** CO decreased by 22% to 5.4 L/min in the standing position (Fig. 3-2). The decrease in CO in the supine position, compared with the lateral recumbent position, is 10% to 30%. **In both the standing and the supine positions, decreased CO results from a fall in SV secondary to decreased blood return to the heart.** In the supine position, the enlarged uterus compresses the inferior vena cava (IVC), which reduces venous return; before 24 weeks, this effect is not observed. In late pregnancy, the IVC is completely occluded in the supine position, and venous return from the lower extremities occurs through the dilated paravertebral collateral circulation. It is worth noting that whereas the original studies of CO were done with invasive testing, the current accepted practice is to estimate CO in pregnancy using echocardiography.[11]

Despite decreased cardiac output, most supine women are not hypotensive or symptomatic because of the compensated rise in systemic vascular resistance (SVR). However, 5% to 10% of gravidas manifest supine hypotension with symptoms of dizziness, lightheadedness, nausea, and even syncope. The women who become symptomatic have a greater decrease in CO and blood pressure (BP) and a greater increase in HR when in the supine position than do asymptomatic women. Interestingly, with engagement of the fetal head, less of an effect on CO is seen. The ability to maintain a normal BP in the supine position may be lost during epidural or spinal anesthesia because of an inability to increase SVR. Clinically, the effects of maternal position on CO are especially important when the mother is clinically hypotensive or in the setting of a nonreassuring fetal heart rate tracing. The finding of a decreased CO in the standing position may give a physiologic basis for the finding of decreased birthweight in working women who stand for prolonged periods.[12] In twin pregnancies, CO is notably 15% higher than in singleton pregnancies. This finding is corroborated with findings of increased left atrial diameter in twin pregnancies, indicating volume overload.

Arterial Blood Pressure and Systemic Vascular Resistance

Blood pressure is the product of cardiac output and systemic vascular resistance (BP = CO × SVR). **Despite the significant increase in cardiac output, the maternal BP is decreased until later in pregnancy as a result of a decrease in SVR that reaches its nadir at midpregnancy and is followed by a gradual rise until term.** Even at full term, SVR remains 21% lower than prepregnancy values in pregnancies not affected by gestational hypertension or preeclampsia.[13] The most obvious cause for the decreased SVR is progesterone-mediated smooth muscle relaxation. However, the exact mechanism for the fall in SVR is poorly understood and likely involves vasorelaxation via the nitric oxide pathway and blunting of vascular responsiveness to vasoconstrictors such as angiotensin II and norepinephrine. **As a result, despite the overall increase in the renin-angiotensin aldosterone system (RAAS), the normal gravida is refractory to the vasoconstrictive effects of angiotensin II. Gant and colleagues[14] showed that nulliparous women who later develop preeclampsia retain their response to angiotensin II before the appearance of clinical signs of preeclampsia.**

Decreases in maternal BP parallel the falling SVR, with initial decreased BP that manifests at 8 weeks' gestation or earlier. Because BP fluctuates with menstruation and is decreased in the luteal phase, it seems reasonable that BP drops immediately in early pregnancy. The diastolic BP and the mean arterial pressure (MAP, [2 × diastolic BP + systolic BP]/3) decrease more than the systolic BP, which changes minimally. The overall decrease in diastolic BP and MAP is 5 to 10 mm Hg (Fig. 3-3).[13] **The diastolic BP and the MAP reach their nadir at midpregnancy and return to prepregnancy levels by term. In most studies, they rarely exceed prepregnancy or postpartum values; however, some investigators have reported that at term, the BP is greater than that in matched nonpregnant controls. They have also found that in the third trimester, the BP is higher than prepregnant values.** As noted previously, pregnancy-induced BP changes happen very early, possibly even before the patient realizes that she is pregnant, and therefore even early pregnancy BP assessments may not be consistent with prepregnancy values.[15]

The position when the BP is taken and what Korotkoff sound is used to determine the diastolic BP are important.

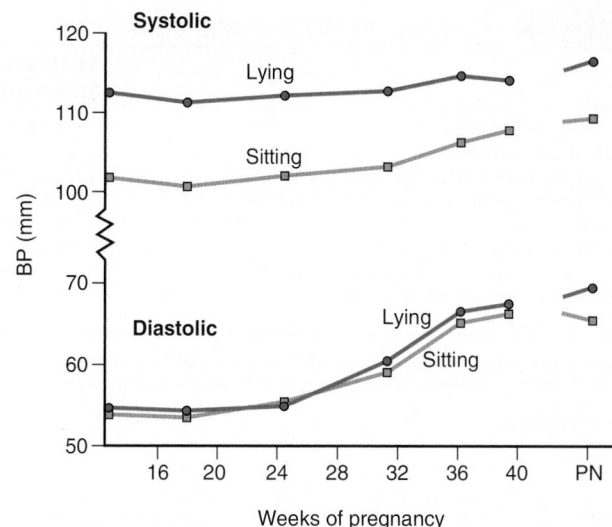

FIG 3-3 Blood pressure (BP) trends (sitting and lying) during pregnancy. Postnatal (PN) measures were performed 6 weeks postpartum. (From MacGillivray I, Rose G, Rowe B. Blood pressure survey in pregnancy. *Clin Sci.* 1969;37:395.)

BP is lowest in the lateral recumbent position, and the BP of the superior arm in this position is 10 to 12 mm Hg lower than that in the inferior arm. In the ambulatory setting, BP should be measured in the sitting position, and the Korotkoff 5 sound should be used. This is the diastolic BP when the sound disappears, as opposed to the Korotkoff 4, when a muffling of the sound is apparent. In a study of 250 gravidas, the Korotkoff 4 sound could only be identified in 48% of patients, whereas the Korotkoff 5 sound could always be determined. The Korotkoff 4 should only be used when the Korotkoff 5 occurs at 0 mm Hg.[16] Automated BP monitors have been compared with mercury sphygmomanometry during pregnancy, and although they tended to overestimate the diastolic BP, the overall results were similar in normotensive women. Of note in patients with suspected preeclampsia, automated monitors appear increasingly inaccurate at higher BPs.

Venous Pressure

Venous pressure in the upper extremities remains unchanged in pregnancy but rises progressively in the lower extremities. Femoral venous pressure increases from values near 10 cm H_2O at 10 weeks' gestation to 25 cm H_2O near term. From a clinical standpoint, this increase in pressure—in addition to the obstruction of the IVC by the expanding uterus—leads to the development of edema, varicose veins, and hemorrhoids and increases the risk for deep venous thrombosis (DVT).

Central Hemodynamic Assessment

Clark and colleagues studied 10 carefully selected normal women at 36 to 38 weeks' gestation and again at 11 to 13 weeks' postpartum with arterial lines and Swan-Ganz catheterization to characterize the central hemodynamics of term pregnancy (Table 3-2). Newer, noninvasive methods of central hemodynamic monitoring are being developed and validated in the pregnant population. As described earlier, CO, HR, SVR,

TABLE 3-2   CENTRAL HEMODYNAMIC CHANGES

	11-12 WEEKS POSTPARTUM	36-38 WEEKS' GESTATION	CHANGE FROM NONPREGNANT STATE
Cardiac output (L/min)	4.3 ± 0.9	6.2 ± 1.0	+43%*
Heart rate (beats/min)	71 ± 10.0	83 ± 10.0	+17%*
Systemic vascular resistance (dyne • cm • sec^{-5})	1530 ± 520	1210 ± 266	−21%*
Pulmonary vascular resistance (dyne • cm • sec^{-5})	119 ± 47.0	78 ± 22	−34%*
Colloid oncotic pressure (mm Hg)	20.8 ± 1.0	18 ± 1.5	−14%*
Mean arterial pressure (mm Hg)	86.4 ± 7.5	90.3 ± 5.8	NS
Pulmonary capillary wedge pressure (mm Hg)	3.7 ± 2.6	3.6 ± 2.5	NS
Central venous pressure (mm Hg)	3.7 ± 2.6	3.6 ± 2.5	NS
Left ventricular stroke work index (g/m/m^2)	41 ± 8	48 ± 6	NS

Modified from Clark S, Cotton D, Lee W, et al. Central hemodynamic assessment of normal term pregnancy. *Am J Obstet Gynecol.* 1989;161:1439.
Data are presented as mean ± standard deviation. Although data on pulmonary artery pressures are not presented, they were not significantly different.
*$P < .05$.
NS, not significant.

and pulmonary vascular resistance (PVR) change significantly with pregnancy. **In addition, clinically significant decreases occur in colloidal oncotic pressure (COP) and in the COP–pulmonary capillary wedge pressure (PCWP) difference, which explains why gravid women have a greater propensity for developing pulmonary edema with changes in capillary permeability or elevations in cardiac preload. The COP can fall even further after delivery, to 17 mm Hg, and if the pregnancy is complicated by preeclampsia, it can reach levels as low as 14 mm Hg.**[17] **When the PCWP is more than 4 mm Hg above the COP, the risk for pulmonary edema increases; therefore pregnant women can experience pulmonary edema at PCWPs of 18 to 20 mm Hg, which is significantly lower than the typical nonpregnant threshold of 24 mm Hg.**

Normal Changes That Mimic Heart Disease

The physiologic adaptations of pregnancy lead to a number of changes in maternal signs and symptoms that can mimic cardiac disease and make it difficult to determine whether true disease is present. Dyspnea is common to both cardiac disease and pregnancy, but certain distinguishing features should be considered. First, the onset of pregnancy-related dyspnea usually occurs before 20 weeks, and 75% of women experience it by the third trimester. **Unlike cardiac dyspnea, pregnancy-related dyspnea does not worsen significantly with advancing gestation. Second, physiologic dyspnea is usually mild, does not stop women from performing normal daily activities, and does not occur at rest. The mechanism for dyspnea of pregnancy is not well characterized but is thought to be secondary to the increased effort of inspiratory muscles.**[18] Other normal symptoms that can mimic cardiac disease include decreased exercise tolerance, fatigue, occasional orthopnea, syncope, and chest discomfort. **Symptoms that should not be attributed to pregnancy and that need a more thorough investigation include hemoptysis, syncope or chest pain with exertion, progressive orthopnea, or paroxysmal nocturnal dyspnea.** Normal physical findings that could be mistaken as evidence of cardiac disease include peripheral edema, mild tachycardia, jugular venous distension after midpregnancy, and lateral displacement of the left ventricular apex.

Pregnancy also alters normal heart sounds. At the end of the first trimester, both components of the first heart sound become louder, and exaggerated splitting is apparent. The second heart sound usually remains normal with only minimal changes. Up to 80% to 90% of gravidas demonstrate a third heart sound (S_3) after midpregnancy because of rapid diastolic filling. Rarely, a fourth heart sound may be auscultated, but typically phonocardiography is needed to detect this. Systolic ejection murmurs along the left sternal border develop in 96% of pregnancies, and increased blood flow across the pulmonic and aortic valves is thought to be the cause. Most commonly, these are midsystolic and less than grade 3. **Diastolic murmurs have been found in up to 18% of gravidas, but their presence is uncommon enough to warrant further evaluation.** A continuous murmur in the second to fourth intercostal space may be heard in the second or third trimester owing to the so-called mammary souffle caused by increased blood flow in the breast (Fig. 3-4).

Troponin 1 and creatinine kinase-MB levels are tests used to assess myocardial injury in acute myocardial infarction. **Uterine contractions can lead to significant increases in the creatinine kinase-MB level, but troponin levels are not affected by pregnancy or labor.**[19]

Effect of Labor and the Immediate Puerperium

The profound anatomic and functional changes in cardiac function reach a crescendo during the labor process. In addition to the dramatic rise in cardiac output with normal pregnancy, even greater increases in cardiac output occur with labor and in the immediate puerperium. In a Doppler echocardiography study[9] of 15 uncomplicated cases without epidural anesthesia, the CO between contractions increased 12% during the first stage of labor (Fig. 3-5). This increase in CO is caused primarily by an increased SV, but HR may also rise. By the end of the first stage of labor, the CO during contractions is 51% above baseline term pregnancy values (6.99 to 10.57 L/min). Increased CO is in part secondary to increased venous return from the 300- to 500-mL autotransfusion that occurs at the onset of each contraction as blood is expressed from the uterus.[20] Paralleling increases in CO, the MAP also rises in the first stage of labor, from 82 to 91 mm Hg in early labor to 102 mm Hg by the beginning of the second stage. MAP also increases with uterine contractions.

Much of the increase in CO and MAP is due to pain and anxiety. With epidural anesthesia, the baseline increase in CO is reduced, but the rise observed with contractions persists. Maternal posture also influences hemodynamics during labor.

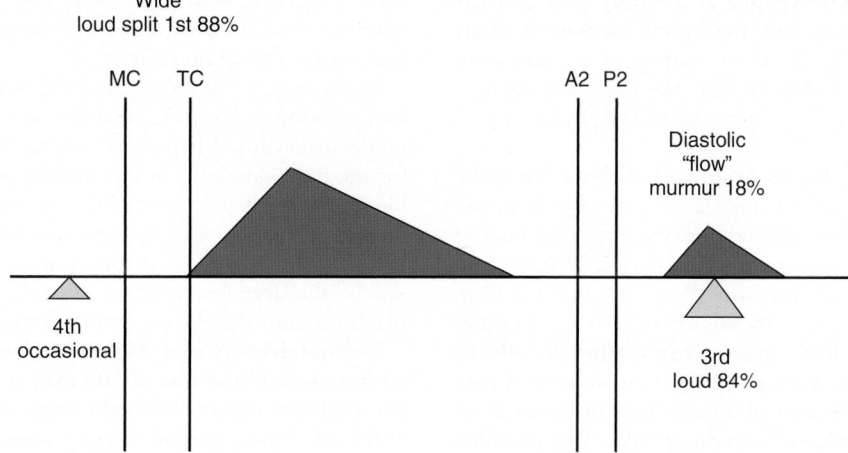

Wide
loud split 1st 88%

MC   TC

A2 P2

Diastolic
"flow"
murmur 18%

4th
occasional

3rd
loud 84%

FIG 3-4 Summary of the findings on auscultation of the heart in pregnancy. MC, mitral closure; TC, tricuspid closure; A2 and P2, aortic and pulmonary elements of the second heart sound. (From Cutforth R, MacDonald C. Heart sounds and murmurs in pregnancy. *Am Heart J.* 1966;71:741.)

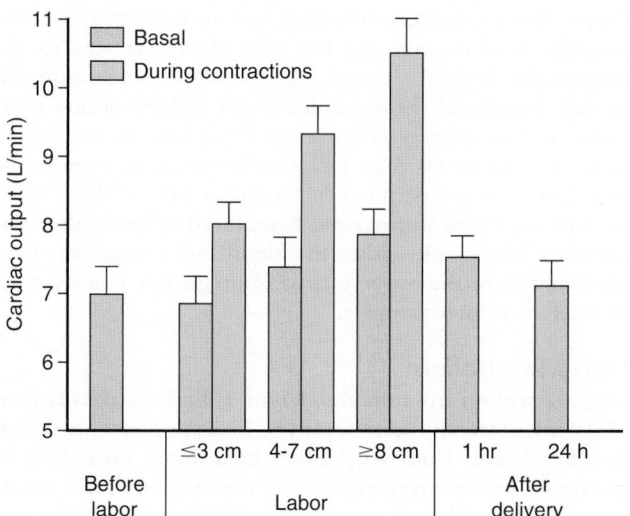

FIG 3-5 Changes in cardiac output during normal labor. (From Hunter S, Robson S. Adaptation of the maternal heart in pregnancy. *Br Heart J* 1992;68:540.)

Changing position from supine to lateral recumbent increases CO. This change is greater than the increase seen before labor and suggests that during labor, CO may be more dependent on preload. Therefore it is important to avoid the supine position in laboring women and to give a sufficient fluid bolus before an epidural to maintain an adequate preload.

In the immediate postpartum period (10 to 30 min after delivery), **with a further rise in cardiac output of 10% to 20%, CO reaches its maximum.** This increase is accompanied by a fall in the maternal HR that is likely secondary to increased SV. Traditionally, this rise was thought to be the result of uterine autotransfusion as described earlier with contractions, but the validity of this concept is uncertain. In both vaginal and elective cesarean deliveries, the maximal increase in the CO occurs 10 to 30 min after delivery and returns to the prelabor baseline 1 hour after delivery. **The increase was 37% with epidural anesthesia and 28% with general anesthesia.** Over the next 2 to 4 postpartum weeks, the cardiac hemodynamic parameters return to near-preconceptional levels.[21]

Cardiac Rhythm

The effect of pregnancy on cardiac rhythm is limited to an increase in HR and a significant increase in isolated atrial and ventricular contractions. In a Holter monitor study,[22] 110 pregnant women referred for evaluation of symptoms of palpitations, dizziness, or syncope were compared with 52 healthy pregnant women. Symptomatic women had similar rates of isolated sinus tachycardia (9%), isolated premature atrial complexes (56%), and premature ventricular contractions (PVCs; 49%) but increased rates of frequent PVCs greater than 10/hour (22% vs. 2%, $P = .03$). A subset of patients with frequent premature atrial complexes or PVCs had comparative Holter studies performed postpartum that revealed an 85% decrease in arrhythmia frequency ($P < .05$). This dramatic decline, with patients acting as their own controls, supports the arrhythmogenic effect of pregnancy. In a study of 30 healthy women placed on Holter monitors during labor, a similarly high incidence of benign arrhythmias was found (93%). Reassuringly, the prevalence of concerning arrhythmias was no higher than expected. An unexpected finding was a 35% rate of asymptomatic bradycardia, defined as an HR of less than 60 beats/min in the immediate postpartum period. Other studies have shown that women with preexisting tachyarrhythmias have an increased incidence of these rate abnormalities during pregnancy. **Whether labor increases the rate of arrhythmias in women with cardiac disease has not been thoroughly studied, but multiple case reports suggest labor may increase arrhythmias in these women.**

HEMATOLOGIC CHANGES
Plasma Volume and Red Cell Mass
Maternal blood volume begins to increase at about 6 weeks' gestation. Thereafter, it rises progressively until 30 to 34 weeks and then plateaus until delivery. The average expansion of blood volume is 40% to 50% (range 20% to 100%). Women with multiple pregnancies have a larger increase in blood volume than those with singletons. Likewise, volume expansion correlates with infant birthweight, but it is not clear whether this is a cause or an effect. The increase in blood volume results from a combined expansion of both plasma volume and red blood cell (RBC) mass. **The plasma volume begins to**

increase by 6 weeks and expands at a steady pace until it plateaus at 30 weeks' gestation; the overall increase is about **50%** (1200 to 1300 mL). The exact etiology of the expansion of the blood volume is unknown, but the hormonal changes of gestation and the increase in nitric oxide (NO) play important roles.

Erythrocyte mass also begins to expand at about 10 weeks' gestation. Although the initial slope of this increase is slower than that of the plasma volume, erythrocyte mass continues to grow progressively until term without plateauing. Without iron supplementation, RBC mass increases about 18% by term, from a mean nonpregnant level of 1400 mL up to 1650 mL. **Supplemental iron increases RBC mass accumulation to 400 to 450 mL, or 30%, and a corresponding improvement is seen in hemoglobin levels. Because plasma volume increases more than the RBC mass, maternal hematocrit falls. This so-called physiologic anemia of pregnancy reaches a nadir at 30 to 34 weeks. Because the RBC mass continues to increase after 30 weeks when the plasma volume expansion has plateaued, the hematocrit may rise somewhat after 30 weeks** (Fig. 3-6). The mean and fifth-percentile hemoglobin concentrations for normal iron-supplemented pregnant women are outlined in Table 3-3. A hemoglobin level that reaches its nadir at 9 to 11 g/dL has

been associated with the lowest rate of perinatal mortality, whereas values below or above this range have been linked to an increased perinatal mortality.[23]

In pregnancy, erythropoietin levels increase twofold to threefold, starting at 16 weeks, and they may be responsible for the moderate erythroid hyperplasia found in the bone marrow and for the mild elevations in the reticulocyte count. The increased blood volume is protective given the possibility of hemorrhage during pregnancy or at delivery. The larger blood volume also helps fill the expanded vascular system created by vasodilation and by the large, low-resistance vascular pool within the utero-placental unit, thereby preventing hypotension.[18]

Vaginal delivery of a singleton infant at term is associated with a mean blood loss of 500 mL; an uncomplicated cesarean delivery, about 1000 mL; and a cesarean hysterectomy, 1500 mL.[24] In a normal delivery, almost all of the blood loss occurs in the first hour. Pritchard and colleagues[24] found that over the subsequent 72 hours, only 80 mL of blood is lost. Gravid women respond to blood loss in a different fashion than in the nonpregnant state. **In pregnancy, the blood volume drops after postpartum bleeding, but no reexpansion to the prelabor level occurs, and less of a change is seen in the hematocrit. Indeed, instead of volume redistribution, an overall diuresis of the expanded water volume occurs postpartum.** After delivery with average blood loss, the hematocrit drops moderately for 3 to 4 days, followed by an increase. By days 5 to 7, the postpartum hematocrit is similar to the prelabor hematocrit. **If the postpartum hematocrit is lower than the prelabor hematocrit, either the blood loss was greater than appreciated, or the hypervolemia of pregnancy was less than normal, as in preeclampsia.**[24]

Iron Metabolism

Iron absorption from the duodenum is limited to its ferrous (divalent) state, the form found in iron supplements. Ferric (trivalent) iron from vegetable food sources must first be converted to the divalent state by the enzyme ferric reductase. If body iron stores are normal, only about 10% of ingested iron is absorbed, most of which remains in the mucosal cells or enterocytes until sloughing leads to excretion in the feces (1 mg/day). Under conditions of increased iron needs, such as during pregnancy, the fraction of iron absorbed increases. After absorption, iron is released from the enterocytes into the circulation, where it is carried bound to transferrin to the liver, spleen, muscle, and bone marrow. In those sites, iron is freed from transferrin and is incorporated into hemoglobin (75% of iron) and myoglobin or is stored as ferritin and hemosiderin. Menstruating women have about half the iron stores of men, with total body iron of 2 to 2.5 g and iron stores of only 300 mg. Before pregnancy, 8% to 10% of women in Western nations have an iron deficiency.

The iron requirements of gestation are about 1000 mg. This includes 500 mg used to increase the maternal RBC mass (1 mL of erythrocytes contains 1.1 mg iron), 300 mg transported to the fetus, and 200 mg to compensate for the normal daily iron losses by the mother. Thus the normal expectant woman needs to absorb an average of 3.5 mg/day of iron. In actuality, the iron requirements are not constant but increase remarkably during the pregnancy from 0.8 mg/day in the first trimester to 6 to 7 mg/day in the third trimester. The fetus receives its iron through active transport via transferrin receptors located on the apical surface of the placental

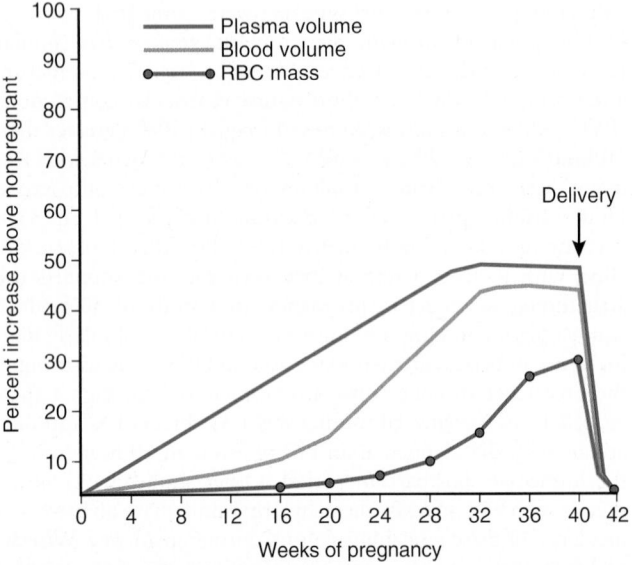

FIG 3-6 Blood volume changes during pregnancy. RBC, red blood cell. (From Scott DE. Anemia in pregnancy. *Obstet Gynecol Annu.* 1972;1:219-244.)

TABLE 3-3   HEMOGLOBIN VALUES IN PREGNANCY

GESTATION (WK)	MEAN HEMOGLOBIN (g/dL)	5TH PERCENTILE HEMOGLOBIN (g/dL)
12	12.2	11.0
16	11.8	10.6
20	11.6	10.5
24	11.6	10.5
28	11.8	10.7
32	12.1	11.0
36	12.5	11.4
40	12.9	11.9

From U.S. Department of Health and Human Services. Recommendations to prevent and control iron deficiency in the United States. *MMWR Morb Mortal Wkly Rep.* 1998;47:1.

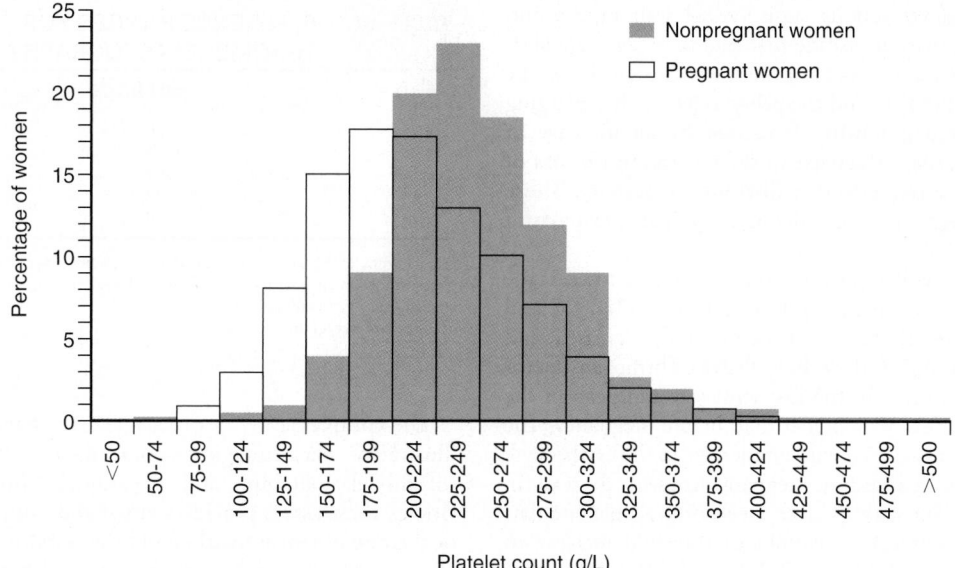

FIG 3-7 Histogram of platelet count of pregnant women in the third trimester (*n* = 6770) compared with nonpregnant women (*n* = 287). (From Boehlen F, Hohlfield P, Extermann P. Platelet count at term pregnancy: a reappraisal of the threshold. *Obstet Gynecol.* 2000;95:29.)

syncytiotrophoblast. Holotransferrin is then endocytosed, and the iron is released and follows a similar pattern to reach the fetal circulation. In the setting of maternal iron deficiency, the number of placental transferrin receptors increases so that more iron is taken up by the placenta; however, the capacity of this compensatory mechanism can be inadequate and can result in fetal iron deficiency. Maternal iron deficiency anemia has also been associated with adverse pregnancy outcomes, such as low birthweight infants and preterm birth.[25] For a review on the use of supplemental iron in pregnancy, see Chapter 44.

Platelets

Before the introduction of automated analyzers, studies of platelet counts during pregnancy reported conflicting results. Even with the availability of automated cell counters, the data on the change in platelet count during pregnancy are still somewhat unclear. Pitkin and colleagues[26] measured platelet counts in 23 women every 4 weeks and found that the counts dropped from $322 \pm 75 \times 10^3/mm^3$ in the first trimester to $278 \pm 75 \times 10^3/mm^3$ in the third trimester. More recent studies confirm a decline in the platelet count during gestation possibly caused by increased destruction or hemodilution. **In addition to the mild decrease in the mean platelet count, Burrows and Kelton[27] demonstrated that in the third trimester, about 8% of gravidas develop gestational thrombocytopenia with platelet counts between 70,000 and 150,000/mm^3. Gestational thrombocytopenia is not associated with an increase in pregnancy complications,[27] and platelet counts return to normal by 1 to 2 weeks postpartum** (see Chapter 44). Many features of gestational thrombocytopenia are similar to those of mild immune thrombocytopenia, so the etiology may be immunologic.[28] Another hypothesis is that gestational thrombocytopenia is due to exaggerated platelet consumption, similar to that seen in normal pregnancy.[27] Consistent with these findings, Boehlen and associates[29] compared platelet counts during the third trimester of pregnancy with those in nonpregnant controls and showed a shift to a lower mean platelet count and an overall shift to the left of the "platelet curve" in the pregnant women

(Fig. 3-7). This study found that only 2.5% of nonpregnant women have platelet counts less than 150,000/mm^3, the traditional value used outside of pregnancy as the cutoff for normal, versus 11.5% of gravid women. **A platelet count of less than 116,000/mm^3 occurred in 2.5% of gravid women; therefore these investigators recommended using this value as the lower limit for normal in the third trimester.** In addition, they suggested that workups for the etiology of decreased platelet count were unneeded at values above this level.[29]

The normal decrease in platelet count is associated with an increase in platelet aggregability. This is evidenced by decreased platelet-function analyzer (PFA-100) values, which signify a decreased time for a platelet plug to occlude an aperture in a collagen membrane and measures the ability of platelets to occlude a vascular breach.[30] **Thus while the number of platelets decreases, platelet function increases to maintain hemostasis.**

Leukocytes

The peripheral white blood cell (WBC) count rises progressively during pregnancy. During the first trimester, the mean WBC count is 8000/mm^3 with a normal range of 5110 to 9900/mm^3. During the second and third trimesters, the mean is 8500/mm^3 with a range of 5600 to 12,200/mm^3.[31] In labor, the count may rise to 20,000 to 30,000/mm^3, and counts are highly correlated with labor progression as determined by cervical dilation. **Because of the normal increase of WBCs in labor, the WBC count should not be used clinically in determining the presence of infection.** The increase in the WBC count is largely due to increases in circulating segmented neutrophils and granulocytes, whose absolute number is nearly doubled at term. The reason for the increased leukocytosis is unclear, but it may be caused by the elevated estrogen and cortisol levels. Leukocyte levels return to normal within 1 to 2 weeks of delivery.

Coagulation System

Pregnancy places women at a fivefold to sixfold increased risk for thromboembolic disease (see Chapter 45). This greater risk is caused by increased venous stasis, vessel wall injury, and changes in the coagulation cascade that lead to hypercoagulability. The increase in venous stasis in the lower extremities is due to compression of the IVC and the pelvic veins by the enlarging uterus. **The hypercoagulability is caused by an increase in several procoagulants, a decrease in the natural inhibitors of coagulation, and a reduction in fibrinolytic activity. These physiologic changes provide defense against peripartum hemorrhage.**

Most of the procoagulant factors from the coagulation cascade are markedly increased, including factors I, VII, VIII, IX, and X. Factors II, V, and XII are unchanged or mildly increased, and levels of factors XI and XIII decline. Plasma fibrinogen (factor I) levels begin to increase in the first trimester and peak in the third trimester at levels 50% higher than before pregnancy. The rise in fibrinogen is associated with an increase in the erythrocyte sedimentation rate. In addition, pregnancy causes a decrease in the fibrinolytic system with reduced levels of available circulating plasminogen activator, a twofold to threefold increase in plasminogen activator inhibitor 1 (PAI-1), and a 25-fold increase in PAI-2. The placenta produces PAI-1 and is the primary source of PAI-2.

Pregnancy has been shown to cause a progressive and significant decrease in the levels of total and free protein S from early in pregnancy, but it has no effect on the levels of protein C and antithrombin III.[32] The activated protein C (APC)/sensitivity (S) ratio, the ratio of the clotting time in the presence and the absence of APC, declines during pregnancy. The APC/S ratio is considered abnormal if it is less than 2.6. In a study of 239 women,[32] the APC/S ratio decreased from a mean of 3.12 in the first trimester to 2.63 by the third trimester. By the third trimester, 38% of women were found to have an acquired APC resistance, with APC/S ratio values below 2.6. Whether the changes in the protein-S level and the APC/S ratio are responsible for some of the hypercoagulability of pregnancy is unknown. **If a workup for thrombophilias is performed during gestation, the clinician should use caution when attempting to interpret these levels if they are abnormal. Ideally the clinician should order DNA testing for the Leiden mutation instead of testing for APC. For protein-S screening during pregnancy, the free protein-S antigen level should be tested, with normal levels in the second and third trimesters being identified as greater than 30% and 24%, respectively.**[33]

Most coagulation testing is unaffected by pregnancy. The prothrombin time (PT), activated partial thromboplastin time (PTT), and thrombin time all fall slightly but remain within the limits of normal nonpregnant values, whereas the bleeding time and whole blood clotting times are unchanged. Testing for von Willebrand disease is affected in pregnancy because levels of factor VIII, von Willebrand factor activity and antigen, and ristocetin cofactor all increase.[34] Levels of coagulation factors normalize 2 weeks postpartum.

Researchers have found evidence to support the theory that during pregnancy, a state of low-level intravascular coagulation occurs. Low concentrations of fibrin degradation products (markers of fibrinolysis), elevated levels of fibrinopeptide A (a marker for increased clotting), and increased levels of platelet factor 4 and β-thromboglobulin (markers of increased platelet activity) have been found in maternal blood. The most likely cause for these findings involves localized physiologic changes needed for maintenance of the uterine-placental interface.

TABLE 3-4	REFERENCE RANGES FOR THROMBOELASTOGRAPHY IN PREGNANCY	
	AVERAGE	**SD**
R	6.19	1.85
K	1.9	0.56
α	69.2	6.55
MA	73.2	4.41
Ly30	0.58	1.83

From Antony K, Mansouri R, Arndt M, et al. Establishing thromboelastography and platelet-function analyzer reference ranges and other measures in healthy term pregnant women. *Am J Perinatol.* 2015;32: 545-554.
SD, standard deviation.

The complex array of procoagulative changes can be further illustrated via emerging point-of-care analyses, such as thromboelastography and rotational thromboelastography. Briefly, these assays provide a visual and numeric representation of the rate of clot formation and the stability of the clot, which allows a detailed analysis of the expected hypercoagulable state and, if indicated, targets for transfusion.[35] Use of these tests in pregnancy requires caution, however, because physiologic values vary in pregnancy compared with a nonpregnant state; these changes reflect a procoagulative state.[36,37] Reference ranges for pregnancy are shown in Table 3-4.

RESPIRATORY SYSTEM
Upper Respiratory Tract
During pregnancy, the mucosa of the nasopharynx becomes hyperemic and edematous with hypersecretion of mucus due to increased estrogen. These changes often lead to marked nasal stuffiness and decreased nasal patency; 27% of women at 12 weeks' gestation report nasal congestion and rhinitis, and this increases to 42% at 36 weeks' gestation. This decreased patency can lead to anesthesia complications; in fact, the Mallampati score is demonstrably increased (see Chapter 16).[38] Epistaxis is also common and may rarely require surgery. Additionally, the placement of nasogastric tubes may cause excessive bleeding if adequate lubrication is not used.[18] Polyposis of the nose and nasal sinuses develops in some individuals but regresses postpartum. **Because of these changes, many gravid women complain of chronic cold symptoms. However, the temptation to use nasal decongestants should be avoided because of the risk for hypertension and rebound congestion.**

Mechanical Changes
The configuration of the thoracic cage changes early in pregnancy, much earlier than can be accounted for by mechanical pressure from the enlarging uterus. Relaxation of the ligamentous attachments between the ribs and sternum may be responsible. The subcostal angle increases from 68 to 103 degrees, the transverse diameter of the chest expands by 2 cm, and the chest circumference expands by 5 to 7 cm. As gestation progresses, the level of the diaphragm rises 4 cm; however, diaphragmatic excursion is not impeded and actually increases 1 to 2 cm. This increased diaphragmatic excursion is the effect of progesterone, which acts at the level of the central chemoreceptors to increase diaphragmatic effort and results in greater negative inspiratory pressures.[39] **Respiratory muscle function is not affected by pregnancy, and maximal inspiratory and expiratory pressures are unchanged.**

Lung Volume and Pulmonary Function

The described alterations in chest wall configuration and in the diaphragm lead to changes in static lung volumes. In a review of studies with at least 15 subjects, compared with nonpregnant controls, Crapo[18] found significant changes (Fig. 3-8, Table 3-5). The elevation of the diaphragm decreases the volume of the lungs in the resting state, thereby reducing total lung capacity (TLC) and the functional residual capacity (FRC). The FRC can be subdivided into *expiratory reserve volume* (ERV) and *residual volume* (RV), and both decrease.

Some spirometric measurements to assess bronchial flow are unchanged in pregnancy, whereas others are altered. Historically, it has been well accepted that the forced expiratory volume in 1 second (FEV_1) does not change, which suggests that the airway function remains stable. However, FEV_1 may indeed decrease across pregnancy under certain circumstances, such as high altitude. Different studies have observed varied effects on the peak expiratory flow. In a longitudinal study of the peak flow in 38 women from the first trimester until 6 weeks postpartum, peak flows had a statistically significant decrease as gestation progressed, but the amount of the decrease was of questionable

clinical significance.[40] Likewise, a small decline in the peak flow was found in the supine position versus the standing or sitting position. In a similar study of 80 women, peak expiratory flow (PEF) was found to increase progressively after 14 to 16 weeks.[41] Notably, these values were also significantly higher at any time point during pregnancy in parous compared with nulliparous women, which may suggest that this change is permanent.[41] An additional finding of this study was that no differences in forced vital capacity (FVC), FEV_1, or PEF were noted based on overweight status or excess gestational weight gain. **In summary, both spirometry and peak flowmeters can be used to diagnose and manage respiratory illness, but the clinician should ensure that measurements are performed in the same maternal position.**[40]

Gas Exchange

Increasing progesterone levels drive a state of chronic hyperventilation, as reflected by a 30% to 50% increase in tidal volume by 8 weeks' gestation. In turn, increased tidal volume results in an overall parallel rise in minute ventilation, despite a stable respiratory rate (minute ventilation = tidal volume × respiratory rate). The rise in minute ventilation, combined with a decrease in FRC, leads to a larger than expected increase in alveolar ventilation (50% to 70%). **Chronic mild hyperventilation results in increased alveolar oxygen (PaO_2) and decreased arterial carbon dioxide ($PaCO_2$) from normal levels** (Table 3-6). The drop in the $PaCO_2$ is especially critical because it drives a more favorable CO_2 gradient between the fetus and mother, which facilitates CO_2 transfer. **The low maternal $PaCO_2$ results in a chronic respiratory alkalosis.** Partial renal compensation occurs through increased excretion of bicarbonate, which helps maintain the pH between 7.4 and 7.45 and lowers the serum bicarbonate levels. Early in pregnancy, the arterial oxygen (PaO_2) increases (106 to 108 mm Hg) as the $PaCO_2$ decreases, but by the third trimester, a slight decrease in the PaO_2 (101 to 104 mm Hg) occurs as a result of the enlarging uterus. This decrease in the PaO_2 late in pregnancy is even more pronounced in the supine position; one study found a further drop of 5 to 10 mm Hg and an increase in the alveolar-to-arterial gradient to 26 mm Hg. Up to 25% of women may exhibit a PaO_2 of less than 90 mm Hg. The mean PaO_2 is lower in the supine position than in the sitting position.[18,42]

As the minute ventilation increases, a simultaneous but smaller increase in oxygen uptake and consumption occurs. Most investigators have found **maternal oxygen consumption to be 20% to 40% above nonpregnant levels. This increase**

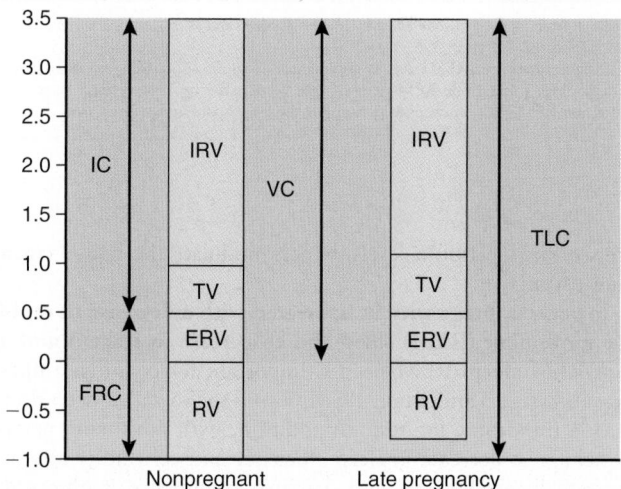

FIG 3-8 Lung volumes in nonpregnant and pregnant women. *ERV,* expiratory reserve; *FRC,* functional residual capacity; *IC,* inspiratory capacity; *IRV,* inspiratory reserve; *RV,* residual volume; *TLC,* total lung capacity; *TV,* tidal volume; *VC,* vital capacity. (From Cruickshank DP, Wigton TR, Hays PM. Maternal physiology in pregnancy. In Gabbe SG, Niebyl JR, Simpson JL, eds. *Obstetrics: Normal and Problem Pregnancies,* 3rd ed. New York: Churchill Livingstone; 1996, p 94.)

TABLE 3-5   LUNG VOLUMES AND CAPACITIES IN PREGNANCY

MEASUREMENT	DEFINITION	CHANGE IN PREGNANCY
Respiratory rate	Number of breaths per minute	Unchanged
Vital capacity (VC)	Maximal amount of air that can be forcibly expired after maximal inspiration (IC + ERV)	Unchanged
Inspiratory capacity (IC)	Maximal amount of air that can be inspired from resting expiratory level (TV + IRV)	Increased 5%-10%
Tidal volume (TV)	Amount of air inspired and expired with a normal breath	Increased 30%-40%
Inspiratory reserve volume (IRV)	Maximal amount of air that can be inspired at the end of normal inspiration	Unchanged
Functional residual capacity	Amount of air in lungs at resting expiratory level (ERV + RV)	Decreased 20%
Expiratory reserve volume (ERV)	Maximal amount of air that can be expired from resting expiratory level	Decreased 15%-20%
Residual volume (RV)	Amount of air in lungs after maximal expiration	Decreased 20%-25%
Total lung capacity	Total amount of air in lungs at maximal inspiration (VC + RV)	Decreased 5%

From Cruickshank DP, Wigton TR, Hays PM. Maternal physiology in pregnancy. In Gabbe SG, Niebyl JR, Simpson JL, eds. *Obstetrics: Normal and Problem Pregnancies,* 3rd ed. New York: Churchill Livingstone; 1996.

TABLE 3-6	BLOOD GAS VALUES IN THE THIRD TRIMESTER OF PREGNANCY

	PREGNANT	NONPREGNANT
PaO_2 (mm Hg)*	101.8 ± 1	93.4 ± 2.04
Arterial hemoglobin saturation (%)†	98.5 ± 0.7	98 ± 0.8
$PaCO_2$ (mm Hg)*	30.4 ± 0.6	40 ± 2.5
pH*	7.43 ± 0.006	7.43 ± 0.02
Serum bicarbonate (HCO_3) (mmol/L)	21.7 ± 1.6	25.3 ± 1.2
Base deficit (mmol/L)*	3.1 ± 0.2	1.06 ± 0.6
Alveolar-arterial gradient $[P(A-a)O_2]$ (mm Hg)*	16.1 ± 0.9	15.7 ± 0.6

*Data from Templeton A, Kelman G. Maternal blood-gases (PAO_2-PaO_2), physiological shunt and VD/VT in normal pregnancy. *Br J Anaesth* 1976;48:1001. Data presented as mean ± standard error of the mean.
†Data from McAuliffe F, Kametas N, Krampl E. Blood gases in prepregnancy at sea level and at high altitude. *Br J Obstet Gynaecol.* 2001;108:980. Data presented as mean ± standard deviation.

TABLE 3-7	CHARACTERISTICS OF SLEEP IN PREGNANCY

STAGE OF PREGNANCY	SUBJECTIVE SYMPTOMS	OBJECTIVE SYMPTOMS (POLYSOMNOGRAPHY)*
First trimester	Increased total sleep time: increase in naps / Increased daytime sleepiness / Increased nocturnal insomnia	Increased total sleep time / Decreased stage 3 and 4 non-REM sleep
Second trimester	Normalization of total sleep time / Increased awakenings	Normal total sleep time / Decreased stage 3 and 4 non-REM sleep / Decreased REM sleep
Third trimester	Decreased total sleep time / Increased insomnia / Increased nocturnal awakenings / Increased daytime sleepiness	Decreased total sleep time / Increased awakenings after sleep onset / Increased stage 1 non-REM sleep / Decreased stage 3 and 4 non-REM sleep / Decreased REM sleep

Modified from Santiago J, Nolledo M, Kinzler W. Sleep and sleep disorders in pregnancy. *Ann Intern Med.* 2001;134:396.
*Rapid eye movement (REM) sleep is important for cognition and makes up 20%-25% of sleep. Stage 1 and 2 non-REM sleep, or light sleep, makes up 55% of sleep. Stage 3 and 4 non-REM sleep, or deep sleep, is important for rest and makes up 20% of sleep.

occurs as a result of the oxygen requirements of the fetus and placenta and the increased oxygen requirement of maternal organs. With exercise or during labor, an even greater rise in both minute ventilation and oxygen consumption takes place.[18,38] During a contraction, oxygen consumption can triple. As a result of the increased oxygen consumption, and because the FRC is decreased, a lowering of the maternal oxygen reserve occurs. Therefore the pregnant patient is more susceptible to the effects of apnea, such as during intubation, when a more rapid onset of hypoxia, hypercapnia, and respiratory acidosis is seen. Indeed, the desaturation time after thorough preoxygenation is shortened from 9 minutes in the nonpregnant state to 3 minutes in pregnancy.

Sleep

Pregnancy causes both an increase in sleep disorders and significant changes in sleep profile and pattern that persist into the postpartum period.[43] Pregnancy causes such significant changes that the American Academy of Sleep Medicine has described a specific pregnancy-associated sleep disorder: diagnostic criteria include a complaint of either insomnia or excessive sleepiness with onset during pregnancy. Sleep disturbances are associated with poor health outcomes in the general population, and emerging evidence suggests that abnormal sleep patterns in pregnancy may contribute to certain complications, such as hypertensive disorders and fetal growth restriction.[39,44] It is well known that hormones and physical discomfort affect sleep (Table 3-7). With the dramatic change in hormone levels and the significant mechanical effects that make women more uncomfortable, it is not difficult to understand why sleep is profoundly affected. Multiple authors have investigated the changes in sleep during pregnancy using questionnaires, sleep logs, and polysomnographic studies. From these studies, investigators have shown that most pregnant women (66% to 94%) report alterations in sleep that lead to the subjective perception of poor sleep quality. Sleep disturbances begin as early as the first trimester and worsen as the pregnancy progresses.[45] During the third trimester, multiple discomforts occur that can impair sleep: urinary frequency, backache, general abdominal discomfort and contractions, leg cramps, restless legs syndrome (RLS), heartburn, and fetal movement. Interestingly, no changes

are seen in melatonin levels, which modulate the body's circadian pacemaker.

In general, pregnancy is associated with a decrease in rapid eye movement (REM) sleep and a decrease in stage 3 and 4 non-REM sleep. REM sleep is important for cognitive thinking, and stage 3 and 4 non-REM sleep is the so-called deep sleep that is important for rest. In addition, with advancing gestational age, a decrease in sleep efficiency and continuity and an increase in awake time and daytime somnolence is observed. By 3 months postpartum, the amount of non-REM and REM sleep recovers, but a persistent decrease in sleeping efficiency and nocturnal awakenings occurs, presumably because of the newborn.[43] Although pregnancy causes changes in sleep, it is important for the clinician to consider other primary sleep disorders that may be unrelated to pregnancy, such as sleep apnea. The physiologic changes of pregnancy also increase the incidence of sleep-disordered breathing, which includes snoring (in up to 35% of women), upper airway obstruction,[38] and potentially obstructive sleep apnea (OSA). The prevalence of sleep apnea in pregnancy is unknown and has been difficult to determine; the screening questionnaires appear to perform poorly in pregnancy, likely due to the frequency of daytime sleepiness and snoring in pregnancy in the absence of OSA.[46] When it is diagnosed or highly suspected based upon symptoms, OSA appears to increase the risk for intrauterine growth restriction (IUGR) and gestational hypertension via endothelial dysfunction.[44] Women with excessive daytime sleepiness, loud excessive snoring, and witnessed apneas should be evaluated for OSA with overnight polysomnography. In addition, individuals with known sleep apnea may need repeat sleep studies to determine whether changes in treatment are necessary to prevent intermittent hypoxia.[47]

Although the majority of gravidas have sleep problems, most do not complain to their providers or ask for treatment. **Treatment options include improving sleep habits by avoiding fluids after dinner, establishing regular sleep hours, avoiding naps and caffeine, minimizing bedroom noises, and using pillow support.** Other options include relaxation techniques, managing back pain, and use of sleep medications such as diphenhydramine (Benadryl) and zolpidem (Ambien).

Another potential cause of sleep disturbances in pregnancy is the development of restless legs syndrome (RLS) and periodic leg movements during sleep. RLS is a neurosensory disorder that typically begins in the evening and can prevent women from falling asleep. Pregnancy can be a cause of this syndrome, and in one study, up to 34% of gravidas reported symptoms of RLS, although the true prevalence of this disorder during pregnancy is unknown.[48] If treatment is needed, options include improving sleep habits, use of an electric vibrator to the calves, and use of a dopaminergic agent such as levodopa or carbidopa.

URINARY SYSTEM
Anatomic Changes
The kidneys enlarge during pregnancy, with the length as measured by intravenous pyelography increasing about 1 cm. This growth in size and weight is due to increased renal vasculature, interstitial volume, and urinary dead space. **The increase in urinary dead space is attributed to dilation of the renal pelvis, calyces, and ureters. Pelvicalyceal dilation by term averages 15 mm (range, 5 to 25 mm) on the right and 5 mm (range, 3 to 8 mm) on the left.**[49]

The well-known dilation of the ureters and renal pelvis begins by the second month of pregnancy and is maximal by the middle of the second trimester, when ureteric diameter may be as much as 2 cm. The right ureter is almost invariably dilated more than the left, and the dilation usually cannot be demonstrated below the pelvic brim. These findings have led some investigators to argue that the dilation is caused entirely by mechanical compression of the ureters by the enlarging uterus and ovarian venous plexus. However, the early onset of ureteral dilation suggests that **smooth muscle relaxation caused by progesterone** plays an additional role. Also supporting the role of progesterone is the finding of ureteral dilation in women with a renal transplant and pelvic kidney. By 6 weeks postpartum, ureteral dilation resolves.[49] A clinical consequence of ureterocalyceal dilation is an increased incidence of pyelonephritis among gravidas with asymptomatic bacteriuria.[50] **In addition, the ureterocalyceal dilation makes interpretation of urinary radiographs more difficult when evaluating possible urinary tract obstruction or nephrolithiasis.**

Anatomic changes are also observed in the bladder. From midpregnancy on, an elevation in the bladder trigone occurs, with increased vascular tortuosity throughout the bladder. This can cause an increased incidence of microhematuria. **Three percent of gravidas have idiopathic hematuria, defined as greater than 1+ on a urine dipstick, and up to 16% have microscopic hematuria.** Because of the increasing size of the uterus, a decrease in bladder capacity develops as pregnancy progresses, accompanied by an increase in urinary frequency, urgency, and incontinence.

Renal Hemodynamics
Renal plasma flow (RPF) increases markedly from early in gestation and may begin to increase during the luteal phase before implantation.[51] Dunlop showed convincingly that **the effective RPF rises 75% over nonpregnant levels by 16 weeks' gestation** (Table 3-8). The increase is maintained until 34 weeks' gestation, when a decline in RPF of about 25% occurs. The fall in RPF has been demonstrated in subjects studied serially in sitting and left lateral recumbent positions. Like RPF, glomerular filtration rate (GFR), as measured by inulin clearance, increases by 5 to 7 weeks. **By the end of the first trimester, GFR is 50% higher than in the nonpregnant state, and this is maintained until the end of pregnancy.** Three months postpartum, GFR values have declined to normal levels. **This renal hyperfiltration seen in pregnancy is a result of the increase in the RPF.** Because the RPF increases more than the GFR early in pregnancy, the filtration fraction falls from nonpregnant levels until the late third trimester. At this time, because of the decline in RPF, the filtration fraction returns to preconceptional values.

Clinically, GFR is not determined by measuring the clearance of infused inulin (inulin is filtered by the glomerulus and is unaffected by the tubules), but rather by measuring endogenous creatinine clearance. This test gives a less precise measure of GFR because creatinine is secreted by the tubules to a variable extent. Therefore endogenous creatinine clearance is usually higher than the actual GFR. **The creatinine clearance in pregnancy is greatly increased to values of 150 to 200 mL/min (normal, 120 mL/min).** As with GFR, the increase in creatinine clearance occurs by 5 to 7 weeks' gestation and normally is maintained until the third trimester. **GFR is best estimated in pregnancy using a 24-hour urine collection for creatinine clearance. Formulas used in patients with renal disease that estimate the GFR using serum collections and clinical parameters (which avoid a 24-hour urine collection) are inaccurate in pregnancy and underestimate the GFR.**

The increase in the RPF and GFR precede the increase in blood volume and may be induced by a reduction in the preglomerular and postglomerular arteriolar resistance. **Importantly, the increase in hyperfiltration occurs without an increase in glomerular pressure, which if it occurred could have the potential for injury to the kidney with long-term consequences.**[51] Recently, the mechanisms that underlie the marked increase in RPF and GFR have been carefully studied. Although numerous factors are involved in this process, nitric oxide (NO) has been demonstrated to play a critical role in the decrease in renal resistance and the subsequent renal hyperemia. During pregnancy, the activation and expression of the NO synthase is enhanced in the kidneys, and inhibition of NO synthase isoforms has been shown to attenuate the hemodynamic changes within the gravid kidney. Finally, the hormone relaxin appears to be important by initiating or activating some of the effects of NO on the kidney. Failure of this crucial adaptation is associated with adverse outcomes such as preeclampsia and fetal growth restriction (FGR).[52]

The clinical consequence of glomerular hyperfiltration is a reduction in maternal plasma levels of creatinine, blood urea nitrogen (BUN), and uric acid. Serum creatinine decreases from a nonpregnant level of 0.8 to 0.5 mg/dL by term. Likewise, BUN falls from nonpregnant levels of 13 to 9 mg/dL by term. Serum uric acid declines in early pregnancy

TABLE 3-8 SERIAL CHANGES IN RENAL HEMODYNAMICS

| | NONPREGNANT | SEATED POSITION (*N* = 25)* | | | LEFT LATERAL RECUMBENT POSITION (*N* = 17)† | |
		16 WK	26 WK	36 WK	29 WK	37 WK
Effective renal plasma flow (mL/min)	480 ± 72	840 ± 145	891 ± 279	771 ± 175	748 ± 85	677 ± 82
Glomerular filtration rate (mL/min)	99 ± 18	149 ± 17	152 ± 18	150 ± 32	145 ± 19	138 ± 22
Filtration fraction	0.21	0.18	0.18	0.20	0.19	0.21

*Data from Dunlop W. Serial changes in renal haemodynamics during normal pregnancy. *Br J Obstet Gynaecol.* 1981;88:1.
†Data from Ezimokhai M, Davison J, Philips P, et al. Nonpostural serial changes in renal function during the third trimester of normal human pregnancy. *Br J Obstet Gynaecol* 1981;88:465.

because of the rise in GFR and reaches a nadir by 24 weeks with levels of 2 to 3 mg/dL. After 24 weeks, the uric acid level begins to rise, and by the end of pregnancy, the levels in most women are essentially the same as before conception. The rise in uric acid levels is caused by increased renal tubular absorption of urate and increased fetal uric acid production. **Patients with preeclampsia have elevated uric acid level concentrations; however, because uric acid levels normally rise during the third trimester, overreliance on this test should be avoided in the diagnosis and management of preeclampsia.**

During pregnancy, urine volume is increased, and nocturia is more common. In the standing position, sodium and water are retained; therefore during the daytime, gravidas tend to retain an increased amount of water. At night, while in the lateral recumbent position, this added water is excreted, which results in nocturia. Later in gestation, renal function is affected by position, and the GFR and renal hemodynamics are decreased with changes from lateral recumbency to supine or standing positions.

Renal Tubular Function and Excretion of Nutrients

Despite high levels of aldosterone, which would be expected to result in enhanced urinary excretion of potassium, **gravid women retain about 300 mmol of potassium.**[53] Most of the excess potassium is stored in the fetus and placenta.[53] The mean potassium concentrations in maternal blood are just slightly below nonpregnant levels. The ability of the kidney to conserve potassium has been attributed to increased progesterone levels.[53] For information on the changes in sodium, see the next section, "Body Water Metabolism."

Glucose excretion increases in almost all pregnant women, and glycosuria is common. Nonpregnant urinary excretion of glucose is less than 100 mg/day, but 90% of gravidas with normal blood glucose levels excrete 1 to 10 g of glucose per day. This glycosuria is intermittent and not necessarily related to blood glucose levels or the stage of gestation. Glucose is freely filtered by the glomerulus, and with the 50% increase in GFR, a greater load of glucose is presented to the proximal tubules. A change may occur in the reabsorptive capability of the proximal tubules themselves, but the old concept of pregnancy leading to an overwhelming of the maximal tubular reabsorptive capacity for glucose is misleading and oversimplified. The exact mechanisms that underlie the altered handling of glucose by the proximal tubules appears to be a reduced threshold for glucose resorption via reduced renal glucose transporter expression combined with increased renal blood flow. Aberrations in this mechanism may play a pathophysiologic role in the development of

TABLE 3-9 COMPARISON OF 24-HOUR URINARY PROTEIN AND ALBUMIN EXCRETION

	≤20 WEEKS (*N* = 95)	>20 WEEKS (*N* = 175)	*P* VALUE
Protein (mg/24 hr)	98.1 ± 62.3	121.8 ± 71	.007
Albumin (mg/24 hr)	9.7 ± 6.2	12.2 ± 8.5	.012

From Higby K, Suiter C, Phelps J, et al. Normal values of urinary albumin and total protein excretion during pregnancy. *Am J Obstet Gynecol.* 1994;171:984.
Values are mean ± standard deviation.

gestational diabetes mellitus, and higher thresholds for glucose resorption have been associated with gestational diabetes mellitus.[54] **Even though glycosuria is common, gravidas with repetitive glycosuria should be screened for diabetes mellitus if they have not already been tested.**

Urinary protein and albumin excretion increase during pregnancy, with an upper limit of 300 mg of proteinuria and 30 mg of albuminuria in a 24-hour period.[54] Higby and associates[54a] found that the amount of proteinuria and albuminuria increases both when compared with nonpregnant levels and as the pregnancy advances. They collected 24-hour urine samples from 270 women over the course of pregnancy and determined the amount of proteinuria and albuminuria; they found that the amount of protein and albumin excreted in urine did not increase significantly by trimester but did increase significantly when compared between the first and second half of pregnancy (Table 3-9). Similarly, the protein/creatinine ratio increases across pregnancy. **In women who did not have preeclampsia, underlying renal disease, or urinary tract infections, the mean 24-hour urine protein across pregnancy was 116.9 mg, with a 95% upper confidence limit of 260 mg.**[54a] These researchers also noted that patients do not normally have microalbuminuria. **In women with preexisting proteinuria, the amount of proteinuria increases in both the second and third trimesters and potentially in the first trimester.** In a study of women with diabetic nephropathy, the amount of proteinuria increased from a mean of 1.74g ± 1.33 g per 24 hours in the first trimester to a mean of 4.82 ± 4.7 g per 24 hours in the third trimester, even in the absence of preeclampsia.[56] The increase in the renal excretion of proteins is due to a physiologic impairment of the proximal tubular function within the kidney and the increase in the GFR.[55]

Other changes in tubular function include an increase in the excretion of amino acids in the urine and an increase in calcium excretion (see Chapter 39). Also, the kidney responds to the respiratory alkalosis of pregnancy by enhanced excretion of bicarbonate; however, renal handling of acid excretion is unchanged.

BODY WATER METABOLISM

The increase in total body water of 6.5 to 8.5 L by the end of gestation represents one of the most significant adaptations of pregnancy. The water content of the fetus, placenta, and amniotic fluid at term totals about 3.5 L. **Additional water is accounted for by expansion of the maternal blood volume by 1500 to 1600 mL, plasma volume by 1200 to 1300 mL, and red blood cells by 300 to 400 mL.** The remainder is attributed to extravascular fluid, intracellular fluid in the uterus and breasts, and expanded adipose tissue. As a result, **pregnancy is a condition of chronic volume overload with active sodium and water retention secondary to changes in osmoregulation and the renin-angiotensin system.** Increase in body water content contributes to maternal weight gain, hemodilution, physiologic anemia of pregnancy, and the elevation in maternal cardiac output. Inadequate plasma volume expansion has been associated with increased risks for preeclampsia and fetal growth restriction.

Osmoregulation

Expansion in plasma volume begins shortly after conception, partially mediated by a change in maternal osmoregulation through altered secretion of arginine vasopressin (AVP) by the posterior pituitary. **Water retention exceeds sodium retention; even though an additional 900 mEq of sodium is retained during pregnancy, serum levels of sodium decrease by 3 to 4 mmol/L.** This is mirrored by decreases in overall plasma osmolality of 8 to 10 mOsm/kg, a change that is in place by 10 weeks' gestation and that continues through 1 to 2 weeks postpartum (Fig. 3-9).[25] Similarly, the threshold for thirst and vasopressin release changes early in pregnancy; during gestational weeks 5 to 8, an increase in water intake occurs and results in a transient increase in urinary volume but a net increase in total body water. Initial changes in AVP regulation may be due to placental signals that involve NO and the hormone relaxin. After 8 weeks of gestation, the new steady state for osmolality has been established with little subsequent change in water turnover, resulting in decreased polyuria. Pregnant women perceive fluid challenges or dehydration normally with changes in thirst and AVP secretion, but this occurs at a new, lower "osmostat."

Plasma levels of AVP remain relatively unchanged despite heightened production, owing to a threefold to fourfold increase in metabolic clearance. **Increased clearance results from a circulating vasopressinase synthesized by the placenta that rapidly inactivates both AVP and oxytocin.** This enzyme increases about 300-fold to 1000-fold over the course of gestation proportional to fetal weight, with the highest concentrations occurring in multiple gestations. **Increased AVP clearance can unmask subclinical forms of diabetes insipidus, presumably because of an insufficient pituitary AVP reserve, and it causes transient diabetes insipidus with an incidence of 2 to 6 per 1000.** Typically presenting with both polydipsia and polyuria, hyperosmolality is usually mild unless the thirst mechanism is abnormal or access to water is limited (see Chapter 43).

Salt Metabolism

Sodium metabolism is delicately balanced and facilitates a net accumulation of about 900 mEq. Sixty percent of the

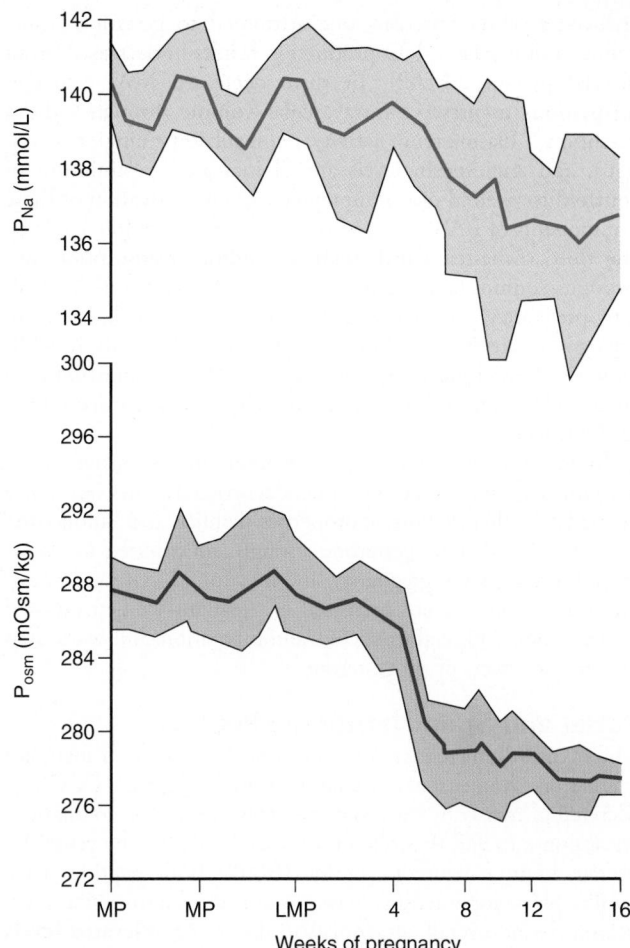

FIG 3-9 Plasma osmolality (P_{osm}) and plasma sodium (P_{Na}) during human gestation ($n = 9$; mean values ± standard deviation). *LMP*, last menstrual period; *MP*, menstrual period. (From Davison JM, Vallotton MB, Lindheimer MD. Plasma osmolality and urinary concentration and dilution during and after pregnancy: evidence that lateral recumbency inhibits maximal urinary concentrating ability. *Br J Obstet Gynaecol.* 1981;88:472.)

additional sodium is contained within the fetoplacental unit, including amniotic fluid, and is lost at birth. By 2 months postpartum, the serum sodium returns to preconceptional levels. Pregnancy increases the preference for sodium intake, but the primary mechanism is **enhanced tubular sodium reabsorption.** Increased glomerular filtration raises the total filtered sodium load from 20,000 to about 30,000 mmol/day; sodium reabsorption must increase to prevent sodium loss. However, the adaptive rise in tubular reabsorption surpasses the increase in filtered load, which results in an additional 2 to 6 mEq of sodium reabsorption per day. **Alterations in sodium handling represent the largest renal adjustment that occurs in gestation.** Hormonal control of sodium balance is under the opposing actions of the renin-angiotensin-aldosterone system (RAAS) and the natriuretic peptides, and both are modified during pregnancy.

Renin-Angiotensin-Aldosterone System

Normal pregnancy is characterized by a marked increase in all components of the RAAS system. In early pregnancy, reduced systemic vascular tone attributed to gestational hormones and increased NO production results in decreased mean arterial pressure (MAP). In turn, decreased MAP activates adaptations to preserve intravascular volume through sodium retention.[57] Plasma renin activity, renin substrate (angiotensinogen), and angiotensin levels are all increased a minimum of fourfold to fivefold over nonpregnant levels. Activation of these components of RAAS leads to doubling of aldosterone levels by the third trimester, which increases sodium reabsorption and prevents sodium loss. Despite the elevated aldosterone levels in late pregnancy, normal homeostatic responses still occur to changes in salt balance, fluid loss, and postural stimuli. In addition to aldosterone, other hormones that may contribute to increased tubular sodium retention include deoxycorticosterone and estrogen.

Importantly, whereas pregnant women are responsive to the sodium-retaining effects of mineralocorticoids, they are fairly refractive to their kaliuretic properties. Erhlich and Lindheimer hypothesized that progesterone strongly contributed to potassium homeostasis in pregnancy, and they found that renal potassium excretion was not increased in pregnant women exposed to exogenous mineralocorticoid administration and attributed this to the effects of progesterone.

Atrial and Brain Natriuretic Peptide

The myocardium releases neuropeptides that serve to maintain circulatory homeostasis. Atrial natriuretic peptide (ANP) is secreted primarily by the atrial myocytes in response to dilation; in response to end-diastolic pressure and volume, the ventricles secrete brain natriuretic peptide (BNP). Both peptides have similar physiologic actions, acting as diuretics, natriuretics, vasorelaxants, and overall antagonists to the RAAS. **Elevated levels of ANP and BNP are found in both physiologic and pathologic conditions of volume overload and can be used to screen for congestive heart failure outside of pregnancy in symptomatic patients.** Because pregnant women frequently present with dyspnea, and many of the physiologic effects of conception mimic heart disease, whether pregnancy affects the levels of these hormones is clinically important. Although ANP levels in pregnancy are variably reported, a meta-analysis[52] showed that ANP levels were 40% higher during gestation and 150% higher during the first postpartum week.

The circulating concentration of BNP is 20% less than that of ANP in normal individuals and has been found to be more useful in the diagnosis of congestive heart failure. Levels of BNP are reported to increase significantly in the third trimester of pregnancy compared with first-trimester levels (21.5 ± 8 pg/mL vs. 15.2 ± 5 pg/mL) and are highest in pregnancies complicated by preeclampsia (37.1 ± 10 pg/mL). In pregnancies with preeclampsia, higher levels of BNP are associated with echocardiographic evidence of left ventricular enlargement. **Whereas the BNP levels are increased during pregnancy, in preeclampsia, the mean values are still lower than the levels used to screen for cardiac dysfunction (>75 to 100 pg/mL). Therefore BNP can be used to screen for congestive heart failure in pregnancy** (see Chapter 37).[58]

Clinical Implications of Pregnancy-Related Renal and Urologic Changes

The normal pregnancy-related changes in the kidneys and urinary tract can have profound clinical implications. From **2%**

to 8% of pregnancies are complicated by asymptomatic bacteriuria, and risk is increased among multiparous women; those of a low socioeconomic class; and women with diabetes, sickle cell disease, and history of previous urinary tract infections. Although this prevalence is approximately equivalent to that in the nonpregnant population, in pregnancy, 30% of these progress to pyelonephritis. This rate is three to four times higher in pregnancy compared with that of nonpregnant controls; overall, 1% to 2% of all pregnancies are complicated by urinary tract infections.[59] For this reason, many providers screen pregnant women for bacteriuria at every clinical encounter. Asymptomatic bacteriuria and symptomatic urinary tract infections are treated to prevent subsequent progression to pyelonephritis and the accompanying maternal and fetal morbidity (see Chapter 54).

Many pregnant women report urinary frequency and nocturnal voiding that start as early as the first trimester, and 60% describe urinary urgency, 10% to 19% develop urge incontinence, and 30% to 60% develop stress incontinence. In a longitudinal cohort study of 241 women, the onset of stress urinary incontinence during the first pregnancy was found to carry an increased risk of long-term symptoms. The rate of urinary incontinence at the 12-year mark was ultimately lower in women who had resolution of their symptoms postpartum (57%) compared with those who did not (91%).[60]

ALIMENTARY TRACT
Appetite
In the absence of nausea or "morning sickness," women who eat according to appetite will increase food intake by about 200 kcal/day by the end of the first trimester. **The recommended dietary allowance calls for an additional 300 kcal/day, although in reality, most women make up for this with decreased activity.** Energy requirements vary depending on the population studied, teenage status, and level of physical activity. The sense of taste may be blunted in some women, which can lead to an increased desire for highly seasoned food. **Pica**, a bizarre craving for strange foods, is relatively common among gravidas, and a history of pica should be sought in those with poor weight gain or refractory anemia. Examples of pica include the consumption of clay, starch, toothpaste, and ice.

Mouth
The pH and the production of saliva are probably unchanged during pregnancy. Ptyalism, an unusual complication of pregnancy, most often occurs in women suffering from nausea and may be associated with the loss of 1 to 2 L of saliva per day. Most authorities believe ptyalism actually represents inability of the nauseated woman to swallow normal amounts of saliva rather than a true increase in the production of saliva. A decrease in the ingestion of starchy foods may help decrease the amount of saliva. No evidence suggests that pregnancy causes or accelerates the course of dental caries; however, the gums swell and may bleed after tooth brushing, giving rise to the so-called gingivitis of pregnancy. At times, a tumorous gingivitis may occur that presents as a violaceous pedunculated lesion at the gum line that may bleed profusely. Called *epulis gravidarum,* or *pyogenic granulomas,* these lesions consist of granulation tissue and an inflammatory infiltrate (see Chapter 51).

Importantly, up to 40% of pregnant women have periodontal disease. Although it has been linked to preterm birth, more recent data and a report by the American College of Obstetricians and Gynecologists (ACOG)[61] suggest evidence is insufficient to show an association between periodontal infection and preterm birth and that no evidence supports improvement in outcomes following dental treatment during pregnancy. However, for general health and well-being, counseling on good oral habits in pregnancy is recommended.

Stomach

In pregnancy, the tone and motility of the stomach and gastroesophageal (GE) sphincter are decreased, probably because of the smooth muscle–relaxing effects of progesterone and estrogen. Nevertheless, scientific evidence in regard to delayed gastric emptying is inconclusive. **Although gastric emptying does not appear to be delayed in pregnancy, compared with nonpregnant controls, an increased delay is seen in labor with the etiology ascribed to the pain and stress of labor.**

Pregnancy reduces the risk for peptic ulcer disease, but it increases GE reflux disease and dyspepsia in 30% to 50% of individuals.[62] This apparent paradox can be partially explained by physiologic changes in the stomach and lower esophagus. The increase in GE reflux disease is multifactorial and is attributed to esophageal dysmotility caused by gestational hormones, gastric compression from the enlarged uterus, and a decrease in the pressure of the GE sphincter. Estrogen may also lead to increased reflux of stomach acids into the esophagus and may be the predominant cause of reflux symptoms. Theories proposed to explain the decreased incidence of peptic ulcer disease include increased placental histaminase synthesis with lower maternal histamine levels; increased gastric mucin production, which protects the gastric mucosa; reduced gastric acid secretion; and enhanced immunologic tolerance of *Helicobacter pylori,* the infectious agent that causes peptic ulcer disease (see Chapter 48).

Intestines

Perturbations in the motility of the small intestines and colon are common in pregnancy and result in an increased incidence of constipation in some and diarrhea in others. Up to 34% of women in one study noted an increased frequency of bowel movements, perhaps related to increased prostaglandin synthesis. The prevalence of constipation appears to be higher in early pregnancy: 35% to 39% of women report constipation in the first and second trimesters, but only 21% report it in the last trimester. The motility of the small intestines is reduced in pregnancy, with increased oral-cecal transit times. No studies on the colonic transit time have been performed, but limited information suggests reduced colonic motility. Although progesterone has been thought to be the primary cause of the decrease in gastrointestinal (GI) motility, newer studies show that estrogen-induced nitric oxide released from nerves that innervate the GI tract results in relaxation of the GI tract musculature.[62] Absorption of nutrients from the small bowel is unchanged, with the exception of increased iron and calcium absorption, but the increased transit time due to decreased motility allows for more efficient absorption. In addition, both water and sodium absorption in the colon are increased.

The enlarging uterus displaces the intestines and, most importantly, moves the position of the appendix. Thus the presentation, physical signs, and type of surgical incision are affected in the management of appendicitis. Portal venous pressure is increased in pregnancy, which leads to dilation wherever there is portosystemic venous anastomosis; this includes not only the GE junction but also the hemorrhoidal veins, the dilation of which results in the common complaint of hemorrhoids.

With the prevalence of obesity in today's society, it is becoming more common to care for women with a history of bariatric surgery. Such surgeries are performed in women with a body mass index (BMI) of 40 kg/m^2 or greater or 35 kg/m^2 with comorbidities. It is important to be aware of the nutritional deficiencies that can accompany such surgery. These include protein, iron, vitamins B_{12} and D, and calcium.[63] Additionally, practitioners should exercise caution when prescribing nonsteroidal antinflammatory drugs (NSAIDs) to patients with smaller gastric pouches because the risk of gastric ulceration increases because of the reduced absorptive surface in these patients.

Gallbladder

Because of progesterone, the rate at which the gallbladder empties is much slower. After the first trimester, the fasting and residual volumes of the gallbladder are twice as great. In addition, the biliary cholesterol saturation is increased, and the chenodeoxycholic acid level is decreased.[64] This change in the composition of the bile fluid favors the formation of cholesterol crystals, and with incomplete emptying of the gallbladder, the crystals are retained and gallstone formation is enhanced. Furthermore, the progesterone acts to inhibit smooth muscle contraction of the gallbladder, thereby predisposing to formation of sludge or gallstones. **By the time they deliver, up to 10% of women have gallstones on ultrasonographic examination;** however, only 1 in 6000 to 1 in 10,000 pregnancies ultimately require cholecystectomy.[65]

Liver

The size and histology of the liver are unchanged in pregnancy. However, many clinical and laboratory signs usually associated with liver disease are present. Spider angiomas and palmar erythema caused by elevated estrogen levels are normal and disappear soon after delivery. **Although total body protein increases, serum albumin and total protein levels fall progressively during gestation as a result of hemodilution. By term, albumin levels are 25% lower than nonpregnant levels. In addition, serum alkaline phosphatase activity rises during the third trimester to levels two to four times those of nongravid women.** Most of this increase is caused by placental production of the heat-stable isoenzyme and not from the liver. The serum concentrations of many proteins produced by the liver increase. These include elevations in fibrinogen, ceruloplasmin, transferrin, and the binding proteins for corticosteroids, sex steroids, and thyroid hormones.

With the exception of alkaline phosphatase, the other liver function tests are unaffected by pregnancy, including serum levels of bilirubin, aspartate aminotransferase (AST), alanine aminotransferase (ALT), γ-glutamyl transferase (GGT), 5′-nucleotidase, creatinine phosphokinase, and lactate dehydrogenase. In some studies, the mean levels of ALT and AST are mildly elevated but still fall within normal values. Levels of creatinine phosphokinase and lactate dehydrogenase can increase with labor, and pregnancy may be associated with mild subclinical cholestasis that results from the high concentrations of estrogen. Reports on serum bile acid concentrations are conflicting: some studies show an increase, whereas others show no change. **The fasting levels are unchanged, and the measurement of a fasting level appears to be the best test for diagnosing cholestasis of pregnancy.**[66] Cholestasis results from elevated levels of bile acids and is associated with significant pruritus, usually mild increases of ALT and AST, and an increased risk for poor fetal outcomes (see Chapter 47).

Nausea and Vomiting of Pregnancy

Nausea and vomiting, or so-called morning sickness, complicates up to 70% of pregnancies. Typical onset is between 4 and 8 weeks' gestation with improvement before 16 weeks; however, 10% to 25% of women still experience symptoms at 20 to 22 weeks' gestation, and some women will have symptoms throughout the gestation.[67] Although the symptoms are often distressing, simple morning sickness seldom leads to significant weight loss, ketonemia, or electrolyte disturbances. The cause is not well understood, although relaxation of the smooth muscle of the stomach probably plays a role. Elevated levels of human chorionic gonadotropin (hCG) may be involved. However, a good correlation between maternal hCG concentrations and the degree of nausea and vomiting has not been observed. Similarly, minimal data exist to show the etiology is associated with higher levels of estrogen or progesterone. Interestingly, pregnancies complicated by nausea and vomiting generally have a more favorable outcome than those without such symptoms.[67] Treatment is largely supportive and consists of reassurance, avoidance of foods found to trigger nausea, and frequent small meals. Eating dry toast or crackers before getting out of bed may be beneficial. **ACOG states that the use of either vitamin B_6 alone or in combination with doxylamine (Unisom) is safe and effective and should be considered a first line of medical treatment.**

A recent review of alternative therapies to antiemetic drugs found that acupressure, wristbands, or treatment with ginger root may be helpful. For details on hyperemesis gravidarum, please see Chapter 6.

ENDOCRINE CHANGES

Thyroid

Thyroid diseases are common in women of childbearing age (see Chapter 42). **However, normal pregnancy symptoms mirror those of thyroid disease, which makes it difficult to know when screening for thyroid disease is appropriate. In addition, the physiologic effects of pregnancy frequently make the interpretation of thyroid tests difficult.** Therefore it is important for the obstetrician to be familiar with the normal changes in thyroid function that occur. Recent data have shown that the correct and timely diagnosis and treatment of thyroid disease is important to prevent both maternal and fetal complications.

Despite alterations in thyroid morphology, histology, and laboratory indices, pregnant women remain euthyroid. The thyroid gland does increase in size but not as much as was commonly believed. **If adequate iodine intake is maintained, the size of the thyroid gland remains unchanged or undergoes a small increase that can be detected only by ultrasound.** The World Health Organization (WHO) recommends that iodine intake be increased in pregnancy from 100 mg/day to 150 to 200 mg/day. In an iodine-deficient state, the thyroid gland is up

to 25% larger, and goiters occur in 10% of women.[68] Histologically, an increase in thyroid vascularity occurs during pregnancy with evidence of follicular hyperplasia. **The development of a clinically apparent goiter during pregnancy is abnormal and should be evaluated.**

During pregnancy, serum iodide levels fall because of increased renal loss. In addition, in the latter half of pregnancy, iodine is also transferred to the fetus, which further decreases maternal levels; these alterations cause the thyroid to synthesize and secrete thyroid hormone actively.[68] However, at least one investigator has reported that in iodine-sufficient regions, the concentration of iodide does not decrease. Although increased uptake of iodine by the thyroid occurs in pregnancy, pregnant women remain euthyroid by laboratory evaluation.

Total thyroxine (TT4) and total triiodothyronine (TT3) levels begin to increase in the first trimester and peak at midgestation as a result of increased production of thyroxine-binding globulin (TBG). The increase in TBG is seen in the first trimester and plateaus at 12 to 14 weeks' gestation. The concentration of TT4 increases by a factor of about 1.5 in parallel with the TBG from a normal range of 5 to 12 mg/dL in nonpregnant women to 9 to 16 mg/dL during pregnancy. **Only a small amount of TT4 and TT3 is unbound, but these free fractions—normally about 0.04% for T4 and 0.5% for T3—are the major determinants of whether an individual is euthyroid.** The extent of change in free T4 and T3 levels during pregnancy has been controversial, and the discrepancies in past studies have been attributed to the techniques used to measure the free hormone levels. **The current best evidence is that the free T4 levels rise slightly in the first trimester and then decrease so that by delivery, the free T4 levels are 10% to 15% lower than in nonpregnant women; however, these changes are small, and in most gravidas, free T4 concentrations remain within the normal nonpregnant range** (Fig. 3-10).[68] In clinical practice, the free T4 level can be measured using either the free thyroxine index (FTI) or estimates of free T4.

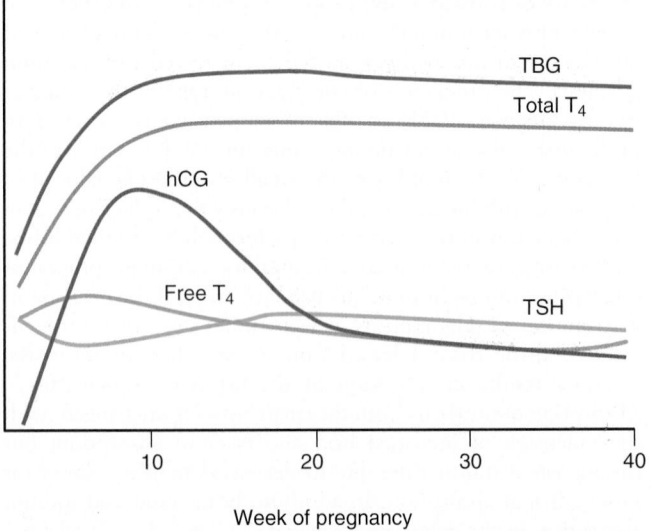

FIG 3-10 Relative changes in maternal thyroid function during pregnancy. *hCG*, human chorionic gonadotropin; T_4, thyroxine; *TBG*, thyroxine-binding globulin; *TSH*, thyroid-stimulating hormone. (From Burrow G, Fisher D, Larsen P. Maternal and fetal thyroid function. *N Engl J Med* 1994;331:1072.)

These tests use immunoassays that do not measure the free T4 directly and may be less accurate in pregnancy because they are TBG dependent. **The FTI is a more accurate method for measuring free T4, and the currently used estimates for free T4 may incorrectly diagnose women as hypothyroid in the second and third trimesters; however, other authors have shown that these free T4 estimates are accurate.**[69] Free T3 levels follow a similar pattern as free T4 levels.

Thyroid-stimulating hormone (TSH) concentrations decrease transiently in the first trimester and then rise to prepregnant levels by the end of this trimester. TSH levels then remain stable throughout the remainder of gestation.[69] **The transient decrease in TSH coincides with the first-trimester increase in free T4 levels, and both appear to be caused by the thyrotropic effects of hCG.** Women with higher peak hCG levels have more TSH suppression. TSH and hCG are structurally very similar, and they share a common α-subunit and have a similar β-unit. **It has been estimated that a 10,000-IU/L increment in circulating hCG corresponds to a mean free T4 increment of 0.6 pmol/L (0.1 ng/dL) and in turn lowers TSH by 0.1 mIU/L.**[68,70] These investigators measured TSH levels during successive trimesters of pregnancy in a large group of women and found that **TSH was suppressed below normal in 18% in the first trimester, 5% during the second trimester, and 2% in the third trimester.** In the first two trimesters, the mean hCG level was higher in women with suppressed TSH levels.[71] It appears that hCG has some thyrotropic activity, but conflicting data on the exact role of hCG in maternal thyroid function remain.[68] **In some women, the thyrotropic effects of hCG can cause a transient form of hyperthyroidism called** *transient gestational thyrotoxicosis* (see Chapter 42).

The influence of maternal thyroid physiology on the fetus appears much more complex than previously thought. Whereas the maternal thyroid does not directly control fetal thyroid function, the systems interact through the placenta, which regulates the transfer of iodine and a small but important amount of thyroxine to the fetus. It was previously thought that little if any transplacental passage of T4 and T3 occurred. **It is now recognized that T4 crosses the placenta, and in early pregnancy, the fetus is critically dependent on the maternal T4 supply for normal neurologic development.**[72] However, as a result of the deiodinase activity of the placenta, a large percentage of T4 is broken down before transfer to the fetus. **The human fetus cannot synthesize thyroid hormones until after 12 weeks' gestation, and any fetal requirement before this time is totally dependent on maternal transfer.** Even after the fetal thyroid is functional, the fetus continues to rely to some extent on a maternal supply of thyroxine. Like T4, thyrotropin-releasing hormone crosses the placenta; TSH does not.

Neonates with thyroid agenesis or a total defect in thyroid hormone synthesis have umbilical cord thyroxine levels between 20% and 50% of those in normal infants, which demonstrates that the placenta is not impermeable to T4. In women who live in iodine-deficient areas, maternal hypothyroidism is associated with neonatal hypothyroidism and defects in long-term neurologic function and mental retardation termed *endemic cretinism.* These abnormalities can be prevented if maternal iodine intake is initiated at the beginning of the second trimester. **Haddow and coworkers**[73] **have found that maternal hypothyroidism during pregnancy results in slightly lower intelligence quotient (IQ) scores in children tested at ages 7 to 9 years. These** findings have resulted in controversy over whether all pregnant women should be screened for subclinical hypothyroidism, which has an incidence of 2% to 5%. Position statements from various organizations are currently contradictory. The Endocrine Society recommends universal screening, whereas ACOG does not support this position (Committee Opinion No. 381). The Maternal-Fetal Medicine Unit Network is currently conducting a randomized trial to investigate the long-term downstream effects (children's intellectual development at 5 years of age) of subclinical hypothyroidism in pregnancy.

Because iodine is actively transported across the placenta and the concentration of iodide in the fetal blood is 75% that of the maternal blood, the fetus is susceptible to iodine-induced goiters when the mother is given pharmacologic amounts of iodine. **Similarly, radioactive iodine crosses the placenta, and if given after 12 weeks' gestation when the fetal thyroid is able to concentrate iodine, profound adverse effects can occur.** These include fetal hypothyroidism, mental retardation, attention-deficit disorder, and a 1% to 2% increase in the lifetime cancer risk.

The American Academy of Pediatrics (AAP) recently released a policy statement urging all pregnant and breastfeeding women to take a supplement with adequate levels of iodine in order to optimize fetal neurocognitive development and to decrease vulnerability to certain environmental pollutants. Even mild iodine deficiency in pregnancy is associated with decreased IQ scores. The National Academy of Sciences and American Thyroid Association recommend 290 µg of daily iodine intake.[74] In order to achieve this, most women require supplementation with 150 µg of iodine daily. Currently, only 15% to 20% of pregnant and breastfeeding mothers take supplemental iodine.

Adrenals

Increased steroid production is essential in pregnancy to meet the need for an increase in maternal production of estrogen and cortisol and the fetal need for reproductive and somatic growth development. **Pregnancy is associated with marked changes in adrenocortical function with increased serum levels of aldosterone, deoxycorticosterone, corticosteroid-binding globulin (CBG), adrenocorticotropic hormone (ACTH), cortisol, and free cortisol, causing a state of physiologic hypercortisolism** (see Chapter 43 and Appendix A).[75] Although the combined weight of the adrenal glands does not increase significantly, expansion of the zona fasciculata, which primarily produces glucocorticoids, is observed. The plasma concentration of CBG doubles because of hepatic stimulation by estrogen by the end of the sixth month of gestation, compared with nonpregnant values; this results in elevated levels of total plasma cortisol. **The levels of total cortisol rise after the first trimester, and by the end of pregnancy, they are nearly three times higher than nonpregnant values and reach levels in the range seen in Cushing syndrome.** The diurnal variations in cortisol levels may be partly blunted but are maintained, and the highest values occur in the morning.

Only free cortisol, the fraction of cortisol not bound to CBG, is metabolically active; however, direct measurements are difficult to perform. Urinary free cortisol concentrations, the free cortisol index, and salivary cortisol concentrations—all of which reflect active free cortisol levels—are elevated after the first trimester. In a study of 21 uncomplicated pregnancies, urinary free cortisol concentration doubled from the first to the third trimester. Although the increase in total cortisol concentrations can be explained by the increase in CBG, this does not explain the higher free cortisol levels. The elevation in free cortisol levels seems to be caused in part by a marked increase in corticotropin-releasing hormone (CRH) during pregnancy, which in turn stimulates the production of ACTH in the pituitary and from the placenta. **Outside of pregnancy, CRH is mainly secreted from the hypothalamus. During pregnancy, CRH is also produced by the placenta and fetal membranes and is secreted into the maternal circulation.** First-trimester values of CRH are similar to prepregnant levels, followed by an exponential rise in CRH during the third trimester predominantly as a result of the placental production. CRH and ACTH concentrations continue to rise in the third trimester despite the increased levels of total and free cortisol levels, which supports the theory that an increase in CRH drives the increased levels of cortisol seen in pregnancy. Furthermore, significant correlation is observed between the rise in CRH levels and maternal ACTH and urinary free cortisol concentrations. Other possible causes for the hypercortisolism include delayed plasma clearance of cortisol as a result of changes in renal clearance, pituitary desensitization to cortisol feedback, or enhanced pituitary responses to corticotropin-releasing factors such as vasopressin and CRH.[75]

Although the levels of cortisol are increased to concentrations observed in Cushing syndrome, little clinical evidence is present for hypercortisolism during pregnancy with the exception of weight gain, striae, hyperglycemia, and tiredness. **The diagnosis of Cushing syndrome during pregnancy is difficult because of these changes; this is discussed further in Chapter 43.**

Like aldosterone, deoxycorticosterone (DOC) is a potent mineralocorticoid. Marked elevations in the maternal concentrations of DOC are present by midgestation and reach peak levels in the third trimester. In contrast to the nonpregnant state, plasma DOC levels in the third trimester do not respond to ACTH stimulation, dexamethasone suppression, or salt intake.[75] These findings suggest that an autonomous source of DOC, specifically the fetoplacental unit, may be responsible for the increased levels. Dehydroepiandrosterone sulfate levels are decreased in gestation because of a marked rise in the metabolic clearance of this adrenal androgenic steroid. Maternal concentrations of testosterone and androstenedione are slightly higher; testosterone is increased because of an elevation in sex hormone–binding protein, and androstenedione rises because of an increase in its synthesis.

Pituitary

The pituitary gland enlarges by approximately one third in pregnancy, principally because of proliferation of prolactin-producing cells in the anterior pituitary (see Chapter 43). **The enlargement of the pituitary gland and subsequent increased intrasellar pressure make it more susceptible to alterations in blood supply and hypotension and increases the risk for postpartum infarction (Sheehan syndrome) should a large maternal blood loss occur.**[76]

Anterior pituitary hormone levels are significantly affected by pregnancy. **Serum prolactin levels begin to rise at 5 to 8 weeks' gestation and by term are 10 times higher.** Consistent with this, the number of lactotroph (prolactin-producing) cells increases dramatically within the anterior lobe of the pituitary from 20% of the cells in nongravid women to 60% in the third trimester. In the second and third trimesters, the decidua is a source of much of the increased prolactin production. Despite the increase, prolactin levels remain suppressible by

bromocriptine therapy.[77] **The principal function of prolactin in pregnancy is to prepare the breasts for lactation** (see Chapter 24). In nonlactating women, the prolactin levels return to normal by 3 months postpartum. In lactating women, the return to baseline levels takes several months, with intermittent episodes of hyperprolactinemia in conjunction with nursing. **Maternal follicle-stimulating hormone (FSH) and luteinizing hormone (LH) are decreased to undetectable levels as a result of feedback inhibition from the elevated levels of estrogen, progesterone, and inhibin.** Maternal pituitary growth hormone production is also suppressed because of the action of the placental growth hormone variant on the hypothalamus and pituitary; however, the serum levels of growth hormone increase as a result of the production of growth hormone from the placenta.

The hormones produced by the posterior pituitary are also altered, and the changes in arginine vasopressin (AVP) were discussed earlier in this chapter under "Osmoregulation." Oxytocin levels increase throughout pregnancy, and they rise dramatically and peak in the second stage of labor.

PANCREAS AND FUEL METABOLISM
Glucose

Pregnancy is associated with significant physiologic changes in carbohydrate metabolism. This allows for the continuous transport of energy, in the form of glucose, from the gravid woman to the developing fetus and placenta. Pregnancy taxes maternal insulin and carbohydrate physiology, and in all pregnancies, some deterioration in glucose tolerance occurs. In most women, only mild changes take place. In others, pregnancy is sufficiently diabetogenic to result in gestational diabetes mellitus. Overall, **pregnancy results in fasting hypoglycemia, postprandial hyperglycemia, and hyperinsulinemia.**[78] To accommodate the increased demand for insulin, hypertrophy and hyperplasia of the insulin-producing β-cells occur within the islets of Langerhans in the maternal pancreas. For a complete review of the physiologic changes in glucose metabolism, please see Chapter 40.

Proteins and Lipids

Amino acids are actively transported across the placenta for the fetus to use for protein synthesis and as an energy source. In late pregnancy, the fetoplacental unit contains about 500 mg of protein.[6,79] During pregnancy, fat stores are preferentially used as a substrate for fuel metabolism, and thus protein catabolism is decreased. Dietary protein is used efficiently in pregnancy as has been shown by measuring nitrogen balance at multiple points throughout gestation and finding an increased nitrogen balance toward the end of pregnancy.

Plasma lipids and lipoproteins increase in pregnancy. A gradual twofold to threefold rise in triglyceride levels occurs by term, and levels of 200 to 300 mg/dL are normal. Total cholesterol and low-density lipoprotein levels are also higher such that by term, a 50% to 60% increase is observed. High-density lipoprotein (HDL) levels initially rise in the first half of pregnancy and then fall in the second half. By term, HDL concentrations are 15% higher than nonpregnant levels. Triglyceride concentrations return to normal by 8 weeks postpartum even with lactation, but cholesterol and low-density lipoprotein (LDL) levels remain elevated (Fig. 3-11). Women with preexisting hyperlipidemia can have a transient worsening of their lipid

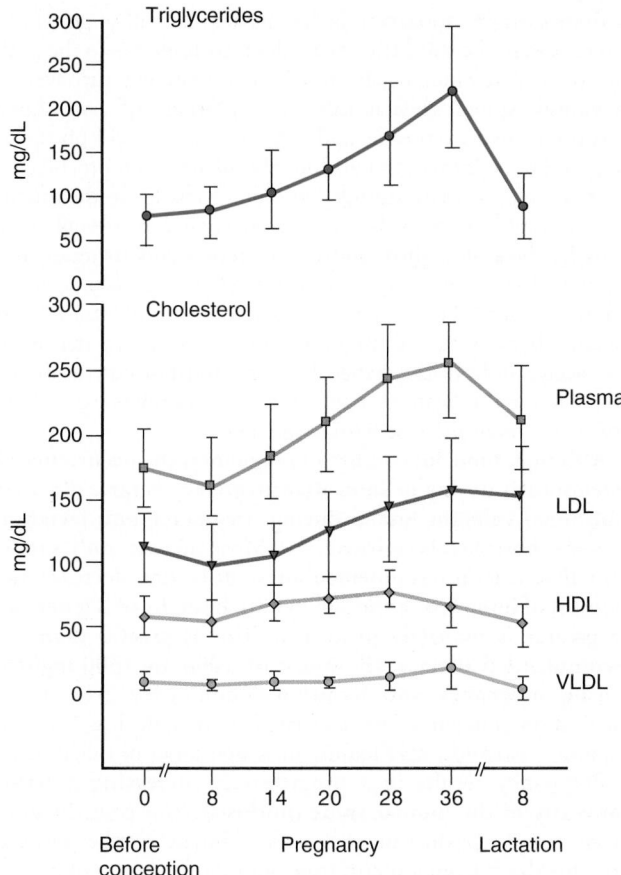

FIG 3-11 Triglycerides (*upper panel*) and cholesterol (*lower panel*) in plasma and in lipoprotein fractions before, during, and after pregnancy. *HDL,* high-density lipoprotein; *LDL,* low-density lipoprotein; *VLDL,* very-low-density lipoprotein. (From Salameh W, Mastrogiannis D. Maternal hyperlipidemia in pregnancy. *Clin Obstet Gynecol.* 1994;37:66.)

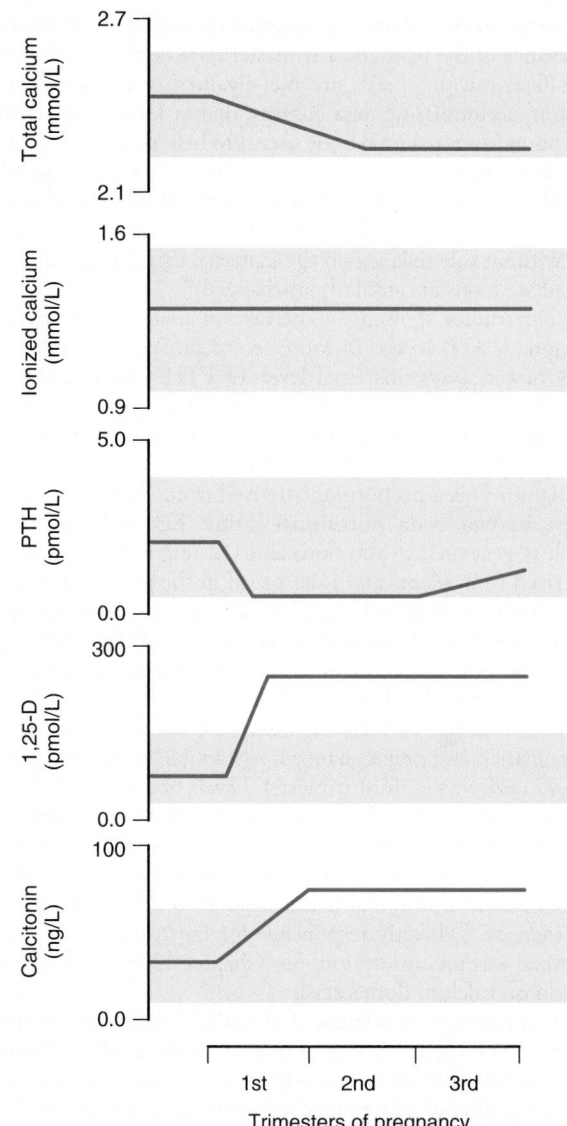

FIG 3-12 The longitudinal changes in calcium and calcitropic hormone levels that occur during human pregnancy. Normal adult ranges are indicated by the *shaded areas. 1,25-D,* 1,25-dihydroxyvitamin D; *PTH,* parathyroid hormone. (From Kovacs CS, Kronenberg HM. Maternal-fetal calcium and bone metabolism during pregnancy, puerperium, and lactation. *Endocr Rev.* 1997;18:832.)

profiles accentuated by the necessity for discontinuing medications such as HMG-CoA reductase inhibitors (statins).

The mechanisms for the pregnancy-induced changes in lipids are not completely understood but appear to be partly caused by the elevated levels of estrogen, progesterone, and human placental lactogen. The rise in LDL is associated with placental steroidogenesis, and the pattern of LDL variation in pregnancy can be used to predict long-term predisposition to atherogenesis.[79] In a study of parity and carotid atherosclerosis in 1005 women over a 6-year period, a significant relationship was found between the progression of carotid atherosclerosis and parity, even after controlling for traditional risk factors. This suggests that pregnancy itself may present an increased risk of subsequent development of atherosclerosis.

SKELETON
Calcium Metabolism

Pregnancy was initially thought to be a state of "physiologic hyperparathyroidism" with maternal skeletal calcium loss needed to supply the fetus with calcium. **However, most fetal calcium needs are met through a series of physiologic changes in calcium metabolism without long-term consequences to the maternal skeleton.**[80] This allows the fetus to accumulate 21 g

(range of 13 to 33 g) of calcium—80% of this during the third trimester, when fetal skeletal mineralization is at its peak. Calcium is actively transported across the placenta. Surprisingly, calcium is excreted in greater amounts by the maternal kidneys so that by term, calciuria is doubled.

Maternal total calcium levels decline throughout pregnancy. The fall in total calcium is caused by the reduced serum albumin levels that result in a decrease in the albumin-bound fraction of calcium. However, the physiologically important fraction, serum ionized calcium, is unchanged and constant (Fig. 3-12).[80] **Therefore the actual maternal serum calcium levels are maintained, and the fetal calcium needs are met mainly through increased intestinal calcium absorption.** Calcium is absorbed through the small intestines, and its absorption is doubled by 12 weeks' gestation, with maximal absorption in the third trimester.[80] The early increase in absorption may allow the maternal skeleton to store calcium in advance of the peak third-trimester fetal demands. Although most fetal calcium needs are met by increased absorption of calcium, accumulating data confirm that at least some calcium resorption from maternal bone occurs to help meet the increased fetal demands in the third trimester. These data are compatible with the hypothesis that physiologic mechanisms exist to ensure an adequate supply of calcium for fetal growth and milk production without sole reliance on the maternal diet. Maternal serum phosphate levels are similarly unchanged.[80]

Older studies showed an increase in maternal parathyroid hormone (PTH) levels. In more recent prospective studies, all using newer assays, maternal levels of PTH were not elevated and actually remained in the low-normal range throughout gestation.[80] Therefore pregnancy is not associated with relative hyperparathyroidism (see Chapter 42).

Vitamin D is a prohormone derived from cholesterol, and it occurs in two main nutritional forms: D3 (cholecalciferol), which is generated in the skin, and D2 (ergocalciferol), which is derived from plants and is absorbed in the gut. **Serum levels of 25-hydroxyvitamin D (25[OH]D) increase in proportion to vitamin D synthesis and intake. Levels of 25[OH]D represent the best indicator of vitamin D status.**[81] 25[OH]D is furthered metabolized to 1,25-dihydroxyvitamin D or active vitamin D. Levels of 1,25-dihydroxyvitamin D increase overall in pregnancy, and prepregnancy levels double in the first trimester and peak in the third trimester. Levels of 25[OH]D do not change in pregnancy unless vitamin D intake or synthesis is changed. The increase in 1,25-dihydroxyvitamin D is secondary to increased production by the maternal kidneys and potentially the fetoplacental unit and is independent of PTH control, and this increase is directly responsible for most of the increase in intestinal calcium absorption. See Chapter 42 for further information on calcium homeostasis.

The estimated prevalence of vitamin D deficiency in pregnancy in the United States may be as high as 50%. Controversy exists over recommendations to institute universal screening during pregnancy by measuring serum levels of 25[OH]D. Levels less than 32 ng/mL indicate vitamin D deficiency, with recommendations to increase vitamin D supplementation if such a deficiency is diagnosed.[81] Results from a cohort study found that maternal vitamin D deficiency was associated with impaired lung development, neurocognitive difficulties, increased risk of eating disorders, and lower peak bone mass. Calcitonin levels also rise by 20% and may help protect the maternal skeleton from excess bone loss.[80]

Skeletal and Postural Changes

The effect of pregnancy on bone metabolism is complex, and evidence of maternal bone loss during pregnancy has been inconsistent, with various studies reporting bone loss, no change, and even gain. Whether pregnancy causes bone loss is not the primary question; instead, the critical question is whether pregnancy and lactation have a long-term risk for causing osteoporosis later in life. **Pregnancy is a period of high bone turnover and remodeling.**[82] **Both pregnancy and lactation cause reversible bone loss, and this loss is increased in women who breastfeed for longer intervals. Studies do not support an association between parity and osteoporosis later in life.** Additionally, in a comparison of female twins discordant for parity, pregnancy and lactation were found to have no detrimental effect on long-term bone loss.

Bone turnover appears to be low in the first half of gestation; it increases in the third trimester, which corresponds to the peak rate of fetal calcium needs, and it may represent turnover of previously stored skeletal calcium.[80] Markers of both bone resorption (hydroxyproline and tartrate-resistant acid phosphatase) and bone formation (alkaline phosphatase and procollagen peptides) are increased during gestation. A change in the microarchitectural pattern of bone with no change in overall bone mass has been described, and this pattern seems to result in a framework more resistant to the bending forces and biomechanical stresses needed to carry a growing fetus. Multiple studies that measure bone density during pregnancy have shown that bone loss occurs only in the trabecular bone and not cortical bone. Older reports indicate that the cortical bone thickness of long bones may even increase with pregnancy.

Although bone loss occurs in pregnancy, the occurrence of osteoporosis during or soon after pregnancy is rare. Whether additional calcium intake during pregnancy and lactation prevents bone loss is controversial. Most current studies indicate that calcium supplementation does not decrease the amount of bone loss, although maternal intake of 2 g per day or greater is modestly protective. This is greater than the recommended dietary allowance of 1000 to 1300 mg/day during pregnancy and lactation. Additionally, women on medications known to be associated with bone loss, such as heparin or steroids, may require increased doses of calcium.[83]

Pregnancy results in a progressively increasing anterior convexity of the lumbar spine (lordosis). This compensatory mechanism keeps the woman's center of gravity over her legs and prevents the enlarging uterus from shifting the center of gravity anteriorly. The unfortunate side effect of this necessary alteration is low back pain in two thirds of women, with the pain described as severe in one third. Because the ligaments of the pubic symphysis and sacroiliac joints loosen, some have hypothesized that this increase in joint laxity is secondary to increased relaxin, whereas others have found no correlation throughout gestation. **Marked widening of the pubic symphysis occurs by 28 to 32 weeks' gestation, with the width increasing from 3 to 4 mm to 7.7 to 7.9 mm.** This commonly results in pain near the symphysis that is referred down the inner thigh with standing and may result in a maternal sensation of snapping or movement of the bones with walking.

SKIN

During pregnancy, physiologic alterations take place in the skin, nails, and hair (see Chapter 51). Increased cutaneous blood flow allows heat to dissipate and is responsible for the "glow" of pregnancy. Hyperpigmentation is also observed in about 90% of women, likely due to increased melanocyte-stimulating hormone and estrogen. This hyperpigmentation accentuates the areola, genital skin, and linea alba in addition to scars and freckles, and it results in melasma, also known as the *mask of pregnancy*. Many women also notice hirsuitism and thickening of scalp hair during pregnancy, which commonly sheds about 1 to 5 months postpartum and is the result of a prolonged anagen phase followed by a large proportion of follicles entering the telogen phase simultaneously.[84] During pregnancy, the nails can develop brittleness, leukonychia, transverse grooving, subungual hyperkeratosis, and distal onycholysis.[84] **The high estrogen state of pregnancy also enhances the appearance of telangectasias and palmar erythema.**[84]

CENTRAL NERVOUS SYSTEM

Whereas central nervous system complaints such as headache and problems with attention are common in pregnancy, few intrinsic changes occur in the central nervous system. Volumetric magnetic resonance imaging (MRI) has demonstrated decreased brain size in healthy women over the course of pregnancy, with a return to baseline by 6 months postpartum; the etiology and significance of these changes are unclear. Volumetric assessment of the pituitary gland, however, reveals that it increases in size and volume, as discussed earlier in this chapter. Changes in vessel-wall integrity predispose to aneurysm rupture; increased relaxin, for example, upregulates collagenase and collagen remodeling.[85] In addition, the risk of subarachnoid hemorrhage is increased fivefold in pregnancy.

EYES

Pregnancy is associated with ocular changes, most of which are transient. The two most significant of these are increased thickness of the cornea and decreased intraocular pressure.[86] Corneal thickening is apparent by 10 weeks' gestation and may cause problems with contact lenses. **Corneal changes persist for several weeks postpartum, and patients should be advised to wait before obtaining a new eyeglass or contact prescription.** Concomitant visual changes are also frequent with a reported incidence of 25% to 89%.[84] The majority of these women had changes in their visual acuity and refractive error, as well as a myopic shift (i.e., they became more far-sighted), from pregravid levels with a return to baseline vision postpartum.[70] Because of these transient alterations in the eye, pregnancy is considered by most to be a contraindication to photorefractive keratectomy, and it has been recommended that pregnancy be avoided for 1 year after such surgery. Intraocular pressure falls by about 10%, and individuals with preexisting glaucoma typically improve.[87] Pregnancy either does not change or minimally decreases visual fields. Therefore any complaints of visual field changes are atypical and need evaluation. Similarly, visual changes such as a loss of vision or "dark floaters" are also atypical and may signify retinal detachment or posterior reversible encephalopathy syndrome, and such changes require evaluation.

BREASTS

Pregnancy-related breast changes begin in the first trimester and continue throughout pregnancy. For a complete review on normal development and physiologic changes of the breast in pregnancy, please see Chapter 24.

LOWER REPRODUCTIVE TRACT
Vagina

Nearly every organ system changes during pregnancy to promote pregnancy maintenance or to prepare for parturition. In the vagina, increased vascularity and hyperemia develop in the skin of the vulva and the mucosa of the vagina, which may cause a bluish discoloration of the vulva, cervix, and vagina as described by Chadwick in 1887 and Jacquemin in 1836.[88] Progesterone increases venous distensibility which, combined with the mechanical effects of the uterus and the increased circulating blood volume, may result in the appearance or worsening of varicose veins in the vulva. The connective tissue underlying the vaginal epithelium also relaxes, and the muscle fibers thicken.[88] The vaginal mucosa itself increases in thickness, and the epithelial cells acquire a characteristic oval form. Estradiol rises across gestation, which leads to increased glycogen levels, namely in the epithelial cells. This glycogen is metabolized into lactic acid, which causes the vaginal pH to decrease. This lactic acid appears to primarily be a byproduct of lactobacilli,[86] which dominate the vaginal flora in pregnancy,[71,89-92] as will be discussed in the microbiome section of this chapter. **Thus it is a combination of hormonal and microbiotic changes that contribute to alterations in the vagina.**

Cervix

During pregnancy, the cervix undergoes a reversible transformation from a closed, rigid, nondistensible structure charged with maintaining a pregnancy to a soft, distensible, nearly indistinguishable ring of tissue capable of stretching to permit the passage of a term fetus. **Unlike the body of the uterus, cervical tissue comprises little smooth muscle; the major component is connective tissue, which consists of collagen, elastin, proteoglycans, and a cellular portion.**[92] Changes in the collagen structure and glycosaminoglycans, which are under hormonal control, contribute to the successful softening and dilation of the cervix.[92] Following delivery, this tissue is repaired to allow subsequent pregnancies.

During pregnancy, the cervix also produces copious amounts of mucus that is thicker and more acidic during pregnancy owing to the effects of progesterone. This mucus is rich in matrix metalloproteinases, which change in composition as pregnancy progresses as their role shifts from cervical remodeling to sentinels against ascending infection.[93] Levels of immunoglobulin G (IgG)—and, to a lesser extent, IgA—increase during pregnancy. IgG levels are highest in the first trimester and subsequently decrease in the second and third trimesters, whereas IgA levels remain relatively constant. Because peak levels of IgG and IgA during all trimesters of pregnancy significantly exceed levels in all phases of the menstrual cycle, it has been postulated that this enhancement may result from increased estrogen and progestin levels. Expression of particular interleukins correlates with immunoglobulin levels but also appears to be influenced by the vaginal microbial composition with decreased *Lactobacillus* species associated with increased cervical interleukin 8 (IL-8), a proinflammatory cytokine.

MICROBIOME

The human microbiome encompasses the totality of the microbes living on and within our bodies. The microbes and their human hosts have co-evolved as a physiologic community comprised of unique, body-site specific niches, meaning that the composition of microbes present at any body site is distinct from other body sites. These microbes generally form a symbiotic relationship with their human hosts, although exceptions do exist. The microbiome of healthy nonpregnant women was described in 2012.[94,95] More recent work has demonstrated that the microbiome of specific body sites change during pregnancy.[71,91,96] **The body site–specific changes in the microbiome during pregnancy may serve to maintain pregnancy, prepare the body for parturition, or establish the neonatal microbiome at the time of parturition.** This emerging field poses exciting questions for the mechanisms of not only

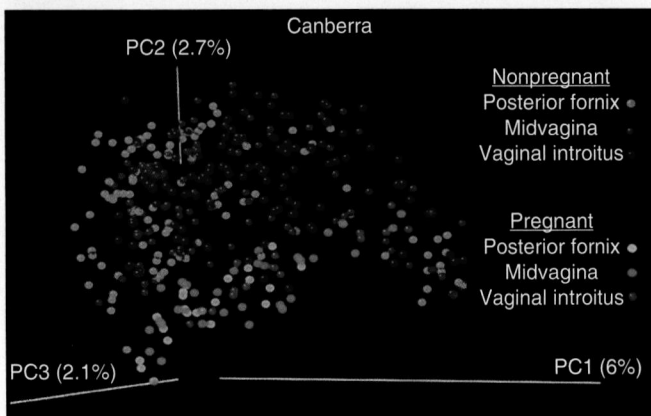

FIG 3-13 This principal coordinate analysis (PCoA) plot demonstrates the degree to which each woman's vaginal microbiome differs from the microbiome of other women's vaginas. Here, nonpregnant women are shown in blue, and pregnant women are shown in green with different vaginal sites indicated by the shades of blue or green. Visually apparent clustering is seen based upon pregnancy status (pregnant vs. nonpregnant), whereas the vaginal site contributed less to cluster formation. (From Aagaard K, Riehle K, Ma J, et al. A metagenomic approach to characterization of the vaginal microbiome signature in pregnancy. *PLoS One.* 2012;7[6]:e36466.)

preterm birth but also the nature of the interaction between microbes and their human hosts in general.

Vaginal Microbiome

As discussed previously in this chapter, the estrogen-induced increase in glycogen is metabolized into lactic acid by *Lactobacillus*, which decreases the pH of the vagina and fosters further *Lactobacillus* growth. The presence of lactobacilli has long been noted to increase as gestational age advances, but since the advent of metagenomics (detailed microbiome analysis), more specific compositional changes have been noted.

The microbiome of the vagina in pregnancy has decreased diversity (alpha diversity) and decreased richness (less different species present).[71] As recently demonstrated, the composition of the microbiome is also different (Fig. 3-13). **Whereas the number of genera and species present decreased, a subsequent dominance by several genera was apparent, notably *Lactobacillus*. The particular species enriched—*L. jensenii*, *L. johnsonii*, or *L. crispatus*—is of probable biologic significance.**[71] For example, *L. jensenii* anaerobically metabolizes glycogen, which is increased with the rising estrogen levels and thereby contributes to the acidic vaginal environment. Additionally, *L. jensenii* may have surface-associated proteins that inhibit sexually transmitted infections, including infection by *Neisseria gonorrhoeae*; thereby *L. jensenii* may help prevent preterm birth. Both *L. jensenii* and *L. crispatus* are strong hydrogen peroxide producers and have been hypothesized to protect against bacterial vaginosis, which has been posited as a risk factor for preterm birth and human immunodeficiency virus (HIV) infection.[97,98]

One of the predominant species in the GI tract of neonates, *L. johnsonii,* is also enriched in the vaginal microbiome during pregnancy. It is able to survive passage through the acidic stomach and can colonize the lower GI tract; it secretes antimicrobial bacteriocins, which can kill *Enterococcus* species[99]; and it is associated with increased mucus thickness in the stomach.[100] Thus it may be important for establishing the neonatal GI microbiome.

Gut Microbiome

Pregnancy is also characterized by changes in the gut microbiota. Over the course of gestation, the bacterial load of the intestines is reported to increase, and the composition also changes. One study found that the diversity within an individual (alpha diversity) decreased with advancing gestation, but diversity between individuals (beta diversity) increased. These changes occurred in parallel with an overall increase in Proteobacteria and a decrease in *Faecalibacterium*. An abundance of Proteobacteria is often associated with inflammatory conditions, and *Faecalibacterium* has antiinflammatory effects; taken together, **the stool in the third trimester of pregnancy resembles stool from inflammatory disease states.** One study innoculated mice with the stool of women in their first and third trimesters of pregnancy and found that stool from the third trimester induced higher levels of inflammation, adiposity, and glucose intolerance in the mice than stool from the first trimester of pregnancy. **Thus pregnancy is associated with changes in the gut microbiome that resemble proinflammatory and prodiabetogenic states.** However, these changes may promote energy storage and fetal growth.

Placental Microbiome

Contrary to the commonly held belief that the upper reproductive tract and placenta are sterile, evidence has been mounting that microbiota are present even in the absence of clinically evident intraamniotic infection.[96,101-103] One recent study that utilized detailed metagenomic analytic methods not only identified bacteria in healthy term deliveries, it found that the **composition of the microbiome was different among women with term versus preterm birth and was also different among women with or without a remote antenatal infection, such as pyelonephritis.**[96] This study also found that the particular composition of the bacteria present in the placenta most closely resembled the oral microbiome and did not resemble the vaginal or skin microbiome. This implies that the bulk of the bacteria isolated were neither contaminants nor ascending infections but may have arrived in the placenta via hematogenous spread from the oral cavity.[96] Together these findings may explain the proposed link between periodontal disease and preterm birth.

SUMMARY

In conclusion, the physiologic changes of pregnancy overall serve to support and maintain the pregnancy in a manner that encompasses almost every organ system from head to toe. Some of these shifts lead to symptoms that can be worrisome to patients, and the role of the practitioner is to discern whether symptoms reflect normal physiologic changes or more concerning pathology. Lastly, the role of microbes in maintaining, or perhaps disrupting, the pregnancy is an emerging field; within a few years, the depth and breadth of the relationship between humans and their microbiomes will likely be further elucidated.

KEY POINTS

- The "healthy" amount of weight to gain during pregnancy is BMI specific.
- Maternal cardiac output increases 30% to 50% during pregnancy. Supine positioning and standing are both

- associated with a fall in cardiac output, which is highest during labor and in the immediate postpartum period.

♦ As a result of the marked fall in systemic vascular resistance and pulmonary vascular resistance, PCWP does not rise despite an increase in blood volume.

♦ Maternal BP decreases early in pregnancy. The diastolic BP and the mean arterial pressure reach a nadir at mid-pregnancy (16 to 20 weeks) and return to prepregnancy levels by term.

♦ Maternal plasma volume increases 50% during pregnancy. Red blood cell volume increases about 18% to 30%, and the hematocrit normally decreases during gestation but not below 30%.

♦ Pregnancy is a hypercoagulable state that is accompanied by increases in the levels of most of the procoagulant factors and decreases in the fibrinolytic system and in some of the natural inhibitors of coagulation.

♦ PaO_2 and $PaCO_2$ fall during pregnancy because of increased minute ventilation. This facilitates transfer of CO_2 from the fetus to the mother and results in a mild respiratory alkalosis.

♦ BUN and creatinine normally decrease during pregnancy as a result of the increased glomerular filtration rate.

♦ Plasma osmolality decreases during pregnancy as a result of a reduction in the serum concentration of sodium and associated anions. The osmolality set points for AVP release and thirst are also decreased.

♦ Despite alterations in thyroid morphology, histology, and laboratory indices, the normal pregnant woman is euthyroid, with levels of free T_4 within nonpregnant norms.

♦ Pregnancy is associated with a peripheral resistance to insulin, primarily mediated by tumor necrosis factor alpha and human placental lactogen. Insulin resistance increases as pregnancy advances; this results in hyperglycemia, hyperinsulinemia, and hyperlipidemia in response to feeding, especially in the third trimester.

♦ Physiologic changes in the vagina interact with the vaginal microbiome to protect against infection and promote pregnancy maintenance.

Acknowledgment

This chapter is based on the contribution by Dr. Michael C. Gordon in the three previous editions.

REFERENCES

1. Committee to Reexamine IOM Pregnancy Weight Guidelines, Institute of Medicine, National Research Council. Rasmussen KM, Yaktine AL, eds. *Weight Gain During Pregnancy: Reexamining the Guidelines.* Washington, D.C.: The National Academies Press; 2009.
2. Gunderson EP, Sternfeld B, Wellons MF, et al. Childbearing may increase visceral adipose tissue independent of overall increase in body fat. *Obesity (Silver Spring).* 2008;16(5):1078-1084.
3. Pitkin R. Nutritional support in obstetrics and gynecology. *Clin Obstet Gynecol.* 1976;19(3):489-513.
4. Abrams B, Selvin S. Maternal weight gain pattern and birth weight. *Obstet Gynecol.* 1995;86(2):163-169.
5. Blomberg M. Maternal and neonatal outcomes among obese women with weight gain below the new Institute of Medicine recommendations. *Obstet Gynecol.* 2011;117(5):1065-1070.
6. Kominiarek MA, Seligman NS, Dolin C, et al. Gestational weight gain and obesity: is 20 pounds too much? *Am J Obstet Gynecol.* 2013;209(3):214 e1-214 e11.
7. Turan OM, De Paco C, Kametas N, Khaw A, Nicolaides KH. Effect of parity on maternal cardiac function during the first trimester of pregnancy. *Ultrasound Obstet Gynecol.* 2008;32(7):849-854.
8. Van Oppen AC, Stigter RH, Bruinse HW. Cardiac output in normal pregnancy: a critical review. *Obstet Gynecol.* 1996;87:310-318.
9. Robson SC, Hunter S, Boys RJ, Dunlop W. Serial study of factors influencing changes in cardiac output during human pregnancy. *Am J Physiol.* 1989;256(4 Pt 2):H1060-H1065.
10. Desai DK, Moodley J, Naidoo DP. Echocardiographic assessment of cardiovascular hemodynamics in normal pregnancy. *Obstet Gynecol.* 2004; 104(1):20-29.
11. Sanghavi M, Rutherford JD. Cardiovascular physiology of pregnancy. *Circulation.* 2014;130(12):1003-1008.
12. Snijder CA, Brand T, Jaddoe V, et al. Physically demanding work, fetal growth and the risk of adverse birth outcomes. The Generation R Study. *Occup Environ Med.* 2012;69(8):543-550.
13. MacGillivray I, Rose GA, Rowe B. Blood pressure survey in pregnancy. *Clin Sci.* 1969;37(2):395-407.
14. Gant NF, Daley GL, Chand S, Whalley PJ, Macdonald PC. A study of angiotensin ii pressor response throughout primigravid pregnancy. *J Clin Invest.* 1973;52(November):2682–2689.
15. Mahendru AA, Everett TR, Wilkinson IB, Lees CC, McEniery CM. A longitudinal study of maternal cardiovascular function from preconception to the postpartum period. *J Hypertens.* 2014;32(4):849-856.
16. De Swiet M. Blood pressure measurement in pregnancy. *Br J Obstet Gynaecol.* 1996;103:862-863.
17. Zinaman M, Rubin J, Lindheimer MD. Serial plasma oncotic pressure levels and echoencephalography during and after delivery in severe preeclampsia. *Lancet.* 1985;1:1245-1247.
18. Crapo R. Normal cardiopulmonary physiology during pregnancy. *Clin Obstet Gynecol.* 1996;39(1):3-16.
19. Roth A, Elkayam U. Acute myocardial infarction associated with pregnancy. *J Am Coll Cardiol.* 2008;52(3):171-180.
20. Lee W, Rokey R, Miller J, Cotton DB. Maternal hemodynamic effects of uterine contractions by M-mode and pulsed-Doppler echocardiography. *Am J Obstet Gynecol.* 1989;161(4):974-977.
21. Robson SC, Boys RJ, Hunter S, Dunlop W. Maternal hemodynamics after normal delivery and delivery complicated by postpartum hemorrhage. *Obstet Gynecol.* 1989;74(2):234-239.
22. Shotan A, Ostrzega E, Mehra A, Johnson J V, Elkayam U. Incidence of Arrhythmias in Normal Pregnancy and Relation to Palpitations. *Am J Cardiol.* 1997;79(8):1061-1064.
23. Little MP, Brocard P, Elliott P, Steer PJ. Hemoglobin concentration in pregnancy and perinatal mortality: a London-based cohort study. *Am J Obstet Gynecol.* 2005;193(1):220-226.
24. Pritchard J, Baldwin R, Dickey J. Blood volume changes in pregnancy and the puerperium, II. Red blood cell loss and changes in apparent blood volume during and following vaginal delivery, cesarean section, and cesarean section plus total hysterectomy. *Am J Obstet Gynecol.* 1962; 84(10):1271.
25. Haider BA, Olofin I, Wang M, Spiegelman D, Ezzati M, Fawzi WW. Anaemia, prenatal iron use, and risk of adverse pregnancy outcomes: systematic review and meta-analysis. *BMJ.* 2013;346(June):f3443.
26. Pitkin R, Witte D. Platelet and Leukocyte Counts in Pregnancy. *J Am Med Assoc.* 1979;242:2696-2698.
27. Burrows R, Kelton J. Incidentally detected thrombocytopenia in healthy mothers and their infants. *N Engl J Med.* 1988;319:142-145.
28. Lescale KB, Eddleman KA, Cines DB, et al. Antiplatelet antibody testing in thrombocytopenic pregnant women. *Am J Obstet Gynecol.* 1996; 174(3):1014-1018.
29. Boehlen F, Hohlfeld P, Extermann P, Perneger TV, de Moerloose P. Platelet count at term pregnancy: a reappraisal of the threshold. *Obstet Gynecol.* 2000;95(1):29-33.
30. Vincelot A, Nathan N, Collet D, Mehaddi Y, Grandchamp P, Julia A. Platelet function during pregnancy: an evaluation using the PFA-100 analyser. *Br J Anaesth.* 2001;87(6):890-893. Available at: <http://www.ncbi.nlm.nih.gov/pubmed/11878692>.
31. Pitkin R, Witte D. Platelet and leukocyte counts in pregnancy. *JAMA.* 1979;242:2696-2698.
32. Clark P, Brennand J, Conkie JA, Mccall F, Greer IA, Walker ID. Activated protein C sensitivity, protein C, protein S and coagulation in normal pregnancy. *Thromb Haemost.* 1998;79:1166-1170.

33. American College of Obstetricians and Gynecologists. Practice Bulletin Number 138: Inherited Thrombophilias in Pregnancy. *Obstet Gynecol.* 2013;122(3):706-717.

34. Molvarec A, Rigó J, Bőze T, et al. Increased plasma von Willebrand factor antigen levels but normal von Willebrand factor cleaving protease (ADAMTS13) activity in preeclampsia. *Thromb Haemost.* 2009;101(2):305-311.

35. Hill JS, Devenie G, Powell M. Point-of-care testing of coagulation and fibrinolytic status during postpartum haemorrhage: developing a thrombelastography®-guided transfusion algorithm. *Anaesth Intensive Care.* 2012;40(6):1007-1015. Available at: <http://www.ncbi.nlm.nih.gov/pubmed/23194210>.

36. Sharma SK, Philip J, Wiley J. Thromboelastographic changes in healthy parturients and postpartum women. *Anesth Analg.* 1997;85:94-98.

37. Karlsson O, Sporrong T, Hillarp A, Jeppsson A, Hellgren M. Prospective longitudinal study of thromboelastography and standard hemostatic laboratory tests in healthy women during normal pregnancy. *Anesth Analg.* 2012;115(4):890-898.

38. Pilkington S, Carli F, Dakin MJ, et al. Increase in Mallampati score during pregnancy. *Br J Anaesth.* 1995;74(6):638-642.

39. Izci B, Riha RL, Martin SE, et al. The upper airway in pregnancy and pre-eclampsia. *Am J Respir Crit Care Med.* 2003;167(2):137-140.

40. Harirah HM, Donia SE, Nasrallah FK, Saade GR, Belfort MA. Effect of gestational age and position on peak expiratory flow rate: a longitudinal study. *Obstet Gynecol.* 2005;105(2):372-376.

41. Grindheim G, Toska K, Estensen M-E, Rosseland L. Changes in pulmonary function during pregnancy: a longitudinal cohort study. *Br J Obstet Gynaecol.* 2012;119(1):94-101.

42. Awe RJ, Nicotra B, Newson TD, Viles R. Arterial oxygenation and alveolar-arterial gradients in term pregnancy. *Obstet Gynecol.* 1979;53:182-186.

43. Lee KA, Zaffke ME, McEnany G. Parity and sleep patterns during and after pregnancy. *Obstet Gynecol.* 2000;95:14-18.

44. Louis JM, Auckley D, Sokol RJ, Mercer BM. Maternal and neonatal morbidities associated with obstructive sleep apnea complicating pregnancy. *Am J Obstet Gynecol.* 2010;202(3):261 e1-261 e5.

45. Facco FL, Kramer J, Ho KH, Zee PC, Grobman WA. Sleep disturbances in pregnancy. *Obstet Gynecol.* 2010;115(1):77-83.

46. Facco FL, Ouyang DW, Zee PC, Grobman W. Development of a pregnancy-specific screening tool for sleep apnea. *J Clin Sleep Med.* 2012;8(4):389-394.

47. Guilleminault C, Palombini L, Poyares D, Takaoka S, Huynh NT, El-Sayed Y. Pre-eclampsia and nasal CPAP: part 1. Early intervention with nasal CPAP in pregnant women with risk-factors for pre-eclampsia: preliminary findings. *Sleep Med.* 2007;9(1):9-14.

48. Uglane MT, Westad S, Backe B. Restless legs syndrome in pregnancy is a frequent disorder with a good prognosis. *Acta Obstet Gynecol Scand.* 2011;90(9):1046-1048.

49. Fried A, Woodring J, Thompson D. Hydronephrosis of pregnancy: a prospective sequential study of the course of dilatation. *J Ultrasound Med.* 1983;2:255.

50. Smaill F, Vazquez J. Antibiotics for asymptomatic bacteriuria in pregnancy (Review). *Cochrane Database Syst Rev.* 2007;18(2):CD000490.

51. Lindheimer M, Davison J, Katz A. The kidney and hypertension in pregnancy: Twenty exciting years. *Semin Nephrol.* 2001;21:173-189.

52. Castro LC, Hobel CJ, Gornbein J. Plasma levels of atrial natriuretic peptide in normal and hypertensive pregnancies: A meta-analysis. *Am J Obstet Gynecol.* 1994;171(December):1642-1651.

53. Lindheimer M, Richardson D, Ehrlich E. Potassium homeostasis in pregnancy. *J Reprod Med.* 1987;32:517.

54. Klein P, Polidori D, Twito O, Jaffe A. Impaired decline in renal threshold for glucose during pregnancy—a possible novel mechanism for gestational diabetes mellitus. *Diabetes Metab Res Rev.* 2014;30(4):140-145.

54a. Higby K, Suiter CR, Phelps JY, Siler-Khodr T, Langer O. Normal values of urinary albumin and total protein excretion during pregnancy. *Am J Obstet Gynecol.* 1994;171(4):984-989.

55. Conrad KP, Stillman IE, Lindheimer MD. The kidney in normal pregnancy and preeclampsia. In: Taylor RN, Roberts JM, Cunningham FG, Lindheimer MD, eds. *Chesley's Hypertensive Disorders in Pregnancy.* 4th ed. New York: Academic Press; 2014:335-378.

56. Gordon M, Landon MB, Samuels P, Hissrich S, Gabbe SG. Perinatal outcome and long-term follow-up associated with modern management of diabetic nephropathy. *Obstet Gynecol.* 1996;87(3):401-409.

57. Duvekot JJ, Cheriex EC, Pieters FA, Menheere PP, Peeters LH. Early pregnancy changes in hemodynamics and volume homeostasis are consecutive adjustments triggered by a primary fall in systemic vascular tone. *Am J Obstet Gynecol.* 1993;169(6):1382-1392.

58. Hameed AB, Chan K, Ghamsary M, Elkayam U. Longitudinal changes in the B-type natriuretic peptide levels in normal pregnancy and postpartum. *Clin Cardiol.* 2009;32(8):E60-E62.

59. Gilstrap LC, Cunningham FG, Whalley PJ. Acute pyelonephritis in pregnancy: an anterospective study. *Obstet Gynecol.* 1981;57(4):409-413.

60. Viktrup L, Rortveit G, Lose G. Risk of stress urinary incontinence twelve years after the first pregnancy and delivery. *Obstet Gynecol.* 2006;108(2):248-254.

61. American College of Obstetricians and Gynecologists. Committee opinion number 569: oral health care during pregnancy and through the lifespan. *Obstet Gynecol.* 2013;122(2):417-422.

62. Shah S, Nathan L, Singh R, Fu YS, Chaudhuri G. E2 and not P4 increases NO release from NANC nerves of the gastrointestinal tract: implications in pregnancy. *Am J Physiol Regul Integr Comp Physiol.* 2001;280:R1546-R1554.

63. The American College of Obstetricians and Gynecologists. ACOG practice bulletin no. 105: bariatric surgery and pregnancy. *Obstet Gynecol.* 2009;113(6):1405-1413.

64. Kern FJ, Everson GT, DeMark B, et al. Biliary lipids, bile acids, and gallbladder function in the human female. *J Clin Invest.* 1981;68:1229-1242.

65. Angelini DJ. Gallbladder and pancreatic disease during pregnancy. *J Perinat Neonatal Nurs.* 2002;15(4):1-12.

66. Arthur C, Mahomed K. Intrahepatic cholestasis of pregnancy: diagnosis and management; a survey of Royal Australian and New Zealand College of Obstetrics and Gynaecology fellows. *Aust N Z J Obstet Gynaecol.* 2014;54(3):263-267.

67. Furneaux EC, Langley-Evans AJ, Langley-Evans SC. Nausea and vomiting of pregnancy. *Obstet Gynecol Surv.* 2001;56(12):775-782.

68. Glinoer D. The regulation of thyroid function in pregnancy: pathways of endocrine adaptation from physiology. *Endocr Rev.* 2014;18(3):404-433.

69. Lee RH, Spencer CA, Mestman JH, et al. Free T4 immunoassays are flawed during pregnancy. *Am J Obstet Gynecol.* 2009;200(3):260.e1-260.e6.

70. Mehdizadehkashi K, Chaichian S, Mehdizadehkashi A, et al. Visual acuity changes during pregnancy and postpartum: a cross-sectional study in Iran. *J Pregnancy.* 2014;2014:675792.

71. Aagaard K, Riehle K, Ma J, et al. A metagenomic approach to characterization of the vaginal microbiome signature in pregnancy. *PLoS ONE.* 2012;7(6):e36466.

72. Calvo RM, Jauniaux E, Gulbis B, et al. Fetal tissues are exposed to biologically relevant free thyroxine concentrations during early phases of development. *J Clin Endocrinol Metab.* 2002;87(4):1768-1777.

73. Haddow JE, Palomaki GE, Allan WC, et al. Maternal thyroid deficiency during pregnancy and subsequent neuropsychological development of the child. *N Engl J Med.* 1999;341(8):549-555.

74. Institute of Medicine Committee on the Scientific Evaluation of Dietary Reference. *Dietary Reference Intakes for Vitamin A, Vitamin K, Arsenic, Boron, Chromium, Copper, Iodine, Iron, Manganese, Molybdenum, Nickel, Silicon, Vanadium, and Zinc.* National Academies Press; 2001.

75. Nolten WE, Lindheimer MD, Oparil S, Ehrlich EN. Desoxycorticosterone in normal pregnancy. I. Sequential studies of the secretory patterns of desoxycorticosterone, aldosterone, and cortisol. *Am J Obstet Gynecol.* 1978;132(4):414-420.

76. Tessnow AH, Wilson JD. The changing face of Sheehan's syndrome. *Am J Med Sci.* 2010;340(5):402-406.

77. Prager D, Braunstein GD. Pituitary disorders during pregnancy. *Endocrinol Metab Clin North Am.* 1995;24(1):1-14.

78. Phelps RL, Metzger BE, Freinkel N. Carbohydrate metabolism in pregnancy. XVII. Diurnal profiles of plasma glucose, insulin, free fatty acids, triglycerides, cholesterol, and individual amino acids in late normal pregnancy. *Am J Obstet Gynecol.* 1981;140(7):730-736.

79. Cunningham FG, Leveno KJ, Bloom SL, Hauth JC, Rouse DJ, Spong CY. *23rd Edition Williams Obstetrics.* New York: McGraw-Hilll; 2010.

80. Kovacs CS, Kronenberg HM. Maternal-fetal calcium and bone metabolism during pregnancy, puerperium, and lactation. *Endocr Rev.* 1997;18(6):832-872.

81. Mulligan ML, Felton SK, Riek AE, Bernal-Mizrachi C. Implications of vitamin D deficiency in pregnancy and lactation. *Am J Obstet Gynecol.* 2010;202(5):429.e1-429.e9.

82. Ensom MH, Liu PY, Stephenson MD. Effect of pregnancy on bone mineral density in healthy women. *Obstet Gynecol Surv.* 2002;57(2):99-111.

83. Nelson-Piercy C, Letsky EA, de Swiet M. Low-molecular-weight heparin for obstetric thromboprophylaxis: experience of sixty-nine pregnancies in sixty-one women at high risk. *Am J Obstet Gynecol.* 1997;176(5):1062-1068.

84. Muallem MM, Rubeiz NG. Physiological and biological skin changes in pregnancy. *Clin Dermatol.* 2006;24(2):80-83.

85. Delfyett WT, Fetzer DT. Imaging of neurologic conditions during pregnancy and the perinatal period. *Neurol Clin.* 2012;30(3):791-822.

86. Millodot M. The influence of pregnancy on the sensitivity of the cornea. *Br J Ophthalmol.* 1977;61:646-649.

87. Horven I, Gjonnaess H. Corneal indentation pulse and intraocular pressure in pregnancy. *Arch Ophthalmol.* 1974;91:92-98.

88. Farage MA, Maibach HI. Morphology and physiological changes of genital skin and mucous membranes. *Curr Probl Dermatol.* 2011;40:9-19.

89. Boskey ER, Cone RA, Whaley KJ, Moench TR. Origins of vaginal acidity: high D/L lactate ratio is consistent with bacteria being the primary source. *Hum Reprod.* 2001;16(9):1809-1813. Available at: <http://www.ncbi.nlm.nih.gov/pubmed/11527880>.

90. Hernández-Rodríguez C, Romero-González R, Albani-Campanario M, Figueroa-Damián R, Meraz-Cruz N, Hernández-Guerrero C. Vaginal microbiota of healthy pregnant Mexican women is constituted by four Lactobacillus species and several vaginosis-associated bacteria. *Infect Dis Obstet Gynecol.* 2011;2011:article 851485.

91. Romero R, Hassan SS, Gajer P, et al. The composition and stability of the vaginal microbiota of normal pregnant women is different from that of non-pregnant women. *Microbiome.* 2014;2(1):4.

92. Leppert P. Anatomy and physiology of cervical ripening. *Clin Obstet Gynecol.* 1995;38(2):267-279.

93. Becher N, Hein M, Danielsen CC, Uldbjerg N. Matrix metalloproteinases in the cervical mucus plug in relation to gestational age, plug compartment, and preterm labor. *Reprod Biol Endocrinol.* 2010;8:113.

94. The Human Microbiome Project Consortium. Structure, function and diversity of the healthy human microbiome. *Nature.* 2012;486(7402):207-214.

95. Aagaard K, Petrosino J, Keitel W, et al. The Human Microbiome Project strategy for comprehensive sampling of the human microbiome and why it matters. *FASEB J.* 2013;27(3):1012-1022.

96. Aagaard K, Ma J, Antony KM, Ganu R, Petrosino J, Versalovic J. The placenta harbors a unique microbiome. *Sci Transl Med.* 2014;6(237):237ra65.

97. Atashili J, Poole C, Ndumbe PM, Adimora AA, Smith JS. Bacterial vaginosis and HIV acquisition: a meta-analysis of published studies. *AIDS.* 2008;22(12):1493-1501.

98. Hillier SL, Nugent RP, Eschenbach DA, et al. Association between bacterial vaginosis and preterm delivery of a low-birth-weight infant. The Vaginal Infections and Prematurity Study Group. *N Engl J Med.* 1995;333(26):1737-1742.

99. Pridmore RD, Berger B, Desiere F, et al. The genome sequence of the probiotic intestinal bacterium Lactobacillus johnsonii NCC 533. *Proc Natl Acad Sci U S A.* 2004;101(8):2512-2517.

100. Pantoflickova D, Corthesy-Theulaz I, Dorta G, et al. Favourable effect of regular intake of fermented milk containing Lactobacillus johnsonii on Helicobacter pylori associated gastritis. *Aliment Pharmacol Ther.* 2003;18:805-813.

101. Stout MJ, Conlon B, Landeau M, et al. Identification of intracellular bacteria in the basal plate of the human placenta in term and preterm gestations. *Am J Obstet Gynecol.* 2013;208(3):226.e1-226.e7.

102. Combs CA, Gravett M, Garite TJ, et al. Amniotic fluid infection, inflammation, and colonization in preterm labor with intact membranes. *Am J Obstet Gynecol.* 2014;210(2):125.e1-125.e15.

103. Fortner KB, Grotegut CA, Ransom CE, et al. Bacteria localization and chorion thinning among preterm premature rupture of membranes. *PLoS ONE.* 2014;9(1):e83338.

See ExpertConsult.com for additional references for this chapter.

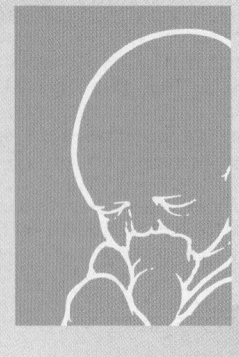

CHAPTER 4

Maternal-Fetal Immunology

KRISTINA M. ADAMS WALDORF

KEY ABBREVIATIONS

Antigen-presenting cell	APC	Microchimerism	Mc
B-cell activating factor of the		Monocyte chemotactic protein 1	MCP-1 or
tumor necrosis factor family	BAFF		CCL2
B-cell receptor	BCR	Natural killer	NK
CC receptor	CCR	NOD-like receptor	NLR
Chemokine (C-C motif) ligand 5	CCL5	Pattern-recognition receptor	PRR
CXC receptor	CXCR	Peripheral T-regulatory cell	pT_{REG}
Decidual natural killer	dNK	Programmed death 1 receptor	PD-1
Dendritic cell	DC	Regulated on activation, normal	RANTES
Fas ligand	FasL	T-cell expressed and secreted	(CCL5)
Graft-versus-host disease	GVHD	Regulatory B cell	B_{REG} or B10
Human chorionic gonadotropin	hCG	Regulatory T cell	T_{REG}
Human immunodeficiency virus	HIV	Rheumatoid arthritis	RA
Human leukocyte antigen	HLA	T-cell receptor	TCR
Indoleamine 2,3 dioxygenase	IDO	T Helper cell type 1	Th1
Immunoglobulin	Ig	T Helper cell type 2	Th2
Interferon-γ	IFN-γ	Thymic T-regulatory cell	tT_{REG}
Interleukin	IL	TNF-related apoptosis-inducing	TRAIL
Kilodalton	kDa	ligand/Apo-2L	
Lipopolysaccharide	LPS	Toll-like receptor	TLR
Lipopolysaccharide binding protein	LBP	Transforming growth factor beta	TGF-β
Major histocompatibility complex	MHC	Tumor necrosis factor alpha	TNF-α
Membrane attack complex	MAC	Vascular endothelial growth factor	VEGF

Pregnancy poses unique immunologic challenges to the mother, who must become tolerant to a genetically foreign fetus yet remain immunocompetent to fight infection. Immunology is one of the fastest moving fields in medical science with many recent advances in the understanding of immunologic changes in pregnancy. The study of maternal-fetal immunology was initially driven by a desire to understand how such a paradoxical feat could occur naturally. Sir Peter Medawar[1] suggested several possibilities to explain fetal tolerance by the mother, including anatomic separation of the fetus and mother, antigenic immaturity of the fetus, and immunologic inertness of the mother. Over time, research has revealed that none of these explanations were adequate for several reasons. First, maternal and fetal cells were discovered to come into contact with each other throughout pregnancy; therefore neither the mother nor the fetus is truly anatomically separated from the other.[2-4] Small populations of fetal cells in the mother and maternal cells in the fetus can persist for decades after pregnancy, which is known as *microchimerism (Mc)*.[5] Secondly, the fetus is not antigenically immature. Fetal immune cells in the skin can elicit potent immune responses.[6] Other fetal immune cells become highly specialized to suppress the fetal immune system and prevent reactivity toward maternal microchimeric cells that enter the fetus.[7] Finally, the mother is not immunologically inert; maintaining the ability to recognize pathogens and fight infection is paramount to her survival during pregnancy. Instead, the maternal immune system has developed an elaborate strategy to become more flexible to what she considers "self" during pregnancy in order to prevent immunologic attack of the fetus.[8,9] The study of pregnancy immunology has revealed many fascinating mechanisms at work to achieve and maintain fetal tolerance during pregnancy while still allowing for normal immune defense.

In this chapter, we focus on describing pregnancy immunology as it relates to normal pregnancy and obstetric complications. In some perinatal conditions, the study of pregnancy immunology is central to the discovery of better diagnostic strategies and therapies. For example, preterm labor associated with infection is characterized by immunologic proteins in the blood, amniotic fluid, and vaginal fluid, which are thought to play a major role in triggering labor.[10-12] Understanding the functions of the immune system and individual immune cells as they relate to maternal tolerance of the fetus, preterm birth, preeclampsia, pregnancy loss, and common perinatal infections will allow the clinician to gain a deeper appreciation for normal and abnormal pregnancy.

IMMUNE SYSTEM OVERVIEW: INNATE AND ADAPTIVE IMMUNITY

The immune system is classically divided into two arms, the innate (Fig. 4-1) and adaptive (Fig. 4-2) immune systems. Each arm of the immune system fights infection by a slightly different and complementary method. Both systems have several important mechanisms to prevent maternal immunity from targeting and killing the fetus, yet the immune system must remain competent to overcome an infection to preserve the mother's life. Achieving a balance between controlling normal immune responses and maintaining immune function is a major challenge of pregnancy.

The innate immune system uses fast, nonspecific methods of pathogen detection to prevent and control an initial infection. Innate immunity consists of immune cells such as macrophages, dendritic cells (DCs), natural killer (NK) cells, eosinophils, and basophils. In pregnancy, these cells have been implicated in preterm labor, preeclampsia, maternal-fetal tolerance, and intrauterine growth restriction (IUGR). Many of these cells identify pathogens through pattern-recognition receptors (PRRs) that recognize common pathogen structures such as lipoteichoic acid and lipopolysaccharide (LPS), constituents of the cell walls of gram-positive and gram-negative bacteria. PRRs include the macrophage mannose receptor and Toll-like receptors (TLRs), a large family of PRRs likely responsible for the earliest immune responses to a pathogen.[13] TLR activation is often triggered by components of bacterial cell walls, which initiate a signaling cascade that leads to release of cytokines. Cytokines are small immunologic proteins implicated in the pathogenesis of preterm labor. Another component of innate immunity is complement, a system of plasma proteins that coat pathogen surfaces with protein fragments to target them for destruction.

In many cases, innate immune defenses are effective in combating pathogens. Sometimes, pathogens may evolve more rapidly than the hosts they infect, or they evade innate immune responses, like seasonal influenza viruses. The adaptive immune system must then act to control infection. Adaptive immunity results in the clonal expansion of lymphocytes (T cells and B cells) and antibodies against a specific antigen. Although slower to respond, adaptive immunity targets specific components of a pathogen and is capable of eradicating an infection that has overwhelmed the innate immune system. Adaptive immunity also requires presentation of antigen by specialized antigen-presenting cells (APCs), production and secretion of stimulatory cytokines, and ultimately, amplification of antigen-specific lymphocyte clones (T cells and B cells). These memory T and B cells provide lifelong immunity to the specific antigen.

INNATE IMMUNITY: FIRST LINE OF HOST DEFENSE

Epithelial surfaces of the body are the first defenses against infection. Mechanical epithelial barriers to infection include ciliary movement of mucus and epithelial cell tight junctions that prevent microorganisms from easily penetrating intercellular spaces. Chemical mechanisms of defense include enzymes (e.g., lysozyme in saliva, pepsin), low pH in the stomach, and antibacterial peptides (e.g., defensins in the vagina) that degrade bacteria.

After a pathogen enters the tissues, it is often recognized and killed by phagocytes, a process mediated by macrophages and neutrophils. TLRs, a family of PRRs on the surface of macrophages and other innate immune and epithelial cells, represent a primary mechanism of pathogen detection. TLR activation results in secretion of cytokines that initiate inflammatory responses. Nucleotide-binding oligomerization domain receptors (NOD-like receptors, NLRs) are also PRRs, and they operate inside the cell to recognize pathogen structures once they have entered the cell through phagocytosis or via pores. NLRs can cooperate with TLRs to initiate or regulate an inflammatory or apoptotic response. Cytokines and chemokines such as interleukin-8 (IL-8) are released after activation of PRRs to recruit neutrophils to sites of inflammation; they also coordinate many immune functions that include cell activation,

INNATE IMMUNITY
- First line of host defense to infection
- Rapid response
- Nonspecific recognition of broad classes of pathogens
- Preexisting effector cell population *(no amplification required)*
- Inability to discriminate self vs. non-self; only recognizes pathogens

A. Cells

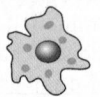 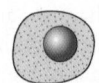 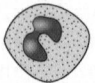

Macrophage   Natural killer   Eosinophil   Basophil
                   (NK cell)

B. Pattern Recognition Receptors: Recognize common microbial patterns and structures

		Example ligand	Origin of ligand
• Toll-like receptors (TLR)	— TLR1	Triacyl lipopeptides	Bacteria & mycobacteria
	— TLR2	Lipoprotein/lipopeptides	Various pathogens
• Macrophage mannose receptor		Peptidoglycan & lipotechoic acid	Gram-positive bacteria
	— TLR3	Double-stranded DNA	Viruses
• Mannan-binding lectin	— TLR4	Lipopolysaccharide	Gram-negative bacteria
	— TLR5	Flagellin	Bacteria
	— TLR6	Diacyl lipopeptides	*Mycoplasma*
	— TLR7 & 8	Single-stranded DNA	Viruses
	— TLR9	CpG-containing DNA	Bacteria and viruses
	— TLR10	Unknown	

C. Complement System: Plasma proteins that cooperate to facilitate destruction of pathogens

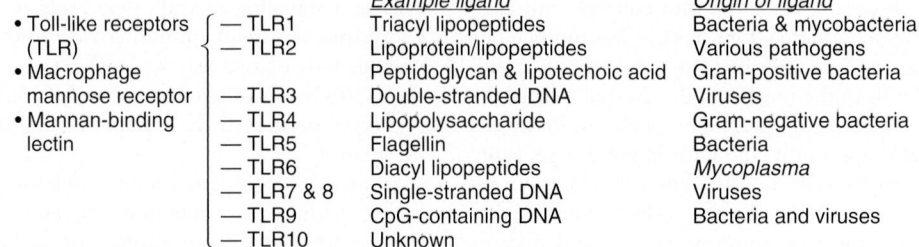

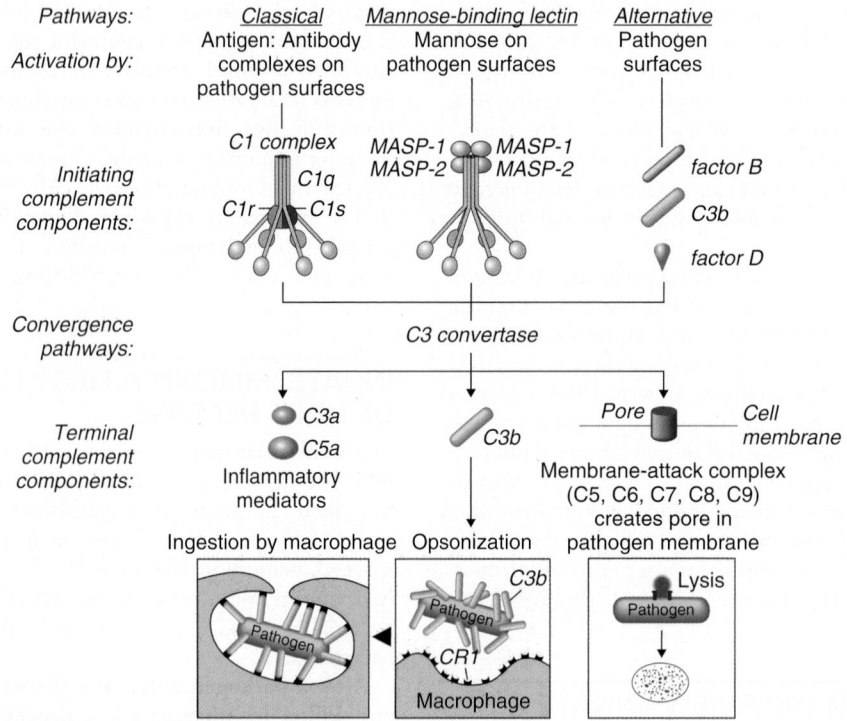

D. Induced Innate Immune Responses

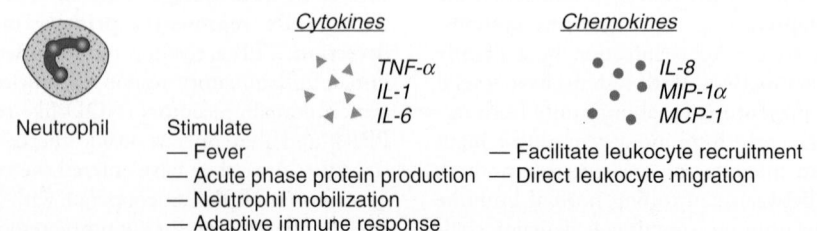

Neutrophil   Stimulate
              — Fever
              — Acute phase protein production
              — Neutrophil mobilization
              — Adaptive immune response

Cytokines
TNF-α
IL-1
IL-6

Chemokines
IL-8
MIP-1α
MCP-1

— Facilitate leukocyte recruitment
— Direct leukocyte migration

FIG 4-1 The innate immune system. This system acts as the first line of host defense and consists of immune cells **(A)**, the pattern-recognition receptors that target common pathogen structures **(B)**, the complement system **(C)**, and induced innate immune responses **(D)**. The toll-like receptors and their common ligands are listed because they act as the principal immune sensors of pathogens **(B)**. Complement activation may occur through three different initiating pathways that converge with production of the C3 convertase and generation of the terminal complement proteins **(C)**. As a result of activation of these components of the innate immune system, neutrophils may be recruited to the site of infection, and cytokines and chemokines may be produced **(D)**.

ADAPTIVE IMMUNITY
- Activated when innate immune defenses overwhelmed
- Delayed response
- Specific recognition of small protein peptides
- Requires amplification of lymphocyte clones
- Ability to discriminate self from non-self

A. B Cells Receptors and Antibodies

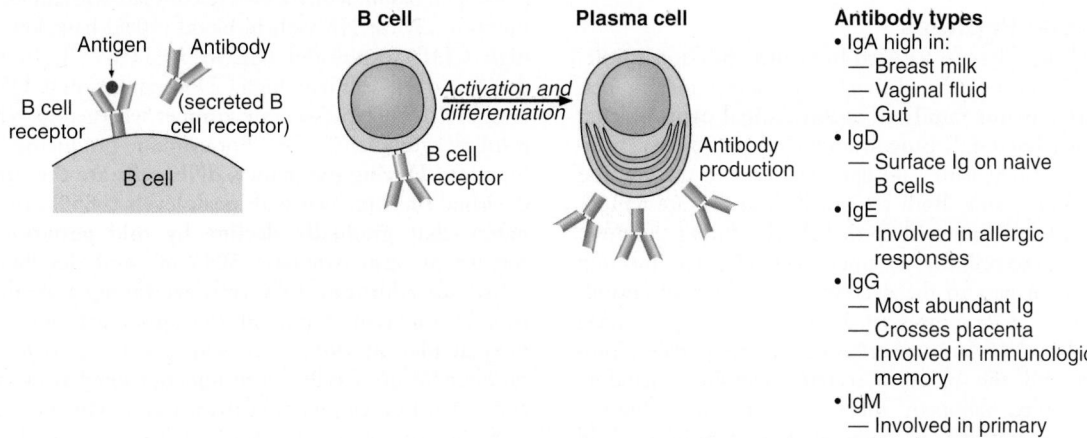

Antibody types
- IgA high in:
  — Breast milk
  — Vaginal fluid
  — Gut
- IgD
  — Surface Ig on naive B cells
- IgE
  — Involved in allergic responses
- IgG
  — Most abundant Ig
  — Crosses placenta
  — Involved in immunologic memory
- IgM
  — Involved in primary B cell responses

B. T Cells and T Cell Receptors

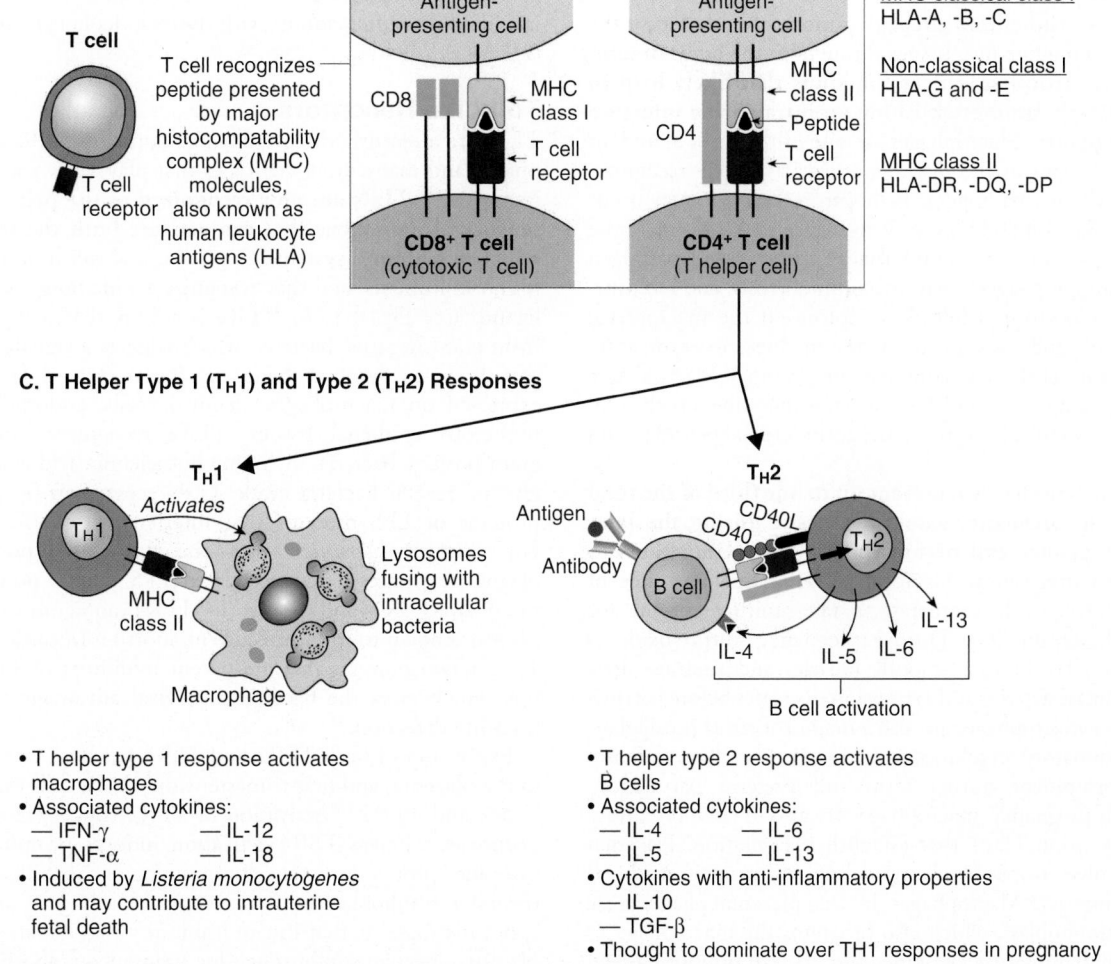

MHC classical class I
HLA-A, -B, -C

Non-classical class I
HLA-G and -E

MHC class II
HLA-DR, -DQ, -DP

C. T Helper Type 1 (T$_H$1) and Type 2 (T$_H$2) Responses

- T helper type 1 response activates macrophages
- Associated cytokines:
  — IFN-γ   — IL-12
  — TNF-α   — IL-18
- Induced by *Listeria monocytogenes* and may contribute to intrauterine fetal death

- T helper type 2 response activates B cells
- Associated cytokines:
  — IL-4   — IL-6
  — IL-5   — IL-13
- Cytokines with anti-inflammatory properties
  — IL-10
  — TGF-β
- Thought to dominate over TH1 responses in pregnancy

FIG 4-2 The adaptive immune system acts to control infection that has overwhelmed the innate immune system and is also important in transplant rejection and tumor killing. B cells secrete antibodies to protect the extracellular spaces of the body from infection and assist in the activation of helper T (CD4$^+$) cells **(A)**. Different classes of antibodies reflect structural variations that allow antibodies to be targeted to different bodily compartments and serve slightly different functions. The first step in T-cell activation occurs when the T-cell receptor recognizes a complex of peptides presented by a major histocompatibility (MHC) molecule **(B)**. A CD4$^+$ T cell recognizes peptide presented by MHC class II, and a CD8$^+$ T cell interacts with peptides presented by MHC class I. Peptides may be presented by many different types of the listed MHC class I or class II molecules. After activation, the CD4$^+$ T cell (or helper T cell) may either activate macrophages through a helper T-cell type 1 response or activate B cells through the helper T-cell type 2 response **(C)**.

replication, and differentiation. **Proinflammatory cytokines have been described in the mother and fetus and in the amniotic fluid of women with preterm labor and intraamniotic infection.**[10,11]

Antimicrobial Peptides

Antimicrobial peptides are secreted by neutrophils and epithelial cells to kill bacteria by damaging pathogen membranes. **Defensins are a major family of antimicrobial peptides that protect against bacterial, fungal, and viral pathogens.** Neutrophils secrete α-defensins, and epithelial cells in the gut and lung secrete β-defensins. Both α- and β-defensins are temporally expressed by endometrial epithelial cells during the menstrual cycle.[14] Susceptibility to upper genital tract infection may be related in part to the decreased expression of antimicrobial peptides in response to hormonal changes during the menstrual cycle. Many other tissues of the female reproductive tract and the placenta secrete defensins, including the vagina, cervix, fallopian tubes, decidua, and chorion. **Elevated concentrations of vaginal and amniotic fluid defensins have been associated with intraamniotic infection and preterm birth.**

Macrophages

Macrophages mature from circulating monocytes that leave the circulation to migrate into tissues throughout the body. **Macrophages have critical scavenger functions that likely help to prevent bacteria from establishing an intrauterine infection during pregnancy.** Macrophages are one of the most abundant immune cell types in the placenta and can directly recognize, ingest, and destroy pathogens. Pathogen recognition may occur through PRRs such as TLRs, scavenger receptors, and mannose receptors. Macrophages also internalize pathogens or pathogen particles through phagocytosis, macropinocytosis, and receptor-mediated endocytosis. Multiple receptors on the macrophage can induce phagocytosis, including the mannose receptor, scavenger receptor, CD14, and complement receptors. Macrophages also release many bactericidal agents after ingesting a pathogen, such as oxygen radicals, nitric oxide, antimicrobial peptides, and lysozyme.

Uterine macrophages represent up to one third of the total leukocytes in pregnancy-associated tissue during the later parts of pregnancy and perform many critical functions to support the pregnancy. Macrophages are a major source of inducible nitric oxide synthetase, a rate-limiting enzyme for nitric oxide production. During pregnancy, nitric oxide is thought to relax uterine smooth muscle, and uterine nitric oxide synthetase activity and expression decreases before parturition. Uterine macrophages are also a major source of prostaglandins, inflammatory cytokines, and matrix metalloproteinases that are prominent during term and preterm parturition. Throughout pregnancy, macrophages are also in close proximity to invading trophoblasts that establish placentation. Placental growth involves trophoblast remodeling and programmed cell death (apoptosis). Macrophages in the placenta phagocytose apoptotic trophoblast, which also programs the macrophage to release antiinflammatory cytokines (e.g., IL-10) promoting fetal tolerance.

Natural Killer Cells

The NK cell has important functions during pregnancy and becomes the most abundant leukocyte in the pregnant uterus.

NK cells differ from T and B cells in that they do not express clonally distributed receptors for foreign antigens and can lyse target cells without prior sensitization. The phenotype of decidual NK (dNK) cells is different from that of NK cells in peripheral blood, which seems to correlate with different primary functions. Most NK cells in blood (90%) have low CD56 and high CD16 expression (CD56^dim/CD16^bright); in the uterine decidua, dNK cells have high CD56 expression (CD56^bright). The level of CD56 expression determines whether an NK cell has a primary cytolytic (CD56^dim) or cytokine-producing (CD56^bright) function. **During pregnancy, dNK cells are the predominant decidual immune cell with peak levels (~85%) in early pregnancy that gradually decline by mid gestation but that remain at approximately 50% of total decidual immune cells.**[15] **In addition, dNK cells are thought to play a major role in the remodeling of the spiral arteries to establish normal placentation.** Mice with genetically defective or low numbers of dNK cells fail to undergo spiral artery remodeling and normal development of the decidua, which are critical processes for normal placentation (see Chapter 1).[16,17] This defect is corrected with administration of interferon-γ (IFN-γ), a prominent NK cell cytokine, which suggests that dNK cells play an important role in the angiogenesis necessary for trophoblast invasion. The cytolytic activity of dNK cells is low and is further inhibited by interactions with human leukocyte antigen G (HLA-G).[18,19]

Toll-Like Receptors

TLRs are a recently discovered large family of PRRs on macrophages and many other cell types that play a key role in innate immunity.[13] **TLRs are now recognized as the principal early sensors of pathogens that can activate both the innate and adaptive immune system.** Ten functional toll homologues are found in humans, and they recognize a wide range of pathogen ligands (see Fig. 4-1, *B*). TLR4 is a TLR that recognizes LPS from gram-negative bacteria, which triggers a signaling cascade that leads to cytokine gene expression (Fig. 4-3). TLR4 is expressed on macrophages, dendritic cells, endothelium, and numerous epithelial tissues. TLR2 recognizes motifs from gram-positive bacteria, including lipoteichoic acid and peptidoglycan. Several bacteria evade TLR recognition by producing proteins or LPS mutants that interfere with TLR signaling. For example, *Yersinia pestis*—the bacteria responsible for plague—expresses a tetraacetylated LPS that is poorly recognized by TLR4 and results in TLR4 antagonism. *Brucella abortus*, known to induce recurrent abortion in cattle, produces at least two proteins that are potent inhibitors of TLR signaling, which gives the bacteria a survival advantage in evading immune detection.[20]

Expression of both TLR2 and TLR4 has been demonstrated in the placenta, and first-trimester trophoblast cells express both TLR2 and TLR4.[21] Activation of TLR2 triggers Fas-mediated apoptosis, whereas TLR4 activation induces proinflammatory cytokine production. The immunologic capability of first-trimester trophoblast cells to recognize pathogens and induce apoptosis suggests that innate immunity may be an important placental mechanism for triggering spontaneous abortion. TLR4 is also expressed in villous macrophages, villous and extravillous trophoblast, and the amniochorion. Expression of TLR4 and TLR2 increases in the chorioamniotic membranes of women with intraamniotic infection and also in term labor. Although intrauterine injection of LPS induces preterm birth in many

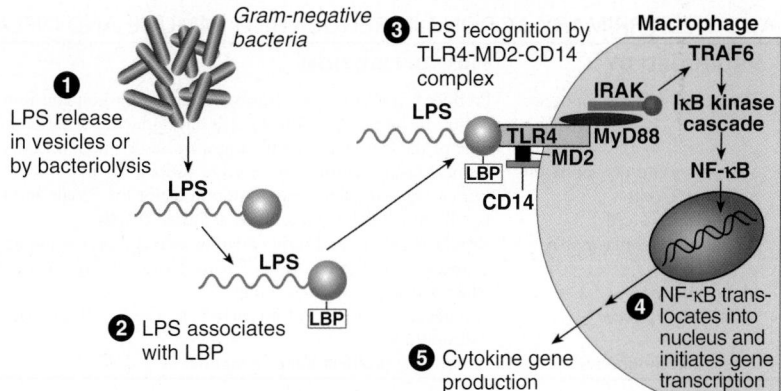

FIG 4-3 Toll-like receptor 4 (TLR4) recognition of lipopolysaccharide (LPS). Recognition of LPS by TLR4 occurs through several steps. *(1)* LPS is released from intact or lysed bacteria. *(2)* LPS binds to LPS-binding protein (LBP). *(3)* The LPS-LBP complex is recognized by a cell surface receptor complex TLR4, CD14, and MD-2. Binding of LPS-LBP to the TLR4–CD14–MD-2 receptor recruits the intracellular adapter molecule, myeloid differentiation factor 88 (MyD88). Binding of MyD88 promotes the association of IL-1 receptor–associated protein kinase 4 (IRAK). Next, tumor necrosis factor receptor–associated kinase 6 (TRAF6) initiates a signaling cascade that results in degradation of Iκ-B, which releases nuclear factor κB (NF-κB), a transcription factor, into the cytoplasm. *(4)* NF-κB translocates into the nucleus and activates cytokine gene expression. Although the figure depicts TLR4 activation in a macrophage, many other immunologic and epithelial cells express TLR4 and induce cytokine production *(5)* through this mechanism.

murine and nonhuman primate models, administration of LPS to TLR4 mutant mice or LPS blockade with a TLR4 antagonist does not result in preterm delivery.[22,23] This finding suggests that TLR4 is required for LPS-induced preterm birth in mice and that it is an important driver of the inflammatory cascade that results from intraamniotic infection.

Maturation of TLR expression in the fetal membranes over time may explain the tendency for infection-associated preterm births to occur no earlier than the late second or early third trimester.[24] Although TLR4 is expressed in the cytoplasm of amniotic epithelium in the first trimester, not until 25 weeks is there TLR4 expression on the apical membrane, which is in contact with amniotic fluid and potential pathogens.[25] A similar ontogeny in TLR4 expression is seen in the fetal lung. When mouse fetal lung is exposed to LPS on fetal day 14 (term is 20 days), TLR4 expression and cytokines are undetectable. By day 17, TLR4 is expressed and an acute cytokine response occurs in fetal lungs. TLR4 likely controls the magnitude of the LPS-induced cytokine response during the perinatal period, and TLR4 placental expression is dependent on gestational age.

Complement System

An important component of the innate immune system is the complement system, which consists of a large number of plasma proteins that cooperate to destroy and facilitate the removal of pathogens (see Fig. 4-1, *C*). Complement proteins are detected in the amniotic fluid during intraamniotic infection, and regulation of complement is necessary to protect placental and fetal tissues from inflammation and destruction. The nature of the initial pathogen trigger determines one of three activation pathways: 1) classic, 2) alternate, and 3) lectin-binding pathways. For example, the *classic pathway* of complement activation is triggered when the complement protein C1q binds to antigen-antibody complexes on the surface of pathogens. This binding then results in a series of activation and amplification steps that result in production of the membrane

attack complex (MAC), which creates a pore in the pathogen membrane and leads to cell lysis. Formation of the MAC is an important mechanism of host defense against *Neisseria* species. Genetic deficiencies in C5-C9 complement proteins have been associated with susceptibility to *N. gonorrhoeae* and *N. meningitidis.*

Regulatory proteins exist to protect cells from the deleterious effects of complement and are expressed on the placental membranes. Placental tissues at the maternal-fetal interface strongly express several negative regulators of complement activation, including CD59 (MAC antagonist), membrane cofactor protein, and decay-accelerating factor (inhibitor of C3 and C5 convertases).[26,27] Whether these regulatory proteins might become overwhelmed during an intraamniotic infection, leading to weakening of the membranes by complement proteins, is unknown.

Cytokines

The release of cytokines and chemokines by macrophages and other immune cells represents an important induced innate immune response (Table 4-1; see Fig. 4-1, *D*). Activated macrophages secrete cytokines—IL-1β, IL-6, IL-12, and tumor necrosis factor alpha (TNF-α)—that initiate inflammatory responses to control infections. **These cytokines are often referred to as *proinflammatory* because they mediate fever, lymphocyte activation, tissue destruction, and shock.** Higher levels of several cytokines and chemokines have been implicated in the increased morbidity and mortality with influenza during pregnancy. In lung homogenates of infected pregnant mice, levels of IL-6 and IL-8; regulated on activation, normal T-cell expressed and secreted (RANTES [CCL5]); and monocyte chemotactic protein 1 (MCP-1 [CCL2]) were higher after infection with the 2009 H1N1 influenza virus strain. Dramatic elevations in IL-6 have also been implicated in deaths, such as in the 1918 influenza virus, with an estimated mortality in pregnancy of 27%.[28] An increase in cytokine levels is likely not the only explanation for increased morbidity and mortality from

TABLE 4-1   CYTOKINES AND THEIR PRIMARY ACTIONS IN REGULATING IMMUNE AND INFLAMMATORY RESPONSE

CYTOKINE	PRODUCED BY	PRIMARY ACTION
Interferons	Monocytes and macrophages	Produced in response to viruses, bacteria, parasites, and tumor cells Action includes killing tumor cells and inducing secretion of other inflammatory cytokines One of the first cytokines to appear during an inflammatory response
Interleukin-1	Monocytes and macrophages	Induces fever; costimulator of CD4+ helper T cells
Interleukin-2	Activated T cells	Primary growth factor and activation factor for T cells and natural killer cells
Interleukin-4	CD4+ helper T cells	B-cell growth factor for antigen-activated B cells
Interleukin-6	Monocytes and macrophages	Regulates growth and differentiation of lymphocytes and growth factor for plasma cells and induces the synthesis of acute-phase reactants by the liver
Interleukin-8	Monocytes	Chemoattractant for neutrophils
Interleukin-10	CD4+ helper T cells	Suppresses production of interferon, suppresses cell-mediated immunity, enhances humoral immunity
Transforming growth factor β	T cells and monocytes	Inhibits the proliferation of lymphocytes

influenza infection during pregnancy. Recently, enhanced NK- and T-cell responses to influenza vaccination in pregnant women were reported, which suggests that robust cellular immune responses also play a role.[29]

During normal pregnancy, many cytokines become repressed with advancing gestation, including IFN-γ, vascular endothelial growth factor (VEGF), MCP-1 (CCL2), and eotaxin. TNF-α and granulocyte colony-stimulating factor (G-CSF) levels increase slightly with advancing gestation, which is surprising because both have been linked to proinflammatory responses, and maintaining uterine quiescence during pregnancy is thought to require repression of inflammation. **Proinflammatory cytokines such as IL-1β, TNF-α, and IL-6 have also been identified in the amniotic fluid, maternal and fetal blood, and vaginal fluid of women with intraamniotic infection at much higher levels than that observed during normal pregnancy.**[10-12,30] **These cytokines not only serve as a marker of intraamniotic infection, they may trigger preterm labor and lead to neonatal complications. The** *fetal inflammatory response syndrome* **describes the connection between elevated proinflammatory cytokines in fetal blood, preterm labor, and increased adverse fetal outcomes (see Chapter 29).**[30]

The relative contribution of individual cytokines and chemokines to preterm labor was studied in a unique nonhuman primate model. Preterm labor was induced by intraamniotic infusions of IL-1β and TNF-α but not by IL-6 or IL-8. IL-1β stimulated preterm labor in all cases and was associated with an intense contraction pattern.[31] TNF-α induced a variable degree of uterine activity characterized as preterm labor in some animals or as a uterine contraction pattern of moderate intensity. Despite prolonged elevations in amniotic fluid levels, neither IL-6 nor IL-8 induced an increase in uterine contractions until near term. **These results suggest a primary role for IL-1β and TNF-α in the induction of infection-associated preterm birth.** Recent data suggest that parturition and prostaglandin mRNA expression was delayed in IL-6 null mutant mice by 1 day compared with wild-type mice.[32] Furthermore, LPS did not induce preterm birth in IL-6–null mutant mice, in contrast to wild-type mice. **Together, these data indicate that IL-6 plays a role in triggering normal parturition, perhaps in activation of labor pathways.**

Investigation of the individual effect of a single cytokine on pregnancy or complications of pregnancy in humans has proved challenging for several reasons. Many cytokines tend to be functionally redundant, with one cytokine compensating for the absence of another. Second, multiple cytokine receptors (i.e., interleukin-1 [IL-1] receptor antagonist, IL-18 binding protein) modulate similar cytokine effects. New families of decoy or silent cytokine receptors and suppressors of cytokine signaling have also been discovered in the placenta and amniotic fluid. Finally, molecular variants of cytokines may act as receptor antagonists. Therefore **individual cytokine effects during pregnancy must be interpreted in the context of cytokine receptors, receptor antagonists, silent cytokine receptors, and suppressors of cytokine signaling.**

Chemokines

Chemokines are a class of cytokines that act primarily as chemoattractants that direct leukocytes to sites of infection. These chemotactic agents constitute a superfamily of small (8 to 10 kDa) molecules that can be divided into three groups—C, CC, and CXC—based on the position of either one or two cysteine residues located near the amino terminus of the protein. IL-8, CCL2 (also known as MCP-1), and RANTES (CCL5) are a few examples of chemokines. CXC chemokines, such as IL-8, bind to CXC receptors (CXCRs) and are important for neutrophil activation and mobilization. **Increases in IL-8 levels have been described in the amniotic fluid, maternal blood, and vaginal fluid with infection-associated preterm birth.**[33] **IL-8 and CCL2 have also been implicated in uterine stretch-induced preterm labor thought to occur in multiple gestation.**[34]

Some chemokine receptors are used as a coreceptor for the viral entry of the human immunodeficiency virus (HIV; see Chapter 53). The two major chemokine co-receptors for HIV are CXCR4 and CCR5, both of which are expressed on activated T cells. CCR5 is also expressed on DCs and macrophages, which allows HIV to infect these cell types. Rare resistance to HIV infection was discovered to correlate with homozygosity for a nonfunctional variant of CCR5 caused by a gene deletion in the coding region. The gene frequency for this CCR5 variant is highest in Northern Europeans but has not been detected in many black or Southeast Asian populations, in whom the prevalence of HIV infection is high. CCR3 is another chemokine coreceptor for HIV that is expressed by microglia, and it can be used by some HIV strains to infect the brain.

ADAPTIVE IMMUNITY

The function of the adaptive immune system is to eliminate infection as the second line of immune defense and to provide increased protection against reinfection through immunologic "memory." Adaptive immunity comprises primarily B cells and T cells (lymphocytes), which differ from innate immune cells in several important respects, including the mechanism for pathogen recognition and lymphocyte activation. Targeting a specific pathogen component in an immune response is a critical feature of the adaptive immune system and is necessary, in most cases, for resolution of the infection. However, achieving this specificity requires generation of an incredible diversity of T-cell receptors (TCRs) and B-cell receptors (BCRs). This creates the potential for self-antigens to be mistakenly targeted, resulting in an autoimmune response. Self-reactive T cells and B cells are thought to either undergo apoptosis in the thymus or to be regulated in the periphery. A small population of regulatory T cells contributes to peripheral regulatory mechanisms to prevent autoimmune responses and is discussed specifically in reference to mechanisms of fetal tolerance.

Major Histocompatibility Complex

Discriminating cells that are "self" from those that are "nonself" is a critical function of the immune system to determine which cells should be destroyed and which to leave alone. In pregnancy, this process must be carefully regulated to prevent the killing of fetal cells, which express paternal genes that appear foreign to the maternal immune system; this in effect expands the maternal immune system's definition of "self" to include the fetus. The ability of a lymphocyte to distinguish self from nonself is based on the expression of unique major histocompatibility complex (MHC) molecules on a cell's surface, which present small peptides from within the cell. MHC molecules are highly polymorphic proteins produced by a cluster of genes on the short arm of chromosome 6. This gene complex is classically divided into two distinct regions referred to as *class I* and *class II*. Class I contains classical transplantation HLA genes (e.g., *HLA-A, -B,* and *-C*) and nonclassical HLA genes distinguished by more limited polymorphism (e.g., *HLA-G, -E,* and *-F*). Class II contains polymorphic genes that are often matched for transplantation, including those of the *HLA-DR, -DQ,* and *-DP* families of genes. Reduced HLA matching is associated with graft rejection after transplantation through activation of T cells. This system differs significantly from the innate immune system, in which recognition of MHC is not necessary for pathogen destruction.

Humoral Immune Responses: B Cells and Antibodies

The function of B cells is to protect the extracellular spaces (e.g., plasma, vagina) in the body through which infectious pathogens usually spread (see Fig. 4-2, *A*). B cells mainly fight infection by secreting antibodies, also called *immunoglobulins.* Many similarities are found between B and T lymphocytes. Like T cells, B cells also undergo clonal expansion after antigen stimulation and can be identified by a variety of specific cell surface markers (e.g., CD19, CD20, and BCR antigens). Activated B cells may proliferate and differentiate into antibody-secreting plasma cells. Antibodies control infection by several mechanisms that include neutralization, opsonization, and complement activation. *Neutralization* of a pathogen refers to the process of antibody binding, which prevents the pathogen from binding to a cell surface and internalizing. Alternatively, antibodies that coat the pathogen may enhance phagocytosis, also referred to as **opsonization.** Antibodies may also directly activate the classical complement pathway. Activation of the B cell drives the B cell to proliferate and differentiate into an antibody-secreting plasma cell.

Recently it was discovered that profound changes occur in many types of B cells during pregnancy.[35] Immature B cells that are the precursors to antigen-specific mature B cells are significantly reduced with advancing gestation in the maternal bone marrow, blood, and spleens of pregnant mice. Lymphopoiesis of B cells is reduced during pregnancy, which may be mediated by the normal pregnancy rise in estradiol.[36] Estradiol reduces levels of IL-17, a critical factor necessary for B-cell production in the bone marrow.[37] This reduction in immature B cells is further potentiated during the second half of pregnancy by the antigen-induced deletion of immature B cells.[38] Although immature B cells are reduced during pregnancy, the number of mature B cells is significantly increased. Surprisingly, an increased number of mature B cells are found in the lymph nodes that drain the uterus.[35] Overall, pregnancy is associated with profound changes in the numbers of B cells in several compartments.

Autoantibodies produced by B cells against angiotensin receptor I, known as *AT1-AA,* are thought to play a role in inducing hypertension and proteinuria in women with preeclampsia and fetal growth restriction.[39,40] AT1-AA is present in 70% to 95% of women with preeclampsia, and antibody titer is correlated with disease severity.[41] AT1-AA can bind to endothelial and placental cells in vitro to induce oxidative stress and cytokine and endothelin production.[42,43] Transfer of these autoantibodies from women with preeclampsia can also induce hypertension and proteinuria in pregnant mice.[39] Although a wide spectrum of immunologic abnormalities is found in preeclampsia, the concept that an autoantibody can cause disease in pregnancy is well established. For example, Graves disease is the most common causes of thyrotoxicosis in pregnancy (see Chapter 42). More than 80% of individuals with Graves disease have anti–thyroid stimulating hormone (TSH) receptor autoantibodies. B cells are likely beneficial in establishing fetal tolerance but may also contribute to the pathogenesis of certain obstetric complications, such as preeclampsia.

Antibody Isotypes

Antibodies share the same general structure produced by the interaction and binding of four separate polypeptides (Fig. 4-4). These include two identical light (L) chains (23 kDa) and two identical heavy (H) chains (55 kDa). The composition of the H chain determines the antibody isotype, function, and distribution in the body. In humans, there are five types of H chains—designated mu (M), delta (D), gamma (G), alpha (A), and epsilon (E)—that correspond to the five major antibody isotypes (immunoglobulin M [IgM], IgD, IgG, IgA, and IgE). To effectively combat extracellular pathogens, antibodies must be specialized to cross epithelia into different bodily compartments. In fact, antibodies are made in several distinct classes or isotypes (i.e., IgM and IgG) that vary in their composition. Naïve B cells express only IgM and IgD. Activated B cells undergo isotype switching, a process that produces different

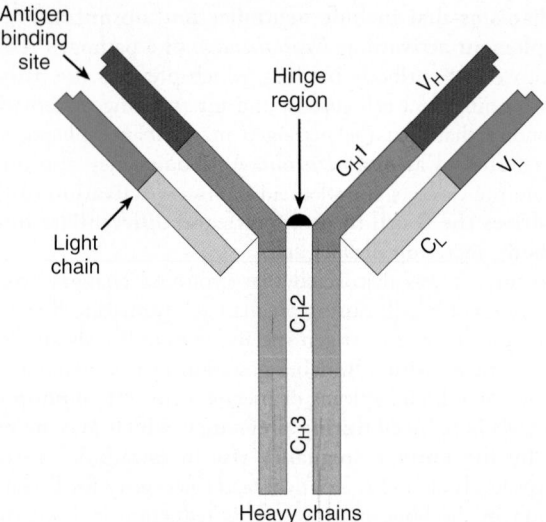

FIG 4-4 Structure of immunoglobulin. Immunoglobulins are produced by B cells to neutralize foreign substances, such as bacteria and viruses. They are large, Y-shaped proteins found in the serum and plasma. CH, constant domain of the heavy chain; CL, constant domain of the light chain; VH, variable domain of the heavy chain; VL, variable domain of the light chain.

antibody isotypes specialized for different functions and areas of the body.

The first antibody to be produced during an immune response is IgM because it is expressed before isotype switching. The serum concentration of IgM is 50 to 400 mg/dL, with a circulation half-life of 5 days. IgM antibodies are low in affinity, but the antibodies form pentamers that compensate by binding at multiple points to the antigen. **IgM is highly efficient at activating the complement system, which is critical during the earliest stages of controlling an infection.** Other isotypes dominate in the later stages of antibody responses.

IgG represents about 75% of serum immunoglobulin in adults and is further divided into four subclasses: IgG1, IgG2, IgG3, and IgG4. Two subtypes of IgG, IgG1 and IgG3, are efficiently transported across the placenta and are important in conferring humoral immune protection for the fetus after birth. The smaller size of IgG and its monomeric structure allows it to easily diffuse into extravascular sites. In mice, the level of IgG3 and IgM increase in early pregnancy but decline as pregnancy advances.[35]

IgA is the predominant antibody class in epithelial secretions from the vagina, intestine, and lung. IgA forms dimers and mainly functions as a neutralizing antibody. As a secreted antibody, IgA is not in close contact with either phagocytes or complement and, therefore, is less efficient in opsonization and complement activation. **IgA is the principal antibody in breast milk, which provides the neonate with humoral immunity from the mother** (see Chapter 24). **Neonates are particularly susceptible to infectious pathogens through their intestinal mucosa, and IgA is highly effective in neutralizing these bacteria and toxins.** Epidemiologic studies indicate that deaths from diarrheal diseases could be reduced between 14- and 24-fold by breastfeeding, owing in part to the maternal-infant transmission of IgA.[44] Levels of IgA rise toward the end of pregnancy in pregnant mice.[35]

IgE has the lowest concentration in serum of all the antibodies but is bound efficiently by mast cell receptors. IgE binding of antibody triggers the mast cell to release granules, which results in an allergic response. Prenatal maternal exposure to allergens may have an effect on IgE in the fetus at birth; concentration of house dust mite allergens has been correlated in a dose-dependent manner with total IgE measured in neonatal heel capillary blood. IgE also plays a prominent role in immune responses to eukaryotic parasites.

T CELLS

When pathogens replicate inside cells (all viruses, some bacteria and parasites), they are inaccessible to antibodies and must be destroyed by T cells. T cells are lymphocytes responsible for the cell-mediated immune responses of adaptive immunity, which require direct interactions between T lymphocytes and cells bearing the antigen that the T cells recognize. Common to all mature T cells is the TCR complex. T cells develop a vast array of antigen specificity through a series of TCR gene rearrangements, and many aspects of TCR rearrangements are similar to those that produce antibody specificity. For example, during viral replication inside a host cell, viral antigen is expressed on the surface of the infected cell. T cells, along with HLA, then recognize these foreign antigens. HLA class I molecules present peptides from proteins in the cytosol, which may include degraded host or viral proteins. HLA class II molecules bind peptides derived from proteins in intracellular vesicles and thus display peptides that originate from pathogens in macrophage vesicles internalized by phagocytic cells and from B cells.

A variety of T cells are recognized based on their expression of different cell surface markers (i.e., CD2, CD3, CD4, CD8). **Cytotoxic T cells kill infected cells directly and express a variety of cell surface antigen and specific receptors, including CD8. Helper T cells activate B cells and express CD4.** Cytotoxic and helper T cells recognize peptides bound to proteins of two different classes of HLA molecules (see Fig. 4-2, B). APCs will present antigen to CD8+ T cells in the context of MHC class I molecules (e.g., HLA-A). In contrast, antigen-presenting cells that present antigens with MHC class II molecules (e.g., HLA-DR) interact with T cells bearing CD4.

HIV uses multiple strategies to disable T-cell responses, mainly by targeting CD4+ T cells. Targeting viral infection to CD4+ T cells allows the virus to control and ultimately destroy this important T-cell subset. HIV destroys CD4+ T cells through direct viral killing, which lowers the apoptosis threshold of infected cells, and through CD8+ T cells that recognize viral peptides on the CD4+ T-cell surface. CD8+ T cells likely contain the infection but are unable to eradicate the virus. Viral mutants produced during one of the earliest steps of viral infection may contribute to the escape of virus-infected cells from CD8+ T-cell killing. HIV also has an error-prone reverse transcriptase that copies the viral RNA genome into DNA, making "mistakes" that lead to production of viral variants. The presentation of peptides from HIV variants by CD4+ T cells may also interfere and downregulate the CD8+ T-cell response to the original (wild-type) virus. Finally, the HIV negative-regulation factor gene *(nef)* downregulates expression of MHC class II and CD4, which decreases the presentation of viral antigens on the cell surface.

Helper T-Cell Subsets

CD4+ T cells were originally classified into T-helper 1 (Th1) and T-helper 2 (Th2) subsets depending on whether their main function involved cell-mediated responses and selective production of IFN-γ (Th1) or humoral-mediated responses with production of IL-4 (Th2). The number of subsets identified continues to expand and now includes regulatory T cells (T$_{REG}$), Th17, follicular helper T cells (T$_{FH}$), Th22, and Th9. The most well-characterized subsets are Th1 and Th2. **The Th1 subset is important in the control of intracellular bacterial infections such as *Mycobacterium tuberculosis* and *Chlamydia trachomatis*.** Intracellular bacteria survive because the vesicles they occupy do not fuse with intracellular lysosomes, which contain a variety of enzymes and antimicrobial substances. Th1 cells activate macrophages to induce fusion of their lysosomes with vesicles that contain the bacteria. Th1 cells also release cytokines and chemokines that attract macrophages to the site of infection, like IFN-γ, TNF-α, IL-12, and IL-18. Th2 immune responses are mainly responsible for activating B cells by providing a critical "second signal." Th2 cells produce cytokines that include IL-4, -5, -6, -10, and -13 and transforming growth factor beta (TGF-β). Although CD4+ T cells can be described in a discrete manner using named subsets like Th1 or Th2, overlap between the functions of these cells is likely.

REGULATORY T CELLS

T$_{REG}$ cells are now recognized as master regulators of the immune system, a feat they accomplish by downregulating antigen-specific T-cell responses to diminish tissue damage during inflammation and to prevent autoimmunity.[45] The most well-defined "naturally occurring" T$_{REG}$ cells express CD4 and CD25 (CD4+, CD25+), but other "suppressor" T cell populations can be generated in vitro (e.g., Tr1, Th3). Although CD4+CD25+ cells were originally thought to also be defined by Forkhead box p3 (Foxp3) expression, this population now appears to be more complex and sometimes expresses other regulatory factors. **T$_{REG}$ cells are unique among the many mechanisms identified to maintain tolerance of the fetus, because fetal antigen-specific T$_{REG}$ cells are maintained in the maternal circulation after delivery, which may benefit the next pregnancy (see "Maternal Tolerance of the Fetus").**[46] Human chorionic gonadotropin (hCG) acts as a chemoattractant for T$_{REG}$ to the maternal-fetal interface, and in the mouse this stimulates T$_{REG}$ frequency and suppressive activity.[47] Similarly, the number of B$_{REG}$ cells and B$_{REG}$ secretion of IL-10 increased when co-cultured with hCG.[48] In this way, hCG may act as an early critical regulator of fetal tolerance by stimulating the populations and suppressive activity of T$_{REG}$ and B$_{REG}$ cells.

The function of T$_{REG}$ cells during pregnancy may be critical for fetal tolerance but could also underlie the unique susceptibility of pregnant women to *Listeria monocytogenes* (see Chapter 54). Pathogen-specific CD8+ T cells confer protection against *L. monocytogenes*. T$_{REG}$ cells act to suppress the function of CD8+ T cells, which is necessary for fetal tolerance, but secondarily disrupt maternal immunity toward *L. monocytogenes*, which is necessary for bacterial eradication.[49,50] Infection also reduces the suppressive activity of T$_{REG}$, which may increase inflammation at the maternal-fetal interface and may promote bacterial invasion into the placenta and the fetus. Although trophoblast cells are resistant to *L. monocytogenes* in vitro, the placenta becomes highly infected in vivo, perhaps because of the immunosuppressive actions of T$_{REG}$ cells. **Once infected, the placenta acts as a reservoir of *L. monocytogenes*, which continually releases bacteria into the maternal circulation and propagates the infection, preventing bacterial clearance until the placenta is expelled.**[51] In contrast, *Plasmodium* infection increases T$_{REG}$ activation and suppressive activity during pregnancy, which may allow for host evasion and further parasite replication. The role of T$_{REG}$ cells in pregnancy may explain the unique susceptibility of pregnant women to certain perinatal infections.

FETAL IMMUNE SYSTEM

Descriptions of the development of the fetal immune system are relatively limited, but sufficient information exists to determine that the fetus, even very early in gestation, has innate immune capacity.[52,53] Acquired immunity, particularly the capacity to produce a humoral response, develops more slowly and is not completely functional until well after birth. Many of the immune protective mechanisms that are present to protect the fetus from both pathogens and maternal immune recognition occur at the maternal-fetal interface. Fortunately, abnormalities of normal immune development are relatively rare. However, when they do occur, they can have profound effects on newborn and child health. Some of the more common immunodeficiencies are listed in Table 4-2.

Fetal thymic development begins with a primordial thymus at about 7 weeks' gestation. The thymus is first colonized with cells from the fetal liver at 8.5 to 9.5 weeks' gestation. These cells express primitive (CD34) and early T-cell surface antigen (CD7). Between 12 and 13 weeks, cells within the fetal liver and spleen express the TCR. By 16 weeks' gestation, the fetal

TABLE 4-2 COMMON IMMUNE DEFECTS

COMMON NAME	DEFECT	CELLS AFFECTED	COMMENTS
X-SCID	Common γ chain of IL-2 receptor	T cells and NK cells	X-linked recessive and most common form of SCID, accounting for about 45%-50% of cases
ADA-SCID	Defect in purine metabolism leading to abnormal accumulation of adenosine	T cells, B cells, and NK cells	Autosomal recessive affecting both male and female infants; accounts for about 20% of SCID cases
Jak-3 deficiency	Mutation on chromosome 19 of Janus kinase 3 activated by cytokine binding to the common γ chain of the IL-2 receptor	T cells and NK cells	Autosomal recessive, affecting both male and female infants; accounts for about 10% of SCID cases
Hyper-IgM syndrome, autosomal recessive	Defect in CD40 ligand (T cell) and CD40 (B cell) signaling, resulting in the inability of immunoglobulin class switching	Elevated IgM	X-linked and autosomal recessive

ADA-SCID, adenosine deaminase severe combined immunodeficiency; *Ig*, immunoglobulin; *IL-2*, interleukin 2; *NK*, natural killer; *X-SCID*, X-linked severe combined immunodeficiency.

thymus has distinct cortical and medullary regions suggestive of functional maturity, and this is confirmed by the brisk response to allogeneic and mitogen stimulation. Functionally, fetal T cells show proliferative capacity very early in gestation. Stimulation by phytohemagglutinin of fetal T cells in vitro can be demonstrated as early as 10 weeks. Allogeneic responses in mixed lymphocyte culture can be detected in cells obtained from fetal liver as early 9.5 weeks and are consistently seen at 12 weeks' gestation. The fetal immune system generates T_{REG} cells within lymph nodes in response to maternal microchimeric cells, which is further evidence that fetal T cells are functional and must be regulated to prevent an immune response.[7]

The ontogeny of fetal B-cell development in many ways parallels the development of T cells, and early pre-B cells (CD19 and CD20) are identified by cell surface markings in the fetal liver by 7 to 8 weeks' gestation.[54] Ultimately, these cells are produced in the fetal bone marrow when the marrow becomes the primary hematopoietic organ in the second trimester. Surface expression of IgM can be noted as early as 9 to 10 weeks. Cells in the fetal circulation express the common B-cell antigens (CD20) by 14 to 16 weeks' gestation, and secretion of IgM has been noted as early as 15 weeks. The level of IgM continues to increase and reaches normal postnatal levels by 1 year of age. The appearance of surface IgG and IgA is noted in fetal B cells at 13 weeks with secretion of IgG at 20 weeks' gestation. Postnatal levels of immunoglobulin are not reached until about 5 years of age.

The neonatal immune system has unique challenges at the time of birth when the newborn is no longer protected from pathogens by the placenta and maternal immune system. A puzzling observation has been that neonatal T cells could become functionally activated in vitro, yet the neonate is profoundly susceptible to systemic infection, as evidenced by the high rates of infection-related neonatal deaths in low- and middle-income countries.[55] To investigate the basis for neonatal susceptibility to infection, a mouse model of *L. monocytogenes* was used in which neonates have diminished survival and bacterial counts are a thousandfold higher than in adults.[56] Interestingly, transfer of adult immune cells from splenocytes into the neonates resulted in diminished cytokine production by the adult cells; when the neonatal immune cells were transferred into the adult, the neonatal cells demonstrated greater cytokine production. These results suggested active suppression of the immune response within the neonate, which was identified to reside within a population of fetal red blood cells (CD71[+]), making an enzyme called *arginase*. Destruction of the CD71[+] cells allowed the neonate to defend itself against *Escherichia coli* and *L. monocytogenes*, but the fetal intestine was found to be inflamed. **CD71[+] cells appear to protect the neonate from excessive inflammation that would occur from commensal microbes during bacterial colonization of the gut at the expense of impairing neonatal immunity to systemic infections.** An understanding of the basis for neonatal susceptibility to infection may allow for therapeutic strategies.

Cord Blood Transplantation

Fetal blood contains a high number of hematopoietic stem cells as well as naïve T cells and NK cells, which makes it an ideal source of cells for hematopoietic cell transplantation. In 1988, the first hematopoietic cell transplant was carried out in a child with Fanconi anemia using a cord blood sample from an HLA-identical sibling. Today, more than 30,000 cord blood transplantations have been performed, and obstetricians are often asked to collect umbilical cord blood remaining in the placenta after cord clamping. Cord blood is typically collected into closed-system bags or syringes that contain anticoagulation additives. The average volume per collection is about 75 mL of cord blood, which is processed to deplete red blood cells and then cryopreserved for later use. Cord blood samples are processed at either private or public cord blood banks. Specimens banked at private cord blood banks will be reserved for the donor family, with an estimated need for use between 1 per 1000 and 1 per 200,000.[57] Samples donated to public cord blood banks are processed, HLA typed, and entered into the National Marrow Donor Program, where they are made available to any individual who requires bone marrow transplantation. The major advantage of public banks is that samples are available to ethnic groups, which traditionally have difficulty finding a suitable HLA-matched donor (e.g., Native Americans, Asian/Pacific Islanders, and African Americans). **The American Congress of Obstetricians and Gynecologists (ACOG) recommends that if a patient requests information regarding collection and banking of umbilical cord blood, balanced and accurate information regarding the advantages and disadvantages of public versus private banking should be provided. Private umbilical cord blood banking is cost effective only for children with a very high likelihood of needing a stem cell transplant.**

Cord blood specimens were initially used only in children because of the reduced number of CD34[+] cells that were present in the donor specimen. As use increased, even in the setting of less than ideal HLA matching, engraftment success was accompanied by a reduction in the frequency of severe (grades 3 and 4) graft-versus-host disease (GVHD). Because of the success noted in children, cord blood specimens are now commonly used in adults. **Double-unit cord blood transplantation is standard practice at many centers and appears to be associated with a lower risk of disease relapse.**[58] After engraftment, usually only one donor source predominates, and the recipient does not develop multisource mixed chimerism. At the present time, the need for autologous cord blood cells is limited. In 2010, more than 450,000 cord blood units were banked worldwide with donor registries present in nearly all regions of the world (47 registries in Europe, 9 in North America, 2 in Africa, 11 in Asia, and 2 in Australia). Umbilical cord blood units are shared internationally, and approximately 40% are matched to a donor across an international border. **The obstetrician-gynecologist can play an important role in improving the availability of cord blood units internationally by encouraging pregnant women to donate to a public cord blood bank.**

MATERNAL TOLERANCE OF THE FETUS

Pregnancy is a unique immunologic phenomenon in which the normal immune rejection of foreign tissues does not occur. The maternal immune system clearly recognizes fetal cells as foreign,[59] and about 30% of primiparous and multiparous women develop antibodies against the inherited paternal HLA of the fetus.[60] The continued presence of these antibodies does not appear to be harmful to the fetus. Persistent fetal cells in the mother may play a role in maintaining the levels of these antibodies because in some women, the antibodies persist, whereas in others they disappear. Formation of IgG antibodies against inherited paternal HLA antigens is associated with the presence of primed cytotoxic T lymphocytes specific for these HLA antigens. Maternal T lymphocytes specific for fetal antigens exist during pregnancy but appear to be hyporesponsive.[9,61] The normal growth and development of the fetus despite maternal immune recognition requires several maternal and fetal adaptations that in most women allow pregnancy to be carried uneventfully to term.

Achieving fetal tolerance requires changes to maternal immunity in multiple locations and by many different cell types because maternal and fetal cells are in direct contact with each other (Fig. 4-5). The syncytiotrophoblast, the outermost layer of chorionic villi, is in direct contact with maternal blood in the intervillous space. Extravillous trophoblast in the decidua is in contact with many different maternal cells, including macrophages, dNK cells, and T cells. Endovascular trophoblast replaces endothelial cells in the maternal spiral arteries and is in direct contact with maternal blood. Fetal and maternal macrophages are also in close contact in the chorion layer of the fetal membranes. **A final and critical interface is within the secondary lymphoid organs (lymph nodes and spleen), where shed fetal trophoblast debris from the placenta comes into contact with maternal immune cells.**[62] A series of studies using a murine model with a unique fetal antigen demonstrated that secondary lymphoid organs are the primary site of fetal and placental alloantigen presentation by maternal, not fetal, APCs.[58,63,64] Maternal recognition of fetal alloantigens likely begins before pregnancy in the lymph nodes that drain the uterus after intercourse with genital tract exposure to seminal fluid.[64] **In summary, the complex nature of the cells and the many locations of the maternal-fetal interface necessitate a number of different immune mechanisms to prevent fetal rejection.** We describe many of the well-known mechanisms of fetal tolerance with a focus on T_{REG} cells because of recent exciting studies that implicate their critical role.

Tolerance Through Regulation of Maternal T Cells

Maternal T cells acquire a state of tolerance for fetal alloantigens during pregnancy. This has been elegantly demonstrated in female mice sensitized to known paternal antigens before pregnancy.[9,61] During pregnancy, the female mice became tolerant to the same paternal antigens expressed by the fetus that were previously recognized and destroyed. **Several mechanisms exist to suppress maternal T-cell responses.** Activated maternal T cells may be deleted, killed, or become anergic in several ways. Suppression of T-cell activation by maternal T_{REG} cells is a focus of this section, but other mechanisms to regulate T-cell activation also occur, including chemokine gene silencing in decidual stromal cells, upregulation of a T-cell immunoinhibitory receptor (programmed death 1 [PD-1]), enzymatic depletion of tryptophan (indoleamine 2,3-dioxygenase [IDO]), and the presence of Fas ligand (FasL) and B7-family molecules (B7-DC, B7-H2, B7-H3) on placental trophoblast.[63,65-67] The importance of suppressing maternal T cells to prevent fetal rejection is evident by the multiple mechanisms used both in the periphery and at the maternal-fetal interface.

T_{REG} cells suppress antigen-specific immune responses and are elevated in the maternal circulation of women and mice during pregnancy.[68] Outside of pregnancy, T_{REG} cells (CD4+, CD25+) act mainly to prevent autoimmune responses from occurring when self-reactive T cells escape from the thymus during normal T-cell development. In mice, depletion of CD25+ T_{REG} cells resulted in fetal resorptions from allogeneic matings.[69,70]

In a mouse model of spontaneous abortion, transfer of T_{REG} cells from mice with a normal pregnancy could also prevent abortion in the mice that were otherwise destined to abort. In women with recurrent spontaneous abortion and preeclampsia, decreased numbers of CD4+CD25+ T_{REG} cells are present, which suggests a connection between these conditions and T_{REG} activity. The mechanism of T_{REG} suppression of T-cell responses is unknown but may involve either direct cell contact or production of anti-inflammatory cytokines such as IL-10 and TGF-β.

Pregnancy selectively drives expansion of maternal T_{REG} cells (>100-fold), which are maintained after delivery and are rapidly expanded in a subsequent pregnancy.[46] This preexisting pool of fetal-specific maternal T_{REG} cells is poised to impart tolerance and benefit the next pregnancy.

T_{REG} cells may be generated through several mechanisms. Before conception, T_{REG} cells may be induced after exposure to seminal fluid.[71] During pregnancy, induction of peripheral T_{REG} cells may occur through immature DC exposure to fetal antigens shed into the maternal circulation from the placenta (see "Amelioration of Rheumatoid Arthritis in Pregnancy").[8,72] Estrogen has also been shown to increase proliferation of T_{REG} cells, and the higher levels of estrogen in pregnancy may drive expansion of this cell population during pregnancy.

A specific gene called *conserved noncoding sequence 1* (CNS1) confers the ability to generate T_{REG} cells in the periphery and has been identified as a critical evolutionary step in allowing for pregnancy to occur in mammals with a placenta.[73] T_{REG} cells can be made in two locations, which are now thought to also inform their function: production in the thymus (thymic T_{REG}; tT_{REG}) mediates tolerance to self-antigens, and induction in the periphery (peripheral T_{REG}; pT_{REG}) occurs in response to commensal bacteria, food, or pregnancy.[74] In a mouse model, pT_{REG} cells specific for a fetal alloantigen were found to accumulate in the placenta.[73] Deletion of the *CNS1* gene in female mice resulted in abortion (fetal resorption) with immune cell infiltration of the placenta and defective remodeling of the uterine spiral arteries. Interestingly, in syngeneic matings (breeding pairs with the same genetic background), deletion of the *CNS1* gene was not associated with fetal abortion. This suggests that pT_{REG} cells are critical in achieving fetal tolerance with maternal-fetal HLA disparity. *CNS1* is highly conserved in eutherian (placental) mammals (i.e., humans, dolphins, elephants) but is absent from noneutherian mammals (platypus, wallaby) and nonmammals (zebrafish) that lack a placenta.[73] **This evidence suggests that *CNS1* is a critical gene that allows for the evolution of a placenta in eutherian mammals.**

Tolerance Through Regulation of Maternal B Cells

Several mechanisms act to protect the fetus from an antibody-mediated attack. First, immature B cells are partially deleted in the spleen and bone marrow during the second half of pregnancy in mice.[38] Secondly, the combination of reduced immature B cells and depletion of the IDO enzyme acts to prevent differentiation of B cells in a mouse model.[75] IDO is also depleted at the maternal-fetal interface, which may have a dual role in suppressing both B- and T-cell responses (see "Maternal Tolerance of the Fetus"). Levels of B-cell activating factor of the tumor necrosis factor family (BAFF) are reduced during pregnancy; BAFF acts to costimulate B cells and to promote proliferation.[35] Finally, a special class of B cells is upregulated during pregnancy;

Maternal T and B cells

- hCG stimulates proliferation of B_{REG} and T_{REG} cells and acts as a chemoattractant for T_{REG} to maternal-fetal interface
- Induction of fetal-specific T_{REG} cells in the uterine draining lymph nodes after exposure to seminal fluid
- Pregnancy induces expansion of maternal T_{REG} cells, which are sustained postpartum and rapidly expanded in the next pregnancy
- Upregulation of PD-1 on maternal T cells
- CNS1 (Foxp3 enhancer) enables generation of maternal T_{REG} in periphery
- B_{REG} (B10) cells produce IL-10

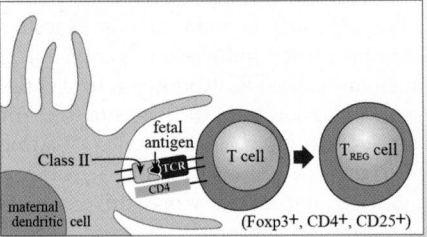

(Foxp3+, CD4+, CD25+)

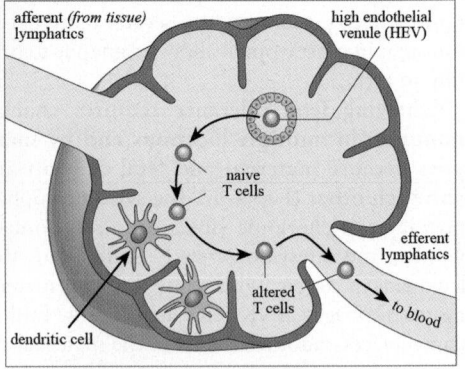

Peripheral Lymphoid Organs

lymph nodes   spleen

Lymph Nodes and Spleen

- Persistent fetal antigen presentation by lymph node resident DC to CD8+ T cells induces tolerance
- Partial deletion of maternal B cells specific for fetal antigens in spleen and bone marrow

Maternal-Fetal Interface, Decidua, Villous and Extravillous Trophoblast

- Limited expression of polymorphic HLA by extravillous trophoblast (e.g. HLA-G, HLA-E)
- B7 family molecules (B7-DC, B7-H2, B7-H3)
- Tryptophan depletion
- Epigenetic silencing of chemokine genes in decidual stromal cells
- Secretion of FasL by villous trophoblast
- Decoy receptors and non-death domain containing TNF receptors
- Syncytiotrophoblast sloughing releases apoptotic cells containing fetal antigens that induce a "tolerogenic" DC phenotype
- Negative regulators of complement activation (e.g. CD59)
- Suppression of Th1 & activation of Th2
- Secretion of IL-10
- Few numbers of DC in decidua
- Cytolyic function of dNK cells is low and further inhibited by HLA-G

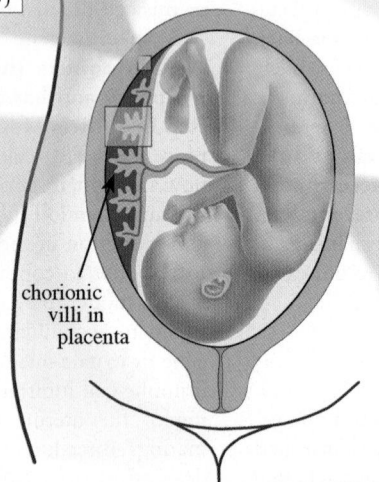

chorionic villi in placenta

Fetal Immunity

- Production of T_{REG} cells in fetal lymph nodes specific for maternal microchimeric cells
- Neonatal CD71+ cells expressing arginase-2 suppress inflammation associated with rapid gut colonization with commensal microbes after birth

Decidua Basalis

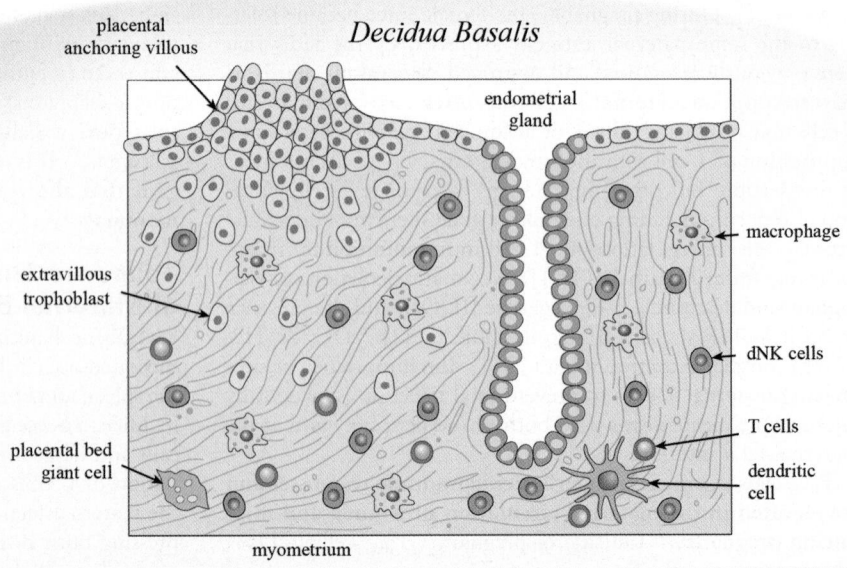

FIG 4-5 Mechanisms that promote maternal-fetal tolerance. Many different mechanisms and cell types have been identified that prevent rejection or dangerous immune responses during pregnancy. We have illustrated some of these mechanisms that operate within the maternal-fetal interface, maternal B- and T-cell populations, secondary lymphoid organs, and the fetus. The term *maternal-fetal interface* may refer to several locations where maternal and fetal cells come into direct contact, including the decidua and the intervillous space.

these are called *regulatory B cells* (B$_{REG}$ or B10), and they act to downregulate immune responses, mainly through the production of antiinflammatory cytokines (e.g., TGF-β, IL-10).[76-79] **An important cofactor for B$_{REG}$ cells is hCG, and the rise of hCG in early pregnancy is likely to stimulate proliferation of B$_{REG}$ cells to support early tolerance of the fetus.**[48]

Tolerance Through Dendritic Cells and Antigen Presentation

Dendritic cells (DCs) present antigen to naïve T cells and initiate T-cell expansion and polarization to foreign antigens, which could represent a problem for fetal tolerance. Fortunately, DCs are relatively rare in the decidua, which would effectively limit the ability to initiate a T-cell response to fetal antigens encountered at this maternal-fetal interface.[80] Despite the scarcity of DCs at the maternal-fetal interface, fetal antigens are detected in mice throughout all secondary lymphoid organs (spleen, lymph nodes). Antigens from the fetus are presented exclusively by maternal APCs; this is quite different than the case of a transplanted organ, in which either donor or host APCs are capable of presenting antigens and initiating T-cell responses.[58] Fetal antigens come mainly from apoptotic trophoblast debris that results from normal placental growth. An interesting mechanism to promote fetal tolerance occurs through the uptake of fetal antigens by follicular DCs that results in a prolonged period (weeks to months) of fetal antigen presentation.[81] Several waves of bone marrow-derived DCs sample the fetal antigens presented by follicular DCs and subsequently represent these antigens to maternal CD8$^+$ T cells, which induces deletion of CD8$^+$ T cells. In this case, tolerance and T-cell deletion is likely induced for two reasons. First, fetal antigens are mainly derived from apoptotic cells, which induce tolerogenic responses after uptake by DCs.[82] Secondly, the continuous nature of fetal antigen presentation mediated by follicular DCs is a powerful signal to induce T-cell tolerance.[83] Although follicular DCs were thought to only play a role in the regulation of B-cell immunity, evidence now suggests that the long-term nature of antigen presentation by these cells is a significant factor in shaping peripheral T-cell tolerance to fetal antigens.

Tolerance Through Human Leukocyte Antigens

Fetal trophoblast cells are in direct contact with maternal blood and should be at risk for maternal immunologic rejection. **The expression of MHC molecules by fetal trophoblast cells is limited to class I antigens—primarily class Ib HLA-G, HLA-E, and HLA-F—all of which have limited polymorphisms.** The exception to this rule of limited genetic variability is the expression of HLA-C, a class Ia molecule that is highly polymorphic, expressed primarily by extravillous trophoblast, and is thought to interact with dNK cells to facilitate uterine spiral artery remodeling.[84] **Expression of HLA-G by fetal trophoblast cells is thought to protect the invasive cytotrophoblast from killing by dNK cells and is also thought to contain placental infection.** HLA-G also inhibits macrophage activation through ILT-4, an inhibitory receptor. Through interactions with dNK cells, HLA-G likely contributes to normal pregnancy by maintenance of immune tolerance at the maternal-fetal interface. However, other mechanisms must also contribute to this process because normal pregnancies in women and fetuses that lack a functional HLA-G gene (HLA-G null) have been described.[85]

Tolerance Through Regulation of Complement, Chemokines, and Cytokines

Local inhibition of complement in the placenta may be important in preventing fetal rejection or preterm labor, particularly in the setting of inflammation or infection. In a murine model of abortion induced by antiphospholipid antibodies, protection against abortion was conferred by antagonizing factor B, an alternative complement component. Defects of placental formation were also observed in a murine model associated with activation of the alternative complement pathway and maternal C3. Finally, several negative regulators of complement are expressed by trophoblast cells, including CD59 (MAC antagonist), membrane cofactor protein, and decay accelerating factor (inhibitors of C3 and C5 convertases).[27] When a negative regulator of murine complement (*Crry*) was genetically ablated, embryo survival was compromised and placental inflammation was observed.[86] C3 activation plays a major role in fetal rejection in this model because the embryos survived when genetically deficient *Crry* mice were mated to C3-deficient mice. **Several studies suggest that inhibition of complement activation may contribute significantly to fetal tolerance, particularly in the setting of inflammation.**

Expression of chemokines and some cytokines at the maternal-fetal interface could be dangerous for the fetus because these small proteins may be inflammatory and may attract immune cells. **Regulation of chemokine expression (CXCL9, CXCL10, CXCL11, CCL5) by decidual stromal cells in mice was found to prevent the accumulation of T cells in the decidua after an inflammatory challenge.**[67] Chemokine expression was effectively silenced by epigenetic changes that involve histone repressor marks on chemokine gene promoters that appeared after transformation of endometrial stromal cells into decidual stromal cells. T cells are known to be relatively rare in decidua, which may be the result of a lack of chemokine production by decidual stromal cells.

Whether a change in the T-helper cytokine profile plays a role in fetal tolerance remains controversial.[87] It was originally thought that a Th2-type immune response might predominate during pregnancy, a theory based on the adverse effects of Th1 cytokines on murine pregnancy and weakened immunity during pregnancy to intracellular infections that require Th1 cytokine activity.[88-90] IL-10 is a Th2 cytokine that is elevated during pregnancy, and it is known to downregulate Th1 cytokine production to prevent fetal resorption in mice genetically predisposed to abortion. In a study of women with a history of recurrent spontaneous abortion, maternal cytokine profiles of stimulated peripheral blood mononuclear cells were compared between women who had a successful pregnancy and those who had a spontaneous abortion. Increased Th2 cytokines were associated with a successful pregnancy, and elevated Th1 cytokines were associated with a spontaneous abortion. Although several studies have reported a Th2-type profile in the blood of healthy pregnant women, not all studies supported the Th2 bias.[91,92] **Most studies have noted suppression of Th1 and activation of Th2 cytokine profiles in the blood of women with a normal pregnancy, and this effect may be more pronounced at the maternal-fetal interface. Interestingly, the Th1 cytokine profile is activated in preterm labor.**

Fetal Rejection

The idea that loss of maternal-fetal tolerance may contribute to unexplained preterm fetal death or spontaneous preterm birth is emerging. **Unexplained preterm fetal death has been linked to a loss of fetal tolerance and chronic chorioamnionitis, which describes an influx of T cells into the fetal membranes.**[93] *Chronic chorioamnionitis* is an unusual pathologic diagnosis in the placenta, and it differs significantly from *acute chorioamnionitis,* which refers to neutrophilic infiltration into the membranes that often occurs in the setting of placental infection. **In chronic chorioamnionitis, a large number of CD3+ and CD8+ T cells are found in the fetal membranes in addition to some CD4+ T cells.** In a case series of 30 women with an unexplained preterm fetal death, chronic chorioamnionitis was diagnosed significantly more often in fetal death cases than in preterm birth controls (60% vs. 38%). In addition, maternal anti-HLA class II seropositivity was significantly higher in women with a fetal death than in women after live birth (36% vs. 11%). A similar pattern of immunologic changes associated with a maternal antifetal response was identified in women with spontaneous preterm birth, which included a significantly higher frequency of chronic chorioamnionitis, maternal anti-HLA class I seropositivity, and complement (C4d) deposition along the umbilical vein endothelium. These observations suggest that a maternal antifetal immune response similar to allograft rejection is common in cases of unexplained fetal death and spontaneous preterm birth. **The conclusion that maternal tolerance of the fetus can be impaired is also supported by recent observations and hypotheses surrounding perinatal infections (e.g., *L. monocytogenes*) through an infection-associated reduction in T_{REG} leading to maternal T-cell infiltration of the placenta.**[50] **Once maternal-fetal tolerance is sufficiently impaired to allow maternal T cells into the placenta, inflammation can then facilitate pathogenic invasion of the fetus and fetal death.**

SOLID ORGAN TRANSPLANTATION IN PREGNANCY

Women with a solid organ transplant present many interesting questions as to how tolerance is maintained for the fetus and the transplanted organ during pregnancy.[94] Although it was classically thought that the placenta served as an impenetrable barrier between mother and fetus, we now know that bidirectional cell trafficking occurs routinely between the mother and the fetus.[3] Thus in nearly every pregnancy, cells that originate from the fetus can be found in the mother, and conversely, cells that originate from the mother can be found in the fetus. The long-term persistence of fetal cells in the mother and maternal cells in her progeny leads to the coexistence of at least two cell populations in a single person and is referred to as *microchimerism (Mc).* **A pregnant woman with a solid organ transplant has at least three, and possibly more, sources of Mc that include fetal Mc, maternal Mc from her own mother's cells that entered when she was a fetus, and cells from the donor allograft.** APCs in the pregnant woman, the donor organ, and the microchimeric cell populations can all present antigens from each other, which results in at least 16 combinations of antigens and APCs.[94]

Maintaining tolerance to all of these cell populations is a formidable task, and in a few instances, it has been documented to fail, which results in transplant rejection during pregnancy or postpartum. In two women with a history of cardiac transplant, HLA class II antibodies to fetal antigens developed during pregnancy and then cross-reacted with the transplanted organ, culminating in graft rejection. In the first case, cardiac rejection occurred 3 months postpartum in a woman who had otherwise been on a stable immunosuppressant regimen for 17 years.[95] HLA typing on the baby and the baby's father determined that paternal antigens presented by the fetus were likely to have triggered rejection. A second case of cardiac rejection linked to pregnancy occurred after an 8-week miscarriage in a woman 6 years after her transplantation.[96] A deeper understanding of the mechanisms of fetal tolerance and allograft rejection during and after pregnancy will lead to further advances in identifying pregnant women at unique risk for rejection during pregnancy.

Remarkably, uterine transplantation has now been performed in at least 11 women, and one live birth has been reported following transplantation.[97] In women with a history of uterine transplantation, menstruation has been reported to resume in the recipient as early as 43 days after transplant. Rejection episodes have been reported and were reversed successfully by corticosteroids. The woman who achieved a live birth underwent single embryo transfer 1 year after transplantation and was maintained on tacrolimus, azathioprine, and corticosteroids throughout pregnancy; corticosteroids were also used to reverse one episode of mild rejection that was diagnosed during the pregnancy. Blood flow through the uterine vessels and fetal growth were both normal throughout the pregnancy; however, preeclampsia developed at 31 weeks' gestation, and a cesarean delivery was performed because of an abnormal fetal heart rate tracing. The infant was born with an appropriate birthweight (1775 g) and excellent Apgar scores (9, 9, 10). Although uterine transplantation was once thought impossible, it has now been shown to withstand the challenge of pregnancy.

AMELIORATION OF RHEUMATOID ARTHRITIS IN PREGNANCY

Pregnancy has a remarkable effect on the disease course of some autoimmune inflammatory diseases, such as rheumatoid arthritis (RA) and multiple sclerosis, that results in a temporary amelioration or remission of symptoms (see Chapter 46).[98] RA is characterized by a symmetric inflammatory arthritis that causes pain, stiffness, and swelling of multiple joints. **Nearly three quarters of pregnant women with RA experience improvement in symptoms during the second and third trimesters with a return of symptoms postpartum.** Early hypotheses to explain this phenomenon focused on the role of sex hormones; cortisol and placental gamma globulin were rejected as potential therapies after studies that tested each could not mimic the effect of pregnancy on RA. Interestingly, the odds that pregnancy will result in amelioration of symptoms are not related to disease severity, duration, maternal age, or rheumatoid factor positivity.[8] Instead, amelioration of RA symptoms was observed significantly more often in women carrying a fetus with different paternally inherited HLA class II antigens from those of the mother.[99] This is strong evidence that fetal genetics and the maternal immune response to paternal (fetal) HLA antigens play a role in the pregnancy-induced remission of RA.

We have previously hypothesized that amelioration of RA occurs as a secondary benefit from the maternal T- and B-cell tolerance that develops to release of fetal antigens during pregnancy, which is coupled to normal placental growth.[8,100] As the placenta grows, apoptotic syncytiotrophoblast cells (the outer epithelial lining of the chorionic villi) are shed into the maternal blood. This process starts in the first trimester and by the third trimester results in gram quantities of fetal debris entering the maternal circulation daily. Fetal antigens are present in this apoptotic debris, including fetal minor histocompatibility antigens.[72] Phagocytosis of this debris by maternal immature DCs would result in presentation of fetal antigens to maternal T cells. As the antigens came from apoptotic cells, the immature DCs would change to a "tolerogenic" phenotype specialized to promote induction of T_{REG}, T-cell deletion, and anergy toward the presented fetal antigen. **Amelioration of RA could occur through the simultaneous presentation of fetal and self HLA (RA-associated) peptides by tolerogenic DCs and downregulation of maternal T-cell immunoreactivity.**

Supportive evidence for this theory comes from studies of both murine and human pregnancy. Murine studies demonstrate maternal T-cell deletion, anergy, and induction of T_{REG} to fetal antigens.[9,46,61] **Maternal-fetal HLA disparity is the strongest predictor of RA amelioration/remission in human pregnancy.**[99] Induction and suppressive activity of T_{REG} cells is impaired in syngeneic versus allogeneic murine pregnancy, which suggests that maternal-fetal HLA disparity is important in the degree of maternal T-cell tolerance achieved. Finally, a significant correlation has been found between levels of human fetal DNA (representing the quantity of placental debris in maternal circulation) and changes in RA activity during pregnancy.[9,99]

SUMMARY

Adaptations of the maternal immune system to tolerate the fetus during pregnancy are remarkable. No other condition in medicine allows foreign tissue to be so readily accepted and tolerated. We have gained tremendous insight into how maternal immunity adapts to the challenge of protecting the fetus from immunologic attack, but further research is necessary to understand how these mechanisms operate during normal and abnormal pregnancy. Preeclampsia and preterm labor are obstetric conditions with known abnormalities of the maternal immune system. The potential to make breakthroughs in these areas through the study of immunology in pregnancy is enormous.

KEY POINTS

◆ The innate immune system uses fast, nonspecific methods of pathogen detection to prevent and control an initial infection and includes macrophages, NK cells, the complement system, and cytokines. Macrophages have critical scavenger functions that likely help to prevent bacteria from establishing an intrauterine infection during pregnancy. Decidual NK (dNK) cells are thought to play a major role in remodeling of the spiral arteries to establish normal placentation.

◆ Proinflammatory cytokines such as IL-1β, TNF-α, and IL-6 have been identified in the amniotic fluid, maternal and fetal blood, and vaginal fluid of women with intraamniotic infection at much higher levels than those observed during normal pregnancy. These cytokines not only serve as a marker of intraamniotic infection, they trigger preterm labor and can lead to neonatal complications.

◆ Adaptive immunity results in the clonal expansion of lymphocytes (T cells and B cells) and an increase in antibodies against a specific antigen. Although slower to respond, adaptive immunity targets specific components of a pathogen and is capable of eradicating an infection that has overwhelmed the innate immune system.

◆ The function of B cells is to protect the extracellular spaces in the body (e.g., plasma, vagina) through which infectious pathogens usually spread by secreting antibodies (immunoglobulins). Antibodies control infection by several mechanisms, including neutralization, opsonization, and complement activation. Autoantibodies produced by B cells against angiotensin receptor I (AT1-AA) are thought to play a role in inducing hypertension and proteinuria in women with preeclampsia and intrauterine fetal growth restriction.

◆ When pathogens replicate inside cells (all viruses, some bacteria and parasites), they are inaccessible to antibodies and must be destroyed by T cells. A variety of T cells are recognized based on their expression of different cell surface markers that include those of CD8+ (effector or cytotoxic T cells), CD4+ (helper T cells), and CD4+CD25+ (T_{REG} cells). CD8+ T cells kill cells directly, whereas helper T cells activate B cells to produce antibodies. T_{REG} cells are now recognized as master regulators of the immune system that work by downregulating antigen-specific T-cell responses to diminish tissue damage during inflammation and to prevent autoimmunity.

◆ The fetal immune system, even very early in gestation, has innate immune capacity. Acquired immunity, particularly the capacity to produce antibodies, develops more slowly and is not completely functional until well after birth. CD71+ cells appear to protect the neonate from excessive inflammation that would occur from commensal microbes during bacterial colonization of the gut at the expense of impairing neonatal immunity to systemic infections.

◆ Fetal blood contains a high number of hematopoietic stem cells, making it an ideal source of cells for hematopoietic stem cell transplantation. The estimated need for the use of privately banked cord blood is between 1 in 1000 and 1 in 200,000, which is cost effective only for children with a very high likelihood of needing a transplant.

◆ Maintaining tolerance to the fetus requires several immunologic mechanisms, both at the maternal-fetal interface and in the maternal periphery. A critical interface is within the secondary lymphoid organs (lymph nodes and spleen), where fetal antigens are presented to maternal immune cells. Some of these mechanisms include generation of paternal-specific T_{REG} and B_{REG} cells in the maternal periphery, T-cell deletion, tryptophan depletion, presence of FasL or TNF-related apoptosis-inducing ligand/Apo-2L (TRAIL) on trophoblast cells, HLA-G expression by the placenta, and inhibition of complement activation by the placenta.

♦ Among the many mechanisms identified to maintain tolerance of the fetus, T_{REG} cells are unique because fetal antigen-specific T_{REG} cells are maintained after delivery, which may benefit the next pregnancy. T_{REG} cells suppress antigen-specific immune responses and are elevated in the maternal circulation of women and mice during pregnancy. Pregnancy selectively drives expansion of maternal T_{REG} cells (>100-fold), which are maintained after delivery and are rapidly expanded in subsequent pregnancies. In addition, hCG acts as a chemoattractant for T_{REG} to the maternal-fetal interface and, in the mouse, stimulates T_{REG} cell numbers and their suppressive activity.

♦ Unexplained preterm fetal death has been linked to a loss of fetal tolerance and chronic chorioamnionitis, which refers to an influx of T cells into the fetal membranes. A related observation in mice connects maternal T-cell infiltration of the placenta with a loss of maternal T_{REG} cells and perinatal death during infection with *L. monocytogenes*.

♦ A pregnant woman with a solid organ transplant has at least three and possibly more sources of small foreign cell populations (Mc) to which she must maintain tolerance: fetal Mc, maternal Mc (her own mother's cells that entered when she was a fetus), and cells from the donor allograft. In a few cases, transplant rejection has been linked to antifetal antibodies that developed during pregnancy.

♦ Remarkably, uterine transplantation has now been performed in at least 11 women with one live birth reported following transplantation.

♦ Pregnancy has a remarkable effect on the disease course of some autoimmune or inflammatory diseases, such as RA and multiple sclerosis, that results in a temporary amelioration or remission of symptoms. Amelioration of RA during pregnancy may occur as a secondary benefit from the maternal T- and B-cell tolerance that develops to fetal antigens during pregnancy.

Acknowledgments

We thank Jan Hamanishi for assistance with graphic design. Portions of this chapter are based on material in the last two editions of this text contributed by Dr. Hilary S. Gammill and Dr. Laurence E. Shields.

REFERENCES

1. Medawar PB. Some immunological and endocrinological problems raised by the evolution of viviparity in vertebrates. *Symp Soc Exp Biol.* 1954;7:320.
2. Maloney S, Smith A, Furst DE, et al. Microchimerism of maternal origin persists into adult life. *J Clin Invest.* 1999;104:41-47.
3. Lo YM, Lau TK, Chan LY, et al. Quantitative analysis of the bidirectional fetomaternal transfer of nucleated cells and plasma DNA. *Clin Chem.* 2000;46:1301-1309.
4. Bianchi DW, Zickwolf GK, Weil GJ, et al. Male fetal progenitor cells persist in maternal blood for as long as 27 years postpartum. *Proc Natl Acad Sci U S A.* 1996;93:705-708.
5. Nelson JL. Your cells are my cells. *Sci Am.* 2008;298:64-71.
6. Elbe-Burger A, Mommaas AM, Prieschl EE, et al. Major histocompatibility complex class II: fetal skin dendritic cells are potent accessory cells of polyclonal T-cell responses. *Immunology.* 2000;101:242-253.
7. Mold JE, Michaelsson J, Burt TD, et al. Maternal alloantigens promote the development of tolerogenic fetal regulatory T cells in utero. *Science.* 2008;322:1562-1565.
8. Adams KM, Yan Z, Stevens AM, Nelson JL. The changing maternal "self" hypothesis: a mechanism for maternal tolerance of the fetus. *Placenta.* 2007;28:378-382.
9. Tafuri A, Alferink J, Moller P, et al. T cell awareness of paternal alloantigens during pregnancy. *Science.* 1995;270:630-633.
10. Romero R, Manogue KR, Mitchell MD, et al. Infection and labor. IV. Cachectin-tumor necrosis factor in the amniotic fluid of women with intraamniotic infection and preterm labor. *Am J Obstet Gynecol.* 1989;161:336-341.
11. Romero R, Brody DT, Oyarzun E, et al. Infection and labor. III. Interleukin-1: a signal for the onset of parturition. *Am J Obstet Gynecol.* 1989;160:1117-1123.
12. Hitti J, Hillier SL, Agnew KJ, et al. Vaginal indicators of amniotic fluid infection in preterm labor. *Obstet Gynecol.* 2001;97:211-219.
13. Kawai T, Akira S. The role of pattern-recognition receptors in innate immunity: update on Toll-like receptors. *Nat Immunol.* 2010;11:373-384.
14. Quayle AJ. The innate and early immune response to pathogen challenge in the female genital tract and the pivotal role of epithelial cells. *J Reprod Immunol.* 2002;57:61-79.
15. Bartmann C, Segerer SE, Rieger L, et al. Quantification of the predominant immune cell populations in decidua throughout human pregnancy. *Am J Reprod Immunol.* 2014;71:109-119.
16. Tirado-Gonzalez I, Barrientos G, Freitag N, et al. Uterine NK cells are critical in shaping DC immunogenic functions compatible with pregnancy progression. *PLoS ONE.* 2012;7:e46755.
17. Ashkar AA, Di Santo JP, Croy BA. Interferon gamma contributes to initiation of uterine vascular modification, decidual integrity, and uterine natural killer cell maturation during normal murine pregnancy. *J Exp Med.* 2000;192:259-270.
18. Ponte M, Cantoni C, Biassoni R, et al. Inhibitory receptors sensing HLA-G1 molecules in pregnancy: decidua-associated natural killer cells express LIR-1 and CD94/NKG2A and acquire p49, an HLA-G1-specific receptor. *Proc Natl Acad Sci U S A.* 1999;96:5674-5679.
19. Bulmer JN, Longfellow M, Ritson A. Leukocytes and resident blood cells in endometrium. *Ann N Y Acad Sci.* 1991;622:57-68.
20. Cirl C, Wieser A, Yadav M, et al. Subversion of Toll-like receptor signaling by a unique family of bacterial Toll/interleukin-1 receptor domain-containing proteins. *Nat Med.* 2008;14:399-406.
21. Abrahams VM, Bole-Aldo P, Kim YM, et al. Divergent trophoblast responses to bacterial products mediated by TLRs. *J Immunol.* 2004;173:4286-4296.
22. Elovitz MA, Wang Z, Chien EK, et al. A new model for inflammation-induced preterm birth: the role of platelet-activating factor and Toll-like receptor-4. *Am J Pathol.* 2003;163:2103-2111.
23. Adams Waldorf KM, Persing D, Novy MJ, et al. Pretreatment with toll-like receptor 4 antagonist inhibits lipopolysaccharide-induced preterm uterine contractility, cytokines, and prostaglandins in rhesus monkeys. *Reprod Sci.* 2008;15:121-127.
24. Harju K, Ojaniemi M, Rounioja S, et al. Expression of Toll-Like Receptor 4 and Endotoxin Responsiveness in Mice during Perinatal Period. *Pediatr Res.* 2005;57(5 Pt 1):644-648.
25. Adams KM, Lucas J, Kapur RP, Stevens AM. LPS induces translocation of TLR4 in amniotic epithelium. *Placenta.* 2007;28:477-481.
26. Vanderpuye OA, Labarrere CA, McIntyre JA. Expression of CD59, a human complement system regulatory protein, in extraembryonic membranes. *Int Arch Allergy Immunol.* 1993;101:376-384.
27. Cunningham DS, Tichenor JR Jr. Decay-accelerating factor protects human trophoblast from complement-mediated attack. *Clin Immunol Immunopathol.* 1995;74:156-161.
28. Kobasa D, Jones SM, Shinya K, et al. Aberrant innate immune response in lethal infection of macaques with the 1918 influenza virus. *Nature.* 2007;445:319-323.
29. Kay AW, Fukuyama J, Aziz N, et al. Enhanced natural killer-cell and T-cell responses to influenza A virus during pregnancy. *Proc Natl Acad Sci U S A.* 2014;111:14506-14511.
30. Romero R, Gomez R, Ghezzi F, et al. A fetal systemic inflammatory response is followed by the spontaneous onset of preterm parturition. *Am J Obstet Gynecol.* 1998;179:186-193.

31. Sadowsky DW, Adams KM, Gravett MG, et al. Preterm labor is induced by intraamniotic infusions of interleukin-1beta and tumor necrosis factor-alpha but not by interleukin-6 or interleukin-8 in a nonhuman primate model. *Am J Obstet Gynecol.* 2006;195:1578-1589.

32. Robertson SA, Christiaens I, Dorian CL, et al. Interleukin-6 is an essential determinant of on-time parturition in the mouse. *Endocrinology.* 2010; 151:3996-4006.

33. Romero R, Ceska M, Avila C, Mazor M, Behnke E, Lindley I. Neutrophil attractant/activating peptide-1/interleukin-8 in term and preterm parturition. *Am J Obstet Gynecol.* 1991;165:813-820.

34. Loudon JA, Sooranna SR, Bennett PR, Johnson MR. Mechanical stretch of human uterine smooth muscle cells increases IL-8 mRNA expression and peptide synthesis. *Mol Hum Reprod.* 2004;10:895-899.

35. Muzzio DO, Soldati R, Ehrhardt J, et al. B cell development undergoes profound modifications and adaptations during pregnancy in mice. *Biol Reprod.* 2014;91:115.

36. Medina KL, Smithson G, Kincade PW. Suppression of B lymphopoiesis during normal pregnancy. *J Exp Med.* 1993;178:1507-1515.

37. Bosco N, Ceredig R, Rolink A. Transient decrease in interleukin-7 availability arrests B lymphopoiesis during pregnancy. *Eur J Immunol.* 2008; 38:381-390.

38. Ait-Azzouzene D, Gendron MC, Houdayer M, et al. Maternal B lymphocytes specific for paternal histocompatibility antigens are partially deleted during pregnancy. *J Immunol.* 1998;161:2677-2683.

39. Zhou CC, Zhang Y, Irani RA, et al. Angiotensin receptor agonistic autoantibodies induce pre-eclampsia in pregnant mice. *Nat Med.* 2008;14: 855-862.

40. Nguyen TG, Ward CM, Morris JM. To B or not to B cells-mediate a healthy start to life. *Clin Exp Immunol.* 2013;171:124-134.

41. Siddiqui AH, Irani RA, Blackwell SC, Ramin SM, Kellems RE, Xia Y. Angiotensin receptor agonistic autoantibody is highly prevalent in preeclampsia: correlation with disease severity. *Hypertension.* 2010;55: 386-393.

42. Parrish MR, Murphy SR, Rutland S, et al. The effect of immune factors, tumor necrosis factor-alpha, and agonistic autoantibodies to the angiotensin II type I receptor on soluble fms-like tyrosine-1 and soluble endoglin production in response to hypertension during pregnancy. *Am J Hypertens.* 2010;23:911-916.

43. Zhou CC, Irani RA, Dai Y, et al. Autoantibody-mediated IL-6-dependent endothelin-1 elevation underlies pathogenesis in a mouse model of pre-eclampsia. *J Immunol.* 2011;186:6024-6034.

44. Brandtzaeg P. Mucosal immunity: integration between mother and the breast-fed infant. *Vaccine.* 2003;21:3382-3388.

45. Hori S, Carvalho TL, Demengeot J. CD25+CD4+ regulatory T cells suppress CD4+ T cell-mediated pulmonary hyperinflammation driven by Pneumocystis carinii in immunodeficient mice. *Eur J Immunol.* 2002;32: 1282-1291.

46. Rowe JH, Ertelt JM, Xin L, Way SS. Pregnancy imprints regulatory memory that sustains anergy to fetal antigen. *Nature.* 2012;490: 102-106.

47. Schumacher A, Heinze K, Witte J, et al. Human chorionic gonadotropin as a central regulator of pregnancy immune tolerance. *J Immunol.* 2013; 190:2650-2658.

48. Rolle L, Memarzadeh Tehran M, Morell-Garcia A, et al. Cutting edge: IL-10-producing regulatory B cells in early human pregnancy. *Am J Reprod Immunol.* 2013;70:448-453.

49. Rowe JH, Ertelt JM, Aguilera MN, et al. Foxp3(+) regulatory T cell expansion required for sustaining pregnancy compromises host defense against prenatal bacterial pathogens. *Cell Host Microbe.* 2011;10:54-64.

50. Rowe JH, Ertelt JM, Xin L, Way SS. Regulatory T cells and the immune pathogenesis of prenatal infection. *Reproduction.* 2013;146:R191-R203.

51. Bakardjiev AI, Theriot JA, Portnoy DA. Listeria monocytogenes traffics from maternal organs to the placenta and back. *PLoS Pathog.* 2006;2:e66.

52. Shields LE, Lindton B, Andrews RG, Westgren M. Fetal hematopoietic stem cell transplantation: a challenge for the twenty-first century. *J Hematother Stem Cell Res.* 2002;11:617-631.

53. Hermann E, Truyens C, Alonso-Vega C, et al. Human fetuses are able to mount an adultlike CD8 T-cell response. *Blood.* 2002;100:2153-2158.

54. Gathings WE, Lawton AR, Cooper MD. Immunofluorescent studies of the development of pre-B cells, B lymphocytes and immunoglobulin isotype diversity in humans. *Eur J Immunol.* 1977;7:804-810.

55. Lawn JE, Cousens S, Zupan J. 4 million neonatal deaths: When? Where? Why? *Lancet.* 2005;365:891-900.

56. Elahi S, Ertelt JM, Kinder JM, et al. Immunosuppressive CD71+ erythroid cells compromise neonatal host defence against infection. *Nature.* 2013;504:158-162.

57. Lubin BH, Shearer WT. Cord blood banking for potential future transplantation. *Pediatrics.* 2007;119:165-170.

58. Erlebacher A, Vencato D, Price KA, et al. Constraints in antigen presentation severely restrict T cell recognition of the allogeneic fetus. *J Clin Invest.* 2007;117:1399-1411.

59. Bonney EA, Matzinger P. The maternal immune system's interaction with circulating fetal cells. *J Immunol.* 1997;158:40-47.

60. Van Rood JJ, Eernisse JG, Van Leeuwen A. Leucocyte antibodies in sera from pregnant women. *Nature.* 1958;181:1735-1736.

61. Jiang SP, Vacchio MS. Multiple mechanisms of peripheral T cell tolerance to the fetal "allograft." *J Immunol.* 1998;160:3086-3090.

62. Taglauer ES, Adams Waldorf KM, Petroff MG. The hidden maternal-fetal interface: events involving the lymphoid organs in maternal-fetal tolerance. *Int J Dev Biol.* 2010;54:421-430.

63. Taglauer ES, Yankee TM, Petroff MG. Maternal PD-1 regulates accumulation of fetal antigen-specific CD8+ T cells in pregnancy. *J Reprod Immunol.* 2009;80:12-21.

64. Moldenhauer LM, Diener KR, Thring DM, Brown MP, Hayball JD, Robertson SA. Cross-presentation of male seminal fluid antigens elicits T cell activation to initiate the female immune response to pregnancy. *J Immunol.* 2009;182:8080-8093.

65. Petroff MG, Perchellet A. B7 family molecules as regulators of the maternal immune system in pregnancy. *Am J Reprod Immunol.* 2010;63: 506-519.

66. Munn DH, Zhou M, Attwood JT, et al. Prevention of allogeneic fetal rejection by tryptophan catabolism. *Science.* 1998;281:1191-1193.

67. Nancy P, Tagliani E, Tay CS, et al. Chemokine gene silencing in decidual stromal cells limits T cell access to the maternal-fetal interface. *Science.* 2012;336:1317-1321.

68. Somerset DA, Zheng Y, Kilby MD, et al. Normal human pregnancy is associated with an elevation in the immune suppressive CD25+ CD4+ regulatory T-cell subset. *Immunology.* 2004;112:38-43.

69. Aluvihare VR, Kallikourdis M, Betz AG. Regulatory T cells mediate maternal tolerance to the fetus. *Nat Immunol.* 2004;5:266-271.

70. Shima T, Sasaki Y, Itoh M, et al. Regulatory T cells are necessary for implantation and maintenance of early pregnancy but not late pregnancy in allogeneic mice. *J Reprod Immunol.* 2010;85:121-129.

71. Robertson SA, Guerin LR, Bromfield JJ, et al. Seminal fluid drives expansion of the CD4+CD25+ T regulatory cell pool and induces tolerance to paternal alloantigens in mice. *Biol Reprod.* 2009;80:1036-1045.

72. Holland OJ, Linscheid C, Hodes HC, et al. Minor histocompatibility antigens are expressed in syncytiotrophoblast and trophoblast debris: implications for maternal alloreactivity to the fetus. *Am J Pathol.* 2012;180: 256-266.

73. Samstein RM, Josefowicz SZ, Arvey A, et al. Extrathymic generation of regulatory T cells in placental mammals mitigates maternal-fetal conflict. *Cell.* 2012;150:29-38.

74. Chen W, Jin W, Hardegen N, et al. Conversion of peripheral CD4+CD25-naive T cells to CD4+CD25+ regulatory T cells by TGF-beta induction of transcription factor Foxp3. *J Exp Med.* 2003;198:1875-1886.

75. Pigott E, Mandik-Nayak L. Addition of an indoleamine 2,3,-dioxygenase inhibitor to B cell-depletion therapy blocks autoreactive B cell activation and recurrence of arthritis in K/BxN mice. *Arthritis Rheum.* 2012;64: 2169-2178.

76. Jensen F, Muzzio D, Soldati R, et al. Regulatory B10 cells restore pregnancy tolerance in a mouse model. *Biol Reprod.* 2013;89:90.

77. Mizoguchi A, Bhan AK. A case for regulatory B cells. *J Immunol.* 2006;176:705-710.

78. Yang M, Rui K, Wang S, Lu L. Regulatory B cells in autoimmune diseases. *Cell Mol Immunol.* 2013;10:122-132.

79. Fettke F, Schumacher A, Costa SD, Zenclussen AC. B cells: the old new players in reproductive immunology. *Front Immunol.* 2014;5:285.

80. Erlebacher A. Immunology of the maternal-fetal interface. *Annu Rev Immunol.* 2013;31:387-411.

81. McCloskey ML, Curotto de Lafaille MA, Carroll MC, Erlebacher A. Acquisition and presentation of follicular dendritic cell-bound antigen by lymph node-resident dendritic cells. *J Exp Med.* 2011;208:135-148.

82. Gleisner MA, Rosemblatt M, Fierro JA, Bono MR. Delivery of alloantigens via apoptotic cells generates dendritic cells with an immature tolerogenic phenotype. *Transplant Proc.* 2011;43:2325-2333.

83. Probst HC, Lagnel J, Kollias G, van den Broek M. Inducible transgenic mice reveal resting dendritic cells as potent inducers of CD8+ T cell tolerance. *Immunity.* 2003;18:713-720.

84. Hiby SE, Walker JJ, O'Shaughnessy KM, et al. Combinations of maternal KIR and fetal HLA-C genes influence the risk of preeclampsia and reproductive success. *J Exp Med.* 2004;200:957-965.

85. Ober C, Aldrich C, Rosinsky B, et al. HLA-G1 protein expression is not essential for fetal survival. *Placenta*. 1998;19:127-132.

86. Xu C, Mao D, Holers VM, et al. A critical role for murine complement regulator crry in fetomaternal tolerance. *Science*. 2000;287:498-501.

87. Chaouat G, Ledee-Bataille N, Dubanchet S, et al. TH1/TH2 paradigm in pregnancy: paradigm lost? Cytokines in pregnancy/early abortion: reexamining the TH1/TH2 paradigm. *Int Arch Allergy Immunol*. 2004;134:93-119.

88. Wegmann TG, Lin H, Guilbert L, Mosmann TR. Bidirectional cytokine interactions in the maternal-fetal relationship: is successful pregnancy a TH2 phenomenon? *Immunol Today*. 1993;14:353-356.

89. Raghupathy R. Th1-type immunity is incompatible with successful pregnancy. *Immunol Today*. 1997;18:478-482.

90. Raghupathy R. Pregnancy: success and failure within the Th1/Th2/Th3 paradigm. *Semin Immunol*. 2001;13:219-227.

91. Shimaoka Y, Hidaka Y, Tada H, et al. Changes in cytokine production during and after normal pregnancy. *Am J Reprod Immunol*. 2000;44:143-147.

92. Matthiesen L, Khademi M, Ekerfelt C, et al. In-situ detection of both inflammatory and anti-inflammatory cytokines in resting peripheral blood mononuclear cells during pregnancy. *J Reprod Immunol*. 2003;58:49-59.

93. Lee J, Romero R, Dong Z, et al. Unexplained fetal death has a biological signature of maternal anti-fetal rejection: chronic chorioamnionitis and alloimmune anti-human leucocyte antigen antibodies. *Histopathology*. 2011;59:928-938.

94. Ma KK, Petroff MG, Coscia LA, et al. Complex chimerism: pregnancy after solid organ transplantation. *Chimerism*. 2013;4:71-77.

95. Ginwalla M, Pando MJ, Khush KK. Pregnancy-related human leukocyte antigen sensitization leading to cardiac allograft vasculopathy and graft failure in a heart transplant recipient: a case report. *Transplant Proc*. 2013;45:800-802.

96. O'Boyle PJ, Smith JD, Danskine AJ, et al. De novo HLA sensitization and antibody mediated rejection following pregnancy in a heart transplant recipient. *Am J Transplant*. 2010;10:180-183.

97. Brännström M, Johannesson L, Bokström H, et al. Livebirth after uterus transplantation. *Lancet*. 2015;385(9968):607-616.

98. Hench PS. The ameliorating effect of pregnancy on chronic atrophic (infectious rheumatoid) arthritis, fibrositis, and intermittent hydrarthrosis. *Mayo Clin Proc*. 1938;13:161-167.

99. Nelson JL, Hughes KA, Smith AG, Nisperos BB, Branchaud AM, Hansen JA. Maternal-fetal disparity in HLA class II alloantigens and the pregnancy-induced amelioration of rheumatoid arthritis. *N Engl J Med*. 1993;329:466-471.

100. Taglauer ES, Adams Waldorf KM, Petroff MG. The hidden maternal-fetal interface: events involving the lymphoid organs in maternal-fetal tolerance. *Int J Dev Biol*. 2010;54:421-430.

Additional references for this chapter are available at ExpertConsult.com.

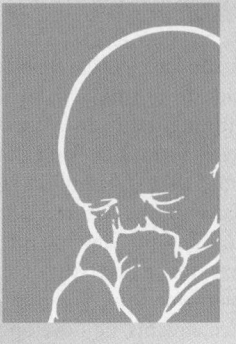

CHAPTER 5

Developmental Origins of Adult Health and Disease

MICHAEL G. ROSS and MINA DESAI

KEY ABBREVIATIONS

11-β-hydroxysteroid dehydrogenase type 1	11β-HSD1	Lipopolysaccharide	LPS
		Magnetic resonance imaging	MRI
11-β-hydroxysteroid dehydrogenase type 2	11β-HSD2	Nonalcoholic fatty liver disease	NAFLD
		Noncoding ribonucleic acids	ncRNA
Attention-deficit/hyperactivity disorder	ADHD	N-methyl-D-aspartate	NMDA
Average for gestational age	AGA	Neuropeptide Y	NPY
Body mass index	BMI	Otoacoustic emissions	OAE
Bisphenol A	BPA	Paired box 2 gene	*PAX2*
Corticotrophin-releasing hormone	CRH	Polychlorinated biphenyl	PCB
C-reactive protein	CRP	Polycystic ovary syndrome	PCOS
Diethylstilbestrol	DES	Pancreatic duodenal homeobox 1 gene	PDX1
Endocrine-disrupter chemical	EDC		
Food and Drug Administration	FDA	Peroxisome proliferator–activated receptor gamma coactivator	PGC-1α
Glial cell–derived neurotropic factor	GDNF		
Glomerular filtration rate	GFR	Peroxisome proliferator–activated receptor	PPAR
Histone deacetylase	HDAC		
Hypoxia inducible factor	HIF	Small for gestational age	SGA
Hypothalamic pituitary adrenal	HPA	NAD-dependent deacetylase sirtuin 1	SIRT1
Interleukin-6	IL-6	Type 2 helper T cells	TH2
Intelligence quotient	IQ	Tumor necrosis factor alpha	TNF-α
Low birthweight	LBW	Vascular endothelial growth factor	VEGF
Large for gestational age	LGA		

Perinatal care has progressed remarkably from its original focus on maternal mortality, which approximated 1% per pregnancy in the early 1900s. Following the tremendous strides in reducing maternal morbidity and mortality, obstetric care has made great advances in regard to optimization of fetal and neonatal health, including the diagnosis, prevention, and treatment of congenital malformations; the reduction in infectious diseases; and improvements in sequelae of prematurity. It is now commonplace to deliver infants who would not have survived childbirth or the neonatal period in previous eras. For example, low birthweight (LBW) premature infants routinely survive beyond a weight of 400 to 500 g. Conversely, large for gestational age (LGA) infants

are often delivered by cesarean section, avoiding the potential trauma of labor. As we now examine the long-term consequences associated with this improved survival, as well as the effects of treatment aimed at improving outcomes (e.g., maternal glucocorticoids), we have begun to recognize long-term health effects of perinatal influences in adults. **An understanding of the developmental origins of adult health and disease provides an appreciation of the critical role of perinatal care and may ultimately guide our treatment paradigms.**

The concept of developmental origins of adult disease should not be surprising to obstetricians. Teratogenesis represents perhaps the most acute consequence of developmental effects.

In the late 1950s, thalidomide was marketed as both a sedative and a morning sickness prescription for pregnant women. Although the drug was not actively marketed in the United States for lack of Food and Drug Administration (FDA) approval, more than 2.5 million tablets were distributed to private physicians in the United States. Thalidomide was widely used in Europe and was included in some 50 over-the-counter products for a diversity of indications. Thalidomide-induced limb malformations are now well recognized. Notably, similar to mechanisms of developmental programming discussed below, thalidomide may induce its teratogenic effects through epigenetic mechanisms. As described by Stephens and colleagues,[1] thalidomide likely binds to promotor sites of insulin-like growth factor and fibroblast growth factor as well as downstream signaling genes that regulate angiogenesis. The resulting inhibition of angiogenesis truncates limbs during development. As will be discussed below, **a variety of mechanisms may "program" the phenotype of the offspring via aberrations in cellular signaling or epigenetic function.**

Whereas the short-term consequences of thalidomide were rapidly recognized, longer-term programming effects of diethylstilbestrol (DES) were slow to be identified. Prior to FDA approval in 1947, DES was used off label to prevent adverse pregnancy outcomes in women with a history of miscarriage. Despite a double-blind trial in the early 1950s that demonstrated no benefit of taking DES during pregnancy,[2] DES continued to be given to pregnant women throughout the 1960s. It was not until 1971 that the FDA advised against the use of DES in pregnant women in response to a report that demonstrated the link between DES and vaginal clear cell adenocarcinoma in girls and young women. Similar to thalidomide, it is now recognized that the oncogenic and teratogenic effects of in utero DES exposure may be mediated via epigenetic mechanisms. As reported by Bromer and colleagues,[3] in utero DES exposure results in hypermethylation of the *HOXA10* gene, which regulates uterine organogenesis. Thus both the short-term anatomic defects associated with thalidomide and the delayed oncogenic effects associated with DES are examples of developmental origins of adult disease mediated via epigenetic effects.

This chapter will review the consequences and mechanisms of these prenatal and neonatal influences on developmental programming. We will primarily focus on the associations demonstrated in human studies, utilizing evidence from case reports, epidemiologic studies, and meta-analyses. We selectively discuss evidence from animal models that confirm the phenotype or suggest pathogenic pathways and potential mechanisms.

EPIGENETICS AND PROGRAMMING

Epigenetics is a genetic process that switches genes on and off in response to external or environmental factors. The essential concept of **"gestational programming" signifies that the nutritional, hormonal, and metabolic environment provided by the mother permanently alters organ structure, cellular responses, and gene expression that ultimately impact the metabolism and physiology of her offspring** (Fig. 5-1). Further, these effects vary and are dependent upon the developmental period, and as such, rapidly growing fetuses and neonates are more vulnerable. The programming events may have immediate effects—for example, impairment of organ growth at a critical stage—whereas other programming effects are deferred until expressed by altered organ function at a later age. In this instance, the question is about how the memory of early events is stored and later expressed despite continuous cellular replication and replacement. This may be mediated through epigenetic

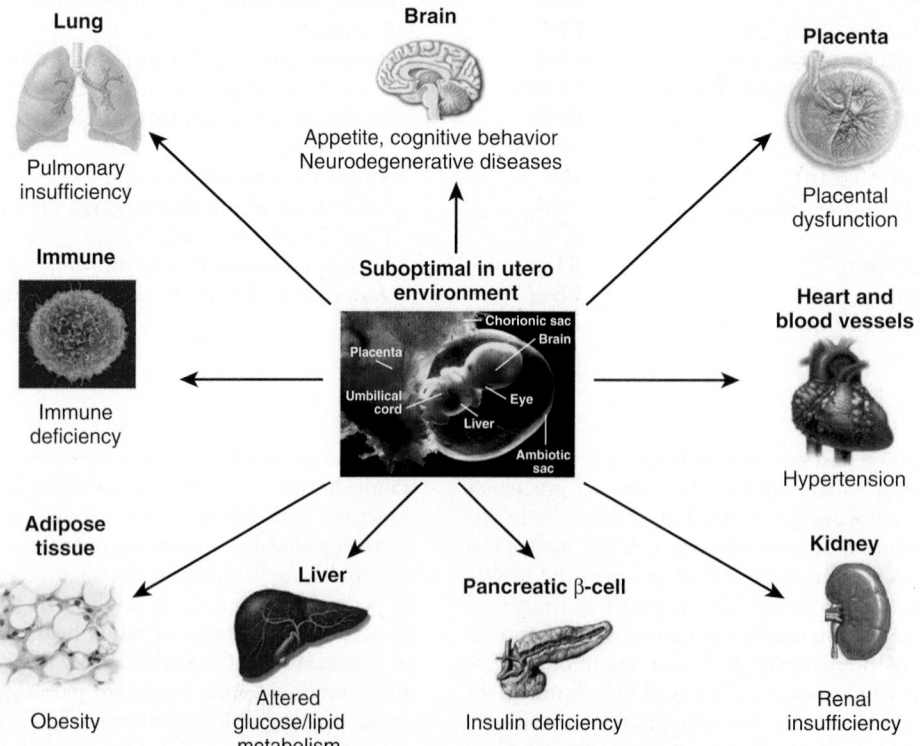

FIG 5-1 Impact of gestational programming on organ systems.

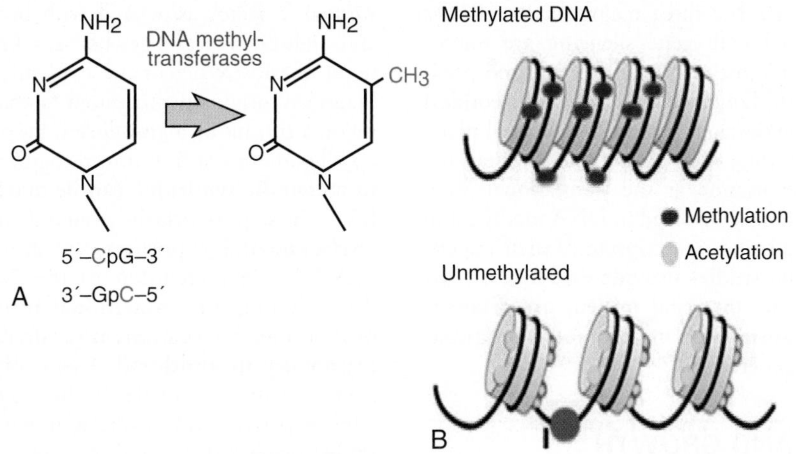

FIG 5-2 DNA methylation. **A,** Methylation by DNA methyltransferases at CpG islands. **B,** DNA demethylation relaxes chromatin structure, which allows histone acetylation and the binding of transcriptional complexes.

control of gene expression, which involves modification of the genome without altering the DNA sequence.

Epigenetic phenomena are fundamental features of mammalian development that cause heritable and persistent changes in gene expression without altering DNA sequence. Epigenetic regulation includes changes in the DNA methylation pattern and modifications of chromatin packaging via posttranslational histone changes.

DNA methylation represents a primary epigenetic mechanism. The DNA of the early embryo is hypomethylated, and with progressive increases in DNA methylation in response to environmental signals, organogenesis and tissue differentiation occur. DNA methylation typically occurs on cytosine bases that are followed by a guanine, termed *CpG dinucleotides.* The methylation by a DNA methyltransferase leads to recruitment of methyl-CpG binding proteins, which induce transcriptional silencing both by blocking transcription factor binding and by recruiting transcriptional corepressors or histone-modifying complexes. Anomalous DNA methylation in normally hypomethylated CpG-rich regions of gene promoters is associated with inappropriate gene silencing (e.g., cancer). It is during embryogenesis and early postnatal life that DNA methylation patterns are fundamentally established and are imperative for silencing of specific gene regions, such as imprinted genes and repetitive nucleic acid sequences. The epigenome is reestablished at specific stages of development, making it a prime candidate as the basis for fetal programming. As such, **changes in epigenetic markers are associated with inflammation and multiple human diseases, including many cancers and neurologic disorders.** Because methylation requires the nutrient supply and enzymatic transfer of methyl groups, it is plausible that in utero nutritional, hormonal, or other metabolic cues alter the timing and direction of methylation patterns during fetal development (Fig. 5-2).

Another essential mechanism of gene expression and silencing is the packaging of chromatin into open (euchromatic) or closed (heterochromatic) states, respectively. Chromatin consists of DNA packaged around histones into a nucleoprotein complex. Posttranslational modification of histone tails through acetylation, methylation, phosphorylation, ubiquitination, and SUMOylation can alter histone interaction with DNA and recruit proteins (e.g., transcriptional factors) that alter chromatin conformation. Histone tail acetylation by histone acetyltransferases promotes active gene expression,

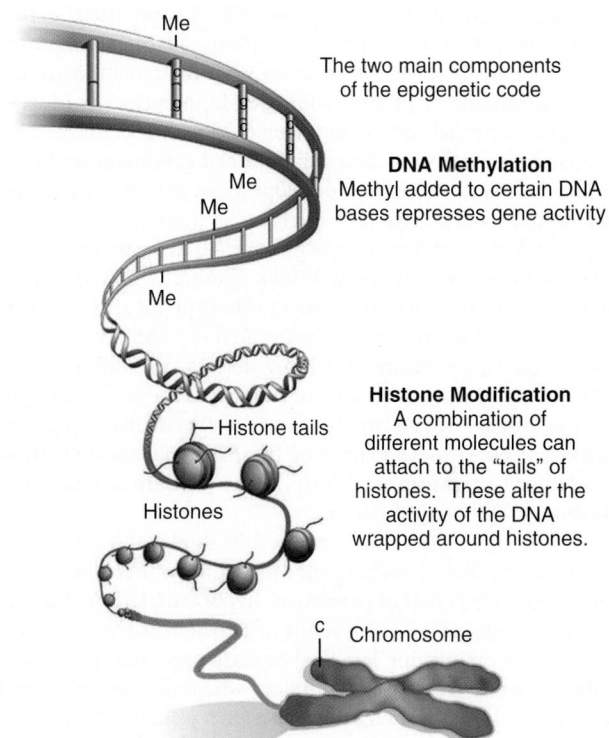

FIG 5-3 DNA methylation, histone modification, and noncoding RNA.

whereas histone tail deacetylation by histone deacetylases (HDACs) is associated with gene silencing (Fig. 5-3). Histone methylation can either repress or activate transcription depending on which lysine is methylated. For example, trimethylation of histone H3 at lysine 4 (H3K4me3) is associated with active gene transcription, whereas dimethylation of histone H3 at lysine 9 (H3K9me2) is associated with transcriptional silencing.[4] Histone modifications and DNA methylation patterns are not exclusively independent, and thus they can reciprocally regulate one another's state.

Finally, noncoding RNAs (ncRNAs) are emerging as a potential third epigenetic mediator. The ncRNAs are transcribed from DNA but are not translated into proteins, and they function to regulate gene expression at the transcriptional and posttranscriptional level. The three major short ncRNAs (<30 nucleotides) associated with gene silencing are microRNAs (miRNAs), short inhibitory RNAs (siRNAs), and piwi-interacting RNAs (piRNAs).[5] Long ncRNAs (>200 nucleotides) play a regulatory role during development and exhibit cell type–specific expression. Whereas these ncRNAs are usually associated with regulation of gene expression at the translational level, recent work suggests they may be involved in DNA methylation as well, thereby further regulating transcription of their targets.

Both human and animal studies provide evidence of epigenomic modulation by the maternal milieu; importantly, they implicate it in the transmission of gestational programming effects to multiple generations.[6]

FETAL NUTRITION AND GROWTH

Nutrition is unquestionably one of the cornerstones of health. More importantly, **good evidence suggests that appropriate nutritional supplementation before conception and during pregnancy may reduce the risk of some birth defects** (see Chapters 6 and 7). Perhaps the most convincing argument that can be made for the need to consider maternal nutrition as a critical modulator of embryonic development is the observation that maternal iodine supplementation has eradicated the occurrence of **iodine deficiency–induced cretinism** and other iodine deficiency–associated developmental defects. In addition, adverse maternal nutrition—which has an immediate and visible impact on the outcome of pregnancy—is seen in the case of **folate deficiency and spina bifida.** Similarly, maternal polymorphisms in the genes of folate metabolism are also associated with intrauterine growth restriction (IUGR) and abnormalities that include cleft palate and heart defects. In addition to its critical role in the conversion of homocysteine to methionine, the functional mechanism for folate likely involves epigenetic effects, because **folate generates the principal methyl donor (s-adenosyl methionine [SAMe]) that participates in methylation of DNA and histones.**

Animal studies have also irrevocably shown the importance of a mother's diet in shaping the epigenome of her offspring. A classic example is that of permanent hypomethylation of certain regions of the genome as a result of deficient folate or choline (methyl donors) during late fetal or early postnatal life. Specifically, in viable yellow agouti mice, when the agouti gene is completely unmethylated, the mouse has a yellow coat color and is obese and prone to diabetes and cancer. When the agouti gene is methylated, as in normal mice, the coat color is brown and the mouse has a low disease risk. Although both the fat yellow and skinny brown mice are genetically identical, the former exhibits an epigenetic "mutation."[7]

Although teratogenesis, structural malformations, and even onogenic risks can be linked to developmental insults, it is only recently that the epidemic of metabolic syndrome has been attributed, in part, to consequences of fetal and newborn development. **Obesity now represents a major public health problem and health epidemic** (see Chapter 41). As recently reported, the adverse consequences of obesity are projected to overwhelm the beneficial effects of reduced smoking in the United States and have resulted in an actual *decline* in life expectancy. In the United States, 69% of adults are *overweight* (body mass index [BMI] from 25 to 30 kg/m^2), and 35% are *obese* (BMI ≥30 kg/m^2). Of concern to obstetricians is a marked and continuing increase in the prevalence of obesity among pregnant

women, a factor associated with both obstetric complications and high-birthweight newborns, a known risk factor for childhood obesity. Whereas the epidemic of obesity in the United States was originally attributed to changes in the work environment, a surplus of high calories, inexpensive food, and a lack of childhood exercise, it is now recognized that **the risks of obesity in metabolic syndrome can be markedly influenced by early life events, particularly prenatal and neonatal growth and environmental exposures.** In the early 1990s, Barker and Hales[8] brought attention to this with epidemiologic studies demonstrating that **nutritional insufficiency during embryonic and fetal development resulted in latent disease, including obesity, in adulthood.** A series of studies have demonstrated a marked increase in deaths from coronary heart disease and adult hypertension in association with small for gestational age (SGA) newborns. In addition, investigators observed impaired glucose tolerance and diabetes in association with LBW.

Whereas the incidence of growth restriction has risen in the United States due in part to medical complications such as hypertension and multiple gestations, an approximate 25% increase in the incidence of high-birthweight (HBW) babies has also been seen during the past decade. Epidemiologic studies have confirmed that **the relationship between birthweight and adult obesity, cardiovascular disease, and insulin resistance is in fact a U-shaped curve, with increasing risks at both the low and high ends of the birthweight spectrum.** Importantly, the sequelae of programming do *not* occur as a threshold response associated with either very low or very high birthweight, rather they represent a continuum of risk for adult disease in relation to variance from an ideal newborn birthweight.

As will be described below, these studies have spawned a burst of epidemiologic and mechanistic studies of the developmental origins of adult diseases. The original focus on cardiovascular disease and metabolic syndrome has been extended to a diversity of adult diseases—including cancer and diseases that affect the kidneys, lungs, and immune system—and also with learning ability, mental health, and aging. Thus **the field of developmental origins of adult disease has grown from considering short-term toxic or teratogenic effects to looking at long-term adult sequelae of low or high birthweight and, more recently, at the impact of environmental toxins** (e.g., bisphenol A [BPA]). In addition to these influences, other factors that include maternal stress, preterm delivery, and maternal glucocorticoid therapy, among others, may significantly impact adult health and disease.

ENERGY-BALANCE PROGRAMMING

As noted above, epidemiologic studies demonstrate that the *metabolic syndrome*—a cluster of conditions that include obesity, hypertension, dyslipidemia, and impaired glucose tolerance—may be a result in part of the effects of LBW. Ultimately, **obesity results from an imbalance in energy intake and expenditure as regulated by appetite, metabolism, adipogenic propensity, and energy utilization.** In 1992, Hales and Barker[8] proposed the **"thrifty phenotype hypothesis"** and suggested that **in response to an impaired nutrient supply in utero, the growing fetus adapts to maximize metabolic efficiency because it will increase survival likelihood in the postnatal environment.** This adaptation would be beneficial in response to environmental cycles of famine and drought, in which reduced maternal—and thus fetal—nutrient supply would likely be replicated in the subsequent extrauterine environment. Numerous studies have demonstrated the **increased risk of obesity associated with LBW.** In addition to obesity, **LBW appears to predispose to excess central adiposity, a phenotype specifically associated with risk for cardiovascular disease.**

Although the long-term effects of LBW are linked to adult obesity, several studies have demonstrated important effects of **newborn or childhood catch-up growth among the LBW infants.** Those infants who are born small and remain small in comparison to their peers exhibit a lower risk of obesity and metabolic syndrome than those born small who catch up and exceed normal weights through infancy or early adolescence. These findings, replicated in animal models, have great significance for neonatal and childhood care. For example, a major goal of the treatment for premature LBW infants is the achievement of a minimum weight satisfactory for hospital discharge at birth. **Contrary to current practice, it may be advisable to limit rapid weight gain in the neonatal period. Importantly, breastfeeding results in a lower obesity risk compared with formula feeding.**[9] Breastfeeding may have advantages over formula feeding in both nutrient and hormone composition as well as in the natural limitations that prevent overfeeding.

As discussed above, programming effects of birthweight simulate a U-shaped curve because LGA infants also are at an increased risk of adult cardiovascular disease and diabetes. Understandably, LGA infants are often born to obese women, who frequently express glucose intolerance or insulin resistance and who often consume high-fat Western diets prior to and throughout pregnancy. Studies demonstrate that each of these risks—**obesity, glucose intolerance, and a high-fat diet—and their outcomes (LGA) may individually contribute to the programming of adult obesity.** When combined with variations in maternal feeding and different childhood diets, it is understandable that epidemiologic studies have not yet determined which of these factors is paramount in programming mechanisms. As discussed below, animal models demonstrate programming effects independently associated with each of these risks.

Animal models of LBW that have used a variety of methods—such as maternal nutrient restriction (global or specific), uterine artery ligation, and glucocorticoid exposure, among others—have effectively demonstrated increased adult adiposity. Similar to human studies, the propensity to obesity is particularly evident in LBW newborns who exhibit postnatal catch-up growth.[10] Studies primarily on rodents and sheep have provided important insights into the underlying mechanisms of programmed obesity, which include lasting changes in proportions of fat and lean body mass, central nervous system appetite control, adiposity structure and function, adipokine secretion and regulation, and energy expenditure.

Animal models of overnutrition mimic the modern dietary intake of high-fat, high-carbohydrate diets. Maternal obesity and high-fat, high-carbohydrate diets also result in increased adult programmed adiposity, notably via mechanisms that impact appetite and adipose tissue.[11]

Programming by Environmental Agents

Increasing human exposure to a wide range of industrial and agricultural chemicals has been well recognized. The Centers for Disease Control and Prevention (CDC) reported significant human exposure to endocrine-disrupter chemicals (EDCs), including those that act via estrogen receptors (eEDCs). BPA is a nearly ubiquitous monomer plasticizer. The consistent findings

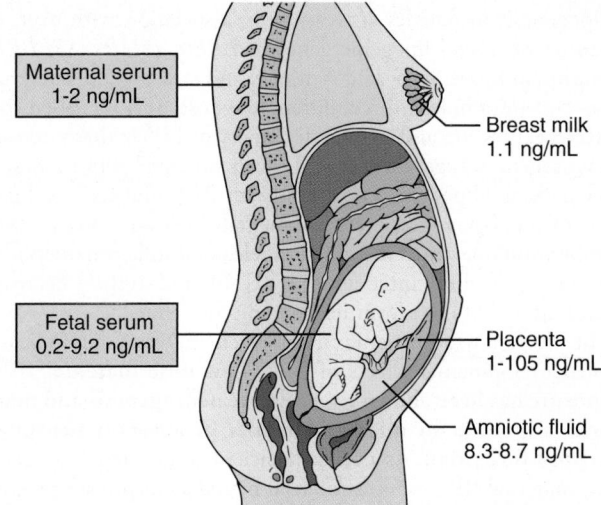

FIG 5-4 Bisphenol A levels during pregnancy.

of elevated BPA levels indicates continued routine exposure of adults and children. BPA is measurable in breast milk (1.1 ng/mL), maternal (1 to 2 ng/mL) and fetal serum (0.2 to 9.2 ng/mL), amniotic fluid (8.3 to 8.7 ng/mL), and placental tissues (1.0 to 104.9 ng/mL; Fig. 5-4).[12] BPA pharmacokinetics are similar in women, female monkeys, and rodents.[13] BPA metabolism includes conjugation and clearance as BPA-glucuronide and BPA-sulfate, with most BPA found recovered in urine. Because the fetus and newborn have reduced conjugation capacity, BPA elimination is likely prolonged. Furthermore, the well-documented fetal swallowing of amniotic fluid recirculates BPA excreted in fetal urine. These findings explain, in part, the elevated fetal serum and amniotic fluid BPA levels.

Higher BPA urinary concentrations are associated with increased adiposity at 9 years of age,[14] **and BPA levels are associated strongly with levels of the adipokines adiponectin and leptin.** Thus BPA exposure and maternal obesity may act synergistically to program obesity in the offspring. Epidemiologic studies support the association of human developmental EDC exposure and obesity in later life. Prenatal and early life polychlorinated biphenyl (PCB) exposure is associated with increased male and female weight at puberty. In utero exposure to hexachlorobenzene is linked to overweight children at age 6 years, and organochlorine pesticides are positively associated with BMI.[15]

The programming effects of BPA exposure are likely diverse; human epidemiologic studies have associated maternal BPA urinary concentrations with hyperactivity, aggression, anxiety, and depression, with effects more apparent in female offspring. Among inner-city children, prenatal BPA exposure is linked to altered emotional behavior such that males were more aggressive and females were less anxious or depressed.[16]

Animal models of BPA exposure indicate that BPA-programmed obesity mechanisms include changes in adipogenesis and neurogenesis. In vitro studies reveal marked embryologic effects of BPA that include alterations in cell differentiation. The proadipogenic effects of environmental obesogens have been well documented; recent studies have demonstrated effects on adipocyte generation that resulted in an increased number, differentiation, and lipogenic function with potential epigenetic effects that traverse generations. In rats, prenatal BPA increased adipogenesis in females at weaning in association with overexpression of several lipogenic genes (*C/EBPα, PPARγ, SREBP1*, lipoprotein lipase, fatty acid synthase, and stearoyl-CoA desaturase-1).[17] In samples from children, low-dose BPA increased the mRNA expression and enzymatic activity of 11β-hydroxysteroid dehydrogenase type 1 (11β-HSD1) in omental adipose tissue and visceral adipocytes, consistent with BPA-induced acceleration of adipogenesis. At environmentally relevant doses, BPA inhibits adiponectin and stimulates release of inflammatory adipokines, including interleukin 6 (IL-6) and tumor necrosis factor alpha (TNFα) from human adipose tissue.

In addition to adipogenic effects, recent EDC studies indicate neurodevelopmental effects of BPA. **Low-dose maternal BPA exposure has been shown to accelerate neurogenesis and neuronal migration in mice and results in aberrant neuronal network formation.** As a consequence of accelerated neurogenesis, maternal BPA reduces the fetal neural stem/progenitor cell population at embryonic day 14.5.[18] Maternal BPA exposure may ultimately program offspring appetite development; BPA upregulates critical mouse embryonic genes associated with appetite pathway neurogenesis, and in vitro BPA stimulates proliferation of neuroprogenitor cells.

BPA effects have been demonstrated both histologically and behaviorally. Prenatal and neonatal BPA exposure induces dysfunction of the hippocampal cholinergic system. Prenatal BPA may also alter development of dopamine and N-methyl-D-aspartate (NMDA) systems in association with offspring anxious behaviors and cognitive deficits as well as serotoninergic systems that regulate mood. **Gender-specific effects are well documented; in utero BPA exposure has been found to alter offspring rat brain structure and behavior, including sexually dimorphic behaviors, with effects more apparent in females than in males.** Male mice offspring demonstrated increased aggression and memory impairment in addition to increased brain expression of estrogen receptors alpha and beta during early life. In studies of primates, prenatal BPA was found to alter male cynomolgus monkey offspring sexual behavior. As noted earlier, these effects have been identified in human offspring as well.[16]

Mechanisms of Programmed Obesity: Appetite and Adiposity

The hypothalamic regulation of appetite and satiety function develops in utero in precocial species, those in which the young are relatively mature as newborns. In the rat and in humans, although neurons that regulate appetite and satiety become detectable in the fetal hypothalamus early in gestation, the functional neuronal pathways form during the second week of postnatal life in the rat and likely during the third trimester in humans. Notably, the obesity gene product leptin, which is synthesized primarily by adipose tissue and the placenta, is a critical neurotrophic factor during development. In contrast to the adult, in which leptin acts as a satiety factor, fetal/neonatal leptin promotes the development of satiety pathways. In leptin-deficient (ob/ob) mice, satiety pathways are permanently disrupted and demonstrate axonal densities one third to one fourth that of controls.[19] Treatment of *adult* ob/ob mice with leptin does not restore satiety projections, but leptin treatment of *newborn* ob/ob mice does rescue the neuronal development,[19] indicating the critical role of leptin during the perinatal period.

Early-life leptin exposure is likely a putative programming mechanism in SGA and LGA human newborns. In LBW

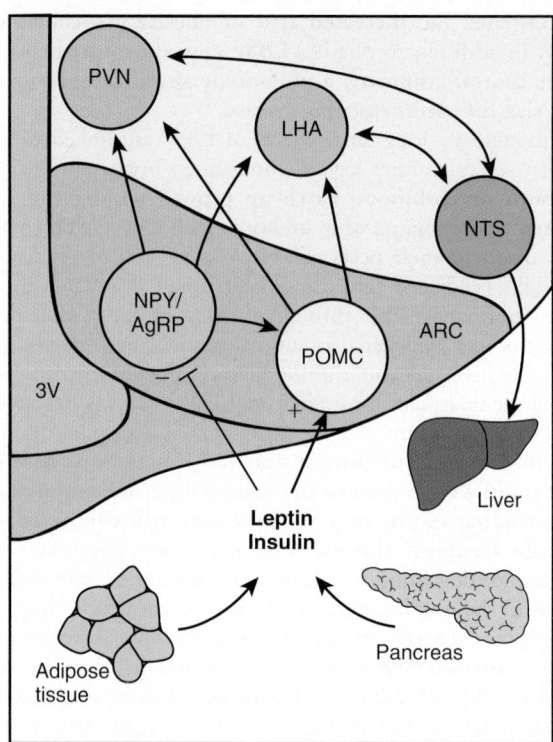

FIG 5-5 Leptin secreted by adipose tissue and insulin secreted by the pancreas suppress neuropeptide Y (NPY) and increase proopiomelanocortin (POMC). 3V, third ventricle; AgRP, agouti gene–related protein; ARC, arcuate nucleus; LHA, lateral hypothalamic area; NTS, nucleus of the solitary tract; PVN, paraventricular nucleus.

human offspring, leptin levels are low at delivery, and cord blood levels reflect neonatal fat mass. In contrast to the low serum levels of leptin in SGA newborns, LGA infants have elevated leptin levels. Obese pregnant mothers further have elevated leptin levels related to maternal adiposity, and breast milk leptin levels also reflect maternal fat mass.

Leptin binding to its receptor activates proopiomelanocortin (POMC) neurons and downstream anorexigenic pathways. Obesity is often associated with leptin resistance, which results in an inability to balance food intake with actual energy needs. The leptin pathway is counterregulated by the orexigenic neuropeptide Y (NPY; Fig. 5-5). Impaired leptin signaling could result in increased expression of NPY, which would promote increased nutrient intake while decreasing overall physical activity. In LBW newborns, appetite dysregulation has been demonstrated as a key predisposing factor for the obese phenotype.[20] Studies on LBW offspring specifically indicate dysfunction at several aspects of the satiety pathway, as evidenced by reduced satiety and cellular signaling responses to leptin.[21] Recent studies have demonstrated an upregulation of the hypothalamic nutrient sensor nicotinamide adenine dinucleotide (NAD)-dependent deacetylase sirtuin 1 (SIRT1), a factor that epigenetically regulates gene transcription of factors critical to neural development. Importantly, neuronal stem cells from rodent SGA fetuses and newborns demonstrate reduced growth and impaired differentiation to neurons and glial cells.[22] Thus impaired neuronal development, and ultimately reduced satiety pathways, may be a consequence of a reduction in neural stem cell growth potential and reduced leptin-mediated neurotrophic stimulation during periods of axonal development.

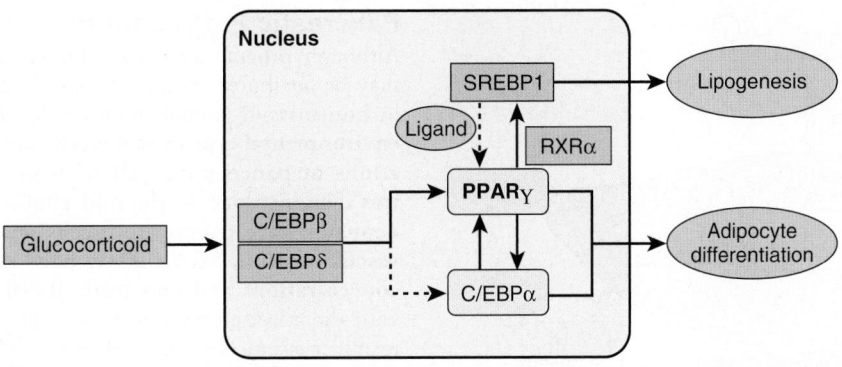

FIG 5-6 Transcriptional regulation of adipogenesis. C/EBP, CCAAT/enhancer binding protein; PPAR: peroxisome proliferator–activated receptor; RXR, retinoic X receptor; SREBP, sterol regulatory element–binding protein.

In addition to appetite/satiety dysfunction, **mechanisms that regulate adipose tissue development and function (lipogenesis) may be a key factor in the development of programmed obesity.** Increase in adipose tissue mass or adipogenesis occurs primarily during prenatal and postnatal development, although some adipogenesis continues throughout adulthood. The process of adipogenesis requires highly organized and precisely controlled expression of a cascade of transcription factors within the preadipocyte (Fig. 5-6), and this process is regulated by hormones, nutrients, and epigenetic factors. Of note, LBW offspring show a paradoxic increased expression of the principal adipogenic transcription factor, peroxisome proliferator–activated receptor gamma (PPARγ), and of hypertrophic adipocytes with increased propensity for fat storage, as evidenced by increased lipogenesis and de novo fatty acid synthesis. **In accordance with this, LBW preadipocytes exhibit early differentiation and premature induction of adipogenic genes.[23,24] Because the signaling pathways of adipogenesis and lipogenesis are upregulated prior to the development of obesity, they may be among the crucial contributory factors that predispose to programmed obesity.** Furthermore, cellular studies indicate that in LBW infants, adipocytes at birth have fundamental traits identical to those seen with thiazolidine (PPAR agonist) treatment; that is, the adipocytes are more insulin sensitive and demonstrate increased glucose uptake and thereby facilitate increased lipid storage within the adipocytes. Thus early activation of PPAR or its downstream targets could promote the storage of lipids and thereby increase the risk of obesity. This concept reverberates with studies on maternal exposure to PPAR agonists, which induces fetal mesenchymal stem cells along the adipocyte lineage and causes a reduction in the osteogenic potential in these cells, resulting in greater fat mass in adult offspring.[25] The role of stem cell precursor programming in metabolic disease pathways in response to maternal nutrient supply is an intriguing area for understanding developmental plasticity and potential preventive therapeutic strategies. Also, **the potential transdifferentiation of white adipose tissue toward a brown-fat phenotype, which can expend energy via thermogenesis, offers an alternative preventive strategy for programmed obesity.**

Offspring born to obese rat dams fed a high-fat diet also demonstrate increased food intake, adiposity, and circulating leptin levels and impaired glucose homeostasis dependent upon the period of exposure.[11] In addition, these offspring have an activated adipose tissue renin-angiotensin system that partly contributes to their hypertensive phenotype.[26] The underlying phenotype appears to be similar to that of LBW infants, with altered appetite regulation, enhanced adipogenesis, and reduced energy expenditure. Nonetheless, salient mechanistic differences exist, such as increased proliferation of appetite-stimulating or orexigenic neurons in the fetus, the inability of elevated leptin to downregulate NPY, and decreased PPARγ corepressors.

Hepatic Programming

In conjunction with the increased incidence of childhood and adolescent obesity, **children and adolescents now have an increased risk of developing nonalcoholic fatty liver disease (NAFLD), or nonalcoholic steatohepatitis, and type 2 diabetes.** Type 2 diabetes has increased tenfold in some regions of the United States during the past decade, and the prevalence is particularly high in adolescent Native Americans, approaching rates of 6%. NAFLD, as determined by elevated serum aminotransferase, may occur in up to 10% of obese adolescents in the United States, although studies using ultrasonographic measures of fatty liver have estimated rates of up to 25% to 50% of obese adolescents. As a reflection of the severity of the metabolic syndrome, **cases of cirrhosis associated with NAFLD in obese children have been described recently.** Further evidence suggests that obesity can potentiate additional insults to the liver, such as with alcohol and hepatitis C infection.

Men and women with reduced abdominal circumference at birth, potentially reflecting reduced hepatic growth during fetal life, have elevated serum cholesterol and plasma fibrinogen. Similarly, **poor weight gain in infancy is associated with altered adult liver function,** reflected by elevated serum total and low-density lipoprotein (LDL) cholesterol and increased plasma fibrinogen concentrations.[27] Although human studies have focused on the diagnosis and consequences of NAFLD in obese children and adolescents, animal studies (described below) indicate the early expression of fatty liver in fetuses exposed to maternal high-fat diets that were not LGA. Consequently, **a heretofore undiagnosed increase in liver adiposity may exist among normal-weight offspring of mothers exposed to Western, high-fat diets.**

Animal models of both maternal nutrient restriction and nutrient excess demonstrate the presence of NAFLD, alterations in liver structure, and changes in key metabolic transcription factors and enzymes involved in glucose-lipid homeostasis in offspring. Specifically, maternal protein restriction during a rat pregnancy shifts the enzyme setting of the liver in favor of

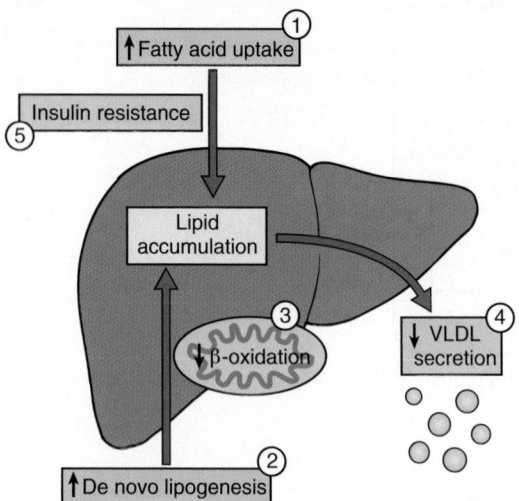

FIG 5-7 Mechanisms for nonalcoholic hepatic steatosis (nonalcoholic fatty liver disease [NAFLD]) include (1) increased fatty acid uptake by the liver and increased triglyceride synthesis; (2) increased de novo lipogenesis; (3) decreased fatty acid oxidation; (4) decreased very-low-density lipoprotein (VLDL) secretion, preventing release of fatty acid from the liver; and (5) hepatic insulin resistance, which promotes lipogenesis and gluconeogenesis and inhibits lipolysis.

glucose production, rather than glucose utilization, as evidenced by increased phosphoenolpyruvate carboxykinase and decreased glucokinase enzyme activities in offspring. Furthermore, these key hepatic enzymes of glucose homeostasis retain the ability to respond to the challenge of a high-fat, high-calorie diet but with an altered "set point" of regulation. Moreover, because these enzymes are predominantly located in different metabolic zones of the liver (glucokinase in the perivenous and phosphoenolpyruvate carboxykinase in the periportal zone), these altered activities have been attributed to clonal expansion of the periportal and contraction of the perivenous cell populations.[28]

Five potential mechanisms lead to abnormal hepatic lipid metabolism and NAFLD (Fig. 5-7). On a molecular level, PPAR transcription factors are implicated in regulating lipid metabolism. PPARα in particular is predominantly expressed in the liver and regulates genes involved in fatty acid oxidation. Although PPARγ is expressed at very low levels in the liver, PPARγ agonists have been shown to ameliorate NAFLD in a rat model.[29] In addition, PPARα and PPARγ modulate the inflammatory response, and PPAR activators have been shown to exert antiinflammatory activities in various cell types by inhibiting the expression of acute-phase proteins, such as C-reactive protein (CRP).[30] CRP is produced by hepatocytes in response to tissue injury, infection, and inflammation and is moderately elevated in obesity, metabolic syndrome, diabetes, and NAFLD. Rat studies have demonstrated NAFLD and elevated hepatic CRP levels in LBW adult offspring associated with reduced expression of hepatic PPARγ and PPARα.[31] PPAR transcription factors and their coregulator peroxisome proliferator–activated receptor gamma coactivator (PGC-1α) are in turn regulated by SIRT1, which is a nutrient sensor that has epigenetic effects. Consistent with reduced PPARα, LBW offspring have reduced hepatic SIRT1 activity and PGC-1α expression, which likely promotes hepatic lipogenesis and suppresses hepatic lipolysis.[32] Similar changes of reduced hepatic SIRT1 activity and PGC-1α expression are observed in offspring from maternal high-fat diet and obese pregnancies.[33]

Pancreatic Programming

Although programmed adult obesity or diet-induced obesity may be attributed to the etiology of insulin resistance, studies in humans and animals indicate that **in utero nutrition and environmental exposures directly impact the pancreas. Alterations of pancreatic β-cell mass by maternal malnutrition was demonstrated in the mid 1960s. Whereas LGA human neonates have pancreatic β-cell hyperplasia and increased vascularization, SGA infants have reduced plasma insulin concentrations and pancreatic β-cell numbers.**[34] Consistent with the adverse effects of rapid catch-up growth, the greatest insulin resistance is observed in individuals who are LBW but develop adult obesity.[35] **In humans, growth in utero is directly associated with fetal insulin levels. Importantly, beyond the regulation of glucose uptake, insulin has important developmental functions in systems that include skeletal and connective tissues and neural development.**

These extremes of weight are critical because the risk of insulin resistance in adult life is twofold greater among men who weighed less than 8.2 kg at 1 year of age and in those who weighed 12.3 kg or more.[36] A link has also been found between reduced early growth and proinsulin concentrations, suggesting that pancreatic tissue or function may be impaired, whereas other studies have suggested that fetal programming may alter the structure or function of insulin-sensitive target tissues.

Dependent upon the prevalence of obesity, **approximately 25% of individuals with normal glucose tolerance have insulin resistance similar to that seen in type 2 diabetes, but they compensate for this with enhanced insulin secretion.** These individuals are at increased risk to develop of overt diabetes. Studies of fetal programming have focused upon the finding that birthweight and newborn plasma glucose levels are directly correlated in normal pregnancies and in those complicated by diabetes. Far less focus has been paid to levels of amino acids in maternal or fetal blood, although amino acids are also major determinants of fetal growth.

In addition to low and high birthweight, recent studies suggest that **antenatal exposure to betamethasone may result in insulin resistance in adult offspring.** A 30-year follow-up of a double-blind, placebo-controlled randomized trial of antenatal betamethasone for the prevention of neonatal respiratory distress syndrome demonstrated **no differences in body size, blood lipids, blood pressure, or cardiovascular disease among those exposed to betamethasone or placebo. However, offspring exposed to betamethasone demonstrated higher plasma insulin concentrations at 30 min in a 75 g oral glucose tolerance test, and lower glucose concentrations were observed at 120 min.**[37] The authors suggest that antenatal exposure to betamethasone may result in insulin resistance in adult offspring. A further study of 20-year-old offspring demonstrated significantly reduced blood pressure in betamethasone-exposed offspring.[38] In view of these findings, the authors recommend that obstetricians utilize a single course, rather than multiple courses, of antenatal glucocorticoids.

Various animal models of maternal diabetes, nutritional manipulation—both underfeeding and overfeeding—and uterine ligation all have reported altered β-cell growth, disturbances in insulin secretion, and long-term effects on insulin sensitivity. **Reduced β-cell growth and insulin secretion have been observed in LBW offspring,**[39] whereas accelerated β-cell mass and excess insulin secretion was observed in offspring of obese pregnant women.[40] Despite differing nutrition and growth, both led to β-cell failure, tissue-specific insulin resistance, and development of diabetes in the adult offspring. This phenomenon has been attributed to developmental epigenetic regulation. The β-cell transcription factor pancreatic duodenal homeobox 1 (*PDX1*) is critical for β-cell development, and progressive silencing of Pdx-1 expression has been observed in β-cells isolated from LBW offspring. Importantly, this silencing corresponds with persistent altered epigenetic regulation of the *PDX1* gene. Additionally, increased circulating lipids can induce β-cell apoptosis via endoplasmic reticulum stress pathways. Interestingly, Pdx-1 is protective against pancreatic endoplasmic reticulum stress in response to high-fat feeding in rodents. Whereas obesity in pregnancy can increase pancreatic fat deposition in rodent models, whether this in turn leads to permanent changes in gene expression as observed in the growth-restricted fetus remains unknown.

The transgeneration diabetogenic effect is evident: maternal gestational diabetes and the resultant intrauterine hyperglycemia can transmit the diabetogenic phenotype to a subsequent generation.[41] Consequently, the incidence of mothers who exhibit gestational diabetes has increased.[42] Similar to humans, rat models of maternal diabetes demonstrate a transgeneration diabetogenic effect. Female offspring of diabetic mothers develop gestational diabetes and induce the effect in their fetuses and thereby in the next generation. Notably, intrauterine hyperglycemia alters imprinted gene expression in sperm.[43]

Cardiac Programming

In addition to the aforementioned glucocorticoid effects on insulin resistance, evidence suggests that maternal betamethasone treatment of preterm infants is associated with long-term adverse cardiac outcomes, including hypertrophic cardiomyopathy.[44] Animal models discussed below confirm the association of fetal cortisol exposure with increased left ventricular cardiomyocyte size. A reduction in cardiomyocyte number through either reduced cellular proliferation or increased apoptosis appears to be a central feature. Because cardiomyocytes are highly differentiated and rarely replicate after birth, their inappropriate prenatal reduction is likely to result in a permanent loss of myocardial functioning units and an increased susceptibility to cardiac hypertrophy and ischemic heart disease. Confounding the direct association, left ventricular hypertrophy also has been reported in growth-restricted infants. Recent studies have suggested that maternal vitamin D deficiency may program long-term vulnerability to cardiovascular disease via effects on the fetal renin-angiotensin system and altered cardiomyocyte growth.

Similar to programming of the metabolic syndrome, extensive epidemiologic data have demonstrated the association of birthweight with adult coronary heart disease. Slow growth during fetal life and infancy followed by accelerated weight gain in childhood predisposes to adult coronary heart disease in both men and women.[45] The association between LBW and coronary heart disease has been replicated among men and women throughout North America, the Indian subcontinent, and Europe.

As a result of similar pathophysiologic mechanisms, a strong interaction of these risk factors exists with stroke. However, the impact of programming is again evident in the marked differences in adult phenotype dependent upon fetal and childhood

environments. In a study of over 2000 people within the Helsinki birth cohort, two different paths of early growth preceded the development of hypertension in adult life.[46] Small body size at birth and low weight gain during infancy followed by a rapid gain in BMI during childhood was associated with an increase in coronary heart disease as adults. In contrast, LBW in utero and throughout infancy followed by a persistent small body size at adolescence resulted in an increased risk of stroke and an atherogenic lipid profile. These two different paths of growth may lead to hypertension via altered biologic processes. Although restriction of rodent weight gain following LBW prevents an obese phenotype, significant atherogenic and pancreatic abnormalities are present, and these offspring exhibit markedly elevated cholesterol levels and insulin deficiency.[47] These results, in both humans and animals, indicate that preventive strategies may be elusive; prevention of LBW, rather than modulation of infant growth rates, is key.

In addition to the effect of fetal nutrient exposure on cardiac development, significant mechanisms of vasculogenesis underlie the programming of hypertension. These may include modifications in arterial elastin and stiffness and in the size of the arterial and capillary beds.[48] Although no direct evidence suggests that elastin synthesis is impaired in the developing large arteries of human fetuses whose growth is restricted, children with a single umbilical artery demonstrate striking asymmetry in the compliance of their iliac arteries at 5 to 9 years of age. Importantly, preterm birth also significantly affects the elastin content and viscoelastic properties of the vascular extracellular matrix in human arteries. Inadequate elastin synthesis during early development may cause a permanent increase in arterial stiffness in adulthood, leading to hypertension and cardiovascular disease.[49]

Although this chapter does not seek to review all toxic teratogenic exposures, prenatal cocaine exposure has been demonstrated to have significant effects on cardiac function in offspring. Cocaine exposure results in an increased rate of neonatal arrhythmia and transient cardiac ST elevations. Although a blinded cross-sectional study did not demonstrate any significant differences in human left ventricular cardiac function, prenatal cocaine exposure did result in changes in diastolic filling in neonates with the degree of change correlated to the degree of cocaine exposure. Some changes persisted to the age of 26 months, particularly in those infants exposed to high levels of cocaine in utero. The mechanisms of these cocaine effects may relate to the inhibition of dopamine, serotonin, and norepinephrine reuptake. In addition to direct effects, the impact of cocaine on the programming of cardiac function may be mediated via the autonomic nervous system. Some studies, although not all, have demonstrated an alteration in resting heart rate and heart rate variability. A well-performed investigation revealed a dose-dependent effect of fetal cocaine on neonatal heart rate at 4 to 8 weeks of age, although the duration of this effect is unknown.[50] Further effects on static stress, renal sympathetic activity, and heart rate variability confirm the effects of cocaine on the developing cardioregulatory systems. Taken in sum, these studies suggest that fetal cocaine exposure has at least a short-term impact, and potentially a longer-term impact, on cardiac function in humans.

Although no clear epidemiologic evidence links prenatal hypoxia and adult cardiovascular disease, animal models suggest an effect of hypoxia on adult cardiac function. Chronic hypoxia during the course of pregnancy also results in LBW newborns with altered myocardial structure and altered heart development.

Antenatal hypoxia causes pulmonary vascular remodeling during fetal life that results in pulmonary vascular disease (i.e., hypertension) in newborns.[51] Hypoxia-mediated responses act in part via hypoxia inducible factor (HIF) regulating multiple genes, including vascular endothelial growth factor (VEGF), and downstream inflammatory responses.[52] Among other effects, prolonged hypoxia in utero suppresses fetal cardiac function, alters cardiac gene expression, increases myocyte apoptosis, and results in a premature exiting of the cell cycle by cardiomyocytes in addition to myocyte hypertrophy.[53]

Osteoporosis Programming

Recent evidence indicates that **fetal and neonatal life may be a critical factor in the development of osteoporosis,** a disease typically associated with aging. In considering the major determinants of bone mass in later life, the most critical issues are 1) peak bone mass achieved during the third decade of life and 2) the rate of bone loss following this period. Thus **bone mass in the elderly is largely determined by peak bone mass that occurs much earlier in life.** Several epidemiologic studies have demonstrated that LBW and weight at 1 year are directly correlated with reduced bone marrow content and bone mineral density.[54] Consistent with these findings, poor childhood growth was associated with an increased risk of hip fracture in elderly adults.

The mechanisms by which the fetal and neonatal period can influence peak bone mineral content include the interaction of vitamin D and calcium and additional factors such as fetal and neonatal growth hormone, cortisol, and insulin-like growth factor 1 (IGF-1). An undernourished fetus deprived of calcium may upregulate vitamin D activity in an attempt to increase calcium availability. Although more than 60% of peak bone mass is gained during puberty, a growing body of evidence suggests that a substantial proportion of peak bone mass is determined by growth earlier in life. Additional maternal factors may influence neonatal bone mineral content. **Low maternal fat stores, maternal smoking or increased physical exercise in late pregnancy, and low maternal birthweight all predict lower whole-body bone marrow content in the neonate.**[55] Breastfed children initially have lower bone mass than bottle-fed children but may ultimately accrue greater bone mass by 8 years. In rats, maternal diet modulation or uterine artery ligation affects the bone structure of offspring. As adults, these offspring had lower serum 25-hydroxy vitamin D levels and lower bone mineral content and bone area, which was also associated with changes in their growth plates. This is consistent with the nutritional programming of the skeletal growth trajectory and complements the epidemiologic evidence for programming of osteoporosis in humans.

Brain Programming

Cerebral function and development during the critical fetal/neonatal window is highly complex; therefore it is understandable that a number of stressors during early life would impact a variety of areas, including cognition and behavior, dysfunction of which could lead to anxiety and even addictive behavior. **In utero exposure to cocaine, and perhaps methamphetamine, demonstrates a number of cerebral effects.**[56] Children exposed to prenatal cocaine evidence a significant impact on behavior (aggression), attention-deficit/hyperactivity disorder (ADHD), substance abuse (e.g., cigarettes), and impaired language.[56] Additional studies have suggested potential impairment of

intelligence quotient (IQ), cognition, motor function, and school performance. Understandably, windows of exposure and dose-dependent responses are difficult to quantify. Nevertheless, a number of studies have suggested that **heavy cocaine use is related to worse outcome in regard to behavior, language, and IQ.**[56] Studies of neuroimaging have demonstrated significant alterations in the specific volumes of brain regions among cocaine-exposed children when assessed as children, adolescents, and adults. Studies of diffusion tensor imaging and functional magnetic resonance imaging (MRI) reveal increased creatine in the frontal white matter, a potential sign of abnormal energy metabolism.[57] Cocaine-exposed children exhibit greater activation in the white inferior frontal cortex and the caudate nucleus during response inhibition, suggesting that **prenatal cocaine may affect the development of brain systems involved in the regulation of attention and response inhibition.**[56]

Considering other substances of abuse, among children exposed to methamphetamine, magnetic resonance spectroscopy demonstrated increases in total creatine in the basal ganglia, again indicative of possible alterations in cellular energy metabolism.[58] Neuroimaging of children exposed to opiates in utero further reveal smaller intracranial and brain volumes, including a smaller cerebral cortex, amygdala, brainstem, and cerebellar white matter among other areas. This is consistent with **animal studies, which indicate that prenatal nicotine or cocaine exposure targets specific neurotransmitter receptors in the fetal brain and elicits abnormalities in cell proliferation and differentiation and thus leads to reduced neurogenesis and altered synaptic activity.**[59] **The underlying mechanism may involve increased apoptosis of neuronal cells.**

MATERNAL STRESS AND ANXIETY

Although the effects of maternal substance abuse may be a direct impact of the specific drug-receptor interaction, the commonality of behavioral effects in the offspring suggests that disruption in the fetal neuroendocrine environment—potentially associated with increased fetal adrenocorticotropic hormone (ACTH)/cortisol—may impact fetal/neonatal brain development. In view of these findings, extensive epidemiologic investigation has been focused on maternal stress and anxiety. During the second trimester, increased maternal anxiety has been associated with lower neonatal dopamine and serotonin levels, greater right frontal electroencephalogram (EEG) activation, and lower vagal tone. In late pregnancy, maternal anxiety has been associated with increased salivary cortisol levels among 10-year-old children, suggesting that maternal anxiety during pregnancy programs the offspring's stress responsiveness. In a recent study, **neonates of mothers with high anxiety demonstrated altered auditory evoked responses, which suggests differences in attention allocation.** In addition to chronic maternal anxiety, acute stress responses during pregnancy may include death of close relatives, natural disasters, and maternal neuropsychiatric conditions. Many of these stress exposures have significant impact, with potential neurodevelopmental consequences for the offspring. **Children of mothers with posttraumatic stress disorder (PTSD) during pregnancy display altered cortisol levels accompanied by signs of behavioral distress during the first 9 months of life.**[60]

The role of the maternal hypothalamic-pituitary-adrenal (HPA) axis is recognized as contributing to maternal stress-mediated effects on fetal development. Although the developing fetus is normally protected from high levels of circulating maternal cortisol by the placental enzyme 11-β-hydroxysteroid dehydrogenase type 2 (11β-HSD2), which metabolizes cortisol to inactive cortisone, downregulation of placental 11β-HSD2 may occur in response to drug exposure, maternal diet, and obstetric conditions that include preeclampsia, preterm birth, and IUGR.[61] **A reduction in placental 11β-HSD2 may thus increase fetal exposure to maternal cortisol levels and may have secondary effects on brain maturation and development.** Among pregnant women who undergo amniocentesis, a strong correlation exists between maternal plasma and amniotic fluid cortisol levels indicative of fetal levels. The correlation with maternal anxiety suggests that measures of amniotic fluid cortisol may serve as an index for fetal hormone exposure.

Psychiatric disorders seen in the offspring of pregnancies associated with maternal stress may be a consequence of cortisol binding to select brain regions during development. Notably, most fetal tissues express glucocorticoid receptors from mid gestation onward. It is well established that steroid hormones in the fetus are involved in organ development and maturation, such as of the brain, heart, lungs, gastrointestinal (GI) tract, and kidneys. Glucocorticoids may impact diverse gene expression via epigenetic mechanisms that include DNA methylation, histone acetylation, and miRNA.[62] Of note, the hippocampus, which is critical for learning and memory, has extensive glucocorticoid receptors. Although not studied in humans, glucocorticoid exposure in rat dams results in a reduction in the volume and number of cells in the nucleus accumbens, a central limbic nucleus critical to reward circuitry.[63] These findings may provide a mechanism by which maternal stress or substance abuse contributes to offspring addictive behavior, which represents a dysfunction of the limbic system.

The effects of maternal stress may extend beyond fetal/neonatal neurologic and behavioral issues. Maternal prenatal anxiety and stress predicted a significant adverse effect on illness in the infant and also predicted antibiotic use,[64] whereas a wide range of prenatal stressors were associated with morbidity in childhood. Specifically, **prenatal anxiety has been associated with childhood asthma, whereas stress-related maternal factors have been linked to increased eczema during early childhood.**

A generational effect of fetal programming and the HPA axis is suggested by findings that LBW babies have elevated cortisol concentrations in umbilical cord blood and have elevated urinary cortisol secretion in childhood.[65] Nilsson and colleagues[66] demonstrated a continuous relationship between size at birth and stress susceptibility, whereas other studies have found that cortisol responses to stress were significantly and inversely related to birthweight. Similarly, in regard to physiologic responses, LBW is associated with increased blood pressure and heart rate responses to psychologic stressors in women but not in men.

In corroboration of the human data, findings from experiments with rodent models show that prenatal stress, such as restraint and administration of exogenous glucocorticoids, not only impairs cognition and increases anxiety and reactivity to stress but also alters brain development.[67] Furthermore, prenatal stress increases sensitivity to nicotine and other addictive drugs. Interestingly, m**aternal nurturing impacts the offspring's epigenome and behavior.** In rats, maternal nurturing behavior altered the offspring epigenome at a glucocorticoid receptor gene

promoter in the hippocampus. As a result, highly nurtured rat pups demonstrated less anxiety than those that received minimal nurturing.

More recent studies of nonhuman primates implicate chronic consumption of a high-fat diet during pregnancy in increased anxious behavior in offspring. This behavior is thought to be caused by perturbations in the fetal brain serotonergic-melanocortin pathways.[68]

GLUCOCORTICOIDS AND PREMATURITY

Although glucocorticoid therapy for the preterm infant has made a significant contribution to the reduction of neonatal respiratory distress syndrome, intraventricular hemorrhage, and infant mortality, the tendency has been for clinicians to utilize multiple courses of glucocorticoids. Studies that have examined the impact of human perinatal glucocorticoid exposure have demonstrated that **children exposed to dexamethasone during preterm gestation who were born at term have increased emotionality, general behavioral problems, and impairments in verbal working memory.**[64] Further, **offspring of women given multiple doses of antenatal glucocorticoids have reduced head circumference and significantly increased aggressive violent behavior and attention deficits.**[69] These findings suggest that fetal exposure to pharmacologic glucocorticoid levels during critical developmental periods, prior to the normal increase seen in the term newborn, may have adverse consequences, including to the programming of the offspring's HPA axis. Preterm babies exposed to antenatal betamethasone had a lower salivary cortisol response to a heel stick than matched controls at 3 to 6 days after delivery.[70] Additional studies demonstrate that antenatal corticosteroids are associated with suppressed cortisol responses to corticotrophin-releasing hormone (CRH) during the immediate neonatal period. Salivary cortisol responses to immunization at 4 months of age were significantly correlated with the mean plasma cortisol in the first 4 weeks of life independent of maternal glucocorticoid exposure. It is notable that preterm infants have a similar spectrum of developmental and behavioral problems as do babies whose mothers have experienced extreme stress or anxiety during pregnancy, and both groups demonstrate increased levels of attention deficit, hyperactivity, anxiety, and depression.

Although premature exogenous glucocorticoid exposure via maternal administration has consequences, **it should be recognized that if actually delivered preterm, infants are exposed to increased endogenous cortisol prior to the time at which they would normally experience this increase—that is, at term.** Several studies demonstrate that LBW is associated with increased resting heart rate and fasting plasma cortisol concentrations in adulthood. Among preterm babies born at less than 32 weeks, newborn plasma cortisol levels are four to seven times higher than the fetal levels would be at the same gestational age. As the elevated levels persist through 4 weeks of age, they likely result from a combination of both the acute antenatal steroids and postnatal endogenous glucocorticoid exposure. Whether a consequence of prematurity or perhaps of premature cortisol exposure, preterm infants—especially those born prior to 28 weeks' gestation—have significant neurologic impairments, including visual-motor coordination when measured at 8 years of age. **In view of these consequences of exogenous and endogenous glucocorticoids, maternal glucocorticoid use**

should be directed only at those infants most likely to benefit and those most likely to deliver preterm.

Whereas the effects of glucocorticoids on programming brain development and organ maturation is well accepted, it is less well recognized that glycyrrhiza—a natural constituent of licorice—may also impact fetal programming by disrupting cortisol metabolism. Glycyrrhiza inhibits placental 11β-HSD2 and thus results in a potential increased transmission of maternal cortisol to the fetal compartment. In a study of Finnish children at 8 years of age, those with **high exposure to glycyrrhiza from maternal licorice ingestion had significant deficits in verbal and visual spatial abilities and in narrative memory, and they had significant increases in externalizing symptoms and in aggression-related problems.** These effects on cognitive performance appear to be related to the degree of licorice consumption.[71] In addition to licorice, glycyrrhiza is often used as a flavoring in candies, chewing gum, herbal teas, alcoholic and nonalcoholic drinks, and herbal medications. Although these results suggest that exposure to glycyrrhiza should be limited during pregnancy, it more importantly indicates the diversity of foods and drugs that can impact fetal development and programming, perhaps through effects on fetal cortisol exposure.

As adults, prematurely born infants also display abnormalities of insulin resistance, elevated blood pressure, and abnormal retinal vasculature. Although much attention has been focused on the effects of LBW on the programming of metabolic syndrome, a study of 49-year-old Swedish men demonstrated that systolic and diastolic blood pressures were inversely correlated with gestational age, rather than birthweight, independent of current BMI. Similar results have been demonstrated in women born preterm. An intergenerational effect may occur because consequences of elevated blood pressure and abnormal vascularization among women may have a subsequent impact on future pregnancies. Thus **women who were born before 37 weeks of gestational age demonstrate a 2.5-fold increased risk of developing gestational hypertension in their own pregnancies.**[72]

In a recent study from western North Carolina, boys and girls aged 9 through 16 were tested for depression in relation to birthweight and additional prenatal and perinatal factors. **LBW predicted depression in adolescent girls** (38.1% vs. 8.4% among girls with normal birthweight) but not boys. In addition, **LBW was associated with an increased risk of social phobia, posttraumatic stress symptoms, and generalized anxiety disorder—all of which were far more common in girls than in boys.**[73] Further studies have demonstrated that LBW is associated with an increased risk of schizophrenia, ADHD, and eating disorders. These findings are consistent with animal studies that indicate gender-specific effects of developmental programming.

IMMUNE FUNCTION

Prenatal stress may influence the developing immune system, particularly as related to asthma and atopic diseases. Maternal nervousness during gestation correlates with elevated immunoglobulin E (IgE) levels in cord blood and may predict atopic diseases in early childhood. Importantly, pregnant women with prenatal stress have elevated proinflammatory cytokine levels,[74] which may impact the risk of allergy in childhood. Although these findings suggest that *enhanced* immunologic responses may occur following maternal stress, LBW may be associated with

reduced inflammatory responses that contribute to increased morbidity. Young adults born during seasonal famine and likely growth restricted were more likely to die of infectious diseases. These infants demonstrated reduced thymic size and altered patterns of T-cell subsets with a lower CD4/CD8 ratio, suggestive of lower thymic output. Interestingly, Hartwig and colleagues[75] reported that the likelihood of asthma and eczema at the age of 14 years was significantly increased in children of mothers who had experienced adverse life events during the second half of gestation, but a greater increase was found if this occurred in mothers without asthma compared with mothers who had asthma. Postpartum maternal influences also may contribute because mothers of these infants express lower levels of maternal breast milk interleukin 7 (IL-7), a putative thymic trophic factor. In support of the impaired inflammation response among LBW infants, antibody **responses to typhoid vaccination are positively associated with birthweight. These findings suggest that atopy-related immune function may be enhanced in either LBW offspring or offspring associated with maternal prenatal stress, although LBW may well result in significant impairment in offspring infectious disease–related immune function.** The consequences of LBW and reduced immune function may be a critical factor that predisposes to infant mortality in developing countries.

Much as perinatal factors can influence immunity, mothers who are allergic have lower interferon-γ responses during pregnancy, which has been postulated to influence the cytokine milieu of the fetus.[76] Similarly, maternal asthma during pregnancy is associated with fetal growth restriction and preterm birth. Placental expression of proinflammatory placental cytokines is significantly increased in pregnancies complicated by mild asthma, although only in the presence of a female fetus.[77] Significant evidence shows that **both the maternal allergic phenotype and the maternal environmental exposures during pregnancy affect the risk of subsequent allergic disease in childhood.** Evidence indicates that maternal allergy is a recognized risk factor for allergic disease. In regard to maternal environmental exposures, a number of factors may influence fetal immune development and allergic outcomes. Although evidence is inconsistent and mechanisms are unclear, several studies have demonstrated that a Mediterranean diet may protect against early childhood wheezing.[78] Other studies have explored the effects of folate supplementation, polyunsaturated fatty acids, antioxidants, and a range of vitamins and micronutrients, although again with a lack of consistency.

Interestingly, recent evidence suggests that **maternal exposure to microbials may influence fetal immune competence.** Exposure in utero to a farming environment has been demonstrated to protect against the development of childhood asthma and eczema.[79] Similar results have demonstrated that farming environments alter the expression of innate immune genes and modify umbilical cord IgE levels. Some studies,[80,81] although not all,[82,83] suggest an association between cesarean delivery and chronic immune disorders, particularly childhood asthma. Because the newborn GI flora is markedly affected by elective cesarean delivery, it is possible that changes in the microbiome may influence early development or maturation of diverse immune systems.

In contrast to the potential beneficial effect of microbial exposure, maternal cigarette smoking increases the risk of asthma in the offspring. This likely occurs via an allergic sensitization rather than by the classic direct pulmonary effects of cigarette smoke. Animal studies also support the premise that innate immune function can be programmed as a result of perinatal challenges to the immune system during development. In rats, administration of bacterial endotoxin, lipopolysaccharide (LPS), to neonates influences the adult neuroimmune response to a second LPS challenge, in part through the HPA axis.[84] In addition, undernutrition—particularly during prenatal and postnatal periods—affects immune competence of offspring by increasing basal inflammation and also reducing cytokine induction in response to inflammatory stimuli.

Potentially confounding the association of cigarette smoking is a finding that children with a smaller head circumference at 10 to 15 days of age had a markedly increased odds ratio for wheezing at 7 years of age. Thus **factors that determine fetal growth may also be associated with wheezing in childhood.** Children with both small and large head circumferences at birth, consistent with both undernutrition and overnutrition, have increased atopic sensitization and elevated serum IgE at ages 5 to 7 years.[85] Large head circumference at birth has previously been reported to be marked by elevated IgG levels in adulthood and a risk of asthma in adolescence. The relationship of developmental origins to childhood asthma is complex because several asthma phenotypes are possible, including those associated with atopy compared with those associated with acute childhood viral infection. Although both of these diseases exhibit childhood wheezing and/or immune modulation, they likely have significant alterations in predisposition. Because asthma is associated with an exaggerated type 2 helper T cell (TH2) response to both allergic and nonallergic stimuli, it has been proposed that genes involved in IgE synthesis and airway remodeling have failed to be silenced during early infancy. In utero programming of these genes may result in the predisposition to allergic responses.

OTHER PROGRAMMING
Endocrine Programming
Low birthweight may also be associated with additional endocrine disorders that affect gonadal and adrenal axes. **Reduced fetal growth results in exaggerated adrenarche, early puberty, and small ovarian size with the subsequent development of ovarian hyperandrogenism.**[86] Children born SGA may have puberty at a normal age or even earlier but appear to exhibit a more rapid progression, which compromises adult ovarian function.[87] Compared with average for gestational age (AGA) girls, SGA girls displayed increased baseline estradiol, stimulated estradiol, and 17-hydroxyprogesterone at the beginning of puberty, whereas LBW is associated with precocious puberty in girls.[86] Among LBW girls, those who demonstrate postnatal catch-up growth have greater fat mass and more central fat. Whether this suggests that early puberty is a consequence of hyperandrogenism or hyperinsulinism associated with the central adiposity is uncertain. Importantly, **children who present with precocious puberty, particularly those with a history of LBW, have an increased risk of developing ovarian hyperandrogenism and other features of polycystic ovary syndrome (PCOS) during or soon after menarche.**[86] Growth restriction may thus program adrenal function and induce permanent changes in ovarian morphology and function in utero, contributing to PCOS in adult life.

Despite the association with PCOS, women born during a famine do not appear to have differences in fertility rates as measured by age at first pregnancy, completed family size, and interpregnancy interval. Recent studies have suggested that the cohort of offspring from the Dutch famine may even have an increased fertility compared with controls.[88] Furthermore, despite the impact on puberty, **LBW does not appear to advance the age of menopause in women.**[89] There is evidence, however, of an increased prevalence of anovulation in adolescent girls born SGA compared with controls (40% vs. 4%),[90] although this may be a consequence of obesity-associated endocrine perturbations. These findings suggest that the effects of maternal nutritional status during pregnancy on reproductive performance of offspring are relatively small.

In the female rat, pubertal timing and subsequent ovarian function is influenced by the animal's nutritional status in utero, with both maternal caloric restriction and a high-fat maternal diet resulting in the early onset of puberty. However, the former leads to a reduction in progesterone levels, whereas the latter causes elevated progesterone concentrations in adult offspring. In sheep, reduced lifetime reproductive capacity has been demonstrated in ewes born to mothers undernourished during late pregnancy or in the first months of life. Similarly, in rodents, maternal undernutrition causes premature reproductive senescence via alteration of the hypothalamic-pituitary-gonadal axis,[91] whereas maternal obesity and a high-fat diet result in increased ovarian apoptosis and follicular growth in the adult offspring.[92] Prenatal exposure to testosterone impairs female reproductive capacity in sheep, and prepubertal administration of estradiol disrupts ovarian cyclicity in adult rats. Furthermore, animals that receive an excess of thyroxine during the neonatal period exhibit changes in the pituitary-hypothalamic responses linked to the secretion of thyroid-stimulating hormone (TSH) in later life.

Sexuality Programming
The following discussion is not meant to imply disease states or opine on issues of normalcy of sexuality but rather to discuss the developmental processes that result in adult sexual orientation. Among males, sexual orientation is largely dichotomous (heterosexual, homosexual), although bisexual orientation among women is likely more prevalent. A genetic component for sexual orientation is evident from studies that demonstrate an increased rate of homosexuality among relatives of homosexuals. Twin studies report moderate hereditability of sexual orientation,[93] although advances have been limited in the identification of specific genetic loci responsible for sexual orientation. **Significant research demonstrates a major role for gonadal steroidal androgens in regulating sexual dimorphism in the brain and subsequent behavior.** Animal studies confirm that hormonal signals that operate during critical periods may have programming effects on sexuality. The classic example of such a phenomenon is the exposure of female rats at a critical period of fetal life to a single exogenous dose of testosterone, which permanently reoriented sexual behavior. A similar dose of testosterone in 20-day-old females had no effect. Thus, a critical time exists at which the animal's sexual physiology is sensitive and can be permanently changed.[94] Based upon early animal models, initial studies resulted in what is likely an oversimplified theory: relative overexposure of females to androgens may contribute to female homosexuality, and underexposure to prenatal androgens in men may contribute to male homosexuality. Using a proxy marker of prenatal hormonal androgen exposure, the ratio of the second to fourth finger lengths, several studies have demonstrated that homosexual women have

significantly masculine measurements compared with heterosexual women, although one study reported no difference. A further proxy marker is otoacoustic emissions (OAEs), which represent sounds emitted by the cochlea, which are more numerous in females than in males. Significant evidence suggests that OAEs are influenced by prenatal androgen exposure, with evidence that females with male co-twins have a masculinized OAE pattern. Despite the tendency for homosexual women to be exposed to more prenatal androgens than heterosexual women, overlap is considerable between the two female groups, indicating that prenatal androgens do not act in isolation.[95] Reports among heterosexual and homosexual men are inconclusive in regard to proxy markers.

In contrast to the stronger correlation of female versus male homosexuality with measures of prenatal androgen exposure, birth order impacts more significantly among males. The *fraternal birth order effect* indicates that homosexual men have a greater number of older brothers than heterosexual men do, with the estimated odds of being homosexual increasing by 33% with each older brother.[95] Of note, homosexual males with older brothers have significantly lower birthweights compared with heterosexual males with older brothers.[96] These findings may suggest an interaction of birthweight and additional developmental factors. Several investigators have proposed a role of immunization of mothers to male-linked androgens, which results in maternal Y-chromosome linked antibodies that may act on male-differentiating receptors within the fetal brain.[91] Further studies demonstrate sexual orientation–related neuronal variation that includes hypothalamic and selected cortical regions. Despite these associations, **little conclusive understanding exists of specific neurodevelopmental mechanisms that produce homosexuality or heterosexuality.** However, emerging evidence suggests that prenatal exposure to EDCs affects neural circuits at the hypothalamus-pituitary axis, impacts fetal testicular development, masculinizes genitalia in females, feminizes yolk production (vitellogenesis) in males, and alters sex and social behavior.[97]

Renal Programming

In humans, the total number of nephrons ranges between approximately 600,000 and slightly over one million, although the factors that determine an individual's glomerular number are unknown. Nephrogenesis occurs up to approximately 36 weeks' gestation, and both genetic and environmental effects alter or regulate the number of nephrons. From a genetic perspective, **select genes that regulate renal signaling and transcription permutation have been associated with renal hypoplasia. Thus most congenital renal anomalies have an inheritable component.**

Environmental exposures and stresses are well demonstrated to alter nephron number. Autopsies of newborns and children have demonstrated a marked association between LBW and reduced nephron number.[98] Importantly, **low glomerular number and high glomerular size have been associated with the development of hypertension, cardiovascular diseases, and an increased susceptibility to renal disease in later life.** Reduced nephron number as a result of developmental programming may result in single nephron glomerular hyperfiltration. The compensatory glomerular hypertrophy, which maintains normal glomerular filtration rate (GFR), ultimately may cause glomerular sclerosis and nephron loss and can contribute to later hypertension and chronic renal disease.

Reduced nephron number beginning in the fetal/neonatal period may have effects different from that of adult nephrectomy. In sheep, fetal unilateral nephrectomy at 110 days gestation leads to subsequent hypertension.[99] Similarly, unilateral nephrectomy in the neonatal rat results in adult hypertension and impaired renal function. These findings differ from observations after human nephrectomy performed in adults (e.g., renal transplant donors), in whom hypertension generally does develop. The mechanisms that contribute to hypertension resulting from reduced glomerular number that occurs during fetal and neonatal life are unclear, but they indicate that **the developmental impact on nephron number may play an important role in programmed hypertension.** These include the role of specific genes and growth factors involved in this process, the paired box 2 gene (*PAX2*) and glial cell–derived neurotropic factor (GDNF) as well as apoptotic markers and signaling pathways.

In view of the contribution of renal disease to hypertension, it is notable that **very LBW infants exhibit a high rate of hypertension during adolescence.**[100] Preterm children also demonstrate a higher prevalence of hypertension, as do AGA and SGA offspring.[101] Among black Americans in the southeastern United States and among Australian aboriginals, LBW is associated with adult-onset renal disease.[98] As a marker of impending renal disease, microalbuminuria is more than twofold greater in SGA offspring at a young adult age than that occurring in AGA offspring, although not all studies demonstrate this effect. Nutritional insults seen in SGA, LBW, and premature births are perhaps associated with excess glucocorticoid exposure and secondarily reduced glomerular number. Paradoxically, autopsy studies indicate that the number of renal podocytes in full-term newborns is significantly lower than in preterm fetuses. It is unknown whether this is a pathologic process related to continued adverse exposures (e.g., drugs, maternal diet) during intrauterine life that results in renal podocyte demise or a normal physiologic process (e.g., apoptosis).

Pregnant patients are also exposed to a variety of **nephrotoxic drugs, including nonsteroidal antiinflammatory drugs (NSAIDs), ampicillin/penicillin, and aminoglycosides. NSAIDs may lead to renal hypoperfusion during critical nephrogenic periods, resulting in cystic changes in developing nephrons**[102] and acute or chronic renal failure in preterm newborns. The impairment in renal development that results from angiotensin-converting enzyme (ACE) inhibitors is well documented, likely a result of the critical role of angiotensin in nephrogenesis.

Although less is known regarding offspring of pregnancies complicated by diabetes, exposure to transiently high blood glucose concentrations may reduce nephron development in rat pups. In humans, increased urinary albumin excretion has been demonstrated in adult offspring of Pima Indian mothers with diabetes, suggesting an early glomerular injury.[103] Notably, individuals with a history of hypertension had only 50% as many nephrons as those without hypertension.[104] The nephron number in adult kidneys is correlated to birthweight, with each kilogram increase in birthweight associated with an additional 250,000 nephrons.[98] However, these studies could not differentiate age or disease-related loss of nephrons compared with developmental origins. Reduced nephron number has been demonstrated in the absence of hypertension, indicating that additional processes of programmed hypertension may occur independently of a reduction in nephron number. **Whether a reduced nephron** number is etiologic of hypertension, a consequence of hypertension, or a coincident finding may depend upon the individual.

SUMMARY

As we continue to learn of the significance and mechanisms of developmental programming of adult health and disease, the critical consequences of developmental windows are increasingly recognized. Programming effects may affect development by altering organ size, structure, or function. Cellular signaling mechanisms and increasingly recognized epigenetic consequences may be highly dependent upon the magnitude of the exposure and the window of exposure during embryogenesis or organogenesis. Most importantly, we are only beginning to recognize how consequences of prophylactic treatments may alter programmed phenotypes. Certainly, it appears there is no single mechanism, nor one single developmental window, that affects each organ or system development. Consequently, the ultimate management of fetuses and newborns is likely to be individualized rather than universal. We hope to develop a greater understanding of the relative risks and benefits of current day obstetric decisions, including repeated doses of maternal glucocorticoids, advantages versus disadvantages of early delivery of SGA fetuses, use of oral hypoglycemic agents that cross the placenta, and many other management dilemmas.

KEY POINTS

- Maternal influences on the in utero environment (nutrition, hormonal, metabolic, stress, environmental toxins, and drugs) are critical determinants of fetal growth and influence a wide variety of metabolic, developmental, and pathologic processes in adulthood.
- Both ends of the growth spectrum (i.e., both low and high birthweight) are associated with increased risk of adult obesity, metabolic syndrome, cardiovascular disease, insulin resistance, and neuroendocrine disorders.
- The mechanisms that link early developmental events to the later manifestation of disease states involve "programmed" changes in organ structure, cellular responses, gene expression, the epigenome, and/or stem cells.
- Gestational programming events may have immediate effects or are deferred and expressed at a later age, with potential transmission to multiple generations.
- Transmission of gestational programming effects to multiple generations may occur via epigenomic modulation that causes heritable and persistent changes in gene expression without altering the DNA sequence.
- Prenatal care is evolving to provide essential goals of optimizing maternal, fetal, and neonatal health to prevent or reduce adult-onset diseases.
- Guiding policy regarding optimal pregnancy nutrition and weight gain, management of low and high fetal-weight pregnancies, use of maternal glucocorticoids, and newborn feeding strategies, among others, have yet to comprehensively integrate the long-term consequences on adult health.

REFERENCES

1. Stephens TD, Bunde CJ, Fillmore BJ. Mechanism of action in thalidomide teratogenesis. *Biochem Pharmacol.* 2000;59(12):1489-1499.
2. Dieckmann WJ, Davis ME, Rynkiewicz LM, Pottinger RE. Does the administration of diethylstilbestrol during pregnancy have therapeutic value? *Am J Obstet Gynecol.* 1953;66(5):1062-1081.
3. Bromer JG, Wu J, Zhou Y, Taylor HS. Hypermethylation of homeobox A10 by in utero diethylstilbestrol exposure: an epigenetic mechanism for altered developmental programming. *Endocrinol.* 2009;150(7):3376-3382.
4. Cosgrove MS. Histone proteomics and the epigenetic regulation of nucleosome mobility. *Expert Rev Proteomics.* 2007;4(4):465-478.
5. Higgs PG, Lehman N. The RNA world: molecular cooperation at the origins of life. *Nat Rev Genet.* 2015;16(1):7-17.
6. Skinner MK. What is an epigenetic transgenerational phenotype? F3 or F2. *Reprod Toxicol.* 2008;25(1):2-6.
7. Waterland RA. Is epigenetics an important link between early life events and adult disease? *Horm Res.* 2009;71(suppl 1):13-16.
8. Hales CN, Barker DJ. Type 2 (non-insulin-dependent) diabetes mellitus: the thrifty phenotype hypothesis. *Diabetologia.* 1992;35(7):595-601.
9. Dewey KG. Is breastfeeding protective against child obesity? *J Hum Lact.* 2003;19(1):9-18.
10. Desai M, Gayle D, Babu J, Ross MG. Programmed obesity in intrauterine growth-restricted newborns: modulation by newborn nutrition. *Am J Physiol Regul Integr Comp Physiol.* 2005;288(1):R91-R96.
11. Desai M, Jellyman JK, Han G, Beall M, Lane RH, Ross MG. Maternal obesity and high-fat diet program offspring metabolic syndrome. *Am J Obstet Gynecol.* 2014;211(3):237.
12. Ranjit N, Siefert K, Padmanabhan V. Bisphenol-A and disparities in birth outcomes: a review and directions for future research. *J Perinatol.* 2010;30(1):2-9.
13. Taylor JA, vom Saal FS, Welshons WV, et al. Similarity of bisphenol A pharmacokinetics in rhesus monkeys and mice: relevance for human exposure. *Environ Health Perspect.* 2011;119(4):422-430.
14. Harley KG, Aguilar SR, Chevrier J, et al. Prenatal and postnatal bisphenol A exposure and body mass index in childhood in the CHAMACOS cohort. *Environ Health Perspect.* 2013;121(4):514-520.
15. Lee DH, Lee IK, Jin SH, Steffes M, Jacobs DR Jr. Association between serum concentrations of persistent organic pollutants and insulin resistance among nondiabetic adults: results from the National Health and Nutrition Examination Survey 1999-2002. *Diabetes Care.* 2007;30(3):622-628.
16. Perera F, Vishnevetsky J, Herbstman JB, et al. Prenatal bisphenol A exposure and child behavior in an inner-city cohort. *Environ Health Perspect.* 2012;120(8):1190-1194.
17. Somm E, Schwitzgebel VM, Toulotte A, et al. Perinatal exposure to bisphenol A alters early adipogenesis in the rat. *Environ Health Perspect.* 2009;117(10):1549-1555.
18. Komada M, Asai Y, Morii M, Matsuki M, Sato M, Nagao T. Maternal bisphenol A oral dosing relates to the acceleration of neurogenesis in the developing neocortex of mouse fetuses. *Toxicology.* 2012;295(1-3):31-38.
19. Bouret SG, Draper SJ, Simerly RB. Trophic action of leptin on hypothalamic neurons that regulate feeding. *Science.* 2004;304(5667):108-110.
20. Yousheng J, Nguyen T, Desai M, Ross MG. Programmed alterations in hypothalamic neuronal orexigenic responses to ghrelin following gestational nutrient restriction. *Reprod Sci.* 2008;15(7):702-709.
21. Desai M, Gayle D, Han G, Ross MG. Programmed hyperphagia due to reduced anorexigenic mechanisms in intrauterine growth-restricted offspring. *Reprod Sci.* 2007;14(4):329-337.
22. Desai M, Li T, Ross MG. Hypothalamic neurosphere progenitor cells in low birth weight rat newborns: neurotrophic effects of leptin and insulin. *Brain Res.* 2011;1378:29-42.
23. Desai M, Guang H, Ferelli M, Kallichanda N, Lane RH. Programmed upregulation of adipogenic transcription factors in intrauterine growth-restricted offspring. *Reprod Sci.* 2008;15(8):785-796.
24. Yee JK, Lee WN, Ross MG, et al. Peroxisome proliferator-activated receptor gamma modulation and lipogenic response in adipocytes of small-for-gestational age offspring. *Nutr Metab (Lond).* 2012;9(1):62.
25. Kirchner S, Kieu T, Chow C, Casey S, Blumberg B. Prenatal exposure to the environmental obesogen tributyltin predisposes multipotent stem cells to become adipocytes. *Mol Endocrinol.* 2010;24(3):526-539.
26. Guberman C, Jellyman JK, Han G, Ross MG, Desai M. Maternal high-fat diet programs rat offspring hypertension and activates the adipose renin-angiotensin system. *Am J Obstet Gynecol.* 2013;209(3):262-268.

27. Barker DJ, Meade TW, et al. Relation of fetal and infant growth to plasma fibrinogen and factor VII concentrations in adult life. *BMJ*. 1992;304(6820):148-152.

28. Burns SP, Desai M, Cohen RD, et al. Gluconeogenesis, glucose handling, and structural changes in livers of the adult offspring of rats partially deprived of protein during pregnancy and lactation. *J Clin Invest*. 1997;100(7):1768-1774.

29. Seo YS, Kim JH, Jo NY, et al. PPAR agonists treatment is effective in a nonalcoholic fatty liver disease animal model by modulating fatty-acid metabolic enzymes. *J Gastroenterol Hepatol*. 2008;23(1):102-109.

30. Kleemann R, Verschuren L, de Rooij BJ, et al. Evidence for anti-inflammatory activity of statins and PPARalpha activators in human C-reactive protein transgenic mice in vivo and in cultured human hepatocytes in vitro. *Blood*. 2004;103(11):4188-4194.

31. Magee TR, Han G, Cherian B, Khorram O, Ross MG, Desai M. Down-regulation of transcription factor peroxisome proliferator-activated receptor in programmed hepatic lipid dysregulation and inflammation in intrauterine growth-restricted offspring. *Am J Obstet Gynecol*. 2008; 199(3):271-275.

32. Wolfe D, Gong M, Han G, Magee TR, Ross MG, Desai M. Nutrient sensor-mediated programmed nonalcoholic fatty liver disease in low birth-weight offspring. *Am J Obstet Gynecol*. 2012;207(4):308.e1-308.e6.

33. Borengasser SJ, Kang P, Faske J, et al. High fat diet and in utero exposure to maternal obesity disrupts circadian rhythm and leads to metabolic programming of liver in rat offspring. *PLoS ONE*. 2014;9(1):e84209.

34. Economides DL, Proudler A, Nicolaides KH. Plasma insulin in appropriate- and small-for-gestational-age fetuses. *Am J Obstet Gynecol*. 1989; 160(5 Pt 1):1091-1094.

35. Phillips DI, Barker DJ, Hales CN, Hirst S, Osmond C. Thinness at birth and insulin resistance in adult life. *Diabetologia*. 1994;37(2):150-154.

36. Hales CN, Barker DJ, Clark PM, et al. Fetal and infant growth and impaired glucose tolerance at age 64. *BMJ*. 1991;303(6809):1019-1022.

37. Dalziel SR, Walker NK, Parag V, et al. Cardiovascular risk factors after antenatal exposure to betamethasone: 30-year follow-up of a randomised controlled trial. *Lancet*. 2005;365(9474):1856-1862.

38. Dessens AB, Haas HS, Koppe JG. Twenty-year follow-up of antenatal corticosteroid treatment. *Pediatrics*. 2000;105(6):E77.

39. Reusens B, Remacle C. Programming of the endocrine pancreas by the early nutritional environment. *Int J Biochem Cell Biol*. 2006;38(5-6):913-922.

40. Ford SP, Zhang L, Zhu M, et al. Maternal obesity accelerates fetal pancreatic beta-cell but not alpha-cell development in sheep: prenatal consequences. *Am J Physiol Regul Integr Comp Physiol*. 2009;297(3):R835-R843.

41. Aerts L, Van Assche FA. Animal evidence for the transgenerational development of diabetes mellitus. *Int J Biochem Cell Biol*. 2006;38(5-6): 894-903.

42. Frantz ED, Peixoto-Silva N, Pinheiro-Mulder A. Endocrine pancreas development: effects of metabolic and intergenerational programming caused by a protein-restricted diet. *Pancreas*. 2012;41(1):1-9.

43. Ding GL, Huang HF. Paternal transgenerational glucose intolerance with epigenetic alterations in second generation offspring of GDM. *Asian J Androl*. 2013;15(4):451-452.

44. Werner JC, Sicard RE, Hansen TW, Solomon E, Cowett RM, Oh W. Hypertrophic cardiomyopathy associated with dexamethasone therapy for bronchopulmonary dysplasia. *J Pediatr*. 1992;120(2 Pt 1):286-291.

45. Barker DJ. Fetal programming of coronary heart disease. *Trends Endocrinol Metab*. 2002;13(9):364-368.

46. Eriksson JG, Forsen TJ, Kajantie E, Osmond C, Barker DJ. Childhood growth and hypertension in later life. *Hypertension*. 2007;49(6): 1415-1421.

47. Desai M, Gayle D, Babu J, Ross MG. The timing of nutrient restriction during rat pregnancy/lactation alters metabolic syndrome phenotype. *Am J Obstet Gynecol*. 2007;196(6):555-557.

48. Khorram O, Momeni M, Ferrini M, Desai M, Ross MG. In utero undernutrition in rats induces increased vascular smooth muscle content in the offspring. *Am J Obstet Gynecol*. 2007;196(5):486-488.

49. Tauzin L. Alterations in viscoelastic properties following premature birth may lead to hypertension and cardiovascular disease development in later life. *Acta Paediatr*. 2015;104(1):19-26.

50. Schuetze P, Eiden RD. The association between maternal cocaine use during pregnancy and physiological regulation in 4- to 8-week-old infants: an examination of possible mediators and moderators. *J Pediatr Psychol*. 2006;31(1):15-26.

51. Papamatheakis DG, Blood AB, Kim JH, Wilson SM. Antenatal hypoxia and pulmonary vascular function and remodeling. *Curr Vasc Pharmacol*. 2013;11(5):616-640.

52. Ramakrishnan S, Anand V, Roy S. Vascular endothelial growth factor signaling in hypoxia and inflammation. *J Neuroimmune Pharmacol*. 2014;9(2):142-160.

53. Patterson AJ, Zhang L. Hypoxia and fetal heart development. *Curr Mol Med*. 2010;10(7):653-666.

54. Cooper C, Eriksson JG, Forsen T, Osmond C, Tuomilehto J, Barker DJ. Maternal height, childhood growth and risk of hip fracture in later life: a longitudinal study. *Osteoporos Int*. 2001;12(8):623-629.

55. Godfrey K, Walker-Bone K, Robinson S, et al. Neonatal bone mass: influence of parental birthweight, maternal smoking, body composition, and activity during pregnancy. *J Bone Miner Res*. 2001;16(9):1694-1703.

56. Lester BM, Lagasse LL. Children of addicted women. *J Addict Dis*. 2010;29(2):259-276.

57. Smith LM, Chang L, Yonekura ML, et al. Brain proton magnetic resonance spectroscopy and imaging in children exposed to cocaine in utero. *Pediatrics*. 2001;107(2):227-231.

58. Smith LM, Chang L, Yonekura ML, Grob C, Osborn D, Ernst T. Brain proton magnetic resonance spectroscopy in children exposed to methamphetamine in utero. *Neurology*. 2001;57(2):255-260.

59. Slotkin TA. Fetal nicotine or cocaine exposure: which one is worse? *J Pharmacol Exp Ther*. 1998;285(3):931-945.

60. Yehuda R, Teicher MH, Seckl JR, Grossman RA, Morris A, Bierer LM. Parental posttraumatic stress disorder as a vulnerability factor for low cortisol trait in offspring of holocaust survivors. *Arch Gen Psychiatry*. 2007;64(9):1040-1048.

61. Dy J, Guan H, Sampath-Kumar R, Richardson BS, Yang K. Placental 11beta-hydroxysteroid dehydrogenase type 2 is reduced in pregnancies complicated with idiopathic intrauterine growth restriction: evidence that this is associated with an attenuated ratio of cortisone to cortisol in the umbilical artery. *Placenta*. 2008;29(2):193-200.

62. Moisiadis VG, Matthews SG. Glucocorticoids and fetal programming part 2: Mechanisms. *Nat Rev Endocrinol*. 2014;10(7):403-411.

63. Mesquita AR, Wegerich Y, Patchev AV, et al. Glucocorticoids and neuro- and behavioural development. *Semin Fetal Neonatal Med*. 2009;14(3): 130-135.

64. Hirvikoski T, Nordenstrom A, Lindholm T, et al. Cognitive functions in children at risk for congenital adrenal hyperplasia treated prenatally with dexamethasone. *J Clin Endocrinol Metab*. 2007;92(2):542-548.

65. Clark PM, Hindmarsh PC, Shiell AW, Law CM, Honour JW, Barker DJ. Size at birth and adrenocortical function in childhood. *Clin Endocrinol (Oxf)*. 1996;45(6):721-726.

66. Nilsson PM, Nyberg P, Ostergren PO. Increased susceptibility to stress at a psychological assessment of stress tolerance is associated with impaired fetal growth. *Int J Epidemiol*. 2001;30(1):75-80.

67. McCormick CM, Mathews IZ, Thomas C, Waters P. Investigations of HPA function and the enduring consequences of stressors in adolescence in animal models. *Brain Cogn*. 2010;72(1):73-85.

68. Sullivan EL, Grayson B, Takahashi D, et al. Chronic consumption of a high-fat diet during pregnancy causes perturbations in the serotonergic system and increased anxiety-like behavior in nonhuman primate offspring. *J Neurosci*. 2010;30(10):3826-3830.

69. French NP, Hagan R, Evans SF, Mullan A, Newnham JP. Repeated antenatal corticosteroids: effects on cerebral palsy and childhood behavior. *Am J Obstet Gynecol*. 2004;190(3):588-595.

70. Davis EP, Townsend EL, Gunnar MR, et al. Effects of prenatal betamethasone exposure on regulation of stress physiology in healthy premature infants. *Psychoneuroendocrinology*. 2004;29(8):1028-1036.

71. Raikkonen K, Pesonen AK, Heinonen K, et al. Maternal licorice consumption and detrimental cognitive and psychiatric outcomes in children. *Am J Epidemiol*. 2009;170(9):1137-1146.

72. Pouta A, Hartikainen AL, Sovio U, et al. Manifestations of metabolic syndrome after hypertensive pregnancy. *Hypertension*. 2004;43(4):825-831.

73. Costello EJ, Worthman C, Erkanli A, Angold A. Prediction from low birth weight to female adolescent depression: a test of competing hypotheses. *Arch Gen Psychiatry*. 2007;64(3):338-344.

74. Coussons-Read ME, Okun ML, Nettles CD. Psychosocial stress increases inflammatory markers and alters cytokine production across pregnancy. *Brain Behav Immun*. 2007;21(3):343-350.

75. Hartwig IR, Sly PD, Schmidt LA, et al. Prenatal adverse life events increase the risk for atopic diseases in children, which is enhanced in the absence of a maternal atopic predisposition. *J Allergy Clin Immunol*. 2014;134(1): 160-169.

76. Breckler LA, Hale J, Taylor A, Dunstan JA, Thornton CA, Prescott SL. Pregnancy IFN-gamma responses to foetal alloantigens are altered by maternal allergy and gravidity status. *Allergy*. 2008;63(11):1473-1480.

77. Scott NM, Hodyl NA, Murphy VE, et al. Placental cytokine expression covaries with maternal asthma severity and fetal sex. *J Immunol.* 2009;182(3):1411-1420.

78. Shaheen SO, Northstone K, Newson RB, Emmett PM, Sherriff A, Henderson AJ. Dietary patterns in pregnancy and respiratory and atopic outcomes in childhood. *Thorax.* 2009;64(5):411-417.

79. Douwes J, Cheng S, Travier N, et al. Farm exposure in utero may protect against asthma, hay fever and eczema. *Eur Respir J.* 2008;32(3):603-611.

80. van Berkel AC, den Dekker HT, Jaddoe VW, et al. Mode of delivery and childhood fractional exhaled nitric oxide, interrupter resistance, and asthma: The Generation R Study. *Pediatr Allergy Immunol.* 2015;26(4):330-336.

81. Sevelsted A, Stokholm J, Bonnelykke K, Bisgaard H. Cesarean section and chronic immune disorders. *Pediatrics.* 2015;135(1):e92-e98.

82. Bruske I, Pei Z, Thiering E, et al. Caesarean section has no impact on lung function at the age of 15 years. *Pediatr Pulmonol.* 2015. [Epub ahead of print].

83. Leung JY, Li AM, Leung GM, Schooling CM. Mode of delivery and childhood hospitalizations for asthma and other wheezing disorders. *Clin Exp Allergy.* 2015;45(6):1109-1117.

84. Spencer SJ, Galic MA, Pittman QJ. Neonatal programming of innate immune function. *Am J Physiol Endocrinol Metab.* 2011;300(1):E11-E18.

85. Bolte G, Schmidt M, Maziak W, et al. The relation of markers of fetal growth with asthma, allergies and serum immunoglobulin E levels in children at age 5-7 years. *Clin Exp Allergy.* 2004;34(3):381-388.

86. Ibáñez L, Potau N, Francois I, de Zegher F. Precocious pubarche, hyperinsulinism, and ovarian hyperandrogenism in girls: relation to reduced fetal growth. *J Clin Endocrinol Metab.* 1998;83(10):3558-3562.

87. Lazar L, Pollak U, Kalter-Leibovici O, Pertzelan A, Phillip M. Pubertal course of persistently short children born small for gestational age (SGA) compared with idiopathic short children born appropriate for gestational age (AGA). *Eur J Endocrinol.* 2003;149(5):425-432.

88. Painter RC, Westendorp RG, de Rooij SR, Osmond C, Barker DJ, Roseboom TJ. Increased reproductive success of women after prenatal undernutrition. *Hum Reprod.* 2008;23(11):2591-2595.

89. Cresswell JL, Egger P, Fall CH, Osmond C, Fraser RB, Barker DJ. Is the age of menopause determined in-utero? *Early Hum Dev.* 1997;49(2):143-148.

90. Ibáñez L, Potau N, Ferrer A, et al. Reduced ovulation rate in adolescent girls born small for gestational age. *J Clin Endocrinol Metab.* 2002;87(7):3391-3393.

91. Khorram O, Keen-Rinehart E, Chuang TD, Ross MG, Desai M. Maternal undernutrition induces premature reproductive senescence in adult female rat offspring. *Fertil Steril.* 2015;103(1):291-298.

92. Cheong Y, Sadek KH, Bruce KD, Macklon N, Cagampang FR. Diet-induced maternal obesity alters ovarian morphology and gene expression in the adult mouse offspring. *Fertil Steril.* 2014;102(3):899-907.

93. Kirk KM, Bailey JM, Dunne MP, Martin NG. Measurement models for sexual orientation in a community twin sample. *Behav Genet.* 2000;30(4):345-356.

94. Angelbeck JH, DuBrul EF. The effect of neonatal testosterone on specific male and female patterns of phosphorylated cytosolic proteins in the rat preoptic-hypothalamus, cortex and amygdala. *Brain Res.* 1983;264(2):277-283.

95. Rahman Q. The neurodevelopment of human sexual orientation. *Neurosci Biobehav Rev.* 2005;29(7):1057-1066.

96. Blanchard R, Zucker KJ, Cavacas A, Allin S, Bradley SJ, Schachter DC. Fraternal birth order and birth weight in probably prehomosexual feminine boys. *Horm Behav.* 2002;41(3):321-327.

97. Schneider JE, Brozek JM, Keen-Rinehart E. Our stolen figures: the interface of sexual differentiation, endocrine disruptors, maternal programming, and energy balance. *Horm Behav.* 2014;66(1):104-119.

98. Hughson M, Farris AB III, Douglas-Denton R, Hoy WE, Bertram JF. Glomerular number and size in autopsy kidneys: the relationship to birth weight. *Kidney Int.* 2003;63(6):2113-2122.

99. Moritz KM, Wintour EM, Dodic M. Fetal uninephrectomy leads to postnatal hypertension and compromised renal function. *Hypertension.* 2002;39(6):1071-1076.

100. Rodriguez-Soriano J, Aguirre M, Oliveros R, Vallo A. Long-term renal follow-up of extremely low birth weight infants. *Pediatr Nephrol.* 2005;20(5):579-584.

101. Puddu M, Podda MF, Mussap M, Tumbarello R, Fanos V. Early detection of microalbuminuria and hypertension in children of very low birthweight. *J Matern Fetal Neonatal Med.* 2009;22(2):83-88.

102. van der Heijden BJ, Carlus C, Narcy F, Bavoux F, Delezoide AL, Gubler MC. Persistent anuria, neonatal death, and renal microcystic lesions after prenatal exposure to indomethacin. *Am J Obstet Gynecol.* 1994;171(3):617-623.

103. Nelson RG, Morgenstern H, Bennett PH. Intrauterine diabetes exposure and the risk of renal disease in diabetic Pima Indians. *Diabetes.* 1998;47(9):1489-1493.

104. Keller G, Zimmer G, Mall G, Ritz E, Amann K. Nephron number in patients with primary hypertension. *N Engl J Med.* 2003;348(2):101-108.

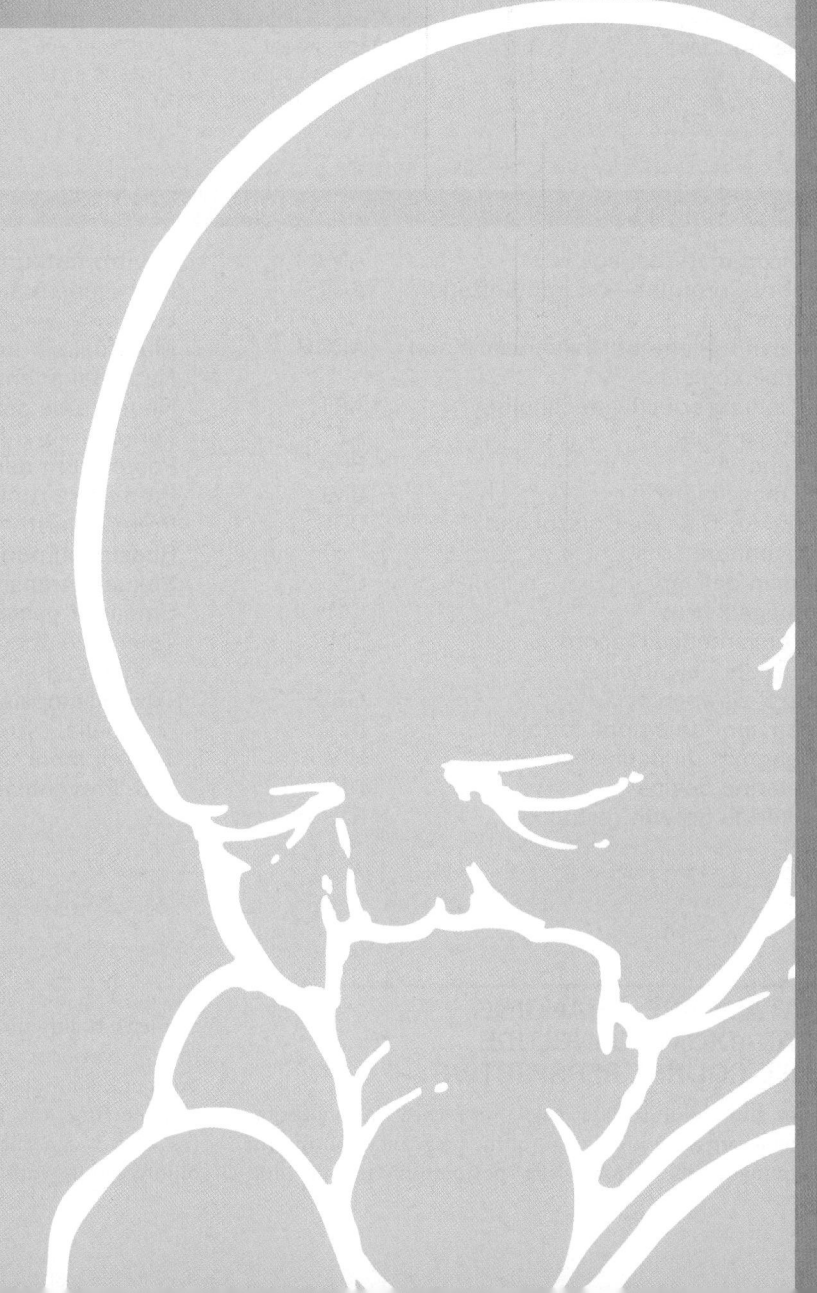

Prenatal Care

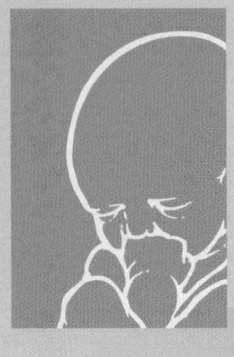

CHAPTER 6

Preconception and Prenatal Care

KIMBERLY D. GREGORY, DIANA E. RAMOS, and ERIC R.M. JAUNIAUX

KEY ABBREVIATIONS

Advanced maternal age	AMA	In vitro fertilization	IVF
Advisory Committee on Immunization Practices	ACIP	Last menstrual period	LMP
		Low birthweight	LBW
American College of Obstetricians and Gynecologists	ACOG	Maternal serum alpha-fetoprotein	MSAFP
		Neonatal intensive care unit	NICU
Artificial reproductive technology	ART	Neural tube defect	NTD
Azidothymidine	AZT	Peripherally inserted central catheter	PICC
Bisphenol A	BPA	Postpartum hemorrhage	PPH
Body mass index	BMI	Premature rupture of the membranes	PROM
Centers for Disease Control and Prevention	CDC	Preterm birth	PTB
		Rhesus immune globulin	RhIG
Cesarean delivery	CD	Sexually transmitted infections	STIs
Cytomegalovirus	CMV	Small for gestational age	SGA
Electronic medical record	EMR	Tolerance-annoyance, cut-down, eye-opener	T-ACE
Fetal alcohol syndrome	FAS		
Group B *Streptococcus*	GBS	Toxoplasmosis, other infections, rubella, cytomegalovirus, herpes	TORCH
Human chorionic gonadotropin	hCG		
Human immunodeficiency virus	HIV	Trial of labor after cesarean	TOLAC
Intrauterine device	IUD	U.S. Preventive Services Task Force	USPSTF
Intrauterine growth restriction	IUGR		

PRENATAL CARE: CHANGING THE PARADIGM TO INCLUDE THE LIFE-COURSE PERSPECTIVE

Pregnancy and childbirth are major life events. Preconception and prenatal care are not only part of the pregnancy continuum that culminates in delivery, the postpartum period, and parenthood, they should also be considered in the context of women's health throughout the life span.[1,2] This chapter will review pertinent considerations for prenatal care using the broader definitions espoused by the U.S. Public Health Service and the American College of Obstetricians and Gynecologists (ACOG).[3,4] Specifically, prenatal care should consist of a series of interactions with caretakers, defined as *visits* and *contacts,* that includes three components: 1) early and continuing risk assessment, 2) health promotion, and 3) medical and psychosocial interventions and follow-up.[5] The overarching objective of prenatal care is to promote the health and well-being not only of the pregnant woman, fetus, and newborn but also of the family. Hence, **the breadth of prenatal care does not end with delivery but rather includes preconception care and postpartum care that extends up to 1 year after the infant's birth.**[4] Importantly, this introduces the concept of interconception care and the notion that almost all health care interactions with reproductive-age women (and men) are opportunities to assess risk; promote healthy lifestyle behaviors; and identify, treat, and optimize medical and psychosocial issues that could impact pregnancy and the lifetime health of the mother and child.

Definition and Goals of Care

National and international societies have recognized the importance of the continuum of preconception, prenatal, and interconception care as a comprehensive public health priority across the life span, beginning as early as adolescence, for multiple reasons.[6-9] **The aim of preconception care is to promote the health of women before conception in order to reduce preventable adverse pregnancy outcomes by facilitating risk screening, health promotion, and effective interventions as part of routine health care.**[6] As defined by the Centers for Disease Control and Prevention (CDC), it includes "interventions that aim to identify and modify biomedical, behavioral, and social risks to a woman's health or pregnancy outcome through prevention and management, emphasizing those factors which must be acted on before conception or early in pregnancy to have maximal impact."[6] *Interconception care* **is defined as care provided between delivery and the beginning of the woman's next pregnancy.** The term *interconception health* has limited familiarity among many medical providers, with *preconception care* being the term used more often in medical circles to refer to care that can maximize parental health *before* pregnancy. The term *interconception health* was coined by the CDC as a strategy to optimize parental health between pregnancies by addressing disease processes, health behaviors, and environmental hazards causally associated with infant mortality and other adverse pregnancy outcomes. **During the interconception period, intensive interventions are provided to women who have had a previous pregnancy that ended in an adverse outcome** (i.e., fetal loss, preterm birth [PTB], low birthweight [LBW], birth defects, or infant death).[10] Many medical conditions among reproductive-age women frequently become apparent during pregnancy and may contribute to negative birth outcomes in the infant. Hence, interconception care typically refers to enhanced interventions after an adverse pregnancy outcome.[11,12] However, for purposes of this discussion, preconception and interconception care are essentially interchangeable.

Evidence and Rationale for Paradigm Shift

The evidence and rationale for providing these services are multiple. First, increasing evidence suggests that human health status in adulthood is dictated by microenvironmental and macroenvironmental conditions around the time of conception (fetal programing of adult disease; see Chapter 5). Hence, the first prenatal visit may be too late to address modifiable behaviors that could optimize not only pregnancy outcome but the

health of the child and future adult.[13-15] A second significant contribution to adverse pregnancy outcome is related to congenital anomalies, PTB, and LBW. Children born with these conditions contribute significantly to neonatal and infant mortality as well as to family and society health care costs. **Patients who present at their first prenatal visit, even as early as the first trimester, are often too late to initiate behaviors or therapeutic interventions to prevent developmental abnormalities or mitigate risk for LBW and potential preterm delivery.** Third, almost half of pregnancies are mistimed, unplanned, or unwanted such that women may not be at optimal health or practicing ideal health behaviors at the time of conception, and this is particularly true for adolescents and/or low-income women.[16-18] Fourth, the proportion of women who delay childbearing or get pregnant with significant medical conditions is increasing, and specific opportunities exist to optimize fertility and pregnancy outcomes as it relates to medication management for those planning pregnancy.[6,15,20-23] **Specifically, for those planning pregnancy, preconception/interconception visits provide an opportunity for teachable moments, and data suggest couples planning pregnancy are more likely to change behaviors.**[12,15,24,25] Hence, although the functional set of services provided during preconception care, prenatal care, and interconception care are distinct and should be individualized for the patient, operationally—and perhaps politically—these clinical visits should be viewed as a continuum of comprehensive women's health services provided across a woman's life span, from menarche to menopause or sterilization.[7,12,26,27] Finally, national surveys reveal that 84% of reproductive-age women (18 to 44 years) have had a health care visit within the past year, which suggests significant opportunity to provide preconception counseling, yet data indicate this is not being done.[27] Although primary care settings and the well-woman visit are an ideal time to provide these services, all health care practitioners—including but not limited to nutritionists, pharmacists, nurses, midwives, physicians in family practice, obstetrician-gynecologists, and medical subspecialists—should approach every health care encounter with a reproductive-age woman as an opportunity to maximize her health and that of her future offspring by asking two simple questions: 1) Are you pregnant or planning to become pregnant? 2) If not, what are you doing to keep from becoming pregnant?

Collectively, these questions are a great segue to the ultimate question: What is your reproductive life plan? The answers to these questions will guide the subsequent health care interaction and appropriate preconception or interconception counseling and any intervention.[11]

Components of Preconception Care and Well-Woman Visits

A pregnancy or the desire to become pregnant is the sentinel event in differentiating preconception, interconception, and well-woman care (Fig. 6-1). **Preconception care is included as a preventive health service in well-woman visits covered by the Patient Protection and Affordable Care Act.**[27] Barriers to more widespread utilization of preconception care include lack of provider knowledge and training about essential components of preconception care across all specialties.[8] Although multiple checklists and online assessments exist, a detailed description provided by the Select Panel on Preconception Care as part of the CDC work groups and the corresponding rationale and evidence rating scale has been published, along with a recent

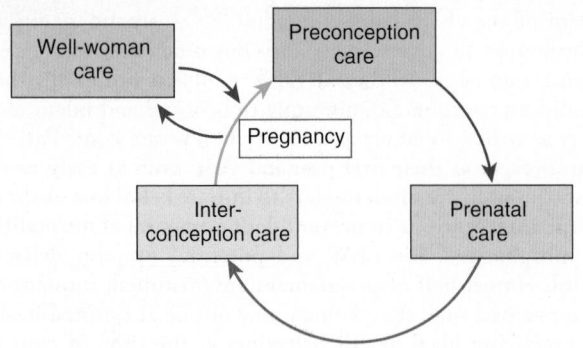

FIG 6-1 The fluid interconnections among preconception care, postpartum/interconception care, and well-woman care.

update of published validated tools.[28,29] The strategy is similar to most health care interactions: the provider asks screening questions in regard to personal and family history and exposures, undertakes health promotion (counseling for risk reduction), and provides treatment and/or intervention if specific conditions are identified. Table 6-1 lists representative examples of potential topic areas pertinent for a preconception care visit, and it gives examples of medical conditions that could be optimized prior to conception, assuming pregnancy is planned. Ideally, a checklist or questionnaire should be completed prior to seeing the clinician, and the patient would raise questions or ask for clarification as required. Online and interactive modules are also available, and inclusion in electronic medical records (EMRs) and sharing across clinical sites should be encouraged.[30] Perhaps

---

TABLE 6-1   PERTINENT TOPICS FOR PRECONCEPTION/INTERCONCEPTION COUNSELING AND OF MEDICAL CONDITIONS THAT CAN BE OPTIMIZED WHEN PREGNANCY IS PLANNED

CLINICAL CONDITION	COMMENT
General Health	
Age	**<18 years:** Teenage pregnancy is associated with adverse maternal and familial consequences and increased risk of preterm birth.
	>18 to 34 years: This is the ideal age group, especially if part of the reproductive life plan.
	>35 years: Increased genetic risks; increase in complications, risk of cesarean delivery, obstetric morbidity, and mortality; general health, not age, should guide recommendations for pregnancy.
Weight	**Underweight:** Advise weight gain before conceiving and/or greater weight gain with pregnancy.
	Overweight: Advise weight loss before conceiving; increased BMI is associated with multiple adverse outcomes that include pregnancy loss, stillbirth, diabetes, preeclampsia, and cesarean delivery.
Psychiatric/ Neurologic	
Depression, anxiety	Adjust medications to those most favorable to pregnancy at the lowest possible dose; counsel about fetal echocardiography and neonatal withdrawal syndrome for some medications; reassure that risk/benefit profile favors treatment.
Seizure disorders	Start folic acid 4 mg when considering pregnancy to decrease risk of NTD; if no seizure in 2 yr, consider trial off medication; adjust medications to those most favorable to pregnancy to avoid risk of dysmorphic structural malformation syndromes; close serum monitoring is required during pregnancy; reassure that risk/benefit profile favors treatment.
Migraines	Migraine pattern can change with pregnancy. Most migraine-specific medications are not contraindicated.
Cardiac	
Congenital cardiac disease or valve disease	Coordinate with cardiologist; pregnancy may be contraindicated with some conditions depending on severity (NYHA classification) or medications needed.
Coronary artery disease	Coordinate with cardiologist.
Hypertension	Adjust medications to optimize blood pressure.
	Discontinue ACE inhibitors and ARBs; these drugs are associated with congenital abnormalities.
Respiratory	
Asthma	Optimize treatment regimen per stepped protocol; if steroid dependent, use early ultrasound to evaluate for fetal cleft; advise patients at increased risk for gestational diabetes that medications, including steroids, are not contraindicated; emphasize that benefits of treatment exceed risks.
Gastrointestinal	
Inflammatory bowel disease	Optimize treatment regimen, advise that it is ideal to conceive while in remission; some medications have absolute versus relative contraindications.
Genitourinary	
Uterine malformations	Coordinate with reproductive endocrinologist if indicated.
Metabolic/Endocrine	
Diabetes	Achieve euglycemia before conception (hemoglobin A <7%); dose-dependent relationship regarding risk of congenital anomalies with medications; with type 1 and longstanding type 2 diabetes, insulin therapy is best; sulfonylureas are usually reserved for gestational diabetes mellitus.
Hematologic	
Sickle cell/thalassemia	Genetic counseling; advise sickle cell patient that crises can be exacerbated by pregnancy, and a risk of preterm birth/low birthweight is present.
History of DVT/PE, known hereditary thrombophilias	Risk of recurrent DVT/PE requires prophylaxis during pregnancy
Infectious	
STIs, TORCH, parvovirus	Establish risk factors, counsel to avoid infection, and treat as appropriate.
Rheumatologic	
SLE	It is ideal to conceive while SLE is in remission; some medications may be contraindicated.
Genetic	
Known genetic disorder in patient or partner	Genetic counseling, medical records to confirm diagnosis, and evaluation are warranted for prenatal diagnosis or assisted reproduction to avoid inheritance risk based on parents preferences and values.

ACE, angiotensin-converting enzyme; *ARB,* angiotensin II receptor blockers; *BMI,* body mass index; *DVT,* deep vein thrombosis; *NTD,* neural tube defect; *NYHA,* New York Hospital Association; *PE,* pulmonary embolism; *STI,* sexually transmitted infection; *SLE,* systemic lupus erythematosus; *TORCH,* toxoplasmosis, other infections, rubella, cytomegalovirus, herpes.

the most essential component of the preconception or well-woman visit that needs more consistent and widespread implementation and dissemination is the development and documentation of an individual's reproductive life plan.

Reproductive Life Plan: Definition

Files and associates[11] have defined a *reproductive life plan* as a **"set of personal goals regarding the conscious decision about whether or not to bear children"** and ideally, such a **plan outlines a strategy to achieve those goals.** Certain key elements should be considered when developing or discussing a reproductive life plan. These include 1) the desire or lack of desire to have children; 2) parental ages; 3) maternal health and coexisting medical conditions; 4) the desired number of children and anticipated spacing of children, taking into consideration ideal birth-spacing intervals, maternal age, and likelihood of fertility; 5) risk tolerance, such as for genetic or medical/obstetric complications; 6) family history; and 7) life context (age, school, career, partner, readiness for childbearing). Importantly, **reproductive life plans should be individualized, iterative, and addressed initially at menarche, confirmed or modified at subsequent health encounters by all care providers, and retired with menopause or sterilization.** Files and colleagues[11] have provided an algorithm and guidelines for developing a reproductive life plan, and convenient online tools have been designed for women contemplating pregnancy.[31-32] Unfortunately, studies indicate that even when women have achieved the pregnancy intention stage of readiness, many are still practicing preconception behaviors associated with poor pregnancy outcomes, such as poor diet (overweight or underweight), smoking, and binge drinking; this suggests a greater need for both one-on-one provider-patient interactions and more pervasive social media messages.[12,26,33] Research has demonstrated that patients want to be told this information from their providers, and many will respond favorably.[34] Further, sharing this information in groups, community settings, and in the presence of the partner has been shown to increase effectiveness.[26] Importantly, reproductive life plans should not be limited to reproductive-age women—the concept is pertinent for adolescent boys and men as well. **If conception is not anticipated within the year, an obvious discussion/intervention includes effective contraception options.**

When specific conditions are detected and pregnancy is not recommended or intended, reliable contraception should be prescribed, and the importance of compliance should be strongly reinforced. Data suggest that many women with complex medical problems who are advised against pregnancy conceive unintentionally and/or do not use contraception because of low perceived risk of conceiving.[33,35] If pregnancy is desired, in addition to screening and encouraging healthy behaviors, interventions to optimize the medical condition and adjust medications to profiles favorable for pregnancy should occur (see Table 6-1 for medical conditions and interventions common for preconception care and pregnancy).

PRECONCEPTION HEALTH COUNSELING

Maternal Age

The average maternal age at first birth has increased steadily over the last three decades in developed countries. **In 1970, the average age of first childbirth was 24.3, compared with 27.8 in 2009, the most recent year for which comparable international data are available.**[36] The United States has one of the lowest average maternal ages at first birth (25 years), whereas British and German women are delaying motherhood longer than anywhere else in the world (30 years). Advanced maternal age (AMA) is a contributing factor to maternal mortality. Maternal mortality is defined and the causes are described in Chapter 57.

Advanced Maternal Age

With advancing maternal age comes an increased likelihood of preexisting chronic medical diseases such as arthritis, hypertension, and diabetes.[37-42] The national Maternity Experiences Survey of the Canadian Perinatal Surveillance System[42] found that nulliparous women aged 35 years and over are significantly more likely to have had a miscarriage or infertility treatment, to request or be offered a cesarean delivery (CD), and to have a higher rate of CD than primiparous women aged 20 to 29 years, but they are not at higher risk for PTB, LBW, or small-for-gestational-age (SGA) infants. Overall, maternal age seems to have little impact on the rate of obstetric complications in women in their fourth decade of life. However, women aged 50 years or more are at increased risk for preeclampsia and gestational diabetes mellitus (GDM), and the vast majority of them can expect to deliver via CD.[37-42] A recent population-based register study found that a maternal age of 30 years or older was associated with the same number of additional cases of fetal deaths as those with comorbid overweight or obesity.[43]

Many nulliparous women age 40 and over require artificial reproductive technology (ART) to become pregnant. For ART singleton pregnancies, most studies have demonstrated a similar age- and parity-adjusted risk of pregnancy-induced hypertension and GDM in in vitro fertilization (IVF) and in controls.[44] In older women, ART techniques may require oocyte donation, which has been associated with increased risks of preeclampsia and premature labor. A recent meta-analysis[45] has found that the overall rate of preeclampsia after oocyte donation is approximately 22%. Furthermore, as a result of ART, the twin birth rate to women aged 40 to 44 nearly doubled between 1990 and 2001, and that of triplets increased fourfold in women 35 years and older between 1975 and 1998.[46] Within this context, in particular in older women with a preexisting medical condition, a multidisciplinary approach involving a maternal-fetal medicine specialist and an obstetrician should be started prior to conception.

Teen Pregnancies

Before the development of effective methods of female contraception, such as oral contraception and intrauterine devices (IUDs), and before access of women to education, late-teenage first pregnancy was common around the world. Not surprisingly, pregnancy in the late teenage years and early twenties is not associated with a major increase in pregnancy complications. A recent Swedish survey has found that adolescents are more likely to be delivered vaginally than older women and that the risks of placenta previa, postpartum hemorrhage (PPH), and perineal rupture are lower for adolescents than for adult women.[47] Neonates of teenage mothers have less fetal distress and meconium aspiration but have greater risk of being delivered prematurely. **This higher risk of prematurity has been consistently reported by other authors and seems to be the only significant obstetric risk of late teen pregnancy.**[48] However, in modern Western societies, adolescent pregnancy is often unplanned and unwanted and has a negative impact on the physical, emotional, educational, and economic condition of the pregnant teenager. In particular, **adolescent parenthood is associated with a range of adverse outcomes for young mothers, including mental health problems such as depression, substance abuse, and posttraumatic stress disorder (PTSD).**[49] Teen mothers are also more likely to be impoverished and to reside in communities and families that are socially and economically disadvantaged, which could be one of the factors that contributes to their higher risk of delivering prematurely.

In middle- and low-income countries, higher risks of preterm delivery have also been demonstrated for adolescent mothers aged 10 to 19 years (see Chapter 57). In addition, their risk of eclampsia, puerperal endometritis, emergency CD, PPH, and systemic infections is higher compared with mothers aged 20 to 24 years.[50] These worldwide consistent trends stress the important role of health care workers not only in providing guidance for teenagers and their parents, but also serving as health policy advocates to influence school and community leadership to ensure that all teenagers receive sound sex education in school programs and that family planning agencies are permitted to counsel teenagers and provide contraception services that include medications and devices.

Body Mass Index

Abnormal maternal weight is an increasingly common complication in developed and developing countries and affects an increasing number of women of reproductive age. Maternal obesity has become a global issue associated with obstetric, surgical, and anesthetic risks and increased risk for acute and chronic diseases, both in the mother and in the child; it also affects the economic productivity of individuals in the society and creates an additional cost burden on the health care system (see Chapter 41). Anorexia and bulimia nervosa, once thought to be rare eating disorders, have also been increasing because of cultural pressure on the drive for thinness in developed countries in contrast to longstanding food deprivation in developing countries.

Weight Gain

Weight gain during pregnancy has been shown to be an important predictor of pregnancy outcome (see Chapter 7). Maternal weight gain correlates with fetal weight gain and is, therefore, closely monitored. Too little weight gain should lead to an evaluation of nutritional factors and an assessment of associated fetal growth. Excess weight gain is one of the first signs of fluid retention, but it may also reflect increased dietary intake or decreased physical activity.

In the United States, the total weight gain recommended in pregnancy is 11 to 16 kg (25 to 35 lb) for women at a healthy weight.[51] Underweight women can gain up to 18 kg (40 lb), but overweight women should limit weight gain to 7 kg (15 lb), although they do not need to gain any weight if they are morbidly obese.[52] At term, the typical woman gains about 3 to 4 kg (7 to 9 lb) from increased tissue fluid volume and fat, 1.5 to 2 kg (3 to 4 lb) from increased blood volume, 0.5 to 1 kg (1 to 2 lb) from breast enlargement, 1 kg (2 lb) from enlargement of the uterus, 1 kg or 1 L (2 lb) from amniotic fluid, 2.7 to 3.6 kg (6 to 8 lb) for the fetus, and 0.5 to 1 kg (1 to 2 lb) of placental weight. Usually, 1.4 to 2.7 kg (3 to 6 lb) are gained in the first trimester, and 0.2 to 0.6 kg (0.5 to 1 lb) per week are gained during the last two trimesters of pregnancy.

If the patient does not show a 4.5 kg (10 lb) weight gain by mid pregnancy, her nutritional status should be reviewed. Inadequate weight gain is associated with an increased risk of an LBW infant. Inadequate weight gain seems to have its greatest effect in woman at a healthy weight or those who are underweight before pregnancy. Underweight mothers must gain more weight during pregnancy to produce infants of normal weight. In overweight and obese women, weight loss or gain of 11 lb (5 kg) or less is associated with increased risk of an SGA infant and decreased neonatal fat mass, lean mass, and head circumference.[53]

When excess weight gain is noted, patients should be counseled to avoid foods that are high in fats and carbohydrates, to limit sugar intake, and to increase their physical activity. Rapid weight gain requires an assessment for fluid retention. Factors that contribute to excessive weight gain during pregnancy include high fat and low fiber intake, high carbohydrate or sugar intake, and decreased physical activity during pregnancy. Several small studies suggest that monitoring weight gain, quantity of food consumed, and physical activity combined with behavioral counseling can limit weight gain during pregnancy and promote postpartum weight loss. However, larger randomized controlled trials are needed to demonstrate long-term effectiveness.[54]

Dietary and lifestyle interventions in pregnancy can reduce maternal gestational weight gain and improve outcomes for both mother and baby.[55] **Among the interventions, those based on diet are the most effective and are associated with reductions in maternal gestational weight gain and improved obstetric outcomes.**

Weight gain and weight retention after pregnancy is a risk factor for subsequent obesity.[23,56] Thus postpartum weight loss should be encouraged. Women who resumed their prepregnancy weight by 6 months postpartum gained only 2.4 kg (5 lb) over the next 10 years compared with 8.3 kg (18 lb) for women who retained weight after delivery.[57] Weight retention between the first and second pregnancy is associated with an increased risk for perinatal complications, even in underweight and normal-weight women.[58]

Stabilizing interpregnancy weight appears to be an important target in order to avoid adverse perinatal outcomes in a second pregnancy. Although clinicians have focused on teaching women that appropriate weight gain is important for pregnancy, the concomitant importance of postpartum weight loss has not been given equal attention.[24,59,60] A recent meta-analysis on the effect of diet, exercise, or both for weight reduction in women after childbirth has found that both diet and exercise together and diet alone help women lose weight after childbirth.[61] The authors also concluded that this needs confirmation in large trials of high methodologic quality.

Overweight and Obesity

Sixty-five percent of Americans are overweight (body mass index [BMI] ≥25 kg/m^2) or obese (BMI ≥30 kg/m^2).[62] Pregestational weight gain or obesity and excessive gestational weight gain are now well-established independent risk factors for maternal-fetal complications and long-term risks in adult life for the child. The selected risks include increased miscarriage, congenital anomalies, hypertensive disorders, GDM, macrosomia, and delivery complications that include instrumental delivery, shoulder dystocia, emergency CD, PPH, venous thromboembolism (VTE), anesthetic complications, and wound infections.[63,64] In overweight and obese women, the adjusted odds ratio (OR) is 2.04 (95% confidence interval [CI], 1.41-2.95) for cesarean delivery for an interpregnancy weight retention of 2 or more BMI units.[65] Being overweight or obese before pregnancy is also associated with a higher risk of fetal loss.[66] In women who are overweight or obese at 18 years, losing 4 kg or more before pregnancy is associated with a lower risk of fetal loss.[66]

Maternal obesity is a key predictor of childhood obesity and metabolic complications in adulthood. The children of women who are overweight or obese during pregnancy are also at increased risk for cognitive deficits, externalizing problems (particularly attention-deficit/hyperactivity disorder), and internalizing psychopathology in childhood and adolescence.[67]

Emerging evidence supports the role of first microbial contacts in promoting and maintaining a balanced immune response in early life, and recent findings suggest that microbial contact begins prior to birth and is shaped by the maternal microbiota (see Chapter 3). Although the mechanisms remain unclear, postnatal maturation of immune regulation seems to be largely driven by exposure to microbes, and the gastrointestinal tract is the largest source of microbial exposure.[68] Early exposures that impact the intestinal microbiota are associated with the development of childhood diseases that may persist into adulthood such as asthma, allergic disorders (atopic dermatitis, rhinitis), chronic immune-mediated inflammatory diseases, type 1 diabetes, obesity, and eczema.[68,69] Breast milk samples from obese mothers tend to contain a different and less diverse bacterial microbiota compared with milk from those at a healthy weight.[70] The gut microbiome can rapidly respond to altered diet, potentially facilitating the diversity of human dietary lifestyles.[65] Alterations in the bacterial composition of the mother have been shown to affect the development and function of the gastrointestinal tract of her offspring.[68,69] Thus prepregnancy strategies to modify the microbiota of future mothers may prove to be a safe and effective target for interventions to decrease the risk of allergic and noncommunicable diseases in future generations.

Underweight

Prepregnancy underweight and insufficient gestational weight gain have been considered as individual risk factors for the occurrence of miscarriage, PTB, intrauterine growth restriction (IUGR), and hypertensive disorders.[71] A recent systematic review and meta-analysis[72] has shown that the birthweight of children of mothers with anorexia nervosa is lower by 0.19 kg compared with children of mothers at a healthy weight. A population study from the same authors has also shown that eating disorders are associated with increased odds of receiving fertility treatment and subsequent twin births.[73] Women with anorexia nervosa were more likely to have an unplanned pregnancy and to have mixed feelings about the unplanned pregnancy.

In underweight women and in those at a healthy weight, the risk for macrosomia can be halved if women lost more than 1 BMI unit between pregnancies, but at the same time, the risk for LBW doubled.[65]

Pregnancy After Bariatric Surgery

Pregnancy after bariatric surgery appears to effectively reduce the risk of complications such as fetal macrosomia, GDM, and hypertensive disorders of pregnancy (see Chapters 25 and 41).[74-77] Women who become pregnant after bariatric surgery may constitute a unique obstetric population with an increased

risk of severe deficiencies in iron, vitamin A, vitamin B$_{12}$, vitamin K, folate, and calcium; these deficiencies can result in both maternal complications such as severe anemia and fetal complications such as congenital abnormalities, IUGR, and failure to thrive.[76] Less invasive techniques, such as laparoscopic adjustable gastric banding, do not appear to increase the rate of small neonates seen with other bariatric surgery procedures.[77] Close supervision before, during, and after pregnancy following bariatric surgery and nutrient supplementation adapted to the patient's individual requirements can help to prevent nutrition-related complications and can improve maternal and fetal health in this high-risk obstetric population.

Infections and Immunizations

Primary care, preventative health, and well-women visits are ideal settings in which to screen and counsel women about sexually transmitted infections (STIs) such as syphilis, gonorrhea, chlamydia, and human immunodeficiency virus (HIV) in addition to toxoplasmosis, other infections, rubella, cytomegalovirus, and herpes (TORCH) infections. It is also an ideal time to confirm and update immunization status (see Chapters 52, 53, and 54). Patients who are sexually active should be counseled about the importance of condoms to prevent STIs (irrespective of other contraceptive methods), and they should be screened for STIs based on age and geographic prevalence as per national guidelines.[78,79]

Toxoplasmosis screening based on risk factors may be indicated at this time because approximately one fourth of the U.S. population is infected.[80] Patients who have negative screens are at risk for congenital toxoplasmosis and should be counseled to avoid risks such as contact with infected cats and ingestion of raw or undercooked meat. Immunocompetent patients who screen positive can be reassured of low risk with regard to fetal loss or stillbirth; although rare, reports of congenital infection after previous infection have been described.[81] A prospective analysis of the population risks and benefits to substantiate routine screening for and education about toxoplasmosis has not been done in the United States. However, proponents argue a theoretic benefit based on treatment availability, extrapolated epidemiologic data from some European countries (France, Belgium, Austria) where screening is widespread, and the prevalence of congenital infection comparable to other congenital diseases that are currently screened for by mandate, such as phenylketonuria and congenital hypothyroidism.[82] The screening for toxoplasmosis could be performed once at the beginning of pregnancy to provide patients with the information on measures to prevent acquiring the infection during pregnancy, such as avoiding raw vegetables and meat or freezing meat before consumption.

Approximately 50% to 80% of reproductive-age women have evidence of prior cytomegalovirus (CMV) infection, and susceptible women (e.g., child care workers and women with small children in day care) should be counseled about the importance of hand hygiene after contact with toys, saliva, and urine as a preventive measure. Risk of vertical transmission is more likely after primary infection, and current treatment options are limited. Routinely screening for CMV to enhance awareness and encourage prevention practices in at-risk mothers is performed in a few European countries (France, Belgium) but is currently not endorsed in the United States.[83] Likewise, women with primary or recurrent herpes should be informed about the benefits of prophylactic antiviral suppression in the third trimester to decrease risk of vertical transmission and the need for cesarean delivery.[84]

All reproductive-age women should be current with immunizations recommended by the Advisory Committee on Immunization Practices (ACIP) and the CDC.[85] This is the time to draw and document protective titers for rubella, varicella, and hepatitis B and to immunize the susceptible patient. Patients should use contraception for up to 3 months following immunizations with live vaccines. If the woman conceives and is expected to deliver during flu season, she should be counseled to receive the influenza vaccine to decrease disease severity for her. She should be given the tetanus, diphtheria, and pertussis (Tdap) vaccine in late pregnancy (27 to 36 weeks) to provide passive immunity for the newborn.[85]

Genetic and Family History

The time to screen appropriate populations for genetic disease-carrier status and multifactorial congenital malformations or familial diseases with major genetic components is *before* pregnancy. If patients screen positive, referral for genetic counseling is indicated, and consideration of additional preconception options may be warranted including donor egg or sperm, ART after preimplantation selection, prenatal genetic testing after conception, or adoption (see Chapter 10).[86] Certain diseases may be related to race/ethnicity or geographic origin. Patients of African, Asian, or Mediterranean descent should be screened for the various heritable hemoglobinopathies (sickle cell disease, α- and β-thalassemia). Patients of Jewish and French-Canadian heritage should be screened for Tay-Sachs disease, Canavan disease, and cystic fibrosis. In the United States, it has been suggested that cystic fibrosis screening be offered to all couples planning a pregnancy or seeking prenatal testing.[87] Resolution of these issues during the preconception period is much easier and less hurried without the time limits placed by an advancing pregnancy. The age of the father is also important because genetic, structural, behavioral, or cognitive risks to the child may exist when the father is older; this emphasizes the importance of a reproductive life plan for men as well as women.[88,89]

Substance Abuse and Other Hazards

In the general population, fetal and neonatal exposures to drugs and other toxins are often the consequence of the lifestyle choices of the parents, with exposure to tobacco smoke and alcohol among the most pervasive and easily documented. **Smoking and use of alcohol and drugs by pregnant women are all harmful to the developing fetus, but because these substances are often used in combination, teasing apart the specific contributions of each substance to adverse child outcomes can prove difficult when analyzing epidemiologic data** (see Chapter 8). **Overall, the risks to the neonate include IUGR, birth defects, altered neuropsychological behavior, and, for some drugs, withdrawal symptoms. Subsequent behavior, development, and neurologic function may also be impaired by behaviors that occurred during the preconception period.** Consideration of socioeconomic inequalities in unplanned pregnancy is important in assessing the impact of a specific toxic substance on the developing fetus, because exposure may precede pregnancy recognition. A U.S. study of reproductive-age nonpregnant women looked at the prevalence of behavioral risk factors individually and in combination.[90] One third of the women had at least one risk factor, and 19% had

two or more risk factors, which confirms the opportunity for preconception care to mitigate outcomes.[90]

Active and Passive Smoking

In many countries, smoking has replaced poverty as the most important risk factor for PTB, IUGR, and sudden infant death syndrome (SIDS).[91] Cigarette smoke contains scores of toxins that exert a direct effect on placental and fetal cell proliferation and differentiation.[92] The use of or exposure to tobacco products by pregnant women is associated more specifically with placenta previa, placental abruption, placenta accreta, pregnancy bleeding of unknown origin, and preterm premature rupture of membranes. Smoking is linked to a reduction of weight, fat mass, and most anthropometric parameters in the fetus; in the placenta, it is linked with alterations in protein metabolism and enzyme activity.[92] The transplacental induction of genetic alterations by tobacco smoke carcinogens and their implication to childhood diseases remain poorly understood.[93] However, epidemiologic studies support a relationship between maternal smoking during pregnancy and adverse neurobehavioral effects for her offspring later in life.[94] Prenatal exposure to tobacco seems to increase the risks for cognitive deficits, attention-deficit/hyperactivity disorder, conduct disorder, criminality in adulthood, and a predisposition in the offspring to start smoking and to abuse alcohol. A direct, specific action on the developing human brain is plausible during the major part of prenatal life because the nicotinic receptors are already present in the brain during the first trimester. The long-term effects of passive and active smoking during pregnancy on childhood or adulthood diseases, including respiratory and cardiovascular disease and cancer, are only starting to emerge from large epidemiologic studies.[93]

In spite of these well-established negative consequences, epidemiologic studies have shown that, depending on the patient population, **20% to 50% of pregnant women smoke or are exposed to passive smoking**. In many industrialized countries, prevalence rates of women actively smoking appear to have peaked and have begun to decline, whereas in other countries, smoking is becoming increasingly common among young women.[91] Smoking during pregnancy has been linked to high health care costs, and it accounted for approximately $250 million in direct medical costs each year in the United States at the end of the last decade.[95,96] The complications with the largest smoking-attributable cost were LBW and lower respiratory tract infection. More than a decade ago, it was calculated that an annual drop of 1 percentage point in smoking prevalence among pregnant women would prevent the delivery of 1300 LBW infants and would save $21 million in direct medical costs during the first year of the program.[96] Smoking during pregnancy has been recognized as the most important modifiable risk factor associated with adverse perinatal outcomes. **Because most of the placental and fetal damage is done in the first trimester of pregnancy, helping women to quit smoking before conceiving should be a primary objective in prepregnancy counseling.**

Alcohol

Alcohol is a well-established teratogen, and alcohol used during pregnancy can lead to fetal alcohol syndrome (FAS), which includes specific morphologic features, such as microcephaly, and long-term abnormal neuropsychological outcomes. The main issue with alcohol use during pregnancy is

that no amount of alcohol consumption has been found to be safe during pregnancy; this can explain the blanket policy advice of many national departments of health that support total alcohol abstinence during pregnancy. There is no doubt that heavy or binge drinking is detrimental to fetal development in utero and that it has long-term negative effects on the offspring's cognition and behavior. A systematic review[97] of obstetric outcomes that included miscarriage, stillbirth, IUGR, prematurity, SGA infants, and birth defects including FAS found no convincing evidence of the adverse effects of prenatal alcohol exposure at low to moderate levels of exposure. A recent systematic review of child neuropsychological outcomes found a detrimental association between moderate prenatal alcohol exposure and child behavior and between mild-to-moderate prenatal alcohol exposure and child cognition.[98] A recent prospective follow-up study has also shown that intake of 15 to 21 drinks per week on average prior to pregnancy is not associated with abnormal neurophysiological outcome at 5 years of age, but intake of 22 or more drinks per week is associated with lower intelligence quotient (IQ) and lower attention scores.[99] These data support the concept of prepregnancy support to reduce or quit alcohol consumption for women planning a pregnancy. Regular screening for alcohol use should be carried out using such tools as the Tolerance-Annoyance, Cut-Down, Eye-Opener (T-ACE) questionnaire[100] (see Chapter 8) or other simple screening tools, and appropriate directed therapy should be made available to those women who screen positive.

Other Substance Abuse

Substance abuse in pregnancy (see Chapter 55) has increased over the past three decades, and it has been recently estimated that approximately 225,000 infants yearly in the United States are exposed prenatally to illicit substances.

Cannabis is the most commonly used illicit substance in the United States, predominantly for its pleasurable physical and psychotropic effects. Four states and the District of Columbia have now made recreational use of *Cannabis* legal, and this topic has gained national attention. It has been shown that *Cannabis* use can lead to IUGR and withdrawal symptoms in the neonate. **A recent case-control study has also found that *Cannabis* use, cigarette smoking, illicit drug use, and apparent exposure to second-hand cigarette smoke separately or in combination during pregnancy were associated with an increased risk of stillbirth.** In longitudinal studies, fetal *Cannabis* exposure has been associated with negative effects on intellectual outcome.

Cocaine use in pregnancy can lead to spontaneous abortion, PTB, placental abruption, and preeclampsia. Although fetal cocaine exposure has been linked to numerous abnormalities in arousal, attention, and neurologic and neurophysiological function, most such effects appear to be self-limited and restricted to early infancy and childhood. Neonatal issues include poor feeding, lethargy, and seizures.

Poor obstetric outcomes can be up to six times higher in patients who abuse opiates such as heroin and methadone. Opiate exposure elicits a well-described withdrawal syndrome that affects central nervous, autonomic, and gastrointestinal systems; this effect is most severe among methadone-exposed infants.

Amphetamine use can lead to congenital anomalies and other poor obstetric outcomes. Methamphetamine use in particular is an escalating problem worldwide because it is the only illegal substance that can be made from legally obtained over-the-counter cold medications. It is a powerful stimulant with a long half-life that crosses the placenta and concentrates in breast milk. Although evidence of an increased risk of congenital anomalies has been inconsistent, studies have consistently demonstrated an association between amphetamines and late/no prenatal care, maternal psychiatric disorders, homelessness, IPV, LBW and SGA infants, IUGR, neonatal intensive care unit (NICU) admissions, and childhood neurodevelopmental abnormalities. Maternal deaths from severe hypertension, tachycardia, and cardiac decompensation have also been reported.

Mothers who use illicit drugs require specialized prenatal care, and the neonate may need extra supportive care. Once recognized, a specialized approach can lead to improved maternal and neonatal outcomes. A similar multidisciplinary approach that includes access to rehabilitation centers is essential to help future mothers with an addiction quit before starting a pregnancy.

Intimate Partner Violence

Violence against women is increasingly recognized as a problem that should be addressed, and reports suggest that abuse occurs during 3% to 8% of pregnancies. Questions that address personal safety and violence should be included during the prenatal period, and tools such as the Abuse Assessment Score are recommended.

Mercury Exposure

Data regarding the accumulation of mercury in fish has led to warnings advising pregnant women to avoid or decrease fish consumption. In the United States, all 50 states have recommended limits on the ingestion of locally caught fish for pregnant women and children. Mercury is neurotoxic and has been associated with a dose-dependent impact on neurologic development. Approximately 5% to 8% of pregnant women may have mercury levels above the recommended amount, and increased awareness of the risks associated with mercury has led to decreased consumption or elimination of fish from the diets of many pregnant women. Unfortunately, the harms of mercury are counterbalanced by the benefits of omega-3 fatty acids found in fish that include decreased LBW and PTB, an increase in visual acuity, and higher performance on developmental tests and higher IQ scores in offspring. It is unclear whether dietary supplements are similarly beneficial because the stability and bioavailability varies and has not been well characterized. The U.S. Environmental Protection Agency (EPA) has attempted to clarify these mixed messages by recommending that reproductive-age women, pregnant women, and children eat a variety of fish two or three times a week (4 to 6 oz per serving) but that they should avoid eating fish with a high mercury content (king mackerel, shark, swordfish, and tilefish).

Occupational Hazards and Environmental Exposures

Occupational hazards should be identified. If a patient works in a laboratory with chemicals or in agriculture around a lot of pesticides, for example, she should be advised to identify potential reproductive toxins and limit her exposure. This is an active area of research, and several online resources are available for information about potential environmental and occupational teratogens. Patients whose occupations require heavy physical exercise or excess stress should be informed that they may need to decrease such activity later in pregnancy because both have been associated with an increased risk of PTB and reduced fetal growth in observational studies.

ENVIRONMENTAL EXPOSURES

A study based on the National Health and Nutrition Examination Survey demonstrated that all pregnant women are exposed to and have detectable levels of chemicals that can be harmful to reproduction or human development. Because exposure to environmental agents can be mitigated or prevented, it is important for women to be made aware of known toxic substances and to be informed as to how to access resources to gain additional information. Environmental contributors to reproductive health begin in utero and are influenced by social, physical, nutritional, and chemical agents. Lead has historical significance, but more recent concerns are related to mercury, phthalates, perchlorates, pesticides, and bisphenol A (BPA; see Chapter 8). These agents are considered endocrine-disrupting chemicals that interfere with cellular proliferation or differentiation and result in altered metabolic, hormonal, or immunologic capabilities. For example, pesticides are used widely in agriculture and household settings, with an estimated 1.2 billion lb per year of active ingredients used in the United States. These chemicals have been associated with impaired cognitive development and fetal growth and increased risk of childhood cancers. BPA is commonly found in plastics used for food and beverage products and packaging and has been associated with recurrent miscarriages and aggression and hyperactivity in girls. Primary care physicians can play an important role by providing guidance to women about how to avoid toxic exposures at home and in the community, and they can help educate patients by referring them to online resources.

Screening for Chronic Disease, Optimizing Care, and Managing Medication Exposure

Clear evidence shows that for some conditions—such as diabetes mellitus, phenylketonuria, and inflammatory bowel disease—medical disease management before conception can positively influence pregnancy outcome. Medical management to normalize the intrauterine biochemical environment should be discussed with the patient, and appropriate management plans should be outlined before conception; advice can also be given about avoiding specific medications in the first trimester (e.g., isotretinoin). Table 6-1 gives examples of general health and medical conditions by organ system that can be optimized by preventing pregnancy until it can be planned and then adjusting medication type or dose to minimize teratogenicity or impact on neonatal development.

PRENATAL CARE

Components of Prenatal Care

Recent guidelines to address the content and efficacy of prenatal care have focused on the medical, psychosocial, and educational aspects of the prenatal care system. **Prenatal care satisfies the definition of primary care from the Institute of Medicine as "integrated, accessible health care services by clinicians who are accountable for addressing a large majority of personal health care needs, developing a sustained partnership with patients, and practicing in the context of family and community."** Prenatal care satisfies other criteria for primary care in that it is comprehensive and continuous and offers coordinated health care. Hence, prenatal care provides additional opportunities to advance wellness and prevention. It is another opportunity to introduce and reinforce habits, knowledge, and life-long skills in self-care, health education, and wellness to inculcate

principles of routine screening, immunization, and regular assessment for psychological, behavioral, and medical risk factors. Phelan[24] argues that clinicians are not taking advantage of pregnancy as a "teachable moment"—a naturally occurring life transition that motivates people to spontaneously adopt risk-reducing behaviors. If health and habits are not optimized during the preconception period, **pregnancy qualifies as a teachable moment because it meets the following criteria proposed by McBride[25] and colleagues:**

- Perception of personal risk and outcome expectancies is increased.
- The perceptions are associated with strong affective or emotional responses.
- The event is associated with a redefinition of self-concept or social role.

Education about pregnancy, childbearing, and childrearing is an important part of prenatal care, as are detection and treatment of abnormalities. However, more recently, contemporary models of prenatal and childbirth education have been criticized because research has not shown a strong association between class attendance and childbirth experiences or parenting expectations. In fact, among first-time mothers, a decline in childbirth class attendance has been observed, from 70% in 2002 to 56% in 2005.

High-Tech Versus Low-Tech Care

Historically, the primary goal of prenatal care was to minimize maternal and neonatal mortality. However, new technology has been introduced to assess the fetus antepartum that includes electronic fetal monitoring, sonography, prenatal diagnosis, and other in utero interventions with the fetus emerging as a patient in utero. **Prevention of morbidity and mortality is now the goal.** This has made the task of prenatal care more complex because mother and fetus now require an increasingly sophisticated level of care. At the same time, pregnancy is basically a physiologic process, and the healthy pregnant patient may not benefit from application of advanced technology; that is, she may receive poor quality care as a result of misuse or overutilization of the health care system.

Prenatal care can be provided at a variety of sites that range from the patient's home to the physician or midwife's private office to a public health or hospital clinic. **Obstetricians must optimize their efforts by resourceful use of other professionals and support groups that include nutritionists, childbirth educators, public health nurses, nurse practitioners, family physicians, nurse midwives, and specialty medical consultants.** Most pregnant women who are healthy and have normal pregnancies can be followed by an obstetric team that includes nurses, nurse practitioners, and nurse-midwives in addition to the obstetrician. These women should be cared for by practitioners who have adequate time to spend on patient education and parenting preparation, while physicians can appropriately concentrate on complicated problems that require their medical skills. This also provides for improved continuity of care, which is recognized as extremely important for patient satisfaction.

No prospective controlled trials have demonstrated the efficacy of prenatal care overall. Two documents that have addressed the content and efficacy of prenatal care have suggested changes in the current prenatal care system. Since publication of these recommendations, several well-designed randomized clinical trials and cost-benefit analyses have been reported using alternative visit schedules. **No difference was evident in outcomes for** patients who underwent a reduced frequency of visits as measured by rates of PTB and LBW, and the reduced frequency model was shown to be cost effective. Although fewer visits were associated with decreased maternal satisfaction with care, as well as increased maternal anxiety, studies support the concept of reduced antenatal visits for selected women.

Efficacy of prenatal care also depends on the quality of care provided by the caretaker. If a blood pressure is recorded as "elevated," and no therapeutic maneuvers are recommended, the outcome will remain unchanged. Recommendations must be made and must be carried out by the patient, whose compliance is essential to alter outcome. Using national survey data, Kogan and colleagues reported that women received only 56% of the procedures and 32% of the advice recommended as part of prenatal care content, whereas poor women and black women received even fewer of the recommended interventions. Site of care was also an important determinant, suggesting that infrastructure must be geared to address population-specific needs.

Risk Assessment

The concept of risk in obstetrics can be examined at many levels. **All the problems that arise in pregnancy, whether common complaints or more hazardous diseases, convey some risk to the pregnancy depending on how they are managed by the patient and her care provider. Risk assessment has received detailed attention in the past. It has been shown that most women and infants who suffer morbidity and mortality will come from a small segment of those with high-risk factors; by reassessing risk factors before pregnancy, during pregnancy, and again in labor, the ability to identify those at highest risk increases.** Most of the emphasis for screening, risk assessment, and associated trials for therapeutic interventions have focused primarily on preeclampsia and PTB prevention. Table 6-2 lists representative examples of other clinical conditions that have been proposed to be included as part of routine screening and risk assessment during the antepartum period since 1989. Although commonly included as part of current routine screening programs, few of these screening programs were implemented as a result of evidence-based criteria, such as those proposed by the U.S. Preventive Services Task Force (USPSTF). Most have been utilized as a result of expert or consensus opinion, cost-benefit, or risk-management decisions.

Initial Prenatal Visit

It is important to individualize patient care and to be thorough. Therefore the initial visit should include a detailed history along with physical and laboratory examinations.

Social and Demographic Risks

Low socioeconomic status should be identified, and attempts to improve nutritional and hygienic measures should be undertaken. Appropriate referral to federal programs—such as for the Special Supplemental Nutrition Program for Women, Infants, and Children (WIC)—and to public health nurses can have real benefits. If a patient has a history of a previous neonatal death, stillbirth, or PTB, records should be carefully reviewed so that the correct diagnosis is made and recurrence risk is appropriately assessed. A history of drug abuse or recent blood transfusion should be elicited. The history of medical illnesses should be detailed, and records should be obtained if possible. A rapid procedure for diagnosing mental disorders in primary care may be useful in pregnancy. If appropriate, patients should be screened and treated for depression.

Medical Risk

Family history of diabetes, hypertension, tuberculosis, seizures, hematologic disorders, multiple pregnancies, congenital abnormalities, and reproductive loss should be elicited. Often, a family history of mental retardation, birth defects, or genetic traits is difficult to elicit without formal genetic counseling or questionnaires; nonetheless, these areas should be emphasized at the initial history. **A better history may be obtained if patients are asked to fill out a preinterview questionnaire or history form.** Any significant maternal cardiovascular, renal, or metabolic disease should be defined. Infectious diseases such as urinary tract disease, syphilis, tuberculosis, or herpes genitalis should be identified. Surgical history with special attention to any abdominal or pelvic operations should be noted. A history of previous cesarean delivery should include indication, type of uterine

TABLE 6-2	COMPARISON OF DIFFERENT RECOMMENDATIONS REGARDING VISIT FREQUENCY AND PROPOSED CLINICAL INTERVENTIONS FOR PRENATAL CARE FOR LOW-RISK WOMEN			
WEEK OF GESTATION	**ACOG 1997**	**EXPERT PANEL NP WOMAN**	**EXPERT PANEL MP WOMAN**	**CLINICAL INTERVENTION**
1-4		X	X	Preconception counseling, dating
5-8	X	X	X	Dating
9-12	X	X		Dating; nuchal translucency; serum marker screening for aneuploidy
13-16	X	X	X	
17-20	X			AFP/multiple marker screening; ultrasound
21-24	X			
25-28	X	X	X	Glucose tolerance test
31-32	X	X	X	Childbirth education, risk assessment
35-36	X	X	X	GBS growth
37	X	X		Risk assessment
38	X	X		Risk assessment
39	X			
40	X	X		Risk assessment
41	X	X	X	Postterm evaluation

Modified from Gregory KD, Davidson E. Prenatal care: who needs it and why? *Clin Obstet Gynecol.* 1999;42:725-736.
AFP, alpha-fetoprotein; *GBS,* group B *Streptococcus; MP,* multiparous; *NP,* nulliparous.

incision, and any complications; in addition, a copy of the surgical report may be informative. Allergies, particularly drug allergies, should be prominent on the problem list.

Obstetric Risk

Previous obstetric and reproductive history is essential to optimizing care in subsequent pregnancies. The gravidity and parity should be noted with the outcome for each prior pregnancy recorded in detail. Previous miscarriages and documentation about the gestational age at the time of the loss is important; these not only confer risk and anxiety for another pregnancy loss, they can be associated with an increased risk for genetic disease and PTB.

Previous preterm delivery is strongly associated with recurrence; therefore it is important to delineate the events that surrounded the PTB. Did the membranes rupture before labor? Were painful uterine contractions present? Was there any bleeding? Were any fetal abnormalities evident? What was the neonatal outcome? All these questions are vital in determining the etiology and prognosis of the condition, although specific recommendations will vary and the efficacy of routine prevention programs is not clear. In patients with a previous premature delivery from preterm labor or premature rupture of the membranes (PROM), progesterone administration reduces the risk of recurrence. Cervical insufficiency and uterine anomalies are all conditions that may be known from a previous pregnancy.

After all the specific inquiries, it is recommended that the patient be asked a few simple questions: What important items haven't I asked? What concerns or questions do you have? Leaving time for open-ended questions is the best way to complete the initial visit.

Physical and Laboratory Evaluation

Physical examination should include a general physical examination and a pelvic examination. Baseline height and weight, prepregnancy weight, and vital signs are recorded. Any physical finding that might have an impact on pregnancy or that might be affected by pregnancy should be defined. It is particularly important to perform and record a complete physical examination at this initial visit because in the absence of specific problems or complaints, less emphasis will be placed on nonobstetric portions of the examination as pregnancy progresses. Documentation of baseline vital signs, cardiac examination, and other physical findings is important prior to the expected physiologic changes that will occur over time.

A pelvic examination should be performed in early pregnancy. Cervical cytology, if indicated, and testing for *Neisseria gonorrhoeae* and *Chlamydia trachomatis* are done. Bacterial vaginosis should be recognized. Bimanual exam should focus on the uterine size and the presence of palpable adnexal masses. The cervix should be carefully palpated, and any deviation from normal should be noted. Clinical pelvimetry should be performed with the clinical impression of adequacy noted (see Chapter 12). The exam may be limited by examiner skill and patient variation (e.g., obesity). Most practitioners perform an ultrasound in the first and/or second trimester, which confirms dating and should also evaluate for the presence of uterine or adnexal pathology. A detailed description of gestational age determination utilizing ultrasound is provided in Chapter 9.

Basic laboratory studies are routinely performed. Some studies need not be repeated if recent normal values have been obtained,

such as at a visit following a preconceptional visit or a recent gynecologic or infertility examination. Blood studies should include Rh type and screening for irregular antibodies, hemoglobin level, or hematocrit and serologic tests for syphilis and rubella. A urine sample should be obtained and tested for abnormal protein and glucose levels. Screening for asymptomatic bacteriuria has been traditionally done by urine culture, but screening may be simplified by testing for nitrites and leukocyte esterase. Tuberculosis screening should also be performed in areas of disease prevalence. Multiple options exist for aneuploidy screening and/or diagnosis depending on when women present for prenatal care (see Chapter 10).

The laboratory evaluations outlined above are the minimum standard tests; specific conditions will require further evaluation. A history of thyroid disease will lead to thyroid function testing. Anticonvulsant therapy requires measurement of blood levels of medication to determine if the appropriate dose is being used. The importance of compliance with dosing and serial evaluation of serum blood levels should be emphasized; for example, both thyroid medications and anticonvulsant levels are sensitive to the physiologic expansion of blood volume and metabolic changes that occur during pregnancy. Adequacy of hormone replacement and/or drug levels will need to be monitored throughout pregnancy. Identification of problems on screening (e.g., anemia, abnormal glucose screen) will mandate further testing. If not done before conception, screening for varicella has been suggested for women with no known history of chickenpox. The ACOG has recommended routine screening of all pregnant women for hepatitis B. In addition, HIV screening should also be offered because maternal therapy with azidothymidine (AZT) can reduce vertical transmission (see Chapter 53). Hepatitis C and CMV screening should be considered for at-risk populations. Recommendations for the content of prenatal care are summarized in Table 6-3. Note that these recommendations are drawn from various sources; most are based on expert opinion, and although similar, they are not entirely in agreement with regard to all recommendations.

Repeat Prenatal Visits

A plan of visits is outlined to the patient. **Traditionally, this has been every 4 weeks for the first 28 weeks of pregnancy, every 2 to 3 weeks until 36 weeks, and weekly thereafter if the pregnancy progresses normally.** The U.S. Public Health Service suggested that this number of visits can be decreased—especially in parous, healthy women—and studies suggest that this can be done safely. If any complications are present, the intervals can be increased appropriately. For example, patients with hypertensive disease or those at risk for preterm delivery may require weekly visits.

At regular visits, the patient is weighed, the blood pressure is recorded, and the presence of edema is evaluated (see "Intercurrent Problems" below). Fundal height is regularly measured with a tape measure, fetal heart tones are recorded, and fetal position is noted. The goal of subsequent pregnancy visits is to assess fetal growth and maternal well-being. **In addition, at each prenatal visit, time should be allowed ask the patient whether she has any problems or questions. Family members should be encouraged to come to prenatal visits, ask questions, and participate to the degree that the patient wishes.**

In patients at risk of prematurity, or in those with a short cervix noted during an ultrasound, frequent cervical checks or sonographic evaluation of cervical length may reveal premature

TABLE 6-3   RECOMMENDATIONS FOR ALL WOMEN FOR PRENATAL CARE

	FIRST VISIT*	WEEK OF GESTATION								
		6-8†	14-16	24-28	32	36	38	39	40	41
History										
Medical, including genetic	X									
Psychosocial	X									
Update medical and psychosocial		X	X	X	X	X	X	X	X	X
Physical Examination										
General	X									
Blood pressure	X	X	X	X	X	X	X	X	X	X
Height	X									
Weight	X	X	X	X	X	X	X	X	X	X
Height and weight profile	X									
Pelvic examination and pelvimetry	X	X								
Breast examination	X	X								
Fundal height			X	X	X	X	X	X	X	X
Fetal position and heart rate			X	X	X	X	X	X	X	X
Cervical examination	X									
Laboratory Tests										
Hemoglobin or hematocrit	X	X		X		X				
Rh factor, blood type	X									
Antibody screen	X			X						
Pap smear	X									
Screen for GDM				X						
MSAFP			X							
Urine										
Dipstick	X									
Protein	X									
Sugar	X									
Culture		X								
Infections										
Rubella titer	X									
Syphilis test	X									
Gonococcal culture	X	X				X				
Hepatitis B	X									
HIV (offered)	X	X								
Toxoplasmosis	X									
Illicit drug screen (offered)	X									
Genetic screen	X									

*Includes preconception visit.
†If preconception care has preceded.
GDM, gestational diabetes mellitus; *HIV,* human immunodeficiency virus; *MSAFP,* maternal serum α-fetoprotein.

dilation or effacement that can be treated with progesterone suppositories or cerclage (see Chapters 28 and 29).

Further laboratory evaluations are routinely performed at 28 weeks, when the hemoglobin or hematocrit, Rh type and screen for antibodies, serologic test for syphilis, and possibly HIV testing can be repeated. If the patient is Rh negative and unsensitized, she should receive Rhesus immune globulin (RhIG) prophylaxis at this time (see Chapter 34). A glucose screening test for diabetes is also appropriately performed at this time (see Chapter 40), and some clinicians advocate routine fetal movement counting using a movement chart (see Chapter 11). At 36 weeks, a repeat hematocrit, especially in those women with anemia or those at risk for peripartum hemorrhage (multipara, repeat CD), may be performed. Group B *Streptococcus* (GBS) screening should be done at 35 to 36 weeks with consideration given to possible intrapartum prophylaxis. Also, appropriate cultures for the pathogens responsible for STIs (*N. gonorrhoeae* and *C. trachomatis*) should be obtained as indicated in the third trimester based on geographic prevalence rates and demographic risk factors.

After 41 weeks from the last menstrual period, the patient should be entered into a screening program for fetal well-being, which may include electronic monitoring tests or ultrasound evaluation (see Chapter 11). If labor has not occurred by 41 to 42 weeks, induction should be recommended (see Chapter 36).

Intercurrent Problems

It is the practice in prenatal care to evaluate the pregnant patient for the development of certain important complications. Inherent in these checks is surveillance for intervening problems, an important one being preeclampsia. Blood pressure will change physiologically in response to pregnancy, but development of hypertension must be recognized so that evaluation, treatment, or hospitalization can be promptly initiated (see Chapter 31).

Dependent edema is physiologic in pregnancy, but generalized or facial edema can be a first sign of disease. It is critical here, as in all areas, for the practitioner to understand the normal changes associated with pregnancy in order to accept and explain these (see Chapter 3) but also to aggressively manage any abnormal changes.

Proteinuria reflects urinary tract disease, generally either from infection or glomerular dysfunction and possibly as a result of preeclampsia. The degree of proteinuria should be quantitated in a 24-hour urine collection. Any urinary tract infection should be treated because **asymptomatic bacteriuria is a risk factor for pyelonephritis and PTB.**

Fetal, placental, or amniotic fluid abnormalities are often first detected by deviation from the clinical expectation. In some conditions, the risk of fetal anomaly will be so high as to prompt baseline screening or testing (e.g., sonography, fetal echocardiography, prenatal karyotype). At other times, risk only becomes evident during the course of prenatal care. Growth restriction and macrosomia can often be suspected clinically, usually on the basis of an abnormality in fundal growth. For the patient who has a history of these conditions or other predisposing factors such as hypertension, renal disease, or diabetes, particular vigilance is in order. Alteration in amniotic fluid, too much or too little, can sometimes be detected clinically based on a uterine size/date discrepancy. In addition to maternal conditions, abnormalities in amniotic fluid volume (see Chapter 35) may be caused by fetal disease that can be defined using sonography and that may alter management of the pregnancy; for example, prompt delivery or therapeutic amnioreduction may be considered.

Common Patient-Centered Issues

Although not exhaustive, this section includes common issues or concerns likely to be raised by the patient at some point during successive prenatal visits. The practitioner should be prepared to address these as part of the health education, promotion, and prevention goals of each patient.

Nutrition During Pregnancy

Chapter 7 provides a detailed description of diet guidelines for weight gain. In addition, iron and vitamin supplementation, including folic acid supplementation, are also discussed in that chapter.

Activity and Employment

Most patients are able to maintain their normal activity levels in pregnancy. Mothers tolerate pregnancy with considerable physical activity, such as looking after small children, working, and routine exercise; however, **heavy lifting and excessive physical activity should be avoided.** Modification of activity level as the pregnancy progresses is seldom needed, except if the mother's job involves physical danger. Recreational exercises should be encouraged, such as those available in prenatal exercise classes. The importance of physical activity cannot be overstressed. Unfortunately, many women are routinely told to decrease their physical activity, even though research on moderate aerobic activity shows no negative impact on pregnancy outcomes. In the absence of medical or obstetric complications, **current ACOG recommendations advocate for 30 minutes or more of moderate exercise daily**. A Cochrane review of aerobic exercise in pregnancy indicated improved maternal fitness, but evidence is insufficient to determine whether maternal or neonatal risks or benefits exist.

Previously sedentary women with no medical contraindications can start with 15 minutes of continuous exercise three times per week and work toward a goal of 30 minutes four times per week. With regard to exercise intensity, a good rule of thumb is the so-called talk test; that is, if the exercising woman cannot maintain a conversation (perceived moderate intensity), she is probably overexercising. Studies suggest that women who engage in regular recreational activity have less GDM, less preeclampsia, and less low back and pelvic pain. The patient should be counseled to discontinue activity whenever she experiences discomfort.

If the job presents hazards no greater than those encountered in daily life, healthy pregnant women may work until their delivery. Strenuous physical exercise, standing for prolonged periods, and work on industrial machines in addition to other adverse environmental factors may be associated with increased risk of poor pregnancy outcome, and these should be modified as necessary.

Travel

A pregnant woman should be advised against prolonged sitting during car or airplane travel because of the risk of venous stasis and possible thromboembolism. The usual recommendation is a maximum of 6 hours per day driving, stopping at least every 2 hours for 10 minutes to allow the patient to walk around and increase venous return from the legs. Hydration and support stockings are also recommended.

The patient should be instructed to wear her seatbelt during car travel but to wear it under the abdomen as pregnancy advances (see Chapter 26). It may also be helpful to take pillows along to increase comfort. If the patient is traveling a significant distance, it might be helpful for her to carry a copy of her medical record with her should an emergency arise in a strange environment. She should also become familiar with the medical facilities in the area or perhaps obtain the name of a local obstetrician should a problem occur.

Nausea and Vomiting in Pregnancy

Nausea and vomiting are common in pregnancy and affect approximately 75% of pregnancies. **Hyperemesis gravidarum is an extreme form characterized by vomiting, dehydration, and weight loss that frequently results in hospitalization.** The exact etiology of hyperemesis gravidarum is unknown, but it is believed to be related to a product of the placenta and is correlated with human chorionic gonadotropin (hCG) and estradiol concentrations. Twin and sibling studies suggest a genetic component, whereas epidemiologic risk factors include younger age, low prepregnancy body mass, female fetus, history of motion sickness or migraines, and *Helicobacter pylori* infection. Smoking and obesity are associated with a *decreased* risk of hyperemesis. If hyperemesis gravidarum occurs in a first pregnancy, the recurrence risk is approximately 15%, although this may be reduced if there is a change in paternity.

Women with hyperemesis gravidarum can have transient laboratory abnormalities that may include suppressed thyroid-stimulating hormone (TSH) or elevated free thyroxine (see Chapter 42). They can also have elevated liver enzymes and bilirubin, higher levels of amylase and lipase, and altered electrolytes (loss of sodium, potassium, and chloride). Women with severe hyperemesis can develop rare, severe complications such as Wernicke encephalopathy, beriberi, central pontine myelinolyis, peripheral neuropathy, and hepatic or renal failure. Similarly, severe vomiting has been associated with Mallory-Weiss tears, esophageal rupture, pneumomediastinum, and retinal detachment.

Fetal effects of hyperemesis gravidarum are unclear. In general, if the problem is corrected or resolves and the patient is able to gain weight, there are no consequences. However, if the woman has poor weight gain (<15 lb), the fetus is at increased risk for LBW and PTB.

Treatment of hyperemesis gravidarum is primarily symptomatic. No evidence is available to support an ideal diet in these cases, but women are frequently advised to eat small meals that favor proteins over carbohydrates and liquids over solids. Women admitted to the hospital typically require intravenous (IV) hydration, and most recommend initial supplementation with thiamine (100 mg) for 3 days to prevent the possibility of Wernicke encephalopathy. Three randomized controlled trials suggest a benefit of vitamin B$_6$ in reducing nausea. If symptoms persist, adding an antihistamine may be beneficial. In addition to antihistamines, benzamides, phenothiazines, butyrophenones, type 3 serotonin receptor antagonists, and corticosteroids have all been used in the treatment of hyperemesis. Although anecdotally successful, the evidence of efficacy from randomized trials is inconclusive. This is important to consider given that some of the agents can cause adverse reactions that include but are not limited to extrapyramidal symptoms, anxiety, and depression. Ginger is an alternative therapy that has been successful in treating the nausea and vomiting of pregnancy.

In rare instances, patients do not respond to treatment, are unable to tolerate oral intake, and cannot maintain their weight or continue to lose weight. **These patients may benefit from enteral or parenteral nutrition,** although significant complications have been described with parenteral nutrition that include thrombophlebitis and death from infection or pericardial tamponade. A recent study by Holmgren and colleagues described maternal and neonatal outcomes from 94 patients admitted with hyperemesis gravidarum and treated with medications, but only as compared with a nasogastric tube (NGT) or a peripherally inserted central catheter (PICC); they found no difference in gestational age, mean birthweight, or Apgar scores, but an increased risk of NICU admissions was reported in the PICC line group (9.1% vs. 4.1% or 0%). Of patients managed with medication, 7% (3/42) had an adverse reaction from the medication that resolved after treatment, whereas 11% (2/19) of patients had the NGT dislodge, and 64% (21/33) of patients with a PICC line required treatment for infection, thromboembolism, or both. Based on their findings and those of others, the authors suggested that PICC lines should be avoided.

Finally, some patients who fail treatment opt to terminate their pregnancy, although the exact incidence is unknown; a web-based survey of over 800 women who agreed to be part of a hyperemesis gravidarum registry noted that 15% had at least one termination, and 6% had more than one termination as a direct or indirect result of severe hyperemesis gravidarum. These women felt they were too sick to care for their family or themselves, or they were concerned about the potential adverse consequences of hyperemesis gravidarum on their baby. Further, these women indicated that health care providers were uncaring or did not appear to understand or acknowledge how sick they were, which suggests that further education within the medical community about the physical and psychological burden of hyperemesis gravidarum is needed.

Heartburn

Heartburn is a common complaint in pregnancy because of relaxation of the esophageal sphincter (see Chapter 3). Overeating contributes to this problem, therefore the patient who experiences postprandial heartburn should be advised to save part of her meal for later and to not eat immediately before lying down. Pillows to prop up the upper body at bedtime may help. If necessary, antacids may be prescribed. Liquid antacids coat the esophageal lining more effectively than do tablets. In a subset of patients, H$_2$ receptor blockers may be helpful (see Chapter 48).

Backache

Back pain is a common complaint in pregnancy that affects over 50% of women. Numerous physiologic changes of pregnancy likely contribute to the development of back pain including ligament laxity related to relaxin and estrogen, weight gain, hyperlordosis, and anterior tilt of the pelvis; these altered biomechanics lead to mechanical strain on the lower back. **Backache can be prevented to a large degree by avoidance of excessive weight gain and a regular exercise program before pregnancy.** Exercises to strengthen back muscles can also be helpful. Posture is important, and sensible shoes should be worn, not high heels. Scheduled rest periods with elevation of the feet to flex the hips may be helpful. Other successful treatment modalities that have been described include nonelastic maternity support binders, acupuncture, aquatic exercises, and pharmacologic regimens that incorporate acetaminophen, narcotics, prednisone, and rarely, antiprostaglandins (if remote from term).

Sexual Activity

Generally speaking, in the absence of any known contraindications, no restrictions need to be placed on sexual intercourse. However, the patient should be advised that pregnancy may cause changes in comfort and sexual desire. Frequently, increased uterine activity is noted after sexual intercourse; it is unclear whether this is due to breast stimulation, female orgasm, or prostaglandins in male ejaculate. In a survey of 425 primiparous women, Fox and colleagues reported that over 60% of women reported sexual activity in the third trimester, and up to one-third engaged in sexual activity within 2 days of delivery. Studies suggest that sexual activity during pregnancy is rarely discussed, although most women feel the need to receive more information. For women at risk for preterm labor or those with a history of previous pregnancy loss and who note increased uterine activity after sex, use of a condom or avoidance of sexual activity may be recommended.

Prepared Parenthood and Support Groups

Routine classes on newborn child care and parenting should be part of the prenatal care program. Many parents are completely unprepared for the myriad changes in their lives, and some idea of what to expect is beneficial. As pregnancy progresses, challenging needs can arise. Support groups for families with genetic or medical conditions, such as Down syndrome or skeletal dysplasias, or preterm infants and maternal support groups for mothers of twins or triplets and for women who have had cesarean delivery have all shown that they can meet the special needs of these parents. Unsuccessful pregnancies lead to special problems and needs for which social workers, clergy, and specialized support groups can be invaluable. Miscarriage, stillbirth, and infant death are particularly devastating events best managed by a team approach with special attention given to the grieving process. Referral to such groups as Compassionate Friends of Miscarriage, Infant Death, and Stillbirth is recommended. Careful evaluation and follow-up for depression should be part of the routine pregnancy postpartum care (see Chapter 23).

Prenatal Record

The prenatal care record should describe the comprehensive care provided and should allow for systematic documentation of coordinated services. One such example is the antepartum record designed by ACOG. Many of the advances in risk assessment and perinatal regionalization result directly from widespread implementation of this record. Most electronic medical record (EMR) systems have attempted to capture the important components, but they are limited in the degree to which different EMR systems can interrelate with each other. Technology allows sophisticated recording, display, and retrieval—often computer based—of prenatal care records, but quality relies on accurate, consistent compiling and concurrent recording of the information. The record must be complete yet simple, directive but flexible, and at the same time legible, transmittable, and able to display necessary data rapidly. Some data exist regarding the quality of documentation in prenatal/intrapartum records as it relates to billing diagnosis, but little data is available regarding the quality of documentation in EMRs. Implementation of the International Classifications of Diseases may help, but this has yet to be determined. European nations often have one record for uniform care, and many health care systems have adopted records to permit internal consistency. Commonly used records accurately reflect the following:

1. Demographic data, obstetric history
2. Medical and family history, including genetic screening
3. Baseline physical examination with emphasis on the gynecologic examination
4. Menstrual history, especially last normal menstrual period (LMP), with documentation of established due date and reference criteria for dating if that was done with something other than LMP
5. Record of individual visits
6. Routine laboratory data (e.g., Rh, GBS, Rapid Plasma Reagin Test [RPR], rubella, hepatitis, and HIV)
7. Problem list
8. Space for special notations and plans (e.g., planned trial of labor after cesarean [TOLAC; see Chapter 20], repeat CD, tubal ligation)

These records must be made available to consultants, and they should be available at the facility where delivery is planned. If transfer is expected, a copy of the prenatal record should accompany the patient.

Prenatal Education

In general, it is believed that patient education leads to better self-care, and pregnancy is no exception. Efforts to improve understanding, involvement, and satisfaction with pregnancy and the perinatal period are increasing. In this area more than any other, the options for paramedical support have expanded. Practitioners and patients have access to a vast array of support personnel (e.g., doulas) and groups to assist and advise in the pregnancy and subsequent parenthood. Group prenatal care has recently been initiated and has been associated with improved patient satisfaction. Patients should be educated about care options and should be allowed to participate in decision making.

POSTPARTUM CARE
Components of the Postpartum Visit

Postpartum care is covered in detail in Chapter 23; however, it should be stressed that a key element in ensuring the optimal interconception period is by encouraging and reinforcing the importance of keeping the postpartum appointment. Most patients should be seen approximately 6 weeks postpartum, sooner for complicated deliveries and cesarean deliveries. The goal of this visit is to evaluate the physical, psychosocial, and mental well-being of the mother; to provide support and referral for breastfeeding; and to initiate or encourage compliance with the preferred family planning option and preconception care for the next pregnancy. Depending on the mother's education and insurance status, the likelihood of attending the postpartum visit ranges from 77% to 95%. Data suggest that maternal health after pregnancy is associated with improved child health, and so increasing compliance with postpartum visits has been identified as both a national and international public health priority.

Birth Spacing

An important goal of the postpartum visit and interconception care is to encourage birth spacing—specifically, to educate women about the importance of waiting at least 24 months to conceive again. This interconception interval has been associated with decreased risk of PTB/LBW and decreased risk for uterine rupture among women attempting a vaginal birth after a cesarean delivery (VBAC).

An estimated one in three pregnancies in the United States occurs within 18 months of a previous birth, 1 in 2 occurs within 18 to 59 months, and 1 in 6 occurs after 60 months or more. *Short birth spacing,* defined as 18 months or less, was found to be strongly linked to unintended pregnancies and age, specifically teenagers (between 15 and 19 years old at the time of conception) and women whose first conception was after the age of 30. For women who do wait the recommended interval, using the most efficacious contraceptive method in light of their medical comorbidities is critical to optimize the interconception period because 49% of pregnancies are unplanned. For example, an estimated 26% to 41% percent of postpartum women have intercourse before their 6-week postpartum visit, 41% by 6 weeks, 65% by 8 weeks, and 78% by 12 weeks. Whether they had complications during the birth was a significant factor in how long they waited. **Educating women on the most appropriate contraception based on medical conditions and discharging patients with an effective contraception method is essential to assist women in achieving the recommended 24-month interval.**

Specific nutritional recommendations such as calcium, folate, or iron supplementation vary during the interconception period depending on whether the woman is breastfeeding or anemic or has had any other complications. In general, most women are nutrient depleted post partum, and a daily prenatal vitamin should be continued for at least 8 weeks after delivery. Further, attention should be directed toward counseling about the common tendency and known hazards of weight retention.

Recent systematic reviews have demonstrated the benefits of postpartum psychosocial support for early detection and prevention of maternal depression as well as for decreased newborn readmissions. Psychosocial support can be provided by clinicians or trained lay personnel.

Counseling Regarding Medical Conditions and Obstetric Complications

Finally, follow-up is needed for medical complications such as heart disease, hypertension, diabetes, and depression—conditions that may have been exacerbated by pregnancy—as well as thyroid disease and epilepsy, conditions in which postpartum medication adjustments may be required. One focus of interconception care is on medical complications that were present during pregnancy. Chronic diseases such as diabetes, hypertension, obesity, and depression may first become apparent during prenatal care. Lack of access to routine well-woman and medical care contribute to a disproportionate number of pregnancy complications among minority women and those of low socioeconomic status. Medical complications during pregnancy may also account for the increasing rate of cesarean delivery and also of LBW/PTB, the most common cause of infant deaths. A history of a previous pregnancy outcome is an important predictor of future reproductive risk. However, **many women with adverse pregnancy outcomes do not receive targeted interventions to reduce risks during future pregnancies.** Women with a history of PTB, preeclampsia, and GDM should be informed that they are at increased risk of recurrence with subsequent pregnancies in addition to being at risk for subsequent development of hypertension and cardiovascular disease. Likewise, women with GDM are at increased risk of developing type 2 diabetes. Patients should be counseled to inform all subsequent health care providers of these prior medical conditions that occurred during pregnancy.

Pregnancy complications, both maternal and fetal/newborn, should be reviewed, and recurrence risk should be discussed along with any potential interventions considered. For example, cesarean delivery has a high likelihood of repeating; therefore the risks, benefits, and alternatives should be addressed, and this discussion should include the type of uterine incision used, any abnormal placentation, and the possibility of a TOLAC. If childbirth was traumatic, the clinician should be alert for signs or symptoms of depression or PTSD. Women with preeclampsia or chronic hypertension should be advised to start a low-dose aspirin regimen after 12 weeks' gestation in their next pregnancy. To prevent recurrence, women with preterm deliveries should be counseled to seek care early to discuss treatment options, which may include progesterone therapy or cerclage based on clinical history.

COMING FULL CIRCLE: COMPONENTS OF INTERCONCEPTION CARE AND WELL-WOMAN VISITS

As noted throughout this chapter, the specific components of preconception, postpartum, and interconception care and the well-woman visit overlap conceptually to the point of redundancy. However, on a pragmatic basis, much work needs to be done relative to dissemination of good information and implementation of quality care. Models to incorporate interconception care into health programs for women are limited but are currently being investigated. The most common settings have focused on low-income and minority populations as a potential intervention to eliminate their disparate maternal and birth outcomes.

One example of the implementation of interconception care was in Chicago among low-income black women with a prior adverse pregnancy outcome. This program, Interconception Care Period (ICCP), focused on the integration of social services, family planning, and medical care provided through a team approach (Table 6-4). The planned delivery of

TABLE 6-4 INTERCONCEPTION CARE RESOURCES

RESOURCE	DESCRIPTION AND LINK
Interconception Care Project of California	The Interconception Care Project is a collection of recommendations to improve and promote the interconception health of women by maximizing care provided during the postpartum visit. A panel of obstetric and health experts developed evidence-based postpartum clinical management algorithms and companion patient education materials based on the 21 most common pregnancy and delivery complications identified using ICD-9 discharge code data in California. The algorithms are designed to guide risk assessment, management, and counseling based on risk of adverse pregnancy outcome and/or maternal/neonatal complications in order to improve the mother's health and reduce risks in future pregnancies. Patient handouts were developed (English and Spanish) that offer explanations of the condition and treatment options; they discuss self-care strategies to improve the health of the woman, her baby, and any future pregnancies (www.everywomancalifornia.org).
Planning for a Healthy Future: Algorithm for Providers Caring for Women of Childbearing Age	Wisconsin Association for Perinatal Care (WAPC) developed a program to put the life course approach to women's health into action. Health care providers can use the algorithm to integrate preconception and interconception care into well-woman care and to identify areas of risk of which a woman may not be aware. Links to other WAPC preconception health resources are also available. http://www.perinatalweb.org/major-initiatives/reducing-infant-mortality/resources
March of Dimes Screening and Counseling Checklist	Patients are given the checklist at the reception desk and are asked to fill it out before seeing the provider. Providers can use this one-page summary to initiate discussions about preconception care. This list offers a series of essential questions that help providers develop good clinical management plans. www.healthteamworks.org/guidelines/preconception.html
Smiles for Life: Women's Oral Health Curriculum	Addresses the importance of oral health before, during, and after pregnancy and includes information on the prevalence of oral disease during pregnancy, its consequences for both mothers and children, and a review of dental treatment guidelines for pregnant women. www.smilesforlifeoralhealth.org/buildcontent.aspx?tut=560&pagekey=61366&cbreceipt=0
Preconception and Interconception Care Guideline	Colorado Department of Public Health developed guidelines designed to assist clinicians providing preconception and interconception care. The guidelines were adapted from the *American Journal of Obstetrics and Gynecology Supplement*, December 2008, and CDC Proceedings of the Preconception Health and Health Care Clinical, Public Health, and Consumer Workgroup Meetings, June 2006. http://www.healthteamworks.org/guidelines/preconception.html
Before, Between, and Beyond Pregnancy	The National Preconception/Interconception Care Clinical Toolkit was designed to help primary care providers, their colleagues, and their practices incorporate preconception health into the routine care of women of childbearing age. http://beforeandbeyond.org/toolkit
Guidelines for Preconception and Interconception Care: Specific Health Conditions	This concise pocket-sized brochure highlights common medical disorders and includes patient counseling recommendations, confirmatory tests, and contraindicated medications (if not using contraception) as well as recommended contraception for high-risk medical diseases. www.everywomancalifornia.org/files.cfm?filesID=531

ICD-9, *International Classification of Diseases*, 9th edition.

interventions based on a woman's unique interconceptional health needs was often replaced by efforts to address the woman's socioeconomic needs. Although medical care remained important, participants viewed themselves as healthy and did not view medical care as a priority; in addition, women's perceptions of contraceptive effectiveness were not always aligned with clinical knowledge.

Since 2005, all 97 federal Healthy Start Programs—initiated in 1991 to address the factors that contribute to the high infant mortality rate in the United States, particularly among populations with disproportionately high rates of adverse perinatal health outcomes—have been required to include an interconception care component. Recommendations for health care providers to address interconception medical conditions have been developed and range from algorithms to toolkits; Table 6-4 gives resources for additional interconception care.

In summary, the traditional approach to improving perinatal outcomes has focused on prenatal care once a woman is already pregnant. **However, the fact is that birth outcomes and maternal outcomes have not significantly improved in the past 40 years. This, coupled with new knowledge that maternal complications during pregnancy and postpartum and newborn complications are associated with long-term health outcomes for both the mother and child, requires that the health care system reframe the approach to providing care to women. Hence, the life-course perspective was proposed.** The improvement of maternal health before conception and in the interconception interval can reduce prematurity and LBW and can subsequently improve the health of infants, and it can maximize the health of mothers and children for generations to come.

KEY POINTS

- The breadth of prenatal care does not end with delivery but rather includes both preconception and postpartum care, which extends up to 1 year after the infant's birth. Importantly, this introduces the concept of interconception care and the principle that almost all health care interactions with reproductive-age women (and men) are opportunities to assess risk, promote healthy lifestyle behaviors, and identify and treat medical and psychosocial issues that could impact pregnancy and the lifetime health of the mother and child.
- *Interconception care* is defined as care provided between the end of a woman's pregnancy to the beginning of her next pregnancy. During the interconception period, intensive interventions are provided to women who have had a previous pregnancy that ended in an adverse outcome (i.e., fetal loss, PTB, LBW, infant death, or birth defect).
- A *reproductive life plan* is a "set of personal goals regarding the conscious decision about whether or not to bear children." Ideally, it outlines a plan to achieve those goals. Reproductive life plans should be individualized, iterative, and addressed initially at menarche, confirmed or modified at subsequent health encounters by all care providers, and retired with menopause or sterilization.
- When specific conditions are detected such that pregnancy is not recommended or intended, reliable contraception should be prescribed, and the importance of compliance should be reinforced. Many women with complex medical problems who are advised against pregnancy conceive unintentionally and/or do not use contraception because of a low perceived risk of conceiving.
- Age, weight (BMI), and changes in weight during pregnancy and over time impact pregnancy outcome and long-term maternal health.
- Primary care, preventative health, and well-women visits are ideal times to screen and counsel patients about STIs and TORCH infections and to confirm and/or update immunization status.
- All reproductive-age women should be current with immunizations as recommended by ACIP and the CDC. This is the time to draw and document protective titers for rubella, varicella, and hepatitis B and to immunize the susceptible patient.
- The time to screen appropriate populations for genetic disease-carrier status, congenital malformations, or familial diseases with major genetic components is *before* pregnancy. If patients screen positive, referral for genetic counseling is indicated because consideration of additional preconception options may be warranted.
- Smoking and alcohol and drug use by pregnant women are all harmful to the developing fetus, but because these substances are often used in combination, teasing apart the specific contributions of each substance to adverse child outcomes can prove difficult. Overall, the risks to the neonate include IUGR, birth defects, altered neuropsychological behavior, and for some drugs, withdrawal symptoms. Subsequent behavior, development, and neurologic function may also be impaired from health problems that started during the preconception period.
- A study based on the National Health and Nutrition Examination Survey demonstrated that all pregnant women are exposed to and have detectable levels of chemicals that can be harmful to reproduction or human development. Because exposure to environmental agents can be mitigated or prevented, it is important for women to be made aware of known toxic substances and to inform them as to how to access resources to gain additional information.
- Clear evidence shows that for some conditions—such as diabetes mellitus, phenylketonuria, and inflammatory bowel disease—medical disease management before conception can positively influence pregnancy outcome. Medical management should be discussed with the patient, and appropriate management plans should be outlined before conception. Advice should also be given about specific medications to avoid during the first trimester (e.g., isotretinoin).
- All the problems that arise in pregnancy, whether common complaints or more hazardous diseases, convey some risk to the pregnancy that will depend on how these problems are managed by the patient and her care provider. It has been shown that most women and infants who suffer morbidity and mortality will come from a small segment of women with high-risk factors; by reassessing risk factors before and during pregnancy

and again in labor, the ability to identify those at highest risk improves.

◆ A key element to ensure the optimal interconception period is to encourage and reinforce the importance of keeping the postpartum appointment. Most patients should be seen approximately 6 weeks post partum, sooner for complicated or cesarean deliveries. The goal of this visit is to evaluate the physical, psychosocial, and mental well-being of the mother; to provide support and referral for breastfeeding; to initiate or encourage compliance with the preferred family planning option; and to initiate preconception care for the next pregnancy.

◆ An important goal of the postpartum visit and interconception care is to encourage birth spacing—specifically, to educate women about the importance of waiting at least 24 months after delivery to conceive again because this interval has been associated with a decreased risk of preterm birth and low birthweight, and it decreases the risk for uterine rupture among women who attempt a vaginal birth after a cesarean delivery.

REFERENCES

1. Misra DP, Guyer B, Allston A. Integrated perinatal health framework. A multiple determinants model with a life span approach. *Am J Prev Med.* 2003;25:65-75.
2. Public Health Service. *Caring for Our Future: The Content of Prenatal Care—A Report of the Public Health Service Expert Panel on the Content of Prenatal Care.* Washington, DC: PHS-DHRS; 1989.
3. *Expert Panel on the Content of Prenatal Care. Caring for our future: T he content of Prenatal Care.* Washington (DC): Public Health Service; 1989.
4. American Academy of Pediatrics, American College of Obstetricians and Gynecologists. *Guidelines for perinatal care.* 4th ed. Elk Grove Village (IL): American Academy of Pediatrics; 1997.
5. Cochrane A. In: Chalmers I, Enkin M, Keirse M, eds. *Effective Care in Pregnancy and Childbirth.* Oxford University Press; 1989.
6. Centers for Disease Control (CDC). Recommendations to improve preconception health and health care—United States: a report of the CDC/ATSDR Preconception Care Work Group and the Select Panel on Preconception Care. *MMWR Recomm Rep.* 2006;55(RR-6).
7. Wise PH. Transformaing preconceptional, prenatal, and interconceptional care into a comprehensive commitment to women's health. *Womens Health Issues.* 2008;18S:S13-S18.
8. Jack BW, Atrash H, Bickmore T, Johnson KJ. The future of preconception care: a clinical perspective. *Womens Health Issues.* 2008;18(suppl 6):S19-S25.
9. World Health Organization. *Preconception care to reduce maternal and childhood mortality and morbidity: Meeting report and packages of interventions.* Available at <http://apps.who.int/iris/bitstream/10665/78067/1/9789241505000_eng.pdf>.
10. Preconception and Interconception Health Status of Women Who Recently Gave Birth to a Live-Born Infant—Pregnancy Risk Assessment Monitoring System (PRAMS), United States, 26 Reporting Areas, 2004. *MMWR Surveill Summ.* 2007;56(SS-10). <http://www.cdc.gov/mmwr/pdf/ss/ss5610.pdf>.
11. Files JA, Frey KA, Paru DS, Hunt KS, Nobel BN, Mayer AP. Developing a reproductive life plan. *J Midwifery Womens Health.* 2011;56:468-474.
12. Floyd LR, Johnson K, Owens JR, Verbiest S, Moore CA, Boyle C. A national action plan for promoting preconception health and health care in the United States (2012-2014). *J Womens Health (Larchmt).* 2013;22:797-802.
13. Barker DJ, Winter PD, Osmond C, Margetts B, Simmonds SJ. Weight in infancy and death from ischaemic heart disease. *Lancet.* 1989;2:577-580.
14. Dover GJ. The Barker Hypothesis: How Pediatricians Will Diagnose and Prevent Common Adult-Onset Diseases. *Trans Am Clin Climatol Assoc.* 2009;120:199-207.
15. Kermack AJ, Macklon N. Preconception care and fertility. *Minerva Ginecol.* 2013;65:253-269.
16. CDC. *Unintended Pregnancy Prevention.* Available at <www.cdc.gov/reproductivehealth/unintendedpregnancy>.
17. Finer LB, Zolna MR. Unintended pregnancy in the United States: incidence and disparities 2006. *Contraception.* 2011;84:478-485.
18. Mosher WD, Jones J, Abma JC. Intended and unintended births in the United States: 1982-2010. *Natl Health Stat Report.* 2012;(55):1-28.
19. Deleted in review.
20. Mathews TJ, Hamilton BE. Delayed Childbearing: More Women are Having Their First Child Later in Life. *NCHS Data Brief.* 2009;21:1-8.
21. Dean SV, Iman AM, Lassi ZS, Bhutta ZA. Importance of intervening in the preconception period to impact pregnancy outcomes. *Nestle Nutr Inst Workshop Ser.* 2013;74:63-73.
22. Kersten I, Lange AE, Haas JP, et al. Chronic diseases in pregnant women: prevalence and birth outcomes based on the SNiP-Study. *BMC Pregnancy Childbirth.* 2014;14:75.
23. Chatterjee S, Kotelchuck M, Sambamoorthi U. Prevalence of chronic illness in pregnancy, access to care and health care costs. Implications for Interconception care. *Womens Health Issues.* 2008;18S:S107-S116.
24. Phelan S. Pregnancy: a "teachable moment" for weight control and obesity prevention. *Am J Obstet Gynecol.* 2010;202:135.e1-135.e8.
25. McBride CM, Emmons KM, Lipkus IM. Understanding the potential of teachable moments: the case of smoking cessation. *Health Educ Res.* 2003;8:156-170.
26. Johnson K, Atrash H, Johnson A. Policy and finance for preconception care: Opportunities for today and the future. *Womens Health Issues.* 2008;18S:S2-S9.
27. IOM (Institute of Medicine). *Clinical Preventive Services for Women: Closing the Gaps.* Washington, DC: The National Academies Press Washington DC; 2011.
28. Jack BW, Atrash H, Coonrod DV, Moos MK, O'Donnell J, Johnson K. The clinical content of preconception care: an overview and preparation of this supplement. *Am J Obstet Gynecol.* 2008;199(6 suppl 2):S267-S279.
29. Humphrey JR, Floyd L. *Preconception Health and Health Care Environmental Scan: Report on clinical screening tools and interventions. National Center of Birth Defects and Developmental Disabilities.* Atlanta: Centers for Disease Control; 2012.
30. Gardiner P, Hempstead MD, Ring L, et al. Reaching women through health information technology: the Gabby preconception care system. *Am J Health Promot.* 2013;273(suppl 3):eS11-eS20.
31. Planning your family: developing a reproductive live plan. *J Midwifery Womens Health.* 2011;56:535-536.
32. *Get ready for pregnancy. March of Dimes.* Available at <www.marchofdimes.com/getready.html>.
33. Delissaint D, McKyer J. A systematic review of factors utilized in preconception health behavior research. *Health Educ Behav.* 2011;38:603-616.
34. Frey KA, Files JA. Preconception healthcare: what women know and believe. *Matern Child Health J.* 2006;10:S73-S77.
35. CDC. *US Medical Eligibility Criteria for Contraceptive Use, 2010: Adapted from the World Health Organization Medical Eligibility Criteria for Contraceptive Use, 4th ed.* MMWR 2010;59(RR04)1-6.
36. Organisation for Economic Co-operation and Development. Available at <www.oecd.org/els/soc/47701118.pdf>.
37. Bayrampour H, Heaman M. Comparison of demographic and obstetric characteristics of Canadian primiparous women of advanced maternal age and younger age. *J Obstet Gynaecol Can.* 2011;33:820-829.
38. Usta IM, Nassar AH. Advanced maternal age. Part I: obstetric complications. *Am J Perinatol.* 2008;25:521-534.
39. Paulson RJ, Boostanfar R, Saadat P, et al. Pregnancy in the sixth decade of life: obstetric outcomes in women of advanced reproductive age. *JAMA.* 2002;288:2320.
40. Chibber R. Child-bearing beyond age 50: pregnancy outcome in 59 cases "a concern"? *Arch Gynecol Obstet.* 2005;271:189-194.
41. Montan S. Increased risk in the elderly parturient. *Curr Opin Obstet Gynecol.* 2007;19:110-112.
42. Franz MB, Husslein PW. Obstetrical management of the older gravida. *Womens Health (Lond Engl).* 2010;6:463-468.
43. Waldenström U, Aasheim V, Nilsen AB, Rasmussen S, Pettersson HJ, Schytt E. Adverse pregnancy outcomes related to advanced maternal age compared with smoking and being overweight. *Obstet Gynecol.* 2014;123(1):104-112.

44. Ludwig AK, Ludwig M, Jauniaux ERM. Singleton pregnancies after assisted reproductive technology: the obstetric perspective. In: Jauniaux ERM, Risk RMB, eds. *Pregnancy after Assisted Reproductive Technology.* Cambridge.: Cambridge University Press; 2012:66-71.

45. Pecks U, Maass N, Neulen J. Oocyte donation: a risk factor for pregnancy-induced hypertension: a meta-analysis and case series. *Dtsch Arztebl Int.* 2011;108:23-31.

46. Jauniaux ERM. Multiple gestation pregnancy after assisted reproductive technology. In: Jauniaux ERM, Risk RMB, eds. *Pregnancy after Assisted Reproductive Technology.* Cambridge.: Cambridge University Press; 2012: 82-92.

47. Tyrberg RB, Blomberg M, Kjølhede P. Deliveries among teenage women—with emphasis on incidence and mode of delivery: a Swedish national survey from 1973 to 2010. *BMC Pregnancy Childbirth.* 2013;13:204.

48. Lao TT, Ho LF. The obstetric implications of teenage pregnancy. *Hum Reprod.* 1997;12(10):2303-2305.

49. Hodgkinson S, Beers L, Southammakosane C, Lewin A. Addressing the mental health needs of pregnant and parenting adolescents. *Pediatrics.* 2014;133(1):114-122.

50. Ganchimeg T, Mori R, Ota E, et al. Maternal and perinatal outcomes among nulliparous adolescents in low- and middle-income countries: a multi-country study. *BJOG.* 2013;120:1622-1630.

51. Food and Nutrition Board Institute of Medicine. *National Academy of Sciences: Nutrition During Pregnancy.* Washington, DC: National Academy Press; 1990:10.

52. Zlatnik FJ, Burmeister LF. Dietary protein in pregnancy: effect on anthropometric indices of the newborn infant. *Am J Obstet Gynecol.* 1983;146:199.

53. Catalano PM, Mele L, Landon MB, et al. Inadequate weight gain in overweight and obese pregnant women: what is the effect on fetal growth? *Am J Obstet Gynecol.* 2014;211(2):137.e1-137.e7.

54. Fitzsimons KJ, Modder J. Setting maternity care standards for women with obesity in pregnancy. *Semin Fetal Neonatal Med.* 2010;15:100-107.

55. Thangaratinam S, Rogozinska E, Jolly K, et al. Effects of interventions in pregnancy on maternal weight and obstetric outcomes: meta-analysis of randomised evidence. *BMJ.* 2012;16:344, e2088.

56. Linne Y, Dye L, Barkeling B, Rossner S. Long-term weight development in women: a 15-year follow-up of the effects of pregnancy. *Obes Res.* 2004;12:1166-1178.

57. Rooney BL, Schauber CW. Excess pregnancy weight gain and long-term obesity: One decade later. *Obstet Gynecol.* 2002;100:245-252.

58. Bogaerts A, Van den Bergh BR, Ameye L, et al. Interpregnancy weight change and risk for adverse perinatal outcome. *Obstet Gynecol.* 2013;122(5):999-1009.

59. Walker DA, Wisger JM, Rossie D. Contemporary childbirth education models. *J Midwifery Womens Health.* 2009;54:469-476.

60. Institute of Medicine (US): Subcommittee on Nutritional Status and Weight Gain during Pregnancy. *Institute of Medicine (US) Subcommittee on Dietary Intake and Nutrient Supplements during Pregnancy. Nutrition during pregnancy: Part I, weight gain; Part II, nutritional supplements.* Washington, DC: National Academy Press; 1990.

61. Amorim Adegboye AR, Linne YM. Diet or exercise, or both, for weight reduction in women after childbirth. *Cochrane Database Syst Rev.* 2013; (7):CD005627.

62. Hedly AA, Ogden CL, Johnson CL, Carroll MD, Curtin LR, Flegal KM. Prevalence of overweight and obesity among US children, adolescents, and adults, 1992-2002. *JAMA.* 2004;291:2847-2850.

63. Athukorala C, Rumbold AR, Willson KJ, Crowther CA. The risk of adverse pregnancy outcomes in women who are overweight or obese. *BMC Pregnancy Childbirth.* 2010;10:56.

64. Avcı ME, Sanlıkan F, Celik M, Avcı A, Kocaer M, Göçmen A. Effects of maternal obesity on antenatal, perinatal, and neonatal outcomes. *J Matern Fetal Neonatal Med.* 2014;20:1-13.

65. David LA, Maurice CF, Carmody RN, et al. Diet rapidly and reproducibly alters the human gut microbiome. *Nature.* 2014;505(7484):559-563.

66. Gaskins AJ, Rich-Edwards JW, Colaci DS, et al. Prepregnancy and early adulthood body mass index and adult weight change in relation to fetal loss. *Obstet Gynecol.* 2014;124(4):662-669.

67. Van Lieshout RJ. Role of maternal adiposity prior to and during pregnancy in cognitive and psychiatric problems in offspring. *Nutr Rev.* 2013;71(suppl 1):S95-S101.

68. Li M, Wang M, Donovan SM. Early development of the gut microbiome and immune-mediated childhood disorders. *Semin Reprod Med.* 2014; 32(1):74-86.

69. Putignani L, Del Chierico F, Petrucca A, Vernocchi P, Dallapiccola B. The human gut microbiota: a dynamic interplay with the host from birth to senescence settled during childhood. *Pediatr Res.* 2014;76(1):2-10.

70. Cabrera-Rubio R, Collado MC, Laitinen K, Salminen S, Isolauri E, Mira A. The human milk microbiome changes over lactation and is shaped by maternal weight and mode of delivery. *Am J Clin Nutr.* 2012;96: 544-551.

71. Triunfo S, Lanzone A. Impact of maternal under nutrition on obstetric outcomes. *J Endocrinol Invest.* 2015;38(1):31-38. [Epub 2014 Sep 7].

72. Solmi F, Sallis H, Stahl D, Treasure J, Micali N. Low birth weight in the offspring of women with anorexia nervosa. *Epidemiol Rev.* 2014;36(1):49-56.

73. Micali N, dos-Santos-Silva I, De Stavola B, et al. Fertility treatment, twin births, and unplanned pregnancies in women with eating disorders: findings from a population-based birth cohort. *BJOG.* 2014;121(4): 408-416.

74. Weintraub AY, Levy A, Levi I, Mazor M, Wiznitzer A, Sheiner E. Effect of bariatric surgery on pregnancy outcome. *Int J Gynaecol Obstet.* 2008;103(3):246-251.

75. Shai D, Shoham-Vardi I, Amsalem D, Silverberg D, Levi I, Sheiner E. Pregnancy outcome of patients following bariatric surgery as compared with obese women: a population-based study. *J Matern Fetal Neonatal Med.* 2014;27(3):275-278.

76. Guelinckx I, Devlieger R, Vansant G. Reproductive outcome after bariatric surgery: a critical review. *Hum Reprod Update.* 2009;15(2): 189-201.

77. Galazis N, Docheva N, Simillis C, Nicolaides KH. Maternal and neonatal outcomes in women undergoing bariatric surgery: a systematic review and meta-analysis. *Eur J Obstet Gynecol Reprod Biol.* 2014;181C:45-53.

78. *Sexually Transmitted Diseases Treatment Guidelines.* Available at <www.cdc.gov/std/treatment/2014/2014-std-guidelines-peer-reviewers-08-20-2014.pdf>.

79. Meyers D, Wolff T, Gregory K, et al. USPSTF. USPSTF recommendations for STI screening. *Am Fam Physician* 2008;77(6):819-824.

80. Adams EM, Bruce C, Shulman MS, et al. The PRAMS Working Group: pregnancy planning and pre-conceptional counseling. *Obstet Gynecol.* 1993;82:955.

81. Jones JL, Schulkin J, Maguire JH. Therapy for common parasitic diseases in pregnancy in the Unites States: a review and a survey of obstetrician/gynecologists' level of knowledge about these diseases. *Obstet Gynecol Surv.* 2005;60:386-393.

82. Boyer KM, Holfels E, Roisen N, et al. Risk factors for Toxoplasma gondii infection in mothers of infants with congenital toxoplasmosis: Implications for prenatal management and screening. *Am J Obstet Gynecol.* 2005;192:564-571.

83. Carlson A, Norwitz ER, Stiller RJ. Cytomegalovirus in pregnancy: should all women be screened? *Rev Obstet Gynecol.* 2010;3:172-179.

84. ACOG Practice Bulletin. Clinical management guidelines for obstetrician-gynecologists. No 82 June 2007. Management of herpes in pregnancy. *Obstet Gynecol.* 2007;109:1489-1498.

85. *Advisory Committee on Immunization Practices (ACIP).* Available at <www.cdc.gov/vaccines/acip/index.html>.

86. Wilson RD, Audibert F, Brock JA, et al. Genetic considerations for a women's preconception evaluation. *J Obstet Gynaecol Can.* 2011;3: 57-64.

87. *Genetic Testing for Cystic Fibrosis. National Institutes of Health Consensus Development Conference Statement, Apr 14-16, 1997.* Available at <https://consensus.nih.gov/1997/1997GeneticTestCysticFibrosis106html.htm>.

88. Toriello HV, Meck JM. Professional Practice and Guidelines Committee. Statement on guidance for genetic counseling in advanced paternal age. *Genet Med.* 2008;10(6):457-460.

89. Zofinat W, Auslender R. Dirnfeld M. Advanced paternal age and reproductive outcome. *Asian J Androl.* 2012;14:69-76.

90. Denny CH, Floyd L, Green PP, Hayes DK. Racial and ethnic disparities in preconception risk factors and preconception care. *J Womens Health (Larchmt).* 2012;21:720-729.

91. Cnattingius S. The epidemiology of smoking during pregnancy: smoking prevalence, maternal characteristics, and pregnancy outcomes. *Nicotine Tob Res.* 2004;6(suppl 2):S125-S140.

92. Jauniaux E, Burton GJ. Morphological and biological effects of maternal exposure to tobacco smoke on the feto-placental unit. *Early Hum Dev.* 2007;83:699-706.

93. Jauniaux E, Greenough A. Short and long term outcomes of smoking during pregnancy. *Early Hum Dev.* 2007;83:697-698.

94. Hellstrom-Lindahl E, Nordberg A. Smoking during pregnancy: a way to transfer the addiction to the next generation? *Respiration.* 2002;69(4): 289-293.

95. Adams EK, Melvin CL. Costs of maternal conditions attributable to smoking during pregnancy. *Am J Prev Med.* 1998;15(3):212-219.

96. Miller DP, Villa KF, Hogue SL, Sivapathasundaram D. Birth and first-year costs for mothers and infants attributable to maternal smoking. *Nicotine Tob Res.* 2001;3(1):25-35.

97. Henderson J, Gray R, Brocklehurst P. Systematic review of effects of low-moderate prenatal alcohol exposure on pregnancy outcome. *BJOG.* 2007;114(3):243-252.

98. Flak AL, Su S, Bertrand J, Denny CH, Kesmodel US, Cogswell ME. The association of mild, moderate, and binge prenatal alcohol exposure and child neuropsychological outcomes: a meta-analysis. *Alcohol Clin Exp Res.* 2014;38(1):214-226.

99. Kesmodel U, Kjaersgaard M, Denny C, et al. The association of pre-pregnancy alcohol drinking with child neuropsychological functioning. *BJOG.* 2014 [Epub ahead of print].

100. Sokol RJ, Martier SS, Ager JW. The T-ACE questions: practical prenatal detection of risk-drinking. *Am J Obstet Gynecol.* 1989;160:863.

Additional references for this chapter are available at ExpertConsult.com.

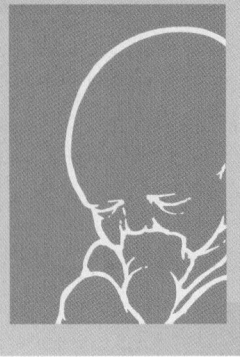

Nutrition During Pregnancy

ELIZABETH HORVITZ WEST, LISA HARK, and PATRICK M. CATALANO

KEY ABBREVIATIONS

American College of Obstetricians and Gynecologists	ACOG
Body mass index	BMI
Centers for Disease Control and Prevention	CDC
Dietary Reference Intakes	DRI
Docosahexaenoic acid	DHA
Eicosapentaenoic acid	EPA
Food and Drug Administration	FDA
Institute of Medicine	IOM
Neural tube defect	NTD
Polyunsaturated fatty acid	PUFA
Recommended Daily Allowance	RDA
Resting metabolic rate	RMR
Small for gestational age	SGA
Thermic effect of energy	TEE
Thermic effect of food	TEF
Upper intake level	UL
World Health Organization	WHO
Women, Infants, and Children Program	WIC

OVERVIEW

In light of the obesity epidemic, the concept of eating for two during pregnancy has come under great scrutiny in recent years. Despite public health efforts to promote weight loss, the number of reproductive-age women who are overweight (body mass index [BMI] >25.0 to 29.9 kg/m^2) has remained stable at approximately 30%. Of more concern is the twofold increase in obesity (BMI $\geq$30 kg/m^2) from 13% to 35% in the same population (Fig. 7-1).[1] **This increase in obesity disproportionately affects minority populations, such as Hispanics and blacks, and especially women.**[2] The increased rates of obesity are attributed to numerous factors that include increased consumption of nonnutritious foods and decreased physical activity. In pregnancy, excessive gestational weight gain increases the risk of higher BMI in a subsequent pregnancy.

Excessive weight gain during pregnancy significantly increases the risk of postpartum weight retention and contributes to the accretion of excess adipose tissue in the fetus. Additionally, obesity poses specific risks to the process of labor and delivery and to fetal outcomes. Obesity, however, is not the only concern in the management of nutrition during pregnancy. The importance of adequate nutrition is also a critical issue during pregnancy, and deficiency or excess of various nutrients can have both short- and long-term consequences to the mother and her fetus. In this chapter we address the specific nutrient requirements during pregnancy, recommendations for weight gain, and other special concerns regarding nutrition and pregnancy.

INTEGRATING NUTRITION INTO THE OBSTETRIC HISTORY

Every woman should have the opportunity to meet with a health care provider for a prepregnancy history and physical examination that includes a nutritional assessment. **The purpose of this assessment is to identify the quality of a patient's diet and to assess any nutritional risk factors that could jeopardize her health or the health of her developing baby.** Adequate intake

Prevalence* of Self-Reported Obesity Among U.S. Adults by State and Territory, BRFSS, 2013

*Prevalence estimates reflect BRFSS methodological changes started in 2011. These estimates should not be compared to prevalence estimates before 2011.

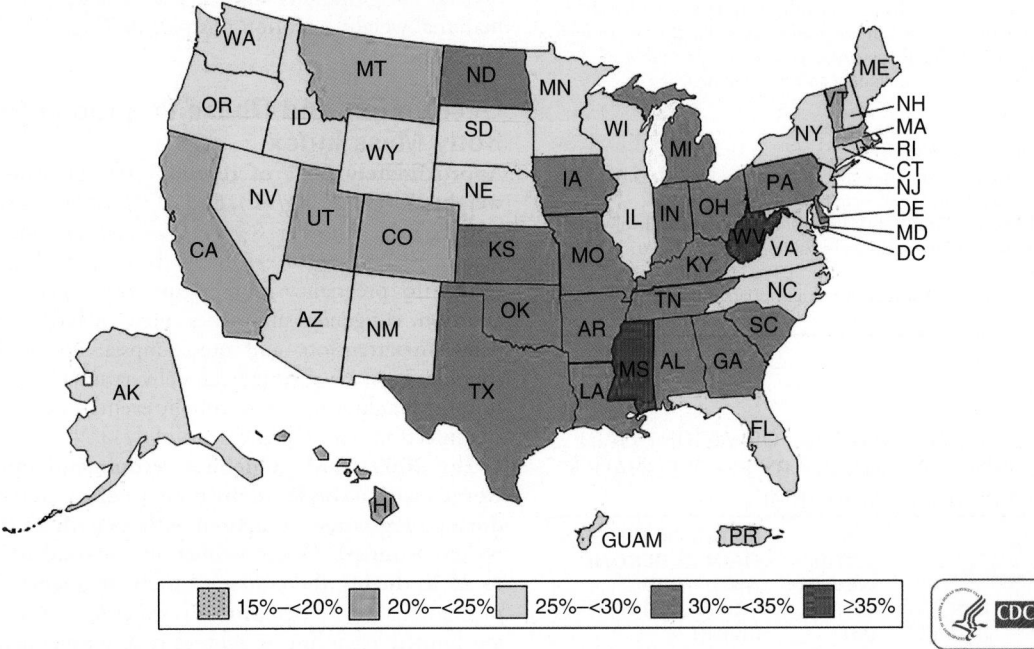

15%–<20%   20%–<25%   25%–<30%   30%–<35%   ≥35%

FIG 7-1 Adult obesity in the United States in 2013. (From Behavioral Risk Factor Surveillance System [BRFSS], Centers for Disease Control and Prevention. Available at http://www.cdc.gov/obesity/data/prevalence-maps.html.)

of nutrients supports the developing fetus, reduces fetal risk, and improves pregnancy outcomes.[3] During the nutritional assessment, the patient's medical history, weight status, dietary intake, and laboratory data should be reviewed. The medical history will identify maternal risk factors for nutritional deficiencies and chronic diseases with nutritional implications (e.g., absorption, eating, and metabolic disorders; infections; inflammatory bowel disease; diabetes mellitus; phenylketonuria; sickle cell trait; and renal disease).

Pertinent dietary information includes appetite, meal patterns, dieting regimens, cultural or religious dietary practices, dietary restrictions, food allergies, cravings, and aversions. Information about abnormal eating practices such as bingeing, purging, laxative or diuretic use, or pica—eating nonfood items (ice, detergent, starch)—should be ascertained.

During the assessment, other relevant information includes the habitual use of caffeine-containing beverages or sugary soft drinks, tobacco, alcohol, recreational drugs, vitamins, and herbal supplements.[4] Specifically asking about nutritional supplements is critically important because many patients do not consider these items to be "medications" and thus will not volunteer that these are being used. **A patient's diet can be assessed by asking about intake over the previous 24 hours or by administering a diet history questionnaire in the waiting room.**

Nutrition-related complications during a prior pregnancy are also important to assess. Gestational weight gain in previous pregnancies and history of hyperemesis, gestational diabetes, anemia, and pica should be determined (see Chapters 6 and 40). **Women with a short interpregnancy interval (e.g., <1 year between pregnancies) may have depleted nutrient reserves,** **which is associated with increased preterm birth, intrauterine growth restriction (IUGR), and maternal morbidity and mortality.**[5,6]

In addition to the medical history, the social history may provide key information regarding the patient's nutritional risk. For example, some work environments adversely impact dietary intake because they may not provide adequate time to eat balanced meals, or they allow access to food that is only marginally nutritious. Women with lower socioeconomic status often need support to obtain nutritious food, and referral to food-assistance programs may be appropriate (e.g., Women, Infants, and Children Program [WIC]).

Many women are receptive to nutritional counseling just prior to or during pregnancy, making this an opportune time to encourage the development of good nutrition and physical activity practices aimed at preventing future medical problems such as obesity, diabetes, hypertension, and osteoporosis.[3] Pregnant women found to be at risk may benefit from a referral to a registered dietitian as shown in Table 7-1.

MATERNAL WEIGHT GAIN RECOMMENDATIONS

In 1990 the Institute of Medicine (IOM) first published recommendations on weight gain during pregnancy.[7] The guidelines were proposed to address many issues regarding the role of nutrition in pregnancy, including the prevention of small-for-gestational-age (SGA) and growth-restricted neonates. As noted previously, the obesity rate has surged in recent decades. As such, in 2009, the IOM updated the 1990 guidelines regarding weight

TABLE 7-1 SITUATIONS IN WHICH CONSULTATION WITH A REGISTERED DIETITIAN IS ADVISABLE

- Pregnancy involves multiple gestations (twins, triplets).
- Gestations are frequent (less than a 3-month interpregnancy interval).
- Tobacco, alcohol, or drug use (chronic medicinal or illicit) is occurring.
- Severe nausea and vomiting (hyperemesis gravidarum) is a problem.
- Eating disorders are present, including anorexia, bulimia, and compulsive eating.
- Weight gain is inadequate during pregnancy.
- Pregnancy occurs in adolescence.
- Eating is restrictive (vegetarianism, macrobiotic, raw food, vegan).
- Food allergies or food intolerances are present.
- Gestational diabetes mellitus (GDM) or history of GDM is involved.
- Patient has a history of low-birthweight babies or other obstetric complications.
- Social factors are present that may limit appropriate intake (e.g., religion, poverty).

Courtesy Lisa Hark, PhD, RD.

TABLE 7-2 RECOMMENDATIONS FOR WEIGHT GAIN DURING PREGNANCY BY PREPREGNANCY BODY MASS INDEX (BMI)

PREGNANCY BMI	BMI (kg/m²)	TOTAL WEIGHT GAIN (lb)	RATES OF WEIGHT GAIN IN SECOND AND THIRD TRIMESTERS (lb/wk)
Underweight	<18.5	28-40	1 (1-1.3)
Normal weight	18.5-24.9	25-35	1 (0.8-1)
Overweight	25.0-29.9	15-25	0.6 (0.5-0.7)
Obese (all classes)	≥30.0	11-20	0.5 (0.4-0.6)

From Composition and compound of gestational weight gain: physiology and metabolism. In Rasmussin KM, Yaktin AL, eds: *Weight Gain During Pregnancy: Reexamining the Guidelines.* Washington, DC: National Academy Press; 2009;77-83.

gain in pregnancy. In contrast to the 1990 recommendations, these guidelines consider both the short- and long-term outcome for the pregnant woman and her child. Additionally, because of the great importance of achieving appropriate pregravid weight, the 2009 guidelines emphasize that women begin pregnancy at a healthy weight. Lastly, the guidelines call for individualized preconceptual, prenatal, and postpartum care to help women attain healthy weight gain and return to a healthy pregravid weight after delivery.[8]

Many general recommendations exist regarding diets for pregnant women to avoid problems such as excessive gestational weight gain and potential complications such as gestational diabetes and fetal overgrowth. These diets vary from those high in complex carbohydrates and low in fats[9] to those low on the glycemic index[10] to diets high in probiotics.[11] Whereas all of these diets may offer some theoretic advantage, presently none can be endorsed as optimal. **Consuming healthy food is the goal to meet the IOM gestational weight guidelines and address the individual needs of the patient.**

Low or Underweight Preconception Body Mass Index

The 2009 IOM guidelines are based upon the World Health Organization (WHO) classifications to define underweight, normal weight, overweight, and obese patients (Table 7-2). *Underweight* is classified as a BMI below 18.5 kg/m². **Based on the available data, there is strong support that women with**

low pregnancy BMI and low gestational weight gain have an increased risk (<10%) for having SGA infants, preterm birth, and perinatal mortality.[12] In contrast, excessive gestational weight gain for women with a low pregravid BMI increases risk of large-for-gestational-age (LGA) neonates and for increased maternal weight retention postpartum (Fig. 7-2; also see Chapters 6 and 41).[13]

Overweight and Obese Prepregnancy Body Mass Index

Approximately 60% of reproductive-age women are overweight (BMI >25 kg/m²), and of these, 50% are obese (BMI >30 kg/m²). Another 8% have severe obesity, with a BMI greater than 40 kg/m². Obesity poses a multitude of threats related to pregnancy: antepartum risks include spontaneous abortion, congenital anomalies, preterm birth, gestational diabetes, hypertension, and preeclampsia; during labor, risk of shoulder dystocia and cesarean delivery are higher; and postpartum risks include thromboembolic events, anemia, and incision-site infections (see Chapters 6 and 41).[14]

The 2009 IOM guidelines recommend that overweight women with a singleton pregnancy gain a total of 15 to 25 lb during pregnancy (compared with 25 with 35 lb for normal-weight women). Obese women are advised to gain only 11 to 20 lb during the course of their pregnancy. These recommendations were based primarily on class I obesity because data are limited regarding weight gain recommendations for each class of obesity. As such, the IOM guidelines do not differentiate between class I obesity (BMI 30 to 34.9 kg/m²), class II obesity (BMI 35 to 39.9 kg/m²), and class III obesity (BMI ≥40 kg/m²).[15,16] The 11 to 20 lb gestational weight gain for obese patients primarily represents the obligatory weight gain of pregnancy. This includes approximately 12 to 14 lb of water, 2 lb of protein, and a variable amount of adipose tissue (Table 7-3).

Some authors have recommended less gestational weight gain for obese class II and III women to decrease neonatal morbidity.[17] Whereas others have noted an increased risk of SGA babies with decreased lean body mass, as well as decreased fat mass, in overweight and obese women with inadequate gestational weight gain.[18]

MATERNAL WEIGHT GAIN RECOMMENDATIONS FOR SPECIAL POPULATIONS

Multiple Gestations

For twin pregnancies, the IOM recommends a gestational weight gain of 37 to 54 lb for women of normal weight, 31 to 50 lb for overweight women, and 25 to 42 lb for obese women (Table 7-4). For triplet and higher-order gestations, the data on ideal gestational weight gain are insufficient; thus no specific recommendations exist for these.[15]

Adolescents

Approximately 17% of teenage girls ages 12 through 19 are obese in America, and these obese teens face the same obstetric risks that adult obese women face. Because 80% of teen pregnancies are unintended, the ability of an obstetrician to discuss preconception nutrition concerns with an obese teen is nearly impossible. Thus efforts should be made during the early prenatal care visits to emphasize the importance of appropriate gestational weight gain and adequate nutrition. Studies have

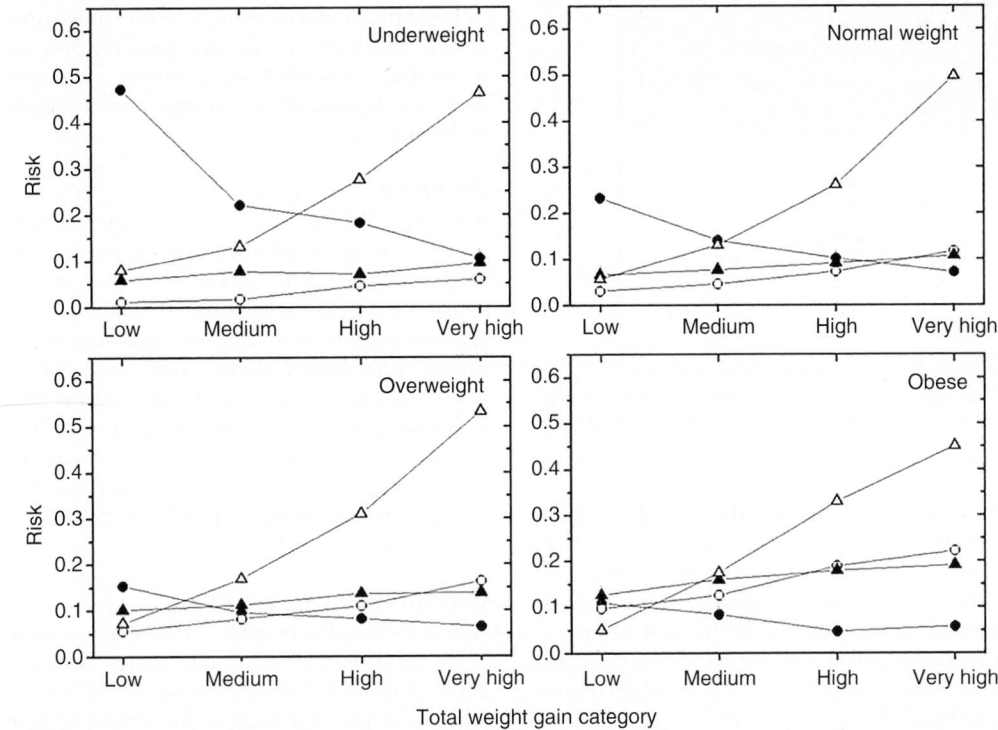

FIG 7-2 Adjusted absolute risks for infants small for gestational age (*solid circle*) and large for gestational age (*open circle)* and for emergency cesarean delivery (*solid triangle*) and postpartum weight retention of ≥5 kg (*open triangle*) according to prepregnancy body mass index (in kg/m²) and gestational weight gain categories of the World Health Organization. Gestational weight gain categories are low (<10 kg), medium (10-19 kg), high (16-19 kg), and very high (≥20 kg). (Modified from Nohr EA, Vaeth M, Baker JL, et al. Combined associations of pre-pregnancy body mass index and gestational weight gain with the outcome of pregnancy. *Am J Clin Nutr.* 2008;87:1750.)

TABLE 7-3	OBLIGATORY COMPONENTS OF WEIGHT GAIN DURING PREGNANCY
	GRAMS
Protein	
Fetus	420
Uterus	170
Blood	140
Placenta	100
Breasts	80
Total	900-1000
Water	
Fetus	2400
Placenta	500
Amniotic fluid	500
Uterus	800
Breasts	300
Maternal blood	1300
Extracellular fluid	1500
Total	7000-8000
Variable Components of Weight Gain	
Carbohydrate	Negligible
Lipids	0-6 kg

From Composition and compound of gestational weight gain: physiology and metabolism. In Rasmussin KM, Yaktin AL, eds: *Weight Gain During Pregnancy: Reexamining the Guidelines.* Washington, DC: National Academy Press; 2009;77-83.

shown that teens who are obese before conceiving are more likely to remain obese postpartum.[19] The IOM recommendations state that adolescents should follow the adult BMI categories to guide their weight gain.

Other Groups
Based on the available evidence, no specific recommendations exist for gestational weight gain in women of short stature, for

TABLE 7-4	PROVISIONAL GUIDELINES FOR WEIGHT GAIN WITH TWIN PREGNANCIES	
PREPREGNANCY BMI	**BMI (kg/m²)**	**TOTAL WEIGHT GAIN (lb)**
Normal weight	18.5-24.9	37-54
Overweight	25.0-29.9	31-50
Obese	≥30.0	25-42

From Composition and compound of gestational weight gain: physiology and metabolism. In Rasmussin KM, Yaktin AL, eds: *Weight Gain During Pregnancy: Reexamining the Guidelines.* Washington, DC: National Academy Press; 2009;77-83. BMI, body mass index.

specific racial or ethnic groups, or in those who smoke cigarettes. The IOM guidelines recognize that each of these special groups may possibly benefit from specific gestational weight gain guidelines, but the available evidence is insufficient to make recommendations.

MATERNAL NUTRIENT NEEDS: CURRENT RECOMMENDATIONS
Energy
Energy expenditure consists of four basic components: (1) resting metabolic rate (RMR); (2) the thermic effect of food (TEF), or diet-induced thermogenesis; (3) the thermic effect of energy (TEE); and (4) adaptive, or facultative, thermogenesis. RMR is the amount of energy, or calories, used at rest and accounts for approximately 60% of total energy expenditure in healthy people. TEF is the caloric cost of eating, digesting, absorbing, resynthesizing, and storing food and accounts for

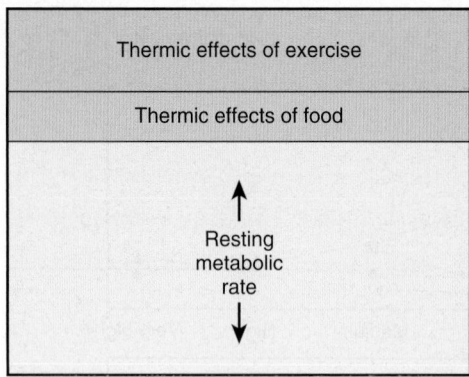

FIG 7-3 Components of energy expenditure. (From Catalano PM, Hollenbeck C. Energy requirements in pregnancy. *Obstet Gynecol Surv.* 1992;47:368.)

about 5% to 10% of total energy expenditure. TEE is quite variable and in sedentary individuals may account for only 15% to 20% of total energy expenditure. *Adaptive thermogenesis,* or *facultative thermogenesis,* refers to adaptations by an organism to adjust to environmental changes, such as overfeeding or underfeeding, as well as to alterations in ambient temperature. Adaptive thermogenesis accounts for no more that 10% of RMR and varies by individual (Fig. 7-3).

The total maternal energy requirement for a full-term pregnancy is estimated at 80,000 kilocalories (kcal). This accounts for the increased metabolic activity of the maternal and fetal tissues as well as for the growth of the fetus and placenta. Maternal energy needs are increased to support the maternal cardiovascular, renal, and respiratory systems. Basal requirements can be determined based on maternal age, stature, activity level, preconception weight, BMI, and gestational weight gain goals. Daily caloric requirements have been estimated by the WHO by dividing the gross energy cost of pregnancy (80,000 kcal) by the approximate duration of pregnancy (250 days after the first month), producing an average additional 300 kcal/day for the entire pregnancy. During the first trimester, total energy expenditure does not change greatly, and weight gain is minimal assuming the woman began her pregnancy without depleted body reserves. Therefore additional energy intake is recommended primarily in the second and third trimesters. During the second trimester, a pregnant woman should consume an additional 340 kcal/day above the nonpregnant energy requirement, and in the third trimester, the additional caloric requirement is 452 kcal/day.[20]

However, a series of prospective studies were conducted in the late 1980s and 1990s to assess energy expenditure in pregnancy. Many of these studies obtained baseline data prior to a planned pregnancy and incorporated measurements such as estimates of body composition, energy intake in the diet, RMR, standard measures of exercise, and activity diaries. These studies showed that the energy cost of pregnancy is much lower than previously estimated.[21-25]

The introduction of the doubly labeled water method has allowed researchers to estimate total energy expenditure in the free-living state. In well-nourished women, RMR usually begins to rise soon after conception and continues to rise until delivery. However, considerable interindividual variation is apparent. In healthy, well-nourished women, the average increases in RMR above prepregnancy values are 4.5%, 10.8%, and 24.0% for the first, second, and third trimesters, respectively.

Pregnancy induces changes in fuel utilization. **Later in pregnancy, the basal or fasting contribution of carbohydrates to oxidative metabolism increases. Fetal growth and lactation are dependent on energy preferentially derived from carbohydrates.**[26]

Proteins

Additional protein is required during pregnancy for fetal, placental, and maternal tissue development. During the course of the pregnancy, an average of 925 g of protein are stored, which is required for the tissue development. **Maternal protein synthesis increases to support expansion of the blood volume, uterus, and breast tissue.** Fetal and placental proteins are synthesized from amino acids supplied by the mother. Protein recommendations are therefore increased from 46 g/day for an adult, nonpregnant woman to 71 g/day during pregnancy. This represents a change in protein recommendation from 0.8 g/kg/day for nonpregnant women to 1.1 g/kg/day during pregnancy.[20]

Omega-3 Fatty Acids

Polyunsaturated fatty acids (PUFAs) are an essential component of neural tissue and are found in high concentrations in membrane phospholipids of the gray matter and the retina. These critically important fatty acids cannot be synthesized by the body and thus must be consumed in the diet as either linoleic or α-linolenic acid. After ingestion, α-linoleic acid is converted to its biologically active forms, eicosapentaenoic acid (EPA) and docosahexaenoic acid (DHA). The amount of fatty acids that are transported to the fetus depends both on maternal dietary intake and placental function. With n-3 PUFA supplementation, randomized, placebo-controlled studies have shown a positive relationship between maternal intake and umbilical cord concentrations.[27]

The best dietary sources for PUFAs are seafood—namely, oily fish such as salmon, sardines, and anchovies—as well as oils from some plants, such as flax seeds and walnuts.[28,29] **The Food and Drug Administration (FDA) recommends that pregnant women consume 200 to 300 mg/day of DHA, which can be achieved by consuming 1 to 2 servings (8 to 12 ounces) of fish per week. However, the average pregnant or lactating woman consumes only 52 mg/day of DHA and 20 mg/day of EPA.**[30] For those women with insufficient seafood consumption, alternate sources of DHA include fish oil supplements (150 to 1200 mg/day), enhanced prenatal vitamins (200 to 300 mg/day), DHA-enriched eggs (up to 150 mg/egg), and the plant oils listed above.[31] Regarding seafood consumption, the American College of Obstetricians and Gynecologists (ACOG) encourages women who are pregnant, planning to become pregnant, or breastfeeding to follow the updated FDA recommendations to **avoid fish with the highest mercury concentration, specifically tilefish, shark, swordfish, and king mackerel. They should also limit consumption of white albacore tuna to 6 oz/week.**[32]

During the third trimester of pregnancy and the first 2 years of infancy, brain development occurs rapidly, and DHA supplementation has been well studied during this period.[33] **The best evidence in support of PUFA supplementation comes from studies that show a positive relationship between PUFA supplementation and neurodevelopmental outcomes in children.**[34,35] Results of randomized, controlled trials have generally supported these findings. For example, one study used cod liver oil supplementation from 18 weeks gestational age until 12 weeks postpartum and found children's mental processing scores at 4 years of age correlated significantly with maternal intake of DHA.[35] However, other randomized, controlled trials have found no difference in cognitive and language scores between offspring of women supplemented with fish oil during pregnancy and those who received placebo.[36] A recently published follow-up study showed that at 18 months of age, children of mothers who were supplemented with 800 mg of DHA during pregnancy showed no difference in mean cognitive, language, or motor scores, although fewer children in the DHA group had delayed development compared with controls.[37]

In addition to the well-studied effects of PUFA on fetal brain development, much interest has been paid to other potential benefits of DHA supplementation during pregnancy. For instance, dietary supplementation with PUFA has been promoted as a means to prolong gestation and prevent prematurity. This hypothesis originated after an epidemiologic study compared the diets of women in Denmark to those of the Faroe Islanders, and researchers noted that the seafood-based diet of the island population was associated with higher birthweight (+225 g) at term.[38] This association spawned subsequent research; however, a **Maternal Fetal Medicine Network trial did not find evidence that fish oil supplementation decreased the risk of preterm delivery in high-risk patients.**[39] However, moderate fish intake of up to three meals/week before 22 weeks gestation was associated with a decreased risk of preterm birth.[40] Although older trials of PUFA supplementation purported an increase in birthweight because of prolonged gestational age,[41] more recent trials have reported a *decrease* in birthweight after adjusting for gestational age.[42,43] Thus at present, evidence is insufficient to recommend PUFA supplementation as a means to reduce the risk of preterm birth.

VITAMIN AND MINERAL SUPPLEMENTATION GUIDELINES

Dietary Reference Intakes

To address the changing nutritional needs of the American population, the Food and Nutrition Board of the IOM established the first Dietary Reference Intakes (DRIs) in 1997. These values moved beyond the traditional Recommended Daily Allowances (RDAs) to focus on the prevention of chronic disease, and **the DRIs provide a range for safe and appropriate intake, as well as tolerable upper limit, based on the available research. The DRIs include four dietary reference values for every life stage and gender group.** These include (1) estimated average requirement, (2) recommended dietary allowance, (3) adequate intake, and (4) tolerable upper intake level (UL). At present, DRIs have been established for vitamin A, the carotenoids, the B vitamins, vitamin C, vitamin D, vitamin K, folate, calcium, choline, chromium, copper, fluoride, iodine, iron, magnesium, manganese, molybdenum, phosphorus, biotin, pantothenic acid, selenium, and zinc. Recommendations regarding the intake of other nutrients will be available over the next decade as the scientific evidence is evaluated (Table 7-5).[44]

Tolerable Upper Intake Level

The UL is the highest level of daily nutrient intake that is unlikely to pose risks of adverse health effects to almost all (97% to 98%) of the individuals in a specified life stage and gender group (see Table 7-5).

Routine vitamin/mineral supplementation for women who report appropriate dietary intake and demonstrate adequate weight gain (without edema) is not mandatory. However, **most health care providers prescribe a prenatal vitamin and mineral supplement because many women do not meet their nutritional requirements during the first trimester, especially with regard to folic acid and iron.**

Vitamins

Vitamin A

Vitamin A is a fat-soluble vitamin that exists in various compounds, including retinal, retinyl esters, retinol, and retinoic acid. Retinoic acid is the most active form of vitamin A. Retinol is considered preformed vitamin A. In plants, vitamin A exists in its precursor forms, such as provitamin A, carotenoids (e.g. beta-carotene), and cryptoxanthin. Vitamin A is required for cell differentiation, regulation of gene expression, and for the development of the vertebrae, spinal cord, limbs, heart, eyes, and ears.

Severe vitamin A deficiency is rare in the United States, and an adequate intake of vitamin A is readily available in a healthy diet. Women with lower socioeconomic status, however, may consume diets with inadequate amounts of vitamin A. Vitamin A deficiency during pregnancy weakens the immune system, increases risk of infection, and has been linked with night blindness. However, increasing dietary intake of vitamin A is advised, rather than supplementation, because excess retinol intake is a known human teratogen. Excess vitamin A causes abnormalities of the cranial neural crest cells, resulting in cardiac and craniofacial defects that include microcephaly.[45]

The DRI for vitamin A during pregnancy is 770 μg/day, and the tolerable UL has been established at 3000 μg/day.[46] **Over-the-counter multivitamin supplements may contain excessive doses of vitamin A and therefore should be discontinued during pregnancy. Additionally, topical creams that contain retinol derivatives, commonly used to treat acne, should be avoided during pregnancy and in women trying to conceive.**

Vitamin D

Vitamin D intake is essential for proper absorption of calcium, normal bone health, and skeletal homeostasis. **During pregnancy, vitamin D is also critically important for fetal growth and development as well as for regulation of genes associated with normal implantation and angiogenesis.** Low maternal vitamin D status has been associated with reduced intrauterine long-bone growth, shorter gestation, congenital rickets, and fractures in the newborn. Low maternal vitamin D status may also have consequences for fetal imprinting that may affect neurodevelopment, immune function, and chronic disease susceptibility soon after birth and later in life.

Maternal vitamin D status may also be an independent risk factor for preeclampsia, and supplementation may be helpful in preventing this complication and in promoting neonatal well-being.[47] However, these data come from observational studies, and prospective cohort studies have not found an association.[48] A recent multicenter European trial examined whether vitamin D supplementation (1600 IU/day) can improve maternal glucose metabolism.[49]

The recommended intake of vitamin D during pregnancy and lactation is 600 IU/day.[50] Recent studies have shown that low maternal vitamin D levels are common during pregnancy, even in patients who take daily prenatal vitamins that contain 400 IU

TABLE 7-5   DIETARY REFERENCE INTAKES: RECOMMENDED DAILY INTAKES FOR INDIVIDUALS

VITAMIN/MINERAL	AGE (YR)	NONPREGNANT	PREGNANT	UPPER INTAKE LEVELS
Vitamin A (µg)	<18	700	750-1200	2800
	19-30	700	770-1300	3000
	31-50	700	770-1300	3000
Vitamin C (mg)	<18	65	80	1800
	19-30	75	85	2000
	31-50	75	85	2000
Vitamin D (µg)	<18	15	15	100
	19-30	15	15	100
	31-50	15	15	100
Vitamin E (mg)	<18	15	15	800
	19-30	15	15	1000
	31-50	15	15	1000
Vitamin K (µg)	<18	75	75	ND
	19-30	90	90	ND
	31-50	90	90	ND
Thiamin (mg)	<18	1.1	1.4	ND
	19-30	1.1	1.4	ND
	31-50	1.1	1.4	ND
Riboflavin (mg)	<18	1.1	1.4	ND
	19-30	1.1	1.4	ND
	31-50	1.1	1.4	ND
Niacin (mg)	<18	14	18	30
	19-30	14	18	35
	31-50	14	18	35
Vitamin B_6 (mg)	<18	1.2	1.9	80
	19-30	1.3	1.9	100
	31-50	1.3	1.9	100
Folate (µg)	<18	400	600	800
	19-30	400	600	1000
	31-50	400	600	1000
Vitamin B_{12} (µg)	<18	2.4	2.6	ND
	19-30	2.4	2.6	ND
	31-50	2.4	2.6	ND
Pantothenic acid (mg)	<18	5	6	ND
	19-30	5	6	ND
	31-50	5	6	ND
Biotin (µg)	<18	25	30	ND
	19-30	30	30	ND
	31-50	30	30	ND
Choline (mg)	<18	400	450	3000
	19-30	425	450	3500
	31-50	425	450	3500
Calcium (mg)	<18	1300	1300	3000
	19-30	1000	1000	2500
	31-50	1000	1000	2500
Chromium (µg)	<18	24	29	ND
	19-30	25	30	ND
	31-50	25	30	ND
Copper (µg)	<18	890	1000	8000
	19-30	900	1000	10000
	31-50	900	1000	10000
Fluoride (mg)	<18	3	3	10
	19-30	3	3	10
	31-50	3	3	10
Iodine (µg)	<18	150	220	900
	19-30	150	220	1100
	31-50	150	220	1100
Iron (mg)	<18	15	27	45
	19-30	18	27	45
	31-50	18	27	45
Magnesium (mg)	<18	360	400	350
	19-30	310	350	350
	31-50	320	360	350

TABLE 7-5   DIETARY REFERENCE INTAKES: RECOMMENDED DAILY INTAKES FOR INDIVIDUALS—cont'd

VITAMIN/MINERAL	AGE (YR)	NONPREGNANT	PREGNANT	UPPER INTAKE LEVELS
Phosphorous (mg)	<18	1250	1250	4000
	19-30	700	700	4000
	31-50	700	700	4000
Selenium (µg)	<18	55	60	400
	19-30	55	60	400
	31-50	55	60	400
Zinc (mg)	<18	9	12	34
	19-30	8	11	40
	31-50	8	11	40

DRIs are included for calcium, phosphorous, magnesium, vitamin D, and fluoride (1997); for thiamin, riboflavin, niacin, vitamins B_6 and B_{12}, folate, pantothenic acid, biotin, and choline (1998); for vitamins C and E, selenium, and the carotenoids (2000); for vitamins A and K, arsenic, boron, chromium, copper, iodine, iron, manganese, molybdenum, nickel, silicon, vanadium, and zinc (2001); and for calcium and vitamin D (2011). Reports were accessed April 24, 2015; available online at http://www.iom.edu/Activities/Nutrition/SummaryDRIs/DRI-Tables.aspx.
ND, not determined.

of vitamin D. Lee and colleagues[51] found that 50% of mothers and 65% of newborns infants were significantly vitamin D deficient at the time of birth despite daily supplementation with 400 IU of vitamin D and drinking two glasses of vitamin D fortified milk. Poor vitamin D status is also significantly more common among black pregnant women.[52,53]

Vitamin D supplementation is advised for women who are strict vegetarians, those with limited exposure to sunlight, and those who avoid dairy foods. To evaluate vitamin D levels during a preconception or prenatal visit, serum 25-hydroxy-D levels should be evaluated. Most experts agree that 20 ng/mL (50 nmol/L) are needed daily for optimal bone health. Supplementation with 1000 to 4000 IU per day of vitamin D is safe during pregnancy.[54]

Vitamin C

Vitamin C, also known as *ascorbic acid,* is a water-soluble vitamin and antioxidant that functions to reduce free radicals and also aids in procollagen formation. Adequate vitamin C is also needed for iron uptake. Women who smoke have an increased need for vitamin C. Current recommendations indicate that pregnant women should consume 85 mg/day rather than the 75 mg/day recommended for nonpregnant adult women. The increased requirement protects against depleted plasma vitamin C levels and ensures that adequate vitamin C is transported to the developing fetus. No human studies have been done to examine the effects of large doses of vitamin C on fetal growth and development. Because it is known that vitamin C is actively transported from the maternal to the fetal circulation, a tolerable upper intake has been set at 1800 to 2000 mg/day.[55]

The hypothesis that oxidative stress contributes to development of preeclampsia has spurred interest in the use of antioxidants for prevention of the disease. **However, several large, randomized placebo-controlled studies and a Cochrane review have shown no benefit.**[56] **Thus supplementation with antioxidant vitamins C and E for the prevention of preeclampsia is *not* recommended.**[57]

Vitamin B_6

Vitamin B_6, also known as *pyridoxine,* is a water-soluble B-complex vitamin that serves as a coenzyme in protein, carbohydrate, and lipid metabolism. Vitamin B_6 is involved in the synthesis of heme compounds and aids in the formation of maternal and fetal red blood cells, antibodies, and neurotransmitters. **Research shows that supplemental vitamin B_6 is**

effective at relieving nausea and vomiting during pregnancy.[58] Whereas a recent Cochrane review of hyperemesis protocols could not draw firm conclusions about the efficacy of vitamin B_6, evidence was sufficient for ACOG to support monotherapy with B_6 as a first-line treatment to reduce nausea and vomiting (10 to 25 mg three times a day).[59,60] Because excessive amounts of vitamin B_6 can cause numbness and nerve damage, the tolerable upper intake level for pregnant women was established at 100 mg/day.

Vitamin K

Vitamin K, a fat-soluble vitamin, is required for synthesis of clotting factors II, VII, IX, and X. Transportation of vitamin K from mother to fetus is limited; nevertheless, significant bleeding problems in the fetus are rare. However, newborn infants are often functionally deficient in vitamin K and receive parenteral supplementation at birth. The DRI for vitamin K is 90 mg for pregnant and nonpregnant women; the tolerable UL has not been established.[55]

Folate

Folate and its metabolically active form tetrahydrofolate function as coenzymes in one-carbon transfer reactions for the synthesis of nucleic acids and several amino acids. **Therefore adequate levels of dietary folate are important for fetal and placental development and are needed to support rapid cell growth, replication, cell division, and nucleotide synthesis.**[61] **Because embryonic neural tube closure is complete by 18 to 28 days after conception, it is critical that pregnant women consume adequate folate before and during the first 4 weeks of embryologic development (6 weeks gestational age by last menstrual period [LMP]).** Demand for folate is also increased during the second and third trimesters to support maternal erythropoiesis.

Unfortunately, folate deficiency is the most prevalent vitamin deficiency during pregnancy.[62] Folate deficiency in humans is attributed to suboptimal dietary intake, behavioral and environmental factors, and genetic defects. Humans cannot synthesize folate and are therefore entirely dependent on dietary sources or supplements to meet their requirements. In 1992, the U.S. Centers for Disease Control and Prevention (CDC) recommended that all women of childbearing age take 400 µg/day of supplemental folate to ensure the presence of adequate folate levels when pregnancy occurs, whether intended or not.[63] **The DRI for folate in women of childbearing age is 400 µg/day;**

for pregnant women it is 600 µg/day. The tolerable UL for folate has been established at 1000 µg/day. Additionally, evidence suggests that the long-term use of oral contraceptives inhibits folate absorption and enhances folate degradation in the liver.[64] Therefore folate stores may be more rapidly depleted in women who have used oral contraceptives, which may lead to a higher incidence of folate deficiency in such women if they become pregnant.

FOLATE AND NEURAL TUBE DEFECTS

Neural tube defects (NTDs) occur in 1.4 to 2 per 1000 pregnancies and are second only to cardiac anomalies in terms of the most common congenital malformations worldwide.[65] Prevalence varies according to race and ethnicity. Hispanic women have the highest rates, whereas black women and Asian women have the lowest rates.[66] Women who have had a previous pregnancy affected by an NTD or who are personally affected by an NTD are at a higher risk (2% to 3%).[67] A family history of a close family member (sibling, niece, or nephew) with an NTD raises a woman's risk of an affected pregnancy to approximately 1%, as does maternal diabetes or the consumption of certain antiseizure medications such as valproic acid or carbamazepine. A higher risk of NTDs is also associated with increased maternal weight.[68] However, 95% of children with NTDs are born to couples without any family history of NTDs.[69]

The etiology of NTDs is thought to be insufficient folate intake coupled with the increased folate demands of pregnancy. A genetic defect in the production of enzymes involved in folate metabolism has also been linked to NTDs.[62] The neural tube is formed very early in pregnancy, between 18 and 28 days post conception. Defects in the formation of the neural tube include the absence of brain formation (anencephaly), defects in the closure of the lower tube (spina bifida), and open NTDs (meningoceles and myoceles). **The early formation and the detrimental effects of folate deficiency on neural tube formation are the basis behind the recommendation that folate supplementation begin prior to conception and be continued at least through the first trimester of pregnancy.**[70]

FOLATE SUPPLEMENTATION

Several randomized, controlled, and observational trials have shown that periconceptional and early pregnancy consumption of folate supplements can reduce a woman's risk for having an infant with an NTD by as much as 50% to 70%.[62] Since the U.S. government began the Folate Fortification Program in 1998, cereals, pastas, rice, and breads have been fortified with folate, and NTD rates have declined.[66] Using data from eight population-based birth defect surveillance systems with prenatal diagnosis of NTDs, the CDC reported that the prevalence of NTDs in the United States declined from an estimated 4000 cases between 1995 and 1996 to 3000 cases from 1999 through 2000.[71] This 26% decrease in NTD-affected pregnancies highlights the success of this public health policy. Using a similar level of folate fortification, a Canadian study showed a 46% reduction in the prevalence of NTDs.[72] The higher baseline rate of NTDs compared with the United States might explain the greater risk reduction.

In women with a previous pregnancy affected by an NTD, research has shown that supplementation with 4000 µg/day (4 mg/day of folate initiated at least 1 month prior to attempting to conceive and continued throughout the first trimester of pregnancy reduced the risk of a repeat NTD

TABLE 7-6   DIAGNOSIS OF ANEMIA IN PREGNANCY

LAB TEST	FIRST TRIMESTER	SECOND TRIMESTER	THIRD TRIMESTER
Hemoglobin (g/dL)	<11	10.5	<11
Hematocrit (%)	<33	32	<33

Data from U.S. Centers for Disease Control and Prevention (www.cdc.gov).

by 72%.[61] **Whereas no definitive evidence proves that other high-risk groups such as close family members of affected individuals, diabetics, or women on antiseizure medications will benefit from higher levels of supplementation, many experts recommend a higher dose of folate—at least 1000 µg/day—before conception and in early pregnancy.** For these women, a separate folate supplement should be prescribed; additional doses of multivitamins should not be used. Additional daily multivitamin consumption could lead to toxicity of other vitamins, particularly vitamin A, which is teratogenic to the developing fetus.[63]

Minerals

Iron

Iron is an essential component of hemoglobin production, and requirements increase significantly during pregnancy. **Additional iron is needed to expand maternal red cell volume by 20% to 30%, and iron is also required for fetal and placental tissue production.** Throughout pregnancy, an additional 450 mg of iron is delivered to the maternal marrow, and 250 mg of iron is depleted from blood loss during delivery. It is estimated that approximately 1000 mg of iron is required during pregnancy. The DRI has been established at 27 mg/day in pregnancy, compared with 18 mg/day for nonpregnant women. The tolerable upper intake for iron has been established at 45 mg/day.[46]

Maintaining adequate iron stores is important but difficult for many women during pregnancy. According to the CDC, screening for anemia should take place prior to pregnancy and during the first, second, and third trimesters in high-risk individuals, as shown in Table 7-6. Iron deficiency anemia increases the risk of maternal and infant death, preterm delivery, and low neonatal birth weight. Anemia also negatively impacts normal infant brain development and function. The prevalence of iron deficiency in pregnancy is higher in black women, low-income women, teenagers, women with less than a high school education, and women with multiple gestations.[73]

As shown in Table 7-6, hemoglobin less than 11 g/dL or hematocrit below 33% in the first or third trimester indicates anemia. Hemoglobin less than 10.5 g/dL or hematocrit below 32% in the second trimester also indicates anemia.

Additional laboratory findings include microcytic hypochromic anemia with evidence of depleted iron stores, low plasma iron levels, high total iron-binding capacity, and low serum ferritin levels. Ferritin levels less than 10 to 15 µg/L have the highest sensitivity and specificity for diagnosing iron deficiency in the anemic patient.

Prenatal care providers generally recommend daily iron supplementation with 30 mg of elemental iron in the form of simple salts beginning around the twelfth week of pregnancy for women who have normal preconception hemoglobin measurements (Table 7-7).[74] For women who are pregnant with multiples or for those with low preconception hemoglobin levels, a supplement of between 60 and 100 mg/day of elemental

TABLE 7-7   ORAL IRON SUPPLEMENTS

ORAL SUPPLEMENT	ELEMENTAL IRON
Ferrous fumarate	106 mg/tablet
Ferrous sulfate	65 mg/tablet
Ferrous gluconate	28-36 mg/tablet

Data from the American College of Obstetricians and Gynecologists. ACOG Practice Bulletin No. 95: Anemia in pregnancy. *Obstet Gynecol.* 2008;112(1):201-207.

iron is recommended until hemoglobin concentrations have normalized, after which supplementation can be decreased to 30 mg/day.[75]

For women with severe iron deficiency, those who cannot tolerate oral iron, or those with malabsorption syndromes, parenteral iron can be used. Parenteral iron is especially valuable for increasing hemoglobin levels faster than oral iron. One randomized, controlled trial of oral versus intravenous (IV) iron sucrose showed that IV iron significantly increased hemoglobin levels after both 5 and 14 days, whereas women treated with an oral supplement showed no improvement. However, by day 40, no significant difference between the hemoglobin levels of the two groups was noted.[76]

Iron supplements may produce gastrointestinal (GI) side effects, namely constipation and nausea, which should be taken into account when prescribing the course of treatment. Deferring supplementation until the second trimester, when iron requirements increase and nausea has waned, may be helpful to improve adherence. Nausea resulting from iron supplements can be minimized by taking the supplement following a meal; however, this may decrease total iron absorption. Recommending bulk laxatives and/or stool softeners when prescribing iron supplements may also improve adherence.

Antacids impair iron absorption and should not be taken concurrently; this is of particular importance during the third trimester, when gastroesophageal reflux is common. Iron is better absorbed if the maternal diet contains adequate amounts of vitamin C. Occasionally, pregnant women develop pica and ingest nonfood substances such as clay, dirt, or ice. Iron deficiency has been postulated to cause pica, but certain cultural influences may also lead to these practices. Pregnant women with iron deficiency should be questioned about ingestion of these nonfood substances, and women experiencing pica should be tested for iron deficiency. Pica is mostly of concern if it prevents the mother from consuming nutrient-rich foods or if the materials she consumes contain toxic components.

Calcium

Large quantities of calcium are essential for the development of the fetal skeleton and tissues and for hormonal adaptations during pregnancy. These include changes in calcium regulatory hormones that affect intestinal absorption, renal reabsorption, and bone turnover of calcium. The presence of $1,25(OH)_2D_3$ stimulates increased intestinal absorption of calcium during the second and third trimesters, which protects maternal bone while meeting fetal calcium requirements. In contrast to maternal iron and folate stores, which are relatively small and easily depleted, maternal calcium stores are large and are mostly stored skeletally, allowing for easy mobilization. Fetal calcium needs are highest during the third trimester, when the fetus utilizes an average of 300 mg/day in response to the increased maternal $1,25(OH)_2D_3$. Studies suggest that inadequate calcium during pregnancy is

associated with gestational hypertension, preterm delivery, and preeclampsia.[77,78]

The DRI for calcium in pregnant women 19 to 50 years old is 1000 mg/day, and it is 1300 mg/day for adolescent females ages 9 to 19. Adolescents may need additional calcium during pregnancy because their own bones still require calcium deposition to ensure adequate bone density. The tolerable upper intake for calcium during pregnancy is 2500 mg/day.[79] Obtaining adequate dietary calcium is difficult for many women before and during pregnancy, and supplementation may be needed, especially for black, Hispanic, and Native American women. Consuming at least three servings of dairy foods every day, including calcium-fortified juices and beverages, can help meet these requirements. Women who limit their intake of dairy foods because of lactose intolerance may be able to tolerate yogurt and cheese on a daily basis but may also require a supplement. Calcium carbonate, gluconate, lactate, or citrate may provide 500 to 600 mg/day of calcium to account for the difference between the amount of calcium required and that consumed. **The standard prenatal vitamin typically contains 150 to 300 mg per tablet.** Multivitamins marketed to the nonpregnant population generally have less than 200 mg per tablet. Calcium is thought to be absorbed in doses of 600 mg at one time, making it unlikely that pregnant women would reach the upper tolerable limit.

The data concerning the role of calcium in preventing pregnancy-induced hypertension or preeclampsia remain controversial. Whereas calcium supplementation has been shown to decrease blood pressure and preeclampsia in smaller studies, larger trials have failed to show an effect.[78,80] Evidence has shown that calcium supplementation reduces the risk of developing hypertension during pregnancy but only in women who did not have adequate calcium intake prior to supplementation.[63] It is prudent to ensure women are meeting their calcium requirements for their age and to stress the importance of adequate calcium intake before and during pregnancy.

Zinc

Zinc is involved in catalytic, structural, and regulatory functions for nucleic acid and protein metabolism. More than 100 enzymes require zinc, and maternal zinc deficiency can lead to prolonged labor, IUGR, teratogenesis, and embryonic or fetal death.[52] The DRI for pregnant women is 11 mg/day and may be higher for vegetarians or vegans because phytates from whole grains and beans bind with zinc and can reduce absorption. The tolerable upper intake for zinc has been established at 40 mg/day for both pregnant and nonpregnant women. Pregnant women who eat well-balanced diets do not typically require zinc supplementation. However, if a woman is prescribed more than 60 mg/day of elemental iron, zinc supplementation is recommended because iron competes with zinc for absorption.

Choline

Choline is an essential nutrient needed for cell signaling and structural cell membrane integrity. It is critical for stem cell proliferation and apoptosis. Demand for choline is high during pregnancy because maternal choline is transported to the fetus to aid in brain and spinal cord development.[81] Adequate choline is needed for normal fetal neural development and function, and it is essential for memory.[82] Choline is derived not only from the diet but also from de novo synthesis. The current recommendation for choline during pregnancy is 450 mg/day, and it is 550 mg/day for breastfeeding mothers. Dietary sources of choline include eggs (126 mg/egg), tofu (100 mg/3 oz), lean beef (67 mg/3 oz), Brussels sprouts (62 mg/cup cooked), cauliflower (62 mg/¾ cup cooked), navy beans (48 mg/½ cup cooked), peanut butter (20 mg/2 tablespoons), and skim milk (38 mg/cup).

NUTRITION-RELATED PROBLEMS DURING PREGNANCY

Nausea and Vomiting

During pregnancy, nausea and vomiting commonly occur between 5 and 18 weeks of gestation and typically improve by 16 to 18 weeks. As many as 15% to 20% of women experience these symptoms until the third trimester, and 5% of women suffer these up until delivery. Between 50% and 90% of women have some degree of nausea with or without vomiting, but only a small percentage of these require hospitalization for severe hyperemesis gravidarum.[83] **Women with hyperemesis may vomit multiple times throughout the day, lose more than 5% of their prepregnancy body weight, and usually require hospitalization for dehydration and electrolyte replacement.**

The causes of pregnancy-related nausea and vomiting are unclear but may be related to increased levels of human chorionic gonadotropin (hCG), which doubles every 48 hours in early pregnancy and peaks at about 12 weeks gestation. Studies show that women are more likely to have nausea or vomiting during pregnancy if they (1) are pregnant with twins or higher multiples; (2) have a history of nausea and vomiting in a previous pregnancy; (3) have a history of nausea or vomiting as a side effect of taking birth control pills; (4) have a history of motion sickness; (5) have a relative (mother or sister) who had morning sickness during pregnancy; or (6) have a history of migraine headaches.

Strategies for managing nausea and vomiting during pregnancy are shown in Box 7-1. **After following these recommendations, vitamin B$_6$ (10 to 25 mg three times daily) can be considered as first-line treatment for nausea and vomiting during pregnancy.** Ginger and acupuncture may also be helpful to treat nausea during pregnancy.[58,84]

Heartburn and Indigestion

Heartburn and indigestion affect two thirds of pregnant women and are usually caused by gastric content reflux that results from both lower esophageal pressure and decreased motility secondary to increased progesterone.[84] Limited gastric capacity due to a shift of organs to accommodate the growing fetus contributes to these symptoms in the third trimester of pregnancy. Strategies for managing heartburn and indigestion are also shown in Box 7-1.

Constipation

Fifty percent of pregnant women experience constipation at some point during their pregnancy, which is often associated with straining, hard stools, and incomplete evacuation rather than infrequent defecation. Constipation during pregnancy is associated with smooth muscle relaxation, an increase in water reabsorption from the large intestine, and slower GI motility. Pregnant women often note overall GI discomfort, a bloated sensation, an increase in hemorrhoids and heartburn, and decreased appetite. Constipation can also be aggravated by iron supplements. Strategies for managing constipation during pregnancy are shown in Box 7-2.

Food Contamination

Both the pregnant woman and her unborn fetus are more susceptible to food poisoning secondary to hormonal changes associated with pregnancy. **Pathogens of special concern during pregnancy include *Listeria monocytogenes*, *Toxoplasma gondii*, *Salmonella* species, and *Campylobacter jejuni*.** These organisms can cross the placenta and therefore pose a risk of foodborne infection to the developing fetus.[85] To avoid listeriosis, pregnant women should be advised to wash vegetables and fruits well; cook all meats to minimum safe internal temperatures; avoid processed, precooked meats (cold cuts, smoked seafood, pâté) and soft cheeses (brie, blue cheese, Camembert, and Mexican *queso blanco* [white cheese]); and only consume dairy products that have been pasteurized. All foods should be handled in a sanitary and appropriate manner to prevent bacterial contamination. Toxoplasmosis can be passed to humans by water, dust, and soil or by eating contaminated foods, and cats are the main host of *T. gondii*. Toxoplasmosis most often results from eating raw or uncooked meat, unwashed fruits and vegetables, and by cleaning a cat's litter box or handling contaminated soil. *Salmonella* and *Campylobacter* can be found in raw, unpasteurized milk; raw or undercooked meat and poultry; eggs,

---

BOX 7-1 STRATEGIES FOR MANAGING NAUSEA, VOMITING, HEARTBURN, AND INDIGESTION IN PREGNANCY

- Eat small, low-fat meals and snacks (fruits, pretzels, crackers, nonfat yogurt).
- Eat slowly and frequently.
- Avoid strong food odors by eating room temperature or cold foods and using good ventilation while cooking.
- Drink fluids between meals rather than with meals.
- Avoid foods that may cause stomach irritation such as spearmint, peppermint, caffeine, citrus fruits, spicy foods, high-fat foods, or tomato products.
- Wait 1-2 hours after eating a meal before lying down.
- Take a walk after meals.
- Wear loose-fitting clothes.
- Brush teeth after eating to prevent symptoms.

Courtesy Lisa Hark, PhD, RD.

BOX 7-2 STRATEGIES FOR MANAGING CONSTIPATION IN PREGNANCY

- Increase fluid intake by drinking water, herbal teas, and noncaffeinated beverages.
- Increase daily fiber intake by eating high-fiber cereals, whole grains, legumes, and bran.
- Use a psyllium fiber supplement (e.g., Metamucil).
- Increase consumption of fresh, frozen, or dried fruits and vegetables.
- Participate in moderate physical activity such as walking, swimming, or yoga.
- Take stool softeners in conjunction with iron supplementation.

Courtesy Lisa Hark, PhD, RD.

salads, cream desserts, and dessert fillings; and untreated water. To avoid infection, pregnant women should wash their hands often, especially after handling animals or working in the garden, and they should avoid undercooked food and unpasteurized juices. All surfaces that come into contact with raw meat, fish, or poultry should also be washed with hot soapy water.[85]

Food contaminated with heavy metals can also produce devastating neurotoxic and teratogenic effects in the developing fetus that may result in miscarriage, stillbirth, premature labor, or other fetal complications.[86] In particular, case reports of teratogenicity or embryotoxicity have been reported with exposure to methyl mercury, lead, cadmium, nickel, and selenium. Mercury can be removed from vegetables by peeling them or by washing them well with soap and water. All dairy foods and juices consumed during pregnancy should be pasteurized.[87-89]

SPECIAL NUTRITIONAL CONSIDERATIONS DURING PREGNANCY

Caffeine

Caffeine is metabolized slowly in pregnancy and passes readily through the placenta to the fetus. **Moderate caffeine intake is common during pregnancy, however, women who are pregnant or trying to become pregnant should limit their caffeine intake to no more than 200 mg/day,** the equivalent of one 12-ounce cup of coffee. Other sources of caffeine include teas, hot cocoa, chocolate, energy drinks, coffee ice cream, and soda. Many studies have looked for a correlation between high caffeine intake and miscarriage, preterm birth, and IUGR. Review of the available literature reveals that moderate caffeine consumption (<200 mg per day) is not a major contributing factor to miscarriage or preterm birth.

Vegetarian and Vegan Diets

Balanced vegetarian diets—those that exclude meat, fish, and poultry but still include dairy and eggs—have not been linked to any significant health effects during pregnancy.[90] Research from vegetarian populations worldwide reveals that macronutrient intake of pregnant vegetarians is similar to that of pregnant nonvegetarians, except that vegetarians consume less protein and more carbohydrates. **Vegan diets—those that exclude all animal products, including eggs and dairy—may provide insufficient iron, essential amino acids, trace minerals (zinc), vitamin B$_{12}$, vitamin D, calcium, and PUFAs to support normal embryonic and fetal development. Thus it is recommended that patients who follow a vegan diet meet with a dietitian early during the pregnancy to analyze their nutritional intake and assess any necessary supplementation that should be added.** For example, fortified vegetarian food products are now widely available and include some nondairy milk with added calcium and vitamin D, meat substitutes that contain protein, and fortified juice and breakfast cereals.[90]

Herbal Supplements

Because of the unregulated nature of herbal supplements, they are generally not recommended for consumption during pregnancy. In addition, data are sparse regarding their use during pregnancy, and the strength and purity of supplements can vary widely among products and manufacturers. Despite this, the consumer market for complementary and alternative treatments continues to grow. Studies have shown that pregnant women often choose herbal supplements because their use represents a holistic approach to health and overall wellness. The best-studied herb in the pregnancy literature is ginger, which has been used for centuries for nausea and vomiting.[91] Experts recommend a trial of 250 mg capsules three times daily or consumption of ginger tea. **Whereas countless other herbs and supplements certainly hold potential benefits, more research is needed before any of these supplements can be safely recommended in pregnancy.**

KEY POINTS

- ◆ Pregnant women may need as much as an additional 300 kcal/day for the entire pregnancy, but requirements may be significantly less and vary among individuals.
- ◆ The Institute of Medicine recommendations for gestational weight gain for women are set by weight category: underweight (BMI <18.5; 28 to 40 lb), normal weight (BMI 18.5 to 24.9; 25 to 35 lb), overweight (BMI 25.0 to 29.9; 15 to 35 lb), and obese (BMI >30; 11 to 20 lb).
- ◆ Protein requirements during pregnancy increase from 0.8 g/kg/day for nonpregnant women to 1.1 g/kg/day during pregnancy.
- ◆ The daily recommended intake for folate in women of childbearing age is 400 µg/day; for pregnant women, it is 600 µg/day. Women whose fetuses are at high risk of a neural tube defect should be prescribed a higher dose of folate (4 mg/day) both before conception and in early pregnancy.
- ◆ Iron supplementation is often prescribed during pregnancy because of the (20% to 30%) expanded maternal red cell mass as well as for fetal and placental tissue production. Iron supplements can cause GI side effects such as constipation.
- ◆ Vitamin D supplementation is often required during pregnancy in women with specific dietary preferences or for those with minimal exposure to sunlight. To evaluate vitamin D concentrations before and during pregnancy, check serum 25(OH)D levels and aim for concentrations of 25(OH)D of greater than 20 nmol/L. The DRI for vitamin D is 600 IU/day in all pregnant and reproductive-age women.
- ◆ The DRI for calcium in nonpregnant and pregnant women 19 to 50 years of age is 1000 mg/day, and it is 1300 mg/day for females 9 to 19 years of age.
- ◆ Many common GI problems during pregnancy—such as heartburn, nausea and vomiting, and constipation— are improved with proper nutritional counseling.

REFERENCES

1. Ogden CL, Carroll MD, Kit BK, Flegal KM. Prevalence of childhood and adult obesity in the United States, 2011-2012. *JAMA.* 2014;311(8): 806-814.
2. *Overweight and Obesity.* Centers for Disease Control and Prevention. Available at: <www.cdc.gov/obesity/>.
3. West E, Hark LA, Deen DD. Nutrition in pregnancy and lactation. In: *Medical Nutrition and Disease.* 5th ed. Malden, MA: Wiley-Blackwell Publishing; 2014.
4. Deen DD, Hark LA. *Feeding the Mother-to-be. The Complete Guide to Nutrition in Primary Care.* Maden, MA: Wiley-Blackwell; 2007.

5. Ehrenberg HM, Iams JD, Goldenberg RL, et al. Maternal obesity, uterine activity, and the risk of spontaneous preterm birth. *Obstet Gynecol.* 2009; 113:48-52.

6. Haider BA, Olofin I, Wang M, Spiegelman D, Ezzati M, Fawzi WW, Nutrition Impact Model Study Group (anaemia). Anaemia, prenatal iron use, and risk of adverse pregnancy outcomes: systematic review and meta-analysis. *BMJ.* 2013;346:f3443.

7. *"Weight Gain During Pregnancy: Reexamining the Guidelines" Institutes of Medicine.* Available at: <iom.nationalacademies.org/en/Reports/2009/ Weight-Gain-During-Pregnancy-Reexamining-the-Guidelines.aspx>.

8. *"Weight Gain During Pregnancy: Reexamining the Guidelines" Institutes of Medicine.* May 28, 2009. Web. July 21, 2014.

9. Hernandez TL, Van Pelt RE, Anderson MA, et al. A higher-complex carbohydrate diet in gestational diabetes mellitus achieves glucose targets and lowers postprandial lipids: a randomized crossover study. *Diabetes Care.* 2014;37(5):1254-1262.

10. Moses RG, Casey SA, Quinn EG, et al. Pregnancy and Glycemic Index Outcomes study: effects of low glycemic index compared with conventional dietary advice on selected pregnancy outcomes. *Am J Clin Nutr.* 2014; 99(3):517-523.

11. Nitert MD, Barrett HL, Foxcroft K, et al. SPRING: an RCT study of probiotics in the prevention of gestational diabetes mellitus in overweight and obese women. *BMC Pregnancy Childbirth.* 2013;13:50.

12. Beyerlein A, Schiessl B, Lack N, von Kries R. Optimal gestational weight gain ranges for the avoidance of adverse birth weight outcomes: a novel approach. *Am J Clin Nutr.* 2009;90:1552-1558.

13. Nohr EA, Vaeth M, Baker JL, Sørensen T, Olsen J, Rasmussen KM. Combined associations of prepregnancy body mass index and gestational weight gain with the outcome of pregnancy. *Am J Clin Nutr.* 2008;87(6): 1750-1759.

14. *"Pregnancy and Weight Gain: How Much Is Too Little?"* American College of Obstetricians and Gynecologists. News Release. December 20, 2012.

15. Institute of Medicine. *Weight gain during pregnancy: reexamining the guidelines.* Washington, DC: National Academies Press; 2009.

16. Weight gain during pregnancy. Committee Opinion No. 548. American College of Obstetricians and Gynecologists. *Obstet Gynecol.* 2013;121: 210-212.

17. Bodnar LM, Siega-Riz AM, Simhan HN, Himes KP, Abrams B. Severe obesity, gestational weight gain, and adverse birth outcomes. *Am J Clin Nutr.* 2010;91(6):1642-1648.

18. Catalano PM, Mele L, Landon MB, et al., Eunice Kennedy Shriver National Institute of Child Health and Human Development Maternal-Fetal Medicine Units Network. Inadequate weight gain in overweight and obese pregnant women: what is the effect on fetal growth? *Am J Obstet Gynecol.* 2014;211(2):137.

19. Joseph NP, Hunkali KB, Wilson B, Morgan E, Cross M, Freund KM. Prepregnancy body mass index among pregnant adolescents: gestational weight gain and long-term post partum weight retention. *J Pediatr Adolesc Gynecol.* 2008;21(4):195-200.

20. Trumbo P, Schlicker S, Yates AA, Poos M. Dietary reference intakes for energy, carbohydrate, fiber, fat, fatty acids, cholesterol, protein and amino acids. Food and Nutrition Board of the Institute of Medicine, The National Academies. *J Am Diet Assoc.* 2002;102(11):1621-1630.

21. Forsum E, Kabir N, Sadurskis A, Westerterp K. Total energy expenditure of healthy Swedish women during pregnancy and lactation. *Am J Clin Nutr.* 1992;56:334.

22. Durnin JVGA, McKillop FM, Grant S, et al. Energy requirements of pregnancy in Scotland. *Lancet.* 1987;2:897.

23. Lawrence M, Lawrence F, Coward WA, et al. Energy requirements of pregnancy in the Gambia. *Lancet.* 1987;2:1072.

24. Van Raaij JMA, Vermat-Miedema SH, Schonk CM, et al. Energy requirements of pregnancy in the Netherlands. *Lancet.* 1987;2:953.

25. Goldberg GR, Prentice AM, Coward WA, et al. Longitudinal assessment of energy expenditure in pregnancy by the doubly labeled water method. *Am J Clin Nutr.* 1993;57:94.

26. Butte NF, Hopkinson JM, Mehta N, Moon JK, Smith EO. Adjustments in energy expenditure and substrate utilization during late pregnancy and lactation. *Am J Clin Nutr.* 1999;69(2):299-307.

27. Escolano-Margarit MV, Campoy C, Ramírez-Tortosa MC, et al. Effects of fish oil supplementation on the fatty acid profile in erythrocyte membrane and plasma phospholipids of pregnant women and their offspring: a randomised controlled trial. *Br J Nutr.* 2013;109:1647-1656.

28. *"Fish: What Pregnant Women and Parents Should Know" US Food and Drug Administration. U.S. Department of Health and Human Services.* Available at: <www.fda.gov/food/foodborneillnesscontaminants/metals/ ucm393070.htm>.

29. Greenberg JA, Bell SJ, Ausdal WV. Omega-3 fatty acid supplementation during pregnancy. *Rev Obstet Gynecol.* 2008;1:162-169.

30. Peyron-Caso E, Quignard-Boulangé A, Laromiguière M, et al. Dietary fish oil increases lipid mobilization but does not decrease lipid storage-related enzyme activities in adipose tissue of insulin-resistant, sucrose-fed rats. *J Nutr.* 2003;133(7):2239-2243.

31. Coletta JM, Bell SJ, Roman AS. Omega-3 Fatty acids and pregnancy. *Rev Obstet Gynecol.* 2010;3(4):163-171.

32. ACOG Practice Advisory. Seafood Consumption During Pregnancy. *Obstet Gynecol.* 2014.

33. Guesnet P, Alessandri JM. Docosahexaenoic acid (DHA) and the developing central nervous system (CNS)—Implications for dietary recommendations. *Biochimie.* 2011;93(1):7-12.

34. Hibbeln JR, Davis JM, Steer C, et al. Maternal seafood consumption in pregnancy and neurodevelopmental outcomes in childhood (ALSPAC study): an observational cohort study. *Lancet.* 2007;369:578-585.

35. Helland IB, Smith L, Saarem K, et al. Maternal supplementation with very-long-chain n-3 fatty acids during pregnancy and lactation augments children's IQ at 4 years of age. *Pediatrics.* 2003;111:e39-e44.

36. Gould JF, Makrides M, Colombo J, Smithers LG. Randomized controlled trial of maternal omega-3 long-chain PUFA supplementation during pregnancy and early childhood development of attention, working memory, and inhibitory control. *Am J Clin Nutr.* 2014;99(4):851-859.

37. Makrides M, Gould JF, Gawlik NR, et al. Four-year follow-up of children born to women in a randomized trial of prenatal DHA supplementation. *JAMA.* 2014;311(17):1802-1804.

38. Olsen SF, Joensen HD. High liveborn birth weights in the Faeroes: a comparison between birth weights in the Faroes and in Denmark. *J Epidemiol Community Health.* 1985;39:27-32.

39. Harper M, Thom E, Klebanoff MA, et al. Omega-3 fatty acid supplementation to prevent recurrent preterm birth: a randomized controlled trial. *Obstet Gynecol.* 2010;115:234.

40. Klebanoff MA, Harper M, Lai Y, et al. Fish consumption, erythrocyte fatty acids, and preterm birth. *Obstet Gynecol.* 2011;117(5):1071-1077.

41. Simopoulos A, Leaf A, Salem N. US Expert Panel: essentiality of and recommended diet intakes for omega-6 and omega-3 fatty acids. *Ann Nutr Metab.* 1999;43:127.

42. Oken E, Kleinman KP, Olsen SF, et al. Associations of seafood and elongated n-3 fatty acid intake with fetal growth and length of gestation: results from a US pregnancy cohort. *Am J Epidemiol.* 2004;160:774.

43. Grandjean P, Bjerve KS, Weihe P, Steuerwald U. Birth weight in a fishing community: significance of essential fatty acids and marine food contaminants. *Int J Epidemiol.* 2001;30:1272.

44. Trumbo P, Schlicker S, Yates AA, Poos M. *Food and Nutrition Board, Institute of Medicine: Dietary Reference Intakes for Energy, Carbohydrate, Fiber, Fat, Fatty Acids, Cholesterol, Protein, and Amino Acids.* Washington, DC: National Academies Press; 2002.

45. Soprano DR, Soprano KJ. Retinoids as teratogens. *Annu Rev Nutr.* 1995;15:111.

46. Trumbo P, Yates AA, Schlicker S, Poos M. *Food and Nutrition Board, Institute of Medicine. Dietary Reference Intakes for Vitamin A, Vitamin K, Arsenic, Boron, Chromium, Copper, Iodine, Iron, Manganese, Molybdenum, Nickel, Silicon, Vanadium, and Zinc.* Washington, DC: National Academy Press; 2001.

47. Bodnar LM, Catov JM, Simhan HN, et al. Maternal vitamin D deficiency increases the risk of preeclampsia. *J Clin Endocrinol Metab.* 2007;92: 3517.

48. Shand AW, Nassar N, Von Dadelszen P, et al. Maternal vitamin D status in pregnancy and adverse pregnancy outcomes in a group at high risk for preeclampsia. *BJOG.* 2010;117:1593.

49. Jelsma JG, van Poppel MN, Galjaard S, et al. Dali: Vitamin D and lifestyle intervention for gestational diabetes mellitus (GDM) prevention: an European multicenter, randomized trial-study protocol. *BMC Pregnancy Childbirth.* 2013;13:142.

50. Institute of Medicine of the National Academies (US). *Dietary reference intakes for calcium and vitamin D.* Washington, DC: National Academy Press; 2010.

51. Lee JM, Smith JR, Philipp BL, et al. Vitamin D deficiency in a healthy group of mothers and newborn infants. *Clin Pediatr.* 2007;46:42.

52. Looker A, et al. Serum 25-hydroxyvitamin D status of the US population: 1988-1994 compared with 2000-2004. *Am J Clin Nutr.* 2008;88:1519.

53. Bodnar LM, Simhan HN. Vitamin D may be a link to black-white disparities in adverse birth outcomes. *Obstet Gynecol Surv.* 2010;65:273.

54. ACOG Committee on Obstetric Practice. ACOG Committee Opinion No. 495: Vitamin D: Screening and supplementation during pregnancy. *Obstet Gynecol.* 2011;118(1):197-198.

55. Food and Nutrition Board, Institute of Medicine. *Dietary Reference Intakes: Vitamin C, Vitamin E, Selenium, and Carotenoids.* Washington, DC: National Academy Press; 2000.

56. Rumbold A, Duley L, Crowther CA, Haslam RR. Antioxidants for preventing preeclampsia. *Cochrane Database Syst Rev.* 2008;(1):CD004227.

57. Roberts J, et al. *Task Force on Hypertension in Pregnancy. "Hypertension in Pregnancy."* The American Congress of Obstetricians and Gynecologists. November 2013.

58. Chittumma P, Kaewkiattikun K, Wiriyasiriwach B. Comparison of the effectiveness of ginger and vitamin B6 for treatment of nausea and vomiting in early pregnancy: a randomized double-blind controlled trial. *J Med Assoc Thai.* 2007;90:15.

59. Matthews A, Dowswell T, Haas DM, Doyle M, O'Mathuna DP. Interventions for nausea and vomiting in early pregnancy. *Cochrane Database Syst Rev.* 2010;CD007575.

60. ACOG (American College of Obstetrics and Gynecology) Practice Bulletin: nausea and vomiting of pregnancy. *Obstet Gynecol.* 2004;103:803-814.

61. Molloy AM, Kirke PN, Brody LC, et al. Effects of folate and vitamin B12 deficiencies during pregnancy on fetal, infant, and child development. *Food Nutr Bull.* 2008;29:101.

62. Blencowe H, Cousens S, Modell B, et al. Folic acid to reduce neonatal mortality from neural tube disorders. *Int J Epidemiol.* 2010;39:110.

63. US Preventive Services Task Force, Agency for Healthcare Research and Quality. Folic acid for the prevention of neural tube defects: US Preventive Services Task Force recommendation statement. *Ann Intern Med.* 2009;150:626.

64. Burau KD, Cech I. Serological differences in folate/vitamin B12 in pregnancies affected by neural tube defects. *South Med J.* 2010;103:419.

65. *The March of Dimes Global Report on Birth Defects: The Hidden Toll of Dying and Disabled Children.* <http://www.marchofdimes.com/glue/files/BirthDefectsExecutiveSummary.pdf>; 2006 Accessed on July 24, 2014.

66. Bentley TG, Willett WC, Weinstein MC, Kuntz KM. Population-level changes in folate intake by age, gender, and race/ethnicity after folic acid fortification. *Am J Public Health.* 2006;96:2040.

67. Nussbaum RL, McInnes RR, Willard HF. Genetics of disorders with complex inheritance. In: *Thompson & Thompson Genetics in Medicine.* 6th ed. Philadelphia (PA): WB Saunders; 2001:289-310.

68. Stothard KJ, Tennant PWG, Bell R, Rankin J. Maternal overweight and obesity and the risk of congenital anomalies: a systematic review and meta-analysis. *JAMA.* 2009;301(6):636-650.

69. Aitken DA, Crossley JA, Spencer K. Prenatal screening for neural tube defects and aneuploidy. In: Rimoin DL, Connor JM, Pyeritz RE, Korf BR, eds. *Emery and Rimoin's principles and practice of medical genetics.* 4th ed. New York: Churchill & Livingstone; 2002:763-801.

70. Neural tube defects. ACOG Practice Bulletin No. 44. American College of Obstetricians and Gynecologists. *Obstet Gynecol.* 2003;102:203-213.

71. Pfeiffer CM, Caudill SP, Gunter EW, et al. Biochemical indicators of B vitamin status in the US population after folic acid fortification: results from the National Health and Nutrition Examination Survey 1999-2000. *Am J Clin Nutr.* 2005;82:442.

72. De Wals P, Tairou F, Van Allen MI, et al. Reduction in neural-neural tube defects after folic acid fortification in Canada. *N Engl J Med.* 2007;357:135.

73. Belfort M, Rifas-Shiman SL, Rich-Edwards JW, et al. Maternal iron intake and iron status during pregnancy and child blood pressure at age 3 years. *Int J Epidemiol.* 2008;37:301.

74. Anemia in Pregnancy. ACOG Practice Bulletin No. 95. American College of Obstetricians and Gynecologists. *Obstet Gynecol.* 2008;112:201-207.

75. Institute of Medicine. *Iron Deficiency Anemia: Recommended Guidelines for the Prevention, Detection, and Management Among U.S. Children and Women of Childbearing Age.* Washington, DC: National Academy Press; 1993.

76. Bhandal N, Russell R. Intravenous versus oral iron therapy for postpartum anaemia. *BJOG.* 2006;113:1248-1252.

77. Hofmeyr GJ, Lawrie TA, Atallah AN, Duley L, Torloni MR. Calcium supplementation during pregnancy for preventing hypertensive disorders and related problems. *Cochrane Database Syst Rev.* 2014;(6):CD001059.

78. Solomon CG, Seely EW. Hypertension in pregnancy. *Endocrinol Metab Clin North Am.* 2006;35:157.

79. Bergman C, Gray-Scott D, Chen JJ, Meacham S. *Food and Nutrition Board, Institute of Medicine. Dietary Reference Intakes for Calcium, Phosphorous, Magnesium, Vitamin D, and Fluoride.* Washington, DC: National Academy Press; 1997.

80. Levine RJ, Hauth JC, Curet LB, et al. Trial of calcium to prevent preeclampsia. *N Engl J Med.* 1997;337:69.

81. Zeisel S. Choline: Critical Role During Fetal Development and Dietary Requirements in Adults. *Annu Rev Nutr.* 2006;26:229-250.

82. Cohen BM, Renshaw PF, Stoll AL, Wurtman RJ, Yurgelun-Todd D, Babb SM. Decreased brain choline up-take in older adults. An in vivo proton magnetic resonance spectroscopy study. *JAMA.* 1995;274:902-907.

83. Dodds L, Fell DB, Joseph KS, et al. Outcomes of pregnancies complicated by hyperemesis gravidarum. *Obstet Gynecol.* 2006;107:285.

84. Jewell D, Young G. Interventions for nausea and vomiting in early pregnancy. *Cochrane Database Syst Rev.* 2003;CD000145.

85. Dean J, Kendall P. *Food safety during pregnancy.* Colorado State University Cooperative Extension. <http://extension.colostate.edu/topic-areas/nutrition-food-safety-health/food-safety-during-pregnancy-9-372/>; Accessed Oct 1, 2010.

86. Olsen SF, Østerdal ML, Salvig JD, et al. Duration of pregnancy in relation to seafood intake during early and mid pregnancy: prospective cohort. *Eur J Epidemiol.* 2006;21:749.

87. Hibbein JR, Davis JM, Steer C, et al. Maternal seafood consumption in pregnancy and neurodevelopmental outcomes in childhood (ALSPAC Study): an observational cohort study. *Lancet.* 2007;269:578.

88. Brender JD, Suarez L, Felkner M, et al. Maternal exposure to arsenic, cadmium, lead, and mercury and neural tube defects in offspring. *Environ Res.* 2006;101:132.

89. US Department of Health and Human Services & US Environmental Protection Agency. *What you need to know about mercury in fish and shellfish.* <http://www.fda.gov/food/resourcesforyou/consumers/ucm110591.htm>; Accessed July 1, 2014.

90. Craig WJ, Mangels AR, American Dietetic Association. Position of the American Dietetic Association: vegetarian diets. *J Am Diet Assoc.* 2009;109:1266.

91. Warriner S, Bryan K, Brown AM. Women's attitude towards the use of complementary and alternative medicines (CAM) in pregnancy. *Midwifery.* 2014;30(1):138-143.

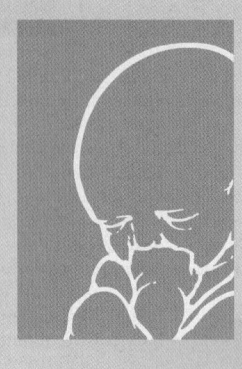

CHAPTER 8

Drugs and Environmental Agents in Pregnancy and Lactation: Teratology, Epidemiology

JENNIFER R. NIEBYL, ROBERT J. WEBER, and GERALD G. BRIGGS

KEY ABBREVIATIONS

Angiotensin-converting enzyme	ACE
Birth defects surveillance monitoring system	BDSMS
Electroencephalogram	EEG
Fetal alcohol syndrome	FAS
Food and Drug Administration	FDA
Glucose-6-phosphate dehydrogenase	G6PD
Neural tube defect	NTD
Propylthiouracil	PTU
Sudden infant death syndrome	SIDS
Saturated solution of potassium iodide	SSKI
Thyroid-stimulating hormone	TSH
Zidovudine	ZDV

OVERVIEW

The placenta allows the transfer of many drugs and dietary substances. Lipid-soluble compounds readily cross the placenta, and water-soluble substances pass less well the greater their molecular weight. The degree to which a drug is bound to plasma protein also influences the amount of drug that is free to cross the placenta. **Virtually all drugs cross the placenta to some degree, with the exception of large molecules such as heparin and insulin.**

Developmental defects in humans may result from genetic, environmental, or unknown causes. Approximately 25% are unequivocally genetic in origin; drug exposure accounts for only 2% to 3% of birth defects. Approximately 65% of defects are of unknown etiology, but most are thought to be combinations of genetic and environmental factors.

The incidence of major malformations in the general population is 2% to 3%.[1] A *major malformation* is defined as one that is incompatible with survival, such as anencephaly; one that requires major surgery for correction, such as cleft palate or congenital heart disease; or one that produces major dysfunction, such as mental retardation. If minor malformations are also included, such as ear tags or extra digits, the rate may be as high as 7% to 10%. The risk of malformation after exposure to a drug must be compared with this background rate.

Species specificity is marked in drug teratogenesis. For example, thalidomide was not found to be teratogenic in rats and mice but is a potent human teratogen. However, it was thought that the original animal studies were flawed because subsequent studies found teratogenicity in mice, rats, rabbits, and monkeys. Animal studies can be used to estimate human risk in about 24% of drugs.

The Teratology Society suggested abandoning the U.S. Food and Drug Administration (FDA) letter classification,[2] and 20 years later, this has finally occurred. The categories implied that risk increases from category A to X. However, the drugs in different categories may pose similar risks but be in different categories based on risk/benefit considerations. The categories create the impression that drugs within a category present similar risks, whereas the category definition permits inclusion in the same category of drugs that vary in type, degree, or extent of risk, depending on potential benefit. The risks and benefits of a drug's use in pregnancy are described in this chapter.

The categories were designed for prescribing physicians and not to address inadvertent exposure. For example, isotretinoin and oral contraceptives were both category X based on lack of benefit for oral contraceptives during pregnancy, yet oral contraceptives do not have any teratogenic risk with inadvertent exposure. When counseling patients or responding to queries from physicians, we recommend using specific descriptions from teratogen information databases (Box 8-1).

The classic teratogenic period is from day 31 after the last menstrual period (LMP) in a 28-day cycle to 71 days from the LMP (Fig. 8-1). **During this critical period, organs are forming, and teratogens may cause malformations that are usually overt at birth.** Timing of exposure is important. Administration of drugs early in the period of organogenesis affects the organs developing at that time, such as the heart or neural tube. Closer to the end of the classic teratogenic period, the ear and palate are forming and may be affected by a teratogen.

BOX 8-1   TERATOGEN INFORMATION DATABASES

- **Micromedex, Inc.** 6200 South Syracuse Way, Suite 300, Greenwood Village, CO 80111-4740; phone 800-525-9083; www.micromedex.com
- **Reproductive Toxicology Center (REPROTOX).** 7831 Woodmont Avenue, Suite 375, Bethesda, MD 20814; phone 301-514-3081; www.reprotox.org
- **Organization of Teratology Information Services (OTIS).** Medical Center, 200 W. Arbor Drive, #8446, San Diego, CA 92103-9981; phone 886-626-6847; www.otispregnancy.org

---

Before day 31, exposure to a teratogen produces an all-or-none effect. With exposure around conception, the conceptus usually either does not survive or survives without anomalies. Because so few cells exist in the early stages, irreparable damage to some may be lethal to the entire organism. If the organism remains viable, however, organ-specific anomalies are not manifested because either repair or replacement will occur to permit normal development. However, a similar insult at a later stage may produce organ-specific defects.

BASIC PRINCIPLES OF TERATOLOGY

To understand the etiology of birth defects, it is important to enumerate the principles of abnormal development, or teratogenesis. **Wilson's six general principles of teratogenesis[3] provide a framework for understanding how structural or functional teratogens may act.** Each principle is covered here.

Genotype and Interaction With Environmental Factors

The first principle is that susceptibility to a teratogen depends on the *genotype of the conceptus* and on the manner in which the genotype interacts with environmental factors. This is perhaps most clearly shown by experiments in which different genetic strains of mice have varied greatly in their susceptibility

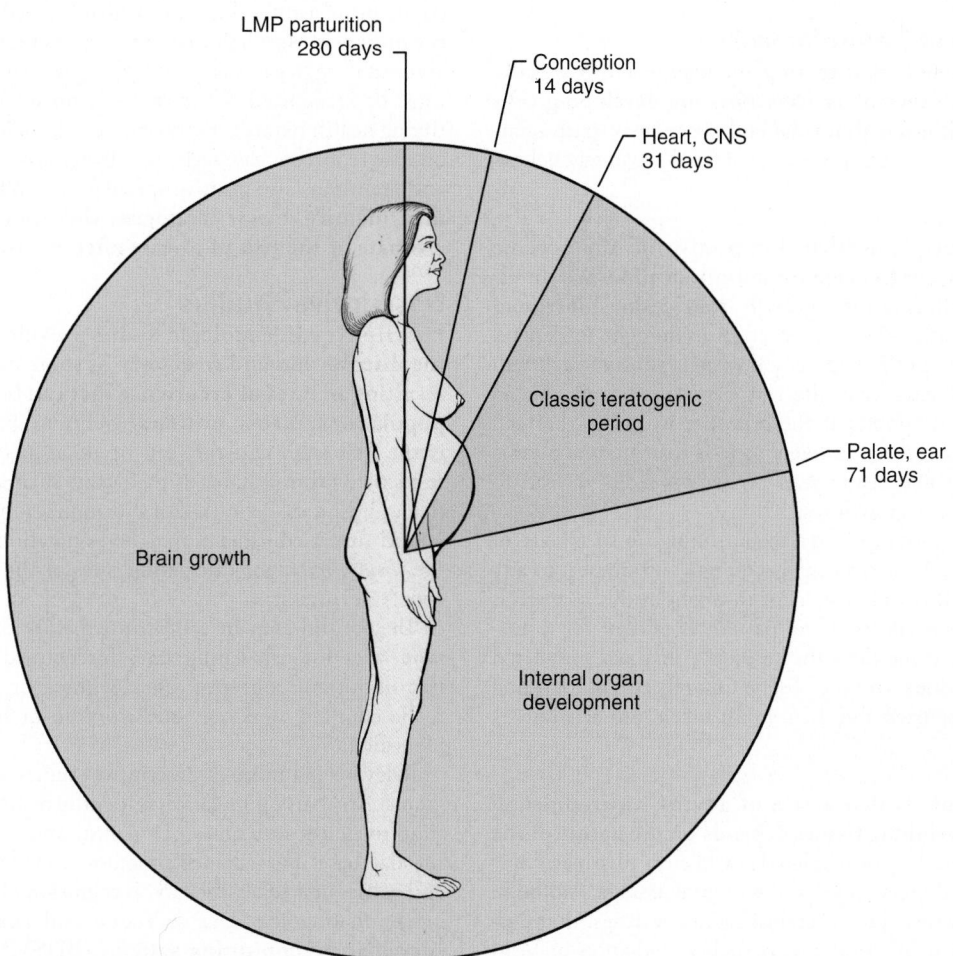

FIG 8-1 Gestational clock showing the classic teratogenic period. *LMP,* last menstrual period. (From Blake DA, Niebyl JR. Requirements and limitations in reproductive and teratogenic risk assessment. In: Niebyl JR, ed. *Drug Use in Pregnancy,* 2nd ed. Philadelphia: Lea & Febiger; 1988:2.)

to teratogens that lead to oral clefts. Some of the variability in responses to human teratogens, such as to anticonvulsant drugs such as valproic acid and hydantoin, probably relates to genotype of the embryo. The increasing complexity of these potential interactions is illustrated by a series of elegant studies by Musselman and colleagues.[4]

Timing of Exposure

The second principle is that susceptibility of the conceptus to teratogenic agents varies with the developmental stage at the time of exposure. This concept of *critical stages of development* is particularly applicable to alterations in structure. **Most structural defects occur during the second to the eighth weeks of development after conception, during the embryonic period.** For such defects, it is believed that a critical stage in the developmental process exists after which abnormal embryogenesis cannot be initiated. For example, neural tube defects (NTDs) result from the failure of the neural tube to close. Given that this process occurs between 22 and 28 days postconception, any exogenous effect on development must be present at or before this time. The neural tube has five distinct closure sites that may respond differentially to agents and may respond differently in timing. Investigations of thalidomide teratogenicity have clearly shown that the effects of the drug differ as a function of the developmental stage at which the pregnant woman took the drug.

Mechanisms of Teratogenesis

The third principle is that teratogenic agents act in specific ways—that is, via specific *mechanisms*—on developing cells and tissues in initiating abnormal embryogenesis (pathogenesis). Teratogenic mechanisms are considered separately below.

Manifestations

The fourth principle is that irrespective of the specific deleterious agent, the final manifestations of abnormal development are malformation, growth restriction, functional disorder, and death. The manifestation is thought to depend largely on the stage of development at which exposure occurred; a teratogen may have one effect if exposure occurs during embryogenesis and another if the exposure is during the fetal period. *Embryonic exposure* is likely to lead to structural abnormalities or embryonic death; *fetal exposure* is likely to lead to functional deficits or growth restriction.

Despite the importance of teratogen timing on specificity of anomalies, a general pattern usually emerges with respect to any given teratogen. This will be evident throughout this chapter as we consider various agents. If no pattern is evident for a purported teratogen, it increases the suspicion that any purported association is spurious, and the observation reflects confounding variables not recognized and, hence, not taken into account.

Agent

The fifth principle is that access of adverse environmental influences to developing tissues depends on the nature of the influence (*agent*). This principle relates to such pharmacologic factors as maternal metabolism and placental passage. Although most clearly understood for chemical agents or drugs, the principle also applies to physical agents such as radiation or heat. For an adverse effect to occur, an agent must reach the conceptus, either indirectly through maternal tissues or directly by traversing the maternal body.

Dose Effect

The final principle is that manifestations of abnormal development increase in degree from the no-effect level to the lethal level as *dosage* increases. This means that the response (e.g., malformation, growth restriction) may be expected to vary according to the dose, duration, or amount of exposure. For most human teratogens, this dose response is not clearly understood, but along with the principle of critical stages of development, these concepts are important in supporting causal inferences about human reproductive hazards. Data regarding in utero exposure to ionizing radiation clearly show the importance of dose on observed effects. The potential complexity of relationships between dose and observed effects for teratogens has been noted.

EPIDEMIOLOGIC APPROACHES TO BIRTH DEFECTS

Teratogens and reproductive toxicants have been identified and are being sought in various ways. Here we enumerate most common approaches, their strengths, and their pitfalls.

Case Reports

Many known teratogens and reproductive toxicants were identified initially through case reports of an unusual number of cases or a constellation of abnormalities. These have often come from astute clinicians who observed something out of the ordinary. Although the importance of astute observations of abnormal aggregations of cases or patterns of malformations must be recognized, we cannot rely on such methods for identifying health hazards. Furthermore, etiologic speculations based on case reports or case series usually do not lead to a causal agent and are often false-positive speculations. **Whereas case reports may identify a new teratogen, they can never provide an estimate of the risk of disease after exposure.**

Descriptive Studies

Descriptive epidemiologic studies provide information about the distribution and frequency of some outcome of interest, resulting in rates of occurrence that can be compared among populations, places, or times. Defining the population at risk is the first step, and this can be done geographically, such as residents within a state, or medically, such as patients at a particular hospital. Definition of the population at risk includes the period under consideration. The population at risk constitutes the *denominator* for calculating rates of the occurrence of outcomes of interest.

The second step in a descriptive study is to determine the *numerator* for calculating rates for comparison. This involves two important concepts: *case definition,* or what defines a case to be counted, and *case ascertainment,* or how cases are to be identified.

Relevant examples of descriptive studies are surveillance programs. An at-risk population is identified and then followed over time to detect outcomes of interest, and cases are included in the database. Surveillance programs can develop baseline data and subsequently permit early recognition of potential problems based on ongoing data collection and analysis. **Birth defect surveillance monitoring systems (BDSMSs) are designed to identify cases that occur in a defined population, usually by reviewing vital records or hospital record abstracts or charts.** In the past 20 years, a dramatic increase has been seen in the number of state-based birth defect surveillance systems, and approximately half the states now have some type of BDSMS. These programs conduct routine reviews of occurrence rates of specific malformations and attempt to identify increases in rates or clusters of cases.

Case-Control Studies

In a case-control study design, groups of individuals (cases) with some outcome or disease of interest (e.g., a congenital malformation) are compared with controls with regard to a history of one or more exposures. This is the most widely used approach in reproductive outcomes research. Controls are ideally as similar as possible to the cases except of course lacking the outcome of interest. After cases and controls have been identified, the hypothesis to be tested is whether these two groups differ in exposure as well as outcome. How accurately exposure and its timing are determined may vary greatly among studies, but in any study, the same methods must be used to establish the exposure of both cases and controls.

Case-control studies are advantageous in testing outcomes of infrequent occurrence. This can be conducted relatively rapidly and inexpensively. A disadvantage is the potential for several important types of bias, including bias in recalling exposure, in selecting appropriate controls, and in ascertaining cases.

These problems can be addressed in part by use of two control groups, one "normal" and the second "abnormal." Any of several abnormal controls seem equally useful (e.g., infants with mendelian or chromosomal disorders as well as infants with no specific malformations).[5] In the former, mothers have incentive to recall, but teratogenesis is not the etiology. Ideally, case-control studies of potential teratogens should follow descriptive studies. After suspecting on the basis of case observations that thalidomide was teratogenic, Lenz[6] conducted a case-control study. **The association between valproic acid use and spina bifida was also verified by case-control studies.**[7]

Cohort Studies

In cohort studies, groups are defined by the presence or absence of exposure to a given factor and then are followed over time and compared for rates of occurrence (i.e., incidence rates) of the outcome of interest. Cohort studies have three advantages: (1) the cohort is classified by exposure before the outcome is determined, thereby eliminating exposure recall bias; (2) incidence rates can be calculated among those exposed; and (3) multiple outcomes can be observed simultaneously.

Cohort studies, often called *prospective studies,* require that groups differing in exposure be followed through time with outcomes observed; therefore these studies tend to be time consuming and expensive. In addition, occurrence rates for many adverse reproductive outcomes, such as congenital malformations, are low; thus large samples must be followed for a considerable period of time. Two main types of cohort studies have been developed, those that identify a cohort and follow it into the future (*concurrent* cohort study) and those that identify a cohort at some time in the past and follow it to the present (*nonconcurrent* or *historical* cohort study). In both cases, risks of adverse outcomes are compared between groups. **Cohort studies enable investigators to calculate incidence rates that provide a measure of risk of an outcome after the exposure.** Risk in the exposed group can be compared with risk in an unexposed group. Most frequently, the ratio of the incidence rate among the exposed to the rate among the unexposed is determined. This

ratio, referred to as *relative risk,* is a measure of how much the presence of exposure increases the risk of the outcome.

In *historical prospective studies,* the study begins by identifying groups who differ in terms of some past exposure, and these are followed to the present to determine outcomes; exposure groups are defined before outcomes are known. A major advantage is that although the time frame is prospective, investigators do not have to follow the cohort into the future and wait for events to occur. A disadvantage is that these studies require the ability to determine exposure status retrospectively.

Clinical Trials

Ideally, analytic studies—case control or cohort—are followed by a randomized clinical trial in which the efficiency of a prevention or treatment regimen is evaluated; that is, subjects are randomly assigned to different treatment groups. The individuals should be as similar as possible in terms of unknown factors that may affect the response before they are randomly assigned to the treatment groups to receive the different regimens.

Clinical trials of both NTD recurrence[8] and occurrence[9] have shown a protective effect of periconceptional folic acid supplementation, findings that have led to key public health recommendations regarding the use of folic acid to reduce the risk of these often devastating defects.

MEDICAL DRUG USE

Patients should be educated about drug alternatives to cope with tension, aches and pains, and viral and other medical illnesses during pregnancy. The risk/benefit ratio should justify the use of a particular drug, and the minimum effective dose should be used. Because long-term effects of drug exposure in utero may not be revealed for many years, caution with regard to the use of any drug in pregnancy is warranted. Also, some drug doses may have a significant effect on the concentrations of analytes routinely used in serum screening for aneuploidy and NTDs.[10] Methadone has been reported to increase screen-positive results for trisomy 18, and screen-positive rates for NTDs were higher for those on corticosteroids, antibiotics, and antidepressants.[10]

Effects of Specific Drugs
Estrogens and Progestins

Studies have not confirmed any teratogenic risk for oral contraceptives or progestins. A meta-analysis of first-trimester sex hormone exposure revealed no association between exposure and fetal genital malformations. However, because of the medicolegal climate and the conflicting past literature, it is wise to exclude pregnancy before giving progestins to an amenorrheic patient.

Androgenic Steroids

Androgens may masculinize a developing female fetus. Danazol has been reported to produce clitoral enlargement and labial fusion when given inadvertently for the first 9 to 12 weeks after conception (Fig. 8-2) in 23 of 57 female infants exposed.

Spermicides

The once touted increased risk of abnormal offspring in mothers who had used spermicides for contraception has not been confirmed. **A meta-analysis of reports of spermicide exposure concludes that the risk of birth defects is not increased.**[11]

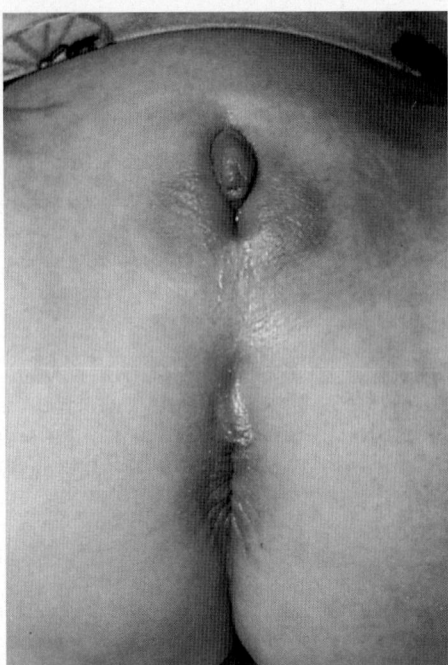

FIG 8-2 Perineum of a female fetus exposed to danazol in utero. (From Duck SC, Katayama KP. Danazol may cause female pseudohermaphroditism. *Fertil Steril.* 1981;35:230.)

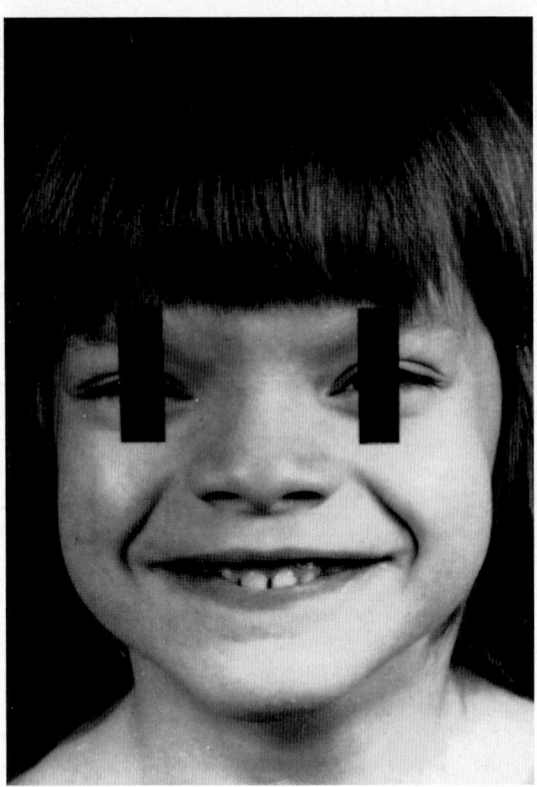

FIG 8-3 Facial features of the fetal hydantoin syndrome. Note broad, flat nasal ridge; epicanthic folds; mild hypertelorism; and wide mouth with prominent upper lip. (Courtesy Dr. Thaddeus Kelly, Charlottesville, VA.)

Antiepileptic Drugs

Women with epilepsy who take antiepileptic drugs (AEDs) during pregnancy have approximately double the general population risk of malformations in offspring. Compared with the general risk of 2% to 3%, the risk of major malformations in women with epilepsy who take AEDs is about 5%, especially cleft lip with or without cleft palate and congenital heart disease. **Valproic acid and carbamazepine each carry approximately a 1% risk of NTDs and other anomalies.** Valproic acid monotherapy significantly increases risk for spina bifida (odds ratio [OR] 12.7), atrial septal defect (2.5), cleft palate (5.2), hypospadias (4.8), polydactyly (2.2), and craniosynostosis (6.8).[12] A high daily dose or a combination of two or three drugs increases the chance of malformations.

Holmes and colleagues[13] screened 128,049 pregnant women at delivery to identify three groups of infants: those exposed to AEDs, those unexposed to AEDs but with a maternal history of seizures, and those unexposed to AEDs with no maternal history of seizures (control group). The infants were examined systematically for the presence of malformations. The combined frequency of anticonvulsant embryopathy was higher in 223 infants exposed to one AED than in 508 control infants (20.6% vs. 8.5%; OR, 2.8; 95% confidence interval [CI], 1.1-9.7). The frequency was also higher in 93 infants exposed to two or more AEDs than in the controls (28.0% vs. 8.5%; OR, 4.2; 95% CI, 1.1-5.1). The greater the number of AEDs, the higher the risk of malformation. The 98 infants whose mothers had a history of epilepsy but who took no AEDs during the pregnancy did not have a higher frequency of abnormalities than the control infants.

Phenytoin decreases folate absorption and lowers serum folate, which has been implicated in birth defects. Therefore folic acid supplementation should be given to these mothers, but this may require adjustment of the AED. Although women with epilepsy were not included in the Medical Research Council study, most authorities would recommend 4 mg/day folic acid for high-risk women. One study suggested that folic acid at doses of 2.5 to 5 mg daily could reduce birth defects in the offspring of women who take AEDs.[14]

Fewer than 10% of offspring show the fetal hydantoin syndrome, which consists of microcephaly, growth deficiency, developmental delays, mental retardation, and dysmorphic craniofacial features (Fig. 8-3). In fact, the risk may be as low as 1% to 2% above background. Although several of these features are also found in other syndromes, such as fetal alcohol syndrome, more common in the fetal hydantoin syndrome are hypoplasia of the nails and distal phalanges (Fig. 8-4) and hypertelorism. Carbamazepine is also associated with an increased risk of a dysmorphic syndrome.[15] A genetically determined metabolic defect in arene oxide detoxification in the infant may increase the risk of a major birth defect. Epoxide hydrolase deficiency may indicate susceptibility to fetal hydantoin syndrome.[16]

In a follow-up study of long-term effects of antenatal exposure to phenobarbital and carbamazepine, no neurologic or behavioral differences were noted between the two groups. However, children exposed in utero to phenytoin scored 10 points lower on IQ tests than children exposed to carbamazepine and nonexposed controls. At 3 years of age, children who had been exposed to valproate in utero had significantly lower IQ scores than those exposed to other antiepileptic drugs; therefore **valproate should not be used as a first-choice drug in women of reproductive age.** Also, prenatal exposure to phenobarbital decreased verbal IQ scores in adult men.

Lamotrigine exposures have been compiled in a voluntary registry established by the manufacturer, GlaxoSmithKline. After 1558 exposures in the first trimester, no increased risk of birth defects overall has been observed.[17] **Of 1532 infant exposures to newer-generation antiepileptic drugs, 1019 were to lamotrigine, and 3.7% had major birth defects. Of 393 infants exposed to oxcarbazepine, the rate was 2.8%, and for 108 exposed to topiramate, the rate was 4.6%. None of these differences were statistically different from controls.** Valproic acid carries significantly higher risks than lamotrigine or carbamazepine.[18] One study suggested a fivefold increased risk of cleft lip and/or cleft palate with use of topiramate.[19] In general, polytherapy exposure is associated with some poorer outcomes in neuropsychological or developmental testing.[20] Minimizing the dose during pregnancy is also critical in preventing birth defects.[21]

Some women may have taken AEDs for a long period without reevaluation of the need for continuation of the drugs. For patients with idiopathic epilepsy who have been seizure free for 2 years and who have a normal electroencephalogram (EEG), it may be safe to attempt a trial of withdrawal of the drug before pregnancy.

Most authorities agree that the benefits of AEDs during pregnancy outweigh the risks of discontinuation of the drug if the patient is first seen during pregnancy. Continuing AEDs depends on the type of seizures, seizure control, adverse effects of the AED regimen, and patient adherence. Adherence can be determined by measuring a serum concentration of the AED. If the level is low or undetected and the patient is seizure free, AED therapy may not be required. Because the albumin concentration falls in pregnancy, the total amount of phenytoin measured is decreased because it is highly protein bound. However, the level of free phenytoin, which is the pharmacologically active portion, is unchanged.

Pediatric care providers need to be notified at birth when a patient has been on anticonvulsants because this therapy can affect vitamin K–dependent clotting factors in the newborn.

Isotretinoin

Isotretinoin is a significant human teratogen. This drug is marketed as Accutane for treatment of cystic acne, and it unfortunately has been taken by women who were not planning pregnancy.[22] Long-acting reversible contraception such as an intrauterine device (IUD) or an etonogestrel implant (Nexplanon) are recommended. Isotretinoin is labeled as contraindicated in pregnancy (FDA category X) with appropriate warnings that a negative pregnancy test is required before therapy. Of 154 exposed human pregnancies, 21 cases of birth defects, 12 spontaneous abortions, 95 elective abortions, and 26 normal infants were reported in women who took isotretinoin during early pregnancy. **The risk of structural anomalies in patients studied prospectively is now estimated to be about 25%, and an additional 25% have mental retardation alone.** The malformed infants have a characteristic pattern of craniofacial, cardiac, thymic, and central nervous system (CNS) anomalies that include microtia/anotia (small/absent ears; Fig. 8-5), micrognathia, cleft palate, heart defects, thymic defects, retinal or

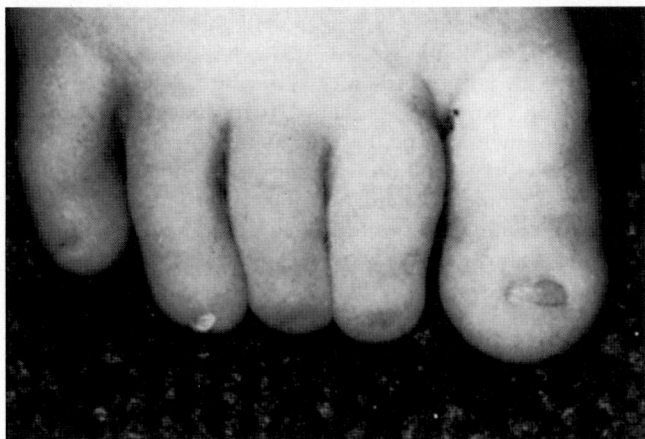

FIG 8-4 Hypoplasia of toenails and distal phalanges. (From Hanson JW, Smith DW. Fetal hydantoin syndrome. *Lancet* 1976;1[7961]:186.)

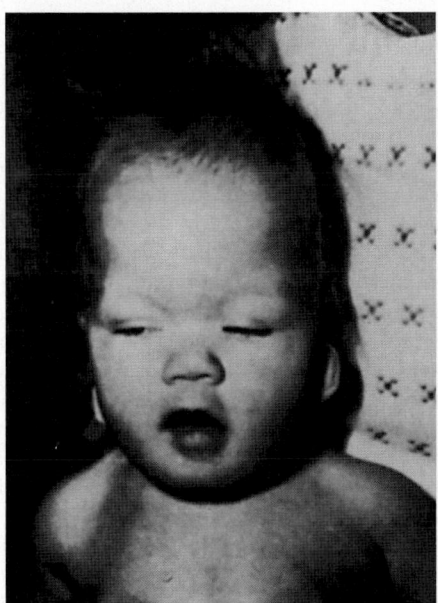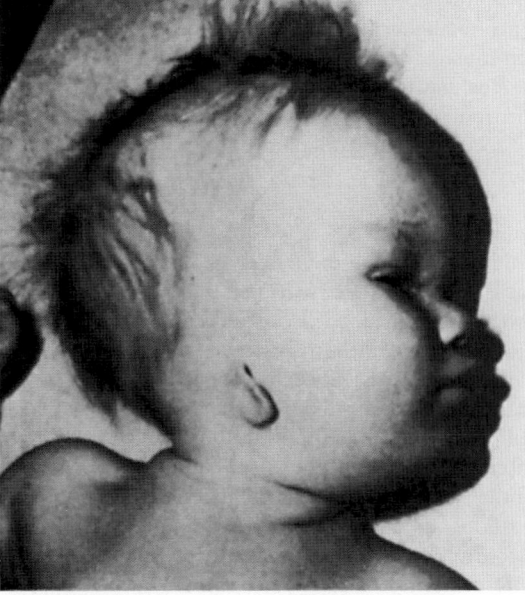

FIG 8-5 Infant exposed to isotretinoin (Accutane) in utero. Note high forehead, hypoplastic nasal bridge, and abnormal ears. (From Lot IT, Bocian M, Pribam HW, Leitner M. Fetal hydrocephalus and ear anomalies associated with use of isotretinoin. *J Pediatr.* 1984;105:598.)

optic nerve anomalies, and CNS malformations that include hydrocephalus.[22] Microtia is rare as an isolated anomaly yet appears commonly as part of the retinoic acid embryopathy. Cardiovascular defects include great vessel transposition and ventricular septal defects (VSDs).

Unlike vitamin A, isotretinoin is not stored in tissue. Therefore a pregnancy after discontinuation of isotretinoin is not at risk because the drug is no longer detectable in serum 5 days after its ingestion. **In 88 pregnancies prospectively ascertained after discontinuation of isotretinoin, no increased risk of anomalies was noted.** Topical tretinoin has not been associated with any teratogenic risk.

Vitamin A

No evidence suggests that vitamin A or β-carotene is teratogenic in normal doses. The vitamin A levels in prenatal vitamins (5000 IU/day) have not been associated with any documented risk. **Eighteen cases of birth defects have been reported after exposure to levels of 25,000 IU or more of vitamin A during pregnancy.** Vitamin A in doses greater than 10,000 IU/day was shown to increase the risk of malformations in one study but not in another.

Psychoactive Drugs

No clear risk has been documented for most psychoactive drugs with respect to overt birth defects. However, effects of chronic use of these agents on the developing brain in humans is difficult to study, and so a conservative attitude is appropriate. Lack of overt defects does not exclude the possibility of behavioral teratogenesis, and neonatal withdrawal may occur. However, untreated depression carries risks also.

TRANQUILIZERS

Conflicting reports of the possible teratogenicity of the various tranquilizers, including meprobamate and chlordiazepoxide, have appeared, but in prospective studies no increased risk of anomalies has been shown.

A fetal benzodiazepine syndrome has been reported in seven infants of 36 mothers who regularly took benzodiazepines during pregnancy. However, the high rate of abnormality occurred with concomitant alcohol and substance abuse and may not have been caused by the benzodiazepine exposure. In most clinical situations, however, the risk/benefit ratio does not justify the use of benzodiazepines in pregnancy. Use of diazepam in labor has been associated with neonatal hypotonia, hypothermia, and respiratory depression.

LITHIUM

In the International Register of Lithium Babies, 217 infants were listed as exposed at least during the first trimester of pregnancy, and 25 (11.5%) were malformed. Eighteen had cardiovascular anomalies, including six cases of the rare Ebstein anomaly, which occurs in only 1 in 20,000 in the nonexposed population. Of 60 unaffected infants who were followed to age 5 years, no increased mental or physical abnormalities were noted compared with unexposed siblings.

However, two other reports suggest bias of ascertainment in the registry and a risk of anomalies much lower than previously thought. A case-control study of 59 patients with Ebstein anomaly showed no difference in the rate of lithium exposure in pregnancy from a control group of 168 children with neuroblastoma.[23] **A prospective study of 148 women exposed to lithium in the first trimester showed no difference in the incidence of major anomalies compared with controls.**[24] One fetus in the lithium-exposed group had Ebstein anomaly, and one infant in the control group had a VSD. The authors concluded that lithium is not a major human teratogen. **Nevertheless, we recommend that women exposed to lithium be offered ultrasound and fetal echocardiography.**

Lithium is excreted more rapidly during pregnancy, thus serum lithium levels should be monitored. Perinatal effects of lithium have been noted and include hypotonia, lethargy, and poor feeding in the infant. Also, complications similar to those seen in adults taking lithium have been noted in newborns, including goiter and hypothyroidism.

Two cases of polyhydramnios associated with maternal lithium treatment have been reported. Because nephrogenic diabetes insipidus has been reported in adults taking lithium, the presumed mechanism of this polyhydramnios is fetal diabetes insipidus. **Polyhydramnios may be a sign of fetal lithium toxicity.**

It is usually recommended that drug therapy be changed in pregnant women taking lithium to avoid fetal drug exposure. Tapering over 10 days delays the risk of relapse. However, discontinuing lithium is associated with a 70% chance of relapse of the affective disorder in 1 year as opposed to 20% in those who remain on lithium. **Discontinuation of lithium may pose an unacceptable risk of increased morbidity in women who have had multiple episodes of affective instability. These women should be offered appropriate prenatal diagnosis with ultrasound, including fetal echocardiography.** Lithium may be withheld for 24 to 48 hours before delivery to reduce neonatal complications and reduce infant hospital stays.[25]

ANTIDEPRESSANTS

Imipramine was the original tricyclic antidepressant (TCA) claimed to be associated with cardiovascular defects, but the number of patients studied remains small. Of 75 newborns exposed in the first trimester, six major defects were observed —three cardiovascular—and neonatal withdrawal has been observed.

Amitriptyline has been more widely used, and the majority of the evidence supports its safety. In the Michigan Medicaid study, 467 newborns had been exposed during the first trimester, with no increased risk of birth defects.

No increased risk of major malformations has been found after first-trimester exposure to fluoxetine in several studies.[26] **However, one recent study showed a twofold increased risk of VSDs.**[27] Chambers and associates found more minor malformations and perinatal complications among infants exposed to fluoxetine throughout pregnancy, but this study is difficult to interpret because the authors did not control for depression. When a group whose mothers received tricyclic agents was used as a control for depression, infants exposed to fluoxetine in utero did not appear to have more minor malformations or perinatal complications. One study suggested an increased risk of low-birthweight infants with higher doses of fluoxetine (40 to 80 mg) throughout pregnancy.

Nulman evaluated the neurobehavioral effects of long-term fluoxetine exposure during pregnancy and found no abnormalities among 228 children aged 16 to 86 months (average age, 3 years). Theoretically, some psychiatric or neurobehavioral abnormality might occur as a result of exposure, but it would be very difficult to ascertain because of all of the confounding variables.

Current data on other selective serotonin reuptake inhibitor (SSRI) exposures show no consistent teratogenic risk.[28] Citalopram is transferred across the placenta the most, followed by fluoxetine. The lowest transfer is found with sertraline, followed by paroxetine,[29] although **two studies found an increased risk of cardiac defects after exposure to paroxetine.**[27] A recent large, population-based cohort study suggested no substantial increased risk of cardiac defects attributable to antidepressant use in the first trimester.[30] One study showed a twofold increased risk of NTDs after citalopram.[27]

Studies have described neonatal withdrawal in the first 2 days after in utero exposure to these drugs.[31] Infants exposed during pregnancy exhibited more tremulousness and sleep changes at 1 to 2 days of age. However, no abnormalities were found when children were examined at ages of 16 to 86 months after prolonged exposure during pregnancy.

A sixfold increased risk of persistent pulmonary hypertension (PPH) in newborns has been reported in infants exposed to SSRIs after 20 weeks of pregnancy,[32] raising the absolute risk from 1 to 2 per 1000 in unexposed infants to 6 to 12 per 1000 in exposed infants. Another study did not confirm this finding but did confirm a fivefold increased risk of PPH with cesarean section before labor.[33] Exposure to SSRIs in the first trimester did not increase the risk of miscarriage.[34] No major malformations have been reported in 133 infants exposed to bupropion.[35]

When considering the use of antidepressant drugs during pregnancy, it should be noted that among women who maintained their medication throughout pregnancy, 26% relapsed compared with 68% who discontinued medication.[36] **Also, fetal alcohol spectrum disorders were 10 times more common in SSRI-exposed offspring than in unexposed offspring.** Therefore controversy exists as to whether the risks of antidepressants outweigh the benefits, and counseling may be as effective as drug therapy.[37]

Anticoagulants

Warfarin has been associated with chondrodysplasia punctata, which is similar to the genetically determined Conradi-Hünermann syndrome. **Warfarin embryopathy occurs in about 5% of exposed pregnancies and includes nasal hypoplasia, bone stippling seen on radiologic examination, ophthalmologic abnormalities including bilateral optic atrophy, and mental retardation** (Fig. 8-6). Ophthalmologic abnormalities and mental retardation may occur even with use only beyond the first trimester. **The risk for pregnancy complications is higher when the mean daily dose of warfarin is more than 5 mg.**

The alternative drugs, heparin and enoxaparin, do not cross the placenta because they are large molecules with a strong negative charge. **Because heparin does not have an adverse effect on the fetus when given in pregnancy, it should be the drug of choice for patients who require anticoagulation, except in women with artificial heart valves.** However, therapy with 20,000 U/day for more than 20 weeks has been associated with bone demineralization, and 36% of patients had more than a 10% decrease from baseline bone density to postpartum values. The risk of spine fractures was 0.7% with low-dose heparin and 3% with a high-dose regimen. Heparin can also cause thrombocytopenia.

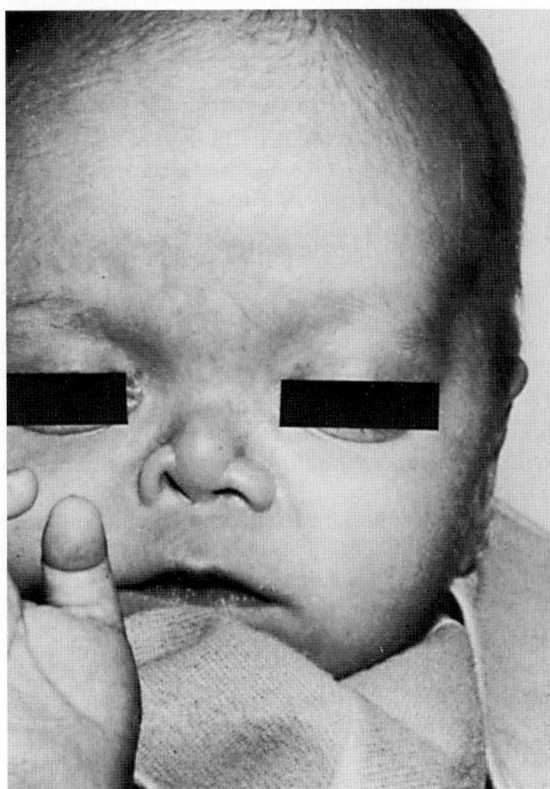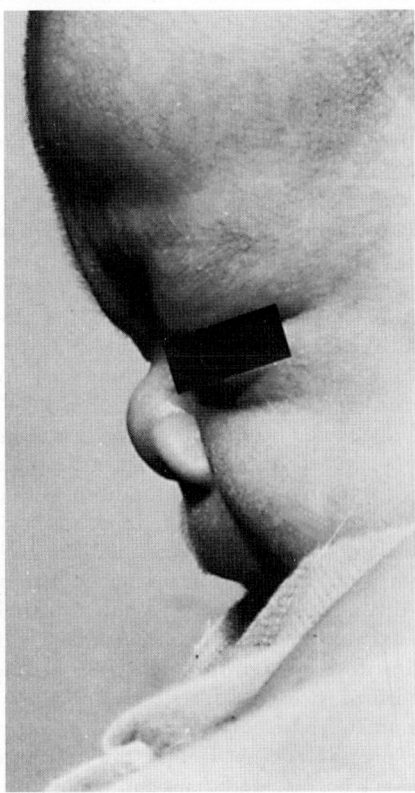

FIG 8-6 Warfarin embryopathy. Note small nose with hypoplastic bridge. (From Shaul W, Hall JG. Multiple congenital anomalies associated with oral anticoagulants. *Am J Obstet Gynecol.* 1977;127:191.)

Low-molecular-weight heparins (LMWHs) may have substantial benefits over standard unfractionated heparin (UFH). The molecules are still relatively large and do not cross the placenta, plus the half-life is longer, which allows for once-daily administration. However, enoxaparin is cleared more rapidly during pregnancy, so twice-daily dosing is advised. LMWHs have a much more predictable dose-response relationship, which obviates the need for monitoring of partial thromboplastin time. The risk of heparin-induced thrombocytopenia and clinical bleeding at delivery is lower, but studies that suggest less risk of osteoporosis are preliminary.

Women with mechanical heart valves, especially the first-generation valves, require warfarin anticoagulation because heparin is neither safe nor effective. Heparin treatment is associated with more thromboembolic complications and more bleeding complications than warfarin therapy.

The risks of heparin during pregnancy may not be justified in patients with only a single remote episode of thrombosis in the past. Certainly, conservative measures should be recommended, such as elastic stockings and avoidance of prolonged sitting or standing.

Thyroid and Antithyroid Drugs

Propylthiouracil (PTU) and methimazole both cross the placenta and may cause some degree of fetal goiter. In contrast, the thyroid hormones triiodothyronine and thyroxine cross the placenta poorly, so that fetal hypothyroidism produced by antithyroid drugs cannot be corrected satisfactorily by administration of thyroid hormone to the mother. Thus the goal of such therapy during pregnancy is to keep the mother slightly hyperthyroid to minimize fetal drug exposure. By the third trimester, 30% of women no longer need antithyroid medication.[38]

Methimazole has been associated with scalp defects in infants and choanal or esophageal atresia[38] as well as a higher incidence of maternal side effects. However, PTU and methimazole are equally effective and safe for therapy of hyperthyroidism. Still, in 2009 the FDA released a black box warning highlighting serious liver injury with PTU treatment, to a greater extent than methimazole. The Endocrine Society is now advocating treatment with PTU only during the first trimester and switching to methimazole for the remainder of the pregnancy.[39,40]

Radioactive iodine (^{131}I or ^{125}I) administered for thyroid ablation or for diagnostic studies is not concentrated by the fetal thyroid until after 12 weeks of pregnancy. Thus with inadvertent exposure before 12 weeks, no specific risk to the fetal thyroid results from ^{131}I or ^{125}I administration.

The need for thyroxine increases in many women with primary hypothyroidism when they are pregnant, as reflected by an increase in serum thyroid-stimulating hormone (TSH) concentrations.[41] Because hypothyroidism in pregnancy may adversely affect the fetus, possibly by increasing prematurity, it is prudent to monitor thyroid function throughout pregnancy and to adjust the thyroid dose to maintain a normal TSH level. It is recommended that women with hypothyroidism increase their levothyroxine dose by approximately 30% as soon as pregnancy is confirmed (two extra doses each week) and then have dosing adjustments based on TSH levels.[41]

Topical iodine preparations are readily absorbed through the vagina during pregnancy, and transient hypothyroidism has been demonstrated in the newborn after exposure during labor.

Digoxin

In 194 exposures, no teratogenicity of digoxin was noted. Blood levels should be monitored in pregnancy to ensure adequate therapeutic maternal levels.

Digoxin-like immunoreactive substances may be mistaken in assays for fetal concentrations of digoxin. In one study of fetuses with cardiac anomalies, no difference was found in the immunoreactive digoxin levels whether the mother had received digoxin or not. In hydropic fetuses, digoxin may not easily cross the placenta.

Antihypertensive Drugs

For treatment of chronic hypertension in pregnancy, α-methyldopa has been widely used. Although postural hypotension may occur, no unusual fetal effects have been noted. Hydralazine is used frequently in pregnancy, and no teratogenic effect has been observed. For more on antihypertensive drugs, see Chapter 31.

SYMPATHETIC BLOCKING AGENTS

Propranolol is a β-adrenergic blocking agent in widespread use for various indications, for which no evidence of teratogenicity has been found. Bradycardia has been reported in the newborn as a direct effect of a dose of the drug given to the mother within 2 hours of delivery.

Several studies of propranolol use in pregnancy show an increased risk of intrauterine growth restriction (IUGR) or at least a skewing of the birthweight distribution toward the lower range. Ultrasound monitoring of exposed patients is prudent. Studies from Scotland suggest improved outcome with the use of atenolol to treat chronic hypertension during pregnancy.

Calcium channel blockers such as nifedipine have been widely used for chronic hypertension in pregnancy without evidence of teratogenicity. Magnesium sulfate should be used with caution in women taking these agents.

ANGIOTENSIN-CONVERTING ENZYME INHIBITORS AND ANGIOTENSIN RECEPTOR BLOCKERS

Fetal exposure to angiotensin-converting enzyme (ACE) inhibitors and angiotensin receptor blockers (ARBs) in the first trimester has not been associated with an increased risk of birth defects. ACE inhibitors such as enalapril and captopril and angiotensin II receptor antagonists such as valsartan can cause fetal renal tubular dysplasia in the second and third trimesters, leading to oligohydramnios, fetal limb contractures, craniofacial deformities, and hypoplastic lung development. Fetal skull ossification defects have also been described. For these reasons, women taking these medications who plan pregnancy should be switched to other agents.

Antineoplastic Drugs and Immunosuppressants

Mycophenolate mofetil carries a moderate teratogenic risk.[42] Frequent features include microtia or anotia, cleft lip and/or palate, heart defects, and dysmorphic facial features. The numbers are too small to determine the actual rate of malformations.

Methotrexate, a folic acid antagonist, appears to be a human teratogen, although experience is limited. Infants of three women known to have received methotrexate in the first trimester of pregnancy had multiple congenital anomalies, including cranial defects and malformed extremities. Of eight women inadvertently treated with methotrexate after misdiagnosis of ectopic pregnancy, two infants were severely malformed, three patients miscarried, and three chose to terminate the pregnancies.[43] Eight normal infants were delivered to seven women treated with methotrexate in combination with other agents after the first trimester. When low-dose oral methotrexate (7.5 mg/week) was used for rheumatoid disease in the first trimester, five full-term infants were normal and three patients experienced spontaneous abortions.

Azathioprine has been used by patients with renal transplants or systemic lupus erythematosus. The frequency of anomalies in 375 women treated in the first trimester was not increased. Some infants had leukopenia, some were small for gestational age (SGA), and the others were normal.

No increased risk of anomalies in fetuses exposed to cyclosporine in utero has been reported. An increased rate of prematurity and growth restriction has been noted, but it is difficult to separate the contributions of the underlying disease and the drugs given to these transplant patients. The B-cell line may be depleted more than the T-cell line, and one author recommends that infants exposed to immunosuppressive agents be followed for possible immunodeficiency.

Eight malformed infants have resulted from first-trimester exposure to cyclophosphamide, but these infants were also exposed to other drugs or radiation. Low birthweight may be associated with use after the first trimester, but this may also reflect the underlying medical problem.

Chloroquine is safe in doses used for malarial prophylaxis, and no increased incidence of birth defects was reported among 169 infants exposed to 300 mg once weekly. However, after exposure to larger antiinflammatory doses (250 to 500 mg/day), two cases of cochleovestibular paresis were reported.[44] No abnormalities were noted in 114 other infants.

No association was found between administration of tumor necrosis factor (TNF) inhibitors infliximab or adalimumab and congenital anomalies.[45]

When cancer chemotherapy must be used during embryogenesis, the rate of spontaneous abortion and major birth defects is increased. Later in pregnancy, the risk of stillbirth and IUGR is greater, and myelosuppression is often present in the infant.

Antiasthmatics
TERBUTALINE
Terbutaline has been widely used in the treatment of preterm labor. It is more rapid in onset, has a longer duration of action than epinephrine, and is preferred for asthma in the pregnant patient. No risk of birth defects has been reported with terbutaline, although long-term use has been associated with an increased risk of glucose intolerance.

CROMOLYN SODIUM
Cromolyn sodium may be administered in pregnancy, and the systemic absorption is minimal. Teratogenicity has not been reported in humans.

ISOPROTERENOL AND METAPROTERENOL
When isoproterenol and metaproterenol are given as topical aerosols for the treatment of asthma, the total dose absorbed is usually not significant. With oral or intravenous (IV) doses, however, the cardiovascular effects of the agents may decrease uterine blood flow. For this reason, they should be used with caution. No teratogenicity has been reported.

CORTICOSTEROIDS
All steroids cross the placenta to some degree, but prednisone and prednisolone are inactivated by the placenta. When prednisone or prednisolone is given to a pregnant woman, the concentration of active compound in the fetus is less than 10% of that in the mother. Therefore these agents are the drugs of choice for treating medical diseases such as asthma. Inhaled corticosteroids are also effective therapy, and very little drug is absorbed. When steroid effects are desired in the fetus to accelerate lung maturity, betamethasone and dexamethasone are preferred because these are minimally inactivated by the placenta. **A meta-analysis of exposure to corticosteroids in the first trimester showed an odds ratio of 3.0 for cleft lip and/or cleft palate.**

IODIDE
Iodide, such as that found in a saturated solution of potassium iodide (SSKI) expectorant, crosses the placenta and may produce a fetal goiter large enough to produce respiratory obstruction in the newborn (Fig. 8-7). Before a pregnant patient is advised to take a cough medicine, the clinician should be sure to ascertain that it does *not* contain iodide.

Antiemetics
Remedies suggested to help nausea and vomiting in pregnancy without pharmacologic intervention include eating crackers at the bedside on first awakening in the morning (before getting out of bed), getting up very slowly, omitting iron tablets, consuming frequent small meals, and eating protein snacks at night. **None of the current medications used to treat nausea and vomiting have been found to be teratogenic except possibly methylprednisolone used before 10 weeks of gestation.**

VITAMIN B$_6$
Vitamin B$_6$ (pyridoxine) 25 mg three times a day has been reported in two randomized placebo-controlled trials to be effective for treating the nausea and vomiting of pregnancy. In several other controlled trials, no evidence of teratogenicity was found.

DOXYLAMINE
Delayed-release doxylamine 10 mg plus pyridoxine 10 mg (Diclegis) is effective and well tolerated.[46] It has been approved by the FDA for NVP.

Doxylamine is an effective antihistamine for nausea and vomiting of pregnancy and can be combined with vitamin B$_6$ to produce a therapy similar to Diclegis. Vitamin B$_6$ (25 mg) and doxylamine (25 mg) at bedtime plus 12.5 mg doxylamine (one-half tablet) with vitamin B$_6$ (25 mg) in the morning and afternoon is an effective combination.

MECLIZINE
In one randomized, placebo-controlled study, meclizine gave significantly better results than placebo, and prospective clinical studies have provided no evidence that meclizine is teratogenic in humans. In 1014 patients in the Collaborative Perinatal Project and in an additional 613 patients from the Kaiser Health Plan, no teratogenic risk was found.

DIMENHYDRINATE
No teratogenicity has been noted with dimenhydrinate, but a 29% failure rate and a significant incidence of side effects, especially drowsiness, has been reported.

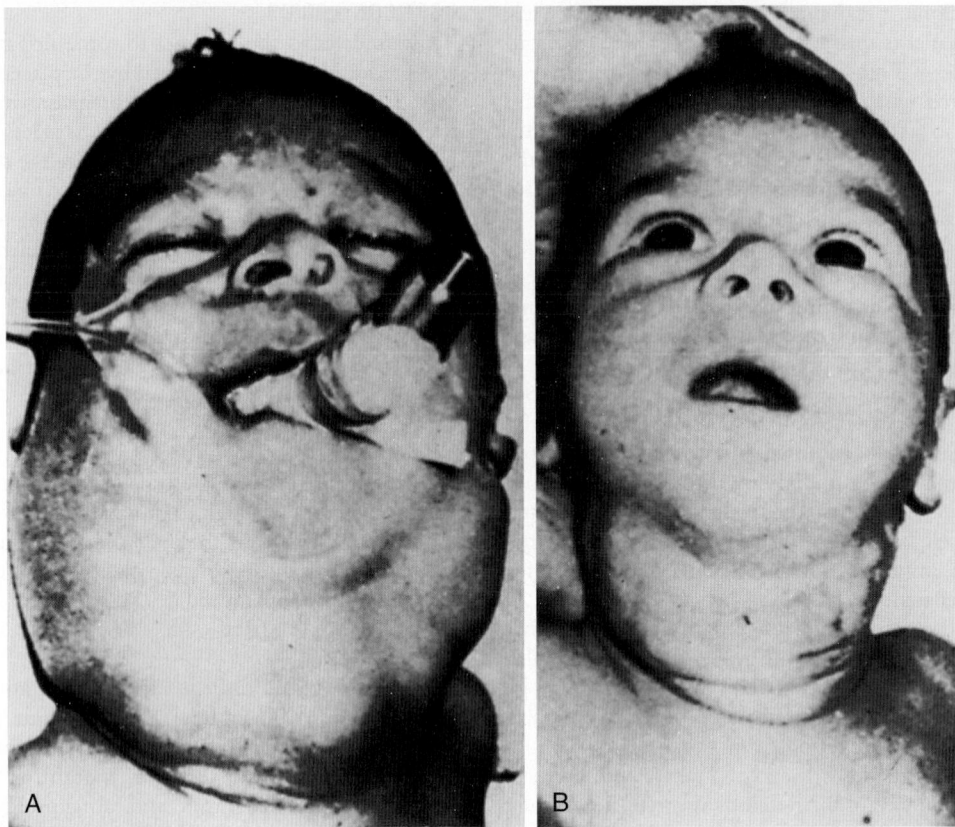

FIG 8-7 Iodide-induced neonatal goiter. **A,** Appearance on the first day of life. **B,** Appearance at 2 months of age. (From Senior B, Chernoff HL. Iodide goiter in the newborn. *Pediatrics.* 1971;47:510.)

DIPHENHYDRAMINE

In 595 patients treated in the Collaborative Perinatal Project, no teratogenicity was noted with diphenhydramine. However, drowsiness can be a problem.

PHENOTHIAZINES

Teratogenicity does not appear to be a problem with the phenothiazines when evaluated as a group. In the Kaiser Health Plan Study, 976 patients were treated, and in the Collaborative Perinatal Project 1309 patients were treated; in both studies, no evidence of association between these drugs and malformations was noted. In 114 mothers treated with promethazine and in 877 mothers given prochlorperazine, no increased risk of malformations was found.

METOCLOPRAMIDE

Of 3458 infants exposed to metoclopramide during the first trimester, no increased risk of malformations, low birthweight, or preterm delivery was reported.[47]

ONDANSETRON

Ondansetron is no more effective than promethazine, but it is less sedating.[48] It has not been associated with a significant risk of adverse fetal outcomes.[49] One study showed no increased risk of birth defects after ondansetron exposure.[49] However, a larger study[50] found a doubling in the prevalence of heart defects in exposed children.

In a double-blind randomized trial, ondansetron and metoclopramide demonstrated similar antiemetic effects, but the overall profile of adverse effects was better with ondansetron.[51]

METHYLPREDNISOLONE

Forty patients with hyperemesis who were admitted to the hospital were randomized to oral methylprednisolone or oral promethazine, and methylprednisolone was more effective.[52] In a larger study in which all patients received promethazine and metoclopramide, methylprednisolone did not reduce the need for rehospitalization. Methylprednisolone should be used only after 10 weeks of pregnancy because of the potential risk of cleft lip and/or cleft palate.

GINGER

Ginger has been used with success for treating nausea, vomiting, and hyperemesis in the outpatient setting. A significantly greater relief of symptoms was found after ginger treatment than with placebo. Patients took 250-mg capsules containing powdered ginger root four times a day.

Acid-Suppressing Drugs

The use of cimetidine, omeprazole, and ranitidine has not been found to be associated with any teratogenic risk in 2261 exposures.[53] Of an additional 3651 infants exposed to proton-pump inhibitors in the first trimester, no increased risk of birth defects was reported.[54] Drugs taken in the study were mostly omeprazole but also included lansoprazole, esomeprazole, and pantoprazole.

Antihistamines and Decongestants

No increased risk of anomalies has been associated with most of the commonly used antihistamines, such as chlorpheniramine. However, in one study, terfenadine was associated with an increased risk of polydactyly. Astemizole did not increase the risk of birth defects in 114 infants exposed in the first trimester. However, an association between exposure to antihistamines during the last 2 weeks of pregnancy and retrolental fibroplasia in premature infants has been reported.

An increased risk of birth defects was noted with phenylpropanolamine exposure in the first trimester, specifically ear defects and pyloric stenosis.[55] In one retrospective study, an increased risk of gastroschisis was associated with first-trimester pseudoephedrine use. Phenylephrine has been associated with endocardial cushion defects.[55] Use of these drugs for trivial indications should be discouraged because long-term effects are unknown. If decongestion is necessary, topical nasal sprays will result in a lower dose to the fetus than systemic medication.

Patients should be educated that antihistamines and decongestants are only symptomatic therapy for the common cold and have no influence on the course of the disease. Other remedies should be recommended, such as use of a humidifier, rest, and fluids. If medications are necessary, combinations with two drugs should not be used if only one drug is necessary. If the diagnosis is truly an allergy, an antihistamine alone will suffice.

Antibiotics and Antiinfective Agents

Because pregnant patients are particularly susceptible to vaginal yeast infections, antibiotics should be used only when clearly indicated. Therapy with antifungal agents may be necessary during or after the course of therapy.

PENICILLINS

Penicillin, ampicillin, and amoxicillin are safe in pregnancy. In the Collaborative Perinatal Project, 3546 mothers took penicillin derivatives in the first trimester of pregnancy with no increased risk of anomalies. Of 86 infants exposed to dicloxacillin in the first trimester, no increase in birth defects was reported.

Clavulanate is added to penicillin derivatives to broaden their antibacterial spectrum. Of 556 infants exposed in the first trimester, no increased risk of birth defects was observed. Amoxicillin/clavulanate was studied in randomized controlled trials (RCTs) as a potential therapy for chorioamnionitis in women with preterm premature rupture of membranes (PPROM). During this trial, amoxicillin/clavulanate was compared with both placebo and erythromycin. An increased incidence of necrotizing enterocolitis was found in the amoxicillin/clavulanate group when compared with both the placebo and erythromycin groups. It has been suggested that amoxicillin/clavulanate selects for specific pathogens, which leads to abnormal microbial colonization of the gastrointestinal tract and ultimately to the initiation of necrotizing enterocolitis. **Therefore amoxicillin/clavulanate should be avoided in women at risk for preterm delivery.**

CEPHALOSPORINS

In a study of 5000 Michigan Medicaid recipients, a suggestion of possible teratogenicity (25% increased birth defects) was found with cefaclor, cephalexin, and cephradine but not with other cephalosporins. However, another study of 308 women exposed in the first trimester showed no increase in malformations, therefore the consensus is that these drugs are safe.

SULFONAMIDES

Among 1455 human infants exposed to sulfonamides during the first trimester, no teratogenic effects were noted. However, the administration of sulfonamides should be avoided in women deficient in glucose-6-phosphate dehydrogenase (G6PD) because dose-related hemolysis may occur.

Sulfonamides cause no known damage to the fetus in utero because the fetus can clear free bilirubin through the placenta. However, these drugs might theoretically have deleterious effects if they were to be present in the blood of the neonate after birth. Sulfonamides compete with bilirubin for binding sites on albumin and thus raise the levels of free bilirubin in the serum and increase the risk of hyperbilirubinemia in the neonate. Although this toxicity occurs with direct administration to the neonate, kernicterus in the newborn following in utero exposure has not been reported.

SULFAMETHOXAZOLE WITH TRIMETHOPRIM

Trimethoprim is often given with sulfa to treat urinary tract infections. However, one unpublished study of 2296 Michigan Medicaid recipients suggested an increased risk of cardiovascular defects after exposure in the first trimester. **In one retrospective study of trimethoprim with sulfamethoxazole, the odds ratio for birth defects was 2.3, whereas in another study it was 2.5 to 3.4.**

NITROFURANTOIN

Nitrofurantoin is used in the treatment of acute uncomplicated lower urinary tract infections, as well as for long-term suppression, in patients with chronic bacteriuria. Nitrofurantoin is capable of inducing hemolytic anemia in patients deficient in G6PD. However, hemolytic anemia in the newborn as a result of in utero exposure to nitrofurantoin has not been reported.

No reports have associated nitrofurantoins with congenital defects. In the Collaborative Perinatal Project, 590 infants were exposed—83 in the first trimester—with no increased risk of adverse effects. In another study[56] in 1334 women exposed in the first trimester, no increase in malformations was reported. Use in the last 30 days before delivery was associated with increased risk of neonatal jaundice.

TETRACYCLINES

Tetracyclines readily cross the placenta and are firmly bound by chelation to calcium in developing bone and tooth structures. This produces brown discoloration of the deciduous teeth, hypoplasia of the enamel, and inhibition of bone growth. The staining of the teeth takes place in the second or third trimesters of pregnancy, whereas bone incorporation can occur earlier. Depression of skeletal growth was particularly common among premature infants treated with tetracycline. **First-trimester exposure to doxycycline is not known to carry any risk. First-trimester exposure to tetracyclines was not found to have any teratogenic risk in 341 women in the Collaborative Perinatal Project or in 174 women in another study. Alternative antibiotics are currently recommended during pregnancy.**

AMINOGLYCOSIDES

Streptomycin and kanamycin have been associated with congenital deafness in the offspring of mothers who took these drugs during pregnancy. Ototoxicity was reported with doses as low as 1 g of streptomycin twice a week for 8 weeks during the first trimester. Of 391 mothers who had received 50 mg/kg of kanamycin for prolonged periods during pregnancy, nine children (2.3%) were found to have hearing loss.

Nephrotoxicity may be greater when aminoglycosides are combined with cephalosporins. Neuromuscular blockade may be potentiated by the combined use of aminoglycosides and curariform drugs. Potentiation of magnesium sulfate–induced neuromuscular weakness has also been reported in a neonate exposed to magnesium sulfate and gentamicin.

Other than ototoxicity, no known teratogenic effect has been associated with aminoglycosides in the first trimester. In 135 infants exposed to streptomycin in the Collaborative Perinatal Project, no teratogenic effects were observed. Among 1619 newborns whose mothers were treated for tuberculosis with multiple drugs, including streptomycin, the incidence of congenital defects was the same as in a healthy control group.

ANTITUBERCULOSIS DRUGS

No evidence suggests any teratogenic effect of isoniazid, para-aminosalicylic acid, rifampin, or ethambutol.

ERYTHROMYCIN

No teratogenic risk of erythromycin has been reported. In 79 patients in the Collaborative Perinatal Project and 260 in another study, no increase in birth defects was noted.

CLARITHROMYCIN

Of 122 first-trimester exposures, no significant risk of birth defects was reported with clarithromycin.

FLUOROQUINOLONES

The quinolones (ciprofloxacin and norfloxacin) have a high affinity for bone tissue and cartilage and may cause arthralgia in children. However, no malformations or musculoskeletal problems were noted in 38 infants exposed in utero in the first trimester, in 132 newborns exposed in the first trimester in the Michigan Medicaid data, or in 200 other first trimester exposures.

METRONIDAZOLE

Studies have failed to show any increase in the incidence of congenital defects among the newborns of mothers treated with metronidazole during early or late gestation. Among 1387 prescriptions filled, no increase in birth defects could be determined. A meta-analysis confirmed lack of teratogenic risk.

Antiviral Agents

The Acyclovir Registry has recorded 756 first-trimester exposures with no increased risk of abnormalities in the infants.[57] Among 1561 pregnancies exposed to acyclovir, 229 exposed to valacyclovir, and 26 exposed to famciclovir—all in the first trimester—no increased risk of birth defects was found.[58] The Centers for Disease Control and Prevention (CDC) recommends that pregnant women with disseminated infection (e.g., herpetic encephalitis or hepatitis or varicella pneumonia) be treated with acyclovir.

LINDANE

After application of lindane to the skin, about 10% of the dose used can be recovered in the urine. Toxicity in humans after use of topical 1% lindane has been observed almost exclusively after misuse and overexposure to the agent. Although no evidence of specific fetal damage is attributable to lindane, the agent is a potent neurotoxin, and its use during pregnancy should be limited. Pregnant women should be cautioned about

shampooing their children's hair because absorption could easily occur across the skin of the hands. An alternate drug for lice is usually recommended, such as pyrethrins with piperonyl butoxide.

Antiretroviral Agents

Zidovudine (ZDV) should be included as a component in the antiretroviral regimen whenever possible because of its record of safety and efficacy. In a prospective cohort study, children exposed to ZDV in the perinatal period through Pediatric AIDS Clinical Trials Group Protocol 076 were studied up to a median age of 4.2 years. No adverse effects were observed in these children. The International Antiretroviral Registry was established in 1989 to detect any major teratogenic effect of the antiretroviral drugs. Through January 2004, more than 1000 pregnancies had first-trimester exposures to ZDV and lamivudine, and no increase in teratogenicity was reported.

Concerns have been raised regarding the use of other antiretroviral therapies. Efavirenz is not recommended during pregnancy because of reports of significant malformations in monkeys who received efavirenz during the first trimester and also three case reports of fetal NTDs in women who received the drug.[59] In 2001, Bristol-Myers Squibb issued a warning advising against the use of didanosine and stavudine in pregnant women after cases of lactic acidosis were reported, some of which were fatal. These two drugs should only be used if no other alternatives are available.

Antifungal Agents

Nystatin is poorly absorbed from intact skin and mucous membranes, and topical use has not been associated with teratogenesis. Clotrimazole or miconazole use in pregnancy is not known to be associated with congenital malformations. However, in one study, a statistically significant increase in risk of first-trimester abortion was noted after use of these drugs, but these findings were considered not to be definitive evidence of risk. Of 2092 newborns exposed in the first trimester in the Michigan Medicaid data, no increased risk of anomalies was found.

Limb deformities were reported in three infants exposed to 400 to 800 mg/day of fluconazole in the first trimester. However, in systematic studies of 460 patients who received a single 150-mg dose of fluconazole, no increased risk of defects was observed.[60] In one registry study,[61] fluconazole was associated with an increased risk of Tetralogy of Fallot.

Drugs for Induction of Ovulation

In more than 2000 exposures, no evidence of teratogenic risk of clomiphene has been noted, and the percentage of spontaneous abortions is close to the expected rate. Although infants are often exposed to bromocriptine in early pregnancy, no teratogenic effects have been observed in more than 1400 pregnancies.

Mild Analgesics

Some pains during pregnancy justify the use of a mild analgesic. However, pregnant patients should be encouraged to use nonpharmacologic remedies such as local heat and rest.

ASPIRIN

No evidence suggests any teratogenic effect of aspirin taken in the first trimester. **Aspirin does have significant perinatal effects, however, because it inhibits prostaglandin synthesis. Uterine contractility is decreased, and patients taking aspirin** in analgesic doses have delayed onset of labor, longer duration of labor, and an increased risk of a prolonged pregnancy.

Aspirin also decreases platelet aggregation, which can increase the risk of bleeding before as well as at delivery. Platelet dysfunction has been described in newborns within 5 days of ingestion of aspirin by the mother. Because aspirin causes permanent inhibition of prostaglandin synthetase in platelets, the only way for adequate clotting to occur is for more platelets to be produced.

Multiple organs may be affected by chronic aspirin use. Of note, prostaglandins mediate the neonatal closure of the ductus arteriosus. In one case report, maternal ingestion of aspirin close to the time of delivery was related to closure of the ductus arteriosus in utero.

ACETAMINOPHEN

Acetaminophen has also shown no evidence of teratogenicity.[62] With acetaminophen, inhibition of prostaglandin synthesis is reversible; thus once the drug has cleared, platelet aggregation returns to normal. In contrast to aspirin, bleeding time is not prolonged with acetaminophen, and the drug is not toxic to the newborn. Thus if a mild analgesic or antipyretic is indicated, acetaminophen is preferred over aspirin.

Patients should be counseled on the risks associated with taking excessive amounts of acetaminophen. Doses of greater than 4 g daily (8 extra strength acetaminophen, 12 regular strength acetaminophen) are associated with liver fibrosis, leading to cirrhosis and liver failure. These deleterious effects are only effectively managed by liver transplantation. Patients should understand the doses of acetaminophen in all the products taken for pain. Combination products that contain acetaminophen may be overlooked in calculating the total daily dose, leading to unintentional overdose.

NONSTEROIDAL ANTIINFLAMMATORY AGENTS

No evidence of teratogenicity has been reported for other nonsteroidal antiinflammatory drugs (NSAIDs such as ibuprofen, naproxen, diclofenac, and piroxicam).[63,64] Chronic use may lead to oligohydramnios, and constriction of the fetal ductus arteriosus or neonatal pulmonary hypertension, as has been reported with indomethacin, might occur.

CODEINE

In the Collaborative Perinatal Project, no increased relative risk of malformations was observed in 563 codeine users. In one recent study, maternal treatment with opioid analgesics was associated with an increased risk of heart defects, spina bifida, and gastroschisis. Codeine can cause addiction and newborn withdrawal symptoms if used to excess perinatally.

SUMATRIPTAN

Of 479 exposures to sumatriptan in the first trimester,[65] 4.6% of infants had birth defects—not significantly different from the nonexposed population. For women whose severe headaches do not respond to other therapy, sumatriptan may be used during pregnancy.[66]

BISPHOSPHONATES

The bisphosphonate drug class represents a group of medications used for treating a variety of bone disorders, including osteoporosis and Paget disease, and for controlling excess blood calcium in the setting of cancer or after chemotherapy administration. A published review of case reports for the bisphosphonate drug class—which includes alendronate, ibandronate, risedronate, etidronate, pamidronate, tiludronate, and zoledronic acid—in both short- and long-term use showed no serious fetal or neonatal adverse effects. Marginal decreases in gestational age, birthweight, and neonatal abnormalities may be attributed to bisphosphonate use. The decision to continue bisphosphonate use in pregnancy is based on the patient's duration and amount of osteopenia or osteoporosis. Patients should also be counseled on appropriate calcium supplementation and the use of vitamin D, which can mitigate the risk of bone-related issues.[67]

DRUGS OF ABUSE

Tobacco and Nicotine Products

Sorting out potential confounding factors is complicated when comparing smokers with nonsmokers. However, smoking is associated with a fourfold increase in small size for gestational age as well as an increased prematurity rate. The higher perinatal mortality rate associated with smoking is attributable to an increased risk of abruptio placentae, placenta previa, premature and prolonged rupture of membranes, and IUGR. The risks of complications and of the associated perinatal loss rise with the number of cigarettes smoked. Discontinuation of smoking during pregnancy can reduce the risk of both pregnancy complications and perinatal mortality, especially in women at high risk for other reasons. Maternal passive smoking was also associated with a twofold risk of low birthweight at term in one study (see Chapter 6).

A positive association has also been found between smoking and sudden infant death syndrome (SIDS) and increased respiratory illnesses in children. In such reports, it is not possible to distinguish between apparent effects of maternal smoking during pregnancy and smoking after pregnancy, but both may play a role.

The spontaneous abortion rate for smokers may be up to twice that of nonsmokers, and abortions associated with maternal smoking tend to have a higher percentage of normal karyotypes and occur later than those with chromosomal aberrations.

Smoking Cessation During Pregnancy

Tobacco smoke contains nicotine, carbon monoxide, and thousands of other compounds. Although nicotine is the mechanism of addiction to cigarettes, other chemicals may contribute to adverse pregnancy outcomes. For example, carbon monoxide decreases oxygen delivery to the fetus, whereas nicotine decreases uterine blood flow.

Nicotine withdrawal may first be attempted with *nicotine fading,* switching to brands of cigarettes with progressively less nicotine over a 3-week period. Exercise may also improve quitting success rates. Nicotine medications are indicated for patients with nicotine dependence, defined as smoking more than one pack per day, smoking within 30 minutes of getting up in the morning, or prior withdrawal symptoms. Nicotine medications are available as patches, gums, or inhalers. Although the propriety of prescribing nicotine during pregnancy might be questioned, cessation of smoking eliminates many other toxins, including carbon monoxide; nicotine blood levels are not increased over that of smokers. In a randomized trial,[68] adding a nicotine patch to behavioral cessation support did not increase the rate of abstinence from smoking until delivery.

Compliance was low, and fewer than 10% of women in both groups used patches for more than 1 month.

Congenital anomalies occurred in five of 188 infants of women treated with bupropion during the first trimester of pregnancy—not a significant difference from the number expected. No data are available on the safety of varenicline use in pregnancy.[69] However, both of these medications have recently had product warnings mandated by the FDA about the risk of psychiatric symptoms and suicide associated with their use.

Alcohol

Fetal alcohol syndrome (FAS) has been reported in the offspring of alcoholic mothers and includes the features of gross physical retardation with onset prenatally and continuing after birth (Fig. 8-8).

In 1980, the Fetal Alcohol Study Group of the Research Society on Alcoholism proposed criteria for the diagnosis of FAS. At least one characteristic from each of the following three categories had to be present for a valid diagnosis of the syndrome:

1. Growth retardation before and/or after birth
2. Facial anomalies including small palpebral fissures; indistinct or absent philtrum; epicanthic folds; flattened nasal bridge; short nose length; thin upper lip; low-set, unparallel ears; and retarded midfacial development
3. Central nervous system dysfunction including microcephaly, varying degrees of mental retardation, or other evidence of abnormal neurobehavioral development such as attention-deficit/hyperactivity disorder (ADHD)

The full syndrome occurs in 6% of infants of heavy drinkers, and less severe birth defects and neurocognitive deficits occur in a larger proportion of children whose mothers drank heavily during pregnancy.

Jones and colleagues compared 23 chronically alcoholic women with 46 controls and compared the pregnancy outcomes of the two groups. Among the alcoholic mothers, perinatal deaths were about eight times more frequent. Growth restriction, microcephaly, and IQ below 80 were considerably more frequent in alcoholic women than among the controls. Overall outcome was abnormal in 43% of the offspring of the alcoholic mothers compared with 2% of the controls.

Ouellette and associates addressed the risks of smaller amounts of alcohol. Nine percent of infants of abstinent or rare drinkers and 14% of infants of moderate drinkers were abnormal—not a significant difference. **In heavy drinkers (average daily intake of 3 oz of 100-proof liquor or more), 32% of the infants had anomalies.** The aggregate pool of anomalies, growth restriction, and an abnormal neurologic examination was found in 71% of the children of heavy drinkers, twice the frequency in the moderate and rarely drinking groups. In this study, an increased frequency of abnormality was not found until 45 mL of ethanol daily (equivalent to three drinks) were exceeded. The study of Mills and Graubard also showed that total malformation rates were not significantly higher among offspring of women who had an average of less than one drink per day or one to two drinks per day than among nondrinkers. Genitourinary malformations increased with increasing alcohol consumption, however, so the possibility remains that for some malformations, no safe drinking level exists.

Heavy drinking remains a major risk to the fetus, and reduction even in midpregnancy can benefit the infant.[70] An occasional drink during pregnancy carries no documentable risk, but no level of drinking is known to be safe (see Chapter 6).

Sokol and colleagues have addressed history taking for prenatal detection of risky drinking. Four questions help differentiate patients who drink sufficiently to potentially injure the fetus (Box 8-2). The patient is considered at risk if more than two drinks are required to make her feel "high." The probability of risky drinking increases to 63% for those who respond positively to all four questions.

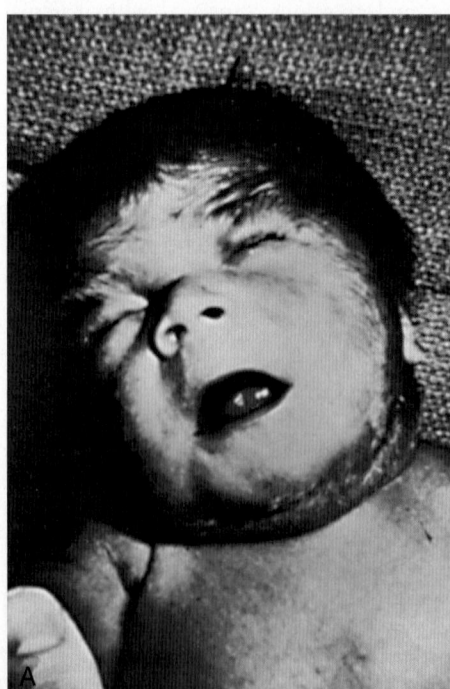
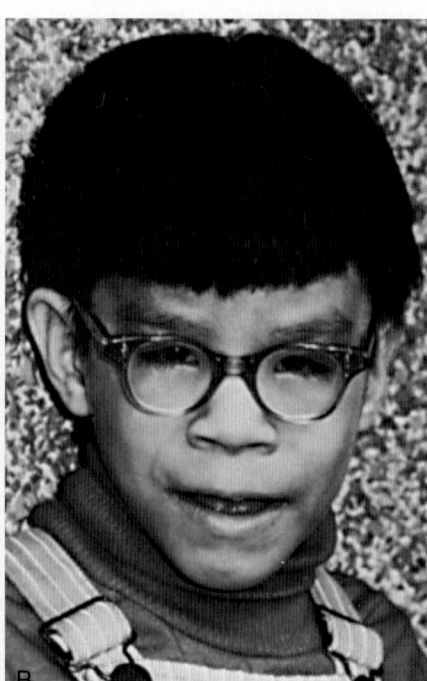
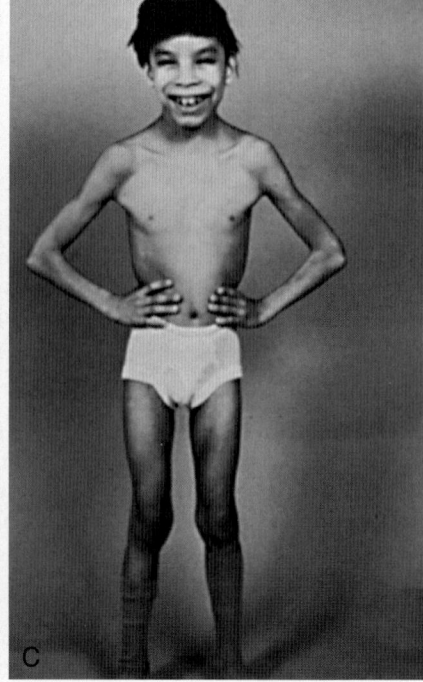

FIG 8-8 Fetal alcohol syndrome. **A,** At birth. **B,** At 5 years. **C,** At 8 years. Note the short palpebral fissures, short nose, hypoplastic philtrum, thinned upper lip vermillion, and flattened midface. (From Streissguth AP. CIBA Foundation Monograph 105. London: Pitman; 1984.)

Cannabis

No significant teratogenic effect of *Cannabis* has been documented, but the data are insufficient to say that no risk is present. One study that found a mean 73-g decrease in birthweight associated with *Cannabis* use validated exposure with urine assays rather than relying on self-reporting. Other studies have not shown an effect on birthweight or length. Behavioral and developmental alterations have been observed in some studies but not in others.

Cocaine

A serious difficulty in defining the effects of cocaine on the infant is the frequent presence of many confounding variables in the population using cocaine. These mothers often abuse other drugs, smoke, have poor nutrition, fail to seek prenatal care, and live under poor socioeconomic conditions. All of these factors are difficult to take into account in comparison groups. Another difficulty is the choice of outcome measures for infants exposed in utero. The neural systems likely to be affected by cocaine are involved in neurologic and behavioral functions not easily quantitated by standard infant development tests.

Cocaine-using women have a higher rate of spontaneous abortion than controls. Other studies have suggested an increased risk of congenital anomalies after first-trimester cocaine use, most frequently those of the cardiac and central nervous systems. In the study of Bingol and colleagues, the malformation rate was 10% in cocaine users, 4.5% in "polydrug users," and 2% in controls. MacGregor and associates reported a 6% anomaly rate compared with 1% for controls.

Cocaine is a CNS stimulant that has local anesthetic and marked vasoconstrictive effects. Not surprisingly, **abruptio placentae has been reported to occur immediately after nasal or IV administration.**[71] Several studies have also noted increased stillbirths, preterm labor, premature birth, and SGA infants with cocaine use.

The most common brain abnormality in infants exposed to cocaine in utero is impairment of intrauterine brain growth as manifested by microcephaly.[72] In one study, 16% of cocaine-exposed newborns had microcephaly compared with 6% of controls. Somatic growth is also impaired, and so the growth restriction may be symmetric or characterized by a relatively low head circumference/abdominal circumference ratio. Multiple other neurologic problems have been reported after cocaine exposure in addition to dysmorphic features and neurobehavioral abnormalities.

Aside from causing congenital anomalies in the first trimester, cocaine has been reported to cause fetal disruption, presumably as a result of interruption of blood flow to various organs. Bowel infarction has been noted with unusual ileal atresia and bowel perforation. Limb infarction has resulted in missing fingers in a distribution different from the usual congenital limb anomalies. CNS bleeding in utero may result in porencephalic cysts.

Narcotics and Methadone

Menstrual abnormalities, especially amenorrhea, are common in heroin abusers, although these symptoms are not associated with the use of methadone. Medical intervention is more likely to involve methadone maintenance, with the goal being a dose of approximately 20 to 40 mg/day. The dose should be individualized at a level sufficient to minimize the use of supplemental illicit drugs, which represent greater risk to the fetus than even the higher doses of methadone required by some patients. Manipulation of the dose in women maintained on methadone should be avoided in the last trimester because of an association with increased fetal complications and deaths attributed to fetal withdrawal in utero. Because management of narcotic addiction during pregnancy requires a host of social, nutritional, educational, and psychiatric interventions, these patients are best managed in specialized programs. Buprenorphine is also an acceptable treatment, and infants exposed to this drug required less morphine and had shorter hospital stays and shorter duration of treatment for neonatal abstinence syndrome than did infants exposed to methadone. However, women on buprenorphine were more likely to discontinue treatment.

The pregnancy of the narcotic addict is at increased risk for abortion, prematurity, and growth restriction. Withdrawal should be watched for carefully in the neonatal period.[73]

Caffeine

No evidence of teratogenic effects of caffeine in humans has been found. The Collaborative Perinatal Project showed no increased incidence of congenital defects in 5773 women taking caffeine in pregnancy, usually in a fixed-dose analgesic medication. The average cup of coffee contains about 100 mg of caffeine, and a 12 oz can of soda contains about 50 mg. Some conflicting evidence exists concerning the association between heavy ingestion of caffeine and increased pregnancy complications. Early studies suggested that the intake of greater than seven to eight cups of coffee per day was associated with low-birthweight infants, spontaneous abortions, prematurity, and stillbirths. However, these studies were not controlled for the concomitant use of tobacco and alcohol. **In one report that controlled for smoking and other habits, demographic characteristics, and medical history, no relationship was found between malformations, low birthweight, or short gestation and heavy coffee consumption.** When pregnant women consumed more than 300 mg of caffeine per day, one study suggested an increase in term low-birthweight infants less than 2500 g at greater than 36 weeks.

Concomitant consumption of caffeine with cigarette smoking may increase the risk of low birthweight. Maternal coffee intake decreases iron absorption and may contribute to maternal anemia.

Two other studies have shown conflicting results. One retrospective investigation that reported a higher risk of fetal loss was biased by ascertainment of the patients at the time of fetal loss because these patients typically have less nausea and would be expected to drink more coffee. A prospective cohort study found no evidence that moderate caffeine use increased the risk of spontaneous abortion or growth restriction. Measurement of serum paraxanthine, a caffeine metabolite, revealed that only extremely high levels are associated with spontaneous abortions.

The American College of Obstetricians and Gynecologists (ACOG) concluded that moderate caffeine consumption (less than 200 mg/day) does not appear to be a major contributing factor in miscarriage or preterm birth, but the relationship to growth restriction remains undetermined.[74] High caffeine intake may or may not be related to miscarriage, and so limiting intake to 200 mg/day seems prudent.[74]

Aspartame

The major metabolite of aspartame is phenylalanine,[75] which is concentrated in the fetus by active placental transport. Sustained high blood levels of phenylalanine in the fetus as seen in maternal phenylketonuria (PKU) are associated with mental retardation in the infant. However, within the usual range of aspartame ingestion in normal individuals, peak phenylalanine levels do not exceed normal postprandial levels, and even with high doses, phenylalanine concentrations are still very far below those associated with mental retardation. These responses have also been studied in women who are obligate carriers of PKU, and their levels are still normal. Thus it seems unlikely that aspartame during pregnancy would cause any fetal toxicity.

DRUGS IN BREAST MILK

Many drugs that are not usually of clinical significance to the infant can be detected in breast milk at low levels. The rate of transfer into milk depends on the lipid solubility, molecular weight, degree of protein binding, degree of ionization of the drug, and the presence or absence of active secretion. Nonionized molecules of low molecular weight, such as ethanol, cross easily. If the mother has unusually high blood concentrations, such as with increased dosage or decreased renal function, drugs may appear in higher concentrations in the milk.

The amount of drug in breast milk is a variable fraction of the maternal blood level, which itself is proportional to the maternal oral dose. Thus the dose to the infant is usually subtherapeutic, approximately 1% to 2% of the maternal dose on average. This amount is usually so trivial that no adverse effects are noted. In the case of toxic drugs, however, any exposure may be inappropriate. Allergy may also exist or may be initiated. Long-term effects of even small doses of drugs may yet be discovered. Also, drugs are eliminated more slowly in the infant with immature enzyme systems. Short-term effects of most maternal medications on breastfed infants are mild and pose little risk to the infants. Because the benefits of breastfeeding are well known, the risk of drug exposure must be weighed against these benefits.

With drug administration in the immediate few days postpartum, before lactation is fully established, the infant receives only a small volume of colostrum; thus little drug is excreted into the milk. It is also helpful to allay the fears of patients undergoing cesarean deliveries that analgesics or other drugs administered at this time might have some adverse effects on the infant because no adverse effects have been shown. For drugs that require daily dosing during lactation, knowledge of pharmacokinetics in breast milk may minimize the dose to the infant. For example, dosing immediately after nursing decreases the neonatal exposure because the blood level will be at its nadir just before the next dose.

Short-term effects, if any, of most maternal medications on breastfed infants are mild and pose little risk to the infants.[76] Of 838 breastfeeding women, 11.2% reported minor adverse reactions in the infants, but these reactions did not require medical attention. In 19%, antibiotics caused diarrhea; in 11%, narcotics caused drowsiness; in 9%, antihistamines caused irritability; and in 10%, sedatives, antidepressants, or antiepileptics caused drowsiness.[76]

The American Academy of Pediatrics has reviewed drugs in lactation[77,78] and now refers providers to LactMed (http://toxnet.nlm.nih.gov) for effects of specific drugs.

Drugs Commonly Listed as Contraindicated During Breastfeeding

Cytotoxic Drugs That May Interfere With Cellular Metabolism of the Nursing Infant

Cyclosporine, doxorubicin, and cyclophosphamide might cause immune suppression in the infant, although data are limited with respect to these drugs. In general, the potential risks of the drugs would outweigh the benefits of continuing nursing.[78]

After oral administration to a lactating patient with choriocarcinoma, methotrexate was found in milk in low but detectable levels. Most individuals would elect to avoid any exposure of the infant to this drug. However, in environments in which bottle feeding is rarely practiced or presents practical or cultural difficulties, therapy with this drug would not in itself appear to constitute a contraindication to breastfeeding.

Drugs of Abuse for Which Adverse Effects on the Infant During Breastfeeding Have Been Reported

Drugs of abuse such as amphetamines, cocaine, heroin, LSD, and phencyclidine are all contraindicated during breast feeding because they are hazardous to the nursing infant and to the health of the mother.[78]

Radioactive Compounds That Require Temporary Cessation of Breastfeeding

The American Academy of Pediatrics[78] suggests consultation with a nuclear medicine physician so that the radionuclide with the shortest excretion time in breast milk can be used for lactating patients. The mother can attempt to store breast milk before the study, and she should continue to pump to maintain milk production but should discard the milk during therapy. The physician may reassure the patient by assessing the radioactivity of the milk before nursing is resumed. Radiopharmaceuticals require variable intervals of interruption of nursing.

Drugs for Which the Effect on Nursing Infants Is Unknown but May Be of Concern

This category includes several classes of psychotropic drugs, amiodarone (associated with hypothyroidism), lamotrigine (potential for therapeutic serum concentration in the infant), metoclopramide (potential dopaminergic blocking, but no reported detrimental effects), and metronidazole.[78]

Antianxiety, antidepressant, and antipsychotic agents are sometimes given to nursing mothers. Although no data are available about adverse effects in infants exposed to these drugs through breast milk, they could theoretically alter CNS function.[78] Some psychoactive drugs have been reported to appear in breast milk in levels that approach clinical significance (10% or more). These include bupropion, fluoxetine, citalopram, sertraline, and venlafaxine.[78] Fluoxetine is excreted in breast milk

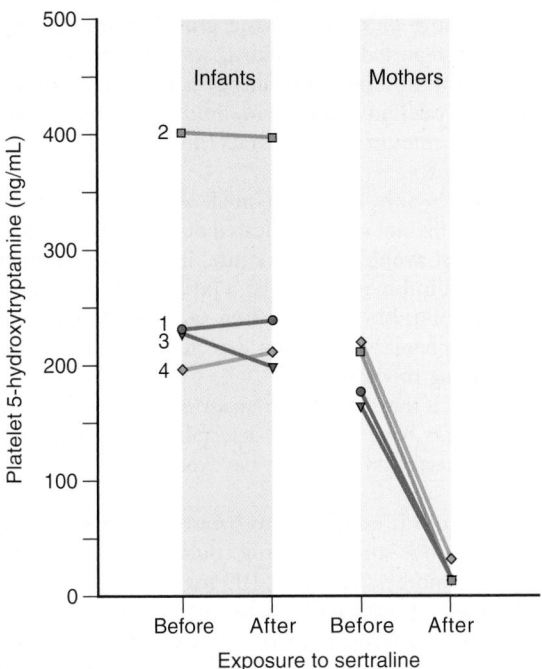

FIG 8-9 Effect of sertraline on platelet 5-hydroxytryptamine levels in four breastfed infants and their mothers. (From Epperson CN, Anderson GM, McDougle CJ. Sertraline and breast-feeding. *N Engl J Med.* 1997;336:1189.)

at low levels, so the infant receives approximately 6.7% of the maternal dose.[79] The level in the breastfed newborn is certainly lower than the level during pregnancy.

Sertraline causes a decline in 5-hydroxytryptamine levels in mothers but not in their breastfed infants.[80] This implies that the small amount of drug the infant ingests in breast milk is not enough to have a pharmacologic effect (Fig. 8-9). **Infants of mothers taking psychotropic drugs should be monitored for sedation during use and for withdrawal after cessation of the drug.**

A bigger problem is postpartum depression exacerbated by fatigue, and **the benefits of nursing should be weighed against the negative effect on bonding that would result from untreated postpartum depression.**

Temporary cessation of breastfeeding after a single dose of metronidazole may be considered. Its half-life is such that interruption of lactation for 12 to 24 hours after single-dose therapy usually results in negligible exposure to the infant. However, no adverse effects in infants have been reported.

Drugs Associated With Significant Effects in Some Nursing Infants That Should Be Given to Nursing Mothers With Caution
BROMOCRIPTINE
Bromocriptine is an ergot alkaloid derivative. Because it has an inhibitory effect on lactation, it should be avoided unless the mother has taken it during the pregnancy.

ERGOTAMINE
Ergotamine is used by some for migraine headache, and it has been associated with vomiting, diarrhea, and convulsions in the infant. Administration of an ergot alkaloid for the treatment of uterine atony does not contraindicate lactation.

LITHIUM
Breast milk levels of lithium are one third to one half of the maternal serum levels, and the infant's serum levels while nursing are much lower than the fetal levels that occur when the mother takes lithium during pregnancy. The benefits of breastfeeding must be weighed against the theoretic effects of small amounts of the drug on the developing brain.[78]

Maternal Medication Usually Compatible With Breastfeeding
NARCOTICS, SEDATIVES, AND ANTICONVULSANTS
In general, no evidence of adverse effect is noted with most of the sedatives, narcotic analgesics, and anticonvulsants. Patients may be reassured that in normal doses, carbamazepine, phenytoin, magnesium sulfate, codeine, morphine, and meperidine do not cause any obvious adverse effects in breastfed infants because the dose detectable in the breast milk is approximately 1% to 2% of the mother's dose, which is sufficiently low to have no significant pharmacologic activity.

Although the short-term use of codeine by a breastfeeding mother appears to be harmless, in one case, a mother was breastfeeding while taking codeine and acetaminophen for episiotomy pain. On day 7, the infant was lethargic and had difficulty feeding, and the infant died on day 13. The mother was an ultra-rapid metabolizer who converted codeine to morphine at a rapid rate. The milk level of morphine was 87 ng/mL, whereas the infant's level was 70 ng/mL.[81] Because a mother's status is rarely known, the use of any codeine product should be restricted to less than 2 days.

With diazepam, the milk/plasma ratio at peak dose is 0.68, with only small amounts detected in the breast milk. In two lactating patients who took carbamazepine while nursing, the concentration of the drug in the breast milk at 4 and 5 weeks postpartum was similar—about 60% of the maternal serum level. Accumulation does not seem to occur, and no adverse effects were noted in either infant.

COLD PREPARATIONS
Although studies are not extensive, no harmful effects have been noted from antihistamines or decongestants. Less than 1% of a pseudoephedrine dose or triprolidine dose ingested by the mother is excreted in the breast milk.

ANTIHYPERTENSIVES
THIAZIDES
After a single 500-mg oral dose of chlorothiazide, no drug was detected in breast milk. In one mother taking 50 mg of hydrochlorothiazide daily, the drug was not detectable in the nursing infant's serum, and the infant's electrolytes were normal. Thiazide diuretics may decrease milk production in the first month of lactation.

β-BLOCKERS
Propranolol is excreted in breast milk, with milk concentrations after a single 40-mg dose less than 40% of peak plasma concentrations. Thus an infant consuming 500 mL/day of milk would ingest an amount that represents approximately 1% of a therapeutic dose, which is unlikely to cause any adverse effect.

Atenolol is concentrated in breast milk to about three times the plasma level. One case was reported in which a 5-day-old term infant had signs of β-adrenergic blockade with bradycardia (80 beats/min) with the breast milk dose calculated to be 9% of the maternal dose. Adverse effects in other infants have not been reported. Because milk accumulation occurs with atenolol, infants must be monitored closely for bradycardia. Propranolol is a safer alternative.

Clonidine concentrations in milk are almost twice the maternal serum levels. Neurologic and laboratory parameters in the infants of treated mothers are similar to those of controls.

ANGIOTENSIN-CONVERTING ENZYME INHIBITORS
Captopril is excreted into breast milk in low levels, and no effects on nursing infants have been observed.

CALCIUM CHANNEL BLOCKERS
Nifedipine is excreted into breast milk at a concentration of less than 5% of the maternal dose, and verapamil is excreted at an even lower level. Neither have caused adverse effects in the infant.

ANTICOAGULANTS
Most mothers who require anticoagulation may continue to nurse their infants with no problems. Heparin does not cross into milk and is not active orally.

At a maternal dose of warfarin of 5 to 12 mg/day in seven patients, no warfarin was detected in breast milk or in infant plasma. This low concentration is probably because warfarin is 98% protein bound, and the milk would contain an insignificant amount of drug to exert an anticoagulant effect.[82] Another report confirmed that warfarin appears only in insignificant quantities in breast milk.[83] The oral anticoagulant bishydroxycoumarin was given to 125 nursing mothers with no effect on the infants' prothrombin times and no hemorrhages. **Thus with careful monitoring of maternal prothrombin time, so that the dosage is minimized, and of neonatal prothrombin times to ensure lack of drug accumulation, warfarin may be safely administered to nursing mothers.**

CORTICOSTEROIDS
Prednisone enters breast milk in an amount not likely to have any deleterious effect. In a study of seven patients, 0.14% of a sample was secreted in the milk in the subsequent 60 hours, a negligible quantity. Even at 80 mg/day, the nursing infant would ingest less than 0.1% of the dose, less than 10% of its endogenous cortisol.

DIGOXIN
Digoxin enters breast milk in a small amount because of significant maternal protein binding. In 24 hours, an infant would receive about 1% of the maternal dose. No adverse effects in nursing infants have been reported.

ANTIBIOTICS
Penicillin derivatives are safe in nursing mothers. With the usual therapeutic doses of penicillin or ampicillin, no adverse effects are noted in the breastfed infants. In susceptible individuals or with prolonged therapy, diarrhea and candidiasis are concerns.

Dicloxacillin is 98% protein bound. If this drug is used to treat breast infections, very little will get into the breast milk, and nursing may be continued.

Cephalosporins appear only in trace amounts in milk. In one study, after cefazolin 500 mg was administered intramuscularly three times a day, no drug was detected in breast milk. After 2 g of cefazolin was administered intravenously, the infant was exposed to less than 1% of the maternal dose.

Tooth staining or delayed bone growth from tetracyclines have not been reported after the drug was taken by a breastfeeding mother. This finding is probably because of the high binding of the drug to calcium and protein, limiting its absorption from the milk. The amount of free tetracycline available is too small to be significant.

Sulfonamides only appear in small amounts in breast milk and are ordinarily not contraindicated during nursing. However, the drug is best avoided in premature, ill, or stressed infants in whom hyperbilirubinemia may be a problem, because the drug may displace bilirubin from binding sites on albumin. On the other hand, sulfasalazine was not detected in the breast milk of a mother taking this drug.[84]

Gentamicin is transferred into breast milk, and half of nursing newborn infants have the drug detectable in their serum. The low levels detected would not be expected to cause clinical effects.

Nitrofurantoin is excreted into breast milk in very low concentrations. In one study, the drug could not be detected in 20 samples from mothers receiving 100 mg four times a day.

Erythromycin is excreted into breast milk in small amounts, although no reports of adverse effects on infants exposed to erythromycin in breast milk have been noted. Azithromycin also appears in breast milk in low concentrations. Clindamycin is excreted into breast milk in low levels, and nursing is usually continued during administration of this drug.

There are no reported adverse effects on the breastfed infant when isoniazid is administered to nursing mothers, and its use is considered to be compatible with breastfeeding.[78]

ACYCLOVIR
Acyclovir is compatible with breastfeeding. If a mother takes 1 g/day, the infant receives less than 1 mg/day—a very low dose.

ANTIFUNGAL AGENTS
No data are available on the effects of nystatin, miconazole, or clotrimazole in breast milk. However, with only small amounts absorbed vaginally and poor oral bioavailability, this would not be expected to be a clinical problem. Infant exposure to ketoconazole in human milk was 0.4% of the therapeutic dose, again unlikely to cause adverse effects.

ORAL CONTRACEPTIVES
Estrogen and progestin combination oral contraceptives cause dose-related suppression of milk production. Oral contraceptives that contain 50 μg or more of estrogen during lactation have been associated with shortened duration of lactation, decreased milk production, decreased infant weight gain, and decreased protein content of the milk. Lactation is inhibited to a lesser degree if the pill is started about 3 weeks postpartum and with lower doses of estrogen than 50 μg. Although the magnitude of the change is low, it still may be of nutritional importance, particularly in malnourished mothers.

An infant who consumes 600 mL of breast milk daily from a mother using an oral contraceptive that contains 50 μg of ethinylestradiol receives a daily dose in the range of 10 ng of the estrogen. The amount of natural estradiol received by infants who consume a similar volume of milk from mothers not using oral contraceptives is estimated at 3 to 6 ng during anovulatory cycles and 6 to 12 ng during ovulatory cycles. No consistent long-term adverse effects on growth and development have been described.

Evidence indicates that norgestrel is metabolized, rather than accumulated, by infants, and to date, no adverse effects have been identified as a result of progestational agents taken by the mother. ACOG recommends placement of the etonogestrel contraceptive implant 4 weeks or more after childbirth. Progestin-only contraceptives do not cause alteration of breast milk composition or volume, making them ideal for the breastfeeding mother. When the infant is weaned, the mother should be switched to combined oral contraceptives for maximum contraceptive efficacy.

ALCOHOL

Alcohol levels in breast milk are similar to those in maternal blood. If a moderate social drinker had two cocktails and had a blood alcohol concentration of 50 mg/dL, the nursing infant would receive about 82 mg of alcohol, which would produce insignificant blood concentrations. No evidence suggests that occasional ingestion of alcohol by a lactating mother is harmful to the breastfed infant. However, one study showed that ethanol ingested chronically through breast milk might have a detrimental effect on motor development but not mental development.[85] Also, alcohol in breast milk has an immediate effect on the odor of the milk, and this may decrease the amount of milk the infant consumes.[86]

PROPYLTHIOURACIL

Propylthiouracil (PTU) is found in breast milk in small amounts. If the mother takes 200 mg of PTU three times a day, the child would receive 149 μg daily, or the equivalent of a 70-kg adult receiving 3 mg/day. Several infants studied up to 5 months of age show no changes in thyroid parameters. **Lactating mothers on PTU can thus continue nursing with close supervision of the infant.** PTU has been preferred over methimazole because of its high protein binding (80%) and lower breast milk concentrations. However, recently it has been observed that liver injury is higher with PTU than with methimazole, but no cases of liver damage in infants of nursing mothers taking PTU have been reported.

H2–RECEPTOR BLOCKERS

In theory, H2-receptor antagonists such as ranitidine and cimetidine might suppress gastric acidity and cause CNS stimulation in the infant, but these effects have not been confirmed. The American Academy of Pediatrics now considers H2-receptor antagonists to be compatible with breastfeeding. Famotidine, nizatidine, and roxatidine are less concentrated in breast milk and may be preferable in nursing mothers.

CAFFEINE

Caffeine has been reported to have no adverse effects on the nursing infant, even if the mother consumes five cups of coffee per day. In one study, the milk level contained 1% of the total dose 6 hours after coffee ingestion, which is not enough to affect the infant. In another report, no significant difference in 24-hour heart rate or sleep time was observed in nursing infants when their mothers drank coffee for 5 days or abstained for 5 days.[87]

TOBACCO

Nicotine and its metabolite cotinine enter breast milk. Infants of smoking mothers achieve significant serum concentrations of nicotine even if they are not exposed to passive smoking; exposure to passive smoking further raises the levels of nicotine. Women who smoke should be encouraged to stop during lactation as well as during pregnancy.

OCCUPATIONAL AND ENVIRONMENTAL HAZARDS
Ionizing Radiation

The general hazards of radiation exposure are well known. To provide counseling in specific clinical situations, key variables are dose, timing, and temporal sequence.

Acute Exposure

Systematic studies of atomic bomb survivors in Japan showed conclusively that in utero exposure to high-dose radiation increased the risk of microcephaly and mental and growth restriction in the offspring. Distance from the hypocenter—the area directly beneath the detonated bomb—and gestational age at the time of exposure were directly related to microcephaly and mental and growth restriction in the infant. **The greatest number of children with microcephaly, mental retardation, and growth restriction were in the group exposed at 15 weeks' gestation or earlier.** Exposures were calculated by the distance of the victims from the epicenter. Microcephaly and mental retardation were associated with ionizing radiation at doses of 50 rads or greater, with 20 rads being the lowest dose at which microcephaly was observed. It is noteworthy that radiation from the atomic bomb blast differs from the low linear transfer of filtered radiation used in diagnostic studies.

Although teratogenic effects have been found in several organ systems of animals exposed to acute, high-dose radiation, the only structural malformations reported among humans exposed prenatally are those mentioned earlier. Using data from animals and from outcomes of reported human exposures at various times during pregnancy, Dekaban[88] constructed a timetable for extrapolating acute, high-dose radiation (>250 rad) to various reproductive outcomes in humans. Similarities between animal and known human effects support Dekaban's proposal.

Effects of chronic low-dose radiation on reproduction have not been identified in animals or humans. Increased risk of adverse outcomes was not detected among animals with continuous low-dose exposure (<5 rad) throughout pregnancy. The National Council for Radiation Protection[89] concluded that exposures less than 5 rads were not associated with increased risk of malformations.

Exposures are expressed in Gray (Gy) increments: 1 Gy equals 1000 mGy equals 100 rads (Table 8-1). Thus 10 mGy equals 1 rad. **Fortunately, virtually no single diagnostic test produces a substantive risk.** Table 8-1 shows mean and maximum fetal exposure. Only multiple computed tomography (CT) scans and fluoroscopies would lead to cumulative exposures of 100 mGy or 10 rads. Internal exposures are 50% less than maternal surface doses.

Female frequent flyers or aircraft crew members may be exposed to radiation during frequent, long, high-altitude flights. The Federal Aviation Administration (FAA) recommends that exposure be limited to 1 mSv (0.1 rad) during the pregnancy.[90]

Therapeutic exposures for maternal thyroid ablation with I[131] are rare, but they can cause fetal thyroid damage after 12 weeks of pregnancy.

TABLE 8-1   APPROXIMATE FETAL DOSES FROM COMMON DIAGNOSTIC PROCEDURES

EXAMINATION	MEAN (mGY)	MAXIMUM (mGY)
Conventional Radiography		
Abdomen	1.4	4.2
Chest	<0.01	<0.01
Intravenous urogram	1.7	10
Lumbar spine	1.7	10
Pelvis	1.1	4
Skull	<0.01	<0.01
Thoracic spine	<0.01	<0.01
Fluoroscopic Examinations		
Barium meal (upper gastrointestinal)	1.1	5.8
Barium enema	6.8	24
Computed Tomography		
Abdomen	8.0	49
Chest	0.06	0.96
Head	<0.005	<0.005
Lumbar spine	2.4	8.6
Pelvis	25	79

From Lowe SA: Diagnostic radiography in pregnancy: risks and reality. *Aust N Z J Obstet Gynaecol.* 2004;44:191.
10 mGY = 1 rad.

Mutagenesis

Mutagenic effects in the offspring of irradiated women may be manifested years after the birth of the infant. Mutagenic effects presumably explain the 50% increased risk of leukemia in children exposed in utero to radiation during maternal pelvimetry examinations compared with nonirradiated controls. However, the clinical consequence is almost nil. The absolute risk is approximately 1 in 2000 for exposed versus 1 in 3000 for unexposed children.

Lowe[89] estimates one additional cancer death per 1700 exposures of 10 mGy (1 rad). If it were to be recommended that pregnancies be terminated whenever exposure from diagnostic radiation occurred because of the increased probability of leukemia in the offspring, 1699 exposed pregnancies would have to be terminated to prevent a single case of leukemia. Radiation exposures should be minimized, but fear of radiation should never preclude a necessary diagnostic procedure. A consent form has been developed for use with pregnant women.[91]

Questions have also been raised about potential risks to children associated with paternal occupational exposure to low-dose radiation. A case-control study by Gardner and colleagues in the area around the Sellafield Nuclear Facility in the United Kingdom found a statistically significant association between paternal preconception radiation dose and childhood leukemia risk. A similar association had been observed between paternal preconception radiation and risk in workers at the Hanford nuclear facility in the United States. The finding regarding childhood leukemia risk is a particularly contentious issue, contradicting studies of the children born to atomic bomb survivors who do not show genetic effects, such as increased risks of childhood cancers. A study in the vicinity of nuclear facilities in Ontario also failed to demonstrate an association between childhood leukemia risk and paternal preconceptional radiation exposure.

Video Display Terminals

Concern about video display terminals (VDTs) linked to adverse reproductive outcomes now seems unwarranted. Early concern grew out of reports of spontaneous abortion clusters among groups of women who used VDTs at work; some reported clusters included birth defects. Since then, numerous reassuring papers have been published on this topic, along with a number of reviews.[92] **VDT use does not increase the risk of adverse reproductive outcomes.**

Lead

Twenty-five years of public health efforts have produced a striking reduction in lead exposure in the United States. The average blood lead level has decreased to less than 20% of levels measured in the 1970s. However, elevated blood lead (>20 μg/dL) has a higher incidence among immigrants to Southern California. In Los Angeles, 25 of the 30 cases of elevated blood lead occurred in immigrants.

High lead concentration in maternal blood is associated with an increased risk of delivery of an SGA infant. The frequency of preterm birth was also almost three times higher among women who had umbilical cord levels greater than or equal to 5.1 μg/dL, compared with those who had levels below that cutoff. One study in Norway found an increased risk of low birthweight and also NTDs.[93]

Lead poisoning was reported after a pregnant woman ingested *Garbhpal ras,* an Asian Indian health supplement that contained extremely high levels of lead.[94]

Asking pregnant women about risk factors for lead exposure can aid in assessing prenatal exposure risk. A questionnaire that gathered information on housing conditions, smoking status, and consumption of canned foods had a sensitivity of 89.2% and a negative predictive value of 96.4%.[95] Consumption of calcium and avoidance of the use of lead-glazed ceramics resulted in lowering of blood lead, especially in pregnant women of low socioeconomic status in Mexico City.

Because the nervous system may be more susceptible to the toxic effects during the embryonic and fetal periods than at any other time of life, and because maternal and cord blood lead concentrations are directly correlated, lead concentrations in blood should not exceed 25 μg/dL in women of reproductive age.[96]

Ideally, the maternal blood lead level should be less than 10 μg/dL to ensure that a child begins life with minimal lead exposure. A dose-response relationship is strongly supported by numerous epidemiologic studies of children showing a reduction in IQ with increasing blood lead concentrations above 10 μg/dL. Of note, these studies measured blood lead concentrations over time (often 2 years or more) and reported averaged values. **Other neurologic impairments associated with increased blood lead concentrations include ADHD, hearing deficits, and learning disabilities; shorter stature has also been noted.** Thus for public health purposes, childhood lead *poisoning* has been defined as a blood lead level of 10 μg/dL or higher.

In occupational settings, federal standards mandate that women should not work in areas where air lead concentrations can reach 50 μg/cm because this can result in blood concentrations above 25 to 30 μg/dL.[97] Subtle but permanent neurologic impairment in children may occur at lower blood lead concentrations.

Mercury in Fish

Fish and shellfish are an important part of a healthy diet, but some large fish contain significant amounts of mercury. **Mercury in high levels may harm an unborn baby or young child's developing nervous system.**[98]

Pregnant women, those who may become pregnant, and nursing mothers should avoid shark, swordfish, king mackerel, and tile fish because they contain high levels of mercury.[99] Consumption of up to 12 oz a week of shrimp, canned light tuna, salmon, pollock, and catfish—all of which are very low in mercury—is considered safe. Albacore (white) tuna and tuna steaks have more mercury than canned light tuna, but 6 oz per week are allowed.

OBSTETRICIAN'S ROLE IN EVALUATING DRUG AND REPRODUCTIVE RISKS IN AND BEYOND THE WORKPLACE

Clinical questions about adverse reproductive outcomes of potential drug teratogens or environmental or occupational exposures are difficult to answer, and answers are seldom as clear cut as the obstetrician would like. Even if the exposure were known, often no study of similar exposure with a sufficient sample size is available. Without this, a physician cannot give a reliable estimate of risk.

For drugs and other exposures discussed in this chapter, the threshold is unknown below which no adverse reproductive outcome can be expected. Except for ionizing radiation, maximum recommended exposure levels are difficult to quantify. When available, epidemiologic studies often have limitations in design, execution, analysis, and interpretation. Thus the questions must often be answered on the basis of reasoned judgments in the face of inadequate data.

In addition to traditional genetic referral sources, a variety of teratology information services and computer databases are available to physicians who counsel pregnant women (see Box 8-1). The options include personal computer software (e.g., Grateful Med) and CD-ROM copies in medical libraries or leased from commercial versions. Information is available from a TOXNET representative through the National Library of Medicine Specialized Information Services (http://sis.nlm.nih.gov/).

The National Library of Medicine (NLM) maintains several files on the TOXNET database system, including reproductive and developmental toxicology information in bibliographic or text form. Examples include Developmental and Reproductive Toxicology, GEN-TOX (genetic toxicology), LactMed, and the Environmental Mutagen Information Center. Other very useful sources are Reprotox (http://reprotox.org) and TERIS (depts. washington.edu/%7Eterisweb/teris/index.html). The book by Briggs and Freeman, *Drugs in Pregnancy and Lactation*, tenth edition (2014), is now available both in print and online. The online version is updated quarterly.

SUMMARY

Many medical conditions during pregnancy and lactation are best treated initially with nonpharmacologic remedies. Before a drug is administered in pregnancy, the indications should be clear and the risk/benefit ratio should justify drug use. If possible, therapy should be postponed until after the first trimester. In addition, patients should be cautioned about the risks of social drug use such as smoking, alcohol, and illicit drug use during pregnancy. Most drug therapy does not require cessation of lactation, because the amount excreted into breast milk is sufficiently small as to be pharmacologically insignificant.

KEY POINTS

- The critical period of organ development extends from day 31 to day 71 after the first day of the last menstrual period.
- Infants of epileptic women taking certain anticonvulsants, such as valproic acid, have double the rate of malformations of unexposed infants; the risk of fetal hydantoin syndrome is less than 10%.
- The risk of malformations after in utero exposure to isotretinoin is 25%, and an additional 25% of infants have mental retardation.
- Heparin is the drug of choice for anticoagulation during pregnancy except for women with artificial heart valves, who should receive coumadin despite the 5% risk of warfarin embryopathy.
- Angiotensin-converting enzyme inhibitors and angiotensin receptor blockers can cause fetal renal failure in the second and third trimesters, leading to oligohydramnios and hypoplastic lungs.
- Vitamin B_6 25 mg three times a day is a safe and effective therapy for first-trimester nausea and vomiting; doxylamine 12.5 mg three times a day is also effective in combination with B_6.
- Most antibiotics are generally safe in pregnancy, although aminoglycosides are known to be ototoxic. Trimethoprim may carry an increased risk in the first trimester, and tetracyclines taken in the second and third trimesters may cause tooth discoloration in offspring.
- Aspirin in analgesic doses inhibits platelet function and prolongs bleeding time, increasing the risk of peripartum hemorrhage.
- Fetal alcohol syndrome occurs in infants of mothers who drink heavily during pregnancy. A safe level of alcohol intake during pregnancy has not been determined.
- Cocaine has been associated with increased risk of spontaneous abortions, abruptio placentae, and congenital malformations, in particular, microcephaly.
- Most drugs are safe during lactation because subtherapeutic amounts, approximately 1% to 2% of the maternal dose, appear in breast milk. Only short-term (<2 days) use of codeine is safe during breastfeeding.
- Only a small amount of prednisone crosses the placenta, so it is the preferred corticosteroid for most illnesses. In contrast, betamethasone and dexamethasone readily cross the placenta and are preferred for acceleration of fetal lung maturity.
- Exposure to high-dose ionizing radiation during gestation causes microcephaly and mental retardation; however, diagnostic exposures below 5 rads do not pose increased teratogenic risks.
- Lead levels in blood have decreased in recent years in all except immigrant populations, making it easier to achieve blood levels below 25 µg/dL in women of reproductive age; this low level minimizes fetal growth restriction.
- Mercury in high levels deleteriously affects the fetal nervous system. For this reason pregnant and nursing women should avoid shark, swordfish, king mackerel, and tile fish; exposures to mercury can further be limited by restricting ingestion of certain other seafood (shrimp, canned tuna, salmon, pollock, catfish) to 12 oz/week.

REFERENCES

1. Wilson JG, Fraser FC. *Handbook of Teratology*. New York: Plenum; 1979.
2. Teratology Society Public Affairs Committee. FDA Classification of drugs for teratogenic risk. *Teratol.* 1994;49:446.
3. Wilson JG. Current status of teratology—general principles and mechanisms derived from animal studies. In: Wilson JG, Fraser FC, eds. *Handbook of Teratology*. New York: Plenum; 1977:47.
4. Musselman AC, Bennett GD, Greer KA, et al. Preliminary evidence of phenytoin-induced alterations in embryonic gene expression in a mouse model. *Reprod Toxicol.* 1994;8:383.
5. Lieff S, Olshan AF, Werler M, et al. Selection bias and the use of controls with malformations in case-control studies of birth defects. *Epidemiology.* 1999;10:238.
6. Lenz W. Thalidomide and congenital abnormalities. *Lancet.* 1962;1:45.
7. Lammer EJ, Sever LE, Oakley GP Jr. Teratogen update: valproic acid. *Teratology.* 1987;35:465.
8. MRC Vitamin Study Research Group. Prevention of neural tube defects: Results of the Medical Research Council Vitamin Study. *Lancet.* 1991; 338:131.
9. Czeizel AE, Dudas I. Prevention of the first occurrence of neural-tube defects by periconceptional vitamin supplementation. *N Engl J Med.* 1992;327:1832.
10. Pekarek DM, Chapman VR, Neely CL, et al. Medication effects on midtrimester maternal serum screening. *Am J Obstet Gynecol.* 2009;201:622, e1-5.
11. Einarson TR, Koren G, Mattice D, et al. Maternal spermicide use and adverse reproductive outcome: A meta-analysis. *Am J Obstet Gynecol.* 1990;162:665.
12. Jentink J, Loane MA, Dolk H, et al. Valproic acid monotherapy in pregnancy and major congenital malformations. *N Engl J Med.* 2010;362: 2185.
13. Holmes LB, Harvey EA, Coull BA, et al. The teratogenicity of anticonvulsant drugs. *N Engl J Med.* 2001;344:1132.
14. Biale Y, Lewenthal H. Effect of folic acid supplementation on congenital malformations due to anticonvulsive drugs. *Eur J Obstet Gynecol Reprod Biol.* 1984;18:211.
15. Jones KL, Lacro RV, Johnson KA, et al. Pattern of malformations in the children of women treated with carbamazepine during pregnancy. *N Engl J Med.* 1989;320:1661.
16. Buehler BA, Delimont D, VanWaes M, et al. Prenatal prediction of risk of the fetal hydantoin syndrome. *N Engl J Med.* 1990;322:1567.
17. GlaxoSmithKline International. *Lamotrigine Pregnancy Registry, Final Report*, July 2010.
18. Campbell E, Kennedy F, Russell A, et al. Malformation risks of antiepileptic drug monotherapies in pregnancy: Updated results from the UK and Ireland epilepsy and pregnancy registers. *J Neurol Neurosurg Psychiatry.* 2014.
19. Margulis AV, Mitchell AA, Gilboa SM, et al. Use of topiramate in pregnancy and risk of oral clefts. *Am J Obstet Gynecol.* 2012;207:405.e1-7.
20. Adab N, Tudur Smith C, Vinten J, et al. *Common antiepileptic drugs in pregnancy in women with epilepsy (Review)*, The Cochrane Collaboration, the Cochrane Library. John Wiley & Sons; 2010, Issue 1.
21. Hesdorffer DC, Tomson T. Adjunctive antiepileptic drug therapy and prevention of SUDEP. *Lancet Neurol.* 2011;10(11):948-949.
22. Lammer EJ, Chen DT, Hoar RM, et al. Retinoic acid embryopathy. *N Engl J Med.* 1985;313:837.
23. Zalzstein E, Koren G, Einarson T, et al. A case-control study on the association between first trimester exposure to lithium and Ebstein's anomaly. *Am J Cardiol.* 1990;65:817.
24. Jacobson SJ, Jones K, Johnson K, et al. Prospective multi-centre study of pregnancy outcome after lithium exposure during first trimester. *Lancet.* 1992;339:530.
25. Newport DJ, Viguera AC, Beach AJ, et al. Lithium placental passage and obstetrical outcome: Implications for clinical management during late pregnancy. *Am J Psychiatry.* 2005;162:2162-2170.
26. Way CM. Safety of Newer Antidepressants in Pregnancy. *Pharmacotherapy.* 2007;27:546.
27. Malm H, Artama M, Gissler M, et al. Selective serotonin reuptake inhibitors and risk for major congenital anomalies. *Obstet Obstet Gynecol.* 2011;118:111.
28. Yonkers KA, Wisner KL, Stewart DE, et al. The management of depression during pregnancy: A report from the American Psychiatric Association and the American College of Obstetricians and Gynecologists. *Obstet Gynecol.* 2009;114:703.
29. Rampono J, Simmer K, Ilett KF, et al. Placental transfer of SSRI and SNRI antidepressants and effects on the neonate. *Pharmacopsychiatry.* 2009;42: 95-100.
30. Huybrechts KF, Palmsten K, Avorn J, et al. Antidepressant use in pregnancy and the risk of cardiac defects. *N Engl J Med.* 2014;370:2397-2407.
31. Zeskind PS, Stephens LE. Maternal selective serotonin reuptake inhibitor use during pregnancy and newborn neurobehavior. *Pediatrics.* 2004;113:368.
32. Chambers CD, Hernandez-Diaz S, Von Marter LJ, et al. Selective serotonin-reuptake inhibitors and risk of persistent pulmonary hypertension of the newborn. *N Engl J Med.* 2006;354:579.
33. Wilson KL, Zelig CM, Harvey JP, et al. Persistent pulmonary hypertension of the newborn is associated with mode of delivery and not with maternal use of selective serotonin reuptake inhibitors. *Am J Perinatol.* 2011;28:19.
34. Andersen JT, Andersen NL, Horwitz H, et al. Exposure to selective serotonin reuptake inhibitors in early pregnancy and the risk of miscarriage. *Obstet Gynecol.* 2014;124(4):655-661.
35. Chun-Fai-Chan B, Koren G, Fayez I, et al. Pregnancy outcome of women exposed to bupropion during pregnancy: A prospective comparative study. *Am J Obstet Gynecol.* 2005;192:932.
36. Cohen LS, Altshuler LL, Harlow BL, et al. Relapse of major depression during pregnancy in women who maintain or discontinue antidepressant treatment. *JAMA.* 2006;295:499-507.
37. McDonagh MS, Matthews A, Phillipi C, et al. Depression drug treatment outcomes in pregnancy and the postpartum period. A systematic review and meta-analysis. *Obstet Gynecol.* 2014;124(3):526-534.
38. Cooper DS. Antithyroid drugs. *N Engl J Med.* 2005;352:905.
39. Cooper DS, Rivkees SA. Putting propylthiouracil in perspective. *J Clin Endocrinol Metab.* 2009;94:1881.
40. De Groot L, Abalovich M, Alexander EK, et al. Management of thyroid dysfunction during pregnancy and postpartum: An Endocrine Society clinical practice guideline. *J Clin Endocrinol Metab.* 2012;97:2543-2564.
41. Alexander EK, Marqusee E, Lawrence J, et al. Timing and magnitude of increases in levothyroxine requirements during pregnancy in women with hypothyroidism. *N Engl J Med.* 2004;351:241.
42. Velinov M, Zellers N. The fetal mycophenolate mofetil syndrome. *Clin Dysmorphol.* 2008;17(1):77.
43. Nurmohamed L, Moretti ME, Schechter T, et al. Outcome following high-dose methotrexate in pregnancies misdiagnosed as ectopic. *Am J Obstet Gynecol.* 2011;205:533.e1-3.
44. Hart CW, Naunton RF. The ototoxicity of chloroquine phosphate. *Arch Otolaryngol.* 1964;80:407.
45. Haagen Nielsen O, Loftus EV Jr, Jess T. Safety of TNF-α inhibitors during IBD pregnancy: A systematic review. *BMC Med.* 2013;11:174.
46. Koren G, Clark S, Hankins GD, et al. Effectiveness of delayed-release doxylamine and pyridoxine for nausea and vomiting of pregnancy: A randomized placebo controlled trial. *Am J Obstet Gynecol.* 2010;203:571, e1-7.
47. Matok I, Gorodischer R, Koren G, et al. The safety of metoclopramide use in the first trimester of pregnancy. *N Engl J Med.* 2009;360:2528.
48. Sullivan CA, Johnson CA, Roach H, et al. A pilot study of intravenous ondansetron for hyperemesis gravidarum. *Am J Obstet Gynecol.* 1996;174: 2565.
49. Pasternak B, Svanstrom H, Hviid A. Ondansetron in pregnancy and risk of adverse fetal outcomes. *N Engl J Med.* 2013;368:814-823.
50. Andersen JT, Jimenez-Solem E, Andersen NL, et al. *Ondansetron use in early pregnancy and the risk of congenital malformations—a register based nationwide cohort study*. Paper presented at: 29th International Conference on Pharmacoepidemiology & Therapeutic Risk Management: August 25-28, 2013; Montreal, Quebec, Canada.
51. Abas MN, Tan PC, Azmi N, et al. Ondansetron compared with metoclopramide for hyperemesis gravidarum. A randomized controlled trial. *Obstet Gynecol.* 2014;123:1272-1279.
52. Safari HR, Fassett MJ, Souter IC, et al. The efficacy of methylprednisolone in the treatment of hyperemesis gravidarum: A randomized, double-blind, controlled study. *Am J Obstet Gynecol.* 1998;179:921.
53. Ruigomez A, Garcia Rodriguez LA, Cattaruzzi C, et al. Use of cimetidine, omeprazole, and ranitidine in pregnant women and pregnancy outcomes. *Am J Epidemiol.* 1999;150:476.
54. Pasternak B, Hviid A. Use of proton pump inhibitors in early pregnancy and the risk of birth defects. *N Engl J Med.* 2010;363:2114.
55. Yau W-P, Mitchell AA, Lin KJ. Use of decongestants during pregnancy and the risk of birth defects. *Am J Epidemiol.* 2013;178(2):198-208.
56. Nordeng H, Lupattelli A, Romoren M, et al. Neonatal outcomes after gestational exposure to nitrofurantoin. *Obstet Gynecol.* 2013;121(2): 306-313.

57. Stone KM, Reiff-Eldridge R, White AD, et al. Pregnancy outcomes following systemic prenatal acyclovir exposure: Conclusions from the international acyclovir pregnancy registry, 1984–1999. *Birth Defects Res A Clin Mol Teratol.* 2004;70:201.

58. Pasternak B, Hviid A. Use of acyclovir, valacyclovir and famciclovir in the first trimester of pregnancy and the risk of birth defects. *JAMA.* 2010;304:859.

59. Perinatal HIV Guidelines Working Group. *Public Health Service Task Force. Recommendations for use of antiretroviral drugs in pregnant HIV-1-infected women for maternal health and interventions to reduce perinatal HIV-1 transmission in the United States.* Available at: <http://AIDSinfo.nih.gov>.

60. Mastroiacovo P, Mazzone T, Botto LD, et al. Prospective assessment of pregnancy outcomes after first-trimester exposure to fluconazole. *Am J Obstet Gynecol.* 1996;175:1645.

61. Molgaard-Nielsen D, Pasternak B, Hviid A. Use of oral fluconazole during pregnancy and the risk of birth defects. *N Engl J Med.* 2013;369:830-839.

62. Feldkamp M, Meyer RE, Krikov S, et al. Acetaminophen use in pregnancy and risk of birth defects: Findings from the National Birth Defects Prevention Study. *Obstet Gynecol.* 2010;115:109.

63. Nezvalova-Henriksen K, Spigset O, Nordeng H. Effects of ibuprofen, diclofenac, naproxen, and piroxicam on the course of pregnancy and pregnancy outcome: A prospective cohort study. *Br J Obstet Gynecol.* 2013;120:948-959.

64. Hernandez RK, Werler MM, Romitti P, et al. Nonsteroidal antiinflammatory drug use among women and the risk of birth defects. *Am J Obstet Gynecol.* 2012;206:228.e.1-8.

65. Cunnington M, Ephross S, Churchill P. The safety of sumatriptan and naratriptan in pregnancy: What have we learned? *Headache.* 2009;49:1414.

66. Loder E. Triptan therapy in migraine. *N Engl J Med.* 2010;363:63.

67. Green SB, Pappas AL. Effects of maternal bisphosphonate use on fetal and neonatal outcomes. *Am J Health Syst Pharm.* 2014;71:2028-2035.

68. Coleman T, Cooper S, Thornton JG, et al. A randomized trial of nicotine-replacement therapy patches in pregnancy. *N Engl J Med.* 2012;366:808-818.

69. ACOG Committee Opinion. Smoking cessation during pregnancy. *Obstet Gynecol.* 2010;116:1241.

70. Waterman EH, Pruett D, Caughey AB. Reducing fetal alcohol exposure in the United States. *Obstet Gynecol Surv.* 2013;68(5):367-378.

71. Acker D, Sachs BP, Tracey KJ, et al. Abruptio placentae associated with cocaine use. *Am J Obstet Gynecol.* 1983;146:220.

72. Volpe JJ. Effect of cocaine use on the fetus. *N Engl J Med.* 1992;327:399.

73. Brown HL, Britton KA, Mahaffey D, et al. Methadone maintenance in pregnancy: A reappraisal. *Am J Obstet Gynecol.* 1998;179:459.

74. ACOG Committee Opinion. Moderate caffeine consumption during pregnancy. *Obstet Gynecol.* 2010;116:467.

75. Sturtevant FM. Use of aspartame in pregnancy. *Int J Fertil.* 1985;30:85.

76. Ito S, Blajchman A, Stephenson M, et al. Prospective follow-up of adverse reactions in breast-fed infants exposed to maternal medication. *Am J Obstet Gynecol.* 1993;168:1393.

77. Sachs HC, Committee on Drugs. The transfer of drugs and therapeutics into human breast milk: An update on selected topics. *Pediatrics.* 2013.

78. Committee on Drugs, American Academy of Pediatrics. The transfer of drugs and therapeutics into human breast milk. *Pediatrics.* 2013;132:e796-e809.

79. Nulman I, Koren G. The safety of fluoxetine during pregnancy and lactation. *Teratology.* 1996;53:304.

80. Epperson CN, Anderson GM, McDougle CJ. Sertraline and breast-feeding. *N Engl J Med.* 1997;336:1189.

81. Koren G, Cairns J, Chitayat D, et al. Pharmacogenetics of morphine poisoning in a breastfed neonate of a codeine-prescribed mother. *Lancet.* 2006;368:704.

82. Orme ME, Lewis PJ, deSwiet M, et al. May mothers given warfarin breast-feed their infants? *Br Med J.* 1977;1:1564.

83. deSwiet M, Lewis PJ. Excretion of anticoagulants in human milk. *N Engl J Med.* 1977;297:1471.

84. Berlin CM Jr, Yaffe SJ. Disposition of salicylazosulfapyridine (Azulfidine) and metabolites in human breast milk. *Dev Pharmacol Ther.* 1980;1:31.

85. Little RE, Anderson KW, Ervin CH, et al. Maternal alcohol use during breastfeeding and infant mental and motor development at one year. *N Engl J Med.* 1989;321:425.

86. Mennella JA, Beauchamp GK. The transfer of alcohol to human milk. Effects on flavor and the infant's behavior. *N Engl J Med.* 1991;325:981.

87. Ryu JE. Effect of maternal caffeine consumption on heart rate and sleep time of breast-fed infants. *Dev Pharmacol Ther.* 1985;8:355.

88. Dekaban AS. Abnormalities in children exposed to x-radiation during various stages of gestation: tentative timetable of radiation injury to the human fetus. *J Nucl Med.* 1968;9:471.

89. Lowe SA. Diagnostic radiography in pregnancy: risks and reality. *Aust N Z J Obstet Gynaecol.* 2004;44:191.

90. Barish RJ. In-flight radiation exposure during pregnancy. *Obstet Gynecol.* 2004;103:1326.

91. El-Khoury GY, Madsen MT, Blake ME, et al. A new pregnancy policy for a new era. *AJR Am J Roentgenol.* 2003;181:335.

92. Blackwell R, Chang A. Video display terminals and pregnancy. A review. *Br J Obstet Gynaecol.* 1988;95:446.

93. Irgens A, Kruger K, Skorve AH, et al. Reproductive outcome in offspring of parents occupationally exposed to lead in Norway. *Am J Ind Med.* 1998;34:431.

94. Shamshirsaz AA, Yankowitz J, Rijhsinghani A, et al. Severe lead poisoning caused by use of health supplements presenting as acute abdominal pain during pregnancy. *Obstet Gynecol.* 2009;114:448.

95. Stefanak MA, Bourguet CC, Benzies-Styka T. Use of the Centers for Disease Control and Prevention childhood lead poisoning risk questionnaire to predict blood lead elevations in pregnant women. *Obstet Gynecol.* 1996;87:209.

96. Centers for Disease Control. *Preventing lead poisoning in young children.* Atlanta, Department of Health and Human Services. Atlanta, Public Health Service, Centers for Disease Control. 1991:7.

97. Needleman HL, Schell A, Bellinger D, et al. The long-term effects of exposure to low doses of lead in childhood. An 11-year follow-up report. *N Engl J Med.* 1990;322:83.

98. Harada M. Congenital minamata disease: Intrauterine methylmercury poisoning. *Teratology.* 1978;18:285.

99. Food and Drug Administration and the U.S. Environmental Protection Agency. *Consumption Advice: Joint Federal Advisory for Mercury in Fish.* Available at: <www.epa.gov/fishadvisories/advice/factsheet.html>.

Additional references for this chapter are available at ExpertConsult.com.

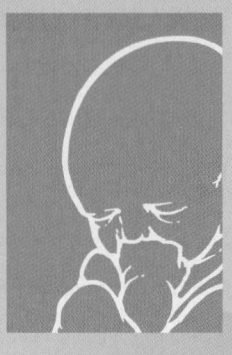

CHAPTER 9

Obstetric Ultrasound: Imaging, Dating, Growth, and Anomaly

DOUGLAS S. RICHARDS

KEY ABBREVIATIONS			
Abdominal circumference	AC	Femur length	FL
American College of Obstetricians and Gynecologists	ACOG	Head circumference	HC
		Human chorionic gonadotropin	hCG
Amniotic fluid index	AFI	Hertz; 1 cycle per second	Hz
American Institute of Ultrasound in Medicine	AIUM	Intrauterine growth restriction	IUGR
		Kilohertz; 1000 cycles per second	kHz
As low as reasonably achievable	ALARA	Last menstrual period	LMP
Biparietal diameter	BPD	Megahertz; 1 million cycles per second	MHz
Congenital pulmonary adenomatoid malformation	CPAM	National Institute of Child Health and Human Development	NICHD
Crown-rump length	CRL	Small for gestational age	SGA
Current procedural terminology	CPT	Society for Maternal-Fetal Medicine	SMFM
Estimated date of delivery	EDD	Spatial-peak temporal-average	SPTA
Estimated fetal weight	EFW	Three dimensional	3-D
Expected date of confinement	EDC	Time-gain compensation	TGC
Food and Drug Administration	FDA		

OVERVIEW

Over the past several decades, the clinical use of ultrasound imaging in obstetrics has expanded remarkably. It is now considered by many to be the most valuable diagnostic tool in the field. Ultrasound was first used clinically in pregnancy in the early 1960s to measure the biparietal diameter (BPD)—the distance between spikes on an oscilloscope screen. Since then, the technology has progressed to the point that even relatively inexpensive ultrasound machines yield detailed real-time images of the fetus. This chapter addresses general aspects of ultrasound in pregnancy as well as the use of ultrasound to diagnose birth defects. More detailed discussions of other specific pregnancy problems that include ultrasound assessment—such as multiple gestation, third-trimester bleeding, and cervical insufficiency—are covered in other chapters.

BIOPHYSICS OF ULTRASOUND

The underlying basis of ultrasound image production relies on the piezoelectric effect: when electrical impulses are applied to certain ceramic crystals, mechanical oscillations are induced. Conversely, induced vibrations of piezoelectric crystals generate a detectable electric current. In diagnostic ultrasound applications, the ultrasound machine sends an electric signal of the desired frequency to piezoelectric crystals embedded in the ultrasound probe. When the probe is placed in contact with a patient's skin, the skin and underlying tissues begin to vibrate, generating a sound or pressure wave. As this pulse of energy encounters an interface between materials of different impedance, a small amount of the energy is reflected as an echo. The pulses that return to the patient's skin cause the crystals in the probe to vibrate, which generates an electric current that is passed back to the ultrasound machine. The pulses of energy emitted are very brief—about 1 μsec. The number of pressure peaks produced in 1 sec is the frequency of the sound waves. **Ultrasound machines used in obstetrics operate at frequencies between about 2 and 9 MHz. Sound frequencies above 20 KHz cannot be detected by the human ear, hence the term *ultrasound*.** Between each emitted sound pulse, the probe "listens" for an echo. **Because of this alternating send-receive function, the piezoelectric crystal serves as both the transmitter and receiver of the ultrasonic waves.**

To produce an image, the ultrasound machine must sense the intensity and the time elapsed from the sending to the receipt of the returning echoes. Highly reflective tissues, such as bone, generate relatively more intense echoes. The deeper an object lies, the longer it will take for the return echo to be registered. Because the velocity of sound in tissues is known, the return time can be used to calculate the distance of the object from the transducer. Intensity and depth characteristics are registered in the machine's computer memory, and this information is then used by the computer to activate pixels on the monitor with the appropriate location and intensity.

Modern ultrasound probes used in obstetrics have a curved face in which are embedded a row of crystals. The linear arrangement of the crystals on the probe allows the mechanical oscillations generated by each crystal to be combined into to a wedge-shaped beam. A two-dimensional (2-D) image of the scan plane is then displayed with the curved shape of the probe face at the top of the screen. With endovaginal probes, the crystals are mounted on a smaller surface with a tighter curvature.

OPTIMIZING THE ULTRASOUND IMAGE
Frequency

As noted above, ultrasound transducers are designed to operate at a certain frequency or over a range of frequencies. Lower-frequency sound waves penetrate tissues better but cannot achieve the same resolution as higher-frequency probes. However, if too high a frequency for a certain patient is used, the lack of penetration severely degrades the images. **Thus the highest frequency probe that allows adequate penetration should be used. This usually depends on the thickness of the patient's** abdominal wall. For obese patients, a lower-frequency probe must be chosen. The frequency used for most general purpose transabdominal obstetric probes is about 3 to 5 MHz. A lower-frequency transducer (2 to 2.25) may be needed to provide adequate resolution in obese patients. When available, a higher-frequency probe that operates at 5 MHz or above is useful in selected patients. Higher-end probes now operate at a range of frequencies, thus one transducer may operate at 2 to 5 MHz and another at 5 to 8 MHz. **Because penetration of the maternal abdominal wall is not an issue, transvaginal probes usually operate at a frequency of 5 to 10 MHz.** Most quality ultrasound machines now have a feature called *tissue harmonic imaging*. With this modality, a standard frequency (e.g., 3 MHz) is transmitted and propagated in the usual manner. Because a relatively low-frequency wave is emitted, good penetration is preserved. However, in the receive part of the cycle, the ultrasound machine listens for the reflection of the first harmonic wave (e.g., 6 MHz). This higher-frequency wave only has to travel one direction, thus some of the resolution benefit of high-frequency scanning is retained. This process also reduces noise in the image by removing various forms of artifact, making cystic structures appear free of echoes. Harmonic imaging often significantly improves image quality and should be used liberally when available.

Power

Ultrasound machines have the capability of delivering varying amounts of voltage to the transducer elements. Increasing the power output increases the amplitude of energy waves in the ultrasound beam and results in stronger returning echoes. This can improve the signal-to-noise ratio and can improve imaging capabilities. However, energy is required to create oscillations in the molecules of insonated tissues. Because this energy is absorbed into the tissues, delivering an unnecessarily high energy dose raises safety concerns. The safety of diagnostic ultrasound will be discussed later in this chapter.

Gain

Signals from the weak echoes returning to the transducer elements must be amplified before being used for display. This amplification process is referred to as *gain*. Because of attenuation, echoes returning from deeper within the body have a lower intensity, and the machine must boost the amplification from these echoes. This built-in processing feature is known as *time-gain compensation* (TGC), meaning that echoes with a greater time delay automatically have greater amplification. The amount of amplification, or gain, can be controlled by the sonographer in two ways, with the gain control knob or the TGC controls. The gain control knob adjusts the overall gain up or down, so the brightness of the image can be changed to optimize visualization of anatomic details. When an image is too bright or too dark, much diagnostic information is lost (Fig. 9-1). Because tissue characteristics vary from patient to patient, penetration of sound waves at different depths may vary, so the gain at different depths may be adjusted. This is done using the TGC controls, a set of sliders on the instrument control panel (Figs. 9-2 and 9-3). A uniform scale across the brightness values should be sought.

Attenuation

Attenuation of ultrasound waves is affected by the medium through which the sound waves pass. Virtually no pulses pass

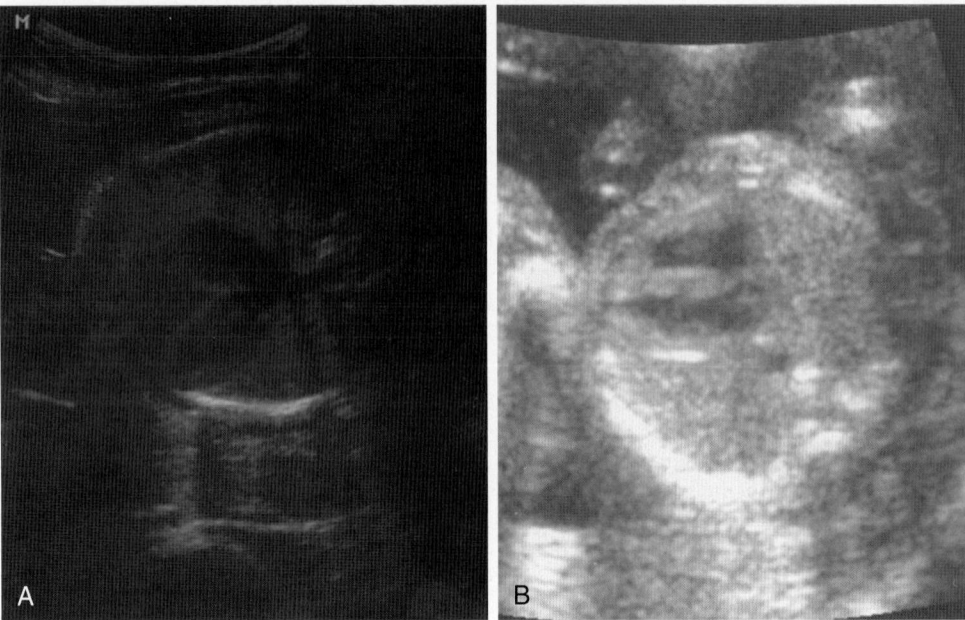

FIG 9-1 A, In this image the overall gain is too low, yielding a dark image. **B,** This image has too much gain. In both cases, diagnostic detail is lost.

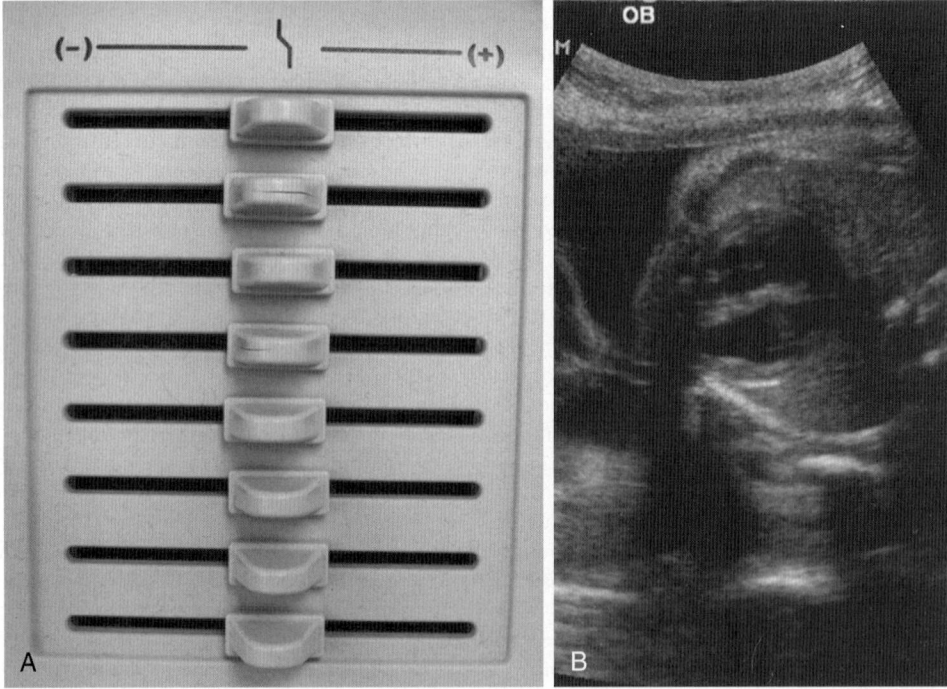

FIG 9-2 A shows the slide bars that comprise the time-gain compensation controls. In this case, the fact they are lined up in the center indicates that no adjustment for different depths was needed **(B)**.

through gas. This is why there must be a coupling agent (e.g., ultrasound gel) applied between the transducer face and the patient's skin. For several reasons, ultrasound waves lose intensity as they pass through tissues. The pressure waves gradually diverge from the central beam and are scattered by reflection from small structures within the tissue, and part of the sound energy is absorbed within tissues. Some tissues, such as bone, strongly attenuate sound waves. The thicker the tissues through which sound waves must pass before arriving at the target, the more the attenuation and the greater the difficulty in retrieving good information from the echoes. **Because of attenuation, obstetric ultrasound imaging is greatly affected if the patient is obese. In patients with a thick, dense abdominal wall, image quality is greatly reduced. In such patients, attention to equipment controls and scanning technique is essential.**

Focus

A linear array transducer makes an ultrasound beam by firing a row of crystals placed along the surface of the probe. When adjacent crystals fire, the pressure waves reinforce one another

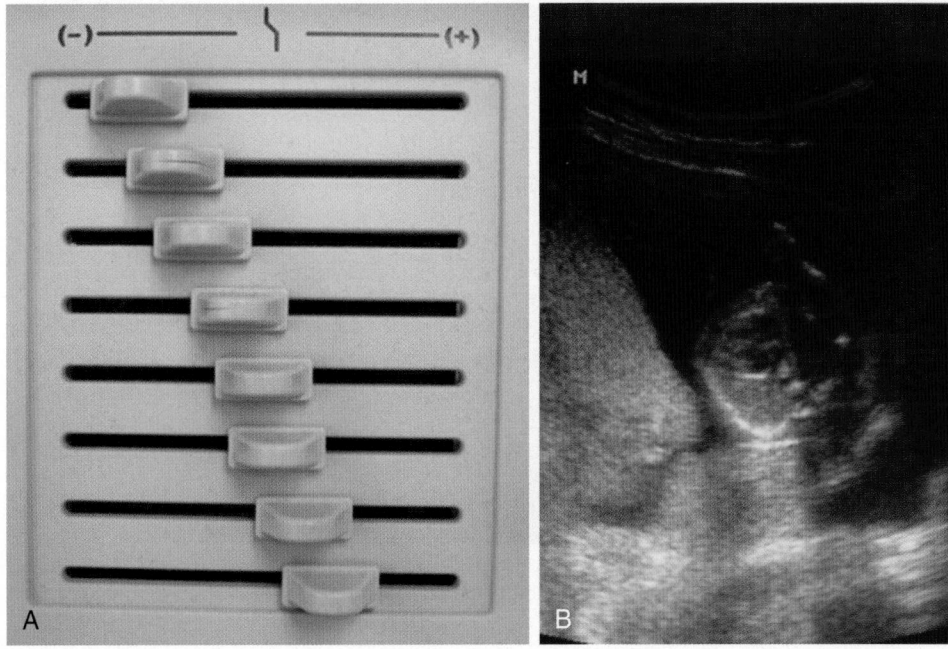

FIG 9-3 Incorrect time-gain compensation settings **(A)**. The slide bars are inappropriately shifted to the left in the near field, making the corresponding area of the image too dark **(B)**.

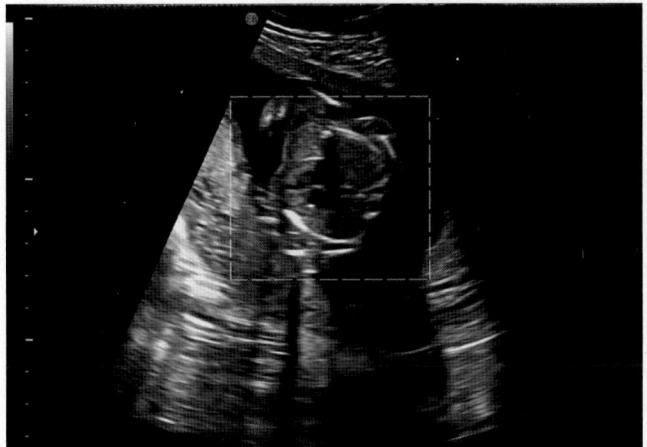

FIG 9-4 Ultrasound image before zoom is applied. The area within the dotted lines should be expanded to fill the entire screen.

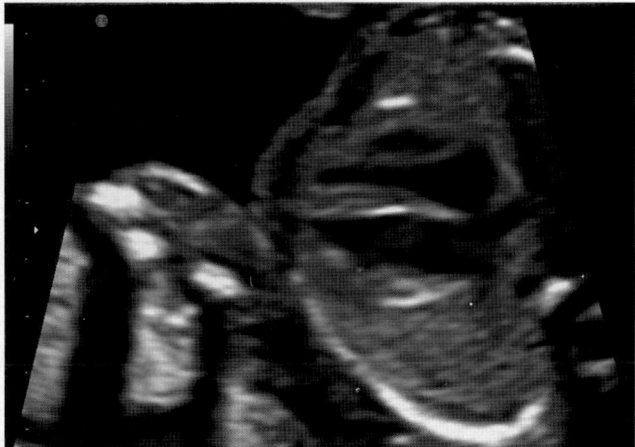

FIG 9-5 Appearance after zoom is applied. Compared with Figure 9-4, the cardiac structures are more easily seen. Additionally, because a smaller area was being scanned, the frame rate increased from 25 to 58 frames per second.

by a process called ***constructive interference***. This phenomenon creates the central ultrasound beam that extends out from the probe. Electronic control of the timing and order that crystals are activated can work to focus this beam at the region of interest within the tissues. **Image resolution is optimal when the structure of interest lies within this zone of optimal focus, which can be adjusted by the sonographer.**

Depth and Zoom

When scanning, the sonographer should strive to cone down the view to best demonstrate important structures without filling the screen with irrelevant material. The depth control can be used to simply crop extraneous structures at the bottom of the image. The zoom control is a little more sophisticated; it magnifies a box within the image rather than just removing information from the bottom of the image (Figs. 9-4 and 9-5).

Proper depth and zoom are important for several reasons. Most importantly, limiting the size of the scanned area allows

a higher frame rate and resolution. Additionally, homing-in on the area of interest draws attention to important detail within that scanned area.

SPECIAL ULTRASOUND MODALITIES

M-Mode

For most obstetric applications, the familiar 2-D gray-scale real-time ultrasound is used. This is formally known as *B-mode ultrasound*. Another ultrasound modality that is available on most machines is referred to as *M-mode ultrasound* ("motion mode"). M-mode ultrasound shows changes along a single ultrasound beam over time. The depth of the echo-producing structures is shown on the y-axis, and time is shown on the x-axis. M-mode is useful for documenting the presence of fetal cardiac

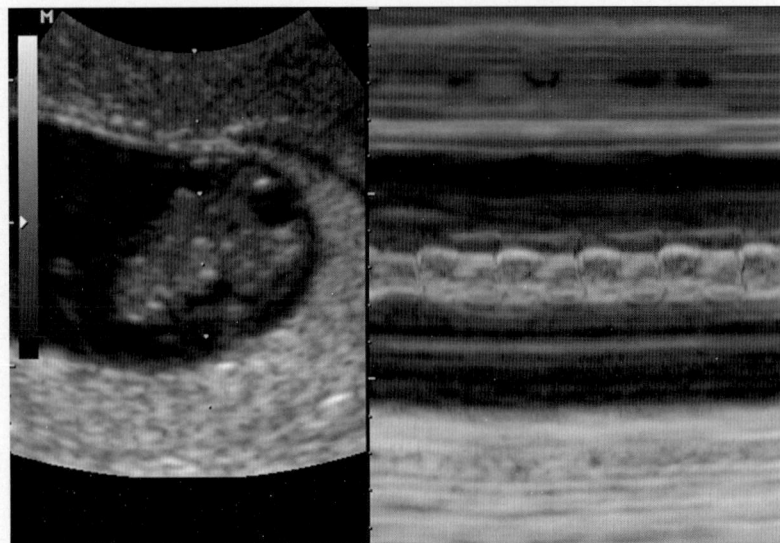

FIG 9-6 M-mode application in an 8-week fetus. The row of dots in the left panel indicates the line of information, in this case cardiac pulsations, being displayed over time in the right panel. M-mode is preferred to Doppler for documenting fetal viability before 10 weeks. Note the prominent brain vesicle in the fetal head, a normal finding.

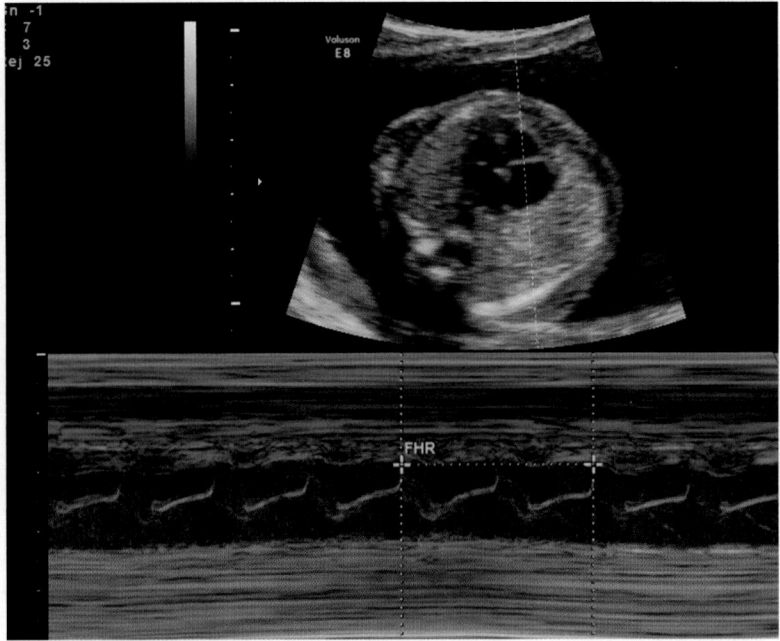

FIG 9-7 M-mode ultrasound with the cursor through the heart valves. In any ultrasound exam, it is important to have a permanent record showing fetal viability. M-mode is convenient for this purpose and can be used to determine the fetal heart rate.

activity (Figs. 9-6 and 9-7), and **M-mode is also sometimes used for specialized echocardiography applications.**

Color and Pulse-Wave Doppler

Over the past 25 years, Doppler ultrasound imaging has assumed a key role in obstetrics. With this modality, the ultrasound machine detects shifts in the frequency of echoes returning from a specific location in the image. **This frequency shift, the Doppler shift, is caused by motion of the insonated material toward or away from the transducer. Doppler ultrasound is primarily used to demonstrate the presence, direction, and velocity of blood flow.** The machine displays moving blood as color superimposed on the 2-D gray-scale image. By convention,

flow toward the ultrasound transducer is displayed in red and flow away is displayed in blue. Pulse-wave Doppler continuously measures the relative velocity of flow within a designated gate inside a vessel. **Flow velocity waveforms are used to calculate the systolic/diastolic (S/D) ratio, the pulsatility index, and the resistance index.**

These indexes are primarily used to assess downstream resistance in the vessel being interrogated. In pregnancies with fetal growth restriction, the flow within the umbilical artery is used to assess placental function (Fig. 9-8). **For some applications, the absolute flow velocity is needed. For example, when screening for fetal anemia, the peak flow velocity in the fetal middle cerebral artery is measured, as this correlates**

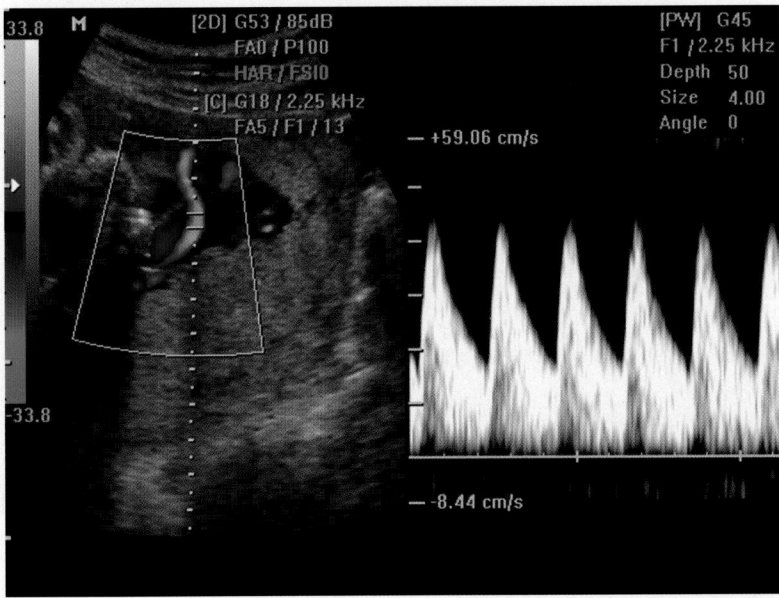

FIG 9-8 Color and spectral Doppler evaluation of the umbilical artery. In the left panel, the coiling arteries and vein are shown. Red indicates flow toward the transducer and blue is flow away. The sample gate for the pulse Doppler is superimposed. On the right is the result of the pulse Doppler, depicting a normal flow velocity waveform.

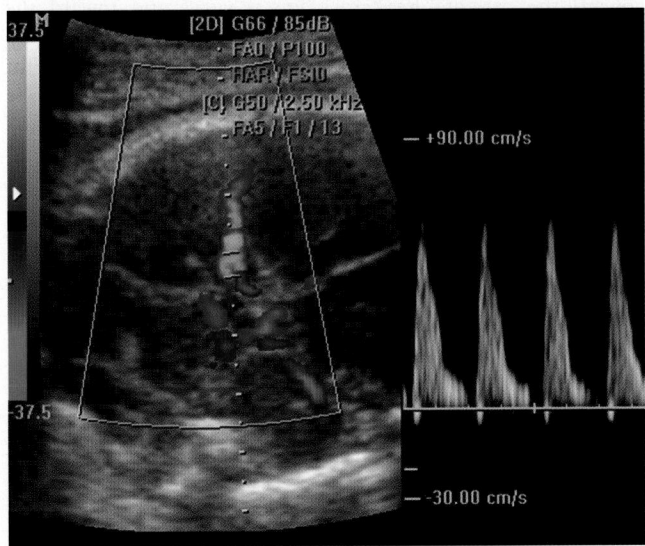

FIG 9-9 Color and spectral Doppler interrogation of the middle cerebral artery. Abnormally high peak velocity is an indicator of moderate to severe fetal anemia. Because the actual velocity is being measured, the angle of insonation should line up with the vessel.

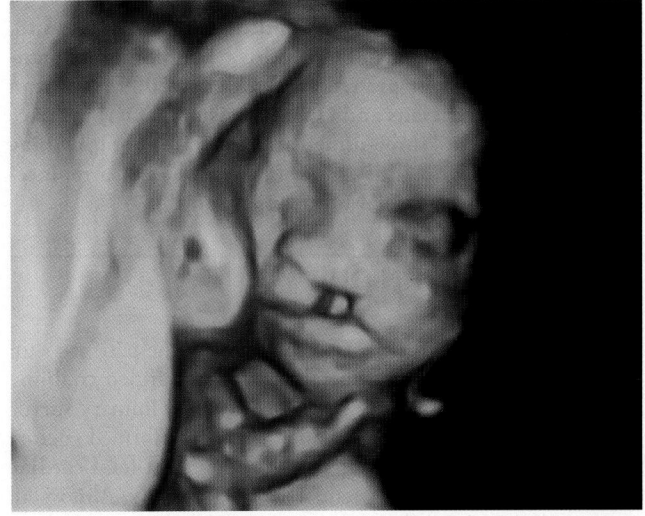

FIG 9-10 Three-dimensional image shows bilateral cleft lip. Images such as this can be helpful for counseling patients.

with the degree of fetal anemia. To give meaningful results, it is absolutely essential that the angle of insonation (θ) must be in line with the direction of blood flow (Fig. 9-9). Most ultrasound machines are equipped with the technology to allow the sonologist to autocorrect the angle of insonation when the optimal angle cannot be obtained.

Three-Dimensional Ultrasound

High-performance computers have allowed the development of ultrasound machines and probes that can acquire, process, and display a three-dimensional (3-D) volume, as opposed to the single plane displayed with 2-D ultrasound. To obtain this volume, the transducer uses an internal mechanical sweep mechanism that summates contiguous 2-D planes. This volume

data can either be stored for analysis or updated and displayed on a continuous basis. Adding a real-time updating of a rendered image is commonly referred to as *four-dimensional ultrasound*.

For diagnosing certain birth defects, 3-D ultrasound may be useful. Information from an acquired volume may be processed in such a way that the fetal surface is displayed in a lifelike manner. Surface abnormalities, such as facial clefts, can be well demonstrated with this approach (Fig. 9-10).[1] In addition, 3-D images can be more readily understood by patients and other professionals who will participate in care of the baby.

Software available for use with 3-D ultrasound machines can manipulate stored volume data off-line to show any desired plane through the scanned area. Some of these planes may be difficult to obtain with standard 2-D imaging. Storage of a volume of data also allows retrospective generation of 2-D images from different planes than were originally recorded. This

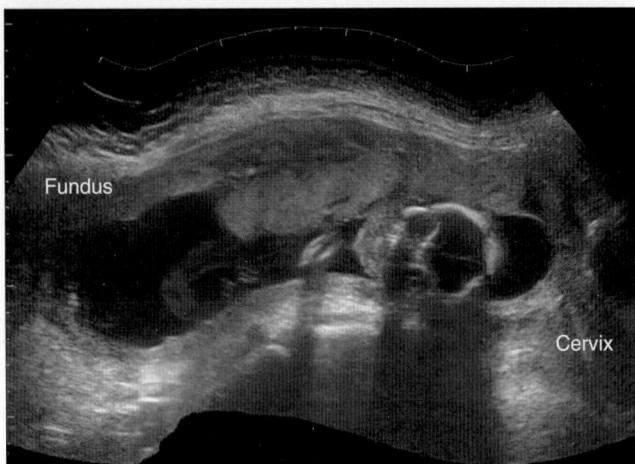

FIG 9-11 Transabdominal sagittal view of the uterus. The uterine fundus and cervix are labeled. By convention, the right side of the ultrasound screen corresponds to the inferior aspect of the patient.

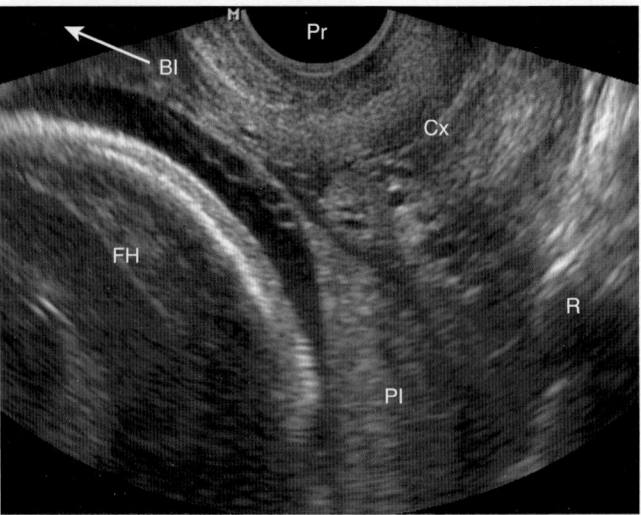

FIG 9-12 Transvaginal sagittal view showing proper orientation. The left of the screen is "up" on the patient, that is, toward the bladder (Bl). The probe tip (Pr), fetal head (FH), cervix (Cx), placenta (Pl), and rectum (R) are labeled. Note how transvaginal ultrasound provides the ultimate "window," showing very clear views of structures close to the vaginal apex. Also note the presence of vasa previa.

could be a powerful tool for review of ultrasound exams. Another feature of 3-D ultrasound is its ability to calculate tissue and fluid volumes. For example, lung volume measurements have been used to predict pulmonary hypoplasia.[2]

Despite the demonstrated capabilities of 3-D ultrasound, no proof exists of an advantage of this technology over standard 2-D imaging for prenatal diagnosis. A 2009 American College of Obstetricians and Gynecologists (ACOG) practice bulletin states that "three-dimensional ultrasonography may be helpful in diagnosis as an adjunct to, but not a replacement for, two dimensional ultrasonography."[3]

SCANNING TECHNIQUE
Orientation

The sonographer starts the exam by exposing the patient's skin over the entire uterus and liberally applying warmed coupling gel. An appropriate probe is selected, and a preliminary survey of the entire uterine contents and adnexa is performed. Before going any further, it is a good idea to **document fetal cardiac activity**. Images are frozen and recorded liberally. Almost all machines have a **cine loop** feature in which a few seconds of sequential images are saved so that the sonographer can scroll backward if the desired image was missed.

Every effort should be made to perform the scan with the sonographer and the patient in standard positions. In most settings, the ultrasound machine and the sonographer are on the patient's right, with the sonographer comfortably seated facing the head of the patient. **The probe is held in such a way that the image on the screen is properly oriented. By convention, the probe surface is shown at the top of the screen. For sagittal views, the right of the screen corresponds to the inferior aspect of the patient** (Fig. 9-11). **For transverse views, the patient's right is shown on the left of the screen.** With transvaginal ultrasound, transverse views also show the patient's right side to the left of the screen. In transvaginal sagittal views, "up" is to the left of the screen (i.e., toward the bladder), and "down" (toward the sacrum) is to the right of the screen (Fig. 9-12). Ultrasound transducers have a notch or ridge that demarcates the side of the probe that will correspond to the left side of the monitor. Thus with transabdominal work, this mark would be

toward the patient's head for sagittal views and toward the patient's right for transverse views. With transvaginal scanning, the mark is up for sagittal views and to the patient's right for transverse views. Thus in going from sagittal to transverse, the probe is always rotated counterclockwise, and the clinician goes clockwise to move from transverse to sagittal.

If the sonographer sits or stands on the wrong side of the patient or holds the probe backward, standard orientation of the images is difficult to maintain. A "backward" image is clearly unacceptable for diagnostics and for documentation. Also, a casual approach to probe orientation will prevent the sonographer from developing the hand-eye coordination needed to quickly and accurately steer the probe.

To establish the position of the fetus, the orientation of the probe must obviously be correct. This is important not only when deciding whether the fetus is cephalic or breech but also when determining the right and left side of the fetus. For example, when the image shows the fetal spine to the right side of the uterus, the fetal left will be up in a cephalic presentation and down with a breech. The sonographer should not depend on the side of the stomach or axis of the heart to define the position of the fetus because these structures are not always in a normal position.

Angle of Insonation

There is often a best angle from which to view aspects of the intrauterine contents and fetal structures. For example, transverse views of the kidneys are best obtained from a directly anterior or posterior direction. With a lateral view, one kidney is shadowed by the spine (Fig. 9-13). Sliding the transducer across the mother's abdomen to change the angle of insonation by 90 degrees corrects this problem. Sometimes, significant pressure with the transducer is needed to get the probe into position for optimal visualization. If the fetal position precludes clear visualization of a structure, a good strategy is to move forward with the examination and come back to the troublesome area. The fetus will often have moved in such a way that adequate views can be obtained.

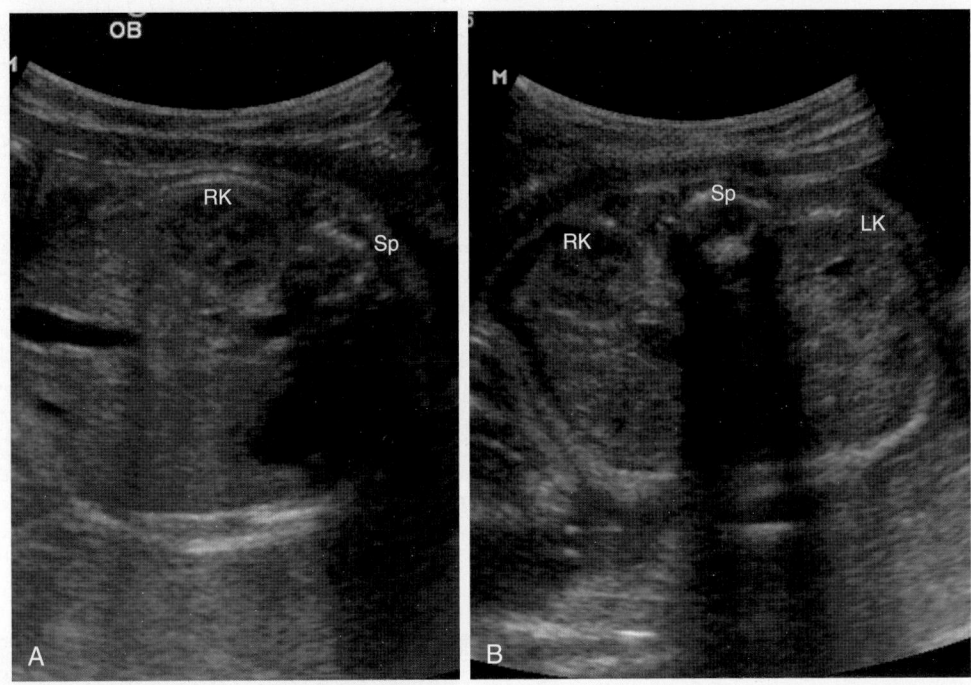

FIG 9-13 A, Shadowing by the spine precludes visualization of the left kidney. **B,** By sliding the transducer to a different location on the maternal abdominal wall, a more favorable angle of insonation is possible. The spine (Sp), right kidney (RK), and left kidney (LK) are labeled.

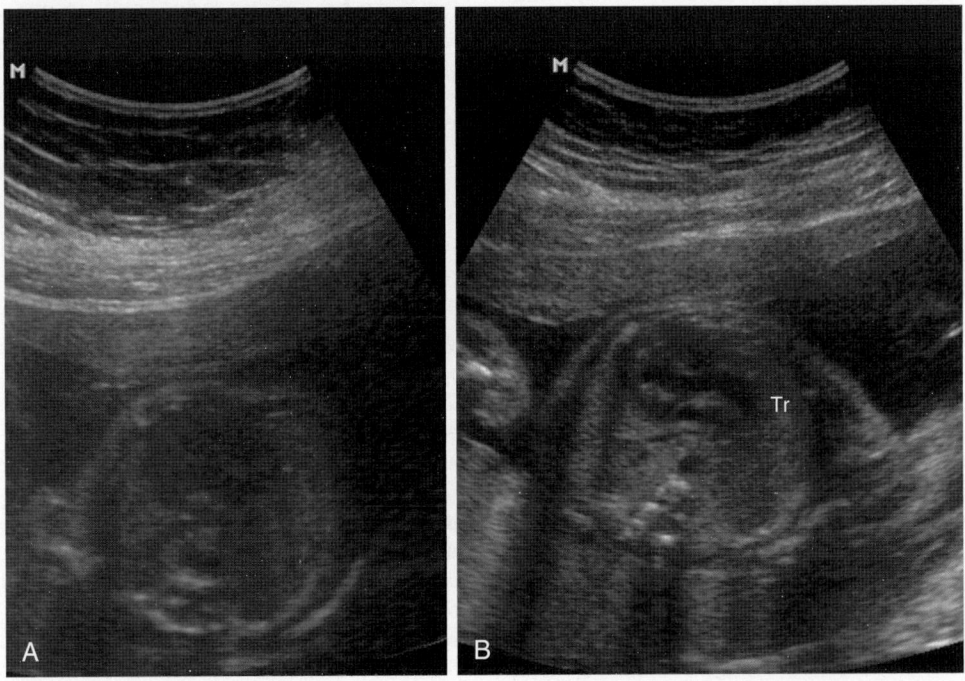

FIG 9-14 A, Scan through the pannus of the abdominal wall. **B,** By moving the probe into the relatively thinner area near the maternal umbilicus, the resolution improved dramatically. A similar result can be obtained when scanning below the pannus in the suprapubic area. Of course, when an object of interest is in the maternal pelvis, transvaginal ultrasound provides an even better window (see Fig. 9-12). This fetus has truncus arteriosus (Tr).

Using Natural Windows

As previously noted, increasing the power of ultrasound impulses can overcome some of the effects of attenuation in maternal tissues. Although it is tempting to use higher-power settings for obese patients, other methods should be attempted first. As a starting point, the proper probe frequency and gain setting should be used. **Even more effective, however, is to avoid** **attenuation altogether by scanning though one of the natural "windows" in the maternal abdominal wall.** The abdominal wall thickness in obese women is substantially less near the umbilicus (Fig. 9-14) and in the suprapubic area. **To a lesser extent, thickness is also decreased lateral to the central pannus.** Using these windows can often improve the quality of images dramatically. Of course, in early pregnancy or when structures of interest are low in the pelvis, the problem of attenuation is reduced considerably by the use of an endovaginal probe (see Fig. 9-12). The reduction of attenuation with transvaginal ultrasound allows the use of a higher-frequency probe, which usually results in excellent resolution. **Another natural window is amniotic fluid, and scanning through amniotic fluid improves the image quality below or deep to the amniotic fluid.** This is especially true for imaging the surface of the fetus. A full bladder provides a window to structures low in the maternal pelvis. However, scanning with a full maternal bladder has significant disadvantages; not only is it uncomfortable for the patient, it also artificially elongates the cervix and may distort the apparent relationship of the cervix and placenta. Fortunately, this is no longer necessary because transvaginal ultrasound can provide superior views to structures in the maternal pelvis.

FIRST-TRIMESTER ULTRASOUND

Transvaginal ultrasound is almost always superior to transabdominal ultrasound for evaluation very early in pregnancy. Because the distance between the probe and pregnancy structures is often just a few centimeters, attenuation of sound waves is minimal, and high-frequency probes may be used. As previously noted, this allows better resolution of detail. Although an acceptable first-trimester scan can usually be completed transabdominally, it is often helpful to use transvaginal ultrasound as a supplement to or replacement for transabdominal ultrasound. **In general, structures are visible one week earlier with transvaginal ultrasound. At about 10 to 12 weeks' gestation, the uterus has grown enough—and the fetus is far enough away from the transducer—that advantages of transvaginal scanning are lost.** Even if a structure of interest is low in the uterus, lack of maneuverability of the probe tip may make it difficult or impossible to obtain images through the desired fetal plane. Because of this limitation and the need for a precise midsagittal plane, measurement of the fetal nuchal translucency as part of the first-trimester aneuploidy screen is almost always done transabdominally.

Transvaginal ultrasound is well accepted by most patients and can be accomplished with minimal discomfort. In some clinics, women are given the option of inserting the probe themselves.

First-Trimester Normal Findings

Both ACOG and the American Institute of Ultrasound Medicine (AIUM) have defined the essential components of a first-trimester scan. Knowledge of the time at which embryonic structures normally appear is important for identifying pathologic pregnancies. For the reasons noted earlier, it will be assumed that transvaginal ultrasound is being used for this discussion.

The gestational sac can usually be seen at 4 weeks, the yolk sac at 5 weeks (Fig. 9-15), and the fetal pole with cardiac activity by 6 weeks. Cardiac activity can be seen simultaneously with the appearance of a fetal pole as a pulsation at the lateral aspect of the yolk sac. **Because pulse or color Doppler carry higher energy, which theoretically could be harmful during embryogenesis (before 10 menstrual weeks),[4] M-mode ultrasound is used to document cardiac activity during this time** (see Fig. 9-6). Starting at 7 weeks, the embryo has grown to the point that recognizable features, such as a cephalic pole, can be seen. As shown in Figure 9-6, a prominent midline brain vesicle can be seen at this time. **The cerebral falx is visible at 9 weeks, and the appearance and disappearance of physiologic gut**

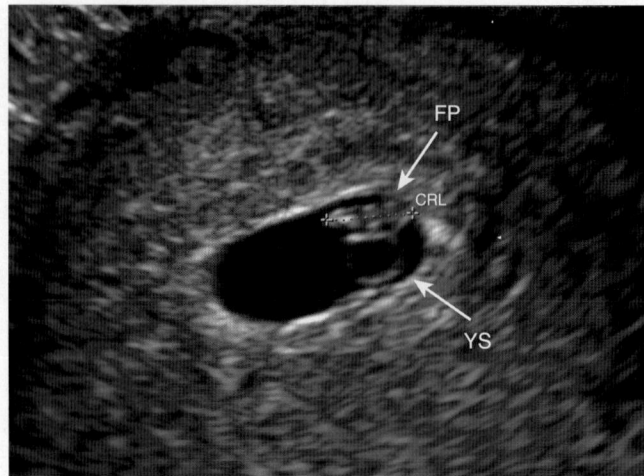

FIG 9-15 This image shows a normal 7-week gestational sac with the yolk sac (YS) and adjacent fetal pole (FP). Calipers show the measurement to establish the gestational age. CRL, crown-rump length.

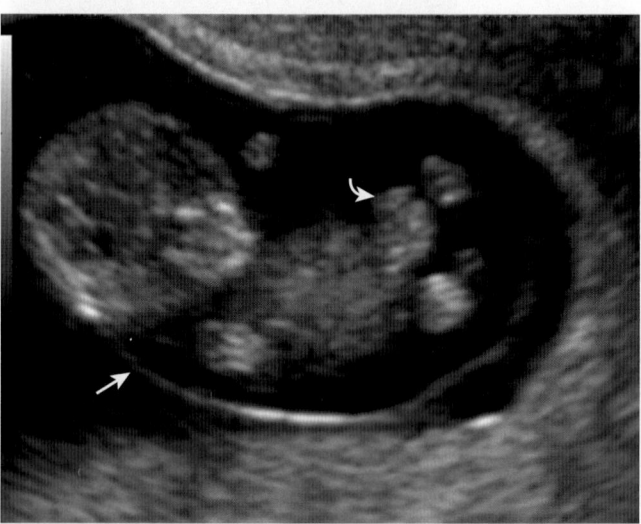

FIG 9-16 Nine-week fetus showing the physiologic gut herniation (*curved arrow*). Note also how the amnion (*straight arrow*) has not yet fused to the chorion at the uterine wall.

herniation are noted between 8 and 11 weeks (Fig. 9-16). **In the course of this physiologic process, the bowel is seen to lie within the umbilical cord and does not float freely. Obviously, the diagnosis of an abdominal wall defect should be made with caution at this age.** The stomach can consistently be seen by 11 weeks. If conditions are favorable, it is often possible to also visualize the bladder and kidneys at 11 weeks. At about 12 weeks, using color Doppler, the two umbilical arteries can often be identified as they course around the bladder. The fetal heart rate is initially quite slow, averaging 110 beats/min at 6 weeks,[5] then it increases steadily to a mean peak of 157 beats/min at 8 weeks. When the fetal position is favorable, transvaginal ultrasound has the potential for giving good views of the fetal cardiac anatomy in most patients at 13 weeks.[6] Until 13 to 16 weeks' gestation, the amnion has not fused to the chorion and is seen as a separate membrane (see Fig. 9-16). **Until 12 weeks, the crown-rump length (CRL) should be measured for gestational age determination.** Care should be taken to measure

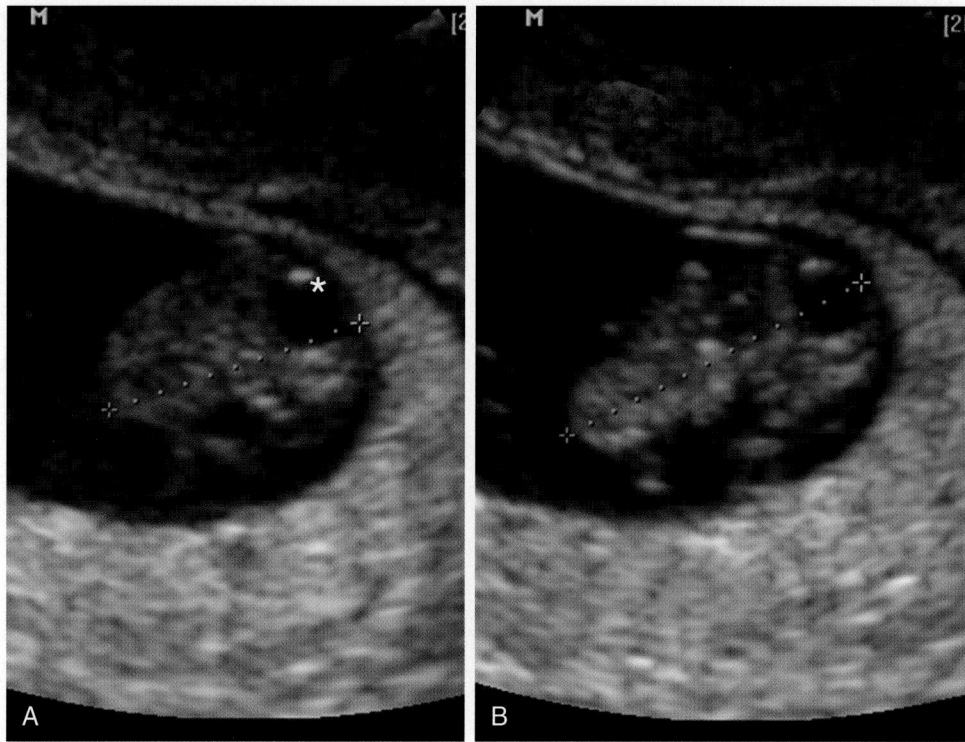

FIG 9-17 **A,** Image of the fetus is cut obliquely, and the crown-rump length is inappropriately short. It is measured correctly in **B.** The difference in the calculated gestational age from these two measurements was 5 days. The normal brain vesicle (asterisk) is noted.

the full length of the fetus. The gestational age can be significantly underestimated if an oblique plane is used (Fig. 9-17).

First-Trimester Abnormal Findings

Spontaneous abortion occurs in 15% of clinically established pregnancies. When cardiac activity has been demonstrated, the miscarriage rate is reduced to 2% to 3% in asymptomatic low-risk women.[7] It is important to note, however, that in some groups at high risk for miscarriage—such as women over the age of 35 years who are undergoing infertility treatments—early visualization of cardiac activity does not provide quite as much reassurance. In one study that involved such women, the miscarriage rate in asymptomatic women was still 16% after a heartbeat was documented.[8] **In younger women who present with bleeding, only 5% miscarry if the ultrasound is normal and shows a live embryo.**[9] If an intrauterine clot is present (Fig. 9-18), coexistent with an otherwise normal-appearing pregnancy, the miscarriage rate is 15%.[9]

In the majority of pregnancies destined to abort, the embryo does not develop, and ultrasound shows an empty gestational sac (Fig. 9-19). Such a pregnancy is termed an *anembryonic gestation.* When a failed pregnancy is suspected based on clinical or sonographic grounds, patients and clinicians alike are anxious to determine viability as soon as possible. However, the potential for great harm is obvious if a pregnancy is incorrectly deemed to be a failed pregnancy, and a desired pregnancy is interrupted. There have been cases in which a premature diagnosis of a failed pregnancy was made, medical evacuation of the uterus was unsuccessfully attempted, and the fetus was subsequently found to be viable. Because no significant medical risk attends waiting for certainty when a failed pregnancy is suspected, a cautious approach is always advisable. **Criteria for deciding that a pregnancy of uncertain viability is in fact a failed pregnancy**

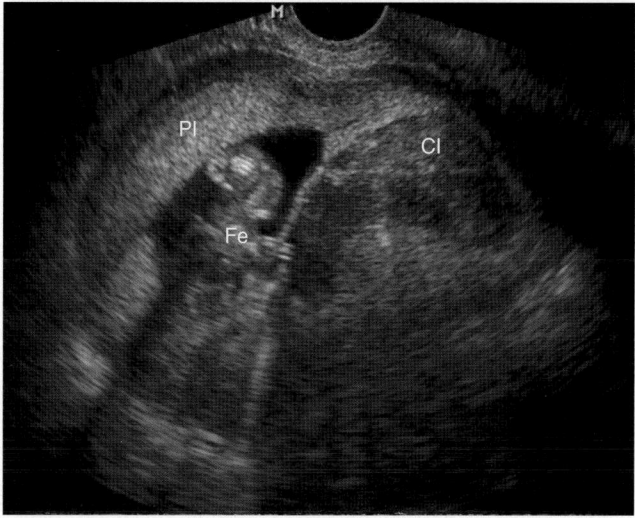

FIG 9-18 This patient presented with vaginal bleeding. A subchorionic clot (CI) was present in the lower uterine segment. This patient carried the pregnancy successfully. The fetus (Fe) and placenta (PI) are shown.

should be set to virtually eliminate the possibility of a false-positive diagnosis. A multispecialty panel from the Society of Radiologists in Ultrasound panel recommended criteria to achieve this end.[10] **These include (1) the presence of a fetus with a CRL of more than 7 mm and no heartbeat, (2) the absence of an embryo when the mean sac diameter is greater than 25 mm, (3) the absence of an embryo with a heartbeat more than 2 weeks after a scan showed a gestational sac without a yolk sac, and (4) the absence of an embryo with a heartbeat more than 11 days after a gestational sac with a**

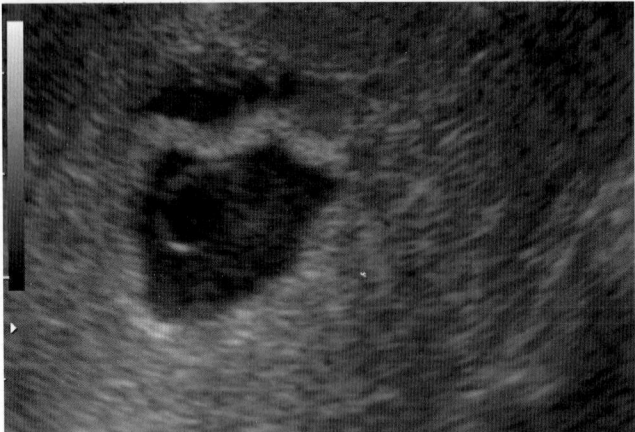

FIG 9-19 Irregular gestational sac from an anembryonic gestation.

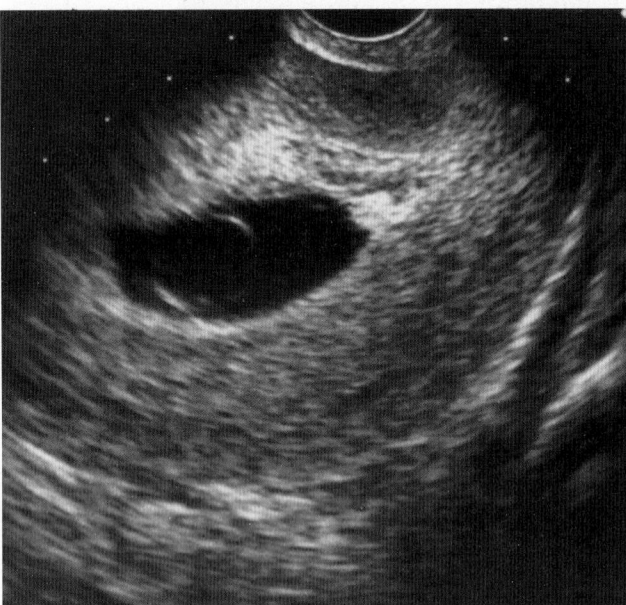

FIG 9-20 Compared with Figure 9-15, the yolk sac in this image is relatively large for the gestational age. An embryo was never seen with this pregnancy.

yolk sac was seen. Similar but less stringent criteria that are suspicious for a pregnancy failure are described in the same report. Other signs that indicate a possible failed pregnancy include an enlarged yolk sac (>7 mm; Fig. 9-20) or less than 5 mm difference between gestational sac diameter and the CRL of the embryo. **If there are borderline findings and uterine evacuation is being considered, it is prudent to repeat the ultrasound in 7 to 10 days to be absolutely sure that a viable pregnancy is not interrupted.**[10] Although a quantitative human chorionic gonadotropin (hCG) value that does not show an appropriate rise may indicate an abnormal pregnancy, a decision to medically or surgically evacuate an intrauterine failed pregnancy should be based on abnormal ultrasound findings.

First-trimester ultrasound findings predictive of a chromosome abnormality include a thick nuchal translucency, absent nasal bone, abnormally fast or slow fetal heart rate, and some structural malformations.[11] The first-trimester aneuploidy screen will be discussed in detail in Chapter 10.

BOX 9-1 SUGGESTED COMPONENTS OF THE STANDARD OBSTETRIC ULTRASOUND PERFORMED IN THE SECOND AND THIRD TRIMESTERS

- Standard biometry
- Fetal cardiac activity (present or absent, normal or abnormal)
- Number of fetuses (if multiples, document chorionicity, amnionicity, comparison of fetal sizes, estimation of amniotic fluid normality in each sac, and fetal genitalia)
- Presentation
- Qualitative or semiquantitative estimate of amniotic fluid volume
- Placental location, especially its relationship to the internal os, and placental cord insertion site
- Evaluation of the uterus that includes fibroids, adnexal structures, and the cervix
- Cervix when clinically appropriate and technically feasible
- Anatomic survey to include:
Head and neck
  - Cerebellum
  - Choroid plexus
  - Cisterna magna
  - Lateral cerebral ventricles
  - Midline falx
  - Cavum septum pellucidum
  - Fetal lip
  - Nuchal skin fold may be helpful for aneuploidy risk
Chest
  - Four-chamber view of the heart
  - Outflow tracts (if possible)
Abdomen
  - Stomach (presence, size, and situs)
  - Kidneys
  - Bladder
  - Umbilical cord insertion into the abdomen
  - Number of umbilical cord vessels
Spine
Extremities (presence or absence of legs and arms)
Gender

Data from American College of Obstetricians and Gynecologists. ACOG Practice Bulletin No. 101: ultrasonography in pregnancy. *Obstet Gynecol.* 2009; 113:451-461; American Institute of Ultrasound in Medicine (AIUM). AIUM practice guidelines for the performance of an antepartum obstetric ultrasound examination. *J Ultrasound Med.* 2003;22:1116-1125; and Reddy UM, Abuhamad AZ, Levine D. Saade GR. Fetal imaging: executive summary of a joint Eunice Kennedy Shriver National Institute of Child Health and Human Development, Society for Maternal-Fetal Medicine, American Institute of Ultrasound in Medicine, American College of Obstetricians and Gynecologists, American College of Radiology, Society for Pediatric Radiology, and Society of Radiologists in Ultrasound Fetal Imaging Workshop. *Obstet Gynecol.* 2014;123:1070-1082.

SECOND- AND THIRD-TRIMESTER ULTRASOUND

Types of Examinations

The AIUM, in conjunction with ACOG and the American College of Radiology (ACR), have defined a set of criteria for standard obstetric ultrasound examinations performed in the second and third trimesters.[3,12] **Components of a standard obstetric examination are shown in** Box 9-1. A complete description of the AIUM and ACOG guidelines can be found in the listed references.

These guidelines recognize that not all ultrasound examinations have the same purpose. For this reason, types of fetal sonographic evaluations have been defined. Components of the first-trimester ultrasound examination were described previously. A *standard* second- or third-trimester examination (current procedural terminology [CPT] code 76805), as defined in Box 9-1, can be performed by any appropriately qualified sonographer. **It is recognized that certain scans, termed *specialized* examinations (CPT code 76811), are more complex than the complete standard examinations performed in the course of routine pregnancy care. This designation and billing code are intended to be used for referral practices with special expertise in the identification of and counseling on fetal anomalies.** Other specialized examinations may include fetal Doppler ultrasonography and fetal echocardiography.[3] Follow-up examinations are needed for many obstetric conditions; these are termed *repeat* examinations (CPT 76816).

Another examination category is the *limited* examination (CPT 76815). **Limited ultrasound examinations, also performed by a trained sonographer, are used to obtain a specific piece of information about the pregnancy.** Examples of this type of examination include the determination of fetal lie or assessment of amniotic fluid volume. **The importance of restricting limited examinations to those cases in which a complete examination has previously been performed should be self-evident.** Consider the consequence if a brief ultrasound is done and critically important information is missed, such as a serious malformation in the fetus. Unfortunately, it is all too common for practitioners to perform limited examinations in a manner inconsistent with good medical practice. For example, in some clinics, practitioners perform an ultrasound at the first prenatal visit to document viability but do not measure the fetus or record the results of the examination. Such a practice can create problems later in pregnancy when the gestational age is in doubt.

All the aspects of the standard obstetric examination listed in Box 9-1 are important for clinical management and should not be neglected. It is clearly unacceptable for an ultrasound exam to miss such conditions as placenta previa, multiple gestation, or an ovarian tumor. The diagnosis and management of these and other conditions are discussed in detail elsewhere in this book, but a brief description of the importance of the components of the standard ultrasound examination will be given here.

Qualifications for Performing and Interpreting Diagnostic Ultrasound Examinations

Most ultrasound exams in the United States are performed by professionals who are credentialed by the American Registry of Diagnostic Medical Sonography (ARDMS). Individuals with these credentials have had extensive education and testing to ensure their competency. A physician then generates a report based on the images and information obtained by the sonographer. When appropriate, the physician may personally perform or repeat parts of the exam. **The AIUM has published guidelines on the training and experience needed for physicians to perform or interpret ultrasound examinations.**[13] In brief, these guidelines recommend that licensed physicians have completed an equivalent of 3 months training dedicated to ultrasound in the context of an approved residency, fellowship, or other postgraduate training. In the absence of a formal training program, physicians can qualify through having 100 American Medical Association (AMA) category I credits dedicated to diagnostic ultrasound. In addition to participation in either a formal training program or by taking postgraduate courses, physicians should

have been involved with the performance, evaluation, and interpretation of at least 300 appropriately supervised sonograms. The full text of the guidelines is in the referenced document.

COMPONENTS OF THE EXAMINATION
Cardiac Activity

Obviously, the presence or absence of cardiac activity should be documented. As noted previously, after about 6 weeks' gestation, the diagnosis of fetal life is rarely difficult. Even though fetal death may be obvious with B-mode imaging, **confirming the absence of a heartbeat with color or pulse-wave Doppler is recommended.** Absence of color signal in the fetal chest, contrasted with the demonstration of flow in the surrounding uterine tissues, can increase the confidence that fetal death has indeed occurred. Throughout pregnancy, an abnormally fast, slow, or irregular heartbeat can be detected by visual inspection with gray-scale ultrasonography. The abnormal rate can be quantified and documented with M-mode or pulse-wave Doppler ultrasound.

Number of Fetuses

When a multiple pregnancy is diagnosed, the number of amnions and chorions should always be determined (see Chapter 32). **Determination of chorionicity is most easily accomplished in early pregnancy. The presence of unlike sex twins, separate placentae, or a thick membrane dividing the sacs with a twin peak or "lambda sign" all indicate the presence of two chorions** (see Fig. 9-3). **It is well-recognized that the level of fetal risk is much higher when fetuses share chorions,** and the risk is extremely high if there is a single amnion.[14] Monochorionic pregnancies require early referral for a specialized ultrasound. **In all twin pregnancies, periodic ultrasound examinations should be performed to assess fetal growth.** Twins are at significantly increased risk for growth abnormalities, and it is not possible to assess the growth of the twins individually by abdominal palpation.

Presentation

The assessment of presentation is not merely a matter of determining whether the fetus is head down or breech. A more precise ultrasound analysis of presentation is important in certain circumstances. If a transverse lie is diagnosed, it is important to diagnose whether the fetus is back down (i.e., back toward the cervix) because this may require a vertical incision for cesarean delivery. If the patient has preterm labor or ruptured membranes, a back-up transverse lie indicates a high risk for cord prolapse. The attitude of the fetal head, especially a face presentation, can be important in assessing progress in labor. In cases of marked caput or molding in late labor, it is often difficult to determine the position of the fetal head by palpation of the cranial sutures. Under these circumstances, ultrasound can be used to readily identify fetal cranial landmarks to clarify the position of the fetal head.[15]

Amniotic Fluid Volume

Every ultrasound examination should include an assessment of the amniotic fluid volume (see Chapter 35). It is acceptable for an experienced examiner to make this determination subjectively.[12] However, to aid in communication and to provide criteria for management protocols, semiquantitative methods have been devised. **A popular method is the amniotic fluid index**

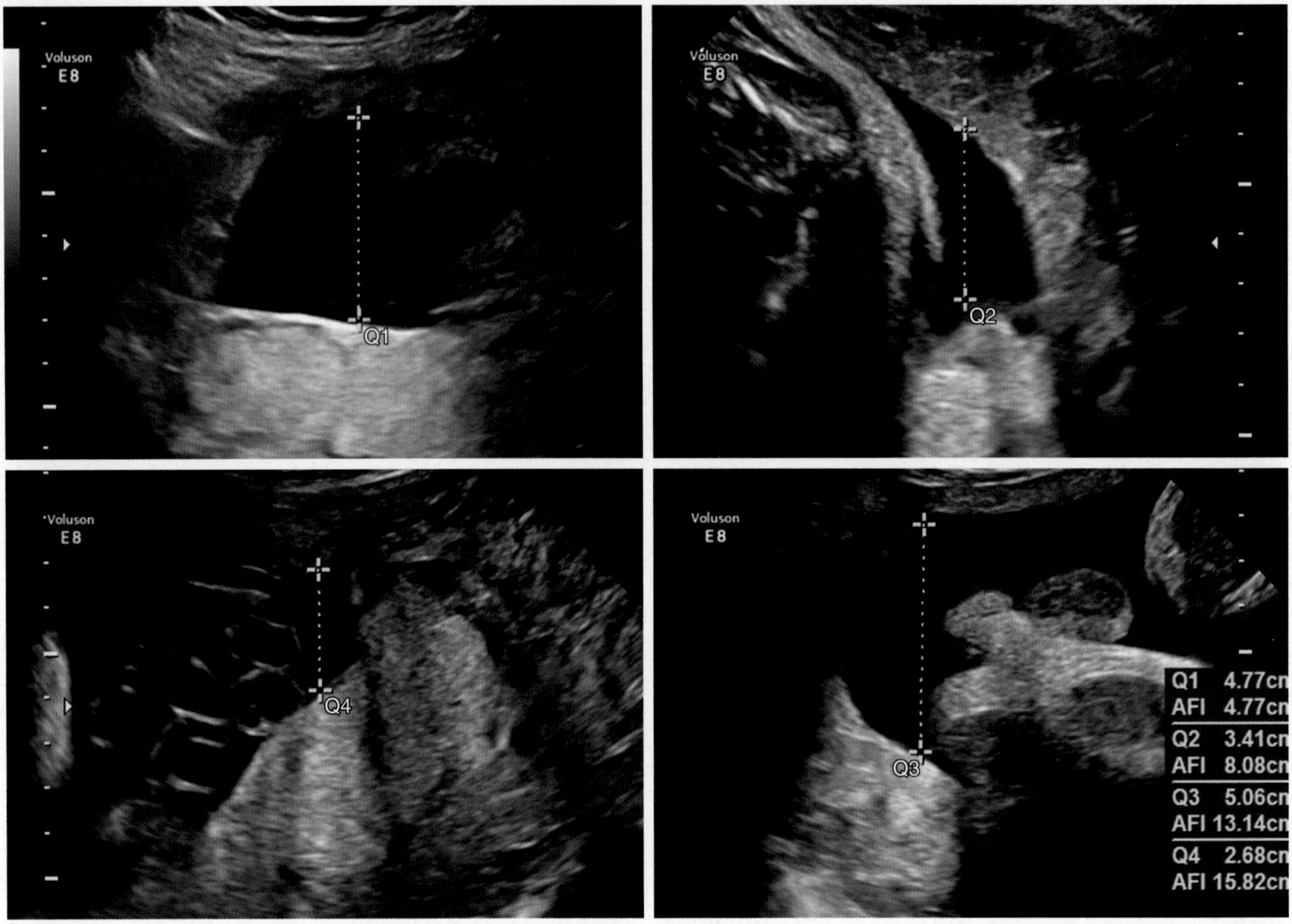

Q1	4.77cm
AFI	4.77cm
Q2	3.41cm
AFI	8.08cm
Q3	5.06cm
AFI	13.14cm
Q4	2.68cm
AFI	15.82cm

FIG 9-21 These sonographic images show the deepest vertical pocket in each of the four quadrants of the uterus. The sum of the measurements of these pockets is the amniotic fluid index.

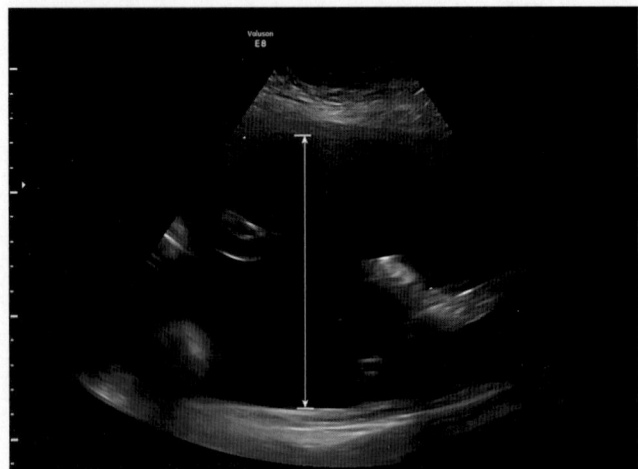

FIG 9-22 An ultrasound image showing polyhydramnios. The distance between the anterior and posterior uterine walls was 9 cm.

(AFI), the sum of the measurements of the deepest vertical pocket of fluid in each of the uterine quadrants (Fig. 9-21). The limits of the quadrants are the maternal midline and a horizontal line through the maternal umbilicus. Each pocket should measure at least 1 cm in width.[16] **The line between the calipers should not cross through loops of cord or fetal parts.**

Polyhydramnios and oligohydramnios can be defined either by an AFI outside of a fixed range, usually defined as greater than 24 cm or less than 5 cm, respectively.[17] A simpler semi-quantitative method is to diagnose *polyhydramnios* when the single deepest pool measures greater than 8 cm (Fig. 9-22)[18] and *oligohydramnios* when the shallowest pool measures less than 2 cm in two dimensions.[16]

The actual volume of amniotic fluid can be determined by dye-dilution techniques performed at the time of amniocentesis. The semiquantitative ultrasound methods described previously correlate somewhat with actual fluid volume, but their accuracy for predicting abnormal fluid volume is limited.[18]

Oligohydramnios

The complete absence of amniotic fluid before labor can indicate fetal malformations, rupture of the membranes, or placental insufficiency. A **deficit of amniotic fluid that occurs before the mid second trimester can result in the oligohydramnios sequence, which includes pulmonary hypoplasia, fetal deformations, and flexion contractures of the extremities.** The outcome with anhydramnios depends on the cause and the gestational age at which it is first present. Fetal malformations that cause absence of fluid usually involve the urinary tract. These may include complete bladder outlet obstruction or bilateral renal anomalies in which no urine is produced. Examples include bilateral renal agenesis, bilateral multicystic dysplastic kidneys, or autosomal-recessive polycystic kidney disease. The development of lethal pulmonary hypoplasia when the cause of mid second trimester oligohydramnios is other than a urinary tract malformation is not as predictable.

For many years, it has been recognized that less extreme alterations of amniotic fluid volume can be important. **Chamberlain and associates[19] found that with less than a 1-cm pocket of fluid, perinatal mortality increased fortyfold. The incidence of intrauterine growth restriction (IUGR) was also much higher when this degree of oligohydramnios was found.** These findings and those of other investigators led to the recognition that oligohydramnios can be an important sign of placental insufficiency, and amniotic fluid volume assessment became part of the biophysical profile (see Chapter 11). Because of the association between oligohydramnios and fetal compromise, it became common practice to deliver the baby when the AFI was less than 5. More recently, it has been shown that isolated ultrasound-diagnosed oligohydramnios is not as predictive of perinatal outcome as was previously thought.[20] **In 2014, ACOG recommended using a deepest vertical pocket of 2 cm or less as the definition of oligohydramnios by which clinical management decisions should be made. This method is simpler than the AFI, and more importantly, it has been shown to reduce the rate of obstetric interventions for oligohydramnios with no difference in perinatal outcomes compared with using an AFI of less than 5.[21]**

Polyhydramnios

Polyhydramnios has been classified as *mild* if the AFI is more than 24 cm, or the deepest pocket is more than 8 cm; it is considered *moderate* with an AFI greater than 30 cm, or when the deepest pocket is more than 12 cm; and it is *severe* when the AFI is greater than 35 cm or the deepest pocket is more than 16 cm.[22] Severe polyhydramnios may be indicative of a fetal problem and requires specialized ultrasound to determine the etiology. It is often caused by malformations that can greatly affect neonatal management or prognosis. For many of these conditions, the excess amniotic fluid is a result of poor fetal swallowing because of neurologic abnormalities, genetic syndromes, or gastrointestinal (GI) malformations. **The chance of a malformation or genetic syndrome being present with mild, moderate, or severe polyhydramnios is approximately 8%, 12%, and 30%, respectively.[23] The chance of a fetus with polyhydramnios having aneuploidy is 10% when other anomalies are present.** Other serious causes of severe polyhydramnios include twin-to-twin transfusion syndrome and fetal hydrops. An association has been found between polyhydramnios and fetal macrosomia, and maternal diabetes mellitus is present in about 5% of cases.[23] Mild polyhydramnios may simply be a variant of normal, and it often resolves spontaneously. **With polyhydramnios, an increase in preterm birth is observed when the patient has diabetes (22%) or the fetus has anomalies (39%) but not when it is idiopathic.[24]** No studies have researched whether antepartum testing is helpful, although polyhydramnios is listed as an indication for antepartum testing in an ACOG technical bulletin.[21] When polyhydramnios persists, follow-up ultrasound exams are appropriate to assess fetal growth and amniotic fluid volume.

Placenta and Umbilical Cord

One of the principal advantages of routine ultrasound is that serious problems of placentation—such as placenta previa,

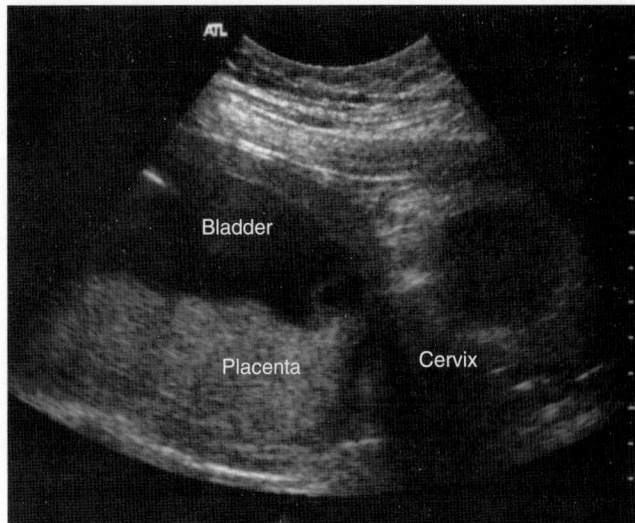

FIG 9-23 Sagittal transabdominal view of the lower uterus and cervix. The relationship between the edge of the placenta and cervix is unclear, and placenta previa cannot be accurately diagnosed.

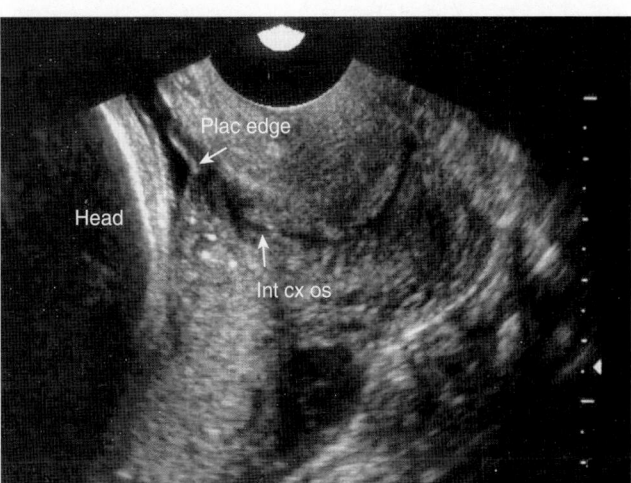

FIG 9-24 Sagittal transvaginal view of the same patient. Marginal placenta is clearly visible, and the edge of the placenta (Plac edge) extends 1.5 cm over the internal os (Int cx os). Calipers are not shown.

placenta accreta, and vasa previa—can be diagnosed in a timely manner (see Chapter 18). At the time of the routine screening ultrasound (beyond 18 weeks), it should be determined whether the placenta covers the internal cervical os. If the placenta and the cervix are not seen clearly, or if it appears that the edge of the placenta is close to the cervix, vaginal ultrasound should be used liberally to clarify this relationship (Figs. 9-23 and 9-24).[25]

The terms *complete* and *partial placenta previa* originated from a time when the relationship of the placenta to the partially dilated cervix was determined by digital examination. Because the internal cervical os is not typically dilated at the time of ultrasound, these definitions are confusing and often uninformative. For this reason, a joint statement by the major ultrasound and obstetric societies in the United States[16] and a policy statement by the Society of Obstetricians and Gynaecologists of Canada[26] recommended a classification that retains only the terms *placenta previa* and *low-lying placenta*. **The distance**

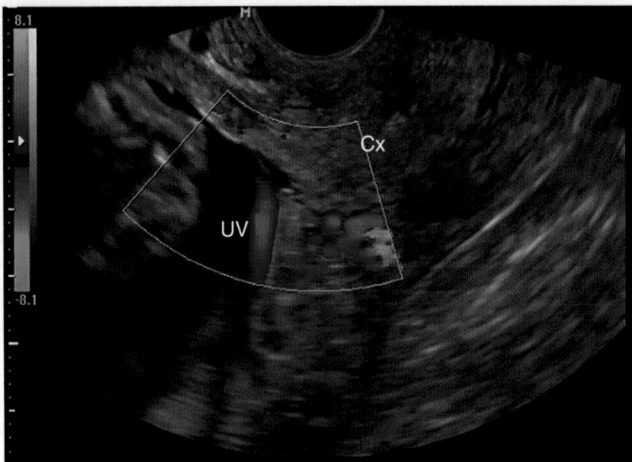

FIG 9-25 Sagittal transvaginal image showing vasa previa. An umbilical vessel (UV) passes over the internal os of the cervix (Cx). In this case, a velamentous cord insertion was evident, and this vessel passed over the cervix running from the cord insertion to the placenta.

that the edge of the placenta covers or ends short of the internal cervical os should be measured and reported. This quantitative description is much more helpful than a report of "complete" or "partial" previa for predicting the future placental position and in planning management. **For pregnancies greater than 16 weeks, if the placental edge ends 2 cm or more from the cervix, the placental location should be reported as normal. If the placental edge is less than 2 cm from the internal os but not covering the internal os, the placenta should be labeled as low lying, and follow-up ultrasonography is recommended at 32 weeks' gestation.**[16]

Between 18 and 23 weeks' gestation, the edge of the placenta extends to or covers the internal os of the cervix in about 2% of patients.[27] However, most cases of placenta previa diagnosed early in pregnancy resolve as pregnancy progresses. The rate of persistence of placenta previa depends on the degree of overlap. When the degree of overlap is 15 mm or greater, 19% persist as placenta previa, whereas if the overlap is 25 mm or greater, 40% remain.[27] Another study found that when placenta previa is present at 15 to 19 weeks, only 12% persist.[28] **The rate of persistence gradually increases as the gestational age advances, up to 73% if placenta previa is present at 32 to 35 weeks.** This study also showed that the degree of overlap was helpful in predicting persistence. These results suggest that **repeated ultrasound examinations should be performed until the placenta moves well away from the cervix or until it becomes clear that the previa will persist.** If the placenta previa persists, ultrasound can be very valuable in planning delivery.

The diagnosis of vasa previa is critical because the recognition of this finding at the time of a screening ultrasound greatly affects the chance of fetal survival.[29] **The fetal mortality rate is high when vasa previa is not diagnosed before labor.** Conversely, early diagnosis and aggressive obstetric management of patients with vasa previa almost always results in a live baby born in good condition. The fetal vessels that cover the cervix may not be readily apparent with a routine transabdominal screening examination; therefore a high index of suspicion should be maintained. Transvaginal color Doppler ultrasound should be strongly considered in any case of velamentous cord insertion, a succenturiate lobe, or when portions of umbilical

cord are noted to be low in the uterus (Fig. 9-25). The sonographer should also be aware that when placenta previa "resolves," branches of the umbilical vessels on the chorionic plate may still course over the cervix as placental villi degenerate beneath them, resulting in vasa previa. Identifying the cord insertion onto the placenta eliminates the possibility of velamentous cord insertion, but it does not exclude vasa previa from the other placentation abnormalities. **Documentation of the cord insertion onto the placenta is good practice, and it is recommended when technically possible.**[16]

In addition to determining the placenta's location, its appearance should be assessed. Many changes observed in the placenta are related to calcification, fibrosis, and infarction. The general trend is for these changes to become more apparent as pregnancy progresses, but their clinical significance is unclear. It has recently been recognized that a "globular" placenta, with a narrow base compared with height, is associated with an increased rate of IUGR, fetal death, and other complications.[30]

The sonographer should confirm that there are two arteries and a vein in the umbilical cord.[16] In late pregnancy, this can be ascertained by looking at a transverse cut of the cord in a free loop. In the second trimester, two umbilical arteries are most easily confirmed by identifying the vessels with color Doppler as they course around the fetal bladder (Fig. 9-26). **A single umbilical artery is present in about 0.5% of all newborns. Because of the increased incidence of associated malformations, especially those that involve the kidneys and heart, this finding should prompt a detailed fetal survey.** Fetuses with a single umbilical artery have a 20% chance of growth restriction. Additionally, the rate of polyhydramnios, abruption, placenta previa, structural placental abnormalities, cesarean delivery, low Apgar scores, and fetal death are all increased.[31]

Uterus and Adnexa

With any obstetric ultrasound, including those performed in the first trimester, the adnexal and uterine morphology should be evaluated. Many women enter pregnancy without being aware that they have fibroids or a müllerian malformation. Fibroids are usually readily apparent with transvaginal or transabdominal ultrasound. **A common pitfall is to confuse uterine contractions, which are commonly present in the second trimester, with fibroids** (Fig. 9-27). **Contractions have a more lenticular shape and blend with the surrounding myometrium, whereas fibroids usually are spherical with distinct borders and a whorled internal echo texture.** Pedunculated fibroids, even large ones, can be missed if the sonographer does not examine areas around the periphery of the uterus. Most studies have shown a higher rate of pregnancy complications when fibroids are present. However, the odds ratios are typically modest and of limited clinical importance.[32] It is difficult to predict how fibroids will affect an individual patient's pregnancy because the number, size, and location can vary markedly. **Ultrasound mapping of fibroids can help in making a delivery plan.** Although large fibroids that fill the pelvis may preclude vaginal birth, it is usually prudent to not predict early in the pregnancy the need for cesarean delivery. Fibroids can rise out of the pelvis, leaving a relatively clear lower uterine segment. **Because multiple fibroids in the lower uterus can greatly complicate the performance of a low transverse cesarean delivery, ultrasound may help predict the need for a classical incision.** Studies with serial ultrasound exams have had conflicting results in regard to the growth of fibroids during pregnancy.[33,34]

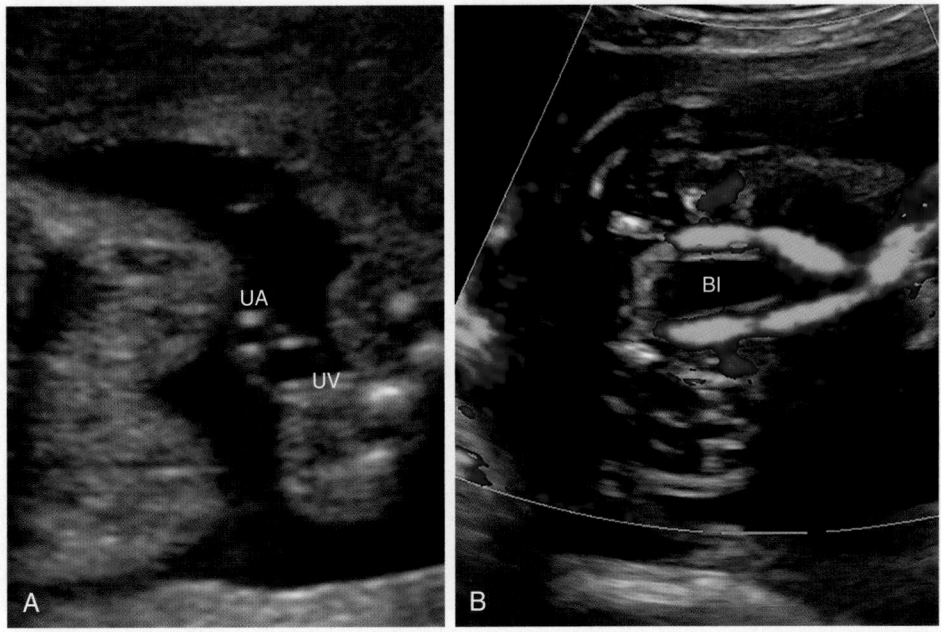

FIG 9-26 A, Umbilical vein (UV) and a single umbilical artery (UA) are shown in a transverse section of a free loop of cord. **B,** A transverse view of the fetal pelvis, using color Doppler, clearly shows the normal paired umbilical arteries coursing around the bladder (Bl). It is often easier to document the umbilical arteries in early pregnancy with this color Doppler method.

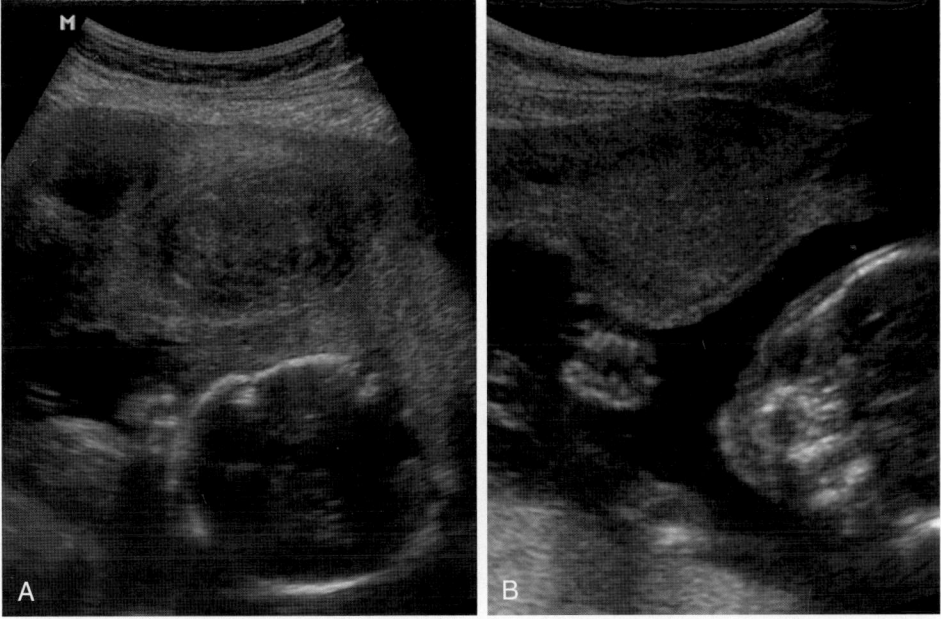

FIG 9-27 A, Two fibroids are shown that are round and well circumscribed. **B,** Uterine contraction is lenticular in shape and does not have a clear border. Contractions such as this are very common in the second trimester.

Cervix

It has been clearly documented that a short cervix, as measured with transvaginal ultrasound, is associated with an increased risk of preterm birth in both high- and low-risk patients (see Chapters 28 and 29). Intervention with a cervical cerclage has been shown to improve outcome in patients with a prior spontaneous preterm birth who have a short cervix in a subsequent pregnancy.[35] **Treatment of low-risk women who have a short cervix with vaginal progesterone has also been shown to reduce the rate of preterm birth.**[36] However, the value of universal screening is unproven, and ACOG currently does not recommend this practice.[3] The lower limit of normal for cervical length in the mid second trimester is 25 mm. When the routine 18- to 20-week transabdominal ultrasound shows a length less than this, referral for a specialized exam is appropriate.

Adnexa

It is important for a complete obstetric ultrasound to include an assessment of the adnexa. Normal-sized ovaries may be difficult or impossible to see in the second or third trimester because of shielding by bowel. In a study of sonographic

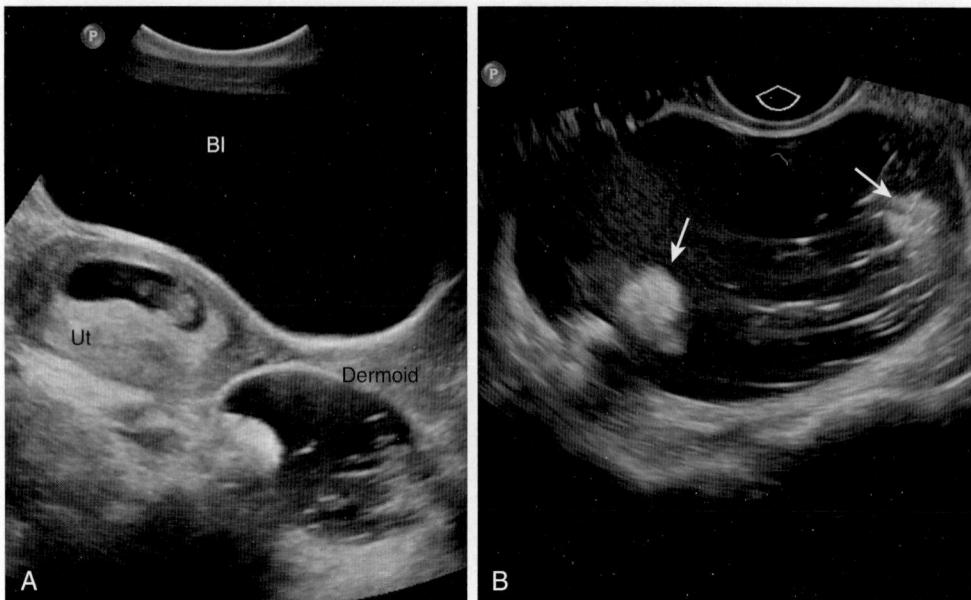

FIG 9-28 Transabdominal and transvaginal images of an ovarian dermoid. **A,** An 8-week pregnancy with the uterus (Ut) demarcated in the transabdominal image. **B,** Using transvaginal ultrasound, the mass fills the entire field of view. Characteristic irregular mixed solid and cystic areas with highly echogenic nodules (*arrows*) are seen within the dermoid. To see the pelvic structures clearly with transabdominal ultrasound, the maternal bladder (Bl) must be very full. Although this provides a good window, the structures of interest are pushed away from the probe, which limits resolution. In contrast, the probe is less than 1 cm from the mass when vaginal ultrasound is used.

visualization of normal ovaries, Shalev and coworkers[37] found that although both ovaries were visible in almost all first-trimester scans, both ovaries were visible in only 16% of second- and third-trimester scans, and in 60% of these, neither ovary was seen. However, in most cases when a significant tumor is present, it will be visible. The sonographic appearance of an adnexal mass discovered during pregnancy guides decision making regarding the need for surgical removal. **Masses that consist of simple cysts usually represent benign processes and do not require removal during pregnancy. Masses with features of malignancy—such as large size, multiple cystic cavities, thick septa, internal papillae, or solid areas—require careful evaluation and may require operative removal.** The most common neoplasms in pregnancy are benign cystic teratomas (Fig. 9-28). These can usually be identified by their sonographic characteristics.

Anatomic Survey

Systematic evaluation of fetal anatomy is critical. It is a good idea to proceed with an examination in a consistent order so that important parts are not forgotten. Although many well-recognized maternal risk factors exist for congenital anomalies, 90% of birth defects occur in fetuses of low-risk women.[3] For this reason, it is important that anyone who performs obstetric ultrasound have familiarity with the appearance of normal fetal anatomy in order to recognize deviations from normal. As mentioned previously, although more advanced detailed sonograms (specialized examinations) are appropriate for patients with identified risk factors, **all standard examinations should include a full anatomic survey.** An overview of some of the more common fetal malformations that can be recognized at the time of a standard ultrasound examination is presented later in this chapter.

When components of the standard second- or third-trimester ultrasound examination cannot be obtained because of maternal obesity, unfavorable fetal position, or other technical factors, this should be documented in the report. In such patients, it is reasonable to repeat the ultrasound in 2 to 4 weeks. If a second attempt is unsuccessful, no further exams to attempt better visualization are necessary.[3,16]

Documentation

A report for any ultrasound exam should list the indication. Documentation of ultrasound findings is important not only for good patient care but also for quality review and legal defense. **AIUM guidelines in regard to record keeping state, "Adequate documentation of the study is essential for high-quality patient care. This should include a permanent record of the sonographic images, incorporating whenever possible … measurement parameters and anatomic findings."[3,12]**

Cleaning and Disinfection of Probes

To avoid transmitting disease from one patient to another, **proper cleansing and disinfecting of probes is important.**[3] With a transabdominal probe, it is sufficient to simply wipe the probe clean with a disposable antiseptic paper towelette. Transvaginal probes should be covered during use with a disposable latex or nonlatex cover. Following the exam, the probe should be cleaned with running water or a damp cloth. It is then important that chemical high-level disinfection be carried out as per the probe manufacturer's recommendations.

ULTRASOUND FOR DETERMINING GESTATIONAL AGE

Determination of the correct gestational age is one of the most important aspects of prenatal care. Making correct management decisions for conditions such as preterm labor, prolonged and postterm pregnancy, and preeclampsia depends heavily on knowledge of the gestational age of the fetus. Without early confirmation of the estimated date of delivery (EDD), it is very difficult to diagnose growth disorders in the fetus. Biochemical screening for open fetal defects and chromosomal anomalies likewise requires accurate dating. **For these and other reasons, it has become routine in developed countries to offer at least one ultrasound examination in the first half of pregnancy to accurately establish the gestational age.**[3]

Standard Measurements

Ian Donald first demonstrated the clinical use of ultrasound in obstetrics in the early 1960s with the measurement of the BPD. Since that time, a large number of publications have correlated this parameter with gestational age. The BPD can first be measured from 12 to 13 weeks' gestation, when the skull has become ossified. Other standard measurements that include the femur length (FL), abdominal circumference (AC), and head circumference (HC) can also be made starting in the late first trimester.

With transvaginal ultrasound, the embryo can be measured when it is only a few millimeters long, between 5 and 6 weeks' gestation. From 6 to 10 weeks' gestation, the maximal length of the embryo is measured. After about 10 weeks, the head, trunk, and extremities are visible, and the measurement is literally from the well-visualized crown to the rump.[38] Views of the CRL such as those shown in Figure 9-29 are obtained. **Because the fetus is often in a flexed position** (Fig. 9-30)**, the CRL becomes less accurate after the first trimester and should not be used after it reaches 84 mm** (14 weeks of gestation).[39]

It is possible to measure virtually any body part of the fetus. However, a standard set of measurements has been accepted as being the most useful for gestational age prediction. After the first trimester, these include the BPD, HC, AC, and FL. Unless these are measured according to standard criteria (Box 9-2), their value in defining the age or growth of a fetus is limited. Optimal views for obtaining measurements are shown in Figures 9-31 to 9-35. Common errors to be avoided are also shown. With practice, a sonographer learns to slide the transducer to the proper position on the maternal abdominal wall then angulate and rotate the transducer until the precise plane for biometry or anatomic assessment is obtained. In time, making these adjustments becomes second nature.

Gestational Age Determination

In very early pregnancy, the gestational sac diameter can give a fairly close approximation of the gestational age. The mean sac diameter increases by about 1 mm per day, and the gestational age (in days) can be figured by adding 30 to the mean sac diameter (in millimeters).[40] Because the range of error in age prediction from sac measurement is significantly greater than for the CRL and other standard measurements, the sac

---

BOX 9-2   DESCRIPTION OF IMAGES FOR FETAL BIOMETRY

Head
- Image is from side not front or back.
- Head is oval rather than round.
- Midline structures are centered not displaced to the side.
- Measure at the level of thalamus and cavum septum pellucidum.
- Image should not include the top of the orbits or any part of the brainstem or cerebellum.
- Measure outer edge of the proximal skull to the inner edge of the distal skull.
- Head circumference is measured at the level of the biparietal diameter, around the outer perimeter of the skull.

Abdomen
- Abdomen is nearly round, not oval or squashed.
- Obtain a true transverse image not oblique.
- Images of ribs should be similar on both sides.
- Measure at the level where the umbilical vein joins the portal sinus.
- Calipers are all the way to the skin surface not at the rib, liver, or spine edge.

Femur
- Femur should be perpendicular to direction of insonation.
- Ends should be sharply visible not tapered or fuzzy.
- The measurement should exclude the distal epiphysis.

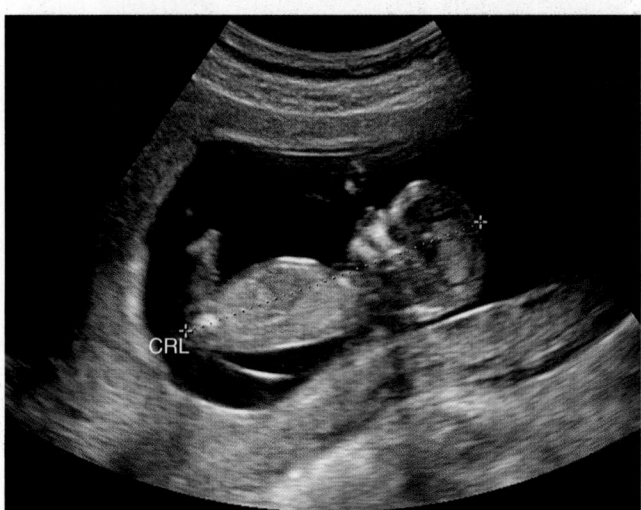

FIG 9-29 Measurement of the crown-rump length (CRL). This is a sagittal view of the fetus with the crown of the head to the right and the rump to the left.

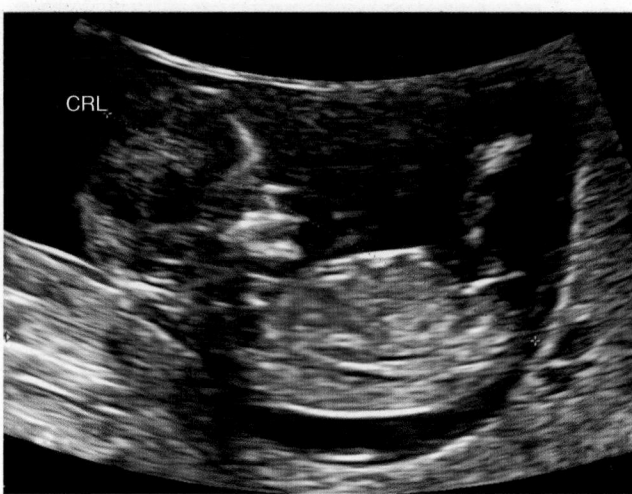

FIG 9-30 This is an inappropriate image for obtaining the crown-rump length (CRL) because the flexed position of the fetus gives a falsely low measurement.

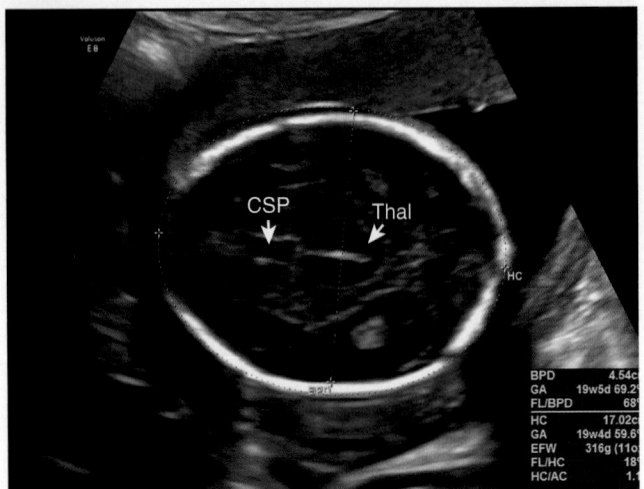

FIG 9-31 Image of the fetal head for biparietal diameter and head circumference measurements. The cavum septum pellucidum (CSP) and the thalami (Thal) are indicated. Criteria for an appropriate image are listed in Box 9-2.

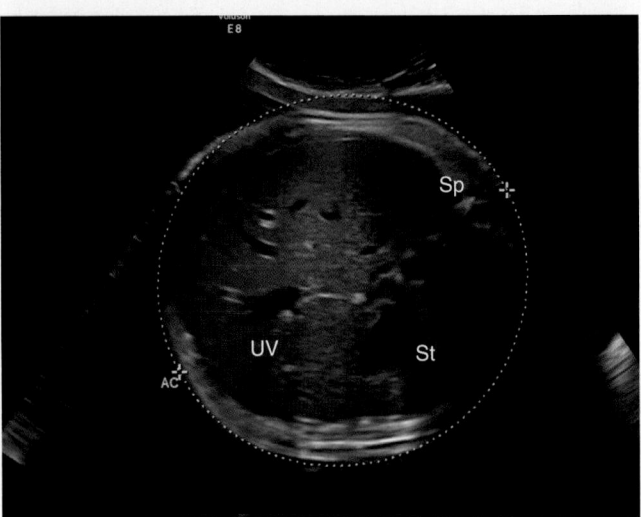

FIG 9-33 Proper image for measurement of the abdominal circumference (AC). Criteria for an appropriate image are listed in Box 9-2. The umbilical vein (UV) is seen at the level of the portal sinus. The stomach (St) and spine (Sp) are also labeled.

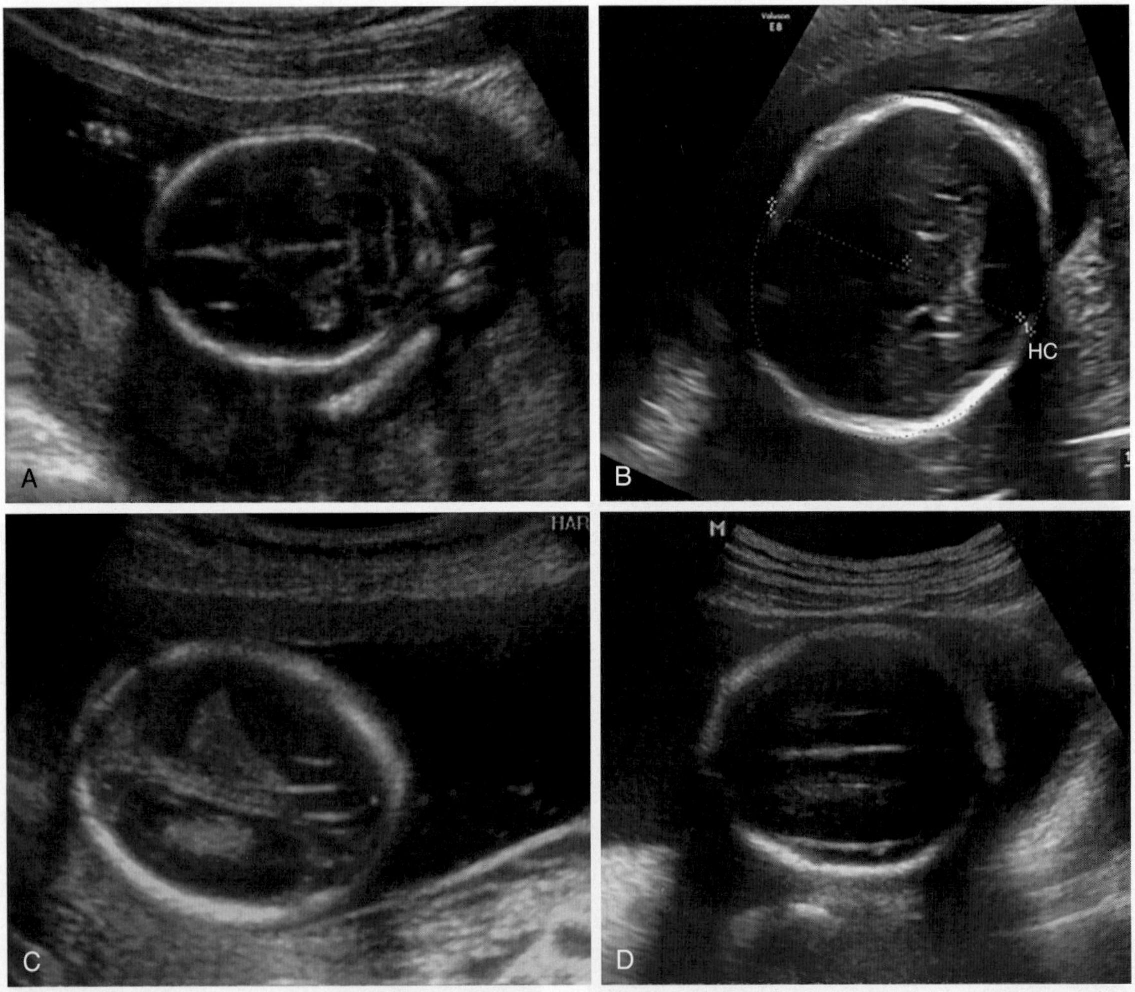

FIG 9-32 Examples of inappropriate head views for biparietal diameter and head circumference (HC) measurements. **A,** The transducer is rotated in such a way that the image includes the cerebellum. **B,** The head is imaged from the back and not from the side. **C,** The scan plane goes though the head obliquely. Note how the brain structures are asymmetric. **D,** This true axial image is too high on the head. The cavum septum pellucidum is not seen.

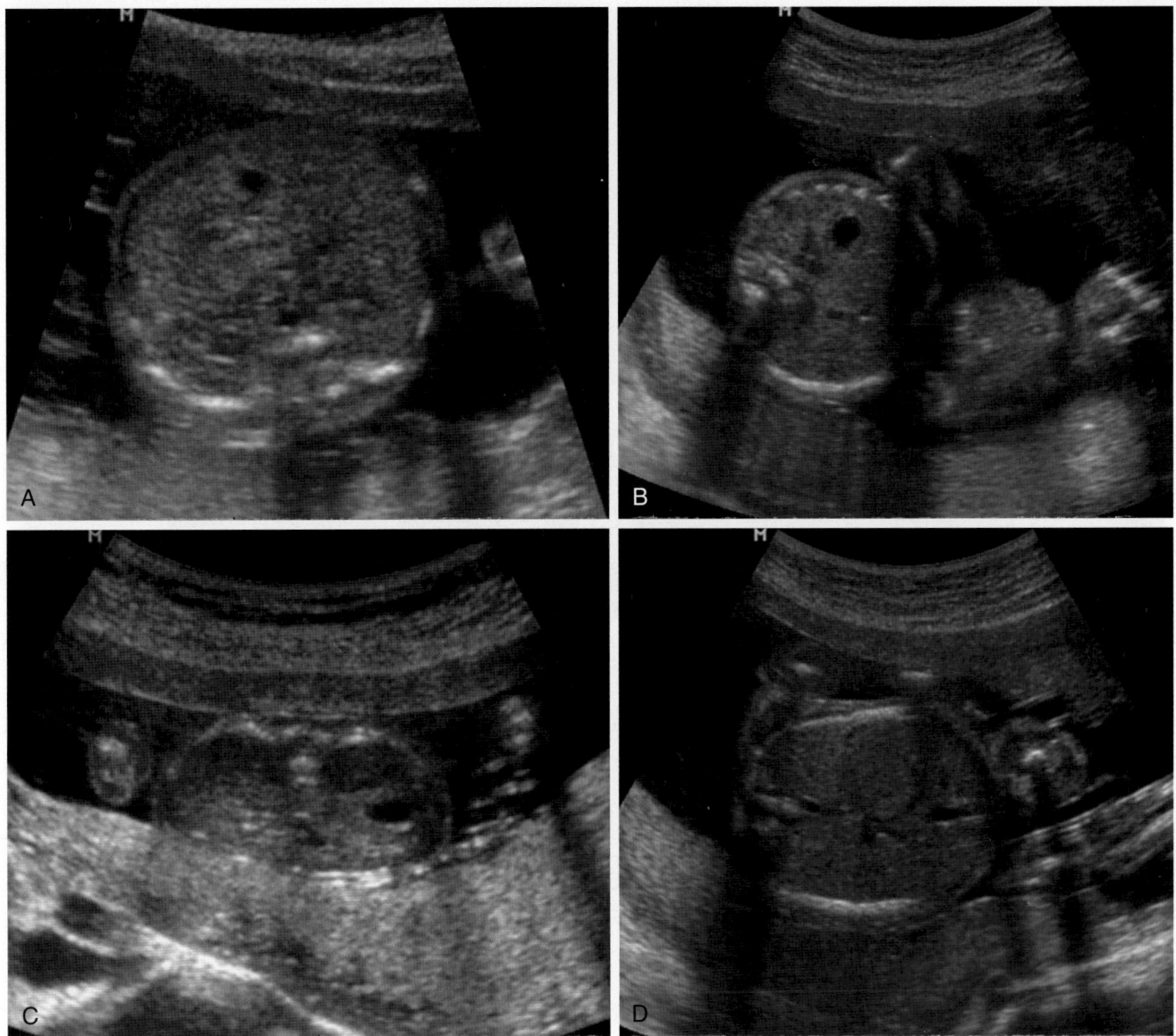

FIG 9-34 Examples of abdominal views that are inappropriate for abdominal circumference measurements. **A,** This true axial image is too low on the abdomen. The umbilical vein is seen close to the anterior abdominal wall. **B,** This is an oblique cut through the abdomen. Note the asymmetric appearance of the ribs. **C,** The abdomen is overly compressed because the sonographer has applied too much pressure to the maternal abdominal wall. **D,** The transducer is rotated in such a way that an oblong view of the abdomen is obtained. This gives an artificially elongated anterior-posterior dimension.

size should not be used as the final gestational age determinant.[3] **The measurement of the early embryo, either as the maximal embryo length or CRL, is commonly accepted as the best sonographic method for gestational age determination.** Using a static scanner in pregnancies dated by "good" menstrual dates, Robinson and Fleming[41] found that the 95% confidence intervals for gestational age prediction using the CRL was ±4.7 days. Later studies, in which gestational age was determined by in vitro fertilization, showed an even smaller random error.[42] **The high accuracy of ultrasound dating of early embryos is explained by their relatively large weekly percentage change in size and the fact that very little variation is seen among early embryos in their growth rates. The variability of gestational age estimations increases with advancing gestation.**[3,39]

The 95% confidence intervals for gestational age prediction using the BPD as a single parameter between 14 and 21 weeks is ±7 days.[43] In a study of pregnancies dated by in vitro fertilization, Chervenak and colleagues[44] found that in this period of pregnancy, all of the single parameters considered (BPD, HC, and FL) performed quite well: 95% confidence intervals for the gestational age ranged between ±7.5 days for the HC and ±8.7 days for the FL. Composite gestational age assessment using mathematic modeling from multiple parameters is now the most accepted method of ultrasound dating after the first trimester.[39] **The studies previously cited show that gestational age calculation using a combination of standard parameters before 22 weeks is accurate to within ±7 days and is comparable to CRL measurement in the first trimester. For this reason, it is not necessary to refer a patient for ultrasound in the first trimester for the sole purpose of obtaining optimal dates.**[45]

As pregnancy progress beyond 22 weeks, variability in fetal size increases considerably, and ultrasound prediction of gestational age becomes progressively less accurate. In

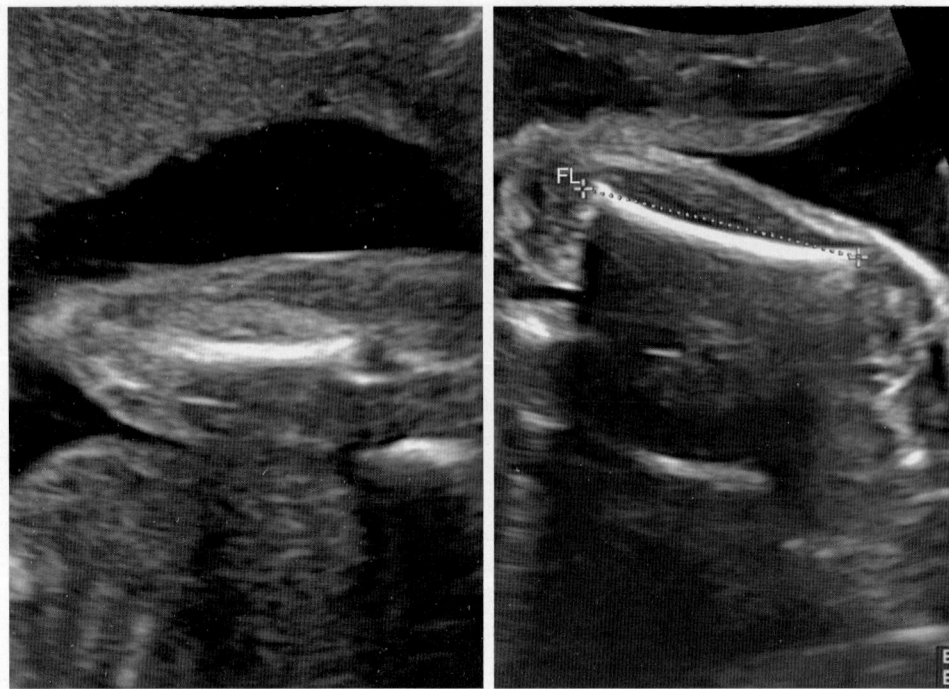

FIG 9-35 In the left image, the entire diaphysis of the femur is not clearly shown. This will give an inappropriately short measurement. The ends should be distinct, as shown in the image on the right. FL, femur length.

one study, the composite gestational age assessment at 24 to 30 weeks had a variability (±2 standard deviations) of 1.8 weeks, and after 30 weeks, the variability was 2 to 3 weeks.[38] These variability figures represent a statistical description of the variability of the gestational age calculations in the studied population. In the third trimester, growth disorders in fetuses are relatively common and can bring about marked size variation. For this reason, **the obstetrician must exercise caution when basing management decisions on third-trimester ultrasound dates.**

When to Use Ultrasound Dating

Since the time of Nägele in the early 1800s, obstetric providers have routinely used menstrual dates for determining the EDD. **Agreement is near universal that in pregnancies in which the menstrual dates are uncertain or thought to be unreliable because of a history of uncertain recall, irregular cycles, recent hormonal contraception use, or an abnormally light last menstrual period (LMP), dates derived from ultrasound biometry are preferred.**[3,16,39] Because variations in timing of ovulation even with a certain LMP have never been shown to be less than the variation in age assessment from ultrasound,[16] it could be argued that dating can be best be established by ultrasound measurements, ignoring menstrual dates. Nevertheless, all recent guidelines on establishing gestational age include references to menstrual dates. **In a 2014 reaffirmation of a 2009 ACOG practice bulletin,[3] it was suggested that ultrasound dates should take precedence over the menstrual dates if an ultrasound performed in the first trimester is more than 7 days different or an ultrasound exam before 20 weeks is discrepant by more than 10 days.** A joint committee opinion issued in 2014 from ACOG, AIUM, and the Society for Maternal-Fetal Medicine (SMFM) entitled "Method for Estimating Due Date" made very specific recommendations that extend through the entire pregnancy (Table 9-1).[39] **Importantly, the committee opinion and the 2009 ACOG practice bulletin**

TABLE 9-1	CIRCUMSTANCE IN WHICH ULTRASOUND GESTATIONAL AGE DETERMINATION SHOULD TAKE PRECEDENCE OVER "GOOD" MENSTRUAL DATES
GESTATIONAL AGE (WEEKS)	**USE ULTRASOUND DATES IF DISCREPANCY IS:**
Less than 8 6/7	>5 days
From 9 0/7 to 15 6/7	>7 days
From 16 0/7 to 21 6/7	>10 days
From 22 0/7 to 27 6/7	>14 days
Greater than 28 0/7	>21 days

From American College of Obstetricians and Gynecologists. Committee opinion no 611: method for estimating due date: *Obstet Gynecol.* 2014;124:863-866.

both note that in the third trimester aberrant growth is relatively common, so changing certain menstrual dates in favor of a late ultrasound date risks missing the presence of a significant growth disorder, and decisions about changing dates require careful consideration and close surveillance.[3,39]

Assessing Fetal Growth

The first ultrasound examination is generally considered to be a dating examination; that is, the measurements are used to determine the gestational age. An accurate knowledge of gestational age determined or confirmed by the first ultrasound examination forms the basis for subsequent clinical and sonographic assessments of fetal growth. **Because insufficient or excessive growth can be associated with significant fetal morbidity, recognition of growth abnormalities is one of the primary aims of prenatal care and is an important aspect of ultrasound examinations.** In most obstetric practices, growth ultrasound examinations are obtained when abdominal palpation and fundal height measurements raise the suspicion of abnormal growth.[46] A lagging fundal height, combined with the knowledge of clinical risk factors for IUGR, is commonly used as a "screening test" for insufficient fetal growth, whereas ultrasound is considered the "diagnostic test." This scheme for the prenatal detection of growth-restricted fetuses has met with mixed results. Although some studies have shown sensitivities for the detection of small for gestational age (SGA) fetuses with fundal height to be as low as 15%,[46] others suggest a 65% to 85% sensitivity and 96% specificity.[47] The positive predictive value of a lagging fundal height for diagnosing IUGR has been reported to be 50%. Schemes for the antenatal diagnosis of small fetuses may perform significantly better if clinical risk factors are taken into account.[48,49]

Serial ultrasound examinations have been shown to be superior to physical examination for diagnosing insufficient growth.[50] For this reason, some have advocated a routine third-trimester ultrasound examination to screen for growth abnormalities even in low-risk pregnancies. Studies have shown, however, that this policy has little or no impact on perinatal morbidity and mortality.[47,51] **Because of the high cost and unproven benefit of such a screening program, routine ultrasound examinations for growth are generally not a part of prenatal care in the United States. However, it is still accepted that ultrasound should be ordered when clinical examination is suspicious and when significant risk factors for a growth abnormality are present.** Such risk factors include diabetes mellitus, maternal hypertension, a previous small or large baby, multiple gestation, or poor maternal weight gain. A risk-based approach is particularly appropriate in cases such as multiple gestation or marked maternal obesity, in which clinical evaluation of fetal size is difficult or impossible.[16,47]

Estimating Fetal Weight

A large number of formulas for calculating the estimated fetal weight (EFW) have been proposed. The most popular of these have been compiled in a review by Nyberg and colleagues.[40] **All incorporate the abdominal circumference because this is the standard measurement most susceptible to the variations in fetal soft tissue mass.** Although the AC alone is a fairly good marker for detecting abnormal fetal growth, the addition of other standard measurements to estimated weight formulas increases their accuracy.[52] **It has been shown that the addition of measurements beyond the standard set (BPD, HC, AC, and FL) does not significantly improve weight estimations. It appears that the error inherent in obtaining the basic measurements, especially the AC, is great enough to obscure any refinement in accuracy that might be gained from additional measurements.**

Many studies have been done to evaluate the accuracy of ultrasound for predicting birthweight.[40] It has been claimed in some publications that one formula is better than another when statistically significant differences in accuracy are seen. However, the differences in accuracy are usually of limited clinical significance, and no formula has been consistently shown to be superior to another.[53]

When scans are done by well-trained sonographers, most studies show a mean absolute error in weight prediction of about 8% to 10% of the actual birthweight. Overall, 74% of infants have a birthweight within 10% of ultrasound estimates.[54] In 5% of cases, the deviation is greater than 20%.[47]

It is often assumed that ultrasound is more objective than clinical examination and that ultrasound estimates of fetal weight are therefore more reliable. Surprisingly, most studies have not shown this to be true. In a review by Sherman and colleagues[53] of 12 studies in which ultrasound was compared with clinical examination for weight estimation, ultrasound was found to be clearly superior in only one, and it involved a subgroup of patients with birthweights less than 2500 g. In three studies, clinical estimates were superior, and in the remaining eight, the two methods either were equivalent or had mixed results depending on the specific formula used. Interestingly, one study[55] showed that a term parous woman in labor is about as accurate in predicting the birthweight as clinical estimation by a physician or a sonographic estimate. Although it has not been proven, it is reasonable to assume that ultrasound measurements, fetal palpation, and maternal characteristics can complement one another. When the discrepancy between modalities is marked, the clinician should be prompted to reassess the results of each method. Strategies aimed at improving the performance of ultrasound for estimating fetal weight—for example, using formulas based on subpopulations of fetuses, such as those who are preterm or are thought to be small or large for gestational age—have not shown a clinically important improvement in the accuracy of weight estimates compared with traditional "one-size-fits-all" formulas.[56]

Diagnosing Abnormal Growth

The most accepted way of diagnosing abnormal growth in a fetus is to calculate the EFW using standard ultrasound measurements and then compare the estimated weight with an accepted standard. Several of these are in common use in currently available ultrasound software.

If the EFW is less than the 10th or greater than the 90th percentile, the fetus is said to be small or large for the gestational age.[47,57] Defining abnormal growth using these percentile cutoffs includes many babies who are healthy but are constitutionally large or small. Using a more restrictive definition, such as a birthweight less than the 3rd or greater than the 97th percentile, is more predictive of a poor neonatal outcome. Of course, using these criteria would fail to detect many less severely affected fetuses. Additionally, some infants have a birthweight within the normal range but have not grown to their genetic potential. For this reason, some investigators have argued that individual birthweight percentile limits that incorporate such characteristics as maternal weight, height, ethnic group, parity, and fetal sex should be used.[58] Claussen and colleagues[59] found that about one fourth of fetuses judged to be abnormally small using conventional limits were within normal limits with adjusted percentiles. Conversely, one fourth of babies identified as small or large with adjusted percentiles would have been missed by conventional assessment. In another study from the same institution, it was demonstrated that the risk for stillbirth, neonatal death, and low Apgar scores can be better predicted by the customized weight percentiles. However, the use of customized formulas has not been shown to improve outcomes and are not in common use.[47]

Growth Restriction

In 1977, Campbell and Thoms[60] described the HC/AC ratio as a useful marker for detecting fetal growth restriction (see Chapter 33). This was based on the observation that growth of the soft tissues in the fetal abdomen is more likely to be compromised than the head when nutritional deprivation is an issue. This understanding led to the concept that *asymmetric growth restriction* is virtually pathognomonic of nutritional deprivation, whereas *symmetric growth restriction* signifies an underlying condition such as aneuploidy. This categorization has some utility, but it should be recognized that a great deal of overlap exists between body ratios of fetuses whose growth is restricted from either nutritional or intrinsic factors. However, because a very high HC/AC ratio is uncommon in normal fetuses, such a ratio points away from constitutional smallness. Additionally, it has been shown in newborns that a low weight/length ratio is associated with an increase in several markers of morbidity even if the birthweight is greater than the 10th percentile; this perhaps indicates these infants also experienced growth restriction.[61] Currently, no consensus has been reached concerning the level of surveillance appropriate for a fetus with a high HC/AC ratio but normal estimated weight.

When a patient presents late for prenatal care and the gestational age is uncertain, diagnosis of a growth disorder is particularly difficult. In these cases, a high or low HC/AC ratio can raise the suspicion of a growth disorder. Other ultrasound findings may be useful to help confirm the suspicion. For example, IUGR is often associated with oligohydramnios, abnormal umbilical artery Doppler flow studies, or an abnormal-appearing placenta. Macrosomic fetuses may demonstrate obviously thickened subcutaneous fat pads. In suspected cases, as long as the fetus is stable, serial ultrasound examinations to evaluate growth are appropriate. **Repeated ultrasound exams for growth should be performed at least 2 to 4 weeks apart.** A shorter interval makes it difficult to tell if apparent trends are due to the real growth or variations in the measurement technique.[3] The rate of growth can be valuable for predicting adverse outcome. Formulas that define rates of normal growth have been published, but most clinicians rely on an observation of progressively increasing or decreasing weight percentiles to evaluate the severity of an ongoing growth disorder.

Macrosomia

The term *macrosomia* implies growth beyond a specific weight, usually 4000 or 4500 g. Morbidity is increased for infants who weigh 4000 to 4500 g compared with the general population, and risks increase sharply above 4500 g. **Large cohort studies support 4500 g as an EFW above which a fetus should be considered macrosomic.[57] The absolute error of ultrasound-estimated fetal weight is increased with macrosomia. When the birthweight exceeds 4500 g, only 50% of fetuses weigh within 10% of the ultrasound-derived estimate.**[54]

It has been hoped by many that ultrasound could aid in the difficult decisions faced by obstetricians when macrosomia is suspected. Because difficult delivery from shoulder dystocia can lead to permanent neurologic injury in the fetus, this is one of the most feared complications in obstetrics (see Chapter 17). Unfortunately, ultrasound for fetal weight estimation has proved to be of limited usefulness for the prevention of shoulder dystocia and other complications associated with fetal macrosomia.

In a review of 4480 deliveries by Gonen and colleagues,[62] ultrasound ordered because of a clinical suspicion of macrosomia only detected 17% of the infants who weighed over 4500 g, and only 1 of the 23 infants who weighed over 4500 g had a brachial plexus injury. Additionally, 93% of infants who had shoulder dystocia weighed less than 4500 g. **For these reasons, clinical investigators have concluded that most cases of injury that result from shoulder dystocia cannot be predicted by ultrasound and that if cesarean delivery were routinely performed when macrosomia was suspected, the rate of cesarean delivery would be increased with very little benefit.**

SAFETY OF ULTRASOUND

Since diagnostic ultrasound was introduced for clinical use, attention has appropriately been given to ensuring its safety. It has been recognized that the energy from sound waves is converted into heat as sound waves are attenuated. **Mechanical energy from the sound waves can cause the formation of microbubbles, resulting in a phenomenon called *cavitation*.** Because cavitation occurs only under high ultrasound intensities where air is present, it is not of significant concern with diagnostic ultrasound of the fetus.

Quantifying Machine Power Output

As of 1976, trials had indicated that no clinically significant biologic effects were apparent from diagnostic ultrasound. It was subsequently recognized that it would be impractical to repeat safety studies for each new generation of ultrasound machines operating with different modalities and power outputs. The U.S. Food and Drug Administration (FDA) decided that approval for equipment marketed after 1976 would require acoustic outputs less than that of equipment that existed at that time, which was 94 mW/cm^2 spatial-peak temporal-average (SPTA). However, it has become apparent that improvements in ultrasound imaging can be obtained in some cases with higher power levels than is allowed under this regulation. The FDA agreed to relax this standard if machines provided users with real-time information that indicates the potential for fetal harm from the higher-power outputs now allowed. An *output display standard* was adopted that showed the required information on the ultrasound monitor. The numbers pertinent to users of obstetric ultrasound are the thermal indexes for soft tissue (TIs) and bone (TIb). **The thermal index denotes the potential for increasing the temperature of tissue being insonated with that power output.** It is determined by the settings and ultrasound modalities being used. A thermal index (TI) of 1.0 indicates that given certain conditions, the temperature of the tissue may be increased by 1° C. Because little bone formation occurs in the first trimester, the TIs is more relevant. Later in pregnancy, as ossification occurs, sound waves have a greater impact on bone, so the TIb becomes more important. If the output display standard is followed, the new regulations allow the ultrasound intensity to be as high as 720 mW/cm^2. Machines that do not have the output display still must operate with a maximal sound intensity of less than 94 mW/cm^2.

A 2008 official statement from the AIUM[63] on ultrasound bioeffects states that no effects have been observed from unfocused beam SPTA intensities below 100 mW/cm^2 or TI values less than 2. In 2009, the World Health Organization (WHO) sponsored a systematic review and meta-analysis to evaluate the safety of human exposure to ultrasonography in pregnancy. This study showed no adverse maternal or perinatal effects, impaired physical or neurologic development, increased risk for malignancy in childhood, subnormal intellectual performance, or mental diseases. This analysis concluded that according to the available evidence, exposure to diagnostic ultrasonography during pregnancy appears to be safe.[64] **Taking into account the many studies that have been done to date, an official statement from the AIUM on prudent use and clinical safety states, "No independently confirmed adverse effects caused by exposure from present diagnostic ultrasound instruments have been reported in human patients in the absence of contrast agents."**[65] Nevertheless, researchers in the field caution about the possibility that unrecognized harm exists. For this reason, the AIUM position remains that ultrasound should be used by qualified health professionals to provide medical benefit to the patient. **In another official statement, the AIUM propounds the ALARA principle (as low as reasonably achievable).**[66] **This means that the potential benefits and risks of each examination should be considered, and equipment controls should be adjusted to reduce as much as the possible the acoustic output from the transducer.**

In general, ultrasound energy and the potential for temperature elevation become progressively greater from B-mode to color Doppler to spectral Doppler. For this reason, M-mode ultrasound is preferred for documenting fetal viability in the first trimester (see Fig. 9-7).[4] However, Doppler modes should be used liberally to confirm fetal death.

ULTRASOUND DIAGNOSIS OF MALFORMATIONS

Over the past few decades, a large number of publications have described the ultrasound diagnosis of fetal malformations. A catalog of the diseases now considered detectable with prenatal ultrasound is beyond the scope of this chapter. This section addresses the use of ultrasound as a general screening test for malformations, discusses the role of ultrasound in aneuploidy screening, and describes the relatively common birth defects that may be diagnosed with a standard ultrasound examination.

Ultrasound as a Screening Tool for Birth Defects

With improvements of ultrasound equipment in the last few decades, many patients and clinicians have come to assume an ultrasound exam will likely detect all serious fetal anomalies. Indeed, in the 1980s and early 1990s, several individual centers reported detection rates of greater than 75% in referral and low-risk patients. **However, serious questions in regard to the sensitivity of routine ultrasound exams in more general settings were raised by a large multicenter randomized trial published in 1993,** the Routine Antenatal Diagnostic Imaging With Ultrasound Study (RADIUS).[67] This randomized trial included standardized ultrasound exams of over 15,000 women between 16 and 20 weeks' gestation and then again at 31 to 33 weeks. Patients were selected to be at low risk for pregnancy complications. In this study, only 17% of major anomalies were diagnosed by ultrasound prior to 24 weeks' gestation, and only 35% were detected overall. **The study's authors concluded that routine ultrasound to screen for birth defects in low-risk women was not efficacious.** A subsequent large study of ultrasound screening for birth defects, the Eurofetus study,[68] included over 200,000 women screened with routine ultrasound in 61 hospital units in 14 European countries. In contrast to the low rate of detection of anomalies in the RADIUS trial, 61% of malformed fetuses were detected. The sensitivity was higher for major malformations (74%), and a significant difference in detection rates was found according to the particular malformation or organ system involved. Defects of the central nervous system and urinary tract were detected 88% of the time, whereas only 18% of cases of cleft lip and palate were diagnosed. Ultrasound identified 18% of minor musculoskeletal malformations and 21% of minor cardiac malformations, and sensitivities were 74% and 39% for major anomalies of these two organ systems.

The nature of the population being screened and the thoroughness of postnatal ascertainment of birth defects also affect the sensitivity of ultrasound for detecting defects. **The detection rate has been shown to be higher in high-risk populations screened at centers with extensive experience at diagnosing birth defects.** In studies that did not include rigorous prospective neonatal evaluation, subtle anomalies may not have been noted, and a sonographic "miss" of these defects would not be counted. This would give a falsely optimistic detection rate. **The gestational age at which ultrasound is performed can influence the sensitivity of anomaly screening.** Whereas many defects can now be recognized in the late first trimester (e.g. anencephaly and large abdominal wall defects), most are not visible until later. Some defects may become more readily apparent late in pregnancy. Although multiple exams in each pregnancy would undoubtedly increase the detection rate of malformations, resource and financial constraints make this impractical.

Summarizing the results of large studies and systematic reviews, the report of the 2014 National Institute of Child Health and Human Development (NICHD) Workshop on Fetal Imaging concluded that the range of detection rates for anomalies overall is wide, from 16% to 44% prior to 24 weeks of gestation, with a detection rate of 84% for major and lethal anomalies.[16]

In the hands of a well-trained examiner, the detection rate of some anomalies should approach 100%. For example, anencephaly, abdominal wall defects, and anomalies that involve an abnormal accumulation of fluid within a body cavity (e.g., hydronephrosis or hydrocephalus) will rarely be missed. The fact that spina bifida, which itself may be difficult to see, is almost always accompanied by easily recognized intracranial findings makes the detection rate of this defect quite high. The growing awareness that a screening ultrasound should include not only the four-chamber view of the heart (Fig. 9-36) but also views of the outflow tracts (Figs. 9-37 and 9-38) has resulted in a significant increase in the detection rate of heart defects. DeVore[69] reviewed three studies from the 1990s in which only the four-chamber view was obtained as part of a screening ultrasound in low-risk populations. Only 8 of 151 cases were identified with the four-chamber screening, giving a detection rate of 5%. In contrast, a 2006 Norwegian study[70] of over 30,000 unselected patients used not only the four-chamber view but also the great vessel views and showed a 57% prenatal detection rate of heart defects. **Because of studies that show the importance of outflow tract visualization for the detection of many heart defects, ACOG and the AIUM now recommend that attempts should be made to obtain these views in all second- and third-trimester scans.**[3,12]

It is well recognized that adequate training is essential to the proper performance and interpretation of obstetric ultrasound exams. In the RADIUS trial, the detection rate for anomalies was almost three times higher when the exams were performed at a tertiary center compared with a general practice setting (13% vs. 35%), presumably because of greater experience of sonographers at the tertiary centers. To maintain acceptable levels of sensitivity, compliance with the AIUM guidelines for training and experience is important.

It is generally agreed that the most cost-effective approach for screening low-risk pregnancies is to perform a standard examination between 18 and 20 weeks. At this gestational age, adequate visualization of major organs is possible for most women. In some, because of an unusually thick or dense maternal abdominal wall or unfavorable fetal position, completion of the anatomic survey is suboptimal, and a follow-up scan may be helpful.[3,16]

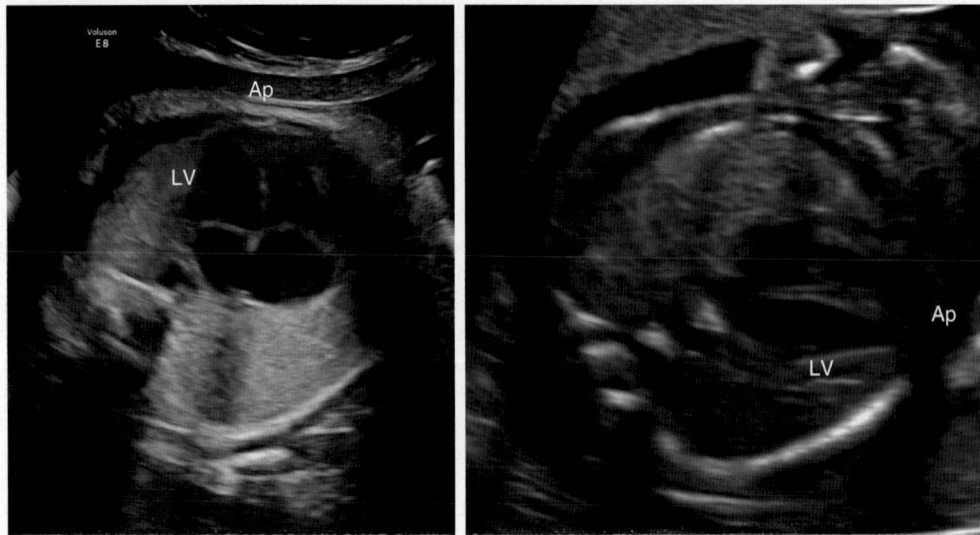

FIG 9-36 Normal four-chamber cardiac images from the apex (*left*) and lateral views (*right*). The apex (Ap) and left ventricle (LV) are labeled.

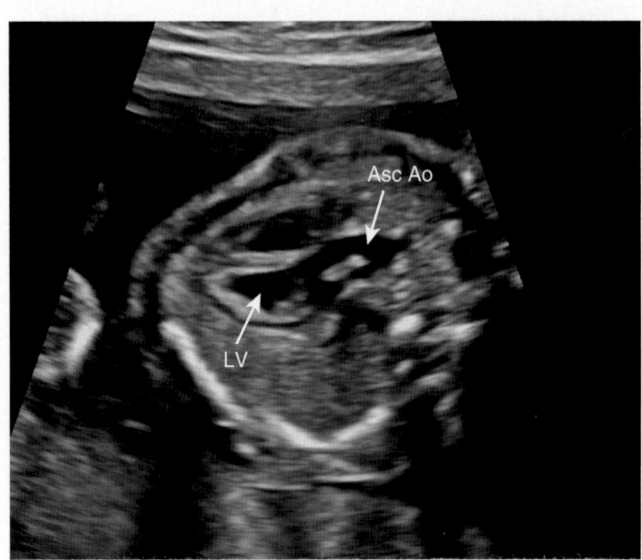

FIG 9-37 Left ventricular outflow tract view. The left ventricle (LV) and ascending aorta (Asc Ao) are indicated.

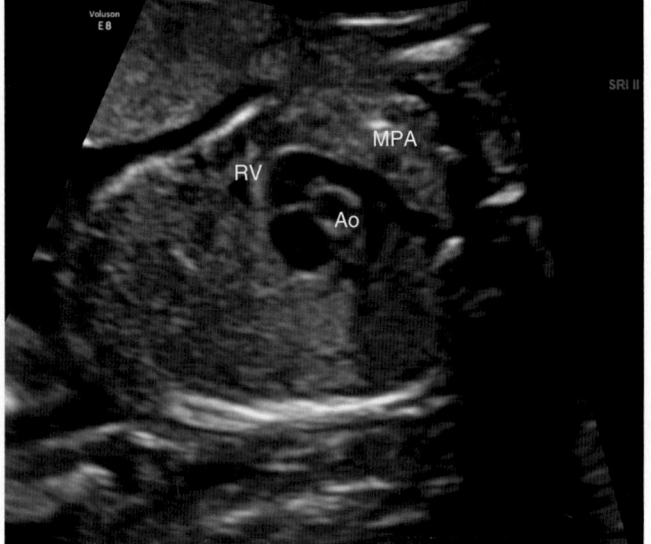

FIG 9-38 Right ventricular outflow tract view. The main pulmonary artery (MPA) arises from the right ventricle (RV) and crosses anterior to the ascending aorta (Ao) before bifurcating.

False-positive results must be taken into account when considering the effectiveness of ultrasound screening for birth defects. **Falsely abnormal results can cause patients and families considerable anguish and result in unnecessary follow-up tests.** Fortunately, in both the RADIUS and the Eurofetus trials, fewer than one in 500 women was erroneously told that her healthy fetus had a malformation.[67,68] However, of the nearly 3000 suspected malformations in the Eurofetus study, 10% were false-positive diagnoses, and 6% involved fetuses in which an initial concern was resolved on a subsequent ultrasound exam.

Screening for Aneuploidy
First Trimester
As has been previously discussed in this chapter, ultrasound assessment is an important part of first-trimester aneuploidy screening (see Chapter 10). **The most important sonographic component of first-trimester screening is the nuchal translucency measurement** (Fig. 9-39). **The presence or absence of a**
visible nasal bone is another important ultrasound finding. Other ultrasound findings have been described, such as reverse ductus venosus flow and tricuspid regurgitation, but they are not in general use.[71] Criteria are rigorous for appropriate nuchal translucency and nasal bone images, and individuals who wish to perform the ultrasound component of the first-trimester screen must be certified to do so.

Second Trimester
As is discussed in Chapter 10, well-established screening tests exist for fetal aneuploidy; however, the role of ultrasound in aneuploidy screening is less straightforward. Starting in 1985, a number of **"soft markers,"** as opposed to actual birth defects, were found to have an association with Down syndrome. **These include a thick nuchal fold, short nasal bone, cerebral ventriculomegaly, short femur or humerus, echogenic intracardiac focus, echogenic bowel, and pelviectasis** (Fig. 9-40, e-Figs. 9-1 and 9-2). It has been shown that these markers

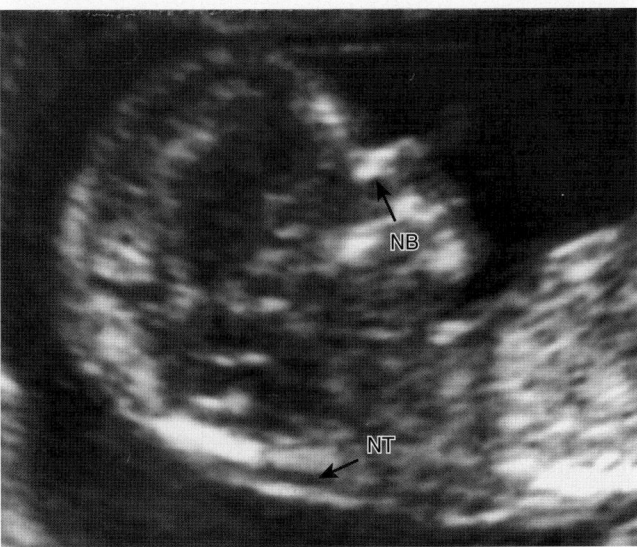

FIG 9-39 Midsagittal view of a 12-week fetus showing the nuchal translucency (NT) and nasal bone (NB).

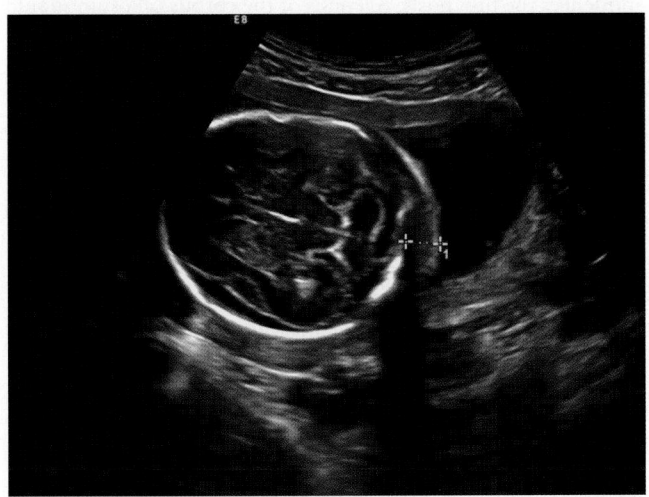

FIG 9-40 Axial image of a fetus with trisomy 21, showing a thick posterior nuchal fold (calipers).

perform poorly as individual predictors of Down syndrome. However, using likelihood ratios for each marker, they can be used in combination to calculate a formal risk adjustment for the presence of trisomy 21.[72] **In spite of the well-documented association between these markers and trisomy 21, the ultrasound at 18 to 20 weeks should not be considered an adequate screening test. A patient who desires such screening should be encouraged to use better-defined and well-established screening methods, which may include first-trimester screening, the quad screen, or cell-free DNA testing.**

Not infrequently, these soft markers are seen incidentally at the time of the screening exam at 20 weeks. The NICHD workshop on fetal imaging made recommendations on how to proceed in this circumstance.[16] It concluded that an echogenic intracardiac focus has such a small likelihood ratio that it does not significantly change the prior risk and can thus be ignored. The presence of other soft markers should prompt referral for a targeted ultrasound and other aneuploidy screening tests. Whenever a structural anomaly is identified, a finding that is not just a soft marker, invasive prenatal diagnosis should be offered.[71]

Screening for Anomalies With the Standard Ultrasound Examination

As previously noted, specific components should be evaluated in the course of a standard ultrasound exam performed in the second or third trimesters (see Box 9-1).[3,16] Careful attention to each of these components will allow detection of many, if not most, serious birth defects. In the following sections, normal structures will be demonstrated, and the alterations expected with different birth defects will be shown. The conditions described are those for which the general obstetrician should have familiarity and that might reasonably be detected with a standard screening ultrasound examination. Ultrasound images of most of these conditions are found in the online version of this book.

Head and Neck
GENERAL APPEARANCE
On axial views, the head should have an oval appearance. Elongation of the head, termed *dolichocephaly*, is often caused by lateral compressive forces associated with oligohydramnios, especially if the fetus is in a breech presentation. An abnormally round shape, termed *brachycephaly*, can be an important indicator of fetal abnormalities, especially holoprosencephaly and aneuploidies (e-Fig. 9-3).

NEURAL TUBE DEFECTS
Anencephaly is often first suspected when a proper image for measuring the BPD cannot be obtained. The absence of the cranial vault can be diagnosed after 10 weeks' gestation. Although the skull is missing, lobulated disorganized brain tissue can be prominent between 9 and 11 weeks. This tissue degenerates by 15 weeks, leaving the characteristic appearance in which there is there is no cortex or cranium and the fetal eyes appear at the top of an intact lower face (e-Figs. 9-4 and 9-5). Meningomyelocele that extends varying distances from the base of the skull down the neck and body may be present along with anencephaly. Fetuses with anencephaly do not swallow normally, so polyhydramnios commonly develops in pregnancies that are allowed to continue.

Whenever a normal calvarium is absent, especially if there are additional clefts or amputations in the fetus, a careful search should be made for strands of membranes attached to the fetus, which are diagnostic of the amniotic band sequence. When major skull deficits are caused by amniotic bands, typically some cerebral cortex remains (e-Fig. 9-6), although this is not the case with anencephaly.

Encephalocele is the least common type of neural tube defect and is manifested by a protrusion of the meninges, and sometimes brain tissue, through a midline defect in the cranium. Ultrasound shows a midline sac protruding though the skull, most often in the occiput (e-Fig. 9-7). The outcome with encephalocele is very poor if brain tissue is present within the encephalocele sac or other significant associated anomalies are apparent. When the defect is isolated with no brain involvement, most children have a good neurologic outcome.

The sensitivity of ultrasound for diagnosing spina bifida increased dramatically in the 1980s when it was discovered that fetuses with this condition have readily apparent secondary changes in the brain and skull.[73] **These include frontal narrowing of the skull (the "lemon" sign; e-Fig. 9-8), ventriculomegaly, and an abnormal cerebellum and posterior fossa. The cerebellum is deformed and drawn backward to obliterate** the posterior fossa. This finding, the Arnold-Chiari type II malformation, is referred to as the *banana sign* (e-Figs. 9-9 and 9-10).

CYSTIC HYGROMA

A **cystic hygroma** is a loculated accumulation of fluid in the skin of posterior neck (e-Fig. 9-11). In fetuses with this finding, edema may be widespread and is often associated with severe hydrops. These fetuses do not survive into the third trimester. **When a cystic hygroma is present, the chance is more than 60% that the fetus has a chromosome abnormality, most commonly Turner syndrome.**[74]

CLEFT LIP AND PALATE

A coronal view of the fetal face is usually readily obtainable (e-Fig. 9-12). e-Figure 9-13 shows the presence of cleft lip, and 3-D views of a cleft lip (see Fig. 9-10) can help patients understand the nature of the fetal deformity. **Approximately two-thirds of those with cleft lip also have cleft palate,** which may be demonstrated with oblique views that show a defect in the maxillary ridge (e-Fig. 9-14). An isolated cleft palate is rarely diagnosed with prenatal ultrasound.

MICROGNATHIA

A midsagittal view of the face is the best for the detection of micrognathia (e-Fig. 9-15), which may be an important marker for genetic syndromes such as trisomy 18. **Severe hypoplasia of the mandible, such as that seen with Pierre-Robin sequence, can cause breathing difficulties at birth; therefore prenatal diagnosis is invaluable in planning proactively for management of the neonate.**

CEREBELLUM AND CISTERNA MAGNA

The cerebellum and posterior fossa should always be visualized to diagnose spina bifida, as described above, and the Dandy-Walker malformation. In the latter condition, a posterior fossa cyst is present that is continuous with the fourth ventricle; also apparent are complete or partial absence of the cerebellar vermis and varying degrees of hydrocephalus (e-Fig. 9-16 and Video 9-1). About 50% of affected fetuses have other intracranial malformations, 35% have extracranial abnormalities, and 15% to 30% have aneuploidy.[75] Many infants with Dandy-Walker syndrome die after birth, usually as a result of associated malformations; the majority of survivors have some degree of mental handicap.

CHOROID PLEXUS

Cysts within the choroid plexus are noted in approximately 1% of normal fetuses (e-Fig. 9-17). They generally are benign and resolve before 26 weeks' gestation without sequelae. Because their presence indicates a sevenfold increase in risk that the fetus has trisomy 18, referral for a specialist ultrasound is indicated.[16] **In a fetus without trisomy 18, a choroid plexus cyst is not considered significant, and no further follow-up is needed.**[16,76]

LATERAL VENTRICLES

Hydrocephalus is a general term used to describe a head in which the cerebral ventricles are dilated. Many causes are possible and include spina bifida; stenosis of the aqueduct of Sylvius; normal pressure hydrocephalus; agenesis of the corpus callosum; fetal toxoplasmosis, other infections, rubella, cytomegalovirus, and herpes simplex (TORCH) infections (see Chapters 52 and 53);

and other serious developmental malformations of the brain. In some cases, particularly those caused by aqueductal stenosis, the head can be markedly enlarged. The lateral and third ventricles may be very dilated with marked thinning of the cerebral cortex (e-Fig. 9-18). **With atraumatic delivery and appropriate neurosurgical treatment, more than half of infants with aqueductal stenosis survive, but about 75% of survivors have moderate to severe developmental delay.**[77] **The degree of hydrocephalus and the thickness of the remaining cerebral cortex are weak predictors of the neurologic outcome.**

The appearance of the choroid plexus can assist in the diagnosis of less obvious hydrocephalus. With hydrocephalus, the choroid plexus—which usually fills this portion of the lateral ventricle from side to side (e-Fig. 9-19)—appears compressed and "dangles" (e-Fig. 9-20). The accepted upper limit of the transverse diameter of the lateral ventricles at the atrium is 10 mm. **When the ventricles measure between 10 and 12 mm, the chance of a normal neurologic outcome is 96%, and it is 86% with a measurement between 12 and 15 mm.**[78] Whenever any degree of hydrocephalus is seen, a careful search for other malformations is essential, because their presence strongly influences the prognosis. Agenesis of the corpus callosum should be considered when modest ventricular dilation is primarily confined to the posterior horns (e-Fig. 9-21). Although fetuses with spina bifida usually have dilation of the lateral ventricles, the head size is usually not increased.[79]

A unilateral cystic lesion adjacent to the cerebral cortex most likely represents an arachnoid cyst (e-Fig. 9-22). These generally are associated with a good prognosis but can reach considerable size and can cause symptoms such as seizures or hydrocephalus. Porencephalic cysts are unilateral cystic lesions in the brain that have a much worse outcome. These arise from intracerebral infarcts or hemorrhages with subsequent liquefaction of the brain tissue or clot (e-Fig. 9-23). The resultant cystic cavity within the brain parenchyma may be in communication with the subarachnoid space or a cerebral ventricle.

MIDLINE FALX

Absence or abnormality of midline structures of the brain should point to a diagnosis of holoprosencephaly. This condition results from incomplete division of the cerebral hemispheres. With the *alobar* form of holoprosencephaly, the head is usually small and brachycephalic. No midline echo divides the cerebral cortex, and a single crescent-shaped ventricle lies anterior to the bulbous-appearing thalamus (e-Fig. 9-24). Many fetuses with holoprosencephaly have facial abnormalities that may include hypotelorism or cyclopia, facial clefts, absent nose or single nostril, and presence of a proboscis above or between the eyes. Chromosome abnormalities, especially trisomy 13, and other malformations are present in one third of these cases. **Regardless of the karyotype or presence of other malformations, alobar holoprosencephaly is associated with a dismal neurologic prognosis, and death almost always occurs either before or shortly after birth.** When partial division of the brain is evident, the fetus may have *semilobar* (e-Fig. 9-25) or *lobar* holoprosencephaly, both of which have a somewhat more favorable prognosis.

Chest
CHEST MASSES

Displacement of the heart away from the midline is often a sign of a diaphragmatic hernia or a lung mass such as congenital pulmonary adenomatoid malformation (CPAM) or pulmonary sequestration. The presence of these conditions can be life threatening because vital chest structures are compressed or displaced. Space-occupying chest lesions can severely impair lung growth. Compression of the esophagus by a lung mass may cause symptomatic polyhydramnios. Similar pressure on the central veins and lymphatics may cause fetal death from generalized hydrops.

With diaphragmatic hernia, the heart is displaced to the side opposite the location of the defect, which is on the left in 75% of cases. The condition can be distinguished from other chest masses by the appearance of bowel, stomach, and other abdominal organs in the chest at the level of the four-chamber view of the heart (e-Fig. 9-26). In the midabdominal view, the stomach is typically not seen with left-sided hernias and is shifted toward the right in right-sided lesions. The intrahepatic umbilical vein is usually shifted toward the side of the defect, and variable amounts of liver will sometimes be seen prolapsed into the chest. Ultrasound does not usually demonstrate significant lung tissue on the affected side. The contralateral lung can be very small. Displacement of the GI tract often results in swallowing abnormalities, and half of such cases develop polyhydramnios.

CPAM appears as a solid or multicystic lung mass (e-Figs. 9-27 and 9-28) that is almost always unilateral and confined to one lobe. Frequently, a shift in the mediastinum is apparent with compression of the contralateral lung. Nonimmune hydrops can develop, and this finding is associated with a poor prognosis. Because an apparently very large CPAM can seem to regress as a pregnancy advances, the clinician should be cautious about predicting a poor outcome.[80] Most affected children require nonemergent surgical resection.

Pulmonary sequestration is a congenital anomaly in which a mass of lung tissue arises from the foregut independently of the normal lung. It does not communicate with the tracheobronchial tree, and it receives its blood supply directly from the aorta (e-Fig. 9-29). Ultrasound shows an echogenic intrathoracic or intraabdominal mass, usually just above or just below the diaphragm. Color Doppler ultrasound can sometimes show the aberrant blood supply, thus distinguishing a pulmonary sequestration from CPAM. A pulmonary sequestration usually must be removed in childhood but rarely causes prenatal complications.[81]

FOUR-CHAMBER VIEW OF THE HEART

In addition to the position of the heart within the chest, the axis should be carefully noted. The sonographer must identify the fetal right and left side based on the position of the fetus, not the position of the organs. Otherwise, abnormalities of sidedness—such as situs inversus—would be missed.

The starting place for diagnosing congenital heart defects is the four-chamber view (e-Fig. 9-30). Examples of defects that present with an abnormal four-chamber view include many septal defects and hypoplastic left heart syndrome. Ventricular septal defects account for 20% to 30% of congenital heart defects. Whereas large defects can often be seen in the four-chamber view (e-Fig. 9-31), small defects are commonly missed even by experienced examiners. Some significant defects are in the anterior, membranous portion and are not visible with the four-chamber view. The most obvious septal defect visible with prenatal ultrasound is an atrioventricular canal defect. With this, a large defect is evident in the atrial and ventricular septum, and a common atrioventricular valve is present (e-Fig. 9-32). This particular lesion has a strong association with Down syndrome, which is present in about half of the cases. In about half of the cases of ventricular septal defects, other more complex malformations are present. It is difficult to distinguish an atrial septal defect from a normal patent foramen ovale.

Hypoplastic left heart syndrome is suspected when the left ventricle, which should be similar in size to the right ventricle, appears very small with a four-chamber view (e-Fig. 9-33). To better characterize such defects, visualizing the outflow tracts is critical (see Figs. 9-37 and 9-38). In hypoplastic left heart syndrome, the ascending aorta and aortic arch are very narrow in comparison with the pulmonary artery and ductus arteriosus.

OUTFLOW TRACTS

Many relatively common serious congenital heart defects may be missed entirely unless the outflow tracts are assessed. One example of such a condition is the tetralogy of Fallot, which consists of a ventricular septal defect (VSD), pulmonary stenosis, and an aorta that overrides the VSD (e-Figs. 9-34 and 9-35). The fourth part of the tetralogy, hypertrophy of the right ventricle, develops postnatally. Transposition of the great arteries may also present with a completely normal four-chamber view. This disorder is recognized with the outflow tract views when the aorta and pulmonary artery run parallel to each other instead of crossing (e-Fig. 9-36). The aorta, which can be recognized from the shape of the arch, arises from the right ventricle and runs anterior to the main pulmonary artery, which arises posteriorly from the left ventricle. A VSD is found in 40% of cases.

Abdomen

The fetal stomach should always be visualized after the first trimester. If the stomach is small or absent and does fill after 30 to 60 minutes of observation, esophageal atresia should be suspected. In most cases, ultrasound also shows polyhydramnios that results from an inability of the fetus to swallow amniotic fluid normally (e-Fig. 9-37 and Video 9-2). An empty stomach in a fetus with anhydramnios is not suggestive of GI pathology but simply reflects the absence of fluid available for the fetus to swallow.

Duodenal atresia is usually easily diagnosed by third-trimester fetal ultrasound. The diagnosis is based on the demonstration of the "double bubble" sign in which adjacent cysts are seen that represent the fluid-filled dilated stomach and proximal duodenum (e-Fig. 9-38). Polyhydramnios is almost always seen in these cases, and trisomy 21 is present in 30%. Small bowel obstruction further along the intestinal tract is less common than duodenal atresia. Ultrasound in these cases shows multiple actively peristalsing loops of distended small bowel (e-Fig. 9-39 and Video 9-3). The degree of polyhydramnios depends on the proximity of the obstruction to the stomach.

Urinary Tract
KIDNEYS

Bilateral renal agenesis is usually first suspected with ultrasound when amniotic fluid is absent and the fetal bladder cannot be visualized (e-Fig. 9-40). The diagnosis is confirmed by the absence of kidneys in the renal fossae (e-Fig. 9-41). The diagnosis is sometimes difficult because the absent amniotic fluid makes adequate visualization of the fetal anatomy challenging and because the discoid-shaped adrenals can be confused with fetal kidneys. Transvaginal scanning can be very helpful because with no amniotic fluid, the fetus is often close to the upper vagina. Bilateral agenesis is invariably associated with pulmonary hypoplasia, which is the cause of death in liveborn infants. In this setting, ultrasound shows a small, bell-shaped chest (e-Fig. 9-42).

Infantile polycystic kidney disease is an autosomal-recessive disorder characterized by bilateral symmetric enlargement of the kidneys. In this condition, normal parenchyma is replaced by dilated collecting tubules that measure less than 2 mm in diameter. These cysts are not seen macroscopically with ultrasound but rather give the kidneys a markedly echogenic appearance (e-Fig. 9-43). In most cases, the kidneys are nonfunctioning in the fetus, and no bladder filling or amniotic fluid production occurs; these neonates die of pulmonary hypoplasia.

Multicystic dysplasia is a disorder with sporadic occurrence characterized by noncommunicating cysts of various sizes scattered randomly through the kidneys. The renal parenchyma between the cyst has an echogenic appearance (e-Fig. 9-44). The disorder can be bilateral, unilateral, or segmental. Affected kidneys may become quite large. **This condition should be differentiated from** *hydronephrosis,* **in which the parenchyma is normal and a dilated renal pelvis communicates with dilated calyces.** In bilateral multicystic dysplasia, urine is not produced, so the bladder is not visualized and no amniotic fluid is present. As with renal agenesis, unilateral disease is associated with normal bladder filling and amniotic fluid volume and has an excellent prognosis.

Varying degrees of dilation of the renal pelvis and calyces are seen with **hydronephrosis** (e-Fig. 9-45). The degree of dilation is recorded as the anterior-posterior (A-P) diameter of the renal pelvis (see e-Fig. 9-2). Mild dilation of the renal pelvis, termed *pyelectasis* or *pelviectasis,* is often a benign physiologic finding. **However, if the A-P diameter is greater than 4 mm, referral for a targeted ultrasound and a follow-up ultrasound at 32 weeks are recommended. If the pelvis measures 7 mm or more beyond 32 weeks, postnatal evaluation is indicated.**[82]

These cutoffs were set in order to ensure a sensitivity of nearly 100% for detecting any postnatal compromise or the need for surgery. Using these cutoffs, 20% to 50% of cases have normal kidneys at postnatal evaluation. Persistent hydronephrosis is most often caused by ureteropelvic junction obstruction or vesicoureteral reflux. Dilated ureters signify the presence of severe vesicoureteral reflux (e-Fig. 9-46), bladder outlet obstruction, or ureterovesical junction obstruction. The latter condition is often associated with a duplicated collecting system. A ureterocele may form at the point of ureteral implantation into the bladder.

BLADDER

Bladder outlet obstruction is most commonly seen in male fetuses and is usually caused by posterior urethral valves. These are membranelike structures in the posterior urethra that cause varying grades of urethral obstruction. More complex malformations that involve the urogenital tract may also cause bladder outlet obstruction and are more common when the affected fetus is a female. Sonographically, bladder outlet obstruction is diagnosed when the bladder is abnormally enlarged and normal emptying is not seen (e-Fig. 9-47). When the obstruction is severe, other findings include oligohydramnios, dilated ureters, hydronephrosis, and cystic dysplasia of the kidneys (e-Figs. 9-48 and 9-49). **When complete urethral obstruction has been present from early in pregnancy, anhydramnios causes lethal pulmonary hypoplasia and ureteral reflux results in irreversible damage to the kidneys.** *Prune belly syndrome* occurs in male fetuses and has the same sonographic appearance as

bladder outlet obstruction. With this condition, however, the impairment of bladder emptying is thought to result from a neuromuscular defect in the bladder and not physical obstruction of the urethra.

Placenta and Umbilical Cord
UMBILICAL CORD INSERTION INTO THE ABDOMEN

Omphalocele is a ventral wall defect characterized by a membrane-covered herniation of the intraabdominal contents into the base of the umbilical cord. Bowel loops, stomach, and liver are the most frequently herniated organs (e-Fig. 9-50). **With omphalocele comes a 75% rate of associated birth defects, and the karyotype is abnormal in 20% of cases.**[83] These other problems account for most of the mortality associated with this condition.

Gastroschisis is a right paraumbilical defect of the anterior abdominal wall associated with evisceration of the abdominal organs. Gastroschisis is distinguished from omphalocele by the fact that the umbilical cord inserts normally into the abdominal wall, and no membrane covers the herniated viscera (e-Fig. 9-51). Most commonly, only bowel loops are involved, but liver, stomach, and bladder may be outside the abdomen. Because of associated atresias or obstruction at the small abdominal wall ring, bowel loops and the stomach may be dilated inside or outside the abdomen. **Gastroschisis is rarely associated with chromosome abnormalities and usually does not involve abnormalities outside of the GI tract.**[84]

NUMBER OF UMBILICAL CORD VESSELS

An attempt should be made to confirm that two arteries and a vein are present in the umbilical cord. In late pregnancy, this can be easily ascertained by looking at a transverse cut of the cord in a free loop (see Fig. 9-26). In the second trimester, two umbilical arteries are most easily confirmed by identifying the vessels as they course around the fetal bladder. These can be seen with gray-scale ultrasound but are made much more obvious with color Doppler ultrasound. **A single umbilical artery is present in 1% of all newborns. Because of the 20% incidence of associated malformations, this finding should prompt a detailed fetal survey. Several studies have suggested an increased risk of growth restriction and stillbirth, so follow-up growth ultrasounds and testing for fetal well-being should be considered.**

Spine

Normal transverse views of the spine show intact skin with the echocenters in an equilateral triangle (e-Fig. 9-52). Coronal views show these same lateral echocenters running parallel to each other (e-Fig. 9-53). With spina bifida, transverse views of the spine show widening of the lateral echocenters. A meningomyelocele sac is usually present (e-Fig. 9-54). In coronal images, the ossification centers, which usually run a parallel course down the back, are widened in the area of the defect (e-Fig. 9-55). The meningomyelocele sac is also seen in a sagittal view (e-Fig. 9-56). **The presence of clubfoot and absence of movement of the lower extremities signify a poor prognosis for motor function of the lower extremities.**

Extremities

In most cases of confirmed skeletal dysplasia, the long bones are obviously abnormal, with measurements that fall far below the normal range. Concern sometimes arises when routine measurement of the femur gives a result several weeks less than expected for the gestational age. **For most long bone nomograms, the lower confidence limit corresponds to "2 weeks behind" up to 28 weeks, and "3 weeks behind" beyond 28 weeks.** For this reason, when the femur is more than 2 or 3 weeks less than expected, a detailed survey of fetal anatomy—especially of the long bones—is advisable. **A femur/foot ratio close to 1 usually implies that the fetus is normal or merely constitutionally small.**

Achondroplasia is the most common form of skeletal dysplasia and is associated with a normal life span. Ultrasound shows severe shortening of the long bones, a relatively large head with a protruding forehead, and polyhydramnios. Although this condition has autosomal-dominant inheritance, 80% of cases result from new mutations.

Thanatophoric dysplasia is the most common lethal skeletal dysplasia. In this condition, extreme shortening of the long bones occurs (e-Figs. 9-57 and 9-58). The femur is often bowed, resembling an old-fashioned telephone receiver (e-Fig. 9-59). The fetus has a small, narrow chest that results in lethal pulmonary hypoplasia (e-Figs. 9-60 and 9-61), and the abdomen and head appear relatively enlarged. In about one in six cases, the head has a "cloverleaf" shape. Hydrocephalus, frontal bossing (e-Fig. 9-62), and polyhydramnios are common.

Over a dozen discrete forms of osteogenesis imperfecta exist, all characterized by abnormalities of the biochemical composition of the bone matrix. The more severe forms are lethal, with hypoplastic lungs (e-Fig. 9-63), very short limbs with multiple fractures (e-Fig. 9-64), and demineralized bones (e-Fig. 9-65). More mild forms may show few or no fractures, bowing of the femurs, and limb lengths close to the normal range.

Clubfoot is best diagnosed with a coronal view of the lower leg, with the tibia and fibula both seen in a lengthwise section. **A normal foot is perpendicular to this plane, but a clubfoot is turned down and in and is seen falling within the coronal plane** (e-Fig. 9-66). It may be very difficult to diagnose clubfoot in the third trimester or in the presence of oligohydramnios.

Hydrops

The term *hydrops* refers to generalized edema in the neonate manifested by skin edema and accumulations of fluid in body cavities, including the pleural spaces, pericardium, and peritoneal cavity (e-Fig. 9-67). Prior to the introduction of Rh immune prophylaxis, most hydrops resulted from erythroblastosis fetalis (see Chapter 34). Currently, the great majority of cases of hydrops are from nonimmune causes. With improvement in diagnostic methods, the etiology of most cases of nonimmune hydrops can be determined. Box 9-3 lists the more common causes of nonimmune hydrops. In recent years it has become apparent that parvovirus infection is responsible for many of the cases of hydrops that were previously classified as "idiopathic" (see Chapter 53).

CLINICAL VALUE OF BIRTH DEFECT SCREENING

It is surprisingly difficult to prove that prenatal ultrasound reduces morbidity or mortality in newborns with birth defects. The RADIUS study demonstrated similar outcomes in the control group and in the group with routine screening.[67] A randomized trial of routine ultrasound conducted in Finland demonstrated a decrease in perinatal mortality when routine

---

BOX 9-3   CAUSES OF HYDROPS FETALIS

- Twin-to-twin transfusion
- Chromosome abnormalities
- Structural heart defects
- Cardiac arrhythmia, especially tachyarrhythmia
- Cardiac tumor
- High-output failure from vascular malformation or tumor
  - Sacrococcygeal teratoma
  - Vein of Galen malformation
  - Placenta chorangioma
  - Twin reverse arterial perfusion sequence
- Fetal anemia
  - Parvovirus infection
  - Alpha-thalassemia
  - Fetomaternal hemorrhage
- Other infection
  - TORCH infections
  - Syphilis
- Chest mass
  - Congenital cystic adenomatoid malformation
  - Pulmonary sequestration

TORCH, toxoplasmosis, other infections, rubella, cytomegalovirus, and herpes simplex.

---

ultrasound was used, but this was because most pregnancies with serious malformations were terminated, not because offspring from continued pregnancies did better.[85] However, studies have shown an improved outcome when congenital heart defects were diagnosed with prenatal ultrasound.[86,87] Although less critical, the prenatal diagnosis of urinary tract malformations can also lead to proper postnatal evaluation and treatment, presumably leading to improved long-term prognosis.[88] **Although definitive proof is scarce for most conditions, it seems self-evident that prenatal diagnosis has its advantages. For one, it gives parents the option of pregnancy termination when serious malformations are diagnosed. Another advantage is that it allows families and caregivers time to gather complete information about the fetal problem so that practical and emotional preparations can be made. Plans can be made for delivery at the proper time at a high-risk perinatal center where the newborn can receive optimal care. When the mother delivers at the tertiary care center, there is no need to transport a potentially unstable newborn, and the mother and baby are not separated.**

Routine ultrasound to screen for birth defects involves significant costs, but the cost per defect diagnosed is not out of line with other accepted screening tests. The cost/benefit ratio is much more favorable when exams are performed by sonographers with good detection rates.[89] Ideally, in offering a screening ultrasound, the obstetrician should inform the patients in general terms of the sensitivity of this test in the setting in which it is to be performed.

"ENTERTAINMENT" ULTRASOUND EXAMINATIONS

As previously noted, when birth defects are suspected, 3-D ultrasound can provide helpful images. In recent years, 3-D ultrasound has been increasingly offered to patients in a nonmedical setting for entertainment or to provide keepsake images of the fetus. **The use of ultrasound for nondiagnostic** purposes has been condemned by the AIUM and the ACOG.[65,90] Concerns raised in their policy statements include possible adverse bioeffects of ultrasound energy, the possibility that an examination could give false reassurance to women, and the fact that abnormalities may be detected in settings where personnel are not prepared to discuss and provide follow-up for concerning findings. The 2007 statement by the AIUM regarding the prudent use of ultrasound in obstetrics states, "**The AIUM advocates the responsible use of diagnostic ultrasound and strongly discourages the nonmedical use of ultrasound for entertainment purposes. The use of ultrasound without a medical indication to view the fetus, obtain a picture of the fetus, or determine the fetal gender is inappropriate and contrary to responsible medical practice. Ultrasound should be used by qualified health professionals to provide medical benefit to the patient.**"[65]

KEY POINTS

- Sonographers should become familiar with the basic physics of ultrasound, equipment controls, and scanning techniques to optimize ultrasound images.
- All of the elements of the standard obstetric ultrasound exam are important for clinical management and should not be neglected.
- Because most birth defects occur in fetuses of low-risk women, all standard exams should include a full anatomic survey.
- Physicians who perform and interpret obstetric ultrasound examinations should have appropriate training and experience.
- Appropriate documentation of ultrasound studies is important for good medical care.
- Pregnancy dating by ultrasound measurements is most accurate early in pregnancy. Guidelines have been established for when ultrasound dates should be used in preference to menstrual dates.
- Ultrasound for fetal weight estimation is of limited usefulness for the prevention of shoulder dystocia and other complications associated with fetal macrosomia.
- The AIUM and ACOG strongly discourage nonmedical use of ultrasound for entertainment purposes.
- It is not expected that all birth defects will be diagnosed by prenatal ultrasound.
- The sensitivity of ultrasound for the detection of birth defects depends on the level of training of examiners and the maintenance of a structured approach to the fetal examination.
- Performance of the first trimester ultrasound component of the aneuploidy screen requires formal training and certification.
- Individuals who perform prenatal sonography should be aware of conditions that can be detected with a standard examination.

REFERENCES

1. Ramos GA, Ylagan MV, Romine LE, et al. Diagnostic evaluation of the fetal face using 3-dimensional ultrasound. *Ultrasound Q.* 2008;24: 215-223.
2. Ruano R, Aubry MC, Barthe B, et al. Ipsilateral lung volumes assessed by three-dimensional ultrasonography in fetuses with isolated congenital diaphragmatic hernia. *Fetal Diagn Ther.* 2008;24:389-394.
3. American College of Obstetricians and Gynecologists. ACOG Practice Bulletin No. 101: ultrasonography in pregnancy. *Obstet Gynecol.* 2009;113: 451-461.
4. Abramowicz JS, Kossoff G, Marsal K, Ter Haar G. Safety Statement, International Society of Ultrasound in Obstetrics and Gynecology. *Ultrasound Obstet Gynecol.* 2003;21:100.
5. Stefos TI, Lolis DE, Sotiriadis AJ, Ziakas GV. Embryonic heart rate in early pregnancy. *J Clin Ultrasound.* 1998;26:33-36.
6. Haak MC, Twisk JW, Van Vugt JM. How successful is fetal echocardiographic examination in the first trimester of pregnancy? *Ultrasound Obstet Gynecol.* 2002;20:9-13.
7. Tongsong T, Srisomboon J, Wanapirak C, et al. Pregnancy outcome of threatened abortion with demonstrable fetal cardiac activity: a cohort study. *J Obstet Gynaecol.* 1995;21:331-335.
8. Smith KE, Buyalos RP. The profound impact of patient age on pregnancy outcome after early detection of fetal cardiac activity. *Fertil Steril.* 1996; 65:35-40.
9. Maso G, D'Ottavio G, De Seta F, et al. First-trimester intrauterine hematoma and outcome of pregnancy. *Obstet Gynecol.* 2005;105:339-344.
10. Doubilet PM, Benson CB, Bourne T, Blaivas M. Diagnostic Criteria for Nonviable Pregnancy Early in the First Trimester. *N Engl J Med.* 2013;369: 1443-1451.
11. Nicolaides KH. Nuchal translucency and other first-trimester sonographic markers of chromosomal abnormalities. *Am J Obstet Gynecol.* 2004;191: 45-67.
12. American Institute of Ultrasound in Medicine. AIUM Practice Guidelines for the performance of an antepartum obstetric ultrasound examination. *J Ultrasound Med.* 2003;22:1116-1125.
13. American Institute of Ultrasound in Medicine. *AIUM Training Guidelines for Physicians Who Evaluate and Interpret Diagnostic Ultrasound Examinations.* Laurel, Md.: 2010.
14. Hack KE, Derks JB, Elias SG, et al. Increased perinatal mortality and morbidity in monochorionic versus dichorionic twin pregnancies: clinical implications of a large Dutch cohort study. *BJOG.* 2008;115:58-67.
15. Rozenberg P, Porcher R, Salomon LJ, et al. Comparison of the learning curves of digital examination and transabdominal sonography for the determination of fetal head position during labor. *Ultrasound Obstet Gynecol.* 2008;31:332-337.
16. Reddy UM, Abuhamad AZ, Levine D, Saade GR, invited participants. Fetal imaging: executive summary of a joint Eunice Kennedy Shriver National Institute of Child Health and Human Development, Society for Maternal-Fetal Medicine, American Institute of Ultrasound in Medicine, American College of Obstetricians and Gynecologists, American College of Radiology, Society for Pediatric Radiology, and Society of Radiologists in Ultrasound Fetal Imaging workshop. *Obstet Gynecol.* 2014;123:1070-1082.
17. Rutherford SE, Phelan JP, Smith CV, et al. The four-quadrant assessment of amniotic fluid volume: an adjunct to antepartum fetal heart rate testing. *Obstet Gynecol.* 1987;70:353-356.
18. Magann EF, Perry KG Jr, Chauhan SP, et al. The accuracy of ultrasound evaluation of amniotic fluid volume in singleton pregnancies: the effect of operator experience and ultrasound interpretative technique. *J Clin Ultrasound.* 1997;25:249-253.
19. Chamberlain PF, Manning FA, Morrison I, et al. Ultrasound evaluation of amniotic fluid volume. I. The relationship of marginal and decreased amniotic fluid volumes to perinatal outcome. *Am J Obstet Gynecol.* 1984;150: 245-249.
20. Ott WJ. Reevaluation of the relationship between amniotic fluid volume and perinatal outcome. *Am J Obstet Gynecol.* 2005;192:1803-1809.
21. American College of Obstetricians and Gynecologists. ACOG Practice bulletin no. 145: antepartum fetal surveillance. *Obstet Gynecol.* 2014;124: 182-192.
22. Sandlin AT, Chauhan SP, Magann EF. Clinical relevance of sonographically estimated amniotic fluid volume. *J Ultrasound Med.* 2013;32:851-863.
23. Dashe JS, McIntire DD, Ramus RM, et al. Hydramnios: anomaly prevalence and sonographic detection. *Obstet Gynecol.* 2002;100:134-139.
24. Many A, Hill LM, Lazebnik N, Martin JG. The association between polyhydramnios and preterm delivery. *Obstet Gynecol.* 1995;86:389-391.
25. Leerentveld RA, Gilberts EC, Arnold MJ, et al. Accuracy and safety of transvaginal sonographic placental localization. *Obstet Gynecol.* 1990;76: 759-762.
26. Oppenheimer L. Society of Obstetricians and Gynaecologists of Canada: Diagnosis and management of placenta previa. *J Obstet Gynaecol Can.* 2007;29:261-273.

27. Taipale P, Hiilesmaa V, Ylöstalo P. Transvaginal ultrasonography at 18-23 weeks in predicting placenta previa at delivery. *Ultrasound Obstet Gynecol.* 1998;12:422-425.

28. Dashe JS, McIntire DD, Ramus RM, et al. Persistence of placenta previa according to gestational age at ultrasound detection. *Obstet Gynecol.* 2002;99:692-697.

29. Oyelese Y, Catanzarite V, Prefumo F, et al. Vasa previa: the impact of prenatal diagnosis on outcomes. *Obstet Gynecol.* 2004;103:937-942.

30. Fisteag-Kiprono L, Neiger R, Sonek JD, et al. Perinatal outcome associated with sonographically detected globular placenta. *J Reprod Med.* 2006;51: 563-566.

31. Hua M, Odibo AO, Macones GA, et al. Single umbilical artery and its associated findings. *Obstet Gynecol.* 2010;115:930-934.

32. Stout MJ, Odibo AO, Graseck AS, et al. Leiomyomas at routine second-trimester ultrasound examination and adverse obstetric outcomes. *Obstet Gynecol.* 2010;116:1056-1063.

33. Rosati P, Exacoustòs C, Mancuso S. Longitudinal evaluation of uterine myoma growth during pregnancy: a sonographic study. *J Ultrasound Med.* 1992;11:511-515.

34. Neiger R, Sonek JD, Croom CS, Ventolini G. Pregnancy-related changes in the size of uterine leiomyomas. *J Reprod Med.* 2006;51:671-674.

35. Berghella V, Rafael TJ, Szychowski JM, et al. Cerclage for short cervix on ultrasonography in women with singleton gestations and previous preterm birth: a meta-analysis. *Obstet Gynecol.* 2011;117:663-671.

36. Parry S, Simhan H, Elovitz M, et al. Universal maternal cervical length screening during the second trimester: pros and cons of a strategy to identify women at risk of spontaneous preterm delivery. *Am J Obstet Gynecol.* 2012; 207:101-106.

37. Shalev J, Blankstein J, Mashiach R, et al. Sonographic visualization of normal-size ovaries during pregnancy. *Ultrasound Obstet Gynecol.* 2000;15: 523-526.

38. Hadlock FP, Shah YP, Kanon DJ, et al. Fetal crown rump length: reevaluation of relation to menstrual age (5-18 weeks) with high-resolution real-time US. *Radiology.* 1992;182:501-505.

39. ACOG Committee opinion no 611: method for estimating due date. *Obstet Gynecol.* 2014;124:863-866.

40. Nyberg DA, Abuhamad A, Ville Y. Ultrasound assessment of abnormal fetal growth. *Semin Perinatol.* 2004;28:3-22.

41. Robinson HP, Fleming JE. A critical evaluation of sonar "crown-rump length" measurements. *Br J Obstet Gynecol.* 1975;82:702-710.

42. Schats R, Van Os HC, Jansen CA, et al. The crown-rump length in early human pregnancy: a reappraisal. *Br J Obstet Gynaecol.* 1991;98:460-462.

43. Hadlock FP, Harrist RB, Martinez-Poyer J. How accurate is second trimester fetal dating? *J Ultrasound Med.* 1991;10:557-561.

44. Chervenak FA, Skupski DW, Romero R, et al. How accurate is fetal biometry in the assessment of fetal age? *Am J Obstet Gynecol.* 1998;178: 678-687.

45. Spong CY. Defining "term" pregnancy. *JAMA.* 2013;309:2445-2446.

46. Sparks TN. Fundal height: a useful screening tool for fetal growth? *J Matern Fetal Neonatal Med.* 2011;24:708-712.

47. ACOG Practice Bulletin number 134: Fetal growth restriction. *Obstet Gynecol.* 2013;121:1122-1133.

48. McDermott JC. Fundal height measurement. In: Wildshut HIJ, Weiner CP, Peter TJ, eds. *When to screen in obstetrics and gynecology.* Philadelphia: Elsevier; 2006:326-343.

49. Deter FL, Harrist RB. Detection of growth abnormalities. In: Chervenak FA, Isaacson GC, Campbell S, eds. *Ultrasound in Obstetrics and Gynecology.* Boston: Little, Brown and Company; 1993:394-395.

50. Kayem G, Grangé G, Bréart G, et al. Comparison of fundal height measurement and sonographically measured fetal abdominal circumference in the prediction of high and low birth weight at term. *Ultrasound Obstet Gynecol.* 2009;34:566-571.

51. Bricker L, Neilson JP, Dowswell T. Routine ultrasound in late pregnancy (after 24 weeks' gestation). *Cochrane Database Syst Rev.* 2008;(8): CD001451.326-343.

52. Hadlock F. Evaluation of fetal weight estimation procedures. In: Deter R, Harist R, Birnholz J, et al., eds. *Quantitative Obstetrical Ultrasonography.* New York: Wiley; 1986:113.

53. Sherman DJ, Arieli S, Tovbin J, et al. A comparison of clinical and ultrasound estimation of fetal weight. *Obstet Gynecol.* 1998;91:212-217.

54. Benacerraf BR, Gelman R, Frigoletto FD Jr. Sonographically estimated fetal weights: accuracy and limitation. *Am J Obstet Gynecol.* 1988;159: 1118-1121.

55. Chauhan SP, Lutton PM, Bailey KJ, et al. Intrapartum clinical, sonographic, and parous patients' estimates of newborn weight. *Obstet Gynecol.* 1992;79:956-958.

56. Robson SC, Gallivan S, Walkinshaw SA, et al. Ultrasonic estimation of fetal weight: use of targeted formulas in small for gestational age fetuses. *Obstet Gynecol.* 1993;82:359-364.

57. *ACOG practice bulletin 22, Fetal Macrosomia,* November 2000, reaffirmed 2013.

58. Gardosi J, Chang A, Kalyan B, et al. Customised antenatal growth charts. *Lancet.* 1992;339:283-287.

59. Clausson B, Gardosi J, Francis A, et al. Perinatal outcome in SGA births defined by customised versus population-based birthweight standards. *Br J Obstet Gynaecol.* 2001;108:830-834.

60. Campbell S, Thoms A. Ultrasound measurement of fetal head to abdomen circumference ratio in the assessment of growth retardation. *Br J Obstet Gynaecol.* 1977;84:165-174.

61. Williams MC, O'Brien WF. A comparison of birth weight and weight/length ratio for gestation as correlates of perinatal morbidity. *J Perinatol.* 1997;17:346-350.

62. Gonen R, Spiegel D, Abend M. Is macrosomia predictable, and are shoulder dystocia and birth trauma preventable? *Obstet Gynecol.* 1996;88: 526-529.

63. American Institute of Ultrasound Medicine. *Official Statement, Mammalian In Vivo Ultrasonic Biological Effects.* Approved November 8, 2008.

64. Torloni MR, Vedmedovska N, Merialdi M, et al., for the ISUOG-WHO Fetal Growth Study Group. Safety of ultrasonography in pregnancy: WHO systematic review of the literature and meta-analysis. *Ultrasound Obstet Gynecol.* 2009;33:599-608.

65. American Institute of Ultrasound in Medicine. *Official Statement, Prudent Use and Clinical Safety, American Institute of Ultrasound in Medicine,* March 2007.

66. American Institute of Ultrasound in Medicine. *Official Statement, As Low As Reasonably Achievable (ALARA) Principle.* Approved March 16, 2008.

67. Ewigman BG, Crane JP, Frigoletto FD, et al. Effect of prenatal ultrasound screening on perinatal outcome. RADIUS Study Group. *NEJM.* 1993; 329:821-827.

68. Grandjean H, Larroque D, Levi S, et al. The performance of routine ultrasonographic screening of pregnancies in the Eurofetus Study. *Am J Obstet Gynecol.* 1999;181:446-454.

69. DeVore GR. Influence of Prenatal Diagnosis on Congenital Heart Defects. *Ann N Y Acad Sci.* 1998;847:46-52.

70. Tegnander E, Williams W, Johansen OJ, Blaas HG, et al. Prenatal detection of heart defects in a non-selected population of 30,149 fetuses–detection rates and outcome. *Ultrasound Obstet Gynecol.* 2006;27:252-265.

71. ACOG Committee Opinion No. 545. Noninvasive prenatal testing for fetal aneuploidy. *Obstet Gynecol.* 2012;120:1532-1534.

72. Nyberg DA, Souter VL. Use of genetic sonography for adjusting the risk for fetal Down syndrome. *Semin Perinatol.* 2003;27:130-144.

73. Nicolaides KH, Campbell S, Gabbe SG, et al. Ultrasound screening for spina bifida: cranial and cerebellar signs. *Lancet.* 1986;2:72-74.

74. Descamps P, Jourdain O, Paillet C, et al. Etiology, prognosis and management of nuchal cystic hygroma: 25 new cases and literature review. *Eur J Obstet Gynecol Reprod Biol.* 1997;71:3-10.

75. Ulm B, Ulm MR, Deutinger J, et al. Dandy-Walker malformation diagnosed before 21 weeks of gestation: Associated malformations and chromosomal abnormalities. *Ultrasound Obstet Gynecol.* 1997;10:167-170.

76. Coco C, Jeanty P. Karyotyping of fetuses with isolated choroid plexus cysts is not justified in an unselected population. *J Ultrasound Med.* 2004;23: 899-906.

77. Levitsky DB, Mack LA, Nyberg DA, et al. Fetal aqueductal stenosis diagnosed sonographically: how grave is the prognosis? *AJR Am J Roentgenol.* 1995;164:725-730.

78. Pilu G, Falco P, Gabrielli S, et al. The clinical significance of fetal isolated cerebral borderline ventriculomegaly: report of 31 cases and review of the literature. *Ultrasound Obstet Gynecol.* 1999;14:320-326.

79. Van den Hof MC, Nicolaides KH, Campbell J, et al. Evaluation of the lemon and banana signs in one hundred thirty fetuses with open spina bifida. *Am J Obstet Gynecol.* 1990;162:322-327.

80. Roggin KK, Breuer CK, Carr SR, et al. The unpredictable character of congenital cystic lung lesions. *J Pediatr Surg.* 2000;35:801-805.

81. Lopoo JB, Goldstein RB, Lipshutz GS, et al. Fetal pulmonary sequestration: a favorable congenital lung lesion. *Obstet Gynecol.* 1999;94: 567-571.

82. Corteville JE, Gray DL, Crane JP. Congenital hydronephrosis: correlation of fetal ultrasonographic findings with infant outcome. *Am J Obstet Gynecol.* 1991;165:384-388.

83. Hwang PJ, Kousseff BG. Omphalocele and gastroschisis: an 18-year review study. *Genet Med.* 2004;6:232-236.

84. Barisic I, Clementi M, Hausler M, et al. Evaluation of prenatal ultrasound diagnosis of fetal abdominal wall defects by 19 European registries. *Ultrasound Obstet Gynecol.* 2001;18:309-316.

85. Saari-Kemppainen A, Karjalainen O, Ylostalo P, et al. Fetal anomalies in a controlled one-stage ultrasound screening trial. A report from the Helsinki Ultrasound Trial. *J Perinat Med.* 1994;22:279-289.

86. Tworetzky W, McElhinney DB, Reddy VM, et al. Improved surgical outcome after fetal diagnosis of hypoplastic left heart syndrome. *Circulation.* 2001;6:1269-1273.

87. Bonnet D, Coltri A, Butera G, et al. Detection of transposition of the great arteries in fetuses reduces neonatal morbidity and mortality. *Circulation.* 1999;23:916-918.

88. Persutte WH, Koyle M, Lenke RR, et al. Mild pyelectasis ascertained with prenatal ultrasonography is pediatrically significant. *Ultrasound Obstet Gynecol.* 1997;10:12-18.

89. DeVore GR. The Routine Antenatal Diagnostic Imaging with Ultrasound Study: another perspective. *Obstet Gynecol.* 1994;84:622-626.

90. American College of Obstetricians and Gynecologists. Nonmedical use of obstetric ultrasound. ACOG Committee Opinion No. 297 (reconfirmed 2012). *Obstet Gynecol.* 2004;104:423-424.

CHAPTER 10

Genetic Screening and Prenatal Genetic Diagnosis

DEBORAH A. DRISCOLL, JOE LEIGH SIMPSON,
WOLFGANG HOLZGREVE, and LUCAS OTAÑO

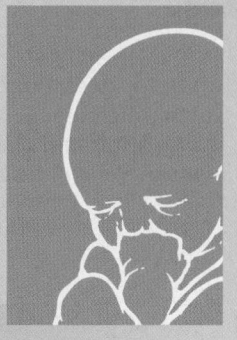

KEY ABBREVIATIONS

Acetylcholinesterase	AchE	Human leukocyte antigen	HLA
Alpha-fetoprotein	AFP	Inhibin A	INHA
Allele dropout	ADO	Intelligence quotient	IQ
American College of Medical Genetics	ACMG	Intracytoplasmic sperm injection	ICSI
American College of Obstetricians and	ACOG	Intrauterine growth restriction	IUGR
Gynecologists		Limb reduction defect	LRD
Assisted reproductive technology	ART	Massively parallel DNA shotgun	MPSS
Biochemistry Ultrasound Nuchal	BUN	sequencing	
Translucency		Maternal serum α-fetoprotein	MSAFP
Cell-free DNA	cfDNA	Mean corpuscular volume	MCV
Chorionic villus sampling	CVS	Microarray analysis	MA
Comparative genomic hybridization	CGH	Multiples of the median	MoM
Confidence interval	CI	Nasal bone	NB
Confined placental mosaicism	CPM	National Institute of Child Health and	NICHD
Congenital bilateral absence of the vas	CBAVD	Human Development	
deferens		Neural tube defect	NTD
Cystic fibrosis	CF	Noninvasive prenatal testing	NIPT
Deoxyribonucleic acid	DNA	Nuchal translucency	NT
Early amniocentesis	EA	Percutaneous umbilical blood sampling	PUBS
First- and Second-Trimester Evaluation	FASTER	Pregnancy-associated plasma protein A	PAPP-A
of Risk		Polymerase chain reaction	PCR
Fluorescence in situ hybridization	FISH	Preimplantation genetic diagnosis	PGD
Genitourinary	GU	Qualitative polymerase chain reaction	QPCR
Human immunodeficiency virus	HIV	Randomized controlled trial	RCT
Human chorionic gonadotropin	hCG	Single nucleotide polymorphism	SNP

Small for gestational age	SGA	Unconjugated estriol	uE$_3$
Spinal muscular atrophy	SMA	Uniparental disomy	UPD
Transabdominal chorionic villus sampling	TA-CVS	Variants of uncertain significance	VOUS
Transcervical chorionic villus sampling	TC-CVS	Whole-genomic amplification	WGA

The goal of genetic screening is to identify individuals or couples at risk for having a child with an inherited condition, chromosome abnormality, or birth defect. Ideally, screening should take place before conception to ensure that couples are fully informed of their reproductive options, including preimplantation genetic screening and diagnosis, or screening should be done as early as possible in pregnancy to allow couples the opportunity to consider aneuploidy screening and prenatal diagnostic testing. Genetic screening begins with a thorough personal and family history, followed by genetic counseling if indicated. **Approximately 3% of liveborn infants will have a major congenital anomaly; about one half of these anomalies are detected at birth and are due to a genetic cause—a chromosome abnormality, single-gene mutation, or polygenic/multifactorial inheritance.** Less frequently, malformations may be due to nongenetic causes or teratogens (see Chapter 8). The detection of many congenital malformations is possible using ultrasonography and fetal echocardiography (see Chapter 9). Screening for aneuploidy, inherited disorders, and structural malformations is an integral part of routine obstetric care. When indicated and desired, amniotic fluid, placental tissue, and cord blood can be readily obtained and analyzed for chromosome abnormalities and genetic disorders. In this chapter, we review genetic history and counseling, common chromosome abnormalities, aneuploidy screening and cytogenetic testing, mendelian disorders, molecular carrier and diagnostic testing, and techniques for prenatal and preimplantation genetic diagnostic testing.

GENETIC HISTORY

Obstetricians/gynecologists should attempt to take a thorough personal and family history to determine whether a woman, her partner, or a relative has a heritable disorder, birth defect, mental retardation, or psychiatric disorder that may increase their risk of having an affected offspring. To address this question, some will find it helpful to elicit genetic information through the use of questionnaires or checklists.

The clinician should inquire into the health status of first-degree relatives (siblings, parents, offspring), second-degree relatives (nephews, nieces, aunts, uncles, grandparents), and third-degree relatives (first cousins, especially maternal). **A positive family history of a genetic disorder may warrant referral to a clinical geneticist or genetic counselor who can accurately assess the risk of having an affected offspring and review genetic screening and testing options.** In some cases, it may be straightforward enough for the well-informed obstetrician to manage. For example, if a birth defect such as a cleft lip and palate or neural tube defect (NTD) exists in a second- or third-degree relative, the risk for that anomaly will usually not prove substantially increased over that of the general population. In contrast, identification of a second-degree relative with an autosomal-recessive disorder such as cystic fibrosis (CF) increases the risk for an affected offspring; therefore more extensive genetic counseling should be considered. Adverse reproductive outcomes such as repetitive spontaneous abortions, stillbirths, and anomalous liveborn infants should be noted. Couples who have such histories should undergo chromosome studies to exclude balanced translocations, which could impact a subsequent pregnancy (see Chapter 27).

Parental ages should be recorded. Advanced maternal age confers an increased risk for aneuploidy.[1,2] A few studies indicate an increased frequency of aneuploidy in sperm in the sixth and seventh decades. However, risks are only marginally increased above background, **and data do not indicate that the risks of having aneuploid liveborns is increased based on paternal age.** A paternal-age effect is associated with a small aggregate increased risk (0.3% to 0.5% or less in men over 40 years of age) for sporadic gene mutations for certain autosomal-dominant conditions such as achondroplasia and craniosynostosis. No specific screening tests exist for anomalies associated with advanced paternal age, although some of these conditions may be detected by ultrasonography (see Chapter 9).

Ethnic origin should also be recorded because certain genetic diseases are increased in selected ethnic groups; this will be discussed in this chapter. Such queries also apply to gamete donors.

GENETIC COUNSELING

Although situations exist in which referral to a clinical geneticist or genetic counselor is indicated, it is impractical for obstetricians to refer all patients with genetic inquiries. **Obstetricians should be able to counsel patients before performing screening tests for aneuploidy and NTDs, carrier screening, and diagnostic procedures such as amniocentesis.** Therefore salient principles of the genetic counseling process are described in this section.

Communication

Pivotal to counseling is communication in terms readily understood by patients. It is useful to preface remarks with a few sentences that recount the major causes of genetic abnormalities, such as cytogenetic, single-gene, polygenic/multifactorial ("complex"), and environmental causes (i.e., teratogens). Writing out unfamiliar words and using tables or diagrams to reinforce important concepts is helpful, and repetition is essential. Allow the couple not only to ask questions but also to talk with one another to formulate their concerns.

Preprinted information, videos, and select Web sites that cover common genetic conditions are useful and have the additional advantage of emphasizing that the couple's problem is not unique. For unique situations, the provision of detailed letters serves as a couple's permanent record, and these help to allay misunderstanding and assist in dealing with relatives.

Irrespective of how obvious a diagnosis may seem, confirmation is always obligatory. Accepting a patient's verbal recollection does not suffice, nor would accepting a diagnosis made by a physician not highly knowledgeable about the condition. Medical records should be requested and reviewed. It may be necessary for an appropriate specialist to examine the affected individual and order confirmatory diagnostic tests; examining first-degree relatives may also be required to detect subtle findings. This is particularly applicable for autosomal-dominant disorders such as neurofibromatosis or Marfan syndrome, for which variable expressivity is expected. **Accurate counseling requires a definitive diagnosis. However, the physician should not hesitate to acknowledge whether a definitive diagnosis cannot be established.**

Nondirective Counseling

In genetic counseling, the clinician should provide accurate genetic information and outline the options for screening and testing without being prescriptive. Of course, completely nondirective counseling is probably unrealistic. Despite the difficulties of remaining truly objective, the clinician should attempt to provide information in a nondirective manner and then support the couple's decision.

Psychological Defenses

If not appreciated, psychological defenses can impede the entire counseling process. Anxiety is low in couples counseled for advanced maternal age or for an abnormality in a distant relative. So long as anxiety remains low, comprehension of information is usually not impeded. However, couples who have experienced a stillborn infant, an anomalous child, or multiple repetitive abortions are inherently more anxious; thus their ability to retain information may be hindered.

Couples who experience abnormal pregnancy outcomes manifest the same five stages of grief that occur after the death of a loved one: (1) denial, (2) anger, (3) bargaining, (4) grief/depression, and (5) acceptance. Deference should be paid to this sequence by not attempting definitive counseling immediately after the birth of an abnormal neonate. The obstetrician should avoid discussing specific recurrence risks for fear of adding to the immediate burden. By 4 to 6 weeks, the couple has begun to cope and is often more receptive to counseling.

An additional psychological consideration is that of parental guilt. A person naturally searches for exogenous factors that might have caused an abnormal outcome. In the process of such a search, guilt may arise. Conversely, a tendency to blame the spouse may be seen. Usually, guilt or blame is not justified, but occasionally the "blame" has a basis in reality (e.g., in autosomal-dominant traits). Fortunately, most couples can be assured that nothing could have prevented a given abnormality in their offspring. Appreciating psychological defenses helps in understanding the failure of ostensibly intelligent and well-counseled couples to comprehend genetic information.

CHROMOSOME ABNORMALITIES

A basic fund of knowledge about common chromosome disorders is essential for the obstetrician who offers genetic screening for aneuploidy or who may encounter an abnormal fetus or infant during pregnancy or at delivery. With increasing utilization of chromosome microarrays for prenatal diagnosis, it is important for obstetricians to be familiar with the clinical significance of both numeric and structural chromosome abnormalities.

The incidence of chromosome aberrations is 1 in 160 newborns. In addition, more than 50% of first-trimester spontaneous abortions and at least 5% of stillborn infants exhibit chromosome abnormalities (see Chapter 27). The chromosome abnormalities that generate the greatest attention are the autosomal trisomies (Table 10-1). Autosomal trisomy usually arises as a result of nondisjunction that produces a gamete with 24 chromosomes, rather than the expected 23 chromosomes; this results in a zygote having 47 chromosomes. **This error most commonly occurs during maternal meiosis and is associated with the well-known maternal-age effect.** Table 10-2 shows the year-to-year (maternal age) increase in frequency of Down syndrome and other aneuploidies.[1] The frequency is about 30% higher in midpregnancy than at term, which reflects lethality throughout pregnancy.[2] Some trisomies—for example, trisomy 16—arise almost exclusively in maternal meiosis, usually

TABLE 10-1	INCIDENCE AND CLINICAL FEATURES OF MAJOR AUTOSOMAL TRISOMIES	
AUTOSOMAL TRISOMY	**INCIDENCE LIVE BIRTHS**	**CLINICAL FEATURES**
Trisomy 21	1 in 800	*Facial features:* brachycephaly; oblique palpebral fissures; epicanthal folds; broad nasal bridge; protruding tongue; small, low-set ears with an overlapping helix and a prominent antihelix; iridial Brushfield spots *Skeletal features:* broad, short fingers (brachymesophalangia); clinodactyly (incurving fifth finger resulting from an abnormality of the middle phalanx); a single flexion crease on the fifth digit; wide space between the first two toes Cardiac defects, duodenal atresia, neonatal hypotonia Increased susceptibility to respiratory infections and leukemia Mean survival extends into the fifth decade Mean IQ is 25 to 70
Trisomy 13	1 in 20,000	Holoprosencephaly, eye anomalies (microphthalmia, anophthalmia, or coloboma), cleft lip and palate, polydactyly, cardiac defects, cutaneous scalp defects, hemangiomata on the face or neck, low-set ears with an abnormal helix, and rocker-bottom feet (convex soles and protruding heels) Intrauterine and postnatal growth restriction Severe developmental retardation
Trisomy 18	1 in 8000	*Facial features:* microcephaly, prominent occiput, low-set and pointed "fawnlike" ears, micrognathia *Skeletal anomalies:* overlapping fingers (V over IV, II over III), short sternum, shield chest, narrow pelvis, limited thigh abduction or congenital hip dislocation, rocker-bottom feet with protrusion of the calcaneum, and a short dorsiflexed hallux ("hammer toe") Cardiac defects, renal anomalies Intrauterine growth restriction, developmental retardation

TABLE 10-2	MATERNAL AGE AND CHROMOSOMAL ABNORMALITIES (LIVE BIRTHS)*	
MATERNAL AGE	RISK FOR DOWN SYNDROME	RISK FOR ANY CHROMOSOME ABNORMALITIES
20	1/1667	1/526[†]
21	1/1667	1/526[†]
22	1/1429	1/500[†]
23	1/1429	1/500[†]
24	1/1250	1/476[†]
25	1/1250	1/476[†]
26	1/1176	1/476[†]
27	1/1111	1/455[†]
28	1/1053	1/435[†]
29	1/1100	1/417[†]
30	1/952	1/384[†]
31	1/909	1/385[†]
32	1/769	1/322[†]
33	1/625	1/317[†]
34	1/500	1/260
35	1/385	1/204
36	1/294	1/164
37	1/227	1/130
38	1/175	1/103
39	1/137	1/82
40	1/106	1/65
41	1/82	1/51
42	1/64	1/40
43	1/50	1/32
44	1/38	1/25
45	1/30	1/20
46	1/23	1/15
47	1/18	1/12
48	1/14	1/10
49	1/11	1/7

Data from Hook EB. Rates of chromosome abnormalities at different maternal ages. *Obstet Gynecol.* 1981;58:282; and Hook EB, Cross PK, Schreinemachers DM. Chromosomal abnormality rates at amniocentesis and in live-born infants. *JAMA.* 1983;249:2034.

*Because sample size for some intervals is relatively small, confidence limits are sometimes relatively large. Nonetheless, these figures are suitable for genetic counseling.
[†]47,XXX excluded for ages 20 to 32 years (data not available).

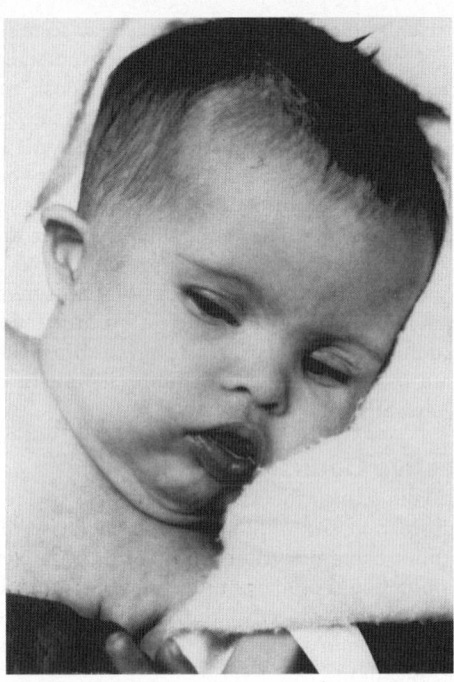

FIG 10-1 An infant with trisomy 21. (From Simpson JL, Elias S. *Genetics in Obstetrics and Gynecology*, ed 3. Philadelphia: WB Saunders; 2003:24.)

Autosomal Trisomy

Trisomy 21

Trisomy 21, or Down syndrome, is the most frequent autosomal chromosome syndrome with characteristic craniofacial features and congenital anomalies (Fig. 10-1; see also Table 10-1). The relationship of Down syndrome to advanced maternal age is well known (see Table 10-2). Approximately 95% of cases arise in maternal meiosis, usually meiosis I, and have 47 chromosomes (47,XX,+21 or 47,XY,+21). Mosaicism for chromosome 21 occurs in 2% to 4% of cases of Down syndrome and usually results in a higher IQ (70 to 80). Women with Down syndrome are usually fertile, and although relatively few trisomic mothers have reproduced, about 30% of their offspring are also trisomic. Men are invariably infertile.

Translocations (sporadic or familial) most commonly associated with Down syndrome involve chromosomes 14 and 21. One parent may have the same translocation, 45t(14q;21q), referred to as a *robertsonian translocation*. **Empiric risks for having an offspring with Down syndrome are approximately 10% for female robertsonian translocation carriers and 2% for male translocation carriers.** A potential concern is that offspring who are diploid (46,XX or 46,XY) actually have uniparental disomy (UPD), a condition in which both chromosomes originate from the same parent. In a study of 65 robertsonian translocation carriers (44t[13q;14q], 11t[14q;21q], 4t[14q;22q], and six others), only one UPD case was observed (0.6%).[3] The authors also surveyed 357 inherited and 102 de novo published cases and concluded that overall risk for UPD 14 or 15 was 3%.

Other structural rearrangements that result in Down syndrome include t(21q;21q) and translocations that involve chromosome 21 and other acrocentric chromosomes (13,15 or 22). In t(21q;21q) carriers, normal gametes do not ordinarily form. Thus only trisomic or monosomic zygotes are produced, and the

maternal meiosis I. For a few chromosomes, the frequency of errors is relatively higher in meiosis II (e.g., trisomy 18), and in yet others, errors in paternal meiosis are not uncommon (e.g., trisomy 2). **Autosomal trisomy can recur and has a recurrence risk of approximately 1% following either trisomy 18 or 21.** This suggests that genetic factors perturb meiosis, a phenomenon that serves as justification for offering prenatal genetic screening or testing after one aneuploid conception.

In addition to numeric abnormalities, structural chromosome abnormalities such as translocations, deletions, and duplications can occur. Individuals with a balanced translocation caused by an interchange between two or more chromosomes are usually phenotypically normal. However, such individuals are at increased risk for offspring with unbalanced gametes, which may result in recurrent pregnancy loss, fetal demise, congenital anomalies, and mental retardation. Small, often submicroscopic deletions and duplications of chromosome material can result in recognizable syndromes, such as the 22q11 deletion syndrome, and may cause structural malformations as well as cognitive, behavioral, and neuropsychological problems.

This section reviews the common autosomal trisomies and sex chromosome abnormalities an obstetrician is likely to encounter, and we discuss the clinical significance of deletions and duplications.

latter presumably appear as preclinical embryonic losses. Parents who have other translocations have a low empiric risk of having offspring with Down syndrome.

Trisomy 13

Trisomy 13 occurs in about 1/20,000 live births. The clinical features of trisomy 13 are summarized in Table 10-1. Most cases are caused by nondisjunction (47,XX,+13 or 47,XY,+13) and are maternal in origin. Robertsonian translocations are responsible for fewer than 20% of cases and are invariably associated with two group D (13 to 15) chromosomes joining at their centromeric regions. If neither parent has a rearrangement, the risk for subsequent affected progeny is not increased. If either parent has a balanced 13q;14q translocation, the recurrence risk for an affected offspring is increased but only to 1% to 2%. The exception is a 13q;13q parental translocation in which no normal gametes are formed; this has the same dire prognosis as a 21q;21q translocation. For live births with trisomy 13, survival beyond 3 years is rare.

Trisomy 18

Trisomy 18 occurs in 1 per 8000 live births (see Table 10-1). Stillbirth is not uncommon. Fetal movement is feeble, and approximately 50% develop nonreassuring fetal status during labor. For live births, mean survival is measured in months, and pronounced developmental and growth retardation is apparent. Approximately 80% of trisomy 18 cases are caused by primary nondisjunction (47,+18). Errors usually arise in maternal meiosis, frequently meiosis II. Recurrence risk is about 1%.

Other Autosomal Trisomies

All autosomes show trisomies, but usually the trisomies other than those described above end in abortuses. In addition to trisomies 13, 18, and 21, only a few other trisomies are detected in liveborns (8, 9, 14, 16, and 22), often as mosaics in conjunction with a normal cell line (46 chromosomes). All exhibit some degree of mental retardation, various structural anomalies, and intrauterine growth restriction (IUGR).

Autosomal Deletions and Duplications

Well-described genetic disorders have been associated with deletions or duplications of a number of chromosomes (Table 10-3). Although some of these may be diagnosed on a routine karyotype, most will only be detected by microarray analysis (MA) capable of detecting deletions and duplications smaller than 5 Mb (5,000,000 base pairs). Over 210 microdeletions and almost 80 microduplications have been reported as a result of the increased utilization of MA.[4] Specific clinical features vary but may include learning difficulties, mental retardation, neurologic and behavioral disorders, psychiatric disorders, and various congenital anomalies. De novo, large (1 Mb or greater) deletions or duplications, also referred to as *copy number variants* (CNVs), may contain dosage-sensitive genes and are more likely to be of clinical significance; however, even small CNVs can be significant. A growing body of literature and registries have compiled data on the outcomes of postnatal and prenatally ascertained CNVs. MA has been recommended as a first-tier test for the postnatal evaluation of individuals with undiagnosed developmental delay, intellectual disabilities, autism spectrum disorder, and/or multiple congenital anomalies based on a review of 33 studies showing that pathogenic CNVs were found in 12.2% of the 21,698 individuals studied (10% higher than with routine karyotype).[5] It is also important to recognize that many CNVs are of no ostensible clinical significance. In some cases, the clinical significance remains unknown; these CNVs are referred to as *variants of uncertain significance* (VOUS).

Most deletions and duplications occur sporadically because of nonallelic homologous recombination mediated by low-copy repetitive sequences of DNA during meiosis or mitosis and are not related to parental age. Hence, although the recurrence risk is low (<1%), it still may be elevated above baseline as a result of germline mosaicism. Thus a couple may be prompted to consider prenatal testing in a future pregnancy. However, CNVs can be familial; therefore parental studies are recommended. If a parent has the same CNV as one child, the risk to subsequent offspring is 50%. **It is important to note that the phenotype of many deletion and duplication syndromes is highly variable, and even within the same family, this can range from mild to severe.** In some cases, a parent may appear phenotypically normal. The inability to accurately predict the outcome can lead to uncertainty and heightened anxiety; thus it is critically important that patients receive the most up-to-date information from an experienced counselor or geneticist.

Sex Chromosome Abnormalities
Monosomy X (45,X)

The incidence of 45,X in liveborn girls is about 1 in 10,000. **Monosomy X, or Turner syndrome, accounts for 10% of all**

TABLE 10-3	COMMON DELETION SYNDROMES	
CHROMOSOME REGION	**SYNDROME**	**CLINICAL FEATURES**
4p16.3	Wolf-Hirschhorn	IUGR, failure to thrive, microcephaly, developmental delay, hypotonia, cognitive deficits, seizures, cardiac defects, GU abnormalities
5p15.2	Cri du chat	Microcephaly, SGA, hypotonia, catlike cry, cardiac defects
7q11.23	Williams	Supravalvular aortic stenosis, hypercalcemia, developmental delay, mild to moderate intellectual disability, social personality, attention-deficit disorder, female precocious puberty
15q11.2q13	Prader-Willi Angelman	*Prader-Willi:* Hypotonia, delayed development, short stature, small hands and feet, childhood obesity, learning disabilities, behavioral problems, delayed puberty *Angelman:* Developmental delay, intellectual disability, impaired speech, gait ataxia, happy personality, seizures, microcephaly
17p11.2	Smith-Magenis	Mild to moderate intellectual disability, delayed speech and language skills, behavioral problems, short stature, reduced sensitivity to pain and temperature, ear and eye abnormalities
20p12	Alagille	Bile duct paucity, peripheral pulmonary artery stenosis, cardiac defects, vertebral and GU anomalies
22q11.2	DiGeorge (velocardiofacial)	Cardiac defects, hypocalcemia, thymic hypoplasia, immune defect, renal and skeletal anomalies, delayed speech, learning difficulties, psychological and behavioral problems

GU, genitourinary; *IUGR,* intrauterine growth restriction; *SGA,* small for gestational age.

first-trimester abortions; therefore it can be calculated that more than 99% of 45,X conceptuses are lost early in pregnancy. The error usually (80%) involves loss of a paternal sex chromosome. Mosaicism is frequent and usually involves a coexisting 45,X cell line.

Common features include primary ovarian failure, absent pubertal development due to gonadal dysgenesis (streak gonads), and short stature (<150 cm). Structural abnormalities of the X chromosome may also result in premature ovarian failure. Both the long arm and the short arm of the X chromosome contain determinants necessary for ovarian differentiation and for normal stature. Various somatic anomalies include renal and cardiac defects, skeletal abnormalities (cubitus valgus and clinodactyly), vertebral anomalies, pigmented nevi, nail hypoplasia, and a low posterior hairline. Performance IQ is lower than verbal IQ, but overall IQ is considered normal. Adult-onset diseases include hypertension, coronary artery disease, hypothyroidism, and type 2 diabetes mellitus.

Low-dose estrogen therapy is needed to induce puberty, and long-term hormone replacement is needed in adulthood. Pregnancy may be achieved with the use of donor eggs but requires careful monitoring of cardiovascular status before and throughout pregnancy and in the postpartum period. Growth hormone treatment increases the final adult height 6 to 8 cm. Comprehensive guidelines for evaluation and clinical management of Turner syndrome are available.[6]

Klinefelter Syndrome

About 1 in 1000 males are born with Klinefelter syndrome, the result of two or more X chromosomes (47,XXY; 48,XXXY; and 49,XXXXY). Characteristic features include small testes, azoospermia, elevated follicle-stimulating hormone (FSH) and luteinizing hormone levels, and decreased testosterone. The most common chromosome complement associated with this phenotype is 47,XXY.

Mental retardation is uncommon in 47,XXY males, but behavioral problems and receptive language difficulties are common. Mental retardation is almost invariably associated with 48,XXXY and 49,XXXXY. Skeletal, trunk, and craniofacial anomalies occur infrequently in 47,XXY but are commonly observed in 48,XXXY and 49,XXXXY. Regardless of the specific chromosome complement, patients with Klinefelter syndrome all have male phenotypes. The penis may be hypoplastic, but hypospadias is uncommon. With intracytoplasmic sperm injection and other assisted reproductive technology (ART), siring a pregnancy is now possible. Simpson and colleagues[7] and Graham and colleagues[8] have provided guidelines on evaluation and clinical management.

Polysomy X in Girls (47,XXX; 48,XXXX; 49,XXXX)

About 1 in 800 liveborn girls has a 47, complement. The IQ of such individuals is 10 to 15 points lower than that of their siblings. The absolute risk for mental retardation does not exceed 5% to 10%, and even then, IQ is usually 60 to 80. Most of these individuals have a normal reproductive system. The theoretic risk of women with the 47, complement delivering an infant who also has an abnormal chromosome complement is 50%, given half of the maternal gametes carry 24 chromosomes (24,XX). Empiric risks are much less. Somatic anomalies are uncommon in those with the 47, complement, but anomalies may occur and have been observed in some prenatally detected cases.[9] However, 48,XXXX and 49,XXXXX individuals are

TABLE 10-4	ANEUPLOIDY SCREENING TESTS	
SCREENING TEST	TRISOMY 21 DETECTION RATE (%)	FALSE-POSITIVE RATE (%)
First-trimester NT, PAPP-A, free β-hCG	82 to 87	5
Second-trimester quad (MSAFP, hCG, uE₃, INHA)	81	5
Sequential (first- and second-trimester quad)	95	5
Serum integrated (PAPP-A, quad screen)	85 to 88	5
cfDNA	99	<1

Data from American College of Obstetricians and Gynecologists Committee on Practice Bulletins: screening for fetal chromosomal abnormalities, ACOG Practice Bulletin 77, 2007.
cfDNA, cell-free DNA; *hCG*, human chorionic gonadotropin; *INHA*, inhibin A; *MSAFP*, maternal serum alpha-fetoprotein; *NT*, nuchal translucency; *PAPP-A*, pregnancy-associated plasma protein A; *uE₃*, unconjugated estriol.

invariably retarded and are more likely to have somatic malformations than individuals with the 47, complement.

Polysomy Y in Boys (47,XYY and 48,XYYY)

Presence of more than one Y chromosome is another frequent chromosome abnormality in liveborn boys (1 in 1000). Those born 47,XYY are more likely than 46,XY boys to be tall and are at increased risk for learning disabilities, speech and language delay, and behavioral and emotional difficulties. These individuals have normal male phenotype and sexual development.

Screening for Aneuploidy

Noninvasive screening for chromosome disorders such as trisomies 21 and 18 is routinely offered to women during pregnancy regardless of maternal age. Several noninvasive approaches to screening are available that utilize maternal serum analytes and/or ultrasonography in the first and second trimesters (Table 10-4). More recently, noninvasive prenatal testing (NIPT) using cell-free DNA (cfDNA) has been introduced into clinical practice and can be performed as early as 10 weeks' gestation. However, screening has limitations that must be taken into consideration when deciding which testing strategy best meets the patient's needs and preferences. That is, *screening* is not equivalent to *testing*, which implies a definitive answer. Pretest counseling should thus remind parents of the possibilities of false-negative or false-positive test results. Women with a positive screening test for aneuploidy should be referred for genetic counseling and offered an invasive diagnostic test.

First-Trimester Screening

First-trimester screening can be performed between 11 and 14 weeks using a combination of biochemical markers, pregnancy-associated plasma protein A (PAPP-A) and free β–human chorionic gonadotropin (β-hCG), and ultrasound measurement of the nuchal translucency (NT), a sonolucent space present in all fetuses behind the fetal neck. The detection rate for trisomy 21 is greater than 80% with a false-positive rate of 5% compared with a 70% detection rate based on NT measurement alone.[10] In trisomy 21, PAPP-A levels are typically reduced, whereas hCG and the NT measurement are increased. First-trimester screening is comparable or

TABLE 10-5	DETECTION RATES IN THE NATIONAL INSTITUTE OF CHILD HEALTH AND HUMAN DEVELOPMENT BIOCHEMISTRY ULTRASOUND NUCHAL TRANSLUCENCY STUDY*

MATERNAL AGE	DETECTION RATE TRISOMY 21 (%)	FALSE-POSITIVE RATE (%)
<35 yr	66.7	3.7
≥35 yr	89.8	15.2
Total	**85.2**	**9.4**
Modeling for U.S. population (mean)	78.7	5
27 yr	63.9	1

From Wapner R, Thom E, Simpson JL, et al. First trimester screening for trisomies 21 and 18. *N Engl J Med*. 2003;349:1405.
*The National Institute of Child Health and Human Development first-trimester only screening (nuchal translucency, pregnancy-associated plasma protein A, free β-human chorionic gonadotropin) cohort of Wapner and colleagues. The sample of 8515 pregnancies prospectively applied a cutoff of 1/270. Detection rate increases with prevalence (increased maternal age) albeit at the cost of more procedures. Because the mean maternal age was 34.5 years, data were then modeled to apply to the U.S. population (whose mean maternal age is 27 years) at a 5% to 1% false-positive rate.

TABLE 10-6	DETECTION RATES IN THE NATIONAL INSTITUTE OF CHILD HEALTH AND HUMAN DEVELOPMENT FIRST- AND SECOND-TRIMESTER EVALUATION OF RISK (FASTER) TRIAL

TESTS*	TRISOMY 21 DETECTION RATE (%)
First Trimester (Free β-hCG, PAPP-A, NT)	
11 weeks	87
12 weeks	85
13 weeks	82
Second Trimester (15 to 18 weeks)	
AFP, uE₃, total hCG ("triple test")	69
AFP, uE₃, total hCG, inhibin A ("quad test")	81
First Plus Second Trimester (PAPP-A, NT, AFP, uE₃, hCG, inhibin A)	
Disclosure of first-trimester results	95
Nondisclosure of first-trimester results	96
Serum screening only	88

From Malone FD, Canick JA, Ball RH, et al. First-trimester or second-trimester screening or both for Down's syndrome. *N Engl J Med*. 2005;353:2001.
*If first-trimester ultrasound revealed septated cystic hygromas, intervention was taken (chorionic villus sampling was offered). Otherwise results were not disclosed until after second-trimester screening. Compiled data were then used to compare detection rates that would have occurred given various approaches, all at 5% false-positive (procedure) rates for each.
AFP, alpha-fetoprotein; *hCG*, human chorionic gonadotropin; *NT*, nuchal translucency; *PAPP-A*, pregnancy-associated plasma protein A; *uE₃*, unconjugated estriol.

superior to second-trimester screening alone and, most importantly, it provides parents with the option of earlier diagnostic testing in the event the screen indicates that the fetus is at high risk for aneuploidy. However, mandatory training and quality assurance for the NT measurement is a critical necessity.

Several large, multicenter, prospective studies have validated the clinical application of first-trimester screening. When comparing studies, it is important to keep in mind that detection rates vary according to sample characteristics. In particular, sensitivity for noninvasive screening is age dependent, and software is constructed such that the proportion of cases detected at a given age is greater for older women than for younger women. Hence the false-positive rate and the related procedure rate also increase with maternal age. Detection rates also depend not just on the trimester but on the week of gestation and on the arbitrarily set false-positive rate. If more procedures are accepted (i.e., the false-positive rate is higher), detection rates increases. The converse is also true.

In the first U.S. large-scale, prospective study of over 5800 women using both ultrasound (NT) and serum analytes (PAPP-A, free β-hCG), the detection rate for trisomy 21 was 87.5% (7 of 8 cases) in women younger than 35 years of age. In women older than 35 years, the detection rate was 92% (23 of 25), albeit with higher false-positive and invasive procedure rates. For trisomy 18, detection rates were 100% in both age groups.[11] **In 2003, an National Institute of Child Health and Human Development (NICHD) multicenter cohort study, the Biochemstry Ultrasound Nuchal Translucency (BUN) Study, reported results in 8514 women screened between 74 and 97 days' gestation** (Table 10-5).[12] Applying the traditional midtrimester screen positive cutoff of 1 in 270, 85.2% of trisomy 21 pregnancies were identified with a false-positive rate of 9.4%. The high false-positive rate was predictable, given the higher mean maternal age of the sample. Stratifying by age, the detection rate for trisomy 21 was 66.7% for patients younger than age 35 years with a 3.7% false-positive rate, and it was 89.8% in patients older than age 35 years with a 15.2% false-positive rate. The detection rate for trisomy 18 was 90.9%. Modeling for the general population (with a lower mean age) and setting a false-positive procedure rate of 5%, sensitivity for trisomy 21 was estimated to be 78.7%; at a false-positive rate of 1%, the sensitivity was estimated to be 63.9%. These findings were consistent with other studies.

Two other large, collaborative studies also have provided results comparable to the NICHD BUN study. The Serum, Urine, and Ultrasound Screening Study (SURUSS) was a 25-center European trial[13] in which 47,000 patients were evaluated in both the first and second trimesters. Using a similar design, Malone and colleagues[14] studied 38,167 women in 15 U.S. centers in the NICHD First- and Second-Trimester Evaluation of Risk (FASTER) trial. Detection rates for Down syndrome were 87% at 11 weeks and 85% at 12 weeks (Table 10-6). In this study, 134 women who had fetuses with a septated cystic hygroma were removed from the cohort; 51% had a chromosome abnormality and 34% had other major abnormalities.[15] The group later stratified their data and found that **NT greater than 4 mm was *never* associated with a normal noninvasive screen; therefore women with an NT that exceeded this threshold should be offered diagnostic testing without needing to undergo further analyte analysis.**[16] In fact, only 8% of pregnancies with NT greater than 3 mm had a screen-negative value.

Nicolaides[10] tabulated that NT, PAPP-A, and hCG detected 87% of 215 trisomy fetuses at a false-positive rate of 5%. Later results of Avgidou and colleagues[17] reported superior results from the same U.K. group. This group screened 30,564 women with NT, PAPP-A, and hCG, providing results the same day and detecting 93% of trisomy 21 cases. The incorporation of the other sonographic markers such as the presence of a nasal bone, reverse ductus venosus flow, and tricuspid regurgitation has been proposed to increase the detection rates further. In general these markers are not utilized except in specialized centers.

When an increased NT measurement is associated with a normal karyotype, fetal loss rates are increased and other fetal anomalies and genetic syndromes are observed, in particular, congenital heart defects.[18] **A targeted ultrasound examination during the second trimester and fetal echocardiography are recommended when the NT measurement is 3.5 mm or greater and the fetal karyotype is normal.**

Second-Trimester Serum Screening

The most widely used second-trimester aneuploidy screening test is the so-called quad screen, which utilizes four biochemical analytes—alpha-fetoprotein (AFP), hCG, unconjugated estriol (uE$_3$), and dimeric inhibin A (INHA). Performed between 15 and 22 weeks' gestation, the detection rate for trisomy 21 is about 75% in women who are less than 35 years of age and over 80% in women 35 years or older, with a false-positive rate of 5%. For trisomy 18, using only the first three markers provides a detection rate of about 70%. Serum screening does not detect other age-related forms of aneuploidy such as Klinefelter syndrome (47,XXY).

Serum hCG and INHA levels are increased in women carrying fetuses with Down syndrome.[19] Levels of AFP and uE$_3$ in maternal serum are lower in pregnancies affected with Down syndrome compared with unaffected pregnancies.[20] Typically, levels of AFP, uE$_3$, and hCG are reduced in trisomy 18. A simple approach to detect trisomy 18 is to offer invasive prenatal diagnostic testing whenever serum screening for each of these three markers falls below certain thresholds (maternal serum α-fetoprotein [MSAFP], 0.6 multiples of the median [MoM]; hCG, 0.55 MoM; uE$_3$, 0.5 MoM).[21] Using these thresholds would detect 60% to 80% of trisomy 18 fetuses with a 0.4% amniocentesis rate. Calculating individual risk estimation on the basis of three markers and maternal age, Palomaki and colleagues[22] reported that 60% of trisomy 18 pregnancies can be detected with a low false-positive rate of 0.2%. The value of individual risk estimates is that one in nine pregnancies identified as being at increased risk for trisomy 18 by serum screening would actually be affected.

Confounding factors influence serum screening, and adjustments for gestational age, maternal weight, ethnicity, diabetes, and number of fetuses are necessary. Weight adjustment is needed because without adjustment, dilutional effects would result in heavier women having a spuriously low value, whereas thinner women would have a spuriously elevated value. In women with type 1 diabetes mellitus, a population at increased risk for NTDs, the median levels of MSAFP, uE$_3$ and hCG are lower than in nondiabetic women. In black women, who have a lower risk for a fetal NTD, the median MSAFP is higher than in other ethnic groups. Maternal smoking increases MSAFP by 3% but decreases maternal serum uE$_3$ and hCG levels by 3% and 23%, respectively.[23] Maternal serum hCG is higher and MSAFP is lower in pregnancies conceived in vitro compared with pregnancies conceived spontaneously.[23] A claim has been made that adjustments should be made for prior aneuploidy; β-hCG is reported to be 10% higher in a pregnancy after aneuploidy, whereas PAPP-A is increased 15% in the first trimester.[24]

First- and Second-Trimester Screening

Several approaches have been proposed using the combination of both first- and second-trimester screening to increase the detection rate over that achieved by screening in either trimester alone, with detection rates of 88% to 96% with false-positive rates of 5% reported. A caveat is that independent screening (i.e., using both first- and second-trimester screening tests to assess the risk separately and independently) is not recommended because of the unacceptably high false-positive rates.

Sequential screening begins with first-trimester screening. A woman is informed of the adjusted risk for aneuploidy based on the first-trimester results. If her risk is high (greater than 1 in 50), she is offered genetic counseling and diagnostic testing. If the risk is low or moderate, a second-trimester screening test is performed with results of both the first- and second-trimester screening tests used to generate a final adjusted risk for trisomies 21 and 18. **This is called the *stepwise approach*. With contingency screening, not all women will proceed to second-trimester screening because this occurs only with an intermediate risk; if the risk is low after the first-trimester screening, no further testing is indicated.** The detection rates of the contingency approach are about 90% with low positive screening rates (2% to 3%). Malone and colleagues[25] compared several different first- plus second-trimester contingent sequential approaches (see Table 10-5). They concluded that the optimal method was contingency screening, in which patients were divided into three groups: (1) women whose calculated (NT, PAPP-A, hCG) first-trimester risk was greater than 1/30 would undergo chorionic villus sampling (CVS); (2) women whose risk was less than 1/1500 would undergo no further testing; and (3) all other women would undergo second-trimester serum testing. Using this approach, only 21.8% of the cohort would need second-trimester testing in order to detect 93% of trisomy 21 cases with a 4.3% false-positive rate; 65% would be detected in the first trimester with only 1.5% of patients having CVS procedures.

Integrated screening has the highest theoretic detection rate (93% to 96%), but with this approach, the first-trimester screening results are withheld until the second-trimester screen is completed. The individual receives only a single adjusted risk for trisomy 21 and trisomy 18 based on the results of both the first- and second-trimester screen. The obvious disadvantage with this approach is that the individual does not have an option of early diagnostic testing in the event that the first-trimester screen would have indicated a high risk for trisomy 21 or 18. Another is that patients may not return for their second-trimester screening. Fortunately, Cuckle and colleagues[26,27] showed that disclosure of first-trimester results could be made with very little loss in sensitivity of integrated screening.

When an NT measurement cannot be obtained, and in communities where NT measurement is not available, serum integrated screening is acceptable. In the FASTER trial, the sensitivity was 88%.[14] With this approach, the first-trimester PAPP-A and the second-trimester serum analytes are used to adjust the risk for trisomy 21, and the individual receives one adjusted risk after the second-trimester screen is completed.

Cell-Free DNA Analysis

The newest screening test for aneuploidy uses maternal cell-free DNA (cfDNA). Maternal plasma contains small fragments of cfDNA (50 to 200 base pairs) derived from the breakdown of both maternal and fetal cells, primarily derived from the placenta. The concept of using cfDNA for prenatal diagnosis is not new; cfDNA has been used successfully to determine fetal sex in pregnancies at risk for X-linked disorders by identifying the Y-chromosome signal. In Europe, noninvasive testing is commonly used to determine fetal Rhesus factor (Rh) status in RhD-negative women using real-time polymerase chain reaction (PCR) amplification. A similar approach can be adapted for the detection of some single-gene disorders. However, to screen for aneuploidy requires a different approach—the use of massively parallel DNA shotgun sequencing (MPSS).

The detection of aneuploidy is more difficult than for single-gene disorders because detecting fetal trisomy must reflect quantitative differences between affected and unaffected pregnancies. With MPSS technology, millions of fragments of maternal and fetal DNA are sequenced simultaneously in a single sample of maternal plasma, which is assigned to a chromosome region and counted. A woman carrying a trisomy 21 fetus will have relatively more chromosome 21 counts than a woman carrying a normal fetus. Alternatively, some laboratories use a targeted approach that sequences specific chromosomes of interest, such as 18 and 21, and adjusts for the proportion of fetal DNA (fetal fraction) to provide a patient-specific risk assessment that takes into account maternal age. An alternative approach is to use single nucleotide polymorphism (SNP)-based sequencing, which allows for the detection of triploidy and some of the common deletion syndromes.

Several studies have demonstrated the ability to detect fetal trisomy 21 using MPSS. A blinded, nested, case-control study of 4664 pregnancies at increased risk for trisomy 21 from 27 prenatal diagnostic centers worldwide validated the use of cfDNA analysis as a screening test for trisomy 21. In this study, 209 of 221 cases of trisomy 21 were detected; sensitivity was 98.6% with a false-positive rate of 0.2%.[28] Subsequently, Palomaki and colleagues[29] reported that all cases of trisomy 18 in this cohort were detected with a false-positive rate of 0.28%, but only 91.7% of the cases of trisomy 13 were detected with a false-positive rate of 0.97%.

Norton and colleagues[30] conducted a multicenter, prospective cohort study—the Noninvasive Chromosomal Evaluation (NICE) study—of over 3200 primarily high-risk women undergoing invasive diagnostic testing. For trisomy 21, the sensitivity was 100% with a false-positive rate of 0.03%, whereas the sensitivity for trisomy 18 was 97.4% and the false-positive rate was 0.07%. Two patients were classified as high risk for trisomy 18 and had a normal karyotype; this highlights the need for confirmatory diagnostic testing when an NIPT is positive or shows high risk for aneuploidy. Further, 29% of the chromosome abnormalities in this cohort were abnormalities other than trisomy 18 and 21 or were sex chromosome abnormalities such as unbalanced translocations, deletions, and duplications.

In a series of 1982 consecutive pregnancies at 12 weeks' gestation or greater referred for NIPT at a center in Hong Kong, 11 pregnancies screened positive for sex chromosome abnormalities, and 85.7% were confirmed to be fetal in origin.[31] Fetal mosaicism was detected in two cases, emphasizing that it is important to counsel patients about this possibility. Maternal mosaicism for 45,X/XX and confined placental mosaicism also lead to false-positive NIPT results, underscoring the importance of confirmatory invasive diagnostic testing.

Another limitation of cfDNA screening is the reported assay failure rate of up to 5%. One of the reasons is a low fetal fraction; a minimum fetal fraction of 4% is required. The ability to detect the small differences between euploid and triploid fetuses depends on the relative proportion of fetal to maternal cfDNA. The average fetal fraction at 10 to 22 weeks' gestation is 10% independent of gestational age, maternal age, race/ethnicity, or

fetal karyotype.[30] Fetal fraction decreases with maternal weight, and if NIPT fails in an obese patient, it may be necessary to repeat the test on a second sample or to offer serum and/or ultrasound screening as an alternative. Further consideration should be given to offering invasive testing because recent studies have reported a higher frequency of aneuploidy when cfDNA testing fails.

The American College of Obstetricians and Gynecologists (ACOG) and the American College of Medical Genetics (ACMG) recommend that women be offered aneuploidy screening, and both acknowledge that NIPT is one of the screening options for women at increased risk for aneuploidy.[32,33] This includes women 35 years or older and those with fetal ultrasound markers and structural anomalies associated with aneuploidy, prior pregnancy with trisomy, positive serum screening test, or a parental robertsonian translocation with risk for trisomy 21 or 13. However, as studies of low-risk women are conducted, we can expect that NIPT will become more widely available. In a cohort study of over 2000 women who presented for routine first-trimester screening (11 to 14 weeks) with a mean maternal age of 31.8 years, Nicolaides and colleagues[34] demonstrated that cfDNA analysis using targeted MPSS is feasible in a lower-risk population. The detection rate for trisomy 21 was 100% with a false-positive rate of 0.1%. Norton and colleagues[35] reported similar results in the international, blinded, prospective multicenter Noninvasive Examination of Trisomy (NEXT) study, which compared cfDNA to first-trimester screening at 10 to 14 weeks' gestation in 15,841 women (mean age 30.7) with a singleton gestation. The positive predictive value was 80.9% (95% confidence interval [CI], 66.7 to 90.9). Although all cases of trisomy 21 and 13 were detected, it is important to note that cfDNA testing did *not* detect one in 10 cases of trisomy 18, nor would it have detected the other forms of aneuploidy found in this study population. Furthermore, the rate of aneuploidy among patients with no cfDNA results was 2.7%, a prevalence of 1 in 38.[35] Hence, careful consideration should be given to offering diagnostic testing to this group of patients.

In the United States, Bianchi and colleagues[36] conducted a multicenter study to compare the false-positive rates of cfDNA analysis to routine first- and second-trimester screening. In 1914 women (mean age 29.6 years), the false-positive rate for trisomy 21 with cfDNA testing was significantly lower, 0.3% compared with 3.6%. All cases of aneuploidy were detected, but this finding should be interpreted cautiously because of the small sample size. **Patients will need to be counseled that a negative cfDNA test does *not* ensure an unaffected pregnancy and cannot provide the diagnostic accuracy of an invasive prenatal diagnostic test, especially if fetal structural anomalies exist or with a family history of a genetic disorder.**

Aneuploidy Screening in Multiple Gestation

In dizygotic pregnancies, each twin has an individual risk for trisomy 21; analysis of the European National Down Syndrome Cytogenetic Registry found that dizygotic pregnancies were one third more likely to have at least one fetus with trisomy 21 than age-adjusted singleton pregnancies.[37] The pregnancy-specific and fetus-specific risks should be the same for monozygotic twins as for singleton pregnancies, although the study found the actual risk to be about a third that of a singleton pregnancy. Unfortunately, **Down syndrome screening using multiple** serum markers is less sensitive in twin pregnancies than in singleton pregnancies. Using singleton cutoffs, one study showed that 73% of monozygotic twin pregnancies but only 43% of dizygotic twin pregnancies with Down syndrome were detected, given a 5% false-positive rate.[38] Decreased sensitivity in detecting trisomy 21 in dizygotic twins reflects the blunting effect of the concomitant presence of one normal and one aneuploid fetus. Thus patients with twins should be informed that the detection rate by serum screening is less than that in singleton pregnancies. First-trimester screening identifies about 70% of Down syndrome pregnancies; NT measurement alone has been shown to be as effective a screening test for higher-order multiple gestation as it is for twin gestations. The addition of the nasal bone (NB) assessment to the NT measurement increased the detection rate to 87% at a screen-positive rate of 5% and to 89% when serum analytes were included in a retrospective study of 2094 twin pregnancies.[39] First-trimester screening further provides the option of early diagnostic testing if the risk is increased and if selective reduction is undertaken.

Experience using cfDNA analysis in multiple gestations is limited, but a few studies suggest that cfDNA has similar sensitivity and specificity rates as in singleton pregnancies.[40,41] For dizygotic twins, a higher fetal fraction (minimum of 8%) may be necessary to detect a quantitative difference. NIPT should be interpreted cautiously in pregnancies with a vanishing twin; the results may be discordant because the vanishing twin may continue to release cfDNA into the maternal circulation. SNP-based NIPT may be helpful in identifying this phenomenon.

Ultrasound Screening for Aneuploidy

Second-trimester ultrasonography may detect anomalies associated with aneuploidy, such as cardiac defects or duodenal atresia (see Chapter 9). In 1985, Benacerraf and colleagues[42] showed a **significant association between the thickness of the fetal nuchal skin fold and the presence of trisomy 21.** For the first time, a "marker," as opposed to an actual birth defect, could be used to assess the likelihood that Down syndrome was present. **Other markers now commonly used in the genetic sonogram include the NB length, short femur or humerus, echogenic intracardiac focus, echogenic bowel, and pyelectasis.** The use of these markers has gradually become common clinical practice. As markers were studied in larger numbers of women, it became possible to assign likelihood ratios to each marker and to do a formal risk adjustment from the a priori risk to an ultrasound-adjusted risk. However, **most of the markers perform poorly as individual predictors of Down syndrome and have a very low sensitivity and a high rate of false-positive results.**[43] Further, the test performance depends on the skill of the examiner and the subjective assessment required for several markers, particularly echogenic intracardiac focus and echogenic bowel. Most women who undergo a genetic sonogram have no markers, but **women should be informed that the absence of markers does _not_ rule out the possibility of Down syndrome or other chromosome abnormalities.**

The incidental finding of "soft markers," minor markers such as echogenic intracardiac focus or pyelectasis, in otherwise low-risk pregnancies can cause a great deal of anxiety in the expectant parents. Opinions vary as to what to do when these soft markers are noted in a low-risk patient. A reasonable approach is to refer such a patient for consultation with an expert to evaluate the presence of other markers in the context of other screening tests (i.e., multiple marker screening or cfDNA).

Prenatal Diagnostic Testing for Chromosome Abnormalities

Every chromosome disorder is potentially detectable in utero with the availability of chromosome microarrays. Thus any pregnant woman could undergo an invasive procedure, if she so desired, to assess the chromosome status of the fetus. However, for most couples, the risks of an invasive procedure outweigh the diagnostic benefits. Many will elect noninvasive screening with the understanding that the sensitivity is less than 100% and that the screen is only intended to identify pregnancies at increased risk for the common trisomies. In the setting of a "positive" screening test, a true test—which requires an invasive diagnostic procedure—is then necessary. In this section, we review the indications for prenatal diagnostic testing for chromosome abnormalities and also discuss the types of tests currently available.

Indications for Prenatal Cytogenetic Testing

In January 2007, ACOG published a new recommendation that all women, regardless of age, should have the option of invasive testing without first having been screened.[44] Prenatal cytogenetic testing can be as basic as a routine G-banded karyotype, or it might include a whole genome microarray. In some cases, a more targeted approach may be desirable and could include either fluorescence in situ hybridization (FISH) for a specific chromosome region of interest or a targeted chromosome microarray.

PREVIOUS CHILD WITH A CHROMOSOME ABNORMALITY

After the birth of one child, stillborn fetus, or abortus with a chromosome abnormality, couples may elect to have prenatal diagnostic testing in subsequent pregnancies. **With autosomal trisomy, the likelihood that subsequent progeny will have an autosomal trisomy is about 1%, even if parental chromosome complements are normal.** The recurrence risk for other de novo chromosome abnormalities is low (1% or less because of the possibility of germline mosaicism), and diagnostic testing can provide reassurance.

PARENTAL CHROMOSOME REARRANGEMENTS

An uncommon but important indication for prenatal cytogenetic studies is presence of a parental chromosome abnormality such as a balanced translocation, inversion, deletion, or duplication. A mother or father with a balanced translocation is at risk for offspring with an unbalanced translocation and, hence, an abnormal phenotype. Fortunately, **empiric data show that theoretic risks for abnormal (unbalanced) offspring are greater than empiric risks, but miscarriages are common.** It is for this reason that preimplantation genetic diagnosis (PGD) can be especially helpful. The risk for having a liveborn infant with an unbalanced chromosome complement varies by rearrangement, sex of the parental carrier, and method of ascertainment.[45] Pooled empiric risks tabulated at CVS or amniocentesis approximate 12% risk for clinically abnormal offspring of either male or female translocation carriers with reciprocal translocations.[46] For robertsonian (centric fusion) translocations, risks vary according to the chromosomes involved as discussed above.

A parent with a deletion or duplication has a 1 in 2 chance of transmitting the abnormal chromosome and having an affected child. Due to the wide phenotypic variability of many of the deletion/duplication syndromes, it can be difficult to predict the phenotype of an affected offspring prenatally.

ASSISTED REPRODUCTION THROUGH INTRACYTOPLASMIC SPERM INJECTION

Intracytoplasmic sperm injection (ICSI) is used in ART when the man is subfertile. Empiric data demonstrate an increased frequency of aneuploidies, mainly sex chromosome anomalies (1% to 2%).[47] The excess risk appears unrelated to the ICSI technique, rather it relates to the underlying male infertility that necessitated ICSI.

CYTOGENETIC TESTING

The gold standard for prenatal cytogenetic testing has been the G-banded karyotype, first introduced in the late 1970s. Karyotyping can detect numeric abnormalities, balanced translocations, and structural abnormalities greater than 5 to 10 Mb (5 to 10 million base pairs). The routine karyotype remains a valid test for those interested in knowing whether the fetus has a major trisomy or for the cytogenetic evaluation of a couple with a history of recurrent pregnancy loss (see Chapter 27). However, with the availability of tests with a higher resolution for detecting chromosome rearrangements of less than 5 Mb, such as chromosome MAs, **ACOG recommends that women who desire an invasive prenatal diagnostic test be offered MAs as an option.**[48] **Recent studies also support the use of MAs for the evaluation of the fetus with a structural malformation.**[46,49-51] When a specific chromosome region is of interest, a more targeted approach using FISH may be utilized.

CHROMOSOME MICROARRAYS

Chromosome MAs allow comprehensive analysis of the entire genome at a finer resolution than a routine karyotype and are capable of detecting trisomies and submicroscopic deletions and duplications of the genome (CNVs). CNVs can be detected using either comparative genomic hybridization (CGH) or SNP arrays (Fig. 10-2). For both, the principle is based on single-stranded DNA annealing (hybridizing) with a complementary single-stranded DNA. To look for CNVs, a sample of test DNA is labeled with a fluorochrome (e.g., red), denatured to single-stranded DNA, and then hybridized to single-stranded copies of DNA of known sequence differentially labeled (e.g., green) and embedded on a platform (array) in an ordered fashion. If equal amounts of control and test DNA are present, the color of the hybridized mixture could be expected to be yellow. If the test DNA were in excess (e.g., trisomy or duplication), the mixture for the relevant chromosome region would be relatively more of the color used to connote test (patient) DNA. This would be red in the previous example. SNP arrays can also detect homozygosity or heterozygosity for regions of DNA and can detect triploidy, UPD, and consanguinity.

Several different commercial platforms are available, but all interrogate sequences of DNA along every chromosome. "Coverage" varies slightly based on sensitivity sought, and all have redundancy—that is, a given region that is interrogated more than once to ensure replicability before making a diagnosis. Targeted arrays contain sequences from the pericentromeric and telomeric regions of the chromosome as well as clinically significant deletion and duplication syndromes. Although less sensitive than a whole-genome array, a targeted MA reduces the likelihood of finding CNVs of uncertain significance.

Several studies have demonstrated that prenatal microarrays are reliable and have several advantages over conventional cytogenetic testing, especially in the fetus with a structural malformation. The NICHD prospective prenatal cytogenetic array

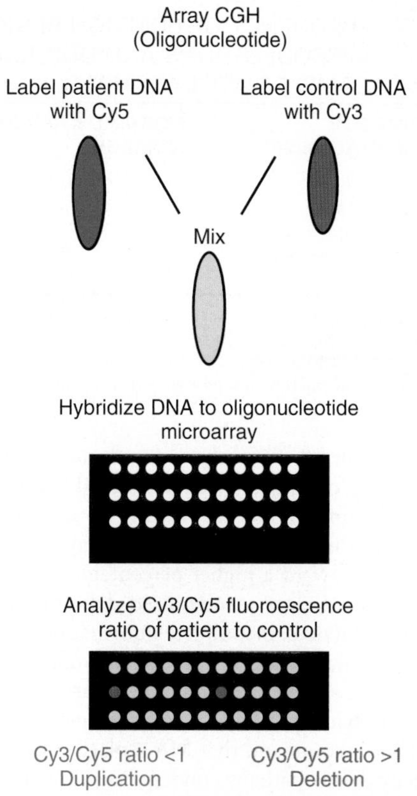

FIG 10-2 Schematic diagram illustrating principles of array comparative genome hybridization (CGH). Patient DNA is labeled in *red* (CY5), whereas references (normal control) are labeled in *green* (Cy3). When denatured into single-stranded DNA, patient DNA and control DNA hybridize with DNA of the same type embedded on a platform (*circles*). The diagram shows only 33 "spots" of similar sequence, whereas in actual practice, a diagnostic platform would consist of thousands of embedded sequences. If the region being interrogated shows equal amounts of patient DNA and control DNA, the signal is *yellow*. A *green* signal indicates deficiency of test DNA (deletion or mosaicism), whereas a *red* signal indicates excess of test DNA (duplication or trisomy). Array CGH detects trisomies just like a karyotype; smaller deletions or duplications (<5 million base pairs) are detected only by array CGH. (Courtesy Ron J. Wapner, Columbia University, New York.)

study of 4401 women with varying indications for prenatal genetic diagnosis detected all of the trisomies, sex chromosome abnormalities, and unbalanced translocations identified by routine karyotype.[49] **In addition, clinically significant CNVs were detected in 6% of the 755 fetuses with a normal karyotype and suspected structural anomalies or growth abnormalities** (Table 10-7). Clinically significant CNVs were also detected in 1.7% of those with advanced maternal age or a positive serum screen result. These chromosome abnormalities were not detected on a routine karyotype. A smaller study that used high-resolution SNP arrays yielded comparable findings (1.6% in cases of advanced maternal age and 6.9% for ultrasound anomalies).[49] Similar results were found in a retrospective analysis of 2858 prenatal samples referred with abnormal sonographic findings, and 6.2% with a known normal karyotype had a clinically significant CNV.[46] The majority of samples in this study were tested using a whole-genome array. The odds of finding a clinically significant CNV increased when anomalies were present in two or more organ systems (9.5%) but were less common in samples referred for isolated growth abnormalities

| TABLE 10-7 | FREQUENCY OF COMMON BENIGN, PATHOGENIC, AND POTENTIALLY CLINICALLY SIGNIFICANT MICRODELETIONS AND DUPLICATIONS ON CHROMOSOME MICROARRAY ANALYSIS OF PRENATAL SAMPLES WITH A NORMAL KARYOTYPE |

INDICATION FOR PRENATAL DIAGNOSIS	NORMAL KARYOTYPE NUMBER	COMMON BENIGN NUMBER (%)	KNOWN PATHOGENIC AND POTENTIAL FOR CLINICAL SIGNFICANCE NUMBER (%) [CI]*
Any	3822	1234 (32.3)	96 (2.5) [2.1-3.1]
Advanced maternal age	1966	628 (31.9)	34 (1.7) [1.2-2.4]
Positive Down syndrome screening	729	247 (33.9)	12 (1.6) [0.9-2.9]
Anomaly on ultrasonography	755	247 (32.7)	45 (6.0) [4.5-7.9]
Other†	372	112 (30.1)	5 (1.3) [0.6-3.1]

From American College of Obstetricians and Gynecologists Committee on Genetics. ACOG Committee Opinion No. 581: the use of chromosomal microarray analysis in prenatal diagnosis. *Obstet Gynecol.* 2013;122:1374-1377.
*All confidence intervals (CIs) are 95%.
†Other indications include family history, previous pregnancy with chromosomal abnormalities, and elective decision.

(2.6%) or so-called soft markers on ultrasound examination (2.6%). Lee and colleagues[51] reported a 10.5% detection rate with a single anomaly and 15.4% with two or more anomalies. A number of factors may explain the differences among studies, including a bias toward a higher percentage of trisomies, types of malformations, lack of standardized definition of anomalies from referring practices, incomplete information on the number and type of anomalies, lack of postnatal confirmation of ultrasound anomalies, sample size, and types of arrays utilized. Based on the current evidence, ACOG and the Society for Maternal-Fetal Medicine recommend that MA replace conventional cytogenetic analysis in patients undergoing invasive diagnostic testing for the evaluation of a fetus with one or more structural abnormalities.[48]

One of the major concerns with this technology is the identification of VOUS. The NICHD study detected VOUS in 3.4% of cases with a normal karyotype, but it is equally important to note that one third were reclassified several years later as pathogenic.[49] As cases are ascertained and followed longitudinally, additional information will provide more accurate information for genetic counseling. The percentage of VOUS reported in the literature will vary with the microarray platform utilized. Shaffer and colleagues[50] reported on their experience with MAs of over 5000 prenatal samples over 7 years. The rate of VOUS was 4.2%; however, if only de novo variants were considered, the rate dropped to 0.39%, the same rate reported using a whole-genome SNP array.[50] Such a low rate may be acceptable in light of the diagnostic yield obtained with MAs.

In addition to identifying clinically significant CNVs in the fetus, prenatal MAs have the potential to identify variants in the parents that may connote increased susceptibility to cancer or adult-onset disorders. MAs may also reveal consanguinity or nonpaternity; therefore it is critical that patients are informed of the limitation and potential test results prior to testing to minimize the anxiety and distress associated with uncertain or unexpected findings.[52]

One disadvantage of array CGH compared with the traditional karyotype is that chromosome MAs cannot distinguish between balanced translocations and normal karyotype; unbalanced (duplication, deficiency) rearrangements are readily detected. Another difficulty is the inability to detect low-level mosaicism in which one of the two cell lines is infrequent. In some platforms, triploidy cannot be excluded. On the other hand, MAs can be performed on uncultured DNA, and this has been shown to be useful in the evaluation of stillbirths in which cell cultures for chromosome abnormalities are not often successful. The NICHD Stillbirth Collaborative Research

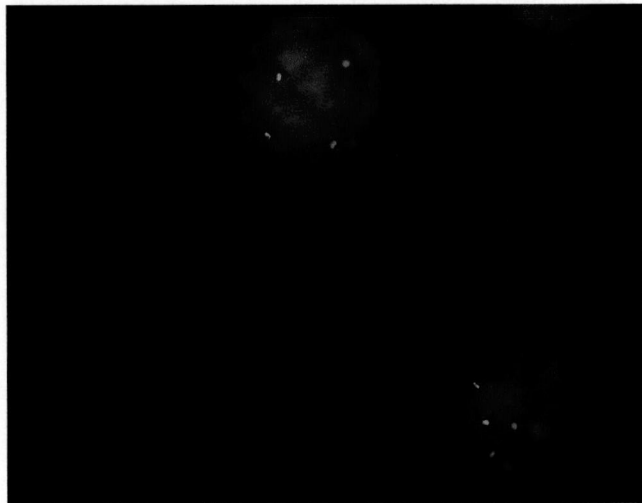

FIG 10-3 Fluorescence in situ hybridization (FISH) performed on interphase nuclei obtained from peripheral blood lymphocytes. Dual-color FISH has been performed using Vysis (Abbot Molecular) locus-specific probes for chromosome 13 (*green*) and chromosome 21 (*red*). Chromosomal DNA is stained with DAPI (*blue*). Two signals for each indicates disomy (normal numbers) for these two chromosomes. (Courtesy Helen Tempest, Florida International University, Miami.)

Network demonstrated a higher success rate with MAs compared with conventional karyotyping (87.4% vs. 70.5%) in the evaluation of 532 stillbirths.[53] The detection rate of chromosome abnormalities was also higher (8.3% vs. 5.8%).

FLUORESCENCE IN SITU HYBRIDIZATION

Prior to the availability of MAs, FISH was a useful adjunct to a karyotype to examine a specific chromosome region or rapidly screen for aneuploidy. FISH is still useful when a parent with a known deletion or a couple with a previous affected child requests prenatal diagnosis for just that specific region.

DNA sequences unique to the chromosome in question are labeled with a fluorochrome and are hybridized to a metaphase chromosome or interphase nuclei (Fig. 10-3). Cells with two copies should show two separate signals; trisomic cells show three signals. One signal is present in the setting of a deletion. Because of geometric vicissitudes (e.g., one chromosome overlying another may not be appreciated in a two-dimensional scan), not every trisomic cell shows three signals; however, the modal count is readily determined. A single cell can be interrogated for up to five chromosomes. **FISH uses**

interphase cells and thus permits rapid or same-day diagnosis of aneuploidy. **This becomes particularly important when a rapid diagnosis is needed to aid in the management of a fetus at high risk, such as one with multiple anomalies detected by ultrasound.** FISH can also be used on preserved tissue (e.g., paraffin blocks) when culture for metaphase analysis is obviously not possible.

QUANTITATIVE FLUORESCENT POLYMERASE CHAIN REACTION

Polymerase chain reaction (PCR) is a widely used test that permits a small amount of DNA (e.g., from one cell) to be amplified to generate an amount sufficient for a diagnostic test. In quantitative PCR (QPCR), the rapidity with which the exponential increase in DNA occurs allows rapid and accurate detection of major numeric chromosome disorders in CVS.[54] This technique can be a powerful adjunct to conventional cytogenetics and in some venues, such as in Europe, it has replaced the traditional karyotype in prenatal diagnosis.

Accuracy of Prenatal Cytogenetic Diagnosis

Although invasive diagnostic testing for routine cytogenetic testing has markedly declined with the availability of noninvasive screening for aneuploidy and higher resolution MA, it is important for the obstetrician/gynecologist to be aware of the common pitfalls associated with analysis of chorionic villi or amniotic fluid cells. One problem is that cells may not grow, or growth may be insufficient for proper analysis (although with MAs, this is not a problem). Uncommonly, there may be maternal cell contamination, which can be minimized by discarding the first 1 to 2 mL of aspirated amniotic fluid during amniocentesis. In CVS, examination under a dissecting microscope allows the clinician to distinguish villi from maternal decidua.

A more vexing concern is that chromosome abnormalities detected in villi or amniotic fluid may not reflect fetal status. Chromosome aberrations may arise in culture (in vitro) or may be confined to placental tissue. This possibility should be suspected when mosaicism (more than one cell line) is restricted to only one of the several culture flasks or to clones initiated from a single amniotic fluid or CVS specimen, or when an abnormal karyotype with a known severely anomalous phenotype does not correlate with a normal ultrasound. Although the reference laboratory and clinical geneticists are naturally expected to have requisite expertise, the obstetrician should be prepared to discuss certain common dilemmas with the patient.

MOSAICISM

Cells that contain at least one additional structurally normal chromosome are not uncommon (1% to 2%) in amniotic fluid or CVS specimens. If these abnormal cells are found in a single culture or clone, the phenomenon is termed *pseudomosaicism* and is usually of no clinical significance. ***True mosaicism* is more likely when the same abnormality is present in more than one clone or culture flask,** and it is confirmed by studies of the abortus or liveborn infant in 70% to 80% of cases[55] and actually can never truly be excluded because the abnormality could be restricted to tissue not readily accessible.

Numeric problems are more frequent in short-term cultures, which can be performed on chorionic villi but not on amniotic fluid cells. Metaphases from the trophoblasts or villi can accumulate within hours of sampling, allowing rapid results. In CVS, discrepancies may arise between short-term trophoblast cultures and long-term cultures, which are initiated from the mesenchymal core of villi.[5] Discrepancies may further exist between CVS preparations and the embryo. If CVS results seem at odds with clinical findings, it is reasonable to track interval growth and, if abnormal, to perform a follow-up amniocentesis. Several rare trisomies in particular (+16, +22, +7) may not be confirmed. **Sometimes mosaicism is present in the placenta but not in the embryo; this is called *confined placental mosaicism* (CPM).** In this circumstance, the likelihood of anomalies is considered low.[56] However, the U.S. NICHD Collaborative CVS trial observed increased late loss rates (8.6%) in pregnancies showing CPM compared with pregnancies without mosaicism (3.4%). **Although CPM usually does not have clinical significance,[57] two potential adverse effects associated with CPM should be considered: IUGR and UPD.** UPD, the inheritance of both homologous chromosomes from a single parent, may result from a reduction to disomy from a trisomic embryo rescue.[58] The phenotypic effect of UPD depends on the chromosome involved.[59] Imprinted genes that have phenotypic effects with regard to UPD include chromosomes 7 (Russell-Silver syndrome), 11 (Beckwith-Wiedemann syndrome), 14 (mental retardation and multiple anomalies), and 15 (Prader-Willi and Angelman syndromes).

Potential technical problems notwithstanding, **amniotic fluid analysis and chorionic villi analysis are highly accurate for the detection of numeric chromosome abnormalities.** The U.S. NICHD Collaborative CVS trial[57] evaluated 11,473 chorionic villus samples by direct methods, long-term culture, or both. There were no incorrect sex predictions. No diagnostic errors occurred among 148 common autosomal trisomies (+13, +18, +21), 16 sex chromosome aneuploidies, and 13 structural aberrations; no normal cytogenetic diagnosis with CVS has ever been followed by birth of a trisomic infant. Overall, accuracy of CVS by karyotype is comparable to that of amniocentesis. However, with MAs, the ability to detect submicroscopic chromosome abnormalities has further increased the accuracy of prenatal diagnosis.

IMPLICATIONS OF DE NOVO STRUCTURAL ABNORMALITIES

If an ostensibly balanced inversion or translocation is detected in the fetus but is not found in either parent, the rearrangement arose de novo. The inversion or translocation may not actually be balanced; genes around breakpoints may be deleted but unappreciated by routine cytogenetic analysis. **The risk for the fetus being abnormal has been tabulated at 6% for a de novo reciprocal inversion and 10% to 15% for a de novo translocation.**[60] Risks are not chromosome specific but represent pooled data that involve many chromosomes. These risks also apply only to anatomic or developmental abnormalities evident at birth, not taking into account abnormalities that become evident only later in life. **Thus when a de novo structural abnormality is present, an MA should be performed to determine whether a gain or loss has occurred at the breakpoint as a result of the abnormality.** This will allow for more precise counseling; if array CGH shows no abnormality, the likelihood of an abnormality is markedly reduced.

Marker chromosomes, also called *supernumerary chromosomes,* by definition cannot be fully characterized on the basis of standard cytogenetic analyses. These small chromosomes usually contain a centromere, a high proportion are derived from the short arms of acrocentric chromosomes (13, 14, 15, 21, and 22), and their significance depends on whether the marker is de novo or familial. In reviewing 15,522 prenatal diagnostic procedures, Hume and colleagues[61] ascertained 19 marker chromosomes, 5 from CVS specimens and 14 from amniotic fluid samples. Monitoring these pregnancies with high-resolution ultrasonography revealed an association between de novo marker chromosomes and anomalies. When ultrasound examination was normal, the likelihood of a phenotypically normal offspring was high. With MA, the origin of the marker chromosomes can usually be established.

SINGLE-GENE OR MENDELIAN DISORDERS

Approximately 1% of liveborn infants are phenotypically abnormal as result of gene mutations, and yet most inherited disorders are rare except in some ethnic groups in which common mutations have been identified. With the sequencing of the human genome and the development of molecular diagnostic testing, it is now possible to identify carriers for some single-gene mutations and to more accurately assess their risk for having an affected offspring. **The risk is 50% for autosomal-dominant disorders like Marfan syndrome or for X-linked disorders such as fragile X syndrome or Duchenne muscular dystrophy. For autosomal recessive disorders like CF or Tay-Sachs disease, if both parents have a mutation, there is a 1 in 4 chance of an affected offspring in each pregnancy.** Individuals and couples at risk with known mutations may elect to have either prenatal or preimplantation genetic testing. Further, with the identification of the common gene mutations for many disorders, especially in some ethnic groups, it is now possible to offer population-based carrier screening. Also, some carriers are ascertained through the birth of an affected child or as a result of state newborn screening programs, which screen for over 30 inherited conditions at birth. In this section, we review carrier screening, newborn screening, and DNA-based molecular diagnosis—the platform for preimplantation and prenatal genetic testing.

Carrier Screening for Heritable Disorders

Carrier screening is performed to determine whether an individual has a mutation in one of two copies (heterozygous carrier) of the gene of interest. Screening is voluntary, and informed consent is recommended. Ideally, individuals should be provided with information about the condition, its prevalence and severity, and treatment options in addition to information about the test, including detection rates and the limitations. When the detection rate is less than 100%, it is important to explain that a negative screening test reduces the likelihood that an individual is a carrier and is at risk for having an affected offspring, but it does not eliminate the possibility. Individuals should also be assured that their test results are confidential. For some individuals, genetic counseling may assist with the decision-making process; therefore it may be helpful to provide individuals with disease-specific educational material. Further, it is prudent to document in the medical record that screening tests were offered and the individual's decision.

ACOG recommends population carrier screening for selected disorders in families amenable to prenatal diagnosis in which no previously affected individual has been born (Table 10-8).[62-66] DNA-based tests also exist for fragile X mental retardation and spinal muscular atrophy (SMA). ACOG does not currently recommend universal screening for fragile X, but testing is recommended with a family history of unexplained

TABLE 10-8   GENETIC SCREENING IN VARIOUS ETHNIC GROUPS

ETHNIC GROUP	DISORDER	SCREENING TEST
All	Cystic fibrosis	DNA analysis of a selected panel of 23 CFTR mutations (alleles present in 0.1% of the general U.S. population)
Blacks	Sickle cell anemia	MCV <80%, followed by hemoglobin electrophoresis
Ashkenazi Jews	Tay-Sachs disease	Decreased serum Hexosaminidase-A or DNA analysis for selected alleles
	Canavan disease	DNA analysis for selected alleles
	Familial dysautonomia	DNA analysis for selected alleles
Cajuns	Tay-Sachs disease	DNA analysis for selected alleles
French-Canadians	Tay-Sachs disease	DNA analysis for selected alleles
Mediterranean (Italians, Greeks)	β-Thalassemia	MCV <80%, followed by hemoglobin electrophoresis if iron deficiency has been excluded
Southeast Asians (Filipino, Chinese, Vietnamese, Laotian, Cambodian) and Africans	α-Thalassemia	MCV <80%, followed by hemoglobin electrophoresis if iron deficiency has been excluded

CFTR, cystic fibrosis transmembrane conductance regulator; *MCV,* mean corpuscular volume.

mental retardation, autism, a motor movement disorder, premature ovarian failure, and, of course, fragile X syndrome itself as well as at the request of the patient.[65] ACOG also does not recommend population screening for SMA, formerly called *Werdnig-Hoffman disease.*[66] On the other hand, the ACMG recommends SMA screening, reasoning that 95% of carriers can be detected for a disorder in which the panethnic population incidence is comparable to that of CF.[67] Individualized testing to assess carrier status is recommended for individuals with a family history of an inherited condition if the gene and the mutation have been identified.

A cost-effective approach to carrier screening begins with testing the partner at risk (e.g., family history of the disease of interest) or the mother. However, it is also acceptable to test both concurrently. If one member of the couple has a mutation for an autosomal recessive disorder, the next step is to test the partner. When both parents are carriers for an autosomal recessive disorder, the risk of having an affected offspring is 25%. Genetic counseling is recommended, and the couple is informed of the availability of prenatal diagnostic testing, PGD, donor gametes (eggs or sperm), and adoption to avoid the risk of having an affected child. In addition, the parents should be informed that their relatives are at risk and should also be informed of the availability of carrier screening. Infrequently, a screening test may identify an individual with two mutations who is so mildly affected that the mutations escaped medical attention. In this situation, the individual may benefit from a referral to a specialist for further evaluation.

TABLE 10-9	GENETIC SCREENING FOR SELECTED DISORDERS IN ASHKENAZI JEWS	
DISORDERS	**CARRIER (HETEROZYGOTE) FREQUENCY**	**CARRIER (HETEROZYGOTE) DETECTION RATE (%)**
Tay-Sachs	1/25	99
Canavan syndrome	1/40	97
Familial dysautonomia	1/35	99.5
Cystic fibrosis	1/25	96
Niemann-Pick disease	1/70	95
Fanconi anemia, type C	1/90	95
Bloom syndrome	1/100	95
Mucolipidosis type IV	1/125	96
Gaucher disease, type I	1/19	95

Ashkenazi Jewish Genetic Diseases

A number of genetic conditions are very prevalent among individuals of Ashkenazi Jewish ancestry (Table 10-9). Heterozygote or carrier detection rates for each condition are 95% to 99%, the sensitivity reflecting that only a few mutations are responsible for each disorder in this specific population. In aggregate, the likelihood of an Ashkenazi Jewish individual being heterozygous for one of the autosomal-recessive disorders listed in this section is 1 in 4.[62] In the United States, Jewish individuals may be uncertain whether they are of Ashkenazic or Sephardic descent (90% are Ashkenazi); thus obstetricians should offer screening to *all* Jewish couples. **ACOG recommends carrier screening for Ashkenazi couples for Tay-Sachs, CF, Canavan disease, and familial dysautonomia and also recommends that couples be made aware of the availability of carrier screening for other less prevalent and less severe diseases.**[61] **These disorders include mucolipidosis IV, Niemann-Pick disease type A, Fanconi anemia type C, Bloom syndrome, and Gaucher disease.** Many laboratories and programs offer expanded carrier screening to Ashkenazi Jews.

Screening usually involves molecular testing for common selected mutations. In all the disorders listed in Table 10-8, screening only a few mutations (alleles for the mutant gene) will detect a very high percentage of heterozygotes. In Tay-Sachs disease, for example, molecular testing in Ashkenazi Jews detects 94% of heterozygotes; screening by the more laborious biochemical methods (based on ratio of hexosaminidase A to total hexosaminidase—A plus B) detects 98%.[62] **If only one partner is Ashkenazi, ACOG[61] suggests screening that individual first.** In low-risk populations (e.g., non-Ashkenazi Europeans), the carrier frequency for Tay-Sachs is only 1 in 300. Given that molecular heterogeneity is so prevalent, biochemical testing is often necessary in testing individuals who are not Ashkenazi Jews.

With the exception of Tay-Sachs disease and CF, the carrier rate and the detection rate applicable for the non-Jewish partner has not been established and, hence, screening is of limited value. It may thus not be possible to provide the couple with an accurate assessment of their risk to have an affected child.

Hemoglobinopathies

Sickle cell disease occurs most commonly among individuals of African origin but is also found in high frequency in Greeks, Italians (Sicilians), Turks, Arabs, Southern Iranians, and Asian Indians. Classic sickle cell disease is caused by homozygosity for a single base-pair mutation in the β-globin gene (hemoglobin S; see Chapter 44). **Approximately 1 in 12 blacks are carriers of a single copy (heterozygous) of the mutation and have sickle cell trait. Hemoglobin electrophoresis is the recommended screening test because it can detect other abnormal forms of hemoglobin and thalassemia.**[63]

Thalassemia is caused by the reduced synthesis of either α- or β-globin (see Chapter 44) and is more common among individuals of Southeast Asian, African, West Indian, Mediterranean (Greek, Italian), Asian, and Middle Eastern origin. **ACOG recommends a complete blood count (mean corpuscular volume [MCV]) and hemoglobin electrophoresis to detect thalassemia.**[63] **MCV values of less than 80% are indicative of either iron deficiency anemia or thalassemia heterozygosity; therefore it is necessary to test for iron deficiency. If a deficiency is not found, an elevated hemoglobin A$_2$ and hemoglobin F will confirm β-thalassemia. DNA-based testing is necessary to detect α-globin deletions, which cause α-thalassemia.**[63]

Cystic Fibrosis

Carrier screening for CF was initially recommended by ACOG and ACMG in 2001.[64,68] **CF is more common in whites of Northern European and Ashkenazi Jewish ancestry and primarily affects pulmonary and pancreatic function.** The disorder usually is manifested early in childhood; 10% to 20% are detected at birth because of meconium ileus. Increasing accumulation of viscous secretions progressively leads to chronic respiratory obstruction. Malnutrition and poor postnatal growth arise secondary to blockage of pancreatic ducts that produce insufficient pancreatic enzymes, which interferes with intestinal absorption. The majority of men with CF have azoospermia, the result of congenital bilateral absence of the vas deferens (CBAVD). Sometimes CBAVD is the only manifestation of CF. In these cases, the mutant alleles are less deleterious than those that cause severe CF. Individuals without pancreatic involvement have a milder course and longer survival (median survival 56 years compared with 30 years).[25] **CF may be diagnosed by the chloride sweat test or suspected on a newborn screening test, but mutation testing or DNA sequencing is used to confirm the diagnosis.** Once a mutation is identified in a given family, genetic studies are indicated to detect other carriers (heterozygotes) and affected relatives.

Since the initial report that localized the gene for CF, over 1500 disease-causing mutations have been identified, but **one mutation—ΔF508, a deletion of phenylalanine (F) at codon 508—accounts for about 75% of CF mutations in whites who are not Ashkenazi Jews.**[69] **ACOG and ACMG recommend using a panethnic panel of 23 mutations as a screening test to identify CF carriers.**[64] Many commercial laboratories offer gene sequencing and/or expanded carrier screening panels that include mutations that are less prevalent in the general population that minimally increase the sensitivity. Neither is recommended for routine carrier screening, although an expanded panel or sequencing may be considered if a family member is affected and routine panels have failed to reveal a mutation. Even if the entire gene is sequenced, not all CF mutations will be identified. Those not identified

TABLE 10-10	DETECTION OF CYSTIC FIBROSIS HETEROZYGOTES*		
ETHNIC GROUP	**CARRIER (HETEROZYGOTES) FREQUENCY**	**PERCENT OF CARRIERS (HETEROZYGOTES) DETECTABLE (%)**	**LIKELIHOOD OF BEING A CARRIER (HETEROZYGOUS) DESPITE NEGATIVE SCREEN**
Ashkenazi Jew	1/24	94	1/380
European non-Hispanic white	1/25	88	1/200
Hispanic white	1/58	72	1/200
Black	1/61	64	1/170
Asian	1/94	49	1/180

Data from American College of Obstetricians and Gynecologists (ACOG) Committee on Obstetrics. ACOG Practice Bulletin No. 78: hemoglobinopathies in pregnancy. *Obstet Gynecol.* 2007;109:229-237 and ACOG Committee Opinion 486 (2011).
*The current panel encompasses 23 mutations.

TABLE 10-11	LIKELIHOOD OF AFFECTED FETUS AFTER CYSTIC FIBROSIS CARRIER SCREENING	
	NON-HISPANIC EUROPEAN WHITE	**ASHKENAZI JEW**
No screening	1/2500	1/2304
Both partners negative	1/173,056	1/640,000
One partner negative, one untested	1/20,800	1/38,400
One partner positive, one negative	1/832	1/1600
One partner positive, other untested	1/100	1/96
Both partners positive	1/4	1/4

These calculations are based on the frequencies shown in Table 10-6.

presumably act in promoter regions or perturb posttranslational modification.

The carrier frequency and detection rates in various ethnic groups is shown in Table 10-10. The likelihood of having an affected offspring when one or both partners are tested and screen positive or negative is shown in Table 10-11. The detection rate varies depending on ethnic origin. Individuals without a family history of CF, an affected partner, or a partner with CBAVD may benefit from genetic counseling, expanded screening, and, possibly, gene sequencing.

Newborn Screening

Screening the neonate is mandated by each state, although parents may decline testing and in some states need to consent. These screening tests may also identify couples who are carriers and who may benefit from genetic counseling to learn about their options in subsequent pregnancies.

The ACMG and the March of Dimes have recommended screening for a core panel of 31 conditions, including inborn errors of metabolism amenable to treatment such as phenylketonuria, galactosemia, and homocystinuria; endocrine conditions such as hypothyroidism and 21-hydroxylase deficiency; sickle cell anemia; and congenital hearing loss. Information by state is available at www.marchofdimes.com/professionals/580.asp or at the National Newborn Screening and Genetics Resource Center's Web site at genes-r-us.uthscsa.edu.

Molecular Approach to Prenatal Diagnosis of Single-Gene Disorders

Sequencing the human genome has revealed approximately 22,000 genes (based on certain established sequencing criteria that define a gene). The function of many genes is still unknown, but increasingly, mendelian disorders of potential prenatal genetic diagnostic interest are being identified, and their molecular perturbations are known. The molecular basis of recognized single-gene disorders varies and includes point mutations that lead to a single nucleotide and hence to a single amino acid change (e.g., sickle cell anemia), premature stop codons that truncate the protein gene products, deletions of three nucleotides that lead to loss of entire amino acids, and deletions of one or two nucleotides that lead to frame shifts that result in an altered reading frame with all subsequent amino acids being coded erroneously.

In a given disorder, it is exceptional for a single molecular perturbation to be responsible for all cases, as is the case in sickle cell anemia and achondroplasia. One or more perturbations may account for a significant proportion within a given ethnic group; however, the molecular basis in the broader population is typically more heterogeneous. An array of mutations may be used for diagnostic or carrier testing as described above, or targeted sequencing of such genes may be performed. Still, the molecular basis may not always be evident for every affected individual, even in well-studied disorders like CF. **If sequencing all coding regions of the gene in question does not reveal a perturbation, the assumption is that the pathogenesis involves the promoter region or posttranscriptional processes (e.g., translation).**

The general approach for detecting single-gene disorders involves the determination of a known molecular perturbation. Alternatively, if the actual mutation is not known, linkage analysis can still be used to identify affected cases if the chromosome location has been determined. Suppose a couple is at risk for a known disorder, but the molecular basis in their family is unknown. In linkage analysis, the clinician relies on polymorphic markers upstream and downstream from the mutation site. These polymorphisms are without clinical significance but can serve as markers (short tandem repeats of nucleotides; SNPs). At every locus, polymorphic or mutant, one marker allele is of paternal origin and one is maternal. A panel of markers can be identified that coexist (in phase) with the chromosome having the mutation, said to be *cis* and in contrast to those markers on the chromosome having the normal allele (*trans*). That is, given two chromosomes, one set of markers will be on the chromosome containing the mutant allele for the disorder in question (dominant or recessive), whereas the other will lie on the "normal" chromosome. Studying affected and unaffected family members will allow the clinician to determine the "phase" of markers unique to that family. If there are no surviving affected family members, the clinician may still be able to deduce phase (*cis* versus *trans*) by analyzing individual sperm, should the disorder have arisen de novo in a male. Regardless, the principle is that a diagnosis can be deduced without knowledge of the precise nucleotide perturbations.

A molecularly based diagnosis can thus be readily achieved for patients at risk for hundreds of disorders. Any nucleated fetal cell—chorionic villus, amniotic fluid cell, or blastomere from an embryo—will suffice. Technical details are beyond the purview of this text, save appreciation that **molecular diagnosis is highly accurate in good laboratories but perfect in none.**

Mendelian Disorders Without Known Molecular Basis

Some disorders remain whose genetic basis is not yet elucidated. If the causative gene is not known and thus cannot be localized, linkage analysis is not applicable. Whether the concern originates in a previously affected child or in the current pregnancy, the clinician may have to resort to imaging (see Chapter 9), assuming cytogenetic findings (including MAs) are normal in the previously affected child, and structural anomalies are present.

MULTIFACTORIAL AND POLYGENIC DISORDERS

It is postulated that some congenital malformations, especially those that involve a single organ system, are the result of the cumulative effects of more than one gene (polygenic) and gene-environment interactions (multifactorial). These include hydrocephaly, anencephaly, and spina bifida (NTDs); facial clefts (cleft lip and palate); cardiac defects; pyloric stenosis; omphalocele; hip dislocation; uterine fusion defects; and club foot (Box 10-1). **After the birth of one child with a defect involving only one organ system, the recurrence risk in subsequent offspring is 1% to 5%.** The frequency is less than would be expected if only a single gene were responsible, but it is still greater than that for the general population. The recurrence risks are similar for offspring of an affected parent.

Many of these congenital anomalies can be diagnosed in utero using ultrasonography or fetal echocardiography (see Chapter 9). A few are associated with elevated AFP levels in the maternal serum and amniotic fluid. In this section, we review the use of serum markers and ultrasound to screen and diagnose NTDs.

BOX 10-1   MULTIFACTORIAL/POLYGENIC TRAITS

Hydrocephaly (except some forms of aqueductal stenosis and Dandy-Walker syndrome)
Neural tube defects (anencephaly, spina bifida, encephalocele)
Cleft lip with or without cleft palate
Cleft lip (alone)
Cardiac anomalies (most types)
Diaphragmatic hernia
Pyloric stenosis
Omphalocele
Renal agenesis (unilateral or bilateral)
Ureteral anomalies
Posterior urethral values
Hypospadias
Müllerian fusion effects
Müllerian aplasia
Limb reduction defects
Talipes equinovarus (clubfoot)

These are relatively common traits considered to be inherited in polygenic/multifactorial fashion. For each, normal parents have recurrence risks of 1% to 5% after one affected child. After two affected offspring, the risk is higher.

Screening for Neural Tube Defects

Maternal serum AFP (MSAFP) is a useful screening test for open NTDs.[70] MSAFP screening for NTD detection should be performed at 15 to 20 weeks' gestation. As with aneuploidy screening, corrections must be made for gestational age, multiple gestations, and presence of diabetes mellitus. Maternal serum values above 2.0 or 2.5 MoM are considered elevated with respect to NTDs. Values above 2.0 MoM are considered elevated in women with type 1 diabetes, whereas in twin gestations, MSAFP is considered abnormal only at 4.5 to 5.0 MoM or greater.

Approximately 3% to 5% of women have an elevated MSAFP depending on the threshold set and accuracy of pregnancy dating; most are false-positive results. If gestational age assessment is determined accurately (e.g., by first-trimester sonogram), the number of women who have an abnormal serum value is relatively lower. If MSAFP is elevated, an ultrasound examination should be performed to look for evidence of an NTD or other anomalies, such as gastroschisis or omphalocele, as well as to confirm gestational age and the number of fetuses. **MSAFP is greater than 2.5 MoM in 90% of pregnancies with anencephaly and in 80% with open spina bifida.**[69] **With ultrasound alone, it is possible to achieve very high detection rates for NTDs (90% or higher in experienced centers), and this has led some centers to utilize ultrasonography as the primary screening test, acknowledging limitations that exist for the detection of small spinal defects.** Some NTDs may be evident on sonogram as early as 11 to 14 weeks' gestation. In some cases, amniocentesis to measure the amniotic fluid AFP and acetylcholinesterase levels may be necessary.

An elevation of MSAFP may not reflect an NTD because of other circumstances, such as (1) underestimated gestational age, inasmuch as MSAFP increases as gestation progresses; (2) unrecognized multiple gestation (60% of twins and almost all triplets with MSAFP values that would be elevated if judged on the basis of singleton values); (3) fetal demise, presumably reflecting fetal blood extravasating into the maternal circulation; (4) Rh isoimmunization, cystic hygroma, and other conditions associated with fetal edema; and (5) other anomalies, mainly abdominal wall defects such as gastroschisis and omphalocele.

The sensitivity for detection of an NTD in twin gestations is predictably lower than in singleton gestations; it is only about 30% for spina bifida given a threshold of 4.5 MoM. The lower sensitivity exists because twins are usually discordant for an NTD. **Ultrasound is recommended in twin gestations for assessment of NTD.**

If aneuploidy screening is performed in the second trimester, an MSAFP value will already be available as part of serum analyte screening for aneuploidy. First-trimester MSAFP is, however, not a sensitive method for detecting NTDs. **If first-trimester aneuploidy screening is done alone, or if cell-free fetal DNA or CVS is performed, second-trimester MSAFP screening or ultrasound is recommended to detect NTDs.**

Obstetric Significance of Unexplained Elevated Maternal Serum Alpha-Fetoprotein

Often, no evident cause is detected after a comprehensive assessment of a patient with an elevated MSAFP. This group of patients has been consistently described to be at higher risk of adverse perinatal outcomes that include spontaneous abortion, preterm birth, small size for gestational age, low birthweight, and infant death. On the other hand, extremely low MSAFP values (<0.25 MoM) have also been associated with increased morbidity that includes spontaneous abortion, preterm birth, stillbirth, and infant death.[71-73]

INDICATIONS FOR PRENATAL GENETIC TESTING

Indications for prenatal genetic studies arise from those clinical situations associated with an increased risk for a diagnosable prenatal genetic condition. These include **maternal age, parental chromosome rearrangements, prior pregnancy with a chromosome abnormality, and carriers for an inheritable condition.** Other risk factors become evident only during the pregnancy. These include positive results for aneuploidy screening, ultrasound detection of fetal structural anomalies, and IUGR.

PROCEDURES FOR PRENATAL GENETIC DIAGNOSIS

Prenatal detection of chromosome abnormalities and many genetic conditions requires an invasive procedure such as amniocentesis or CVS to obtain fetal cells or placental tissue for chromosome and genetic testing. Less frequently, cordocentesis is performed to obtain fetal blood. In this section, we review these techniques and their safety.

As a common feature of any prenatal invasive procedure, the patient should receive genetic counseling and should be fully informed about the nature of the procedure, and the patient and her spouse must provide informed consent. Information about the nature, accuracy, and possible results of the test; how, when, and by whom it is performed; safety of the procedure; culture failure rates; reporting time; and postprocedure recommendations should be communicated to the patient.

Amniocentesis

Genetic amniocentesis was first performed in the 1950s. Analytes such as AFP can be measured in the amniotic fluid, and amniocytes can be cultured for cytogenetic and molecular analyses. **Genetic amniocentesis is usually performed after 15 weeks' gestation. Early amniocentesis (EA) before 14 weeks' gestation, especially before 13 weeks' gestation, should be avoided because of higher rates of pregnancy loss, amniotic fluid leakage, and talipes equinovarus.**[74]

A 20- or 22-gauge spinal needle with a stylet is introduced percutaneously into the amniotic cavity under continuous ultrasound guidance, taking care to avoid the fetus and umbilical cord. A local anesthetic may be given at the puncture site. Approximately 20 to 30 mL of amniotic fluid is aspirated, and the first 1 or 2 mL is usually discarded to avoid maternal-cell contamination. Rh immune globulin should be administered to the Rh-negative, Du-negative, unsensitized patient who has an Rh-positive fetus or a fetus whose Rh status is unknown.

Continuous visualization of the needle by ultrasound significantly reduces the incidence of bloody amniotic fluid, dry taps, and the need for multiple insertions. Bloody amniotic fluid is occasionally aspirated; however, the blood is almost always maternal in origin and does not adversely affect amniotic cell growth. Brown, dark red, or wine-colored amniotic fluid indicates that intraamniotic bleeding has occurred earlier in the pregnancy, and hemoglobin breakdown products are persistent in the fluid; pregnancy loss eventually occurs in about one third

of such cases. If the abnormally colored fluid is associated with an elevated amniotic AFP level, the outcome is almost always unfavorable (fetal demise or fetal abnormality). Greenish amniotic fluid is the result of meconium staining and apparently is not associated with poor pregnancy outcome.

After amniocentesis, the patient may resume all normal activities. Common sense dictates that strenuous exercise such as jogging or aerobic exercise is deferred for a day or so. Deferring sexual activity for 24 to 48 hours also seems prudent. The patient should report persistent uterine cramping, vaginal bleeding, leakage of amniotic fluid, or fever; however, physician intervention is almost never required, unless, of course, overt abortion occurs.

Amniocentesis in Twin Pregnancies

In multiple gestations, amniocentesis can usually be performed on all fetuses. It is important to assess and record chorionicity, placental location, fetal viability, anatomy, and gender and to carefully identify each sac, should selective termination be desired at a later date. A simple and reliable technique to ensure that the same sac is not sampled twice is to inject 2 to 3 mL of indigo carmine following aspiration of amniotic fluid from the first sac, before the needle is withdrawn. A second amniocentesis is then performed at a site determined after visualizing the membranes that separate the two sacs. Aspiration of clear fluid confirms that the second (new) sac was entered. Gestations greater than two can be managed similarly, sequentially injecting dye into successive sacs. Cross-contamination of fetal cells in multiple gestations appears rare, but confusion may sometimes arise in interpreting amniotic fluid acetylcholinesterase (AchE) or AFP results. Some obstetricians aspirate the second sac without dye injection, use a single-puncture technique, or perform simultaneous visualization of the two inserted needles in each sac.

If only one fetus in a multiple gestation is abnormal, parents should be prepared to choose between aborting all fetuses or continuing the pregnancy with one or more normal fetuses and one abnormal fetus. Selective termination in the second trimester is possible but is associated with a higher rate of complications (fetal loss and prematurity) than if it is done in the first trimester; therefore **CVS should be considered the preferred test for multiple gestations.**

Safety of Amniocentesis

The risk of amniocentesis is very low in experienced hands: approximately 1 in 300 to 500 procedure-related losses or less.[74] The risk for pregnancy loss has decreased since the large collaborative studies to assess safety were first done in the 1970s. In none of these early collaborative studies was quality ultrasonography, as defined by today's standards, available, nor was concurrent ultrasonography universally applied. By contrast, studies conducted within the past decade universally use quality ultrasound and have shown no statistical difference in outcomes for women who did and did not undergo amniocentesis. The risk does not appear to increase when amniocentesis is performed in twins.

Maternal risks are low, and symptomatic amnionitis occurs only rarely (0.1%). Minor maternal complications such as transient vaginal spotting or minimal amniotic fluid leakage occur in 1% or less of cases, but these complications are almost always self-limited in nature. Other complications include intraabdominal viscus injury or hemorrhage. The most serious is fulminant

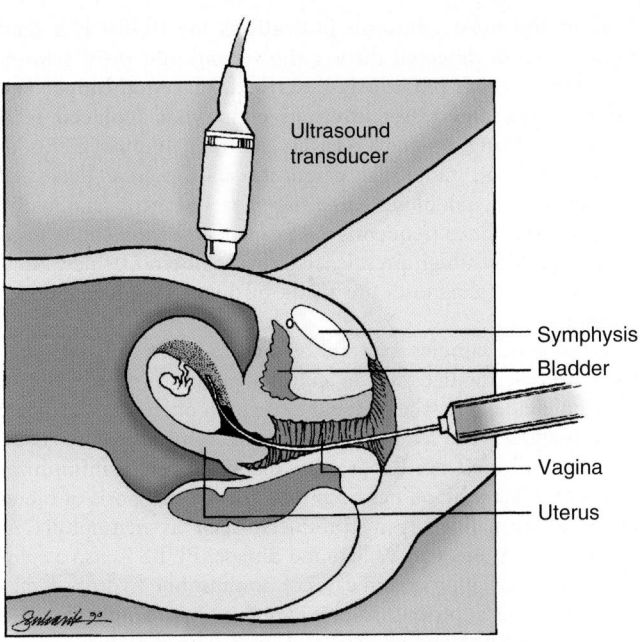

FIG 10-4 Transcervical chorionic villus sampling.

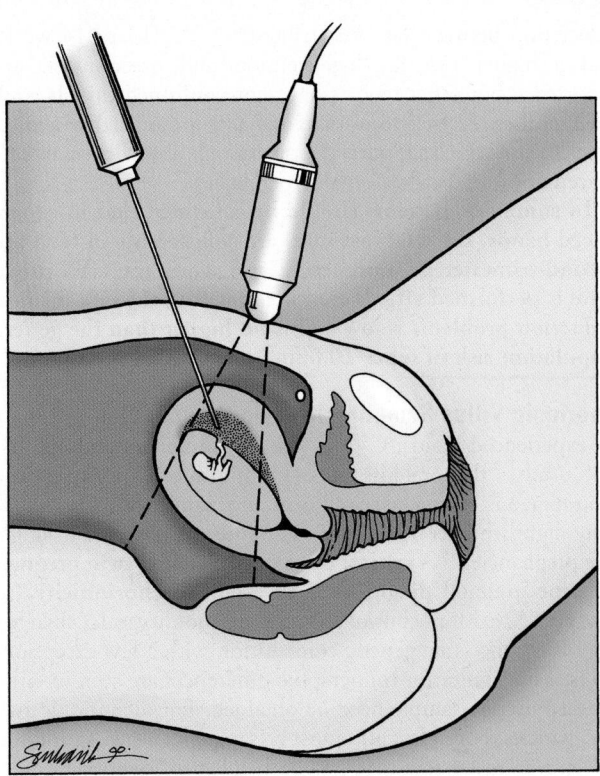

FIG 10-5 Transabdominal chorionic villus sampling.

sepsis (such as with *Escherichia coli* or clostridial species) that results in maternal mortality, but this is extraordinarily rare.

Chorionic Villus Sampling

Chorionic villus sampling (CVS) allows genetic diagnosis in the first trimester of pregnancy. If desired, pregnancy termination can be performed earlier, when it is safer for the mother. For example, the maternal death rate is 1 per 100,000 early in pregnancy compared with 7 to 10 per 100,000 in mid pregnancy.[75] Early diagnosis also makes it feasible to perform selective fetal reduction in multiple gestations, when the risks are less than in the second trimester. Early termination also protects patient privacy. Both chorionic villi analysis and amniotic fluid cell analysis offer the same information concerning chromosome status, enzyme levels, and gene mutations. CVS is not useful for the few assays that require amniotic fluid liquor, such as AFP for the detection of NTDs.

CVS is performed between 10 and 13 weeks' gestation by either a transcervical (*TC*-CVS) or transabdominal (*TA*-CVS) approach (Figs. 10-4 and 10-5). TC-CVS is usually performed with a flexible polyethylene catheter with a metal obturator, which is introduced through the cervical canal toward the placenta under direct ultrasonographic visualization. After withdrawal of the obturator, 10 to 25 mg of villi is aspirated by negative pressure into a 20- or 30-mL syringe that contains tissue culture media. TA-CVS is performed by introducing an 18- or 20-gauge spinal needle percutaneously into the long axis of the placenta under ultrasound guidance. After removal of the stylet, villi are aspirated into a 20-mL syringe that contains about 5 mL of tissue culture media, keeping negative pressure and performing a gentle, longitudinal, back-and-forth movement of the needle. TA-CVS can be performed later in gestation for rapid fetal karyotyping or when there is oligohydramnios and a fluid pocket is not accessible. After the first trimester, this procedure is better known as *late CVS* or *placental biopsy*. Placental biopsy has now replaced cordocentesis for rapid fetal karyotyping during the second and third trimesters in many centers,

given that it carries a lower risk, is technically easier, and can yield cytogenetic results within 24 to 48 hours.

In many cases, either TA-CVS or TC-CVS is acceptable. However, one approach may be preferable in certain situations. For example, cervical myomas or sharply angulated uteri may preclude transcervical passage of the catheter, whereas TA-CVS would permit sampling. The transabdominal approach is preferable in the presence of genital herpes, cervicitis, or bicornuate uteri. With either approach, Rh immune globulin should be administered to the Rh-negative, Du-negative, unsensitized patient unless the fetus is known to be Rh negative. Sampling women sensitized to red blood cell antigens should be deferred until later in gestation when amniocentesis can be performed.

Safety of Chorionic Villus Sampling

CVS is a relatively safe procedure. Several studies, including randomized studies in the United States and Italy, reported that the risk for pregnancy loss is similar to that of second-trimester amniocentesis.[76,77] However, a systematic review to assess comparative safety between TA-CVS and TC-CVS and EA and second-trimester amniocentesis concluded that second-trimester amniocentesis and TA-CVS are safer than TC-CVS and EA.[78] A simple comparison to amniocentesis may not be valid when CVS is performed because of an increased NT measurement, a cystic hygroma, or any other anomaly in which the risk for miscarriage is increased.

The prevalence of IUGR, placental abruption, and premature delivery is no higher in women who undergo CVS than in the general population. In the early 1990s, controversy about the safety of CVS focused on the risk for limb reduction defects (LRDs). **The consensus of most studies was that LRD is not a major concern when CVS is performed by experienced individuals at 10 to 13 weeks of gestation.**[74] A possible association between late first-trimester CVS (13 to 14 weeks) and a higher risk for hypertension and preeclampsia was reported,[24] but other reports have not confirmed this. It could be hypothesized that focal placental disruption is the involved mechanism, which supports the theory that disturbances of early placentation lead to maternal hypertension.

In summary, patients should be informed that in experienced hands, the fetal loss rates are comparable in CVS and second-trimester amniocentesis; and when the CVS procedure is performed after 9 completed weeks, the risk for limb reduction problems is low and is no higher than the general population risk of 6 per 10,000.[74]

Chorionic Villus Sampling in Twin Pregnancies

In experienced hands, CVS is safe in multiple gestations. In a U.S. study,[79] the total loss rate of chromosomally normal fetuses (spontaneous abortions, stillborns, neonatal deaths) was 5%, only slightly higher than the 4% absolute rate observed in singleton pregnancies.[16] **A critical issue in counseling twin pregnancies for prenatal diagnosis is to establish chorionicity** (see Chapter 32). Monochorionic twins are monozygotic; therefore they carry the same genetic constitution with a few exceptions. Thus if no significant sonographic differences are seen in either fetus, only one sample need be obtained. For dichorionic twin pregnancies, both placentas must be sampled. When the placentas appear to be fused, it can be helpful to identify the cord insertion sites to avoid the cross-contamination of chorionic tissue, leading to either false-positive or false-negative results. Alternatively, amniocentesis may be the preferred test.

CVS is widely used before selective reduction in multiple gestations. Here, it is especially desirable to sample the inferiorly lying fetus (usually retained to minimize risk for ascending infection) as well as at least two or three of the other fetuses potentially slated to be retained.

Invasive Diagnostic Testing in Women With Hepatitis B, Hepatitis C, and Human Immunodeficiency Virus

Bloodborne viruses constitute a risk factor for maternal-fetal transmission. Available evidence is limited, but the risk for transmission for hepatitis B seems to be very low.[80] Knowledge of the maternal hepatitis B "e" antigen status is valuable in the counseling of risks associated with amniocentesis. Less information is available about hepatitis C, but to date there is no evidence that transmission is increased following amniocentesis.[80] **Invasive prenatal testing can be carried out in women who carry hepatitis B or C; however, the patient should be informed of the limited data on transmission.**

In HIV-positive women, noninvasive testing is preferable, and invasive testing should be avoided, particularly in the third trimester when the relative risk for transmission is fourfold when an invasive procedure is performed.[80,81] Some authors have suggested that procedures early in pregnancy would carry a very low risk, provided that antiretroviral therapy is administered and the maternal viral load is low. For those who insist on an invasive test, amniocentesis is the preferred test, and every effort should be made to avoid traversing the placenta.

Fetal Blood Sampling

Ultrasound-directed percutaneous umbilical blood sampling (PUBS), also termed *cordocentesis* or *funipuncture,* can be used to obtain fetal blood for cytogenetic or molecular analyses.

One of the most common indications for PUBS is a fetal malformation detected during the second and third trimesters. However, as previously described, placental biopsy is a safer, easier, and faster alternative that has replaced fetal blood sampling in many centers. Further, improvements in cytogenetic and molecular diagnostic testing have decreased the need for fetal blood sampling. For instance, fetal blood sampling was once frequently performed for diagnostic reasons in regions with a high prevalence of hemoglobinopathies. Now, most of those diagnoses are made by DNA-based analysis of chorionic villi.

Fetal blood samples may still be used to help clarify chromosome mosaicism detected in cultured amniotic fluid cells or chorionic villi or for the prenatal evaluation of fetal hematologic abnormalities. The fetal hematocrit can be measured to assess anemia resulting from Rh or other blood antigen isoimmunization states. Fetal blood has been used for the diagnosis of blood factor abnormalities (gene products) such as hemophilia A, hemophilia B, and von Willebrand disease. PUBS is also a valuable diagnostic approach in cases of nonimmune hydrops fetalis because a single procedure provides the opportunity to assess different hematologic, genetic, and infectious etiologies.

Technique

Cordocentesis is usually performed from 18 weeks onward, although successful procedures have been reported as early as 12 weeks. Ultrasonographic examination before the procedure is necessary to assess fetal viability, placental and umbilical cord location, fetal position, and presence or absence of fetal or placental anomalies. Color-flow Doppler imaging is an important tool in evaluating the cord and placenta. Maternal sedation is not usually required, but oral benzodiazepine before the procedure may be of benefit. Although there is no good evidence, many centers use prophylactic antibiotics.

Under continuous ultrasound guidance, a 21- or 22-gauge spinal needle with a stylet is inserted percutaneously and is directed into the umbilical vein. The needle may be inserted using a freehand technique or with a needle-guiding device fixed to the transducer. Most experienced maternal-fetal medicine specialists use the freehand technique. **The umbilical vein is preferred over the artery because the vein is larger and is less likely to be associated with fetal bradycardia and significant hemorrhage when punctured.** Puncture of the umbilical cord at the placental insertion site is technically easier but is associated with a higher rate of maternal blood contamination. Free loops of cord and the intrahepatic vein are alternatives.

Once the needle is positioned in the umbilical vein, the stylet is removed, and a small amount of blood is aspirated into a heparin-coated syringe. It is crucial to confirm that the sample is fetal in origin, thus a small amount is used for a complete blood count to assess the MCV. **Fetal blood cells (140 fL) are larger than maternal cells (80 fL). The MCV of a sample of fetal blood should be higher than 100.** A useful alternative when a complete blood analysis cannot be performed at once is the Apt test, or hemoglobin alkaline denaturation test, especially before 28 weeks of gestation. Based on the ability of fetal hemoglobin to resist denaturation in alkaline conditions, the Apt test is a rapid, inexpensive, and simple bedside alternative.

Fetal movements can interfere with the procedure and can sometimes dislodge the needle, which increases the risk of complications (bleeding, cord hematoma) and the necessity of further cord punctures. In some situations, it may be helpful to perform a fetal neuromuscular blockade as is done in therapeutic cordocentesis. An intravascular injection as part of the cordocentesis or intramuscular administration of pancuronium bromide (0.1 to 0.3 mg/kg of estimated fetal weight) can achieve fetal paralysis.[82]

In at least 1% of pregnancies, a single umbilical artery is present, which is usually larger in diameter than normal umbilical cord arteries. The fetal loss risk associated with puncture of a single umbilical artery (two-vessel cord) appears to be no different from that with a normal three-vessel cord. Nevertheless, the use of Doppler color-flow mapping to guide the procedure and an experienced operator is recommended.

Safety of Fetal Blood Sampling

Loss rates for patients undergoing PUBS vary greatly by indication and by operator experience, more so than with amniocentesis or CVS. No randomized clinical trial has been reported. **Collaborative data from 14 North American centers sampling 1600 patients at varying gestational ages for a variety of indications found an uncorrected fetal loss rate of 1.6%.**[83] Tongsong and associates[83] compared a cohort of 1281 women with a singleton gestation without a fetal anomaly and undergoing cordocentesis between 16 and 24 weeks of gestational age with a control group matched for maternal and gestational age; the fetal loss rate was 3.2% in the study group compared with 1.8% in the controls. In another series of 2010 cordocentesis procedures in singleton pregnancies, the procedure-related fetal loss rates within 2 weeks were 1% when performed before 24 weeks and 0.8% after 24 weeks.[84] Cordocentesis can be successfully performed in multifetal gestation; limited data suggest higher overall fetal loss rates (10.5%) with no increase in the procedure-related loss rates.[85]

Bleeding from the cord puncture is the most common complication and may be seen in 30% to 41% of cases.[86] Duration of bleeding is significantly longer after arterial than after umbilical vein puncture. However, usually the blood loss is not clinically significant in either case. Van Kamp and coworkers[87] also describe bleeding from the puncture site significantly more often and of longer duration after transamniotic cord puncture than after transplacental puncture. Transient fetal bradycardia occurs in approximately 10% of procedures. Both umbilical artery puncture and severe, early-onset growth restriction were associated with increased rates of bradycardia. Finally, the extent of fetomaternal hemorrhage or transfusion depends on the duration of the procedure, bleeding time, puncture site, and use of a transplacental approach.

Maternal complications are rare but include amnionitis and transplacental hemorrhage.[87] In general, these complications do not significantly compromise maternal health status. However, there are case reports of severe sepsis.[39]

PREIMPLANTATION GENETIC DIAGNOSIS

Preimplantation genetic diagnosis (PGD) is not simply "earlier" prenatal genetic diagnosis but an additional approach with novel applications. **PGD allows diagnosis within 6 days of conception, when implantation occurs.**

Obtaining Embryonic and Gamete DNA

There are three potential approaches for obtaining embryonic DNA for PGD as a part of ART: (1) polar body biopsy, prior to or at the time of fertilization; (2) blastomere biopsy (aspiration) from the 3-day six- to eight-cell cleaving embryo; and (3) trophectoderm biopsy from the 5- to 6-day blastocyst.

Initial work in most centers involved blastomere biopsy, the zona pellucida being traversed by mechanical or laser means to remove a blastomere. A pitfall is that removal of a blastomere reduces embryo survival by 10%; removal of two cells reduces the pregnancy rate further and is generally not performed.[88]

Polar bodies are extruded at both the first and second meiotic divisions, as the number of chromosomes is first reduced (46 to 23) in meiosis I, and then each chromosome is divided into single chromatids in meiosis II. Diagnosis is by deduction given that the oocyte per se is not tested. As an example, if the first polar body shows *no* chromosome 21, the oocyte can safely be presumed to have *two* 21 chromosomes and, hence, once fertilized, the embryo would be trisomic. The same deductive reasoning can be applied in single-gene disorders. If a polar body from a heterozygous female shows a mutant allele, the nondisturbed oocyte can be deduced to be genetically normal.

The obvious disadvantage of polar body biopsy is the inability to assess paternal genotype, which precludes application if the father has an autosomal-dominant disorder and makes analysis less efficient in managing couples at risk for autosomal-recessive traits. However, 95% of chromosome abnormalities arise from maternal meiotic errors, thus polar body approaches are almost always applicable. The reader can refer to the work of Simpson[89] or Kuliev and colleagues[90] for additional details, in particular concerning how to handle recombination observed in the first polar body.

At present, the preferred approach for PGD involves biopsy of the trophectoderm in the 5- to 6-day blastocyst. Given 120 or more total cells, more cells can be safely removed at biopsy, which facilitates diagnosis. Another advantage is that the trophectoderm forms the placenta, thus cells removed were not destined to be in the embryo (inner cell mass). The additional 2 to 3 days in culture for blastocysts beyond that required for an eight-cell embryo further allows self-selection against nonthriving embryos. Approximately one third of embryos with chromosome abnormalities are selected against (lost) between days 3 and 5; however, PGD is still necessary to exclude the remaining aneuploidies. The value of trophectoderm biopsy has been enhanced by the ability to cryopreserve a biopsied embryo. This allows transfer at a later time, when the endometrium should be more receptive after the effects of ovulation stimulation have dissipated.

Novel Indications Addressed Only by Preimplantation Genetic Diagnosis
To Avoid Pregnancy Termination

PGD is the only prenatal genetic diagnostic approach available for couples who wish to avoid an abnormal fetus yet are opposed to pregnancy termination for religious or other reasons. In fact, PGD using only the first polar body allows preconceptional diagnosis—that is, before fertilization has even occurred and an embryo has been formed. The second polar body is, however, not extruded until the mature oocyte is fertilized, thus its analysis would not truly be preconceptional.

Nondisclosure of Parental Genotype

Suppose a person at risk for an adult-onset disorder wishes to remain unaware of his or her genotype yet not transmit any mutation present to his or her offspring. Prototypic indications involve Huntington disease and autosomal-dominant early-onset Alzheimer disease. PGD is the only practical prenatal diagnostic approach because multiple embryos can be screened and only unaffected embryos transferred; the patient volitionally remains oblivious to diagnostic results and whether he or she is or is not destined to develop the conditions. A caveat is that the scenario must be repeated in subsequent cycles, even if the (undisclosed) patient proves unaffected. Otherwise, any at-risk patients would readily deduce their genotype.

Human Leukocyte Antigen–Compatible Embryos for Umbilical Cord Blood Stem Cell Transplantation

Given a couple at risk for certain single-gene disorders that affect bone marrow (e.g., β-thalassemia), it may be desirable to avoid having another genetically abnormal child. Having the transferred embryo be a human leukocyte antigen (HLA)–compatible sibling would be invaluable if an older, moribund sibling has a lethal disease that could be treated by stem cell transplantation to repopulate his or her bone marrow. Stem cell transplantation using cord blood is very successful (95%) if the cord blood is HLA compatible but much less so (65%) if not HLA compatible. PGD allows selection of the one in four embryos that are HLA compatible with a liveborn sibling.

This strategy is practical only with PGD because if the pregnancy is at risk for an autosomal-recessive disorder, the likelihood of a genetically normal, HLA-compatible embryo is only 3 in 16—that is, the odds are 1 in 4 for the desired HLA-compatible embryo, multiplied by the 3 in 4 likelihood of also being unaffected, or 3 in 16. Experience using the above approach has paralleled predictions.

In the United States and Turkey, testing for HLA-compatible embryos *without* risk for genetic disease is also well accepted. The prime indication is an older sibling with leukemia. In the United States, approximately one third of HLA PGD cases are performed for this purpose; this indication is uncommon in the United Kingdom.

Preimplantation Genetic Diagnosis for Chromosomal Indications
METHODOLOGY

Because it is not possible to reliably obtain a karyotype on a single cell, preimplantation cytogenetic analysis (numeric or structural) must rely on other methods. Initially, this involved FISH using chromosome-specific probes.[91]

Array CGH now allows interrogation of all chromosomes and some microdeletions and microduplications, whereas FISH can only evaluate 9 to 12 chromosomes. Of note, the type of array CGH used in PGD is different from that used in chorionic villi or amniotic fluid cells; it has lower resolution and was principally designed only for aneuploidy detection. Thus the dilemma of disclosing or not disclosing CNVs of uncertain clinical significance arises only rarely in PGD. An alternative approach that allows interrogation of all 24 chromosomes uses SNP "karyomapping" or "comprehensive screening."

NUMERIC CHROMOSOME ABNORMALITIES

Excluding aneuploidy in couples at increased risk who also wish to avoid clinical pregnancy termination uniquely requires PGD. Ordinarily, excluding aneuploidy definitively would not be accomplished by PGD but rather by CVS or amniocentesis. However, PGD would be more logical if a couple must undergo ART for infertility, and PGD offers the added benefit of transferring only euploid embryos. Indeed, an inverse relationship exists

between the ART pregnancy rate and frequency of miscarriages. That ART success declines precipitously beginning late in the fourth decade is not due to endometrial factors, as witnessed by successful pregnancies following use of donor oocytes for women in their sixth decade and beyond. However, miscarriage of aneuploid embryos increases with age. Thus an obvious strategy would be to perform PGD, transfer euploid embryos, and increase the proportion of potentially viable pregnancies.

By 2000, larger PGD and ART centers in the United States and Europe were thus offering PGD to improve pregnancy rates in older women, using FISH with a limited number of (5 to 9) chromosome-specific probes. Despite these experienced centers not being able to conduct a randomized controlled trial (RCT), impressive results were observed.[89,91] However, RCTs in smaller centers later failed to show salutary benefits. Although these RCTs had methodologic flaws, lack of an RCT showing benefit understandably impeded acceptance. By 2012, however, new approaches were being applied. First, trophectoderm biopsy became the principal method, rather than cleavage-stage embryo biopsy, which is subject to mosaicism and can sometimes be technically demanding. Second, most importantly array- or SNP-based 24-chromosome aneuploidy testing became possible, as noted. In 2012, RCTs from several U.S. labs showed a 20% improvement in blastocyst-transfer pregnancy rates when comparing transfer of a single PGD euploid pregnancy to a single nonbiopsied embryo.[92,93] **Although encouraging, the use of PGD has not yet clearly demonstrated the ability to improve the frequency of liveborn neonates in RCTs.**

PGD aneuploidy testing also has the potential to reduce multiple gestations in ART, given that multiple embryos are often transferred on the assumption that not all embryos will generate viable pregnancies. But if they do, multiple gestations can arise. Forman and colleagues[94] performed an RCT of women at a mean age of approximately 35 years who were undergoing ART. There were two arms: transfer of two blastocysts without PGD versus transfer of one blastocyst known to be euploid by PGD. Pregnancy rates were not statistically different (65% vs. 61%), but the rate of twins was impressively different (55% vs. 0%).

STRUCTURAL CHROMOSOME ABNORMALITIES

PGD is applicable for detecting unbalanced translocations. In Chapter 27 we describe how translocations predispose to unbalanced gametes that often yield miscarriages. This unavoidably delays the time needed to achieve a normal pregnancy. In couples with a translocation, the mean time to achieve a natural liveborn pregnancy is 5 years, much greater than in couples without a translocation.[95] Therefore PGD can shorten the amount of time it takes to achieve a liveborn delivery for those with a translocation. One caveat when using array CGH in PGD is that genetically normal embryos cannot be distinguished from those that are translocation carriers because in both, the same (normal) amount of DNA is present.

Preimplantation Genetic Diagnosis for Single-Gene Disorders

Approximately one fourth of PGD cases are performed for couples at risk for one or more single-gene disorders. Like other forms of single-gene prenatal genetic diagnosis, PGD can be performed when the chromosomal location of the gene with the disorder is known, even if the causative mutation is not. Over 300 different conditions have been tested by PGD worldwide, the most frequent being hemoglobinopathies, CF, fragile X syndrome, and Duchenne muscular dystrophy. Kuliev and colleagues[90] enumerated experience with PGD for single-gene disorders at their center in 2982 cycles that involved 1685 patients. This yielded 1095 pregnancies and 1118 live births; 47 pregnancies were still ongoing at the time of publication.

The major technical pitfall in single-gene PGD is the small amount of DNA that must be amplified to provide a sufficient amount for diagnostic tests. The technology for whole-genome amplification (WGA) is imperfect, such that 5% to 10% of alleles are not amplified sufficiently even in the most experienced hands.[90] This results in the phenomenon of allele dropout (ADO), which probably reflects stochastic phenomena (i.e., failure of probes to locate and anneal with patient DNA) and likely is exacerbated if embryo damage occurs during biopsy. Linkage data are thus obligatory in single-gene PGD analysis to limit the chance of erroneous or noninformative results that could arise if only the mutant allele were interrogated.

Another indication for PGD involves adult-onset mendelian conditions. PGD is most frequently performed for pregnancies at risk for adult-onset cancers, such as with the presence of *BRCA1,* Li-Fraumeni syndrome, multiple endocrine neoplasia (MEN), familial adenomatous polyposis (FAP), retinoblastoma, and von Hippel-Lindau syndrome.[96] In the United States, relatively little controversy now exists for testing for these conditions, but reticence remains in Europe.

Safety of Preimplantation Genetic Diagnosis

Removal of an embryonic cell logically might decrease survival or prevent implantation, and hence it would reduce pregnancy rates. This appears true at least with respect to removal of blastomeres[88]; **viability is reduced by 10% when a single blastomere is removed.** Viability aside, the totipotential nature of embryonic cells means, at least theoretically, that biopsy will not cause anomalies in liveborn infants. The reason is that loss of one or more cells prior to irrevocable differentiation into a specific embryologic developmental pathway should not confer organ-specific damage if another cell has the capacity to accomplish the same purpose.

Indeed, available data indicate no increased rate of birth defects in liveborn infants who had been subjected as embryos to PGD.[97] In addition, no differences are apparent between offspring that result from single-gene PGD testing for single-gene mutations versus PGD testing for aneuploidy.

INTACT FETAL CELLS

Intact fetal cells exist in maternal blood at an esimated ratio of one intact fetal cell per million to 10 million maternal cells. Noninvasive diagnosis based on intact fetal cells is very attractive because genetic information derived from a single nucleated fetal cell would be considerably greater than that currently attainable by cell-free fetal DNA methods. If feasible and not overly expensive, the recovery of intact fetal cells noninvasively would likely be the optimal method of prenatal genetic diagnosis.

Enriching for nucleated fetal red blood cells and interrogating FISH with chromosome-specific probes, Price and colleagues[98] were the first to detect fetal aneuploidy (trisomy 18) in maternal blood. This advance soon was followed by noninvasive detection of trisomy 21 by others.[99] The major problem became that the expected number of fetal cells was not recovered, presumably

having been lost in processing. An NICHD collaborative study assessed the accuracy of intact fetal cell recovery in four centers that used two different methods. Overall, 74% of aneuploidies were detected (32 of 43 cases).[100] However, this method was laborious and was hindered by lack of consistent cell recovery. Noninvasive prenatal testing thereafter began to focus on cell-free fetal DNA, as discussed above. However, several biotech groups have continued to pursue recovery of intact fetal cells, including nucleated red blood cells. None currently offers clinical testing.

At present the most promising approach appears to involve recovery of fetal trophoblasts in maternal blood. Paterlini-Brechot and colleagues initially demonstrated proof of principle for recovering individual trophoblasts on a filter. Fetal origin was confirmed based on paternal polymorphisms, and fetal genotype was determined. A 2012 study[101] of 63 consecutive cases of CF and SMA showed clinically useful sensitivity and specificity.

In summary, ability to recover, transport, and analyze intact fetal cells in maternal blood would be transformative and would likely replace all other approaches used to obtain fetal DNA. However, additional development is still necessary before clinical utility will exist.

KEY POINTS

- About 3% of liveborn infants have a major congenital anomaly due to a chromosome abnormality, single-gene mutation or multifactorial/polygenic inheritance, or exogenous factors (teratogens).
- Noninvasive screening tests for the common autosomal trisomies should be offered at any age, providing patient-specific aneuploidy risks. First-trimester screening using serum analytes (free hCG and PAPP-A) and an NT measurement has a detection rate of 85% to 87% with a false-positive rate of 5%. For women at high risk for trisomy 21, cfDNA analysis is available as early as 10 weeks' gestation, with a detection rate of greater than 99%; however, confirmatory invasive diagnostic testing is recommended.
- Second-trimester noninvasive screening with four analytes—hCG, AFP, uE₃, and inhibin A—has an 80% detection rate and can be performed in conjunction with first-trimester screening to yield a higher detection rate of 95%.
- Invasive prenatal diagnosis with chromosome microarrays allows comprehensive analysis of the entire genome at a finer resolution than a routine karyotype and is capable of detecting trisomies and unbalanced translocations as well as submicroscopic deletions and duplications of the genome (CNVs). It has several advantages over conventional cytogenetic testing, especially in the fetus with a structural malformation. Clinically significant CNVs were detected in 6% of the fetuses with a normal karyotype and suspected structural anomalies or growth abnormalities.
- Screening for carriers for β-thalassemia and α-thalassemia can be inexpensively performed on the basis of an MCV less than 80% followed by hemoglobin electrophoresis, once iron deficiency has been excluded.

- CF is found in all ethnic groups, but the heterozygote frequency is higher in non-Hispanic whites of northern European (1 in 25) or Ashkenazi Jewish origin (1 in 24) than in other ethnic groups (black 1/61, Hispanic 1/58, Asian 1/94). More than 1500 mutations have been identified in the gene for CF, but carrier screening is obligatory only for a specified panel of 23 mutations. In northern European white and Ashkenazi Jewish individuals, the heterozygote detection rate using the specified panel is 88% and 94%, respectively. In other ethnic groups, detection rates are lower (64% in blacks, 72% in Hispanics, and 49% in Asian Americans).

- Most single-gene disorders can now be detected by molecular methods if fetal tissue is available, given that the location of the causative mutant gene is known for most disorders. Linkage analysis can be applied if the gene has been localized but not yet sequenced or if the mutation responsible for the disorder in a given family remains unknown despite sequencing. This option represents a transformational improvement over previous methods, which relied on a number of different indirect approaches.

- Amniocentesis (15 weeks or later) and CVS (10 to 13 weeks) are equivalent in safety (1 in 300 to 500 loss rate) and diagnostic accuracy. Amniocentesis before 13 weeks is not recommended because of an unacceptable risk for pregnancy loss and clubfoot (talipes equinovarus).

- Congenital malformations that involve a single organ system (e.g., spina bifida, facial clefts, cardiac defects) are considered multifactorial or polygenic. After the birth of one child with a birth defect that involves only one organ system, the recurrence risk in subsequent offspring is 1% to 5%. Many of these congenital anomalies can be diagnosed in utero using ultrasonography or fetal echocardiography.

- Neural tube defects may be detected by either ultrasonography or MSAFP screening in the second trimester.

- PGD requires removal of one or more cells (polar body blastomere, trophectoderm) from the embryo. Diagnosis uses molecular techniques to detect single-gene disorders and either FISH or chromosome array CGH to detect chromosome abnormalities (e.g., trisomy). PGD also allows for avoidance of clinical pregnancy termination, fetal (embryonic) diagnosis without disclosure of parental genotype (e.g., Huntington disease), and selection of HLA-compatible embryos.

REFERENCES

1. Hook EB. Rates of chromosome abnormalities at different maternal ages. *Obstet Gynecol.* 1981;58:282.
2. Hook EB, Cross PK, Schreinemachers DM. Chromosomal abnormality rates at amniocentesis and in live-born infants. *JAMA.* 1983;249:2034.
3. Ruggeri A, Dulcetti F, Miozzo M, et al. Prenatal search for UPD 14 and UPD 15 in 83 cases of familial and de novo heterologous robertsonian translocations. *Prenat Diagn.* 2004;24:997.
4. Weise A, Mrasek K, Klein E, et al. Microdeletion and microduplication syndromes. *J Histochem Cytochem.* 2012;60:346-358.
5. Miller DT, Adam MP, Aradhya S, et al. Consensus statement: chromosomal microarray is a first-tier clinical diagnostic test for individuals with developmental disabilities or congenital anomalies. *Am J Hum Genet.* 2010;86:749-764.
6. Bondy CA, Turner Syndrome Study Group. Care of girls and women with Turner syndrome: a guideline of the Turner Syndrome Study Group. *J Clin Endocrinol Metab.* 2007;92:10.
7. Simpson JL, de La Cruz F, Swerdloff RS, et al. Klinefelter syndrome: expanding the phenotype and identifying new research directions. *Genet Med.* 2003;5:460.
8. Graham JM, Simpson JL, Samango-Sprouse C. Klinefelter syndrome. In: Cassidy SB, Allanson J, eds. *Management of Genetic Syndromes.* 2nd ed. Hoboken, NJ: John Wiley & Sons; 2005:323.
9. Haverty CE, Lin AE, Simpson E, et al. 47, XXX associated with malformations. *Am J Med Genet A.* 2004;125:108.
10. Nicolaides KH. Nuchal transparency and other first trimester sonographic markers of chromosomal abnormalities. *Am J Obstet Gynecol.* 2004;191:45.
11. Krantz DA, Hallahan TW, Orlandi F, et al. First-trimester Down syndrome screening using dried blood biochemistry and nuchal translucency. *Obstet Gynecol.* 2000;96:207.
12. Wapner R, Thom E, Simpson JL, et al. First trimester screening for trisomies 21 and 18. *N Engl J Med.* 2003;349:1405.
13. Wald NJ, Rodeck C, Hackshaw AK, et al. First and second trimester antenatal screening for Down's syndrome: the results of the serum, urine and ultrasound screening study (SURUSS). *J Med Screen.* 2003;10:56.
14. Malone FD, Canick JA, Ball RH, et al. First-trimester or second-trimester screening or both for Down's syndrome. *N Engl J Med.* 2005;353:2001.
15. Malone FD, Ball RH, Nyberg DA, et al. First-trimester septated cystic hygroma: prevalence, natural history and pediatric outcome. *Obstet Gynecol.* 2005;106:288.
16. Comstock CH, Malone FD, Ball RH, et al. Is there a nuchal translucency millimeter measurement above which there is no added benefit from first trimester serum screening? *Am J Obstet Gynecol.* 2006;195:843.
17. Avgidou K, Papageorghiou A, Bindra R, et al. Prospective first-trimester screening for trisomy 21 in 30,564 pregnancies. *Am J Obstet Gynecol.* 2005;192:1761.
18. Souka AP, Krampl E, Bakalis S, et al. Outcome of pregnancy in chromosomally normal fetus with increased nuchal translucency in the first trimester. *Ultrasound Obstet Gynecol.* 2001;18:9.
19. Bogart MH, Pandian MR, Jones OW. Abnormal maternal serum chorionic gonadotropin levels in pregnancies with fetal chromosome abnormalities. *Prenat Diagn.* 1987;7:623.
20. Canik JA, Knight GI, Palomaki GE, et al. Low second trimester maternal serum unconjugated oestriol in pregnancies with Down's syndrome. *Br J Obstet Gynaecol.* 1988;95:330.
21. Palomaki GE, Knight GJ, Haddow JE, et al. Prospective intervention trial of a screening protocol to identify fetal trisomy 18 using maternal serum alpha-fetoprotein, unconjugated oestrial and human chorionic gonadotropin. *Prenat Diagn.* 1992;12:925.
22. Palomaki GE, Haddow JE, Knight GJ, et al. Risk-based prenatal screening for trisomy 18 using alpha-fetoprotein, unconjugated oestriol and human chorionic gonadotrophin. *Prenat Diagn.* 1995;15:713.
23. Palomaki GE, Knight GJ, Haddow JE, et al. Cigarette smoking and levels of maternal serum alpha-fetoprotein, unconjugated estriol, and hCG: impact on Down syndrome screening. *Obstet Gynecol.* 1993;81:675.
24. Cuckle HS, Spenser K, Nicolaides KH. Down syndrome screening marker levels in women with a previous aneuploidy pregnancy. *Prenat Diagn.* 2005;25:47.
25. Malone FD, Cuckle H, Ball RH, et al. Contingent screening for trisomy 21 results from a general population screening trial. *Am J Obstet Gynecol.* 2005;193:S29.
26. Cuckle H. Integrating antenatal Down's syndrome screening. *Curr Opin Obstet Gynecol.* 2001;13:175.
27. Cuckle H, Arbuzova S. Multimarkers maternal serum screening for chromosomal abnormalities. In: Milunsky A, ed. *Genetic Disorders and the Fetus.* 5th ed. Baltimore: Johns Hopkins University Press; 2004:795.
28. Palomaki GE, Kloza EM, Lambert-Messerlian GM, et al. DNA sequencing of maternal plasma to detect Down syndrome: an international clinical validation study. *Genet Med.* 2011;13:913-920.
29. Palomaki GE, Deciu C, Kloza EM, et al. DNA sequencing of maternal plasma reliably identifies trisomy 18 as well as Down syndrome: an international collaborative. *Genet Med.* 2012;14:296-305.
30. Norton ME, Brar H, Weiss J, et al. Non-invasive chromosomal evaluation (NICE) study: results of a multicenter prospective cohort study for detection of fetal trisomy 21 and 18. *Am J Obstet Gynecol.* 2012;207:137.e1-137.e8.
31. Lau TK, Cheung SW, Lo PS, et al. Non-invasive prenatal testing for fetal chromosomal abnormalities by low-coverage whole-genome sequencing of

maternal plasma DNA: review of 1982 consecutive cases in a single center. *Ultrasound Obstet Gynecol.* 2014;43:254-264.

32. American College of Obstetricians and Gynecologists Committee on Genetics and the Society for Maternal Fetal Medicine Publications Committee: Noninvasive prenatal testing for fetal aneuploidy, ACOG Committee Opinion 545 (Dec 2012). *Obstet Gynecol.* 2012;120:1532-1534.

33. Gregg AH, Gross SJ, Best RG, et al. ACMG statement on noninvasive prenatal screening for fetal aneuploidy. *Genet Med.* 2013;15:395-398.

34. Nicolaides KH, Syngelaki A, Ashoor G, et al. Noninvasive prenatal testing for fetal trisomies in a routinely screened first-trimester population. *Am J Obstet Gynecol.* 2012;207:374.e1-374.e6.

35. Norton ME, Jacobsson B, Swamy GK, et al. Cell-free DNA analysis for noninvasive examination of trisomy. *New Engl J Med.* 2015;372:1589-1597.

36. Bianchi DW, Parker RL, Wentworth J, et al. DNA sequencing versus standard prenatal aneuploidy. *N Engl J Med.* 2014;370:799-808.

37. Boyle B, Morris JK, McConkey E, et al. Prevalence and risk of Down syndrome in monozygotic and dizygotic multiple pregnancies in Europe: implications for prenatal screening. *BJOG.* 2014;121:809-820.

38. Nicolaides KH, Brizot ML, Snijders RJ. Fetal nuchal translucency: ultrasound screening for fetal trisomy in the first trimester of pregnancy. *Br J Obstet Gynaecol.* 1994;101:782.

39. Cleary-Goldman J, Rebarber J, Krantz D, et al. First-trimester screening with nasal bone in twins. *Am J Obstet Gynecol.* 2008;199:e1-283.e3.

40. Canick JA, Kloza EM, Lambert-Messerlian GM, et al. DNA sequencing of maternal plasma to identify Down syndrome and other trisomies in multiple gestation. *Prenat Diagn.* 2012;32:730-734.

41. Grömminger S, Smerdka P, Ehrich M, et al. Fetal aneuploidy detection by cell-free DNA sequencing for multiple pregnancies and quality issues with vanishing twins. *J Clin Med.* 2014;3:679-692.

42. Benacerraf BR, Barss VA, Laboda LA. A sonographic sign for the detection in the second trimester of the fetus with Down's syndrome. *Am J Obstet Gynecol.* 1985;151:1078.

43. Smith-Bindman R, Hosmer W, Feldstein VA, et al. Second-trimester ultrasound to detect fetuses with Down syndrome: a meta-analysis. *JAMA.* 2001;285:1044.

44. American College of Obstetricians and Gynecologists Committee on Practice Bulletins: screening for fetal chromosomal abnormalities, ACOG Practice Bulletin 77 (Jan 2007). *Obstet Gynecol.* 2007;109:217.

45. Daniel A, Hook EB, Wulf G. Risks of unbalanced progeny at amniocentesis to carriers of chromosome rearrangements: data from United States and Canadian laboratories. *Am J Med Genet.* 1989;33:14.

46. Shaffer LG, Dabel MP, Fisher AJ, et al. Experience with microarray-based comparative genomic hybridization for prenatal diagnosis in over 5000 pregnancies. *Prenat Diagn.* 2012;32:976-985.

47. Simpson JL, Lamb DJ. Genetic effects of intracytoplasmic sperm injection. *Semin Reprod Med.* 2001;19:239.

48. American College of Obstetricians and Gynecologists Committee on Genetics. ACOG Committee Opinion No. 581: the use of chromosomal microarray analysis in prenatal diagnosis. *Obstet Gynecol.* 2013;122:1374-1377.

49. Wapner RJ, Martin CL, Levy B, et al. Chromosomal microarray versus karyotyping for prenatal diagnosis. *N Engl J Med.* 2012;367:2175-2184.

50. Oneda B, Baldinger R, Reissmann R, et al. High-resolution chromosomal microarrays in prenatal diagnosis significantly increase diagnostic power. *Prenat Diagn.* 2014;34:525-533.

51. Lee C-N, Lin SY, Lin CH, et al. Clinical utility of array comparative genomic hybridization for prenatal diagnosis: a cohort study of 3171 pregnancies. *BJOG.* 2012;119:614-625.

52. Bernhardt BA, Soucier D, Hanson K, et al. Women's experiences receiving abnormal prenaatal chromosomal microarray testing results. *Genet Med.* 2013;15:139-145.

53. Reddy UM, Page GP, Saade GR, et al. Karyotype versus microarray testing for genetic abnormalities after stillbirth. *N Engl J Med.* 2012;367:2185-2193.

54. Pertl B, Kopp S, Kroisel PM, et al. Rapid detection of chromosome aneuploidies by quantitative fluorescence PCR: first application on 247 chorionic villus samples. *J Med Genet.* 1999;36:300.

55. Hsu LY. Prenatal diagnosis of chromosome abnormalities through amniocentesis. In: Milunsky A, ed. *Genetic Disorders and the Fetus.* 3rd ed. Baltimore: The Johns Hopkins University Press; 1986:155.

56. Stetten G, Escallon CS, South ST, et al. Reevaluating confined placental mosaicism. *Am J Med Genet A.* 2004;131:232.

57. Ledbetter DH, Zachary JM, Simpson JL, et al. Cytogenetic results from the U.S. Collaborative Study on CVS. *Prenat Diagn.* 1992;12:317.

58. Hahnemann JM, Vejerslev LO. European collaborative research on mosaicism in CVS (EUCROMIC): fetal and extrafetal cell lineages in 192 gestations with CVS mosaicism involving single autosomal trisomy. *Am J Med Genet.* 1997;70:179.

59. Kotzot D. Abnormal phenotypes in uniparental disomy (UPD): fundamental aspects and a critical review with bibliography of UPD other than 15. *Am J Med Genet.* 1999;82:265.

60. Warburton D. De novo balanced chromosome rearrangements and extra marker chromosomes identified at prenatal diagnosis: clinical significance and distribution of breakpoints. *Am J Med Genet.* 1991;49:995.

61. Hume RF Jr, Drugan A, Ebrahim SA, et al. Role of ultrasonography in pregnancies with marker chromosome aneuploidy. *Fetal Diagn Ther.* 1995;10:182.

62. ACOG Committee on Genetics. Committee Opinion No. 442: Prenatal and Preconceptional Carrier Screening for Genetic Diseases in Individuals of Eastern European Jewish Descent. *Gynecol Obstet.* 2009;114:950-953.

63. American College of Obstetricians and Gynecologists Committee on Obstetrics. ACOG Practice Bulletin No. 78: hemoglobinopathies in pregnancy. *Obstet Gynecol.* 2007;109:229-237.

64. American College of Obstetricians and Gynecologists Committee on Genetics. ACOG Committee Opinion No. 486: update on carrier screening for cystic fibrosis. *Obstet Gynecol.* 2011;117:1028-1031.

65. American College of Obstetricians and Gynecologists Committee on Genetics. ACOG Committee Opinion No. 469: carrier screening for fragile X syndrome. *Obstet Gynecol.* 2010;116:1008.

66. ACOG Committee on Genetics. ACOG Committee Opinion no. 432: spinal muscular atrophy. *Obstet Gynecol.* 2009;113:1194.

67. Prior TW. Carrier screening for spinal muscular atrophy. *Genet Med.* 2008;10:840.

68. Grody WW, Cutting GR, Klinger KW, et al. Laboratory standards and guidelines for population-based cystic fibrosis carrier screening. *Genet Med.* 2001;3:149.

69. Abeliovich D, Lavon IP, Lerer I, et al. Screening for five mutations detects 97% of cystic fibrosis (CF) chromosomes and predicts a carrier frequency of 1:29 in the Jewish Ashkenazi population. *Am J Hum Genet.* 1992;51:951.

70. ACOG Practice Bulletin. *Neural tube defects. Number 44.* Washington, DC: American College of Obstetricians and Gynecologists; 2003.

71. Simpson JL, Palomaki GE, Mercer B, et al. Associations between adverse perinatal outcome and serially obtained serum. *Am J Obstet Gynecol.* 1995;173:1742.

72. Krause TG, Christens P, Wohlfahrt J, et al. Second-trimester maternal serum alpha-fetoprotein and risk of adverse pregnancy outcome (1). *Obstet Gynecol.* 2001;97:277.

73. Smith GC, Wood AM, Pell JP, et al. Second-trimester maternal serum levels of alpha-fetoprotein and the subsequent risk of sudden infant death syndrome. *N Engl J Med.* 2004;351:978.

74. American College of Obstetricians and Gynecologists. ACOG Practice Bulletin No. 88: Invasive Prenatal Testing for Aneuploidy. *Obstet Gynecol.* 2007;110:1459-1467.

75. Lawson HW, Frye A, Atrash HK, et al. Abortion mortality, United States, 1972 through 1987. *Am J Obstet Gynecol.* 1994;171:1365.

76. Rhoads GG, Jackson LG, Schlesselman SE, et al. The safety and efficacy of chorionic villus sampling for early prenatal diagnosis of cytogenetic abnormalities. *N Engl J Med.* 1989;320:609.

77. Jackson LG, Zachary JM, Fowler SE, et al. A randomized comparison of transcervical and transabdominal chorionic-villus sampling. The U.S. National Institute of Child Health and Human Development Chorionic-Villus Sampling and Amniocentesis Study Group. *N Engl J Med.* 1992;327:594.

78. Alfirevic Z, Sundberg K, Brigham S. Amniocentesis and chorionic villus sampling for prenatal diagnosis. *Cochrane Database Syst Rev.* 2003;CD003252.

79. Pergament E, Schulman JD, Copeland K, et al. The risk and efficacy of chorionic villus sampling in multiple gestations. *Prenat Diagn.* 1992;12:377.

80. Davies G, Wilson RD, Desilets V, et al. Amniocentesis and women with hepatitis B, hepatitis C, or human immunodeficiency virus. *JOGC.* 2003;25:145.

81. Maiques V, Garcia-Tejedor A, Perales A, et al. HIV detection in amniotic fluid samples: Amniocentesis can be performed in HIV pregnant women? *Eur J Obstet Gynaecol.* 2003;108:137.

82. Copel JA, Grannum PA, Harrison D, Hobbins JC. The use of intravenous pancuronium bromide to produce fetal paralysis during intravascular transfusion. *Am J Obstet Gynecol.* 1988;158:170.

83. Tongsong T, Wanapirak C, Kunavikatikul C, et al. Fetal loss rate associated with cordocentesis at midgestation. *Am J Obstet Gynecol.* 2001;184:719.
84. Liao C, Wei J, Li Q, et al. Efficacy and safety of cordocentesis for prenatal diagnosis. *Int J Gynaecol Obstet.* 2006;93:13.
85. Tongprasert F, Tongsong T, Wanapirak C, et al. Cordocentesis in multifetal pregnancies. *Prenat Diagn.* 2007;27:1100.
86. Weiner CP, Wenstrom KD, Sipes SL, Williamson RA. Risk factors for cordocentesis and fetal intravascular transfusion. *Am J Obstet Gynecol.* 1991;165:1020.
87. Van Kamp IL, Klumper FJ, Oepkes D, et al. Complications of intrauterine intravascular transfusion for fetal anemia due to maternal red-cell alloimmunization. *Am J Obstet Gynecol.* 2005;192:171.
88. Cohen J, Wells D, Munné S. Removal of two cells from cleavage stage embryos is likely to reduce the efficacy of chromosomal test employed to enhance implantation rates. *Fertil Steril.* 2007;87:496-503.
89. Simpson JL. Preimplantation Genetic Diagnosis at 20 years. *Prenat Diagn.* 2010;30:682-695.
90. Kuliev A, Rechitsky S, Verlinsky O. *Atlas of Preimplantation Genetic Diagnosis.* Third ed. CRC Press; 2014.
91. Munné S, Fragouli E, Colls P, et al. Improved detection of aneuploid blastocysts using a new 12-chromosome FISH test. *Reprod Bio Med Online.* 2010;20:92-97.
92. Scott RT Jr, Ferry K, Su J, et al. Comprehensive chromosome screening is highly predicative of the reproductive potential of human embryos: a prospective, blinded nonselection study. *Fertil Steril.* 2012;97:870-875.
93. Yang Z, Liu J, Collins GS, et al. Selection of single blastocysts for fresh transfer via standard morphology assessment alone and with array CGH for good prognosis IVF patients: results from a randomized pilot study. *Mol Cytogenet.* 2012;5:24-31.
94. Forman EJ, Hong KH, Ferry KM, et al. In vitro fertilization with single euploid blastocyst transfer: a randomized controlled trial. *Fertil Steril.* 2013;100(1):100-107.
95. Stephenson MD, Sierra S. Reproductive outcomes in recurrent pregnancy loss associated with a parental carrier of a structural chromosome rearrangement. *Hum Reprod.* 2006;21:1076-1082.
96. Rechitsky S, Verlinsky O, Christokhina A, et al. Preimplantation genetic diagnosis for cancer predisposition. *Reprod Bio Med Online.* 2002;5:148-155.
97. Liebaers I, Desmyuttere S, Verposet W, et al. Report on a consecutive series of 581 children born after blastomere biopsy for preimplantation diagnosis. *Hum Reprod.* 2010;25:275-282.
98. Price JO, Elias S, Wachtel SS, et al. Prenatal diagnosis with fetal cells isolated from maternal blood by multiparameter flow cytometry. *Am J Obstet Gynecol.* 1991;165:1731-1737.
99. Simpson JL, Elias S. Isolating fetal cells from maternal blood: advances in prenatal diagnosis through molecular technology. *JAMA.* 1993;270:2357-2361.
100. Bianchi DW, Simpson JL, Jackson LG, et al. Fetal gender and aneuploidy detection using fetal cells in maternal blood: analysis of NIFTY I data. National Institute of Child Health and Development Fetal Cell Isolation Study. *Prenat Diagn.* 2002;22:609-615.
101. Mouawia H, Saker A, Jais J-P, et al. Circulating trophoblastic cells provide genetic diagnosis in 63 fetuses at risk for cystic fibrosis or spinal muscular atrophy. *Reprod Biomed Online.* 2012;25:508-520.

CHAPTER 11

Antepartum Fetal Evaluation

MARA B. GREENBERG and MAURICE L. DRUZIN

KEY ABBREVIATIONS

American College of Obstetricians and Gynecologists	ACOG
Amniotic fluid index	AFI
Antiphospholipid antibody syndrome	APLAS
Assisted reproductive technology	ART
Biophysical profile	BPP
Body mass index	BMI
Central nervous system	CNS
Contraction stress test	CST
Deepest vertical pocket	DVP
Fetal breathing movement	FBM
Fetal movement counting	FMC
Human chorionic gonadotropin	hCG
Intrauterine growth restriction	IUGR
Lecithin/sphingomyelin ratio	L/S ratio
Modified biophysical profile	mBPP
Multiples of the median	MoM
National Center for Health Statistics	NCHS
National Institute for Child Health and Human Development	NICHD
Nonstress test	NST
Perinatal mortality rate	PMR
Phosphatidylglycerol	PG
Pregnancy-associated plasma protein A	PAPP-A
Rapid eye movement	REM
Respiratory distress syndrome	RDS
Systemic lupus erythematosus	SLE
Vibroacoustic stimulation	VAS
World Health Organization	WHO

Antepartum fetal evaluation is an ever growing and changing science. **The goal of evidence-based antepartum fetal evaluation is to decrease perinatal mortality and permanent neurologic injury through judicious use of reliable and valid methods of fetal assessment without acting prematurely to modify an otherwise-healthy pregnancy or providing a false sense of well-being in cases of impending morbidity.** The opportunity for obstetric care providers to participate in this delicate balance has been made possible by continued advances in our ability to assess the physiologic well-being of the fetus, concurrent with great improvement in neonatal care and survival.[1] However, despite these advances in antepartum fetal surveillance and the widespread use of antepartum testing programs, the ability of these techniques to prevent intrauterine injury or death remains unproved in many cases.[2] The focus of this chapter is on antepartum evaluation in the United States and similarly technologically advanced and resource-rich countries, noting that the worldwide problem of stillbirth is a vast and compelling area of international interest.[3]

DEFINING THE PROBLEM OF PERINATAL MORTALITY

Identification of fetuses at risk for perinatal mortality has historically been the goal of antepartum fetal assessment. Our emerging understanding that long-term neurologic disability is an integrally related and often competing entity to perinatal mortality makes this goal more complex.[2]

The National Center for Health Statistics (NCHS) provides two different definitions for perinatal mortality, acknowledging that variation in definitions and reporting rates both among states in the United States and throughout different countries worldwide makes comparisons difficult; an agenda to develop a classification consensus has been the focus of a number of international committees, including the National Institute for Child Health and Human Development (NICHD).[3] The NCHS National Vital Statistics Report (NVSR) on fetal and perinatal mortality describes two different definitions for *perinatal mortality rate* (PMR). *Definition I* includes deaths of infants of less than 7 days of age and fetal deaths of 28 weeks of gestation or more per 1000 live births plus fetal deaths, whereas *definition II* is more comprehensive and includes infant deaths of less than 28 days of age and fetal deaths of 20 weeks or more per the same denominator.[4,5] The definitions of PMR provided by the World Health Organization (WHO) and the American College of Obstetricians and Gynecologists (ACOG) differ slightly and include the number of fetuses and live births weighing at least 500 g rather than using a gestational age cutoff.[6,7] According to the NCHS, "Fetal death means death prior to the complete expulsion or extraction from its mother of a product of human conception, irrespective of the duration of pregnancy and which is not an induced termination of pregnancy. The death is indicated by the fact that after such expulsion or extraction, the fetus does not breathe or show any other evidence of life such as beating of the heart, pulsation of the umbilical cord, or definite movement of voluntary muscles."[4] The term *fetal death* is used in these definitions and hereafter in this chapter rather than *stillbirth, spontaneous abortion,* or *miscarriage.*

In 2006, about 26,000 fetal deaths occurred in the United States. **Although the PMR has fallen steadily in the United States since 1965, the number of fetal deaths has not changed substantially in the past decade** (Fig. 11-1).[4,5,8] Using NCHS definition I, the PMR reported in 2006 was 6.5 per 1000, and fetal deaths accounted for about 50% of all perinatal mortality in the United States.[4] The PMR varies greatly by maternal race and ethnicity (Fig. 11-2). In 2006, rates (per 1000) were lowest for Asian/Pacific Islander women (4.83), followed by non-Hispanic white (5.34), Hispanic (5.76), and Native American/Alaskan Native women (6.72). The rate for non-Hispanic black women (11.76) was the highest among the racial and ethnic

groups and was more than twice the rate for non-Hispanic white women. The significantly greater PMR in blacks results from higher rates of *both* neonatal and fetal deaths.[4]

Characteristics of Fetal Death

Another way to consider the contribution of fetal events on PMR is to look at the infant mortality rate (Fig. 11-3).[4] Although the infant mortality rate includes all deaths of infants younger than 1 year of age, 50% of all infant deaths occur in the first week of life, and 50% of these losses result during the first day of life.[7] The infant mortality rate has fallen progressively and even more steeply over time than the fetal death rate, from 47 per 1000 in 1940 to 6.14 per 1000 in 2010.[6,9-11] In 2010 about 24,500 infant deaths (6.14 per 1000 live births) were reported, which included 16,200 neonatal deaths (4.05 per 1000 live births), and 12,900 of these were in the first week of life.[6,9-11] In

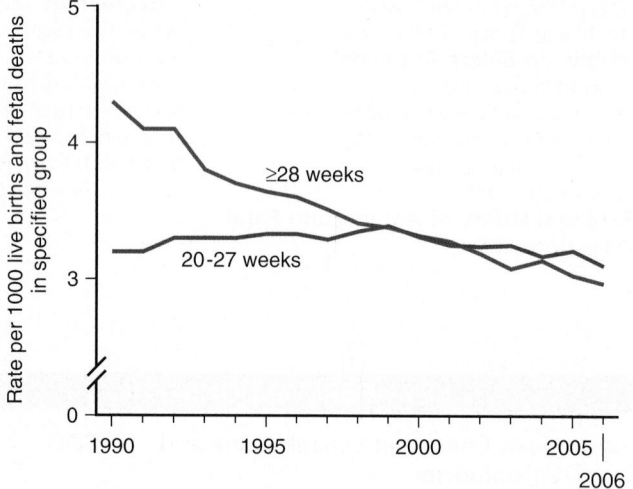

FIG 11-1 U.S. trends in fetal mortality rates over time by period of gestation, 1990 through 2006. (Data from the Centers for Disease Control and Prevention/National Center for Health Statistics, National Vital Statistics System, August 2012.)

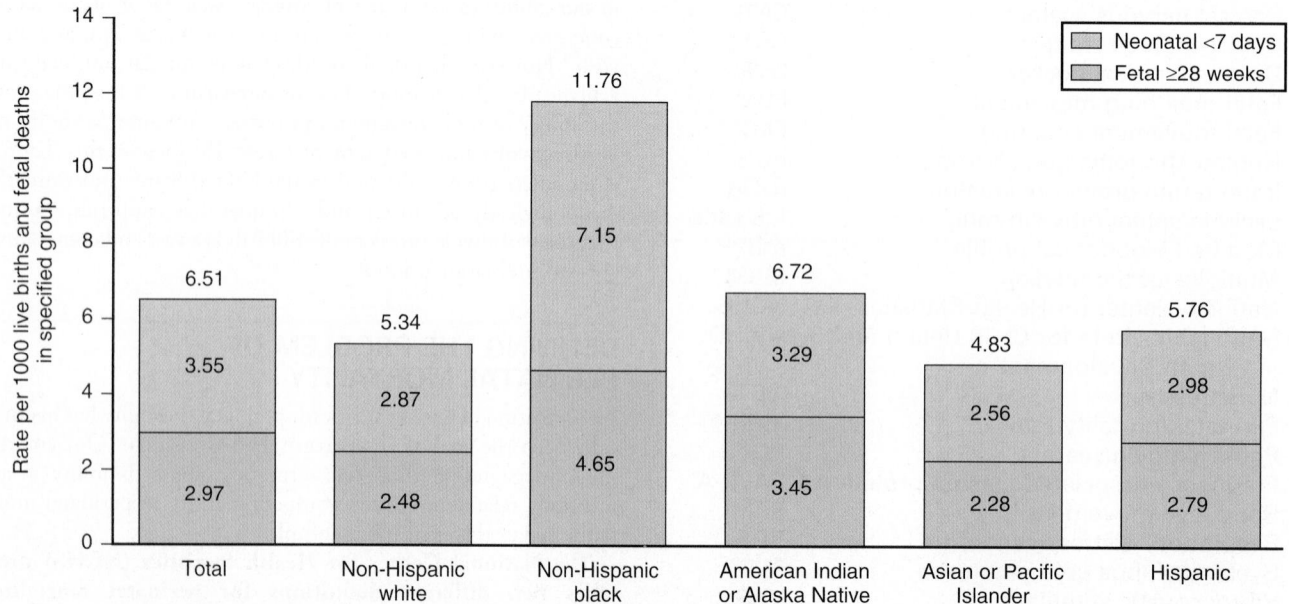

FIG 11-2 U.S. fetal mortality rates by maternal race and ethnicity, 2006. (Data from the Centers for Disease Control and Prevention/National Center for Health Statistics, National Vital Statistics System, August 2012.)

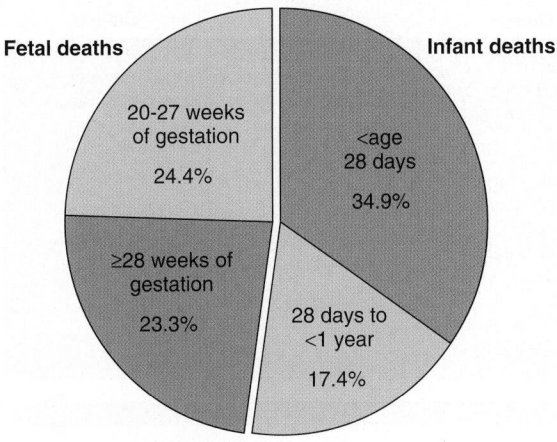

Fetal deaths

20-27 weeks
of gestation
24.4%

≥28 weeks of
gestation
23.3%

Infant deaths

<age
28 days
34.9%

28 days to
<1 year
17.4%

FIG 11-3 Relative magnitude of components of fetal and infant mortality, United States 2006. (Data from the Centers for Disease Control and Prevention/National Center for Health Statistics, National Vital Statistics System, August 2012.)

2010, the leading causes of infant mortality were congenital malformations, deformations, and chromosome abnormalities (21%); disorders related to short gestation and low birthweight, not elsewhere classified (17%); sudden infant death syndrome (8%); and maternal complications of pregnancy (6%). Together, these leading causes accounted for over 50% of all infant deaths in the United States in 2010.[10] Clearly, **perinatal events play an important role in infant mortality.**

Causes of Fetal Death

In addition to declining frequency in PMR over time, the overall pattern of perinatal deaths in the United States has changed considerably during the past 40 years. Manning and associates[12] suggest that antepartum deaths may be divided into four broad categories: (1) chronic asphyxia of diverse origin; (2) congenital malformations; (3) superimposed complications of pregnancy, such as Rh isoimmunization, placental abruption, and fetal infection; and (4) deaths of unexplained cause. Fretts and colleagues[13,14] analyzed the causes of deaths, confirmed by autopsy, in fetuses weighing more than 500 g in 94,346 births at the Royal Victoria Hospital in Montreal from 1961 to 1993. The population studied was predominantly white, participated in prenatal care, and included patients from all socioeconomic groups. Overall, the fetal death rate in this group declined by 70%, from 11.5 per 1000 in the 1960s to 3.2 per 1000 during 1990 to 1993.[14] The decline in the fetal death rate in this cohort was attributed to the prevention of Rh sensitization, antepartum and intrapartum fetal surveillance, improved detection of intrauterine growth restriction (IUGR) and fetal anomalies with ultrasound, and improved care of maternal diabetes mellitus and preeclampsia. The role of antenatal diagnosis and management of congenital malformations and aneuploidy is obviously critical to a goal of reducing perinatal morbidity and mortality and will be discussed separately (see Chapters 9, 10, and 27).

Fretts and colleagues[13,14] noted that most of the deaths in the Canadian cohort occurred between 28 and 36 weeks' gestation and that the diagnosis of IUGR was rarely identified before death. In addition to IUGR, leading causes of fetal death after 28 weeks' gestation included abruptio placentae and unexplained antepartum losses. Despite a marked fall in unexplained fetal deaths, from 38.1 to 13.6 per 1000, this category was used for more than 25% of all stillbirths. Fetal to maternal hemorrhage

may occur in 10% to 15% of cases of unexplained fetal deaths. Fetal deaths caused by infection, most often associated with premature rupture of the membranes (PROM) before 28 weeks' gestation, did not decline over the 30 years of the study and accounted for about 19% of fetal deaths. Further population-based analyses of the causes of fetal death have confirmed these findings, including a 2011 evaluation by the Stillbirth Collaborative Research Network, which utilized rigorous methods to classify as many "unexplained" fetal deaths as possible.[15]

In summary, based on available data, about 30% of antepartum fetal deaths may be attributed to asphyxia (IUGR, prolonged gestation), 30% to maternal complications (placental abruption, hypertension, preeclampsia, and diabetes mellitus), 15% to congenital malformations and chromosome abnormalities, and 5% to infection. At least 20% of fetal deaths have no obvious fetal, placental, maternal, or obstetric etiology, and this percentage increases with advancing gestational age. Late-gestation stillbirths are more likely to have no identifiable etiology.[6] The ability of our current methods of surveillance to make an impact on the perinatal mortality will depend on the ability of available tests to predict and predate injury and on use of obstetric interventions to prevent adverse outcomes. In one British series,[16] obstetric and pediatric assessors reviewed the circumstances surrounding each case of perinatal death to identify any *avoidable* factors that may have contributed to the death. Of the 309 perinatal deaths in this population (half fetal and half in the first week of life), 59% were considered to have had avoidable factors, including 74% of normal-birthweight infants with no fetal abnormalities and no maternal complications. Most avoidable factors were found to be obstetric rather than pediatric or maternal and social. The failure to respond appropriately to abnormalities during pregnancy and labor—including results from the monitoring of fetal growth or intrapartum fetal well-being, significant maternal weight loss, or reported reductions in fetal movement—constituted the largest groups of avoidable factors. This characterization of avoidable factors that contribute to perinatal death has been confirmed in additional studies.

Timing of Fetal Death

Another way to classify fetal deaths may be to differentiate those that occur during the antepartum period and those that occur during labor, or *intrapartum deaths.* **Antepartum fetal death is much more common than intrapartum fetal death, and unexplained fetal death occurs far more commonly than unexplained infant death.**[4,11,17] In a population-based study in the United States in 2007, the antepartum fetal death rate was 3.7 per 1000, compared with 0.6 per 1000 intrapartum fetal deaths.[17] Although most fetal deaths occur before 32 weeks' gestation, in planning a strategy for antepartum fetal monitoring, the risk for fetal death must be examined in the population of women who are still pregnant at that point in pregnancy.[18] When this approach is taken, the data would suggest that fetuses at 40 to 41 weeks are at a threefold greater risk and those at 42 or more weeks are at a twelvefold greater risk for intrauterine death than fetuses at 28 to 31 weeks. The risks are even higher in multiple gestations as pregnancy progresses. For twin gestations, the optimal time for delivery to prevent late-gestation perinatal deaths is by 39 weeks, and for triplets, 36 weeks.[19] The issue of timing is also illustrated by a recent cohort study of over 75,000 singleton pregnancies with fetal growth restriction, the focus of which was to find the point at which the competing

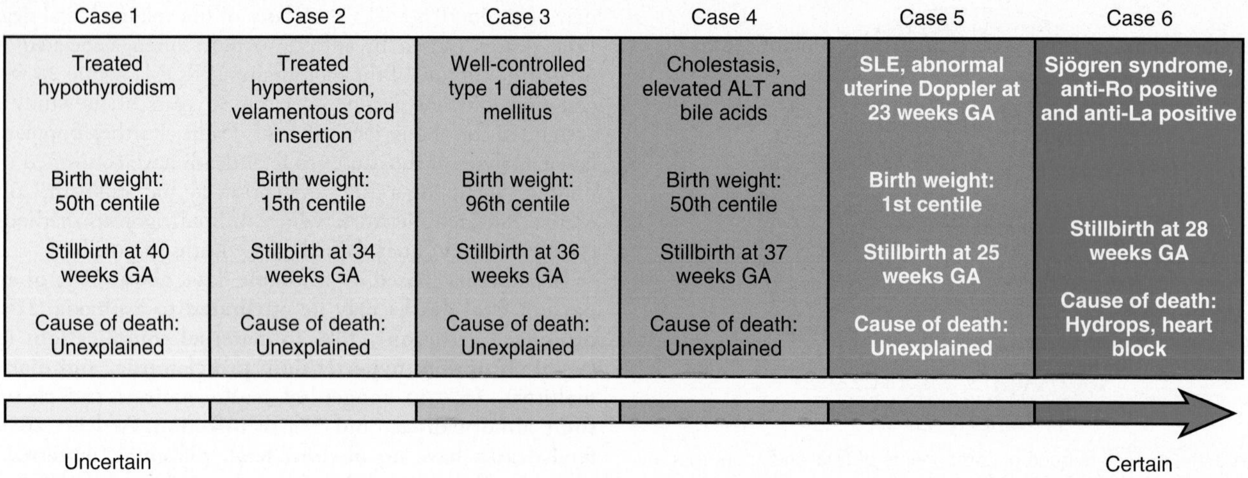

Case 1	Case 2	Case 3	Case 4	Case 5	Case 6
Treated hypothyroidism	Treated hypertension, velamentous cord insertion	Well-controlled type 1 diabetes mellitus	Cholestasis, elevated ALT and bile acids	SLE, abnormal uterine Doppler at 23 weeks GA	Sjögren syndrome, anti-Ro positive and anti-La positive
Birth weight: 50th centile	Birth weight: 15th centile	Birth weight: 96th centile	Birth weight: 50th centile	Birth weight: 1st centile	
Stillbirth at 40 weeks GA	Stillbirth at 34 weeks GA	Stillbirth at 36 weeks GA	Stillbirth at 37 weeks GA	Stillbirth at 25 weeks GA	Stillbirth at 28 weeks GA
Cause of death: Unexplained	Cause of death: Unexplained	Cause of death: Unexplained	Cause of death: Unexplained	Cause of death: Unexplained	Cause of death: Hydrops, heart block

Uncertain   Certain

FIG 11-4 Continuum of certainty in pathophysiology of cause of fetal death. Progressing from left to right on the continuum, levels of certainty increase as to the role of the pathophysiology of a particular condition in causing the fetal death. *ALT,* alanine aminotransferase; *GA,* gestational age; *SLE,* systemic lupus erythematosus. (Courtesy Professor Gordon Smith. Modified from Reddy UM, Goldenberg R, Silver R, et al. Stillbirth classification: developing an international consensus for research. Executive summary of a National Institute of Child Health and Human Development workshop. Stillbirth Classification of Cause of Death. *Obstet Gynecol.* 2009;114:901-914.)

risks of fetal death and neonatal death were in balance, in order to inform delivery decisions. In this cohort, the balance point was 32 to 34 weeks.[20]

Identifying Those at Risk

Some risk factors have a clear etiologic relationship to fetal compromise and death, such as exposures to teratogens or maternal conditions that alter the fetal environment or blood supply or content. Other risk factors—such as epidemiologic factors that include maternal age, race, and body habitus—have a perhaps more complex and less well-understood link to fetal death risk (Fig. 11-4).[3] Common risk factors for fetal death in the United States are listed in Table 11-1.[2,21] Many of these conditions can coexist in individual patients, which makes assessment of the contribution of each factor to perinatal mortality a challenge. A recent concept of looking at individual risk factors as part of a "triple risk model" may prove useful in making sense of this challenge, similar to that used to understand contributors to sudden infant death syndrome (SIDS). In this model, proposed by Warland and Mitchell,[22] an interplay exists among maternal, fetal, and placental factors and a stressor. They posit that whereas these factors in isolation may be insufficient to cause fetal death, they may prove lethal in combination (Fig. 11-5). Also necessary to consider is the contribution of these conditions to fetal injury that results in liveborn children with permanent neurologic compromise; this has yet to be determined but is an important alternative outcome to perinatal mortality that deserves further study.[2]

DETAILS ON SELECT ANTENATAL CONDITIONS
Maternal Characteristics
Maternal Age

Multiple investigators[2,14,23] have found that after controlling for risk factors such as multiple gestation, hypertension, diabetes mellitus, placenta previa and placental abruption, previous abortion, and prior fetal death, women 35 years of age or older have a greater risk for fetal death than women younger than 30 years, and women 40 years or older have an even further increased risk.

A J-shaped curve relationship exists between maternal age and fetal deaths, with the highest rates in teenagers and women older than 35 years (Fig. 11-6). The interplay of fetal death, maternal age, and gestational age was demonstrated in a population-based 2006 study in the United States of almost 5.5 million births.[24] In this cohort, compared with their counterparts aged 30 to 34 years at 41 weeks of gestation, women older than 35 to 39 years had the same risk for fetal death at 40 weeks, and women older than 40 years had the same risk at 39 weeks. Only 10% of the women older than 35 years had medical comorbidities, and the results of this study did *not* change when those women were excluded; this highlights the point that the increase in fetal death risk exists in otherwise healthy older gravidas compared with younger women.

Maternal Race

The variation in fetal death risk in the United States by maternal race is complex, which makes ascertainment of biologic risk factors related to race difficult.[21] Factors that contribute to increased rates of fetal death among black women compared with white women include disparities in socioeconomic status, access to health care, and preexisting medical conditions.[25] A 2009 population-based study of more than 5 million U.S. births demonstrated that the greatest black-and-white disparity is in preterm perinatal death, with a hazard ratio at 20 to 23 weeks of 2.75, which decreases to 1.57 at 39 to 40 weeks. Lower education levels and higher rates of medical, pregnancy, and labor complications contributed more to the adverse outcomes in blacks than in whites, with congenital anomalies more contributory in whites.[26]

Socioeconomic Factors, Prenatal Care, and Substance Abuse

Poor access to prenatal care and poor underlying health and nutrition have been linked to increased risk for fetal death both in developing and developed nations. As with other sociodemographic risk factors, these potential influences on fetal death risk are difficult to quantify and may be additive to other high-risk conditions.[27] Smoking and abuse of alcohol or illicit drugs, along with obesity, represent potentially modifiable risk factors for

TABLE 11-1	COMMON RISK FACTORS FOR FETAL DEATH IN THE UNITED STATES	
RISK FACTOR	**PREVALENCE (%)**	**ODDS RATIO**
All pregnancies	—	1.0
Low-risk pregnancies	80	0.86
Obesity:		
BMI 25-29.9	21-24	1.4-2.7
BMI >30	20-34	2.1-2.8
Nulliparity compared with second pregnancy	40	1.2-1.6
Fourth child or greater compared with second	11	2.2-2.3
Maternal age (reference: <35 yr):		
35-39 yr	15-18	1.8-2.2
≥40 yr	2	1.8-3.3
Multiple gestation:		
Twins	2.7	1.0-2.2
Triplets or greater	0.14	2.8-3.7
Oligohydramnios	2	4.5
Assisted reproductive technologies (all)	1-3	1.2-3.0
Abnormal serum markers:		
First-trimester PAPP-A <5%	5	2.2-4.0
Two or more second-trimester markers	0.1-2	4.2-9.2
Intrahepatic cholestasis	<0.1	1.8-4.4
Renal disease	<1	2.2-30
Systemic lupus erythematosus	<1	6-20
Smoking	10-20	1.7-3.0
Alcohol use (any)	6-10	1.2-1.7
Illicit drug use	2-4	1.2-3.0
Low education and socioeconomic status	30	2.0-7.0
Fewer than four antenatal visits*	6	2.7
Black (reference: white)	15	2.0-2.2
Hypertension	6-10	1.5-4.4
Diabetes	2-5	1.5-7.0
Large for gestational age (>97% without diabetes)	12	2.4
Fetal growth restriction (%):		
<3	3.0	4.8
3-10	7.5	2.8
Previous growth-restricted infant	6.7	2.0-4.6
Previous preterm birth with growth restriction	2	4.0-8.0
Decreased fetal movement	4-8	4.0-12.0
Previous stillbirth	0.5	2.0-10.0
Previous cesarean section	22-25	1.0-1.5
Postterm pregnancy compared with 38-40 wk		2.0-3.0
41 wk	9	1.5
42 wk	5	2.0-3.0

Modified from Signore C, Freeman RK, Spong CY. Antenatal testing: a reevaluation. Executive Summary of a Eunice Kennedy Shriver National Institute of Child Health and Human Development Workshop. *Obstet Gynecol.* 2009;113:687-701; and Fretts RC. Stillbirth epidemiology, risk factors, and opportunities for stillbirth prevention. *Clin Obstet Gynecol.* 2010;53:588-596.
BMI, body mass index; *PAPP-A,* pregnancy associated plasma protein A.
*For stillbirths, 37 weeks' gestation.

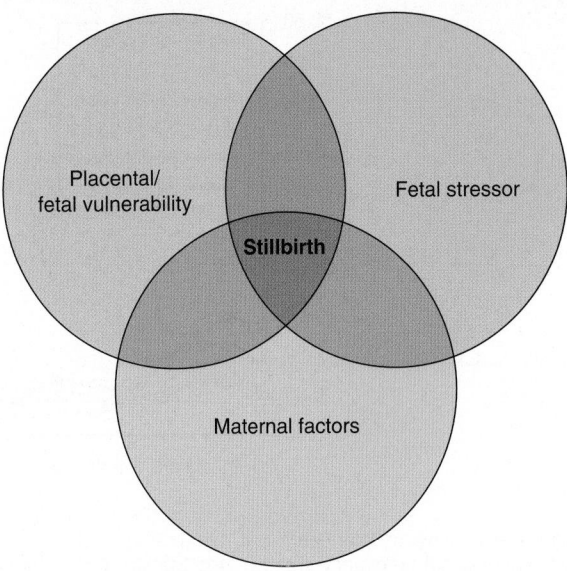

FIG 11-5 Triple risk model in which an interplay of maternal factors, fetal/placental factors, and a stressor contribute to fetal death. Whereas these factors in isolation may be insufficient to cause fetal death, they may prove lethal in combination. (From Warland J, Mitchell EA. A triple risk model for unexplained late stillbirth. *BMC Pregnancy Childbirth.* 2014;14:142.)

Maternal Comorbidities

Obesity
Prepregnancy obesity is associated with increased perinatal mortality, especially in late gestation. This has been demonstrated in several large series, including a meta-analysis of 38 studies that included more than 3 million women.[28] The connection between obesity and fetal death is still under investigation and is made more complex by the frequent comorbidities encountered in patients with prepregnancy obesity. Theoretic contributors to adverse perinatal outcomes in this group include placental dysfunction, sleep apnea, metabolic abnormalities, and difficulty in clinical assessment of fetal growth.[21] The strength of the association increases with advancing body mass index (BMI) and with advancing gestational age.

Diabetes Mellitus
Although historically, insulin-dependent diabetes has been a major risk factor for fetal death, the fetal death rate in women with optimal glycemic control now approaches that of women without diabetes.[2,29] However, the relationship between glycemic control and fetal death remains uncertain. Poor glycemic control is associated with increased perinatal mortality, in large part as a result of congenital anomalies; indicated preterm deliveries; and sudden, unexplained fetal death. A recent population-based study of over 1 million births in Ontario, Canada, revealed an odds ratio (OR) of 2.3 for fetal death among women with pregestational diabetes compared with those without diabetes.[29] No evidence suggests that gestational diabetes controlled by diet alone is associated with increased rates of intrauterine fetal death.[2,30]

Hypertensive Disorders
Studies have shown conflicting evidence regarding whether fetal death rates with well-controlled preexisting hypertension are comparable to those in the general population or increased. The increased risk for perinatal mortality associated with

fetal death. Although these behaviors are attractive candidates for fetal death prevention through counseling and modification of intake, prospective trials of behavior modification strategies have generally been underpowered to detect a difference in fetal death with these interventions.[21]

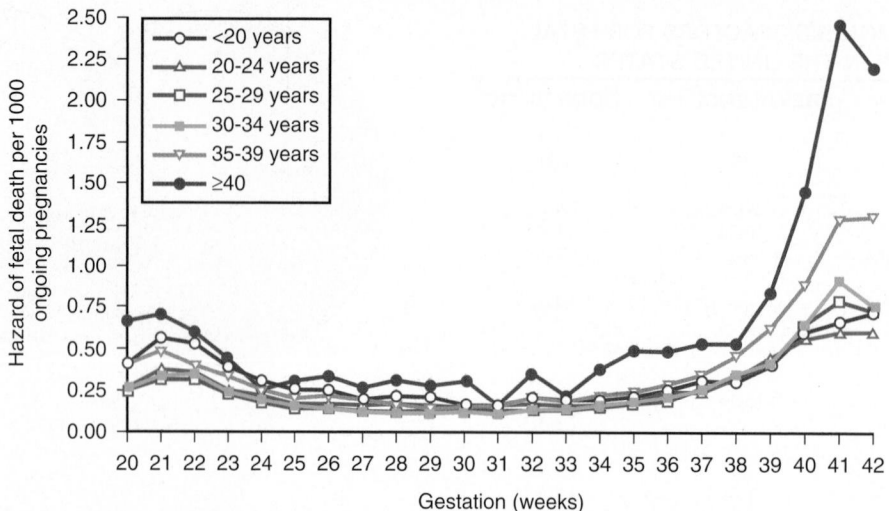

FIG 11-6 Relationship of fetal death and maternal age across gestation. (From Reddy UM, Ko CW, Willinger M. Maternal age and the risk of stillbirth throughout pregnancy in the United States. *Am J Obstet Gynecol.* 2006;195:764-770.)

hypertension is most often related to complicated hypertension, with sequelae of placental insufficiency that include IUGR and oligohydramnios. Proteinuric hypertension, especially preeclampsia with severe features or eclampsia, may be associated with fetal death through placental and coagulation-related pathways, including placental abruption.[3,31]

Thrombophilia

In general, no demonstrable link has been found between inherited thrombophilia and risk for fetal death.[3,32] Although initial reports seemed to support an association between fetal death and thrombophilia, such as factor V Leiden mutation and prothrombin gene mutation, large prospective trials have failed to substantiate this association. The presence of circulating maternal antiphospholipid antibodies—in particular lupus anticoagulant, anticardiolipin antibodies, and anti–β_2-glycoprotein I antibodies—in the antiphospholipid antibody syndrome (APLAS) have been associated with a variety of adverse pregnancy outcomes, including fetal loss.[33] The mechanism of these adverse outcomes remains unclear but likely includes inflammation, thrombosis, and placental infarction.[3] However, the link between fetal death and these antibodies or the presence of APLAS is still under investigation, but evidence is insufficient to conclude that an increased risk exists for fetal death.[34]

Intrahepatic Cholestasis

The cause of fetal death in women with gestational cholestasis remains unknown, and timing and predictive features of impending fetal death remain unpredictable. Fetal deaths in these pregnancies are not preceded by signs of placental insufficiency such as growth restriction or abnormal placental pathology, and normal fetal heart rate tracings proximal to fetal death (i.e., within 24 hours) have often been reported. It has also not been established whether maternal serum levels of bile acids, liver enzymes, or pharmacologic therapy modify or predict the risk of fetal death.[35]

Renal Disease and Systemic Lupus Erythematosus

With chronic maternal renal disease, perinatal outcome is largely associated with the degree of renal dysfunction and the presence of coexisting hypertension or diabetes. Although data are limited by lack of prospective studies with appropriate control groups, the greatest risk for fetal death appears to be in mothers with severe renal impairment (i.e., serum creatinine levels >2.4-2.8 mg/dL).[36] As with maternal renal disease, the prognosis for fetal outcome in women with systemic lupus erythematosus (SLE) is dependent on disease state and comorbid conditions, including hypertension, circulating autoantibodies, and renal involvement.[37] Prognosis for fetal survival in pregnancies complicated by both maternal renal disease and maternal SLE has improved over time with advances in therapies that promote disease quiescence for both of these conditions.

Obstetric Factors

Fertility History and Assisted Reproductive Technology

Multiple aspects of a woman's obstetric and fertility history may contribute to risk for fetal death in a current pregnancy, including parity, use of assisted reproductive technology (ART), and history of prior adverse obstetric outcomes. Both nulliparity and high parity are associated with an increased risk for fetal death compared with low multiparity (one, two, or three prior births).[38] This association is likely mediated through a variety of sociodemographic risk factors related to overall health and interconception health status, although studies have confirmed the association between parity and fetal death after controlling for several social and medical comorbidities. History of prior adverse pregnancy outcomes—including fetal growth restriction, preterm birth, and fetal death—marks a current pregnancy at risk for fetal death. However, the association with preventable recurrent fetal death is complex and is modified by coexistence of other high-risk conditions. Recurrence risk for fetal death in particular has received recent scrutiny because rates vary dramatically by study population and presence of other risk factors. Given that many fetal deaths occur in pregnancies with no identifiable risk factors and that well-designed studies with appropriate comparison groups (i.e., low-risk women without identifiable risk factors) are lacking, clinician and patient perception of increased risk in a pregnancy subsequent to a fetal death will likely continue to drive management of these patients.[39] Regarding use of ART and risk for fetal death, several systematic reviews have confirmed an independent association between the use of in vitro fertilization in particular and fetal death.

However, whether the association is mediated through the technologies themselves or the underlying infertility or through other undetermined mechanisms remains unclear.[40]

PARITY

Nulliparity and high parity have both been associated with fetal death in contrast to women having their second child. This association has not been fully explored and may be subject to significant confounding influences, including advanced maternal age, related conditions in nulliparous women with delayed childbearing in developed nations, and other medical and socioeconomic comorbidities in women with high parity.[8,21]

MULTIPLE GESTATIONS

The higher rate of perinatal mortality in multiple gestations compared with singletons is related both to complications unique to multiple gestations, such as twin-to-twin transfusion syndrome, and to more general complications, such as fetal abnormalities and growth restriction.[21,41] Additionally, many women who carry more than one fetus have maternal risk factors for increased perinatal mortality, including advanced maternal age and use of ART, and are subject to development of complications such as preeclampsia and preterm delivery.[2,42] Optimal timing of delivery between 37 and 38 weeks has been considered for twins, compared with 39 to 40 weeks among singletons, because of increased rate of late fetal death in this group.[43] Chorionicity is of paramount importance in determining fetal risk, and rates of adverse outcomes are higher among monochorionic twins.[2,42]

Early Pregnancy Markers

First- and second-trimester serum markers for aneuploidy, when abnormally low or elevated, have been associated to varying degrees with adverse perinatal outcomes even in the absence of aneuploidy. Biophysical uterine factors have also been studied in this light. Regarding fetal death after 24 weeks, markers of interest include first-trimester levels of pregnancy-associated plasma protein A (PAPP-A) of less than the fifth percentile (0.415 multiples of the median [MoM]); second-trimester free β-human chorionic gonadotropin (free β-hCG), α-fetoprotein (AFP), and inhibin A of more than 2 MoM; and uterine artery pulsatility index above the 90th percentile. The sensitivity and positive predictive value of these markers for fetal death are still under investigation. The pathophysiologic link between these markers and adverse outcomes is unclear and likely variable but most plausibly involves abnormal placental attachment or function.[44]

Amniotic Fluid Abnormalities

The predictive value of either oligohydramnios or polyhydramnios for adverse pregnancy outcomes, in particular fetal death, typically lies in their association with other abnormal conditions, such as maternal diabetes mellitus, hypertensive disorders, rupture of membranes, fetal growth restriction, or fetal anomalies. Isolated oligohydramnios and polyhydramnios have not been conclusively linked to increased risk for fetal death; nevertheless, evaluation of amniotic fluid volume as a marker of long-term fetal health status is a mainstay of antepartum fetal evaluation.[2,45]

Fetal Growth Restriction

IUGR is a well-known risk factor for perinatal death that has historically been underrecognized before fetal death. Placental dysfunction is commonly implicated in nonmalformed and chromosomally normal IUGR fetuses. This topic is reviewed in further detail in Chapter 33.

Postterm Pregnancy

The definition of *postterm pregnancy* has been reevaluated in the past decade based on reappraisal of the peak time of fetal risk in relation to the 40-week mark (see Chapter 36). The pathophysiology of increased fetal death risk in the postterm pregnancy is thought to be mediated by impaired placental oxygen exchange and is often associated with oligohydramnios. Traditionally oligohydramnios has been used as a marker for increased risk in the postterm pregnancy for which intervention in the form of delivery is thought to be necessary, although as described previously, whether oligohydramnios is independently associated with fetal death in pregnancies after 40 weeks' gestation is unproven.[46]

Fetal Malformations

Pregnancies complicated by major fetal anomalies are at increased risk of stillbirth, independent of coexisting fetal growth restriction, as demonstrated recently in a large retrospective cohort study.[47] The overall stillbirth rate among fetuses with a major anomaly was 55 per 1000 compared with 4 per 1000 in non-anomalous fetuses with an adjusted odds ratio of 15. The rate of stillbirth was highest in fetuses with congenital cardiac defects. The authors caution that in this group of at-risk fetuses in particular, "health care practitioners caring for these patients should weigh the competing risks of postnatal mortality with antenatal death."

Conclusions

The best use of available antenatal testing modalities may vary according to the risk profile of each individual pregnancy. Discussion of condition to specific testing will be undertaken after review of the individual testing modalities described later.

POTENTIAL UTILITY OF ANTEPARTUM FETAL TESTING

Can antepartum fetal deaths and injury be prevented? Before using antepartum fetal testing, the obstetrician must ask several important questions:

1. Does the test provide information not already known by the patient's clinical status?
2. Can the information be helpful in managing the patient?
3. If an abnormality is detected, is a treatment available for the problem?
4. Could an abnormal test result lead to increased risk for the mother or fetus?
5. Will the test ultimately decrease perinatal morbidity and mortality?

A large body of clinical and research experience suggests that antepartum fetal assessment can have a significant impact on the frequency and causes of antenatal fetal deaths.[1] However, according to several reviews of the benefits and costs of antenatal testing, "strong evidence for the efficacy of antepartum testing is lacking."[48] **Unfortunately, few of the antepartum tests commonly used in clinical practice today have been subjected to large-scale prospective and randomized evaluations that can speak to the true efficacy of testing.**[32,49] In most cases, the test has been applied and good perinatal outcomes have been observed; therefore the test has gained further acceptance and has been used more widely. In such cases, it is uncertain whether the information provided by the test has accurately led to the improved outcomes or the total program of care has made the difference. When prospective randomized investigations are conducted, large numbers of patients must be studied because many adverse outcomes, such as intrauterine death, are uncommon even in high-risk populations. For example, although several controlled trials have failed to demonstrate improved outcomes with nonstress testing, the study populations ranged from only 300 to 530 subjects.

To determine the clinical application of antepartum diagnostic testing, the predictive value of the tests must be considered. The *sensitivity* of the test is the probability that the test will be positive or abnormal when the disease is present; the *specificity* of the test is the probability that the test result will be negative when the disease is *not* present. Note that the sensitivity and specificity refer not to the actual numbers of patients with a positive or abnormal result but to the proportion or probability of these test results. The predictive value of an abnormal test would be that fraction of patients with an abnormal test result who have the abnormal condition, and the predictive value of a normal test would be the fraction of patients with a normal test result who are normal.

Antepartum fetal tests may be used to screen a large obstetric population to detect fetal disease. In this setting, a test of high sensitivity is preferable to minimize the risk of missing a patient whose fetus might be compromised. It would be prudent to be willing to overdiagnose the problem—that is, to accept some false-positive diagnoses. In further evaluating the patient whose fetus may be at risk, and when attempting to confirm the presence of disease, a test of high specificity is preferable. It is best not to intervene unnecessarily and deliver a fetus that was doing well. In this setting, multiple tests may be helpful. When multiple test results are normal, they tend to exclude disease; however, when all are abnormal, they tend to support the diagnosis of fetal disease.

The prevalence of the abnormal condition has great impact on the predictive value of antenatal fetal tests and the number needed to evaluate with testing and to treat with interventions (delivery) to presumably prevent fetal death. The impact of these parameters on the utility of testing was illustrated in a decision analysis of the risks and benefits of antepartum testing late in pregnancy for women 35 years or older using the McGill Obstetric/Neonatal Database (MOND) to obtain risk estimates.[50] In this model, as in practice, the relative benefit of antenatal testing lies in the balance of the number of fetal deaths prevented with the number and type of interventions required to prevent them. At an estimated risk for unexplained fetal death of 5.2 per 1000 pregnancies (nulliparas ≥35 years of age in the McGill cohort), 863 additional antenatal tests, 71 additional inductions of labor, and 14 additional cesarean deliveries would be required to prevent one additional fetal death using this model. Comparatively, using the same model at an estimated risk of 1 to 2 per 1000 pregnancies, 2862 additional antenatal tests, 233 additional inductions, and 44 additional cesarean deliveries would be required to prevent one additional fetal death. Thus **the number needed to evaluate and treat to prevent one fetal death decreases as risk for fetal death increases in the population being tested.**

In interpreting the results of studies of antepartum testing, the obstetrician must consider the application of that test to

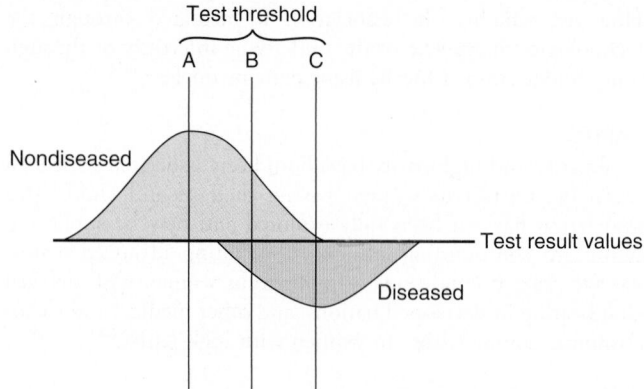

FIG 11-7 Hypothetical distribution of test results in a normal and diseased population demonstrating the differences in test sensitivity and specificity with a change in test threshold. Making it more difficult for the fetus to pass the test by raising the test threshold (*A*) will increase the sensitivity but decrease the specificity of the test. On the other hand, making the test easier to pass by decreasing the test threshold (*C*) will increase the specificity of the test but decrease the sensitivity. (Modified from Carpenter M, Coustan D. Criteria for screening tests for gestational diabetes. *Am J Obstet Gynecol.* 1982;144:768.)

his or her own population. If the study has been done in a population of patients at great risk, it is more likely that an abnormal test will be associated with an abnormal fetus. If the obstetrician is practicing in a community with patients who are, in general, at low risk, an abnormal test result will more likely be associated with a false-positive diagnosis.

For most antepartum diagnostic tests, a cutoff point used to define an abnormal result must be arbitrarily established. The cutoff point is selected to maximize the separation between the normal and diseased populations (Fig. 11-7). Changing the cutoff will have a great impact on the predictive value of the test. For example, suppose that 10 accelerations in 10 minutes were required for a fetus to have a reactive nonstress test (NST; threshold A). The fetus that fulfilled this rigid definition would almost certainly be in good condition. However, many fetuses that failed to achieve 10 accelerations in 10 minutes would also be in good condition but would be judged to be abnormal using this cutoff. In this instance, the test would have many abnormal results; it would be highly sensitive and capture all of the abnormal fetuses, but it would have a low specificity. If the number of accelerations required to pass an NST were lowered to one in 10 min, it would decrease the sensitivity of the test (threshold C). That is, the clinician might miss a truly sick fetus. At the same time, however, the specificity of the test or its ability to predict that percentage of patients who are normal would improve. Using the criterion of two accelerations of the fetal heart rate in 20 min for a reactive NST (threshold B), it is hoped that the test will have both high sensitivity and high specificity.

WHAT DO THESE TESTS TELL US ABOUT THE FETUS?

Fetal State

To be able to diagnose suspected fetal compromise using tests of fetal biophysical state, blood flow, and heart rate, we must be able to appreciate how these parameters appear under normal conditions and in response to suboptimal conditions.

Regarding fetal biophysical characteristics, it must be appreciated that during the third trimester, the normal fetus can exhibit marked changes in its neurologic state.[51] Four fetal states have been identified. The near-term fetus spends about 25% of its time in a *quiet sleep state* (state 1F) and 60% to 70% in an *active sleep state* (state 2F). Active sleep is associated with rapid eye movement (REM). In fetal lambs, electrocortical activity during REM sleep is characterized by low-voltage, high-frequency waves. The fetus exhibits regular breathing movements and intermittent abrupt movements of its head, limbs, and trunk. The fetal heart rate in active sleep (state 2F) exhibits increased variability and frequent accelerations with movement. During quiet, or non-REM, sleep, the fetal heart rate slows, and heart rate variability is reduced. The fetus may make infrequent breathing and startled movements. Electrocortical activity recordings at this time reveal high-voltage, low-frequency waves. Near term, periods of quiet sleep may last 20 minutes, and those of active sleep, about 40 minutes.[51] The mechanisms that control these periods of rest and activity in the fetus are not well established. External factors such as the mother's activity, her ingestion of drugs, and her nutrition may play a role. Specific factors that may decrease fetal movement in the third trimester include fetal anomalies, particularly central nervous system (CNS) anomalies; maternal exposures, including corticosteroids, sedatives, smoking, and anxiety; low amniotic fluid volume; and decreased placental blood flow due to placental insufficiency.[52]

When evaluating fetal condition using the NST or the biophysical profile (BPP), the clinician must consider whether a fetus who is not making breathing movements or showing accelerations of its baseline heart rate is in a quiet sleep state or is neurologically compromised. In such circumstances, prolonging the period of evaluation usually allows a change in fetal state, and more normal parameters of fetal well-being will appear.

Regarding regulation of fetal heart rate and blood flow, **fetal adaptation to hypoxemia is mediated through changes in heart rate and redistribution of cardiac output.** However, changes in fetal cardiac output are generally observed during hypoxemia only with coexisting acidemia. In response to sudden hypoxemia, fetal heart rate slowing and increased variability can be observed initially through vagally mediated chemoreceptor responses. With prolonged hypoxemia (30-60 min), increasing levels of circulating adrenergic agonists and modulation of vagal activity by endogenous opiates lead to a fetal heart rate return to or rise from the previous baseline.[53] Development of acidemia on top of hypoxemia can accelerate the rate of fetal deterioration and amplify the hypoxemia by a shift of the oxyhemoglobin dissociation curve to the right, which further reduces the oxygen-carrying capacity of fetal blood and eventually leads to a redistribution of cardiac output that can be appreciated as a "brain-sparing" effect in the evaluation of fetal blood flow. Redistribution of blood flow in the compromised fetus preferentially preserves perfusion not only to the brain but also to the heart and adrenal glands.[53]

Fetal movement is a more indirect indicator of fetal oxygen status and CNS function, and decreased fetal movement is noted in response to hypoxemia.[2] However, gestational development of fetal movement must be considered when evaluating fetal well-being as marked by fetal activity. Periods of absent fetal movement become more prolonged as gestation advances, and normal fetuses progressively exhibit longer periods of quiescence as the late second and third trimesters advance. Up to and perhaps longer than 40 minutes of fetal inactivity at 40 weeks

may be a normal finding, compared with less than 10 minutes at 20 weeks and less than 20 minutes at 32 weeks.[53] Keeping these trends in mind, an abnormal degree or absence of fetal movement can be an appropriate marker for fetal hypoxemia. However, fetal activity levels have been seen in animal studies to adapt to inducement of hypoxemia with a resumption of fetal breathing and body movements after a prolonged period of hypoxemia, especially if induced gradually. Therefore observation of these fetal states during antenatal testing does not guarantee a normoxic fetus.

BIOPHYSICAL TECHNIQUES OF FETAL EVALUATION

Descriptions of the predictive value of several commonly performed antenatal tests of fetal well-being are presented in Table 11-2, and details on each methodology are given in the sections that follow.

Maternal Assessment of Fetal Activity

Studies performed using real-time ultrasonography have demonstrated that during the third trimester, the human fetus spends 10% of its time making gross fetal body movements and that 30 such movements are made each hour.[54] Periods of active fetal body movement last about 40 minutes, whereas quiet periods last about 20 minutes. Patrick and colleagues[54] noted that the longest period without fetal movements in a normal fetus was about 75 minutes. The mother is able to perceive about 70% to 80% of gross fetal movements. The fetus does make fine body movements such as limb flexion and extension, hand grasping, and sucking; these probably reflect more coordinated CNS function, although the mother is generally unable to perceive these fine movements. Fetal movement appears to peak between 9:00 PM and 1:00 AM, a time when maternal glucose levels are falling.[51,54] In a study in which maternal glucose levels were carefully controlled with an artificial pancreas, Holden and coworkers found that hypoglycemia was associated with increased fetal movement. Fetal activity does not increase after meals or after maternal glucose administration,[55] but it may increase during exposure to music, as was demonstrated in one novel randomized trial.[56]

The decrease in fetal movement with hypoxemia makes maternal assessment of fetal activity a potentially simple and widely applicable method of monitoring fetal well-being. However, prospective trials of this method for prevention of perinatal mortality have failed to conclusively show benefit.[2] Neldam demonstrated a 73% reduction in avoidable fetal deaths in a prospective trial of more than 1500 women instructed to count fetal movements. In contrast, a subsequent international

TABLE 11-2	COMPARISON OF SELECTED ANTENATAL TESTS	
TEST	**FALSE-NEGATIVE RATE (%)**	**FALSE-POSITIVE RATE (%)**
Contraction stress test	0.04	35-65
Nonstress test	0.2-0.8	55-90
Biophysical profile	0.07-0.08	40-50
Modified biophysical profile	0.08	60

Modified from Signore C, Freeman RK, Spong CY. Antenatal testing: a reevaluation. Executive Summary of a Eunice Kennedy Shriver National Institute of Child Health and Human Development Workshop. *Obstet Gynecol*. 2009;113:687-701.

trial[57] of more than 68,000 women randomized to routine fetal movement assessment versus no formal assessment of fetal activity failed to show a significant reduction in fetal deaths in the group randomized to routine movement counting. Significant differences were noted in the method of fetal movement counting (FMC), the definition of "abnormal" fetal movements, patient compliance with the intervention, and provider response to patients who presented to care as a result of an abnormal fetal movement count in the latter, compared with the former, trial and throughout the literature on this topic. This illustrates the difficulties in validating and reproducing the results of these trials and the uncertain clinical benefit that may be derived from introducing maternal assessment of fetal movement into routine clinical practice. A 2007 Cochrane review[58] of four trials that involved more than 71,000 women concluded that evidence is insufficient to recommend routine FMC to prevent fetal death.

Despite these results, this type of fetal assessment may offer some advantages. Although the range in fetal activity will be wide but normal, with FMC, each mother and her fetus serve as his or her own control.[18] Factors that affect maternal perception of fetal movement are not well understood. Fetal and placental factors that may contribute include placental location, the length and type of fetal movements, and amniotic fluid volume (AFV), although whether AFV affects maternal perception or actual fetal movement is unclear.[52] Maternal factors that may influence the evaluation of fetal movement include maternal activity, parity, obesity, medications, and psychological factors, including anxiety. Studies of these associations have demonstrated conflicting results.[52] **About 80% of all mothers are able to comply with a program of counting fetal activity.**[18]

Several methods have been used to monitor fetal activity in research and clinical practice. These methods include FMC over a prescribed time period, such as 30 to 60 minutes one to three times daily, or conversely a target number of fetal movements to be counted over a variable time range. A variety of "normal" and "abnormal" FMC results or thresholds have been proposed, to which the patient should be instructed to respond by presenting for further evaluation of the condition of the fetus (Fig. 11-8). These potential triggers for further evaluation include fewer than three movements in 1 hour or no movements for 12 hours, Sadovsky's "movement alarm signal"; fewer than three movements an hour for 2 consecutive days; or inability to count 10 movements in a 12-hour period, the Cardiff "count-to-10" method advocated by Pearson and Weaver. The count-to-10 method has received wide scrutiny and is used perhaps most frequently in clinical practice. The use of this technique as a screening tool has most recently been reexamined by Froen and associates.[59] In a cohort of 1200 women instructed to start their fetal movement count at the first convenient time of the day,

they found that the mean time to count to 10 was less than 10 minutes, compared with significantly longer and more variable average times reported in previous investigations. Noting the variation in defining normal and abnormal patterns and maternal perception of fetal movement as mentioned previously, Froen and associates concluded that significant research is needed to better define the changes in fetal activity patterns and perception associated with good and adverse perinatal outcomes.

Potential negative impacts of maternal assessment of fetal activity include maternal anxiety and a potential increase in utility of other testing modalities and antepartum admissions.[60] However, given the likely low impact of false-positive FMC results, and the fact that this has been the only form of antenatal testing to be compared with no testing and found to have a favorable impact on fetal death, it seems reasonable to continue to prescribe some form of maternal assessment of fetal movement to patients until more conclusive evidence can be generated. As stated by Froen and associates[59] in a 2008 review, "The fact that FMC versus no counting seems to be beneficial irrespective of the chosen definition of decreased fetal movement (DFM) would support the hypothesis that benefit was derived from increased maternal vigilance regarding FM. When awareness, vigilance, and fetal movement counting is to be promoted, we have suggested that a maternal perception of significant and sustained reduction in fetal activity should remain the main definition of DFM. Any alarm limits, as '10 FM in 2 hours,' should only be for guidance as a 'rule of thumb.'"

Contraction Stress Test

The *contraction stress test* (CST), also known as the *oxytocin challenge test* (OCT), was the first biophysical technique widely applied for antepartum fetal surveillance. It was well known that uterine contractions produced a reduction in blood flow to the intervillous space. Analyses of intrapartum fetal heart rate monitoring had shown that a fetus with inadequate placental respiratory reserve would demonstrate recurrent late decelerations in response to hypoxia, in particular a fetal arterial oxygen pressure below 20 mm Hg (see Chapter 15). As noted earlier, this drop in fetal heart rate in response to transient hypoxia is mediated by a vagal response to transient systemic fetal vascular reactivity provoked by hypoxia. The CST extended these observations to the antepartum period. The response of the fetus at risk for uteroplacental insufficiency to uterine contractions formed the basis for this test.

To perform the CST, the patient is placed in the semi-Fowler position at a 30- to 45-degree angle with a slight left tilt to avoid the supine hypotensive syndrome. Continuous external fetal heart rate and uterine contraction monitoring is recorded, and a baseline is obtained before stimulating uterine activity. Maternal blood pressure is determined every 5 to 10 minutes to detect maternal hypotension. In some cases, adequate uterine activity occurs spontaneously, and additional uterine stimulation is unnecessary. An adequate CST requires uterine contractions of moderate intensity that last about 40 to 60 seconds with a frequency of three in 10 minutes. These criteria were selected to approximate the stress experienced by the fetus during the first stage of labor. If uterine activity is absent or inadequate, intravenous oxytocin is begun to initiate contractions, and it is increased until adequate uterine contractions have been achieved.[32] Several methods of nipple stimulation have been used to induce adequate uterine activity, and the success rate at achieving adequate contractions and test results is comparable

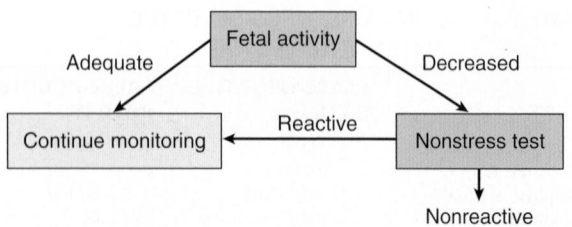

FIG 11-8 Maternal assessment of fetal activity is a valuable screening test for fetal condition. Should the mother report decreased fetal activity, a nonstress test is performed. In this situation, most nonstress tests are reactive.

to that of oxytocin infusion.[32,42] After the CST has been completed, the patient should be observed until uterine activity has returned to its baseline level. Contraindications to the test include a high risk for premature labor, such as in patients with PROM, multiple gestations, and cervical incompetence, although the CST has not been associated with an increased incidence of premature labor.[61] The CST should also be avoided in conditions in which uterine contractions may be dangerous, such as placenta previa and a previous classic cesarean delivery or uterine surgery.

Most clinicians use the definitions proposed by Braly and Freeman and colleagues[61,62] to interpret the CST (detail in Table 11-3):

Negative: No late or significant variable decelerations
Positive: Late decelerations with at least 50% of contractions
Suspicious: Intermittent late or variable decelerations
Hyperstimulation: Decelerations with contractions longer than 90 seconds' duration or a greater than 2-minute frequency
Unsatisfactory: Fewer than three contractions per 10 minutes or an uninterpretable tracing

Predictive Value of the Contraction Stress Test

A negative CST has been consistently associated with good fetal outcome. Studies have shown the incidence of perinatal death within 1 week of a negative CST (i.e., the false-negative rate) to be less than 1 per 1000.[2,42,63,64] Many of these deaths, however, can be attributed to cord accidents, malformations, placental abruption, and acute deterioration of glucose control in patients with diabetes. Thus **the CST, like most methods of antepartum fetal surveillance, cannot predict acute fetal compromise.** If the CST is negative and reactive, a repeat study is usually scheduled in 1 week (Fig. 11-9). A negative but nonreactive CST is not suggestive of acute fetal compromise but cannot be seen as constituting the same low false-negative rate over the course of 1 week as a negative reactive CST. A negative nonreactive CST is usually repeated in 24 hours (Fig. 11-10). Changes in the patient's clinical condition may warrant more frequent studies. A positive CST has been associated with an increased incidence of intrauterine death, late decelerations in labor, low 5-minute Apgar scores, IUGR, and meconium-stained amniotic fluid (Fig. 11-11)[63] with an overall likelihood of perinatal death after a positive CST ranging from 7% to 15%.

TABLE 11-3 INTERPRETATION OF CONTRACTION STRESS TEST

FINDING	DESCRIPTION	INCIDENCE (%)
Negative	No late decelerations appear anywhere on the tracing with adequate uterine contractions (three in 10 min).	80
Positive	Late decelerations that are consistent and persistent present with the majority (>50%) of contractions without excessive uterine activity; if persistent late decelerations are seen before the frequency of contractions is adequate, the test is interpreted as positive.	3-5
Suspicious	Decelerations are late and inconsistent.	5
Hyperstimulation	Uterine contractions closer than every 2 min or lasting more than 90 sec or five uterine contractions in 10 min; if no late decelerations are seen, the test is interpreted as negative.	5
Unsatisfactory	The quality of the tracing is inadequate for interpretation or adequate uterine activity cannot be achieved.	5

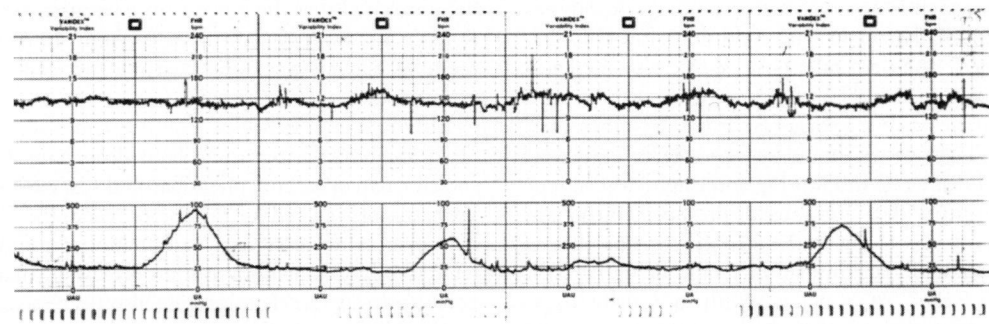

FIG 11-9 A reactive and negative contraction stress test. With this result, the test would ordinarily be repeated in 1 week.

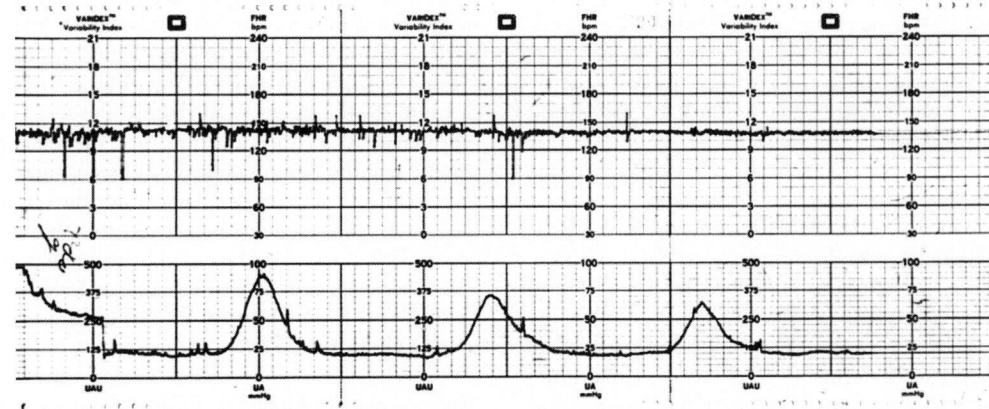

FIG 11-10 A nonreactive and negative contraction stress test. After this result, the test would ordinarily be repeated in 24 hours.

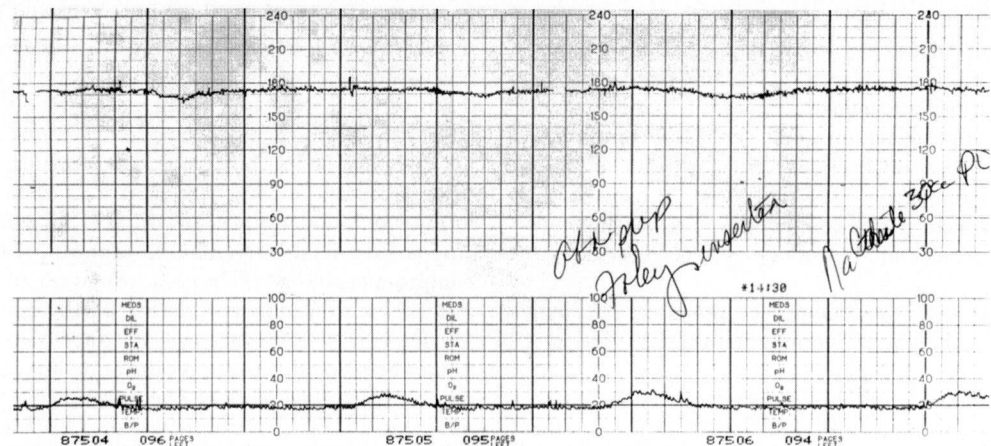

FIG 11-11 A nonreactive and positive contraction stress test with fetal tachycardia. At 34 weeks, a poorly compliant patient with type 1 diabetes mellitus reported decreased fetal activity. The nonstress test revealed a fetal tachycardia of 170 beats/min and was nonreactive. The CST was positive, and a biophysical profile score was 2. The patient's cervix was unfavorable for induction. The patient underwent a low transverse cesarean delivery of a 2200-g male infant with Apgar scores of 1 and 3. The umbilical arterial pH was 7.21.

On the other hand, the incidence of false-positive CSTs has been significant; depending on the end point used, it can be between 35% and 65%.[2,64] The positive CST is more likely to be associated with fetal compromise if the baseline heart rate lacks accelerations and the latency period between the onset of the uterine contractions and the onset of the late deceleration is less than 45 seconds.

The high incidence of false-positive CSTs is one of the greatest limitations of this test because such results could lead to unnecessary premature intervention. False-positive CSTs may be attributable to misinterpretation of the tracing; supine hypotension, which decreases uterine perfusion; uterine hyperstimulation, which is not appreciated using the tocodynamometer; or an improvement in fetal condition after the CST has been performed. The high false-positive rate also indicates that a patient with a positive CST need not necessarily require an elective cesarean delivery. If a trial of labor is to be undertaken after a positive CST, the cervix should be favorable for induction so that direct fetal heart rate monitoring and careful assessment of uterine contractility with an intrauterine pressure catheter can be performed. A suspicious or equivocal CST or one that is unsatisfactory or shows hyperstimulation should be repeated in 24 hours. In one series, 7.5% of patients with an initially suspicious CST exhibited positive tests on further evaluation, 53.7% became negative, and 38.8% remained suspicious.[65] In follow-up studies of children who demonstrated a positive CST, few have exhibited abnormalities in neurologic and psychological development.[66] A potential determinant in the long-term outcome for these children may have been the early recognition of nonreassuring fetal heart rate patterns that enabled the prevention of intrapartum compromise.

Nonstress Test

Observations made in the mid twentieth century that **accelerations of the fetal heart rate in response to fetal activity, uterine contractions, or stimulation reflect fetal well-being formed the basis for the nonstress test (NST).** The NST is the most widely applied technique for antepartum fetal evaluation despite the uncertainty regarding its reliability and reproducibility as a test of fetal assessment. The basic technology that underlies its performance and application has changed little since its introduction and wide acceptance into antenatal practice.[67]

In late gestation, the healthy fetus exhibits an average of 34 accelerations above the baseline fetal heart rate each hour.[68] These accelerations, which average 20 to 25 beats/min in amplitude and about 40 seconds in duration, require intact neurologic coupling between the fetal CNS and the fetal heart.[68] Fetal hypoxia disrupts this pathway. At term, fetal accelerations are associated with fetal movement more than 85% of the time, and more than 90% of gross movements are accompanied by accelerations. Fetal heart rate accelerations may be absent during periods of quiet fetal sleep. Studies by Patrick and associates[68] demonstrated that the longest time between successive accelerations in the healthy term fetus is about 40 minutes. However, the fetus may fail to exhibit heart rate accelerations for up to 80 minutes and still be normal.

Although an absence of fetal heart rate accelerations is most often attributable to a quiet fetal sleep state, CNS depressants such as narcotics and phenobarbital, as well as the β-blocker propranolol, can reduce heart rate reactivity. Chronic smoking is known to decrease fetal oxygenation through an increase in fetal carboxyhemoglobin and a decrease in uterine blood flow. Fetal heart rate accelerations are also decreased in smokers.

The NST is usually performed in an outpatient setting. In most cases, only 10 to 15 minutes are required to complete the test. It has virtually no contraindications, and few equivocal test results are observed. The patient may be seated in a reclining chair, with care taken to ensure that she is tilted to the left to avoid the supine hypotensive syndrome.[32] The patient's blood pressure should be recorded before the test is begun and then repeated at 5- to 10-minute intervals. The fetal heart rate is monitored using the Doppler ultrasound transducer, and the tocodynamometer is applied to detect uterine contractions or fetal movement. Fetal activity may be recorded by the patient using an event marker, or it may be noted by the staff performing the test.

Fetal Heart Rate Patterns Observable on the Nonstress Test
REACTIVE
The most widely applied definition of a reactive test requires that at least two accelerations of the fetal heart rate, each with a peak

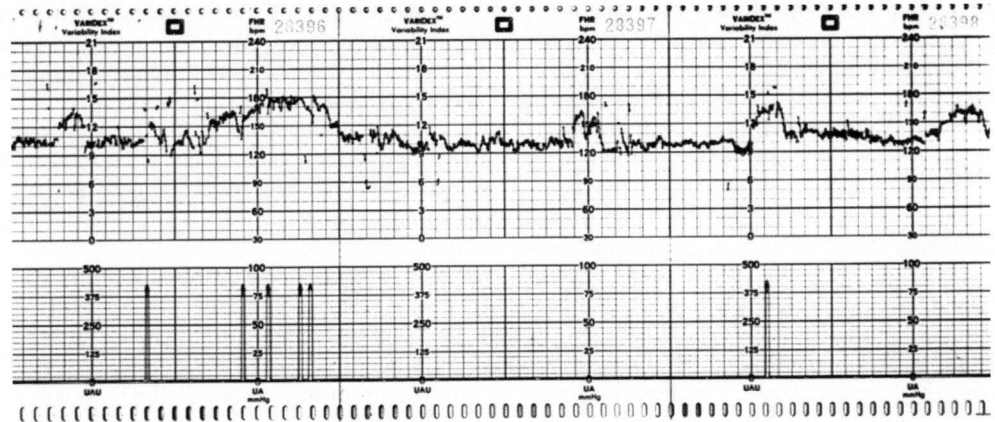

FIG 11-12 A reactive nonstress test. Accelerations of the fetal heart greater than 15 beats/min and that last longer than 15 sec can be identified. When the patient appreciates a fetal movement, she presses an event marker on the monitor, which creates arrows on the lower portion of the tracing.

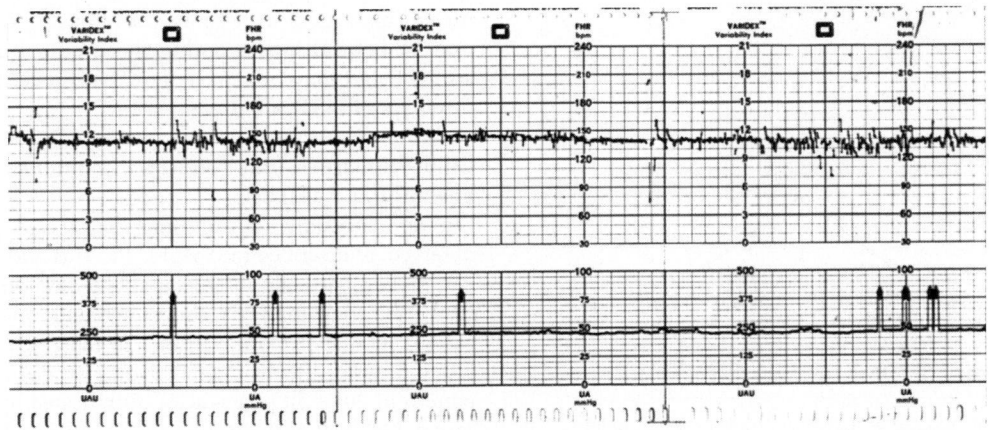

FIG 11-13 A nonreactive nonstress test. No accelerations of the fetal heart rate are observed. The patient has perceived fetal activity as indicated by the arrows in the lower portion of the tracing.

amplitude of 15 beats/min and total duration of 15 seconds, be observed in 20 minutes of monitoring (Fig. 11-12).[69] Gestational age affects reactivity criteria because sympathetic and parasympathetic influences on fetal heart rate change with advancing gestational age. Compared with the early third trimester, increased frequency and amplitude of fetal heart rate accelerations are seen after 30 weeks of gestation; although half of normal fetuses demonstrate accelerations with fetal movements at 24 weeks, nearly all fetuses will do so after 30 weeks. Similarly, before 30 to 32 weeks' gestation, acceptable criteria for a reactive fetal heart rate tracing include accelerations with a peak of only 10 beats/min amplitude and 10 seconds' duration rather than the widely applied 15-and-15 definition for reactivity described above.[69]

NONREACTIVE

If the criteria for reactivity are not met, the test is considered nonreactive (Fig. 11-13). The most common cause for a nonreactive test is a period of fetal inactivity or quiet sleep. Therefore the test may be extended for an additional 20 minutes with the expectation that the fetal state will change and reactivity will appear. Keegan and colleagues[70] noted that about 80% of tests that were nonreactive in the morning became reactive when repeated later the same day. In an effort to change the fetal state, some clinicians have manually stimulated the fetus or attempted

to increase fetal glucose levels by giving the mother orange juice. No evidence suggests that such efforts will increase fetal activity.[71,72] If the test has been extended for 40 minutes, and reactivity has not been seen, a BPP or CST should be performed. Of those fetuses that exhibit a nonreactive NST, about 25% will have a positive CST on further evaluation.[73-75] Reactivity that occurs during preparations for the CST has proved to be a reliable index of fetal well-being.

Overall, on initial testing, 85% of NSTs are reactive and 15% are nonreactive (Fig. 11-14).[73] Fewer than 1% of NSTs prove unsatisfactory because of inadequately recorded fetal heart rate data.

The likelihood of a nonreactive test is substantially increased early in the third trimester. Between 24 and 28 weeks' gestation, about 50% of NSTs are nonreactive, and 15% of NSTs remain nonreactive between 28 and 32 weeks.[76] After 32 weeks, the incidences of reactive and nonreactive tests is comparable to that seen at term. **In summary, when accelerations of the baseline heart rate are seen during monitoring in the late second and early third trimesters, the NST has been associated with fetal well-being.**

When nonreactive, the NST is extended in an attempt to distinguish the fetus in a period of prolonged quiet sleep from those who are hypoxemic or asphyxiated. **Most fetuses that exhibit a nonreactive NST are not compromised but simply**

fail to exhibit heart rate reactivity during the 40-minute period of testing. Malformed fetuses also exhibit a significantly higher incidence of nonreactive NSTs.[77] Vibroacoustic stimulation (VAS) may be used to change the fetal state from quiet to active sleep (Fig. 11-15). Auditory brainstem response appears to be functional in the fetus at 26 to 28 weeks' gestation. Thus VAS may significantly increase the incidence of reactive NSTs after 26 weeks' gestation and may reduce the testing time, making this a potentially useful adjunct to antepartum fetal testing.[76,78] Most studies of VAS have used an electronic artificial larynx that generates sound pressure levels measured at 1 meter in air of 82 dB with a frequency of 80 Hz and a harmonic of 20 to 9000 Hz. Whether it is the acoustic or vibratory component of this stimulus that alters fetal state is unclear. VAS may produce a significant increase in the mean duration and amplitude of heart rate accelerations, fetal heart rate variability, and

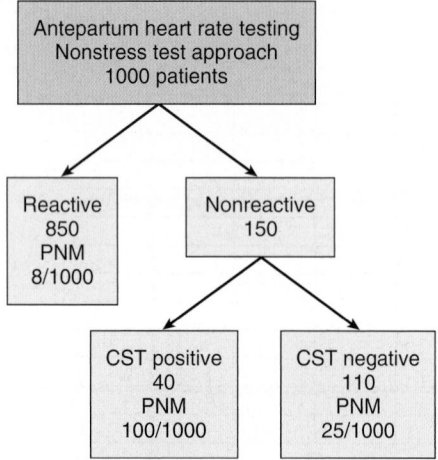

FIG 11-14 Results of nonstress testing in 1000 high-risk patients. In general, 85% of tests are reactive, and 15% are nonreactive. Of those patients with a nonreactive nonstress test (NST), about 25% have a positive contraction stress test (CST) on further evaluation. The highest perinatal mortality (PNM) is observed in patients with a nonreactive NST and a positive CST. Patients with a nonreactive NST and a negative CST have a PNM rate higher than that found in patients whose NST is initially reactive. (PNM rates are based on data from Evertson L, Gauthier R, Schifrin B, et al. Antepartum fetal heart rate testing. I. Evolution of the nonstress test. *Am J Obstet Gynecol.* 1979;133:29.)

gross fetal body movements within 3 minutes of stimulation.[79] Several studies using VAS have shown a decreased incidence of nonreactive NSTs from 13% to 14% down to 6% to 9%. A reactive NST after VAS stimulation appears to be as reliable an index of fetal well-being as spontaneous reactivity.[79] However, those fetuses that remain nonreactive even after VAS may be at increased risk for poor perinatal outcome, with increased rates of intrapartum fetal distress and growth restriction and low Apgar scores.

In most centers that use VAS, the baseline fetal heart rate is first observed for 5 minutes. If the pattern is nonreactive, a stimulus of 3 seconds or less is applied near the fetal head. If the NST remains nonreactive, the stimulus is repeated at 1-minute intervals up to three times. If the fetus still does not respond, further evaluation should be carried out with a BPP or CST. Studies have confirmed the safety of VAS use during pregnancy, and no long-term evidence of hearing loss has been found in children followed in the neonatal period and up to 4 years of age.[80] Other interventions to safely shorten NST time have been investigated, most with equivocal results.[81] **In summary, VAS may be helpful in shortening the time required to perform an NST and may be especially useful in centers where large numbers of NSTs are done.**

Other Nonstress Test Patterns or Findings
SINUSOIDAL PATTERN
On rare occasions, a sinusoidal heart rate pattern may be observed, as described in Chapter 15. This undulating heart rate pattern with virtually absent variability has been associated with fetal anemia and asphyxia, congenital malformations, and medications such as narcotics. In one of the earliest reports on the use of the NST, Rochard and coworkers[82] described a sinusoidal pattern in 20 of 50 pregnancies complicated by Rh isoimmunization. One half of these pregnancies ended in a perinatal death, and 40% of the surviving infants required prolonged hospitalization. Only 10% of the babies with a sinusoidal pattern had an uncomplicated course.

BRADYCARDIA
Before 27 weeks' gestation, the normal fetal heart rate response to fetal movement may in fact be a bradycardia. However, in settings with a high a priori risk of fetal compromise, such as

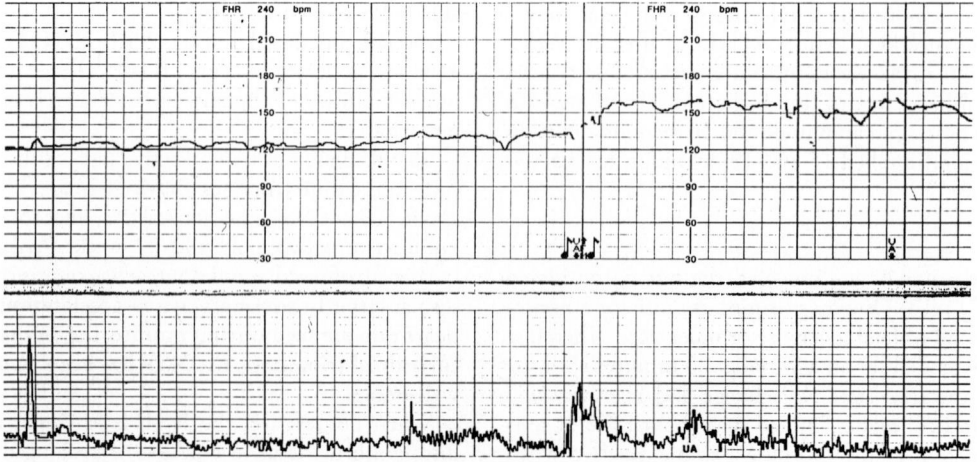

FIG 11-15 Reactive nonstress test after vibroacoustic stimulation. The stimulus was applied at the point marked by the musical notes, and a sustained fetal heart rate acceleration was produced.

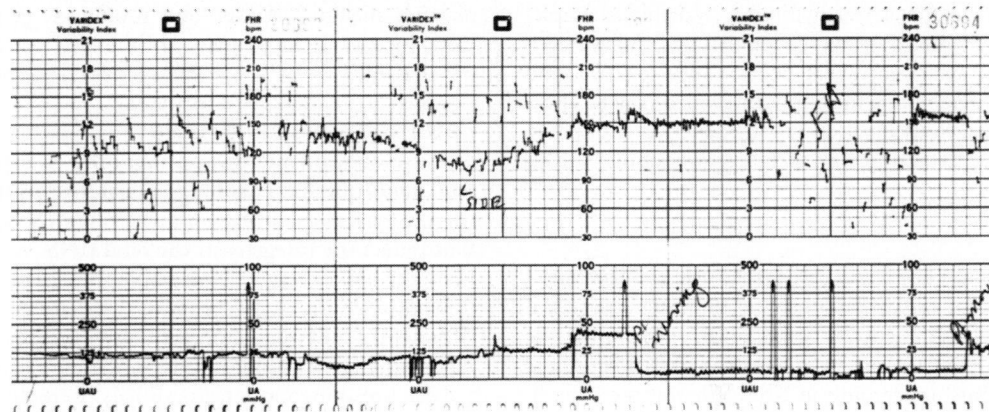

FIG 11-16 A nonstress test in this primigravid patient of 43 weeks' gestation reveals a spontaneous bradycardia. The fetal heart rate has fallen from a baseline of 150-100 beats/min. Upon induction of labor, the patient required cesarean delivery for fetal distress associated with severe variable decelerations. The amniotic fluid was decreased in amount and was meconium stained.

IUGR associated with antiphospholipid syndrome, bradycardia at a gestational age of 26 to 28 weeks may be a predictor of impending fetal death. In these challenging cases, the entire clinical situation needs to be evaluated and discussed in full with the parents; this should include a neonatology consultation, initiated before intervention and delivery of a very preterm fetus exhibiting fetal heart rate decelerations.

Significant fetal heart rate bradycardias have been observed in 1% to 2% of all NSTs, defined as a fetal heart rate of 90 beats/min or a fall in the fetal heart rate of 40 beats/min below the baseline for 2 minutes or longer (Fig. 11-16). In a review of 121 cases, bradycardia was associated with increased perinatal morbidity and mortality, particularly antepartum fetal death, cord compression, IUGR, and fetal malformations.[83] Although about one half of the NSTs associated with bradycardia were reactive, the incidence of a nonreassuring fetal heart rate pattern in labor that led to emergency delivery in this group was identical to that of patients who exhibited nonreactive NSTs. Clinical management decisions should be based on the finding of bradycardia *not* on the presence or absence of reactivity. Bradycardia has a higher positive predictive value for fetal compromise (fetal death or fetal intolerance of labor) than does the nonreactive NST. In this setting, antepartum fetal death is most likely due to a cord accident.

If a bradycardia is observed, an ultrasound examination should be performed to assess amniotic fluid volume and to detect the presence of anomalies. Expectant management in the setting of a bradycardia has been associated with a PMR of 25%. Therefore several reports have recommended that delivery be undertaken if the fetus is mature. When the fetus is premature, the physician might elect to administer corticosteroids to accelerate fetal lung maturation before delivery. Continuous fetal heart rate monitoring is necessary if expectant management is followed.

TACHYCARDIA

The fetal heart rate baseline evaluation must also take gestational age into account, as with fetal heart rate reactivity. Vagal activity has a greater influence on fetal heart rate at baseline as gestation advances; thus baseline fetal heart rate will decrease from an average of 155 beats/min at 20 weeks to 145 beats/min at 30 weeks. **The most common etiology of fetal tachycardia is maternal-fetal fever secondary to maternal-fetal infection**

such as chorioamnionitis. Other causes include chronic hypoxemia, maternal hyperthyroidism, and fetal tachyarrhythmia. Fetal heart rates above 200 beats/min, and certainly above 220 beats/min, should increase the index of suspicion of fetal tachyarrhythmia and lead to further fetal cardiac evaluation with a targeted fetal echocardiogram. For fetal heart rates between 160 and 180 beats/min, the presence or absence of baseline variability is an important indicator of fetal acid-base status. Fetal acidosis is more likely if baseline variability is absent.[69]

ARRHYTHMIA

Among fetal arrhythmias, most (approximately 90%) are tachyarrhythmias. Fetal tachyarrhythmia is most often diagnosed when the fetal ventricular heart rate is faster than 180 beats/min. Common causes of fetal tachyarrhythmias are paroxysmal supraventricular tachycardia and atrial flutter. The administration of antiarrhythmic therapy to the pregnant mothers of fetuses with sustained supraventricular tachycardia represented the first examples of successful prenatal cardiac therapy. Multiple publications describe treatment protocols for this arrhythmia. Characteristics of fetuses who may need treatment include hydrops fetalis in the face of a sustained arrhythmia and a gestational age too early to preclude safe delivery and postnatal treatment. In such cases, therapy is best initiated with medications that have a relatively broad therapeutic margin and a low risk for proarrhythmia (unwanted precipitation or exacerbation of the arrhythmia) for the fetus and the mother. Digoxin is the most commonly used first-line agent but is rarely effective in the presence of fetal hydrops, for which sotalol or flecainide are typical first-line choices.[84]

Fetal bradyarrhythmia is diagnosed when the fetal ventricular heart rate is slower than 100 beats/min, mainly because of atrioventricular block. About half of all cases are caused by fetal cardiac anomalies, and of the remaining cases with normal cardiac structure, many are related to maternal antibodies. These antibodies, which include SS-A and SS-B, may directly target the fetal atrioventricular node or the myocardium, resulting in heart block and myocarditis. Fetuses with bradyarrhythmia may develop hydrops fetalis, particularly with sustained bradycardia at a rate less than 55 beats/min. In utero heart failure with congenital heart block, with or without congenital heart disease, represents an indication for electrical pacemaker therapy in surviving neonates. This condition is less often successfully treated antenatally than fetal tachyarrhythmia. Available therapies include maternal administration of β-agonists, which have been shown to increase fetal ventricular rate by 10% to 20%, and steroid or immunoglobulin administration, which may be effective in cases of fetal heart block caused by maternal antibodies. Potential improved fetal outcome includes reversal of hydrops in several reports.[84]

DECELERATION

In most cases, mild variable decelerations are not associated with poor perinatal outcome. Meis and associates[85] reported that variable decelerations of 20 beats/min or more below the baseline heart rate but lasting less than 10 seconds were noted in 50.7% of patients undergoing an NST. Whereas these decelerations were more often associated with a nuchal cord, they were not predictive of IUGR, a nonreassuring fetal heart rate pattern, or more severe variable decelerations during labor. When mild variable decelerations are observed, even if the NST is reactive, an ultrasound examination should be performed to rule out oligohydramnios. A low amniotic fluid index (AFI) and mild variable decelerations increase the likelihood of a cord accident. If late decelerations in response to contractions are observed in the performance of an NST, criteria for interpretation of a CST should then be used.

Predictive Value of the Nonstress Test

The NST is most predictive when it is normal or reactive. The reported false-negative rate over multiple studies ranges from 0.2% to 0.8%, which corresponds to a fetal death rate of 3 to 8 per 1000 within 1 week of a reactive NST. The false-positive rate is considerably higher and ranges from 50% to more than 90% in various studies.[2,42]

A 2012 Cochrane review[67] integrated the results of six randomized controlled trials that included 2105 women; four studies with 1636 women compared nonstress testing (or NST with results revealed) to no NST (or NST with results concealed), and two studies with 469 women compared NST with computerized analysis to traditional (visually analyzed) NST. The six included studies only recruited high-risk women, and none provided information about singleton and multiple pregnancies. Of note, all four of the studies that compared NST with no NST were performed in the 1980s. In the studies that compared NST with no NST, no significant differences were identified in the risk for perinatal mortality (risk ratio [RR], 2.05; 95% confidence interval [CI], 0.95-4.42; 2.3% vs. 1.1%). In addition, no differences were identified in rates of cesarean delivery, "potentially preventable perinatal mortality," Apgar scores, neonatal intensive care unit (NICU) admissions, gestational age at birth, or neonatal seizures. However, in the two studies that compared computerized analysis to visual analysis, a significant reduction was seen in perinatal mortality with computerized analysis (RR, 0.20; 95% CI, 0.04-0.88; 0.9% vs. 4.2%).[67] The authors concluded that the analysis was underpowered to detect possible important differences in perinatal mortality and pointed out that many aspects of antenatal and postnatal care may have changed since the included trials were performed. They called for new studies to assess the effects of the traditional and computer-analyzed NST in order to assess the true impact on perinatal mortality and other outcomes.

In selected high-risk pregnancies, the false-negative rate associated with a weekly NST may be unacceptably high, especially in those pregnancies complicated by pregestational

diabetes mellitus, IUGR, and prolonged gestation. In these cases, increasing the frequency of the NST to twice weekly may be advisable.[86,87]

Fetal Biophysical Profile

The use of real-time ultrasonography to assess antepartum fetal condition has enabled the obstetrician to perform an in utero physical examination and evaluate dynamic functions that reflect the integrity of the fetal CNS.[88] As emphasized by Manning and colleagues,[89] "fetal biophysical scoring rests on the principle that the more complete the examination of the fetus, its activities, and its environment, the more accurate may be the differentiation of fetal health from disease states."

Fetal breathing movements (FBMs) were the first biophysical parameter to be assessed using real-time ultrasonography. It is thought that the fetus exercises its breathing muscles in utero in preparation for postdelivery respiratory function. With real-time ultrasonography, FBM is evidenced by downward movement of the diaphragm and abdominal contents and by an inward collapsing of the chest. FBMs become regular at 20 to 21 weeks and are controlled by centers on the ventral surface of the fourth ventricle of the fetus.[90] They are observed about 30% of the time, are seen more often during REM sleep, and demonstrate intact neurologic control when present. Although the absence of FBMs may reflect fetal asphyxia, this finding may also indicate that the fetus is in a period of quiet sleep.[51] Several factors other than fetal state and hypoxia can influence the presence of FBM. As maternal glucose levels rise, FBM becomes more frequent, and during periods of maternal hypoglycemia, FBM decreases. Maternal smoking reduces FBM, probably as a result of fetal hypoxemia. Narcotics that depress the fetal CNS also decrease FBM.

Regarding other observable fetal states as markers of fetal oxygen status and well-being, Vintzileos and coworkers[90] stressed that **fetal biophysical activities that are present earliest in fetal development are the last to disappear with fetal hypoxia.** The fetal tone center in the cortex begins to function at 7.5 to 8.5 weeks, therefore fetal tone would be the last fetal parameter to be lost with worsening fetal condition. The fetal movement center in the cortex nuclei is functional at 9 weeks and would be more sensitive than fetal tone. As noted earlier, FBM becomes regular at 20 to 21 weeks. Finally, fetal heart rate control, which resides within the posterior hypothalamus and medulla, becomes functional at the end of the second trimester and early in the third trimester. An alteration in fetal heart rate would theoretically be the earliest sign of fetal compromise.

Using these principles, Manning and colleagues[91] developed the concept of the fetal BPP score. These researchers elected to combine the NST with four parameters that could be assessed using real-time ultrasonography: FBM, fetal movement, fetal tone, and amniotic fluid volume (AFV). FBM, fetal movement, and fetal tone are mediated by complex neurologic pathways and should reflect the function of the fetal CNS at the time of the examination. On the other hand, AFV should provide information about the presence of chronic fetal asphyxia. Finally, the ultrasound examination performed for the BPP has the added advantage of detecting previously unrecognized major fetal anomalies. A BPP score was developed that is similar to the Apgar score used to assess the condition of the newborn.[91] The presence of a normal parameter, such as a reactive NST, was awarded 2 points, whereas the absence of that parameter was scored as 0. The highest score a fetus can receive is 10, and the

TABLE 11-4   CRITERIA OF BIOPHYSICAL PROFILE SCORING

BIOPHYSICAL VARIABLE (SCORE = 0)	NORMAL (SCORE = 2)	ABNORMAL
Fetal breathing movements	At least one episode of ≥30 sec duration in 30-min observation	Absent or no episode of ≥30 sec duration in 30 min
Gross body/limb movement	At least three discrete body/limb movements in 30 min (episodes of active continuous movement considered a single movement)	Up to two episodes of movements in 30 min
Fetal tone	At least one episode of active extension with return-flexion of fetal limb or trunk, with opening and closing of the hand considered to reflect normal tone	Either slow extension with return-partial flexion, movement of limb in full extension, or absent fetal movement
Reactive fetal heart rate	At least two episodes of acceleration of ≥15 beats/min and 15 sec duration associated with fetal movement in 20 min*	Fewer than two accelerations or acceleration <15 beats/min in 20 min
Amniotic fluid volume	At least one pocket of amniotic fluid measuring ≥2 cm in two perpendicular planes	Either no amniotic fluid pockets or a pocket <2 cm in two perpendicular planes

Modified from Manning FA. Biophysical profile scoring. In Nijhuis J (ed): *Fetal Behaviour*. New York, Oxford University Press; 1992:241.
*For gestational age >30 weeks.

TABLE 11-5   MANAGEMENT BASED ON BIOPHYSICAL PROFILE

SCORE	INTERPRETATION	MANAGEMENT
10	Normal; low risk for chronic asphyxia	Repeat testing at weekly to twice-weekly intervals.
8	Normal; low risk for chronic asphyxia	Repeat testing at weekly to twice-weekly intervals.
6	Suspect chronic asphyxia	If ≥36-37 wk gestation or <36 wk with positive testing for fetal pulmonary maturity, consider delivery; if <36 wk and/or fetal pulmonary maturity testing is negative, repeat biophysical profile in 4-6 hr; deliver if oligohydramnios is present.
4	Suspect chronic asphyxia	If ≥36 wk gestation, deliver; if <32 wk gestation, repeat score.
0-2	Strongly suspect chronic asphyxia	Extend testing time-120 min; if persistent score is 4 or less, deliver regardless of gestational age.

Modified from Manning FA, Harman CR, Morrison I, et al. Fetal assessment based on fetal biophysical profile scoring. *Am J Obstet Gynecol.* 1990;162:703; and Manning FA. Biophysical profile scoring. In Nijhuis J, ed: *Fetal behaviour*. New York, Oxford University Press; 1992:241.

lowest score is 0. The BPP may be used as early as 26 to 28 weeks' gestation. The time required for the fetus to achieve a satisfactory BPP score is closely related to fetal state, with an average of only 5 minutes if the fetus is in a 2F state but over 25 minutes if it is in a 1F state.[92]

The criteria proposed by Manning and colleagues[91] are shown in Table 11-4, and the clinical actions recommended in response to these scores are presented in Table 11-5. A low score on the BPP does not prohibit attempted vaginal delivery if other obstetric factors are favorable.

In a prospective blinded study of 216 high-risk patients, no perinatal deaths were observed when all five variables described earlier were normal, but a PMR of 60% was seen in fetuses with a score of zero.[91] Fetal deaths were increased fourteenfold with the absence of fetal movement, and the PMR was increased eighteenfold if FBM was absent. Any single test was associated with a significant false-positive rate that ranged from 50% to 79%. However, combining abnormal variables significantly decreased the false-positive rate to as low as 20%. The false-negative rate—that is, the incidence of babies who were compromised but who had normal testing—was low and ranged from a PMR of 6.9 per 1000 for infants with normal amniotic fluid volume to 12.8 per 1000 for fetuses with a reactive NST. These investigators found that in most cases, the ultrasound-derived BPP parameters and NST could be completed within a relatively short time; each requires about 10 minutes.

Manning and colleagues[93] presented their experience with 26,780 high-risk pregnancies followed with the BPP. In their protocol, a routine NST is not performed if all of the ultrasound parameters are found to be normal for a score of 8. An NST is performed when one ultrasound finding is abnormal. The corrected PMR in this series was 1.9 per 1000 with fewer than 1 fetal death per 1000 patients within 1 week of a normal profile. Of all patients tested, almost 97% had a score of 8, which means

that only 3% required further evaluation for scores of 6 or less. In a study of 525 patients with scores of 6 or less, poor perinatal outcome was most often associated with either a nonreactive NST and absent fetal tone or a nonreactive NST and absent FBM.[94] A significant inverse linear relationship was observed between the last BPP score and both perinatal morbidity and mortality (Figs. 11-17 and 11-18).[95] Depending on the end point used, the false-positive rate ranged from 75% for a score of 6 to less than 20% for a score of 0. Manning has summarized the data reported in eight investigations using the BPP for fetal evaluation. Overall, 23,780 patients and 54,337 tests were reviewed. The corrected PMR, excluding lethal anomalies, was 0.77 per 1000.

The BPP correlates well with fetal acid-base status. Vintzileos and associates[90] studied 124 patients undergoing cesarean birth *before* the onset of labor. Deliveries were undertaken for severe preeclampsia, elective repeat cesarean delivery, growth restriction, breech presentation, placenta previa, and fetal macrosomia. *Acidosis* was defined as an umbilical cord arterial pH less than 7.20. The earliest manifestations of fetal acidosis were a nonreactive NST and loss of FBM. With scores of 8 or more, the mean arterial pH was 7.28, and only 2 of 102 fetuses were acidotic. Nine fetuses with scores of 4 or less had a mean pH of 6.99, and all were acidotic.

Some studies have demonstrated that antenatal corticosteroid administration may have an effect on the BPP, decreasing the profile score. Because corticosteroids are used in cases of anticipated premature delivery (24-34 weeks), any false-positive results on biophysical testing may lead to inappropriate intervention and delivery. Kelly and coworkers reported that BPP scores were decreased in more than one third of the fetuses tested at 28 to 34 weeks' gestation. This effect was seen within 48 hours of corticosteroid administration. Neonatal outcome was not affected. Repeat BPPs within 24 to 48 hours were normal in

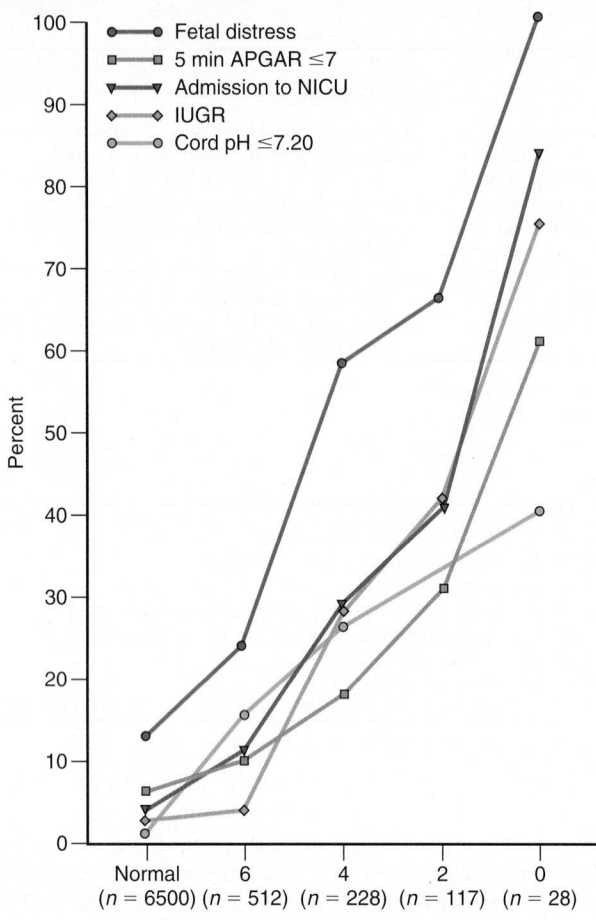

FIG 11-17 The relationship between five indexes of perinatal morbidity and last biophysical profile (BPP) score before delivery. A significant inverse linear correlation is observed for each variable. *IUGR,* intrauterine growth restriction; *NICU,* neonatal intensive care unit. (From Manning FA, Harman CR, Morrison I, et al. Fetal assessment based on fetal biophysical profile scoring. *Am J Obstet Gynecol.* 1990;162:703.)

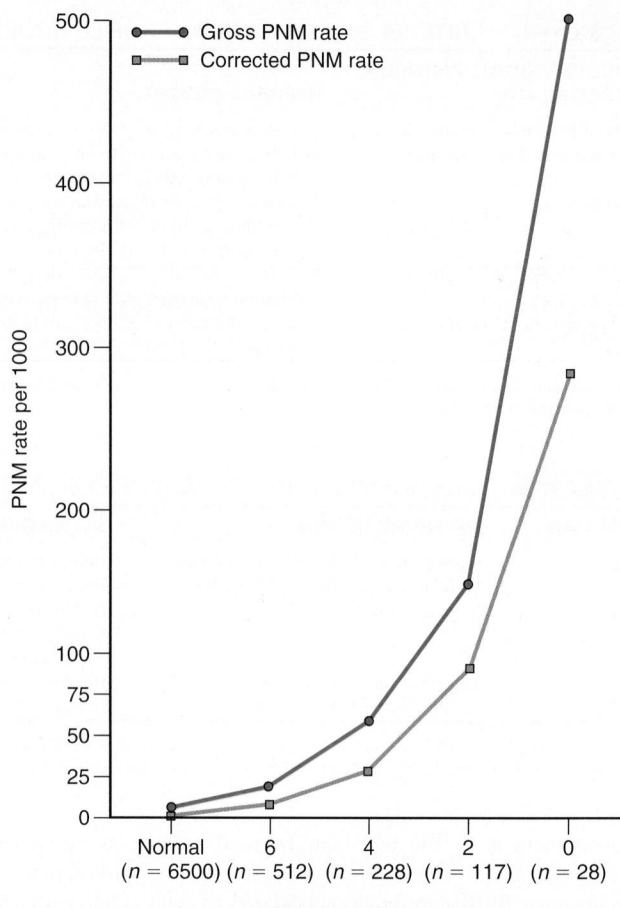

FIG 11-18 The relationship between perinatal mortality (PNM), both total and corrected for major anomalies, and the last biophysical profile (BPP) score before delivery. A highly significant inverse and exponential relationship is observed. (From Manning FA, Harman CR, Morrison I, et al. Fetal assessment based on fetal biophysical profile scoring. *Am J Obstet Gynecol.* 1990;162:703.)

cases in which the BPP score had decreased by 4 points. The most commonly affected variables were FBM and the NST. Other investigators have reported transient suppression of FBM and heart rate reactivity after corticosteroid administration at less than 34 weeks' gestation, with return of these parameters to normal by 48 to 96 hours after corticosteroid treatment. This effect must be considered at institutions where daily BPPs are used to evaluate the fetus in cases of preterm labor or preterm premature rupture of the membranes (PPROM).

Some controversy concerns the utility of the BPP in predicting chorioamnionitis in pregnancies complicated by preterm labor or PPROM. Sherer and colleagues reported that the absence of FBM is associated with histologic evidence of fetal inflammation and intrauterine infection in patients with preterm labor and intact membranes before 32 weeks' gestation. However, they recommend that this finding not be used to guide clinical management because of the low positive predictive value of absent FBM. Lewis and associates performed a randomized trial of daily NSTs versus BPP in the management of PPROM. They concluded that neither daily NSTs nor BPPs had high sensitivity in predicting infectious complications in these patients. Daily BPPs increased cost without apparent benefit.

Manning and colleagues have described the correlation between biophysical scoring and the incidence of cerebral palsy in Manitoba. In patients referred for a BPP, an inverse, exponential, and highly significant relationship was found between last BPP score and the incidence of cerebral palsy. Scores of 6 or less had a sensitivity of 49%. The more abnormal the last BPP, the greater the risk for cerebral palsy. Gestational age, birthweight, and assumed timing of the injury were not related to the incidence of cerebral palsy, which ranged from 0.7 per 1000 live births for a normal BPP score to 13.1 per 1000 live births for a score of 6 to 333 per 1000 live births for a score of 0.

Several drawbacks of the BPP should be considered. Unlike the NST and CST, an ultrasound machine is required, and unless the BPP is videotaped, it cannot be reviewed. If the fetus is in a quiet sleep state, the BPP can require a long period of observation. The present scoring system does not consider the impact of hydramnios. For example, in a pregnancy complicated by diabetes mellitus, the presence of excessive amniotic fluid may be an indicator of fetal risk.

Predictive Value of the Biophysical Profile

To summarize the results of multiple studies, the false-negative rate of a normal BPP is less than 0.1%, or less than

1 fetal death per 1000 within 1 week of a normal BPP.[2] The false-positive rate of a particular test has always been of concern because of the possibility of unnecessary intervention (usually delivery) and subsequent iatrogenic complications. The BPP was developed in part to address the issue of the high false-positive rate of the CST and the NST. Little attention has been paid to the possible false-positive rate of the abnormal or equivocal BPP. This is particularly relevant because the BPP is most commonly used as the final back-up test in the NST and CST sequence of testing and is critically important when dealing with the premature fetus. As noted earlier, the false-positive rate of a score of 0 is less than 20%, but for a score of 6, it is up to 75%. Inglis and coworkers used VAS to define fetal condition with BPP scores of 6 or less in 81 patients at 28 to 42 weeks. Obstetric and neonatal outcomes of 41 patients whose score improved to normal after VAS were compared with those of 238 patients who had normal scores without VAS. The obstetric and neonatal outcomes were not significantly different between the two groups. VAS improved the BPP in about 80% of cases. Use of VAS for an equivocal BPP did not increase the false-negative rate and may reduce the likelihood of unnecessary obstetric intervention.

A 2008 Cochrane review[96] included evaluation of 2829 women randomized to BPP versus NST. The majority were term pregnancies. No differences were found in perinatal mortality, cesarean delivery rate, Apgar scores, or admission to the NICU. As with the 2012 Cochrane review[67] of the NST mentioned earlier, this analysis was underpowered to detect a significant difference in perinatal mortality among BPP and other modalities. The authors also note that "it is regrettable that since the introduction of the BPP in the 1980s, and following reports of observational studies of tens of thousands of pregnancies, less than 3000 women have been enrolled into randomized trials."

Modified Biophysical Profile

In an attempt to simplify and reduce the time necessary to complete testing, a variety of modifications of the full BPP have been evaluated by focusing on the components of the BPP that are most predictive of perinatal outcome. The NST, an indicator of present fetal condition, may be combined with assessment of AFV (see Chapter 35), a marker of long-term status, in a modified BPP (mBPP). In this setting, a deepest vertical pocket (DVP) of amniotic fluid greater than 2 by 1 cm is usually considered normal, although different criteria have been applied. **Multiple investigations,** including a trial by Miller an colleagues of 56,617 antepartum tests in 15,482 women, **have demonstrated comparable results of the mBPP to the full BPP, namely a false-negative rate (or rate of fetal death within 1 week of a normal mBPP) of 0.8 per 1000.** Nageotte and associates[97] demonstrated that the mBPP was as good a predictor of adverse fetal outcome as a negative CST. Additional evaluation for an abnormal mBPP is required in about 10% of patients. If the NST is nonreactive despite VAS or extended monitoring, or if the AFV is abnormal, either a full BPP or CST is performed. The CST as a back-up test is associated with a higher rate of intervention for an abnormal test than the use of a complete BPP as a back-up test. Overall, the mBPP has a false-positive rate comparable to that of the NST but higher than that of the CST and full BPP. The low false-negative rate and ease of performance of the mBPP make it an excellent approach for the evaluation of large numbers of high-risk patients. As such,

although potentially still a useful test, the CST has become less frequently used in current practice.

Whether to use a full AFI for AFV assessment or an abbreviated measure, the DVP, has undergone investigation. Chauhan and colleagues performed a randomized trial of more than 1000 women and found that the AFI led to more diagnoses of oligohydramnios, a higher rate of intervention, and more iatrogenic prematurity but offered no advantage in detecting or preventing adverse outcomes. Similarly, a 2009 Cochrane review[98] of five trials that included more than 3200 women concluded that no differences were apparent in perinatal outcomes. However, the use of AFI did result in an increased rate of diagnosis of oligohydramnios and an increased rate of induction of labor compared with DVP. This review could not comment on the relative ability of AFI, compared with DVP, for prevention of perinatal death because no deaths were reported in the included trials. Based on these data, more recent endorsement of DVP as the primary fluid to assessment strategy has been proposed.[32]

Doppler Ultrasound

The advent of Doppler ultrasound has permitted noninvasive assessment of the fetal, maternal, and placental circulations. With Doppler ultrasound, we can obtain information about uteroplacental blood flow and resistance, which may be markers of fetal adaptation and reserve. **This method of fetal assessment has only been demonstrated to be of value in reducing perinatal mortality and unnecessary obstetric interventions in fetuses with suspected IUGR and possibly other disorders of uteroplacental blood flow.**[2] A detailed description of the underlying principles and use of Doppler ultrasound for fetal assessment of IUGR is available in Chapter 33. For the purposes of this chapter on antenatal fetal assessment, Doppler interrogation of fetal vascular flow and resistance can be conceptualized as a follow-up test to determine fetal reserve in cases of suspected IUGR and not as a primary method of antenatal fetal surveillance for either high- or low-risk pregnancies.

Perhaps ironically, however, Doppler ultrasound has been more stringently evaluated in randomized trials than other antenatal testing methods, as has been summarized in an editorial by Divon and Ferber. The most recent summary of the available evidence comes from a 2013 Cochrane review of 18 randomized trials that included more than 10,000 high-risk women, in which the use of Doppler ultrasound was associated with decreased perinatal deaths (RR, 0.71; 95% CI, 0.52-0.98) and significantly fewer inductions of labor and cesarean deliveries. Studies of low-risk pregnancies have not shown a benefit from the use of Doppler ultrasound, as has been most recently described in a 2010 systematic review of five studies that included more than 14,000 women.

CLINICAL APPLICATION OF TESTS OF FETAL WELL-BEING

Our ability to detect and prevent impending fetal death or injury depends not only on the predictive value of the tests used and the population selected for testing but also on our ability to respond to abnormal test results. To have an impact on testing outcomes and the overall fetal death rate, we must consider available strategies to deal with abnormal test results. These strategies would ideally include a series of antenatal evaluations and interventions short of premature delivery, with premature delivery ultimately reserved for cases when it is ascertained

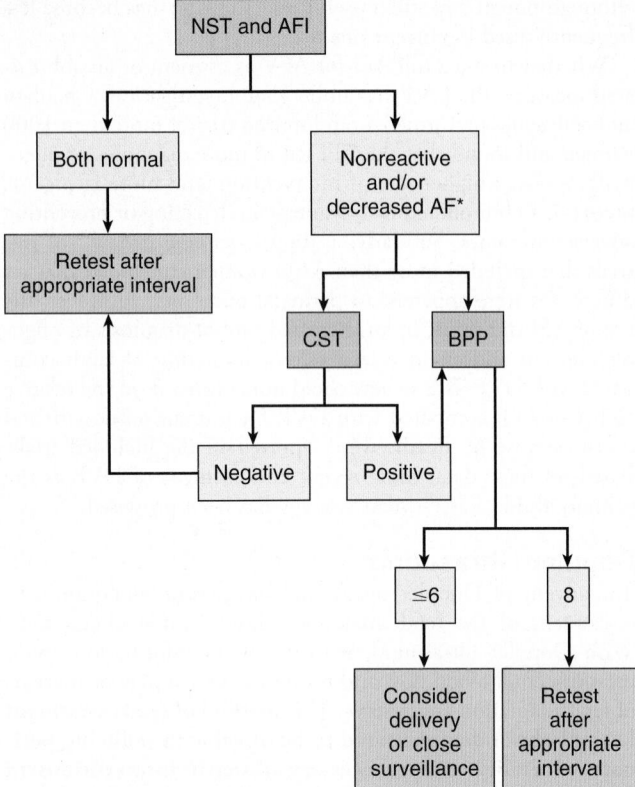

FIG 11-19 Flow chart for antepartum fetal surveillance in which the nonstress test (NST) and amniotic fluid index (AFI) are used as the primary methods for fetal evaluation. A nonreactive NST and decreased AFI are further evaluated using either the contraction stress test (CST) or the biophysical profile (BPP). Further details regarding the use of the BPP are provided in Table 11-6. *If the fetus is mature and amniotic fluid volume is reduced, delivery should be considered before further testing is undertaken. (Modified from Finberg HJ, Kurtz AB, Johnson RL, et al. The biophysical profile: a literature review and reassessment of its usefulness in the evaluation of fetal well-being. *J Ultrasound Med.* 1990;9:583.)

that intrauterine injury or death can no longer be delayed or prevented. Figure 11-19 presents a practical testing scheme that has been used successfully by several centers.[88] This strategy would include using combinations of antepartum tests in an organized sequence to evaluate the fetus further; administration of antenatal steroids; potentially modified maternal activity level; and correction of maternal metabolic, cardiopulmonary, or other medical disorders. In some cases, fetal therapy may be indicated, such as intrauterine transfusion for anemia, removal of fluid from body cavities, diagnostic procedures, and direct administration of medication to the fetus.

Testing can be initiated at early gestational ages in high-risk pregnancies (25-26 weeks) to identify the fetus at risk. Maternal and fetal interventions can then be considered. Obviously, safe prolongation of intrauterine life is the primary goal, and better understanding of the pathophysiology of the premature fetus and the use of combinations of tests will allow this to be accomplished.

The question of routine antepartum fetal surveillance must be carefully examined. Antepartum fetal testing can more accurately predict fetal outcome than antenatal risk assessment using an established scoring system. Patients judged to be at high risk based on known medical factors but whose fetuses demonstrate normal antepartum fetal evaluation have a lower PMR than patients considered at low risk whose fetuses have abnormal antepartum testing results. Routine antepartum fetal evaluation would be necessary to detect the considerable proportion of fetuses destined for fetal death or injury with no identifiable risk factors. It would therefore seem reasonable to consider extending some form of antepartum fetal surveillance to all obstetric patients, such as maternal assessment of fetal activity as described previously.

The question is how best to combine antenatal tests in clinical practice and in which patients. **The approach to prescribing testing modalities must take into account gestational age, medical comorbidities, and sociodemographic risk factors** described in this chapter in order to prevent fetal injury or death without causing iatrogenic prematurity or an excess of testing and worry. According to a summary by Fretts and Duru[23] in 2008, "The best opportunity for stillbirth reduction is to identify patients who have an increased risk of stillbirth late in pregnancy, where the downside of antepartum testing and early delivery, if warranted, can be minimized."

The condition to specific use of antenatal testing may be illustrated by the following examples. In a prolonged pregnancy, a **parallel testing scheme** would be used. In this situation, the obstetrician is not concerned with fetal maturity but rather with fetal well-being. Several tests are performed at the same time, such as antepartum fetal heart rate testing and the BPP. It is acceptable in this high-risk situation to intervene when a single test is abnormal. It seems prudent to accept a false-positive test result to avoid the intrauterine death of a mature and otherwise healthy fetus. In most other high-risk pregnancies, such as those complicated by diabetes mellitus or hypertension, it is preferable to allow the fetus to remain in utero as long as possible. In these situations, a **branched testing scheme** is used to decrease the likelihood of unnecessary premature intervention, the obstetrician uses a series of tests and, under most circumstances, would only deliver a premature infant when all parameters suggest fetal compromise. In this situation, the physician must consider the likelihood of neonatal respiratory distress syndrome (RDS) and review these risks with colleagues in neonatology.

The comparable performance of the various available antenatal tests, along with their utility in series, has been illustrated by numerous investigators (see Table 11-2). Maternal assessment of fetal activity would appear to be a reasonable first-line screening test for both high- and low-risk patients. The use of this approach may decrease the number of unexpected intrauterine deaths in so-called normal pregnancies. The NST and mBPP remain the primary methods used for antepartum fetal evaluation in high-risk patients at most centers, with full BPP and CST to assess fetal condition in patients who exhibit a persistently nonreactive NST or abnormal mBPP. This sequential approach may be particularly valuable in avoiding unnecessary premature intervention. The NST and mBPP can be quickly performed in an outpatient setting and are easily interpreted. In contrast, the CST is usually performed near the labor and delivery suite, it may require an intravenous infusion of oxytocin and may be more difficult to interpret. However, the ability of the CST to stress the fetus and evaluate its response to intermittent interruptions in intervillous blood flow may provide an earlier warning of fetal compromise than the NST or mBPP.

The frequency with which to use specific tests will depend on a number of features, including the predictive value of the test and the underlying condition prompting the test. Most tests described previously have relatively reliable risk profiles over the course of a week when normal, with decreased intervals between tests recommended for abnormal results. Regarding the underlying condition contributing to risk for adverse outcomes, consideration must be given to whether that condition is stable, worsening, or improving. The gestational age at which to initiate testing has not been clearly defined for most high-risk conditions. **Initiating testing at 32 to 34 weeks of gestation has historically been prescribed for most high-risk pregnancies, with earlier testing recommended for cases with multiple comorbidities or particularly worrisome features.**

In considering the pros and cons of testing in the preterm period, it is worthwhile to return to the question of potential harms of testing, from increases in preterm birth and cesarean delivery rates to maternal anxiety and financial costs. Although no evidence exists of improved outcomes from any one testing strategy, as a counterpoint some authors have begun to study whether the implementation of testing increases the chances of induction of labor or cesarean delivery rates. In addition, it is reasonable to question whether a program of antenatal testing contributes to maternal anxiety or other indirect costs that are difficult to quantify. Kafali and colleagues[56] demonstrated increased maternal anxiety scores after an NST session and a decrease in anxiety scores in women randomized to administration of music during the NST. Taking patient-specific risk factors, and perhaps maternal preferences, into account when considering an individualized testing plan is most likely to contribute to optimal outcomes.

On behalf of the Eunice Kennedy Shriver National Institute of Child Health and Human Development Workshop, Signore and coworkers[2] have proposed a series of guidelines for condition-specific antenatal testing based on the available evidence (Table 11-6). In their 2009 publication, they stress that **"the basis for antepartum testing relies on the premise that the fetus whose** oxygenation in utero is challenged will respond with a series of detectable physiologic adaptive or decompensatory signs as hypoxemia or frank metabolic academia develop," hence the recommendation for the use of antenatal tests in series to follow the changes in observable measures of fetal response to a suboptimal intrauterine environment. Although this proposed strategy is certainly not comprehensive, it is hoped that future research into specific testing strategies stratified by risk category will enhance our ability to prescribe these tests effectively and safely.

Evidence for Condition-Specific Testing

For most of the conditions identified as constituting an increased risk for fetal death, insufficient studies exist to permit an evidence-based recommendation for a particular testing scheme. In addition to this limitation, condition-specific testing is problematic as a general strategy for prevention of fetal death, given the many fetal deaths that occur in pregnancies otherwise categorized as low risk or without identifiable risk factors.[2] However, it is incumbent on care providers to consider all conditions associated with an increased risk for fetal death or other adverse outcomes as a potential indication for some form of antenatal surveillance[2,32] and to individualize antenatal testing plans based on specific underlying conditions. This strategy is outlined in an excellent summary by Kontopoulos and Vintzileos,[99] in which they explore several pathophysiologic mechanisms as potentially distinct etiologies for risk of fetal death in different populations. **The authors acknowledge that no ideal single test or testing strategy exists for all high-risk pregnancies but that clinician judgment and logic, as well as evidence from observational trials, should guide testing strategies for each patient.**

Difficulty in generating evidence-based recommendations for condition-specific testing schemes in cases of identified risk factors can be illustrated by considering the example of

TABLE 11-6	PROPOSED INITIAL TESTING STRATEGY BY SELECTED ANTENATAL CONDITION		
RISK FACTOR	**TEST**	**FREQUENCY**	**START**
All pregnancies	FMC	Daily	24-28 wk
Low-risk pregnancies	FMC	Daily	24-28 wk
Insulin-treated diabetes:			
Uncomplicated pregestational or gestational	mBPP	Twice weekly	32 wk
With hypertension, renal disease, or IUGR	As above, plus consider CST	Weekly	26-28 wk
Hypertensive disorders:			
Uncomplicated	mBPP	Twice weekly	32 wk
With comorbidities	mBPP	Twice weekly	26-28 wk
IUGR	mBPP/Doppler	Once or twice weekly	At diagnosis
Multiple gestation:			
Twins			
Concordant growth	mBPP	Weekly	32 wk
Discordant growth or AFV	mBPP	Twice weekly	At diagnosis
Triplets or greater	mBPP	Twice weekly	28 wk
Oligohydramnios	mBPP	Twice weekly	At diagnosis
Intrahepatic cholestasis	mBPP	Weekly	34 wk
Renal disease	mBPP	Weekly	30-32 wk
Decreased fetal movement	mBPP	PRN	At diagnosis
Previous fetal death	mBPP	Once or twice weekly	32-34 wk or 1 wk before previous fetal death
	Alternative: BPP or CST	Weekly	
Postterm pregnancy	mBPP	Once or twice weekly	≥41 wk
SLE	mBPP	Weekly	26 wk
Renal disease	mBPP	Once or twice weekly	30-32 wk
Intrahepatic cholestasis	mBPP	Weekly	34 wk

Modified from Signore C, Freeman RK, Spong CY. Antenatal testing: a reevaluation. Executive Summary of a Eunice Kennedy Shriver National Institute of Child Health and Human Development Workshop. *Obstet Gynecol* 2009;113:687-701.

AFV, amniotic fluid volume; *BPP*, biophysical profile; *CST*, contraction stress test; *FMC*, fetal movement counting; *IUGR*, intrauterine growth restriction; *mBPP*, modified biophysical profile; *PRN*, *pro re nata* (as needed); SLE, systemic lupus erythematosus.

hypertensive disorders. Well-designed prospective trials that provide evidence for any specific testing strategy are not available despite the very frequent use of a variety of antenatal testing schemes used in clinical practice for hypertensive disorders. The heterogeneity of pathophysiologic mechanisms at play in the general category of hypertensive disorders contributes to the difficulty in generating specific recommendations. Freeman[37] summarized the situation in a 2008 review and noted that despite previous testing guidelines that recommended a wider application of antenatal testing in women with varying degrees of hypertension, the most recent expert recommendations do not support antepartum fetal testing for mild to moderate blood pressure abnormalities, nor do they support it in the absence of preeclampsia or IUGR. However, for many practitioners, the evidence that all forms of chronic hypertension constitute an increased risk for fetal death and adverse outcomes prompts broad use of testing modalities for these patients.

Another challenge in the implementation of condition-specific testing may lie in the appreciation and acknowledgment of individual patient characteristics as risk factors for fetal death, in particular certain demographic risk factors without clear pathophysiologic links. For example, the condition of advanced maternal age has garnered a great deal of investigation into associations with fetal death and other adverse pregnancy outcomes and related management strategies. However, the same cannot be said for other demographic risk factors such as obesity and black race, which have equal or greater relative risks of fetal death yet are arguably less accepted in the community as being risks for adverse outcomes.

ASSESSMENT OF FETAL PULMONARY MATURATION

This section reviews those techniques that enable the obstetrician to predict the risks of RDS for the infant who requires premature delivery. The risk of iatrogenic prematurity for the neonate balanced against the risk of continued antepartum assessment of the potentially compromised fetus determines ultimate management strategies. As one marker of fetal maturity that can be assessed antenatally, incorporation of the discussion of fetal pulmonary maturity assessment with that of antepartum assessment is critical.

RDS is caused by a deficiency of pulmonary surfactant, an antiatelectasis factor that is able to maintain a low stable surface tension at the air-water interface within alveoli. Surfactant decreases the pressure needed to distend the lung and prevents alveolar collapse (see Chapter 22). The type 2 alveolar cell is the major site of surfactant synthesis. Surfactant is packaged in lamellar bodies, discharged into the alveoli, and carried into the amniotic cavity with pulmonary fluid.

Phospholipids account for more than 80% of the surface to active material within the lung, and more than 50% of this phospholipid is dipalmitoyl lecithin. The latter is a derivative of glycerol phosphate and contains two fatty acids and the nitrogenous base choline. Other phospholipids contained in the surfactant complex include phosphatidylglycerol (PG), phosphatidylinositol, phosphatidylserine, phosphatidylethanolamine, sphingomyelin, and lysolecithin. PG is the second most abundant lipid in surfactant and significantly improves its properties.

Important differences in neonatal adaptation, including development of RDS, have been demonstrated not only between preterm and term neonates but also with each advancing gestational week from 37 to 39 weeks. This places even more responsibility on the physician to judiciously assess indications for and timing of delivery before 39 weeks. In weighing the risks and benefits of effecting delivery as a result of antenatal testing results before 39 weeks, assessment of fetal pulmonary maturity may in some cases be indicated. At the same time, it is important to recognize that many perinatal processes contribute to the prognosis for neonatal respiratory function, including surfactant deficiency, immaturity, and intrapartum complications—all prime factors in determining the pathogenesis of RDS that may not be predicted by fetal pulmonary maturity testing.

Tests of Fetal Pulmonary Maturity

Available methods for evaluating fetal pulmonary maturity rely generally on either presence or quantitation of components of pulmonary surfactant or measurement of surfactant function. The former category has become the most common and reliable in current practice, although no data show that one method is preferable to the others with regard to prediction of pulmonary maturity. **In general, a test that is positive for fetal pulmonary maturity will much more** accurately predict the absence of RDS than a negative test will predict the presence of RDS.

With the exception of amniotic fluid specimens obtained from the vaginal pool, the evaluation of fetal pulmonary maturation requires that a sample of amniotic fluid be obtained by amniocentesis. This is generally a low-risk procedure with few potential adverse outcomes, including unsuccessful amniocentesis (1.6%-4.4%) and complications that require same-day delivery (0.7%-3.3%).

Quantitation of Pulmonary Surfactant

Methods of quantifying pulmonary surfactant include the lecithin/sphingomyelin (L/S) ratio, presence of PG, visual inspection of fluid, and surfactant/albumin ratio.

The L/S ratio was the first reliable assay for the assessment of fetal pulmonary maturity. The amniotic fluid concentration of lecithin increases markedly at about 35 weeks' gestation, whereas sphingomyelin levels remain stable or decrease. Amniotic fluid sphingomyelin exceeds lecithin until 31 to 32 weeks, when the L/S ratio reaches 1. Lecithin then rises rapidly, and an L/S ratio of 2 is observed at about 35 weeks. Wide variation in the L/S ratio at each gestational age has been noted. Nevertheless, a ratio of 2 or greater has repeatedly been associated with pulmonary maturity. Note that the presence of blood or meconium in the amniotic fluid sample can cause erroneous results.

PG, which does not appear until 35 weeks' gestation and increases rapidly between 37 and 40 weeks, is a marker of completed pulmonary maturation. A rapid immunologic semiquantitative agglutination test (AmnioStat-FLM; Irvine Scientific, Santa Ana, CA) can be used to determine the presence of PG within 30 min and requires only 1.5 mL of amniotic fluid. Presence of blood and meconium do not interfere with PG assessment.

Visual inspection of amniotic fluid can give some information about the presence of pulmonary surfactant components. During the first and second trimesters, amniotic fluid is yellow and clear. It becomes colorless in the third trimester. By 33 to 34 weeks' gestation, cloudiness and flocculation are noted, and as term approaches, vernix appears. Amniotic fluid with obvious vernix or fluid so turbid it does not permit the reading of newsprint through it will usually have a mature L/S ratio.

The ratio of the surfactant-albumin in amniotic fluid was previously a popular test run on an automated fluorescence polarimeter that was easy to use, low in cost, and had high reproducibility. Currently the device is not commercially available for use, although newer platforms may be in development.

Measurements of Surfactant Function

Lamellar bodies are the storage form of surfactant released by fetal type 2 pneumocytes into the amniotic fluid. A lamellar body count requires less than 1 mL of amniotic fluid and takes only 15 minutes to perform using a commercial cell counter. A count greater than 30,000 to 55,000/µL is highly predictive of pulmonary maturity, whereas a count below 10,000/µL suggests a significant risk for RDS. Neither meconium nor blood has a significant effect on the lamellar body count. The ease and relatively low cost of this test have contributed to its popularity, although poor concordance among various instruments for the assay of lamellar body counts has been noted.

Determination of Fetal Pulmonary Maturation in Clinical Practice

As data have been assimilated in recent years related to lung maturity assessment and its role in high-risk pregnancy management, new important paradigms are emerging. Traditionally, lung maturity tests have been interpreted in categorical fashion, usually as either "positive," indicating lung maturity and a low risk for RDS, or "negative," indicating the absence of maturity and a higher risk for RDS. However, the presence of RDS in neonates is associated with both gestational age and lung maturity assessments. As further information has been gathered, it is now possible to stratify risk for RDS based on both gestational age and lung maturity assessment. This represents a more appropriate use of the lung maturity tests. **In assessing the risk for RDS complicating subsequent delivery, results from fetal lung maturity testing are most appropriately correlated with the gestational age at the time of fluid retrieval.**

An even more recent paradigm shift that has taken place over the last several years has seen a decrease in the frequency with which fetal lung maturity testing is recommended and used. Both ACOG and the NICHD[32,100] have endorsed increased stringency of indications for late preterm and early term births, which if followed stand to decrease the opportunities for clinical uncertainty around need for delivery and thus decrease the need for fetal lung maturity testing. As noted in the 2011 NICHD publication on this topic, "If significant maternal or fetal risk exists, delivery should occur regardless of biochemical maturity, and if delivery could be deferred owing to the absence of pulmonary maturity, there is not a stringent indication for prompt delivery. Additionally, it is recognized that a mature fetal lung profile denoting the presence of pulmonary surfactant does not necessarily translate to maturity of other organ systems."[100]

we assume that by testing and intervening with delivery for abnormal test results we are contributing to a good outcome, as Scifres and Macones[48] stated in their 2008 review of costs and benefits of antenatal testing, "In the absence of data we cannot be assured that our interventions, even if they prevent stillbirth, may not involve a tradeoff between long-term neurologic dysfunction and fetal death." Additionally, aside from potential unknown medical sequelae of antenatal testing and interventions, monetary, time, and psychological costs must also be considered, but these are difficult to quantify in both research settings and in practice.

As clinicians aim to implement evidence-based strategies to screen for and prevent fetal injury and death, the limitations of existing research must be considered. Because it is in many ways impractical and perhaps unethical to carry out placebo-controlled trials of antenatal testing methodologies in high-risk pregnancies, we must acknowledge that this type of rigorous evidence is not likely to be imminently forthcoming.[2] Nevertheless, we propose that biologic plausibility and clinician judgment prevail over therapeutic nihilism in clinical practice and that future research efforts embrace a creative approach to both condition-specific and apparently unpredictable fetal death and injury.

SUMMARY

We must be aware of our limited understanding of the pathophysiology of fetal death and injury in many situations, and we must attempt judicious use of antenatal testing measures with the hope of preventing some adverse outcomes and with the goal of doing no harm. Although

KEY POINTS

♦ Although the PMR has fallen steadily in the United States since 1965, the number of fetal deaths has not changed substantially in the past decade.
♦ Perinatal events play an important role in infant mortality and long-term disability of survivors in addition to their contribution to fetal death.
♦ At least 20% of fetal deaths have no obvious fetal, placental, maternal, or obstetric etiology, and this percentage increases with advancing gestational age.
♦ The prevalence of an abnormal condition (i.e., fetal death) has great impact on the predictive value of antepartum fetal tests.
♦ Few of the antepartum tests commonly used in clinical practice today have been subjected to large-scale prospective and randomized evaluations that can speak to the true efficacy of testing.
♦ Fetal adaptation to hypoxemia is mediated by changes in heart rate and redistribution of cardiac output.
♦ The decrease in fetal movement with hypoxemia makes maternal assessment of fetal activity a potentially simple and widely applicable method of monitoring fetal well-being. However, prospective trials of this method for prevention of perinatal mortality have failed to conclusively show benefit.
♦ The CST has a low false-negative rate but a high false-positive rate and is cumbersome to perform and thus is used less frequently in common practice than other testing modalities.
♦ The observation that accelerations of the fetal heart rate in response to fetal activity, uterine contractions, or stimulation reflect fetal well-being is the basis for the NST.

- Use of VAS for a nonreactive NST or equivocal BPP does not increase the false-negative rate and may reduce the likelihood of unnecessary obstetric intervention.
- The NST has a low false-negative rate, although higher than that of CST, and a high false-positive rate.
- Fetal biophysical activities can be evaluated with real-time ultrasonography by BPP, and those fetal biophysical activities that are present earliest in fetal development are the last to disappear with fetal hypoxia.
- The mBPP performs comparably to the full BPP. Both modalities have a false-negative rate, or rate of fetal death within 1 week of a normal test, of 0.8 per 1000.
- Most amniotic fluid tests of fetal pulmonary maturation accurately predict pulmonary maturity, but results should be taken in context with anticipated total neonatal maturity as indicated by gestational age.
- Condition-specific testing involves modifying the frequency, type, and initiation of antenatal tests according to maternal high-risk conditions.
- Both costs and benefits should be considered when using a particular testing strategy, taking into account competing risks of fetal death and postnatal morbidity.

REFERENCES

1. Manning FA. Antepartum fetal testing: a critical appraisal. *Curr Opin Obstet Gynecol.* 2009;21:348.
2. Signore C, Freeman RK, Spong CY. Antenatal testing: a reevaluation. Executive Summary of a Eunice Kennedy Shriver National Institute of Child Health and Human Development Workshop. *Obstet Gynecol.* 2009;113:687.
3. Reddy UM, Goldenberg R, Silver R, et al. Stillbirth classification: developing an international consensus for research. Executive Summary of a National Institute of Child Health and Human Development Workshop. *Obstet Gynecol.* 2009;114:901.
4. MacDorman MF, Kirmeyer SE, Wilson EC. Fetal and perinatal mortality, United States. In: *National Vital Statistics Reports*, Vol. 60, no, 8. Hyattsville, MD: National Center for Health Statistics; 2006:2012.
5. Fretts RC. Etiology and prevention of stillbirth. *Am J Obstet Gyncecol.* 1923;193:2005.
6. World Health Organization: The OBSQUID Project: quality development in perinatal care, final report. *Publ Eur Surv* 1995; WHO Regional Publication Series.
7. American College of Obstetricians and Gynecologists. Perinatal and infant mortality statistics. *Committee Opinion.* 1995;167.
8. MacDorman M, Kirmeyer S. The challenge of fetal mortality. In: *NCHS Data Brief, no. 16.* Hyattsville, MD: National Center for Health Statistics; 2009.
9. MacDorman MF, Hoyert DL, Mathews TJ. *Recent declines in infant mortality in the United States, 2005–2011. NCHS data brief, no 120.* Hyattsville, MD: National Center for Health Statistics.; 2013.
10. Mathews TJ, MacDorman MF. *Infant mortality statistics from the 2010 period linked birth/infant death data set. National vital statistics reports*, Vol. 62 no 8. Hyattsville, MD: National Center for Health Statistics.; 2013.
11. Martin JA, Hsiang-Ching K, Mathews TJ, et al. Annual summary of vital statistics. *Pediatrics.* 2006;121(788):2008.
12. Manning FA, Lange IR, Morrison I, Harman CR. Determination of fetal health: methods for antepartum and intrapartum fetal assessment. In: Leventhal J, ed. *Current Problems in Obstetrics and Gynecology.* Chicago: Year Book Medical Publishers; 1983.
13. Fretts RC, Boyd ME, Usher RH, Usher H. The changing pattern of fetal death, 1961-1988. *Obstet Gynecol.* 1992;79:35.
14. Fretts RC, Schmittdiel J, McLean FH, et al. Increased maternal age and the risk of fetal death. *N Engl J Med.* 1995;333:953.
15. Stillbirth Collaborative Research Network Writing Group. Causes of death among stillbirths. *JAMA.* 2011;306:2459-2468.
16. Mersey Region Working Party on Perinatal Mortality. Perinatal health. *Lancet.* 1982;1:491.
17. Getahun D, Ananth CV, Kinzler WL. Risk factors for antepartum and intrapartum stillbirth: a population-based study. *Am J Obstet Gynecol.* 2007;196:499.
18. Grant A, Elbourne D. Fetal movement counting to assess fetal well-being. In: Chalmers I, Enkin M, Keirse MJ, eds. *Effective Care in Pregnancy and Childbirth.* Oxford: Oxford University Press; 1989:440.
19. Kahn B, Lumey LH, Zybert PA, et al. Prospective risk of fetal death in singleton, twin, and triplet gestations: implications for practice. *Obstet Gynecol.* 2003;102:685.
20. Trudell AS, Tuuli MG, Cahill AG, Macones GA, Odibo AO. Balancing the risks of stillbirth and neonatal death in the early preterm small-for-gestational-age fetus. *Am J Obstet Gynecol.* 2014;211:295.e1-295.e7.
21. Fretts RC. Stillbirth epidemiology, risk factors, and opportunities for stillbirth prevention. *Clin Obstet Gynecol.* 2010;53:588.
22. Warland J, Mitchell EA. A triple risk model for unexplained late stillbirth. *BMC Pregnancy Childbirth.* 2014;14:142.
23. Fretts RC, Duru UA. New indications for antepartum testing: making the case for antepartum surveillance or timed delivery for women of advanced maternal age. *Semin Perinatol.* 2008;32:312.
24. Reddy UM, Chia-Wen K, Willinger M. Maternal age and the risk of stillbirth throughout pregnancy in the United States. *Am J Obstet Gynecol.* 2006;195:764.
25. Rowland Hogue CJ, Silver RM. Racial and ethnic disparities in United States: stillbirth rates: trends, risk factors, and research needs. *Semin Perinatol.* 2011;35:221-233.
26. Willinger M, Chia-Wen K, Reddy UM. Racial disparities in stillbirth across gestation in the United States. *Am J Obstet Gynecol.* 2009;201:469.e1.
27. Smith GCS, Fretts RC. Stillbirth. *Lancet.* 2007;370:1715.
28. Aune D, Saugstad OD, Henriksen T, Tonstad S. Maternal body mass index and the risk of fetal death, stillbirth, and infant death: a systematic review and meta-analysis. *JAMA.* 2014;311:1536-1546.
29. Feig DS, Hwee J, Shah BR, Booth GL, Bierman AS, Lipscombe LL. Trends in incidence of diabetes in pregnancy and serious perinatal outcomes: a large, population-based study in Ontario, Canada, 1996-2010. *Diabetes Care.* 2014;37:1590-1596.
30. Nageotte MP. Antenatal testing: diabetes mellitus. *Semin Perinatol.* 2008;32:269.
31. Freeman RK. Antepartum testing in patients with hypertensive disorders in pregnancy. *Semin Perinatol.* 2008;32:271.
32. Practice bulletin. Antepartum Fetal Surveillance, Number 145. (Replaces Practice Bulletin Number 9, October 1999). American College of Obstetricians and Gynecologists. *Obstet Gynecol.* 2014;124:182-192.
33. Practice bulletin. Antiphospholipid syndrome, Number 132. American College of Obstetricians and Gynecologists. *Obstet Gynecol.* 2012;120:1514-1521.
34. Inherited thrombophilias in pregnancy. Practice Bulletin No. 138 American College of Obstetricians and Gynecologists. *Obstet Gynecol.* 2013;122:706-717.
35. Geenes V, Chappell LC, Seed PT, Steer PJ, Knight M, Williamson C. Association of severe intrahepatic cholestasis of pregnancy with adverse pregnancy outcomes: a prospective population-based case-control study. *Hepatology.* 2014;59:1482-1491.
36. Vidaeff AC, Yeomans ER, Ramin SM. Pregnancy in women with renal disease. I. General principles. *Am J Perinatol.* 2008;25:385.
37. Adams D, Druzin ML, Edersheim T, et al. Condition-specific antepartum testing: systemic lupus erythematosus and associated serologic abnormalities. *Am J Reprod Immunol.* 1992;28:159.
38. Bai J, Wong FW, Bauman A, et al. Parity and pregnancy outcomes. *Am J Obstet Gynecol.* 2002;186:274.
39. Weeks JW. Antepartum testing for women with previous stillbirth. *Semin Perinatol.* 2008;32:301.
40. Allen VM, Wilson RD, Cheung A, for the Genetics Committee of the Society of Obstetricians and Gynaecologists of Canada (SOGC) and the Reproductive Endocrinology Infertility Committee of the Society of Obstetricians and Gynaecologists of Canada (SOGC). Pregnancy outcomes after assisted reproductive technology. *J Obstet Gynaecol Can.* 2006;28:220.
41. Salihu HS, Aliyu MH, Rouse DJ, et al. Potentially preventable excess mortality among higher-order multiples. *Obstet Gynecol.* 2003;102:679.
42. Devoe LD. Antenatal fetal assessment: contraction stress test, nonstress test, vibroacoustic stimulation, amniotic fluid volume, biophysical profile, and modified biophysical profile: an overview. *Semin Perinatol.* 2008;32:247.

43. Wood S, Tang S, Ross S, Sauve R. Stillbirth in twins, exploring the optimal gestational age for delivery: a retrospective cohort study. *Br J Obstet Gynaecol.* 2014;121:1284-1293.

44. Conde-Agudelo A, Bird S, Kennedy SH, Villar J, Papageorghiou A. First- and second-trimester tests to predict stillbirth in unselected pregnant women: a systematic review and meta-analysis. *Br J Obstet Gynaecol.* 2015;122:41-55.

45. Harman CR. Amniotic fluid abnormalities. *Semin Perinatol.* 2008;32:288.

46. Divon MY, Feldman-Leidner N. Postdates and antenatal testing. *Semin Perinatol.* 2008;32:295.

47. Frey HA, Odibo AO, Dicke JM, Shanks AL, Macones GA, Cahill AG. Stillbirth risk among fetuses with ultrasound-detected isolated congenital anomalies. *Obstet Gynecol.* 2014;124:91-98.

48. Scifres CM, Macones GA. Antenatal testing: benefits and costs. *Semin Perinatol.* 2008;32:318.

49. Divon MY, Ferber A. Evidence-based antepartum fetal testing. In: *Prenatal and Neonatal Medicine.* New York: Parthenon; 2000.

50. Fretts RC, Elkin EB, Myers ER, Heffner LJ. Should older women have antepartum testing to prevent unexplained stillbirth? *Obstet Gynecol.* 2004;104:56.

51. Van Woerden EE. VanGeijn HP: Heart-rate patterns and fetal movements. In: Nijhuis J, ed. *Fetal Behaviour.* New York: Oxford University Press; 1992:41.

52. Hijazi ZR, East CE. Factors affecting maternal perception of fetal movement. *Obstet Gynecol Surv.* 2009;64:489.

53. Martin CB. Normal fetal physiology and behavior, and adaptive responses with hypoxemia. *Semin Perinatol.* 2008;32:239.

54. Patrick J, Campbell K, Carmichael L, et al. Patterns of gross fetal body movements over 24-hour observation intervals during the last 10 weeks of pregnancy. *Am J Obstet Gynecol.* 1982;142:363.

55. Druzin ML, Foodim J. Effect of maternal glucose ingestion compared with maternal water ingestion on the nonstress test. *Obstet Gynecol.* 1982;67:4.

56. Kafali H, Derbent A, Keskin E. Simavli S, Gözdemir E. Effect of maternal anxiety and music on fetal movements and fetal heart rate patterns. *J Matern Fetal Neonatal Med.* 2011;24:461-464.

57. Grant A, Valentin L, Elbourne D, Alexander S. Routine formal fetal movement counting and risk of antepartum late death in normally formed singletons. *Lancet.* 1989;2:345.

58. Mangesi L, Hofmeyr GJ. Fetal movement counting for assessment of fetal wellbeing. *Cochrane Database Syst Rev.* 2007;(24):CD004909.

59. Froen JF, Heazell AEP, Holm Tveit JP, et al. Fetal movement assessment. *Semin Perinatol.* 2008;32:243.

60. Mikhail MS, Freda MC, Merkatz RB, et al. The effect of fetal movement counting on maternal attachment to fetus. *Am J Obstet Gynecol.* 1991; 165:988.

61. Braly P, Freeman R, Garite T, et al. Incidence of premature delivery following the oxytocin challenge test. *Am J Obstet Gynecol.* 1981;141:5.

62. Freeman R. The use of the oxytocin challenge test for antepartum clinical evaluation of uteroplacental respiratory function. *Am J Obstet Gynecol.* 1975;121:481.

63. Freeman R, Anderson G, Dorchester W. A prospective multi-institutional study of antepartum fetal heart rate monitoring. I. Risk of perinatal mortality and morbidity according to antepartum fetal heart rate test results. *Am J Obstet Gynecol.* 1982;143:771.

64. Freeman R, Anderson G, Dorchester W. A prospective multi-institutional study of antepartum fetal heart rate monitoring. II. CST vs NST for primary surveillance. *Am J Obstet Gynecol.* 1982;143:778.

65. Bruce S, Petrie R, Yeh S-Y. The suspicious contraction stress test. *Obstet Gynecol.* 1978;51:415.

66. Beischer N, Drew J, Ashton P, et al. Quality of survival of infants with critical fetal reserve detected by antenatal cardiotocography. *Am J Obstet Gynecol.* 1983;146:662.

67. Grivell RM, Alfirevic Z, Gyte GM, Devane D. Antenatal cardiotocography for fetal assessment. *Cochrane Database Syst Rev.* 2012;(12):CD007863.

68. Patrick J, Carmichael L, Chess L, Staples C. Accelerations of the human fetal heart rate at 38-40 weeks' gestational age. *Am J Obstet Gynecol.* 1984;148:35.

69. Macones GA, Hankins GD, Spong CY, et al. The 2008 National Institute of Child Health and Human Development workshop report on electronic fetal monitoring: update on definitions, interpretation, and research guidelines. *Obstet Gynecol.* 2008;112:661.

70. Keegan K, Paul R, Broussard P, et al. Antepartum fetal heart rate testing. V. The nonstress test: an outpatient approach. *Am J Obstet Gynecol.* 1980; 136:81.

71. Tan KH, Sabapathy A. Maternal glucose administration for facilitating tests of fetal wellbeing. *Cochrane Database Syst Rev.* 2012;(4):CD003397.

72. Tan KH, Sabapathy A, Wei X. Fetal manipulation for facilitating tests of fetal wellbeing. *Cochrane Database Syst Rev.* 2013;(4):CD003396.

73. Lavery J. Nonstress fetal heart rate testing. *Clin Obstet Gynecol.* 1982; 25:689.

74. Keegan K, Paul R. Antepartum fetal heart rate testing. IV. The nonstress test as a primary approach. *Am J Obstet Gynecol.* 1980;136:75.

75. Evertson L, Gauthier R, Schifrin B, et al. Antepartum fetal heart rate testing. I. Evolution of the nonstress test. *Am J Obstet Gynecol.* 1979;133:29.

76. Druzin ML, Edersheim TG, Hutson JM, et al. The effect of vibroacoustic stimulation on the nonstress test at gestational ages of thirty-two weeks or less. *Am J Obstet Gynecol.* 1661;1476:1989.

77. Phillips W, Towell M. Abnormal fetal heart rate associated with congenital abnormalities. *Br J Obstet Gynaecol.* 1980;87:270.

78. Gagnon R, Hunse C, Foreman J. Human fetal behavioral states after vibratory stimulation. *Am J Obstet Gynecol.* 1989;161:1470.

79. Tan KH, Smyth RD, Wei X. Fetal vibroacoustic stimulation for facilitation of tests of fetal wellbeing. *Cochrane Database Syst Rev.* 2013;(12):CD002963.

80. Arulkumaran S, Skurr B, Tong H, et al. No evidence of hearing loss due to fetal acoustic stimulation test. *Obstet Gynecol.* 1991;78:2.

81. Esin S. Factors that increase reactivity during fetal nonstress testing. *Curr Opin Obstet Gynecol.* 2014;26:61-66.

82. Rochard F, Schifrin B, Goupil F, et al. Nonstressed fetal heart rate monitoring in the antepartum period. *Am J Obstet Gynecol.* 1976;126:699.

83. Druzin ML. Fetal bradycardia during antepartum testing, further observations. *J Reprod Med.* 1989;34:47.

84. Maeno J. Fetal arrhythmia: prenatal diagnosis and perinatal management. *Obstet Gynaecol Res.* 2009;35:623.

85. Meis P, Ureda J, Swain M, et al. Variable decelerations during non-stress tests are not a sign of fetal compromise. *Am J Obstet Gynecol.* 1994;154: 586.

86. Boehm FH, Salyer S, Shah DM, et al. Improved outcome of twice weekly nonstress testing. *Obstet Gynecol.* 1986;67:566.

87. Barss V, Frigoletto F, Diamond F. Stillbirth after nonstress testing. *Obstet Gynecol.* 1985;65:541.

88. Finberg HJ, Kurtz AB, Johnson RL, et al. The biophysical profile: a literature review and reassessment of its usefulness in the evaluation of fetal well-being. *J Ultrasound Med.* 1990;9:583.

89. Manning FA, Morrison I, Lange IR, et al. Fetal assessment based on fetal biophysical profile scoring: experience in 12,620 referred high-risk pregnancies. *Am J Obstet Gynecol.* 1985;151:343.

90. Vintzileos AM, Gaffney SE, Salinger LM, et al. The relationship between fetal biophysical profile and cord pH in patients undergoing cesarean section before the onset of labor. *Obstet Gynecol.* 1987;70:196.

91. Manning F, Platt L, Sipos L. Antepartum fetal evaluation: development of a fetal biophysical profile. *Am J Obstet Gynecol.* 1980;136:787.

92. Pillai M, James D. The importance of behavioral state in biophysical assessment of the term human fetus. *Br J Obstet Gynaecol.* 1990;97:1130.

93. Manning FA, Morrison I, Lange IR, et al. Fetal biophysical profile scoring: selective use of the nonstress test. *Am J Obstet Gynecol.* 1987;156:709.

94. Manning FA, Morrison I, Harman CR, et al. The abnormal fetal biophysical profile score. V. Predictive accuracy according to score composition. *Am J Obstet Gynecol.* 1990;162:918.

95. Manning FA, Harman CR, Morrison I, et al. Fetal assessment based on fetal biophysical profile scoring. *Am J Obstet Gynecol.* 1990;162:703.

96. Lalor JG, Fawole B, Alfirevic Z, Devane D. Biophysical profile for fetal assessment in high risk pregnancies. *Cochrane Database Syst Rev.* 2008;(1): CD000038.

97. Nageotte MP, Towers CV, Asrat T, Freeman RK, Dorchester W. The value of a negative antepartum test: contraction stress test and modified biophysical profile. *Obstet Gynecol.* 1994;84:231-234.

98. Nabhan AF, Abdelmoula YA. Amniotic fluid index versus single deepest vertical pocket as a screening test for preventing adverse pregnancy outcome. *Cochrane Database Syst Rev.* 2009;(16):CD006593.

99. Kontopoulos EV, Vintzileos AM. Condition-specific antepartum fetal testing. *Am J Obstet Gynecol.* 1546;191:2004.

100. Spong CY, Mercer BM, D'alton M, Kilpatrick S, Blackwell S, Saade G. Timing of indicated late-preterm and early-term birth. *Obstet Gynecol.* 2011;118:323-333.

Additional references for this chapter are available at ExpertConsult.com.

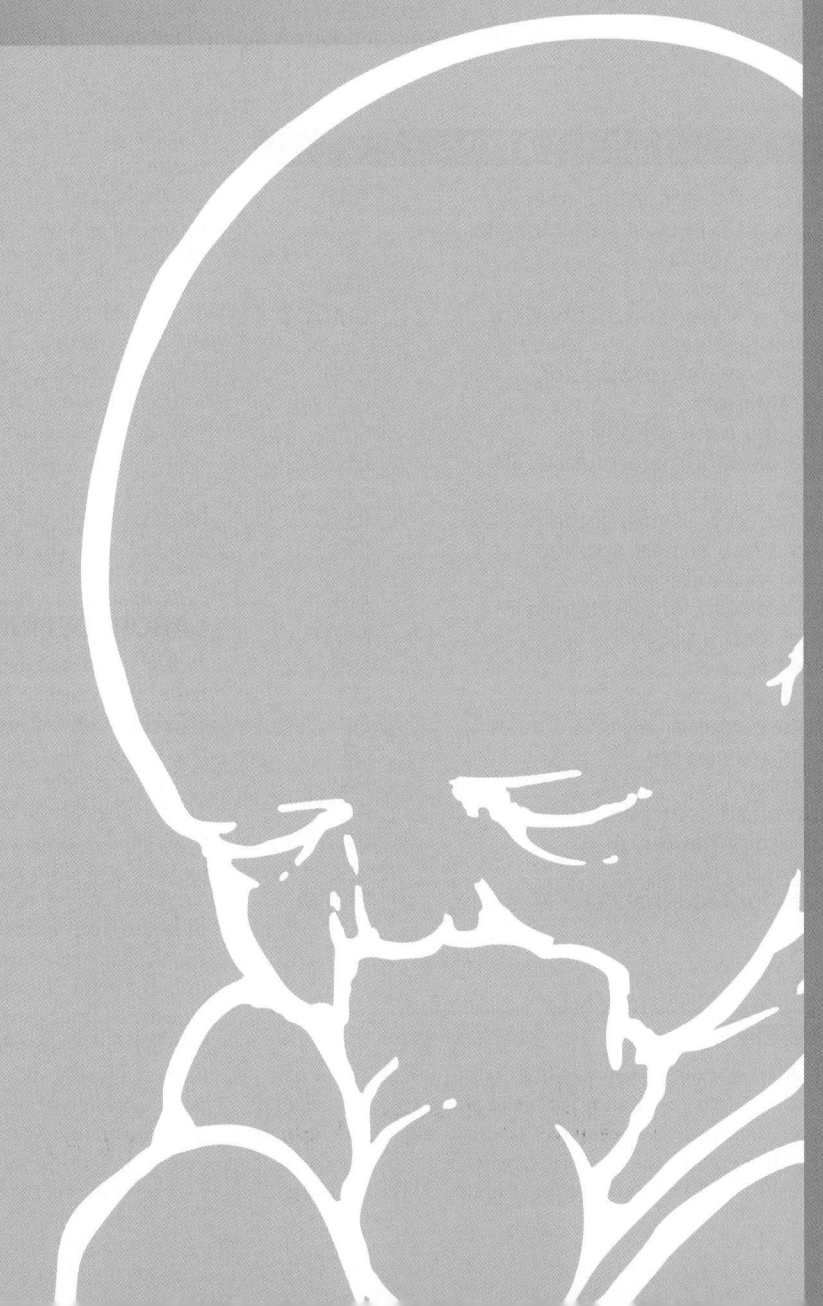

Intrapartum Care

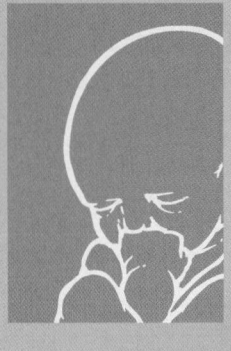

CHAPTER 12

Normal Labor and Delivery

SARAH KILPATRICK and ETOI GARRISON

KEY ABBREVIATIONS

American Academy of Pediatrics	AAP
American College of Obstetricians and Gynecologists	ACOG
Body mass index	BMI
California Maternal Quality Care Collaborative	CMQCC
Cephalopelvic disproportion	CPD
Cervical length	CL
Computed tomography	CT
Dehydroepiandrosterone sulfate	DHEAS
Fetal heart rate	FHR
Intrauterine pressure catheter	IUPC
Intraventricular hemorrhage	IVH
Left occiput anterior	LOA
Magnetic resonance imaging	MRI
Montevideo unit	MVU
Normal saline	NS
Occiput anterior	OA
Occiput posterior	OP
Occiput transverse	OT
Prostaglandin	PG
Randomized controlled trial	RCT
Right occiput anterior	ROA
Skin-to-skin contact	SSC
Society for Maternal-Fetal Medicine	SMFM

OVERVIEW

The initiation of normal labor at term requires endocrine, paracrine, and autocrine signaling between the fetus, uterus, placenta, and the mother. Although the exact trigger for human labor at term remains unknown, it is believed to involve conversion of fetal dehydroepiandrosterone sulfate (DHEAS) to estriol and estradiol by the placenta. These hormones upregulate transcription of progesterone, progesterone receptors, oxytocin receptors, and gap junction proteins within the uterus, which helps to facilitate regular uterine contractions. The *latent phase* of labor is characterized by a slower rate of cervical dilation, whereas the *active phase* of labor is characterized by a faster rate of cervical dilation and does not begin for most women until the cervix is dilated 6 cm. The duration of the second stage of labor can be affected by a number of factors including epidural use, fetal position, fetal weight, ethnicity, and parity. This chapter will review the characteristics and physiology of normal labor at term. Factors that affect the average duration of the first and second stage of labor progress will be reviewed, and an evidence-based evaluation of strategies to support the mother during labor and facilitate safe delivery of the fetus will be presented.

LABOR: DEFINITION AND PHYSIOLOGY

Labor is defined as the process by which the fetus is expelled from the uterus. More specifically, labor requires regular, effective contractions that lead to dilation and effacement of the cervix. This chapter describes the physiology and normal characteristics of term labor and delivery.

The physiology of labor initiation has not been completely elucidated, but the putative mechanisms have been well reviewed by Liao and colleagues.[1] Labor initiation is species specific, and the mechanisms of human labor are unique. **The four phases of labor from quiescence to involution are outlined in** Figure 12-1.[2] The first phase is **quiescence,** which represents that time in utero before labor begins, when uterine activity is suppressed by the action of progesterone, prostacyclin, relaxin, nitric oxide, parathyroid hormone–related peptide, and possibly other hormones. During the **activation phase**, estrogen begins to facilitate expression of myometrial receptors for prostaglandins (PGs) and oxytocin, which results in ion channel activation and increased gap junctions. This increase in the gap junctions between myometrial cells facilitates effective contractions. In

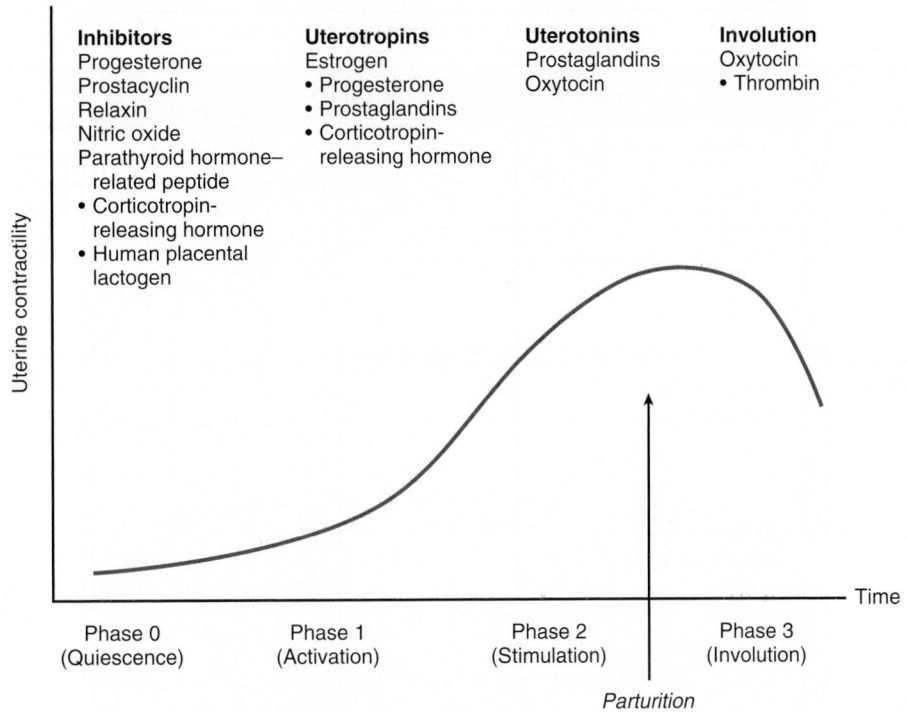

FIG 12-1 Regulation of uterine activity during pregnancy and labor. (Modified from Challis JRG, Gibb W. Control of parturition. *Prenat Neonat Med.* 1996;1:283.)

essence, the activation phase readies the uterus for the subsequent **stimulation phase**, when uterotonics—particularly PGs and oxytocin—stimulate regular contractions. In the human, this process at term may be protracted, occurring over days to weeks. The final phase, **uterine involution**, occurs after delivery and is mediated primarily by oxytocin. The first three phases of labor require endocrine, paracrine, and autocrine interaction between the fetus, membranes, placenta, and mother.

The fetus has a central role in the initiation of term labor in nonhuman mammals; in humans, the fetal role is not completely understood (Fig. 12-2).[2-5] In sheep, term labor is initiated through activation of the fetal hypothalamic-pituitary-adrenal (HPA) axis, with a resultant increase in fetal adrenocorticotropic hormone (ACTH) and cortisol.[4,5] Fetal cortisol increases production of estradiol and decreases production of progesterone by a shift in placental metabolism of cortisol dependent on placental 17α-hydroxylase. The change in the circulating progesterone/estradiol concentration stimulates placental production of oxytocin and PG, particularly $PGF_{2\alpha}$, which in turn promotes myometrial contractility.[4] If this increase in fetal ACTH and cortisol is blocked, progesterone levels remain unchanged, and parturition is delayed.[5] In contrast, humans lack placental 17α-hydroxylase, maternal and fetal levels of progesterone remain elevated, and no trigger exists for parturition because of an increase in fetal cortisol near term. Rather, in humans, evidence suggests that **placental production of corticotropin-releasing hormone (CRH) near term activates the fetal hypothalamic-pituitary axis and results in increased production of dehydroepiandrostenedione by the fetal adrenal gland.**[6] Fetal dehydroepiandrostenedione is converted in the placenta to estradiol and estriol. Placenta-derived estriol potentiates uterine activity by enhancing the transcription of maternal (likely decidual) $PGF_{2\alpha}$, PG receptors, oxytocin receptors, and gap-junction proteins.[6-8] **In**

humans, no documented decrease in progesterone has been observed near term, and a fall in progesterone is not necessary for labor initiation. However, some research suggests the possibility of a **functional progesterone withdrawal** in humans. Labor is accompanied by a decrease in the concentration of progesterone receptors and a change in the ratio of progesterone receptor isoforms A and B in both the myometrium[9-11] and the membranes.[12] During labor, increased expression of nuclear and membrane progesterone receptor isoforms serve to enhance genomic expression of contraction-associated proteins, increase intracellular calcium, and decrease cyclic adenosine monophosphate (cAMP).[13] More research is needed to elucidate the precise mechanism through which the human parturition cascade is activated. Fetal maturation might play an important role as might maternal cues that affect circadian cycling. Most species have distinct diurnal patterns of contractions and delivery, and in humans, the majority of contractions occur at night.[2,14]

Oxytocin is commonly used for labor induction and augmentation, and a full understanding of the mechanism of oxytocin action is important. **Oxytocin is a peptide hormone synthesized in the hypothalamus and released from the posterior pituitary in a pulsatile fashion. At term, oxytocin serves as a potent uterotonic agent capable of stimulating uterine contractions at intravenous (IV) infusion rates of 1 to 2 mIU/min.[15] Oxytocin is inactivated largely in the liver and kidney, and during pregnancy, it is degraded primarily by placental oxytocinase. Its biologic half-life is approximately 3 to 4 minutes, but it appears to be shorter when higher doses are infused.** Concentrations of oxytocin in the maternal circulation do not change significantly during pregnancy or before the onset of labor, but they do rise late in the second stage of labor.[15,16] Studies of fetal pituitary oxytocin production and the umbilical arteriovenous differences in plasma oxytocin strongly suggest that the fetus secretes oxytocin that reaches the maternal side of

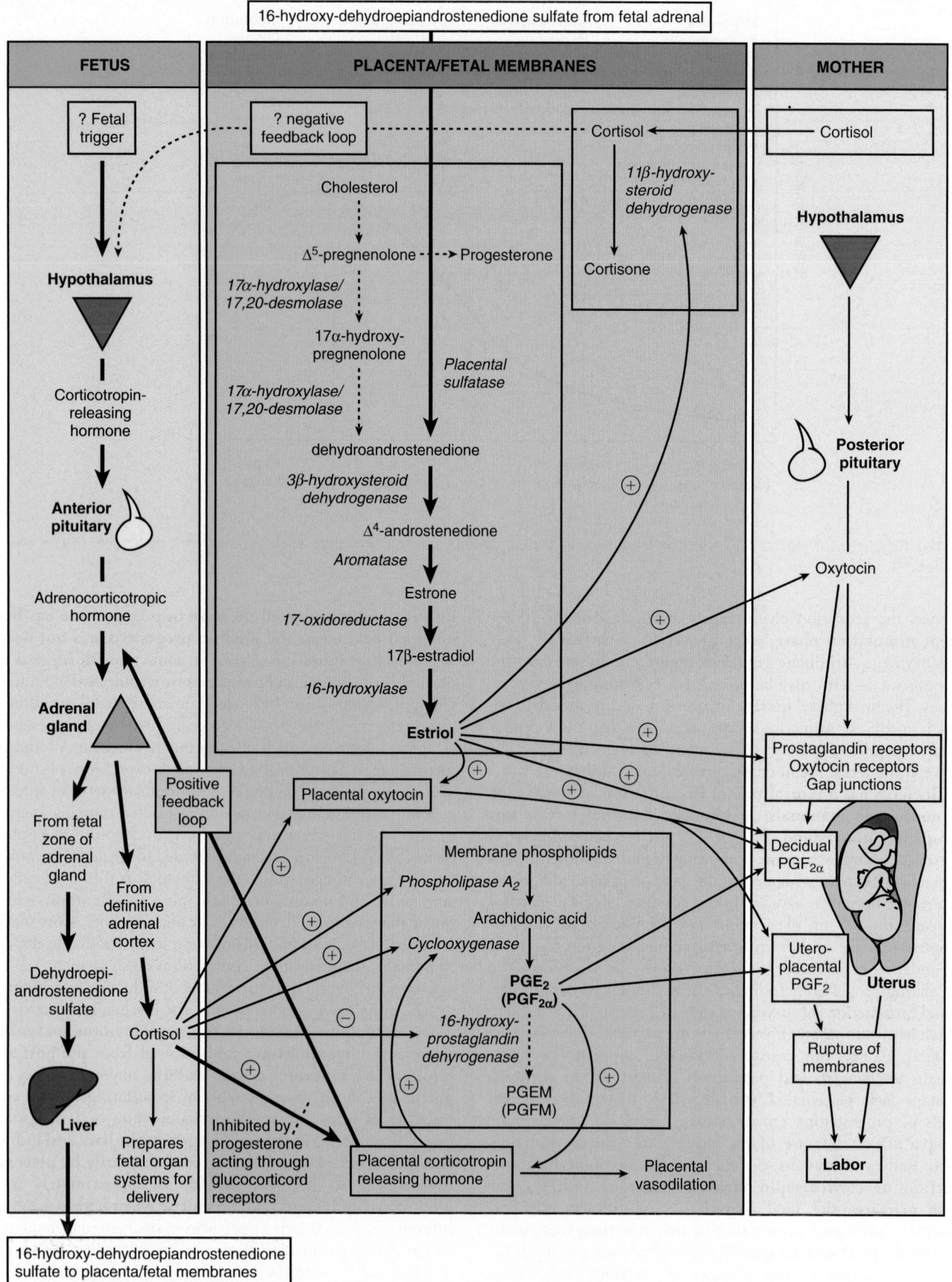

FIG 12-2 Proposed "parturition cascade" for labor induction at term. The spontaneous induction of labor at term in the human is regulated by a series of paracrine/autocrine hormones acting in an integrated parturition cascade responsible for promoting uterine contractions. PGE$_2$, prostaglandin E$_2$; PGEM, 13,14-dihydro-15-keto-PGE$_2$; PGF$_{2\alpha}$, prostaglandin F$_{2\alpha}$; PGFM, 13, 14-dihydro-15keto-PGF$_{2\alpha}$. (Modified from Norwitz ER, Robinson JN, Repke JT. The initiation of parturition: a comparative analysis across the species. *Curr Prob Obstet Gynecol Fertil.* 1999;22:41.)

the placenta.[15,17] **The calculated rate of active oxytocin secretion from the fetus increases from a baseline of 1 mIU/min before labor to around 3 mIU/min after spontaneous labor.**

Significant differences in myometrial oxytocin receptor distribution have been reported, with large numbers of fundal receptors and fewer receptors in the lower uterine segment and cervix.[18] Myometrial oxytocin receptors increase on average by 100- to 200-fold during pregnancy and reach a maximum during early labor.[15,16,19,20] This rise in receptor concentration is paralleled by an increase in uterine sensitivity to circulating oxytocin. Specific high-affinity oxytocin receptors have also been isolated from human amnion and decidua parietalis but not decidua vera.[15,18] **It has been suggested that oxytocin plays a dual role in parturition. First, through its receptor, oxytocin directly stimulates uterine contractions. Second, oxytocin may act indirectly by stimulating the amnion and decidua to produce PG.**[18,21-23] **Indeed, even when uterine contractions are adequate, induction of labor at term is successful only when oxytocin infusion is associated with an increase in PGF production.**[18]

Oxytocin binding to its receptor activates phospholipase C.[24] In turn, phospholipase C increases intracellular calcium both by stimulating the release of intracellular calcium and by promoting the influx of extracellular calcium. Oxytocin stimulation of phospholipase C can be inhibited by increased levels of cAMP.[24] Increased calcium levels stimulate the calmodulin-mediated activation of myosin light-chain kinase. Oxytocin may also stimulate uterine contractions via a calcium-independent pathway by inhibiting myosin phosphatase, which in turn increases myosin phosphorylation. These pathways (of $PGF_{2\alpha}$ and intracellular calcium) have been the target of multiple tocolytic agents: indomethacin, calcium channel blockers, β-mimetics (through stimulation of cAMP), and magnesium.

MECHANICS OF LABOR

Labor and delivery are not passive processes in which uterine contractions push a rigid object through a fixed aperture. The ability of the fetus to successfully negotiate the pelvis during labor and delivery depends on the complex interactions of three variables: uterine activity, the fetus, and the maternal pelvis. This complex relationship has been simplified in the mnemonic *powers, passenger, passage.*

Uterine Activity (Powers)

The *powers* refer to the forces generated by the uterine musculature. **Uterine activity is characterized by the frequency, amplitude (intensity), and duration of contractions.** Assessment of uterine activity may include simple observation, manual palpation, external objective assessment techniques (such as external tocodynamometry), and direct measurement via an intrauterine pressure catheter (IUPC). **External tocodynamometry** measures the change in shape of the abdominal wall as a function of uterine contractions and, as such, is qualitative rather than quantitative. Although it permits graphic display of uterine activity and allows for accurate correlation of fetal heart rate (FHR) patterns with uterine activity, external tocodynamometry does not allow measurement of contraction intensity or basal intrauterine tone. **The most precise method for determination of uterine activity is the direct measurement of intrauterine pressure with an IUPC.** However, this procedure should not be performed unless indicated given the small but finite associated risks of uterine perforation, placental disruption, and intrauterine infection.

Despite technologic improvements, the definition of "adequate" uterine activity during labor remains unclear. **Classically, three to five contractions in 10 minutes has been used to define adequate labor; this pattern has been observed in approximately 95% of women in spontaneous labor.** In labor, patients usually contract every 2 to 5 minutes, with contractions becoming as frequent as every 2 to 3 minutes in late active labor and during the second stage. Abnormal uterine activity can also be observed either spontaneously or as a result of iatrogenic interventions. *Tachysystole* **is defined as more than five contractions in 10 minutes averaged over 30 minutes. If tachysystole occurs, documentation should note the presence or absence of FHR decelerations. The term** *hyperstimulation* **should no longer be used.**[25]

Various units of measure have been devised to objectively quantify uterine activity, the most common of which is the *Montevideo unit* **(MVU)**, a measure of average frequency and amplitude above basal tone (the average strength of contractions in millimeters of mercury multiplied by the number of contractions per 10 min). Although 150 to 350 MVU has been described for adequate labor, 200 to 250 MVU is commonly accepted to define adequate labor in the active phase.[26,27] No data identify adequate forces during latent labor. Although it is generally believed that optimal uterine contractions are associated with an increased likelihood of vaginal delivery, data are limited to support this assumption. **If uterine contractions are "adequate" to effect vaginal delivery, one of two things will happen: either the cervix will efface and dilate, and the fetal head will descend, or caput succedaneum (scalp edema) and molding of the fetal head (overlapping of the skull bones) will worsen without cervical effacement and dilation. The latter situation suggests the presence of cephalopelvic disproportion (CPD),** which can be either *absolute*, in which the fetus is simply too large to negotiate the pelvis, or *relative*, in which delivery of the fetus through the pelvis would be possible under optimal conditions but is precluded by malposition or abnormal attitude of the fetal head.

Fetus (Passenger)

The passenger, of course, is the fetus. Several fetal variables influence the course of labor and delivery. **Fetal size** can be estimated clinically by abdominal palpation or ultrasound or by asking a multiparous patient about her best estimate, but all of these methods are subject to a large degree of error. *Fetal macrosomia* **is defined by the American College of Obstetricians and Gynecologists (ACOG) as birthweight greater than or equal to the 90th percentile for a given gestational age or greater than 4500 g for any gestational age,**[28] and it is associated with an increased likelihood of planned cesarean delivery, labor dystocia, cesarean delivery after a failed trial of labor, shoulder dystocia, and birth trauma.[29] **Fetal** *lie* **refers to the longitudinal axis of the fetus relative to the longitudinal axis of the uterus.** Fetal lie can be longitudinal, transverse, or oblique (Fig. 12-3). In a singleton pregnancy, only fetuses in a longitudinal lie can be safely delivered vaginally.

Presentation **refers to the fetal part that directly overlies the pelvic inlet.** In a fetus presenting in the longitudinal lie, the presentation can be cephalic (vertex) or breech. *Compound presentation* refers to the presence of more than one fetal part overlying the pelvic inlet, such as a fetal hand and the vertex. *Funic* *presentation* refers to presentation of the umbilical cord and is rare at term. In a cephalic fetus, the presentation is classified according to the leading bony landmark of the skull, which can be either the occiput (vertex), the chin (mentum), or the brow (Fig. 12-4). *Malpresentation*, a term that refers to any presentation other than vertex, is seen in approximately 5% of all term labors (see Chapter 17).

Attitude **refers to the position of the head with regard to the fetal spine (the degree of flexion and/or extension of the fetal head).** Flexion of the head is important to facilitate *engagement* of the head in the maternal pelvis. When the fetal chin is optimally flexed onto the chest, the **suboccipitobregmatic diameter** (9.5 cm) presents at the pelvic inlet (Fig. 12-5). This is the smallest possible presenting diameter in the cephalic presentation. As the head deflexes (extends), the diameter presenting to the pelvic inlet progressively increases even before the malpresentations of brow and face are encountered (see Fig. 12-5) and may contribute to failure to progress in labor. The

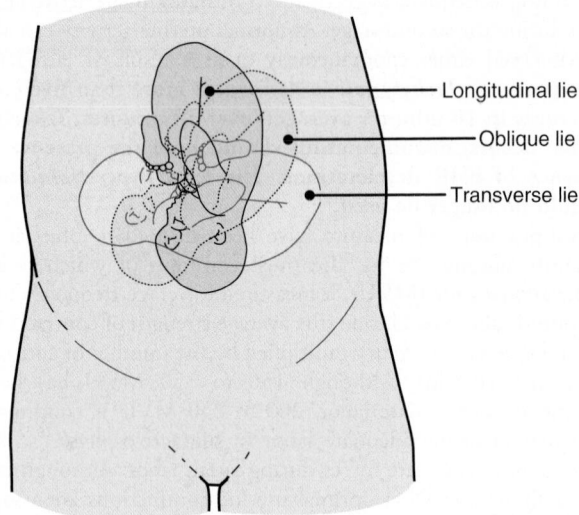

FIG 12-3 Examples of fetal lie.

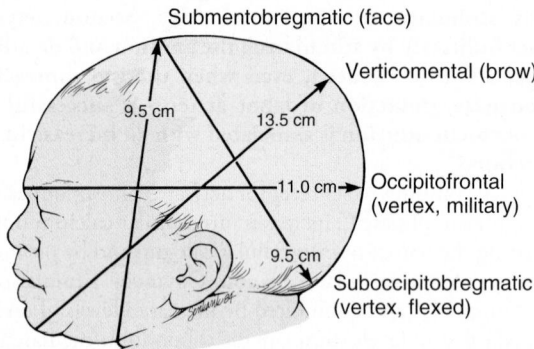

FIG 12-5 Presenting diameters of the average term fetal skull.

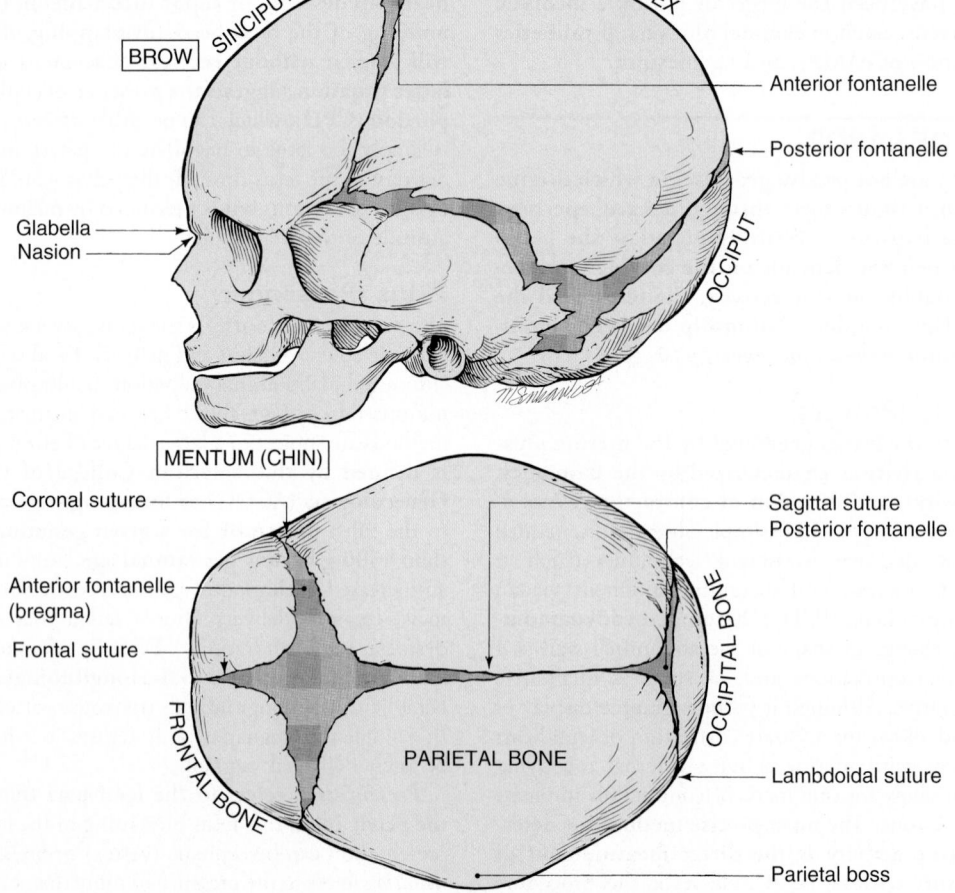

FIG 12-4 Landmarks of fetal skull for determination of fetal position.

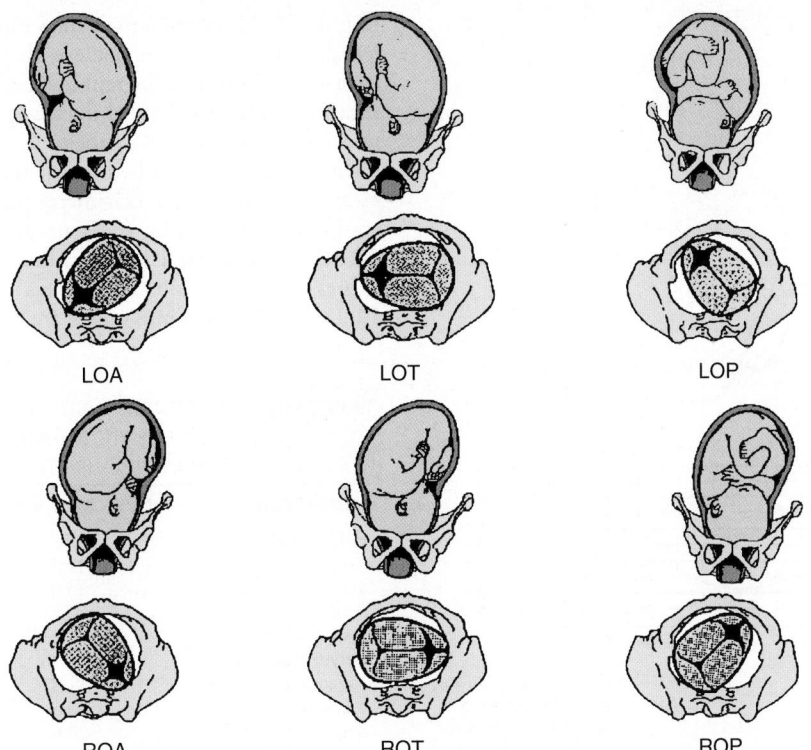

FIG 12-6 Fetal presentations and positions in labor. LOA, left occiput anterior; LOP, left occiput posterior; LOT, left occiput transverse; ROA, right occiput anterior; ROT, right occiput transverse; ROP, right occiput posterior. (Modified from Norwitz ER, Robinson J, Repke JT. The initiation and management of labor. In Seifer DB, Samuels P, Kniss DA, eds. *The Physiologic Basis of Gynecology and Obstetrics*. Philadelphia: Lippincott, Williams & Wilkins; 2001.)

architecture of the pelvic floor along with increased uterine activity may correct deflexion in the early stages of labor.

Position of the fetus refers to the relationship of the fetal presenting part to the maternal pelvis, and it can be assessed most accurately on vaginal examination. For *cephalic presentations*, the fetal occiput is the reference: if the occiput is directly anterior, the position is occiput anterior (OA); if the occiput is turned toward the mother's right side, the position is right occiput anterior (ROA). In the *breech presentation*, the sacrum is the reference (right sacrum anterior). The various positions of a cephalic presentation are illustrated in Figure 12-6. In a *vertex presentation*, position can be determined by palpation of the fetal sutures: the sagittal suture is the easiest to palpate, but palpation of the distinctive lambdoid sutures should identify the position of the fetal occiput; the frontal suture can also be used to determine the position of the front of the vertex.

Most commonly, the fetal head enters the pelvis in a transverse position and then, as a normal part of labor, it rotates to an OA position. Most fetuses deliver in the OA, left occiput anterior (LOA), or ROA position. *Malposition* refers to any position in labor that is not in the above three categories. In the past, fewer than 10% of presentations were occiput posterior (OP) at delivery.[30] However, epidural analgesia may be an independent risk factor for persistent OP presentation in labor. In an observational cohort study, OP presentation was observed in 12.9% of women with epidurals compared with 3.3% of controls ($P = .002$).[31] In a Cochrane meta-analysis of four randomized controlled trials (RCTs), malposition was 40% more likely for women with an epidural compared with controls; however, this difference was not statistically significant, and more RCTs are needed (odds ratio [OR] 1.40; 95% confidence interval [CI],

0.98 to 1.99).[32] *Asynclitism* occurs when the sagittal suture is not directly central relative to the maternal pelvis. If the fetal head is turned such that more parietal bone is present posteriorly, the sagittal suture is more anterior; this is referred to as *posterior asynclitism*. In contrast, *anterior asynclitism* occurs more parietal bone presents anteriorly. The occiput transverse (OT) and OP positions are less common at delivery and are more difficult to deliver.

Station is a measure of descent of the bony presenting part of the fetus through the birth canal (Fig. 12-7). The current standard classification (−5 to +5) is based on a quantitative measure in centimeters of the distance of the leading bony edge from the ischial spines. The *midpoint* (0 station) is defined as the plane of the maternal ischial spines. The ischial spines can be palpated on vaginal examination at approximately 8 o'clock and 4 o'clock. For the right-handed person, they are most easily felt on the maternal right.

An abnormality in any of these fetal variables may affect both the course of labor and the route of delivery. For example, OP presentation is well known to be associated with longer labor, operative vaginal delivery, and an increased risk of cesarean delivery.[31,33]

Maternal Pelvis (Passage)

The passage consists of the bony pelvis—composed of the sacrum, ilium, ischium, and pubis—and the resistance provided by the soft tissues. The bony pelvis is divided into the *false* (greater) and *true* (lesser) pelvis by the pelvic brim, which is demarcated by the sacral promontory, the anterior ala of the sacrum, the arcuate line of the ilium, the pectineal line of the pubis, and the pubic crest culminating in the symphysis

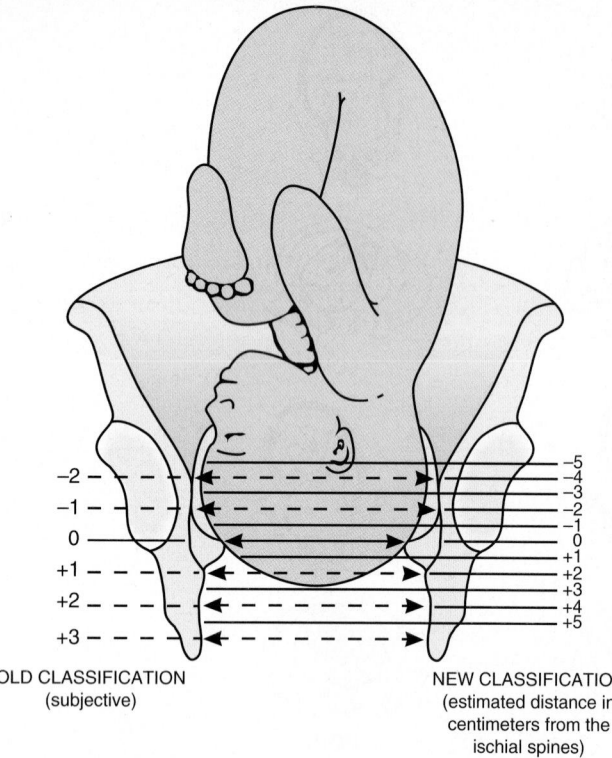

OLD CLASSIFICATION
(subjective)

NEW CLASSIFICATION
(estimated distance in
centimeters from the
ischial spines)

FIG 12-7 The relationship of the leading edge of the presenting part of the fetus to the plane of the maternal ischial spines determines the station. Station +1/+3 (old classification), or +2/+5 (new classification), is illustrated.

(Fig. 12-8). Measurements of the various parameters of the bony female pelvis have been made with great precision, directly in cadavers and using radiographic imaging in living women. Such measurements have divided the true pelvis into a series of planes that must be negotiated by the fetus during passage through the birth canal, which can be broadly termed the *pelvic inlet, mid-pelvis,* and *pelvic outlet.* Pelvimetry performed with radiographic computed tomography (CT) or magnetic resonance imaging (MRI) has been used to determine average and **critical limit values** for the various parameters of the bony pelvis (Table 12-1).[34,35] Critical limit values are measurements that may be

TABLE 12-1	AVERAGE AND CRITICAL LIMIT VALUES FOR PELVIC MEASUREMENTS BY X-RAY PELVIMETRY		
DIAMETER	**AVERAGE VALUE**	**CRITICAL LIMIT***	
Pelvic Inlet			
Anteroposterior (cm)	12.5	10.0	
Transverse (cm)	13.0	12.0	
Sum (cm)	25.5	22.0	
Area (cm²)	145.0	123.0	
Pelvic Midcavity			
Anteroposterior (cm)	11.5	10.0	
Transverse (cm)	10.5	9.5	
Sum (cm)	22.0	19.5	
Area (cm²)	125.0	106.0	

Modified from O'Brien WF, Cefalo RC. Labor and delivery. In: Gabbe SG, Niebyl JR, Simpson JL, eds. *Obstetrics: Normal and Problem Pregnancies,* ed 3. New York: Churchill Livingstone; 1996;377.
*The critical limit values cited imply a high likelihood of cephalopelvic disproportion.

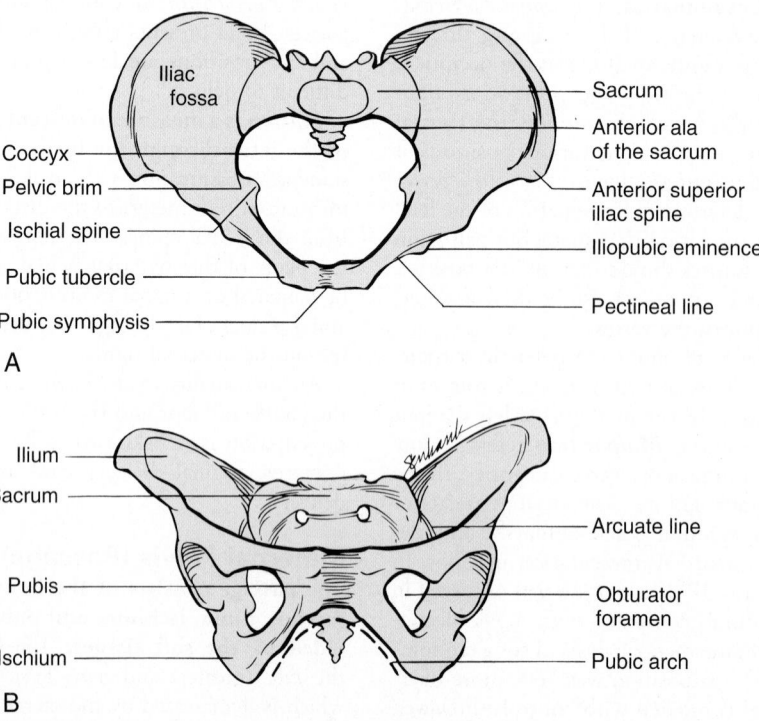

FIG 12-8 Superior **(A)** and anterior **(B)** view of the female pelvis. (From Repke JT. *Intrapartum Obstetrics.* New York: Churchill Livingstone; 1996;68.)

associated with a significant probability of CPD depending upon fetal size and gestational age.[34] However, subsequent studies were unable to demonstrate threshold pelvic or fetal cutoff values with sufficient sensitivity or specificity to predict CPD and the subsequent need for cesarean delivery prior to the onset of labor.[36,37] **In current obstetric practice, radiographic CT and MRI pelvimetry are rarely used given the lack of evidence of benefit and some data that show possible harm (increased incidence of cesarean delivery); instead, a clinical trial of the pelvis (labor) is used.** The remaining indications for radiography, CT pelvimetry, or MRI are evaluation for vaginal breech delivery or evaluation of a woman who has suffered a significant pelvic fracture.[38]

Clinical pelvimetry is currently the only method of assessing the shape and dimensions of the bony pelvis in labor.[36] A useful protocol for clinical pelvimetry is detailed in Figure 12-9 and involves assessment of the pelvic inlet, midpelvis, and pelvic outlet. Reported average and critical-limit pelvic diameters may be used as a historical reference during the clinical examination to determine pelvic shape and assess risk for CPD. The inlet of the true pelvis is largest in its transverse diameter and averages 13.5 cm.[36] The *diagonal conjugate,* the distance from the sacral promontory to the inferior margin of the symphysis pubis as assessed on vaginal examination, is a clinical representation of the anteroposterior (AP) diameter of the pelvic inlet. The *true conjugate, or obstetric conjugate,* of the pelvic inlet is the distance from the sacral promontory to the superior aspect of the symphysis pubis. The obstetric conjugate has an average value of 11 cm and is the smallest diameter of the inlet. It is considered to be contracted if it measures less than 10 cm.[36] The obstetric conjugate cannot be measured clinically but can be estimated by subtracting 1.5 to 2.0 cm from the *diagonal conjugate,* which has an average distance of 12.5 cm.

The limiting factor in the midpelvis is the transverse interspinous diameter (the measurement between the ischial spines), which is usually the smallest diameter of the pelvis but should be greater than 10 cm. The pelvic outlet is rarely of clinical significance, however. The average pubic angle is greater than 90 degrees and will typically accommodate two fingerbreadths.[36] The AP diameter from the coccyx to the symphysis pubis is approximately 13 cm in most cases, and the transverse diameter between the ischial tuberosities is approximately 8 cm and will typically accommodate four knuckles (see Fig. 12-9).

The shape of the female bony pelvis can be classified into four broad categories: gynecoid, anthropoid, android, and platypelloid (Fig. 12-10). This classification is based on the radiographic studies of Caldwell and Moloy[39] and separates those with more favorable characteristics (gynecoid, anthropoid) from those less favorable for vaginal delivery (android, platypelloid). In reality, however, many women fall into intermediate classes, and the distinctions become arbitrary. The *gynecoid* pelvis is the classic female shape. The *anthropoid* pelvis— with its exaggerated oval shape of the inlet, largest AP diameter, and limited anterior capacity—is more often associated with delivery in the OP position. The *android* pelvis is male in pattern and theoretically has an increased risk of CPD, and the broad and flat *platypelloid* pelvis theoretically predisposes to a transverse arrest. Although the assessment of fetal size, along with pelvic shape and capacity, is still of clinical utility, it is a very inexact science. **An adequate trial of labor is**

the only definitive method to determine whether a fetus will be able to safely negotiate through the pelvis.

Pelvic soft tissues may provide resistance in both the first and second stages of labor. In the first stage, resistance is offered primarily by the cervix, whereas in the second stage, it is offered by the muscles of the pelvic floor. In the second stage of labor, the resistance of the pelvic musculature is believed to play an important role in the rotation and movement of the presenting part through the pelvis.

CARDINAL MOVEMENTS IN LABOR

The *cardinal movements* refer to changes in the position of the fetal head during its passage through the birth canal. Because of the asymmetry of the shape of both the fetal head and the maternal bony pelvis, such rotations are required for the fetus to successfully negotiate the birth canal. **Although labor and birth comprise a continuous process, seven discrete cardinal movements are described: (1) engagement, (2) descent, (3) flexion, (4) internal rotation, (5) extension, (6) external rotation or restitution, and (7) expulsion** (Fig. 12-11).

Engagement

Engagement **refers to passage of the widest diameter of the presenting part to a level below the plane of the pelvic inlet** (Fig. 12-12). In the cephalic presentation with a well-flexed head, the largest transverse diameter of the fetal head is the biparietal diameter (9.5 cm). In the breech, the widest diameter is the bitrochanteric diameter. Clinically, engagement can be confirmed by palpation of the presenting part both abdominally and vaginally. **With a cephalic presentation, engagement is achieved when the presenting part is at zero station on vaginal examination.** Engagement is considered an important clinical prognostic sign because it demonstrates that, at least at the level of the pelvic inlet, the maternal bony pelvis is sufficiently large to allow descent of the fetal head. In nulliparas, engagement of the fetal head usually occurs by 36 weeks' gestation; however, in multiparas engagement can occur later in gestation or even during the course of labor.

Descent

Descent **refers to the downward passage of the presenting part through the pelvis. Descent of the fetus is not continuous; the greatest rates of descent occur in the late active phase and during the second stage of labor.**

Flexion

Flexion of the fetal head occurs passively as the head descends owing to the shape of the bony pelvis and the resistance offered by the soft tissues of the pelvic floor. Although flexion of the fetal head onto the chest is present to some degree in most fetuses before labor, complete flexion usually occurs only during the course of labor. **The result of complete flexion is to present the smallest diameter of the fetal head (the suboccipitobregmatic diameter) for optimal passage through the pelvis.**

Internal Rotation

Internal rotation **refers to rotation of the presenting part from its original position as it enters the pelvic inlet (usually OT) to the AP position as it passes through the pelvis.** As with flexion, internal rotation is a passive movement that results from the shape of the pelvis and the pelvic floor musculature.

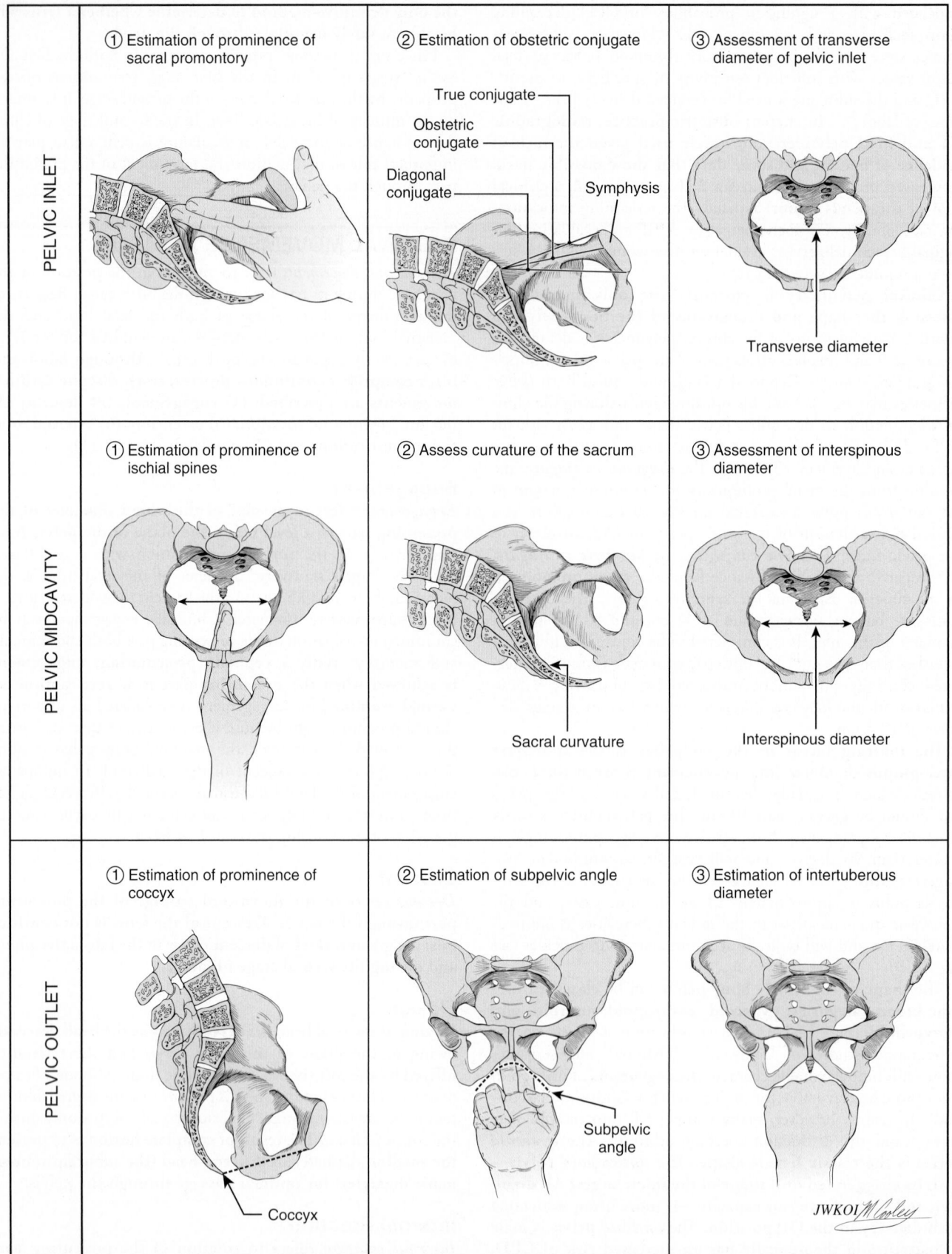

FIG 12-9 A protocol for clinical pelvimetry.

		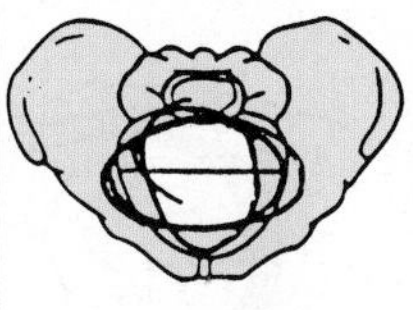 Gynecoid	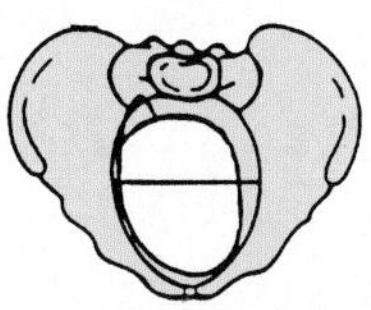 Anthropoid	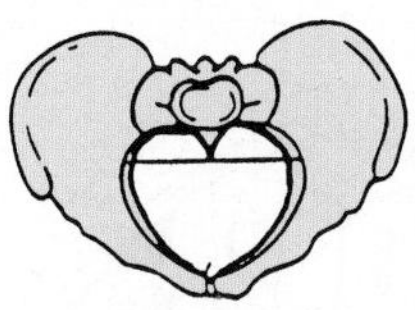 Android	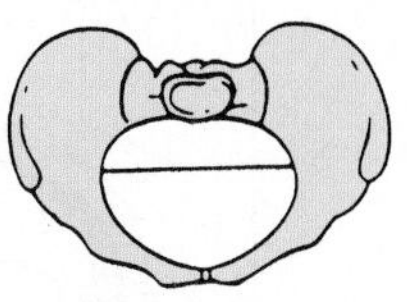 Platypelloid
Pelvic inlet 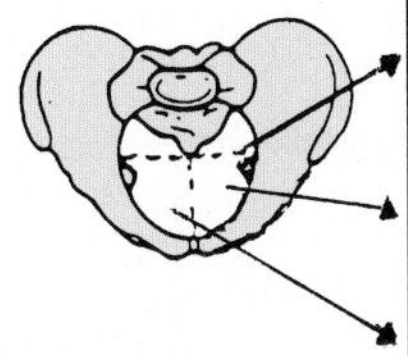	Widest transverse diameter of inlet	12 cm	<12 cm	12 cm	12 cm
	Anteroposterior diameter of inlet	11 cm	>12 cm	11 cm	10 cm
	Forepelvis	Wide	Divergent	Narrow	Straight
Pelvic midcavity 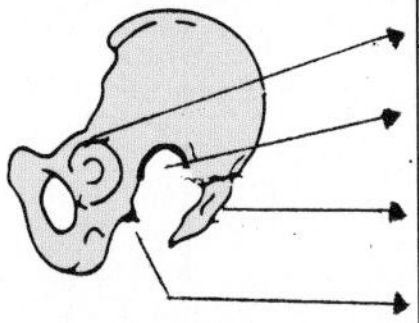	Side walls	Straight	Narrow	Convergent	Wide
	Sacrosciatic notch	Medium	Backward	Narrow	Forward
	Inclination of sacrum	Medium	Wide	Forward (lower third)	Narrow
	Ischial spines	Not prominent	Not prominent	Not prominent	Not prominent
Pelvic outlet 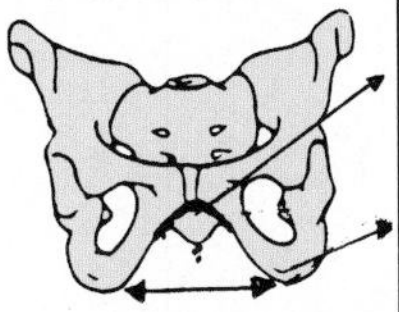	Subpubic arch	Wide	Medium	Narrow	Wide
	Transverse diameter of outlet	10 cm	10 cm	<10 cm	10 cm

FIG 12-10 Characteristics of the four types of female bony pelvis. (Modified from Callahan TL, Caughey AB, Heffner LJ, eds. *Blueprints in Obstetrics and Gynecology.* Malden, MA: Blackwell Science; 1998;45.)

The pelvic floor musculature, including the coccygeus and ileo-coccygeus muscles, forms a V-shaped "hammock" that diverges anteriorly. As the head descends, the occiput of the fetus rotates toward the symphysis pubis—or, less commonly, toward the hollow of the sacrum—thereby allowing the widest portion of the fetus to negotiate the pelvis at its widest dimension. Owing to the angle of inclination between the maternal lumbar spine and pelvic inlet, the fetal head engages in an asynclitic fashion (i.e., with one parietal eminence lower than the other). With uterine contractions, the leading parietal eminence descends and is first to engage the pelvic floor. As the uterus relaxes, the pelvic floor musculature causes the fetal head to rotate until it is no longer asynclitic.

Extension

Extension occurs once the fetus has descended to the level of the introitus. This descent brings the base of the occiput into contact with the inferior margin at the symphysis pubis. At this point, the birth canal curves upward. The fetal head is delivered by extension and rotates around the symphysis pubis. The forces responsible for this motion are the downward force exerted on the fetus by the uterine contractions along with the upward forces exerted by the muscles of the pelvic floor.

External Rotation

External rotation, also known as *restitution*, refers to the return of the fetal head to the correct anatomic position in relation to the fetal torso. This can occur to either side

depending on the orientation of the fetus; this is again a passive movement that results from a release of the forces exerted on the fetal head by the maternal bony pelvis and its musculature and mediated by the basal tone of the fetal musculature.

Expulsion

***Expulsion* refers to delivery of the rest of the fetus.** After delivery of the head and external rotation, further descent brings the anterior shoulder to the level of the symphysis pubis. **The anterior shoulder is delivered in much the same manner as the head, with rotation of the shoulder under the symphysis pubis.** After the shoulder, the rest of the body is usually delivered without difficulty.

NORMAL PROGRESS OF LABOR

Progress of labor is measured with multiple variables. With the onset of regular contractions, the fetus descends in the pelvis as the cervix both effaces and dilates. With each vaginal examination to judge labor progress, the clinician must assess not only cervical effacement and dilation but fetal station and position. This assessment depends on skilled digital palpation of the maternal cervix and the presenting part. As the cervix dilates in labor, it thins and shortens—or becomes more *effaced*—over time. Cervical *effacement* refers to the length of the remaining cervix and can be reported in length or as a percentage. If percentage is used, 0% effacement at term refers to at least a 2 cm long or a very thick

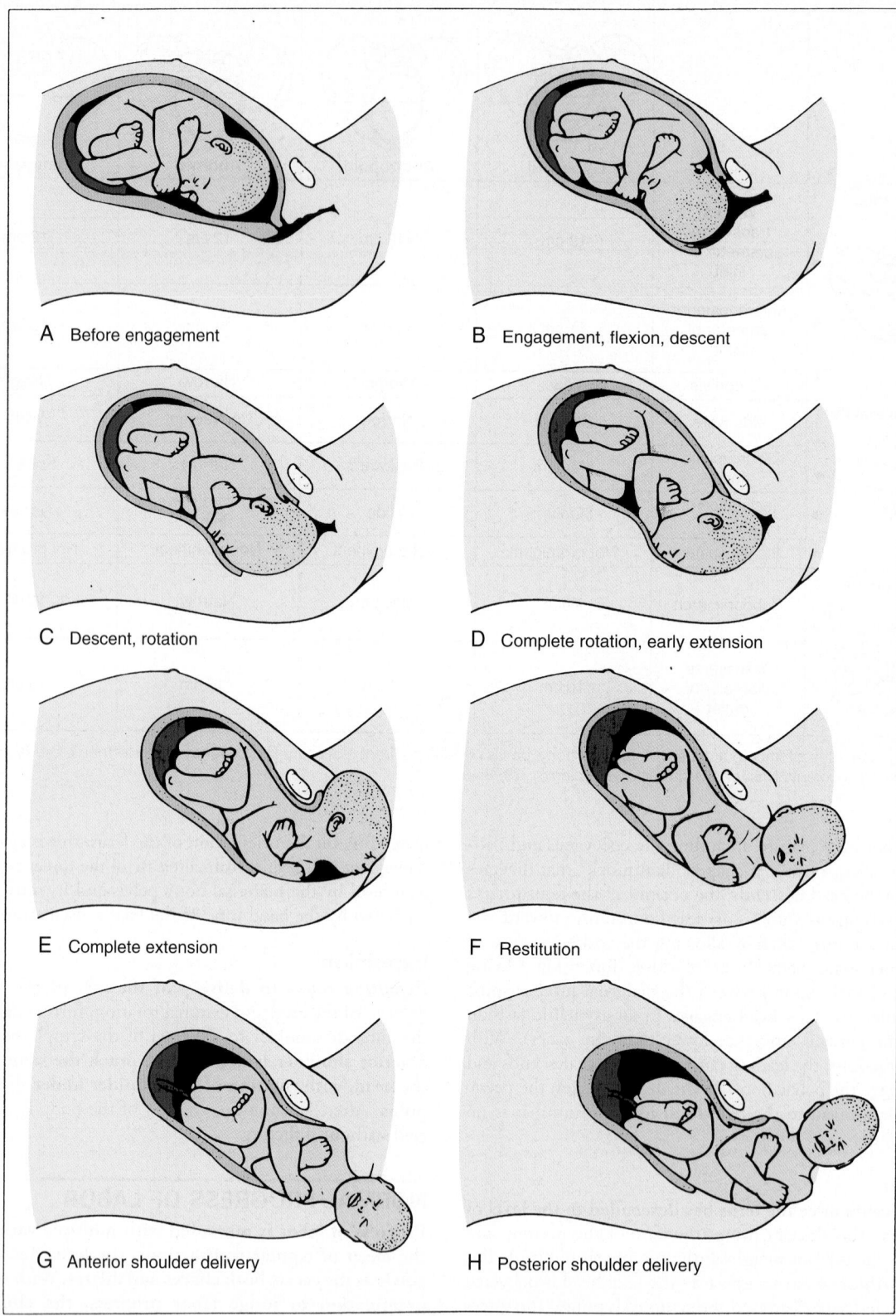

A   Before engagement

B   Engagement, flexion, descent

C   Descent, rotation

D   Complete rotation, early extension

E   Complete extension

F   Restitution

G   Anterior shoulder delivery

H   Posterior shoulder delivery

FIG 12-11 Cardinal movements of labor.

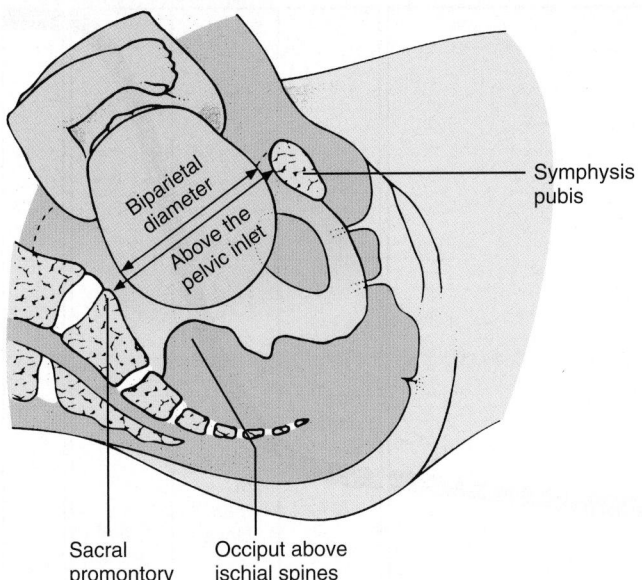

Sacric

FIG 12-12 Engagement of the fetal head.

cervix, and 100% effacement refers to no length remaining or a very thin cervix. Most clinicians use percentages to follow cervical effacement during labor. Generally, 80% or greater effacement is observed in women who are in active labor. Dilation, perhaps the easiest assessment to master, ranges from closed (no dilation) to complete (10 cm dilated). For most women, a cervical dilation that accommodates a single index finger is equal to 1 cm, and two index fingers' dilation is equal to 3 cm. If no cervix can be palpated around the presenting part, the cervix is 10 cm or completely dilated. The assessment of station, discussed earlier, is important for documentation of progress, but it is also critical when determining if an operative vaginal delivery is feasible. Fetal head position should be regularly determined once the woman is in active labor; ideally, this should occur before significant caput has developed, which obscures the sutures. Like station, knowledge of the fetal position is critical before performing an operative vaginal delivery (see Chapter 14).

Labor occurs in three stages: the *first stage* is from labor onset until full dilation of the cervix; the *second stage* is from full cervical dilation until delivery of the baby; and the *third stage* begins with delivery of the baby and ends with delivery of the placenta. The first stage of labor is divided into two phases: the first is the *latent phase,* and the second is the *active phase.* The *latent phase* begins with the onset of labor and is characterized by regular, painful uterine contractions and a slow rate of cervical change. When the rate of cervical dilation is accelerated, latent labor ends and active labor begins. Labor onset is a retrospective diagnosis that is difficult to identify objectively. It is defined by the initiation of regular painful contractions of sufficient duration and intensity to result in cervical dilation or effacement. Women are frequently at home during this time; therefore the identification of labor onset depends on patient memory and the timing of contractions in relation to the cervical examination. The *active phase* of labor is defined as the period in which the greatest rate of cervical dilation occurs. Identification of the point at which labor transitions from the latent to the active phase will depend upon the frequency of cervical examinations and retrospective

examination of labor progress. **Historically, based upon Friedman's[40] seminal data on cervical dilation and labor progress from the 1950s and 1960s, active labor required 80% or more effacement and 4 cm or greater dilation of the cervix.** He analyzed labor progress in 500 nulliparous and multiparous women and reported normative data that have been used for more than half a century to define our expectations of normal and abnormal labor.[40,41]

Friedman revolutionized our understanding of labor because he was able to plot static observations of cervical dilation against time and successfully translate the dynamic process of labor into a sigmoid-shaped curve (Fig. 12-13). Friedman's data popularized the use of the labor graph, which first depicted only cervical dilation and was then later modified to include fetal descent.[42] Four-centimeter cervical dilation marks the transition from the latent to the active phase because it corresponds to the flexion point on the averaged labor curve generated from a review of 500 individual labor curves in the original Friedman dataset.[40] **Rates of 1.5 and 1.2 cm dilation per hour in the active phase for multiparous and nulliparous women, respectively, represent the 5th percentile of normal.**[41] These data have led to the general concept that in active labor, a rate of dilation of at least 1 cm per hour should occur.

More recent analysis of contemporary labor from several studies challenges our understanding of the cervical dilation at which active labor occurs and suggests that the transition from the latent phase to the active phase of labor is a more gradual process.[43] An analysis of labor curves for 1699 multiparous and nulliparous women who presented in spontaneous labor at term and underwent a vaginal delivery determined that only half of the women with a cervical dilation of 4 cm were in the active phase.[44] By 5 cm of cervical dilation, 75% of the women were in the active phase, and by 6 cm cervical dilation, 89% of the women were in the active phase.[44] Zhang and colleagues[45] reviewed data from the National Collaborative Perinatal Project, a historic cohort of 26,838 term parturients in spontaneous labor from 1959 through 1966. This study used a repeated measures analysis to construct labor curves for parturients whose intrapartum management was similar to those studied by Friedman in the 1950s. The cesarean delivery rate was 5.6%, and only 20% of nulliparas and 12% of multiparas received oxytocin for labor augmentation. **This study determined that labor progress in nulliparous women who ultimately had a vaginal delivery is in fact slower than previously reported until 6 cm of cervical dilation.**[45] Specifically, most nulliparous women were not in active labor until approximately 5 to 6 cm of cervical dilation, and the slope of labor progress did not increase until after 6 cm. These findings were confirmed in an analysis[46] of contemporary data collected prospectively by the Consortium on Safe Labor, which enrolled and followed 62,415 singleton term parturients who presented in spontaneous labor at 19 institutions from 2002 through 2007. This dataset included a greater percentage of women with oxytocin augmentation (45% to 47%) and epidural analgesia (71% to 84%) compared with those studied by Friedman in the 1950s. Zhang and colleagues[45] reported the median and 95th percentile of time to progress from one centimeter to the next and confirmed that labor may take more than 6 hours to progress from 4 to 5 cm and more than 3 hours to progress from 5 to 6 cm regardless of parity (Table 12-2). Multiparas had a faster rate of cervical dilation compared with nulliparas only after 6 cm of cervical dilation had been reached. **These data suggest that it**

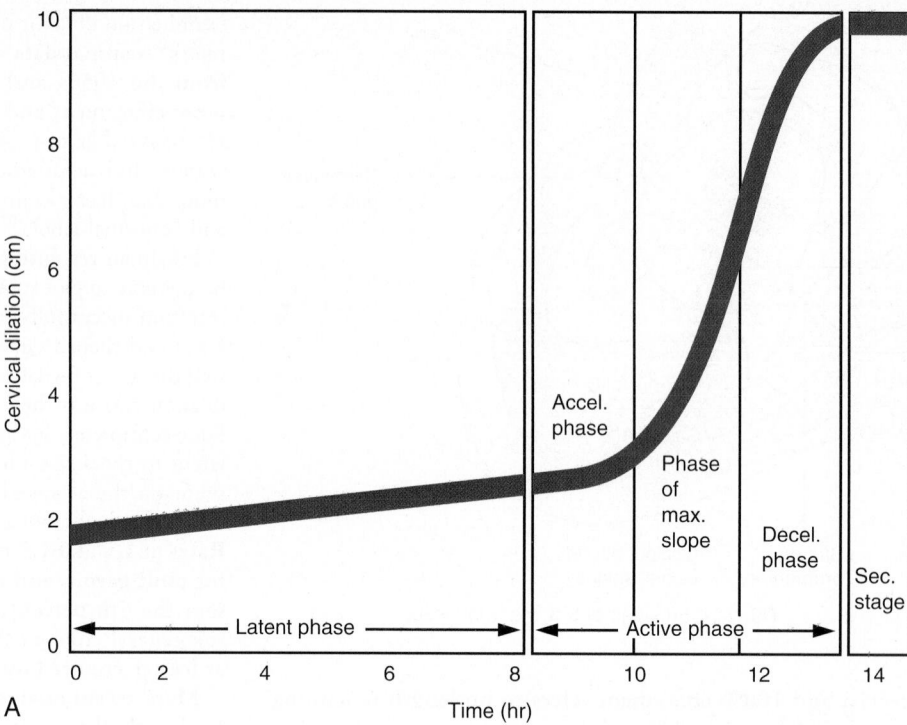

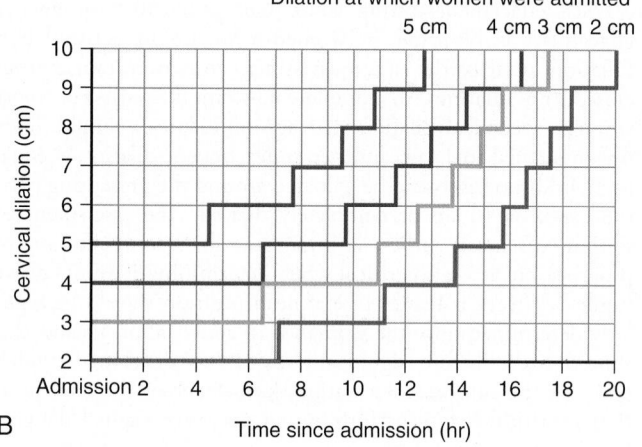

FIG 12-13 **A,** Modern labor graph. Characteristics of the average cervical dilation curve for nulliparous labor. **B,** Zhang labor partogram. The 95th percentiles of cumulative duration of labor from admission among singleton term nulliparous women with spontaneous onset of labor. *Accel.,* acceleration; *Decel.,* deceleration; *Max.,* maximum; *Sec.,* seconds. (**A,** Modified from Friedman EA. *Labor: Clinical Evaluation and Management,* ed 2. Norwalk, CT: Appleton-Century-Crofts; 1978. **B,** From Zhang J, Landy H, Branch D, et al; the Consortium on Safe Labor. Contemporary patterns of spontaneous labor with normal neonatal outcomes. *Obstet Gynecol.* 2010;1116:1281.)

TABLE 12-2	MEDIAN DURATION OF TIME ELAPSED IN HOURS FOR EACH CENTIMETER OF CHANGE IN CERVICAL DILATION IN SPONTANEOUS LABOR STRATIFIED BY PARITY

CERVICAL DILATION (cm)	PARITY 0*	PARITY 1	PARITY ≥2
3-4	1.8 (8.1)	–	–
4-5	1.3 (6.4)	1.4 (7.3)	1.4 (7.0)
5-6	0.8 (3.2)	0.8 (3.4)	0.8 (3.4)
6-7	0.6 (2.2)	0.5 (1.9)	0.5 (1.8)
7-8	0.5 (1.6)	0.4 (1.3)	0.4 (1.2)
8-9	0.5 (1.2)	0.3 (1.0)	0.3 (0.9)
9-10	0.5 (1.8)	0.3 (0.9)	0.3 (0.8)

Modified from Zhang J, Landy H, Branch D, et al. Consortium on safe labor: Contemporary patterns of spontaneous labor with normal neonatal outcomes. *Obstet Gynecol.* 2010;116:1281.
*Median elapsed time in hours (95th percentile). An interval-censored regression model was used to estimate the distribution of time for progression from one centimeter to the next with the assumption of log normal distribution of the labor data.

would be more appropriate to utilize a threshold of 6 cm cervical dilation to define active phase labor onset and that the rate of cervical dilation for nulliparas at the 95th percentile of normal may be greater than the 1 cm per hour previously expected. These are important findings that suggest clinicians using the Friedman dataset to determine the threshold for active labor may be diagnosing active phase arrest prematurely, which could result in unnecessary cesarean deliveries (see Chapter 13).[3,42,45,46]

The labor partogram commonly in use today was based upon the graph introduced in 1964 by Schulman and Ledger,[47] in which labor progression focused on latent and active phase only. Another and perhaps better approach, based upon contemporary data from the Consortium on Safe Labor,[46] is shown in Figure 12-13, along with the modified Friedman curve. **The Zhang partogram (see Fig. 12-13, *B*) graphically depicts the 95th percentile of the duration of labor in hours stratified by cervical dilation on admission. Cervical dilation is not recorded as a continuous measure, and as a result, interval**

| TABLE 12-3 | SUMMARY OF MEANS AND 95TH PERCENTILES FOR DURATION OF FIRST- AND SECOND-STAGE LABOR | |

PARAMETER	MEAN	95TH PERCENTILE
Nulliparas		
Latent labor	7.3-8.6 hr	17-21 hr
First stage	6-13.3 hr	16.6-30 hr
Second stage	36-57 min	122-197 min
Second stage, epidural	79 min	336 min
Multiparas		
Latent labor	4.1-5.3 hr	12-14 hr
First stage	5.7-7.5 hr	12.5-13.7 hr
Second stage	17-19 min	57-81 min
Second stage, epidural	45 min	255 min

Data from references 40-41, 46, and 52-55.

cervical change over time is depicted in a stair-step pattern. The Zhang partogram may be more appropriate for the identification of those parturients with a duration of labor that exceeds the 95th percentile of normal. Its clinical utility, however, has yet to be confirmed and validated.

Factors that affect the duration of labor include parity, maternal body mass index (BMI), fetal position, maternal age, and fetal size. Longer labors are associated with increased maternal BMI,[48] fetal position other than OA,[49] and older maternal age.[5,50,51] Data conflict in regard to the effect of epidural use on the duration of the first stage of labor. Retrospective cohort studies have suggested that epidural use may significantly increase the duration of the first stage of labor.[47,52,53] However, **a Cochrane meta-analysis of 11 RCTs did not identify a statistically significant difference in the mean length of the first stage of labor in women randomized to epidural analgesia compared with those who went without** (average mean difference [MD] 18.51 min; 95% CI, −12.91 to 49.92).[32] Additional studies are needed to confirm the effect of epidural use on the 95th percentile duration for the first stage of normal labor. Table 12-3 summarizes the means and 95th percentile duration of first- and second-stage labor that have been reported.[40,41,46,47,52-55]

Factors significantly associated with a prolonged second stage included induced labor, chorioamnionitis, older maternal age, OP position, delayed pushing, nonblack ethnicity, epidural analgesia, and parity of five or more.[50,56] Of note, Friedman's second-stage lengths are somewhat artificial because most nulliparous women in that era had a forceps delivery once the duration of the second stage reached 2 hours. More recent labor duration data that evaluated women in spontaneous labor without augmentation or operative delivery from multiple countries report similar mean labor durations, which suggests that these normative data are reliable and useful (see Table 12-3). A Cochrane meta-analysis[32] of 13 RCTs confirmed that **epidural use significantly increased the mean duration of the second stage** compared with no epidural (average MD in second stage length with an epidural, 13.66 min; 95% CI, 6.67 to 20.66 min). According to the ACOG/Society for Maternal-Fetal Medicine (SMFM) obstetric care consensus,[57] it is important to consider not just the mean or median duration of the second stage with epidural analgesia but also the 95th percentile duration. In a recent large retrospective cohort study of 33,239 women with term spontaneous vaginal deliveries, **an epidural was associated with an increase in the 95th percentile duration of the second stage in nulliparous women by 94 minutes** (P < .001).[54] **For multiparous women with a spontaneous vaginal delivery, an**

epidural increased the 95th percentile duration of the second stage by 102 minutes (P < .001; see Chapter 16).[54] Determination of the upper limits of time for normal second-stage labor that incorporates epidural use and other more contemporary labor interventions are helpful in identifying normative values for labor duration that are associated with the lowest risk of maternal and neonatal morbidity.[52,53,58]

The third stage of labor is generally short. **In a case series of nearly 13,000 singleton vaginal deliveries at greater than 20 weeks' gestation, the median third-stage duration was 6 minutes and exceeded 30 minutes in only 3% of women.**[59] **However, third stages lasting greater than 30 minutes were associated with significant maternal morbidity that included an increased risk of blood loss greater than 500 mL, a decrease in postpartum hematocrit by greater than or equal to 10%, need for dilation and curettage, and a sixfold increased risk of postpartum hemorrhage.**[59,60] **These data suggest that if spontaneous separation does not occur, manual removal and/or extraction of the placenta should be considered after 30 minutes to reduce the risk of maternal hemorrhage.** The factors associated with a prolonged third stage of labor include preterm delivery, preeclampsia, labor augmentation, nulliparity, maternal age over 35 years, and a second-stage labor duration greater than 2 hours.[61,62] Several strategies to minimize the risk of postpartum hemorrhage for women in the third stage of labor have been recommended and include early administration of a uterotonic agent after delivery of the anterior fetal shoulder, early cord clamping, controlled traction on the umbilical cord, and fundal massage to facilitate early placental separation.[63,64] A Cochrane meta-analysis[63] of seven randomized to quasi-randomized controlled studies found that for a heterogeneous population of women at mixed risk of bleeding, active management of the third stage of labor was associated with a significant reduction in blood loss over 1000 mL (relative risk [RR], 0.34; 95% CI, 0.14 to 0.87) and a lower risk of anemia (hemoglobin [Hgb], <9 g/dL; average RR, 0.50; 95% CI, 0.30 to 0.83). However, a significant reduction in neonatal birthweight was reported, likely due to early cord clamping and reduced time for placental transfusion. In women at low risk for postpartum hemorrhage, active management of labor was not associated with a significant reduction in the risk of maternal hemorrhage (blood loss >500 mL) or maternal anemia (Hgb <9 g/dL) compared with women who were expectantly managed.[63]

Interventions That Affect Normal Labor Outcomes

Various interventions have been suggested to promote normal labor progress, including maternal ambulation and upright maternal positioning during active labor.[65,66] A well-designed randomized trial[65] of over 1000 low-risk women in early labor at 3- to 5-cm cervical dilation compared ambulation with usual care and found no differences in the duration of the first stage, need for oxytocin, use of analgesia, neonatal outcomes, or route of delivery. These results suggest that given appropriate staffing resources and fetal surveillance protocols, walking in the first stage of labor is an option that may be considered for low-risk women. A Cochrane review of 25 randomized to quasi RCTs of considerable heterogeneity found that in low-risk nulliparous women, **upright rather than recumbent positioning during labor was associated with a significantly shorter first stage of labor by 1 hour and 22 minutes** (average MD, −1.36; 95% CI, −2.22 to −0.51), **less epidural use, and** a reduction in the risk of cesarean delivery by 30% (RR, 0.71; 95% CI, 0.54 to 0.94).[66] Women should be encouraged to consider upright positioning in labor, and the potential benefits should be discussed to facilitate informed decision making. In a Cochrane review[67] of 22 trials that involved 15,288 low-risk women randomized to continuous labor support (doula) compared with routine care, **the presence of a labor doula was associated with a significant reduction in the use of analgesia, oxytocin, and operative vaginal delivery** (RR, 0.90; 95% CI, 0.85 to 0.96) **or cesarean delivery** (RR, 0.78; 95% CI, 0.67 to 0.91) **and an increase in personal satisfaction.** These data were compelling enough for doula support to receive an A rating, meaning that it should be recommended for use during labor.[68] Other models of **continuous labor support with a friend or family member should be encouraged** if a doula is unavailable.

The benefits of IV hydration in labor have been less well studied. The use of IV fluids is a routine practice in many labor and delivery units, although its benefit compared with oral hydration has not been well elucidated, and the volume and type of IV fluid that may promote optimal progress in labor is unclear. A Cochrane review[69] of nine randomized trials included studies of considerable heterogeneity. Two trials compared women randomized to receive up to 250 mL/hr of Ringer's lactate solution and oral intake versus oral intake alone. No difference was found in the cesarean delivery rate. However, a reduced duration of labor was reported for women with a vaginal delivery who received Ringer's lactate (MD, −28.86 min; 95% CI, −47.41 to −10.30). Four trials compared rates of IV fluids (125 mL/hr vs. 250 mL/hr) in women whose oral intake was restricted, and a significant reduction in the duration of labor was reported in women who received IV fluid at 250 mL/hr.[69] With regard to the type of IV fluid, in a randomized trial of nulliparas in active labor, IV administration at 125 mL/min of dextrose in normal saline (NS) was associated with a significant reduction in labor length and in second-stage length compared with normal saline.[70] Although **the available data suggest that IV fluid is beneficial in labor,** additional studies are needed to determine the risks and benefits of appropriate oral hydration. Furthermore, the optimal volume of fluid replacement in labor from all sources, oral and IV, is unclear.

Active Management of Labor

Dystocia refers to a lack of progress of labor for any reason, and it is the most common indication for cesarean delivery (CD) in nulliparous women and the second most common indication for CD in multiparous women. In the late 1980s, in an effort to reduce the rapidly rising rate of CD, active management of labor was popularized in the United States based on findings in Ireland, where the routine use of active management was associated with very low rates of CD.[71] **Protocols for active management included (1) admission only when labor was established, evidenced by painful contractions and spontaneous rupture of membranes, 100% effacement, or passage of blood-stained mucus; (2) artificial rupture of membranes on diagnosis of labor; (3) aggressive oxytocin augmentation for labor progress of less than 1 cm/hr with high-dose oxytocin (6 mIU/min initial dose, increased by 6 mIU/min every 15 min to a maximum of 40 mIU/min); and (4) patient education.**[71] Observational data suggested that this management protocol was associated with rates of CD of 5.5% and delivery within 12 hours in 98% of women.[71] Only 41% of the nulliparas

actually required oxytocin augmentation. Multiple nonrandomized studies were subsequently published that attempted to duplicate these results in the United States and Canada.[72-75] Two of these reported a significant reduction in cesarean delivery when compared with historical controls.[72,74] However, in two of three RCTs, no significant decrease in the rate of cesarean delivery was observed with active compared with routine management of labor.[76-77] In the third RCT, the overall CD rate was not significantly different. However, when confounding variables were controlled, CD was significantly lower in the actively managed group.[75] In all randomized trials, labor duration was significantly decreased by a range of 1.7 to 2.7 hours, and neonatal morbidity was not different between groups. **In a recent Cochrane review,[78] a meta-analysis of 11 trials (7753 women) concluded that early oxytocin augmentation in women with spontaneous labor was associated with a significant decrease in CD** (RR, 0.87; 95% CI, 0.77 to 0.99). A meta-analysis of eight trials (4816 women) determined that early amniotomy and oxytocin augmentation was associated with a significantly shortened duration of labor (average MD, 1.28 hr; 95% CI, −1.97 to −0.59).[78] Of note, amniotomy alone did not affect labor length or the rate of CD. This reduction in labor duration has significant cost and bed-management implications, especially for busy labor and delivery units. **Perhaps the most important factor in active management is delaying admission until active labor has been established.**

Second Stage of Labor

Abnormal progress in fetal descent is the dystocia of the second stage. A wide range of mean and 95th percentile second-stage labor durations have been reported for vaginal deliveries and are influenced by parity, presence or absence of epidural analgesia, and local or regional practice patterns (see Table 12-3). According to the summary of a National Institutes of Health (NIH)–sponsored workshop on prevention of the first cesarean, **no specific threshold maximum second-stage duration exists beyond which all women should undergo operative vaginal delivery.**[79] **However, a direct correlation has been found between second-stage duration, adverse maternal outcomes (hemorrhage, infection, perineal lacerations), and the likelihood of a successful vaginal delivery.**[80] A secondary analysis[42] of a multicenter study on fetal pulse oximetry compared second-stage duration with maternal and perinatal outcomes in 4126 nulliparous women. Chorioamnionitis (overall rate, 3.9%), third- and fourth-degree lacerations (overall rate, 8.7%), and uterine atony (overall rate, 3.9%; combined OR, 1.31 to 1.60; 95% CI, 1.14 to 1.86) were significantly increased with longer second-stage duration. Adverse maternal outcomes with longer labor duration in multiparous women have also been reported.[81,82] In regard to the correlation between adverse neonatal outcomes and longer second-stage lengths, the reports are mixed; one study reported a lack of association between neonatal outcomes and the duration of the second stage of labor in nulliparous women.[80,83-85] However, in a study of 43,810 nulliparas in the second stage of labor, **second-stage lengths of greater than 3 hours were associated with increased maternal and neonatal morbidity.**[86] In nulliparous women with an epidural who had a nonoperative vaginal delivery, a prolonged second stage greater than 3 hours was associated with an increased risk of a shoulder dystocia (adjusted OR, 1.62; 95% CI, 1.17 to 1.65), 5-minute Apgar score less than 4 (adjusted OR, 2.58; 95% CI, 1.07 to 6.17), increased risk of neonatal intensive care unit (NICU)

TABLE 12-4	RECOMMENDATIONS FOR 95TH PERCENTILE DURATION FOR THE SECOND STAGE OF LABOR	
		95TH PERCENTILE
Multiparas		
Second stage without an epidural		2 hours
Second stage with an epidural		3 hours
Nulliparas		
Second stage without an epidural		3 hours
Second stage with an epidural		4 hours

Modified from Spong C, Berghella V, Wenstrom K, et al. Preventing the first cesarean delivery: Summary of a joint Eunice Kennedy Shriver National Institute of Child Health and Human Development, Society for Maternal-Fetal Medicine, and American College of Obstetricians and Gynecologists Workshop. *Obstet Gynecol.* 2012;120(5):1181.

admission (adjusted OR, 1.25; 95% CI, 1.02 to 1.53), and neonatal sepsis (adjusted OR, 2.01; 95% CI, 1.39 to 2.91).[86] It should be noted that although these results are significant, the absolute incidence of each event is extremely low. **These findings suggest that the benefits of vaginal delivery with second-stage prolongation must be weighed against possible small but significant increases in neonatal risk.**[80] **Although less frequent, adverse neonatal outcomes for multiparous women with a prolonged second-stage duration have also been reported.**[80-82]

Based upon the available evidence, a workshop convened by the Eunice Kennedy Shriver National Institute of Health Child Health and Human Development (NICHD), ACOG, and SMFM recommend at **least a 3- to 4-hour second-stage duration for nulliparous women and at least a 2- to 3-hour second-stage duration for multiparas, if maternal and fetal conditions permit.**[79] Documentation of patient progress and individualization of care is paramount because longer durations of pushing may also be appropriate. Epidural use or fetal malposition, for example, may prolong the duration of the second stage. Recommended guidelines to identify those with abnormal prolongation of the second stage stratified by parity and epidural use are detailed in Table 12-4. These limits should not be used arbitrarily to justify ending the second stage. They can, however, be used to identify a subset of women who require further evaluation.[83]

As with active labor, poor progress in the second stage may be related to inadequate contractions; therefore initiating oxytocin in the second stage may be effective to facilitate descent if contraction frequency is diminished. If malposition is diagnosed, rotation to OA—either manually or by forceps—may also be indicated in the second stage to facilitate descent. For women with a prolonged second-stage duration, arbitrary time cutoffs are unnecessary if steady progress is observed and fetal status is reassuring.[87-91] Whereas evidence suggests maternal morbidity is significantly higher in women with a prolonged second stage,[83,92] it is important to note that the decision to proceed with an operative vaginal delivery or cesarean delivery simply to shorten the second stage must be based upon weighing the risks of operative delivery against the risks associated with a prolonged second stage and the likelihood of a successful vaginal delivery (see Chapters 13 and 14). **Multiple factors influence the duration of the second stage; these include epidural analgesia, nulliparity, older maternal age, maternal BMI, longer active phase, greater birthweight, and excess maternal weight gain.**[83,92] Modifiable factors that have been evaluated in management of the second

stage include maternal position, decreasing or discontinuation of epidural analgesia (see Chapter 16), and delayed pushing. A Cochrane review of five RCTs that studied the risks and benefits of discontinuation of second-stage epidural analgesia found no difference in route of delivery, operative vaginal delivery rate, or second-stage duration.[93-96] However, a Cochrane review of 38 RCTs to evaluate epidural versus no epidural in labor found that epidural analgesia was clearly associated with an increased duration of the second stage of labor (MD, 13.66 min; 95% CI, 6.67 to 20.66) and rate of operative delivery (OR, 1.42; 95% CI, 1.28 to 1.57).[32,95,97] A recent retrospective review[98] of second-stage durations for 4605 women reported a 60-minute increase in the median duration of second-stage labor for nulliparas with an epidural compared with those without. In women who had a vaginal delivery, the 95th percentile duration of the second stage was 95 minutes longer for nulliparas with an epidural and 101 minutes longer for multiparas with an epidural compared with those who went without an epidural ($P < .001$). Delayed pushing was compared with immediate pushing in the second stage in nulliparas with epidural analgesia to determine whether this strategy would reduce the need for operative delivery.[97,99-101] It has been suggested that delaying pushing until the woman feels the urge to push would maximize maternal pushing efforts, reduce maternal exhaustion, and decrease the risk of operative vaginal delivery.

A meta-analysis of 12 RCTs found that delayed pushing was associated with an increased rate of vaginal delivery. However, this benefit was not statistically significant among the quality studies reviewed.[97,99-102] Delayed pushing prolonged the duration of the second stage (weighted MD, 56.92 min; 95% CI, 42.19 to 71.64) and shortened the duration of active pushing (weighted MD, 21.98 min; 95% CI, −31.29 to −12.68).[102] However, no significant difference was found in the operative vaginal delivery rate.[102] Only one trial reported a significant decrease in midpelvic operative deliveries.[99] Risks associated with delayed pushing have also been reported. In a retrospective evaluation of 5290 term multiparous and nulliparous women, delayed pushing was associated with a statistically significant increase in cesarean and operative delivery rates, increased maternal fever, and a significant decrease in arterial cord pH.[103,104] **Data suggest that delayed pushing is not associated with fewer cesarean or operative deliveries and may have maternal risks. Additional studies are needed to determine whether delayed pushing is associated with increased neonatal risk.**

Finally, the effect of maternal position in the second stage has been evaluated.[105,106] A Cochrane review[107] of five RCTs evaluated the effect of any upright position compared with recumbent positioning in the second stage of labor on route of delivery and duration of labor. No statistically significant difference between groups was observed for operative delivery, duration of second stage, or neonatal outcome.[107] A significant increase in the percent of women with an intact perineum in the upright group was identified[106]; therefore **nonrecumbent positioning in the second stage should be considered.**

SPONTANEOUS VAGINAL DELIVERY

Preparation for delivery should take into account the patient's parity, the progression of labor, fetal presentation, and any labor complications. Among women for whom delivery complications are anticipated (risk factors for shoulder dystocia or multiple gestation), transfer to a larger and better equipped delivery room, removal of the foot of the bed, and delivery in the lithotomy position may be appropriate. If no complications are anticipated, delivery can be accomplished with the mother in her preferred position. Common positions include the lateral (Sims) position or the partial sitting position.

The goals of clinical assistance at spontaneous delivery are the reduction of maternal trauma, prevention of fetal injury, and initial support of the newborn. When the fetal head crowns and delivery is imminent, gentle pressure should be used to maintain flexion of the fetal head and to control delivery, potentially protecting against perineal injury. Once the fetal head is delivered, external rotation (restitution) is allowed. If a shoulder dystocia is anticipated, it is appropriate to proceed directly with gentle downward traction of the fetal head before restitution occurs. During restitution, nuchal umbilical cord loops should be identified and reduced; in rare cases in which simple reduction is not possible, the cord can be doubly clamped and transected. The anterior shoulder should then be delivered by gentle downward traction in concert with maternal expulsive efforts; the posterior shoulder is delivered by upward traction. These movements should be performed with the minimal force possible to avoid perineal injury and traction injuries to the brachial plexus.

No evidence shows that DeLee suction reduces the risk of meconium aspiration syndrome in the presence of meconium; thus this should not be performed.[108] For a vigorous infant, the ACOG Committee on Obstetric Practice and the American Academy of Pediatrics (AAP) no longer recommend routine suctioning in the presence of meconium. If the infant is depressed, and meconium staining is evident, intubation and visualization of meconium or other foreign material below the vocal cords is recommended and should be performed by appropriately trained providers per AAP guidelines.[109]

The timing of cord clamping is usually dictated by convenience and is commonly performed immediately after delivery. However, an ongoing debate exists about the benefits and risks to the newborn of late cord clamping. A Cochrane review of 15 RCTs that compared late (>2 minutes) and immediate cord clamping in term infants showed a significant increase in infant hematocrit, ferritin, and stored iron at 2 to 6 months with no significant increase in the risk of maternal hemorrhage.[110,111] However, a significant increase was also seen in neonatal polycythemia and treatment for neonatal jaundice in the delayed group. A Cochrane review[112] of 15 RCTs to compare late (>30 seconds) to immediate cord clamping in preterm infants (<37 weeks' gestation) showed significant decreases in anemia that required transfusion, intraventricular hemorrhage (IVH), and necrotizing enterocolitis in infants with delayed clamping. Those infants who had their cords clamped later were also noted to have a higher bilirubin levels. No significant difference was reported in the risk of grade 3 or 4 IVH or interventricular leukomalacia, primarily due to considerable heterogeneity among the studies.[112] In 2012, ACOG issued a committee opinion affirming the practice of delayed cord clamping for preterm infants in light of the up to 50% reduction in the risk of IVH reported for these infants when delayed cord clamping is performed.[113] However, for term infants, ACOG determined that evidence was insufficient to either confirm or refute the benefits of delayed cord clamping. Additional studies are needed to determine barriers to implementation of delayed cord clamping in preterm infants and to further determine the benefits and risks of this practice for term infants in resource-rich locations.[114]

If possible, the steps described here are best done with the infant on the mother's abdomen. Initially, the infant should be wiped dry and kept warm while any mucus remaining in the airway is suctioned. Keeping the infant warm is particularly important, and because heat is lost quickly from the head, placing a hat on the infant is appropriate. After clamping of the cord, the vigorous term infant should be placed on the mother's bare skin if at all possible. Early *skin-to-skin contact* (SSC) refers to the placement of the naked infant in a prone position onto the mother's bare chest and abdomen near the breast with the infant's side and back covered by blankets or towels.[115] Early SSC is recommended for the healthy term newborn immediately after vaginal delivery and as soon as possible after cesarean delivery by ACOG, the AAP, and the Baby-Friendly Health Initiative developed by the World Health Organization.[116,117] Meta-analysis of data from RCTs (13 trials, 702 participants) suggests that immediate or early SSC increases the likelihood of breastfeeding initiation at 1 to 4 months (RR 1.27; 95% CI, 1.06 to 1.53) and results in higher blood glucose at 75 to 90 min of life compared with standard care (MD, 10.56 mg/dL; 95% CI, 8.40 to 12.72).[118] Positive effects of SSC on maternal-infant bonding, breastfeeding duration, cardiorespiratory stability, and body temperature have also been demonstrated.[118-120] The term *Kangaroo care* refers to a model of postdelivery care that includes continuous SSC contact and exclusive breastfeeding for low birthweight (LBW) infants, and it was originally promoted as an alternative to incubators in resource-poor settings. A meta-analysis of the RCTs identified a significant reduction in neonatal mortality, nosocomial infection and sepsis, and hypothermia as well as improvements in measures of infant growth, breastfeeding, and mother-infant attachment with kangaroo care compared with conventional methods for LBW infants.[121] Additional prospective RCTs are needed to further characterize the benefits and limitations, if any, of SSC and kangaroo care in term and stable LBW infants; in resource-rich, compared with resource-poor, settings; and after cesarean delivery.

DELIVERY OF THE PLACENTA AND FETAL MEMBRANES

The third stage of labor can be managed either passively or actively. *Passive management* is characterized by clamping of the cord once spontaneous pulsations have ceased and delivery of the placenta by gravity or spontaneously, without manipulation of the uterus or traction on the cord. Placental separation is heralded by lengthening of the umbilical cord and a gush of blood from the vagina, signifying separation of the placenta from the uterine wall. With passive management, uterotonic medications are not given until after delivery of the placenta. With *active management* of the third stage, uterotonic medication is administered shortly after delivery of the baby but prior to delivery of the placenta. Controlled umbilical cord traction and countertraction are used to support the uterus until the placenta separates and is delivered, followed by uterine massage after delivery of the placenta. Two techniques of controlled cord traction are commonly used to facilitate separation and delivery of the placenta: in the *Brandt-Andrews maneuver*, a hand pressed against the abdomen secures the uterine fundus to prevent uterine inversion, while the other hand exerts sustained downward traction on the umbilical cord; with the *Créde maneuver,* the cord is fixed with the lower hand, and while the uterine fundus is secured and sustained, upward traction is applied by a hand pressed against the abdomen. Care should be taken to avoid evulsion of the cord.

Implementation of active management strategies in the third stage of labor can significantly decrease the risk of postpartum hemorrhage. In a meta-analysis of three RCTs to compare active to expectant management, subjects randomized to active management were 66% less likely to have postpartum hemorrhage (estimated blood loss [EBL] ≥1000 mL; RR, 0.34; 95% CI, 0.14 to 0.87).[122,123] Active management of the third stage of labor is recommended by ACOG District II and the California Maternal Quality Care Collaborative (CMQCC) as an integral component of multifaceted perinatal quality initiatives to reduce the severe maternal morbidity and mortality that results from obstetric hemorrhage. Active management of the third stage of labor specifically includes administration of dilute IV oxytocin or 10 units of intramuscular oxytocin after delivery of the fetus and prior to delivery of the placenta (ACOG District II). In the CMQCC obstetric hemorrhage protocol, additional components of the active management strategy include umbilical cord clamping at or prior to 2 minutes after delivery, controlled cord traction to facilitate delivery of the placenta, followed by fundal massage to facilitate uterine involution (CMQCC).

After delivery, the placenta, umbilical cord, and fetal membranes should be examined. Placental weight (excluding membranes and cord) varies with fetal weight, with a ratio of approximately 1:6. Abnormally large placentae are associated with such conditions as hydrops fetalis and congenital syphilis. **Inspection and palpation of the placenta should include the fetal and maternal surfaces and may reveal areas of fibrosis, infarction, or calcification.** Although each of these conditions may be seen in the normal term placenta, extensive lesions should prompt histologic examination. Adherent clots on the maternal placental surface may indicate recent placental abruption; however, their absence does not exclude the diagnosis. A missing placental cotyledon or a membrane defect suggestive of a missing succenturiate lobe also suggests retention of a portion of placenta and should prompt further clinical evaluation. **Routine manual exploration of the uterus after delivery is unnecessary unless retained products of conception or a postpartum hemorrhage is suspected.**

The site of insertion of the umbilical cord into the placenta should be noted. Abnormal insertions include *marginal insertion,* in which the cord inserts into the edge of the placenta, and *membranous insertion,* in which the vessels of the umbilical cord course through the membranes before attachment to the placental disc. The cord should be inspected for length; the correct number of umbilical vessels, normally two arteries and one vein; true knots; hematomas; and strictures. The average cord length is about 50 to 60 cm. A single umbilical artery discovered on pathologic examination is associated with an increased risk of fetal growth restriction and up to a 6.77-fold higher risk of one or more major congenital anomalies (OR, 6.77; 95% CI, 5.7 to 8.06).[124-127] Therefore this finding should be relayed to the attending neonatologist or pediatrician, and any abnormalities of the placenta or cord should be noted in the mother's chart.

EPISIOTOMY AND PERINEAL INJURY AND REPAIR

Following delivery of the placenta, the vagina and perineum should be carefully examined for evidence of injury. If a laceration is seen, its length and position should be noted and repair should be initiated. Adequate analgesia, either regional or local, is essential for repair. Special attention should be paid to repair of the perineal body, the external anal sphincter, and the rectal mucosa (see Chapter 18). Failure to recognize and repair rectal injury can lead to serious long-term morbidity, most notably fecal incontinence. The cervix should be inspected for lacerations if an operative delivery was performed or when bleeding is significant with or after delivery.

Perineal injuries, either spontaneous or with the episiotomy, are the most common complications of spontaneous or operative vaginal deliveries. **A *first-degree tear* is defined as a superficial tear confined to the epithelial layer; it may or may not need to be repaired depending on size, location, and amount of bleeding. A *second-degree tear* extends into the perineal body but not into the external anal sphincter. A *third-degree tear* involves superficial or deep injury to the external anal sphincter, whereas a *fourth-degree tear* extends completely through the sphincter and the rectal mucosa. All second-, third-, and fourth-degree tears should be repaired** (see Chapter 18). Significant morbidity is associated with third- and fourth-degree tears, including risk of flatus and stool incontinence, rectovaginal fistula, infection, and pain (see Chapter 14). Primary approximation of perineal lacerations affords the best opportunity for functional repair, especially if rectal sphincter injury is evident. The external anal sphincter should be repaired by direct apposition or overlapping the cut ends and securing them using interrupted sutures.

Episiotomy is an incision into the perineal body made during the second stage of labor to facilitate delivery. It is by definition at least a second-degree tear. Episiotomy can be classified into two broad categories, midline and mediolateral. **With a *midline episiotomy,* a vertical midline incision is made from the posterior fourchette toward the rectum** (Fig. 12-14). After adequate analgesia has been achieved, either local or regional, straight Mayo scissors are generally used to perform the episiotomy. Care should be taken to displace the perineum from the fetal head. The size of the incision depends on the length of the perineum but is generally approximately half of the length of the perineum and should be extended vertically up the vaginal mucosa for a distance of 2 to 3 cm. Every effort should be made to avoid direct injury to the anal sphincter. **Complications of midline episiotomy include increased blood loss, especially if the incision is made too early; fetal injury; and localized pain. With a *mediolateral episiotomy,* an incision is made at a 45-degree angle from the inferior portion of the hymeneal ring** (Fig. 12-15). The length of the incision is less critical than with midline episiotomy, but longer incisions require lengthier repair. The side to which the episiotomy is performed is usually dictated by the dominant hand of the practitioner. **Because such incisions appear to be moderately protective against severe perineal trauma, if an episiotomy is needed, the mediolateral episiotomy is the procedure of choice for women with inflammatory bowel disease** (see Chapter 48) **because of the critical need to prevent rectal injury.** Historically, it was believed that episiotomy improved outcome by reducing pressure on the fetal head, protecting the maternal perineum from

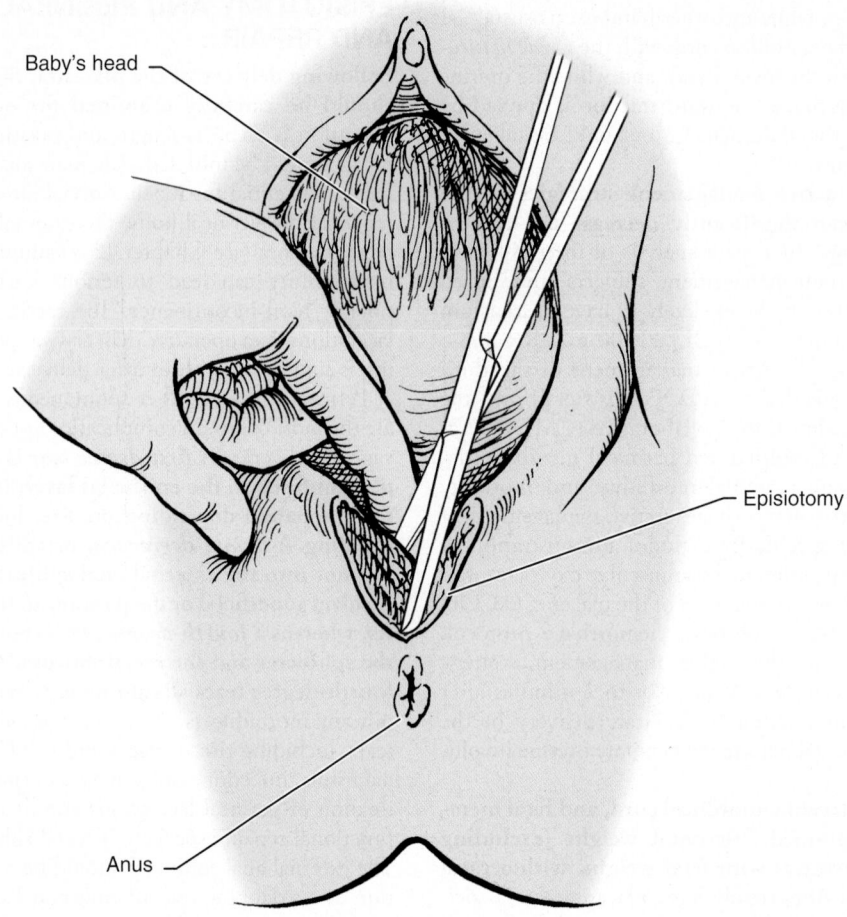

Baby's head

Episiotomy

Anus

FIG 12-14 Cutting a midline episiotomy.

extensive tearing and preventing subsequent pelvic relaxation. However, consistent data since the late 1980s confirm that *midline episiotomy* does not protect the perineum from further tearing, and data do not show that episiotomy improves neonatal outcome.[128,129] **Midline episiotomy was associated with a significant increase in third- and fourth-degree lacerations in spontaneous vaginal delivery in nulliparous women with both spontaneous and operative vaginal delivery.[128-135] Episiotomy had the highest odds ratio (OR, 3.2; CI, 2.73 to 3.80) for anal sphincter laceration in a large study of nulliparous women when compared with other risk factors, including forceps delivery.[136]** Few papers reported that midline episiotomy was associated with no difference in fourth-degree tears compared with no episiotomy.[137] Randomized trials that compared routine to indicated use of episiotomy report a 23% reduction in perineal lacerations that required repair in the indicated group (11% to 35%).[138] Finally, **a recent Cochrane review of eight RCTs that compared restrictive to routine use of episiotomy showed a significant reduction of severe perineal tears, suturing, and healing complications in the restrictive group.[139]** Although the restrictive episiotomy group had a significantly higher incidence of anterior tears, no difference was found in pain measures between the groups. All of these findings were similar whether midline or mediolateral episiotomy was used. **Based on the lack of consistent evidence that episiotomy is of benefit, routine episiotomy has no role in modern obstetrics.[128,129,139-141]** In fact, a recent evidence-based review recommended that episiotomy should be avoided if possible, based on U.S. Preventive Task Force quality of evidence.[68] Based on these data and the ACOG recommendations,[141] rates of midline episiotomy have decreased, although episiotomies are performed in 10% to 17% of deliveries, which suggests that elective episiotomy continues to be performed.[131-138] In one study, decreasing episiotomy rates from 87% in 1976 to 10% in 1994 were associated with a parallel decrease in the rates of third- or fourth-degree lacerations (9% to 4%) and an increase in the incidence of an intact perineum (10% to 26%).[131]

The relationship of episiotomy to subsequent pelvic relaxation and incontinence has been evaluated, and no studies suggest that episiotomy reduces risk of incontinence. Fourth-degree tears are clearly associated with future incontinence,[142] and neither midline nor mediolateral episiotomy is associated with a reduction in incontinence.[143] **No data suggest that episiotomy protects the woman from later incontinence; therefore avoidance of fourth-degree tearing should be a priority.**

If an episiotomy is deemed indicated, the decision of which type to perform rests on their individual risks. It does appear that mediolateral episiotomy is associated with fewer

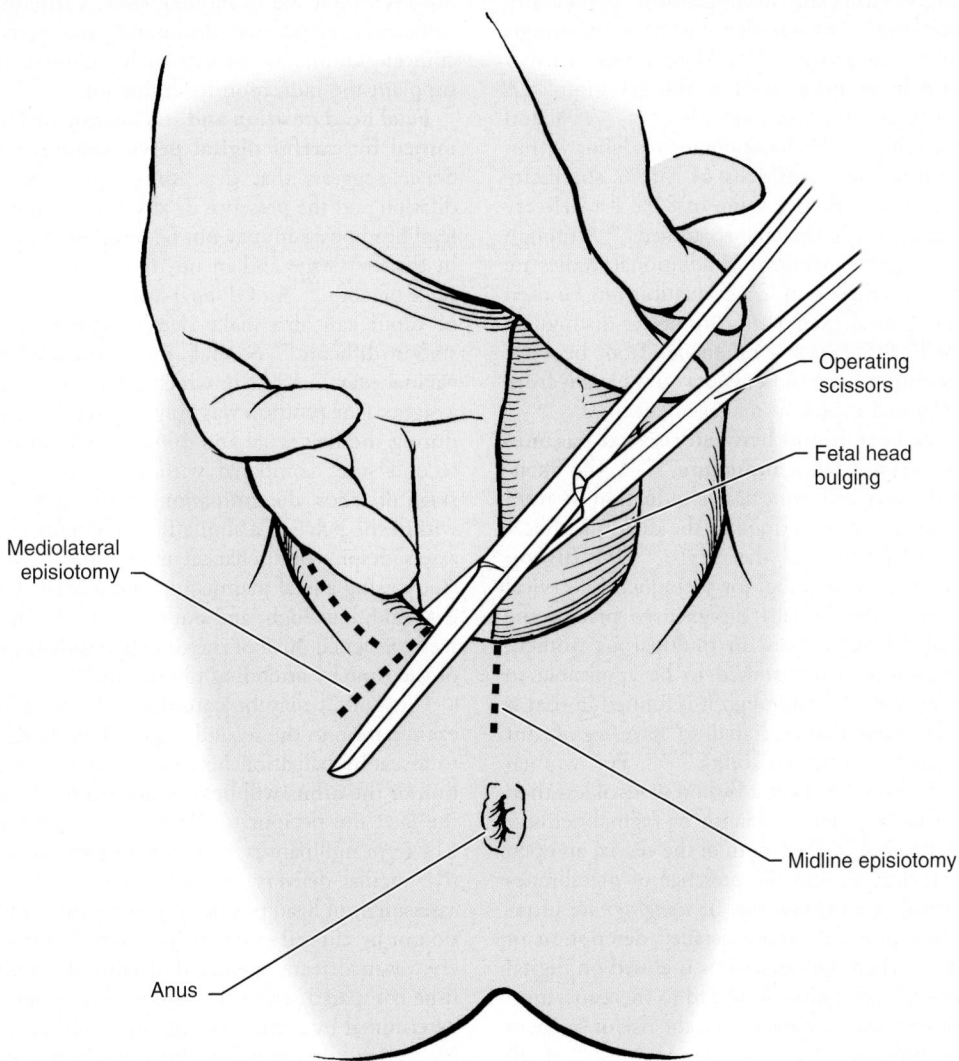

FIG 12-15 Cutting a mediolateral episiotomy.

fourth-degree tears compared with midline episiotomy.[144-146] However, other studies do not show benefit of mediolateral over midline episiotomy for future prolapse.[143] Chronic complications such as unsatisfactory cosmetic results and inclusions within the scar may be more common with mediolateral episiotomies, and blood loss is greater. Finally, it must be remembered that neither episiotomy type has been shown to reduce severe perineal tears compared with no episiotomy.

Although there is no role for *routine* episiotomy, *indicated* episiotomy should be performed in select situations, and providers should receive training in the skill.[137] Potential indications for episiotomy include the need to expedite delivery in the setting of FHR abnormalities or for relief of shoulder dystocia.

ULTRASOUND IN LABOR AND DELIVERY

Ultrasound is a useful adjunct to the clinical examination in the peripartum period. Sonographic findings may be used to confirm the clinical impression of fetal lie and presentation and gestational age when needed. In women with vaginal bleeding, ultrasound can identify placental location and rule out placenta previa prior to a digital examination of the cervix. In women with twins, ultrasound estimation of fetal lie and weight are an integral component of patient counseling regarding mode of delivery for the first and second twin. In women with a breech-presenting fetus at term, ultrasound can be used to confirm presentation, placental location, and amniotic fluid volume prior to patient counseling and performance of a breech version. In the third stage of labor, ultrasound may be used to assist with removal of the placenta for those with a prolonged third stage and/or to better facilitate uterine evacuation during a postpartum hemorrhage.

The association between sonographic cervical length (CL) at term and labor outcome has also been studied. An evaluation of weekly CL measurements between 37 and 40 weeks in term nulliparous women found that cervical shortening could only be documented in 50% of the participants prior to onset of spontaneous labor and that 25% of the participants had a CL of more than 30 mm within the last 48 hours prior to delivery.[147] CL measurements obtained between 37 and 38 weeks' gestation were found to have a low sensitivity and negative predictive value for spontaneous labor prior to 41 weeks' gestation. In an evaluation of a more ethnically heterogeneous population, however, a significant correlation was identified between a single CL measurement obtained between 37 and 40 weeks, delivery within 7 days, and delivery prior to 41 weeks' gestation.[148] A term cervical length of 25 mm had a sensitivity of 77.5% and a negative predictive value 84.7% for spontaneous labor within 7 days. A CL of 30 mm had a sensitivity of 73.1%, specificity of 40.7%, and a positive predictive value of 81% for delivery prior to 41 weeks' gestation in the cohort studied.[148] Although these data are interesting and encouraging, additional studies are needed to determine whether term CL evaluation can be used as an adjunct to the clinical examination to better distinguish those who are most likely to have spontaneous labor between 37 and 40 weeks' gestation from those who would benefit from reassurance and continued expectant management.

An association has been found between cervical parameters at term and successful labor induction.[149-151] The likelihood of a vaginal delivery following labor induction at term depends in part upon maternal parity and the dilation, effacement, consistency, and position of the cervix.[149] The **Bishop score** is the most commonly used tool for preinduction cervical assessment. Although it was initially designed to predict the likelihood of vaginal delivery success in multiparous women, the Bishop score has been demonstrated to be applicable to nulliparous women as well,[149-150] although it is limited in that it is subjective and has been demonstrated to have significant interobserver and intraobserver variability.[151-153] For women undergoing labor induction, however, a Bishop score of less than 6 has been reported to be a poor predictor of vaginal delivery and labor induction success.[151] The length of the cervix, an open or closed internal cervical os, and the presence of membranes within the endocervical canal (*funneling*, or *wedging*) are ultrasound parameters that provide a more detailed description of the cervix, particularly when the external os is closed on digital examination. However, data conflict in regard to the association between sonographic cervical parameters and the risk of cesarean delivery with labor induction.[151,154] A meta-analysis[155] of 20 prospective trials that evaluated the association between preinduction CL and successful labor induction found that a shorter CL was associated with successful induction (likelihood ratio of a positive test, 1.66; 95% CI, 1.20 to 2.31), and a longer CL was associated with a failed induction (likelihood ratio of a negative test, 0.51; 95% CI, 0.39 to 0.67). However, subgroup analysis of seven studies found that a specific preinduction CL of less than 30 mm was not predictive of vaginal delivery. A subgroup analysis of 10 studies found that CL was equivalent to Bishop score with regard to prediction of labor induction success, route of delivery, vaginal delivery within 24 hours, and achievement of the active stage of labor. A more recent meta-analysis[156] of 31 studies, including 12 studies published after 2006, found that in nulliparous women undergoing induction of labor, a CL of more than 30 mm best identified those at high risk for cesarean delivery, with a sensitivity of 0.70, specificity of 0.74, positive likelihood ratio of 2.7, and a negative likelihood ratio of 0.40. CL of more than 30 mm performed as well as a Bishop score less than 6 with regard to its sensitivity and specificity in nulliparous women.[150] A long cervix (>30 mm) and the absence of funneling were found to approximately double the odds of failed induction, whereas a short cervix and funneling decreased the odds of failed induction by up to 50%. CL and the assessment of wedging (funneling) can be easily performed and can provide a more objective description of the cervix;

however, these are of limited value. Currently, we do not have sufficient evidence that ultrasound parameters should replace the clinical examination or that such parameters should be used to supplant the indication for induction.

Fetal head position and station during labor are best determined by careful digital pelvic examination. However, evidence suggests that depending upon the degree of cervical dilation and the presence or absence of caput, an assignment of fetal head position may not be possible in up to 61% of patients in the first stage and in up to 31% of patients in the second stage of labor.[157] An OP fetal head presentation and the presence of caput can also make determination of fetal position and station difficult.[158] Several studies reported that during digital vaginal examinations in which a fetal head position is clinically assigned, the position was only accurate 50% to 60% of the time during the first stage and 30% to 40% of the time during the second stage compared with ultrasound.[158-161] In the second stage of labor, determination of the station of the fetal head within the pelvis is a similarly challenging clinical parameter to assess despite our reliance upon bony pelvic landmarks. In a study using a fetal mannequin and a pelvic trainer, it was found that mid, low, high, and outlet pelvic classifications were incorrectly assigned 30% of the time by resident physicians and 34% of the time by attending physicians.[162]

Ultrasound may be considered as an adjunct to the clinical examination in the second stage, when head position is difficult to assess by palpation because of caput. Sonographic visualization of the orbits will help to determine the general position of the face and occiput within the maternal pelvis. In a study of 514 term nulliparous women who required second-stage operative vaginal delivery, subjects were randomized to predelivery assessment of head position by ultrasound and clinical examination or by clinical examination alone.[163] Head position at delivery was incorrectly predicted by clinical examination 20% of the time compared with a 1.6% error rate when head position was determined by clinical examination and ultrasound ($P < .001$). No statistically significant difference was found between groups in the maternal or neonatal outcomes studied. Additional trials are needed to determine whether ultrasound-based evaluations of fetal position and station have sufficient sensitivity to influence clinical decision making regarding second-stage labor and route of delivery.[156,158,163,164]

KEY POINTS

◆ Labor is a clinical diagnosis that includes regular painful uterine contractions and progressive cervical effacement and dilation.

◆ The fetus likely plays a key role in determining the onset of labor, although the precise mechanism by which this occurs is not clear.

◆ Labor has three stages: the first stage is from labor onset until full dilation of the cervix, the second stage is from full cervical dilation until delivery of the baby, and the third stage begins with delivery of the baby and ends with delivery of the placenta. The first stage of labor is divided into two phases: the first is the *latent phase* and the second is the *active phase*.

◆ Active labor is diagnosed as the time when the slope of cervical change increases, which is more difficult to identify in nulliparas and may not occur until at least 6 cm dilation.

♦ The ability of the fetus to successfully negotiate the pelvis during labor and delivery is dependent on the complex interaction of three variables: uterine force, the fetus, and the maternal pelvis.

♦ Labor length is affected by many variables that include parity, epidural use, fetal position, fetal size, and maternal BMI.

♦ Upright, rather than recumbent, positioning during labor was associated with a significantly shorter first stage of labor, less epidural use, and a reduction in the risk of cesarean delivery by 30%.

♦ The presence of a labor doula was associated with a significant reduction in the use of analgesia, oxytocin, and operative vaginal delivery or cesarean delivery and an increase in patient satisfaction.

♦ Routine midline episiotomy is associated with a significant increase in the incidence of severe perineal trauma and should be avoided.

♦ Active management of the third stage of labor was associated with a significant reduction in blood loss greater than1000 mL and therefore a lower risk of maternal anemia.

♦ Ultrasound may be a useful adjunct to the clinical examination in the peripartum period.

REFERENCES

1. Liao J, Buhimschi C, Norwitz E. Normal labor: mechanism and duration. *Obstet Gynecol Clin North Am.* 2005;32:145.
2. Challis J, Gibb W. Control of parturition. *Prenat Neonat Med.* 1996;1:283.
3. Garfield R, Blennerhassett M, Miller S. Control of myometrial contractility: role and regulation of gap junctions. *Oxf Rev Reprod Biol.* 1988;10:436.
4. Liggins G. Initiation of labour. *Neonatology.* 1989;55:366.
5. Nathanielsz P. Comparative studies on the initiation of labor. *Eur J Obstet Gynecol Reprod Biol.* 1998;78:127.
6. Lockwood C. The initiation of parturition at term. *Obstet Gynecol Clin North Am.* 2004;31(4):935.
7. Makino S, Zaragoza D, Mitchell B, et al. Prostaglandin F2alpha and its receptor as activators of human decidua. *Semin Reprod Med.* 2007;25(1):60.
8. Beshay V, Carr B, Rainey W. The human fetal adrenal gland, corticotropin-releasing hormone, and parturition. *Semin Reprod Med.* 2007;25(1):14.
9. Pieber D, Allport V, Hills F, et al. Interactions between progesterone receptor isoforms in myometrial cells in human labour. *Mol Hum Reprod.* 2001;7:875.
10. Mesiano S, Chan E, Fitter J, et al. Progesterone withdrawal and estrogen activation in human parturition are coordinated by progesterone receptor A expression in the myometrium. *J Clin Endocrinol Metab.* 2002;87:2924.
11. Zakar T, Hertelendy F. Progesterone withdrawal: key to parturition. *Am J Obstet Gynecol.* 2007;196(4):289.
12. Oh S, Kim C, Park I, et al. Progesterone receptor isoform (A/B) ratio of human fetal membranes increases during term parturition. *Am J Obstet Gynecol.* 2005;193:1156.
13. Messano S. Myometrial progesterone responsiveness. *Semin Reprod Med.* 2007;25:5-13.
14. Honnebier M, Nathanielsz P. Primate parturition and the role of the maternal circadian system. *Eur J Obstet Gynecol Reprod Biol.* 1994;55:193.
15. Zeeman G, Khan-Dawood F, Dawood M. Oxytocin and its receptor in pregnancy and parturition: current concepts and clinical implications. *Obstet Gynecol.* 1997;89:873.
16. Fuchs A, Fuchs F. Endocrinology of human parturition: a review. *Br J Obstet Gynaecol.* 1984;9:948.
17. Dawood M, Wang C, Gupta R, et al. Fetal contribution to oxytocin in human labor. *Obstet Gynecol.* 1978;52:205.
18. Fuchs A. The role of oxytocin in parturition. In: Huszar G, ed. *The Physiology and Biochemistry of the Uterus in Pregnancy and Labour.* Boca Raton, FL: CRC Press; 1986:163.
19. Fuchs A, Fuchs F, Husslein P, et al. Oxytocin receptors and human parturition: a dual role for oxytocin in the initiation of labor. *Obstet Gynecol Surv.* 1982;37:567.
20. Fuchs A, Fuchs F, Husslein P, Soloff M. Oxytocin receptors in the human uterus during pregnancy and parturition. *Am J Obstet Gynecol.* 1984; 150:734.
21. Husslein P, Fuchs A, Fuchs F. Oxytocin and the initiation of human parturition. I. Prostaglandin release during induction of labor by oxytocin. *Am J Obstet Gynecol.* 1981;141:688.
22. Fuchs A, Husslein P, Fuchs F. Oxytocin and the initiation of human parturition. II. Stimulation of prostaglandin production in human decidua by oxytocin. *Am J Obstet Gynecol.* 1981;141:694.
23. Blanks AM, Thornton S. The role of oxytocin in parturition. *Br J Obstet Gynecol.* 2003;110(suppl 20):46.
24. Blanks AM, Shmygol A, Thornton S, et al. Regulation of oxytocin receptors and oxytocin receptor signaling. *Semin Reprod Med.* 2007;25(1): 52-59.
25. Macones G, Hankins G, Spong C, et al. The 2008 National Institute of Child Health and Human Development workshop report on electronic fetal monitoring: update on definitions, interpretation, and research guidelines. *Obstet Gynecol.* 2008;112:661.
26. Caldeyro-Barcia R, Sica-Blanco Y, Poseiro J, et al. A quantitative study of the action of synthetic oxytocin on the pregnant human uterus. *J Pharmacol Exp Ther.* 1957;121:18.
27. Miller F. Uterine activity, labor management, and perinatal outcome. *Semin Perinatol.* 1978;2:181.
28. American College of Obstetricians and Gynecologists. *Fetal Macrosomia.* Washington, DC: American College of Obstetricians and Gynecologists; 2000.
29. Rossi A, Mullin P, Prefumo F. Prevention, management, and outcomes of macrosomia: a systematic review of literature and meta-analysis. *Obstet Gynecol Surv.* 2013;68(10):702.
30. Friedman E, Kroll B. Computer analysis of labor progression. II. Distribution of data and limits of normal. *J Reprod Med.* 1971;6:20.
31. Cheng Y, Shaffer B, Caughey A. Associated factors and outcomes of persistent occiput posterior position: a retrospective cohort study from 1976 to 2001. *J Matern Fetal Neonatal Med.* 2006;19(9):563.
32. Anim-Somuah M, Smyth R, Jones L. Epidural versus non-epidural or no analgesia in labour. *Cochrane Database Syst Rev.* 2011;(12):Art. No.: CD000331.
33. Piper J, Bolling D, Newton E. The second stage of labor: factors influencing duration. *Am J Obstet Gynecol.* 1991;165:976.
34. Joyce D, Giwa-Osagie F, Stevenson G. Role of pelvimetry in active management of labour. *Br Med J.* 1975;4:505.
35. Morris C, Heggie J, Acton C. Computed tomography pelvimetry: accuracy and radiation dose compared with conventional pelvimetry. *Australas Radiol.* 1993;37:186.
36. Maharaj D. Assessing cephalopelvic disproportion: back to the basics. *Obstet Gynecol Surv.* 2010;65(6):387.
37. Zaretsky M, Alexander J, McIntire D, et al. Magnetic resonance imaging pelvimetry and the prediction of labor dystocia. *Obstet Gynecol.* 2005;106(5 Pt 1):919.
38. Jeyabalan A, Larkin R, Landers D. Vaginal breech deliveries selected using computed tomographic pelvimetry may be associated with fewer adverse outcomes. *J Matern Fetal Neonatal Med.* 2005;17:381.
39. Caldwell W, Moloy H. Anatomical variations in the female pelvis and their effect in labor, with a suggested classification. *Am J Obstet Gynecol.* 1933;26:479.
40. Friedman E. Primigravid labor. *Obstet Gynecol.* 1955;6:567.
41. Friedman E. Labor in multiparas; a graphicostatistical analysis. *Obstet Gynecol.* 1956;8:691.
42. Rouse D, Owen J, Savage K, et al. Active phase labor arrest: revisiting the 2-hour minimum. *Obstet Gynecol.* 2001;98:550.
43. Zhang J, Troendle JF, Yancey MK. Reassessing the labor curve in nulliparous women. *Am J Obstet Gynecol.* 2002;187:824.
44. Peisner DB, Rosen MG. Transition from latent to active labor. *Obstet Gynecol.* 1986;68:441.
45. Zhang J, Troendle J, Mikolajczyk R, et al. The natural history of the normal first stage of labor. *Obstet Gynecol.* 2010;115:705.
46. Zhang J, Landy H, Branch D, et al. Consortium on Safe Labor. Contemporary patterns of spontaneous labor with normal neonatal outcomes. *Obstet Gynecol.* 2010;116:1281.

47. Schulman H, Ledger W. Practical applications of the graphic portrayal of labor. *Obstet Gynecol.* 1964;23:442.

48. Vahratian A, Zhang J, Troendle J, et al. Maternal prepregnancy overweight and obesity and the pattern of labor progression in term nulliparous women. *Obstet Gynecol.* 2004;104:943.

49. Sheiner E, Levy A, Feinstein U, et al. Risk factors and outcome of failure to progress during the first stage of labor: a population based study. *Acta Obstet Gynecol Scand.* 2002;81:222.

50. Greenberg MB, Cheng YW, Sullivan M, et al. Does length of labor vary by maternal age? *Am J Obstet Gynecol.* 2007;197:428.

51. Dencker A, Berg M, Bergqvist L, Lilja H. Identification of latent phase factors associated with active labor duration in low-risk nulliparous women with spontaneous contractions. *Acta Obstet Gynecol Scand.* 2010;89:1034.

52. Albers L, Schiff M, Gorwoda J. The length of active labor in normal pregnancies. *Obstet Gynecol.* 1996;87:355.

53. Kilpatrick S, Laros R Jr. Characteristics of normal labor. *Obstet Gynecol.* 1989;74:85.

54. Cheng Y, Shaffer B, Nicholson J, et al. Second stage of labor and epidural use: A larger effect than previously suggested. *Obstet Gynecol.* 2014;123:527.

55. Cheng Y, Shaffer B, Bryant A, et al. Length of the first stage of labor and associated perinatal outcomes in nulliparous women. *Obstet Gynecol.* 2010;116(5):1127.

56. Greenberg M, Cheng Y, Hopkins L, et al. Are there ethnic differences in the length of labor? *Am J Obstet Gynecol.* 2006;195:743.

57. Obstetrics Care Consensus No. 1: Safe prevention of the primary cesarean delivery. *Obstet Gynecol.* 2014;123(3):693.

58. Duignan N, Sudd J, Hughes A. Characteristics of normal labour in different racial groups. *Br J Obstet Gynecol.* 1975;82:593.

59. Combs C, Laros R Jr. Prolonged third stage of labor: morbidity and risk factors. *Obstet Gynecol.* 1991;77:863.

60. Magann E, Lanneau G. Third Stage of Labor. *Obstet Gynecol Clin North Am.* 2005;32(2):323.

61. Magann E, Doherty D, Briery C, et al. Obstetric characteristics for a prolonged third stage of labor and risk for postpartum hemorrhage. *Gynecol Obstet Invest.* 2008;65(3):201.

62. Dombrowski M, Bottoms S, Saleh A, et al. Third stage of labor: analysis of duration and clinical practice. *Am J Obstet Gynecol.* 1995;172:1279.

63. Begley C, Gyte G, Devane D, et al. Active versus expectant management for women in the third stage of labour. *Cochrane Database Syst Rev.* 2011;(11):CD007412.

64. Andersson O, Hellström-Westas L, Andersson D, et al. Effects of delayed compared with early umbilical cord clamping on maternal postpartum hemorrhage and cord blood gas sampling: a randomized trial. *Acta Obstet Gynecol Scand.* 2013;92(5):567.

65. Bloom S, McIntire D, Kelly M, et al. Lack of effect of walking on labor and delivery. *N Engl J Med.* 1998;339:76.

66. Lawrence A, Lewis L, Hofmeyr G, et al. Maternal positions and mobility during first stage labour. *Cochrane Database Syst Rev.* 2013;(8):CD003934.

67. Hodnett E, Gates S, Hofmeyr G, Sakala C. Continuous support for women during childbirth. *Cochrane Database Syst Rev.* 2013;(7):CD003766.

68. Berghella V, Baxter J, Chauhan S. Evidence-based labor and delivery management. *Am J Obstet Gynecol.* 2008;199:445.

69. Dawood F, Doswell T, Quenby S. Intravenous fluids for reducing the duration of labour in low risk nulliparous women. *Cochrane Database Syst Rev.* 2013;(6):CD007715.

70. Shrivastava V, Garite T, Jenkins S, et al. A randomized, double-blinded, controlled trial comparing parenteral normal saline with and without dextrose on the course of labor in nulliparas. *Am J Obstet Gynecol.* 2009; 200:379.

71. O'Driscoll K, Foley M, MacDonald D. Active management of labor as an alternative to cesarean section for dystocia. *Obstet Gynecol.* 1984;63:485.

72. Akoury H, Brodie G, Caddick R, et al. Active management of labor and operative delivery in nulliparous women. *Am J Obstet Gynecol.* 1988; 158:255.

73. Akoury H, MacDonald F, Brodie G, et al. Oxytocin augmentation of labor and perinatal outcome in nulliparas. *Obstet Gynecol.* 1991;78:227.

74. Boylan P, Frankowski R, Rountree R, et al. Effect of active management of labor on the incidence of cesarean section for dystocia in nulliparas. *Am J Perinatol.* 1991;375:389.

75. López-Zeno J, Peaceman A, Adashek J, Socol M. A controlled trial of a program for the active management of labor. *N Engl J Med.* 1992;326:450.

76. Frigoletto F, Lieberman E, Lang J, et al. A clinical trial of active management of labor. *N Engl J Med.* 1995;333:745.

77. Rogers R, Gilson G, Miller A, et al. Active management of labor: does it make a difference? *Am J Obstet Gynecol.* 1997;177:599.

78. Wei S, Wo B, Qi H, et al. Early amniotomy and early oxytocin for prevention of, or therapy for, delay in first stage spontaneous labour compared with routine care. *Cochrane Database Syst Rev.* 2013;(8):CD006794.

79. Spong C, Berghella V, Wenstrom K, et al. Preventing the first cesarean delivery: Summary of a joint Eunice Kennedy Shriver National Institute of Child Health and Human Development, Society for Maternal-Fetal Medicine, and American College of Obstetricians and Gynecologists Workshop. *Obstet Gynecol.* 2012;120(5):1181.

80. American College of Obstetricians and Gynecologists (College); Society for Maternal-Fetal Medicine, Caughey A, Cahill A, Guise J, et al. Safe prevention of the primary cesarean delivery. *Am J Obstet Gynecol.* 2014;210(3):179-193.

81. Cheng Y, Hopkins L, Laros R, et al. Duration of the second stage of labor in multiparous women: maternal and neonatal outcomes. *Am J Obstet Gynecol.* 2007;196(6):585.e1.

82. Allen V, Baskett T, O'Connell C, et al. Maternal and perinatal outcomes with increasing duration of the second stage of labor. *Obstet Gynecol.* 2009;113:1248.

83. Rouse D, Weiner S, Bloom S, et al. Second-stage labor duration in nulliparous women: relationship to maternal and perinatal outcomes. *Am J Obstet Gynecol.* 2009;201:357.

84. Le Ray C, Audibert F, Goffinet F, et al. When to stop pushing: effects of duration of second-stage expulsion efforts on maternal and neonatal outcomes in nulliparous women with epidural analgesia. *Am J Obstet Gynecol.* 2009;201:361.e1.

85. Cheng YW, Hopkins LM, Caughey AB. How long is too long: Does a prolonged second stage of labor in nulliparous women affect maternal and neonatal outcomes? *Am J Obstet Gynecol.* 2004;191:933.

86. Laughon S, Berghella V, Reddy U, et al. Neonatal and maternal outcomes with prolonged second stage of labor. *Obstet Gynecol.* 2014; 124(1):57.

87. Cohen W. Influence of the duration of second stage labor on perinatal outcome and puerperal morbidity. *Obstet Gynecol.* 1977;49:266.

88. Deiham R, Crowhurst J, Crowther C. The second stage of labour: durational dilemmas. *Aust N Z J Obstet Gynaecol.* 1991;31:31.

89. Menticoglou S, Manning F, Harman C, et al. Perinatal outcome in relation to second-stage duration. *Am J Obstet Gynecol.* 1995;173:906.

90. Moon J, Smith C, Rayburn W. Perinatal outcome after a prolonged second stage of labor. *J Reprod Med.* 1990;35:229.

91. Myles T, Santolaya J. Maternal and neonatal outcomes in patients with a prolonged second stage of labor. *Obstet Gynecol.* 2003;102:52.

92. Sizer A, Evans J, Bailey S, Wiener J. A second-stage partogram. *Obstet Gynecol.* 2000;96:678.

93. Chestnut D, Bates J, Choi W. Continuous infusion epidural analgesia with lidocaine: efficacy and influence during the second stage of labor. *Obstet Gynecol.* 1987;69:323.

94. Chestnut D, Laszewski L, Pollack K, et al. Continuous epidural infusion of 0.0625% bupivacaine-0.0002% fentanyl during the second stage of labor. *Anesthesiology.* 1990;72:613.

95. Chestnut D, Vandewalker G, Owen C, et al. The influence of continuous epidural bupivacaine analgesia on the second stage of labor and method of delivery in nulliparous women. *Anesthesiology.* 1987;66:774.

96. Sng B, Leong W, Zeng Y, et al. Early versus late initiation of epidural analgesia for labour. *Cochrane Database Syst Rev.* 2014;(10):CD007238.

97. Manyonda I, Shaw D, Drife J. The effect of delayed pushing in the second stage of labor with continuous lumbar epidural analgesia. *Acta Obstet Gynecol Scand.* 1990;69:291.

98. Worstell T, Ahsan AD, Cahill AG, Caughey AB. Length of the second stage of labor: What is the effect of an epidural? *Obstet Gynecol.* 2014; 123(suppl 1):84S.

99. Fraser W, Marcoux S, Krauss I, et al. Multicenter, randomized, controlled trial of delayed pushing for nulliparous women in the second stage of labor with continuous epidural analgesia. *Am J Obstet Gynecol.* 2000; 182:1165.

100. Hansen S, Clark S, Foster J. Active pushing versus passive fetal descent in the second stage of labor: a randomized controlled trial. *Obstet Gynecol.* 2002;99:29.

101. Plunkett B, Lin A, Wong C, et al. Management of the second stage of labor in nulliparas with continuous epidural analgesia. *Obstet Gynecol.* 2003;102:109.

102. Tuuli M, Frey H, Odibo A, Macones G, Cahill A. Immediate compared with delayed pushing in the second stage of labor: a systematic review and meta-analysis. *Obstet Gynecol.* 2012;120(3):660.

103. Frey H, Tuuli M, Cortez S, et al. Does delayed pushing in the second stage of labor impact perinatal outcomes? *Am J Perinatol.* 2012;29(10):807.

104. Frey H, Tuuli M, Cortez S, et al. Medical and nonmedical factors influencing utilization of delayed pushing in the second stage. *Am J Perinatol.* 2013;30(7):595.

105. Gardosi J, Hutson N. Randomised, controlled trial of squatting in the second stage of labour. *Lancet.* 1989;334:74.

106. Gardosi J, Sylvester S, B-Lynch C. Alternative positions in the second stage of labour: a randomized controlled trial. *Br J Obstet Gynaecol.* 1989;96:1290.

107. Kemp E, Kingswood CJ, Kibuka M, Thornton JG. Position in the second stage of labour for women with epidural anaesthesia. *Cochrane Database Syst Rev.* 2013;(1):CD008070.

108. ACOG Committee Obstetric Practice. ACOG Committee Opinion Number 346, October 2006: amnioinfusion does not prevent meconium aspiration syndrome. *Obstet Gynecol.* 2006;108:1053.

109. Committee on Obstetric Practice, American College of Obstetricians and Gynecologists. (ACOG) Committee Opinion No. 379: Management of delivery of a newborn with meconium-stained amniotic fluid. *Obstet Gynecol.* 2007;110(3):739.

110. Hutton E, Hassan E. Late vs early clamping of the umbilical cord in full-term neonates: systematic review and meta-analysis of controlled trials. *JAMA.* 2007;297:1241.

111. McDonald S, Middleton P, Dowswell T, et al. Effect of timing of umbilical cord clamping of term infants on maternal and neonatal outcomes. *Cochrane Database Syst Rev.* 2013;(7):CD004074.

112. Rabe H, Diaz-Rossello J, Duley L, et al. Effect of timing of umbilical cord clamping and other strategies to influence placental transfusion at preterm birth on maternal and infant outcomes. *Cochrane Database Syst Rev.* 2012;(8):CD003248.

113. Committee on Obstetric Practice, American College of Obstetricians and Gynecologists. Committee Opinion No. 543: Timing of umbilical cord clamping after birth. *Obstet Gynecol.* 2012;120:1522-1526.

114. McAdams RM. Time to implement delayed cord clamping. *Obstet Gynecol.* 2014;123(3):549.

115. UNICEF. (2011) *How to Implement Baby-Friendly Standards: A Guide for Maternity Settings.* Available at <www.unicef.org.uk%2FDocuments%2FBaby_Friendly%2FGuidance%2FImplementation%2520Guidance%2FImplementation_guidance_maternity_web.pdf&ei=zUYmU6ykKMW8kQXr-4DgCg&usg=AFQjCNFR80z33R_cvkB5kaMhn4NQO0ucdg&bvm=bv.62922401,d.dGI>.

116. World Health Organization & UNICEF. (2009) *Baby-Friendly Hospital Initiative. Revised, Updated and Expanded for Integrated Care. Section 3: Breastfeeding Promotion and Support in a Baby-Friendly Hospital: A 20-Hour Course for Maternity Staff.* Available at <http://whqlibdoc.who.int/publications/2009/9789241594981_eng.pdf?ua=1>.

117. American College of Obstetricians and Gynecologists. *(ACOG) Guidelines for Perinatal Care,* Seventh Edition, October 2012.

118. Moore ER, Anderson GC, Bergman N, Dowswell T. Early skin-to-skin contact for mothers and their healthy newborn infants. *Cochrane Database Syst Rev.* 2012;(5):CD003519.

119. Mori R, Khanna R, Pledge D, Nakayama T. Meta-analysis of physiological effects of skin-to-skin contact for newborns and mothers. *Pediatr Int.* 2010;52:161-2009.

120. Stevens J, Schmied V, Burns E, et al. Immediate or early skin-to-skin contact after a Cesarean Section: a review of the literature. *Matern Child Nutr.* 2014;10:456.

121. Conde-Agudelo A, Diaz-Rossello J. Kangaroo mother care to reduce morbidity and mortality in low birthweight infants. *Cochrane Database Syst Rev.* 2014;(4):CD002771.

122. Rogers J, Wood J, McCandlish R, et al. Active versus expectant management of third stage of labour: the Hinchingbrooke randomised controlled trial. *Lancet.* 1998;351:693.

123. Begley M, Gyte G, Devane D, McGuire W, Weeks A. Active versus expectant management for women in the third stage of labour. *Cochrane Database Syst Rev.* 2011;(11):CD007412.

124. Prucka S, Clemens M, Craven C, McPherson E. Single umbilical artery: what does it mean for the fetus? A case-control analysis of pathologically ascertained cases. *Genet Med.* 2004;6:54.

125. Thummala M, Raju T, Langenberg P. Isolated single umbilical artery anomaly and the risk for congenital malformations: a meta-analysis. *J Pediatr Surg.* 1998;33:580.

126. Hua M, Odibo A, Macones G, et al. Single umbilical artery and its associated findings. *Obstet Gynecol.* 2010;115(5):930.

127. Murphy-Kaulbeck L, Dodds L, Joseph K, et al. Single umbilical artery risk factors and pregnancy outcomes. *Obstet Gynecol.* 2010;116(4):843.

128. Thorp JH Jr, Bowes WA Jr. Episiotomy: can its routine use be defended? *Am J Obstet Gynecol.* 1989;160:1027.

129. Shiono P, Klebanof M, Carey J. Midline episiotomies: more harm than good? *Obstet Gynecol.* 1990;75:765.

130. Angioli R, Gómez-Marín O, Cantuaria G, O'Sullivan M. Severe perineal lacerations during vaginal delivery: the University of Miami experience. *Am J Obstet Gynecol.* 2000;182:1083.

131. Bansal R, Tan W, Ecker J, et al. Is there a benefit to episiotomy at spontaneous vaginal delivery? A natural experiment. *Am J Obstet Gynecol.* 1996;175:897.

132. Robinson J, Norwitz E, Cohen A, et al. Epidural analgesia and the occurrence of third and fourth degree obstetric laceration in nulliparas. *Obstet Gynecol.* 1999;94:259.

133. Helwig J, Thorp J Jr, Bowes W Jr. Does midline episiotomy increase the risk of third- and fourth-degree lacerations in operative vaginal deliveries? *Obstet Gynecol.* 1993;82:276.

134. Ecker J, Tan W, Bansal R, et al. Is there a benefit to episiotomy at operative vaginal delivery? Observations over ten years in a stable population. *Am J Obstet Gynecol.* 1997;176:411.

135. Robinson J, Norwitz E, Cohen A, et al. Episiotomy, operative vaginal delivery, and significant perineal trauma in nulliparous women. *Am J Obstet Gynecol.* 1999;181:1180.

136. Baumann P, Hammoud AO, McNeeley SG, et al. Factors associated with anal sphincter laceration in 40,923 primiparous women. *Int Urogynecol J Pelvic Floor Dysfunct.* 2007;18:985.

137. Eason E, Labrecque M, Wells G, Feldman P. Preventing perineal trauma during childbirth: a systematic review. *Obstet Gynecol.* 2000;95:464.

138. Clemons J, Towers G, McClure G, O'Boyle A. Decreased anal sphincter lacerations associated with restrictive episiotomy use. *Am J Obstet Gynecol.* 2005;192:1620.

139. Carroli G, Belizan J. Episiotomy for vaginal birth. *Cochrane Database Syst Rev.* 2009;(1):CD000081.

140. Hartmann K, Viswanathan M, Palmieri R, et al. Outcomes of routine episiotomy: a systematic review. *JAMA.* 2005;293:2141.

141. American College of Obstetricians and Gynecologists. *ACOG Practice Guidelines on Episiotomy.* Washington, DC: American College of Obstetricians and Gynecologists; 2006.

142. Fenner D, Genberg B, Brahma P, et al. Fecal and urinary incontinence after vaginal delivery with anal sphincter disruption in an obstetrics unit in the United States. *Am J Obstet Gynecol.* 2003;189:1543.

143. Sartore A, De Seta F, Maso G, et al. The effects of mediolateral episiotomy on pelvic floor function after vaginal delivery. *Obstet Gynecol.* 2004;103:669.

144. Riskin-Mashiah S, O'Brian Smith E, Wilkins I. Risk factors for severe perineal tear: can we do better? *Am J Perinatol.* 2002;19:225.

145. Signorello L, Harlow B, Chekos A, Repke J. Midline episiotomy and anal incontinence: retrospective cohort study. *BMJ.* 2000;320:86.

146. De Leeuw J, Vierhout M, Struijk P, et al. Anal sphincter damage after vaginal delivery: functional outcome and risk factors for fecal incontinence. *Acta Obstet Gynecol Scand.* 2001;80:830.

147. Meijer-Hoogeveen M, Van Holsbeke C, Van Der Tweel I, et al. Sonographic longitudinal cervical length measurements in nulliparous women at term: prediction of spontaneous onset of labor. *Ultrasound Obstet Gynecol.* 2008;32:652.

148. Tolaymat L, Gonzalez-Quintero V, Sanchez-Ramos L, et al. Cervical length and the risk of spontaneous labor at term. *J Perinatol.* 2007;27:749.

149. Bishop EH. Pelvic scoring for elective induction. *Obstet Gynecol.* 1964;24:266.

150. Vrouenraets F, Roumen F, Dehing C, et al. Bishop score and risk of cesarean delivery after induction of labor in nulliparous women. *Obstet Gynecol.* 2005;105:690.

151. Kolkman DG, Verhoeven CJ, Brinkhorst SJ, et al. The Bishop score as a predictor of labor induction success: a systematic review. *Am J Perinatol.* 2013;30:625.

152. Jackson GM, Ludmir J, Bader T. The accuracy of digital examination and ultrasound in the evaluation of cervical length. *Obstet Gynecol.* 1992;79:214.

153. Watson WJ, Stevens D, Welter S, et al. Factors predicting successful labor induction. *Obstet Gynecol.* 1996;88:990.

154. Boozarjomehri F, Timor-Tritsch I, Chao C, et al. Transvaginal ultrasonographic evaluation of the cervix before labor: presence of cervical wedging is associated with shorter duration of induced labor. *Am J Obstet Gynecol.* 1994;171:1081.

155. Hatfield A, Sanchez-Ramos L, Kaunitz A. Sonographic cervical assessment to predict the success of labor induction: a systematic review with meta-analysis. *Am J Obstet Gynecol.* 2007;197(2):186.

156. Verhoeven C, Opmeer B, Oei S, et al. Transvaginal sonographic assessment of cervical length and wedging for predicting outcome of labor induction at term: a systematic review and meta-analysis. *Ultrasound Obstet Gynecol.* 2013;42:500.

157. Souka AP, Haritos T, Basayiannis K, et al. Intrapartum ultrasound for the examination of the fetal head position in normal and obstructed labor. *J Matern Fetal Neonatal Med.* 2003;13:59.

158. Molina F, Nicolaides K. Ultrasound in labor and delivery. *Fetal Diagn Ther.* 2010;27(2):61.

159. Sherer DM, Miodovnik M, Bradley K, et al. Intrapartum head position I: comparison between transvaginal digital examination and transabdominal ultrasound assessment during the active stage of labor. *Ultrasound Obstet Gynecol.* 2002;19:258.

160. Sherer D, Miodovnik M, Bradley K, et al. Intrapartum head position II: comparison between transvaginal digital examination and transabdominal ultrasound assessment during the second stage of labor. *Ultrasound Obstet Gynecol.* 2002;19:264.

161. Akmal S, Tsoi E, Kametos N, et al. Intrapartum sonography to determine head position. *J Matern Fetal Neonatal Med.* 2002;12:172.

162. Dupuis O, Silveira R, Zentner A, et al. Birth Simulator: reliability of transvaginal assessment of fetal head station as defined by the American College of Obstetricians and Gynecologists classification. *Am J Obstset Gynecol.* 2005;192:868.

163. Ramphul M, Ooi PV, Burke G. Instrumental delivery and ultrasound: a multicenter randomized controlled trial of ultrasound assessment of the head position versus standard care as an approach to prevent morbidity at instrumental delivery. *Br J Obstet Gynecol.* 2014;121(8):1029.

164. Tutschek B, Torkildsen E, Eggebø T. Comparison between ultrasound parameters and clinical examination to assess fetal head station in labor. *Ultrasound Obstet Gynecol.* 2013;41:425.

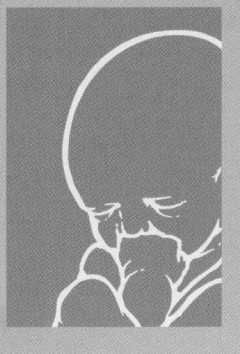

CHAPTER 13

Abnormal Labor and Induction of Labor

LILI SHEIBANI and DEBORAH A. WING

KEY ABBREVIATIONS	
American College of Obstetricians and Gynecologists	ACOG
Body mass index	BMI
Consortium on Safe Labor	CSL
Cephalopelvic disproportion	CPD
Confidence interval	CI
Electronic fetal monitoring	EFM
Food and Drug Administration	FDA
Group B *Streptococcus*	GBS
Intrauterine pressure catheter	IUPC
National Collaborative Perinatal Project	NCPP
National Institute of Child Health and Human Development	NICHD
Neonatal intensive care unit	NICU
Occiput posterior	OP
Odds ratio	OR
Premature rupture of membranes	PROM
Prostaglandin	PG
Prostaglandin E1 (misoprostol)	PGE_1
Prostaglandin E2 (dinoprostone)	PGE_2
Relative risk	RR
Society for Maternal-Fetal Medicine	SMFM
Trial of labor after cesarean delivery	TOLAC

OVERVIEW

Labor is the physiologic process by which a fetus is expelled from the uterus to the outside world. A switch from *contractures* (long-lasting, low-frequency activity) to *contractions* (frequent, high-intensity, high-frequency activity) occurs before progressive cervical effacement and dilation of the cervix and regular uterine contractions.[1] The timing of the switch varies from patient to patient. The exact trigger for the onset of labor is unknown, but considerable evidence suggests that the fetus provides the stimulus through complex neuronal-hormonal signaling (see Chapter 12).

The mean duration of a human singleton pregnancy is 280 days or 40 weeks from the first day of the last menstrual period assuming a normal 28-day menstrual cycle. In 2012, **an American College of Obstetricians and Gynecologists (ACOG) and Society for Maternal-Fetal Medicine (SMFM) working group[2] convened and recommended that the conventional "term" be replaced by the designations *early term* (37 0/7 to 38 6/7 weeks of gestation), *full term* (39 0/7 weeks of gestation to 40 6/7 weeks of gestation), *late term* (41 0/7 weeks to 41 6/7 weeks of gestation), and *postterm* (42 0/7 weeks of gestation and beyond).** These new gestational age designations are intended to improve data reporting, delivery of health care, and research.

DIAGNOSIS

Labor is a clinical diagnosis defined as uterine contractions that result in progressive cervical effacement and dilation, often accompanied by a bloody discharge referred to as *bloody show,* followed by birth of the baby. The diagnosis of bona fide labor is often elusive, and wide variations exist in the clinical spectrum of normal labor in addition to many opinions of the definitions for normal and abnormal labor progress. To gain an understanding of abnormal labor progress and induction of labor, a fundamental understanding of normal spontaneous labor is needed.

ABNORMAL LABOR AT TERM

The original guidelines for normal human labor progress are derived from Friedman's[1] clinical observations of women in labor in the 1950s. Friedman characterized a sigmoid pattern for labor when graphing cervical dilation against time (Fig. 13-1). He divided labor into three functional divisions: preparatory,

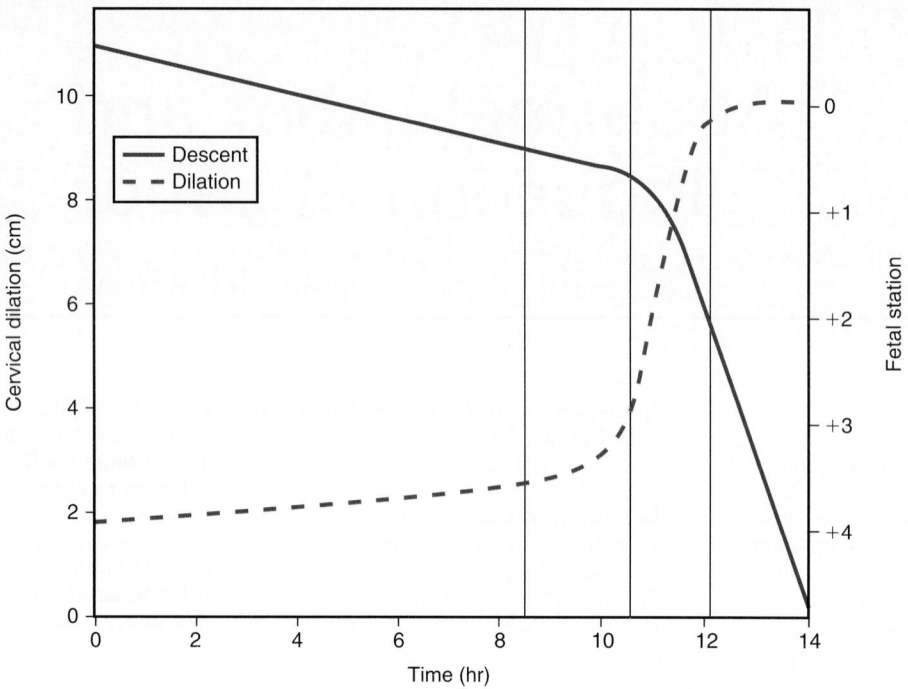

FIG 13-1 Characteristics of the average cervical dilation curve for nulliparous labor. (Modified from Friedman EA. *Labor: clinical evaluation and management,* 2nd ed. Norwalk, CT, Appleton-Century-Crofts; 1978.)

dilational, and pelvic. The *preparatory division* is better known as the *latent phase,* during which little cervical dilation occurs but considerable changes are taking place in the connective tissue components of the cervix, and the *dilational division*—or *active phase*—is when dilation proceeds at its most rapid rate to complete cervical dilation; these two phases together make up the *first stage of labor.* The *pelvic division,* or *second stage, of labor* refers to the time of full cervical dilation to the delivery of the infant. The *third stage of labor* refers to the time from the delivery of the infant to expulsion of the placenta.

Subsequent observations challenge Friedman's original labor curves. Between 1959 and 1966, the National Collaborative Perinatal Project (NCPP) prospectively observed labor progression along with several other factors possibly associated with cerebral palsy. This large multicenter project gathered data at a time when natural labor progress could be evaluated more easily than current obstetric practices allow. Using these data, Zhang and colleagues[3] derived a labor curve from this cohort of women and compared it to labor curves from the more recent Consortium on Safe Labor (CSL). Differences between these two labor curves are apparent, most notably that the nulliparous women in the NCPP had a more gradual transition to the active phase and that the active phase in the multiparous women began around 5 cm dilation (Figs. 13-2 and 13-3). Further, the rate of cervical dilation was slower in both nulliparous and multiparous women compared with that described by Friedman,[1] especially from 4 to 6 cm, with an acceleration point that suggests an active phase that occurs around 6 cm. Beyond 6 cm, cervical dilation was more rapid in multiparous than in nulliparous women.[4]

Since the 1960s, maternal characteristics and obstetric practices have changed significantly. Women have an older mean age and a higher mean body mass index (BMI), and oxytocin and epidural anesthesia are more frequently used,[5] all of which can affect the length of labor. Yet even after adjusting for maternal

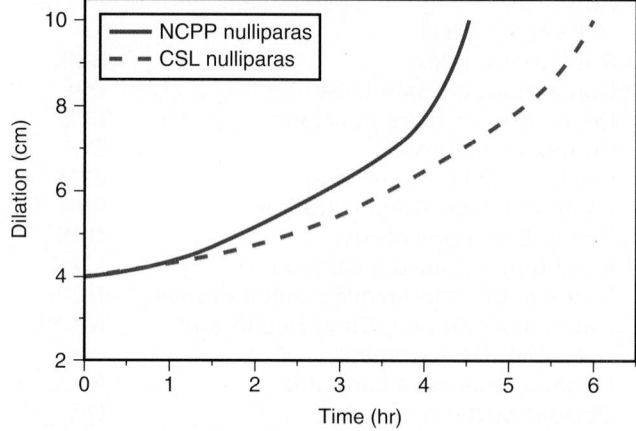

FIG 13-2 Average labor curves for nulliparas. NCPP, National Collaborative Perinatal Project; CSL, Consortium on Safe Labor. (Modified from Laughon KS, Branch DW, Beaver J, et al. Changes in labor patterns over 50 years. *Am J Obstet Gynecol.* 2012;206:419.e1-e9.)

and obstetric characteristics, the longer overall median differences in the first stage of labor persisted in the more recent data. This is likely because of changes in contemporary obstetric practice. Regardless of the differing results of these two investigations, a **graduated approach for diagnosis of labor protraction and arrest should be considered based on the level of cervical dilation** (Table 13-1).

Disorders of the Latent Phase

Historically, the first stage of labor has been divided into the *latent phase* and the *active phase* based on the work by Friedman in the 1950s. The onset of latent labor is considered to be the point at which regular uterine contractions are perceived. Friedman found that the mean duration of latent labor was 6.4 hours for nulliparas and 4.8 for multiparas, and the 95th percentile

TABLE 13-1	LABOR AT TERM (ZHANG)		
CERVICAL DILATION (CM)	**PARITY 0**	**PARITY 1**	**PARITY 2+**
From 3 to 4	1.2 (6.6)		
From 4 to 5	0.9 (4.5)	0.7 (3.3)	0.7 (3.5)
From 5 to 6	0.6 (2.6)	0.4 (1.6)	0.4 (1.6)
From 6 to 7	0.5 (1.8)	0.4 (1.2)	0.3 (1.2)
From 7 to 8	0.4 (1.4)	0.3 (0.8)	0.3 (0.7)
From 8 to 9	0.4 (1.3)	0.3 (0.7)	0.2 (0.6)
From 9 to 10	0.4 (1.2)	0.2 (0.5)	0.2 (0.5)
From 4 to 10	3.7 (16.7)	2.4 (13.8)	2.2 (14.2)

Data from Zhang J, Troendle J, Mikolajczyk R, et al. The natural history of the normal first stage of labor. *Obstet Gynecol.* 2010;115(4):705.
Data presented in hours as median (95th percentile).

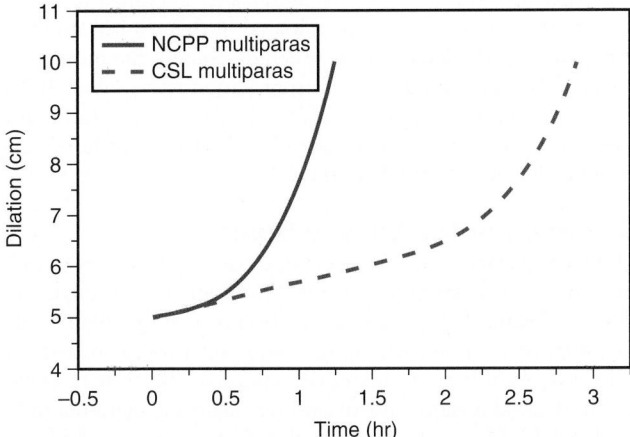

FIG 13-3 Average labor curves for multiparas. NCPP, National Collaborative Perinatal Project; CSL, Consortium on Safe Labor. (Modified from Laughon KS, Branch DW, Beaver J, et al. Changes in labor patterns over 50 years. *Am J Obstet Gynecol.* 2012;206:419.e1-e9.)

TABLE 13-2	PROGRESSION OF SPONTANEOUS LABOR AT TERM (FRIEDMAN)	
PARAMETER	**MEDIAN**	**95TH PERCENTILE**
Nulliparas		
Total duration	10.1 hr	25.8 hr
Stages:		
First	9.7 hr	24.7 hr
Second	33.0 min	117.5 min
Third	5.0 min	30 min
Latent phase (duration)	6.4 hr	20.6 hr
Maximal dilation (rate)	3.0 cm/hr	1.2 cm/hr
Descent (rate)	3.3 cm/hr	1.0 cm/hr
Multiparas		
Total duration	6.2 hr	19.5 hr
Stages:		
First	8.0 hr	18.8 hr
Second	8.5 min	46.5 min
Third	5.0 min	30 min
Latent phase (duration)	4.8 hr	13.6 hr
Maximal dilation (rate)	5.7 cm/hr	1.5 cm/hr
Descent (rate)	6.6 cm/hr	2.1 cm/hr

Data from Friedman EA. Primigravid labor: a graphicostatistical analysis. *Obstet Gynecol.* 1955; 6:567; Friedman EA. Labor in multiparas: a graphicostatistical analysis. *Obstet Gynecol.* 1956;8:691; and Cohen W, Friedman EA (eds). *Management of Labor.* Baltimore, University Park Press; 1983.

for maximum length in latent labor was 20 hours for nulliparous women and 14 hours for multiparous women (Table 13-2). The definitions of prolonged latent phase are still based on the data from Friedman, and modern investigators have not focused on the latent phase of labor.

Because the duration of latent labor is highly variable, even in the setting of a prolonged latent phase, expectant management is appropriate because most women will ultimately enter the active phase. Some women can spend days in latent labor; provided no indication exists for delivery, awaiting active labor is appropriate. With few exceptions, women who do not enter the active phase will either stop contracting or they will achieve the active phase following amniotomy, oxytocin administration, or both.

Another option is to administer "therapeutic rest," especially if contractions are painful or the patient is exhausted, with an analgesic agent such as morphine to abate or alleviate painful contractions and allow the patient to rest comfortably until active labor begins.

Disorders of the Active Phase

Active labor demarcates a rapid change in cervical dilation. Active-phase abnormalities can be divided into either *protraction disorders* (slower progress than normal) or *arrest disorders* (complete cessation of progress). **Based on Friedman's work, the active phase begins once cervical dilation progresses at a minimum rate of 1.2 cm/hr for nulliparous women and**

1.5 cm/hr for multiparous women. Labor is considered protracted if less than these minimum rates of change are seen. Rates of cervical dilation varied greatly in Friedman's report[1] and ranged from 1.2 to 6.8 cm/hr.

Active-phase arrest traditionally has been defined as the absence of cervical change for 2 hours or more in the presence of adequate uterine contractions and cervical dilation of at least 4 cm. However, revisions in the definitions of *labor progress* have been made using data from the CSL. **The threshold for the active phase of labor is now cervical dilation of 6 cm.** Before this dilation is achieved, standards of active-phase progress should not be applied. Thus neither a protracted active phase nor arrest of dilation should be diagnosed in a nullipara before 6 cm cervical dilation, and the lower limit of normal active-phase dilation is about 0.5 cm/hr rather than the 1.0 or 1.2 cm/hr reported by Friedman and others.

Several studies have evaluated the optimal duration of oxytocin augmentation in labor protraction or arrest of labor. In a study of more than 500 women, Rouse and colleagues[6] found that extending the minimum period of oxytocin augmentation for active-phase labor arrest from 2 to at least 4 hours allowed the majority of women who had not progressed at the 2-hour mark to deliver vaginally without an adverse effect on neonatal outcome. Thus as long as fetal and maternal status are reassuring, **the diagnosis of arrest (i.e., no cervical change) in the first stage of labor should be reserved for women at or beyond 6 cm cervical dilation with membrane rupture and one of the following: 4 hours or more of adequate contractions (e.g., more than 200 Montevideo units) or 6 hours or more of inadequate contractions.**[7]

The most common cause of a protraction disorder is inadequate uterine activity. External tocodynamometry is used to evaluate the duration of and time interval between contractions but cannot be used to evaluate the strength of uterine contractions. The external monitor is held against the abdominal wall and records a relative measurement of uterine contraction intensity, which reflects the monitor's movement as the uterine shape changes. More precise measurements of uterine activity must be obtained with an *intrauterine pressure catheter* (IUPC). After amniotomy, an IUPC can be placed into the uterus to measure the pressure generated during a uterine contraction. **An IUPC is frequently used when inadequate uterine activity is suspected owing to a protraction or arrest disorder. It can also be used to titrate oxytocin augmentation of labor to the desired effect, particularly when an external monitor cannot effectively record contractions.** The lower limit of contraction pressure required to dilate the cervix has been observed to be 15 mm Hg over baseline. Normal spontaneous contractions often exert pressures up to 60 mm Hg.

Once inadequate uterine activity is diagnosed with an IUPC in the setting of a protraction or arrest disorder, oxytocin is usually administered. Typically, the dose is increased until labor progresses normally with adequate contractions that occur at 2- to 3-minute intervals and last 60 to 90 seconds, with a peak intrauterine pressure of 50 to 60 mm Hg and a resting tone of 10 to 15 mm Hg (i.e., uterine activity equal to 150 to 350 Montevideo units).

Another common cause of protraction disorders is abnormal positioning of the fetal presenting part. Some examples of malpresentation are an extended, rather than flexed, fetal head; brow or face presentation; and occiput posterior (OP) position. When persistent OP position is present, labor is reported to be prolonged an average of 1 hour in multiparous women and 2 hours in nulliparous women. In one series, sonography showed OP position in 35% of women in early active labor, indicating that this may contribute to prolongation of labor in many women. In another investigation,[8] the prevalence of persistent OP position at the time of vaginal delivery regardless of parity was 5.5% (7.2% in nulliparas and 4.0% in multiparas). The OP position was found to be associated with longer first and second stages and a lower rate of vaginal delivery (26% for nulliparas and 57% for multiparas) when compared with the occiput anterior (OA) position (74% for nulliparas and 92.3% for multiparas).[8] Most fetuses in the OP position undergo spontaneous anterior rotation during the course of labor, and expectant management is generally indicated.

Cephalopelvic disproportion (CPD) refers to the size disproportion of the fetus relative to the mother, and it can be the cause of a protraction or arrest disorder. This is a diagnosis of exclusion that is often made when a protracted labor course is observed. Most frequently, malposition of the fetal presenting part is the culprit rather than true CPD. Unfortunately, despite past efforts, there is no way to accurately predict CPD. In a decision analysis,[9] it has been estimated that thousands of unnecessary cesarean deliveries would need to be performed in low-risk pregnancies to prevent one diagnosis of true CPD.

Evaluation of arrest of the first stage of labor includes an assessment of uterine activity with an IUPC; performance of clinical pelvimetry; and evaluation of fetal presentation, position, station, and estimated fetal weight. Amniotomy and oxytocin therapy can be initiated if uterine activity is found to be inadequate. The majority of gravidas respond to this intervention, resume progression of cervical dilation, and achieve vaginal delivery.

Electromechanical Classification

An alternative classification system for disorders of the active phase of labor is based on the electromechanical state of the uterus and regard uterine tone. This classification reflects an understanding of the propagation of electrical signals through the myometrium. In normal labor, a gradient of myometrial activity sweeps from the fundus and propagates toward the cervix through the excitation of cellular gap junctions. *Hypotonic dysfunction* reflects an inefficient generation and propagation of these action potentials through the myometrium or a lack of contractile response of myometrial cells to the initial stimulus. Hypotonic uterine contractions are infrequent, of low amplitude, and are accompanied by low or normal baseline intrauterine pressures. Maternal discomfort is minimal.

Hypertonic dysfunction is primarily a condition of primiparas and usually occurs in early labor. It is characterized by the presence of regular uterine contractions that fail to effect cervical effacement and dilation. Frequent contractions of low amplitude are often associated with an elevated basal intrauterine pressure. Maternal discomfort is usually significant. Therapeutic rest or expectant management can be initiated in this clinical situation if the patient is in latent labor. When diagnosed, the most likely scenario is that the patient will soon enter active labor. If the patient is in active labor and is found to have hypertonic dysfunction, amniotomy can be performed with or without concomitant oxytocin administration.

Disorders of the Second Stage

The second stage of labor begins once the cervix becomes fully dilated and ends with the delivery of the neonate. Although fetal descent begins before the cervix becomes fully dilated, the majority of fetal descent occurs once full cervical dilation is achieved. At this time, maternal expulsion efforts may begin. Parity, delayed pushing, use of epidural analgesia, maternal BMI, birthweight, OP position, and fetal station at completed dilation all have been shown to affect the length of the second stage of labor.[10]

In an effort to define a normal second stage of labor, multiple investigators have studied the relationship between the duration of the second stage of labor and adverse maternal and neonatal outcomes. In one secondary analysis of a multicenter randomized study of fetal pulse oximetry in which 4126 nulliparous women were examined, none of the following outcomes were related to the duration of the second stage: 5-minute Apgar score of less than 4, umbilical artery pH less than 7, intubation in the delivery room, need for admission to the neonatal intensive care unit (NICU), or neonatal sepsis.[11] Fewer investigators have examined the duration of the second stage of labor and the relationship to neonatal outcomes in multiparous women. In one study of 5158 multiparous women, when second stage exceeded 3 hours, the risk of 5-minute Apgar scores of less than 7, admissions to the NICU, and composite neonatal morbidity were all increased.[12]

With appropriate monitoring, however, the absolute risks for adverse fetal or neonatal consequences of increasing second-stage duration appear to be, at worst, low and incremental. Although the risk of a 5-minute Apgar score below 7 and neonatal depression at birth were statistically increased when the second stage was longer than 2 hours, in a study of 58,113 multiparous women, the absolute risk of these outcomes was low (<1.5%) with a second-stage labor duration less than 2 hours, and it did not double even with durations greater than 5 hours.[13] Given the findings in these studies, the absolute permissible maximum length of time spent in the second stage of labor has not been identified.

Protraction of descent is defined as descent of the presenting part during the second stage of labor that occurs at less than

1 cm/hr in nulliparous women and less than 2 cm/hr in multiparous women. *Arrest (failure) of descent* refers to no progress in descent. Both diagnoses require evaluation of five factors: (1) uterine activity, (2) maternal expulsive efforts, (3) fetal heart rate status, (4) fetal position, and (5) clinical pelvimetry. Decisions then may be made regarding interventions, such as increasing or initiating oxytocin infusion to improve maternal expulsive efforts or proceeding with operative vaginal or cesarean delivery. **Management of the second stage of labor can be difficult, and decisions regarding intervention must be individualized.**

The median duration of the second stage is 50 to 60 minutes for nulliparas and 20 to 30 minutes for multiparas, but the range of second-stage duration is highly variable.[13,14] Janakiraman and colleagues compared the second stage in 3139 induced women to that of 11,588 women in spontaneous labor. No differences in the length of the second stage or in the risk of a prolonged second stage were noted between the groups, although the induced nulliparas appeared to be at increased risk for postpartum hemorrhage and cesarean delivery (4.2% vs. 2.0%, odds radio [OR] 1.62; 95% confidence interval [CI], 1.02 to 2.58; and 10.9% vs. 7.2%, OR 1.32; 95% CI, 1.01 to 1.71, respectively).

In classic obstetric teaching, the upper limit for the duration of the second stage of labor was considered to be 2 hours. In the available literature, before diagnosing arrest of labor in the second stage—and if maternal and fetal conditions permit—it suggests at least 2 hours of pushing should be allowed with multiparous women, and at least 3 hours should be allowed with nulliparous women. Longer durations may be appropriate on an individualized basis (e.g., with epidural analgesia or with fetal malposition) as long as progress is documented.[15] The labor guidelines from the Eunice Kennedy Shriver National Institute of Child Health and Human Development (NICHD)[16] suggest allowing at least 1 additional hour if an epidural is present (i.e., at least 3 hours in multiparous and at least 4 hours in nulliparous women) before diagnosing second-stage arrest. **A specific absolute maximum length of time spent in the second stage of labor beyond which all women should undergo operative delivery has not been identified.**

Many authors have studied the perinatal and maternal effects of a prolonged second stage. Several studies found no increase in infant morbidity or mortality with a second stage lasting longer than 2 hours,[17] although the rate of vaginal delivery decreased after 3 hours in the second stage. However, a recent population-based cohort study by Allen and colleagues[13] examined 63,404 nulliparous women and found increased risks of low 5-minute Apgar score, birth depression, and admission to the NICU with increasing duration of the second stage greater than 3 hours. This study is the largest thus far to evaluate neonatal and maternal outcomes with a prolonged second stage. **In this study, as well as others, evidence shows that maternal morbidities—including perineal trauma, chorioamnionitis, instrumental delivery, and postpartum hemorrhage—increase with prolonged second stages that last greater than 2 hours.**

Disorders of the Third Stage

The third stage of labor is the period from delivery of the infant to the expulsion of the placenta. Separation of the placenta is the consequence of continued uterine contractions. Signs of placental separation include a gush of blood, lengthening of the umbilical cord, and change in shape of the uterine fundus from discoid to globular with elevation of the fundal height. **The interval between delivery of the infant and delivery of the placenta and fetal membranes is usually less than 10 minutes and is complete within 15 minutes in 95% of deliveries.**[18] The most important risk associated with a prolonged third stage is hemorrhage; this risk increases proportionally with increased duration.[19] **Because of the associated increased incidence of hemorrhage after 30 minutes, most practitioners diagnose retained placenta after this time interval has elapsed.** Interventions to expedite placental delivery are usually undertaken at this point.

Management of the third stage of labor may be expectant or active. *Expectant management* refers to the delivery of the placenta without cord clamping, cord traction, or the administration of uterotonic agents such as oxytocin. *Active management* consists of some combination of early cord clamping, controlled cord traction, and administration of a uterotonic agent. Oxytocin is the usual uterotonic agent given, but others have been used, such as misoprostol or other prostaglandin compounds. **Compared with expectant management of the third stage, active management has been associated with a reduced risk of postpartum hemorrhage.**[20] Cochrane reviewers evaluated five trials that comprised 6486 women and compared active and expectant management. They confirmed that active management reduced the risk of maternal hemorrhage (relative risk [RR], 0.34; 95% CI, 0.14 to 0.87) but that significant increases in maternal diastolic blood pressure, afterpains, and analgesia use occurred as well. These adverse events may reflect the side effects of the various uterotonic medications used in different countries.

Some debate exists regarding the timing of oxytocin administration when active management of the third stage is practiced—that is, whether it should be after the placenta has delivered or after the anterior shoulder of the fetus has delivered. A randomized controlled trial (RCT) that included 1486 women compared the effects of oxytocin administration upon delivery of the anterior shoulder to administration after delivery of the placenta and showed no significant differences in blood loss or retained placenta between the groups.[21]

Retained placenta can usually be treated with measures such as manual removal or sharp curettage. Attempting manual removal can be performed under regional anesthesia or conscious sedation. If this is not successful, a sharp curettage can be performed under sonographic guidance. Prophylactic broad-spectrum antimicrobial agents are often administered when manual removal of the placenta is performed, although little evidence supports or refutes their use.[22]

Anesthesia Effects on Labor Progress

Conduction epidural anesthesia's effect on the rate of cervical change remains controversial, (see Chapter 16). Unfortunately, RCTs have several limitations, mainly that there cannot be a placebo group. Thus multiple randomized trials have investigated cesarean delivery rates between women who received epidural anesthesia versus those who received systemic analgesia in labor. A 2005 Cochrane review[23] that involved 20 studies reported no increase in cesarean delivery rates between women who received epidural anesthesia versus those who received systemic analgesia for labor (RR, 1.07; 95% CI, 0.93 to 1.23). A more recent meta-analysis[24] that involved 15 RCTs and included 4619 patients also compared the effects of epidural anesthesia to parenteral opioids. The incidence of cesarean delivery was the same between the groups, although the incidence of operative vaginal delivery was increased in the conduction anesthesia group [OR, 1.92; 95% CI, 1.52 to 1.22). It has been difficult to establish whether this increase in operative vaginal delivery was due to a direct effect of the epidural analgesia on the progress of labor or an indirect effect, such as greater opportunities for resident training. No difference in the duration of the first stage was noted; however, the second stage was prolonged by approximately 16 minutes (95% CI, 10 to 23 minutes). This statistically significant finding lacks clinical relevance.[24]

It has also been suggested that receiving epidural anesthesia during latent labor, as opposed to during the active phase, results in prolongation of the labor. Accordingly, many practitioners refrain from administering epidural analgesia until the patient reaches 4 cm or more dilation. In one investigation, 12,693 nulliparas were randomized to receive early epidural analgesia (at first request if cervical dilation was at least 1 cm) or late epidural analgesia (parenteral meperidine until cervical dilation of 4 cm was achieved). The median cervical dilation at the time of epidural placement was 1.6 cm for the early group and 5.1 for the late group. These researchers found no difference in the incidence of cesarean birth, operative vaginal delivery, or length of the first or second stages of labor.

MANAGEMENT OF ABNORMAL LABOR AND DELIVERY

Pharmacologic Augmentation

When the first stage of labor is protracted or an arrest disorder is diagnosed, an evaluation of uterine activity; clinical pelvimetry; and fetal position, station, and estimated weight should be performed. If uterine activity is found to be suboptimal, the most common remedy is oxytocin augmentation. Various oxytocin dosing regimens have been described in the obstetric literature. Local protocols for oxytocin administration should include the dose of oxytocin being delivered (mU/min) as opposed to the volume of fluid being infused (mL/min) and should specify initial dose, incremental increases with time, and maximum permissible dose. Although oxytocin currently is used in a majority of labors in the United States, it is important for clinicians to recognize that it is also the medication implicated in approximately half of all paid obstetric litigation claims, and it is the medication most commonly associated with preventable adverse events during childbirth.[25]

Misoprostol solution given orally has been proposed as an alternative augmentation agent. Ho and colleagues[26] randomized 231 women to a solution of 20 µg misoprostol, prepared by dissolving one 200-µg tablet of misoprostol in 200 mL tap water, or to intravenous (IV) oxytocin. The results of this admittedly small study revealed similar rates of vaginal delivery between the two groups, and no difference was noted in side effects or neonatal outcomes.

Side Effects

One of the advantages of oxytocin administration is that if uterine overactivity is encountered, the infusion can quickly be stopped, and **the half-life of oxytocin is approximately 3 minutes.** The most frequently encountered complication of oxytocin or prostaglandin administration is uterine overactivity. However, until an NICHD workshop attempted to provide standardized nomenclature for uterine activity and electronic fetal heart monitoring,[27] no uniform definitions existed for terms like *hyperstimulation* and *tachysystole*. These guidelines define *tachysystole* as more than five contractions in 10 minutes averaged over a 30-minute window, and they recommend abandoning the terms *hyperstimulation* and *hypercontractility*.[27]

Because oxytocin is structurally and functionally related to vasopressin, one of its side effects is, in rare instances, water intoxication and hyponatremia. Historically, bolus injections of oxytocin were thought to cause hypotension, and the current practice for labor management is administration by infusion pump or slow drip. Some investigators[28] have suggested that a 10-IU bolus of oxytocin given in the third stage of labor is not associated with adverse hemodynamic responses compared with oxytocin given as an infusion. However, Jonsson and colleagues found that an IV bolus was associated with ST depressions seen on the electrocardiogram. **Given that no advantage has been found with the use of IV boluses of oxytocin, and given the potential hemodynamic adverse consequences, this form of administration is not recommended.** Finally, uterine rupture is rare and in most instances occurs in women who have had a prior uterine surgery, such as a cesarean delivery or myomectomy.

Recent investigations have shed light on the question of labor augmentation and induction for women attempting a trial of labor after cesarean delivery (TOLAC; see Chapter 20). Whereas no randomized trials have been done, a large prospective investigation[29] evaluated more than 17,000 women attempting TOLAC. The incidence of uterine rupture was 0.4% for those subjects who spontaneously labored versus 0.9% for those who received augmentation and 1.0% for subjects who underwent induction. Other complications of attempting TOLAC are illustrated in Table 13-3. **ACOG currently recommends the use of oxytocin in augmentation and induction of women undergoing a TOLAC.[30]**

INDUCTION OF LABOR

Induction of labor refers to the iatrogenic stimulation of uterine contractions before the onset of spontaneous labor to accomplish vaginal delivery, and it is one of the most commonly performed obstetric procedures in the United States.[31] *Augmentation of labor* refers to increasing the frequency and intensity of existing uterine contractions to accomplish vaginal delivery in a patient who is in labor but is not progressing adequately.

Indications and Contraindications

Induction of labor should be undertaken when the benefits of delivery to either mother or fetus outweigh the risks of pregnancy continuation.[31] Many accepted medical and obstetric indications for labor induction exist (Table 13-4). Contraindications include those that preclude vaginal delivery (Table 13-5).

With regard to induction of labor versus expectant management for gestational hypertension or preeclampsia without severe features, investigators in the Netherlands performed a trial in which 756 patients were randomized to receive induction (*n* = 377) or expectant monitoring (*n* = 379). Of women who were randomized to induction of labor, 117 (31%) experienced poor maternal outcome compared with the 166 (44%) allocated to expectant management (RR, 0.71; 95% CI, 0.59 to 0.86; *P* = .0001). No cases of maternal or neonatal death or eclampsia were recorded.[32] Thus in women with gestational hypertension or preeclampsia without severe features, induction of labor is associated with improved maternal outcome, and it should be advised at 37 weeks' gestation.

TABLE 13-3   MATERNAL COMPLICATIONS ASSOCIATED WITH TRIAL OF LABOR AFTER PREVIOUS CESAREAN

COMPLICATION	TRIAL OF LABOR (N = 17,898)	ELECTIVE REPEATED CESAREAN DELIVERY (N = 15,801)	ODDS RATIO (95% CI)	P VALUE
Uterine rupture	124 (0.7%)	0	—	<.001
Uterine dehiscence	119 (0.7%)	76 (0.5%)	1.38 (1.04-1.85)	.03
Hysterectomy	41 (0.2%)	47 (0.3%)	0.77 (0.51-1.17)	.22
Thromboembolic disease (DVT, PE)	7 (0.04%)	10 (0.1%)	0.62 (0.24-1.62)	.32
Transfusion	304 (1.7%)	158 (1.0%)	1.71 (1.41-2.08)	<.001
Endometritis	517 (2.9%)	285 (1.8%)	1.62 (1.40-1.87)	<.001
Maternal death	3 (0.02%)	7 (0.04%)	0.38 (0.10-1.46)	.21
Other maternal adverse events*	64 (0.4%)	52 (0.3%)	1.09 (0.75-1.57)	.66
One or more of the above	978 (5.5%)	563 (3.6%)	1.56 (1.41-1.74)	<.001

Data from Landon MB, Hauth JC, Leveno KJ, et al. for the National Institute of Child Health and Human Development Maternal-Fetal Medicine Units Network. Maternal and perinatal outcomes associated with a trial of labor after prior cesarean delivery. *N Engl J Med.* 2004;351(25):2581.
*Other adverse events include broad-ligament hematoma, cystotomy, bowel injury, and ureteral injury.
CI, confidence interval; *DVT,* deep venous thrombosis; *PE,* pulmonary embolism.

TABLE 13-4   ACCEPTED INDICATIONS FOR LABOR INDUCTION

Hypertensive disorders
- Preeclampsia/eclampsia
- Gestational hypertension

Maternal medical conditions
- Diabetes mellitus
- Renal disease
- Chronic pulmonary disease
- Cholestasis of pregnancy

Premature rupture of membranes
Chorioamnionitis
Abruptio placentae
Fetal compromise
- Fetal growth restriction
- Isoimmunization
- Nonreassuring antepartum fetal testing
- Oligohydramnios
- Multiple gestations

Fetal demise (≥41 wk)

TABLE 13-5   ACCEPTED ABSOLUTE CONTRAINDICATIONS TO LABOR INDUCTION

Prior classic uterine incision or transfundal uterine surgery (other high-risk cesarean incision)
Prior uterine rupture
Active genital herpes infection
Placenta or vasa previa
Umbilical cord prolapse
Transverse or oblique fetal lie
Absolute cephalopelvic disproportion (as in women with pelvic deformities)
Category III fetal heart rate tracing

TABLE 13-6   EVALUATION BEFORE INDUCTION OF LABOR

PARAMETER	CRITERIA
Maternal	Confirm the indication for induction. Review contraindications to labor and/or vaginal delivery. Perform clinical pelvimetry to assess the shape and adequacy of the bony pelvis. Assess the cervical condition (assign Bishop score). Review risks, benefits, and alternatives of induction of labor with the patient.
Fetal/neonatal	Confirm gestational age. Assess the need to document fetal lung maturity status. Estimate fetal weight, either by clinical or ultrasound examination. Determine fetal presentation and lie. Confirm fetal well-being.

Examination of the maternal and fetal condition is required before undertaking labor induction (Table 13-6). Indications and contraindications for induction should be reviewed along with the alternatives. Risks and benefits of labor induction should be discussed with the patient, including the risks of cesarean delivery (discussed later). Confirmation of gestational age is critical, and evaluation of fetal lung maturity status should be performed if indicated (Table 13-7).[31] Fetal weight should be estimated, clinical pelvimetry should be performed, and fetal presentation should be confirmed; in addition, a cervical examination should be performed and documented, and labor induction should be performed at a location where personnel are available who are familiar with the process and its potential complications. Uterine activity and electronic fetal monitoring (EFM) are recommended for any gravida receiving uterotonic medications.

Prolonged Pregnancy

In a joint Committee Opinion,[2] the ACOG and SMFM discourage the use of the label *term pregnancy* and instead have replaced it with the labels *early term, full term, late term,* and *postterm.* **Postterm pregnancy (≥42 weeks of gestation) is associated with increased risks for the fetus and mother** (see Chapter 36). According to a large epidemiologic study by Hilder and colleagues,[34] the perinatal mortality rate—which combines stillbirths (fetal death after 20 weeks' gestation) and early neonatal deaths (death of a liveborn infant within the first 28 days of life)—at greater than 42 weeks of gestation is approximately twice that at term (4 to 7 deaths vs. 2 to 3 deaths per 1000

"Impending" macrosomia, a favorable cervix, patients considered to be at increased risk for preeclampsia (such as having a prior history of preeclampsia), or concerns about intrauterine growth restriction (e.g., a fetus with an estimated weight at the 19th percentile) are *not* accepted medical indications for induction. Additionally, preterm or early-term induction is not medically indicated for maternal anxiety or discomfort related to normal pregnancy, previous pregnancy with labor abnormalities such as rapid labor or shoulder dystocia, or simply because the mother lives far from the hospital. Currently, experts concur that elective induction should not be performed before 39 weeks of gestation; however, insufficient data are available to recommend for or against induction of labor at 39 or more weeks of gestation.[33]

TABLE 13-7	CRITERIA FOR CONFIRMATION OF GESTATIONAL AGE AND/OR FETAL PULMONARY MATURITY
	PARAMETERS
Confirmation of gestational age	Fetal heart tones have been documented as present for ≥30 weeks by Doppler ultrasound.
	At least 36 weeks have elapsed since a positive serum or urine human chorionic gonadotropin pregnancy test.
	Ultrasound measurement at less than 20 weeks' gestation supports gestational age of 39 weeks or more.
Fetal pulmonary maturity	If term gestation cannot be confirmed by two or more of the above obstetric clinical or laboratory criteria, amniotic fluid analysis can be used to provide evidence of fetal lung maturity. A variety of tests are available. The parameters for evidence of fetal pulmonary maturity include:
	1. Lecithin/sphingomyelin (L/S) ratio greater than 2.1
	2. Presence of phosphatidylglycerol
	3. TDx-FLM assay shows ≥70 mg surfactant per gram of albumin
	4. Presence of saturated phosphatidylcholine (SPC) 500 ng/mL or more in nondiabetic patients (≥1000 ng/mL for pregestational diabetic patients)
	5. Lamellar body count exceeds 30,000/µL

Data from Induction of Labor. ACOG Practice Bulletin No 107. American College of Obstetricians and Gynecologists. *Obstet Gynecol.* 2009;114:386; and Fetal Lung Maturity. ACOG Practice Bulletin No. 97. American College of Obstetricians and Gynecologists. *Obstet Gynecol.* 2008;112:717.

deliveries) and increases more than sixfold at 43 weeks of gestation and beyond.

Two more recent studies[35,36] consisted of prospective cohort evaluations of singleton pregnancies based on ultrasound dating. Nakling and Backe[35] found the incidence of postterm pregnancies to be 7.6% in the cohort, with 0.3% of pregnancies progressing to 301 days (43 weeks' gestation) if inductions were not permitted prior to 43 weeks. This investigation found a significantly increased rate of perinatal mortality after 41 weeks' gestation. In contrast, Heimstad and colleagues[36] found an increased trend toward intrauterine fetal demise at 42 weeks' gestation compared with that at 38 weeks, but this study allowed inductions prior to 43 weeks and did not calculate the perinatal mortality rates. Factors that may contribute to the increased rate of perinatal deaths are uteroplacental insufficiency, meconium aspiration, intrauterine growth restriction (IUGR), and intrauterine infection.[37] For these reasons, common practice has been to deliver patients by 42 0/7 weeks.

Postterm pregnancy is also associated with increased risks for the pregnant woman, including an increase in labor dystocia (9% to 12% vs. 2% to 7% at term) and an increase in severe perineal injury (3.3% vs. 2.6% at term).[36,38-40]

Overall, comparisons of induction of labor to expectant management in observational studies have found no difference in, or a decreased risk of, cesarean delivery among women who are induced.[41-44] This is also true for women with an unfavorable cervix.[45] For example, a meta-analysis revealed that women at less than 42 0/7 weeks' gestation who underwent induction of labor had a lower cesarean section delivery rate than those who received expectant management.[46] In this meta-analysis, 11 RCTs and 25 observational studies were included and overall, expectant management of pregnancy was associated with a higher odds of cesarean delivery than was induction of labor (OR, 1.22; 95% CI, 1.07 to 1.39). Also, in a 2012 Cochrane meta-analysis of three smaller studies of induction of labor at 41 0/7 weeks, a reduction in the rate of cesarean delivery was demonstrated.[47] Thus the evidence base suggests that labor inductions at 41 0/7 weeks should be performed to reduce the risk of cesarean delivery and the risk of perinatal morbidity and mortality.

Elective Induction of Labor

The rate of induction of labor more than doubled from 1990 through 2010, from 9.6% to 23.8%. Induction rates were at least twice as high in 2010 compared with 1990 for women at

all gestational ages except for those in the post term, whose rate of induction rose 90%.[48] Reasons for the general increase over time in inductions include the availability of better cervical ripening agents, patient and provider desire for a more convenient time of delivery, and more acceptance of a variety of indications for induction. Nevertheless, the overall induction rate declined slightly in 2011, to 23.7% (from 23.8% in 2010), and then it declined again in 2012, to 23.3%.[48] Induction rates were lower for all gestational age categories.

Elective induction of labor refers to the initiation of labor for convenience in an individual with a term pregnancy who is free of medical or obstetric indications. Although elective induction at or after 39 weeks of gestation is not recommended or encouraged, it may be appropriate in specific instances, such as for women with a history of very short labors or those who live a great distance from the hospital.[31] Also, a patient who has experienced a prior stillbirth at or near term may request labor induction to ease anxiety and fears about the loss of a subsequent pregnancy. In addition, certain maternal medical conditions require multispecialty participation, in which the benefit of a planned delivery in order to have experienced personnel readily available is most appropriate, such as when a fetal anomaly is present.

Some concerns have been raised that induction of labor increases the rate of cesarean delivery and increases health care costs. Seyb and colleagues noted in their investigation that the mean time spent on labor and delivery was almost twice as long, and postpartum stays were prolonged for those induced. The total cost associated with hospitalization for elective induction was also 17.4% higher than for those in spontaneous labor. These findings were confirmed in investigations by Maslow and Sweeney and Cammu and colleagues.[49]

However, these results are based on the faulty comparison of women who are induced with those in spontaneous labor.[40] In fact, most observational studies that compare induction of labor to expectant management—which is the actual clinical alternative to labor induction—have found either no difference or a decreased risk of cesarean delivery among women who are induced.[41] Because these studies are retrospective in nature, they should be interpreted with caution.

In addition, several RCTs have been recently undertaken. In a meta-analysis by Caughey and colleagues,[46] nine RCTs were evaluated. These trials utilized patients undergoing expectant management, rather than spontaneous labor, as the comparison group for the patients being electively induced, and the meta-analysis revealed a decreased risk of cesarean delivery in the induction group compared with the group managed expectantly (RR, 1.17; 95% CI, 1.05 to 1.29). Similarly, Cochrane reviewers[50] examined 19 trials that included 7984 women and found that women induced at 37 to 40 completed weeks were less likely to have a cesarean delivery than those in the expectant management group (RR, 0.58; 95% CI, 0.34 to 0.99). Caughey and colleagues[51] also examined the risk of cesarean delivery for each week of gestational age ranging from 38 to 41 weeks. In their retrospective study, which again compared induction to expectant management, cesarean delivery was decreased in the induction groups.

With regard to perinatal outcomes, it appears that compared with infants who undergo spontaneous labor, fewer electively induced infants have meconium passage and therefore likely have a reduced incidence of meconium aspiration syndrome.[46] Macrosomia also may be reduced, as noted in an ecological study performed by Zhang and colleagues.[52] This study revealed that the increased induction rate between 1992 and 2003 (14% to 27%) was significantly associated with reduced mean fetal birth weight ($r = -0.54$; 95% CI, -0.71 to -0.29) and rate of macrosomia ($r = -0.55$; 95% CI, -0.74 to -0.32).

The risk of respiratory morbidity associated with labor induction was illustrated in a retrospective review of infants admitted to the NICU following elective delivery at term.[53] These results support delaying elective delivery until 39 weeks' gestation (Table 13-8). In further support of these findings, Clark and colleagues[54] performed a prospective observational study of 27 hospitals that included 17,794 deliveries. Of these, 14,955 (84%) occurred at 37 weeks or greater; 6562 (44%) of them were planned deliveries, rather than spontaneous. Among the planned deliveries, 4645 (71%) were elective. The percentage of the electively delivered infants admitted to the NICU was 17.8% (n = 43) at 37 to 38 weeks, 8% (n = 118) at 38 to 39 weeks, and 4.6% (n = 135) at 39 weeks. These studies reiterate the importance of considering neonatal morbidity with elective induction prior to 39 weeks' gestation. After 39 weeks, however, one study[55] has suggested that infants of electively induced mothers were less likely to receive ventilatory support, become septic, or be admitted to the NICU.

One other concern regarding elective induction is the cost. Kaufman and colleagues[56] studied the economic consequences of elective induction of labor at term. Using decision analysis, these researchers examined a hypothetic cohort of 100,000 pregnant patients for whom an initial decision was made to either induce labor at 39 weeks or follow the patient expectantly through the remainder of the pregnancy. All patients in this model underwent induction at 42 weeks' gestation if they were not yet delivered. Using baseline estimates, the investigators concluded that elective induction would result in more than 12,000 excess cesarean deliveries and would impose an annual cost to the medical system of nearly $100 million. A policy of induction at any gestational age, regardless of parity or cervical ripeness, requires economic expenditures by the medical system. Although they never were cost saving, inductions in this study were less expensive at later gestational ages, for multiparous patients, and for those women with a favorable cervix. The inductions most costly to the health care system were those performed in nulliparas with unfavorable cervices at 39 weeks. That said, this model incorporated the assumption that labor induction increased the risk of cesarean delivery. When all outpatient and inpatient costs are considered, it remains uncertain whether labor induction is more costly than expectant management.

Prediction of Labor Induction Success

In observational studies, characteristics associated with successful induction include multiparity, tall stature (over 5 feet 5 inches), nonobese maternal weight or BMI, and infant birthweight less than 3.5 kg.[53,57] However, these characteristics are predictive of success even in spontaneous labors. Success can vary widely depending on the characteristics of the population being induced (e.g., intact or ruptured membranes, parity, baseline cervical exam), induction methods, and choice of end points (delivery within 24 or 48 hr, dose/duration of oxytocin infusion, route of delivery, and maternal and neonatal morbidity).

Some researchers[58] have tried to identify, with varying success, biochemical and biophysical assays to predict the probability of vaginal delivery following labor induction. These measures include digital evaluation of the cervix, ultrasonographic cervical length measurements, and use of fetal fibronectin before labor induction.

Cervical status is one of the most important factors for predicting the likelihood of success in induction of labor. The modified Bishop score is the system most commonly used in clinical practice in the United States to evaluate the cervix prior to induction. This system tabulates a score based upon the station of the presenting part and four characteristics of the cervix: (1) dilation, (2) effacement, (3) consistency, and (4) position (Table 13-9).[59] If the Bishop score is *high,* variously defined but often considered to be a score of 8 or higher, the likelihood of vaginal delivery is similar whether labor is spontaneous or induced.[60] In contrast, a low Bishop score, variously defined but

TABLE 13-8   NEONATAL RESPIRATORY MORBIDITY

GESTATIONAL AGE (WEEKS)	FREQUENCY OF NICU ADMISSION PER 1000 DELIVERIES	ODDS RATIO (95% CI)
After Vaginal Delivery		
37 0/7 to 37 6/7	12.6 (7.6-19.6)	2.5 (1.5-4.2)
38 0/7 to 38 6/7	7.0 (4.6-10.2)	1.4 (0.8-2.2)
39 0/7 to 39 6/7	3.2 (1.8-4.5)	0.6 (0.4-1.0)
After Cesarean Delivery		
37 0/7 to 37 6/7	57.7 (26.7-107.1)	11.2 (5.4-13.1)
38 0/7 to 38 6/7	9.4 (1.9-27.2)	1.8 (0.6-5.9)
39 0/7 to 39 6/7	16.2 (5.9-35.5)	3.2 (1.4-7.4)

Morrison JJ, Rennie JM, Milton PJ. Neonatal respiratory morbidity and mode of delivery at term: influence of timing of elective caesarean section. *Br J Obstet Gynaecol.* 1995;102:101.
CI, confidence interval; *NICU,* neonatal intensive care unit.

TABLE 13-9   MODIFIED BISHOP SCORE

PARAMETER	SCORE 0	1	2	3
Dilation (cm)	Closed	1-2	3-4	≥5
Effacement (%)	0-30	40-50	60-70	≥80
Length* (cm)	>4	2-4	1-2	1-2
Station	−3	−2	−1 or 0	+1 or +2
Consistency	Firm	Medium	Soft	
Cervical position	Posterior	Midposition	Anterior	

From Bishop EH. Pelvic scoring for elective induction. *Obstet Gynecol.* 1964;24:266.
*Modification by Calder AA, Brennand JE. Labor and normal delivery: induction of labor. *Curr Opin Obstet Gynecol.* 1991;3:764. This modification replaces percent effacement as one of the parameters of the Bishop score.

often considered to be 6 or lower, increases the likelihood that induction will fail to result in vaginal delivery.[31] These relationships are stronger in nulliparous women.[61,62] As an example, a study[61] of 4635 spontaneous and 2647 induced labors in nulliparous women at term reported that the cesarean delivery rates were almost doubled for women with induced labors with Bishop scores below 5 compared with those with Bishop scores of 5 or higher (32% vs. 18%). Of note, the relationship between a low Bishop score and failed induction, prolonged labor, and a high cesarean birth rate was first described prior to widespread use of cervical ripening agents.[63] However, this relationship has persisted even after introduction of these agents.

Sonographic assessment of cervical length for predicting the outcome of labor induction has been evaluated in numerous studies. A systematic review[64] of 20 prospective studies found that short cervical length was associated with successful induction (likelihood ratio of a positive test, 1.66; 95% CI, 1.20 to 2.31) and failed induction (likelihood ratio of a negative test, 0.51; 95% CI, 0.39 to 0.67). The results of the study are limited by the fact that the trials that were included used different cervical length cutoff values (16.5 to 35 mm). Additionally, subgroup analysis on the seven trials that used a cervical length cutoff of 30 mm demonstrated that cervical length did not accurately predict any single specific outcome. Sonographic cervical length performed poorly for predicting vaginal delivery within 24 hours (sensitivity 59%, specificity 65%), vaginal delivery (sensitivity 67%, specificity 58%), or achievement of active labor (sensitivity 57%, specificity 60%), and it did not perform significantly better than the Bishop score for predicting a successful induction. In another systematic review[65] of 31 prospective studies that comprised 5029 women, cervical length did not perform better than Bishop score for predicting a successful induction. Thus **the role of ultrasound examination as a tool for selecting women likely to have a successful induction is uncertain, and more data are needed before this test can be recommended in choosing candidates for induction.**

The presence of an elevated fetal fibronectin (fFN) concentration in cervicovaginal secretions also has been used to try to predict success of induction, and fFN is thought to represent a disruption or inflammation of the chorionic-decidual interface. In some studies,[66] women with a positive fFN result had a significantly shorter interval before delivery than those with a negative fFN result, and a reduction was seen in the frequency of cesarean delivery. However, other investigations[67] have not confirmed these findings.

Bailit and colleagues[68] used a decision analysis to determine whether the vaginal delivery rate is increased in nulliparous women who undergo elective labor induction following fFN testing. In this model, three management strategies were evaluated: (1) no elective induction of labor for any candidate until 41 weeks' gestation (expectant management), (2) induction only of those patients with a positive fFN result at 39 weeks, and (3) elective induction for every woman at 39 weeks' gestation without performance of an fFN test. These investigators found that the expectant management strategy had the highest rate of vaginal delivery, and they concluded that the best approach to improve vaginal delivery rates was to avoid elective induction in nulliparous women.

Thus the role of fFN testing as a tool for selecting women likely to have a successful induction is uncertain. More data are needed before this test can be recommended for choosing candidates for induction.

TABLE 13-10	METHODS OF CERVICAL RIPENING
PHARMACOLOGIC	**MECHANICAL**
Oxytocin	Membrane stripping
Prostaglandins	Amniotomy
• E₂ (dinoprostone, Prepidil gel and Cervidil time-released vaginal insert)	Mechanical dilators
	• *Laminaria* tents
	• Dilapan
• E₁ (misoprostol)	• Lamicel
Estrogen	• Transcervical balloon catheters
Relaxin	• With extraamniotic saline infusion
Hyaluronic acid	
Progesterone receptor antagonists	• With concomitant oxytocin administration

Cervical Ripening

As discussed earlier, the condition of the cervix greatly influences the success of inducing labor. Cervical ripening is a complex process that results in physical softening and distensibility of the cervix and ultimately leads to partial cervical effacement and dilation.[69] Remodeling of the cervix involves enzymatic dissolution of collagen fibrils, increase in water content, and chemical changes. These changes are induced by hormones (estrogen, progesterone, relaxin), cytokines, prostaglandin, and nitric oxide synthesis enzymes.[69] Cervical ripening methods fall into two main categories: *pharmacologic* and *mechanical* (Table 13-10). **Because the state of the cervix plays such a crucial role in labor induction, a cervical examination is essential before determining which, if any, method to use for labor induction.**

Failed Induction

Vaginal delivery is the goal of the induction process; however, this occurs less often than when women labor spontaneously. It is important for the clinician to recall that cervical ripening itself can take some time, and that the development of an active labor pattern should be achieved prior to the determination that the induction has failed. **No universal standard exists for what constitutes a failed induction.** The key principle is to allow adequate time for cervical ripening and development of active labor before diagnosing a failed induction. The importance of allowing enough time to progress from the latent phase of labor to the active phase is illustrated by a number of reports.

In one large prospective study,[60] the mean duration of the *latent phase* of labor—defined as the interval from initiation of induction with either prostaglandins or oxytocin to a cervical dilation of 4 cm—in women with a Bishop score of 0 to 3 was 12 hours in multiparas and 16 hours in nulliparas. In another study,[70] requiring a minimum of 12 hours of oxytocin administration after membrane rupture before diagnosing failed labor induction led to vaginal deliveries in 75% of nulliparas and eliminated failed labor induction as an indication for cesarean delivery in parous women. A third series[71] found that 73% of women who ultimately delivered vaginally had a latent phase of up to 18 hours. *Latent phase* was defined as the interval from initiation of oxytocin or amniotomy to the beginning of the active phase (i.e., cervical dilation of 4 cm with 80% effacement or 5 cm dilation).

In a retrospective cohort study,[72] the duration of the *first stage*—defined as cervical dilation from 4 to 10 cm—was significantly longer in induced labor than in spontaneous labor: the median (95th percentile) for induced versus spontaneous labor in nulliparas was 5.5 hours (16.8 hr) versus 3.8 hours

(11.8 hours); and for multiparas, it was 4.4 hours (16.2 hours) versus 2.4 hours (8.8 hours). Although the short (≤1 hour) *active phase*, defined as cervical dilation from 6 to 10 cm, was similar for induced and spontaneous labors, each centimeter of dilation between 3 and 5 cm could take 8 to 10 hours (95th percentile) in induced labor, and dilating from 5 to 6 cm could take 4 to 6 hours (95th percentile).

The workshop convened by the NICHD, SMFM, and ACOG[16] proposed that *failed induction* be defined as failure to generate regular contractions approximately every 3 minutes and failure of the cervix to change after at least 24 hours of oxytocin administration. If safe and feasible, membranes should also be artificially ruptured. Of note, the time for cervical ripening is not included in calculating the length of induction or diagnosing a failed induction.

Lin and Rouse[73] proposed that *failed induction* be defined as the inability to achieve cervical dilation of 4 cm and 80% effacement or 5 cm (regardless of effacement) after a minimum of 12 to 18 hours of both oxytocin administration and membrane rupture. They also specified that uterine contractile activity should reach five contractions in 10 minutes or 250 Montevideo units, which is the minimum level achieved by most women whose labor is progressing normally.

Beckman[74] evaluated a group of 978 nulliparous women after either artificial or spontaneous rupture of membranes to determine factors that could predict failed induction. After membrane rupture and 10 hours of oxytocin administration, the 8% of women not in the active phase of labor had an approximately 75% chance of being delivered by cesarean section for failed induction; after 12 hours of oxytocin administration, the chance of cesarean delivery was almost 90%. Multivariate analysis showed that short maternal stature and use of pharmacologic or mechanical methods of cervical ripening contributed to an increased probability of cesarean delivery. Similarly, a linear relationship was found between lack of cervical dilation and cesarean delivery. The authors concluded that the continuation of oxytocin after amniotomy for women who had not yet reached at least 4 cm dilation was not unreasonable, but that beyond 12 hours, the benefit was unclear.

Membrane rupture and oxytocin administration should in most cases be a prerequisite before diagnosis of failed induction of labor. Additionally, experts have proposed waiting at least 24 hours in the setting of both oxytocin and ruptured membranes before diagnosing failed induction of labor.[16]

TECHNIQUES FOR CERVICAL RIPENING AND LABOR INDUCTION

Oxytocin

Oxytocin is a polypeptide hormone produced in the hypothalamus and secreted from the posterior lobe of the pituitary gland in a pulsatile fashion. It is identical to its synthetic analogue, which is among the most potent uterotonic agents known. Synthetic oxytocin is an effective means of labor induction.[75] Exogenous oxytocin administration produces periodic uterine contractions first demonstrable at approximately 20 weeks' gestation, with increasing responsiveness with advancing gestational age primarily due to an increase in myometrial oxytocin binding sites. Little change occurs in myometrial sensitivity to oxytocin from 34 weeks to term; however, **once spontaneous labor begins, the uterine sensitivity to oxytocin increases rapidly.**

This physiologic mechanism makes oxytocin more effective in augmenting labor than in inducing it, and it is even less successful as a cervical ripening agent.

Oxytocin is most often given intravenously. It cannot be given orally because the polypeptide is degraded to small, inactive forms by gastrointestinal enzymes. **The plasma half-life is short, estimated at 3 to 6 minutes, and steady-state concentrations are reached within 30 to 40 minutes of initiation or dose change. Synthetic oxytocin is generally diluted by placing 10 units in 1000 mL of an isotonic solution, such as normal saline, yielding an oxytocin concentration of 10 mU/ mL. It is given by infusion pump to allow continuous, precise control of the dose administered.**

Although oxytocin is an effective means of labor induction in women with a favorable cervix, as noted earlier, it is less effective as a cervical ripening agent. Many RCTs that have compared oxytocin with various prostaglandin (PG) formulations and other methods of cervical ripening confirm this observation. Lyndrup and colleagues compared the efficacy of labor induction with vaginal PGE$_2$ with continuous oxytocin infusion in 91 women with an unfavorable cervix (Bishop score <6). They found PGE$_2$ more efficacious for labor induction with fewer women undelivered at 24 hours. However, they also found no difference in vaginal delivery rates after 48 hours between the two groups. In a larger study that involved 200 women with an unfavorable cervix undergoing labor induction, vaginally applied PGE$_2$ was compared with continuous oxytocin infusion. These investigators found a shorter time interval to active labor, a significantly greater change in Bishop score, fewer failed inductions, and fewer multiple-day inductions with PGE$_2$ compared with oxytocin. No difference in the rate of cesarean delivery was found between the groups overall. In a Cochrane review[75] of 110 trials that included more than 11,000 women and compared oxytocin with any vaginal PG formulation for labor induction, oxytocin alone was associated with an increase in unsuccessful vaginal delivery within 24 hours (52% vs. 28%; RR, 1.85; 95% CI, 1.41 to 2.43). No difference was found in the rate of cesarean delivery between the groups. When intracervical PGs were compared with oxytocin alone for labor induction, oxytocin alone was associated with an increase in unsuccessful vaginal delivery within 24 hours (51% vs. 35%; RR, 1.49; 95% CI, 1.12 to 1.99) and an increase in cesarean delivery (19% vs. 13%; RR, 1.42; 95% CI, 1.11 to 1.82).

In the setting of *premature rupture of membranes* (PROM) at term, defined as rupture of membranes before the onset of labor, labor induction is recommended if spontaneous labor does not ensue within a certain amount of time because as the time between rupture of membranes and the onset of labor increases, so may the risk of maternal and fetal infection.[76] A series of systematic reviews examined the outcomes of pregnancies with PROM at or near term.[76] One trial accounts for most of the patients included in the analysis. Hannah and colleagues studied 5041 women with PROM at term. Subjects were randomly assigned to receive IV oxytocin, vaginal PGE$_2$ gel, or expectant management for up to 4 days. Those randomized to the expectant management group were induced if complications such as chorioamnionitis developed. The rates of neonatal infection and cesarean delivery were not statistically different between the groups. Rates of clinical chorioamnionitis were lower in the group that received IV oxytocin. When Cochrane reviewers[75] compared oxytocin alone with vaginal PGs in 14 trials for labor induction after PROM, both medications

| TABLE 13-11 | LABOR STIMULATION WITH OXYTOCIN: EXAMPLES OF LOW- AND HIGH-DOSE OXYTOCIN DOSING REGIMENS |

REGIMEN	STARTING DOSE (mU/MIN)	INCREMENTAL INCREASE (mU/MIN)	DOSAGE INTERVAL (MIN)
Low dose	0.5-1.0	1	30-40
Alternative low dose	1-2	2	15-30
High dose	6	6*	15-40
Alternative high dose	4	4	15

From Induction of Labor. ACOG Practice Bulletin No 107. American College of Obstetricians and Gynecologists. *Obstet Gynecol.* 2009;114:386.
*The incremental increase should be reduced to 3 mU/min if tachysystole is present and should be reduced to 1 mU/min for recurrent tachysystole.

| TABLE 13-12 | STANDARDIZED OXYTOCIN REGIMEN |

1. Dilution: 10 U oxytocin in 1000 mL normal saline for a resultant concentration of 10 mU oxytocin/mL
2. Infusion rate: initial dose 2 mU/min (infusion rate 12 mL/hr)
3. Incremental increase: 2 mU/min or 12 mL/hr every 45 min until contraction frequency is adequate
4. Maximum dose: 16 mU/min or 96 mL/hr

From Hayes EJ, Weinstein L. Improving patient safety and uniformity of care by a standardized regimen for the use of oxytocin. *Am J Obstet Gynecol.* 2008;198(6):622.e1-7. Epub 2008 Mar 20.

were found to be equally efficacious. Thus both can be used in this clinical setting.

The optimal regimen for oxytocin administration is debatable, although success rates for varying protocols are similar. Protocols differ as to the initial dose, incremental time period, and steady-state dose (Table 13-11).[31] A maximum oxytocin dose has not been established, but most protocols do not exceed 42 mU/min.

Low-dose protocols mimic endogenous maternal physiology and are associated with lower rates of uterine tachysystole. Low-dose oxytocin is initiated at 0.5 to 1 mU and is increased by 1 mU/min at 30- to 40-minute intervals. An alternative low dose begins at 1 to 2 mU/min increased by 2 mU/min with shorter incremental time intervals of 15 to 30 minutes.

High-dose oxytocin regimens are often used in active management of labor protocols. These regimens are largely used for labor augmentation, rather than for labor induction, and often start with an initial oxytocin dose of 6 mU/min[77] that is increased by 6 mU/min at 15- to 40-minute intervals or start at 4 mU/min with 4 mU/min incremental increases every 15 minutes. A prospective study[78] that involved nearly 5000 women at Parkland Hospital compared low- and high-dose oxytocin regimens for labor induction, and augmentation was undertaken. The high-dose protocol provided for reduction of the dosage to 3 mU/min in the presence of uterine tachysystole. The results indicated that subjects given the high-dose regimen had a significantly shorter mean admission to delivery time, fewer failed inductions, fewer forceps deliveries, fewer cesarean deliveries for failure to progress, less chorioamnionitis, and less neonatal sepsis than subjects given the low-dose regimen. Notably, these subjects had a higher rate of cesarean delivery performed for "fetal distress," but no differences in neonatal outcomes were noted. Merrill and Zlatnik[79] conducted a randomized, double-blind trial that included 1307 patients and compared high-dose oxytocin (4.5 mU/min initially increased by 4.5 mU/min every 30 minutes) with a low-dose regimen (1.5 mU/min initially, increased by 1.5 mU/min every 30 minutes) for augmentation and induction of labor. Oxytocin solutions were prepared by a central pharmacy, and infusion volumes were identical to ensure double masking. In the group that received high-dose oxytocin, labor was significantly shortened whether the drug was used for induction (8.5 vs. 10.5 hours, $P < .001$) or for augmentation (4.4 vs. 5.1 hours, $P = .3$). No significant difference was reported in the rates of cesarean delivery between the two regimens (15% vs. 11.3%, $P = .17$). However, more decreases or discontinuations of oxytocin were seen in the high-dose group both for

uterine tachysystole and fetal heart rate abnormalities, yet neonatal outcomes were observed to be similar in both groups.

Satin and colleagues[78] studied the differences in outcomes when oxytocin was used to *augment,* as opposed to *induce,* labor. The low-dose regimen consisted of a starting dose of 1 mU/min with incremental increases of 1 mU/min at 20-min intervals until 8 mU/min then 2 mU/min increases up to a maximum of 20 mU/min. The high-dose regimen consisted of a starting dose of 6 mU/min with increases of 6 mU/min at 20-minute intervals up to a maximum dose of 42 mU/min. Labor augmentation was more than 3 hours shorter in the high-dose group, and high-dose augmentation resulted in fewer cesarean deliveries for labor dystocia and fewer failed inductions when compared with the low-dose regimen. A literature review of randomized clinical trials of high- versus low-dose oxytocin regimens published from 1966 to 2003 revealed that high-dose oxytocin decreased the time from admission to vaginal delivery but did not decrease the incidence of cesarean delivery compared with low-dose therapy. The only double-blinded randomized trial that has been published had similar findings.[79] In a 2014 Cochrane review of nine trials, high-dose oxytocin reduced the induction to delivery interval in high-quality trials but did not decrease the frequency of cesarean delivery compared with a low-dose regimen. In this review, high-dose regimens were associated with a higher rate of tachysystole, with similar maternal and neonatal complications in both regimens.

Oxytocin Dosing Intervals and Protocols

Several experts have suggested that implementation of a standardized protocol is desirable to minimize errors in oxytocin administration.[80-82] Clark and colleagues[82] implemented an oxytocin checklist-based protocol at a tertiary facility and evaluated outcomes in 100 women prior to utilization of the protocol versus another 100 women after the protocol was put into practice. In the checklist-managed group, the maximum dose of oxytocin used to achieve delivery was significantly lower. No differences were noted before or after the protocol in the length of labor, total time of oxytocin administration, or rate of operative vaginal or abdominal delivery. When the protocol was then implemented throughout the Hospital Corporation of America system (125 obstetric facilities in 20 states), the rate of cesarean delivery decreased from 23.6% to 21.0%, and Apgar scores below 8 and newborn complications requiring NICU admission also decreased. Hayes and Weinstein[80] defined a standardized protocol for oxytocin administration based on a literature review and also described the specific pharmacokinetics of oxytocin (Table 13-12). **However, at this time, no protocol has demonstrated its superiority in both efficacy and safety over another.**

Limited data are available to guide how long the oxytocin infusion should be maintained once an adequate contraction pattern has been achieved. One noninferiority study[83] involved

138 subjects and compared the strategy of continuing oxytocin until delivery versus discontinuing oxytocin at onset of active labor, and it suggested discontinuation of prolonged labor. The authors of a meta-analysis[84] assessed the effect of discontinuation of oxytocin after onset of the active phase of labor. Eight studies were included and involved 1232 subjects, and these researchers observed decreased cesarean delivery in subjects who had oxytocin discontinued (OR, 0.51; 95% CI, 0.35 to 0.74). Similarly, cases of nonreassuring fetal heart patterns were less likely among women who did not receive oxytocin after the establishment of the active phase of labor (OR, 0.63; 95% CI, 0.41 to 0.97).

Prostaglandins

Administration of PG results in dissolution of collagen bundles and an increase in submucosal water content of the cervix. These changes in cervical connective tissue at term are similar to those observed in early labor. PGs are endogenous compounds found in the myometrium, decidua, and fetal membranes during pregnancy. The chemical precursor is arachidonic acid. PG formulations have been used since they were first synthesized in the laboratory in 1968, and PG analogues were originally given intravenously and by oral routes. Later, local administration of PGs in the vagina or the endocervix became the route of choice because of fewer side effects and acceptable clinical response. Side effects of all PG formulations and routes may include fever, chills, vomiting, and diarrhea.

The efficacy of locally applied PG (vaginal or intracervical) for cervical ripening and labor induction has been demonstrated in a Cochrane review that involved more than 10,000 women. For example, vaginal PGE_2 reduced the likelihood of vaginal delivery not being achieved within 24 hours, the risk of the cervix remaining unfavorable or unchanged, and the need for oxytocin. In addition, no difference was found between cesarean delivery rates, although there was a trade-off with PGE_2 use because the risk of uterine tachysystole with fetal heart rate changes was increased.

The various administration vehicles for PG (tablet, gel, and timed-release pessary) appear to be equally efficacious. The optimal route, frequency, and dose of PGs of all types and formulations for cervical ripening and labor induction have not been determined. Also, PG formulations of any kind should be avoided in women with a prior uterine scar, such as a prior cesarean delivery or myomectomy, because their use has been associated with an increased risk of uterine rupture.[85] Uterine activity and fetal heart rate monitoring are indicated for 0.5 to 2 hours after administration of prostaglandins for cervical ripening and should be maintained as long as regular uterine activity is present.[31]

Prostaglandin E₂

One of the first RCTs to use intravaginal PG was conducted in 1979 by Liggins. Eighty-four term women with singleton pregnancies were randomly assigned to three groups that received either placebo or a 0.2 mg or 0.4 mg PGE_2 compound. Labor was established in 48 hours in 9.3% of women who received a placebo, 65.4% of women who received 0.2 mg PGE_2, and 85.7% of women who received 0.4 mg PGE_2. Rayburn summarized the experience with more than 3313 pregnancies representing 59 prospective clinical trials in which either intracervical or intravaginal PGE_2 was used for cervical ripening before the induction of labor. He concluded that **local administration of PGE_2 is effective in enhancing cervical effacement and dilation thus reducing the failed induction rate, shortening the induction-to-delivery interval, and reducing oxytocin use and cesarean delivery for failure to progress.** These findings were confirmed in a meta-analysis of 44 trials performed worldwide using various PG compounds and dosing regimens. Because no difference in clinical outcomes are apparent when comparing intravaginal or intracervical PGE_2 preparations, and for ease of administration and patient satisfaction, vaginal administration is recommended.[86] A sustained-release vaginal pessary for PGE_2 has been developed whose use eliminates the need for repeated dosing. Although data are limited, when comparing the efficacy of the intravaginally applied PGE_2 to the sustained-release suppository, no difference is apparent in rates of vaginal delivery, fetal heart rate abnormalities, or uterine tachysystole.

Currently, two PGE_2 preparations have been approved by the United States Food and Drug Administration (FDA) for cervical ripening. Although not approved by the FDA for cervical ripening, a variety of other PGE_2 compounds are available—such as suppositories in the United States and tablets in Europe and other parts of the world. PGE_2 was originally manufactured as a 20-mg vaginal suppository. However, to prepare the medication in smaller doses for induction of labor at term, pharmacists resuspend the suppository into small amounts of methylcellulose gel. The preparation is then frozen in plastic syringes in various doses.

Prepidil contains dinoprostone, 0.5 mg per 3-g syringe (2.5 mL gel) for intracervical administration. The dose can be repeated in 6 to 12 hours if cervical change is inadequate and uterine activity is minimal following the first dose. The manufacturer recommends that the maximum cumulative dose of dinoprostone not exceed 1.5 mg (three doses) within a 24-hour period. Oxytocin should not be initiated until 6 to 12 hours after the last dose because of the potential for uterine tachysystole with concurrent oxytocin and prostaglandin administration.

Cervidil is a vaginal insert that contains 10 mg of dinoprostone in a timed-release formulation. The vaginal insert administers the medication at 0.3 mg/hr and may be left in place for up to 12 hours. An advantage of the vaginal insert over the gel formulation is that the insert may be removed with the onset of active labor, rupture of membranes, or with the development of uterine tachysystole. This abnormality of uterine contractions is more often defined as six or more contractions in 10 minutes for a total of 20 minutes and may be associated with concurrent fetal heart rate tracing abnormalities. Per the manufacturer's recommendations, oxytocin may be initiated 30 to 60 minutes after removal of the insert.

These two preparations are relatively expensive, require refrigerated storage, and become unstable at room temperature.

Prostaglandin E₁

Misoprostol is a synthetic PGE_1 analogue available as 100-μg and 200-μg tablets. The current FDA approved use for misoprostol is for the treatment and prevention of peptic ulcer disease related to chronic nonsteroidal antiinflammatory drug (NSAID) use. **Administration of misoprostol for preinduction cervical ripening is considered a safe and effective off-label use by ACOG.**[87] Misoprostol is inexpensive and is also stable at room temperature, and it can be administered orally or placed vaginally with few systemic side effects. Although not scored, the tablets may be divided to provide 25- or 50-μg doses.

Multiple studies suggest that misoprostol tablets placed vaginally are either superior to or equivalent in efficacy compared with intracervical PGE_2 gel.[88] More recently, a meta-analysis of

70 trials revealed the following points regarding the use of misoprostol compared with other methods of cervical ripening and labor induction. Misoprostol improved cervical ripening compared with placebo and was associated with a reduced failure to achieve vaginal delivery within 24 hours (RR, 0.36; 95% CI, 0.19 to 0.68). Compared with other vaginal prostaglandins for labor induction, vaginal misoprostol was more effective in achieving vaginal delivery within 24 hours (RR, 0.80; 95% CI, 0.73 to 0.87). Compared with vaginal or intracervical PGE_2, oxytocin augmentation also was less common with misoprostol (RR, 0.65; 95% CI, 0.57 to 0.73). However, uterine tachysystole with fetal heart rate changes (RR, 2.04; 95% CI, 1.49 to 2.80) and meconium-stained amniotic fluid (RR, 1.42; 95% CI, 1.11 to 1.81) were more common with misoprostol. Most studies suggested that restricting the dose of misoprostol to 25 µg every 4 hours significantly reduced the risk of uterine tachysystole with and without fetal heart rate changes and meconium passage. Most important, regardless of misoprostol dose, no significant differences were reported in immediate neonatal outcomes.

Although based on its review of the existing evidence, ACOG recommends 25 µg dosing every 3 to 6 hours with vaginally applied misoprostol, the optimal dose and timing interval is not known.[31] If necessary, oxytocin may be initiated 4 hours after the final misoprostol dose. A meta-analysis that compared 25-µg with 50-µg dosing reported that 50-µg dosing resulted in a higher rate of vaginal delivery within 24 hours with higher rates of uterine tachysystole and meconium passage but without compromising neonatal outcomes. A higher frequency of *fetal acidosis,* defined as an umbilical arterial pH of less than 7.16, was found in infants born to mothers given 50 µg of intravaginally applied misoprostol every 3 hours compared with those born to mothers given 25 µg every 3 hours. In their Committee Opinions on the use of misoprostol for labor induction, ACOG concludes that safety using the higher 50-µg (every 6 hours) dosing could not be adequately evaluated, may be associated with uterine tachysystole with fetal heart rate decelerations, and suggests the higher doses should only be used in select circumstances.

A misoprostol vaginal insert (MVI) that contains a controlled-release retrievable polymer chip for gradual delivery of 200 µg over 24 hours has been developed and is available in some countries in Western Europe, but it is currently not available in the United States.[89,90] The 200 µg dose is released at a mean rate of approximately 7 µg/hr while the insert remains in place, allowing a constant dosing to occur over a 24-hour period with the benefit of rapid and easy removal if needed.

Oral misoprostol for cervical ripening has also been studied. This route of administration has promise for offering more patient comfort, satisfaction, and convenience. Most trials compared oral misoprostol dosages of 20 to 50 µg with similar vaginal misoprostol dosing regimens, such as 25 to 50 µg. This oral dosing regimen appears to be no more effective than vaginal administration for achieving vaginal delivery, but it may be associated with less uterine tachysystole. A clear, positive dose-response relationship exists between the dosage of oral misoprostol and the frequency of tachysystole.[91]

Some investigators have described titrating oral misoprostol to its desired effect.[92] This method appears to achieve vaginal delivery rates similar to vaginally administered misoprostol with less uterine tachysystole. Low doses of oral misoprostol were achieved by making a solution (e.g., dissolving a 200 µg tablet in 200 mL tap water) because this was believed to provide more accurate dosing than simply cutting the tablet into pieces. Because oral dosing has a short (2 hr) duration of action, administration was repeated at 2-hour intervals.

In a Cochrane review of 76 RCTs that included 14,412 women, oral misoprostol appeared to be at least as effective as current methods of induction. In 12 trials (3859 women) that compared oral misoprostol with vaginal dinoprostone, women given misoprostol were less likely to need cesarean delivery (21% compared with 26% of women), although the time in labor was longer. The 37 trials (6417 women) that compared oral and vaginal misoprostol reported similar effectiveness, but those taking oral misoprostol had better neonatal outcomes at birth and less postpartum hemorrhage. Nine trials[93] that comprised 1282 women showed that oral misoprostol was equivalent to IV oxytocin but resulted in significantly fewer cesarean deliveries. The authors of this Cochrane review recommend that if clinicians choose to use oral misoprostol, a dose of 20 to 25 µg in solution is preferred for both the safety considerations and the imprecision of dividing misoprostol tablets for recommended dosages. However, concerns have been raised that the pharmacy and nursing administration needed for dose titration adds a layer of complexity, and more data are needed to shed light on the optimal dosing, safety, and cost-effectiveness of oral misoprostol for cervical ripening and labor induction.

Other novel methods of administration for misoprostol that have been assessed include buccal and sublingual routes. The theory is that avoiding first-pass hepatic circulation from oral administration will lead to bioavailability similar to that achieved with vaginal administration. In an RCT that included 250 women admitted for labor induction, 50 µg of sublingual misoprostol was compared with 100 µg of orally administered misoprostol given every 4 hours to a maximum of five doses. Sublingual misoprostol appeared to have the same efficacy as orally administered misoprostol to achieve vaginal delivery within 24 hours with no increase in uterine tachysystole. In another RCT, 152 women received either buccal misoprostol (200 µg for first two doses, then 300 µg to total 1600 µg) or vaginal (50 µg for first two doses, then 100 µg to total 500 µg). No statistically significant difference was noted in time to vaginal delivery, the rate of vaginal delivery, or the rate of uterine tachysystole. Based on only three small trials included in the Cochrane meta-analysis, sublingual misoprostol appears to be at least as effective as the same dose administered orally, although data are inadequate to comment on the relative complications and side effects. Therefore more data are needed to clarify not only the safety but the efficacy of buccal and sublingual misoprostol.

Alternative Methods

Researchers have evaluated several other methods and compounds as mechanical and pharmacologic alternatives for cervical ripening and labor induction in term pregnancies (Table 13-13). Some of the advantages of the mechanical techniques include low cost, low risk of tachysystole, and few systemic side

TABLE 13-13	ALTERNATIVE METHODS FOR INDUCTION
PHARMACOLOGIC	**MECHANICAL**
Mifepristone	Stripping (sweeping) fetal membranes
Estrogen	Amniotomy
Relaxin	Hygroscopic dilators
Hyaluronic acid	Foley balloon catheter above internal os

effects. The disadvantages of mechanical methods include a small increase in risk of infection from introduction of a foreign body, the potential for disruption of a low-lying placenta, and some maternal discomfort upon manipulation of the cervix. **All of these methods likely work, at least in part, by causing the release of prostaglandin F2-alpha from the decidua and adjacent membranes or PGE$_2$ from the cervix.** Also, the dilators (e.g., laminaria) and balloon catheter physically cause gradual cervical dilation with minimal discomfort to the patient.

Stripping or sweeping of the fetal membranes refers to digital separation of the chorioamniotic membrane from the wall of the cervix and lower uterine segment by inserting the examiner's finger beyond the internal cervical os and then rotating the finger circumferentially along the lower uterine segment. Investigations[94] have studied routine membrane stripping at 38 or 39 weeks to either prevent prolonged pregnancies or decrease the frequency of more formal inductions after 41 weeks. Two randomized trials compared outcomes of women who underwent membrane stripping or no membrane stripping at initiation of labor induction with oxytocin. The results of these trials suggested that membrane stripping increased the rate of spontaneous vaginal delivery and shortened the induction to delivery interval. However, differences in study design and heterogeneous management of induction preclude definitive conclusions. None of these trials reported harmful side effects that could be attributed to the procedure.

Although the existing meta-analysis on the use of membrane stripping[95] did not reveal an increase in either maternal or neonatal infection associated with the procedure, it is unclear whether these studies included carriers of Group B *Streptococcus* (GBS). Only one small study evaluated GBS colonization associated with sweeping membranes, and whereas no additional risk was found in women with sweeping, the study was too small to exclude an effect. GBS colonization is not a contraindication to membrane stripping because no direct evidence of harm exists, but given the limited data for the procedure in known GBS carriers, the potential benefits and risks should be carefully weighed before performing the procedure in known carriers.[96]

Another commonly used method for cervical ripening is the **transcervical balloon catheter**, which appears to be as effective for preinduction cervical ripening as PGE$_2$ gel and intravaginal misoprostol. The combination of a balloon catheter plus administration of a prostaglandin does not appear to be more effective than prostaglandins alone.

MIDTRIMESTER INDUCTION

In particular circumstances, such as when a fetus has died in utero or in cases of termination of pregnancy, a woman may choose to have an induction of labor to effect delivery of the fetus. Although in the case of an intrauterine demise, some women would prefer expectant management in order to avoid an induction of labor, this approach raises concerns regarding the development of a consumptive coagulopathy and/or intrauterine infection. Some studies[97] report that 80% to 90% of women will spontaneously labor within 2 weeks of a fetal demise, but the latency period may be longer.

Options for delivery in the case of intrauterine demise or pregnancy termination in the mid second trimester include induction of labor and dilation and evacuation (D&E; Table 13-14). The decision for which mode of delivery to choose must

TABLE 13-14 SECOND-TRIMESTER TERMINATION METHODS

SURGICAL	MEDICAL
Dilation and evacuation	Intravenous oxytocin
Laparotomy	Intraamniotic hyperosmotic fluid
Hysterotomy	20% saline
Hysterectomy	30% urea
	Prostaglandins E2, F2-alpha, E1, and analogues
	Mifepristone
	Various combinations of above

be individualized by practitioner experience, gestational age, and a patient's desires. The emotional and psychological factors vary with each patient, with one advantage of induction being the delivery of an intact fetus, whereas an advantage of D&E may be avoiding a prolonged induction.

Most of the research available regarding modes of midtrimester delivery is extrapolated from the investigations performed on second trimester abortions. One study compared patients undergoing surgical termination between 14 and 24 weeks of gestation with women undergoing labor induction and revealed an overall lower rate of complications in those undergoing D&E (4% vs. 29%). Cochrane reviewers[98] recently concluded that D&E is superior to intraamniotic instillation of prostaglandin F2-alpha and may be favored over mifepristone and misoprostol, but larger randomized studies are necessary to confirm the latter finding. At this time, both methods of delivery are considered reasonably safe.

Several methods of labor induction have been utilized, but no single protocol is currently accepted as best practice. More recent protocols have implemented regimens with gemeprost or misoprostol, both PGE$_1$ analogues; however, a meta-analysis of randomized trials to compare the two medications reported that misoprostol suppositories were associated with a reduced need for narcotic analgesia and surgical evacuation of the uterus. The application of gemeprost is limited secondary to its expense and instability at room temperature. It is also not currently available in the United States. At this time, the World Health Organization (WHO) also recommends the use of mifepristone prior to PGE$_1$ analogues for expeditious and safe second trimester abortions. As an antiprogestin, mifepristone increases uterine sensitivity to prostaglandins, which permits lower doses and minimizes side effects. However, current studies[99] do not reveal any advantage of pretreatment with mifepristone for induction in second-trimester fetal demise.

When planning an induction of labor, gestational age plays a significant role regarding the methods of induction. When the gestational age is less than 28 weeks, the uterus is less sensitive to oxytocin and therefore prostaglandins or mechanical devices may be required to commence labor. Current induction protocols vary by dose, route, and gestational age (Table 13-15). It is important to keep in mind that although side effects (uterine tachysystole, nausea, vomiting, diarrhea) and safety remain important considerations for the patient in these circumstances, fetal well-being is no longer an issue.

Women with a prior cesarean delivery are candidates for induction of labor with PG in these circumstances as well. A recent review by Berghella and colleagues reported an incidence of uterine rupture of 0.4%, hysterectomy 0%, and transfusion 0.2% for women undergoing second-trimester misoprostol terminations.

TABLE 13-15   SUGGESTED PROTOCOLS FOR STILLBIRTH DELIVERY

DILATION AND EVACUATION FOR UTERUS 13- TO 22-WK SIZE	INDUCTION OF LABOR
• Admit to hospital, day operating room, or clinic. • Obtain hematocrit and type and screen. • Give doxycycline 100 mg orally 1 hr before procedure and 200 mg after procedure or postoperative metronidazole 500 mg orally twice a day for 5 days.	• Admit to labor and delivery. • Obtain complete blood count and type and screen; consider fibrinogen if the fetus has been dead for more than 4 wk.
TO FACILITATE CERVICAL DILATION	**INDUCTION PROTOCOLS**
• Administer misoprostol 200 µg in the posterior fornix 4 hr before the procedure (may be placed by patient). • Place *Laminaria* in cervix (usually carried out in the office on the afternoon before the procedure).	• For uterus <28 wk: misoprostol 200 to 400 µg vaginally or orally every 4 hr until delivery of fetus. • For uterus >28 wk: misoprostol 25 to 50 µg vaginally or orally every 4 hr or oxytocin infusion per usual protocol. • Consider transcervical Foley catheter or *Laminaria* for cervical ripening.
OPERATIVE	**INTRAPARTUM**
• Perform dilation and evacuation under ultrasound guidance.	• To minimize risk of retained placenta, allow for spontaneous placental delivery, avoid pulling on the umbilical cord, and consider further doses of misoprostol or high-dose oxytocin. • Monitor vital signs per the routine for labor and delivery. • Pain management includes epidural or intravenous narcotics via patient-controlled analgesia or intermittent doses. • Parents should be encouraged to spend time with the infant and should be offered keepsake items such as pictures and handprints or footprints.
POSTPROCEDURE INSTRUCTIONS	**POSTPROCEDURE INSTRUCTIONS**
• Discharge home after anesthesia has worn off and vaginal bleeding is minimal. • Administer RhD immune globulin if patient is Rh negative. • Schedule a follow-up visit in 2 wk. • Prescribe NSAIDs or mild narcotics. • Offer bereavement services.	• Discharge home in 6 to 24 hr if vital signs are stable and bleeding is appropriate. • Consider postpartum care on a nonmaternity ward. • Administer RhD immune globulin if patient is Rh negative. • Follow-up visit in 2 to 6 wk. • Offer bereavement services.

Modified from Silver RM, Heuser CC. Stillbirth workup and delivery management. *Clin Obstet Gynecol.* 2010;53(3):681.
NSAIDs, nonsteroidal antiinflammatory drugs.

SUMMARY

Induction of labor is one of the most commonly performed procedures in obstetrics and can be undertaken for a variety of medical and obstetric indications. The likelihood for success in the induction of labor has been studied with focus on a number of clinical, biochemical, and radiographic approaches. Cervical dilation at the time of induction is the factor most associated with success, but no single factor has been shown to be a good predictor. A variety of pharmacologic and mechanical methods for cervical ripening are available. The most commonly used approaches include prostaglandins, such as dinoprostone and misoprostol, and transcervical Foley balloon catheter placement. Augmentation of labor is usually accomplished with IV oxytocin, which can be administered using either low- or high-dose infusion protocols. In the case of a midtrimester induction, either induction of labor or dilation and evacuation is considered a safe approach.

KEY POINTS

• *Labor* is a clinical diagnosis defined as uterine contractions that result in progressive cervical effacement and dilation, often accompanied by a bloody discharge referred to as *bloody show,* that results in birth of the baby.

• The diagnosis of labor protraction and arrest should account for the level of cervical dilation.

• Because the duration of latent labor is highly variable, expectant management is most appropriate.

• The most common causes of protraction or arrest disorders are inadequate uterine activity and abnormal positioning of the fetal presenting part.

• Under new guidelines, neither a protracted active phase nor arrest of dilation should be diagnosed in a nullipara before 6 cm cervical dilation.

• Before a diagnosis of arrest of active-phase arrest is made, rupture of membranes should have occurred and the cervix must be dilated at least 6 cm, with either 4 hours or more of adequate contractions (e.g., more than 200 Montevideo units) or 6 hours or more of inadequate contractions and no cervical change.

• Induction of labor should be undertaken when the benefits of delivery to either mother or fetus outweigh the risks of pregnancy continuation.

• Studies have demonstrated that routine induction of labor at 41 weeks' gestation is not associated with an increased risk of cesarean delivery regardless of parity, state of the cervix, or method of induction.

• If elective induction is undertaken for nonmedical reasons, women should have pregnancies of 39 weeks' gestation or more.

• It is important for the clinician to recall that cervical ripening itself can take some time and that the development of an active labor pattern should be achieved prior to the determination that the induction has failed.

◆ Induction of labor with IV oxytocin, intravaginal prostaglandin compounds, and expectant management (with defined time limits) are all reasonable options for women and their infants in the face of PROM at term because they result in similar rates of neonatal infection and cesarean delivery.

◆ Options of delivery for midtrimester stillbirth or induction for pregnancy termination include induction of labor and dilation and evacuation. The decision for which mode of delivery to choose must be individualized by practitioner experience, gestational age, and a patient's desires.

REFERENCES

1. Friedman E. An objective approach to the diagnosis and management of abnormal labor. *Bull N Y Acad Med.* 1972;48:842.
2. Spong CY. Defining "term" pregnancy: recommendations from the Defining "Term" Pregnancy Workgroup. *JAMA.* 2013;309:2445-2446.
3. Zhang J, Troendle J, Mikolajczyk R, et al. The natural history of the normal first stage of labor. *Obstet Gynecol.* 2010;115:705.
4. Zhang J, Landy HJ, Branch DW, et al. Contemporary patterns of spontaneous labor with normal neonatal outcomes. *Obstet Gynecol.* 2010;116: 1281-1287.
5. Zhang J, Troendle J, Reddy UM, et al. Contemporary cesarean delivery practice in the United States. *Am J Obstet Gynecol.* 2010;203:326.e1-326.e10.
6. Rouse DJ, Owen J, Hauth JC. Active-phase labor arrest: Oxytocin augmentation for at least 4 hours. *Obstet Gynecol.* 1999;93:323.
7. American College of Obstetricians and Gynecologists. Safe prevention of the primary cesarean delivery. Obstetric Care Consensus No. 1. *Obstet Gynecol.* 2014;123:693-711.
8. Ponkey SE, Cohen AP, Heffner LJ, Lieberman E. Persistent fetal occiput posterior position: obstetric outcomes. *Obstet Gynecol.* 2003;101:915.
9. Rouse DJ, Owen J, Goldenberg RL, Cliver SP. The effectiveness and costs of elective cesarean delivery for fetal macrosomia diagnosed by ultrasound. *JAMA.* 1996;276:1480.
10. Piper JM, Bolling DR, Newton ER. The second stage of labor: factors influencing duration. *Am J Obstet Gynecol.* 1991;165:976.
11. Rouse DJ, Weiner SJ, Bloom SL, Varner MW, Spong CY, Ramin SM, et al. Second-stage labor duration in nulliparous women: relationship to maternal and perinatal outcomes. Eunice Kennedy Shriver National Institute of Child Health and Human Development. Maternal-Fetal Medicine Units Network. *Am J Obstet Gynecol.* 2009;201:357.e1-357.e7.
12. Cheng YW, Hopkins LM, Laros RK Jr, Caughey AB. Duration of the second stage of labor in multiparous women: maternal and neonatal outcomes. *Am J Obstet Gynecol.* 2007;196:585.e1-585.e6, -.
13. Allen VM, Baskett TF, O'Connell CM, et al. Maternal and perinatal outcomes with increasing duration of the second stage of labor. *Obstet Gynecol.* 2009;113:1248-1258.
14. Kilpatrick SJ, Laros RK. Characteristics of normal labor. *Obstet Gynecol.* 1989;74:85.
15. American College of Obstetricians and Gynecologists. Dystocia and augmentation of labor. ACOG Practice Bulletin No. 49. *Obstet Gynecol.* 2004; 102:1445.
16. Spong CY, Berghella V, Wenstrom KC, Mercer BM, Saade GR. Prevention of the fist cesarean delivery: Eunice Kennedy Shriver National Institute of Child Health and Development, Society for Maternal-Fetal Medicine, and American College of Obstetricians and Gynecologists Workshop. *Obstet Gynecol.* 2012;120:1181-1193.
17. Myles TD, Santolaya J. Maternal and neonatal outcomes in patients with a prolonged second stage of labor. *Obstet Gynecol.* 2003;102:52.
18. Dombrowski MP, Bottoms SF, Saleh AA, et al. Third stage of labor: Analysis of duration and clinical practice. *Am J Obstet Gynecol.* 1995;172:1279.
19. Magann EF, Evans S, Chauhan SP, et al. The length of the third stage of labor and the risk of postpartum hemorrhage. *Obstet Gynecol.* 2005;105:290.

20. Begley CM, Gyte GM, Murphy DJ, et al. Active versus expectant management for women in the third stage of labour. *Cochrane Database Syst Rev.* 2010;(7):CD007412.
21. Jackson KW, Allbert JR, Schemmer GK, et al. A randomized controlled trial comparing oxytocin administration before and after placental delivery in the prevention of postpartum hemorrhage. *Am J Obstet Gynecol.* 2001; 185:873.
22. American College of Obstetricians and Gynecologists. Prophylactic antibiotics in labor and delivery. *Obstet Gynecol.* 2003;102:875.
23. Anim-Somuah M, Smyth R, Howell C. Epidural versus non-epidural or no analgesia in labor. *Cochrane Database Syst Rev.* 2005;(4):CD000331.
24. Halpern SH, Abdallah FW. Effect of labor analgesia on labor outcome. *Curr Opin Anaesthesiol.* 2010;23:317.
25. Clark S, Simpson KR, Knox GE, Garite TJ. Oxytocin: New perspectives on an old drug. *Am J Obstet Gynecol.* 2009;200:35.e1.
26. Ho M, Cheng SY, Tsai-Chung L. Titrated oral misoprostol solution compared with intravenous oxytocin for labor augmentation. *Obstet Gynecol.* 2010;116:612.
27. Robinson B, Nelson L. A review of the proceedings from the 2008 NICHD workshop on standardized nomenclature for cardiotocography. *Rev Obstet Gynecol.* 2008;1:186.
28. Davies GA, Tessier JL, Woodman MC, et al. Maternal hemodynamics after oxytocin bolus compared with infusion in the third stage of labor: A randomized controlled trial. *Obstet Gynecol.* 2005;105:294.
29. Landon MB, Hauth JC, Leveno KJ, et al. and NICHD Maternal Fetal Medicine Unit Network. Maternal and perinatal outcomes associated with a trial of labor after prior cesarean delivery. *N Engl J Med.* 2004;351:2581.
30. American College of Obstetricians and Gynecologists. Vaginal birth after previous cesarean delivery. ACOG Practice Bulletin No. 115. *Obstet Gynecol.* 2010;116:450.
31. American College of Obstetricians and Gynecologists. Induction of labor. ACOG Practice Bulletin No. 107. *Obstet Gynecol.* 2009;114:386.
32. HYPITAT Study Group. Induction of labour versus expectant monitoring for gestational hypertension or mild pre-eclampsia after 36 weeks' gestation (HYPITAT): a multicenter, open-label randomized controlled trial. *Lancet.* 2009;374(9694):979-988.
33. American College of Obstetricians and Gynecologists. ACOG Committee Opinion no. 561: Nonmedically indicated early-term deliveries. *Obstet Gynecol.* 2013;121:911.
34. Hilder L, Costeloe K, Thilaganathan B. Prolonged pregnancy: Evaluating gestation-specific risks of fetal and infant mortality. *Br J Obstet Gynecol.* 1998;105:169.
35. Nakling J, Backe B. Pregnancy risk increases from 41 weeks gestation. *Acta Obstet Gynecol Scand.* 2006;85:663.
36. Heimstad R, Romundstad PR, Eik-Nes SH, Salvesen KA. Outcomes of pregnancy beyond 37 weeks gestation. *Obstet Gynecol.* 2006;108:500.
37. Hannah ME. Postterm pregnancy: Should all women have labour induced? A review of the literature. *Fetal Matern Med Review.* 1993;5:3.
38. Alexander JM, McIntire DD, Leveno KJ. Forty weeks and beyond: Pregnancy outcomes by week of gestation. *Obstet Gynecol.* 2000;96:291.
39. Caughey AB, Stotland NE, Washington AE, et al. Maternal obstetric complications of pregnancy are associated with increasing gestational age at term. *Am J Obstet Gynecol.* 2007;196(155):e1.
40. Caughey AB, Bishop J. Maternal complications of pregnancy increase beyond 40 weeks of gestation in low-risk women. *J Perinatol.* 2006;26:540.
41. Stock SJ, Ferguson E, Duffy A, et al. Outcomes of elective induction of labour compared with expectant management: population based study. *BMJ.* 2012;344:e2838.
42. Cheng YW, Kaimal AJ, Snowden JM, et al. Induction of labor compared to expectant management in low-risk women and associated perinatal outcomes. *Am J Obstet Gynecol.* 2012;207:502.e1-502.e8.
43. Darney BG, Snowden JM, Chen YW, et al. Elective induction of labor at term compared with expectant management: maternal and nenonatal outcomes. *Obstet Gynecol.* 2013.
44. Osmundson SS, Ou-Yang RJ, Grobman WA. Elective induction compared with expectant management in nulliparous women with a favorable cervix. *Obstet Gyencol.* 2010;116:601-605.
45. Osmundson S, Ou-Yang RJ, Grobman WA. Elective induction compared with expectant management in nulliparous women with a unfavorable cervix. *Obstet Gynecol.* 2011;117:583-587.
46. Caughey AB, Sundaram V, Kaimal AJ, et al. Systematic review: Elective induction of labor versus expectant management of pregnancy. *Ann Intern Med.* 2009;151:252.
47. Guzmezoglu AM, Crowther CA, Middleton P, Heatley E. Induction of labor for improving birth outcomes for women at or beyond term. *Cochrane Database Syst Rev.* 2012;(6):Art No. CD004945.

48. Osterman MJ, Martin JA. Recent declines in induction of labor by gestational age. *NCHS Data Brief.* 2014;155:1-8.

49. Cammu H, Martens G, Ruyssinck G, Amy JJ. Outcome after elective labor induction in nulliparous women: A matched cohort study. *Am J Obstet Gynecol.* 2002;186:240.

50. Gulmezoglu AM, Crowther CA, Middleton P. Induction of labour for improving birth outcomes for women at or beyond term. *Cochrane Database Syst Rev.* 2006;(4):CD004945.

51. Caughey AB, Nicholson JM, Cheng YW, et al. Induction of labor and cesarean delivery by gestational age. *Am J Obstet Gynecol.* 2006;195:700.

52. Zhang X, Joseph KS, Kramer MS. Decreased term and postterm birthweight in the US: Impact of labor induction. *Am J Obstet Gynecol.* 2010;124:e1.

53. Pevzner L, Rayburn WF, Rumney P, Wing DA. Factors predicting successful labor induction with dinoprostone and misoprostol vaginal inserts. *Obstet Gynecol.* 2009;114:261.

54. Clark SL, Miller DD, Belfort MA, et al. Neonatal and maternal outcomes associated with elective term delivery. *Am J Obstet Gynecol.* 2009;200:156.e1.

55. Bailit JL, Gregory KD, Reddy UM, et al. Maternal and neonatal outcomes by labor onset type and gestational age. *Am J Obstet Gynecol.* 2010;202:245.e1.

56. Kaufman KE, Bailit JL, Grobman W. Elective induction: An analysis of economic and health consequences. *Am J Obstet Gynecol.* 2002;187:858.

57. Crane JM. Factors predicting labor induction success: a critical analysis. *Clin Obstet Gynecol.* 2006;49:573.

58. Chandra S, Crane JM, Hutchens D, Young DC. Transvaginal ultrasound and digital examination in predicting successful labor induction. *Obstet Gynecol.* 2001;98:2.

59. Calder AA, Brennand JE. Labor and normal delivery: Induction of labor. *Curr Opin Obstet Gynecol.* 1991;3:764.

60. Xenakis EM, Piper JM, Conway DL, Langer O. Induction of labor in the nineties: Conquering the unfavorable cervix. *Obstet Gynecol.* 1997;90:235.

61. Johnson DP, Davis NR, Brown AJ. Risk of cesarean delivery after induction at term in nulliparous women with an unfavorable cervix. *Am J Obstet Gynecol.* 2003;188:1565.

62. Vrouenraets FP, Roumen FJ, Dehing CJ, et al. Bishop score and risk of cesarean delivery after induction of labor in nulliparous women. *Obstet Gynecol.* 2005;105:690.

63. Arulkumaran S, Gibb DM, TambyRaja RL, et al. Failed induction of labour. *Aust N Z J Obstet Gynaecol.* 1985;25:190.

64. Hatfield AS, Sanchez-Ramos L, Kaunitz AM. Sonographic cervical assessment to predict the success of labor induction: A systematic review with meta-analysis. *Am J Obstet Gynecol.* 2007;197:186.

65. Verhoeven CJ, Opmeer BC, Oei SG, et al. Transvaginal sonographic assessment of cervical length and wedging for predicting outcome of labor induction at term: a systematic review and meta-analysis. *Ultrasound Obstet Gynecol.* 2013;42:500.

66. Sciscione A, Hoffman MK, Deluca S, et al. Fetal fibronectin as a predictor of vaginal birth in nulliparas undergoing preinduction cervical ripening. *Obstet Gynecol.* 2005;106:980.

67. Reis FM, Gervasi MT, Florio P, et al. Prediction of successful induction of labor at term: Role of clinical history, digital examination, ultrasound assessment of the cervix, and fetal fibronectin assay. *Am J Obstet Gynecol.* 2003;189:1361.

68. Bailit JL, Downs SM, Thorp JM. Reducing the caesarean delivery risk in elective inductions of labour: A decision analysis. *Paediatr Perinat Epidemiol.* 2002;16:90.

69. Maul H, Mackay L, Garfield RE. Cervical ripening: Biochemical, molecular, and clinical considerations. *Clin Obstet Gynecol.* 2006;49:551.

70. Rouse DJ, Owen J, Hauth JC. Criteria for failed labor induction: Prospective evaluation of a standardized protocol. *Obstet Gynecol.* 2000;96:671.

71. Simon CE, Grobman WA. When has an induction failed? *Obstet Gynecol.* 2005;105:705.

72. Harper LM, Caughey AB, Odibo AO, et al. Normal progress of induced labor. *Obstet Gynecol.* 2012;119:1113.

73. Lin MG, Rouse DJ. What is a failed labor induction? *Clin Obstet Gynecol.* 2006;49:585.

74. Beckmann M. Predicting a failed induction. *Aust N Z J Obstet Gynaecol.* 2007;47:394.

75. Kelly AJ, Tan B. Intravenous oxytocin alone for cervical ripening and induction of labour. *Cochrane Database Syst Rev.* 2001;(3):CD003246.

76. Tan BP, Hannah ME. Oxytocin for preterm labor rupture of membranes at or near term. *Cochrane Database Syst Rev.* 2000;(2):CD000157.

77. O'Driscoll K, Foley M, MacDonald D. Active management of labor as an alternative to cesarean section for dystocia. *Obstet Gynecol.* 1984;63:485.

78. Satin AJ, Leveno KJ, Sherman ML, et al. High- versus low-dose oxytocin for labor stimulation. *Obstet Gynecol.* 1992;80:111.

79. Merrill DC, Zlatnik FJ. Randomized double-masked comparison of oxytocin dosage in induction and augmentation of labor. *Obstet Gynecol.* 1999;94:455.

80. Hayes EJ, Weinstein L. Improving patient safety and uniformity of care by a standardized regimen for the use of oxytocin. *Am J Obstet Gynecol.* 2008;198:622.

81. Freeman RK, Nageotte M. A protocol for use of oxytocin. *Am J Obstet Gynecol.* 2007;197:445.

82. Clark S, Belfort M, Saade G, et al. Implementation of a conservative checklist-based protocol for oxytocin administration: maternal and newborn outcomes. *Am J Obstet Gynecol.* 2007;197:480.

83. Girard B, Vardon D, Creveuil C, et al. Discontinuation of oxytocin in the active phase of labor. *Acta Obstet Gynecol Scand.* 2009;88:172.

84. Vlachos DE, Pergialiotis V, Papantonious N, et al. Oxytocin discontinuation after the active phase of labor is established. *J Matern Fetal Neonatal Med.* 2014;1-7.

85. Lydon-Rochelle M, Holt VL, Easterling TR, Martin DP. Risk of uterine rupture during labor among women with a prior cesarean delivery. *N Engl J Med.* 2001;345:3.

86. Kelly AJ, Kavanagh J, Thomas J. Vaginal prostaglandin (PGE2 and PGF2a) for induction of labour at term. *Cochrane Database Syst Rev.* 2003;(4):CD003101.

87. American College of Obstetricians and Gynecologists. New U.S. Food and Drug Administration labeling on Cytotec (misoprostol) use and pregnancy. ACOG Committee Opinion No. 283. *Obstet Gynecol.* 2003;101:1049.

88. Wing DA, Rahall A, Jones MM, et al. Misoprostol: An effective agent for cervical ripening and labor induction. *Am J Obstet Gynecol.* 1995;172:1811.

89. Wing DA. Misoprostol vaginal insert compared with dinoprostone vaginal insert: a randomized controlled trial. *Obstet Gynecol.* 2008;112(4):801-812.

90. Wing DA, Brown R, Plante LA, et al. Misoprostol vaginal insert and time to vaginal delivery: a randomized controlled trial. *Obstet Gynecol.* 2013;122 (2 Pt 1):201-209.

91. Alfirevic Z, Weeks A. Oral misoprostol for induction of labour. *Cochrane Database Syst Rev.* 2006;(2):CD001338.

92. Hofmeyr GJ, Alfirevic Z, Matonhodze B, et al. Titrated oral misoprostol solution for induction of labour: A multi-centre, randomised trial. *Br J Obstet Gynecol.* 2001;108:952.

93. Alfirevic Z, Aflaifel N, Weeks A. Oral misoprostol for induction of labour. *Cochrane Database Syst Rev.* 2014;(6):Art. No.: CD001338.

94. Neilson JP. Mifepristone for induction of labour. *Cochrane Database Syst Rev.* 2000;(4):CD002865.

95. Boulvain M, Kelly AJ, Lohse C, et al. Mechanical methods for induction of labour. *Cochrane Database Syst Rev.* 2001;(4):CD001233.

96. Verani JR, McGee L, Schrag SJ. Prevention of perinatal group B streptococcal disease—revised guidelines from CDC, 2010. Division of Bacterial Diseases, National Center for Immunization and Respiratory Diseases, Centers for Disease Control and Prevention (CDC). *MMWR Recomm Rep.* 2010;59(RR–10):1-36.

97. Silver RM, Heuser CC. Stillbirth workup and delivery management. *Clin Obstet Gynecol.* 2010;53:681.

98. Lohr PA, Hayes JL, Gemzell-Danielsson K. Surgical versus medical methods for second trimester induced abortion. *Cochrane Database Syst Rev.* 2008;(1):CD006714.

99. Wagaarachchi PT, Ashok PW, Narvekar NN, et al. A medical management of late intrauterine death using a combination of mifepristone and misoprostol. *Br J Obstet Gynaecol.* 2002;109:443.

Additional references for this chapter are available at ExpertConsult.com.

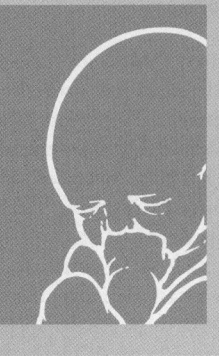

CHAPTER 14

Operative Vaginal Delivery

PETER E. NIELSEN, SHAD H. DEERING, and HENRY L. GALAN

KEY ABBREVIATIONS

American College of Obstetricians and Gynecologists	ACOG
Anteroposterior	AP
Biparietal diameter	BPD
Body mass index	BMI
Confidence interval	CI
Disseminated intravascular coagulation	DIC
Food and Drug Administration	FDA
Intracranial hemorrhage	ICH
Intelligence quotient	IQ
Left occiput anterior	LOA
Left occiput posterior	LOP
Neonatal intensive care unit	NICU
Occiput anterior	OA
Occiput posterior	OP
Occiput transverse	OT
Odds ratio	OR
Randomized controlled trial	RCT
Relative risk	RR
Right occiput anterior	ROA

Obstetric forceps are the one instrument that makes the practice of obstetric care unique to obstetricians. The proper use of these instruments has afforded safe and timely vaginal delivery to those whose abnormal labor course and/or urgent need for delivery required their use.

Following the introduction of forceps by Chamberlin during the 1600s, much discussion about the proper use and timing of forceps application ensued. After Smellie's retirement from practice in 1760, forceps began to be used more frequently, resulting in an increase in both maternal and neonatal injury owing to the application techniques common at the time. In his 1788 text entitled "An Introduction to the Practice of Midwifery," Thomas Denman[1] stated that "the head of the child shall have rested for 6 hours as low as the perineum before the forceps are applied though the pains should have ceased during that time." Denman's law then became widely accepted as the standard of this time. However, after the news of Princess Charlotte's death following the birth of a stillborn Prince on November 6, 1817, a review of Denman's law ensued with much public discussion regarding the timely use of forceps. Princess Charlotte's labor had been managed by one of Denman's students and son-in-law, Sir Richard Croft, whose second-stage labor management during this delivery came into question. Croft had permitted the second stage to last 24 hours, including 6 hours on the perineum, as Denman's law had advised. However, the Princess delivered a 9 lb stillborn male heir, and within 24 hours of delivery, the Princess herself died of a massive postpartum hemorrhage. Disturbed with depression and despair at the blame for the death of both the Princess and the heir to the British throne, Croft shot himself 3 months later. During a lecture delivered at the Royal College of Obstetricians and Gynaecologists (RCOG) on September 28, 1951, Sir Eardley Holland[2] named his lecture on these events "A Triple Obstetric Tragedy" in which he described a mother, baby, and accoucheur all dead, victims of a mistaken system. In a subsequent text in 1817, Denman[3] wrote: "Care is also to be taken that we do not, through an aversion to the use of instruments, too long delay that assistance we have the power of affording them." The debate regarding the use of these instruments continued into the twentieth century with prophylactic forceps delivery advocated by DeLee[4] in 1920. This clinical management strategy resulted in forceps delivery rates in excess of 65% by 1950.

With these lessons in mind, a review of operative vaginal delivery in modern obstetric practice is extremely important and timely. **Rates of cesarean delivery have risen in both the United States and the United Kingdom,[5,6] increasing 60% between 1996 and 2009 in the United States, when the rate reached 32.9%—the highest rate ever reported—and increasing 100% between 1990 and 2008** (12% to 24%) **in the United Kingdom. Between 2009 and 2013, the rate of cesarean delivery in the United States has declined only slightly to 32.7%. In contrast, rates of forceps and vacuum extraction to assist delivery have decreased dramatically from 9% in 1990 to 3.4% in 2012.[7] Forceps have been used for fewer than 1% of all births in the United States since 2005** (0.59% in 2013).[7] However, most residency training programs in the United States still expect proficiency in outlet and low forceps delivery (less than or greater than a 45-degree rotation), whereas less than 40% expect proficiency in midforceps delivery.[8] **However, to make education and teaching of these procedures even more challenging, new resident work hour restrictions have resulted in a decline in resident experience with both primary cesarean delivery and vacuum-assisted vaginal delivery despite increased institutional volumes of these procedures.** In a study by Blanchard and colleagues,[9] the decrease in experience was shown to be dramatic: they noted a 54% decline in experience with primary cesarean delivery and a 56% decline in vacuum-assisted vaginal delivery. Because both forceps and vacuum extractors are acceptable and safe instruments for operative vaginal delivery, operator experience is the determining factor in deciding which instrument should be used in a specific clinical situation.[10] Declining use and resident experience may make it difficult to provide the level of operator skills required for proficiency of this obstetric art. However, because most women prefer a vaginal delivery, focused experience with the use of these instruments during residency training is crucial to ensure safe, timely, and effective vaginal delivery. Furthermore, women are more likely to achieve a spontaneous vaginal delivery in a subsequent pregnancy after forceps delivery than after cesarean delivery (78% vs. 31%).[11-14] The challenge, therefore, is to ensure that women who experience second-stage labor abnormalities are afforded all options for a safe and timely delivery.

OPERATIVE VAGINAL DELIVERY
Classification, Prerequisites, and Indications

The use of a well-defined and consistent classification system for operative vaginal deliveries facilitates the comparison of maternal and neonatal outcomes among spontaneous delivery, cesarean delivery, and operative vaginal delivery as well as instruction in these techniques. It is intuitive that not all operative vaginal deliveries are the same with respect to degree of difficulty or maternal and fetal risk; therefore classification systems have been developed and modified over time. In 1949, Titus created a classification system that permitted general practitioners to perform operative vaginal delivery without consultation from a specialist. This system divided the pelvis into thirds from the ischial spines to the inlet and, in the opposite direction, in thirds to the outlet. Dennen[15] proposed an alternative classification system in 1952 that was based on the four major obstetric planes of the pelvis with the following definitions: *high forceps* is the biparietal diameter (BPD) in the plane of the inlet but above the ischial spines; *midforceps* is the BPD just at or below the ischial spines and the sacral hollow not filled; *low midforceps* is the BPD below the ischial spines, the leading bony part within

a fingerbreadth of the perineum between contractions, and the hollow of the sacrum filled; and *outlet forceps* is the BPD below the level of the ischial spines, the sagittal suture in the anteroposterior diameter, and the head visible at the perineum during a contraction.

In 1965, the American College of Obstetricians and Gynecologists (ACOG) created a classification system[16] that defined *midforceps* extremely broadly, from the ischial spines to the pelvic floor and any rotation. This category clearly included many forceps operations that ranged from delivery of a straightforward anteroposterior position of the fetal vertex to complex rotations. The broad category for these operations led many practicing clinicians to question whether the classification should be narrowed to reflect the clinically significant differences between deliveries such as these.

In 1988, ACOG revised the classification[17] of forceps operations to address two significant shortcomings of the previous system: that *midforceps* was too widely defined and *outlet forceps* was too narrowly defined. This system was validated in 1991 by Hagadorn-Freathy and colleagues,[18] who demonstrated that 25% of deliveries in this study that would have been previously classified as midforceps but were reclassified into the low forceps (greater than 45-degree rotation) and midforceps categories were associated with 41% of episiotomy extensions and 50% of the lacerations in the cohort. Clearly, the outcomes of these operations confounded the relatively low-risk group of low-forceps operations with up to 45-degree rotation, which would also have been classified as midforceps by the previous system. **In short, these investigators validated the 1988 ACOG classification scheme by demonstrating that the higher station and more complex deliveries carried a greater risk of maternal and fetal injury compared with those that were more straightforward.** This differentiation was lost in the 1965 classification scheme owing to the broad definition of *low forceps*. It is extremely important to appropriately classify operative vaginal delivery based on this system, including accurate determination of fetal station and position. The 1988 classification scheme for operative vaginal delivery is shown in Box 14-1.

With respect to operative vaginal delivery of the vertex, *station* is defined as the relationship of the estimated distance in centimeters between the leading bony portion of the fetal head and the level of the maternal ischial spines, and *position* refers to the relationship of the occiput to a denominating location on the maternal pelvis. Operative vaginal delivery with a fetus in the left occiput anterior (LOA) position with the leading bony portion of the vertex 3 cm below the ischial spines (+3 station) would be classified as low forceps, less than 45-degree rotation delivery. It is also important to note that this classification system applies to both forceps and vacuum extraction instruments and that the precise position and station must be known before the placement of either instrument.

In addition to precise evaluation of the position and station, several other extremely important data are necessary before performing an operative vaginal delivery. **The prerequisites for application of either forceps or vacuum extractor are listed in** Table 14-1. **When these prerequisites have been met, the following two indications are appropriate for consideration of either forceps delivery or vacuum extraction: (1) prolonged second stage** (for nulliparous women, lack of continuing progress for 3 hours with regional analgesia or 2 hours without regional analgesia; for multiparous women, lack of continuing progress for 2 hours with regional analgesia or 1 hour

TABLE 14-1	PREREQUISITES FOR FORCEPS OR VACUUM EXTRACTOR APPLICATION

- Fetal vertex is engaged.
- Membranes have ruptured.
- Cervix is fully dilated.
- Position is precisely known.
- Assessment of maternal pelvis reveals adequacy for the estimated fetal weight.
- Adequate maternal analgesia is available.
- Bladder is drained.
- Operator is knowledgeable.
- Operator is willing to abandon the procedure if necessary.
- Informed consent has been obtained.
- Necessary support personnel and equipment are present.

without regional analgesia) and **(2) suspicion of immediate or potential fetal compromise** (nonreassuring fetal heart rate tracing or shortening of the second stage of labor for maternal benefit [i.e., maternal exhaustion, maternal cardiopulmonary or cerebrovascular disease]).

OPERATIVE VAGINAL DELIVERY INSTRUMENTS

Forceps Instruments

Invention and modification have led to a description and use of more than 700 varieties of forceps instruments. Most of them are of historic interest only, but many common features remain among those still in use. **Except when used at cesarean delivery, forceps are paired instruments and are broadly categorized according to their intended use as** *classic forceps,* *rotational forceps,* **and** *specialized forceps* **designed to assist vaginal breech deliveries.** Each forceps type consists of two

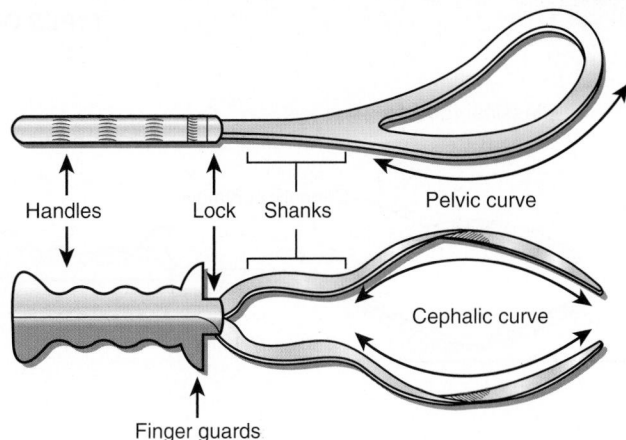

FIG 14-1 Anatomy of the forceps.

halves joined by a lock, which may be sliding or fixed. The key structures of forceps include the blade, shank, lock, finger guards, and handle (Fig. 14-1). The *toe* refers to the tip of the blade, and the *heel* is the end of the blade that is attached to the shank at the posterior lip of the fenestration (if present). The *cephalic curve* is defined by the radius of the two blades when in opposition, and the *pelvic curve* is defined by the upward—or reverse, as in the case of Kielland and Piper forceps—curve of the blades from the shank. The handles transmit the applied force, the screw or lock represents the fulcrum, and the blades transmit the load (Fig. 14-2).[19]

The pelvic curve permits ease of application along the maternal pelvic axis (Fig. 14-3). **Forceps have two functions, traction and rotation, both of which can only be accomplished by some degree of compression on the fetal head. The cephalic curvature of the blade is designed to aid in the even distribution of force about the fetal parietal bone and malar eminence.** Blades may be solid (Tucker-McLane), fenestrated (Simpson), or pseudofenestrated (Luikart-Simpson). The pseudofenestration modification can be applied to the design of any type of forceps and is known as the *Luikart modification.* In general, use of solid or pseudofenestrated blades results in less risk of maternal soft tissue injury, especially during rotation, but fenestrated blades provide improved traction in comparison to solid blades.

Classic Forceps

Classic forceps instruments are typically used when rotation of the vertex is not required for delivery. However, they may be used for rotations such as the Scanzoni-Smellie maneuver. All classic forceps have a cephalic curve, a pelvic curve, and an English lock, in which the articulation is fixed in a slot into which the shank of the opposite blade fits. The type of classic forceps instrument is determined by its shank, whether overlapping or parallel. Examples of classic forceps with parallel shanks include Simpson, DeLee, Irving, and Hawks-Dennen forceps. Classic forceps with overlapping shanks include Elliott and Tucker-McLane. **Because these instruments have a more rounded cephalic curve than the Simpson forceps, they are often used for assisting delivery of the unmolded head, such as that commonly encountered in the multiparous patient. In addition, because the Tucker-McLane forceps have a shorter, solid blade and overlapping shanks, they are more often used for rotations than other classic instruments.**

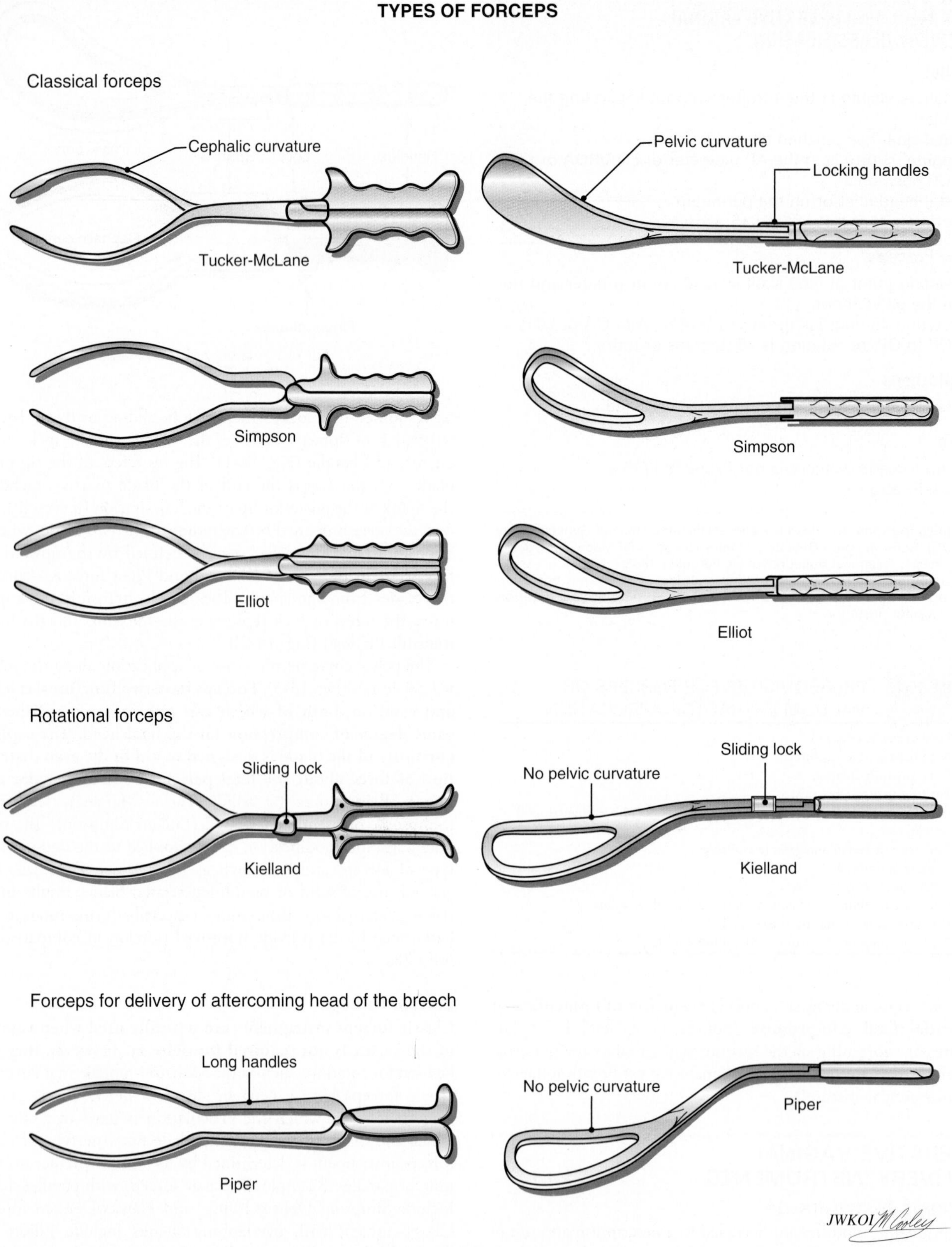

TYPES OF FORCEPS

Classical forceps

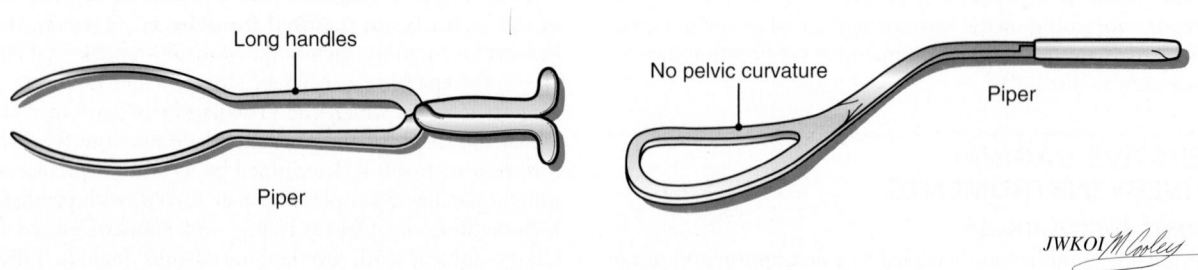

Rotational forceps

Forceps for delivery of aftercoming head of the breech

JWKOL McCooley

FIG 14-2 Classification of forceps.

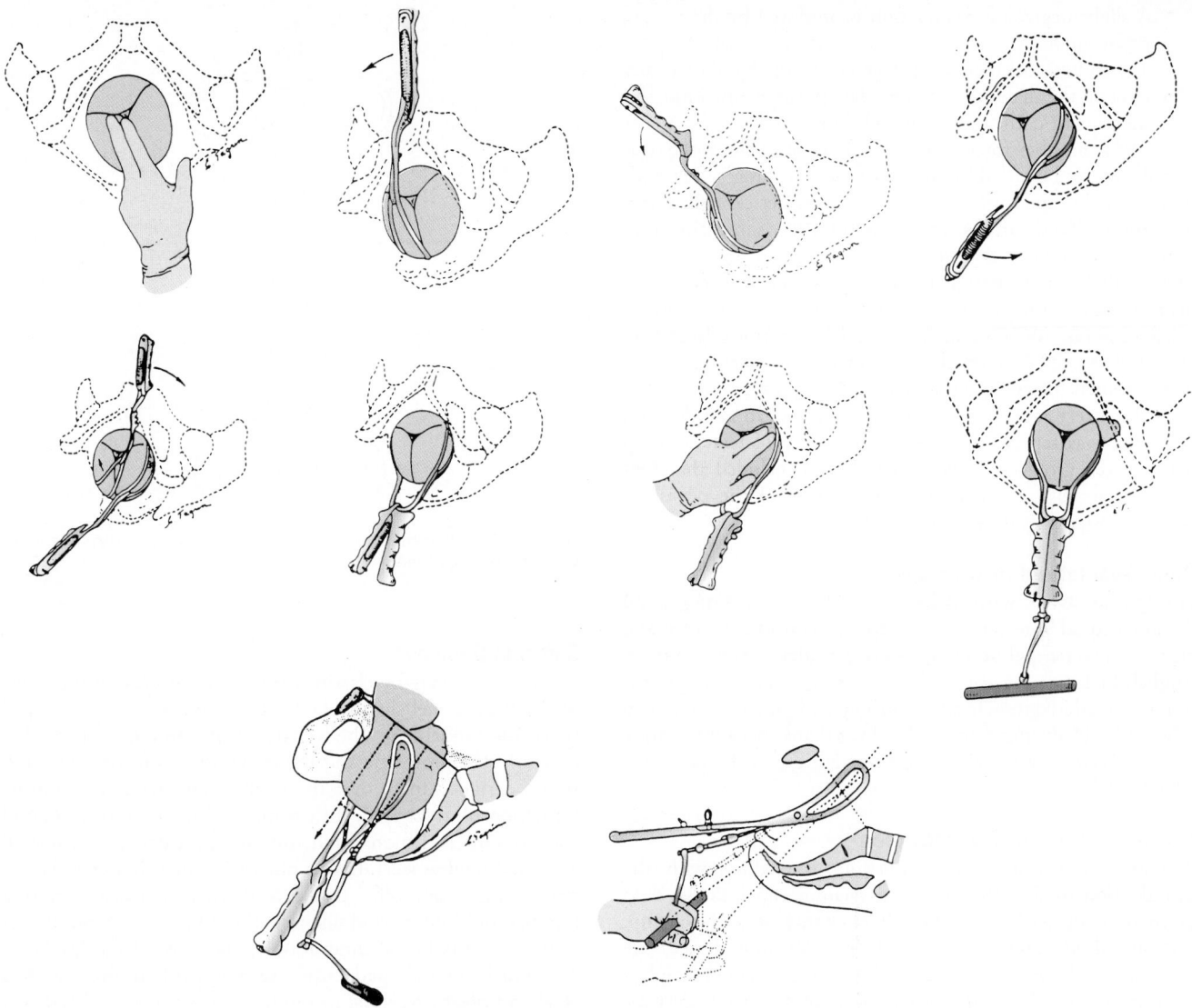

FIG 14-3 Stepwise approach to application of obstetric forceps.

Rotational Forceps

Forceps instruments used for rotation are characterized as having a cephalic curve amenable to application to the molded vertex and either only a slight pelvic curve or none at all. The absence of a pelvic curve in these instruments facilitates rotation of the vertex without moving the handles of the instrument through a wide arc, as is necessary when using one of the classic instruments to accomplish rotation. Forceps that may be used for rotation include some of the classic instruments (e.g., Tucker-McLane) and those with minimal pelvic curvature (e.g., Kielland and Leff). In 1916, Christian Kielland of Norway described the rationale for the introduction of his new forceps[20]:

When the head is high, it has to be pulled through a greater length of the birth canal, which is incompletely prepared. The child's head is in such a position that it cannot be grasped by the blades of the forceps in the way that is possible when the head is low and completely rotated. The forceps do not hold the head in the biparietal diameter but over the occipital and frontal areas, which cannot withstand much pressure. These factors are responsible for the difficulties that occur in such a delivery, but they do not

entirely explain the amount of force required nor the resistance encountered. In the search for an explanation of the chief cause for the remarkable amount of force that had to be used, it was thought that traction might be in the wrong direction, because the blade of the ordinary forceps is curved to correspond with the birth canal. This type of forceps cannot be depressed sufficiently low against the perineum without the risk of damaging it or losing the good position on the fetal head when an attempt is made to exert traction in the pelvic axis.

After their introduction, **Kielland forceps** have become a frequently used instrument for rotation of the vertex (see Fig. 14-1). These forceps have a slightly backward pelvic curve with overlapping shanks and a sliding lock. The advantages of the Kielland forceps, compared with the classic instruments for rotation, include the following:

- The straight design places the handle and shanks in the same plane as the long axis of the fetal head, permitting the toe to travel through a very small arc during rotation.
- The distance between the heel and the intersecting point of the shanks is long, which accommodates heads of various shapes and sizes, associated with unusual molding.

- A slight degree of axis traction is produced by the reverse pelvic curve.
- The sliding lock permits placement of the handles at any level on the shank to accommodate the asynclitic head and subsequent correction of asynclitism.

In 1955, another forceps used for rotation of the vertex was introduced by Leff.[21] These forceps have a locking shank with short, straight, and narrow blades and a smaller cephalic curve than the Kielland forceps. In a series of 104 consecutive rotational forceps deliveries (>90 degrees) using Leff forceps, compared with 163 nonrotational forceps deliveries with traditional instruments, Feldman and colleagues[22] demonstrated a lower episiotomy rate (66% vs. 82%) and a lower perineal laceration rate (16% vs. 23%) with the Leff forceps compared with the nonrotational forceps group, attributed to a 40% spontaneous vaginal delivery rate after Leff forceps rotation. In addition, no difference was reported in the low incidence of fetal bruising between the groups (3% in each). They concluded that Leff forceps were also a safe option for rotation of the persistent occiput posterior (OP) fetal position.

Other Specialized Instruments

Forceps to assist with delivery of the aftercoming head during vaginal breech delivery (Piper forceps) have a cephalic curve, a reverse pelvic curve, long parallel shanks, and an English lock (see Fig. 14-2). This design provides easy application to the aftercoming head, stabilizing and protecting the fetal head and neck during delivery. The long shanks permit the body of the breech to rest against it during delivery of the head (see Chapter 17).

Vacuum Extraction Devices

Swedish obstetrician Tage Malmström is credited with the introduction of the first successful vacuum cup into the field of modern obstetrics in 1953. It consisted of a metal cup, suction tubing, and a traction chain.[23] Vacuum devices are classified by the material used to make the cup, either stainless steel or plastic (silicone). So-called soft (plastic) cups are used much more commonly in the United States than the stainless steel cups owing to the lower rates of scalp trauma associated with these devices,[24] which consist of **a cup connected to a handle grip with tubing that connects them both to a vacuum source** (Fig. 14-4). **The vacuum generated through this tubing attaches the fetal scalp to the cup and allows traction on the vertex. The vacuum force can be generated either from wall suction or by a handheld device with a pumping mechanism.**

Stainless Steel Devices

The Malmström device is the most commonly used instrument for vacuum extraction in the world.[25] This device consists of a mushroom-shaped stainless steel cup, two vacuum hoses, a traction chain and attached metallic disk, a traction handle, and a vacuum source. The cup is available in 40, 50, and 60 mm diameter sizes and is designed such that the diameter of the opening is smaller than the internal diameter of the cup. Therefore when vacuum is established, the fetal scalp fills the internal dimension of the cup, and an artificial caput succedaneum is formed (the "chignon"). This allows for the appropriate traction force to be applied to the vertex without a "pop-off" or detachment.

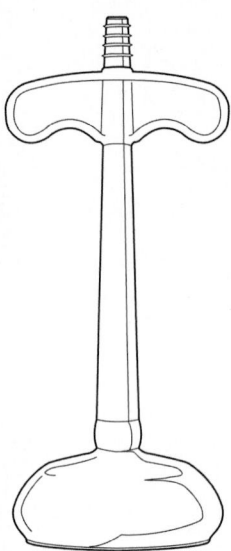

FIG 14-4 "M"-style mushroom vacuum extractor cup with a centrally located stem and handle.

Soft-Cup Devices

These devices may be classified into three groups by the shape of the cup: funnel shaped, bell shaped, and mushroom shaped (Figs. 14-5 and 14-6). The Kobayashi style funnel-shaped Silastic cup is the prototype and the largest cup available (65 mm). It was designed to fit over the fetal occiput without requiring formation of a chignon. This feature results in a lower rate of scalp trauma and more rapid time to effect delivery compared with the stainless steel devices but with a slightly higher failure rate owing to pop-off.[24] Bell-shaped cups are available from a number of vendors and include the MityVac (Prism Enterprises), Kiwi (Clinical Innovations), and CMI (Utah Medical). **The mushroom-shaped cups are a hybrid of the stainless steel and plastic devices.** Examples of these devices include the M-cup (MityVac), OmniCup (Kiwi), and Flex Cup (CMI). The maneuverability of these devices is superior to either the funnel-shaped or bell-shaped devices owing to their smaller size and increased flexibility of the traction stem relative to the cup. However, like other vacuum devices, they are still limited in their use for either OP or occiput transverse (OT) positions owing to an inability to achieve the proper median flexing application. Advances to the Kiwi product have resulted in a style of cup in which the stem is completely collapsible against the cup (see Fig. 14-5), thus allowing placement of the vacuum on the point of flexion of the head that is asynclitic or in the OP position.

OPERATIVE VAGINAL DELIVERY TECHNIQUES

Classic Forceps: Application for Occiput Anterior and Occiput Posterior Positions

Forceps blades are labeled *left* and *right* based on the maternal side into which they are placed. For example, the *left blade* refers to the maternal left side, and its handle is held in the operator's left hand for placement (see Fig. 14-3).[26] The posterior blade is conventionally placed first because it provides a splint for the fetal head to prevent rotation from the occiput

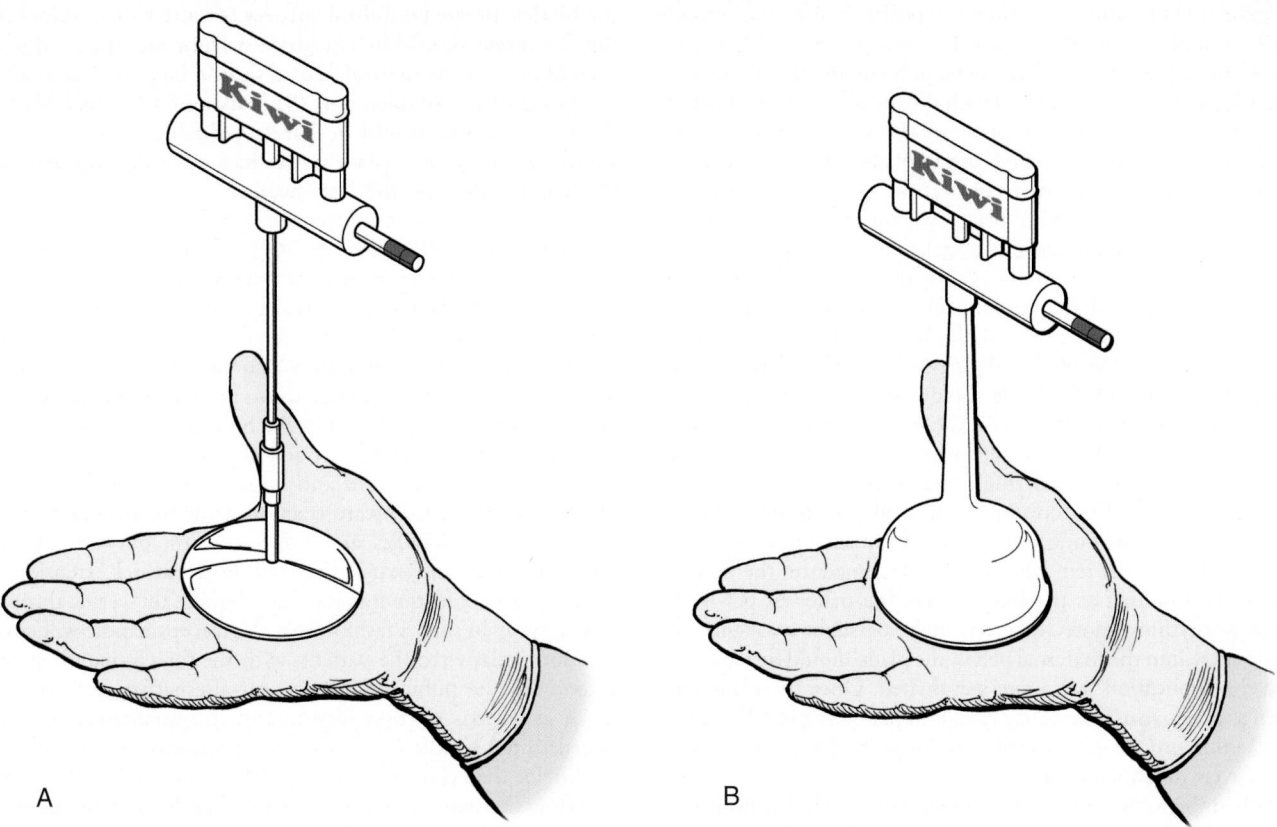

FIG 14-5 Two Kiwi vacuum devices demonstrating the handheld pump and pressure gauge device. Unlike the cup in **B,** the stem on the cup in **A,** the OmniCup, is flexible and can be laid flat against the cup. (From Vacca A. *Handbook of Vacuum Delivery in Obstetric Practice.* Albion, Australia: Vacca Research Pty. Ltd.; 2003.)

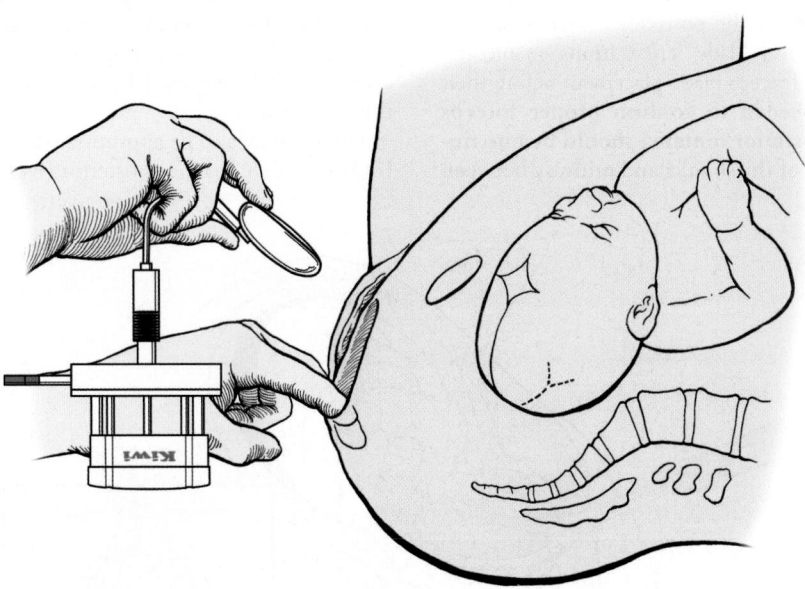

FIG 14-6 Placement of the OmniCup with flexible stem at the point of flexion of a fetus in the occiput posterior position; this is difficult to accomplish with traditional vacuum devices. (From Vacca A. *Handbook of Vacuum Delivery in Obstetric Practice.* Albion, Australia: Vacca Research Pty, Ltd.; 2003.)

anterior (OA) position to a more OP position when the second blade is applied. Therefore when the fetus is OA to LOA, the left blade is placed first. The operator holds the handle of the left blade in his or her left hand with the toe of the blade directed toward the floor. With the plane of the shank perpendicular to the floor, the cephalic curve of the blade is to be applied to the curve of the fetal head. To protect the vaginal sidewalls, the fingers of the right hand are placed within the left vagina with the palm of the hand facing the fetal skull. The cephalic curve of the blade should lie evenly against the fetal skull as the toe of the blade is placed at approximately 6 o'clock. The operator's right thumb guides the heel of the blade and the right index finger guides the toe of the blade gently over the left parietal bone. The handle of the blade should be held lightly with the left thumb and index finger. As the blade is inserted into the pelvis, its shank and handle are to be rotated counterclockwise toward the right maternal thigh and then inward toward the maternal midline. This movement will guide the toe of the blade over the left parietal bone and onto the left malar eminence. The force applied by the left thumb and index finger on the handle should be minimal as the blade enters the maternal pelvis. If there is anything more than very light or slight resistance to blade entry into the maternal pelvis, the blade should be removed and the application technique reevaluated. Once the blade has been applied, an assistant may hold it in place. To place the right blade, this process is repeated with opposite hands doing the maneuvers described earlier.

When the fetus is in a right occiput anterior (ROA) position, the right fetal parietal bone is located in the posterior maternal pelvis so the posterior blade will be the right blade, and this is placed first. Once both blades are in place, if the handles do not lock easily, the application is incorrect. The blades should have a bimalar, biparietal placement when applied properly (Fig. 14-7). Once the handles are locked, proper blade location must be confirmed. Identification of the posterior fontanel, sagittal suture, lambdoid sutures, and blade fenestrations enable the operator to confirm proper forceps blade placement before their use. **The three criteria needed to confirm proper forceps application are (1) the posterior fontanel should be one fingerbreath above the plane of the shanks and midway between** the blades, or the lambdoid sutures (or anterior fontanel for the OP fetus) should be equidistant from the upper edge of each blade; (2) the sagittal suture should be perpendicular to the plane of the shanks; and (3) if using fenestrated blades, the fenestrations should be barely palpable.[26] **The operator should not be able to place more than one fingertip between the fenestration and the fetal head.**

The direction of traction on the fetal head is determined by the station of the BPD (see Fig. 14-3). For example, higher fetal stations require a steeper angle of traction below the horizontal. The shape of the maternal pelvis may be visualized as the terminal end of the letter "J." As the fetal head descends within the pelvis, the axis of traction follows a curved line upward from the floor. The axis of traction rises above the horizontal as the fetal head crowns and extends just as the head does in a spontaneous vaginal delivery. With the axis traction principle, force is directed in two vectors—downward and outward. One hand holds the shanks and exerts downward traction while the operator's other hand holds the handles and exerts traction outward. As the vertex descends and exits, there will be a natural extension of the fetal head, and the forceps should guide the vertex through this pathway in such a fashion that the forceps handle will curve anteriorly relative to the patient, with the forceps handle nearly anterior to the pubic symphysis. An alternative method is to use it as an axis traction instrument; this attachment may be joined to the handle to facilitate traction below the handles in the line of the pelvic axis (see Fig. 14-3) and allows the forceps to follow the natural extension of the fetal head. **Forceps traction should begin with the uterine contraction and should coincide with maternal pushing efforts until the contraction ends. Fetal heart tones should be monitored. Descent should occur with each pull, and if no descent occurs after two to three pulls, the operative delivery should be halted and measures should be taken to proceed with cesarean delivery.** (See Video 14-1 for an example of the technique of forceps application and delivery.) Switching to a vacuum should be done very cautiously (see "Sequential Use of Vacuum and Forceps" later in this chapter).

Forceps may also be appropriate for OP, left occiput posterior (LOP), or right occiput posterior (ROP) positions if the station

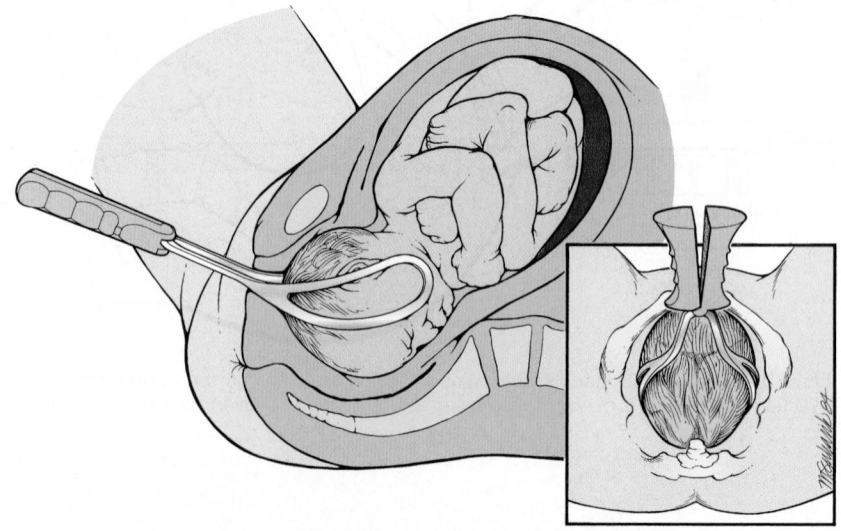

FIG 14-7 Proper application of obstetric forceps. (From O'Brien WF, Cefalo RC. Labor and delivery. In Gabbe SG, Niebyl JR, Simpson JL, eds. *Obstetrics: Normal and Problem Pregnancies*, ed 3. New York: Churchill Livingstone; 1996:377.)

of the bony part of the head is truly at least +2 station. **Infants in persistent OP position represent a unique challenge. With a deflexed or extended head, a wider diameter presents through the pelvic outlet, which requires more force for descent of the fetal head. Proper assessment of fetal station can be made complex by extension and molding of the head.**[26] **With fetal molding, the widest diameter of the fetal head may be at a much higher station than the leading bony part, thus making traction within the proper pelvic axis difficult to ascertain. The tendency is to overestimate station in OP positions, so the operator must be confident in their station assessment.**

Rotational Forceps: Application for Occiput Transverse Positions

Rotation must be accomplished from the OT position before delivery of the fetal head. This may happen spontaneously, with manual assistance, or with use of forceps when appropriate. The reader is referred to *Dennen's Forceps Deliveries* for a more extensive review of forceps rotation techniques.[26] **Forceps rotations should be attempted only with an experienced operator.**

Classic Forceps
For left occiput transverse (LOT) positions, the posterior left blade should be applied first. The toe of the blade is placed at 6 o'clock, and the cephalic curve is applied to the fetal head. The handle is lowered to facilitate blade entry into the posterior pelvis and rests below the horizontal, the degree of which will be determined by fetal station. **The anterior right blade is known as the *wandering blade,*** and it is inserted with the right hand posteriorly at approximately 7 o'clock. Upward pressure on the blade is exerted with the fingers of the left hand as the right hand moves the handle in a clockwise arc across the left thigh toward the floor. The toe of the blade "wanders" from posterior to anterior, around the frontal bone, to rest anterior to the right ear. Elevation of the handle of the right blade permits movement of the blade further into the pelvis beyond the symphysis and articulation at the handles. The proper attitude of flexion is created by moving the handles toward the pelvic midline. Rotation of the fetal head is accomplished by counterclockwise rotation of the handles in a wide arc across the left thigh toward 12 o'clock. With classic forceps, a wide rotational arc at the handles produces the desired smaller arc of rotation at the toe of the blades. Once the OA position is reached, the blades may be readjusted before the generation of traction. This same procedure may be used for the right occiput transverse (ROT) position with classic forceps. In this instance, however, the right blade is posterior and should be applied first.

Kielland Forceps
Kielland forceps were originally designed for delivery of the fetal head in deep transverse arrest.[20] **They are now also used for rotation of the fetal head from OP or OT positions.** The advantage of Kielland forceps lies in the reverse pelvic curve, which permits placement of the blades in the direct OT position without elevation of the fetal head and loss of station. Unlike classic forceps, with Kielland forceps the anterior blade is applied first. **Three methods of Kielland forceps application have been described: (1) the inversion method, or classic application, (2) the wandering method, and (3) the direct method.**[26]

The *inversion method* may be used in OT and LOP or ROP positions. In an LOT position, the right anterior blade is gently guided below the symphysis with assistance from the operator's left hand. With this application, the cephalic curve is facing up and beyond the symphysis, the handle is dropped below the horizontal, and the blade is rotated 180 degrees toward the midline until the cephalic curve rests on the parietal bone and malar eminence. If resistance is met with the inversion technique, the wandering technique may be used.

The *wandering method* for Kielland forceps is similar to that used for classic forceps. It requires initial placement of the anterior blade onto the posterior parietal bone with the cephalic curve directly applied to the fetus. The blade is then gently advanced around the face and frontal bone until it rests above the anterior fetal ear.

The *direct method* of application is preferred when the head is at low fetal station near the pelvic outlet. If the anterior ear is palpable beyond the symphysis, the forceps may be directly applied, often with less difficulty than with the other two methods. With the cephalic curve facing the fetus, the blade is applied by lowering the handle toward the floor. The toe is then gently advanced with guidance from the operator's opposite hand, and the posterior blade is inserted at 6 o'clock with the cephalic curve facing the fetal skull; the operator's free hand is inserted into the posterior pelvis palm side up, and the blade is gently guided into position over the posterior ear. The sliding lock will permit closure of the blades and correction of asynclitism, when the axis of the fetal head is oriented obliquely to the axial planes of the pelvis (see Chapter 12). Unlike rotation with classic forceps, the reverse pelvic curve of Kielland forceps permits rotation directly on the axis of the shanks.[26] The shanks and handles are rotated around the midline point of application and should be held during rotation in a plane perpendicular to the plane of the fetal BPD. In some instances, the fetal head may need to be elevated and even disengaged to accomplish the rotation. This is performed by keeping the handles of the Kielland forceps well below the horizontal plane, pushing the forceps in an anterior-cephalad direction with respect to the maternal pelvis (e.g., toward the maternal umbilicus). Failure to angle in such a direction will result in the forceps making contact with the sacral promontory and an inability to achieve the room needed for rotation. During the rotation, one finger should follow the sutures to ensure that the forceps and fetal head move as a single unit. Generally speaking, use of one hand should provide sufficient force to complete the rotation and is a good guide for avoiding excess force. After successful rotation, proper forceps placement should be confirmed before downward traction is applied. Alternatively, the Kielland forceps could be removed, and classic forceps can be placed before traction. (See Video 14-2 for a demonstration of Kielland forceps application and delivery.)

Forceps Rotation: Application for the Occiput Posterior Position

The fetal head may be rotated from OP to OA by use of the Scanzoni-Smellie technique using classic forceps.[27] The posterior blade should be applied first and then appropriate placement of forceps should be confirmed. Minimal elevation of the fetal head upward within the pelvis will facilitate rotation. Movement of the handles in a wide arc toward the fetal back will enable rotation from the LOP position to OA. After rotation of the handles in a wide arc, the toe of the blades will be upside down with respect to the fetal malar eminence. They must then be removed and replaced properly before traction on the fetal head. Rotation from OP may also be accomplished with Kielland forceps. After successful rotation, traction can be applied for delivery of the fetal head.

Vacuum Extraction

As with forceps, successful use of the vacuum extractor is determined by proper application on the fetal head and traction within the pelvic axis.[28] The leading point of the fetal head is the ideal position for vacuum cup placement. It is labeled the *flexion point,* or *pivot point,* and is located on the sagittal suture 2 to 3 cm below the posterior fontanel for the OA position and 2 to 3 cm above the posterior fontanel for the OP position.[28] Placement of the vacuum cup over the pivot point maintains the attitude of flexion for a well-flexed head and creates flexion in a deflexed head if traction is applied correctly. Incorrect placement on an asynclitic head results in unequal distribution of force and increases the risk of neonatal intracranial injury and scalp lacerations.[28,29] Therefore knowledge of exact fetal position is important for efficacious vacuum placement. The force generated by vacuum suction is substantial, with recommended pressures ranging from 550 to 600 mm Hg (11.6 psi).[30] After initial placement of the cup, correct application must be confirmed, which includes determining that no vaginal tissue is caught beneath the vacuum cup before the vacuum pressure is raised to the desired level. Just as with forceps, traction should begin with each contraction and should coincide with maternal pushing efforts. Routine traction between contractions should be avoided. In the absence of maternal pushing, traction alone increases the force required for fetal descent and increases the risk of cup detachment.[28] Twisting or rocking of the vacuum cup to facilitate descent of the fetal head is not recommended because of an increased risk of scalp laceration and intracranial hemorrhage (ICH).[28,31] With correct application, traction in the pelvic axis often results in flexion and autorotation, depending on fetal station and the vacuum cup selected.[29]

Detachment of the vacuum cup during traction should be viewed as an indication for reevaluation of the site of application, direction of axis traction, and fetal maternal pelvic dimensions. The rapid decompression that results from cup detachment for the soft and rigid vacuum cups has been associated with scalp injury, and it should not be viewed as a safety mechanism that is without potential for fetal risk.[29,32] Data are limited to provide evidence-based support for the maximum duration of safe vacuum application, the maximum number of pulls required before delivery of the fetal head, and the maximum number of pop-offs or cup detachments before abandonment of the procedure.[28,29,33,34] There is a general consensus, however, that descent of the fetal bony vertex should occur with each pull, and if no descent occurs after three pulls, the operative attempt should be stopped. Most authorities have recommended that the maximum number of cup detachments (pop-offs) be limited to two or three and that the duration of vacuum application before abandonment of the procedure be limited to a maximum of 20 to 30 minutes.[34,35] A randomized controlled trial (RCT) compared maintenance of suction of 600 mm Hg throughout the operative delivery to reduction of suction to 100 mm Hg between contractions and found no differences in duration of operative delivery or in neonatal outcome.[36] Finally, vacuum cup selection may play a role in the likelihood of successful vaginal delivery. The soft cup instruments used in modern practice are associated with less scalp trauma but have a higher failure rate than rigid metal vacuum cups.[35] A meta-analysis of nine RCTs of soft versus rigid vacuum extractor cups determined that the average failure rates were 16% and 9% for the soft and metal cups, respectively, and the detachment rates were 22% and 10% for the soft and metal cups, respectively. Higher failure rates with the soft cup may be secondary to difficulties associated with proper placement and traction, particularly if the fetus is deflexed, malpositioned, or at higher station.[27,35]

RISKS AND BENEFITS OF OPERATIVE VAGINAL DELIVERY

Benefits of Operative Vaginal Delivery

Most women desire a vaginal delivery.[14] Therefore the safe and effective application of instrumental delivery during the second stage of labor is crucial. In addition, acknowledging the benefits of operative vaginal delivery and the maternal views following these interventions is an important component to enhance counseling. In a cohort study of 393 women who had either a "difficult" operative vaginal delivery performed in the operating suite or a cesarean delivery for an arrest disorder in the second stage of labor, an equal proportion of patients in both groups desired future pregnancy (51% vs. 54%) when asked before hospital discharge. However, women who had an operative vaginal delivery were much more likely to desire a subsequent vaginal delivery compared with women delivered by cesarean section when asked immediately postpartum (79% vs. 39%)[11] and when asked again 3 years later (87% vs. 33%).[12] In addition, of those patients who achieved pregnancy within 3 years of the index delivery in this cohort, substantially more women who had an operative vaginal delivery achieved subsequent vaginal delivery compared with those who had a prior cesarean delivery (78% vs. 31%).[12] Johanson and colleagues[37] followed patients 5 years after a randomized trial that compared forceps delivery with vacuum extraction and demonstrated that more than 75% achieved a spontaneous vaginal delivery with a larger fetus in their second pregnancy.

Because women report fear of childbirth as a common reason for avoiding future pregnancies,[12] patients who had an operative delivery were asked about their views on this procedure, including preparation for this type of delivery. Most women felt that their birth plan or antenatal classes had not properly prepared them for the possibility of an operative delivery in the second stage of labor.[13] In addition, most had difficulty understanding the need for the intervention despite a review of the indications by the medical staff before discharge. These patients desired more focused antenatal information on operative delivery and a postdelivery debriefing by their delivering physician or midwife focused on the reasons for the intervention and their future pregnancy and delivery implications.[13]

Maternal Risks

The focus of recent attention regarding operative vaginal delivery has been the risk of perineal trauma and subsequent pelvic floor dysfunction. The principle risks appear to be those of urinary and fecal incontinence. However, the difficulty in establishing the precise risks of this dysfunction in patients who have had an operative vaginal delivery compared with those who have not is confounded by many factors, including the indication for the operative delivery, number of deliveries, maternal weight, neonatal birthweight and head circumference, perineal body length, episiotomy, and the effects of maternal aging.[38] We will examine three aspects of maternal risk associated with operative vaginal delivery: significant perineal trauma (third- and fourth-degree lacerations), urinary incontinence, and fecal incontinence.

Perineal Trauma

Significant perineal trauma is generally defined as a third-degree laceration that involves the anal sphincter or a fourth-degree laceration that involves the rectal mucosa (see Chapter 18). Estimated frequencies of these injuries vary based on multiple maternal factors that include parity, birthweight, type of delivery, and use of episiotomy. **In a large, population-based retrospective study of more than 2 million vaginal deliveries, the frequency of severe perineal injury was noted to be 11.5% in nulliparous patients, 13.8% in patients with a successful vaginal birth after cesarean delivery, and 1.8% in multiparous patients.**[39] Increased risks of anal sphincter injuries were found to be associated with primiparity, macrosomia, shoulder dystocia, maternal diabetes mellitus, prolonged pregnancy, nonreassuring fetal heart rate patterns, and operative vaginal delivery. In contrast to other studies that demonstrated a much larger risk of severe perineal injury as a result of forceps and vacuum delivery (sevenfold to eightfold), the study by Handa and colleagues[39] observed an odds ratio (OR) of only 1.4 for forceps delivery and 2.3 for vacuum delivery, suggesting that operative vaginal delivery may be associated with a much lower risk of third- and fourth-degree lacerations than was previously thought. In addition, these researchers found that episiotomy was associated with a 10% decrease in anal sphincter laceration. Other studies have also observed that episiotomy associated with forceps use either did not increase the risk of third- or fourth-degree lacerations[40] or it reduced their risk.[41] Reduction in episiotomy use has also been associated with fewer severe perineal lacerations in two different studies that evaluated a total of more than 7000 consecutive deliveries.[42,43] Whether more liberal use of episiotomy affects the rate of severe perineal lacerations remains to be evaluated in a prospective randomized trial.

Urinary Incontinence

Stress urinary incontinence is defined as the involuntary leakage of urine during effort or exertion and occurs at least once weekly in one third of adult women.[44] **Both pregnancy and the interval following pregnancy predispose women to urinary incontinence.** Viktrup and Lose[45] observed that **32% of nulliparous women developed urinary incontinence during pregnancy and 7% developed it after delivery. One year following delivery, only 3% reported incontinence; however, 5 years later, 19% of women asymptomatic following delivery had incontinence.** The Norwegian Epidemiology of Incontinence in the County of Nord-Trøndelag (EPINCONT) study, with an 80% response rate to a survey of more than 11,000 nulliparous patients, observed a 24% prevalence of urinary incontinence and increased urinary incontinence symptoms with increasing age, body mass index (BMI), and number of years since delivery.[46] In addition, incontinence was significantly associated with birthweight greater than 4000 g and fetal head circumference greater than 38 cm. Having at least one vacuum or forceps delivery in this cohort did not affect the risk of developing urinary incontinence. In a prospective study of the short- and long-term effects of forceps delivery compared with spontaneous vaginal delivery, which included both patient survey and clinical examination data, Meyer and colleagues[47] observed a similar incidence of urinary incontinence at both 9 weeks (32% vs. 21%) and 10 months (20% vs. 15%). In addition, bladder neck and urethral sphincter function and intravaginal pressures were similar between the groups. The only difference noted was an increased incidence of a weak pelvic floor in the forceps group (20% vs. 6%) at the 10-month examination. In a 5-year follow-up study of patients randomized to either forceps or vacuum delivery, Johanson and colleagues[48] observed no difference in the incidence of urinary dysfunction between these groups. However, in a prospective observational study that used patient survey data, Arya and colleagues[49] reported that urinary incontinence after forceps delivery was more likely to persist at 1 year compared with spontaneous vaginal delivery or vacuum delivery (11% vs. 3%). In a nulliparous cohort of more than 1100 women who were continent prior to pregnancy, only those who had a cesarean delivery had significantly reduced odds of reporting persistent incontinence at 18 months postpartum, whereas those whose vaginal births were assisted with either forceps or vacuum reported no difference in persistent incontinence compared with those who had a spontaneous vaginal delivery.[50] In addition, a study by Macleod and colleagues[51] reported that performance of an episiotomy was found to be protective against stress incontinence in those patients who were randomized to routine episiotomy versus restrictive episiotomy.

The only prospective randomized trial to assess urinary incontinence symptoms after planned elective cesarean delivery compared with planned vaginal delivery is the Term Breech Trial.[52] At 3 months postpartum, women randomized to cesarean delivery reported less urinary incontinence compared with those in the planned vaginal delivery group (4.5% vs. 7.3%; relative risk [RR], 0.62; 95% confidence interval [CI], 0.41 to 0.93). Finally, in a long-term (34-year) follow-up study of patients following either forceps, spontaneous vaginal delivery, or an elective cesarean delivery without labor, urinary incontinence was found more frequently in those women who had a spontaneous vaginal delivery compared with those who had a forceps delivery (19% vs. 7%). In addition, the total number of vaginal deliveries was the only risk factor attributed to urinary incontinence in this cohort (OR, 19.5; 95% CI, 4.01 to 34.8; $P = .001$).[53] **The precise association between mode of vaginal delivery (spontaneous, forceps, or vacuum) and urinary incontinence remains unclear at this time in light of the many other factors that appear to contribute to this condition. However, forceps delivery appears to have little if any effect on the subsequent development of urinary incontinence; therefore it is reasonable to counsel patients that the use of forceps or vacuum for an appropriate obstetric indication likely has no increased long-term effect on urinary incontinence compared with spontaneous vaginal delivery.**

Fecal Incontinence

Overall rates of anal sphincter injury noted at the time of vaginal delivery in nulliparous patients are reported to be between 7% and 11.5%.[39,54,55] **Operative vaginal delivery has been associated with an increased risk of perineal injury, specifically third- and fourth-degree lacerations.**[39,40] However, what is not clear is the precise incidence of occult anal sphincter injury in patients who deliver vaginally and the resulting effect on fecal incontinence. In the largest prospective study to evaluate the prevalence of anal sphincter injury after forceps delivery

TABLE 14-2   PREVALENCE OF ANAL SPHINCTER INJURY AFTER FORCEPS DELIVERY

REFERENCE	FORCEPS DELIVERIES (*N*)	IAS INJURY (*N*)	EAS INJURY (*N*)	IAS AND EAS INJURY (*N*)	TOTAL ANAL INJURY (%)
Sultan[57]	26	7	3	11	81
Sultan[60]	19	MD	MD	MD	79
Abramowitz[58]	35	MD	MD	MD	63
Belmonte-Montes[59]	17	0	11	2	76
Fitzpatrick[61]	61	0	34	0	56
De Parades[56]	93	0	11	1	13

EAS, external anal sphincter; *IAS,* internal anal sphincter; *MD,* missing data.

in nulliparous women using endoanal ultrasound, de Parades and colleagues[56] examined 93 patients 6 weeks after delivery and found a 13% prevalence of anal sphincter injury. These findings are in contrast to other studies that have evaluated fewer patients each but found a higher prevalence of anal sphincter injury shortly following forceps delivery (Table 14-2).[56-61]

The difficulty with many of the studies noted in Table 14-2 is the extremely low number of patients who return for the endoanal ultrasound following delivery. For example, even though Sultan and colleagues[60] recruited patients from a previous RCT of forceps and vacuum delivery, only 44 of the original 313 patients (14%) were assessed. Because not all patients were evaluated, it is possible that significant selection bias occurred and that the actual prevalence of anal sphincter injury was lower because those patients most symptomatic would be likeliest to return for endoanal ultrasound. Indeed, in the largest randomized trial to date to evaluate anal sphincter function following forceps or vacuum extraction, Fitzpatrick and colleagues[61] were able to follow up on all 61 patients randomized to forceps delivery and demonstrated a much lower rate of anal sphincter injury than previously reported (56%). Even though in this study, more patients who delivered by forceps described altered fecal continence compared with those who had vacuum delivery (59% vs. 33%), no differences were seen in endoanal ultrasound defects or in anal manometry results. In addition, no differences were reported in symptom scores between the groups, and the degree of disturbance to continence was low in both groups; the most common symptom was occasional flatal incontinence.

However, de Parades and colleagues[56] found lower rates of anal sphincter injury (13%) and complaints of altered fecal continence (30%) following forceps delivery. Most symptomatic patients complained of persistence of incontinence of flatus (17 of 28), as noted in the study by Fitzpatrick.[61] In addition, a significant increase in the daily number of stools was associated with anal sphincter defects visible on endoanal ultrasound, but the development of altered fecal continence symptoms was not.[56]

Even though it appears that immediate complaints of altered fecal continence and evidence of anal sphincter injury may be as high as 60% immediately following operative vaginal delivery, data from long-term follow-up does not bear this figure out. For example, Johanson and colleagues[48] followed patients 5 years after randomization to either forceps or vacuum delivery and found no significant difference in complaints of altered fecal continence between the groups (15% vs. 26%). In addition, most patients in the forceps and vacuum groups who noted altered fecal continence had occasional incontinence of flatus or diarrhea as their only symptom (70% and 68%, respectively). In addition, 34-year follow-up data on 42 patients delivered by forceps, compared with 41 patients

delivered by spontaneous vaginal delivery, demonstrated a higher rate of anal sphincter injury on ultrasonography in the forceps group (44% vs. 22%), but no difference was apparent in the rate of altered fecal continence (14% vs. 10%).[53] **These data suggest that forceps delivery is a risk for sphincter injury but not for long-term fecal incontinence. In fact, logistic regression revealed that greater neonatal birthweight, and not forceps delivery, was the contributing risk for significant fecal incontinence in this study.**[53] However, in a large longitudinal study that surveyed 3763 women up to 12 years after delivery, 6% self-reported persistent fecal incontinence from either their 3-month or 6-year follow-up survey. Logistic regression analysis demonstrated that any forceps delivery, maternal age between 30 and 34 years, and obesity as defined by BMI were all independently associated with persistent fecal incontinence.[62] Therefore, based on these studies, anal sphincter injury rates in women who deliver by forceps may be higher, and outcome data regarding the effect of forceps delivery on long-term rates of fecal incontinence are in conflict; thus further study of these outcomes is required to adequately assess this risk. These observations could reflect the body's ability to heal and compensate for anal sphincter injury over time and may also be the basis for questioning the importance and validity of early outcome assessments of anal incontinence.

Fetal Risks

The focus of possible fetal injury associated with operative vaginal delivery includes craniofacial/intracranial injury and neurologic/cognitive effects. The risks of fetal injury are generally instrument specific, and vacuum deliveries account for significantly higher rates of cephalohematoma and subgaleal and retinal hemorrhages, and forceps deliveries account for a nonsignificantly higher rate of scalp and facial injuries.[63] **In addition, the sequential use of vacuum and forceps requires particular attention because use in this manner is associated with a maternal and neonatal risk that is greater than the sum of the individual risks of these instruments.**[55]

Craniofacial and Intracranial Injury
CEPHALOHEMATOMA AND SUBGALEAL HEMORRHAGE
Rates of subperiosteal cephalohematoma in vacuum-assisted vaginal deliveries are higher than rates for either forceps or spontaneous vaginal delivery (112/1000, 63/1000, and 17/1000, respectively).[64,65] However, the most clinically significant and potentially life-threatening injury in this category is a subgaleal hemorrhage (see Chapter 22). This "false cephalohematoma" was first described by Nägele in 1819 to differentiate it from a true subperiosteal cephalohematoma.[66] **Subgaleal hemorrhage occurs when blood collects in the loose areolar tissue in the**

space between the galea aponeurotica and the periosteum. If the veins that connect the dural sinus and the scalp rupture in this layer due to shear forces, the potential space within this loosely applied connective tissue in the subgaleal space may expand with blood well beyond the limits of the suture lines (unlike a subperiosteal cephalohematoma, which is limited to blood and fluid collections within the margins of the suture lines). This space has the potential volume of several hundred milliliters of blood, which can produce profound neonatal hypovolemia, leading to hypoxia, disseminated intravascular coagulation (DIC), end-organ injury, and death.[67] Older literature cites several causes of subgaleal hemorrhage, along with the source: for vacuum extraction, it was 48%; spontaneous vaginal delivery, 28%; forceps, 14%; and cesarean delivery, 9%.[66] Although this is older literature reported in an era when a "low forceps" delivery was broadly defined by the 1965 ACOG classification scheme, it is most important to note that these potentially life-threatening bleeds can also occur with spontaneous vaginal deliveries.

More recent data suggest that subgaleal hemorrhage occurs nearly exclusively with the vacuum device[68-70] with an incidence of subgaleal bleeding of 26 to 45 per 1000.[71] Benaron[72] reported an incidence of 1 per 200 with soft silicone vacuum cups. Subgaleal hemorrhage has an estimated incidence of approximately 4 per 10,000 spontaneous vaginal deliveries.[66] In a 30-month prospective study, Boo[73] evaluated more than 64,000 neonates and found that the incidence per live birth was much higher for vacuum extraction than for other modes of delivery (41/1000 vs. 1/1000). Both the type of cup and the duration of its use are predictors of scalp injury. Soft cups are more likely to be associated with a decreased incidence of scalp injuries but may not be less likely to result in a subgaleal hemorrhage.[4] In one study, vacuum application duration of more than 10 minutes was the best predictor of scalp injury.[74]

In May 1998, the Food and Drug Administration (FDA) issued a public health advisory[31] regarding the use of vacuum-assisted delivery devices. The advisory cited a fivefold increase in the rate of deaths and serious morbidity during the previous 4 years, compared with the past 11 years, and recommended use of these devices only when a specific obstetric indication is present. Other recommendations included the following:

- Persons who use vacuum devices for assisted delivery should be versed in their use and aware of the indications, contraindications, and precautions supported in the accepted literature and current device labeling.
- The recommended use for all these products is to apply steady traction in the line of the birth canal. Rocking movements or applying torque to the device may be dangerous. Because the instructions may be different for each device type or style, it is important to use the instructions provided by the manufacturer of the particular product being used.
- Alert those who will be responsible for the infant's care that a vacuum-assisted delivery device has been used so that they can monitor the infant for signs of complications.
- Educate the neonatal care staff about the complications of vacuum-assisted delivery devices that have been reported to the FDA and in the literature. They should watch for the signs of these complications in any infant in whom a vacuum-assisted delivery device was used.
- Report reactions associated with the use of vacuum-assisted delivery devices to the FDA.

Despite the fact that many recommend allowing no more than three pop-offs before successful delivery, no clear evidence suggests that three applications are safe; if the cup slips during traction without descent of the vertex, neonatal scalp injury may still occur.[74] For example, Benaron[72] demonstrated that the risk of injury and bleeding is increased in nulliparous patients and in those with severe dystocia, malposition, and forceful, prolonged vacuum extractor use. Therefore caution must be taken with the use of vacuum extractor devices to avoid prolonged (>30 minutes) or forceful use.

INTRACRANIAL HEMORRHAGE
Rates of clinically significant intracranial hemorrhage for vacuum, forceps, and cesarean delivery during labor are similar (1/860, 1/664, and 1/907, respectively) but are higher than those for cesarean delivery without labor (1/2750) and for spontaneous vaginal delivery (1/1900).[75] Because cesarean delivery following abnormal labor was associated with the same rate of ICH as forceps and vacuum in this study, it is likely that the common risk factor for any increased risk of ICH is abnormal labor, not the type of operative vaginal delivery performed. In fact, because the prevalence of clinically silent subdural hemorrhage is approximately 6% following uncomplicated spontaneous vaginal delivery, the presence of this hemorrhage in an otherwise asymptomatic neonate does not necessarily indicate excessive birth trauma and again reflects the natural history of labor and delivery.[76] In these neonates, the silent subdural hemorrhages all resolved within 4 weeks of delivery.

NEUROLOGIC AND COGNITIVE EFFECTS
Vacuum-assisted vaginal deliveries increase the risk of neonatal retinal hemorrhages by approximately twofold compared with forceps deliveries.[63] Despite this finding, data on the long-term consequences of these hemorrhages do not demonstrate any significant effect. Johanson and colleagues[48] followed a cohort of children 5 years following an RCT of forceps versus vacuum extraction and found a 13% rate of visual problems in the group. However, no difference was found between those delivered by forceps compared with those delivered by vacuum extraction (12.8% vs. 12.5%). Seidman and colleagues[77] were also unable to detect any increased risk of vision abnormalities in a cohort of 1747 individuals delivered by vacuum extraction compared with more than 47,000 individuals delivered by spontaneous vaginal delivery and examined at age 17 years by the Israeli Defense Forces draft board.

In addition, no long-term effect of operative vaginal delivery on cognitive development is apparent. Seidman and colleagues[77] demonstrated that mean intelligence scores at age 17 years were no different between those delivered by forceps or vacuum extraction compared with those delivered by spontaneous vaginal delivery. However, the mean intelligence scores for those delivered by cesarean delivery were significantly lower than those of the spontaneous delivery group. Similarly, in a 1993 report from patients within the Kaiser system in Oakland, CA, Wesley and colleagues[78] were unable to detect a difference in cognitive development by measuring IQ in 1192 children delivered by forceps, compared with 1499 who delivered spontaneously, who were examined at age 5 years. Furthermore, of the 1192 forceps deliveries, 114 were midforceps deliveries, and no differences in IQ were seen at age 5 compared with 1500 controls. Finally, no association between forceps delivery and epilepsy in adulthood is apparent. Murphy and colleagues[79] evaluated a cohort of more than 21,000 individuals and found forceps delivery was not associated with an increased risk of epilepsy or anticonvulsant therapy when compared with other methods of delivery.

Regarding long-term neurologic outcomes, in a 5-year follow-up of a prospective cohort of 264 women with term, singleton, cephalic pregnancies that required a second-stage operative delivery from 1999 to 2000, neonates delivered by forceps were found to have no significant differences in neurodevelopmental outcome compared with those delivered by cesarean section.[80]

Evidence also suggests that forceps-assisted vaginal births may be protective against outcomes associated with poor long-term neurologic consequences. A retrospective review[81] of neonatal outcomes from more than 1 million singleton births between 1995 and 2003 revealed that when compared with vacuum–assisted vaginal delivery or cesarean delivery, forceps-assisted vaginal deliveries were associated with a reduced risk of adverse neurologic outcomes, including seizures and 5-minute Apgar scores less than 7.

Complex Operative Vaginal Delivery Procedures
Rotations Greater Than 45 Degrees

The correct application and delivery technique using forceps is critical to the safe performance of this procedure. The outcomes of forceps delivery are often directly compared and contrasted with those of spontaneous vaginal delivery. When these comparisons are made, forceps deliveries are associated with a higher rate of maternal injury than spontaneous vaginal deliveries. However, the comparison of these two modes of delivery is not appropriate because forceps applications require an indication for use that confounds the clinical outcome when compared with spontaneous vaginal delivery. A more appropriate comparison to forceps delivery, or to operative vaginal delivery in general, is cesarean delivery for second-stage arrest disorder. Unfortunately, no prospective randomized trials directly compare these two modes of delivery. However, **numerous retrospective studies that have compared midcavity and rotational forceps delivery with cesarean delivery demonstrate no increased risk of fetal/neonatal adverse outcomes including Apgar score, umbilical cord blood gas values, birth trauma, and neonatal intensive care unit (NICU) admission.**[82-85] Specifically, the rates of neonatal morbidity associated with Kielland forceps rotation are similar to cesarean delivery, including rates of cephalohematoma (9% to 17%), facial bruising (13% to 18%), facial nerve injury (1% to 5%), neonatal encephalopathy (<1%), and brachial plexus injury (<1%).[85-87] Interestingly, rates of maternal morbidity (intraoperative and postoperative complications, blood loss, and length of stay) have been found to be higher in patients delivered by cesarean delivery compared with those delivered by midcavity forceps delivery.[82,83]

The outcomes of rotational forceps deliveries have also been evaluated and compared with nonrotational forceps delivery. Healy and colleagues[88] evaluated 552 Kielland forceps rotations, 95 Scanzoni-Smellie maneuvers with classic instruments, and 160 manual rotations followed by delivery with a classic instrument and found no difference in neonatal outcomes between the groups. Krivac and colleagues[89] compared 55 Kielland forceps rotations with 213 nonrotational forceps deliveries and found that 15 of the rotations were greater than 90 degrees, and 40 were less than 90 degrees but greater than 45 degrees.

They found that the Kielland forceps–rotation group had both a longer labor and longer second stage than the nonrotational group and a higher rate of 1-minute Apgar scores less than 6 and meconium at delivery. However, the nonrotational forceps group had a greater incidence of postpartum hemorrhage (14% vs. 7%) and a higher rate of third- and fourth-degree lacerations (24% vs. 14%). No other differences in maternal or neonatal morbidity were noted, which included no difference in rates of nerve compromise (<1%), facial bruising (7%), shoulder dystocia (1%), or NICU admissions. Hankins and colleagues[90] performed a retrospective case-controlled study that compared 113 forceps deliveries greater than 90 degrees compared with 167 forceps deliveries less than 45 degrees. **No differences in major fetal injury were demonstrated between these two groups.** *Major fetal injury* was defined as skull fracture, subdural hematoma and brachial plexus or facial nerve injury, and fetal acidemia (pH less than 7.0). Finally, Feldman and colleagues[91] compared 104 rotational forceps deliveries using Leff forceps for persistent OP position with 163 nonrotational forceps deliveries and found lower rates of episiotomy (66% vs. 82%) and perineal lacerations (16% vs. 23%) in the forceps-rotation group and no differences in the rates of neonatal morbidity between the groups. **These data suggest that when properly applied and used, forceps deliveries that require more than a 45-degree rotation may be safely accomplished without increased risk of maternal or neonatal morbidity, therefore it should remain a management option for women with second-stage labor abnormalities.**

Midpelvic Cavity Delivery

Like rotational forceps deliveries, delivery of the fetus from a 0 or +1 station (midpelvic or midforceps) requires a specific set of skills and precautions. **In 1988, ACOG reported on required conditions for a midforceps delivery that included (1) an experienced person performing or supervising the procedure, (2) adequate anesthesia, (3) assessment of maternal-fetal size, and (4) willingness to abandon the attempt at delivery.** This information should be taken together with the prerequisites set forth by Richardson and colleagues[92]: **the midforceps procedure (1) must rationally be needed as an alternative method of delivery to cesarean delivery, (2) must be associated with demonstrably less maternal morbidity than cesarean delivery, and (3) should not result in fetal harm.** Several studies that have compared cesarean delivery with midforceps procedures show that midforceps delivery is not associated with more adverse neonatal outcomes including cord blood gases, Apgar scores, NICU admissions, and birth trauma.[82,83,93] In 1997, Revah and colleagues[93] reported their findings of a retrospective chart review of 401 cesarean deliveries over a 7-year period in which a trial of operative delivery (forceps or vacuum) was conducted in 75 cases. No differences were reported for any maternal or fetal outcome between cesarean delivery with a trial of operative delivery versus no operative delivery attempt. **Although the outcomes of these studies are reassuring, because of the technical skills required, it is most reasonable to abide by the guidance set forth in the ACOG practice bulletin[71] published in 2000, which states, "Unless the preoperative assessment is highly suggestive of successful outcome, trial of operative vaginal delivery is best avoided."** In short, following the ACOG statement and the previously stated prerequisites provides the skilled practitioner with guidelines and support for attempting a safe midpelvic cavity delivery.

Sequential Use of Vacuum and Forceps

The sequential use of these instruments appears to increase the likelihood of adverse maternal and neonatal outcomes more than the sum of the relative risks of each instrument.[55,65] Compared with spontaneous vaginal delivery, deliveries by sequential use of vacuum and forceps are associated with significantly higher rates of ICH (RR, 3.9; 95% CI, 1.5 to 10.1), brachial plexus injury (RR, 3.2; 95% CI, 1.6 to 6.4), facial nerve injury (RR, 3.0; 95% CI, 4.7 to 37.7), neonatal seizures (RR, 13.7; 95% CI, 2.1 to 88.0), requirement for mechanical ventilation of the neonate (RR, 4.8; 95% CI, 2.1 to 11.0), severe perineal lacerations (RR, 6.2; 95% CI, 6.4 to 20.1), and postpartum hemorrhage (RR, 1.6; 95% CI, 1.3 to 2.0).[55] Therefore **care should be taken to avoid the sequential use of these instruments to reduce maternal and neonatal morbidity.** Such switching of instruments should be limited to situations in which application of one type of instrument fails, and it should be performed by individuals skilled and experienced with operative vaginal delivery procedures.

Trial of Operative Vaginal Delivery

Historically, an unsuccessful operative vaginal delivery has been associated with a high maternal and neonatal morbidity and up to a 38% fetal mortality rate and 2% maternal mortality rate.[94] Reports of increased morbidity and mortality in these cases led to the development of the concept of a trial of forceps in which immediate cesarean delivery was performed if, following correction of malposition and gentle traction, further descent of the fetal vertex was not noted.[95] These attempts were often performed in the operating room instead of the delivery room, permitting rapid transition to cesarean delivery. **Following implementation of this concept, rates of morbidity and mortality have fallen, documenting no difference in neonatal or maternal outcomes associated with a failed forceps or vacuum attempts in the absence of a nonreassuring fetal heart rate tracing.**[96]

Vacuum Delivery and the Preterm Fetus

No quality data support firm recommendations in regard to a gestational age limit below which the vacuum extractor should not be used. Two studies have reported the use of soft cups without adverse outcomes in preterm fetuses; however, these studies were small and lacked power to demonstrate significance. No RCTs have compared forceps with vacuums or different vacuum types to pass judgment on a gestational age cutoff. **ACOG reports that most experts in operative vaginal delivery limit the vacuum procedure to fetuses beyond 34 weeks' gestation.**[71] This is a reasonable cutoff given that the premature head is likely at greater risk for compression-decompression injuries simply because of the pliability of the preterm skull and the more fragile soft tissues of the scalp.

COUNSELING: FORCEPS, VACUUM, OR CESAREAN DELIVERY

The increasing use of vacuum extraction over forceps has resulted in numerous publications that have compared efficacy and morbidity between methods. Table 14-3 provides a summary of the disadvantages associated with both methods. In a Cochrane meta-analysis[97] that included 10 RCTs of vacuum and forceps use, **vacuum extraction had a greater failure rate than that of forceps but was associated with less maternal trauma,**

TABLE 14-3	COMPARATIVE MORBIDITIES ASSOCIATED WITH FORCEPS DELIVERY AND VACUUM EXTRACTION	
FORCEPS	**VACUUM EXTRACTION**	
Greater third- and fourth-degree and vaginal lacerations	Higher failure rate than forceps	
Greater maternal discomfort postpartum	Increased risk of neonatal injury	
Greater duration of training needed	Minor: cephalohematoma, retinal hemorrhage	
Increased risk of neonatal facial nerve injury	Major: subarachnoid hemorrhage, subgaleal hemorrhage	
	Less need for maternal anesthesia	

Modified from Johanson RB, Menon BK. Vacuum extraction versus forceps for assisted vaginal delivery. *Cochrane Database Syst Rev.* 2000;(2):CD000224.

including third- and fourth-degree extensions and vaginal lacerations, than forceps use. Less maternal regional and general anesthesia was used for vacuum extractions, and no differences were found in significant neonatal injury between the two groups. Despite small sample sizes, vacuum extraction was associated with an increased risk of cephalohematoma and retinal hemorrhage when compared with forceps use.** Cephalohematoma formation with vacuum extraction was reported to have a mean incidence of 6%, with no difference between soft or rigid vacuum cups, and it is considered to be a finding of little significance.[29,97] More information on the long-term effects of retinal hemorrhage related to vacuum delivery is needed.

Unless a patient is willing to undergo cesarean delivery before the onset of advanced labor, there does not appear to be any advantage to avoiding operative vaginal delivery in an attempt to reduce the long-term risks of incontinence. **The effects of both forceps and vacuum delivery on the risk of developing urinary incontinence appear to be the same as those of spontaneous vaginal delivery:** between 5% and 20% of women develop long-term persistent urinary incontinence regardless of vaginal delivery method. In addition, despite evidence that the anal sphincter injury rate in women who deliver by forceps is higher, **it is not clear whether the long-term rates of fecal incontinence in these women is any different than in those who deliver spontaneously.** Approximately 10% to 30% of women develop some degree of altered fecal continence following vaginal delivery, and cesarean delivery before the onset of labor is the only reliable means of reducing this risk.

The greatest risk for urinary incontinence appears to be the total number of vaginal deliveries, and the greatest risk for subsequent development of fecal incontinence appears to be related to the effect of the largest neonate delivered vaginally, irrespective of mode of delivery. Regarding fetal risks, vacuum deliveries appear to increase the incidence of cephalohematoma and subgaleal and retinal hemorrhages compared with forceps or spontaneous vaginal deliveries. Forceps deliveries increase the risk of facial bruising and transient facial nerve palsies compared with vacuum or spontaneous vaginal deliveries. However, no evidence suggests that these immediate neonatal morbidities result in any long-term visual, neurologic, or cognitive developmental abnormalities. Finally, patients delivered by cesarean delivery in the second stage have a higher risk of intraoperative and postoperative complications, higher rates of blood loss, and longer hospital stays than those delivered by operative vaginal delivery.

Patients should also be informed that substantially more women who have an operative vaginal delivery achieve

subsequent vaginal delivery in the next pregnancy compared with those who have a cesarean delivery (78% vs. 31%). Therefore it is reasonable to counsel patients that the options for second-stage assisted delivery include both forceps and vacuum when appropriate, because the proper application of these instruments and execution of these deliveries can avoid the maternal morbidity associated with cesarean delivery and increase the likelihood of a subsequent vaginal delivery for the next pregnancy without additional long-term maternal or neonatal risk.

In a Cochrane review[64] of 10 randomized studies that compared the use of forceps to vacuum extraction for assisted vaginal delivery, vacuum devices were found to be more likely to fail than forceps, as noted above. However, vacuum use was also more likely to result in vaginal delivery, probably because failed vacuum extraction led to the use of forceps and subsequent vaginal delivery due to a lower forceps failure rate. A lower failure rate is not the only reason to consider forceps. **Forceps may be the only acceptable instrument to effect an operative vaginal delivery in some circumstances. Some examples of these clinical situations include delivery of the head at assisted breech delivery, assisted delivery of a preterm infant younger than 34 weeks' gestation, delivery with a face presentation with mentum anterior, suspected coagulopathy or thrombocytopenia in the fetus, and instrumental delivery for maternal medical conditions that preclude pushing.**[14] Because the specific clinical situation and operator experience are the key factors that contribute to the choice of instrument, it is critical that students of obstetrics be thoroughly familiar with the use of both instruments. Finally, **an attempt at counseling patients on the risks, benefits, and alternatives of operative vaginal delivery should take place during prenatal visits.** This is because it is not ideal to counsel patients in the second stage of labor when they are generally experiencing pain and exhaustion and may be under the influence of narcotics. This counseling should also be documented in the medical record.

SIMULATION AND RESIDENCY TRAINING IN OPERATIVE VAGINAL DELIVERY

The overall incidence of operative vaginal delivery has remained stable over the past 15 years. Interestingly, over this same time span, vacuum extraction procedures have overtaken forceps procedures as the method of choice (Fig. 14-8). In a review of operative vaginal delivery, Yeomans[98] strongly advocates that residency training programs incorporate detailed instructions in forceps techniques and that simulation training precede clinical work to enhance understanding of the mechanics. Bahl and colleagues[99] reviewed video recordings to establish critical components of nonrotational vacuum deliveries, and they defined key technical skills required for the evaluation of clinical competence of trainees in this technique. Further detailed studies are needed to ensure that both vacuum and forceps techniques can be taught and evaluated first with the use of simulation and then in the clinical setting.

A 1992 report of a survey conducted by Ramin and colleagues[100] of U.S. residency training programs reported that most programs use the 1988 classification scheme and that 86% taught midforceps delivery. It should be noted that even though a large percentage of programs teach the complex forceps procedures, the number of such procedures to reach proficiency has not been elucidated. In short, the overall decline in forceps

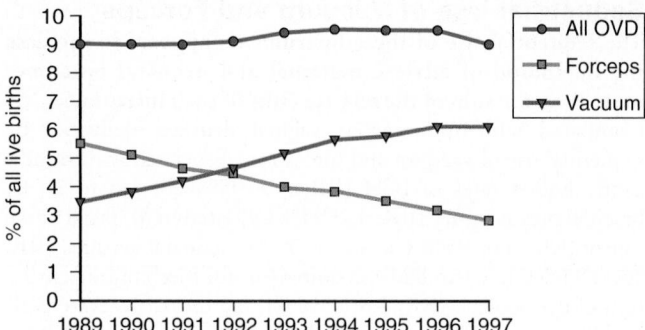

FIG 14-8 The overall incidence of operative vaginal delivery (OVD) has remained stable over the last 15 years. Interestingly, over this same time span, vacuum extraction procedures have overtaken forceps procedures as the method of choice. (Modified from Miksovsky P, Watson WJ. Obstetric vacuum extraction: state of the art in the new millennium. *Obstet Gynecol Surv.* 2001;56:736.)

TABLE 14-4	MODES OF DELIVERY AND BIRTH OUTCOMES BEFORE AND AFTER INITIATION OF DEDICATED OBSTETRICS STAFF LOCATED ON LABOR AND DELIVERY		
	BEFORE	**AFTER**	***P* VALUE**
Births	3481	4338	.0001
Cesarean section	888 (26%)	1183 (27%)	NS
Operative vaginal delivery	394 (11%)	461 (11%)	NS
Forceps	172 (5%)	337 (8%)	.00001
Vacuum	222 (6%)	124 (3%)	.00001
Third- or fourth-degree lacerations	126 (4%)	134 (3%)	NS
Birth injury	8 (0.2%)	13 (0.3%)	NS
Apgar score <7 at 5 min	67 (2%)	104 (2%)	NS

NS, not significant.

procedures performed, the complexity of midpelvic cavity deliveries, and the shift from complex rotational deliveries to vacuum extraction and cesarean deliveries by younger faculty—as shown by Tan and colleagues[86] and Jain and colleagues[101]—may make the midforceps procedure obsolete in the near future.[100] In response to these types of concerns, Solt and associates[102] conducted a unique study to determine whether the rates of vacuum extraction and forceps procedures could be reversed without an increase in morbidity in a residency program. This retrospective study compared outcomes 2 years before and 2 years after an obstetrics faculty member was dedicated to the labor floor from Monday through Thursday, 7 AM to 5 PM. Table 14-4 **depicts how such a dedicated instructor can increase the number of forceps deliveries relative to vacuum extractions without increasing third- or fourth-degree lacerations or adverse neonatal outcomes. In fact, the number of events of fetal pH less than 7.1 was reduced during the teaching period.**[99]

Although the early 1990s report by Ramin and colleagues[100] provided encouraging information regarding the use of the 1988 classification scheme, a 2004 study by Carollo and others[103] is unsettling. This study conducted a survey of several teaching hospitals in the Denver area and asked the following important questions: (1) How do you define fetal station? (2) How do you think a majority of your colleagues define fetal station? (3) How do you think ACOG defines fetal station? and (4) How important do you think these distinctions are? What makes this study additionally unique is that these questions were asked of both attendings and residents in obstetrics and gynecology as well as nurses. **Approximately 35% of attending physicians still defined station by dividing the pelvis into thirds, as set forth in the old 1965 ACOG classification scheme, rather than using centimeters.** In addition, nearly 15% used the BPD, rather than the presenting part, as the landmark on the fetus to define station. These percentage numbers were higher for nurses and residents. The percent of correctly used techniques for defining station was highest at the university teaching hospital. These data suggest that although we do fairly well at teaching proper technique for determining station, we do poorly in disseminating information into practice. **Operative vaginal deliveries will be more difficult and dangerous if misunderstandings in defining fetal station persist.**

KEY POINTS

- Obstetric forceps are the one instrument that makes the practice of obstetric care unique to obstetricians. The proper use of these instruments has afforded safe and timely vaginal delivery to those whose abnormal labor course and urgent need for delivery require their use.
- Rates of cesarean delivery have risen in the United States, reaching a rate of approximately 25% of all deliveries, whereas rates of forceps deliveries have declined from 17.7% in 1980 to 4% in 2000.
- Resident work hour restrictions have resulted in a decline in resident experience with both primary cesarean delivery and vacuum-assisted vaginal delivery.
- Treat the vacuum extractor with the same respect as the forceps. The prerequisites for application of forceps or vacuum extractor are identical.
- When using vacuum extraction, descent of the fetal head should occur with each pull. If no descent occurs after three pulls, the operative attempt should be stopped.
- It appears that forceps delivery has little if any effect on the subsequent development of urinary incontinence.
- The rate of anal sphincter injury in women who deliver by forceps may be higher; however, long-term rates of fetal incontinence appear to be no different than those in women who deliver spontaneously.
- The risks of fetal injury associated with operative vaginal delivery are generally instrument specific: vacuum deliveries account for higher rates of cephalohematoma and subgaleal and retinal hemorrhages, and forceps deliveries account for a nonsignificantly higher rate of scalp and facial injuries.
- Numerous retrospective studies that have compared midcavity and rotation forceps delivery with cesarean delivery demonstrate no increased risk of fetal or neonatal adverse outcomes, including Apgar score, umbilical cord blood gas values, trauma, and NICU admission.
- When properly applied and used, forceps deliveries that require greater than 45 degrees rotation may be safely accomplished without increased risk of maternal or neonatal morbidity and therefore should remain a

management option for women with second-stage labor abnormalities.
- The sequential use of vacuum extraction and forceps increases the likelihood of adverse maternal and neonatal outcomes more than the sum of the relative risks of each instrument.

REFERENCES

1. Denman T. *An Introduction to the Practice of Midwifery.* 1st ed. London: 1788.
2. Holland E. The Princess Charlotte of Wales: a triple obstetric tragedy. *J Obstet Gynaecol Br Emp.* 1951;58:905.
3. Denman T. *Aphorisms on the Application and Use of the Forceps.* 6th ed. London: 1817.
4. DeLee JB. The prophylactic forceps operation. *Am J Obstet Gynecol.* 1920;1:34.
5. Martin JA, Hamilton BE, Osterman MJ. Births in the United States, 2013. *NCHS Data Brief.* 2014;175:1-8.
6. Thomas J, Paranjoth S. *National sentinel caesarean section audit report.* London: Royal College of Obstetricians and Gynaecologists Clinical Effectiveness Support Unit; 2001.
7. Martin JA, Hamilton BE, Osterman MJ, Curtin SC, Mathews TJ. Births: Final Data for 2013. *Natl Vital Stat Rep.* 2015;64:1-65.
8. Hankins GD, Uckan E, Rowe TF, Collier S. Forceps and vacuum delivery: expectations of residency and fellowship training program directors. *Am J Perinatol.* 1999;16:23.
9. Blanchard MH, Amini SB, Frank TM. Impact of work hour restrictions on resident case experience in an obstetrics and gynecology residency program. *Am J Obstet Gynecol.* 2004;191:1746.
10. *American College of Obstetricians and Gynecologists Practice Bulletin Number 17. Operative Vaginal Delivery.* June 2000.
11. Murphy DJ, Liebling RE. Cohort study of maternal views on future mode of delivery following operative delivery in the second stage of labor. *Am J Obstet Gynecol.* 2003;188:542.
12. Bahl R, Strachan B, Murphy DJ. Outcome of subsequent pregnancy three years after previous operative delivery in the second stage of labour: cohort study. *BMJ.* 2004;328:311.
13. Murphy DJ, Pope C, Frost J, Liebling RE. Women's views on the impact of operative delivery in the second stage of labour—qualitative study. *BMJ.* 2003;327:1132.
14. Patel RR, Murphy DJ. Forceps delivery in modern practice. *BMJ.* 2004;328:1302.
15. Dennen EH. A classification of forceps operations according to station of head in pelvis. *Am J Obstet Gynecol.* 1952;63:272.
16. American College of Obstetricians and Gynecologists. *Manual of Standards of Obstetric-Gynecologic Practice: American College of Obstetricians and Gynecologists.* 2nd ed. Washington, DC: ACOG; 1965.
17. American College of Obstetricians and Gynecologists, Committee on Obstetrics, Maternal and Fetal Medicine: *Obstetric Forceps. Technical Bulletin No. 59,* February 1988.
18. Hagadorn-Freathy AS, Yeomans ER, Hankins GD. Validation of the 1988 ACOG forceps classification system. *Obstet Gynecol.* 1991;77:356.
19. Laube DW. Forceps delivery. *Clin Obstet Gynecol.* 1986;29:286.
20. Kielland C: *The application of forceps to the unrotated head. A description of a new type of forceps and a new method of insertion. Translated from the original article in Monafs schrift fur Geburshilfe und Gynakologie 43:48,* 1916.
21. Leff M. An obstetric forceps for rotation of the fetal head. *Am J Obstet Gynecol.* 1955;70:208.
22. Feldman DM, Borgida AF, Sauer F, Rodis JF. Rotational versus nonrotational forceps: maternal and neonatal outcomes. *Am J Obstet Gynecol.* 1999;181:1185.
23. Malmström T. The vacuum extractor: an obstetrical instrument. *Acta Obstet Gynecol Scand.* 1957;36:5.
24. Kuit JA, Eppinga HG, Wallenburg HC, Hiukeshoven FJ. A randomized comparison of vacuum extraction delivery with a rigid and a pliable cup. *Obstet Gynecol.* 1993;82:280.
25. Hillier CE, Johanson RB. Worldwide survey of assisted vaginal delivery. *Int J Gynecol Obstet.* 1994;47:109.

26. Hale RW, ed. *Dennen's Forceps Deliveries*. 4th ed. Washington, DC: American College of Obstetrics and Gynecology; 2001.

27. Scanzoni FW. *Lehrbuch der Geburtshulfe*. 3rd ed. Vienna: Seidel; 1853:838.

28. Mikovsky P, Watson WJ. Obstetric vacuum extraction: state of the art in the new millennium. *Obstet Gynecol Surv*. 2001;56:736.

29. Vacca A. Vacuum assisted delivery. *Best Pract Res Clin Obstet Gynecol*. 2002;16:17.

30. Vacca A. *Handbook of Vacuum Extraction in Obstetrical Practice*. London: Edward Arnold; 1992.

31. Center for Devices and Radiological Health. FDA Public Health Advisory. *Need for caution when using vacuum assisted delivery devices*. Rockville, MD: Food and Drug Administration Available at: <www.fda.gov/MedicalDevices/Safety/AlertsandNotices/PublicHealthNotifications/ucm062295.htm.

32. Plauche WC. Fetal cranial injuries related to delivery with the Malmstrom vacuum extractor. *Obstet Gynecol*. 1979;53:750.

33. O'Grady JP, Pope CS, Patel SS. Vacuum extraction in modern obstetric practice: a review and critique. *Curr Opin Obstet Gynecol*. 2000;12:475.

34. Bofill JA, Rust OA, Schorr SJ, et al. A randomized prospective trial of obstetric forceps versus the m-cup vacuum extractor. *Am J Obstet Gynecol*. 1996;175:1325.

35. Johanson R, Menon V. Soft versus rigid vacuum extractor cups for assisted vaginal delivery. *Cochrane Database Syst Rev*. 2000;(2):CD000446.

36. Bofill JA, Rust OA, Schorr SJ, et al. A randomized trial of two vacuum extraction techniques. *Obstet Gynecol*. 1997;89:758.

37. Johanson RB, Heycock E, Carter J, et al. Maternal and child health after assisted vaginal delivery: five-year follow up of a randomized controlled study comparing forceps and ventouse. *Br J Obstet Gynaecol*. 1999;106:544.

38. Handa VL, Harris TA, Ostergard DR. Protecting the pelvic floor: obstetric management to prevent incontinence and pelvic organ prolapse. *Obstet Gynecol*. 1996;88:470.

39. Handa VL, Danielsen BH, Gilbert WM. Obstetric anal sphincter lacerations. *Obstet Gynecol*. 2001;98:225.

40. Robinson JN, Norwitz ER, Cohen AP, et al. Episiotomy, operative vaginal delivery, and significant perineal trauma in nulliparous women. *Am J Obstet Gynecol*. 1999;181:1180.

41. Gill L, El Nashar S, Garrett AT, Famuyide AO. Predictors of third- and fourth-degree lacerations in forceps-assisted delivery: a case-control study. *Obstet Gynecol*. 2014;123:145S-146S.

42. Clemons JL, Towers GD, McClure GB, O'Boyle AL. Decreased anal sphincter lacerations associated with restrictive episiotomy use. *Am J Obstet Gynecol*. 2005;192:1620-1625.

43. Ecker JL, Tan WM, Bansal RK, et al. Is there a benefit to episiotomy at operative vaginal delivery? Observations over ten years in a stable population. *Am J Obstet Gynecol*. 1997;176:411.

44. Nygaard IE, Heit M. Stress urinary incontinence. *Obstet Gynecol*. 2004;104:607.

45. Viktrup L, Lose G. The risk of stress incontinence 5 years after first delivery. *Am J Obstet Gynecol*. 2001;185:82.

46. Rortveit G, Daltveit AK, Hannestad YS, Hunskaar S. Vaginal delivery parameters and urinary incontinence: the Norwegian EPINCONT study. *Am J Obstet Gynecol*. 2003;189:1268.

47. Meyer S, Hohlfeld P, Achtare C, et al. Birth trauma: short and long term effects of forceps delivery compared with spontaneous delivery on various pelvic floor parameters. *Br J Obstet Gynaecol*. 2000;107:1360.

48. Johanson RB, Heycock E, Carter J, et al. Maternal and child health after assisted vaginal delivery: five-year follow up of a randomized controlled study comparing forceps and ventouse. *Br J Obstet Gynaecol*. 1999;106:544.

49. Arya LA, Jackson ND, Myers DL, Verma A. Risk of new-onset urinary incontinence after forceps and vacuum delivery in primiparous women. *Am J Obstet Gynecol*. 2001;185:1318.

50. Gartland D, Donath S, MacArthur C, Brown SJ. The onset, recurrence and associated obstetric risk factors for urinary incontinence in the first 18 months after a first birth: an Australian nulliparous cohort study. *Br J Obstet Gynaecol*. 2012;119:1361-1369.

51. Macleod M, Goyder K, Howarth L, Bahl R, Strachan B, Murphy DJ. Morbidity experienced by women before and after operative vaginal delivery: prospective cohort study nested within a two-centre randomized controlled trial of restrictive versus routine use of episiotomy. *Br J Obstet Gynaecol*. 2013;120:1020-1026.

52. Hannah ME, Hannah WJ, Hodnett ED, et al. Outcomes at 3 months after planned cesarean versus planned vaginal delivery for breech presentation at term: the International Randomized Term Breech Trial. *JAMA*. 2002;287:1822.

53. Bollard RC, Gardiner A, Duthie GS. Anal sphincter injury, fetal and urinary incontinence: a 34-year follow-up after forceps delivery. *Dis Colon Rectum*. 2003;46:1083.

54. Richter HE, Brumfield CG, Cliver SP, et al. Risk factors associated with anal sphincter tear: a comparison of primiparous patients, vaginal births after cesarean deliveries and patients with previous vaginal delivery. *Am J Obstet Gynecol*. 2002;187:1194.

55. Gardella G, Taylor M, Benedetti T, et al. The effect of sequential use of vacuum and forceps for assisted vaginal delivery on neonatal and maternal outcomes. *Am J Obstet Gynecol*. 2001;185:896.

56. deParades V, Etienney I, Thabut D, et al. Anal sphincter injury after forceps delivery: myth or reality? *Dis Colon Rectum*. 2004;47:24.

57. Sultan AH, Kamm MA, Bartram CI, Hudson CN. Anal sphincter trauma during instrumental delivery. *Int J Gynecol Obstet*. 1993;43:263.

58. Abramowitz L, Sobhani I, Ganansia R, et al. Are sphincter defects the cause of anal incontinence after vaginal delivery? Results of a prospective study. *Dis Colon Rectum*. 2000;43:590.

59. Belmonte-Montes C, Hagerman G, Vega-Yepez PA, et al. Anal sphincter injury after vaginal delivery in primiparous females. *Dis Colon Rectum*. 2001;44:1244.

60. Sultan AH, Johanson RB, Carter JE. Occult anal sphincter trauma following randomized forceps and vacuum delivery. *Int J Gynecol Obstet*. 1998;61:113.

61. Fitzpatrick M, Behan M, O'Connell PR, O'Herlihy C. Randomised clinical trial to assess anal sphincter function following forceps or vacuum assisted vaginal delivery. *BJOG*. 2003;110:424.

62. MacArthur C, Wilson D, Herbison P, et al. Feacal incontinence persisting after childbirth: a 12 year longitudinal study. *Br J Obstet Gynaecol*. 2013;120:169-179.

63. Johanson RB, Menon V. Vacuum extraction versus forceps for assisted vaginal delivery. [revised 23 Nov 2001]. In: *The Cochrane Pregnancy and Childbirth Database. The Cochrane Collaboration*, Issue 1. Oxford: Update Software; 2002.

64. Caughey AB, Sandberg PL, Zlatnik MG, Thiet MP, Parer JT, Laros RK. Forceps compared with vacuum. *Obstet Gynecol*. 2005;106:908-912.

65. Demissie K, Rhoads GG, Smulian JC, et al. Operative vaginal delivery and neonatal and infant adverse outcomes: population based retrospective analysis. *BMJ*. 2004;329:24.

66. Plauche WC. Subgaleal haematoma: a complication of instrumental delivery. *JAMA*. 1980;244:1597.

67. Eliachar E, Bret AJ, Bardiaux M, et al. Cranial subcutaneous hematoma in the newborn. *Arch Fr Pediatr*. 1963;20:1105.

68. Schaal JP, Equy V, Hoffman P. Comparison of vacuum extractor versus forceps. *J Gynecol Obstet Biol Reprod*. 2008;37:S231-S243.

69. Ngan HY, Miu P, Ko L, Ma HK. Long-term neurological sequelae following vacuum extractor delivery. *Aust N Z J Obstetr Gynaecol*. 1990;30:111.

70. Chadwick LM, Pemberton PJ, Kurinczuk JJ. Neonatal subgaleal haematoma: associated risk factors, complications and outcome. *J Paediatr Child Health*. 1996;32:228.

71. *ACOG Practice Bulletin, No 17, June 2000; or ACOG Compendium of Selected Publications*, 2005, p 640.

72. Benaron DA. Subgaleal hematoma causing hypovolemic shock during delivery after failed vacuum extraction: case report. *J Perinatol*. 1993;12:228.

73. Boo N. Subaponeurotic haemorrhage in Malaysian neonates. *Singapore Med J*. 1990;31:207.

74. Teng FY, Sayer JW. Vacuum extraction: does duration predict scalp injury? *Obstet Gynecol*. 1997;89:281.

75. Towner D, Castro MA, Eby-Wilkens E, Gilbert WM. Effect of mode of delivery in nulliparous women on neonatal intracranial injury. *N Engl J Med*. 1999;341:1709.

76. Whitby EH, Griffiths PD, Rutter S, et al. Frequency and natural history of subdural haemorrhages in babies and relation to obstetric factors. *Lancet*. 2004;363:846.

77. Seidman DS, Laor A, Gale R, et al. Long-term effects of vacuum and forceps deliveries. *Lancet*. 1991;337:15835.

78. Wesley BD, van den Berg BJ, Reece EA. The effect of forceps delivery on cognitive development. *Am J Obstet Gynecol*. 1993;169:1091.

79. Murphy DJ, Libby G, Chien P, et al. Cohort study of forceps delivery and the risk of epilepsy in adulthood. *Am J Obstet Gynecol*. 2004;191:392.

80. Bahl R, Patel RR, Swingler R, et al. Neurodevelopmental outcome at 5 years after operative vaginal delivery in the second stage of labor: a cohort study. *Am J Obstet Gynecol*. 2007;197:147.e1.

81. Werner EF, Janevic TM, Illuzzi J, Funai EF, Savitz DA, Lipkind HS. Mode of delivery in nulliparous women and neonatal intracranial injury. *Obstet Gynecol*. 2011;118:1239-1246.

82. Bashore RA, Phillips WH Jr, Brickman CR 3rd. A comparison of the morbidity of midforceps and cesarean delivery. *Am J Obstet Gynecol*. 1990; 162:1428.

83. Traub AI, Morrow RJ, Ritchie JW, et al. A continuing use for Kielland's forceps? *Br J Obstet Gynaecol*. 1984;91:894.

84. Murphy DJ, Liebling RE, Verity L, et al. Early maternal and neonatal morbidity associated with operative delivery in the second stage of labour: a cohort study. *Lancet*. 2001;358:1203.

85. Stock SJ, Josephs K, Farquharson S, et al. Maternal and neonatal outcomes of successful Kielland's rotational forceps delivery. *Obstet Gynecol*. 2013; 121:1032-1039.

86. Tan KH, Sim R, Yam KL. Kielland's forceps delivery: is it a dying art? *Singapore Med J*. 1992;33:380.

87. Hankins GD, Rowe TF. Operative vaginal delivery—year 2000. *Am J Obstet Gynecol*. 1996;175:275.

88. Healy DL, Quinn MA, Pepperell RJ. Rotational delivery of the fetus: Kielland's forceps and two other methods compared. *Br J Obstet Gynaecol*. 1982;89:501.

89. Krivac TC, Drewes P, Horowitz GM, et al. Kielland vs. nonrotational forceps for the second stage of labor. *J Reprod Med*. 1999;44:511.

90. Hankins GD, Leicht T, Van Hook J, Uckan EM. The role of forceps rotation in maternal and neonatal injury. *Am J Obstet Gynecol*. 1999;180:231.

91. Feldman DM, Borgida AF, Sauer F, Rodis JF. Rotational versus nonrotational forceps: maternal and neonatal outcomes. *Am J Obstet Gynecol*. 1999;181:1185.

92. Richardson DA, Evans MI, Cibils LA. Midforceps delivery: a critical review. *Am J Obstet Gynecol*. 1983;145:621.

93. Revah A, Ezra Y, Farine D, Ritchie K. Failed trail of vacuum or forceps-maternal and fetal outcome. *Am J Obstet Gynecol*. 1997;176:200.

94. Freeth HD. The cause and management of failed forceps cases. *BMJ*. 1950;2:18.

95. Douglass LH, Kaltreider DF. Trial forceps. *Am J Obstet Gynecol*. 1953; 65:889.

96. Alexander JM, Leveno KJ, Hauth JC, et al. Failed operative vaginal delivery. *Obstet Gynecol*. 2009;114:1017.

97. Johanson R, Menon V. Vacuum extraction vs. forceps delivery. Cochrane Pregnancy and Childbirth Group. *Cochran Database Syst Rev*. 2005;2.

98. Yeomans ER. Operative vaginal delivery. *Obstet Gynecol*. 2010;115: 645.

99. Bahl R, Murphy DJ, Strachan B. Qualitative analysis by interviews and video recordings to establish the components of a skilled low-cavity nonrotational vacuum delivery. *BJOG*. 2009;116:319.

100. Ramin SM, Little BB, Gilstrap LC 3rd. Survey of forceps delivery in North America in 1990. *Obstet Gynecol*. 1993;81:307.

101. Jain V, Guleria K, Gopalan S, Narang A. Mode of delivery in deep transverse arrest. *Int J Gynecol Obstet*. 1993;43:129.

102. Solt I, Jackson S, Moore T, Rotmensch S, Kim MJ. Teaching forceps: the impact of proactive faculty. *Am J Obstet Gynecol*. 2011;204:448.e1-448.e4.

103. Carollo TC, Reuter JM, Galan HL, Jones RO. Defining fetal station. *Am J Obstet Gynecol*. 2004;191:1793.

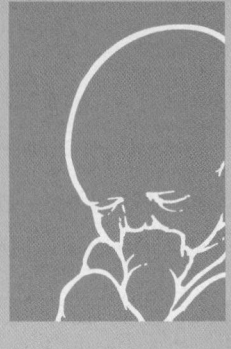

CHAPTER 15

Intrapartum Fetal Evaluation

DAVID ARTHUR MILLER

KEY TERMS

Acidemia	Increased hydrogen ion concentration in blood	**Hypoxia**	Decreased oxygen concentration in tissue
Acidosis	Increased hydrogen ion concentration in tissue	**pH**	Negative log of hydrogen ion concentration (e.g., $7.4 = 1 \times 10^{-7.4}$)
Asphyxia	Hypoxia with metabolic acidosis	PO_2	Partial pressure of oxygen
Base deficit	Buffer base content below normal	PaO_2	Partial pressure of oxygen dissolved in arterial blood
Hypoxemia	Decreased oxygen concentration in blood	PCO_2	Partial pressure of carbon dioxide

KEY ABBREVIATIONS

Acute respiratory distress syndrome	ARDS	Association of Women's Health, Obstetric and Neonatal Nurses	AWHONN
Adenosine triphosphate	ATP		
American College of Nurse Midwives	ACNM	Beats per minute	beats/min
American College of Obstetricians and Gynecologists	ACOG	Central nervous system	CNS
		Cerebral palsy	CP
American Academy of Pediatrics	AAP	Diphosphoglycerate	DPG

Electrocardiogram	ECG	Intermittent auscultation	IA
Electronic fetal heart rate monitoring	EFM	Intrauterine pressure catheter	IUPC
Fetal heart rate	FHR	Millimeters of mercury	mm Hg
Human immunodeficiency virus	HIV	National Institute of Child Health and	NICHD
Herpes simplex virus	HSV	Human Development	
Hypoxic-ischemic encephalopathy	HIE	Systemic lupus erythematosus	SLE

OVERVIEW

Normal human labor is characterized by rhythmic uterine contractions that intermittently interrupt the transplacental passage of oxygen from the mother to the fetus. These brief episodes of transient interruption of oxygenation are tolerated without consequence by almost all fetuses. In a very small subset, however, severe fetal oxygen deficiency can lead to hypoxic injury or even death. Many possible causes of fetal or neonatal injury are not directly related to fetal oxygenation, including conditions such as infection, congenital anomalies, and meconium aspiration. However, intrapartum interruption of fetal oxygenation is the condition for which conservative and/or operative interventions have the greatest potential to prevent injury or death. To that end, intrapartum fetal monitoring is intended to assess the adequacy of fetal oxygenation during labor. Evidence of interrupted fetal oxygenation demonstrated by the monitor can alert the clinician to the need for further evaluation and possible conservative interventions to ameliorate oxygen deficiency, such as administration of supplemental oxygen or maternal position changes. If conservative measures are not successful, the monitor can help determine the frequency, duration, and severity of interrupted oxygenation so that appropriately informed decisions can be made regarding the optimal timing and method of delivery to avoid the potential consequences of fetal hypoxia.

BRIEF HISTORY OF FETAL MONITORING

Auscultation of the fetal heart was described in the medical literature as early as the eighteenth century.[1,2] In 1822, Le Jumeau de Kergaradec proposed that auscultation of the fetal heart could be useful in confirming pregnancy, diagnosing multiple gestations, determining fetal position, and judging the state of fetal health or disease by changes in strength and frequency of the heart tones.[2] Later, others described fetal heart rate (FHR) changes associated with changes in fetal oxygenation, umbilical cord compression, fetal head compression, "fetal distress," and "asphyxic intoxication."[1,2] These observations were made using the stethoscope (*mediate auscultation*) or with the ear of the examiner placed directly upon the maternal abdomen (*immediate auscultation*). In 1917, Hillis described the modified stethoscope known today as the *DeLee-Hillis fetoscope*.

In 1906, Cremer recorded the first fetal electrocardiogram (ECG). By placing one electrode on the maternal abdomen and another in the vagina, he observed small fetal electrical impulses among the higher-voltage maternal signals. For decades, the clinical usefulness of the abdominal fetal ECG was limited by unreliable signal quality. Recent technological advances that have improved the accuracy and reliability of abdominal fetal ECG will be discussed later in this chapter.

The concept of direct application of the ECG electrode to the fetus in utero was introduced in the 1950s. During the 1960s, Hon[3] in the United States, Caldeyro-Barcia and colleagues[4] in Uruguay, and Hammacher[5] in Germany pioneered the development of electronic fetal monitoring (EFM). The first practical clinical FHR monitor became available in the United States in 1968, and throughout the 1970s, FHR monitoring became increasingly incorporated into obstetric practice. The introduction of Doppler ultrasound technology permitted FHR monitoring in patients with intact membranes. By 2002, EFM was used in approximately 85% of all births in the United States.[6] Today, most women who give birth in the United States have EFM during labor.

INSTRUMENTATION

The fetal monitor tracing is a continuous paper strip comprising two Cartesian graphs. The upper graph displays an instantaneous recording of the FHR; time is shown on the x-axis, and heart rate is shown on the y-axis. On the x-axis, fine vertical lines represent intervals of 10 seconds, and heavy vertical lines represent 1-minutes intervals. Fine horizontal lines on the y-axis represent intervals of 10 beats/min with a range of 30 to 240 beats/min. Uterine activity is displayed on the lower graph, time is on the x-axis, and pressure is on the y-axis. Fine vertical lines represent intervals of 10 seconds, and heavy vertical lines represent 1-minutes intervals. On the y-axis, fine horizontal lines represent intervals of 5 mm Hg with a range of 0 to 100 mm Hg. Heart rate and uterine activity are plotted separately on the heat-sensitive paper by thermal pens. Standard paper speed is 3 cm/min in the United States and 1 cm/min in most other countries.

Direct Fetal Heart Rate and Uterine Activity Monitoring

Direct FHR monitoring involves transcervical application of an ECG electrode to the fetus, dilation of the cervix, rupture of the membranes, and access to the fetal presenting part. These requirements limit the use of direct monitoring to the intrapartum period. The bipolar fetal ECG electrode is attached directly to the fetal presenting part by gently screwing a small spiral metal wire into the skin. When one pole of the electrode is applied to the fetal presenting part and the other pole is bathed in vaginal fluid to complete the electrical circuit, the ECG electrode detects electrical impulses that originate in the fetal heart; amplified signals are processed by a cardiotachometer (Fig. 15-1). Computer logic compares each incoming fetal QRS complex with the one immediately preceding it. The time interval between the two complexes is measured electronically and is

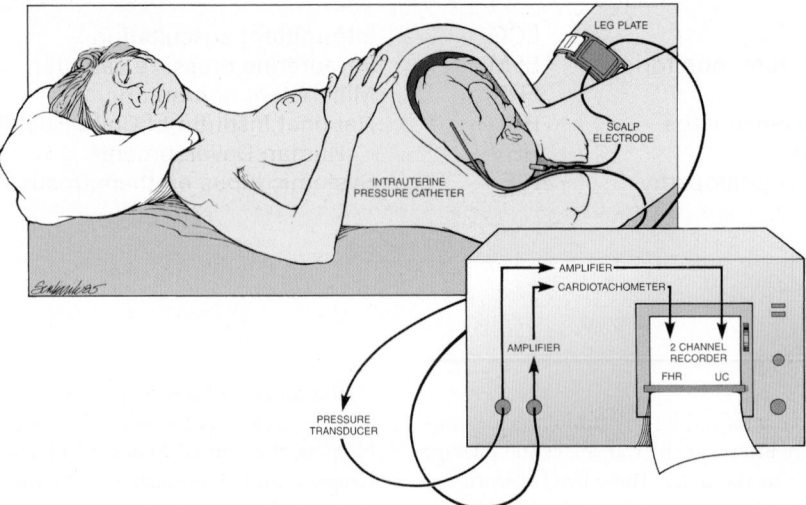

FIG 15-1 Techniques used for direct monitoring of fetal heart rate (FHR) and uterine contractions (UC). The fetal electrocardiogram is obtained by direct application of the scalp electrode, which is then attached to a leg plate on the mother's thigh. The signal is transmitted to the monitor, where it is amplified, counted by the cardiotachometer, and then recorded. Uterine contractions are assessed with an intrauterine pressure catheter connected to a pressure transducer. This signal is then amplified and recorded.

used to calculate a heart rate, which is plotted as a point on the FHR graph located on the upper channel of the paper chart. This process is repeated with each cardiac cycle to produce a series of closely spaced individual points that appear on the paper chart as an irregular line that represents a graphic instantaneous display of the FHR.

Direct assessment of uterine activity uses a thin, flexible intrauterine pressure catheter (IUPC) placed transcervically into the amniotic cavity. Intrauterine pressure is transmitted from the amniotic fluid through the fluid-filled catheter to an external pressure transducer. The transducer converts pressure measurements into electrical signals to permit the continuous display of pressure readings on the uterine activity graph located on the lower channel of the paper chart. Newer catheters use closed systems with a strain gauge or sensors in the catheter tip that relay signals to a strain gauge located at the base of the catheter. A second port can be used to infuse saline into the amniotic cavity (*amnioinfusion*) to relieve variable FHR decelerations caused by umbilical cord compression. **An appropriately calibrated IUPC permits accurate assessment of the frequency, duration, and intensity of uterine contractions as well as the baseline uterine tone between contractions**.

Indirect Fetal Heart Rate and Uterine Activity Monitoring

Indirect (external) monitoring does not require the transcervical placement of electrodes or catheters. Consequently, external FHR monitoring uses an ultrasound transducer applied with straps to the maternal abdomen and can be performed prior to labor. Ultrasound waves produced by the transducer are transmitted to the maternal skin through coupling gel; these waves penetrate maternal and fetal tissues and are reflected by moving tissue interfaces. Waves reflected from moving structures of the fetal heart return to the transducer for processing. Fetal heart structures moving *toward* the transducer reflect ultrasound waves at a *higher* frequency than the outgoing signal, whereas structures moving *away* from the transducer reflect ultrasound waves at a *lower* frequency. These changes in frequency, known as *Doppler shift* or *Doppler effect,* produce phasic signals that are

converted into a graphic display of the FHR in a process similar to that used in direct monitoring (Fig. 15-2). The raw signals produced by an external ultrasound transducer are more prone to artifact than those produced by a direct fetal ECG electrode. However, with improved computer processing and application of the autocorrelation technique, FHR tracings produced by modern external monitors are comparable to those produced by a direct fetal ECG electrode.

Indirect assessment of uterine activity is performed with a pressure transducer (tocodynamometer) applied tightly to the maternal abdomen over the uterine fundus. Uterine contractions change the shape and rigidity of the uterus and anterior abdominal wall, which generates pressure changes that are transmitted to the sensor located in the tocodynamometer transducer. Changes in pressure are converted into electrical signals and are plotted on the lower channel of the paper chart as a continuous display of uterine activity. **When properly positioned on the maternal abdomen, the external tocodynamometer permits assessment of the relative frequency and duration of uterine contractions. However, it does not directly measure intrauterine pressure and therefore does not provide a reliable assessment of uterine contraction intensity or resting tone between contractions**. When external uterine activity monitoring is used, contraction intensity and baseline uterine tone usually are assessed by palpation. Contraction strength is graded as *mild, moderate,* or *strong* depending upon the degree to which the uterine fundus can be indented by palpation with the fingertips during the peak of a uterine contraction. During mild contractions, the fundus is easily indented by the fingertips; during strong contractions, the fundus cannot be indented. If the fundus can be indented by intermediate pressure, the contraction strength is moderate.

PHYSIOLOGIC BASIS FOR ELECTRONIC FETAL HEART RATE MONITORING

The objective of intrapartum FHR monitoring is to prevent fetal injury that might result from interruption of normal fetal oxygenation during labor. The underlying assumption is that

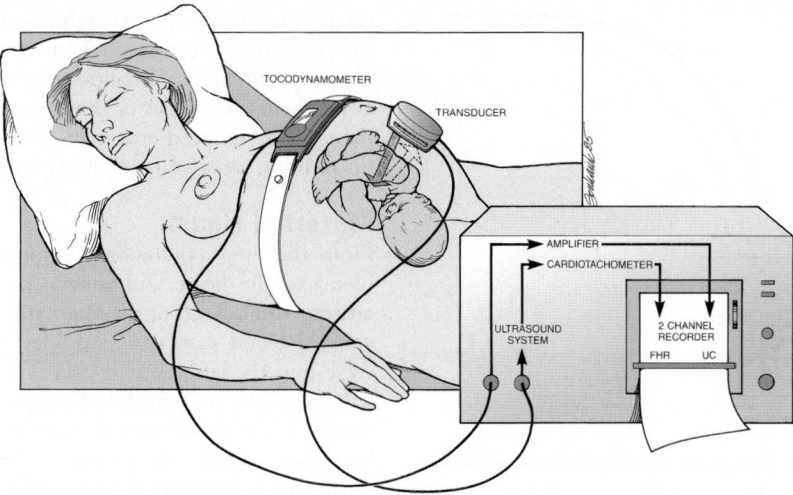

FIG 15-2 Instrumentation for external monitoring. Fetal heart rate (FHR) is monitored using the Doppler ultrasound transducer, which both emits and receives the reflected ultrasound signal that is then counted and recorded. Uterine contractions (UC) are detected by the pressure-sensitive tocodynamometer and are then amplified and recorded.

interruption of fetal oxygenation leads to characteristic physiologic changes that can be detected by changes in the FHR. The role of intrapartum FHR monitoring in assessing the fetal physiologic changes caused by interrupted oxygenation can be summarized in two key points. Fetal oxygenation involves (1) the transfer of oxygen from the environment to the fetus, and (2) the fetal response to interruption of oxygen transfer. Specific FHR patterns provide reliable information regarding these two aspects of fetal oxygenation.

TRANSFER OF OXYGEN FROM THE ENVIRONMENT TO THE FETUS

Oxygen is transferred from the environment to the fetus by maternal and fetal blood along a pathway that includes the maternal lungs, heart, vasculature, uterus, placenta, and umbilical cord. The "oxygen pathway" is illustrated in Figure 15-3. Interruption of oxygen transfer can occur at any or all of the points along this pathway.

External Environment

Oxygen comprises approximately 21% of inspired air. Therefore in inspired air, the partial pressure exerted by oxygen gas (PO_2) is approximately 21% of total atmospheric pressure (760 mm Hg) minus the pressure exerted by water vapor (47 mm Hg). At sea level, this translates to approximately 150 mm Hg. As oxygen is transferred from the external atmosphere to maternal blood and then to fetal blood, the partial pressure progressively declines. **By the time oxygen reaches fetal umbilical venous blood, the partial pressure may be as low as 30 mm Hg. After oxygen is delivered to fetal tissues, the PO_2 of deoxygenated blood in the umbilical arteries returning to the placenta is approximately 15 to 25 mm Hg.**[7-9] The sequential transfer of oxygen from the environment to the fetus and potential causes of interruption at each step are described below.

Maternal Lungs

Inspiration carries oxygenated air from the external environment to the distal air spaces of the lungs, the alveoli. On the way to the alveoli, inspired air mixes with less oxygenated air leaving

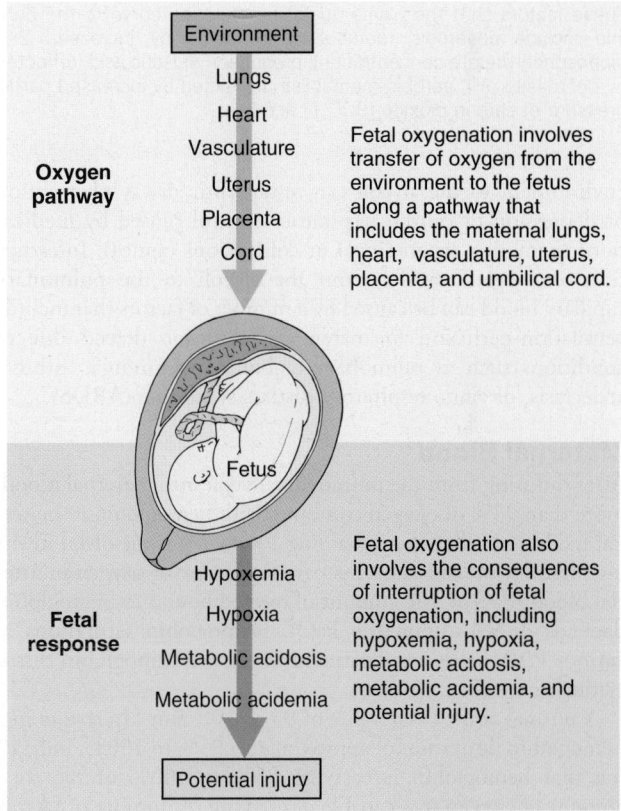

FIG 15-3 The oxygen pathway.

the lungs. As a result, the PO_2 of air within the alveoli is lower than that in inspired air. At sea level, alveolar PO_2 is approximately 100 to 105 mm Hg. From the alveoli, oxygen diffuses across a thin blood-gas barrier into the pulmonary capillary blood. This pulmonary blood-gas barrier consists of three layers: a single-cell layer of alveolar epithelium and basement membrane, a layer of extracellular matrix (interstitium), and a single-cell layer of pulmonary capillary endothelium and basement membrane. Interruption of oxygen transfer from the

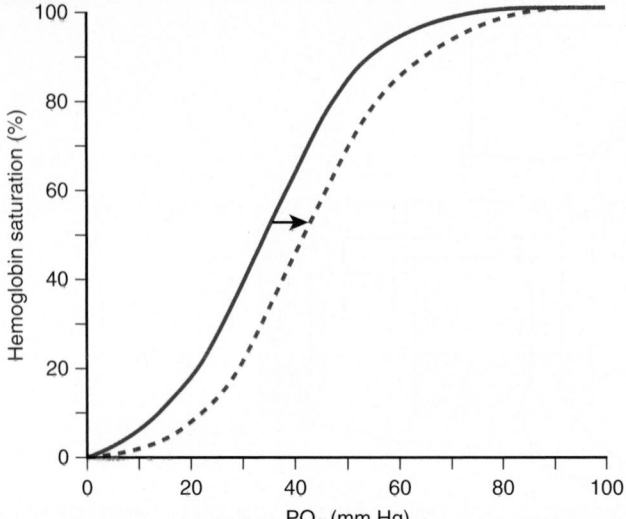

FIG 15-4 Maternal oxygen dissociation curve. The tendency for hemoglobin to release oxygen is increased by factors that signal an increased requirement for oxygen. Specifically, oxygen release is enhanced by factors that indicate active cellular metabolism. These factors shift the oxyhemoglobin saturation curve to the right and include anaerobic metabolism (reflected by increased 2,3-diphosphoglycerate concentration), production of lactic acid (reflected by decreased pH), aerobic metabolism (reflected by increased partial pressure of carbon dioxide [PCO_2]), and heat.

environment to the alveoli can result from airway obstruction or depression of central respiratory control caused by medications (narcotics, magnesium) or convulsions (apnea). Interruption of oxygen transfer from the alveoli to the pulmonary capillary blood can be caused by a number of factors that include ventilation-perfusion mismatch and diffusion defects due to conditions such as pulmonary embolus, pneumonia, asthma, atelectasis, or acute respiratory distress syndrome (ARDS).

Maternal Blood

After diffusing from the pulmonary alveoli into maternal blood, more than 98% of oxygen combines with hemoglobin in maternal red blood cells. The remaining 1% to 2% is dissolved in the blood and is measured by the partial pressure of oxygen in arterial blood (PaO_2). The amount of oxygen bound to hemoglobin depends directly upon the PaO_2. Hemoglobin saturations at various PaO_2 levels are illustrated by the oxyhemoglobin dissociation curve (Fig. 15-4).

A normal adult PaO_2 value of 95 to 100 mm Hg results in a hemoglobin saturation of approximately 95% to 100%, indicating that hemoglobin is carrying 95% to 100% of the total amount of oxygen it is capable of carrying. A number of factors affect the affinity of hemoglobin for oxygen and can shift the oxyhemoglobin dissociation curve to the left or right. **In general, the tendency for hemoglobin to release oxygen is increased by factors that signal an increased requirement for oxygen.** Specifically, oxygen release is enhanced by factors that indicate active cellular metabolism. These factors shift the oxyhemoglobin saturation curve to the right and include by-products of anaerobic metabolism (reflected by increased 2,3-diphosphoglycerate [DPG] concentration), production of lactic acid (reflected by decreased pH), by-products of aerobic metabolism (reflected by increased partial pressure of carbon dioxide [PCO_2]), and heat. Interruption of oxygen transfer from

the environment to the fetus due to abnormal maternal oxygen-carrying capacity can result from severe anemia or from hereditary or acquired abnormalities that affect oxygen binding, such as hemoglobinopathies or methemoglobinemia. In an obstetric population, reduced maternal oxygen-carrying capacity is an uncommon cause of interrupted fetal oxygenation.

Maternal Heart

From the lungs, pulmonary veins carry oxygenated maternal blood to the heart. Pulmonary venous blood enters the left atrium with a PaO_2 of approximately 95 to 100 mm Hg. Oxygenated blood passes from the left atrium through the mitral valve into the left ventricle and out the aorta for systemic distribution. Normal transfer of oxygen from the environment to the fetus is dependent upon normal cardiac function, reflected by cardiac output—the product of heart rate and stroke volume. Heart rate is determined by intrinsic cardiac pacemakers (sino-atrial node, atrioventricular node), the cardiac conduction system, autonomic regulation (sympathetic, parasympathetic), intrinsic humoral factors (catecholamines), extrinsic factors (medications), and local factors (calcium, potassium). Stroke volume is determined by preload, contractility, and afterload. *Preload* is the amount of stretch on myocardial fibers at the end of diastole when the ventricles are full of blood, and it is dependent on the volume of venous blood returning to the heart. *Contractility* is the force and speed with which myocardial fibers shorten during systole to expel blood from the heart. *Afterload* is the pressure that opposes the shortening of myocardial fibers during systole and is estimated by the systemic vascular resistance or systemic blood pressure.

Interruption of oxygen transfer from the environment to the fetus at the level of the maternal heart can be caused by any condition that reduces cardiac output, including altered heart rate (arrhythmia), reduced preload (hypovolemia, compression of the inferior vena cava), impaired contractility (ischemic heart disease, diabetes, cardiomyopathy, congestive heart failure), or increased afterload (hypertension). In addition, structural abnormalities of the heart and great vessels (valvular stenosis, valvular insufficiency, pulmonary hypertension, coarctation of the aorta) may impede its ability to pump blood. **In a healthy obstetric patient, the most common cause of reduced cardiac output is reduced preload resulting from hypovolemia or compression of the inferior vena cava by the gravid uterus.**

Maternal Vasculature

Oxygenated blood leaving the heart is carried by the systemic vasculature to the uterus. The vascular path includes the aorta, common iliac artery, internal iliac (hypogastric) artery, anterior division of the internal iliac artery, and the uterine artery. From the uterine artery, oxygenated blood travels through the arcuate, radial, and finally the spiral arteries before exiting the maternal vasculature and entering the intervillous space of the placenta. **Interruption of oxygen transfer from the environment to the fetus at the level of the maternal vasculature commonly results from hypotension caused by regional anesthesia, hypovolemia, impaired venous return, impaired cardiac output, or medication.** Alternatively, it may result from vasoconstriction of distal arterioles in response to endogenous vasoconstrictors or medications. Conditions associated with chronic vasculopathy—such as chronic hypertension, long-standing diabetes, collagen vascular disease, thyroid disease, or renal disease—may result in chronic suboptimal transfer of

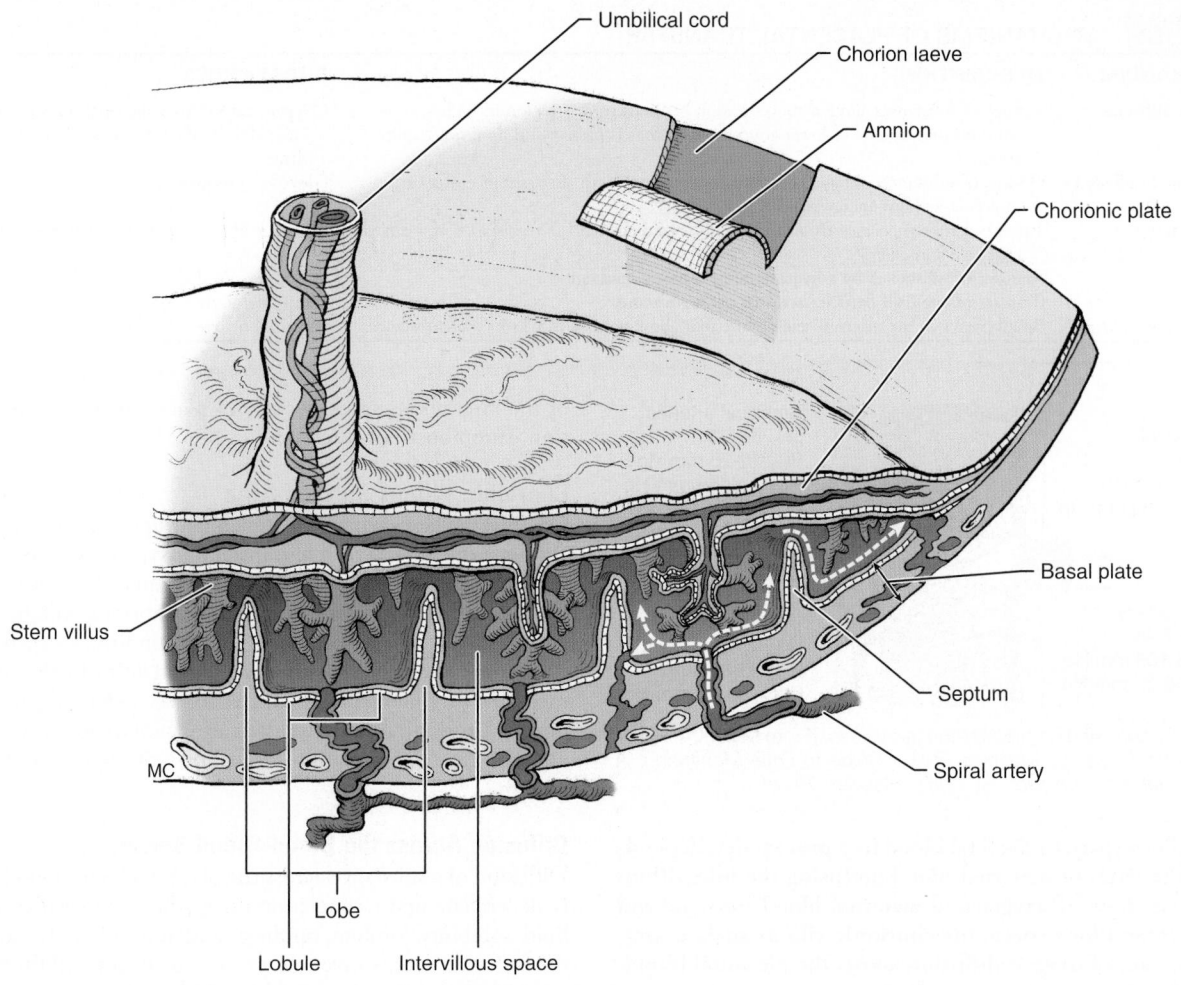

FIG 15-5 Placental blood flow.

oxygen and nutrients to the fetus at the level of the maternal vasculature. Preeclampsia is associated with abnormal vascular remodeling at the level of the spiral arteries and can impede perfusion of the intervillous space. Acute vascular injuries (trauma, aortic dissection) are rare. In a healthy obstetric patient, transient hypotension is the most common cause of interrupted oxygen transfer at the level of the maternal vasculature. Chronic vascular conditions can exacerbate this interruption and should be considered in the course of thorough evaluation.

Uterus

Between the maternal uterine arteries and the intervillous space of the placenta, the arcuate, radial, and spiral arteries and their corresponding veins traverse the muscular wall of the uterus. **Interruption of oxygen transfer from the environment to the fetus at the level of the uterus commonly results from uterine contractions that compress intramural blood vessels and impede the flow of blood.** Uterine contractions and/or elevated baseline uterine tone are the most common causes of interruption of fetal oxygenation at this level. Uterine rupture is less common but must be considered in the appropriate clinical context.

Placenta

The placenta facilitates the exchange of gases, nutrients, wastes, and other molecules—for example antibodies, hormones, and medications—between maternal blood in the intervillous space and fetal blood in the villous capillaries. On the maternal side of the placenta, oxygenated blood exits the spiral arteries and enters the intervillous space to surround and bathe the chorionic villi. On the fetal side of the placenta, paired umbilical arteries carry blood from the fetus through the umbilical cord to the placenta. **At term, the umbilical arteries receive 40% of fetal cardiac output**. Upon reaching the placental cord insertion site, the umbilical arteries divide into multiple branches that fan out across the surface of the placenta. As illustrated in Figure 15-5, at each cotyledon, placental arteries dive beneath the surface en route to the chorionic villi.

The chorionic villi are microscopic branches of trophoblast that protrude into the intervillous space. Each villus is perfused by a fetal capillary bed that represents the terminal distribution of an umbilical artery. At term, fetal villous capillary blood is separated from maternal blood in the intervillous space by a thin blood-blood barrier similar to the blood-gas barrier in the maternal lung. The placental blood-blood barrier is comprised of a layer of placental trophoblast and a layer of fetal capillary endothelium with intervening basement membranes separated by a layer of villous stroma. Substances are exchanged between maternal and fetal blood by a number of mechanisms, including simple diffusion, facilitated diffusion, active transport, bulk flow, pinocytosis, and leakage. Examples of these mechanisms are summarized in Table 15-1. **Oxygen is transferred from the**

TABLE 15-1   MECHANISMS OF PLACENTAL TRANSFER

MECHANISM	DESCRIPTION	SUBSTANCES
Simple diffusion	Passage of substances along a concentration gradient from a region of higher concentration to one of lower concentration that is passive and does not require energy	Oxygen, carbon dioxide, small ions (sodium chloride), lipids, fat-soluble vitamins, many drugs
Facilitated diffusion	Passage of substances along a concentration gradient with the assistance of a carrier molecule without energy requirement	Glucose, carbohydrates
Active transport	Passage of substances against a concentration gradient with the assistance of a carrier molecule and energy	Amino acids, water-soluble vitamins, large ions
Bulk flow	Transfer of substances by a hydrostatic or osmotic gradient	Water, dissolved electrolytes
Pinocytosis	Transfer of engulfed particles across a cell membrane	Immunoglobulins, proteins
Breaks and leakage	Small breaks in the placental membrane that allow passage of plasma and substances	Maternal or fetal blood cells

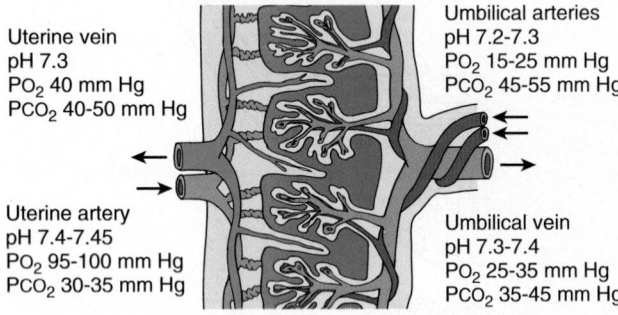

Uterine vein
pH 7.3
PO_2 40 mm Hg
PCO_2 40-50 mm Hg

Uterine artery
pH 7.4-7.45
PO_2 95-100 mm Hg
PCO_2 30-35 mm Hg

Umbilical arteries
pH 7.2-7.3
PO_2 15-25 mm Hg
PCO_2 45-55 mm Hg

Umbilical vein
pH 7.3-7.4
PO_2 25-35 mm Hg
PCO_2 35-45 mm Hg

FIG 15-6 Uterine and umbilical blood gas values. (From Miller LA, Miller DA, Martin Tucker S. *Mosby's Pocket Guide to Fetal Monitoring: A Multidisciplinary Approach*. St. Louis: Elsevier; 2012.)

intervillous space to the fetal blood by a process that depends upon the PaO_2 of maternal blood perfusing the intervillous space, the flow of oxygenated maternal blood into and out of the intervillous space, the chorionic villous surface area, and the rate of oxygen diffusion across the placental blood-blood barrier.

Intervillous Space PaO_2

Oxygenated maternal blood leaves the maternal heart with a partial pressure of oxygen dissolved in arterial blood (PaO_2) of approximately 95 to 100 mm Hg. Exiting the spiral arteries to perfuse the intervillous space of the placenta, oxygenated maternal blood has a PaO_2 of approximately 95 to 100 mm Hg. Oxygen is released from maternal hemoglobin and diffuses across the placental blood-blood barrier into fetal blood, where it combines with fetal hemoglobin. As a result, maternal blood in the intervillous space becomes relatively oxygen depleted and exits the intervillous space via uterine veins with a PaO_2 of approximately 40 mm Hg (Fig. 15-6).

The average PaO_2 of maternal blood in the intervillous space is between the PaO_2 of blood entering the intervillous space (95 to 100 mm Hg) and the PaO_2 of blood exiting the intervillous space (40 mm Hg). **The average intervillous space PaO_2 is in the range of 45 mm Hg.** Interruption of fetal oxygenation can result from conditions that reduce the PaO_2 of maternal blood entering the intervillous space. These conditions have been discussed previously.

Intervillous Space Blood Flow

At term, uterine perfusion accounts for 10% to 15% of maternal cardiac output, or approximately 700 to 800 mL/min. Much of this blood is located in the intervillous space of the placenta surrounding the chorionic villi. Conditions that can reduce the volume of the intervillous space include collapse or destruction of the intervillous space because of placental abruption, infarction, thrombosis, or infection.

Chorionic Villous Surface Area

Optimal oxygen exchange is dependent upon normal chorionic villous surface area. Normal transfer of oxygen from the environment to the fetus at the level of the placenta can be interrupted by conditions that limit or reduce the chorionic villous surface area available for gas exchange. These conditions can be acute or chronic and include primary abnormalities in the development of the villous vascular tree or secondary distortion of normal chorionic villous architecture by infarction, thrombosis, hemorrhage, inflammation, infection, or abnormal vascular growth.

Diffusion Across the Blood-Blood Barrier

Diffusion of a substance across the placental blood-blood barrier is dependent upon concentration gradient, molecular weight, lipid solubility, protein binding, and ionization. In addition, the diffusion rate is inversely proportional to the diffusion distance. **At term, the placental blood-blood barrier is very thin, and the diffusion distance is short.** Under normal circumstances, oxygen and carbon dioxide diffuse readily across this thin barrier; however, normal diffusion can be impeded by conditions that increase the distance between maternal and fetal blood. These conditions can be acute, subacute, or chronic and include villous hemorrhage, inflammation, thrombosis, infarction, edema, fibrosis, and excessive cellular proliferation characterized by the presence of syncytial knots.[10]

Interruption of Placental Blood Vessels

For the sake of completeness, fetal blood loss caused by injury to blood vessels at the level of the placenta warrants discussion. Damaged chorionic vessels can allow fetal blood to leak into the intervillous space, leading to fetal-maternal hemorrhage. This may be a consequence of abdominal trauma but can also occur in association with placental abruption or invasive procedures, and a specific cause is not always identified. Ruptured vasa previa is a rare cause of fetal hemorrhage. Vasa previa is a placental vessel traversing the chorioamniotic membrane in close proximity to the cervical os. Such a vessel may be damaged by normal cervical change during labor, or it can be injured inadvertently during membrane rupture or digital exam.

Summary of Placental Causes of Interrupted Oxygenation

Many conditions can interfere with the transfer of oxygen across the placenta. Those that involve the microvasculature frequently are diagnosed by histopathologic examination after delivery. Clinically detectable causes, such as placental abruption or bleeding placenta previa or vasa previa, should be considered but may not be amenable to conservative corrective measures.

Fetal Blood

After oxygen has diffused from the intervillous space across the placental blood-blood barrier and into fetal blood, the venous PO_2 is in the range of 30 mm Hg, and fetal hemoglobin saturation is between 50% and 70%. **Although fetal PO_2 and hemoglobin saturation values are low in comparison to adult values, adequate delivery of oxygen to the fetal tissues is maintained by a number of compensatory mechanisms.** For example, fetal cardiac output per unit weight is greater than that of the adult. Hemoglobin concentration and affinity for oxygen are greater in the fetus as well, resulting in increased oxygen-carrying capacity. Finally, oxygenated blood is directed preferentially toward vital organs by way of laminar blood flow and anatomic shunts at the level of the ductus venosus and foramen ovale. Conditions that can interrupt the transfer of oxygen from the environment to the fetus at the level of the fetal blood are uncommon but may include fetal anemia and reduced oxygen-carrying capacity secondary to alloimmunization, hemoglobinopathy, glucose-6-phosphate dehydrogenase (G6PD) deficiency, viral infections, fetomaternal hemorrhage, methemoglobinemia, or bleeding vasa previa.

Umbilical Cord

After oxygen binds to fetal hemoglobin in the villous capillaries, oxygenated blood returns to the fetus by way of villous veins that coalesce to form placental veins on the surface of the placenta. Placental surface veins unite to form a single umbilical vein within the umbilical cord. **Interruption of the transfer of oxygen from the environment to the fetus at the level of the umbilical cord can result from simple mechanical compression.** Other uncommon causes may include vasospasm, thrombosis, atherosis, hypertrophy, hemorrhage, inflammation, or a true "knot." From the environment to the fetus, maternal and fetal blood carries oxygen along the oxygen pathway illustrated in Figure 15-3. Examples of causes of interrupted oxygen transfer at each step along the pathway are summarized in Table 15-2.

Gas exchange also involves the transfer of carbon dioxide in the opposite direction, from the fetus to the environment. Any condition that interrupts the transfer of oxygen from the environment to the fetus has the potential to interrupt the transfer of carbon dioxide from the fetus to the environment. However, carbon dioxide diffuses across the placental blood-blood barrier more rapidly than does oxygen; therefore any interruption of the pathway is likely to impact oxygen transfer to a greater extent than it does carbon dioxide transfer.

FETAL RESPONSE TO INTERRUPTED OXYGEN TRANSFER

Depending upon frequency, degree, and duration, interruption of oxygen transfer at any point along the oxygen pathway may result in progressive deterioration of fetal oxygenation. The cascade begins with hypoxemia, defined as decreased oxygen content in the blood. At term, hypoxemia is characterized by an umbilical artery PaO_2 below the normal fetal range of approximately 15 to 25 mm Hg. Recurrent or sustained hypoxemia can lead to decreased delivery of oxygen to the tissues and reduced tissue oxygen content, termed *hypoxia*.

TABLE 15-2	EXAMPLES OF CAUSES OF INTERRUPTED OXYGEN TRANSFER AT EACH STEP IN THE OXYGEN PATHWAY
OXYGEN PATHWAY	**CAUSES OF INTERRUPTED OXYGEN TRANSFER**
Lungs	Respiratory depression (narcotics, magnesium)
	Seizure (eclampsia)
	Pulmonary embolus
	Pulmonary edema
	Pneumonia/acute respiratory distress syndrome
	Asthma
	Atelectasis
	Pulmonary hypertension (rarely)
	Chronic lung disease (rarely)
Heart	Reduced cardiac output
	Hypovolemia
	Compression of the inferior vena cava
	Regional anesthesia (sympathetic blockade)
	Cardiac arrhythmia
	Congestive heart failure (rarely)
	Structural cardiac disease (rarely)
Vasculature	Hypotension
	Hypovolemia
	Compression of the inferior vena cava
	Regional anesthesia (sympathetic blockade)
	Medications (hydralazine, labetalol, nifedipine)
	Vasculopathy (chronic hypertension, SLE, preeclampsia)
	Vasoconstriction (cocaine, methylergonovine)
Uterus	Excessive uterine activity
	Uterine stimulants (prostaglandins, oxytocin)
	Uterine rupture
Placenta	Placental abruption
	Vasa previa (rarely)
	Fetal-maternal hemorrhage (rarely)
	Placental infarction, infection (usually confirmed retrospectively)
Umbilical cord	Cord compression
	Cord prolapse
	True "knot"

SLE, systemic lupus erythematosus.

Normal homeostasis requires an adequate supply of oxygen and fuel in order to generate the energy required by basic cellular activities. When oxygen is readily available, aerobic metabolism efficiently generates energy in the form of adenosine triphosphate (ATP). By-products of aerobic metabolism include carbon dioxide and water. **When oxygen is in short supply, tissues may be forced to switch from aerobic to anaerobic metabolism, which generates energy less efficiently and results in the production of lactic acid. Accumulation of lactic acid in the tissues results in metabolic acidosis.** Lactic acid accumulation can lead to utilization of buffer bases, primarily bicarbonate, to help stabilize tissue pH. If the buffering capacity is exceeded, tissue pH and eventually blood pH may begin to fall, leading to metabolic acidemia.

Acidemia is defined as increased hydrogen ion content (decreased pH) in the blood. Recurrent or sustained hypoxia and acidosis in the peripheral tissues can lead to loss of peripheral vascular smooth muscle contraction, reduced peripheral vascular resistance, hypotension, and potential hypoxic-ischemic injury to critical tissues and organs, including the brain and heart. With respect to fetal physiology, **it is critical to distinguish between *respiratory acidemia*, caused by accumulation of CO_2, and *metabolic acidemia*, caused by accumulation of lactic acid in excess of buffering capacity. Respiratory acidemia is relatively common and clinically benign.**[9] Conversely, metabolic acidemia is uncommon and may be a marker of clinically significant interruption of fetal oxygenation.[11]

Mechanisms of Injury

If interruption of fetal oxygenation progresses to the stage of metabolic acidemia and hypotension, as described above, multiple organs and systems—including the brain and heart—can suffer hypoperfusion, reduced oxygenation, lowered pH, and reduced delivery of fuel for metabolism. These changes can contribute to a cascade of cellular events that include altered enzyme function, protease activation, ion shifts, altered water regulation, abnormal neurotransmitter metabolism, free radical production, and phospholipid degradation. Disruption of normal cellular metabolism can to lead to cellular and tissue dysfunction, injury, and even death.

Injury Threshold

The relationship between fetal oxygen deprivation and neurologic injury is complex. Electronic FHR monitoring was introduced with the hope that it would reduce the incidence of neurologic injury in the form of cerebral palsy (CP) caused by intrapartum interruption of fetal oxygenation. Subsequently, **it has become apparent that most cases of CP are unrelated to intrapartum events and therefore cannot be prevented by modification of intrapartum management, including FHR monitoring.** Nevertheless, some cases of CP may be linked to events during labor and delivery; therefore it is important to understand, to the extent possible, the relationship between intrapartum fetal oxygenation and the subsequent development of CP. In 1999, the International Cerebral Palsy Task Force published a consensus statement[12] identifying essential criteria to establish intrapartum interruption of fetal oxygenation as a possible cause of CP. In January of 2003, The American College of Obstetricians and Gynecologists (ACOG) and the American Academy of Pediatrics (AAP) Cerebral Palsy Task Force published a monograph[11] entitled "Neonatal Encephalopathy and Cerebral Palsy: Defining the Pathogenesis and Pathophysiology," which summarized the literature regarding the relationship between intrapartum events and neurologic injury. Agencies and professional organizations that endorsed the ACOG-AAP task force report include the Centers for Disease Control and Prevention (CDC), the Child Neurology Society, the March of Dimes Birth Defects Foundation, the National Institute of Child Health and Human Development (NICHD), the Royal Australian and New Zealand College of Obstetricians and Gynecologists, the Society for Maternal-Fetal Medicine (SMFM), and the Society of Obstetricians and Gynaecologists of Canada.

The consensus report established four essential criteria to define an acute intrapartum hypoxic event sufficient to cause CP (Box 15-1). The first criterion identified significant umbilical artery metabolic acidemia at birth (pH <7.0 and base deficit ≥12 mmol/L) as an essential prerequisite to establish a possible link between intrapartum interruption of fetal oxygenation and the later diagnosis of CP. **It is important to recognize that even when significant metabolic acidemia is present, neonatal encephalopathy and fetal neurologic injury are uncommon.** Respiratory acidemia without a metabolic component is not a significant risk factor for fetal neurologic injury.[9]

The second criterion emphasized that in the absence of moderate to severe neonatal encephalopathy, intrapartum interruption of fetal oxygenation is very unlikely to result in CP. Neonatal encephalopathy has many possible causes. Hypoxic-ischemic

---

BOX 15-1   ESSENTIAL CRITERIA TO DEFINE AN ACUTE INTRAPARTUM EVENT SUFFICIENT TO CAUSE CEREBRAL PALSY

1. Umbilical cord arterial blood pH <7 and base deficit ≥12 mmol/L
2. Early onset of severe or moderate neonatal encephalopathy in infants born at 34 or more weeks of gestation
3. Cerebral palsy of the spastic quadriplegic or dyskinetic type
4. Exclusion of other identifiable etiologies such as trauma,* coagulation disorders, infectious conditions, or genetic disorders

*Does not refer to fetal injury potentially related to the mechanical forces of labor or maternal expulsive efforts.

BOX 15-2   CRITERIA THAT COLLECTIVELY SUGGEST THE EVENT OCCURRED WITHIN 48 HOURS OF BIRTH

1. A sentinel hypoxic event immediately before or during labor
2. A sudden and sustained fetal bradycardia, or the absence of fetal heart rate variability in the presence of persistent late or variable decelerations, usually after a hypoxic sentinel event when the pattern was previously normal
3. Apgar scores of 0 to 3 beyond 5 min
4. Onset of multisystem involvement within 72 hr of birth
5. Early imaging study showing evidence of acute nonfocal cerebral abnormality

---

encephalopathy (HIE) resulting from intrapartum interruption of fetal oxygenation represents only a small subset of neonatal encephalopathy, and most cases of HIE do not result in permanent neurologic injury.

The third criterion acknowledged that different subtypes of CP have different potential origins. The spastic quadriplegic subtype of CP caused by injury to the parasagittal cortex is characterized by abnormal motor control of all four extremities. The dyskinetic subtype of CP associated with injury to the basal ganglia involves disorganized, choreoathetoid movements. Although the presence of these CP subtypes does not constitute conclusive evidence of intrapartum hypoxic injury, they are the only subtypes that have been linked to hypoxic-ischemic neurologic injury at term. Other CP subtypes such as spastic diplegia, hemiplegia, ataxia, and hemiparetic CP are unlikely to result from acute intrapartum hypoxia. **Conditions such as epilepsy, mental retardation, and attention-deficit/hyperactivity disorder do not result from intrapartum fetal hypoxia in the absence of CP.**[11]

The fourth criterion highlighted the fact that hypoxic-ischemic injury due to intrapartum interruption of fetal oxygenation is a potential cause of a relatively small subset of all cases of CP. Other identifiable etiologies include trauma, coagulation disorders, vascular accidents, infectious conditions, and genetic disorders. The 2003 ACOG-AAP Cerebral Palsy Task Force report[11] further identified five criteria to help establish the timing of injury, emphasizing that these criteria are not specific to hypoxic-ischemic injury. These criteria are summarized in Box 15-2.

In 2014, the ACOG-AAP Neonatal Encephalopathy Task Force revisited the scientific evidence linking intrapartum events, neonatal encephalopathy and subsequent neurologic outcome. The resulting monograph, *Neonatal Encephalopathy and Neurologic Outcome* (Second Edition), reaffirmed the concept that the pathway from intrapartum hypoxic-ischemic injury to subsequent CP must progress through neonatal encephalopathy.[13] The report also reaffirmed the conclusion that spastic quadriplegia and dyskinetic CP are the subtypes most likely to be associated with hypoxic intrapartum injury at term. These conditions were *not* identified as absolute requirements for the diagnosis of intrapartum hypoxic neurologic injury. **The 2014 report further concluded that "unless the newborn has accumulated significant metabolic acidemia, the likelihood of subsequent neurologic and cardiovascular morbidities attributable to perinatal events is low," and "in a fetus exhibiting either moderate variability or accelerations of the FHR, damaging degrees of hypoxia-induced metabolic acidemia can reliably be excluded."** Unlike its predecessor, the 2014 task force report did not identify metabolic acidemia as an absolute requirement to diagnose intrapartum hypoxic neurologic injury.

PATTERN RECOGNITION AND INTERPRETATION

The clinical application of electronic FHR monitoring (EFM) consists of three interdependent elements: (1) *definition,* that is, the words used to describe the FHR observations; (2) *interpretation,* or the physiologic significance of the FHR observations; and (3) *management,* or the clinical response to the FHR observations.

EVOLUTION OF STANDARDIZED FETAL HEART RATE DEFINITIONS

Electronic FHR monitoring was introduced into clinical practice before consensus was reached regarding standardized definitions of FHR patterns. This resulted in wide variations in the descriptions and interpretations of common FHR observations, and this lack of standardization was a major impediment to effective communication. In 1995 and 1996, the NICHD convened a workshop to develop "standardized and unambiguous definitions for fetal heart rate tracings."[14] However, the NICHD recommendations were not incorporated rapidly into clinical practice, and wide variations persisted. In May, 2005, ACOG endorsed the 1997 NICHD recommendations in Practice Bulletin #62 (subsequently updated in December 2005 in Practice Bulletin #70).[15] Shortly thereafter, the NICHD definitions were endorsed by the Association of Women's Health, Obstetric and Neonatal Nurses (AWHONN) and the American College of Nurse Midwives (ACNM).

2008 NATIONAL INSTITUTE OF CHILD HEALTH AND HUMAN DEVELOPMENT CONSENSUS REPORT

A second NICHD consensus panel was convened in 2008 to review and update the standardized definitions published in 1997 and to seek consensus regarding basic principles of FHR interpretation.[16] The standardized NICHD definitions published in 2008 are summarized in Table 15-3.

In addition to clarifying and reiterating the standardized FHR definitions proposed by the 1997 NICHD consensus statement, the 2008 report recommended a simplified, objective system

TABLE 15-3	STANDARD FETAL HEART RATE DEFINITIONS
PATTERN	**DEFINITION**
Baseline	Mean FHR rounded to increments of 5 beats/min in a 10-min window, excluding accelerations, decelerations, and periods of marked FHR variability (>25 beats/min). There must be at least 2 min of identifiable baseline segments (not necessarily contiguous) in any 10-min window or the baseline for that period is indeterminate. • Normal baseline FHR range 110 to 160 beats/min • *Tachycardia* is defined as an FHR baseline >160 beats/min • *Bradycardia* is defined as an FHR baseline <110 beats/min
Variability	Fluctuations in the FHR baseline are irregular in amplitude and frequency and are visually quantitated as the amplitude of the peak to the trough in beats per minute. • Absent—amplitude range undetectable • Minimal—amplitude range detectable but ≤5 beats/min • Moderate (normal)—amplitude range 6 to 25 beats/min • Marked—amplitude range >25 beats/min
Accelerations	Abrupt increase (onset to peak <30 sec) in the FHR from the most recently calculated baseline. At ≥32 weeks, an acceleration peaks ≥15 beats/min above baseline and lasts ≥15 sec but <2 min. At <32 weeks, acceleration peaks ≥10 beats/min above baseline and lasts ≥10 sec but <2 min. Prolonged acceleration lasts ≥2 min but <10 min. Acceleration ≥10 min is a baseline change.
Early	Gradual (onset to nadir ≥30 sec) decrease in FHR during a uterine contraction. Onset, nadir, and recovery of the deceleration occur at the same time as the beginning, peak, and end of the contraction, respectively.
Late	Decrease in FHR is gradual (onset to nadir ≥30 sec) during a uterine contraction. Onset, nadir, and recovery of the deceleration occur after the beginning, peak, and end of the contraction, respectively.
Variable	Decrease in the FHR is abrupt (onset to nadir <30 sec) and ≥15 beats/min below the baseline and lasting ≥15 sec but less than 2 min.
Prolonged	Deceleration is ≥15 beats/min below baseline and lasts ≥2 min or more but <10 min. Deceleration ≥10 min is a baseline change.
Sinusoidal pattern	Pattern in FHR baseline is smooth, sine wave–like, and undulating with a cycle frequency of 3 to 5/min that persists for at least 20 min.

FHR, fetal heart rate.

for classifying FHR tracings. The 2008 NICHD classification system replaced subjective terms such as *fetal distress, fetal stress, reassuring fetal status, nonreassuring fetal status,* and *fetal intolerance to labor*—all of which are defined inconsistently in the literature.

As summarized in Box 15-3, the three-tier system groups FHR tracings into one of three categories. *Category I* includes tracings with a normal baseline rate (110 to 160 beats/min); moderate variability; and no variable, late, or prolonged decelerations. *Category III* includes tracings with at least one of the following four traits: (1) absent variability with recurrent late decelerations, (2) absent variability with recurrent variable decelerations, (3) absent variability with bradycardia for at least 10 minutes, or (4) a sinusoidal pattern for at least 20 minutes. *Category II* includes all tracings that do not meet criteria for

BOX 15-3   FETAL HEART RATE CATEGORIES

Category I requires *all* of the following:
- Baseline rate: 110 to 160 beats/min
- Variability: Moderate
- Accelerations: Present or absent
- Decelerations: No late, variable, or prolonged decelerations

Category II
- Any fetal heart rate tracing that does not meet criteria for classification in category I or III

Category III requires at least *one* of the following:
- Absent variability with recurrent late decelerations
- Absent variability with recurrent variable decelerations
- Absent variability with bradycardia for at least 10 min
- Sinusoidal pattern for at least 20 min

BOX 15-4   STRATIFICATION OF SCIENTIFIC EVIDENCE ACCORDING TO THE METHOD OUTLINED BY THE U.S. PREVENTIVE SERVICES TASK FORCE

Level I: Evidence obtained from at least one properly designed randomized controlled trial

Level II-1: Evidence obtained from well-designed controlled trials without randomization

Level II-2: Evidence obtained from well-designed cohort or case-control analytic studies, preferably from more than one center or research group

Level II-3: Evidence obtained from multiple time series with or without the intervention; dramatic results in uncontrolled experiments also could be regarded as this type of evidence.

Level III: Opinions of respected authorities, based on clinical experience, descriptive studies, or reports of expert committees

classification as category I or category III. The proposed FHR categories provide a summary method of defining FHR tracings, but they do not replace complete description of baseline rate, variability, accelerations, decelerations, sinusoidal pattern, and changes or trends over time.

The 2008 NICHD consensus report also addressed uterine activity. *Normal uterine contraction frequency* was defined as five or fewer contractions in a 10-minute window averaged over 30 minutes. Contraction frequency of more than 5 in 10 minutes averaged over 30 minutes was defined as *tachysystole*,[16] a term that applies to both spontaneous and stimulated labor.[16,17] Equally important aspects of uterine activity include contraction intensity, contraction duration, resting time between contractions, and resting uterine tone between contractions. The terms *hyperstimulation* and *hypercontractility* are defined inconsistently in the literature; therefore the consensus report recommended they be abandoned. The recommendations of the 2008 NICHD consensus report were subsequently published in ACOG Practice Bulletins 106 and 116.[17,18]

The physiology underlying common FHR patterns has been the subject of scientific investigation for decades; however, most theories regarding the physiologic significance of specific FHR patterns have not been substantiated by appropriately controlled scientific research. In an area as critical as intrapartum FHR monitoring, it is imperative to distinguish between concepts based on scientific evidence and those based on unsubstantiated theories. Scientific evidence can be stratified according to the method outlined by the U.S. Preventive Services Task Force as summarized in Box 15-4.[19]

Level I evidence is considered the most robust, and level III is the least so. Only level I and level II analytic evidence is capable of establishing statistically significant relationships. Level III descriptive evidence can be used to generate theories, but is not capable of proving them.

Definitions and General Considerations

The standardized definitions proposed by the NICHD in 1997 and reiterated in 2008 apply to the interpretation of FHR patterns, produced either by a direct fetal electrode that detects the fetal ECG or by an external Doppler device that detects fetal cardiac motion using the autocorrelation technique, a computerized method of minimizing the artifact associated with Doppler ultrasound calculation of the FHR, a feature incorporated in all modern FHR monitors. **Other important general considerations are as follows:**

- Patterns are categorized as *baseline, periodic,* or *episodic.*
- Baseline patterns include baseline rate and variability.
- Periodic and episodic patterns include FHR accelerations and decelerations.
- *Periodic* patterns are those associated with uterine contractions.
- *Episodic* patterns are those *not* associated with uterine contractions.
- *Deceleration onset* is defined as abrupt if the onset to nadir (lowest point) is less than 30 seconds and gradual if the onset to nadir is 30 seconds or greater.
- Although terms such as *beat-to-beat variability, short-term variability,* and *long-term variability* are used frequently in clinical practice, the NICHD panel recommended that no distinction be made between short-term or beat-to-beat variability and long-term variability because in actual practice, they are visually determined as a unit.
- A number of FHR characteristics are dependent upon gestational age, so gestational age must be considered in the full evaluation of the pattern.
- In addition, the FHR tracing should be evaluated in the context of maternal medical condition, prior results of fetal assessment, medications, and other factors.
- FHR patterns do not occur alone and generally evolve over time. Therefore a full description requires a qualitative and quantitative assessment of baseline rate, variability, accelerations, decelerations, sinusoidal pattern, and changes or trends over time.

Specific Fetal Heart Rate Patterns

Understanding the common FHR patterns and characteristics is fundamental to the interpretation of these as they relate to intrapartum care. As decribed above, intrapartum FHR monitoring is critical to ensuring fetal and maternal well-being.

BASELINE RATE

DEFINITION

Baseline FHR is defined as the approximate mean FHR rounded to increments of 5 beats/min during a 10-minutes segment excluding accelerations, decelerations, and periods of marked variability. In any 10-minute window, the minimum baseline duration must be at least 2 minutes—not necessarily contiguous—or the baseline for that period is deemed

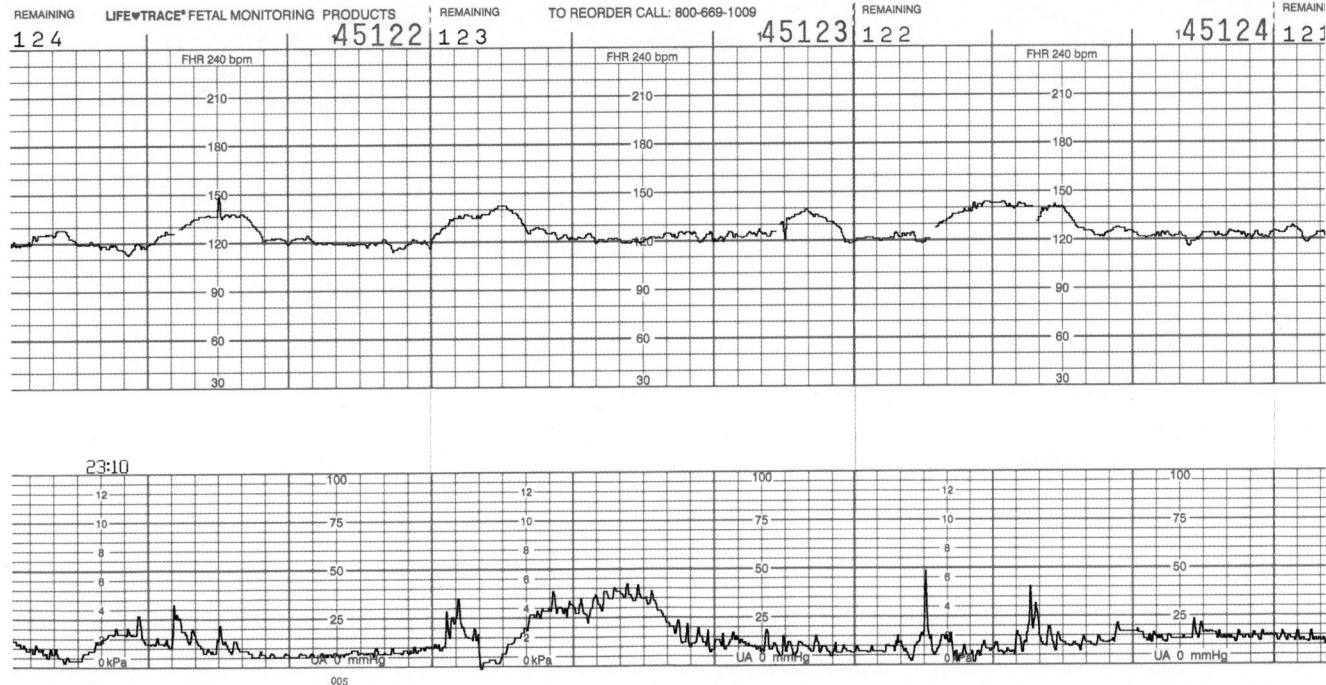

FIG 15-7 Baseline fetal heart rate (FHR) is the mean FHR rounded to increments of 5 beats/min in a 10-minute window excluding accelerations, decelerations, and periods of marked FHR variability (>25 beats/min). At least 2 minutes of identifiable baseline segments, not necessarily contiguous, must be present in any 10-minute window or the baseline for that period is indeterminate. In this tracing, the baseline heart rate is 120 beats/min with accelerations.

indeterminate. If the baseline during any 10-minute segment is deemed indeterminate, it may be necessary to refer to any previous 10-minute segments for determination of the baseline (Fig. 15-7).

PHYSIOLOGY
Baseline FHR is regulated by intrinsic cardiac pacemakers (sinoatrial node, atrioventricular node), cardiac conduction pathways, autonomic innervation (sympathetic, parasympathetic), intrinsic humoral factors (catecholamines), extrinsic factors (medications), and local factors (calcium, potassium). Sympathetic innervation and plasma catecholamines increase baseline FHR, whereas parasympathetic innervation reduces the baseline rate. Autonomic input regulates the FHR in response to fluctuations in the partial pressure of oxygen (PO_2), partial pressure of carbon dioxide (PCO_2), and blood pressure detected by chemoreceptors and baroreceptors located in the aortic arch and carotid arteries. **A normal FHR baseline of 110 to 160 beats/min is consistent with normal neurologic regulation of the FHR.** *Fetal tachycardia is defined as a baseline rate above 160 beats/min for at least 10 minutes.* Conditions potentially associated with fetal tachycardia are summarized in Box 15-5.

Fetal bradycardia is defined as a baseline rate below 110 beats/min for at least 10 minutes. Box 15-6 summarizes conditions associated with fetal bradycardia.

VARIABILITY
DEFINITION
Variability is defined as fluctuations in the baseline FHR that are irregular in amplitude and frequency. Variability is measured from the peak to the trough of the fluctuations and is quantitated in beats per minute. No distinction is made between short-term (beat-to-beat) variability and long-term variability

BOX 15-5   CONDITIONS POTENTIALLY ASSOCIATED WITH FETAL TACHYCARDIA

Maternal fever
Infection
Medications/drugs
• Sympathomimetics
• Parasympatholytics
• Caffeine
• Theophylline
• Cocaine
• Methamphetamine
Fetal anemia

Hyperthyroidism
Arrhythmia
• Sinus tachycardia
• Supraventricular tachycardia
• Atrial fibrillation
• Atrial flutter
• Ventricular arrhythmia
Metabolic acidemia

BOX 15-6   CONDITIONS POTENTIALLY ASSOCIATED WITH FETAL BRADYCARDIA

Medications
• Sympatholytics
• Parasympathomimetics
Cardiac pacing and conduction abnormalities
• Heart block
• Sjögren antibodies
• Heterotaxy syndrome
Structural cardiac defects
Viral infections (e.g., cytomegalovirus)
Fetal heart failure
Maternal hypoglycemia
Maternal hypothermia
Interruption of fetal oxygenation

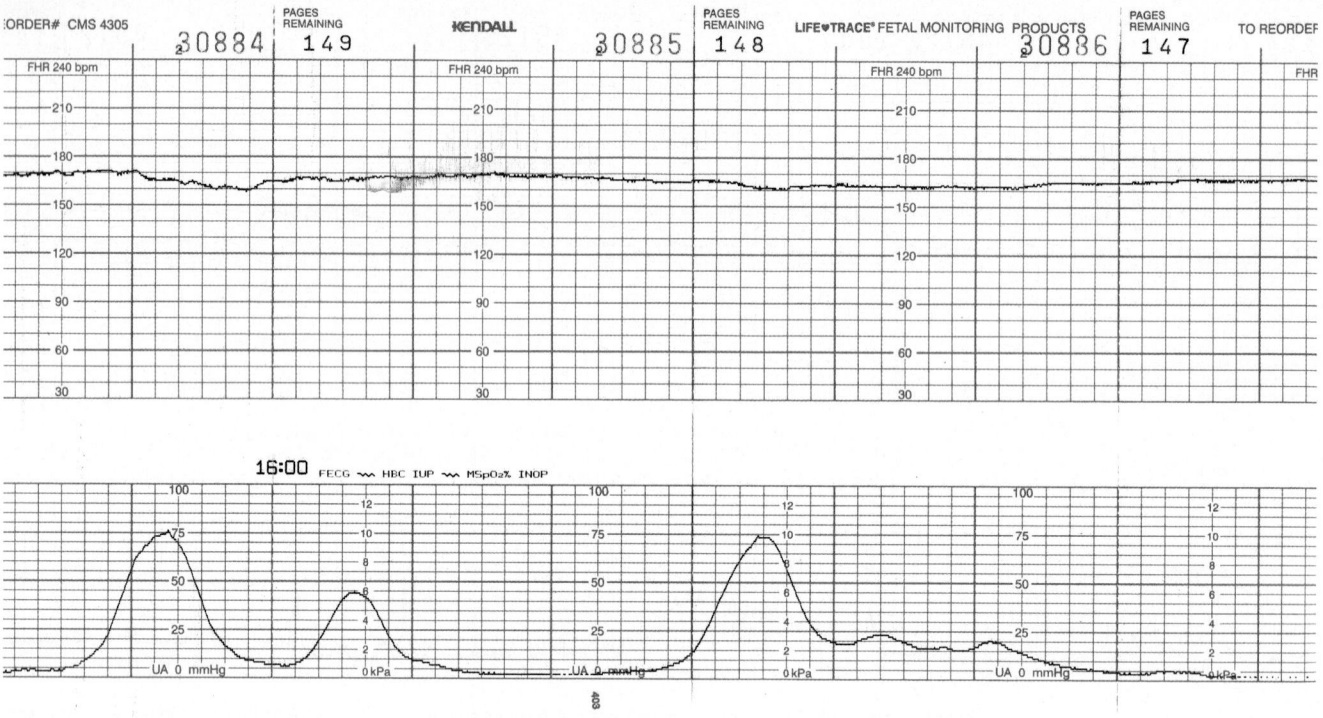

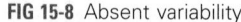

FIG 15-8 Absent variability.

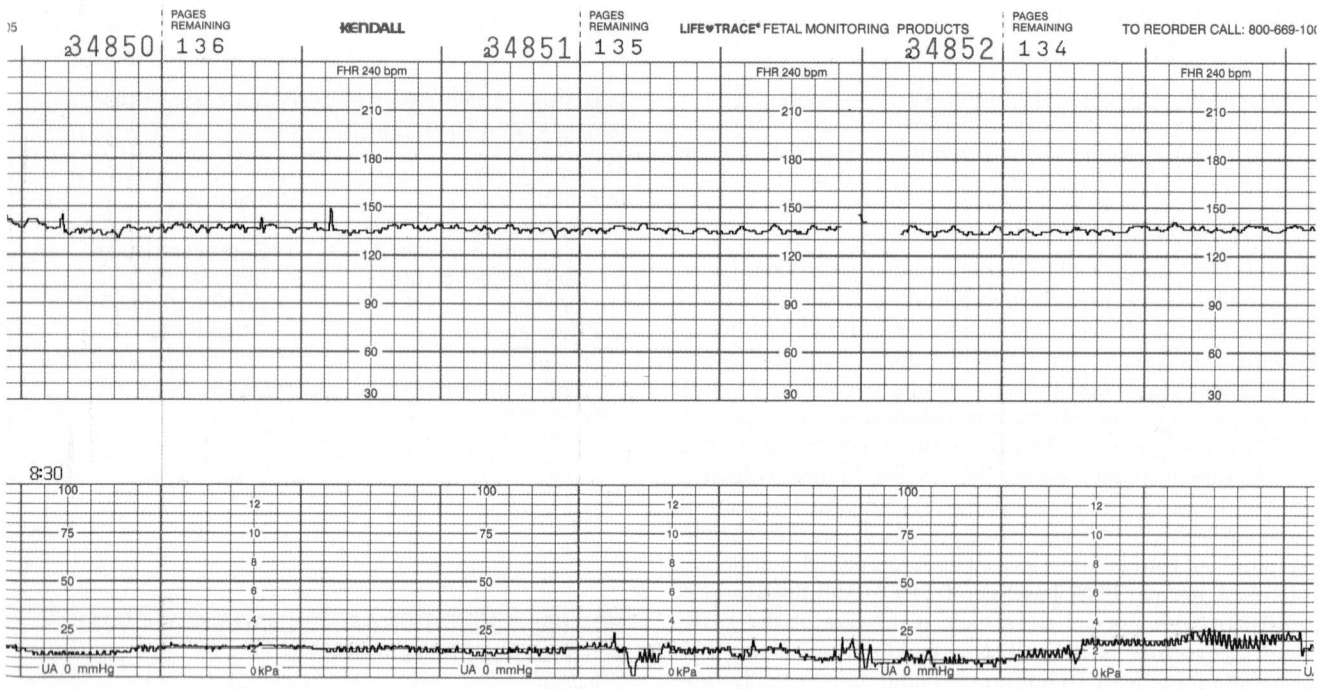

FIG 15-9 Minimal variability.

because in actual practice, they are visually determined as a unit. In addition, there is no consensus that beat-to-beat differences in rate can be quantitated accurately with the unaided eye. Standardized NICHD nomenclature classifies variability as absent, minimal, moderate, or marked. As depicted in Figure 15-8, variability is defined as *absent* when the amplitude range of the FHR fluctuations is undetectable to the unaided eye. Variability is defined as *minimal* when the amplitude range is visually detectable but is less than or equal to 5 beats/min, as illustrated in Figure 15-9. When the amplitude range of the

FHR fluctuations is 6 to 25 beats/min, variability is defined as *moderate,* as illustrated in Figure 15-10. Variability is defined as *marked* when the amplitude range of the FHR fluctuations is greater than 25 beats/min (Fig. 15-11).

PHYSIOLOGY

Many factors interact to regulate FHR variability, including intrinsic cardiac pacemakers (sinoatrial node, atrioventricular node), cardiac conduction pathways, autonomic innervation (sympathetic, parasympathetic), intrinsic humoral factors

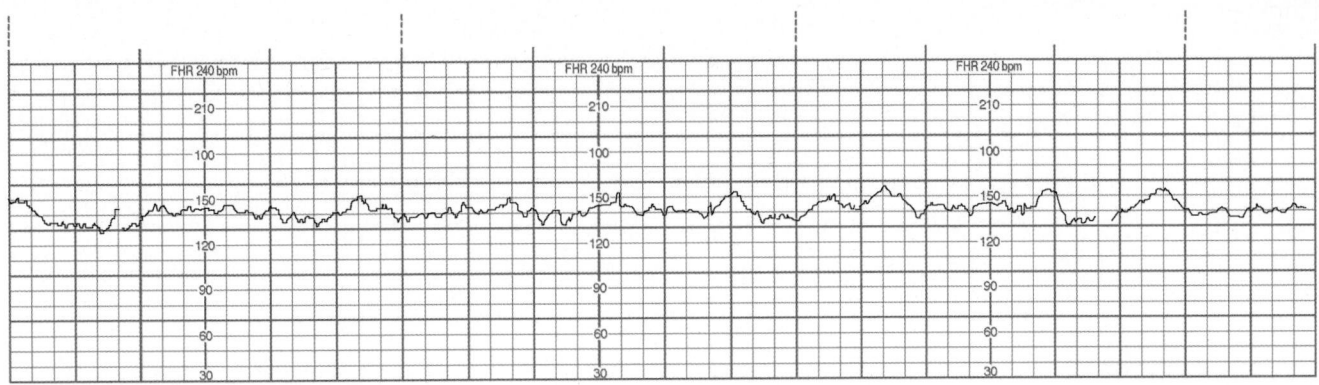

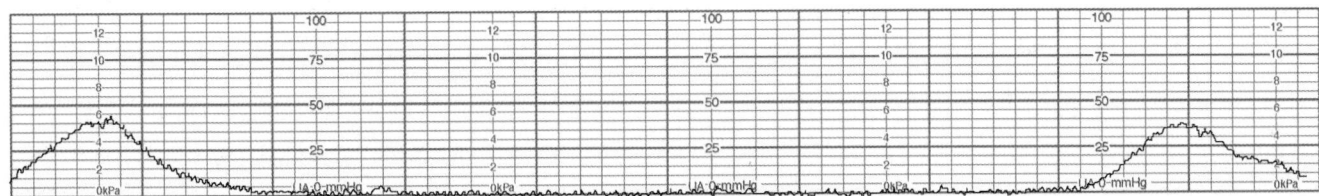

FIG 15-10 Moderate variability.

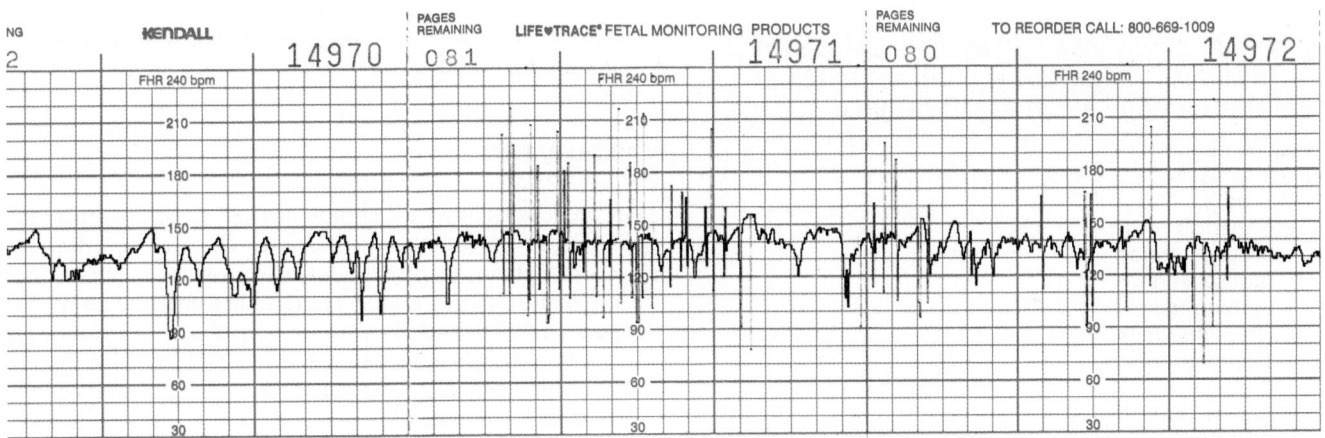

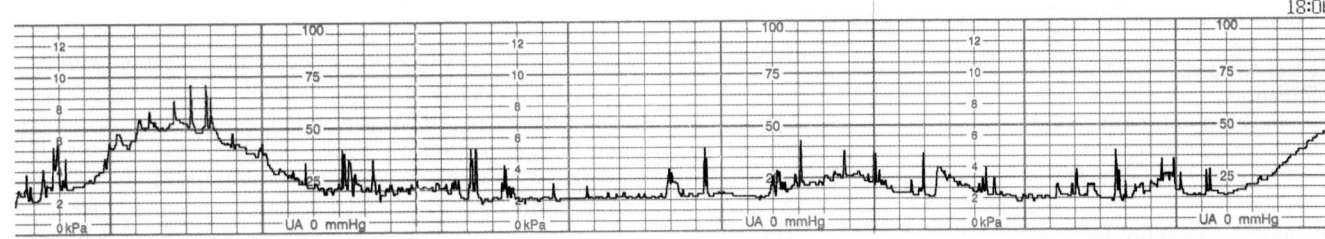

FIG 15-11 Marked variability.

(catecholamines), extrinsic factors (medications), and local factors (calcium, potassium). Fluctuations in PO_2, PCO_2, and blood pressure are detected by chemoreceptors and baroreceptors located in the aortic arch and carotid arteries. Signals from these receptors are processed in the medullary vasomotor center, likely with regulatory input from higher centers in the hypothalamus and cerebral cortex. Sympathetic and parasympathetic signals from the medullary vasomotor center modulate the FHR in response to moment-to-moment changes in fetal PO_2, PCO_2, and blood pressure. With every heartbeat, slight fluctuations in

heart rate help to optimize fetal cardiac output and distribution of oxygenated blood to the fetal tissues. These fluctuations are referred to as *fetal heart rate variability* and are displayed graphically on the FHR tracing as an irregular horizontal line. The 2008 NICHD consensus report concluded that moderate variability reliably predicts the absence of fetal metabolic acidemia at the time it is observed.[16] **However, the converse is not true; minimal or absent variability does *not* confirm the presence of fetal metabolic acidemia or ongoing hypoxic injury.**[16] Other conditions potentially associated with minimal

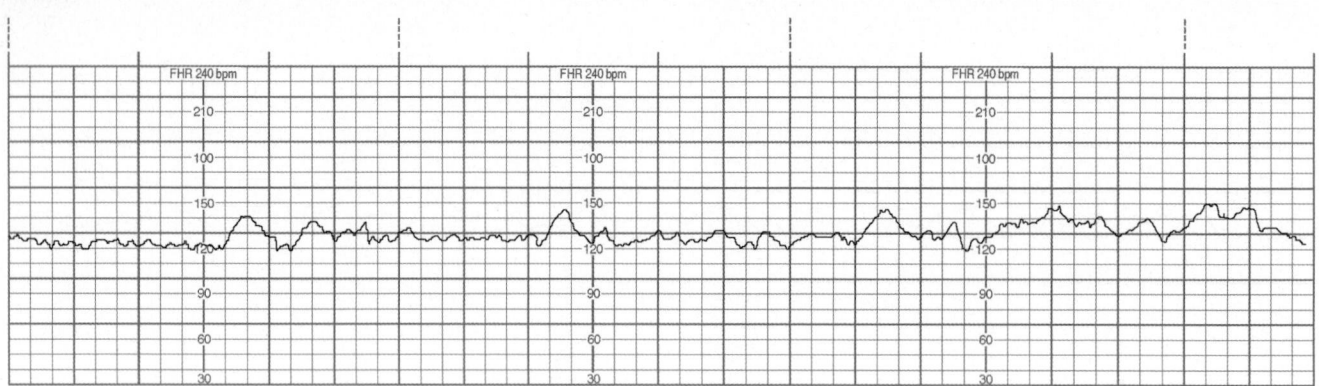

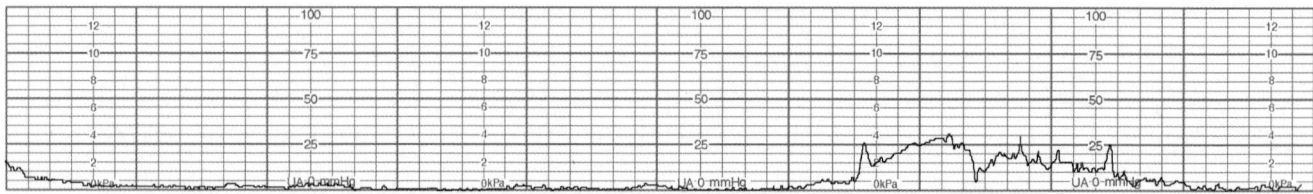

FIG 15-12 Accelerations. (From Clark SL, Nageotte MP, Garite TJ, et al. Intrapartum management of category II fetal heart rate tracings: towards standardization of care. *Am J Obstet Gynecol.* 2013;209[2]:89-97.)

BOX 15-7 CONDITIONS POTENTIALLY ASSOCIATED WITH MINIMAL TO ABSENT FETAL HEART RATE VARIABILITY AND ABSENT ACCELERATIONS

Fetal sleep cycle
Fetal tachycardia
Medications
- Narcotics
- Corticosteroids
- Butorphanol
- Barbiturates
- Phenothiazines
- Tranquilizers
- Cocaine
- General anesthetics
- Atropine
- Phenothiazines
Prematurity
Congenital anomalies
Fetal anemia
Fetal cardiac arrhythmia
Infection
Preexisting neurologic injury
Fetal metabolic acidemia

---

or absent variability are summarized in Box 15-7. **The 2014 Neonatal Encephalopathy Task Force consensus report**[13] **identified moderate variability as one of the features of the FHR tracing that reliably excludes "damaging degrees of hypoxia-induced metabolic acidemia."** Most of the literature regarding "decreased" FHR variability does not differentiate between *absent variability,* when the amplitude range is undetectable, and *minimal variability,* when the amplitude range is detectable but is 5 beats/min or less. Therefore it is not possible to draw valid conclusions regarding the relative clinical significance of these two categories; the significance of marked variability has not been established.[16] Possible explanations include a normal variant or an exaggerated autonomic response to early

stages of interrupted fetal oxygenation. Box 15-7 summarizes some conditions potentially associated with minimal or absent variability.

ACCELERATION

DEFINITION

An *acceleration* is as an abrupt increase (onset to peak <30 seconds) in FHR above the baseline. The peak is at least 15 beats/min above the baseline, and the acceleration lasts at least 15 seconds from the onset to return to baseline, as illustrated in Figure 15-12. Before 32 weeks of gestation, an *acceleration* is defined as having a peak at least 10 beats/min above the baseline and a duration of at least 10 seconds. An acceleration that lasts at least 2 minutes but less than 10 minutes is defined as a *prolonged acceleration.* An acceleration that lasts 10 minutes or longer is defined as a *baseline change.*

PHYSIOLOGY

Accelerations in FHR frequently occur in association with fetal movement, possibly as a result of stimulation of peripheral proprioceptors, increased catecholamine release, and autonomic stimulation of the heart. Another possible mechanism of FHR acceleration is transient compression of the umbilical vein, which results in decreased fetal venous return and a reflex rise in heart rate. The 2008 NICHD consensus report concluded that accelerations reliably predict the absence of fetal metabolic acidemia at the time they are observed.[16] **However, the converse is not true. The absence of accelerations does *not* confirm the presence of fetal metabolic acidemia or ongoing hypoxic injury.**[16] Other conditions potentially associated with the absence of accelerations are summarized in Table 15-4.[17] **The 2014 Neonatal Encephalopathy Task Force concluded that the presence of FHR accelerations reliably excludes "damaging degrees of hypoxia-induced metabolic academia."**[16] In the absence of spontaneous accelerations, fetal stimulation can provoke fetal movement and FHR accelerations. **Accelerations can be provoked with a variety of methods that**

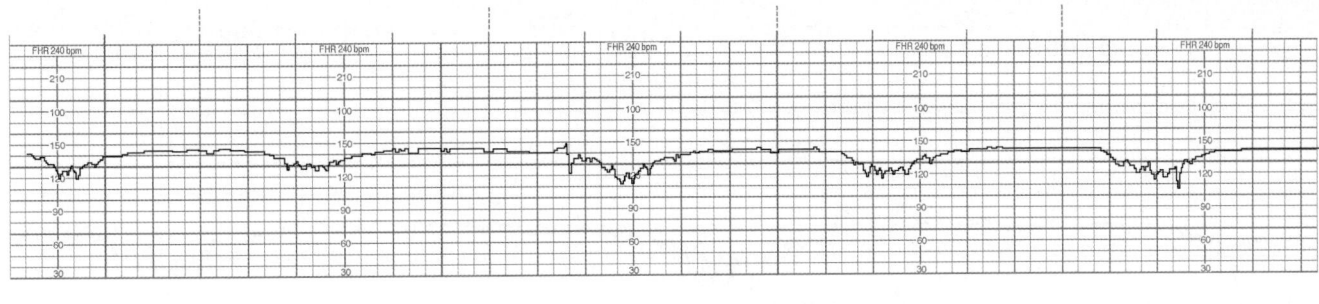
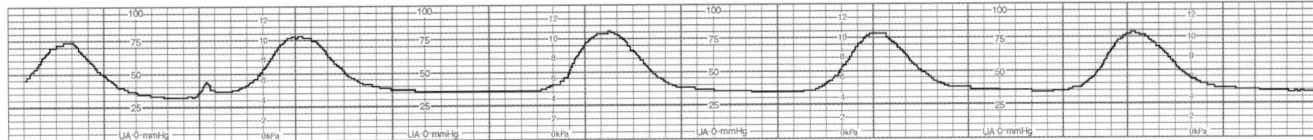

FIG 15-13 Early decelerations.

TABLE 15-4	MATERNAL AND FETAL FACTORS THAT CAN INFLUENCE THE FETAL HEART RATE TRACING BY MECHANISMS NOT SPECIFICALLY RELATED TO FETAL OXYGENATION

FACTOR	REPORTED FETAL HEART RATE ASSOCIATIONS
Fever/infection	Increased baseline rate, decreased variability
Medications	Effects depend upon specific medication and may include changes in baseline rate, frequency and amplitude of accelerations, variability and sinusoidal pattern[17]
Hyperthyroidism	Tachycardia, decreased variability
Prematurity	Increased baseline rate, decreased variability, reduced frequency and amplitude of accelerations
Fetal anemia	Sinusoidal pattern, tachycardia
Heart block	Bradycardia, decreased variability
Tachyarrhythmia	Variable degrees of tachycardia, decreased variability
Congenital anomaly	Decreased variability, decelerations
Preexisting injury	Decreased variability, absent accelerations
Sleep cycle	Decreased variability, reduced frequency and amplitude of accelerations

include vibroacoustic stimulation (VAS), transabdominal halogen light stimulation, and direct fetal scalp stimulation. Accelerations provoked by external stimuli have the same clinical significance as spontaneous accelerations.[16]

DECELERATIONS

Decelerations in the FHR are categorized as early, late, variable, or prolonged and are quantitated by depth in beats per minute below the baseline and duration in minutes and seconds. An abrupt deceleration reaches its nadir within 30 seconds from the time it starts. A gradual deceleration will reach its nadir in 30 seconds or more. Decelerations that occur with at least 50% of uterine contractions in a 20-minute window are defined as *recurrent*. Decelerations that occur with fewer than 50% of contractions in a 20-minute period are defined as *intermittent*. Classification of decelerations as mild, moderate, or severe has not been shown to correlate with metabolic acidemia or newborn outcome independent of other FHR characteristics such as moderate variability, accelerations, frequency of decelerations, duration of decelerations, or total number of decelerations. Therefore

such classification is not included in standardized NICHD terminology.[16]

EARLY DECELERATION

DEFINITION

Early deceleration is defined as a gradual decrease (onset to nadir <30 seconds) in FHR from the baseline and a subsequent return to baseline associated with a uterine contraction (Fig. 15-13). In most cases the onset, nadir, and recovery of the deceleration occur at the same time as the beginning, peak, and end of the contraction, respectively.

PHYSIOLOGY

Although the precise physiologic mechanism is not known, early decelerations are considered to represent a fetal autonomic response to changes in intracranial pressure and/or cerebral blood flow caused by intrapartum compression of the fetal head during uterine contractions. *Early decelerations are not associated with interruption of fetal oxygenation or adverse neonatal outcome and are considered clinically benign.* No level I or level II analytic evidence in the literature supports the notion that mechanical compression of the fetal head by uterine contractions and/or maternal expulsive efforts can cause local cerebral ischemia and neurologic injury in the absence of global hypoxia and neonatal encephalopathy. Furthermore, no scientific evidence suggests that mechanical compression of the fetal head by the forces of labor is a predictable or preventable cause of perinatal stroke. On the contrary, a consensus report from the National Institute of Neurologic Disorders and Stroke and the NICHD in 2007 concluded "there are no reliable predictors of perinatal ischemic stroke upon which to base prevention or treatment strategies."[20] Despite the absence of scientific merit, these theories have become increasingly popular in the legal arena. Unless such theories can be validated and replicated by appropriately controlled analytic studies, they play no meaningful role in intrapartum management decisions.

LATE DECELERATION

DEFINITION

Late deceleration of the FHR is defined as a gradual decrease (onset to nadir ≥30 seconds) of the FHR from the baseline and subsequent return to the baseline associated with a uterine contraction, as illustrated in Figure 15-14. In most cases the onset,

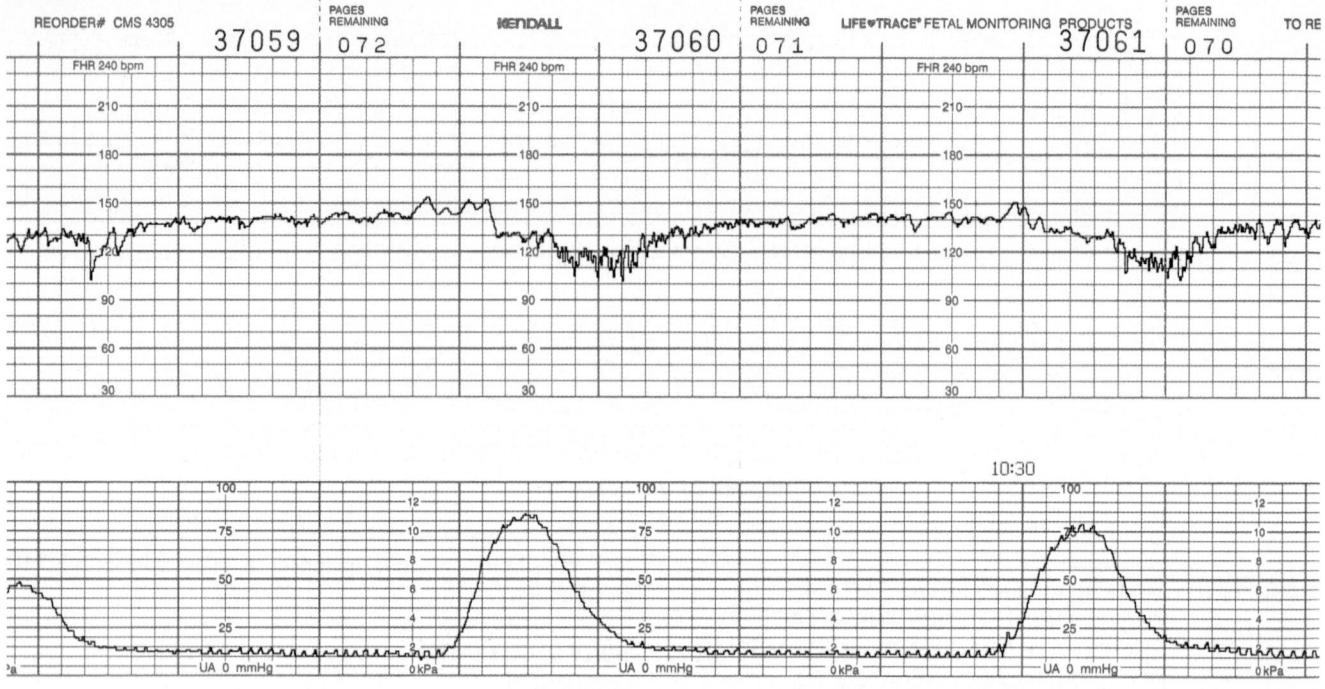

FIG 15-14 Late decelerations.

nadir, and recovery of the deceleration occur after the beginning, peak, and ending of the contraction, respectively.

PHYSIOLOGY

A *late deceleration* is a reflex fetal response to transient hypoxemia during a uterine contraction. Myometrial contractions can compress maternal blood vessels that traverse the uterine wall and reduce maternal perfusion of the intervillous space of the placenta. Reduced delivery of oxygenated blood to the intervillous space can reduce the diffusion of oxygen into the fetal capillary blood in the chorionic villi, leading to a decline in fetal PO_2. If the fetal PO_2 falls below the normal range (approximately 15 to 25 mm Hg in the umbilical artery), chemoreceptors detect the change and signal the medullary vasomotor center in the brainstem to initiate a protective autonomic reflex response. Initially, sympathetic outflow causes peripheral vasoconstriction and shunts oxygenated blood flow away from nonvital vascular beds and toward vital organs such as the brain, heart, and adrenal glands. The resulting increase in fetal blood pressure is detected by baroreceptors that trigger a parasympathetic reflex slowing of the heart rate to reduce cardiac output and return the blood pressure to normal. After the contraction, fetal oxygenation is restored, autonomic reflexes subside, and the FHR gradually returns to baseline. This combined sympathetic-parasympathetic reflex response to transient interruption of fetal oxygenation, summarized in Figure 15-15, has been confirmed in animal studies.[21] **If interruption of fetal oxygenation is sufficient to result in metabolic acidemia, a late deceleration may result from direct hypoxic myocardial depression during a contraction,** as illustrated in Figure 15-15.[21] Because the latter mechanism requires metabolic acidemia, it is virtually excluded by the observation of moderate variability or accelerations. Late decelerations classically have been attributed to "uteroplacental insufficiency." However, this term is potentially misleading because it can be interpreted to indicate that interruption of fetal oxygenation is limited to the uterus and placenta. In reality,

interruption of the oxygen pathway at any point can contribute to a late deceleration. For example, conditions such as maternal hypoxemia, decreased cardiac output, or hypotension can result in late decelerations even with mild uterine contractions and a normally functioning placenta. *Regardless of the underlying mechanism, all late decelerations reflect interruption of oxygen transfer from the environment to the fetus at one or more points along the oxygen pathway.* Supporting evidence is level II-1 and II-2.

As illustrated in Figure 15-16, common causes of late deceleration include a relative increase in uterine contraction intensity or baseline tone and/or a relative lowering of maternal blood pressure.

VARIABLE DECELERATION

DEFINITION

Variable deceleration of the FHR is defined as an abrupt decrease (onset to nadir <30 seconds) in FHR below the baseline (Fig. 15-17). The decrease is at least 15 beats/min below the baseline, the deceleration lasts at least 15 seconds, and fewer than 2 minutes pass from onset to return to baseline. Variable decelerations can occur with or without uterine contractions.

PHYSIOLOGY

A variable deceleration represents a fetal autonomic reflex response to transient mechanical compression or stretch of the umbilical cord.[22] Initially, compression of the umbilical cord occludes the thin-walled, compliant umbilical vein; decreases fetal venous return; and triggers a baroreceptor-mediated reflex rise in FHR, sometimes described as a "shoulder." Further compression occludes the umbilical arteries and causes an abrupt increase in fetal peripheral resistance and blood pressure. Baroreceptors detect the abrupt rise in blood pressure and signal the medullary vasomotor center in the brainstem, which in turn triggers an increase in parasympathetic outflow and an abrupt decrease in heart rate. As the cord is decompressed, this sequence

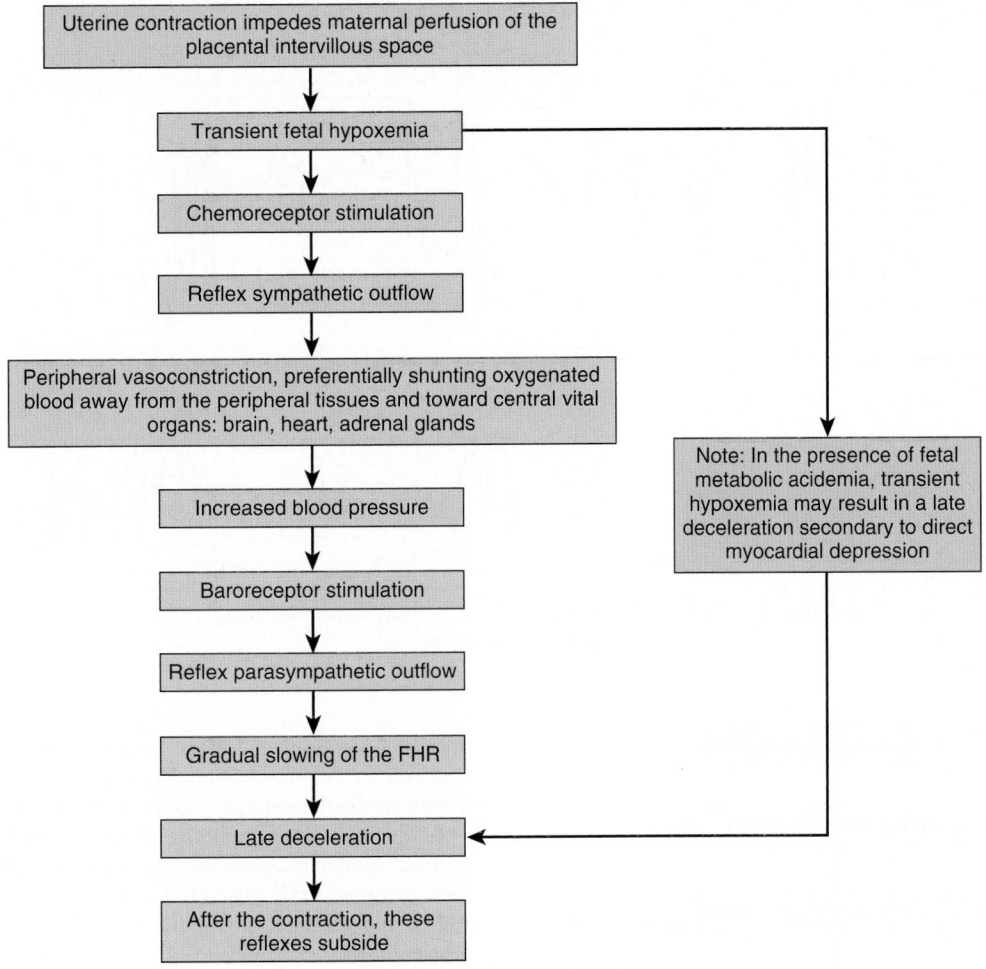

FIG 15-15 Mechanism of late deceleration. FHR, fetal heart rate.

EFFECTS OF HYPERTONUS AND MATERNAL HYPOTENSION

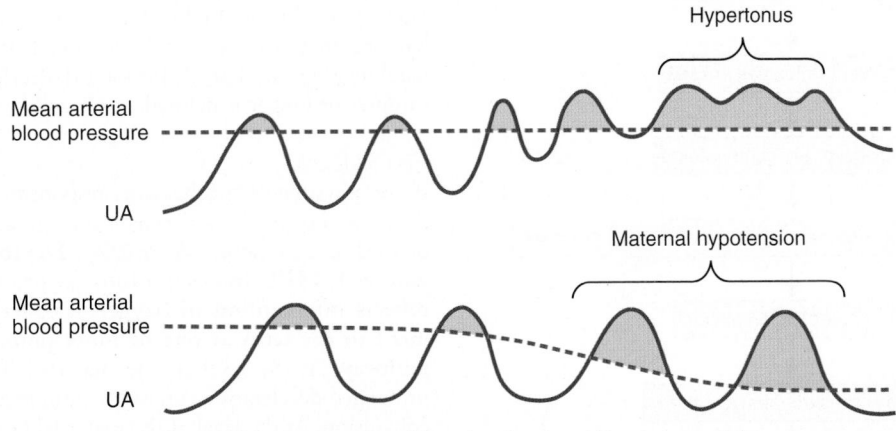

FIG 15-16 Common causes of late deceleration. UA, uterine activity.

of events occurs in reverse; this mechanism is summarized in Figure 15-18. Umbilical cord compression can coincide with interruption at any or all of the other points along the oxygen pathway; therefore the observation of a variable deceleration does not preclude interruption of the oxygen pathway at the level of the maternal lungs, heart, vasculature, uterus or placenta. *For the purposes of standardized FHR interpretation, a variable deceleration reflects interruption of oxygen transfer from the environment* *to the fetus at one or more points along the oxygen pathway.* Supporting evidence is level II and III. The 2008 NICHD Consensus Report identified several additional features of variable decelerations, the clinical significance of which requires further research investigation.[16] Examples include a slow return of the FHR after the end of the contraction, sometimes called *variable with a late component;* biphasic or *W-shaped decelerations;* tachycardia following variable decelerations; accelerations

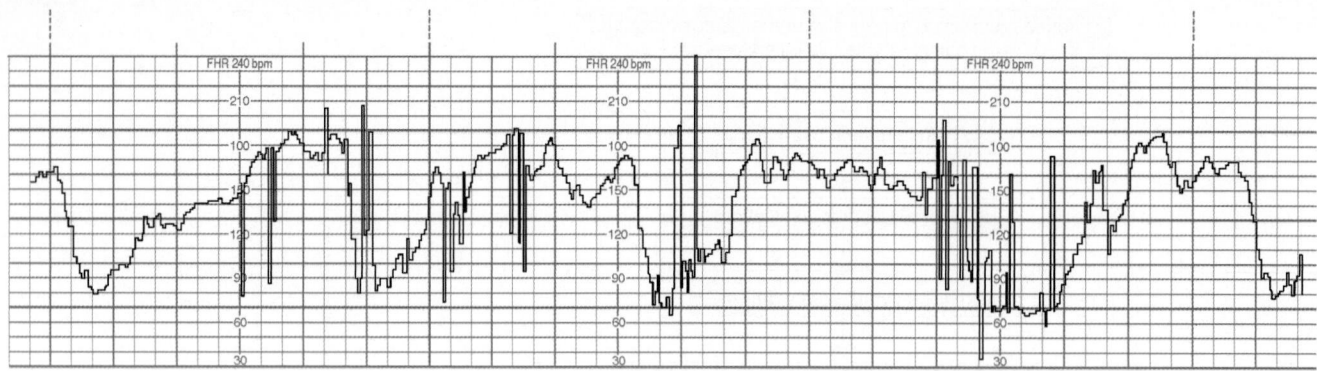

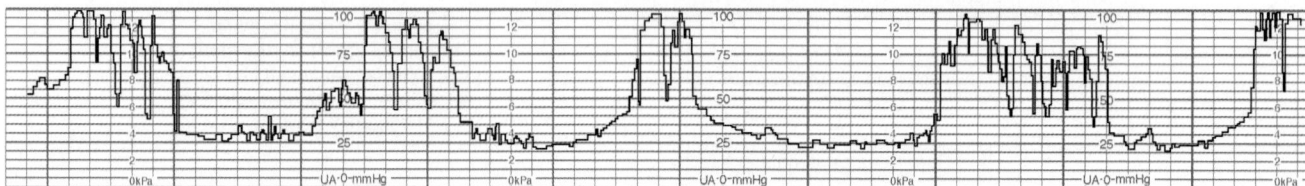

FIG 15-17 Variable decelerations.

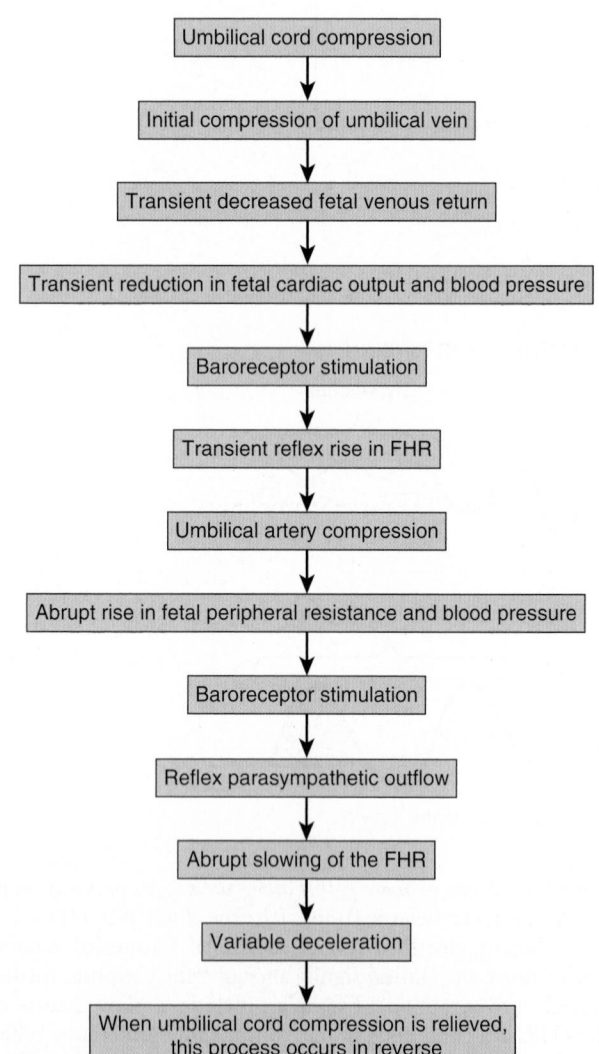

FIG 15-18 Mechanism of a variable deceleration. FHR, fetal heart rate.

that precede and/or follow decelerations, sometimes called *shoulders* or *overshoots;* and fluctuations in the FHR in the trough of the deceleration, sometimes termed *variability within a deceleration.* The predictive value of grading decelerations as mild, moderate, or severe has not been established independent of other FHR characteristics such as baseline rate, variability, and accelerations or frequency, duration, or number of decelerations.

PROLONGED DECELERATION

DEFINITION

Prolonged deceleration of the FHR is defined as a decrease, either gradual or abrupt, in FHR at least 15 beats/min below the baseline that lasts at least 2 minutes from onset to return to baseline (Fig. 15-19). A prolonged deceleration that lasts 10 minutes or longer is defined as a *baseline change.*

PHYSIOLOGY

If the physiologic mechanisms responsible for late or variable decelerations persist, a deceleration can last long enough to be defined as a *prolonged deceleration.* **For the purposes of standardized FHR interpretation, a prolonged deceleration reflects interruption of oxygen transfer from the environment to the fetus at one or more points along the oxygen pathway.** At the level of the maternal lungs, for example, a prolonged deceleration can result from maternal apnea during a convulsion. At the level of the maternal heart, a cardiac arrhythmia can compromise cardiac output and cause a prolonged FHR deceleration. At the level of the vasculature, the oxygen pathway can be interrupted by maternal hypotension associated with regional anesthesia or compression of the great vessels by the gravid uterus. Examples of interruption of the oxygen pathway at the level of the uterus include excessive uterine activity or uterine rupture; at the level of the placenta, they include abruption or bleeding placenta previa; finally, at the level of the umbilical cord, examples include cord compression, stretch, or prolapse.

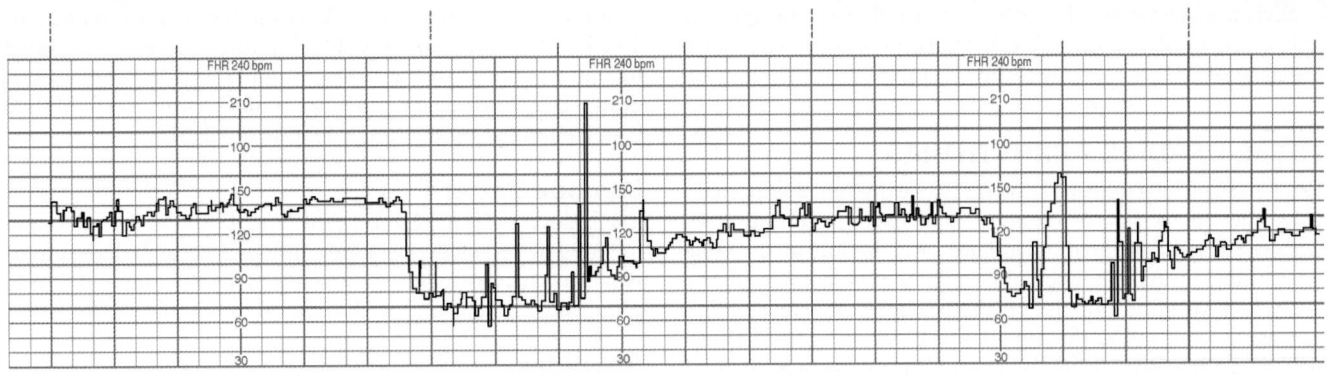

FIG 15-19 Prolonged deceleration.

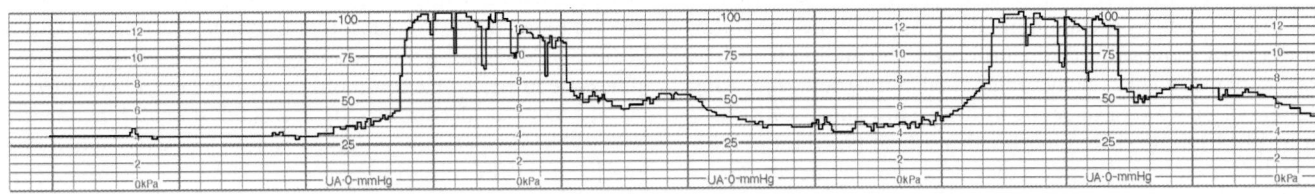

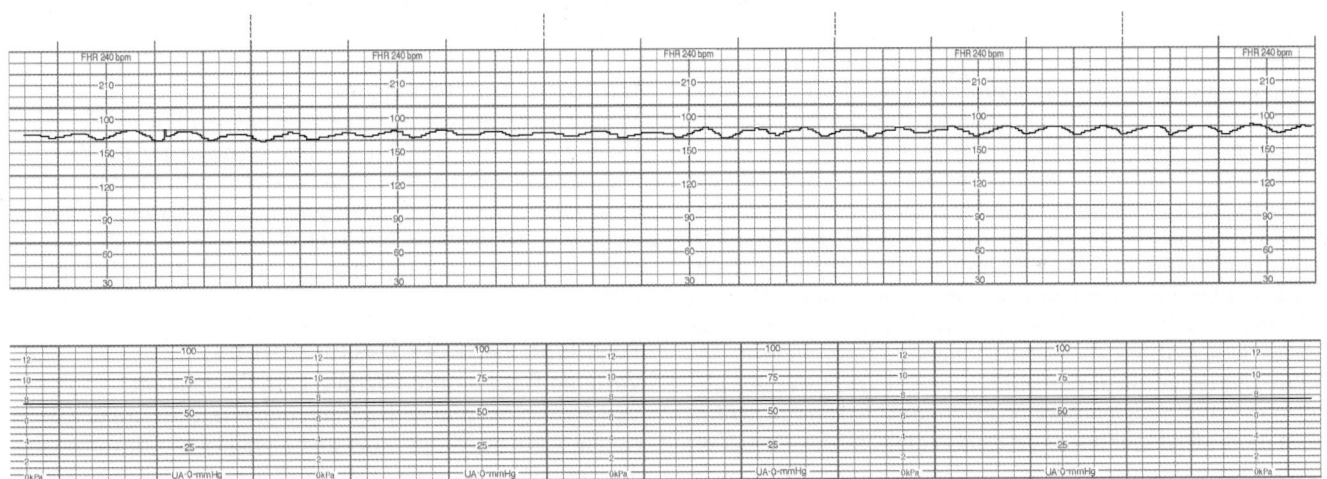

FIG 15-20 Sinusoidal pattern.

SINUSOIDAL PATTERN

DEFINITION

The sinusoidal pattern, illustrated in Figure 15-20, is a smooth, sine wave–like undulating pattern in FHR baseline with a frequency of 3 to 5 cycles/min that persists for at least 20 minutes. The sinusoidal pattern is excluded from the definition of variability and can be distinguished from variability because it is characterized by fluctuations in the baseline that are regular in amplitude in frequency.

PHYSIOLOGY

Although the pathophysiologic mechanism is not known, this pattern is classically associated with severe fetal anemia. Variations of the pattern have been described in association with chorioamnionitis, fetal sepsis, or administration of narcotic analgesics. Scientific evidence regarding associated factors is level II-2 to level III, and evidence regarding pathophysiology is level III.

STANDARDIZED FETAL HEART RATE INTERPRETATION

Intrapartum FHR interpretation can be summarized in two evidence-based central principles that reflect consensus in the medical literature. These two principles can be applied to an FHR tracing to produce a factually accurate, logical, and consistent interpretation that can help guide management.

1. Variable, late, and prolonged decelerations signal interruption of oxygen transfer from the environment to the fetus at one or more points along the oxygen pathway.
2. Moderate variability and/or accelerations reliably exclude ongoing hypoxic injury at the time they are observed.

Several maternal and fetal factors can influence the appearance of an FHR tracing by mechanisms not directly related to oxygenation. These are summarized in Table 15-4.

FETAL CARDIAC ARRHYTHMIAS

Precise characterization of fetal cardiac arrhythmias can challenge the clinical skill of the most experienced specialist, even with the benefit of direct, magnified visualization of the fetal heart using advanced sonography equipment with color, pulse-wave, and M-mode Doppler capabilities; therefore any attempt to classify fetal cardiac rhythm abnormalities using EFM alone will yield a tentative diagnosis at best. This imprecision is compounded by the fact that rates above 240 beats/min (the upper limit of the FHR graph on standard paper) may be halved or not printed at all by the monitor. This critically limits the ability of the FHR monitor to distinguish between conditions such as fetal supraventricular tachycardia, atrial fibrillation, and atrial flutter, all of which can result in heart rates above 240 beats/min. EFM cannot determine whether a fetal heartbeat is initiated by an electrical impulse that originates in the atrium or in the ventricle. In other words, the electronic monitor cannot reliably distinguish an atrial arrhythmia from a ventricular arrhythmia. Nevertheless, EFM can offer some clues to the presence of an abnormal fetal heart rhythm. For example, dropped beats might appear on the FHR monitor as sharp downward spikes with a nadir at approximately half of the baseline rate. A premature beat with a compensatory pause might appear as a sharp upward spike followed immediately by a downward spike. Bradycardia as a result of 2:1 (atrioventricular) heart block can appear persistently or intermittently as a baseline rate that is approximately half of the normal rate. Sinus bradycardia should be suspected if the baseline rate is lower than 110 beats/min but higher than half of the normal rate. Any FHR less than 110 beats/min requires thorough evaluation before it can be attributed to a benign condition. If the fetal heart is not generating electrical activity, as in the case of fetal demise, a fetal scalp electrode may detect the electrical impulses from the maternal heart and record the maternal heart rate. If any question exists as to the clinical significance of any unusual fetal heart rhythm seen on the fetal monitor or detected audibly, further evaluation with other modalities, such as ultrasound, is necessary to establish an accurate diagnosis.

PATTERNS NOT DEFINED BY THE NATIONAL INSTITUTE OF CHILD HEALTH AND HUMAN DEVELOPMENT

Several terms and concepts that are not defined by the NICHD may be encountered in clinical practice. The 2008 NICHD consensus report[16] states that FHR characteristics such as overshoot, shoulders, FHR fluctuations within a deceleration, variable deceleration with a slow return to baseline, and biphasic decelerations require further research investigation to determine clinical significance. These and other undefined terms are discussed below.

Wandering Baseline

An FHR baseline that is within the normal range (110 to 160 beats/min) but that is not stable at a single rate long enough to define a mean has been described as a "wandering baseline." Absent variability and absent accelerations are characteristic features of the pattern, and decelerations may be present or absent. This combination of FHR findings has been suggested to indicate preexisting neurologic injury and impending fetal death. The physiologic mechanism is not known, and published data are limited to descriptive reports (level III).

Lambda Pattern

The lambda FHR pattern is characterized by a brief acceleration followed by a small deceleration. Although the underlying physiologic mechanism is not known, this pattern is common during early labor and has no specific clinical significance.[23]

Shoulder

As discussed previously, variable decelerations result from transient mechanical compression of umbilical blood vessels within the umbilical cord. Initial compression of the umbilical vein reduces fetal venous return and triggers a baroreceptor-mediated reflex rise in FHR that commonly is described as a "shoulder."[22] As the cord is decompressed, a second shoulder frequently follows the deceleration and likely reflects the same underlying mechanism. This observation has no known association with adverse newborn outcome. On the other hand, no evidence suggests conclusively that such shoulders imply the same ability to exclude ongoing hypoxic injury as do spontaneous or stimulated FHR accelerations. The clinical significance of a shoulder requires further research investigation.[16] Supporting evidence is level II and III.

Uniform Accelerations

Various terms have been used to describe FHR accelerations. Examples include *uniform sporadic accelerations, variable sporadic accelerations, uniform periodic accelerations, variable periodic accelerations,* and *crown accelerations.* These terms are not included in standardized NICHD definitions, and no basis for such subclassification has been established. Available evidence is level III.

Atypical Variable Decelerations
Variable Deceleration With a Late Component

Variable deceleration with a "late component" describes a deceleration with an abrupt onset and a gradual return to baseline. The abrupt onset suggests that the deceleration begins as a reflex autonomic response to an abrupt rise in blood pressure caused by umbilical cord compression (the variable component of the pattern). The gradual return to baseline suggests a gradual reduction of autonomic outflow upon resolution of transient hypoxemia, as occurs in a late deceleration (the late component of the pattern). A plausible explanation of the pattern is initial umbilical cord compression that causes an abrupt reflex fall in FHR and a transient decline in fetal PO_2. A drop in fetal PO_2 below the normal range may trigger the reflex sympathetic outflow, peripheral vasoconstriction, elevation of blood pressure, and reflex parasympathetic slowing of the fetal heart that is characteristic of a late deceleration. Decompression of the umbilical cord results in rapid resolution of the parasympathetic outflow that accompanies a variable deceleration. However, the physiologic mechanism responsible for late deceleration resolves more gradually, which causes the FHR to return gradually to the previous baseline. Although this explanation is plausible, the specific physiologic mechanism has not been studied systematically. In regard to neonatal outcome, no level I or level II evidence has demonstrated that a variable deceleration with a late component confers a different prognosis than a variable deceleration without a late component. Scientific evidence regarding the underlying physiologic mechanism is limited to level III evidence. Second-stage variable decelerations with slow recovery have been reported to increase the likelihood of operative delivery; however, no consistent impact on newborn outcome has been described.

Overshoot

The term *overshoot* has been used to describe an FHR pattern that consists of a variable deceleration followed by a smooth, prolonged rise in the FHR above the previous baseline with gradual return.[24-27] The essential elements of this uncommon pattern include the persistent absence of variability and the absence of accelerations. The overshoot pattern has been attributed to a range of conditions that include preexisting neurologic injury, "chronic fetal distress," "repetitive transient central nervous system ischemia," and "mild fetal hypoxia above the deceleration threshold."[25-28] These claims have not been substantiated by level I or level II evidence, and the physiologic mechanism responsible for the overshoot pattern is unknown. Because of the wide variation in reported associations and the absence of agreement in the literature regarding the definition, visual appearance, or clinical significance of overshoot, it is advisable to avoid the term in favor of standard NICHD nomenclature. All evidence regarding the overshoot pattern in humans is descriptive (level III), and this pattern is not included in standardized NICHD terminology.

V- and W-Shaped Variable Decelerations

The visual appearance of a variable deceleration has been suggested to predict the underlying cause. For example, a V-shaped variable deceleration has been suggested to indicate umbilical cord compression due to oligohydramnios, whereas a W-shaped variable deceleration has been suggested to reflect umbilical cord compression due to a nuchal cord. Such atypical features have not been demonstrated to predict outcome independent of known confounding factors such as baseline rate, variability, and accelerations or frequency, duration, or number of decelerations. These terms are not included in standardized NICHD terminology.

Variability Within a Deceleration

At the nadir of a variable or late deceleration, the FHR frequently appears irregular, similar to the appearance of moderate variability. The visual similarity has led some to suggest that FHR fluctuations during a deceleration have the same clinical significance as baseline variability. Whereas the notion is not implausible, it has not been confirmed. In addition, it is inconsistent with standard NICHD terminology. Variability is a characteristic of the FHR baseline; it is not a characteristic of periodic or episodic decelerations that interrupt the baseline. In the absence of supporting evidence, the most appropriate approach is to avoid assigning undue significance to this observation. Evidence regarding these patterns is limited to level III.

Mild, Moderate, and Severe Variable Decelerations

The depth and duration of variable decelerations have been suggested to predict newborn outcome. Kubli and colleagues[28] proposed three categories of variable decelerations based upon these characteristics. According to this classification system, a *mild variable deceleration* was defined by a duration of less than 30 seconds regardless of depth, a depth no lower than 80 beats/min, or a depth of 70 to 80 beats/min that lasts less than 60 seconds. A *moderate variable deceleration* was defined by a depth of less than 70 beats/min that lasts 30 to 60 seconds or a depth of 70 to 80 beats/min that lasts more than 60 seconds. A *severe deceleration* was defined as a deceleration below 70 beats/min that lasts more than 60 seconds. No level I or level II evidence in the literature confirms that the depth of any type of deceleration—early, variable, late, or prolonged—is predictive of fetal metabolic acidemia, fetal hypoxia, or newborn outcome independent of other important FHR characteristics such as baseline rate, variability, accelerations and frequency, duration, and number of decelerations. Therefore mild, moderate, and severe categories are not included in standard NICHD definitions of FHR decelerations. The 2008 NICHD report[16] states that such classification requires further research investigation to determine clinical significance. Consistent with NICHD terminology, decelerations are quantitated by depth in beats per minute and duration in minutes and seconds.

STANDARDIZED MANAGEMENT DECISION MODEL

Evolving consensus regarding FHR definitions and interpretation facilitates the development of a standardized, evidence-based approach to intrapartum FHR management. Standardized FHR management does not replace individual clinical judgment. On the contrary, standardized management encourages the timely application of individual clinical judgment. By serving as a forcing function, standardized intrapartum FHR management helps to identify and avoid potential sources of preventable error in an organized, systematic fashion. A *forcing function* is a critical step in an algorithm that prevents the user from taking a subsequent action without consciously considering information relevant to that action. By forcing conscious attention upon the action, it helps to reduce the risk of error and increase the likelihood that the action will be reasonable. The management decision support model described in this chapter uses the standardized FHR definitions and categories proposed by the NICHD in 1997 and 2008.[14,16] It does not include adjunctive tests of fetal status such as fetal scalp blood sampling, fetal pulse oximetry, and fetal ECG analysis, which currently are unavailable for general clinical use in the United States. These techniques are reviewed later in the chapter.

Standard of Care

Standard of care is a legal concept that typically is defined as the level of care expected of a reasonable, competent clinician under similar circumstances. In order for care to be deemed reasonable, the underlying rationale must be credible. **Credibility requires factual accuracy and the ability to articulate clearly and understandably. Standard FHR definitions and interpretation facilitate factual accuracy. A standardized, simplified approach to FHR management provides an organized, evidence-based framework that can be articulated clearly and understandably.**

Initiation of Monitoring

Intrapartum monitoring is intended to assess the adequacy of fetal oxygenation and uterine activity during labor so that appropriate measures can be taken to avoid hypoxic fetal injury, ensure appropriate labor progress, and optimize the likelihood of safe vaginal delivery. **Effective intrapartum monitoring requires**

		"A" assess oxygen pathway	"B" begin corrective measures *if indicated*		"C" clear obstacles to rapid delivery	"D" determine decision to delivery time
Lungs		☐ Respiration	☐ Oxygen	Facility	Consider ☐ OR availability ☐ Equipment	Consider ☐ Facility response time
Heart		☐ Heart rate	☐ Position changes ☐ Fluid bolus ☐ Correct hypotension	Staff	Consider notifying ☐ *Obstetrician* ☐ *Surgical assistant* ☐ *Anesthesiologist* ☐ *Neonatologist* ☐ *Pediatrician* ☐ *Nursing staff*	Consider ☐ *Availability* ☐ *Training* ☐ *Experience*
Vasculature		☐ Blood pressure		Mother	Consider ☐ *Informed consent* ☐ *Anesthesia options* ☐ *Laboratory tests* ☐ *Blood products* ☐ *Intravenous access* ☐ *Urinary catheter* ☐ *Abdominal prep* ☐ *Transfer to OR*	☐ Surgical considerations *(prior abdominal or* *uterine surgery)* ☐ Medical considerations *(obesity, hypertension,* *diabetes, SLE)* ☐ Obstetric considerations *(parity, pelvimetry,* *placental location)*
Uterus		☐ Contraction strength ☐ Contraction frequency ☐ Contraction duration ☐ Baseline uterine tone ☐ Exclude uterine rupture	☐ Reduce stimulant ☐ Consider relaxant	Fetus	Consider ☐ *Fetal number* ☐ *Estimated fetal weight* ☐ *Gestational age* ☐ *Presentation* ☐ *Position* ☐ *Anomalies*	Consider ☐ *Fetal number* ☐ *Estimated fetal weight* ☐ *Gestational age* ☐ *Presentation* ☐ *Position* ☐ *Anomalies*
Placenta		☐ Check for bleeding				
Cord		☐ Exclude cord prolapse	☐ Consider amnioinfusion	Labor	☐ *Confirm that monitoring* *is adequate to allow* *appropriately informed* *management decisions*	Consider factors such as: ☐ *Protracted labor* ☐ *Previous uterine relaxant* ☐ *Remote from delivery* ☐ *Poor expulsive efforts*

FIG 15-21 "ABCD" approach to fetal heart rate management. OR, operating room; SLE, systemic lupus erythematosus.

reliable information; therefore it is essential to confirm that the monitor is recording the FHR and uterine activity adequately to permit appropriately informed management decisions (Fig. 15-21). If external monitoring does not provide adequate information for accurate definition and interpretation, internal monitoring with a fetal scalp electrode and/or IUPC should be considered. Under certain circumstances, the FHR monitor can inadvertently record the maternal heart rate. **If the fetus is not alive, an internal fetal scalp electrode can detect the maternal ECG and record the maternal heart rate. An external Doppler device can record the maternal heart rate even if the fetus is alive.** Particularly in the setting of maternal tachycardia, the maternal heart rate can appear deceptively similar to a normal FHR pattern, including normal-appearing baseline rate and variability. A widely recognized pattern that warrants particular attention is the observation of maternal heart rate accelerations during uterine contractions that can be mistaken for FHR accelerations. Heart rate accelerations that coincide with uterine contractions should prompt further evaluation to exclude this phenomenon. At times, the external Doppler monitor can alternate between the fetus and the mother. When switching from one to the other, the tracing will not necessarily demonstrate visual discontinuity; therefore visual continuity of the tracing alone cannot be relied upon to exclude this phenomenon. Some newer systems will alert the user to the presence of "signal coincidence" or "signal ambiguity" when the monitor's computer logic determines that the maternal heart rate derived from a maternal ECG or pulse oximetry transducer is the same as the presumed FHR derived from the Doppler transducer or scalp electrode. Suspected signal coincidence or ambiguity should prompt further evaluation to confirm the source of the heart rate signal. Unless the monitor is recording the FHR, it cannot be used to assess fetal oxygenation; therefore it is essential to distinguish between maternal and fetal heart rates. If any question exists, other methods should be used as needed, including ultrasound, palpation of the maternal pulse, fetal scalp electrode, or maternal pulse oximetry.

Evaluation of Fetal Heart Rate Components

Thorough, systematic evaluation of the FHR tracing includes assessment of uterine activity along with the FHR components defined by the NICHD: baseline rate, variability, accelerations, decelerations, sinusoidal pattern, and changes or trends in the tracing over time. **After assessing all components, the tracing can be placed into one of the three FHR categories introduced in the 2008 NICHD consensus report** (see Fig. 15-21).

If all FHR components are normal (category I), the FHR tracing reliably predicts the absence of interruption of oxygenation by the absence of variable, late, or prolonged decelerations and reliably predicts the absence of ongoing hypoxic neurologic

TABLE 15-5	NORMAL UMBILICAL CORD BLOOD VALUES			
VESSEL	**pH**	**PCO₂**	**PO₂**	**BASE DEFICIT**
Artery	7.2-7.3	45-55	15-25	<12
Vein	7.3-7.4	35-45	25-35	<12

injury by the presence of moderate variability with or without accelerations. In low-risk patients, ACOG Practice Bulletin 116 and ACOG-AAP *Guidelines for Perinatal Care* recommend that the FHR tracing should be reviewed at least every 30 minutes during the active phase of the first stage of labor and at least every 15 minutes during the second stage.[18,29] In patients who are not deemed to be low risk, the FHR tracing should be reviewed at least every 15 minutes during the active phase of the first stage of labor and at least every 5 minutes during the second stage (see Fig. 15-21). Documentation should be performed periodically at reasonable intervals in accordance with institutional policies and procedures.

A Standardized "ABCD" Approach to Fetal Heart Rate Management

If assessment of the FHR indicates that the tracing is not in category I, further evaluation is warranted. A practical, systematic "ABCD" approach to management begins with "A"—*assess* the oxygen pathway (see Fig. 15-21).

Assess the Oxygen Pathway

Rapid, systematic assessment of the pathway of oxygen transfer from the environment to the fetus can identify potential sources of interrupted oxygenation (Table 15-5). **Initial assessment of the maternal lungs, heart, and vasculature usually is accomplished by reviewing the vital signs, including respiratory rate, heart rate, and blood pressure. Uterine activity is assessed by palpation or by review of the information provided by a tocodynamometer or IUPC. Suspected uterine rupture or placental abruption requires immediate attention and targeted evaluation. Finally, umbilical cord prolapse usually can be excluded by visualization or examination. If rapid evaluation of these steps suggests that further investigation is warranted, it should be undertaken as necessary. As summarized in Figure 15-21, several maternal and fetal factors can influence the appearance of the FHR tracing by mechanisms other than direct interruption of fetal oxygenation. If FHR changes are thought to be due to any of these conditions, individualized assessment and management should be directed at the specific cause. Some examples include a sinusoidal pattern in the setting of severe fetal anemia, bradycardia due to fetal heart block, or tachycardia due to fever, infection, or medications or cardiac arrhythmia.**

Begin Corrective Measures as Indicated

If assessment of the oxygen pathway suggests interruption at one or more points, corrective measures are initiated as indicated. Specific measures are summarized in Figure 15-21. **The choice of appropriate corrective measures is based on interpretation of the FHR tracing as a whole. Interpretation of individual components out of context provides an incomplete clinical picture and is discouraged. Selection of the most appropriate corrective measures can be refined by acknowledging some specific associations. For example, in the setting of variable** decelerations, initial attention may focus on umbilical cord compression or prolapse. In the setting of late decelerations, initial attention may focus on maternal cardiac output, blood pressure, and uterine activity.

CONSERVATIVE CORRECTIVE MEASURES
SUPPLEMENTAL OXYGEN

Fetal oxygenation is dependent upon the oxygen content of maternal blood perfusing the intervillous space of the placenta. Administration of supplemental oxygen can increase the PO₂ of inspired air, increasing both the partial pressure of oxygen dissolved in maternal blood and the amount of oxygen bound to hemoglobin. This can increase the oxygen concentration gradient across the placental blood-blood barrier and can lead to increased fetal PO₂ and oxygen content. Several studies have reported resolution of FHR decelerations and improvement of variability after administration of supplemental oxygen to the mother, providing indirect evidence of improved fetal oxygenation.[30-32] Direct evidence is provided by fetal pulse oximetry studies that demonstrate increased fetal hemoglobin saturation following maternal administration of oxygen.[30-32] Higher saturation values may persist for 30 minutes after oxygen is discontinued. Evidence regarding the optimal duration of oxygen administration is inconsistent. The potential for fetal free radical production argues in favor of the use of supplemental oxygen in clinical settings in which there is a reasonable expectation of benefit.[32] Although the optimal method and duration of oxygen administration have not been established, available data support the use of a nonrebreather face mask to administer oxygen at a rate of 10 L/min for approximately 15 to 30 minutes.[30]

MATERNAL POSITION CHANGES

There are sound physiologic reasons to avoid the supine position during labor. In the supine position, the pressure of the gravid uterus on the inferior vena cava can impair venous return, cardiac output, and perfusion of the uterus and placenta. Pressure on the aorta and/or iliac arteries may impede the delivery of oxygenated blood to the uterus and placenta. Lateral maternal positioning (right or left) appears to have a more beneficial impact on fetal oxygen status than does the supine position.[30,33] In the setting of suspected umbilical cord compression, maternal position changes may result in fetal position changes and relief of pressure on the umbilical cord.

INTRAVENOUS FLUID ADMINISTRATION

Uteroplacental perfusion is dependent upon cardiac output and intravascular volume. Normal blood pressure does not necessarily reflect optimal intravascular volume, venous return, preload, or cardiac output. An intravascular bolus of isotonic fluid can improve cardiac output by increasing circulating volume, venous return, left ventricular end diastolic pressure, ventricular preload, and ultimately stroke volume in accordance with the Frank-Starling mechanism. Consequently, an increase in intravascular volume may have a significant impact on cardiac output and uteroplacental perfusion.[34] An intravenous (IV) fluid bolus of 500 to 1000 mL can result in improved fetal oxygenation even in an apparently euvolemic patient.[30,31] Caution must be exercised in patients at risk for volume overload and pulmonary edema. The optimal rate of IV fluid administration during labor is not known. Potential maternal and fetal complications argue against administering large-volume IV boluses of glucose-containing fluids.

CORRECT MATERNAL HYPOTENSION

A number of factors predispose laboring women to transient episodes of hypotension, including inadequate hydration, supine position resulting in compression of the inferior vena cava, decreased venous return and reduced cardiac output, and peripheral vasodilation due to sympathetic blockade during regional anesthesia. Maternal hypotension can reduce uteroplacental perfusion and fetal oxygenation. Maternal position changes and IV hydration usually correct the blood pressure. However, if these measures do not achieve the desired result, medication may be necessary. Ephedrine is a sympathomimetic amine with weak α- and β-agonist activity. The primary mechanism of action is the release of norepinephrine from presynaptic vesicles, which results in stimulation of postsynaptic adrenergic receptors.[34]

REDUCE UTERINE ACTIVITY

Excessive uterine activity is a common cause of interrupted fetal oxygenation. A number of terms used to describe excessive uterine activity—including *hyperstimulation, hypercontractility,* and *tetanic contraction*—are defined inconsistently in the literature. The 2008 NICHD consensus statement[16] recommended using the term *tachysystole* to describe uterine contraction frequency in excess of five contractions in 10 minutes averaged over 30 minutes. Normal contraction frequency is defined as five or fewer contractions in 10 minutes averaged over 30 minutes. Other important features of uterine activity include contraction intensity, duration, resting tone, and time between contractions. If an abnormal FHR pattern is thought to be related to excessive uterine activity, options include discontinuing uterine stimulants, reducing the dose of uterine stimulants, and/or administering uterine relaxants such as terbutaline.

AMNIOINFUSION

Intrapartum amnioinfusion involves the instillation of isotonic fluid through an intrauterine catheter into the amniotic cavity to restore the amniotic fluid volume to normal or near-normal levels. The procedure is intended to relieve intermittent umbilical cord compression, variable FHR decelerations, and transient episodes of interrupted fetal oxygenation. The impact of amnioinfusion on late decelerations is not known. Routine amnioinfusion for meconium-stained amniotic fluid without variable decelerations is not recommended.[35]

ALTER SECOND-STAGE PUSHING AND BREATHING TECHNIQUE

During the second stage of labor, maternal expulsive efforts can be associated with FHR decelerations. Suggested corrective approaches include open-glottis, rather than Valsalva-style, pushing; fewer pushing efforts per contraction; shorter individual pushing efforts; pushing with every other or every third contraction; and pushing only with perceived urge.[30,31] A systematic approach to FHR management does not require the use of all of these measures in every situation. It simply helps to ensure that important considerations are not overlooked and that decisions are made in a timely manner. In addition, it provides a framework to help clinicians articulate an organized, clear, and understandable plan of management—a key element of credibility, reasonableness, and the standard of care.

REEVALUATE THE FETAL HEART RATE TRACING

After assessing the oxygen pathway and beginning corrective measures deemed appropriate, the tracing is reevaluated. The time frame for reevaluation is based on clinical judgment and usually ranges from 5 to 30 minutes in accordance with ACOG-AAP guidelines and applicable institutional policies.[29] If the FHR tracing returns to category I and labor progress is adequate, continued surveillance is appropriate. The decision to perform routine or heightened surveillance is based on clinical judgment, taking into account the entire clinical situation. If the FHR tracing progresses to category III despite appropriate conservative corrective measures, delivery usually is expedited as rapidly as safely and reasonably feasible. Tracings that remain in category II warrant additional evaluation.

Category II is extremely broad and includes FHR tracings for which continued surveillance is appropriate. However, it also includes tracings that warrant preparation for rapid delivery. If a category II FHR tracing demonstrates moderate variability or accelerations and does not demonstrate clinically significant decelerations, continued surveillance is reasonable (Fig. 15-22). Category II tracings that do not meet these criteria require additional attention. If any question remains regarding the presence of moderate variability or accelerations or the clinical significance of any decelerations, a reasonable approach is to take the next step in the ABCD management model.

Clear Obstacles to Rapid Delivery

If conservative corrective measures do not correct the FHR tracing to the satisfaction of the clinician, it is reasonable to plan ahead by clearing common obstacles to rapid delivery. **This does not constitute a commitment to a particular time or method of delivery. Instead, this step serves as a forcing function to systematically address common sources of unnecessary delay so that important factors are not overlooked and decisions are made in a timely manner. This is accomplished by considering information relevant to the next action and communicating proactively with other members of the team. Potential sources of unnecessary delay can be grouped into major categories. Organized in nonrandom order from largest to smallest, these categories include the facility, staff, mother, fetus, and labor. Standardized intrapartum FHR management does not mandate that every possible corrective measure should be carried out. It simply provides a practical checklist of common factors that should be considered in order to optimize team communication, encourage timely decision making, and minimize preventable errors.**

Determine Decision-to-Delivery Time

When weighing the risks and benefits of continued expectant management versus expeditious delivery, the anticipated decision-to-delivery time must be taken into consideration. **After appropriate conservative measures have been implemented, it is reasonable to make a good-faith estimate of the time needed to accomplish delivery in the event of a sudden deterioration of the FHR. This step can be facilitated by systematically considering individual characteristics of the facility, staff, mother, fetus, and labor.**

Management steps in the ABCD model are amenable to standardization and represent the majority of decisions that must be made during labor. However, once they are exhausted, further management decisions require the individual judgment of the clinician, who ultimately will assume responsibility for the safety of the mother and the fetus in the event that operative delivery becomes necessary.

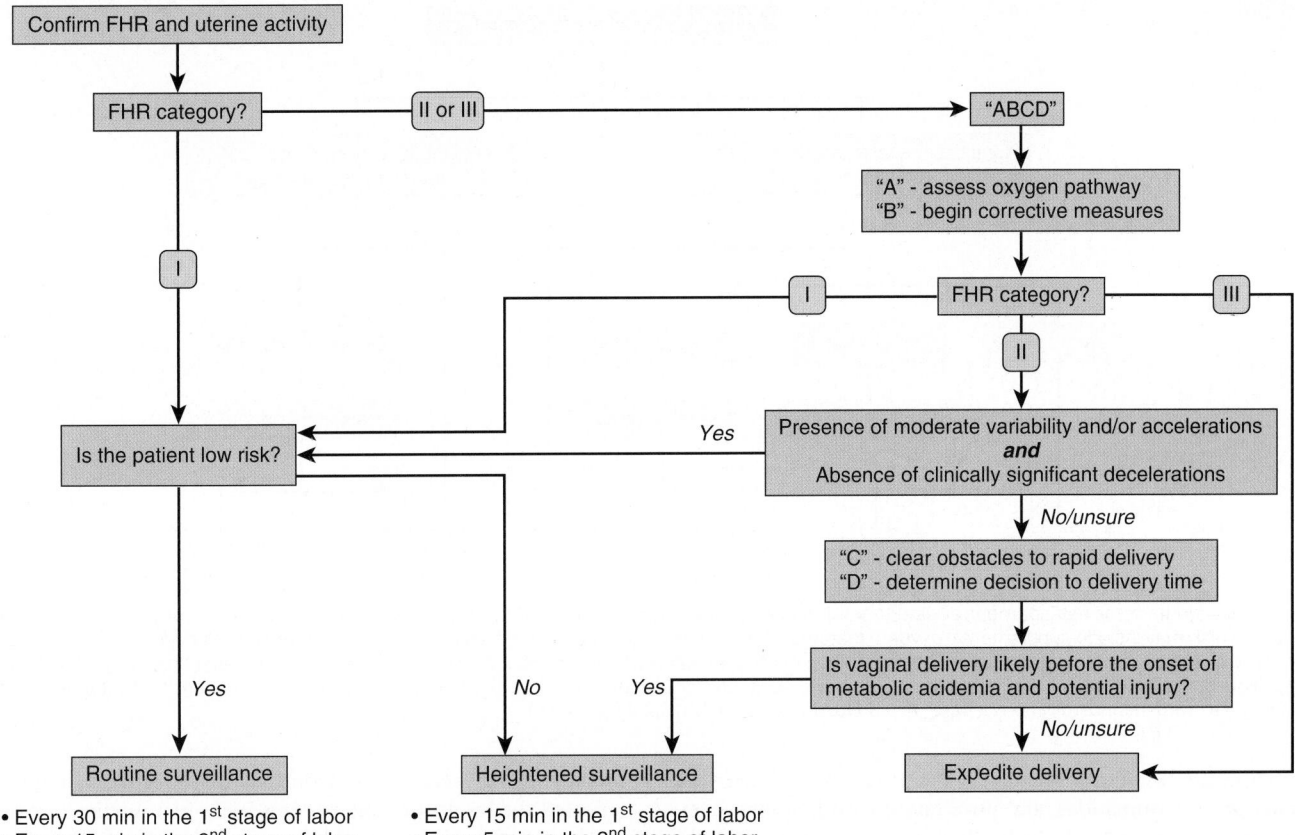

FIG 15-22 Intrapartum fetal heart rate (FHR) management decision model.

Expectant Management Versus Delivery

If conservative measures do not correct a persistent category II FHR tracing, the clinician must decide whether to continue to await spontaneous vaginal delivery or to proceed with operative delivery. **The decision balances the likelihood of safe vaginal delivery against the potential for fetal hypoxic injury. In 2013, Clark and colleagues[36] proposed a standardized approach to the management of persistent category II FHR tracings.** As illustrated in Figure 15-23, the algorithm emphasizes the reliability of moderate variability or accelerations to exclude ongoing hypoxic injury.[36]

For the purposes of this algorithm, *significant decelerations* are defined as late decelerations or variable decelerations that last more than 60 seconds. **Recommended management of prolonged decelerations includes discontinuation of the algorithm and initiation of appropriate corrective measures. In the setting of moderate variability or accelerations and normal progress in the active phase or second stage of labor, the algorithm permits continued expectant management with close observation in most cases, regardless of the presence of decelerations. One exception is the scenario in which conservative measures fail to correct recurrent significant decelerations remote from delivery. Another is the setting in which vaginal bleeding and/or previous cesarean section introduce the risks of placental abruption or uterine rupture. In such situations, further evaluation may be necessary, and adherence to the algorithm should be individualized. On the other side of the algorithm, if moderate variability and accelerations are absent, and recurrent significant decelerations fail to respond to corrective measures for 30 minutes,** delivery should be considered regardless of the stage of labor. **If moderate variability and accelerations are absent for 30 minutes *without* recurrent decelerations, the algorithm permits observation for an hour, beyond which time persistence of the pattern warrants consideration of delivery. This algorithm reflects the consensus of 18 authors regarding one reasonable approach to persistent category II FHR patterns. No single approach to such patterns has been demonstrated to be superior to all others. However, a growing body of evidence supports the concept that the adoption of one appropriate management plan, by virtue of standardization alone, will yield results superior to those achieved by random application of several individually equivalent approaches.**[36,37]

Other Methods of Evaluating Fetal Status

One of the primary shortcomings of electronic FHR monitoring is the high rate of false-positive results. Even the most abnormal FHR patterns are poorly predictive of neonatal morbidity. **Consequently, alternative methods of evaluating fetal status have been explored and include fetal scalp pH and lactate determination, fetal stimulation, computer analysis of FHR, fetal pulse oximetry, and ST-segment analysis. In assessing the immediate condition of the newborn, umbilical cord acid-base determination can serve as an adjunct to the Apgar score.**

Intrapartum Fetal Scalp pH and Lactate Determination

Intermittent sampling of fetal scalp blood for pH determination was described in the 1960s and was studied extensively in the 1970s. However, its use has been limited by many factors, including the requirements for cervical dilation and membrane

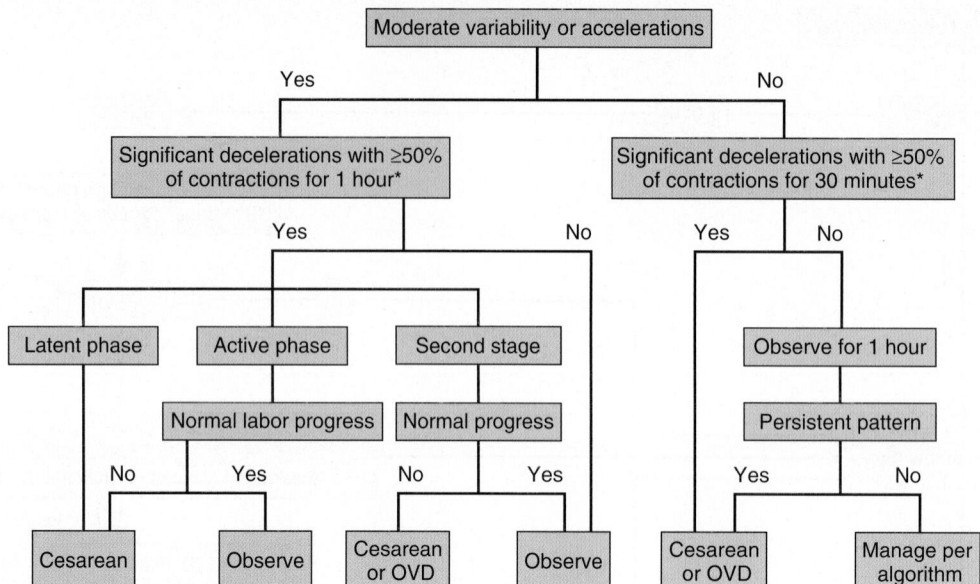

FIG 15-23 Algorithm for management of category II fetal heart rate tracings. *Have not resolved with appropriate conservative corrective measures, which may include supplemental oxygen, maternal position changes, intravenous fluid administration, correction of hypotension, reduction or discontinuation of uterine stimulation, administration of uterine relaxant, amnioinfusion, and/or changes in second-stage breathing and pushing techniques. OVD, operative vaginal delivery. (Clark SL, Nageotte MP, Garite TJ, et al. Intrapartum management of category II fetal heart rate tracings: towards standardization of care. *Am J Obstet Gynecol.* 2013;209[2]:89-97.)

rupture, the technical difficulty of the procedure, the need for serial pH determinations, and uncertainty regarding interpretation and application of results. It is used infrequently in the United States but remains a common practice in many other countries. A recent meta-analysis[38] compared fetal scalp pH determination to fetal scalp lactate determination and found no differences in maternal, fetal, neonatal, or infant outcomes. Goodwin and colleagues[39] reported that the elimination of fetal scalp pH determination in a large clinical service resulted in no increase in the rates of cesarean delivery for fetal distress, low Apgar scores requiring neonatal intensive care unit (NICU) admission, or the clinical diagnosis of perinatal asphyxia.

Fetal Scalp Stimulation and Vibroacoustic Stimulation

A number of studies have reported that FHR accelerations in response to fetal scalp stimulation or vibroacoustic stimulation (VAS) are highly predictive of normal scalp blood pH.[40,41] A literature review and meta-analysis by Skupski and colleagues[42] confirmed the utility of various methods of intrapartum fetal stimulation, including scalp puncture, atraumatic stimulation with an Allis clamp, VAS, and digital stimulation. Fetal scalp stimulation, VAS, and halogen light stimulation can be used to provoke FHR accelerations in order to exclude the presence of fetal metabolic acidemia.[42] Accelerations provoked by fetal stimulation have the same prognostic significance as spontaneous FHR accelerations.[16] Fetal stimulation should be performed at times when the FHR is at baseline. The utility of fetal stimulation during FHR decelerations or bradycardia has not been established.

Computer Analysis of Fetal Heart Rate

Visual analysis of the FHR has been plagued by reports of poor interobserver and intraobserver reliability. In an attempt to overcome these limitations, Dawes and others[43,44] derived an objective system of numeric FHR analysis. Computer analysis of intrapartum FHR records has been reported to be more precise than visual assessment but has not been shown to improve

prediction of neonatal outcome.[45] Keith and colleagues[46] reported the results of a multicenter trial of an intelligent computer system that used clinical data in addition to FHR data. In 50 cases analyzed, the system's performance was indistinguishable from that of 17 expert clinicians. The authors reported that the system was highly consistent, recommended no unnecessary intervention, and performed better than all but two of the experts.

Fetal Pulse Oximetry

Intrapartum reflectance fetal pulse oximetry is a modification of transmission pulse oximetry that indirectly measures the oxygen saturation of hemoglobin in fetal blood. An intrauterine sensor placed in contact with fetal skin uses the differential absorption of red and infrared light by oxygenated and deoxygenated fetal hemoglobin to provide a continuous estimation of fetal oxygen saturation. Several studies have examined the utility of intrapartum fetal pulse oximetry.[47-52] Although the studies reported a reduction in the incidence of cesarean delivery for fetal indications, no consistent impact on overall cesarean rates or newborn outcomes has been demonstrated. The results of a number of randomized trials led the manufacturer to announce that it would no longer distribute the sensors in the United States, effectively withdrawing the product from the market.

P-R and ST-Segment Analysis

P-R and ST-segment analysis study of the fetal ECG has produced varying results. In animal studies, FHR decelerations that accompany hypoxemia have been observed in association with characteristic changes in the fetal P-R interval. Strachan and colleagues[53] compared standard EFM to EFM plus P-R interval analysis in 1038 women. The groups demonstrated statistically similar rates of operative intervention for presumed fetal distress and the authors reported no differences in newborn outcomes. The ST segment of the fetal ECG reflects myocardial repolarization. Myocardial hypoxia can lead to elevation of the ST segment and T wave secondary to catecholamine release, β-adrenoceptor activation, glycogenolysis, and tissue metabolic acidosis.[54-58] These observations have led to the development of technology to analyze the fetal ECG plus the ST waveform (STAN; Neoventa Medical). One randomized trial[59] in 2434 patients demonstrated a 46% reduction in operative intervention for fetal distress when ST-segment analysis was added to standard EFM. Operative interventions for dystocia and other indications were not increased. Fewer cases of metabolic acidemia and low 5-minute Apgar scores were observed in the group with EFM plus ST-segment analysis; however, these differences did not reach statistical significance. Another trial[60] that used newer technology included 4966 women randomized to EFM alone versus EFM plus ST-segment analysis. When analyzed according to intention to treat, the incidence of umbilical artery acidemia was 53% lower in the group who had EFM plus ST-segment analysis, but cesarean delivery rates were not different. A large multicenter trial[61] randomized 5681 women to intrapartum EFM alone versus EFM plus ST-segment analysis. No significant difference was observed in the primary outcome of *metabolic acidosis,* defined as an umbilical artery pH below 7.05 with a base deficit of more than 12 mmol/L in the extracellular fluid. In the group with EFM plus ST analysis, statistically fewer cases were reported of fetal blood sampling during labor (10.6% vs. 20.4%), umbilical artery pH below 7.05 and base deficit greater than 12 mmol/L in the blood (1.6% vs. 2.6%), and umbilical artery pH below 7.05 (1.9% vs. 2.7%). Cesarean deliveries, instrumented vaginal deliveries, and total operative deliveries occurred with statistically similar frequency in both groups, with no differences in operative deliveries for fetal distress. No other statistically significant differences were reported in newborn outcome. A 2013 meta-analysis[62] of five studies that included 15,338 women concluded that adjunctive ST-segment analysis resulted in fewer fetal scalp samples, fewer operative vaginal deliveries, and fewer NICU admissions. However, no significant differences were found in the rate of cesarean births, low Apgar scores, metabolic acidemia at birth, neonatal intubation, or neonatal encephalopathy.

The Eunice Kennedy Shriver NICHD Maternal Fetal Medicine Units Network recently completed analysis of data from a Phase III trial (NCT01131260) of the safety and efficacy of fetal ECG ST-segment and T-wave analysis (STAN) as an adjunct to electronic FHR monitoring. The study[63] randomized 11,108 women to undergo standard intrapartum FHR monitoring alone or standard FHR monitoring plus STAN. No significant differences were found between the groups in the primary outcome—a composite of one or more of intrapartum fetal death, neonatal death, Apgar score of 3 of lower at 5 minutes, neonatal seizure, umbilical cord artery pH of 7.05 or lower plus base deficit of at least 12 mmol/L, intubation for ventilation at delivery, and neonatal encephalopathy. Moreover, no differences were reported between the groups in operative vaginal deliveries, cesarean deliveries, NICU stay, meconium aspiration, or shoulder dystocia. The authors concluded that the use of STAN as an adjunct to conventional intrapartum electronic FHR monitoring did not improve perinatal outcomes, nor did it decrease operative deliveries in hospitals in the United States.[63]

Abdominal Fetal Electrocardiogram

A noninvasive abdominal fetal ECG (fECG) monitoring system, the Monica AN24 (Monica Healthcare, Nottingham, UK) has been approved for clinical practice.[64] The system uses five ECG electrodes placed around the maternal abdomen. The electrodes detect the fetal ECG, as well as the uterine electromyogram, to provide a continuous display of FHR and uterine activity. Prospective observational studies have demonstrated that FHR detection using abdominal fECG was more reliable and accurate than Doppler ultrasound during the first stage of labor and was equivalent to Doppler during the second stage.[64] Abdominal fECG was less likely than Doppler ultrasound to display the maternal heart rate in place of the fetal heart rate. Another study demonstrated that Doppler ultrasound detection of FHR degraded with increasing maternal body mass index (BMI); however, maternal habitus did not affect the accuracy and reliability of the abdominal fECG.[65]

Umbilical Cord Blood Gas Determination

Umbilical cord blood gas and pH assessment is a useful adjunct to the Apgar score in assessing the immediate condition of the newborn. **No contraindications exist to obtaining cord gases. The ACOG Committee on Obstetric Practice recommends that physicians should attempt to obtain umbilical venous and arterial blood samples in the following situations**[66]:

- Cesarean delivery for fetal compromise
- Low 5-minute Apgar score
- Severe growth restriction
- Abnormal fetal heart rate tracing
- Maternal thyroid disease
- Intrapartum fever
- Multifetal gestations

Immediately after delivery of the neonate, a segment of umbilical cord should be double-clamped and divided. A clamped segment of cord will remain stable for pH, PO_2, and PCO_2 analysis for at least 60 minutes.[65] A cord blood sample in a heparin-flushed syringe is stable for up to 60 minutes.[64] Base-deficit values may increase by 1.2 mmol/L in 20 minutes and by 4.5 mmol/L in 60 minutes.[13,65] Lactate values can increase by 40% within 20 minutes and by 245% in 60 minutes, therefore if warranted by the condition of the neonate, blood should be drawn from an artery and a vein in the clamped cord segment and should be sent to the laboratory for blood gas analysis, including pH, PO_2, PCO_2, and base deficit, preferably within 20 minutes. If blood gas analysis is expected to take longer than 20 minutes, the syringe should be stored on ice. In all such cases, base deficit and lactate values should be interpreted with caution.[13] Umbilical arterial values reflect the metabolic status of fetal tissues before placental gas exchange, whereas umbilical venous values reflect metabolic status after gas and acid transfer in the placenta. Normal umbilical arterial results preclude significant fetal hypoxia or acidemia around the time of delivery. An attempt should be made to obtain paired arterial and venous specimens to help ensure that at least one artery is sampled and to minimize debate over whether a true arterial specimen was obtained. If it is not possible to draw blood from the umbilical cord, blood may be obtained from the surface of the placenta, where umbilical arteries cross over veins. Blood gas values can change significantly over time when the sample is obtained from the placenta via an unclamped vessel. Therefore such samples should be analyzed as promptly as possible and interpreted with appropriate caution. Exposure of arterial or venous samples to air tends to increase the PO_2 and decrease the PCO_2 toward atmospheric values.[13] Approximate normal values for cord blood are summarized in Table 15-5.[7,8,13]

The base deficit reflects utilization of buffer bases (primarily bicarbonate) to help stabilize pH, usually in the setting of peripheral tissue hypoxia, anaerobic metabolism, and production and accumulation of lactic acid. An umbilical artery pH less than 7.20 usually is considered to define acidemia. **A much lower pH (7.0) has been defined as the threshold of potential injury. Acidemia is categorized as respiratory, metabolic, or mixed. Isolated *respiratory acidemia* is diagnosed when the umbilical artery pH is less than 7.20, the PCO$_2$ is elevated, and the base deficit is less than 12 mmol/L. This reflects interrupted exchange of blood gases, usually as a transient phenomenon related to umbilical cord compression. Isolated respiratory acidemia is not associated with fetal neurologic injury.**[9] **Isolated *metabolic acidemia* is diagnosed when the pH is less than 7.20, the PCO$_2$ is normal, and the base deficit is at least 12 mmol/L. Metabolic acidemia can result from recurrent or prolonged interruption of fetal oxygenation that has progressed to the stage of peripheral tissue hypoxia, anaerobic metabolism, and lactic acid production in excess of buffering capacity.** Although most cases of fetal metabolic acidemia do not result in injury, the risk is increased in the setting of significant metabolic acidemia (umbilical artery pH <7.0 and base deficit ≥12 mmol/L).[11,12] **Mixed acidemia (respiratory and metabolic) is diagnosed when the pH is below 7.20, the PCO$_2$ is elevated, and the base deficit is 12 mmol/L or greater. The clinical significance of mixed acidemia is similar to that of isolated metabolic acidemia. The categories of acidemia are summarized in** Table 15-6.

ALTERNATIVES TO ELECTRONIC FETAL MONITORING
Electronic Fetal Monitoring Versus Traditional Auscultation

As early as the nineteenth century, certain audible FHR patterns were observed to be associated with poor newborn outcome. In the 1960s, the introduction of EFM and fetal scalp blood sampling provided additional tools to evaluate the fetus. In 1967, Hon and Quilligan[67] proposed a system for classifying FHR decelerations. In 1969, Kubli and Hon[28] explored the relationship between the type and severity of FHR deceleration and the

fetal scalp blood pH. They reported that fetuses with no decelerations, early decelerations, or mild variable decelerations had average scalp pH values greater than 7.29, whereas those with severe variable or late decelerations had pH values below 7.15. Investigators have demonstrated the importance of FHR variability and FHR accelerations as indicators of the absence of metabolic acidemia and ongoing hypoxic injury.[40,41] When intrapartum EFM replaced the traditional practice of intermittent auscultation (IA) in the 1970s, a series of studies reported significantly lower perinatal mortality rates in electronically monitored patients. These studies were nonrandomized and used nonconcurrent controls. Critics have cited rapidly improving neonatal care and falling perinatal mortality rates as possible sources of bias. During the time of these studies, hospitals that were not using EFM experienced improvements in perinatal outcome similar to those seen in hospitals that were using EFM.[68] Nevertheless, these studies had the effect of validating the use of EFM. In 1976, the first of a series of randomized controlled trials was published that compared EFM to IA during labor. To date, 12 such studies have been published.[69-80] These trials are summarized in Table 15-7.

Randomized Controlled Trials of Electronic Fetal Monitoring Versus Auscultation

In 1976, Haverkamp and associates[69] reported the first prospective randomized study of 483 high-risk obstetric patients to compare EFM to IA in labor. In the EFM group, a scalp electrode was placed as soon as possible. Auscultation in the control (IA) group was performed every 15 minutes in the first stage of labor and every 5 minutes in the second stage, for 30 seconds after uterine contractions. Electronic monitoring was used in both groups but was blinded in the IA group. In the EFM group, FHR patterns were evaluated using the criteria of Kubli and Hon.[28] In patients with late decelerations or severe variable decelerations that persisted after 15 minutes of corrective measures (oxygen, positional changes, correction of hypotension), delivery was accomplished. "Fetal distress" in the IA group was diagnosed by the presence of bradycardia to 100 beats/min after three or more consecutive contractions. Delivery was accomplished if the pattern was not relieved within 15 minutes. No significant differences were reported between the EFM and control groups in the outcomes of perinatal mortality, Apgar scores, cord blood pH values, neurologic signs in the neonate, or neonatal nursery morbidity. The monitored group, however, had significantly higher rates of cesarean delivery overall (16.5%

TABLE 15-6	CATEGORIES OF UMBILICAL ARTERY ACIDEMIA		
VALUE	**RESPIRATORY**	**METABOLIC**	**MIXED**
pH	<7.20	<7.20	<7.20
PCO$_2$	Elevated	Normal	Elevated
Base deficit	<12 mmol/L	≥12 mmol/L	≥12 mmol/L

TABLE 15-7	RANDOMIZED TRIALS OF ELECTRONIC FETAL MONITORING VERSUS INTERMITTENT AUSCULTATION				
STUDY	**YEAR**	**N**	**PERINATAL MORBIDITY**	**PERINATAL MORTALITY**	**CESAREAN RATE**
Haverkamp[69]	1976	483	No difference	No difference	Higher in EFM group
Renou[70]	1976	350	See text	No difference	Higher in EFM group
Kelso[71]	1978	504	No difference	No difference	Higher in EFM group
Haverkamp[72]	1979	690	No difference	No difference	Higher in EFM group
Wood[73]	1981	989	No difference	No difference	No difference
MacDonald[74]	1985	12,964	Lower in EFM group*	No difference	No difference
Neldam[75]	1986	969	No difference	No difference	No difference
Leveno[76]	1986	14,618	No difference	No difference	Not reported†
Luthy[77]	1987	246	No difference	No difference	No difference
Vintzileos[78]	1993	1428	No difference	Lower in EFM group‡	No difference
Herbst[79]	1994	4044	No difference	No difference	No difference
Madaan[80]	2006	100	No difference	No difference	No difference

*Fewer neonatal seizures were reported in the electronic fetal monitoring (EFM) group, but no difference was found at 4 years of age.
†The cesarean rate for fetal indications was higher in the EFM group, but overall cesarean rates were not reported.
‡The study ended after the third quarterly review because of a statistically significant fivefold decrease in perinatal mortality in the EFM group.

vs. 6.8%) and higher rates of cesarean delivery for "fetal distress" (7.4% vs. 1.2%).

The second study, by Renou and colleagues[70] in 1976, randomized 350 patients to undergo intrapartum fetal monitoring with EFM or IA. Continuous EFM was performed in the study group, and scalp pH was measured if the FHR tracing was judged to be abnormal. The protocol for auscultation in the IA group was not reported. No significant differences were found between the groups with respect to perinatal mortality, Apgar scores, or maternal or neonatal infection; however, patients in the monitored group had significantly higher cord blood pH values and significantly lower rates of NICU admission, neonatal neurologic signs and symptoms, and neonatally diagnosed brain damage (not further defined). The cesarean section rate was significantly higher in the monitored group than in the control group (22.3% vs. 13.7%), but the rates of cesarean delivery for suspected fetal compromise were not reported.

In 1978, Kelso and colleagues published the third randomized controlled trial (RCT) to compare EFM and IA in 504 patients.[71] Continuous EFM was used in study patients, and a fetal scalp electrode was placed as early as possible. Auscultation in the IA group was performed at least every 15 minutes for 1 minutes during and immediately following a contraction. Crossover was not permitted, and scalp pH determination was not utilized. No significant differences were reported between the groups with respect to perinatal mortality, low Apgar scores, cord blood pH values, NICU admissions or lengths of stay, neonatal or maternal infections, or abnormal neonatal neurologic findings. The only significant difference between the groups was an increase in the incidence of cesarean birth in the monitored group (9.5% vs. 4.4%); however, no significant difference was found in the incidence of cesarean delivery for fetal distress (EFM 1.6%, control 1.2%).

In 1979, Haverkamp and associates[72] published another RCT that included additional measures of infant status and the option to perform fetal scalp pH determination during labor. A total of 690 high-risk patients were randomized into three groups: in the first group, fetal assessment during labor was accomplished by IA; the second group had continuous EFM alone; and the third group had continuous EFM with the option to measure scalp blood pH as needed. Among the three groups, no significant differences were seen in perinatal mortality, Apgar scores, cord blood pH values, maternal or neonatal infectious morbidity, NICU admissions, or neonatal neurologic abnormalities. A significant increase in the incidence of cesarean birth was demonstrated in the group monitored with EFM alone (EFM alone, 18%; EFM with the option to scalp sample, 11%; IA, 6%). The option to perform scalp sampling resulted in an intermediate cesarean delivery rate that was not significantly different from either of the other groups. Analyzed together, electronically monitored patients had a significantly higher incidence of cesarean delivery for fetal distress than did controls (5.2% vs. 0.43%).

The fifth trial was published in 1981 by Wood and colleagues,[73] wherein a total of 989 patients were randomized to undergo EFM or IA during labor. Monitored patients had placement of a fetal scalp electrode as early as possible. The protocol for auscultated patients was not described. Scalp pH measurements were performed as needed, and no significant differences were found between the groups in perinatal mortality, Apgar scores, cord blood pH values, NICU admissions, or neonatal neurologic abnormalities. In this study, the overall rate of operative intervention (including forceps) was significantly higher in

the monitored group, but the cesarean delivery rates were not significantly different (4% in the EFM group and 2% in the IA group). Rates of cesarean delivery for fetal distress were not reported.

In 1985, MacDonald and colleagues[74] published a randomized controlled trial that compared EFM to IA in 12,964 pregnancies. It was the first study to calculate prospectively the sample size needed to demonstrate statistically significant differences between the groups. Prior to initiation of the study, estimates were made of the anticipated frequencies of intrapartum stillbirths, neonatal deaths, neonatal seizures in survivors, and other severe abnormal neurologic characteristics. The authors calculated that 13,000 patients would be needed to demonstrate a 50% reduction in the combined incidence of intrapartum stillbirths, neonatal deaths, and neonatal seizures in survivors (power 75%, $P = .05$). A trial of that size would have a 50% chance of detecting a 50% reduction in the rate of seizures alone. In the EFM group, a fetal scalp electrode was applied as early as possible, and scalp pH measurements were performed as needed. Criteria for evaluation of the FHR tracings were similar to those of Kubli and Hon.[28] Suspicious or ominous tracings were those with marked tachycardia or bradycardia, moderate tachycardia or bradycardia with decreased variability, absent to minimal variability, late decelerations, moderate to severe variable decelerations, and other difficult-to-interpret patterns. In the first stage of labor, a scalp pH evaluation was performed if such patterns persisted for at least 10 minutes. A scalp pH below 7.20 was an indication for delivery. If the fetal scalp pH was between 7.20 and 7.25 with persistent suspicious or ominous FHR patterns, or if it was less than 7.20 regardless of the FHR pattern, delivery was accomplished. If the scalp pH was greater than 7.25 but the tracing remained suspicious or ominous, the scalp pH was repeated within 30 to 60 minutes. In the second stage of labor, delivery was accomplished if FHR abnormalities persisted for at least 10 minutes. In the control group, IA was performed every 15 minutes for 60 seconds in the first stage of labor and between each contraction during the second stage. If the FHR was less than 100 beats/min or greater than 160 beats/min during three contractions and could not be corrected with conservative measures, a scalp pH was measured and managed as above, or delivery was expedited, depending on the stage of labor. Blood sampling also was performed at unspecified intervals in the control group when labor exceeded 8 hours, and no significant differences were found between the groups in perinatal mortality, low Apgar scores, neonatal trauma, resuscitation requirement, NICU admissions, or infectious morbidity. Among the 28 perinatal deaths, asphyxia was considered to be the primary cause in seven patients in each group. Significantly more cases of neonatal seizures and persistent neurologic abnormalities (>1 week) were present in the control group. However, follow-up at 4 years of age revealed three cases of CP in each group.[81] Labor was significantly shorter in the EFM group, and analgesia was required less often. Twice as many fetuses with low scalp pH (<7.20) were identified in the EFM group, and scalp sampling was used more frequently (EFM 4.4%, control 3.5%). The cesarean delivery rate in the EFM group (2.4%) was not significantly different from that in the auscultated group (2.2%). Overall rates of operative delivery were higher in the EFM group (10.6% vs. 8.5%) because of an increased use of forceps (8.2% vs. 6.3%). Rates of cesarean delivery for fetal distress were not significantly different (EFM 0.4%, IA 0.2%). In this study, the largest to date, EFM was associated with no increase in maternal morbidity.

In 1986, Neldam and colleagues[75] reported a randomized controlled trial of EFM versus IA in 969 patients. In the EFM group, monitoring was initiated when patients no longer desired to ambulate. A scalp electrode was placed as soon as possible thereafter. In the IA group, fetal heart tones were auscultated twice an hour for at least 15 seconds at cervical dilation less than 5 cm, every 15 minutes from 5 cm until the second stage of labor, and for 30 seconds after each contraction or at least every 5 minutes during the second stage. Scalp pH sampling was optional and was performed only five times (EFM three, control two). No statistical differences were detected between the groups with respect to perinatal mortality, low Apgar scores, seizures, NICU admissions, or lengths of stay. Significantly more abnormal FHR patterns were detected in the EFM group, however, no difference was reported in the incidence of cesarean delivery.

In 1986, Leveno and colleagues[76] published a prospective trial that included 14,618 patients randomized to EFM or IA during alternate months. Perinatal mortality, 5-minute Apgar scores, NICU admissions, ventilator requirement, and neonatal seizures were similar in the two groups. More abnormal FHR patterns were observed in the monitored group, which led to significantly more cesarean sections for "fetal distress" (9% vs. 4%). However, overall cesarean rates were not reported.

The ninth study, by Luthy and colleagues[77] in 1987, compared EFM and IA in 246 patients with preterm labor. In the EFM group, external monitoring was used until advanced cervical dilation (7 cm) had been attained, at which time amniotomy was performed and a scalp electrode was placed. In those with ruptured membranes, a scalp electrode was placed once delivery was inevitable. Fetal scalp blood sampling was used as clinically indicated in both groups. The groups did not differ with respect to the use of tocolytics, corticosteroids, oxytocin, or regional anesthesia. No differences were found in perinatal mortality, low Apgar scores, cord pH values, neonatal seizures, respiratory distress syndrome, or intracranial hemorrhage. Cesarean section rates were not statistically different (EFM 15.6%, controls 15.2%), and no difference was found in the incidence of cesarean delivery for "fetal distress" (EFM 8.2%, controls 5.6%).

In 1993, Vintzileos and colleagues[78] published a randomized trial that was conducted in Greece to compare EFM and IA in 1428 patients in a population with high baseline perinatal mortality rates (20.4 to 22.6 per 1000). The relatively high incidence of perinatal death markedly improved the likelihood of detecting a statistically significant effect of EFM. The authors prospectively calculated that in a sample of 2210 patients, they would have an 80% chance of detecting a 67% reduction in perinatal mortality at a 0.05 level of significance. Reviews were conducted every 3 months, and the study was ended after the third review in light of a statistically significant fivefold decrease in perinatal mortality in the EFM group, in which external monitoring was used as long as satisfactory tracings were obtained. Scalp electrodes were placed as needed. In the control group, IA was performed every 15 minutes during the first stage of labor and every 5 minutes during the second stage. Fetal scalp blood sampling was not used in either group, and crossover was not permitted. Significantly fewer perinatal deaths occurred in the EFM group than in the controls (2.6 vs. 13 per 1000), and no hypoxia-related perinatal deaths were reported in the EFM group, whereas 6 such deaths occurred in the auscultation group (0.9%). This difference was statistically significant. The groups did not differ significantly with respect to low Apgar scores, NICU admissions or lengths of stay, ventilator requirements,

neonatal HIE, intraventricular hemorrhage, seizures, hypotonia, necrotizing enterocolitis, or respiratory distress syndrome. The incidence of cesarean delivery for fetal distress was significantly higher in the EFM group (5.3% vs. 2.3%), but the overall incidence of cesarean birth was not significantly different between the EFM and IA groups (9.5% vs. 8.6%).

In Sweden in 1994, Herbst and Ingemarsson[79] randomized 4044 patients to receive continuous EFM or intermittent EFM with IA during labor. In the latter group, EFM was used for 10 to 30 minutes every 2 to 2.5 hours during the first stage of labor with intermittent auscultation every 15 to 30 minutes between recording periods. No statistically significant differences were found between the groups in the rates of cesarean delivery, cesarean delivery for fetal distress, low umbilical artery pH values, low Apgar scores, or admissions to the NICU.

In India in 2006, Madaan and Trivedi[80] randomized 100 patients with one previous low transverse cesarean delivery to either continuous EFM or IA during labor and found no differences between the groups in maternal or neonatal morbidity or in rates of vaginal, forceps, or cesarean delivery.

Summary of Randomized Trials of Electronic Fetal Monitoring Versus Intermittent Auscultation

Randomized trials have demonstrated, with some caveats, that IA and EFM can perform similarly with respect to perinatal morbidity and mortality without contemporary evidence of a significant impact on cesarean delivery rates. It is important to note that the randomized trials compared EFM with IA combined with one-on-one nursing and frequent auscultation of fetal heart sounds. This level of individualized nursing care may be available in some settings, however, most obstetric units will find the personnel requirements to be impractical and cost prohibitive. Although FHR decelerations and accelerations can be detected with IA, no evidence suggests that IA can confirm the presence of moderate variability—an FHR characteristic that has emerged as one of the most reliable measures of adequate fetal oxygenation, and one that is used by clinicians on a daily basis to ensure that it is safe to continue labor. Thus in most of the randomized trials, an abnormal FHR observed during IA warranted a change to EFM. The safety of managing an abnormal FHR pattern with IA alone has not been established. The AGOC-AAP *Guidelines for Perinatal Care*[29] indicate that EFM or IA may be used to determine fetal status during labor. When IA is used, obstetric unit guidelines should clearly delineate the procedures to be followed, including the consistent use of standard NICHD definitions of FHR. In the absence of risk factors, a standard approach is to determine, evaluate, and record the FHR every 30 minutes in the active phase of the first stage of labor and at least every 15 minutes in the second stage.[29] If risk factors are present, the FHR should be determined, evaluated, and recorded at least every 15 minutes during the active phase of the first stage of labor, preferably before, during, and after a uterine contraction. During the second stage, the FHR should be determined, evaluated, and recorded at least every 5 minutes.[29]

POTENTIAL RISKS OF ELECTRONIC FETAL MONITORING

Infection

Early concerns regarding the potential for maternal or neonatal bacterial infections in electronically monitored patients appear to have been unfounded. One randomized trial demonstrated an increased risk of maternal infectious morbidity in patients randomized to EFM.[69] However, these results are difficult to interpret in light of the fact that fetal scalp electrodes were used in both the EFM and IA groups (FHR tracings were recorded in the IA group, but clinicians were blinded to them). The largest randomized trial to date revealed no increased infectious morbidity in electronically monitored patients.[74] Nevertheless, **disruption of the integrity of fetal skin with a fetal scalp electrode should be avoided in patients at risk for vertical perinatal transmission of viral infections, including human immunodeficiency virus (HIV), herpes simplex virus (HSV), and hepatitis.**

Operative Intervention

Meta-analyses of the randomized trials of EFM versus IA have reported higher rates of operative intervention in monitored patients compared with controls.[82,83] A Cochrane review[84] that spanned three decades reported a 15% higher rate of instrumental vaginal delivery in electronically monitored patients (risk ratio [RR], 1.15; 95% confidence interval [CI], 1.01 to 1.33). The same review reported a 63% higher rate of cesarean delivery in electronically monitored patients (RR, 1.63; 95% CI, 1.29 to 2.07).[84] However, published data from the most contemporary randomized trials suggest that the effect of EFM on cesarean delivery rates is minimal. Four randomized trials that included a total of 2027 subjects were published before 1980, during the first decade of clinical use of EFM.[69-72] All of these studies reported significantly higher rates of cesarean delivery in electronically monitored patients. However, as summarized in Table 15-7, seven of the eight randomized trials published after 1980, which included more than 10 times the number of subjects (20,740), failed to replicate this observation.[73-75,77-80] The eighth trial[76] did not report overall cesarean delivery rates. **Although historically EFM has been considered to contribute to higher cesarean rates, an alternative explanation of the most contemporary data is that the early impact of EFM on cesarean delivery rates has been mitigated by refinements in FHR interpretation and management that have accompanied decades of clinical experience with the technology.**

BENEFITS OF ELECTRONIC FETAL MONITORING

Nonrandomized studies in the 1970s reported significantly lower perinatal mortality rates in electronically monitored patients. In subsequent years, only one randomized trial was able to replicate these observations.[78] Despite a lack of consensus on many points, EFM has been demonstrated to be at least as effective in preventing perinatal morbidity and mortality as the previous practice of IA.

LIMITATIONS OF ELECTRONIC FETAL MONITORING
Prediction and Prevention of Hypoxic Injury

Despite early hopes, EFM has not proven to be a reliable predictor of fetal or neonatal metabolic acidemia, neonatal encephalopathy, or long-term neurologic impairment in the form of CP. The reported false-positive rate of EFM for detecting CP is 99.8%, yielding a positive predictive value of 1 in 500.[17,85] To provide context for this figure, the prevalence of CP in the general population is approximately 1 in 500.[85] The failure of EFM to predict hypoxic neurologic injury is largely due to the

fact that EFM is *not a diagnostic test for hypoxic neurologic injury*. Instead, it is a *screening test* that detects transient intrapartum interruption of fetal oxygenation as an early precursor to hypoxic neurologic injury. When used as a screening test, the negative predictive value of EFM is excellent. Normal EFM results virtually preclude intrapartum interruption of fetal oxygenation sufficient to cause hypoxic injury; however, the converse is not true. Abnormal EFM results rarely predict the presence of hypoxic injury. Instead, abnormal EFM results usually reflect transient interruption of fetal oxygenation, a common feature of normal labor that rarely leads to hypoxic injury. This is particularly true when abnormal EFM results trigger conservative measures that alter the natural progression of oxygen deficiency. After decades of research, it is clear that EFM is a reliable screening test with exceptional negative predictive value. Normal screening results confirm the safety of continued expectant management. Abnormal screening results should prompt additional investigation, heightened surveillance, and initiation of conservative measures as needed to improve fetal oxygenation. Definitive intervention in the form of operative delivery is ideally reserved for cases in which conservative measures are unsuccessful and ongoing hypoxic injury cannot be excluded. No single EFM finding or combination of findings has been found to be a reliable predictor of long-term neurodevelopmental impairment in the form of CP. Consequently, any attempt to use EFM for its positive predictive value as a diagnostic test for CP is destined to yield unsatisfactory results. When EFM replaced the traditional practice of IA in the 1970s, nonrandomized trials reported significantly lower perinatal mortality rates in electronically monitored patients. In subsequent years, only one randomized trial—conducted in a setting with high baseline perinatal mortality rates of 20.4 to 22.6 per 1000—was able to replicate this observation. A recent meta-analysis[84] of published randomized trials that included more than 33,000 patients demonstrated no significant reduction in perinatal mortality in electronically monitored patients compared with those monitored with IA. In fact, data derived from all of the randomized trials combined have failed to demonstrate the ability of EFM to reduce the risk of fetal metabolic acidemia, neonatal HIE, CP, or perinatal death compared with IA conducted with one-on-one nursing under strict research protocols.[84] This has led some to conclude that EFM has failed as a public health screening program.[86] An alternative interpretation is that in appropriately selected patients, EFM and IA conducted with vigilance commensurate with that applied in the randomized trials can be expected to perform similarly with respect to maternal and perinatal morbidity and mortality.

Prediction and Prevention of Fetal Stroke

As old EFM polemics gradually give way to evidence-based consensus, new controversies are arising. For example, a recent meta-analysis of four studies reported a possible relationship between abnormal intrapartum FHR patterns and the later diagnosis of perinatal arterial ischemic stroke (PAIS).[87] One of the four studies included only preterm deliveries and did not report the specific FHR abnormalities observed in the control and study groups.[88] The other three studies included only term deliveries, and none of these demonstrated an independent link between FHR abnormalities and PAIS.[89-91] No published evidence supports a causal relationship between FHR abnormalities and PAIS at any gestational age. Moreover, no published evidence suggests that intrapartum EFM is capable of detecting or predicting PAIS or that any form of obstetric intervention is capable of preventing PAIS. No level I or II evidence exists that links PAIS independently with any measure of uterine activity or labor duration.[13] This is consistent with the 2007 consensus report of the National Institute of Neurologic Disorders and Stroke and the NICHD, which concluded that "there are no reliable predictors of perinatal ischemic stroke upon which to base prevention or treatment strategies."[20]

Fetal Head Compression

Early deceleration of the FHR has long been recognized as a benign reflex response to transient compression of the fetal head during a uterine contraction. The innocuous nature of this phenomenon is underscored by the fact that early decelerations are included in NICHD category I, indicating normal fetal oxygenation.[16] However, some have suggested that intrapartum fetal head compression can cause hypoxic-ischemic brain injury, even in a normally oxygenated fetus.[92] This theory suggests that uterine contractions compress the fetal head against the maternal pelvis with such force that fetal intracranial pressure exceeds cerebral perfusion pressure, reducing intracranial blood flow to the point of regional cerebral ischemia and focal hypoxic-ischemic injury. Descriptive studies have reported that fetal head pressures during uterine contractions can be more than twice as high as intraamniotic pressures.[93] Other studies have demonstrated changes in fetal cerebral perfusion pressure, cerebral blood flow, and cerebral oxygen consumption during fetal head pressure.[94-96] However, no published level I or level II evidence has demonstrated that these changes translate to histologic neuropathology or clinical neurologic impairment. On the contrary, observations in fetal sheep suggest that the reflex Cushing response to head compression could be protective against such injury.[97,98] Level II evidence in the form of case-control studies has identified several perinatal risk factors for CP that include prematurity, infection, maternal thyroid disease, and congenital malformations.[99] However, no level I or II evidence has demonstrated a link between any measure of uterine activity and the later development of CP. The notion that fetal brain injury can be caused by the mechanical forces of labor is further challenged by level II evidence from a large cohort study that included more than 380,000 spontaneous vaginal deliveries and more than 33,000 cesarean deliveries without labor.[100] Neonates exposed to uterine contractions of sufficient frequency, intensity, and duration to result in spontaneous vaginal delivery had no higher rates of mechanical brain injury in the form of intracranial hemorrhage than did neonates who were exposed to no uterine contractions at all. This theory is not supported by analytic evidence in the literature. Consequently, it should not be used as a foundation for intrapartum management decisions.

SUMMARY

Evolving standardization and evidence-based consensus regarding EFM definitions, interpretation, and management are gradually supplanting the controversy and confusion that characterized EFM for decades. **Intrapartum FHR decelerations—variable, late, and prolonged—reliably identify transient episodes of interruption of fetal oxygenation. Moderate variability or accelerations confirm the absence of ongoing hypoxic neurologic**

---

injury with an extremely high degree of reliability, and the negative predictive value of EFM is near 100%. A test that is virtually always right is the ideal foundation for rational decision making. Conversely, if EFM is relied upon for its positive predictive value to detect hypoxic neurologic injury, it will be wrong approximately 499 times out of 500.[85] Reasonable management decisions cannot be based on the results of a test that is virtually always wrong. The standardized EFM definitions proposed by the NICHD and endorsed by ACOG, AWHONN, and ACNM should be used consistently. Standardized interpretation should eschew unproven theories in favor of evidence-based principles derived from appropriately controlled scientific research. Together, standardized definitions and evidence-based principles of interpretation help ensure factual accuracy. A standardized, simplified approach to EFM management provides a framework to help clinicians formulate a thoughtful, systematic plan of action that can be articulated clearly and understandably.

KEY POINTS

- The goal of intrapartum FHR monitoring is to assess the adequacy of fetal oxygenation during labor so that timely and appropriate steps can be taken when necessary to avoid fetal hypoxic injury.
- Fetal oxygenation involves the transfer of oxygen from the environment to the fetus. Oxygen is transported by maternal and fetal blood along the oxygen pathway, which includes the maternal lungs, heart, vasculature, uterus, placenta, and umbilical cord.
- The consequences of interruption of fetal oxygenation can lead sequentially to fetal hypoxemia (low oxygen content in the blood), fetal hypoxia (low oxygen content in the tissues), metabolic acidosis (accumulation of lactic acid in the tissues), metabolic acidemia (accumulation of lactic acid in the blood), and eventually injury or death.
- The FHR monitor provides reliable information regarding interruption of the oxygen pathway. The observation of an FHR deceleration that reaches its nadir in less than 30 seconds (variable deceleration) suggests compression of the umbilical cord. However, the mere fact that a deceleration reaches its nadir in less than 30 seconds does not exclude interruption of the oxygen pathway at other points, such as the lungs (hypoxemia), heart (poor cardiac output), vasculature (acute hypotension), uterus (uterine rupture, uterine contraction), or placenta (placental abruption). A late deceleration, by definition, reaches its nadir in 30 seconds or more. Historically, late decelerations have been attributed to uteroplacental insufficiency, which suggests interruption of the oxygen pathway at the level of the uterus or placenta. However, the fact that a deceleration takes 30 seconds to reach its nadir does not exclude the possibility of interruption of the oxygen pathway at other points, such as the maternal lungs (hypoxemia), heart

(poor cardiac output), or vasculature (hypotension). A prolonged deceleration can result from interruption of the oxygen pathway at any point. For the purposes of practical FHR interpretation, all clinically significant FHR decelerations that have any potential impact on fetal oxygenation (variable, late, or prolonged decelerations) have the same common trigger: interruption of the oxygen pathway *at one or more points*. This unifying concept helps reduce conflict and controversy and offers the additional benefits of standardization, simplicity, factual accuracy, and ease of articulation.

♦ In addition to providing practical information regarding interruption of the oxygen pathway, the FHR monitor provides useful information regarding the adequacy of fetal oxygenation. Moderate FHR variability or accelerations reliably exclude fetal hypoxic injury at the time they are observed; however, the converse is not true. The absence of moderate variability and/or accelerations does not indicate the presence of hypoxic injury.

♦ The negative predictive value of electronic FHR monitoring is excellent. A normal test virtually precludes fetal hypoxic injury at the time it is observed.

♦ The positive predictive value of electronic FHR monitoring is poor. Abnormal FHR monitoring accurately predicts CP approximately one time out of 500, yielding a false-positive rate above 99%. Except in extreme cases, no FHR pattern or combination of patterns has been demonstrated to predict hypoxic neurologic injury with a meaningful degree of accuracy.

♦ Even in the setting of abnormal FHR monitoring, the pathway from intrapartum hypoxic-ischemic injury to subsequent CP must progress through neonatal encephalopathy. The absence of neonatal encephalopathy is inconsistent with hypoxic-ischemic neurologic injury near the time of delivery.

♦ No randomized controlled trials, cohort studies, case-control studies, or other peer-reviewed studies in the literature support the hypothesis that fetal head compression caused by uterine contractions or maternal pushing efforts can cause local cerebral ischemia and hypoxic-ischemic injury in the absence of the established mechanism of global hypoxia. Similarly, no predictors of perinatal ischemic stroke are known upon which to base prevention strategies, and no known relationship exists between FHR monitoring and local cerebral hypoxic injury or stroke that can be used to identify, predict, or prevent such injuries.

♦ In the United States, standard FHR terminology has been proposed by the NICHD and is endorsed by virtually all major organizations that represent providers of obstetric care. Consistent use of standard terminology helps to ensure effective communication and optimize outcomes.

REFERENCES

1. Gültekin-Zootzmann B. The history of monitoring the human fetus. *J Perinat Med*. 1975;3(3):135-144.
2. Goodlin RC. History of fetal monitoring. *Am J Obstet Gynecol*. 1979; 133(3):323-352.
3. Hon EH. The electronic evaluation of the fetal heart rate. *Am J Obstet Gynecol*. 1958;75:1215.
4. Caldeyro-Barcia R, Mendez-Bauer C, Posiero JJ, et al. Control of the human fetal heart rate during labor. In: Cassels DE, ed. *The heart and circulation of the newborn and infant*. New York: Grune and Stratton; 1966:7-36.
5. Hammacher K. The diagnosis of fetal distress with an electronic fetal heart monitor. In: Horsky J, Stembera ZK, eds. *Intrauterine dangers to the fetus*. Amsterdam: Excerpta Medica; 1967.
6. Martin JA, Hamilton BE, Sutton PD, Ventura SJ, Menacker F, Munson ML. Births: final data for 2002. *Natl Vital Stat Rep*. 2003;52:1-113.
7. Helwig JT, Parer JT, Kilpatrick SJ, Laros RK. Umbilical cord blood acid-base state: What is normal? *Am J Obstet Gynecol*. 1996;174(6): 1807-1812.
8. Victory R, Penava D, Da Silva O, Natale R, Richardson B. Umbilical cord pH and base excess values in relation to adverse outcome events for infants delivering at term. *Am J Obstet Gynecol*. 2004;191(6):2021-2028.
9. Low JA, Panagiotopoulos C, Derrick EJ. Newborn complications after intrapartum asphyxia with metabolic acidosis in the term fetus. *Am J Obstet Gynecol*. 1994;170:1081-1087.
10. Arabin B, Jimenez E, Vogel M, Weitzel HK. Relationship of utero- and fetoplacental blood flow velocity wave forms with pathomorphological placental findings. *Fetal Diagn Ther*. 1992;7(3–4):173-179.
11. *American College of Obstetricians and Gynecologists Task Force on Neonatal Encephalopathy and Cerebral Palsy, American College of Obstetricians and Gynecologists, American Academy of Pediatrics 2003 Neonatal encephalopathy and cerebral palsy: Defining the pathogenesis and pathophysiology ACOG*, AAP: Washington, DC.
12. MacLennan A. A template for defining a causal relation between acute intrapartum events and cerebral palsy: International consensus statement. *BMJ*. 1999;319(7216):1054-1059.
13. *Neonatal Encephalopathy and Neurologic Outcome, Second Edition, American College of Obstetricians and Gynecologists, American Academy of Pediatrics 2014*.
14. Electronic fetal heart rate monitoring: research guidelines for interpretation. National Institute of Child Health and Human Development Research Planning Workshop. *Am J Obstet Gynecol*. 1997;177: 1385-1390.
15. American College of Obstetricians and Gynecologists. ACOG Practice Bulletin No. 70. December 2005 (replaces practice bulletin number 62, May 2005). Intrapartum fetal heart rate monitoring. *Obstet Gynecol*. 2005;106:1453-1461.
16. Macones GA, Hankins GD, Spong CY, Hauth J, Moore T. The 2008 National Institute of Child Health and Human Development workshop report on electronic fetal monitoring: update on definitions, interpretation, and research guidelines. *Obstet Gynecol*. 2008;112(3):661-666.
17. American College of Obstetricians and Gynecologists. ACOG Practice Bulletin No. 106 Intrapartum fetal heart rate monitoring: Nomenclature, Interpretation, and General management principles. *Obstet Gynecol*. 2009;114:192-202.
18. American College of Obstetricians and Gynecologists. ACOG Practice Bulletin No. 116. Management of intrapartum fetal heart rate tracings. *Obstet Gynecol*. 2010;116:1232-1240.
19. United States Preventive Services Task Force. *Guide to Clinical Preventative Services. Report of the US Preventive Services Task Force 2d ed*. Williams and Wilkins; 1996.
20. Raju T, Nelson K, Ischemic Perinatal Stroke, et al. Summary of a Workshop Sponsored by the National Institute of Child Health and Human Development and the National Institute of Neurological Disorders and Stroke. *Pediatrics*. 2007;120(3):609-616.
21. Martin CB Jr, de Haan J, van der Wildt B, Jongsma HW, Dieleman A, Arts TH. Mechanisms of late decelerations in the fetal heart rate. A study with autonomic blocking agents in fetal lambs. *Eur J Obstet Gynecol Reprod Biol*. 1979;9(6):361-373.
22. Itskovitz J, LaGamma EF, Rudolph AM. Heart rate and blood pressure responses to umbilical cord compression in fetal lambs with special reference to the mechanism of variable deceleration. *Am J Obstet Gynecol*. 1983;147:451-457.
23. Brubaker K, Garite TJ. The lambda fetal heart rate pattern: an assessment of its significance in the intrapartum period. *Obstet Gynecol*. 1988;72: 881-885.
24. Goodlin RC, Lowe EW. A functional umbilical cord occlusion heart rate pattern. The significance of overshoot. *Obstet Gynecol*. 1974;43: 22-30.
25. Schifrin BS, Hamilton-Rubinstein T, Shield JR. Fetal heart rate patterns and the timing of fetal injury. *J Perinatol*. 1994;14:174-181.

26. Shields JR, Schifrin BS. Perinatal antecedents of cerebral palsy. *Obstet Gynecol.* 1988;71:899.

27. Westgate JA, Bennet L, de Haan HH, Gunn AJ. Fetal heart rate overshoot during repeated umbilical cord occlusion in sheep. *Obstet Gynecol.* 2001;97:454-459.

28. Kubli FW, Hon EH, Khazin AF, Takemura H. Observations on heart rate and pH in the human fetus during labor. *Am J Obstet Gynecol.* 1969;104: 1190-1206.

29. American Academy of Pediatrics, American College of Obstetricians and Gynecologists. *Guidelines for Perinatal Care.* 7th ed. Washington, DC; 2012. Riley LE, Stark AR, Kilpatrick SJ, Papile LA, eds.

30. Simpson KR, James DC. Efficacy of intrauterine resuscitation techniques in improving fetal oxygen status during labor. *Obstet Gynecol.* 2005;105: 1362-1368.

31. Simpson KR. Intrauterine Resuscitation During Labor: Review of Current Methods and Supportive Evidence. *J Midwifery Womens Health.* 2007;52: 229-237.

32. Simpson KR. Intrauterine resuscitation during labor: should maternal oxygen administration be a first-line measure? *Semin Fetal Neonatal Med.* 2008;13:362-367.

33. Carbonne B, Benachi A, Leveque ML, Cabrol D, Papiernik E. Maternal position during labor: effects on fetal oxygen saturation measured by pulse oximetry. *Obstet Gynecol.* 1996;88:797-800.

34. Freeman RK, Garite TJ, Nageotte MP. *Fetal heart rate monitoring.* 3rd ed. Philadelphia: Lippincott, Williams & Wilkins; 2003.

35. Amnioinfusion does not prevent meconium aspiration syndrome. ACOG Committee Opinion No. 346. American College of Obstetricians and Gynecologists. *Obstet Gynecol.* 2006;108:1053-1055.

36. Clark SL, Nageotte MP, Garite TJ, et al. Intrapartum Management of Category II Fetal Heart Rate Tracings: Towards Standardization of Care. *Am J Obstet Gynecol.* 2013;209(2):89-97.

37. Institute of Medicine. *To err is human: building a safer health care system.* Washington, DC: National Academy Press; 2000.

38. East CE, Leader LR, Sheehan P, Henshall NE, Colditz PB. Intrapartum fetal scalp lactate sampling for fetal assessment in the presence of a non-reassuring fetal heart rate trace. *Cochrane Database Syst Rev.* 2010;(3):Art. No.:CD006174.

39. Goodwin TM, Milner-Masterson L, Paul RH. Elimination of fetal scalp blood sampling on a large clinical service. *Obstet Gynecol.* 1994;83: 971-974.

40. Clark SL, Gimovsky ML, Miller FC. Fetal heart rate response to scalp blood sampling. *Am J Obstet Gynecol.* 1982;144(6):706-708.

41. Smith CV, Nguyen HN, Phelan JP, Paul RH. Intrapartum assessment of fetal well-being: a comparison of fetal acoustic stimulation with acid-base determinations. *Am J Obstet Gynecol.* 1986;155(4):726-728.

42. Skupski DW, Rosenberg CR, Eglington GS. Intrapartum fetal stimulation tests: A meta-analysis. *Obstet Gynecol.* 2002;99(1):129-134.

43. Dawes GS. Computerised analysis of the fetal heart rate. *Eur J Obstet Gynecol Reprod Biol.* 1991;42(suppl):S5-S8.

44. Dawes GS, Moulden M, Sheil O, Redman CW. Approximate entropy, a statistic of regularity, applied to fetal heart rate data before and during labor. *Obstet Gynecol.* 1992;80(5):763-768.

45. Pello LC, Rosevear BM, Dawes GS, Moulden M, Redman CW. Computerized fetal heart rate analysis in labor. *Obstet Gynecol.* 1991;78(4): 602-610.

46. Keith RD, Beckley S, Garibaldi JM, Westgate JA, Ifeachor EC, Greene KR. A multicentre comparative study of 17 experts and an intelligent computer system for managing labour using the cardiotocogram. *Br J Obstet Gynaecol.* 1995;102(9):688-700.

47. Bloom SL, Spong CY, Thom E, et al. National Institute of Child Health and Human Development Maternal-Fetal Medicine Units Network: Fetal pulse oximetry and cesarean delivery. *N Engl J Med.* 2006;355(21): 2195-2202.

48. Dildy GA, van den Berg PP, Katz M, Clark SL, Jongsma HW, Nijhuis JG, et al. Intrapartum fetal pulse oximetry: fetal oxygen saturation trends during labor and relation to delivery outcome. *Am J Obstet Gynecol.* 1994;171(3):679-684.

49. East CE, Brennecke SP, King JF, Chan FY, Colditz PB. The effect of intrapartum fetal pulse oximetry, in the presence of a nonreassuring fetal heart rate pattern, on operative delivery rates: A multicenter, randomized, controlled trial (the FOREMOST trial). *Am J Obstet Gynecol.* 2006;194(3): 606.e1-606.e16.

50. Garite TJ, Dildy GA, McNamara H, et al. A multicenter controlled trial of fetal pulse oximetry in the intrapartum management of nonreassuring fetal heart rate patterns. *Am J Obstet Gynecol.* 2000;183(5): 1049-1058.

51. Klauser CK, Christensen EE, Chauhan SP, Bufkin L, Magann EF, Bofill JA, et al. Use of fetal pulse oximetry among high-risk women in labor: A randomized clinical trial. *Am J Obstet Gynecol.* 2005;192(16): 1810-1819.

52. Kuhnert M, Seelbach-Goebel G, Butterwegge M. Predictive agreement between the fetal arterial oxygen saturation and fetal scalp pH: Results of the German multicenter study. *Am J Obstet Gynecol.* 1998;178(2): 330-335.

53. Strachan BK, van Wijngaarden WJ, Sahota D, Chang A, James DK. Cardiotocography only versus cardiotocography plus PR-interval analysis in intrapartum surveillance: A randomized, multicentre trial. *Lancet.* 2000;355(9202):456-459.

54. Nijland R, Jongsma HW, Nijhuis JG, van den Berg PP, Oeseburg B. Arterial oxygen saturation in relation to metabolic acidosis in fetal lambs. *Am J Obstet Gynecol.* 1995;172(3):810-819.

55. Oeseburg B, Ringnalda BEM, Crevels J, et al. Fetal oxygenation in chronic maternal hypoxia: What's critical? *Adv Exp Med Biol.* 1992;317: 499-502.

56. Hökegård KH, Eriksson BO, Kjellemer I, Magno R, Rosén KG. Myocardial metabolism in relation to electrocardiographic changes and cardiac function during graded hypoxia in the fetal lamb. *Acta Physiol Scand.* 1981;113(1):1-7.

57. Rosén KG, Dagbjartsson A, Henriksson BA, Lagercrantz H, Kjellmer I. The relationship between circulating catecholamine and ST waveform in the fetal lamb electrocardiogram during hypoxia. *Am J Obstet Gynecol.* 1984;149(2):190-195.

58. Widmark C, Jansson T, Lindecrantz K, Rosén KG. ECG waveform, short-term heart rate variability and plasma catecholamine concentrations in response to hypoxia in intrauterine growth retarded guinea pig fetuses. *J Dev Physiol.* 1991;15(3):161-168.

59. Westgate J, Harris M, Curnow JS, Greene KR. Plymouth randomized trial of cardiotocogram only versus ST waveform plus cardiotocogram for intrapartum monitoring in 2400 cases. *Am J Obstet Gynecol.* 1993;169(5): 1151-1160.

60. Amer-Wåhlin I, Hellsten C, Norén H, et al. Cardiotocography only versus cardiotocography plus ST analysis of fetal electrocardiogram for intrapartum fetal monitoring: A Swedish randomised controlled trial. *Lancet.* 2001;358(9281):534-538.

61. Westerhuis ME, Visser GH, Moons KG, et al. Cardiotography plus ST analysis of fetal electrocardiogram compared with cardiotocography only for intrapartum monitoring: A randomized trail. *Obstet Gynecolol.* 2010;115:1173-1180.

62. Neilson JP. Fetal electrocardiogram (ECG) for fetal monitoring during labour. *Cochrane Database Syst Rev.* 2013;(5):Art. No.: CD000116.

63. Belfort MA, Saade GR, Thom E, et al. A randomized trial of intrapartum fetal ECG ST-segment analysis. *N Engl J Med.* 2015;373(7):632-641.

64. Reinhard J, Hayes-Gill BR, Schiermeier S, Hatzmann W, Herrmann E, Henrich TM, et al. Intrapartum signal quality with external fetal heart rate monitoring: a two-way trial of external Doppler CTG ultrasound and the abdominal fetal electrocardiogram. *Arch Gynecol Obstet.* 2012;286(5): 1103-1107.

65. Graatsma EM, Miller J, Mulder EJ, Harman C, Baschat AA, Visser GH. Maternal body mass index does not affect performance of fetal electrocardiography. *Am J Perinatol.* 2010;27(7):573-577.

66. American College of Obstetricians and Gynecologists. ACOG Committee Opinion No. 348. Umbilical cord blood gas and acid—base analysis. *Obstet Gynecol.* 2006;108(5):1319-1322.

67. Hon EH, Quilligan EJ. The classification of fetal heart rate. II. A revised working classification. *Conn Med.* 1967;31:779-784.

68. MacDonald D, Grant A. Fetal surveillance in labour - the present position. In: Bonnar J, ed. *Recent advances in obstetrics and gynaecology 15.* London: Churchill Livingstone; 1987:83-100.

69. Haverkamp AD, Thompson HE, McFee JG, Cetrullo C. The evaluation of continuous fetal heart rate monitoring in high-risk pregnancy. *Am J Obstet Gynecol.* 1976;125:310-320.

70. Renou P, Chang A, Anderson I, Wood C. Controlled trial of fetal intensive care. *Am J Obstet Gynecol.* 1976;126:470-476.

71. Kelso IM, Parsons RJ, Lawrence GF, Arora SS, Edmonds DK, Cooke ID. An assessment of continuous fetal heart rate monitoring in labor: a randomized trial. *Am J Obstet Gynecol.* 1978;131:526-532.

72. Haverkamp AD, Orleans M, Langendoerfer S, McFee J, Murphy J, Thompson HE. A controlled trial of the differential effects of intrapartum fetal monitoring. *Am J Obstet Gynecol.* 1979;134:399-408.

73. Wood C, Renou P, Oats J, Farrell E, Bleischer N, Anderson I. A controlled trial of fetal heart rate monitoring in a low-risk obstetric population. *Am J Obstet Gynecol.* 1981;141:527-534.

74. MacDonald D, Grant A, Sheridan-Pereira M, Boylan P, Chalmers I. The Dublin randomized controlled trial of intrapartum fetal heart rate monitoring. *Am J Obstet Gynecol.* 1985;152:524-539.

75. Neldam S, Osler M, Hansen PK, Nim J, Smith SF, Hertel J. Intrapartum fetal heart rate monitoring in a combined low- and high-risk population: a controlled clinical trial. *Eur J Obstet Gynecol Reprod Biol.* 1986;23: 1-11.

76. Leveno KJ, Cunningham FG, Nelson S, et al. A prospective comparison of selective and universal electronic fetal monitoring in 34,995 pregnancies. *NEJM.* 1986;315:615-619.

77. Luthy DA, Kirkwood KS, van Belle G, et al. A randomized trial of electronic fetal monitoring in preterm labor. *Obstet Gynecol.* 1987;69: 687-695.

78. Vintzileos AM, Antsaklis A, Varvarigos I, Papas C, Sofatzis I, Montgomery JT. A randomized trial of intrapartum electronic fetal heart rate montoring versus intermittent auscultation. *Obstet Gynecol.* 1993;81:899-907.

79. Herbst A, Ingemarsson I. Intermittent versus continuous electronic monitoring in labour: a randomised study. *Br J Obstet Gynaecol.* 1994;101: 663-668.

80. Madaan M, Trivedi SS. Intrapartum electronic fetal monitoring vs. intermittent auscultation in postcesarean pregnancies. *Int J Gynecol Obstet.* 2006;94:123-125.

81. Grant A, O'Brien N, Joy MT, Hennessy E, MacDonald D. Cerebral palsy among children born during the Dublin randomized trial of intrapartum monitoring. *Lancet.* 1989;2:1233-1236.

82. Vintzileos AM, Nochimson DJ, Guzman ER, Knuppel RA, Lake M, Schifrin BS. Intrapartum electronic fetal heart rate monitoring versus intermittent auscultation: a meta-analysis. *Obstet Gynecol.* 1995;85: 149-155.

83. Thacker SB, Stroup DF. Continuous electronic heart rate monitoring versus intermittent auscultation for assessment during labor. Cochrane Review. In: *The Cochrane Library, 3.* Oxford: Update Software; 1999.

84. Alfirevic Z, Devane D, Gyte GML. Continuous cardiotocography (CTG) as a form of electronic fetal monitoring (EFM) for fetal assessment during labour. *Cochrane Database Syst Rev.* 2013;(5):Art. No.: CD006066.

85. Nelson KB, Dambrosia JM, Ting TY, Grether JK. Uncertain value of electronic fetal monitoring in predicting cerebral palsy. *NEJM.* 1996; 334(10):613-618.

86. Grimes DA, Peipert JF. Electronic fetal monitoring as a public health screening program: the arithmetic of failure. *Obstet Gynecol.* 2010;116: 1397-1400.

87. Luo L, Chen D, Qu Y, Wu J, Li X, Mu D. Association between Hypoxia and Perinatal Arterial Ischemic Stroke: A Meta-Analysis. *PLoS ONE.* 2014;9(2):e90106.

88. Benders MJ, Groenendaal F, Uiterwaal CS, et al. Maternal and infant characteristics associated with perinatal arterial stroke in the preterm infant. *Stroke.* 2007;38(6):1759-1765.

89. Lee J, Croen LA, Backstrand KH, et al. Maternal and infant characteristics associated with perinatal arterial stroke in the infant. *JAMA.* 2005; 293(6):723-729.

90. Darmency-Stamboul V, Chantegret C, Ferdynus C, et al. Antenatal factors associated with perinatal arterial ischemic stroke. *Stroke.* 2012;43(9): 2307-2312.

91. Harteman JC, Groenendaal F, Kwee A, Welsing PM, Benders MJ, de Vries LS. Risk factors for perinatal arterial ischaemic stroke in full-term infants: a case-control study. *Arch Dis Child Fetal Neonatal Ed.* 2012;97(6): F411-F416.

92. Schifrin BS, Ater S. Fetal hypoxic and ischemic injuries. *Curr Opin Obstet Gynecol.* 2006;18:112-122.

93. Svenningsen L, Lindemann R, Eidal K. Measurements of fetal head compression pressure during bearing down and their relationship to the condition of the newborn. *Acta Obstet Gynecol Scand.* 1988;67(2):129-133.

94. Mann LI, Carmichael A, Duchin S. The effect of head compression on FHR, brain metabolism, and function. *Obstet Gynecol.* 1972;39: 721-726.

95. O'Brien WF, Davis SE, Grissom MP, Eng RR, Golden SM. Effect of cephalic pressure on fetal cerebral blood flow. *Am J Perinat.* 1984;1: 223-226.

96. Aldrich CJ, D'Antona D, Spencer JA, et al. The effect of maternal pushing on fetal cerebral oxygenation and blood volume during the second stage of labour. *Br J Obstet Gynaecol.* 1995;102:448-453.

97. Harris AP, Koehler RC, Gleason CA, Jones MD Jr, Traystman RJ. Cerebral and peripheral circulatory responses to intracranial hypertension in fetal sheep. *Circ Res.* 1989;64(5):991-1000.

98. Harris AP, Helou S, Traystman RJ, Jones MD Jr, Koehler RC. Efficacy of the Cushing response in maintaining cerebral blood flow in premature and near-term fetal sheep. *Pediatr Res.* 1998;43(1):50-56.

99. Nelson KB, Ellenberg JH. Antecedents of cerebral palsy. Multivariate analysis of risk. *N Engl J Med.* 1986;315(2):81-86.

100. Towner D, Castro MA, Eby-Wilkens E, Gilbert WM. Effect of mode of delivery in nulliparous women on neonatal intracranial injury. *N Engl J Med.* 1999;341:1709-1714.

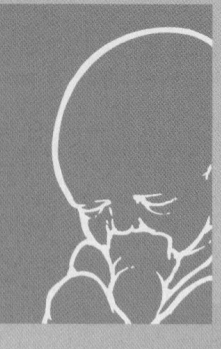

CHAPTER 16

Obstetric Anesthesia

JOY L. HAWKINS and BRENDA A. BUCKLIN

KEY ABBREVIATIONS

Advanced cardiovascular life support	ACLS
American College of Obstetricians and Gynecologists	ACOG
American Society of Anesthesiologists	ASA
Basic life support	BLS
Confidence interval	CI
Central nervous system	CNS
Combined spinal-epidural	CSE
Induction-to-delivery interval	I-D
Laryngeal mask airway	LMA
N-methyl-D-aspartate receptor	NMDA receptor
Odds ratio	OR
Para-aminobenzoic acid	PABA
Patient-controlled analgesia	PCA
Patient-controlled epidural analgesia	PCEA
Postanesthesia care unit	PACU
Postdural puncture headache	PDPH
Randomized controlled trial	RCT
Relative risk	RR
Society of Obstetric Anesthesia and Perinatology	SOAP
Uterine incision–to-delivery interval	U-D

Obstetric anesthesia encompasses all techniques used by anesthesiologists and obstetricians to alleviate the pain associated with labor and delivery: this includes general anesthesia, neuraxial anesthesia (spinal or epidural), local anesthesia (local infiltration, paracervical block, pudendal block), and parenteral analgesia. **Pain relief during labor and delivery is an essential part of good obstetric care.** Unique clinical considerations guide anesthesia provided for obstetric patients; physiologic changes of pregnancy and increases in certain complications must be considered. This chapter reviews the various methods that can be used for obstetric analgesia and anesthesia as well as their indications and complications.

PERSONNEL

In larger hospitals in the United States, anesthesiologists—working either independently or supervising a team of residents—along with anesthesiologist assistants and certified nurse anesthetists provide anesthesia for 98% of obstetric procedures.[1] Nurse anesthetists working independent of anesthesiologists rarely provide anesthesia for obstetric cases in larger hospitals but provide anesthesia for 34% of obstetric procedures in hospitals with fewer than 500 births per year.[1] The American Society of Anesthesiologists (ASA) partnered with the American College of Obstetricians and Gynecologists (ACOG) to issue a Joint Statement on the Optimal Goals for Anesthesia Care in Obstetrics,[2] which recommends that a qualified anesthesiologist assume responsibility for anesthetics in every hospital that provides obstetric care. The statement notes: "There are many obstetric units where obstetricians or obstetrician-supervised nurse anesthetists administer labor anesthetics. **The administration of general or neuraxial anesthesia requires both medical judgment and technical skills.** Thus a physician with privileges in anesthesiology should be readily available."[2] To provide optimal care for the parturient, the ASA also states in their Practice Guidelines for Obstetric Anesthesia that "**A communication system should be in place to encourage early and ongoing contact between obstetric providers, anesthesiologists, and other members of the multidisciplinary team.**"[3]

PAIN PATHWAYS

Pain during the first stage of labor results from a combination of uterine contractions and cervical dilation. Painful sensations travel from the uterus through visceral afferent (sympathetic)

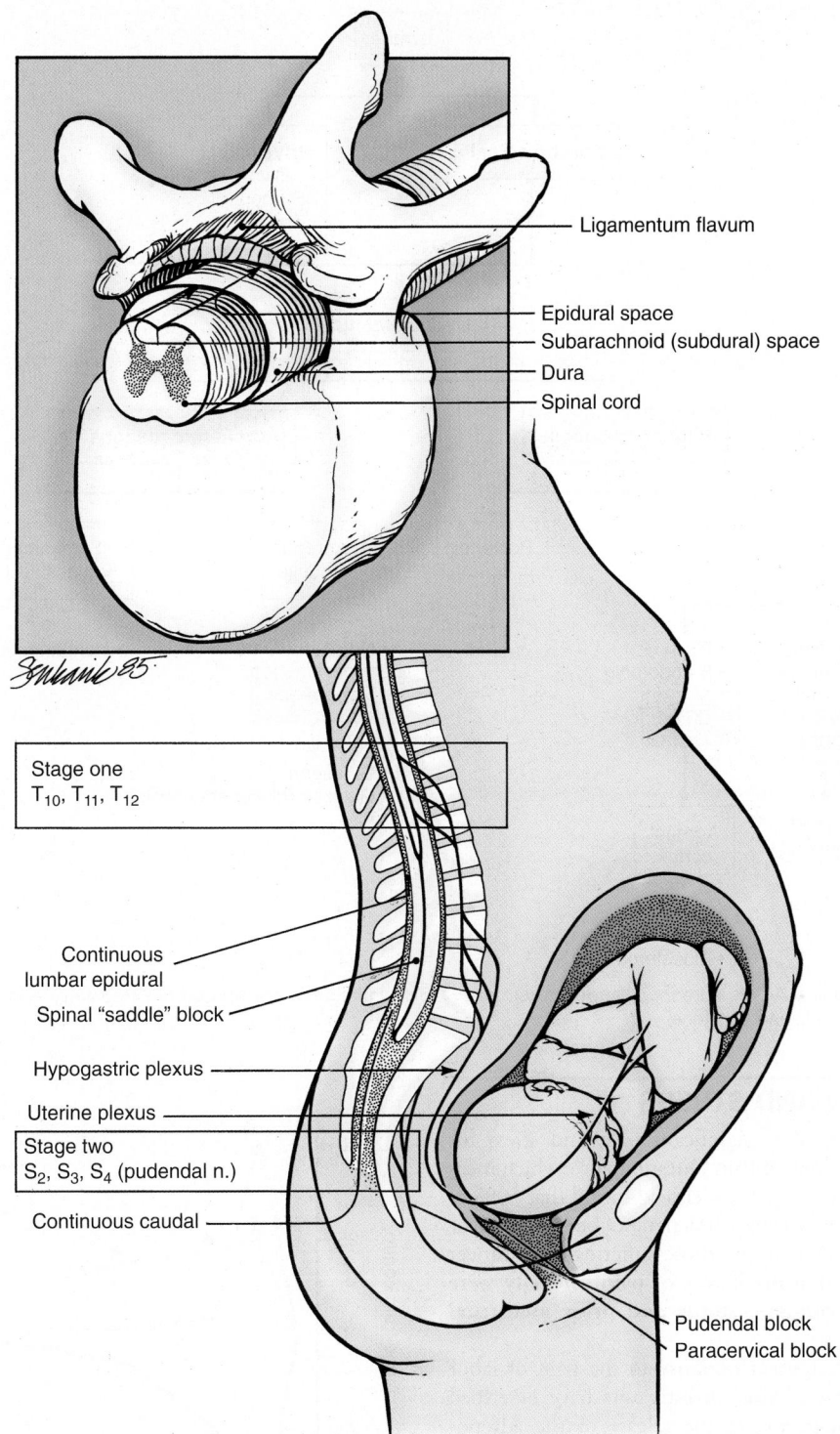

Ligamentum flavum

Epidural space
Subarachnoid (subdural) space
Dura
Spinal cord

Stage one
T₁₀, T₁₁, T₁₂

Continuous
lumbar epidural

Spinal "saddle" block

Hypogastric plexus

Uterine plexus

Stage two
S₂, S₃, S₄ (pudendal n.)

Continuous caudal

Pudendal block
Paracervical block

FIG 16-1 Pain pathways of labor and delivery and nerves blocked by various anesthetic techniques.

nerves that enter the spinal cord through the posterior segments of thoracic spinal nerves 10, 11, and 12 (Fig. 16-1). During the second stage of labor, additional painful stimuli are added as the fetal head distends the pelvic floor, vagina, and perineum. The sensory fibers of sacral nerves 2, 3, and 4 (i.e., the pudendal nerves) transmit painful impulses from the perineum to the spinal cord during the second stage and during any perineal repair (see Fig. 16-1). **During cesarean delivery, although the incision is usually around the thoracic spinal nerve 12 (T-12) dermatome, anesthesia is required to the level of thoracic spinal nerve 4 (T-4) to completely block peritoneal discomfort, especially during uterine exteriorization.** Pain after cesarean delivery is due to both incisional pain and uterine involution.

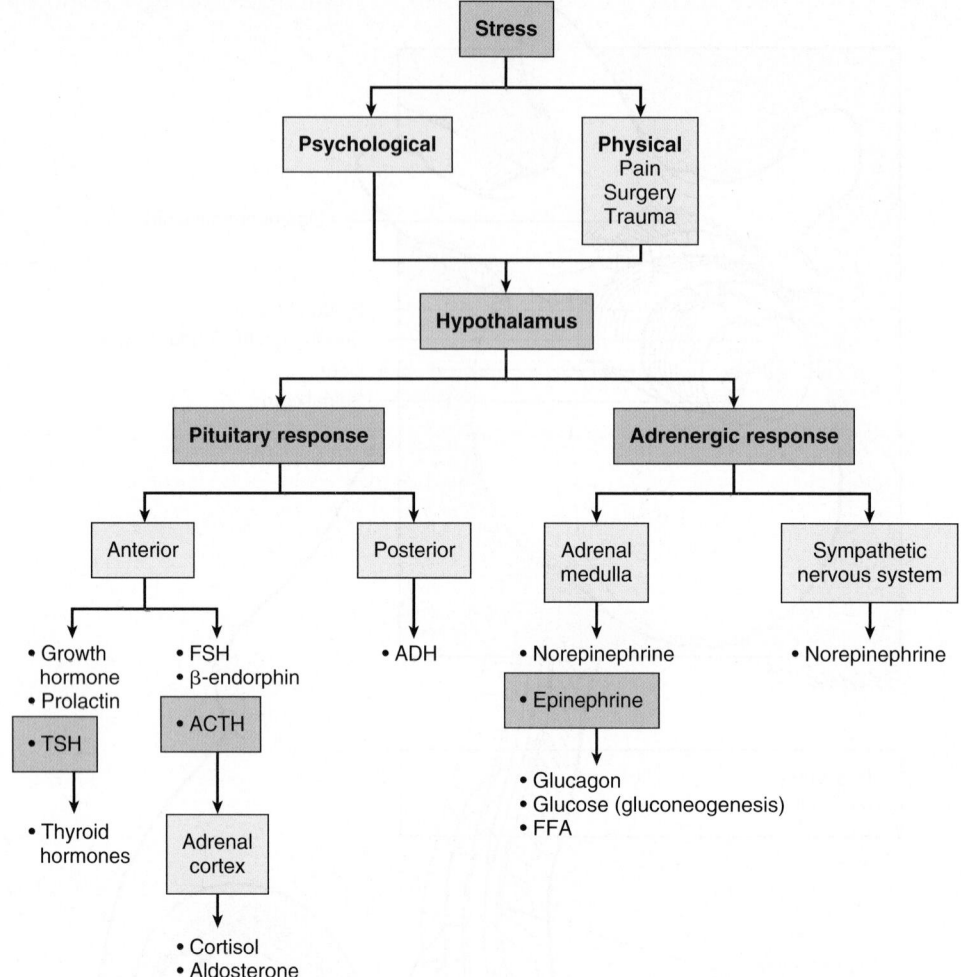

FIG 16-2 The stress response. ACTH, adrenocorticotropic hormone; ADH, antidiuretic hormone; FFA, free fatty acid; FSH, follicle-stimulating hormone; TSH, thyroid-stimulating hormone.

EFFECTS OF PAIN AND STRESS

The process of labor involves significant pain and stress for most women. Using the McGill Pain Questionnaire, which measures intensity and quality of pain, Melzack[4] found that 59% of nulliparous and 43% of parous women described their labor pain in terms more severe than did those suffering from cancer pain. **The most substantial predictors of pain intensity were ultimately low socioeconomic status and prior menstrual difficulties.**

The maternal and fetal stress response to the pain of labor has been difficult to assess. Most investigators have described and quantified stress in terms of the release of the adrenocorticotropic hormone (ACTH) cortisol, catecholamines, and β-endorphins (Fig. 16-2). Furthermore, **animal studies indicate that both epinephrine and norepinephrine can decrease uterine blood flow in the absence of maternal heart rate and blood pressure changes, which contributes to occult fetal asphyxia.** As demonstrated in baboons and monkeys, maternal psychological stress (induced by bright lights or toe clamping) can detrimentally affect uterine blood flow and fetal acid-base status.[5] In pregnant sheep, catecholamines increase and uterine blood flow decreases after painful stimuli and after nonpainful stimuli such as loud noises induce fear and anxiety, as evidenced by struggling (Fig. 16-3).

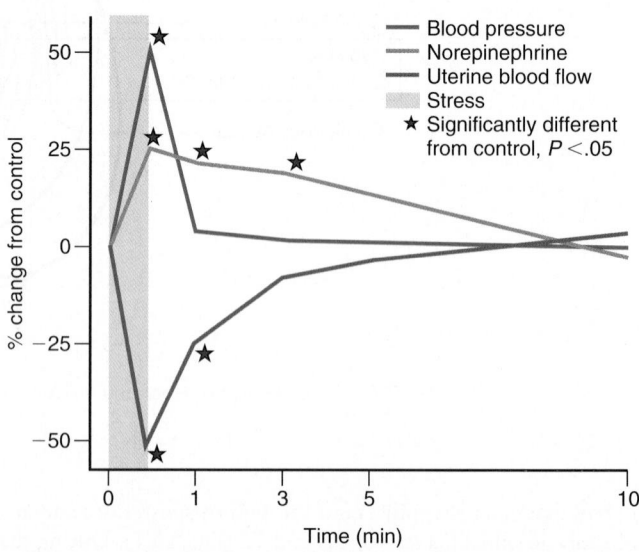

FIG 16-3 Effects of electrically induced stress (30 to 60 seconds) on maternal mean arterial blood pressure, plasma norepinephrine levels, and uterine blood flow. (Modified from Shnider SM, Wright RG, Levinson G, et al. Uterine blood flow and plasma norepinephrine changes during maternal stress in the pregnant ewe. *Anesthesiology.* 1979;50:524.)

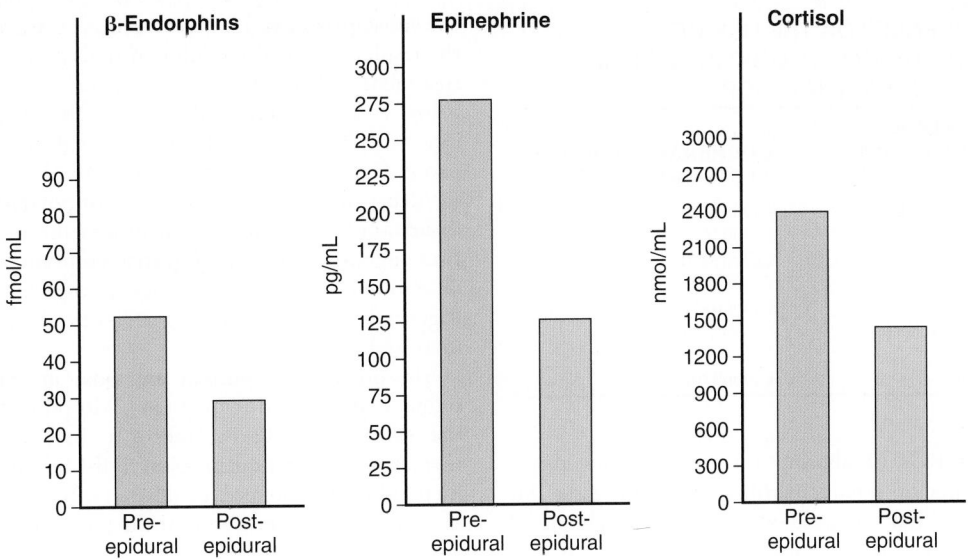

FIG 16-4 Effects of epidural analgesia on the response to stress.

TABLE 16-1   ANALGESIC PROCEDURES USED FOR LABOR PAIN RELIEF IN 2001 ACCORDING TO SIZE OF DELIVERY SERVICE

HOSPITAL SIZE (BIRTHS/YEAR)	NO ANESTHESIA (%)	NARCOTICS, BARBITURATES, TRANQUILIZERS (%)	PARACERVICAL BLOCK (%)	SPINAL OR EPIDURAL BLOCK (%)
<500	12	37	3	57
500-1499	10	42	3	59
>1500	6	34	2	77

Modified from Bucklin BA, Hawkins JL, Anderson JR, Ullrich FA. Obstetric anesthesia workforce survey. *Anesthesiology.* 2005;103:645.

Although some of the physiologic stress of labor is unavoidable, analgesia and anesthesia may reduce stress responses secondary to pain. Postpartum women suffer objective deficits in cognitive and memory function when compared with nonpregnant women, and intrapartum analgesia does not exacerbate but rather *lessens* the cognitive defect compared with unmedicated parturients.[6] Epidural analgesia is associated with a decreased risk of postpartum depression. In one study, depression occurred in 14% of parturients who received epidural labor analgesia and in 34.6% of those who did not.[7] Analgesia also reduces paternal anxiety and stress, increases fathers' feelings of helpfulness, and enhances their involvement and satisfaction with the childbirth experience.[8] Epidural analgesia prevents increases in both cortisol and 11-hydroxycorticosteroid levels during labor, but systemically administered opioids do not. Epidural analgesia also attenuates elevations of epinephrine and norepinephrine and endorphin levels (Fig. 16-4).[9] **Assuming any hypotension is rapidly treated and that perfusion is preserved by preventing aortocaval compression with uterine displacement, fetal acid-base status (as measured by base deficit) of human infants whose mothers receive epidural anesthesia during the first stage of labor is altered less than that of infants of mothers who receive systemic opioid analgesia.**

ANALGESIA FOR LABOR

Table 16-1 presents the frequency with which the various forms of analgesia are used during labor. The data are from a large survey of hospitals in the United States, stratified by the size of their delivery service.[1]

Psychoprophylaxis and Nonpharmacologic Analgesia Techniques

Psychoprophylaxis is any nonpharmacologic method that minimizes the perception of painful uterine contractions. Relaxation, concentration on breathing, gentle massage, and partner or doula participation contribute to effectiveness. One of the method's most valuable contributions is that it is often taught in prepared childbirth classes, where parents tour the labor and delivery suite and learn about the normal processes of labor and delivery, which in many instances mitigates their fear of the unknown.[10]

Although psychoprophylactic techniques can be empowering, the majority of women will still ultimately blend them with pharmacologic methods.[1] Because the majority of first-time mothers choose epidural analgesia, teaching that use of drug-induced pain relief represents failure or will harm the child are counterproductive and can heighten fear and anxiety during labor.

Nonpharmacologic techniques for labor analgesia may be used alone or in conjunction with parenteral or neuraxial techniques. Table 16-2 shows frequently used techniques and the evidence that supports their use. A systematic review of acupuncture concluded that the evidence for efficacy is promising but few data are available.[11] From the three randomized controlled trials (RCTs) they reviewed, the authors suggest that acupuncture alleviates labor pain and reduces use of both epidural analgesia and parenteral opioids. Acupuncture may be helpful for patients who feel strongly about avoiding epidural analgesia in labor, although arranging to have a qualified and credentialed acupuncturist available at the time of delivery may

TABLE 16-2	EVIDENCE FOR THE USE OF NONPHARMACOLOGIC ANALGESIC TECHNIQUES IN LABOR	
NONPHARMACOLOGIC ANALGESIC TECHNIQUES FOR LABOR	**COCHRANE DATABASE SYSTEMATIC REVIEWS**	
Continuous support (e.g., doula)	CD003766	
Alternative therapies	CD003521	
Massage, reflexology	CD009290	
Acupuncture, acupressure	CD009232	
Immersion in water	CD000111	
Transcutaneous electrical nerve stimulation	CD007214	
Sterile water injection	CD009107	

be challenging. An RCT of laboring in water found no advantage in labor outcome or in reducing the need for analgesia, but the request for epidural analgesia was delayed by about 30 minutes.[12] The ACOG has expressed concerns about *delivering* in water because of the lack of trials to demonstrate safety and the rare but reported unusual complications, such as infection or asphyxia.[13] They state that "the safety and efficacy of immersion in water during the second stage of labor have not been established, and immersion in water during the second stage of labor has not been associated with maternal or fetal benefit. Given these facts and case reports of rare but serious adverse effects in the newborn, the practice of immersion in the second stage of labor (underwater delivery) should be considered an experimental procedure that should only be performed within the context of an appropriately designed clinical trial with informed consent."

Intradermal sterile water injections at four sites in the lower back were once thought to have a similar gating mechanism as acupuncture and are simple to perform, but little evidence exists for their efficacy (see Table 16-2). A number of studies have examined transcutaneous electrical nerve stimulation (TENS) during labor. Patients tend to rate the device as helpful despite the fact that it does not decrease pain scores or the use of additional analgesics. As one study noted, TENS units do not appear to change the degree of pain but may have somehow made the pain less disturbing (see Table 16-2). **Although the efficacy of these techniques is largely unproven because of a lack of RCTs, no serious safety concerns exist with any of these techniques, which is attractive to patients and their caregivers.** Women expect to have choices and a degree of control during childbirth, and their caregivers should provide analgesic options for them to choose from, including nonpharmacologic methods.

Systemic Opioid Analgesia

Opioids can be given in intermittent doses by intramuscular (IM) or intravenous (IV) routes at the patient's request, or the patient can self-administer with patient-controlled analgesia (PCA). **All opioids provide sedation and a sense of euphoria, but their analgesic effect in labor is limited, and their primary mechanism of action is sedation.**[14] Opioids can also produce nausea and respiratory depression in the mother, the degree of which is usually comparable for equipotent analgesic doses. Also, **all opioids freely cross the placenta to the newborn and decrease beat-to-beat variability in the fetal heart rate (FHR). They can increase the likelihood of significant respiratory depression in the newborn at birth and can increase**

the subsequent need for treatment. A meta-analysis aggregated the results of several randomized trials and revealed that opioid treatment is associated with an increased risk of Apgar scores below 7 at 5 minutes (odds ratio [OR], 2.6; 95% confidence interval [CI], 1.2 to 5.6), and increased need for neonatal naloxone (OR, 4.17; 95% CI, 1.3 to 14.3), although the overall incidence of both was low.[15] **An important and significant disadvantage of opioid analgesia is the prolonged effect of these agents on maternal gastric emptying.** When parenteral or epidural opioids are used, gastric emptying is prolonged, and if general anesthesia becomes necessary, the risk of aspiration is increased.[16]

The opioids in common use today are meperidine, nalbuphine, fentanyl, and remifentanil. Morphine fell out of favor in the 1960s to 1970s because of a single study that reported increased respiratory depression in the newborn compared with meperidine, but no recent study has compared the relative safety of opioids for the newborn in the setting of modern practice.

Patient-Controlled Analgesia

IV patient-controlled analgesia (PCA) is often used for women who have a contraindication to neuraxial analgesia (e.g., severe thrombocytopenia). The infusion pump is programmed to give a predetermined dose of drug upon patient demand. The physician will program the pump to include a lockout interval to limit the total dose administered per hour. Advantages of this method include the sense of autonomy, which patients appreciate, and elimination of delays in treatment while the patient's nurse obtains and administers the dose. In general, PCA results in a decreased total dose of opioid during labor.[17] Fentanyl, remifentanil,[18] and meperidine are the opioids most commonly used with this technique.

Meperidine (Demerol)

Meperidine is a synthetic opioid, and 100 mg is roughly equianalgesic to morphine 10 mg but has been reported to have a somewhat less depressive effect on respiration. Usually, 25 to 50 mg are administered intravenously; it may also be used intramuscularly or in a PCA pump to deliver 15 mg of meperidine every 10 minutes as needed until delivery.[19] Intravenously, the onset of analgesia begins almost immediately and lasts approximately 1.5 to 2 hours. Side effects may include tachycardia, nausea and vomiting, and delayed gastric emptying.

Normeperidine is an active metabolite of meperidine and potentiates meperidine's depressant effects in the newborn. Normeperidine concentrations increase slowly; therefore it exerts its effect on the newborn during the second hour after administration. Multiple doses of meperidine result in greater accumulation of both meperidine and normeperidine in fetal tissues[20]; thus administration of large doses of meperidine in the first stage of labor, rather than during the second stage, leads to high doses accumulated in the fetus. A randomized controlled study using intravenous PCA with meperidine for labor analgesia found that 3.4% of infants required naloxone at delivery (vs. 0.8% with epidural analgesia).[21] Normeperidine accumulation in the fetus can result in prolonged neonatal sedation and neurobehavioral changes.[22] These neurobehavioral changes are evident into day 2 and day 3 of life.

Nalbuphine (Nubain)

Nalbuphine is a synthetic agonist-antagonist opioid, meaning it has opioid-blocking properties as well as analgesic properties. Its analgesic potency is similar to that of morphine when compared on a milligram-per-milligram basis, and usual doses are 5 to 10 mg intravenously every 3 hours. A reported advantage of nalbuphine is its ceiling effect for respiratory depression,[23] that is, respiratory depression from multiple doses appears to plateau. One limitation of nalbuphine is that its antagonist activity may also limit the analgesia it can produce, and it may interfere with spinal and epidural opioids given as part of a neuraxial technique. Nalbuphine causes less maternal nausea and vomiting than meperidine, but it tends to produce more maternal sedation, dizziness, and dysphoria and increases the risk of opioid withdrawal in susceptible patients.

Fentanyl

Fentanyl is a fast-onset, short-acting synthetic opioid with no active metabolites. In a randomized comparison with meperidine, fentanyl 50 to 100 μg every hour provided equivalent analgesia with fewer neonatal effects and less maternal sedation and nausea. The main drawback of fentanyl is its short duration of action, which requires frequent redosing or the use of a patient-controlled IV infusion pump. A sample PCA setting for fentanyl is a 50 μg incremental dose with a 10-minute lockout and no basal rate.[17]

Remifentanil

Remifentanil is an even faster-onset, shorter-acting synthetic opioid with no active metabolites; it is metabolized by plasma esterases and is not affected by impaired renal or hepatic function.[18] It should be administered as PCA because of its half-life of only 3 minutes. The ideal dosing regimen has not been determined, but a sample PCA setting might be 0.5 μg/kg boluses every 2 to 3 minutes with no basal rate. Sedation and hypoventilation with oxygen desaturations are more common than with other opioids; therefore respiratory monitoring is required. Placental transfer occurs, but in the neonate it appears to be rapidly metabolized or redistributed.

Sedatives

Sedatives such as barbiturates, phenothiazines, and benzodiazepines do not possess analgesic qualities. All sedatives and hypnotics cross the placenta freely, and except for the benzodiazepines, they have no known antagonists. Sedation is rarely desirable during the childbirth experience.

Promethazine may actually impair the analgesic efficacy of opioids. In a randomized double-blind trial, women received placebo, metoclopramide, or promethazine as an antiemetic with meperidine analgesia.[24] Analgesia after placebo or metoclopramide was significantly better than that after promethazine as measured by pain scores and need for supplemental analgesics. Metoclopramide 10 mg has also been shown to improve PCA analgesia during second-trimester termination of pregnancy.[25] In two randomized double-blind studies, the group that received metoclopramide (vs. saline) used 54% and 66% less IV morphine.

Two major disadvantages of benzodiazepines are that they cause undesirable maternal amnesia[26] and may disrupt thermoregulation in newborns, which renders them less able to maintain an appropriate body temperature.[27] Presumably this can occur with any of the benzodiazepines. As with many drugs, beat-to-beat variability of the FHR can be reduced even with a single IV dose, although these changes do not reflect alterations in the acid-base status of the newborn. Flumazenil, a specific

benzodiazepine antagonist, can reliably reverse benzodiazepine-induced sedation and ventilatory depression.

Inhaled Nitrous Oxide (N₂O)

Nitrous oxide, an inhaled anesthetic gas commonly used during general anesthesia and dental care, has been used in many parts of the world for labor analgesia.[28] It is administered in a 50:50 mix with oxygen using a blender device and a mask held by the mother. A one-way valve allows her to inhale nitrous oxide before and during contractions. Patients report that nitrous oxide does not completely relieve pain, but in many women, it diminishes the perception of pain. Nitrous oxide is safe for the mother and the fetus and does not diminish uterine contractility; the main side effects are nausea and dizziness. It can also be used for short painful procedures such as perineal repair or manual removal of the placenta.[29]

Placental Transfer

Essentially, all analgesic and anesthetic agents except highly ionized muscle relaxants cross the placenta freely (Box 16-1).[30] The limited transfer of muscle relaxants such as succinylcholine enables anesthesiologists to use general anesthesia for cesarean delivery without causing fetal paralysis.

Because the placenta has the properties of a lipid membrane, most drugs and all anesthetic agents cross by simple diffusion. Thus the amount of drug that crosses the placenta increases as concentrations in the maternal circulation and total area of the placenta increase. **Diffusion is also affected by the properties of the drug itself, including molecular weight, spatial configuration, degree of ionization, lipid solubility, and protein binding.** For example, bupivacaine is highly protein bound, a characteristic that some believe explains why fetal blood concentrations are so much lower than with other local anesthetics. On the other hand, bupivacaine is also highly lipid soluble. The more lipid soluble a drug is, the more freely it passes through a lipid membrane. Furthermore, once in the fetal system, lipid solubility enables the drug to be taken up by fetal tissues rapidly (i.e., redistribution), which again contributes to the lower blood concentration of the agent.

BOX 16-1 FACTORS THAT INFLUENCE PLACENTAL TRANSFER FROM MOTHER TO FETUS

Drug
- Molecular weight
- Lipid solubility
- Ionization, pH of blood
- Spatial configuration

Maternal
- Uptake into bloodstream
- Distribution via circulation
- Uterine blood flow: amount, distribution (myometrium vs. placenta)

Placental
- Circulation: intermittent spurting arterioles
- Lipid membrane: Fick's law of simple diffusion

Fetal
- Circulation: ductus venosus, foramen ovale, ductus arteriosus

The degree of ionization of a drug is also important. Most drugs exist in both an ionized and nonionized state, and the nonionized form more freely crosses lipid membranes. The degree of ionization is influenced by the pH; this may become relevant when there is a significant pH gradient between the mother (normal pH of 7.40) and an acidotic infant (pH <7.2). For example, local anesthetics are more ionized at a lower pH, so the nonionized portion of the drug in the maternal circulation (normal pH) crosses to the acidotic fetus, becomes ionized, and thus remains in the fetus, potentially leading to higher local anesthetic concentrations in the fetus/newborn. Whether this has relevant adverse clinical effects on the fetus is unknown.

Neuraxial Analgesic and Anesthetic Techniques

Neuraxial analgesic and anesthetic techniques—spinal, epidural, or a combination—use local anesthetics to provide sensory blockade, as well as various degrees of motor blockade, over a specific region of the body. In obstetrics, neuraxial and other regional analgesic techniques include major blocks, such as lumbar epidural and spinal, and minor blocks, such as paracervical, pudendal, and local infiltration (see Fig. 16-1).

Lumbar Epidural Analgesia/Anesthesia

Epidural blockade is a neuraxial anesthetic used to provide *analgesia* **during labor or surgical** *anesthesia* **for vaginal or cesarean delivery.**[31] **Epidural analgesia offers the most effective form of pain relief**[32] **and is used by the majority of women in the United States.**[1] In most obstetric patients, the primary indication for epidural analgesia is the patient's desire for pain relief. Medical indications for epidural analgesia during labor may include anticipated difficult intubation due to morbid obesity or other causes, a history of malignant hyperthermia, selected forms of cardiovascular and respiratory disease, and prevention or treatment of autonomic hyperreflexia in parturients with a high spinal cord lesion. The technique uses a large-bore needle (16, 17, or 18 gauge) to locate the epidural space. Next, a catheter is inserted through the needle, and the needle is removed over the catheter. After aspirating the catheter, a test dose of local anesthetic with a "marker" such as epinephrine may be given first to be certain the catheter has not been unintentionally placed in the subarachnoid (spinal) space or in a blood vessel. Intravascular placement will lead to maternal tachycardia because of the epinephrine, and rapid onset of sensory and motor block will occur if the local anesthetic is injected into the spinal fluid. Once intravascular and intrathecal placement have been ruled out, local anesthetic is injected through the catheter, which remains taped in place to the mother's back to enable subsequent injections throughout labor (Fig. 16-5; see also Fig. 16-1). Thus it is often called *continuous epidural analgesia.* Anesthesiologists also use a technique described as *segmental epidural analgesia* (Fig. 16-6), in which low concentrations of local anesthetic[3] (<0.25% bupivacaine) are injected at L2 to L5 and affect the small, easily blocked sympathetic nerves that mediate early labor pain but spare the sensation of pressure and motor function of the perineum and lower extremities. The patient should be able to move about in bed and perceive the impact of the presenting part on the perineum.

A dilute local anesthetic combined with an opioid such as fentanyl is administered for maintenance of epidural analgesia. Although the administration may be by continuous infusion at a rate of 5 to 15 mL/hr, patient-controlled epidural analgesia

(PCEA) allows for patient-controlled epidural boluses combined with a continuous infusion. More recently, programmed epidural boluses have been combined with patient-controlled boluses as supplements.[33] Patients vary in their responses to local anesthetics, and infusions may need to be adjusted to a lower rate or concentration if the patient develops excessive motor block. If perineal anesthesia is needed for delivery, a larger volume of local anesthetic can be administered at that time through the catheter (see Fig. 16-6). Alternatively, for perineal anesthesia, the obstetrician can perform a pudendal block or provide local infiltration of the perineum.

A variant of the epidural technique involves passing a small-gauge pencil-point spinal needle through the epidural needle before catheter placement. This combined spinal-epidural (CSE) technique provides more rapid onset of analgesia using a very small dose of opioid or a local anesthetic and opioid combination. An RCT in a private practice setting compared CSE and traditional epidural analgesia in 800 term parturients.[34] They found that patients who received CSE had better pain scores during the first stage of labor and required fewer top-ups by the anesthesiologist, an important consideration when anesthesia manpower is limited. Some practitioners have used this technique to allow parturients to ambulate during labor (the "walking epidural") because there is little or no interference with motor function. Because the dose of drug used in the subarachnoid space is much smaller than that used for epidural analgesia, the risks of local anesthetic toxicity or high spinal block are avoided. Side effects of spinal opioids are usually mild and easily treated and include pruritus and nausea.

Nonreassuring fetal heart rate changes may occur more often in patients who receive combined spinal-epidural analgesia than in those who receive epidural analgesia alone.[35] Although the incidence of hypotension is similar between the two techniques, the etiology of fetal bradycardia after spinal analgesia may relate more to uterine hypertonus than to hypotension. Maternal endogenous catecholamines, specifically the β-agonist epinephrine, decrease rapidly with the onset of spinal analgesia. Loss of β-agonist activity may result in uterine hypertonus, especially in the presence of exogenous oxytocin infusions. Fortunately, these nonreassuring FHR changes do not seem to affect labor outcome. In a review of 2380 deliveries in a community hospital, no increase was found in emergency cesarean delivery in the 1240 patients who received neuraxial analgesia for labor (98% of which were CSE) compared with the 1140 patients who received systemic or no medication.[36] A systematic review of randomized comparisons of intrathecal opioid analgesia versus epidural or parenteral opioids in labor found that the use of intrathecal opioids significantly increased the risk of fetal bradycardia (OR, 1.8; 95% CI, 1.0 to 3.1).[37] However, the risk of cesarean delivery for FHR abnormalities was similar in the two groups (6.0% vs. 7.8%). FHR should be monitored during and after the administration of either epidural or intrathecal medications to allow for timely intrauterine resuscitation.[3]

Complications of Neuraxial Blocks

The Serious Complication Repository Project of the Society of Obstetric Anesthesia and Perinatology (SOAP) reported that high neuraxial block, respiratory arrest in labor and delivery, and unrecognized spinal catheters were the most frequently reported serious complications in more than 257,000 anesthesia procedures over a 5-year study period (Table 16-3).[38] Other side effects of epidural or CSE analgesia include hypotension, local

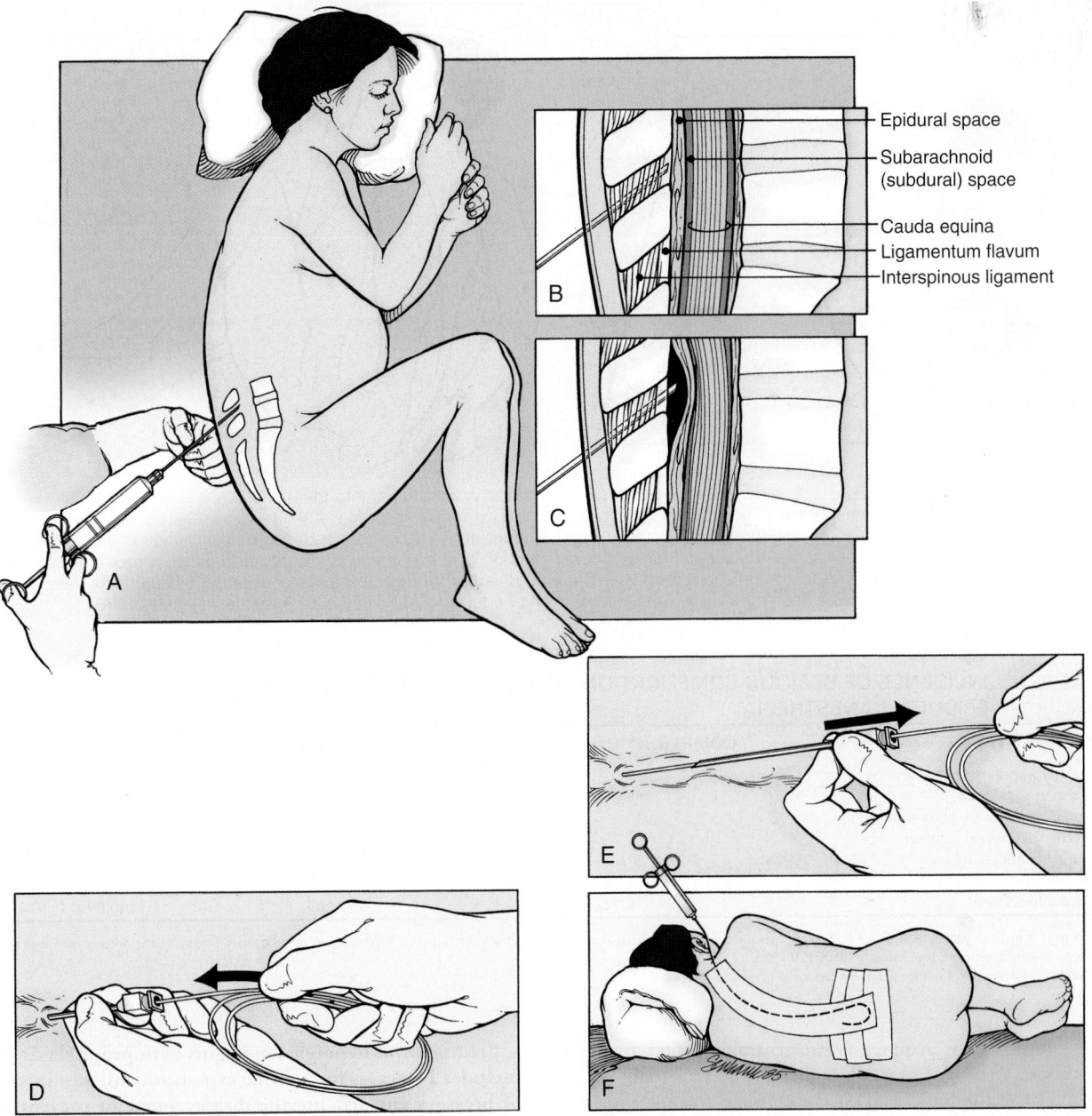

FIG 16-5 Technique of lumbar epidural puncture by the midline approach. **A,** This side view shows the left hand held against the patient's back with the thumb and index finger grasping the hub. Attempts to inject solution while the point of the needle is in the interspinous ligament meet resistance. **B,** The point of the needle is in the ligamentum flavum, which offers marked resistance and makes it almost impossible to inject solution. **C,** Entrance of the needle's point into the epidural space is discerned by sudden lack of resistance to injection of saline. Force of injected solution pushes dura-arachnoid away from the point of the needle. **D,** Catheter is introduced through needle. Note that the hub of the needle is pulled caudad toward the patient, increasing the angle between the shaft of the needle and the epidural space. Also note the technique of holding the tubing, which is wound around the right hand. **E,** Needle is withdrawn over the tubing and is held steady with the right hand. **F,** Catheter is immobilized with adhesive tape. Note the large loop made by the catheter to decrease risk of kinking at the point where the tube exits from the skin. (From Bonica JJ. *Obstetric Analgesia and Anesthesia.* Amsterdam: World Federation of Societies of Anesthesiologists; 1980.)

anesthetic toxicity, allergic reaction, neurologic injury, and post-dural puncture headache. In addition, epidural analgesia use may increase the rate of intrapartum fever and can lengthen the second stage of labor. The effect of epidural analgesia on labor progression is discussed in detail below.

Because epidural anesthesia is associated with side effects and complications, some of which are dangerous, those who administer it must be thoroughly familiar not only with the technical

aspects of its administration but also with the signs and symptoms of complications and their treatment. Specifically, the ASA and ACOG have stated: "Persons administering or supervising obstetric anesthesia should be qualified to manage the infrequent but occasionally life-threatening complications of major regional anesthesia such as respiratory and cardiovascular failure, toxic local anesthetic convulsions, or vomiting and aspiration. Mastering and retaining the skills and knowledge necessary to manage

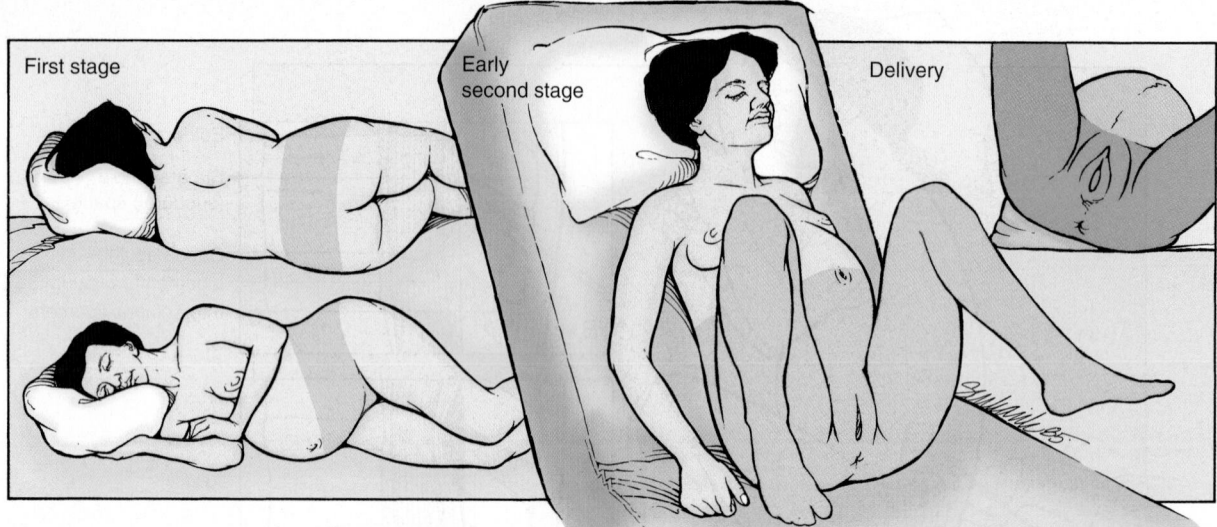

FIG 16-6 Segmental epidural analgesia for labor and delivery. A single catheter is introduced into the epidural space and is advanced so that its tip is at L2. Initially, small volumes of low concentrations of local anesthetic are used to produce segmental analgesia. For the second stage, the analgesia is extended to the sacral segments by injecting a larger amount of the same concentration of local anesthetic with the patient in the semirecumbent position. After internal rotation, a higher concentration of local anesthetic is injected to produce motor block of the sacral segments and thus achieve perineal relaxation and anesthesia. The wedge under the right buttocks causes the uterus to displace to the left. (From Bonica JJ. *Obstetric Analgesia and Anesthesia.* Amsterdam: World Federation of Societies of Anesthesiologists; 1980.)

TABLE 16-3   INCIDENCE OF SERIOUS COMPLICATIONS RELATED TO NEURAXIAL (SPINAL OR EPIDURAL) ANESTHESIA

COMPLICATION	COMPLICATIONS (N)	INCIDENCE	95% CI
Postdural puncture headache	1647	1:144	1:137, 1:151
High neuraxial block	58	1:4336	1:3356, 1:5587
Respiratory arrest in labor suite	25	1:10,042	1:6172, 1:16,131
Unrecognized spinal catheter	14	1:15,435	1:9176, 1:25,634
Serious neurologic injury	27	1:35,923	1:17,805, 1:91,244
Epidural abscess/meningitis	4	1:62,866	1:25,074, 1:235,620
Epidural hematoma	1	1:251,463	1:46,090, 1:10,142,861

Data from D'Angelo R, Smiley RM, Riley E, Segal S. Serious complications related to obstetric anesthesia. The serious complication repository project of the Society for Obstetric Anesthesia and Perinatology. *Anesthesiology.* 2014;120:1505.
CI, confidence interval; *N,* number of complications.

these complications requires adequate training and frequent application."[2] The ASA practice guidelines also state that "When a neuraxial technique is chosen, appropriate resources for the treatment of complications (e.g., hypotension, systemic toxicity, high spinal anesthesia) should be available."[3]

HYPOTENSION

Hypotension is defined variably but most often as a systolic blood pressure less than 100 mm Hg or a 20% decrease from baseline. It occurs after approximately 10% of spinal or epidural blocks given during labor.[39] Hypotension occurs primarily as a result of the effects of local anesthetic agents on sympathetic fibers, which normally maintain blood vessel tone. Vasodilation results in decreased venous return of blood to the right side of the heart, with subsequent decreased cardiac output and hypotension. A secondary mechanism may be decreased maternal endogenous catecholamines following pain relief. Hypotension threatens the fetus by decreasing uterine blood flow. However, when recognized promptly and treated effectively, few if any untoward effects result in either mother or fetus. Special care should be taken to avoid or promptly treat hypotension, especially when acute or chronic fetal compromise is suspected.

Treatment of hypotension begins with prophylaxis, which includes IV access for volume expansion and administration of pressors and left uterine displacement to prevent aortocaval compression by the gravid uterus and to maintain cardiac preload and cardiac output. Isotonic crystalloid boluses should not contain dextrose because of the association with subsequent neonatal hypoglycemia. Proper treatment of hypotension depends on immediate diagnosis; therefore the individual administering the anesthesia must be present and attentive. **Once diagnosed, hypotension is corrected by increasing the rate of IV fluid infusion and exaggerating left uterine displacement. If these simple measures do not suffice, a vasopressor is indicated.**

The vasopressor of choice has evolved from ephedrine given in 5- to 10-mg doses to phenylephrine in 50- to 100-μg increments. Ephedrine is a mixed α- and β-agonist and was thought to be less likely to compromise uteroplacental perfusion than the pure α-agonists, but ephedrine has been associated with fetal tachycardia. **Recent clinical studies have suggested that phenylephrine may be given to safely treat hypotension during neuraxial anesthesia for cesarean delivery and that it leads to higher umbilical artery pH values in the fetus and results in** less maternal nausea and vomiting. When compared with phenylephrine for treatment of hypotension following neuraxial analgesia in multiple randomized trials, ephedrine was associated with higher degrees of fetal acidosis.[40] The β-agonist action of ephedrine may increase fetal oxygen requirements and can lead to hypoxia in cases of uteroplacental insufficiency. Phenylephrine corrects maternal hypotension, apparently without causing clinically significant uterine artery vasoconstriction or decreased placental perfusion even in extremely high doses. Rather than causing abnormal increases in systemic vascular resistance, these doses may simply return vascular tone to normal after spinal anesthesia. It is also possible that constricting peripheral arteries may preferentially shunt blood to the uterine arteries. The parturient has decreased sensitivity to all vasopressors, and that may also protect the fetus from excessive vasoconstriction. The α-adrenergic agents, such as methoxamine and phenylephrine, cause reflex bradycardia that may be useful when a parturient is excessively tachycardic in association with hypotension, or if tachycardia associated with ephedrine would be detrimental. Ephedrine may be preferable if the patient's heart rate is below 70 at baseline.

LOCAL ANESTHETIC TOXICITY

The incidence of systemic local anesthetic toxicity (high blood concentrations of local anesthetic) after obstetric lumbar epidural analgesia is less than 1 in 250,000.[38] Cases of local anesthetic toxicity were absent from the most recent review of the ASA Closed Claims Project database.[41] Toxicity occurs when the local anesthetic is injected into a blood vessel, rather than into the epidural space, or when too much is administered even though injected properly. **These reactions can also occur during placement of pudendal or paracervical blocks. All local anesthetics have maximal recommended doses, and these should not be exceeded.** For example, the maximum recommended dose of lidocaine is 4 mg/kg when used without epinephrine and 7 mg/kg when used with epinephrine. Epinephrine delays and decreases the uptake of local anesthetic into the bloodstream. Package inserts for all local anesthetics contain appropriate dosing information (Table 16-4).

Local anesthetic reactions have two components, central nervous system (CNS) and cardiovascular. Usually, the CNS component precedes the cardiovascular component. Prodromal symptoms of the CNS reaction include excitation, bizarre behavior, ringing in the ears, and disorientation. These symptoms may culminate in convulsions, which are usually brief. After the convulsions, cognitive depression follows, manifested by the postictal state. The *cardiovascular component* of the local anesthetic reaction usually begins with hypertension and tachycardia but is soon followed by hypotension, arrhythmias, and in some instances, cardiac arrest. Thus the cardiovascular

component also has excitant and depressant characteristics. Often the CNS component occurs without the more serious cardiovascular component, although bupivacaine may represent an exception to this principle. **Resuscitation of patients who receive an intravascular injection of bupivacaine is extremely challenging, likely owing to the prolonged blocking effect on sodium channels.** Laboratory evidence supports bupivacaine's increased cardiotoxicity over equianalgesic doses of other amide local anesthetics such as ropivacaine and lidocaine.[42] The manufacturers of bupivacaine have recommended that the 0.75% concentration not be used in obstetric patients or for paracervical block. However, use of a more dilute concentration does not guarantee safety; **bupivacaine and all local anesthetics should be administered by slow, incremental injection.**

Adverse events due to local anesthetic toxicity have decreased because of greater emphasis on incremental dosing and use of a test dose, typically one containing 15 μg of epinephrine, to exclude unintentional IV or subarachnoid catheter placement. Others have questioned the lack of specificity of test doses during labor and the potential harm to the fetus or hypertensive mother.[43] Intravascular injection of 15 μg epinephrine produces maternal tachycardia, which may be difficult to differentiate from that seen during a contraction. Nonreassuring fetal heart tones due to decreased uterine blood flow may also occur after administration of intravascular epinephrine, especially when the fetus is already compromised.

Treatment of a local anesthetic reaction depends on recognizing the signs and symptoms. Prodromal symptoms should trigger the immediate cessation of the injection of local anesthetic. If convulsions have already occurred, treatment is aimed at maintaining proper oxygenation and preventing the patient from harming herself. Convulsions use considerable amounts of oxygen, which results in hypoxia and acidosis. Should the convulsions continue for more than a brief period, small IV doses of propofol (30 to 50 mg) or a benzodiazepine (2 to 5 mg midazolam) are useful. The cardiac and respiratory depressant effects of these agents add to the depressant phase of the local anesthetic reaction; therefore appropriate equipment and personnel must be available to maintain oxygenation and a patent airway and to provide cardiovascular support. Rarely, succinylcholine is needed for paralysis to prevent the muscular activity and to facilitate ventilation and perhaps intubation. In cases of complete cardiac collapse, delivery of the infant may facilitate maternal resuscitation. **IV lipid emulsion may be an effective therapy for cardiotoxic effects of lipid-soluble local anesthetics such as bupivacaine or ropivacaine.[44] Intralipid should be available wherever regional anesthesia is provided.**

The SOAP developed a consensus statement on the management of cardiac arrest in pregnancy that aims to improve maternal resuscitation by providing health care providers critical

TABLE 16-4	MAXIMAL RECOMMENDED DOSES OF COMMON LOCAL ANESTHETICS				
	WITH EPINEPHRINE*		**WITHOUT EPINEPHRINE**	
LOCAL ANESTHETIC	**mg/kg**	**DOSE (mg/70 kg)**	**mg/kg**	**DOSE (mg/70 kg)**
Bupivacaine	3.0	210	2.5	175
Chloroprocaine	14.0	980	11.0	770
Etidocaine	5.5	385	4.0	300
Lidocaine	7.0	490	4.0	300
Mepivacaine	–	–	5.0	350
Tetracaine	–	–	1.5	105

*All epinephrine concentrations are 1:200,000.

information relevant to maternal cardiac arrest.[45] The document includes key cognitive and technical interventions to be undertaken that include immediate basic life support (BLS) and calls for help, chest compressions monitored by capnography if possible, manual left uterine displacement while supine on a backboard, defibrillation, airway management and ventilation, IV access to administer drugs per current advanced cardiovascular life support (ACLS) guidelines, and perimortem cesarean or operative vaginal delivery. Delivery should be performed as soon as possible, striving to make the skin incision for cesarean delivery at 4 minutes after the start of cardiac arrest.

ALLERGY TO LOCAL ANESTHETICS

The two classes of local anesthetics are *amides* and *esters*. **A true allergic reaction to an amide-type local anesthetic (e.g., lidocaine, bupivacaine, ropivacaine) is extremely rare. Allergic reactions to the esters (2-chloroprocaine, procaine, tetracaine) are also uncommon but can occur** and are often associated with a reaction to para-aminobenzoic acid (PABA) in skin creams or suntan lotions. When a patient reports that she is "allergic" to local anesthetics, she is frequently referring to a normal reaction to the epinephrine that is occasionally added to local anesthetics, particularly by dentists. Epinephrine can cause increased heart rate, pounding in the ears, and nausea—symptoms that may be interpreted as an allergic reaction. Therefore it is important to document the situation in which the reaction occurred.

HIGH SPINAL OR "TOTAL SPINAL" ANESTHESIA

This complication occurs when the level of anesthesia rises dangerously high and results in paralysis of the respiratory muscles, including the diaphragm (C3-C5). The incidence of total spinal anesthesia after neuraxial blocks is 1 in 4336 (see Table 16-3).[38] This is the most frequent complication encountered secondary to spinal or epidural anesthesia. Total spinal anesthesia can result from a miscalculated dose of drug or unintentional subarachnoid injection during an epidural block. The ASA Closed Claims Project analysis of obstetric anesthesia liability claims found that the most common cause of maternal death or brain damage in neuraxial anesthesia claims was high block; 80% were associated with dosing epidural anesthesia and 20% involved spinal anesthesia.[41] The accessory muscles of respiration are paralyzed earlier, and their paralysis may result in apprehension and anxiety and a feeling of dyspnea. The patient usually can breathe adequately as long as the diaphragm is not paralyzed, but treatment must be individualized. Dyspnea, real or imagined, should always be considered an effect of paralysis until proved otherwise. Cardiovascular effects, including hypotension and even cardiovascular collapse, may accompany total spinal anesthesia.

Treatment of total spinal anesthesia includes rapidly assessing the true level of anesthesia; therefore individuals who administer major regional anesthesia should be thoroughly familiar with dermatome charts (Fig. 16-7) and should also be able to recognize what a certain sensory level of anesthesia means with regard to innervation of other organs or systems. For example, a T4 sensory level may represent total sympathetic nervous system blockade. **Numbness and weakness of the fingers and hands indicates that the anesthesia has reached the cervical level (C6-C8), which is dangerously close to the innervation of the diaphragm.** If the diaphragm is not paralyzed, the patient is breathing adequately, and cardiovascular stability is maintained, administration of oxygen and reassurance may suffice. If the patient remains anxious or if the level of anesthesia seems to involve the diaphragm, assisted ventilation is indicated, and endotracheal intubation will be necessary to protect the airway. In addition, cardiovascular support is provided as necessary. Delay in treatment due to inadequate monitoring, absence of the anesthesia provider, lack of airway equipment or emergency drugs in the labor room, or delay in resuscitation during transfer of the patient to the operating room for delivery will worsen outcome.[46] With prompt and adequate treatment, serious sequelae should be extremely rare.

NERVE INJURY

Paralysis after either epidural or spinal anesthesia is extremely rare; even minor injuries such as foot-drop and segmental loss of sensation are uncommon. **However, the ASA Closed Claim Project analysis of liability claims notes that the incidence of claims for nerve injury has increased in their most recent review and is now the most common cause of liability in obstetric anesthesia.**[41] Serious neurologic injury occurs with an incidence of 1 in 35,923 (see Table 16-3).[38] Most postpartum neurologic complications are caused by nerve compression during delivery, and both anesthesiologists and obstetricians should be able to recognize common manifestations of these neuropathies.[47] With commercially prepared drugs, ampules, and disposable needles, infection and caustic injury rarely occur. **When nerve damage follows neuraxial analgesia during obstetric or surgical procedures, the anesthetic technique must be suspected, although causation is rare. Other potential etiologies include incorrectly positioned stirrups, difficult forceps applications, or abnormal fetal presentations.** During abdominal procedures, overzealous or prolonged application of pressure with retractors on sensitive nerve tissues may also result in injury. Fortunately, most neurologic deficits after labor and delivery are minor and transient; however, if they are prolonged or worsen, consultation with a neurologist or neurosurgeon should be considered.

A systematic review of serious adverse events among 1.37 million women who received epidural analgesia during labor found the risks of epidural hematoma and epidural abscess were 1 case per 168,000 women and 1 per 145,000 respectively.[48] The risk of persistent neurologic injury was one case per 240,000 women, and the risk of transient neurologic injury was one per 6700. In contrast, the SOAP Serious Complication Registry found the incidence of anesthesia-related epidural hematoma was 1 in 251,463 and the incidence of epidural abscess or meningitis was 1 in 62,866 (see Table 16-3).[38] One of the more dramatic and correctable forms of nerve damage follows compression of the spinal cord by a hematoma that has formed during the administration of spinal or epidural anesthesia, presumably from accidental puncture of an epidural vessel. If the condition is diagnosed early, usually with the aid of a neurologist or neurosurgeon, the hematoma can be removed by laminectomy and the problem will resolve without permanent damage. Fortunately, this is a rare complication. Nonetheless, spinal and epidural blocks are contraindicated if the patient has a coagulopathy or is pharmacologically anticoagulated. Hemolysis, elevated liver enzymes, and low platelets (HELLP) syndrome may be a particularly strong risk factor because of multifactorial sources for coagulation defects.[49] Any significant motor or sensory deficit after neuraxial anesthesia should be investigated immediately and thoroughly (see Fig. 16-7).

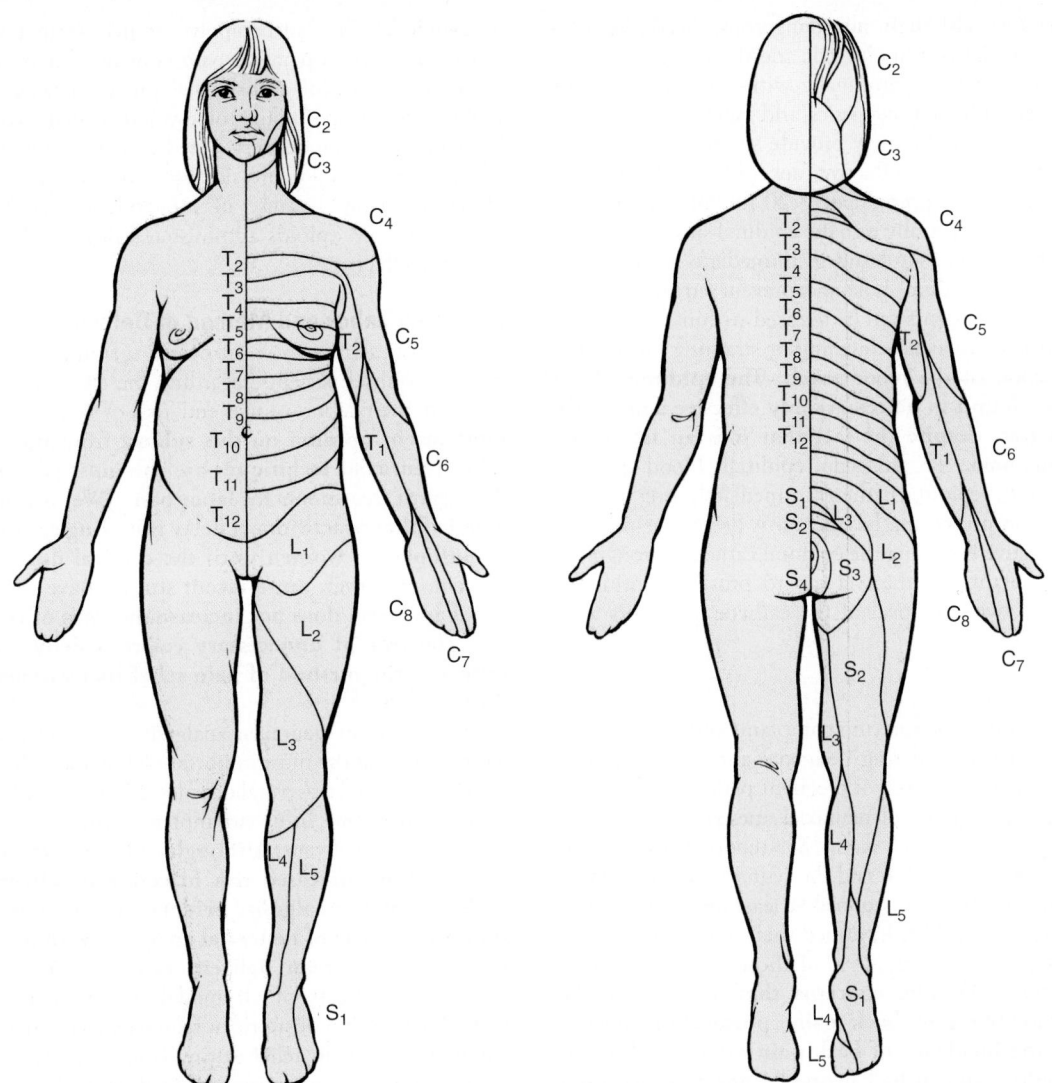

FIG 16-7 Dermatome chart. (Modified from Haymaker L, Woodhall B. *Peripheral Nerve Injuries*. Philadelphia: WB Saunders; 1945.)

Although the incidence of neuraxial infection such as spinal meningitis or epidural abscess is rare, when it occurs it is an important cause of significant maternal morbidity and mortality. In 2009, the Centers for Disease Control and Prevention (CDC) reviewed five cases of bacterial meningitis linked to intrapartum spinal anesthesia in which one woman died.[50] A common denominator in these cases was that either the anesthesiologist who performed the block or visitors in the room were not wearing masks. **Both the American Society of Regional Anesthesia (ASRA) and the ASA have published guidelines on prevention of infection during neuraxial anesthesia that include recommendations to remove jewelry, wash hands, wear a fresh face mask, and disinfect the patient's back using 2% chlorhexadine in alcohol.**[51,52]

SPINAL HEADACHE

Spinal headache rarely follows uncomplicated spinal anesthesia but usually occurs when, during the process of administering an epidural block, the dura is punctured with a large-bore needle ("wet tap"). The incidence of this complication varies between 1% and 3%, and its occurrence depends on the experience of the person performing the epidural block.[53] The risk of postdural puncture headache following CSE is no different than that with epidural analgesia alone, approximately 1.5%.

Once a wet tap occurs, a spinal headache results in as many as 70% of patients. The incidence is much less following spinal anesthesia, because smaller atraumatic (pencil-point) needles are used. **Characteristically, a spinal headache is more severe in the upright position and is relieved by the supine position. A differential diagnosis should include migraine, pneumocephalus from the loss of resistance to air technique, infection, cortical vein thrombosis, preeclampsia, and intracerebral or subarachnoid hemorrhage.**[54] All epidurals are placed using a loss of resistance technique. The loss of resistance can be discerned with either air or saline in the syringe (see Fig. 16-8, *A*). A spinal headache is thought to be caused by loss of cerebrospinal fluid, which causes the brain to settle and thus causes the meninges and vessels to stretch. Hydration, bed rest, abdominal binders, and the prone position have all been advocated as prophylactic measures after known dural puncture. However, most anesthesiologists now agree that these actions are of little value.[55]

When a patient develops a postdural puncture headache (PDPH), she should be counseled about the cause and potential treatment options, which range from conservative to aggressive. Close follow-up, reassurance, and treatment if required is important, because although not dangerous, headache is a common cause of a lawsuit in obstetric anesthesia.[41] If the headache is mild and interferes minimally with activity, treatment may be initiated with oral analgesics and caffeine, which is a cerebral vasoconstrictor that may provide symptomatic relief.[55] If simple measures prove ineffective, an epidural blood patch should be considered. Approximately 20 mL of the patient's own blood is placed aseptically into the epidural space to provide a tamponade effect that may result in immediate relief. It may also coagulate over the dural hole and prevent further cerebrospinal fluid leakage. Patients can be released within an hour and should be instructed to avoid coughing or straining for the first day after insertion of the blood patch. **The epidural blood patch has been found to be remarkably effective and nearly complication free, despite the fact that it is an iatrogenic epidural hematoma.** Prophylactic epidural blood patches inserted through the epidural catheter immediately after delivery are not effective in preventing headaches. A preventive measure that may be effective is passing the epidural catheter through the dural hole at the time of the wet tap to provide continuous spinal anesthesia, with removal of the catheter 24 hours after delivery.[56]

BACK PAIN

Back pain is a common peripartum complaint and is a common concern for women considering neuraxial anesthesia for their delivery. An antepartum survey of pregnant patients before their delivery and before any use of neuraxial anesthesia found that 69% of patients reported back pain, 58% reported sleep disturbances due to back pain, 57% said the pain impaired activities of daily living, and 30% had stopped at least one daily activity because of pain.[57] Only 32% informed their obstetric providers they had back pain, and only 25% of those providers recommended treatment. **Despite concerns that using neuraxial anesthesia contributes to back pain, postpartum surveys indicate that the incidence of back pain after childbirth is the same whether women had neuraxial analgesia for their delivery or not, approximately 40% to 50% at 2 and 6 months postpartum.**[58,59] Despite these reassuring findings, liability for back pain claims is increasing for obstetric anesthesiologists.[41]

BREASTFEEDING ISSUES

Breastfeeding has been recognized as an important public health initiative because of the short- and long-term advantages for mothers and newborns. The Joint Commission has introduced obstetric quality indicators (e.g., breastfeeding) that set expectations for minimum performance on accountability measures for delivery of perinatal care.[60] Some patients and providers are concerned that neuraxial analgesia may hinder the newborn's ability to breastfeed effectively.[61] Observational studies that show an association between difficult breastfeeding and anesthetic use during labor do not account for obstetric events such as prolonged labor or operative delivery, factors that can cause difficulty with early breastfeeding. **Factors that contribute to successful breastfeeding include lactation consultation services, maternal motivation, and support from obstetricians and pediatricians.**[62]

No randomized trials have compared breastfeeding outcomes in patients who received epidural analgesia to those who received no medication.[62] Large doses of epidural fentanyl (>150 μg) given during the course of labor may interfere with early breastfeeding success; thus high concentrations and boluses should

be avoided.[63] Not surprisingly, women treated with epidural analgesia for postoperative pain control after cesarean delivery are more successful at breastfeeding than those treated with systemic opioids.[64] Infants of women treated with intravenous PCA after cesarean delivery were less alert and had more neonatal neurobehavioral depression after meperidine than after morphine, probably because of meperidine's active metabolites; presumably, IV opioids administered during labor would have the same effect.

Effects on Labor and Method of Delivery

In the past, significant controversy surrounded how to appropriately counsel patients regarding the effect of neuraxial analgesia on their labor course and risk of cesarean delivery. **The most recent opinion on this subject from the ACOG states that "Neuraxial techniques are the most effective and least depressant treatments for labor pain. [We] previously recommended that practitioners delay initiating epidural analgesia in nulliparous women until the cervical dilatation reached 4-5 cm. However, more recent studies have shown that epidural analgesia does not increase the risks of cesarean delivery. The fear of unnecessary cesarean delivery should not influence the method of pain relief that women can choose during labor."**[65]

The impact of neuraxial analgesia on cesarean delivery rates has been one of the most important labor and delivery outcomes studied over the last several decades. Multiple studies have evaluated this outcome in an attempt to identify factors associated with cesarean delivery. **Although older observational studies suggested an increased risk of cesarean delivery associated with neuraxial analgesia, evidence from recent RCTs now supports the use of neuraxial analgesia without a significant increase in cesarean delivery rates.** A Cochrane Review[66] assessed the effects of all modalities of neuraxial analgesia, including CSE, on obstetric outcome when compared with nonepidural or no pain relief during labor. Twenty-one RCTs that involved 6664 women were included, and all the studies except one compared epidural analgesia with opiates. The authors concluded that epidural analgesia was effective in reducing pain during labor without evidence of a significant difference in the risk of cesarean delivery (relative risk [RR], 1.07; 95% CI, 0.93 to 1.23; 20 trials, 6534 women).[66]

Other studies[67-69] of early labor versus late initiation of neuraxial analgesia further support the ACOG committee opinion that states no increase in cesarean delivery rate results when epidural analgesia is initiated early in labor (<4 cm dilated). A Cochrane Review on early versus late initiation of epidural analgesia for labor concluded that quality evidence suggests early and late initiation of epidural analgesia for labor have similar effects on all measured outcomes.[70]

STUDY DESIGN

Multiple prospective randomized studies of epidural analgesia have been performed both in nulliparous populations and in mixed populations. However, the poor quality of analgesia provided by systemic opioids typically leads to high rates of crossover of control patients into the epidural analgesia arm. Neither intent-to-treat analysis nor actual-use analysis are entirely satisfactory in this situation. Studies with the lowest crossover rates have accomplished their goal through the use of substantial doses of parenteral opioids, which has resulted in higher than expected rates of neonatal resuscitation in the opioid groups.[19,21] Nonrandomized studies provide interesting observational data;

however, careful analysis of potential confounders is critical because patients who self-select epidural analgesia are clearly different from patients who avoid it. Of concern, randomized studies are often conducted in academic centers where operative delivery rates in low-risk patients may be significantly different than in community hospitals. Finally, neuraxial analgesia techniques vary, and modifications in technique occur continuously. More modern techniques use lower concentrations of local anesthetic and titrate the dose to the specific needs of the patient, potentially lowering the risk of operative delivery.[3]

PROGRESS OF LABOR AND CESAREAN DELIVERY RATE

Management of epidural analgesia and timing of administration should be individualized to the patient's needs and level of pain. Attention should be focused on minimizing local anesthetic concentrations while still providing adequate pain control and avoiding administration of epidural analgesia until the obstetrician is committed to delivery. A concern has been a possible dose-response effect—that is, more dense analgesia could result in an increased cesarean delivery rate. Several RCTs have evaluated traditional epidural analgesia with 0.25% bupivacaine compared with low-dose bupivacaine/fentanyl epidural techniques and have found no differences in the rate of cesarean delivery.[71] **Although epidural analgesia does not increase the risk of cesarean delivery, management of neuraxial analgesia should be individualized to the patient's needs and level of pain with a focus on minimizing local anesthetic concentrations and motor block while still providing adequate pain control.**

The potential for prolonged labor, increased oxytocin use, and increased risk of instrumental delivery have been additional considerations for clinicians and their patients who receive neuraxial analgesia. Although the relative risk of oxytocin treatment after initiation of epidural analgesia varies considerably depending on obstetric practice (i.e., rates of induction and active management of labor), systematic reviews[66,72] that have evaluated this outcome demonstrate that **epidural analgesia is associated with a significant increase in the use of oxytocin after the initiation of epidural analgesia**. Epidural analgesia also exerts some effect on the length of active labor. **Although neuraxial analgesia may shorten first-stage labor in some women and lengthen it in others, there is little doubt that effective neuraxial analgesia prolongs the second stage of labor by 15 to 30 minutes.**[72] However, when asked their preferences, women prefer a lower intensity and longer duration of pain during labor to higher intensity, shorter duration labor pain.[73] Although few obstetricians in the past would allow the second stage to continue for more than 2 hours, most agree that a delay in the second stage does not adversely affect maternal or neonatal outcome provided (1) electronic fetal monitoring confirms reassuring fetal status, (2) maternal hydration and analgesia are adequate, and (3) progress is ongoing in the descent of the fetal head. A retrospective study of 42,268 women, half of whom had epidural analgesia, found that both nulliparous and multiparous women who had epidural analgesia had longer second stages of labor.[74] However the 95th percentile threshold for second-stage labor was more than 2 hours longer in women with epidural analgesia compared with women who did not receive epidural analgesia. Adopting this longer time period might prevent some unnecessary interventions. ACOG has stated that if progress is being made, the duration of the second stage alone does not mandate intervention. In such cases, **potential strategies for decreasing the risk of instrument-assisted delivery include reduced density of neuraxial analgesia during the second stage, delayed pushing, and avoiding arbitrary definitions of a prolonged second stage.**

Any analysis of the relationship between neuraxial analgesia and instrument-assisted vaginal delivery is complicated by the strong influence of obstetric practice and the obstetrician's attitude toward operative vaginal delivery. Also, obstetricians may be more likely to perform elective instrument-assisted delivery in patients with effective analgesia. Three systematic reviews have evaluated the effect of neuraxial analgesia on mode of vaginal delivery.[71,72,75] These trials included nearly 10,000 patients, and the results suggested that epidural analgesia was associated with an increased risk of instrumented vaginal delivery. However, operator bias is an important consideration. In clinical practice, indications vary widely among obstetricians, and it is often difficult to distinguish between *indicated* and *elective* instrumented deliveries. Although most obstetricians are more likely to perform such deliveries in women with adequate pain relief, another factor that affects the rate of instrumented vaginal deliveries is whether these deliveries are conducted in teaching institutions. Such deliveries are more likely to be performed in patients with adequate analgesia for the purposes of teaching; residents in obstetrics need to perform a minimum number of instrumented vaginal deliveries to graduate from training. Minimizing the risk of instrumented vaginal delivery while maximizing analgesia requires attention by the anesthesiologist to the individual needs of the patient. Modern neuraxial techniques use lower concentrations of local anesthetic and a titrated dose, factors that likely contribute to lowering the risk of operative delivery in such patients.

In a given population, the risk of cesarean delivery may vary depending on the patient population, obstetric management, protocols for oxytocin augmentation, the obstetric provider, patient attitudes toward cesarean delivery, and provider comfort with instrument-assisted vaginal delivery as well as additional risk factors. Neuraxial analgesia alone does not increase the risk of cesarean delivery.

FEVER

Epidural analgesia during labor is associated with an increase in maternal temperature compared with women who receive no analgesia or systemic opioids alone.[76] In a well-designed study with a low crossover rate (6%), Sharma and colleagues[75] reported a 33% rate of intrapartum fever greater than 37.5°C in nulliparous patients randomized to epidural analgesia compared with 7% in those who received parenteral opioids. The more than fourfold increased risk of fever occurred despite relatively minor prolongations in the mean duration of labor (50 minutes). Similarly, Yancey and colleagues[77] also described an eighteenfold increase in the rate of intrapartum fever in nulliparous patients (from 0.6% to 11%) in a single year following the introduction of an epidural analgesia service in their hospital.

The etiology of this febrile response is not well understood; possible mechanisms include noninfectious inflammatory activation, changes in thermoregulation, and acquired intrapartum infection. Intrapartum fever after epidural analgesia is associated with increased serum levels of inflammatory cytokines in the mother and fetus, but no mechanism in which epidural blockade might cause inflammation has been elucidated. Thermoregulation may be altered because epidural analgesia leads to decreased sweating (by providing sympathetic blockade) and less hyperventilation after relief of pain in labor. Both sweating and hyperventilation would otherwise provide heat dissipation. **No study has found an increased rate of infection associated with epidural analgesia for labor.**

Acetaminophen, the standard therapy used to ameliorate hyperthermia, is not effective in preventing fever secondary to epidural analgesia. High-dose maternal corticosteroids given to parturients with epidural analgesia blocks the febrile response but also substantially increases the risk of bacteremia in exposed babies.[78] A randomized trial of prophylactic cefoxitin versus placebo did not prevent fever in nulliparous women who requested epidural analgesia.[79]

Despite the lack of infectious morbidity, intrapartum exposure to hyperthermia may not be benign for the neonate. A retrospective review of low-risk women who received epidural analgesia found maternal temperature greater than 99.5°F was associated with adverse neonatal outcomes such as hypotonia, assisted ventilation, low Apgar scores, and early-onset seizures.[80] Without temperature elevation, epidural use was not associated with adverse neonatal outcomes, but the rate of adverse outcomes increased directly with maximum maternal temperature. An animal study indicates that the presence of hyperthermia during an ischemic event increases susceptibility to hypoxic-ischemic insult.[81] Although the absolute risk is low, maternal temperature greater than 38°C is associated with 9.3-fold increased risk of cerebral palsy in term infants (95% CI, 2.7 to 31). **It is important to clarify that no evidence suggests that epidural analgesia is associated with infection, encephalopathy, or cerebral palsy.** Active cooling measures such as decreasing room temperature, removing blankets from the mother, and use of cool IV fluids should be used for all febrile parturients.

Paracervical Block

Paracervical block analgesia is a simple and effective procedure when performed properly (see Table 16-1). Commonly, 5 to 6 mL of a dilute solution of local anesthetic without epinephrine (e.g., 1% lidocaine or 1% or 2% 2-chloroprocaine) is injected into the mucosa of the cervix at the 3 and 9 o'clock positions (Fig. 16-8). The duration of analgesia depends on the local anesthetic used. This technique has fallen out of favor owing to its association with the fetal bradycardia that follows in 2% to 70% of applications. Occurring within 2 to 10 minutes and persisting from 3 to 30 minutes, these bradycardias are usually benign; however, cases of fetal acidosis and death have been reported. A significant decrease in pH and a rise in base deficit occur only in those fetuses with bradycardia that persists more than 10 minutes.[82] **Although no consensus has been reached regarding the mechanism of paracervical block bradycardia, this block should be used cautiously at all times and should not be used at all in the presence of nonreassuring fetal heart rate monitoring or suspected uteroplacental insufficiency.**

ANESTHESIA FOR INSTRUMENTED VAGINAL DELIVERY OR PERINEAL REPAIR

The goal of pain relief for vaginal delivery is to match the patient's wishes with the requirements of the delivery without subjecting either mother or fetus to unnecessary risk.

Local Anesthesia

In the form of perineal infiltration, local anesthesia is widely used and very safe. Spontaneous vaginal delivery, episiotomy, and perhaps outlet vacuum deliveries can be accomplished

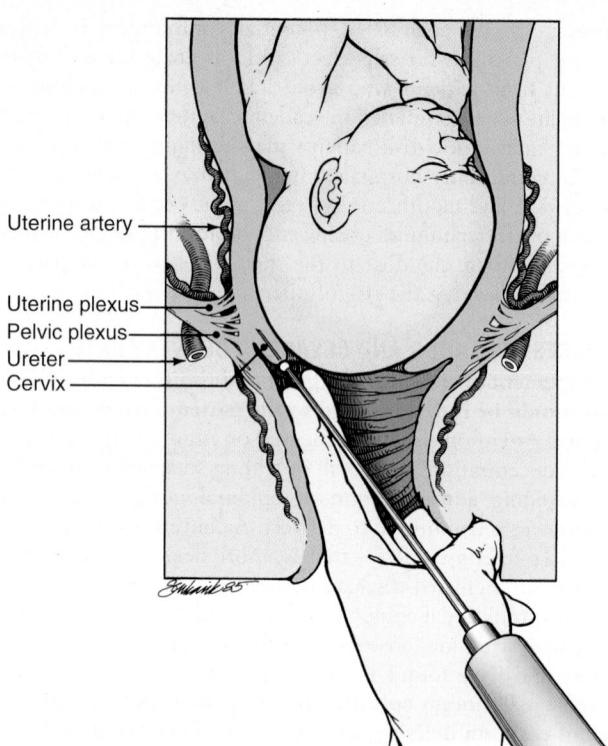

FIG 16-8 Technique of paracervical block. Schematic coronal section (*enlarged*) of lower portion of cervix and upper portion of vagina shows relation of needle to paracervical region. (Modified from Bonica JJ. *Principles and Practice of Obstetric Analgesia and Anesthesia.* Philadelphia: FA Davis; 1967:234.)

TABLE 16-5	LIDOCAINE CONCENTRATIONS IN MATERNAL PLASMA AND UMBILICAL CORD VEIN AT DELIVERY AFTER PERINEAL INFILTRATION

	CONCENTRATION (ng/mL)	
SAMPLE (*N* = 15)	**MEAN ± SD**	**RANGE**
Maternal plasma		
Peak concentration	648 ± 666	60-2400
At delivery	548 ± 468	33-1474
Umbilical cord vein	420 ± 406	45-1380
Fetal/maternal ratio*	1.32 ± 1.46	0.05-4.66

From Philipson EH, Kuhnert BR, Syracuse CD. Maternal, fetal, and neonatal lidocaine levels following local perineal infiltration. *Am J Obstet Gynecol.* 1984;149:403.
*Ratio of level in cord vein to level in maternal vein at delivery (mean of individual ratios, not ratio of means).
SD, standard deviation.

with this simple technique. Local anesthetic toxicity may occur if large amounts of local anesthetic are used or if an inadvertent intravascular injection occurs. Usually, 5 to 15 mL of 1% lidocaine suffices. Rapid and significant transfer of lidocaine to the fetus occurs after perineal infiltration. The concentration of lidocaine at delivery was greater in the umbilical vein than in the mother in 5 of 15 infants (Table 16-5).

Pudendal Nerve Block

Pudendal nerve block is a minor regional block that is also reasonably effective and very safe. Using an Iowa trumpet and a 20-gauge needle, the obstetrician injects 5 to 10 mL of local anesthetic just below the ischial spine. Because the hemorrhoidal nerve may be aberrant in 50% of patients, some physicians prefer to inject a portion of the local anesthetic somewhat posterior to the spine (Fig. 16-9). Although a transperineal approach to the ischial spine is possible, most prefer the transvaginal approach, for which 1% lidocaine or 2% 2-chloroprocaine can be used.

Pudendal block is generally satisfactory for all spontaneous vaginal deliveries and episiotomies and for some outlet or low operative vaginal deliveries, but it may not be sufficient for deliveries that require additional manipulation. **The potential for local anesthetic toxicity is higher with pudendal block, compared with perineal infiltration, because of large vessels proximal to the injection site** (see Fig. 16-9). Therefore aspiration of the needle before injection is particularly important. When perineal and labial infiltration are required in addition to pudendal block, it is critically important to closely monitor the total amount of local anesthetic given.

Monitored Anesthesia Care With Sedation

For urgent or unanticipated instrumented deliveries, an anesthesiologist, anesthesiologist assistant, or nurse anesthetist may administer nitrous oxide or IV analgesia while maintaining protective laryngeal and cough reflexes. The obstetrician should add local infiltration or a pudendal block. The combined effects are additive and are satisfactory for most operative vaginal deliveries, shoulder dystocias, and head entrapments. The anesthesiologist frequently questions the patient to determine the level of anesthesia and to ensure that deeper planes of anesthesia are avoided. Such precautions are important because if the patient becomes unconscious, all of the hazards associated with general anesthesia are possible, including airway obstruction, hypoxia, and aspiration. Because continual assessment of the patient's state of consciousness is required and is sometimes difficult, only anesthesiologists, anesthesiologist assistants, or nurse anesthetists should administer inhalation analgesia. Furthermore, in the United States, this technique may require use of the anesthesia machine, misuse of which can prove disastrous. The anesthesiologist may use 50% nitrous oxide or, for IV analgesia, ketamine 0.25 to 0.5 mg/kg. This latter agent may be particularly effective in the labor room when an anesthesia machine is not available or for the patient who cannot or will not tolerate an anesthetic face mask. Inhalation or IV analgesia renders some patients amnesic of the event, which may be undesirable for the mother.

Spinal (Subarachnoid) Block

A saddle block is a spinal block in which the level of anesthesia is limited to little more than the perineum. Spinal anesthesia is reasonably easy to perform and usually provides total pain relief in the blocked area; therefore spontaneous

and forceps deliveries, perineal repairs, and more complicated deliveries can all be accomplished without pain for the mother. The patient's ability to push may be compromised somewhat by diminished motor strength and significant sensory block. Left uterine displacement should be maintained after the local anesthetic has been injected to maintain venous return and prevent excess hypotension.

Other techniques such as initiation of epidural anesthesia (assuming it is not already in place for labor analgesia) or general anesthesia are rarely if ever used in modern practice.

ANESTHESIA FOR CESAREAN DELIVERY

In the United States, general anesthesia is used for about 10% of cesarean births (depending on the size of the hospital), and spinal, epidural, or CSE anesthetics are used for approximately 90% of these deliveries (Table 16-6).[1] Local anesthesia for cesarean delivery is possible but is rarely used or taught anymore. Although neuraxial anesthesia may have benefits for the mother, neuraxial or general anesthesia results in similar fetal outcomes as ascertained by Apgar scores and blood gas measurements (Table 16-7).

Premedication

Premedication using sedative or opioid agents is usually omitted because these agents cross the placenta and can depress the newborn. Sedation should be unnecessary if the procedure is explained well and the patient is reassured.

Aspiration and Aspiration Prophylaxis

Aspiration is a serious and potentially fatal complication of general anesthesia and therefore deserves specific attention. When aspiration does occur, the consequences are worse if gastric volume is high and if the acidity of the aspirate is low. Pregnant patients are at higher risk for aspiration because the enlarged uterus increases intraabdominal pressure and thus intragastric pressure; the gastroesophageal sphincter is distorted by the enlarged uterus, making it less competent and possibly explaining the high incidence of heartburn that occurs during pregnancy. Increased progesterone levels affect smooth muscle, which delays gastric emptying and relaxes the gastroesophageal sphincter. Labor itself delays gastric emptying, primarily when patients have received opioids.[16]

The severity of lung damage and rates of morbidity after aspiration vary and depend on the type of material aspirated. Less acidic aspirates (pH >2.5) fill the alveoli and decrease PaO_2 without a significant destructive or inflammatory effect. Aspirates with a pH of less than 2.5 cause hemorrhage, inflammatory exudates, and edema and result in lower PaO_2. **Aspiration of partially digested food produces the most severe physiologic and histologic alterations.** PaO_2 decreases more than with any

TABLE 16-6	ANESTHETIC PROCEDURES USED FOR CESAREAN DELIVERY IN 2001 ACCORDING TO SIZE OF DELIVERY SERVICE					
HOSPITAL SIZE	**EPIDURAL BLOCK (%)**		**SPINAL BLOCK (%)**		**GENERAL ANESTHESIA (%)**	
(BIRTHS/YEAR)	ELECTIVE	EMERGENT	ELECTIVE	EMERGENT	ELECTIVE	EMERGENT
<500	14	14	80	59	3	25
500-1499	17	21	75	48	5	30
>1500	22	36	67	45	3	15

Modified from Bucklin BA, Hawkins JL, Anderson JR, Ullrich FA. Obstetric anesthesia workforce survey. *Anesthesiology.* 2005;103:645.

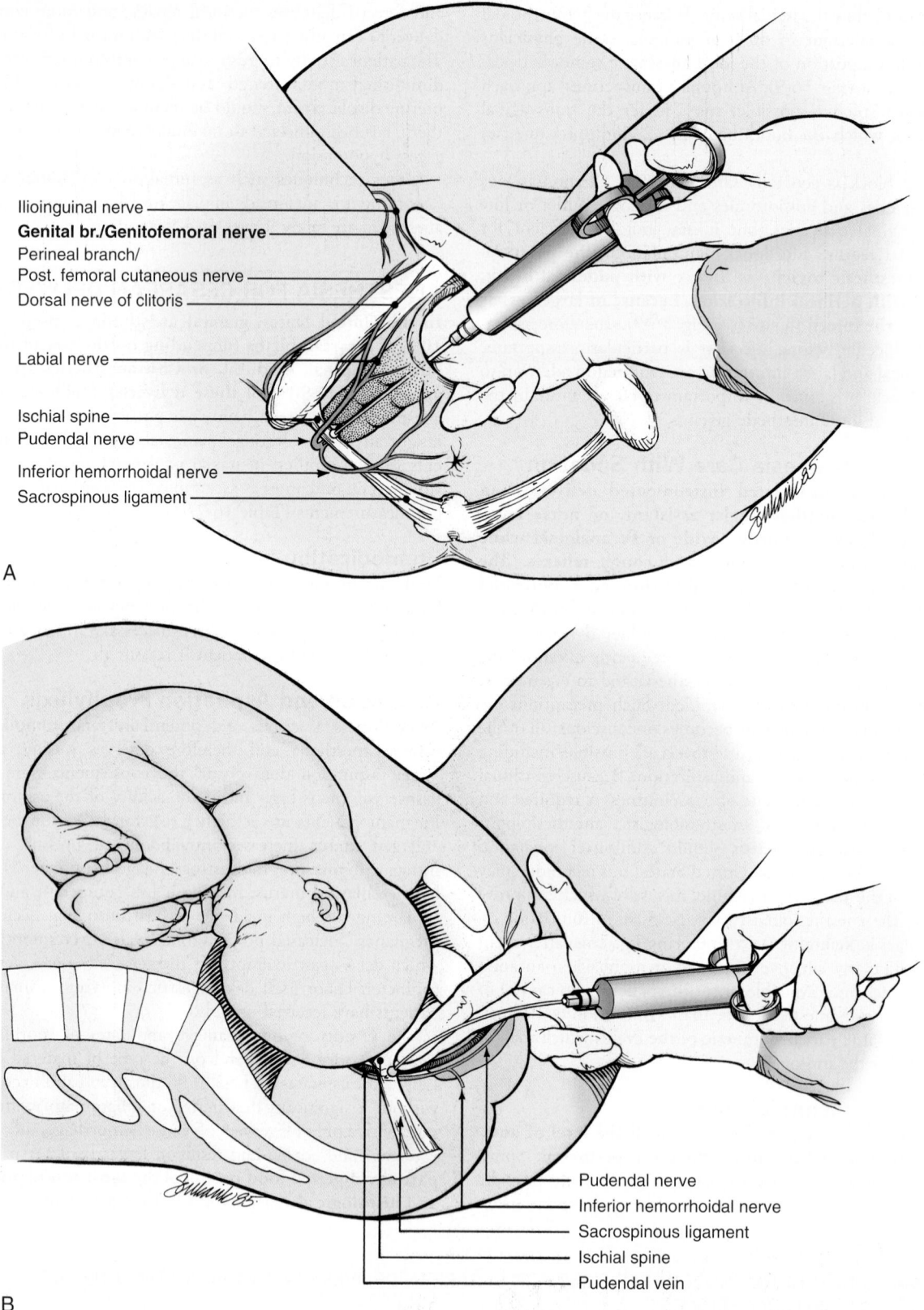

Ilioinguinal nerve

Genital br./Genitofemoral nerve

Perineal branch/
Post. femoral cutaneous nerve

Dorsal nerve of clitoris

Labial nerve

Ischial spine

Pudendal nerve

Inferior hemorrhoidal nerve

Sacrospinous ligament

A

Pudendal nerve

Inferior hemorrhoidal nerve

Sacrospinous ligament

Ischial spine

Pudendal vein

B

FIG 16-9 Anatomy of the pudendal nerve and techniques of pudendal block.

TABLE 16-7   ELECTIVE CESAREAN DELIVERY BLOOD GAS AND APGAR SCORES

	GENERAL ANESTHESIA* (N = 20)	EPIDURAL ANESTHESIA* (N = 15)	SPINAL ANESTHESIA[†] (N = 15)
Umbilical Vein			
pH	−7.38	−7.359	−7.34
PO_2 (mm Hg)	35	36	37
PCO_2 (mm Hg)	38	42	48
Apgar <6			
1	−1	−0	−0
5	−0	−0	−0
Umbilical Artery			
pH	−7.32	−7.28	−7.28
PO_2 (mm Hg)	22	18	18
PCO_2 (mm Hg)	47	55	63
BE (mEq/L)	−1.80	−1.60	−1.40

*Data from James FM III, Crawford JS, Hopkinson R, et al. A comparison of general anesthesia and lumbar epidural analgesia for elective cesarean section. *Anesth Analg.* 1977;56:228.
[†]Data from Datta S, Brown WU. Acid-base status in diabetic mothers and their infants following general or spinal anesthesia for cesarean section. *Anesthesiology.* 1977;47:272.
BE, base excess.

TABLE 16-8   ARTERIAL BLOOD GAS TENSIONS AND pH OF DOGS 30 MINUTES AFTER ASPIRATION OF 2 mL/kg OF VARIOUS MATERIALS

ASPIRATE COMPOSITION	pH	RESPONSE PO_2 (mm Hg)	PCO_2 (mm Hg)	pH
Saline	5.9	61	34	7.37
Hydrochloride	1.8	41	45	7.29
Food particles	5.9	34	51	7.19
Food particles	1.8	23	56	7.13

From Gibbs CP, Modell JH. Management of aspiration pneumonitis. In: Miller RD ed. *Anesthesia.* 3rd ed. New York: Churchill Livingstone; 1990:1293.

other type of aspiration, and lung damage is considerably more destructive (Table 16-8).

Although acidic stomach contents can be neutralized safely and effectively with clear antacids or an H_2-receptor antagonist, antacids cannot ameliorate the risks of aspiration after food intake. Aspiration of partially digested food causes significant hypoxia and lung damage, even at a pH level as high as 5.9. To decrease aspiration risk in cases of unplanned cesarean delivery, oral intake during labor should be limited to modest amounts of clear liquids or ice chips.[3]

Use of a clear antacid is considered routine for all parturients prior to surgery. Additional aspiration prophylaxis using an H_2-receptor blocking agent and metoclopramide may be given to parturients with risk factors such as morbid obesity, diabetes mellitus, or a difficult airway or for those who have previously received opioids. As soon as it is known that the patient requires cesarean delivery, be it with neuraxial or general anesthesia, 30 mL of a clear, nonparticulate antacid—such as 0.3 M sodium citrate, Bicitra (citric acid and sodium citrate), or Alka Seltzer, 2 tablets in 30 mL water—is administered to decrease gastric acidity and ameliorate the consequences of aspiration, should it occur. The chalky white particulate antacids are avoided because they can produce lung damage if aspirated (Fig. 16-10).[83]

Left Uterine Displacement

As during labor, the uterus may compress the inferior vena cava and the aorta during cesarean delivery, leading to reduced venous return to the heart, reduced cardiac output, and reduced

BOX 16-2   **ADVANTAGES AND DISADVANTAGES OF GENERAL ANESTHESIA FOR CESAREAN DELIVERY**

Advantages
- Patient does not have to be awake during a major operation.
- General anesthesia provides total pain relief.
- Operating conditions are optimal.
- The mother can be given 100% oxygen if needed.

Disadvantages
- Patients will not be awake during cesarean delivery, but there is a small risk of undesirable awareness.
- A slight risk of fetal depression exists immediately after birth.
- Intubation causes hypertension and tachycardia, which may be particularly dangerous in severely preeclamptic patients.
- Intubation can be difficult or impossible.
- Aspiration of stomach contents is possible.

uteroplacental perfusion. **Aortocaval compression is detrimental to both mother and fetus.** The duration of anesthesia has little effect on neonatal acid-base status when left uterine displacement is practiced; however, when patients remain supine, Apgar scores decrease as time of anesthesia increases.[84]

General Anesthesia

The term *balanced general anesthesia* refers to a combination of various agents—including hypnotic agents to induce sleep, inhalation agents, opioids, and muscle relaxants—as opposed to high concentrations of potent inhalation agents alone. It is preferred for obstetric applications (Box 16-2).

Failure to intubate and aspiration continue to cause anesthesia-related maternal mortality, and as a result, many anesthesiologists, obstetricians, and patients now prefer neuraxial anesthesia over general anesthesia.[1] To understand how these complications may arise, the obstetrician should be aware of the sequence of events during general anesthesia.

Preoxygenation

Preoxygenation is especially important in pregnant patients, who have decreased functional residual capacity and are more likely than nonpregnant patients to rapidly become

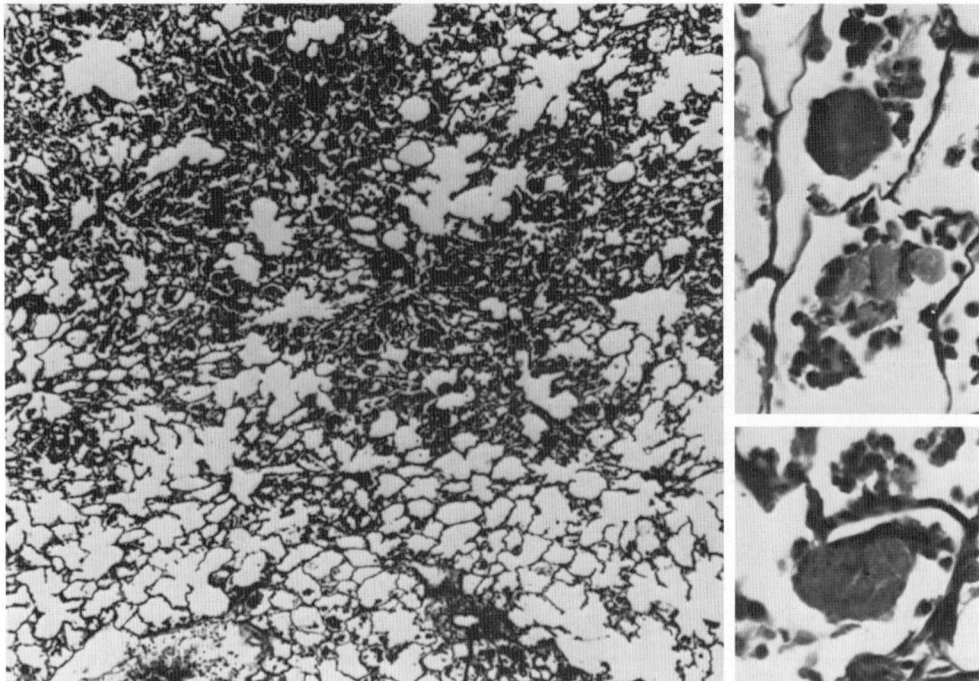

FIG 16-10 Lung after aspiration of particulate antacid. Note marked extensive inflammatory reaction. The alveoli are filled with polymorphonuclear leukocytes and macrophages in approximately equal numbers. Insets at right show large and small intraalveolar particles surrounded by inflammatory cells (48 hours). Later, the reaction changed to an intraalveolar cellular collection of clusters of large macrophages with abundant granular cytoplasm, some of which contained small amphophilic particles similar to those seen in the insets. No fibrosis or other inflammatory reaction was seen (28 days). (From Gibbs CP, Schwartz DJ, Wynne JW, et al. Antacid pulmonary aspiration in the dog. *Anesthesiology*. 1979;51:380.)

hypoxemic if difficult intubation accompanied by apnea occurs. Before starting induction, 100% oxygen should be administered through a face mask for 2 to 3 minutes. In situations of dire emergency, four vital-capacity breaths of 100% oxygen through a tight-circle system will provide similar benefit.[85]

Induction

The anesthesiologist administers a short-acting induction agent to render the patient unconscious. An appropriate dose of any of these agents has little effect on the fetus. **Induction agents that may be used are propofol,[86] etomidate,[87] and ketamine,[88] all of which are rapidly redistributed in both mother and fetus.** Women who receive ketamine for induction require less analgesic medications in the first 24 hours after their cesarean delivery compared with those who received thiopental.[89] Ketamine antagonism of N-methyl-D-aspartate (NMDA) receptors may prevent central hypersensitization and provide preemptive analgesia.

Although obstetricians are often concerned about the *induction-to-delivery interval* (I-D) during general anesthesia, the *uterine incision-to-delivery interval* (U-D) is more predictive of neonatal status.[84,90] With a prolonged I-D interval, there is fetal uptake of the inhaled anesthetic and depressed Apgar scores (i.e., sleepy babies), but fetal acid-base status is normal, and effective ventilation is all that is needed. A prolonged U-D interval greater than 3 minutes leads to depressed Apgar scores with neuraxial or general anesthesia and is associated with elevated fetal umbilical artery norepinephrine concentrations and associated fetal acidosis.[90]

Immediately after the induction agent, the anesthesiologist gives a muscle relaxant to facilitate intubation. Succinylcholine—a rapid-onset, short-acting muscle relaxant—remains the agent of choice in most patients.

During rapid-sequence induction, as the induction agent begins to take effect and the patient approaches unconsciousness, an assistant applies pressure to the cricoid cartilage just below the thyroid cartilage and does not release the pressure until an endotracheal tube is placed, the cuff is inflated, and its position is verified by end-tidal carbon dioxide measurement and bilateral breath sounds. **Pressure on the cricoid compresses the esophagus and is extremely important in preventing aspiration should regurgitation or vomiting occur.** In most instances, aspiration can be prevented by using cricoid pressure at induction of anesthesia.

Intubation

In most cases, intubation proceeds smoothly. However, in approximately 1 in 533 obstetric patients, it is difficult, delayed, or impossible.[38] The incidence of failed intubation in obstetric patients is more common than in patients in the general operating room (1 in 533 in obstetric patients vs. 1 in 2230 in surgical patients).[38,91] When the delay is prolonged or the intubation is impossible, **the critical factors include delivering oxygen to the now unconscious and paralyzed patient and preventing aspiration.** Delay in intubation is associated with escalating aspiration risk; therefore it is particularly important during a difficult intubation that the person applying cricoid pressure not release that pressure until told to do so by the anesthesiologist.

The patient at risk for a difficult or impossible intubation can often be identified before surgery. Examination of the airway is a critical part of the preanesthetic evaluation (Fig. 16-11). The anesthesiologist will assess four factors: (1) the ability to visualize oropharyngeal structures (Mallampati classification[92]); (2) range of motion of the neck; (3) presence of a receding mandible, which indicates the depth of the submandibular space; and (4) whether protruding maxillary incisors are present. It is important to know that airway patency can worsen significantly over the course of labor. One study found significant increases in the Mallampati score and the incidence of class III and class IV airways along with a decrease in oral volume and pharyngeal areas when they compared prelabor and postlabor airway examinations.[93] The worsening airways were unrelated to labor duration or fluid intake. These changes would make endotracheal intubation more difficult; thus a careful airway examination is essential just before administering anesthesia rather than relying on prelabor information. **Obstetricians should be alert to the**

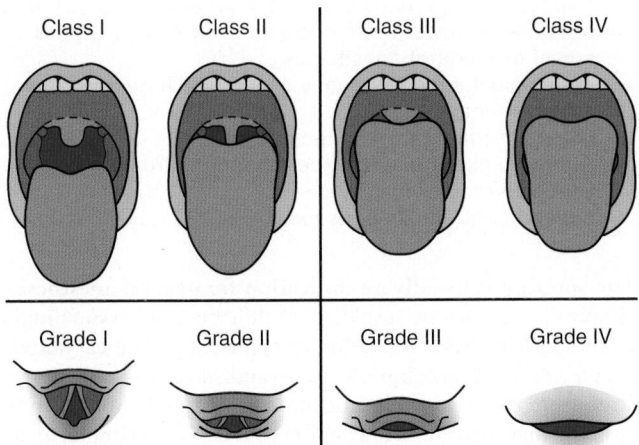

FIG 16-11 Mallampati airway classifications with corresponding laryngoscopic view of the vocal cords. (Modified from Hughes SC, Levinson G, Rosen MA, eds. *Shnider and Levinson's Anesthesia for Obstetrics,* 4th ed. Philadelphia: Lippincott Williams & Wilkins; 2002.)

presence of obesity, severe edema, and anatomic abnormalities of the face, neck, or spine that include those from trauma or surgery, abnormal dentition, difficulty opening the mouth, extremely short stature, short neck or arthritis of the neck, or goiter. When the obstetrician recognizes airway abnormalities, patients should be referred for an early preoperative evaluation by the anesthesiologist.

Before surgery begins, the anesthesiologist must ensure that the endotracheal tube is properly positioned using capnography and auscultation. The operation should not proceed until the airway is secure because the patient cannot be allowed to awaken after the abdomen is opened.

FAILED INTUBATION

When intubation cannot be accomplished and cesarean delivery is not urgent, the decision to delay the operation and allow the mother to awaken is easy. However, if the operation is being done because of rapidly worsening fetal condition or maternal hemorrhage, allowing the mother to awaken may further jeopardize the fetus or mother. Rarely, in situations of dire fetal compromise, the anesthesiologist and obstetrician may jointly decide to proceed with cesarean delivery while the anesthesiologist provides oxygenation, ventilation, and anesthesia by face mask ventilation or laryngeal mask airway (LMA), with an additional person maintaining continuous cricoid pressure. In these emergent situations, it may be necessary to have additional trained personnel to provide assistance. After delivery, the obstetrician may need to obtain temporary hemostasis and then halt surgery while the anesthesiologist secures the airway by fiberoptics or other methods.

An algorithm for management of failed intubation in the obstetric patient is shown in Figure 16-12. Nursing staff should also be familiar with the difficult airway algorithm in case they are called upon to assist during an airway emergency.[94] Videolaryngoscopy is a valuable tool in the emergency setting,[95] and supraglottic devices such as the LMA should always be immediately available for rescue in the case of difficult or failed intubation.[94]

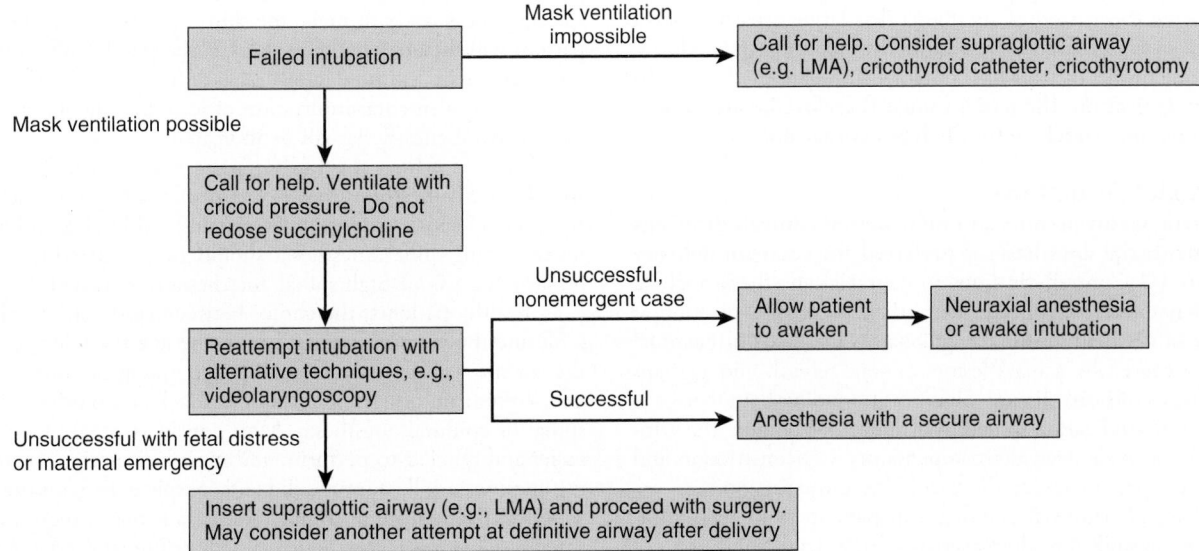

FIG 16-12 An algorithm for the management of failed intubation in the obstetric patient. LMA, laryngeal mask airway.

Agents
NITROUS OXIDE AND OXYGEN
Once the endotracheal tube is in place, a 50:50 mixture of nitrous oxide and oxygen—which is safe for both mother and fetus—is usually added to provide analgesia and amnesia.

VOLATILE HALOGENATED AGENT
In addition to nitrous oxide, a low concentration of a volatile halogenated agent (e.g., isoflurane, sevoflurane, or desflurane) is added to provide maternal amnesia and additional analgesia. In low concentrations, these agents are not harmful to mother or fetus. **Uterine relaxation does not result from low concentrations of these agents, and bleeding should not be increased secondary to their addition. Proceeding without a potent inhalation agent results in an unacceptably high incidence of maternal awareness and recall.** Even with the use of one of these agents, maternal awareness and recall occasionally occur.[96] Therefore it is important that all operating room personnel use discretion in conversation and conduct themselves as if the patient were awake.

Post Delivery
The concentration of nitrous oxide can be increased after delivery if the mother tolerates a lower inspired concentration of oxygen. In addition, the volatile halogenated agent is continued at a low concentration, and pain relief is supplemented with an opioid such as fentanyl or morphine. Other IV agents such as benzodiazepines may be added to ensure maternal amnesia. Oxytocin is infused intravenously to improve uterine tone; however, large bolus injections are avoided because they can cause a drop in systemic vascular resistance, hypotension, and tachycardia. **Maternal deaths have been reported following IV bolus oxytocin in the setting of hypovolemia or pulmonary hypertension.**[97]

Extubation
Because the patient can aspirate while awakening and during emergence, extubation is not done until the patient is awake and can respond appropriately to commands. Coughing and bucking do not necessarily indicate that the patient is awake, merely that she is in the second stage—the excitement stage—of anesthesia. It is during this period of anesthesia that laryngospasm is most likely to occur should any foreign body, including the endotracheal tube or bits of stomach contents, stimulate the larynx. **To prevent aspiration, the patient must therefore be awake and conscious, not merely active, before extubation.**

Neuraxial Anesthesia
If the fetal status permits and no maternal contraindications exist, neuraxial anesthesia is preferred for cesarean delivery (Box 16-3).[1] Contraindications to neuraxial anesthesia include hemodynamically significant hemorrhage or sepsis, infection at the site of needle insertion, coagulopathy, increased intracranial pressure caused by a mass lesion, patient refusal, and perhaps some forms of heart disease. Significant ongoing hemorrhage is a firm contraindication to neuraxial anesthesia because the sympathetic blockade overrides compensatory vasoconstriction and potentially precipitates cardiovascular decompensation.

The use of neuraxial anesthesia in patients with fetal compromise depends on the severity of the fetal condition. **If the situation is severe and acute, do not delay delivery to perform a neuraxial technique de novo. Ongoing acute fetal**

BOX 16-3   ADVANTAGES AND DISADVANTAGES OF NEURAXIAL ANESTHESIA

Advantages
- The patient is awake and can participate in the birth of her child.
- There is little risk of drug depression or aspiration and no intubation difficulties.
- Newborns generally have good neurobehavioral scores.
- The father is more likely to be allowed in the operating room.
- Postoperative pain control using neuraxial opioids may be superior to intravenous patient-controlled anesthesia.

Disadvantages
- Patients may prefer not to be awake during major surgery.
- A block that provides inadequate anesthesia may result.
- Hypotension, perhaps the most common complication of neuraxial anesthesia, occurs during 25% to 85% of spinal or epidural anesthetics.
- Total spinal anesthesia may occur, which necessitates airway management.
- Local anesthetic toxicity may occur.
- Although extremely rare, permanent neurologic sequelae may occur.
- Several contraindications exist.

---

deterioration is usually an indication for general anesthesia. However, a history or suspicion of difficult intubation should prompt either awake intubation or neuraxial anesthesia, despite the presence of fetal compromise, because of the risk of maternal death from unsuccessful intubation. Lesser degrees of fetal compromise may permit neuraxial anesthesia. For example, if an epidural catheter has been placed earlier, a partial level of anesthesia already exists, and the patient is hemodynamically stable, extension of epidural anesthesia may be appropriate for cesarean delivery. The anesthesiologist can give additional local anesthetic while the urethral catheter is inserted and the abdomen is prepared and draped. Often, anesthesia will be satisfactory when the surgeon is ready to make the skin incision. If not, the FHR pattern will dictate whether a delay is acceptable. When partial but inadequate epidural anesthesia results, the clinician may consider supplemental infiltration of local anesthetic, but most often general anesthesia will be indicated.

In cases in which the FHR tracing is not critical, de novo spinal or CSE anesthesia may be performed for cesarean delivery. In cases in which extension of existing epidural anesthesia is unsuccessful, spinal anesthesia should be placed with caution because the risk of high spinal anesthesia is increased.[38]

In healthy patients, the choice between epidural, spinal, and CSE anesthesia primarily rests with the anesthesiologist. With the recent availability of small-gauge spinal needles with a pencil-point tip design, the risk of headache is no different after spinal or epidural anesthesia. Most consider spinal block to be easier and quicker to perform, and most believe that the resulting anesthesia will be more solid and complete. Perhaps the most significant advantage of spinal anesthesia is that it requires considerably less local anesthetic, and therefore, the potential for local anesthetic toxicity is reduced. A CSE technique provides the benefits of spinal anesthesia plus the ability to prolong the anesthetic if needed by dosing the epidural catheter; however, any of these techniques is satisfactory and should provide safe, effective anesthesia for the mother and the fetus.

Postoperative Care

If spinal or epidural anesthesia was used for cesarean delivery, excellent postoperative analgesia can be obtained by addition of preservative-free morphine to the local anesthetic solution. The more lipid-soluble opioids such as fentanyl or sufentanil are used to improve the quality of intraoperative anesthesia but have a short duration of 2 to 4 hours. They may be used postoperatively in combination with a local anesthetic in a continuous or patient-controlled epidural infusion. In contrast, morphine is hydrophilic, which gives it a prolonged duration of up to 24 hours, and it can be given as a single dose at the time of cesarean delivery. Unfortunately, its water solubility also gives morphine a long onset time and a higher incidence of side effects. The most common side effects of spinal and epidural opioids are itching and nausea; respiratory depression is a rare but serious complication. **Several studies have shown that spinal or epidural opioids provide superior pain relief when compared with parenteral (intramuscular or intravenous PCA) opioids with a trend toward earlier hospital discharge and lower cost.**[3]

If general anesthesia was used, or neuraxial opioids provide inadequate pain control, an intravenous PCA can be used for postoperative pain management. Morphine, hydromorphone, and fentanyl have all been used successfully. When intravenous PCA is used, the pump settings include an incremental dose of 1 to 2 mg morphine, 0.2 to 0.4 mg hydromorphone, or 25 µg fentanyl and a lockout interval of 6 to 10 minutes. Basal rates are rarely necessary for pain control and only increase maternal sedation and side effects. Using PCA provides better patient satisfaction by allowing the patient to control her pain medication.

The addition of nonsteroidal antiinflammatory drugs (NSAIDs) significantly improves pain scores with neuraxial morphine and reduces use of PCA opioids.[98] IV ketorolac, rectal indomethacin, or oral ibuprofen can be used depending on the patient's ability to tolerate oral intake. Contraindications for NSAID use include renal insufficiency or low urine output, use of gentamicin or similar drugs with renal toxicity, coagulopathy, and uterine atony. Although the package insert for ketorolac states that it is contraindicated for use in breastfeeding mothers, the American Academy of Pediatrics approves its use while women are breastfeeding. IV or oral acetaminophen should also be used as part of a multimodal analgesic regimen.

In most cases, postoperative care is uneventful in obstetric patients. However, **recent reports suggest that the postoperative period can be an important time for anesthetic-related maternal mortality.** In a state review of maternal deaths in Michigan from 1985 through 2003, 8 of 855 maternal deaths were found to be anesthesia related and occurred during emergence or recovery from general anesthesia.[99] Hypoventilation or airway obstruction occurred in these cases, and obesity and black race were factors associated with these deaths. These cases raise important questions about appropriate postanesthesia care unit (PACU) management after general anesthesia for cesarean delivery and point out the need for additional monitoring in obese patients at risk for obstructive sleep apnea. A recent survey of obstetric anesthesiology directors of North American academic institutions found that 45% of institutions (28 of 62) had no

specific postanesthesia recovery training for nursing staff who provide postcesarean care for patients recovering from neuraxial or general anesthesia.[100] In addition, 43% of respondents (29 of 67) rated the recovery care provided to cesarean delivery patients as lower quality than care given to general surgical patients. Results from this survey suggest that in many cases, the level of care provided for postanesthesia recovery from cesarean delivery may not meet guidelines established by the ASA Task Force on Postanesthetic Care and the American Society of Perianesthesia Nurses. However, the ASA Practice Guidelines for Obstetric Anesthesia[3] emphasize that labor and delivery units should have the same staffing and equipment as surgical operating and recovery rooms to reduce risks associated with emergence after general anesthesia for cesarean delivery and to reduce the risk associated with obesity and obstructive sleep apnea.

KEY POINTS

- Analgesia during labor can reduce or prevent potentially adverse stress responses to the pain of labor, including postpartum depression.
- Parenteral opioids for labor analgesia work primarily by sedation and, except at high doses, result in minimal reduction of maternal pain. Side effects include maternal nausea and respiratory depression in both the mother and newborn. The routine use of promethazine in conjunction with opioids should be avoided.
- Placental transfer of a drug between mother and fetus is governed by the characteristics of the drug, including its size, lipid solubility, and ionization; maternal blood levels and uterine blood flow; placental circulation; and the fetal circulation.
- Continuous neuraxial (epidural or spinal) analgesia is the most effective form of intrapartum pain relief currently available and has the flexibility to provide additional anesthesia for spontaneous or instrumented delivery, cesarean delivery, and postoperative pain control.
- Spinal opioids as part of a CSE technique provide excellent analgesia during much of the first stage of labor, and they decrease or avoid the risks of local anesthetic toxicity, high spinal anesthesia, and motor block. Most patients need additional analgesia with epidural local anesthetics later in labor and during the second stage.
- Side effects and complications of neuraxial anesthesia include hypotension, local anesthetic toxicity, total spinal anesthesia, neurologic injury, and spinal headache. Personnel who provide anesthesia must be competent and available to treat these problems.
- Epidural analgesia does not increase the rate of cesarean delivery but may increase oxytocin use and the rate of instrument-assisted vaginal deliveries. The duration of the second stage is increased by 15 to 30 minutes. Maternal-fetal factors and obstetric management are the most important determinants of the cesarean delivery rate.
- Epidural analgesia is associated with an increased rate of maternal fever during labor, although the mechanism is unknown. This does not alter the rate of documented neonatal sepsis. Other neonatal implications are unclear.

◆ General anesthesia is used for less than 5% of elective and roughly 25% of emergent cesarean deliveries. Although safe for the newborn, general anesthesia can be associated with failed intubation and aspiration, causes of anesthesia-related maternal mortality.

◆ Aspiration of gastric contents is most detrimental when food particles are present or the pH is less than 2.5; therefore patients should be encouraged not to eat during labor, and acid-neutralizing medications should be used before operative deliveries.

◆ The use of neuraxial anesthesia is not absolutely contra-indicated in cases of nonreassuring fetal testing; the method of anesthesia should be chosen based on the degree of fetal compromise and maternal safety.

REFERENCES

1. Bucklin BA, Hawkins JL, Anderson JR, Ullrich FA. Obstetric anesthesia workforce survey. *Anesthesiology*. 2005;103:645.
2. Optimal goals for anesthesia care in obstetrics. ACOG Committee Opinion No. 433. American College of Obstetricians and Gynecologists and American Society of Anesthesiologists. *Obstet Gynecol*. 2009;113:1197.
3. American Society of Anesthesiologists Task Force on Obstetric Anesthesia. Practice guidelines for obstetric anesthesia. *Anesthesiology*. 2016. Epub ahead of print.
4. Melzack R. The myth of painless childbirth (the John J. Bonica Lecture). *Pain*. 1984;19:321.
5. Morishima HO, Yeh M-N, James LS. Reduced uterine blood flow and fetal hypoxemia with acute maternal stress: experimental observation in the pregnant baboon. *Am J Obstet Gynecol*. 1979;134:270.
6. Eidelman AI, Hoffmann NW, Kaitz M. Cognitive deficits in women after childbirth. *Obstet Gynecol*. 1993;81:764.
7. Ding T, Dong-Xin W, Qu Y, Chen Q, Zhu SN. Epidural labor analgesia is associated with a decreased risk of postpartum depression: a prospective cohort study. *Anesthesiology*. 2014;119:383.
8. Campogna G, Camorcia M, Stirparo S. Expectant fathers' experience during labor with or without epidural analgesia. *Int J Obstet Anesth*. 2007;16:110.
9. Reynolds F, Sharma SK, Seed PT. Analgesia in labour and fetal acid-base balance: a meta-analysis comparing epidural with systemic opioid analgesia. *Br J Obstet Gynaecol*. 2002;109:1344.
10. Maimburg RD, Vaeth M, Durr J, et al. Randomized trial of structured antenatal training sessions to improve the birth process. *Br J Obstet Gynaecol*. 2010;117:921.
11. Lee H, Ernst E. Acupuncture for labor pain management: a systematic review. *Am J Obstet Gynecol*. 2004;191:1573.
12. Cluett ER, Pickering RM, Getliffe K, St. George Saunders NJ. Randomised controlled trial of labouring in water compared with standard of augmentation for management of dystocia in first stage of labour. *BMJ*. 2004;328:314.
13. Immersion in water during labor and delivery. Committee Opinion No. 594. American College of Obstetricians and Gynecologists. *Obstet Gynecol*. 2014;123:912.
14. Olofsson C, Ekblom A, Ekman-Ordeberg G, Hjelm A, Irestedt L. Lack of analgesic effect of systemically administered morphine or pethidine on labour pain. *Br J Obstet Gynaecol*. 1996;103:968.
15. Halpern SH, Leighton BL, Ohlsson A, et al. Effect of epidural vs parenteral opioid analgesia on the progress of labor: a meta-analysis. *JAMA*. 1998;280:2105.
16. O'Sullivan GM, Sutton AJ, Thompson SA, et al. Noninvasive measurement of gastric emptying in obstetric patients. *Anesth Analg*. 1987;66:505.
17. Campbell DC. Parenteral opioids for labor analgesia. *Clin Obstet Gynecol*. 2003;46:616.
18. Stocki D, Matot I, Einav S, Eventov-Friedman S, Ginosar Y, Weiniger CF. A randomized controlled trial of the efficacy and respiratory effects of patient-controlled intravenous remifentanil analgesia and patient-controlled epidural analgesia in laboring women. *Anesth Analg*. 2014;118:589.
19. Sharma SK, Alexander JM, Messick G, et al. A randomized trial of epidural analgesia versus intravenous meperidine analgesia during labor in nulliparous women. *Anesthesiology*. 2002;96:546.
20. Kuhnert BR, Kuhnert PM, Philipson EH, Syracuse CD. Disposition of meperidine and normeperidine following multiple doses during labor. II Fetus and neonate. *Am J Obstet Gynecol*. 1985;151:410.
21. Sharma SK, Sidawi JE, Ramin SM, et al. A randomized trial of epidural versus patient-controlled meperidine analgesia during labor. *Anesthesiology*. 1997;87:487.
22. Wittels B, Glosten B, Faure EA, et al. Postcesarean analgesia with both epidural morphine and intravenous patient-controlled analgesia: neurobehavioral outcomes among nursing neonates. *Anesth Analg*. 1997;85:600.
23. Romagnoli A, Keats AS. Ceiling effect for respiratory depression by nalbuphine. *Clin Pharmacol Ther*. 1980;27:478.
24. Vella L, Francis D, Houlton P, Reynolds F. Comparison of the antiemetics metoclopramide and promethazine in labour. *BMJ*. 1985;290:1173.
25. Rosenblatt WH, Cioffi AM, Sinatra R, Silverman DG. Metoclopramide-enhanced analgesia for prostaglandin-induced termination of pregnancy. *Anesth Analg*. 1992;75:760.
26. Camann W, Cohen MB, Ostheimer GW. Is midazolam desirable for sedation in parturients? *Anesthesiology*. 1986;65:441.
27. Owen JR, Irani SF, Blair AW. Effect of diazepam administered to mothers during labour on temperature regulation of neonate. *Arch Dis Child*. 1972;47:107.
28. Likis FE, Andrews JC, Collins MR. Nitrous oxide for the management of labor pain: a systematic review. *Anesth Analg*. 2014;118:153.
29. Barbieri RL, Camann W, McGover C. Nitrous oxide for labor pain. *OBG Manag*. 2014;26:10.
30. Zakowski MI, Geller A. The Placenta: Anatomy, Physiology, and Transfer of Drugs. In: Chestnut DH, Wong CA, Tsen LC, Warwick DNK, Beilin Y, Mhyre JM, eds. *Chestnut's Obstetric Anesthesia: Principles and Practice*. 5th ed. Philadelphia: Elsevier; 2014:55.
31. Hawkins JL. Epidural analgesia for labor and delivery. *N Engl J Med*. 2010;362:1503.
32. Pain relief during labor. ACOG Committee Opinion No. 295. American College of Obstetricians and Gynecologists. *Obstet Gynecol*. 2004;104:213.
33. George RB, Allen TK, Habib AS. Intermittent epidural bolus compared with continuous epidural infusions for labor analgesia: a systematic review and meta-analysis. *Anesth Analg*. 2013;116:133.
34. Gambling D, Berkowitz J, Farrell TR, Pue A, Shay D. A randomized controlled comparison of epidural analgesia and combined spinal-epidural analgesia in a private practice setting: pain scores during first and second stages of labor and at delivery. *Anesth Analg*. 2013;116:636.
35. Abrão KC, Francisco RP, Miyadahira S, Cicarelli DD, Zugaib M. Elevation of uterine basal tone and fetal heart rate abnormalities after labor analgesia. *Obstet Gynecol*. 2009;113:41.
36. Albright GA, Forster RM. Does combined spinal-epidural analgesia with subarachnoid sufentanil increase the incidence of emergency cesarean delivery? *Reg Anesth*. 1997;22:400.
37. Mardirosoff C, Dumont L, Boulvain M, Tramer MR. Fetal bradycardia due to intrathecal opioids for labor analgesia: a systematic review. *Br J Obstet Gynaecol*. 2002;109:274.
38. D'Angelo R, Smiley RM, Riley E, Segal S. Serious complications related to obstetric anesthesia. The serious complication repository project of the Society for Obstetric Anesthesia and Perinatology. *Anesthesiology*. 2014; 120:1505.
39. Simmons SW, Taghizadeh N, Dennis AT, Hughes D, Cyna AM. Combined spinal-epidural versus epidural analgesia in labour. *Cochrane Database Syst Rev*. 2012;CD003401.
40. Ngan Kee WD, Khaw KS, Tan PE, Ng FF, Karmakar MK. Placental transfer and fetal metabolic effects of phenylephrine and ephedrine during spinal anesthesia for cesarean delivery. *Anesthesiology*. 2009;111:506.
41. Davies JM, Posner KL, Lee LA, Cheney FW, Domino KB. Liability associated with obstetric anesthesia. *Anesthesiology*. 2009;110:131.
42. Groban L, Deal DD, Vernon JC, et al. Cardiac resuscitation after incremental overdosage with lidocaine, bupivacaine, levobupivacaine, and ropivacaine in anesthetized dogs. *Anesth Analg*. 2001;92:37.
43. Leighton BL, Norris MC, Sosis M, et al. Limitations of epinephrine as a marker of intravascular injection in laboring women. *Anesthesiology*. 1987;66:688.
44. Neal JM, Bernards CM, Butterworth JF, et al. ASRA practice advisory on local anesthetic systemic toxicity. *Reg Anesth Pain Med*. 2010;35:152.
45. Lipman S, Cohen S, Einav S, et al. The Society for Obstetric Anesthesia and Perinatology consensus statement on the management of cardiac arrest in pregnancy. *Anesth Analg*. 2014;118:1003.

46. Leighton BL. Why obstetric anesthesiologists get sued. *Anesthesiology*. 2009;110:8.

47. O'Neal MA, Chang LY, Salajegheh MK. Postpartum spinal cord, root, plexus and peripheral nerve injuries involving the lower extremities: a practical approach. *Anesth Analg*. 2015;120:141.

48. Ruppen W, Derry S, McQuay H, Moore RA. Incidence of epidural hematoma, infection and neurologic injury in obstetric patients with epidural analgesia/anesthesia. *Anesthesiology*. 2006;105:394.

49. Moen V, Dahlgren N, Irestedt L. Severe neurological complications after central neuraxial blockades in Sweden 1990–1999. *Anesthesiology*. 2004;101:950.

50. de Fijter S, DiOrio M, Carmean J. Bacterial meningitis after intrapartum spinal anesthesia – New York and Ohio, 2008-2009. *CDC Morb Mortal Wkly Rep*. 2010;59:65.

51. Hebl JR. The importance and implications of aseptic techniques during regional anesthesia. *Reg Anesth Pain Med*. 2006;31:311.

52. American Society of Anesthesiologists Task Force on Infectious Complication Associated with Neuraxial Techniques. Practice advisory for the prevention, diagnosis, and management of infectious complications associated with neuraxial techniques. *Anesthesiology*. 2010;112:530.

53. Sachs A, Smiley R. Post-dural puncture headache: The worst common complication in obstetric anesthesia. *Semin Perinatol*. 2014;38:386.

54. Stella CL, Jodicke CD, How HY, Harkness UF, Sibai BM. Postpartum headache: is your work-up complete? *Am J Obstet Gynecol*. 2007;196:318.e1.

55. Month RC. Postdural puncture headache and the arduous quest to teach old docs new tricks. *J Clin Anesth*. 2011;23:347.

56. Heesen M, Klohr S, Rossaint R, Walters M, Straube S, van de Velde M. Insertion of an intrathecal catheter following accidental dural puncture: a meta-analysis. *Int J Obstet Anesth*. 2013;22:26.

57. Wang SM, Dezinno P, Maranets I, et al. Low back pain during pregnancy: prevalence, risk factors, and outcomes. *Obstet Gynecol*. 2004;104:65.

58. Howell CJ, Dean T, Lucking L, et al. Randomised study of long term outcome after epidural versus non-epidural analgesia during labour. *BMJ*. 2002;325:357.

59. Loughnan BA, Carli F, Romney J, et al. Epidural analgesia and backache: a randomized controlled comparison with intramuscular meperidine for analgesia during labour. *Br J Anaesth*. 2002;89:466.

60. The Joint Commission. Questions and answers: The perinatal care core measure set. *Jt Comm Perspect*. 2013;33:12-14. Available at: <http://www.jointcommission.org/assets/1/6/s11.pdf>.

61. Wiklund I, Norman M, Uvnas-Moberg K, Ransjo-Arvidson AB, Andolf E. Epidural analgesia: breast-feeding success and related factors. *Midwifery*. 2009;25:e31.

62. Szabo A. Intrapartum neuraxial analgesia and breastfeeding outcomes: limitations of current knowledge. *Anesth Analg*. 2013;116:399.

63. Beilin Y, Bodian CA, Weiser J, et al. Effect of labor epidural analgesia with and without fentanyl on infant breast-feeding: a prospective, randomized, double-blind study. *Anesthesiology*. 2005;103:1211.

64. Hirose M, Hara Y, Hosokawa T, Tanaka Y. The effect of postoperative analgesia with continuous epidural bupivacaine after cesarean section on the amount of breast feeding and infant weight gain. *Anesth Analg*. 1996;82:1166.

65. Analgesia and cesarean delivery rates. ACOG Committee Opinion No. 339. American College of Obstetricians and Gynecologists. *Obstet Gynecol*. 2006;107:1487.

66. Anim-Somuah M, Smyth R, Howell C. Epidural versus non-epidural or no analgesia in labour. *Cochrane Database Syst Rev*. 2005;(4):CD000331.

67. Wong CA, Scavone BM, Peaceman AM, et al. The risk of cesarean delivery with neuraxial analgesia given early versus late in labor. *N Engl J Med*. 2005;352:655.

68. Ohel G, Gonen R, Vaida S, Barak S, Gaitini L. Early versus late initiation of epidural analgesia in labor: does it increase the risk of cesarean section? A randomized trial. *Am J Obstet Gynecol*. 2006;194:600.

69. Marucci M, Cinnella G, Perchiazzi G, Brienza N, Fiore T. Patient-requested neuraxial analgesia for labor: impact on rates of cesarean and instrumental vaginal delivery. *Anesthesiology*. 2007;106:1035.

70. Sng BL, Leong WL, Zeng Y, et al. Early versus late initiation of epidural analgesia for labour. *Cochrane Database Syst Rev*. 2014;(10):CD007238.

71. Comparative Obstetric Mobile Epidural Trial (COMET) Study Group UK. Effect of low-dose mobile versus traditional epidural techniques on mode of delivery: a randomised controlled trial. *Lancet*. 2001;358:19.

72. Liu EH, Sia AT. Rates of caesarean section and instrumental vaginal delivery in nulliparous women after low concentration epidural infusions or opioid analgesia: systematic review. *BMJ*. 2004;328:1410.

73. Carvalho B, Hilton G, Wen L, Weiniger CF. Prospective longitudinal cohort questionnaire assessment of laboring women's preference both pre-and post-delivery for either reduced pain intensity for a longer duration or greater pain intensity for a shorter duration. *Br J Anaesth*. 2014;113:468.

74. Cheng YW, Shaffer BL, Nicholson JM, Caughey AB. Second stage of labor and epidural use. *Obstet Gynecol*. 2014;123:527.

75. Sharma SK, McIntire DD, Wiley J, Leveno KJ. Labor analgesia and cesarean delivery. *Anesthesiology*. 2004;100:142.

76. Goetzl L. Epidural fever in obstetric patients: it's a hot topic. *Anesth Analg*. 2014;118:494.

77. Yancey MK, Zhang J, Schwarz J, Dietrich CS, Klebanoff M. Labor epidural analgesia and intrapartum maternal hyperthermia. *Obstet Gynecol*. 2001;98:763.

78. Goetzl L, Zighelboim I, Badell M, et al. Maternal corticosteroids to prevent intrauterine exposure to hyperthermia and inflammation: a randomized, double-blind, placebo-controlled trial. *Am J Obstet Gynecol*. 2006;195:1031.

79. Sharma SK, Rogers BB, Alexander JM, McIntire DD, Leveno KJ. A randomized trial of the effects of antibiotic prophylaxis on epidural-related fever in labor. *Anesth Analg*. 2014;118:604.

80. Greenwell EA, Wyshak G, Ringer SA, Johnson SC, Rivkin MJ, Liberman E. Intrapartum temperature elevation, epidural use, and adverse outcome in term infants. *Pediatrics*. 2012;129:e447.

81. Wu YW, Escobar GJ, Grether JK, et al. Chorioamnionitis and cerebral palsy in term and near term infants. *JAMA*. 2003;290:2677.

82. Freeman RK, Gutierrez NA, Ray ML, et al. Fetal cardiac response to paracervical block anesthesia. Part I. *Am J Obstet Gynecol*. 1972;113:583.

83. Gibbs CP, Schwartz DJ, Wynne JW, et al. Antacid pulmonary aspiration in the dog. *Anesthesiology*. 1979;51:380.

84. Datta S, Ostheimer GW, Weiss JB, et al. Neonatal effect of prolonged anesthetic induction for cesarean section. *Obstet Gynecol*. 1981;58:331.

85. Norris MC, Dewan DM. Preoxygenation for cesarean section: a comparison of two techniques. *Anesthesiology*. 1985;62:827.

86. Gin T. Propofol during pregnancy. *Acta Anaesthesiol Sin*. 1994;32:127.

87. Gregory MA, Davidson DG. Plasma etomidate levels in mother and fetus. *Anaesthesia*. 1991;46:716.

88. Bernstein K, Gisselsson L, Jacobsson T, Ohrlander S. Influence of two different anaesthetic agents on the newborn and the correlation between foetal oxygenation and induction-delivery time in elective caesarean section. *Acta Anaesthesiol Scand*. 1985;29:157.

89. Ngan Kee WD, Khaw KS, Ma ML, Mainland PA, Gin T. Postoperative analgesic requirement after cesarean section: a comparison of anesthetic induction with ketamine or thiopental. *Anesth Analg*. 1997;85:1294.

90. Bader AM, Datta S, Arthur GR, et al. Maternal and fetal catecholamines and uterine incision-to-delivery interval during elective cesarean. *Obstet Gynecol*. 1990;75:600.

91. Samsoon GL, Young JR. Difficult tracheal intubation: a retrospective study. *Anaesthesia*. 1987;42:487.

92. Mallampati SR, Gatt SP, Gugino LD, et al. A clinical sign to predict difficult tracheal intubation: a prospective study. *Can Anaesth Soc J*. 1985;32:429.

93. Kodali BS, Chandrasekhar S, Bulich LN, Topulos GP, Datta S. Airway changes during labor and delivery. *Anesthesiology*. 2008;108:357.

94. An updated report by the American Society of Anesthesiologists Task Force on Difficult Airway Management: Practice guidelines for management of the difficult airway. *Anesthesiology*. 2013;118:251.

95. Aziz MF, Kim D, Mako J, Hand K, Brambrink AM. A retrospective study of the performance of video laryngoscopy in an obstetric unit. *Anesth Analg*. 2012;115:904.

96. Pandit JJ, Andrade J, Bogod DG, et al. 5th national audit project (NAP5) on accidental awareness during general anaesthesia: summary of main findings and risk factors. *Br J Anaesth*. 2014;113:549.

97. Thomas TA, Cooper GM. Maternal deaths from anaesthesia. An extract from Why Mothers Die 1997–1999, the confidential enquiries into maternal deaths in the United Kingdom. *Br J Anaesth*. 2002;89:499.

98. Lowder JL, Shackelford DP, Holbert D, Beste TM. A randomized, controlled trial to compare ketorolac tromethamine versus placebo after cesarean section to reduce pain and narcotic usage. *Am J Obstet Gynecol*. 2003;189:1559.

99. Mhyre JM, Riesner MN, Polley LS, Naughton NN. A series of anesthesia-related maternal deaths in Michigan, 1985-2003. *Anesthesiology*. 2007;106:1096.

100. Wilkins KK, Greenfield ML, Polley LS, Mhyre JM. A survey of obstetric perianesthesia care unit standards. *Anesth Analg*. 2009;108:1869.

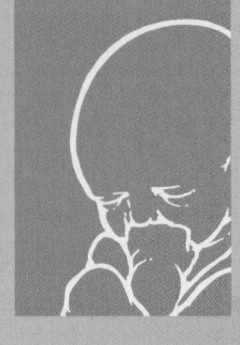

CHAPTER 17

Malpresentations

SUSAN M. LANNI, ROBERT GHERMAN, and BERNARD GONIK

KEY ABBREVIATIONS

Abdominal diameter	AD
American College of Obstetricians and Gynecologists	ACOG
Amniotic fluid index	AFI
Anteroposterior	AP
Biparietal diameter	BPD
Cerebral palsy	CP
Combined spinal-epidural	CSE
Computed tomography	CT
Confidence interval	CI
External cephalic version	ECV
Ex utero intrapartum treatment	EXIT
Fetal heart rate	FHR
Internal podalic version	IPV
Magnetic resonance imaging	MRI
Occipitofrontal diameter	OFD
Odds ratio	OR
Perinatal mortality rate	PMR
Periventricular leukomalacia	PVL
Preterm premature rupture of the membranes	PPROM
Relative risk	RR
Term breech trial	TBT

Near term or during labor, the fetus normally assumes a vertical orientation, or *lie,* and a cephalic presentation, with the flexed fetal vertex presenting to the pelvis (Fig. 17-1). However, in about 3% to 5% of singleton gestations at term, an abnormal lie, presentation, or flexed attitude occurs; such deviations constitute fetal malpresentations. **The word *malpresentation* suggests the possibility of adverse consequences, and malpresentation is often associated with increased risk to both the mother and the fetus.** In the early twentieth century, malpresentation often led to a variety of maneuvers intended to facilitate vaginal delivery, including destructive operations leading, predictably, to fetal death. Later, manual or instrumented attempts to convert the malpresenting fetus to a more favorable orientation were devised. Internal podalic version (IPV) followed by a complete breech extraction was once advocated as a solution to many malpresentation situations. However, like with most manipulative efforts to achieve vaginal delivery, IPV was associated with high fetal and maternal morbidity and mortality rates and has been largely abandoned. **In contemporary practice, cesarean delivery has become the recommended mode of delivery in the malpresenting fetus.**

CLINICAL CIRCUMSTANCES ASSOCIATED WITH MALPRESENTATION

Generally, factors associated with malpresentation include (1) diminished vertical polarity of the uterine cavity, (2) increased or decreased fetal mobility, (3) obstructed pelvic inlet, (4) fetal malformation, and (5) prematurity. The association of great parity with malpresentation is presumably related to laxity of maternal abdominal musculature and resultant loss of the normal vertical orientation of the uterine cavity. Placentation either high in the fundus or low in the pelvis (Fig. 17-2) is another factor that diminishes the likelihood of a fetus assuming a longitudinal axis. Uterine myomata, intrauterine synechiae, and müllerian duct fusion abnormalities such as a septate uterus or uterine didelphys are similarly associated with a higher than expected rate of malpresentation. Because both prematurity and polyhydramnios permit increased fetal mobility, the probability of a noncephalic presentation is greater if preterm labor or rupture of the membranes occurs. Furthermore, preterm birth involves a fetus that is small relative to the maternal pelvis; therefore engagement and descent with labor or rupture of the membranes can occur despite a malpresentation. In contrast, conditions such as chromosomal aneuploidies, congenital myotonic dystrophy, joint contractures from various

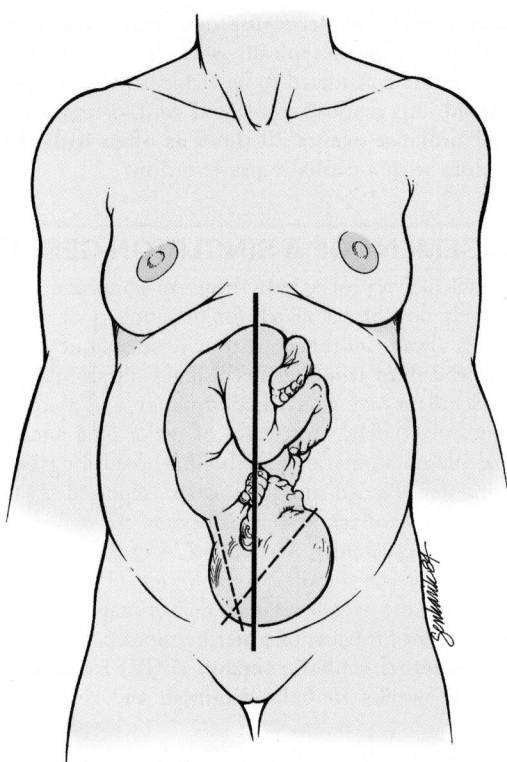

FIG 17-1 Frontal view of a fetus in a longitudinal lie with fetal vertex flexed on the neck.

etiologies, arthrogryposis, oligohydramnios, and fetal neurologic dysfunction that result in decreased fetal muscle tone, strength, or activity are also associated with an increased incidence of fetal malpresentation. Finally, the cephalopelvic disproportion associated with severe fetal hydrocephalus or with a contracted maternal pelvis may be implicated as an etiology of malpresentation because normal engagement of the fetal head is prevented.

ABNORMAL AXIAL LIE

The fetal *lie* indicates the orientation of the fetal spine relative to the spine of the mother. The normal fetal lie is longitudinal and by itself does not indicate whether the presentation is cephalic or breech. If the fetal spine or long axis crosses that of the mother, the fetus may be said to occupy a *transverse* or *oblique lie* (Fig. 17-3), which may cause an arm, foot, or shoulder to be the presenting part (Fig. 17-4). The lie may be termed *unstable* if the fetal membranes are intact and fetal mobility is increased, which results in frequent changes of lie and/or presentation.

Abnormal fetal lie is diagnosed in approximately 1 in 300 cases, or 0.33% of pregnancies at term. Prematurity is often a factor, with abnormal lie reported to occur in about 2% of pregnancies at 32 weeks' gestation—six times the rate found at term. Persistence of a transverse, oblique, or unstable lie beyond 37 weeks' gestation requires a systematic clinical assessment and a plan for management; this is because rupture of the membranes without a fetal part filling the inlet of the pelvis poses an increased risk of cord prolapse, fetal compromise, and maternal morbidity if neglected.

As noted, great parity, prematurity, contraction or deformity of the maternal pelvis, and abnormal placentation are

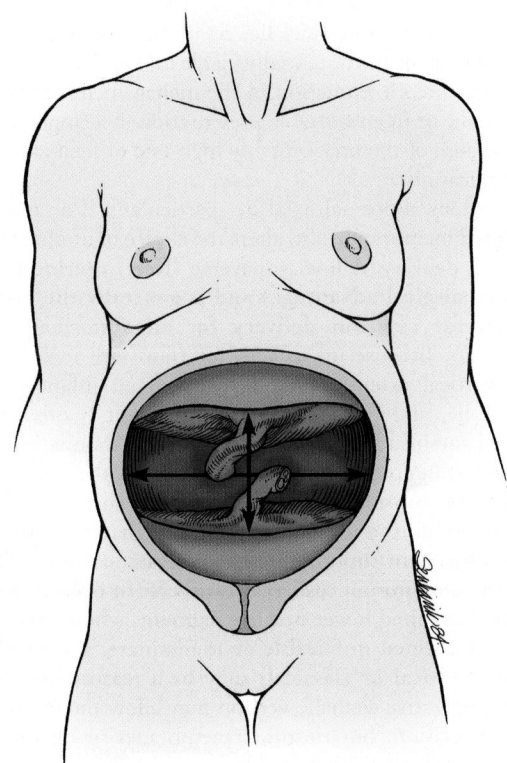

FIG 17-2 Either the high fundal or low implantation of the placenta, as illustrated here, would normally be in the vertical orientation of the intrauterine cavity and increase the probability of a malpresentation.

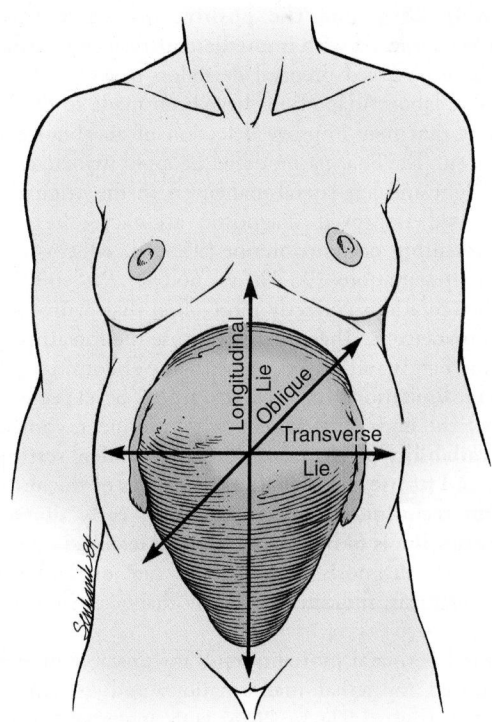

FIG 17-3 A fetus may lie on a longitudinal, oblique, or transverse axis, as illustrated. The lie does not indicate whether the vertex or the breech is closest to the cervix.

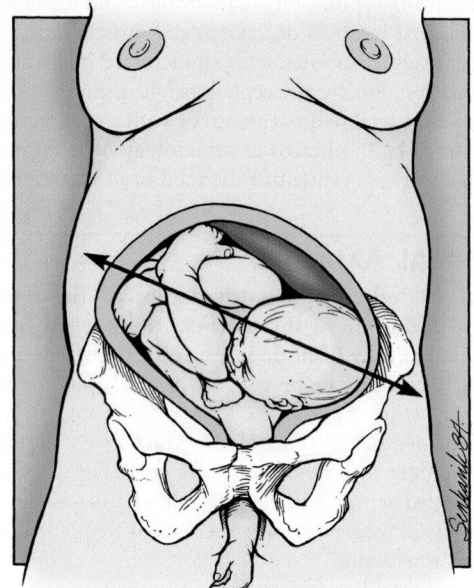

FIG 17-4 This fetus lies in an oblique axis with an arm prolapsing.

the most commonly reported clinical factors associated with abnormal lie; however, it often happens that none of these factors are present. In fact, any condition that alters the normal vertical polarity of the intrauterine cavity will predispose to abnormal lie.

Diagnosis of the abnormal lie may be made by palpation using Leopold maneuvers or by vaginal examination verified by ultrasound. Whereas routine use of Leopold maneuvers may be helpful, Thorp and colleagues[1] found **the sensitivity of Leopold maneuvers for the detection of malpresentation to be only 28%, and the positive predictive value was only 24% compared with immediate ultrasound verification.** Others have observed prenatal detection in as few as 41% of cases before labor. Adaptations have been made to the Leopold maneuvers that may improve detection of an abnormal lie or presentation. The Sharma modified Leopold maneuver and the Sharma right and left lateral maneuvers in the original report[2] demonstrated improved diagnostic accuracy; they detected vertex presenting occipitoanterior (95% vs. 84.4%, $P = .04$), posterior presentations (96.3% vs. 66.6%, $P = .00012$), and breech presentations correctly more often than with traditional Leopold maneuvers. These maneuvers use the forearms in addition to the hands and fingers. As with any abdominal palpation technique, limitations on accuracy are to be expected in the obese patient and in a patient with uterine myomata. **The ready availability of ultrasound in most clinical settings is of benefit, and its use can obviate the vagaries of the abdominal palpation techniques. In all situations, early diagnosis of malpresentation is of benefit**. A reported fetal loss rate of 9.2% with an early diagnosis, versus a loss rate of 27.5% with a delayed diagnosis, indicates that early diagnosis improves fetal outcome.

Reported perinatal mortality rates for unstable or transverse lie (corrected for lethal malformations and extreme prematurity) vary from 3.9% to 24%, with maternal mortality as high as 10%. Maternal deaths are usually related to infection after premature rupture of membranes (PROM), hemorrhage secondary to abnormal placentation, complications of operative intervention for cephalopelvic disproportion, or traumatic delivery. Fetal loss of phenotypically and chromosomally normal gestations at ages considered to be viable is primarily associated with delayed interventions, prolapsed cord, or traumatic delivery. **Cord prolapse occurs 20 times as often with abnormal lie as it does with a cephalic presentation.**

MANAGEMENT OF A SINGLETON GESTATION

Safe vaginal delivery of a fetus from an abnormal axial lie is not generally possible. A search for the etiology of the malpresentation is always indicated. A transverse/oblique or unstable lie late in the third trimester necessitates ultrasound examination to exclude a major fetal malformation and abnormal placentation. Fortunately, most cases of major fetal anomalies or abnormal placentation can now be diagnosed long before the third trimester. Phelan and colleagues[3] reported 29 patients with transverse lie diagnosed at or beyond 37 weeks' gestation and managed expectantly, and 83% (24 of 29) spontaneously converted to breech (9 of 24) or vertex (15 of 24) before labor; however, the overall cesarean delivery rate was 45%, with two cases of cord prolapse, one uterine rupture, and one neonatal death. **External cephalic version (ECV) is recommended at 36 to 37 weeks to help diminish the risk of adverse outcome.**

In cases of an abnormal lie, the risk of fetal death varies with the obstetric intervention. Fetal mortality should approach zero for cesarean birth but has been reported to be as high as 10% in older reports and between 25% and 90% when IPV and breech extraction are performed. **ECV has been found to be safe and relatively efficacious**[4] and is further discussed later in this chapter. If external version is unsuccessful or unavailable, if spontaneous rupture of the membranes occurs, or if active labor has begun with an abnormal lie, cesarean delivery is the treatment of choice for the potentially viable infant. There is no place for IPV and breech extraction in the management of transverse or oblique lie or in an unstable presentation in a singleton pregnancy because of the unacceptably high rate of fetal and maternal complications.

A persistent abnormal axial lie, particularly if accompanied by ruptured membranes, also alters the choice of uterine incision at cesarean delivery. **A low transverse (Kerr) uterine incision has many surgical advantages and is generally the preferred approach for cesarean delivery for an abnormal lie** (see Chapter 19). Because up to 25% of transverse incisions may require vertical extension for delivery of an infant from an abnormal lie, and the lower uterine segment is often poorly developed and insufficiently broad such that a traumatic delivery of the presenting part is made more difficult, other uterine incisions may be considered. A "J" or "T" extension of the low transverse incision results in a uterine scar that is more susceptible to subsequent rupture due to poor vascularization. **Therefore in the uncommon case of a transverse or oblique lie with a poorly developed lower uterine segment, when a transverse incision is deemed unfeasible or inadequate, a vertical incision (low vertical or classical) may be a reasonable alternative.** Intraoperative cephalic version may allow the use of a low transverse incision, but ruptured membranes or oligohydramnios may make this difficult. Uterine relaxing agents such as inhalational anesthetics or intravenous (IV) nitroglycerin may improve success of these maneuvers if the difficulty is attributable to a contracted uterine fundus.

DEFLECTION ATTITUDES

Attitude refers to the position of the fetal head in relation to the neck. The normal attitude of the fetal head during labor is one of full flexion with the fetal chin against the upper chest. Deflexed attitudes include various degrees of deflection or even extension of the fetal neck and head (Fig. 17-5), leading to, for example, face or brow presentations. Spontaneous conversion to a more normal, flexed attitude or further extension of an intermediate deflection to a fully extended position commonly occurs as labor progresses owing to resistance exerted by the bony pelvis and soft tissues. **Although safe vaginal delivery is possible in many cases, experience indicates that cesarean** delivery may be the most appropriate alternative when arrest of progress is observed.

FACE PRESENTATION

A face presentation is characterized by a longitudinal lie and full extension of the fetal neck and head with the occiput against the upper back (Fig. 17-6). **The fetal chin (mentum) is chosen as the point of designation during vaginal examination.** For example, a fetus presenting by the face whose chin is in the right posterior quadrant of the maternal pelvis would be called a *right mentum posterior* (Fig. 17-7). The reported incidence of face presentation ranges from 0.14% to 0.54% and averages about 0.2%, or 1 in 500 live births overall.[5,6] The reported perinatal mortality rate, corrected for nonviable malformations and extreme prematurity, varies from 0.6% to 5% and averages about 2% to 3%.

All clinical factors known to increase the general rate of malpresentation have been implicated in face presentation; many infants with a face presentation have malformations. Anencephaly, for instance, is found in about one third of cases of face presentation. Fetal goiter and tumors of the soft tissues of the head and neck may also cause deflexion of the head. Frequently observed maternal factors include a contracted pelvis or cephalopelvic disproportion in 10% to 40% of cases. In a review of face presentation, Duff[6] found that one of these etiologic factors was found in up to 90% of cases.

Early recognition of the face presentation is important, and the diagnosis can be suspected when abdominal palpation finds the fetal cephalic prominence on the same side of the maternal abdomen as the fetal back (Fig. 17-8); however, **face presentation is more often discovered by vaginal examination.** In practice, fewer than 1 in 20 infants with face presentation is diagnosed by abdominal examination. In fact, only half of these infants are found by any means to have a face presentation before the second stage of labor, and half of the remaining cases are

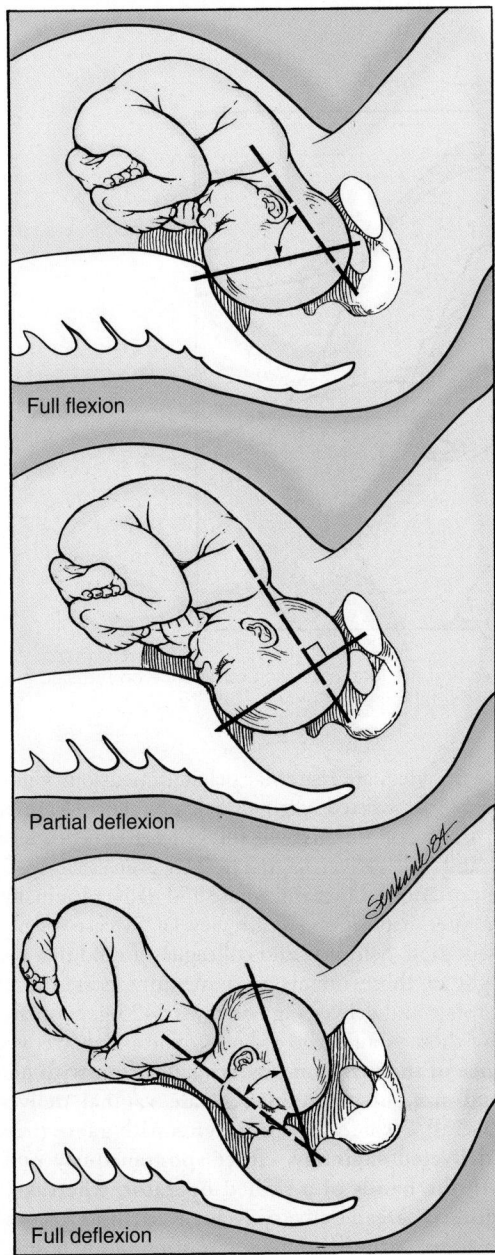

FIG 17-5 The normal "attitude" (*top*) shows the fetal vertex flexed on the neck. Partial deflexion (*middle*) shows the fetal vertex intermediate between flexion and extension. Full deflexion (*lower*) shows the fetal vertex completely extended with the face presenting.

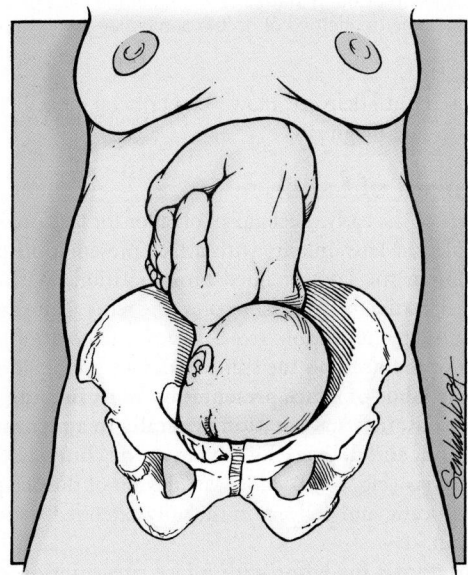

FIG 17-6 This fetus with the vertex completely extended on the neck enters the maternal pelvis in a face presentation. The cephalic prominence would be palpable on the same side of the maternal abdomen as the fetal spine.

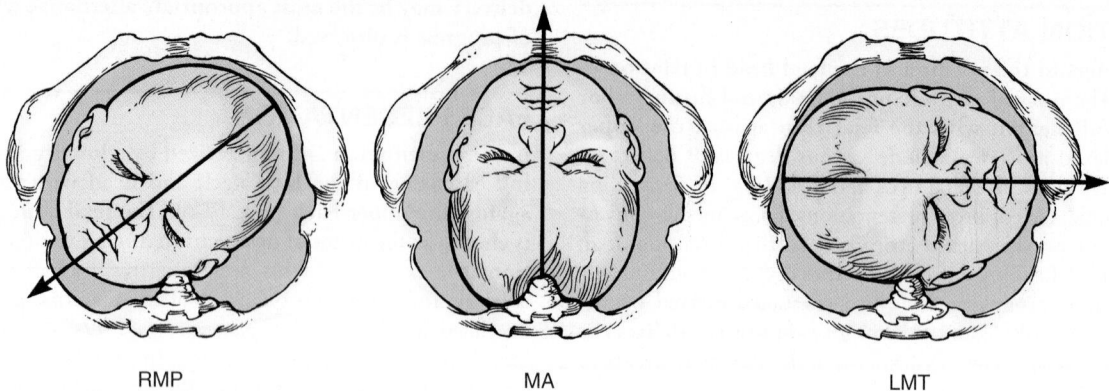

RMP   MA   LMT

FIG 17-7 The point of designation from digital examination in the case of a face presentation is the fetal chin relative to the maternal pelvis. *Left,* right mentum posterior (RMP); *middle,* mentum anterior (MA); *right,* left mentum transverse (LMT).

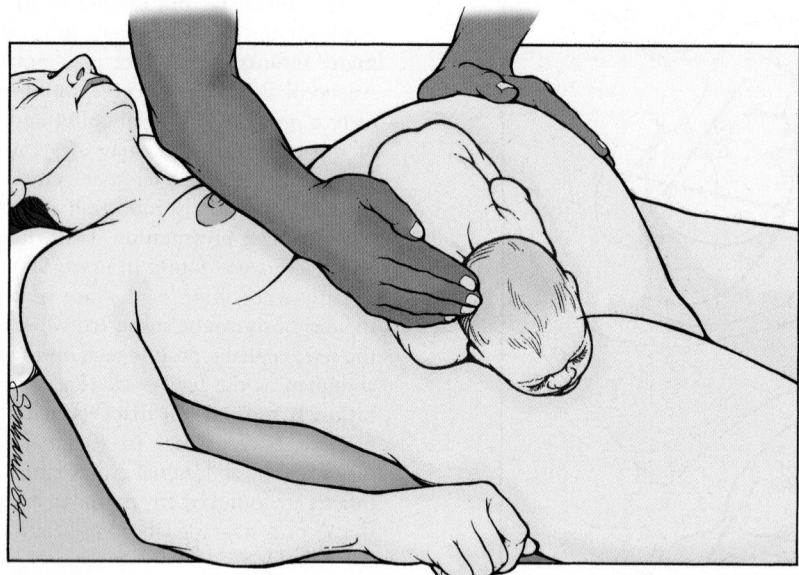

FIG 17-8 Palpation of the maternal abdomen in the case of a face presentation should find the fetal cephalic prominence on the side *away* from the fetal small parts, instead of on the same side, as in the case of a normally flexed fetal neck and head.

undiagnosed until delivery. However, perinatal mortality may be higher with late diagnosis.

Mechanism of Labor

Knowledge of the early mechanism of labor for face presentation is incomplete. Many infants with a face presentation probably begin labor in the less extended brow position. With descent into the pelvis, the forces of labor press the fetus against maternal tissues; subsequent flexion (to a vertex presentation) or full extension of the head on the spine (to a face presentation) then occurs. **The labor of a face presentation must include engagement, descent, internal rotation generally to a mentum anterior position, and delivery by flexion as the chin passes under the symphysis** (Fig. 17-9). However, flexion of the occiput may not always occur, and delivery in the fully extended attitude may be common.

The prognosis for labor with a face presentation depends on the orientation of the fetal chin. At diagnosis, 60% to 80% of infants with a face presentation are mentum anterior,[6] 10% to 12% are mentum transverse,[7] and 20% to 25% are mentum posterior.[7] Almost all average-sized infants presenting mentum

anterior with adequate maternal pelvic dimensions will achieve spontaneous or assisted vaginal delivery. Furthermore, most mentum transverse infants will rotate to the mentum anterior position and will deliver vaginally, and even 25% to 33% of mentum posterior infants will rotate and deliver vaginally in the mentum anterior position. In a review of 51 cases of persistent face presentation, Schwartz and colleagues[7] found that the mean birthweight of those infants in a mentum posterior position who did rotate and deliver vaginally was 3425 g, compared with 3792 g for those infants who did not rotate and deliver vaginally. **Persistence of the mentum posterior position with an infant of normal size, however, makes safe vaginal delivery less likely. Overall, 70% to 80% of infants with a face presenting can be delivered vaginally, either spontaneously or by low forceps in the hands of a skilled operator, whereas 12% to 30% require cesarean delivery.** Manual attempts to convert the face to a flexed attitude or to rotate a posterior position to a more favorable mentum anterior position are rarely successful and increase both maternal and fetal risks.[5] Again, IPV and breech extraction for face presentation historically are associated with unacceptably high fetal loss rates. Maternal deaths from

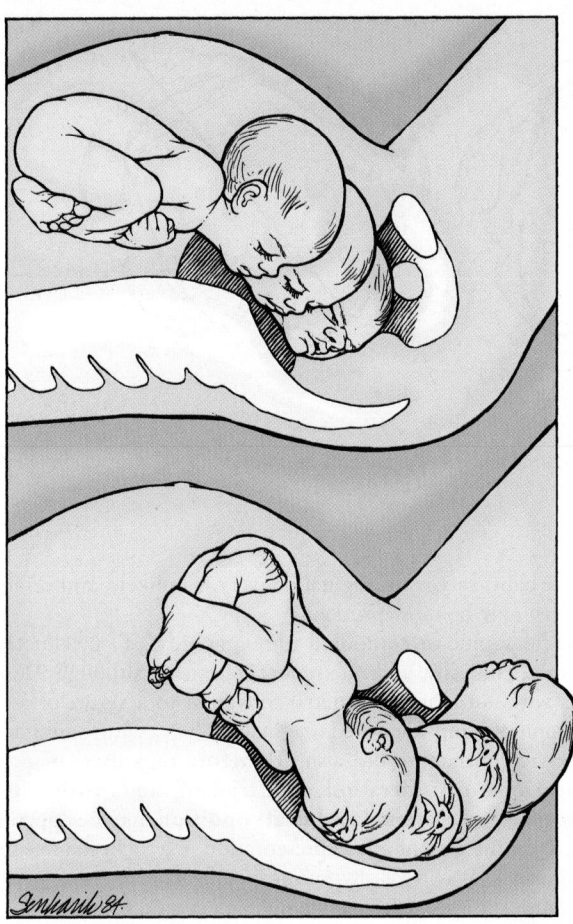

FIG 17-9 Engagement, descent, and internal rotation remain cardinal elements of vaginal delivery in the case of a face presentation, but successful vaginal delivery of a term-size fetus presenting a face generally requires delivery by flexion under the symphysis from a mentum anterior position, as illustrated here.

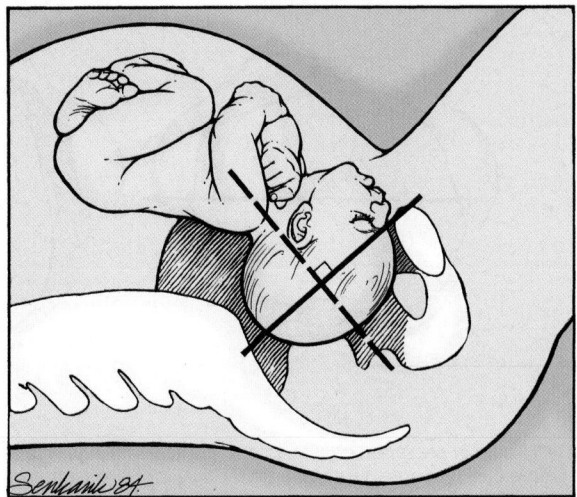

FIG 17-10 This fetus is in a brow presentation in a frontum anterior position. The head is in an intermediate deflexion attitude.

uterine rupture and trauma have also been documented. Thus contemporary management through spontaneous delivery and cesarean delivery for other obstetric indications as necessary are the preferred routes for both maternal and fetal safety.[5]

Prolonged labor is a common feature of face presentation and has been associated with an increased number of intrapartum deaths; therefore prompt attention to an arrested labor pattern is recommended. In the case of an average or small fetus, an adequate pelvis, and hypotonic labor, oxytocin may be considered. No absolute contraindication to oxytocin augmentation of hypotonic labor in face presentations exists, but an arrest of progress despite adequate labor should call for cesarean delivery.

Worsening of the fetal condition in labor is common. Salzmann and colleagues observed a **tenfold increase in fetal compromise with face presentation.** Several other observers have also found that abnormal fetal heart rate (FHR) patterns occur more often with face presentation.[5,6] Continuous intrapartum electronic FHR monitoring of a fetus with face presentation is considered mandatory, but extreme care must be exercised in the placement of an electrode because ocular or cosmetic damage is possible. **If external Doppler heart rate monitoring is inadequate and an internal electrode is recommended, placement of the electrode on the fetal chin is often preferred.**

Contraindications to vaginal delivery of a face presentation include macrosomia, nonreassurance of FHR monitoring even without arrested or protracted labor, or an inadequate maternal pelvis; cesarean delivery has been reported in as many as 60% of cases of face presentation for these reasons.[6] If cesarean delivery is warranted, care should be taken to flex the head gently, both to accomplish elevation of the head through the hysterotomy incision as well as to avoid potential cervical nerve damage to the neonate. Forced flexion may also result in fetal injury, especially with fetal goiter or neck tumors.

Fetal laryngeal and tracheal edema that results from the pressure of the birth process might require immediate nasotracheal intubation. Nuchal tumors or simple goiters, fetal anomalies that might have caused the malpresentation, require expert neonatal management, including the possibility of an ex utero intrapartum treatment (EXIT) procedure, which establishes a fetal/neonatal airway before the umbilical cord is clamped. Identification of and planning for these particular circumstances in the prelabor setting are ideal.

BROW PRESENTATION

A fetus in a brow presentation occupies a longitudinal axis with a partially deflexed cephalic attitude midway between full flexion and full extension (Fig. 17-10). **The frontal bones are the point of designation.** If the anterior fontanel is on the mother's left side, with the sagittal suture in the transverse pelvic axis, the fetus would be in a left frontum transverse position (Fig. 17-11). The reported incidence of brow presentation varies widely, from 1 in 670 to 1 in 3433, **averaging about 1 in 1500 deliveries.** Brow presentation is detected more often in early labor before flexion occurs to a normal attitude. Less frequently, further extension results in a face presentation.

In 1976, the perinatal mortality rate corrected for lethal anomalies and very low birthweight varied from 1% to 8%.[8] In a study of 88,988 deliveries, corrected perinatal mortality rates for brow presentations depended on the mode of delivery; a loss rate of 16%, the highest in this study, was associated with manipulative vaginal birth.

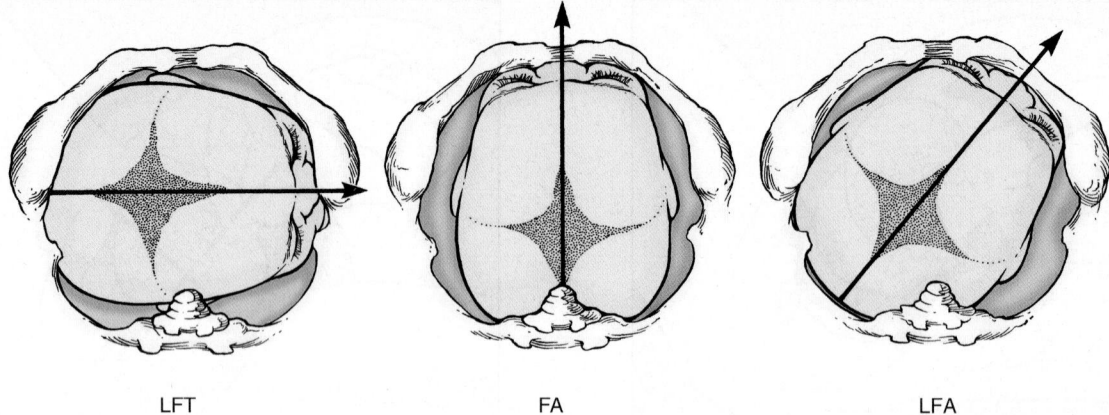

LFT   FA   LFA

FIG 17-11 In brow presentation, the anterior fontanel (frontum) relative to the maternal pelvis is the point of designation. *Left,* fetus in left frontum transverse (LFT); *middle,* frontum anterior (FA); *right,* left frontum anterior (LFA).

In general, factors that delay engagement are associated with persistent brow presentation. Cephalopelvic disproportion, prematurity, and high parity are often found and have been implicated in more than 60% of cases of persistent brow presentation.

Detection of a brow presentation by abdominal palpation is unusual in practice. More often, a brow presentation is detected on vaginal examination. As in the case of a face presentation, diagnosis in labor is more likely. **Fewer than 50% of brow presentations are detected before the second stage of labor, and most of the remainder are undiagnosed until delivery.** Frontum anterior is reportedly the most common position at diagnosis, occurring about twice as often as either transverse or posterior positions. Although the initial position at diagnosis may be of limited prognostic value, the cesarean delivery rate is higher with frontum transverse or frontum posterior than with frontum anterior positioning.

A persistent brow presentation requires engagement and descent of the largest (mento-occipital) diameter of the fetal head. This process is possible only with a large pelvis or a small infant, or both. However, most brow presentations convert spontaneously by flexion or further extension to either a vertex or a face presentation and are then managed accordingly. The earlier the diagnosis is made, the more likely conversion will occur spontaneously. Fewer than half of fetuses with persistent brow presentations undergo spontaneous vaginal delivery, but in most cases, a trial of labor is not contraindicated.[8]

Prolonged labors have been observed in 33% to 50% of brow presentations, and secondary arrest is not uncommon. Forced conversion of the brow to a more favorable position with forceps is contraindicated, as are attempts at manual conversion. One unexpected cause of persistent brow presentation may be an open fetal mouth pressed against the vaginal wall, splinting the head and preventing either flexion or extension (Fig. 17-12). Although this is rare in phenotypically normal fetuses, it needs to be considered in anomalous conditions of the fetus such as epignathus, a rare oropharyngeal teratoma.

Similar to face presentations, minimal manipulation yields the best results if the FHR pattern remains reassuring. Expectant management may be justified, preferably with a relatively large pelvis in relation to fetal size and adequate labor progress, according to one large study.[9] If a brow presentation persists with a large baby, successful vaginal delivery is unlikely, and cesarean delivery may be most prudent.

Radiographic or computed tomographic (CT) pelvimetry is not used clinically, and one report states that although 91% of cases with adequate pelvimetry converted to a vertex or a face presentation and delivered vaginally, 20% with some form of pelvic contracture did also. **Therefore regardless of pelvic dimensions, consideration of a trial of labor with careful monitoring of maternal and fetal condition may be appropriate.** As in the case of a face presentation, oxytocin may be used cautiously to correct hypotonic contractions, but prompt resumption of progress toward delivery should follow.

COMPOUND PRESENTATION

Whenever an extremity, most commonly an upper extremity, is found prolapsed beside the main presenting fetal part, the situation is referred to as a *compound presentation* (Fig. 17-13). **The reported incidence ranges from 1 in 377 to 1 in 1213 deliveries.**[8] **The combination of an upper extremity and the vertex is the most common.**

This diagnosis should be suspected with any arrest of labor in the active phase or failure to engage during active labor. Diagnosis is made on vaginal examination by discovery of an irregular mobile tissue mass adjacent to the larger presenting part. Recognition late in labor is common, and as many as 50% of persisting compound presentations are not detected until the second stage. Delay in diagnosis may not be detrimental because it is likely that only the persistent cases require intervention.

Although maternal age, race, parity, and pelvic size have been associated with compound presentation, prematurity is the most consistent clinical finding. The very small premature fetus is at great risk of persistent compound presentation. In late pregnancy, ECV of a fetus in breech position increases the risk of a compound presentation.

Older, uncontrolled studies report elevated perinatal mortality rates with a compound presentation, with an overall rate of 93 per 1000. Higher loss rates of 17% to 19% have been reported when the foot prolapses. As with other malpresentations, fetal risk is directly related to the method of management. A fetal mortality rate of 4.8% has been noted if no intervention is required compared with 14.4% with intervention other than cesarean delivery. A 30% fetal mortality rate has been observed

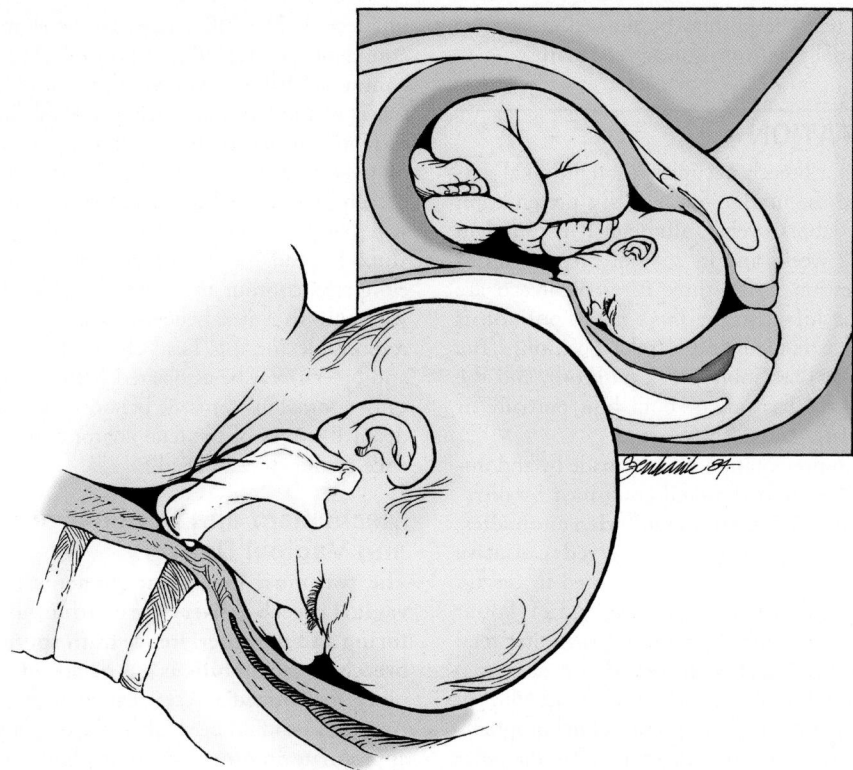

FIG 17-12 The open fetal mouth against the vaginal sidewall may brace the head in the intermediate deflexion attitude as shown here.

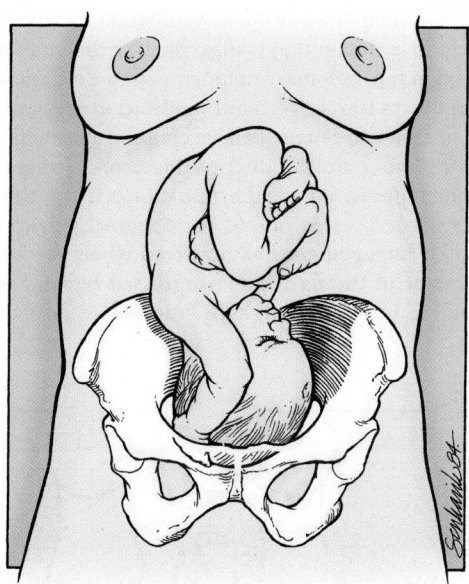

FIG 17-13 The compound presentation of an upper extremity and the vertex illustrated here most often spontaneously resolves with further labor and descent.

with IPV and breech extraction. These figures may demonstrate selection bias because it is possible that more often, the difficult cases were chosen for manipulative intervention. **When intervention is necessary, cesarean delivery appears to be the only safe choice.**

Fetal risk in compound presentation is specifically associated with birth trauma and cord prolapse. **Cord prolapse occurs in 11% to 20% of cases, and it is the most frequent complication of this malpresentation.** Cord prolapse probably occurs because the compound extremity splints the larger presenting part and results in an irregular fetal aggregate that incompletely fills the pelvic inlet. In addition to the hypoxic risk of cord prolapse, common fetal morbidity includes neurologic and musculoskeletal damage to the involved extremity. Maternal risks include soft tissue damage and obstetric laceration. Again, although laboring is not proscribed, **the prolapsed extremity should not be manipulated. However, it may spontaneously retract as the major presenting part descends.** Seventy-five percent of vertex/upper extremity combinations deliver spontaneously. Occult or obscured cord prolapse is possible, and therefore continuous electronic FHR monitoring is recommended.

The primary indications for surgical intervention (i.e., cesarean delivery) are cord prolapse, nonreassuring FHR patterns, and arrest of labor. **Cesarean delivery is the only appropriate clinical intervention for cord prolapse and nonreassuring FHR patterns because both version extraction and repositioning the prolapsed extremity are associated with adverse outcome and should be avoided.** From 2% to 25% of compound presentations require cesarean delivery. Protraction of the second stage of labor and dysfunctional labor patterns have been noted to occur more frequently with persistent compound presentations. As in other malpresentations, spontaneous resolution occurs more often, and surgical intervention is less frequently necessary in those cases diagnosed early in labor. Small or premature fetuses are more likely to have persistent compound presentations but are also more likely to have a successful vaginal delivery. **Persistent compound presentation with parts other than the vertex and hand in combination in a term-sized infant has a poor prognosis for safe vaginal delivery, and cesarean delivery is usually necessary.** However, a simple compound presentation (e.g., hand) may be allowed to labor, if labor is progressing normally with reassuring fetal status.

BREECH PRESENTATION

The infant presenting as a breech occupies a longitudinal axis with the cephalic pole in the uterine fundus. This presentation occurs in 3% to 4% of labors overall, although it is found in 7% of pregnancies at 32 weeks and in 25% of pregnancies of less than 28 weeks' duration.[10] The three types of breech are noted in Table 17-1. The infant in the *frank breech* position is flexed at the hips with extended knees (pike position). The *complete breech* is flexed at both joints (tuck position), and the *footling* or *incomplete breech* has one or both hips partially or fully extended (Fig. 17-14).

The diagnosis of breech presentation may be made by abdominal palpation or vaginal examination and confirmed by ultrasound. **Prematurity, fetal malformation, müllerian anomalies, and polar placentation are commonly observed causative factors.** High rates of breech presentation are noted in certain fetal genetic disorders, including trisomies 13, 18, and 21; Potter syndrome; and myotonic dystrophy. Conditions that alter fetal muscular tone and mobility—such as increased and decreased amniotic fluid, for example—also increase the frequency of breech presentation. The breech head appears dolichocephalic on ultrasound, and for that reason, the biparietal diameter (BPD) appears small. However, the head circumference remains

unaffected. This difference may be as much as 16+ days (95% confidence interval [CI], 14.3 to 18.1; *P* = .001).[11] Whereas the contracted BPD may affect ultrasound-determined weight estimates of the fetus, an occipitofrontal diameter (OFD) to BPD ratio of greater than 1.3 in the absence of other indicators of growth delay signals the deformation characteristic of the breech-presenting fetus. Approximately 80% of breech fetuses will have a dolichocephalic contour, previously termed the "breech head."[12] The fundus of the uterus assumes a more elongated contour than the bowl-like developed lower uterine segment. Thus it is believed that forces external to the fetus are responsible for this head shape. Because both dolichocephaly and breech *may* be associated with a genetically and phenotypically anomalous fetus, it behooves the sonologist to perform a detailed survey of the fetal anatomy prior to assuming the presence of the "breech head."

Mechanism and Conduct of Labor and Vaginal Delivery

The two most important elements for the safe conduct of vaginal breech delivery are continuous electronic FHR monitoring and noninterference until spontaneous delivery of the breech to the umbilicus has occurred. Early in labor, the capability for immediate cesarean delivery should be established. Anesthesia should be available, the operating room readied, and appropriate informed consent obtained (discussed later). Two obstetricians should be in attendance in addition to a pediatric team. Appropriate training and experience with vaginal breech delivery are fundamental to success. Although experience is becoming infinitely less common, simulation of breech deliveries will help to maintain these skills. The instrument table should be prepared in the customary manner, with the addition of Piper forceps and extra towels. No contraindication exists to epidural analgesia in labor, and many believe epidural anesthesia to be an asset in the control and conduct of the second stage.

The infant presenting in the frank breech position usually enters the pelvic inlet in one of the diagonal pelvic diameters (Fig. 17-15). **Engagement has occurred when the bitrochanteric diameter of the fetus has progressed beyond the plane of the pelvic inlet, although by vaginal examination, the**

TABLE 17-1	BREECH CATEGORIES		
TYPE	**OVERALL % OF BREECHES**	**RISK OF PROLAPSE (%)[†]**	**PREMATURE (%)[‡]**
Frank	48-73[*†‡]	0.5	38
Complete	4.6-11.5[†‡]	4-6	12
Footling	12-38[‡]	15-18	50

*Data from Collea JV, Chein C, Quilligan EJ. The randomized management of term frank breech presentation: a study of 208 cases. *Am J Obstet Gynecol.* 1980;137:235-244.
[†]Data from Gimovsky ML, Wallace RL, Schifrin BS, Paul RH. Randomized management of the nonfrank breech presentation at term: a preliminary report. *Am J Obstet Gynecol.* 1983;146:34-40.
[‡]Data from Brown L, Karrison T, Cibils LA. Mode of delivery and perinatal results in breech presentation. *Am J Obstet Gynecol.* 1994;171:28-34.

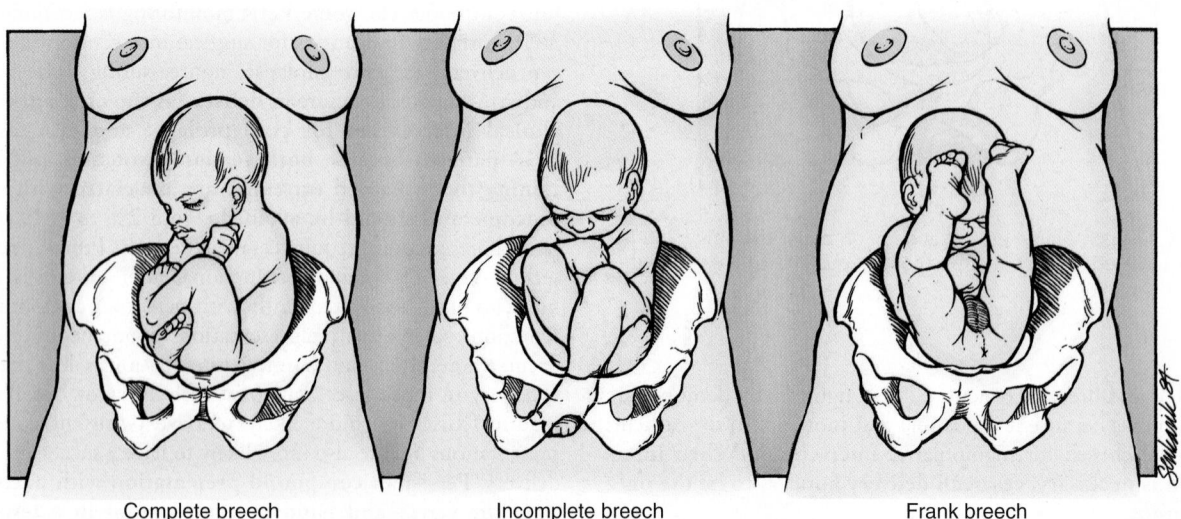

Complete breech   Incomplete breech   Frank breech

FIG 17-14 The *complete breech* is flexed at the hips and flexed at the knees. The *incomplete breech* shows incomplete deflexion of one or both knees or hips. The *frank breech* is flexed at the hips and extended at the knees.

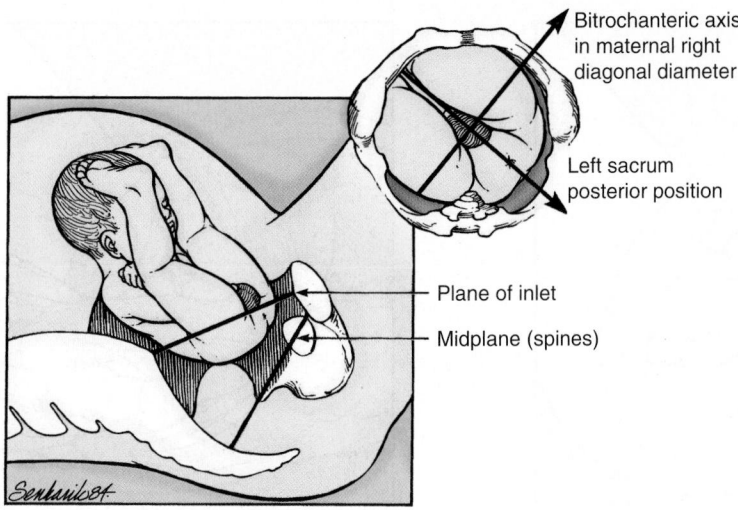

FIG 17-15 The breech typically enters the inlet with the bitrochanteric diameter aligned with one of the diagonal diameters, with the sacrum as the point of designation in the other diagonal diameter. This illustrates a left sacrum posterior alignment.

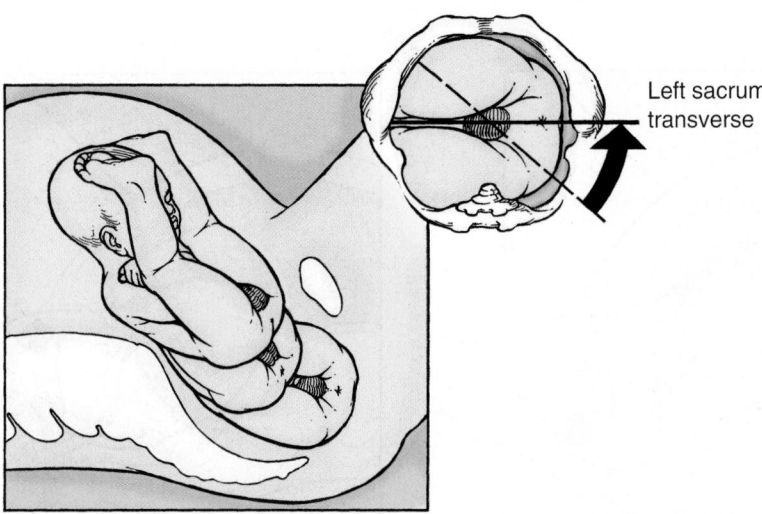

FIG 17-16 With labor and descent, the bitrochanteric diameter generally rotates toward the anteroposterior axis, and the sacrum rotates toward the transverse axis.

presenting part may be palpated only at a station of −2 to −4 (out of 5). As the breech descends and encounters the levator ani muscular sling, internal rotation usually occurs to bring the bitrochanteric diameter into the anteroposterior (AP) axis of the pelvis. **The point of designation in a breech labor is the fetal sacrum**; therefore when the bitrochanteric diameter is in the AP axis of the pelvis, the fetal sacrum will lie in the transverse pelvic diameter (Fig. 17-16).

If normal descent occurs, the breech will present at the outlet and will begin to emerge, first as sacrum transverse, then rotating to sacrum anterior. This direction of rotation may reflect the greater capacity of the hollow of the posterior pelvis to accept the fetal chest and small parts. Crowning occurs when the bitrochanteric diameter passes under the pubic symphysis. It is important to emphasize that operator intervention is not yet needed or helpful, other than possibly to perform the episiotomy if indicated and to encourage maternal expulsive efforts.

Premature or aggressive intervention may adversely affect the delivery in at least two ways. First, complete cervical dilation must be sustained for sufficient duration to retard retraction of the cervix and entrapment of the aftercoming fetal head. Rushing the delivery of the trunk may result in cervical retraction. Second, the safe descent and delivery of the breech infant must be the result of uterine and maternal expulsive forces only in order to maintain neck flexion. Any traction by the provider in an effort to speed delivery would encourage deflexion of the neck and result in the presentation of the larger occipitofrontal fetal cranial profile to the pelvic inlet (Fig. 17-17). **Such an event could be catastrophic. Rushed delivery also increases the risk of a nuchal arm, with one or both arms trapped behind the head above the pelvic inlet.** Entrapment of a nuchal arm makes safe vaginal delivery much more difficult because it dramatically increases the aggregate size of delivering fetal parts that must egress vaginally. Safe breech delivery of an average-sized infant, therefore, depends predominantly on maternal expulsive forces and patience, *not* traction, from the provider.

As the frank breech emerges further, the fetal thighs are typically flexed firmly against the fetal abdomen, often splinting and protecting the umbilicus and cord. **The Pinard maneuver**

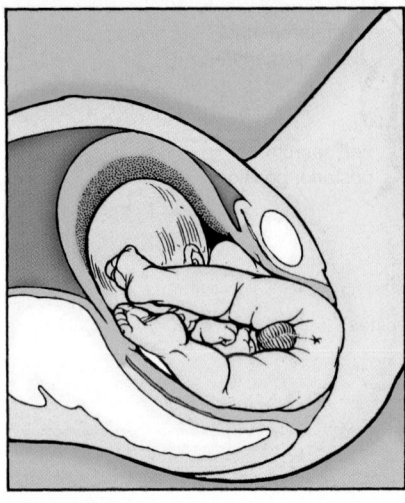
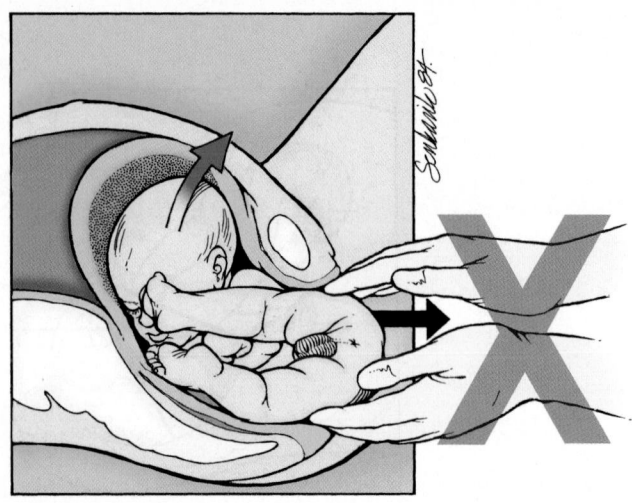

A Spontaneous expulsion   B Undesired deflexion

FIG 17-17 The fetus emerges spontaneously **(A)**, whereas uterine contractions maintain cephalic flexion. Premature aggressive traction **(B)** encourages deflexion of the fetal vertex and increases the risk of head entrapment or nuchal arm entrapment.

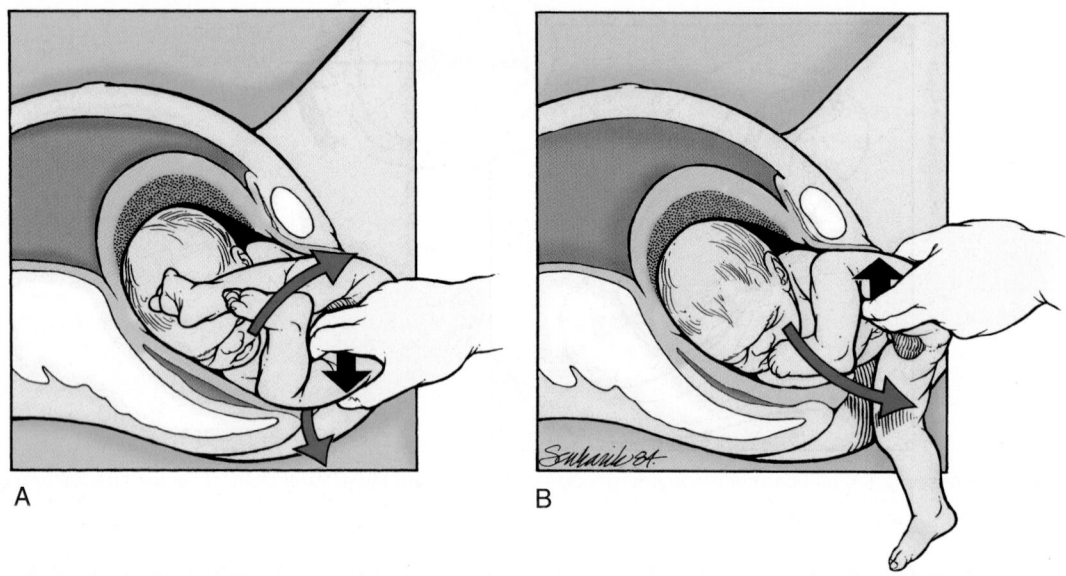

A   B

FIG 17-18 After spontaneous expulsion to the umbilicus, external rotation of each thigh **(A)** combined with opposite rotation of the fetal pelvis results in flexion of the knee and delivery of each leg **(B)**.

may be needed to facilitate delivery of the legs in a frank breech presentation. After delivery to the umbilicus has occurred, pressure is applied to the medial aspect of the knee, which causes flexion and subsequent delivery of the lower leg. Simultaneous to this, the fetal pelvis is rotated away from that side (Fig. 17-18). This results in external rotation of the thigh at the hip, flexion of the knee, and delivery of one leg at a time. The dual movement of counterclockwise rotation of the fetal pelvis as the operator externally rotates the right thigh and clockwise rotation of the fetal pelvis as the operator externally rotates the fetal left thigh is most effective in facilitating delivery. The fetal trunk is then wrapped with a towel to provide secure support of the body while further descent results from expulsive forces from the mother. The operator primarily facilitates the delivery of the fetus by providing support and guiding the body through the introitus. The operator is not applying outward

traction on the fetus, which might result in deflexion of the fetal head or nuchal arm.

When the scapulae appear at the introitus, the operator may slip a hand over the fetal shoulder from the back (Fig. 17-19); follow the humerus; and, with movement from medial to lateral, sweep first one and then the other arm across the chest and out over the perineum. Gentle rotation of the fetal trunk counterclockwise assists delivery of the right arm, and clockwise rotation assists delivery of the left arm (turning the body "into" the arm). This accomplishes delivery of the arms by drawing them across the fetal chest in a fashion similar to that used for delivery of the legs (Fig. 17-20). These movements cause the fetal elbow to emerge first, followed by the forearm and hand. Once both arms have been delivered, if the vertex has remained flexed on the neck, the chin and face will appear at the outlet, and the airway may be cleared and suctioned (Fig. 17-21).

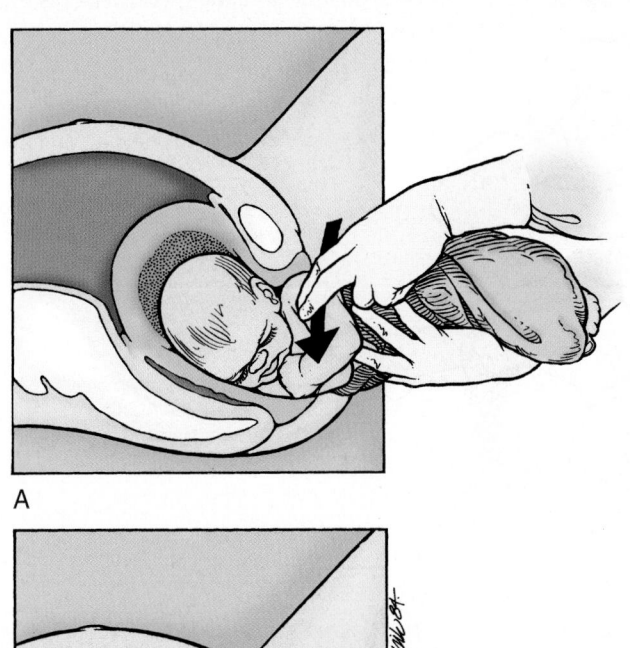

A

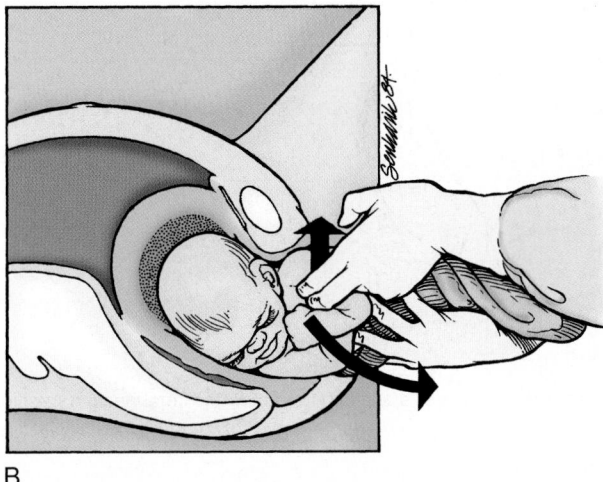

B

FIG 17-19 When the scapulae appear under the symphysis, the operator reaches over the left shoulder, sweeps the arm across the chest **(A)**, and delivers the arm **(B)**.

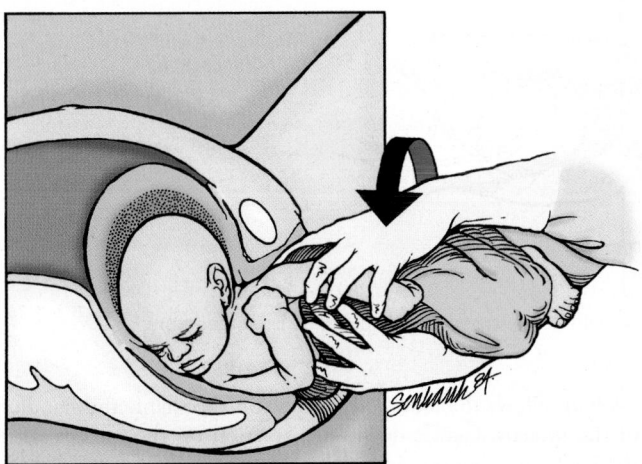

FIG 17-20 Gentle rotation of the shoulder girdle facilitates delivery of the right arm.

With further maternal expulsive forces alone, spontaneous controlled delivery of the fetal head often occurs. If not, delivery may be accomplished with a simple manual effort to maximize flexion of the vertex using pressure on the fetal maxilla (not the mandible), the Mauriceau-Smellie-Veit maneuver, using gentle

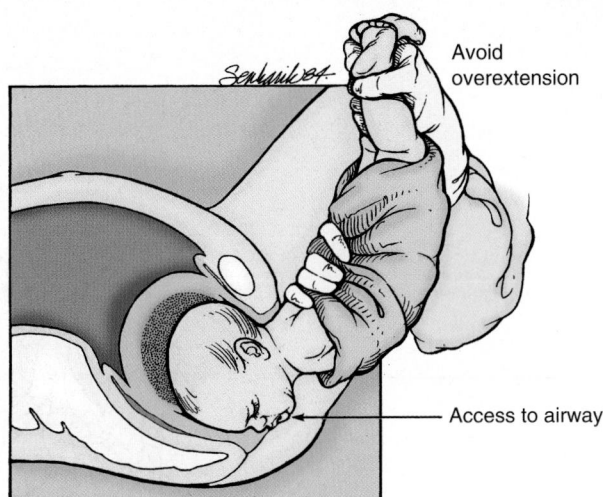

Avoid overextension

Access to airway

FIG 17-21 Following delivery of the arms, the fetus is wrapped in a towel for control and is slightly elevated. The fetal face and airway may be visible over the perineum. Excessive elevation of the trunk is avoided.

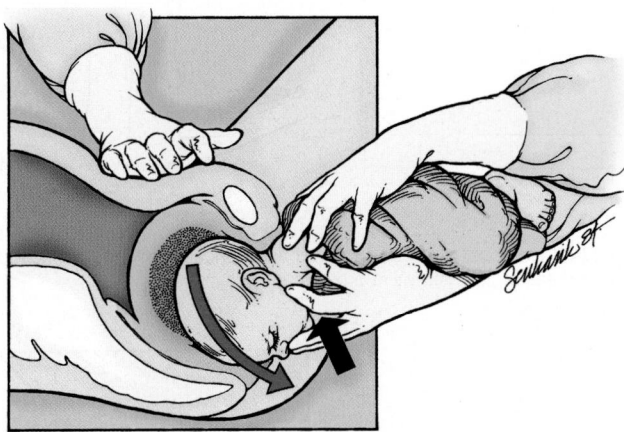

FIG 17-22 Cephalic flexion is maintained by pressure (*black arrow*) on the fetal maxilla, *not* the mandible. Often, delivery of the head is easily accomplished with continued expulsive forces from above and gentle downward traction.

downward traction along with suprapubic pressure (Credé maneuver; Fig. 17-22). Although maxillary pressure facilitates flexion, the main force effecting delivery remains the mother.

Alternatively, the operator may apply Piper forceps to the aftercoming head. The application requires *very slight* elevation of the fetal trunk by the assistant, while the operator kneels and applies the Piper forceps from beneath the fetus directly to the fetal head in the pelvis. Delivery of the breech presenting fetus, therefore, should occur on a table/bed capable of allowing the operators to correctly position themselves for the application of forceps. Direct access to the perineum is required. If a delivery bed is used, merely dropping the foot of the bed will be inadequate. The position of the operator for applying the forceps is depicted in Figure 17-23, which also demonstrates how *excessive* elevation by the assistant may potentially cause harm to the neonate. Hyperextension of the fetal neck from excessive elevation of the fetal trunk, shown in Figure 17-23, should be avoided because of the potential for spinal cord injury.

Piper forceps are characterized by absence of pelvic curvature. This modification allows *direct* application to the fetal head and

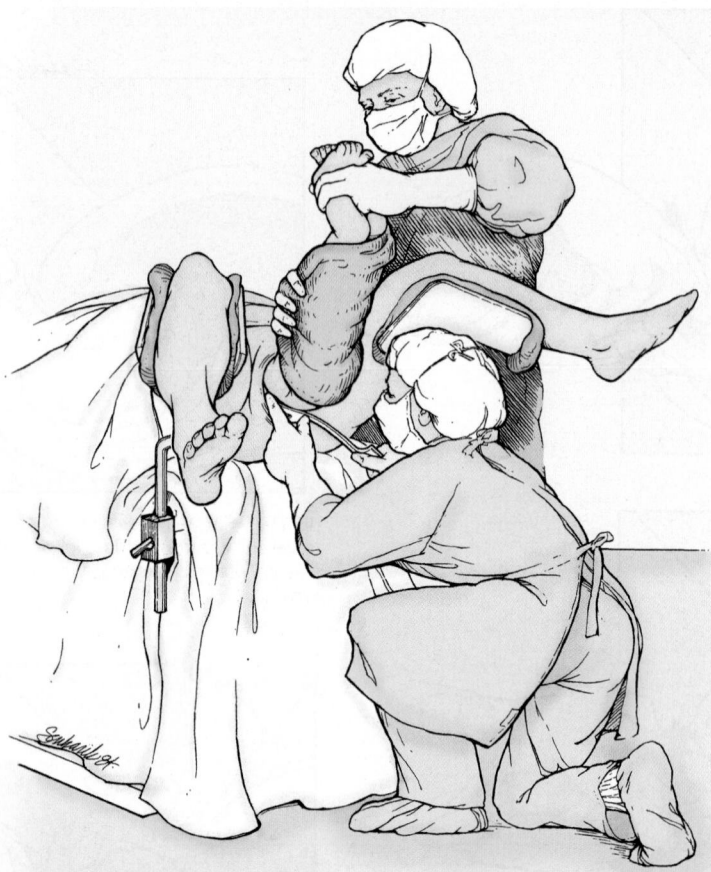

FIG 17-23 Demonstration of *incorrect* assistance during the application of Piper forceps. The assistant hyperextends the fetal neck, a position that increases the risk for neurologic injury.

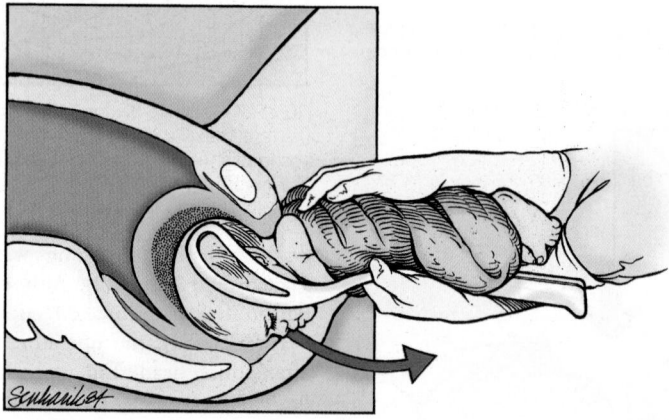

FIG 17-24 The fetus may be laid on the forceps and delivered with gentle downward traction, as illustrated here.

avoids conflict with the fetal body that would occur with the application of standard instruments from below. The assistant maintains control of the fetal body while the forceps are inserted into the vagina from beneath the fetus by the primary operator. The blade to be placed on the maternal left is held by the handle in the operator's left hand; the blade is inserted with the operator's right hand in the vagina along the left maternal sidewall and is placed against the right fetal parietal bone. The handle of the right blade is then held in the operator's right hand and is inserted by the left hand along the right maternal sidewall and placed against the left fetal parietal bone. At this point, the

assistant allows the fetal body to rest on the shank and handles of the forceps. Gentle downward traction on the forceps with the fetal trunk supported on the forceps shanks results in controlled delivery of the vertex (Fig. 17-24). Forceps application controls the fetal head and prevents extension of the head on the neck. Application of Piper forceps to the aftercoming head may be advisable both to ensure control of the delivery and to maintain optimal operator proficiency in anticipation of deliveries that may require their use.

Arrest of spontaneous progress in labor with adequate uterine contractions necessitates consideration of cesarean

delivery. Any evidence of fetal compromise or sustained cord compression on the basis of continuous electronic FHR monitoring also requires consideration of cesarean delivery. Vaginal interventions directed at facilitating delivery of the breech complicated by an arrest of spontaneous progress are discouraged because fetal and maternal morbidity and mortality are both greatly increased. However, if labor is deemed to be hypotonic by internally monitored uterine pressures, oxytocin is not contraindicated.[13,14]

Mechanisms of descent and delivery of the incomplete and the complete breech are not unlike those used for the frank breech described earlier; at least one leg may not require attention. The risk of cord prolapse or entanglement is greater, and hence the possibility of emergency cesarean delivery is increased. Furthermore, incomplete and complete breeches may not be as effective as cervical dilators as either the vertex or the larger aggregate profile of the thighs and buttocks of the frank breech. Thus the risk of entrapment of the aftercoming head is increased, and as a result, **primary cesarean delivery is often advocated for nonfrank breech presentations.** However, the randomized trial of Gimovsky and colleagues[15] found vaginal delivery of the nonfrank breech to be reasonably safe.

Contemporary Management of the Term Breech

Debate has largely diminished about the proper management of the term breech. Much of the older data were derived from relatively few studies of varied methodologies, patient populations, and multiple retrospective cohort analyses, which are subject to bias. These reports indicated that the perinatal mortality rate for the vaginally delivered breech appears to be greater than for its cephalic counterpart, but much of the reported perinatal mortality rate associated with breech presentation was largely due to lethal anomalies and complications of prematurity, both of which are found more frequently among breech infants. Excluding anomalies and extreme prematurity, the corrected perinatal mortality reported by some investigators approached zero regardless of the method of delivery, whereas others found that even with exclusion of these factors, the term breech infant has been found to be at higher risk for birth trauma and asphyxia.[16] To date, only three randomized trials have been reported.[13,15] Although conclusions regarding the safety of breech vaginal delivery from a fetal standpoint may continue to vary, **the practical reality today is that intentional vaginal breech delivery is rare.** A summary of some of the reported complications is listed in Table 17-2. **Overall, consideration of a potential breech vaginal delivery must be mutually agreed on by the patient and the physician after complete informed consent is obtained.**

Further Discussion of Delivery for the Term Frank or Complete Breech

The cesarean delivery rate for breech presentation approached 90% in some centers in the mid-1970s without a consequent proportionate drop in the perinatal mortality rate. Maternal mortality is clearly higher with cesarean delivery and ranges from 0.2% to 0.43%.[10] With an older, more obese, sicker maternal population who have more chronic medical problems and have sustained more cesarean deliveries, we can expect this rate to further increase. Maternal morbidity is also higher with cesarean delivery. Some institutions reported a 50% incidence of post-cesarean maternal morbidity compared with as little as 5% with

TABLE 17-2	INCIDENCE OF COMPLICATIONS SEEN WITH BREECH PRESENTATION
COMPLICATION	**INCIDENCE**
Intrapartum fetal death	Increased 16-fold[23]
Perinatal mortality	1.3%[20]
Intrapartum asphyxia	Increased 3.8-fold[31]
Cord prolapse	Increased 5- to 20-fold[14,15]
	1.3%[20]
Birth trauma	Increased 13-fold[14]
	1.4%[20]
Dystocia, difficulty delivering head	4.6%[20] to 8.8%[14]
Spinal cord injuries with extended head	21%
Major anomalies	6% to 18%[31]
Prematurity	16% to 33%[22,25]
Hyperextension of head	5%
Fetal heart rate abnormalities	15.2%[20]

TABLE 17-3	ZATUCHNI-ANDROS SYSTEM		
FACTOR	**0**	**1**	**2**
Parity	Nullipara	Multipara	Multipara
Gestational age	39	38	37
Estimated fetal weight	8 lb	7-8 lb	7 lb
Previous breech	No	One	Two
Dilation (cm)	2	3	≥4
Station	−3 or greater	−2	−1 or less

From Zatuchni GI, Andros GJ. Prognostic index for vaginal delivery in breech presentation at term. *Am J Obstet Gynecol.* 1965;93:237.

vaginal delivery.[10,15] **In an attempt to balance both maternal and fetal risks, plans were proposed to select appropriate candidates for a trial of labor.**

In 1965, **Zatuchni and Andros**[17] retrospectively analyzed 182 breech births, of which 25 infants had poor outcomes. These investigators devised a score based on six clinical variables at the time of admission (Table 17-3) that identified those patients destined to manifest difficulties in labor, for whom prompt and appropriate interventions could be made. **The score used parity, gestational age, estimated weight, prior successful breech vaginal delivery, dilation, and station to ascertain likelihood of successful vaginal delivery.** However, the parturient could increase the score by presenting later in labor; other factors that affect the score are less modifiable. At least three subsequent prospective studies applied the Zatuchni-Andros system and found it to be both sensitive and accurate in selecting candidates for successful vaginal delivery.[18] **A Zatuchni-Andros score of less than 4 in these studies accurately predicted poor outcomes in patients with infants presenting as a breech.** Furthermore, in applying the scoring system, only 21% to 27% of patients failed to qualify for a trial of labor.[18] Previous breech delivery, one of the items scored in the Zatuchni-Andros system, has a significant odds ratio (OR) for recurrence of breech (4.32; 95% CI, 4.08 to 4.59) after one breech delivery, and the OR jumps up to 28.1 after three (95% CI, 12.2 to 64.8). However, this study did not control for recurrent causes of breech presentation such as uterine malformations and abnormal placentation.[19]

Because most reports of breech delivery are level II to III evidence, their validity and, most importantly, their universal applicability may be questioned. Many data were gathered before electronic FHR monitoring became commonplace. Until the year 2000, only one randomized trial (level I evidence) had examined term frank breech and method of delivery.[13] Improved perinatal survival had been reported for breeches delivered by cesarean section, and some evidence, although inconsistent, suggests that the method of delivery may also have an impact on the quality of survival.[16] Functional neurologic defects were found by 2 years of age in 24% of breech infants born vaginally but only in 2.5% of those breech weight- and age-matched infants born by cesarean delivery.[20] However, in comparing 175 breech infants with a 94% cesarean delivery rate with 595 historic controls with a 22% rate of abdominal delivery, Green and colleagues[21] found no significant differences in outcome. Neurologic outcomes were reviewed for 239 of 348 infants delivered from breech position.[22] Examinations performed at 3 to 10 years of age showed no statistically significant neurologic differences between neonates delivered by vaginal breech versus matched vertex controls. Thus, **these authors concluded that breech outcomes relate to degree of prematurity, maternal pregnancy complications, and fetal malformations as well as to birth trauma or asphyxia.** A 2009 Norwegian study[23] demonstrated that breech presentation *and* breech delivery are significant risk factors for cerebral palsy and represent a trend toward increasing risk for cerebral palsy among singletons born at term in breech by vaginal delivery (nearly fourfold). This adds to the body of literature that demonstrates that **breech-presenting fetuses are already at increased risk for neurologic adversity, even when controlled for birth order, prematurity, smallness for gestational age, assisted reproduction, sex, and route of delivery.**

Pelvimetry is frequently used when deciding whether to allow a trial of labor in a breech presenting fetus. Clinical pelvimetry is an acceptable technique that can be used to determine the dimensions of the mid pelvis, the outlet, and the inlet by way of surrogate measurement (the obstetric conjugate). The reader is referred to the Intrapartum Care section and Chapter 12, on normal labor and delivery, for discussion and demonstration of clinical pelvimetry. **Radiographic pelvimetry has been included in the management of the breech presentation with little objective validation.** Regardless, it is expected to predict successful vaginal delivery when adequate pelvic dimensions are present. At least four techniques for pelvimetry are commonly used worldwide: these include (1) conventional plain-film radiography, using up to three films; (2) CT with up to three views that include lateral, AP, and axial slice; (3) magnetic resonance imaging (MRI); and (4) digital fluorography, which is not presently used in the United States. MRI is the only technique not associated with radiation exposure, and CT pelvimetry using a single lateral view results in the lowest exposure dose; air-gap technique with conventional radiography will lower the radiation dosage, and current trends show a move toward the lower-dose CT techniques of up to three images.

The clinician must possess the necessary training and experience to offer a patient with a persistent breech presentation a trial of labor. Furthermore, the relationship between the patient and the clinician should be well established, and the discussions of risks and benefits must be objective and nondirective with accurate documentation of the discussion. If any of these factors are lacking, cesarean delivery becomes the safer choice. However, even if a clinician has made the choice that he or she will *never* prospectively offer a patient with breech presentation a trial of labor, the burden of responsibility to know and understand the mechanism and management of a breech delivery is not relieved. No one active in obstetrics will avoid the occasional emergency breech delivery. Regular review of principles and practice with

---

BOX 17-1   MANAGEMENT OF BREECH PRESENTATION

A trial of labor may be considered if the following conditions are met:
- EFW is between 2000 and 3800 g
- Presentation is a frank breech
- Maternal pelvis is adequate
- Fetal neck and head are flexed
- Fetal monitoring is used
- Zatuchni-Andros score is ≥4
- Rapid cesarean delivery is possible
- Good progress is maintained in labor
- Experience and training are available
- Informed consent is possible
  Cesarean delivery may be prudent if:
- EFW is <1500 g or >4000 g
- Fetus is in a footling presentation
- Parturient has a small pelvis
- Fetal neck and head are hyperextended
- Zatuchni-Andros score is <4
- Expertise in breech delivery is absent
- A nonreassuring FHR pattern is present
- Arrest of progress has occurred

EFW, estimated fetal weight; FHR, fetal heart rate.

---

simulations using a mannequin and model pelvis with an experienced colleague can increase the skills and improve the performance of anyone facing such an emergency. A 2006 study[24] of resident skill before and after simulation training showed universal improvement in technique and performance of key maneuvers required for vaginal delivery of a breech fetus when such maneuvers were performed in mock emergency settings using a Noelle pelvic trainer (Gaumard Scientific). Maintenance of skill is particularly important as breech vaginal delivery becomes less frequently encountered in routine obstetric practice (this is discussed in greater detail below, in regard to the Term Breech Trial).

Factors that affect the decision to deliver a breech vaginally or by cesarean delivery are listed in Box 17-1. The obvious implication of the dramatically diminished experience in training programs with vaginal breech delivery is that inexperience will constitute an indication for cesarean delivery. Certainly, **in no case should a woman with an infant presenting as a breech be allowed to labor unless (1) anesthesia coverage is immediately available, (2) cesarean delivery can be undertaken promptly, (3) continuous FHR monitoring is used, and (4) the delivery is attended by a pediatrician and two obstetricians, of whom at least one is experienced with vaginal breech birth.**

TERM BREECH TRIAL

One of the most influential publications was the multicenter prospective study known as the *Term Breech Trial* (TBT). The impetus for this investigation was a series of retrospective studies that demonstrated increased morbidity and mortality of neonates after vaginal breech delivery, which included neonatal intensive care unit admissions, hyperbilirubinemia, bone fractures, intracranial hemorrhage, neonatal depression,[25] convulsions, and death.[26] Other studies, however, found that emergent cesarean delivery was also associated with poor neonatal outcomes. Irion and colleagues[27] reported similarly poor neonatal outcomes from cesarean deliveries of 705 singleton breeches and concluded that as a result of the increased *maternal* morbidity associated with cesarean birth, delivery of the breech by cesarean section was not firmly indicated. This opinion was supported by Brown and colleagues[14] in their prospective case series, noting that the corrected perinatal mortality rate did not differ for neonates who weighed 1500 g or more.

In October 2000, the first results from the TBT were published.[16] Overall, 2088 patients from 121 centers in 26 countries with varied national perinatal mortality statistics, according to the World Health Organization (WHO), were enrolled in the study. Assignment was random, with 1041 to the planned cesarean delivery group and 1042 to the planned vaginal delivery group. The data were analyzed by the intention-to-treat method, and 941 of 1041 (90.4%) and 591 of 1042 (56.7%) delivered by their intended route of delivery, cesarean delivery and vaginal birth, respectively. Intrapartum events, including cord prolapse and FHR abnormalities, occurred at rates similar to prior studies. Maternal and fetal/neonatal short-term (immediate, 6 weeks, and 3 months) and long-term (2 year) outcome data were presented in this and subsequent reports. **For countries with both low and high perinatal mortality rates (PMRs), the occurrence of perinatal mortality or serious neonatal morbidity (defined within the report) was significantly lower in the planned cesarean delivery group than in the planned vaginal delivery group (relative risk [RR], 0.33; 95% CI, 0.19 to 0.56; $P < .0001$). In countries with an already low PMR, a proportionately greater risk reduction in PMR was found in the planned cesarean delivery. The effects of operator experience and prolonged labor did not affect the direction of the risk reduction and only marginally affected the amplitude. No differences existed in maternal mortality or serious maternal morbidity between the groups.**[16]

The effects on the correlation between labor and delivery factors were assessed in a separate regression analysis that used only delivery mode in one regression and only labor factors—including all other variables such as fetal monitoring, length of labor, and medications—in the other. **Mode of delivery and birth weight were both significantly associated with adverse fetal outcome without a significant degree of interaction of these variables. Essentially, smaller infants (less than 2800 g) were at greatest risk (OR, 2.13; 95% CI, 1.2 to 3.8; $P = .01$).** Neonates with birthweights greater than 3500 g showed a trend toward more adverse outcomes, but the trend did not reach significance. The analysis of the labor data shows a "dose-response relationship between the progression of labor and the risk of adverse perinatal outcome," such that **a prelabor cesarean delivery is associated with the lowest rates of adverse outcome compared with vaginal breech delivery.**[28] Maternal outcomes at 3 months showed a reduced rate of urinary incontinence (RR, 0.62; 95% CI, 0.41 to 0.93) in the planned cesarean delivery group,[29] but 2 years after delivery, no differences were found in urinary incontinence or breastfeeding, medical, sexual, social, pain, or reproductive issues.[30] Neonatal outcomes at 2 years showed no difference in mortality rates or neurodevelopmental delay between the planned cesarean delivery and planned vaginal delivery groups.[31] **To summarize the TBT, if a trial of labor is attempted and is successful, babies born by planned vaginal delivery have a small but significant risk of dying or sustaining a debilitating insult in the short term compared with a planned cesarean delivery. If they survive, no difference is seen in the mortality rate or in the presence of developmental delay when compared with children born by planned cesarean delivery.**

The worldwide repercussions of the TBT are still being realized. Eighty of the collaborating centers in 23 of 26 countries responded to a follow-up questionnaire regarding change in practice patterns after the results of the TBT were published. A plurality stated that practice had changed (92.5%), and 85% of respondents reported that an analysis of relative costs would not affect the continued implementation of a policy of planned cesarean delivery for the breech at term.[32]

A Dutch study examined the effects on delivery statistics and outcomes following the TBT and showed an increase in the cesarean delivery rate for the term breech from 50% to 80%, which was associated with a concomitant reduction in perinatal mortality rate from 0.35% to 0.18%.[33]

The total U.S. cesarean delivery rate peaked in 2009 at 32.9% of all births, rising from a low of 20.7% in 1996. A modest decline to 32.8% occurred in 2010, and this rate has been maintained through 2012. The 1981 National Institutes of Health Consensus Report found that 12% of cesarean deliveries in 1978 were performed for breech presentation and that this indication contributed 10% to 15% to the overall rise in the rate of cesarean births. At least a portion of the increase in cesarean delivery rates is a response to the perceived risk of morbidity and mortality associated with the breech presentation.[16,21] **Currently, 17% of cesarean deliveries are performed for breech.**[34] **In the United States, the cesarean delivery rate for breech presentation increased from 11.6% to 86.9% in 2002 and stood at 85% as of 2003.**[21,35,36] **Comparing the U.S. cesarean delivery rates from 1998 and 2011, before and after the TBT's publication, a marked increase is apparent in the rates for cesarean delivery: 21.2% of all live births in 1998, compared with 26.1% in 2002, and up to 32.8% currently.** Rates of both primary and repeat cesarean deliveries increased. This may be in part because of the staggering number of multiple births and their related degree of prematurity, the relative reduction in vaginal birth after cesarean delivery,[35] and the self-fulfilling prophecy of lack of experience owing to increasing trends toward cesarean delivery for breech, which leaves a void of experienced operators to perform breech vaginal deliveries (see Chapter 20). Currently, the American College of Obstetricians and Gynecologists (ACOG) has released statements that place emphasis on reducing the cesarean delivery rate; one of the recommendations is to offer ECV for the persistent breech at term and for a trial of labor with twins when the first twin is in a cephalic presentation. Both of these bear continued consideration with each pregnancy. The implications for future pregnancies have been studied: maternal morbidity and mortality rates are significantly increased with cesarean birth compared with vaginal delivery (8.6% vs. 9.2%),[37] in particular repeat cesarean delivery, for which breech presentation has become an inarguable cause, perhaps unnecessarily.

Even though greater risks appear to face the breech infant, many still believe that complete abandonment of vaginal delivery for the breech is not yet justified. The TBT also has its detractors, who state that inclusion of fetuses with estimated weights up to 4 kg and less than 2500 g, procedural aberrations in labor assessment and adequacy (length of time permitted for first and second stage of labor, liberal use of induction and augmentation of labor), and worldwide differences in standards of obstetric care and its providers make the trial's results not generalizable. No study is perfect in its methodology or results;

this trial has been criticized for its statistical methodology, the ascertainment of expertise, inclusion of both fetal deaths and anomalous fetuses, and the absence of ultrasound from some participating centers, among other transgressions.[38] However flawed it may, the TBT adds to the body of literature on breech vaginal delivery but as such may not be the final answer to the question of the safety of vaginal breech delivery.

Since that time, a large prospective cohort analysis was performed at 174 centers in France and Belgium, two countries where the TBT has had only a modest effect on vaginal breech delivery rates. Termed the PREMODA trial (*Presentation et Mode d'Accouchement*, [Presentation and Mode of Delivery]), it evaluated pregnancy and delivery data—a composite of morbidities, similar to the TBT—from women who gave birth to a fetus, alive or not, from 37 or more weeks. An expert committee not blinded to the mode of delivery evaluated each birth outcome as to whether an elective cesarean delivery at 39 weeks would have prevented the particular outcome. They found that 6 of the 22 fetal deaths and 17 of the 18 neonatal or postneonatal deaths before discharge were due to lethal anomalies; only one death occurred among phenotypically normal fetuses, and this was deemed sudden and unexpected at 15 days of life. In sum, this study noted a global fetal or neonatal mortality risk of 1.59% (95% CI, 1.33 to 1.89); this was not significantly different from the population delivered by planned cesarean. The mortality and serious morbidity rate was significantly less than that of countries with a low PMR rate in the TBT (1.59% vs. 5.7%). Thus in these countries with an already low PMR, excess neonatal morbidity and mortality are not attributed to breech vaginal delivery. However, these results may not be applicable to the United States because the expertise for performing breech vaginal delivery is unfortunately not as available in this country.[39]

Special Clinical Circumstances and Risks: Preterm Breech, Hyperextended Head, and Footling Breech

The various categories of breech presentation clearly demonstrate dissimilar risks, and management plans might vary among these situations. **The premature breech, the breech with a hyperextended head, and the footling breech are categories that have high rates of fetal morbidity or mortality. Complications associated with incomplete dilation and cephalic entrapment may be more frequent. For these three breech situations, in general, cesarean delivery appears to optimize fetal outcome and is therefore recommended.**

Low birthweight (<2500 g) is a confounding factor in about one third of all breech presentations.[17] Whereas the benefit of cesarean delivery for the breech infant weighing 1500 to 2500 g remains controversial,[13] some studies have shown improved survival with cesarean delivery in the 1000- to 1500-g weight group.[40,41] A multicenter study of long-term outcomes of vaginally delivered infants at 26 to 31 weeks' gestation found no differences in rates of death or developmental disability within 2 years of follow-up.[42] Traumatic morbidity is reportedly decreased in both weight groups by the use of cesarean delivery, including a lower rate of both intraventricular and periventricular hemorrhage. Although some advocate a trial of labor in the frank breech infant weighing over 1500 g, others recommend labor only when the infant exceeds 2000 grams. Proportionately fewer frank breech presentations occur in the low-birthweight group. **In fact, most infants who weigh less than 1500 g and present as a breech are footling breeches.** Although

most deaths in those with a very low birthweight are due to prematurity or lethal anomalies, cesarean delivery has been shown by some to decrease corrected perinatal mortality in this weight group compared with that in similar-sized vertex presentations.[43] Other authors suggest that improved survival in these studies relates to improved neonatal care of the premature infant when compared with the outcomes of historic controls. However, when vaginal delivery of the preterm breech is chosen or is unavoidable, older studies have demonstrated reduced fetal morbidity and mortality when conduction anesthesia and forceps for the delivery of the aftercoming head are used; neither are commonplace in modern obstetrics. A study of neonates at 26 to 29 weeks 6 days gestational age born by planned breech versus planned cesarean delivery showed no difference in mortality rate.[44] Although in this study, premature rupture of the membranes (PROM) at a gestational age less than 24 weeks, head entrapment, and a gestational age between 26 to 27 weeks 6 days were all independently associated with neonatal death.

Preterm premature rupture of the fetal membranes (PPROM) is associated with prematurity and chorioamnionitis, both of which have been found to be independent risk factors for the development of cerebral palsy (CP). PPROM is associated with a high rate of malpresentation because of prematurity and decreased amniotic fluid. Knowing the association of chorioamnionitis with periventricular leukomalacia (PVL), a lesion found to precede development of CP in the premature neonate, Baud and colleagues[45] correlated the mode of delivery with PVL and subsequent CP in breech preterm deliveries. **The authors found that in the presence of chorioamnionitis, delivery by planned cesarean section was associated with a dramatic decrease in the incidence of PVL.**

Hyperextension of the fetal head during vaginal breech delivery has been consistently associated with a high (21%) risk of spinal cord injury. It is important to differentiate simple deflexion of the head from clear hyperextension, given that Ballas and colleagues demonstrated that simple deflexion carries no excess risk. Deflexion of the fetal vertex, as opposed to hyperextension, is similar to the relationship between the occipito-frontal cranial plane and the axis of the fetal cervical spine illustrated in Figure 17-5. Often, as labor progresses, spontaneous flexion will occur in response to fundal forces.

Finally, the footling breech carries a prohibitively high (16% to 19%) risk of cord prolapse during labor. In many cases, cord prolapse manifests only late in labor, after commitment to vaginal delivery may have been made. Cord prolapse necessitates prompt cesarean delivery. Furthermore, the footling breech is a poor cervical dilator, and cephalic entrapment becomes more likely.

Breech Second Twin

Approximately one third of all twin gestations present as cephalic/breech—that is, first twin is a cephalic presentation and the second is a breech (see also Chapter 32, Multiple Gestations). **The management alternatives in the case of the cephalic/breech twin pregnancy in labor include cesarean delivery, vaginal delivery of the first twin, and either attempted ECV or IPV and breech extraction of the second twin. Blickstein and colleagues compared the obstetric outcomes of 39 cases of vertex/breech twins with the outcomes of 48 vertex/vertex twins.** Although the breech second twin had a higher incidence of low birthweight and a longer hospital stay, the authors found no basis for elective cesarean delivery in this clinical circumstance. The outcomes of another study[46] of 136 pairs of cephalic/noncephalic twins weighing more than 1500 g allows us to conclude that breech extraction of the second twin appears to be a safe alternative to cesarean delivery. Laros and Dattel[47] studied 206 twin pairs and similarly found no clear advantage to arbitrary cesarean delivery because of a specific presentation. When comparing outcomes of 390 vaginally delivered second twins (207 delivered vertex, 183 delivered breech), with 95% of the breech deliveries being total breech extractions, it is noted that no significant differences existed between the cephalic and breech infants even when stratified by birthweight.[48] These outcomes assume the skills and experience required to perform a successful breech extraction. A recent Danish retrospective evaluation[49] of IPV for a noncephalic second twin demonstrated that although it occurs only rarely, IPV is associated with fewer asphyxiated neonates than second twins delivered by cesarean delivery after a vaginal delivery of the first twin; in addition, a trend was seen toward higher cord pH and higher Apgar scores in the IPV group. The disturbing trend highlighted by this study is the very high chance of the vaginal and cesarean combination delivery.

The Twin Birth Study,[50] a multicenter randomized trial, showed that cesarean delivery of twins demonstrated neither a decrease nor an increase in the rate of fetal or neonatal death or morbidity compared with vaginal delivery. The authors of this study advocate that patients seek out providers who are skilled in the vaginal birth of the second twin. For any clinician uncomfortable with the prospective vaginal delivery of a singleton breech, however, cesarean delivery may be a safer option for the pregnancy with a noncephalic-presenting second twin.

Vaginal delivery of the first twin followed by external version of the second is a viable alternative, using ultrasound in the delivery room to directly visualize the fetus. Often a transient decrease in uterine activity occurs after the delivery of the first infant, which can be used to advantage in the performance of a cephalic version. Description of experience with 30 noncephalic second twins (12 transverse and 18 breech) shows that version after birth of the first twin was successful in 11 of the 12 infants in a transverse lie and in 16 of the 18 breech infants.[51] These twins were all older than 35 weeks' gestation, with intact membranes of the second twin after delivery of the first, no evidence of anomalies, and normal amniotic fluid volume.

If IPV/extraction of the second twin is to be performed, it can be facilitated by ultrasonic guidance. A hand is inserted into the uterus, both fetal feet are identified and grasped with the membranes intact, and traction is applied to bring the feet into the pelvis and out the introitus, with maternal expulsive efforts remaining the major force in effecting descent of the fetus. The membranes are left intact until both feet are at the introitus. Once the membranes are ruptured, the delivery is subsequently managed as a footling breech delivery. If the operator has difficulty identifying the fetal feet, intrapartum ultrasound may be of assistance.

During breech extraction, and perhaps more often with a breech extraction of a smaller twin, the fetal head can become entrapped in the cervix. In such cases, the operator's entire hand is placed in the uterus, the fetal head is cradled, and as the hand is withdrawn, the head is protected.[52] This splinting technique has also been used for the safe extraction of the breech head at the time of cesarean delivery. Head entrapment may also occur

because of increased uterine tone or contractions. In this case, a uterine relaxing agent may be used, with nitroglycerin 50 to 200 μg intravenously being one of the fastest acting, safest agents in appropriately selected patients. Terbutaline, ritodrine, or inhalational anesthesia may also be used.

External Cephalic Version

External cephalic version (ECV) is recommended for the breech fetus at 36 to 37 weeks' gestation.[4,53] Many have found that ECV significantly reduces the incidence of breech presentation in labor and is associated with few complications such as cord compression or placental abruption.[4] Reported success with ECV varies from 60% to 75%, and a similar percentage of these remain vertex at the time of labor.[4] Although many infants in breech presentation before 34 weeks' gestation will convert spontaneously to a cephalic presentation, the percentage that spontaneously convert decreases as term approaches. Repetitive external version applied weekly after 34 weeks' gestation in one report was successful in converting more than two thirds of cases and reducing their breech presentation rate by 50%. In another randomized trial[53] of ECV in low-risk pregnancies between 37 and 39 weeks' gestation, success was achieved in 68% of 25 cases in the version group, whereas only 4 of the 23 controls converted to a vertex spontaneously before labor. All of those in whom external version was successful presented in labor as a vertex. In another prospective, controlled study of ECV performed weekly between 33 weeks' gestation and term, 48% of the study group was vertex in labor compared with only 26% of controls. Another experience with 112 patients demonstrated a 49% success rate with ECV. The cesarean delivery rate was 17% among those patients with successful ECV compared with 78% among those with an unsuccessful version attempt.

The timing of ECV has been evaluated in the early ECV2 trial,[54] published in 2011. Whereas a greater percentage of ECVs performed early (34 weeks to 35 weeks 6 days gestational age), as opposed to those performed late (at or beyond 37 weeks' gestation), were cephalic at the time of delivery, no difference was found in the rate of cesarean delivery between the two groups. The additional detractor from doing an early ECV is that the rate of late preterm births did increase. The study noted that the success rate of early versus late ECV was greater, but the authors did not comment on the significance of this difference.

Outcomes of pregnancies after ECV prove that it is a safe and effective intervention.[4] Successful version was reported more often in parous than in nulliparous women and more often between 37 and 39 weeks' gestation than after 40 weeks. Fetal complications include abruption, a nonreassuring FHR pattern, rupture of the membranes, cord prolapse, spontaneous conversion back to breech, and fetomaternal hemorrhage. Maternal complications include a high rate of cesarean delivery—up to 64% in one study, and a twofold to fourfold risk in another—primarily for dystocia, despite successful conversion.[55]

Gentle, constant pressure applied in a relaxed patient with frequent FHR assessments are elements of success stressed by all investigators.[53] Methodology varies, although the "forward roll" is more widely supported than the "back flip" (Fig. 17-25).[53] The mechanical goal is to squeeze the fetal vertex gently out of the fundal area to the transverse and finally the lower segment of the uterus.

A number of factors predict success of ECV with reliability. A study in 2010 by Burgos and colleagues[56] demonstrated

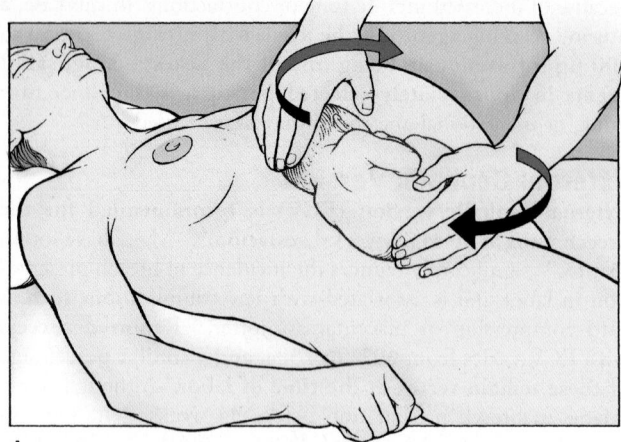

A

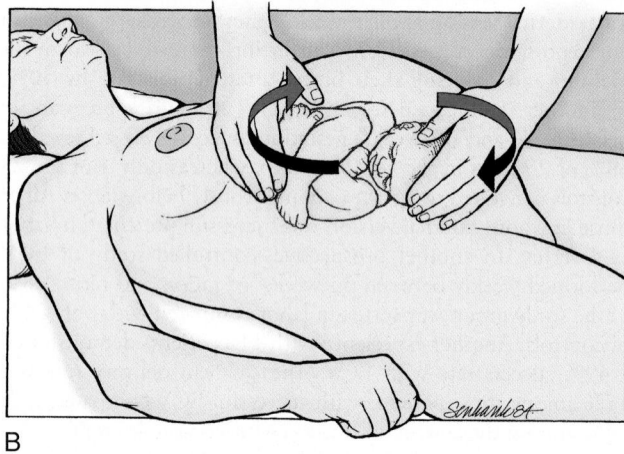

B

FIG 17-25 External cephalic version is accomplished by gently "squeezing" the fetus out of one area of the uterus and into another. Illustrated here is the popular "forward roll."

increased rates of successful ECV at approximately 37 weeks' gestation with parity greater than two (OR, 3.74; 95% CI, 2.37 to 5.9), posterior placental location (OR, 2.85; 95% CI,1.87 to 4.36), and double footling breech as opposed to frank breech (OR, 2.77; 95% CI, 1.16 to 6.62). Complete breech also showed increased odds of success, but not to the extent that the double-footling breech did. Relative assessment of amniotic fluid volume was also made, and both "normal" and "abundant" fluid volumes showed improved successes. Two studies[57,58] demonstrated better results when the amniotic fluid index (AFI) exceeded 7 cm.

Tocolysis, regional anesthesia, and ultrasound during ECV may also be helpful. Use of a number of tocolytics has been reported; however, considerable experience has been reported using IV ritodrine, which has been voluntarily withdrawn from the U.S. market by the manufacturer. Other agents that have been used include hexoprenaline, salbutamol (albuterol), nitroglycerin, and terbutaline, which now carries a Food and Drug Administration (FDA) black-box warning. A randomized trial[59] of 103 nulliparous patients found that the success rate with subcutaneous terbutaline was 52%, compared with 27% in the control group, and no adverse maternal effects resulting from the drug were found. A randomized trial of 58 patients at 37 to 41 weeks' gestation with breech presentation found no benefit from β-mimetic tocolysis, with success rates of approximately two thirds in each group.

The use of regional anesthesia for ECV has also been controversial. Many believe that operators might apply excessive pressure to the maternal abdomen when epidural anesthesia is used, which might make fetal compromise more likely, as indicated by FHR decelerations and possibly related to placental abruption. However, a randomized trial[60] of ECV in 69 women using epidural anesthesia demonstrated a better than twofold increase in the success of the procedure when an epidural was used. Disparate results are demonstrated when combined spinal-epidural (CSE) analgesia or spinal anesthesia is used. A randomized study[61] of nulliparas undergoing ECV showed a fourfold improvement in the success of ECV and a reduced visual analog pain score with spinal anesthesia compared with no anesthetic. Another randomized trial[62] of CSE anesthesia at analgesic doses versus systemic opioids showed no difference in the rates of successful ECV. This trial had an overall low rate of successful ECV (39%) and a low rate in each arm (47% in the CSE and 31% in the opioid arms, respectively), and the participation of 47 physicians suggests the possibility of highly varied skill levels across the providers. This trial specifically aimed to determine whether analgesia, as opposed to anesthesia, improves success. It appears that **the relationship of ECV success may be dose dependent as far as neuraxial anesthetic use is concerned because other trials that have used large anesthetic doses favor improved ECV success rates.**

A Cochrane database study[63] of the effects of tocolysis, regional anesthesia, vibroacoustic stimulation (VAS), and transabdominal amnioinfusion for ECV was performed and reported in 2012. It reviewed 25 studies with data on 2548 women. Tocolytics, in particular β-mimetics, increased the rate of cephalic presentation at term (RR, 1.38; 95% CI, 1.03 to 1.85) and reduced the cesarean delivery rate (RR, 0.82; 95% CI, 0.71 to 0.94). No difference was noted between success rates in nulliparas and multiparas with a cephalic presentation in labor or cesarean delivery; **therefore terbutaline before ECV is recommended.**

Regional anesthesia *in combination with tocolysis* demonstrated more successful ECVs than the tocolytic drug alone (RR, 0.67; 95% CI, 0.51 to 0.89), but no difference was noted in either the rate of cesarean delivery or cephalic presentation in labor, and no difference in the occurrence of fetal bradycardia was observed. Data were insufficient to determine the efficacy of VAS, amnioinfusion, opioids, nitric oxide donors, or calcium channel blockers for improving ECV success rate.[14]

On the adverse side, factors associated with failure of ECV included obesity, deep pelvic engagement of the breech, oligohydramnios, and posterior positioning of the fetal back. Fetomaternal transfusion has been reported to occur in up to 6% of patients undergoing external version[64]; thus **Rh-negative unsensitized women should receive RhD immune globulin.** Quantitation of fetomaternal hemorrhage with the Kleihauer-Betke (acid elution) or flow cytometry test will determine the number of vials of RhOD immune globulin to be administered.

In the case of the gravida with a previous cesarean delivery, ECV has also been controversial. Studies of limited sample size have concluded that ECV is safe for mother and fetus and that it results in increased rates of vaginal delivery. Success rates of up to 82% in patients with a previous cesarean delivery have been reported.[65] Use of IV ritodrine tocolysis in 11 patients with a history of a previous low cervical transverse cesarean delivery resulted in no uterine dehiscences found clinically or at the time of cesarean delivery.[66]

A 2009 study by Sela and colleagues[67] that included a review of the world literature (of singleton fetuses without anomalies at 36 or more weeks' gestation, all retrospective studies) found ECV success rates in multiparas that ranged between 65.8% and 100% (mean 76.6%) in patients with a single prior cesarean delivery. Prior successful vaginal delivery was predictive of higher success rates for ECV overall, and no excess morbidity/mortality or asymptomatic scar dehiscence was noted in these patients. The largest study of complication rates from ECV included patients with a prior cesarean delivery, but neither the success nor complication rates for this subgroup were reported; descriptions of overall complications included no case of overt uterine rupture or scar dehiscence.[68] Although these are now limited recommendations for patients with two prior cesarean deliveries to attempt a trial of labor after cesarean (TOLAC; see Chapter 20), data are not available regarding success rates and complications of ECV in this population.

Acupuncture and moxibustion of acupoint BL 67 (Zhiyin, which lies beside the outer corner of the fifth toenail) have been studied in relation to converting the noncephalic presenting fetus, and a Cochrane review[69] on this topic was recently published. Although early studies demonstrated benefit of these therapies, this review of eight studies with data on 1346 women showed that moxibustion alone did not reduce noncephalic presentation compared with no treatment. In comparison to acupuncture, however, moxibustion proved to be superior (RR, 0.25; 95% CI, 0.09 to 0.72), but in *combination* with acupuncture, a reduction was noted in both noncephalic presentations (RR, 0.73; 95% CI, 0.57 to 0.94) and cesarean deliveries (RR, 0.79; 95% CI, 0.64 to 0.98). The increasing role of complementary and alternative medicine and traditional techniques in modern medicine remain to be further examined.

SHOULDER DYSTOCIA

In a normal delivery, after expulsion of the fetal head, external rotation occurs and returns the head to a right-angle position in relation to the shoulder girdle. The fetal shoulder during descent is in an oblique pelvic diameter; however, after expulsion and restitution, the anterior fetal shoulder should emerge from the oblique axis under the pubic ramus. **Shoulder dystocia occurs when the fetal shoulders are obstructed at the level of the pelvic inlet. Shoulder dystocia results from a size discrepancy between the fetal shoulders and the pelvic inlet, which may be absolute or relative, because of malposition.** A persistent anterior-posterior location of the fetal shoulders at the pelvic brim occurs when increased resistance is present between the fetal skin and the vaginal walls, such as with accelerated fetal growth; a large fetal chest relative to the biparietal diameter, seen in infants of diabetic gravidas; and when truncal rotation does not occur, as with precipitous labor. Shoulder dystocia typically occurs when the descent of the anterior shoulder is obstructed by the symphysis pubis. It can also result from impaction of the posterior shoulder on the maternal sacral promontory.[70]

Unfortunately, the ultimate diagnosis of this obstetric emergency will not occur until after the fetal head has emerged from the vagina (Fig. 17-26). The *turtle sign,* in which there is retraction of the fetal head against the maternal perineum, is suggestive but not diagnostic of the presence of shoulder dystocia. Shoulder dystocia is therefore most commonly diagnosed upon

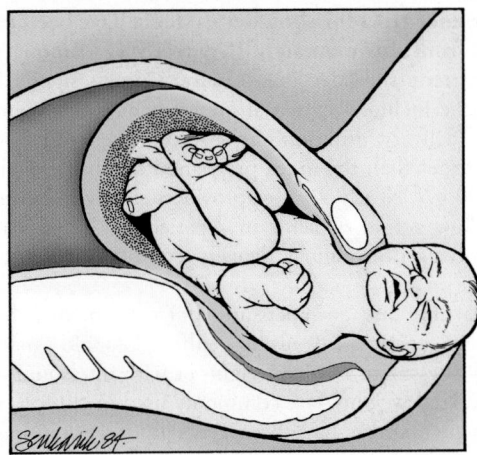

FIG 17-26 When delivery of the fetal head is not followed by delivery of the shoulders, the anterior shoulder often becomes caught behind the symphysis, as illustrated. The head may retract toward the perineum, and desperate traction on the fetal head is not likely to facilitate delivery and may lead to trauma.

failure of delivery of the fetal shoulder(s) after initial attempts at extraction-oriented manual traction and when ancillary obstetric maneuvers are required. Although other definitions have been reported in the literature, these are not commonly used in daily clinical practice. Two studies have proposed defining *shoulder dystocia* as a prolonged head-to-body delivery interval of 60 seconds (the mean plus two standard deviations) and/or use of ancillary obstetric maneuvers.[71,72] In Hoffman's multicenter study,[73] however, only two (0.01%) among the 2018 reported shoulder dystocias documented such a head-to-body time in the delivery notes.

Shoulder dystocia has been reported to complicate 0.2% to 3% of all vaginal deliveries.[73] This wide range has been attributed to the inherent subjectivity of the clinician's definition of *shoulder dystocia,* the degree of reporting, and differences in defining the study population. The risk of shoulder dystocia rises with increasing fetal birthweight; in these instances, the trunk—and in particular, the chest—grow larger relative to the head. **The percentage of deliveries complicated by shoulder dystocia for unassisted births not complicated by diabetes was 5.2% for infants weighing 4000 to 4250 g, 9.1% for those between 4250 and 4500 g, 14.3% for those 4500 and 4750 g, and 21.1% for those 4750 to 5000 g.**[74] **It must be remembered that approximately 50% to 60% of shoulder dystocias occur in infants who weigh less than 4000 g. Moreover, even if the birthweight of the infant is over 4000 g, shoulder dystocia will complicate only 3.3% of the deliveries.**[70]

In addition to being generally poor predictors for shoulder dystocia, historic clinical risk factors such as maternal obesity, prolonged second stage, previous birth of an infant weighing more than 4000 g, gestational diabetes mellitus, prolonged second stage of labor, prolonged deceleration phase (8 to 10 cm), prolonged and postterm pregnancy, increased maternal age, excess maternal weight gain, male fetus, and epidural analgesia/anesthesia are also not readily amenable to interventions that can alter fetal outcome. A trivariate analysis of labor induction, oxytocin use, and a birthweight greater than 4500 g only showed a sensitivity of 12.4% and a positive predictive value of 3.4% for the prediction of shoulder dystocia.[75]

Recurrence risks for shoulder dystocia have been reported to range from approximately 10% to 25%.[76] Among patients with recurrent shoulder dystocia, statistically significant risk factors have included maternal prepregnancy weight, maternal weight at delivery, duration of the second stage of labor, birthweight greater than the index pregnancy, and birthweight more than 4000 g.[70] Nearly 40% of providers surveyed in one study would allow a trial of labor in a patient with a documented history of a prior vaginal delivery complicated by shoulder dystocia.[77]

Antepartum and intrapartum efforts to predict postnatal birthweight—performed using either Leopold maneuvers, maternal assessment of birthweight, or with ultrasound-derived estimated fetal weight—are commonly used in clinical practice, although such efforts have been generally disappointing in the prediction and prevention of shoulder dystocia. The American College of Obstetricians and Gynecologists recommends that planned cesarean delivery *may be considered* with estimated fetal weights that exceed 5000 g in women without diabetes and 4500 g in women with diabetes.[78] Mean error rates for late third trimester ultrasound, however, have been reported to approximate 10% to 15%.[79] The fetal vertex is often too deeply engaged in the pelvis to allow accurate measurement of head circumference. Maternal body habitus and the presence of oligohydramnios are also contributing factors to this inability to accurately estimate fetal weight.

The concept of prophylactic cesarean delivery as a means to prevent shoulder dystocia and therefore avoid brachial plexus injury has not been supported by either clinical or theoretic data. The model of Rouse and associates[80] compared policies of management 1) without ultrasound; 2) with ultrasound and elective cesarean delivery for an estimated fetal weight over 4000 g; and 3) with ultrasound and elective cesarean delivery for an estimated fetal weight over 5000 g. It was found that 2345 to 3695 cesarean deliveries would need to be performed to prevent one permanent brachial plexus injury among nondiabetic women, with additional costs of $4.9 to $8.7 million. Using decision analysis techniques, Herbst[81] compared three strategies for an infant with an estimated fetal weight of 4500 g. She similarly found that expectant treatment was the preferred strategy at a cost of $4104.33 per injury-free child, compared with planned cesarean delivery at a cost of $5212.06 and an induction cost of $5165.08.

A few authors have retrospectively evaluated the fetal abdominal diameter–biparietal diameter difference (AD-BPD) as a predictor for shoulder dystocia. These studies have been limited by their retrospective nature, difficulty in measuring the fetal abdominal outline at advanced gestational ages, small sample size, and lack of applicability to the general population. Among infants of diabetic mothers whose estimated fetal weights were 3800 to 4200 grams, Cohen and colleagues[82] found that shoulder dystocia occurred in 6 of 20 patients (30%) in whom the AD-BPD difference was at least 2.6 cm but in none of 11 patients in whom it was less than 2.6 cm ($P = .05$). In nondiabetic women with suspected *macrosomia,* defined as an estimated fetal weight above 4000 g, the adjusted odds ratio of shoulder dystocia in the group with an AD-BPD difference of 2.6 cm or more was 3.67 (95% CI, 1.44 to 9.36).[83] In a study by Miller and colleagues,[84] those patients with shoulder dystocia had an increased AD-BPD difference (2.9 vs. 1.97, $P = .0002$), and when the difference was 2.6 cm or more, the risk of dystocia was 25% for unselected patients and 38.5% for patients with

diabetes. Overall, an OR of 5.88 (95% CI, 1.18 to 19.09) for presence of dystocia was noted in all patients and carried a sensitivity of 35.7% and a specificity of 91.4%. For patients with diabetes, an OR of 7.19 for shoulder dystocia (95% CI, 1.58 to 32.67) was found.

Postpartum hemorrhage and the unintentional extension of the episiotomy or laceration into the rectum are the most common maternal complications associated with shoulder dystocia. In a study by Gherman and associates,[85] these occurred in 11% and 3.8%, respectively, of the described shoulder dystocias.

A large multicenter study that evaluated 2018 cases of shoulder dystocia included 60 cases of Erb-Duchenne paralysis, four with Klumpke paralysis, 41 clavicular or humeral fractures, and six episodes of hypoxic-ischemic encephalopathy (HIE).[73] Unilateral brachial plexus palsies are the most common neurologic injury sustained by the neonate. The right arm is typically affected owing to the fact that the left occiput anterior presentation is more common. Most (80%) of the brachial plexus palsies have been located within the C5-C6 nerve roots (Erb-Duchenne paralysis). Other types of brachial plexus palsies that have been described include Klumpke paralysis (C8-T1), an intermediate palsy, and complete palsy of the entire brachial plexus. Diaphragmatic paralysis, Horner syndrome, and facial nerve injuries have occasionally been reported to accompany brachial plexus paralysis. Approximately one third of brachial plexus palsies will be associated with a concomitant bone fracture, most commonly of the clavicle (94%).[86]

Using computer modeling, the forces applied to the fetal brachial plexus during shoulder dystocia—and also with the addition of release maneuvers—were estimated by Grimm and colleagues.[87] All maneuvers resulted in less stretch to the brachial plexus than with standard lithotomy delivery alone. Delivery of the posterior arm showed a 71% reduction in stretch applied to the anterior nerve plexus and was the maneuver that required the least force to deliver the anterior shoulder. In the past, it had been empirically deduced that brachial plexus injury resulted exclusively from operator-induced excess traction in the setting of shoulder dystocia. In addition to research within the obstetric community, the pediatric, orthopedic, and neurologic literature now stresses that the existence of brachial plexus paralysis does not constitute a priori proof that exogenous forces were the cause of the injury.[88] Maternal endogenous forces have been shown to exceed clinician-applied exogenous forces. It has been consistently reported that approximately 50% of brachial plexus paralysis occurs in the absence of clinically recognized shoulder dystocia. Gherman and colleagues[89] showed that neonates who experienced brachial plexus palsy without shoulder dystocia were of lower birthweight and had an increased rate of clavicular fractures, and these paralyses were more likely to be persistent at 1 year of life.

The use of an exogenous force (traction) by the delivering provider is inherent in the management of the majority of vaginal deliveries and in the management of shoulder dystocia cases. Clinical diagnosis of shoulder dystocia results from failure of delivery of the fetal shoulder(s) after an initial traction attempt. A few authors have empirically advocated proceeding directly to maneuvers for attempted delivery of the fetal shoulders (i.e., avoidance of initial diagnostic traction) in order to maintain the forward momentum of the fetus. Others support a short delay in the delivery of the shoulders and advocate observation alone, arguing that the endogenous rotational

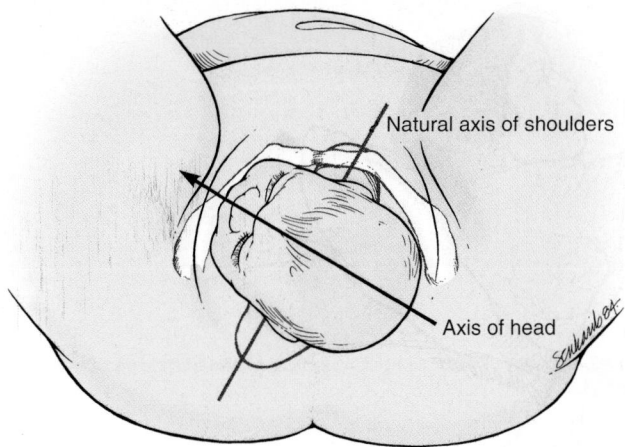

FIG 17-27 After delivery of the head, *restitution* results in the long axis of the head reassuming its normal orientation to the shoulders as seen here.

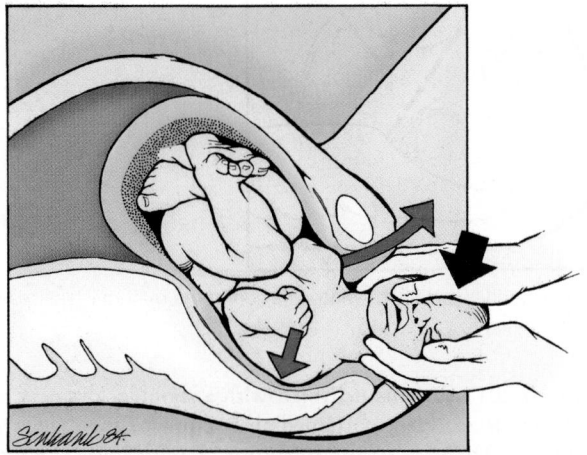

FIG 17-28 Gentle, symmetric pressure on the head will move the posterior shoulder into the hollow of the sacrum and will encourage delivery of the anterior shoulder. Care should be taken not to "pry" the anterior shoulder out asymmetrically because this might lead to trauma to the anterior brachial plexus.

mechanics of the second stage may spontaneously alleviate the obstruction.

When shoulder dystocia is clinically diagnosed, the first order of business should be to stop all endogenous and exogenous forces until an attempt is made to alleviate the obstruction. The patient should be instructed to stop pushing, although it must be recognized that most likely, the gravida will continue to involuntarily exert endogenous expulsive forces because uterine contractions do not spontaneously abate once the head emerges from the vagina. Maternal expulsive efforts will need to be restarted after the fetal shoulders have been converted to the oblique diameter—that is, as a diagnostic step to prove that a maneuver has been successful—in order to complete the delivery (Fig. 17-27).

Whenever extraction (exogenous) forces are applied by the delivering clinician, the fetal head should be maintained in an axial position, and rotation of the head should be avoided. By following the natural curve of the maternal pelvis, axially derived traction does by definition have a downward component (Fig. 17-28). Axial traction is traction applied in alignment with

TABLE 17-4	MANEUVERS FOR THE ALLEVIATION OF SHOULDER DYSTOCIA

McRoberts maneuver
Suprapubic pressure
Rubin maneuver
Woods corkscrew maneuver
Extraction of the posterior arm
Gaskin maneuver
Zavanelli maneuver
Symphysiotomy

the fetal cervicothoracic spine. Traction applied in the plane of the fetal cervicothoracic spine is typically along a vector estimated to be 20 to 25 degrees below the horizontal plane when the woman in labor is in a lithotomy position.[88] Thus while axial traction is also downward, it is applied without lateral bending of the fetal neck (i.e., bending the neck toward the floor or the ceiling). Laterally derived traction should not be used as the sole maneuver to effect delivery in the absence of ancillary obstetric maneuvers. Among the four cases in which this occurred in the series by Leung and associates,[90] three (75%) brachial plexus injuries and one (25%) clavicular fracture were reported.

No randomized clinical trials have been undertaken to guide physicians as to the order of the maneuvers that are to be performed (Table 17-4). The most effective preventive measure is to be familiar with the normal mechanism of labor and to be prepared to deal with the potential for shoulder dystocia in any vaginal delivery. Attendants should refrain from applying fundal pressure as a maneuver for the alleviation of shoulder dystocia, because pushing on the fundus serves only to further impact the anterior shoulder behind the symphysis pubis. Fundal pressure can be used to assist with delivery of the fetal body, but only if the shoulder dystocia has already been alleviated.

The McRoberts maneuver is a simple, logical, and effective measure and is typically considered as the first-line treatment for shoulder dystocia. The McRoberts maneuver and suprapubic pressure are appropriate first-line techniques because they are noninvasive, easy to learn, and can be performed quickly. In a retrospective review, Gherman and colleagues[85] found that the McRoberts maneuver was the only step required in 42% of 236 cases. The McRoberts maneuver involves hyperflexion of the maternal legs onto the abdomen, which results in flattening of the lumbar spine and ventral rotation of the maternal pelvis and symphysis (Fig. 17-29). Care should be taken to avoid prolonged or overly aggressive application of the McRoberts maneuver because the fibrocartilaginous articular surfaces of the symphysis pubis and surrounding ligaments may be unduly stretched.[91]

It is reasonable to consider performing delivery of the posterior shoulder/arm as the next maneuver in this sequence (Fig. 17-30). The ultimate decision for this, however, should be based on provider experience and the clinical situation. Several techniques to deliver the posterior shoulder have been described, but the most widely used method is extraction of the posterior fetal arm. To approach the posterior arm, the delivering clinician's hand is placed in the vagina, and the humerus of the posterior fetal arm is traced from the shoulder to the elbow. Once the forearm is grasped, it is swept across the fetal chest, and the arm is pulled out of the vagina. If the forearm is not accessible, pressure can be placed on the antecubital fossa to flex the elbow. If this allows access to the forearm, delivery of the posterior arm is accomplished as described above. If the forearm

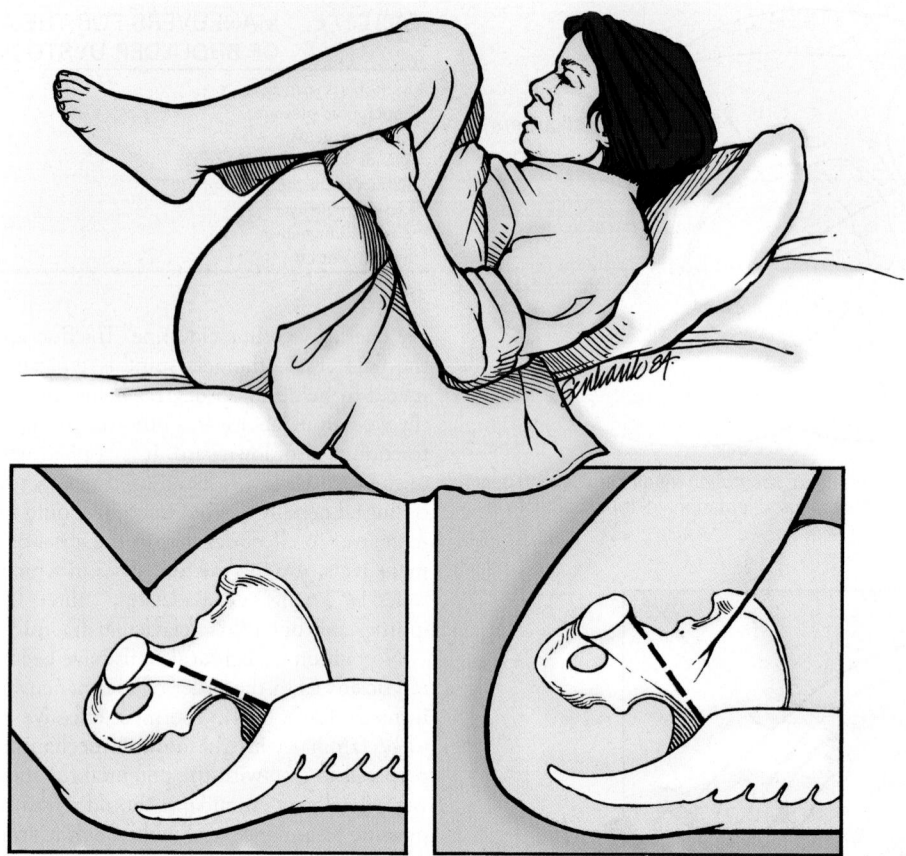

FIG 17-29 The least invasive maneuver to disimpact the shoulders is the McRoberts maneuver. Sharp ventral flexion of the maternal hips results in ventral rotation of the maternal pelvis and an increase in the useful size of the outlet.

is still not accessible, attempts are then made to deliver the posterior shoulder or to make the posterior arm accessible using posterior axillary traction methods. Menticoglou[92] described a technique of using the fingers to accomplish axillary traction. The technique starts by having an assistant hold the fetal head up, avoiding traction. Then, the operator's two middle fingers are positioned from each side of the posterior fetal shoulder and into the axilla. Downward and outward traction is then placed on the posterior shoulder to follow the curve of the sacrum. As the shoulder comes into view, the posterior arm is delivered as previously described. Another method of performing axillary traction is with the use of a sling. Hofmeyr and Cluver[93] described a technique of applying axillary traction using a sling fashioned from a 12- to 14-French suction catheter. In this technique, the suction catheter is passed over the shoulder and around the axilla. The two free ends of the catheter are clamped, and downward traction is used until the shoulder descends enough to allow for delivery of the posterior arm.

In the computer modeling evaluation of Grimm and colleagues,[87] **posterior arm delivery required the least exogenous force to effect delivery and resulted in the lowest brachial plexus stretch.** This decreases the impacted diameter from the bisacromial diameter to the axilloacromial diameter. The end point of posterior arm extraction is to substitute the axilloacromial diameter for the bisacromial diameter, with the former being approximately 3 cm shorter than the latter. Geometric analysis[94] has revealed that posterior arm delivery reduces shoulder dystocia more than twice as often relative to the McRoberts maneuver. Hoffman and associates[73] completed a cohort study

in which 2018 patients delivered with a shoulder dystocia had their records analyzed by trained abstractors for the maneuvers performed. **Delivery of the posterior shoulder was the most successful maneuver (84.4%) to alleviate shoulder dystocia, and the Woods maneuver (72%), Rubin maneuver (66%), and suprapubic pressure (62.2%) also showed high rates of delivery.** Multiple logistic regression analysis revealed a higher risk of neonatal injury with the Rubin (OR 1.54) and Woods (OR 2.22) maneuvers than with delivery of the posterior shoulder (OR 1.36). Leung and colleagues[90] found that among cases in which the McRoberts maneuver was unsuccessful, subsequent rotational methods and posterior arm delivery were similarly successful (72% vs. 63.6%) without a statistically significant increase in the rate of brachial plexus injury.

Suprapubic pressure is applied either directly downward onto the anterior presenting shoulder or by using a rocking motion from the fetal back toward the front. The aim of this maneuver is to decrease the bisacromial diameter by adducting the anterior shoulder and to deflect the bisacromial diameter to an oblique plane.

Rotational maneuvers routinely performed include the Rubin or Woods corkscrew maneuvers. The *Rubin maneuver* is performed by placing a hand into the vagina and applying pressure to the posterior aspect of the most accessible fetal shoulder (Fig. 17-31). The shoulder is then pushed toward the anterior surface of the fetal chest. The proposed mechanism of this maneuver is via adduction of the fetal shoulder, which reduces the bisacromial diameter and allows for the anterior shoulder to be rotated and dislodged from behind the pubic symphysis. The

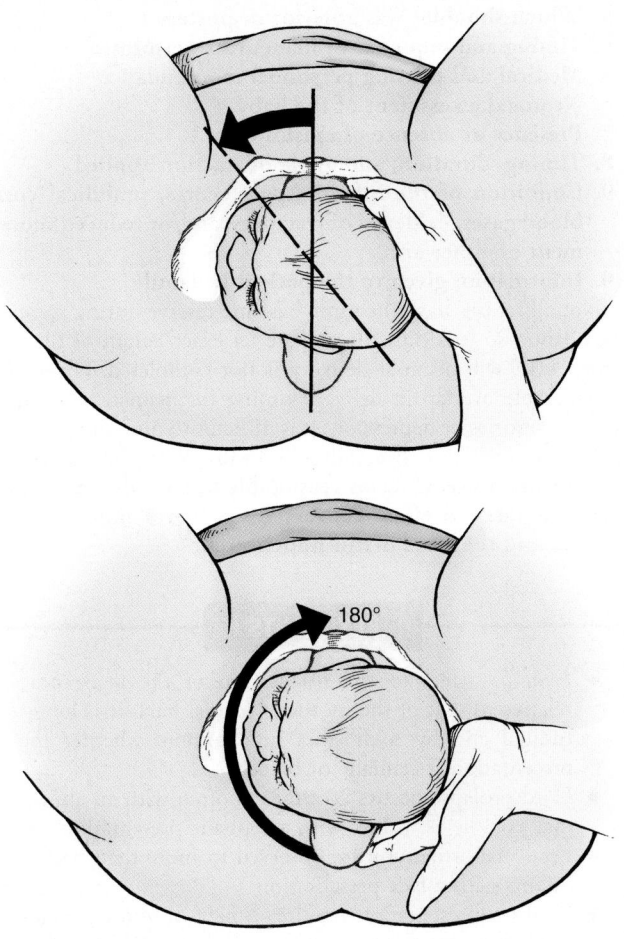

Alternative method

FIG 17-30 Rotation of the anterior shoulder forward through a small arc or of the posterior shoulder forward through a larger one will often lead to descent and delivery of the shoulders. Forward rotation is preferred, because it tends to compress and diminish the size of the shoulder girdle, whereas backward rotation would open the shoulder girdle and increase its size.

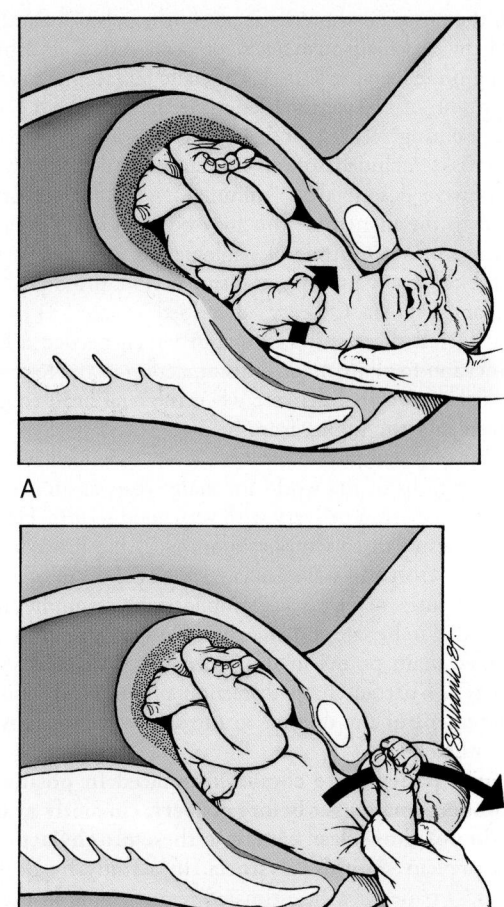

A

B

FIG 17-31 The operator here inserts a hand and sweeps the posterior arm across the chest and over the perineum. Care should be taken to distribute the pressure evenly across the humerus to avoid unnecessary fracture.

Woods corkscrew maneuver is performed by placing the fingers on the anterior aspect of the posterior fetal shoulder and rotating the shoulder toward the fetal back. The suggested mechanism for this maneuver relates to an attempt at rotation of the fetal torso in a 180-degree fashion to allow descent with rotation, much like the movement of a threaded screw when rotated.

Change of maternal position into an "all fours" position (*Gaskin maneuver*) may help to disimpact the fetal shoulder(s) to allow gravitational forces to push the posterior shoulder anteriorly. This maneuver has not been tested prospectively nor has it been compared with the traditional shoulder dystocia–relieving maneuvers, and it may be impractical for some patients. Fetal monitors and IV lines may hinder the patient's mobility, and neuraxial anesthesia with concomitant motor blockade may reduce strength, making this maneuver difficult. A series of 82 consecutive cases of shoulder dystocia managed with the all-fours maneuver showed no increased maternal or neonatal morbidity or mortality and only one case of humerus fracture, noted in a fetus whose weight exceeded 4500 g.[95]

The use of routine episiotomy in the management of all shoulder dystocia cases has been advocated in the past but with little scientific evidence in support of this practice. From a theoretic standpoint, it does not seem probable that an incision into the soft tissue of the vagina and perineum would be helpful in resolving an impaction of the bony structures of the fetal shoulders in the bony construct of the maternal pelvis. **The need for cutting a generous episiotomy must be based on clinical circumstances, such as a narrow vaginal fourchette in a nulliparous patient. Episiotomy can allow for greater access to the vagina for the performance of the internal manipulations necessary for the rotational maneuvers or for delivery of the posterior shoulder.**[96]

Two techniques rarely used in the United States for the management of shoulder dystocia are vaginal replacement of the fetal head with subsequent cesarean delivery (Zavanelli maneuver) and subcutaneous symphysiotomy. These should be considered as heroic, last resort maneuvers to be performed after consideration of potentially significant maternal and fetal risks. **In the Zavanelli maneuver, the fetal head is rotated back to a direct occiput anterior position and then subsequently flexed. Constant, firm pressure is used to push the head back into the vagina.** Tocolytic agents or uterine-relaxing general anesthesia may be administered during the maneuver and in preparation for cesarean delivery. Use of the Zavanelli maneuver may be considered when impaction of the fetal shoulder on the sacral promontory has occurred, for bilateral shoulder dystocia, or when the posterior shoulder is not in the pelvis.[97] Sandberg[98] reviewed the Zavanelli maneuver for both vertex- and breech-presenting undeliverable fetuses. Cephalic replacement was successful in 84 of 92 vertex-presenting fetuses; in 11 of 11 breech-presenting fetuses, podalic replacement was successful. Maternal risks included soft tissue trauma and sepsis, but the fetal risks were described as "minimal," with no fetal injuries attributed to the maneuver; this may be misleading because of the presence of a multitude of etiologies for permanent injury or death, likely from attempts at disimpaction, prolonged delivery time, and hypoxia. O'Leary[99] described 35 cases, 31 of which were considered successful and one of which needed a hysterotomy incision to allow manual disimpaction of the fetal shoulders to facilitate vaginal delivery when the fetal head could not be replaced into the vagina from below.

Subcutaneous symphysiotomy has been practiced in underdeveloped regions of the world for many years as an expedient alternative to cesarean delivery with very good results. However, in a case series of three symphysiotomies,[100] the procedure was used as a last resort and was associated with the death of all three neonates because of hypoxic complications. Symphysiotomy was concluded to be safe and effective as long as attention is paid to the three main points in the procedure: 1) lateral support of the legs, 2) partial sharp dissection of the symphysis, and 3) displacement of the urethra to the side with an indwelling urinary catheter.

Although patients are commonly placed in position for the McRoberts maneuver before delivery, currently available studies do not show clear benefit to these prophylactic measures to prevent shoulder dystocia. In a study by Beall and colleagues,[101] patients with estimated fetal weights in excess of 3800 g were randomized to undergo a prophylactic McRoberts maneuver and suprapubic pressure before delivery of the fetal head or to undergo maneuvers only after delivery of the head, if necessary. No differences were reported between the two groups in the average head-to-body time, the proportion of patients with head-to-body time greater than 60 seconds, and the proportion of identified shoulder dystocias. Patients in the prophylactic group had a significant increase in the risk of cesarean delivery (31/90 [34%] vs. 11/95 [12%], $P < .001$). In a study by Poggi and associates,[102] multiparous patients were randomized to delivery in the lithotomy position or were positioned for the McRoberts maneuver after the fetal head was delivered. The peak force for delivery of the anterior shoulder, the peak force rate, and head-to-body delivery interval were not statistically different between the two groups. Similar numbers of clinical shoulder dystocias (one per group) were encountered in each study group.

Shoulder dystocia should be viewed as an obstetric emergency because of the short period of time required to relieve the obstruction prior to the onset of hypoxic brain injury. **Contemporaneous documentation of the management of shoulder dystocia is recommended to record significant facts, findings, and observations about the shoulder dystocia event and its sequelae. Although no standard has been defined as to what exactly should be documented, a useful guideline is the ACOG Patient Safety Checklist (e-Fig. 17-1).[103] Many electronic health records also allow easy documentation of the following suggested items:**

1. **Type of delivery; if instrumented, document station and indication**
2. **Time interval between delivery of the fetal head and body**
3. **Which shoulder was anterior or posterior**
4. **Timing and sequence of maneuvers performed**
5. **Medical and nursing personnel in attendance**
6. **Neonatal assessment of the baby**
7. **Presence or absence of episiotomy**
8. **Timing, duration, and angle of traction applied**
9. **Condition of the infant: Apgar scores, umbilical cord blood gases, evidence of fractures, and/or reduced movement of either arm**
10. **Information given to the patient or family**

Not all fetuses have the same baseline reserve during second-stage labor, so it is difficult to state an exact length of time in which HIE will occur if delivery is not completed. Given the considerable overlap in delivery timing for neonates with and without injuries or depression, it is difficult to pinpoint an exact time within which delivery should ideally occur. **Based on the current literature, it seems reasonable to consider extraordinary measures to effect delivery once 4 to 5 minutes have elapsed and the fetus is still undelivered.[70]**

KEY POINTS

- *Fetal lie* refers to the orientation of the fetal spine relative to that of the mother. Normal fetal lie is longitudinal and by itself does not connote whether the presentation is cephalic or breech.
- Cord prolapse occurs 20 times as often with an abnormal axial lie as it does with a cephalic presentation.
- Fetal malformations are observed in more than half of infants with a face presentation.
- Fetal malpresentation requires timely diagnostic exclusion of major fetal or uterine malformations and/or abnormal placentation.
- A closely monitored labor and vaginal delivery is a safe possibility with face or brow malpresentations. However, cesarean delivery is the only acceptable alternative if normal progress toward spontaneous vaginal delivery is not observed.
- External cephalic version of the infant in breech presentation near term is a safe and often successful management option. Use of tocolytics and epidural anesthesia may improve success.
- Appropriate training and experience is a prerequisite to the safe vaginal delivery of selected infants in breech presentation.
- In experienced hands, women with twins presenting vertex/nonvertex can undergo a trial of labor because this management has similar maternal and perinatal outcomes to a planned cesarean delivery.
- A simple compound presentation may be permitted a trial of labor as long as labor progresses normally with reassuring fetal status. However, compression or reduction of the fetal part may result in injury.

REFERENCES

1. Thorp JM Jr, Jenkins T, Watson W. Utility of Leopold maneuvers in screening for malpresentation. *Obstet Gynecol.* 1991;78:394-396.
2. Sharma JB. Evaluation of Sharma's modified Leopold's maneuvers: a new method for fetal palpation in late pregnancy. *Arch Gynecol Obstet.* 2009; 279:481-487.

3. Phelan JP, Boucher M, Mueller E, McCart D, Horenstein J, Clark SL. The nonlaboring transverse lie. A management dilemma. *J Reprod Med.* 1986;31:184-186.

4. Zhang J, Bowes WA Jr, Fortney JA. Efficacy of external cephalic version: a review. *Obstet Gynecol.* 1993;82:306-312.

5. Benedetti TJ, Lowensohn RI, Truscott AM. Face presentation at term. *Obstet Gynecol.* 1980;55:199-202.

6. Duff P. Diagnosis and management of face presentation. *Obstet Gynecol.* 1981;57:105-112.

7. Schwartz Z, Dgani R, Lancet M, Kessler I. Face presentation. *Aust N Z J Obstet Gynaecol.* 1986;26:172-176.

8. Levy DL. Persistent brow presentation: a new approach to management. *Southern Med J.* 1976;69:191-192.

9. Ingolfsson A. Brow presentations. *Acta Obstet Gynecol Scand.* 1969;48:486-496.

10. Collea JV. Current management of breech presentation. *Clin Obstet Gynecol.* 1980;23:525-531.

11. Lubusky M, Prochazka M, Langova M, Vomackova K, Cizek L. Discrepancy in ultrasound biometric parameters of the head (HC–head circumference, BPD–biparietal diameter) in breech presented fetuses. *Biomed Pap Med Fac Univ Palacky Olomouc Czech Repub.* 2007;151:323-326.

12. Kasby CB, Poll V. The breech head and its ultrasound significance. *Br J Obstet Gynaecol.* 1982;89:106-110.

13. Collea JV, Chein C, Quilligan EJ. The randomized management of term frank breech presentation: a study of 208 cases. *Am J Obstet Gynecol.* 1980;137:235-244.

14. Brown L, Karrison T, Cibils LA. Mode of delivery and perinatal results in breech presentation. *Am J Obstet Gynecol.* 1994;171:28-34.

15. Gimovsky ML, Wallace RL, Schifrin BS, Paul RH. Randomized management of the nonfrank breech presentation at term: a preliminary report. *Am J Obstet Gynecol.* 1983;146:34-40.

16. Hannah ME, Hannah WJ, Hewson SA, Hodnett ED, Saigal S, Willan AR. Planned caesarean section versus planned vaginal birth for breech presentation at term: a randomised multicentre trial. Term Breech Trial Collaborative Group. *Lancet.* 2000;356:1375-1383.

17. Zatuchni GI, Andros GJ. Prognostic index for vaginal delivery in breech presentation at term. *Am J Obstet Gynecol.* 1965;93:237-242.

18. Bird CC, McElin TW. A six-year prospective study of term breech deliveries utilizing the Zatuchni-Andros Prognostic Scoring Index. *Am J Obstet Gynecol.* 1975;121:551-558.

19. Albrechtsen S, Rasmussen S, Dalaker K, Irgens LM. Reproductive career after breech presentation: subsequent pregnancy rates, interpregnancy interval, and recurrence. *Obstet Gynecol.* 1998;92:345-350.

20. Westgren M, Ingemarsson I, Svenningsen NW. Long-term follow up of pre-term infants in breech presentation delivered by caesarean section. *Dan Med Bull.* 1979;26:141-142.

21. Green JE, McLean F, Smith LP, Usher R. Has an increased cesarean section rate for term breech delivery reduced in incidence of birth asphyxia, trauma, and death? *Am J Obstet Gynecol.* 1982;142:643-648.

22. Faber-Nijholt R, Huisjes HJ, Touwen BC, Fidler VJ. Neurological follow-up of 281 children born in breech presentation: a controlled study. *Br Med J (Clin Res Ed).* 1983;286:9-12.

23. Andersen GL, Irgens LM, Skranes J, Salvesen KA, Meberg A, Vik T. Is breech presentation a risk factor for cerebral palsy? A Norwegian birth cohort study. *Dev Med Child Neurol.* 2009;51:860-865.

24. Deering S, Brown J, Hodor J, Satin AJ. Simulation training and resident performance of singleton vaginal breech delivery. *Obstet Gynecol.* 2006;107:86-89.

25. Diro M, Puangsricharern A, Royer L, O'Sullivan MJ, Burkett G. Singleton term breech deliveries in nulliparous and multiparous women: a 5-year experience at the University of Miami/Jackson Memorial Hospital. *Am J Obstet Gynecol.* 1999;181:247-252.

26. Roman J, Bakos O, Cnattingius S. Pregnancy outcomes by mode of delivery among term breech births: Swedish experience 1987-1993. *Obstet Gynecol.* 1998;92:945-950.

27. Irion O, Hirsbrunner Almagbaly P, Morabia A. Planned vaginal delivery versus elective caesarean section: a study of 705 singleton term breech presentations. *Br J Obstet Gynaecol.* 1998;105:710-717.

28. Su M, McLeod L, Ross S, et al. Factors associated with adverse perinatal outcome in the Term Breech Trial. *Am J Obstet Gynecol.* 2003;189:740-745.

29. Hannah ME, Hannah WJ, Hodnett ED, et al. Outcomes at 3 months after planned cesarean vs planned vaginal delivery for breech presentation at term: the international randomized Term Breech Trial. *JAMA.* 2002;287:1822-1831.

30. Hannah ME, Whyte H, Hannah WJ, et al. Maternal outcomes at 2 years after planned cesarean section versus planned vaginal birth for breech presentation at term: the international randomized Term Breech Trial. *Am J Obstet Gynecol.* 2004;191:917-927.

31. Whyte H, Hannah ME, Saigal S, et al. Outcomes of children at 2 years after planned cesarean birth versus planned vaginal birth for breech presentation at term: the International Randomized Term Breech Trial. *Am J Obstet Gynecol.* 2004;191:864-871.

32. Hogle KL, Kilburn L, Hewson S, Gafni A, Wall R, Hannah ME. Impact of the international term breech trial on clinical practice and concerns: a survey of centre collaborators. *J Obstet Gynaecol Can.* 2003;25:14-16.

33. Rietberg CC, Elferink-Stinkens PM, Visser GH. The effect of the Term Breech Trial on medical intervention behaviour and neonatal outcome in The Netherlands: an analysis of 35,453 term breech infants. *BJOG.* 2005;112:205-209.

34. Barber EL, Lundsberg LS, Belanger K, Pettker CM, Funai EF, Illuzzi JL. Indications contributing to the increasing cesarean delivery rate. *Obstet Gynecol.* 2011;118:29-38.

35. Lee HC, El-Sayed YY, Gould JB. Population trends in cesarean delivery for breech presentation in the United States, 1997-2003. *Am J Obstet Gynecol.* 2008;199:59.e1-59.e8.

36. Croughan-Minihane MS, Petitti DB, Gordis L, Golditch I. Morbidity among breech infants according to method of delivery. *Obstet Gynecol.* 1990;75:821-825.

37. Caughey AB, Cahill AG, Guise JM, Rouse DJ. Safe prevention of the primary cesarean delivery. *Am J Obstet Gynecol.* 2014;210:179-193.

38. Lawson GW. The term breech trial ten years on: primum non nocere? *Birth.* 2012;39:3-9.

39. Goffinet F, Carayol M, Foidart JM, et al. Is planned vaginal delivery for breech presentation at term still an option? Results of an observational prospective survey in France and Belgium. *Am J Obstet Gynecol.* 2006;194:1002-1011.

40. Ulstein M. Breech delivery. *Ann Chir Gynaecol.* 1980;69:70-74.

41. Demirci O, Tugrul AS, Turgut A, Ceylan S, Eren S. Pregnancy outcomes by mode of delivery among breech births. *Arch Gynecol Obstet.* 2012;285:297-303.

42. Wolf H, Schaap AH, Bruinse HW, Smolders-de Haas H, van Ertbruggen I, Treffers PE. Vaginal delivery compared with caesarean section in early preterm breech delivery: a comparison of long term outcome. *Br J Obstet Gynaecol.* 1999;106:486-491.

43. Duenhoelter JH, Wells CE, Reisch JS, Santos-Ramos R, Jimenez JM. A paired controlled study of vaginal and abdominal delivery of the low birth weight breech fetus. *Obstet Gynecol.* 1979;54:310-313.

44. Kayem G, Baumann R, Goffinet F, et al. Early preterm breech delivery: is a policy of planned vaginal delivery associated with increased risk of neonatal death? *Am J Obstet Gynecol.* 2008;198:289.e1-289.e6.

45. Baud O, Ville Y, Zupan V, et al. Are neonatal brain lesions due to intrauterine infection related to mode of delivery? *Br J Obstet Gynaecol.* 1998;105:121-124.

46. Gocke SE, Nageotte MP, Garite T, Towers CV, Dorcester W. Management of the nonvertex second twin: primary cesarean section, external version, or primary breech extraction. *Am J Obstet Gynecol.* 1989;161:111-114.

47. Laros RK Jr, Dattel BJ. Management of twin pregnancy: the vaginal route is still safe. *Am J Obstet Gynecol.* 1988;158:1330-1338.

48. Fishman A, Grubb DK, Kovacs BW. Vaginal delivery of the nonvertex second twin. *Am J Obstet Gynecol.* 1993;168:861-864.

49. Jonsdottir F, Henriksen L, Secher NJ, Maaloe N. Does internal podalic version of the non-vertex second twin still have a place in obstetrics? A Danish national retrospective cohort study. *Acta Obstet Gynecol Scand.* 2015;94:59-64.

50. Barrett JF, Hannah ME, Hutton EK, et al. A randomized trial of planned cesarean or vaginal delivery for twin pregnancy. *New Engl J Med.* 2013;369:1295-1305.

51. Tchabo JG, Tomai T. Selected intrapartum external cephalic version of the second twin. *Obstet Gynecol.* 1992;79:421-423.

52. Druzin ML. Atraumatic delivery in cases of malpresentation of the very low birth weight fetus at cesarean section: the splint technique. *Am J Obstet Gynecol.* 1986;154:941-942.

53. Van Dorsten JP, Schifrin BS, Wallace RL. Randomized control trial of external cephalic version with tocolysis in late pregnancy. *Am J Obstet Gynecol.* 1981;141:417-424.

54. Hutton EK, Hannah ME, Ross SJ, et al. The Early External Cephalic Version (ECV) 2 Trial: an international multicentre randomised controlled trial of timing of ECV for breech pregnancies. *BJOG.* 2011;118:564-577.

55. Vezina Y, Bujold E, Varin J, Marquette GP, Boucher M. Cesarean delivery after successful external cephalic version of breech presentation at term: a comparative study. *Am J Obstet Gynecol.* 2004;190:763-768.

56. Burgos J, Melchor JC, Pijoan JI, Cobos P, Fernandez-Llebrez L, Martinez-Astorquiza T. A prospective study of the factors associated with the success rate of external cephalic version for breech presentation at term. *Int J Gynaecol Obstet.* 2011;112:48-51.

57. Tasnim N, Mahmud G, Khurshid M. External cephalic version with salbutamol - success rate and predictors of success. *J Coll Physicians Surg Pak.* 2009;19:91-94.

58. Ben-Meir A, Erez Y, Sela HY, Shveiky D, Tsafrir A, Ezra Y. Prognostic parameters for successful external cephalic version. *J Matern Fetal Neonatal Med.* 2008;21:660-662.

59. Fernandez CO, Bloom SL, Smulian JC, Ananth CV, Wendel GD Jr. A randomized placebo-controlled evaluation of terbutaline for external cephalic version. *Obstet Gynecol.* 1997;90:775-779.

60. Schorr SJ, Speights SE, Ross EL, et al. A randomized trial of epidural anesthesia to improve external cephalic version success. *Am J Obstet Gynecol.* 1997;177:1133-1137.

61. Weiniger CF, Ginosar Y, Elchalal U, Sharon E, Nokrian M, Ezra Y. External cephalic version for breech presentation with or without spinal analgesia in nulliparous women at term: a randomized controlled trial. *Obstet Gynecol.* 2007;110:1343-1350.

62. Sullivan JT, Grobman WA, Bauchat JR, et al. A randomized controlled trial of the effect of combined spinal-epidural analgesia on the success of external cephalic version for breech presentation. *Int J Obstet Anesth.* 2009;18:328-334.

63. Hofmeyr GJ, Kulier R. External cephalic version for breech presentation at term. *Cochrane Database Syst Rev.* 2012;(10):CD000083.

64. Marcus RG, Crewe-Brown H, Krawitz S, Katz J. Feto-maternal haemorrhage following successful and unsuccessful attempts at external cephalic version. *Br J Obstet Gynaecol.* 1975;82:578-580.

65. Flamm BL, Fried MW, Lonky NM, Giles WS. External cephalic version after previous cesarean section. *Am J Obstet Gynecol.* 1991;165:370-372.

66. Schachter M, Kogan S, Blickstein I. External cephalic version after previous cesarean section–a clinical dilemma. *Int J Gynaecol Obstet.* 1994;45:17-20.

67. Sela HY, Fiegenberg T, Ben-Meir A, Elchalal U, Ezra Y. Safety and efficacy of external cephalic version for women with a previous cesarean delivery. *Eur J Obstet Gynecol Reprod Biol.* 2009;142:111-114.

68. Collins S, Ellaway P, Harrington D, Pandit M, Impey LW. The complications of external cephalic version: results from 805 consecutive attempts. *BJOG.* 2007;114:636-638.

69. Coyle ME, Smith CA, Peat B. Cephalic version by moxibustion for breech presentation. *Cochrane Database Syst Rev.* 2012;(5):CD003928.

70. Gherman RB, Chauhan S, Ouzounian JG, Lerner H, Gonik B, Goodwin TM. Shoulder dystocia: the unpreventable obstetric emergency with empiric management guidelines. *Am J Obstet Gynecol.* 2006;195:657-672.

71. Spong CY, Beall M, Rodrigues D, Ross MG. An objective definition of shoulder dystocia: prolonged head-to-body delivery intervals and/or the use of ancillary obstetric maneuvers. *Obstet Gynecol.* 1995;86:433-436.

72. Beall MH, Spong C, McKay J, Ross MG. Objective definition of shoulder dystocia: a prospective evaluation. *Am J Obstet Gynecol.* 1998;179:934-937.

73. Hoffman MK, Bailit JL, Branch DW, et al. A comparison of obstetric maneuvers for the acute management of shoulder dystocia. *Obstet Gynecol.* 2011;117:1272-1278.

74. Nesbitt TS, Gilbert WM, Herrchen B. Shoulder dystocia and associated risk factors with macrosomic infants born in California. *Am J Obstet Gynecol.* 1998;179:476-480.

75. Ouzounian JG, Gherman RB. Shoulder dystocia: are historic risk factors reliable predictors? *Am J Obstet Gynecol.* 2005;192:1933-1935, discussion 1935-1938.

76. Bingham J, Chauhan SP, Hayes E, Gherman R, Lewis D. Recurrent shoulder dystocia: a review. *Obstet Gynecol Survey.* 2010;65:183-188.

77. Gherman RB, Chauhan SP, Lewis DF. A survey of central association members about the definition, management, and complications of shoulder dystocia. *Obstet Gynecol.* 2012;119:830-837.

78. American College of Obstetricians and Gynecologists. *Fetal macrosomia. Practice Bulletin 22.* Washington, DC: ACOG; 2000.

79. Chauhan SP, Parker D, Shields D, Sanderson M, Cole JH, Scardo JA. Sonographic estimate of birth weight among high-risk patients: feasibility and factors influencing accuracy. *Am J Obstet Gynecol.* 2006;195:601-606.

80. Rouse DJ, Owen J, Goldenberg RL, Cliver SP. The effectiveness and costs of elective cesarean delivery for fetal macrosomia diagnosed by ultrasound. *JAMA.* 1996;276:1480-1486.

81. Herbst MA. Treatment of suspected fetal macrosomia: a cost-effectiveness analysis. *Am J Obstet Gynecol.* 2005;193:1035-1039.

82. Cohen B, Penning S, Major C, Ansley D, Porto M, Garite T. Sonographic prediction of shoulder dystocia in infants of diabetic mothers. *Obstet Gynecol.* 1996;88:10-13.

83. Rajan PV, Chung JH, Porto M, Wing DA. Correlation of increased fetal asymmetry with shoulder dystocia in the nondiabetic woman with suspected macrosomia. *J Reprod Med.* 2009;54:478-482.

84. Miller RS, Devine PC, Johnson EB. Sonographic fetal asymmetry predicts shoulder dystocia. *J Ultrasound Med.* 2007;26:1523-1528.

85. Gherman RB, Goodwin TM, Souter I, Neumann K, Ouzounian JG, Paul RH. The McRoberts' maneuver for the alleviation of shoulder dystocia: how successful is it? *Am J Obstet Gynecol.* 1997;176:656-661.

86. Gherman RB, Ouzounian JG, Goodwin TM. Obstetric maneuvers for shoulder dystocia and associated fetal morbidity. *Am J Obstet Gynecol.* 1998;178:1126-1130.

87. Grimm MJ, Costello RE, Gonik B. Effect of clinician-applied maneuvers on brachial plexus stretch during a shoulder dystocia event: investigation using a computer simulation model. *Am J Obstet Gynecol.* 2010;203:339.e1-339.e5.

88. Executive summary: Neonatal brachial plexus palsy. Report of the American College of Obstetricians and Gynecologists' Task Force on Neonatal Brachial Plexus Palsy. *Obstet Gynecol.* 2014;123:902-904.

89. Gherman RB, Ouzounian JG, Miller DA, Kwok L, Goodwin TM. Spontaneous vaginal delivery: a risk factor for Erb's palsy? *Am J Obstet Gynecol.* 1998;178:423-427.

90. Leung TY, Stuart O, Suen SS, Sahota DS, Lau TK, Lao TT. Comparison of perinatal outcomes of shoulder dystocia alleviated by different type and sequence of manoeuvres: a retrospective review. *BJOG.* 2011;118:985-990.

91. Gherman RB, Ouzounian JG, Incerpi MH, Goodwin TM. Symphyseal separation and transient femoral neuropathy associated with the McRoberts' maneuver. *Am J Obstet Gynecol.* 1998;178:609-610.

92. Menticoglou SM. A modified technique to deliver the posterior arm in severe shoulder dystocia. *Obstet Gynecol.* 2006;108:755-757.

93. Hofmeyr GJ, Cluver CA. Posterior axilla sling traction for intractable shoulder dystocia. *BJOG.* 2009;116:1818-1820.

94. Poggi SH, Spong CY, Allen RH. Prioritizing posterior arm delivery during severe shoulder dystocia. *Obstet Gynecol.* 2003;101:1068-1072.

95. Bruner JP, Drummond SB, Meenan AL, Gaskin IM. All-fours maneuver for reducing shoulder dystocia during labor. *J Reprod Med.* 1998;43:439-443.

96. Gurewitsch ED, Donithan M, Stallings SP, et al. Episiotomy versus fetal manipulation in managing severe shoulder dystocia: a comparison of outcomes. *Am J Obstet Gynecol.* 2004;191:911-916.

97. Gherman RB, Ouzounian JG, Chauhan S. Posterior arm shoulder dystocia alleviated by the Zavanelli maneuver. *Am J Perinatol.* 2010;27:749-751.

98. Sandberg EC. The Zavanelli maneuver: 12 years of recorded experience. *Obstet Gynecol.* 1999;93:312-317.

99. O'Leary JA. Cephalic replacement for shoulder dystocia: present status and future role of the Zavanelli maneuver. *Obstet Gynecol.* 1993;82:847-850.

100. Goodwin TM, Banks E, Millar LK, Phelan JP. Catastrophic shoulder dystocia and emergency symphysiotomy. *Am J Obstet Gynecol.* 1997;177:463-464.

101. Beall MH, Spong CY, Ross MG. A randomized controlled trial of prophylactic maneuvers to reduce head-to-body delivery time in patients at risk for shoulder dystocia. *Obstet Gynecol.* 2003;102:31-35.

102. Poggi SH, Allen RH, Patel CR, Ghidini A, Pezzullo JC, Spong CY. Randomized trial of McRoberts versus lithotomy positioning to decrease the force that is applied to the fetus during delivery. *Am J Obstet Gynecol.* 2004;191:874-878.

103. Shoulder dystocia. ACOG Practice Bulletin No. 40. American College of Obstetricians and Gynecologists. *Obstet Gynecol.* 2002;100:1045-1050.

Additional references for this chapter are available at ExpertConsult.com.

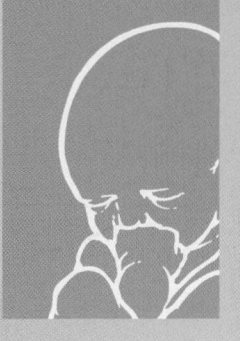

CHAPTER 18

Antepartum and Postpartum Hemorrhage

KARRIE E. FRANCOIS and MICHAEL R. FOLEY

KEY ABBREVIATIONS

Bilevel positive airway pressure	BiPAP
Continuous positive airway pressure	CPAP
Fresh frozen plasma	FFP
Packed red blood cells	pRBCs

Obstetric hemorrhage is one of the leading causes of maternal morbidity and mortality throughout the world. Hemorrhage following delivery is the leading reason for an obstetric admission to the intensive care unit (ICU), and it is responsible for one third of all pregnancy-related deaths in both high- and low-income countries.[1] Therefore it is critical for the obstetrician to have a thorough understanding of the hemodynamic changes that accompany pregnancy, the maternal adaptations that occur with excessive blood loss, and the management principles for obstetric hemorrhage.

PREGNANCY-RELATED HEMODYNAMIC CHANGES

Pregnancy is associated with five significant hemodynamic changes (see Chapter 3). The first of these changes is plasma volume expansion. The average singleton pregnancy is accompanied by a 40% to 50% increase in plasma volume by the thirtieth week of gestation. This increase in plasma volume occurs along with the second change, an increase in red blood cell (RBC) mass. With appropriate substrate availability, RBC mass can be expected to increase 20% to 30% by the end of pregnancy. Third, maternal cardiac output rises with normal pregnancy owing to both increased stroke volume and increased heart rate. According to consensus, the average rise in cardiac output is 30% to 50% above nonpregnant levels, and the peak occurs in the early third trimester. Fourth, systemic vascular resistance falls in parallel with this rise in cardiac output and blood volume expansion. Fifth, fibrinogen and the majority of

procoagulant blood factors (II, VII, VIII, IX, and X) increase during pregnancy. These five changes are protective of maternal hemodynamic status and thus allow for certain physiologic adaptations that accompany obstetric hemorrhage.

PHYSIOLOGIC ADAPTATION TO HEMORRHAGE

During pregnancy and the puerperium, a defined sequence of physiologic adaptations occurs with hemorrhage (Fig. 18-1). When 10% of the circulatory blood volume is lost, vasoconstriction occurs in both the arterial and venous compartments in order to maintain blood pressure and to preserve blood flow to essential organs. As blood loss reaches 20% or more of the total blood volume, increases in systemic vascular resistance can no longer compensate for the lost intravascular volume, and blood pressure decreases with a commensurate rise in heart rate. Cardiac output falls in parallel because of a loss in preload that results in poor end-organ perfusion. If the intravascular volume is not appropriately replaced, shock will ensue.

In severe preeclampsia (PE), these physiologic adaptations are altered. Unlike in most pregnant women, the protective mechanism of blood volume expansion is diminished with severe PE. It is estimated that plasma volume expansion is 9% lower in the setting of PE. In addition, because of the significant vasoconstriction that accompanies PE, blood loss in these patients may be underestimated because blood pressure is often maintained in the normotensive range. Finally, oliguria may not be as reliable an indicator of poor end-organ perfusion secondary to hemorrhage because reduced urine output is often a manifestation of the severity of PE.

CLASSIFICATION OF HEMORRHAGE

A standard classification for acute blood loss is illustrated in Table 18-1. Understanding the physiologic responses that accompany varying degrees of volume deficit can assist the clinician when caring for hemorrhaging patients.

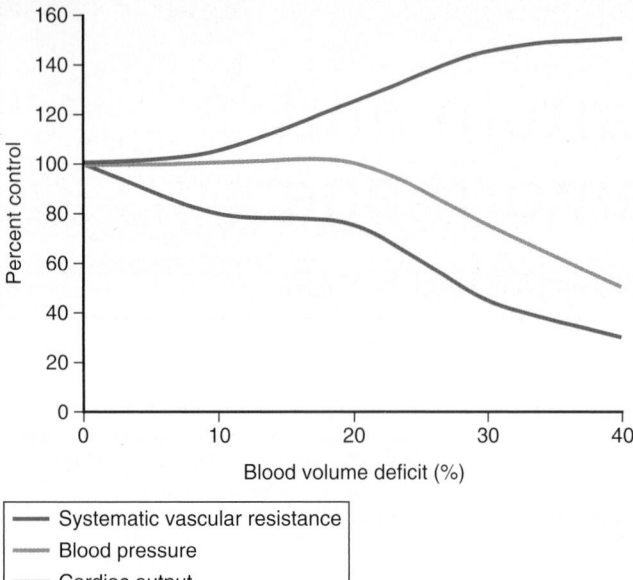

FIG 18-1 Relationships among systemic vascular resistance, blood pressure, and cardiac output in the face of progressive blood volume deficit.

TABLE 18-1	HEMORRHAGE CLASSIFICATION AND PHYSIOLOGIC RESPONSE		
CLASS	ACUTE BLOOD LOSS (mL)	% LOST	PHYSIOLOGIC RESPONSE
1	1000	15	Dizziness, palpitations, minimal blood pressure change
2	1500	20-25	Tachycardia, tachypnea, sweating, weakness, narrowed pulse pressure
3	2000	30-35	Significant tachycardia and tachypnea, restlessness, pallor, cool extremities
4	≥2500	40	Shock, air hunger, oliguria or anuria

Modified from Baker RJ. Evaluation and management of critically ill patients. *Obstet Gynecol Annu.* 1977;6:295; and Bonnar J. Massive obstetric haemorrhage. *Baillieres Best Pract Res Clin Obstet Gynaecol.* 2000;14:1.

Determination of the hemorrhage class reflects the volume deficit, which may not be the same as the volume loss. **The average 70-kg pregnant woman maintains a blood volume of 6000 mL by 30 weeks of gestation (85 mL/kg).**

Class 1 hemorrhage **corresponds to approximately 1000 mL of blood loss.** This blood loss correlates to a **15% volume deficit.** Women with this amount of volume deficit exhibit mild physiologic changes such as dizziness and palpitations owing to the hemodynamic adaptations that accompany normal pregnancy.

Class 2 hemorrhage **is characterized by 1500 mL of blood loss, or a 20% to 25% volume deficit.** Early physical changes that occur during a hemorrhage of this class include **tachycardia and tachypnea.** Although tachycardia is usually recognized as a compensatory mechanism to increase cardiac output, the significance of tachypnea is unclear and is often unappreciated clinically. Tachypnea can represent a sign of impending clinical decompensation. **Narrowing of the pulse pressure** is another

sign of a class 2 hemorrhage. The pulse pressure represents the difference between the systolic and diastolic blood pressures. Systolic blood pressure is a good representation of stroke volume and β_1 stimulation. Diastolic blood pressure is a reflection of systemic vasoconstriction; therefore the pulse pressure represents the interrelationship between these entities. With a class 2 volume deficit, the sympathoadrenal system is activated, which results in a diversion of blood away from nonvital organs (skin, muscle, and kidney) and a redistribution of the circulation to vital body organs, including the brain and heart. The end result is increased vasoconstriction, increased diastolic blood pressure, maintenance of systolic blood pressure, and a narrowing of the pulse pressure. With greater narrowing of the pulse pressure, more compensatory vasoconstriction occurs to accommodate for a loss in stroke volume. A final physiologic response of class 2 hemorrhage is **orthostatic hypotension.** Although blood pressure comparisons can be made in the supine, sitting, and standing positions to document this response, a practical approach is to assess the time needed to refill a blanched hypothenar area on the patient's hand. Typically, a patient with normal volume status can reperfuse this area within 1 to 2 seconds after pressure is applied. A patient with a class 2 hemorrhage and orthostatic hypotension will have significant reperfusion delay.

Class 3 hemorrhage **is defined as a blood loss of 2000 mL and corresponds to a volume deficit of 30% to 35%.** Within this hemorrhage class, the physiologic responses noted in class 2 hemorrhage are exaggerated. Patients demonstrate significant **tachycardia** (120 to 160 beats/min), **tachypnea** (30 to 50 breaths/min), **overt hypotension, restlessness, pallor, and cool extremities.**

Class 4 hemorrhage **is characterized by more than 2500 mL of blood loss.** This amount of blood loss exceeds **40% of the patient's total blood volume.** The clinical manifestations of this volume deficit include **absent distal pulses, shock, air hunger, and oliguria or anuria.** When significant hemorrhage occurs, renal blood flow is reduced and is redirected from the outer renal cortex to the juxtamedullary region. In this region, increased water and sodium absorption occur and result in decreased urine volume, lower urinary sodium concentration, and increased urine osmolarity. A urine sodium concentration less than 10 to 20 mEq/L or a urine/serum osmolar ratio greater than 2 indicates significantly reduced renal perfusion in the face of hemorrhage.

ANTEPARTUM HEMORRHAGE
Placental Abruption
Definition and Pathogenesis

Placental abruption, or *abruptio placentae,* **refers to the premature separation of a normally implanted placenta from the uterus prior to delivery of the fetus.** The diagnosis is typically reserved for pregnancies at greater than 20 weeks of gestation. Abruption is characterized by defective maternal vessels in the decidua basalis, which rupture and cause the separation. On rare occasions, the separation may be caused by a disruption of the fetal-placental vessels. These damaged vessels cause bleeding, which results in a decidual hematoma that may promote placental separation, destruction of placental tissue, and a loss of maternal-fetal surface area for nutrient and gas exchange.

Whereas some placental abruptions may occur acutely after a sudden mechanical event (e.g., blunt trauma, sudden uterine decompression, or motor vehicle accident), most

cases result from more chronic processes.[2] Abnormal development of the spiral arteries can lead to decidual necrosis, inflammation, infarction, and bleeding due to vascular disruption.[3-6] Thrombin, which is released in response to decidual hemorrhage or hypoxia, appears to play an active role in the pathogenesis of placental abruption. Thrombin acts as a direct uterotonic, enhances the action of matrix metalloproteinases, upregulates apoptosis genes, increases the expression of inflammatory cytokines, triggers the coagulation cascade, and initiates functional progesterone withdrawal.[7-9] These thrombin-mediated events initiate a cyclic pathway of vascular disruption, hemorrhage, inflammation, contractions, and rupture of membranes.[5]

Incidence

The overall incidence of placental abruption is approximately 1 in 100 births; however, a range of 1 in 80 to 1 in 250 deliveries has been reported.[10,11] The range in incidence likely reflects variable criteria for diagnosis as well as an increased recognition in recent years of milder forms of abruption. About one third of all antepartum bleeding can be attributed to placental abruption, which peaks in the third trimester; 40% to 60% of abruptions occur prior to 37 weeks of gestation.[10]

Clinical Manifestations

Several factors determine the clinical manifestations of placental abruption. These factors include (1) the temporal nature of the abruption (acute vs. chronic), (2) clinical presentation (overt vs. concealed), and (3) severity. An acute, overt abruption typically presents with vaginal bleeding, abdominal pain, and uterine contractions. As the placental separation worsens, uterine tenderness, tachysystole, fetal heart rate (FHR) patterns consistent with hypoxia, and fetal death may occur. The amount of vaginal bleeding correlates poorly with the extent of placental separation and its potential for fetal compromise. In fact, concealed abruption occurs in 10% to 20% of cases.[12] With severe abruptions, more than 50% of the placental surface area separates. With extensive abruption, a significant risk for fetal death exists, and maternal compromise in the form of consumptive coagulopathy may result from the triggering of the clotting cascade by hemorrhage and extensive thrombin deposition.

Chronic abruption may be insidious in its presentation and is often associated with ischemic placental disease.[13] Typically, these cases present with intermittent, light vaginal bleeding and evidence of chronic placental inflammation and dysfunction, such as oligohydramnios, fetal growth restriction, preterm labor, premature preterm rupture of membranes (PPROM), and PE.

Risk Factors

Although the exact etiology of placental abruption is unclear, a variety of risk factors have been identified (Box 18-1).

INCREASING PARITY AND MATERNAL AGE

Several studies have noted a higher incidence of placental abruption with increasing parity. Among primigravid women, the frequency of placental abruption is less than 1%; however, 2.5% of grand multiparas experience placental abruption. Theories suggest that damaged endometrium, impaired decidualization, and aberrant vasculature may have causal roles with increasing parity or age.

Maternal age is often cited as an associated risk factor for placental abruption. Although a 15-year population-based

---

BOX 18-1   RISK FACTORS FOR PLACENTAL ABRUPTION

Increasing parity and maternal age
Maternal substance use
- Cigarette smoking
- Cocaine abuse
Trauma
Maternal diseases
- Hypertension
- Hypothyroidism
- Asthma
Preterm premature rupture of membranes
Rapid uterine decompression associated with multiple gestation and polyhydramnios
Uterine and placental factors
- Anomalies
- Synechiae
- Fibroids
- Cesarean scar
- Abnormal placental formation
- Chronic ischemia
Prior abruption
Hyperhomocysteinemia

---

study in Norway was able to demonstrate a strong relationship between maternal age and placental abruption for all levels of parity, others studies suggest that there is no increased risk for placental abruption among older women when parity and hypertensive disease are excluded.

MATERNAL SUBSTANCE ABUSE

Cigarette smoking is associated with a significantly increased incidence of placental abruption and fetal death. There appears to be a dose-response relationship with the number of cigarettes smoked and the risks for placental abruption and fetal loss. Compared with nonsmokers, smokers have a 40% increased risk for fetal death from placental abruption with each pack of cigarettes smoked. In addition, smoking and hypertensive disease appear to have an additive effect on the likelihood of placental abruption. Proposed etiologies include placental hypoperfusion with resulting decidual ischemia and necrosis.

Cocaine abuse in the third trimester has been associated with as high as a 10% placental abruption rate. The pathogenesis appears to be related to cocaine-induced vasospasm with subsequent decidual ischemia, reflex vasodilation, and vascular disruption within the placental bed.

TRAUMA

Blunt or penetrating trauma to the gravid abdomen has been associated with placental abruption. After a minor trauma, the risk for placental abruption is between 7% and 9%, whereas the risk may be as high as 13% after severe injury.[14] The two most common causes of maternal trauma are motor vehicle crashes and domestic abuse. With motor vehicle crashes, uterine stretch, direct penetration, and placental shearing from acceleration-deceleration forces are the primary etiologies of trauma-related placental abruption (see Chapter 26).

MATERNAL DISEASES

Maternal hypertension has been the most consistently identified risk factor for placental abruption.[13] This relationship has been observed with both chronic and pregnancy-related hypertensive disease. Compared with normotensive women, hypertensive women have a fivefold increased risk for placental abruption. Unfortunately, antihypertensive therapy has not been shown to reduce the risk for placental abruption in women with chronic hypertension.

Maternal subclinical hypothyroidism and asthma have also been associated with placental abruption in some studies.[15,16]

PRETERM PREMATURE RUPTURE OF MEMBRANES

Placental abruption occurs in 2% to 5% of pregnancies with PPROM. Intrauterine infection and oligohydramnios significantly increase the risk for placental abruption, and nonreassuring FHR patterns occur in nearly half of these pregnancies.

It is unclear whether placental abruption is the cause or consequence of PPROM. Hemorrhage and associated thrombin generation may stimulate cytokine and protease production, which results in membrane rupture. Alternatively, the cytokine-protease cascade that follows ruptured membranes may cause damage to the decidual vasculature, which predisposes the placenta to separation.

RAPID UTERINE DECOMPRESSION ASSOCIATED WITH MULTIPLE GESTATIONS AND POLYHYDRAMNIOS

Rapid decompression of an overdistended uterus can precipitate an acute placental abruption. This may occur in the setting of multiple gestations or with polyhydramnios. Compared with singletons, twins have been reported to have nearly a threefold increased risk for placental abruption. Although the exact timing of placental abruption in multiple gestations is difficult to ascertain, it has been attributed to rapid decompression of the uterus after the delivery of the first twin. Likewise, rapid loss of amniotic fluid in pregnancies complicated by polyhydramnios has been implicated in placental abruption. This can occur with spontaneous rupture of membranes or may follow therapeutic amniocentesis. For this reason, controlled artificial rupture of membranes with induction of labor may be advisable if significant polyhdramnios complicates pregnancy.

UTERINE AND PLACENTAL FACTORS

Suboptimal placental implantation in patients with uterine anomalies, synechiae, fibroids, and cesarean scars is associated with abruption.[17] In addition, abnormal placental formation (e.g., circumvallate placenta) or chronic ischemia associated with PE and fetal growth restriction have been implicated in placental abruption.[18]

PRIOR ABRUPTION

Women who have had a previous abruption are at significant risk for recurrent abruption. **After one abruption, the recurrence risk is 5% to 15%, whereas the risk increases to 20% to 25% after two abruptions.**[19] **The risk of recurrence is greater after a severe abruption. When an abruption is associated with fetal demise, there is a 7% incidence of the same outcome in a future gestation.**

THROMBOPHILIA

Inconsistent data exist regarding an association among thrombophilias and placental abruptions.[20,21] Hyperhomocysteinemia (a fasting homocysteine level >15 μmol/L) may be associated with recurrent abruption.

Diagnosis

Placental abruption is primarily a clinical diagnosis that is supported by radiographic, laboratory, and pathologic studies. Any findings of vaginal bleeding, uterine contractions, abdominal and/or back pain, or trauma should prompt an investigation for potential placental abruption. Vaginal bleeding may range from mild to severe. Unfortunately, bleeding may be underestimated because it can be retained behind the placenta. The typical abruption contraction pattern is high frequency and low amplitude; however, it may simulate labor in some circumstances.

RADIOLOGY

Although early studies that evaluated the use of **ultrasound** for the diagnosis of placental abruption identified less than 2% of cases, recent advances in imaging and its interpretation have improved detection rates. Early hemorrhage is typically hyperechoic or isoechoic, whereas resolving hematomas are hypoechoic within 1 week and sonolucent within 2 weeks of the abruption. Acute hemorrhage may be misinterpreted as a homogeneous thickened placenta or fibroid.

Ultrasound can identify **three predominant locations for placental abruption.** These are **subchorionic** (between the placenta and the membranes), **retroplacental** (between the placenta and the myometrium), and **preplacental** (between the placenta and the amniotic fluid). Figure 18-2 illustrates the classification of hematomas in relation to the placenta. Figure 18-3 demonstrates a sonographic representation of a subchorionic abruption.

The location and extent of the placental abruption identified on ultrasound examination is of clinical significance. **Retroplacental hematomas are associated with a worse prognosis for fetal survival than subchorionic hemorrhage.** The size of the hemorrhage is also predictive of fetal survival. Large retroplacental hemorrhages (>60 mL) have been associated with a 50% or greater fetal mortality, whereas similarly sized subchorionic hemorrhages are associated with a 10% mortality risk.[22]

Magnetic resonance imaging (MRI) has been used occasionally for the diagnosis of placental abruption when sonography is equivocal.[23,24]

LABORATORY FINDINGS

Few laboratory studies assist in the diagnosis of placental abruption. **Hypofibrinogenemia and evidence of consumptive coagulopathy may accompany severe abruption**; however, clinical correlation is necessary. Moreover, most abruptions are not accompanied by maternal coagulopathy.

Abnormal serum markers early in pregnancy, such as an unexplained elevated maternal serum α-fetoprotein (MSAFP) or human chorionic gonadotropin (hCG) and decreased pregnancy-associated plasma protein A (PAPP-A) or estriol, have been associated with an increased risk for subsequent placental abruption.[18,25]

PATHOLOGIC STUDIES

Macroscopic inspection of the placenta may demonstrate adherent clot and depression of the placental surface. Fresh or acute placental abruptions may not have any identifiable evidence on gross pathologic examination, but histologic analysis may show preservation of the villous stroma, eosinophilic degeneration of the syncytiotrophoblast, and scattered neutrophils with villous agglutination.[5] Chronic abruptions may demonstrate histologic signs of chronic deciduitis, maternal floor decidual necrosis, villitis, decidual vasculopathy, infarction,

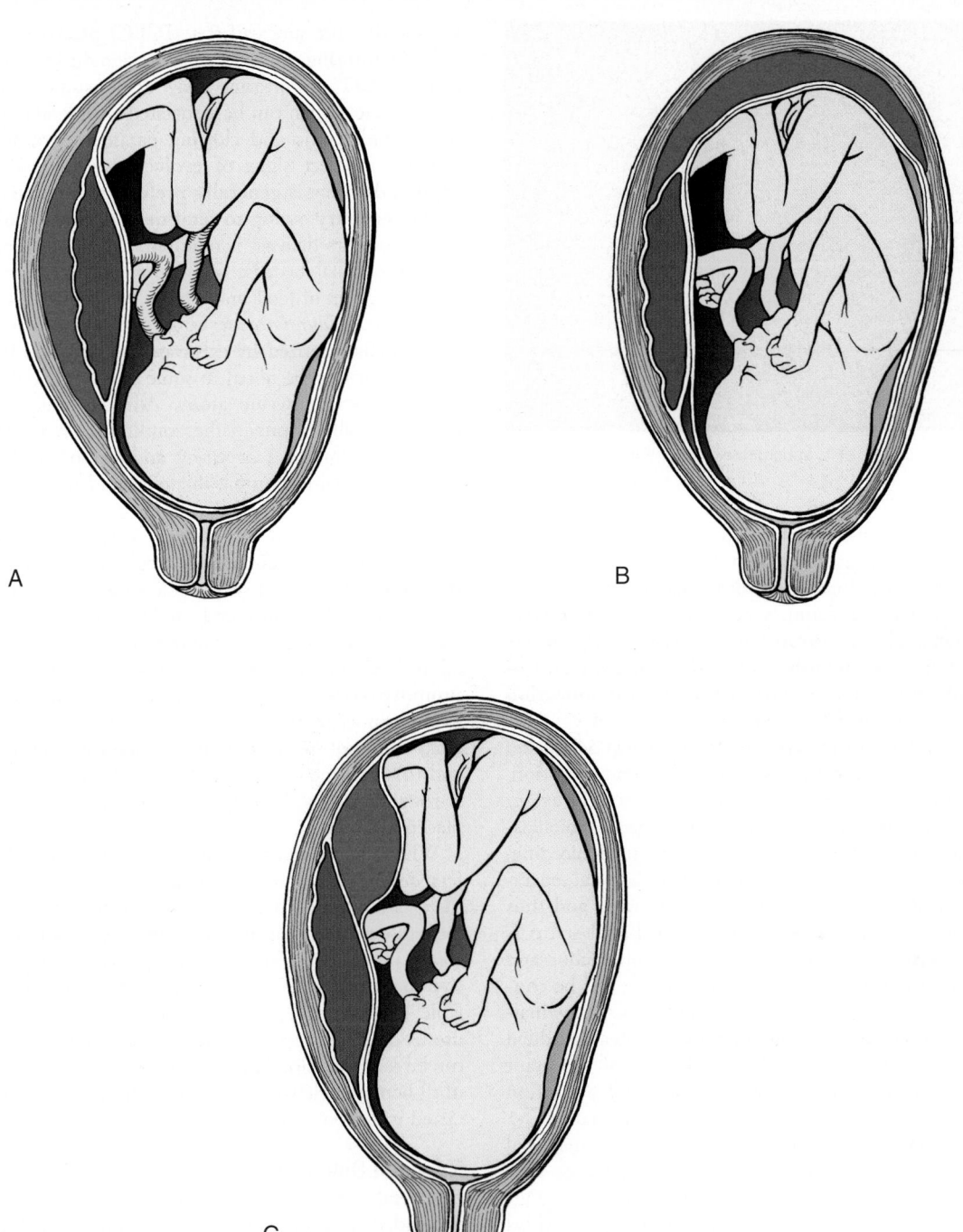

FIG 18-2 The classification system of placental abruption. **A,** Retroplacental abruption. The bright red area represents a blood collection behind the placenta (*dark red*). **B,** Subchorionic abruption. The bright red area represents subchorionic bleeding, which is observed to dissect along the chorion. **C,** Preplacental abruption. The bright red area represents a blood collection anterior to the placenta within the amnion and chorion (subamniotic). (From Trop I, Levine D. Hemorrhage during pregnancy: sonography and MR imaging. *AJR Am J Roentgenol.* 2001;176:607.)

intervillous thrombosis, villous maldevelopment, and hemosiderin deposition.[9]

Management

Both maternal and fetal complications may occur with placental abruption. Maternal complications include blood loss, consumptive coagulopathy, need for transfusion, endorgan damage, cesarean delivery, and death. Fetal complications include intrauterine growth restriction (IUGR), **oligohydramnios, prematurity, hypoxemia, and stillbirth.** Although maternal complications are related to the severity of the abruption, fetal complications are related to both the severity and timing of the hemorrhage.[12]

Despite its relative frequency, no randomized trials and few studies have examined management approaches for placental abruption.[26] **Typically, management of placental abruption depends on the severity, gestational age, and maternal-fetal status.** Once the diagnosis of placental abruption has been

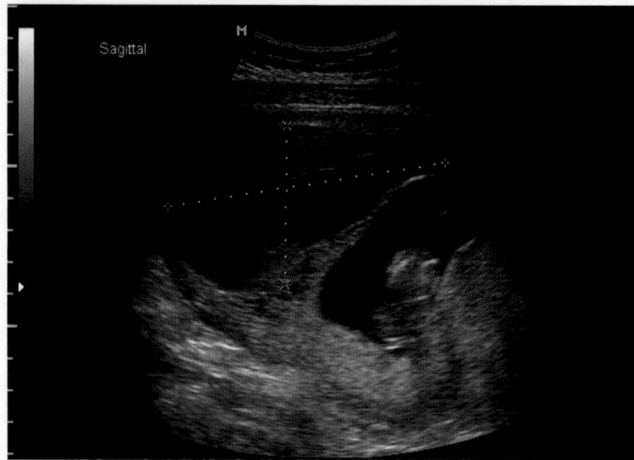

FIG 18-3 Ultrasonic image of a subchorionic abruption. (Courtesy K. Francois.)

made, precautions should be taken to anticipate the possible life-threatening consequences for both mother and fetus. These precautions include baseline **laboratory assessment** (hemoglobin, hematocrit, platelet count, type and screen, fibrinogen, and coagulation studies), **appropriate intravenous (IV) access** (large-bore catheter), **availability of blood products, continuous FHR and contraction monitoring, and communication with operating room (OR) and neonatal personnel.**

Small placental abruptions remote from term (<34 weeks) may be managed expectantly. With cases of chronic abruption, clinical circumstances that include gestational age and the extent of the abruption influence the need for prolonged hospitalization until delivery. In many cases, a cyclic event of bleeding, thrombin generation, contractions, and further placental separation occurs. Tocolysis may help prevent contractions and thus may break the abruption cycle. If the maternal-fetal status is stable, a trial of tocolysis for documented preterm labor and administration of antenatal corticosteroid therapy can be considered. Whereas the choice of tocolysis should be individualized, magnesium sulfate administration may confer an added benefit of fetal neuroprotection. Reported series of expectant management in preterm gestations with placental abruption have shown a significant prolongation of the pregnancy (>1 week) in more than 50% of patients without adverse maternal or fetal outcomes. In a large series of preterm patients who presented with placental abruption and received tocolysis, about one third delivered within 48 hours of admission, one third delivered within 7 days, and one third delivered more than 1 week from initial presentation. No cases of intrauterine demise were reported in women who presented with a live fetus. Although these results are encouraging, the clinician must always keep in mind that placental abruption can result in both maternal and fetal morbidity. Any attempt to arrest preterm labor in a known or suspected placental abruption must be weighed against the likelihood of neonatal survival and morbidity, the severity of the abruption, and the safety of the mother.

Women who present at or near term with a placental abruption should undergo delivery. Induction or augmentation of labor is not contraindicated in the setting of an abruption; however, close surveillance for any evidence of maternal or fetal compromise is advised. Continuous FHR monitoring is recommended because 60% of fetuses may exhibit intrapartum heart rate patterns consistent with hypoxia.

Intrauterine pressure catheter (IUPC) placement and internal FHR monitoring can assist the clinician during the intrapartum course. IUPC monitoring may demonstrate elevated uterine resting tone, which can be associated with fetal hypoxia. Maternal hemodynamic and clotting parameters must be followed closely to detect signs of evolving coagulopathy. **Although vaginal delivery is generally preferable, operative delivery is often necessary owing to fetal or maternal decompensation.** When cesarean delivery is required, a rapid decision-to-delivery time is optimal because an interval of less than 20 minutes from the onset of fetal bradycardia is associated with improved outcomes. A *Couvelaire uterus,* also known as *uteroplacental apoplexy,* is characterized by extravasation of blood into the myometrium; it may be noted in some cases and is often associated with significant uterine atony. Administration of uterotonic therapy usually improves the condition. Hysterectomy should be reserved for cases of atony and hemorrhage unresponsive to conventional uterotonic therapies and replacement of blood products.

The management of women with consumptive coagulopathy and fetal demise requires a thorough knowledge of the natural history of severe placental abruption. Nearly five decades ago, Pritchard and Brekken noted several clinically important observations: (1) about 40% of patients with placental abruption and fetal demise will demonstrate signs of consumptive coagulopathy; (2) within 8 hours of initial symptoms, hypofibrinogenemia will be present; (3) severe hypofibrinogenemia will not recover without blood product replacement; and (4) the time course for recovery from hypofibrinogenemia is roughly 10 mg/dL per hour after delivery of the fetus and placenta.

When managing women with severe placental abruptions and fetal demise, maintenance of maternal volume status and replacement of blood products is essential. Although operative delivery may appear to lead to the most rapid resolution of the problem, it may pose significant risks to the patient. Unless the consumptive coagulopathy is corrected, surgery can result in uncontrollable bleeding and an increased need for hysterectomy. The uterus does not need to be evacuated before coagulation status can be restored. Blood product replacement and delayed delivery until hematologic parameters have improved are generally associated with good maternal outcomes.

Neonatal Outcome

Placental abruption is associated with increased perinatal morbidity and mortality. When compared with normal pregnancies, pregnancies complicated by abruption have a **tenfold increased risk for perinatal death.** A case-control study has also shown a **greater risk for adverse long-term neurobehavioral outcomes** in infants delivered after placental abruption. Neonates at risk for abnormal outcomes had higher incidences of abnormal FHR tracings (45%) and emergency cesarean deliveries (53%) compared with controls (10% and 10%, respectively). **Finally, hypoxia-associated periventricular leukomalacia and sudden infant death syndrome (SIDS) are more common in newborns delivered after placental abruptions.**

Placenta Previa
Definition and Pathogenesis

Placenta previa **is defined as the presence of placental tissue over or adjacent to the cervical os.** Traditionally, four variations of placenta previa were recognized: 1) complete, 2) partial,

3) marginal, and 4) low lying.[27] Although *complete placenta previa* has been the term used to refer to the total coverage of the internal cervical os by placental tissue, the differences among the terms *partial* (placental edge partially covering the internal cervical os), *marginal* (placental edge at the margin of the internal cervical os), and *low lying* (placental edge within 2 cm of the interval cervical os) were often subtle and varied by the timing and method of diagnosis. Improved ultrasound technology and precision have allowed for more accurate assessments of the placental location in relation to the cervical os. **Recent revised classification of placenta previa consists of two variations: true *placenta previa,* in which the internal cervical os is covered by placental tissue, and *low-lying placenta,* in which the placenta lies within 2 cm of the cervical os but does not cover it.**[27] Although not a true placenta previa, low-lying placentas are associated with increased risks for bleeding and other adverse pregnancy events.[28]

Incidence

The overall reported incidence of placenta previa at delivery is 1 in 200 births. In the second trimester, placenta previa may occur in up to 6% of pregnancies.[29] The term *placental migration* **has been used to explain this "resolution" of placenta previa that is noted near term. Three theories have been suggested to account for this phenomenon.** The first hypothesis proposes that as the pregnancy advances, the stationary lower placental edge relocates away from the cervical os with the development of the lower uterine segment. Indeed, the lower uterine segment has been noted to increase from 0.5 cm at 20 weeks to more than 5 cm at term. Secondly, the placenta-free uterine wall has been proposed to grow at a faster rate than the uterine wall covered by the placenta. A final hypothesis suggests that *trophotropism,* the growth of trophoblastic tissue away from the cervical os toward the fundus, results in resolution of the placenta previa.[30]

Clinical Manifestations

Placenta previa typically presents as painless vaginal bleeding in the second or third trimester. The bleeding is believed to occur from disruption of placental blood vessels in association with the development and thinning out of the lower uterine segment. **Between 70% and 80% of patients with placenta previa will have at least one bleeding episode.** About 10% to 20% of patients present with uterine contractions before bleeding, and fewer than 10% remain asymptomatic until term. Of those with bleeding, **one third of women will present before 30 weeks of gestation, one third between 30 and 36 weeks, and one third after 36 weeks.** Early-onset bleeding (<30 weeks) carries with it the greatest risk for blood transfusion and associated perinatal morbidity and mortality.

Risk Factors

Several risk factors for placenta previa have been noted (Box 18-2). Additionally, some reports have documented a higher association of fetal malpresentation, preterm labor, PPROM, IUGR, congenital anomalies, and amniotic fluid embolism with placenta previa.[31]

INTRINSIC MATERNAL FACTORS

Studies have reported **more cases of placenta previa with increasing parity.** Grand multiparas have been reported to have a 5% risk for placenta previa compared with 0.2% among

---

BOX 18-2   RISK FACTORS FOR PLACENTA PREVIA

Intrinsic maternal factors
- Increasing parity
- Advanced maternal age
- Maternal race

Extrinsic maternal factors
- Cigarette smoking
- Cocaine use
- Residence at higher elevation
- Infertility treatments

Fetal factors
- Multiple gestations
- Male fetus

Prior placenta previa
Prior uterine surgery and cesarean delivery

---

nulliparous women. **Maternal age also seems to influence the occurrence of placenta previa.** Women older than 35 years of age have more than a fourfold increased risk for placenta previa, and women older than 40 years of age have a ninefold greater risk. Finally, **maternal race has been associated with placenta previa.** In a large population-based cohort,[32] the rate of placenta previa among white, black, and other races was 3.3, 3, and 4.5 per 1000 births, respectively. Asian women appear to have the highest rates of placenta previa.

EXTRINSIC MATERNAL FACTORS

Cigarette smoking has been associated with as high as a threefold increased risk for previa formation. Likewise, a case-control study has demonstrated that **maternal cocaine use increases the risk of placenta previa fourfold.** Residence at higher elevations may also contribute to previa development. The need for increased placental surface area secondary to decreased uteroplacental oxygenation may play a role in this association. Finally, prior **infertility treatment is statistically associated with higher rates of placenta previa.**[33]

FETAL FACTORS

Controversy exists regarding an increased risk for placenta previa with multiple gestations. Although some studies have shown a higher incidence of placenta previa among twins, others have not documented a significantly increased risk.[34] A consistently **higher proportion of offspring in women with placenta previa are male.** This association is unexplained; however, two theories suggest larger placental sizes among male fetuses and delayed implantation of the male blastocyst in the lower uterine segment.

PRIOR PLACENTA PREVIA

Having had a prior placenta previa increases the risk for the development of another previa in a subsequent pregnancy. This association has been reported to be as high as an eightfold relative risk. The exact etiology for this increased risk is unclear.

PRIOR UTERINE SURGERY AND PRIOR CESAREAN DELIVERY

Prior uterine surgery has been associated with placenta previa formation. Although a history of curettage and/or myomectomy attends a slightly elevated previa risk, prior cesarean delivery has been the most consistent risk factor. **In the pregnancy following a cesarean delivery, the risk for placenta previa has been reported to range from 1% to 4%.**[35,36] A **linear increase is seen in placenta previa risk with the number**

of prior cesarean deliveries. Placenta previa occurs in 0.9% of women with one prior cesarean delivery, in 1.7% of women with two prior cesarean deliveries, and in 3% of those with three or more cesarean deliveries.[37] In patients with four or more cesarean deliveries, the risk for placenta previa has been reported to be as high as 10%.[35] Endometrial scarring is thought to be the etiologic factor for this increased risk.

Diagnosis

The timing of the diagnosis of placenta previa has undergone significant change in the past four decades. Painless third-trimester bleeding was a common presentation for placenta previa in the past, whereas **most cases of placenta previa are now detected antenatally with ultrasound** prior to the onset of significant bleeding.

RADIOLOGY

Transabdominal and transvaginal ultrasound provide the best means for diagnosing placenta previa. Although transabdominal ultrasound can detect at least 95% of placenta previa cases, transvaginal ultrasound has a reported diagnostic accuracy that approaches 100%. Typically, a combined approach can be used in which transabdominal ultrasound is the initial diagnostic modality, followed by transvaginal ultrasound for uncertain cases. Transvaginal ultrasound is safe and is not contraindicated in these circumstances. Of note, quality images can be obtained using transvaginal ultrasound without the probe contacting the cervix (Fig. 18-4).

If a placenta previa or low-lying placenta is diagnosed in the second trimester, repeat sonography should be obtained in the early third trimester at 32 weeks.[27] **More than 90% of the cases of placenta previa diagnosed in the second trimester resolve by term. The potential for placenta previa resolution is dependent on the timing of the diagnosis, extension over the cervical os, and placental location.** For example, one study of 714 women with an ultrasound diagnosis of placenta previa noted that the earlier the diagnosis, the more likely the previa would resolve by term (Table 18-2). In addition, complete placenta previa diagnosed in the second trimester will persist into the third trimester in 26% of cases, whereas a low-lying placenta will persist in only 2.5% of cases. Finally, anterior placenta previa is less likely to migrate away from the cervical os than posterior placement.

Occasionally, MRI may be used to diagnose placenta previa. MRI is particularly helpful with posterior placenta previa identification and assessment of invasive placentation (see below).

Management

General management principles for patients with placenta previa in the third trimester include serial ultrasounds to assess placental location and fetal growth, avoidance of cervical examinations and intercourse, activity restrictions, counseling regarding labor symptoms and vaginal bleeding, dietary and nutrient supplementation to avoid maternal anemia, and early medical attention if any vaginal bleeding occurs.

ASYMPTOMATIC PLACENTA PREVIA

A recent working group has given specific recommendations for management of asymptomatic placenta previa at varying gestational ages.[27] For pregnancies at greater than 16 weeks of gestation with a low-lying placenta (placental edge within 2 cm from

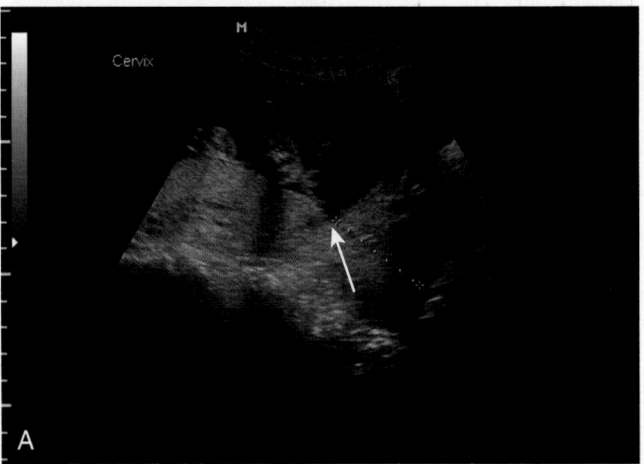

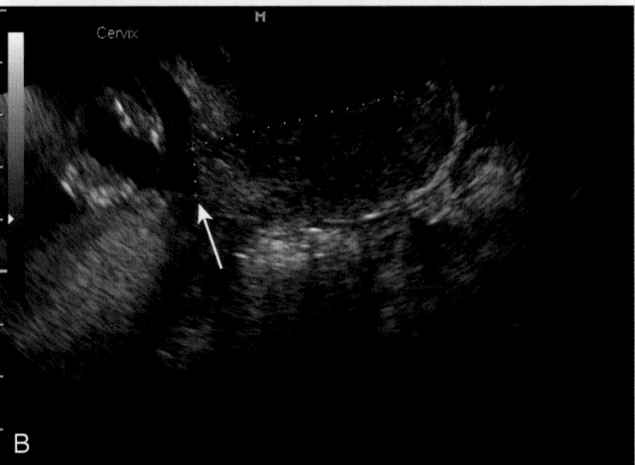

FIG 18-4 Transabdominal and transvaginal ultrasounds of low-lying placenta. Arrows identify the placental edge. (Courtesy K. Francois.)

TABLE 18-2	POTENTIAL FOR PLACENTA PREVIA AT TERM BY GESTATIONAL AGE AT DIAGNOSIS
GESTATIONAL AGE AT DIAGNOSIS (WK)	**PREVIA AT TERM (%)**
15-19	12
20-23	34
24-27	49
28-31	62
32-35	73

From Dashe JS, McIntire DD, Ramus RM, et al. Persistence of placenta previa according to gestational age at ultrasound detection. *Obstet Gynecol.* 2002;99:692.

the internal cervical os) or a placenta previa, repeat ultrasound to assess placental location is recommended at 32 weeks. If a low-lying placenta or placenta previa persists at 32 weeks, repeat sonography is again obtained at 36 weeks.

Asymptomatic women with placenta previa may be managed expectantly as outpatients. Although some sonographic features have been associated with a higher likelihood of bleeding—such as complete placental coverage of the cervical os, a thickened placental edge, echo-free placental space over the cervical os, and cervical length less than 3 cm—it is not possible to predict all cases of bleeding that result from placenta previa.[30] With this in mind, asymptomatic patients should be instructed to avoid activities that may stimulate uterine contractions and/or cervical irritation, such as strenuous exercise, intercourse, and digital cervical examinations. Several studies have documented the safety, efficacy, and cost savings of outpatient management for asymptomatic placenta previa. **Candidates for outpatient management must (1) be compliant, (2) live within a short commute from the hospital, (3) have 24-hour emergency transportation to the hospital, and (4) verbalize a thorough understanding of the risks associated with placenta previa.**

BLEEDING PLACENTA PREVIA

Women with placenta previa who present with acute vaginal bleeding require hospitalization and immediate evaluation to assess maternal-fetal stability. They should initially be managed in a labor and delivery unit with hemodynamic surveillance of the mother and continuous FHR monitoring. Large-bore IV access and baseline laboratory studies (hemoglobin, hematocrit, platelet count, blood type and screen, and coagulation studies) should be obtained. **If the pregnancy is less than 34 weeks of gestation, administration of antenatal corticosteroids should be undertaken** as well as an assessment of the facility's emergency resources for both the mother and the neonate. In some cases, maternal transport and consultation with a maternal-fetal medicine specialist and a neonatologist may be warranted. **Finally, tocolysis may be used if the vaginal bleeding is preceded by or associated with uterine contractions.** Whereas various agents have been used, magnesium sulfate is often preferred as a first-line agent because of its limited potential for hemodynamic-related maternal side effects and its added benefit for fetal neuroprotection.[30]

Once stabilized, most women with symptomatic placenta previa can be maintained on hospitalized bed rest and expectantly managed. In several observational studies, 50% of women with bleeding placenta previa were undelivered in 4 weeks, including those with initial bleeding episodes of more than 500 mL. Minimizing maternal anemia by using blood conservation techniques is recommended. Although some patients may require transfusion, many patients can be supplemented with iron replacement (oral or IV), vitamin C to enhance oral iron absorption, and B vitamins. Erythropoietin may be used in selected cases to hasten red cell formation. Lastly, autologous donation may be considered in patients with hemoglobin concentrations greater than 11 g/dL.[38,39]

Although maternal hemorrhage is of the utmost concern, **fetal blood can also be lost during the process of placental separation with a bleeding placenta previa. Rh0(D) immune globulin should be given to all Rh-negative unsensitized women with third-trimester bleeding from placenta previa.** A Kleihauer-Betke preparation of maternal blood should be considered. Occasionally, a fetomaternal hemorrhage of greater than 30 mL occurs that necessitates additional doses of Rh0(D) immune globulin. One study noted that 35% of infants whose mothers received an antepartum transfusion were also anemic and required a transfusion following delivery.

DELIVERY

Cesarean delivery is indicated for all women with sonographic evidence of placenta previa and most women with low-lying placenta. When the placental distance is between 1 and 20 mm from the internal cervical os, the rate of cesarean delivery ranges from 40% to 90%.[40] If a vaginal trial of labor is attempted for a low-lying placenta, precautions should be taken for the possibility of an emergent cesarean delivery and need for blood transfusion.

A consensus panel has given delivery-timing guidelines for uncomplicated placenta previa,[22] which includes cases with normal fetal growth and no other pregnancy-associated complications. **Cesarean delivery of asymptomatic placenta previa should occur between $36^{0/7}$ and $37^{0/7}$ weeks of gestation. In cases of complicated placenta previa, delivery should occur immediately regardless of gestational age. Complicated placenta previa includes bleeding associated with a nonreassuring fetal heart pattern despite resuscitative measures, life-threatening maternal hemorrhage, and/or refractory labor.**[30]

When performing a cesarean delivery for placenta previa, the surgeon should be aware of the potential for rapid blood loss during the delivery process. Blood products that are cross-matched should be readily available for delivery. In addition, before incising the lower uterine segment, the surgeon should assess the vascularity of this region. Although a low transverse incision is not contraindicated in patients with placenta previa, performing a vertical uterine incision may be preferable in some cases. This is particularly true with an anterior placenta previa. Ideally, the placenta should not be disrupted when entering the uterus. If disruption occurs, expedited delivery is essential. Given the potential for invasive placentation, the physician should allow the placenta to spontaneously deliver. If it does not separate easily, precautions should be taken for placenta accreta management (see below). Once the placenta separates, bleeding is controlled by the contraction of uterine myometrial fibers around the spiral arterioles. Because the lower uterine segment often contracts poorly, significant bleeding may occur from the placental implantation site. Aggressive uterotonic therapy, surgical intervention, and/or tamponade techniques should be undertaken to rapidly control bleeding. Finally, some studies have shown reduced bleeding at the placental site with the injection of subendometrial vasopressin after delivery of the fetus.[41]

Associated Conditions

Placenta Accreta

DEFINITION AND PATHOGENESIS

Placenta accreta represents the abnormal attachment of the placenta to the uterine lining due to an absence of the decidua basalis and an incomplete development of the fibrinoid layer. Variations of placenta accreta include placenta increta and placenta percreta, in which the placenta extends to or through the uterine myometrium, respectively (Fig. 18-5).

INCIDENCE AND RISK FACTORS

The overall incidence of placenta accreta or one of its variations is 3 per 1000 deliveries. Based on histologic diagnosis, placenta accreta is the most common form of invasive placentation (79%) followed by placenta increta (14%) and placenta percreta (7%), respectively. **The two most significant risk factors for placenta accreta are placenta previa and prior cesarean delivery.** The risk for placenta accreta in patients with placenta previa and an unscarred uterus is approximately 3%.[35] This risk dramatically increases with one or more cesarean deliveries (Table 18-3). Even without a coexisting placenta previa, placenta accreta is more common in women with a prior cesarean delivery.[37]

Other reported risk factors include increasing parity and maternal age, submucosal uterine fibroids, prior uterine surgery, cesarean scar, and endometrial defects.[42,43] Unlike

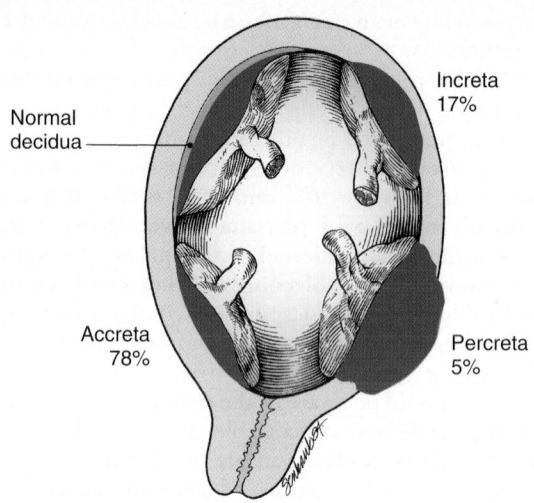

FIG 18-5 Uteroplacental relationships found with invasive placentation.

TABLE 18-3	RISK OF PLACENTA ACCRETA WITH PLACENTA PREVIA AND PRIOR CESAREAN DELIVERY

NO. OF PRIOR CESAREAN DELIVERIES	PLACENTA ACCRETA RISK (%)
0	3
1	11
2	40
3	61
≥4	67

From Silver RM, Landon MB, Rouse DJ, et al. Maternal morbidity associated with multiple repeat cesarean deliveries. *Obstet Gynecol.* 2006;107:1226.

placenta previa, a **female fetus is more common with invasive placentation.**

CLINICAL MANIFESTATIONS

The clinical manifestations of placenta accreta are often similar to those of placenta previa; however, **profuse bleeding usually follows attempted manual placental separation. Hematuria can be a feature of placenta percreta with bladder invasion.**

DIAGNOSIS

Most cases of placenta accreta are now diagnosed antenatally by advanced radiographic techniques. Prenatal diagnosis has been shown to improve maternal outcomes, resulting in less blood loss and decreased transfusion requirements.[44]

RADIOGRAPHIC TECHNIQUES

Ultrasound is the preferred radiographic modality for the diagnosis of placenta accreta. Findings suggestive of placenta accreta include a loss of the normal hypoechoic retroplacental-myometrial zone, thinning and disruption of the uterine serosa–bladder wall interface, focal exophytic masses within the placenta, and numerous intraplacental vascular lacunae (Fig. 18-6).[45] A recent systemic review and meta-analysis of 23 studies that used prenatal sonographic identification of placenta accreta demonstrated a sensitivity of 90%, a specificity of 97%, a positive likelihood ratio of 11, and a negative likelihood ratio of 0.16.[46]

Color Doppler ultrasound is also useful as an adjunctive tool in diagnosing placenta accreta. Specific color Doppler findings that differentiate placenta accreta from normal placentation

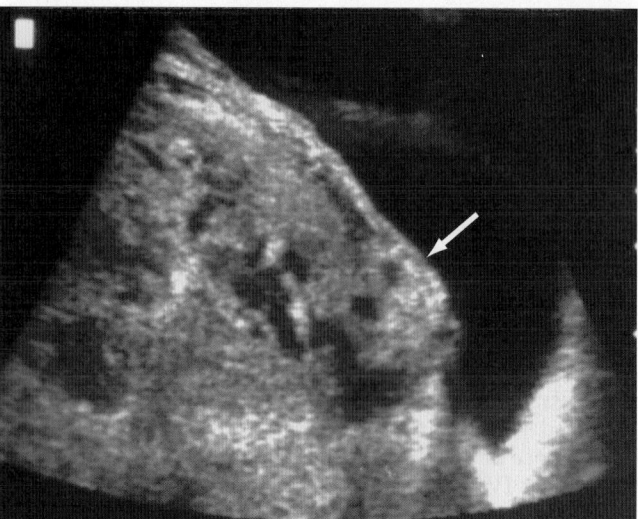

FIG 18-6 Ultrasonic image of focal placenta accreta (*arrow*). An area at the uterine-placental interface demonstrates loss of the normal hypoechoic zone, thinning and disruption of the uterine serosa–bladder interface, and a focal exophytic mass within the placenta.

include diffuse and focal intraparenchymal placental lacunar blood flow, hypervascularity of the bladder and uterine serosa, prominent subplacental venous complexes, and loss of subplacental Doppler vascular signals.[47] Some color-flow mapping studies suggest that a myometrial thickness less than 1 mm with large intraplacental venous lakes is highly predictive of invasive placentation (sensitivity, 100%; specificity, 72%; positive predictive value, 72%; and negative predictive value, 100%).

In addition to the above ultrasound modalities, three-dimensional ultrasound has been used successfully to identify invasive placentation.[48,49] Diagnostic criteria include irregular intraplacental vascularization and hypervascularity of the uterine serosa–bladder wall interface.

Finally, **MRI can be used in conjunction with sonography to assess abnormal placental invasion.** MRI is particularly helpful when ultrasound findings are equivocal, the placenta is in a posterior location, and for determination of the extent of placental invasion within surrounding tissue, such as the parametrium and bladder. In a review and meta-analysis[50] of 1010 pregnancies at risk for placenta accreta, MRI had a diagnostic sensitivity of 94% and a specificity of 84%.

LABORATORY FINDINGS

Placenta accreta has been associated with unexplained elevations in maternal serum α-fetoprotein (MSAFP).

PATHOLOGIC STUDIES

Placenta accreta is confirmed by the pathologic examination of a hysterectomy specimen. Histologic evaluation demonstrates placental villi within the uterine myometrium and absence of a decidual plate. In focal accreta cases in which the uterus is not removed, curettage specimens may show myometrial cells adherent to the placenta.[51]

MANAGEMENT

Because of its associated risk for massive postpartum hemorrhage, **placenta accreta accounts for a large percentage of peripartum hysterectomies.[52] A multidisciplinary team approach is the ideal way to manage these cases.** Preoperative assessments by **maternal-fetal medicine specialists, neonatologists, blood conservation teams, anesthesiologists, advanced pelvic surgeons, and urologists**—especially for a suspected placenta percreta—are recommended. Timing of delivery depends upon clinical circumstances; however, **most authorities favor delivery at 34$^{0/7}$ to 35$^{6/7}$ weeks** with or without antenatal corticosteroid administration.[38] Ideally, the delivery should be scheduled at a time with optimal personnel availability at a facility prepared to manage significant obstetric hemorrhage. **Adequate IV access with two large-bore catheters and ample blood product availability are mandatory.** Cell-saver technology, donor-directed or autologous blood donation, and recombinant VIIa should be considered. Placement of ureteral stents preoperatively or intraoperatively can assist in maintaining urinary tract integrity. When performing the surgery, **it is recommended that the uterus be incised above the placental attachment site and that the placenta be left in situ after clamping the cord because disruption of the implantation site may result in rapid blood loss.** Finally, adjuvant use of aortic and/or internal iliac artery balloon occlusion catheters with postsurgical embolization has been shown to reduce blood loss, transfusion requirements, and duration of surgery in some studies.[53]

In specific circumstances, uterine conservation may be attempted. These situations include focal accreta, desired future fertility, and fundal or posterior placenta accreta. Uterine conservation techniques typically include leaving the placenta in situ at the delivery with subsequent expectant management, delayed manual placental removal, wedge resection or oversewing of the placental implantation site, tamponade of the lower uterine segment, curettage, uterine artery embolization, hemostatic sutures, arterial ligation, and/or administration of methotrexate.[54] Although each of these techniques has reported success, each is also associated with potential complications, including delayed hemorrhage, infection, fistula formation, subsequent surgery and/or hysterectomy, uterine necrosis, and even death.[55] Data are limited regarding long-term reproductive outcomes in women treated conservatively for invasive placentation. Although most women are able to conceive after conservative management, they remain at risk for spontaneous abortion, uterine synechiae and rupture, preterm delivery, recurrent placenta accreta, and peripartum hysterectomy.[54,56-58]

Vasa Previa
DEFINITION AND PATHOGENESIS
Vasa previa is defined as the presence of fetal vessels over the cervical os. Typically, these fetal vessels lack protection from Wharton jelly (velamentous cord insertion) and are prone to rupture and compression. When the vessels rupture, the fetus is at high risk for exsanguination. **Velamentous cord insertion may occur without vasa previa and can occasionally exist as fetal vessels that run between a bilobed or succenturiate-lobed placenta.**

INCIDENCE AND RISK FACTORS
The overall incidence of vasa previa is **1 in 2500 deliveries;** however, data have shown a range from 1 in 2000 to 1 in 5000 deliveries.[59] **Reported risk factors for vasa previa include bilobed and succenturiate-lobed placentas; pregnancies that result from assisted reproductive technology (ART); multiple gestations; and history of second-trimester placenta previa or low-lying placenta.**[59-61]

CLINICAL MANIFESTATIONS
In the past, most cases of vasa previa presented after rupture of membranes with acute onset of vaginal bleeding from a lacerated fetal vessel. If immediate intervention was not provided, fetal bradycardia and subsequent fetal death occurred. Today, many cases of vasa previa are diagnosed antenatally by ultrasound. In rare cases, **pulsating fetal vessels may be palpable in the membranes that overlie the cervical os.**

DIAGNOSIS
Vasa previa is often diagnosed antenatally by **ultrasound with color and pulsed Doppler mapping.** Transabdominal and transvaginal approaches are most often used. **The diagnosis is confirmed by documenting umbilical vessels over the cervical os using color and pulsed Doppler imaging** (Fig. 18-7).

MANAGEMENT
When diagnosed antenatally, vasa previa should be managed similarly to placenta previa. Some authorities have recommended twice-weekly nonstress testing at 28 to 30 weeks of gestation to assess for cord compression; others have favored

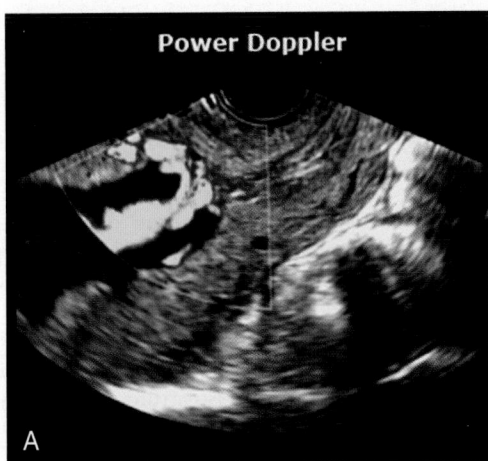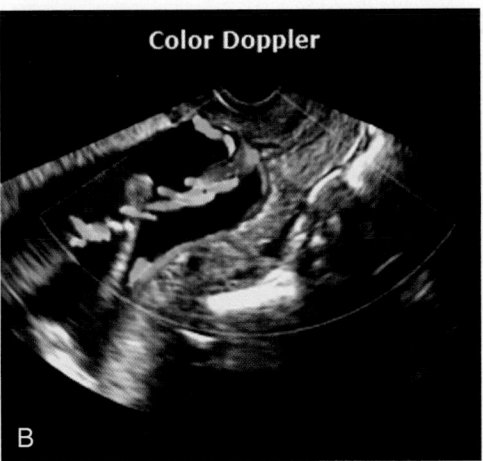

FIG 18-7 Transvaginal ultrasound images showing vasa previa and velamentous cord. The placenta is posterior with an anterior succenturiate lobe. (From Lockwood CJ, Russo-Steiglitz K. *Velamentous umbilical cord insertion and vasa previa,* www.uptodate.com, July 17, 2015.)

hospitalization in the third trimester with administration of antenatal corticosteroids, serial antepartum testing, and **cesarean delivery between $34^{0/7}$ to $36^{0/7}$ weeks of gestation**.[62,63] If an intrapartum diagnosis of vasa previa is made, expeditious delivery is needed. Immediate neonatal blood transfusion is often required in these circumstances.

POSTPARTUM HEMORRHAGE

Postpartum hemorrhage is an obstetric emergency that complicates between 1 in 20 and 1 in 100 deliveries. In the past decade, reported postpartum hemorrhage has increased 26% within the United States.[64] Because it is a major cause of maternal morbidity and mortality, obstetricians need to have a clear understanding of normal delivery-related blood loss so that postpartum hemorrhage can be efficiently recognized and managed.

Normal Blood Loss and Postpartum Hemorrhage

Normal delivery-related blood loss depends on the type of delivery. Based on objective data, the mean blood losses for a vaginal delivery, cesarean delivery, and cesarean hysterectomy are 500, 1000, and 1500 mL, respectively.[65] These values are often underestimated and unappreciated clinically owing to the significant blood volume expansion that accompanies normal pregnancy.

Postpartum hemorrhage has been variably defined in the literature. Definitions have included subjective assessments greater than the standard norms, a 10% decline in hemoglobin concentration, and the need for blood transfusion. A more practical definition is excessive delivery-related blood loss that causes the patient to be hemodynamically symptomatic and/or hypovolemic.

Postpartum Hemorrhage Etiologies

The etiologies of postpartum hemorrhage can be categorized as primary (early) or secondary (late). *Primary postpartum hemorrhage* refers to excessive bleeding that occurs within 24 hours of delivery, whereas *secondary postpartum hemorrhage* refers to bleeding that occurs from 24 hours until 12 weeks after delivery. Box 18-3 lists the most common causes of primary and secondary postpartum hemorrhage. Because primary postpartum hemorrhage is more common than the

---

BOX 18-3   ETIOLOGIES OF POSTPARTUM HEMORRHAGE

Early

Uterine atony
Lower genital tract lacerations (perineal, vaginal, cervical, periclitoral, periurethral, rectum)
Upper genital tract lacerations (broad ligament)
Lower urinary tract lacerations (bladder, urethra)
Retained products of conception (placenta, membranes)
Invasive placentation (placenta accreta, placenta increta, placenta percreta)
Uterine rupture
Uterine inversion
Coagulopathy

Late

Infection
Retained products of conception
Placental site subinvolution
Coagulopathy

---

secondary kind, the remainder of this discussion focuses on its etiology and management (Fig. 18-8).

Uterine Atony
DEFINITION AND PATHOGENESIS
Uterine atony, or the inability of the uterine myometrium to contract effectively, is the most common cause of primary postpartum hemorrhage. At term, blood flow through the placental site averages 500 to 700 mL per minute. After placental delivery, the uterus controls bleeding by contracting its myometrial fibers in a tourniquet fashion around the spiral arterioles. If inadequate uterine contraction occurs, rapid blood loss can ensue.

INCIDENCE AND RISK FACTORS
Uterine atony complicates 1 in 20 deliveries and is responsible for 80% of postpartum hemorrhage cases. Risk factors for uterine atony include **uterine overdistention** (multiple gestation, polyhydramnios, fetal macrosomia), **labor induction, rapid or prolonged labor, grand multiparity, uterine infection, uterine inversion, retained products of conception, abnormal placentation, and use of uterine-relaxing agents** (tocolytic therapy, halogenated anesthetics, nitroglycerin).

CLINICAL MANIFESTATIONS AND DIAGNOSIS
Uterine atony is diagnosed clinically by rapid uterine bleeding associated with a lack of myometrial tone and an absence of other etiologies for postpartum hemorrhage. Typically, bimanual palpation of the uterus confirms the diagnosis.

PREVENTION AND MANAGEMENT
By recognizing risk factors for uterine atony and quickly initiating a treatment cascade, the clinician can minimize blood loss. Three preventive methods for atonic postpartum hemorrhage are 1) active management of the third stage of labor, 2) spontaneous placental separation during cesarean delivery, and 3) prolonged postpartum oxytocin infusion. Active management of the third stage of labor includes early cord clamping, controlled cord traction, uterine massage, and administration of uterotonic therapy before placental separation. A systematic review[66] of seven studies that compared active to expectant management of the third stage of labor showed significant reductions in maternal blood loss, postpartum hemorrhage, prolonged third stage of labor, and the need for additional uterotonic therapies. Whereas controversy exists regarding the timing of uterotonic administration, a recent systematic review[67] suggested that giving uterotonic therapy before delivery of the placenta results in less blood loss and fewer postpartum transfusions.

A second strategy to minimize uterine atony is to allow spontaneous placental separation during cesarean delivery. In one controlled study, spontaneous placental separation reduced blood loss by 30% and reduced postpartum endometritis sevenfold compared with manual removal.

A final preventive approach for atonic postpartum hemorrhage is prolonged postpartum oxytocin infusion. A recent clinical trial[68] assessed two postpartum oxytocin regimens following delivery: a bolus of oxytocin after delivery versus a bolus of oxytocin followed by a 4-hour IV infusion of oxytocin. A significant reduction was seen in uterine atony and need for additional uterotonic therapy in the women who received the prolonged oxytocin infusion. Additional evidence-based review

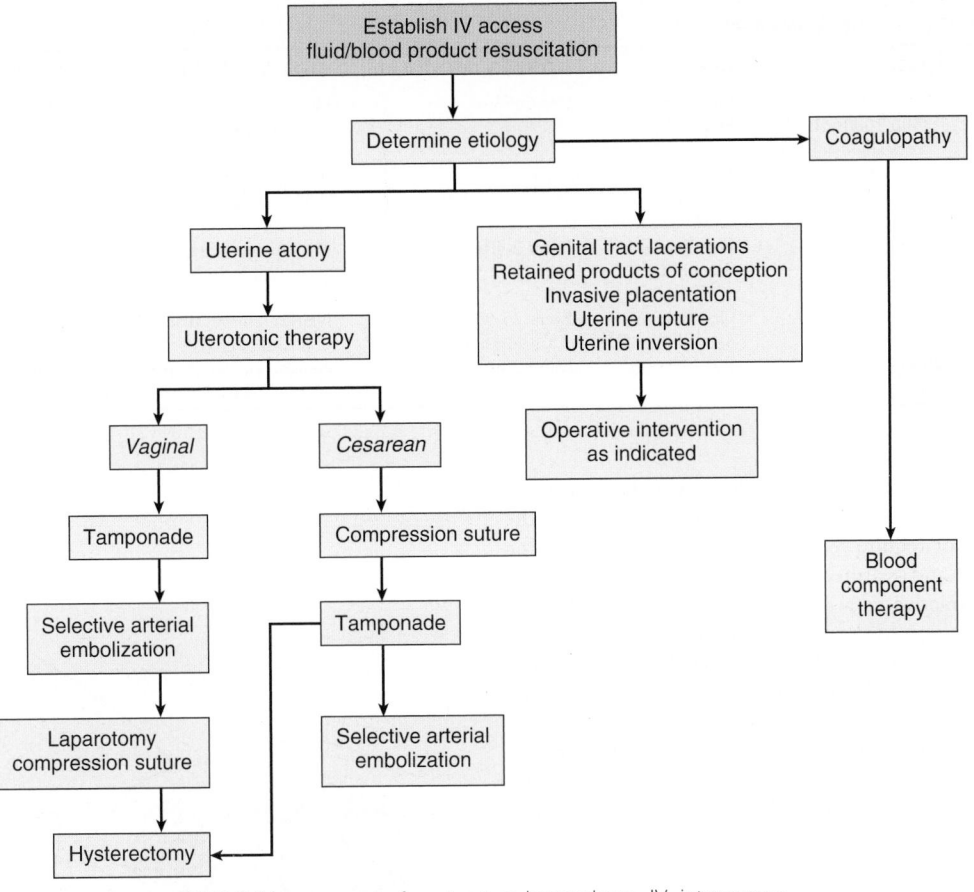

FIG 18-8 Management of postpartum hemorrhage. IV, intravenous.

data support prolonged (4 to 8 hours) oxytocin administration after delivery.[69]

If preventive measures are unsuccessful, medical management for uterine atony should be initiated. This treatment includes bimanual uterine massage and uterotonic therapy.

BIMANUAL UTERINE MASSAGE

To provide effective bimanual uterine massage, **the uterus should be compressed between the external, fundally placed hand and the internal, intravaginal hand** (Fig. 18-9). **Care must be taken to avoid aggressive massage that can injure the large vessels of the broad ligament.**

UTEROTONIC THERAPY

Uterotonic medications represent the mainstay of drug therapy for postpartum hemorrhage secondary to uterine atony. Table 18-4 lists available uterotonic agents with their dosages, side effects, and contraindications. **Oxytocin** is usually given as a first-line agent. IV therapy is the preferred route of administration, but intramuscular and intrauterine dosing is possible. Initial treatment starts with 10 to 30 units of oxytocin in 500 to 1000 mL of crystalloid solution. Higher doses (80 units in 500 to 1000 mL) have proved safe and efficacious, with a 20% reduction in the need for additional uterotonic therapy and reduced composite hemorrhage treatment (uterotonic drugs, transfusion, tamponade, embolization, surgery).[70]

When oxytocin fails to produce adequate uterine tone, second-line therapy must be initiated. Currently, a variety of additional uterotonic agents are available. The choice of a second-line agent depends on its side-effect profile as well as its

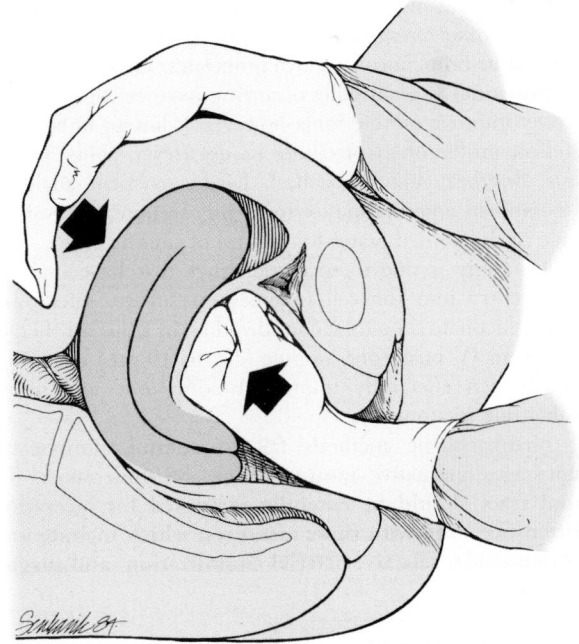

FIG 18-9 Bimanual uterine massage.

TABLE 18-4	UTEROTONIC THERAPIES				
AGENT	**DOSE**	**ROUTE**	**DOSING INTERVAL**	**SIDE EFFECTS**	**CONTRAINDICATIONS**
Oxytocin (Pitocin)	10 to 80 U in 500-1000 mL crystalloid solution	First line: IV Second line: IM or IU	Continuous	Nausea, emesis, water intoxication	None
Misoprostol (Cytotec)	600-1000 μg	First line: PR Second line: PO or SL	Single dose	Nausea, emesis, diarrhea, fever, chills	None
Methylergonovine (Methergine)	0.2 mg	First line: IM Second line: IU or PO	Every 2-4 hr	Hypertension, hypotension, nausea, emesis	Hypertension, migraines, scleroderma, Raynaud syndrome
Prostaglandin $F_{2\alpha}$ (Hemabate)	0.25 mg	First line: IM Second line: IU	Every 15-90 min (maximum of 8 doses)	Nausea, emesis, diarrhea, flushing, chills	Active cardiac, pulmonary, renal, or hepatic disease
Prostaglandin E_2 (Dinoprostone)	20 mg	PR	Every 2 hr	Nausea, emesis, diarrhea, fever, chills, headache	Hypotension

IM, intramuscular; *IU*, intrauterine; *IV*, intravenous; *PO*, per os; *PR*, per rectum; *SL*, sublingual.

contraindications. **Misoprostol, a synthetic prostaglandin E_1 analogue,** is a safe, inexpensive, and efficacious uterotonic medication that does not require refrigeration. It has been used for both the prevention and treatment of postpartum hemorrhage.[71-73] Misoprostol is attractive as a second-line agent in that it has multiple administration routes that can be combined. Although higher doses (600 to 1000 μg) have traditionally been used rectally, the sublingual route allows for lower dosing (400 μg) with higher bioavailability.[71] Although helpful in some settings, **methylergonovine** has limited usefulness for acute postpartum hemorrhage because of its relatively long half-life and potential for worsening hypertension in patients with preexisting disease.

Prostaglandins are highly effective uterotonic agents. Both natural and synthetic prostaglandin formulations are available. Intramuscular and intrauterine administration of **prostaglandin $F_{2\alpha}$** can be used for control of atony. Recurrent doses (0.25 mg) may be administered as often as every 15 minutes to a maximum of eight doses (2 mg total dose). It is important to note that asthma is a *strong contraindication* to the use of prostaglandin $F_{2\alpha}$ because of its bronchoconstrictive properties. **Prostaglandin E_2 (dinoprostone)** is a naturally occurring oxytocic that can dramatically improve uterine tone; however, it has an unfavorable side-effect profile often precludes its use (fever, chills, nausea, emesis, diarrhea, and headaches). Lastly, oxytocin analogues and combined ergometrine-oxytocin preparations are available outside of the United States for control of uterine atony.

When atony is due to tocolytic drugs that have impaired calcium entry into the cell (magnesium sulfate, nifedipine), calcium gluconate should be considered as an adjuvant therapy. Given as an IV push, one ampule (1 g in 10 mL) of calcium gluconate can effectively improve uterine tone and resolve bleeding due to atony.

If pharmacologic methods fail to control atony-related hemorrhage, alternative measures must be undertaken. **The genital tract should be carefully inspected for lacerations before proceeding with these measures, which include uterine tamponade, selective arterial embolization, and surgical intervention.**

UTERINE TAMPONADE

Uterine packing is a safe, simple, and effective way to control postpartum hemorrhage by providing tamponade to the bleeding uterine surface. Although packing techniques vary, a few basic principles should be followed. The pack should be made of long, continuous gauze (e.g., Kerlix) rather than multiple small sponges. Some authorities have had success with

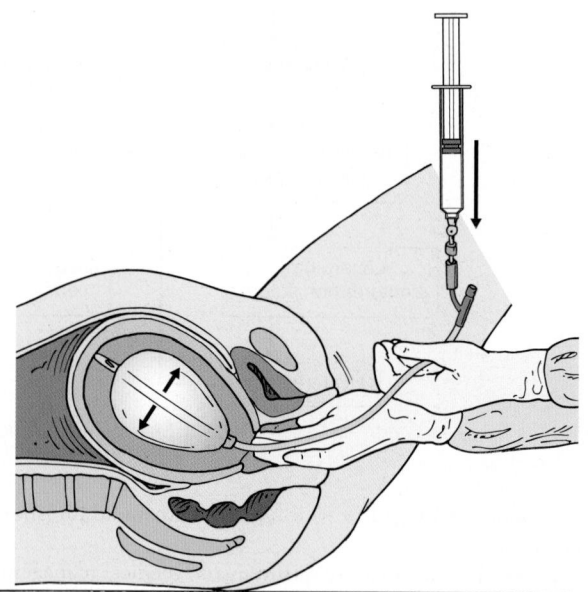

FIG 18-10 The Bakri tamponade balloon. (From Bakri YN, Arulkumaran S. *Intrauterine balloon tamponade for control of postpartum hemorrhage,* www.uptodate.com, July 7, 2015.)

the use of thrombin-impregnated or chitosan-covered gauze.[74] When packing the uterus, placement should begin at the fundus and progress downward in a side-to-side fashion to avoid dead space for blood accumulation. Transurethral Foley catheter placement and prophylactic antibiotic use should be considered to prevent urinary retention and infection, respectively. Finally, prolonged packing should be avoided (not more than 12 to 24 hours), and close attention should be paid to the patient's vital signs and blood indices while the pack is in place in order to minimize unrecognized ongoing bleeding.

In recent years, **intrauterine tamponade balloons** have largely replaced traditional uterine packing. Multiple balloon types have been used and include the Bakri tamponade balloon, the BT-Cath, the Belfort-Dildy Obstetrical Tamponade System, the Sengstaken-Blakemore tube, and the #24 Foley catheter with 30 mL balloon. The **Bakri tamponade balloon**, the **BT-Cath**, and the **Belfort-Dildy Obstetrical Tamponade System** were all developed specifically for postpartum hemorrhage management. The Bakri tamponade balloon (Cook Women's Health; Fig. 18-10) consists of a silicone balloon attached to a catheter. The catheter is inserted into the uterus either manually or under

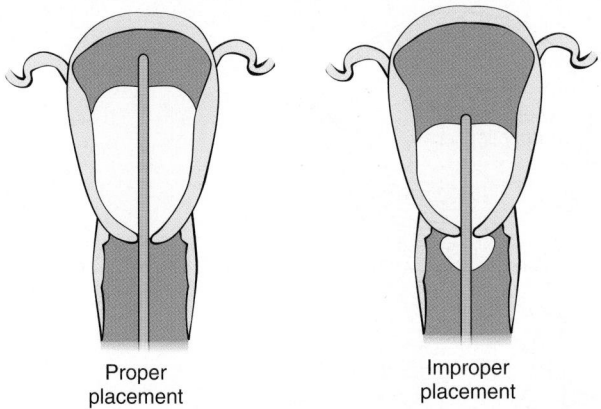

Proper placement   Improper placement

FIG 18-11 Proper placement of the Bakri tamponade balloon. (Courtesy Cook Women's Health.)

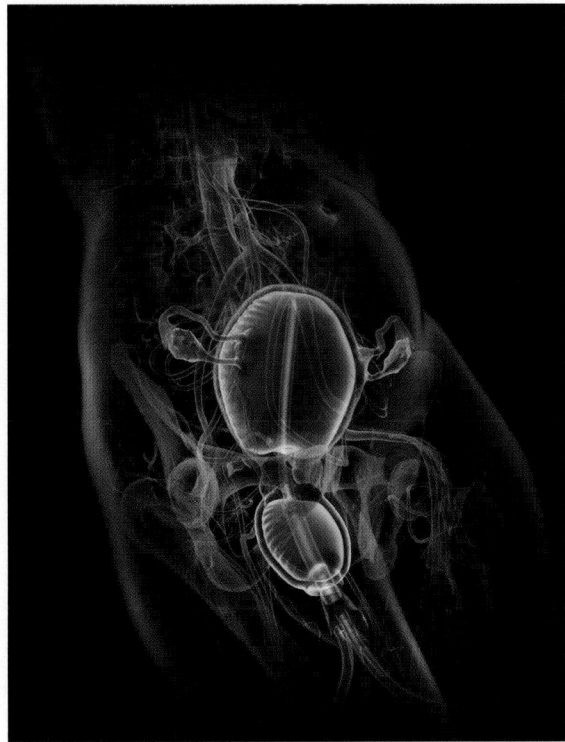

FIG 18-12 The Belfort-Dildy obstetrical tamponade system. (Courtesy Glenveigh Medical.)

ultrasound guidance, and the silicone balloon is subsequently inflated with sterile saline (maximum of 500 mL). Once inflated, the balloon should adapt to the uterine configuration to provide tamponade to the endometrial surface. The intraluminal catheter allows drainage from within the uterus so that ongoing assessment of blood loss can occur. Proper placement of the balloon is essential to provide adequate tamponade (Fig. 18-11). Like the Bakri tamponade balloon, the BT-Cath (Utah Medical Products) is a silicone balloon; however, it is shaped like an inverted pear. This tamponade balloon also has a double-lumen catheter that allows saline filling of the balloon as well as drainage of blood from within the uterus. Finally, the Belfort-Dildy Obstetrical Tamponade System (Glenveigh Medical) incorporates both intrauterine and intravaginal polyurethane balloons that conform to these cavities, respectively (Fig. 18-12).[75] The uterine balloon can be rapidly inflated from a saline bag to a larger volume of 750 mL when the smaller balloons are inadequate (e.g., with multiple gestations). Like the other balloons, this system has a drainage port to assess for ongoing bleeding; however, unlike the others, it also has an infusion port to irrigate the uterus.

SELECTIVE ARTERIAL EMBOLIZATION

Selective arterial embolization is an increasingly common therapeutic option for hemodynamically stable patients with postpartum hemorrhage. The procedure can be performed alone or after failed surgical intervention.[76] Diagnostic pelvic angiography is used to visualize bleeding vessels, and gelatin (e.g., Gelfoam]) pledgets are placed into the vessels for occlusion. **Cumulative success rates of 90% to 97% have been reported.**[76]

Selective arterial embolization has several advantages over surgical intervention. First, it allows for selective occlusion of bleeding vessels. This can be extremely valuable in circumstances of aberrant pelvic vasculature, such as uterine arteriovenous malformations. Second, the uterus and potential future fertility are preserved. Case series[76] have reported successful pregnancies after pelvic embolization. Finally, the procedure has minimal morbidity, enables the physician to forego or delay surgical intervention, and can be performed in coagulopathic patients, which allows more time for blood and clotting factor replacement. Procedure-related complications occur in 3% to 6% of cases.[76] Reported complications include postembolization fever, infection, ischemic pain, vascular perforation, and tissue necrosis. A relative disadvantage of the procedure is its limited availability. Timely coordination of services between the obstetric team and interventional radiology personnel, as well as a hemodynamically stable patient, are necessary to provide this treatment option.

SURGICAL INTERVENTION

When uterine atony is unresponsive to conservative management, surgical intervention by laparotomy is necessary. Possible interventions include arterial ligation, uterine compression sutures, and hysterectomy.

The goal of arterial ligation is to decrease uterine perfusion and subsequent bleeding. Success rates have varied from 40% to 95% in the literature depending on which vessels are ligated. Arterial ligation may be performed on the ascending uterine arteries, the uteroovarian arteries, the infundibulopelvic ligament vessels, and the internal iliac (hypogastric) arteries. Because internal iliac arterial ligation can be technically challenging and time consuming, it is not advised as a first-line technique unless the surgeon is extremely skilled in performing the procedure. Instead, a stepwise progression of uterine vessel ligation is recommended.

Nearly five decades ago, O'Leary described a technique of bilateral uterine artery ligation for control of postpartum hemorrhage. Today, it is still considered the initial ligation technique given its ease in performance and the accessibility of the uterine artery. To perform the procedure, the ascending uterine artery should be located at the border of the upper and lower uterine segment. Absorbable suture is passed through the uterine myometrium at the level of the lower uterine segment and laterally around the uterine vessels through a clear space in the broad ligament. The suture is then tied to compress the vessels against the uterine wall (Fig. 18-13). Because the suture is placed fairly high in the lower uterine segment, ureteral injury is avoided;

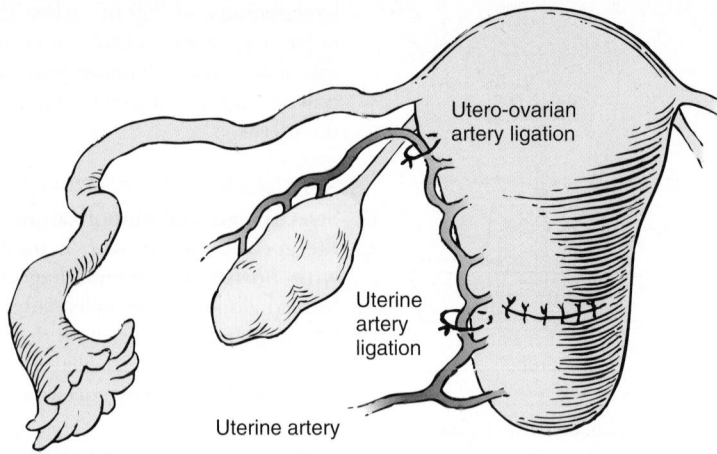

FIG 18-13 Uterine artery ligation.

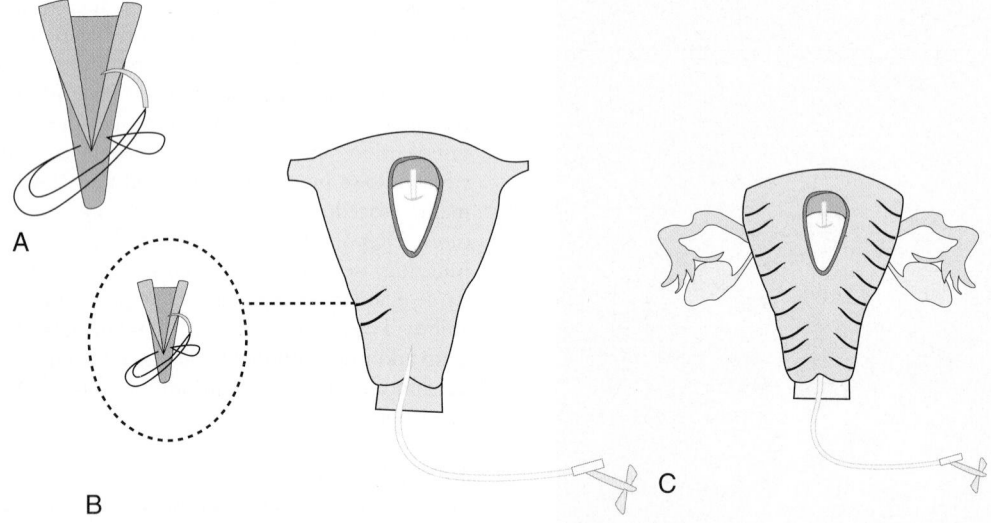

FIG 18-14 Bilateral looped uterine vessel sutures. (From Bakri YN, Arulkumaran S. *Intrauterine balloon tamponade for control of postpartum hemorrhage,* www.uptodate.com, July 7, 2015.)

therefore the bladder does not need to be mobilized. Unilateral artery ligation will control hemorrhage in 10% to 15% of cases, whereas bilateral ligation will control hemorrhage in over 90% of cases.

If bleeding persists, the uteroovarian and infundibulopelvic vessels should be ligated. The uteroovarian arteries can be ligated similarly to what has been described for the ascending uterine vessels. If this measure is unsuccessful, interruption of the infundibulopelvic vessels can be undertaken. Although the ovarian blood supply may be decreased with an infundibulopelvic vessel ligation, successful pregnancy has been reported following this procedure.

Bakri has described a newer technique for bilateral uterine artery ligation in combination with tamponade balloon placement (Fig. 18-14). The procedure, termed ***Bilateral Looped Uterine Vessel Sutures*** (B-LUVS), incorporates absorbable sutures looped bilaterally through the myometrium around the uterine vessels from the lower segment up to the corneal region. Once the sutures are tied, a Bakri tamponade balloon is placed within the uterine cavity to provide internal tamponade. A small series has had high success with this combined ligation-tamponade approach.

In addition to arterial ligation, **uterine compression sutures** have been described for atony control. Several techniques have evolved over the past two decades, including the **B-Lynch suture, Hayman vertical sutures, Pereira transverse and vertical sutures, and multiple square sutures.**[77,78] To place a compression suture, the patient should lie in the dorsal lithotomy position to facilitate assessment of vaginal bleeding. Large absorbable suture is typically anchored within the uterine myometrium both anteriorly and posteriorly. It is passed in a continuous or intermittent fashion around or through the external surface of the uterus and tied firmly so that adequate uterine compression occurs. Figures 18-15 to 18-18 demonstrate proper placements of these sutures. Like arterial ligation, uterine compression sutures can be combined with tamponade balloons for refractory bleeding. The "uterine sandwich" technique refers to placement of a B-Lynch suture followed by a Bakri tamponade balloon within the uterine cavity.[79] Typically, the tamponade balloon is inflated to a lesser volume (median of 100 mL) in these cases. Small series[79] have demonstrated high success rates for this combined approach.

The final surgical intervention for refractory bleeding due to atony is hysterectomy, which provides definitive therapy.

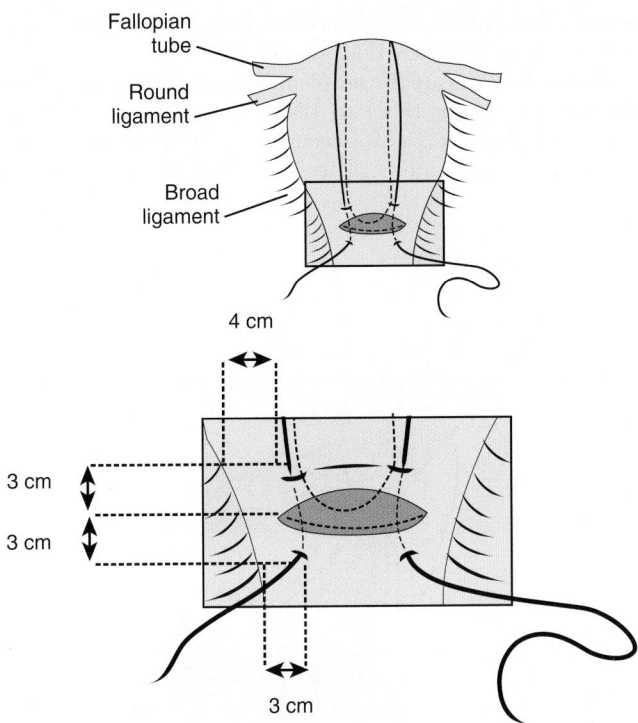

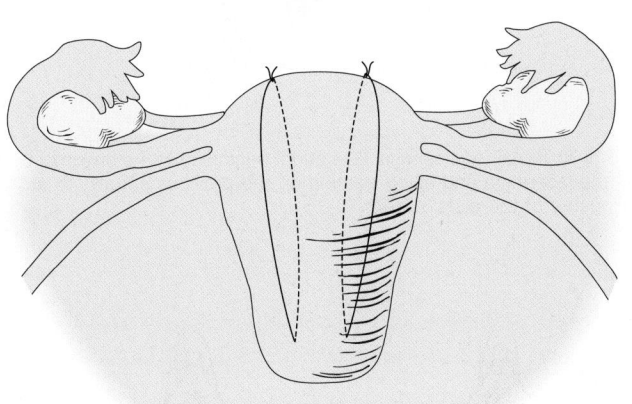

FIG 18-15 B-Lynch compression suture. (From Belfort MA. Management of postpartum hemorrhage at cesarean delivery, www.uptodate.com, June 26, 2015.)

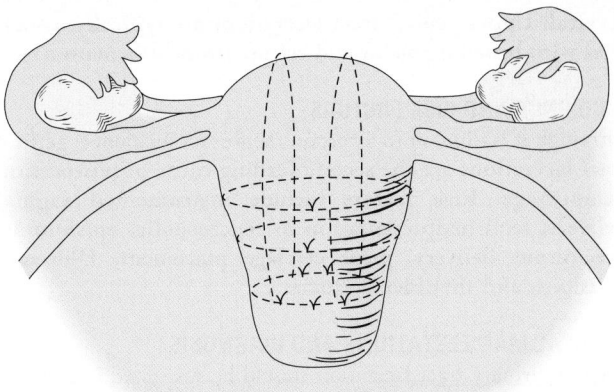

FIG 18-17 Pereira transverse and vertical sutures (From Belfort MA. *Management of postpartum hemorrhage at cesarean delivery,* www.uptodate.com, June 26, 2015.)

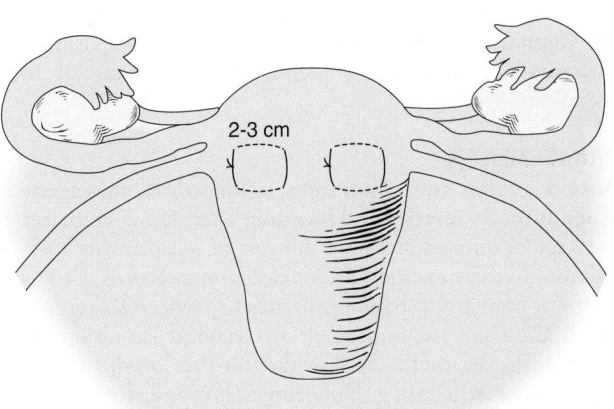

FIG 18-18 Multiple square sutures. (From Belfort MA. *Management of postpartum hemorrhage at cesarean delivery,* www.uptodate.com, June 26, 2015.)

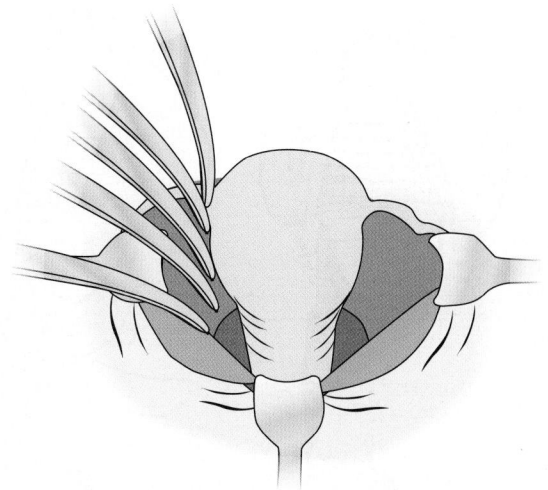

FIG 18-16 Hayman vertical sutures. (From Belfort MA. *Management of postpartum hemorrhage at cesarean delivery,* www.uptodate.com, June 26, 2015.)

FIG 18-19 Clamp-cut-drop technique for hysterectomy. (From Wright JD, Bonanno C, Shah M, et al. Peripartum hysterectomy. *Obstet Gynecol.* 2010;116:429-434.)

Because blood loss may be severe, it is often prudent to modify the surgical approach by using the "clamp-cut-drop" technique (Fig. 18-19), performing a supracervical hysterectomy, or both.[80] These considerations are especially important when the patient is hemodynamically unstable (Video 18-1).

Genital Tract Lacerations
DEFINITION AND PATHOGENESIS
Genital tract lacerations may occur with both vaginal and cesarean deliveries. These lacerations involve the maternal soft tissue structures and can be associated with large hematomas and rapid blood loss if unrecognized. **The most common lower genital tract lacerations are perineal, vulvar, vaginal, and**

cervical. Upper genital tract lacerations are typically associated with broad ligament and retroperitoneal hematomas.

INCIDENCE AND RISK FACTORS

Although it is difficult to ascertain their exact incidence, **genital tract lacerations are the second leading cause of postpartum hemorrhage. Risk factors include instrumented vaginal delivery, fetal malpresentation or macrosomia, episiotomy, precipitous delivery, prior cerclage placement, Dührssen incisions, and shoulder dystocia.**

CLINICAL MANIFESTATIONS AND DIAGNOSIS

A genitourinary tract laceration should be suspected if bleeding persists after delivery despite adequate uterine tone. Occasionally, the bleeding may be masked because of its location, such as with the broad ligament. In these circumstances, large amounts of blood loss may occur in an unrecognized hematoma. Pain and hemodynamic instability are often the primary presenting symptoms.

For diagnosis, it is best to evaluate the lower genital tract superiorly from the cervix and to progress inferiorly to the vagina, perineum, and vulva. Adequate exposure and retraction are essential for identification of many of these lacerations.

MANAGEMENT

Once a genital tract laceration is identified, management depends on its severity and location. Lacerations of the cervix and vaginal fornices are often difficult to repair owing to their position. In these circumstances, relocation to an OR with anesthesia assistance for better pain relief, pelvic relaxation, and visualization are recommended. For cervical lacerations, it is important to secure the apex of the tear because this is often a major source of bleeding. Unfortunately, exposure of this angle can be difficult. A helpful technique for these scenarios is to start suturing the laceration at its proximal end, thereby using the

suture for traction to expose the more distal portion of the cervix until the apex is in view (Fig. 18-20).

Perineal repairs are the most common types of genital tract lacerations. Figures 18-21 to 18-23 illustrate second-, third-, and fourth-degree perineal lacerations and techniques for their repair. If the laceration is adjacent to the urethra, the use of a

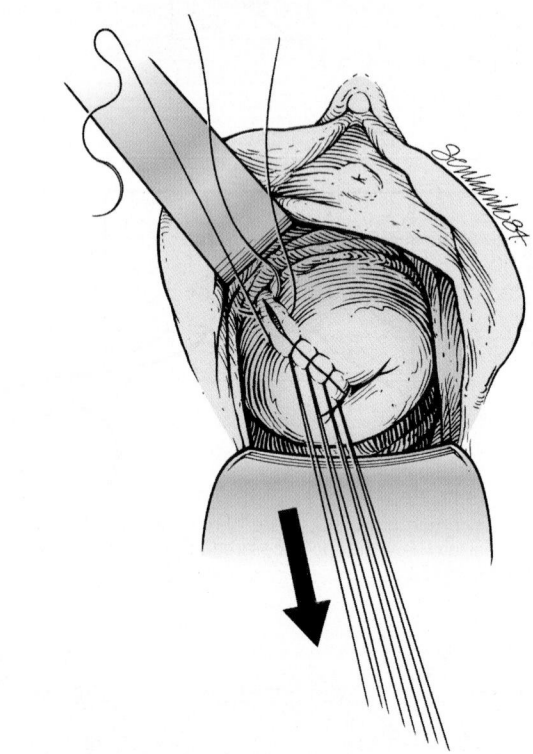

FIG 18-20 Repair of a cervical laceration, beginning at the proximal part of the laceration and using traction on the previous sutures to aid in exposure of the distal defect.

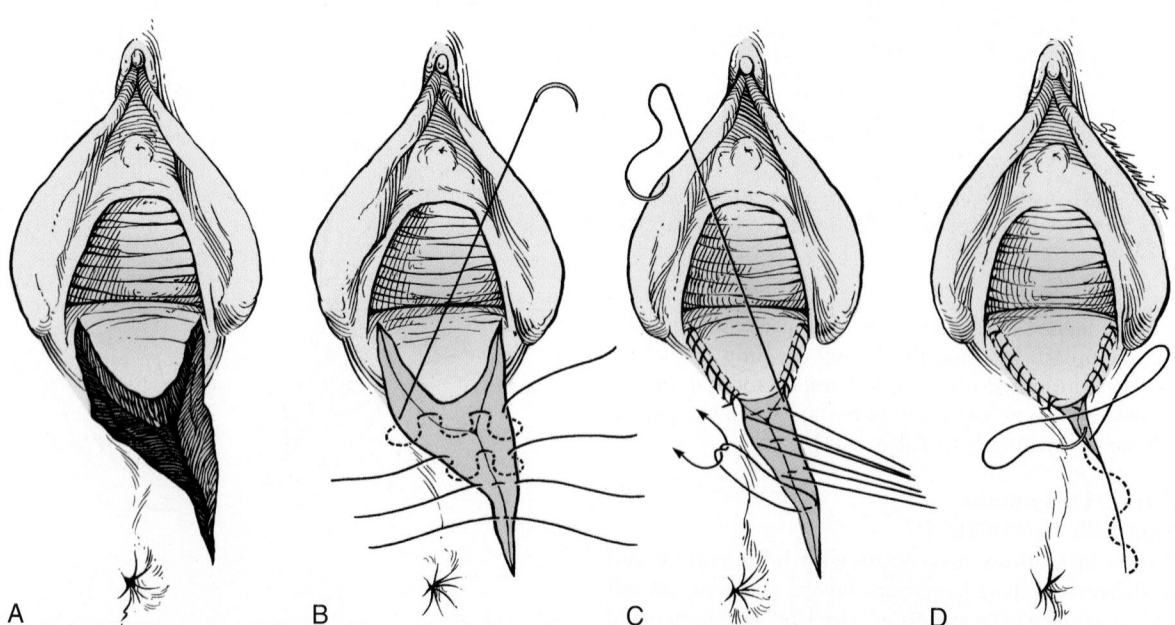

FIG 18-21 Repair of a second-degree laceration. A first-degree laceration involves the fourchette, the perineal skin, and the vaginal mucous membrane. A second-degree laceration also includes the muscles of the perineal body. The rectal sphincter remains intact.

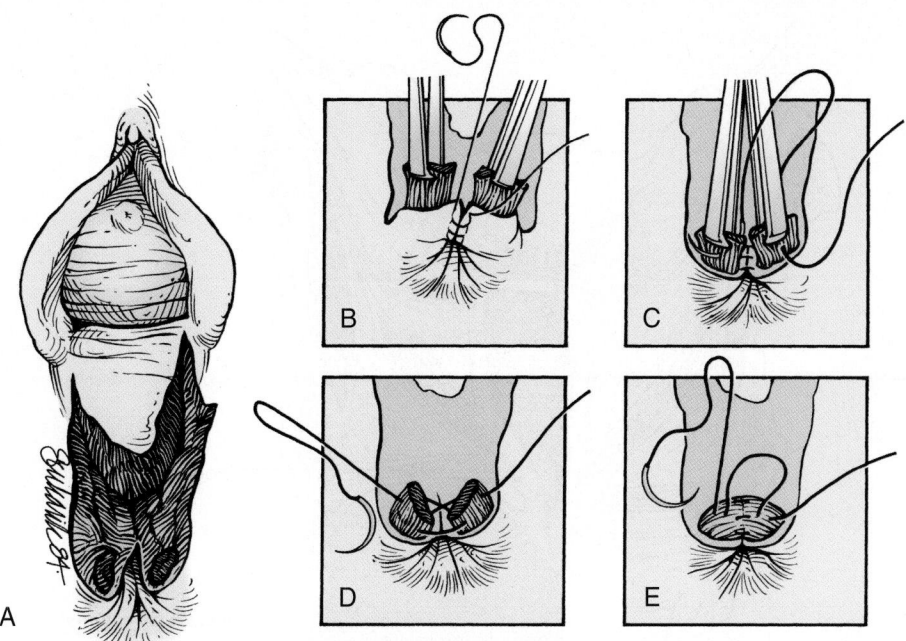

FIG 18-22 Repair of the sphincter after a third-degree laceration. A third-degree laceration extends not only through the skin, mucous membrane, and perineal body but includes the anal sphincter. Interrupted figure-of-eight sutures should be placed in the capsule of the sphincter muscle.

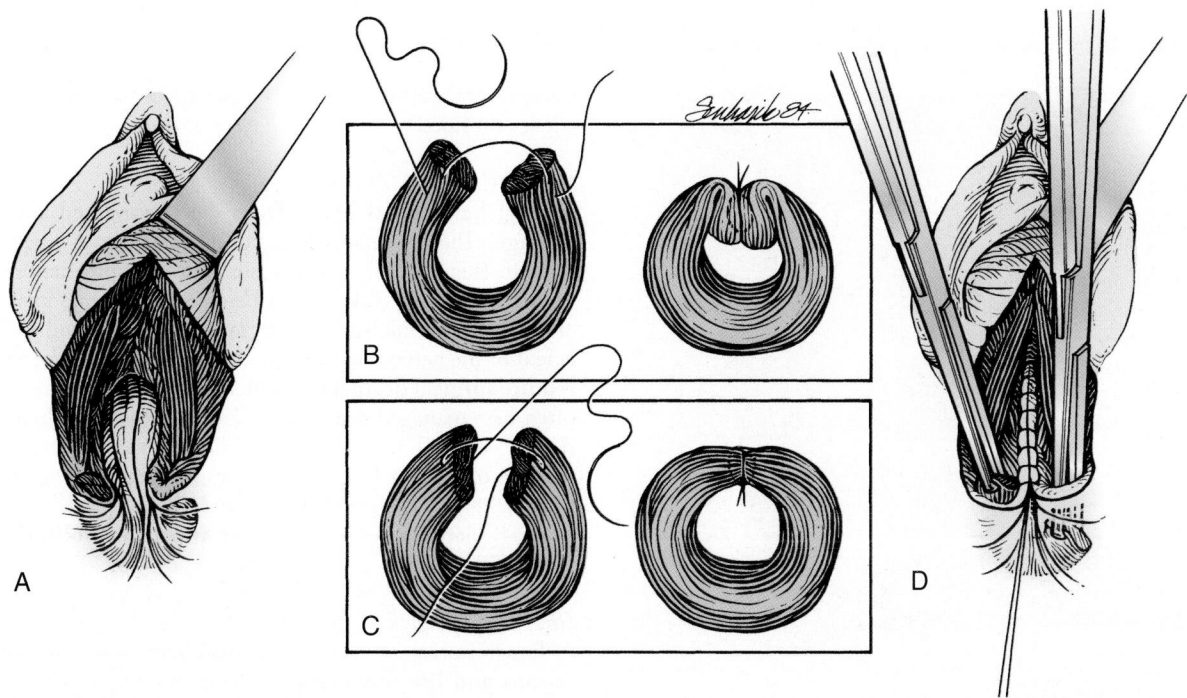

FIG 18-23 Repair of a fourth-degree laceration. This laceration extends through the rectal mucosa. **A,** The extent of this laceration is shown with a segment of the rectum exposed. **B,** Approximation of the rectal submucosa. This is the most commonly recommended method for repair. **C,** Alternative method of approximating the rectal mucosa in which the knots are actually buried inside the rectal lumen. **D,** After closure of the rectal submucosa, an additional layer of running sutures may be placed. The rectal sphincter is then repaired.

transurethral catheter can aid in a more efficient repair and can protect uninjured organs. Digital rectal exam is recommended after repair of third- and fourth-degree lacerations in order to ensure proper integrity of the rectum.

On occasion, a blood vessel laceration may lead to the formation of a pelvic hematoma in the lower or upper genital tract.

The three most common locations for a pelvic hematoma are vulvar, vaginal, and retroperitoneal.

VULVAR HEMATOMA

Vulvar hematomas usually result from lacerated vessels in the superficial fascia of the anterior or posterior pelvic triangle.

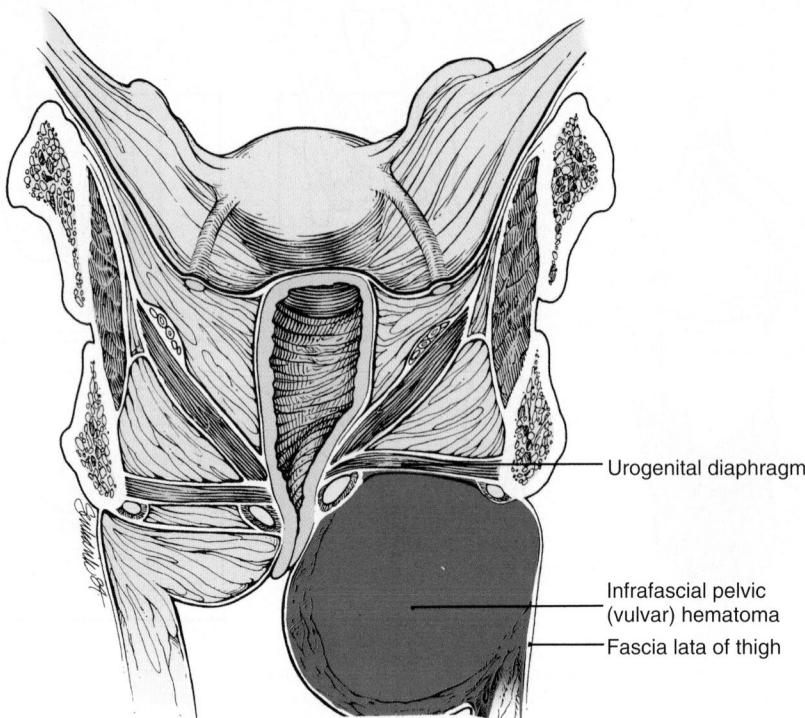

FIG 18-24 Vulvar hematoma fascial boundaries.

Urogenital diaphragm

Infrafascial pelvic
(vulvar) hematoma

Fascia lata of thigh

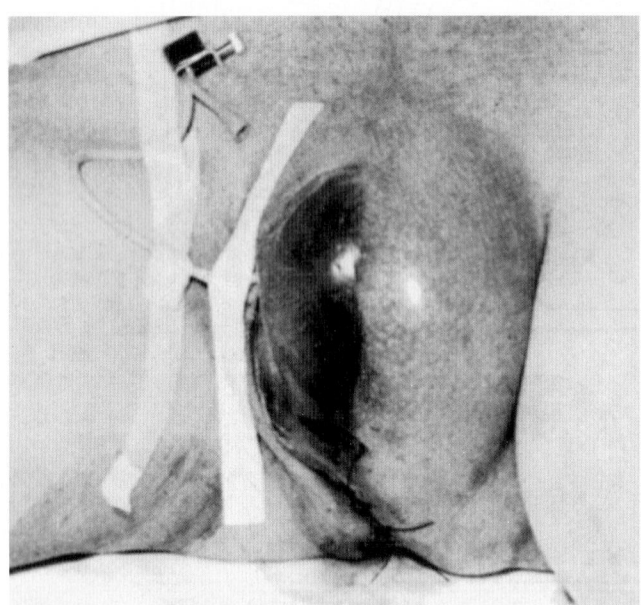

FIG 18-25 Large vulvar hematoma.

Blood loss is tamponaded by Colles fascia, the urogenital dia-phragm, and anal fascia (Fig. 18-24). Because of these fascial boundaries, the mass will extend to the skin, and a visible hema-toma results (Fig. 18-25).

Surgical drainage is the primary treatment for vulvar hematomas. A wide linear incision through the skin is recom-mended. Typically, the bleeding is due to multiple small vessels; hence, vessel ligation is not possible. Once the hematoma is evacuated, the dead space should be closed in layers with absorb-able suture, and a sterile pressure dressing should be applied. A transurethral catheter should be placed until significant tissue edema subsides.

VAGINAL HEMATOMA

Vaginal hematomas result from delivery-related soft tissue damage. These hematomas accumulate above the pelvic dia-phragm (Fig. 18-26), and occasionally, they protrude into the vaginal-rectal area. Like vulvar hematomas, vaginal hematomas are due to multiple small vessel lacerations. Depending on the extent of the hemorrhage, **vaginal hematomas may or may not require surgical drainage.** Small, nonexpanding hematomas are often best managed expectantly. Larger, expanding hematomas require surgical intervention. Unlike vulvar hematomas, the incision of a vaginal hematoma does not require closing, rather a vaginal pack or tamponade device should be placed on the raw edges. If bleeding persists, **selective arterial embolization may be considered.**

RETROPERITONEAL HEMATOMA

Although infrequent, **retroperitoneal hematomas are the most serious and life threatening.** The early symptoms of a retro-peritoneal hematoma are often subtle, with the hematoma being unrecognized until the patient is hemodynamically unstable from massive hemorrhage. **These hematomas usually occur after a vessel laceration from the internal iliac (hypogastric) arterial tree** (Fig. 18-27). Such lacerations may result from instrumented vaginal delivery, inadequate hemostasis of the uterine arteries at the time of cesarean delivery, or uterine rupture during a trial of labor after cesarean delivery (TOLAC). **Treatment of a retroperitoneal hematoma typically involves laparotomy, hematoma evacuation, and arterial ligation. In some situations, selective arterial embolization may be used as a primary or adjunctive treatment.**

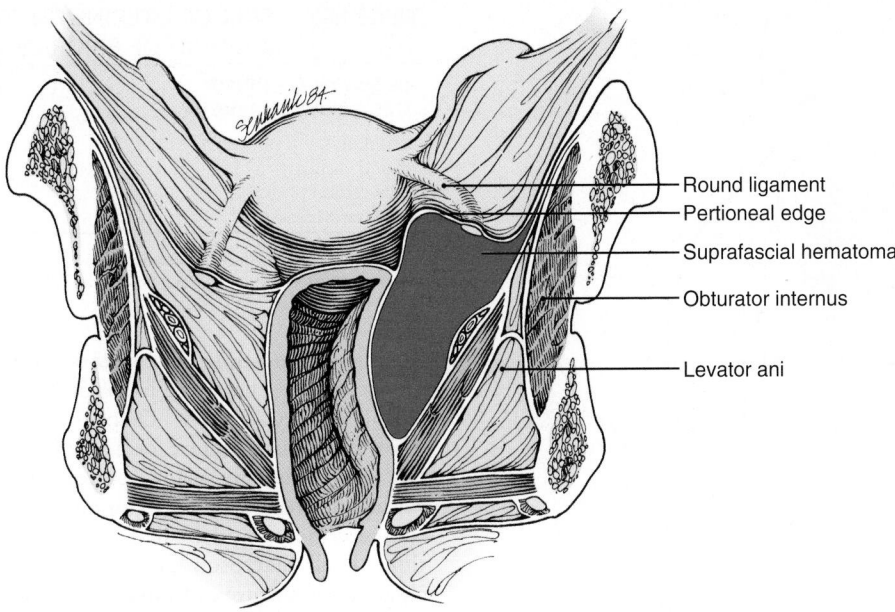

Round ligament
Pertioneal edge
Suprafascial hematoma
Obturator internus
Levator ani

FIG 18-26 Vaginal hematoma.

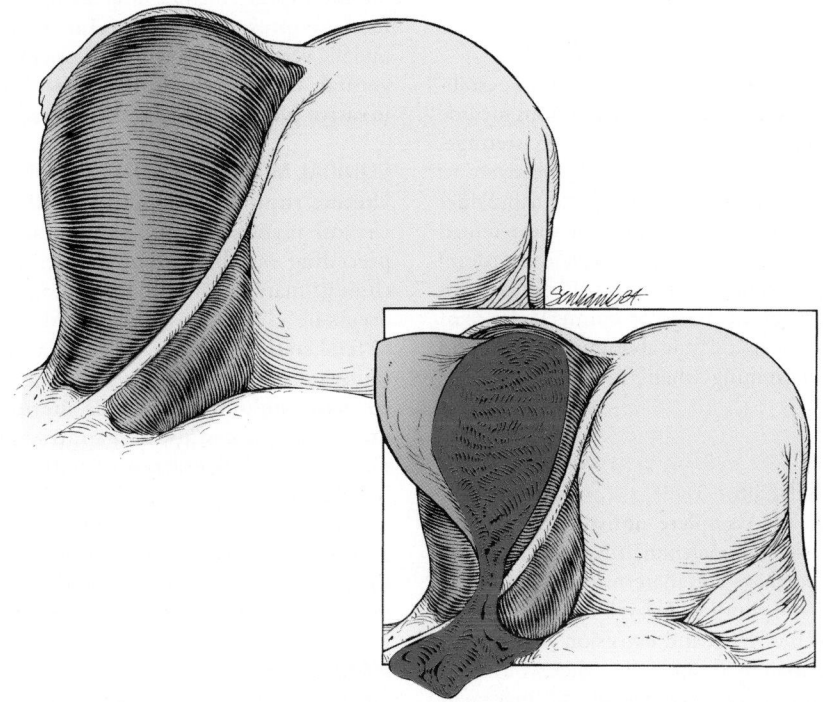

FIG 18-27 Retroperitoneal hematoma.

Retained Products of Conception
DEFINITION AND PATHOGENESIS
Retained products of conception, namely placental tissue and amniotic membranes, can inhibit the uterus from adequate contraction and can result in hemorrhage. The diagnosis is made when spontaneous expulsion of the tissue has not occurred within 30 to 60 minutes of delivery.

INCIDENCE AND RISK FACTORS
Retained products of conception complicate 0.5% to 1% of deliveries. Risk factors include midtrimester delivery, chorioamnionitis, and accessory placental lobes.

CLINICAL MANIFESTATIONS AND DIAGNOSIS
Retained products of conception typically present with uterine bleeding and associated atony. To assess the uterus for retained products of conception, the uterine cavity needs to be explored. Manual exploration is not only diagnostic but is also often therapeutic (Fig. 18-28). By wrapping the examination hand with moist gauze, removal of retained placental fragments and amniotic membranes can be facilitated. If manual access to the uterine cavity is difficult or limited owing to maternal body habitus or inadequate pain relief, **transabdominal or transvaginal ultrasound may be used to determine whether retained placental fragments are present.**[81]

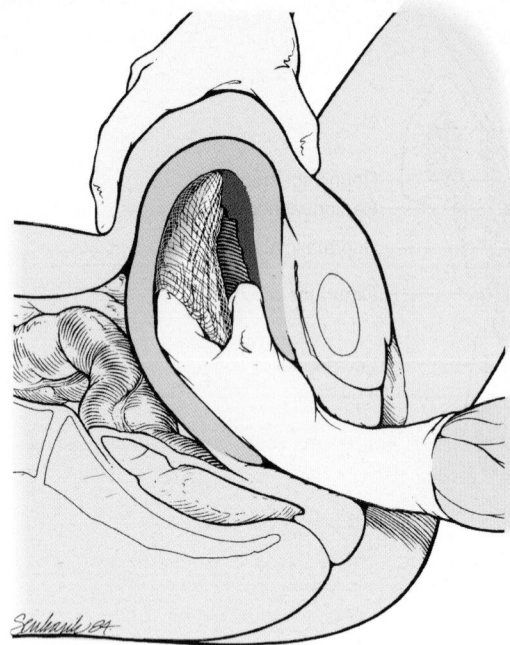

FIG 18-28 Manual uterine exploration.

MANAGEMENT

Once a diagnosis of retained products of conception is established, removal must be undertaken. Therapeutic options include **manual extraction,** as noted previously, or **uterine curettage.** Nitroglycerin (50 to 200 μg IV) has been used effectively to assist with manual placental extraction. Nitroglycerin provides rapid uterine relaxation to assist with removal of the retained tissue. Uterine curettage may be performed in a delivery room; however, excessive bleeding mandates that an OR be used for the procedure. Either a large blunt (Banjo or Hunter) curette or vacuum suction curette can be used. Transabdominal ultrasound guidance is helpful in determining when tissue evacuation is complete.

Uterine Rupture
DEFINITION AND PATHOGENESIS

Uterine rupture refers to the complete nonsurgical disruption of all uterine layers—endometrium, myometrium, and serosa. The severity of hemorrhage and maternal-fetal morbidity depends on the extent of the rupture. A large rupture may be associated with massive hemorrhage and extrusion of the fetus and/or placenta into the maternal abdomen; whereas a small rupture may have minimal bleeding and insignificant maternal-fetal consequences. *Uterine dehiscence* refers to an incomplete or occult uterine scar separation, in which the uterine serosa remains intact. Typically, no adverse obstetric outcomes are associated with a dehiscence.

INCIDENCE AND RISK FACTORS

The overall incidence of uterine rupture (scarred and unscarred uteri) is 1 in 2000 deliveries. Uterine rupture is most common in women with a scarred uterus, including those with prior cesarean delivery and myomectomy. The incidence of uterine rupture in women with prior cesarean delivery varies from 0.3% to 1%.[82] The location of the previous hysterotomy affects the uterine rupture risk. For prior cesarean deliveries, the risk of uterine rupture is illustrated in Table 18-5.

TABLE 18-5	RISK OF UTERINE RUPTURE BASED ON INCISION OF PRIOR CESAREAN DELIVERY
INCISION OF PRIOR CESAREAN DELIVERY	**UTERINE RUPTURE RISK (%)**
Classical	2-6
T or J shaped	2-6
Low vertical	2
Low transverse	0.5-1

From Landon MB, Hauth JC, Leveno KJ, et al. Maternal and perinatal outcomes associated with a trial of labor after prior cesarean delivery. *N Engl J Med.* 2004;351(25):2581.

Although **multiple risk factors** have been associated with uterine rupture, no single factor or combination of factors can reliably predict all cases.[83] Despite this, consistent data demonstrate strong associations for TOLAC and one or more of the following: **multiple prior cesarean deliveries, no previous vaginal delivery, induced or augmented labor, term gestation, thin uterine scar identified by ultrasound, multiple gestation, fetal macrosomia, postcesarean delivery infection, single-layer closure of hysterotomy incision, and short interpregnancy interval.**[84] Uterine rupture associated with TOLAC is discussed in Chapter 20. Other reported risk factors for uterine rupture include **increasing maternal age, multiparity, fetal malpresentation, uterine manipulation** (e.g., internal podalic version), **mid- to high-operative vaginal delivery, congenital uterine malformations, Ehlers-Danlos syndrome, invasive placentation, and trauma.**[85]

CLINICAL MANIFESTATIONS AND DIAGNOSIS

Uterine rupture is associated with both fetal and maternal clinical manifestations. Fetal bradycardia with or without preceding variable or late decelerations is the most common clinical manifestation of symptomatic uterine rupture and occurs in 33% to 70% of cases.[86] In some circumstances, a **loss of fetal station in labor** may occur. **Maternal clinical manifestations** are variable and may include **acute vaginal bleeding, constant abdominal pain or uterine tenderness, change in uterine shape, cessation of contractions, hematuria** (if extension into the bladder has occurred), and **signs of hemodynamic instability.**

Uterine rupture is suspected clinically but confirmed surgically. Laparotomy will demonstrate complete disruption of the uterine wall with hemoperitoneum and partial or complete extravasation of the fetus into the maternal abdomen.

MANAGEMENT

Once the fetus and placenta are delivered, the **site of rupture should be assessed to determine whether it can be repaired. If feasible, the defect should be repaired in multiple layers with absorbable suture.** Adjacent structures (e.g., bladder and adnexa) should be assessed for damage and repaired accordingly. Hysterectomy is reserved for cases of massive hemorrhage, irreparable uterine defects, and/or maternal hemodynamic instability.

Uterine Inversion
DEFINITION AND PATHOGENESIS

Uterine inversion refers to the collapse of the fundus into the uterine cavity, and it is classified by degree and timing. **With regard to degree, uterine inversion may be first degree (incomplete), second degree (complete), third degree**

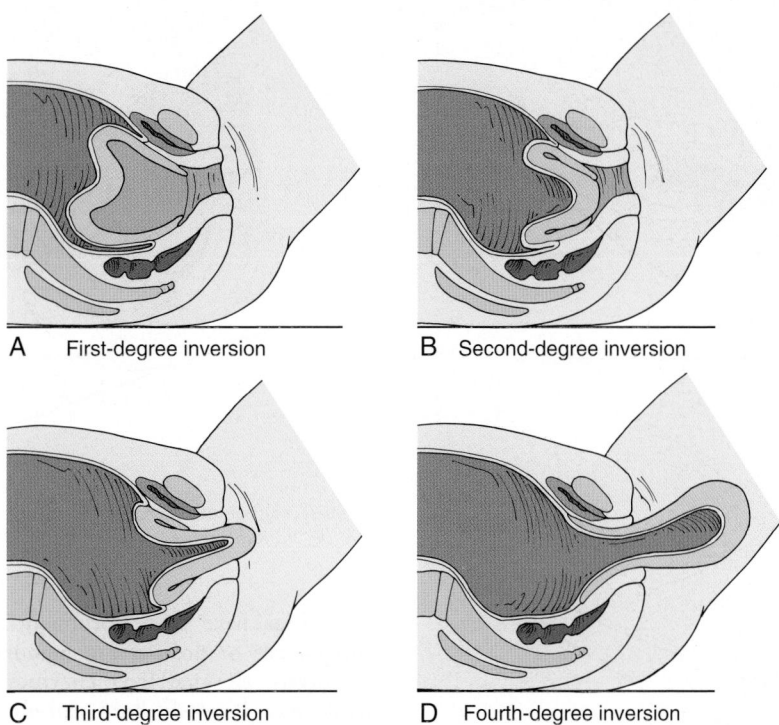

A   First-degree inversion   B   Second-degree inversion

C   Third-degree inversion   D   Fourth-degree inversion

FIG 18-29 Classification of uterine inversion. (From Repke JT. *Puerperal uterine inversion,* www.uptodate.com, Dec 8, 2004.)

(prolapsed), or fourth degree (total; Fig. 18-29). *First-degree uterine inversion* represents a partial extrusion of the fundus into the uterine cavity. In *second-degree uterine inversion,* the internal lining of the fundus crosses through the cervical os, forming a rounded mass in the vagina with no palpable fundus abdominally. *Third-degree uterine inversion* refers to the entire uterus prolapsing through the cervix with the fundus passing out of the vaginal introitus. *Fourth-degree uterine inversion* represents both total uterine and vaginal prolapse through the vaginal introitus. Uterine inversion timing is classified as *acute* **(within 24 hours of delivery),** *subacute* **(>24 hours postpartum but <4 weeks), or** *chronic* **>1 month postpartum).**

The two most commonly proposed etiologies for uterine inversion include excessive umbilical cord traction with a fundally attached placenta and fundal pressure in the setting of a relaxed uterus. However, a causal relationship between active management of the third stage of labor and uterine inversion remains unproven.

INCIDENCE AND RISK FACTORS

Uterine inversion is a rare event that complicates about 1 in 1200 to 1 in 57,000 deliveries.[87] Proposed **risk factors** include **uterine overdistention, fetal macrosomia, rapid labor and delivery, congenital uterine malformations, uterine fibroids, invasive placentation, retained placenta, short umbilical cord, use of uterine-relaxing agents, nulliparity, manual placental extraction, and Ehlers-Danlos syndrome.**[87]

CLINICAL MANIFESTATIONS AND DIAGNOSIS

The clinical presentation of uterine inversion varies by its degree and timing. Whereas incomplete uterine inversion may be subtle in its clinical findings, complete uterine inversion often presents with **brisk vaginal bleeding, inability to palpate the fundus abdominally, and maternal hemodynamic instability.** It may

occur before or after placental detachment. The diagnosis is made clinically with bimanual examination, during which the uterine fundus is palpated in the lower uterine segment or within the vagina. Sonography can be used to confirm the diagnosis if the clinical examination is unclear.[88]

MANAGEMENT

Once diagnosed, uterine inversion requires rapid intervention in order to restore maternal hemodynamic stability and control hemorrhage. Maternal fluid resuscitation through a large-bore IV catheter is recommended. The uterus must be replaced to its proper orientation to resolve the hemorrhage, which is best accomplished in an OR with the assistance of an anesthesiologist. The uterus and cervix should initially be relaxed with nitroglycerin (50 to 500 μg), a tocolytic agent (magnesium sulfate or β-mimetic), or an inhaled anesthetic. Once relaxed, gentle manual pressure is applied to the uterine fundus to return it to its proper abdominal location (Fig. 18-30). Uterotonic therapy should then be given to assist with uterine contraction and to prevent recurrence of the inversion.

If manual repositioning is unsuccessful, other options include hydrostatic reduction and surgical correction. With hydrostatic reduction, warmed sterile saline is infused into the vagina. The physician's hand or a Silastic ventouse cup is used as a fluid retainer to generate intravaginal hydrostatic pressure and resultant correction of the inversion (Fig. 18-31). Surgical options include the Huntington and Haultain procedures, laparoscopic-assisted repositioning, and cervical incisions with manual uterine repositioning.[89] The Huntington procedure involves a laparotomy with serial clamping and upward traction of the round ligaments to restore the uterus to its proper position. If this technique fails, the Haultain procedure can be attempted, which includes a vertical incision within the inversion and subsequent repositioning of the fundus. As with manual repositioning, uterotonic

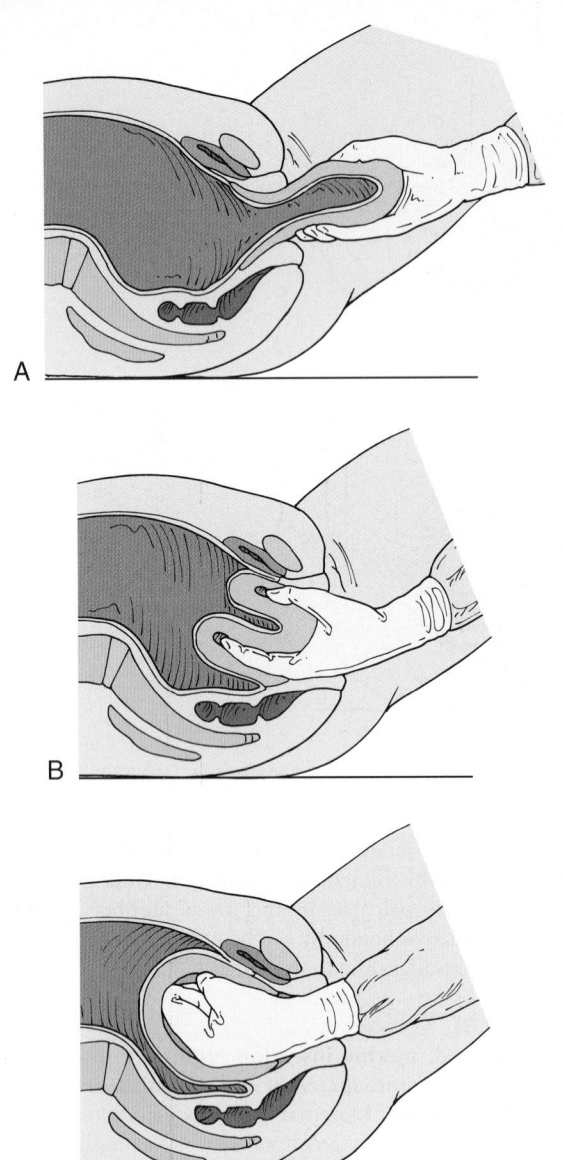

FIG 18-30 Manual replacement of uterine inversion. (From Repke JT. *Puerperal uterine inversion,* www.uptodate.com, Dec 8, 2004.)

therapy should be administered immediately after uterine replacement in order to prevent reinversion.

Coagulopathy

DEFINITION AND PATHOGENESIS

Coagulopathy represents an imbalance between the clotting and fibrinolytic systems. This imbalance may be hereditary or acquired in origin. *Hereditary coagulopathies* are relatively rare and have variable etiologies. Although *acquired coagulopathy* can be iatrogenic, such as that associated with anticoagulant administration, it is **usually the result of clotting factor consumption.** Figure 18-32 demonstrates the pathophysiology of consumptive coagulopathy and its association with hemorrhage.

INCIDENCE AND RISK FACTORS

The overall incidence of coagulopathy in the obstetric population has not been reported; however, several **associated clinical**

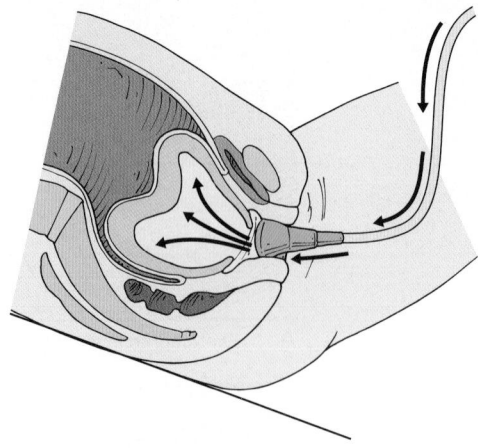

FIG 18-31 Hydrostatic reduction for uterine inversion. (From Repke JT. *Puerperal uterine inversion,* www.uptodate.com, Dec 8, 2004.)

conditions have been documented. These include **massive antepartum or postpartum hemorrhage; sepsis; severe PE; hemolysis, elevated liver enzymes, low platelets (HELLP) syndrome; amniotic fluid embolism; fetal demise; placental abruption; septic abortion; and acute fatty liver of pregnancy.**

CLINICAL MANIFESTATIONS AND DIAGNOSIS

The primary clinical manifestations of consumptive coagulopathy include bleeding, hypotension out of proportion to blood loss, microangiopathic hemolytic anemia, acute lung injury, acute renal failure, and ischemic end-organ tissue damage.

Consumptive coagulopathy is a clinical diagnosis that is confirmed with laboratory data, such as evidence of thrombocytopenia, hemolytic changes on the peripheral blood smear, decreased fibrinogen, elevated fibrin degradation products, and prolonged prothrombin time (PT) and activated partial thromboplastin time (aPTT). When timely laboratory assessment is unavailable, drawing 5 mL of maternal blood into an empty red-topped tube and watching for clot formation will provide the clinician with a rough estimate of the degree of existing coagulopathy. If a clot is not visible within 6 minutes or forms and lyses within 30 minutes, the fibrinogen level is usually less than 150 mg/dL.

MANAGEMENT

The most important factor in the successful treatment of coagulopathy is identifying and correcting the underlying etiology. For most obstetric causes, **delivery of the fetus initiates resolution of the coagulopathy.** In addition, rapid replacement of blood products and clotting factors should occur simultaneously. The patient should **have two large-bore IV catheters for fluid and blood component therapy, and laboratory studies should be drawn serially every 4 hours until resolution** of the coagulopathy is evident. The obstetrician should attempt to achieve a hematocrit greater than 21%, a platelet count greater than 50,000/mm^3, a fibrinogen level greater than 100 mg/dL, and PT and aPTT less than 1.5 times control. It also is important **to maintain adequate oxygenation and normothermia.** Finally, adjuvant therapies should be

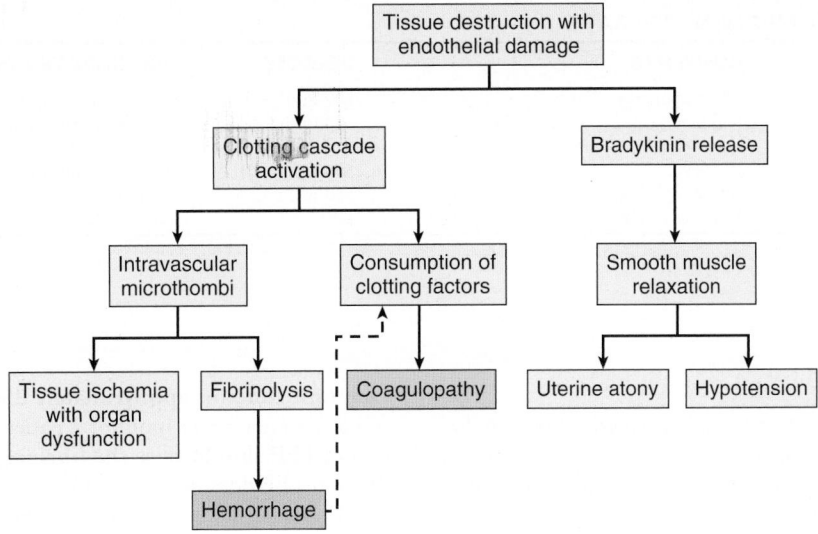

FIG 18-32 Pathophysiology and clinical manifestations of consumptive coagulopathy.

considered such as vitamin K, recombinant activated factor VII, fibrinogen concentrate, prothrombin complex concentrate, tranexamic acid, and hemostatic agents.

VITAMIN K
Factors II, VII, IX, and X are vitamin K–dependent clotting factors. In consumptive coagulopathy, these clotting factors are consumed. Administration of vitamin K (5 to 10 mg) by subcutaneous, intramuscular, or IV routes can assist with endogenous replenishment of these procoagulants.

RECOMBINANT ACTIVATED FACTOR VII
Factor VII is a precursor for the extrinsic clotting cascade. When massive procoagulant factor consumption occurs, replacement is necessary. **Human recombinant factor VIIa has been used successfully in cases of consumptive coagulopathy attributed to postpartum hemorrhage.**[90] The dosage of this IV therapy has ranged from 16.7 to 120 µg/kg.[90] An important advantage of this therapy is its rapid bioavailability (10 to 40 minutes) for reversal of coagulopathy; however, disadvantages include a relatively short half-life (2 hours), cost (approximately $1 per microgram), and thromboembolism risk. Recombinant activated factor VIIa should be considered in cases of refractory coagulopathy or when blood component replacement is delayed.

FIBRINOGEN CONCENTRATE
A human fibrinogen concentrate (RiaStap [CSL Behring]) has been approved by the U.S. Food and Drug Administration (FDA). Each vial of fibrinogen concentrate contains 900 to 1300 mg fibrinogen and 400 to 700 mg human albumin. Fibrinogen concentrate can be used alone or in combination with cryoprecipitate. It has been used successfully in Europe for the treatment of massive obstetric hemorrhage due to consumptive coagulopathy.[91]

PROTHROMBIN COMPLEX CONCENTRATE
Prothrombin complex concentrate (Kcentra [CSL Behring]) contains factors II, VII, IX, and X and proteins C and S. It can be used as an alternative to fresh frozen plasma (FFP).

Advantages to its use include no need for thawing or blood group typing and decreased risks of volume overload, transfusion-related acute lung injury (TRALI), and allergic reactions.

TRANEXAMIC ACID
Tranexamic acid is an IV antifibrinolytic drug that may be used for the prevention and treatment of hemorrhage. In a small multicenter trial, tranexamic acid reduced postpartum hemorrhage and transfusion requirements.[92]

HEMOSTATIC AGENTS
A variety of topical hemostatic agents are available for control of coagulopathic surface bleeding. These agents have different clotting factors and mechanisms of action. Examples include oxidized regenerated cellulose (e.g., Surgicel [Ethicon]), fibrin sealants (e.g., Tisseal [Baxter]), microporous polysaccharide spheres (e.g., Arista [Bard Davol]), microfibrillar collagen (e.g. Avitene [Bard Davol]), hemostatic matrices (e.g., Floseal [Baxter]), gelatin matrices (e.g., Gelfoam), and topical thrombin. These agents may be used alone or in combination.

Fluid Resuscitation and Transfusion
All obstetricians will encounter antepartum and postpartum hemorrhage. In most instances, **fluid resuscitation and blood component therapy are life-saving.** Therefore every physician should have a thorough understanding of appropriate volume resuscitation, transfusion therapy, and alternative treatment options and their risks.

Volume Resuscitation
Initial management of a hemorrhaging patient requires appropriate volume resuscitation. Two large-bore IV catheters are recommended. **Warmed crystalloid solution in a 3 : 1 ratio to the estimated blood loss should be rapidly infused.** Goals of therapy are to maintain an adequate maternal blood pressure (systolic blood pressure >90 mm Hg) and urine output (at least 30 mL/hr). If the hemorrhage is easily controlled, this may be the only therapy needed. The patient should have serial assessments of her vital signs and hematologic profiles to confirm hemodynamic stability.

TABLE 18-6   BLOOD COMPONENT THERAPY

PRODUCT	CONTENTS	VOLUME	ANTICIPATED EFFECT (PER UNIT)
Whole blood	All components	500 mL	Used only in emergencies*
Packed red blood cells	Red blood cells	300 mL	Increase hemoglobin by 1 g/dL
			Increase hematocrit by 3%
Platelets (single donor pooled)	Platelets	300 mL (6 U)	Increase platelet count by 30,000 to 60,000/mm^3
Fresh frozen plasma	All clotting factors	250 mL	Increase fibrinogen by 5-10 mg/dL
Cryoprecipitate	Fibrinogen, vWF, factors VIII and XIII	10-15 mL	Increase fibrinogen by 5-10 mg/dL

vWF, von Willebrand factor.

COLLOID SOLUTIONS

Colloid solutions contain larger particles, *colloids*, which are less permeable across vascular membranes. These solutions provide a greater increase in colloid oncotic pressure and plasma volume; however, they are more expensive than crystalloids and may be associated with anaphylactoid reactions. Examples of colloid solutions include albumin, hetastarch, and dextran.

Blood Component Therapy
WHOLE BLOOD

Whole blood contains red blood cells (RBCs), clotting factors, and platelets. Whole blood is rarely used in modern obstetrics because of its many disadvantages, including a short storage life (24 hr), large volume (500 mL per unit), and potential for hypercalcemia.

PACKED RED BLOOD CELLS

Packed red blood cells (pRBCs) are the most appropriate therapy for patients who require RBC replacement because of hemorrhage. They are the only blood product to provide oxygen-carrying capacity. **Each pRBC unit contains approximately 300 mL of volume (250 mL RBCs and 50 mL of plasma). In a 70-kg patient, one unit of pRBCs will raise the hemoglobin by 1 g/dL and the hematocrit by 3%.** Transfusion of pRBCs should be considered in any gravida with hemoglobin less than 8 g/dL or with active hemorrhage and associated coagulopathy.

PLATELET CONCENTRATES

Platelets are separated from whole blood and are stored in plasma. Because 1 unit of platelets provides an increase of only approximately 7500/mm^3, platelet concentrates of 6 to 10 units need to be transfused. Platelet concentrates can be derived from multiple donors or single donors. The single-donor concentrates are preferred because they expose the patient to fewer potential antigenic and immunologic risks. Transfusion of a single-donor platelet concentrate will increase the circulating platelet count by 30,000 to 60,000/mm^3. Because sensitization can occur, it is important for platelets to be ABO and Rh specific. **Transfusion of platelets should be considered when the platelet count is less than 20,000/mm^3 after a vaginal delivery or less than 50,000/mm^3 after a cesarean delivery, or when coagulopathy is evident.**

FRESH FROZEN PLASMA

FFP is plasma that is extracted from whole blood. FFP primarily contains fibrinogen, antithrombin, and clotting factors V, XI, and XII. Transfusing FFP not only assists with coagulation but also provides the patient with volume resuscitation because each unit contains approximately 250 mL. Typically, fibrinogen levels are used to monitor a patient's response to FFP. Each unit of **FFP should raise the fibrinogen level by 5 to 10 mg/dL, and FFP does not need to be ABO or Rh compatible. FFP should be considered for hemorrhaging patients with evidence of consumptive coagulopathy, coagulopathic liver disease, and for warfarin reversal.**

CRYOPRECIPITATE

Cryoprecipitate is the precipitate that results from thawed FFP. It is rich in fibrinogen, von Willebrand factor, and factors VIII and XIII. Like FFP, **cryoprecipitate can be measured clinically by the fibrinogen response, which should increase by 5 to 10 mg/dL per unit. Unlike FFP, each unit of cryoprecipitate provides minimal volume (10 to 15 mL),** so it is an ineffective agent for volume resuscitation. Cryoprecipitate is indicated for patients with coagulopathy and concerns of volume overload, hypofibrinogenemia, factor VIII deficiency, and von Willebrand disease.

Table 18-6 contains a summary of the available blood component therapies.

MASSIVE TRANSFUSION PROTOCOLS

Although no universally accepted guidelines exist for blood product replacement, expert opinion derived from trauma and military experience suggests that more aggressive replacement of coagulation factors with pRBCs improves outcomes and survival.[93-95] A variety of protocols have been recommended, most of which aim for an equal ratio of pRBCs, FFP, and platelets. **A commonly adopted massive transfusion protocol is 6 units of pRBCs to 4 units of FFP to 1 unit of platelet concentrate (6:4:1).**[93] Some centers have added **6 to 10 units of cryoprecipitate** to this regimen.

TRANSFUSION RISKS AND REACTIONS
METABOLIC ABNORMALITIES AND HYPOTHERMIA

When pRBCs are stored, leakage of potassium and ammonia can occur into the plasma. This may result in hyperkalemia and high ammonia concentrations in patients who require massive transfusion. In addition, because most pRBC units are stored in a citrate solution, hypocalcemia may occur. Serial assessments of metabolic profiles with ionized calcium levels can assist the clinician in managing these changes.

In addition to metabolic abnormalities, hypothermia may complicate the clinical course of massive transfusion and result in cardiac arrhythmias. Hypothermia can be prevented by warming pRBC units before transfusion and by providing alternative heating devices to the patient (e.g., Bair Hugger anesthesia warmer [3M]).

TABLE 18-7 TRANSFUSION-RELATED
INFECTION RISKS

INFECTION	TRANSMISSION RISK
HIV-1, HIV-2	1 in 1.4-4.7 million
Hepatitis B	1 in 100,000-400,000
Hepatitis C	1 in 1.6 to 3.1 million
HTLV-I and -II	1 in 500,000 to 3 million
Bacterial contamination:	
Red blood cells	1 in 28,000-143,000
Platelets	1 in 2000-8000

From Hall NR, Martin SR. Transfusion of blood components and derivatives in the obstetric intensive care patient. In: Foley MR, Strong TH Jr, Garite TJ, eds: *Obstetric Intensive Care Manual,* 4th ed. New York: McGraw-Hill; 2014.
HIV, human immunodeficiency virus; *HTLV,* human T-cell lymphotropic virus.

IMMUNOLOGIC REACTIONS

Transfusions introduce interactions between inherited or acquired antibodies and the foreign antigens of the transfused blood products; the most common immunologic reactions are febrile nonhemolytic transfusion reactions. Cytokines are believed to be the primary cause of these reactions. Retrospective cohort studies suggest that transfusion of leukoreduced blood products may decrease the frequency of these reactions; however, randomized controlled trial (RCT) data are limited. Less common immunologic complications include acute or delayed hemolytic transfusion reactions, anaphylaxis, urticarial reactions, posttransfusion purpura, and graft-versus-host disease.

INFECTION RISKS

All blood products have the potential to transmit viral and bacterial infections. Although transmission rates have substantially decreased in the past two decades, they are still a potential risk that must be disclosed when a transfusion is needed. Table 18-7 lists current transfusion-associated infection risks.[96]

TRANSFUSION-ASSOCIATED VOLUME/CIRCULATORY OVERLOAD AND TRANSFUSION-RELATED ACUTE LUNG INJURY

Transfusion-associated volume/circulatory overload (TACO) refers to pulmonary edema that results from excessively large infusions of fluids and blood products. Symptoms include dyspnea, orthopnea, tachycardia, wide pulse pressure, hypertension, and hypoxemia. TACO typically is associated with elevated brain natriuretic peptide (BNP), central venous pressure, and pulmonary artery wedge pressure. TACO is usually treated with diuresis and supplemental oxygen.

Transfusion-related acute lung injury (TRALI) refers to a rare but potentially life-threatening form of acute lung injury that can result from blood product administration. TRALI is thought to result from a "two-hit" mechanism that involves neutrophil sequestration/priming and activation.[97] TRALI is characterized by sudden onset of hypoxemic respiratory insufficiency during or within 6 hours of blood product administration. Additional findings include noncardiogenic pulmonary edema, hypotension, fever, tachypnea, tachycardia, and cyanosis. Treatment is twofold and includes transfusion discontinuation and supportive care with oxygen administration, ventilatory support (continuous positive airway pressure [CPAP], bilevel positive airway pressure [BiPAP], or mechanical ventilation), hemodynamic stabilization (fluid resuscitation and/or vasoactive agents), and possible steroid administration.

Blood Conservation Approaches
Preoperative Autologous Blood Donation and Transfusion

Preoperative autologous blood donation and transfusion refers to the collection of the patient's own RBCs prior to surgery and reinfusion of those cells intraoperatively or postoperatively. Although it is unreasonable to have all pregnant individuals consider autologous blood donation, patients at high risk for transfusion (e.g., those with placenta previa or placenta accreta) may be good candidates. Guidelines for autologous blood donation include a minimum predonation hemoglobin of 11 g/dL, first donation within 6 weeks of anticipated delivery (because of the pRBC storage life of 42 days), a week-long interval between donations, and no donation within 2 weeks of anticipated delivery.[96]

Autologous transfusion should be used selectively. Not only is it significantly more expensive than homologous transfusion, but also the risks for bacterial contamination and subsequent homologous transfusion are not completely eliminated.

Acute Normovolemic Hemodilution

Acute normovolemic hemodilution refers to a blood conservation technique in which blood is removed from the patient preoperatively and is replaced by a crystalloid or colloid solution to maintain normovolemia. During surgery, the blood loss is diluted. The patient is reinfused with her more concentrated blood postoperatively. Acute normovolemic hemodilution can be considered for patients with good initial hemoglobin concentrations who are expected to have a blood loss of at least 1000 mL during surgery (e.g., placenta accreta).

Intraoperative Blood Salvage

Intraoperative blood salvage refers to collecting the patient's blood during surgery, filtering the blood, and then reinfusing the red cells back to the patient. Cell-Saver technology is the most widely used blood-salvage system. In the past, theoretic concerns regarding the risks for infection and amniotic fluid embolism limited the use of blood-salvage technology in obstetrics; however, **several studies have documented its safety and effectivenes.**[98] Intraoperative blood salvage has many advantages over homologous transfusion. It eliminates the risk for infectious disease transmission, alloimmunization, and immunologic transfusion reactions. It is a cost-effective procedure that avoids wastage of blood and thereby reduces the need for homologous transfusion. In addition, it can rapidly provide the patient with RBCs (1 unit of pRBCs per 3-minute interval). Finally, many Jehovah's Witnesses will accept intraoperative blood salvage because the blood remains in a continuous circuit and does not leave the OR.

Alternative Oxygen Carriers

Because some patients refuse to accept blood products (e.g., Jehovah's Witnesses) or are unable to be transfused owing to a lack of blood compatibility, oxygen carriers have been developed as alternatives to transfusion therapy. The two primary products are hemoglobin-based oxygen carriers and perfluorocarbons. Hemoglobin-based oxygen carriers use hemoglobin derived from animals or outdated human blood. The hemoglobin is separated from the red cell stroma and undergoes multiple filtration and polymerization processes before use. Perfluorocarbons are inert compounds that can dissolve gases, including oxygen.

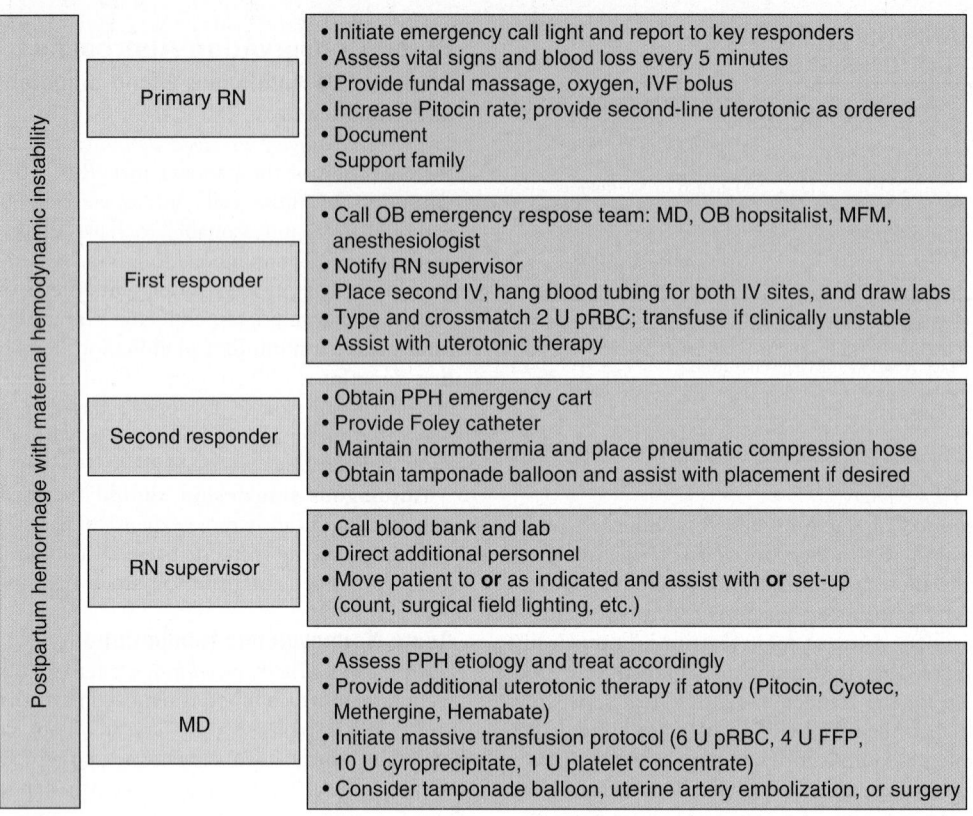

Postpartum hemorrhage with maternal hemodynamic instability

Primary RN
- Initiate emergency call light and report to key responders
- Assess vital signs and blood loss every 5 minutes
- Provide fundal massage, oxygen, IVF bolus
- Increase Pitocin rate; provide second-line uterotonic as ordered
- Document
- Support family

First responder
- Call OB emergency respose team: MD, OB hopsitalist, MFM, anesthesiologist
- Notify RN supervisor
- Place second IV, hang blood tubing for both IV sites, and draw labs
- Type and crossmatch 2 U pRBC; transfuse if clinically unstable
- Assist with uterotonic therapy

Second responder
- Obtain PPH emergency cart
- Provide Foley catheter
- Maintain normothermia and place pneumatic compression hose
- Obtain tamponade balloon and assist with placement if desired

RN supervisor
- Call blood bank and lab
- Direct additional personnel
- Move patient to **or** as indicated and assist with **or** set-up (count, surgical field lighting, etc.)

MD
- Assess PPH etiology and treat accordingly
- Provide additional uterotonic therapy if atony (Pitocin, Cyotec, Methergine, Hemabate)
- Initiate massive transfusion protocol (6 U pRBC, 4 U FFP, 10 U cyroprecipitate, 1 U platelet concentrate)
- Consider tamponade balloon, uterine artery embolization, or surgery

FIG 18-33 Postpartum hemorrhage treatment protocol. FFP, fresh frozen plasma; IV, intravenous; IVF, intravenous fluids; MD, physician; MFM, maternal-fetal medicine; OB, obstetric; PPH, postpartum hemorrhage; pRBC, packed red blood cells; RN, registered nurse. (Courtesy K. Francois.)

Both products have high oxygen-carrying capacities. Unfortunately, cost, supply problems, lack of FDA approval, and poor side-effect profiles have limited the usefulness of these agents.

Hemorrhage Prevention and Protocols

Because obstetric hemorrhage is such a widespread problem, it is important for institutions to develop standardized management protocols and to conduct hemorrhage drills. Multiple organizations have developed guidelines for the diagnosis, management, and prevention of postpartum hemorrhage. The use of obstetric rapid response teams, massive transfusion protocols, and prescriptive checklists is vital to program success. In addition, simulation-based teaching models have been helpful to identify knowledge deficits, improve accuracy of blood loss estimation, and instill provider confidence in the clinical management of postpartum hemorrhage.[99-102] Figure 18-33 provides a modified postpartum hemorrhage treatment protocol from the author's institution.

KEY POINTS

- Hemorrhage is a major cause of obstetric morbidity and mortality throughout the world. It is responsible for one third of all pregnancy-related deaths in both high- and low-income countries.
- Understanding the hemodynamic changes of pregnancy and the physiologic responses that occur with hemorrhage assists in appropriate management. Clinicians should recognize the four classes of hemorrhage to allow for rapid intervention.

- Placental abruption is diagnosed primarily by clinical findings and is confirmed by radiographic, laboratory, and pathologic studies. Management of placental abruption is dependent on the severity, gestational age, and maternal-fetal status.
- Placenta previa is typically diagnosed with sonography. Placenta previa remote from term can be expectantly managed, and outpatient management is possible in selected cases.
- Placenta previa in association with a prior cesarean delivery is a major risk factor for placenta accreta. Additional radiographic surveillance should be attempted in these cases to provide antenatal diagnosis of placenta accreta.
- Placenta accreta is best managed with a multidisciplinary approach that includes maternal-fetal medicine specialists, neonatologists, blood-conservation teams, anesthesiologists, advanced pelvic surgeons, and urologists. Scheduled preterm delivery at 34 to 35 weeks of gestation is recommended.
- Antenatal detection of vasa previa is possible with sonography and significantly improves perinatal outcomes.
- Postpartum hemorrhage complicates 1 in 20 to 1 in 100 deliveries. Every obstetrician and birth attendant needs to have a thorough understanding of normal delivery-related blood loss in order to recognize postpartum hemorrhage.
- Management of uterine atony should follow a rapidly initiated sequenced protocol that may include bimanual

massage, uterotonic therapy, uterine tamponade, selective arterial embolization, or surgical intervention.
- Coagulopathy mandates treatment of the initiating event and rapid replacement of consumed blood products. Transfusion of blood components should not be delayed, and replacement protocols should be followed.
- Blood conservation approaches should be considered if clinically appropriate.
- Standardized obstetric hemorrhage management protocols, checklists, and drills have been shown to improve outcomes.

REFERENCES

1. Prata N, Gerdts C. Measurement of postpartum blood loss. *BMJ.* 2010;340:c555.
2. Melamed N, Aviram A, Sliver M, et al. Pregnancy course and outcome following blunt trauma. *J Matern Fetal Neonatal Med.* 2012;25(9):1612-1617.
3. Anath CV, Getahun D, Peltier MR, et al. Placental abruption in term and preterm gestations: evidence for heterogeneity in clinical pathways. *Obstet Gynecol.* 2006;107(4):785.
4. Anath CV, Oyelese Y, Prasas V, et al. Evidence of placental abruption as a chronic process: associations with vaginal bleeding in pregnancy and placental lesions. *Eur J Obstet Gynecol Reprod Biol.* 2006;128(1-2):15.
5. Elsasser DA, Anath CV, Prasad V, et al. Diagnosis of placental abruption: relationship between clinical and histopathological findings. *Eur J Obstet Gynecol Reprod Biol.* 2010;148(2):125-130.
6. Avagliano L, Bulfamante GP, Morabito A, et al. Abnormal spiral artery remodeling in the decidual segment during pregnancy: from histology to clinical correlation. *J Clin Pathol.* 2011;64(12):1064-1068.
7. Buhimschi CS, Schatz F, Krikun G, et al. Novel insights into molecular mechanisms of abruption-induced preterm birth. *Expert Rev Mol Med.* 2010;12:e35.
8. Thachil J, Toh CH. Disseminated intravascular coagulation in obstetric disorders and its acute haematological management. *Blood Rev.* 2009;23(4):167.
9. Lockwood CJ, Kayisli UA, Stocco C, et al. Abruption-induced preterm delivery is associated with thrombin-mediated functional progesterone withdrawal in decidual cells. *Am J Pathol.* 2012;181(6):2138.
10. Tikkanen M. Placental abruption: epidemiology, risk factors and consequences. *Acta Obstet Gynecol Scand.* 2011;90(2):140-149.
11. Parienta G, Wiznitzer A, Sergienko R, et al. Placental abruption: clinical analysis of risk factors and perinatal outcomes. *J Matern Fetal Neonatal Med.* 2011;24(5):698-702.
12. Oyelese Y, Ananth CV. Placental abruption. *Obstet Gynecol.* 2006;108:1005.
13. Ananth CV, Peltier MR, Kinzler WL, et al. Chronic hypertension and risk of placental abruption: is the association modified by ischemic placental disease? *Am J Obstet Gynecol.* 2007;197:273.
14. Harris CM. Trauma and pregnancy. In: Foley MR, Strong TH Jr, Garite TJ, eds. *Obstetric Intensive Care Manual.* 4th ed. New York: McGraw-Hill; 2014:230.
15. Breathnach FM, Donnelly J, Cooley SM, et al. Subclinical hypothyroidism as a risk factor for placental abruption: evidence from a low-risk primigravid population. *Aust N Z J Obstet Gynaecol.* 2013;53(6):553.
16. Mendola P, Luaghon SK, Mannisto TI, et al. Obstetric complications among women with asthma. *Am J Obstet Gynecol.* 2013;208(2):127.e1.
17. Jackson S, Fleege L, Fridman M, et al. Morbidity following primary cesarean delivery in Danish National Birth Cohort. *Am J Obstet Gynecol.* 2012;206(2):139.e1.
18. Tikkanen M, Hamalainen E, Nuutila M, et al. Elevated maternal second-trimester serum alpha-fetoprotein as a risk factor for placental abruption. *Prenat Diagn.* 2007;27:240.
19. Tikkanen M, Nuutila M, Hiilesmaa V, et al. Pregnancy risk factors for placental abruption. *Acta Obstet Gynecol Scand.* 2006;85(1):40.
20. Said JM, Higgins JR, Moses EK, et al. Inherited thrombophilia polymorphisms and pregnancy outcomes in nulliparous women. *Obstet Gynecol.* 2010;115(1):5.
21. Silver RM, Zhao Y, Spong CY, et al. Prothrombin gene G20210A mutation and obstetric complications. *Obstet Gynecol.* 2010;115(4):14.
22. Spong CY, Merceer BM, D'Alton M, et al. Timing of indicated late-preterm and early-term birth. *Obstet Gynecol.* 2011;188(2 Pt1):323.
23. Masselli G, Brunelli R, Di Tola M, et al. MR imaging in the evaluation of placental abruption: correlation with sonographic findings. *Radiology.* 2011;259(1):222.
24. Linduska N, Dekan S, Messerschmidt A, et al. Placental pathologies in fetal MRI with pathohistological correlation. *Placenta.* 2009;30(6):555.
25. Blumenfeld YJ, Baar RJ, Druzin ML, et al. Association between maternal characteristics, abnormal serum aneuploidy analytes, and placental abruption. *Am J Obstet Gynecol.* 2014;211(2):144.e1.
26. Neilson JP. Interventions for treating placental abruption. *Cochrane Database Syst Rev.* 2012.
27. Reddy UM, Abuhamad AZ, Levine D, et al. Executive summary of a joint Eunice Kennedy Shriver National Institute of Child Health and Human Development, Society of Maternal-Fetal Medicine, American Institute of Ultrasound in Medicine, American College of Obstetricians and Gynecologists, American College of Radiology, Society for Pediatric Radiology, and Society of Radiologists in Ultrasound Fetal Imaging Workshop. *Obstet Gynecol.* 2014;123(5):1070.
28. Magann EF, Doherty DA, Turner K. Second trimester placental location as a predictor of an adverse pregnancy outcome. *J Perinatol.* 2007;27:9.
29. Oyelese Y, Smulian JC. Placenta previa, placenta accreta, and vasa previa. *Obstet Gynecol.* 2006;107(4):927.
30. Lockwood CJ, Russa-Stieglitz K. *Clinical features, diagnosis, and course of placenta previa.* Available at: <http://www.uptodate.com>.
31. Abenhaim HA, Azoulay L, Kramer MS. Incidence and risk factors of amniotic fluid embolisms: a population-based study on 3 million births in the United States. *Am J Obstet Gynecol.* 2008;199:49.e1-49.e8.
32. Yang Q, Wu Wen S, Caughey S. Placenta previa: its relationship with race and the country of origin among Asian women. *Acta Obstet Gynecol Scand.* 2008;87:612.
33. Rosenberg T, Pariente G, Sergienko R, et al. Critical analysis of risk factors and outcome of placenta previa. *Arch Gynecol Obstet.* 2011;284(1):47.
34. Francois K, Johnson J, Harris C. Is placenta previa more common in multiple gestations? *Am J Obstet Gynecol.* 2003;188:1226.
35. Silver RM, Landon MB, Rouse DJ, et al. Maternal morbidity associated with multiple repeat cesarean deliveries. *Obstet Gynecol.* 2006;107:1226.
36. Gurol-Urganci I, Cromwell DA, Edozien LC, et al. Risk of placenta previa in second birth after first birth cesarean section: a population-based study and meta-analysis. *BMC Pregnancy Childbirth.* 2011;11:95.
37. *National Institutes of Health Consensus Development Conference Statement: NIH Consensus Development Conference. Vaginal Birth After Cesarean: New Insights.* March 8-10, 2010.
38. Watanabe N, Suzuki T, Ogawa K, et al. Five-year study assessing the feasibility and safety of autologous blood transfusion in pregnant Japanese women. *J Obstet Gynaecol Res.* 2011;37(12):1773.
39. Yamamoto Y, Yamashita T, Tsuno NH, et al. Safety and efficacy of preoperative autologous blood donation for high-risk pregnant women: experience of a large university hospital in Japan. *J Obstet Gynaecol Res.* 2014;40(5):1308.
40. Vergani P, Ornaghi S, Pozzi I, et al. Placenta previa: distance to internal os and mode of delivery. *Am J Obstet Gynecol.* 2009;201(3):266.
41. Kato S, Tanabe A, Kanki K, et al. Local injection of vasopressin reduces the blood loss during cesarean section in placenta previa. *J Obstet Gynaecol Res.* 2014;40(5):1249-1256.
42. Nageotte MP. Always be vigilant for placenta accreta. *Am J Obstet Gynecol.* 2014;211(2):87.
43. Timor-Tritsch IE, Monteagudo A, Cali G, et al. Cesarean scar pregnancy is a precursor of morbidly adherent placenta. *Ultrasound Obstet Gynecol.* 2014;44(3):346.
44. Warshak CR, Ramos GA, Eskander R, et al. Effect of predelivery diagnosis in 99 consecutive cases of placenta accrete. *Obstet Gynecol.* 2010;115:65.
45. Bowman ZS, Eller AG, Kennedy AM, et al. Accuracy of ultrasound for the prediction of placenta accreta. *Am J Obstet Gynecol.* 2014;211(2):177.
46. D'Antonio F, Iacovella C, Bhide A. Prenatal identification of invasive placentation using ultrasound: systemic review and meta-analysis. *Ultrasound Obstet Gynecol.* 2013;42(5):509.
47. Chou MM, Ho ES, Lee YH. Prenatal diagnosis of placenta previa accreta by transabdominal color Doppler ultrasound. *Ultrasound Obstet Gynecol.* 2000;15:28.
48. Shih JC, Palacios-Jaraquemada JM, Su YN, et al. Role of three-dimensional power Doppler in the antenatal diagnosis of placenta accreta: comparison

with gray-scale and color Doppler techniques. *Ultrasound Obstet Gynecol.* 2009;33(2):193.

49. Cai G, Giambanco L, Puccio G, et al. Morbidly adherent placenta: evaluation of ultrasound diagnostic criteria and differentiation of placenta accreta from percreta. *Ultrasound Obstet Gynecol.* 2013;41(4):406.

50. D'Antonio F, Iacovella C, Palacios-Jaraquemada JM, et al. Prenatal identification of invasive placentation using magnetic resonance imaging: systemic review and meta-analysis. *Ultrasound Obstet Gynecol.* 2014; 44(1):8.

51. Resnick R. *Clinical features and diagnosis of placenta accreta, increta, and percreta.* Available at: <http://www.uptodate.com>.

52. Glaze S, Ekwalanga P, Roberts G, et al. Peripartum hysterectomy: 1999 to 2006. *Obstet Gynecol.* 2008;111:732.

53. Ballas J, Hull AD, Saenz C, et al. Preoperative intravascular balloon catheters and surgical outcomes in pregnancies complicated by placenta accreta: a management paradox. *Am J Obstet Gynecol.* 2012;207(3):216.

54. Steins-Bisschop CN, Schaap TP, Vogelvang TE, et al. Invasive placentation and uterus-preserving treatment modalities: a systemic review. *Arch Gynecol Obstet.* 2011;284(2):491.

55. Sentilhes L, Ambroselli C, Kayem G, et al. Maternal outcome after conservative treatment of placenta accreta. *Obstet Gynecol.* 2011;115:526.

56. Sentilhes L, Kayem G, Ambroselli C, et al. Fertility and pregnancy outcomes following conservative treatment for placenta accreta. *Hum Reprod.* 2010;25(11):2803.

57. Provansal M, Courbiere B, Agostini A, et al. Fertility and obstetric outcome after conservative management of placenta accreta. *Int J Gynaecol Obstet.* 2011;09(2):147.

58. Eshkoli T, Weintraub AY, Sergienko R, et al. Placenta accreta: risk factors, perinatal outcomes, and consequences for subsequent births. *Am J Obstet Gynecol.* 2013;208(3):219.

59. Bronsteen R, Hitten A, Balasubramanian M, et al. Vasa previa: clinical presentations, outcomes, and implications for management. *Obstet Gynecol.* 2013;122(2Pt1):352.

60. Baulies S, Maiz N, Muñoz A, et al. Prenatal ultrasound diagnosis of vasa previa and analysis of risk factors. *Prenat Diagn.* 2007;27(7):595.

61. Hasegawa J, Farina A, Nakamura M, et al. Analysis of the Ultrasonographic findings predictive of vasa previa. *Prenat Diagn.* 2010;30(12-13): 1121.

62. Gagnon R, Morin L, Bly S, et al. Guidelines for the management of vasa previa. *J Obstet Gynaecol Can.* 2009;31:748.

63. Robinson BK, Grobman WA. Effectiveness of timing strategies for delivery of individuals with vasa previa. *Obstet Gynecol.* 2011;177(3):542.

64. Callaghan WM, Kuklina EV, Berg CJ. Trends in postpartum hemorrhage: United States, 1994-2006. *Am J Obstet Gynecol.* 2010;202(4):353.

65. Stafford I, Dildy GA, Clark SL. Visually estimated and calculated blood loss in vaginal and cesarean delivery. *Am J Obstet Gynecol.* 2008;199:519.

66. Begely CM, Gyte GM, Devane D, McGuire W, Weeks A. Active versus expectant management for women in the third stage of labour. *Cochrane Database Syst Rev.* 2011;(11):CD007412.

67. Westhoff G, Cotter AM, Tolosa JE. Prophylactic oxytocin for the third stage of labour to prevent postpartum hemorrhage. *Cochrane Database Syst Rev.* 2013;(10):CD0001808.

68. Sheehan SR, Montgomery AA, Carey M, et al. Oxytocin bolus versus oxytocin bolus and infusion for control of blood loss after elective cesarean section: double blind placebo controlled randomized trial. *BMJ.* 2011;343: d4661.

69. Dahlke JD, Mendez-Figueroa H, Rouse DJ, et al. Evidence-based surgery for cesarean delivery: an updated systemic review. *Am J Obstet Gynecol.* 2013;209(4):294.

70. Tita AT, Szychowski JM, Rouse DJ, et al. Higher-dose oxytocin and hemorrhage after vaginal delivery: a randomized controlled trial. *Obstet Gynecol.* 2012;119(2Pt1):293.

71. Hofmeyr GJ, Gulmezoglu AM, Novikova N, et al. Misoprostol to prevent and treat postpartum haemorrhage: a systematic review and meta-analysis of maternal deaths and dose-related effects. *Bull World Health Org.* 2009;87:666.

72. Tang J, Kapp N, Dragoman M, et al. WHO recommendations for misoprostol use for obstetric and gynecologic indications. *Int J Gynaecol Obstet.* 2013;121(2):186.

73. Tuncalp O, Hofmeyr GJ, Gulmezoglu AM. Prostaglandins for preventing postpartum hemorrhage. *Cochrane Database Syst Rev.* 2012;(8):CD000494.

74. Schmid BC, Rezniczek GA, Rolf N, et al. Uterine packing with chitosan-covered gauze for control of postpartum hemorrhage. *Am J Obstet Gynecol.* 2013;209(3):225.

75. Dildy GA, Belfort MA, Adair CD, et al. Initial experience with a dual-balloon catheter for the management of postpartum hemorrhage. *Am J Obstet Gynecol.* 2014;210(2):136.

76. Sentilhes L, Gromez A, Clavier E, et al. Predictors of failed pelvic arterial embolization for severe postpartum hemorrhage. *Obstet Gynecol.* 2009; 113:992.

77. Kayem G, Kurinczuk JJ, Alfirevic Z, et al. Uterine compression sutures for the management of severe postpartum hemorrhage. *Obstet Gynecol.* 2011;117(1):14.

78. Ghezzi F, Cromi A, Uccella S, et al. The Hayman technique: a simple method to treat postpartum haemorrhage. *BJOG.* 2007;114:362.

79. Nelson WL, O'Brien JM. The uterine sandwich for persistent uterine atony: combining the B-Lynch compression suture and an intrauterine Bakri balloon. *Am J Obstet Gynecol.* 2007;196(5):e9.

80. Wright JD, Bonanno C, Shah M, et al. Peripartum hysterectomy. *Obstet Gynecol.* 2010;116:429.

81. Lousquy R, Morel O, Soyer P, et al. Routine use of abdominopelvic ultrasonography in severe postpartum hemorrhage: retrospective evaluation of 125 patients. *Am J Obstet Gynecol.* 2011;104(3):232e1.

82. National Institutes of Health Consensus Development Conference Panel. National Institutes of Health Consensus Development conference statement: vaginal birth after cesarean: new insights March 8-10, 2010. *Obstet Gynecol.* 2010;115(6):1279.

83. Grobman WA, Lai Y, Landon MB, et al. Prediction of uterine rupture associated with attempted vaginal birth after cesarean delivery. *Am J Obstet Gynecol.* 2008;199:30.e1-30.e5.

84. Mercer BM, Gilbert S, Landon MB, et al. Labor outcomes with increasing number of prior vaginal births after cesarean delivery. *Obstet Gynecol.* 2008;111:285.

85. Walsh CA, Baxi LV. Rupture of the primigravid uterus: a review of the literature. *Obstet Gynecol Surv.* 2007;62:327.

86. Zwart JJ, Richters JM, Ory F, et al. Uterine rupture in the Netherlands: a nationwide population-based cohort study. *BJOG.* 2009;116:1069.

87. Witteveen T, van Stralen G, Zwart J, et al. Puerperal uterine inversion in the Netherlands: a nationwide cohort study. *Acta Obstet Gynecol Scand.* 2013;92(3):334.

88. Pethani NR, et al. Sonography of postpartum uterine inversion from acute to chronic stage. *J Clin Ultrasound.* 2009;37(1):53.

89. Sardeshpande NS, Sawant RM, Sardeshpande SN, et al. Laparoscopic correction of chronic uterine inversion. *J Minim Invasive Gynecol.* 2009; 16:646.

90. Phillips LE, McLintock C, Pollack W, et al. Recombinant factor VII in obstetric hemorrhage: experiences from Australian and New Zealand Haemostasis Registry. *Anesth Analg.* 2009;109(6):1908.

91. Ahmed S, Harrity C, Johnson S, et al. The efficacy of fibrinogen concentrate compared with cryoprecipitate in major obstetric haemorrhage: an observational study. *Transfus Med.* 2012;22(5):344.

92. Ducloy-Bouthors AS, Jude B, Duhamel A, et al. High-dose Tranexamic acid reduces blood loss in postpartum hemorrhage. *Crit Care.* 2011;15(2): R117.

93. Burtelow M, Riley E, Druzin M, et al. How we treat: management of life-threatening primary postpartum hemorrhage with a standardized massive transfusion protocol. *Transfusion.* 2007;47:1564.

94. Holcomb JB, Wade CE, Michalek JE, et al. Increased plasma and platelet to red blood cell ratios improves outcome in 466 massively transfused civilian trauma patients. *Ann Surg.* 2008;24:447.

95. Shaz BH, Dente CJ, Nicholas J, et al. Increased number of coagulation products in relationship to red blood cell products transfused improves mortality in trauma patients. *Transfusion.* 2010;50:493.

96. Hall NR, Martin SR. Transfusion of blood components and derivatives in the obstetric intensive care patient. In: Foley MR, Strong TH Jr, Garite TJ, eds. *Obstetric Intensive Care Manual.* 4th ed. New York: McGraw-Hill; 2014:15-27.

97. Bux J, Sachs UJ. The pathogenesis of transfusion-related acute lung injury (TRALI). *Br J Haematol.* 2007;136(6):788.

98. Elagamy A, Abdelaziz A, Ellaithy M. The use of cell salvage in women undergoing cesarean hysterectomy for abnormal placentation. *Int J Obstet Anesth.* 2013;22(4):289.

99. Maslovitz S, Barkai G, Lessing JB, et al. Recurrent obstetric management mistakes identified by simulation. *Obstet Gynecol.* 2007;109(6):1295.

100. Deering SH, Chinn M, Hodor J, et al. Use of postpartum hemorrhage simulator for instruction and evaluation of residents. *J Grad Med Educ.* 2009;1(2):260.

101. Zuckerwise LC, Pettker CM, Illuzzi J, et al. Use of a novel visual aid to improve estimation of obstetric blood loss. *Obstet Gynecol.* 2014;123(5):982.

102. Birch L, Jones N, Doyle PM, et al. Obstetric skills drills: evaluation of teaching models. *Nurse Educ Today.* 2007;27(8):915.

Additional references for this chapter are available at ExpertConsult.com.

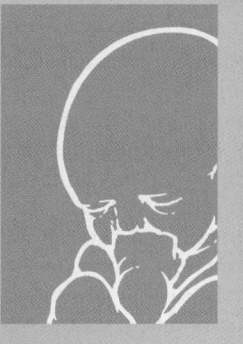

CHAPTER 19

Cesarean Delivery

VINCENZO BERGHELLA, A. DHANYA MACKEEN, and ERIC R.M. JAUNIAUX

KEY ABBREVIATIONS

American College of Obstetricians and Gynecologists	ACOG
Cephalopelvic disproportion	CPD
Cesarean delivery	CD
Computed tomography	CT
Delayed cord clamping	DCC
Deep venous thrombosis	DVT
Fetal heart rate	FHR
Hypoxic-ischemic encephalopathy	HIE
National Institutes of Health	NIH
Pulmonary embolism	PE
Randomized controlled trial	RCT
Relative risk	RR
Trial of labor after cesarean	TOLAC
Vaginal birth after cesarean	VBAC
Venous thromboembolism	VTE

DEFINITIONS

Cesarean delivery (CD) is defined as birth of a fetus from the uterus through an abdominal incision.[1] The terms *cesarean delivery* or *cesarean birth* are preferred as opposed to *cesarean section*. *Primary cesarean* refers to a CD done in a woman without a prior cesarean birth, whereas *repeat cesarean* refers to a CD done in a woman who had a cesarean birth in a previous pregnancy.[1] This chapter reviews the history, incidence, indications, techniques, and complications of CD as well as tubal sterilization.

HISTORY OF CESAREAN DELIVERY

CD has been described since ancient times, and evidence exists from both early Western and non-Western societies of this surgical procedure being performed.[2] The evolution of the term *cesarean* has been debated over time. Although originally believed to have been derived from the birth of Julius Caesar, it is unlikely that his mother, Aurelia, would have survived the operation; her knowledge of her son's invasion of Europe many years later indicates that she survived childbirth. In Caesar's time, surgical delivery was reserved for when the mother was dead or dying. Roman law under Numa Pompilius the first ("Lex Regia"), then renamed after Caesar ("Lex Cesarea"), specified surgical removal of the fetus before burial of the deceased pregnant woman; religious edicts required separate burial for the infant and mother. The term *cesarean* may also refer to patients being cut open, because the Latin verb *caedare* means to cut. *Cesarean operation* was the preferred term before the 1598 publication of Guillimeau, who introduced the term *section*.

Although sporadic reports of heroic life-saving efforts through cesarean childbirth existed for hundreds of years, it was not until the latter part of the nineteenth century that the operation became established as part of obstetric practice. This coincided with the gradual transition of childbirth as primarily a midwife-attended event, often in rural settings, to an urban hospital experience. The wide emergence of hospitals laid the foundation for establishing obstetrics as a hospital-based specialty. As new methods for anesthesia emerged, CD for obstructed labor gained popularity over destructive procedures, such as craniotomy, that accompanied difficult vaginal births. Despite the dangers that still existed with CD, the operation was viewed as preferable to a difficult high forceps delivery, which was associated with fetal injury and deep pelvic lacerations. Although refinements in anesthesia techniques allowed the operation to be performed, mortality rates remained very high, with sepsis and peritonitis as leading causes of postoperative deaths. Primitive surgical techniques and lack of antisepsis clearly contributed to morbidity. Surgeons attempted to complete the operation without closing the uterus, fearing that the suture material itself would promote infection and that the uterus would best heal by secondary intention. As a result, women were placed at risk for both hemorrhage and infection.

Lebas first advocated suturing the uterus after CD in 1769. Traditionally, sutures were not used inside the abdomen or pelvis because they were considered impossible to remove once the cavity was closed. In 1876, Eduardo Porro advocated for supracervical hysterectomy and bilateral salpingo-oopherectomy during CD to control bleeding and to prevent postoperative infection. Shortly thereafter, surgeons gained experience with internal suturing because silver-wire stitches were developed by the gynecologist J. Marion Sims, who had perfected the use of these sutures in the treatment of vesicovaginal fistulae resulting from obstructed labors. In the early 1880s, two German obstetricians, Ferdinand Adolf Kehrer (1837-1914) and Max Sänger (1853-1903), both independently proposed a transverse incision of the lower segment of the uterus, at the level of the internal cervical os, and developed two-layer uterine closure methods with the sutures used by J. Marion Sims. Another pivotal contribution was made in 1900 by Hermann Johannes Pfannenstiel (1862-1909), a German gynecologist who described a transverse suprapubic incision, or pelvic skin incision.

As gynecologic surgeons performed more CDs and the outcomes improved, greater attention was placed on technique, including the site of the uterine incision. Between 1890 and 1925, more and more surgeons began using transverse incisions of the uterus. John Martin Munro Kerr (1868-1960), a professor of Obstetrics Midwifery at the University of Glasgow, popularized the Pfannenstiel skin incision and lower segment uterine incision and is considered the "father" of the modern CD. It was noted that such incisions reduced the rate of infection and the risks of incisional hernia and rupture with subsequent pregnancies compared with the vertical incisions. However, before the advent of antibiotics, owing to the risk for peritonitis, extraperitoneal cesarean was advocated by Frank (1907), Veit and Fromme (1907), and Latzko (1909) and was popularized by Beck (1919) in the United States. Interestingly, the vertical opening of the abdomen was still the main technique used in the 1970s, although it was known from the beginning of the twentieth century to be associated with higher rates of long-term postoperative complications, such as wound dehiscence and abdominal incision hernia, and it is also cosmetically less pleasing.

The introduction of penicillin in 1940 dramatically reduced the risk for peripartum infections. As antibiotic therapy emerged, the need for extraperitoneal dissection diminished. As technology developed, including improved anesthesia, and the medical management of pregnancy and childbirth accelerated, CD became more commonplace in obstetrics. Given its current safety and effectiveness, a liberalized approach to using cesarean childbirth has emerged in developed countries over the past 40 years.

INCIDENCE

The CD *rate* describes the proportion of women undergoing CD of all women giving birth during a specific time period. The CD rate may be further subdivided into primary and repeat CD

> ## BOX 19-1 SELECTED FACTORS RESPONSIBLE FOR INCREASED CESAREAN DELIVERY RATES
>
> **Obstetric Factors**
>
> Increased primary CD rate
>   Failed induction, increased use of induction
>   Decreased use of operative vaginal delivery
>   Increased macrosomia, CD for macrosomia
>   Decline in vaginal breech delivery
> Increased repeat CD rate
>   Decreased use of vaginal birth after CD
>
> **Maternal Factors**
>
> Increased proportion of women >35 yr
> Increased proportion of NP women
> Increased primary CDs on maternal request
>
> **Physician Factors**
>
> Malpractice litigation concerns
>
> ---
>
> *CD,* cesarean delivery; *NP,* nulliparous.

---

rates, both as a proportion of the entire obstetric population. **CD rates have risen in the United States in a dramatic fashion from less than 5% in the 1960s to 32.7% by 2013, with stable rates around 32% to 33% in the last 5 years or so.**[3] CD accounts for more than 1 million major operations performed annually in the United States. It is the most common major surgical procedure undertaken today in the United States and around the world. **Among the reasons for this increase are (1) a continued increase in primary CDs for dystocia, failed induction, and malpresentation; (2) an increase in the proportion of women with obesity, diabetes mellitus, and multiple gestation, which predispose to CD; (3) increased practice of CD on maternal request; and (4) limited use of a trial of labor after cesarean (TOLAC) delivery due to both safety and medicolegal concerns.** Factors responsible for increased cesarean rates are shown in Box 19-1.

A recent increase in international CD rates has also been documented. Rates of about 25% to 30% are reported in some European countries, such as the United Kingdom; they are over 40% in Italy, over 50% in China, and even higher in places like Brazil and Egypt. The rise in CD rates has prompted increased interest in the indications, complications, and techniques involved with this procedure.

The World Health Organization (WHO) has proposed an incidence of CD between 10% and 15% as a target to optimize maternal and perinatal health. However, it is not possible to determine an optimal CD rate because any ideal rate must be a function of multiple clinical factors that vary in each population and are influenced by the level of obstetric care provided. Further complicating this issue is the absence of complete and accurate data that focus on both maternal and infant outcomes. Hence, although **CD rates** can be considered a measure of a specific health care process (mode of delivery), these rates **are not appropriate outcome measures** because they do not indicate whether cesarean or vaginal birth results in optimal perinatal outcomes. **Maternal and perinatal morbidity and mortality should be the outcomes monitored to ensure best quality of care.** Higher CD rates (e.g., 15% to 20% compared with <5% to 10%) have been associated with better perinatal outcomes in several studies.[4] So **instead of setting goals or limits for overall CD rates, it is most important to monitor maternal**

and perinatal health outcomes. We would all agree with a 0% or 100% CD rate if either of these were associated with the lowest incidences of complications for mother or baby. The optimal CD rate in the early twenty-first century is in between these extremes and depends on the population. For example, Robson[5] has suggested a helpful classification of different populations to compare cesarean rates. Class I is the most common class in most centers and includes singleton term vertex gestations admitted in spontaneous labor. Only by comparing data for similar Robson classes, or at least a similar case mix, can data regarding CD rates really be objectively evaluated. Moreover, institutions involved in tertiary obstetric care that manage a large number of preterm deliveries and maternal complications of pregnancy should have higher cesarean rates than primary care facilities. Two populations often targeted for comparison include **nulliparous women with a singleton vertex gestation at 37 weeks or greater without other complications and women with one prior low transverse CD delivering a single vertex fetus at 37 weeks or greater without other complications.**[6] The use of these simple case-mix adjusted rates should make comparative evaluation of CD rates and their comparison to maternal and perinatal outcomes more meaningful. As data become more unified and methodologically sound, the quality of obstetric care can be better assessed.

In 2014, the American College of Obstetricians and Gynecologists (ACOG) and the Society for Maternal-Fetal Medicine (SMFM) published an obstetric care consensus document on the safe prevention of primary CD in which several interventions were suggested to prevent unnecessary CDs (Box 19-2).[7] Institutions can indeed safely reduce cesarean birth rates through quality-improvement initiatives.[8]

INDICATIONS FOR CESAREAN DELIVERY

CD can be performed for maternal-fetal, fetal, and maternal indications. The most common current indications are, in order of frequency, (1) failure to progress, also called *cephalopelvic disproportion* (CPD) or *dystocia* (about 30%); (2) prior cesarean (30%); (3) nonreassuring fetal heart rate (FHR) patterns (10%); and (4) fetal malpresentation (10%). Indications are listed by category in Box 19-3. Looking at just the first CD, the common indications are shown in percentages in Figure 19-1.

Maternal-Fetal Indications

Most CDs are performed for conditions that might pose a threat to both mother and fetus if vaginal delivery occurred. Complete placenta previa and placental abruption with the potential for hemorrhage are clear examples. Dystocia presents a risk for both direct fetal and maternal trauma, and it may also compromise fetal oxygenation and metabolic status. **The suggestions for definitions of *arrest* of labor in the first and second stage and *failed induction*, shown in Box 19-2, should be followed for management as long as maternal and fetal conditions are reassuring.**

Fetal Indications

Fetal indications are primarily recognized by nonreassuring FHR testing with the potential for long-term consequences of metabolic acidosis. Continuous FHR monitoring is associated with a significant reduction in neonatal seizures and remains the most commonly used modality for fetal monitoring in labor. Scalp stimulation can be used to ameliorate the high

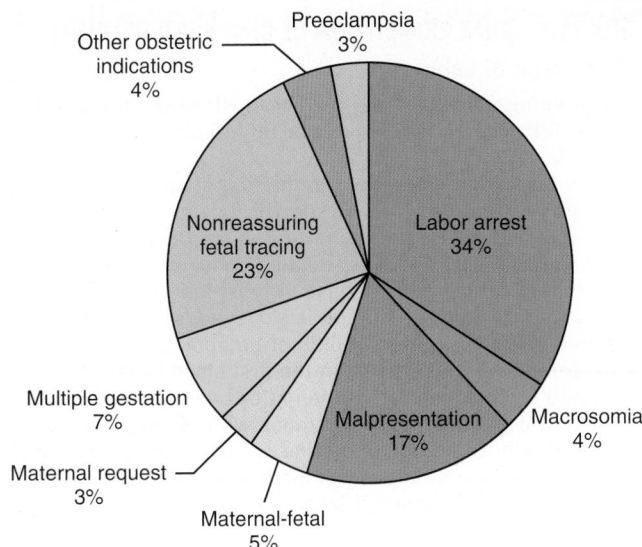

FIG 19-1 Indications for primary cesarean delivery. (Data from Barber EL, Lundsberg LS, Belanger K, Pettker CM, Funai EF, Illuzzi JL. Indications contributing to the increasing cesarean delivery rate. *Obstet Gynecol.* 2011;118:29-38.)

false-positive rate of continuous FHR monitoring (see Box 19-2). Unfortunately, pulse oximetry, ST-segment monitoring, and other modalities have not been shown to affect neonatal outcomes or CD rates (see Chapter 15).

Other fetal indications for CD include malpresentation, such as a breech orientation, and more than 90% of these babies in singleton gestations are delivered by cesarean.[9] Active maternal herpes infection would be an indication for CD to reduce the risk for transmission of infection. Suspected macrosomia or the potential for fetal trauma are indications for CD only in rare circumstances (see Box 19-2). Fetuses with certain birth defects, such as hydrocephalus with macrocephaly and neural tube defects, have traditionally undergone CD; however, insufficient data exist to make this an absolute indication. Babies with fetal abdominal wall defects, such as omphalocele and gastroschisis, can be delivered safely vaginally, if there are no obstetric indications for cesarean.

Maternal Indications

Maternal indications for CD are relatively few and can be considered as medical or mechanical in nature (see Box 19-3). Most of these indications are not based on evidence from randomized controlled trials (RCTs). Certain maternal cardiac conditions, such as a dilated aortic root with Marfan syndrome, are indications for CD. Central nervous system abnormalities in which increased intracranial pressure would be undesirable, such as accompanies the second stage of labor, have also led to recommendations for CD.

Alterations in the capacity of the maternal pelvis can be indications for CD. Mechanical vaginal obstruction as a result of pelvic masses such as lower segment myomata are examples. Finally, women with massive condylomata may also require CD, but this is rare.

Cesarean Delivery on Maternal Request

As CD has become safer, women have occasionally voiced their wish for a cesarean *without* a medical indication. This clinical scenario has been recently called "cesarean delivery on maternal

BOX 19-2 SAFE PREVENTION OF CESAREAN DELIVERY

First Stage of Labor

- A prolonged latent phase (>20 hr in NP women and >14 hr in MP women) should not be an indication for CD. (Grade 1B)
- Slow but progressive labor in the first stage rarely should be an indication for CD. (Grade 1B)
- As long as fetal and maternal status are reassuring, cervical dilation of 6 cm should be considered the threshold for the active phase in most laboring women. Thus before 6 cm of dilation is achieved, standards of active-phase progress should not be applied. (Grade 1B)
- CD for active-phase arrest in the first stage of labor should be reserved for women at or beyond 6 cm of dilation with ruptured membranes who fail to progress despite 4 hr of adequate uterine activity or at least 6 hr of oxytocin administration with inadequate uterine activity and no cervical change. (Grade 1B)

Second Stage of Labor

- A specific absolute maximum length of the second stage of labor above which all women should be delivered operatively has not been identified. (Grade 1C)
- Before diagnosing arrest of labor in the second stage, if the maternal and fetal conditions permit, allow for the following:
  - At least 2 hr of pushing in MP women (Grade 1B)
  - At least 3 hr of pushing in NP women (Grade 1B)
  Longer durations may be appropriate on an individualized basis (e.g., with the use of epidural analgesia or with fetal malposition) as long as progress is being documented. (Grade 1B)
- Operative vaginal delivery in the second stage of labor should be considered an acceptable alternative to CD. Training in, and ongoing maintenance of, practical skills related to operative vaginal delivery should be encouraged. (Grade 1B)
- Manual rotation of the fetal occiput in the setting of fetal malposition in the second stage of labor is a reasonable alternative to operative vaginal delivery or CD. To safely prevent CD in the setting of malposition, it is important to assess fetal position throughout the second stage of labor. (Grade 1B)

Fetal Heart Rate Monitoring

- Amnioinfusion for repetitive variable fetal heart rate decelerations may safely reduce the CD rate. (Grade 1A)
- Scalp stimulation can be used as a means of assessing fetal acid-base status when abnormal or indeterminate (*nonreassuring*) fetal heart patterns (e.g., minimal

variability) are present, and it is a safe alternative to CD in this setting. (Grade 1C)

Induction of Labor

- Induction of labor generally should be performed based on maternal and fetal medical indications and after informed consent is obtained and documented. Inductions at 41 0/7 weeks of gestation and beyond should be performed to reduce the risk of CD and the risk of perinatal morbidity and mortality. (Grade 1A)
- Cervical ripening methods should be used when labor is induced in women with an unfavorable cervix. (Grade 1B)
- If the maternal and fetal status allow, CDs for failed induction of labor in the latent phase can be avoided by allowing longer durations of the latent phase (up to 24 hr or longer) and requiring that oxytocin be administered for at least 18 hr after membrane rupture before deeming the induction a failure. (Grade 1B)

Fetal Malpresentation

- Fetal presentation should be assessed and documented beginning at 36 0/7 weeks of gestation to allow for external cephalic version to be offered. (Grade 1C)

Suspected Fetal Macrosomia

- CD to avoid potential birth trauma should be limited to estimated fetal weights of at least 5000 g in women without diabetes and at least 4500 g in women with diabetes. The prevalence of birthweight of 5000 g or more is rare, and patients should be counseled that estimates of fetal weight, particularly late in gestation, are imprecise. (Grade 2C)
- Women should be counseled about the IOM maternal weight guidelines in an attempt to avoid excessive weight gain. (Grade 1B)

Twin Gestations

- Perinatal outcomes for twin gestations in which the first twin is in cephalic presentation are not improved by CD. Thus women with either cephalic/cephalic–presenting twins or cephalic/noncephalic-presenting twins should be counseled to attempt vaginal delivery. (Grade 1B)

Other

- Individuals, organizations, and governing bodies should work to ensure that research is conducted to provide a better knowledge base to guide decisions regarding CD and to encourage policy changes that safely lower the rate of primary CD. (Grade 1C)

Modified from the American College of Obstetricians and Gynecologists , Society for Maternal-Fetal Medicine, Caughey AB, Cahill AG, Guise JM, Rouse DJ. Safe prevention of the primary cesarean delivery. *Am J Obstet Gynecol.* 2014;210(3):179-193.
CD, cesarean delivery; *IOM,* Institute of Medicine; *MP,* multiparous; *NP,* nulliparous.

BOX 19-3 SELECTED INDICATIONS FOR CESAREAN DELIVERY BY CATEGORY

Maternal-Fetal

Cephalopelvic disproportion
Placental abruption
Placenta previa
Repeat cesarean delivery
Cesarean delivery on maternal request

Maternal

Specific cardiac disease (e.g., Marfan syndrome with dilated aortic root)

Fetal

Nonreassuring fetal status
Breech or transverse lie
Maternal herpes

request." The lack of specificity of the term "elective" suggests the most reasonable and prudent course of action is to not use it, but rather to document the specific indication—whether medical or nonmedical—for the intervention or procedure (i.e., CD on maternal request).[10] At times, physicians have also advocated cesarean as the preferred mode of delivery, even in the absence of accepted indications as described previously. We would term this scenario "cesarean delivery on physician request."

The decision to plan a cesarean or a vaginal birth should be based on the best literature available with which to compare these choices. Cases in which cesarean (or vaginal) delivery is for accepted indications as described previously should be excluded from this comparison. The National Institutes of Health (NIH) and ACOG have carefully reviewed the literature on this topic.[11,12] Both have reported that no quality evidence has compared planned cesarean to planned vaginal delivery because no randomized studies exist for the majority of women—those with a singleton gestation in vertex presentation at term. Moderate-quality evidence shows that planned cesarean is associated with less postpartum hemorrhage, more mild neonatal respiratory morbidity, longer maternal hospital stay, and possibly greater complications in subsequent pregnancies (Box 19-4).[11,12] Women who desire several children should be advised against non–medically indicated CD because of the direct association with an increasing number of CDs and increasing life-threatening complications such as placenta previa, placenta accreta, and the need for cesarean hysterectomy.[12] Unfortunately, at times CD is performed on maternal request because of a fear of excessive pain and fear of damage to the vagina and perineum. Fear of childbirth is present in about 3% to 8% of women, who should be reassured of adequate maternal pain relief in labor and counseled regarding TOLAC. Increased maternal risks attributed to vaginal delivery also include urinary and fecal incontinence, pelvic prolapse, and sexual dysfunction. The precise contribution of vaginal delivery versus pregnancy and labor to these complications remains difficult to ascertain, and many epidemiologic studies do stratify data according to variables such as gestational age, maternal age, parity, and fetal weight.

All remaining comparisons, which will be discussed later, are based on weak evidence and should not decisively sway clinical decisions. **Perinatal mortality has been reported to be several times lower with a planned CD compared with labor and vaginal birth.** Additionally, hypoxic-ischemic encephalopathy (HIE) of the newborn related to intrapartum events—including abruption, cord prolapse, and progressive asphyxia—occurs in approximately 1 in 3000 to 5000 births. Many of these cases presumably would be prevented by planned CD, as would unexplained stillbirths that occur beyond 39 weeks' gestation. Traumatic birth injuries such as intracranial hemorrhage, fractures, and brachial plexus injury are also reduced with CD.

Overall, the maternal risks of CD have been considered marginal compared with those of vaginal delivery. Excluding indicated cesarean deliveries, rates of maternal mortality are comparable with those of vaginal delivery. Sachs and colleagues[13] reported a CD-associated mortality rate of 22.3 per 100,000 compared with 10.9 per 100,000 for vaginal delivery; however, the rates were comparable excluding medical complications.

CD does increase maternal morbidity. Compared with vaginal birth, the rate of endometritis is increased (3.0% vs. 0.4%), yet rates of postpartum hemorrhage, transfusion, and deep venous thrombosis (DVT) are comparable. Other reports confirm increased risks for these morbidities with CD, including major complication rates as high as 4.5%. **CD also presents a risk for future placental abnormalities, including placenta previa and placenta accreta. These risks increase with the increasing number of CDs performed for each woman and are substantial with more than three operations. Thus the decision to undergo CD on request must include thoughtful consideration of future childbearing plans.**

When a planned CD is performed without accepted indications, at the request of either the patient or the physician, it should be performed at 39 weeks.[11,12,14] After appropriate counseling, if the woman still insists on a CD, implementing her request is ethically permissible. Less than 10% of women prefer a CD based solely on their own desires.

TECHNIQUE OF CESAREAN DELIVERY

Because more than 1.3 million CDs are performed in the United States every year,[15] and about 20 million are done worldwide, it is extremely important to adhere to the safest, most effective technique associated with the lowest perinatal and maternal complications. Each aspect of CD should be evaluated individually, optimally by RCT, because it is impossible to evaluate the benefit of a specific technical aspect if multiple aspects are studied together. Proper universal surgical precautions aimed at preventing blood loss and infection should be used. Preferred technical aspects of CD are shown in Table 19-1.

Precesarean Antibiotics

Prophylactic preoperative antibiotics are of clear benefit in reducing the frequency of postcesarean endomyometritis and wound infection in both laboring and nonlaboring CDs.[5] The timing, agents, and dosages of prophylactic antibiotics have been extensively studied.[16,17] Prophylactic antibiotics should be given approximately 30 to 60 minutes before the skin incision to allow for adequate tissue concentrations; pharmacokinetic studies of cefazolin demonstrate that adequate concentration in maternal and amniotic fluid samples are attained 30 minutes after administration.[17-19] The preferred agent for prophylaxis

TABLE 19-1   EVIDENCE-BASED RECOMMENDATIONS FOR CESAREAN DELIVERY TECHNIQUES

STEP	EVIDENCE SUPPORTS IT: DO THIS	EVIDENCE REFUTES IT: DO *NOT* DO THIS	CAN BE CONSIDERED
Antibiotic prophylaxis with IV first-generation cephalosporin or ampicillin	Administer 30 to 60 min before cesarean incision.	Administer at neonatal cord clamp.	
Thromboprophylaxis	Use mechanical prophylaxis with graduated compression stockings or a pneumatic compression device during and after CD.		
Lateral tilt	Consider a lateral tilt.		
Bladder catheterization			Intraoperative catheterization is not mandatory; consider removal immediately after operation.
Vaginal povidone-iodine preparation			This can be considered.
Hair removal	Hair does not need to be removed, but if it is, use hair clippers the morning of the surgery.	Shave preoperatively.	
Site preparation	Use chlorhexidine-alcohol.		
Drapes	Use nonadhesive drapes.	Use adhesive drapes.	
Prevent needle sticks	Consider blunt needles.	Consider not using sharp needles.	
Skin incision	Use a transverse skin incision.		
Bladder flap	Do not develop a bladder flap.		
Uterine incision	Make a low transverse uterine incision unless a vertical incision is indicated (see Box 19-5).	Make a vertical uterine incision.	
Uterine expansion	Use blunt uterine incision expansion with cephalad-caudad traction.	Use sharp uterine extension; use transverse traction.	
Cord clamping	Delay cord clamping for 30 to 120 sec for infants younger than 37 wk.		
Prevention of postpartum hemorrhage	Use oxytocin 10 to 80 IU in 1 L crystalloid.	Use misoprostol in lieu of oxytocin.	Tranexamic acid and carbetocin may be considered.
Placental delivery	Deliver the placenta spontaneously with gentle cord traction.	Deliver the placenta manually.	
Abdominal irrigation		Use intraabdominal irrigation with NS to decrease maternal morbidity.	
Uterine exteriorization			This is suggested to facilitate better visualization.
Cervical dilation	Do *not* manually or surgically dilate the cervix.	Manually or surgically dilate the cervix.	
Uterine repair	Use a single layer if the patient has completed childbearing (e.g., bilateral tubal ligation performed concurrently with CD). Consider a double layer otherwise.		
Subcutaneous space closure	Close subcutaneous space if 2 cm or larger.	Routinely use subcutaneous drains.	
Skin closure	Close the transverse skin incision with suture.	Close the transverse skin incision with staples.	

CD, cesarean delivery; *IV,* intravenous; *NS,* normal saline.

is either a first-generation cephalosporin (e.g., cefazolin) or ampicillin.[20-23] For women who have an anaphylactic allergic reaction to penicillin, either metronidazole or clindamycin and gentamicin can be used. No apparent advantage has been shown with more broad-spectrum antibiotic prophylaxis (e.g., azithromycin or metronidazole), except perhaps for women who do not get antibiotic prophylaxis for CD.[20-25] Single-dose therapy is as effective as multidose therapy[26] and is therefore preferred.

For women with clinical chorioamnionitis, treatment with combination antibiotic therapy (e.g., ampicillin sodium/sulbactam sodium) **supplants the need for prophylaxis if given within the appropriate time frame of cesarean skin incision.** This therapy should be instituted promptly upon diagnosis of chorioamnionitis, and it should be continued until the patient exhibits a clinical response.

Precesarean Thromboprophylaxis
Because venous thromboembolism (VTE) is the leading cause of maternal mortality in developed countries, and CD increases this risk, thromboprophylaxis should be considered in all CDs. Because the incidence of clinically significant thrombosis is 0.9%,[27] an insufficient number of women have been randomized to mechanical prophylaxis, heparin, low-molecular-weight heparin, or no anticoagulation to assess safety and efficacy of these treatment regimens in comparison to one another.[16,28-31] We recommend mechanical prophylaxis with graduated compression stockings or a pneumatic compression device[32,33] during and after every CD until ambulation resumes.[34] Women with additional risk factors such as morbid obesity, prior VTE, or immobility may benefit from medical thromboprophylaxis after cesarean (e.g., with prophylactic heparin).

Other Prophylactic Precesarean Interventions
A lateral tilt of about 15 degrees is suggested to elevate the mother's right side to avoid vena caval compression and supine hypotension syndrome. However, left lateral tilt, head-up or head-down position, the use of wedges and cushions, flexion of the table, and use of a mechanical displacer have been insufficiently studied to provide any strong recommendation for routine clinical use.[35]

Vaginal preparation immediately before CD with povidone-iodine solution significantly reduces the incidence of postcesarean endometritis (from 8.3% in those who received placebo preparations to 4.3%), especially in women with ruptured membranes (17.9% reduced to 4.3%) and those in labor (13.0% reduced to 7.4%).[36] Although antibiotics were administered prophylactically for CD in these trials, at least one trial administered antibiotics at cord clamping, and two trials did not specify the timing of antibiotic administration. Therefore it is unclear whether vaginal preparation reduces morbidity in women who receive antibiotic prophylaxis for CD preoperatively as is currently recommended.

Fixing an indwelling urethral catheter (e.g., Foley) is routinely performed for planned and emergency CD in most countries around the world. The drainage tube is inserted when analgesia is established and is then left in situ for 12 to 24 hours until the patient is able to mobilize. This tube is connected to a closed collection system to evacuate urine and decompress the urinary bladder. This may improve visualization of the lower uterine segment, which could minimize bladder injury. However, one RCT has shown that the incidence of urinary tract infection, time to patient ambulation, time to first postoperative voiding, requirement for oral rehydration, intestinal movement, and duration of hospital stay are all significantly reduced in the uncatheterized group with no increase in intraoperative complications or urinary retention.[37] It should be noted that the study was not powered to assess for differences in bladder or ureteral injury.[37] Alternatively, immediate postoperative removal of a urethral catheter after planned CD may be associated with a lower risk of urinary infection, although the difference was nonsignificant.[38] **Urinary bladder catheterization for CD is prudent until evidence can delineate that eliminating this practice will not result in an increase in bladder or ureteral injury.** For those who choose not to place an indwelling catheter for CD, the patient should void immediately prior to the operation.[39] Indwelling catheter placement in hemodynamically unstable women is recommended to monitor urine output and evaluate fluid balance.

Site Preparation

Preparation of the skin is performed to reduce the risk for wound infection by decreasing the amount of skin flora and contaminants at the incision site. **Hair does not have to be removed from the operative site.** Removal with a razor may actually increase the risk for infection by breaks in the skin that allow entry of bacteria.[40] For this reason, some advocate clipping of the hair on the morning of surgery.[40] Only enough hair should be removed to allow good approximation of skin edges.

Incision-site preparation is accomplished in the operating room through application of a surgical scrub. CD wounds are considered to be clean contaminated. Chlorhexidine-alcohol scrub has been associated with a lower incidence of wound infection compared with povidone-iodine scrub.[41] In addition, **drapes should not be adhesive** because such drapes have been associated with a higher rate of wound infection compared with nonadhesive drapes.[42-44]

Abdominal Skin Incision and Abdominal Entry

In general, universally accepted good surgical techniques aimed at avoiding excessive blood loss and tissue trauma should be used. Compared with sharp needles, the use of blunt needles during CD is associated with a decrease in the rate of

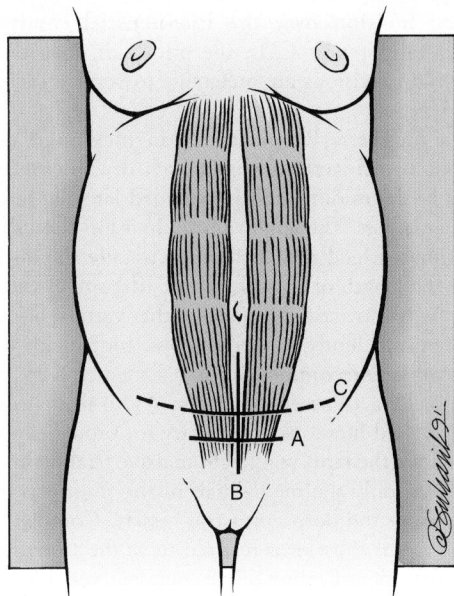

FIG 19-2 The Pfannenstiel abdominal incision is the most common for cesarean delivery **(A)**. The midline **(B)** and Maylard **(C)** incisions are much less common. Hatched lines indicate possible extension. (Modified from Baker C, Shingleton HM. Incisions. *Clin Obstet Gynecol.* 1988;31:701.)

surgeon glove perforation but also with a decrease in surgeon satisfaction.[45]

The surgeon has a choice of a transverse or vertical skin incision, with the transverse Pfannenstiel being the most common incision type in the United States (Fig. 19-2). **Factors that influence the type of incision include the urgency of the delivery, placental disorders such as anterior complete placenta previa and placenta accreta, prior incision type, and the potential need to explore the upper abdomen for nonobstetric pathology. Although some still prefer a vertical incision in emergency situations, a Pfannenstiel incision actually adds only 1 minute of extra operative time in primary and 2 minutes in repeat cesareans, differences that are not associated with improved neonatal outcome compared with that of a vertical incision.**[46] Vertical incisions have been performed very rarely in the United States and Europe for routine CDs since the 1980s. A survey of obstetricians in the United Kingdom found that more than 80% use the Pfannenstiel abdominal entry.[47] The remaining 20% use the incision and abdominal entry described by Joel-Cohen.[48] A survey of obstetric residents in the United States found that 77% use a horizontal skin incision for urgent or emergency CD.[49] Overall, the Pfannenstiel incision is currently the preferred technique around the world and is used for more than 90% of CDs in the United States. The Joel-Cohen incision was described for gynecologic surgical procedures such as abdominal hysterectomy, and it allows similar access to the pelvis and lower abdomen as a vertical incision but is more cosmetic and less painful postoperatively. In the early 1990s, the Joel-Cohen incision (Video 19-1) was integrated by Stark and colleagues[50,51] into a minimalist cesarean technique now called the *Misgav Ladach method.* Thus far, studies reporting the benefits of the Joel-Cohen incision include multiple aspects of the CD technique, not just the skin incision[16]; therefore they are not clinically helpful in determining the benefit of the individual CD steps.[52] **Given this, we do not recommend the**

Joel-Cohen incision over the Pfannenstiel cesarean technique. For most repeat CDs, the prior skin incision is used. Transverse skin incisions are preferable to vertical incisions (see Table 19-1).

When a transverse Pfannenstiel skin incision is used, it is made about two fingerbreadths (1 inch or 2.5 cm) above the symphysis in the midline and is extended laterally in a slightly curvilinear manner. The length of the incision should be based on the estimated fetal size; at term, it usually should be about 15 cm, or the length of an Allis clamp. The site of the incision, either below or above the pannus or either vertical or transverse, has not been sufficiently studied in obese individuals to provide an evidence-based recommendation.

Occasionally, a transverse incision of the rectus sheath and muscles (Maylard incision) is necessary for proper exposure and room to deliver the fetus (e.g., with massive fetal hydrocephaly). In these cases, only the medial half of the muscle is incised to avoid lacerating the deep epigastric vessels. Complete transection of the rectus muscles is referred to as the *Cherney incision,* which requires identification of the epigastric vessels and ligation bilaterally.

Following the skin incision, the subcutaneous tissue is then bluntly pushed away to identify the underlying fascia. In repeat operations, sharp dissection of the subcutaneous adipose tissue may be required. The fascia is incised and dissected or is bluntly extended in a mild curvilinear manner bilaterally. It should be tented with the surgeon's forceps to separate it from the underlying muscle and to identify perforating vessels, which may require ligation or coagulation. Curvilinear extension is essential because direct transverse extension often leads to inadvertent muscle incisions and bleeding.

Once the fascial incision is completed, the fascia is then grasped in the midline bilaterally and is separated from the underlying rectus muscles superiorly and inferiorly by blunt and sharp dissection from the median raphe. The rectus muscles can be separated bluntly in the midline to reveal the posterior rectus sheath and peritoneum, which can also be entered bluntly with the fingers to avoid trauma to the underlying bowel. The point of entry should be as superior as possible to avoid bladder injury, particularly in repeat operations in which the bladder may be adherent superiorly.

Bladder Flap

Creation of a bladder flap versus a direct uterine incision above the bladder fold has been compared in four randomized trials of 581 women.[53] **Bladder flap development was associated with a longer incision-to-delivery interval of 1.27 minutes without any differences in bladder injury, total operating time, blood loss, or hospital length of stay.**[53] **It is important to note that emergency CDs were excluded from the studies, and the majority of pregnancies were over 32 weeks' gestation. Overall, the populations were heterogeneous: two of the four trials were of poor methodologic quality, and one was unpublished.**[53] Because there does not appear to be any direct advantage gained from creating a bladder flap, we do not develop a bladder flap.

Should the obstetrician elect to create a bladder flap, the vesicouterine serosa is picked up with smooth forceps and is incised in the midline with Metzenbaum scissors. The incision is carried out laterally in a curvilinear manner. The vesicouterine fold is then tented with forceps or a pair of hemostats, which allows direct visualization as the bladder flap is bluntly created using the index and middle fingers. Sharp dissection may be necessary, particularly in repeat operations. The surgeon then bluntly sweeps out laterally on each side to allow just enough room for insertion of the bladder blade. A Richardson retractor is then inserted laterally, and continuous suction is made available in preparation for the uterine incision.

Uterine Incision

Following full entry into the peritoneal cavity, the surgeon should palpate the uterus for fetal presentation and alignment and then place a bladder retractor to expose the lower uterine segment. The uterus is often dextrorotated, and its position must be appreciated to plan the incision site. The safety and efficacy of using special retractors, especially in obese women, has been insufficiently studied.

The low transverse uterine incision replaced the vertical uterine incision at the beginning of the twentieth century. The low transverse incision is preferred to a vertical incision because it is associated with less blood loss, is easier to perform and repair, and provides for the option of subsequent TOLAC because the rate of subsequent rupture is lower than with incisions that incorporate the upper uterine segment.[54]

In cases of a low transverse incision, the incision is begun at least 2 cm above the bladder margin (Fig. 19-3) and suction is applied. Tamponade with sponges superiorly and inferiorly can be performed if considerable bleeding is encountered. This technique allows better visualization and minimizes the chance of fetal laceration. Once the uterine cavity is confirmed, typically by visualization of the amniotic membranes or fetus, the incision is extended laterally and superiorly at the angles by blunt spreading using the index fingers. Randomized trials have compared blunt versus sharp extension of the uterine incision. Sharp extension is associated with increased blood loss and the need for transfusion compared with blunt extension.[55] Blunt uterine incision extension can be done preferably with cephalad-caudad traction because transverse expansion is associated with more unintended extension and more blood loss.[56] As for the skin and the fascial incisions, adequate exposure for an easy extraction of the fetus should be obtained. At term, this is usually more than 15 cm.

Vertical uterine incisions are now rarely performed (Box 19-5). When a vertical incision is used, it is either *low* (involving mostly the low uterine segment) or *classical* (involving the upper uterine segment) and should have clear indications. **A vertical uterine incision may need to be performed if the lower uterine segment is poorly developed** (e.g., at 23 to 25 weeks' gestation); **if the fetus is in a back-down transverse lie; in cases of an anterior placenta previa or accreta, often in combination with a hysterectomy** (Chapter 21); **or if leiomyomas obstruct the lower segment.** Other, even less common

---

BOX 19-5 POTENTIAL INDICATIONS FOR VERTICAL UTERINE INCISION

- Lower uterine segment is poorly developed (e.g., at 23 to 25 weeks gestation).
- Fetus is in a back-down transverse lie.
- An anterior leiomyoma obstructs the lower uterine segment.
- Complete anterior placenta previa or placenta accreta is present.

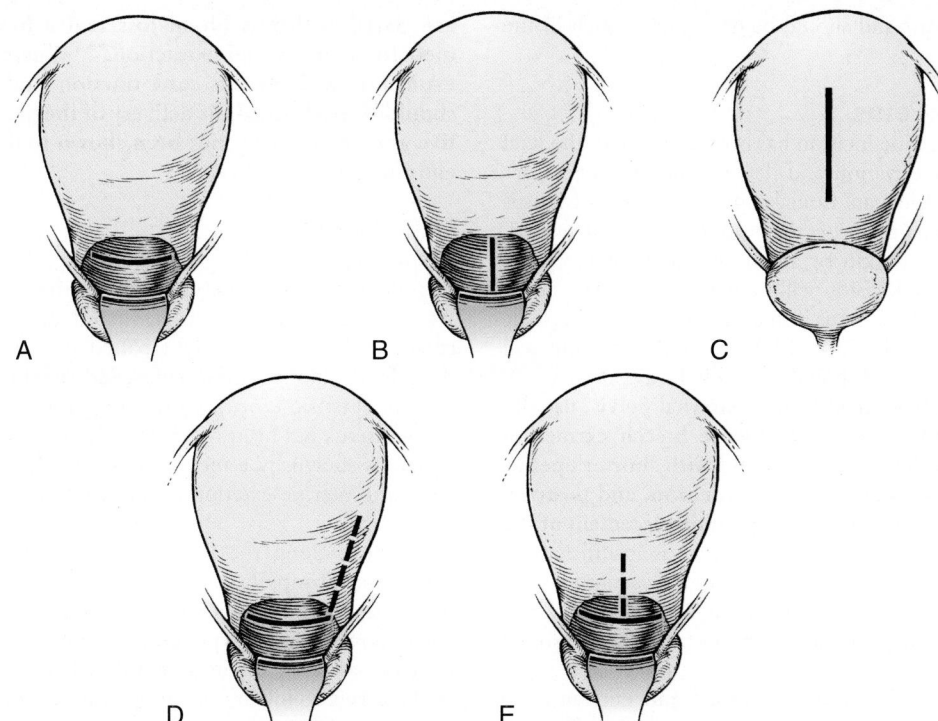

FIG 19-3 Uterine incisions for cesarean delivery. **A,** In the *low transverse incision* (performed in >90% of cesarean deliveries) the incision is made in the lower uterine segment, curving gently upward. If the lower segment is poorly developed, the incision can also curve sharply upward at each end to avoid extending into the ascending branches of the uterine arteries. **B,** The *low vertical incision* is made vertically in the lower uterine segment, avoiding extension into the bladder below. If more room is needed, the incision can be extended upward into the upper uterine segment. **C,** The *classical incision* is entirely within the upper uterine segment and can be at the level shown or in the fundus. **D,** With the *J incision,* if more room is needed when an initial transverse incision has been made, either end of the incision can be extended upward into the upper uterine segment and parallel to the ascending branch of the uterine artery. **E,** With the *T incision,* more room can be obtained in a transverse incision by an upward midline extension into the upper uterine segment.

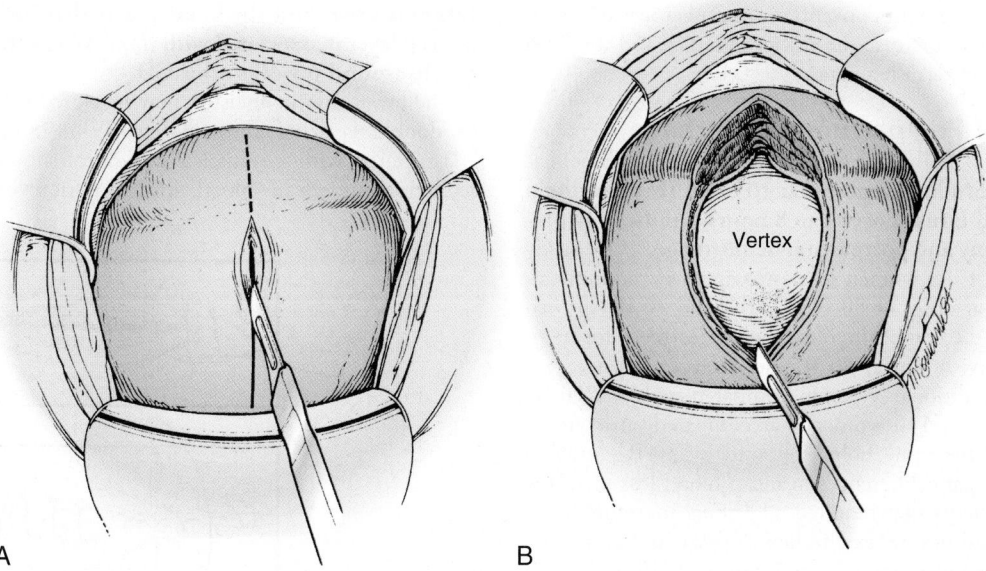

FIG 19-4 Low vertical incision. **A,** Ideally, a vertical incision is contained entirely in the lower uterine segment. **B,** Extension into the upper uterine segment, either inadvertently or by choice, is common.

indications may include certain fetal abnormalities such as massive hydrocephalus, a very large sacrococcygeal teratoma, or to deliver conjoined twins. The disadvantages of a classical incision are its tendency for greater adhesion formation and greater risk for uterine rupture with subsequent pregnancy. The low

vertical incision depends on the downward displacement of the bladder to confine the incision to the true lower segment (Fig. 19-4). The incision is begun as inferiorly as possible and is extended cephalad with the fingers or bandage scissors. If the thick myometrium of the upper segment is incised, the incision becomes a classical one and should be described as such in the operative report.

Delivery of the Fetus

Once an adequate uterine incision has been completed, the fetal head is extracted by elevation and flexion using the operator's hand as a fulcrum. Adequate fundal pressure by the assistant is often critical to obtain delivery. If the head is not easily delivered, the uterine incision (or skin or abdominal incisions) may be extended. Rarely, a tee incision will be made to facilitate delivery; for example, when the fetus is in a back-down transverse lie and cannot be rotated. The use of forceps and/or vacuum will be needed in few cases and should generally be avoided.

When the vertex is wedged in the maternal pelvis, usually in advanced second-stage arrest, reverse breech extraction (the "pull" method) has been associated with shorter operating time, less extension of the uterine incision, and postpartum endometritis compared with vaginal displacement of the presenting part upward,[57] but the evidence is insufficient to make a strong recommendation. As noted above, vacuum extraction or short Simpson forceps should in general be avoided because they are rarely necessary if the previously mentioned steps are taken.

Following delivery, the cord is clamped and cut, and the infant is passed from the field to the pediatric team. Delayed cord clamping (DCC) for 30 to 120 seconds and/or or umbilical cord milking has been shown to increase placental transfusion, which leads to an increase in neonatal blood volume at birth of approximately 30%. In preterm neonates, increasing evidence suggests that DCC significantly decreases the need for blood transfusions, the incidence of necrotizing enterocolitis, and the risks of intraventricular hemorrhage and late-onset sepsis.[58,59] Therefore **DCC is recommended for all CDs done before 37 weeks**. No such strong evidence exists for term newborns: DCC increases early hemoglobin concentrations and iron stores, but it may also adversely increase the risk of jaundice and the need for phototherapy in term neonates.[60]

Prevention of Postpartum Hemorrhage

Following delivery of the infant, intravenous (IV) oxytocin is started as a drip. **Studies suggest that 10 to 80 IU of oxytocin in 1 L crystalloid infused over 4 to 8 hours significantly prevents uterine atony and postpartum hemorrhage.**[16] One study that randomized 1798 women to postcesarean IV administration of oxytocin at doses of 80 IU, 40 IU, and 10 IU showed no differences in the composite outcome of treatment for hemorrhage and atony; however, 80 IU did decrease the need for treatment with additional oxytocin compared with the 10 IU dose.[61] One study of 110 women that compared an oxytocin 5-IU bolus with the same bolus followed by 30-IU infusion revealed no significant differences in mean blood loss or in the percentage of patients that required additional uterotonics.[61,62] Misoprostol should not be used in lieu of oxytocin.[16]

Preincision administration of tranexamic acid (10 mg/kg IV) has been shown to decrease blood loss and the need for uterotonics.[16,63] Postdelivery administration of carbetocin (100 μg) resulted in a decrease in the need for uterotonics and uterine massage.[64]

Placental Extraction

Removal of the placenta by spontaneous expulsion with gentle cord traction has been shown by several RCTs to be associated with less blood loss and a lower rate of endometritis than manual extraction.[65-67] Therefore spontaneous expulsion with gentle cord traction and uterine massage should be performed for delivery of the placenta. Intraoperative glove change has not been shown to decrease the risk of endometritis after CD.[66]

Uterine Repair

Uterine repair may be greatly facilitated by lifting the fundus and delivering the uterus through the abdominal incision. Uterine exteriorization can facilitate better visualization of the extent of the incision to be repaired and can provide a view of the adnexa. No significant increased risk for blood loss, infection, hypotension, or nausea and vomiting with exteriorization of the uterus has been reported compared with intraabdominal repair, as shown by a meta-analysis of 11 trials.[68] The decision regarding uterine exteriorization can be based on the surgeon's preference.

Bleeding along the incision line is temporarily controlled using ring clamps because they are less traumatic than other instruments. The uterus is then manually curetted with a moistened sponge, and all placental fragments or membranes are teased away from the uterine wall. Manual or surgical dilation of the cervix following placental removal is not associated with any benefit.[16,69]

The uterine incision should be well inspected before closure. Any inferior extensions of the incision should be visualized and repaired separately before closure.

The first layer of uterine closure is performed using continuous suturing. This technique is associated with less operating time and reduced blood loss compared with interrupted sutures.[70] The locking of the primary layer of closure facilitates hemostasis but may not be necessary if the incision is fairly hemostatic before closure. Size 1-0 or 0-0 synthetic suture is used. Full-thickness repair that includes the endometrial layer is associated with improved healing as evidenced by ultrasound 6 weeks after CD.[55,71]

The lower uterine incision may be closed with either a single or double layer of sutures (Fig. 19-5). Single-layer closure is associated with a statistically significant but clinically small reduction in mean blood loss, duration of the operative

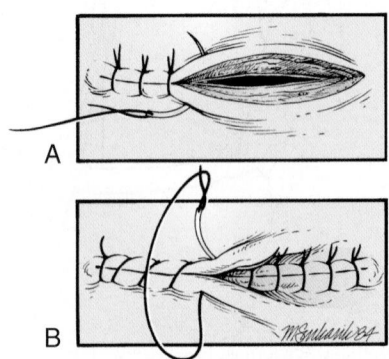

FIG 19-5 Closure of low transverse incision. **A,** The first layer can be either continuous (recommended) or interrupted. Despite its reputed hemostatic abilities, a continuous locking suture is less desirable because it may interfere with incision vasculature and, hence, with healing and scar formation. **B,** A second inverted layer is created using a continuous Lembert or Cushing stitch. Inclusion of too much tissue produces a bulky mass that may delay involution and can interfere with healing.

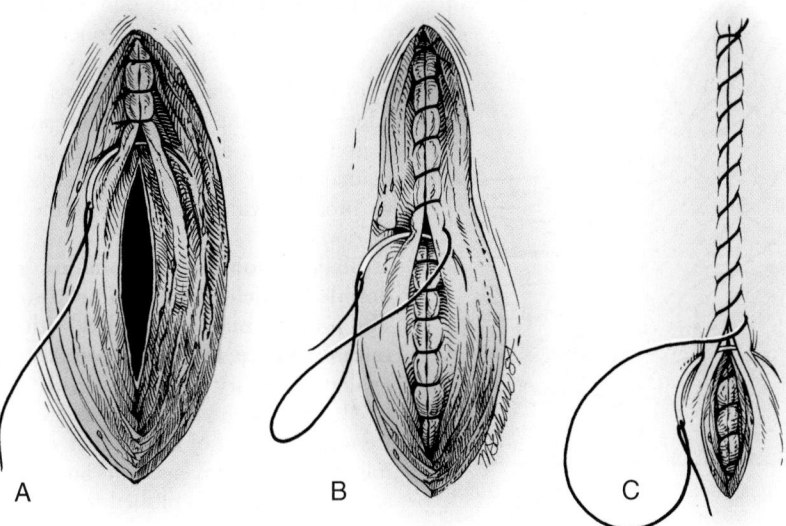

FIG 19-6 Repair of a classical incision. Three-layer closure of a classical incision, including inversion of the serosal layer to discourage adhesion formation. The knot at the superior end of the incision of the second layer can be buried by medial-to-lateral placement of the suture from within the depth of the incision and subsequent lateral-to-medial reentry on the opposing side with resultant knot placement within the incision.

procedure, and presence of postoperative pain compared with a double-layer closure.[72] Controversy surrounds whether an increased risk for subsequent uterine rupture or placenta accreta accompanies the single-layer closure technique (Chapter 20). In women who receive a tubal ligation at the time of CD, we usually perform a single-layer closure if excellent hemostasis is achieved. Otherwise, we prefer a double-layer closure; however, randomized trials that have assessed one- versus two-layer uterine closure have reported mostly short-term outcomes with insufficient evidence to assess long-term outcomes, in particular, uterine rupture with a TOLAC in a future pregnancy.[16]

A vertical uterine incision generally requires at least a double-layer, but more often a triple-layer, closure technique (Fig. 19-6) with a baseball stitch used on the uterine serosa.

The uterine incision is carefully inspected for hemostasis before returning the uterus to the peritoneal cavity. Individual bleeding points are cauterized or ligated using as little suture material as possible. The adnexa are inspected, and tubal ligation is performed if so desired. Following return of the uterus inside the pelvis, sponge and needle counts are then performed before abdominal closure. Intraabdominal irrigation does not reduce intrapartum or postpartum maternal morbidity.[73]

Abdominal Closure

The parietal and visceral peritoneum are not reapproximated because spontaneous closure will occur within days, and non-closure has been associated in several RCTs with less operative time, less fever, reduced hospital stay, and less need for analgesia compared with closure.[74] Some limited non–level 1 data suggest that closure of the parietal peritoneum may decrease the risk of future adhesions,[75] but this has not been confirmed by better data.

No trials have evaluated the technical aspects of fascial closure at CD. The rectus fascia is usually closed with a continuous nonlocking technique, but some prefer interrupted sutures. Because the fascia is not as vascular, this layer is not locked so as not to cause strangulation of the fascia, which could

increase the risk of fascial dehiscence. A suture with good tensile strength and relatively delayed absorption is preferred. Synthetic braided or monofilament sutures are best to use. In most instances, a running continuous monofilament propylene suture will suffice for a transverse incision. In closing the fascia, placement of the sutures should be at a minimum 1 cm from the margin of the incision; sutures are placed at about 1-cm intervals. In most cases of wound disruption, the suture remains intact but has cut through the fascia as a result of placement too close to the cut margin. Patients at risk for wound disruption may benefit from either the Smead-Jones technique or interrupted figure-of-eight suturing, both using delayed-absorption suture material such as monofilament polyglycolic acid. The Smead-Jones closure technique is preferred for vertical incisions in high-risk cases (Fig. 19-7). To accomplish this technique, a suture is made with either far-near or near-far placement that passes through the lateral side of the anterior rectus fascia and adjacent subcutaneous adipose tissue; then, it crosses the midline of the incision to pick up the medial edge of the rectus fascia, then catches the near side of the opposite rectus sheath before returning to the far margin of the opposite rectus sheath and subcutaneous fat.

The subcutaneous tissue is closed if it will facilitate skin closure or if the fat thickness is at least 2 cm. Closure of the subcutaneous tissue of at least 2 cm with sutures is associated with fewer wound complications—such as a hematoma, seroma, wound infection, or wound separation—compared with no closure.[76] Prophylactic wound drainage is not associated with benefits and should therefore not be performed routinely.[77-79] Occasionally, when hemostasis is not adequate either intraabdominally or subcutaneously, drains can be used, but there are no level 1 data that prove their effectiveness.

The transverse cesarean skin incision should be closed with subcuticular suture, rather than staples, because suture closure significantly decreases by 57% the risks of wound complications (from 10.6% to 4.9%) and specifically wound separation (from 7.4% to 1.6%).[80,81] Staple closure

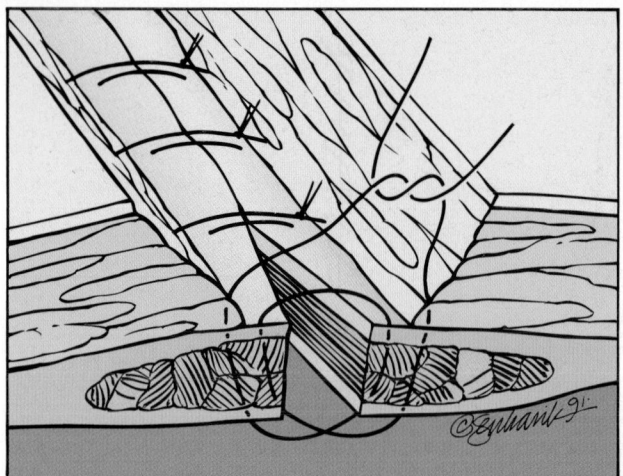

FIG 19-7 Modification of far-near, near-far Smead-Jones suture. Suture passes deeply through the lateral side of the anterior rectus fascia and adjacent fat, crosses the midline of the incision to pick up the medial edge of the rectus fascia, then catches the near side of the opposite rectus sheath; finally, it returns to the far margin of the opposite rectus sheath and subcutaneous fat. (Modified from American College of Obstetricians and Gynecologists. Prologue. In: *Gynecologic Oncology and Surgery.* Washington, DC: American College of Obstetricians and Gynecologists; 1991, p 187.)

is approximately 7 minutes faster than suture closure.[82] Evidence is insufficient to make a recommendation for closure method for CDs performed using vertical skin incisions.[80,81]

COMPLICATIONS OF CESAREAN DELIVERY
Intraoperative Complications

Women undergoing CD are at risk for several intraoperative complications, including hemorrhage and injury to adjacent organs. Injury to the bowel, bladder, and ureters is uncommon; however, the obstetrician must be familiar with management of these problems. The key element is to recognize and define the extent of these injuries and to promptly institute repair. Consultation with a urologist, general surgeon, or gynecologic oncologist may be necessary depending on the skill level of the obstetrician and the complexity of the injury encountered.

Uterine Lacerations

Lacerations of the uterine incision most commonly involve extension of a low transverse incision following arrest of descent in the second stage or with delivery of a large fetus. **Most lacerations are myometrial extensions that can be closed with a running locking suture independently or in conjunction with closure of the primary uterine incision. High lateral extensions may require unilateral ascending uterine artery branch ligation.** In cases that extend laterally and inferiorly, care must be taken to avoid ureteral injury. On occasion, if the extension involves bleeding into the broad ligament, opening this space and identifying the ureters before suture placement may be helpful. On rare occasions, retrograde ureteral stent placement may be necessary. Opening the dome of the bladder is the preferred technique for retrograde stent placement.

Bladder Injury

Minor injury to the bladder from vigorous retraction and bruising with resultant hematuria is common. More significant injury, such as a bladder dome laceration, is infrequent but can occur on entering the peritoneum, particularly with multiple repeat operations. Bladder injury is also encountered with development of the bladder flap in cases in which scarring increases adherence to the lower anterior uterine wall. This is another reason that we do not routinely perform a bladder flap. If the bladder is very adherent and is tacked high, it may be advisable to proceed with a vertical uterine incision to avoid bladder disruption.

Bladder dome lacerations are generally repaired with a double-layer closure technique using 2-0 or 3-0 Vicryl suture. The mucosa may be avoided with closure, although this is not imperative. If any question exists regarding possible trigone or ureteral injury before repair, IV indigo carmine is administered, and the ureteral orifices are visualized for dye spillage. Retrograde filling of the bladder with sterile milk may be useful following closure to ensure its integrity. Continuous Foley drainage should be accomplished for several days following repair of a bladder injury.

Ureteral Injury

Ureteral injury has been reported to occur in about 1 in 1000 CDs. The frequency of injury increases with cesarean hysterectomy. **Most ureteral injuries follow attempts to control bleeding from lateral extensions into the broad ligament. As described previously, opening the broad ligament before suture placement may reduce the risk for this complication.** If the integrity of the ureter is in doubt, IV indigo carmine can be administered, with visualization of spillage in the bladder by cystoscope (usually performed by a urologic consultant). The ureteral orifices are visualized for dye spillage, which signifies ureteral patency. If ureteral injury is recognized postoperatively, cystoscopy with stent placement or nephrostomy with radiologic imaging may define the extent of injury and can help in planning appropriate management.

Gastrointestinal Tract Injury

Bowel injury during CD is rare. Most cases involve incidental enterotomy on entering the abdomen for a repeat laparotomy, especially if scissors or a scalpel are used. This is another reason why we use blunt dissection with fingers for peritoneal entry. Defects in the bowel serosa are closed with interrupted suture of fine silk using an atraumatic needle. If the lumen of the small bowel is lacerated, closure is accomplished in two layers. A 3-0 absorbable suture is preferred for the mucosa, followed by interrupted silk sutures for the serosa.

Large defects of the small bowel or injuries of the colon generally require consultation with a general surgeon or gynecologic oncologist. Small defects may be closed primarily; however, large defects with fecal contamination may require a temporary colostomy. Broad-spectrum antibiotic coverage is recommended for such cases, which must include administration of an aminoglycoside in addition to metronidazole or clindamycin.

Uterine Atony

A more complete review of the management of uterine atony is found in Chapter 18. Uterine atony can be controlled in most cases by a combination of uterine massage and uterotonic agents. IV oxytocin in dosages up to 80 IU/L running wide open is attempted initially. If this fails to result in uterine contraction, either 0.2 mg of methergonovine maleate is administered intramuscularly or 0.25 mg of 15-methylprostaglandin F2-alpha is

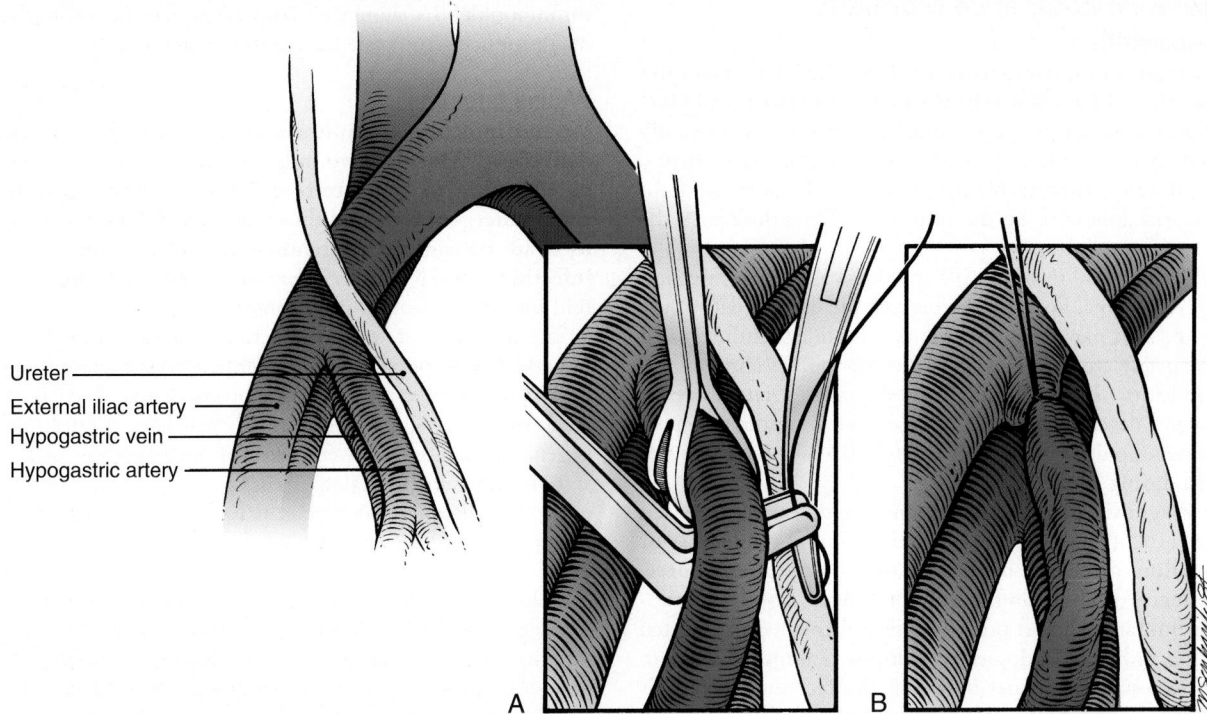

Ureter
External iliac artery
Hypogastric vein
Hypogastric artery

A   B

FIG 19-8 Hypogastric artery ligation. Approach to the hypogastric artery through the peritoneum, parallel and just lateral to the ovarian vessels, exposing the interior surface of the posterior layer of the broad ligament. The ureter will be found attached to the medial leaf of the broad ligament. The bifurcation of the common iliac artery into its external and internal (hypogastric) branches is exposed by blunt dissection of the loose overlying areolar tissues. Identification of these structures is essential. **A** and **B,** To avoid traumatizing the underlying hypogastric vein, the hypogastric artery is elevated by means of a Babcock clamp before passing an angled clamp to catch a free tie. (Modified from Breen J, Cregori CA, Kindierski JA. *Hemorrhage in Gynecologic Surgery*. Hagerstown, MD: Harper & Row; 1981; 438.)

administered intramuscularly or directly into the myometrium. Several successive doses of 15-methylprostaglandin F2-alpha every 10 to 15 minutes may be tried (up to 1 mg) if necessary. Most individuals respond to one or two doses. Misoprostol, up to 1000 μg per rectum, can be administered. Packing or use of a uterine balloon is also beneficial in these cases if medical management is not fully effective. In most cases of uterine atony, medical management is successful if used promptly and correctly.

In the rare cases in which nonsurgical management does not control bleeding, a surgical approach should be used. The initial surgical approach is bilateral ascending uterine artery branch ligation, especially if future fertility is desired. If this fails, hypogastric artery ligation or hysterectomy may be undertaken (Fig. 19-8). Hypogastric artery ligation is effective in less than 50% of cases.

Placenta Previa and Placenta Accreta

The incidence of placenta previa and placenta accreta has increased in frequency with rising CD rates, and in some series of cesarean hysterectomy, placenta accreta is the most common indication. The risk for placenta accreta increases with each repeat CD and is substantially increased by the presence of placenta previa. The management of placenta accreta is presented in Chapter 21. Specific surgical and additional procedures have also been described for CD for placenta previa (not accreta). A recent study that compared transecting to avoiding incision of the anterior placenta previa during CD has found that avoiding incision by circumventing the placenta and passing a hand around its margin reduces the frequency of maternal

blood transfusion during and after CD.[83] Another technique had been described that uses insertion of interrupted circular suture at the placental separation site via the lower segment uterine incision.[84] The vessels are ligated using interrupted 2- to 3-cm sutures at 1-cm intervals in a circle around the bleeding area on the external (serosal) surface of the uterus. The sutures are placed as deeply as possible in order to reach the endometrium, which leads to a marked decrease in intraoperative bleeding. Similarly, anteroposterior compressive suture of the lower uterine segment has been shown to successfully control the bleeding in CD for placenta previa.[85,86] The local injection of vasopressin into the placental implantation site[87] or the use of a Bakri balloon[88] can also reduce the blood loss without increasing the morbidity.

Maternal Mortality

The attributable maternal death rate has ranged from 6 to 22 per 100,000. In a study of 250,000 deliveries, Lilford and colleagues[89] reported the relative risk (RR) for maternal death from CD, compared with vaginal birth, to be about sevenfold higher when preexisting medical conditions were excluded. In contrast, Lydon-Rochelle and associates[90] noted **similar rates of maternal death among women delivered by CD versus those delivered vaginally when adjusting for maternal age and the presence of severe preeclampsia.**

Anesthesia-related morbidity and mortality have been substantially reduced through the expanded use of regional anesthesia and awake intubation for patients who require general anesthesia who may have a difficult airway for standard intubation.

Maternal Postoperative Morbidity

Endomyometritis

Postcesarean endomyometritis remains the most common complication of CD. With the use of appropriate prophylactic antibiotics as described previously, its frequency is usually less than 5%,[25,91] much reduced from preantibiotic times. Prolonged labor, rupture of membranes, and lower socioeconomic status appear to be the factors that most influence the rate of this complication.

Most cases of endomyometritis arise from ascending infection from cervicovaginal flora. Infections past the deepest part of the uterine incision may extend to the uterine musculature and, if not adequately treated, may produce peritonitis, abscess, and septic phlebitis. Using antibiotic prophylaxis, pelvic abscesses are rare and develop in 0.47% of cases following the diagnosis of chorioamnionitis compared with only 0.1% if fever was not observed during labor.

The diagnosis of postpartum endomyometritis is based on fever (100.4° F or more) with either fundal tenderness or foul-smelling discharge in the absence of any other source. The presence of chorioamnionitis, prolonged labor, and ruptured membranes should prompt early treatment in suspected cases. The utility of endometrial cultures is limited owing to contamination with vaginal flora and the fact that therapy is rarely guided by these results. Treatment is primarily based on clinical findings, including uterine tenderness and fever.

Parenteral antibiotics that use a regimen directed against possible anaerobic infection are the preferred therapeutic agents. **A regimen of clindamycin and an aminoglycoside such as gentamicin is associated with better safety and efficacy compared with other regimens.** An alternative is a single-agent penicillin-based regimen using β-lactamase inhibition to allow for anaerobic coverage (e.g., ampicillin and sulbactam). These antibiotics should be continued for at least 24 hours after the patient has defervesced. Once uncomplicated endometritis has clinically improved with IV therapy, oral therapy is not needed.

For women who fail to respond to antibiotic therapy over 2 to 3 days, an alternative source for the fever such as a wound infection, deep abscess, hematoma (Fig. 19-9), or septic pelvic thrombophlebitis should be considered. On occasion, mastitis may produce significant temperature elevations.

Wound Infection

Wound infection complicates about 1% to 5% of cesarean deliveries.[92] Most CD wounds are considered clean contaminated owing to the interface with the lower reproductive tract. Emergent CDs and those associated with chorioamnionitis are considered contaminated and have higher wound infection rates. Morbidly obese women have a twofold to fourfold increase in wound infections.[93]

The diagnosis of wound infection is usually straightforward in patients who present with tenderness, erythema, or discharge. Early wound infection (first two postoperative days) is often a result of streptococcal infection, whereas later wound infection is generally caused by overgrowth of *Staphylococcus* or a mixed aerobic-anaerobic infection.

Wound discharge may be sent for culture before instituting therapy. The infected portion of the wound should be opened, inspected, irrigated, and debrided as necessary. In most cases, this alone will suffice for therapy. A wound abscess may require drainage (Fig. 19-10). Antibiotic coverage, which is rarely necessary for simple wound infections, should be instituted promptly for advanced serious wound disruptions. Wound closure once the infection has resolved can be accomplished either surgically or by secondary intention. Reclosure of disrupted laparotomy wounds is safe and is successful in more than 80% of patients,

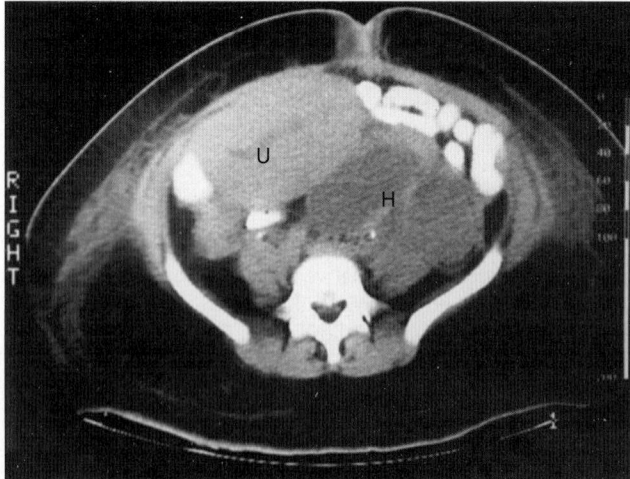

FIG 19-9 Computed tomographic scan of pelvis 6 days after a cesarean section showing left-sided broad ligament hematoma (H). The uterus (U) is displaced to the right. The patient responded to antibiotics. (Courtesy Dr. Michael Blumenfeld, Department of Obstetrics and Gynecology, Ohio State University–Columbus.)

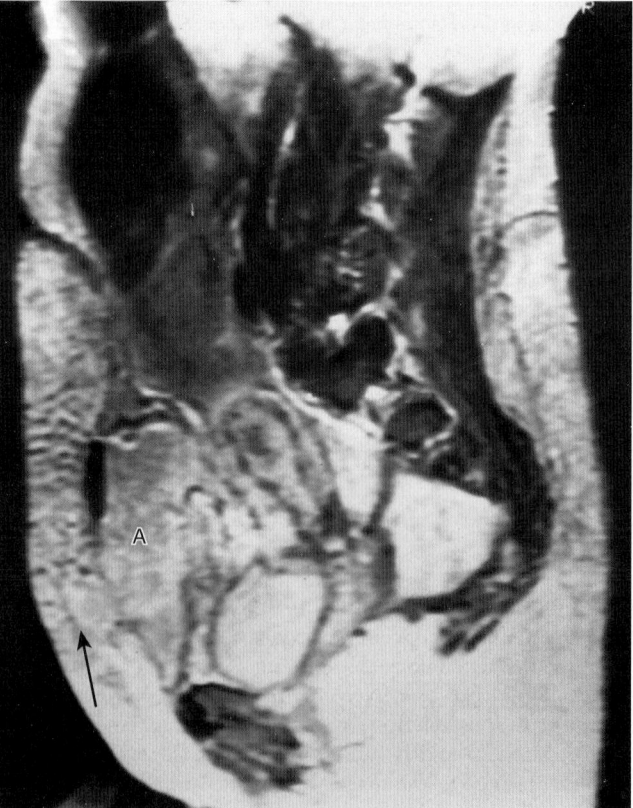

FIG 19-10 Magnetic resonance image of abdominal wall abscess. This patient presented 1 week after a cesarean delivery with fever and an abdominal mass. The differential diagnosis included an intraperitoneal infection with extension or a wound abscess. This image shows a wound abscess (A) above fascia that extended to the abdominal wall (*arrow*). The abscess responded to drainage and antibiotics.

and it decreases healing times compared with healing by secondary intention.

Extreme wound discoloration, extensive infection, gangrene, bullae, or anesthesia of the surrounding tissue should prompt consideration of necrotizing fasciitis, a life-threatening surgical emergency that has been reported to develop in 1 in 2500 women undergoing primary CD. In these cases, the wound should be debrided under general anesthesia. Examination of histologic specimens may aid in the diagnosis of necrotizing infection. In such cases, all nonviable tissue should be removed, and consultation with an experienced surgeon is recommended. Antibiotic coverage should be instituted promptly.

Thromboembolic Disease

Venous thromboembolism (VTE) occurs more commonly during pregnancy secondary to higher levels of clotting factors and venous stasis (see Chapter 45), and it is the leading cause of maternal death in developed countries. Risk factors are also the puerperal period, CD, immobility, obesity, advanced age, and parity. **The incidence of DVT was reported at 0.17%, and that of pulmonary embolism (PE) at 0.12%, in women undergoing CD.**

The diagnosis of DVT is suggested by the presence of unilateral leg pain and swelling. A significant difference in the calf or thigh diameter may be present; however, error with this measurement is possible. The presence of Homans sign, pain with foot dorsiflexion, is often observed if the calf is involved. Many cases of DVT present as PE, particularly in the postoperative patient. Tachypnea, dyspnea, tachycardia, and pleuritic pain are the classic symptoms, with cough and specific pulmonary auscultatory findings less common.

If DVT is suggested, Doppler studies may be useful for proximal disease but are less sensitive for calf thrombosis. Impedance plethysmography is also helpful in detecting proximal disease but it is of limited value in the diagnosis of pelvic thrombosis. If DVT is highly suspected and previous studies were inconclusive, a venogram should be obtained.

The workup for suspected PE includes an arterial blood gas and chest film followed by a ventilation-perfusion study or spiral computed tomography (CT) study. Oxygen should be administered and heparin begun if a clinical PE appears likely. An indeterminate perfusion scan requires pulmonary angiography to establish or rule out the diagnosis of PE.

Septic Pelvic Thrombophlebitis

Probably less than 1% of women with endomyometritis develop septic pelvic thrombophlebitis; however, accurate figures for the frequency of this condition in current practice are lacking.

Septic pelvic thrombophlebitis is most often a diagnosis of exclusion established in refractory cases of women being treated for endomyometritis. A pelvic CT scan may aid in the diagnosis, although the sensitivity and specificity of this technique are clearly difficult to establish. In practice, a febrile patient who has undergone CD and fails to respond to appropriate broad-coverage antibiotic therapy for suspected uterine infection for several days, usually more than 5 to 7 days, may be started on full-dose heparin therapy. The evidence for this practice is very limited. Long-term anticoagulation is not prescribed. Patients with septic pelvic phlebitis may present with spiking nocturnal fever and chills. However, these findings

may be absent, and a persistent febrile state may be all that is present. When anticoagulation therapy elicits no response, imaging studies that include pelvic CT are indicated to rule out an abscess or hematoma.

TUBAL STERILIZATION

The surgical approach to tubal sterilization is influenced by whether the procedure is being performed on a postpartum or interval basis. Advantages to the postpartum approach include the use of one anesthesia for labor, delivery, and sterilization and only one hospitalization. Tubal ligations after vaginal delivery are performed through a minilaparotomy incision at the level of the uterine fundus, usually subumbilically. The same surgical techniques are applied if tubal ligation is performed at the time of CD.

Modified Pomeroy

The method of tubal occlusion used by Pomeroy was described in 1930, and it is the most popular means of postpartum tubal ligation because of its simplicity. **The Pomeroy technique as originally described included grasping the fallopian tube at its midportion, creating a small knuckle, and then ligating the loop of tube with a double strand of catgut suture.** It is critical that the fallopian tube be conclusively identified. Visualizing the fimbriated portion of the tube and identifying the round ligament as a separate structure can accomplish this. Absorbable sutures are used so that the tubal ends will separate quickly after surgery, leaving a gap between the proximal and distal ends. In performing the procedure, care should be taken to make the loop of fallopian tube sufficient in size to ensure that complete transection of the tubal lumen will occur. After the loop of fallopian tube is ligated, the mesosalpinx of the ligated loop should be perforated using scissors, and then the knuckle of the tube is transected (Fig. 19-11). It is important not to resect the fallopian tube so close to the suture that the remaining portion of the fallopian tube slips out of the ligature and causes delayed bleeding.

Parkland Procedure

The Parkland procedure was designed to avoid close approximation of the cut ends of the fallopian tube accompanying the Pomeroy procedure. An avascular segment of midposition

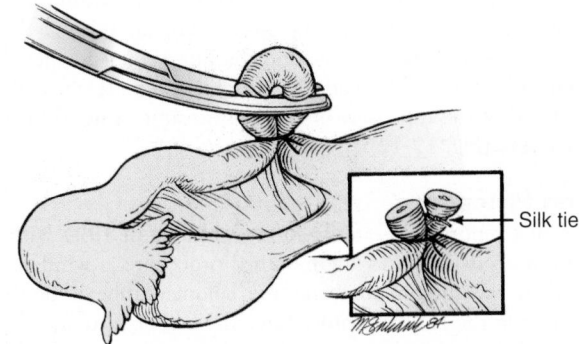

FIG 19-11 Pomeroy sterilization. A knuckle of tube is ligated with absorbable suture, and a small segment is excised. Note that the ligation is performed at a site that will favor reanastomosis, should that become desirable. Some surgeons place an extra tie of nonabsorbable suture around the proximal stump as added protection against recanalization.

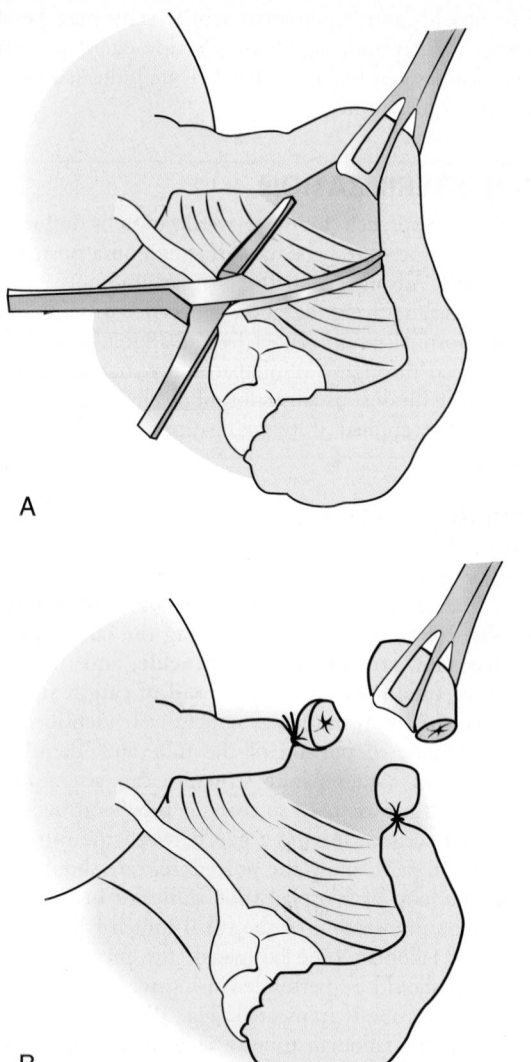

A

B

FIG 19-12 Parkland tubal ligation. The avascular mesosalpinx is opened by blunt dissection. A 2-cm midsegment of tube is ligated with 0-0 chromic suture and is divided between the sutures. (Modified from Cunningham FG, Leveno KJ, Bloom SL, et al [eds]. *Williams Obstetrics*, 22nd ed. New York: McGraw-Hill; 2005.)

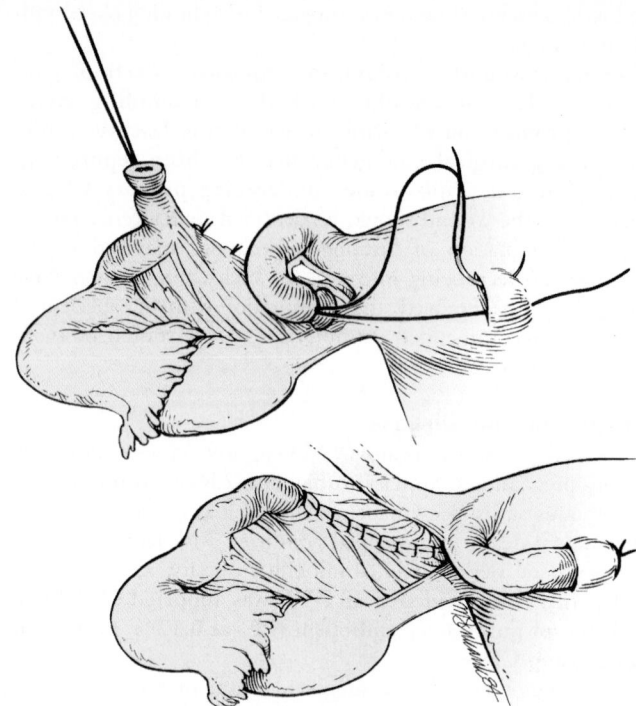

FIG 19-13 Irving sterilization. The tube is transected 3 to 4 cm from its insertion, and a short tunnel is created by means of a sharp-nosed hemostat in either the anterior or posterior uterine wall. The cut end of the tube can then be buried in the tunnel, and if necessary, it can be further secured by an interrupted suture at the opening of the tunnel. The distal cut end is buried between the leaves of the broad ligament.

mesosalpinx is identified, and a hemostat or coagulation can be used to create an opening. The freed fallopian tube is then ligated proximally and distally, and the intervening segment is excised and submitted for pathologic examination. The proximal ligated end of the tube may be left free or can be buried in the mesosalpinx (Fig. 19-12).

Irving Procedure

Irving first reported his sterilization technique in 1924 with a modification in 1950. In the modified procedure, a window is created in the mesosalpinx and the fallopian tube is doubly ligated, as in the Parkland procedure. The fallopian tube is then transected about 4 cm from the uterotubal portion; the two free ends of the ligation stitch on the proximal tubal segment are held long. The proximal portion of the fallopian tube is dissected free from the mesosalpinx and is then buried into an incision in the myometrium of the posterior uterine wall, near the uterotubal junction. This is accomplished by first creating a tunnel

about 2 cm in length with a mosquito clamp in the uterine wall. The two free ends of the ligation stitch on the proximal tubal segment are then brought deep into the myometrial tunnel and are brought out through the uterine serosa. Traction is then placed on the sutures to draw the proximal tubal stump into the myometrial tunnel; tying the free sutures fixes the tube in that location. No treatment of the distal tubal stump is necessary, but some choose to bury the segment in the mesosalpinx (Fig. 19-13). **Although this technique is slightly more complicated than the others, it has the lowest failure rate.**

Uchida Procedure

In the Uchida sterilization procedure, the muscular portion of the fallopian tube is separated from its serosal cover and is grasped about 6 to 7 cm from the uterotubal junction. Saline solution is injected subserosally, and the serosa is then incised. The muscular portion of the fallopian tube is grasped with a clamp and divided. The serosa over the proximal tubal segment is bluntly dissected toward the uterus, exposing about 5 cm of the proximal tubal segment. The tube is then ligated with chromic suture near the uterotubal junction, and about 5 cm of the tube is resected. The shortened proximal tubal stump is allowed to retract into the mesosalpinx. The serosa around the opening in the mesosalpinx is sutured in a purse-string fashion with a fine absorbable stitch; when the suture is tied, the mesosalpinx is gathered around the distal tubal segment (Fig. 19-14). **Some surgeons choose to excise only 1 cm of fallopian tube, rather than the recommended 5 cm, in case the patient wishes to have a tubal reanastomosis in the future.**

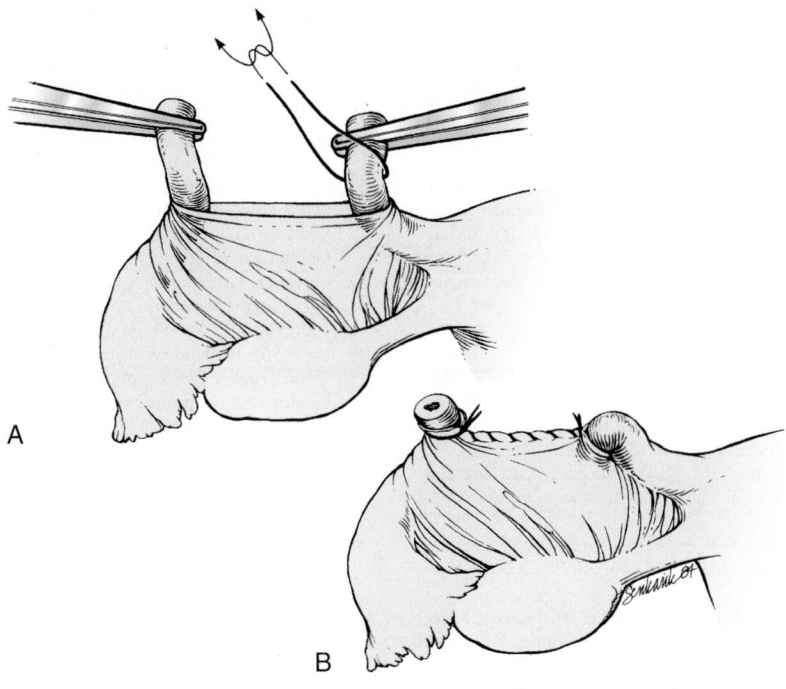

FIG 19-14 Uchida sterilization. The leaves of the broad ligament and peritubal peritoneum are infiltrated with saline so that the tube can be easily isolated from these structures, divided **(A),** and ligated **(B).** The broad ligament is then closed, and the proximal stump is buried between the leaves and includes the distal stump in the line of closure.

KEY POINTS

- In 1970, the CD rate was about 5%. By 2008, it had reached 32.8%, the highest rate ever recorded in the United States. Vaginal birth after cesarean (VBAC) rates have plummeted, from a peak of 28.3% in 1996 to 8.5% in 2008, contributing to the rise in CD. Most recently, CD rates have stabilized around 31% to 32% in the United States.
- Factors that have contributed to the rise in CD during the past decades include (1) continued increase in primary CDs for dystocia, failed induction, and abnormal presentation; (2) an increase in the proportion of women with obesity, diabetes mellitus, and multiple gestations; (3) increased use of planned CD; and (4) limited use of TOLAC after CD because of both safety and medicolegal concerns.
- Single-dose, preoperative prophylactic antibiotics are of clear benefit in reducing the frequency of postcesarean endomyometritis and wound infection.
- Mechanical prophylaxis with graduated compression stockings or a pneumatic compression device during and after all cesarean deliveries should be considered.
- Horizontal skin incision is preferred because vertical skin incision is associated with long-term postoperative complications, such as wound dehiscence and abdominal incisional hernia, and it is also cosmetically less pleasing.
- A low transverse uterine incision is preferred for almost all CDs.
- Blunt uterine extension is associated with decreased blood loss and is therefore preferred.

- Delayed cord clamping should be done for 30 to 120 seconds for all infants delivered at less than 37 weeks' gestation.
- IV oxytocin, 10 to 80 IU in 1 L crystalloid, should be given prophylactically after the baby is delivered in all CDs.
- Several RCTs have demonstrated greater blood loss and a higher rate of endometritis with manual extraction of the placenta at CD. Thus spontaneous expulsion of the placenta with gentle cord traction is preferred.
- The uterine incision can be repaired in a single layer if the patient has completed child-bearing, such as a bilateral tubal ligation performed concurrently with CD. Consider double-layer closure otherwise.
- When closing the abdomen after a CD, the subcutaneous tissue is closed if its thickness exceeds 2 cm. This approach significantly reduces the risk for wound disruption.
- The skin should be closed with sutures, not staples.
- Postcesarean endomyometritis remains the most common complication of CD. With the use of appropriate prophylactic antibiotics as described previously, its frequency is usually less than 5%.

REFERENCES

1. American College of Obstetricians and Gynecologists (ACOG). *reVITALize Obstetric Data Definitions.* Available at: <www.acog.org/about-ACOG/ACOG-departments/patient-safety-and-quality-improvement/reVITALize-obstetric-data-definitions>.
2. West M, Irvine L, Jauniaux E. *A Modern Textbook of Cesarean Section.* Oxford, UK: Oxford University Press; 2015.

3. Martin J, Hamilton B, Osterman M. Births in the United States, 2013. *NCHS Data Brief*. 2014;175.

4. Matthews TG, Crowley P, Chong A, McKenna P, McGarvey C, O'Regan M. Rising caesarean section rates: a cause for concern? *BJOG*. 2003;110(4):346-349.

5. Robson M. Can we reduce the caesarean section rate? *Best Pract Res Clin Obstet Gynaecol*. 2001;15:179-194.

6. American College of Obstetricians and Gynecologists. ACOG executive summary: evaluation of cesarean delivery. *ACOG*. 2000;Updated.

7. American College of Obstetricians and Gynecologists (College); Society for Maternal-Fetal Medicine, Caughey AB, Cahill AG, Guise JM, Rouse DJ. Safe prevention of the primary cesarean delivery. *Am J Obstet Gynecol*. 2014;210(3):179-193.

8. Myers SA, Gleicher N. A successful program to lower cesarean-section rates. *N Engl J Med*. 1988;319(23):1511-1516.

9. Hannah ME, Hannah WJ, Hewson SA, Hodnett ED, Saigal S, Willan AR. Planned caesarean section versus planned vaginal birth for breech presentation at term: a randomised multicentre trial. term breech trial collaborative group. *Lancet*. 2000;356(9239):1375-1383.

10. Berghella V, Blackwell SC, Ramin SM, Sibai BM, Saade GR. Use and misuse of the term "elective" in obstetrics. *Obstet Gynecol*. 2011; 117(2 Pt 1):372-376.

11. National Institutes of Health state-of-the-science conference statement. Cesarean delivery on maternal request. March 27-29, 2006. *Obstet Gynecol*. 2006;107(6):1386-1397.

12. American College of Obstetricians and Gynecologists. ACOG committee opinion no. 386 November 2007: Cesarean delivery on maternal request. *Obstet Gynecol*. 2007;110(5):1209-1212.

13. Sachs BP, Yeh J, Acker D, Driscoll S, Brown DA, Jewett JF. Cesarean section-related maternal mortality in Massachusetts, 1954-1985. *Obstet Gynecol*. 1988;71(3 Pt 1):385-388.

14. Tita AT, Landon MB, Spong CY, et al. Timing of elective repeat cesarean delivery at term and neonatal outcomes. *N Engl J Med*. 2009;360(2): 111-120.

15. Martin JA, Hamilton BE, Ventura SJ, Osterman MJ, Wilson EC, Mathews TJ. Births: final data for 2010. *Natl Vital Stat Rep*. 2012;61(1): 1-72.

16. Dahlke JD, Mendez-Figueroa H, Rouse DJ, Berghella V, Baxter JK, Chauhan SP. Evidence-based surgery for cesarean delivery: an updated systematic review. *Am J Obstet Gynecol*. 2013;209(4):294-306.

17. Mackeen AD, Packard RE, Ota E, Berghella V, Baxter JK. Timing of intravenous prophylactic antibiotics for preventing postpartum infectious morbidity in women undergoing cesarean delivery. *Cochrane Database Syst Rev*. 2014;(12):CD009516.

18. Fiore MT, Pearlman MD, Chapman RL, Bhatt-Mehta V, Faiz RG. Maternal and transplacental pharmacokinetics of cefazolin. *Obstet Gynecol*. 2001;98(6):1075-1079.

19. Elkomy MH, Sultan P, Drover DR, Epshtein E, Galinkin JL, Carvalho B. Pharmacokinetics of prophylactic cefazolin in parturients undergoing cesarean delivery. *Antimicrob Agents Chemother*. 2014;58(6):3504-3513.

20. Ziogos E, Tsiodras S, Matalliotakis I, Giamarellou H, Kanellakopoulou K. Ampicillin/sulbactam versus cefuroxime as antimicrobial prophylaxis for cesarean delivery: A randomized study. *BMC Infect Dis*. 2010;10:341.

21. Alekwe LO, Kuti O, Orji EO, Ogunniyi SO. Comparison of ceftriaxone versus triple drug regimen in the prevention of cesarean section infectious morbidities. *J Matern Fetal Neonatal Med*. 2008;21(9):638-642.

22. Rudge MV, Atallah AN, Peracoli JC, Tristão Ada R, Mendonça Neto M. Randomized controlled trial on prevention of postcesarean infection using penicillin and cephalothin in Brazil. *Acta Obstet Gynecol Scand*. 2006;85(8):945-948.

23. Mackeen AD, Packard RE, Ota E, Speer L. Antibiotic regimens for postpartum endometritis. *Cochrane Database Syst Rev*. 2015;(2):CD001067.

24. Costantine MM, Rahman M, Ghulmiyah L, et al. Timing of perioperative antibiotics for cesarean delivery: a metaanalysis. *Am J Obstet Gynecol*. 2008;199(3):301.e1-301.e6.

25. Tita AT, Rouse DJ, Blackwell S, Saade GR, Spong CY, Andrews WW. Emerging concepts in antibiotic prophylaxis for cesarean delivery: a systematic review. *Obstet Gynecol*. 2009;113(3):675-682.

26. Faro S, Martens MG, Hammill HA, Riddle G, Tortolero G. Antibiotic prophylaxis: is there a difference? *Am J Obstet Gynecol*. 1990;162(4):900-907, discussion 907-909.

27. Lindqvist P, Dahlbäck B, Marsál K. Thrombotic risk during pregnancy: A population study. *Obstet Gynecol*. 1999;94(4):595-599.

28. Tooher R, Gates S, Dowswell T, Davis LJ. Prophylaxis for venous thromboembolic disease in pregnancy and the early postnatal period. *Cochrane Database Syst Rev*. 2010;(5):CD001689.

29. Burrows RF, Gan ET, Gallus AS, Wallace EM, Burrows EA. A randomised double-blind placebo controlled trial of low molecular weight heparin as prophylaxis in preventing venous thrombolic events after caesarean section: A pilot study. *BJOG*. 2001;108(8):835-839.

30. Hill NC, Hill JG, Sargent JM, Taylor CG, Bush PV. Effect of low dose heparin on blood loss at caesarean section. *Br Med J (Clin Res Ed)*. 1988;296(6635):1505-1506.

31. Gates S, Brocklehurst P, Ayers S, Bowler U, Thromboprophylaxis in Pregnancy Advisory Group. Thromboprophylaxis and pregnancy: two randomized controlled pilot trials that used low-molecular-weight heparin. *Am J Obstet Gynecol*. 2004;191(4):1296-1303.

32. Casele H, Grobman WA. Cost-effectiveness of thromboprophylaxis with intermittent pneumatic compression at cesarean delivery. *Obstet Gynecol*. 2006;108(3 Pt 1):535-540.

33. Davis SM, Branch DW. Thromboprophylaxis in pregnancy: who and how? *Obstet Gynecol Clin North Am*. 2010;37(2):333-343.

34. Publications Committee, Society for Maternal-fetal Medicine, MW Varner. Thromboprophylaxis for cesarean delivery. *Contemporary Ob/Gyn*. 2011.

35. Cluver C, Novikova N, Hofmeyr GJ, Hall DR. Maternal position during caesarean section for preventing maternal and neonatal complications. *Cochrane Database Syst Rev*. 2010;(6):CD007623.

36. Haas DM, Morgan S, Contreras K. Vaginal preparation with antiseptic solution before cesarean section for preventing postoperative infections. *Cochrane Database Syst Rev*. 2014;(12):CD007892.

37. Nasr AM, ElBigawy AF, Abdelamid AE, Al-Khulaidi S, Al-Inany HG, Sayed EH. Evaluation of the use vs nonuse of urinary catheterization during cesarean delivery: a prospective, multicenter, randomized controlled trial. *J Perinatol*. 2009;29(6):416-421.

38. Onile TG, Kuti O, Orji EO, Ogunniyi SO. A prospective randomized clinical trial of urethral catheter removal following elective cesarean delivery. *Int J Gynaecol Obstet*. 2008;102(3):267-270.

39. Li L, Wen J, Wang L, Li YP, Li Y. Is routine indwelling catheterisation of the bladder for caesarean section necessary? A systematic review. *BJOG*. 2011;118(4):400-409.

40. Alexander JW, Fischer JE, Boyajian M, Palmquist J, Morris MJ. The influence of hair-removal methods on wound infections. *Arch Surg*. 1983; 118(3):347-352.

41. Darouiche RO, Wall MJ Jr, Itani KM, et al. Chlorhexidine-alcohol versus povidone-iodine for surgical-site antisepsis. *N Engl J Med*. 2010;362(1): 18-26.

42. Ward HR, Jennings OG, Potgieter P, Lombard CJ. Do plastic adhesive drapes prevent post caesarean wound infection? *J Hosp Infect*. 2001;47(3): 230-234.

43. Cordtz T, Schouenborg L, Laursen K, et al. The effect of incisional plastic drapes and redisinfection of operation site on wound infection following caesarean section. *J Hosp Infect*. 1989;13(3):267-272.

44. Berghella V, Baxter JK, Chauhan SP. Evidence-based surgery for cesarean delivery. *Am J Obstet Gynecol*. 2005;193:1607-1617.

45. Sullivan S, Williamson B, Wilson LK, Korte JE, Soper D. Blunt needles for the reduction of needlestick injuries during cesarean delivery: a randomized controlled trial. *Obstet Gynecol*. 2009;114(2 Pt 1): 211-216.

46. Wylie BJ, Gilbert S, Landon MB, et al. Comparison of transverse and vertical skin incision for emergency cesarean delivery. *Obstet Gynecol*. 2010;115(6):1134-1140.

47. Tully L, Gates S, Brocklehurst P, McKenzie-McHarg K, Ayers S. Surgical techniques used during caesarean section operations: results of a national survey of practice in the UK. *Eur J Obstet Gynecol Reprod Biol*. 2002; 102(2):120-126.

48. Joel-Cohen S. Abdominal and vaginal hysterectomy: New techniques based on time and motion studies. Philadelphia: Lippincott; 1977: 18-23.

49. Dandolu V, Raj J, Harmanli O, Lorico A, Chatwani AJ. Resident education regarding technical aspects of cesarean section. *J Reprod Med*. 2006; 51(1):49-54.

50. Stark M, Finkel AR. Comparison between the Joel-Cohen and Pfannenstiel incisions in cesarean section. *Eur J Obstet Gynecol Reprod Biol*. 1994; 53(2):121-122.

51. Stark M, Chavkin Y, Kupfersztain C, Guedj P, Finkel AR. Evaluation of combinations of procedures in cesarean section. *Int J Gynaecol Obstet*. 1995;48(3):273-276.

52. Hofmeyr GJ, Mathai M, Shah A, Novikova N. Techniques for caesarean section. *Cochrane Database Syst Rev*. 2008;(1):CD004662.

53. O'Neill HA, Egan G, Walsh CA, Cotter AM, Walsh SR. Omission of the bladder flap at caesarean section reduces delivery time without increased

morbidity: a meta-analysis of randomised controlled trials. *Eur J Obstet Gynecol Reprod Biol.* 2014;174:20-26.

54. American College of Obstetricians and Gynecologists. ACOG practice bulletin no. 115: Vaginal birth after previous cesarean delivery. *Obstet Gynecol.* 2010;116(2 Pt 1):450-463.

55. Dodd JM, Anderson ER, Gates S, Grivell RM. Surgical techniques for uterine incision and uterine closure at the time of caesarean section. *Cochrane Database Syst Rev.* 2014;(7):CD004732.

56. Cromi A, Ghezzi F, Di Naro E, Siesto G, Loverro G, Bolis P. Blunt expansion of the low transverse uterine incision at cesarean delivery: a randomized comparison of 2 techniques. *Am J Obstet Gynecol.* 2008;199(3):292.e1-292.e6.

57. Fasubaa OB, Ezechi OC, Orji EO, et al. Delivery of the impacted head of the fetus at caesarean section after prolonged obstructed labour: a randomised comparative study of two methods. *J Obstet Gynaecol.* 2002;22(4):375-378.

58. Rabe H, Diaz-Rossello JL, Duley L, Dowswell T. Effect of timing of umbilical cord clamping and other strategies to influence placental transfusion at preterm birth on maternal and infant outcomes. *Cochrane Database Syst Rev.* 2012;(8):CD003248.

59. Backes CH, Rivera BK, Haque U, et al. Placental transfusion strategies in very preterm neonates: a systematic review and meta-analysis. *Obstet Gynecol.* 2014;124(1):47-56.

60. McDonald SJ, Middleton P, Dowswell T, Morris PS. Effect of timing of umbilical cord clamping of term infants on maternal and neonatal outcomes. *Cochrane Database Syst Rev.* 2013;(7):CD004074.

61. Roach MK, Abramovici A, Tita AT. Dose and duration of oxytocin to prevent postpartum hemorrhage: a review. *Am J Perinatol.* 2013;30(7):523-528.

62. Murphy DJ, MacGregor H, Munishankar B, McLeod G. A randomised controlled trial of oxytocin 5IU and placebo infusion versus oxytocin 5IU and 30IU infusion for the control of blood loss at elective caesarean section—pilot study. ISRCTN 40302163. *Eur J Obstet Gynecol Reprod Biol.* 2009;142(1):30-33.

63. Simonazzi G, Bisulli M, Saccone G, Moro E, Marshall A, Berghella V. Tranexamic acid for preventing postpartum blood loss after cesarean delivery: A pooled meta-analysis of randomized controlled trials. *Obstet Gynecol.* 2015;(In press).

64. Su LL, Chong YS, Samuel M. Carbetocin for preventing postpartum haemorrhage. *Cochrane Database Syst Rev.* 2012;(4):CD005457.

65. Magann EF, Dodson MK, Allbert JR, McCurdy CM Jr, Martin RW, Morrison JC. Blood loss at time of cesarean section by method of placental removal and exteriorization versus in situ repair of the uterine incision. *Surg Gynecol Obstet.* 1993;177(4):389-392.

66. Atkinson MW, Owen J, Wren A, Hauth JC. The effect of manual removal of the placenta on post-cesarean endometritis. *Obstet Gynecol.* 1996;87(1):99-102.

67. Anorlu RI, Maholwana B, Hofmeyr GJ. Methods of delivering the placenta at caesarean section. *Cochrane Database Syst Rev.* 2008;(3):CD004737.

68. Walsh CA, Walsh SR. Extraabdominal vs intraabdominal uterine repair at cesarean delivery: a metaanalysis. *Am J Obstet Gynecol.* 2009;200(6):625.e1-625.e8.

69. Ahmed B, Abu Nahia F, Abushama M. Routine cervical dilatation during elective cesarean section and its influence on maternal morbidity: a randomized controlled study. *J Perinat Med.* 2005;33(6):510-513.

70. Hohlagschwandtner M, Chalubinski K, Nather A, Husslein P, Joura EA. Continuous vs interrupted sutures for single-layer closure of uterine incision at cesarean section. *Arch Gynecol Obstet.* 2003;268(1):26-28.

71. Yazicioglu F, Gökdogan A, Kelekci S, Aygün M, Savan K. Incomplete healing of the uterine incision after caesarean section: Is it preventable? *Eur J Obstet Gynecol Reprod Biol.* 2006;124(1):32-36.

72. Dodd JM, Anderson ER, Gates S. Surgical techniques for uterine incision and uterine closure at the time of caesarean section. *Cochrane Database Syst Rev.* 2008;(3):CD004732.

73. Harrigill KM, Miller HS, Haynes DE. The effect of intraabdominal irrigation at cesarean delivery on maternal morbidity: a randomized trial. *Obstet Gynecol.* 2003;101(1):80-85.

74. Bamigboye AA, Hofmeyr GJ. Closure versus non-closure of the peritoneum at caesarean section. *Cochrane Database Syst Rev.* 2003;(4):CD000163.

75. Shi Z, Ma L, Yang Y, et al. Adhesion formation after previous caesarean section-a meta-analysis and systematic review. *BJOG.* 2011;118(4):410-422.

76. Anderson ER, Gates S. Techniques and materials for closure of the abdominal wall in caesarean section. *Cochrane Database Syst Rev.* 2004;(4):CD004663.

77. Gates S, Anderson ER. Wound drainage for caesarean section. *Cochrane Database Syst Rev.* 2005;(1):CD004549.

78. Hellums EK, Lin MG, Ramsey PS. Prophylactic subcutaneous drainage for prevention of wound complications after cesarean delivery–a meta-analysis. *Am J Obstet Gynecol.* 2007;197(3):229-235.

79. CAESAR study collaborative group. Caesarean section surgical techniques: a randomised factorial trial (CAESAR). *BJOG.* 2010;117(11):1366-1376.

80. Mackeen AD, Khalifeh K, Fleisher J, et al. Suture compared with staple skin closure after cesarean delivery: a randomized controlled trial. *Obstet Gynecol.* 2014;123(6):1169-1175.

81. Mackeen AD, Berghella V, Larsen ML. Techniques and materials for skin closure in caesarean section. *Cochrane Database Syst Rev.* 2012;(11):CD003577.

82. Mackeen AD, Schuster M, Berghella V. Suture versus staples for skin closure after cesarean: a metaanalysis. *Am J Obstet Gynecol.* 2015;212(5):621.e1-621.e10.

83. Verspyck E, Douysset X, Roman H, Marret S, Marpeau L. Transecting versus avoiding incision of the anterior placenta previa during cesarean delivery. *Int J Gynaecol Obstet.* 2015;128(1):44-47.

84. Cho JY, Kim SJ, Cha KY, Kay CW, Kim MI, Cha KS. Interrupted circular suture: bleeding control during cesarean delivery in placenta previa accreta. *Obstet Gynecol.* 1991;78(5 Pt 1):876-879.

85. Penotti M, Vercellini P, Bolis G, Fedele L. Compressive suture of the lower uterine segment for the treatment of postpartum hemorrhage due to complete placenta previa: a preliminary study. *Gynecol Obstet Invest.* 2012;73(4):314-320.

86. Matsubara S, Kuwata T, Baba Y, et al. A novel 'uterine sandwich' for haemorrhage at caesarean section for placenta praevia. *Aust N Z J Obstet Gynaecol.* 2014;54(3):283-286.

87. Kato S, Tanabe A, Kanki K, et al. Local injection of vasopressin reduces the blood loss during cesarean section in placenta previa. *J Obstet Gynaecol Res.* 2014;40(5):1249-1256.

88. Beckmann MM, Chaplin J. Bakri balloon during cesarean delivery for placenta previa. *Int J Gynaecol Obstet.* 2014;124(2):118-122.

89. Lilford RJ, van Coeverden de Groot HA, Moore PJ, Bingham P. The relative risks of caesarean section (intrapartum and elective) and vaginal delivery: a detailed analysis to exclude the effects of medical disorders and other acute pre-existing physiological disturbances. *Br J Obstet Gynaecol.* 1990;97(10):883-892.

90. Lydon-Rochelle M, Holt VL, Easterling TR, Martin DP. Cesarean delivery and postpartum mortality among primiparas in Washington state, 1987-1996(1). *Obstet Gynecol.* 2001;97(2):169-174.

91. Tita AT, Hauth JC, Grimes A, Owen J, Stamm AM, Andrews WW. Decreasing incidence of postcesarean endometritis with extended-spectrum antibiotic prophylaxis. *Obstet Gynecol.* 2008;111(1):51-56.

92. Gibbs RS, Sweet RL, Duff WP. Maternal and fetal infectious disorders. In: Creasy RK, Resnik R, eds. *Maternal-Fetal Medicine: Principles and Practice.* 5th ed. Philadelphia: Saunders; 2004:752.

93. Stamilio DM, Scifres CM. Extreme obesity and postcesarean maternal complications. *Obstet Gynecol.* 2014;124(2 Pt 1):227-232.

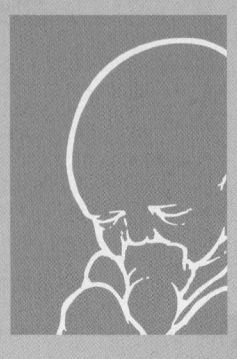

CHAPTER 20

Vaginal Birth After Cesarean Delivery

MARK B. LANDON and WILLIAM A. GROBMAN

KEY ABBREVIATIONS

American College of Obstetricians and Gynecologists	ACOG
Body mass index	BMI
Cephalopelvic disproportion	CPD
Fetal heart rate	FHR
Hypoxic-ischemic encephalopathy	HIE
Lower uterine segment	LUS
Maternal-fetal medicine units	MFMU
National Institute of Child Health and Human Development	NICHD
National Institutes of Health	NIH
Odds ratio	OR
Relative risk	RR
Trial of labor after cesarean	TOLAC
Vaginal birth after cesarean	VBAC

VAGINAL BIRTH AFTER CESAREAN DELIVERY
Trends

In a review of contemporary cesarean delivery practice, Zhang and colleagues[1] concluded that one of the most important contributors to the rising cesarean delivery rate in the United States was the decline in vaginal birth after cesarean delivery (VBAC). Specifically, after a steady increase in the overall U.S. cesarean delivery rate beginning in the early 1960s, a modest decline in this rate was observed that reached a nadir of 21% in 1996, largely because of an increased rate of allowing a trial of labor after cesarean delivery (TOLAC) that was estimated to exceed 50% (Fig. 20-1). However, by 2006 the TOLAC rate had plummeted to approximately 15%, and the rate of successful TOLAC has also had declined. Given that **it has been suggested that about two thirds of women with a prior cesarean delivery are** actually candidates for a TOLAC, most planned repeat operations are influenced by physician discretion and patient choice. A comparison of TOLAC rates between the United States and several European nations, where TOLAC rates vary between 50% and 70%, suggest significant underuse of TOLAC in this country. Given this information and the fact that 10% of the obstetric population has had a previous cesarean delivery, more widespread use of TOLAC has the potential to decrease the overall rate of cesarean delivery.

The evolution in management of the woman with a prior cesarean delivery can be traced through several American College of Obstetricians and Gynecologists (ACOG) documents and key studies over the past 25 years. In 1988, ACOG published "Guidelines for Vaginal Delivery after a Previous Cesarean Birth," recommending TOLAC and VBAC as it became clear that this procedure was safe and did not appear to be associated with excess perinatal morbidity compared with repeat cesarean delivery. They recommended that each hospital develop its own protocol for the management of VBAC patients and that in the absence of a contraindication such as a prior classical incision, women who had undergone one prior low transverse cesarean section should be counseled and encouraged to attempt labor. This recommendation was supported by several large case series that attested to the safety and effectiveness of TOLAC. With this information, TOLAC rates exceeded 50% in many institutions. Some third-party payers and managed care organizations began to mandate a TOLAC for women with a prior cesarean delivery. Feeling institutional pressure to lower cesarean rates, physicians began to offer a TOLAC liberally and likely included less-than-optimal candidates. With the rise in VBAC experience, a number of reports appeared in the literature suggesting a possible increase in uterine rupture and its maternal and fetal consequences. Descriptions of uterine rupture with hysterectomy and adverse perinatal outcomes, including fetal death and neonatal brain injury, set the stage for the precipitous decline in VBAC rates during the past 20 years.[2,3]

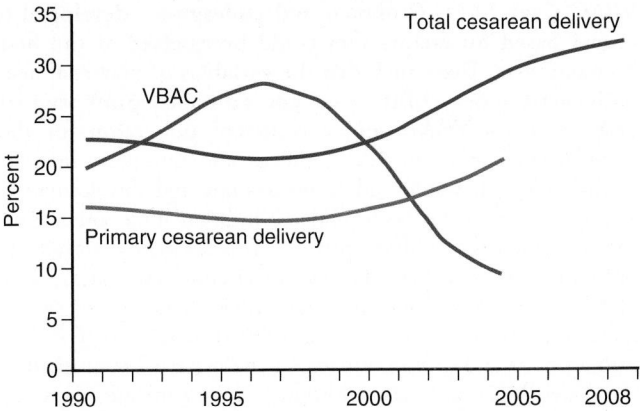

FIG 20-1 United States total cesarean delivery rate from 1990 through 2008 and the primary cesarean delivery and vaginal birth after cesarean (VBAC) rates from 1990 through 2004. (Modified from MacDorman M, DeClercq E, Menacker F. Recent trends and patterns in cesarean and vaginal birth after cesarean deliveries in the United States. *Clin Perinatol.* 2011;38;179-192.)

In 1999, ACOG issued a practice bulletin[5] acknowledging that while the risks of TOLAC were apparently small in magnitude, clinically significant risks of uterine rupture did exist, with poor outcomes for both women and their infants. It was also recognized that such adverse events during a TOLAC could lead to malpractice suits.[4] ACOG thus recommended that TOLAC be conducted in settings in which a physician capable of performing a cesarean delivery was "immediately available" and that institutions be equipped to respond to emergencies such as uterine rupture. The language in the 1999 document also suggested that instead of "encouraging" TOLAC, women with prior low transverse cesarean deliveries should be "offered" TOLAC.[5] A more conservative approach to TOLAC then followed with recognition of the need to reevaluate VBAC recommendations.

In the aftermath of the 1999 document, many hospitals began to no longer offer planned TOLAC. The role of nonclinical factors in the declined utilization of TOLAC has been reviewed by Korst and colleagues.[6] These authors noted five factors that seem to have influenced VBAC rates: (1) recommendations of opinion leaders and professional guidelines, (2) hospital facilities and cesarean delivery availability, (3) reimbursement, (4) medical liability, and (5) patient-level factors. Among patient-level factors is the consideration that patients are becoming more risk averse and are thus more comfortable with choosing planned repeat cesarean delivery. The question remains as to whether women are less convinced on their own that VBAC is a reasonable option or whether they are being dissuaded by the health care system. Nonetheless, the 2010 ACOG practice bulletin—consistent with prior publications—concludes that most women with one previous cesarean delivery via a low transverse incision are candidates for TOLAC and should be counseled about and offered a TOLAC.[7]

In response to a growing body of evidence that indicates restriction of a women's access to TOLAC-VBAC, despite two recent large-scale contemporary multicenter studies that attest to their relative safety,[8,9] the National Institutes of Health (NIH) held a consensus development conference concerning VBAC in 2010. The panel at that conference concluded that TOLAC is a reasonable birth option for many women with a previous cesarean delivery. The panel also

found that existing practice guidelines and the medical liability climate were restricting access to TOLAC-VBAC and that these factors need to be addressed.[10] A specific concern raised was the low level of evidence for the requirement for "immediately available" surgical and anesthesia personnel in existing guidelines and the need to reassess this recommendation with reference to other obstetric complications of comparable risk given limited physician and nursing resources.

The ACOG 2010 practice bulletin[7] acknowledged a background of limited access to TOLAC-VBAC evolving over time as well as the recommendation by the NIH panel to facilitate access. Although again recommending that TOLAC-VBAC be undertaken in facilities with staff immediately available to provide emergency care, ACOG recognized that resources for immediate cesarean delivery may not be available in smaller institutions. In such cases, the decision to offer and pursue TOLAC should be carefully considered by patients and their health care providers. It was recommended that the best alternative may be to refer patients to a facility with available resources.

Candidates for a Trial of Labor After Cesarean

The optimal candidates for planned TOLAC are those women in whom the balance of risks (i.e., as low as possible) and chances of success (i.e., as high as possible) are acceptable to the patient and health care provider.[7] Most women who have had a low transverse uterine incision with a prior cesarean delivery and have no contraindications to vaginal birth should be considered candidates for a TOLAC. **The following are selection criteria suggested by ACOG[7] for identifying candidates for TOLAC:**

- One or two previous low transverse cesarean deliveries
- Clinically adequate pelvis
- No other uterine scars or previous rupture
- Physicians immediately available throughout active labor capable of monitoring labor and performing an emergency cesarean delivery

It should be noted that these criteria identify women who are likely to be reasonable candidates and do not exclude women with any other clinical situation from the option of TOLAC. For example, several studies indicate that it may be reasonable to offer a TOLAC to women with macrosomia, gestation beyond 40 weeks, previous low vertical incision, unknown uterine scar type, and twin gestation.[8,11-14]

Conversely, a TOLAC is contraindicated in women at high risk for uterine rupture. **A TOLAC should *not* be attempted in the following circumstances:**

- Previous classical or T-shaped incision or extensive transfundal uterine surgery
- Previous uterine rupture
- Medical or obstetric complications that preclude vaginal delivery

Success Rates for a Trial of Labor After Cesarean

The overall success rate for a population of women undergoing TOLAC appears to be in the 60% to 80% range,[7] although some data suggest this rate may be lower in contemporary practice. A cross-sectional analysis study[15] that utilized National Hospital Discharge Survey information noted that TOLAC success rates had fallen from nearly 70% in 2000 to 40% to 50% by 2009.

Predictors of successful TOLAC are well described.[16-24] The ability to predict successful TOLAC is important because maternal morbidity is lowest among women who achieve VBAC and is greatest among women who fail TOLAC and require a repeat operation. The prior indication for cesarean delivery clearly affects the likelihood of successful TOLAC because women with "recurrent" indications (i.e., labor arrest disorders) are less likely to achieve VBAC. Also, a history of prior vaginal birth is associated with the highest success rates for VBAC (Table 20-1). **Several authors have developed models for predicting**

TABLE 20-1	SUCCESS RATES FOR TRIAL OF LABOR AFTER CESAREAN DELIVERY	
		VBAC SUCCESS (%)
Prior Indication		
CPD/FTP		63.5
NRFWB		72.6
Malpresentation		83.8
Prior Vaginal Delivery		
Yes		86.6
No		60.9
Labor Type		
Induction		67.4
Augmented		73.9
Spontaneous		80.6

Modified from Landon MB, Leindecker S, Spong CY, et al. Factors affecting the success of trial of labor following prior cesarean delivery. *Am J Obstet Gynecol.* 2005;193:1016. *CPD,* cephalopelvic disproportion; *FTP,* failure to progress; *NRFWB,* nonreassuring fetal well-being; *VBAC,* vaginal birth after cesarean.

VBAC (Fig. 20-2). **Grobman and colleagues[25] developed a model based on factors that could be assessed at the first prenatal visit. These included the variables of maternal age, body mass index (BMI), race and ethnicity, prior vaginal delivery, prior VBAC, and a recurrent indication for the cesarean delivery.** After development and internal validation of the model, it was found to be accurate and discriminating and subsequently has been validated in populations other than that in which it was developed.[26-29] The calculator is available online at mfmu.bsc.gwu.edu. Because circumstances at the time of admission for delivery may affect the chance of successful TOLAC, a second calculator was created to take these factors into account and is also available at the maternal-fetal medical units (MFMU) site. The additional factors include maternal BMI at delivery, cervical status, need for induction, and the presence or absence of preeclampsia.[30] A simple admission model and scoring system for the prediction of VBAC success that incorporates cervical status, history of vaginal birth, maternal age, prior indication for cesarean delivery, and maternal BMI has also been investigated by Metz and colleagues.[31]

A summary of factors associated with VBAC in the setting of TOLAC is summarized in the following sections.

Maternal Demographics

Race, age, BMI, and insurance status have all been demonstrated to be associated with the success of TOLAC.[16] In a multicenter

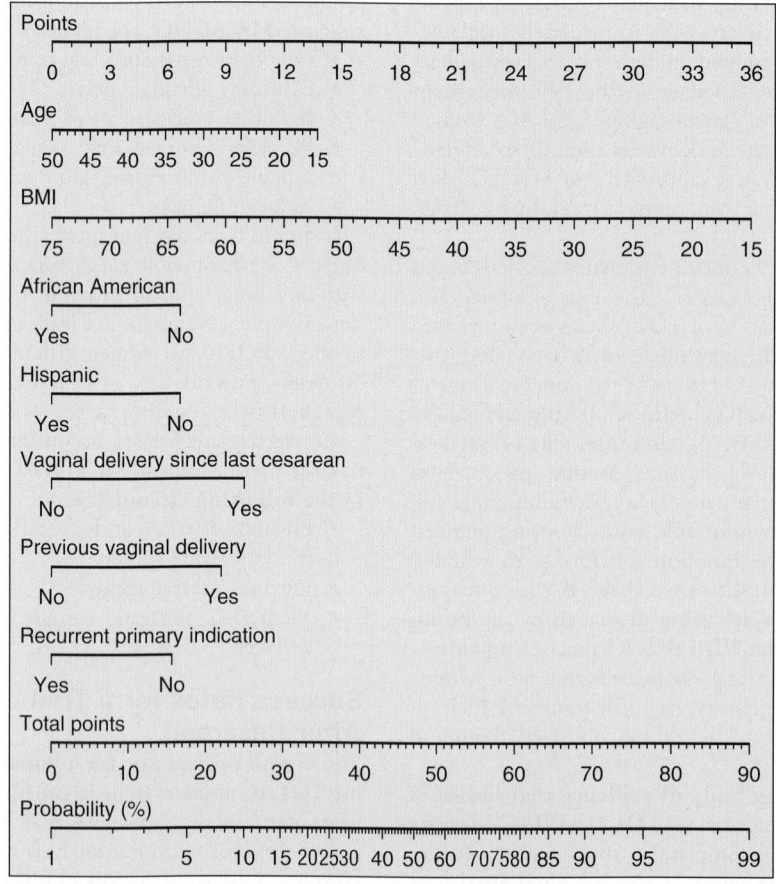

FIG 20-2 Graphic nomogram used to predict probability of vaginal birth after cesarean (VBAC). The nomogram is used by locating each patient characteristic and finding the number of points on the uppermost scale to which that characteristic corresponds. The sum of total points predicts the probability of VBAC on the lower scale. BMI, body mass index. (Modified from Grobman WA, Lai Y, Landon MB, et al, for the National Institute of Child Health and Human Development [NICHD] Maternal Fetal Medicine Units Network [MFMU]. Development of a nomogram for prediction of vaginal birth after cesarean delivery. *Obstet Gynecol.* 2007;109:806-812.)

study of 14,529 term pregnancies in which TOLAC was attempted, white women had a 78% success rate, compared with 70% in nonwhite women.[16] Obese women are more likely to fail a TOLAC, as are women older than 40 years.[16] Conflicting data exist with regard to payer status.[32]

Prior Indication for Cesarean Delivery

Success rates for women whose first cesarean delivery was performed for a nonrecurring indication (breech, nonreassuring fetal well-being) are similar to vaginal delivery rates for nulliparous women. Prior cesarean delivery for a breech presentation is associated with a reported success rate of 89%.[16] In contrast, **prior cesarean delivery for cephalopelvic disproportion (CPD) or failure to progress (FTP) has been associated with success rates that range from 50% to 67%.**

Prior Vaginal Delivery

Prior vaginal delivery, including prior VBAC, is one of the greatest predictors for successful TOLAC. In one series,[16] **women with a prior vaginal delivery had an 87% TOLAC success rate, compared with a 61% success rate in women without a prior vaginal delivery.** Caughey and colleagues[17] reported that for patients with a prior VBAC, the success rate was 93%, compared with 85% in women with a vaginal delivery before their cesarean birth but who had not had a successful VBAC. Mercer and colleagues[18] noted that the success rate increased from 87.6% with one prior vaginal delivery to 90.0% in those with two prior successful attempts.

Birthweight

Increased birthweight is associated with a lower likelihood of a successful VBAC.[11,19] **Birthweight greater than 4000 g in particular is associated with a higher risk for failed VBAC.**[33] Although some report success rates below 50%, others have documented that as many as 60% to 70% of women who attempt VBAC with a macrosomic fetus are successful. Peaceman and colleagues[20] reported a 34% success rate when the second pregnancy birthweight exceeded the first by 500 g and the prior indication was dystocia, compared with a 64% success rate with other prior indications. It should be noted that although birthweight has been associated with the success of VBAC, this factor cannot be known with precision prior to undertaking TOLAC, and it has not been demonstrated to what degree estimated fetal weight is associated with VBAC.

Labor Status and Cervical Examinations

Both labor status and cervical examination on admission influence the success of a TOLAC. Flamm and Geiger[21] reported **an 86% success rate in women who presented in labor with cervical dilation greater than 4 cm. Conversely, the VBAC success rate dropped to 67% if the cervix was dilated less than 4 cm on admission.**

Not surprisingly, women who undergo induction of labor are at higher risk for repeat cesarean delivery compared with those who enter spontaneous labor.[16,22] Data from the National Institute of Child Health and Human Development (NICHD) MFMU Cesarean Registry demonstrated a **67.4% success rate in women who underwent induction versus 80.5% in those who underwent spontaneous labor.**[22] In a study of 429 women undergoing induction with a prior cesarean delivery, Grinstead and Grobman[23] reported an overall 78% success rate. These authors noted several factors related to the labor induction as

TABLE 20-2 SUCCESS RATES FOR TRIAL OF LABOR AFTER TWO PRIOR CESAREAN DELIVERIES

STUDY	SUBJECTS (N)	SUCCESS RATE (%)
Miller et al[42]	2936	75.3
Caughey et al[43]	134	62.0
Macones et al[34]	1082	74.6
Landon et al[45]	876	67.0

determinants of VBAC success, including indication for induction and the need for cervical ripening. Grobman and colleagues[22] have also reported a VBAC success rate of 83% in 1208 women with a prior cesarean delivery and prior vaginal delivery undergoing induction of labor.

Previous or Unknown Incision Type

Previous incision type cannot be ascertained in certain patients. Nevertheless, it appears that **women whose previous incision type is unknown have VBAC success rates similar to those of women with documented prior low transverse incisions.**[16] Similarly, **women with previous low vertical incisions do not appear to have lower VBAC success rates.**[24]

Multiple Prior Cesarean Deliveries

Women with more than one prior cesarean delivery have been demonstrated to have a lower likelihood of achieving VBAC (Table 20-2). Caughey and colleagues[17] reported a 75% success rate for women with one prior cesarean delivery compared with 62% in women with two prior operations. In contrast, a larger multicenter study[34] of 13,617 women undergoing a TOLAC revealed a 75.5% success rate for women with two prior cesarean deliveries, which was not statistically different from the 75% success rate in women with one prior operation.

Postterm Pregnancy

TOLAC success rates may be lower for women at or beyond 40 weeks of gestation when compared with those who have yet to reach 40 weeks. Nevertheless, the chance of success for women who are at or beyond 40 weeks of gestation has been demonstrated to be approximately 70%,[12] and a gestational age beyond a woman's due date should not preclude TOLAC.

Twin Gestation

Two large-scale contemporary studies[9,16] of women attempting VBAC indicate that success rates for women undergoing TOLAC with twins are not different than for those with singleton gestations.

RISKS ASSOCIATED WITH A TRIAL OF LABOR AFTER CESAREAN

Uterine Rupture

The principal risk associated with TOLAC is uterine rupture. This complication is directly attributable to TOLAC because symptomatic rupture is rarely observed in planned repeat operations.[8,35-39] **It is important to differentiate between *uterine rupture* and *uterine scar dehiscence*. This distinction is clinically relevant because dehiscence most often represents an occult scar separation observed at laparotomy in women with a prior cesarean delivery.** With uterine dehiscence, the serosa of the uterus is intact and hemorrhage, with its potential for

TABLE 20-3 RISK FOR UTERINE RUPTURE BASED ON INCISION TYPE

PRIOR INCISION TYPE	RUPTURE RATE (%)
Low transverse	0.5-1.0
Low vertical	0.8-1.1
Classic or T shaped	4-9

TABLE 20-4 RISK FOR PERINATAL DEATH RELATED TO UTERINE RUPTURE

STUDY		PERINATAL DEATHS/ RUPTURES WITH TOLAC
Guise et al[38] (pooled data)	74	0.14/1000
Landon et al[8]	123	0.11/1000
Chauhaun et al[39] (pooled data)	880	0.40/1000

TOLAC, trial of labor after cesarean delivery.

TABLE 20-5 PERINATAL OUTCOMES AFTER UTERINE RUPTURE IN TERM PREGNANCIES

OUTCOME	TERM PREGNANCIES WITH UTERINE RUPTURE (*N* = 114)
Intrapartum stillbirth	0
Hypoxic-ischemic encephalopathy	7 (6.1%)
Neonatal death	2 (1.8%)
Admission to the neonatal intensive care unit	46 (40.4%)
Five-minute Apgar score ≤5	16 (14.0%)
Umbilical artery blood pH ≤7.0	23 (20.2%)

Modified from Landon MB, Hauth JC, Leveno KJ, et al, for the National Institute of Child Health and Human Development Maternal-Fetal Medicine Units Network: Maternal and perinatal outcomes associated with a trial of labor after prior cesarean section. *N Engl J Med* 2004;351:2581.

fetal and maternal sequelae, is absent. In contrast, uterine rupture is a through-and-through disruption of all uterine layers, with potential consequences of nonreassuring fetal status and perinatal mortality along with severe maternal morbidity, hemorrhage, and mortality. Terminology, definitions, and ascertainment for uterine rupture vary significantly in the existing VBAC literature.[37] A review[38] of four observational studies reported the risks of symptomatic uterine rupture in the TOLAC group and elective repeat cesarean group to be 0.47% (95% confidence interval [CI], 0.28% to 0.77%) and 0.026% (95% CI, 0.009% to 0.082%), respectively. **The large multicenter MFMU Network Study[8] reported a 0.69% frequency of uterine rupture, with 124 symptomatic ruptures occurring in 17,898 women undergoing TOLAC.**

The rate of uterine rupture depends both on the type and location of the previous uterine incision (Table 20-3). Uterine rupture rates are highest with a previous classical or T-shaped incision, with a range reported between 4% and 9%. The risk for rupture with a previous low vertical incision has been difficult to estimate owing to imprecision with the diagnosis and the uncommon use of this incision type. Naif and colleagues[40] reported a 1.1% risk for rupture in 174 women with a prior low vertical scar undergoing TOLAC, whereas Shipp and associates[41] reported a 0.8% (3 of 377) risk for rupture with a prior low vertical incision. On the basis of these two studies, the authors concluded that **women with a prior low vertical uterine incision are not at significantly increased risk for rupture compared with women with a prior low transverse incision.**

Women with an unknown incision type do not appear to be at increased risk for uterine rupture. Among 3206 women with an unknown scar in the MFMU Network Cesarean Registry, uterine rupture occurred in 0.5% of women undergoing TOLAC.[13] Nevertheless, this frequency is a reflection of the fact that in a contemporary setting, most women with unknown scars will have had a prior low transverse incision. **In counseling women with an unknown scar, the physician should attempt to understand whether a prior cesarean delivery had been performed under circumstances in which it was more likely that a different type of incision had been used.** For example, a history of preterm cesarean delivery should warrant caution, especially in the setting of malpresentation, because the incision may have involved an undeveloped muscular portion of the uterus, or it may have been a classical incision. For these reasons, if the clinician suspects that the prior delivery occurred under circumstances in which an incision that extended into the muscular portion of the uterus was used, we generally proceed with repeat cesarean delivery.

The most serious sequelae of uterine rupture include perinatal death, hypoxic-ischemic encephalopathy (HIE), and hysterectomy. Citing six perinatal deaths in 74 uterine ruptures among 11 studies, Guise and colleagues[38] calculated 0.14 additional perinatal deaths per 1000 TOLACs. This figure is remarkably similar to that from the NICHD MFMU Network study by Landon and colleagues,[8] in which there were two neonatal deaths among 124 ruptures, for **an overall rate of rupture-related perinatal death of 0.11 per 1000 TOLACs.** An all-inclusive review[39] of 880 maternal uterine ruptures in studies of varying quality during a 20-year period showed a rate of 0.4 per 1000 (Table 20-4).

Perinatal hypoxic brain injury is another recognized adverse outcome related to uterine rupture. However, estimates of the frequency of perinatal "asphyxia" have varied in the literature because it has been inconsistently defined in TOLAC studies, and variables such as cord blood gas levels and Apgar scores are reported in only a fraction of cases. Landon and colleagues[8] found a significant increase in the rate of HIE related to uterine rupture among the offspring of women who underwent a TOLAC at term compared with the children of women who underwent a planned repeat cesarean delivery (0.46 per 1000 vs. 0 cases, respectively). **In this study of 114 cases of uterine rupture at term, seven infants (6.1%) sustained HIE, and two of these infants died in the neonatal period** (Table 20-5).

Maternal hysterectomy also may be a complication of uterine rupture if the defect cannot be repaired or is associated with uncontrollable hemorrhage. In five studies[37] that reported on hysterectomies related to rupture, seven cases occurred in 60 symptomatic ruptures (13%; range, 4% to 27%), indicating that 3.4 per 10,000 women electing a TOLAC sustain a rupture that necessitates hysterectomy. Five of 124 women (4%) included in the NICHD MFMU Network study[8] experienced hysterectomy following rupture. However, hysterectomy also can occur in the setting of a planned repeat cesarean, and some evidence suggests that it is no more likely during a TOLAC than during a planned repeat cesarean delivery. Guise and colleagues,[38] for example, reported that the risk for hysterectomy in women attempting TOLAC was not significantly different than that in those undergoing planned repeat cesareans.

Risk Factors for Uterine Rupture

Rates of uterine rupture vary significantly depending on a variety of associated risk factors. In addition to the type of

uterine scar, characteristics of the obstetric history that include the number of prior cesarean and vaginal deliveries, the interdelivery interval, and the uterine closure technique have been reported to be associated with the risk for uterine rupture. Similarly, factors related to labor management, including induction and the use of oxytocin augmentation, have been studied.

Number of Prior Cesarean Deliveries

In a large single-center study of more than 1000 women with multiple prior cesarean deliveries undergoing TOLAC, Miller and colleagues[42] reported uterine rupture in 1.7% of women with two or more previous cesarean deliveries compared with 0.6% in those with one prior cesarean (odds ratio [OR], 3.06; 95% CI, 1.95 to 4.79). Interestingly, the risk for uterine rupture was not increased further for women with three prior cesarean deliveries. Caughey and colleagues[43] conducted a smaller study of 134 women with two prior cesarean deliveries and controlled for labor characteristics as well as obstetric history. These authors reported a rate of uterine rupture of 3.7% among these 134 women, compared with 0.8% in the 3757 women with one previous scar (OR, 4.5; 95% CI, 1.18 to 11.5). Macones and colleagues[34] reported a rate of uterine rupture of 1.8% (20 of 1082) in women with two prior cesarean deliveries compared with 0.9% (113 of 12,535) in women with one prior operation (adjusted OR, 2.3; 95% CI, 1.37 to 3.85). A meta-analysis also suggested a nearly threefold increased risk for uterine rupture with two previous cesarean deliveries (1.59% vs. 0.72%).[44] In contrast, the analysis of Landon and colleagues[45] from the MFMU Network Cesarean Registry found no significant difference in rupture rates in women with one prior cesarean (115 of 16,916 [0.7%]) versus multiple prior cesareans (9 of 975 [0.9%]). **It thus appears that even if having had more than one prior cesarean section is associated with an increased risk for uterine rupture, the magnitude of any additional risk is fairly small** (Table 20-6). **ACOG considers it reasonable to offer TOLAC to women with more than one prior cesarean delivery and to counsel such women based on the combination of other factors that affect their probability of achieving a successful VBAC.**[7]

Prior Vaginal Delivery

Prior vaginal delivery, either before or after a prior cesarean delivery, appears to be highly protective against uterine rupture in the setting of TOLAC. In a study of 3783 women undergoing a TOLAC, Zelop and colleagues[46] noted that the rate of uterine rupture among women with a prior vaginal birth was 0.2% (2 of 1021), compared with 1.1% (30 of 2762) among women with no prior vaginal deliveries. After controlling for demographic differences and labor characteristics, women who had one or more vaginal deliveries had a rate of uterine rupture that was one fifth that of women who did not have a prior vaginal birth (adjusted OR, 0.2; 95% CI, 0.04 to 0.8). A similar protective effect of prior vaginal birth has been reported in two large multicenter studies.[8,9]

Uterine Closure Technique

Over the past 20 years, the single-layer closure technique has gained popularity because it has appeared to be associated with shorter operating time and comparable short-term complications compared with the traditional two-layer technique. In a randomized trial, Chapman and colleagues[47] compared the frequency of uterine rupture in 145 women who received either one- or two-layer closure at their primary cesarean delivery. Following TOLAC, no cases of uterine rupture were found in either group; however, the study was underpowered to detect a potential difference. A larger observational study[48] identified an approximately fourfold increased rate (3.1% vs. 0.5%) of rupture following a single-closure technique when compared with a previous double-layer closure. In a 2010 case-control study,[49] the same group suggested an increased risk for uterine rupture in women with a history of a single-layer closure (OR, 2.69; 95% CI, 1.57 to 5.28) compared with a two-layer closure. Further, single-layer uterine closure was the only significant variable associated with adverse neonatal outcome, yet it has been postulated that single-layer closure may have been used in some cases when the lower uterine segment was thin and not amenable to a two-layer closure or that other aspects of the closure, such as suture type or locking technique, may be confounding the apparent association. Indeed, in another study by Durnwald and Mercer,[50] no association between the number of layers closed and uterine rupture was found. Thus it remains unclear whether the single-layer closure technique increases the risk for rupture.

Interpregnancy Interval

Several studies have addressed whether TOLAC after a short interpregnancy interval may be associated with an increased risk for uterine rupture. Shipp and colleagues[51] reported an incidence of rupture of 2.3% (7 of 311) in women with an interdelivery interval less than 18 months compared with 1.1% (22 of 2098) with a longer interdelivery interval. After controlling for demographic characteristics and oxytocin use, women with a shorter interpregnancy interval were three times more likely to experience uterine rupture. Using a multivariable approach, Bujold and associates[52] reported an interdelivery interval of less than 24 months to be associated with an almost threefold increased risk for uterine rupture. In their study, the rate of rupture was 2.8% in women with a short interval versus 0.9% in women when it had been more than 2 years since the prior cesarean birth. Yet in a study of 1185 women undergoing a TOLAC, Huang and colleagues[53] found no increased risk for uterine rupture with an interdelivery interval of less than 18 months.

Induction of Labor

Induction of labor may be associated with an increased risk for uterine rupture when compared with spontaneous labor.[54,55] **In a population-based cohort analysis, Lydon-Rochelle and colleagues[54] reported a rate of uterine rupture of 24 of 2326**

TABLE 20-6	RISK FOR UTERINE RUPTURE FOLLOWING MULTIPLE PRIOR CESAREAN DELIVERIES			
		RUPTURE RATE		
STUDY	**N**	**SINGLE PRIOR (%)**	**MULTIPLE PRIOR (%)**	**RR (CI)**
Miller et al[42]	3728	0.6	1.7	3.1 (1.9-4.8)
Caughey et al[43]	134	0.8	3.7	4.5 (1.2-11.5)
Macones et al[34]	1082	0.9	1.8	2.3 (1.4-3.9)
Landon et al[45]	975	0.7	0.9	1.4 (0.7-2.7)

CI, confidence interval; *N*, number of women with multiple prior cesarean sections attempting vaginal birth after cesarean; *RR*, relative risk.

(1.0%) for women undergoing induction compared with 56 of 10,789 (0.5%) in women who had spontaneous onset of labor. Landon and colleagues[8] noted the risk for uterine rupture to be elevated nearly threefold (OR, 2.86; 95% CI, 1.75 to 4.67), although the attributable risk of rupture related to labor induction was relatively small (1.0% vs. 0.4%). In an analysis[22] from this study of women (n = 11,778), those with only one prior low transverse cesarean delivery showed an increase in uterine rupture in those undergoing induction who had no prior vaginal delivery but did not reveal any increased risk of uterine rupture with labor induction among women who had a TOLAC with a history of prior vaginal delivery. In this study, the need for cervical ripening did not appear to affect the frequency of uterine rupture. Conversely, in another investigation,[56] women with a favorable cervix undergoing induction had a similar risk for uterine rupture as women entering labor spontaneously, whereas those being induced with an unfavorable cervix had a fourfold increased risk of uterine rupture. Despite these analyses, it remains unclear whether induction increases the risk for uterine rupture in comparison to expectant management—the clinical alternative for women who desire a TOLAC. Based on the cumulative data, ACOG considers induction of labor for maternal or fetal indications to be an option for women undergoing TOLAC.

Conflicting data have also been reported concerning whether various induction methods increase the risk for uterine rupture (Table 20-7). The study of Lydon-Rochelle and colleagues[54] suggests an increased risk for uterine rupture with the use of prostaglandins for labor induction. Uterine rupture was noted in 15 of 1960 women (0.8%) induced without prostaglandins, compared with 9 of 366 women (2.5%) induced with prostaglandin. Unfortunately, these authors could not determine which specific prostaglandin agent was used. In the study of Dekker and associates,[55] the risk for rupture with oxytocin alone was 0.54% compared with 0.68% with prostaglandins and 0.88% when the combined agents were used.

Neither Landon's group[8] nor that of Macones[9] confirmed the findings of Lydon-Rochelle and colleagues[54] of an increased risk for rupture associated with the use of prostaglandin agents alone for induction. Macones and colleagues[9] did report an increased risk for rupture in women undergoing induction but only if they received both prostaglandins *and* oxytocin, and the methodology in this study allowed the authors to distinguish between induction methods. Interestingly, in the MFMU Network study of Landon and associates,[8] no cases of uterine rupture were reported when prostaglandin alone was used for induction, including 52 cases in which misoprostol was used. Nevertheless, the safety of this medication, which is popular for cervical

ripening and labor induction (see Chapter 13), has been challenged for women attempting VBAC. Plaut and colleagues[32] reported a uterine rupture rate of 5.6% (5 of 89) in women who received misoprostol for labor induction. However, as in other series, it is unclear whether these women received oxytocin as well. The timing (delay) of uterine rupture in relation to misoprostol administration also calls into question cause and effect. Following several case reports of uterine rupture with misoprostol use, Wing and colleagues[33] conducted a randomized trial of intravaginal misoprostol versus oxytocin in women attempting VBAC in which 17 women received misoprostol and 21 women received oxytocin. The study was stopped prematurely because two emergency cesarean deliveries were performed with uterine disruption in patients who received misoprostol.

Unfortunately, many VBAC studies fail to specify the prostaglandin used for labor induction. In the largest report of women who received prostaglandins for labor induction attempting VBAC, Smith and colleagues[57] reported a 0.87% risk for uterine rupture among 4475 women who received unspecified prostaglandins, compared with 0.29% in 4429 women who did not receive this class of medication. Although the relative risk associated with prostaglandin use was elevated, the absolute risk increase for rupture was low. At present, based on the limited data that do exist, ACOG suggests that misoprostol (prostaglandin E$_1$) not be used for third-trimester cervical ripening or labor induction in women who have had a cesarean delivery and that sequential use of prostaglandin E$_2$ and oxytocin be avoided in women undergoing TOLAC. This recommendation has thus limited the induction options for women undergoing TOLAC and in need of cervical ripening, primarily in regard to oxytocin or mechanical methods with or without oxytocin. Small studies[58] of women with prior cesarean delivery undergoing induction with a transcervical Foley catheter suggest that uterine rupture rates are similar to those of women entering spontaneous labor attempting VBAC.

Labor Augmentation

Data conflict as to whether oxytocin used for labor augmentation during TOLAC in contemporary obstetric practice is associated with an increased risk of uterine rupture. In a case-control study, Leung and colleagues[59] reported an OR of 2.7 for uterine rupture in women who received oxytocin augmentation. However, it is possible that the dysfunctional labor may be the risk factor responsible for rupture. In contrast to the data of Leung and associates, Zelop and others[60] found that labor augmentation with oxytocin did not significantly increase the risk for rupture. Cahill and colleagues[61] reported a dose-response relationship between maximal oxytocin dose and the risk for rupture among women who attempt TOLAC. A limitation of this report is that it includes both women undergoing induction and those receiving oxytocin augmentation. At their maximal dose of oxytocin (>20 mU/min), these authors noted the risk for uterine rupture to be 2.07%. From these data, it appears that oxytocin may be used in women undergoing TOLAC, although higher infusion rates should be used with caution.

Sonographic Evaluation of the Uterine Scar

To better identify women at risk for uterine rupture undergoing TOLAC, the thickness of the lower uterine segment (LUS) prior to labor has been assessed with ultrasound. Ultrasound measurement of the thickness of residual myometrium in the LUS

TABLE 20-7	RISK FOR UTERINE RUPTURE AFTER LABOR INDUCTION		
	STUDY		
	LYDON-ROCHELLE ET AL[54]	**LANDON ET AL[8]**	**DEKKER ET AL[55]**
All inductions	24/2326 (1.0)	48/4708 (1.0)	16/1867 (0.9)
Spontaneous	56/10,789 (0.5)	24/6685 (0.4)	16/8221 (0.2)
Prostaglandins	9/366 (2.5)	0/227 (0.0)	4/586 (0.7)
Prostaglandin and oxytocin	—	13/926 (1.4)	4/226 (1.8)

TABLE 20-8	COMPARISON OF MATERNAL COMPLICATIONS IN A TRIAL OF LABOR AFTER CESAREAN VERSUS PLANNED REPEAT CESAREAN DELIVERY

COMPLICATION	TRIAL OF LABOR (N = 17,898)	PLANNED REPEAT CESAREAN (N = 15,801)	ODDS RATIO (98% CI)
Uterine rupture	124 (0.7%)	0	—
Hysterectomy	41 (0.2%)	47 (0.3%)	0.77 (0.51-1.17)
Thromboembolic disease	7 (0.04%)	10 (0.1%)	0.62 (0.24-1.62)
Transfusion	304 (1.7%)	158 (1.0%)	1.71 (1.41-2.08)
Endometritis	517 (2.9%)	285 (1.8%)	1.62 (1.40-1.87)
Maternal death	3 (0.02%)	7 (0.04%)	0.38 (1.10-1.46)
One or more of the above	978 (5.5%)	563 (3.6%)	1.56 (1.41-1.74)

Modified from Landon MB, Hauth JC, Leveno KJ, et al, for the National Institute of Child Health and Human Development Maternal-Fetal Medicine Units Network. Maternal and perinatal outcomes associated with a trial of labor after prior cesarean section. *N Engl J Med.* 2004;351:2581.
CI, confidence interval.

TABLE 20-9	MATERNAL COMPLICATIONS ACCORDING TO THE OUTCOME OF A TRIAL OF LABOR AFTER CESAREAN DELIVERY

COMPLICATION	FAILED VAGINAL DELIVERY (N = 4759) (%)	SUCCESSFUL VAGINAL DELIVERY (N = 13,139) (%)	ODDS RATIO (95% CI)	P VALUE
Uterine rupture	110 (2.3)	14 (0.1)	22.18 (12.70-38.72)	<.001
Uterine dehiscence	100 (2.1)	19 (0.1)	14.82 (9.06-24.23)	<.001
Hysterectomy	22 (0.5)	19 (0.1)	3.21 (1.73-5.93)	<.001
Thromboembolic disease*	4 (0.1)	3 (0.02)	3.69 (0.83-16.51)	<.09
Transfusion	152 (3.2)	152 (1.2)	2.82 (2.25-3.54)	<.001
Endometritis	365 (7.7)	152 (1.2)	7.10 (5.86-8.60)	<.001
Maternal death	2 (0.04)	1 (0.01)	5.52 (0.50-60.92)	<.17
Other adverse events†	63 (1.3)	1 (0.01)	176.24 (24.44-127.05)	<.001
One or more of the above	669 (14.1)	309 (2.4)	6.81 (5.93-7.83)	<.001

Modified from Landon MB, Hauth JC, Leveno KJ, et al, for the National Institute of Child Health and Human Development Maternal-Fetal Medicine Units Network. Maternal and perinatal outcomes associated with a trial of labor after prior cesarean section. *N Engl J Med.* 2004;351:2581.
*Thromboembolic disease includes deep venous thrombosis or pulmonary embolism.
†Other adverse events include broad ligament hematoma, cystotomy, bowel injury, and ureteral injury.
CI, confidence interval.

has been assessed, as has the width, depth, and length of the hypoechoic interface at the site of the prior cesarean delivery.[62] However, these measurements may change with gestational age, and at present, there appears to be no value for any measurement that performs well enough for use in clinical practice to predict the integrity of the uterine scar during labor. In one systematic review[63] of 21 studies of the use of sonographic LUS thickness to predict the risk of a uterine scar defect during a TOLAC, no ideal cutoff value for use in clinical practice could be found.

Other Risks Associated With a Trial of Labor After Cesarean Delivery

In the absence of randomized controlled trials, the observational data that exist to inform women and health care providers about the variety of adverse outcomes that may be associated with a TOLAC, compared with a planned repeat cesarean delivery, do not provide certainty with regard to these risks because there may be a lack of comparability between women undergoing a TOLAC and those having a planned repeat cesarean delivery.[36-38]

Based on the data, it has been generally accepted that vaginal delivery is associated with lower morbidity and mortality than cesarean delivery. Landon and colleagues[8] found an increased risk for both postpartum endometritis and blood transfusion in women undergoing a TOLAC compared with those undergoing planned repeat cesarean delivery without labor (Table 20-8). However, the exclusion of women who presented in early labor, who subsequently underwent a repeat operation that had been intended, may have lowered the risk for complications in the

planned repeat cesarean group. Gilbert and colleagues[64] attempted to produce a more minimally biased cohort by performing propensity analysis to determine more precisely the comparative risks of spontaneous labor and planned cesarean delivery. They found that the rates of endometritis and operative injury were lower and the rates of hysterectomy and wound complication were higher among women who underwent a planned repeat cesarean delivery.

It should be noted that these comparisons are for entire populations of women and may not hold for a given individual. It is well accepted that most of the excess adverse events that accompany a TOLAC are attributable to the group of women who require a repeat cesarean operation in labor (Table 20-9).[65] Thus when considering the balance of risks between TOLAC and planned repeat cesarean delivery, it is important to consider the chance that a woman who is undertaking a TOLAC will achieve a vaginal birth. In one analysis, if a woman undergoing a TOLAC had a greater than 60% to 70% chance of VBAC, her chance of having major or minor morbidity was no greater than that of a woman undergoing a planned repeat cesarean delivery.[66]

An increased risk for maternal mortality in the context of cesarean delivery in general has been extrapolated to women undergoing a planned repeat operation versus a planned TOLAC, although the data to support this association are limited. Guise and colleagues[38] evaluated 24 maternal deaths among 402,833 patients with prior a cesarean delivery and noted that the overall risk for maternal death associated with TOLAC was significantly lower (RR, 0.33; 95% CI, 0.13 to 0.88) than with a repeat operation. Nevertheless, the infrequency of maternal death, confounding variables such as maternal disease, and the classification of a planned or unplanned procedure complicate mortality estimates and comparisons. **Maternal death attributable to uterine rupture is exceedingly rare, and in the population of the MFMU Cesarean Registry, maternal death was not significantly more common with planned repeat cesarean delivery.**[8] However, the study was not powered to detect a difference between this group and women attempting a TOLAC.

Management of a Trial of Labor after Cesarean

The optimal management of labor in women undergoing a TOLAC is based not on randomized trials but primarily on opinion. Women attempting VBAC should be encouraged to contact their health care provider promptly when labor begins or rupture of the membranes occurs. Continuous electronic fetal monitoring is recommended, although the need for routine internal monitoring with fetal scalp or intrauterine pressure catheters has not been established. **Studies that have examined fetal heart rate (FHR) patterns before uterine rupture consistently report that nonreassuring signs, particularly prolonged decelerations or bradycardia, are the most common finding accompanying uterine rupture.**[67,68]

Uterine rupture can be catastrophic, sudden, and unpredictable.[69] Personnel who care for women undergoing TOLAC should be familiar with electronic FHR patterns that may be associated with uterine rupture as well as the potential need for emergent delivery. Despite the presence of adequate personnel to conduct an emergency cesarean delivery, prompt and appropriate intervention does not always prevent fetal neurologic injury or death (Fig. 20-3).[70] In the study of Leung and colleagues,[67] significant neonatal morbidity occurred when 18 minutes or longer elapsed between the onset of FHR deceleration and delivery. In contrast to Leung's findings, Bujold and Gauthier[70] reported that fewer than 18 minutes elapsed between prolonged decelerations and delivery in two of three neonates diagnosed with HIE in 23 cases of uterine rupture.

Epidural analgesia is not contraindicated in the setting of TOLAC and does not appear to affect success rates.[16] Epidural analgesia also does not mask the signs and symptoms of uterine rupture. In fact, women may manifest evidence of abdominal pain and may respond by attempting to have their epidural dosed more frequently when a uterine rupture occurs.[71] As has been discussed previously, neither oxytocin induction nor augmentation is contraindicated, and it is reasonable when indicated to consider modest doses of oxytocin.

Performance of the vaginal delivery itself is not altered by a history of prior cesarean birth. Most obstetricians do not routinely explore the uterus to detect asymptomatic scar dehiscences. However, excessive vaginal bleeding or maternal hypotension should be promptly evaluated, which includes assessment for possible uterine rupture. Of 124 cases of uterine rupture accompanying 17,898 trials of labor, 14 (11%) were identified following vaginal delivery.[8]

Counseling for a Trial of Labor After Cesarean

Because uterine rupture may be a catastrophic event, ACOG continues to recommend that it is optimal to attempt TOLAC in institutions equipped to respond to emergencies with physicians immediately available to provide emergency care, and they recognize that referral may be appropriate if a facility has inadequate resources to offer TOLAC.[7] ACOG further recommends

---

BOX 20-1   RISKS ASSOCIATED WITH TRIAL OF LABOR AFTER CESAREAN DELIVERY

Uterine Rupture and Related Morbidity

Uterine rupture (0.5-1.0/100)
Perinatal death and/or encephalopathy (0.5/1000)
Hysterectomy (0.3/1000)

Increased Maternal Morbidity With Failed TOLAC

Transfusion
Endometritis
Length of stay

Other Risks With TOLAC

Potential risk for perinatal asphyxia with labor (cord prolapse, abruption)
Potential risk for antepartum stillbirth beyond 39 weeks' gestation

TOLAC, trial of labor after cesarean.

BOX 20-2   RISKS ASSOCIATED WITH PLANNED REPEAT CESAREAN DELIVERY

- Increased maternal morbidity compared with successful trial of labor
- Increased length of stay and recovery
- Increased risks for abnormal placentation and hemorrhage with successive cesarean deliveries

---

that when resources for immediate cesarean delivery are not available, health care providers and patients considering TOLAC should discuss the hospital's resources and the availability of staff. The decision to pursue TOLAC in such a setting should be carefully considered by patients and their health care providers.

Regardless of the approach to delivery, a pregnant woman with a previous cesarean delivery is at risk for both maternal and perinatal complications. Complications associated with both procedures should be discussed, and an attempt should be made to include an individualized risk assessment for the likelihood of successful VBAC (Box 20-1) and the corresponding comparative risk of maternal and perinatal morbidity. Such an estimate may be obtained from prior prediction models that have been developed, such as those by Grobman and associates.[25,30] Whereas no prediction model can provide an individual risk of uterine rupture that is as accurate and reliable as that of the prediction of VBAC, a consideration of individual-specific factors associated with uterine rupture should also be considered. Lastly, plans for future childbearing and the risks for multiple cesarean deliveries, including the risks for placenta previa and placenta accreta, should also be considered (Box 20-2).[72,73]

It is essential to make an effort to obtain records of the prior cesarean delivery to ascertain the previous uterine incision type. This is particularly relevant to cases in which it is more likely that a non–low transverse uterine incision was used. If previous uterine incision type is unknown, the implications of that missing information should be discussed.

Following informed consent detailing the most relevant risks and benefits for the individual woman, the delivery plan should be formulated using a shared decision-making process by both the patient and physician. There should be clear recognition that this plan may change depending on clinical circumstances, including events during the labor process. It is inappropriate to mandate TOLAC because many women desire a planned repeat

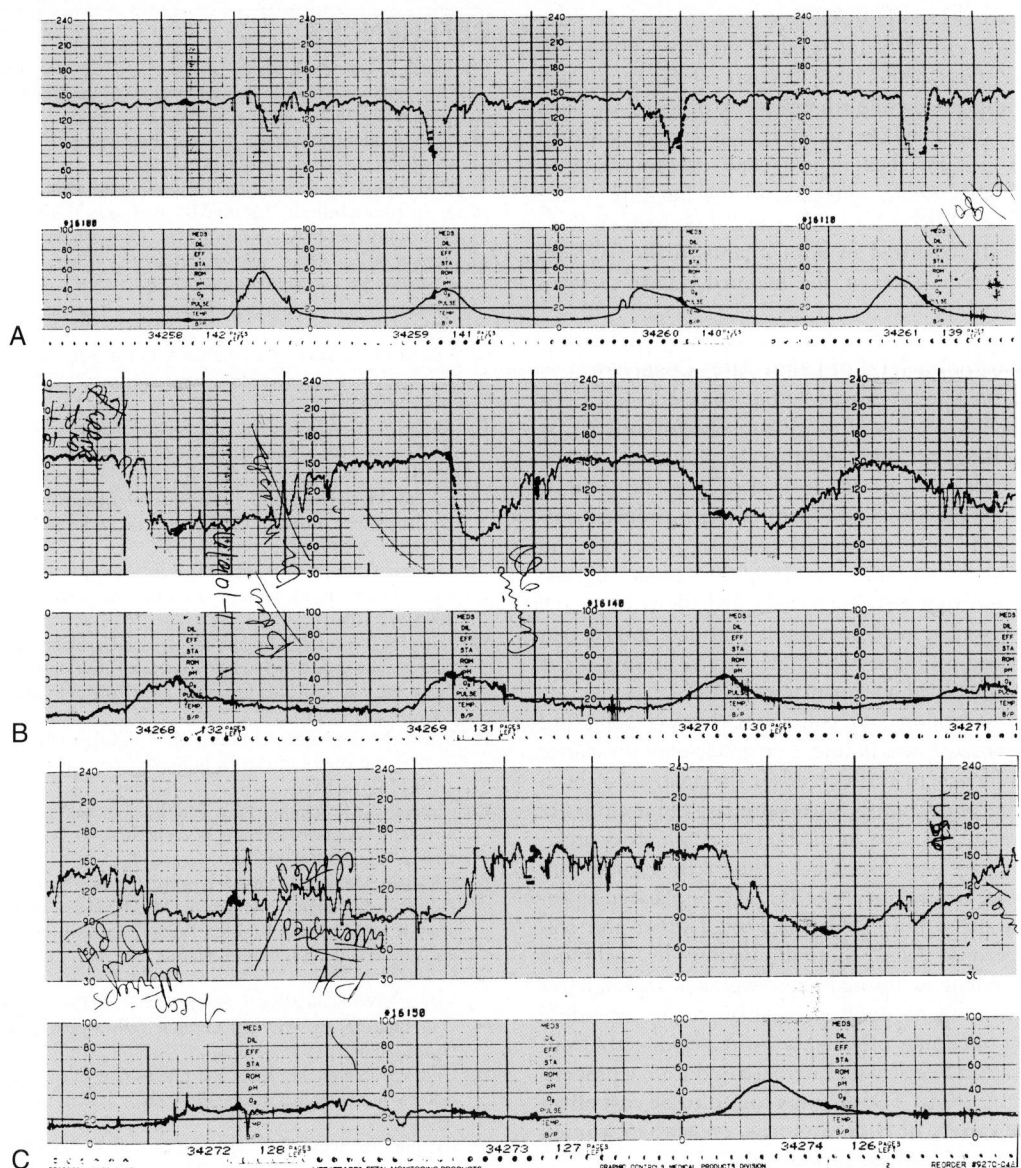

FIG 20-3 A, This 37-year-old patient (gravida 7, para 3, ab 3) presented for induction of labor at 41 weeks' gestation. She had had two prior vaginal deliveries, but her last baby was born at 33 weeks by low transverse cesarean section for nonimmune hydrops caused by a cardiac malformation. The patient's induction was begun with prostaglandin gel. Her cervix changed from fingertip dilated, 50% effaced to 1-cm dilated, 70% effaced with a cephalic presentation at −2 station. Oxytocin was then begun at 1 mU/min. The patient progressed well, and epidural anesthesia was administered at 4 to 5 cm dilation, 90% effaced, and 0 station. The patient was at 6 cm dilation with a tracing that demonstrated normal heart rate variability and variable decelerations. **B,** Thirty minutes after the above tracing was recorded, the fetal heart rate pattern changed to severe variable decelerations. **C,** The tracing then demonstrated prolonged decelerations at 90 beats/min. The patient was taken to the operating room for an emergency cesarean delivery, and it was found that rupture had occurred along the site of the previous uterine incision. A female fetus weighting 3200 g with Apgar scores of 7 and 8 was delivered; umbilical arterial pH was 7.17 and venous pH was 7.22. The uterine incision had not extended and was easily closed, and the baby did well.

operation after thorough counseling. Similarly, patient autonomy requires that practitioners document informed consent regarding TOLAC and attempt to enable women who desire TOLAC to achieve their goal. Korst and colleagues[6] have noted the reported high frequency of lack of informed consent regarding TOLAC-VBAC and have questioned the extent to which women are able to truly choose TOLAC as opposed to being dissuaded by the health care system. Because facilities, resources, and policies vary widely among health care institutions, it has been suggested that health care organizations and physicians consider making public their TOLAC policies and VBAC rates as well as their plans for responding to obstetric emergencies.[10] This transparency in data would no doubt help inform women

with prior cesarean deliveries in choosing both their planned approach to delivery and an appropriate facility for their childbirth.

Based on the available evidence, TOLAC should continue to remain an option for most women with a prior cesarean delivery, particularly when the low absolute risks that accompany TOLAC are considered. The attributable risk for a serious adverse perinatal outcome (perinatal death or HIE) at term appears to be about 1 per 2000 TOLACs. Combining an independent risk for hysterectomy attributable to uterine rupture at term with the risk for newborn HIE indicates the chance of one of these adverse events occurring to be about 1 in 1250 cases.

The decision to elect a TOLAC may also increase the risk for perinatal death and HIE unrelated to uterine rupture. For women awaiting spontaneous labor beyond 39 weeks, a small possibility of unexplained stillbirth exists that might have been avoidable had a scheduled repeat operation been performed at 39 weeks. A risk for fetal hypoxia and its sequelae may also accompany labor events unrelated to the integrity of the uterine scar. In the MFMU Network study,[8] five cases of non–rupture-related HIE occurred in term infants in the TOLAC group compared with none in the planned repeat cesarean population.

Cost-Effectiveness of a Trial of Labor After Cesarean

Several investigators have assessed whether and under what circumstances TOLAC is a cost-effective strategy. An analysis by Grobman and colleagues[74] suggested that the choice of planned repeat cesarean delivery, instead of TOLAC, at the time of a second pregnancy prevented one major adverse neonatal outcome but required 1591 additional cesarean deliveries and cost an additional $2.4 million per 100,000 women. Chung and associates[75] incorporated quality-adjusted life-years as the measure of effectiveness in their analysis and determined that TOLAC in a second pregnancy was cost-effective as long as the chance of VBAC exceeded approximately 74%.

The analysis by Chung and colleagues, however, did not account for the consequences in future pregnancies of the choice regarding the approach to delivery. Also, the analyses of both groups, Grobman's and Chung's, used summary point estimates from the observational studies in the literature, which as previously noted, may have been biased as a result of the nonrandom nature of the choice to attempt either TOLAC or planned repeat cesarean delivery. In a more recent analysis, Gilbert and colleagues[76] attempted to rectify both limitations by including probabilities of outcomes throughout a woman's reproductive life that were contingent upon her initial choice regarding TOLAC and by obtaining probability estimates directly from the MFMU Cesarean Registry that were derived from a propensity analysis. In this study, **TOLAC was found to be cost effective over a wide variety of circumstances, even when women had a probability of VBAC as low as 43%.**

KEY POINTS

- VBAC rates have plummeted from a peak of approximately 30% in 1996 to 5% in 2010.
- Most women with a prior low transverse cesarean delivery are candidates for TOLAC and should be counseled about and offered this option.
- The success rate for TOLAC is influenced by prior indication for cesarean delivery, history of vaginal delivery, demographic characteristics such as maternal age and BMI, the occurrence of spontaneous labor, and cervical status at admission.
- Oxytocin may be used for induction, as well as augmentation, of labor in women undergoing TOLAC.
- The use of misoprostol for cervical ripening is contraindicated in women undergoing TOLAC.
- The most consistent sign associated with uterine rupture is fetal heart rate abnormalities that include prolonged variable decelerations and bradycardia.

REFERENCES

1. Zhang J, Troendle J, Reddy UM, et al., for the Consortium on Safe Labor. Contemporary cesarean delivery practice in the United States. *Am J Obstet Gynecol.* 2010;303:326e1-326e10.
2. Scott J. Mandatory trial of labor after cesarean delivery: an alternative viewpoint. *Obstet Gynecol.* 1991;77:811.
3. Pitkin RM. Once a cesarean? *Obstet Gynecol.* 1991;77:939.
4. Sachs BP, Kobelin C, Castro MA, Frigoletto F. The risks of lowering the cesarean-delivery rate. *N Engl J Med.* 1990;340:54.
5. *Vaginal birth after previous cesarean delivery: clinical management guidelines for obstetricians-gynecologists.* ACOG practice bulletin no. 5. Washington, DC: American College of Obstetricians and Gynecologists; 1999.
6. Korst LM, Gregory KD, Fridman M, Phelan JP. Nonclinical factors affecting women's access to trial of labor after cesarean delivery. *Clin Perinatol.* 2011;38:193.
7. *ACOG Practice Bulletin No. 115: Vaginal birth after previous cesarean delivery.* Washington, DC: American College of Obstetricians and Gynecologists; 2010.
8. Landon MB, Hauth JC, Leveno KJ, et al. Maternal and perinatal outcomes associated with a trial of labor after prior cesarean delivery. *N Engl J Med.* 2004;351:2581.
9. Macones G, Peipert J, Nelson D, et al. Maternal complications with vaginal birth after cesarean delivery: a multicenter study. *Am J Obstet Gynecol.* 2005;193:1656.
10. National Institutes of Health Consensus Development Conference Panel. National Institutes of Health Consensus Development Conference Statement. Vaginal Birth after Cesarean: New Insights, March 8-10, 2010. *Obstet Gynecol.* 2010;115:1279.
11. Jastrow N, Roberge S, Gauthier RJ, et al. Effect of birth weight on adverse obstetric outcomes in vaginal birth after cesarean delivery. *Obstet Gynecol.* 2010;115:338-343.
12. Coassolo KM, Stamilio DM, Paré E, et al. Safety and efficacy of vaginal birth after cesarean attempts at or beyond 40 weeks of gestation. *Obstet Gynecol.* 2005;106:700-706.
13. Hickman MA for the Eunice Kennedy Shriver National Institute of Child Health and Human Development, MFMU Network, Bethesda, Maryland. The MFMU Cesarean Registry: Risk of uterine rupture in women attempting VBAC with an unknown uterine scar. *Am J Obstet Gynecol.* 2008;199: S36(#81).
14. Varner MW, Leindecker S, Spong CY, et al. The Maternal-Fetal Medicine Unit cesarean registry: trial of labor with a twin gestation. *Am J Obstet Gynecol.* 2005;193:135-140.
15. Uddin SF, Simon AE. Rates and success rates of trial of labor after cesarean delivery in the United States, 1990-2009. *Matern Child Health J.* 2013;17: 1309-1314.
16. Landon MB, Leindecker S, Spong CY, et al. The MFMU Cesarean Registry: factors affecting the success and trial of labor following prior cesarean delivery. *Am J Obstet Gynecol.* 2005;193:1016.
17. Caughey AB, Shipp TD, Repke JT, et al. Trial of labor after cesarean delivery: the effects of previous vaginal delivery. *Am J Obstet Gynecol.* 1998;179: 938.
18. Mercer BM, Gilbert S, Landon MB, et al. Labor outcomes with increasing number of prior vaginal births after cesarean delivery. *Obstet Gynecol.* 2008; 111:285.
19. Elkousy MA, Samuel M, Stevens E, et al. The effect of birthweight on vaginal birth after cesarean delivery success rates. *Am J Obstet Gynecol.* 2003; 188:824.
20. Peaceman AM, Genoviez R, Landon MB, et al. *Am J Obstet Gynecol.* 2005; 195:1127.
21. Flamm BL, Geiger AM. Vaginal birth after cesarean delivery: an admission scoring system. *Obstet Gynecol.* 1997;90:907.
22. Grobman WA, Gilbert S, Landon MB, et al. Outcome of induction of labor after one prior cesarean. *Obstet Gynecol.* 2007;109:262-269.
23. Grinstead J, Grobman WA. Induction of labor after one prior cesarean: predictors of vaginal delivery. *Obstet Gynecol.* 2004;103:534.
24. Rosen MG, Dickinson JC. Vaginal birth after cesarean: a meta-analysis of indicators for success. *Obstet Gynecol.* 1990;76:865.
25. Grobman WA, Lai Y, Landon MB, et al. Development of a normogram for prediction of vaginal birth after cesarean delivery. *Obstet Gynecol.* 2007;109: 806.
26. Costantine MM, Fox K, Byers BD, et al. Validation of the prediction model to predict success of vaginal birth after cesarean. *Obstet Gynecol.* 2009;114: 1029-1033.

27. Chaillet N, Bujold E, Dube E, Grobman WA. Validation of a Prediction Model for Vaginal Birth after Cesarean. *J Obstet Gynaecol Can.* 2013;35: 119-124.

28. Yokoi A, Ishikawa K, Miyazaki K, et al. Validation of the prediction model for success of vaginal birth after cesarean delivery in Japanese women. *Int J Med Sci.* 2012;9:488-491.

29. Schoorel E, Melman S, van Kuijk S, et al. Predicting successful intended vaginal delivery after previous caesarean section: external validation of two predictive models in a Dutch nationwide registration-based cohort with a high intended vaginal delivery rate. *BJOG.* 2014;121:840-847.

30. Grobman WA, Lai Y, Landon MB, et al. Does information available at admission for delivery improve prediction of vaginal birth after cesarean? *Am J Perinatol.* 2009;26:693-701.

31. Metz TD, Stoddard GJ, Henry E, et al. Simple, validated vaginal birth after cesarean delivery prediction model for use at the time of admission. *Obstet Gynecol.* 2013;122:571.

32. Plaut MM, Schwartz ML, Lubarsky SL. Uterine rupture associated with the use of misoprostol in the gravid patient with a previous cesarean section. *Am J Obstet Gynecol.* 1999;180:1535.

33. Wing DA, Lovett K, Paul RH. Disruption of prior uterine incision following misoprostol for labor induction in women with previous cesarean delivery. *Obstet Gynecol.* 1998;91:828.

34. Macones GA, Cahill A, Para E, et al. Obstetric outcomes in women with two prior cesarean deliveries: is vaginal birth after cesarean delivery a viable option? *Am J Obstet Gynecol.* 2005;192:1223.

35. Kieser KE, Baskett TF. A 10-year population-based study of uterine rupture. *Obstet Gynecol.* 2002;100:749.

36. Mozurkewich EL, Hutton EK. Elective repeat cesarean delivery versus trial of labor: a meta-analysis of the literature from 1989 to 1999. *Am J Obstet Gynecol.* 2000;183:1187.

37. *Vaginal Birth after Cesarean (VBAC). Rockville, MD: Agency for Health Care Research and Quality.* 2003 (AHRQ publication no. 03-E018).

38. Guise JM, Berlin M, McDonagh M, Osterweil P, Chan B, Helfand M. Safety of vaginal birth after cesarean: a systematic review. *Obstet Gynecol.* 2004;103:420-429.

39. Chauhan SP, Martin JN, Henrichs CE, et al. Maternal and perinatal complications with uterine rupture in 142,075 patients who attempted vaginal birth after cesarean delivery: a review of the literature. *Am J Obstet Gynecol.* 2003;189:408.

40. Naif RW, Ray MA, Chauhan SP, et al. Trial of labor after cesarean delivery with a lower-segment, vertical uterine incision: is it safe? *Am J Obstet Gynecol.* 1995;172:1666.

41. Shipp TD, Zelop CM, Repke TJ, et al. Intrapartum uterine rupture and dehiscence in patients with prior lower uterine segment vertical and transverse incisions. *Obstet Gynecol.* 1999;94:735.

42. Miller DA, Diaz FG, Paul RH. Vaginal birth after cesarean: a 10 year experience. *Obstet Gynecol.* 1994;84:255.

43. Caughey AB, Shipp TD, Repke JT, et al. Rate of uterine rupture during a trial of labor in women with one or two prior cesarean deliveries. *Am J Obstet Gynecol.* 1999;181:872.

44. Tahseen S, Griffiths M. Vaginal birth after two caesarean sections (VBAC-2): a systematic review with meta-analysis of success rate and adverse outcomes of VBAC-2 versus VBAC-1 and repeat (third) caesarean section. *BJOG.* 2010;117:5.

45. Landon MB, Spong CY, Thom E, et al. Risk of uterine rupture with a trial of labor in women with multiple and single prior cesarean delivery. *Obstet Gynecol.* 2006;108:12.

46. Zelop CM, Shipp TD, Repke JT, et al. Uterine rupture during induced or augmented labor in gravid women with one prior cesarean delivery. *Am J Obstet Gynecol.* 1999;181:882.

47. Chapman SJ, Owen J, Hauth JC. One-versus two-layer closure of a low transverse cesarean: the next pregnancy. *Obstet Gynecol.* 1997;89:16.

48. Bujold E, Bujold C, Hamilton EF, et al. The impact of a single-layer or double-layer closure on uterine rupture. *Am J Obstet Gynecol.* 2002;186: 1326.

49. Bujold E, Goyet M, Marxouz S, et al. The role of uterine closure in the risk of uterine rupture. *Obstet Gynecol.* 2010;116:143.

50. Durnwald C, Mercer B. Uterine rupture, perioperative and perinatal morbidity after single-layer and double-layer closure at cesarean delivery. *Am J Obstet Gynecol.* 2003;189:925-929.

51. Shipp TD, Zelop CM, Repke JT, et al. Interdelivery interval and risk of symptomatic uterine rupture. *Obstet Gynecol.* 2001;97:175.

52. Bujold E, Mehta SH, Bujold C, Gauthier RJ. Interdelivery interval and uterine rupture. *Am J Obstet Gynecol.* 2002;187:199.

53. Huang WH, Nakashima DK, Rumney PJ, et al. Interdelivery interval and the success of vaginal birth after cesarean delivery. *Obstet Gynecol.* 2002; 99:41.

54. Lydon-Rochelle M, Holt V, Easterling TR, Martin DP. Risk of uterine rupture during labor among women with a prior cesarean delivery. *N Engl J Med.* 2001;345:36.

55. Dekker GA, Chan A, Luke CG, et al. Risk of uterine rupture in Australian women attempting vaginal birth after one prior cesarean section: a retrospective population-based cohort study. *BJOG.* 2010;117:1358.

56. Harper LM, Cahill AG, Boslaugh S, et al. Association of induction of labor and uterine rupture in women attempting vaginal birth after cesarean: a survival analysis. *Am J Obstet Gynecol.* 2012;206:51.e1.

57. Smith GC, Peil JP, Pasupathy D, et al. Factors predisposing to perinatal death related to uterine rupture during attempted vaginal birth after cesarean section: retrospective cohort study. *BMJ.* 2004;329:359.

58. Bujold E, Blackwell SC, Gauthier RJ. Cervical ripening with transcervical Foley catheter and the risk of uterine rupture. *Obstet Gynecol.* 2004;103: 18-23.

59. Leung AS, Famer RM, Leung EK, et al. Risk factors associated with uterine rupture during trial of labor after cesarean delivery: a case-control study. *Am J Obstet Gynecol.* 1993;168:1358-1363.

60. Zelop CM, Shipp TD, Repke JT, Cohen A, Caughey AB, Lieberman E. Uterine rupture during induced or augmented labor in gravid women with one prior cesarean delivery. *Am J Obstet Gynecol.* 1999;181:882.

61. Cahill AG, Waterman BM, Stamilio DM, et al. Higher maximum doses of oxytocin are associated with an unacceptably high risk of uterine patients attempting vaginal birth after cesarean delivery. *Am J Obstet Gynecol.* 2008;199:41.

62. Bujold E, Jastrow N, Simoneau J, et al. Prediction of complete uterine rupture of sonographic evaluation of the lower uterine segment. *Am J Obstet Gynecol.* 2009;201:320.e1-320.e6.

63. Kok N, Wiersma IC, Opmeer BC, et al. Sonographic measurement of lower uterine segment thickness to predict uterine rupture during a trial of labor in women with previous Cesarean section: a meta-analysis. *Ultrasound Obstet Gynecol.* 2013;42:132.

64. Gilbert SA, Grobman WA, Landon MB, et al. Elective repeat cesarean delivery compared with spontaneous trial of labor after a prior cesarean delivery: a propensity score analysis. *Am J Obstet Gynecol.* 2012;206:311.e1-311.e9.

65. McMahon MJ, Luther ER, Bowes WA, Olshan AF. Comparison of a trial of labor with an elective second cesarean section. *N Engl J Med.* 1996; 335:689.

66. Grobman WA, Lai Y, Landon MB, et al. Can a predictive model for vaginal birth after cesarean also predict the probability of morbidity related to a trial of labor? *Am J Obstet Gynecol.* 2009;200:56.e1-56.e6.

67. Leung AS, Leung EK, Paul RH. Uterine rupture after previous cesarean delivery: maternal and fetal consequences. *Am J Obstet Gynecol.* 1993; 169(4):945-950.

68. Ouzounian JG, Quist-Nelson J, Miller DA, Korst LM. Maternal and fetal signs and symptoms associated with uterine rupture in women with prior cesarean delivery. *J Matern Fetal Neonatal Med.* 2014;1-8.

69. Grobman WA, Lai Y, Landon MB, et al. Prediction of uterine rupture associated with attempted vaginal birth after cesarean. *Am J Obstet Gynecol.* 2008;199:30.e1-e5.

70. Bujold E, Gauthier RJ. Neonatal morbidity associated with uterine rupture: what are the risk factors. *Am J Obstet Gynecol.* 2002;186(2):311-314.

71. Cahill AG, Odibo AO, Allsworth JE, Macones GA. Frequent epidural dosing as marker for impending uterine rupture in patients who attempt vaginal birth after cesarean section. *Am J Obstet Gynecol.* 2010;202:335.e1-335.e5.

72. Silver RM, Landon MB, Rouse DJ, et al. Maternal morbidity associated with multiple repeat cesarean deliveries. *Obstet Gynecol.* 2006;107:1226.

73. Grobman WA, Lai Y, Landon MB, et al. Pregnancy outcomes for women with placenta previa in relation to the number of prior cesareans. *Obstet Gynecol.* 2007;110:1249-1255.

74. Grobman WA, Peaceman AM, Socol ML. Elective cesarean delivery after one prior low transverse cesarean birth: A cost-effectiveness analysis. *Obstet Gynecol.* 2000;95:745-751.

75. Chung A, Macario A, El-Sayed YY, Riley ET, Duncan B, Druzin ML. Cost effectiveness of a trial of labor after previous cesarean. *Obstet Gynecol.* 2001;97:932-941.

76. Gilbert SA, Grobman WA, Landon MB, et al. Cost-Effectiveness of Trial of Labor After Previous Cesarean in a Minimally Biased Cohort. *Am J Perinatol.* 2013;30:11-20.

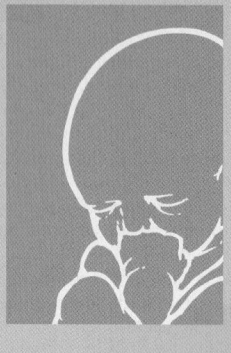

CHAPTER 21

Placenta Accreta

ERIC R.M. JAUNIAUX, AMAR BHIDE, and JASON D. WRIGHT

KEY ABBREVIATIONS	
Cesaean delivery scar defect	CDSD
Magnetic resonance imaging	MRI
Odds ratio	OR
Placenta accreta	PA
Postpartum hemorrhage	PPH
Randomized controlled trial	RCT
Trial of labor after cesarean	TOLAC

Placenta accreta (PA) refers to different grades of morbid placental attachment to the uterine wall secondary to invasion of the trophoblast into the myometrium beyond the uteroplacental interface. **The term *placenta increta* is used to describe deep myometrial invasion by trophoblast villi, and *placenta percreta* refers to villi perforating through the full thickness of the myometrium and uterine serosa with possible involvement of adjacent organs.[1-3] The difference between placenta accreta, increta, and percreta is related to the extent of invasion, and the umbrella term *disorders of invasive placentation* is used to encompass all three** (Fig. 21-1).

PA has also been categorized as total, partial, or focal depending on the amount of placental tissue involved. This subclassification has been used less frequently because microscopic examination of the hysterectomy specimen is rarely complete, and attempts at manual removal often distort the placental anatomy.[2] However, with increasing numbers of cases of PA being diagnosed antenatally, and with greater expertise in conservative therapeutic procedures, this classification might become more useful.

The first detailed description of a PA[1] **appeared within 20 years of major changes in the surgical techniques for, and more common use of, cesarean delivery (CD). It was not reported by the prominent pathologists of the eighteenth and nineteenth centuries, which may indicate the direct relationship between the increased use of CD and morbid placental adherence.**[4] Although PA remains a relatively uncommon obstetric pathology, it has become a complication that an obstetrician with a practice of average volume is likely to encounter more commonly, compared with the once or twice in a lifetime encounter of two decades ago. PA has also become a major cause of life-threatening obstetric complications worldwide.

When PA is present, the failure of the entire placenta to separate normally from the uterine wall after delivery is typically accompanied by severe postpartum hemorrhage (PPH; see Chapter 18). Attempts to remove the adherent tissue may provoke further bleeding and a cascade of ongoing hemorrhage, shock, and coagulation disorders that require complex clinical management (Box 21-1). This chapter reviews the pathogenesis, epidemiology, antenatal diagnosis, and management of this obstetric disease.

PATHOGENESIS

Unlike many other placental disorders—such as hydatidiform moles, which have been known for centuries—PA was only recently described, in 1937 by Irving and Hertig.[1] Before the nineteenth century, few successful attempts had been made at performing CDs.[5] CD was a surgical procedure of last resort, and the operation was essentially performed to save the baby's life. It is only when surgeons started to remove and subsequently to suture the uterus after delivery that the maternal death rate following CD started to improve. By the 1920s, the combination of surgical improvements by Kehrer (uterine closure), Pfannenstiel (suprapubic transverse entry), and Munro Kerr (lower segment uterine incision) and developments in anesthesia and microbiology had brought down the maternal mortality from 70% in the 1850s to less than 10%. The introduction of uterotonic agents, blood transfusions, and antibiotics just before and after the Second World War further reduced the complication rate of CD.[5] These changes made the technique safer and allowed mothers not only to survive the surgical procedure but also to have one or more subsequent pregnancies (see Chapter 19).

Total or partial absence of decidua is the characteristic histologic feature of PA and is relatively clear cut in cases of implantation on a uterine scar.[2] **This results in the absence of the normal plane of cleavage above the decidua basalis,**

BOX 21-1 CRITERIA FOR THE DIAGNOSIS OF CLINICALLY SIGNIFICANT PLACENTA ACCRETA

1. Placenta does not separate and is expelled spontaneously, fully, or partially after delivery of the baby.
2. Attempt at removal of the placenta leads to brisk hemorrhage.
3. Histopathology confirms myometrial fibers in apposition with trophoblasts at the suspected site of invasive placentation if partial or complete excision of the uterus has been performed.

BOX 21-2 PRIMARY AND SECONDARY UTERINE PATHOLOGIES ASSOCIATED WITH PLACENTA ACCRETA

Primary Uterine Pathology

Major uterine anomalies
Adenomyosis
Submucous uterine fibroids
Myotonic dystrophy

Secondary Uterine Pathology

Cesarean delivery
Uterine curettage
Manual removal of the placenta
Cavity-entering myomectomy
Hysteroscopic surgery (endometrial resection)
In vitro fertilization procedures
Uterine artery embolization
Chemotherapy and radiotherapy

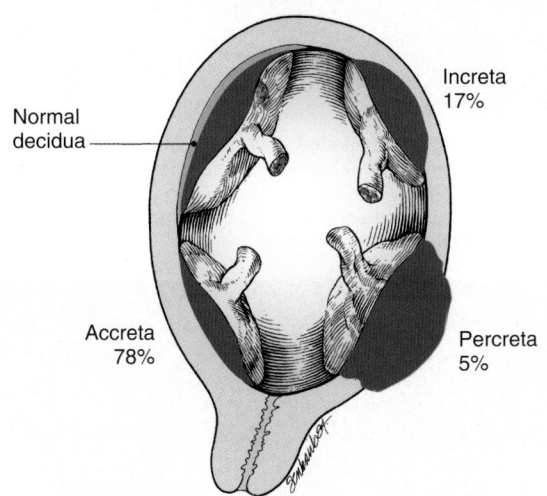

FIG 21-1 Uteroplacental relationships found with invasive placentation.

thus preventing placental separation after delivery. Myometrium does not actually heal by regenerating muscle fibers, rather it forms "foreign" substances, including collagen. The resulting fibrous tissue is weaker, less elastic, and more prone to injury than the original muscle. Myofiber disarray, tissue edema, inflammation, and elastosis have all been observed in uterine wound healing after surgery.[6] Experiments in mice have indicated that differences in regenerative ability translate into histologic, proliferative, and functional differences in biomechanical properties of the scarred myometrium after CD.[7]

Several concepts have been proposed to explain the abnormal placentation in PA including (1) a primary defect of trophoblast function; (2) a secondary decidua basalis defect as the result of a failure of normal decidualization; and, more recently, (3) abnormal vascularization and tissue oxygenation of the scar area.[4] The strongest risk factor for placenta previa is a prior caesarean delivery, which indicates that a failure of decidualization in the area of a previous uterine scar can have an impact on both implantation and placentation. These findings suggest that the decidual defect following a uterine scar may have an adverse effect on early implantation by creating conditions for preferential attachment of the blastocyst to scar tissue and facilitating abnormally deep invasion of the extravillous trophoblast.

Comparison of the ultrasound features of the uterine cesarean scar with histologic findings has shown that large and deep myometrial defects are often associated with absence of reepithelialization of the scar area.[8] These findings support the concept of a primary defect in PA, exposing the deep vasculature of the myometrium below the junctional zone to the migrating trophoblast. The loss of this normal plane of cleavage

and the excessive vascular remodeling of the radial and arcuate arteries can explain the antenatal findings and the clinical consequences of PA. A recent study[9] of the uterine circulation in women with a previous CD has shown that uterine artery resistance is increased, and the volume of uterine blood flow is decreased, as a fraction of maternal cardiac output compared with women with a previous vaginal birth. These data suggest a possible relationship between a poorly vascularized uterine scar area and an increase in the resistance to uterine blood flow with a secondary impact on reepithelialization of the scar area and subsequent decidualization. Overall, these data support the concept that abnormal decidualization and deep invasion of the placental bed by the trophoblast in PA are often secondary to the presence of a myometrial scar.[4]

Fragments of myometrium are found in the products of conception in approximately one third of uterine curettages after miscarriage.[10] The fact that it does not have a clear correlation with clinical PA in a subsequent pregnancy suggests that the trauma to the myometrium and the surface of the endometrial damage is often limited in a curettage procedure compared with that of a CD or other major uterine surgery. By contrast, severely deficient uterine scars with complete loss of large areas of the myometrium could explain rare reports of placenta percreta leading to uterine rupture in the first half of pregnancy.[11-15] Although this is an extremely rare complication of placentation, the mechanism of uterine rupture due to a placenta percreta is likely to be similar to that of a tubal rupture in an ectopic placentation. These findings emphasize the pivotal role of the superficial myometrium in modulating normal uterine placentation.

EPIDEMIOLOGY

Any primary or secondary alterations of the uterine endometrial-myometrial integrity have been associated with the development of PA. **With the rapid increase in the incidence of CD over the last several decades, this procedure has become associated with most cases of PA, whereas other factors are now responsible for a relatively small proportion of PA** (Box 21-2). CD is now the most commonly performed major operation around the world, with more than 1 million procedures performed each year in the United States alone (see Chapter 19). Not surprisingly, a substantial increase has been seen in the occurrence of PA over the last 50 years with as much as a tenfold rise in its incidence in most Western countries. Studies in the United States have indicated an overall incidence of PA of approximately 1 in 533 deliveries.[16,17] A recent meta-analysis has shown a calculated summary odds ratio (OR) of 1.96 for PA after one CD.[18] A recent case-control study has shown that, compared with primary intrapartum CD, primary prelabor CD significantly increased the risk of PA in a subsequent pregnancy in the presence of placenta previa.[19] **Overall, the data from epidemiologic studies consistently indicate that prior CD is the most important factor associated with subsequent PA and that the risk of PA increases with the number of prior CDs.**

Placenta Previa With Accreta

Epidemiologic studies have also indicated that **CD is associated with an increased risk of placenta previa** (see Chapter 18) **in subsequent pregnancies.**[17,18,20,21] A recent meta-analysis of five cohort and 11 case-control studies published between 1990 and 2011 revealed that after a CD, the calculated summary OR is 1.47 for placenta previa.[18] The risk of previa is higher with an increasing number of prior CDs.[16] Following a single CD, a 50% increase is seen in the risk of placenta previa in a subsequent singleton pregnancy. For women with two CDs, there is a twofold increase in the risk of placenta previa compared with women with a history of two vaginal deliveries.[17]

PA complicates about 5% of pregnancies with placenta previa.[22] The risk of PA in the setting of placenta previa increases with the number of prior CDs. Thus among women with placenta previa, 40% of those with two previous CDs and 61% of those with three prior CDs develop a PA.[23] This risk is independent of other maternal characteristics such as parity, body mass index (BMI), tobacco use, and coexisting hypertension or diabetes. It has been recently estimated that if the CD rate continues to rise as it has in recent years, by 2020, there will be an additional 6236 placenta previas, 4504 PAs, and 130 maternal deaths annually.[22]

Cesarean Delivery Scar Defects

With the increasing use of transvaginal ultrasound, a uterine cesarean delivery defect (CDSD), or "niche," is a condition that has been described recently. Much of the focus has been on identifying ultrasound criteria of CDSD during pregnancy that may indicate a higher risk of scar dehiscence and/or uterine rupture during a trial of labor after caesarean (TOLAC) in subsequent pregnancies.[24] Yet ultrasound imaging, including three-dimensional (3-D) imaging and sonohysterography, have been increasingly used to investigate uterine scars in nonpregnant women (Fig. 21-2). CDSDs have been seen in between 20% and 65% of women undergoing transvaginal ultrasound with a previous CD.[24-28] A CDSD is described as a tethering of the endometrium that can serve as a reservoir for blood and fluid, and it can be associated with clinical gynecologic symptoms such as intermenstrual and postmenstrual spotting and dysmenorrhea. A CDSD may range from a small defect of the superficial myometrium to a larger defect with a direct communication between the endometrial cavity and the visceral serosa (Fig. 21-3). Studies have demonstrated that a history of multiple CDs and uterine retroflexion are significantly associated with larger CDSDs, and larger CDSDs are more likely to be associated with symptoms such as intermenstrual spotting and pelvic pain.[25-27]

A recent retrospective cohort study has shown that a clinically evident uterine scar dehiscence in a previous pregnancy is a potential risk factor for preterm delivery, low birthweight, and peripartum hysterectomy in the following pregnancy.[28]

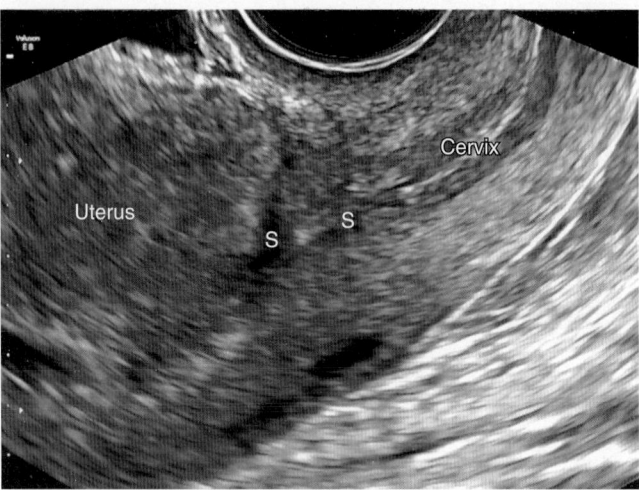

FIG 21-2 Transvaginal ultrasound view of the uterus in a 5-week pregnancy after two previous elective cesarean deliveries. Note the two small defects through the uterine wall at the junction between the lower and upper uterine segment corresponding to the scar (S) of the previous cesarean delivery incisions.

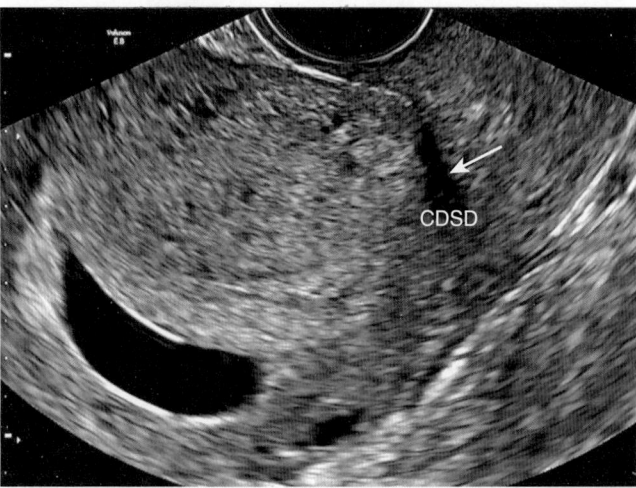

FIG 21-3 Transvaginal ultrasound view of the uterus in a 6-week pregnancy after a previous emergency cesarean delivery. A large cesarean delivery scar defect (CDSD) creates a niche at the junction between lower and upper uterine segment (*arrow*).

Interestingly, in this study, previous uterine scar dehiscence did not increase the risk of uterine rupture, PA, or adverse perinatal outcomes, such as low Apgar scores at 5 minutes and perinatal mortality. A recent series of 14 women (20 pregnancies) with a prior uterine rupture and 30 women (40 pregnancies) with a prior uterine dehiscence has shown that these women can have excellent outcomes in subsequent pregnancies if managed in a standardized manner, including CD before the onset of labor or immediately at the onset of spontaneous preterm labor.[29]

Theoretically, uterine scar surgical repair could prevent recurrent cesarean scar pregnancies and could also prevent PA (Fig. 21-4). A recent systematic review of studies reporting on hysteroscopic and laparoscopic CDSD resection has found that abnormal uterine bleeding improved in the vast majority (i.e., 87% to 100%) of patients after these interventions.[30] However, the methodologic quality of the reviewed papers was considered to be moderate to poor, and therefore data were insufficient to make firm conclusions. Until surgical interventions are evaluated in a prospective trial, the benefits and efficacy of surgical repair when a CDSD is observed should be considered unknown. A recent

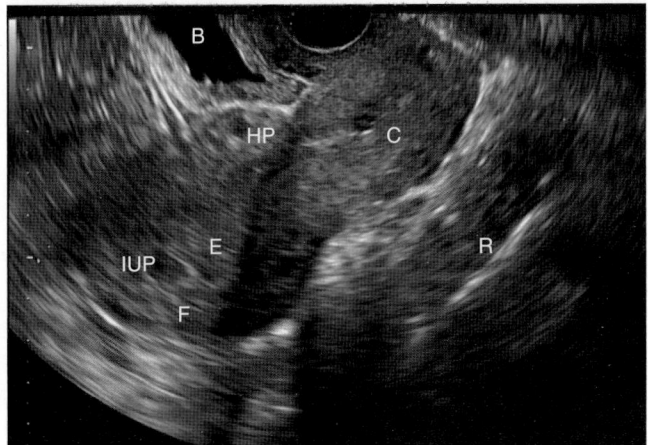

FIG 21-4 A 28-year-old gravida 4, para 1 patient with a history of prior low transverse cesarean delivery, presented for a routing ultrasound at 5-6 weeks' gestation. She had no complaints. The transvaginal ultrasound revealed a heterotopic pregnancy in the uterine scar (HP) and a normal intrauterine pregnancy (IUP). The bladder (B), endometrium (E), cervix (C), uterine fundus (F), and rectum (R) can be seen. The heterotopic pregnancy was surgically excised at laparotomy, and the pregnancy continued. (Courtesy Christopher Lang, MD, Maternal-Fetal Medicine, Mount Carmel St. Ann's Hospital, Columbus, Ohio.)

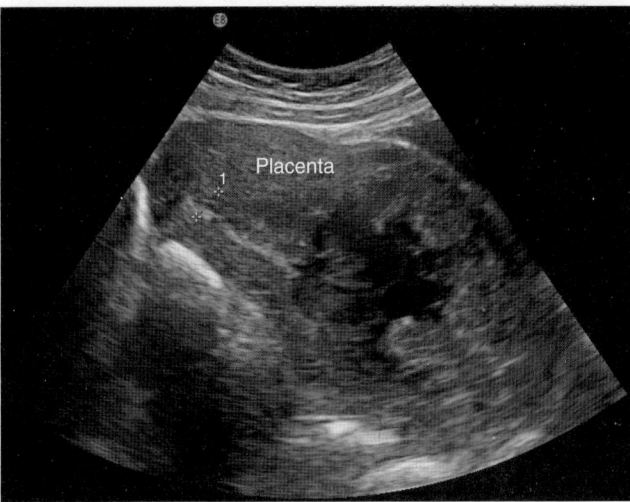

FIG 21-5 Transabdominal grayscale ultrasound longitudinal view of the lower uterine segment at 10 weeks' gestation in a patient with placenta previa major covering the cervix. The basal plate is missing, over an area of 3 cm in diameter, and the placental tissue above it is distorted by a large intervillous lake or lacuna.

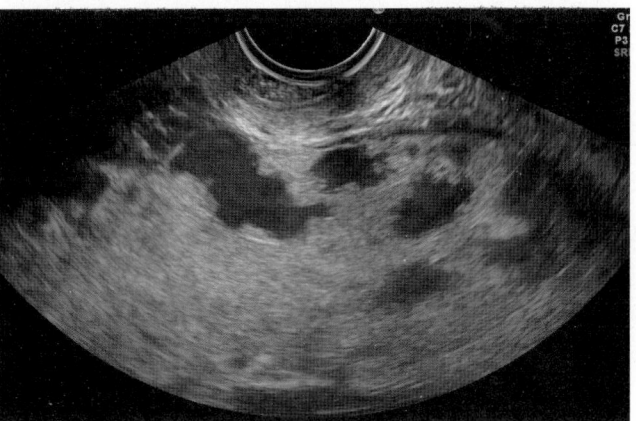

FIG 21-6 Transvaginal grayscale ultrasound longitudinal view of the lower uterine segment at 22 weeks' gestation in a patient with placenta previa major covering the cervix. The basal plate is missing, and the placental anatomy is distorted by large intervillous lakes, or lacunae, which gives the placenta a "moth-eaten" appearance.

small retrospective study[31] found that the use of monofilament suture for hysterotomy closure at the time of CD significantly reduced the chance of having placenta previa in the subsequent pregnancy. However, these data have not been replicated, and there is a need for properly designed, quality randomized controlled trials (RCTs) with larger sample sizes to evaluate the impact of different suture materials on uterine scar defects and risk of uterine rupture during TOLAC and on the development of placenta previa/accreta in subsequent pregnancies.

PRENATAL DIAGNOSIS

Before the development of newer imaging techniques, it was not possible prenatally to assess the depth of placental invasion or, in many cases, to even assess the existence of a PA. Consequently, many publications on PA report what can be considered a mixture of the conditions of accreta, increta, and percreta as well as antenatally suspected and pathologically diagnosed PA, which makes it difficult to assess the results of management for each individual pathologic entity and clinical situation. At present, however, prenatal diagnosis of PA has become a useful tool for a better understanding of the pathophysiology of an abnormally adherent placenta and its appropriate management.

Ultrasound Imaging

Ultrasound has become the primary screening tool for women at risk of PA. Gray-scale ultrasound features suggestive of PA include the loss of the myometrial interface or retroplacental clear space, reduced myometrial thickness, and chaotic intraplacental blood flow and intraplacental lacunae (Figs. 21-5 to 21-8). *Placenta increta* may be suggested by an examination of the border between the bladder and myometrium, which is normally echogenic and smooth.[4] In *placenta percreta*, the placenta often is seen bulging into the bladder. In rare cases, frank placental invasion into the bladder, which appears as exophytic masses, can be seen.

Much attention has been focused on the presence of "intraplacental lacunae" as a marker of PA.[15] These sonolucent spaces contain slow-moving maternal blood on gray-scale imaging and have been described as intraplacental "lakes."[21] The mere presence of some lacunae, however, does *not* signify the presence of a PA. When they involve a small area of the placenta or are found in an area of low villous tissue density, such as in the center of the cotyledons or under the chorionic plate, these lakes may be normal variants and have no clinical significance. Conversely, when a PA is present, the lacunae are extensive and create a "moth-eaten" appearance of the placenta (see Figs. 21-5 and 21-6).

The most common sonographic finding associated with PA is the loss of myometrial interface with enlargement of the underlying uterine vasculature.[32] The addition of color or power Doppler evaluation has been valuable in improving the screening capacity of ultrasound for PA.[32-40] Doppler features that suggest PA include chaotic intraplacental blood flow, the presence of increased blood flow in the retroplacental space, and aberrant vessels crossing between placental surfaces (see Figs. 21-7 and 21-8). In at-risk women, gray-scale ultrasound is moderately sensitive (70% to 90%), although this sensitivity may be

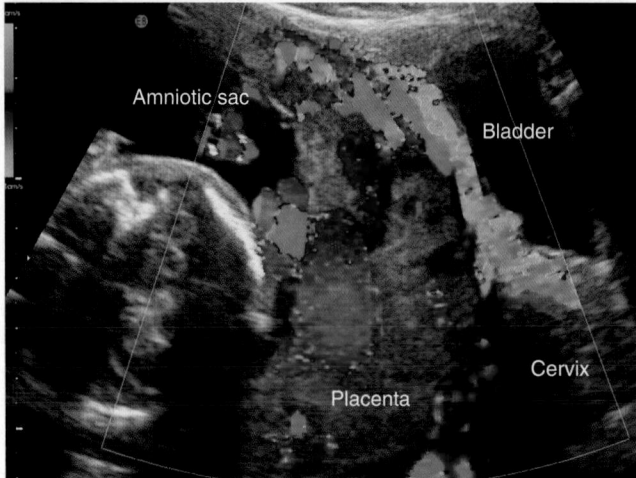

FIG 21-7 Transabdominal color mapping ultrasound longitudinal view of the lower uterine segment at 20 weeks' gestation in a patient with anterior placenta previa covering the cervix after previous cesarean delivery and a delivery defect detected before pregnancy showing chaotic intraplacental blood flow, the presence of altered blood flow in the retroplacental space, and aberrant vessels crossing between placental surfaces.

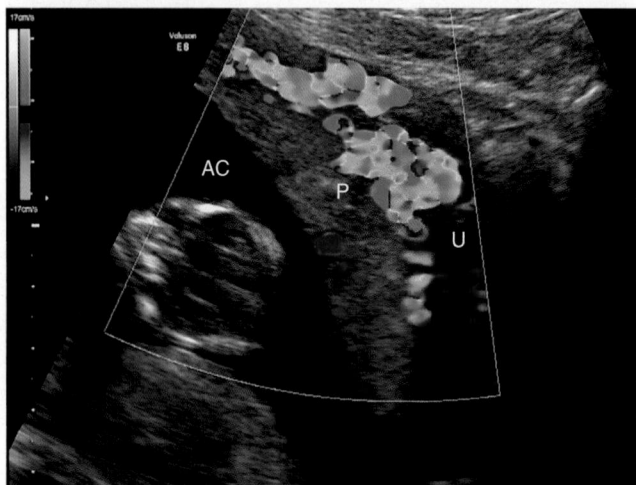

FIG 21-8 Transabdominal color mapping ultrasound longitudinal view of the lower uterine segment at 38 weeks' gestation in a patient with anterior placenta previa after previous cesarean delivery showing the presence of altered blood flow in the retroplacental space and aberrant vessels crossing between placental surfaces. AC, amniotic cavity; P, placenta; U, uterus.

improved by color flow mapping. A recent meta-analysis[41] of 22 studies that included a total of 3641 pregnancies at risk of invasive placentation indicated that the overall sensitivity of ultrasound in diagnosing PA antenatally is around 90%. Quality assessment of the studies showed that the study quality was generally high. The negative predictive value (NPV) of other recent studies ranged between 95% and 100% (Box 21-3). However, not all studies have yielded sensitivities and specificities that were quite as high. For example, a recent prospective study[40] has shown that the sensitivity, specificity, positive predictive value (PPV), and NPV were 53.5%, 88.0%, 82.1%, and 64.8%, respectively. Moreover, it should be noted that most of these values come from studies of high-risk women, and the predictive values among lower risk women (e.g., those without a placenta previa) would be expected to be lower.

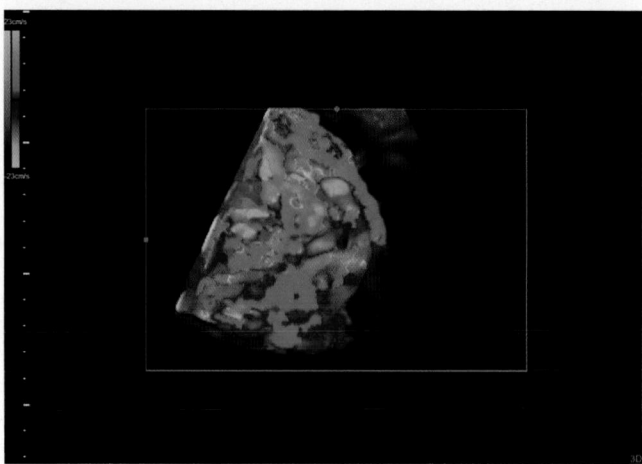

FIG 21-9 Transabdominal color mapping ultrasound longitudinal view of the lower uterine segment at 12 weeks' gestation in a patient with anterior low-lying placenta after previous cesarean delivery showing dilated uteroplacental vessels but no disruption of the basal plate.

BOX 21-3 PERFORMANCE OF ULTRASOUND IN THE PRENATAL DETECTION OF PLACENTA ACCRETA IN 3641 PREGNANCIES AT RISK FOR ABNORMALLY INVASIVE PLACENTATION

Presence of Lacunae

Sensitivity: 77.8% (95% CI, 70.7-83.6)
Specificity: 96.5% (95% CI, 95.6-97.1)

Loss of Hypoechoic Space Between Myometrium and Placenta

Sensitivity: 63.9% (95% CI, 55.1-71.9)
Specificity: 97.3% (95% CI, 96.6-97.9)

Color Doppler Imaging

Sensitivity: 91.2% (95% CI, 87.2-96.7)
Specificity: 91.9% (95% CI, 88.8-94.2)

Ultrasound Overall

Sensitivity: 90.8% (95% CI, 87.0-93.5)
Specificity: 96.9% (95% CI, 96.2-97.4)
Positive predictive value: 74.8% (95% CI, 70.2-78.8)
Negative predictive value: 99.0% (95% CI, 98.6-99.3)

CI, confidence interval.
Modified from D'Antonio F, Iacovella C, Bhide A. Prenatal identification of invasive placentation using ultrasound: systematic review and meta-analysis. *Ultrasound Obstet Gynecol.* 2013;42:509-517.

Disruption of the normal appearance of continuous color flow that results in a gap in myometrial blood flow can also be seen in cases of PA. This gap represents the site of placental invasion into the myometrium and can be diagnosed as early as the first trimester of pregnancy.[42-46] Within this context, it is possible that the suspicion for PA may even be heightened (see Fig. 21-5) or lessened (Fig. 21-9) at the time of an ultrasound examination at 11 to 14 weeks of gestation.[47]

In cases of a placenta in the lower segment, a transvaginal scan will help evaluate the uteroplacental interface near the internal os of the uterine cervix, and it may assist in assessing the degree of placental invasion.[48,49] For example, the degree of excess vascularity of the lower uterine segment assessed by ultrasound

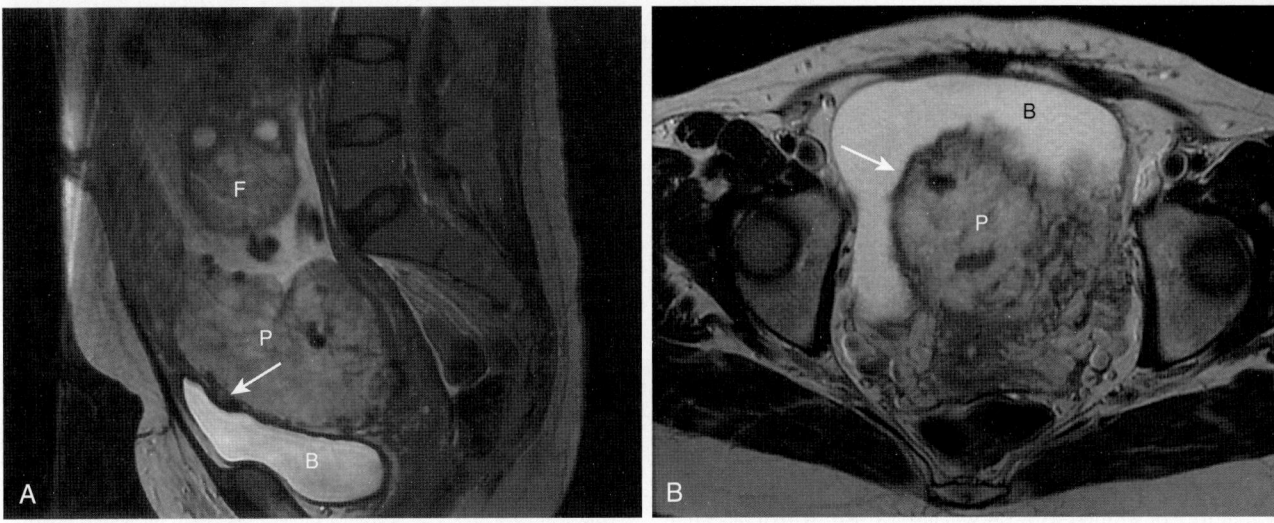

FIG 21-10 **A,** Sagittal magnetic resonance image (MRI) with the fetus (F) in vertex position at 25 weeks' gestation. The placenta (P) is anterior and low lying with loss of the normal myometrial dark signal. Prominent vessels (*arrow*) between the uterus and the bladder (B) are concerning for involvement of the bladder wall by placenta percreta. **B,** Axial MRI demonstrates placental tissue (P) abutting the left posterior aspect of the urinary bladder (B) with loss of the dark myometrial signal, preserved on the right side of the placenta (*arrow*). Findings are suggestive of invasion of the bladder by placenta percreta. Abnormal placentation was confirmed on pathologic examination. (Courtesy Dr. Zarine Shah, Department of Radiology, Ohio State University Wexner Medical Center.)

TABLE 21-1 SUMMARY ESTIMATES OF SENSITIVITY, SPECIFICITY, AND DIAGNOSTIC ODDS RATIO OF MRI FOR DETECTION OF PRESENCE, DEGREE, AND TOPOGRAPHY OF PLACENTAL INVASION AND FOR COMPARISON BETWEEN MRI AND ULTRASOUND FOR DETECTION OF INVASIVE PLACENTATION

PARAMETER	NO. OF STUDIES	TOTAL SAMPLE (N)	SENSITIVITY (%) (95% CI)	SPECIFICITY (%) (95% CI)	DOR (95% CI)
MRI					
Detection of invasive placentation	18*	1010	94.4 (86.0-97.9)	84.0 (76.0-89.8)	89.0 (22.8-348.1)
Depth of placental invasion	3†	62	92.9 (72.8-99.5)	97.6 (87.1-99.9)	44.2 (1.95-1001)
Topography of placental invasion	2†	428	99.6 (98.4-100)	95.0 (83.1-99.4)	803 (9.0-71,411)
Direct Comparison: MRI vs. US					
All studies	8*	255			
MRI			90.2 (81.3-95.1)	88.2 (76.7-94.4)	68.8 (19.7-239.8)
US			85.7 (77.2-91.4)	88.6 (73.0-95.7)	46.5 (13.4-161.0)
Studies with blinding‡	4*	164			
MRI			92.9 (82.4-97.3)	93.5 (82.2-97.8)	186.0 (40.0-864.5)
US			87.8 (75.8-94.3)	96.3 (74.4-99.6)	189.2 (15.8-2269)

Modified from Al-Khan A, Gupta V, Illsley NP, et al. Maternal and fetal outcomes in placenta accreta after institution of team-managed care. *Reprod Sci.* 2014;21(6):761-771.
*Computations based on hierarchical summary receiver–operating characteristics model.
†Computations based on the DerSimonian–Laird random-effect model.
‡Studies in which radiologist was blinded to both ultrasound findings and final diagnosis.
CI, confidence interval; *DOR,* diagnostic odds ratio; *MRI,* magnetic resonance imaging; *US,* ultrasound.

correlates with disease severity.[50] A recent study using logistic regression modeling has shown that the use of formal mathematical modeling to predict PA may have a better PPV than qualitative assessment of ultrasound alone.[51] Therefore **integrating PA screening into the 11- to 14-week and/or midgestation obstetric ultrasound examination of women with a previous cesarean scar who present with a low anterior placenta can be helpful in the management of PA.**

Magnetic Resonance Imaging

Magnetic resonance imaging (MRI) has recently been introduced as a tool that can be used to evaluate the possibility of PA. Controversy exists as to its usefulness, although some authors have suggested that MRI is better than ultrasound in defining areas of abnormal placentation and assessing the depth of myometrial invasion, particularly in cases of posterior placentae (Fig. 21-10).[52-54] A recent meta-analysis of 18 studies that involved 1010 pregnancies at risk for invasive placentation has indicated that the sensitivity and specificity of MRI in diagnosing PA antenatally were 94.4% and 84.0%, respectively.[55] MRI was also useful in assessing both the depth and topography of placental invasion (Table 21-1). Focal interruption of the myometrium and the presence of dark intraplacental bands on T2-weighted sequences showed the best sensitivity (92.0%), whereas tenting of the bladder and uterine bulging had the best specificity (98.6%). The prevalence of PA in the cohort under review was nearly 75%, which suggests that women included in these studies were highly selected and at very high risk. Therefore, the diagnostic accuracy of MRI in a more general population is difficult to ascertain, and it has not yet been shown that the addition of MRI to ultrasound results in improved clinical outcomes.

Studies that have compared MRI and ultrasound have not found a consistent difference in either the sensitivity or the specificity for the diagnosis of PA between the two techniques.

However, in several of these studies, MRI was carried out only on a proportion of women referred for ultrasound, and in most of the studies to assess the diagnostic performance of MRI, the radiologists were not blinded to the ultrasound findings.[55] Thus the value of MRI used alone without knowledge of sonographic findings is uncertain. This issue may not be of great relevance in clinical practice, where MRI images are often read with the knowledge of ultrasound findings.

Large population-based studies are needed to assess what MRI can add to ultrasound in predicting the depth and topography of placental invasion. Even if MRI may be able to add information in some limited instances, the cost and limited access of MRI compared with ultrasound makes it an impractical screening technique for PA in routine clinical practice.

MANAGEMENT

The majority of women with PA will also present with a placenta previa and are therefore at a substantial risk of bleeding and preterm delivery. Each episode of antenatal vaginal bleeding is associated with an increased risk of unscheduled delivery.[56] Therefore antenatal corticosteroid injections to advance fetal lung maturity should be timed according to the maternal symptoms and need for delivery. A decision analysis suggested that **delivery at approximately 34 weeks of gestation among women with a placenta previa and suspected PA, even without confirmation of fetal lung maturity, was the gestational age associated with optimal overall maternal and perinatal outcomes.**[57]

The worst clinical outcomes arise when PA is unsuspected at the time of delivery and the operator attempts to remove the adherent villous tissue.[58] **Women with placenta accreta, increta, or percreta for whom no attempt is made to remove any part of their placenta have reduced levels of hemorrhage and a reduced need for blood transfusion.**[59,60] When the presence of a PA is suspected, careful preoperative planning can minimize maternal morbidity. Thus attempted prenatal diagnosis of morbidly adherent villous tissue is pivotal in the management of PA. Nevertheless, it should be recognized that sonography and MRI are screening tests, and no diagnostic imaging techniques exist that can always be relied on.

Clear clinical evidence shows that **women with PA managed by a multidisciplinary care team,** compared with standard obstetric care, **are less likely to require large-volume blood transfusion and reoperation within 7 days of delivery for bleeding complications.** They are also less likely to experience prolonged admission to the intensive care unit, and they have less coagulopathy and fewer urinary tract injuries.[60-63] Referral of all women diagnosed antenatally with PA to a tertiary care center with experience in the management of PA and use of a multidisciplinary care team is therefore recommended by professional organizations, including the American College of Obstetricians and Gynecologists (ACOG), the American Society of Anesthesiologists (ASA), the Royal College of Anesthetists (RCA), and the Royal College of Obstetricians and Gynaecologists (RCOG).

Over the last decade, conservative management has been described in which the placenta is left in situ in the uterus after delivery of the neonate. **The main aim of conservative management of PA is to reduce operative injury and blood loss and to increase the chance that a hysterectomy can be avoided.** Often adjuvant procedures, including uterine artery embolization, are performed by interventional radiology.[64,65] These

TABLE 21-2	PREPARATION FOR SURGICAL MANAGEMENT OF PLACENTA ACCRETA
INTERVENTION	**COMMENT**
Treatment at a referral center	Availability of multidisciplinary team that includes pelvic surgeons, anesthesiologist, vascular/trauma surgeons, interventional radiologist, neonatologist
Preoperative imaging	Ultrasound evaluation of placenta
Timing of delivery	Approximately 34 weeks (with placenta previa)
Delivery location	Consider main OR or have all available equipment on labor and delivery. OR staff must be trained in advanced pelvic surgical procedures.
Anesthesia	Consider general anesthesia.
Vascular access	Central line, arterial line
Ureteral stents	Consider retrograde ureteral stent placement prior to laparotomy.
Cell salvage	Cell salvage availability
Rapid infusion	Availability of rapid infusion device
Interventional radiology	Consider catheter placement for uterine artery embolization and/or balloon occlusion catheter placement.
Blood bank preparedness	Packed red cells (10-20 U), fresh frozen plasma (10-20 U), platelets (12 U)
Uterine incision	Fundal or posterior hysterotomy as needed to avoid placental disruption

OR, operating room.

attempts, however, also have been associated with instances of significant delayed bleeding and infection. Consequently, the role of adjuvant procedures in the management of PA remains uncertain. RCTs and large cohort studies to compare primary surgical management and conservative management of placenta accreta are lacking. Management decisions must account for the hemodynamic status of the patient, the desire to preserve fertility, and the resource availability and expertise (Table 21-2; see also Table 21-1).

Surgical Management

Hysterectomy remains the most commonly performed procedure for the control of PPH (see Chapter 20). When massive bleeding is anticipated, appropriate equipment for major gynecologic surgery should be available in the operating room, including a self-retaining retractor and instrumentation to perform a major laparotomy. In many tertiary care centers, these surgeries are performed in the main operating room, as opposed to in the labor and delivery units, to ensure the availability of appropriate equipment; nursing staff trained in advanced abdominal surgery; a multidisciplinary team of surgeons, obstetric anesthesiologists, and interventional radiologists; and blood bank support.[66]

Prior to skin incision, blood products should be made available; this includes red blood cells, fresh frozen plasma, and platelets if possible (see Chapter 18). Early blood product replacement with consideration given to volume, oxygen-carrying capacity, and coagulation factors can reduce perioperative complications. Autologous transfusion of salvaged red cells can be used to minimize transfusion of banked blood in women undergoing cesarean hysterectomy.[67] When transfusion is required, infusion of adequate platelets and fresh-frozen plasma in relation to red blood cells (often a 1 : 1 ratio) has been associated with improved outcomes in cases of trauma, although this strategy has not been evaluated in cases of PA.[68,69] Regional anesthesia may limit the ability to manipulate the abdominal contents for retractor placement; therefore general anesthesia may be preferable for patients with a high risk of requiring a hysterectomy and in cases of placenta percreta that involves the bladder or the bowel. Prior to initiation of the surgical procedure, adequate vascular access should be ensured. This often includes central venous access as well as an arterial line. The availability of a rapid infusion device to rapidly reinstall blood products is essential if massive blood loss ensues (see Table 21-2).

The role of interventional radiology at the time of primary CD and hysterectomy remains uncertain. As described below, uterine artery embolization catheters can be placed preoperatively, and balloon occlusion catheters in the internal iliac vessels can be considered. Although these techniques may facilitate hemostasis in some women, both interventions carry risks.

Once the abdomen has been entered, the entire pelvis is inspected. The most common site of placental invasion is through the anterior uterine wall, but the placenta may invade laterally and may encroach upon the parametrium. Lateral placental invasion may hinder identification of the ureters and make isolation of the uterine vasculature difficult.[66,70] The myometrium under and around the abnormally implanted villous tissue is typically very thin and friable, and it is surrounded by dilated vascular channels (Fig. 21-11). The placental location may be mapped out with sonography and the uterine incision site chosen, preferably away from the placenta. This approach may require a fundal or even posterior uterine wall incision, which can be technically challenging and may result in a delay in delivery of the fetus, which highlights the importance of an attempt to accurately diagnosis PA to avoid unnecessarily exposing mothers without PA and their newborns to surgical procedures with a high perioperative morbidity.[71]

If a hysterectomy is required, it can be performed after closing the uterine incision. After the hysterotomy has been closed, the

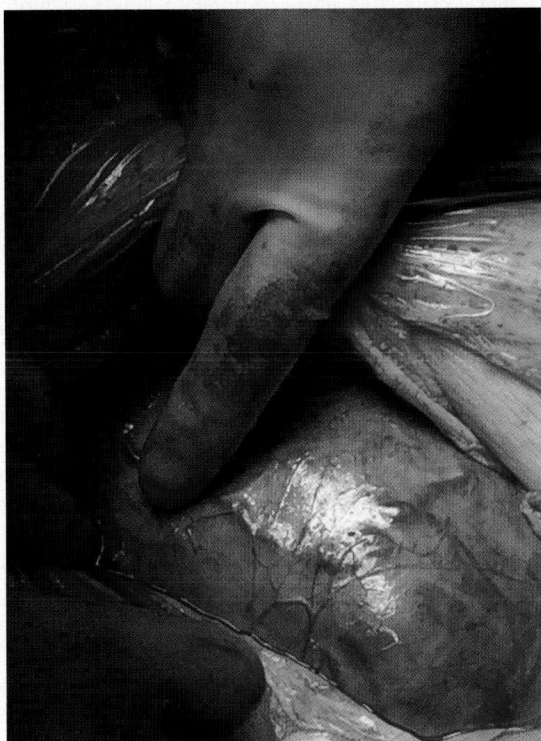

FIG 21-11 Intraoperative view of placenta accreta in the patient from Figure 21-6 shows part of the placentation site. The uterine wall is almost transparent, and an area of the abnormally implanted villous tissue is very thin and friable and surrounded by dilated vascular channels. (Courtesy Dr. Edwin Chandraharan, St. George's University Hospital Foundation Trust.)

round ligament is divided and the retroperitoneum is opened widely. The ureters are visualized, the uteroovarian ligaments are divided, and the ovaries are packed away. The vesicouterine peritoneum is then gently opened, and the bladder is dissected away from the uterus to the extent possible without placental disruption. The uterine artery and its collateral channels are then ligated, again attempting to avoid disrupting the wall of the uterus if it is thinned and friable.[70]

Placement of clamps along the lateral wall of the uterus can result in disruption of the placenta and can lead to significant bleeding. To limit bleeding, the surgeon can attempt to ligate other vasculature running to the uterus.[66,70] The use of ancillary procedures such as prophylactic ligation of the internal iliac artery is of little benefit because of the extensive collateral circulation. After the major vascular channels are divided, dissection should be continued until below the placental tissue; this typically requires additional dissection of the plane between the bladder and uterus/placenta. It is sometimes necessary to perform a cystotomy to fully separate the bladder from the uterus.

Given that PA often occurs in the context of placenta previa, removal of the entire cervix is often required to obtain hemostasis. Placement of a ring forceps on the cervix has also been described to facilitate the identification of the cervix and to limit vaginal blood loss.[72] After the uterus and placenta have been completely removed, the entire pelvis should be reinspected. Multiple, small vascular channels often run along the posterior wall of the bladder, and these must be cauterized or ligated to limit bleeding.

The genitourinary tract is at substantial risk for injury during these procedures.[66] Bladder and ureteral injuries are relatively common. If the villous tissue invades into the parametrium, ureteral identification can be difficult. **Retrograde ureteral stents can be placed via cystoscopy to facilitate ureteral identification.** These can be placed after induction of anesthesia and prior to opening the abdomen. Data are limited on the use of ureteral stents to reduce the risk of ureteral injury; therefore further evaluation is required before considering routine use for all women with PA.

Postoperatively, febrile complications and bowel dysfunction are relatively frequent. Reoperation is required in up to one third of women who undergo peripartum hysterectomy.[66] Among women who require reexploration, approximately three quarters require the procedure to control bleeding. The remainder are mostly done to repair operative injuries, mainly of the genitourinary tract.

Conservative Management

The surgical approach to management of PA is associated with significant maternal morbidity, even when carried out in a tertiary center by an experienced multidisciplinary team.[73] Within this context, conservative (uterine-sparing) approaches for the management of PA have been described. **The conservative surgical approach often involves the use of a fundal/classical incision to deliver the fetus without disturbing the placenta. The uterine incision is closed after delivery, and the placenta is left in situ.** This approach has been combined with additional procedures such as uterine artery embolization, methotrexate therapy, hemostatic sutures, pelvic devascularization, and balloon tamponade with varying rates of success reported in case reports or series (Table 21-3; see Chapter 18).

Few data are available to help select which patients are best served with conservative management and which form of conservative management, if any, is preferable. Routine use of

TABLE 21-3	PREPARATION FOR CONSERVATIVE MANAGEMENT OF PLACENTA ACCRETA
INTERVENTION	**COMMENT**
Treatment at referral center	Availability of multidisciplinary team including pelvic surgeons, anesthesiologist, vascular/trauma surgeons, interventional radiologist, neonatologist
Preoperative preparation	Preparation as above for primary surgical management if bleeding ensues
Delivery location	Consider main OR or have all available equipment on labor and delivery. OR staff must be trained in advanced pelvic surgical procedures.
Interventional radiology	Preoperative uterine artery catheter placement for uterine artery embolization
Vascular access	Central line, arterial line
Uterine incision	Fundal or posterior hysterotomy as needed to avoid placental disruption
Blood bank preparedness	Packed red cells (10-20 U), fresh frozen plasma (10-20 U), platelets (12 U)

OR, operating room.

methotrexate in conservatively managed patients is no longer advocated because it has shown little benefit in enhancing placental reabsorption and can be associated with life-threatening complications.[60,66,74] By contrast, in case series, conservative management combined with pelvic artery embolization has been associated with success rates that range between 85% and 95%.[75] Other more controversial approaches to uterine conservation have also been described. A protocol that consists of preventive radiologic catheterization of the descending aorta, CD, use of Affronti endouterine square hemostatic sutures, and placement of an intrauterine Bakri balloon in conjunction with B-Lynch suture was successfully performed in nine women with placenta previa and PA.[76] More recently, a "Triple-P procedure" was described in four women with placenta percreta.[77] With this technique, the uterine blood supply is reduced with arterial balloon occlusion catheters, the myometrial wall underlying the placental bed is excised, and the defect is closed. A recent review of 119 cases of placenta percreta noted that local resection, compared with hysterectomy or leaving the placenta in situ, was associated with fewer complications within 24 hours postoperatively.[78] Nevertheless, the data about conservative techniques are derived from case reports and series, and the number of women managed with these various conservative techniques is small. In addition, evidence suggests that conservative management is associated with severe long-term complications of hemorrhage and infection, which includes a 58% risk of delayed hysterectomy. Therefore when conservative management is chosen, follow-up should include ultrasound to assess the spontaneous or induced regression of placental tissue as well as careful monitoring of the patient's signs (e.g., temperature) and symptoms. Human chorionic gonadotropin (hCG) levels have not been shown to correlate with the rate of placental resorption.

Pelvic artery embolization performed using minimally invasive interventional radiology techniques has been demonstrated in some but not all reports to reduce intraoperative blood loss, the need for transfusion, and hysterectomy.[66,79,80] After delivery, embolization can performed either in the operating room or in an interventional radiology suite.[66,75] Pelvic artery embolization is also useful in women who continue to bleed after hysterectomy. However, complications of embolization include thrombosis and necrosis of embolized tissue.

The second interventional radiologic modality that may be of use in women with PA is the placement of intraarterial balloon occlusion catheters.[66,81,82] Occlusion catheters contain small balloons that can be inflated to occlude the lumen of a vessel. Balloon occlusion catheters can be placed under fluoroscopic guidance prior to hysterectomy, and placement within the internal iliac artery is the most common site. At the time of hysterectomy, the balloons can be inflated either prophylactically or only after heavy bleeding is encountered.

Both embolization and balloon occlusion incur risks that include thrombosis, tissue necrosis, and vascular dissection. Accordingly, **the utility of embolization and balloon occlusion catheters remains controversial, and it has not been demonstrated that the routine use of these interventions has benefits that outweigh the risks.**

Reproductive Outcomes Following Placenta Accreta

Although data are limited, conservative treatment for PA may be followed by a subsequent pregnancy,[83] although that subsequent pregnancy **is at increased risk for adverse maternal outcomes that include recurrent PA, uterine rupture, PPH, and peripartum hysterectomy.**[84-87] Estimated risks have been reported for recurrent PA (22%[87] to 29%[84]), early PPH (8.6%[83,87]), uterine rupture (3.3%), peripartum hysterectomy (3.3%), and blood transfusions (16.7%).[84] Long-term complications include intrauterine synechiae and secondary amenorrhea.[83]

SUMMARY

Placenta accreta (PA) refers to different grades of morbid placental attachment to the uterine wall secondary to deep invasion of villous tissue into the myometrium. Although any primary or secondary alterations of the uterine endometrial-myometrial integrity have been associated with the development of PA, the rapid increase in the frequency of CD over the last several decades has led to PA becoming an increasingly common obstetric complication. The failure of the entire placenta to separate normally from the uterine wall after delivery in PA is typically accompanied by severe PPH. Therefore accurate prenatal diagnosis is important in the outcome of PA, and along with planned management of the condition through the use of a multidisciplinary team, this has been associated with a reduced rate of maternal morbidity. Women diagnosed antenatally with PA should be referred to a tertiary care center and managed by a multidisciplinary team that includes surgeons, obstetric anesthesiologists, interventional radiologists, and hematologists.

KEY POINTS

◆ Prior CD is the most important factor associated with PA, and the risk of PA increases with the number of prior CDs.

◆ All women with placenta previa who have had a previous CD are at risk of PA, and each additional CD is associated with an increased risk of PA.

- Suspected PA on prenatal imaging allows planned management of the condition and has been associated with a reduced rate of maternal morbidity.
- Ultrasound imaging is superior to MRI for routine screening of PA in at-risk women, but the degree of invasion to adjacent pelvic tissues and organs may be better ascertained with MRI.
- The optimum time for planned delivery for a woman with suspected PA and placenta previa is approximately 34 weeks, following a course of corticosteroid injections.
- When a PA is suspected, it is best to avoid disturbing the placenta and to leave it attached at the time of cesarean delivery.
- Women diagnosed antenatally with PA should be referred to a tertiary care center and managed by a multidisciplinary team that includes surgeons, obstetric anesthesiologists, interventional radiologists, and hematologists.
- The role of interventional radiology at the time of primary caesarean delivery and hysterectomy remains uncertain.
- A pregnancy following a previous PA that was treated with conservative management is at increased risk for adverse maternal outcomes such as recurrent PA, uterine rupture, PPH, and peripartum hysterectomy.

REFERENCES

1. Irving C, Hertig AT. A study of placenta accreta. Surgery. *Gynecol Obstet.* 1937;64:178-200.
2. Fox H. Abnormalities of placentation. In: *Pathology of the Placenta.* 2nd ed. London: Saunders; 1997:54-76.
3. Benirschke K, Burton GJ, Baergen RN, eds. *Pathology of the Human Placenta. Pathology of Trophoblast Invasion.* 6th ed. New York: Springer; 2013:205-211.
4. Jauniaux E, Jurkovic D. Placenta accreta: pathogenesis of a 20th century iatrogenic uterine disease. *Placenta.* 2012;33(4):244-251.
5. West MJ, Irvine LM, Jauniaux E. Caesarean section: from antiquity to the 21st century. In: Jauniaux E, Grobman W, eds. *A Modern Textbook of Cesarean Section.* Oxford UK: Oxford University Press; 2015.
6. Roeder HA, Cramer SF, Leppert PC. A look at uterine wound healing through a histopathological study of uterine scars. *Reprod Sci.* 2012;19(5):463-473.
7. Buhimschi CS, Zhao G, Sora N, Madri JA, Buhimschi IA. Myometrial wound healing post-Cesarean delivery in the MRL/MpJ mouse model of uterine scarring. *Am J Pathol.* 2010;177(1):197-207.
8. Ben-Nagi J, Walker A, Jurkovic D, Yazbek J, Aplin JD. Effect of cesarean delivery on the endometrium. *Int J Gynaecol Obstet.* 2009;106(1):30-34.
9. Flo K, Widnes C, Vårtun Å, Acharya G. Blood flow to the scarred gravid uterus at 22-24 weeks of gestation. *BJOG.* 2014;121(2):210-215.
10. Beuker JM, Erwich JJ, Khong TY. Is endomyometrial injury during termination of pregnancy or curettage following miscarriage the precursor to placenta accreta? *J Clin Pathol.* 2005;58(3):273-275.
11. Liang HS, Jeng CJ, Sheen TC, Lee FK, Yang YC, Tzeng CR. First-trimester uterine rupture from a placenta percreta. A case report. *J Reprod Med.* 2003;489(6):474-478.
12. Fleisch MC, Lux J, Schoppe M, Grieshaber K, Hampl M. Placenta percreta leading to spontaneous complete uterine rupture in the second trimester. Example of a fatal complication of abnormal placentation following uterine scarring. *Gynecol Obstet Invest.* 2008;65(2):81-83.
13. Patsouras K, Panagopoulos P, Sioulas V, Salamalekis G, Kassanos D. Uterine rupture at 17 weeks of a twin pregnancy complicated with placenta percreta. *J Obstet Gynaecol.* 2010;30(1):60-61.
14. Jang DG, Lee GS, Yoon JH, Lee SJ. Placenta percreta-induced uterine rupture diagnosed by laparoscopy in the first trimester. *Int J Med Sci.* 2011;8(7):424-427.
15. Hornemann A, Bohlmann MK, Diedrich K, et al. Spontaneous uterine rupture at the 21st week of gestation caused by placenta percreta. *Arch Gynecol Obstet.* 2011;284(4):875-878.
16. Wu S, Kocherginsky M, Hibbard JU. Abnormal placentation: twenty-year analysis. *Am J Obstet Gynecol.* 2005;192(5):1458-1461.
17. Getahun D, Oyelese Y, Salihu HM, Ananth CV. Previous cesarean delivery and risks of placenta previa and placental abruption. *Obstet Gynecol.* 2006;107(4):771-778.
18. Klar M, Michels KB. Cesarean section and placental disorders in subsequent pregnancies–a meta-analysis. *J Perinat Med.* 2014;42(5):571-583.
19. Kamara M, Henderson JJ, Doherty DA, Dickinson JE, Pennell CE. The risk of placenta accreta following primary elective caesarean delivery: a case-control study. *BJOG.* 2013;120(7):879-886.
20. Yang Q, Wen SW, Oppenheimer L, et al. Association of caesarean delivery for first birth with placenta praevia and placental abruption in second pregnancy. *BJOG.* 2007;114(5):609-613.
21. Gurol-Urganci I, Cromwell DA, Edozien LC, et al. Risk of placenta previa in second birth after first birth cesarean section: a population-based study and meta-analysis. *BMC Pregnancy Childbirth.* 2011;11:95.
22. Solheim KN, Esakoff TF, Little SE, Cheng YW, Sparks TN, Caughey AB. The effect of cesarean delivery rates on the future incidence of placenta previa, placenta accreta, and maternal mortality. *J Matern Fetal Neonatal Med.* 2011;24(11):1341-1346.
23. Bowman ZS, Eller AG, Bardsley TR, Greene T, Varner MW, Silver RM. Risk factors for placenta accreta: a large prospective cohort. *Am J Perinatol.* 2014;31(9):799-804.
24. Jastrow N, Chaillet N, Roberge S, Morency AM, Lacasse Y, Bujold E. Sonographic lower uterine segment thickness and risk of uterine scar defect: a systematic review. *J Obstet Gynaecol Can.* 2010;32(4):321-327.
25. Ofili-Yebovi D, Ben-Nagi J, Sawyer E, et al. Deficient lower-segment cesarean section scars: prevalence and risk factors. *Ultrasound Obstet Gynecol.* 2008;31(1):72-77.
26. Wang CB, Chiu WW, Lee CY, Sun YL, Lin YH, Tseng CJ. Cesarean scar defect: correlation between cesarean section number, defect size, clinical symptoms and uterine position. *Ultrasound Obstet Gynecol.* 2009;34(1):85-89.
27. Vikhareva Osser OV, Valentin L. Clinical importance of appearance of cesarean hysterotomy scar at transvaginal ultrasonography in nonpregnant women. *Obstet Gynecol.* 2011;117(3):525-532.
28. Baron J, Weintraub AY, Eshkoli T, Hershkovitz R, Sheiner E. The consequences of previous uterine scar dehiscence and cesarean delivery on subsequent births. *Int J Gynaecol Obstet.* 2014;126(2):120-122.
29. Fox NS, Gerber RS, Mourad M, et al. Pregnancy outcomes in patients with prior uterine rupture or dehiscence. *Obstet Gynecol.* 2014;123(4):785-789.
30. van der Voet LF, Vervoort AJ, Veersema S, et al. Minimally invasive therapy for gynaecological symptoms related to a niche in the caesarean scar: a systematic review. *BJOG.* 2014;121(2):145-156.
31. Chiu TL, Sadler L, Wise MR. Placenta praevia after prior caesarean section: an exploratory case-control study. *Aust N Z J Obstet Gynaecol.* 2013;53(5):455-458.
32. Jauniaux E, Toplis PJ, Nicolaides KH. Sonographic diagnosis of a non-previa placenta accreta. *Ultrasound Obstet Gynecol.* 1996;7(1):58-60.
33. Twickler DM, Lucas MJ, Balis AB, et al. Color flow mapping for myometrial invasion in women with a prior cesarean delivery. *J Matern Fetal Med.* 2000;9(6):330-335.
34. Chou MM, Ho ES, Lee YH. Prenatal diagnosis of placenta previa accreta by transabdominal color Doppler ultrasound. *Ultrasound Obstet Gynecol.* 2000;15(1):28-35.
35. Warshak CR, Eskander R, Hull AD, et al. Accuracy of ultrasonography and magnetic resonance imaging in the diagnosis of placenta accreta. *Obstet Gynecol.* 2006;108(3):573-581.
36. Wong HS, Cheung YK, Strand L, et al. Specific sonographic features of placenta accreta: tissue interface disruption on gray-scale imaging and evidence of vessels crossing interface- disruption sites on Doppler imaging. *Ultrasound Obstet Gynecol.* 2007;29(2):239-240.
37. Woodring TC, Klauser CK, Bofill JA, Martin RW, Morrison JC. Prediction of placenta accreta by ultrasonography and color Doppler imaging. *J Matern Fetal Neonatal Med.* 2011;24(1):118-121.
38. Esakoff TF, Sparks TN, Kaimal AJ, et al. Diagnosis and morbidity of placenta accreta. *Ultrasound Obstet Gynecol.* 2011;37(3):324-327.

39. Chalubinski KM, Pils S, Klein K, et al. Prenatal sonography can predict degree of placental invasion. *Ultrasound Obstet Gynecol.* 2013;42(5):518-524.

40. Bowman ZS, Eller AG, Kennedy AM, et al. Accuracy of ultrasound for the prediction of placenta accreta. *Am J Obstet Gynecol.* 2014;211(2):177, e1-7.

41. D'Antonio F, Iacovella C, Bhide A. Prenatal identification of invasive placentation using ultrasound: systematic review and meta-analysis. *Ultrasound Obstet Gynecol.* 2013;42(5):509-517.

42. Chen YJ, Wang PH, Liu WM, Lai CR, Shu LP, Hung JH. Placenta accreta diagnosed at 9 weeks' gestation. *Ultrasound Obstet Gynecol.* 2002;19(6):620-622.

43. Shih JC, Cheng WF, Shyu MK, Lee CN, Hsieh FJ. Power Doppler evidence of placenta accreta appearing in the first trimester. *Ultrasound Obstet Gynecol.* 2002;19(6):623-625.

44. Comstock CH, Lee W, Vettraino IM, Bronsteen RA. The early sonographic appearance of placenta accreta. *J Ultrasound Med.* 2003;22(1):19-23.

45. Ben Nagi J, Ofili-Yebovi D, Marsh M, Jurkovic D. First-trimester cesarean scar pregnancy evolving into placenta previa/accreta at term. *J Ultrasound Med.* 2005;24(11):1569-1573.

46. Yang JI, Kim HY, Kim HS, Ryu HS. Diagnosis in the first trimester of placenta accreta with previous Cesarean section. *Ultrasound Obstet Gynecol.* 2009;34(1):116-118.

47. Stirnemann JJ, Mousty E, Chalouhi G, Salomon LJ, Bernard JP, Ville Y. Screening for placenta accreta at 11-14 weeks of gestation. *Am J Obstet Gynecol.* 2011;205(6):547, e1-6.

48. Wong HS, Cheung YK, Williams E. Antenatal ultrasound assessment of placental/myometrial involvement in morbidly adherent placenta. *Aust N Z J Obstet Gynaecol.* 2012;52(1):67-72.

49. Chalubinski KM, Pils S, Klein K, et al. Prenatal sonography can predict degree of placental invasion. *Ultrasound Obstet Gynecol.* 2013;42(5):518-524.

50. Al-Khan A, Gupta V, Illsley NP, et al. Maternal and fetal outcomes in placenta accreta after institution of team-managed care. *Reprod Sci.* 2014;21(6):761-771.

51. Weiniger CF, Einav S, Deutsch L, Ginosar Y, Ezra Y, Eid L. Outcomes of prospectively-collected consecutive cases of antenatal-suspected placenta accreta. *Int J Obstet Anesth.* 2013;22(4):273-279.

52. McLean LA, Heilbrun ME, Eller AG, Kennedy AM, Woodward PJ. Assessing the role of magnetic resonance imaging in the management of gravid patients at risk for placenta accreta. *Acad Radiol.* 2011;18(9):1175-1180.

53. Elhawary TM, Dabees NL, Youssef MA. Diagnostic value of ultrasonography and magnetic resonance imaging in pregnant women at risk for placenta accreta. *J Matern Fetal Neonatal Med.* 2013;26(14):1443-1449.

54. Allen BC, Leyendecker JR. Placental evaluation with magnetic resonance. *Radiol Clin North Am.* 2013;51(6):955-966.

55. D'Antonio F, Iacovella C, Palacios-Jaraquemada J, Bruno CH, Manzoli L, Bhide A. Prenatal identification of invasive placentation using Magnetic Resonance Imaging (MRI): systematic review and meta-analysis. *Ultrasound Obstet Gynecol.* 2014;44(1):8-16.

56. Bowman ZS, Manuck TA, Eller AG, Simons M, Silver RM. Risk factors for unscheduled delivery in patients with placenta accreta. *Am J Obstet Gynecol.* 2014;210(3):e1-e6.

57. Robinson BK, Grobman WA. Effectiveness of timing strategies for delivery of individuals with placenta previa and accreta. *Obstet Gynecol.* 2010;116(4):835-842.

58. Warshak CR, Ramos GA, Eskander R, et al. Effect of predelivery diagnosis in 99 consecutive cases of placenta accreta. *Obstet Gynecol.* 2010;115(1):65-69.

59. Fitzpatrick K, Sellers S, Spark P, Kurinczuk J, Brocklehurst P, Knight M. The management and outcomes of placenta accreta, increta, and percreta in the UK: a population-based descriptive study. *BJOG.* 2014;121(1):62-71.

60. Sentilhes L, Goffinet F, Kayem G. Management of placenta accreta. *Acta Obstet Gynecol Scand.* 2013;92(10):1125-1134.

61. Eller AG, Bennett MA, Sharshiner M, et al. Maternal morbidity in cases of placenta accreta managed by a multidisciplinary care team compared with standard obstetric care. *Obstet Gynecol.* 2011;117(2):331-337.

62. Beilin Y, Halpern SH. Placenta accreta: successful outcome is all in the planning. *Int J Obstet Anesth.* 2013;22(4):269-271.

63. Shamshirsaz AA, Fox KA, Salmanian B, et al. Maternal morbidity in patients with morbidly adherent placenta treated with and without a standardized multidisciplinary approach. *Am J Obstet Gynecol.* 2015;212(2):218, e1-9.

64. Esakoff TF, Handler SJ, Granados JM, Caughey AB. PAMUS: placenta accreta management across the United States. *J Matern Fetal Neonatal Med.* 2012;25(6):761-765.

65. Guleria K, Gupta B, Agarwal S, Suneja A, Vaid N, Jain S. Abnormally invasive placenta changing trends in diagnosis and management. *Acta Obstet Gynecol Scand.* 2013;92(4):461-464.

66. Perez-Delboy A, Wright J. Surgical management of placenta accreta: to leave or remove the placenta? *BJOG.* 2014;121(2):163-170.

67. Elagamy A, Abdelaziz A, Ellaithy M. The use of cell salvage in women undergoing cesarean hysterectomy for abnormal placentation. *Int J Obstet Anesth.* 2013;22(4):289-293.

68. Brown LM, Aro SO, Cohen MJ, et al. A high fresh frozen plasma: packed red blood cell transfusion ratio decreases mortality in all massively transfused trauma patients regardless of admission international normalized ratio. *J Trauma.* 2011;71(2 suppl 3):S358-S363.

69. Rowell SE, Barbosa RR, Diggs BS, et al. Effect of high product ratio massive transfusion on mortality in blunt and penetrating trauma patients. *J Trauma.* 2011;71(2 suppl 3):S353-S357.

70. Wright JD, Bonanno C, Shah M, Gaddipati S, Devine P. Peripartum hysterectomy. *Obstet Gynecol.* 2010;116(6):429-434.

71. Jauniaux E, Jurkovic D. Transverse uterine fundal incision for anterior placenta praevia accreta: more harm than good? *BJOG.* 2014;121(6):771.

72. Matsubara S, Kuwata T, Usui R, et al. Important surgical measures and techniques at cesarean hysterectomy for placenta previa accreta. *Acta Obstet Gynecol Scand.* 2013;92(4):372-377.

73. Grace Tan SE, Jobling TW, Wallace EM, McNeilage LJ, Manolitsas T, Hodges RJ. Surgical management of placenta accreta: a 10-year experience. *Acta Obstet Gynecol Scand.* 2013;92(4):445-450.

74. Steins Bisschop CN, Schaap TP, Vogelvang TE, Scholten PC. Invasive placentation and uterus preserving treatment modalities: a systematic review. *Arch Gynecol Obstet.* 2011;284(2):491-502.

75. Timmermans S, van Hof AC, Duvekot JJ. Conservative management of abnormally invasive placentation. *Obstet Gynecol Surv.* 2007;62(8):529-539.

76. Arduini M, Epicoco G, Clerici G, Bottaccioli E, Arena S, Affronti G. B-Lynch suture, intrauterine balloon, and endouterine hemostatic suture for the management of postpartum hemorrhage due to placenta previa accreta. *Int J Gynaecol Obstet.* 2010;108(3):191-193.

77. Chandraharan E, Rao S, Belli AM, Arulkumaran S. The triple-P procedure as a conservative surgical alternative to peripartum hysterectomy for placenta percreta. *Int J Gynaecol Obstet.* 2012;117(2):191-194.

78. Clausen C, Lönn L, Langhoff-Roos J. Management of placenta percreta: a review of published cases. *Acta Obstet Gynecol Scand.* 2014;93(2):138-143.

79. Bouvier A, Sentilhes L, Thouveny F, et al. Planned caesarean in the interventional radiology cath lab to enable immediate uterine artery embolization for the conservative treatment of placenta accreta. *Clin Radiol.* 2012;67(11):1089-1094.

80. Chung MY, Cheng YK, Yu SC, Sahota DS, Leung TY. Nonremoval of an abnormally invasive placenta at cesarean section with postoperative uterine artery embolization. *Acta Obstet Gynecol Scand.* 2013;92(11):1250-1255.

81. Tan CH, Tay KH, Sheah K, et al. Perioperative endovascular internal iliac artery occlusion balloon placement in management of placenta accreta. *AJR Am J Roentgenol.* 2007;189(5):1158-1163.

82. Clausen C, Stensballe J, Albrechtsen CK, Hansen MA, Lönn L, Langhoff-Roos J. Balloon occlusion of the internal iliac arteries in the multidisciplinary management of placenta percreta. *Acta Obstet Gynecol Scand.* 2013;92(4):386-391.

83. Sentilhes L, Kayem G, Ambroselli C, et al. Fertility and pregnancy outcomes following conservative treatment for placenta accreta. *Hum Reprod.* 2010;25(11):2803-2810.

84. Sentilhes L, Ambroselli C, Kayem G, et al. Maternal outcome after conservative treatment of placenta accreta. *Obstet Gynecol.* 2010;115(3):526-534.

85. Kabiri D, Hants Y, Shanwetter N, et al. Outcomes of subsequent pregnancies after conservative treatment for placenta accreta. *Int J Gynaecol Obstet.* 2014;127(2):206-210.

86. Eshkoli T, Weintraub AY, Sergienko R, Sheiner E. Placenta accreta: risk factors, perinatal outcomes, and consequences for subsequent births. *Am J Obstet Gynecol.* 2013;208(3):219, e1-7.

87. Kabiri D, Hants Y, Shanwetter N, et al. Outcomes of subsequent pregnancies after conservative treatment for placenta accreta. *Int J Gynaecol Obstet.* 2014;127(2):206-210.

Postpartum Care

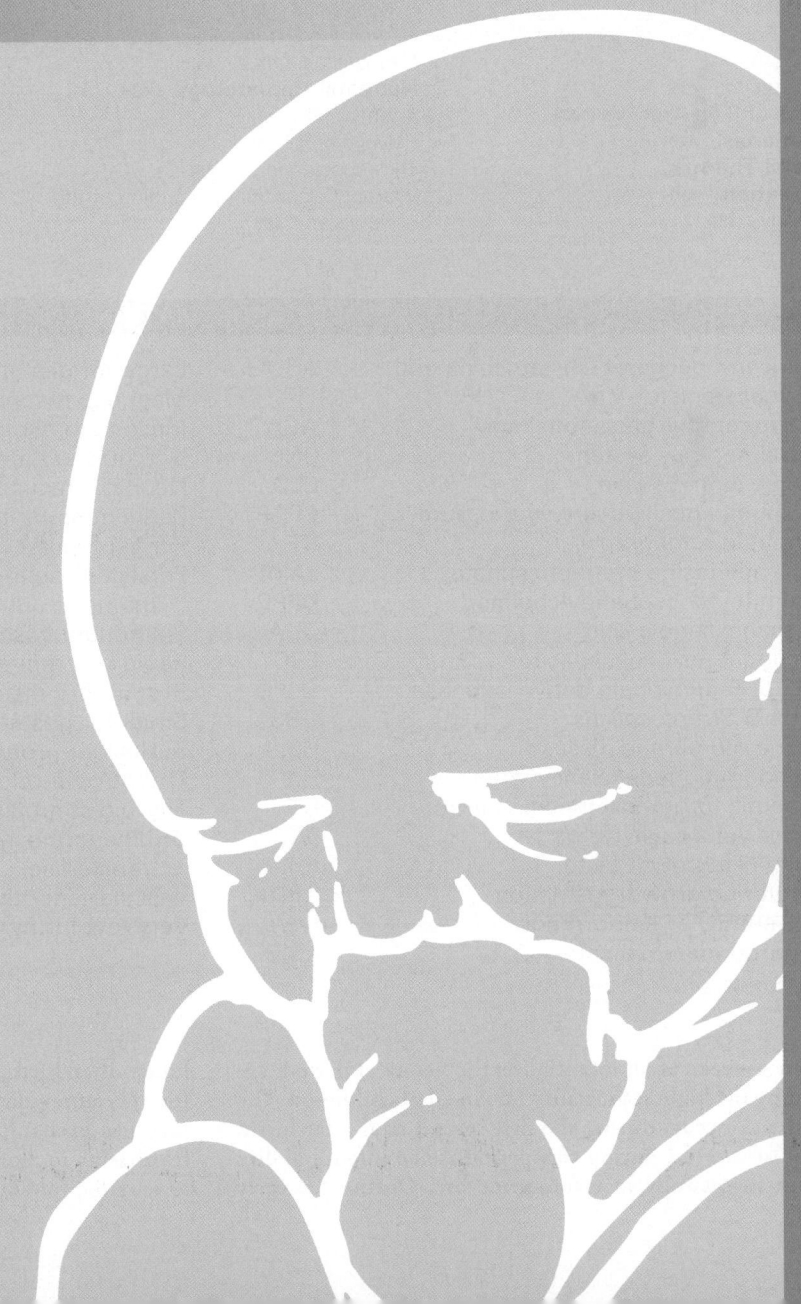

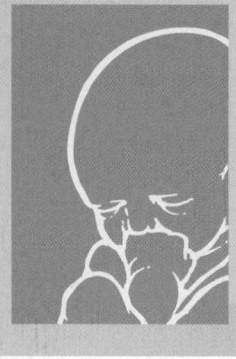

The Neonate

PAUL J. ROZANCE and ADAM A. ROSENBERG

KEY ABBREVIATIONS

American College of Obstetricians and Gynecologists	ACOG	Large for gestational age	LGA
		Magnetic resonance imaging	MRI
Appropriate for gestational age	AGA	Meconium aspiration syndrome	MAS
Central nervous system	CNS	Necrotizing enterocolitis	NEC
Chronic lung disease	CLD	Neonatal resuscitation program	NRP
Continuous positive airway pressure	CPAP	Periventricular hemorrhage	PVH
Computed tomography	CT	Periventricular leukomalacia	PVL
Cyclic adenosine monophosphate	cAMP	Persistent pulmonary hypertension of the newborn	PPHN
Dipalmitoylphosphatidylcholine	DPPC		
Docosahexaenoic acid	DHA	Pulmonary vascular resistance	PVR
Functional residual capacity	FRC	Rapid eye movement	REM
Glucose-6-phosphate dehydrogenase	G6PD	Respiratory distress syndrome	RDS
Group B *Streptococcus*	GBS	Small for gestational age	SGA
Hyaline membrane disease	HMD	Surfactant protein	SP
Human immunodeficiency virus	HIV	Thyrotropin-releasing hormone	TRH
Idiopathic thrombocytopenic purpura	ITP	Thyroid-stimulating hormone	TSH
Inferior vena cava	IVC	Uridine diphosphoglucuronosyl transferase	UDPGT
Insulin-like growth factor 1	IGF-1		
Intrauterine growth restriction	IUGR	Vascular endothelial growth factor	VEGF
Intraventricular hemorrhage	IVH	Very low birthweight	VLBW
Kangaroo maternal care	KMC		

The first 4 weeks of an infant's life, the neonatal period, are marked by the highest mortality rate in all of childhood. The greatest risk occurs during the first several days after birth. Critical to survival during this period is the infant's ability to adapt successfully to extrauterine life. During the early hours after birth, the newborn must assume responsibility for thermoregulation, metabolic homeostasis, and respiratory gas exchange and must also undergo the conversion from fetal to postnatal circulatory pathways. This chapter reviews the physiology of a successful transition as well as the implications of circumstances that disrupt this process. Implicit in these considerations is the understanding that the newborn reflects the sum total of its genetic and environmental past, which includes any minor or major insults to which it was subjected during gestation and parturition. The period of neonatal adaptation is then most meaningfully viewed as continuous with fetal life.

CARDIOPULMONARY TRANSITION
Pulmonary Development

Lung development and maturation require a carefully regulated interaction of anatomic, physiologic, and biochemical processes. The outcome of these events provides an organ with adequate surface area, sufficient vascularization, and the metabolic capability to sustain oxygenation and ventilation during the neonatal period. **Five stages of morphologic lung development have been identified in the human fetus**[1]: (1) the *embryonic period,* from 0 to 6 weeks postconception; (2) the *pseudoglandular period,* from 6 to 16 weeks; (3) the *canalicular period,* from 16 to 24 weeks; (4) the *saccular period,* from 24 to 38 weeks; and (5) the *alveolar period,* from 36 weeks' gestation to 2 years of age.

The lung arises as a ventral diverticulum from the foregut during the fourth week of gestation, in the *embryonic period.* During the ensuing weeks, in the *pseudoglandular period,* branching of the diverticulum occurs and forms a tree of narrow tubes with thick epithelial walls composed of columnar cells. Molecular mechanisms involved in lung development include expression of transcription factors important for specification of the foregut endoderm, endogenous secretion of polypeptides important for pattern formation, and the production of growth and differentiation factors critical to cell development. By 16 weeks, the conducting portion of the tracheobronchial tree up to and including the terminal bronchioles has been established. The vasculature derived from the pulmonary circulation develops concurrently with the conducting airways, and by 16 weeks, preacinar blood vessels are formed. The *canalicular period* is characterized by differentiation of the airways, with widening of the airways and thinning of epithelium. In addition, primitive respiratory bronchioles begin to form, marking the start of the gas-exchanging portion of the lung. Vascular proliferation continues, along with a relative decrease in mesenchyme, which brings the vessels closer to the airway epithelium. The *saccular period* is marked by the development of the gas-exchanging portion of the tracheobronchial tree (acinus) composed of respiratory bronchioles, alveolar ducts, terminal saccules, and finally, alveoli. During this stage, the pulmonary vessels continue to proliferate with the airways and surround the developing air sacs. The final phase of prenatal lung development, the *alveolar period,* is marked by the formation of thin secondary alveolar septa and the remodeling of the capillary bed.

Throughout these periods, mesenchymal and epithelial cell cross-talk directs the normal processes of lung alveolarization and vascularization.[2] **Several million alveoli will form before birth, which emphasizes the importance of the last few weeks of pregnancy to pulmonary adaptation.** Postnatal lung growth is characterized by generation of alveoli, and over 85% of alveolarization takes place after birth.[1]

The critical determinants of extrauterine survival are the formation of the thin air-blood barrier and production of surfactant. By birth, the epithelial lining of the gas-exchanging surface is thin and continuous with two alveolar cell types: *type I cells* are thin and contain few subcellular organelles, whereas *type II cells* contain subcellular organelles that aid in the production of surfactant (Fig. 22-1). Surfactant lipids and surfactant proteins B and C are secreted by exocytosis as lamellar bodies and unravel into tubular myelin. The other surfactant proteins (SPs), SP-A and SP-D, are secreted independently of the lamellar bodies. Tubular myelin is a loose lattice of phospholipids and surfactant-specific proteins. The surface active component of surfactant then adsorbs at the alveolar interface between air and water in a monolayer. With repetitive expansion and compression of the surface monolayer, material is extruded that is either cleared by alveolar macrophages through endocytic pathways or is taken up by the type II cell for recycling back into lamellar bodies.[3]

Because of the development of high surface forces along the respiratory epithelium when breathing begins, the availability of surfactants in terminal airspaces is critical to postnatal lung function. Just as surface tension acts to reduce the size of a bubble in water, it also acts to reduce lung inflation, which promotes atelectasis. This is described by the LaPlace law, which states that within a sphere the pressure (P) is directly proportional to surface tension (T) and is inversely proportional to the radius (r) of curvature (Fig. 22-2). **Surfactant has the physical property of variable surface tension dependent on the degree of surface area compression. In other words, as the radius of the alveolus decreases, surfactant serves to reduce surface tension, which prevents collapse of the alveolus.** If this property is extrapolated to the lung, smaller alveoli will remain more stable than larger alveoli because of their lower surface tension. This feature is emphasized in Figure 22-3, which compares pressure-volume curves from surfactant-deficient and surfactant-treated preterm rabbits. **Surfactant deficiency is characterized by high opening pressure, low maximal lung volume, and lack of deflation stability at low pressures.**

Natural surfactant contains mostly lipids, phospholipids specifically, and some protein (Fig. 22-4).[3] **Approximately half of the protein is specific for surfactant.** The principal classes of phospholipids are:

- Saturated phosphatidylcholine compounds, the surface tension-reducing component of surfactant, 45%—more than 80% of which is dipalmitoylphosphatidylcholine (DPPC)
- Unsaturated phosphatidylcholine compounds, 25%
- Phosphatidylglycerol, phosphatidylinositol, and phosphatidylethanolamine, 10%

Saturated phosphatidylcholine is found in lung tissue of the human fetus earlier in gestation than in other species. Surfactant is released from storage pools into fetal lung fluid at a basal rate during late gestation and is stimulated by labor and the initiation of air breathing. Four unique surfactant-associated proteins have been identified, and all are synthesized and secreted by type II alveolar cells. **Surfactant protein A (SP-A)** functions cooperatively with the other surfactant proteins and lipids to enhance the biophysical activity of the surfactant, but its most important role is in the innate host defense of the lung. **SP-B and SP-C** are lipophilic proteins that facilitate the adsorption and spreading of lipid to form the surfactant monolayer. SP-B deficiencies are associated with neonatal pulmonary complications and death, whereas SP-C deficiencies are associated with interstitial lung disease that presents at a more variable age. **SP-D** plays a

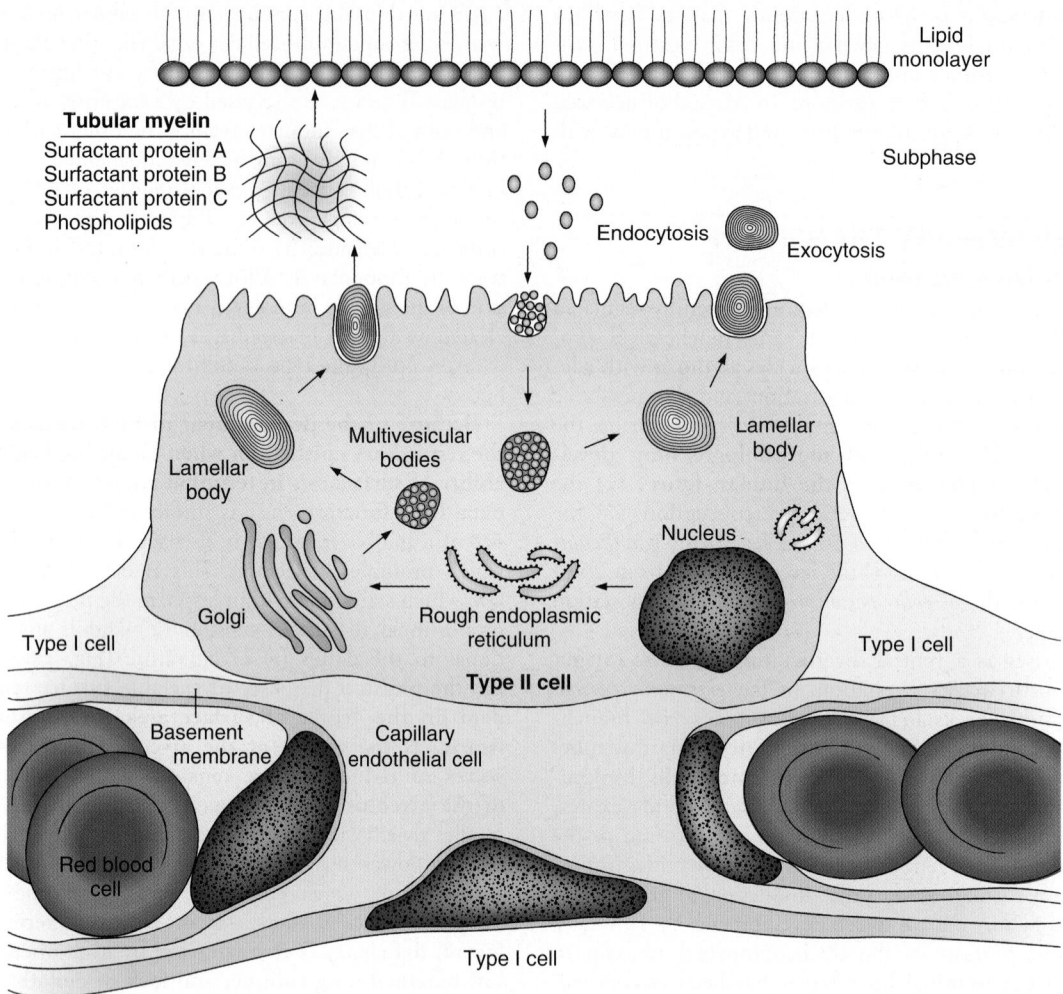

FIG 22-1 Metabolism of surfactant. Surfactant phospholipids are synthesized in the endoplasmic reticulum, transported through the Golgi apparatus to multivesicular bodies, and finally packaged in lamellar bodies. After lamellar body exocytosis, phospholipids are organized into tubular myelin before aligning in a monolayer at the air-fluid interface in the alveolus. Surfactant phospholipids and proteins are taken up by type II cells and are either catabolized or reused. Surfactant proteins are synthesized in polyribosomes and are modified in endoplasmic reticulum, Golgi apparatus, and multivesicular bodies. (Modified from Whitsett JA, Pryhuber GS, Rice WR, et al. Acute respiratory disorders. In Avery GB, Fletcher MA, MacDonald MG [eds]: *Neonatology: Pathophysiology and Management of the Newborn*, 5th ed. Philadelphia: Lippincott, Williams & Wilkins; 1999:485.)

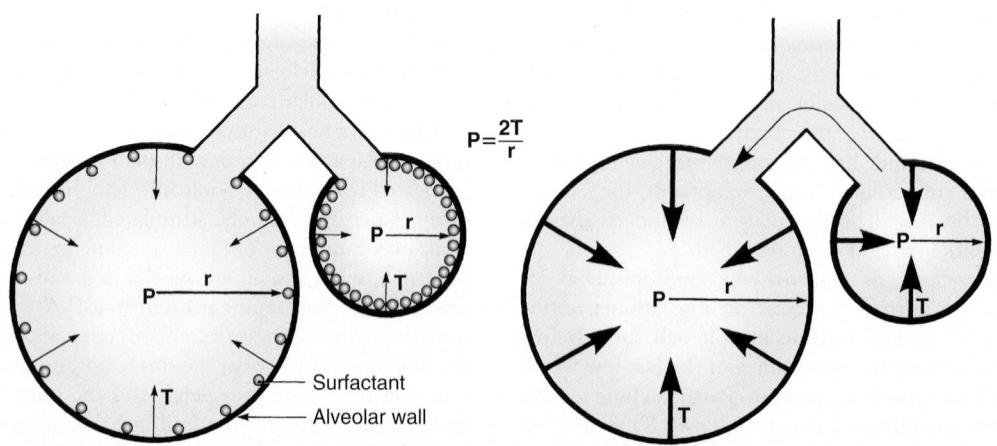

FIG 22-2 LaPlace's law. The pressure (*P*) within a sphere is directly proportional to surface tension (*T*) and is inversely proportional to the radius of curvature (*r*). In the normal lung, as alveolar size decreases, surface tension (*thin arrows*) is reduced because of the presence of surfactant. This serves to decrease the collapsing pressure that must be opposed and maintains equal pressures in the small and large interconnected alveoli. (Modified from Netter FH. *The Ciba Collection of Medical Illustrations. The Respiratory System,* Vol 7. Summit, NJ: Ciba-Geigy; 1979.)

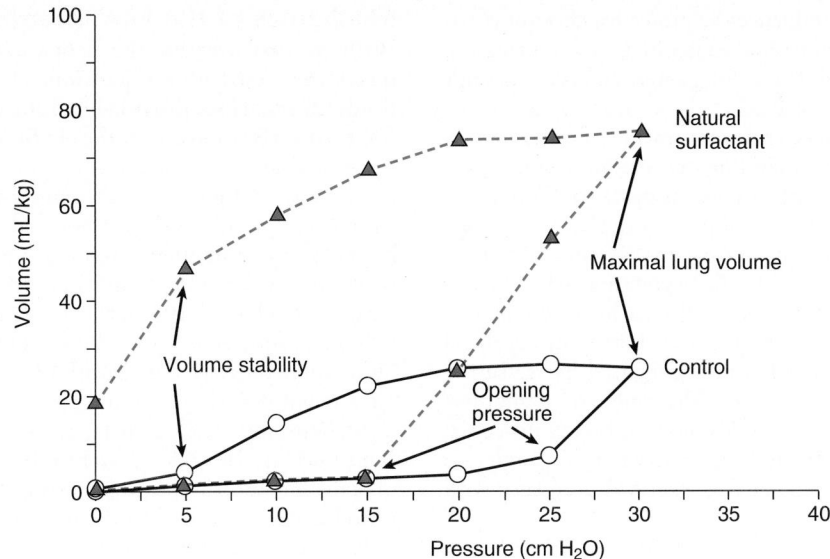

FIG 22-3 Pressure-volume relationships for the inflation and deflation of surfactant-deficient and surfactant-treated (*red line*) preterm rabbit lungs. Surfactant deficiency (*black line*) is indicated by high opening pressure, low maximal volume at a distending pressure of 30 cm of water, and lack of deflation stability at low pressures on deflation. (Modified from Jobe AH. Lung development and maturation. In Fanaroff AA, Martin RJ [eds]: *Neonatal-Perinatal Medicine: Diseases of the Fetus and Infant,* 7th ed. St. Louis: Mosby; 2002:973.)

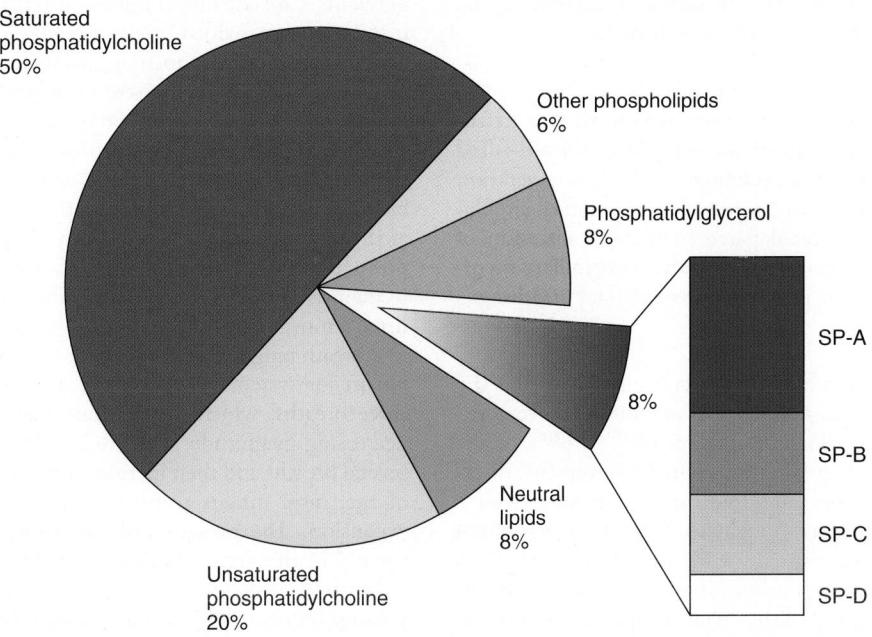

FIG 22-4 Composition of pulmonary surfactant. SP, surfactant protein. (Modified from Jobe AH. Lung development and maturation. In Fanaroff AA, Martin RJ [eds]: *Neonatal-Perinatal Medicine: Diseases of the Fetus and Infant,* 7th ed. St Louis: Mosby; 2002:973.)

role in the regulation of surfactant lipid homeostasis, inflammatory responses, and host defense mechanisms.[3]

Several hormones and growth factors contribute to the regulation of pulmonary phospholipid metabolism and lung maturation: glucocorticoids, thyroid hormone, thyrotropin-releasing hormone, retinoic acid, epidermal growth factor, and others. **Glucocorticoids are the most important and are used clinically to augment the synthesis of surfactant and accelerate morphologic development.**[4] Pregnant women with anticipated preterm delivery have received corticosteroid treatment since 1972. Numerous controlled trials have since been performed. Based on a meta-analysis,[5] **a significant reduction of about 50% in the incidence of respiratory distress syndrome (RDS) is seen in infants born to mothers who received antenatal corticosteroids.** In a secondary analysis, a 70% reduction in RDS was seen among babies born between 24 hours and 7 days after corticosteroid administration. In addition, evidence suggests reductions in mortality and RDS even with treatment started less than 24 hours before delivery. Although most babies in the trials were between 30 and 34 weeks' gestation, clear reduction in RDS was evident when the population of babies less than 31 weeks was examined, and given the impact on neonatal morbidity and mortality, **prenatal steroid use can be recommended in pregnancies as early as 23 weeks' gestation.**[6]

Gender and race do not influence the protective effect of corticosteroids. In the population of patients with preterm premature rupture of the membranes (PPROM), antenatal corticosteroids also reduce the frequency of RDS.

Corticosteroids also accelerate maturation of other organs in the developing fetus, including the cardiovascular, gastrointestinal (GI), and central nervous systems. Corticosteroid therapy reduces the chances of periventricular hemorrhage (PVH) and intraventricular hemorrhage (IVH) in addition to necrotizing enterocolitis (NEC).[5] The significant reductions in serious neonatal morbidity are also reflected in a reduction in the risk of early neonatal mortality. The short-term beneficial effects of antenatal corticosteroids are enhanced by reassuring reports about long-term outcome. The children of mothers treated with antenatal corticosteroids show no lag in intellectual or motor development, no increase in learning disabilities or behavioral disturbances, and no effect on growth compared with untreated infants.[7,8]

Since the advent of antenatal steroids for the prevention of RDS, other therapies have been introduced that decrease mortality and morbidity. **Surfactant replacement therapy to treat specifically the surfactant deficiency that is the cause of RDS has been shown to decrease mortality and the severity of RDS.**[9] **The effects of antenatal corticosteroids and postnatal surfactant appear to be additive in terms of decreasing the severity of RDS and the mortality caused by it.**[10]

First Breaths

A critical step in the transition from intrauterine to extrauterine life is the conversion of the lung from a fluid-filled organ to one capable of gas exchange. This requires aeration of the lungs, establishment of an adequate pulmonary circulation, ventilation of the aerated parenchyma, and diffusion of oxygen and carbon dioxide through the alveolar-capillary membranes. This process has its origins in utero as fetal breathing.

Fetal Breathing

Fetal respiratory activity is initially detectable at 11 weeks. The most prevalent pattern is rapid, small-amplitude movements (60 to 90 per minute), which are present 60% to 80% of the time. Less commonly, irregular low-amplitude movements interspersed with slower, larger amplitude movements are seen.[11] Initially, fetal breathing was thought to depend on behavioral influences. However, subsequent work has shown responses to chemical stimuli and other agents. Acute hypercapnea stimulates breathing. Hypoxia abolishes fetal breathing, whereas an increase in oxygen tension to levels above 200 mm Hg induces continuous fetal breathing. Although peripheral and central chemoreflexes—as well as vagal afferent reflexes—can be demonstrated in the fetus, their role in spontaneous fetal breathing appears to be minimal. The role of fetal breathing in the continuum from fetal to neonatal life is still not completely understood. **Fetal respiratory activity is probably essential to the development of chest wall muscles, including the diaphragm, and serves as a regulator of lung fluid volume and thus lung growth.**

The mechanism responsible for the transition from intermittent fetal to continuous neonatal breathing is unknown. Prostaglandins may be involved in addition to other factors that surround birth, including blood gas changes and various sensory stimuli. Another possibility is the "release" from a placental inhibitory factor that is removed after cord occlusion.

Mechanics of the First Breath

With its first breaths, the neonate must overcome several forces that resist lung expansion: (1) viscosity of fetal lung fluid, (2) resistance provided by lung tissue itself, and (3) the forces of surface tension at the air-liquid interface.[12-14] Viscosity of fetal lung fluid is a major factor as the neonate attempts to displace fluid present in the large airways. As the passage of air moves toward small airways and alveoli, surface tension becomes more important. Resistance to expansion by the lung tissue itself is less significant. The process begins as the infant passes through the birth canal; the intrathoracic pressure caused by vaginal squeeze is up to 200 cm H_2O. With delivery of the head, approximately 5 to 28 mL of tracheal fluid is expressed. Subsequent delivery of the thorax causes an elastic recoil of the chest. With this recoil, a small passive inspiration (no more than 2 mL) occurs. This is accompanied by glossopharyngeal forcing of some air into the proximal airways (*frog breathing*) and the introduction of some blood into pulmonary capillaries. This pulmonary vascular pressure may have a role in producing continuous surfaces throughout the small airways of the lung, into which surfactant can deploy.

The initial breath is characteristically a short inspiration, followed by a more prolonged expiration.[13] The initial breath begins with no air volume and no transpulmonary pressure gradient. Considerable negative intrathoracic pressure during inspiration is provided by diaphragmatic contraction and chest wall expansion. An opening pressure of about 25 cm H_2O usually is necessary to overcome surface tension in the smaller airways and alveoli before air begins to enter. The volume of this first breath varies between 30 and 67 mL and correlates with intrathoracic pressure. The expiratory phase is prolonged, because the infant's expiration is opposed by intermittent closure at the pharyngolaryngeal level with the generation of significant positive intrathoracic pressure. This pressure serves to aid both in maintenance of a functional residual capacity (FRC) and with fluid removal from the air sacs. The residual volume after this first breath ranges between 4 and 30 mL, averaging 16 to 20 mL. No major systematic differences are apparent among the first three breaths, which demonstrate similar pressure patterns of decreasing magnitude. The FRC rapidly increases with the first several breaths and then increases more gradually. By 30 minutes of age, most infants attain a normal FRC with uniform lung expansion. **The presence of functional surfactant is instrumental in the accumulation of an FRC.**

In utero, alveoli are open and stable at a nearly neonatal lung volume because they are filled with fetal lung liquid, probably produced by ultrafiltration of pulmonary capillary blood as well as by secretion by alveolar cells. Transepithelial chloride secretion appears to be a major factor responsible for the production of luminal liquid in the fetal lung. **Normal expansion and aeration of the neonatal lung is dependent on removal of fetal lung liquid. Liquid is removed by a combination of mechanical drainage and absorption across the lung epithelium.**[15] **This process begins before a normal term birth because of decreased fluid secretion and increased absorption. Once labor is initiated, a reversal of liquid flow occurs across the lung epithelium.** Active transcellular sodium absorption drives liquid from the lumen to the interstitial space, where it is drained through the pulmonary circulation and lymphatics.[16] In normal circumstances, the process is complete within 2 hours of birth. Cesarean-delivered infants without benefit of labor and premature infants have delayed lung fluid clearance. In both

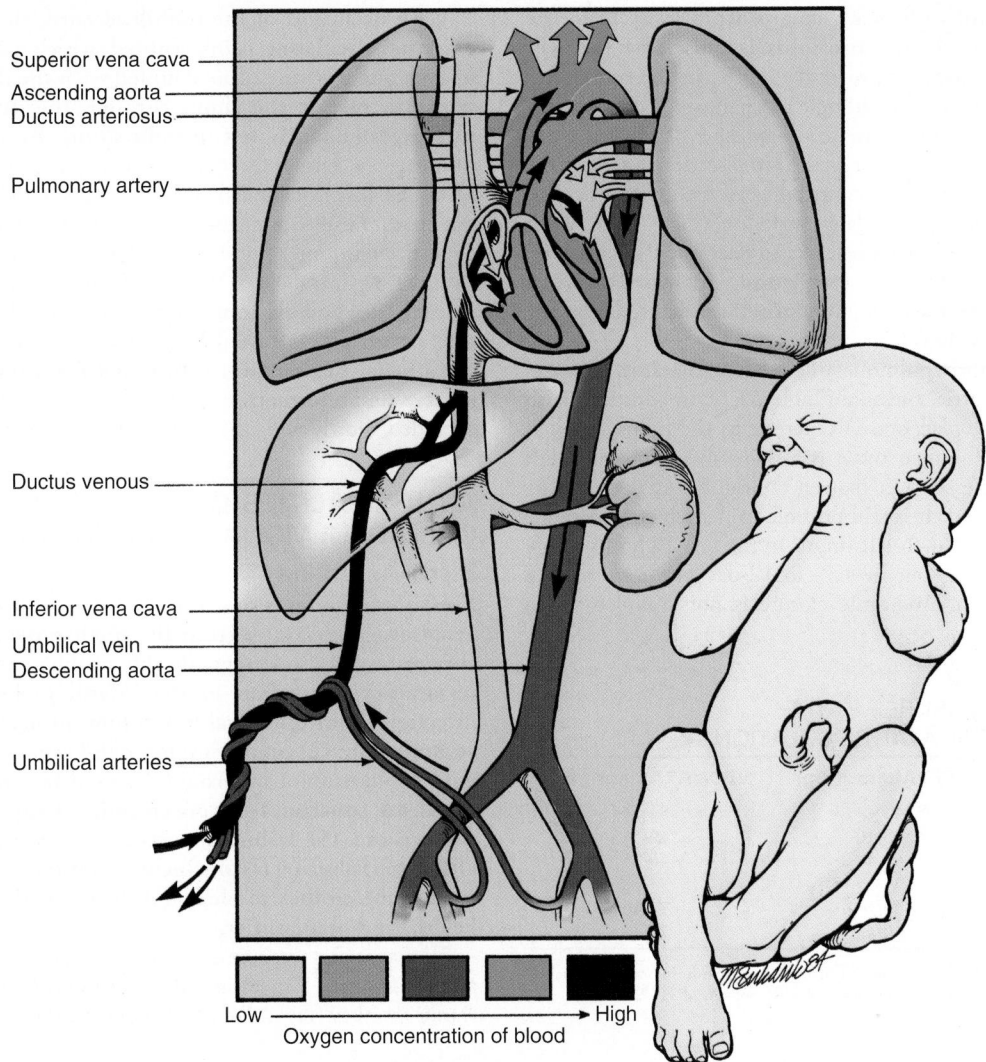

Superior vena cava
Ascending aorta
Ductus arteriosus

Pulmonary artery

Ductus venous

Inferior vena cava
Umbilical vein
Descending aorta

Umbilical arteries

Low ——————————————→ High
Oxygen concentration of blood

FIG 22-5 The fetal circulation.

groups, the prenatal decrease in lung water does not occur. In addition, in the premature neonate, fluid clearance is diminished by increased alveolar surface tension, increased left atrial pressure, and hypoproteinemia.

Circulatory Transition

The circulation in the fetus (Fig. 22-5) **has been studied in a variety of species using several techniques** (see Chapter 2).[17,18] Umbilical venous blood returning from the placenta has a PO_2 of about 30 to 35 mm Hg. Because of the left-shifted fetal hemoglobin-oxyhemoglobin disassociation curve, this corresponds to a saturation of 80% to 90%. About 60% of this blood perfuses the liver, mainly to the middle and left lobes, and it ultimately enters the inferior vena cava (IVC) through the hepatic veins. The remainder (40% in mid-gestation, 20% at term) bypasses the hepatic circulation through the ductus venosus and empties directly into the IVC. Because of streaming in the IVC, the more oxygenated blood from the ductus venosus and left hepatic vein, as it enters the heart, is deflected by the crista dividens through the foramen ovale to the left atrium. The remainder of left atrial blood is the small amount of venous return from the pulmonary circulation. The less oxygenated IVC

blood from the lower body and the renal, mesenteric, and right hepatic veins streams across the tricuspid valve to the right ventricle. Almost all the return from the superior vena cava (SVC) and the coronary sinus passes through the tricuspid valve to the right ventricle, with only 2% to 3% crossing the foramen ovale. In the near-term fetus, the combined ventricular output is about 450 mL/kg/min; two thirds from the right ventricle and one third from the left ventricle. The blood in the left ventricle has a PO_2 of 25 to 28 mm Hg (saturation of 60%) and is distributed to the coronary circulation, brain, head, and upper extremities with the remainder (10% of combined output) passing into the descending aorta. The major portion of the right ventricular output (60% of combined output) is carried by the ductus arteriosus to the descending aorta, with only 7% of combined output going to the lungs. Thus 70% of combined output passes through the descending aorta, with a PO_2 of 20 to 23 mm Hg (saturation of 55%) to supply the abdominal viscera and lower extremities. Forty-five percent of combined output goes through the umbilical arteries to the placenta. **Thus blood of a higher PO_2 supplies the critical coronary and cerebral circulations, and umbilical venous blood is diverted to where oxygenation is critical.**

The diversion of right ventricular output away from the lungs through the ductus arteriosus is caused by the very high pulmonary vascular resistance (PVR) in the fetus. This high PVR is maintained by multiple mechanisms. With advancing gestational age, an increase in the number of small pulmonary vessels occurs that increases the cross-sectional area of the pulmonary vasculature. This contributes to the gradual decline in PVR that begins during later gestation (Fig. 22-6). **With delivery, a variety of factors interact to decrease PVR acutely; these include mechanical ventilation, increased oxygen tension, and the production of endothelium-derived relaxing factor or nitric oxide (NO).**[19]

With the increase in pulmonary flow, left atrial return increases with a rise in left atrial pressure (Table 22-1). In addition, with the removal of the placenta, IVC return to the right atrium is diminished. The foramen ovale is a flap valve, and when left atrial pressure increases over that on the right side, the opening is functionally closed. It is still possible to demonstrate patency with insignificant right-to-left shunts in the first 12 hours of life in a human neonate, but in a 7- to 12-day newborn, such a shunt is rarely seen. Anatomic closure is not complete for a longer time.

TABLE 22-1	PRESSURES IN THE PERINATAL CIRCULATION	
	FETAL (mm Hg)	**NEONATAL (mm Hg)**
Right atrium	4	5
Right ventricle	65/10	40/5
Pulmonary artery	65/40	40/25
Left atrium	3	7
Left ventricle	60/7	70/10
Aorta	60/40	70/45

Modified from Nelson NM. Respiration and circulation after birth. In Smith CA, Nelson NM (eds): *The Physiology of the Newborn Infant,* 4th ed. Springfield, IL: Charles C. Thomas; 1976:117.

With occlusion of the umbilical cord, the low-resistance placental circulation is interrupted, which causes an increase in systemic pressure. This coupled with the decrease in PVR serves to reverse the shunt through the ductus arteriosus to a predominantly left-to-right shunt. By 15 hours of age, shunting in either direction is physiologically insignificant. Although functionally closed by 4 days, the ductus arteriosus is not anatomically occluded for 1 month. The role of an increased oxygen environment and prostaglandin metabolism in ductal closure is well established. **Ductal closure occurs in two phases: constriction and anatomic occlusion. Initially, the muscular wall constricts, followed by permanent closure achieved by endothelial destruction, subintimal proliferation, and connective tissue formation.**[20] The ductus venosus is functionally occluded shortly after the umbilical circulation is interrupted.

ABNORMALITIES OF CARDIOPULMONARY TRANSITION
Birth Asphyxia
Even normal infants may experience some limitation of oxygenation (asphyxia) during the birth process. A variety of circumstances can exaggerate this problem and can result in respiratory depression in the infant, including (1) acute interruption of umbilical blood flow, as occurs during cord compression; (2) premature placental separation; (3) maternal hypotension or hypoxia; (4) any of the above-mentioned problems superimposed on chronic uteroplacental insufficiency; and (5) failure to execute a proper resuscitation. Other contributing factors include anesthetics and analgesics used in the mother, mode and difficulty of delivery, maternal health, and prematurity.

The neonatal response to asphyxia follows a predictable pattern. Dawes[21] investigated the responses of the newborn rhesus monkey (Fig. 22-7). After delivery, the umbilical cord was

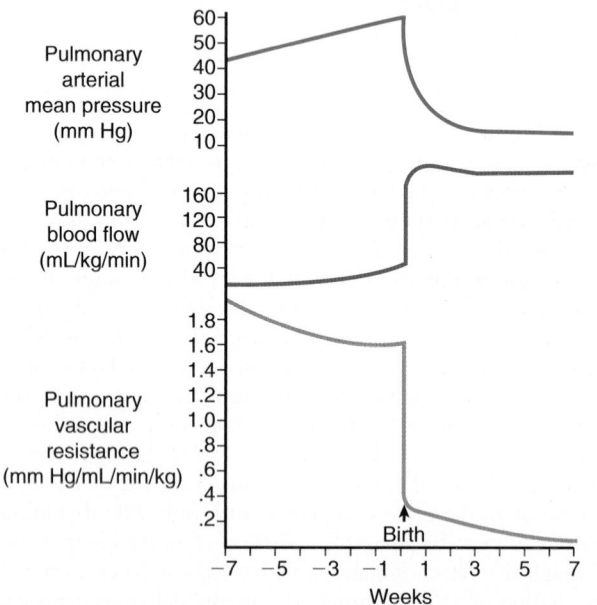

FIG 22-6 Representative changes in pulmonary hemodynamics during transition from the late-term fetal circulation to the neonatal circulation. (Modified from Rudolph AM. Fetal circulation and cardiovascular adjustments after birth. In Rudolph CD, Rudolph AM, Hostetter MK, et al [eds]: *Rudolph's Pediatrics,* 21st ed. New York: McGraw-Hill; 2003:1749.)

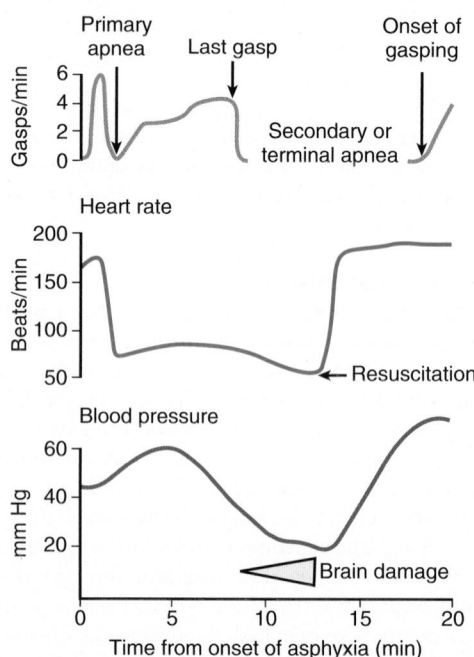

FIG 22-7 Schematic depiction of changes in rhesus monkeys during asphyxia and on resuscitation by positive-pressure ventilation. (Modified from Dawes GS. *Foetal and Neonatal Physiology.* Chicago: Year Book; 1968.)

tied, and the monkey's head was placed in a saline-filled plastic bag. Within about 30 seconds, a short series of respiratory efforts began. These were interrupted by a convulsion or a series of clonic movements accompanied by an abrupt fall in heart rate. The animal then lay inert with no muscle tone. Skin color became progressively cyanotic and then blotchy because of vasoconstriction in an effort to maintain systemic blood pressure. This initial period of apnea lasted about 30 to 60 seconds. The monkey then began to gasp at a rate of three to six breaths per minute. The gasping lasted for about 8 minutes, becoming weaker terminally. The time from onset of asphyxia to last gasp could be related to postnatal age and maturity at birth; the more immature the animal, the longer the time. Secondary or terminal apnea followed, and if resuscitation was not quickly initiated, death ensued. As the animal progressed through the phase of gasping and then on to terminal apnea, heart rate and blood pressure continued to fall, which indicated hypoxic depression of myocardial function. As the heart failed, blood flow to critical organs decreased and resulted in organ injury.

The response to resuscitation is qualitatively similar in many species, including humans. During the first period of apnea, almost any physical or chemical stimulus causes the animal to breathe. If gasping has already ceased, the first sign of recovery with initiation of positive-pressure ventilation is an increase in heart rate. The blood pressure then rises, rapidly if the last gasp has only just passed, but more slowly if the duration of asphyxia has been longer. The skin then becomes pink, and gasping ensues. Rhythmic spontaneous respiratory efforts become established after a further interval. For each minute past the last gasp, 2 minutes of positive-pressure breathing is required before gasping begins, and it takes 4 minutes to reach rhythmic breathing. Later, the spinal and corneal reflexes return. Muscle tone gradually improves over the course of several hours.

Delivery Room Management of the Newborn

A number of situations during pregnancy, labor, and delivery place the infant at increased risk for asphyxia: (1) maternal diseases, such as diabetes mellitus and hypertension, in addition to third-trimester bleeding and prolonged rupture of membranes; (2) fetal conditions, such as prematurity, multiple gestation, growth restriction, fetal anomalies, and rhesus isoimmunization; and (3) conditions related to labor and delivery, including fetal distress, meconium staining, breech presentation, and administration of anesthetics and analgesics.

When an asphyxiated infant is expected, a resuscitation team should be in the delivery room. The team should comprise at least two people, one to manage the airway and one to monitor heart rate and provide whatever assistance is needed. The necessary equipment for an adequate resuscitation is listed in Table 22-2. The equipment should be checked regularly and should be in a continuous state of readiness. **The steps in the resuscitation process[22] are outlined in the algorithm in** Figure 22-8. **Some key points of the algorithm follow.**

1. Do not allow the infant to become hyperthermic under the warmer.
2. The best criteria to use for assessing the infant's condition are respiratory effort—whether it is apneic, gasping, or regular—and heart rate (>100 or <100; Table 22-3).
3. **Most neonates can be effectively resuscitated with a bag and face mask.** The proper bagging devices are pictured in Figure 22-9. In addition, a T-piece resuscitator can be used.

TABLE 22-2   EQUIPMENT FOR NEONATAL RESUSCITATION

CLINICAL NEEDS	EQUIPMENT
Thermoregulation	Radiant heat source with platform, mattress covered with warm sterile blankets, servo control heating, temperature probe
Airway management	Suction: Bulb suction, meconium aspirator, wall vacuum suction with sterile catheters
	Ventilation: Manual infant resuscitation bag connected to a pressure manometer capable of delivering 100% oxygen, appropriate masks for term and preterm infants, oral airways, stethoscope, gloves, compressed air source with oxygen blender, pulse oximeters, and probe (optional)
	Intubation: Neonatal laryngoscope with #0 and #1 blades; extra bulbs and batteries; endotracheal tubes 2.5, 3.0, 3.5, and 4.0 mm OD with stylet; scissors and tape; and end-tidal CO_2 detection device
Gastric decompression	Nasogastric tube, 8 Fr with 20-mL syringe
Administration of drugs/volume	Sterile gloves and sterile umbilical catheterization tray with scalpel or scissors, antiseptic prep solution, umbilical tape, three-way stopcock, umbilical catheters (3.5 and 5 Fr), volume expanders (normal saline), drug box with appropriate neonatal vials and dilutions (see Table 22-5), sterile syringes and needles
Transport	Warmed transport isolette with an oxygen source

TABLE 22-3   THE APGAR SCORING SYSTEM

SIGN	0	1	2
Heart rate	Absent	<100 beats/min	>100 beats/min
Respiratory effort	Apneic	Weak, irregular gasping	Regular
Reflex irritability*	No response	Some response	Facial grimace, sneeze, cough
Muscle tone	Flaccid	Some flexion of arms and legs	Good flexion
Color	Blue, pale hands and blue feet	Body pink	Pink

Modified from Apgar V. A proposal for a new method of evaluation of the newborn infant. *Anesth Analg.* 1953;32:260.
*Elicited by suctioning the oropharynx and nose.

For the initial inflations, pressures of 30 to 40 cm H_2O may be necessary to overcome surface active forces in the lungs. Adequacy of ventilation is assessed by observing expansion of the infant's chest with bagging and watching for a gradual improvement in color, perfusion, and heart rate. Rate of bagging should be 40 to 60 beats/min. If the infant does not initially respond to bag and mask ventilation, try to reposition the head in slight extension, reapply the mask to achieve a good seal, consider suctioning the mouth and oropharynx, and try ventilating with the mouth open. It may be necessary to increase the pressure used. However, if no favorable response is seen in 30 to 40 seconds, proceed to intubation (Fig. 22-10).

4. Failure to respond to intubation and ventilation can result from mechanical causes or severe asphyxia. The mechanical causes listed in Table 22-4 should quickly be ruled out.
5. It is very unusual for a neonatal resuscitation to require either cardiac massage or drugs, and almost all newborns respond to ventilation with supplemental oxygen. If compressions are

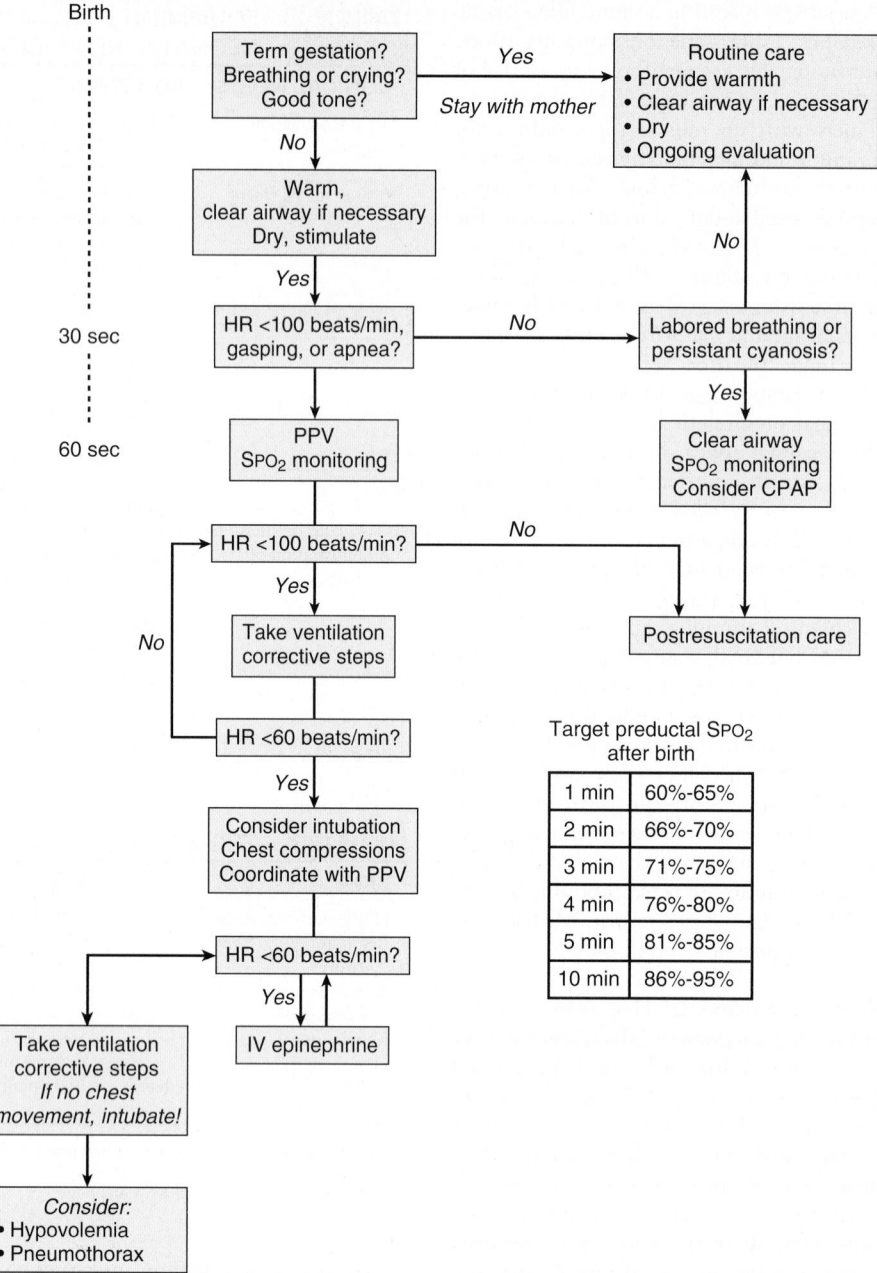

FIG 22-8 Delivery room management of the newborn. CPAP, continuous positive airway pressure; HR, heart rate; IV, intravenous; PPV, positive pressure ventilation; SPO2, peripheral capillary oxygen saturation. (From the American Heart Association and American Academy of Pediatrics. *Neonatal Resuscitation Textbook*, Elk Grove, IL; 2011.)

TABLE 22-4 MECHANICAL CAUSES OF FAILED RESUSCITATION

CATEGORY	EXAMPLES
Equipment failure	Malfunctioning bag, oxygen not connected or running
Endotracheal tube malposition	Esophagus, right mainstem bronchus
Occluded endotracheal tube	
Insufficient inflation pressure to expand lungs	
Space-occupying lesions in the thorax	Pneumothorax, pleural effusions, diaphragmatic hernia
Pulmonary hypoplasia	Extreme prematurity, oligohydramnios

required, they need to be coordinated with bagging at a 3 : 1 ratio (90 compressions to 30 breaths/min). It is even less common to need medications (Table 22-5). The optimal delivery route is through an umbilical venous line.

6. The appropriateness of continued resuscitative efforts should always be reevaluated in an infant who fails to respond to all of the previously mentioned efforts. Today, resuscitative efforts are made even in "apparent stillbirths," that is, infants whose 1-min Apgar scores are 0 to 1. However, efforts should not be sustained in the face of little or no improvement despite an appropriate resuscitation over a reasonable period of time (i.e., 10 to 15 minutes).[22]

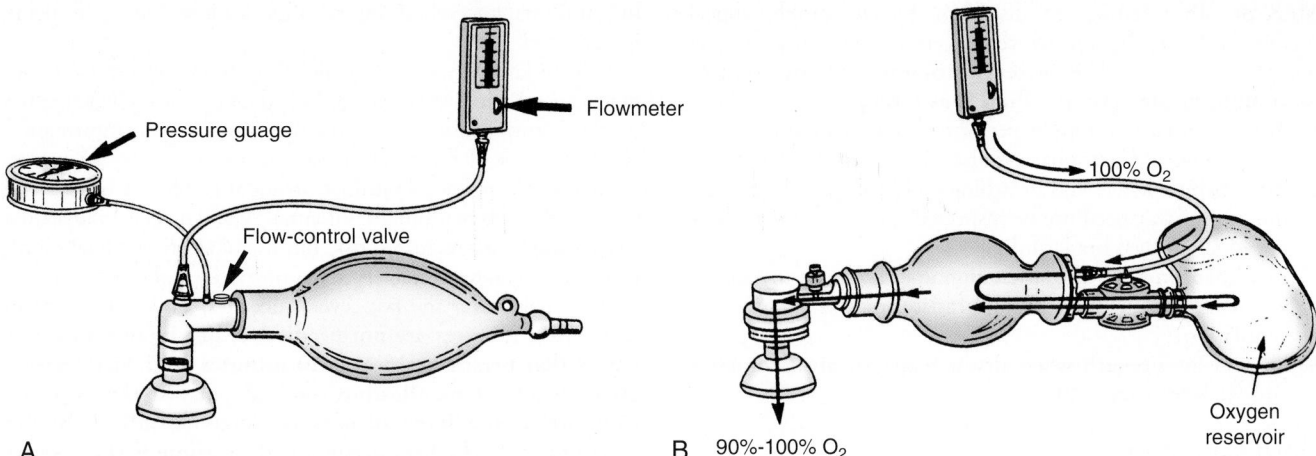

FIG 22-9 Bags used for neonatal resuscitation. **A,** A flow-inflating bag with a pressure manometer and flow-control valve. **B,** A self-inflating bag with an oxygen reservoir to maintain 90% to 100% oxygen. (From the American Heart Association and American Academy of Pediatrics. *Neonatal Resuscitation Textbook,* Elk Grove, IL; 2000.)

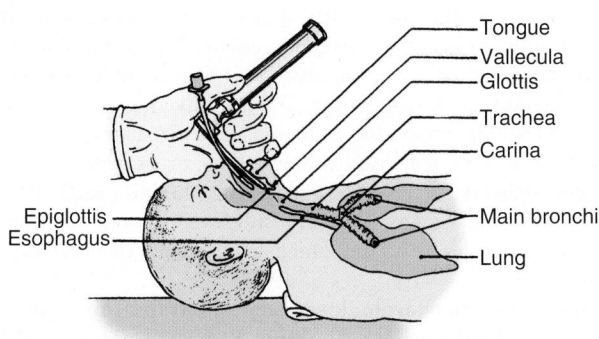

FIG 22-10 Anatomy of laryngoscopy for endotracheal intubation. (From the American Heart Association and American Academy of Pediatrics. *Neonatal Resuscitation Textbook,* Elk Grove, IL 2000.)

TABLE 22-5	NEONATAL DRUG DOSES		
DRUG	**DOSE**	**ROUTE**	**HOW SUPPLIED**
Epinephrine	0.1 to 0.3 mL/kg	IV or ET	1:10,000 dilution
Sodium bicarbonate*	1 to 2 mEq/kg	IV	0.5 mEq/mL (4.2% solution)
Normal saline, whole blood†	10 mL/kg	IV	
Naloxone‡	0.1 mg/kg	IV, ET	1 mg/mL IM, SC¶

Modified from the American Heart Association and American Academy of Pediatrics. *Neonatal Resuscitation Textbook.* American Heart Association and American Academy of Pediatrics; 2006.
*For correction of metabolic acidosis only after adequate ventilation has been achieved; give slowly over several minutes. There is no evidence to support routine use.
†Infuse slowly over 5 to 10 minutes.
¶Insufficient evidence to support safety and efficacy of subcutaneous dose.
‡Use after proceeding with proper airway management and other resuscitative techniques.
ET, endotracheal; *IM,* intramuscular; *IV,* intravenous; *SC,* subcutaneous.

Resuscitation of term newborns should begin with room air because of the potential harmful effects of 100% oxygen, in particular the generation of oxygen free radicals.[23,24] Oxygen should be used and titrated to achieve normal saturations for age in minutes (see Fig. 22-8).[22] If resuscitation is started with room air and no improvement is seen, supplemental oxygen can be given. **Normal healthy term infants require approximately 10 to 15 minutes to achieve oxygen saturations above 90%.**[25]

A few special circumstances merit discussion at this point. Infants in whom respiratory depression secondary to narcotic administration is suspected may be given naloxone, although evidence to support efficacy is limited. However, this should not be done until the airway has been managed and the infant is resuscitated in the usual fashion. In addition, naloxone should not be given to the infant of an addicted mother because it will precipitate withdrawal.

A second special group are the **preterm infants**. Minimizing heat loss improves survival, so prewarmed towels should be available, and the environmental temperature of the delivery suite should be raised. The infant should be placed in a plastic covering after birth to minimize evaporative heat loss.[26] In the infant with an extremely low birthweight (<1000 g), proceed quickly to administration of continuous positive airway pressure (CPAP) and consider early intubation for surfactant administration. Volume expanders should be infused slowly to avoid rapid swings in blood pressure. Resuscitation in preterm infants should begin with 21% to 30% oxygen.[24,27]

A third special circumstance is the presence of **meconium-stained amniotic fluid**. Meconium aspiration syndrome (MAS) is a form of aspiration pneumonia that occurs most often in term or postterm infants who have passed meconium in utero (7% to 20% of all deliveries).[28] **Overall, 2% to 9% of children born through meconium-stained fluid are diagnosed with MAS.**[28] Delivery room management of meconium in the amniotic fluid has been historically based on the notion that aspiration takes place with the initiation of extrauterine respiration and that the pathologic condition is related to the aspirated contents, which resulted in the practice of oropharyngeal suction on the perineum after delivery of the head, followed by airway visualization and suction by the resuscitator after delivery. However, both of the foregoing assumptions are not entirely true. In utero aspiration has been induced in animal models and confirmed in autopsies of human stillbirths. In addition, the combined suction approach has not been uniformly successful in decreasing the incidence of MAS. These data have been confirmed by a large multicenter, prospective, randomized controlled trial (RCT) that assessed selective intubation of apparently vigorous meconium-stained infants.[29] Compared with expectant management, intubation and tracheal suction did not result in a decreased incidence of

MAS or other respiratory disorders. Finally, oropharyngeal suction on the perineum before delivery of the shoulders does not prevent MAS.[30] **The current recommended approach to meconium in the amniotic fluid is as follows:**

1. The obstetrician carefully performs bulb suctioning of the oropharynx and nasopharynx after delivery of the baby.
2. If the baby is active and breathing and requires no resuscitation, the airway need not be inspected, thus avoiding the risk of inducing vagal bradycardia.
3. Any infant in need of resuscitation does not need the airway inspected and suctioned before instituting positive-pressure ventilation.
4. Suction the stomach when airway management is complete and vital signs are stable.

Cord Clamping

Although delayed cord clamping is not currently part of the Neonatal Resuscitation Program (NRP), the practice is now recommended for both term and preterm births. Historically, clamping and cutting of the umbilical cord took place within seconds; however, it has been found that delaying this separation of the newborn from the placental circulation for 30 to 60 seconds results in (1) a more gradual perinatal transition after birth, (2) transfusion of placental blood to the newborn, and (3) a variety of improved outcomes, in particular, for preterm newborns.[31-33] This practice is now endorsed for preterm births by the American College of Obstetricians and Gynecologists (ACOG), although specific patient populations and situations require further study.[33]

Sequelae of Birth Asphyxia

The incidence of birth asphyxia is about 0.1% in term infants, with an increased incidence in infants at lower gestational ages.[34] The acute sequelae that need to be managed in the neonatal period are listed in Table 22-6**.** With asphyxia, widespread organ injury is evident. Management focuses on supportive care and treatment of specific abnormalities; this includes careful fluid management, blood pressure support, intravenous (IV) glucose, and treatment of seizures. Phenobarbital (40 mg/kg) given 1 to 6 hours after the event as neuroprotective therapy is associated with an improved neurologic outcome. **Especially if started within the first 6 hours of life, hypothermia (whole body or selective head cooling) improves outcomes at 6 to 7 years of age.[35-37]** The roles of oxygen free-radical scavengers, excitatory amino acid antagonists, and calcium channel blockers in minimizing cerebral injury after asphyxia are still being investigated.

If the infant survives, the major long-term concern is permanent central nervous system (CNS) damage. The challenge lies in the identification of criteria that can provide information about the risk of future problems for a given infant. A variety of markers have been examined to identify birth asphyxia and risk for adverse neurologic outcome. Marked fetal bradycardia is associated with increased risk, but use of electronic fetal monitoring and cesarean delivery have not altered the incidence of cerebral palsy over the last several decades. **Low Apgar scores at 1 and 5 minutes are not predictive, but infants with low scores that persist at 15 and 20 minutes after birth have a 50% chance of manifesting cerebral palsy if they survive. Cord pH is predictive of adverse outcome only if the pH is less than 7. The best predictor of outcome is the severity of the neonatal neurologic syndrome.[38]** Infants with mild encephalopathy survive and are normal on follow-up examination. Moderate encephalopathy carries a 25% to 50% risk of severe handicap or death, whereas the severe syndrome carries a greater than 75% risk of death or disability. Although outcomes are improved with hypothermia initiated in the first 6 hours of life, these patients remain at high risk for poor neurodevelopment.[35-37] Diagnostic aids that include electroencephalograms and magnetic resonance imaging (MRI) scans can also aid in predicting outcome. The circulatory response to hypoxia is to redistribute blood flow to provide adequate oxygen delivery to critical organs (e.g., brain, heart) at the expense of other organs. Thus an insult severe enough to damage the brain should be accompanied by evidence of other organ dysfunction.

The long-term neurologic sequelae of intrapartum asphyxia are cerebral palsy with or without associated cognitive deficits and epilepsy. Although cerebral palsy can be related to intrapartum events, the large majority of cases are of unknown causes. Furthermore, cognitive deficits and epilepsy, unless associated with cerebral palsy, cannot be related to asphyxia or to other intrapartum events. **To attribute cerebral palsy to peripartum asphyxia, there must be an absence of other demonstrable causes, substantial or prolonged intrapartum asphyxia (fetal heart rate abnormalities, fetal acidosis), and clinical evidence during the first days of life of neurologic dysfunction in the infant** (Box 22-1).[39]

BIRTH INJURIES

Birth injuries are those sustained during labor and delivery. **Factors that predispose to birth injury include macrosomia, cephalopelvic disproportion, shoulder dystocia, prolonged or difficult labor, precipitous delivery, abnormal presentations (including breech), and use of operative vaginal delivery.**[40] Injuries range from minor, requiring no therapy, to life threatening (Table 22-7).

Soft tissue injuries are most common. Most are related to dystocia and to the use of operative vaginal delivery. Accidental lacerations of the scalp, buttocks, and thighs may be inflicted with the scalpel during cesarean delivery. Cumulatively, these injuries are of a minor nature and respond well to therapy. Hyperbilirubinemia, particularly in the premature infant, is the major neonatal complication related to soft tissue bruising.

A **cephalohematoma** occurs in 0.2% to 2.5% of live births. Caused by rupture of blood vessels that traverse from the skull

TABLE 22-6	ACUTE SEQUELAE OF ASPHYXIA
SYSTEM	**MANIFESTATIONS**
Central nervous	Cerebral edema, seizures, hemorrhage, hypoxic-ischemic encephalopathy
Cardiac	Papillary muscle necrosis, transient tricuspid insufficiency, cardiogenic shock
Pulmonary	Aspiration syndromes (meconium, clear fluid), acquired surfactant deficiency, persistent pulmonary hypertension, pulmonary hemorrhage
Renal	Acute tubular necrosis with anuria or oliguria
Adrenal	Hemorrhage with adrenal insufficiency
Hepatic	Enzyme elevations, liver failure
Gastrointestinal	Necrotizing enterocolitis, feeding intolerance
Metabolic	Hypoglycemia, hypocalcemia
Hematologic	Coagulation disorders, thrombocytopenia

BOX 22-1   RELATIONSHIP OF INTRAPARTUM EVENTS AND CEREBRAL PALSY

Neonatal Signs Consistent With an Acute Peripartum or Intrapartum Event

- Evidence of a metabolic acidemia in fetal umbilical cord arterial blood obtained at delivery (pH <7.00 and base deficit ≥12 mmol/L)
- Apgar score of less than 5 at 5 and 10 min
- Neuroimaging evidence of acute brain injury seen on brain magnetic resonance imaging or magnetic resonance spectroscopy consistent with hypoxia-ischemia
- Presence of multisystem organ failure consistent with hypoxic-ischemic encephalopathy

Type and Timing of Contributing Factors Consistent With an Acute Peripartum or Intrapartum Event

- Sentinel hypoxic or ischemic event occurring immediately before or during labor and delivery such as a severe placental abruption
- Fetal heart rate monitor patterns consistent with an acute peripartum or intrapartum event
- Timing and type of brain injury patterns based on imaging studies consistent with an etiology of an acute peripartum or intrapartum event
- No evidence of other proximal or distal factors that could be contributing factors

Developmental Outcome Is Spastic Quadriplegia or Dyskinetic Cerebral Palsy

Modified from American College of Obstetricians and Gynecologists (ACOG), American Academy of Pediatrics (AAP). Neonatal Encephalopathy and Neurologic Outcome. Washington DC: ACOG; 2014.

TABLE 22-7   BIRTH INJURIES

CLASSIFICATION	EXAMPLE
Soft tissue injuries*	Lacerations, abrasions, fat necrosis
Extracranial bleeding	Cephalohematoma,* subgaleal bleed
Intracranial hemorrhage	Subarachnoid, subdural, epidural, cerebral, cerebellar
Nerve injuries	Facial nerve,* cervical nerve roots (brachial plexus palsies,* phrenic nerve, Horner syndrome), recurrent laryngeal nerve (vocal cord paralysis)
Fractures	Clavicle,* facial bones, humerus, femur, skull, nasal bones
Dislocations	Extremities, nasal septum
Eye injuries	Subconjunctival* and retinal hemorrhages, orbital fracture, corneal laceration, breaks in Descemet membrane with corneal opacification
Torticollis†	
Spinal cord injuries	
Visceral rupture	Liver, spleen
Scalp laceration*	Fetal scalp electrode, scalpel
Scalp abscess	Fetal scalp electrode

*More common occurrences.
†Secondary to hemorrhage into the sternocleidomastoid muscle.

to the periosteum, the bleeding is subperiosteal and is therefore limited by suture lines; the most common site of bleeding is over the parietal bones. Associations include prolonged or difficult labor and mechanical trauma from operative vaginal delivery. Linear skull fractures beneath the hematoma have been reported

in 5.4% of cases but are of no major consequence except in the unlikely event that a leptomeningeal cyst develops. Most cephalohematomas are reabsorbed in 2 weeks to 3 months. **Subgaleal bleeds**, which are not limited by suture lines, can occur in association with vacuum extraction alone—especially with multiple pop-offs and prolonged traction—in combination with the use of forceps or with difficult forceps deliveries, and they can result in life-threatening anemia, hypotension, or consumptive coagulopathy. Depressed skull fractures are also seen in neonates, but most do not require surgical elevations.

Intracranial hemorrhages related to trauma include epidural, subdural, subarachnoid, and intraparenchymal bleeds.[41] With improvements in obstetric care, subdural hemorrhages fortunately are now rare. Three major varieties of **subdural bleeds** have been described: (1) posterior fossa hematomas due to tentorial laceration with rupture of the straight sinus, vein of Galen, or transverse sinus or due to occipital osteodiastasis (a separation between the squamous and lateral portions of the occipital bone); (2) falx laceration, with rupture of the inferior sagittal sinus; and (3) rupture of the superficial cerebral veins. The clinical symptoms are related to the location of bleeding. With tentorial laceration, bleeding is infratentorial, leading to brainstem signs and a rapid progression to death. Falx tears cause bilateral cerebral signs (e.g., seizures and focal weakness) until blood extends infratentorially to the brainstem. Subdural hemorrhage over the cerebral convexities can cause several clinical states that range from an asymptomatic newborn to one with seizures and focal neurologic findings. Infants with lacerations of the tentorium and falx have a poor outlook. In contrast, the prognosis for rupture of the superficial cerebral veins is much better, and the majority of survivors are normal. **Primary subarachnoid hemorrhage is the most common variety of neonatal intracranial hemorrhage.**[41] Clinically, these infants are often asymptomatic, although they may present with a characteristic seizure pattern that begins on day 2 of life, and the infants are "well" between convulsions. In general, the prognosis for subarachnoid bleeds is good.

Trauma to peripheral nerves produces another major group of birth injuries. **Brachial plexus injuries are caused by stretching of the cervical roots during delivery, usually when shoulder dystocia is present. Upper arm palsy (Erb-Duchenne paralysis), the most common brachial plexus injury, is caused by injury to the fifth and sixth cervical nerves; lower arm paralysis (Klumpke paralysis) results from damage to the eighth cervical and first thoracic nerves. Damage to all four nerve roots produces paralysis of the entire arm.** Outcome for these injuries is variable, and some infants are left with significant residual damage. Horner syndrome as a result of damage to sympathetic outflow through nerve root T1 may accompany Klumpke paralysis, and approximately 5% of patients with Erb paralysis have an associated phrenic nerve paresis. Facial palsy is another fairly common injury caused either by pressure from the sacral promontory or fetal shoulder as the infant passes through the birth canal or by operative vaginal delivery. Most of these palsies resolve, although in some infants, paralysis is persistent.

The majority of bone fractures that result from birth trauma involve the clavicle and result from shoulder dystocia or breech extractions that require vigorous manipulations. Clinically, many of these fractures are asymptomatic, and when present, symptoms are mild. Prognosis for both clavicular and limb fractures is uniformly good. The most commonly fractured long bone is the humerus.

Spinal cord injuries are a relatively infrequent but often severe form of birth injury. Accurate incidence is difficult to assess, because symptoms mimic other neonatal diseases and autopsies often do not include a careful examination of the spine. Depressed tone, hyporeflexia, and respiratory failure are clues to this diagnosis. Excessive longitudinal traction and head rotation during forceps delivery predispose to spinal injury, and hyperextension of the head in a footling breech is particularly dangerous. Outcomes include death or stillbirth caused by high cervical or brainstem lesions, long-term survival of infants with paralysis from birth, and minimal neurologic symptoms or spasticity.

NEONATAL THERMAL REGULATION

Physiology

The range of environmental temperatures over which the neonate can survive is narrower than that of an adult as a result of the infant's inability to dissipate heat effectively in warm environments and, more critically, to maintain temperature in response to cold. This range narrows with decreasing gestational age.

Although some increases in activity and shivering have been observed, **nonshivering thermogenesis is the most important means of increased heat production in the cold-stressed newborn.**[42] It can be defined as an increase in total heat production without detectable (visible or electrical) muscle activity. The site of this increased heat production is brown fat located between the scapulae; around the muscles and blood vessels of the neck, axillae, and mediastinum; between the esophagus and trachea; and around the kidneys and adrenal glands. Brown fat cells contain more mitochondria and fat vacuoles and have a richer blood and sympathetic nerve supply compared with white fat cells.

Heat loss to the environment is dependent on both an *internal temperature gradient*, from within the body to the surface, and an *external temperature gradient*, from the surface to the environment. The infant can change the *internal gradient* by altering vasomotor tone and, to a lesser extent, by postural changes that decrease the amount of exposed surface area. The *external gradient* is dependent on purely physical variables. **Heat transfer from the surface to the environment involves four routes: radiation, convection, conduction, and evaporation.** *Radiant heat loss,* heat transfer from a warmer to a cooler object that is not in contact, depends on the temperature gradient between the objects. Heat loss by *convection* to the surrounding gaseous environment depends on air speed and temperature. *Conduction,* heat loss to a contacting cooler object, is minimal in most circumstances. Heat loss by *evaporation* is cooling secondary to water loss at the rate of 0.6 cal/g water evaporated and is affected by relative humidity, air speed, exposed surface area, and skin permeability. In infants in excessively warm environments, such as those under overhead radiant heat sources, or in very immature infants with thin, permeable skin, evaporative losses increase considerably. Table 22-8 summarizes the neonate's efforts to maintain a stable core temperature in the face of cold or heat stress. It is advantageous to maintain an infant in a neutral thermal environment (Fig. 22-11). The neutral thermal environment for a given infant depends on size, gestational age, and postnatal age.[43] **In general, maintaining the abdominal skin temperature at 36.5° C minimizes energy expenditure.**

TABLE 22-8	NEONATAL RESPONSE TO THERMAL STRESS		
STRESSOR	**RESPONSE**	**TERM**	**PRETERM**
Cold	Vasoconstriction	++	++
	↓Exposed surface area (posture change)	±	±
	↑Oxygen consumption	++	+
	↑Motor activity, shivering	+	−
Heat	Vasodilation	++	++
	Sweating	+	−

++, Maximum response; +, intermediate; ±, may have a role; −, no response.

CLINICAL APPLICATIONS

Delivery Room

In utero, fetal thermoregulation is the responsibility of the placenta and is dependent on maternal core temperature; fetal temperature is 0.5° C higher than maternal temperature. At birth, the infant's core temperature drops rapidly from 37.8° C because of evaporation from its wet body and radiant and convective losses to the cold air and walls of the room. Even with an increase in oxygen consumption to the maximum capability of the newborn (15 mL/kg/min), the infant can produce only 0.075 cal/kg/min and will rapidly lose heat. **Measures taken to reduce heat loss after birth depend on the clinical situation. For the well term infant, drying the skin and wrapping the baby with warm blankets is sufficient. When it is necessary to leave an infant exposed for close observation or resuscitation, the infant should be dried and placed under a radiant heat source. Room temperature can be elevated as an added precaution for the low-birthweight infant.**

Nursery

Babies are cared for in the newborn nursery wrapped in blankets in bassinets (cot-nursed), in isolettes, or under a radiant heat source. Healthy full-term infants (>2.5 kg) need only be clothed and placed in a bassinet under a blanket. Infants weighing 2 to 2.5 kg who are either slightly premature or growth restricted should be allowed 12 to 24 hours to stabilize in an isolette and should then be advanced to a bassinet. Lower-birthweight babies (<2 kg) will require care in either isolettes or under radiant heat sources. **Adequate thermal protection of the low-birthweight (LBW) infant is essential. This is especially important for the very-low-birthweight (VLBW) infant (<1.5 kg), who often does not behave like a mature homeotherm.** These neonates can react to a small change in environmental temperature with a change in body temperature rather than a change in oxygen consumption. In addition, warmer environments hasten growth of the premature infant.

The isolette, which heats by convection, is the most commonly used heating device for the LBW nude infant. The major source of heat loss while in a neutral thermal environment is radiant to the walls of the isolette. The magnitude of this loss is predictable if room temperature is known, and losses can be minimized using double-walled isolettes in which the inner wall temperature is very close to the air temperature within the isolette. Once clinical status has been stabilized, the infant can be dressed, which will afford increased thermal stability.

Radiant warmers can also be used to ensure thermal stability of both LBW and full-sized infants. Radiant warmers are used most effectively for short-term warming during initial

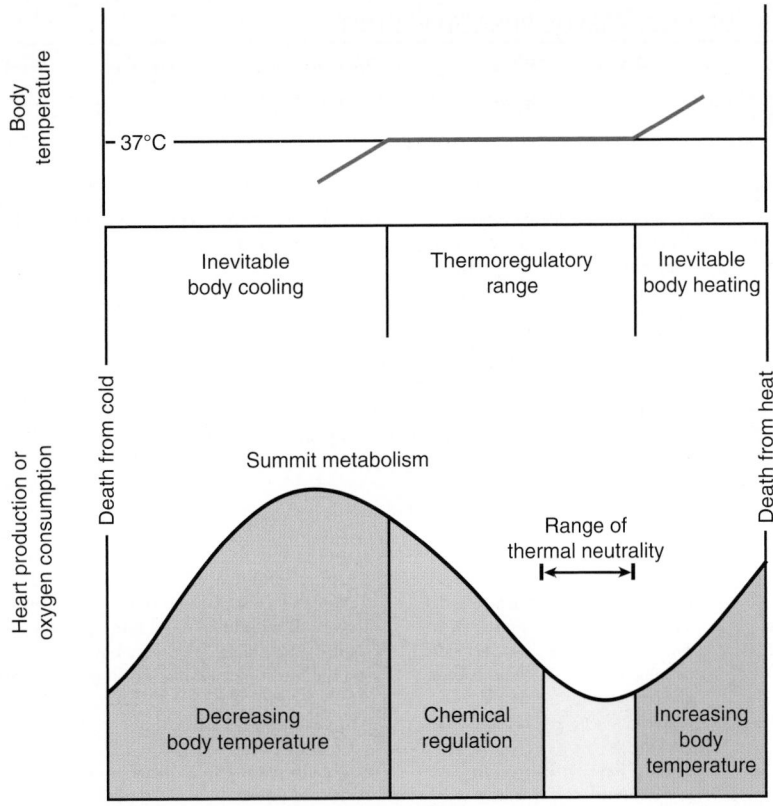

FIG 22-11 Effect of environmental temperature on oxygen consumption and body temperature. (Modified from Klaus MH, Fanaroff AA. The physical environment. In Klaus MH, Fanaroff AA [eds]: *Care of the High-Risk Neonate,* 5th ed. Philadelphia: WB Saunders; 2001:130.)

resuscitation and stabilization and for performing procedures. They provide easy access to the infant while ensuring thermal stability. The main heat losses are convection, which can be significant because of variable air speed in a room, and evaporation. **Evaporative heat loss that results in significant fluid losses is a major concern for the VLBW premature infant cared for under a radiant warmer.** Placing a plastic shield over the infant or covering the skin with a semipermeable membrane can minimize these fluid losses.

The most economical means of thermal support for the LBW infant is skin-to-skin contact with a parent.[44]

NEONATAL NUTRITION AND GASTROENTEROLOGY

At birth, the newborn infant must assume various functions performed by the placenta during fetal life. Cardiopulmonary transition and thermoregulation have already been discussed. The final critical task for the newborn is the assimilation of calories, water, and electrolytes.

Infant Feeding

For the well term or slightly preterm infant, institution of oral feedings within the first 2 to 4 hours of life is reasonable practice. For infants who are small for gestational age (SGA) or large for gestational age (LGA), earlier feedings may be indicated to avoid hypoglycemia. Premature infants (<34 weeks' gestation) who are unable to nipple feed present a more complex set of circumstances. In addition to an inability to suck and swallow

efficiently, such infants face a number of problems: (1) relatively high caloric demand; (2) small stomach capacity; (3) incompetent esophageal-cardiac sphincter that leads to gastroesophageal reflux; (4) poor gag reflex, which creates a tendency for aspiration; (5) decreased digestive capability, especially for fat; and (6) slow gastric emptying and intestinal motility. These infants can initially be supported adequately with parenteral nutrition, followed by institution of nasogastric tube feedings when their cardiopulmonary status is stable.

Although a wide range of infant formulas satisfy the nutritional needs of most neonates, breast milk remains the standard on which formulas are based (see Chapter 24). The distribution of calories in human milk is 7% protein, 55% fat, and 38% carbohydrate. The whey/casein ratio is 70:30, which enhances ease of protein digestion and gastric emptying, whereas fat digestion is augmented by the presence of a breast milk lipase. Despite the low levels of several vitamins and minerals, bioavailability is high. **In addition to the nutritional features, breast milk's immunochemical and cellular components provide protection against infection.**[45]

The growth demands of the LBW infant exceed what can be provided by human milk in terms of protein, calcium, phosphorus, sodium, zinc, copper, and possibly other nutrients. These shortcomings can be addressed through the addition of human milk fortifiers to mother's preterm breast milk.[46] Advantages of breast milk for the premature infant include its antiinfective properties, possible protection against NEC, and its role in enhancing neurodevelopmental outcome.[47] The importance of breast milk for the preterm infant has been emphasized with

TABLE 22-9   GUIDELINES FOR SUCCESSFUL BREASTFEEDING

	FIRST 8 HR	8 TO 24 HR	DAY 2	DAY 3	DAY 4	DAY 5	DAY 6 ON
Milk supply	You may be able to express a few drops of milk.		Milk *should* come in between days 2 and 4.			Milk should be in. Breasts may be firm and may leak milk.	Breasts should feel softer after nursing.
Baby's activity	Baby is usually wide awake in the first hour of life and should be put to the breast within 30 min.	Wake up your baby. Babies may not wake up on their own to feed.	Baby should be more cooperative and less sleepy.	Look for early feeding cues such as rooting, lip smacking, and hands to the face.			Baby should appear satisfied after feedings.
Feeding routine	Baby may go into a deep sleep 2 to 4 hours after birth.	Use a chart to write down each feeding time. Feed your baby every 1 to 4 hr or as often as the baby wants to nurse but at least 8 to 12 times a day.				Baby may go one longer interval (up to 5 hr between feeds) in a 24-hour period.	
Breastfeeding	Baby will wake up and be alert and responsive for several more hours after initial sleep.	As long as the mother is comfortable, nurse at both breasts as long as the baby is actively sucking.	Try to nurse on both sides at each feeding, aiming at 10 min per side. Expect some nipple tenderness.	Consider hand expressing or pumping a few drops of milk to soften the nipple if the breast is too firm for the baby to latch on.	Nurse a minimum of 10 to 30 min per side every feeding for the first few weeks of life. Once milk supply is well established, allow baby to finish the first breast before offering the other one.		Mother's nipple tenderness is improving or is gone.
Baby's urine output		Baby must have a minimum of one wet diaper in the first 24 hr.	Baby must have at least one wet diaper every 8 to 11 hr.	You should see an increase in wet diapers (four to six) in 24 hr.	Baby's urine should be light yellow.	Baby should have six to eight wet diapers per day of colorless or light yellow urine.	
Baby's stools		Baby may have a very dark (meconium) stool.	Baby may have a second very dark (meconium) stool.	Baby's stools should be in transition from black green to yellow.		Baby should have three to four yellow, seedy stools a day.	The number of stools may decrease gradually after 4 to 6 weeks.

Courtesy Beth Gabrielski, RN, The Children's Hospital, Denver, Colorado.

the use of donor banked human milk as a bridge until the mother is producing an adequate amount of milk for her infant.[48,49]

Few contraindications to breastfeeding exist. Infants with galactosemia should not ingest lactose-containing milk. Infants with other inborn errors of metabolism such as phenylketonuria may ingest some human milk with close monitoring of the amount. The presence of environmental pollutants has been documented in breast milk, but to date no serious side effects have been reported. Most drugs do not contraindicate breastfeeding, but a few exceptions do exist (see Chapter 8). Transmission of some viral infections via breast milk is a concern as well. Mothers who are human immunodeficiency virus (HIV) positive should not breastfeed if safe and effective alternatives to breast milk are available. The nursery staff must be aware of problems associated with breastfeeding, and lactation consultants should be available to deal with poor infant latch-on, sore nipples, poor milk supply, and excessive hyperbilirubinemia. The obstetrician and pediatrician should serve as a source of knowledge and, most importantly, support. Table 22-9 illustrates what a mother can expect as she breastfeeds her infant.

Neonatal Hypoglycemia

Glucose is a major fetal fuel transported by facilitated diffusion across the placenta. After birth, before an appropriate supply of exogenous calories is provided, the newborn must maintain blood glucose through endogenous sources. Hepatic glycogen stores are almost entirely depleted within the first 12 hours after birth in the healthy term neonate and even more rapidly in the preterm or stressed infant if no other glucose source is available. Fat and protein stores are then used for energy, and glucose levels are maintained by hepatic gluconeogenesis.

In the healthy unstressed neonate, glucose falls over the first 1 to 2 hours after birth, stabilizes at a minimum of about 40 mg/dL, and then rises to 50 to 80 mg/dL by 3 hours of life.[50] *Low glucose* concentrations can be defined as less than 45 mg/dL. Infants at risk for low blood glucose concentrations and in whom glucose should be monitored include preterm infants, SGA infants, hyperinsulinemic infants (infant of a diabetic mother [IDM]), LGA infants, and infants with perinatal stress or asphyxia. As in term babies, blood glucose drops after birth in preterm babies, but they are less able to mount a counterregulatory response. In addition, the presence of respiratory distress, hypothermia, and other factors

BOX 22-2   ETIOLOGIES OF NEONATAL HYPOGLYCEMIA

I. Transient neonatal hypoglycemia
   A. Preterm and IUGR infants
   B. Transient hyperinsulinism (IDM)
   C. Perinatal stress (hypoxia, RDS)
II. Persistent neonatal hypoglycemia
   A. Hyperinsulinism
      1. Potassium-ATP channel
      2. Glucokinase hyperinsulinism
      3. Glutamate dehydrogenase hyperinsulinism
      4. Beckwith-Wiedemann syndrome
   B. Counterregulatory hormone deficiency
      (hypopituitarism)
   C. Inborn errors of metabolism
      1. Glycogenolysis disorders
      2. Gluconeogenesis disorders
      3. Fatty acid oxidation disorders

ATP, adenosine triphosphate; *IDM*, infant of a diabetic mother; *IUGR*, intrauterine growth restriction; *RDS*, respiratory distress syndrome.

can increase glucose demand and exacerbate hypoglycemia. **SGA infants are at risk for hypoglycemia resulting from rapidly utilized glycogen stores and impaired gluconeogenesis and ketogenesis.** Onset of hypoglycemia in SGA and preterm infants usually occurs at 2 to 6 hours of life. Hyperinsulinemia occurs in IDMs and in babies with other rare conditions, including Beckwith-Weidemann syndrome and congenital hyperinsulinism. Onset of hypoglycemia in these infants can be in the first 30 to 60 minutes after birth. In the case of perinatal asphyxia, hypoglycemia is the result of excessive glucose demand and occasionally transient hyperinsulinism.[51,52] Infants with recurrent hypoglycemia over 3 to 4 days should be evaluated for endocrine disorders (hyperinsulinism, decreased counterregulatory hormones—cortisol, growth hormone, and glucagon) and inborn errors of metabolism (Box 22-2).

Symptoms of hypoglycemia include jitteriness, seizures, cyanosis, respiratory distress, apathy, hypotonia, and eye rolling.[50] However, many infants, particularly premature infants, are asymptomatic. **Because of the risk of subsequent brain injury, hypoglycemia should be aggressively treated. However, the single best treatment is prevention by identifying infants at risk, including premature, SGA, IDM, LGA, and stressed infants.** These newborns should have blood glucose screened with a bedside glucose meter. All values less than or equal to 45 mg/dL should be confirmed with a laboratory measurement. Treatment is initiated by early institution of feedings or an IV glucose bolus (2 mL/kg of $D_{10}W$ solution) followed by a glucose infusion at a rate of 6 mg/kg/min.[53]

Congenital Gastrointestinal Surgical Conditions

Several congenital surgical conditions of the GI tract interfere with a normal transition to neonatal life. Many of these conditions can be diagnosed with antenatal ultrasound to allow transfer of the mother to a perinatal center for delivery. Examples include tracheoesophageal fistula and esophageal atresia, duodenal atresia, abdominal wall defects (gastroschisis and omphalocele), and congenital diaphragmatic hernia (CDH). CDH infants are ideally delivered in centers with access to advanced therapies such as extracorporeal membrane oxygenation (ECMO).

Necrotizing Enterocolitis

NEC is the most common acquired GI emergency in the neonatal intensive care unit (NICU). This disorder predominantly affects premature infants, with higher incidences present with decreasing gestational age, although it is seen in term infants with polycythemia, congenital heart disease, and birth asphyxia. The pathogenesis is multifactorial, with intestinal ischemia, infection, provision of enteral feedings, and gut maturity playing roles to varying degrees in individual patients.[54] Recent research has suggested a critical role for the neonatal intestinal microbiome in the pathogenesis of this complication of prematurity. Use of probiotics appears to be a potentially promising preventative therapy, but data are still insufficient for a general recommendation for their use.[55] **Presumably related to changes in intestinal circulation, tocolysis with indomethacin has been associated with an increased incidence of NEC, whereas antenatal betamethasone may decrease the incidence.**

Clinically, the spectrum of disease varies from a mild GI disturbance to a rapid fulminant course characterized by intestinal gangrene, perforation, sepsis, and shock. The hallmark symptoms are abdominal distension, ileus, delayed gastric emptying, and bloody stools. The radiographic findings are bowel wall edema, pneumatosis intestinalis, biliary free air, and free peritoneal air. Associated symptoms include apnea, bradycardia, hypotension, and temperature instability. Surgical resection of bowel may be necessary with resulting short bowel syndrome in survivors. In addition, severe NEC has a negative impact on neurodevelopmental outcome.[56]

Neonatal Jaundice

The most common problem encountered in a term nursery population is jaundice. Neonatal hyperbilirubinemia occurs when the normal pathways of bilirubin metabolism and excretion are altered. Figure 22-12 demonstrates the metabolism of bilirubin. The normal destruction of circulating red cells accounts for about 75% of the newborn's daily bilirubin production. The remaining sources include ineffective erythropoiesis and tissue heme proteins. Heme is converted to bilirubin in the reticuloendothelial system with carbon monoxide (CO) produced as a by-product. Unconjugated bilirubin is lipid soluble and is transported in the plasma reversibly bound to albumin. Bilirubin enters the liver cells by dissociation from albumin in the hepatic sinusoids. Once in the hepatocyte, bilirubin is conjugated with glucuronic acid in a reaction catalyzed by uridine diphosphoglucuronosyl transferase (UDPGT). The water-soluble conjugated bilirubin is excreted rapidly into the bile canaliculi and into the small intestine. The enzyme β-glucuronidase is present in the small bowel and hydrolyzes some of the conjugated bilirubin. This unconjugated bilirubin can be reabsorbed into the circulation, adding to the total unconjugated bilirubin load (enterohepatic circulation). **Major predisposing factors of neonatal jaundice are (1) increased bilirubin load because of increased red cell volume with decreased cell survival, increased ineffective erythropoiesis, and the enterohepatic circulation; and (2) decreased hepatic uptake, conjugation, and excretion of bilirubin.** These factors result in the presence of clinically apparent jaundice in approximately two thirds of newborns during the first week of life, and in most it is considered physiologic.[57] Infants whose bilirubin levels are above the 95th percentile for age in hours and infants in high-risk groups to develop hyperbilirubinemia require close follow-up (Fig. 22-13 and Box 22-3).[58,59]

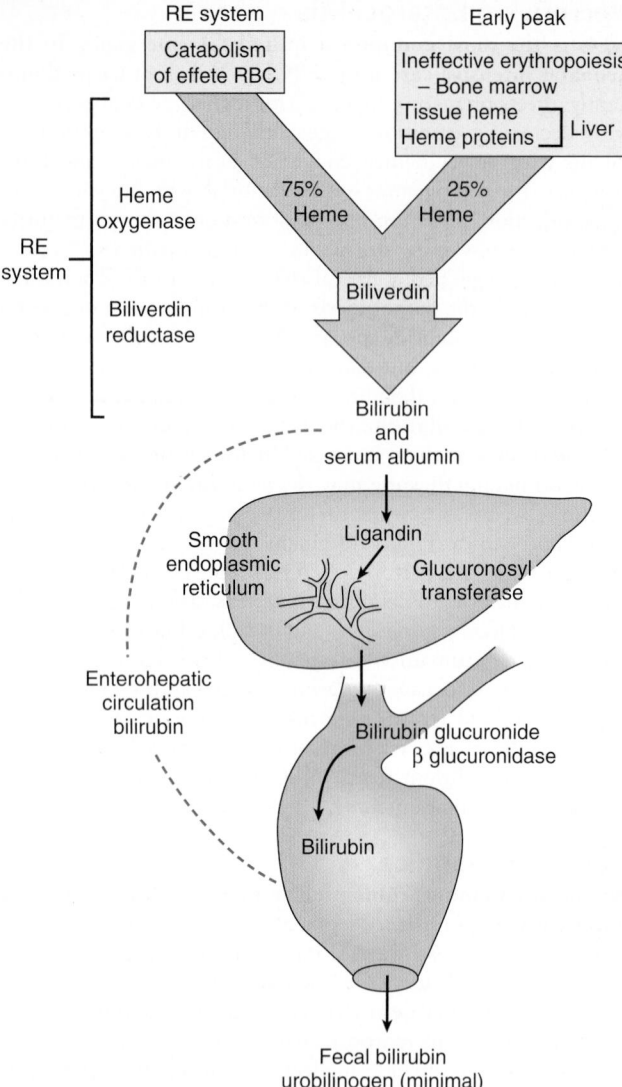

FIG 22-12 Neonatal bile pigment metabolism. RBC, red blood cell; RE, reticuloendothelial. (Modified from Maisels MJ. Jaundice. In Avery GB, Fletcher MA, MacDonald MG, eds. *Neonatology: Pathophysiology and Management of the Newborn,* 5th ed. Philadelphia: Lippincott, Williams & Wilkins; 1999:765.)

BOX 22-3 RISK FACTORS FOR SIGNIFICANT HYPERBILIRUBINEMIA

Jaundice observed at <24 hr
Blood group incompatibility with positive direct Coombs test
Other hemolytic disease (G6PD deficiency)
Gestational age <35 to 36 wk
Previous sibling needing phototherapy
Cephalohematoma, subgaleal blood collection, bruising
Exclusive breastfeeding, especially if it is not going well
East Asian race

Modified from American Academy of Pediatrics Subcommittee on Hyperbilirubinemia. Management of hyperbilirubinemia in the newborn infant 35 or more weeks gestation. *Pediatrics.* 2004;114:297.
G6PD, glucose-6-phosphate dehydrogenase.

Pathologic jaundice during the early neonatal period is indirect hyperbilirubinemia, usually caused by overproduction of bilirubin. The leading cause in this group of patients is hemolytic disease, of which fetomaternal blood group incompatibilities—ABO, Rh, and other minor antibodies—are the most common (see Chapter 34). Other causes of hemolysis include genetic disorders: specifically, hereditary spherocytosis and nonspherocytic hemolytic anemias, such as glucose-6-phosphate dehydrogenase (G6PD) deficiency. Other etiologies of bilirubin overproduction include extravasated blood (bruising, hemorrhage), polycythemia, and exaggerated enterohepatic circulation of bilirubin because of mechanical GI obstruction or reduced peristalsis from inadequate oral intake. Disease states that involve decreased bilirubin clearance must be considered in patients in whom no cause of overproduction can be identified. Causes of indirect hyperbilirubinemia in this category include familial deficiency of UDPGT (Crigler-Najjar syndrome), Gilbert syndrome, breast milk jaundice, and hypothyroidism. Mixed and direct hyperbilirubinemia are rare during the first week of life.

A strong association exists between breastfeeding and neonatal hyperbilirubinemia. The syndrome of breast milk jaundice is characterized by full-term infants who have jaundice that persists into the second and third weeks of life with maximal bilirubin levels of 10 to 30 mg/dL. If breastfeeding is continued, the levels persist for 4 to 10 days and then decline to normal by 3 to 12 weeks. Interruption of breastfeeding is associated with a prompt decline in 48 hours. **In addition to this syndrome, breastfed infants as a whole have higher bilirubin levels over the first 3 to 5 days of life than their formula-fed counterparts (Fig. 22-14). Rather than interrupting breastfeeding, this early jaundice is responsive to increased frequency of breastfeeding.** Suggested mechanisms for breastfeeding-associated jaundice include decreased early caloric intake, inhibitors of bilirubin conjugation in breast milk, and increased intestinal reabsorption of bilirubin. In some patients, overlap is considerable in these described syndromes.

The overriding concern with neonatal hyperbilirubinemia is the development of bilirubin toxicity that causes the pathologic entity of kernicterus, the staining of certain areas of the brain—basal ganglia, hippocampus, geniculate bodies, various brainstem nuclei, and cerebellum—by bilirubin. Neuronal necrosis is the dominant histopathologic feature at 7 to 10 days of life. The early symptoms of bilirubin encephalopathy consist of lethargy, hypotonia, and poor feeding that progresses to a high-pitched cry, hypertonicity, and opisthotonos. Survivors usually suffer sequelae that include athetoid cerebral palsy, high-frequency hearing loss, paralysis of upward gaze, and dental dysplasia.[60,61] **The risk of bilirubin encephalopathy is not well defined except in those infants with Rh isoimmunization in whom a level of 20 mg/dL has been associated with an increased risk of kernicterus.** This observation has been extended to the management of other neonates with hemolytic disease, although no definitive data exist regarding these infants. The risk is probably small for term infants without hemolytic disease even at levels higher than 20 mg/dL. **Recent descriptions of bilirubin encephalopathy in breastfed infants, and in late preterm infants in particular, with dehydration and hyperbilirubinemia in whom an adequate supply of breast milk has not been established mandates close follow-up of all breastfeeding mothers.**[60] The true risk for nonhemolytic hyperbilirubinemia to produce brain damage in the preterm

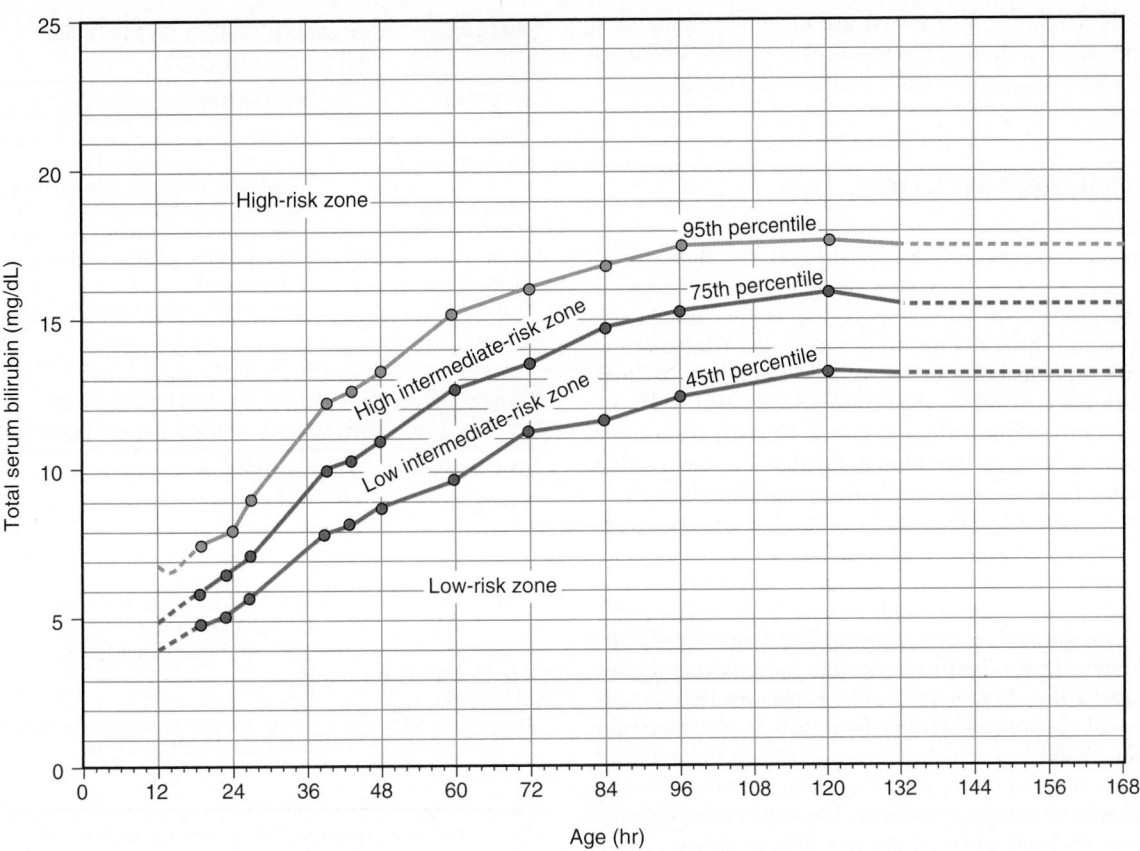

FIG 22-13 Risk of developing significant hyperbilirubinemia in term and near-term infants based on hour-specific bilirubin determinations. (From Bhutani VK, Johnson L, Sivieri EM. Predictive ability of a predischarge hour-specific serum bilirubin for subsequent significant hyperbilirubinemia in healthy term and near-term newborns. *Pediatrics.* 1999;103:6.)

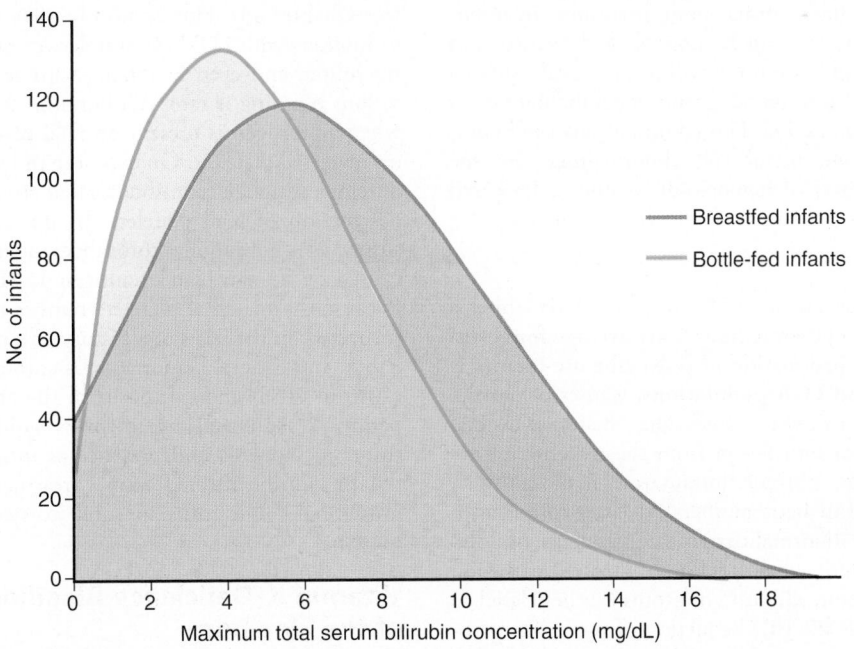

FIG 22-14 Distribution of maximum serum bilirubin concentrations in white infants who weigh more than 2500 g. (Modified from Maisels MJ, Gifford KL. Normal serum bilirubin levels in the newborn and the effect of breast-feeding. *Pediatrics.* 1986;78:837.)

infant in the current era of liberal use of phototherapy that prevents marked elevation of severe bilirubin in these infants is unknown. However, most currently available data would suggest this risk is low.

NEONATAL HEMATOLOGY
Anemia

Early hematopoietic cells originate in the yolk sac. By 8 weeks' gestation, erythropoiesis is taking place in the liver, which remains the primary site of erythroid production through the early fetal period. By 6 months of gestation, the bone marrow becomes the principal site of red cell development. **Normal hemoglobin levels at term range from 13.7 to 20.1 g/dL. In the very preterm infant, values as low as 12 g/dL are acceptable.** Anemia at birth or appearing in the first few weeks of life is the result of blood loss, hemolysis, or underproduction of erythrocytes.[62] Blood loss that results in anemia can occur prenatally, at the time of delivery, or postnatally. In utero blood loss can be the result of fetomaternal bleeding, twin-to-twin transfusion, or blood loss resulting from trauma (maternal trauma, amniocentesis, external cephalic version). **The diagnosis of fetomaternal hemorrhage significant enough to cause anemia can be made using flow cytometry or the Kleihauer-Betke technique of acid elution to identify fetal cells in the maternal circulation.** Blood loss at delivery can be caused by umbilical cord rupture, incision of the placenta during cesarean delivery, placenta previa, or abruptio placentae. Internal hemorrhage can occur in the newborn, often related to a difficult delivery. Sites include intracranial, cephalohematomas, subgaleal, retroperitoneal, liver capsule, and ruptured spleen. When blood loss has been chronic (e.g., fetomaternal), infants will be pale at birth but well compensated and without signs of volume loss. The initial hematocrit will be low. Acute bleeding will present with signs of hypovolemia (tachycardia, poor perfusion, hypotension). The initial hematocrit can be normal or decreased, but after several hours of equilibration, it will be decreased. Anemia caused by hemolysis from blood group incompatibilities is common in the newborn period. Less common causes of hemolysis include erythrocyte membrane abnormalities, enzyme deficiencies, and disorders of hemoglobin synthesis. Impaired erythrocyte production is a rare cause of neonatal anemia.

Polycythemia

Elevated hematocrits occur in 1.5% to 4% of live births. **Although 50% of polycythemic infants are average for gestational age (AGA), the proportion of polycythemic infants is greater in the SGA and LGA populations.** Causes of polycythemia include twin-to-twin transfusion, maternal-to-fetal transfusion, intrapartum transfusion from the placenta associated with fetal distress, chronic intrauterine hypoxia (SGA infants, LGA infants of diabetic mothers), delayed cord clamping, and chromosomal abnormalities. The consequence of polycythemia is hyperviscosity, which results in impaired perfusion of capillary beds. Therefore clinical symptoms can be related to any organ system (Table 22-10). Reduction of venous hematocrit to less than 60% may improve acute symptoms, but it has not been shown to improve long-term neurologic outcome.[63]

Thrombocytopenia

Neonatal thrombocytopenia can be isolated or it can occur associated with deficiency of clotting factors. A differential

TABLE 22-10	ORGAN-RELATED SYMPTOMS OF HYPERVISCOSITY
SYSTEM	**SYMPTOMS**
Central nervous system	Irritability, jitteriness, seizures, lethargy
Cardiopulmonary	Respiratory distress caused by congestive heart failure or persistent pulmonary hypertension
Gastrointestinal	Vomiting, heme-positive stools, abdominal distension, necrotizing enterocolitis
Renal	Decreased urine output, renal vein thrombosis
Metabolic	Hypoglycemia
Hematologic	Hyperbilirubinemia, thrombocytopenia

TABLE 22-11	DIFFERENTIAL DIAGNOSIS OF NEONATAL THROMBOCYTOPENIA
DIAGNOSIS	**COMMENTS**
Immune	Passively acquired antibody (e.g., idiopathic thrombocytopenic purpura, systemic lupus erythematosus, drug induced) Alloimmune sensitization to HPA-1a antigen
Infectious	Bacterial and congenital viral infections (e.g., cytomegalovirus, rubella)
Syndromes Giant hemangioma Thrombosis	Absent radii; Fanconi anemia
High-risk infant with RDS, pulmonary hypertension, and so forth	Disseminated intravascular coagulation Isolated thrombocytopenia

HPA-1a, human platelet antigen 1a; *RDS,* respiratory distress syndrome.

diagnosis is presented in Table 22-11. The immune thrombocytopenias have implications for perinatal care. In idiopathic thrombocytopenic purpura (ITP), maternal antiplatelet antibodies that cross the placenta lead to destruction of fetal platelets (see Chapter 44). However, only 10% to 15% of infants born to mothers with ITP have platelet counts less than 100,000 per microliter, and even in infants with severe thrombocytopenia, serious bleeding is rare. Alloimmune thrombocytopenia occurs when an antigen is present on fetal platelets but is not present on maternal platelets. On exposure to fetal platelets, the mother develops antiplatelet antibodies that cross the placenta and cause destruction of fetal platelets. In the largest series of cases of suspected alloimmune thrombocytopenia, the majority were caused by human platelet antigen 1a (HPA-1a) alloantibodies. Because the maternal platelet count is normal, the diagnosis is suspected on the basis of a history of a previously affected pregnancy. Intracranial hemorrhage is common with this condition (10% to 20%) and can occur in the antenatal or intrapartum periods.[64] Antenatal treatment is guided by the severity of thrombocytopenia and presence of intracranial hemorrhage in the previously affected fetus. Treatment options include IV immunoglobulin infusions and corticosteroids given to the mother.[64]

Vitamin K–Deficiency Bleeding of the Newborn

Vitamin K₁ oxide (1 mg) should be given intramuscularly to all newborns to prevent hemorrhagic disease caused by a deficiency in vitamin K–dependent clotting factors (II, VII, IX, X).[65] Babies born to mothers who are on anticonvulsant medication are particularly at risk of having vitamin K deficiency. Bleeding occurs in 0.25% to 1.4% of newborns who do

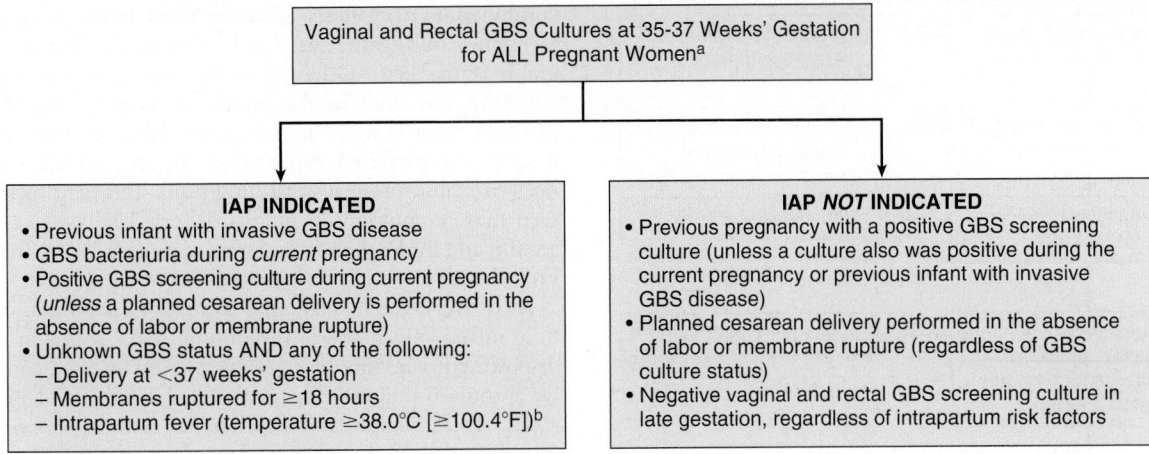

FIG 22-15 Indications for intrapartum antimicrobial prophylaxis to prevent early onset of disease from Group B *Streptococcus* (GBS) using a universal prenatal culture screening strategy at 35 to 37 weeks' gestation for all pregnant women. IAP, intrapartum antimicrobial prophylaxis. (From Verani JR, McGee L, Schrag SJ; Division of Bacterial Diseases, National Center for Immunization and Respiratory Diseases, Centers for Disease Control and Prevention. Prevention of perinatal group B streptococcal disease—revised guidelines from CDC, 2010. *MMWR Recomm Rep.* 2010;59[RR-10]:1-36.)

not receive vitamin K prophylaxis, generally in the first 5 days to 2 weeks but sometimes as late as 12 weeks. Oral vitamin K has been shown to be effective in raising vitamin K levels, but it is not as effective in preventing late hemorrhagic disease of the newborn, which most commonly occurs in breastfed infants whose courses have been complicated by diarrhea.

PERINATAL INFECTION

Early-Onset Bacterial Infection

The unique predisposition of the neonate to bacterial infection is related to defects in both innate and acquired immune responses.[66] The incidence of bacterial infection in infants younger than 5 days of age is 1 to 2 per 1000 live births. **Maternal colonization with group B *Streptococcus* (GBS), rupture of membranes for more than 12 to 18 hours, and the presence of chorioamnionitis increase the risk of infection.**[67,68] Maternal fever from other etiologies (e.g., epidural anesthesia) does not increase the risk of neonatal infection and merits only close observation of the newborn. Irrespective of membrane rupture, infection rates are higher in preterm infants. **The majority of early-onset bacterial infections present on day 1 of life, with respiratory distress the most common presenting symptom.** These infections are most often caused by GBS and gram-negative enteric pathogens. The algorithm for prevention of early-onset GBS infections is presented in Figure 22-15 with the approach to the newborn shown in Figure 22-16. Other etiologies of infection in the newborn are covered in Chapters 52, 53, and 54.

RESPIRATORY DISTRESS

The establishment of respiratory function at birth is dependent on expansion and maintenance of air sacs, clearance of lung fluid, and adequate pulmonary perfusion. In many premature and other high-risk infants, developmental deficiencies or unfavorable perinatal events hamper a smooth respiratory transition. **The presentation of respiratory distress is among the most common symptom complexes seen in the newborn and may be secondary to both noncardiopulmonary and cardiopulmonary etiologies** (Table 22-12). The symptom complex includes an elevation of the respiratory rate to greater than 60 per minute with or without cyanosis, nasal flaring, intercostal and sternal retractions, and expiratory grunting. The retractions are the result of the neonate's efforts to expand a lung with poor compliance using a very compliant chest wall. The expiratory grunt is caused by closure of the glottis during expiration in an effort to increase expiratory pressure to help maintain FRC. The evaluation of such an infant requires use of history, physical examination, and laboratory data to arrive at a diagnosis. It is important to consider causes other than those related to the heart and lungs, because the natural tendency is to focus immediately on the more common cardiopulmonary etiologies.

Cardiovascular Causes

Cardiovascular causes of respiratory distress in the neonatal period can be divided into two major groups—those with structural heart disease and those with persistent right-to-left shunting through fetal pathways and a structurally normal heart. **The two presentations of serious structural heart disease in the first week of life are cyanosis and congestive heart failure.**[69] Examples of cyanotic heart disease include transposition of the great vessels, tricuspid atresia, certain types of truncus arteriosus, total anomalous pulmonary venous return, and right-sided outflow obstruction including tetralogy of Fallot and pulmonary stenosis or atresia. Infants with congestive heart failure generally have some form of left-sided outflow obstruction (e.g., hypoplastic left heart syndrome, coarctation of the aorta). **It is now recommended that all newborns have pulse oximetry screening at 24 hours to identify critical heart disease.**[70]

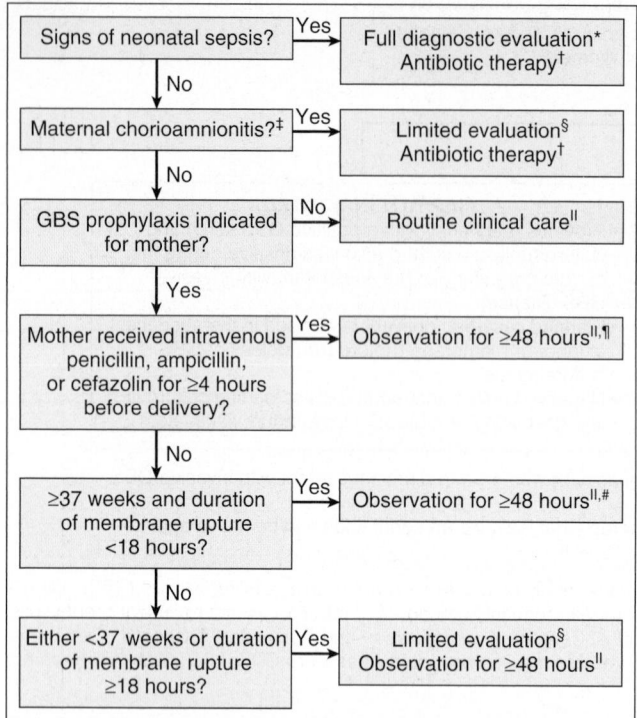

* Full diagnostic evaluation includes a blood culture, a complete blood count (CBC) including white blood cell differential and platelet counts, chest radiograph (if respiratory abnormalities are present), and lumbar puncture (if patient is stable enough to tolerate procedure and sepsis is suspected).

† Antibiotic therapy should be directed toward the most common cause of neonatal sepsis, including intravenous ampicillin for GBS and coverage for other organisms (including *Escherichia coli* and other gram-negative pathogens) and should take into account local antibiotic resistance patterns.

‡ Consultation with obstetric providers is important to determine the level of clinical suspicion for chorioamnionitis. Chorioamnionitis is diagnosed clinically and some of the signs are nonspecific.

§ Limited evaluation includes blood culture (at birth) and CBC with differential and platelets (at birth and/or at 6-12 hours of life).

‖ If signs of sepsis develop, a full diagnostic evaluation should be conducted and antibiotic therapy initiated.

¶ If ≥37 weeks' gestation, observation may occur at home after 24 hours if other discharge criteria have been met, access to medical care is readily available, and a person who is able to comply fully with instructions for home observation will be present. If any of these conditions is not met, the infant should be observed in the hospital for at least 48 hours and until discharge criteria are achieved.

Some experts recommend a CBC with differential and platelets at age 6-12 hours.

FIG 22-16 Algorithm for secondary prevention of early-onset Group B streptococcal disease among newborns. (From Verani JR, McGee L, Schrag SJ; Division of Bacterial Diseases, National Center for Immunization and Respiratory Diseases, Centers for Disease Control and Prevention. Prevention of perinatal group B streptococcal disease—revised guidelines from CDC, 2010. *MMWR Recomm Rep.* 2010; 59[RR-10]:1-36.)

Pulmonary Causes

Of the causes of respiratory distress related to the airways and pulmonary parenchyma listed in Table 22-12, **the differential diagnosis in a term infant includes transient tachypnea, aspiration syndromes, congenital pneumonia, and spontaneous pneumothorax.**[71] The syndrome of transient tachypnea presents as respiratory distress in nonasphyxiated term infants or slightly preterm infants. The clinical features include various combinations of cyanosis, grunting, nasal flaring, retracting, and tachypnea during the first hours after birth. The chest radiograph is the key to the diagnosis, with prominent perihilar streaking and fluid in the interlobar fissures. The symptoms generally subside in 12 to 24 hours, although they can persist longer. The preferred explanation for the clinical features is delayed reabsorption of fetal lung fluid. Transient tachypnea is seen more commonly in infants delivered by elective cesarean section and in the slightly preterm infant (see "Mechanics of the First Breath").

At delivery, the neonate may aspirate clear amniotic fluid or fluid mixed with blood or meconium. MAS occurs in full-term or postmature infants. The perinatal course is often complicated by chronic intrauterine hypoxia, fetal distress, and low Apgar scores. These infants exhibit tachypnea, retractions, cyanosis, an overdistended and barrel-shaped chest, and coarse breath sounds. Chest radiography reveals coarse, irregular pulmonary densities with areas of diminished aeration or consolidation. The incidence of air leaks is high, and many of the infants exhibit persistent pulmonary hypertension.

The lungs represent the most common primary site of infection in the neonate. Both bacterial and viral infections can be acquired before, during, or after birth. The most common route of infection, particularly for bacteria, is ascending from the genital tract before or during labor. Infants with congenital pneumonia present with respiratory distress very early in life. The chest radiograph pattern is often indistinguishable from other causes of respiratory distress, particularly hyaline membrane disease (HMD).

Spontaneous pneumothorax occurs in 1% of all deliveries, but a much lower percentage results in symptoms. The risk is increased by manipulations such as positive-pressure ventilation. Respiratory distress is usually present from shortly after birth, and breath sounds may be diminished on the affected side. The majority of these air leaks resolve spontaneously without specific therapy.

HMD remains the most common etiology for respiratory distress in the neonatal period. Initial reports of Avery and Mead[72] demonstrated a high surface tension in extracts of lungs from infants dying of RDS, which led to the present understanding of the role of surfactant in the pathogenesis of HMD. The deficiency of surfactant in the premature infant increases alveolar surface tension and, according to LaPlace's law (see Fig. 22-2), increases the pressure necessary to maintain patent alveoli. The end result is poor lung compliance, progressive atelectasis, loss of FRC, alterations in ventilation-perfusion mismatch, and uneven distribution of ventilation. HMD is further complicated by the weak respiratory muscles and compliant chest wall of the premature infant. Hypoxemia and respiratory and metabolic acidemia contribute to increased pulmonary vascular resistance, right-to-left ductal shunting, and worsening ventilation-perfusion mismatch that exacerbate hypoxemia. Hypoxemia and hypoperfusion result in alveolar epithelial damage with increased capillary permeability and leakage of plasma into alveolar spaces. Leakage of protein into airspaces serves to inhibit surfactant function, which exacerbates the disease process. **The materials in plasma and cellular debris combine to form the characteristic hyaline membrane seen pathologically.** The recovery phase is characterized by regeneration of alveolar cells, including type II cells, with an increase in surfactant activity.

Clinically, neonates with HMD demonstrate tachypnea, nasal flaring, subcostal and intercostal retractions, cyanosis, and

TABLE 22-12 RESPIRATORY DISTRESS IN THE NEWBORN

NONCARDIOPULMONARY	CARDIOVASCULAR	PULMONARY
Hypothermia or hyperthermia	Left-sided outflow obstruction	Upper airway obstruction
Hypoglycemia	Hypoplastic left heart	Choanal atresia
Metabolic acidosis	Aortic stenosis	Vocal cord paralysis
Drug intoxications, withdrawal	Coarctation of the aorta	Meconium aspiration
Polycythemia	Cyanotic lesions	Clear fluid aspiration
Central nervous system insult	Transposition of the great vessels	Transient tachypnea
Asphyxia	Total anomalous pulmonary venous return	Pneumonia
Hemorrhage	Tricuspid atresia	Pulmonary hypoplasia
Neuromuscular disease	Right-sided outflow obstruction	Primary
Werdnig-Hoffman disease		Secondary
Myopathies		Hyaline membrane disease
Phrenic nerve injury		Pneumothorax
Skeletal abnormalities		Pleural effusions
Asphyxiating thoracic dystrophy		Mass lesions
		Lobar emphysema
		Cystic adenomatoid malformation

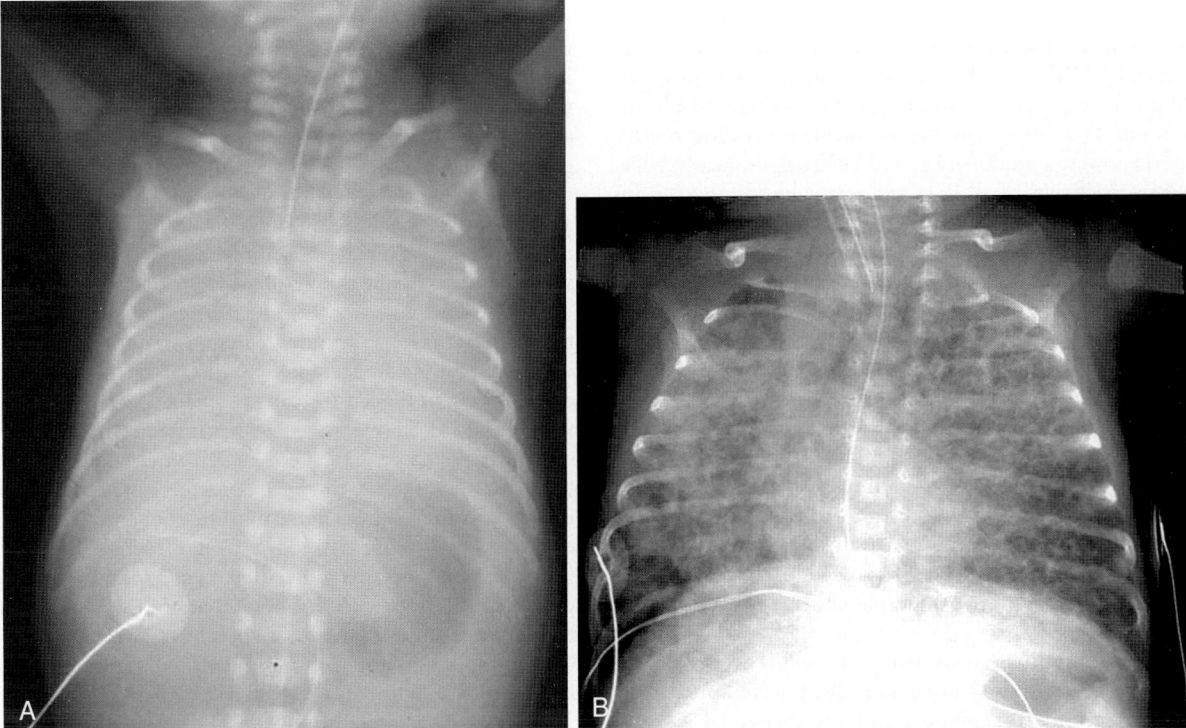

FIG 22-17 A, Chest radiograph demonstrates findings consistent with hyaline membrane disease (respiratory distress syndrome) including extensive atelectasis with homogeneous ground-glass appearance to the lung fields and air bronchograms and elevated diaphragm. **B,** Chest radiographs demonstrate changes consistent with bronchopulmonary dysplasia, including heterogeneous areas of atelectasis and hyperlucency.

expiratory grunting. The radiologic appearance of the lungs is consistent with an extensive atelectatic process (Fig. 22-17). The infiltrate is diffuse and has a ground-glass appearance, and major airways are air filled and contrast with the atelectatic alveoli to create the appearance of air bronchograms. The diaphragm is elevated because of profound hypoexpansion. Acute complications of HMD include infection, air leaks, and persistent patency of the ductus arteriosus.

Of more concern than acute complications are the long-term sequelae suffered by infants with HMD. The major long-term consequences are chronic lung disease (CLD) that requires prolonged ventilator and oxygen therapy and includes bronchopulmonary dysplasia and significant neurologic impairment. The incidence is especially high in infants born at less than 800 g. The severity is variable and ranges from very mild pulmonary insufficiency to severe disease with prolonged mechanical ventilation, frequent readmissions for respiratory exacerbations after nursery discharge, and a higher incidence of neurodevelopmental sequelae compared with VLBW controls. Although pulmonary function improves over time and most children do well, long-term pulmonary sequelae are evident. Factors involved in the etiology of CLD are gestational age, elevated inspired oxygen concentration, ventilator volutrauma, severity of underlying disease, inflammation, and infection.

TABLE 22-13	CLASSIFICATION OF INTRAVENTRICULAR HEMORRHAGE
GRADE	**DEFINITION**
I	Subependymal hemorrhage
II	Intraventricular hemorrhage without ventricular dilatation
III	Intraventricular hemorrhage with ventricular dilatation
IV	Intraventricular hemorrhage with associated parenchymal hemorrhage

Modified from Papile LA, Burstein J, Burstein R, Koffler H. Incidence and evolution of subependymal and intraventricular hemorrhage: a study of infants with birth weights less than 1500 g. *J Pediatr.* 1978;92:529.

NEONATAL NEUROLOGY

Intraventricular Hemorrhage and Periventricular Leukomalacia

Periventricular/intraventricular hemorrhage (PVH/IVH) and periventricular leukomalacia (PVL) are the most common neurologic complications of prematurity. The overall incidence of PVH/IVH is 20% to 30% in infants weighing less than 1500 g or at less than 31 weeks' gestation with severe bleeds (grades 3 and 4) at 10%. The highest incidence is observed in babies of the lowest gestational age and birthweight; nearly 50% and 25%, respectively, of all IVH and severe bleeds are seen in babies born at less than 700 g.[73] Bleeds are graded according to severity as indicated in Table 22-13, and diagnosis is confirmed with ultrasound. PVL is reported in about 2% to 4% of infants younger than 32 weeks' gestation,[73] but the cystic PVL reported likely underestimates the full spectrum of PVL.

Cystic PVL comprises multifocal areas of necrosis with cyst formation in deep periventricular white matter. It has been well characterized by ultrasound, and the expanded use of MRI scans in preterm infants has identified infants—especially among those of lower gestational age—with diffuse white matter injury often accompanied by ventricular dilation. These findings are far more common in the preterm population than cystic PVL and represent part of the spectrum of PVL. The other important clinical correlate with PVL is maternal chorioamnionitis and neonatal infection.

The neurodevelopmental outcome of infants with IVH is related to the severity of the original bleed, development of posthemorrhagic hydrocephalus, and the degree of associated parenchymal injury. Although cranial ultrasound is the primary modality used to diagnose IVH and PVL, it is not a sensitive predictor of outcome. In extremely low-birthweight infants with no abnormalities on cranial ultrasound, nearly one third will have some degree of neurodevelopmental handicap (cerebral palsy or cognitive delays).[74] Infants with grade I or II IVH are at slightly greater risk for handicap.[75] School-aged children who had mild IVH display a variety of neurologic and cognitive abnormalities, including motor incoordination, hyperactivity, attention and learning deficits, and visual motor difficulties.[76] Infants with progressive ventricular dilatation (grade III) or periventricular hemorrhagic infarction (grade IV) are at higher risk for major neurodevelopmental handicap as well as less severe neurologic and cognitive disabilities.[77,78] The presence of severe cystic PVL carries a guarded prognosis with a high risk of cerebral palsy and associated cognitive deficit.

Although the incidence and severity of intracranial hemorrhage have progressively decreased as a result of advances in both obstetric and neonatal care, the therapeutic focus continues to be on strategies to prevent this complication of prematurity. Both antenatal and postnatal approaches have been developed. For the most part, postnatal pharmacologic strategies have not had a major effect in decreasing the incidence, severity, and neurodevelopmental outcomes of IVH. **Because IVH and PVL are likely perinatal events, antenatal prevention holds the most promise. Although not used specifically to decrease the incidence of IVH and PVL, antenatal corticosteroids decrease the frequency of these complications and likely represent the most important antenatal strategy to prevent intracranial hemorrhage.**[5] Furthermore, antenatal magnesium sulfate also is used for neuroprotection of the newborn prior to preterm delivery, although long-term benefits are unclear.[79,80]

CLASSIFICATION OF NEWBORNS BY GROWTH AND GESTATIONAL AGE

In assessing the risk for mortality or morbidity in a given neonate, evaluation of birthweight and gestational age together provide the clearest picture. When large populations are considered, maternal dates remain the single best determinant of gestational age. Early obstetric ultrasound is a very useful adjunct (see Chapter 9). However, in the individual neonate, especially when dates are uncertain, a reliable postnatal assessment of gestational age is necessary. A scoring system that appraises gestational age on the basis of physical and neurologic criteria was developed by Dubowitz and colleagues and later simplified and updated by Ballard and associates (Fig. 22-18).[81] The Ballard examination is less accurate before 28 weeks' gestation, but additional features can be examined to aid in the determination of an accurate gestational age. The anterior vascular capsule of the lens reveals complete coverage of the lens by vessels at 27 to 28 weeks. Foot length (from the heel to the tip of the largest toe) is 4.5 cm at 25 weeks and increases by 0.25 cm/wk. Using growth parameters and gestational age, infants can then be classified by means of intrauterine growth curves such as those developed by Lubchenco and colleagues (Fig. 22-19).[82] **Infants born between 37 and 42 weeks are classified as *term infants*; less than 37 weeks is *preterm*; and greater than 42 weeks is *postterm*** (see Chapter 36). In each grouping, infants are then identified according to growth; *AGA* if birthweight falls between the 10th and 90th percentiles, *SGA* if birthweight is below the 10th percentile, and *LGA* if birthweight is above the 90th percentile. Knowledge of a baby's birthweight in relation to gestational age is helpful in anticipating neonatal problems.

The causes of growth restriction are numerous (see Chapter 33). Those operative early in pregnancy such as chromosomal aberrations, congenital viral infections, and some drug exposures induce symmetric restriction of weight, length, and head circumference. In most cases, the phenomenon occurs later in gestation and leads to more selective restriction of birthweight alone. Such factors include hypertension or other maternal vascular disease and multiple gestation. Neonatal problems in addition to chromosomal abnormalities and congenital viral infections common in SGA infants include birth asphyxia, hypoglycemia, polycythemia, and hypothermia. In addition, congenital malformations are seen more frequently among undergrown infants.[83]

The most common identifiable conditions that lead to excessive infant birthweight are maternal diabetes and maternal

Neuromuscular Maturity

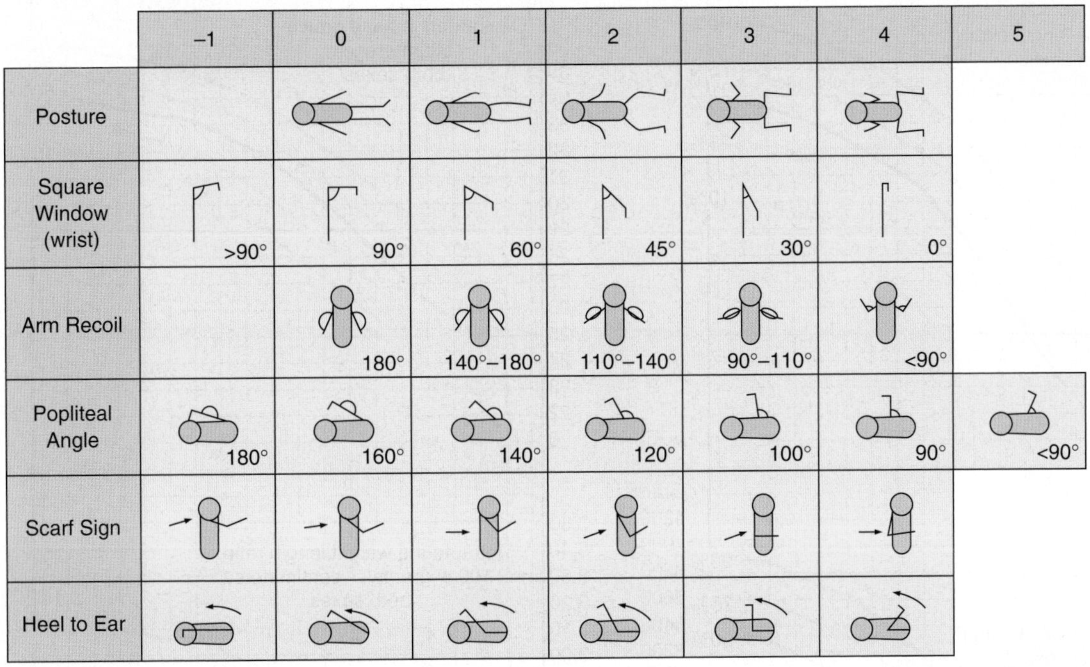

	−1	0	1	2	3	4	5
Posture							
Square Window (wrist)	>90°	90°	60°	45°	30°	0°	
Arm Recoil		180°	140°–180°	110°–140°	90°–110°	<90°	
Popliteal Angle	180°	160°	140°	120°	100°	90°	<90°
Scarf Sign							
Heel to Ear							

Physical Maturity

Skin	sticky, friable, transparent	gelatinous, red, translucent	smooth pink, visible veins	superficial peeling and/or rash, few veins	cracking pale areas, rare veins	parchment, deep, cracking, no vessels	leathery, cracked, wrinkled
Lanugo	none	sparse	abundant	thinning	bald areas	mostly bald	
Plantar Surface	heel-toe 40-50 mm: −1 <40 mm: −2	>50 mm, no crease	faint red marks	anterior transverse crease only	creases ant. 2/3	creases over entire sole	
Breast	imperceptible	barely perceptible	flat areola no bud	stippled areola, 1-2 mm bud	raised areola, 3-4 mm bud	full areola, 5-10 mm bud	
Eye/Ear	lids fused loosely: −1 tightly: −2	lids open, pinna flat and stays folded	slight curved pinna, soft, slow recoil	well-curved pinna, soft but ready recoil	formed and firm, instant recoil	thick cartilage, ear stiff	
Genitals Male	scrotum flat, smooth	scrotum empty, faint rugae	testes in upper canal, rare rugae	testes descending, few rugae	testes down, good rugae	testes pendulous, deep rugae	
Genitals Female	clitoris prominent, labia flat	prominent clitoris, small labia minora	prominent clitoris, enlarging minora	majora and minora equally prominent	majora large, minora small	majora cover clitoris and minora	

Maturity Rating

Score	Weeks
−10	20
−5	22
0	24
5	26
10	28
15	30
20	32
25	34
30	36
35	38
40	40
45	42
50	44

FIG 22-18 Assessment of gestational age. ant., anterior. (From Ballard JL, Khoury JC, Wedig K, et al. New Ballard Score, expanded to include extremely premature infants. *J Pediatr.* 1991;119:417.)

obesity. Other conditions associated with macrosomia are erythroblastosis fetalis, other causes of fetal hydrops, and Beckwith-Wiedemann syndrome. LGA infants are at risk for hypoglycemia, polycythemia, congenital anomalies, cardiomyopathy, hyperbilirubinemia, and birth trauma.

NURSERY CARE

Nurseries are classified on the basis of the level of care provided (Box 22-4). *Level I nurseries* care for infants presumed healthy, with an emphasis on screening and surveillance. *Level II nurseries* can care for infants at more than 32 weeks'

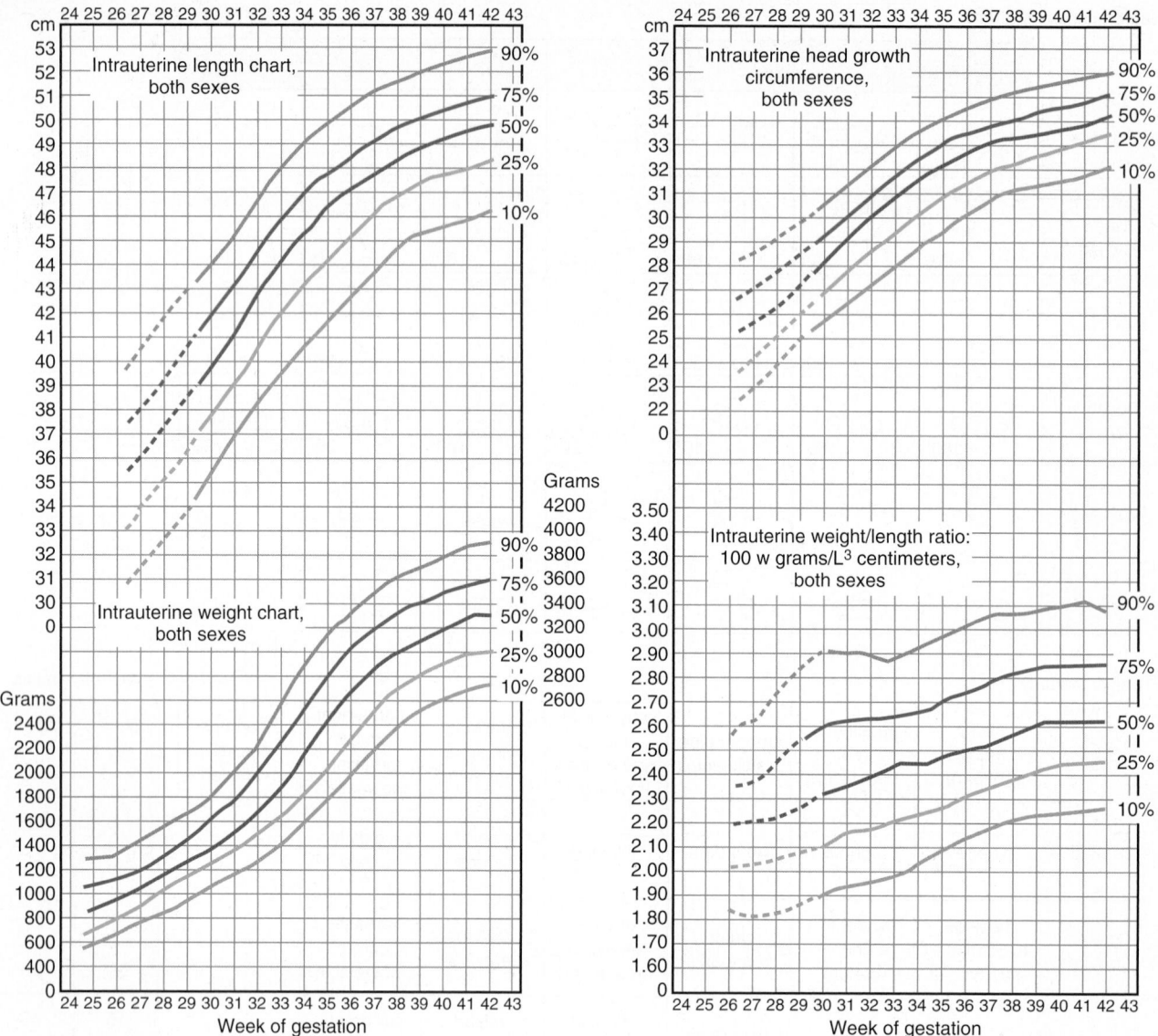

FIG 22-19 Intrauterine growth curves for weight, length, and head circumference for singleton births in Colorado. *100 w grams/L³ centimeters,* weight in grams divided by 100, with the quotient divided by the length cubed. (From Lubchenco LO, Hansman C, Boyd E. Intrauterine growth in length and head circumference as estimated from live births at gestational ages from 26 to 42 weeks. *Pediatrics.* 1966;37:403.)

BOX 22-4   LEVELS OF NURSERY CARE

Level 1: A nursery with personnel and equipment to perform neonatal resuscitation, evaluate and provide newborn care for healthy infants, stabilize and provide care for infants born at 35 to 37 weeks' gestation who remain physiologically stable, and stabilize ill infants and those at less than 35 weeks' gestation before transport to a higher-level facility.

Level 2: A facility able to provide care to infants born at more than 32 weeks' gestation weighing more than 1500 g who have physiologic immaturity, are moderately ill with problems expected to resolve quickly, and do not need urgent subspecialty care; and they can provide convalescent care for infants after intensive care.

  2A: Does *not* do mechanical ventilation or nasal CPAP

  2B: Can do short-term (<24 hr) ventilation.

Level 3: Provides care for the sickest and most complex infants.

  3A: Provides care for infants beyond 28 weeks and 1000 g who are in need of conventional mechanical ventilation.

  3B: Can provide care for infants at less than 28 weeks and 1000 g, including high-frequency ventilation, inhaled nitric oxide, on-site subspecialists, advanced imaging, on-site or nearby pediatric surgeons, and anesthesiologists.

  3C: Can provide ECMO and repair of complex congenital heart disease.

Modified from the American Academy of Pediatrics Committee on Fetus and Newborn. Levels of neonatal care. *Pediatrics.* 2004;114:1341. *CPAP,* continuous positive airway pressure; *ECMO,* extracorporeal membrane oxygenation.

gestation who weigh at least 1500 g but who require special attention but will probably not need subspecialty services. *Level III nurseries* care for all newborn infants who are critically ill regardless of the level of support required.[84] A perinatal center encompasses both high-risk obstetric services and level III nursery services. Survival for VLBW infants is improved with delivery at centers with a higher volume (>100) of VLBW deliveries per year and a higher-level nursery.[85] This survival advantage may extend to moderately preterm newborns as well.[86]

Care of the normal newborn involves observation of transition from intrauterine to extrauterine life, establishing breast or bottle feedings, noting normal patterns of stooling and urination, and surveillance for neonatal problems. Signs suggestive of illness include temperature instability, change in activity, refusal to feed, pallor, cyanosis, jaundice, tachypnea and respiratory distress, delayed (>24 hr) passage of the first stool or void, and bilious vomiting. In addition, the following laboratory screens should be performed: (1) blood type and direct and indirect Coombs test on infants born to mothers with type O or Rh-negative blood; (2) glucose screen in infants at risk for hypoglycemia; (3) hematocrit in infants with signs and symptoms of anemia or polycythemia; and (4) mandated screening for inborn errors of metabolism, such as phenylketonuria (PKU) and galactosemia, sickle cell disease, hypothyroidism, cystic fibrosis, and congenital adrenal hyperplasia. Many states now mandate or offer expanded newborn screening by tandem mass spectroscopy that looks for a variety of other inborn metabolic errors. **All newborns should also have an initial hearing screen performed before discharge.** Finally, babies routinely receive 1 mg of vitamin K intramuscularly to prevent vitamin K–deficient hemorrhagic disease of the newborn, and erythromycin ointment is used to prevent gonococcal ophthalmia neonatorum. Hepatitis B vaccine should be given to all newborns, and hepatitis B immunoglobulin is also administered to infants born to HB$_s$Ag-positive mothers (see Chapter 52). Infants should be positioned supine for sleep to minimize the risk of sudden infant death syndrome (SIDS).[87]

Discharge of the normal newborn is safe provided all criteria are met in Box 22-5. The initial follow-up visit needs to occur 48 to 72 hours after discharge.[88]

Circumcision is an elective procedure to be performed only in healthy, stable infants. The procedure probably has medical benefits that include prevention of phimosis, paraphimosis, and balanoposthitis as well as a decreased incidence of cancer of the penis, cervical cancer in partners of circumcised men, sexually transmitted diseases (including HIV), and urinary tract infection in male infants. Most parents, however, make the decision regarding circumcision for nonmedical reasons. The risks of the procedure include local infection, bleeding, removal of too much skin, and urethral injury. The combined incidence of these complications is less than 1%. **Local anesthesia** (dorsal penile nerve block or circumferential ring block) **with 1% lidocaine without epinephrine is safe and effective and should always be used.** Techniques that allow visualization of the glans throughout the procedure (Plastibell and Gomco clamp) are preferred to a "blind" technique (Mogen clamp) because of occasional amputation of the glans with the latter. Circumcision is contraindicated in infants with genital abnormalities. In infants with a family history of bleeding disorders, appropriate laboratory evaluation should be performed before the procedure.

Care of the Parents

Klaus and Kennell[89] have outlined the steps in maternal-infant attachment: (1) planning the pregnancy; (2) confirming the pregnancy; (3) accepting the pregnancy; (4) noting fetal movement; (5) accepting the fetus as an individual; (6) going through labor; (7) giving birth; (8) hearing and seeing the baby; (9) touching, smelling, and holding the baby; (10) caretaking; and (11) accepting the infant as a separate individual. Numerous influences can affect this process. A mother's and father's actions and responses are derived from their own genetic endowment and their own interfamily relationships, cultural practices, past experiences with this or previous pregnancies, and, most important, how they were raised by their parents. Also critical is the in-hospital experience surrounding the birth—how doctors and nurses act, separation from the baby, and hospital practices.

The 60- to 90-minute period after delivery is a very important time. The infant is alert, active, and able to follow with his or her eyes, allowing meaningful interaction to transpire between infant and parents. The infant's array of sensory and motor abilities evokes responses from the mother and initiates communication that may be helpful for attachment and induction of reciprocal actions. Whether a critical period for these initial interactions exists is unclear, but improved mothering behavior does seem to occur with increased contact over the first 3 postpartum days. **The practical implications of this information are that labor and delivery should pose as little anxiety as possible for the mother, and parents and baby should have time together immediately after delivery if the baby's medical condition permits.**

Mothers with high-risk pregnancies are at increased risk for subsequent parenting problems. It is important for both obstetrician and pediatrician alike to be involved prenatally to allow time to prepare the family for anticipated aspects of the baby's care and to provide reassurance that the odds are heavily in favor of a live baby who will ultimately be healthy. If it is possible before birth to anticipate the need for neonatal intensive care, such as with a known congenital anomaly or with refractory premature labor, maternal transport to a center with a unit that can care for the baby should be planned. Before delivery, it is also very helpful to allow the parents to tour the unit their baby will occupy.

The basic principle in dealing with parents of a sick infant is to provide essential information clearly and accurately to both parents, preferably when they are together. With improved survival rates, especially in premature infants, most babies will do well despite early problems. Therefore it is reasonable in most circumstances to be positive about the outcome. There is also no reason to emphasize problems that might occur in the future or to deal with individual worries of the physician. If asked, questions need to be answered honestly, but the list of parents' worries does not need to be voluntarily increased.

Before the parents' initial visit to the unit, a physician or nurse should describe what the baby and the equipment look like. When they arrive in the nursery, this can again be reviewed in detail. If a baby must be moved to another hospital, the mother should be given time to see and touch her infant before the transfer. The father should be encouraged to meet the baby at the receiving hospital so he can become comfortable with the intensive care unit. He can serve as a link between baby and mother with information and photographs.

BOX 22-5   INFANT CRITERIA FOR EARLY DISCHARGE

1. The newborn is term, defined as an infant born between 37 and 41 completed weeks of gestation.
2. No abnormalities are present that require continued hospitalization.
3. Vital signs are documented as being within normal ranges with appropriate variations based on physiologic state and stable for the 12 hours preceding discharge.
4. The infant has urinated regularly and has passed stool spontaneously.
5. The infant has completed at least two successful consecutive feedings.
6. No significant bleeding is present at the circumcision site.
7. The clinical risk of development of subsequent hyperbilirubinemia has been assessed, and appropriate management and/or follow-up plans have been instituted.
8. The infant has been adequately evaluated and monitored for sepsis on the basis of maternal risk factors and in accordance with current guidelines for prevention of perinatal Group B streptococcal disease.
9. Maternal blood test and screening results are available and have been reviewed, including those for maternal syphilis, hepatitis B surface antigen status, and a test for HIV in accordance with state regulations.
10. Infant blood tests are available and have been reviewed, such as cord or infant blood type and direct Coombs test results as clinically indicated.
11. Newborn metabolic and hearing screenings have been completed per hospital protocol and state regulations.
12. The mother's knowledge, ability, and confidence to provide adequate care for her infant have been assessed for competency regarding:
    • Breastfeeding or bottle feeding (the breastfeeding mother and infant should be assessed by trained staff regarding breastfeeding position, latch-on, and adequacy of swallowing)
    • The importance and benefits of breastfeeding for both mother and infant
    • Appropriate urination and defecation frequency for the infant

• Cord, skin, and genital care for the infant, including circumcision care
• The ability to recognize signs of illness and common infant problems, particularly jaundice
• Infant safety (such as use of an appropriate car safety seat, supine positioning for sleeping, maintaining a smoke-free environment, and room sharing)

13. Family, environmental, and social risk factors have been assessed, and the mother and her other family members have been educated about safe home environment. These risk factors include but are not limited to:
    • Untreated parental substance abuse or positive urine toxicology results in the mother or newborn
    • History of child abuse or neglect
    • Mental illness in a parent who is in the home
    • Lack of social support, particularly for single and first-time mothers
    • Mothers who live in a shelter, a rehabilitation home, or on the street
    • History of domestic violence, particularly during this pregnancy
    • Communicable illness in a parent or other members of the household
    • Adolescent mother, particularly if other above-listed conditions apply
14. A medical home for continuing medical care for the infant has been identified, and a plan for timely communication of pertinent clinical information to the medical home is in place. For newborns discharged less than 48 hours after delivery, an appointment should be made for the infant to be examined by a licensed health care professional, preferably within 48 hours of discharge based on risk factors but no later than 72 hours in most cases.
15. Barriers to adequate follow-up care for the newborn— such as lack of transportation to medical care services, lack of easy access to telephone communication, and non–English-speaking parents—have been assessed and, whenever possible, assistance has been given to the family to make suitable arrangements to address them.

The birth of an infant with a congenital malformation provides another situation in which staff support is essential. Parents' reactions to the birth of a malformed infant follow a predictable course. For most, there is initial shock and denial, a period of sadness and anger, gradual adaptation, and finally an increased satisfaction with and the ability to care for the baby. The parents must be allowed to pass through these stages and, in effect, to mourn the loss of the anticipated normal child.

The death of an infant or a stillborn is a highly stressful family event. This fact has been emphasized by Cullberg,[90] who found that psychiatric disorders developed in 19 of 56 mothers studied 1 to 2 years after the deaths of their neonates. One of the major predispositions was a breakdown of communication between parents. The health care staff needs to encourage the parents to talk with each other, discuss their feelings, and display emotion. The staff should talk with the parents at the time of

death and then several months later to review the findings of the autopsy, answer questions, and see how the family is doing.

Kangaroo Care

As a baby's course proceeds, the nursery staff can help the parents become comfortable with their infant. This can include participation in caretaking as well as skin-to-skin contact with the infant (kangaroo maternal care [KMC]). **In addition to benefits for thermoregulation, in the LBW population (<2500 g), KMC improves rates of mortality, nosocomial infection/ sepsis, and length of hospital stay.** A benefit also may exist for infant growth and breastfeeding rates.[44] Individualized developmentally based care has also shown some benefit for high-risk infants.[91] It is also important for the staff to discuss among themselves any problems that parents may be having as well as to keep a record of visits and phone calls. This approach will allow early intervention to deal with potential problems.

OUTCOME OF NEONATAL INTENSIVE CARE AND THRESHOLD OF VIABILITY

More sophisticated neonatal care has resulted in improved survival of VLBW (<1500 g) infants, in particular those less than 1000 g (Fig. 22-20). Current survival rates are 90% or greater for infants greater than 1000 g and 28 weeks' gestation, 85% at 800 to 1000 g and 26 to 27 weeks' gestation, and nearly 70% to 75% for infants at 700 to 800 g and 25 weeks' gestation, with a considerable drop in survival below 700 g and at less than 25 weeks.[92,93] **Predictions of survival can be significantly improved by consideration of clinical data in addition to birthweight and gestational age.** These data include an appropriate course of antenatal steroids, sex of the baby, and whether the pregnancy is a singleton gestation. It is important to note that survival in terms of best obstetric estimate is greater at very low gestational ages than survival in terms of postnatal assessment of gestational age. **The numbers in terms of best obstetric estimate based on data at the institution of birth should be referred to for antenatal counseling. Alternatively, data from the National Institute of Child Health and Human Development (NICHD) can be referenced as well.** It is critically important when making decisions at the thresholds of viability that a shared understanding is reached among neonatology, obstetrics, and the family. Paramount to that discussion is that improved survival comes with a price, because a variety of morbidities are seen in these infants. **The rate of severe neurologic disability is fairly constant at 10% of all VLBW**

survivors from 1000 to 1500 g. The number increases from 10% to 25% in infants of extremely low birthweight (<1000 g) and is particularly troubling for infants born at less than 25 weeks' gestation. In these infants, approximately half of the survivors have moderate or severe neurosensory disability (Fig. 22-21).[92] **In addition to the increase in severe disability, these infants have an increased rate of lesser disabilities that include deficits in academic achievement, behavior and attention problems, and the need for special education in school** (see Fig. 22-20).[94-96] **Finally, recent information has begun to demonstrate an increase in autism spectrum disorders in preterm infant survivors.[97]** Risk factors for neurologic morbidity include seizures, major intracranial hemorrhage or PVL, severe intrauterine growth restriction (IUGR), NEC, chorioamnionitis in the mother, neonatal infection, need for mechanical ventilation, chronic lung disease (CLD), poor early head growth, retinopathy of prematurity, and low socioeconomic class.

In addition, other morbidities need to be considered. Because the number of survivors weighing less than 1000 g has increased, a reemergence of **retinopathy of prematurity** has been seen. This disorder is caused by retinal vascular proliferation that leads to hemorrhage, scarring, retinal detachment, and blindness. It is triggered by low concentrations of insulin-like growth factor 1 (IGF-1) and relative hyperoxia in the early postnatal period, which leads to delayed retinal vessel growth. Later increases in IGF-1 allow vascular endothelial growth factor (VEGF)–induced angiogenesis and result in an abnormal vascular proliferation.[98]

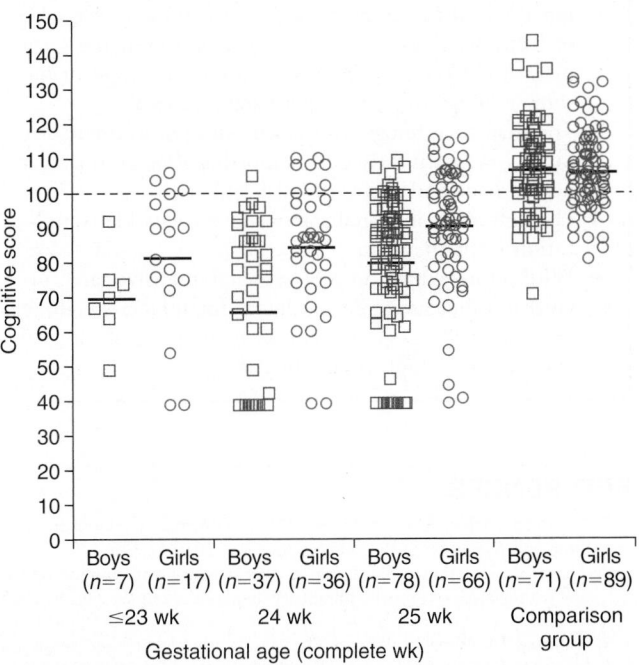

FIG 22-20 Cognitive scores according to sex and completed weeks of gestation at birth for 241 extremely preterm children and 160 age-matched classmates who were full term at birth. The scores are the Kaufman Assessment Battery for Children scores for the Mental Processing Composite or developmental scores according to the Griffiths Scales of Mental Development and NEPSY (a developmental neuropsychological assessment). *Bars* indicate mean scores, and the *dashed line* is the mean of a standardized population. (From Marlow N, Wolke D, Bracewell MA, et al: Neurologic and developmental disability at six years of age after extremely preterm birth. *N Engl J Med.* 2005;352:9.)

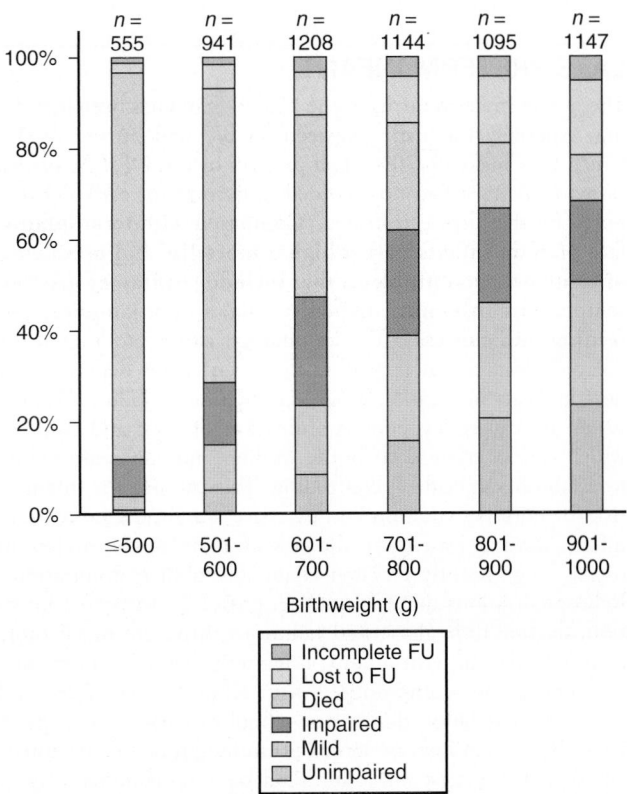

FIG 22-21 Outcomes at 18 and 22 months by birthweight in extremely-low-birthweight infants. FU, follow-up. (From Gargus RA, Vohr BR, Tyson JE, et al. Unimpaired outcomes for extremely low birth weight infants at 18 to 22 months. *Pediatrics.* 2009;124:112.)

Incidence of acute proliferative retinopathy by birthweight is less than 10% in infants who weigh more than 1250 g, 20% in those 1000 to 1250 g, 50% to 60% in those 750 to 1000 g, and 70% in those less than 750 g.[73] Severe retinopathy is evident in 5% of the infants 1000 to 1250 g, in 10% of infants 750 to 1000 g, and in 25% to 40% of infants less than 750 g. Of the infants with severe retinopathy, 10% (4% of the total population) will go on to have severe visual problems. The other major neurosensory morbidity is hearing loss, which occurs in 2% of NICU survivors. Other sequelae of neonatal intensive care include CLD, growth failure, short gut, and need for postdischarge rehospitalization.

The information presented earlier on outcome is relevant to discussions about obstetric and neonatal intervention at the threshold of viability. **If the end point of survival without major disability is considered, this occurs in 0% at 22 weeks, less than 10% at 23 weeks, approximately 20% to 25% at 24 weeks, and approximately 45% to 50% at 25 weeks.**[92,93] With this information in mind, most neonatologists believe that care is clearly beneficial beyond 25 completed weeks, whereas less than half believe that care is beneficial at 24 to 24 6/7 weeks, and even fewer feel care is beneficial at less than 24 completed weeks. That said, more than half would intervene on behalf of an infant beyond 23 weeks' gestation. These discussions need to be modified depending on circumstances. For instance, morbidity and mortality would increase in the face of overt infection or severe IUGR. **A reasonable approach would seem to be to encourage interventions on behalf of a fetus or newborn beyond 25 completed weeks' gestation and to not intervene at less than 23 weeks' gestation. The range between 23 and 25 weeks should be evaluated on a case-by-case basis.**

LATE PRETERM INFANT

The rate of preterm births in the United States has been increasing, especially for births between 34 0/7 and 36 6/7 weeks, which now make up 70% of all preterm births. Of these births, as many as 23% had no recorded indication for early delivery noted on the birth certificate.[99] **Compared with term infants, late preterm infants have a higher mortality and prevalence of acute neonatal problems that include respiratory distress, temperature instability, hypoglycemia, apnea, jaundice, and feeding difficulties.**[97] The respiratory issues are caused by delayed clearance of fetal lung fluid, surfactant deficiency, or both and can on occasion progress to respiratory failure. Feeding issues are caused by poor coordination of suck and swallow, which can interfere with bottle feeding and can cause failure to establish successful breastfeeding. This can put the infant at risk for both dehydration and excessive jaundice. Late preterm infants have at least twice the risk of an infant born at term to have significantly elevated serum bilirubin concentrations. Rehospitalizations due to jaundice, proven or suspected infection, feeding difficulties, and failure to thrive are much more common than in term infants. Long-term neurodevelopmental outcome is also compromised with reports of cognitive and emotional regulation difficulties, school problems, and slightly lower IQs.[100] An increase in deficits in lung function are apparent that may persist into adulthood because of immaturity of the respiratory system at birth.[101]

Late preterm infants, even if similar in size to their term counterparts, should be considered preterm, rather than near term, and need close in-hospital monitoring for potential

complications. Discharge of these babies should be delayed until they have demonstrated reliable oral intake and resolution of any acute neonatal problems. The initial outpatient follow-up visit should occur within 48 to 72 hours of discharge.

KEY POINTS

♦ Surfactant maintains lung expansion on expiration by lowering surface tension at the air-liquid interface in the alveolus.

♦ Respiratory distress syndrome in premature infants is in part caused by a deficiency of surfactant and can be treated with surfactant replacement therapy.

♦ Antenatal corticosteroids accelerate fetal lung maturation and decrease neonatal mortality and respiratory distress syndrome in preterm infants. In addition, corticosteroids are associated with a decrease in intracranial hemorrhage and necrotizing enterocolitis.

♦ Transition from intrauterine to extrauterine life requires removal of fluid from the lungs, switching from fetal to neonatal circulation, and establishment of a normal neonatal lung volume.

♦ The most important step in neonatal resuscitation is to achieve adequate expansion of the lungs.

♦ Meconium aspiration syndrome is likely the result of intrauterine asphyxia with mortality related to associated persistent pulmonary hypertension.

♦ The best predictor of neurologic sequelae of birth asphyxia is the presence of hypoxic ischemic encephalopathy in the neonatal period. The neurologic sequelae of birth asphyxia is cerebral palsy. However, the great majority of cerebral palsy is of unknown origin or has some etiology other than perinatal asphyxia.

♦ The major neurologic complications seen in premature infants are periventricular hemorrhage/intraventricular hemorrhage and periventricular leukomalacia.

♦ Hypoglycemia is a predictable and preventable complication in the newborn.

♦ With improved methods of neonatal intensive care, survival has increased—in particular for infants weighing less than 1000 g—but it comes at the price of medical and neurodevelopmental sequelae.

REFERENCES

1. Smith LJ, McKay KO, van Asperen PP, et al. Normal development of the lung and premature birth. *Pediatr Respir Rev.* 2010;11:135.
2. Stenmark KR, Abman SH. Lung vascular development: implications for the pathogenesis of bronchopulmonary dysplasia. *Annu Rev Physiol.* 2005; 67:623.
3. Whitsett JA, Wert SE, Weaver TE. Alveolar surfactant homeostasis and the pathogenesis of pulmonary disease. *Annu Rev Med.* 2010;61:105.
4. Gross I, Ballard PL. Hormonal therapy for prevention of respiratory distress syndrome. In: Polin RA, Fox WW, Abman SH, eds. *Fetal and Neonatal Physiology.* 3rd ed. Philadelphia: WB Saunders; 2004:1069.
5. Crowley PA. Antenatal corticosteroid therapy: a meta-analysis of the randomized trials, 1972-1994. *Am J Obstet Gynecol.* 1995;173:322.
6. Tyson JE, Parikh NA, Langer J, et al. Intensive care for extreme prematurity—moving beyond gestational age. *N Engl J Med.* 2008;358: 1672.
7. Schmand B, Neuvel J, Smolders-de-Haas H, et al. Psychological development of children who were treated antenatally with corticosteroids to prevent respiratory distress syndrome. *Pediatrics.* 1990;86:58.

8. Smolders-de-Haas H, Neuvel J, Schmand B, et al. Physical development and medical history of children who were treated antenatally with corticosteroids to prevent respiratory distress syndrome: a 10- to 12-year follow-up. *Pediatrics.* 1990;86:65.

9. Engle WA, the AAP Committee on Fetus and Newborn. Surfactant-replacement therapy for respiratory distress in the preterm and term neonate. *Pediatrics.* 2008;121:419.

10. Jobe AH, Mitchell BR, Gunkel JH. Beneficial effects of the combined use of prenatal corticosteroids and postnatal surfactant on preterm infants. *Am J Obstet Gynecol.* 1993;168:508.

11. Kaplan M. Fetal breathing movements, an update for the pediatrician. *Am J Dis Child.* 1983;137:177.

12. Agostoni E, Taglietti A, Agostoni AF. Setnikar I: Mechanical aspects of the first breath. *J Appl Physiol.* 1958;13:344.

13. Milner AD, Vyas H. Lung expansion at birth. *J Pediatr.* 1982;101:879.

14. Arjan B, Pas TE, Davis PG, et al. From liquid to air: breathing after birth. *J Pediatr.* 2008;152:607.

15. Barker PM, Southern KW. Regulation of liquid secretion and absorption by the fetal and neonatal lung. In: Polin RA, Fox WW, Abman SH, eds. *Fetal and Neonatal Physiology.* 3rd ed. Philadelphia: WB Saunders; 2004:822.

16. Helve O, Pitkanen O, Janer C, Andersson S. Pulmonary fluid balance in the human newborn infant. *Neonatology.* 2009;95:347.

17. Rudolph AM. Fetal circulation and cardiovascular adjustments after birth. In: Rudolph CD, Rudolph AM, Hostetter MK, et al., eds. *Rudolph's Pediatrics.* 21st ed. New York: McGraw-Hill; 2003:1749.

18. Adamson SL, Myatt L, Byrne BMP. Regulation of umbilical flow. In: Polin RA, Fox WW, Abman SH, eds. *Fetal and Neonatal Physiology.* 3rd ed. Philadelphia: WB Saunders; 2004:748.

19. Steinhorn RH. Neonatal pulmonary hypertension. *Pediatr Crit Care Med.* 2010;11:S79.

20. Hamrick SEG, Hansmann G. Patent ductus arteriosus of the preterm infant. *Pediatrics.* 2010;125:1020.

21. Dawes GS. *Foetal and Neonatal Physiology.* Chicago: Year Book; 1968.

22. American Heart Association and American Academy of Pediatrics. *Neonatal Resuscitation Textbook.* American Academy of Pediatrics and American Heart Association, Elk Grove, IL; 2011.

23. Saugstad OD, Ramji S, Soll RF, Vento M. Resuscitation of newborn infants with 21% or 100% oxygen: an updated systematic review and meta-analysis. *Neonatology.* 2008;94:176.

24. Vento M, Saugstad OD. Resuscitation of the term and preterm infant. *Semin Fetal Neonatal Med.* 2010;15:216.

25. Mariani G, Brener P, Ezquer A. Pre-ductal and post-ductal O2 saturation in healthy term neonates after birth. *J Pediatr.* 2007;150:418.

26. Trevisanuto D, Doglioni N, Cavallin F, et al. Heat loss prevention in very preterm infants in delivery rooms: a prospective, randomized trial of polyethylene caps. *J Pediatr.* 2010;156:914.

27. Nuntnarumit P, Rojnueangnit K, Tangnoo A. Oxygen saturation trends in preterm infants during the first 15 minutes after birth. *J Perinatol.* 2010;30:399.

28. Velaphi S, Vidyasagar D. Intrapartum and postdelivery management of infants born to mothers with meconium-stained amniotic fluid: evidence-based recommendations. *Clin Perinatol.* 2006;33:29.

29. Wiswell TE, Gannon CM, Jacob J, et al. Delivery room management of the apparently vigorous meconium-stained neonate: results of the multi-center international collaborative trial. *Pediatrics.* 2000;105:1.

30. Vain NE, Szyld EG, Wiswell TE, et al. Oropharyngeal and nasopharyngeal suctioning of meconium-stained neonates before delivery of their shoulders: multicentre, randomized controlled trial. *Lancet.* 2004;364:597.

31. Rabe H, Diaz-Rossello JL, Duley L, Dowswell T. Effect of timing of umbilical cord clamping and other strategies to influence placental transfusion at preterm birth on maternal and infant outcomes. *Cochrane Database of Syst Rev.* 2013;(7):CD004074.

32. McDonald SJ, Middleton P, Dowswell T, Morris PS. Effect of timing of umbilical cord clamping of term infants on maternal and neonatal outcomes. *Cochrane Database Syst Rev.* 2013;(7):CD004074.

33. Committee on Obstetric Practice, American College of Obstetricians and Gynecologists. Committee Opinion No. 543: Timing of umbilical cord clamping after birth. *Obstet Gynecol.* 2012;120:1522.

34. Bailit JL, Gregory KD, Reddy UM, et al. Maternal and neonatal outcomes by labor onset type and gestational age. *Am J Obstet Gynecol.* 2010;202:245e1.

35. Azzopardi D, Strohm B, Marlow N, et al. Effects of Hypothermia for Perinatal Asphyxia on Childhood Outcomes. *N Engl J Med.* 2014;371:140.

36. Shankaran S, Pappas A, McDonald SA, et al. Childhood Outcomes after Hypothermia for Neonatal Encephalopathy. *N Engl J Med.* 2012;366:2085.

37. Jacobs SE, Berg M, Hunt R, et al. Cooling newborns with hypoxic ischaemic encephalopathy. *Cochrane Database Syst Rev.* 2013;(1):CD003311.

38. Flidel-Rimon O, Shinwell ES. Neonatal aspects of the relationship between intrapartum events and cerebral palsy. *Clin Perinatol.* 2007;34:439.

39. American College of Obstetricians and Gynecologists. *American Academy of Pediatrics: Neonatal encephalopathy and neurologic outcome.* Washington, DC: ACOG; 2014.

40. Rosenberg AA. Traumatic birth injury. *Neoreviews.* 2003;4:e273.

41. Volpe JJ, ed. Intracranial hemorrhage: subdural, primary subarachnoid, intracerebellar, intraventricular (term infant) and miscellaneous. In: *Neurology of the Newborn.* 4th ed. Philadelphia: WB Saunders; 2001:397.

42. Sahni R, Schulze K. Temperature control in newborn infants. In: Polin RA, Fox WW, Abman SH, eds. *Fetal and Neonatal Physiology.* 3rd ed. Philadelphia: WB Saunders; 2004:548.

43. Scopes JW. Metabolic rate and temperature control in the human body. *Br Med Bull.* 1966;22:88.

44. Conde-Agudelo A, Diaz-Rossello JL. Kangaroo mother care to reduce morbidity and mortality in low birthweight infants. *Cochrane Database Syst Rev.* 2014;(4):CD002771.

45. Heinig MJ. Host defense benefits of breast feeding for the infant: effect of breast-feeding duration and exclusivity. *Pediatr Clin North Am.* 2001;48:105.

46. Heiman H, Schanler RJ. Enteral nutrition for premature infants: the role of human milk. *Semin Fetal Neonatal Med.* 2007;12:26.

47. Patel AL, Meier PP, Engstrom JL. The evidence for use of human milk in very low-birthweight preterm infants. *Neoreviews.* 2007;8:e459.

48. Sullivan S, Schanler RJ, Kim JH, et al. An exclusively human milk-based diet is associated with a lower rate of necrotizing enterocolitis than a diet of human milk and bovine milk-based products. *J Pediatr.* 2010;156:562.

49. Cristofalo EA, Schanler RJ, Blanco CL, et al. Randomized trial of exclusive human milk versus preterm formula diets in extremely premature infants. *J Pediatr.* 2013;163:1592.

50. McGowan J. Neonatal hypoglycemia. *NeoReviews.* 1999;20:e6.

51. Collins JE, Leonard JV. Hyperinsulinism in asphyxiated and small-for-dates infants with hypoglycemia. *Lancet.* 1984;8398:311.

52. Hoe FM, Thornton PS, Wanner LA, et al. Clinical features and insulin regulation in infants with a syndrome of prolonged neonatal hyperinsulinism. *J Pediatr.* 2006;148:207.

53. Rozance P, Hay WW. Hypoglycemia in newborn infants: features associated with adverse outcomes. *Biol Neonate.* 2006;90:74.

54. Neu J, Walker WA. Necrotizing enterocolitis. *N Engl J Med.* 2011;364:255.

55. Abrahamsson TR, Rautava S, Moore AM, et al. The time for a confirmative necrotizing enterocolitis probiotics prevention trial in the extremely low birthweight infant in North America is now! *J Pediatr.* 2014;165:389.

56. Murthy K, Yanowitz TD, DiGeronimo R, et al. Short-term outcomes for preterm infants with surgical necrotizing enterocolitis. *J Perinatol.* 2014;34:736.

57. Cashore WJ. Bilirubin metabolism and toxicity in the newborn. In: Polin RA, Fox WW, Abman SH, eds. *Fetal and Neonatal Physiology.* 3rd ed. Philadelphia: WB Saunders; 2004:1199.

58. American Academy of Pediatrics Subcommittee on Hyperbilirubinemia. Management of hyperbilirubinemia in the newborn infant 35 or more weeks of gestation. *Pediatrics.* 2004;114:297.

59. Maisals MJ, Bhutani VK, Bogen D. Hyperbilirubinemia in the newborn infant ≥ 35 weeks gestation: an update with clarifications. *Pediatrics.* 2009;124:1193.

60. Watchko JF. Hyperbilirubinemia and bilirubin toxicity in the late preterm infant. *Clin Perinatol.* 2006;33:839.

61. Watchko JF, Tiribelli C. Bilirubin-induced neurologic damage—mechanisms and management approaches. *N Engl J Med.* 2013;369:2012.

62. Widness JA. Pathophysiology, diagnosis, and prevention of neonatal anemia. *Neoreviews.* 2000;1:e61.

63. Schimmel MS, Bromiker R, Soll RF. Neonatal polycythemia: is partial exchange transfusion justified? *Clin Perinatol.* 2004;31:545.

64. Bussel JB, Sola-Visner M. Current approaches to the evaluation and management of the fetus and neonate with immune thrombocytopenia. *Semin Perinatol.* 2009;33:35.

65. American Academy of Pediatrics Committee on the Fetus and Newborn. Controversies concerning vitamin K and the newborn. *Pediatrics.* 2003;112:191.

66. Wynn JL, Levy O. Role of innate host defenses in susceptibility to early-onset neonatal sepsis. *Clin Perinatol.* 2010;37:307.

67. Verani JR, Schrag SJ. Group B streptococcal disease in infants: progress in prevention and continued challenges. *Clin Perinatol.* 2010;37:375.

68. vanDyke MK, Phares CR, Lynfield R, et al. Evaluation of universal antenatal screening for group B Streptococcus. *N Engl J Med.* 2009;360:25.

69. Silberbach M, Hannan D. Presentation of congenital heart disease in the neonate and young infant. *Pediatr Rev.* 2007;28:123.

70. Mahle WT, Martin GR, Beekman RH, et al. Endorsement of Health and Human Services Recommendation for Pulse Oximetry Screening for Critical Congenital Heart Disease. *Pediatrics.* 2012;129:190.

71. Reuter S, Moser C, Baack M. Respiratory distress in the newborn. *Pediatr Rev.* 2014;35:417.

72. Avery ME, Mead J. Surface properties in relation to atelectasis and hyaline membrane disease. *Am J Dis Child.* 1959;97:517.

73. Vermont Oxford Neonatal Network. *Vermont Oxford Network Annual VLBW Database Summary 2003.* Burlington: Vermont Oxford Network; 2004.

74. Laptook AR, et al. Adverse neurodevelopmental outcome among extremely low birth weight infants with normal head ultrasound: prevalence and antecedents. *Pediatrics.* 2005;115:673.

75. Patra K, Wilson-Costello D, Taylor HG, et al. Grades I-II intraventricular hemorrhage in extremely low birth weight infants: effects on neurodevelopment. *J Pediatr.* 2006;149:169.

76. Lowe J, Papille LA. Neurodevelopmental performance of very-low-birth-weight infants with mild periventricular, intraventricular hemorrhage. Outcome at 5 to 6 years of age. *Am J Dis Child.* 1990;144:1242.

77. Brouwer A, et al. Neurodevelopmental outcome of preterm infants with severe intraventricular hemorrhage and therapy for post-hemorrhagic ventricular dilation. *Pediatrics.* 2008;152:648.

78. Bolisetty S, Dhawan A, Abdel-Latif M, et al. Intraventricular hemorrhage and neurodevelopmental outcomes in extreme preterm infants. *Pediatrics.* 2014;133:55.

79. Doyle LW, Crowther CA, Middleton P, et al. Magnesium sulphate for women at risk of preterm birth for neuroprotection of the fetus. *Cochrane Database Syst Rev.* 2009;(1):Art. No.: CD004661.

80. Doyle LW, Anderson PJ, Haslam R, et al. School-age Outcomes of Very Preterm Infants After Antenatal Treatment With Magnesium Sulfate vs Placebo. *JAMA.* 2014;312:1105.

81. Ballard JL, Khoury JC, Wedig K, et al. New Ballard Score, expanded to include extremely premature infants. *J Pediatr.* 1991;119:417.

82. Lubchenco LO, Hansman C, Boyd E. Intrauterine growth in length and head circumference as estimated from live births at gestational ages from 26 to 42 weeks. *Pediatrics.* 1966;37:403.

83. Rosenberg A. The IUGR newborn. *Semin Perinatol.* 2008;32:219.

84. Stark AR. American Academy of Pediatrics Committee on Fetus and Newborn: Levels of neonatal care. *Pediatrics.* 2004;114:1341.

85. Phibbs CS, Baker LC, Caughey AB, et al. Level and Volume of Neonatal Intensive Care and Mortality in Very-Low-Birth-Weight Infants. *N Engl J Med.* 2007;356:2165.

86. Lorch SA, Baiocchi M, Ahlberg CE, Small DS. The Differential Impact of Delivery Hospital on the Outcomes of Premature Infants. *Pediatrics.* 2012;130:270.

87. American Academy of Pediatrics Task Force on Sudden Infant Death Syndrome. The changing concept of sudden infant death syndrome: diagnostic coding shifts, controversies regarding the sleeping environment, and new variables to consider in reducing risk. *Pediatrics.* 2005;116:1245.

88. American Academy of Pediatrics Committee on Fetus and Newborn. Policy statement—hospital stay for healthy term newborns. *Pediatrics.* 2010;125:405.

89. Klaus MH, Kennel JH. Care of the parents. In: Klaus MH, Fanaroff AA, eds. *Care of the High-Risk Neonate.* 5th ed. Philadelphia: WB Saunders; 2001:195.

90. Cullberg J. Mental reactions of women to perinatal death. In: Morris N, ed. *Psychosomatic Medicines in Obstetrics and Gynecology.* New York: S Karger; 1972:326.

91. Peters KL, Rosychuk RJ, Hendson L, et al. Improvement of short- and long-term outcomes for very low birth weight infants: Edmonton NIDCAP trial. *Pediatrics.* 2009;124:1009.

92. Gargus RA, Vohr BR, Tyson JE, et al. Unimpaired outcomes for extremely low birth weight infants at 18-22 months. *Pediatrics.* 2009;124:112.

93. Stoll BJ, Hansen NI, Bell EF, et al. Neonatal outcomes of extremely preterm infants from the NICHD neonatal research network. *Pediatrics.* 2010;126:443.

94. Aarnoudse-Moens CS, Weisglas-Kuperus N, van Goudoever JB, Oosterlaan J. Meta-analysis of neurobehavioral outcomes in very preterm and/or very low birth weight children. *Pediatrics.* 2009;124:717.

95. Hutchinson EA, DeLuca CR, Doyle LW. School-age outcomes of extremely preterm or extremely low birth weight children. *Pediatrics.* 2013;131:e1053.

96. Lampi PM, Lehtonen L, Tran PL, et al. Risk of autism spectrum disorders in low birth weight and small for gestational age infants. *J Pediatr.* 2012; 161:830.

97. Ananth CV, Friedman AM, Gyamfi-Bannerman C. Epidemiology of moderate preterm, late preterm and early term delivery. *Clin Perinatol.* 2013; 40:601.

98. Fleck BW, McIntosh N. Retinopathy of prematurity: recent developments. *Neoreviews.* 2009;10:e20.

99. Reddy UM, Ko CW, Raju TN, Willinger M. Delivery indications at late-preterm gestations and infant mortality rate in the United States. *Pediatrics.* 2009;124:234.

100. vanBaar AL, Vermaas J, Knots E, et al. Functioning at school age of moderately preterm children born at 32 to 36 weeks gestational age. *Pediatrics.* 2009;124:251.

101. Colin AA, McEvoy C, Castile RG. Respiratory morbidity and lung function in preterm infants of 32 to 36 weeks gestational age. *Pediatrics.* 2010;126:115.

Additional references for this chapter are available at ExpertConsult.com.

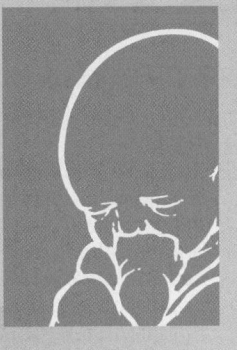

CHAPTER 23

Postpartum Care and Long-Term Health Considerations

MICHELLE M. ISLEY and VERN L. KATZ

KEY ABBREVIATIONS

Bone mineral density	BMD
Combination oral contraceptive	COC
Combined hormonal contraception	CHC
Deep venous thrombosis	DVT
Depot medroxyprogesterone acetate	DMPA
Emergency contraception	EC
Edinburgh postnatal depression scale	EPDS
Etonogestrel	ETG
Follicle-stimulating hormone	FSH
Human immunodeficiency virus	HIV
Intrauterine device	IUD
Levonorgestrel	LNG
Long-acting reversible contraception	LARC
Pelvic floor muscle training	PFMT
Postpartum thyroiditis	PPT
Postpartum depression	PPD
Progestin-only oral contraception	POP
Pulmonary embolus	PE
Sexually transmitted infections	STIs
Venous thromboembolism	VTE

The postpartum period is associated with as much tradition and superstition as any other rite of passage in life because the health of a new infant is so important to the survival of any family or clan. In order to support the successful recovery of the mother and a healthy transition through the neonatal period, customs, taboos, and rituals have developed in most cultures. Indeed, many of the current medical recommendations for the puerperium have developed from adaptations of socially acceptable traditions rather than from science. For example, the 6-week postpartum checkup approximates the end of the 40 days of rest and sexual separation required in traditional societies.

Cultures throughout the world have specific postpartum traditions that include both restrictions on activity and prescribed activities, different foods for the newly delivered mother, and particular and unique taboos regarding postpartum care (Box 23-1, e-Fig. 23-1). For example, bathing after delivery is taboo in some cultures. Because women often cherish these rituals, it is essential for physicians, midwives, and nurses to be sensitive to these customs even though a woman's place of delivery may be far from her native country.

This chapter examines the normal physiologic changes of the puerperium and the transitions to prepregnancy physiology. With respect to these changes, we evaluate the principles and practices of postpartum care and the role of the provider in helping the patient through the transition. We will also discuss the major puerperal disease states, health maintenance postpartum, and pregnancy prevention.

POSTPARTUM INVOLUTION

Uterus

The crude weight of the pregnant uterus at term—excluding the fetus, placenta, membranes, and amniotic fluid—is about 1000 g, approximately 10 to 20 times heavier than the nonpregnant uterus.[1] **The specific time course of uterine involution**

The postpartum period, also called the *puerperium,* lasts from delivery of the placenta until 6 to 12 weeks afterward. Most of the physiology that has changed in pregnancy will have returned to its prepregnancy state by 6 weeks. However, **many of the cardiovascular changes and psychological changes may persist for many more months; and some, such as changes in the pelvic musculature and cardiac remodeling, will last for years.**

BOX 23-1   EXAMPLES OF POSTPARTUM RITUALS

Cultural practices in regard to postpartum activity are found worldwide:

- In the rural Philippines, the mother, who works until she goes into labor, is prohibited from working after delivery, and she is given a new name. The maternal grandmother visits daily and does the housework and cooking for 8 weeks. The mother is bathed by the grandmother daily. When the umbilical cord falls off the infant, a feast is prepared, and the cord is blessed at the feast. The new father is prohibited from building stone walls and from driving nails for 6 months. For 2 months, relatives tend the fields.

Postpartum taboos related to *hot and cold* are found worldwide:

- In some Asian, African, and Latin American cultures, heat and cold must be maintained in balance to promote health and prevent disease. Because blood, which is "hot," is lost during delivery, the parturient must replenish her "heat" by staying bundled and drinking warm liquids.
- In several traditional Middle Eastern areas, it is believed that exposure to cold creates a vulnerability to disease. Bathing is often taboo for traditional women, and sponge baths may be substituted.
- In parts of rural India, the new mother returns to her mother's house for 16 weeks. She is given a hot bath every day. Cold baths are taboo because cold water is associated with disease.

Many cultures have rituals regarding treatment of the placenta and umbilical cord:

- The placenta may be dried and turned to powder for its "medicinal" powers.
- The umbilical cord was hung in a nearby tree by some eastern Native American tribes.
- In Eastern European tradition, in order to ensure prosperity, the cord was buried under specific corners of the house.

has not been fully elucidated, but within 2 weeks after birth, the uterus has usually returned to the pelvis, and by 6 weeks, it is usually normal size as estimated by palpation. The gross anatomic and histologic characteristics of the involutional process are based on the study of autopsy, hysterectomy, and endometrial biopsy specimens.[2] The decrease in the size of the uterus and cervix during the puerperium has been demonstrated with serial magnetic resonance imaging (MRI).[3] The findings are consistent with those of serial sonography and computed tomography (CT).

Immediately after delivery, the rapidly decreasing endometrial surface area facilitates placental shearing at the decidual layer. The average diameter of the placenta is 18 cm; in the immediate postpartum uterus, the average diameter of the site of placental attachment measures 9 cm. In the first 3 days after delivery, the placental site is infiltrated with granulocytes and mononuclear cells, a reaction that extends into the endometrium and superficial myometrium. By the seventh day, the regeneration of endometrial glands is evident, and they often appear atypical with irregular chromatin patterns, misshapen and enlarged nuclei, pleomorphism, and increased cytoplasm. By the end of the first week, regeneration of the endometrial stroma is also evident, and mitotic figures are noted in gland epithelium; by postpartum day 16, the endometrium is fully restored.

Decidual necrosis begins on the first day, and by the seventh day, a well-demarcated zone can be seen between necrotic and viable tissue. An area of viable decidua remains between the necrotic slough and the deeper endomyometrium. Sharman[2] described how the nonnecrotic decidual cells participate in the reconstruction of the endometrium, a likely role given their original role as endometrial connective tissue cells. By the sixth week, decidual cells are rare. The immediate inflammatory cell infiltrate of polymorphonuclear leukocytes and lymphocytes persists for about 10 days and presumably serves as an antibacterial barrier. The leukocyte response diminishes rapidly after day 10, and plasma cells are seen for the first time. The plasma cell and lymphocyte response may last as long as several months. In fact, endometrial stromal infiltrates of plasma cells and lymphocytes are a sign, and they may be the only sign, of a recent pregnancy.

Hemostasis immediately after birth is accomplished by arterial smooth muscle contraction and compression of vessels by the involuting uterine muscle. Vessels in the placental site are characterized during the first 8 days by thrombosis, hyalinization, and endophlebitis in the veins and by hyalinization and obliterative fibrinoid endarteritis in the arteries. The mechanism for hyalinization of arterial walls, which is not completely understood, may be related to the previous trophoblastic infiltration of arterial walls that occurs early in pregnancy. Many of the thrombosed and hyalinized veins are extruded with the slough of the necrotic placental site, but hyalinized arteries remain for extended periods as stigmata of the placental site. Restoration of the endometrium in areas other than the placental site occurs rapidly, a process that is complete by day 16 after delivery. The gland epithelium does not undergo the reactivity, nor does it take on the pseudoneoplastic appearance noted in glands at the placental site.

The postpartum uterine discharge, or *lochia,* begins as a flow of blood that lasts several hours, then rapidly diminishes to a reddish brown discharge through the third or fourth day postpartum. This is followed by a transition to a mucopurulent, somewhat malodorous discharge called *lochia serosa,* which requires several perineal pad changes per day. The median duration of lochia serosa is 22 to 27 days.[4,5] However, 10% to 15% of women will have lochia serosa at the time of the 6-week postpartum examination. In most patients, the lochia serosa is followed by a yellow-white discharge, called *lochia alba.* Breastfeeding or the use of oral contraceptive agents does not affect the duration of lochia. **Frequently, a sudden but transient increase is observed in uterine bleeding between 7 and 14 days postpartum.** This corresponds to the slough of the eschar over the site of placental attachment. Myometrial vessels greater than 5 mm in diameter are present for up to 2 weeks postpartum and account for the dramatic bleeding that can occur with this phenomenon.[5] **Although it can be profuse, this bleeding episode is usually self-limited and requires nothing more than reassurance of the patient.** If it does not subside within 1 or 2 hours, the patient should be evaluated for possible retained placental tissue.

Ultrasound may be helpful in the management of abnormal postpartum bleeding. The empty uterus with a clear midline echo can often be distinguished from the uterine cavity expanded by clot (sonolucent) or retained tissue (echo dense; Fig. 23-1).[6] Serial ultrasound examinations of postpartum patients showed that in 20% to 30%, some retained blood or tissue was apparent within 24 hours after delivery. By the fourth postpartum day,

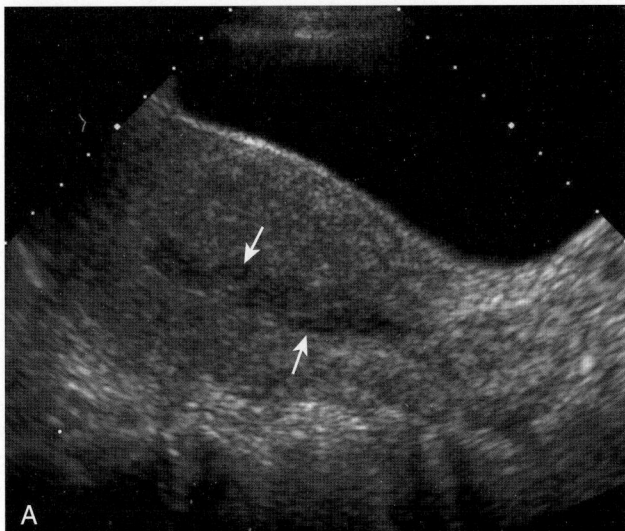

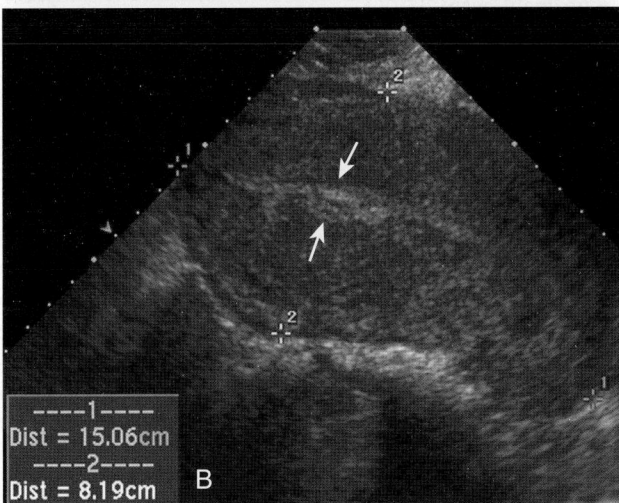

```
----1----
Dist = 15.06cm
----2----
Dist = 8.19cm
```

FIG 23-1 A, Sonogram of a normal postpartum uterus. **B,** Postpartum uterus with retained tissue. (From Poder L. Ultrasound evaluation of the Uterus. In Callen PW: *Ultrasonography in Obstetrics and Gynecology,* 5th ed. Philadelphia: Saunders; 2000:939, 940.)

only about 8% of patients showed endometrial cavity separation, a proportion of whom eventually had abnormal postpartum bleeding because of retained placental tissue.[7] **In cases of abnormal postpartum bleeding, ultrasound examination may be a useful adjunct in detecting patients who have retained tissue or clot and who will therefore benefit from uterine evacuation and curettage.** Those who have an empty uterine cavity may respond to therapy with oxytocin or methylergonovine.[8]

Cervix

During pregnancy, the cervical epithelium increases in thickness, and the cervical glands show both hyperplasia and hypertrophy. Within the stroma, a distinct decidual reaction occurs. These changes are accompanied by a substantial increase in the vascularity of the cervix. Colposcopic examination performed after delivery has demonstrated ulceration, laceration, and ecchymosis of the cervix. Regression of the cervical epithelium begins within the first 4 days after delivery, and by the end of the first week, edema and hemorrhage within the cervix are minimal. Vascular hypertrophy and hyperplasia persist throughout the first week postpartum. By 6 weeks, most of the antepartum

changes have resolved, although round cell infiltration and some edema may persist for several months.

Fallopian Tube

The epithelium of the fallopian tube during pregnancy is characterized by a predominance of nonciliated cells, a phenomenon maintained by the balance between the high levels of progesterone and estrogen. After delivery, in the absence of progesterone and estrogen, further extrusion of nuclei from nonciliated cells occurs along with diminution in height of both ciliated and nonciliated cells. The number and height of ciliated cells can be increased in the puerperium by treatment with estrogen.

Fallopian tubes removed between postpartum days 5 and 15 demonstrate inflammatory changes of acute salpingitis in 38% of cases, but no bacteria are found. The specific cause of the inflammatory change is unknown. Furthermore, no correlation has been found between the presence of histologic inflammation in the fallopian tubes and puerperal fever or other clinical signs of salpingitis.

Ovarian Function

Most women who breastfeed their infants are amenorrheic for extended periods of time, often until the infant is weaned. Using a variety of methods to indicate ovulation, several studies have demonstrated that **ovulation occurs as early as 27 days after delivery, with the mean time being about 70 to 75 days in nonlactating women.**[9] **Among women who are breastfeeding their infants, the mean time to ovulation is about 6 months.**

Menstruation resumes by 12 weeks postpartum in 70% of women who are not lactating. The mean time to the first menstruation is 7 to 9 weeks. Depending on the population, as well as social and nutritional factors of the lactating woman, regular menstruation may be delayed as long as 36 months. The duration of anovulation depends on the frequency of breastfeeding, the duration of each feed, and the proportion of supplementary feeds.[10] **In a woman exclusively breastfeeding, the likelihood of ovulation within the first 6 months postpartum is 1% to 5%.**

The hormonal basis for puerperal ovulation suppression in lactating women appears to be the persistence of elevated serum prolactin levels. Prolactin levels fall to the normal range by the third week postpartum in nonlactating women but remain elevated into the sixth week in lactating women. Estrogen levels fall immediately after delivery in both lactating and nonlactating women and remain depressed in lactating patients. In those who are not lactating, estrogen levels begin to rise 2 weeks after delivery and are significantly higher than in lactating women by postpartum day 17. Follicle-stimulating hormone (FSH) levels are identical in breastfeeding and nonbreastfeeding women, which suggests that the ovary does not respond to FSH stimulation in the presence of increased prolactin levels.

Weight Loss

One of the most welcome changes for most women who have recently given birth is the loss of the weight that was gained during pregnancy. The immediate loss of 10 to 13 lb is attributed to the delivery of the infant, placenta, and amniotic fluid and to blood loss. However, most women will not manifest that loss until 1 to 2 weeks after delivery because of postpartum fluid retention. The physiologic stress of labor and delivery induces hormonal changes, including increased antidiuretic hormone, that lead to a short period of sodium and water retention. With operative birth or epidural anesthesia with fluid boluses, the total body water increases dramatically. Mild pedal edema is also common as the extra fluid moves temporarily into the third space. Women may be reassured that this temporary dependent edema is secondary to this fluid retention. The short period of weight gain from fluid retention that occurs immediately after delivery is sometimes referred to as the *ebb phase* of physiologic response. The diuresis at 4 to 7 days is sometimes called the *flow phase*. It is not uncommon to have a newly delivered mother express mild anxiety about "gaining weight "after delivery.

For most women, weight loss postpartum does not tend to compensate for weight gain during gestation. By 6 weeks postpartum, only 28% of women will have returned to their prepregnant weight. The remainder of any weight loss occurs from 6 weeks postpartum until 6 months after delivery, with most weight loss concentrated in the first 3 months. **Women with excess weight gain in pregnancy (>35 lb) are likely to have a net gain of 11 lb.** Breastfeeding has relatively little effect on postpartum weight loss. With a program of diet and exercise, weight loss of about 0.5 kg/week between 4 and 14 weeks in overweight breastfeeding women did not affect the growth of their infants.[11] Similarly, aerobic exercise has no adverse effect on lactation.[12] In a longitudinal study of pregnancy weight gain, 540 women were followed for 5 to 10 years (mean, 8.5 years) after their index pregnancy. Women who returned to their prepregnancy weight by 6 months after delivery were much more likely to have gained less weight at the 5- to 10-year follow-up compared with women who retained their pregnant weight gains. In this cohort, breastfeeding and aerobic exercise were associated with a significantly lower weight gain over time.[13] A study of 1656 deliveries in a retrospective cohort found that pregnant weight gain greater than the recommended amount was directly related to the increased weight of women 1 year later.[14] Postpartum exercise programs improve long-term effects on health and risks for chronic disease.[15,16] Phelan[17] emphasized that pregnancy and the postpartum period are "teachable moments," ideal for counseling women about weight control. Given the epidemic of obesity in Western society, dietary counseling—along with recommendations for exercise—is an important addition to health maintenance. However, interventions are, as might be expected, more effective for postpartum weight loss and retention of weight loss.[18] A Cochrane Review analyzed literature on weight-loss programs and found that **diet and diet plus exercise are most effective for postpartum weight loss.**[19]

Thyroid Function

Thyroid size and function (see Chapter 42) throughout pregnancy and the puerperium have been quantitated with ultrasonography and thyroid hormone levels.[20] Thyroid volume increases about 30% during pregnancy and regresses to normal gradually over a 12-week period. Thyroxine and triiodothyronine, both elevated throughout pregnancy, return to normal within 4 weeks postpartum. For women taking thyroid medications, it is appropriate to check thyroid levels at 6 weeks postpartum to adjust dosing. It is now recognized that the postpartum period is associated with an increased risk for the development of a transient autoimmune thyroiditis that may in some cases evolve into permanent hypothyroidism. The relationship between subclinical thyroid dysfunction and postpartum depression (PPD) is controversial.[21-23]

Postpartum thyroiditis (PPT) is an autoimmune disease that may present with hyperthyroid or hypothyroid symptoms, and it occurs in 2% to 17% of women with a mean incidence of about 10%. PPT will occur in up to 25% of women with type 1 diabetes. Women with gestational and type 2 diabetes also have a slightly increased risk. Only that subset of women who develop symptoms should be treated. Puerperal hypothyroidism often presents with symptoms that include mild dysphoria; consequently, thyroid function studies are suggested in the evaluation of patients with suspected PPD that occurs 2 to 3 months after delivery. Hyperthyroid symptoms are best treated with β-blockers, and hypothyroid symptoms with thyroid supplementation. Both are acceptable with breastfeeding. Methimazole and propylthiouracil are also safe during lactation. **From 5% to 30% of women with PPT eventually develop hypothyroidism.** If a woman becomes symptomatic and is treated, it is reasonable to stop medications after 1 year and reevaluate thyroid status before the patient considers becoming pregnant again.[21-23]

Cardiovascular System, Immunity, and Coagulation

Blood volume increases throughout pregnancy to levels in the third trimester that are about 35% above nonpregnant values. The greatest proportion of this increase consists of an expansion in plasma volume that begins in the first trimester and amounts to an additional 1200 mL of plasma, which represents a 50% increase by the third trimester. Red blood cell volume increases by about 250 mL.

Immediately after delivery, plasma volume is diminished by about 1000 mL secondary to blood loss. By the third postpartum day, the plasma volume is replenished by a shift of extracellular fluid into the vascular space. In contrast, the total blood volume declines by 16% of the predelivery value, which suggests a relative and transient anemia. By 8 weeks postpartum, the red cell mass has rebounded and the hematocrit is normal in most women. As total blood volume normalizes, venous tone also returns to baseline. In a prospective evaluation of 42 women, at 4 and 42 days postpartum, significant reduction in deep vein vessel size and a concomitant increase in venous flow velocity in the lower extremities were observed.[24]

Pulse rate increases throughout pregnancy, as does stroke volume and cardiac output. Immediately after delivery, these remain elevated or rise even higher for 30 to 60 minutes. Following delivery, a transient rise of about 5% occurs in both diastolic and systolic blood pressures throughout the first 4 days postpartum. Data are scant regarding the rate at which cardiac hemodynamics return to prepregnancy levels. Early studies suggested cardiac output had returned to normal when measurements were made 8 to 10 weeks postpartum. Clapp and Capeless[25] performed longitudinal evaluations of cardiac function at bimonthly intervals in 30 healthy women using M-mode ultrasound before pregnancy; during gestation; and at 12, 24, and 52 weeks postpartum. Cardiac output and left ventricular volume peaked at 24 weeks' gestation, with a slow return to prepregnancy values over the year of the study. However, **even 1 year after delivery, a significantly higher cardiac output was observed in both nulliparous and multiparous women compared with prepregnancy values**. The authors suggested that this "cardiac remodeling" from pregnancy may last for an extended time in healthy women. Anecdotally, elite athletes have tried to take advantage of this physiologic boost to cardiac function by planning pregnancies a year before major sporting events.

Pregnancy is known to be a time of significantly increased coagulability that persists into the postpartum period (see Chapter 45).[26] The greatest level of coagulability is observed immediately after delivery and for the following 48 hours. Fibrinogen concentrations gradually diminish over the first 2 weeks postpartum. Compared with antepartum values, a rapid decrease in platelets is observed in some patients, whereas no change or an increase is seen in others. Within 2 weeks after delivery, the platelet count rises, possibly as a marker of increased bone marrow output as red cell mass is replaced. Fibrinolytic activity increases in the first 1 to 4 days after delivery and returns to normal in 1 week as measured by levels of plasminogen activation inhibitor 1. D-dimer levels are increased over pregnancy levels and are a poor marker of thrombus formation. Protein-S levels and activated protein-C resistance are decreased for up to 6 weeks or longer. In general, tests for thrombophilia and hemostasis should be delayed if possible for 10 to 12 weeks. The changes in the coagulation system, together with vessel trauma and immobility, account for the increased risk for thromboembolism noted in the puerperium, especially when an operative delivery has occurred. **A large multicenter study[27] over a 4½-year period in California found that in 1,688,000 primiparous deliveries, the incidence of thrombotic events was higher in the first 6 weeks after delivery compared with the same period 1 year later** (odds ratio [OR], 10.8; 95% confidence interval [CI], 7.8 to 15.1). **However, the authors noted that the risk remained increased between 7 and 12 weeks postpartum** (OR, 2.2; 95% CI, 1.5 to 3.1). **The risk of a thrombotic event increased to 22.1 per 100,000 deliveries from delivery to 6 weeks postpartum and was increased by 3.0 per 100,000 from 7 through 12 weeks.**

The immune system, which is mildly suppressed during pregnancy—particularly cellular-mediated immunity—rebounds after delivery. This rebound may lead to "flare-ups" of autoimmune disease and latent infections with inflammatory reactions. The inflammatory reactions are what often produce the clinical symptoms. **Autoimmune thyroiditis, multiple sclerosis, and lupus erythematosus are examples of some of the diseases that may show an increase in disease activity in the first few months postpartum.**[28] Large cross-sectional studies of population databases have noted hospital admission rates after delivery to be higher than expected for age-matched controls; readmissions are related to infections such as pneumonia, cholecystitis, and appendicitis. **Overall, postpartum readmission rates vary from 0.8% to 1.5% for vaginal delivery and 1.8% to 2.7% for cesarean birth.**[29-31]

Urinary Tract and Renal Function

It is generally accepted that the urinary tract becomes dilated during pregnancy, especially the renal pelvis and the ureters above the pelvic brim. These findings, demonstrated 70 years ago, show that the collecting system of the right kidney is affected more than that of the left, and this dilation is caused by compression of the ureters by the adjacent vasculature and enlarged uterus, combined with the effects of progesterone. Ultrasound studies of the urinary tract also document the enlargement of the collecting system throughout pregnancy. A study of serial ultrasound examinations of the urinary tract in 20 women throughout pregnancy included a single postpartum examination 6 weeks after delivery. The overall trend was that

of dilation of the collecting system throughout pregnancy, estimated by measurements of the separation of the pelvicaliceal echo complex, from a mean of 5 mm (first trimester) to 10 mm (third trimester) in the right kidney and from 3 to 4 mm in the collecting system for the left kidney. Measurements in all but two patients had returned to prepregnancy status at the time of the 6-week postpartum examination.

Serial nephrosonography on 24 patients throughout pregnancy and the puerperium[32] demonstrated that more than half of the patients at 12 weeks postpartum had persistence of urinary stasis, described as a slight separation of the renal pelvis. This finding is evidence of hyperdistensibility and suggests that pregnancy has a permanent effect on the size of the upper renal tract. Intravenous urography studies also suggest that subtle anatomic changes take place in the ureters that persist long after the pregnancy has ended. Ureteral tone above the pelvic brim, which in pregnancy is higher than normal, returns to nonpregnant levels immediately after cesarean delivery.

Studies in which water cystometry and uroflowmetry were performed within 48 hours of delivery and again 4 weeks postpartum demonstrated a slight but significant decrease in bladder capacity (from 395.5 to 331 mL) and volume at first void (from 277 to 224 mL) in the study interval. Nevertheless, all the urodynamic values studied were within normal limits on both occasions. The results were not affected by the weight of the infant or by an episiotomy; however, prolonged labor and the use of epidural anesthesia appeared to diminish postpartum bladder function transiently.

The most detailed study of renal function in normal pregnancy is that of Sims and Krantz,[33] who studied 12 patients with serial renal function tests throughout pregnancy and for up to 1 year after delivery. Glomerular filtration, which increased by 50% early in pregnancy and remained elevated until delivery, returned to normal nonpregnant levels by postpartum week 8. Endogenous creatinine clearance, similarly elevated throughout pregnancy, also returned to normal by the eighth postpartum week. Renal plasma flow increased by 25% early in pregnancy, gradually diminished in the third trimester (even when measured in the lateral recumbent position), and continued to decrease to below-normal values in the postpartum period for up to 24 weeks. Normal values were finally established by 50 to 60 weeks after delivery. The reason for the prolonged PPD of renal plasma flow is not clear.

Because of the variable changes in renal clearance, mothers who take medications whose dosages have been changed because of the physiologic adaptations of pregnancy will need to have medication levels rechecked. This should be done at 4 to 6 weeks postpartum.

Hair Growth and Bone Loss

Hair growth is altered in pregnancy and postpartum. After delivery, a more rapid hair turnover is seen for up to 3 months. As a greater percentage of hair begins to undergo the growth phase, more hair falls out with combing and brushing. The loss is in a diffuse, not balding, pattern. **This transient phenomenon is called *telogen effluvium,* and the patient may be reassured that her hair growth will return to normal within a few months and that the excess hair lost in the comb or brush will regrow.**

Several investigators have reported on bone mineral changes with lactation and the associated amenorrhea. After delivery, a generalized decrease in bone mineralization is seen that is temporary and resolves by 12 to 18 months postpartum in most women.[34] Bone loss appears to be greater in the femoral neck than in other areas of the skeleton.[35,36] Calcium supplementation does not seem to ameliorate the bone loss because it is not a problem of inadequate calcium stores, and exercise does not prevent it.[37] For almost all women, the bone loss is self-limited and reversible. Recent investigations have found that postpartum aerobic exercises decrease the bone loss associated with lactation.[38]

Management of the Puerperium

For most parturients, the immediate puerperium is spent in the hospital or birthing center. The ideal duration of hospitalization for patients with uncomplicated vaginal births has been controversial and culturally determined. During World War II, early discharge with nurse follow-up was initiated to support the "war bride" baby boom.[39] In the 1950s, the lying-in period after delivery was 8 to 14 days.[40] Today, most women stay in the hospital 24 to 48 hours after a vaginal birth. For patients with an uncomplicated postoperative course following cesarean delivery, the postpartum stay is 2 to 4 days. The optimal time is dependent on a patient's needs and home support. About 3% of women who have vaginal deliveries and 9% of women who have cesarean deliveries have at least one childbirth-related complication that requires longer hospitalization after delivery or readmission to the hospital.[41] Studies that have evaluated the safety and outcomes of discharge before 48 hours have relied on nurse or midwife home visits. Unfortunately, most insurers do not cover this service.

In one study, 1249 randomly selected patients were questioned 8 weeks after delivery about health problems that occurred during the puerperium.[42] Eighty-five percent reported at least one problem during their hospitalization, and 76% noted at least one problem that persisted for 8 weeks. Many types of problems were reported by the patients, including a painful perineum, difficulty with breastfeeding, urinary tract infection, urinary and fecal incontinence, and headache. Three percent of the patients had been rehospitalized, most commonly for abnormal bleeding or infection. This study draws attention to a substantial amount of symptomatic morbidity that occurs during the puerperium. Although longer hospitalization may not improve perineal pain or incontinence, open lines of communication with patients between discharge and the 6-week visit affect patient self-care and promote a more positive patient experience. A study[43] of 597,000 women from New Zealand who delivered over an 8-year period documented that shorter postpartum hospital stays had no effect on readmission rates. **In this study, lactation/breast problems, delayed postpartum hemorrhage, and post–cesarean delivery wound infections were the major causes of readmission.**

In particular, lactation consultation may help to improve effective breastfeeding, and consideration should be given to postponing discharge in primiparas until this service can be performed. As is obvious, home visits and interventions improve lactation effectiveness and duration, postpartum weight loss, and psychological well-being after pregnancy loss.

If a patient has adequate support at home (i.e., help with housekeeping and meal preparation), an extended hospital stay is of little value, provided the mother is adequately educated about infant care and feeding and in the identification of danger signs in either the infant or herself. **Except for an increased incidence of rehospitalization of some neonates for**

hyperbilirubinemia, postpartum hospitalization of less than 48 hours has few disadvantages for many patients.[44-47] For mothers who do not have adequate support at home and who are insecure about infant care and feeding, extending the hospital stay will provide time for them to gain adequate education and some measure of self-confidence. Written and video presentations are also efficient means of patient education. To be most helpful, educational material should be presented before delivery, sometime in the late third trimester, and at the postpartum discharge. **Home nursing visits can be helpful in providing support, education, and advice to mothers in selected situations.** Written materials or handouts are particularly necessary because memory is temporarily affected by the sleep deprivation that is the rule in the first few days after delivery.

Before discharge, women should be offered any vaccines that may be necessary to protect immunity. The measles, mumps, and rubella (MMR) vaccine should be given to rubella-nonimmune mothers. Hepatitis B; tetanus, diphtheria, and pertussis (Tdap); MMR; and influenza vaccines are the four most common vaccines given. All are safe with breastfeeding.[48] **As recommended in 2012 by the Centers for Disease Control and Prevention (CDC), Tdap should be administered during pregnancy to all pregnant women, regardless of the interval since the last Tdap.[49] If Tdap was not given during pregnancy, it should be given immediately after delivery. The varicella vaccine should be initiated postpartum in those with a negative varicella titer.[48]**

The time from delivery until complete physiologic involution and psychological adjustment has been called "the fourth trimester."[50] Patients should understand that lochia will persist for 3 to 8 weeks and that on days 7 to 14, there is often an episode of heavy vaginal bleeding, which occurs when the placental eschar sloughs. Tampons are permissible if they are comfortable upon insertion and are changed frequently and if there are no perineal, vaginal, or cervical lacerations that preclude insertion of a tampon until healing has occurred. **Physical activity such as walking up and down stairs, lifting moderately heavy objects, riding in or driving a car, and performing muscle-toning exercises can be resumed without delay if the delivery has been uncomplicated.** Minig and associates[51] reviewed the scientific evidence behind many postpartum recommendations and noted that very few if any of the traditional recommendations are evidence based. Lifting, sexual activity, driving, and exercise do not need to be overly restricted, even for women after cesarean births. Instructions regarding exercise are patient specific. Studies have found that postpartum exercise has no effect on lactation but may decrease anxiety levels and symptoms of PPD.[52-54] As such, exercise may have benefits beyond the mother's desire to "get back into shape." The most troublesome postpartum symptoms are lethargy and fatigue. Consequently, every task or activity should be a brief one in the first few days of the puerperium. Mothers whose lethargy persists beyond several weeks must be evaluated, especially for thyroid dysfunction and PPD.

Sexual activity may be resumed when the perineum is comfortable and when bleeding has diminished. The desire and willingness to resume sexual activity in the puerperium varies greatly among women, depending on the site and state of healing of perineal or vaginal incisions and lacerations, the amount of vaginal atrophy secondary to breastfeeding, and the return of libido,[55] which is greatly affected by sleep patterns among other new issues. Although the median time to vaginal intercourse after delivery is 6 weeks, 90% of women resume sexual activity by 3 months.[56] Nevertheless, as many as 80% of women have sexual problems at 8 to 12 weeks, including painful intercourse,[56,57] and a substantial proportion have dyspareunia that lasts for a year or more.[58,59] Signorello and coworkers[60] noted a 2.5-fold increased risk for dyspareunia 6 months after operative vaginal delivery compared with other subsets of postpartum women. For all women, breastfeeding at 6 months is associated with a more than fourfold increase in dyspareunia. Similarly, a large review of studies examining postpartum sexuality noted the greatest incidence of sexual dysfunction to be associated with operative vaginal delivery.[61] **Cesarean delivery is associated with a decreased incidence of dyspareunia compared with vaginal birth only for the first 6 months, after which the rates become similar.** In contrast, 25% of all women reported a heightened sexual pleasure 6 months after delivery.

Postpartum dyspareunia is not always related to vulvar trauma and occurs in some women who have a cesarean delivery. Dyspareunia has also been observed in women who use oral contraceptives and do not breastfeed, suggesting that lack of estrogen effect on the vagina is not the major cause of postpartum dyspareunia. In a study of 50 parturients, Ryding[62] found that 20% had little desire for sexual activity 3 months after delivery, and an additional 21% had complete loss of desire or aversion to sexual activity. This variation in attitude, desire, and willingness must be acknowledged when counseling women about the resumption of sexual activity. Women who breastfeed tend to begin intercourse later than the average, and women who have had a cesarean delivery tend to begin sooner.[63] Clinicians commonly advise pregnant women on the use of vaginal lubricants for sexual activity in the first few months postpartum because of the decreased natural lubrication with lower estrogen levels. This may be included in the written handouts given to patients when they go home. Astroglide gel and Comfort gel are more commonly recommended lubricants; KY Jelly is typically too dry. If patients are using barrier contraception, they should be advised against the use of petroleum-based lubricants such as Vaseline. If dyspareunia persists, a small amount of estrogen cream applied daily to the vagina may be helpful in breastfeeding women with atrophic changes. Clinicians may also counsel women about using different sexual positions if deeper penetration with male partners is uncomfortable.[51]

Many patients return to work situations outside the home after their pregnancies. Frequently, the physician must complete insurance or employer forms to establish maternity leave for patients. As mentioned earlier, the 6-week return in the United States is derived from tradition, and 8 weeks are often allowed after a cesarean delivery. Women will often experience discomfort, tiredness, and breast soreness well beyond 6 weeks. **Similar to the return to exercise and sexual activity, the return to work should be individualized.** Other nations and cultures have different standards for returning to prepregnancy routines. In China, 30 days is common, whereas in Western Europe and Canada, maternity leave from several months to a year is common.

HEALTH MAINTENANCE

The postpartum visit is scheduled at the time of discharge and routinely occurs 4 to 6 weeks after delivery. Some women may benefit from a visit sooner, such as women at risk for depression, those with a more complicated labor and **delivery, and women who underwent a cesarean section for delivery.** At this visit, breastfeeding can be addressed along with incisional checks and assessment of mood. Studies have shown that a routine postpartum visit to the physician 1 or 2 weeks after delivery or a home visit by a nurse midwife does little to reduce maternal or infant morbidity.[64,65] However, for the patient with antepartum or intrapartum difficulties, this early postpartum visit or home visit by a nurse or nurse midwife is more productive in detecting problems and providing support for the mother. Thus the need for this visit should be individualized.[66] Late puerperal infections, PPD, and problems with infant care and feeding often occur before the 6-week postpartum visit. Open-ended questions should be asked to detect problems.

At the routine postpartum visit, questions regarding depression, energy, sexuality, contraception, and future pregnancies should be addressed. Unfortunately, some women skip their 6-week postpartum check, deferring questions of contraception. A copy of the Edinburgh postnatal depression scale (EPDS) is provided in Box 23-2. It may be used as a fast, reliable, and user-friendly tool to screen for depression. It is helpful to solicit questions about how women feel after the delivery because they may be hesitant to ask questions spontaneously, especially with regard to sexuality and incontinence. If health issues need to be addressed, such as blood glucose or thyroid level assessment, they may be performed or scheduled at this visit.

Women with chronic medical diseases such as collagen vascular disease, autoimmune disorders, and neurologic conditions should be considered for visits at closer intervals because many patients with these disorders experience flare-ups of their symptoms after delivery. Ideally, these visits should be scheduled in advance with the patient's primary care or subspecialty physician. Prophylactic therapy is not recommended for women with systemic lupus erythematosus or multiple sclerosis. However, warning patients to be attuned to signs and symptoms that reflect a flare-up of their illness allows for early and more effective interventions. For women with epilepsy, special attention to medication doses with the changing renal clearance is necessary. Additionally, increased postpartum sleep deprivation may induce a lower seizure threshold.

Perineal and Pelvic Care

Many women who give birth have lacerations of the perineum or vagina. When an episiotomy is performed in the United States, it is often performed as a midline, rather than as a mediolateral, incision. In the absence of hematoma or extensive ecchymosis, and provided that the incision or laceration does not extend beyond the transverse perineal muscle, if a satisfactory repair has been accomplished, there is little need for perineal care beyond routine cleansing with a bath or shower. Analgesia can be accomplished in most patients with nonsteroidal antiinflammatory drugs (NSAIDs) such as ibuprofen or naproxen sodium. These drugs are superior to acetaminophen or propoxyphene for episiotomy pain and uterine cramping. Furthermore, because of a low milk/maternal plasma drug concentration ratio, a short half-life, and transformation into glucuronide metabolites, ibuprofen is safe for nursing mothers.

A patient who has had a mediolateral episiotomy, third- or fourth-degree perineal laceration, periurethral lacerations, or extensive perineal bruising may experience considerable perineal pain.[67] Occasionally, the pain and periurethral swelling prevent

BOX 23-2 EDINBURGH POSTNATAL DEPRESSION SCALE

In the past 7 days:

1. I have been able to laugh and see the funny side of things.
   __ As much as I always could
   __ Not quite so much now
   __ Definitely not so much now
   __ Not at all

2. I have looked forward with enjoyment to things.
   __ As much as I ever did
   __ Rather less than I used to
   __ Definitely less than I used to
   __ Hardly at all

3. I have blamed myself unnecessarily when things went wrong.
   __ Yes, most of the time
   __ Yes, some of the time
   __ Not very often
   __ No, never

4. I have been anxious or worried for no good reason.
   __ No, not at all
   __ Hardly ever
   __ Yes, sometimes
   __ Yes, very often

5. I have felt scared or panicky for no good reason.
   __ Yes, quite a lot
   __ Yes, sometimes
   __ No, not much
   __ No, not at all

6. Things have been getting on top of me.
   __ Yes, most of the time I haven't been able to cope at all.

   __ Yes, sometimes I haven't been coping as well as usual.
   __ No, most of the time I have coped quite well.
   __ No, I have been coping as well as ever.

7. I have been so unhappy that I have had difficulty sleeping.
   __ Yes, most of the time
   __ Yes, sometimes
   __ Not very often
   __ No, not at all

8. I have felt sad or miserable.
   __ Yes, most of the time
   __ Yes, quite often
   __ Not very often
   __ No, not at all

9. I have been so unhappy that I have been crying.
   __ Yes, most of the time
   __ Yes, quite often
   __ Only occasionally
   __ No, never

10. The thought of harming myself has occurred to me.
    __ Yes, quite often
    __ Sometimes
    __ Hardly ever
    __ Never

Response categories are scored 0, 1, 2, and 3 according to increased severity of the symptom. Items 3 and 5 through 10 are reverse scored (3, 2, 1, 0). The total score is calculated by adding together the scores for each of the 10 items.

From Cox JL, Holden JM, Sagovsky R. Detection of postnatal depression: development of the 10-item Edinburgh Postnatal Depression Scale. *Br J Psychiatry.* 1987;150:782.

the patient from voiding, making urethral catheterization necessary. When a patient complains of inordinate perineal pain, the first and most important step is to reexamine the perineum, vagina, and rectum in an effort to detect and drain a hematoma or to identify a perineal infection. **Perineal pain may be the first symptom of the rare but potentially fatal complications of angioedema, necrotizing fasciitis, or perineal cellulitis.**

In cases of moderate perineal pain, sitz baths will provide additional pain relief. Although hot sitz baths have long been customary therapy for perineal pain, **there is rationale for using cold or "iced" sitz baths.** This therapy is similar to that for the treatment of athletic injuries, for which considerable success has been achieved with cold therapy. Cold provides immediate pain relief as a result of decreased excitability of free nerve endings and decreased nerve conduction. Further pain relief comes from local vasoconstriction, which reduces edema, inhibits hematoma formation, and decreases muscle irritability and spasm. Patients who have alternated using hot and cold sitz baths usually prefer the cold. The technique for administering a cold sitz bath is to first have the patient sit in a tub of room-temperature water to which ice cubes are then added; this avoids the sensation of sudden immersion in ice water. The patient remains in the ice water for 20 to 30 minutes. Patients with perineal incisions or lacerations should be advised to postpone sexual intercourse until perineal discomfort has abated. The application of a perineal ice pack beyond the customary 6 to 8 hours may also be considered. Tampons may be inserted whenever the patient is

comfortable doing so. However, to avoid any risk for toxic shock syndrome, the use of tampons should be confined to daytime to prevent leaving a tampon in the vagina for prolonged periods.

Frequently, what appears to be severe perineal pain is in fact the pain of prolapsed hemorrhoids. Witch hazel compresses, suppositories that contain corticosteroids, or local anesthetic sprays or emollients may be helpful. Occasionally, a thrombus occurs in a prolapsed hemorrhoid. When performed by an obstetrician or a general surgeon trained in this procedure, it is a simple task to remove the thrombus through a small scalpel incision using local anesthesia. Dramatic relief of pain usually follows this procedure. Stool softeners, laxatives, or both should be discussed for women with hemorrhoids. Some women suffer from prolonged pelvic girdle pain. Predictors of this type of pain include a history of low back pain, pelvic girdle pain during pregnancy, and painful postures at their place of employment.[68]

Urinary and anal incontinence is a significant problem in women after delivery.[69] Weidner and colleagues[70] studied 58 primiparous women after delivery and found levator ani neuropathy in 14 of 58 women (24.1%) at 6 weeks. Nine women recovered by 6 months. Seventeen of the 58 women had the neuropathy unresolved at 6 months postpartum, which included 12 newly identified injuries. Elective cesarean delivery was protective for neuropathy in this series, yet labor with subsequent cesarean delivery was not protective. About one third of women at 8 weeks and 15% of women at 12 weeks had urinary incontinence. As would be expected, incontinence has a very detrimental effect on quality of life.[71] A strong predictor for incontinence after delivery is a history of prior urinary incontinence or new-onset incontinence during the index pregnancy. In addition to urinary incontinence, 3% to 10% of women have anal incontinence 3 months after vaginal birth, and most experience flatal, rather than fecal, incontinence.[69,72,73] Forceps-assisted, but not vacuum-assisted, vaginal delivery is associated with a twofold increased risk for fecal incontinence in primiparas.[74] Similarly, anal sphincter disruption in nulliparas is associated with a 2.3-fold increase in anal incontinence 5 years after delivery.[75] Nulliparous women with sphincter disruption or operative vaginal delivery should be screened specifically for symptoms at follow-up visits.

Perineal exercises were developed by Kegel in 1948 and involve voluntary contraction of the pelvic floor. These exercises and consequent refinements are termed *pelvic floor muscle training* (PFMT). The exercises are best taught by a trained instructor in a comfortable environment. PFMT may be initiated before delivery or after, and exercises are performed several times a day. Multiple well-designed studies and reviews have evaluated data from over 10,000 women to assess the value of PFMT for both prevention and treatment.[69,76-79] The results of PFMT appear mixed. In summary, training begun antepartum and reinforced after delivery shows significant benefits for prevention of urinary incontinence up to 6 months postpartum. Counseling and handouts are significantly inferior to instructor training with biofeedback; the more intense the program, the more effective. PFMT begun postpartum for a mixed population of symptomatic and asymptomatic women is minimally effective. However, **symptomatic women experience significant improvement when PFMT is begun postpartum with instructor training and reinforcement.** Long-term (10-year) benefits for incontinence and pelvic prolapse are minimal, although symptom rates are mildly decreased in women who performed PFMT. All studies emphasize the value of hands-on interventions and follow-up as well as the difficulty of studying mixed populations with varying degrees of vaginal disruption.[69-75]

If symptoms of either urinary or flatal incontinence persist for more than 6 months, evaluation should be undertaken to define the specific neuromuscular or anatomic abnormality so that the appropriate treatment can be initiated. Women should be counseled regarding this plan at their postpartum visit so that they can return if symptoms persist. If possible, antepartum PFMT should be offered to primiparous women.

Delayed Postpartum Hemorrhage and Postpartum Anemia

The causes and management of immediate postpartum hemorrhage are discussed in Chapter 18. **Delayed postpartum uterine bleeding of sufficient volume to require medical attention occurs in 1% to 2% of patients. One of the most common causes of postpartum hemorrhage seen 2 to 5 days after delivery is von Willebrand disease.** Von Willebrand factor increases in pregnancy, and thus excessive bleeding usually does not occur in the first 48 hours after birth. Women who present with bleeding more than 48 hours after delivery should be screened for this condition.

Delayed bleeding occurs most frequently between days 8 and 14 of the puerperium.[80] Significant bleeding may require treatment with uterotonic agents or curettage. When suction evacuation and curettage are performed, retained gestational products—usually in small amounts—will be found in about 40% of cases.[81,82] Whether small placental remnants are the cause is unknown. **In the management of patients with heavy delayed bleeding, ultrasound examination can be used to help determine whether a significant amount of retained material is present, although it is sometimes difficult to distinguish between blood clot and retained placental fragments** (see Fig. 23-1). Suction evacuation of the uterus is successful in arresting the bleeding in almost all cases regardless of whether histologic confirmation of retained gestational products is obtained. If curettage is required at this time, especially if a sharp curette is used, a course of broad-spectrum antibiotics with anaerobic coverage should be initiated before surgery for their possible benefit in reducing the formation of uterine synechiae and the sequelae of Asherman syndrome. The curettage should be performed with care because the postpartum uterine wall is soft and easy to perforate. In those rare instances in which delayed postpartum hemorrhage does not respond to the use of oxytocic agents and curettage, selective arterial embolization may be effective in controlling the bleeding. Women with postpartum hemorrhage and subsequent anemia often have excessive fatigue in the postpartum period. Some investigators have advocated the use of recombinant erythropoietin and parenteral iron as alternatives to transfusion for symptomatic women with anemia.

Significant postpartum hemorrhage may lead to problems with mother-infant interactions and lactation both immediately after delivery and in the first few weeks postpartum, particularly with fatigue or readmission. Early and continued attention to this issue is important. A study of 206 women with postpartum hemorrhage of 1500 mL or greater found that, other than more readmissions for infection and recurrent bleeding, this cohort of women did not manifest a greater frequency of PPD or other health complications.[83]

Postpartum Infection

Although the standard definition of postpartum febrile morbidity is a temperature of 38° C (100.4° F) or higher on any two of the first 10 days after delivery, exclusive of the first 24 hours, most clinicians do not wait two full days to begin evaluation and treatment of patients who develop a fever in the puerperium. **The most common cause of postpartum fever is endometritis, which occurs after vaginal delivery in about 2% of patients and after cesarean delivery in about 10% to 15%.** The differential diagnosis includes urinary tract, lower genital tract, wound, and pulmonary infections in addition to thrombophlebitis and mastitis. The diagnosis and management of postpartum infection are discussed in detail in Chapters 53 and 54. Almost all antibiotics are safe during lactation, and these are discussed in Chapter 8.

Maternal-Infant Attachment

Klaus and colleagues[84] were among the first investigators to study maternal-infant attachment and to bring attention to the importance of the first few hours of maternal-infant association. Their studies, as well as those of others, have contributed substantially to major changes in hospital policies for dealing with patients during labor and delivery and in the postpartum period. **It is now recognized that constant opportunities should be provided for parents to be with their newborns, particularly from the first few moments after birth and as frequently as possible during the first days thereafter. Immediate**

skin-to-skin contact is recommended. Separation of the mother and her infant in the first hours after birth has been shown to diminish or delay the development of characteristic mothering behaviors,[85] a problem that is intensified when medical, obstetric, or newborn complications require intensive care for either the mother or her newborn infant.

Robson and Powell[86] summarized the literature on early maternal attachment and emphasized how difficult it is to perform valid research studies about this phenomenon because of the multiple confounders. Although it is generally agreed that early association of the mother and infant is beneficial and should not be interfered with unnecessarily, doubts continue to surround the long-term implications, if any, of a lack of early maternal-infant association. In their monograph summarizing their investigations about parent-infant attachment, Klaus and Kennel[87] warn against drawing far-reaching conclusions. Although favoring the theory of a "sensitive period" soon after birth, during which close parent-infant interaction facilitates subsequent attachment and beneficial parenting behavior, these investigators concur that humans are highly adaptable and state that "there are many fail-safe routes to attachment." Many hospitals and birth centers have recognized the importance of, and have placed emphasis on, the mother-baby interactions in the first several hours after delivery. **Delaying the first bath, eliminating well-baby nurseries, putting the baby onto the mother's chest in skin-to-skin contact (even during cesarean delivery), and keeping the baby in the room with the mother during the first pediatric evaluation are all steps to support and promote that interaction.**

The modern maternity unit should enhance and encourage parent-infant attachment by such policies as free visiting hours for the other parent, encouragement of the other parent to room in with the mother and baby whenever possible, encouragement of the mother to have the infant room in with her, and strong support of breastfeeding. These policies also allow the nursing staff to observe parenting behavior and to identify inept, inexperienced, or inappropriate behavior toward the infant. Some situations may call for more intensive follow-up by visiting nurses, home health visitors, or social workers to provide further support for the family during the posthospital convalescence. The role of postpartum home visits in enhancing parenting behavior is controversial, and Gray and colleagues[88] found this approach beneficial. Conversely, when Siegel and coworkers[89] studied the effect of early and prolonged mother-infant contact in the hospital and a postpartum visitation program on attachment and parenting behavior, they found that early and prolonged maternal-infant contact in the hospital had a significant effect on enhancing subsequent parenting behavior, but the postpartum home visitations had no impact.

The development of the qualities associated with good parenting depends on many factors. Certainly, it does not depend solely on what transpires in the few hours surrounding the birth experience. Evidence suggests that specific identification of an infant with its mother's voice begins in utero during the third trimester. Furthermore, the parents' own experiences as children, as well as their intellectual and emotional attitudes about children, play a significant role in their own parenting behavior. Areskog and associates[90] showed that women who expressed fear of childbirth during the antenatal period had more complications and more pain in labor and also had more difficulties in attachment to their infants. Consequently, the peripartum period provides opportunities to enhance parenting behavior

and to identify families for which follow-up after birth may be necessary to ensure the most favorable child development. For example, adolescents, particularly primiparous adolescents, are a particularly high-risk group because rates of domestic abuse are especially high in adolescent mothers.

In summary, **the postpartum unit should be an environment that provides parents ample opportunity to interact with their newborn infant.** Personnel—including nurses, nurses' aides, and physicians caring for mothers and infants—should be alert to signs of abnormal parenting (e.g., refusal of the mother to care for the infant, use of negative or abusive names in describing or referring to the infant, inordinate delay in naming the infant, or obsessive and unrealistic concerns about the infant's health). These or other signs that maternal-infant attachment is delayed or endangered are as deserving of frequent follow-up during the postpartum period as are any of the traditional medical or obstetric complications.

Lactation and breastfeeding are reviewed in detail in Chapter 24. All cultures have emphasized the importance of breastfeeding, and multiple steps should be taken during the postpartum period to promote and enhance breastfeeding. The use of audiovisual aids, telephone hotlines, and in-service training for personnel have been shown to increase the incidence of successful breastfeeding. The addition of home visits and active phone interventions cannot be underestimated (see Chapter 24).

PREGNANCY PREVENTION

Postpartum contraception use can decrease unintended pregnancy and provides women with a method to control the timing of their pregnancies. **A recent meta-analysis found that birth intervals shorter than 18 months are significantly associated with small size for gestational age, preterm birth, and infant death in the first year of life.**[91] The ideal timing of family planning advice and education about contraception has not been determined. Although antenatal contraceptive counseling is important, and women value the opportunity to discuss contraception during this time, several studies have demonstrated that antenatal education had very little effect on postpartum contraceptive use or subsequent pregnancy rates.[92,93] **Discussion about contraception has become a standard component of postpartum care.** Lopez and colleagues[94] conducted a systematic review to examine randomized trials that evaluated the effectiveness of postpartum education about contraceptive use. They identified and included 10 trials in their review and found that about half of the postpartum interventions led to fewer repeat pregnancies or births and more contraceptive use. One study found that written material given at the time of hospitalization plus a discussion is most helpful to mothers. **Whereas the ideal method and timing of providing contraceptive education postpartum has not been identified, its importance cannot be disputed.**

The percentage of women who choose to breastfeed is increasing. In the United States in 2010, the percentage of women who began breastfeeding after delivery was 77%. The percentage of women still breastfeeding at 6 months was 49%, up from 35% in 2000; at 12 months, it was 27%, up from 16%.[95] Elevated levels of prolactin encountered during breastfeeding act at the level of the pituitary and the ovary to produce lactational amenorrhea and anovulation.[96] The contraceptive efficacy of lactation is dependent on the nutritional status of the mother, the intensity of suckling, and the amount of supplemental food added to the infant diet.[97] **If a woman is exclusively breastfeeding on** demand both day and night, is amenorrheic, and the infant is less than 6 months old, the contraceptive efficacy of lactational amenorrhea is 98%.[98,99] Bleeding or spotting during the first 6 to 8 weeks postpartum in a fully breastfeeding woman is normal and is not due to ovulation. If suckling intensity and/or frequency is reduced, the contraceptive efficacy of lactational amenorrhea is reduced. After 6 months, even fully breastfeeding mothers have a need for contraception as infants start taking in other sources of nutrition. Women who pump breast milk do not do so at the same frequency as on-demand nursing, and pumping does not produce the same intensity that suckling produces; therefore a mother who pumps breast milk cannot rely on lactational amenorrhea to be 98% effective.

In nonbreastfeeding women, prolactin levels return to baseline by the third to fifth postpartum week. In two series, women did not ovulate prior to 25 days postpartum.[98,100] Therefore in nonbreastfeeding women, birth control is needed as soon as 3 weeks postpartum. An argument could be made for a postpartum visit scheduled earlier than 6 weeks because of this observation. Traditionally, women are told not to have intercourse prior to 6 weeks. However, studies demonstrate that many couples have already resumed intercourse prior to this.

A patient should be made aware of the various options for pregnancy prevention in terms that she and her partner can understand. This may be done by individual instruction from nurses, physicians, or midwives or by a variety of films or videos. The decision about family planning methods depends on the patient's motivation, number of children, state of health, whether she is breastfeeding, and the religious background of the couple. It cannot be assumed that because a woman has used a method of contraception effectively before the current pregnancy, she will need no counseling thereafter. More than half of patients change contraceptive techniques between pregnancies. Table 23-1 lists contraceptive options, failure rates, and continuation rates by method.

Long-Acting Reversible Contraception

Long-acting reversible contraception (LARC) methods, which include intrauterine devices (IUDs) and contraceptive implants, are the most effective reversible methods available to women, with failure rates of less than 1%. They are convenient methods, especially for new mothers, because they require little of the patient other than coming in for insertion. In addition to their ease of use, LARC methods are cost effective, and fertility returns immediately after removal, so they are good methods to use for women in their childbearing years. LARC is also very safe, well studied, and has few contraindications (Table 23-2). LARC methods are also safe for women to use while breastfeeding.

The hormonal IUD contains the progestin levonorgestrel (LNG), which is released at an initial rate of 20 µg/day and lasts for up to 5 years.[101] The LNG IUD prevents pregnancy primarily by thickening the cervical mucus so that sperm cannot reach the upper genital tract. This IUD also thins the lining of the uterus but does not reliably inhibit ovulation. The main side effects are related to menstrual bleeding changes. Women should be counseled about irregular bleeding and/or spotting for several months after insertion. This typically improves over time and by 1 year, approximately 30% to 40% of women will be amenorrheic.[102-104] For others, the amount of bleeding will be approximately 90% less than their normal periods.[102-104]

The nonhormonal IUD contains copper and can be used for 10 to 12 years. Copper ions are released into the uterine cavity and cause spermicidal actions. The main side effects to discuss with patients regarding the copper IUD are related to menstrual bleeding changes. With the copper IUD, women need to be counseled about possible heavier periods, worsened dysmenorrhea, and longer periods by approximately 1.5 days. The copper IUD may not be a first choice for women with a history of heavy, painful periods.

The final LARC method is the single-rod implant, usually placed in the inner aspect of the nondominant arm. The contraceptive implant contains etonogestrel and acts primarily by inhibiting ovulation; it also causes changes to bleeding patterns, with irregular spotting or bleeding or amenorrhea. The bleeding patterns for this device are more unpredictable. The implant can be used for up to 3 years. Continuation rates for all three LARC methods are high (see Table 23-1).

LARC methods can be placed immediately after delivery or at another time. If IUDs are placed postpartum, the best practice is to place the device within 10 minutes of placental delivery. Insertion of an IUD is not recommended if intrauterine infection is present. Devices placed immediately after delivery have an up to 20% risk for expulsion; those placed at the time of cesarean delivery versus vaginal delivery have a lower risk of expulsion.[105] **The use of a single-rod implant in postpartum women does not result in changes in milk volume,**

TABLE 23-1	CONTRACEPTIVE EFFECTIVENESS: PERCENTAGE OF WOMEN WHO EXPERIENCE AN UNINTENDED PREGNANCY DURING THE FIRST YEAR OF TYPICAL AND PERFECT CONTRACEPTIVE METHOD USE AND PERCENTAGE OF CONTINUING USE AT 1 YEAR*		
METHOD	**TYPICAL USE**	**PERFECT USE**	**USE AT 1 YEAR**
LNG IUD	0.2	0.2	80
Copper IUD	0.8	0.6	78
ETG Implant	0.05	0.05	84
DMPA	6	0.3	56
Ring	9	0.3	68
Patch	9	0.3	68
COCs, POPs	9	0.3	68
Male condom	15	2	49

*Includes users who fail to use a method consistently or correctly.
COC, combination oral contraception; DMPA, depot medroxyprogesterone acetate; ETG, etonogestrel; IUD, intrauterine device; LNG, levonorgestrel; POP, progestin-only contraception.

TABLE 23-2	ABSOLUTE CONTRAINDICATIONS TO AN INTRAUTERINE DEVICE
DEVICE	**CONTRAINDICATION**
Levonorgestrel IUD	Current breast cancer
Copper IUD	Copper allergy (Wilson disease)
Both IUDs	Pregnancy, puerperal sepsis, current gonorrhea or *Chlamydia* infection, purulent cervicitis, immediately postseptic abortion, current PID, known uterine anomaly or distorted uterine cavity, endometrial or cervical carcinoma, unevaluated unexplained vaginal bleeding, persistently elevated β-hCG levels or malignant disease in a setting of GTD, pelvic tuberculosis

GTD, gestational trophoblastic disease; hCG, human chorionic gonadotropin; IUD, intrauterine device; PID, pelvic inflammatory disease.

milk constituents, or infant growth rates. Although package labeling advises initiating the implant at 6 weeks postpartum, clinical experience and limited randomized trial data with immediate postpartum initiation is reassuring, and placement at this time may be in the patient's best interest for the prevention of a rapid repeat pregnancy. Gurtcheff and colleagues[106] randomized women to receive the implant 1 to 2 days postpartum, versus 4 to 8 weeks, and found no difference between groups in lactation failure, time to lactogenesis stage II, use of formula supplementation, and milk composition at 6 weeks.

Injectable Contraception

Depot medroxyprogesterone acetate (DMPA) is an injectable progestin-only contraceptive given every 3 months. It is available in intramuscular and subcutaneous formulas and has a typical use failure rate of 6%. The mechanism of action of DMPA is to block the luteinizing hormone (LH) surge to prevent ovulation. DMPA is compatible with breastfeeding and can be given immediately after delivery. When initiated immediately or at 6 weeks postpartum, DMPA has not been shown to decrease the duration of lactation or to affect infant weight gain.[107] The main side effects of DMPA are irregular bleeding or amenorrhea, breast tenderness, weight gain, and depression. The side effect most likely related to discontinuation of the method is bleeding changes, which includes both irregular bleeding and amenorrhea.[108] Irregular bleeding decreases with increased length of time used. During the first year of use, the incidence of irregular bleeding is 70%, compared with 10% thereafter. Amenorrhea rates increase with increased duration of use as well. At 1 year, 50% of users are amenorrheic; after 5 years, amenorrhea rates reach 80%. Counseling about the expected bleeding profile is important at the initiation of DMPA because many women will not return for a second injection because of frustrations with bleeding. It is also important to counsel women about the delayed return to fertility after discontinuation of DMPA. The average delay to conception after the last injection of DMPA is 9 months, and the duration of DMPA use does not affect the return to conception.[109]

Limited evidence suggests that some caution should be used when prescribing DMPA in Hispanic women with a history of gestational diabetes. Some evidence suggests that in this group of women, DMPA use is associated with increased risk of type 2 diabetes. Much of this increased risk can be explained by clinical characteristics that placed the women at an increased risk for type 2 diabetes before starting DMPA.[110] Both the World Health Organization (WHO) and the Centers for Disease Control and Prevention (CDC) give all progestin-only methods a category 1 rating in women with a history of gestational diabetes, meaning no restrictions are suggested for use of the method.

Concern has also been expressed about DMPA causing mood changes and worsening depression, but findings from clinical trials have been reassuring, with no worsening of depression symptoms even in those women with high depression scores at baseline.[111,112] **Use of DMPA immediately after delivery does not result in higher rates of PPD.**[113]

Because DMPA inhibits ovarian function, estradiol levels are reduced, which leads to a temporary bone loss during use of DMPA. This bone loss is greatest during the first 2 years of use and declines thereafter. Reassuringly, bone mineral density (BMD) levels return to baseline with discontinuation of DMPA.[114,115] Cross-sectional studies that have demonstrated that BMD in former DMPA users is similar to that of never

users have provided reassurance that loss of BMD associated with DMPA is likely transient.[116,117] The clinical outcome of interest is whether DMPA use causes fracture risk, but no quality data are available to help answer this question. The American College of Obstetricians and Gynecologists (ACOG), American Academy of Pediatrics (AAP), and the WHO acknowledge that DMPA is an effective and convenient contraceptive method, and although providers should inform patients of the potential effects on bone, DMPA use should not be restricted or limited. In addition, BMD testing in DMPA users is not indicated.

Combined Hormonal Contraception

Combined hormonal contraception (CHC) includes oral, transdermal, and vaginal estrogen- and progestin-containing contraception. All of these methods have a typical use failure rate of 9%. The progestin component inhibits the LH surge and blocks ovulation, whereas the estrogen component inhibits FSH and dominant follicle formation; the added estrogen also results in a more regular bleeding pattern, which many women prefer. Before prescribing CHC, appropriate screening of the patient must occur because the estrogen component carries a slightly increased risk of venous thromboembolism (VTE) in healthy reproductive-age women. Box 23-3 provides a list of contraindications to estrogen. During the postpartum period, the risk of VTE is also increased 22-fold to 84-fold compared with that of nonpregnant, nonpostpartum reproductive-age women.[118] This risk is highest during the first weeks postpartum and decreases with time, and the VTE risk returns to baseline by 42 days postpartum (see Chapter 45). Adding estrogen-containing birth control during this timeframe may increase the VTE risk

---

BOX 23-3 ABSOLUTE CONTRAINDICATIONS TO ESTROGEN

- Age ≥35 years and smoking ≥15 cigarettes per day
- Multiple risk factors for arterial cardiovascular disease (older age, smoking, diabetes, hypertension)
- Blood pressure ≥160 mm Hg systolic or ≥100 mm Hg diastolic
- Hypertension with vascular disease
- Acute DVT/PE
- Higher risk for recurrent DVT/PE or history of recurrent DVT/PE
- Prolonged immobilization
- Known thrombogenic mutations
- Ischemic heart disease or a history of ischemic heart disease
- Stroke
- Complicated valvular heart disease
- <6 months since peripartum cardiomyopathy
- Moderately or severely impaired cardiac function
- Positive (or unknown) antiphospholipid antibodies
- Migraine with aura
- Current breast cancer
- Diabetes with end-organ vascular disease or duration >20 years
- Severe acute viral hepatitis
- Severe cirrhosis
- Hepatocellular adenoma
- Liver carcinoma
- Complicated solid-organ transplantation

DVT, deep venous thromboembolism; *PE,* pulmonary embolism.

even more; thus caution must be exercised when using CHC in postpartum women. In nonbreastfeeding women, CHC should not be used prior to 21 days postpartum.[119] In women without additional risk factors for VTE, CHC can be used after 21 days. In postpartum women with additional risk factors for VTE—such as age 35 or older, smoking, or recent cesarean delivery—CHC should not be used until after 42 days postpartum, when VTE risk returns to baseline. In breastfeeding women, initiation of CHC should be delayed until after 30 days because of evidence of its detrimental effects on lactation, such as decreased duration of breastfeeding, declines in milk production, and the need for increased supplementation for the newborn.[120] Breastfeeding women who have additional risk factors for VTE should delay initiation of CHC until after 42 days postpartum.

Progestin-Only Oral Contraception

Often called the *mini pill*, progestin-only pills (POPs) contain a low dose of progestin and are taken daily. The mechanism of action is thickening of the cervical mucus to block sperm entry into the upper genital tract. Because the hormone dose is low and the effects on the cervical mucus begin wearing off after 22 hours, POPs are less forgiving if taken late. Typical use failure rate for POPs is 9%. POPs are safe to take while breastfeeding and have no effect on milk volume or infant growth and development.[120] Immediate initiation of POPs has not been shown to adversely affect breastfeeding, so they can be started immediately after delivery.[121] Like DMPA, evidence is limited that suggests in overweight or obese Hispanic women with prior gestational diabetes who are breastfeeding, POPs tripled the risk for type 2 diabetes.[122]

Emergency Contraception

Emergency contraception (EC) is used after unprotected sex or after known contraceptive failure. Available options include the levonorgestrel-containing progestin-only method—known as the *Yuzpe method*, in which combination estrogen-progestin birth control pills are used—and the copper IUD. These EC options can be used up to 5 days after unprotected sex, but they are more effective the sooner they are used. Ulipristal acetate is the newest EC option. It is a progestin receptor agonist/antagonist and can also be used up to 5 days after unprotected sex. Ulipristal acetate is different in that it is as effective on the fifth day as on the first,[123] although women who are breastfeeding should not take it.

Sterilization

Male and female sterilization are the most frequently used methods of contraception in the United States, used by 37% of all contraceptive users. In women who desire sterilization, the puerperium is a convenient time for tubal ligation procedures because they can be performed at the time of a cesarean delivery or within the first 24 to 48 hours after vaginal delivery. In some hospitals, the operation is performed immediately after delivery in uncomplicated patients, especially when epidural anesthesia is given for labor analgesia. With the use of a small paraumbilical incision, the procedure seldom prolongs the patient's hospitalization.

The 10-year failure rate of postpartum partial salpingectomy is 0.75%.[124] Several modifications of this procedure include the Pomeroy, Parkland, Uchida, and Irving techniques. Because of the relaxed abdominal wall and the easy accessibility of the fallopian tubes, the mini-laparotomy has the advantages of convenience and speed without the possible risks for visceral injury that might occur with the trocar of the laparoscope.

Postpartum female sterilization can also be performed as an interval procedure unrelated to a pregnancy. One method is laparoscopic tubal ligation, which can be performed with titanium clips, Silastic bands, or cautery. Because of the newly discovered role the fallopian tube may play in the development of ovarian cancer, laparoscopic sterilization may also be chosen to be accomplished with bilateral salpingectomy.[125] A second type of interval sterilization is hysteroscopic transcervical sterilization, in which the tubal ostia are identified hysteroscopically and cannulated with titanium and nickel coils. Over 3 months, ingrowth of the tubes into the coils occurs and the tubes become occluded. One advantage of hysteroscopic sterilization is that it may be performed with or without anesthesia in an outpatient setting. One disadvantage is that the woman is not sterilized the day of the procedure and must continue to use a reliable method of contraception until a hysterosalpingogram is performed 3 months later to confirm tubal occlusion. All interval methods of tubal sterilization can be accomplished with a minimum of morbidity as outpatient procedures.

Whether performed in the puerperium or as an interval procedure, the risks of tubal ligation procedures include the short-term problems of anesthetic accidents; injury to bowel, bladder, or blood vessels; and infection. Hysteroscopic sterilization also carries the risk of uterine perforation and failure of cannulization of the tubal ostia. The overall risk for complication is 1.6%. Independent risk factors for complications are general anesthesia, diabetes, previous abdominal or pelvic surgery, and obesity. One to two deaths per 100,000 procedures occur and most often are attributed to anesthesia.

Obstetricians must remember that vasectomy is often a more advisable and desirable alternative for a couple considering sterilization.[126] It can be performed as an outpatient procedure under local anesthesia with an insignificant loss of time from work or family. Furthermore, **almost all failures—about 3 to 4 per 1000 procedures—can be detected by a postoperative semen analysis. This is a decided advantage over tubal ligation, in which failures are discovered only when a pregnancy occurs.** The azoospermia rate at 3 months is 60%, and it is 98% to 99% at 6 months. Interval contraception is required until azoospermia is confirmed. Vasectomy is less expensive and overall is associated with fewer complications than female sterilization; it has no sexual effects, and studies of long-term health effects found no evidence of an increased risk for atherosclerotic heart disease or other chronic illnesses.[126]

Most women who choose sterilization do not regret their decision. In the U.S. Collaborative Review of Sterilization study,[127] the cumulative risk for sterilization regret over 14 years was 12.7%. Age was a risk factor for regret. For women older than 30, risk for regret was 5.9%. In contrast, women 30 and younger had a risk of regret of 20.3%. Other factors that contribute to regret of sterilization are having incomplete information about the procedure; having less access to information about, or less support for use of, alternative birth control methods; and having made the decision for sterilization because of pressure from a spouse or because of a medical condition. Comprehensive counseling is important when couples are considering sterilization.

Tubal ligation can be reversed but it is expensive and is often not covered by insurance; therefore a patient should not undergo sterilization if she is contemplating reversal. Success, as measured by the occurrence of pregnancy after tubal reanastomosis, varies from 40% to 85%, depending on the type of tubal ligation performed and on the length of functioning tube that remains. Success rates for vas reanastomosis vary from 37% to 90%, and higher success rates are associated with shorter intervals from the time of vas ligation.

Barrier Methods

Barrier methods of contraception and vaginal spermicides were long used in Europe and England before they were manufactured in this country beginning in the 1920s. The diaphragm was the first woman-controlled contraceptive method available in the United States. The typical use failure rate for the diaphragm is 16%, with a range of 2% to 23%. Because this method of contraception requires substantial motivation, instruction, and experience, it is more effective in older women who are familiar with the technique. However, younger women may also be successful users with appropriate counseling. A diaphragm fits behind the pubic bone and completely covers the cervix. To get the appropriately sized diaphragm, a fitting with a gynecologic provider is required. **Because of the physical changes of pregnancy and delivery, a diaphragm should not be fitted until 6 weeks postpartum**. Even if a woman was previously using a diaphragm, she requires a refitting. In women who are breastfeeding, anovulation leads to vaginal dryness and tightness, which may make the proper fitting of a diaphragm more difficult. The diaphragm should be used with one of the spermicidal lubricants, all of which contain nonoxynol-9.

Condoms are an effective contraceptive method and also provide protection from sexually transmitted infections (STIs). The various types of condoms available include latex and nonlatex varieties, such as polyurethane, silicone rubber, and natural membrane condoms. It is important to note that whereas natural membrane condoms prevent sperm penetration, they do not protect well against STIs. Spermicide is no longer advocated for use with condoms because of the vaginal irritation and microtears in the vaginal mucosa that can result in—and increase the risk for—infection, especially human immunodeficiency virus (HIV). The typical use failure rate for condoms is 17%, but it can be as low as 2%, depending on the age and motivation of the population studied.

The female condom is more expensive and more awkward to use than the male condom, but it has the advantage of being controlled by the woman. It has a typical use failure rate of 27%.

Natural Family Planning Methods

Natural family planning (NFP) methods, also known as *periodic abstinence* or *fertility awareness* methods, involve women having a great knowledge of their own menstrual cycles and being keyed in to signs and symptoms of the fertile phase of the cycle, during which time they abstain from intercourse. To use these methods with success, a woman must have a regular menstrual cycle in addition to commitment from her partner. Postpartum women should not rely on NFP methods until regular menstrual cycles have resumed.

Several NFP methods can be used and include the *rhythm method*, or *calendar method,* in which the fertile period of one month can be predicted by the timing of the past cycle. The *cervical mucus method* requires a woman to monitor her cervical mucus for estrogen-related changes. The *symptothermal method* typically combines cervical mucus monitoring with basal body temperature monitoring. The *standard days* method has the lowest failure rate of the NFP methods because it has the greatest number of abstinence days. A 26- to 32-day cycle is required for this method, and intercourse is avoided on days 8 through 19. When used perfectly, the pregnancy rate for the first year of use was 3.1%.[128] **Typical use failure rates for NFP methods range from 12% to 25%.** NFP methods are unforgiving if the rules of periodic abstinence are not followed.

POSTPARTUM PSYCHOLOGICAL REACTIONS

The psychological reactions experienced following childbirth include the common, relatively mild physiologic and transient "maternity blues" (occurring in 50% to 70% of women), true depression (occurring in 8% to 20% of women), and frank puerperal psychosis (occurring in 0.14% to 0.26% of women).

Overall, anxiety is the most common emotional symptom in the puerperium. These problems are discussed in Chapter 55. In patients with underlying depression or a history of PPD and in those who report symptoms that develop during the immediate postpartum period, it is essential that a postpartum visit be scheduled sooner than the traditional 6 weeks. Other risk factors for PPD include a family history of depression, a mother with PPD, a poor social situation, and prolonged separation from the infant. The moderately depressed mother often experiences such guilt and embarrassment secondary to her sense of failure in her mothering role that she is unable to call her physician or admit the symptoms of her depression. Consequently, ample time must be set aside to explore in depth even the slightest symptoms or signs of depression. Home visits in this situation may be appropriate to assess the patient. **When a patient calls with a seemingly innocuous question, she should be asked two or three open-ended questions about her general status.** Such questions allow the patient to open up if underlying depression is an issue, and she feels too guilty or afraid to express herself spontaneously. Examples of sample questions are:

1. How do you feel things are going?
2. How are things with the baby?
3. Are you feeling how you expected to feel?

Because nursing staff often triage phone calls for physicians and midwives, it is important that such personnel be instructed to be alert to this protocol. Additionally, we recommend that both parents be warned before hospital discharge that if the maternity blues seem to be lasting longer than 2 weeks or become too tough to handle, either partner should call. An easy screening depression scale, the EPDS, is shown in Box 23-2. Puerperal thyroid disease will often present with symptoms such as mild dysphoria; consequently, thyroid function studies are suggested in the evaluation of patients with suspected PPD that occurs 2 to 3 months after delivery.

MANAGING PERINATAL GRIEVING

For the most part, perinatal events are happy ones and are occasions for rejoicing. **When a patient and her family experience a loss associated with a pregnancy, special attention must be given to the grieving patient and her family.**

The most obvious cases of perinatal loss are those in which a fetal or neonatal death has occurred. Other, more subtle losses can be associated with a significant amount of grieving, such as the birth of a critically ill or malformed infant, an unexpected hysterectomy performed for intractable postpartum hemorrhage, or even a planned postpartum sterilization procedure. **Grief occurs with any significant loss, whether it is the actual death of an infant or the loss of an idealized child in the case of the birth of an infant with an illness or potential disability.**

The clinical signs and symptoms of grief and their psychological ramifications as they relate to loss suffered by women during their pregnancies have been given special consideration in recent years. In studying the relatives of servicemen who died in World War II, Lindemann recognized five manifestations of *normal grieving.* These include somatic symptoms of sleeplessness, fatigue, digestive symptoms, and sighing respirations; preoccupation with the image of the deceased; feelings of guilt; feelings of hostility and anger toward others; and disruption of the normal pattern of daily life. He also described the characteristics of what is now recognized as *pathologic grieving,* which may occur if acute mourning is suppressed or interrupted. Some of the manifestations of this so-called morbid grief reaction are overactivity without a sense of loss; appearance or exacerbations of psychosomatic illness; alterations in relationships with friends and relatives; furious hostility toward specific persons; lasting loss of patterns of social interaction; activities detrimental to personal, social, and economic existence; and agitated depression.

Kennel and associates[129] studied the reaction of 20 mothers to the loss of their newborn infants. Characteristic signs and symptoms of mourning occurred in all the patients, even when the infant was nonviable. Similar grief reactions occurred in most of the parents of 101 critically ill infants who survived after referral to a regional neonatal intensive care unit, showing that separation from a seriously ill newborn is sufficient to provoke a typical grief reaction. **Interestingly, studies over the last 15 years have found that women who do not see their stillborn infant actually have less depression; this suggests that best practice is to give mothers the choice of seeing and holding their infant after delivery but not to necessarily encourage them to do it.**

It is important that the characteristics of a grieving patient be recognized and understood by the health professionals who care for them; otherwise, substantial misunderstanding and mismanagement of the patient will occur. For example, if the patient's reaction of anger and hostility is unanticipated, a nurse or physician may take personally the hostile statements or actions of the patient or her family and may avoid contact at the very time the grieving patient most needs consolation and support. Because of their own discomfort with the implications of death, physicians, nurses, and others on the postpartum unit often find it difficult to deal with patients whose fetus or infant has died. As a consequence, reluctance to discuss the death with the patient is understandable, as is the tendency is to rely on the use of sedatives or tranquilizers to deal with the patient's symptoms of grief. **What is actually beneficial at such a time is a sympathetic listener and an opportunity for the patient to express and discuss feelings of guilt, anger, and hopelessness and to allow the other symptoms of mourning.**

It is not surprising that PPD is more common and more severe in families that have suffered a perinatal loss. In one study, the prolonged grief response occurred more often in those women who became pregnant within 5 months of the death of the infant. This finding suggests that in counseling women after the loss of an infant, it is best to ignore the traditional advice of encouraging the family to embark soon on another pregnancy as a "replacement" for the infant who died. Just how long the normal grief reaction lasts is unknown, and surely it varies with different families. Lockwood and Lewis[130] studied 26 patients who had suffered a stillbirth, and they followed several patients for as long as 2 years. Their data suggest that grief in this situation is usually resolved within 18 months, invariably with a resurgence of symptoms at the first anniversary of the loss.

Somatic symptoms of grief—such as anorexia, weakness, and fatigue—are now well recognized. Spontaneous abortion and infertility increase among couples who attempt to conceive after the loss of an infant. Physical changes that occur with grieving may account for this increase in poor reproductive success. Although the most intense suppression is noted within the first month after a loss, a modified response may last for as long as 14 months.

The regionalization of perinatal health care has resulted in a large proportion of the perinatal deaths occurring in tertiary centers. In some of these centers, teams of physicians, nurses, social workers, and pastoral counselors have evolved to aid specifically in the management of families that suffer a perinatal loss. Although this approach ensures an enlightened, understanding, and consistent approach to bereaved families, it suggests that the support of a grieving patient is a highly complex endeavor that can be accomplished only by a few specially trained individuals who care for postpartum patients. Enlightened and compassionate counseling of parents who have suffered a perinatal loss may be accomplished by any of the mother's health care professionals by using the guidelines listed in Box 23-4. Clearly, management of grief is not solely a postpartum responsibility, and this is particularly true when a prenatal diagnosis is made of fetal death or abnormality. A continuum of support is essential as the patient moves from the prenatal setting, to labor and delivery, to the postpartum ward, and finally to her home. Relaxation of many of the traditional hospital routines may be necessary to provide the type of support these families need. For example, allowing a loved one to remain past visiting hours, providing a couple a private setting in which

---

BOX 23-4   GUIDELINES FOR MANAGING PERINATAL LOSS

Keep parents informed; be honest and forthright.
Recognize and facilitate anticipatory grieving.
Inform parents about the grieving process.
Encourage the support person to remain with the mother throughout labor.
Encourage the mother to make as many choices about her care as possible.
Support parents in seeing, touching, or holding the infant.
Describe the infant in detail, especially for couples who choose not to see the infant.
Allow photographs of the infant.
Prepare the couple for hospital paperwork, such as autopsy requests.
Discuss funeral or memorial services.
Assist the couple in the process of informing siblings, relatives, and friends.
Discuss subsequent pregnancy.
Liberal use of follow-up home or office visits.

Modified from Kowalski K. Managing perinatal loss. *Clin Obstet Gynecol.* 1980;23:1113.

to be with their deceased infant, or allowing unusually early discharge with provisions for frequent phone calls and follow-up visits often facilitates the resolution of grief.

It is also important to realize that after the death of a fetus or neonate, fathers have somewhat different grief responses than do mothers. In a study of 28 fathers who had lost infants, grief was primarily characterized by self-blame, feelings of diminished self-worth, a need to keep busy with increased work, and limited ability to ask for help. Stoic responses are typical of men and may obstruct the normal resolution of grief.

Postpartum Posttraumatic Stress Disorder

Posttraumatic stress disorder (PTSD) may occur after any physical or psychological trauma. The disorder commonly occurs after a labor and delivery experience in which a woman is confronted with circumstances (pain, loss, trauma) that her defenses or sense of well-being cannot overcome. Thus some women develop PTSD from an experience that other women will cope with easily or that a clinician may find fairly unremarkable.

PTSD may lead to behavioral sequelae that include flashbacks, avoidance, and inability to function. Emergency operative deliveries, both vaginal and abdominal, and severe unexpected pain have been reported to produce posttraumatic stress. The reaction may lead to fear of a subsequent delivery that may become incapacitating as well as more generalized symptoms of this disorder. **Whenever an emergency procedure is indicated, debriefing afterward—both early and a few weeks later—may help to decrease the incidence of this problem.** Women with adverse outcomes frequently experience transference of their previous experience as the next delivery approaches. If anxiety is a predominant symptom at the postpartum visit, discussions of a PTSD reaction may be indicated. The symptom complex of PTSD is less severe and is sometimes eliminated with early intervention. Thus if a woman seems to express psychological symptoms out of proportion to her labor and delivery experience, referral for further evaluation is appropriate.

KEY POINTS

- By 6 weeks postpartum, only 28% of women have returned to their prepregnant weight.
- About 50% of parturients experience diminished sexual desire during the 3 months that follow delivery.
- Postpartum uterine bleeding of sufficient quantity to require medical attention occurs in 1% to 2% of parturients. Of patients who require curettage, 40% will be found to have retained placental tissue.
- LARC methods are the most effective contraceptive available and are safe methods for postpartum women, including those who are breastfeeding.
- In nonbreastfeeding postpartum women, combined hormonal contraceptive methods (pill, patch, ring) should not be used prior to 21 days because of the risk of venous thromboembolism; in postpartum women with additional risk factors, combined hormonal contraceptives should not be used until after 42 days.
- Breastfeeding results in 98% contraceptive protection when the woman is exclusively breastfeeding on demand both day and night, is amenorrheic, and the infant is less than 6 months old.
- Progestin-only contraceptives do not diminish lactation performance.
- Postpartum major depression occurs in 8% to 20% of parturients; if possible, risk factors should be considered to identify patients for increased screening and surveillance.
- Puerperal hypothyroidism often presents with symptoms that include mild dysphoria; consequently, thyroid function studies are suggested in the evaluation of patients with suspected PPD that occurs 2 to 3 months after delivery.

REFERENCES

1. Hytten FE, Cheyne GA. The size and composition of the human pregnant uterus. *J Obstet Gynaecol Br Commonw.* 1969;76:400.
2. Sharman A. Postpartum regeneration of the human endometrium. *J Anat.* 1953;87:1.
3. Willms AB, Brown ED, Kettritz UI, et al. Anatomic changes in the pelvis after uncomplicated vaginal delivery: evaluation with serial MR imaging. *Radiology.* 1995;195:91.
4. Oppenheimer LS, Sheriff EA, Goodman JDS, et al. The duration of lochia. *Br J Obstet Gynaecol.* 1986;93:754.
5. Visness CM, Kennedy KI, Ramos R. The duration and character of postpartum bleeding among breast-feeding women. *Obstet Gynecol.* 1997;89:159.
6. Poder L. Ultrasound evaluation of the uterus. In: Callen PW, ed. *Ultrasonography in Obstetrics and Gynecology.* 5th ed. Philadelphia: Saunders; 2000:939-940.
7. Lipinski JK, Adam AH. Ultrasonic prediction of complications following normal vaginal delivery. *J Clin Ultrasound.* 1981;9:17.
8. Chang YL, Madrozo B, Drukker BH. Ultrasonic evaluation of the postpartum uterus in management of postpartum bleeding. *Obstet Gynecol.* 1981;58:227.
9. Perex A, Uela P, Masnick GS, et al. First ovulation after childbirth: the effect of breast feeding. *Am J Obstet Gynecol.* 1972;114:1041.
10. Gray RH, Campbell ON, Apelo R, et al. Risk of ovulation during lactation. *Lancet.* 1990;335:25.
11. Lovelady CA, Garner KE, Thoreno KL, et al. The effect of weight loss in overweight, lactating women on the growth of their infants. *N Engl J Med.* 2000;342:449.
12. Dewey KG, Lovelady CA, Nommsen-Rivers LA, et al. A randomized study of the effects of aerobic exercise by lactating women on breast-milk volume and composition. *N Engl J Med.* 1994;330:449.
13. Rooney BL, Schauberger CW. Excess pregnancy weight gain and long-term obesity: one decade later. *Obstet Gynecol.* 2002;100:245.
14. Vesco KK, Dietz PM, Rizzo J, et al. Excessive gestational weight gain and postpartum weight retention among obese women. *Obstet Gynecol.* 2009;114:1069.
15. Davenport MH, Giroux I, Sopper MM, Mottola A. Postpartum exercise regardless of intensity improves chronic disease risk factors. *Med Sci Sports Exerc.* 2011;43:951-958.
16. Vega SR, Kleinart J, Sulprizio M, Hollmann W, Bloch W. Strüder HK. Responses of serum neurotrophic factors to exercise in pregnant and postpartum women. *Psychoneuroendocrinology.* 2011;36:220-227.
17. Phelan S. Pregnancy: A "teachable moment" for weight control and obesity prevention. *Am J Obstet Gynecol.* 2010;135:e1.
18. Phelan S, Phipps MG, Abrams B, et al. Does behavioral prevention in pregnancy reduce postpartum weight retention? Twelve-month outcomes of the Fit for Delivery randomized trial. *Am J Clin Nutr.* 2014;99:302-311.
19. Adegboye AR, Linne YM. Diet or exercise, or both for weight reduction in women after childbirth. *Cochrane Database Syst Rev.* 2013;7:CD005627.
20. Rasmusen NG, Hornnes PJ, Hegedus L. Ultrasonographically determined thyroid size in pregnancy and postpartum: the goitrogenic effect of pregnancy. *Am J Obstet Gynecol.* 1989;160:1216.

21. Kent GN, Stuckey BG, Allen JR, Lambert T, Gee V. Postpartum thyroid dysfunction: clinical assessment and relationship to psychiatric affective morbidity. *Clin Endocrinol (Oxf)*. 1999;51:429.

22. Pedersen CA, Stern RA, Pate J, et al. Thyroid and adrenal measures during late pregnancy and the puerperium in women who have been major depressed or who become dysmorphic postpartum. *J Affect Disord*. 1993;29:201.

23. Stagnaro-Green A. Postpartum thyroiditis. *Best Pract Res Clin Endocrinol Metab*. 2004;18:303.

24. Macklon NS, Greer IA. The deep venous system in the puerperium: an ultrasound study. *Br J Obstet Gynaecol*. 1997;104:198.

25. Clapp JF 3rd, Capeless E. Cardiovascular function before, during, and after the first and subsequent pregnancies. *Am J Cardiol*. 1997;80:1469.

26. Hellgren M. Hemostasis during normal pregnancy and puerperium. *Semin Thromb Hemost*. 2003;29:125.

27. Kamel H, Navi BB, Sriram N, Hovsepian DA, Deveraux RB, Elkind MS. Risk of a thrombotic event after the 6-week postpartum period. *N Engl J Med*. 2014;370:1307-1315.

28. Singh N, Perfect JR. Immune reconstitution syndrome and exacerbation of infections after pregnancy. *Clin Infect Dis*. 2007;45:1192.

29. Belfort MA, Clark SL, Saade GR, et al. Hospital readmission after delivery: evidence for an increased incidence of nonurogenital infection in the immediate postpartum period. *Am J Obstet Gynecol*. 2010;202:35.e1.

30. Liu S, Heaman M, Joseph KS, et al. Risk of maternal postpartum readmission associated with mode of delivery. *Obstet Gynecol*. 2005;105:836.

31. Thung SF, Norwitz ER. Postpartum care: we can and should do better. *Am J Obstet Gynecol*. 2010;202:1.

32. Cietak KA, Newton JR. Serial qualitative maternal nephrosonography in pregnancy. *Br J Radiol*. 1985;58:399.

33. Sims EA, Krantz KE. Serial studies of renal function during pregnancy and the puerperium in normal women. *J Clin Invest*. 1958;37:1764.

34. Polatti F, Capuzzo E, Viazzo F, et al. Bone mineral changes during and after lactation. *Obstet Gynecol*. 1999;94:52.

35. Holmberg-Marttila D, Sievanen H. Prevalence of bone mineral changes during postpartum amenorrhea and after resumption of menstruation. *Am J Obstet Gynecol*. 1999;180:537.

36. Lasky MA, Prentice A. Bone mineral changes during and after lactation. *Obstet Gynecol*. 1999;94:608.

37. Little KD, Clapp JF 3rd. Self-selected recreational exercise has no impact on early postpartum lactation-induced bone loss. *Med Sci Sports Exerc*. 1998;30:831.

38. Lovelady CA, Bopp MJ, Collerar HL, Mackick K, Wideman L. Effect of exercise training on loss of bone mineral density during lactation. *Med Sci Sports Exerc*. 2009;41:1902-1907.

39. Temkin E. Driving through: postpartum care during World War II. *Am J Public Health*. 1999;89:587.

40. Brown S, Small R, Faber B, et al. Early postnatal discharge from hospital for healthy mothers and term infants. *Cochrane Database Syst Rev*. 2002;3:CD002958.

41. Hebert PR, Reed G, Entman SS, et al. Serious maternal morbidity after childbirth: prolonged hospital stays and readmissions. *Obstet Gynecol*. 1999;94:942.

42. Glazener CM, Abdalla M, Stroud P, Naji S, Templeton A, Russell IT. Postnatal maternal morbidity: extent, causes, prevention and treatment. *Br J Obstet Gynaecol*. 1995;102:282.

43. Ford JB, Algert CS, Morris JM, Roberts CL. Decreasing length of maternal hospital stay is not associated with increased readmission rates. *Aust N Z J Public Health*. 2012;36:430-434.

44. Liu LL, Clemens CJ, Shay DK, et al. The safety of early newborn discharge: the Washington state experience. *JAMA*. 1997;278:293.

45. Mandl KD, Brennan TA, Wise PH, et al. Maternal and infant health: effects of moderate reductions in postpartum length of stay. *Arch Pediatr Adolesc Med*. 1997;151:915.

46. Britton JR, Britton HL, Gronwaldt V. Early perinatal hospital discharge and parenting during infancy. *Pediatrics*. 1999;104:1070.

47. Brumfield CG. Early postpartum discharge. *Clin Obstet Gynecol*. 1998;41:611.

48. Bohlke K, Galil K, Jackson L, et al. Postpartum varicella vaccination: Is the vaccine virus excreted in breast milk? *Obstet Gynecol*. 2003;102:970.

49. Center for Disease Control and Prevention (CDC). Updated recommendations for use of tetanus toxoid, reduced diphtheria toxoid, and acellular pertussis vaccine (Tdap) in pregnant women. Advisory Committee on Immunization Practices 2012. *MMWR Morb Mortal Wkly Rep*. 2013;62:131-135.

50. Jennings B, Edmundson M. The postpartum periods. After confinement: the fourth trimester. *Clin Obstet Gynecol*. 1980;23:1093.

51. Minig L, Trimble EL, Sarsotti C, et al. Building the evidence base for postoperative and postpartum advice. *Obstet Gynecol*. 2009;114:892.

52. Koltyn KF, Schultes SS. Psychological effects of an aerobic exercise session and a rest session following pregnancy. *J Sports Med Phys Fitness*. 1997;37:287.

53. Sampselle CM, Seng J, Yeo S, et al. Physical activity and postpartum well-being. *J Obstet Gynecol Neonatal Nurs*. 1999;28:41.

54. Norman E, Sherburn M, Osborne RH, et al. An exercise and education program improves well-being of new mothers: a randomized controlled trial. *Phys Ther*. 2010;90:348.

55. Reamy K, White SE. Sexuality in pregnancy and the puerperium: a review. *Obstet Gynecol Surv*. 1985;40:1.

56. Leeman LM, Rogers RG. Sex after childbirth. *Obstet Gynecol*. 2012;118:647-655.

57. McDonald EA, Brown SJ. Does method of birth make a difference to when women resume sex after childbirth? *BJOG*. 2013;120:823-830.

58. Glazener CM. Sexual function after childbirth: women's experiences, persistent morbidity and lack of professional recognition. *Br J Obstet Gynaecol*. 1997;104:330.

59. Goetsch MF. Postpartum dyspareunia: an unexplored problem. *J Reprod Med*. 1999;44:963.

60. Signorello L, Harlow B, Chekos A, et al. Postpartum sexual functioning and its relationship to perineal trauma: a retrospective cohort study of primiparous women. *Am J Obstet Gynecol*. 2001;184:881.

61. Hicks TL, Forester-Goodall S, Quattrone EM, et al. Postpartum sexual functioning and method of delivery: summary of the evidence. *Am Coll Nurse Midwives*. 2004;49:430.

62. Ryding E-L. Sexuality during and after pregnancy. *Acta Obstet Gynecol Scand*. 1984;63:679.

63. Byrd JE, Shibley-Hyde J, DeLamater J, et al. Sexuality during pregnancy and the year postpartum. *J Fam Pract*. 1998;47:305.

64. Gagnon AJ, Edgar L, Kramer MS, et al. A randomized trial of a program of early postpartum discharge with nurse visitation. *Am J Obstet Gynecol*. 1997;176:205.

65. Gunn J, Lumley S, Chondros P, Young D. Does an early postnatal check-up improve maternal health: results from a randomized trial in Australian general practice. *Br J Obstet Gynaecol*. 1998;105:991.

66. Lu MC, Kotelchuck M, Culhane JF, et al. Preconception care between pregnancies: the content of internatal care. *Matern Child Health J*. 2006;10:S107.

67. Connolly AM, Thorp JM Jr. Childbirth-related perineal trauma: clinical significance and prevention. *Clin Obstet Gynecol*. 1999;42:820.

68. Stomp-van den Berg SG, Hendriksen IJ, Bruinvels DJ, Twisk JW, van Mechelen W, van Poppel MN. Predictors for postpartum pelvic girdle pain in working women: the Mom@Work cohort study. *Pain*. 2012;153:2370-2379.

69. Boyle R, Hay-Smith EJ, Cody JD, Mørkved S. Pelvic floor muscle training for prevention and treatment of urinary and faecal incontinence in antenatal and postnatal women. *Cochrane Database Syst Rev*. 2012;10:CD007471.

70. Weidner AC, Jamison MG, Branham V, et al. Neuropathic injury to the levator ani occurs in 1 in 4 primiparous women. *Am J Obstet Gynecol*. 2006;195:1851.

71. Handa VL, Zyczynski HM, Burgio KL, et al. The impact of fecal and urinary incontinence on quality of life 6 months after childbirth. *Am J Obstet Gynecol*. 2007;197:636, e1.

72. Chaliha C, Kalia V, Stanton S, et al. Antenatal prediction of postpartum fecal incontinence. *Obstet Gynecol*. 1999;94:689.

73. Harvey MA. Pelvic floor exercises during and after pregnancy: a systematic review of their role in preventing pelvic floor dysfunction. *J Obstet Gynaecol Can*. 2003;25:487.

74. MacArthur C, Glazener C, Lancashire R, et al. Faecal incontinence and mode of first and subsequent delivery: a six-year longitudinal study. *Br J Obstet Gynaecol*. 2005;112:1075.

75. Pollack J, Nordenstam J, Brismar S, et al. Anal incontinence after vaginal delivery: a five-year prospective cohort study. *Obstet Gynecol*. 2004;104:1397.

76. Kocaoz S, Eroglu K, Sivaslioglu AA. Role of pelvic floor muscle exercises in the prevention of stress urinary incontinence during pregnancy and the postpartum period. *Gynecol Obstet Invest*. 2013;75:34-40.

77. Hilde G, Stær-Jensen J, Siafarikas F, Ellström Engh M, Bø K. Postpartum pelvic floor muscle training and urinary incontinence: a randomiozed controlled trial. *Obstet Gynecol*. 2013;122:1231-1238.

78. Peirce C, Murphy C, Fitzpatrick M, et al. Randomized controlled trial comparing early home biofeedback physiotherapy with pelvic floor exercises for the treatment of third degree tears (EBAPT Trial). *BJOG*. 2013;120:1240-1247.

79. Glazener CM, MacArthur C, Hagen S, et al. Twelve year follow-up of conservative management of postnatal urinary and faecal incontinence and prolapse outcomes: randomised controlled trial. *BJOG*. 2014;121: 112-120.

80. King PA, Duthie SJ, Dip V, et al. Secondary postpartum hemorrhage. *Aust N Z J Obstet Gynaecol*. 1989;29:394.

81. Boyd BK, Katz VL, Hansen WF. Delayed postpartum hemorrhage: a retrospective analysis. *J Matern Fetal Med*. 1995;4:19.

82. Hoveyda F, MacKenzie IZ. Secondary postpartum haemorrhage: Incidence, morbidity and current management. *Br J Obstet Gynaecol*. 2001; 108:927.

83. Thompson JF, Roberts CL, Ellwood DA. Emotional and physical health outcomes after significant primary post-partum hemorrhage: A multicenter cohort study. *Aust N Z J Obstet Gynaecol*. 2011;51:365-371.

84. Klaus MH, Jerauld R, Kreger NC, et al. Maternal attachment: importance of the first postpartum days. *N Engl J Med*. 1972;286:460.

85. McClellan MS, Cabianca WC. Effects of early mother-infant contact following cesarean birth. *Obstet Gynecol*. 1980;56:52.

86. Robson KM, Powell E. Early maternal attachment. In: Brickington IF, Kumar R, eds. *Motherhood and Mental Illness*. San Diego: Academic Press; 1982:155.

87. Klaus M, Kennel J. *Parent-Infant Bonding*. St. Louis: CV Mosby; 1982.

88. Gray J, Butler C, Dean J, et al. Prediction and prevention of child abuse and neglect. *Child Abuse Neglect*. 1977;1:45.

89. Siegel E, Cauman KE, Schaefer ES, et al. Hospital and home support during infancy: impact on maternal attachment, child abuse and neglect and health care utilization. *Pediatrics*. 1980;66:183.

90. Areskog B, Uddenberg N, Kjessler B. Experience of delivery in women with and without antenatal fear of childbirth. *Gynecol Obstet Invest*. 1983;16:1.

91. Kozuki N, Lee AC, Silveira MF, et al. The association of birth intervals with small-for-gestational-age, preterm, and neonatal and infant mortality: a meta-analysis. *BMC Public Health*. 2013;13(suppl 3):S3.

92. Miller VL, Laken MA, Ager J, Essenmacher L. Contraceptive decision making among Medicaid-eligible women. *J Community Health*. 2000;25: 473-480.

93. Smith KB, van der Spuy ZM, Cheng L, et al. Is postpartum contraceptive advice given antenatally of value? *Contraception*. 2002;65:237-243.

94. Lopez LM, Hiller JE, Grimes DA, Chen M. Education for contraceptive use by women after childbirth. *Cochrane Database Syst Rev*. 2012;8: CD001863.

95. *Breastfeeding Report Card, United States/2013. National Center for Chronic Disease Prevention and Health Promotion, Division of Nutrition, Physicial Activity, and Obesity*. CDC national Immunization Surveys 2011 and 2012, Provisional Data, 2010 births. <http://www.cdc.gov/breastfeeding/data/NIS_data/index.htm>.

96. Tyson JE, Carter JN, Andreassen B, Huth J, Smith B. Nursing mediated prolactin and luteinizing hormone secretion during puerperal lactation. *Fertil Steril*. 1978;30:154-162.

97. Wasalathanthri S, Tennekoon KH. Lactational amenorrhea/anovulation and some of their determinants: a comparison of well-nourished and undernourished women. *Fertil Steril*. 2001;76:317-325.

98. Campbell OM, Gray RH. Characteristics and determinants of postpartum ovarian function in women in the United States. *Am J Obstet Gynecol*. 1993;169:55-60.

99. Labbok MH, Hight-Laukaran V, Peterson AE, Fletcher V, von Hertzen H, Van Look PF. Multicenter study of the lactational amenorrhea method (LAM): I. Efficacy, duration, and implications for clinical application. *Contraception*. 1997;55:327-336.

100. Gray RH, Campbell OM, Zacur HA, Labbok MH, MacRae SL. Postpartum return of ovarian activity in nonbreastfeeding women monitored by urinary assays. *J Clin Endocrinol Metab*. 1987;64:645-650.

101. Luukkainen T, Allonen H, Haukkamaa M, Lahteenmake P, Nilsson CG, Toivonen J. Five years' experience with levonorgestrel-releasing IUDs. *Contraception*. 1986;33:139-148.

102. Andersson J, Rybo G. Levonorgestrel-releasing intrauterine device in the treatment of menorrhagia. *Br J Obstet Gynaecol*. 1990;97:690-694.

103. Baldszti E, Wimmer-Puchinger B, Loschke K. Acceptability of the long-term contraceptive levonorgestrel-releasing intrauterine system (Mirena): a 3-year follow up study. *Contraception*. 2003;76:87-91.

104. Hidalgo M, Bahamondes L, Perrotti M, Diaz J, Dantas-Monteiro C, Petta C. Bleeding patterns and clinical performance of the levonorgestrel-releasing intrauterine system (Mirena) up to two years. *Contraception*. 2002;65:129-132.

105. Kapp N, Curtis KM. Intrauterine device insertion during the postpartum period: a systematic review. *Contraception*. 2009;80:327-336.

106. Gurtcheff SE, Turok DK, Stoddard G, Murphy PA, Gibson M, Jones KP. Lactogenesis after early postpartum use of the contraceptive implant: a randomized controlled trial. *Obstet Gynecol*. 2011;117:1114-1121.

107. Singhal S, Sarda N, Gupta S, Goel S. Impact of injectable progestogen contraception in early puerperium on lactation and infant health. *J Clin Diagn Res*. 2014;8:69-72.

108. Cromer BA, Smith RD, Blair JM, Dwyer J, Brown RT. A prospective study of adolescents who choose among levonorgestrel implant (Norplant), medroxyprogesterone acetate (Depo-Provera), or the combined oral contraceptive pill as contraception. *Pediatrics*. 1994;94:687-694.

109. Schwallie P, Assenza J. The effect of depo medroxyprogesterone acetate on pituitary and ovarian function, and the return of fertility following its discontinuation: a review. *Contraception*. 1974;10:181-202.

110. Xiang AH, Kawakubo M, Kjos SL, Buchanan TA. Long-acting injectable progestin contraception and risk of type 2 diabetes in Latino women with prior gestational diabetes mellitus. *Diabetes Care*. 2006;29:613-617.

111. Westhoff C, Truman C, Kalmuss D, et al. Depressive symptoms and Depo-Provera. *Contraception*. 1998;57:237-240.

112. Gupta N, O'Brien R, Jacobsen LJ, et al. Mood changes in adolescents using depot-medroxyprogesterone acetate for contraception: a prospective study. *J Pediatr Adolesc Gynecol*. 2001;14:71-76.

113. Tsai R, Schaffir J. Effect of depot medroxyprogesterone acetate on postpartum depression. *Contraception*. 2010;82:174-177.

114. Clark MK, Sowers M, Levy B, Nichols S. Bone mineral density loss and recovery during 48 months in first-time users of depot medroxyprogesterone acetate. *Fertil Steril*. 2006;86:1466-1476.

115. Berenson AB, Breitkopt CR, Grady JJ, Rickert VI, Thomas A. Effects of hormonal contraception on bone mineral density after 24 months of use. *Obstet Gynecol*. 2004;103:899-906.

116. Petitti DB, Piaggio G, Mehta S, Cravioto MC, Meirik O. Steroid hormone contraception and bone mineral density: a cross-sectional study in an international population. The WHO Study of Hormonal Contraception and Bone Health. *Obstet Gynecol*. 2000;95:736-744.

117. Orr-Walker JM, Cundy T, Reid IR. The effect of past use of the injectable contraceptive depot medroxyprogesterone acetate in normal postmenopausal women. *Clin Endocrinol (Oxf)*. 1998;49:615-618.

118. Jackson E, Curtis K, Gaffield M. Risk of venous thromboembolism during the postpartum period: a systematic review. *Obstet Gynecol*. 2011;117: 691-703.

119. MMWR. Update to CDC's *U.S. Medical Eligibility Criteria for Contraceptive Use, 2010*: revised recommendations for the use of contraceptive methods during the postpartum period. *MMWR*. 2011;60:878-883.

120. Tankeyoon M, Dusitsin N, Chalapati S, et al. Effects of hormonal contraceptives on milk volume and infant growth. WHO Special Programme of Research, Development, and Research Training in Human Reproduction, Task Force on Oral Contraceptives. *Contraception*. 1984;30: 505-522.

121. Halderman LD, Nelson AL. Impact of early postpartum administration of progestin-only hormonal contraceptives compared with nonhormonal contraceptives on short-term breast-feeding patterns. *Am J Obstet Gynecol*. 2002;186:1250-1256.

122. Kjos SL, Peters RK, Xiang A, Thomas D, Schaefer U, Buchanan TA. Contraception and the risk of type 2 diabetes in Latino women with prior gestational diabetes. *JAMA*. 1998;280:533-538.

123. Glasier AF, Cameron ST, Fine PM, et al. Ulipristal acetate versus levonorgestrel for emergency contraception: a randomized non-inferiority trial and meta-anlaysis. *Lancet*. 2010;375:555-562.

124. Peterson HB, Xia Z, Hughes JM, Wilcox LS, Tylor LR, Trussell J. The risk of pregnancy after tubal sterilization: findings from the U.S. Collaborative Review of Sterilization. *Am J Obstet Gynecol*. 1996;174:1161-1168.

125. Erickson BK, Conner MG, Landen CN. The role of the fallopian tube in the origin of ovarian cancer. *Am J Obstet Gynecol*. 2013;209:409-414.

126. Peterson HB, Huber DH, Belker AM. Vasectomy: an appraisal for the obstetrician-gynecologist. *Obstet Gynecol*. 1990;76:568.

127. Hillis SD, Marchbanks PA, Tylor LR, Peterson HB. Poststerilization regret: findings from the United States Collaborative Review of Sterilization. *Obstet Gynecol*. 1999;93:889-895.

128. World Health Organization (WHO). A prospective multicentre trial of the ovulation method of family planning. II. The effectiveness phase. *Fertil Steril*. 1981;36:591-598.

129. Kennel JH, Slyter H, Klaus MH. The mourning response of parents to the death of a newborn infant. *N Engl J Med*. 1970;83:344.

130. Lockwood S, Lewis IC. Management of grieving after stillbirth. *Med J Aust*. 1980;2:308.

Additional references for this chapter are available at ExpertConsult.com.

Lactation and Breastfeeding

EDWARD R. NEWTON

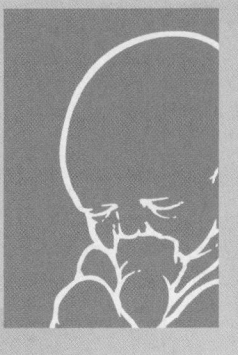

KEY ABBREVIATIONS

Agency for Healthcare Research and Quality	AHRQ
Baby-Friendly Hospital Initiative	BFHI
Centers for Disease Control and Prevention	CDC
Confidence interval	CI
Daily recommended intake	DRI
Food and Drug Administration	FDA
Human immunodeficiency virus	HIV
Hypothalamic-pituitary-adrenal (axis)	HPA
Immunoglobulin A	IgA
Infant Feeding Practices Study	IFPS
Lactational amenorrhea method	LAM
Long-chain polyunsaturated fatty acid	LCPUFA
Luteinizing hormone	LH
Maternal, Infant, and Child Health	MICH
Messenger RNA	mRNA
Methicillin-resistant *Staphylococcus aureus*	MRSA
Odds ratio	OR
Potassium hydroxide	KOH
Purified protein derivative	PPD
Recommended daily allowance	RDA
Secretory immunoglobulin A	sIgA
United Nations Children's Fund	UNICEF
World Health Organization	WHO

Breastfeeding and breast milk are the global standard for infant feeding in undeveloped and developed countries. The World Health Organization (WHO), the U.S. Surgeon General, the American Academy of Pediatrics (AAP),[1] the American College of Obstetricians and Gynecologists (ACOG),[2] the American Academy of Family Practice, and the Academy of Breastfeeding Medicine have endorsed this recommendation for over two decades. **They recommend exclusive breastfeeding for the first 6 months and continued breastfeeding at least through 12 months with subsequent weaning as a mutual decision by the mother and infant dyad in the subsequent months and years. Historic and physioanthropologic data suggest that except for the last century, humans have breastfed their children 3 to 4 years throughout history.**

Unfortunately, the United States has failed to meet the exclusivity and duration goals set out by world and national health organizations. Figure 24-1 describes the historic trends in breastfeeding behaviors in the United States. The latest estimates (2011) of breastfeeding performance (http://www.healthypeople.gov/2020) are that 79.2% of women initiate breastfeeding in the hospital, and only 49.4% of those are still breastfeeding at 6 months. Approximately 26.7% of American infants meet the standard of breastfeeding 1 year or more. Only 40.7% and 18.8% of American infants are exclusively breastfeeding at 3 and 6 months, respectively, and more than 19.4% received supplemental formula in the first 48 hours of life.

Specific populations are at greater risk for failure to initiate and continue breastfeeding. **Women of lower socioeconomic status, those with less education, and teenagers initiate breastfeeding at about half to two thirds the rate of mature high school graduates of middle and upper socioeconomic statuses. Black women tend to have lower rates of initiation and maintenance of breastfeeding than other cultural and**

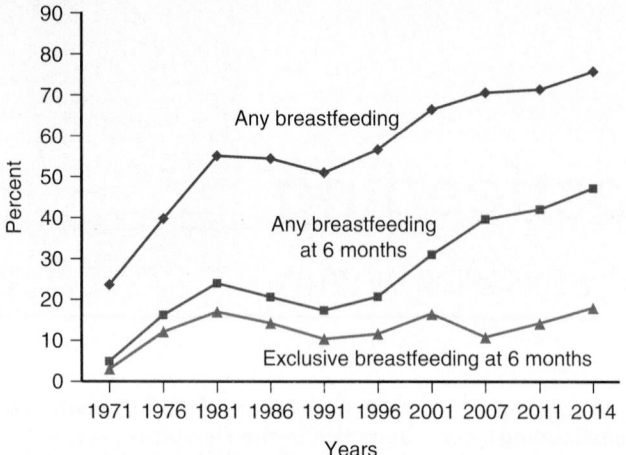

FIG 24-1 Incidence of breastfeeding in the hospital, any breastfeeding at 6 months, and exclusive breastfeeding at 6 months.

ethnic populations.[3] **Fortunately, since 1989, more women at greatest risk for feeding their infants artificial breast milk are initiating breastfeeding in the hospital.**

A recent prospective study has clarified breastfeeding behaviors in the first year after birth.[4] In the Centers for Disease Control and Prevention (CDC) and U.S. Food and Drug Administration (FDA)–sponsored Infant Feeding Practices Study II, 1147 women initiated breastfeeding and stopped breastfeeding during the study period (2005 through 2007). All women were recruited in the third trimester. Approximately 60% of mothers did not meet their personal plans for the duration of breastfeeding; the mean duration of breastfeeding in women who met their intention for breastfeeding was 7.8 months, and it was 3.8 months in those who did not meet their intention. In the multivariable analysis, women who failed to meet their desired duration of breastfeeding had initial challenges with latch-on and nipple pain or injury, perceived that the baby was not getting enough nutrition, or needed to take medications for a maternal illness.

Cultural attitudes underlie the desired duration of breastfeeding and affect the failure to breastfeed through the first year. In an effort to mobilize mothers to increase breastfeeding rates, the U.S. Surgeon General has set goals for the country. The Healthy People 2020 Maternal, Infant, and Child Health (MICH) objectives are (1) any breastfeeding, 81.9%; (2) any breastfeeding at 6 months, 60.6%; (3) any breastfeeding at 12 months, 34.1%; (4) exclusive breastfeeding at 3 months, 46.2%; (5) exclusive breastfeeding at 6 months, 25.5%; and (6) to reduce the number of infants who receive supplemental formula in the first 48 hours to 14.2%. MICH 22 sets a goal that 38% of employers have a worksite lactation support program, and MICH 24 sets a goal that 81% of live births occur in facilities that provide recommended care for the breastfeeding dyad.

Although dysfunctional cultural and familial attitudes are outside the direct control of medicine, these attitudes may directly affect the care delivered by physicians. The normal function of the breasts, to produce breast milk, is muted by three cultural attitudes. First is the association of breasts with sexual attraction; the media is replete with examples that show beautiful, well-formed breasts as a sexual ideal. A corollary of this attitude is that breastfeeding will cause the breasts to sag and lose their sex appeal. Second, an opposing cultural attitude is

that breastfeeding restricts self-fulfillment; mothers who stay at home to breastfeed and care for their babies are considered poor examples of the modern, independent professional woman. Finally, the attitude or myth is prevalent that artificial breast milk, formula, and bottle-feeding are an equivalent source of nutrition to breastfeeding, although research has proven this is not the case.

The latter attitudes are exacerbated by a lack of lay public and health care provider knowledge about breastfeeding and breast milk. The normal function of the breasts is excluded from the curriculum of primary and secondary schools on the basis of the connection between breasts and sex. After completion of their education, few women experience any examples of successful breastfeeding—that is, any breastfeeding for longer than 1 year. Between 1970 and 1990, when they gave birth, only 30% to 50% of today's grandmothers initiated breastfeeding, and less than a quarter breastfed for more than a few weeks. **The lack of exposure to successful, experienced breastfeeding mothers seriously compromises the chances of success for today's women who attempt to breastfeed.**

Physicians are products of the same culture as the women they serve. Unfortunately, many have the same cultural biases as their patients and the same lack of primary and secondary education regarding the normal physiology of breastfeeding. Although the curricula of medical school and residency training programs have improved in the last 5 years, the general lack of didactic education and clinical exposure to successfully breastfeeding mother-infant dyads contribute to the lack of breastfeeding knowledge. Most physicians who reflect on their own education will identify neither a structured curriculum nor practical experiences with successfully breastfeeding mother-infant dyads. On obstetric rotations, medical students and obstetrics residents rarely see normal breastfeeding dyads longer than 1 to 3 days postpartum. On pediatric rotations, students often see the baby only in the nursery and rarely see the normal mother breastfeed as an inpatient or at newborn visits. Although pediatric residents observe and support the mother who nurses or pumps milk for her growing preterm infant, the exposure is often negative. As a result, serious gaps exist in physicians' knowledge as they attempt to serve the over 3 million newborns and mothers per year who initiate breastfeeding. In fact, the most commonly cited resource for physicians is another nonmedical individual or a breastfeeding spouse.

The purpose of this chapter is to begin the educational process through which obstetricians will adopt the lactating mother as their patient. **In order to support the breastfeeding mother, the obstetrician must be convinced of the biologic superiority of breastfeeding and human breast milk over formula.** This chapter reviews breast anatomy and the physiology of lactation in a framework pertinent to breastfeeding management. This chapter describes the vast differences between breast milk and formula, a difference directly related to unique needs and the short- and long-term health of the infant and mother. Specific issues related to the obstetrician and other health care providers will be addressed, including the role of the obstetrician in preconception counseling, prenatal care, delivery room management, and postpartum care for the breastfeeding mother.

BREAST ANATOMY AND DEVELOPMENT

The size and shape of the breast vary greatly by stage of development, physiologic state, and phenotype. Usually, the breast projects into each axilla and thus forms the *tail of Spence.* The mature breast weighs about 200 g in the nonpregnant state; during pregnancy, 500 g; and during lactation, 600 to 800 g. As long as glandular tissue and the nipple are present, the size or shape of the breast has little to do with the functional success of the breast. **The adequacy of glandular tissue for breastfeeding is ascertained by inquiring whether a woman's breasts have enlarged during pregnancy. If the breast fails to enlarge as the result of pregnancy, especially if associated with minimal breast tissue on examination, the clinician should be wary of primary failure of lactation.**

The areola is a circular pigmented area that darkens during pregnancy; the nipple, or *papilla mammae,* is a conical elevation in the middle of the areola, or *areola mammae.* The contrast between the areola and the fairer skin of the rest of the body provides a visual cue for a newborn attempting to latch-on. The areola contains multiple small elevations called *Montgomery tubercles,* which enlarge during pregnancy and lactation. These tubercles contain multiple ductular openings of sebaceous and sweat glands that secrete lubricating and antiinfective substances (immunoglobulin A [IgA]) that protect the nipple and areola during nursing. When the breasts and nipples are washed with soap or alcohol-containing compounds, these substances are washed away, which leaves the nipple prone to cracking and infection.

Unlike the dermis of the body of the breast, which includes fat, the areola and nipple contain smooth muscle and collagenous and elastic tissue. With light touch or anticipation of nursing, these muscles contract, and the nipple erects to form a teat. The contraction pulls the lactiferous sinuses into the nipple-areola complex, which allows the infant to withdraw the breast milk from these reservoirs.

The tip of the nipple contains the openings (0.4 to 0.7 mm diameter) of 15 to 20 milk ducts (2 to 4 mm diameter). Each of the milk ducts empties one tubuloalveolar gland, embedded in the fat of the body of the breast. A sphincter mechanism at the opening of the duct limits the ejection of milk from the breast, although the competency of this mechanism varies. About 80% of women demonstrate milk ejection from the contralateral breast when milk ejection is stimulated. If milk leakage is demonstrated from the contralateral breast during nursing, it is indicative of an intact let-down reflex and is highly suggestive of milk transfer to the infant.

The milk ducts widen (5 to 8 mm) into the lactiferous sinuses 5 to 10 mm from their outlet (Fig. 24-2). These sinuses are pulled into the teat during nursing, and the infant uses its tongue, facial muscles, and mouth to squeeze the milk from the sinuses into its oropharynx. The tubuloalveolar glands (15 to 20) form lobi, which are arranged in a radial fashion from the central nipple-areola complex. The lobi and lactiferous ducts extend into the tail of Spence. Ten to 40 lactiferous ducts connect to each lactiferous sinus, and each forms a lobulus. Each lobulus arborizes into 10 to 100 alveoli that become the tubulosaccular secretory units. **The alveoli are the critical units in the production and ejection of milk: a sac of alveolar cells is surrounded by a basket of myoepithelial cells, and the alveolar cells are stimulated by prolactin to produce milk.** The myoepithelial cells are stimulated by oxytocin to contract and eject the milk into the lactiferous ducts, lactiferous sinuses, and beyond.

The radial projection of lactiferous ducts prompts important considerations relative to breast surgery on women who are breastfeeding or who will breastfeed. **Surgical skin incisions parallel to the circumareolar line, especially at the circumareolar line, have better cosmetic healing and are often chosen by surgeons. However, if the incision is taken deep into the parenchyma, the lactiferous ducts may be compromised; a superficial, parallel skin incision and a radial deep incision are preferred. In women who intend to breastfeed, a circumareolar incision should be avoided because it compromises breastfeeding in three ways: (1) by occlusion of lactiferous ducts, (2) by restriction of the formation of a teat during nursing, and (3) by injury to the lateral cutaneous branch of the fourth intercostal nerve.**

Surgical disruption of the lateral cutaneous branch of the fourth intercostal nerve can have devastating effects on the success of breastfeeding. This nerve is critical to the production and ejection of breast milk. Furthermore, the nerves provide organ-specific control of regional blood flow, and a tremendous increase in mammary blood flow occurs during a nursing episode. Disruption of this autonomic control may severely compromise lactation performance. The rate of breastfeeding failure is two to three times higher when a circumareolar incision has been performed; therefore the obstetrician needs to be alert to old surgical incisions when a pregnant patient expresses a desire to breastfeed or when a breast biopsy is anticipated in a reproductive-age woman.

As mammals, humans have the potential to develop mammary tissue (glandular or nipple tissue) anywhere along the milk line, also called the *galactic band.* The milk line extends from the axilla and inner upper arm down the abdomen along the midclavicular line to the upper lateral mons and upper inner thigh. When accessory glands occur, this is termed *hypermastia,* which may involve accessory glandular tissue, supernumerary nipples, or both. Two to 6% of women have hypermastia, and the response to pregnancy and lactation is variable. **The most common site for accessory breast tissue is the axilla. These women may present at 2 to 5 days postpartum, at initiation of galactogenesis, with painful enlargements in the axilla. Ice and symptomatic therapy for 24 to 48 hours is sufficient treatment. Supernumerary nipples (*polythelia*) are associated with renal abnormalities (11%).**

PHYSIOLOGY OF LACTATION

The best and most extensive research concerning the physiology of lactation focuses on the production of milk and has its roots in the research conducted by the multibillion-dollar dairy industry. Good milk-producing cattle, whose milk composition (i.e., fat percentage) can be controlled, create a competitive advantage in the marketplace. The translation of dairy research to human research plus the expected interest of pediatricians in infant nutrition has led to a preponderance of data on maternal milk production and delivery and its impact on neonatal and childhood outcomes. With the exception of hypothalamic hypogonadism in the breastfeeding mother and its effect on menses and child spacing, very little is understood about the physiologic changes during the breastfeeding episode, such as vascular adaptation to the rapid production (10 to 30 minutes) of 100 to 200 mL of an extremely complex liquid. **Most maternal and child benefits of breastfeeding are accrued in a dose-dependent fashion; the longer (>12 months) and the more intense (exclusive breastfeeding), the better the outcomes in terms of, for example, premenopausal breast cancer or**

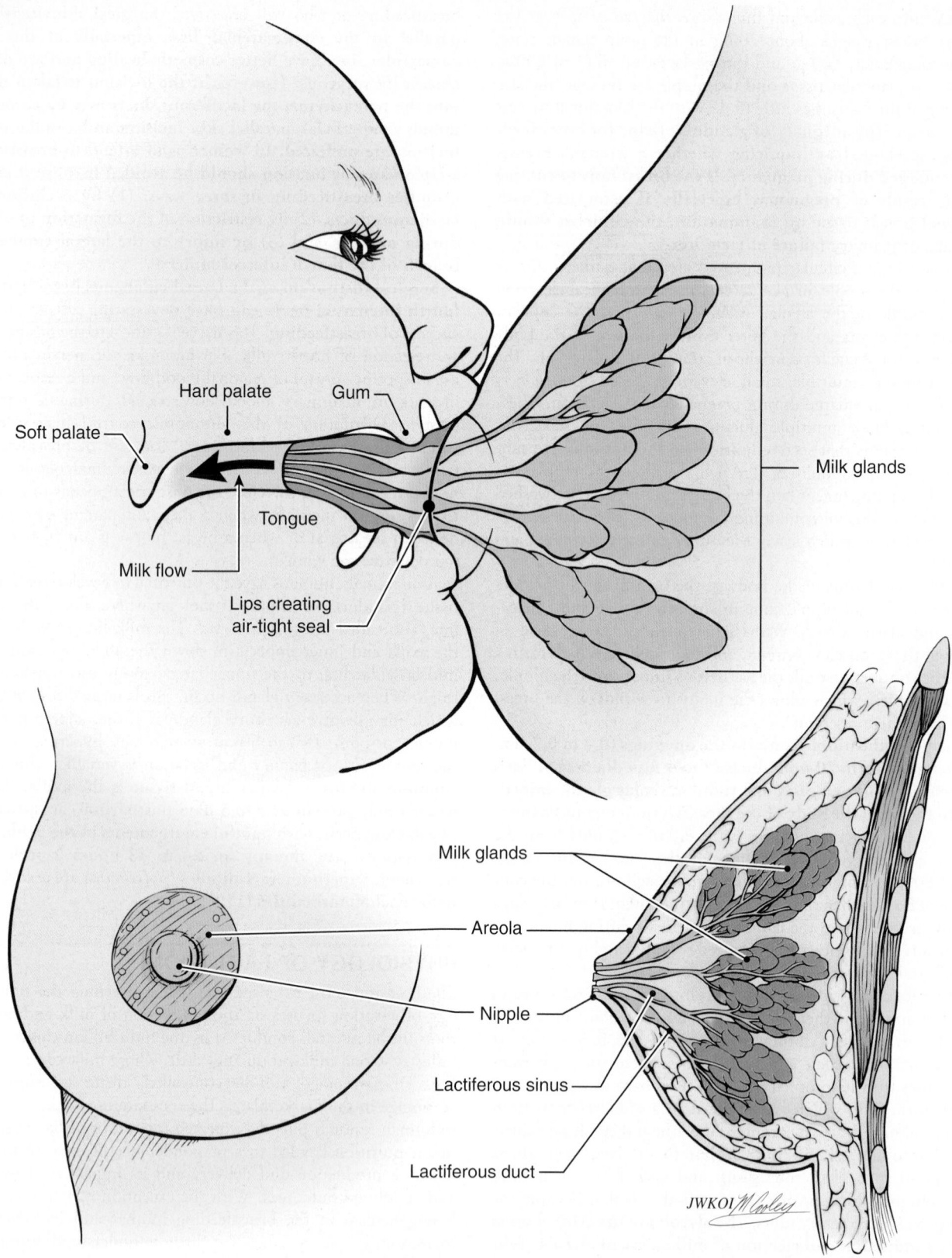

Soft palate

Hard palate

Gum

Milk glands

Tongue

Milk flow

Lips creating
air-tight seal

Milk glands

Areola

Nipple

Lactiferous sinus

Lactiferous duct

JWKOI M Cooley

FIG 24-2 Anatomy of the breast.

cardiovascular disease. We are beginning to ask the questions "why" and "how." Are the benefits of breastfeeding to the mother's health related to the duration of the hormonal changes? Are they from the "antistress" effects of oxytocin? Or do they result from changes in gastrointestinal (GI) absorption of substrates? Does the intense pair-bonding that occurs between a mother and her breast-fed children affect allostatic load later in life? The answers to these questions will greatly improve our knowledge of the human breastfeeding experience.

The physiology of lactation has three major components: (1) the stages of lactogenesis, (2) endocrinology of lactogenesis, and (3) nursing behavior/milk transfer. The following sections summarize what is known about the physiology of human lactation.[5] The composition of mature human breast milk will also be described, with a focus on the differences between breast milk and formula.

Stages of Lactogenesis

Full alveolar development and maturation of the breast must await the hormones of pregnancy—progesterone, prolactin, and human placental lactogen (hPL)—for completion of the developmental process at delivery. This is termed *lactogenesis stage I.* By midpregnancy, the gland is competent to secrete milk (colostrum), although full function is not attained until the tissues are released from the inhibition of high levels of circulating progesterone.

Lactogenesis stage II occurs as the progesterone levels fall after delivery of the placenta, during the subsequent 7 days. During the first 2 to 4 days after delivery, incremental secretion of colostrum occurs (50 to 400 mL/day). Until lactogenesis stage II has fully developed, the breasts secrete colostrum, which is very different from mature milk in volume and constituents. **Colostrum has more protein, especially secretory immunoglobulins, and more lactose; it also has a lower fat content than mature milk.** Prolactin and glucocorticoids play important promoter roles in this stage of development.

At 2 to 5 days postpartum, a dramatic increase occurs in mammary blood flow and oxygen/glucose uptake by the breast. **The secretion of milk is copious, 500 to 700 mL/day when "the milk comes in." This is the most common time for engorgement if the breasts are not drained by efficient, frequent nursing.**

After *lactogenesis stage II,* which occurs from 3 to 7 days postpartum, lactation enters an indefinite period of milk production formerly called *galactopoiesis,* now termed *lactogenesis stage III.* The duration of this stage is dependent on the continued production of breast milk and the efficient transfer of breast milk to the infant. **Prolactin appears to be the single most important *galactopoietic* hormone because selective inhibition of prolactin secretion by bromocriptine disrupts lactogenesis; oxytocin appears to be the major *galactokinetic* hormone.** Stimulation of the nipple and areola and infant behavioral cues cause a reflex contraction of the myoepithelial cells that surround the alveoli and trigger ejection of milk from the breast.

The final stage of lactation, *lactogenesis stage IV,* is involution and cessation of breastfeeding. As the frequency of breastfeeding is reduced to less than six episodes in 24 hours, and the produced milk volume is less than 400 mL in 24 hours, prolactin levels fall in proportion to the frequency of nipple stimulation, which ultimately leads to a total cessation of milk production. After 24 to 48 hours of no transfer of breast milk to the infant, increasing intraductal pressure and production of **lactation inhibitory**

factor from the alveolar epithelium appear to initiate apoptosis of the secretory epithelial cells and proteolytic degradation of the basement membrane. Lactation inhibitory factor is a protein secreted in the milk, and its increasing concentration in the absence of milk drainage appears to decrease milk production by the alveolar cells. It counterbalances pressures to increase milk supply (i.e., increased frequency of nursing) and allows for the day-to-day adjustment in infant demands.

Endocrinology of Lactogenesis

Prolactin is the major hormone that promotes milk production, and thyroid hormones selectively enhance the secretion of lactalbumin. Cortisol, insulin, parathyroid hormone, and growth hormone are supportive metabolic hormones in the production of carbohydrates and lipids in breast milk. Ovarian hormones are not required for the maintenance of established milk production and are suppressed by high levels of prolactin.

The alveolar cell is the principal site for the production of milk. Neville[5] describes five pathways for milk synthesis and secretion in the mammary alveolus, including four major transcellular and one paracellular pathway: (1) exocytosis (merocrine secretion) of milk protein and lactose in Golgi-derived secretory vesicles; (2) milk fat secretion via milk fat globules (apocrine secretion); (3) secretion of ions and water across the apical membrane; (4) pinocytosis-exocytosis of immunoglobulins; and (5) a paracellular pathway for plasma components and leukocytes. During lactation, as opposed to during pregnancy, very few of the constituents of breast milk are transferred directly from maternal blood. The junctions between cells, also known as *tight junctions,* are closed. As weaning occurs, the tight junctions are released and sodium and other minerals easily cross to the milk, which changes the taste of the milk. The change in taste may affect the interest of the infant to continue to breastfeed.

The majority of milk is produced de novo by the breast, rather than by direct absorption from the maternal gut or from manufacture by maternal organs such as the liver, kidneys, and so on. The substrates for milk production are primarily absorbed from the maternal gut or are produced in elemental form by the maternal liver. **Glucose is the major substrate for milk production.** It serves as the main source of energy for other reactions and is a critical source of carbon. The synthesis of fat from carbohydrates plays a predominant role in fat production in human milk, whereas proteins are built from free amino acids derived from plasma.

A sizable proportion of breast milk is produced during the nursing episode. In order to supply the substrates for milk production, blood flow increases to the mammary glands (20% to 40%), GI tract, and liver. Cardiac output is increased by 10% to 20% during a nursing episode. The vasodilation of the regional vascular beds is under the control of the autonomic nervous system, and oxytocin may play a critical role in directing the regional distribution of maternal cardiac output through an autonomic, parasympathetic action.

Given that milk is produced during the nursing episode, variation in content during a feed is expected. During a feeding episode, the lipid content of milk rises by more than twofold to threefold (1% to 5%) with a corresponding 5% fall in lactose concentration. The protein content remains relatively constant. At the extreme, there can be a 30% to 40% difference in the volume obtained from each breast. Likewise, intraindividual variations have been observed in lipid and lactose concentrations.

The rising lipid content during a feed has practical implications in breastfeeding management. **If a woman limits feedings to less than 4 minutes but nurses more frequently, the calorie density of the milk is lower, and the infant's hunger may not be satiated.** As a result, the infant wishes to feed sooner, and the frequency of nursing accelerates; this stimulates more milk production and creates a scenario of a hungry infant despite apparent good volume and milk transfer. **Lengthening the nursing episode or using one breast for each nursing episode often solves the problem.**

The volume and concentration of constituents also vary during the day. The volume per feed increases by 10% to 15% in the late afternoon and evening. Nitrogen content peaks in the late afternoon and falls to a nadir at 5:00 AM. Fat concentrations peak in the early morning and reach a nadir at 9:00 PM. Lactose levels stay relatively stable throughout the day. The variation in milk volume and content in working women who nurse only when at home has not been studied. The variation in volume and content is preserved if the woman pumps breast milk adequately (every 2 to 3 hours) during the day.

Does diet affect the volume and constitution of breast milk? For the average American woman with the range of diets from teenagers to mature, health-conscious adults, the answer is *no*. No convincing evidence suggests that the macronutrients in breast milk—protein, fats, and carbohydrates—vary across the usual range of American diets, although volume may vary in the extremes. In developing countries where starvation is widespread and daily calorie intake is less than 1600 kcal/day during prepregnancy and pregnancy, the mother's milk volume and its caloric density are only minimally decreased (5% to 10%) in underweight breastfeeding women.[6] In a controlled experiment,[7] well-nourished European women reduced their calorie intake by 33% for 1 week. Milk volume was not reduced when the diet was maintained at greater than 1500 kcal/day. If the daily energy intake was less than 1500 kcal, milk volume was reduced by 15%. **Moderate dieting and weight loss postpartum (4.5 lb/month) are not associated with changes in milk volume, nor does aerobic exercise have any adverse effect.[8,9]**

In the first year of life, the infant undergoes tremendous growth: infants double their birthweight in 180 days. Infants fed artificial breast milk (formula) lose up to 5% of their birthweight during the first week of life, and breast milk–fed infants lose about 7% of their birthweight. A maximum weight loss of 10% of birthweight is tolerated in the first week of life in breast-fed infants. If this threshold is exceeded, the breastfeeding dyad needs immediate intervention by a trained health care provider. Although supplementation with donor breast milk or artificial breast milk may be a necessary part of the intervention, the key focus of intervention is establishing good breast milk transfer by ensuring adequate production, correct nursing behavior, correct latch-on, and adequate frequency. Once *lactogenesis stage III* occurs, "the milk has come in"; the term infant will gain about 0.75 to 1 oz/day with adequate breast milk transfer. **By 14 days, the breast-fed infant should have returned to its birthweight.**

Food intake and energy needs are not constant. The infant's need for energy and fluids can vary daily or weekly because of growth spurts; greater activity; immunologic challenges, such as when fighting an illness; or with greater fluid losses, as in hot weather. Mammals have developed an extremely efficient mechanism to adjust milk supply within 24 to 48 hours, depending on demand, via oxytocin and the let-down reflex (Fig. 24-3) and

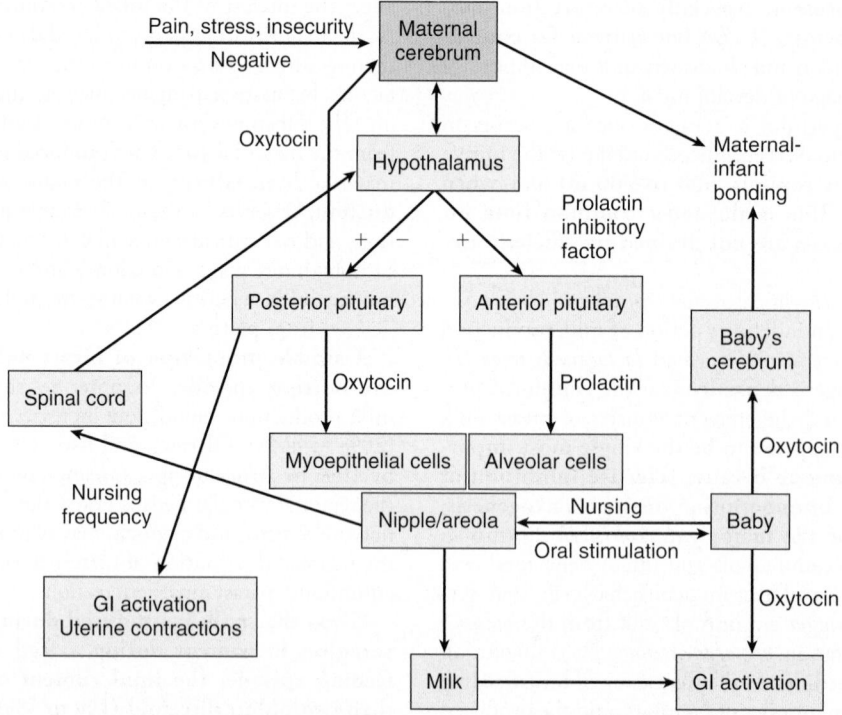

FIG 24-3 Oxytocin and the let-down reflex. The major reflex includes feedback stimulation from the nipple/areola to the hypothalamus to increase/decrease the release of oxytocin from the posterior pituitary and prolactin inhibitor factor (PIF, dopamine). The PIF affects the release of prolactin, which increases milk production; oxytocin causes milk ejection, and the release of both hormones is affected by positive or negative influences from the upper central nervous system (CNS). Oxytocin has three different target sites: the gastrointestinal (GI) tract (motility), uterus (contractions), and the upper CNS (mother-infant bonding). Oral stimulation in the infant initiates oxytocin release to improve GI function and maternal-infant bonding.

prolactin production. **The prolactin and oxytocin travel to their target cells: prolactin goes to the alveolar epithelium in the breast, and oxytocin goes to the myoepithelial cells that shroud the alveolar epithelium.** In lactating women, baseline prolactin levels are 200 ng/mL at delivery, 75 ng/mL between 10 and 90 days postpartum, 50 ng/mL between 90 and 180 days postpartum, and 35 ng/mL after 180 days postpartum. Maternal serum prolactin levels rise by 80% to 150% of baseline levels within seconds of nipple stimulation. **As long as nursing frequency is maintained at more than eight episodes a day for 10 to 20 minutes with each episode, the serum prolactin levels will suppress the luteinizing hormone (LH) surges and ovarian function. Serum oxytocin levels also rise with nipple stimulation.** However, the oxytocin response is much more affected by operant conditioning, and its response may precede the rise in prolactin levels. The maternal cerebrum is influenced by exposure to nursing cues and to the influences of nipple stimulation. The cerebrum either stimulates or inhibits the hypothalamus to increase or decrease the production of prolactin inhibitory factor (dopamine) and, subsequently, this drives the release of oxytocin from the posterior pituitary. Cerebral influences have a lesser effect on the release of prolactin. Positive sights, sounds, or smells related to nursing often stimulate the production of oxytocin, which in turn causes the myoepithelial cells to contact and allows milk to leak from the breasts. This observation is a good clinical clue to indicate an uninhibited let-down reflex.

In a classic series of experiments in 1958, Newton and Egli[10] demonstrated the power of noxious influences to inhibit the release of oxytocin and reduce milk transfer to the infant. The baseline milk production per feed was measured in controlled situations at about 160 g per feed. During a consecutive feed, a noxious event (i.e., saline injection) was administered during the feed. The amount of milk produced was cut in half, to 80 to 100 g per feed. Subsequently, the milk production was measured in a trial in which a noxious event was administered and intranasal oxytocin was given concomitantly. The milk production was restored to almost 90% of baseline production, 130 to 140 g. A wide variety of noxious events elicited the same decrease in milk production, including placing the mother's feet in ice water, applying electric shocks to her toes, having her trace shapes while looking only through a mirror, or requiring her to proofread a document in a timed fashion. These observations have important implications concerning the management of breastfeeding. **Pain, anxiety, and insecurity may be hidden reasons for breastfeeding failure through inhibition of the let-down reflex.**

In contrast, the playing of a soothing motivational/educational audio tape to women who were pumping milk for their premature infants has improved milk yields. These observations have been confirmed by measuring the inhibition of oxytocin release by psychological stress. The positive and negative influences of the cerebrum are further highlighted by the observation that 75% of women who had a positive attitude during pregnancy were likely to be successful at breastfeeding. In contrast, 75% of women who had a negative attitude during pregnancy had an unsuccessful breastfeeding experience. When the mother's attitude was good or very good and family was present, the exclusive breastfeeding rate was 20% at 6 months; if the mother's attitude was fair, the breastfeeding rate at 6 months was 5%.

Oxytocin has additional target cells in the mother (see Fig. 24-3), and **the effect of oxytocin on uterine activity is well known. Uterine involution is enhanced with breastfeeding.** Animal and human research suggests that oxytocin is a neurohormone associated with an anti–fight/flight response in the autonomic nervous system, better toleration of stress by the mother, and improved maternal-infant bonding.[11]

In addition to the antistress effect, surges in oxytocin levels are associated with the release of GI hormones and increased GI motility. In the mother, these actions enhance the absorption of substrates necessary for lactogenesis, and a growing body of knowledge indicates similar associations with oxytocin surges in infants. Skin-to-skin contact and the oral stimulation of nursing stimulate a parasympathetic, anti–fight/flight response in the infant. So-called kangaroo care of premature newborns, with skin-to-skin contact, is associated with a physiologically stable state, improved stress responses, and improved weight gain.[12] Oxytocin appears to mediate this response. Breastfeeding is associated with far more skin-to-skin contact and maternal behaviors than bottle feeding.

Whereas the central nervous system (CNS) locus for imprinting is unknown, imprinting immediately after birth is an important predictor of breastfeeding success. The survival of lambs depends on nursing within an hour after birth. If the lamb has not nursed during the critical period, maternal-infant bonding becomes dysfunctional, and the lamb suffers failure to thrive. In humans, the consequences are not nearly as drastic. **Several trials with random assignment of subjects to early nursing (delivery room) or late nursing (2 hours after birth) demonstrated a 50% to 100% higher number of breastfeeding mothers at 2 to 4 months postpartum among those who had nursed in the delivery room. One of the keys to obstetric management is have the mother nurse her newborn in the delivery room within 30 to 60 minutes of birth.**

Milk Transfer

Milk transfer to the infant is a key physiologic principle in lactation.[13] The initial step of milk transfer is a good latch-on. With light tactile stimulation of the infant's cheek and lateral angle of the mouth, the infant reflexively turns its head and opens its mouth, as in a yawn (Fig. 24-4). The nipple is tilted slightly downward using a "C-hold," or *palmar grasp*. In this hand position, the fingers support the breast from underneath and the thumb lightly grasps the upper surface 1 to 2 cm above the areola-breast line. The infant is brought firmly to the breast by the supporting arm, being careful not to push the back of the baby's head (Fig. 24-5). The nipple and areola are drawn into the mouth as far as the areola-breast line. The posterior areola may be less visible than the anterior areola, and the lower lip of the infant is often curled out. The infant's lower gum lightly fixes over the lactiferous sinuses.

The mechanics of normal breastfeeding behaviors relative to oropharyngeal movements and intraoral pressures have been eloquently demonstrated by transbuccal ultrasound.[14,15] A slight negative pressure exerted by the infant's oropharynx and mouth holds the length of the teat and breast in place and reduces the "work" to refill the lactiferous sinuses after they are drained. **The milk is extracted not by negative pressure but by a peristaltic wave from the tip to the base of the tongue.** There is no stroking or friction, and little in-and-out motion of the teat is apparent; the action is more undulating. The buccal mucosa and tongue mold around the teat, leaving no space.

The peristaltic movement of the infant's tongue is most frequent in the first 3 minutes of a nursing episode; the mean latency from latch-on to milk ejection is 2.2 minutes. After milk flow is established, the frequency of sucking falls to a much slower rate. **The change in cadence is recognizable as *suck-suck-swallow-breath*. Audible swallowing of milk is a good sign of milk transfer.** At the start of a feeding, the infant obtains 0.10 to 0.20 mL per suck. As infants learn how to suck, they become more efficient at obtaining more milk in a shorter period of time. **From 80% to 90% of the milk is obtained in the first 5 minutes the infant nurses on each breast, but the fat-rich and calorie-dense hind milk is obtained in the remainder of the time sucking at each breast, usually less than 20 minutes total.** A bottle-feeding infant sucks steadily in a linear fashion and receives about 80% of the artificial breast milk in the first 10 minutes.

Sucking on a bottle is mechanically very different from nursing on the human teat (Figs. 24-6 and 24-7).[16] The relatively inflexible artificial nipple resists the milking motion of the infant's tongue and mouth. The diameter of the artificial nipple

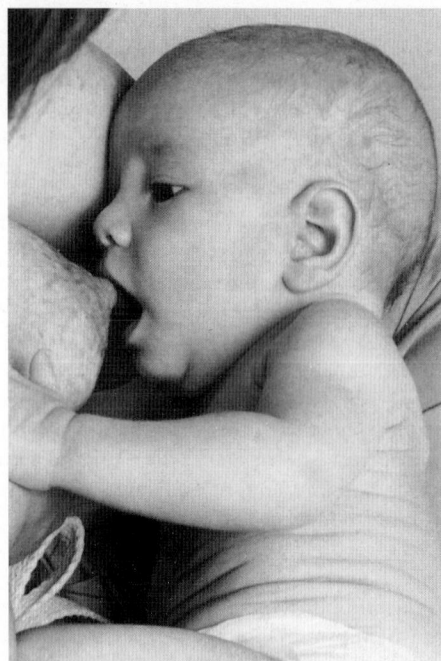

FIG 24-4 The latch-on reflex.

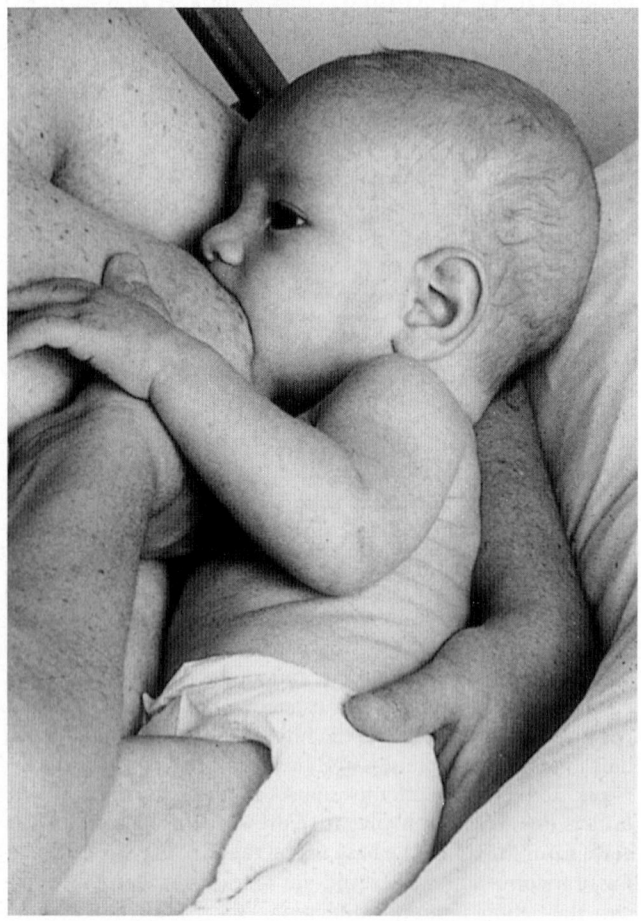

FIG 24-5 The successful C-hold with appropriate latch-on.

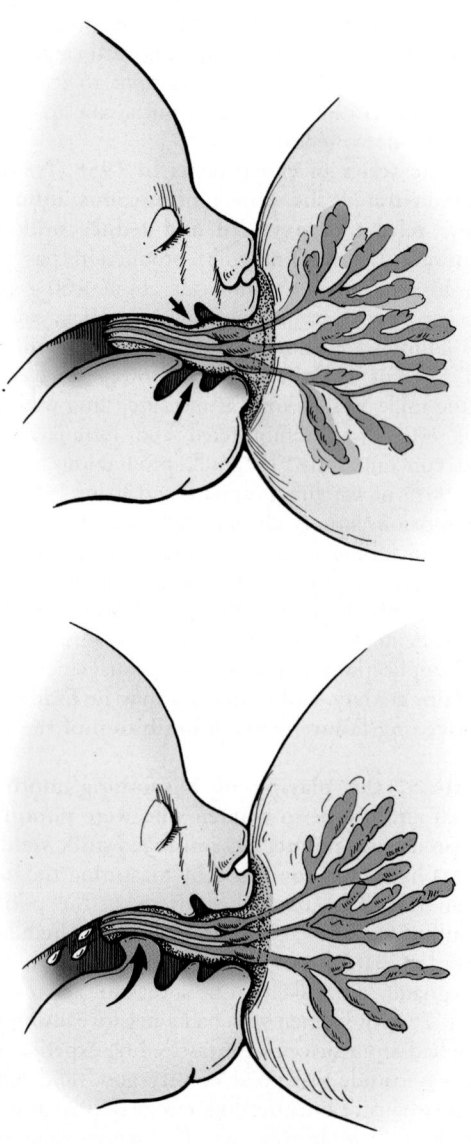

FIG 24-6 The mechanics of breastfeeding.

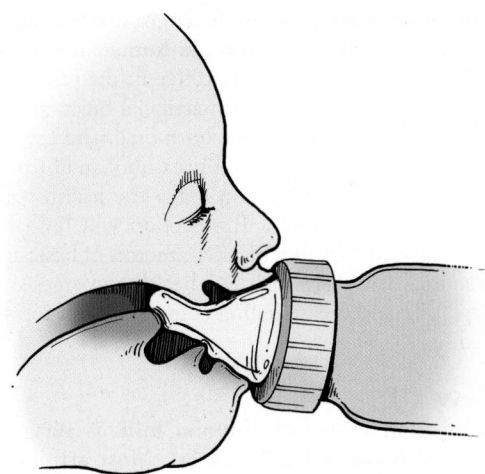

FIG 24-7 The mechanics of bottle feeding.

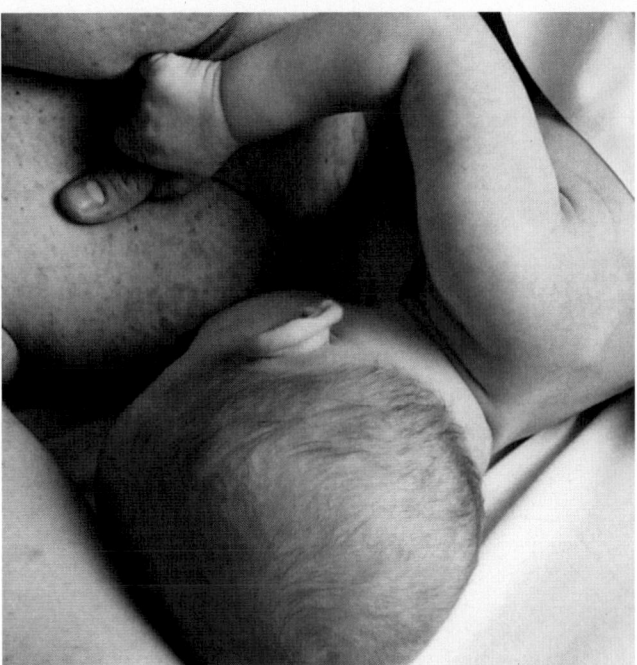

FIG 24-8 Side-lying nursing.

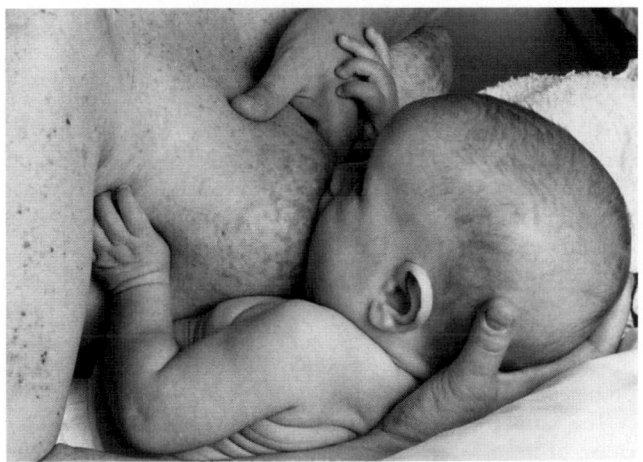

FIG 24-9 The football hold.

expands during a suck, whereas the human teat collapses during the milk flow. The infant who is sucking on a bottle learns to generate strong negative pressures (>100 mm Hg) in order to suck the milk out of the bottle. Because rapid flow from the bottle can gag the infant, he or she quickly learns to use the tongue to regulate flow. **When the infant who has learned to bottle feed is put to the breast, the stopper function of the tongue may abrade the tip of the nipple and force it out of the infant's mouth.** The efficiency of milk transfer falls drastically, and the hungry infant becomes frustrated and angry. A similar rejection may occur 4 to 8 weeks postpartum, when the exclusively breastfeeding infant is given a bottle in preparation for the mother's return to work.

Milk transfer is made more efficient by proper positioning of the infant to the breast, which places the infant and mother chest-to-chest. The infant's ear, shoulder, and hip are in line. The most common maternal positions are the cradle hold, chest to-chest, side-lying, or the football hold (Figs. 24-8 and 24-9). Each has its advantages. Rotating positions for nursing allows improved drainage of different lobules, which is important in the management of a "plugged" duct or mastitis. **Maternal comfort and convenience are the major reasons for changing nursing positions; the football hold and side-lying positions are more comfortable when the mother has an abdominal incision.**

The neonate should be fed every 2 to 3 hours or 8 to 12 times a day on demand. One of the important educational keys is for the mother to recognize the signs of a hungry baby before the baby is crying, angry, or stressed. The signs include lip smacking, hand movement to the mouth, restlessness, and vocalizations.

Baseline prolactin levels appear to be the major determinant of the maternal hormonal state during lactation, a state of high prolactin and low estrogen and progesterone levels. **As the frequency of nursing decreases below eight in 24 hours, the baseline prolactin levels drop below a level at which ovulation is suppressed (35 to 50 ng/mL), LH levels rise, and menstrual cycling is initiated.**[5] The intensity (adjusted odds ratio [OR]) of factors that initiate the onset of menses are the duration of sucking episodes less than 7 minutes (OR 2.4), night feedings less than four per 24 hours (OR 2.3), maternal age 15 to 24 years (OR 2.1), maternal age 25 to 34 years (OR 1.7),

and day feedings less than seven per 24 hours (OR 1.6).[17] In women who feed their infants exclusively artificial breast milk, serum prolactin levels drop to prepregnant levels (8 to 14 ng/mL) within days. In summary, **the total number of nursing episodes per day (more than eight per 24 hours) and night nursings are critical to the successful management of breastfeeding.**

One of the major determinants of nursing frequency is the introduction of substitute nutriment sources for the infant, artificial breast milk, or solids. **Breast milk has the nutritional content to satisfy the growth needs of the infant for at least 6 months postpartum.** In the first 6 months, feeding with artificial breast milk (i.e., formula) affects the physiology of successful lactation in three ways: (1) it reduces proportionally the nutriment requirements from breast milk; (2) it increases the gastric emptying time (digestion is slower than with breast milk), with a subsequent decrease in frequency of nursing episodes; and

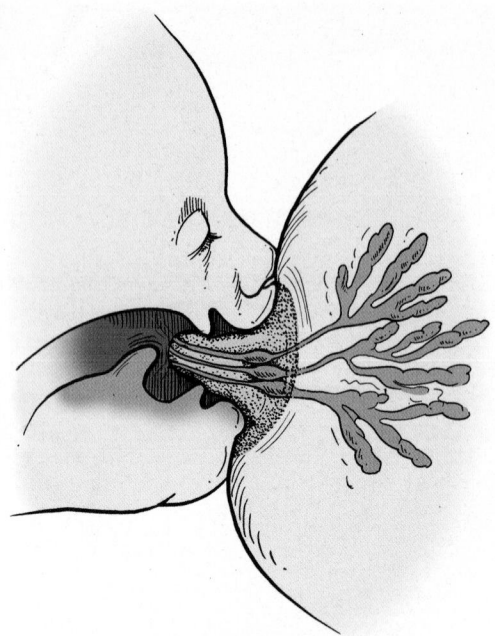

FIG 24-10 Breastfeeding and engorgement. The firm, swollen breast parenchyma pushes the newborn's face away, and she is unable to pull the teat into her mouth. Her tongue abrades the tip of the nipple.

(3) it reduces the efficiency of nursing from use of an opposing sucking technique on the artificial nipple.

Starting the infant on solid foods (e.g., eggs, cereals, pureed food) has a similar effect on the hormonal milieu of the lactating woman, and **one of the errors in Western child care is the early, forced introduction of solids. In most cases, the infant's gut is filled with slowly digesting food with less nutritional value than breast milk, the long-term result of which may be childhood and adolescent obesity.** The most logical time to start solid food substitution is when the infant has reached the neurologic maturity to grasp and bring food to its mouth from its mother's plate, which usually occurs at about 6 months. As the infant matures, his or her ability to feed improves, and the proportion of the diet supplied by solid food gradually increases.

The failure to develop good milk transfer is the major cause of lactation failure and breast pain, especially in the neonatal period. Inhibition of the let-down reflex and failure to empty the breasts completely leads to ductal distension and parenchymal swelling from extravascular fluid. This is termed *engorgement,* **and it compromises the mechanics of nursing (Fig. 24-10); alveolar distension reduces secretion of milk by the alveolar cells.** Without adequate transfer of milk to the infant, lactation is doomed to fail. Distension of the alveoli by retained milk causes a rapid (6 to 12 hours) decrease in milk secretion and enzyme activity by the alveolar epithelium. The decreased production of milk is explained by pressure inhibition and by an inhibitor secreted in breast milk. Distension of the alveoli inhibits secretion directly, rather than indirectly, by a decrease in nutriment or hormonal access.

BREAST MILK: THE GOLD STANDARD

One of the most common misconceptions by physicians and the lay public, and one that is heavily marketed by the formula industry, is that modern "formulas" are equivalent to breast milk. The age-old reality remains: human breast milk is uniquely suited to our biologic needs and remains the best source of nutrition for the human infant. Human breast milk has a composition very different than that of bovine milk or soybean plants from which artificial breast milk is produced.[17] Nutritional, host-defense, hormonal, and psychophysiologic differences between human breast milk and breastfeeding versus formula and bottle feeding make the health benefits of breastfeeding understandable. This section will link the latter differences to a summary of a massive amount of basic and clinical research that demonstrates better health outcomes associated with breast milk and breastfeeding compared with formula and bottle feeding.

Overview

The composition of mature human milk is very different from artificial breast milk (formula). Most artificial breast milk products use bovine milk or soybean constituents as a substrate. Minerals, vitamins, proteins, carbohydrates, and fats are added to pasteurized bovine milk for perceived nutritional needs, as well as marketing aims, to make a product that will successfully compete with human breast milk. For example, human breast milk appears "thinner" than bovine milk. **Artificial breast milk manufacturers add constituents (e.g., palm- or coconut-based oils) to make artificial breast milk appear rich and creamy,** thereby creating a product that is more easily marketed to the American public.

Extensive research describes the unique composition of human milk. The infant formula industry has produced even greater volumes of data concerning their attempts to exactly reproduce human milk. In 1980, the U.S. Congress passed the Infant Formula Act (with revisions in 1985) as the result of severe health consequences when artificial breast milk failed to include key vitamins and minerals in new formula compositions. This law now requires that all formulas for artificial breast milk contain minimum amounts of essential nutrients, vitamins, and minerals. Although life-threatening omissions are unlikely, **current formulas have major differences in the total quantities and qualities of proteins, carbohydrates, minerals, vitamins, and fats when compared with human milk.** The reader is reminded that the recommended daily allowance (RDA) is the amount needed to prevent a deficiency disease, not the amount needed for the best health.

Breast milk promotes optimal somatic growth and metabolic competence. Human breast milk has evolved to ensure the most efficient digestion by the human infant, which is not the case with bovine or soybean-derived formulas.[18] Gastric emptying is faster in neonates fed breast milk versus formula, 1 to 2 hours versus 3 to 4 hours, respectively. The greater speed of digestion with breast milk relates to differences in casein/whey protein ratio, fatty acid content, fatty acid attachment to the glycerol backbone, and presence of GI enzymes and GI hormones to facilitate digestion, motility, and function. Bovine formulas contain only limited and degraded hormones and enzymes appropriate for calves, and none of these important constituents is found in formulas that use a soybean base. In addition, the bioavailability of naturally supplied vitamins and minerals in breast milk is 20% to 50% higher than that of the vitamins and minerals added to artificial breast milk.

The nutritional differences between formula and human milk are reflected in differences in the growth patterns of infants who are exclusively breastfed for 4 to 6 months and infants who are fed artificial breast milk. **In general, breast-fed infants have**

TABLE 24-1	EFFECTS OF INFANT FEEDING ON SOMATIC GROWTH AND CARDIOVASCULAR PATHOPHYSIOLOGY IN DEVELOPED COUNTRIES	
	BENEFIT OF BREASTFEEDING ADJUSTED OR (95% CI)	RISK OF "FORMULA" ADJUSTED OR (95% CI)
Childhood obesity	0.81 (0.77-0.84)	1.23 (1.14-1.3)
Child type 2 diabetes	0.61 (0.44-0.85)	1.64 (1.18-2.27)
Maternal cardiovascular disease	0.72 (0.53-0.97)	1.39 (1.03-1.89)
Maternal hypertension	0.87 (0.82-0.92)	1.15 (1.09-1.22)
Maternal vascular calcifications	0.19 (0.05-0.68)	5.26 (1.47-20.0)
Maternal myocardial infarction	0.77 (0.62-0.94)	1.3 (1.06-1.61)
Maternal type 2 diabetes	0.84 (0.78-0.91)	1.19 (1.10-1.28)

In general, odds ratio (OR) was adjusted for age, parity, race, and socioeconomic status. CI, confidence interval.

faster linear and head growth, whereas formula-fed infants tend to have greater weight gain and fat deposition. The greater deposition in fat may relate in part to the earlier introduction of solid foods in the infants fed formula, a factor that has not been adequately controlled in current studies.

Regardless of the cause, formula has important adverse effects on the metabolic competence of the child, adolescent, and future adult (Table 24-1). Since 2007, when the extensive evidence-based reviews were published by the Agency for Healthcare Research and Quality (AHRQ)[19-26]—and after follow-up analysis by Ip and colleagues[20] in 2009—these findings have been verified, proving a dose-response relationship and providing an improved understanding of the physiologic and endocrine causes for the benefits seen with prolonged breastfeeding.[22-26]

Breastfeeding enhances cognitive development. Human breast milk has superior capacity to enhance the development of the infant's brain and its integrative capacity through many defined and undefined differences between human breast milk and formula. The currently identified constituents of human breast milk that enhance integrative capacity include growth hormones, oligosaccharides, nucleotides, glycoproteins, and long-chain polyunsaturated fatty acids (LCPUFAs). **In high-risk, premature neonates, human breast milk given by gavage enhances the infant's later intelligence quotient (IQ) and performance on psychometric testing in a dose-dependent fashion after controlling for maternal intelligence, family education, and socioeconomic status.**[27] A recent large cohort study that compared very-low-birthweight infants[14] demonstrated that for every 10 mL/kg/day increment of breast milk fed to these high-risk neonates, neurodevelopmental outcomes improved.[28]

Although the effect is most dramatic among high-risk infants, smaller effects on IQ are seen in term infants (adjusted increment [95% CI], 3.16 points [2.35 to 3.98] vs. low birthweight infants, 5.18 points [3.59 to 6.77]).[29] A population-based birth cohort was launched in 1982 in Pelotas, Brazil among 5914 neonates.[30] Initiation, exclusivity, and duration of breastfeeding was recorded between 19 and 42 months. At 30 years of age, 3701 of the enrollees (68% follow-up) underwent ascertainment of their IQ, educational achievement, and family income. In the confounder-adjusted analysis, those who were breastfeed 12

months or more had higher IQ scores (+3.76; 95% CI, 2.20 to 5.33), more years of education (+0.91 years; 95% CI, 0.41 to 1.40), and higher monthly income than those who were breastfed for less than 1 month.[30]

The information regarding breastfeeding, LCPUFAs, and improved intelligence has been powerful enough for formula companies to change their concoctions to include more LCPUFAs. However, just adding LCPUFAs does not change the other deficiencies in formula. Another recent example of neurodevelopmental enhancement with breastfeeding is the strong association found between breastfeeding and enhanced visual acuity. Conversely, infants fed LCPUFA-enhanced formula had similar deficiencies in high-grade foveal stereoacuity (adjusted OR, 2.5; 95% CI, 1.4 to 4.5), as did those infants fed standard formula.[31]

Breastfeeding enhances infant responses to infection and reduces allergic disease. At birth, the fetus enters an unsterile world with a naïve and immature immune system. Full development of the immune system may take up to 6 years. **Breast milk has a wide array of antiinfective properties that will support the developing immune system. The major mechanisms for the protective properties of breast milk include active leukocytes, antibodies, antibacterial products, competitive inhibition, enhancement of nonpathogenic commensal organisms, and suppression of proinflammatory immune responses.**[32-34]

A critical event in host resistance is the recognition of pathogenic agents in the environment and the production of an antigen-specific adaptive immune response. Breastfeeding provides a unique system to help the infant fight infection with an adaptive antigen-specific response. Through breast milk, the neonate takes advantage of maternal recognition of these infectious agents (Fig. 24-11). This important mechanism was described by Slade and Schwartz.[35] An antigen or infectious agent—such as a virus, bacterium, fungus, or protozoan—stimulates the activity of leukocytes in the GI or respiratory tract of the mother. Lymphocytes encoded with the antigen signature travel to the nearest lymph node and stimulate lymphoblasts to develop cytotoxic T cells, helper T cells, and plasma cells programmed to destroy the initiating antigen through phagocytosis or complement/immunoglobulins produced by the B cells. The response is amplified by the migration of committed helper lymphocytes to other sites of white blood cell production, the spleen and bone marrow, where they stimulate the production of antigen-specific committed white blood cells. Some of the committed, antigen-specific helper lymphocytes travel to the mucosa of the breast in the lactating mother. Plasma cells, which produce secretory immunoglobulin A (sIgA), constitute 50% to 80% of the leukocytes in the breast submucosa. They may migrate into the breast milk (macrophages) or may produce immunoglobulins (sIgA, IgG—lymphocytes or plasma cells). Both are uniquely programmed to fight the specific infectious agent that challenges the mother. **Active leukocytes are completely eliminated by pasteurization (formula) and freezing (stored, pumped breast milk).**

Immunoglobulins are a unique component of breast milk that are absent in artificial breast milk. In contrast to *monomeric serum* IgA, the *secretory* IgA (sIgA) in breast milk is dimeric or polymeric; polymerization improves transport across the maternal alveolar cells into the breast milk. The immunoglobulins in breast milk appear to be fully functional. The sIgA is produced locally by plasma cells and does not activate complement or promote opsonic complement subfragments. As a

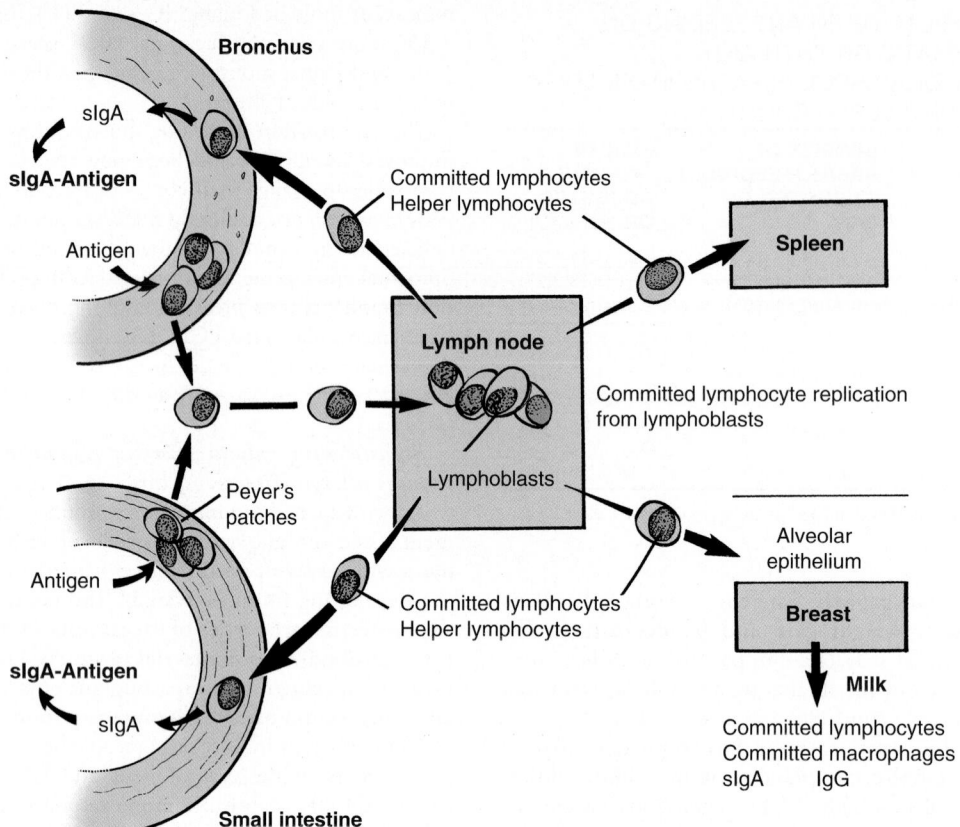

FIG 24-11 The adaptive immunology of the breast. IgG, immunoglobulin G; sIgA, secretory immunoglobulin A.

consequence, sIgA is not bactericidal. It appears that sIgA blocks the mucosal receptors (adhesins) on the infectious agent. The virulence of pathogens is related to their ability to use adhesins capable of interacting with complementary gut epithelial cell-surface receptors. When the antigen-specific sIgA attaches, the pathogen is effectively neutralized.

In the last 5 to 10 years, an increasing amount of research has focused on critical imprinting between neonatal gut flora and future immune responses.[33-38] The neonate is an antigen-naïve organism whose adaptive response is delayed by a lack of exposure. In addition, the cytokine response to TOLL-like receptor (TLR) stimulation appears to be exaggerated, especially in the preterm infant in whom injury is partly cytokine mediated (i.e., periventricular leukomalacia, necrotizing enterocolitis, and bronchopulmonary dysplasia). The adaptive immune system takes between 4 and 8 days to develop an effective defense; **the neonate bombarded by new antigens/organisms during the birth process must rely on an innate host defense system to provide an immediate but controlled response during the first critical 7 days of breastfeeding.**

Human breast milk actively limits pathogenic microbes (e.g., *Escherichia coli*) and promotes the growth of nonpathogenic, commensal microbes (e.g., *Bifidobacterium bifidum* and other species). **One of the most important breast milk constituents in the innate host defense system are human-specific oligosaccharides.** Oligosaccharides are indigestible complex carbohydrate structures that have a microbe (genus)-specific ability to bind to cell-surface receptors of the microbe. The unique oligosaccharide binding to the surface receptor blocks the binding of the microbe to the infant's mucosal receptors, thereby limiting microbe virulence. On the other hand, human milk contains an oligosaccharide homologous to the infant's mucosal receptors. The oligosaccharide-mucosal receptor complex allows specific attachment of *Bifidobacterium* species to the intestinal mucosa, further competitively inhibiting the attachment of pathogenic organisms.

A similar attachment of *B. bifidum* to dendritic cells, which interdigitate through the intestinal epithelial cells, allows for a critical modulation of the developing neonatal immune system. The interaction upregulates the antiinflammatory cytokine system—interleukin (IL)-10, soluble IL-1 receptor antagonist, and so on—and orchestrates the conversion of naive T-helper cells into a mature, balanced response. These early imprinting interactions may have profound effects on the incidence of inflammatory diseases in the adult, intrinsic bowel disease, asthma, rheumatoid arthritis, and perhaps cardiovascular diseases. In addition to the crosstalk between commensal gut bacteria and the immune system of the neonate, human colostrum contains large quantities of a *soluble* form of the bacterial pattern recognition receptor, cluster of differentiation 14 (sCD14). CD14 is a known modulator of host response to bacterial lipopolysaccharides (LPSs). In particular, CD14 binds to TLR-4 receptors and limits the binding of LPS from gram-negative rods. The failure to activate the TLR-4 receptor reduces the exaggerated immature cytokine response possible in neonates. Recent therapeutic interventions have used the immune-modulating qualities of the commensal bacteria–host interactions to successfully treat several important human diseases: necrotizing enterocolitis, inflammatory bowel disease, *Clostridium difficile*–associated colitis, acute gastroenteritis, and atopic dermatitis.

Known and unknown constituents of human breast milk inhibit the growth of and actively destroy pathogenic organisms;

TABLE 24-2	REDUCTION OF INFECTION AND ALLERGIC DISEASE WITH BREASTFEEDING	
OUTCOME	**BENEFIT OF BREASTFEEDING ADJUSTED OR (95% CI)**	**RISK OF "FORMULA" ADJUSTED OR (95% CI)**
Acute otitis media	0.77 (0.64-0.94)	1.30 (1.06-1.56)
Gastrointestinal infections	0.36 (0.32-0.41)	2.78 (2.44-3.12)
	0.54 (0.36-0.80)	1.85 (1.25-2.78)
Lower respiratory infections	0.28 (0.14-0.54)	3.57 (1.85-7.14)
Asthma	0.73 (0.59-0.92)	1.37 (1.09-1.69)
Atopic dermatitis	0.58 (0.41-0.92)	1.72 (1.09-2.44)
Type 1 diabetes	0.70 (0.56-0.87)	1.43 (1.15-1.77)
Childhood leukemia	0.81 (0.71-0.91)	1.23 (1.10-1.41)
Sudden infant death syndrome	0.64 (0.51-0.81)	1.56 (1.23-1.96)

In general, odds ratio (OR) was adjusted for age, parity, race, and socioeconomic status. *AHRQ,* Agency for Healthcare Research and Quality; *CI,* confidence interval.

formula has none of these constituents. Certain vitamins and minerals are essential for the growth of pathogenic bacteria, and a major mechanism by which breast milk protects the infant is the competition for "essential" nutriments for pathogenic bacteria. **Iron and vitamin B$_{12}$ are two essential nutriments for pathogenic bacteria that have been studied relative to breast milk. Breast milk contains lactoferrin, an iron-binding glycoprotein, in large quantities (5.5 mg/mL in the colostrum to 1.5 mg/mL in mature milk); this is absent in artificial breast milk. The free-iron form of lactoferrin competes with siderophilic bacteria for ferric iron and thus disrupts the proliferation of these organisms. The binding of iron to lactoferrin also enhances iron absorption; less iron is required in breast milk in order to satisfy the iron needs of the infant.** The antibacterial role of lactoferrin is more complex than simple competition for ferric iron.[39] Lactoferrin causes a release of LPS molecules from the bacterial cell wall. This appears to sensitize the bacterial cell wall to attack by lysozyme, and lactoferrin and lysozyme work together to destroy the pathogenic organisms.

Table 24-2 describes the effects of breastfeeding on the adaptive and innate host defenses. The cause of sudden infant death syndrome (SIDS) is not clear, but a current theory includes an aberrant immune response.

The hormonal changes of lactation—low estrogen, low progesterone, and hyperprolactinemic amenorrhea—favor a reduction in maternal reproductive cancers, but the relationship is undefined, and the relationship between the maternal immune system and the mother's experience with breastfeeding has not been adequately explored. However, in a dose-dependent fashion, breastfeeding reduces breast cancer per year of cumulative breastfeeding by 4.3% (95% CI, 2.9% to 5.8%). Likewise, breastfeeding for greater than 12 months in the mother's lifetime reduces ovarian cancer (adjusted OR, 0.72; 95% CI, 0.54 to 0.97); conversely, exclusive feeding with formula is associated with an enhanced risk of ovarian cancer (adjusted OR, 1.39; 95% CI, 1.03 to 1.85).[19-21]

Breastfeeding enhances mother-infant bonding and reduces poor social adaptation. The human newborn infant is born entirely dependent on the mother for transportation, food, warmth, and social conditioning. Survival depends on a unique bond between mother and infant to enhance maternal protective behaviors. **Like all other mammals, humans have a critical imprinting period (0.5 to 1 hour) for the establishment of**

mother-infant bonding. The most visible manifestation of the new bond is the duration of breastfeeding. Numerous studies with random assignment of breastfeeding dyads to early (<1 hour) or later (>2 hours) initiation of breastfeeding demonstrate a significantly higher incidence of any breastfeeding or exclusive breastfeeding at 2 to 4 months after birth in those dyads who initiated breastfeeding early.

A 2007 review by Moore and colleagues[12] in the Cochrane Database of Systematic Reviews supports the benefits of early skin-to-skin contact. Their conclusions from a review of 30 studies that involved 1925 mother-infant dyads were that early skin-to-skin contact was associated with babies who interacted more with their mothers, stayed warmer, and cried less. **Babies were more likely to be breastfed, and to breastfeed longer, if they had early skin-to-skin contact.** More recently, a study with random assignment of subjects to immediate skin-to-skin contact or not—with timing of first feeding being mother directed and independently recorded—suggested that **early skin-to-skin contact was a better predictor of duration of exclusive breastfeeding than the timing of the first sucking episode.**[40] This observation complements the success of so-called kangaroo care in the performance of high-risk neonates in the neonatal intensive care unit (NICU).

Recent human studies based on robust animal data[41] suggest that continued skin-to-skin contact and breastfeeding greatly affect the responsiveness to stress in the infant and mother. Experimental physiologic and psychological stressors produce measured stress-induced changes in adrenocorticotropic hormone and cortisol and in autonomic responses in breastfeeding women versus women feeding their infants formula exclusively. In keeping with numerous animal studies, **the breastfeeding mothers had a significantly blunted response of the hypothalamic-pituitary-adrenal (HPA) axis, also known as "fight or flight response," to the experimental stressors.**[41,42] A reciprocal relationship is apparent in the breastfeeding infant, who has greater parasympathetic tone and a blunted HPA-axis response compared with a similar infant fed formula. These observations may be partially explained by a decrease in skin-to-skin contact in infants fed formula. Whereas kangaroo care has a salutary effect on breastfeeding incidence, the positive effects on weight gain and the blunted stress response are independently associated with the amount of skin-to-skin contact.[12,42,43]

The association between breastfeeding and better psychosocial outcomes has been the topic of much epidemiologic research over many decades. Critics have repeatedly pointed out the selection bias inherent with these studies. However, improved epidemiologic research design has confirmed the lifelong value for the breastfeeding dyad in subsequent stressful situations. Two powerful studies illustrate the risk of not breastfeeding. In the first study, **Strathearn and colleagues[44] explored whether breastfeeding was protective against maternal-perpetrated child maltreatment.** The study design monitored prospectively 7223 Australian mother-infant pairs (identified at first prenatal visit) and followed them over a 15-year period after birth. The primary outcome was substantiated maltreatment reports by a governmental child protection agency. Maternally perpetrated substantiated abuse or neglect was identified in 313 pairs (4.3% of the cohort). The analysis adjusted for the 18 confounding variables, which included five sociodemographic variables; four prenatal behaviors/attitudes (i.e., substance abuse, anxiety, attitude toward pregnancy); four infant factors, including NICU admission; seven postnatal behaviors/attitudes (i.e., mother-infant separation, maternal stimulation/teaching the baby, maternal depression). **The adjusted OR for maternal maltreatment cases among children fed exclusively formula was 2.2 (95% CI, 1.5 to 3.2) versus any breastfeeding, and it was 3.8 (95% CI, 2.1 to 7.0) versus exclusive breastfeeding for 4 months or longer.**

In a second study, the response of the child was measured. Montgomery and colleagues[45] used data collected in the 1970 British Cohort Study, in which subjects were followed for 10 years; 8958 (71%) had complete data and were used in the analysis. The study analyzed childhood anxiety associated with parental divorce or separation as reported by their teachers on an analog scale of 0 to 50 related to the question, "Was (the subject) worried and anxious about many things?" **Exclusive feeding with formula, after adjustment for many factors, was associated with a dramatic increase in perceived childhood anxiety** (adjusted OR, 8.8; 95% CI, 5.3 to 12.2), **whereas breastfeeding at entry had no significant effect on childhood anxiety associated with divorce** (adjusted OR, 1.3; 95% CI, −3.6 to 6.1).

Breastfeeding is cost effective for the family and society. The nonmedical costs of artificial breast milk (formula) feeding are considerably higher than for breastfeeding.[46] The direct cost of artificial breast milk feeding includes the cost of the artificial formula (900 mL/day), bottles, and supplies. In eastern North Carolina (April 2015), the average retail cost of 900 mL of brand name prepared formula was about $8.00 daily ($2920 yearly); of brand name concentrate, about $5.50 daily ($2008 yearly); and of powdered formula, about $4.65 daily ($1697 yearly). Store brands cost about two thirds of the price of brand names. Special formulas—including soy-based, LCPUFA-enhanced, and hypoallergenic formulas—cost 50% to 200% more. A major indirect cost of artificial breast milk feeding is the environmental impact of large dairy herds to supply the bovine milk substrate and the mountains of packaging material discarded in landfills or incinerated.

Breastfeeding provides the right amount of a superior product at precisely the right time and at the right temperature. The nonmedical costs of breastfeeding include the cost of increased dietary calorie and protein needs ($2 to $3 daily), nursing bras and breast pads, and an increased number of diapers in the first 2 to 3 months. If a rented electric breast pump is used when the woman returns to work, the cost of breastfeeding will increase $2 to $4 per day.

Increase in acute medical diseases will manifest as increased costs of medical care for those families who choose to feed their infant artificial breast milk or formula.[45-49] Among Medicaid populations in Colorado and California and in health maintenance organizations (HMOs) in Arizona, the medical cost of artificial breast milk feeding amounts to $350 to $600 per year per infant. Among patients who belonged to a large HMO in Tucson, Arizona, **the excess yearly medical costs of 1000 never–breast-fed infants versus 1000 infants who were exclusively breastfed for at least 3 months was $331,041** (Table 24-3).[49]

The health care benefits are also reflected in the reduction of medical leave taken by the working mother to care for the sick child. **The data demonstrate fewer days for sick leave in women who work and continue to breastfeed than working women who formula feed.**

A cost analysis by Bartick and Reinhold[47] calculated the excess pediatric costs with U.S. breastfeeding initiation rates in 2005

TABLE 24-3 EXCESS MEDICAL COST AMONG 1000 NEVER-BREASTFED VERSUS 1000 EXCLUSIVELY (>3 MONTHS) BREASTFED INFANTS

	EXCESS SERVICES PER YEAR PER 1000 NEVER BREASTFED	TOTAL EXCESS COST
Office visits	1693	$111,315
Follow-up visits	340	$22,355
Medications*	609	$7669
Chest radiography	51	$1836
Days of hospitalization†	212	$187,866
Total excess cost per year		$331,041

Modified from Ball TM, Wright AL. Health care costs of formula-feeding in the first year of life. *Pediatrics.* 1999;103:870.
*Lower respiratory infection, otitis media.
†Lower respiratory infection, gastroenteritis.

TABLE 24-4 EXCESS PEDIATRIC COSTS AND DEATHS WITH THE FAILURE TO EXCLUSIVELY BREASTFEED FOR 6 MONTHS IN 80% OF DYADS

	EXCESS COST (DEATHS) COMPARED WITH 80% COMPLIANCE*
Total	$10,491,841,489 (714)
Sudden infant death syndrome	$3,722,074,013 (352)
Necrotizing enterocolitis deaths	$2,218,109,495 (210)
Pneumonia deaths	$1,557,915,767 (146)
Otitis media	$765,766,295
Atopic dermatitis	$497,497,274
Childhood obesity	$404,195,504
Pneumonia hospitalization	$381,578,219
Childhood asthma	$229,194,255
Necrotizing enterocolitis hospitalization	$219,843,084
Childhood asthma deaths	$148,022,294 (14)
Gastroenterocolitis	$162,076,307
Childhood leukemia deaths	$133,422,239 (13)
Childhood type 1 diabetes deaths	$64,999,258 (6)
Type 1 diabetes	$5,717,067
Childhood leukemia	$1,430,416

Modified from Bartick M, Reinhold A. The burden of suboptimal breastfeeding in the United States: a pediatric cost analysis. *Pediatrics.* 2010;125:1048.
*In 2007 U.S. dollars.

(74%) and exclusive breastfeeding rates at 6 months (12.3%) compared with 80% exclusive breastfeeding for 6 months using the published AHRQ analysis.[19-20] The total excess cost amounted to almost $10.5 billion and 714 deaths per year (Table 24-4). Their estimates do not account for the excess burden of chronic disease in the mother and child, obesity, type 2 diabetes, and cardiovascular disease; therefore the true burden is many times greater than just the pediatric costs. A recent similar study[48] in the United Kingdom based on 2009 and 2010 data showed that support for women who are exclusively breastfeeding at 1 week to continue to exclusively breastfeed until 4 months will reduce the incidence of gastroenteritis, lower respiratory infections, and otitis media with a savings of at least £11 million. Similarly, doubling the proportion of women currently breastfeeding for a total of 7 to 18 months is likely to reduce the incidence of maternal breast cancer and will save at least £31 million over a lifetime based on 2009/2010 values.[48]

In the past, the failure to correctly reproduce human milk led to significant infant disease. In 1980, the U.S. Congress passed the Infant Formula Act, with subsequent revisions in 1985, as the result of severe health consequences when artificial breast milk failed to include key vitamins and minerals in new formula compositions. This law now requires that all formulas for artificial breast milk contain minimum amounts of essential nutrients, vitamins, and minerals. Although life-threatening omissions are unlikely, **current formulas have major differences in the total quantities and qualities of proteins, carbohydrates, minerals, vitamins, and fats when compared with human milk.** The reader is reminded that the recommended daily allowance (RDA) is the amount needed to prevent a deficiency disease, not the amount needed for the best health.

ROLE OF THE OBSTETRICIAN AND GYNECOLOGIST

The gynecologist plays a primary role in support of breastfeeding.[21,50,51] Between 50% and 70% of women make a decision regarding how they will feed their infants *before* their pregnancies. The gynecologist needs to start promotion before the first pregnancy. When the reproductive-age woman seeks initial family planning advice and contraception, the likelihood is high that she will become pregnant in the next 2 to 5 years. **The breast examination is a regular part of the family planning visit;** it is used extensively to screen for breast cancer despite its rare occurrence at the ages of usual pregnancies (<35 years). **This visit is a good opportunity to reassure the woman of her normal breast anatomy and build her self-confidence for lactation success through vocal and visible support of breastfeeding.**

The obstetrician/gynecologist amplifies support for breastfeeding by community advocacy, office environment, and personal choices. The office environment needs to be "breastfeeding friendly." **Visible, active support of breastfeeding includes the presence of breastfeeding mothers, patient educational programs on breastfeeding, a quiet area for nursing mothers, an absence of material supplied by formula companies, and visible support for office personnel who choose to breastfeed.** In a trial with random assignment of a prenatal education packet produced by formula companies versus an educational packet produced by a breastfeeding-friendly pediatrician, the formula company packets resulted in less initiation and shorter duration of breastfeeding.[52] The physician, especially a female obstetrician/gynecologist, can be a positive role model for patients. Women will ask the female gynecologist whether and how long she breastfed her children, and her answers will have a powerful influence.

An important role of the obstetrician is to identify early in pregnancy those women who cannot breastfeed or who may have challenges (Table 24-5). The liberal use of galactagogues and tube feeding devices and having lactation consultants as case managers can mediate challenges related to breast milk production or breast milk transfer. The World Health Organization (WHO) has valuable guidelines regarding the use of formula when breastfeeding is contraindicated.[54]

In the second and third trimester, the obstetrician plays a major role in directing and supporting prenatal patient education about breastfeeding. Patient education has been shown to increase the initiation and maintenance of breastfeeding. A review[55] by the U.S. Preventive Service Task Force of 38 well-conducted trials with **random assignment of subjects to primary care interventions to promote breastfeeding versus**

TABLE 24-5	IDENTIFICATION OF WOMEN AT HIGH RISK FOR UNSUCCESSFUL BREASTFEEDING OUTCOMES		
CONDITION	RISK ASSESSMENT	MANAGEMENT
HIV in United States	Contraindicated	Formula feeding
Untreated active tuberculosis	Contraindicated	Neonatal antibiotic treatment, resume breastfeeding after 2 weeks of maternal therapy if mother asymptomatic
Herpes of nipple	Contraindicated on infected side	Isolate lesions, treat mother and infant systemically
Maternal antineoplastic medications	Contraindicated	Formula feeding
Neonatal galactosemia	Breast milk and "formula" contraindicated	Lactose-free supplement
Breast-reduction surgery	High risk	Prenatal consultation with lactation consultant and pediatrician
Breast augmentation	Moderate risk	Prenatal consultation with lactation consultant and pediatrician
Failure of breasts to enlarge during pregnancy, small tubular breasts	Moderate to high risk	Prenatal consultation with lactation consultant and pediatrician
Unsuccessful breastfeeding with prior child	Moderate risk	Identify issues, prenatal education, prenatal consultation with lactation consultant

HIV, human immunodeficiency virus.

"usual care" demonstrated significantly increased rates of short-term (1 to 3 months) and long-term (6 to 8 months) exclusive breastfeeding. In subgroup analysis, a combined prenatal and postnatal intervention had a greater effect on increasing breastfeeding duration than a prenatal or postnatal intervention alone. **Interventions that included individual-level professional support and lay counselors had the most impact.** At the 36-week visit, the obstetrician readdresses the mother's choice and knowledge regarding breastfeeding. Simple concepts of breastfeeding physiology are reinforced: early feeds (<1 hour postpartum), frequent feeds (>10 per day), a supportive environment, and no supplementation unless directed by a pediatrician. The obstetrician reinforces the appropriate way to get the baby to latch on to the breast and ensures that the increase in the mother's breast size reflects hormonal readiness for breastfeeding. The patient is warned of hospital policies and attitudes that interfere with breastfeeding success. **The 36-week visit is also a good time to address the appropriateness of medications and breastfeeding.**

The delivery experience has a tremendous impact on the initiation and maintenance of breastfeeding.[51,52] Obstetric and pediatric care providers, including the nursing team, adapt to maternal, fetal, and neonatal health to enhance or reduce the success of breastfeeding. In the 1980s, international professional organizations recognized that several primarily hospital-based behaviors enhance the initiation and maintenance of breastfeeding. **In 1989, the essential 10 steps (Box 24-1) in protecting, promoting, and supporting breastfeeding were published in**

BOX 24-1   10 STEPS TO SUCCESSFUL BREASTFEEDING

1. Have a written policy to support breastfeeding.
2. Train all health care providers in Baby-Friendly Hospital Initiative protocols.
3. Inform all pregnant women about the benefits of breastfeeding.
4. Initiate breastfeeding within 1 hour after birth.
5. Show mothers how to express breast milk and maintain lactation even if they are separated from their infants.
6. Give newborn infants no food or drink other than breast milk unless medically indicated.
7. Allow mothers and infants to remain together 24 hours a day (i.e., rooming in).
8. Encourage breastfeeding on demand.
9. Give no artificial teats or pacifiers.
10. Foster the establishment of breastfeeding support groups and refer mothers to them on discharge from the hospital or clinic.

Modified from WHO/UNICEF. Protecting, promoting, and supporting breastfeeding: the special role of maternity services, a joint WHO/UNICEF statement. Geneva, World Health Organization, 1989.

a joint statement by the WHO and the United Nations Children's Fund (UNICEF).

The WHO Ten Steps have become institutionalized in the Baby-Friendly Hospital Initiative (BFHI) and accreditation process. **These steps are well founded on evidence-based medicine that demonstrates improvement in breastfeeding success.**[51,55-57]

Newer population research designs demonstrate increased breastfeeding rates and improved population health while reducing the self-selection bias that confuses much epidemiologic research in breastfeeding. Cluster-randomized trials of breastfeeding promotion interventions modeled on the WHO/UNICEF Baby-Friendly Hospital Initiative (see Box 24-1) have been used in at least two separate populations. In these studies, maternity clinics and hospitals are assigned randomly to receive intensive educational programs to increase breastfeeding rates. The outcomes of interest are breastfeeding rates and short-term neonatal morbidities (infections, atopic dermatitis, etc.) In both studies, breastfeeding rates were improved significantly ($P <$ .001) with exclusive breastfeeding at 3 months, 43.4% versus 6.4% in Belarus and 79% versus 48% in India. The interventions were associated with a 30% to 50% lower prevalence of GI infections and atopic dermatitis and better infant growth in their respective populations.

Unfortunately, the United States is far behind the rest of the world in designating their maternity facilities as "baby friendly"; in 2014, only 7.79% of live births occurred in a BFHI-designated facility. In 2008, the CDC started reporting breastfeeding-related maternity practices and outcomes (see http://cdc.gov/breastfeeding/data).[58] These data are used to grade and compare the quality of care given by hospitals and their providers related to breastfeeding support. **The obstetrician is a key player in quality improvement related to breastfeeding and in the application of the essential 10 steps, that is, the BFHI.**

A hospital's BFHI designation does not absolve the obstetric care provider from advocacy and action to support breastfeeding. Support for obstetric quality initiatives such as no elective delivery prior to 39 weeks and initiatives to reduce the primary

cesarean delivery rate will reduce the number of neonates starting the process of learning to breastfeed with additional challenges—that is, more hyperbilirubinemia in early term birth and more transient tachypnea of the newborn delivered by cesarean.

As the "captain of the ship" in the delivery room, the delivering provider is instrumental in getting the baby skin-to-skin with the mother and breastfeeding within 30 minutes.[55,59] In a multivariate analysis of 300 consecutive term patients in a BFHI-certified tertiary care hospital, the four variables that predicted exclusive breastfeeding in the last 24 hours prior to postpartum discharge were at least partially under the control of the obstetric care provider. They included prenatal desire to breastfeed (positive predictor), cesarean delivery (negative predictor), neonate to the breast within 1 hour (positive predictor), and supplementation within the first 48 hours (negative predictor).[60]

As the result of obstetric interventions, health care providers often want to supplement the neonate with 1 to 2 bottles of formula to "allow the mother to recover." In a prospective cohort study, one or more bottles of formula were given to neonates during the postpartum hospitalization whose mothers wished to exclusively breastfeed in the prenatal clinic.[61] Early supplementation had a significant impact on the duration of both breastfeeding and exclusive breastfeeding. No supplementation versus early supplementation resulted in a rate of *not* exclusively breastfeeding at 60 days of 37% versus 68% and of breastfeeding cessation by day 60 of 11% versus 33%, respectively. In addition, the use of one or two bottles of cow's milk–based formula will provide primary sensitization to cow's milk proteins in neonates at risk for atopy.

After postpartum discharge, the obstetrician is primarily focused on maternal concerns about breastfeeding: maternal diet, breast symptoms and signs, hormonal function postpartum, contraception, maternal medications, and a breastfeeding advocate when the mother is referred to other specialists (see Chapter 23). A secondary but equally important focus is the growth and development of the infant. Traditionally, the obstetrician sees the mother at 4 to 6 weeks postpartum, but often the obstetrician and the mother communicate before that visit. By inquiring about the growth and feeding of her infant, the obstetrician provides both reinforcement of the mother's decision to breastfeed and a screen for the pediatrician regarding the growth and feeding of the infant; both are important. The obstetrician can identify critical or developing problems for the pediatrician regarding infant growth and feeding, so the obstetrician must know the indicators of adequate infant growth and clinical indicators that milk is being produced and transferred. **When the obstetrician remains a verbal participant in the mother's breastfeeding experience at the 4- to 6-week postpartum visit, the likelihood that the mother will continue to breastfeed at 16 weeks is almost doubled.**

During the interpregnancy interval, the obstetrician/gynecologist can identify the challenges, myths, and obstacles when a woman has not met her goals for breastfeeding in the last lactation period and can help correct them for any subsequent lactation period. During this interval, the obstetric care provider improves breastfeeding success in the next lactation cycle through an appropriate delay in pregnancy (>18 months), identification of type 2 diabetes or impaired glucose tolerance by glucose screening in women with gestational diabetes, and control and loss of pregnancy weight gain. These foci will reduce adverse pregnancy outcomes and will subsequently improve breastfeeding success in the next lactation cycle. Good long-term reversible contraception to allow for a planned pregnancy is a key feature of this interval.

FOCUSED ISSUES IN THE SUCCESSFUL MANAGEMENT OF BREASTFEEDING

The successful management of breastfeeding requires the active cooperation of the mother, her support group, the obstetric care provider, and the infant care provider; in our current culture, a lactation consultant often becomes an active participant in the care of the breastfeeding dyad. Numerous reliable resources are available for additional information (Table 24-6).

Several issues are in the domain of the obstetric care provider: anatomic abnormalities of the breast, the impact of breast surgeries, labor and delivery management, breast milk expression, breast and nipple pain, maternal nutrition and exercise during lactation, mastitis and breast abscess and masses, milk transfer and infant growth, galactogogues, maternal disease, back-to-work issues, contraception, and weaning.

ANATOMIC ABNORMALITIES OF THE BREAST

The relationship between breast anatomy and lactation should be addressed during the well-woman or family-planning visits in women who anticipate future pregnancy. During pregnancy, infant feeding becomes a major focus, and the woman needs this issue addressed because she often has hidden questions and concerns regarding her adequacy to breastfeed. The breast examination at the first prenatal visit is an excellent opportunity to address infant feeding concerns and myths relative to breast

TABLE 24-6	RESOURCES FOR BREASTFEEDING MANAGEMENT
RESOURCE	**COMMENT**
Print Sources	
Schanler RJ, Krebs NF, Mass SB, eds. *Breastfeeding Handbook for Physicians,* AAP and ACOG; 2014.	Excellent shelf resource on how to support breastfeeding as a part of a team
ACOG Clinical Review. Breastfeeding: Maternal and Infant Aspects. *Obstet Gynecol.* 2007;12(1 Suppl):1S-16S.	Succinct review of management of the breastfeeding mother for the obstetrician
ACOG Committee Opinion. Breastfeeding in underserved women: Increasing initiation and continuation of breastfeeding. Number 570, *Obstet Gynecol.* 2013;122:421.	Focus on underserved women with an update on benefits of breastfeeding
ACOG Committee Opinion. Breastfeeding: Maternal and Infant Aspects, Number 361. *Obstet Gynecol.* 2007;109:479.	States the ACOG position on breastfeeding
AAP: Policy Statement—Breastfeeding and the use of human milk. *Pediatrics.* 2012;129:e827.	States the AAP position on breastfeeding
Lawrence RA, Lawrence RM, eds. *Breastfeeding: A Guide for the Medical Profession,* 8th ed. St. Louis: Elsevier; 2015.	The standard textbook for physicians interested in breastfeeding
Infant and young child feeding: Model chapter for textbooks for medical students and allied health professionals	www.who.int/maternal_child_adolescent/en/ WHO publication
AAP. The transfer of drugs and therapeutics into human breastmilk: An update on selected topics. *Pediatrics.* 2013;132:1.	Clinical report on drugs and medications in human milk
Hale TW, Rowe HE, eds. *Medications and Mothers' Milk,* 16th ed. Plano, TX: Hale Publishing;2014.	A manual of lactational pharmacology
Cadwell K, Turner-Maffei C, eds. *Continuity of Care in Breastfeeding: Best Practice in Maternity Settings.* Sudberry, MA: Jones and Bartlett; 2009.	Manual of application of the WHO 10 Steps
Organizations	
Academy of Breastfeeding Medicine Official journal: *Breastfeeding Medicine* (www.liebertpub.com/bfm)	A physicians-only international professional organization founded by obstetricians, pediatricians, and family medicine physicians dedicated to physician education and clinical research on breastfeeding. Excellent clinical protocols online at bfmed.org.
International Lactation Consultant Association Official journal: *Journal of Human Lactation*	www.ilca.org Certifying examination
Online Training	
American Academy of Pediatrics, Breastfeeding Residency Curriculum	www.aap.org/breastfeeding/curriculum Multidisciplinary input, excellent
Well Start International	www.wellstart.org Oldest and most experienced organization in breastfeeding education
University of Virginia	www.breastfeedingtraining.org
Other Internet Sources	
Academy of Breastfeeding Medicine	www.bfmed.org
American Academy of Family Physicians	www.aafp.org www.familydoctor.org
American College of Obstetricians and Gynecologists	www.acog.org
Business Case for Breastfeeding (Office on Women's Health)	www.womenshealth.gov/breastfeeding/government-in-action/business-case.html
Centers for Disease Control and Prevention	www.cdc.gov
Human Lactation Center, University of Rochester Medical Center	www.urmc.rochester.edu/childrens-hospital/neonatology/lactation.aspx
International Lactation Consultant Association	www.ilca.org
La Leche League International	www.lalecheleague.org
LactMed-Drugs and Lactation Database	www.toxnet.nlm.nih.gov/newtoxnet/lactmed.htm
U.S. Breastfeeding Committee	www.usbreastfeeding.org

AAP, American Association of Pediatrics; *ACOG,* American College of Obstetricians and Gynecologists; *WHO,* World Health Organization.

anatomy. Self-doubt concerning the size or shape of the breasts should be addressed, and the patient should be reassured that fewer than 5% of lactation failures are caused by faulty anatomy.

Excluding inverted nipples, congenital abnormalities of the breasts are rare and occur in fewer than 1 in 1000 women. The most significant defect is glandular hypoplasia, in which abnormal or no development of one or both breasts is apparent during sexual maturation. Women with no development of the breasts often have normally shaped and sized nipples and areolas, and they may have sought consultation from a plastic surgeon. One manifestation of abnormal development is referred to as the *tubular breast.* The nipple and areola—which are often normal in size, shape, and appearance—are attached to a tube of fibrous cords. **Whatever the shape or size of the breasts in a nonpregnant woman, the final evaluation of adequate glandular tissue must await the expected growth during pregnancy.** The size of the average breast will grow from 200 to 600 g during pregnancy; most women will easily recognize this growth. **A routine screening question at the 36-week prenatal visit should be, "Have your breasts grown during pregnancy?" If the response is negative in a woman with unusually small or abnormally shaped breasts, lactation failure is a possibility, and prenatal consultation with a lactation expert is recommended.** Unilateral abnormalities are usually not a problem except for increased asymmetry because the normal breast can usually produce more than enough milk for the infant. The texture of the breast and tethering of the nipple are also assessed. An inelastic breast gives the impression that the skin is fixed to dense underlying tissue, whereas the elastic breast allows elevation of the skin and subcutaneous tissue from the parenchyma. Lack of elasticity may complicate nursing because of increased rigidity with engorgement. Massage of the periareolar tissue four times a day for 10 minutes is recommended. Engorgement should be assiduously avoided in the postpartum period by early, frequent nursing.

Congenital tethering of the nipple to underlying fascia is diagnosed by squeezing the outer edge of the areola (Fig. 24-12); normally, the nipple will protrude. **Severe tethering is manifested by an inverted nipple.** The most severe forms of tethering occur in fewer than 1% of women. Although successful breastfeeding is possible in these severe cases, prenatal consultation and close follow-up are very important to identify and treat poor milk transfers. Flat or inverted nipples are much less likely to preclude successful breastfeeding. Three prenatal methods of treating tethered nipples have been described: (1) nipple pulling, (2) Hoffman exercises, and (3) nipple cups, or shells. **A controlled trial[62] failed to demonstrate efficacy of either shells or Hoffman exercises and recommended that these should be abandoned.**

In the early neonatal period, a breast pump may help women with flat or inverted nipples; the breast is gently pumped at low settings until the teat is drawn out, and the infant is immediately offered that breast. The same procedure is performed on the other side; usually this is only required for a few days. Unfortunately, no controlled trials support their efficacy.

Modern clothing, especially protective brassieres, prevents friction that toughens the skin and also helps protect the nipple from cracking during early lactation. **However, washing with harsh soaps; buffing the nipple with a towel; and using alcohol, benzoin, or other drying agents is not helpful and may increase the incidence of cracking. Normally, the breast**

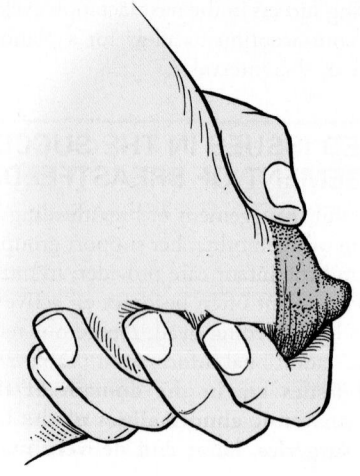

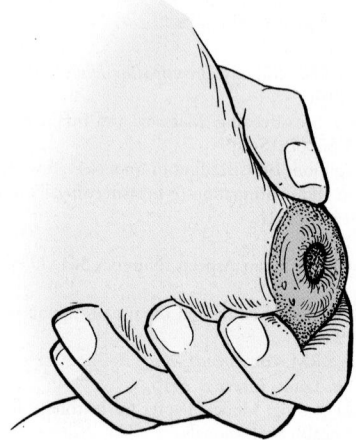

FIG 24-12 Assessment of nipple tethering.

is washed with clean water and should be left to air dry. A cautiously used sunlamp or hair dryer may facilitate drying. Trials involving application of breast cream or expression of colostrum have not shown a reduction in nipple trauma or sensitivity when compared with untreated nipples.[63]

Previous Breast Surgeries

Previous breast surgery may have significant adverse effects on breastfeeding success. The major issues are loss of sensation in the nipple or areola by nerve injury or compromise of the lactiferous ducts. Women who have had breast biopsy or breast or chest surgery, including augmentation, have a threefold higher incidence of unsuccessful breastfeeding.[64,65] Circumareolar skin incisions—which are used for cosmetic considerations in breast biopsies, reductions, and augmentations—may compromise both the nerve and ducts.

Breast augmentation has significant potential to disrupt breastfeeding.[64,65] In a carefully conducted prospective series, **64% of women** (27 of 42) **who exclusively breastfed after preconceptional breast augmentation had insufficient lactation,** and the infant growth rate was less than 20 g/day; **a circumareolar incision was the dominant predictor of insufficient lactation.** One half of women with a submammary or axillary incision had insufficient lactation, whereas 11

women who had a circumareolar incision for breast augmentation all had lactation failure. Compromise of the lactiferous ducts and loss of nipple sensation contribute to lactational insufficiency. Loss of nipple sensation occurs in one third to half of patients after a circumareolar incision. If a woman has had a silicone implant, she can be reassured that no evidence suggests that breastfeeding places her infant at any risk. The concentration of silicone in artificial breast milk (formula) is 5 to 10 times higher than that of breast milk from women who have silicone implants. **Large epidemiologic studies of infants who have nursed from breasts with silicone implants have not shown excess adverse events.**[66]

Reduction mammoplasty is always associated with lactation insufficiency if exclusive breastfeeding is relied upon for infant nutrition. If the reduction involves the removal of greater than 500 g per breast or the procedure uses the free nipple graft technique, the production of even a nominal amount of breast milk is rare. If the nipple and areola are relocated on a pedicle of vascular tissue and ducts, partial breastfeeding is remotely possible. **In any case of reconstructive surgery of the breast, the breastfeeding dyad is considered at high risk for lactation failure.** This observation was confirmed by a controlled study.[67] The control and reduction mammoplasty groups reported rates of any breastfeeding at 1 month of 94% and 58%, respectively. Similarly, the rate of exclusive breastfeeding at 1 month was 70% and 21% in the respective groups. Prenatal referral to an expert on lactation is appropriate for women who have had reconstructive surgery.

LABOR AND DELIVERY MANAGEMENT

Approximately 15% of women who state they wish to breastfeed at the onset of term labor are discharged either completely feeding their infant artificial breast milk (formula) or giving formula at the majority of the infant's feedings. A combination of obstetric management, hospital policies, and pediatric management contribute to this attrition. Obstetric interventions are often critical for the health of the mother or infant, and they may affect the success of lactation.[55-56] Few if any interventions directly inhibit the physiology of lactation. Most obstetric interventions reduce the success of lactation by indirect interference with physiology. Induction of labor is not associated with lactation failure, but a long, tiring induction and labor will reduce the likelihood that the mother will get appropriate amounts of infant contact in the delivery room and in the first 24 hours after birth. Cesarean delivery reduces the incidence of breastfeeding by 10% to 20% in the first week after birth. **After most cesarean deliveries and difficult vaginal deliveries, the infant is not put to the breast immediately after birth, nor will the mother breastfeed her infant more than eight times in the first 24 hours.** Well-meaning nurses become concerned for the baby's nutrition and give the infant formula until the mother "recovers." In 2011, in the United States, one in five breastfeeding neonates was given a bottle of formula in the first 24 hours. That 15% of women desiring to breastfeed are discharged exclusively formula feeding reflects, in part, the mismanagement and/or lack of support for the breastfeeding dyad during their peripartum hospitalization.

Labor analgesia (i.e., meperidine and promethazine) has long been associated with poor breastfeeding success. Intrapartum narcotics appear to adversely affect the infant's ability to nurse effectively. **Epidural anesthesia with local anesthetic agents** seems to be better for breastfeeding than parenteral narcotics. Epidural anesthesia with local anesthetics does not appear to have a major effect. On the other hand, an epidural with intrathecal narcotics has been shown to decrease correct sucking behavior and to reduce lactation success. The **presence of a doula,** or a labor companion other than family, appears to be an effective method to reduce the need for epidural anesthesia and operative deliveries. An added benefit is earlier initiation and longer duration of breastfeeding.[68]

Postsurgical pain control is best achieved with morphine rather than meperidine, which adversely affects neonatal behavior. Obstetric and pediatric protocols can be very effective in separating mother and baby. Several prominent examples include magnesium sulfate therapy for preeclampsia, intravenous antibiotics for a positive maternal group B *Streptococcus* culture, maternal fever workup, and diabetes mellitus/hypoglycemia protocols. All of these medical interventions produce major barriers to nursing in the delivery room and to an adequate frequency of nursing in the first 24 to 48 hours.

The peripartum period is critical for achieving successful lactation. During this time, the obstetrician must attend to the five basic principles of lactation physiology: (1) early imprinting, (2) frequent nursing, (3) good latch-on, (4) a confident and comfortable mother, and (5) no supplementation unless medically indicated. Nursing should be initiated within 30 minutes after birth, preferably in the delivery room. Contraindications include a heavily medicated mother, an infant with a 5-minute Apgar score less than 7, or a premature infant at less than 34 to 36 weeks' gestation.

The instructor, perhaps the obstetric care provider, should pay special attention to the mother's position during the first feeding; she should be relaxed and comfortable. With skin-to-skin contact, the infant is presented to the breast with its ventral surface to the mother's ventral surface with the neonate's ear, shoulder, and hip in a line. A dry neonate, skin-to-skin contact, and supplemental radiant heating will prevent neonatal cold stress. **Routine eye prophylaxis should be delayed because it can disrupt the important family bonding process.**

In the recovery room and on the postpartum floor, the best place for the neonate is with the mother. This maximizes mother-infant bonding and allows on-demand feeding every 1 to 2 hours. Rooming in allows the mother to participate in the care of her baby and gives her an opportunity to ask questions. **The mother should be encouraged to sleep when the neonate sleeps.** Because the usual adult diurnal pattern in the hospital may not foster a restful environment for the mother, she should be discharged as early as safely possible so she can rest at home.

The frequency of early feeding is proportional to milk production and weight gain in neonates[69]; therefore supplementation with glucose or formula should be discouraged. Supplementation decreases milk production through both a reduction in nursing frequency by satiation of the neonate and slower digestion of formula. Supplementation also undermines the mother's confidence about the adequacy of her lactation. Nipple and breast pain may cause the mother not to reach her breastfeeding goals. Improper positioning and poor latch-on are the major causes of nipple trauma, breast pain, and incomplete emptying. **In the early postpartum period, nursing technique should be evaluated in three areas: (1) presentation and latching on, (2) maternal-infant positioning, and (3) breaking of the suction.** The infant should not have to turn its head to nurse.

A ventral surface–ventral surface presentation is necessary (see Fig. 24-4). When latching on to the nipple, the neonate should take as much of the areola as possible into its mouth. This is facilitated by gently stimulating the baby's cheek to elicit a yawn-like opening of its mouth and rapid placement of the breast into it. A supporting hand on the breast helps; the C-hold involves four fingers cupping and supporting the weight of the breast, which is especially important in the weak or premature neonate, whose lower jaw may be depressed by the weight of the breast. The thumb rests above and 1 to 2 cm away from the areolar edge and points the nipple downward (see Fig. 24-5). Retraction by the thumb will pull the areola away from the mouth and will cause an incorrect placement. Any position that is comfortable and convenient, while allowing the appropriate mouth-areola attachment, should be encouraged; the sitting position is the most common in patients who have had a cesarean delivery because pressure on the abdomen is uncomfortable. Therefore a side-lying or football hold may be better. **A rotation of positions is recommended to reduce focal pressure on the nipple and to ensure complete emptying.** Removal of the nursing infant can be a problem because the neonate can injure the nipple if suction is not broken prior to disengagement. **A finger inserted between the baby's lips and the breast will break the suction.**

The single most difficult management issue is the control of routines and hospital attitudes detrimental to lactation, and the genesis in step 1 of the WHO/UNICEF Ten Steps is a standard written hospital policy that supports breastfeeding. Policies that work against the physiology of lactation include formula distribution and supplementation without a medical indication, constant questioning of the mother about breastfeeding, preprinted orders for lactation suppression medication, a requirement for pediatric clearance prior to the first feeding, limited maternal access to the infant, and little educational material for new mothers or staff.

When providers are not well informed or are apathetic about lactation, successful lactation is unlikely. This theme underscores the role of the obstetrician as an opinion leader in the education of patients, nursing staff, and support personnel about the physiology and benefits of lactation (step 2 of the WHO/UNICEF Ten Steps is to train *all* health care providers).

Breast Milk Expression

When an unexpected separation of the mother and baby for longer than 4 to 6 hours occurs, breast milk expression may be critical to prevent stage IV of lactogenesis from occurring prematurely—that is, to avoid reduced production of milk. Despite the ready availability of mechanical breast pumps, in an emergency, the lactating mother may be unable to obtain one within 12 to 24 hours. Her knowledge on how to manually express milk will reduce her anxiety and the pain of acute breast engorgement.

Manual expression of breast milk is a relatively easy technique for the obstetric care team to teach the new mother. The mother's hands are washed with mild soap and warm water prior to manual or mechanical expression. The flow of milk can be improved by placing the mother in a quiet, relaxed, and comfortable environment. The breast is massaged in a spiral fashion, starting at the top and moving toward the areola; the fingers are moved in a circular fashion from one spot to another, much like a breast examination. After the massage and while the woman leans forward, the breast is stroked from the top of the breast to the nipple with a light stroke and is shaken. Once milk starts to flow, manual expression is begun.

Manual expression is performed by holding the thumb and first two fingers on either side of the areola in a half circle, but the breast should not be cupped. The hand pushes the breast straight into the chest wall, as the thumb and fingers are rolled forward. Large, pendulous breasts may need lifting prior to this. The maneuver is repeated in all four quadrants of the areola to drain as many reservoirs as possible. The procedure is repeated rhythmically and gently; squeezing, sliding, or pulling may injure the breast. The sequence of massage, stroke, shake, and express is useful to provide milk immediately for the vigorous infant; it allows an improved latch-on by reducing periareolar engorgement, and it reduces high suction pressures on a traumatized nipple. Manual expression may take 20 to 30 minutes to drain both breasts. The expressed milk is drained into a clean, dry cup and is fed to the neonate if possible. A video that demonstrates this technique can be found online at http://newborns.stanford.edu/Breastfeeding/HandExpression.html.

The mechanical, preferably electric breast pump is a critically important adaptation when breastfeeding is expected to be difficult or impossible. Breast pumps have allowed women and their children to get through the difficult times, and it lets a woman successfully feed her infant breast milk for a prolonged period. These women will accrue much of the benefit of breastfeeding—a much better choice than formula feeding. In most peripartum cases, such as with a preterm delivery or a severely ill mother, the hospital-grade electric breast pump will used by the hospital staff. After the delivery of the placenta, stage II of lactogenesis evolves with the loss of progesterone inhibition. Early drainage of the breast is critical to a healthy evolution to full milk production, whether the drainage occurs with an infant sucking or from using an electric breast pump.

The delay in early drainage is often prolonged when a neonate with very low birthweight is admitted to the NICU. One recent study[70] randomly assigned mothers with neonates of very low birthweight to initiate breast pumping within 1 hour or breast pumping between 1 and 6 hours after birth. The treatment effect was significant despite a very small sample size of 10 women in each arm. When breast pumping was started within 1 hour, women produced almost twice as much milk at 7 days and twice as much daily milk at 3 weeks and 6 weeks. It was found that they experienced earlier maturation of lactogenesis stage II (when "the milk comes in") than those who initiated pumping within 1 to 6 hours after birth. Clearly, the obstetrician plays a major role in getting the mother to the breast pump within 1 hour in these high-risk situations.

Proper fitting and hygiene is an important safety issue when expressing and storing breast milk (Boxes 24-2 and 24-3). Breast milk expression with portable or stationary hospital-grade mechanical breast pumps is increasingly used for the convenience of bottle feeding human milk, particularly for working mothers rather than in emergency situations. A series of recent publications have focused on the results of an FDA and CDC study from May 2005 to June 2007, the Infant Feeding Practices Study II (IFPS II). A broad, national sample included mothers identified in their third trimester who were at least 18 years old and who gave birth to healthy infants born at 35 weeks' or more gestation that weighed more than 2.25 kg. The mothers completed 10 surveys at monthly intervals until 12 months. A key focus was the method of feeding in the previous week[71]: breastfed only, breastfed and human milk by bottle, breastfed and

BOX 24-2   KEY POINTS IN USING AN ELECTRIC BREAST PUMP

1. Have the mother and the principal support individual learn from an expert how to assemble and disassemble the pump apparatus.
2. As in manual expression, a soothing, quiet, and comfortable environment is optimal for milk let-down.
3. The mother should wash her hands before each use of the breast pump.
4. A double-pumping system improves prolactin response and increases milk production.
5. The flange should be wide enough to allow the nipple to move in and out without pain yet not so large as to compromise a pressure seal. A poorly fitted flange can be a major source of nipple trauma and discomfort.
6. Each mother should use only her own collection kit and labeled storage containers.
7. After each use, the pump collection kit should be rinsed to remove milk residue; cleansed with hot, soapy water; and air-dried. Dishwasher cleaning is adequate; however, always follow manufacturer's instructions regarding cleaning.
8. In general, pumping should last about 10 minutes per side and should occur at least every 3 hours.

BOX 24-3   KEY POINTS IN BREAST MILK STORAGE

1. Milk storage containers should be washed with warm, soapy water before and after each use.
2. Hard plastic containers of polycarbonate or polypropylene are recommended for long-term storage of expressed human milk. Label milk containers with the date and time the milk was expressed, and use the oldest milk first.
3. Maximum duration of human milk storage by temperature: Room temperature (<25° C), 4 hours; refrigerator (<4° C), 96 hours; previously thawed refrigerated milk, 24 hours; refrigerator freezer/deep freezer (−20° C), 6 months.
4. Frozen milk should be thawed in a waterless warmer or in a container of tepid, not hot, water. Do not thaw frozen milk in the microwave. The thawed milk should be stored in the refrigerator and should be used within 24 hours.

nonhuman milk by bottle, human milk and nonhuman milk by bottle, human milk by bottle, or nonhuman milk by bottle. Analyses were conducted on three groups of infants at 1.5 to 4.5 months (n = 1564); 4.6 to 6.5 months (n = 1128); and 6.6 to 9.5 months (n = 914). In the youngest group, 85% of mothers had successfully expressed milk since their child was born, more than half in the first week after birth, and 25% expressed breast milk on a regular basis. The adjusted odds ratios for working mothers to express breast milk in a regular fashion in each infant age group ranged from 3.99 to 5.94, and all were highly significant.

In observational surveys, many of these women will report themselves as exclusively breastfeeding when they are actually partially breastfeeding and partially feeding breast milk obtained through a breast pump, often frozen and fed by bottle at a later time. Pumping and bottle-feeding the breast milk later upsets the delicate supply-and-demand relationship in the dyad and reduces skin-to-skin contact. Freezing may affect the nutritional

and antiinfective qualities of stored breast milk, and the use of bottles can increase acute otitis media and may negate the positive benefits seen in breastfeeding dyads; bottle-feeding is a strong predictor of acute otitis media. **Research is limited on the quality of stored breast milk, health outcomes relative to breastfeeding versus bottle-feeding breast milk, and the behavioral impacts of bottle-feeding.**[72] Data from the IFPS II demonstrate that feeding breast milk from a bottle is associated with faster weight gain during the first year of life than feeding infants by breast only. Data showed that infants who received breast milk only by bottle gained about 89 g/month more than infants who were exclusively breastfed. Infants fed human milk from a bottle in more than 66% of their feedings were more likely to finish their bottle and consumed about 10% more milk every day than infants who received a bottle of breast milk in more than 33% of feedings.[73] This suggests that bottle-fed infants have weaker self-regulation of food intake than breast-fed infants. Clearly, this area is a great opportunity for further research.

MATERNAL NUTRITION AND EXERCISE DURING LACTATION

The efficiency of conversion of maternal foodstuff to milk is about 80% to 90%. **If the average milk volume per day is 900 mL, and milk has an average energy content of 75 kcal/dL, the mother must consume an extra 794 kcal/day unless stored energy is used. During pregnancy, most women store an extra 2 to 5 kg (19,000 to 48,000 kcal) in tissue, mainly as fat, in physiologic preparation for lactation.** These calories and nutrients supplement the maternal diet during lactation. As a result, the required dietary increases are easily attainable in healthy mothers and infants.

In lactation, most vitamins and minerals should be increased 20% to 30% over nonpregnant requirements. However, folic acid should be doubled; and calcium, phosphorus, and magnesium should be increased by 40% to 50%, especially in the teenager who is lactating. In practical terms, these needs can be supplied by the following additions to the diet: 2 cups of milk, 2 oz of meat or peanut butter, a slice of enriched or whole wheat bread, a citrus fruit, a salad, and an extra helping ($\frac{1}{2}$ to $\frac{3}{4}$ cup) of a dark green or yellow vegetable. **The appropriate intake of vitamins can be ensured by continuing prenatal vitamins with 1 mg of folic acid throughout lactation.** The mother should drink at least 1 L of extra fluid every day to make up for the fluid lost through breastfeeding.

Calcium and vitamin D are of special importance in women whose infants are breastfeeding exclusively. The daily diet and a lack of sunlight exposure creates baseline deficiencies in many American women. Almost all of the calcium in a pregnant woman and her fetus is located in the bones and teeth. Lactation, like pregnancy, is associated with increased bone turnover to meet these needs. The calcium secreted in breast milk appears to be from a net removal of calcium from trabecular bone and by a reduction in the amount of calcium excreted in the urine. Consuming additional calcium does not appear to prevent bone loss, and after weaning or resumption of menstruation, calcium absorption returns to normal. This may not be true for women who have marginal or low dietary calcium intake, therefore ensuring a woman obtains adequate calcium before, during, and after lactation is important for her health.

There is widespread consensus about the role of vitamin D in bone health, and great interest has been paid to its role in other conditions. Current research links newborn and infant vitamin D deficiency with various clinical outcomes that include rickets, failure to thrive, type 1 diabetes, allergic disease, lower respiratory tract infections, wheezing and asthma, and other immune-related diseases. Breast-fed infants are at risk of developing a deficiency if the mother's milk contains inadequate levels of 25-hydroxyvitamin D for infant nutrition. It has been demonstrated that when sunlight exposure is limited or restricted, intensified vitamin D supplementation of lactating mothers and infants is needed to improve vitamin D status. In 2008, the American Academy of Pediatrics (AAP) recommended 400 IU of vitamin D supplementation for all infants; however, the level of adherence with this recommendation has been low, and women report reluctance to adding supplements to their breast milk. **Except for those that have been fortified, relatively few foods are good sources of vitamin D, therefore leading breastfeeding advocates recommend that women be supplemented for prevention of vitamin D deficiency in themselves and in their breastfeeding infants.** Although the daily recommended intake (DRI) for vitamin D remains unchanged at 15 μg/day (600 IU) in lactation, two recent randomized controlled trials (RCTs) have questioned this level because a growing body of evidence points to the potential role of vitamin D in immune function, which affects maternal and child health. To achieve circulating serum levels greater than 20 ng/mL, a level considered sufficient by the Institute of Medicine, at least 2000 IU/day was required, and 4000 IU/day improved physiologic optimization of active vitamin D without adverse effects. Further research is required to establish the need, safety, and efficacy of supplementation, especially at these dosages or higher during lactation. Women with limited sun exposure and those with darker skin are at an increased risk for maternal and infant vitamin D deficiency.

Vegetarianism has become increasingly more common, and if the nursing mother is a vegetarian, dietary deficiencies may include B vitamins (especially B_{12}), total protein, and the full complement of essential amino acids. In these patients, the clinician should take a good dietary history with a focus on protein, iron, calcium, vitamin D, and the B vitamins. Nutrition should include supplementation with soy flour, molasses, or nuts with use of complementary vegetable protein combinations and avoidance of excess phytate and bran.

Many women are concerned about losing weight postpartum. Investigators[6-8] have examined the effects of diet and exercise on maternal weight, breast milk volume and composition, and infant growth through random assignment of affluent, highly motivated, and exclusively breastfeeding women to intervention and control groups. The exercise group had training to reach a level of 45 minutes at 60% to 70% of heart rate reserve four to six times a week for 12 weeks. The target diet was individually adjusted to reduce calories and maintain protein intake. In these controlled populations, **the women lost 1.0 to 1.5 kg/week, and no significant changes were seen in the volume or composition of their breast milk.** The infant grew approximately 2000 g in both the intervention and control groups. On a practical level, if 700 to 1200 kcal are used daily to nourish an infant, a mother could lose weight by not increasing her caloric intake, but a thoughtful selection of food groups and the elimination of "empty calories" are necessary. A reduction of total calories (<25 kcal/kg) and total protein (<0.6 g/kg) may reduce the daily milk volume by 20% to 30%, but it does not affect the milk quality unless the mother is more than 10% below her ideal body weight. **Because dieting mobilizes fat stores that may contain environmental toxins, women with high exposure to such toxins should not lose weight during lactation** (see Chapters 5 and 8).

BREAST AND NIPPLE PAIN

Breast and nipple pain is one of the most frequent complaints of lactating mothers and a leading cause for women not to meet their intended durations of breastfeeding. Among the enrollees in the IFPS II study, 60% of 1177 women failed to achieve their desired duration of breastfeeding. **Breast pain, nipple injury, and/or breast infection were the cited reasons in the majority of women who stopped breastfeeding early.** The frequency of breast and nipple pain is related to failure in the initial management of lactation related to a late first feeding, decreased frequency of feedings, poor nipple grasp, and/or poor positioning. The differential diagnosis of breast pain includes problems with latching on, engorgement, nipple trauma, mastitis, and occasionally the let-down reflex.

Symptoms and the infant's personality help make the differential diagnosis. In some cases, the nipple and breast pain starts with latching on and diminishes with let-down. Women describe the let-down reflex as painful; this occurs after the first minute of sucking and usually lasts only a minute or two as the ductal swelling is relieved by nursing. Classically, this pain pattern is associated with an anxious, vigorous infant who sucks strongly against empty ducts until the let-down occurs. Contact pain suggests nipple trauma, and pain can persist as long as the nipple is manipulated. The nipple-confused infant who chews on the nipple and abrades the tip with its tongue is associated with this pattern.

Engorgement causes a dull, generalized discomfort in the whole breast that gets worse just before a feeding and is then relieved by it. Localized, unilateral, and continuous pain in the breast may be caused by mastitis. A physical examination and observation of nursing technique can confirm the impression left by a good history. Through observation of a nursing episode, an infant's personality and nursing technique can be assessed. The whole of the nipple and much of the areola should be in the infant's mouth. An examination of the nipple may reveal a fissure or blood blister; bilateral breast firmness and tenderness may indicate engorgement that may be peripheral, periareolar, or both. Mastitis is characterized by fever, malaise, localized erythema, heat, tenderness, and induration (see below).

Infection may be a cofactor associated with the pain of nipple injury. When the microbiology of the nipple and milk of 61 lactating women with nipple pain was compared with that of 64 lactating women without nipple pain and 31 nonlactating women, *Candida albicans* (19%) and *Staphylococcus aureus* (30%) were more common in women with pain and nipple fissures than in controls (3% to 5%).[74] Unfortunately, current data suggest that antibiotics are ineffective in the treatment of nipple pain and trauma.[63]

The management of breast pain consists of general and specific steps, and prevention is a key component. Appropriate nursing technique and positioning will prevent, or significantly decrease, the incidence of nipple trauma, engorgement, and mastitis. Rotation of the nursing position will reduce the suction pressure on the same part of the nipple and will ensure complete emptying of all lobes of the breast, and frequent nursing will reduce engorgement and milk stasis. **The use of soaps, alcohol, and other drying agents on the nipples tends to increase nipple trauma and pain. The nipples should be air dried for a few minutes after each feeding; clean water is sufficient to cleanse the breast, if necessary.** Some experts recommend that fresh breast milk be applied to the nipples and allowed to dry after each feeding.

Stimulating a let-down response for manual expression of milk is useful in the management of many breast problems. The let-down produced by manual expression is never as complete as a normally elicited one; however, an effective let-down can be elicited by initiating nursing on the side without nipple trauma or mastitis. This will effectively reduce breast pain.

In the first 5 days after birth, about 35% of the nipples of breastfeeding mothers show damage, and 69% of mothers have nipple pain.[75] The management of painful, tender, or injured nipples includes prefeeding manual expression, correction of latching on, rotation of positions, and initiation of nursing on the less painful side first, with the affected side exposed to air. Drying is facilitated by the cautious application of dry heat, such as with a hair dryer on a low setting, for 20 minutes four times per day. Aspirin or codeine (15 to 30 mg) given half an hour before nursing may be helpful in severe cases. Engorgement can be avoided, but if it occurs, feeding frequency should be maintained or increased by pumping. **A wide variety of preparations have been applied to traumatized nipples, including lanolin, A&D ointment, white petrolatum, antibiotics, vitamin E oil, and used tea bags, but few of these have been evaluated scientifically, and systematic review fails to show any benefit.[63] Soap and alcohol have been shown to injure nipples.** Nipple shields should be used only as a last resort because they are associated with a 20% to 60% reduction in milk consumption. Thin latex shields may be better than the traditional red rubber ones, although milk flow is still reduced by 22%.[75]

Engorgement of the breast occurs when drainage of milk is inadequate.[76] Swollen, firm, and tender breasts are caused by distension of the ducts and increased extravascular fluid. Aside from the discomfort, engorgement leads to dysfunctional nursing behavior and nipple trauma (see Fig. 24-10). The firm breast tissue pushes the infant's face away from the nipple, the widened base of the nipple disrupts the attachment, and the infant's thrusting tongue abrades the tip. This leads to further engorgement, decreased milk production, and in some cases, early termination of breastfeeding.

The best treatment is prevention, but when this has not occurred, management is centered on symptomatic support and relief of distension. Proper elevation of the breasts is important. The mother should wear a firm-fitting nursing brassiere with neither thin straps nor a plastic lining. A warm shower or bath with manual expression before feeding is effective. Frequent suckling every 1 to 2 hours is the most effective mechanism to relieve engorgement, and postfeeding electric pumping of both breasts may be helpful. In selected cases, intranasal oxytocin may be given just prior to each feeding if let-down seems to be inhibited.

MASTITIS AND BREAST ABSCESS

Mastitis is a common condition in lactating women. Estimates of incidence from prospective studies range from 3% to 20%, depending on the method of ascertainment, case definition, and duration of follow-up. A practical case definition of *mastitis* is an infectious process of the breast characterized by high fever (>38.5° C), localized erythema, tenderness, induration, and palpable heat over the area.[77] Signs and symptoms of a systemic cytokine release, shaking chills (rigor), malaise, flulike symptoms, a white cell count below 4000 or above 12,000 cells/mL, and nausea and vomiting differentiate mastitis from other inflammatory processes of the lactating breast (i.e., plugged ducts or severe engorgement). Antibiotic therapy should not be delayed in patients who meet the above case definition; septic shock, toxic shock syndrome, and abscess formation are possible serious outcomes with delayed antibiotic therapy. Patients with a temperature above 38.5° C and no systemic signs or symptoms can be managed with aggressive breast drainage, especially with the involved lobules and with correction of latch-on. Mastitis occurs most frequently in the first 2 to 4 weeks postpartum. Risk factors include maternal fatigue, poor nursing technique, nipple trauma, rapid reduction in nursing frequency, constrictive clothing, and epidemic *Staphylococcus aureus.* The most common organisms associated with mastitis are *S. aureus,* which includes methicillin-resistant *S. aureus* (MRSA); *S. epidermidis*; streptococci; and occasionally gram-negative rods.

Until recently, the management of mastitis has been directed by retrospective clinical reviews of experience. In most cases, this consisted of bed rest, continued lactation, and antibiotics and came with an 80% to 90% cure rate, a 10% abscess rate, a 10% recurrence rate, and a 50% cessation of breastfeeding. Starting in the 1980s, several important articles were published concerning the pathophysiology, diagnosis, and treatment of mastitis. **The diagnosis and prognosis of inflammatory symptoms of the breast could be established by counts of leukocytes and bacteria in breast milk.** This is obtained after careful washing of the mother's hands and breasts with warm, soapy water. The milk is manually expressed, and the first 3 mL are discarded. A microscopic analysis is performed on an unspun specimen. **When the leukocyte count was greater than 10^6 leukocytes/mL, and the bacterial count was less than 10^3 bacteria/mL, the diagnosis was noninfectious inflammation of the breast.** With no treatment, the inflammatory symptoms lasted 7 days; 50% developed mastitis, and only 21% returned to normal lactation. When the breast was emptied frequently by continued lactation, the symptoms lasted 3 days, and 96% returned to normal lactation.

If the breast milk showed greater than 10^6 leukocytes/mL and greater than 10^3 bacteria/mL, the diagnosis was mastitis. Delay in therapy resulted in abscess formation in 11%, and only 15% returned to normal lactation. Frequent emptying of the infected breast by continued nursing eliminated abscess formation, but only 51% returned to normal lactation. Additional antibiotic therapy increased the return to normal lactation in 97% with resolution of symptoms in 2.1 days.

In summary, the management of mastitis includes (1) breast support, (2) an appropriate intake of fluids, (3) assessment of nursing technique, (4) nursing initiated on the uninfected side first to establish let-down, (5) the infected side emptied by nursing with each feeding (occasionally, a breast pump helps to ensure complete drainage), and (6) dicloxacillin 250 mg every 6 hours for 14 days. Erythromycin may be used in patients allergic to penicillin. It is important to continue antibiotics for a full 14 days because abscess formation

is more likely with shorter courses of treatment. In the hospital and at home, maternal hand washing before each feeding reduces infection rates. In the hospital, hand washing and the use of antiseptic gels by health care workers reduces nosocomial infection rates and, more importantly, reduces MRSA-associated mastitis. In the era before universal hand washing by hospital personnel, rooming in did not reduce the acquisition of hospital strains of *S. aureus,* nor did it reduce infection rates. In the more infection-conscious environment of today, isolation (rooming in) and early discharge may add to the benefits of hand washing by reducing the rates of MRSA-associated mastitis and abscess.[78]

Breast abscess will occur in about 10% of women who are treated for bacterial mastitis. The signs include a high fever (>39° C) and a localized area of erythema, tenderness, and induration. A fluctuant area may be present in the center, but it is difficult to palpate. The patient feels sick, like she "has the flu." Abscesses usually occur in the upper outer quadrants, and *S. aureus* is usually cultured from the abscess cavity.

The management of a breast abscess is similar to that for mastitis except that drainage of the abscess is indicated, and breastfeeding should be limited to the uninvolved side during the initial therapy. The infected breast should be mechanically pumped every 2 hours and with every let-down. Serial percutaneous needle aspirations under ultrasound guidance are the standard and best method to drain the abscess, although occasionally, surgical drainage is required. The skin incision should be made over the fluctuant area in a manner parallel to and as far as possible from the areolar edge. Whereas the skin incision follows skin lines, the deeper extension should be made bluntly in a radial direction. Sharp dissection perpendicular to the lactation ducts increases blood loss, the risk of a fistula, and the risk of ductal occlusion. Once the abscess cavity is entered, all loculations are bluntly reduced, and the cavity is irrigated with saline. American surgeons pack the wound open for drainage and secondary closure, whereas British surgeons advocate removal of the abscess wall and primary closure. In either case, wide closure sutures should be avoided because they may compromise the ducts. Patients have a protracted recovery of 18 to 32 days, and recurrent abscess formation occurs in 9% to 15% of patients. Breastfeeding from the involved side may be resumed if skin erythema and underlying cellulitis have resolved, which may occur in 4 to 7 days.

C. albicans infection is considered a common cause of breast pain, and ***Candida* infection of the breast is commonly diagnosed by clinical presentation: women describe severe pain when the infant nurses, "like a red hot poker being driven through my chest."** Often the patient has received antibiotics recently and has diabetes, or the infant has evidence of oral thrush or diaper rash (*C. albicans*). The areola and nipple are erythematous with a scaly sheen to the nipple. Unfortunately, the clinical presentation of candidal infection of the breast is not as specific or as accurate as a prudent clinician needs it to be. The differential diagnosis includes let-down pain, poor latch-on, nipple trauma, an allergic reaction, Raynaud phenomenon of the nipple, and early bacterial mastitis.

Often the mother is given strong antifungal agents for symptoms not amenable to antifungal agents. In a study by Hale and colleagues,[79] only 1 of 21 patients with a "classic" presentation of *Candida* mastitis had a breast milk specimen positive for yeast. **Given the nonspecificity of the clinical diagnosis, a focused physical examination and biologic confirmation** of *Candida* is prudent. **Biologic confirmation is obtained through a microscopic examination and culture of a midstream sample of breast milk.** First, the nipples and areola are gently cleaned with warm water. Next, a let-down of breast milk is induced and a sample of the milk is obtained after the first 3 mL have been discarded. A potassium hydroxide (KOH) smear can confirm the diagnosis. A drop of the midstream milk is combined with a drop of 10% KOH and is examined under high-power light microscopy. A typical pattern of hyphae and spores will be visualized. The remainder of the sample is sent for culture and isolation of bacteria and fungi. In cases in which multiple antibiotics and antifungal agents have been used, a sensitivity panel on the fungal isolates may be helpful. A fungal culture may take 7 to 10 days for isolation and identification, longer than for antibiotic sensitivities. **Given the intensity of maternal symptoms and the risk of discontinuing breastfeeding, empiric therapy is warranted prior to the availability of culture results.**

The initial treatment is to massage nystatin cream or miconazole oral gel into both nipples after each feeding and in the infant's mouth three times a day for 2 weeks. Recurrent or persistent *Candida* mastitis can be treated by swabbing the infant's mouth with gentian violet liquid (0.5%) and immediately latching the baby to the breast; this should be done twice a day for 3 days. The major disadvantage of this therapy is the permanent staining associated with gentian violet. An alternative therapy in severe cases is oral fluconazole in a 200-mg loading dose followed by 100 mg/day for no more than 14 days.

MILK TRANSFER AND INFANT GROWTH

When is an exclusive diet of breast milk insufficient to supply the nutritional needs of the growing infant? Women who wean in the first 8 weeks most often say that insufficient milk is the reason for quitting, and well-meaning family members often ask, "When are you going to start feeding your baby *real* food?"

Correct answers are not readily available. Many nondietary factors affect the growth of infants, and poor growth is associated with high birth order (more than four living children), lower maternal age, low maternal weight, poor maternal nutrition during pregnancy, short birth interval, birthweight less than 2.4 kg, multiple gestation, infection, death of either of the infant's parents, or their divorce or separation.

In addition, inconsistencies exist in older standard reference charts for growth and nutritional needs. Most older growth charts are based on formula-fed infants, who often receive solid food supplementation earlier and in greater proportion than comparable breast-fed infants. The WHO and the CDC recognized the weakness and have developed appropriate infant growth charts (http://www.cdc.gov/growth chart).[80] Because milk volume is a quantitative measure of nutrition, variations in volume and concentrations of constituents caused by individual variation and different methods of collection confound the interpretation.

Despite the latter concerns, it is apparent that **a healthy and successfully breastfeeding mother can supply enough nutrition through breast milk alone for 6 months.** The clinical markers for adequate breast milk transfer include an alert, healthy appearance; good muscle tone; good skin turgor; six wet diapers per day; eight or more nursing episodes per day; three or four loose stools per day; consistent evidence of a let-down with operant conditioning; and consistent weight gain (0.75 to 1.0 oz/day after lactogenesis stage III has started; that is, when engorgement occurs, or the "milk comes in").

The term *failure to thrive* **has been used loosely to include all infants who show any degree of growth failure. For the breastfeeding mother, it may just be a matter of comparing the growth of her infant to growth charts compiled from formula-fed infants.** This loosely applied term can seriously undermine the mother's confidence, and ill-advised supplementation further compromises milk volume and may mask other important underlying causes. The infant should be evaluated for failure to thrive or slowed growth if (1) it continues to lose weight after 7 days of life, (2) it does not regain birthweight by 2 weeks, or (3) it gains weight at a rate below the 10th percentile beyond the first months of age. If the mother or the maternal care provider recognize jaundice after the first 7 to 10 days of life, the neonate needs to have a serum bilirubin test and should be seen by the care provider in an emergent fashion (<12 hours). If the infant is premature, ill, or small for gestational age, other growth measurements (ponderal index, height, skinfold thickness, etc.) can be used to define adequate growth. The causes of failure to thrive are often complex and are beyond the scope of this chapter.

JAUNDICE IN THE NEWBORN

Jaundice is one of the more common neonatal markers for prompt intervention; most often, a major focus on breast milk transfer is the solution. Ten to 15% of breast-fed neonates will have jaundice, defined by a peak serum bilirubin greater than 12 mg/dL in term infants.[81] Pediatric concerns include hemolysis, liver disease, or infection as underlying causes and kernicterus as a consequence. **Unconjugated serum bilirubin greater than 20 mg/dL, or 15 mg/dL for high-risk neonates, is considered the critical level for the development of kernicterus in healthy term infants because the risk of permanent brain injury is markedly increased.** When the serum bilirubin is greater than 5 mg/dL in the first 24 hours, a serious disease process such as hemolysis may be present, and intervention is appropriate.

The focus on breastfeeding as related to neonatal jaundice results from the characterization of two syndromes, **breastfeeding jaundice syndrome**, described above, **and breast milk jaundice syndrome.** In the early 1960s, 5% to 10% of lactating women were found to have a steroid metabolite of progesterone—5β-pregnane-3(α), 20(β)-diol—in their icterogenic milk, but the compound was not found in the milk of women whose infants were normal (breast milk jaundice syndrome). This metabolite is associated with an inhibition of glucosyl transferase in the liver, differences in the metabolism of long-chain unsaturated fatty acids, and/or increased resorption of bile acids in jaundiced infants.

In breast milk jaundice syndrome, the neonates are healthy and active. The hyperbilirubinemia develops after the fourth day of life and may last several months, with a gradual fall in the bilirubin level. When breastfeeding is stopped for 24 to 48 hours, a 30% to 50% decline in bilirubin level is observed. With resumption of nursing, serum levels will rise slightly (1 to 2 mg/dL), reach a plateau, and then start to fall slowly regardless of feeding method. **After excluding other causes of jaundice, and with careful monitoring of serum bilirubin, breastfeeding can continue.**

Unfortunately, the focus on rare breast milk jaundice cases, the concern about kernicterus, and the increased bilirubin in many breast-fed neonates between 2 and 7 days old has led to routine supplementation of infants with water, glucose, and formula even when bilirubin concentrations were in the moderate range of 8 to 12 mg/dL. The cause of the elevated bilirubin, reduced feeding frequency, or low milk transfer is often unrecognized. **It has been clearly demonstrated that feeding frequency greater than eight feedings per 24 hours is associated with lower bilirubin levels. Likewise, water supplementation studied in a controlled fashion does not decrease the peak serum bilirubin.** Management consists of prevention by improvement in the quality and frequency of nursing. Rooming in and night feedings should be encouraged. If the mother, family, or obstetrician recognizes jaundice in an infant more than 7 days old, an immediate referral should be made to the child's physician, and a serum bilirubin level should be obtained; this is a pediatric emergency.

GALACTOGOGUES: DRUGS TO IMPROVE MILK PRODUCTION

Obstetricians may interface with the breastfeeding dyad when there is a question of adequate milk production and transfer by the mother. The mother and/or the pediatrician often ask for a galactogogue to be prescribed by the obstetrician.[82]

Numerous agents have been shown to increase prolactin production in nonpregnant women, and galactorrhea is a relatively common clinical issue for women on phenothiazines or metoclopramide. It is reasonable that these drugs might be used where milk supply seems insufficient. The most understandable clinical scenarios include glandular hypoplasia, reduction mammoplasty, premature delivery that requires mechanical pumping, and relactation (nursing an adoptive child). The most common clinical presentation is perceived poor milk supply or inhibited milk let-down (oxytocin inhibition). Clinical trials with random assignment of subjects have demonstrated the effectiveness of metoclopramide, sulpiride, and domperidone. When let-down (milk ejection) is obstructed, nasal oxytocin is given to increase milk ejection.[82]

Metoclopramide (Reglan) is used to promote GI tone; however, a secondary effect is to increase prolactin levels. Most studies demonstrate a manifold increase in basal prolactin levels and a 60% to 100% increase in milk volume. The effects of metoclopramide are very dose dependent; the usual dose is 10 to 15 mg orally three times a day, but the side effects—gastric cramping, diarrhea, and depression—often limit its use. The incidence of depression increases with long-term use, therefore treatment should be tapered over time and limited to less than 4 weeks. There appears to be little effect on the infant. The dose that the infants receive is much less than the amount used therapeutically to treat esophageal reflux, regardless of the time postpartum. The U.S. Food and Drug Administration has issued a black box warning concerning the association of tardive dyskinesia and the use of metoclopramide for more than 3 months.

Domperidone, an agent similar to metoclopramide, blocks the dopamine receptors in the gut and brainstem but with fewer of the psychoneurologic side effects. Domperidone is used in Canada as an antiemetic, but it is not FDA approved in the United States. **In placebo-controlled trials in mothers with decreased milk supply, domperidone increased prolactin** levels and milk supply twofold to threefold. The usual dose to improve milk supply is 10 to 20 mg three to four times a day. Slow tapering (reduce by 10 mg/week) is suggested because acute withdrawal rapidly diminishes milk supply. The relatively high protein binding in maternal serum limits transfer to the neonate, and the relative infant dose is 0.04%. Recently, the FDA issued a warning against use of domperidone because of a risk of cardiac arrhythmias. These potentially life-threatening reactions occurred in older patients with hypokalemia who were receiving chemotherapy for cancer, in whom intravenous domperidone was used in high doses as an antiemetic.

Sulpiride is a selective dopamine antagonist used in Europe as an antidepressant and antipsychotic. Smaller doses (50 mg twice daily) do not produce neuroleptic effects in the mother, but prolactin and milk production are increased significantly. Clinical studies suggest an increase in milk production (20% to 50%) but less than that seen with metoclopramide. In a placebo-controlled study with random assignment of 130 subjects, sulpiride 50 mg twice daily for the first 7 days postpartum increased the total milk yield from 916 mL (±66) in the control group to 1211 mL (±65) in the sulpiride-treated group. The transfer of sulpiride to the breast milk was minimal, and no adverse effects were seen in the infants. Sulpiride is not available in the United States.

Intranasal oxytocin substitutes for endogenous oxytocin to contract the myoepithelial cells and cause milk let-down. In theory, its use is to overcome an inhibited let-down reflex. Oxytocin is destroyed by GI enzymes and is not given orally. Until recently, oxytocin was available as an intranasal spray, but it has been taken off the market. A pharmacist can prepare an intranasal spray with a concentration of 2 IU per drop. The let-down dose is a spray (3 drops) to each nostril; the total let-down dose is approximately 12 IU, taken within 2 or 3 minutes of each nursing episode. The suggested duration of therapy is unclear. Underlying causes for an inhibited let-down reflex need to be identified and controlled.

Few clinical trials have used oxytocin alone to improve milk production. In a double-blind group sequential trial, intranasal oxytocin alone was used to enhance milk production in women during the first 5 days after delivery of a premature infant. The cumulative volume of breast milk obtained between the second and fifth days was 3.5 times greater in primiparas given intranasal oxytocin than in primiparas given placebo. This benefit accrues from more complete emptying of the breast with each feed. Because of oxytocin's complementary mechanism to prolactin-stimulating medications, they are often used in combination.

Although metoclopramide, domperidone, sulpiride, and oxytocin appear to be effective and relatively safe for the mother and infant, they are only secondary support interventions. The primary focus should be to enhance prolactin and oxytocin through natural mechanisms—that is, with appropriate and frequent stimulation of the nipple and areola. Galactagogues should only be used for a short duration (2 to 4 weeks) and in conjunction with hands-on counseling by an individual with the time, energy, and knowledge to enhance the "natural" production of breast milk.

MATERNAL DISEASE

In the vast majority of cases of lactating mothers with intercurrent disease, no medical reason exists to stop breastfeeding. However, appropriate management requires individualizing the care of the nursing dyad in order to preserve the supply-and-demand relationship of lactation. For example, a hospitalized nursing mother should have her nursing baby with her in the hospital for on-demand feedings. This situation stretches the flexibility of hospital administrators and nursing services, but the problem can be overcome by education.

The first principle is to maintain lactation. An acute hospitalization for a surgical procedure is a common complication. If breast milk was the neonate's only source of nutrition, an acute reduction in nursing may lead to breast engorgement, a confusing postoperative fever, and mastitis. The infant should be put to the breast just before premedication, and the breasts should be emptied in the recovery room. The most effective way is to have the mother nurse. Although some anesthetic may be present in the milk, most are compatible with lactation. If there is legitimate concern or if the mother cannot communicate (because she is on a ventilator, for example), the breasts should be pumped mechanically in the recovery room and subsequently emptied every 2 to 3 hours by nursing or pumping.

The second principle is to adjust for the special nutritional requirements of nursing mothers. This principle is especially pertinent when intake is restricted postoperatively and when maternal diet must be manipulated. In the postoperative period, the surgeon must account for the calories and fluid required for lactation. Until oral intake is established, a lactating mother needs an additional 800 mL of fluid per day. Early return to a balanced diet is essential to offset the additional energy and protein requirements of lactation and wound healing.

The third principle is to ensure that the maternal disease will not harm the infant. This is most pertinent with infectious disease, but it is equally important in cases in which a mother's judgment is in question, such as with severe mental disease, substance abuse, or a history of physical abuse. The benefits of breastfeeding in the latter situations must be carefully evaluated using the resources of the patient, her family, and social services.

Infection is the most common condition in which breastfeeding is questioned. In general, the necessary exposure of the infant to the mother in day-to-day care is such that breastfeeding does not add to the risk. This recommendation assumes that appropriate therapy is being given to both mother and infant. Isolation of infected areas should still be practiced, such as with a mask in the case of respiratory infection and lesion isolation in herpes. The four acute infections in which breastfeeding is contraindicated are (1) herpes simplex lesions of the breast; (2) acute maternal varicella in the first 3 days of the neonate's life (only until the neonate has received varicella-zoster immunoglobulin [VZIG]); (3) untreated active tuberculosis (chest x-ray positive with documented presence of Mycobacterium, not just purified protein derivative [PPD] positive); and (4) human immunodeficiency virus (HIV) disease when it occurs in developed countries.

The fourth principle is to evaluate adequately the need and type of medication used for therapy (see Chapter 8). The drug management of chronic hypertension illustrates this principle. First, the need for medication must be scrutinized, and considerable controversy exists in the literature as to whether to treat patients with mild chronic hypertension (diastolic blood pressure 90 to 100 mm Hg). The desire of a mother with mild hypertension to breastfeed may change the risk/benefit ratio such that antihypertensive drug therapy should be delayed until after lactation. Second, the medication should be evaluated for its effect on milk production. **In the first 3 to 4 months of therapy, diuretics reduce intravascular volume and, subsequently, milk volume.** On the other hand, if a patient has been on low doses of thiazide diuretics for more than 6 months, the effect on milk volume is minimal as long as adequate oral intake is maintained. Third, the medication should be evaluated for its secretion in breast milk and its possible effects on the infant. Thiazide diuretics, ethacrynic acid, and furosemide also cross into breast milk in small amounts. These agents have the potential to displace bilirubin, and their use during lactation is of concern when the infant is less than 1 month old or is jaundiced. In general, most other antihypertensive drugs are compatible with breastfeeding. Although new drugs come onto the market often, it is wise to use drugs that have had a long history of clinical use.

A **fifth principle and a constant challenge is the blanket proscription by radiologists and x-ray technicians to "pump and dump" breast milk for 24 to 48 hours when contrast agents are used. Most agents have very poor oral bioavailability, and the effective infant dose is less than 0.1%.** The guidelines of the American College of Radiology (2004) reviewed the use of contrast media in breastfeeding mothers. On a practical level, the mother should feed her infant just before the injection of the contrast media. The delay of 2 to 3 hours until the next feeding allows the mother to clear the agent before potential infant exposure; the half-life of many of these agents is less than 2 to 3 hours. If the mother is comfortable with expression or pumping, stored breast milk is an alternative for interim feeds for two to three half-lives.

DRUGS IN BREAST MILK

Most medications taken by the mother appear in the breast milk, but the calculated doses consumed by the nursing infant range from 0.001% to 5% of the standard therapeutic doses and are tolerated by infants without toxicity (see Table 24-6 and Chapter 8).

The following guidelines are helpful:

1. Evaluate the therapeutic benefit of medication. Are drugs really necessary, and are there safer alternatives? Diuretics given for ankle swelling provide very different benefits from diuretics used for congestive heart failure. Choose the drugs most widely tested and with the lowest milk/maternal plasma ratio.
2. Choose drugs with the lowest oral bioavailability.
3. Select the least toxic drug with the shortest half-life.
4. Avoid long-acting forms. Usually, these drugs are detoxified by the liver or are bound to protein.
5. Schedule doses so that the smallest amount gets into the milk. The rate of maternal absorption and the peak maternal serum concentration are helpful in scheduling dosage. Usually, it is best for the mother to take the medication immediately after a feeding.
6. Monitor the infant during the course of therapy. Many pharmacologic agents for maternal use are also used for infants. This implies the availability of knowledge about therapeutic doses and the signs and symptoms of toxicity.

BREAST MASSES DURING LACTATION

Breast cancer is the most common cancer of the reproductive organs of the female. Whereas the risk of breast cancer increases tremendously after the age of 40, 1% to 3% of all breast cancers occur during pregnancy and lactation (see Chapter 50). Breast cancer diagnosed during lactation may have its origin before or during pregnancy. As a result of this assumption and the small numbers of pregnant or lactating women, most studies have lumped these populations together. Researchers in Japan have analyzed breast cancer in age-matched controls ($n = 192$), women who were pregnant at diagnosis ($n = 72$), and women who were lactating at diagnosis ($n = 120$). **The prognosis for breast cancer diagnosed during pregnancy or lactation is poorer than for breast cancer diagnosed at other times.** The 10-year survival for age-matched controls without lymph node metastasis was 93%; for women who were diagnosed during pregnancy or lactation, the survival was 85%. When the lymph nodes were involved, the 10-year survival was 62% in controls and 37% in women who were diagnosed during pregnancy or lactation. The difference in survival is partially explained by a longer duration of symptoms prior to diagnosis (6.3 vs. 5.4 months), tumor size on palpation (4.6 vs. 3.0 cm), and tumor size on cut surface (4.3 vs. 2.6 cm) in lactating women versus controls, respectively. **The delay in diagnosis and the greater size at diagnosis in lactating women is a failure of the obstetric care provider and/or the lactating woman to aggressively pursue the evaluation of a breast mass.**

The lactating woman is most likely to recognize a breast mass through her daily manipulations of her breasts. In her framework of reference, she usually considers this mass a "plugged duct." She should be encouraged to report a plugged duct that persists more than 2 weeks despite efforts to initiate drainage of that lobule. Her provider faces an expanded differential diagnosis; the most common diagnosis is that of a dilated milk duct, a completely benign diagnosis. Fibromas and fibroadenomas are more common in young women; these solid tumors are rubbery, nodular, and mobile, and they may grow rapidly with the hormonal stimulation of pregnancy. A needle aspiration of the mass is the mainstay of diagnosis. **Percutaneous fine-needle aspiration is performed in the same manner as in nonpregnant women.** The use of local anesthetic is optional; infiltration of the area around a small lesion may increase the likelihood of a nondiagnostic aspiration. The area over the mass is swabbed with iodine or alcohol and, using sterile techniques, the lesion is fixed between the thumb and fingers of the nondominant hand. Using a 22-gauge needle attached to a 20-mL syringe, the center of the lesion is probed. Initial aspiration usually reveals the nature of the lesion. If milk or greenish fluid (fibrocystic disease) is found and the lesion disappears, no further diagnostic procedures need to be performed. If the tumor is solid or fails to disappear completely after aspiration, the needle is passed several times through the lesion under strong negative pressure. The aspirated tissue fluid is air-dried on a slide and sent for cytologic evaluation. The pathology requisition should note the age and lactating status. **Fine-needle aspiration biopsy appears to have the same accuracy in pregnancy and lactation as in the nonpregnant, nonlactating woman.** In a study of 214 fine-needle aspirations during pregnancy and lactation, eight (13.7%) were cancer, and the sensitivity, specificity, and positive predictive values were 100%, 81%, and 61%, respectively.

Ultrasound is an accurate method of determining the cystic nature of a breast mass in lactating women. Mammography is more difficult to interpret during lactation. Young breasts are generally more dense, and the massive increase in functioning glands may obscure small cancers. However, the accuracy is still good if the films are interpreted by experienced radiologists. In general, mammography is a secondary diagnostic modality.

A core biopsy using ultrasound or radiographic guidance is a reasonable option to avoid a surgical procedure. If a surgical biopsy is required, the surgeon will usually need guidance regarding the management of lactation. Most breast biopsies can be performed under local anesthesia. If the mother nurses just before the procedure, she will empty the breast—which makes the surgery easier—and will allow 3 to 4 hours to pass before the next feeding. Local anesthetics are not absorbed orally and pose no risk to the infant, so the mother should be allowed to nurse on demand. Most anesthetics used for general anesthesia enter the breast milk in small amounts (1% to 3%) of the maternal dose, and minimal behavioral effects in infants have been observed. In most cases, the mother can nurse within 4 hours of the anesthetic. The mother's breasts should be pumped 3 to 4 hours after the last feeding regardless of the anesthetic status; she will begin to feel the discomfort of engorgement, and the fever of engorgement may confuse the postoperative picture as early as 8 or 10 hours. Failure to empty the breasts within 6 to 8 hours will begin to adversely affect milk supply.

Surgical biopsy usually has little effect on breastfeeding performance unless the procedure is done in the periareolar area or the nerves that supply the nipple are compromised. Circumareolar incisions are to be avoided if possible. Milk fistulae are an uncommon risk (5%) of central biopsy, although fistulae are usually self-limited and will spontaneously heal over several weeks. Prohibiting breastfeeding does not change the likelihood of ultimate healing.

BACK-TO-WORK ISSUES

In 2009, according to the CDC, about 50% of women in the workplace had a child at home younger than 12 months old. One third returned to work within 3 months of birth, and two thirds returned within 6 months. The IFPS II study prospectively surveyed employed breastfeeding mothers ($n = 810$) over the first 12 months after birth for strategies that combined employment and breastfeeding.[83] The important findings were that the average age of the infant when the mother returned to work was a mean of 11.4 weeks, the median hours of work per week was 24.8, and the median duration of breastfeeding after return to paid work was 25.6 weeks. The strategies used to continue breastfeeding in the first month after the mother returned to work included to (1) feed directly from the breast (31.3%), (2) pump and feed directly from the breast (9.4%), (3) pump only and bottle feed breast milk only (43.4%), and (4) neither pump nor feed directly during the day. Directly breastfeeding and a pump-and-feed strategy resulted in the longest durations of breastfeeding after returning to work: 31.4 weeks ($n = 250$) and 32.4 weeks ($n = 75$), respectively. Pumping and bottle-feeding breast milk only averaged 26.3 weeks ($n = 346$), and neither pumping nor feeding breast milk during the work day averaged 14.3 weeks ($n = 128$) and had a significantly shortened duration of breastfeeding. The obstetric provider

should support breastfeeding, and if breastfeeding is not possible during the day, the provider should suggest that the mother pump breast milk to provide bottles for the child care giver to supply to her infant during the work day.

Safe and clean storage of pumped breast milk is critical to the breastfeeding working mother (see the earlier section, "Breast Milk Expression," and also Boxes 24-2 and 24-3). The Academy of Breastfeeding Medicine has a specific protocol to help mothers safely store their milk.[84]

As a consequence of these findings, the CDC, other national organizations, and state legislatures have enhanced or initiated major campaigns to support breastfeeding in the workplace. The CDC has guidelines for workplace safety for working mothers who wish to express breast milk (http://www.cdc.gov/breastfeeding/promotion/employment.htm). In March 2011, federal law amended Section 7 of the Fair Labor Standards Act to require employers to provide "reasonable break time for an employee to express breast milk for her nursing child for 1 year after the child's birth each time such employee has need to express the milk."

The separation between mother and infant adversely affects the psychology and physiology of lactation through breast engorgement, a decrease in the frequency of nursing, and unsatisfied needs of the baby. The anxiety and fatigue associated with the combination of employment and lactation inhibits the let-down reflex, weakens maternal host defenses, and disrupts family dynamics. The infant must adapt to another caregiver, a new sucking technique, and unfamiliar infectious agents found in day care settings. Therefore it is not surprising that formula feeding is viewed as an improvement in mothers' lives, even though it creates feelings of inadequacy and guilt in some women. Fortunately, the rapid increase in breast pump options and technology allows many working mothers (70%) to provide bottled human breast milk to their infant during the work day.

Breastfeeding during employment is both possible and fulfilling. Preparation, milk storage, and choice of child care are the cornerstones to easy adaptation to employment. Preparation involves preemployment change in lifestyle to accommodate the increased stresses. Lactation should be well established with frequent nursing (10 to 14 times per day) and no supplementation prior to return to work. Return to full-time work prior to 4 months has a greater negative impact than return to work after 4 months. Part-time work lessens the impact. About 2 weeks prior to work, the mother should change her nursing schedule at home. During the workday, she should express or pump her breasts two or three times a day, while increasing her nursing with short, frequent feedings before and after work times. The infant should be fed bottles of stored breast milk by a different person in a different place to allow easier adaptation.

During the 2 weeks prior to employment, the day care arrangements should be carefully selected and observed. In addition to references, several questions are pertinent to the selection of the day care setting. Is the sitter a mother herself, and does the sitter have experience with nursing babies? Is the mother welcome to use the child care site for a midday nursing? Does the day care center provide in-arm feeding, or are high chairs and propped bottle-feedings used? Is the time and activity of the center highly structured and rigid, or is it flexible to the needs and requests of the mother and infant? Does the staff treat the parents and children with respect? Many of these questions can be answered by an extended (1- to 2-hr) observation of the center and its children.

Fatigue is the number one enemy of the working mother, and emotional and physical support of the mother is critical. Some helpful suggestions include bringing the infant's bed into the parent's room or construction of a temporary extension to the parents' bed; use of labor-saving devices, division of domestic chores, and the elimination of less important household chores to reduce the workload; and taking naps and frequent rest periods to conserve energy.

Continued stimulation of the breast during working hours is important. Pumping not only improves milk supply, it also supplies human milk for the infant. Manual expression and/or mechanical pumping should be performed more frequently (two to three times during the workday) in the first 6 months postpartum. After 6 months, the workday frequency can be reduced and eliminated as the infant's diet is complemented by fluids or solids during the day.

CONTRACEPTION

Adequate family planning—that is, intentional pregnancy at an appropriate interpregnancy interval (>18 months)—is a critical medical and social principle. Both a shortened interpregnancy interval (<18 months) and unintended pregnancy significantly increase adverse pregnancy outcomes. Having two children in diapers adds considerable social and fiscal stress to the family. The discussion of contraception during breastfeeding is the unique responsibility of the obstetric care provider. Prenatal discussion of contraceptive choices are critically important in a woman who is anticipating breastfeeding, especially a first mother who may have concerns about the effects of hormonal contraception on her breastfeeding infant.

The key issues of contraceptive education are delaying pregnancy at least 18 months and making the next pregnancy intentional. Most women return to sexual relations by 4 to 8 weeks postpartum; if they have had more than two consecutive days of vaginal ("menstrual") bleeding after 56 days postpartum, they are at risk for an often unintended pregnancy. A corollary of the two key contraception educational issues is to provide contraception that does not complicate or potentially affect the success of breastfeeding; or, the converse, to make patients aware that breastfeeding may affect the efficacy of the contraceptive method. A tired, stressed mother with poor support may not be as effective in remembering to use daily (oral hormonal contraceptives) or episodic contraceptives (barrier methods).

Permanent sterilization (i.e., postpartum tubal ligation) is the most effective contraceptive, with a pregnancy rate of 3 to 7 per 1000 woman-years. Postpartum sterilization, even if delayed until after the first 4 hours (for first feeding, skin-to-skin contact, and mother/family bonding), can be performed and completed using the same labor epidural within a short period of time and with minimal impact on breastfeeding. Male sterilization can be performed as an outpatient procedure before delivery with similar effectiveness, as long as postprocedure sperm analysis shows no sperm, usually after 15 ejaculations.

If more children are desired, effective child spacing occurs with lactational amenorrhea. This contraceptive effect has been quantified since the early 1970s.[85] The lactational amenorrhea method (LAM) of birth control utilizes the normal physiology of lactation—a low-estrogen/progesterone, high-prolactin state. If the mother is exclusively breastfeeding, is less than 6 months

postpartum, and has no menses—that is, no bleeding perceived by the mother as menses that occurs after 56 days postpartum or any consecutive 2 days of bleeding—the unintended pregnancy rate is 0.5 to 2 per 100 woman-years. If these conditions are not met, an additional contraceptive is needed. In the first 6 months postpartum, LAM is as effective as the mini pill, or progesterone-only hormonal contraception pill.

When LAM is deemed to be unreliable or the strict conditions are not met, other contraception is needed to prevent unintended pregnancy during the lactation period. The copper intrauterine device (IUD) is very effective, with a pregnancy rate of 3 to 8 per 1000 woman-years, and does not pose concerns related to hormonal exposure to the lactating breasts and neonate. Heavy menses and copper sensitivity are uncommon side effects. Of note, emergency contraception with levonorgestrel is the preferred option, rather than combined oral contraceptives, because it has fewer side effects; in addition, levonorgestrel comes with none of the concerns of high-dose estrogen, which includes reduction of milk volume. Generally, levonorgestrel has little effect on lactation.

In many cases, progesterone-only contraceptives, progestin-releasing IUDs, injections (depot medroxyprogesterone acetate [DMPA]), or implants are the contraception of choice for lactating women who want or need more protection than LAM after the onset of lactogenesis stage III on days 5 to 7 postpartum. Although unproven, a theoretic concern exists for disruption of lactogenesis with a pharmacologic dose of progesterone (i.e., DMPA) when withdrawal of progesterone with placental removal might initiate lactogenesis stage II.

In 2010, the Contraceptive CHOICE Project[86] analysis impacted the recommendations for contraception among lactating women. Long-acting reversible contraception (LARC) addresses the key issues related to contraception during lactation. LARC in this study included the levonorgestrel intrauterine system (LNG-IUD), the copper IUD (Cu-IUD), and the etonogestrel (ETG) implant. Non-LARC methods included all other methods of contraception, such as daily hormonal contraceptive pills, hormonal patches and vaginal rings, and DMPA. Continuation rates at 2 years for LARC methods and non-LARC methods were 71% versus 41%, respectively. **Non-LARC users were 22 times more likely to have an unintended pregnancy than LARC users.** In the prenatal clinic, the obstetric care provider needs to address the very clear implications of this population study to their patients who intend to breastfeed. **LARC methods are far better for achieving a 2-year interpregnancy interval and for reducing unintended pregnancy than non-LARC methods that included oral contraceptives, patches, injectables, and rings.**

WEANING

The AAP recommends exclusive breastfeeding for the first 6 months of life and continuation beyond the first 12 months of life. Breastfeeding is a biologic process modified by cultural expectations. The culture of the United States feels increasingly more uncomfortable when a mother breastfeeds more than a year. From a broader biologic and historic perspective, the U.S. experience reflects cultural bias, not biologic reality. In a remarkable review, **Dettwyler[87] makes a very cogent argument for the "natural" age of weaning in the human to be 3 to 4 years.** She has several arguments, the first being that traditional and prehistoric societies have always weaned between the third and fourth year. Based on weaning when the infant weight is four times its birthweight, similar to other primates, weaning should occur between 2 and 3 years. If weaning corresponds to attainment of one third the adult weight, weaning would occur between 3 and 4 years. If humans behaved like chimpanzees or gorillas and weaned at six times the gestational period, humans would wean at 4.5 years. The dental, neurologic, and immunologic systems are still developing until 6 years of age, and breastfeeding and breast milk provide unique support for these systems up to 4 to 6 years. Developmentally, the infant is able to place solid food in its mouth at 6 months; but if left to the infant's own skills, this intake would not reach a significant proportion of the nutritional requirements until 18 to 24 months. The ability to drink from a cup occurs close to the second year. As the infant supplements an increasing proportion of its nutritional needs with solid or liquid food, the mother will begin to ovulate, and subsequent pregnancy is increasingly more likely. **Through its suppression of gonadal function, breastfeeding can maintain a birth interval of 3 to 4 years. Breastfeeding into the third year is a cultural exception in the United States, but prolonged breastfeeding does *not* constitute abnormal or deviant behavior, an attitude expressed by many so-called modern Americans.** As we learn more about the benefits of long-term lactation, our culture may return to more reasonable expectations for the duration of breastfeeding.

KEY POINTS

- The World Health Organization, the U.S. Surgeon General, the American Academy of Pediatrics, the American Academy of Family Practice, the American College of Obstetricians and Gynecologists, and the Academy of Breastfeeding Medicine endorse breastfeeding as the gold standard for infant feeding.
- Breastfeeding accrues many health benefits for the infant, including protection against infection, fewer allergies, better growth, better neurologic development, and lower rates of chronic diseases, such as type 1 diabetes and childhood cancer.
- Breastfeeding accrues more health benefits for the mother, including faster postpartum involution, improved postpartum weight loss, less premenopausal breast cancer, lower rates of cardiovascular disease, less type 2 diabetes mellitus, and better mother-infant bonding. Breastfeeding also decreases the economic burden.
- Formula lacks key components of breast milk, including defenses against infection, hormones and enzymes to aid digestion, polyunsaturated fatty acids necessary for optimal brain growth, and adequate composition for efficient digestion.
- Prolactin is the major promoter of milk synthesis, and oxytocin is the major initiator of milk ejection. The release of prolactin and oxytocin results from the stimulation of the sensory nerves that supply the areola and nipple.
- Oxytocin released from the posterior pituitary can be operantly conditioned and is influenced negatively by pain, stress, or loss of self-esteem.

- Contact with the breast within 30 minutes of birth increases the duration of breastfeeding. Correct positioning of the nursing infant and correct latch-on promote efficient milk transfer and reduce the incidence of breast pain and nipple injury. A frequency of nursing greater than eight feedings per 24 hours, night nursing, and a duration of nursing longer than 15 minutes are needed to maintain adequate prolactin levels and milk supply.
- The nursing actions on a human teat versus on an artificial teat are very different. Poor lactation is the major cause of nipple injury and poor milk transfer. Perceived or real lack of milk transfer is the major reason for the discontinuation of nursing.
- Milk production is reduced by an autocrine pathway through a protein that inhibits milk production by the alveolar cells and by distension and pressure against the alveolar cells.

REFERENCES

1. AAP. Policy Statement-Breastfeeding and the use of human milk. *Pediatrics.* 2012;129:e827-e841.
2. ACOG Committee Opinion-Breastfeeding. Maternal and Infant Aspects, Number 361. *Obstet Gynecol.* 2007;109:479-480.
3. Scanlon KS, Grummer-Strawn L, Chen J, et al. Racial and ethnic differences in breastfeeding initiation and duration, by state. *Am J Clin Nutr.* 1999;69:959.
4. Odom EC, Li R, Scanlon KS, Perrine CG, Grummer-Strawn L. Reasons for earlier than desired cessation of breastfeeding. *Pediatrics.* 2012;131:e726-e732.
5. Neville MC. Physiology of lactation. *Clin Perinatol.* 1999;26:251.
6. Rasmussen KM. Maternal nutritional status and lactational performance. *Clin Nutr.* 1988;7:147.
7. Strode MA, Dewey KG, Lonnerdal B. Effects of short-term caloric restriction on lactational performance of well-nourished women. *Acta Paediatr Scand.* 1986;75:222.
8. McCrory MA, Nommsen-Rivers LA, Mole PA, et al. Randomized trial of the short-term effects of dieting compared with dieting plus aerobic exercise on lactation performance. *Am J Clin Nutr.* 1999;69:959.
9. Lovelady CA. The impact of energy restriction and exercise in lactating women. *Adv Exp Med Biol.* 2004;554:115.
10. Newton M, Egli GE. The effect of intranasal administration of oxytocin on the let-down of milk in lactating women. *Am J Obstet Gynecol.* 1958;76:103.
11. Uvnas-Moberg K. Oxytocin linked antistress effects—the relaxation and growth response. *Acta Physiol Scand Suppl.* 1997;640:38.
12. Moore ER, Anderson GC, Bergman N. Early skin-to-skin contact for mothers and their healthy newborn infants. *Cochrane Database Sys Rev.* 2007;(3):CD003519.
13. Neifert M. Breastmilk Transfer: Positioning, latch-on, and screening for problems in milk transfer. *Clin Obstet Gynecol.* 2004;47:656.
14. Weber F, Woolridge MW, Baum JD. An ultrasonographic study of the organization of sucking and swallowing by newborn infants. *Dev Med Child Neurol.* 1986;28:19.
15. Geddes DT, Sakakalidis VS, Hepworth AR. Tongue movement and intra-oral vacuum of term infants during breastfeeding and feeding from an experimental teat that released milk under vacuum only. *Early Hum Dev.* 2012;88:443-449.
16. Lucas A, Lucas PI, Baum JD. Differences in the pattern of milk intake between breast and bottle fed infants. *Early Hum Dev.* 1981;5:195.
17. Jones RE. A hazards model analysis of breastfeeding variables and maternal age on return to menses postpartum in rural Indonesian women. *Hum Biol.* 1988;60:853.
18. Newton ER. Breastmilk: The Gold Standard. *Clin Obstet Gynecol.* 2004;47:632.

19. Agency for Healthcare Research and Quality. *Breastfeeding and Maternal and Infant Health Outcomes in Developed Countries—Evidence Report/Technological Assessment.* AHRQ Publication No. 07-E007, 2007.

20. Ip S, Chung M, Raman G, Trikkalinos TA, Lau J. A summary of the Agency for Healthcare Research and Quality's evidence report on breastfeeding in developing countries. *Breastfeed Med.* 2009;4:S17.

21. American Academy of Pediatrics, American College of Obstetricians and Gynecologists. *Breastfeeding Handbook for Physicians.* 2nd ed. 2014.

22. Schwarz EB. Infant feeding in America: Enough to break a mother's heart? *Breastfeed Med.* 2013;8:454.

23. Aune D, Norat T, Romundstad P, Vatten LJ. Breastfeeding and the maternal risk of Type II diabetes: A systematic review and dose-response meta-analysis of cohort studies. *Nutr Metab Cardiovasc Dis.* 2014;24:107.

24. Gunderson EP. Impact of breastfeeding on maternal metabolism: Implications for women with gestational diabetes. *Curr Diab Rep.* 2014;14:460.

25. Savino F, Benetti S, Liguori SA, Sorrenti M, Di Montezemolo LC. Advances on human milk hormones and protection against obesity. *Cell Mol Biol.* 2013;59:89.

26. Ramos-Romain MA. Prolactin and lactation as modifiers of diabetes risk in gestational diabetes. *Horm Metab Res.* 2011;43:593.

27. Lucas A, Morely R, Cole TJ. Randomized trial of early diet in preterm babies and later intelligence quotient. *BMJ.* 1999;31:1481.

28. Vohr BR, Poindexter BB, Dusick AM, et al. Persistent beneficial effects of breast milk ingested in the neonatal intensive care unit on outcomes of extremely low birth weight infants at 30 months of age. *Pediatrics.* 2007;120:e953.

29. Anderson JW, Johnstone BM, Remley DT. Breast-feeding and cognitive development: a meta-analysis. *Am J Clin Nutr.* 1999;70:525.

30. Victora CG, Horta BL, de Mola CL, et al. Association between breastfeeding and intelligence, educational attainment, and income at 30 years of age: a prospective birth cohort study from Brazil. *Lancet Glob Health.* 2014;3:e199-e205.

31. Singhal A, Morley R, Cole T, et al. Infant nutrition and stereoacuity at age 4-6 y. *Am J Clin Nutr.* 2007;85:152.

32. Hanson LA. Human milk and host defense: immediate and long-term effects. *Acta Paediatr Suppl.* 1999;88:42.

33. Kaplan JL, Shi HN, Walker WA. The role of microbes in the developmental immunologic programming. *Pediatr Res.* 2011;69:465.

34. Iyengar SR, Walker WA. Immune factors in breastmilk and the development of atopic disease. *JPGN.* 2012;55:641.

35. Slade HB, Schwartz SA. Mucosal immunity: the immunology of breast milk. *J Allergy Clin Immunol.* 1987;80:346.

36. Schultz C, Temming P, Bucsky P, et al. Immature anti-inflammatory response in neonates. *Clin Exp Immunol.* 2004;135:130.

37. Walker WA. Mechanisms of action of probiotics. *Clin Infect Dis.* 2008;46:S87.

38. Broekaert IJ, Walker WA. Probiotics and chronic disease. *J Clin Gastroenterol.* 2006;40:270.

39. Legrand D, Pierce A, Elass E, et al. Lactoferrin structure and functions. *Adv Exp Med Biol.* 2008;606:163.

40. Vaidya K, Sharma A, Dhungel S. Effect of early mother-baby close contact over the duration of exclusive breastfeeding. *Nepal Med Coll J.* 2005;7:138.

41. Walker CD, Deschamps S, Proulx K, et al. Mother to infant or infant to mother? Reciprocal regulation of responsiveness to stress in rodents and the implications for humans. *J Psychiatry Neurosci.* 2004;29:364.

42. Uvnas-Moberg K. Oxytocin linked antistress effects—the relaxation and growth response. *Acta Physiol Scand Suppl.* 1997;640:38.

43. Mikiel-Kostyra K, Mazur J, Boltruszko I. Effect of early skin-to-skin contact after delivery on duration of breastfeeding: a prospective cohort study. *Acta Paediatr.* 2002;91:1301.

44. Strathearn L, Abdullah A, Mamun J, et al. Does breastfeeding protect against substantiated child abuse and neglect? A 15-year cohort study. *Pediatrics.* 2009;123:483.

45. Montgomery SM, Ehlin A, Sacker A. Breast-feeding and resilience against psychosocial stress. *Arch Dis Child.* 2006;91:990.

46. Ball TM, Bennett DM. The economic impact of breastfeeding. *Pediatr Clin North Am.* 2001;48:253.

47. Bartick M, Reinhold R. The burden of suboptimal breastfeeding in the United States: A pediatric cost analysis. *Pediatrics.* 2010;125:e1048.

48. Pokhrel S, Quigley MA, Fox-Rushby J, et al. Potential economic impacts from improving breastfeeding rates in the UK. *Arch Dis Child.* 2015;100:334-340.

49. Ball TM, Wright AL. Health care costs of formula-feeding in the first year of life. *Pediatrics.* 1999;103:870.

50. Wood J, Hineman E, Meyers D. Academy of Breastfeeding Protocol Committee. Clinical Protocol Number 19: Breastfeeding promotion in the prenatal setting. *Breastfeed Med.* 2009;4:43.

51. Holmes AV, McLeod AY, Bunik M. Academy of Breastfeeding Medicine Protocol Committee. ABM Clinical Protocol #5: Peripartum breastfeeding Management for the healthy mother and infant at term. *Breastfeed Med.* 2013;8:469.

52. Howard C, Howard F, Lawrence R, et al. Office prenatal formula advertising and its effect on breast-feeding patterns. *Obstet Gynecol.* 2000;95:296.

53. WHO/UNICEF. *Protesting, promoting, and supporting breastfeeding: The special role of maternity services, a joint WHO/UNICEF statement.* Geneva: World Health Organization; 1989.

54. Chung M, Rowan G, Trikalinos T, et al. Interventions in primary care to promote breastfeeding: evidence for the U.S. Preventive Task Force. *Ann Intern Med.* 2008;149:565.

55. Cadwell K, Turner-Maffei C. *Continuity of Care in Breastfeeding: Best Practices in Maternity, Settings.* Sudbury, MA: Jones & Bartlett; 2009.

56. DiGirolano AM, Grummer-Strawn LM, Fein SB. Effect of maternity care practices on breastfeeding. *Pediatrics.* 2008;122:s43.

57. Cramton R, Zain-Ul-Abideen M, Whalen B. Optimizing successful breastfeeding in the newborn. *Curr Opin Pediatr.* 2009;21:386.

58. CDC. Breastfeeding-related maternity practices at hospitals and birth centers—United States, 2007. *MMWR.* 2008;57:621.

59. Dewey KG, Nommsen-Rivers LA, Heinig MJ, et al. Risk factors for suboptimal infant breastfeeding behavior, delayed onset of lactation, and excess neonatal weight loss. *Pediatrics.* 2003;112:607.

60. Molina H, Reynolds B, Hodson C, Newton ER, Jackson S. Predictors of exclusive breastfeeding at postpartum discharge in term infants. *Breastfeed Med.* 2014;9:s11.

61. Chantry CJ, Dewey KG, Peerson JM, Wagner EA, Nommensen-Rivers LA. In-hospital formula use increases early breastfeeding cessation among first-time mothers intending to exclusively breastfeed. *J Pediatr.* 2014;164:1339.

62. Alexander JM, Grant AM, Campbell MJ. Randomized controlled trial of breast shells and Hoffman's exercises for inverted and non-protractile nipples. *BMJ.* 1990;304:1030.

63. Dennis CL, Jackson K, Watson J. Interventions for treating painful nipples among breastfeeding women. [Review]. *Cochrane Database Syst Rev.* 2014;12:CD007366.

64. Hurst NM. Lactation after augmentation mammoplasty. *Obstet Gynecol.* 1996;87:30.

65. Kjoller K, McLaughlin JK, Friis S, et al. Health outcomes in offspring of mothers with breast implants. *Pediatrics.* 1998;102:1112.

66. Semple JL, Lugowski SJ, Baines CJ, et al. Breast milk contamination and silicone implants: preliminary results using silicon as a proxy measurement for silicone. *Plast Reconstr Surg.* 1998;102:528.

67. Souto GC, Giugliani ER, Giugliani C, Schneider MA. The impact of breast reduction surgery on breastfeeding performance. *J Hum Lact.* 2003;19:43.

68. Zhang J, Bernasko JW, Leybovich E, et al. Continuous labor support from labor attendant for primiparous women: a meta-analysis. *Obstet Gynecol.* 1996;88:739.

69. Egli GE, Egli NS, Newton M. The influence of the number of breastfeedings on milk production. *Pediatrics.* 1961;27:314.

70. Parker LA, Sullivan S, Krueger C, Kelechi T, Mueller M. Effect of early breastmilk expression on milk volume and timing of lactogenesis Stage II among mothers of very low birth weight infants. *J Perinatol.* 2012;32:205.

71. Labiner-Wolfe J, Fein SB, Shealy KR, Wang C. Prevalence of breast milk expression and associated factors. *Pediatrics.* 2008;122(2):S63-S68.

72. Johns HM, Forster DA, Amir LH, McLachlan HL. Prevalence and outcomes of breast milk expressing in women with healthy term infants: a systematic review. *BMC Pregnancy Childbirth.* 2013;13:212.

73. Li R, Fein SB, Grummer-Strawn LM. Do infants fed from bottles lack self-regulation of milk intake compared with directly breastfed infants? *Pediatrics.* 2010;125:e1386-e1393.

74. Livingston V, Stringer LJ. The treatment of *Staphylococcus* infected sore nipples: A randomized comparative study. *J Hum Lact.* 1999;15:241.

75. McKechnie AC, Eglash A. Nipple shields: A review of the literature. *Breastfeeding Med.* 2010;5:309-314.

76. Berens P, Academy of Breastfeeding Medicine Protocol Committee. ABM Clinical Protocol #20: Engorgement. *Breastfeed Med.* 2009;4(2):111-113.

77. Academy of Breastfeeding Medicine Protocol Committee. ABM Clinical Protocol #4: Mastitis. *Breastfeed Med.* 2014;9(5):239-243.

78. Berens P, Swaim L, Peterson B. Incidence of methicillin-resistant *Staphylococcus aureus* in postpartum breast abscesses. *Breastfeed Med.* 2010;5:113.

79. Hale TW, Bateman TL, Finkelman MA, Berens PD. The absence of *Candida albicans* in milk samples of women with clinical symptoms of ductal candidiasis. *Breastfeed Med.* 2009;4:57.

80. Grummer-Strawn LM, Reinold C, Krebs NF, Centers for Disease Control and Prevention. Use of WHO/CDC growth charts for children 0-59 months. *MMWR.* 2010;59(RR09):1-15.

81. Gartner L, Maisel J, Newman T. Academy of Breastfeeding Medicine Protocol Committee. Guidelines for jaundice in the breastfeeding infant born equal to or greater than 35 weeks. *Breastfeed Med.* 2010;5:87-93.

82. Eglash A, Academy of Breastfeeding Medicine Protocol Committee. ABM clinical protocol #9: Use of galactogogues in initiating or augmenting the rate of maternal milk secretion. *Breastfeed Med.* 2011;6:41.

83. Fein SB, Mandal B, Roe BE. Success of strategies for combining employment and breastfeeding. *Pediatrics.* 2008;122:S56-S62.

84. Powers NG, Montgomery AM, Academy of Breastfeeding Medicine Protocol Committee. ABM Clinical Protocol #8: Human milk storage information for home use for full-term infants. *Breastfeed Med.* 2010;5(3):127-130.

85. Berens P, Labbok M, Academy of Breastfeeding Medicine Protocol Committee. ABM Clinical Protocol #13: Contraception during breastfeeding. *Breastfeed Med.* 2015;10(1):1-10.

86. McNicholas C, Madden T, Segura G, Peipert JF. The Contraceptive CHOICE Project round up: What we did and what we learned. *Clin Obstet Gynecol.* 2014;57:635-643.

87. Dettwyler KA. A time to wean: the hominid blueprint for the natural age of weaning in modern human populations. In: Stuart-MacAdam P, Dettwyler KA, eds. *Breastfeeding: Biocultural Perspectives.* New York: Aldine de Gruyter; 1995.

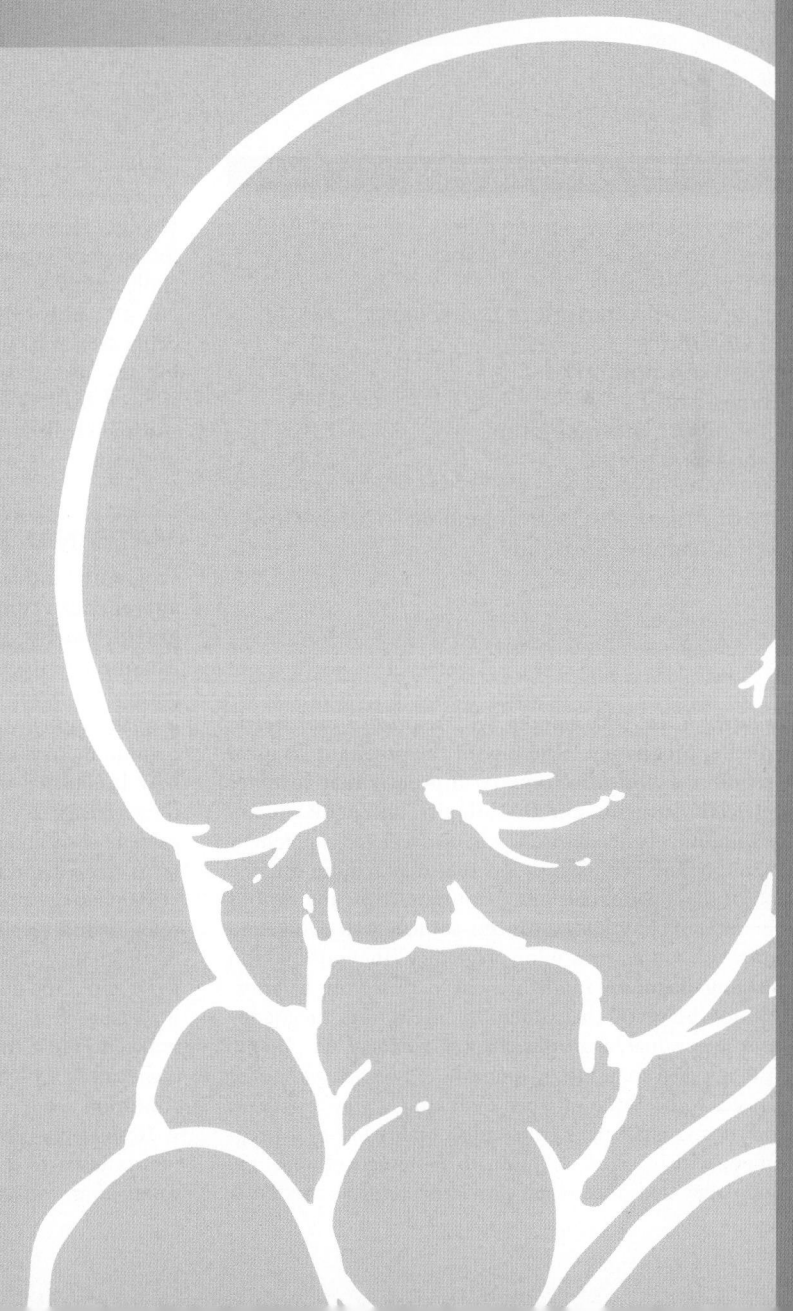

Complicated Pregnancy

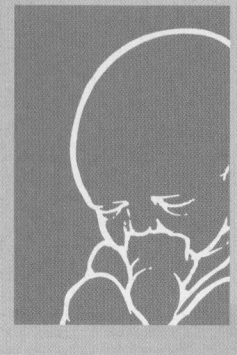

CHAPTER 25

Surgery During Pregnancy

NADAV SCHWARTZ and JACK LUDMIR

KEY ABBREVIATIONS

As low as reasonably achievable	ALARA
American College of Obstetricians and Gynecologists	ACOG
Association of Professors of Gynecology and Obstetrics	APGO
Computed tomography	CT
Fetal heart rate	FHR
Intrauterine growth restriction	IUGR
Last menstrual period	LMP
Magnetic resonance imaging	MRI
Society of American Gastrointestinal and Endoscopic Surgeons	SAGES

Approximately 1 in 500 women will require nonobstetric surgery during pregnancy.[1] The care of the pregnant surgical patient requires a multidisciplinary approach that involves the obstetrician, surgeon, anesthesiologist, and pediatrician. Numerous unique challenges arise when caring for a pregnant woman who presents with symptoms that may require surgery. Evaluation of these patients is often confounded by the various changes in maternal physiology, concern for fetal well-being, and the potential risk to the continuing pregnancy. The introduction of new imaging diagnostic modalities has increased our diagnostic capabilities; however, their safety for use during pregnancy continues to be evaluated. In this chapter, we focus on (1) specific physiologic and anatomic adaptations to pregnancy that the clinician needs to be aware of when evaluating a gravid patient; (2) the diagnostic challenges concerning evaluation of a pregnant woman, with specific attention to radiologic studies; (3) the unique issues that arise when providing surgical anesthesia

during pregnancy; and (4) the potential risks to the pregnancy that are assumed when nonobstetric surgery becomes necessary. Finally, although some of the more common indications for surgery in pregnancy—such as trauma, appendicitis, and cholecystitis—are addressed in more detail elsewhere (Chapters 26, 47, and 48), we address clinical circumstances that are being seen with increasing frequency during pregnancy, including the use of laparoscopy, the evaluation and treatment of adnexal masses, issues related to obesity and bariatric surgery, and the challenges associated with cardiac and neurosurgery in pregnancy.

MATERNAL PHYSIOLOGY

Pregnancy-induced changes in maternal physiology and anatomy can confuse the clinical picture when evaluating the gravid patient who presents with abdominal symptoms. Abdominal discomfort, nausea, vomiting, diarrhea, and constipation are often encountered in pregnancy in the absence of intraabdominal pathology. Furthermore, laboratory changes commonly seen as abnormal in the nonpregnant surgical patient may be normal in the gravid state. Therefore familiarity with these changes is essential when evaluating pregnant women who present with abdominal discomfort and gastrointestinal symptoms (see Chapter 3).

Pregnancy causes profound changes in cardiovascular, hematologic, and respiratory physiology. Cardiovascular adaptations to pregnancy include a significant increase in cardiac output, heart rate, and intravascular volume.[2,3] Because the heart rate increases by up to 15 to 20 beats/min compared with the nongravid state, it may be difficult to determine whether a mild tachycardia is physiologic or related to an underlying pathologic condition.

Respiratory physiology is also altered in pregnancy. The gravid uterus leads to a decrease in functional residual capacity and total lung capacity. In addition, the stimulatory effect of progesterone on respiratory drive leads to an increase in tidal volume and minute ventilation. Of note, the respiratory rate remains unchanged. As a result, pregnancy is associated with a state of relative hyperventilation and mild respiratory alkalosis.

The physical examination of the pregnant abdomen may present a unique challenge. The enlarging gravid uterus becomes an abdominal organ after 12 weeks' gestation and may displace or compress other intraabdominal organs, making localization of pain difficult. For example, progressive upward displacement of the appendix occurs, and the appendix does not return to its original position until 1 to 2 weeks postpartum.[4] **However, despite the altered location, the most consistent and reliable symptom in pregnant women with appendicitis remains right lower quadrant pain.**[5,6] Many other classic signs and symptoms of appendicitis—such as nausea, vomiting, and leukocytosis—may be normal findings in pregnancy. Similarly, physical examination findings of rebound and guarding may not be reliable indicators of intraperitoneal inflammation in pregnancy.[7,8] In addition, abdominal tenderness may be a sign of a pregnancy-specific complication, such as chorioamnionitis or placental abruption. Thus the evaluation of abdominal pain in pregnancy can present a challenging diagnostic dilemma.

The gravid uterus may also limit diagnostic imaging of abdominal organs. After the first trimester, the maternal adnexa are displaced cephalad and may be difficult to image with ultrasound. Some anatomic changes related to the growing uterus may confound the interpretation of diagnostic imaging. For example, mild to moderate hydroureter is commonly encountered in pregnancy secondary to compression of the distal ureters by the uterus and progesterone-induced smooth muscle relaxation. Because the incidence of both pyelonephritis and nephrolithiasis is increased in pregnancy, it is important to recognize that a degree of dilation of the upper urinary tract is often a normal finding.

Laboratory values are also altered in normal pregnancy (see Chapter 58). Maternal blood volume is increased out of proportion to the increase in red blood cell mass. This leads to a dilutional anemia of pregnancy, especially in the later stages. This physiologic anemia may be mistaken for occult blood loss in the patient being evaluated for a surgical abdomen. Pregnancy is also associated with a progressive rise in peripheral white blood cell count, with a mean value of 14,000 cells/mm³ during the second trimester. This physiologic leukocytosis, in conjunction with tachycardia and anemia, may confound the clinical picture and lead to an incorrect diagnosis. Other laboratory values—such as D-dimer, serum creatinine, and alkaline phosphatase—are significantly altered in pregnancy, which limits their role in the diagnostic evaluation of the pregnant patient.

These significant changes in normal maternal physiology and diagnostic evaluation can complicate the evaluation of the pregnant patient who presents with concerning symptoms. The utmost vigilance is necessary to identify true pathology and arrive at the correct diagnosis in a timely fashion so that the appropriate management can be implemented.

DIAGNOSTIC IMAGING

A common concern that arises when evaluating a pregnant woman is the safety of diagnostic radiologic tests. When considering the potential risks related to imaging, it is important to balance any potential for harm against the significant risks associated with an erroneous or delayed diagnosis. It is important to

TABLE 25-1	FETAL EFFECTS OF RADIATION EXPOSURE BY GESTATIONAL AGE	
GESTATIONAL AGE (FROM LMP)	**ADVERSE EFFECT**	**ESTIMATED MINIMUM RADIATION DOSE**
Weeks 3-4 (first 2 weeks post-conception)	Embryonal demise (all or none)	5-20 cGy
Weeks 5-8	Death, congenital anomalies, IUGR	20-50 cGy
Weeks 9-15*	IUGR, microcephaly, severe mental retardation†	6-50 cGy
Weeks 16-25	Mental retardation	25-150 cGy

Data from Brent RL. Saving lives and changing family histories: appropriate counseling of pregnant women and men and women of reproductive age, concerning the risk of diagnostic radiation exposures during and before pregnancy. *Am J Obstet Gynecol.* 2009;200:4-24; and Patel SJ, Reede DL, Katz DS, et al. Imaging the pregnant patient for nonobstetric conditions: algorithms and radiation dose considerations. *Radiographics.* 2007;27:1705-1722.
*Period of neuronal development that is most sensitive to radiation damage.
†Exposure to 1 Gy of radiation during this period has been associated with a loss of 30 IQ points.
IUGR, intrauterine growth restriction; *LMP,* last menstrual period.

recognize that failure to accurately diagnose a serious condition in a timely manner can cause significant harm to the woman and her fetus.

Ionizing Radiation

The overwhelming concern related to diagnostic imaging is exposure of the developing fetus to ionizing radiation. The critical factors that determine the risk to the fetus are the dose of radiation to which the fetus is exposed and the gestational age at the time of the exposure (Table 25-1; see Chapter 8). Very early in gestation, within the first 2 weeks of conception, any significant cell damage caused by radiation is generally believed to result in miscarriage. This is believed to be an "all or none" phenomenon; that is, if the fetus remains viable after this early exposure, no adverse effects are expected. Radiation doses greater than 50 to 100 mGy (5 to 10 rad [1 mGy = 0.1 rad]) are likely necessary to cause embryonic death. Postconception weeks 2 through 8 are particularly sensitive to teratogenicity because this is the period of organogenesis. At this stage, the embryo is more resistant to radiation-induced death, and doses of more than 250 to 500 mGy (25 to 50 rad) are necessary to cause fetal demise.[9,10]

The fetal central nervous system is sensitive to radiation damage between 8 and 25 weeks and particularly during weeks 8 to 15 because this is a period of rapid neuronal development. However, increasingly high doses of radiation are necessary to result in any significant damage. After 25 weeks, the fetus is fairly resistant to radiation-induced abnormalities.[9,10]

In addition to teratogenic risk, a concern remains for potential carcinogenic effects of ionizing radiation to the developing fetus. Some authors have estimated that the incidence of childhood leukemia and other cancers may increase by about 0.06% from baseline with each centigray of exposure.[11] Given the low background risk, diagnostic doses of radiation do not appear to significantly increase the absolute risk to the fetus.[9,12] Also, the causative link between fetal exposure to diagnostic radiation and childhood leukemia has been called into question.[9]

Table 25-2 shows the estimated doses of fetal radiation exposure from various commonly used diagnostic imaging examinations.[12-14] It is important to note that the amount of

TABLE 25-2	ESTIMATED FETAL EXPOSURE TO RADIATION FROM COMMON DIAGNOSTIC RADIOLOGIC STUDIES

RADIOLOGIC STUDY	ESTIMATED FETAL DOSE* (CGY)
Chest radiograph (posteroanterior, lateral)	0.0002
Abdominal radiograph	0.1-0.3
Head CT	0.0005
Chest CT	0.002-0.02
Abdominal CT	0.4-0.8
Abdominopelvic CT	2.5-3.5
Abdominopelvic CT (stone protocol)	1
Ventilation scan	0.007-0.05
Perfusion scan	0.04
Intravenous pyelography	0.6-1.0
Bone scan	0.3-0.5
Positron emission scan	1.0-1.5
Thyroid scan	0.01-0.02
Mammography	0.007-0.02
Small bowel series	0.7
Barium enema	0.7

*Fetal dose can vary significantly based on a variety of patient and imaging parameters. If necessary, more precise estimates can be obtained through consultation with a radiation safety officer or radiation physicist.
CT, computed tomography.

radiation exposure from any of these diagnostic studies is well below the dose threshold for teratogenic risk. **Therefore when evaluating a pregnant woman who presents with significant symptoms, the patient should be reassured that the radiation exposure to the fetus from diagnostic imaging does not confer a significant risk for fetal harm.**[15,16] It is important for the clinician to be familiar with the relative radiation doses delivered by commonly ordered tests because this information may aid in the decision to choose one modality over another. When clinically appropriate, consideration should be given to other diagnostic modalities, such as ultrasound or magnetic resonance imaging (MRI), that do not involve ionizing radiation. The general principle of **ALARA** (as low as reasonably achievable) applies to both mother and baby. Optimization of computed tomography (CT) scan protocols, appropriate shielding, and judicious use of radiation-based imaging remains an important principle.

Although much attention is given to potential risks of fetal exposure, it is thought that the pregnant woman may have an increased sensitivity to radiation compared with other adults. For example, when evaluating a pregnant woman for a suspected pulmonary embolus, current recommendations often favor a ventilation-perfusion study over a CT scan in patients with normal chest radiographs. Despite similarly low fetal radiation exposures, the exposure to the maternal breasts and lungs is significantly higher with a CT scan.[17] **Therefore, although patients should be counseled that no single diagnostic test should be considered harmful to the fetus, justification of the need for imaging should be confirmed with respect to maternal benefit.**

Fluoroscopy, which uses real-time radiography, has been increasingly used in numerous diagnostic and therapeutic procedures. For example, cardiovascular comorbidities are increasingly common in pregnancy, and diagnostic cardiac catheterization, electrophysiology studies, ablation procedures, and cardiac valve interventions all use fluoroscopic guidance. The absolute fetal exposure varies greatly among procedures, but most can be safely performed during pregnancy.[18] Numerous

variables can be controlled for in order to limit the maternal and fetal exposure to radiation and to comply with the ALARA principle during pregnancy.[19]

Overall, the use of diagnostic radiation in pregnant women requires adequate patient counseling to allay concerns of fetal harm and to balance any small potential risk against the need to arrive at an accurate and timely diagnosis. According to the American College of Obstetricians and Gynecologists (ACOG), "Women should be counseled that x-ray exposure from a single diagnostic procedure does not result in harmful fetal effects. **Specifically, exposure to less than 50 mGy (5 rads) has not been associated with an increase in fetal anomalies or pregnancy loss.**"[12]

Ultrasound

Ultrasound remains the initial imaging modality of choice in the evaluation of the pregnant woman who presents with acute abdominal pain. Ultrasound involves the use of sound waves and is not a form of ionizing radiation. Although ultrasound does have the potential to transfer energy to the tissues being imaged,[20] no confirmed adverse fetal effects of diagnostic ultrasound procedures have been reported. Nonetheless, attention should be given to the thermal and mechanical indices in pregnancy. **Overall, the safety and versatility of ultrasonography makes it the first-line diagnostic tool during pregnancy whenever appropriate to address the clinical question at hand.**

Magnetic Resonance Imaging

There are numerous advantages to MRI use during pregnancy. Like ultrasound, MRI does not use ionizing radiation, and no harmful effects to the mother or fetus have been reported. In recent years, the use of MRI has expanded greatly as the image quality and availability have increased. For example, MRI has proved useful for evaluation of pathologies such as adrenal tumors, uterine and ovarian masses, gastrointestinal lesions, and retroperitoneal space evaluation while avoiding the radiation exposure associated with CT scanning.[21]

Contrast in Pregnancy

Commonly used radiocontrast, such as low-osmolarity iodinated contrast media, is known to cross the placenta and be excreted in the fetal urine. Overall, the small quantities and transient exposure is not believed to have any teratogenic effects on the fetus. Theoretic effects on fetal thyroid function have not been observed using clinical doses, and no specific neonatal surveillance is warranted for fetuses exposed to these agents in pregnancy.[22]

No known adverse effects have been observed using gadolinium-based contrast in pregnancy. In addition, the limited data from exposed pregnancies have not revealed any proven harm; therefore gadolinium can be considered in clinical scenarios where the potential exists for significant benefit to the patient or fetus that outweighs the theoretic harms. However, given that gadolinium can concentrate in the amniotic fluid with a potentially long half-life, current recommendations do not support routine use of gadolinium in pregnancy.[22]

ANESTHESIA DURING NONOBSTETRIC SURGERY

When anesthesia is required during pregnancy, the concern for possible adverse effects exists. However, it is also important to consider the physiologic changes of pregnancy that affect the delivery of safe and effective anesthesia.

Anesthesia and Teratogenicity

As is the case when examining the potential teratogenicity of any prenatal exposure, much of the data are limited to retrospective information from case series and registries. However, because prospective research focused on the teratogenicity of a medication is not ethically or logistically feasible, patients must be counseled based on the existing data, with acknowledgment of the inherent limitations.

Several early studies raised the possibility that exposure to anesthesia in the first trimester may be associated with an increased risk for central nervous system malformations.[23,24] However, the methodologies used to arrive at these conclusions have been challenged and are not supported by subsequent studies.[25]

Most studies have been reassuring and have concluded that a significant risk for congenital malformations is unlikely when surgery is performed during the first trimester.[25,26] For example, Mazze and Kallen[26] described 5405 women from the Swedish Birth Registry who underwent nonobstetric surgery during pregnancy, 40% of which occurred during the first trimester. They found no significant difference in the rate of congenital malformations compared with women who had no exposure to surgery during pregnancy. Furthermore, a more recent systematic review of the literature identified more than 12,000 pregnancies exposed to nonobstetric surgery and reported an overall 2% incidence of congenital malformations, 3.9% when surgery occurred in the first trimester.[27] Although no control group was available in this review, the observed rate of malformations falls within the expected range in the general population. Whereas the best available data support the lack of a significantly increased risk for malformations among pregnancies exposed to nonobstetric surgery and anesthesia, **it may be preferable to defer most surgical interventions until the second trimester, when the theoretic risk of teratogenicity— as well as the established risk of spontaneous miscarriage—is further decreased.**

Anesthesia and Pregnancy Physiology

As discussed earlier (see Chapter 16), many significant physiologic changes occur in pregnancy that can have a profound impact on the delivery of safe and effective anesthesia in pregnancy. For example, several physiologic changes contribute to the increased risk for aspiration in pregnant women who undergo general anesthesia. Gastric emptying time is prolonged in pregnancy, especially in the third trimester and in obese women.[28] In addition, progesterone-mediated diminished tone is present at the gastroesophageal junction. **Therefore strategies to decrease the risk for aspiration are essential, such as preoperative fasting, antacid prophylaxis (e.g., 30 mL of sodium citrate), and airway protection.** In some situations, administration of a histamine 2 (H_2) blocker or a gastric motility agent such as metoclopramide, or both, should be considered as well.

Oropharyngeal edema and narrowing of the opening of the glottis are common in pregnancy and can affect the safe access to the airway in a pregnant patient, especially in an emergency situation. **The Mallampati airway examination is often used to assess the airway and predict the degree of difficulty of intubation, with progression from low-risk airways (class I) to high-risk airways (class IV; Fig. 25-1).**[29] **A 34% increase in**

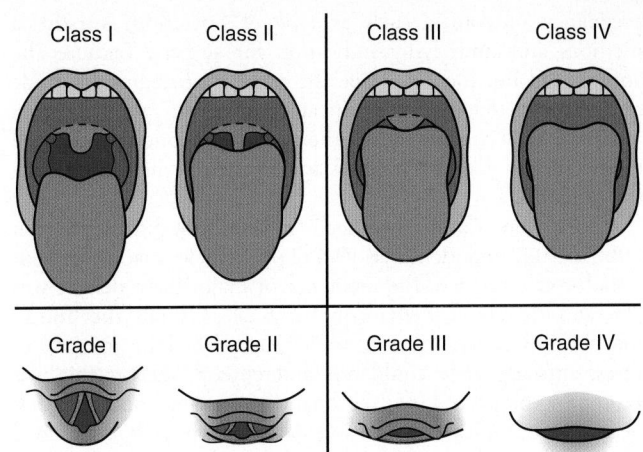

FIG 25-1 Mallampati airway classifications with corresponding laryngoscopic view of the vocal cords. (Modified from Hughes SC, Levinson, G, Rosen MA [eds]. *Shnider & Levinson's Anesthesia for Obstetrics,* 4th ed. Philadelphia, Lippincott Williams & Wilkins, 2002.)

the frequency of class IV Mallampati airways is seen at term compared with the first trimester.[30] **These changes are more pronounced in the third trimester, in obese women, and in women with preeclampsia.**

One of the most significant physiologic phenomena in pregnancy is related to aortocaval compression by the gravid uterus, especially in the supine position. In the latter half of pregnancy, this leads to a decreased preload and cardiac output with a resultant decrease in uterine and placental perfusion. In addition, venous stasis in the lower extremities increases the risk for venous thromboembolism. Thus it is essential for pregnant women who undergo a surgical procedure to be positioned with a lateral tilt to relieve some of this compression by displacing the gravid uterus to the side. This can often be accomplished by placing a wedge under the right hip.

NONOBSTETRIC SURGERY AND PREGNANCY OUTCOME

The largest study to explore pregnancy outcomes in women undergoing nonobstetric surgery was based on the Swedish Birth Registry. Mazze and Kallen[26] identified 5405 nonobstetric surgeries from more than 720,000 births between 1973 and 1981, a prevalence of 0.75%. The nonobstetric surgeries included 1331 abdominal surgeries, 1008 genitourinary or gynecologic procedures, and 868 laparoscopies. Out of 2929 procedures (54% of all cases) performed under general anesthesia, the type of anesthesia was documented for only 68% of cases. The authors found no increased risk for congenital malformations or stillbirth compared with a control population. However, the rates of low birthweight (<2500 g) and very low birthweight (<1500 g) were significantly higher in the surgical group, with odds ratios of 2.0 and 2.2, respectively. The authors noted that the observed reduced birthweight was due to both fetal growth restriction and prematurity. The incidence of preterm birth was increased in the surgery group (7.5% vs. 5.1%; P <.001). Another significant finding was an increased rate of neonatal death within 7 days (incidence, 1%; odds ratio [OR], 2.1; 95% confidence interval [CI], 1.6 to 2.7). However, it is difficult to separate the multiple confounding factors that could potentially play a causative role in the development of these adverse pregnancy outcomes, such as type of operation, anesthesia method, and underlying indication for surgery. Because the authors did not identify a specific surgical procedure or mode of anesthesia that had a significantly increased rate of adverse outcome, they concluded that the underlying condition that led to the surgery likely played an important role in determining the outcome.

Cohen-Kerem and coworkers[27] reviewed the literature from 1966 to 2002 and identified 12,452 pregnancies that underwent nonobstetric surgery. The incidence of major birth defects was 2%, and the rate of prematurity was 8.2%. Overall, they found that surgical intervention led to delivery of the fetus in 3.5% of cases, although they could not differentiate whether this was caused by the procedure itself or the underlying condition that necessitated surgical intervention. Although the lack of matched controls limits the interpretation of their data, it does support the conclusion that most pregnancies that undergo nonobstetric surgery will have favorable outcomes.

Taken together, it would seem reasonable to reassure pregnant patients faced with the need for surgery in pregnancy that the rate of adverse perinatal outcome is relatively low. In addition, although the risk for low birthweight, preterm birth, and neonatal demise may be increased, these risks may be associated with complications related to the underlying indication for surgery. In cases of semielective surgery, such as for an enlarged adnexal mass or refractory biliary colic, it is still prudent to defer surgery until after the first trimester, when the risk for spontaneous miscarriage is decreased and the theoretic concerns of teratogenicity are avoided. Similarly, surgery in the late-second and third trimesters may affect intraoperative visibility and lead to an increased risk for preterm birth. Therefore **the early second trimester is considered the optimal time for elective surgery that cannot be safely deferred until after the pregnancy.**

FETAL MONITORING

The question of whether continuous intraoperative fetal monitoring should be used when a pregnant woman requires nonobstetric surgical intervention is a matter of debate.[31,32] Factors in favor of monitoring include the potential for changes in fetal heart rate (FHR) and uterine activity during the surgery, the potential for fetal well-being to serve as an indicator of maternal status, and the potential to intervene in a case of persistently nonreassuring fetal status. On the other hand, interpretation of the FHR tracing may be particularly unreliable in the very preterm fetus. In addition, the changes in FHR tracing occasionally seen—such as a decreased variability and lower baseline heart rate—are often transient and are not necessarily an indication of fetal compromise. Thus continuous intraoperative fetal monitoring may lead to an unnecessary emergent cesarean delivery with significant risk for both maternal and neonatal morbidity. Furthermore, performing an emergent cesarean delivery can significantly complicate the nonobstetric surgery being conducted and has the potential to significantly increase maternal morbidity. A recent survey of the Association of Professors of Gynecology and Obstetrics (APGO) found that most respondents do not routinely perform intraoperative fetal monitoring but simply monitor the fetus before and after the procedure.[33] **Accordingly, the American College of Obstetricians and Gynecologists (ACOG) recommends that at a minimum, fetal monitoring should be conducted before and after the**

procedure in cases with a viable fetus. However, in select cases, intraoperative monitoring may be performed after consultation with an obstetrician who can properly counsel the pregnant woman facing surgery and individualize the decision based on factors such as gestational age, type of surgery, and facilities available.[34,35]

LAPAROSCOPY IN PREGNANCY

Although the safety of laparoscopy in pregnancy is widely accepted, several important considerations specific to pregnancy must be considered. Pneumoperitoneum further decreases functional residual capacity and can cause ventilation-perfusion mismatch and hypercapnia. These effects can be further exacerbated by Trendelenburg positioning. Bhavani-Shankar and colleagues[36] prospectively demonstrated that end-tidal carbon dioxide pressures correlate well with arterial PCO_2 and that maintaining an end-tidal CO_2 of about 32 mm Hg and a systolic blood pressure within 20% of baseline was effective in preventing respiratory acidosis during laparoscopy. Once again, a left lateral maternal position is essential to displace the gravid uterus and helps to relieve aortocaval compression and also optimizes cardiac output.

The intraabdominal pressure required to obtain adequate laparoscopic visualization during surgery can have significant physiologic effects for both the pregnant woman and the fetus. Early animal studies showed that cardiac output decreases with increasing intraperitoneal pressure. Reedy and colleagues[37] performed laparoscopic baboon studies and compared intraabdominal pressures of 10 and 20 mm Hg. At the higher pressure, a significant increase was seen in pulmonary capillary wedge pressure, central venous pressure, pulmonary artery pressure, and peak airway pressure. In addition, a significant increase in ventilator rate was required to maintain oxygenation and end-tidal CO_2. A pressure of 20 mm Hg was also associated with an increased risk for respiratory acidosis. **Similar studies have shown significant changes in both maternal and fetal physiology at pressures greater than 15 mm Hg.**[36] Therefore although lower insufflation pressures may lead to limited surgical visualization, it is important to try and keep insufflation pressures below 15 mm Hg. If higher pressures are required to safely complete the procedure, it would be advisable to periodically release the pneumoperitoneum to allow for physiologic recovery. This is particularly important in obese patients, who often require higher pressures to counteract the weight of the anterior abdominal wall. Although various techniques, such as gasless laparoscopy[38,39] and mechanical lift retractors,[40] have been proposed to avoid high intraabdominal pressures during laparoscopy, they are not widely utilized.

Laparoscopic Entry Techniques in Pregnancy

Although the conventional entry approach has been using a Veress needle, a variety of other closed and open techniques have been proposed in an effort to decrease the incidence of entry complications in nonobstetric laparoscopic procedures. However, review of the literature fails to support a significant difference in complications between the various approaches.[41,42] Nonetheless, accidental placement of a Veress needle into a 21-week uterus with subsequent pneumoamnion and pregnancy loss has been reported.[43] Thus it may be prudent to use an open approach in the latter half of pregnancy. The Society of American Gastrointestinal and Endoscopic Surgeons (SAGES) guidelines support laparoscopic entry with any technique provided that the location of the entry is adjusted to account for the gravid uterus (Box 25-1).[44] Procedures performed in the later stages of pregnancy may require a left upper quadrant insertion of the initial trocar. The upper limit of gestational age up to which a laparoscopic approach can be performed safely in pregnancy has not been determined. Concerns related to the space occupied by the gravid uterus have led some to recommend that laparoscopy be avoided in the third trimester.[45] However, current practice guidelines do not impose such a limitation, and the decision regarding the optimal surgical approach should therefore be individualized.[44]

Laparoscopy and Pregnancy Outcome

Laparoscopy has become increasingly prevalent in both pregnant and nonpregnant populations. The minimally invasive nature of laparoscopy allows for an easier recovery with less pain, earlier return of bowel function, and shorter hospital stay. Furthermore, earlier postoperative ambulation helps reduce the potential for venous stasis and deep venous thrombosis, which is especially important in a pregnant population already at increased risk for such complications.

The safety of laparoscopy in pregnancy is supported by the analysis of the Swedish Birth Registry. Reedy and coworkers[46] compared fetal outcomes of 2181 pregnancies that underwent laparoscopy between 4 and 20 weeks' gestation to 1522 pregnancies that underwent laparotomy. No differences were noted in any of the fetal outcomes considered. Several other series have further supported the safety of laparoscopy in pregnancy.[47-52] Nevertheless, several reports and case series have been published that raise concerns over the possible increased risk for adverse outcomes when laparoscopy is performed during pregnancy.[53]

Walsh and coworkers[54] performed a systematic review of the literature and concluded that an open appendectomy may be safer than a laparoscopic approach when managing appendicitis. This conclusion was based on the 5.8% incidence of fetal loss following a laparoscopic appendectomy compared with a 3.1% incidence reported after open appendectomy ($P = .001$). However, multiple potential confounders—such as severity of the appendicitis, gestational age at the time of surgery, background rate of miscarriage, and reporting bias—may have significantly affected their results. Furthermore, open appendectomy was associated with a significant increase in preterm delivery (8.1% vs. 2.1%; $P < .0001$). **In summary, no definitive data support a significantly increased risk for adverse pregnancy outcome using the laparoscopic approach for appendectomy during pregnancy.**

McGory and colleagues[55] identified more than 3000 cases of appendectomy in pregnancy using the California Inpatient File and found that after controlling for several potential confounders, laparoscopic appendectomy was associated with an increased risk for fetal loss compared with open appendectomy (OR, 2.31; 95% CI, 1.51 to 3.55). However, the gestational age at the time of surgery was not available. Furthermore, they defined *fetal loss* as the presence of a diagnosis code for spontaneous abortion or intrauterine death or of a procedure code for a dilation and curettage associated with the same hospital admission as the appendectomy. The limitations and potential inaccuracies of this method of data collection must be considered.

Finally, in the largest review and meta-analysis to date of laparoscopic versus open appendectomy in pregnancy, which involved a review of 11 studies with a total of 3145 patients, the rate of fetal loss with the laparoscopic approach was almost two

BOX 25-1 RELEVANT GUIDELINES FOR LAPAROSCOPY IN PREGNANCY FROM THE SOCIETY OF AMERICAN GASTROINTESTINAL AND ENDOSCOPIC SURGEONS

- Diagnostic laparoscopy is safe and effective when used selectively in the workup and treatment of acute abdominal processes in pregnancy.
- Laparoscopic treatment of acute abdominal processes has the same indications in pregnant and nonpregnant patients.
- Laparoscopy can be safely performed during any trimester of pregnancy.
- Gravid patients should be placed in the left lateral recumbent position to minimize compression of the vena cava and the aorta.
- Initial access can be safely accomplished with open (Hassan), Veress needle, or optical trocar technique if the location is adjusted according to fundal height, previous incisions, and experience of the surgeon.
- CO_2 insufflation of 10 to 15 mm Hg can be safely used for laparoscopy in the pregnant patient. Intraabdominal pressure should be sufficient to allow for adequate visualization.
- Intraoperative CO_2 monitoring by capnography should be used during laparoscopy in the pregnant patient.
- Intraoperative and postoperative pneumatic compression devices and early postoperative ambulation are recommended prophylaxis for deep venous thrombosis in the gravid patient.
- Laparoscopic cholecystectomy is the treatment of choice in the pregnant patient with gallbladder disease regardless of trimester.
- Laparoscopic appendectomy may be performed safely in pregnant patients with suspicion of appendicitis.
- Laparoscopic adrenalectomy, nephrectomy, and splenectomy are safe procedures in pregnant patients when indicated, and standard precautions are taken.
- Laparoscopy is safe and effective treatment in gravid patients with symptomatic adnexal cystic masses. Observation is acceptable for all other adnexal cystic lesions provided ultrasound is not worrisome for malignancy and tumor markers are normal. Initial observation is warranted for most adnexal cystic lesions smaller than 6 cm.
- Laparoscopy is recommended for both diagnosis and treatment of adnexal torsion unless clinical severity warrants laparotomy.
- Fetal heart monitoring should occur before and after operation in the setting of urgent abdominal surgery during pregnancy.
- Obstetric consultation can be obtained before and after operation based on the acuteness of the patient's disease, gestational age, and availability of the consultant.
- Tocolytics should not be used prophylactically but should be considered perioperatively, in coordination with obstetric consultation, when signs of preterm labor are present.

From Yumi H; Guidelines Committee of the Society of American Gastrointestinal and Endoscopic Surgeons. Guidelines for diagnosis, treatment, and use of laparoscopy for surgical problems during pregnancy. *Surg Endosc.* 2008;22:849-861.

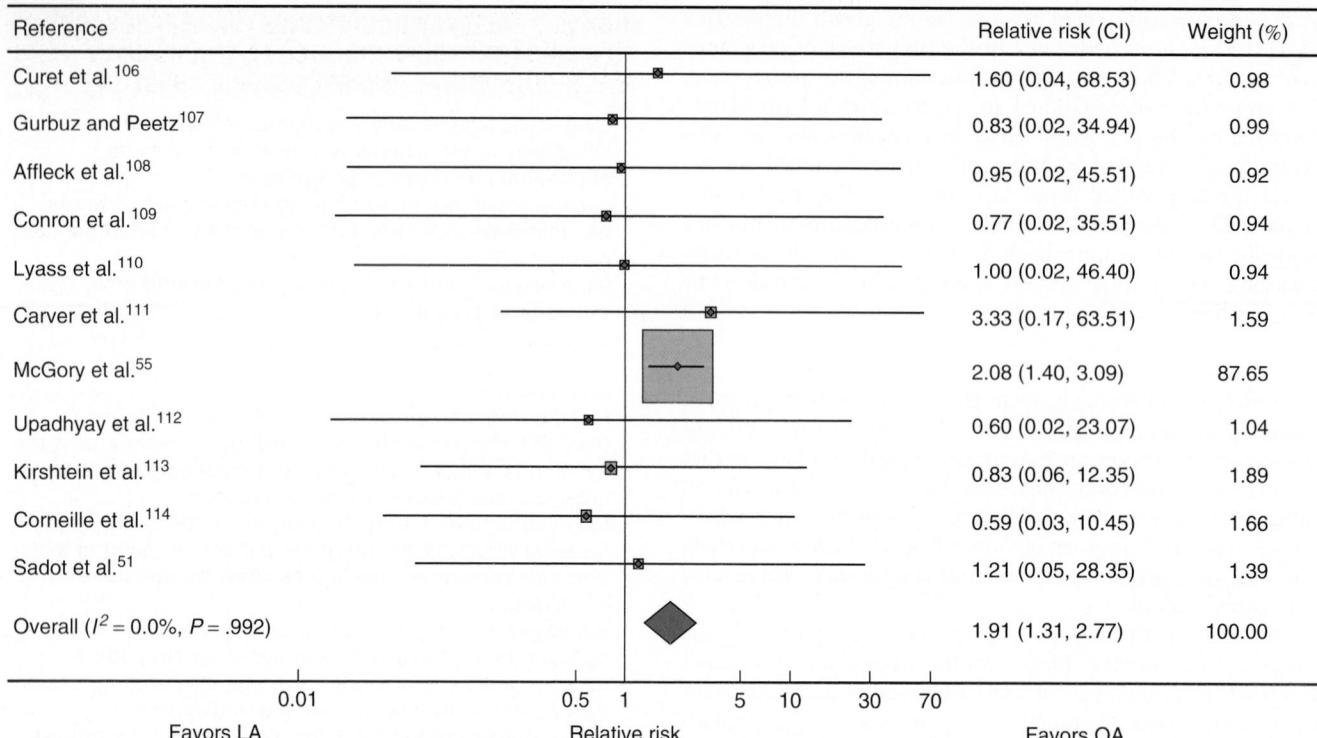

Reference		Relative risk (CI)	Weight (%)
Curet et al.[106]		1.60 (0.04, 68.53)	0.98
Gurbuz and Peetz[107]		0.83 (0.02, 34.94)	0.99
Affleck et al.[108]		0.95 (0.02, 45.51)	0.92
Conron et al.[109]		0.77 (0.02, 35.51)	0.94
Lyass et al.[110]		1.00 (0.02, 46.40)	0.94
Carver et al.[111]		3.33 (0.17, 63.51)	1.59
McGory et al.[55]		2.08 (1.40, 3.09)	87.65
Upadhyay et al.[112]		0.60 (0.02, 23.07)	1.04
Kirshtein et al.[113]		0.83 (0.06, 12.35)	1.89
Corneille et al.[114]		0.59 (0.03, 10.45)	1.66
Sadot et al.[51]		1.21 (0.05, 28.35)	1.39
Overall ($I^2 = 0.0\%$, $P = .992$)		1.91 (1.31, 2.77)	100.00

0.01　　　　0.5　1　　5　10　30　70

Favors LA　　　　Relative risk　　　　Favors OA

FIG 25-2 Meta-analysis of pregnancy outcome. Fetal loss after laparoscopic appendectomy (LA) versus open appendectomy (OA). *CI,* confidence interval. (From Wilasrusmee C, Sukrat B, McEvoy M, Attia J, Thakkinstian A. Systematic review and meta-analysis of safety of laparoscopic versus open appendicectomy for suspected appendicitis in pregnancy. *Br J Surg.* 2012;99:1470-1478.)

times greater than in cases of open appendectomy. No significant differences were observed between the groups in the rate of preterm delivery, Apgar score, or wound infection after surgery (Fig. 25-2). Although the results of this meta-analysis should be interpreted with caution because most studies reviewed were observational, the significantly higher rate of fetal loss associated with laparoscopy warrants caution and further study.[56] **In conclusion, if a laparoscopic procedure is considered in pregnancy, the SAGES practice guidelines should be used until further recommendations are made by national societies based on new data** (see Table 24-3).[44]

ADNEXAL MASSES IN PREGNANCY

The increased use of prenatal ultrasound, the high prevalence of physiologic cysts related to ovulation, and the use of ovulation induction in the treatment of infertility make the evaluation of an adnexal mass in pregnancy commonplace in obstetric practice. The reported prevalence of adnexal masses in pregnancy ranges from less than 1% to 25% and is dependent on a variety of factors, such as gestational age and the criteria used to characterize an adnexal finding as a mass rather than a simple ovarian follicle.[57]

Fortunately, most adnexal masses encountered in pregnancy are benign and spontaneously resolve during the course of pregnancy. In fact, rates of spontaneous resolution have been reported to be as high as 72% to 96%.[57] Most of these cysts are simple follicular cysts—thin-walled, unilocular cysts that contain anechoic fluid. Alternatively, a corpus luteum cyst may develop that contains varying amounts of hemorrhage within the thick-walled and unilocular cyst (Fig. 25-3). These are also benign and transient findings, which generally resolve by the second trimester and rarely require further surveillance.

In women who have undergone ovulation induction for the treatment of infertility, thin-walled multicystic ovaries that contain anechoic fluid and lack internal septations or papillae may be encountered. These usually resolve during the course of the pregnancy, although they can cause patient discomfort if they are particularly enlarged (see Fig. 25-3). *Theca lutein cysts* are multicystic ovarian masses related to significant elevations of β-human chorionic gonadotropin, such as in gestational trophoblastic disease and multiple gestation. They appear as thick-walled multicystic masses with no papillae. Although they generally contain anechoic fluid, internal hemorrhage can occur, especially in large masses (see Fig. 25-3). These usually persist throughout the gestation, although they generally resolve on their own postpartum (see Fig. 25-3, *E*).

Although most benign masses encountered in pregnancy are physiologically related to the gestation, it is not uncommon to incidentally detect other benign ovarian masses, such as mature cystic teratomas (i.e., dermoid cysts), cystadenomas, or endometriomas. *Dermoids* can contain a variety of tissue types and have a variable appearance on ultrasound. Often, a hyperechoic area known as a *Rokitansky tubercle* can help confirm the nature of these masses, which are benign and persist throughout the pregnancy. Fortunately, malignant degeneration is exceedingly rare, especially in women of childbearing age, therefore increased surveillance and surgical intervention are rarely necessary in an asymptomatic woman. As with all sizable masses, the patient should be counseled about the risk for ovarian torsion and must be educated about the typical presenting symptoms. *Cystadenomas* often contain thin internal septations and may exhibit a small mural nodule (Fig. 25-4, *B*). These masses are generally hypovascular and may contain anechoic fluid (serous cystadenomas) or fluid with low-level echoes (mucinous cystadenomas (see Fig. 25-4, *C*). *Endometriomas,* benign ovarian masses that

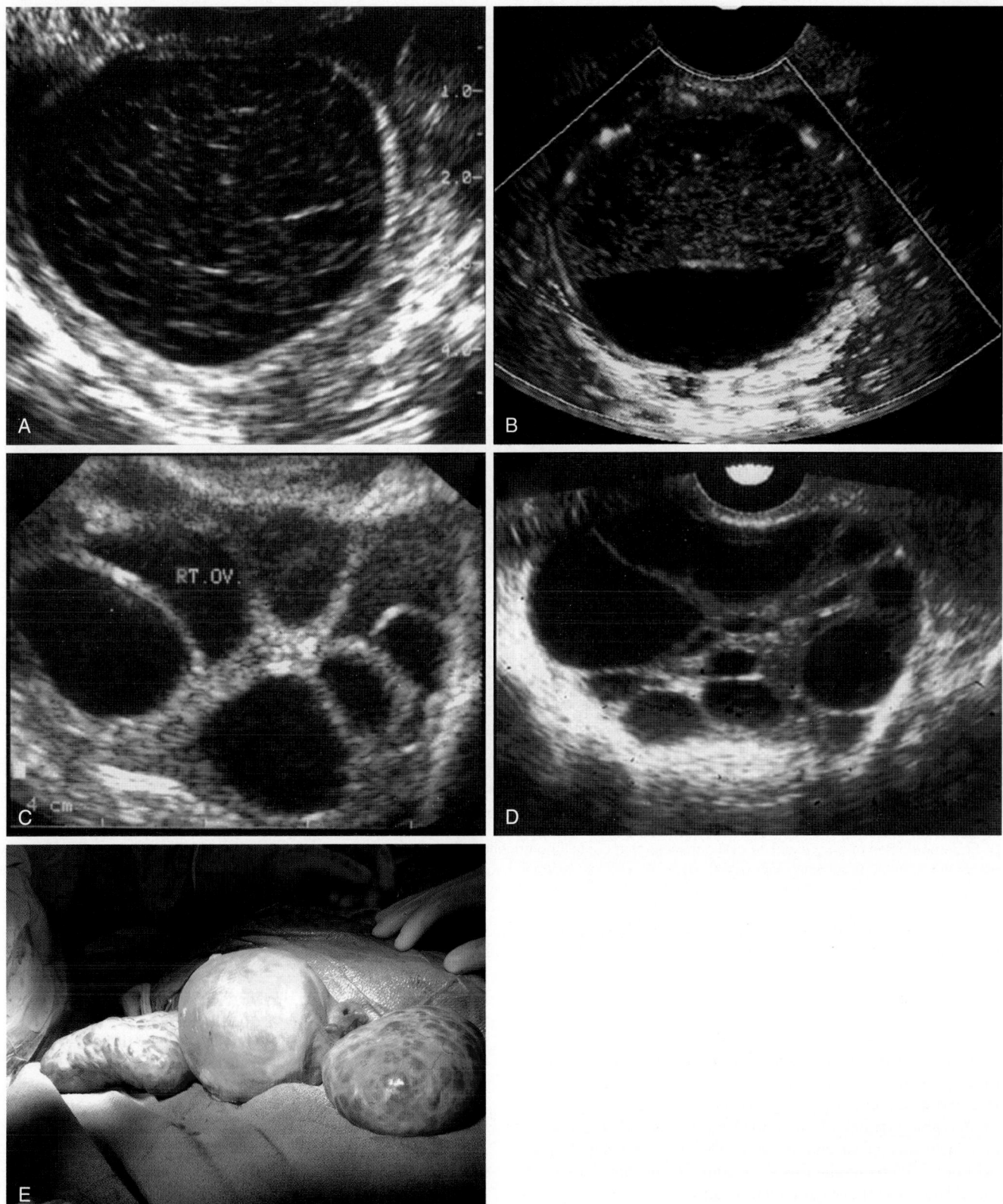

FIG 25-3 A and **B,** Variable appearance of a corpus luteum. The layered echogenicity represents hemorrhage within the cyst. Circumferential vascularity on power Doppler imaging is a typical finding. **C,** A theca lutein cyst is seen as a thick-walled and multiloculated cyst with anechoic fluid. **D,** Typical appearance of a stimulated ovary with multiple follicular cysts after infertility treatment. **E,** Bilateral theca lutein cysts at time of cesarean delivery. (**D,** From Schwartz N, Timor-Tritsch IE, Wang E. Adnexal masses in pregnancy. *Clin Obstet Gynecol.* 2009;52:570-585.)

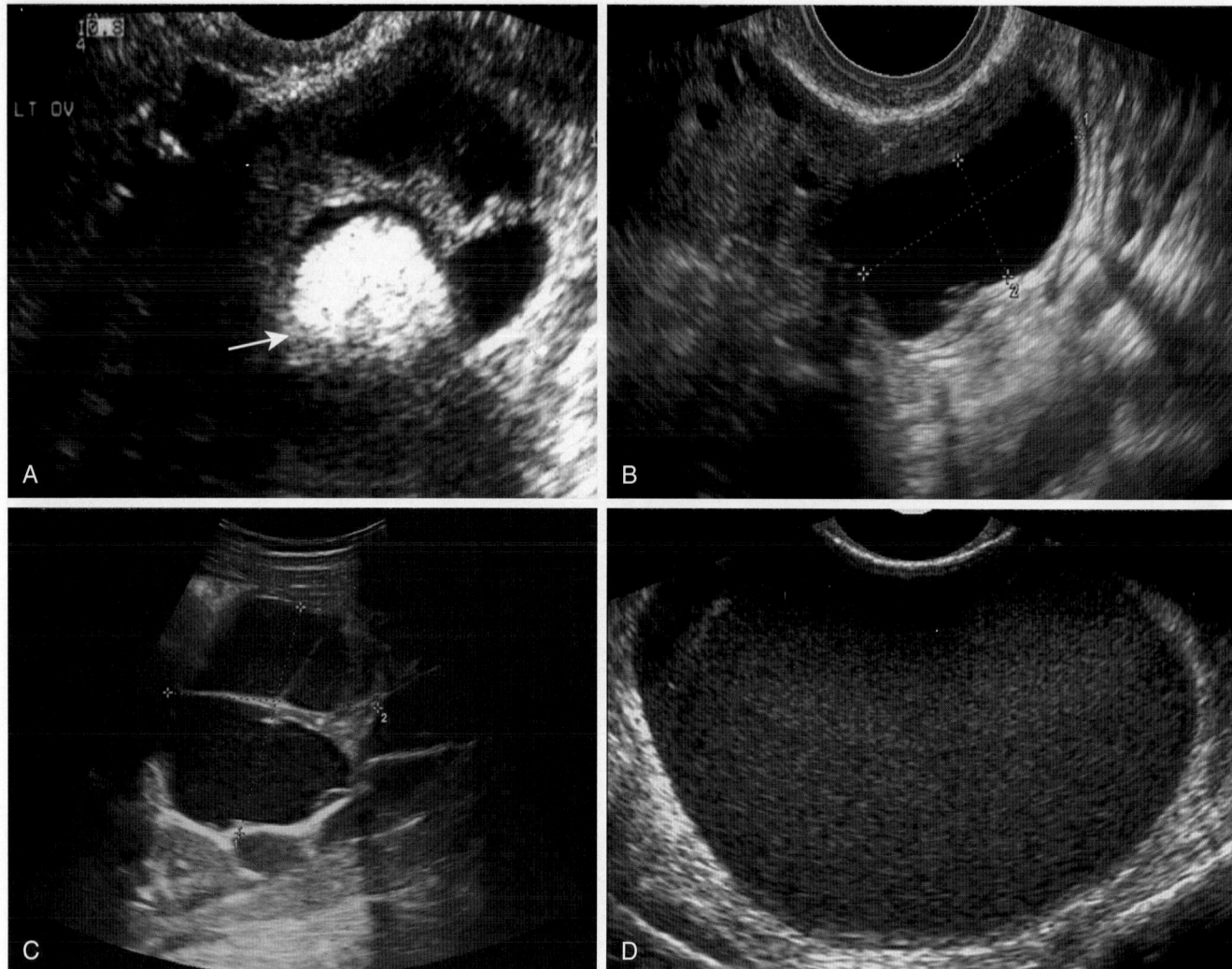

FIG 25-4 A, Dermoid cyst with heterogeneous contents and a typical Rokitansky nodule (*arrow*). **B,** Benign serous cystadenoma presenting as an anechoic cyst with a small mural nodule. **C,** This cystic mass with thin internal septations was shown to be a mucinous cystadenoma. **D,** Endometriomas often present as cystic masses that contain homogeneous low-level echoes. (From Schwartz N, Timor-Tritsch IE, Wang E. Adnexal masses in pregnancy. *Clin Obstet Gynecol.* 2009;52:570-585.)

contain ectopic endometrial tissue, most often display a characteristic appearance with diffuse, low-level echoes (see Fig. 25-4, *D*). Affected patients often have a history of endometriosis or dysmenorrhea. These masses generally persist throughout pregnancy without a significant change in size. Occasionally, an endometrioma can undergo decidualization during pregnancy as the endometrial tissue responds to the hormonal changes. In these cases, the mass may appear heterogeneous with increased vascularization and papillary projections, sharing many of the sonographic features of an ovarian malignancy (Fig. 25-5). A known history of an endometrioma before pregnancy may be helpful in differentiating this mass from a malignancy, but close surveillance and thorough patient counseling are necessary.

Although most adnexal masses encountered in pregnancy are benign, the rare possibility of malignancy should not be discounted. In fact, between 1% and 3% of masses removed in pregnancy are found to be malignant.[58,59] However, these data are confounded by the indication for surgery and likely represent a high-risk group of patients. In the largest series of adnexal masses in pregnancy, Leiserowitz and coworkers[58] identified 9375 adnexal masses associated with pregnancy, of which

87 (0.93%) were found to be malignant. In their population, the incidence of ovarian cancer was 1 per 56,000 deliveries. An additional 115 cases (1.25%) were found to be borderline tumors. Taken together, the prevalence of clinically significant ovarian tumors was 1 in 23,800 deliveries. In addition to being extremely rare, ovarian cancer in pregnancy is associated with more favorable characteristics, such as lower stage and a higher proportion of germ cell tumors (see Chapter 50).[58,59] This is likely because of the younger patient population and the incidental detection of these masses in asymptomatic women.

Although other imaging modalities, such as MRI, may be helpful in some cases—for example, when a thorough evaluation of the mass is difficult because of the gravid uterus—ultrasound examination remains the diagnostic tool of choice when evaluating the adnexa. **Several sonographic features have been associated with an increased risk for malignancy, such as size greater than 7 cm, heterogeneity with solid and cystic components, papillary excrescences or mural nodules, thick internal septations, irregular borders, increased vascularity, and low-resistance blood flow.** However, the specificity of any of these findings remains limited, and no single high-risk feature

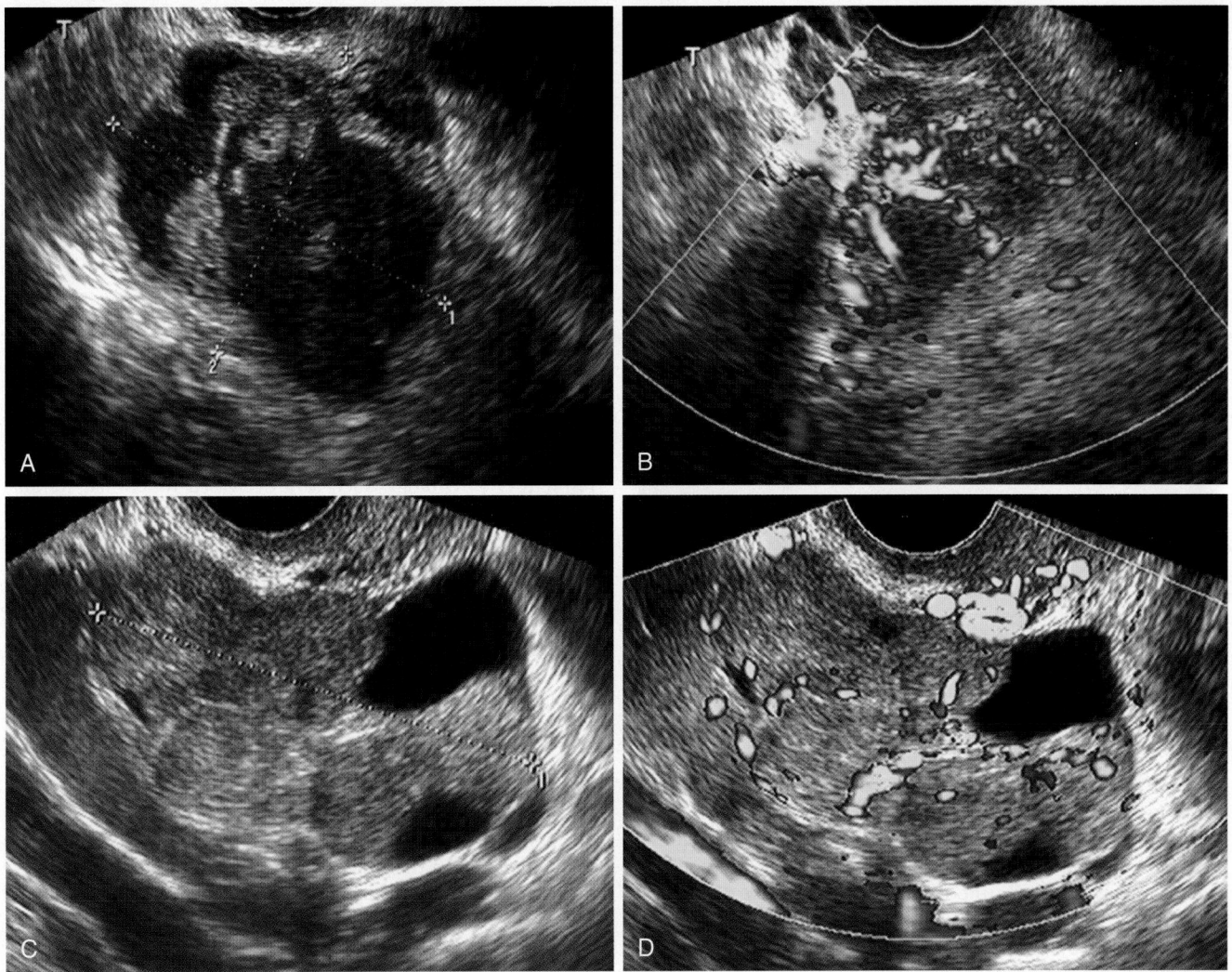

FIG 25-5 **A** and **B,** Complex and heterogeneous mass with thickened septations and increased vascularity in a patient with a known endometrioma. The sonographic features were suspicious for malignancy, which led to surgical excision in the second trimester. Pathology showed it to be a decidualized endometrioma. **C** and **D,** A similar-appearing heterogeneous mass with increased vascularity. This was also excised and was shown to be a stage I cystadenocarcinoma. (From Schwartz N, Timor-Tritsch IE, Wang E. Adnexal masses in pregnancy. *Clin Obstet Gynecol.* 2009;52:570-585.)

is pathognomonic for malignancy. For example, in a retrospective review of 126 pregnancies with a persistent ovarian mass of 5 cm or more, 69 of which underwent surgical excision during or after pregnancy, no cases of malignancy were reported.[60] Rather, overall pattern recognition by experienced sonographers is likely the most accurate diagnostic approach.[61-63] Surgical resection may become necessary when the degree of suspicion is high.

Another potential complication of an adnexal mass is ovarian torsion, which is estimated to occur in up to 7% of adnexal masses in pregnancy; 60% of torsions occur in the first trimester.[64,65] Concern for this complication often leads to the recommendation to electively resect masses in pregnancy. However, Lee and colleagues[64] compared 36 cases of emergency surgery for torsion in pregnancy with 53 cases of electively removed adnexal masses and found no difference in pregnancy outcomes, which indicates that reserving intervention for acute torsion may not necessarily put the patient at increased risk for complications. Thus because nonobstetric surgery in pregnancy is not without risk, preventive surgical intervention may not be

appropriate in most cases. **Rather, patients with persistent adnexal masses in pregnancy should be counseled about the signs and symptoms of ovarian torsion, with surgical resection reserved for symptomatic patients and those in whom there is a suspicion of malignancy.**

When ovarian torsion is confirmed during surgery, a question exists as to whether detorsion plays a role in ovarian conservation when no extensive necrosis is apparent (Fig. 25-6). Some evidence lends support to this approach in nonpregnant women.[66-68] **Although pregnancy data are more limited, several reports are available of successful management of ovarian torsion in pregnancy with preservation of the ovary.**[69-71] However, a case of ovarian necrosis that required a repeat operation 2 days after a detorsion in pregnancy has also been noted.[72] In addition, the potential for recurrence must be taken into account when deciding to preserve the twisted ovary. Some authors recommend performing an oophoropexy to stabilize the ovary in the hope of minimizing recurrence, although this cannot be recommended as a routine approach. If a discrete ovarian cyst or mass is noted, excision of the mass should reduce

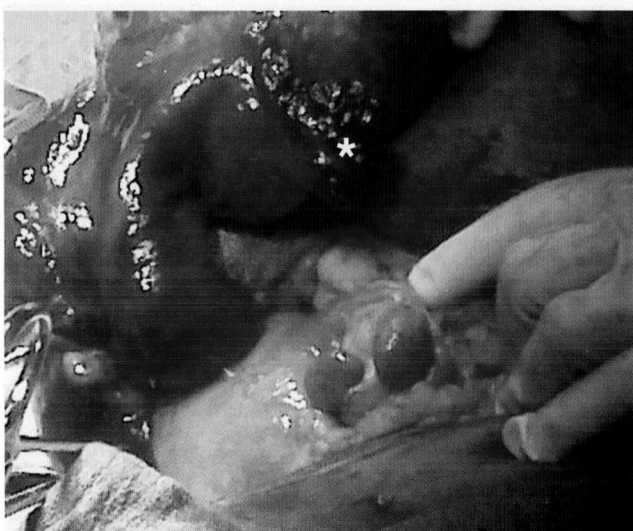

FIG 25-6 Intraoperative photograph of an ovarian torsion at 11 weeks' gestation. A 9-cm adnexal mass (upper left) was torsed around an edematous vascular pedicle. The mass was removed by laparotomy because of concern for necrosis of the fimbria (*asterisk*). The normal-appearing left ovary and tube are seen on the right; the gravid uterus is in the center. Pathology confirmed a dermoid cyst with areas of necrosis. (Courtesy Stephanie Jean, MD.)

the chance of recurrence, especially if there is any concern for potential malignancy. **Ultimately, the decision to untwist and preserve the torsed ovary should be individualized based on intraoperative findings and risk factors for recurrence.**

Overall, when presented with an adnexal mass that requires surgical resection, the decision to proceed with laparoscopy or laparotomy is based on the same approach taken outside of pregnancy. Laparoscopy has been shown to be a safe and effective method to remove adnexal masses in pregnancy,[73-75] although laparotomy may be preferred in certain scenarios, such as in patients with prior abdominal surgeries or large masses and in those who present late in pregnancy, when visualization may be compromised. In general, although some have reported the safe aspiration of large simple cysts in pregnancy, this method runs the risk for leakage of cyst contents into the abdomen, which would be especially harmful if an unsuspected malignancy were present. In addition, cytologic analysis of the cyst contents may not be an accurate method to determine the pathology of the mass.[76] For this reason, cyst aspiration cannot be considered a standard approach for managing adnexal masses in pregnancy. Regardless of the surgical approach, it is important to remember that prior to 8 weeks' gestation, the corpus luteum is the primary source of progesterone for the pregnancy. Therefore progesterone supplementation should be administered to women who undergo adnexal surgery before 8 to 10 weeks' gestation.

OBESITY, BARIATRIC SURGERY, AND PREGNANCY

Maternal obesity is an increasingly common condition in pregnancy and is discussed in greater detail in Chapter 41. In 2010, over a third of adults in the United States were considered obese.[77] Obesity is associated with an increased risk for numerous significant medical comorbidities that include diabetes, hypertension, cardiac disease, and respiratory conditions. Furthermore, maternal obesity is an independent risk factor for

several pregnancy-related complications that include gestational diabetes, preeclampsia, cesarean delivery, infectious morbidity, and thromboembolism. An increase has also been noted in fetal complications such as congenital malformations, macrosomia, and stillbirth.[78-80] **Bariatric surgery is an increasingly common and effective treatment for obesity and has been associated with a significant improvement in overall health and a reduction in adverse pregnancy outcomes.**[81,82] For this discussion, it is important to review the special considerations related to surgery in the obese pregnant patient as well as the implications of prior bariatric surgery in pregnancy.

Obesity presents unique management challenges in the perioperative period and is a risk factor for a multitude of adverse outcomes related to both general anesthesia and surgery.[80-86] Intubation is often more difficult in obese patients, and preoperative assessment of the airway using the Mallampati classification is essential.[87-89] Furthermore, gestational changes in respiratory physiology, such as a decreased functional residual capacity and increased work of breathing, can lead to impaired ventilation and an increase in adverse respiratory events in obese pregnant patients who undergo anesthesia. In addition, the aortocaval compression seen in pregnancy may be exacerbated by maternal body habitus. For these reasons, many authors recommend various maneuvers, such as adjusting patient positioning and preoperative hyperoxygenation, when caring for the obese patient.

Another consideration unique to obese patients undergoing anesthesia is related to the altered pharmacokinetics of anesthetic drugs and to the volume of distribution and concentration of lipophilic drugs in the adipose tissues. Therefore care must be taken when dosing anesthetic agents for the obese patient and when monitoring the recovery from anesthesia after surgery.[90,91] **Regional anesthesia should be considered if possible to avoid some of these risks, although the type of surgery and difficulty accomplishing regional anesthesia may not allow for this approach in some cases.**

Obesity is also an independent risk factor for venous thromboembolism in the postoperative period; therefore early ambulation should be encouraged. Prophylaxis with pneumatic compression devices should be undertaken until full ambulation is achieved. Subcutaneous heparin should also be considered. In addition, given the increased risk for wound infection and dehiscence in obese patients, adequate antibiotic prophylaxis is recommended.[86]

Significant weight loss before pregnancy is the most effective means of reducing the medical risks related to obesity, including pregnancy-related risks.[81,82] One of the most successful treatments for obesity is bariatric surgery, which is becoming an increasingly common procedure in the United States. Thus it is imperative for obstetric providers to be familiar with some of the unique concerns that arise in pregnant patients who have previously undergone bariatric surgery. Furthermore, clinical guidelines for the perioperative nutritional, metabolic, and nonsurgical support of the bariatric surgical patient have been recently updated with a total of 74 recommendations.[83]

In general, bariatric surgery can be divided into *restrictive procedures,* such as gastric banding, and *malabsorptive procedures,* such as gastric bypass. Restrictive procedures are less invasive and can often be accomplished laparoscopically. This approach does not result in the dramatic weight reduction seen with malabsorptive procedures, but they are associated with a lower risk for nutrient deficiencies and other complications related to malabsorption. The gastric band can be adjusted to lessen the degree of gastric restriction and allow for adequate food intake in pregnancy.

The most commonly performed malabsorptive procedure is the Roux-en-Y gastric bypass, in which a proximal stomach pouch is created and most of the stomach and proximal small bowel is bypassed. This often leads to rapid and significant weight loss, especially in the first 1 to 2 years. In fact, some recommend that pregnancy be delayed until 1 to 2 years after the procedure to avoid having rapid weight loss during pregnancy, and thus thorough contraception counseling is imperative.[92,93] Conception rates shortly after bariatric surgery appear to be increased,[93,94] which may be related to poor absorption of oral contraceptives, resumption of regular menstrual cycles, and inadequate contraceptive counseling. **The reduced absorptive capacity of the stomach and proximal small bowel often leads to deficiencies in several essential nutrients, including iron, vitamins B_{12} and D, folate, and calcium. Unfortunately, long-term compliance with vitamin supplementation is poor among bariatric surgery patients.**[95,96] **Obtaining a baseline evaluation of these nutrients before conception or early in pregnancy is recommended. In addition, consultation with a nutritionist should be considered.**[97]

Although no evidence suggests that pregnancy increases the risk for postoperative complications related to prior bariatric surgery, these problems may occur during gestation.[98-99] It is important, therefore, for obstetric providers to be familiar with the possible complications so that the bariatric surgeon can be notified. Some known complications include anastomotic leaks, bowel obstruction, internal hernias, and erosion or migration of gastric bands. **Many of these complications first manifest with symptoms commonly experienced during normal pregnancy—such as nausea, vomiting, and abdominal discomfort—so the potential exists for accurate diagnosis of these complications to be delayed in a pregnant patient, and maternal deaths have been reported.**[100,101] Therefore clinicians should have a high degree of suspicion when these patients present with significant abdominal complaints.[97] Another complication that can be encountered in pregnant patients with a history of malabsorptive bariatric surgery is *dumping syndrome,* in which the consumption of simple sugars can lead to significant fluid shifts into the small intestine, causing cramping, nausea, vomiting, and diarrhea. In severe cases, the patient can become tachycardic and diaphoretic and may complain of palpitations. Consideration should be given to monitoring maternal blood glucose levels because hypoglycemia can result from the relative hyperinsulinemia observed in pregnancy. Patients sensitive to sugar intake may not tolerate the glucose load used to test for gestational diabetes. Having the patient monitor fasting and postprandial glucose levels for 1 to 2 weeks may be a reasonable screening approach in sensitive patients.[102]

Overall, bariatric surgery and successful weight loss may improve pregnancy outcomes by reducing some of the medical complications seen with morbid obesity. However, in the largest population-based matched cohort study done in Sweden,[103] bariatric surgery was associated with a greater risk for preterm birth, both spontaneous and medically indicated (OR, 1.7; 95% CI, 1.4 to 2.0) and a greater risk for infants who are small for gestational age (OR, 2.0; 95% CI, 1.5 to 2.5) compared with control patients starting pregnancy with a body mass index (BMI) below 35. This large population study did not address the reason for these differences, but a micronutrient deficiency

can be speculated to be a contributing factor. A more recent study of the Swedish Medical Birth Register of 670 pregnancies after bariatric surgery noted a decreased risk for gestational diabetes and infants large for gestational age in these patients.[104] **With the increasing prevalence of surgical treatment of obesity among young women, clinicians should familiarize themselves with some of the unique concerns that arise when managing these patients during pregnancy, and they should educate and monitor such patients for potential preterm delivery and intrauterine growth restriction (IUGR).**

CARDIAC SURGERY IN PREGNANCY

As mentioned above, cardiac comorbidities are increasingly common in pregnancy. Many diagnostic and therapeutic procedures are minimally invasive and can be safely performed in pregnancy when indicated with attention to minimization of fetal radiation exposure during fluoroscopy. However, invasive cardiac procedures that require cardiopulmonary bypass represent a unique clinical scenario because the profound changes in maternal perfusion can impact fetal oxygenation. Nonpulsatile blood flow, low perfusion pressures and pump flow, hypothermia, and acid-base disturbances are all critical factors that can affect fetal well-being. Optimizing each of these variables may help limit the fetal risk during these procedures. In fact, cardiopulmonary bypass may be a circumstance in which continuous intraoperative fetal monitoring can help optimize perfusion to the benefit of both mother and fetus.[105]

NEUROSURGERY IN PREGNANCY

Neurosurgical anesthesia often involves several techniques aimed at regulating cerebral blood flow, but these may also impact uteroplacental perfusion. For example, controlled hypotension can lead to reduced placental perfusion and transient FHR abnormalities. Similarly, whereas pregnancies can usually tolerate hypothermia, hyperventilation, and diuresis, potential fetal effects cannot be disregarded.[104] In most cases, maternal health should be the primary focus and should supersede potential fetal effects. Nonetheless, a basic understanding of these effects can help the obstetrician guide the surgical and anesthesia teams caring for the patient.

KEY POINTS

- Care of the pregnant surgical patient requires a multidisciplinary approach with an understanding of the physiologic changes that accompany normal pregnancy.
- Expansion of maternal blood volume during pregnancy may mask signs of maternal hemorrhage, and clinically significant blood loss can occur before hemodynamic changes are evident.
- Delay in surgical intervention can result in increased maternal and fetal morbidity and mortality, which significantly increases the risk for preterm labor and fetal loss.
- Diagnostic doses of radiation (<5 cGy) from radiographs and CT scans are unlikely to pose any significant harm to the developing fetus. MRI and ultrasound can

be safely used when appropriate to further minimize radiation exposure.

♦ No significant increased risk is apparent for congenital malformations in women who require nonobstetric surgery during pregnancy. Although the risk for preterm birth, low birthweight, and neonatal death may be increased, this may be due to the underlying illness rather than the surgical procedure.

♦ Although laparoscopy as a first approach to abdominal surgery in pregnancy seems reasonable, its safety continues to be studied. Abdominal insufflation pressures should be kept below 15 mm Hg whenever possible, and the SAGES guidelines should be followed. The use of a laparoscopic approach in the latter stages of pregnancy should be individualized based on indications and experience of the surgeon.

♦ Adnexal masses are commonly encountered in pregnancy, although most ovarian masses are benign. Pregnant women diagnosed with an adnexal mass should be counseled about the signs and symptoms of ovarian torsion. Surgical resection can generally be reserved for symptomatic women or for masses suspicious for malignancy.

♦ Data are lacking to recommend routine continuous fetal heart rate monitoring during surgery in pregnant women. In most cases, preoperative and postoperative FHR monitoring is appropriate.

♦ Preoperative corticosteroid administration to promote fetal lung maturity should be based on gestational age and the nature and risks of the planned surgery.

♦ Thromboembolic prophylaxis with pneumatic compression devices should be considered for all gravid surgical patients.

♦ Obesity presents unique management considerations during the perioperative period, most notably related to anesthesia risk, intraoperative risk, antibiotic prophylaxis, and thromboembolic prophylaxis. Early ambulation should be encouraged. If early ambulation is not possible, subcutaneous heparin prophylaxis should be considered.

♦ Bariatric surgery with subsequent weight loss may reduce the risk for medical complications in pregnancy. However, it may increase the risk for preterm delivery and intrauterine growth restriction. Women who have undergone bariatric surgery should be evaluated for nutritional deficiencies.

♦ The gravid patient with a history of bariatric surgery who presents with vague abdominal complaints should be critically evaluated because delay in diagnosis of internal hernias, bowel obstruction, or anastomosis leaks can often lead to catastrophic events.

REFERENCES

1. Kilpatrick CC, Monga M. Approach to the acute abdomen in pregnancy. *Obstet Gynecol Clin North Am.* 2007;34:389.
2. Capeless EL, Clapp JF. Cardiovascular changes in early phase of pregnancy. *Am J Obstet Gynecol.* 1989;161:1449.
3. Clapp JF 3rd, Seaward BL, Sleamaker RH, Hiser J. Maternal physiologic adaptations to early human pregnancy. *Am J Obstet Gynecol.* 1988;159:1456.
4. Baer JL, Reis RA, Arens RA. Appendicitis in pregnancy with changes in position and axis of the normal appendix in pregnancy. *JAMA.* 1932;52:1359.
5. Mourad J, Elliott JP, Erickson L, Lisboa L. Appendicitis in pregnancy: new information that contradicts long-held clinical beliefs. *Am J Obstet Gynecol.* 2000;182:1027.
6. Yilmaz HG, Akgun Y, Bac B, Celik Y. Acute appendicitis in pregnancy. Risk factors associated with principal outcomes: a case control study. *Int J Surg.* 2007;5:192.
7. Sharp HT. The acute abdomen during pregnancy. *Clin Obstet Gynecol.* 2002;45:405.
8. Wagner JM, McKinney WP, Carpenter JL. Does this patient have appendicitis? *JAMA.* 1996;276:1589.
9. Brent RL. Saving lives and changing family histories: appropriate counseling of pregnant women and men and women of reproductive age, concerning the risk of diagnostic radiation exposures during and before pregnancy. *Am J Obstet Gynecol.* 2009;200:4.
10. Patel SJ, Reede DL, Katz DS, et al. Imaging the pregnant patient for nonobstetric conditions: algorithms and radiation dose considerations. *Radiographics.* 2007;27:1705.
11. Lee CI, Haims AH, Monico EP, et al. Diagnostic CT scans: assessment of patient, physician, and radiologist awareness of radiation dose and possible risks. *Radiology.* 2004;231:393.
12. ACOG Committee Opinion. No. 299, September 2004 (replaces No. 158, September 1995). Guidelines for diagnostic imaging during pregnancy. *Obstet Gynecol.* 2004;104:647.
13. Goldstone K, Yates SJ. Radiation issues governing radiation protection and patient doses in diagnostic imaging. In: Adam A, ed. *Grainger & Allison's Diagnostic Radiology.* 5th ed. New York: Churchill Livingstone; 2008.
14. McCollough CH, Schueler BA, Atwell TD, et al. Radiation exposure and pregnancy: when should we be concerned? *Radiographics.* 2007;27:909.
15. Nijkeuter M, Geleijns J, De Roos A, et al. Diagnosing pulmonary embolism in pregnancy: rationalizing fetal radiation exposure in radiological procedures. *J Thromb Haemost.* 2004;2:1857.
16. Winer-Muram HT, Boone JM, Brown HL, et al. Pulmonary embolism in pregnant patients: fetal radiation dose with helical CT. *Radiology.* 2002;224:487.
17. Leung AN, Bull TM, Jaeschke R, et al.; ATS/STR Committee on Pulmonary Embolism in Pregnancy. An official American Thoracic Society/Society of Thoracic Radiology clinical practice guideline: evaluation of suspected pulmonary embolism in pregnancy. *Am J Respir Crit Care Med.* 2011;184(10):1200-1208.
18. Picano E, Vañó E, Rehani MM, et al. The appropriate and justified use of medical radiation in cardiovascular imaging: a position document of the ESC Associations of Cardiovascular Imaging, Percutaneous Cardiovascular Interventions and Electrophysiology. *Eur Heart J.* 2014;35(10):665-672.
19. Dauer LT, Thornton RH, Miller DL, et al. Radiation management for interventions using fluoroscopic or computed tomographic guidance during pregnancy: a joint guideline of the Society of Interventional Radiology and the Cardiovascular and Interventional Radiological Society of Europe with Endorsement by the Canadian Interventional Radiology Association. *J Vasc Interv Radiol.* 2012;23(1):19-32.
20. Nelson TR, Fowlkes JB, Abramowicz JS, Church CC. Ultrasound biosafety considerations for the practicing sonographer and sonologist. *J Ultrasound Med.* 2009;28:139.
21. De Wilde JP, Rivers AW, Price DL. A review of the current use of magnetic resonance imaging in pregnancy and safety implications for the fetus. *Prog Biophys Mol Biol.* 2005;87:335.
22. American College of Radiology. *Manual on Contrast Media, Version 10.1,* 2015. Available at: <http://www.acr.org/Quality-Safety/Resources/Contrast-Manual>.
23. Kallen B, Mazze RI. Neural tube defects and first trimester operations. *Teratology.* 1990;41:717.
24. Sylvester GC, Khoury MJ, Lu X, Erickson JD. First-trimester anesthesia exposure and the risk of central nervous system defects: a population-based case-control study. *Am J Public Health.* 1994;84:1757.
25. Czeizel AE, Pataki T, Rockenbauer M. Reproductive outcome after exposure to surgery under anesthesia during pregnancy. *Arch Gynecol Obstet.* 1998;261:193.
26. Mazze RI, Kallen B. Reproductive outcome after anesthesia and operation during pregnancy: a registry study of 5405 cases. *Am J Obstet Gynecol.* 1989;161:1178.
27. Cohen-Kerem R, Railton C, Oren D, et al. Pregnancy outcome following non-obstetric surgical intervention. *Am J Surg.* 2005;190:467.
28. Chiloiro M, Darconza G, Piccioli E, et al. Gastric emptying and orocecal transit time in pregnancy. *J Gastroenterol.* 2001;36:538.

29. Mallampati SR, Gatt SP, Gugino LD, et al. A clinical sign to predict difficult tracheal intubation: a prospective study. *Can Anaesth Soc J.* 1985; 32:429.

30. Pilkington S, Carli F, Dakin MJ, et al. Increase in Mallampati score during pregnancy. *Br J Anaesth.* 1995;74:638.

31. Horrigan TJ, Villarreal R, Weinstein L. Are obstetrical personnel required for intraoperative fetal monitoring during nonobstetric surgery? *J Perinatol.* 1999;19:124.

32. Kendrick JM, Neiger R. Intraoperative fetal monitoring during nonobstetric surgery. *J Perinatol.* 2000;20:276.

33. Kilpatrick CC, Puig C, Chohan L, et al. Intraoperative fetal heart rate monitoring during nonobstetric surgery in pregnancy: a practice survey. *South Med J.* 2010;103:212.

34. ACOG Committee Opinion. Nonobstetric surgery in pregnancy. Committee Opinion No. 474. American College of Obstetricians and Gynecologists. *Obstet Gynecol.* 2011;117:420-421. Reaffirmed 2013.

35. ACOG. Practice bulletin no. 100: critical care in pregnancy. *Obstet Gynecol.* 2009;113:443.

36. Bhavani-Shankar K, Steinbrook RA, Brooks DC, Datta S. Arterial to end-tidal carbon dioxide pressure difference during laparoscopic surgery in pregnancy. *Anesthesiology.* 2000;93:370.

37. Reedy MB, Galan HL, Bean-Lijewski JD, et al. Maternal and fetal effects of laparoscopic insufflation in the gravid baboon. *J Am Assoc Gynecol Laparosc.* 1995;2:399.

38. Akira S, Yamanaka A, Ishihara T, et al. Gasless laparoscopic ovarian cystectomy during pregnancy: comparison with laparotomy. *Am J Obstet Gynecol.* 1999;180:554.

39. Schmidt T, Nawroth F, Foth D, et al. Gasless laparoscopy as an option for conservative therapy of adnexal pedicle torsion with twin pregnancy. *J Am Assoc Gynecol Laparosc.* 2001;8:621.

40. Stany MP, Winter WE 3rd, Dainty L, et al. Laparoscopic exposure in obese high-risk patients with mechanical displacement of the abdominal wall. *Obstet Gynecol.* 2004;103:383.

41. Ahmad G, Duffy JM, Phillips K, Watson A. Laparoscopic entry techniques. *Cochrane Database Syst Rev.* 2008;(2):CD006583.

42. Vilos GA, Ternamian A, Dempster J, Laberge PY, for the Society of Obstetricians and Gynaecologists of Canada. Laparoscopic entry: a review of techniques, technologies, and complications. *J Obstet Gynaecol Can.* 2007;29:433.

43. Friedman JD, Ramsey PS, Ramin KD, Berry C. Pneumoamnion and pregnancy loss after second-trimester laparoscopic surgery. *Obstet Gynecol.* 2003;99:512.

44. Yumi H, Guidelines Committee of the Society of American Gastrointestinal and Endoscopic Surgeons. Guidelines for diagnosis, treatment, and use of laparoscopy for surgical problems during pregnancy: this statement was reviewed and approved by the Board of Governors of the Society of American Gastrointestinal and Endoscopic Surgeons (SAGES), September 2007. It was prepared by the SAGES Guidelines Committee. *Surg Endosc.* 2008;22:849.

45. Fatum M, Rojansky N. Laparoscopic surgery during pregnancy. *Obstet Gynecol Surv.* 2001;56:50.

46. Reedy MB, Kallen B, Kuehl TJ. Laparoscopy during pregnancy: a study of five fetal outcome parameters with use of the Swedish Health Registry. *Am J Obstet Gynecol.* 1997;177:673.

47. Abuabara SF, Gross GW, Sirinek KR. Laparoscopic cholecystectomy during pregnancy is safe for both mother and fetus. *J Gastrointest Surg.* 1997;1:48, discussion, 52.

48. Barone JE, Bears S, Chen S, et al. Outcome study of cholecystectomy during pregnancy. *Am J Surg.* 1999;177:232.

49. Cosenza CA, Saffari B, Jabbour N, et al. Surgical management of biliary gallstone disease during pregnancy. *Am J Surg.* 1999;178:545.

50. Daradkeh S, Sumrein I, Daoud F, et al. Management of gallbladder stones during pregnancy: conservative treatment or laparoscopic cholecystectomy? *Hepatogastroenterology.* 1999;46:3074.

51. Sadot E, Telem DA, Arora M, et al. Laparoscopy: a safe approach to appendicitis during pregnancy. *Surg Endosc.* 2010;24:383.

52. Shalev E, Peleg D. Laparoscopic treatment of adnexal torsion. *Surg Gynecol Obstet.* 1993;176:448.

53. Amos JD, Schorr SJ, Norman PF, et al. Laparoscopic surgery during pregnancy. *Am J Surg.* 1996;171:435.

54. Walsh CA, Tang T, Walsh SR. Laparoscopic versus open appendicectomy in pregnancy: a systematic review. *Int J Surg.* 2008;6:339.

55. McGory ML, Zingmond DS, Tillou A, et al. Negative appendectomy in pregnant women is associated with a substantial risk of fetal loss. *J Am Coll Surg.* 2007;205:534.

56. Wilasrusmee C, Sukrat B, McEvoy M, Attia J, Thakkinstian A. Systematic review and meta-analysis of safety of laparoscopic *versus* open appendicectomy for suspected appendicitis in pregnancy. *Br J Surg.* 2012;99(11): 1470-1478.

57. Schwartz N, Timor-Tritsch IE, Wang E. Adnexal masses in pregnancy. *Clin Obstet Gynecol.* 2009;52:570.

58. Leiserowitz GS, Xing G, Cress R, et al. Adnexal masses in pregnancy: how often are they malignant? *Gynecol Oncol.* 2006;101:315.

59. Whitecar MP, Turner S, Higby MK. Adnexal masses in pregnancy: a review of 130 cases undergoing surgical management. *Am J Obstet Gynecol.* 1999;181:19.

60. Goh WA, Rincon M, Bohrer J, et al. Persistent ovarian masses and pregnancy outcomes. *J Matern Fetal Neonatal Med.* 2013;26(11):1090-1093.

61. Ameye L, Valentin L, Testa AC, et al. A scoring system to differentiate malignant from benign masses in specific ultrasound-based subgroups of adnexal tumors. *Ultrasound Obstet Gynecol.* 2009;33:92.

62. Bromley B, Benacerraf B. Adnexal masses during pregnancy: accuracy of sonographic diagnosis and outcome. *J Ultrasound Med.* 1997;16:447.

63. Chiang G, Levine D. Imaging of adnexal masses in pregnancy. *J Ultrasound Med.* 2004;23:805.

64. Lee GS, Hur SY, Shin JC, et al. Elective vs. conservative management of ovarian tumors in pregnancy. *Int J Gynaecol Obstet.* 2004;85:250.

65. Schmeler KM, Mayo-Smith WW, Peipert JF, et al. Adnexal masses in pregnancy: surgery compared with observation. *Obstet Gynecol.* 2005;105: 1098.

66. Cohen SB, Oelsner G, Seidman DS, et al. Laparoscopic detorsion allows sparing of the twisted ischemic adnexa. *J Am Assoc Gynecol Laparosc.* 1999;6:139.

67. Pansky M, Abargil A, Dreazen E, et al. Conservative management of adnexal torsion in premenarchal girls. *J Am Assoc Gynecol Laparosc.* 2000; 7:121.

68. Wang JH, Wu DH, Jin H, Wu YZ. Predominant etiology of adnexal torsion and ovarian outcome after detorsion in premenarchal girls. *Eur J Pediatr Surg.* 2010;20:298.

69. Djavadian D, Braendle W, Jaenicke F. Laparoscopic oophoropexy for the treatment of recurrent torsion of the adnexa in pregnancy: case report and review. *Fertil Steril.* 2004;82:933.

70. Gorkemli H, Camus M, Clasen K. Adnexal torsion after gonadotrophin ovulation induction for IVF or ICSI and its conservative treatment. *Arch Gynecol Obstet.* 2002;267:4.

71. Rackow BW, Patrizio P. Successful pregnancy complicated by early and late adnexal torsion after in vitro fertilization. *Fertil Steril.* 2007;87: 697.

72. Pryor RA, Wiczyk HP, O'Shea DL. Adnexal infarction after conservative surgical management of torsion of a hyperstimulated ovary. *Fertil Steril.* 1995;63:1344.

73. Andreoli M, Servakov M, Meyers P, Mann WJ Jr. Laparoscopic surgery during pregnancy. *J Am Assoc Gynecol Laparosc.* 1999;6:229.

74. Moore RD, Smith WG. Laparoscopic management of adnexal masses in pregnant women. *J Reprod Med.* 1999;44:97.

75. Soriano D, Yefet Y, Seidman DS, et al. Laparoscopy versus laparotomy in the management of adnexal masses during pregnancy. *Fertil Steril.* 1999;71:955.

76. Higgins RV, Matkins JF, Marroum MC. Comparison of fine-needle aspiration cytologic findings of ovarian cysts with ovarian histologic findings. *Am J Obstet Gynecol.* 1999;180:550.

77. Ogden CL, Carroll MD, Kit BK, et al. Prevalence of obesity in the United States, 2009. *NCHS Data Brief.* 2012;82:1-8.

78. Baeten JM, Bukusi EA, Lambe M. Pregnancy complications and outcomes among overweight and obese nulliparous women. *Am J Public Health.* 2001;91:436.

79. Cedergren MI. Maternal morbid obesity and the risk of adverse pregnancy outcome. *Obstet Gynecol.* 2004;103:219.

80. Weiss JL, Malone FD, Emig D, et al. Obesity, obstetric complications and cesarean delivery rate: a population-based screening study. *Am J Obstet Gynecol.* 2004;190:1091.

81. Karmon A, Sheiner E. Pregnancy after bariatric surgery: a comprehensive review. *Arch Gynecol Obstet.* 2008;277:381.

82. Maggard MA, Yermilov I, Li Z, et al. Pregnancy and fertility following bariatric surgery: a systematic review. *JAMA.* 2008;300:2286.

83. Mechanick JI, Youdim A, Jones DB, et al. Clinical practice guidelines for the perioperative nutritional, metabolic, and nonsurgical support of the bariatric surgery patient—2013 update: cosponsored by American Association of Clinical Endocrinologists, the Obesity Society, and American Society for Metabolic &; Bariatric Surgery. *Obesity (Silver Spring).* 2013; 21(suppl 1):S1-S27.

84. Abir F, Bell R. Assessment and management of the obese patient. *Crit Care Med.* 2004;32:S87.

85. Bryson GL, Chung F, Cox RG, et al. Patient selection in ambulatory anesthesia: an evidence-based review. II. *Can J Anaesth.* 2004;51:782.

86. King DR, Velmahos GC. Difficulties in managing the surgical patient who is morbidly obese. *Crit Care Med.* 2010;38:S478.

87. Juvin P, Lavaut E, Dupont H, et al. Difficult tracheal intubation is more common in obese than in lean patients. *Anesth Analg.* 2003;97:595.

88. Lavi R, Segal D, Ziser A. Predicting difficult airways using the intubation difficulty scale: a study comparing obese and non-obese patients. *J Clin Anesth.* 2009;21:264.

89. Lundstrøm LH, Møller AM, Rosenstock C, et al. High body mass index is a weak predictor for difficult and failed tracheal intubation: a cohort study of 91,332 consecutive patients scheduled for direct laryngoscopy registered in the Danish Anesthesia Database. *Anesthesiology.* 2009;110:266.

90. Cheymol G. Effects of obesity on pharmacokinetics implications for drug therapy. *Clin Pharmacokinet.* 2000;39:215.

91. Servin F. Ambulatory anesthesia for the obese patient. *Curr Opin Anaesthesiol.* 2006;19:597.

92. Apovian CM, Baker C, Ludwig DS, et al. Best practice guidelines in pediatric/adolescent weight loss surgery. *Obes Res.* 2005;13:274.

93. Martin LF, Finigan KM, Nolan TE. Pregnancy after adjustable gastric banding. *Obstet Gynecol.* 2000;95:927.

94. Roehrig HR, Xanthakos SA, Sweeney J, et al. Pregnancy after gastric bypass surgery in adolescents. *Obes Surg.* 2007;17:873.

95. Dixon JB, Dixon ME, O'Brien PE. Elevated homocysteine levels with weight loss after Lap-Band surgery: higher folate and vitamin B12 levels required to maintain homocysteine level. *Int J Obes Relat Metab Disord.* 2001;25:219.

96. Rand CS, Macgregor AM. Adolescents having obesity surgery: a 6-year follow-up. *South Med J.* 1994;87:1208.

97. ACOG. Practice bulletin no. 105: bariatric surgery and pregnancy. *Obstet Gynecol.* 2009;113:1405.

98. Patel JA, Patel NA, Thomas RL, et al. Pregnancy outcomes after laparoscopic Roux-en-Y gastric bypass. *Surg Obes Relat Dis.* 2008;4:39.

99. Wax JR, Cartin A, Wolff R, et al. Pregnancy following gastric bypass surgery for morbid obesity: maternal and neonatal outcomes. *Obes Surg.* 2008;18:540.

100. Loar PV 3rd, Sanchez-Ramos L, Kaunitz AM, et al. Maternal death caused by midgut volvulus after bariatric surgery. *Am J Obstet Gynecol.* 2005;193:1748.

101. Moore KA, Ouyang DW, Whang EE. Maternal and fetal deaths after gastric bypass surgery for morbid obesity. *N Engl J Med.* 2004;351:721.

102. American Diabetes Association. Gestational diabetes mellitus. *Diabetes Care.* 2004;27:S88.

103. Roos N, Neovius M, Cnattingius S, et al. Perinatal outcomes after bariatric surgery: nationwide population based matched cohort study. *BMJ.* 2013;347:f6460.

104. Johnsson K, Cnyattingius S, Nashlund I, et al. Outcomes of Pregnancy after Bariatric Surgery. *N Engl J Med.* 2015;372:814.

105. Reitman E, Flood P. Anaesthetic considerations for non-obstetric surgery during pregnancy. *Br J Anaesth.* 2011;107(suppl 1):i72-i78.

106. Curet MJ, Allen D, Josloff RK, et al. Laparoscopy during pregnancy. *Arch Surg.* 1996;131:546-550.

107. Gurbuz AT, Peetz ME. The acute abdomen in the pregnant patient. Is there a role for laparoscopy? *Surg Endosc.* 1997;11:98-102.

108. Affleck DG, Handrahan DL, Egger MJ, Price RR. The laparoscopic management of appendicitis and cholelithiasis during pregnancy. *Am J Surg.* 1999;178:523-529.

109. Conron RW Jr, Abbruzzi K, Cochrane SO, Sarno AJ, Cochrane PJ. Laparoscopic procedures in pregnancy. *Am Surg.* 1999;65:259-263.

110. Lyass S, Pikarsky A, Eisenberg VH, Elchalal U, Schenker JG, Reissman P. Is laparoscopic appendectomy safe in pregnant women? *Surg Endosc.* 2001;15:377-379.

111. Carver TW, Antevil J, Egan JC, Brown CVR. Appendectomy during early pregnancy: what is the preferred surgical approach? *Am Surg.* 2005;71:809-812.

112. Upadhyay A, Stanten S, Kazantsev G, Horoupian R, Stanten A. Laparoscopic management of a nonobstetric emergency in the third trimester of pregnancy. *Surg Endosc.* 2007;21:1344-1348.

113. Kirshtein B, Perry ZH, Avinoach E, Mizrahi S, Lantsberg L. Safety of laparoscopic appendectomy during pregnancy. *World J Surg.* 2009;33:475-480.

114. Corneille MG, Gallup TM, Bening T, et al. The use of laparoscopic surgery in pregnancy: evaluation of safety and efficacy. *Am J Surg.* 2010;200:363-367.

CHAPTER 26

Trauma and Related Surgery in Pregnancy

HAYWOOD L. BROWN

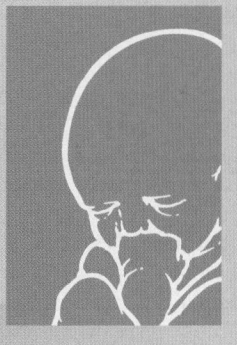

KEY ABBREVIATIONS

100 cGy or 100 rads	1 Gray
Centigray	cGy
Computerized tomography	CT
Focused abdominal sonography for trauma	FAST
Kleihauer-Betke test	KB
Magnetic resonance imaging	MRI
Motor vehicle crash	MVC
Radiation absorbed dose	rad

INCIDENCE OF TRAUMA IN PREGNANCY

Because of underreporting, the actual incidence of trauma during pregnancy is unknown. However, traumatic injury has been reported to complicate 6% to 8% of all pregnancies and is the leading cause of nonobstetric maternal death.[1-3] Approximately 30,000 pregnant women in the United States sustain treatable injuries each year as a result of trauma.

Worldwide, trauma is responsible for at least 1 million deaths annually and is the leading cause of death in individuals under 40 years of age in the United States.[4]

The risk of maternal death is related to injury severity. In a large California database study of women hospitalized for trauma between 1991 and 1997, El Kady and colleagues[5] found that intraabdominal injuries are the most common type of injury leading to maternal death, and intracranial injury resulting from trauma was the second most common cause of maternal death.

In addition to risk for maternal morbidity and mortality, traumatic injuries can have significant fetal effects that include an increased risk for fetal death and other adverse outcomes.[4] The incidence of spontaneous abortion (SAB), preterm birth, preterm premature rupture of membranes (PPROM), uterine rupture, cesarean delivery, placental abruption, and stillbirth are all increased.

A 3-year, 16-state fetal death certificate review calculated the rate of fetal death from maternal trauma at 2.3 per 100,000 live births, and placental abruption was the leading contributing factor.[6,7] Based on a review of Pennsylvania fetal death certificates, it is estimated that motor vehicle crashes (MVCs) result in between 90 and 367 fetal deaths in the United States annually.[6]

However, because of nonstandardized reporting of fetal death or injury resulting from maternal trauma, the exact magnitude of disease burden to the fetus from trauma is believed to be underestimated.[4] Factors associated with an increased risk for traumatic injury during pregnancy include young maternal age, African-American or Hispanic ethnicity, domestic violence, lack of seatbelt use, and drug or alcohol use.[1,8]

In 2002 in the United States, 4.1 injury-related hospitalizations of pregnant women occurred per 1000 deliveries; and of those hospitalizations, it was estimated that 1 in 3 pregnant women admitted to the hospital for trauma underwent delivery during that hospitalization.[9] Alcohol may be involved in as many as 45% of MVCs that involve pregnant women, and the use of illicit substances has been implicated frequently in maternal trauma during pregnancy.[8]

Traumatic injuries may be categorized according to type and include blunt trauma, penetrating trauma, fractures, and thermal injuries. An updated systematic review reported prevalence rates for the various mechanisms of trauma.[10] MVCs had an estimated incidence of 207 per 100,000 live births,[10,11] and the incidence of domestic violence (DV) or intimate partner violence (IPV) was 8307 per 100,000 live births compared with an incidence outside of pregnancy of 5239 per 100,000 women.[10,12] Falls, burns, homicide, suicide, and toxic exposure are also major contributors to traumatic injury.[10] Gunshot wounds and burns account for 4% and 1% of maternal trauma respectively.[13] The most common obstetric complications following maternal trauma are those associated with blunt trauma and include abruptio placentae, preterm labor, and fetal loss.[14]

ANATOMIC AND PHYSIOLOGIC CHANGES OF PREGNANCY

The importance of maternal physiologic changes during pregnancy and an understanding of fetal physiology are critical to effective resuscitation of the injured pregnant woman. This is especially important relative to the maternal response to stress and hypovolemia in the setting of trauma. Fundamental differences exist in the physiologic responses as a result of pregnancy, and a working knowledge of these differences is important to trauma resuscitation.

Fetal Physiology

Several factors are important in determining the impact of a traumatic event on pregnancy outcome. These include gestational age, type and severity of trauma, and the extent of disruption of normal maternal and fetal physiology.[15,16]

In the first week following conception, the nonimplanted embryo is relatively resistant to noxious stimuli. During the first trimester, the uterus resides relatively safely within the confines of the bony pelvis and has reached just above the pubic symphysis by 13 to 14 weeks' gestation. As such, the uterus is protected to a large degree from direct trauma. At any gestational age after implantation, however, maternal hypovolemia may have a significant impact on the developing embryo/fetus. Pregnancy loss in the first trimester is not likely related to direct uterine injury but more so from physiologic cardiovascular changes that occur with maternal hypovolemia and associated hypotension, which results in hypoperfusion of the uterus and the developing fetus. Uterine blood flow is not autoregulated and is maximally dilated in the normal physiologic state. Maternal hypovolemia may result in vasoconstriction in vascular beds, including the uterine vessels. In experimental hypovolemic shock, pregnant sheep will decrease uterine blood flow at rates greater than would be expected with a decrease in maternal blood pressure alone. Even in the absence of uterine artery vasoconstriction, decreases in maternal blood pressure as a result of hypovolemia will result in decreased uterine blood flow. These phenomena underlie the importance of maintaining adequate maternal blood volume as an initial step in fetal resuscitation. The third-trimester fetus can adapt to decreased uterine blood flow and oxygen delivery by redistributing blood flow to the heart, brain, and adrenal glands. Furthermore, because fetal hemoglobin has a greater affinity for oxygen than adult hemoglobin, fetal oxygen consumption does not decrease until oxygen delivery is reduced by 50%.[17]

The leading cause of blunt abdominal trauma in pregnancy is motor vehicle accidents. Penetrating trauma is typically the result of gunshot and stab injuries. Both blunt and penetrating trauma may result in rupture of the amniotic membranes. In the mid second trimester, rupture with oligohydramnios may result in pulmonary hypoplasia or orthopedic deformity. Injury to the placenta may precipitate placental abruption and lead to fetal anemia, hypoxemia, or hypovolemia. **Maternal mortality risk with penetrating trauma is more favorable than with blunt trauma because nonreproductive viscera are provided some protection by the gravid uterus, which absorbs the projectile objects.[18,19]**

Maternal Anatomic and Physiologic Changes

Nearly every maternal organ system undergoes anatomic or physiologic changes during pregnancy. The description that follows emphasizes consideration of these changes that affect trauma management.

A major concern in the management of trauma victims is internal hemorrhage and hypovolemia. The sentinel findings on examination are vital sign abnormalities, typically hypotension and tachycardia. Consideration should be given to the normal decrease in systemic vascular resistance that results in a decrease in mean blood pressure of 10 to 15 mm Hg and an increase in pulse of 5 to 15 beats/min, particularly in the second trimester. These changes can be accentuated if the trauma victim is placed in the supine position (e.g., strapped to a long board to secure the cervical spine). The resultant potential decrease in venous return from the lower extremities can reduce central venous volume and result in a diminished cardiac output by as much as 30%. Simple manual displacement of the uterus to the left or placement of a rolled towel under the backboard while ensuring that the spine remains secure alleviates most of this effect.

Blood volume increases by a mean of 50% in the singleton gestation. This is usually maximal by 28 to 30 weeks' gestation. Red blood cell mass increases to a lesser degree than does plasma volume, resulting in a slight decrease in hemoglobin concentration and a decrease in hematocrit. Iron-deficiency anemia is also common during pregnancy, and together with the normal dilution, hemoglobin concentrations may often be as low as 9 to 11 g/dL. These hematologic changes have two potential implications: anemia may be confused with active bleeding and hypovolemia, and blood volume estimates should be adjusted upward during fluid resuscitation.

Several major pregnancy-induced changes in the gastrointestinal tract are also important for trauma management. Compartmentalization of the bowel upward serves to protect it during lower abdominal trauma but increases the risk of injury when penetrating trauma to the upper abdomen occurs late in pregnancy. Complex injuries to the small bowel can be encountered with multiple entry and exit wounds as a result of its being crowded and compacted into the upper abdomen. Decreased gastric motility results in a prolonged gastric emptying time thereby increasing the risk of aspiration associated with general anesthesia. Rebound tenderness and guarding may be less apparent in later gestation because of stretching and attenuation of the abdominal musculature and peritoneum.

The dramatic increase in uterine blood flow, up to 600 mL/ min, may result in rapid exsanguination in the event of an avulsion or injury to the uterine vasculature or rupture of the uterus. Retroperitoneal hemorrhage from remarkably hypertrophied pelvic vasculature is a common complication of pelvic fracture.

BLUNT TRAUMA

Enlargement of the uterus makes it susceptible to direct abdominal trauma. Injury to the uterus (uterine laceration or rupture), its contents (abruptio placentae or direct fetal injury), or adjacent organs (bladder rupture) are more likely during pregnancy, especially in the second half of gestation. Although some of these complications are associated with more direct and violent trauma—for example, direct fetal injury or uterine rupture—some injuries, such as abruptio placentae, can occur following relatively minor trauma.

Blunt trauma to the maternal abdomen is an important cause of abruptio placentae. This is because blunt trauma exposes the gravid uterus to acceleration-deceleration forces that have a differential effect on the uterus and the attached placenta. By changing its shape, the myometrial tissue can stretch and adapt to these forces, but the placenta is relatively inelastic. This mismatch between myometrial and placental ability to stretch creates a shearing force at the uteroplacental interface that, if sufficient, can result in separation of the placenta from its myometrial attachments (i.e., placental abruption).[4,14,18] Placental abruption leads to a compromise in fetal oxygen transfer and has the potential for fetal death depending on severity. Because amniotic fluid is noncompressible, impact against the uterine wall results in amniotic fluid displacement and uterine distension. **As such, seemly minor or nonseverely injured pregnant women are at increased risk for placental abruption. Abruption may occur immediately after the abdominal impact or may be delayed for several hours after the trauma episode.** Maternal trauma may also result in intramyometrial bleeding that leads to increased uterine contractile activity through activation of thrombin, lysosomal enzymes, cytokines, and prostaglandins.[14] Severe blunt trauma may also lead to maternal splenic, hepatic, and retroperitoneal injuries that result in maternal hemorrhage and hemodynamic instability.[14]

Motor Vehicle Crashes

A number of human factors are related to traffic-related injuries and fatalities in the United States. For many reasons, drivers have become more distracted while driving. According to the National Highway Transportation Safety Administration (NHTSA) report for 2012, a motor vehicle crash (MVC) occurs every 14 seconds, an injury every 14 seconds, and a death on average every 16 minutes in the United States.[19] **MVCs are the most common cause of trauma-associated fetal loss in the United States.**[4] **The likelihood that an MVC will result in fetal loss is directly related to crash severity and to the severity of the maternal injury.**[4,16] **For example, estimates based on case series would suggest that only about 1% of minor MVCs will result in abruptio placentae, whereas clinically evident abruption occurs in as many as 40% to 50% of cases of severe blunt maternal trauma.**[14] In addition, lack of seatbelt use has been found to be associated with fetal loss, particularly if the mother has experienced ejection from the vehicle and head trauma.[16,20] However, even a nonsevere MVC without substantial maternal injury may result in placental abruption and fetal loss because of exposure to the shearing acceleration-deceleration forces described earlier.[2,4,16]

Falls

Because pregnancy changes the center of gravity and results in postural instability, loss of balance is not uncommon, and the likelihood of a significant fall is increased.[21-23] A retrospective study **found that as many as a quarter of pregnant women experience a fall at some time during pregnancy.**[21] Like

MVCs, falls expose the placenta to the shearing forces associated with blunt trauma. However, compared with MVCs, the likelihood that a fall may result in placental abruption and fetal death is low, accounting for only 3% of trauma-associated fetal deaths in one series.[6] In a more recent prospective cohort study that involved 153 women who experienced falls during pregnancy, no instances of placental abruption were reported.[24] Nonetheless, compared with pregnant women who did not experience a fall-related hospitalization during pregnancy, women hospitalized for falls remain at increased risk for adverse outcomes of pregnancy. One retrospective cohort study of 693 women hospitalized for falls during pregnancy, most of whom were in the third trimester, found that these women were at increased risk for preterm labor, placental abruption, cesarean delivery, "fetal distress," and fetal hypoxia.[23]

Domestic Violence and Intimate Partner Violence

Pregnant women are at increased risk to suffer violent assault compared with nonpregnant women.[25] **The period prevalence of intimate partner violence (IPV) during pregnancy has been reported to range from 6% to 22%, and up to 45% of pregnant women report a history of domestic abuse at some time during their lifetime.**[25] The rates of suicide and homicide in pregnancy have been reported as approximately 2.0 per 100,000 and 2.9 per 100,000 live births, respectively.[26] Black women account for nearly half (44.6%) of pregnancy-related homicides but only 17.7% of live births, and 45.3% were associated with IPV. Victims of suicide were more likely to be older and white, and 54.3% of pregnancy-associated suicides involved IPV.[26] Common methods of self-inflicted attempted suicide are drug overdose and poisoning with a corrosive substance.[27] In one study,[28] murder was the most frequent cause of death during pregnancy and in the subsequent year, and the majority of the perpetrators were found to be current or former intimate partners. **This analysis of pregnancy-associated homicides found that intimate partner homicides were most likely to occur during the first 3 months of pregnancy. In a United States study, 5% of female homicide victims were pregnant.**[29] **Although domestic violence occurs in all ethnic and socioeconomic groups, black and Native American women and women from households with lower incomes are at increased risk.**[25] Intentional trauma during pregnancy has a 2.7-fold risk (95% confidence interval [CI], 1.3 to 5.7) for preterm birth and a 5.3-fold risk (95% CI, 3.99 to 7.3) for low birthweight.[30] According to a California database study[31] of maternal discharge records between 1991 and 1999, assaults were significantly associated with uterine rupture and conferred significant risks for placental abruption and low birthweight, even if the victim was not delivered during the initial hospitalization.

SPECIFIC INJURIES
Fractures

Fractures are the most common type of maternal injury to require hospitalization during pregnancy, and the lower extremities are the most common site of fractures that complicate pregnancy.[3] Although pelvic fractures are less frequent than fractures of the extremities, pelvic fractures are most likely to result in adverse outcomes of pregnancy, including placental abruption and perinatal and infant

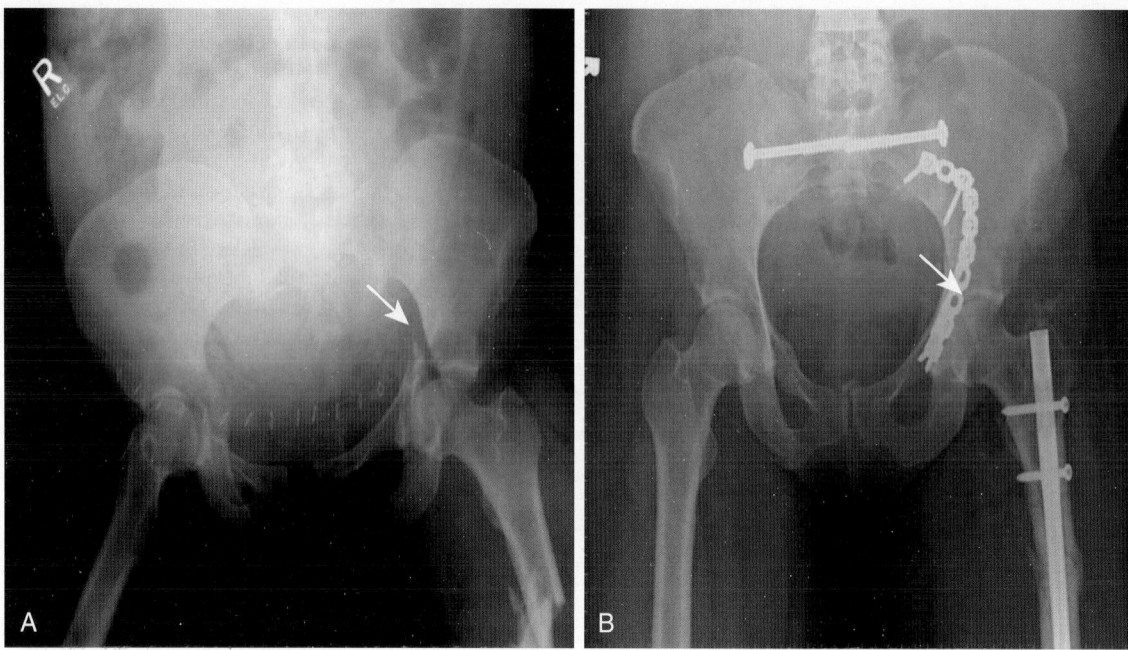

FIG 26-1 The arrow points to a pelvic fracture before **(A)** and after **(B)** fixation in a pregnancy in the late third trimester that resulted in fetal death. (From Brown, Haywood L. Trauma in pregnancy. *Obstet Gynecol.* 2009;114[1]:147-160.)

mortality (Fig. 26-1).[3] Leggon and colleagues[32] reported on a total of 101 pelvic or acetabular fractures in pregnant women, and the three most common reasons for injury were motor vehicle accidents (73%), falls (14%), and pedestrian struck by an automobile (13%). The overall fetal mortality rate in pelvic and acetabular fractures was 35% compared with 9% maternal mortality. Thus pelvic fractures are thought to be an independent risk factor for adverse fetal outcome.[32] Pelvic fractures may also be associated with significant maternal hemorrhage and shock as a result of significant hypertrophy of the pelvic retroperitoneal vasculature and subsequent laceration of these vessels because of sharp bone fragments.[33] **Pelvic fractures may also be associated with bladder and urethral trauma.[1] Pelvic fractures are not a contraindication to vaginal delivery unless the fracture results in obstruction of the birth canal or if the pelvic fracture is unstable; more than 80% of women who have sustained pelvic fractures can deliver vaginally.[33]**

Penetrating Trauma

Gunshot and stab wounds are the most frequent types of penetrating trauma during pregnancy.[4,20] Penetrating trauma in a pregnant woman is less likely to result in death than penetrating trauma in a nonpregnant individual owing to the protective effect of the gravid uterus when penetrating wounds occur in the upper abdomen. However, penetrating trauma poses major risk for complex maternal bowel injury because of the compartmentalization of the bowel in the upper abdomen by the enlarged uterus.[20] Gunshot wounds to the abdomen require exploratory surgery to determine the degree of abdominal viscera injury and debridement of damaged tissues. A stab wound in a pregnant woman should be managed the same as in a nonpregnant woman. Bowel injury with spillage of the intestinal contents increases the risk for peritonitis and pregnancy loss from infection. Penetrating trauma to the uterus is strongly associated with poor fetal outcome.[4,14] Fetal death is dependent upon the degree of

placental or umbilical cord disruption. The risk of fetal death has been reported to be as high as 71% after gunshot wounds and as high as 42% following stabbings.[20]

Thermal Injuries (Burns)

Maternal and fetal prognosis after thermal injury is a reflection of the percentage of body surface involved.[33,34] Minor burns that involve 10% or less of the body surface area are unlikely to result in maternal or fetal compromise and do not always require hospitalization.[14] **Significant burns of 50% or more of the body surface have been associated with high maternal and fetal mortality.[34]** In the past, delivery of the fetus was recommended in an attempt to improve maternal prognosis.[33] **More recent studies have suggested that maternal prognosis after severe thermal injury is not different between pregnant and nonpregnant individuals.[33] However, because of maternal physiologic changes associated with pregnancy, a pregnant woman with a severe burn will require more aggressive fluid resuscitation than a nonpregnant individual.** Major burns may result in maternal hypovolemia and cardiovascular instability in addition to sepsis, respiratory distress, renal failure, and liver failure.[14] Because of the decreased colloid osmotic pressure and increased body surface area associated with pregnancy, pregnant individuals who sustain burns are at risk for increased fluid loss compared with nonpregnant individuals.[34] Preterm labor may result from maternal hypovolemia, which can also result in decreased uteroplacental perfusion. Aggressive fluid resuscitation is critical to forestall this complication.[14,34]

Individuals who suffer from major burns may also sustain inhalation injuries, which carry higher maternal mortality and fetal risk.[14,35] In particular, carbon dioxide freely crosses the placenta and is highly bound by fetal hemoglobin, thus increasing the risk for fetal cardiac failure.[14] Administration of oxygen to the mother is recommended to reduce the half-life of carboxy-hemoglobin.[14]

Direct Fetal Injuries

Direct fetal injuries are uncommon because of the protection by the uterus and amniotic fluid. Fetal injury complicates fewer than 1% of pregnancies with blunt trauma[36] but are most likely to occur with both direct and severe abdominal or pelvic impact and also in later pregnancy, when the fetal head is engaged in the maternal pelvis.[4,14] Direct injury has been reported to result in rupture of the fetal spleen, fracture of the fetal skull, fetal intracranial hemorrhage, and cerebral edema.[4] Near term the fetal head is in the maternal pelvis, thereby increasing the risk for fetal skull fracture and brain injury with maternal pelvic fractures. Blunt trauma due to violence can lead directly to fetal injury.[37] These injuries have been reported to result in long-term developmental disabilities that result from vascular infarctions, global cerebral damage, and periventricular leukomalacia.[4]

PATHOPHYSIOLOGY OF FETAL LOSS RESULTING FROM MATERNAL TRAUMA

Maternal hypotension and hypovolemia associated with trauma are important predictors of poor fetal outcome.[6,16,20] Fetal loss may result from placental hypoperfusion due to maternal hemorrhagic shock.[13] In the instance of severe blood loss that results from maternal trauma, maternal blood is redistributed away from the uterus via uterine artery vasoconstriction, thereby allowing continued perfusion of the heart and brain. Fetal mortality in the setting of maternal hemorrhagic shock has been estimated at 80%.[38]

PREDICTORS OF FETAL MORTALITY

Abruptio placentae is by far the leading cause of fetal death in published series and accounts for between 50% and 70% of all fetal losses due to trauma.[33] Placental abruption will complicate about 1% to 2% of cases of maternal trauma with low injury severity scores and up to 40% of severe maternal abdominal trauma.[20] If a placental abruption occurs, the risk of fetal mortality has been reported to be as high as 50% to 80%.[4] Maternal death has been reported as the next most frequent cause of fetal death after placental abruption, accounting for about 10% of losses.[14] In a large California database study, gestational age at delivery was the strongest predictor of fetal, neonatal, or infant death.[5] MVCs (82%) are the most frequent mechanism of injury leading to fetal death, followed by gunshot wounds (6%) and falls (3%).[4] In particular, lack of seatbelt use is a substantial risk factor for poor fetal outcome, morbidity, and mortality.[20,39,40]

Schiff and colleagues[41,42] used the injury severity score to categorize the severity of maternal injuries. The risk for adverse maternal, fetal, and neonatal outcomes was greatest among the women with severe injuries but was also increased for women with mild injuries compared with uninjured controls. They found that injury severity scoring had limited predictive accuracy for placental abruption and fetal death and that even relatively minor injuries can result in these adverse fetal outcomes.[41,42] Because minor injuries are much more common than severe injuries, they are responsible for 60% to 70% of fetal losses attributable to trauma, even though a severe injury is much more likely to result in fetal loss than a nonsevere injury.[4]

MANAGEMENT CONSIDERATIONS
Initial Approach

The most important initial step in the management of the pregnant trauma victim is a thorough evaluation and stabilization for transport to a trauma center. This initial evaluation is typically provided by on-site emergency medical technicians (EMTs). Most EMT personnel are familiar with the designated trauma units in the community equipped to deal with cases of severe trauma. This is especially important for the pregnant trauma victim, for whom both maternal and fetal survival is a priority. **The Centers for Disease Control and Prevention (CDC) has provided published guidelines for first responders and emergency medical personnel who provide care in the field to injured pregnant women.**[43] *Guidelines for emergency medical personnel include displacing the uterus from the inferior vena cava by positioning the mother in the lateral decubitus position.*[38] *During the initial evaluation, the spine immobilization board may be tilted leftward by 15 degrees by placing a 6-inch rolled towel under the long board to achieve the same result.*[38] *The CDC panel recommended that if possible, women with a pregnancy of at least 20 weeks' gestation be transported to a trauma center with access to obstetric care.* If a pregnant trauma victim must be transported to a closer facility than a designated trauma center because of concerns for maternal survival, the emergency team at that facility must be prepared to make the acute management decisions, stabilize, and then transport to a higher level center.

Improved outcomes can be expected by following a coordinated approach among emergency medicine physicians, trauma surgeons, and obstetricians. **Regardless of gestational age, all pregnant women who sustain or who are suspected to have sustained serious injuries should be first evaluated in the emergency department (ED) with the principle that maternal well-being is prioritized over fetal concerns.** Maternal and fetal survival will depend on this coordinated team effort, which should begin as soon as the ED is notified that a pregnant trauma victim is being transported. **Stabilization of the mother with identification of the maternal injury is the initial priority. Fetal evaluation and interventions can be conducted in the ED as needed.** Pregnancy should not delay the decision to intubate, especially with the likelihood that surgical intervention will become necessary. The fetus is vulnerable to hypoxia, neurologic injury, or death; therefore all pregnant trauma victims should be provided with supplemental oxygen and avoidance of hypotension even if intubation is not required.

A suggested algorithm for care of the pregnant trauma patient is presented in Figure 26-2.

Evaluation on Labor and Delivery

After clearance for severe maternal injury has been completed in the ED, the obstetrics team should provide a more thorough physical and obstetric assessment. A thorough physical examination should look for old and new ecchymosis and bruises over the entire body in the event the injuries might suggest violence as an origin. The vaginal examination can detect bleeding, rupture of membranes, and vaginal lacerations that can occur if there has been a pelvic fracture. An ultrasonographic examination should be performed early in the assessment to document fetal heart activity, viability, and gestational age. **Depending on the labor and delivery gestational age criteria for assumption of care at the facility, the stable patient with**

EMERGENCY DEPARTMENT MANAGEMENT: TRAUMA IN PREGNANCY

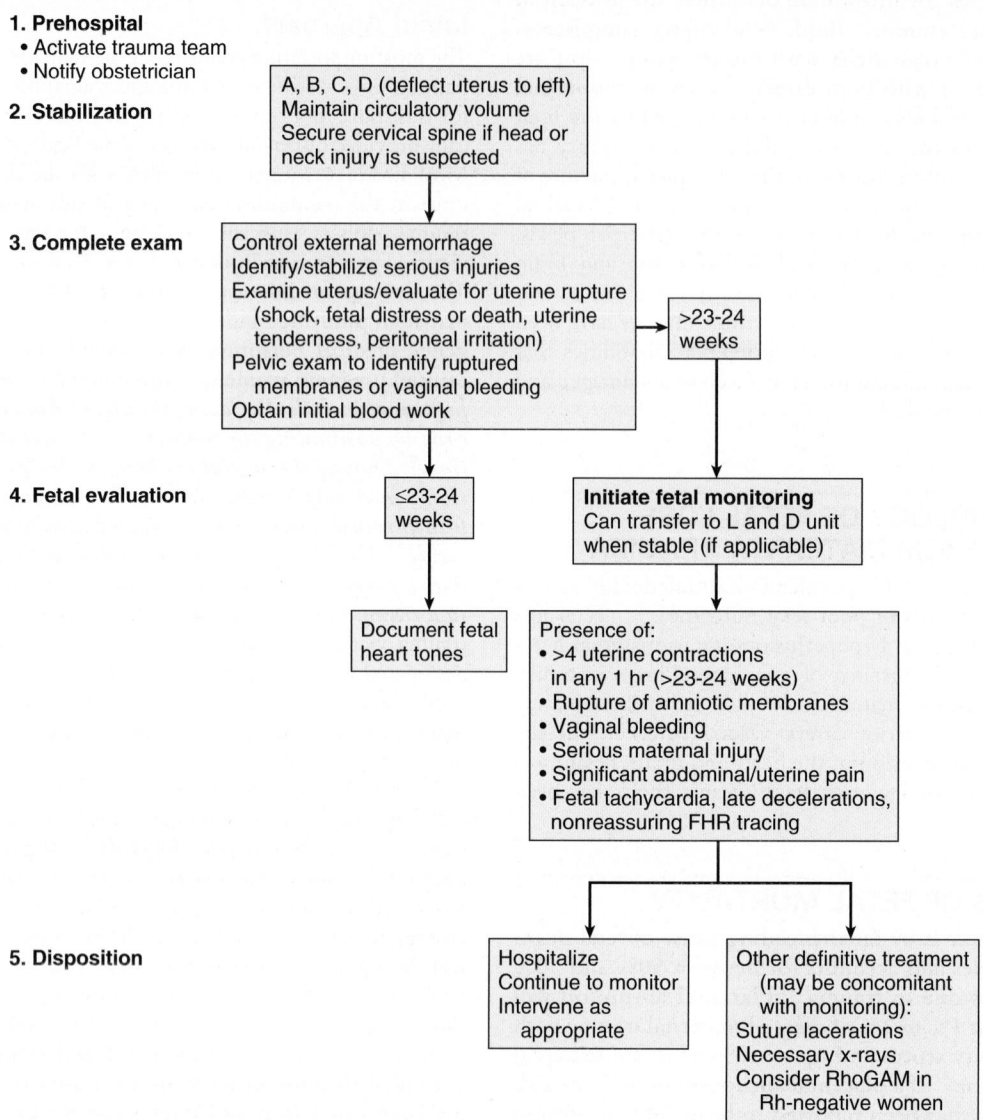

1. Prehospital
- Activate trauma team
- Notify obstetrician

2. Stabilization

A, B, C, D (deflect uterus to left)
Maintain circulatory volume
Secure cervical spine if head or
neck injury is suspected

3. Complete exam

Control external hemorrhage
Identify/stabilize serious injuries
Examine uterus/evaluate for uterine rupture
    (shock, fetal distress or death, uterine
    tenderness, peritoneal irritation)
Pelvic exam to identify ruptured
    membranes or vaginal bleeding
Obtain initial blood work

>23-24 weeks

4. Fetal evaluation

≤23-24 weeks

Initiate fetal monitoring
Can transfer to L and D unit
when stable (if applicable)

Document fetal heart tones

Presence of:
- >4 uterine contractions
  in any 1 hr (>23-24 weeks)
- Rupture of amniotic membranes
- Vaginal bleeding
- Serious maternal injury
- Significant abdominal/uterine pain
- Fetal tachycardia, late decelerations,
  nonreassuring FHR tracing

5. Disposition

Hospitalize
Continue to monitor
Intervene as
    appropriate

Other definitive treatment
    (may be concomitant
    with monitoring):
Suture lacerations
Necessary x-rays
Consider RhoGAM in
    Rh-negative women

FIG 26-2 Algorithm with suggested care plan for pregnant women who experience trauma. FHR, fetal heart rate; L and D, labor and delivery.

trauma at or beyond 23 weeks' gestation (the threshold of fetal viability) should be admitted to labor and delivery for further observation and monitoring for signs and symptoms of placental abruption and preterm labor. Women at fewer than 20 weeks' gestation or prior to fetal viability can be evaluated for fetal life in the ED but do not necessarily require admission to labor and delivery. Based on the patient's clinical presentation and uterine contraction frequency, the patient is observed for 4 to up to 24 hours prior to hospital discharge.

Fetal Monitoring
Fetal and uterine contraction monitoring is the most sensitive method for detecting abruptio placentae following trauma. In pregnant women who are beyond 23 to 24 weeks' gestation, frequent uterine contractions are nearly always present in women who develop placental abruption following trauma.[44,45] Moreover, a nonreassuring fetal heart rate (FHR) pattern may reflect maternal hemorrhagic shock or hypotension.[18] Uterine contraction monitoring is unquestionably

more sensitive than ultrasound in detecting placental abruption, and ultrasound detects only about 40% of abruptio placentae in the setting of trauma.[18,20,46] Although several authors have recommended incorporating assessment of fetal status into the standard focused abdominal sonography for trauma (FAST) exam, it should not replace fetal monitoring.[14,47] The standard FAST exam is performed to evaluate for intraperitoneal hemorrhage and has replaced diagnostic peritoneal lavage in many centers because of its excellent sensitivity (80% to 83%) for detection of intraperitoneal fluid.[47] A fetal biophysical profile test and middle cerebral artery Doppler studies may be performed at the time of the FAST exam for further information regarding fetal well-being, although its ability to predict fetal outcome in the setting of trauma has not been thoroughly assessed.[14,47] The FHR tracing has been called the "fifth vital sign" because it may provide the earliest evidence of maternal hypovolemia or hypotension (Fig. 26-3).[14] Likewise, frequent uterine contractions provide the most reliable warning sign of placental abruption or preterm labor.[15,46,48]

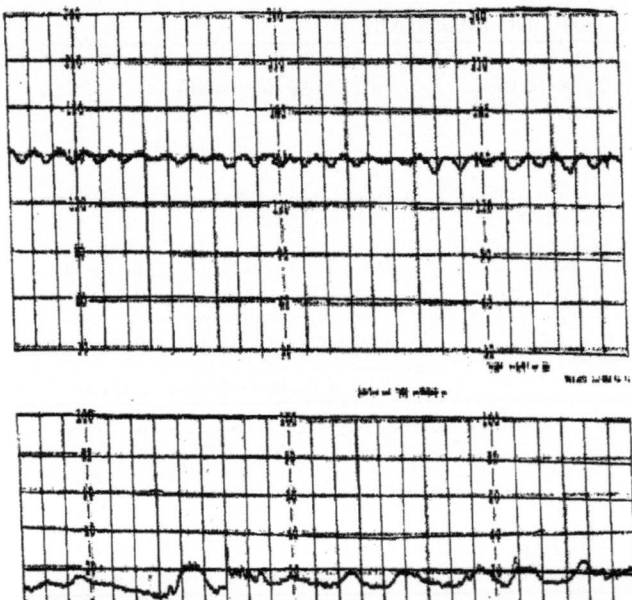

FIG 26-3 Tracing shows a sinusoidal pattern in a woman with fetal-maternal hemorrhage at 30 weeks' gestation after an automobile accident. The infant was severely anemic at birth. (From Brown, Haywood L. Trauma in pregnancy. *Obstet Gynecol.* 2009;114[1]: 147-160.)

The time within which a pregnant woman with trauma should receive fetal monitoring is variable. The rationale for a prolonged period of monitoring is the concern for delayed abruption, which has been reported up to 6 days after a traumatic event.[49] If uterine contractions occur less frequently than every 15 minutes over 4 hours of observation, placental abruption is unlikely to occur.[15,45,46] In fact, delayed placental abruption is unlikely if contraction frequency is less than every 10 minutes with normal fetal heart activity over a 4- to 6-hour period of observation. Adverse outcomes directly related to trauma has a reported negative predictive value of 100% when monitoring was normal and the early warning symptoms of bleeding and abdominal pain were absent.[50] Therefore if the fetus is at or beyond 24 weeks' gestation, the recommended minimal time for monitoring is at least 4 hours from the occurrence of the trauma. Monitoring should be continued if uterine tenderness, contractions, or irritability; abnormal fetal heart activity; or vaginal bleeding are evident. If deteriorating fetal status is apparent, delivery is indicated at a viable gestational age even if placental abruption is not clinically evident. If frequent contractions are noted (every 15 minutes or more often) even though no other signs and symptoms for abruption are present, 24 hours of monitoring is recommended because delayed abruptio placentae has been reported up to 48 hours or longer after maternal trauma.[14,18,46]

Laboratory Testing

Laboratory tests that may be helpful in the evaluation of trauma include a complete blood count with platelets, type, and Rhesus factor (Rh) testing; evaluation of coagulation function if abruptio placentae is a concern; and a Kleihauer-Betke (KB) test in the Rh-negative woman.[14] The KB test is an acid elution test designed to quantify the amount of fetal blood in the maternal circulation.[51] Fetal-maternal hemorrhage can be a complication of maternal trauma that leads to fetal anemia, exsanguination, hypoxia, and fetal death. This increase in fetomaternal hemorrhage appears to be most important in ensuring that Rh-negative women are adequately protected against isoimmunization.

The KB test may be used to determine whether additional vials of Rh immune globulin are required to prevent sensitization in Rh-negative women who experience trauma.[13,46] For approximately 90% of pregnant women who experience trauma, fetal-maternal hemorrhage will be less than 30 mL, and 1 vial of Rh immune globulin will be sufficient to prevent sensitization.[18] Some controversy surrounds the utility of this test among Rh-positive women. Based on a series of 71 women, Muench and colleagues[52] recommended its use as a predictor of risk for preterm labor after trauma. These authors found that the KB test had a 100% sensitivity for the prediction of preterm labor.[52] Other studies have not supported the routine use of this test as a predictor of adverse fetal outcome.[48,53] These reports acknowledge that KB testing has utility for determining those *few Rh-negative women who require additional Rh immune globulin* to protect against isoimmunization but has little predictive value of other adverse pregnancy outcomes such as abruptio placentae, preterm birth, or fetal hypoxemia. Moreover, the use of fetal monitoring is much more likely to provide a timely diagnosis of these complications of pregnancy than KB testing.

When gestational age is less than 20 weeks, 300 μg of Rh immune globulin should be sufficient to cover a fetal-maternal bleed because the expected fetal blood volume is not likely to exceed that covered with a standard dose of 300 μg. It is reasonable to provide Rh immune globulin within 72 hours for all nonsensitized Rh-negative women who experience abdominal trauma irrespective of KB status. Coagulation studies that include prothrombin time (PT), partial thromboplastin time (PTT), platelets, and fibrinogen may be useful in the presence of evidence or suspicion of abruptio placentae or if the patient is experiencing massive hemorrhage that may result in dilutional coagulopathy. A urinalysis may be obtained as well. Hematuria on urinalysis may be associated with pelvic fractures or renal tract injury.[20] Given the strong association of drug and alcohol use with traumatic injuries, a urine toxicology screen may be clinically indicated, especially if the woman has injuries that might require nonobstetric or obstetric surgical intervention.[20]

DIAGNOSTIC IMAGING

Ultrasound

Ultrasound may be used to assess fetal well-being without exposing the fetus to ionizing radiation. Additionally, abdominal ultrasound may be a useful tool in the evaluation of the pregnant trauma victim for free intraperitoneal fluid, with reported sensitivity between 61% and 83% but specificity between 94% and 100%.[54] Ultrasound is not particularly sensitive for detecting abruptio placentae, with reported identification in approximately 40% of cases. No clear guidelines have been established as to whether further imaging is necessary in the event of a negative ultrasound study in a hemodynamically stable patient. The Food and Drug Administration (FDA) has arbitrarily established a safe upper limit for energy exposure during ultrasonography at 94 mW/cm.[2,55]

TABLE 26-1   BIOLOGIC EFFECTS OF IN UTERO EXPOSURE TO IONIZING RADIATION

MENSTRUAL OR GESTATIONAL AGE	CONCEPTION AGE	<50 mGy (<5 rad)	50-100 mGy (5-10 rad)	>100 mGy (>10 rad)
0-2 weeks (0-14) days	Prior to conception	None	None	None
Weeks 3 and 4 (15-28) days	Weeks 1 and 2 (1-14) days	None	Probably none	Possible spontaneous abortion
Weeks 5 and 10 (29-70) days	Weeks 3 and 8 (15-56) days	None	Potential effects are scientifically uncertain and probably too subtle to be clinically detectable	Possible malformations increase in likelihood as dose increases
Weeks 11 and 17 (71-119) days	Weeks 9 and 15 (57-105) days	None	Potential effects are scientifically uncertain and probably too subtle to be clinically detectable	Increased risk of deficits in IQ or mental retardation that increase in frequency and severity with increasing dose
Weeks 18 and 27 (120-189) days	Weeks 16 and 25 (106-175) days	None	None	IQ deficits are not detectable at diagnostic doses
>27 weeks (>189 days)	>25 weeks (>175 days)	None	None	None applicable to diagnostic medicine

Modified from American College of Radiology. *Practice Guidelines for Imaging Pregnant or Potentially Pregnant Adolescents and Women with Ionizing Radiation.* American College of Radiology Practice Parameter, amended 2014 (Resolution 39). Available at: www.acr.org/guidelines.

Ionizing Radiation

Because of concerns about fetal exposure to ionizing radiation, clinicians may be hesitant to order indicated diagnostic tests in the setting of maternal trauma. However, maternal radiologic studies that include radiographs, magnetic resonance imaging (MRI), and computed tomography (CT) should not be deferred over concerns for the fetus if they are required for thorough assessment of the pregnant woman, and certainly if the pregnancy is at a previable gestational age. Concerns regarding exposure to ionizing radiation involve both risk for teratogenesis and risk for development of cancer in later life.[56] The most significant risk for fetal malformation involves microcephaly and mental retardation, which has been observed after human exposure to doses of 100 to 200 cGy. Exposure to ionizing radiation in utero may elevate the risk of childhood leukemia from a background of 1 in 3000 to a risk after exposure to 1 in 2000.[55,57] Similarly, exposure to 50 mGy (5 rads) ionizing radiation during pregnancy may be associated with a 2% lifetime attributable risk for development of malignancy.[58] The risk of teratogenesis or carcinogenesis with exposure to ionizing radiation is dose dependent.[58] According to the American College of Radiology (ACR), no single diagnostic procedure provides a radiation dose sufficient to threaten the well-being of the developing embryo or fetus, especially in the mid to late weeks of gestation.[59] **Both the ACR and the American College of Obstetricians and Gynecologists (ACOG) have published imaging guidelines for the use of diagnostic radiologic techniques during pregnancy.**[55,58] **However, in the setting of maternal trauma, the risk to the fetus for morbidity or mortality from untreated maternal injury far outweighs theoretic concerns for risks of development of malignancy in later life.** Table 26-1 summarizes effects of in utero exposure to ionizing radiation during different stages of pregnancy; radiation doses associated with common diagnostic tests are listed in Table 26-2.

Magnetic Resonance Imaging

MRI may be an attractive option because it does not involve the use of ionizing radiation, although less evidence is available to show the efficacy and safety of its use during pregnancy than for other, more established methods. Currently, the FDA states that the safety of MRI for the fetus "has not been established."[57] However, no evidence exists from studies of children exposed to MRI in utero of any teratogenic effects or of any long-term

TABLE 26-2   RADIATION DOSES ASSOCIATED WITH COMMON DIAGNOSTIC PROCEDURES

PROCEDURE	FETAL DOSE
Single-phase CT of abdomen and pelvis and lumbar spine	3.5 rad
Hip film (single view)	200 mrad
Chest radiograph	0.02-0.07 mrad
CT of head or chest	<1 rad
Diagnostic fluoroscopy of abdomen and pelvis	<10 rad

Modified from ACOG Committee on Obstetric Practice: ACOG Committee Opinion 299: Guidelines for Diagnostic Imaging During Pregnancy and American College of Radiology (ACR) Practice Guidelines for Imaging Pregnant or Potentially Pregnant Adolescents and Women with Ionizing Radiation.
ACOG, American College of Obstetricians and Gynecologists; *CT,* computed tomography.

adverse developmental consequences.[39,42] The ACR described guidelines for the safe use of MRI and provided support for the use of MRI during all trimesters of pregnancy if necessary for accurate diagnosis.[54,60] **The precise role for the use of MRI in the management of trauma in pregnancy has not yet been clearly established but may have benefit in the evaluation of soft tissue injury and spaces of the maternal pelvis.**

Contrast Agents

Iodinated contrast agents cross the placenta via simple diffusion.[61] Because they are taken up by the fetal thyroid and may pose a theoretic risk for fetal hypothyroidism, iodinated contrast images are generally avoided during pregnancy unless clearly necessary for diagnosis.[55,61] **However, no cases of fetal goiter or abnormal neonatal thyroid function have been reported after clinical use of iodinated contrast agents.**[61] Neonates whose mothers have received iodinated contrast media during pregnancy should be screened for hypothyroidism, an already standard practice.[57] A recent guideline for use of CT and MRI during pregnancy has posited that the use of iodinated contrast agents during pregnancy is preferable to the patient receiving repetitive CT studies because of the suboptimal nature of studies performed without contrast agents.[57]

The use of gadolinium for MRI in pregnancy is controversial. Gadolinium crosses the placenta and accumulates in amniotic fluid,[61] although it has not been found to be teratogenic or carcinogenic in doses used clinically.[20,61] However, administration of gadolinium to children and adults with underlying renal insufficiency has resulted in a syndrome known as *nephrogenic*

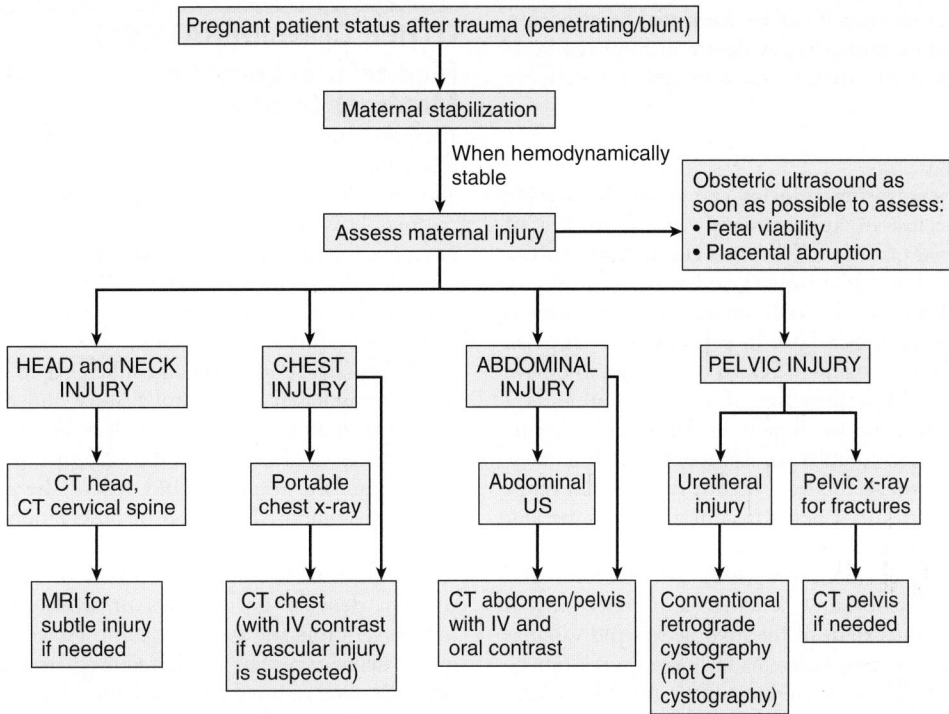

FIG 26-4 Algorithm with suggested plan for diagnostic imaging studies for pregnant women who experience trauma. CT, computed tomography; IV, intravenous; MRI, magnetic resonance imaging; US, ultrasound. (Modified from Patel SJ, Reede DL, Katz DS, et al. Imaging the pregnant patient for nonobstetric conditions: algorithms and radiation dose considerations. *Radiographics*. 2007;27:1719.)

systemic fibrosis in rare cases, which raises a theoretic concern of toxicity after fetal exposure.[57,62] Thus the use of gadolinium should be avoided in patients with acute or chronic renal insufficiency.

Suggested Guidelines for Radiologic Evaluation of Trauma

A recent evidence-based guideline and additional report on use of diagnostic imaging after maternal trauma has recommended the use of ultrasound as the initial modality but recommend the use of CT as the preferred method of evaluation when visceral injuries or injuries of the chest, aorta, mediastinum, spine, bones, bowel, or bladder are suspected (Fig. 26-4).[54,57]

EXPLORATORY SURGERY FOR TRAUMATIC INJURIES DURING PREGNANCY

When nonobstetric surgery is necessary in a pregnant woman, attention to adequate maternal oxygenation, blood volume, and uterine perfusion is important in providing an environment to prevent fetal hypoxia. Penetrating trauma is the most common indication for nonobstetric surgery for traumatic injuries during pregnancy.[14] Historically, surgical exploration was recommended for evaluation and repair of abdominal injuries that resulted from penetrating trauma; however, given the differing pattern of abdominal injuries that result from penetrating trauma during pregnancy, the decision for expectant management or surgery should be individualized.[14] Muench and Canterino[14] recommend an individualized approach to penetrating trauma depending on whether the wound is in the upper or lower abdomen. Because of the significantly increased risk for bowel injury after penetrating trauma to the upper abdomen, women with such wounds should

undergo surgical exploration. Because the gravid uterus provides some protection from visceral injury, pregnant women who sustain penetrating wounds to the lower abdomen may be managed conservatively if they are hemodynamically stable. Penetrating wounds to the gravid uterus increase risk for direct fetal injury but may be managed conservatively if they do not extend past the myometrium.[14] Conservative management may include diagnostic peritoneal lavage, which may be undertaken safely in all trimesters using an open direct-visualization technique through a supraumbilical incision under ultrasound guidance.[14,20] **Indications for surgical exploration include penetrating trauma to the upper abdomen, gunshot wounds to the abdomen, clinical evidence of active intraabdominal hemorrhage, or suspicion for bowel injury.**

The surgical team should not allow the enlarged uterus to compromise adequate surgical exploration and management. If exploratory laparotomy is undertaken, care should be taken to minimize traction on the gravid uterus, and the nature and extent of any injuries should be evaluated.[14] Exploratory laparotomy is not a reflex indication for delivery of the fetus.[20] **In the event that fetal death has occurred prior to surgical exploration, vaginal delivery after induction of labor may be a preferable approach, although Brown recommends surgical uterine evacuation while the mother is under a current anesthetic if there is abruption and potential for coagulopathy.**[20] Coagulopathy further complicates the hemorrhagic picture and leads to a more complicated perioperative course, which includes acute respiratory distress in the mother. In some circumstances, delivery of the fetus may be necessary to adequately explore the abdomen or to facilitate surgical repair of injured viscera.

If the pregnancy is at or beyond 24 weeks, fetal monitoring should be carried out intermittently during the surgical procedure. If nonreassuring fetal status is detected during the

procedure, in most instances it can be alleviated by attention to and correction of maternal hypovolemia or hypoxemia. If these supportive measures are not effective, cesarean delivery may be necessary.[20]

Uterine Rupture

Both blunt and penetrating injuries can result in uterine rupture, which occurs in approximately 0.6% to 1% of instances of maternal trauma.[20,46] Uterine rupture most often results from direct abdominal impact and may occur at any gestational age, although the risk increases as the uterus becomes an abdominal organ later in pregnancy.[1,63] The risk for uterine rupture is particularly increased for women who have experienced assault.[31] Most instances of uterine rupture as a result of maternal trauma are fundal in location.[46] Uterine rupture may also result in complete avulsion of the uterine arteries and massive hemorrhage.[1] Signs of uterine rupture may range from FHR abnormalities in a hemodynamically stable patient to maternal cardiovascular instability and hypovolemic shock.[46] Uterine rupture carries a poor prognosis for the fetus and requires immediate laparotomy. Whether a hysterectomy is required depends on the extent of the myometrial and vascular injury and to what extent the surgeon feels the uterus can be repaired expeditiously. Because uterine rupture may be associated with massive maternal hemorrhage because of the increased uterine vascularity associated with pregnancy; aggressive replacement of red cells and clotting factors is recommended.[20] Maternal mortality has been reported to be as high as 10% following traumatic uterine rupture.[4]

Implications of Cardiac Arrest and Perimortem Cesarean Section

In instances of severe maternal injury and maternal cardiac arrest, cardiopulmonary resuscitation may be less successful because of maternal physiologic alterations associated with pregnancy. The gravid uterus may interfere with systemic perfusion by compression of the inferior vena cava and interference with venous return. The use of left lateral tilt to reduce the impact of aortocaval compression on utero placental perfusion compromises cardiopulmonary resuscitation (CPR) efforts and efficacy of chest compressions; therefore emptying the uterus should facilitate more effective maternal resuscitation. **The chance of maternal survival after cardiac arrest despite aggressive attempts at resuscitation is significantly diminished compared with the nonpregnant state. Long-term outcomes for children born after maternal cardiac arrest are more likely to be favorable if the child is delivered within 5 minutes of cessation of maternal circulation.[38] Perimortem cesarean should be considered early in the resuscitation process in the trauma victim. If the pregnancy has extended beyond an acceptable gestation of viability, the decision to perform a perimortem cesarean should be immediate and decisive. Therefore if the pregnancy is at or beyond fetal viability (23 to 24 weeks' gestation), perimortem cesarean delivery should commence within 4 minutes after maternal cardiac arrest if resuscitation has not restored maternal circulation.[14]**

The incision should be midline from xiphoid to the pubis through all abdominal wall layers and through a midline vertical uterine incision. Once the neonate is delivered, resuscitation efforts can continue, and if successful, the patient can be transferred to the operating theater for closure of the uterus and abdominal wound and to ensure adequate hemostasis.

OTHER CONSIDERATIONS

Medical and Legal Implications After Maternal Trauma

Accurate and careful documentation of all history, physical examination findings, clinical care, and follow-up for the mother and fetus is critical for the pregnant woman who has suffered trauma. It is highly likely, particularly if there is an adverse outcome for the pregnancy, that these records will be revisited if legal action is pursued. The clinicians involved in the initial and follow-up care of the woman will likely have to offer a medical opinion as to causation.

The obstetric evaluation and adherence to monitoring recommendations based on clinical history and clinical observation for up to 4 hours after an accident or injury is necessary as a critical assessment period for maternal and fetal well-being. A documented record should reflect the maternal and fetal status throughout the period of observation. For example, the timing of an emergency cesarean or placental abruption relative to the time of the traumatic event or preterm labor and/or preterm delivery in the days or weeks following the event may have implications to causation. However, labor and subsequent delivery several weeks removed from a traumatic event, when all observational documentation revealed normal findings, is unlikely to be directly related to the acute event.

For all trauma in pregnancy, it is therefore important for all care providers to document throughout the course of care from the ED, labor room, and surgical suite through discharge and follow-up.

Long-Term Effects of Trauma

In some reports, up to 38% of women who experience trauma during pregnancy will require delivery in the same hospitalization,[20] although in most published experiences, the great majority of pregnant women who experience trauma will be discharged undelivered.[4,44] Although most placental abruptions that result from maternal trauma will occur within the first 24 hours after the event, some reports suggest that women who have experienced trauma remain at risk for other complications that include fetal growth restriction, intrauterine fetal demise, "fetal distress," placental abruption, and a higher risk of cesarean delivery.[3,4,64] By contrast, a prospective controlled study demonstrated that pregnancy outcomes beyond 48 hours in injured women are similar to those in the uninjured controls.[44] Suggested discharge instructions are shown in Box 26-1.

Prevention of Trauma

A Canadian study suggests that pregnancy, particularly in the second trimester, is associated with a 42% relative increase in a serious MVC compared with the nonpregnant state. The crash rate was equal to 4.55 events per 1000 individuals, about twice the population average of 2 crashes per 1000 drivers annually.[65] The factors that surround this statistical increase during the second trimester are highly subjective. **Education and reinforcement of seatbelt use during pregnancy should be undertaken as a routine part of prenatal education and care.** In a primate model of motor vehicle impact trauma and its fetal effects, three-point restraints significantly reduced fetal mortality compared with two-point restraints.[2] In a recent study of MVCs that involved 43 pregnant women between 1996 and 1999, Klinich and colleagues[16] from the Times New Romanity of Michigan demonstrated that proper use of seatbelts was significantly associated with good fetal outcome. The authors speculated that proper seatbelt use could prevent as many as 84% of adverse fetal outcomes. Proper counseling by the obstetric care provider for seatbelt usage has also been shown to significantly improve compliance with seatbelt use during pregnancy.[66]

Because of reasonable evidence that restraint use reduces both maternal and fetal morbidity and mortality, ACOG recommends seatbelt use in pregnancy to reduce the chances of

maternal and fetal morbidity and mortality.[67] **The NHTSA recommends that pregnant women wear their seatbelts with the shoulder harness portion positioned over the collarbone between the breasts and the lap belt portion under the pregnant abdomen as low as possible on the hips and across the upper thighs and not above or over the abdomen.** Placement of the lap belt over the dome of the uterus increases pressure transmission and the risk of uterine injury during a significant crash. Restraint use in pregnancy is inconsistent, and the relative risk for perinatal death with lack of restraint use has been reported as high as 5.2 : 1.[68]

Airbags can be life saving in automobile crashes. However, airbags detonate with more than 1200 lb of force at speeds that can exceed 230 mph. No evidence suggests that the effect of airbag deployment during the third trimester increases risk for fetal injury; however, minor maternal injuries from airbag deployments have been reported. **The NHTSA recommends that when a pregnant woman rides in front of an airbag, the airbag should be at least 10 inches away from the dashboard or steering wheel and the seat should be moved back from the gravid uterus as the pregnant abdomen grows. Although some have expressed concern about possible harmful effects of airbag deployment in the event of an MVC during pregnancy, the NHTSA and ACOG do not recommend disabling airbags during pregnancy.**[46,69] Indeed, a retrospective cohort study of pregnant women involved in MVCs in the state of Washington between 2002 and 2005 concluded that airbags do not increase the risk for adverse outcomes of pregnancy.[70] The forces that lead to placental abruption after motor vehicle trauma are depicted in Figure 26-5, and proper use of seatbelt restraints is depicted in Figure 26-6.

BOX 26-1   SUGGESTED DISCHARGE INSTRUCTIONS FOR PREGNANT WOMEN HOSPITALIZED FOR OBSERVATION AFTER TRAUMA

- Discharge after 24 hours of observation.
- Discharge may be indicated in the absence of signs or symptoms of labor, abruption, rupture of membranes, fetal compromise, or maternal compromise.
- Health education
  - After discharge, the woman should be instructed to call Labor and Delivery with decreased fetal movement, vaginal bleeding, rupture of membranes, abdominal pain, or more than three uterine contractions per hour.
  - Advise fetal movement count twice daily.
  - Advise follow-up with provider within the week.
  - Advocate correct seatbelt use: shoulder belt between breasts and uterine fundus, lap belt under the uterus and across the spines of the pelvis.
  - If domestic violence is suspected, order social work consult.

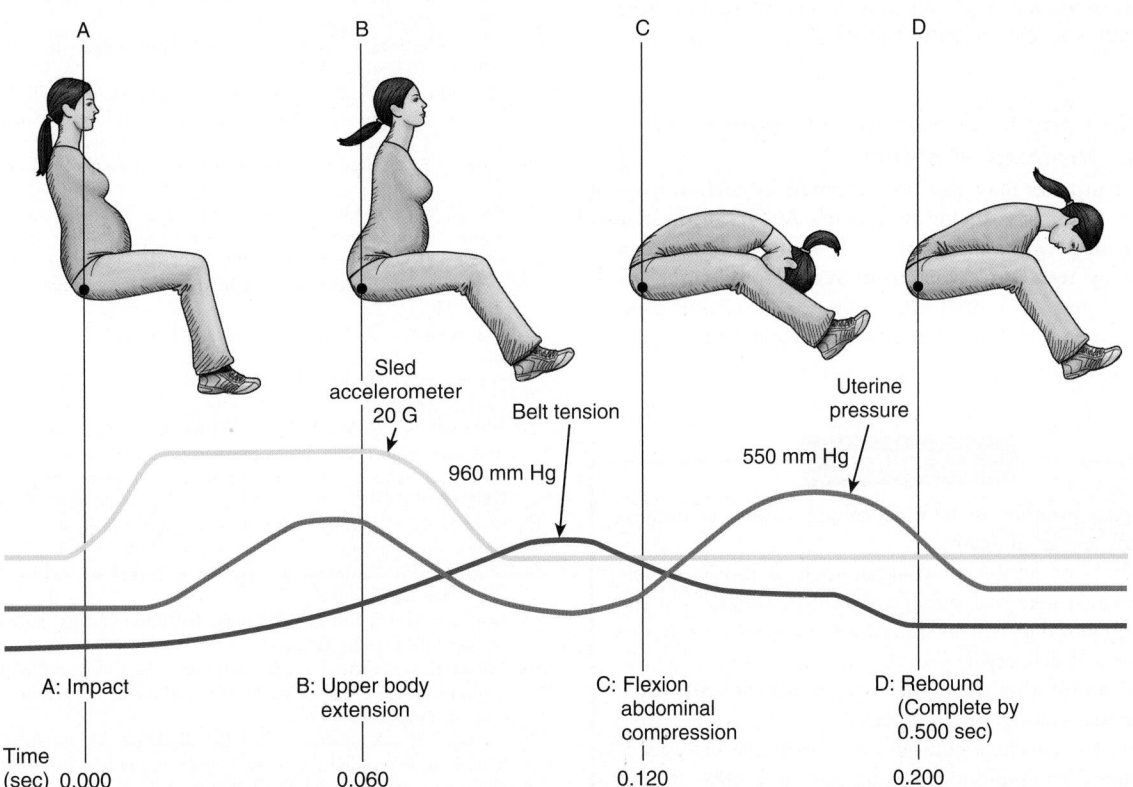

FIG 26-5 Impact sequence. Relationship between body motion, uterine pressure, and belt tension. (Modified from Hankins CVD. *Operative Obstetrics.* Stamford, CT: Appleton & Lange, 1995, Fig. 35-3, p 655.)

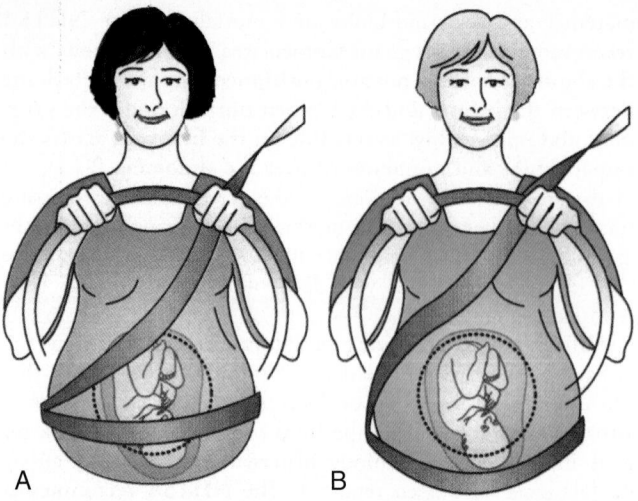

FIG 26-6 **A,** Improper use of a lap belt in pregnancy showing placement across the abdominal dome. **B,** Lap belt appropriately placed below the abdominal dome. (Illustration by John Yanson. Modified from Brown, Haywood L. Trauma in pregnancy. *Obstet Gynecol.* 2009; 114[1]:147-160.)

♦ Following cases of blunt trauma, fetal monitoring is recommended for a period of 4 to 24 hours depending on the findings.
♦ Placental abruption is the most frequent cause of fetal death after trauma.
♦ Most abruptions occur within 24 hours of an accident, but delayed abruption can occur.
♦ Rhogam should be administered to Rh-negative women who experience trauma.
♦ Kleihauer-Betke testing is recommended for Rh-negative women who experience trauma beyond 20 weeks of gestation.
♦ Concerns about fetal effects of ionizing radiation should not delay imaging necessary to care for pregnant trauma victims.
♦ Seatbelt use may reduce adverse fetal outcome resulting from trauma by as much as 84%.
♦ All pregnant women should be screened for domestic violence during each trimester.

BOX 26-2   SUGGESTED DOMESTIC VIOLENCE SCREENING QUESTIONS

Because violence is so common in many women's lives and because there is help available for women being abused, I now ask every patient about domestic violence:

1. Within the past year or since you have been pregnant, have you been hit, slapped, kicked, or otherwise physically hurt by anyone?
2. Are you in a relationship with a person who threatens or physically hurts you?
3. Has anyone forced you to have sexual activities that made you feel uncomfortable?

Screening and Identification of Women at Risk for Domestic Violence

Traumatic injuries may also be prevented by early screening and detection of IPV during pregnancy. ACOG recommends screening all pregnant women for IPV at the first prenatal visit and at least once per trimester of pregnancy. They recommend use of a brief three-question screening tool to identify women at risk for domestic violence during pregnancy (Box 26-2).[71]

KEY POINTS

♦ Maternal trauma is the most frequent cause of nonobstetric maternal death.
♦ In cases of significant trauma, such as motor vehicle accidents, maternal stabilization and evaluation in the emergency department should occur prior to transfer to labor and delivery.
♦ Fetal monitoring should occur as soon as possible while maternal evaluation takes place.
♦ Abruptio placentae complicates 1% to 2% of cases of minor blunt abdominal trauma and up to 40% of cases of severe abdominal trauma.

REFERENCES

1. Mirza FG, Devine PC, Gaddipati S. Trauma in pregnancy: a systematic approach. *Am J Perinatol.* 2010;27:579.
2. Pearlman MD. Motor vehicle crashes, pregnancy loss and preterm labor. *Int J Gynaecol Obstet.* 1997;57:127.
3. El Kady D, Gilbert WM, Xing G, et al. Association of maternal fractures with adverse perinatal outcomes. *Am J Obstet Gynecol.* 2006;195:711.
4. El Kady D. Perinatal outcomes of traumatic injuries during pregnancy. *Clin Obstet Gynecol.* 2007;50:582.
5. El Kady D, Gilbert WM, Anderson J, et al. Trauma during pregnancy: an analysis of maternal and fetal outcomes in a large population. *Am J Obstet Gynecol.* 2004;190:1661.
6. Weiss HB, Songer TJ, Fabio A. Fetal deaths related to maternal injury. *JAMA.* 2001;286:1863.
7. Shah KH, Simons RK, Holbrook T, Fortlage D, Winchell RJ, Hoyt DB. Trauma in pregnancy: maternal and fetal outcomes. *J Trauma.* 1998;45: 83-86.
8. Oxford CM, Ludmir J. Trauma in pregnancy. *Clin Obstet Gynecol.* 2009;52: 611.
9. Kuo C, Jamieson DJ, McPheeters ML. Injury hospitalizations of pregnant women in the United States, 2002. *Am J Obstet Gynecol.* 2007;196.
10. Mendez-Figueroa H, Dahlke HD, Vrees RA, Rouse DJ. Trauma during pregnancy: an updated systematic review. *Am J Obstet Gynecol.* 2013; 209:1-10.
11. Kvarnstrand L, Milsom I, Lekander T, Druid H, Jacobsson B. Maternal fatalities, fetal and neonatal deaths related to motor vehicle crashes during pregnancy: a national population based study. *Acta Obstet Gynecol Scand.* 2008;87:946-952.
12. Silverman JG, Decker MR, Reed E, Raj A. Intimate partner violence victimization prior to and during pregnancy among women residing in 26 US States: associations with maternal and neonatal health. *Am J Obstet Gynecol.* 2006;195:140-148.
13. Chames MC, Pearlman MD. Trauma during pregnancy: outcomes and clinical management. *Clin Obstet Gynecol.* 2008;51:398.
14. Muench MV, Canterino JC. Trauma in pregnancy. *Obstet Gynecol Clin North Am.* 2007;34:555.
15. Pearlman MD, Tintinalli JE, Lorenz RP. Blunt trauma during pregnancy. *N Engl J Med.* 1990;323:609.
16. Klinich KD, Flannagan CA, Rupp JD, et al. Fetal outcome in motor-vehicle crashes: effects of crash characteristics and maternal restraint. *Am J Obstet Gynecol.* 2008;198:450.e1.
17. Iwamoto HS, Kaufman T, Keil LC, Rudolph AM. Responses to acute hypoxemia in fetal sheep at 0.6-0.7 gestation. *Am J Physiol.* 1989;256:H613.
18. Williams J, Mozurkewich E, Chilimigras J, et al. Critical care in obstetrics: pregnancy-specific conditions. *Best Pract Res Clin Obstet Gynaecol.* 2008; 22:825.

19. US Department of Transportation, National Highway Traffic Safety Administration. *2012 Motor Vehicle Crashes: An overview, DOT HS 811 856,* Washington, DC.

20. Brown HL. Trauma in pregnancy. *Obstet Gynecol.* 2009;114:147.

21. Dunning K, LeMasters G, Levin L, et al. Falls in workers during pregnancy: risk factors, job hazards, and high risk occupations. *Am J Ind Med.* 2003;44:664.

22. Butler EE, Colon I, Druzin ML, et al. Postural equilibrium during pregnancy: decreased stability with an increased reliance on visual cues. *Am J Obstet Gynecol.* 2006;195:1104.

23. Schiff MA. Pregnancy outcomes following hospitalization for a fall in Washington State from 1987 to 2004. *BJOG.* 2008;115:1648.

24. Cahill AG, Bastek JA, Stamilio DM, et al. Minor trauma in pregnancy—is the evaluation unwarranted? *Am J Obstet Gynecol.* 2008;198:208.e1.

25. Gunter J. Intimate partner violence. *Obstet Gynecol Clin North Am.* 2007; 34:367, ix.

26. Palladino CL, Singh V, Campbell J, Flynn H, Gold KJ. Homicide and suicide during the perinatal period: findings from the national violent death reporting system. *Obstet Gynecol.* 2011;118:1056-1063.

27. Ghandi SG, Gilbert WM, McElvy SS, et al. Maternal and neonatal outcomes after attempted suicide. *Obstet Gynecol.* 2006;107:984-990.

28. Cheng D, Horon IL. Intimate-partner homicide among pregnant and postpartum women. *Obstet Gynecol.* 2010;115:1181.

29. McFarlane J, Campbell JC, Sharps P, Watson K. Abuse during pregnancy and femicide: urgent implications for women's health. *Obstet Gynecol.* 2002;100:27.

30. Wiencrot A, Nannini A, Manning SE, Kennelly J. Neonatal outcomes and mental illness, substance abuse, and intentional injury during pregnancy. *Matern Child Health J.* 2012;16:979-988.

31. El Kady D, Gilbert WM, Xing G, et al. Maternal and neonatal outcomes of assaults during pregnancy. *Obstet Gynecol.* 2005;105:357.

32. Leggon RE, Wood GC, Indeck MC. Pelvic fractures in pregnancy: factors influencing maternal and fetal outcomes. *J Trauma.* 2002;53:796-804.

33. Gunter J, Pearlman MD. Emergencies during pregnancy: trauma and non-obstetric surgical conditions. In: Ling F, Duff P, eds. *Obstetrics and Gynecology: Principles for Practice.* New York: McGraw-Hill; 2001:253.

34. Pacheco LD, Gei AF, VanHook JW, et al. Burns in pregnancy. *Obstet Gynecol.* 2005;106:1210.

35. Maghsoudi H, Samnia R, Garadaghi A, et al. Burns in pregnancy. *Burns.* 2006;32:246.

36. van Hook JW. Trauma in pregnancy. *Clin Obstet Gynecol.* 2002;45: 414-424.

37. Ellestad SC, Shelton S, James AH. Prenatal diagnosis of trauma-related fetal epidural hematoma. *Obstet Gynecol.* 2004;104:1298-1300.

38. Tsuei BJ. Assessment of the pregnant trauma patient. *Injury.* 2006;37:367.

39. Curet MJ, Schermer CR, Demarest GB, et al. Predictors of outcome in trauma during pregnancy: identification of patients who can be monitored for less than 6 hours. *J Trauma.* 2000;49:18.

40. Pak LL, Reece EA, Chan L. Is adverse pregnancy outcome predictable after blunt abdominal trauma? *Am J Obstet Gynecol.* 1998;179:1140.

41. Schiff MA, Holt VL. The injury severity score in pregnant trauma patients: predicting placental abruption and fetal death. *J Trauma.* 2002;53:946.

42. Schiff MA, Holt VL, Daling JR. Maternal and infant outcomes after injury during pregnancy in Washington State from 1989 to 1997. *J Trauma.* 2002;53:939.

43. Sasser SM, Hunt RC, Faul F, et al. Guidelines for field triage of injured patients: recommendations of the National Expert Panel on Field Triage, 2011. *MMWR Recomm Rep.* 2012;61:1.

44. Pearlman MD, Tintinalli JE, Lorenz RP. A prospective controlled study of outcome after trauma during pregnancy. *Am J Obstet Gynecol.* 1990;162:1502.

45. Williams JK, McClain L, Rosemurgy AS, et al. Evaluation of blunt abdominal trauma in the third trimester of pregnancy: maternal and fetal considerations. *Obstet Gynecol.* 1990;75:33.

46. ACOG Educational Bulletin. Obstetric Aspects of Trauma Management. *Int J Gynaecol Obstet.* 1999;64:87.

47. Cusick SS, Tibbles CD. Trauma in pregnancy. *Emerg Med Clin North Am.* 2007;25:861.

48. Dahmus MA, Sibai BM. Blunt abdominal trauma: are there any predictive factors for abruptio placentae or maternal-fetal distress? *Am J Obstet Gynecol.* 1993;169:1054.

49. Higgins SD, Garite TJ. Late abruption placenta in trauma patients: implications for monitoring. *Obstet Gynecol.* 1984;63:10S.

50. Connolly AM, Katz VL, Bash KL, et al. Trauma in pregnancy. *Am J Perinatol.* 1997;14:331.

51. Grossman NB. Blunt trauma in pregnancy. *Am Fam Physician.* 2004;70:1303.

52. Muench MV, Baschat AA, Reddy UM, et al. Kleihauer-Betke testing is important in all cases of maternal trauma. *J Trauma.* 2004;57:1094.

53. Goodwin TM, Breen MT. Pregnancy outcome and fetomaternal hemorrhage after noncatastrophic trauma. *Am J Obstet Gynecol.* 1990;162:665.

54. Patel SJ, Reede DL, Katz DS, et al. Imaging the pregnant patient for non-obstetric conditions: algorithms and radiation dose considerations. *Radiographics.* 2007;27:1705.

55. ACOG Committee on Obstetric Practice. ACOG Committee Opinion #299: Guidelines for Diagnostic Imaging During Pregnancy. *Obstet Gynecol.* 2004;104:647.

56. Gjelsteen AC, Ching BH, Meyermann MW, et al. CT, MRI, PET, PET/CT, and ultrasound in the evaluation of obstetric and gynecologic patients. *Surg Clin North Am.* 2008;88:361.

57. Chen MM, Coakley FV, Kaimal A, et al. Guidelines for computed tomography and magnetic resonance imaging use during pregnancy and lactation. *Obstet Gynecol.* 2008;112:333.

58. *ACR practice guidelines for imaging pregnant or potentially pregnant adolescents and women with ionizing radiation.* American College of Radiology Practice Parameter, amended 2014 (Resolution 39). Available at: <www.acr.org/guidelines.

59. Hall EJ. Scientific view of low level radiation risks. *Radiographics.* 1991; 11:509-518.

60. Kanal E, Barkovich AJ, Bell C, et al. ACR Guidance Document for Safe MR Practices: 2007. *AJR Am J Roentgenol.* 2007;188:1447.

61. Lee SI, Chew FS. Use of IV iodinated and gadolinium contrast media in the pregnant or lactating patient: self-assessment module. *AJR Am J Roentgenol.* 2009;193:S70.

62. Marckmann P, Skov L. Nephrogenic systemic fibrosis: clinical picture and treatment. *Radiol Clin North Am.* 2009;47:833.

63. Augustin G, Majerovic M. Non-obstetrical acute abdomen during pregnancy. *Eur J Obstet Gynecol Reprod Biol.* 2007;13:4.

64. Weiss HB, Sauber-Schatz EK, Cook LJ. The epidemiology of pregnancy-associated emergency department injury visits and their impact on birth outcomes. *Accid Anal Prev.* 2008;40:1088.

65. Redelmeier DA, May SC, Thiruchelvam D, Barrett J. Pregnancy and risk of a traffic crash. *Can Med Assoc J.* 2014;186:1169.

66. Pearlman MD, Phillips ME. Safety belt use during pregnancy. *Obstet Gynecol.* 1996;88:1026.

67. National Highway Transportation Safety Administration. *Should Pregnant Women Wear Seat Belts? Answers to an expectant mother's common questions about traffic safety.* DOT HS 809-506, September 2002. Available at: <www.nhta.dot.gov>.

68. American College of Obstetricians and Gynecologists. *Aspects of Trauma Management. ACOG Educational Bulletin 251.* Washington (DC: ACOG; 1998.

69. Luley T, Brown HL, Fitzpatrick FB, Hocker M. Trauma during pregnancy: restraint use and perinatal outcome after motor vehicle accidents. *Obstet Gynecol.* 2008;111:1S.

70. Schiff M, Mack CD, Kaufman RP, et al. The effect of air bags on pregnancy outcomes in Washington State: 2002-2005. *Obstet Gynecol.* 2010;115: 85.

71. The American Congress of Obstetricians and Gynecologists (AGOG). *Screening tools—domestic violence.* Available at: <http://www.acog.org/About-ACOG/ACOG-Departments/Violence-Against-Women/Screening-Tools–Domestic-Violence>.

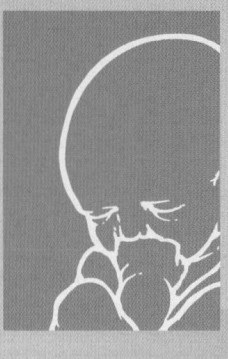

CHAPTER 27

Early Pregnancy Loss and Stillbirth

JOE LEIGH SIMPSON and ERIC R.M. JAUNIAUX

KEY ABBREVIATIONS			
American College of Obstetricians and Gynecologists	ACOG	Luteal phase deficiency	LPD
Anticardiolipin	aCL	National Institute of Child Health and Human Development	NICHD
Antiphospholipid antibody	aPL	Preimplantation genetic diagnosis	PGD
Assisted reproductive technology	ART	Recurrent early pregnancy loss	REPL
β-Human chorionic gonadotropin	β-hCG	Recurrent miscarriage	RM
Bacterial vaginosis	BV	Royal College of Obstetricians and Gynaecologists	RCOG
Cesarean delivery	CD		
Comparative genomic hybridization	CGH	Small for gestational age	SGA
Confidence interval	CI	Standard deviation	SD
Fluorescence in situ hybridization	FISH	Three-dimensional	3-D
Human chorionic gonadotropin	hCG	Thyroid receptor beta	TR-β
In vitro fertilization	IVF	Thyroid-stimulating hormone	TSH
Low birthweight	LBW	Very low birthweight	VLBW
Lupus anticoagulant	LAC	Very preterm delivery	VPTD

Not all conceptions result in a live-born infant, and human reproduction is extremely inefficient compared with that of other mammal species.[1] **About 50% to 70% of spontaneous conceptions are lost before completion of the first trimester, most before implantation or during the first month after the last menstrual period. These losses are often not recognized as conceptions. Of clinically recognized pregnancies, 10% to 15% are lost.** Although epidemiologic data are limited on animals living in the wild, such as monkeys, laboratory rodents are known to have postimplantation pregnancy loss rates of less than 10%.[1] Among married women in the United States, 4% have experienced two fetal losses, and 3% have experienced three or more.[2] A subset of women manifest repetitive spontaneous miscarriages, as opposed to randomly having repeated untoward events. This chapter considers the frequency and timing of pregnancy losses, the causes of fetal wastage, and the management of couples who experience repetitive losses.

FREQUENCY AND TIMING OF PREGNANCY LOSS

Embryos implant 6 days after conception, although physical signs are not generally appreciated until 5 to 6 weeks after the last menstrual period. **Fewer than half of preimplantation embryos persist, as witnessed by assisted reproductive technology (ART) success rates rarely exceeding 30% to 40% of cycles initiated; even after implantation, judged preclinically by the presence of β-human chorionic gonadotropin (β-hCG), about 30% of pregnancies are lost.**[1] **After clinical recognition, 10% to 12% are lost. Most clinical pregnancy losses occur before 8 weeks.** Before widespread availability of ultrasound, embryonic demise was often not appreciated until 9 to 12 weeks' gestation, at which time bleeding and passage of tissue (products of conception) occurred. With widespread availability of ultrasound, it has been shown that fetal demise actually occurs weeks before overt clinical signs are manifested. This conclusion was reached on the basis of cohort studies that showed that only 3% of viable pregnancies are lost after 8 weeks' gestation[3]; studies involving obstetric registrants reached similar conclusions. Fetal viability thus ceases weeks before maternal symptoms of pregnancy loss. That almost all losses are retained in utero for some time before clinical recognition means that virtually all losses could be considered "missed abortions," thus this once widely used term is actually archaic.

After the first trimester, pregnancy losses occur at a slower rate. **Loss rates are only 1% in women confirmed by ultrasound to have viable pregnancies at 16 weeks.** Two confounding factors that influence clinical pregnancy loss rates are clinically relevant: **maternal age is positively correlated with pregnancy loss rates,** and a 40-year-old woman has twice the risk of a 20-year-old woman. This occurs in euploid and aneuploid pregnancies, as discussed later. **Prior pregnancy loss also increases loss rates, but far less than once believed.** Among nulliparous women who have never experienced a loss, the likelihood of pregnancy loss is only 5% to 10% (Table 27-1). After one loss, the risk of another is increased but does not exceed 30% to 40% even for women with three or more losses.[4] These risks apply not only to those women whose losses were recognized at 9 to 12 weeks' gestation but also to those whose pregnancies were ascertained in the fifth week of gestation.[5] Of clinical relevance, no scientific evidence suggests that women with three losses are etiologically distinct from those with two

losses or even one loss. The situation may be different if four or more losses have occurred, and different etiologic factors may exist in this uncommon subgroup.

The clinical consequence of the above information is that in order to be judged efficacious in preventing recurrent first-trimester spontaneous abortions, therapeutic regimens must show success rates substantially greater than 70%. Essentially no therapeutic regimen can make this claim.

PLACENTAL ANATOMIC CHARACTERISTICS OF SUCCESSFUL AND UNSUCCESSFUL PREGNANCIES

As judged by adult tissue criteria, the human fetus develops in a low-oxygen environment. Development of the human placenta is modulated heavily by the intrauterine environment.[6-9] During the first trimester, development takes place in a low-oxygen environment supported by histotrophic nutrition from the endometrial glands. Consequently, the rate of growth of the chorionic sac is almost invariable across this period and is remarkably uniform among individuals. **Toward the end of the first trimester, the intrauterine environment undergoes radical transformation in association with onset of the maternal arterial circulation and the switch to hemotrophic nutrition** (Chapter 1). The accompanying rise in intraplacental oxygen concentration poses a major challenge to placental tissues, and extensive villous remodeling takes place at this time.

The human gestational sac is designed to minimize the flux of oxygen (O_2) from maternal blood to the fetal circulation.[1,6] In particular, the extravillous trophoblast that migrates inside the uterine tissue to anchor the pregnancy creates a cellular shell with plugs inside the tip of the uteroplacental arteries.[2,9] This additional barrier keeps most of the maternal circulation outside the placenta and thus reduces the chemical activity of free oxygen radicals inside the placenta during most of the first trimester of the human pregnancy.[6,7] In normal pregnancies, the onset of the maternal circulation is a progressive phenomenon that starts at about 9 weeks at the periphery of the placenta and gradually extends toward the center.[2,7,9] This process correlates closely with the pattern of trophoblast invasion across the placental bed (Fig. 27-1).

TABLE 27-1 APPROXIMATE RECURRENCE RISK FIGURES USEFUL FOR COUNSELING WOMEN WITH REPEATED SPONTANEOUS ABORTIONS

	PRIOR SPONTANEOUS ABORTIONS	RISK (%)
Women with liveborn infant	0	5-10
	1	20-25
	2	25
	3	30
	4	30
Women without liveborn infant	3	30-40

Data from Regan L. A prospective study on spontaneous abortion. In: Beard RW, Sharp F (eds). *Early Pregnancy Loss: Mechanisms and Treatment.* London: Springer-Verlag; 1988, p 22; Warburton D, Fraser FC. Spontaneous abortion risks in man: data from reproductive histories collected in a medical genetic unit. *Am J Hum Genet.* 1964;16:1; and Poland BJ, Miller JR, Jones DC, et al. Reproductive counseling in patients who have had a spontaneous abortion. *Am J Obstet Gynecol.* 1977;127:685.
Recurrence risks are slightly higher for older women.

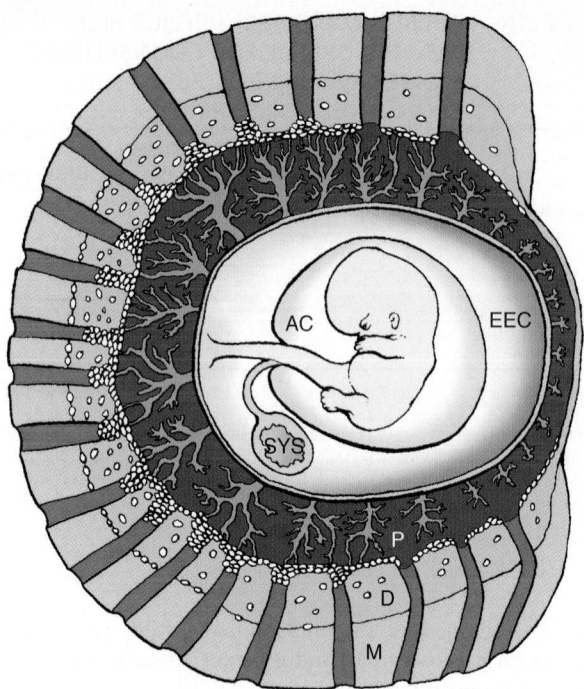

FIG 27-1 A gestational sac at the end of the second month (8 to 9 weeks) showing the myometrium (M), decidua (D), placenta (P), exocoelomic cavity (EEC), amniotic cavity (AC), and secondary yolk sac (SYS). (From Jauniaux E, Cindrova-Davies T, Johns T, et al. Distribution and transfer pathways of antioxidant molecules inside the first trimester human gestational sac. *J Clin Endocrinol Metab.* 2004;89: 1452.)

In about two thirds of early pregnancy failures, anatomic evidence of defective placentation is apparent, which is mainly characterized by a thinner and fragmented trophoblast shell and reduced cytotrophoblast invasion of the lumen at the tips of the spiral arteries.[2,10-12] This is associated with premature onset of the maternal circulation throughout the placenta in most cases of miscarriages.[2,9,10-12] These defects are similar in euploid and in most aneuploid miscarriages but are more pronounced in hydatidiform moles (Fig. 27-2). In vivo ultrasound and histopathologic data indicate that in most early pregnancy losses, the onset of the intervillous circulation is premature and widespread owing to incomplete transformation and plugging of the uteroplacental arteries.[7,10,11] **In about 80% of missed miscarriages, the onset of the maternal placental circulation is both precocious and generalized throughout the placenta.** This occurs independent of the karyotype of the conceptus,[11] leading to higher O_2 concentrations during early pregnancy, widespread trophoblastic oxidative damage, and placental degeneration. Although in vitro studies have demonstrated the ability of damaged syncytium to regenerate from the underlying cytotrophoblast, it is likely that in the face of extensive damage, this ability will be overwhelmed, leading to complete pregnancy failure.[2,12]

NUMERICAL CHROMOSOMAL ABNORMALITIES: THE MOST FREQUENT CAUSE OF EARLY PREGNANCY LOSS

Chromosomal abnormalities are the major cause of both preimplantation and clinically recognized pregnancy loss. Of

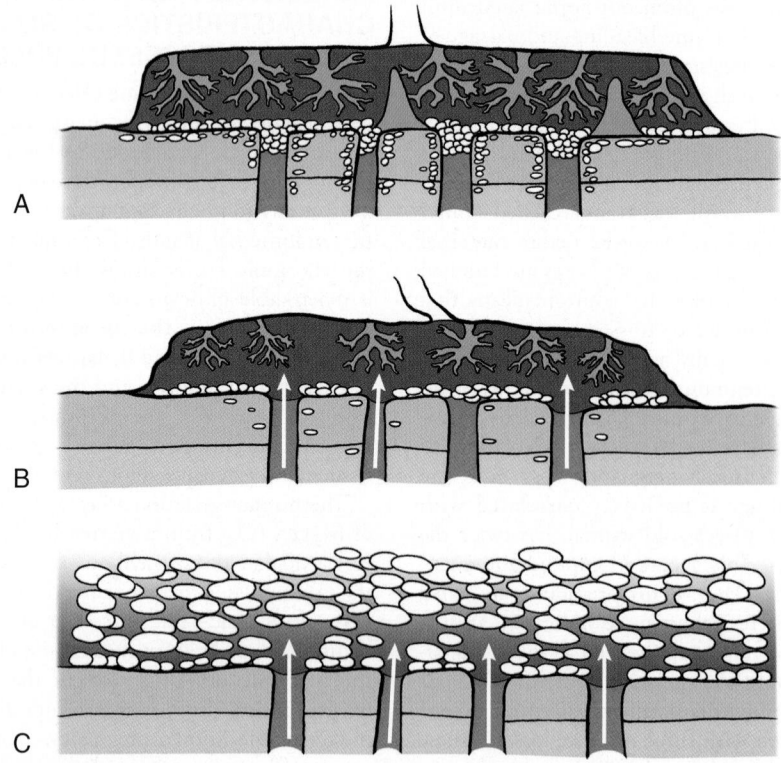

FIG 27-2 Placentation in a normal ongoing pregnancy **(A),** in an early pregnancy failure **(B),** and in a complete hydatidiform mole **(C). A,** Note the continuous trophoblastic shell, the plugs in the lumens of the spiral arteries, and the interstitial migration of the extravillous trophoblast through the decidua down to the superficial layer of the myometrium. **B,** Note the discontinuous trophoblastic shell, the absence of plugs, and the reduced migration of extravillous trophoblastic cells. **C,** Note the absence of trophoblastic plugs and interstitial migration. (From Jauniaux E, Burton GJ. Pathophysiology of histological changes in early pregnancy loss. *Placenta.* 2005;26:114.)

all morphologically *normal* embryos, 25% to 50% show chromosomal abnormalities (aneuploidy or polyploidy).[13] The highest figure occurs in women over age 45, and a more generalizable figure is 25% in the third decade increasing to 50% by late in the fourth decade. The frequency of chromosomal abnormalities in morphologically abnormal embryos is even higher. The high aneuploidy rate in morphologically normal embryos is consistent with 5% to 10% aneuploidy in sperm of ostensibly normal men and 20% aneuploidy in oocytes (deduced from polar bodies) of women undergoing ART.

Not surprisingly, at least 50% of *clinically recognized pregnancy losses* result from a chromosomal abnormality.[14] The frequency is probably higher, because if chorionic villi recovered by chorionic villus sampling (CVS) are analyzed immediately after ultrasound diagnosis of fetal demise, rather than culturing spontaneously expelled products, the chromosomal abnormalities are detected in 75% to 90%.[15] However, these cohorts were older than the general population.

Among second-trimester and third-trimester losses, chromosomal abnormalities are more similar in type to those observed in live-born infants: trisomies 13, 18, and 21; monosomy X; and sex chromosomal polysomies. This also holds true among losses after 20 gestational weeks (stillborn infants), for which the frequency of chromosomal abnormalities detected by karyotype has traditionally been cited as approximately 5%. The frequency is over 20% if anatomic abnormalities are present and chromosomal microarray (comparative genomic hybridization [CGH]) is used because cell culture is not needed to obtain information.[16] The American College of Obstetricians and Gynecologists (ACOG) now recommends array CGH for this purpose.[17] Of stillborn infants, 8.3% show cytogenomic abnormalities such as aneuploidy, microdeletions or microduplication based on array CGH, and copy number variants versus 5.8% by karyotype.[17] Overall, the frequency of demonstrable abnormalities is much less than that observed in earlier abortuses but is much higher than that found among liveborn infants (0.6%). Formal recommendations for the management of couples who have had a stillborn infant is undertaken later in this chapter.

Types of Numerical Chromosomal Abnormalities

Autosomal Trisomy

Autosomal trisomies represent the largest single class (about 50%) **of chromosomal complements in cytogenetically abnormal spontaneous abortions.** That is, 25% of all abortuses are aneuploid, given half of all abortuses have a chromosomal abnormality. Frequencies of various trisomies are listed in Table 27-2. Trisomy for every chromosome has been observed, but the most common is trisomy 16, which is lethal and is not observed in liveborn infants. Most trisomies show a maternal age effect, but the effect varies markedly among chromosomes. The increased maternal age effect is especially impressive for double trisomies.

Trisomies incompatible with life predictably show slower growth than those compatible with life (e.g., trisomies 13, 18, 21); but otherwise, usually no features distinguish the two groups. Abortuses from the former group may show anomalies consistent with those found in full-term, liveborn trisomic infants. Malformations present have been said to be more severe than those observed in induced abortuses following prenatal diagnosis.

TABLE 27-2 CHROMOSOMAL COMPLETION IN SPONTANEOUS ABORTIONS RECOGNIZED CLINICALLY IN THE FIRST TRIMESTER

CHROMOSOMAL COMPLEMENT	FREQUENCY	PERCENT
Normal 46,XX or 46,XY		54.1
Triploidy:		7.7
69,XXX	2.7	
69,XYX	0.2	
69,XXY	4.0	
Other	0.8	
Tetraploidy:		2.6
92,XXX	1.5	
92,XXYY	0.55	
Not stated	0.55	
Monosomy X		18.6
Structural abnormalities		1.5
Sex chromosome polysomy:		0.2
47,XXX	0.05	
47,XXY	0.15	
Autosomal monosomy (G)		0.1
Autosomal trisomy for chromosomes:		22.3
1	0	
2	1.11	
3	0.25	
4	0.64	
5	0.04	
6	0.14	
7	0.89	
8	0.79	
9	0.72	
10	0.36	
11	0.04	
12	0.18	
13	1.07	
14	0.82	
15	1.68	
16	7.27	
17	0.18	
18	1.15	
19	0.01	
20	0.61	
21	2.11	
22	2.26	
Double trisomy		0.7
Mosaic trisomy		1.3
Other abnormalities or not specified		0.9
		100.0

Data from Simpson JL, Bombard AT. Chromosomal abnormalities in spontaneous abortion: frequency, pathology and genetic counseling. In: Edmonds K (ed). *Spontaneous Abortion*. London: Blackwell; 1987.

Attempts have been made to correlate placental morphologic abnormalities with specific trisomies, but these relationships are imprecise. Comparison of ultrasound findings and placental histology indicates that villous changes following in utero fetal demise could explain the low predictive value of placental histology in identifying aneuploidy or another nonchromosomal etiology. By contrast, the histologic features of complete and partial hydatidiform molar gestations are so distinctive that most molar miscarriages can be correctly diagnosed by histologic examination alone.

Aneuploidy usually results from errors at maternal meiosis I, and these are associated with advanced maternal age.[18,19] Once thought to involve mostly missegregation of whole chromosomes, it is now clear that chromatid errors are an equally prevalent cause of maternal meiotic errors.[20] The cytologic mechanism involves decreased or absent meiotic recombination.

The cytologic origin is not the same for all chromosomes. In trisomy 13 and trisomy 21, 90% to 95% of these maternal cases arise at meiosis I; almost all trisomy 16 cases arise in maternal meiosis I.[18] In trisomy 18, two thirds of the 90% of maternal meiotic cases arise at meiosis II.[18]

One practical consequence of the maternal origin of aneuploidy is that deducing the chromosomal status of oocytes is possible by analysis of the polar bodies. In preimplantation genetic diagnosis, the most common approach is now blastocyst biopsy (5-day embryo), but diagnosis based on the first polar body uniquely allows preconception assessment, which in certain cultures or venues is the only option (Chapter 10). **Errors in *paternal* meiosis account for 10% of acrocentric (13, 14, 15, 21, and 22) trisomies.**[18] Among nonacrocentric chromosomes, paternal contribution is uncommon.

Polyploidy

In polyploidy, more than two haploid chromosomal complements are present. Nonmosaic triploidy (3n = 69) and tetraploidy (4n = 92) are common in abortuses. Triploid abortuses are usually 69,XXY or 69,XXX as a result of dispermy. An association exists between diandric (paternally inherited) triploidy and hydatidiform mole, a "partial" mole said to exist if molar tissue and fetal parts coexist. The more common "complete" (classic) hydatidiform mole is 46,XX; androgenetic in origin; and composed exclusively of villous tissue. Pathologic findings in diandric triploid and tetraploid placentae include a disproportionately large gestational sac, focal (partial) hydropic degeneration of placental villi, and trophoblast hyperplasia. Placental hydropic changes are progressive and may be difficult to identify in early pregnancy. By contrast, placental villi often undergo hydropic degeneration after fetal demise. This can occur in all types of miscarriage; thus histologic and cytogenetic

investigations are essential to differentiate between true mole and pseudomole because only a true mole can be associated with persistent trophoblastic disease. Fetal malformations associated with triploid miscarriage include neural tube defects and omphaloceles, anomalies reminiscent of those observed in triploid conceptuses that survive to term. Facial dysmorphia and limb abnormalities have also been reported. Tetraploidy is uncommon and rarely progresses beyond 2 to 3 weeks of embryonic life. This chromosomal abnormality can also be associated with persistent trophoblastic disease and thus needs to be identified in order to offer human chorionic gonadotropin (hCG) follow-up.

Sex Chromosome Polysomy (X or Y)

The complements 47,XXY and 47,XYY have long been stated to occur in about 1 per 800 liveborn male births; 47,XXX occurs in 1 per 800 female births. X and Y polysomies are only slightly more common in abortuses than in live-born infants. Recent work based on cell-free fetal DNA for detection of certain autosomal trisomies and sex chromosome polysomies indicates the incidence of the latter may be less than traditionally stated.[21] Irrespective, the group is not a major contributor to spontaneous abortion.

Monosomy X

Monosomy X is the single most common chromosomal abnormality among spontaneous abortions, accounting for 15% to 20% of abnormal specimens (see Table 27-2). Monosomy X embryos usually consist of only an umbilical cord stump. Later in gestation, anomalies characteristic of Turner syndrome may be seen, such as cystic hygromas and generalized edema (Fig. 27-3). Unlike adult 45,X individuals, 45,X abortuses show germ cells; however, most germ cells in abortuses do

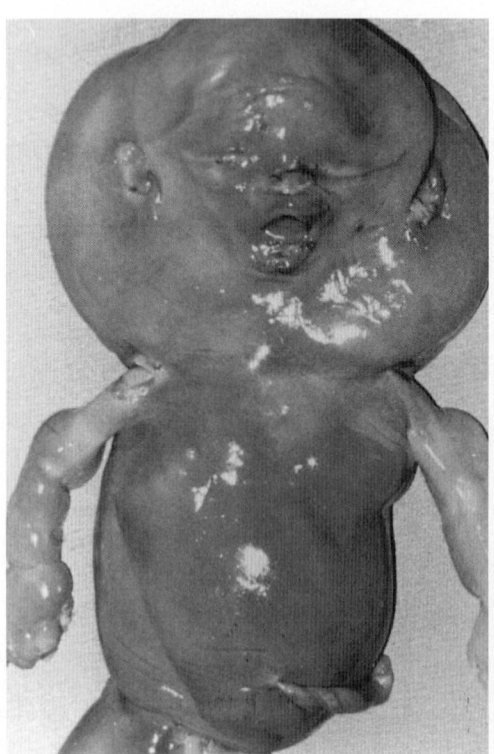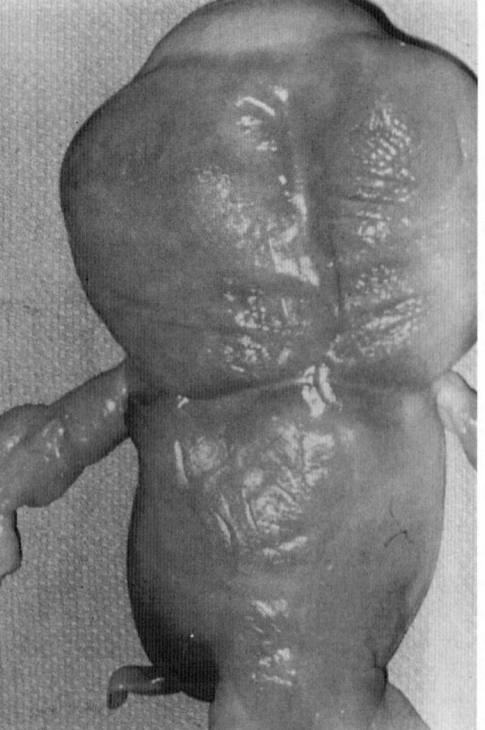

FIG 27-3 Photograph of a 45,X abortus. (From Simpson JL, Bombard AT. Chromosomal abnormalities in spontaneous abortion: frequency, pathology and genetic counseling. In Edmonds K, Bennett MJ [eds]: *Spontaneous Abortion*. London: Blackwell; 1987:51.)

TABLE 27-3	RECURRENT ANEUPLOIDY: RELATIONSHIP BETWEEN KARYOTYPES OF SUCCESSIVE ABORTUSES					
COMPLEMENT OF FIRST ABORTUS	**COMPLEMENT OF SECOND ABORTUS**					
	NORMAL	**TRISOMY**	**MONOSOMY**	**TRIPLOIDY**	**TETRAPLOID**	**DE NOVO REARRANGEMENT**
Normal	142	18	5	7	3	2
Trisomy	31	30	1	4	3	1
Monosomy X	7	5	3	3	0	0
Triploidy	7	4	1	4	0	0
Tetraploidy	3	1	0	2	0	0
De novo rearrangement	1	3	0	0	0	0

From Warburton D, Kline J, Stein Z, et al. Does the karyotype of a spontaneous abortion predict the karyotype of a subsequent abortion? Evidence from 273 women with two karyotyped spontaneous abortions. *Am J Hum Genet.* 1987;41:465.

not develop beyond the primordial germ cell stage. The pathogenesis of 45,X germ cell failure thus involves not so much failure of germ cell development as more rapid attrition in 45,X compared with 46,XX embryos.[24,25] Monosomy X usually occurs (80%) as a result of paternal sex chromosome loss, consistent with lack of a maternal age effect.

Relationship Between Recurrent Losses and Numerical Chromosomal Abnormalities

In both preimplantation and first-trimester abortions, recurrent aneuploidy occurs more often than would be expected by chance. Recurrent aneuploidy is a frequent explanation, at least until the number of losses reaches or exceeds four. **In a given family, successive abortuses are likely to be either recurrently normal or recurrently abnormal.** Table 27-3 shows that if the complement of the first abortus is abnormal,[26,27] recurrence usually involves aneuploidy, although not necessarily of the same chromosome. Further supporting recurrent aneuploidy as a genuine phenomenon is the occurrence of trisomic preimplantation embryos in successive ART cycles.[28,29]

The concept of recurrent aneuploidy implies certain corollaries, one of which has often been the subject of controversy. One is that in recurrent losses, couples should either be experiencing repetitive chromosomally abnormal abortuses or repetitive euploid (chromosomally normal) abortuses. Given that 50% of all abortuses are abnormal cytogenetically, aneuploidy should be as likely to be detected in a randomly karyotyped abortus as in a sporadic abortus. Among 420 abortuses obtained from women with repeated losses, Stephenson and colleagues[31] found 46% had chromosomal abnormalities; 31% of the original sample was trisomic. Their comparison was unselected pooled data, which showed 48% of abortuses to be abnormal; 27% of the original sample was trisomic.

In contrast to these data, a fetal loss—recurrent or not—is much more likely to be cytogenetically normal (85%) when it occurs after the first trimester. Carp and coworkers[32] found that among women with three or more abortions, the likelihood that the abortus would have an abnormal karyotype was only 29%. However, in that series, inclusion criteria extended to 20 weeks' gestation, a time at which there is less reason to expect recurrent aneuploidy than recurrence of other etiologies.

Genetic Counseling and Management for Recurrent Aneuploidy

Couples predisposed to recurrent aneuploidy are at increased risk not only for aneuploid abortuses but also for aneuploid livebornneonates. The trisomic autosome in a subsequent pregnancy might be compatible with life (e.g., trisomy 21). Indeed, the risk for liveborn trisomy 21 following an aneuploid abortus is considered clinically to be about 1% (see Chapter 10). A 1% recurrence risk is considered similar following other autosomal aneuploidies. Bianco and associates[34] provided a useful counseling algorithm applicable following a prior abortion of unknown karyotype. If abortions are recurrent but no information is available on the chromosomal status, the odds ratio can be used to derive a patient-specific risk. For example, if the a priori Down syndrome risk is 1 in 300 and the odds ratio is 1.5, a woman's calculated risk after three abortions would be 1/300 × 1.5, or 1 in 200.

If no information is available concerning the chromosomal status of prior abortions, paraffin blocks of archived products of conception can be retrieved to detect aneuploidy using array CGH, given that array CGH requires only DNA and not the cultured cells needed for a karyotype. Paraffin block or results of other archived DNA showing a prior trisomy confers increased risk for liveborn trisomy in subsequent pregnancies. If no information can be obtained, it is arguable whether prenatal genetic diagnosis is appropriate. The absolute risk for aneuploid offspring can, however, be calculated as shown by Bianco and associates.[34] The small but finite risk for amniocentesis or CVS is troublesome to couples who have had difficulty achieving a live birth. At present, noninvasive cell-free DNA approaches (see Chapter 10) are typically the chosen option. However, sensitivity for detecting aneuploidy by noninvasive methods is not the nearly 100% possible with CVS or amniocentesis. Preimplantation genetic diagnosis (PGD; see Chapter 10) is another option, and it is the only one if the couple eschews clinical pregnancy termination. Selective transfer of euploid embryos clearly decreases the rate of clinical abortions in couples who experience repeated losses.[35,36] When avoiding another loss is paramount, PGD should be offered.

CHROMOSOMAL REARRANGEMENTS
Translocations

Structural chromosomal abnormalities are an unequivocal explanation for repetitive abortions. The most common structural rearrangement encountered is a translocation, **found in about 5% of couples who experience repeated losses.** Individuals with balanced translocations are phenotypically normal, but their offspring—abortuses and abnormal liveborn infants— may show chromosomal duplications or deficiencies as a result of normal meiotic segregation. Among couples with repetitive abortions, about 60% of translocations are reciprocal and 40% are robertsonian. **Women are about twice as likely as men to show a balanced translocation.**[37]

The clinical consequences of a balanced translocation vary depending on the chromosome involved and the type of translocation. If a child has Down syndrome as result of a centric fusion (robertsonian) translocation, the rearrangement will have originated de novo in 50% to 75% of cases. That is, a balanced translocation will not exist in either parent. The likelihood of Down syndrome recurring in subsequent offspring is minimal. On the other hand, the recurrence is significant when an offspring has Down syndrome as result of transmission of a parental translocation. The theoretic risk for having a child with Down syndrome is 33%, but empiric risks are considerably less. The risk is only 2% if the father carries the translocation; the risk is 10% if the mother carries the translocation.[38,39] If robertsonian (centric fusion) translocations involve chromosomes other than 21, liveborn empiric risks are lower; this reflects embryonic lethality. In t(13q;14q), the risk for liveborn trisomy 13 is 1% or less.

Reciprocal translocations involve not centromeric fusion but rather interchanges between two or more chromosomes. Empiric data for specific translocations are usually not available, but generalizations can be made on the basis of pooled data derived from many different translocations.[40] Again, theoretic risks for abnormal offspring (unbalanced reciprocal translocations) are far greater than empiric risks applicable to liveborn infants or even prenatal genetic diagnosis. **Overall, the risk is 12% for offspring of either female heterozygotes or male heterozygotes.**[38,39] Detecting a chromosomal rearrangement thus profoundly affects subsequent pregnancy management. Antenatal cytogenetic studies should be offered. The frequency of unbalanced fetuses is lower if parental balanced translocations are ascertained through repetitive abortions (3%) rather than through anomalous liveborn infants (nearly 20%).[38] Presumably more unbalanced products are lethal.

PGD of embryos from couples who have a balanced translocation reveals that most embryos are unbalanced: 58% in robertsonian translocations and 76% in reciprocal translocations. This means almost all these conceptuses would be lost preclinically. When a balanced translocation is detected in a couple who experiences recurrent abortions, the *cumulative* prognosis for a liveborn infant differs little from that if a translocation had not been detected.[42] However, the length of time to achieve pregnancy is greatly increased (mean, 4 to 6 years). Thus a more realistic strategy is to use PGD to identify and transfer only the few balanced embryos, thereby increasing the statistical likelihood of conception.[43] This strategy is most attractive when the prospective mother is in her fourth or early fifth decade. Using array CGH, an unbalanced embryo can be readily excluded; however, unlike fluorescence in situ hybridization (FISH), array CGH does not distinguish a balanced (translocation heterozygote) from a normal embryo lacking the translocation.

Rarely, a translocation precludes normal liveborn infants. This occurs when a translocation involves homologous, acrocentric chromosomes (e.g., t[13q13q] or t[21q21q]). If the father carries such a structural rearrangement, artificial insemination may be appropriate. If the mother carries the rearrangement, donor oocytes or donor embryos and ART should be considered.

Inversions

Inversions are uncommon parental chromosomal rearrangements but are responsible for repetitive pregnancy losses analogous to translocations. **In inversions, the order of the genes is reversed.** Individuals heterozygous for an inversion should be normal if their genes are merely rearranged. However, individuals with inversions suffer untoward reproductive consequences as a result of normal meiotic phenomena.[44] Crossing over that involves the inverted segment yields unbalanced gametes. Pericentric inversions are present in perhaps 0.1% of women and 0.1% of men who experience repeated spontaneous abortions. Paracentric inversions are even rarer.

Women with a *pericentric* inversion have a 7% risk for abnormal liveborn infants; men carry a 5% risk.[40] Pericentric inversions ascertained through phenotypically normal probands are less likely to result in abnormal liveborn infants. Inversions that involve only a small portion of the total chromosomal length paradoxically are less significant clinically because large duplications or deficiencies arise following crossing over, which usually confers lethality. By contrast, inversions that involve only 30% to 60% of the total chromosomal length are relatively more likely to be characterized by duplications or deficiencies compatible with survival. Prenatal cytogenetic studies should be offered.

Paracentric inversions should carry less risk for unbalanced products than pericentric inversions because nearly all paracentric recombinants should in theory be lethal. However, abortions and abnormal liveborn infants have rarely been observed within the same kindred, and the risk for unbalanced viable offspring has been tabulated at 4%.[45] Prenatal cytogenetic studies should thus still be offered.

MENDELIAN AND POLYGENIC/MULTIFACTORIAL ETIOLOGY

That 30% to 50% of first-trimester abortuses show no chromosomal abnormalities does not mean genetic causation is excluded. Fetal demise may have occurred as a result of other genetic etiologies. Specifically, neither mendelian nor polygenic/multifactorial disorders show chromosomal abnormalities, and these etiologies account for more congenital anomalies than do chromosomal abnormalities. It would thus be naïve to assume that mendelian and polygenic/multifactorial factors do not play pivotal roles in embryonic mortality. The difficulty is that it is challenging to identify developmental genes expressed only during embryogenesis. Most likely to be mendelian or polygenic in etiology are abortuses that demonstrate isolated structural anomalies. Cytogenetic data are often lacking on dissected specimens, making it nearly impossible to determine the relative role of cytogenetic versus mendelian or polygenic mechanisms in early embryonic maldevelopment. However, Philipp and Kalousek[46] correlated cytogenetic status of missed abortuses with morphologic abnormalities at embryoscopy. Embryos with chromosomal abnormalities usually showed one or more external anomalies, although some euploid embryos also showed anatomic anomalies.

In addition to traditional single-gene perturbations (mendelian etiology), novel nonmendelian forms of inheritance probably play a greater role in embryonic loss than in liveborn abnormalities. **Mosaicism may be restricted to the placenta, the embryo per se being normal. This phenomenon is termed** *confined placental mosaicism*.

LUTEAL PHASE DEFECTS

Implantation in an inhospitable endometrium is a plausible explanation for pregnancy loss. Progesterone deficiency in particular could result in the estrogen-primed endometrium being unable to sustain implantation. Luteal phase deficiency (LPD) has long been hypothesized, specifically caused by inadequate progesterone secreted by the corpus luteum.

Once almost universally accepted as a common cause of fetal wastage, LPD is now generally considered an uncommon explanation. One pitfall is that endometrial histology identical to that observed with luteal phase "defects" is observed in fertile women. Efficacy of treatment has also never been proved—no randomized studies exist. Indeed, meta-analysis has shown[47] no beneficial effect of progesterone treatment. **The current consensus is that LPD is either an arguable entity or not proved to be treated successfully with progesterone or progestational therapy.**

Luteal phase abnormalities that arise during ovulation stimulation and necessitated during ART could be a different phenomenon. It is considered standard to administer progesterone until about 9 weeks' gestation. In this circumstance, the cells that surround the oocyte, which would ordinarily contribute to the corpus luteum, may have been removed when the oocyte was aspirated.

THYROID ABNORMALITIES

Decreased conception rates and increased fetal losses are logically associated with overt hypothyroidism or hyperthyroidism (see Chapter 42). The role of subclinical thyroid dysfunction is less clear and is not generally considered an explanation for repeated losses. However, Negro and colleagues[48] reported that pregnancy loss was higher in thyroid peroxidase–negative women whose thyroid-stimulating hormone (TSH) level was 2.5 to 4 mIU/L compared with those whose TSH level was less than 2.5 mIU/L (6.1% vs. 3.6%). Increased frequency of thyroid antibodies has in addition been observed in several series, and some consider autoimmune thyroid disease a significant cause.[49] The value of treatment in such circumstances is unproved.

Elevations of maternal thyroid hormone per se are clearly deleterious. This effect was shown by a family from the Azores, in whom a gene that conferred resistance to thyroid hormone was segregating.[50] Family members with an autosomal dominant mutation in the thyroid receptor beta (TR-β) gene *Arg243Gln* secreted large amounts of TSH to compensate for end-organ resistance. During pregnancy, the fetus of such a mother becomes unavoidably exposed to high levels of maternal TSH because TSH and thyroxine readily cross the placenta. Loss rates were 22.8% in pregnancies of mothers who had the *Arg243Gln* mutation, 2% in those of normal mothers whose male partner had the mutation, and 4.4% when neither parent had the mutation.

DIABETES MELLITUS

Women whose diabetes mellitus is poorly controlled are at increased risk for fetal loss. Mills and colleagues[51] showed in a National Institute of Child Health and Human Development (NICHD) collaborative study that women whose glycosylated hemoglobin (HgB) level was greater than 4 standard deviations

(SDs) above the mean had higher pregnancy loss rates than women with lower glycosylated HgB levels. This finding is consistent with that of many retrospective studies.[52] Poorly controlled diabetes mellitus should be considered one cause for early pregnancy loss. On the other hand, well-controlled or subclinical diabetes should not be considered a cause of early miscarriage. Neither the Royal College of Obstetricians and Gynaecologists (RCOG) nor ACOG recommend testing for occult diabetes mellitus.

INTRAUTERINE ADHESIONS (SYNECHIAE)

Intrauterine adhesions could interfere with implantation or early embryonic development. Adhesions may follow intrauterine surgery (e.g., myomectomy), endometritis, or overzealous uterine curettage during the postpartum period. Curettage is the usual explanation, with adhesions most likely to develop when the procedure is performed 3 or 4 weeks after delivery. Individuals with uterine synechiae usually manifest hypomenorrhea or amenorrhea, but perhaps 15% to 30% have repeated spontaneous abortions. If adhesions are detected in a woman who experiences repetitive losses, lysis under direct hyperoscopic visualization should be performed. Postoperatively, an intrauterine device (IUD) or inflated Foley catheter temporarily placed postoperatively in the uterus discourages reapposition of healing uterine surfaces. Estrogen administration should also be initiated. About 50% of patients conceive after surgery, but the frequency of pregnancy losses remains high.

MÜLLERIAN FUSION DEFECTS

Müllerian fusion defects are an accepted cause of *second-trimester* losses and pregnancy complications. Low birthweight, breech presentation, and uterine bleeding are the most common abnormalities associated with müllerian fusion defects compared with pregnancies in women who have hysterosalpingogram-proven normal uteri.[53] However, reports typically lack controls.

Losses are more likely to be associated with a uterine septum than a bicornuate uterus.[54] In 509 women with recurrent losses studied by three-dimensional (3-D) ultrasound, Salim and associates[55] found greater uterine distortion in women who recounted a history of losses. However, the major problem in attributing cause and effect for second-trimester complications and uterine anomalies is that uterine anomalies are frequent in the general population; thus adverse outcomes could merely be coincidental. For example, in the Salim study, 23.8% of women with recurrent miscarriage had some uterine anomalies on 3-D ultrasound.[55] In another study, unsuspected bicornuate uteri were found in 1.2% of 167 women undergoing laparoscopic sterilization; 3.6% had a severely septate uterus, whereas 15.3% had fundal anomalies.[56] In another series, müllerian defects were found in 22 of 679 fertile women (3.2%), and 20 of the 22 defects were septate.[57]

Treatment has traditionally involved surgical correction, namely metroplasty. Ludmir and colleagues[58] wondered whether aggressive nonsurgical treatment could be just as efficacious. A total of 101 women with an uncorrected malformation were tracked longitudinally. After first being followed without surgery and without a defined nonsurgical regimen, the same women underwent a surgically conservative but medically aggressive protocol that consisted of decreased physical activity and tocolysis. However, fetal survival rates in both bicornuate and septate groups were not significantly different before (52% and 53%, respectively) or after (58% and 65%, respectively) the change in management.

In conclusion, early first-trimester abortions may be caused by müllerian fusion defects, but other explanations are more likely even when such a defect is found. Septate uteri are most plausibly causative, with implantation occurring on a poorly vascularized and inhospitable surface. Abortions that occur after ultrasonographic confirmation of a viable pregnancy— say, at 8 or 9 weeks—may more properly be attributed to uterine fusion defects. Women who experience second-trimester losses could benefit from uterine reconstruction, but reconstructive surgery is not necessarily advisable if losses are restricted to the first trimester.

LEIOMYOMAS

Although leiomyomas are common, relatively few women develop symptoms that require medical or surgical therapy. That leiomyomas cause first- or second-trimester pregnancy wastage per se, rather than obstetric complications such as prematurity, is plausible but probably uncommon. Analogous to uterine anomalies, the coexistence of two common phenomena— uterine leiomyomas and reproductive losses—need not necessarily imply a causal relationship. Hartmann and Herring[59] correlated ultrasonographically detected leiomyomas with pregnancy outcome in a cohort of North Carolina women. Of 1313 women studied early in pregnancy, the 131 with leiomyomas as ascertained by ultrasound had an increased prior spontaneous abortion rate (odds ratio [OR], 2.17). One pitfall is that uterine contractions can mimic fibroids on ultrasound.

Location of leiomyomas is probably more important than size. Submucous leiomyomas are more likely to cause abortion than subserous leiomyomas. Postulated mechanisms that lead to pregnancy loss include (1) thinning of the endometrium over the surface of a submucous leiomyoma, predisposing to implantation in a poorly decidualized site; (2) rapid growth caused by the hormonal milieu of pregnancy, compromising the blood supply of the leiomyoma and resulting in necrosis ("red degeneration") that in turn leads to uterine contractions and eventually fetal expulsion; and (3) encroachment of leiomyomas on the space required for the developing fetus, leading to premature delivery through mechanisms presumably analogous to those operative in incomplete müllerian fusion. In pregnancies that are not lost, the relative lack of space can also lead to fetal deformations (i.e., positional abnormalities that arise in a genetically normal fetus).

Surgical procedures to reduce leiomyomas may occasionally be warranted in women who experience repetitive second-trimester abortions. **More often, however, leiomyomas have no etiologic relationship to pregnancy loss. Surgery should be reserved for women whose abortuses were both phenotypically and karyotypically normal and in whom viability until at least 9 to 10 weeks was documented.**

CERVICAL INSUFFICIENCY

A functionally intact cervix and lower uterine cavity are obvious prerequisites for a successful pregnancy. Characterized by painless dilation and effacement, *cervical incompetence*—now preferably called *cervical insufficiency*—usually occurs during the middle second or early third trimester and usually follows traumatic events such as cervical amputations, lacerations, or conization or forceful cervical dilation. However, the etiology may be genetic; for example, perturbation of a connective tissue gene (e.g., collagen, fibrillin). Indications for surgery and techniques to correct cervical incompetence are discussed in Chapter 28.

INFECTIONS

Infections are a known cause of late fetal losses and a logical cause of early fetal losses. Along with vaccinia, microorganisms associated with spontaneous abortion include variola, *Salmonella typhi, Campylobacter fetus (Vibrio fetus bacterin)*, malaria, cytomegalovirus, *Brucella, Toxoplasma gondii, Mycoplasma hominis, Chlamydia trachomatis,* and *Ureaplasma urealyticum*. Transplacental infection occurs with each of these microorganisms, following which sporadic losses could logically result. However, **infection as a cause of *repetitive* losses is much less likely.**

Of the many organisms implicated in repetitive abortion, *U. urealyticum* and *M. hominis* seem most plausibly related to repetitive spontaneous abortions because they fulfill two important prerequisites: first, the putative organism can persist in an asymptomatic state; second, virulence is not always so severe as to cause infertility as a result of fallopian tube occlusion and, hence, it does not preclude the opportunity for pregnancy. Studies have also suggested a relationship between bacterial vaginosis (BV), presumed to be *Gardnerella vaginalis,* and spontaneous abortion. However, the latter is more typically, if not exclusively, associated with complications (premature delivery) in the second and third trimesters. A recent systematic review and meta-analysis[60] on the risks associated with BV in infertile patients has shown that it is associated with a significantly elevated risk of preclinical pregnancy loss but is not associated with an increased risk of first-trimester miscarriage.

Given lack of evidence for causality for recurrent losses, it could be questioned whether the infectious agents discussed previously actually cause fetal losses or merely arise after fetal demise from other causes. Cohort surveillance for infections can best shed light on the true role of infections in early pregnancy loss. The frequency of clinical infections was assessed prospectively in 386 diabetic subjects and 432 control subjects seen weekly or every other week beginning early in the first trimester.[61] Infection occurred no more often in the 112 subjects who experienced pregnancy loss than in the 706 who experienced successful pregnancies. This held true both for the 2-week interval in which a given loss was recognized clinically and the prior 2-week interval. Similar findings were observed in both control and diabetic subjects and were substantiated when data were stratified into ascending genital infections only versus systemic infection only.

In conclusion, infections doubtless explain some early pregnancy losses and certainly many later losses. However, in the first trimester, attributable risk is low even in sporadic cases, and in recurrent losses, infections are much less likely.

ACQUIRED THROMBOPHILIAS

An association between *second-trimester* pregnancy loss and certain autoimmune diseases is well accepted[16] (see Chapter 46). **For first-trimester losses, consensus holds that a less**

significant relationship exists. The spectrum of antibodies found in women with pregnancy loss encompasses nonspecific antinuclear antibodies as well as antibodies against individual cellular components such as phospholipids, histones, and single- or double-stranded DNA. The primary antigenic determinant is β_2-glycoprotein, which has an affinity for negatively charged phospholipids.[62] The **antiphospholipid syndrome** encompasses lupus anticoagulant (LAC) antibodies, anticardiolipin (aCL) antibody, or anti–β_2-glycoprotein. Values for the latter two should be greater than the 99th percentile of moderate or higher titers, with two positive results obtained 12 weeks apart. Descriptive studies in the 1980s initially seemed to show increased aCLs in women with first-trimester pregnancy losses; however, a pitfall proved to be selection bias because it only studied couples following spontaneous abortions. That antibodies did not arise until *after* the pregnancy loss was also not excluded. To address this, Simpson and associates[63] analyzed sera obtained prospectively from women within 21 days of conception. A total of 93 women who later experienced pregnancy loss were matched 2 to 1 with 190 controls who subsequently had a normal liveborn offspring. No association was observed between pregnancy loss and presence of either aPL or aCL.

In the most recent ACOG bulletin on the topic,[62] three or more losses before the tenth week of pregnancy is considered to fulfill diagnostic criteria for antiphospholipid syndrome in the sense of justifying prophylactic heparin therapy. It was stated that this assumes neither anatomic or hormonal abnormalities, nor paternal or maternal chromosomal abnormalities. However, ACOG provided the caveat that such an increase neither explains many losses nor confers a greatly increased risk for another loss. Given this, treatment regimens should be judicious, perhaps with aspirin and heparin if embarked on at all. Control groups of fertile women showed similar loss frequencies.

INHERITED THROMBOPHILIAS

Inherited maternal hypercoagulable states are unequivocally associated with increased fetal losses in the second trimester but less convincingly in the first trimester (see Chapter 45). Postulated associations include factor V Leiden (Q1691G→A), prothrombin 2021G→A, and homozygosity for 677C→T in the methylenetetrahydrofolate reductase gene *MTHFR*. A meta-analysis[64] of 31 studies published in 2003 revealed **associations between recurrent (two or more) fetal losses earlier than 13 weeks for thrombophilias related to factor V Leiden (G1691A), activated protein-C resistance, prothrombin (*20210A0* gene), and protein-S deficiency.** No associations were found between deficiencies of *MTHFR,* protein C, and antithrombin and recurrent pregnancy loss. A second meta-analysis of 16 studies published by Kovalesky and coworkers[65] reported an association between *recurrent pregnancy loss*, defined as two or more losses in the first two trimesters, and maternal heterozygosity for either factor V Leiden or prothrombin 20210G7→A.

Evidence is less strong for an association between inherited thrombophilias and recurrent early pregnancy loss (REPL) before 10 weeks of gestation. Most authors recommend testing for factor V Leiden, activated protein-C resistance, fasting homocysteine, antiphospholipid antibodies (aPLs), and the prothrombin gene. Pending salutary results in randomized controlled trials (RCTs), treatment for recurrent first-trimester losses with heparin or other antithrombotic or anticoagulant therapies should be initiated with caution.

EXOGENOUS AGENTS

Various exogenous agents have been implicated in fetal losses, although studies fail to stratify these by sporadic and recurrent losses (see Chapter 8). Of course, every pregnant woman is exposed to low doses of ubiquitous agents, and data are rarely adequate to determine with confidence the role these exogenous factors play in early pregnancy losses.

Outcomes following exposures to exogenous agents can usually be derived only on the basis of case-control studies. In such studies, women who experienced an adverse event (e.g., spontaneous abortion) recalled exposure to the agent in question more often than controls. However, case-control studies have inherent biases. The primary bias is accuracy of recall because controls have less incentive to recall antecedent events than subjects who experience an abnormal outcome. Employers also naturally attempt to limit exposure to women of reproductive age; thus exposures to potentially dangerous chemicals are usually unwitting and, hence, poorly documented. Pregnant women are also exposed to many agents concurrently, making it nearly impossible to attribute adverse effects to a single agent. Given these caveats, **physicians should be cautious about attributing pregnancy loss to exogenous agents.** On the other hand, common sense dictates that exposure to potentially noxious agents should be minimized.

Radiation and Chemotherapeutic Agents

Irradiation and antineoplastic agents in high doses are acknowledged abortifacients. Of course, therapeutic radiographs or chemotherapeutic drugs are administered during pregnancy only to seriously ill women whose pregnancies often must be terminated for maternal indications. More frequently encountered, pelvic x-ray exposure of up to perhaps 10 cGy places a woman at little to no increased risk. The exposure is usually to far lower doses (1 to 2 cGy). **It is also prudent for pregnant hospital workers to avoid handling chemotherapeutic agents and to minimize radiation exposures during diagnostic imaging.**

Alcohol

Alcohol consumption should be avoided during pregnancy for reasons independent of pregnancy loss (see Chapters 6 and 8). However, alcohol probably increases pregnancy loss only slightly. Some authors found a slightly increased risk for spontaneous abortion in women who drank in the first trimester, whereas others[66] found alcohol consumption to be nearly identical in women who did and did not experience an abortion: 13% of women who aborted and 11% of control women drank on average three to four drinks per week, and other investigations have reached a similar conclusion. Armstrong and colleagues[67] found the odds ratio to be 1.82 with 20 drinks or more per week.

Abstinence from alcohol should not be expected to prevent pregnancy loss, and evaluation for other causes is still in order. Thus **women should not attribute a loss to social alcohol exposure during early gestation.**

Caffeine

In data gathered in cohort fashion, Mills and colleagues[68] showed that the odds ratio for association between pregnancy loss and caffeine (coffee and other dietary forms) was only 1.15 (95% confidence interval [CI], 0.89 to 1.49). Women exposed to much higher levels may, however, be at greater risk. Klebanoff and coworkers[69] reported an association between pregnancy losses and caffeine ingestion greater than 300 mg daily (a 1.9-fold increase). A confounding problem with investigating caffeine is difficulty in taking into account the effects of nausea, which is believed to be more common in successful pregnancies. **In general, reassurance can be given concerning moderate caffeine exposure and pregnancy loss.**

Contraceptive Agents

Conception with an IUD in place increases the risk for fetal loss and can result in second-trimester sepsis characterized by a flulike syndrome, albeit rarely. If the device is removed before pregnancy, there is no increased risk for spontaneous miscarriage. **Oral contraceptive use before or during pregnancy is not associated with fetal loss.** The same applies for injectable or implantable contraceptives. No evidence suggests increased pregnancy loss after spermicide exposure before or after conception.

Chemicals

Limiting exposure to potential toxins in the workplace is prudent for pregnant women. The difficulty lies in first defining the precise effect of lower exposures and then attributing a specific risk. False alarms concerning potential toxins are frequent. **Various chemical agents have been claimed to be associated with fetal losses, but only a few are accepted as potentially causative.**[70] These include anesthetic gases, arsenic, aniline dyes, benzene, solvents, ethylene oxide, formaldehyde, pesticides, and certain divalent cations (lead, mercury, cadmium). Workers in rubber industries, battery factories, and chemical production plants are among those at potential risk.

Cigarette Smoking

Active and passive maternal smoking has a damaging effect in every trimester of human pregnancy. Cigarette smoke contains scores of toxins that exert a direct effect on the placental and fetal cell proliferation and differentiation and can explain the increased risk for miscarriage, fetal growth restriction (FGR), stillbirth, preterm birth, and placental abruption reported by epidemiologic studies.[71] Smoking during pregnancy is often claimed to cause miscarriage, but in available studies, confounding variables are rarely excluded. Increased miscarriage rates reported in smokers do, however, appear to be independent of maternal age and alcohol consumption[72]; based on urinary cotinine levels, 400 women with spontaneous abortions were compared with 570 who experienced ongoing pregnancies. Women with urinary cotinine had increased risk for miscarriage, but the odds ratio was only 1.8 (95% CI, 1.3 to 2.6). A recent systematic review and meta-analysis[73] has shown that any active smoking is associated with increased risk of miscarriage (relative risk ratio [RR], 1.23; 95% CI, 1.16 to 1.30) and that the risk increases with the amount smoked (1% increase in RR per cigarette smoked per day). Furthermore, **secondhand (passive) smoke exposure during pregnancy increases the risk of miscarriage by 11%.**

Smoking is associated, from early pregnancy, with a thickening in the placenta of the trophoblastic basement membrane, an increase in collagen content of the villous mesenchyme, and a decrease in vascularization. These anatomic changes are associated with changes in placental enzymatic and synthetic functions. In particular, nicotine depresses active amino acid uptake by human placental villi and trophoblast invasion, and cadmium decreases the expression and activity of 11β-hydroxysteroid dehydrogenase type 2, which is causally linked to FGR.[71] Within this context, direct damage to placental tissue could explain the higher rate of miscarriage in heavy smokers.

TRAUMA

Women commonly attribute pregnancy losses to trauma, such as a fall or blow to the abdomen (see Chapter 26). Actually, fetuses are well protected from external trauma by intervening maternal structures and amniotic fluid. The temptation to attribute a loss to minor traumatic events should be avoided. A nested case-control study of 392 cases and 807 controls showed no relationship between physical violence and miscarriage.[74]

PSYCHOLOGICAL FACTORS

That impaired psychological well-being predisposes to early fetal losses has been claimed but never proven. Certainly, mentally ill women experience losses, but so do normal women. Whether the frequency of losses is higher in the mentally ill is less certain because potential confounding variables have not been taken into account, nor have confounding genetic factors been considered. Mental illness in pregnancy is discussed in detail in Chapter 55.

Investigations most frequently cited as showing a benefit of psychological well-being are those of Stray-Pedersen and Stray-Pedersen.[75] Pregnant women who previously experienced repetitive spontaneous abortions received increased attention but no specific medical therapy ("tender loving care"). These women ($n = 16$) were more likely (85%) to complete their pregnancy than women ($n = 42$) not offered such close attention (36%). One pitfall was that only women living close to the university were eligible to be placed in the increased-attention group. Women who lived farther away served as controls; however, these women may have differed from the experimental group in other ways as well. Other studies have also reported a beneficial effect of psychological well-being.[75,76] Again, pitfalls exist in study design, and the biologic explanation for this salutary effect remains obscure.

COMMON MEDICATIONS

Nonsteroidal antiinflammatory drugs (NSAIDs) are widely used during pregnancy. A recent cohort of 65,457 women found no increased risk of early pregnancy loss for specific NSAID drugs except for a significantly increased risk with exposure to indomethacin.[77]

A large Danish epidemiologic study of 22,061 pregnancies exposed to antidepressants found a slightly increased risk of miscarriage.[78] Among women with a diagnosis of depression, antidepressants in general, and individual selective serotonin reuptake inhibitors (SSRIs) in particular, are not associated with miscarriage. In a similar study from Denmark, women taking antiepileptic drugs were not at a higher risk of early pregnancy loss.[79]

MANAGEMENT OF RECURRENT EARLY PREGNANCY LOSS

Although some epidemiologic, clinical, and biochemical risk factors are clearly associated with REPL, a specific etiology in most cases remains unknown. **Two main concepts have dominated the literature on this topic in the last two decades: (1) that REPL is mainly caused by aneuploid conceptions and other genetic errors and that the recurrence rate can be explained by the combination of chance and increased risk and (2) that maternal thrombophilic, endocrine, or immune system abnormalities play a main role in causing loss of euploid conceptions.**

Faced with a couple who has experienced a miscarriage, the obstetrician has several immediate obligations that are to (1) provide the couple information on the overall frequency of fetal wastage (10% to 12% of clinically recognized pregnancies[80] and many more unrecognized) and likely etiology (genetic and especially cytogenetic); (2) provide them with individual applicable recurrence risks (see Table 27-2); and (3) determine the necessity for a formal clinical evaluation that includes ultrasound screening for uterine anomalies and laboratory screening of parental chromosomes and maternal aPLs. Fulfilling the responsibility to inform patients can be facilitated by summarizing the salient facts cited in this chapter, emphasizing common etiologies responsible for fetal losses. Explicitly worth citing is the positive correlation between loss rates and both maternal age and prior losses. The maternal age effect is not solely the result of increased aneuploid conception but is also reflective of endometrial vascular, endocrinologic, and immunologic factors.

When Is Formal Evaluation Necessary?

A couple who experiences even one loss should be counseled and provided with recurrence risk rates. However, not every couple needs formal assessment and a battery of tests. Infertile couples in which the female partner is in her late thirties or older may choose to be evaluated formally after only two losses and may opt for PGD aneuploidy testing if they require in vitro fertilization (IVF). After three losses, couples have traditionally been directed to formal evaluation. **Although a firm scientific basis for waiting until three losses is lacking, this is the benchmark for the RCOG and the European Society of Human Reproduction and Embryology (ESHRE).**[80] **The ACOG defines *recurrent loss* as either two or three consecutive losses.** This 2001 ACOG guideline[81] is perhaps more defensible scientifically, but the "consecutive" part is arguable.

A couple being evaluated should undergo all the tests used by a given practitioner. Little rationale exists for pursuing certain studies after two losses yet deferring others until three or more losses. **Any couple who has a stillborn or anomalous liveborn infant should undergo cytogenetic studies unless the stillborn was known to have a normal chromosomal complement.** Parental chromosomal (conventional metaphase) rearrangements (i.e., translocations or inversions) should be excluded. If chromosomal studies on the stillborn were unsuccessful, common aneuploidies can still be ruled out by performing FISH on stored deparaffined tissue.

Recommended Evaluation

Couples who experience only one first-trimester spontaneous abortion should receive relevant information but not necessarily a formal evaluation. They should be apprised of the relatively high (10% to 15%) pregnancy loss rate in the general population and also the beneficial effects of miscarriage in eliminating abnormal conceptuses. The clinician can also provide relevant recurrence risks; usually 20% to 25% of subsequent losses occur to couples who had a prior liveborn infant, and this statistic is only slightly higher in the absence of a prior liveborn infant (see Table 27-1). However, risks are higher for older women than younger women. If a specific medical illness exists, treatment is obviously necessary. If present, intrauterine adhesions should be lysed. Otherwise, no further evaluation need be undertaken, even if uterine anomalies or leiomyomas are present.

Investigation may or may not be necessary after two spontaneous abortions, depending on the patient's age and personal desires; after three, evaluation is usually indicated. If not done previously, the clinician should (1) obtain a detailed family history, (2) perform a complete physical examination, (3) discuss recurrence risks, and (4) order selected tests enumerated in this chapter. Occurrence of a stillborn or liveborn infant with anomalies warrants genetic evaluation irrespective of the number of pregnancy losses.

Parental chromosomal studies should be undertaken on all couples who experience repetitive losses. Antenatal chromosomal studies should be offered if a balanced chromosomal rearrangement is detected in either parent or if autosomal trisomy occurred in any previous abortus.

Although it is perhaps impractical to karyotype all abortuses, cytogenetic information on abortuses is valuable. Detection of a trisomic abortus suggests recurrent aneuploidy, which justifies prenatal cytogenetic studies in future pregnancies. Performing invasive prenatal cytogenetic studies solely on the basis of repeated losses is more arguable but not unreasonable among women aged 30 years and older.

Endocrine causes for repeated fetal losses include poorly controlled diabetes mellitus, overt thyroid dysfunction, and elevated maternal TSH levels. Subclinical diabetes or subclinical thyroid disease (TSH >2.5 mIU/L) should not be considered firm explanations.[82] Luteal phase defects are also no longer considered a likely explanation, although luteal support (progesterone) is still prescribed in pregnancies achieved with IVF. Progesterone supplementation is safe for both mother and baby, but data are insufficient to support its routine use in women with REPL. Larger trials are currently underway to inform treatment for this group of women.

Of infectious agents, only *C. trachomatis* and *U. urealyticum* seem equally plausible because these two agents generate chronic infections and potentially repetitive losses, whereas others are more likely to cause only sporadic losses. The endometrium could be cultured for *U. urealyticum*. Alternatively, a couple could be treated empirically with doxycycline. The prevalence of chronic endometritis is 7% in REPL, and the live birth rate is increased after antibiotic therapy; this suggests a subgroup of REPL may benefit from this management approach.[83]

If spontaneous abortion occurs after 8 to 10 weeks' gestation, a uterine anomaly should be considered a potential cause, and the uterine cavity should be explored by hysteroscopy or hysterosalpingography. Intrauterine adhesions should be lysed. If a müllerian fusion defect (septate or bicornuate uterus) is detected in a woman who has experienced one or more second-trimester spontaneous abortions, surgical correction may be warranted.

Women with either acquired or inherited thrombophilias appear to have a slightly increased risk for first-trimester pregnancy loss. Thrombophilias explain at best only a small portion of first-trimester losses. The likelihood is much greater that thrombophilias are the cause of a second-trimester loss. Anticoagulant agents such as aspirin and heparin have been shown to increase the chance of live birth in subsequent pregnancies in women with REPL associated with antiphospholipid syndrome.[84] Whether antithrombotic therapy increases the chances of live birth in women with inherited thrombophilia remains unknown. RCTs have consistently shown no beneficial effect of antithrombotic therapy in women with unexplained REPL.[85,84]

The clinician should discourage exposure to cigarettes and alcohol yet not necessarily ascribe cause and effect in an individual case. Similar counsel should apply for exposures to other potential toxins. Identification of substance abuse and environmental history during the preconception period provides an opportunity to assist women in reducing major health risks in addition to reducing early pregnancy loss (see Chapters 6 and 8).

Idiopathic secondary REPL may be associated with an abnormal maternal immune response to subsequent pregnancies, and some authors have proposed that women with REPL should be investigated for autoimmune and cellular immune abnormalities. It is speculated that in women, an elevation of natural killer (NK) cells may have an effect on reproductive performance, and NK cell levels in blood are currently being used as a diagnostic test to guide the initiation of therapies in both infertile women[86] and in those who present with REPL. A recent meta-analysis of studies that evaluated peripheral NK cell percentages and numbers in women with recurrent miscarriage (RM) versus controls showed significantly higher NK cell percentages in women with RM.[86] Several immunotherapies have been used to treat women with otherwise unexplained losses. Paternal cell immunization, third-party donor leukocytes, trophoblast membranes, and intravenous immunoglobulin provide no significant beneficial effect over placebo in improving the live birth rate.[87,88]

LATE PREGNANCY LOSS (STILLBIRTH)

Stillbirth **is the term used to describe pregnancy loss at 20 weeks' gestation or greater.** By weight, the definition is 350 g, the 50th percentile at that week of gestation. The frequency of stillbirths in the United States is 1 in 160 deliveries, or 25,000 annually. Stillbirths are increased in a large number of conditions whose management is discussed elsewhere in this text (see Chapter 11). These conditions include obesity, multiple gestations with or without prematurity, infections (e.g., parvovirus-B19), advanced maternal age, and a host of systemic maternal diseases that include but are not limited to diabetes mellitus, chronic and gestational hypertension, autoimmune diseases, and renal and thyroid diseases. Passive and active smoking and illicit drug use during pregnancy separately or in combination are associated with an increased risk of stillbirth (OR 1.94).[89] Table 27-4 shows prevalence and estimated rates compiled in 2005 by Fretts[90] and reproduced in 2009 by ACOG.[16]

Pregnancy loss after 20 weeks is higher overall in blacks (11 per 1000) than in other ethnic groups (6 per 1000), which include Hispanics and Native Americans.[16]

Recurrence

Recurrence reflects disease severity and ability to treat; thus no single risk factor is necessarily appropriate. However, a few risk

TABLE 27-4   ESTIMATES OF MATERNAL RISK FACTORS AND RISK FOR STILLBIRTH

CONDITION	PREVALENCE AMONG STILLBORNS	ODDS RATIO
General population	—	1.0
Previous growth-restricted infant (<10%)	7%	2-4.6
Previous stillbirth	1%	1.4-3.2
Multiple gestation:		
Twins	3%	1.0-2.8
Triplets	0.1%	2.8-3.7
Low-risk pregnancies	80%	0.86
Hypertensive disorders:		
Chronic hypertension	6%-10%	1.5-2.7
Pregnancy-induced hypertension		
Mild	6%-8%	1.2-4.0
Severe	1%-3%	1.8-4.4
Diabetes:		
Treated with diet	3%-5%	1.2-2.2
Treated with insulin	2.4%	1.7-7.0
Systemic lupus erythematosus	<1%	6 to 20
Renal disease	<1%	2.2-30
Thyroid disorders	0.2%-2%	2.2-3.0
Thrombophilia	1%-5%	2.8-5.0
Cholestasis of pregnancy	<0.1%	1.8-4.4
Smoking >10 cigarettes daily	10%-20%	1.7-3.0
Obesity (prepregnancy):		
Body mass index 25-29.9 kg/m²	21%	1.9-2.7
Body mass index >30	20%	2.1-2.8
Advanced maternal age (reference <35 yr):		
35-39 years	15%-18%	1.8-2.2
≥40 years	2%	1.8-3.3
Black women compared with white women	15%	2.0-2.2
Low educational attainment (<12 yr vs. ≥12 yr)	30%	1.6-2.0

Modified from the American College of Obstetricians and Gynecologists (ACOG). Practice Bulletin: Management of Stillbirth. No. 102:1. Washington, DC: ACOG; 2009.

factors are broadly applicable. Maternal age is positively correlated with stillborn risk. This reflects not only the predictable known fetal etiologies (e.g., chromosomal abnormalities) but also maternal complications that are simply age related.

Stillbirth occurs more often in primiparous women of a given age than in multiparous women of comparable age. This may correlate to difficulty in achieving pregnancy, which is of greatest relevance to women who require ART. Women who are subfertile (increased time to pregnancy) but never require ART have an increased risk for birth defects compared with women who achieve pregnancy in less than 1 year.[91] **Offspring of both ART couples and subfertile couples who do not require ART have 20% to 30% more birth defects (OR 1.2 to 1.3) than offspring of women who previously became pregnant within 12 months of attempting.**[91]

Risks for stillbirth are highest (twofold) in women delivered of a growth-restricted infant earlier than 32 weeks' gestation.[92,93] This risk is, incidentally, independent of mode of delivery (cesarean or vaginal). Using Scottish morbidity records (1981 to 2000), the odds ratio for stillbirth recurring in the *second* pregnancy was 1.94.[94] A recent systematic review and meta-analysis indicated that compared with vaginal birth, women with a previous cesarean delivery (CD) are at higher risk of unexplained stillbirth.[95] The etiology behind the higher rates of stillbirth in subsequent pregnancies after CD remains unknown, but a higher incidence of placental abruption after CD suggests impaired placentation.

Genetic Factors

Genetic factors for stillbirths are receiving increased recognition by the ACOG, which has provided specific management recommendations. **Chromosomal abnormalities or significant copy number variants (microdeletions, microduplications) are detected in 8% to 13% of stillbirths.**[17,96,97] **Thus special effort should be made to determine chromosomal status of a stillborn.** It is now recognized that the traditional approach of obtaining fetal tissue after a stillborn infant has been delivered is suboptimal. Cell culture often fails and leads to no results in perhaps 50% to 75% of cases. **Successful culture for chromosomal analysis occurs in 80% when amniocentesis is used to obtain cells.** It is tempting to eschew an invasive procedure in an already stressed patient, but this would not be in her long-term best interest. Alternatively, as discussed earlier, array CGH does not require cultured cells and further detects microdeletions and microduplications not detectable by a karyotype.

Detecting even trisomies clinically by examination of a stillbirth is unexpectedly difficult because maceration occurs within days of fetal demise. Thus medical records that state lack of dysmorphia should be suspect, save for obvious structural defects (e.g. cleft lip, myelomeningocele). Ultrasound results obtained when the pregnancy was still viable are probably more reliable. If amniocentesis cannot be performed or if cultures fail, an attempt should be made to obtain FISH results to exclude common trisomies. This can be done on placental tissues, umbilical cord segments, or internal (noncontaminated) tissues such as connective tissue.

The major yield of autopsy for a stillborn fetus is detection of an unrecognized mendelian explanation. This obviously alters management in subsequent pregnancies, for which reason a major effort should be exerted. Whole-body photographs and whole-body radiographs are appropriate, as is placental examination by a physician with requisite expertise. Considerable progress has been made in particular in diagnosing skeletal dysplasia, often an autosomal-recessive disorder that can recur in subsequent pregnancies. Other disorders may be autosomal-dominant disorders that arise as a result of de novo mutations. Distinguishing between these two possibilities is important because the recurrence risk should be almost nil if the etiology is a de novo autosomal dominant disorder. If parents refuse autopsy, the provider should attempt to obtain as much information as possible: photographs, radiographs or magnetic resonance images, ultrasound, and examination by a geneticist. A head-sparing autopsy is preferable to no autopsy and may be acceptable to the parents.

Polygenic/Multifactorial Disorders

The frequency of virtually any isolated birth defect is higher among stillborn fetuses than among neonates. This reflects adverse selection in utero, a phenomenon recognized for years in ultrasound surveillance. If an isolated, organ-specific defect occurs (e.g., cardiac), polygenic/multifactorial etiology and recurrence risks (2% to 5%) usually apply. On the other hand, such a defect may be merely the only one evident but is actually a component of a multiple-malformation complex. Ability to distinguish between these possibilities is a major reason for

---

autopsy. **The multiple malformation syndrome could indicate mendelian etiology.**

Maternal Evaluation

Certain maternal laboratory tests are recommended by ACOG (Box 27-1). Of course, a mother whose pregnancies have medical complications has already undergone many tests, and the cause of the stillbirth may seem obvious (e.g., diabetes mellitus). It is prudent, however, to order all these laboratory tests because the ostensible diagnosis may prove erroneous. Of note, ACOG does not recommend testing for antinuclear antibodies and certain serologies (toxoplasmosis, rubella, cytomegalovirus, herpes simplex virus), nor do they recommend genetic tests other than a karyotype. However, it is likely in the foreseeable future that array CGH (see Chapter 10), a panel of organ-specific mutations (e.g., skeletal dysplasias), or other genetic tests will prove practical. Caution is necessary before concluding that a stillbirth was caused by a condition signified by a positive laboratory test (e.g., thrombophilia), and such a finding does not obviate the need for fetal autopsy and fetal genetic tests.

Management in Subsequent Pregnancies

Quality ultrasound and vigilant fetal surveillance are universally recommended. Induction is recommended at 38 weeks, but before that time, only with demonstrated fetal lung maturity. Management otherwise will focus on any specific maternal factors identified (e.g., diabetes mellitus). In some pregnancies, management will differ little from that of the general obstetric patient. In others, prenatal genetic diagnosis will be necessary.

OBSTETRIC OUTCOME AFTER EARLY PREGNANCY COMPLICATIONS

Most early pregnancy complications occur before 12 weeks of gestation and involve placentation and early placental development. Increasing evidence shows that many failures of placentation are associated with an imbalance of free radicals, which will further affect placental development and function and may subsequently have an influence on both the fetus and the mother but are often ignored by clinicians.[2]

Complications that include miscarriage, threatened miscarriage with or without an intrauterine hematoma, and vanishing twin are extremely common in early pregnancy throughout the world. Very little is known about the short- and long-term consequences of these complications on ongoing and, in particular, subsequent pregnancies. Most data available are derived from small retrospective series of many different complications and pathologies or large series that describe specific pathology but with wide variations in the definitions of the pathophysiology.

Recent meta-analysis and reviews have indicated an increased risk for adverse outcome in ongoing pregnancies after an early pregnancy event. Clinically relevant associations of adverse outcome in the *subsequent* pregnancy with an odds ratio higher than 2 after complications in a previous pregnancy are the risk for perinatal death after a single previous miscarriage; the risk for very preterm delivery (VPTD) after two or more miscarriages; and the risk for placenta previa, premature preterm rupture of membranes (PPROM), VPTD, and low birthweight (LBW) after recurrent miscarriage.[98] Clinically relevant associations of adverse obstetric outcome in the *ongoing* pregnancy with an odds ratio higher than 2 after complications in the index pregnancy are the risks for preterm delivery (PTD), VPTD, placental abruption, small for gestational age (SGA), LBW, and very low birthweight (VLBW) after a threatened miscarriage episode; pregnancy-induced hypertension, preeclampsia, placental abruption, PTD, SGA, and low 5-minute Apgar score following the detection of an intrauterine hematoma; and VPTD, VLBW, and perinatal death after a vanishing twin phenomenon.[99] These data indicate a link between early pregnancy complications that involve the placenta and subsequent adverse obstetric and perinatal outcomes.

Heterogeneity is observed among most studies, and many of the older controlled studies did not make adjustments for relevant confounders for adverse obstetric outcome—such as age, ART, economic status, education level, ethnicity, height, marital status, parity, previous obstetric outcome, prolonged infertility, smoking, and maternal weight—or they did not stratify for other first-trimester complications.[98,99] However, overall more recent large meta-analyses and controlled population-based prospective studies have confirmed previous data that indicate a strong association between specific early pregnancy events and subsequent late obstetric complications in the subsequent or ongoing pregnancy.[99] **In particular, the risk for PTD and VPTD is increased after most first-trimester complications.** This suggests that early detection of these risk factors could improve the screening of women at high risk for specific obstetric complications in ongoing and subsequent pregnancies. Furthermore, the antenatal identification of these parameters during the first half of pregnancy should enable better management protocols and new therapeutic guidelines aimed at improving the perinatal outcome in these groups of women at higher risk for abnormal pregnancy outcome.

- About 50% to 70% of conceptions are lost, most in the first trimester. Losses in preimplantation embryos are especially high: 25% to 50% of morphologically normal and 50% to 75% of morphologically abnormal embryos.
- Pregnancy loss is age dependent, and 40-year-old women have twice the loss rate of 20-year-old women. Most of these pregnancies are lost before 8 weeks' gestation.
- At least 50% of clinically recognized pregnancy losses show a chromosomal abnormality, and those in abortuses differ from those found in liveborn infants, although autosomal trisomy still accounts for 50% of abnormalities. A balanced translocation is present in 5% of couples with REPL.
- Many nongenetic causes of REPL have been proposed, but few are proven. Efficacy of treatment often remains uncertain.
- Uterine anomalies are accepted causes of second-trimester losses, but their role in first-trimester losses is less clear. Couples who experience a second-trimester loss may benefit from metroplasty or hysteroscopic resection of a uterine septum.
- Drugs, toxins, and physical agents are uncommon causes of early pregnancy loss, especially repetitive loss. It should not be assumed that exposures to toxicants explain repetitive losses. Passive and active smoking and illicit drug use are associated with higher rates of both early pregnancy loss and stillbirth.
- Antiphospholipid syndrome (antibodies to LAC, aPL, and anti–β_2-glycoprotein) is an accepted cause of second-trimester losses; its role in first-trimester losses is arguable. Strict ACOG criteria exist for applying the diagnosis of antiphospholipid syndrome to a woman who had had repeated first-trimester REPL.
- In REPL, prognosis is good even without therapy. The live birth rate is 60% to 70% even with up to four losses and no prior liveborn infants. An efficacious therapeutic regimen should show success rates greater than these expected background rates, or these should be assessed in an RCT. Women who have had more than four losses are less likely to have a cytogenetic explanation and may have a different prognosis.
- The frequency of chromosomal abnormalities in stillbirths (losses after 20 weeks' gestation or weighing at least 350 g) is underappreciated, as are nonchromosomal genetic factors (e.g., syndromes). Tissue for cytogenetic studies should be obtained by amniocentesis or chorionic villus sampling; cultures initiated from postdelivery products often lead to unsuccessful culture.
- A major effort should be exerted to obtain full autopsy and imaging on all stillbirths because findings can alter management in future pregnancies. If a couple declines an autopsy, whole-body radiographs, magnetic resonance imaging, and other noninvasive imaging should be pursued.
- Adverse first-trimester events or complications in a current or previous pregnancy may interfere with normal placentation and increases the risks for specific later obstetric complications.

REFERENCES

1. Jauniaux E, Poston L. Placental-related diseases of pregnancy: involvement of oxidative stress and implications in human evolution. *Hum Reprod Update*. 2006;12:747.
2. U.S. Department of Health and Human Services. *Reproductive Impairments among Married Couples*. U.S. Vital and Health Statistics Series 23, No. 11, Hyattsville, MD, 1982, p 5.
3. Simpson JL, Mills JL, Holmes LB, et al. Low fetal loss rates after ultrasound-proved viability in early pregnancy. *JAMA*. 1987;258:2555.
4. Regan L. A prospective study on spontaneous abortion. In: Beard RW, Sharp F, eds. *Early Pregnancy Loss: Mechanisms and Treatment*. London: Springer-Verlag; 1988.
5. Simpson JL, Gray RH, Queenan JT, et al. Risk of recurrent spontaneous abortion for pregnancies discovered in the fifth week of gestation. *Lancet*. 1994;344:964.
6. Jauniaux E, Gulbis B. The human first trimester gestational sac limits rather than facilitates oxygen transfer to the foetus: a review. *Placenta*. 2003; 24:S86.
7. Jauniaux E, Hempstock J, Greenwold N, et al. Trophoblastic oxidative stress in relation to temporal and regional differences in maternal placental blood flow in normal and abnormal early pregnancies. *Am J Pathol*. 2003; 162:115.
8. Burton GJ, Jauniaux E. The influence of the intrauterine environment on human placental development. *Int J Dev Biol*. 2010;54:303.
9. Burton GJ, Woods AW. Rheological and physiological consequences of conversion of the maternal spiral arteries for uteroplacental blood flow during human pregnancy. *Placenta*. 2009;30:473.
10. Hustin J, Jauniaux E. Histological study of the materno-embryonic interface in spontaneous abortion. *Placenta*. 1990;11:477.
11. Jauniaux E, Greenwold N, Hempstock J, et al. Comparison of ultrasonographic and Doppler mapping of the intervillous circulation in normal and abnormal early pregnancies. *Fertil Steril*. 2003;79:100.
12. Hempstock J, Jauniaux E, Greenwold N, et al. The contribution of placental oxidative stress to early pregnancy failure. *Hum Pathol*. 2003;34:1265.
13. Munne S, Alikani M, Tomkin G, et al. Embryo morphology, development rates, and maternal age are correlated with chromosome abnormalities. *Fertil Steril*. 1995;64:382.
14. Simpson JL, Bombard AT. Chromosomal abnormalities in spontaneous abortion: frequency, pathology and genetic counseling. In: Edmonds K, ed. *Spontaneous Abortion*. London: Blackwell; 1987:51.
15. Sorokin Y, Johnson MP, Uhlmann WR, et al. Postmortem chorionic villus sampling: correlation of cytogenetic and ultrasound findings. *Am J Med Genet*. 1991;39:314.
16. ACOG Practice Bulletin. Management of stillbirth. *Obstet Gynecol*. 2009; 102:1.
17. ACOG Committee Opinion No. 581. *Obstet Gynecol*. 2013;122:6.
18. Hassold T, Hunt P. Maternal age and chromosomally abnormal pregnancies: what we know and what we wish we knew. *Curr Opin Pediatr*. 2009;21:703.
19. Fragouli E, Wells D. Chromosome abnormalities in the human oocyte. *Cytogenet Genome Res*. 2011;133:107.
20. Kuliev A, Zlatopolsky Z, Kirillova I, et al. Meiosis errors in over 20,000 oocytes studied in the practice of preimplantation aneuploidy testing. *Reprod Biomed Online*. 2011;22:2.
21. Tempest HG. Meiotic recombination errors, the origin of sperm aneuploidy and clinical recommendations. *Syst Biol Reprod Med*. 2011;57:93.
22. Deleted in review.
23. Deleted in review.
24. Singh RP, Carr DH. The anatomy and histology of XO human embryos and fetuses. *Anat Rec*. 1966;155:369.
25. Jirasek JE. Principles of reproductive embryology. In: Simpson JL, ed. *Disorders of Sex Differentiation: Etiology and Clinical Delineation*. San Diego: Academic Press; 1976:51.
26. Warburton D, Kline J, Stein Z, et al. Does the karyotype of a spontaneous abortion predict the karyotype of a subsequent abortion? Evidence from 273 women with two karyotyped spontaneous abortions. *Am J Hum Genet*. 1987;41:465.
27. Warburton D, Dallaire L, Thangavelu M, et al. Trisomy recurrence: a reconsideration based on North American data. *Am J Hum Genet*. 2004;75:376.
28. Rubio C, Simon C, Vidal F, et al. Chromosomal abnormalities and embryo development in recurrent miscarriage couples. *Hum Reprod*. 2003;18:182.
29. Munné S, Sandalinas M, Magli C, et al. Increased rate of aneuploid embryos in young women with previous aneuploid conceptions. *Prenat Diagn*. 2004;24:638.
30. Deleted in review.
31. Stephenson MD, Awartani KA, Robinson WP. Cytogenetic analysis of miscarriages from couples with recurrent miscarriage: a case-control study. *Hum Reprod*. 2002;17:446.
32. Carp H, Toder V, Aviram A, et al. Karyotype of the abortus in recurrent miscarriage. *Fertil Steril*. 2001;75:678.
33. Deleted in review.
34. Bianco K, Caughey AB, Shaffer BL, et al. History of miscarriage and increased incidence of fetal aneuploidy in subsequent pregnancy. *Obstet Gynecol*. 2006;107:1098.
35. Munne S, Fischer J, Warner A, et al. Preimplantation genetic diagnosis significantly reduces pregnancy loss in infertile couples: a multi-center study. *Fertil Steril*. 2006;85:326.
36. Munne S, Escudero T, Colls P, et al. Predictability of preimplantation genetic diagnosis of aneuploidy and translocations on prospective attempts. *Reprod Biomed Online*. 2004;9:645.
37. Simpson JL, Meyers CM, Martin AO, et al. Translocations are infrequent among couples having repeated spontaneous abortions but no other abnormal pregnancies. *Fertil Steril*. 1989;51:811.
38. Boué A, Gallano P. A collaborative study of the segregation of inherited chromosome structural rearrangements in 1,356 prenatal diagnoses. *Prenat Diagn*. 1984;4:45.
39. Daniel A, Hook EB, Wulf G. Risks of unbalanced progeny at amniocentesis to carriers of chromosome rearrangements: data from United States and Canadian laboratories. *Am J Med Genet*. 1989;33:14.
40. Gardner RJM, Sutherland GR, Shaffer LG. *Chromosome abnormalities and genetic counseling*. 4th ed. New York: Oxford; 2012.
41. Deleted in review.
42. Stephenson MD, Sierra S. Reproductive outcomes in recurrent pregnancy loss associated with a parental carrier of a structural chromosome rearrangement. *Hum Reprod*. 2006;21:1076.
43. Verlinsky Y, Tur-Kaspa I, Cieslak J, et al. Preimplantation testing for chromosomal disorders improves reproductive outcome of poor-prognosis patients. *Reprod Biomed Online*. 2005;11:219.
44. Simpson JL, Elias S. *Genetics in Obstetrics and Gynecology*. 3rd ed. Philadelphia: WB Saunders; 2003.
45. Pettenati MJ, Rao PN, Phelan MC, et al. Paracentric inversions in humans: a review of 446 paracentric inversions with presentation of 120 new cases. *Am J Med Genet*. 1995;55:171.
46. Philipp T, Kalousek DK. Generalized abnormal embryonic development in missed abortion: embryoscopic and cytogenetic findings. *Am J Med Genet*. 2002;111:43.
47. Karamardian LM, Grimes DA. Luteal phase deficiency: effect of treatment on pregnancy rates. *Am J Obstet Gynecol*. 1992;167:1391.
48. Negro R, Schwartz A, Gismondi R, et al. Increased pregnancy loss rate in thyroid antibody negative women with TSH levels between 2.5 and 5.0 in the first trimester of pregnancy. *J Clin Endocrinol Metab*. 2010;95:E44.
49. Stagnaro-Green A. Thyroid autoimmunity and the risk of miscarriage. *Best Pract Res Clin Endocrinol Metab*. 2004;18:167.
50. Anselmo J, Cao D, Karrison T, et al. Fetal loss associated with excess thyroid hormone exposure. *JAMA*. 2004;292:691.
51. Mills JL, Simpson JL, Driscoll SG, et al. Incidence of spontaneous abortion among normal women and insulin-dependent diabetic women whose pregnancies were identified within 21 days of conception. *N Engl J Med*. 1988;319:1617.
52. Miodovnik M, Mimouni F, Tsang RC, et al. Glycemic control and spontaneous abortion in insulin-dependent diabetic women. *Obstet Gynecol*. 1986;68:366.
53. Ben Rafael Z, Seidman DS, Recabi K, et al. Uterine anomalies: a retrospective, matched-control study. *J Reprod Med*. 1991;36:723.
54. Proctor JA, Haney AF. Recurrent first trimester pregnancy loss is associated with uterine septum but not with bicornuate uterus. *Fertil Steril*. 2003; 80:1212.
55. Salim R, Regan L, Woelfer B, et al. A comparative study of the morphology of congenital uterine anomalies in women with and without a history of recurrent first trimester miscarriage. *Hum Reprod*. 2003;18:162.
56. Stampe Sørenson S. Estimated prevalence of müllerian anomalies. *Acta Obstet Gynecol Scand*. 1988;67:441.
57. Simon C, Martinez L, Pardo F, et al. Müllerian defects in women with normal reproductive outcome. *Fertil Steril*. 1991;56:1192.
58. Ludmir J, Samuels P, Brooks S, et al. Pregnancy outcome of patients with uncorrected uterine anomalies managed in a high-risk obstetric setting. *Obstet Gynecol*. 1990;75:906.
59. Hartmann KE, Herring AH. Predictors of the presence of uterine fibroids in the first trimester of pregnancy: a prospective cohort study. *J Soc Gynecol Invest*. 2004;11:340A.

60. van Oostrum N, De Sutter P, Meys J, Verstraelen H. Risks associated with bacterial vaginosis in infertility patients: a systematic review and meta-analysis. *Hum Reprod.* 2013;28:1809-1815.
61. Simpson JL, Mills JL, Kim H, et al. Infectious processes: an infrequent cause of first trimester spontaneous abortions. *Hum Reprod.* 1996;11:668.
62. ACOG Practice Bulletin. Antiphospholipid syndrome. *Obstet Gynecol.* 2011;117:192.
63. Simpson JL, Carson SA, Chesney C, et al. Lack of association between antiphospholipid antibodies and first-trimester spontaneous abortion: prospective study of pregnancies detected within 21 days of conception. *Fertil Steril.* 1998;69:814.
64. Rey E, Kahn SR, David M, et al. Thrombophilic disorders and fetal loss: a meta-analysis. *Lancet.* 2003;361:901.
65. Kovalesky G, Gracia CR, Berlin JA, et al. Evaluation of the association between hereditary thrombophilias and recurrent pregnancy loss. *Arch Intern Med.* 2004;164:558.
66. Halmesmaki E, Valimaki M, Roine R, et al. Maternal and paternal alcohol consumption and miscarriage. *Br J Obstet Gynaecol.* 1989;96:188.
67. Armstrong BG, McDonald AD, Sloan M. Cigarette, alcohol, and coffee consumption and spontaneous abortion. *Am J Public Health.* 1992;82:85.
68. Mills JL, Holmes LB, Aarons JH, et al. Moderate caffeine use and the risk of spontaneous abortion and intrauterine growth retardation. *JAMA.* 1993;269:593.
69. Klebanoff MA, Levine RJ, DerSimonian R, et al. Maternal serum paraxanthine, a caffeine metabolite, and the risk of spontaneous abortion. *N Engl J Med.* 1999;341:1639.
70. Savitz DA, Sonnenfeld NL, Olshan AF. Review of epidemiologic studies of paternal occupational exposure and spontaneous abortion. *Am J Ind Med.* 1994;25:361.
71. Jauniaux E, Burton GJ. Morphological and biological effects of maternal exposure to tobacco smoke on the feto-placental unit. *Early Hum Dev.* 2007;83:699.
72. Ness RB, Grisso JA, Hirschinger N, et al. Cocaine and tobacco use and the risk of spontaneous abortion. *N Engl J Med.* 1999;340:333.
73. Pineles BL, Park E, Samet JM. Systematic review and meta-analysis of miscarriage and maternal exposure to tobacco smoke during pregnancy. *Am J Epidemiol.* 2014;179(7):807-823.
74. Nelson DB, Grisso JA, Joffe MM, et al. Violence does not influence early pregnancy loss. *Fertil Steril.* 2003;80:1205.
75. Stray-Pedersen B, Stray-Pedersen S. Recurrent abortion: the role of psychotherapy. In: Beard RW, Sharp F, eds. *Early Pregnancy Loss: Mechanism and Treatment.* London: Royal College of Obstetricians and Gynecologists; 1988:433.
76. Liddell HS, Pattison NS, Zanderigo A. Recurrent miscarriage—outcome after supportive care in early pregnancy. *Aust N Z J Obstet Gynaecol.* 1991;31:320.
77. Daniel S, Koren G, Lunenfeld E, Bilenko N, Ratzon R, Levy A. Fetal exposure to nonsteroidal anti-inflammatory drugs and spontaneous abortions. *CMAJ.* 2014;186(5):E177-E182.
78. Kjaersgaard MI, Parner ET, Vestergaard M, et al. Prenatal antidepressant exposure and risk of spontaneous abortion - a population-based study. *PLoS ONE.* 2013;8(8):e72095.
79. Bech BH, Kjaersgaard MI, Pedersen HS, et al. Use of antiepileptic drugs during pregnancy and risk of spontaneous abortion and stillbirth: population based cohort study. *BMJ.* 2014;349:g5159.
80. Jauniaux E, Farquharson RG, Christiansen OB, Exalto N. Evidence-based guidelines for the investigation and medical treatment of recurrent miscarriage. *Hum Reprod.* 2006;21:2216.
81. ACOG. Practice bulletin: management of recurrent pregnancy loss. Number 24. *Int J Gynaecol Obstet.* 2002;78:179.
82. Bernardi LA, Cohen RN, Stephenson MD. Impact of subclinical hypothyroidism in women with recurrent early pregnancy loss. *Fertil Steril.* 2013;100(5):1326-1331.
83. McQueen DB, Bernardi LA, Stephenson MD. Chronic endometritis in women with recurrent early pregnancy loss and/or fetal demise. *Fertil Steril.* 2014;101(4):1026-1030.
84. de Jong PG, Kaandorp S, Di Nisio M, Goddijn M, Middeldorp S. Aspirin and/or heparin for women with unexplained recurrent miscarriage with or without inherited thrombophilia. *Cochrane Database Syst Rev.* 2014;(7):CD004734.
85. De Jong PG, Goddijn M, Middeldorp S. Antithrombotic therapy for pregnancy loss. *Hum Reprod Update.* 2013;19(6):656-673.
86. Seshadri S, Sunkara SK. Natural killer cells in female infertility and recurrent miscarriage: a systematic review and meta-analysis. *Hum Reprod Update.* 2014;20(3):429-438.
87. Wong LF, Porter TF, Scott JR. Immunotherapy for recurrent miscarriage. *Cochrane Database Syst Rev.* 2014;(10):CD000112.
88. Christiansen OB, Larsen EC, Egerup P, Lunoee L, Egestad L, Nielsen HS. Intravenous immunoglobulin treatment for secondary recurrent miscarriage: a randomised, double-blind, placebo-controlled trial. *BJOG.* 2015;122(4):500-508.
89. Varner MW, Silver RM, Rowland Hogue CJ, et al. Association between stillbirth and illicit drug use and smoking during pregnancy. *Obstet Gynecol.* 2014;123(1):113-125.
90. Fretts R. Etiology and prevention of stillbirth. *Am J Obstet Gynecol.* 2005;193:1923.
91. Hansen M, Boower C, Milne E, et al. Assisted reproductive technologies and the risk of birth defects: a systematic review. *Hum Reprod.* 2005;29:328.
92. Surkan PJ, Stephansson O, Dickman PW, Cnattingius S. Previous preterm and small-for-gestational-age births and the subsequent risk of still birth. *N Engl J Med.* 2004;350:777.
93. Getahum D, Ananth CV, Kinzler WL. Risk factors for antepartum and intrapartum stillbirth: a population-based study. *Am J Obstet Gynecol.* 2007;196:499.
94. Bhattacharya S, Prescott GJ, Black M, Shetty A. Recurrence risk of stillbirth in a second pregnancy. *BJOG.* 2010;117:1243.
95. O'Neill SM, Kearney PM, Kenny LC, et al. Caesarean delivery and subsequent stillbirth or miscarriage: systematic review and meta-analysis. *PLoS ONE.* 2013;8(1):e54588.
96. Laury A, Sanchez-Lara PA, Pepkowitz S, Graham JM Jr. A study of 534 fetal pathology cases from prenatal diagnosis referrals analyzed from 1989 through 2000. *Am J Med Genet.* 2007;143A:3107.
97. Korteweg FJ, Bouman K, Erwich JJ, et al. Cytogenetic analysis after evaluation of 750 fetal deaths: proposal for diagnostic workup. *Obstet Gynecol.* 2008;111:865.
98. van Oppenraaij RH, Jauniaux E, Christiansen OB, et al., for the ESHRE Special Interest Group for Early Pregnancy (SIGEP). Predicting adverse obstetric outcome after early pregnancy events and complications: a review. *Hum Reprod Update.* 2009;15:409.
99. Jauniaux E, Van Oppenraaij RH, Burton GJ. Obstetric outcome after early placental complications. *Curr Opin Obstet Gynecol.* 2010;22:452.

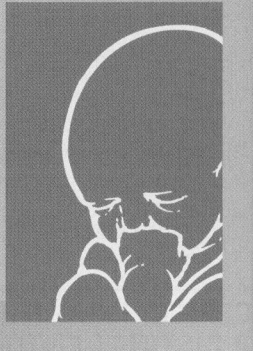

CHAPTER 28

Cervical Insufficiency

JACK LUDMIR, JOHN OWEN, and VINCENZO BERGHELLA

KEY ABBREVIATIONS

17-α-hydroxyprogesterone	17-OH-P
American College of Obstetricians and Gynecologists	ACOG
Cervical insufficiency	CI
Cervical intraepithelial neoplasia	CIN
Cervical length	CL
Diethylstilbestrol	DES
Intramuscular	IM
Interquartile range	IQR
Intraamniotic infection	IAI
Large loop excision of the transformation zone	LLETZ
Loop electrosurgical excision procedure	LEEP
National Institutes of Child Health and Human Development	NICHD
Preterm birth	PTB
Preterm premature rupture of the membranes	PPROM
Randomized controlled trial	RCT
Receiver operating characteristic curve	ROC
Royal College of Obstetricians and Gynaecologists	RCOG
Society for Maternal-Fetal Medicine	SMFM
Spontaneous preterm birth	sPTB
Transabdominal ultrasound	TAU
Translabial ultrasound	TLU
Transvaginal ultrasound	TVU

OVERVIEW

Since the initial description in 1658 of the cervix being "so slack that it cannot keep in the seed" by Cole and Culpepper,[1] few subjects in obstetrics have generated as much controversy as the term *cervical incompetence,* now more correctly termed **cervical insufficiency.** The competent or "sufficient" human uterine cervix is a complex organ that undergoes extensive changes throughout gestation and parturition. It is a key structure responsible for keeping the fetus and membranes inside the uterus until the end of gestation and for undergoing significant changes to allow the delivery of the baby during spontaneous or induced labor.

The cervix is primarily fibrous connective tissue composed of an extracellular matrix that consists of collagen types I and II, elastin, proteoglycans, and a cellular portion that consists of smooth muscle and blood vessels. A complex remodeling process of the cervix occurs during gestation that involves timed biochemical cascades, interactions between the extracellular and cellular compartments, and cervical stromal infiltration by inflammatory cells.[2] Any disarray in this timed interaction could result in early cervical ripening, cervical insufficiency, and preterm birth (PTB) or miscarriage.

The incidence of cervical insufficiency in the general obstetric population is reported to vary between approximately 1/100 and 1/2000.[3] *If women with a singleton gestation, a prior spontaneous preterm birth (sPTB), and a current transvaginal ultrasound (TVU) cervical length (CL) less than 25 mm are labeled as having cervical insufficiency, the incidence is about 3% to 4%.*[4] Wide variations in estimating the incidence are likely due to real biologic differences among study populations, the criteria used to establish the diagnosis, and reporting bias between general practitioners and referral centers. Once considered a discrete entity reserved for patients with a history of midtrimester loss associated with painless cervical dilation, in the last few years, this diagnosis has become a component of the spontaneous preterm birth syndrome (see Chapter 29). Strategies that include the identification of a short cervix in the index gestation have been developed with different management protocols utilized to reduce the rate of PTB.

CERVICAL INSUFFICIENCY: A DISTINCT ENTITY OR EVIDENCE OF PRETERM PARTURITION?

In 1962, Danforth and Buckingham[5] suggested that cervical incompetence was not an all-or-none phenomenon; rather it comprised degrees of insufficiency, and combinations of factors could cause "cervical failure." These classic investigations demonstrated that unlike the uterine corpus, the normal cervix is composed predominantly of connective tissue. This fibrous band is the chief mechanical barrier against the loss of the enlarging products of conception. The cervix and mucous glands also play an important immunologic role in preventing vaginal flora from ascending into the normally sterile intrauterine environment.

In a subsequent report, these investigators analyzed cervical biopsies taken from postpartum women and compared them with hysterectomy specimens from nonpregnant patients.[6] Pregnancy was associated with increased water content, a marked decline in collagen and glycoprotein, and increased glycosaminoglycans. **The cellular and biochemical changes suggested that cervical dilation in pregnancy is a dynamic process,** and this might explain why a woman could have a pregnancy outcome consistent with cervical insufficiency in one pregnancy but then, without treatment, have a subsequent term birth. Presumably, the factors that incite the pathologic cervical changes might vary among pregnancies. Women with a more muscular cervix might have heightened susceptibility to factors that lead to cervical changes and PTB.

These earlier observations were enlarged by Leppert and colleagues,[7] who reported an absence of elastic fibers in the cervix of women with clinically well-characterized cervical insufficiency on the basis of their reproductive history. Conversely, cervical biopsy specimens from women with normal pregnancies showed normal amounts and orientation of these elastic fibers. It is unknown whether these microstructural and biochemical phenomena were congenital, acquired from previous trauma, or the result of other pregnancy-associated pathologic conditions. Collectively, these biochemical and ultrastructural findings support the variable, and often unpredictable, clinical course of women with a history of cervical insufficiency.[8]

Whereas the traditional paradigm depicted the cervix as either competent or incompetent, both clinical data[9,10] and interpretative reviews[11,12] suggest that, **as with most other biologic processes, cervical "competence" is rarely an all-or-none phenomenon.** The term *cervical insufficiency* has been historically thought to represent a defect inherent in the cervix itself that leads to an inability to retain a pregnancy. Initial treatment, as we will discuss later, was aimed at preventing pregnancy loss by reinforcing the structural integrity of the cervix and repairing the defect in the cervical stroma. However, as we have gained more insight into the various surgical, mechanical, and biochemical modalities used to treat cervical pathology, investigators have questioned whether abnormal cervical anatomy is the dominant cause or whether, at times, other factors play a major role.

Cervical insufficiency, **as classically defined, is recurrent painless cervical dilation that leads to three or more midtrimester births.**[13] However, painful contractions are not a prominent feature of early cervical change, with the magnitude of contraction-related pain inversely proportional to the extent of cervical ripening prior to their onset.[14] In contrast to a proposed mechanism of defective cervical tissue, although some patients may have tangible anatomic evidence of poor cervical integrity, most women with a clinical diagnosis of cervical insufficiency have ostensibly normal cervical anatomy. Knowing whether cervical integrity was compromised by a primary mechanical deficiency, versus other local or systemic factors, would help to define the optimal therapy. **In a proposed model of cervical competence as a continuum, a poor obstetric history attributed to cervical insufficiency likely results from a process of premature cervical ripening induced by myriad underlying processes that include infection, inflammation, local or systemic hormonal effects, or even genetic predisposition.** If and when cervical integrity is compromised, other processes may be stimulated (e.g., premature membrane rupture, preterm labor) and appear clinically as the spontaneous preterm parturition syndrome, which may also contain features related to the uterus and chorioamnion.[15] Thus the term *cervical insufficiency* may be increasingly considered a clinically convenient label to describe a complex and poorly understood process of premature cervical ripening and the midtrimester onset of parturition. Given this, we recognize that newer approaches to the management of cervical insufficiency have been included within the broader topic of PTB prevention.

SHORT CERVIX

Traditionally, *cervical insufficiency* (CI) has been defined by criteria based solely on obstetric history: painless cervical dilation that leads to recurrent second-trimester births in the absence of other causes. The modern approach allows the diagnosis of CI to be made in primigravidas or in multigravidas without multiple prior pregnancy losses. **This new description defines CI by the presence of *both* (1) TVU cervical length less than 25 mm and/or cervical changes detected on physical examination before 24 weeks of gestation and (2) prior sPTB at less than 37 weeks.** Regarding this second criterion, some limit it to sPTB up to 34 weeks.[4] TVU screening is the gold standard for evaluation of the CL for prediction of PTB. CL can also be measured with transabdominal ultrasound (TAU) or translabial ultrasound (TLU), but these techniques should not be used clinically for prediction of PTB because TVU is superior in many ways. The TAU CL measurement is less sensitive in detecting a short CL, is noted to overestimate CL and underdiagnose short CL,[16] and has several additional limitations: (1) a full bladder is needed; (2) the cervix maybe obscured by the fetal parts; and (3) the image is of poorer quality because of the distance from the abdominal probe to the cervix.[17] TVU CL screening has been shown to have superior cost-effectiveness compared with TAU because TVU is associated with better prevention of PTB.[18] All major guidelines that have described CL screening have clearly recommended TVU, including the Society for Maternal-Fetal Medicine (SMFM),[19] American College of Obstetricians and Gynecologists (ACOG),[20] and the Royal College of Obstetricians and Gynaecologists (RCOG).[21]

TLU is also less sensitive and less predictive than TVU.[17,21] Given this evidence, TAU or TLU should not be used for CL screening. Moreover, TVU has been shown to be more predictive of sPTB compared with digital manual examination of the cervix.[22]

TVU CL screening should be done using the technique described by the Cervical Length Education and Review (CLEAR) program[23] and the SMFM through its Perinatal Quality Foundation. The CLEAR program provides an official education program on TVU CL screening with examination and continuing image review to certify perinatologists, obstetricians, residents/fellows in training, and sonographers. TVU CL screening should be performed in clinical practice only after this program has been completed.

TVU CL measurement is a safe, acceptable, and reliable screening test that is now widely used to screen women for their risk for PTB.[24] TVU CL screening is done after the patient has emptied her bladder. Then, a sterile transvaginal probe is inserted into the anterior vaginal fornix. Initially the probe is withdrawn until the image blurs to reduce compression from the transducer, then just enough pressure is reapplied to create the best image. The TVU image of the cervix should occupy 75% of the screen, and the lower tip of the bladder should also be visible. The anterior width of cervical thickness should be equal to the posterior cervical thickness, and there should be no increased echogenicity in the cervix because of excessive pressure. Prior to the measurement, the internal and external os and the entire endocervical canal should be identified. The calipers should be correctly placed to measure the distance from the internal to the external os (Fig. 28-1). Three measurements of CL are usually obtained, then mild fundal pressure is applied for about 15 seconds to watch for funneling and/or cervical shortening. It is advisable to reduce probe pressure while fundal or suprapubic pressure is applied. The total time for TVU CL screening should be no less than approximately 5 minutes. With proper technique, the intraobserver and interobserver variabilities are both less than 10%. The population studied can affect the performance of CL screening. These include singleton versus multiple gestations, symptomatic versus asymptomatic women, intact membranes versus ruptured membranes, and prior PTB versus no prior PTB, as well as many others.[24-30] Because TVU

CL has different predictive characteristics in these different patient populations, they should be evaluated separately. Currently, the most appropriate groups to be considered for TVU CL screening are[24]:

- Asymptomatic singleton pregnancies without prior PTB
- Asymptomatic singleton pregnancies with prior PTB
- Asymptomatic multiple pregnancies
- Symptomatic singleton pregnancies

The sensitivity and positive predictive value (PPV) of a short CL is very different, for example, in women with or without a prior PTB. In singleton gestations with no history of sPTB, the sensitivity of a short CL for subsequent PTB is approximately 35% to 45%[10,25] and the PPV is approximately 20% to 30%, which means that the majority of women with a short cervical length will deliver at 35 weeks or later.[10] The sensitivity of TVU CL is also approximately 35% in twins.[27] However, **the sensitivity of a short CL is much higher, about 70%, in a singleton pregnancy with a prior sPTB.**[26]

RISK FACTORS FOR CERVICAL INSUFFICIENCY

Based largely on the epidemiologic associations between the clinical diagnosis of cervical insufficiency and antecedent historic factors, numerous risk factors for CI have been suggested. **Risk factors include prior cervical destructive surgery (i.e., trachelectomy, loop electrosurgical excision procedure [LEEP], large loop excision of the transformation zone [LLETZ], laser conization, or cold-knife cone biopsy), in utero diethylstilbestrol (DES) exposure, prior induced or spontaneous first- and second-trimester abortions, uterine anomalies, multiple gestations, or even prior sPTBs that did not meet typical clinical criteria for cervical insufficiency.** Because DES usage was effectively abandoned in the early 1970s, this congenital risk factor is now only of historic interest.

Conversely, forced cervical dilation, which generally accompanies midtrimester dilation and evacuation, has been associated with midtrimester spontaneous loss in older studies. A review by Atrash and colleagues[31] of literature published prior to 1987 indicated a nominal relative risk of 3. The authors appropriately recognized the limitations of older investigations that did not include proper control groups or consider important confounders. Particularly unclear was whether and to what extent the recorded spontaneous abortions were characterized by clinical circumstances consistent with CI. Women whose first pregnancy was terminated by an induced abortion, generally by vacuum aspiration, do not appear to have a significant risk for CI but do have a risk of PTB.[31,32] A recent series of midtrimester surgical abortion after cervical dilation with osmotic dilators up to 24 weeks' gestation did not confirm the risks observed in the older literature[33]; however, the investigators speculate that their primary use of osmotic dilators, as opposed to mechanical dilators, may have diminished the associated risks.

Because trachelectomy is now rarely performed in reproductive-age women, the associated risks in contemporary practice are difficult to ascertain; however, older series confirm an appreciable risk of early PTB.[34] Whether LEEP, LLETZ, and cervical conization (cold knife or laser) are significant risk factors for CI is still debated because the relevant outcome data are both contradictory for a significant pregnancy effect and investigators have generally focused on the risk of PTB and not CI per se. These associations are further confounded by the presence of and risk factors for intraepithelial neoplasia in addition to the type

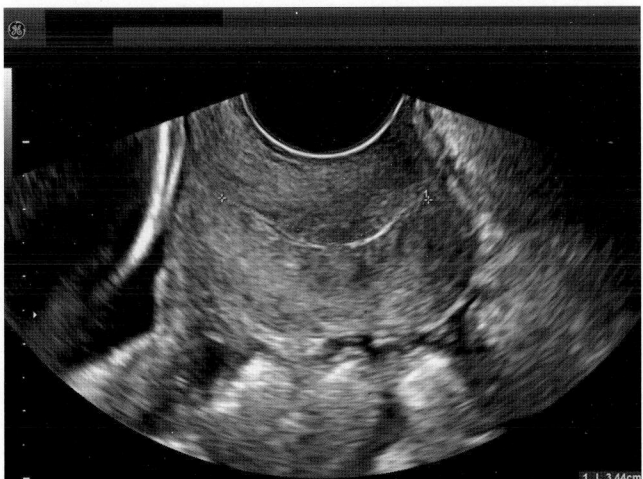

FIG 28-1 Normal cervical length as measured by transvaginal ultrasound.

of procedure used; the amount of cervical tissue removed, especially after repeat procedures; and the residual CL. Moreover, because almost all studies are retrospective and subject to considerable bias, existing evidence must be cautiously interpreted. Given the increasingly widespread use of LEEP/LLETZ and the obvious public health concerns, defining its associated risk is of particular importance.[35-37]

Most but not all investigators have reported an increased risk of PTB before 37 weeks after LEEP or conization. In a meta-analysis that incorporated data from 27 studies, cold knife conization was associated with a 2.6-fold increased risk of PTB before 37 weeks (95% confidence interval [CI], 1.80 to 3.72). Women with prior LEEP were found to have a 1.7-fold increased risk of PTB (95% CI, 1.24 to 2.35) and a nearly threefold increased risk of preterm premature rupture of membranes (PPROM; 95% CI, 1.62 to 4.46); no increased risk was observed after laser ablation. A subgroup analysis that controlled for age, parity, and smoking also revealed an increased relative risk for preterm delivery after LEEP (relative risk [RR], 2.10; 95% CI, 1.34 to 2.69).[38] Two studies that utilized large Finnish registries reported an increased risk of PTB after LEEP or conization.[39,40] The first one reported a nearly threefold increased risk for PTB after repeat LEEP,[39] consistent with other literature. **The second noted a 2.9 relative risk** (95% CI, 2.2 to 3.7) **of very preterm delivery** (28 to 31 weeks) **and a 2.1 relative risk** (95% CI, 1.47 to 2.99) **of extremely preterm delivery** (<28 weeks) **following cervical conization in a population of over 25,000 women who had undergone surgical treatment of cervical intraepithelial neoplasia** (CIN).[40] Possibly the most compelling association between surgical treatment of intraepithelial neoplasia and midtrimester birth comes from a recent systematic review and meta-analysis.[41] These investigators identified 14 studies that reported early pregnancy outcomes, eight of which included midtrimester births. Although seven of these did not individually report a significant association, the inclusion of a large population-based study from Norway[42] confirmed a highly significant association with a pooled risk ratio of 2.6 (95% CI, 1.5 to 4.7). The authors suggested that this increased risk was the result of cervical insufficiency after proportionally large excisions but could not confirm that other components of the sPTB syndrome were excluded.

Analogous to the findings of Sadler and colleagues,[43] several investigators have studied the effect of actual specimen size from LEEP or conization as a better predictor of PTB. Leiman[44] concluded that the risk of PTB was increased only when the maximum cone height was greater than 2 cm or the volume was greater than 4 mL. Raio and colleagues[45] performed a matched cohort study of 64 women who had undergone prior laser conization and observed no difference in the incidence of PTB compared with their controls (9.4% vs. 4.7%). They further reported statistically similar birthweights and gestational ages at delivery. However, in a secondary analysis, a laser cone height greater than 10 mm was a significant independent risk factor for PTB. In a more recent retrospective study[46] of 321 pregnancies following LEEP, a threefold increase in PTB at less than 37 weeks was observed if the excision volume exceeded 6 mL (95% CI, 1.45 to 5.92) or if the thickness of the excised tissue was greater than 12 mm (95% CI, 1.27 to 7.01).

Some investigators have proposed that PTB risk increases merely in the presence of cervical dysplasia, suggesting that the indication for the procedure—rather than the surgical procedure itself—is the more important biologic risk factor. In a recent

meta-analysis that compared 6589 patients with a history of LEEP to over 1 million patients without a history of excision, Conner and associates[47] reported a modestly increased risk of PTB before 37 weeks following LEEP (RR, 1.61; 95% CI, 1.35 to 1.92). However, on further analysis, those with prior LEEP had a risk of PTB similar to those with known dysplasia who had never undergone surgical excision. In a recent retrospective study[39] that utilized a Finnish registry of approximately 450,000 patients, prior LEEP was associated with a 1.61-fold increased risk for preterm delivery before 37 weeks, but the severity of CIN did not increase this risk. Instead, the investigators reported a twofold increased risk (95% CI, 1.5 to 2.9) of PTB in those who underwent LEEP for non-CIN lesions confirmed on histopathology (e.g., condyloma acuminatum); these data suggest that surgery does pose an independent risk.

Poon and colleagues[48] performed a secondary analysis of data from a clinical trial of PTB prevention and suggested that the risk of PTB from prior LEEP may be better reflected by a midgestation CL. In the study, 26,867 women undergoing routine prenatal care had transvaginal sonographic CL screening performed between 20 and 24 6/7 weeks of gestation. In 473 women who had a previous LEEP, the rate of preterm delivery before 34 weeks was increased (3.4% vs. 1.3%, P = .0002), and the median CL was significantly shorter (32 mm; interquartile range [IQR], 27 to 38 mm) versus 34 mm (IQR, 30 to 39 mm; P < .0001). After controlling for cervical length, prior LEEP was not a significant predictor of PTB.

Regarding history-indicated "prophylactic" treatment of presumptive insufficiency following cervical surgery, Kuoppala and Saarikoski[49] retrospectively reviewed 62 women who had undergone cone biopsy and an equal number of matched control patients. The pregnancy outcomes of the 22 who underwent history-indicated cerclage were similar to those managed without cerclage, with fetal salvage rates of 97% and 100%, respectively. On the basis of their findings and a review of seven other published reports, they concluded that history-indicated cerclage should not be routinely recommended for this possible risk factor. Of note, in the largest published randomized trial[34] of history-indicated cerclage for risk factors, summarized later, women with one or more cone biopsies or cervical amputations had an overall PTB rate before 33 weeks of 35%; however, in this population, no benefit was reported from history-indicated cerclage placement.

In summary, the weight of available evidence confirms an association between the surgical treatment of CIN and spontaneous PTB. However, it should be noted that these data do not confirm a disproportionate incidence of midtrimester loss with a clinical presentation consistent with the clinical diagnosis of cervical insufficiency. Women who have had a large cone specimen removed that included cervical amputations and those who have undergone multiple LEEP or conization procedures are the ones most at an increased risk of sPTB and presumably earlier deliveries. Whether history-indicated cerclage would be an effective preventive strategy in these at-risk women remains speculative. Because the available clinical trial data do not suggest a benefit from history-indicated cerclage, these women may be followed for evidence of premature cervical changes suggestive of insufficiency. **Women with a history of prior cervical surgery and recurrent spontaneous midtrimester loss that suggests a clinical diagnosis of insufficiency should be considered for a history-indicated cerclage in future pregnancies. Those with a history of LEEP or conization without**

a history of prior spontaneous midtrimester loss may be considered as candidates for clinical surveillance.

TESTS FOR CERVICAL INSUFFICIENCY

Because cervical insufficiency is likely part of a broader preterm parturition syndrome, there are few proven objective criteria other than perhaps a rare, gross cervical defect. For this reason, along with the greater research initiatives into PTB prevention, considerable effort has been devoted to developing objective and reproducible criteria for cervical insufficiency.

Most of the earlier reported tests for cervical insufficiency were based on the physiology of the internal os in the nonpregnant state and are of historic interest. Attempts at objective assessments include passage of a #8 Hegar dilator into the nonpregnant cervical canal without resistance,[50] diminished force required to dislodge a Foley catheter whose balloon was placed above the internal os and filled with 1 mL of saline solution,[51] and assessment of cervical elastic properties.[52]

All such attempts at providing an objective diagnosis of cervical insufficiency failed because the tests were not evaluated with regard to standard characteristics (e.g., sensitivity, specificity) against some reference standard for the diagnosis. Moreover, none of these tests could reasonably predict pregnancy-associated conditions that would lead to premature ripening and cervical dilation (i.e., *functional* insufficiency). **Finally, because no universally applicable standard exists for the diagnosis of cervical insufficiency, and because the results of such tests were never evaluated and linked to a proven effective treatment, their clinical utility was at best theoretic. Because no test for cervical insufficiency in the nonpregnant patient has been validated, none of these tests are in common use today.**

Although the literature devoted to screening for cervical insufficiency has been dominated by cervical length measurements, there is far more of importance beyond length in assessing the pregnant cervix.[53] Multiple approaches have been described to assess the cervical microstructure, encompassing techniques to evaluate tissue hydration, collagen structure, and tissue elasticity. In a recent review by Feltovich and colleagues,[53] several of these techniques were designated as having high clinical promise in assessment of the cervix, including Raman spectroscopy, backscattered power loss, and shear wave speed. Currently, these innovative modalities are still in the early stages of development. However, they may ultimately improve our understanding of the physiology of the cervix and may have a role in the clinical prediction of premature cervical ripening.

CLINICAL DIAGNOSIS OF CERVICAL INSUFFICIENCY

Patient History

Cervical insufficiency has primarily been a clinical diagnosis characterized by a history of recurrent painless dilation and spontaneous midtrimester (16 to 24 weeks) birth of a nonanomalous living fetus that usually suffers neonatal death or serious long-term morbidities from extreme prematurity. The diagnosis is usually retrospective and made only after poor obstetric outcomes have occurred. On occasion, a patient will be seen who has experienced painless cervical dilation before delivery. In such cases, careful documentation of what has happened is essential. In most cases, however, a careful history and

---

review of the past obstetric records are crucial to the diagnosis. However, in many instances, the records are incomplete or unavailable, and many women cannot provide a reliable history. Even with excellent records and accurate history, clinicians might disagree except in the most classic cases. Confounding factors in the history, records, or physical examination might be used to either support or refute the diagnosis based on their perceived importance.

As noted above, **the physician managing a patient who experiences a spontaneous midtrimester birth is in the optimal position to assess and document whether the clinical criteria for cervical insufficiency were met** (e.g., hourglassing membranes without painful regular uterine contractions) **and to rule out other causes of midtrimester birth** (e.g., placental abruption, antecedent fetal death, or fetal anomaly). However, because the preterm parturition syndrome includes other anatomic components, it is possible that some cases of cervical insufficiency are preceded by premature chorioamnion rupture or develop clinically apparent uterine activity. Although intrauterine infection might conceivably exclude the diagnosis, if cervical ripening and occult dilation have caused loss of the mucus plug, the normal barrier between the vaginal flora and chorioamnion is disrupted, and infection might be the presenting clinical event.[54] Although insufficiency is generally considered a diagnosis of exclusion, precisely how other causes of PTB should be excluded has never been explicitly defined.

Because cervical insufficiency is generally a retrospective diagnosis that depends on a history of poor outcomes, clinicians have sought criteria that might lead to a prospective and more objective diagnosis. In women considered to be at risk for cervical insufficiency based on an atypical history, prior cerclage for questionable historic indications, or because of other identified risk factors as mentioned above, serial examinations may be performed to detect progressive shortening and dilation, leading to a presumptive diagnosis of insufficiency, which may then be amenable to therapeutic intervention (Box 28-1). Use of cerclage merely for the presence of various risk factors, as described above, is not recommended.

SONOGRAPHIC DIAGNOSIS OF CERVICAL INSUFFICIENCY

Over the past several decades, numerous investigators have suggested that cervical insufficiency can be diagnosed by midtrimester sonographic evaluation of the cervix. Various sonographic findings that include CL, funneling at the internal os, and dynamic response to provocative maneuvers (e.g., fundal pressure) have been proposed (Fig. 28-2). In these earlier reports, the sonographic evaluations were not blinded, which led to uncontrolled interventions and difficulty determining their value. Diagnostic criteria were disparate and, in some cases, were not described in a quantitative or reproducible manner.

Later, large, blinded observational studies that used reproducible methods were published.[10,22,26] These investigators reported

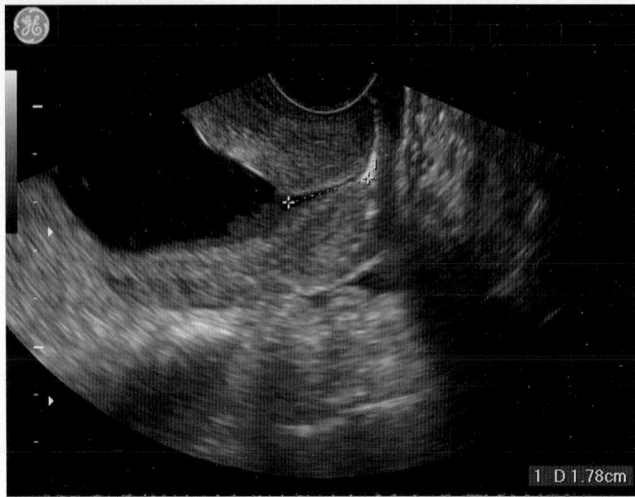

FIG 28-2 Short cervix (calipers) by transvaginal sonogram at 20⁵ᐟ⁷ weeks' gestation. Note the presence of a biofilm (sludge) that has been associated as a potential marker for subclinical infection. (From Romero R, Kusamovic JP, Espinoza J, et al. What is amniotic fluid "sludge"? *Ultrasound Obstet Gynecol.* 2007;30:793-798.)

BOX 28-2   CRITERION FOR THE SONOGRAPHIC DIAGNOSIS OF CERVICAL INSUFFICIENCY

• Shortened cervical length (<25 mm) detected by midtrimester sonography in women with singletons and a history of spontaneous preterm birth at <34-37 weeks

a preponderance of midtrimester births occurred at less than 27 weeks in this group.[55]

These reports[10,26] support the concept of shortened CL as a surrogate measure of cervical competence, but the actual identification of an appropriate CL cutoff that should lead to clinical intervention and confirmation of the potential contribution of related cervical sonographic findings (e.g., funneling at the internal os) **remains problematic. Clearly, cervical sonography has a lower sensitivity** (about 30% to 40%) **as a screening test in low-risk women** (i.e., singleton gestations without prior sPTB),[10] **but it appears to have significant utility for identifying clinically significant cervical pathology in women with a prior early sPTB.[26,56]**

Although some investigators have included women with various risk factors in their study populations composed primarily of women with previous sPTB, the results could not be subcategorized because of small sample sizes.[56] However, in a recent series of 64 women with various uterine anomalies, the authors observed an overall preterm delivery rate at less than 35 weeks of 11% and found a significant relationship between CLs of less than 25 mm and PTB,[30] with summary predictive values similar to those of other high-risk populations.[26]

Use of cervical ultrasound in twin gestations has also been reported.[57] However, the screening test characteristics, especially sensitivity and PPV (<40%), appear to be generally lower than for women with a prior early sPTB. A systematic review[58] summarized the predictive value of vaginal sonography for PTB in 46 published series of both asymptomatic and symptomatic gravidas carrying singleton or twin gestations. Eleven series of asymptomatic women with twins were included. The relationship between cervical shortening and PTB was much stronger in the singleton, as opposed to the twin, populations in both receiver operator curve and meta-analytic assessment of likelihood ratios. Because the management of twins with shortened CL has been particularly problematic, it is unclear how we should be using CL measurements in multiple gestations outside of clinical trials (Box 28-2).

the relationship between midtrimester cervical sonographic findings and PTB and sought to identify cervical changes that indicated a dominant cervical etiology and the possibility for intervention. The Eunice Kennedy Shriver National Institutes of Child Health and Human Development (NICHD) Maternal-Fetal Medicine Units (MFMU) Network[10] completed a study of 2915 unselected women with a singleton pregnancy who underwent a blinded cervical sonographic evaluation at 22 to 24 weeks' gestation: **the relative risk of sPTB increased steadily as the measured CL shortened. In spite of this highly significant relationship, as a test for predicting spontaneous PTB at less than 35 weeks, a CL cutoff of less than 26 mm** (the population 10th percentile) **had low sensitivity (37%) and poor PPV (18%).** Midtrimester birth consistent with cervical insufficiency was not specifically reported, but examination of the survival curve suggests that less than 5% of women with a CL of 25 mm or less at 22 to 24 weeks delivered prior to 28 weeks. Moreover, the circumstances of these early births were not reported, so clinical criteria for insufficiency could not be assessed. Thus in an unselected population, shortened CL at 22 to 24 weeks appeared to be a very ineffective tool for identifying women with cervical insufficiency.

In a subsequent study, the NICHD MFMU Network[26] examined the utility of cervical ultrasound as a predictor of sPTB at less than 35 weeks in high-risk women, defined as those having at least one prior sPTB at less than 32 weeks. Women with a clinical diagnosis of cervical insufficiency were excluded. Beginning at 16 to 18 weeks of gestation, 183 gravidas underwent serial, biweekly sonographic evaluations until the 23rd week of gestation. The study design permitted analysis of the shortest observed CL over time, which also included any fundal pressure–induced or spontaneously occurring CL shortening. As in the previous study,[10] a highly significant inverse relationship was found between CL and spontaneous PTB. However, in this high-risk population, at a CL cutoff of less than 25 mm, the sensitivity increased to 69%, and the PPV increased to 55%. Importantly, a secondary analysis of the data suggested that these high-risk women with a shortened CL might have a clinically significant *component* of diminished cervical competence because

DIAGNOSIS OF CERVICAL INSUFFICIENCY ON PHYSICAL EXAMINATION

Uncommonly, a patient in the midtrimester will present with vague pelvic symptoms such as increased pressure and vaginal discharge with increased urinary frequency but without other symptoms of urinary tract infection. Physical exam with a speculum reveals a relatively uneffaced but dilated cervix (at least 1 to 2 cm but generally less than 5 cm) and membranes visible at or beyond the level of the external os. **Fetal parts or the umbilical cord might be seen behind the membranes or even contained in the prolapsing sac.** Significant uterine contractions and clinical evidence of intrauterine infection (e.g., fever, uterine tenderness) are absent, and a period of observation and monitoring for overt infection and labor are generally performed to establish a diagnosis. **This is termed *acute cervical insufficiency*. Presumably, these findings were antecedent events in most if not all cases of midtrimester birth later attributed to cervical insufficiency based on historic criteria. However, this presentation provides a unique clinical opportunity to witness the natural history of cervical insufficiency, explore possible etiologies, and consider the effectiveness of different interventions** (Box 28-3).

TREATMENT: CERCLAGE

The contemporary mainstay of treatment has been a surgical approach using one of the classic cerclage procedures, although both medical treatments and other mechanical supportive therapies have been used.

Cerclage Technique

The proper placement of a suture in the uterine cervical stroma and/or around its perimeter to treat cervical insufficiency or prevent preterm delivery has been the subject of debate because of the lack of proper randomized studies to assess different perioperative strategies.[59] Techniques based on indications are described below.

History-Indicated Cerclage

Women with a history of recurrent midtrimester losses characterized by painless cervical dilation in the absence of overt labor or placental abruption are considered candidates for history-indicated cerclage. This may also be utilized in women with a

---

prior history of cerclage placement secondary to painless cervical dilation in the midtrimester; that is, those with a prior cerclage based on findings on physical examination.[60] History-indicated cerclage placement is generally performed at 12 to 15 weeks of gestation to avoid the complications of early spontaneous loss often attributable to chromosomal abnormalities.[61]

In 1950, Lash and Lash[62] described repair of the cervix in the nonpregnant state that involved partial excision of the cervix to remove the area of presumed weakness. Unfortunately, this technique was associated with a high incidence of subsequent infertility. In 1955, Shirodkar[63] reported successful management of cervical insufficiency with the use of a submucosal band. Initially, he used catgut as suture material, and later he used Mersilene (Ethicon, Somerville, NJ) placed at the level of the internal cervical os. The procedure required anterior displacement of the bladder in an attempt to place the suture as high as possible at the level of cervical internal os. This type of procedure resulted in a greater number of patients being delivered by cesarean delivery because of the difficulty in removing the suture buried under the cervical surface, and it often required leaving the suture in place postpartum. Several years later, McDonald[64] described a suture technique in the form of a purse string that did not require cervical dissection and that was easily placed during pregnancy. This technique involves taking four or five bites as high as possible in the cervix, trying to avoid injury to the bladder or the rectum, with placement of a knot anteriorly to facilitate removal (Fig. 28-3). Most randomized studies of cerclage have used the McDonald technique. A randomized controlled trial (RCT) based in Europe utilizing the Shirodkar technique did not demonstrate benefit.[65] Therefore, **owing to its simplicity and effectiveness, a McDonald technique is recommended as the first-line procedure.**

Several types of suture material have been used, and no randomized studies had been done to compare the different types of cerclage suture and/or the preferable type of needle to use.[66] We have been successful in using a Mersilene tape. However, the use of thinner suture material, such as Prolene (Ethicon) or other synthetic nonabsorbable sutures like Ethibond (Ethicon), is advocated by others with the argument that the width of the

---

> **BOX 28-3   CRITERIA FOR THE DIAGNOSIS OF CERVICAL INSUFFICIENCY ON PHYSICAL EXAMINATION**
>
> - Midtrimester cervical dilation and membranes visible at or beyond the external os in the absence of clinically defined antecedent labor or overt intrauterine infection
> - Significant (serial) asymptomatic cervical dilation detected by palpation at midtrimester

---

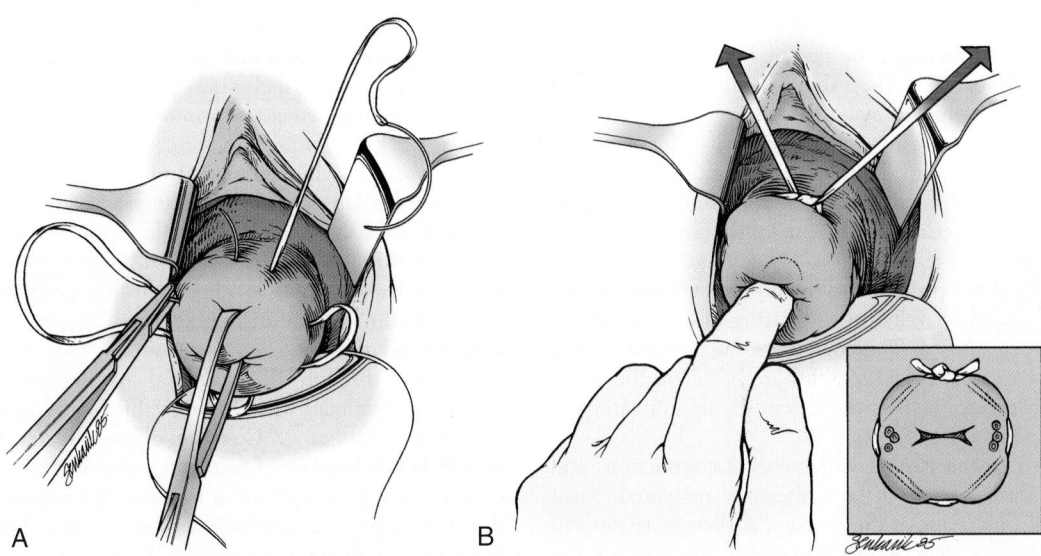

FIG 28-3 Placement of sutures for McDonald cerclage. **A,** Double-headed Mersilene band with four bites in the cervix, avoiding the vessels. **B,** The suture is placed high up in the cervix, close to the cervicovaginal junction, approximately at the level of the internal os.

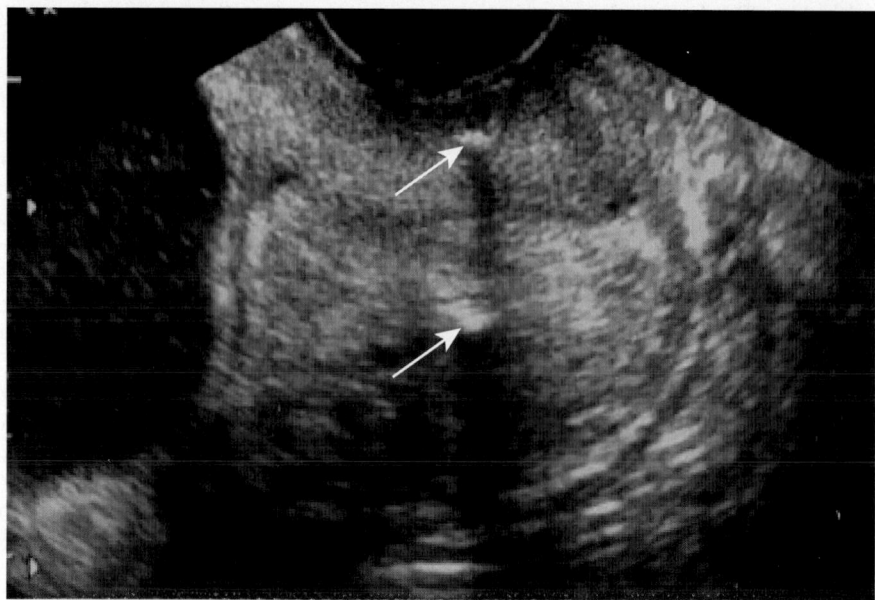

FIG 28-4 Transvaginal sonogram of the cervix after cerclage placement. The internal os is closed, and no funneling is evident. Echogenic spots in the cervix correspond to cerclage (*arrows*).

Mersilene tape places the patient at greater risk for infection.[67-68] **Currently, no evidence suggests that placing two sutures results in better outcomes than placing one.** A recent large retrospective study did not show a difference in PTB rates between the two- versus one-stitch groups.[69] Furthermore, placement of a second occlusive suture at the level of the external os to keep the mucous plug in place has not shown benefit in a recent RCT.[70]

Preoperative patient preparations that include the use of prophylactic antibiotics or tocolytics have not been proven to be of benefit, and evidence is insufficient to recommend their use. The value of performing cultures before the cerclage procedure has not been properly studied, and this practice—as well as giving perioperative antibiotics—should be individualized. Similarly, the use of amniocentesis prior to cerclage has not been subjected to RCTs. **It appears that for a history-indicated cerclage, the rate of subclinical intraamniotic infection (IAI) is very low, and amniocentesis does not seem justifiable.** However, for ultrasound-indicated cerclage, the rate of subclinical IAI could be as high as 1% to 2%.[71] The value of amniocentesis in this setting needs to be evaluated by an RCT.[59]

The choice of anesthesia for cerclage varies.[72] Chen and colleagues[73] did not observe a difference in outcome between general versus regional anesthesia. In our experience, a short-acting regional anesthetic is sufficient, and spinal anesthesia appears to be the preferred anesthesia for cerclage.

The value of bed rest postoperatively has been questioned and even criticized,[74] and its value in the setting of cerclage placement has not been studied. Decisions regarding physical activity and intercourse are individualized and are based on the status of the cervix as determined by outpatient digital evaluation or sonographic findings (Fig. 28-4).

The approach to the patient with preterm contractions and a cerclage in place has not been sufficiently evaluated. Most authorities will only remove the cerclage if there is tension in the suture because of the concern for cervical lacerations if the suture is left behind. **The suture is usually removed electively at 36 to 37 weeks.** Systematic review of the literature showed that planned removal of cervical cerclage before the onset of labor at 36 to 37 weeks is associated with a 28% nonsignificant reduction in the incidence of cervical lacerations compared with removal in labor (6.4% vs. 11.4%; RR, 0.72; 95% CI, 0.35 to 1.49). The mean interval between cerclage removal and spontaneous delivery is 14 days.[75]

In patients with a prior failed vaginal cerclage, an abdominal cerclage has been recommended.[76] A prior history-indicated vaginal cerclage resulting in an sPTB before 33 weeks (i.e., a failed cerclage) is currently the only indication proven by controlled studies to show benefit from a transabdominal cerclage compared with a repeat transvaginal cerclage. This procedure is usually done either in pregnancy between 11 and 12 weeks gestation or prior to conception.[77] The procedure can be done either with a laparotomy or using a laparoscopic or robotic approach. A bladder flap may or may not be created. The procedure requires the placement of a Mersilene tape at the level of the junction between the lower uterine segment and the cervix lateral to the uterus and medial to the uterine vessels (Fig. 28-5). Greater morbidity, including injury to the uterine vessels, requires expertise when performing this procedure. In our experience, we have found it helpful to have an assistant provide fundal traction, while the surgeon grasps the uterine vessels and retracts them laterally to expose an avascular space between the artery and the cervix. A right-angle clamp is passed anterior to posterior through this avascular space, tenting and incising the posterior leaf of the broad ligament and grasping a Mersilene tape brought back through the space. The same procedure is repeated on the opposite side, and the tape is tied anteriorly (Figs. 28-6 through 28-9). Several investigators have reported extensive experience with this procedure with low morbidity and favorable outcomes.[77,78] **Cesarean delivery is necessary, and the suture is left in place if future fertility is desired.**

In cases of pregnancy complications that require midtrimester delivery, we have either performed a posterior colpotomy, cutting the tape and allowing for vaginal delivery, or a laparotomy and hysterotomy, leaving the suture intact. In most of the reported series of abdominal cerclage, including ours, this surgical

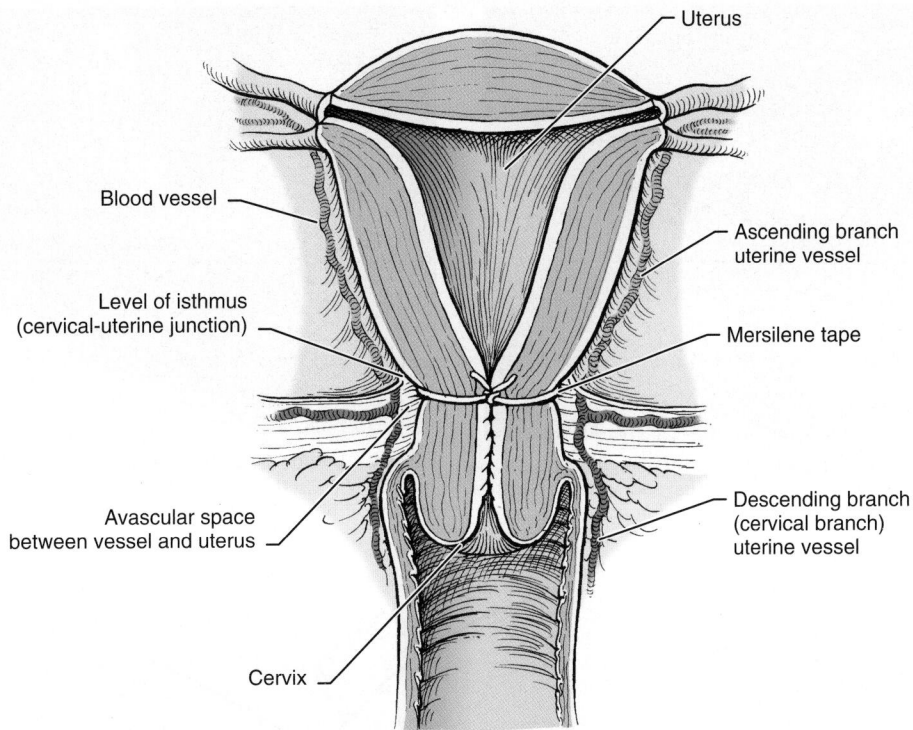

FIG 28-5 Abdominal cerclage. Surgical placement of circumferential Mersilene tape around uterine isthmus and medial to uterine vessels. Knot is tied anteriorly.

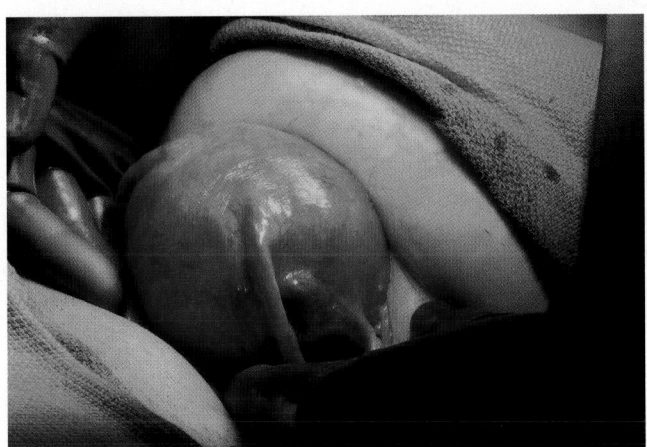

FIG 28-6 Abdominal cerclage at 12 weeks' gestation. Uterus is exteriorized.

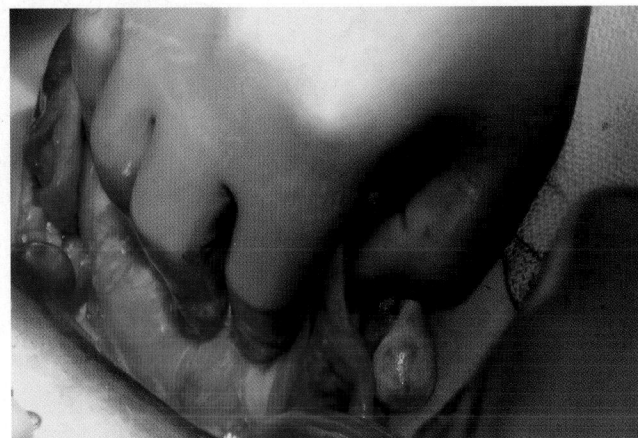

FIG 28-7 Abdominal cerclage. A bladder flap has been created, and the surgeon identifies and palpates the uterine vessel.

procedure was performed during gestation.[78] However, Groom and colleagues[77] described this procedure as an interval cerclage in the nonpregnant state with subsequent good pregnancy outcome. Advantages of an interval procedure include avoidance of laparotomy in pregnancy and less bleeding morbidity. Disadvantages include the inability to become pregnant, and for the clinician, the difficulties of pregnancy management arise if the gestation results in a first-trimester miscarriage. No studies have compared preconception versus abdominal cerclage during gestation that would enable us to make specific recommendations about timing of the procedure.

In the last few years, a laparoscopic abdominal approach to the cervix has been described using the same principles as an abdominal cerclage.[79] The procedure has been described

primarily in the nonpregnant state with subsequent good pregnancy outcome. Cho and colleagues[80] performed laparoscopic abdominal cerclage during pregnancy in 20 patients with minimal morbidity and reported a successful outcome in 19 of them. In a review[81] of the literature that encompassed 31 studies—6 reporting a laparoscopic approach and 26 using laparotomy, either interval or during pregnancy—both approaches were associated with favorable outcomes. A total of 78.5% of those with a laparoscopic abdominal cerclage and 84.8% of those with an abdominal cerclage placed by laparotomy delivered a viable infant after 34 weeks. Midtrimester loss occurred in 8.1% of those using the laparoscopic approach and in 7.8% with laparotomy. Recently, robotic-assisted laparoscopic placement of transabdominal cerclage during pregnancy has been

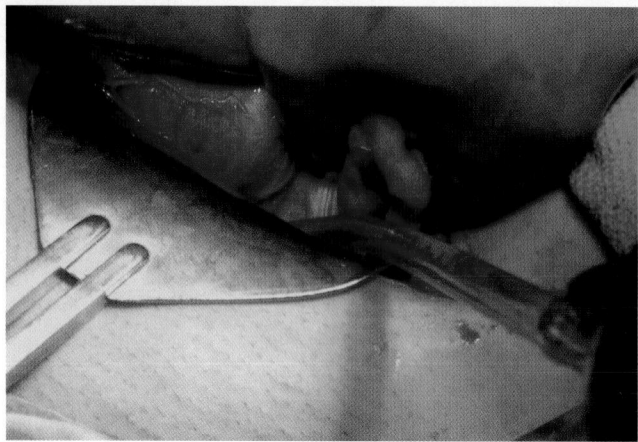

FIG 28-8 Abdominal cerclage. Surgeon retracts uterine vessel laterally to create an avascular space between uterus and vessel, before passing a right angle clamp with Mersilene tape through this space.

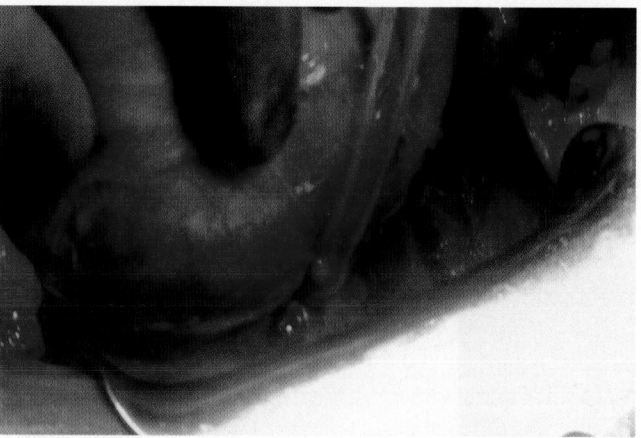

FIG 28-9 Abdominal cerclage. Mersilene tape has been placed circumferentially around the uterine isthmus and tied anteriorly. Notice ballooning of the lower uterine segment above the suture.

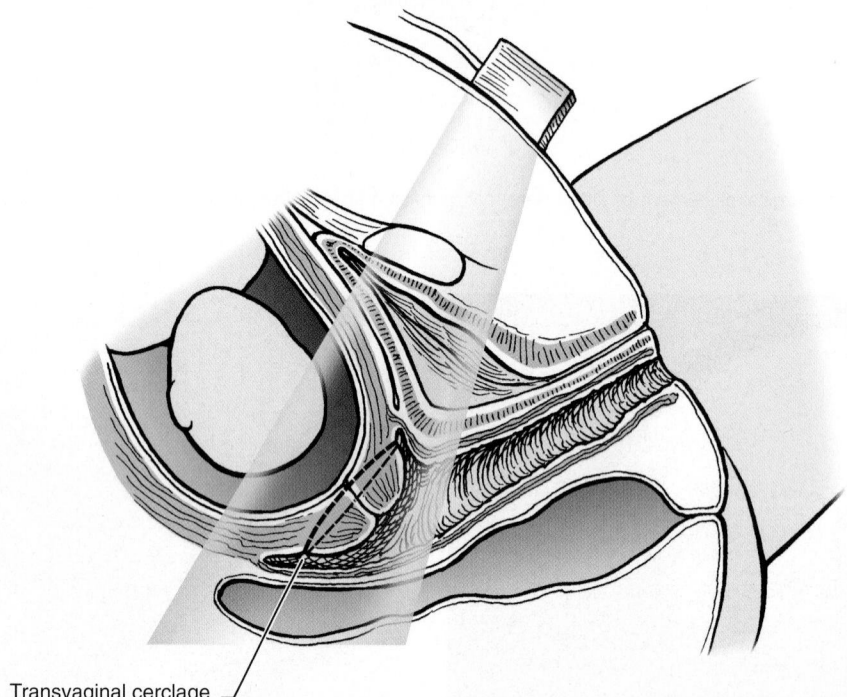

Transvaginal cerclage

FIG 28-10 Transvaginal cerclage under ultrasound guidance. (Modified from Ludmir J, Jackson GM, Samuels P. Transvaginal cerclage under ultrasound guidance in cases of severe cervical hypoplasia. *Obstet Gynecol.* 1991;75:1067.)

described by Wolfe and colleagues,[82] and we have started to use this technique in selected cases. Because of the lack of proper evaluation of these newer modalities of cerclage placement, recommendations based on evidence cannot be made. **Randomized trials are needed to evaluate these newer techniques in nonpregnant and pregnant states and to compare laparoscopic techniques with a vaginal approach to determine the best management of patients with a history of failed cerclage or an extremely short cervix that prevents a vaginal approach.**

To avoid an abdominal procedure in selected patients, we have described the placement of a transvaginal cerclage in cases of a hypoplastic cervix or when the cervix is flush against the vaginal wall.[83] Under ultrasound guidance, the supravaginal portion of the cervix is dissected away from the bladder, and

a suture is placed either in a purse-string fashion or in a cross configuration from 12 to 6 o'clock and 3 to 9 o'clock (Fig. 28-10). We have performed this procedure in 32 patients, avoiding an abdominal procedure, with successful pregnancy outcomes: 50% of our patients have had a cesarean delivery, and the rest delivered vaginally after the suture was cut through a small posterior colpotomy incision.

Physical Examination–Indicated Cerclage

Patients who demonstrate cervical change either by ultrasound or by digital evaluation may benefit from a cerclage.[84] However, the gestational age limit for cerclage placement is poorly defined. **Although some clinicians offer this therapeutic modality up to 28 weeks, we do not advocate the use of cerclage beyond**

24 weeks' gestation because of our concerns about fetal viability should the procedure contribute to a preterm delivery.[85] The perioperative management of these patients has not been subject to rigorous study, and recommendations based on evidence cannot be given.[59] IAI is present in approximately 13% to 50% of patients with acute cervical insufficiency. As discussed below,[85] the value of amniocentesis to rule out IAI is currently being assessed in an RCT.

When the cervix has dilated enough to allow visualization of the membranes, or the membranes have prolapsed into the vagina, placing a cerclage may be difficult but should be considered.[86] Amnioreduction has been suggested to facilitate cerclage placement; in a European study,[87] this procedure was associated with prolonged gestation. Several techniques have been described to reduce the prolapsing membranes that include placing the patient in the Trendelenburg position, using a pediatric Foley catheter to tease the membranes into the endocervical canal, and instilling 1 L of saline into the bladder with upper displacement of the lower uterine segment (Fig. 28-11).[88] The efficacy of antibiotics and tocolytics have not been properly studied in this setting. **Although clinicians have been reluctant to offer cerclage in patients with protruding membranes, some reports have suggested a salvage rate in excess of 70% despite advanced cervical dilation, with only 40% delivering before 35 weeks.**[89] Cerclage may be effective at up to 4-cm dilation, but in the face of advanced cervical dilation and bulging membranes, the correct assessment of cervical dilation is difficult; however, cerclage should be considered even in cases of advanced dilation.

Risks of Cerclage

Cervical lacerations at the time of delivery are one of the most common complications from a cerclage and occur in 1% to 13% of patients.[90] Three percent of patients require cesarean delivery because of the inability of the cervix to dilate secondary to cervical scarring and dystocia.[90] Although the risk of infection is minimal with a history-indicated cerclage, the risk increases significantly in cases of advanced dilation with exposure of membranes to the birth canal.[91] However, this infectious morbidity may be the result of subclinical chorioamnionitis. Cervical cerclage displacement occurs in a small number of patients. We have not performed revision of the cerclage during the index pregnancy, although small series have reported successful surgical treatment of a failed cerclage. At this time, evidence is insufficient to recommend the placement of a reinforcing suture.[92]

Cerclage in the Presence of Premature Rupture of Membranes or Preterm Labor

When the clinician is faced with premature rupture of membranes (PROM) distant from term in a patient with cerclage, the decision to remove or leave the suture in place is controversial. Our own data suggest that with suture retention, the latency period is increased at the expense of an increased risk for neonatal sepsis and mortality.[93] These data have been challenged by reports from Jenkins and colleages,[94] which suggest an increased latency period (244 vs. 119 hours) without an increase in neonatal morbidity in cases of retained cerclage, and by McElrath and colleagues,[95] who did not find differences in latency or neonatal outcome in patients when the suture was left in situ after rupture of the membranes. A recent randomized study[96] that was not completed because of inability to recruit patients showed no difference in latency, infection, or neonatal outcome

in those patients managed with immediate cerclage removal versus suture retention. However, less infectious morbidity was seen with cerclage removal. **Decisions to remove the suture at the time of ruptured membranes should be individualized until more information becomes available.** In the face of preterm contractions, the decision to remove the cerclage should be individualized based on findings such as tension or cervical tearing, although the subject has not been studied appropriately. Finally, even though cerclage placement is considered a benign procedure, a maternal death secondary to sepsis in a patient with retained cerclage has been reported.[97] Because of associated risks and questionable effectiveness, the liberal use of this surgical procedure is discouraged, and the decision should be carefully balanced against potential harm, in particular for patients in whom the indications for cerclage are unclear.

CERCLAGE EFFECTIVENESS BASED ON EVIDENCE

History-Indicated Cerclage

Four randomized trials have been done that included women with various risk factors for sPTB and *possible* cervical insufficiency whose managing physicians did not believe they required a prophylactic cerclage for a typical history of cervical insufficiency.[34,98-100] Three of the trials were relatively small and were based on a scoring system,[98] twin gestation,[99] and recurrent sPTB.[100] None of these trials showed a benefit to cerclage, but together they generally confirmed a higher rate of hospitalizations and medical interventions in the cerclage groups. The largest randomized trial of cerclage was conducted by the RCOG between 1981 and 1988.[34] A total of 1292 women were enrolled in 12 countries because of uncertainty on the part of their managing physicians as to whether a history-indicated cerclage was warranted. As anticipated, these patients comprised a heterogeneous group with at least six distinct risk-factor subgroups identified on the basis of their dominant history or physical examination findings. Although women assigned to cerclage had a significantly lower rate of PTB earlier than 33 weeks (13% vs. 17%, P = .03), the investigators estimated that approximately 25 cerclage procedures would be required to prevent one such birth. Moreover, women assigned to cerclage received more tocolytic medications and spent more time in the hospital. Puerperal fever was significantly more common in the cerclage group. Of interest is the finding in a secondary analysis that only the subgroup of women with multiple pregnancies affected—defined as at least three prior sPTBs, including midtrimester losses—appeared to benefit from cerclage with lower rates of PTB (15% vs. 32%; P = .02). This secondary analysis emphasized the importance of assessing clinical history in considering the diagnosis and treatment of cervical insufficiency.

Data on the efficacy of history-indicated transvaginal cerclage have been varied. As above, in a subgroup analysis of the RCOG RCT, cerclage was found to be beneficial and was associated with a small reduction in PTB (<33 weeks) if placed in the setting of a history of three or more prior PTBs (RR, 0.75; 95% CI, 0.58 to 0.98). A more recent meta-analysis does not support this finding and reports no overall reduction in pregnancy loss or PTB rates in the setting of history-indicated cerclage.[101] When compared with ultrasound-indicated cerclage, multiple studies have noted no change in perinatal outcome but roughly double the number of cerclage procedures performed in the history-indicated group.[60,102] A meta-analysis of the four RCTs that

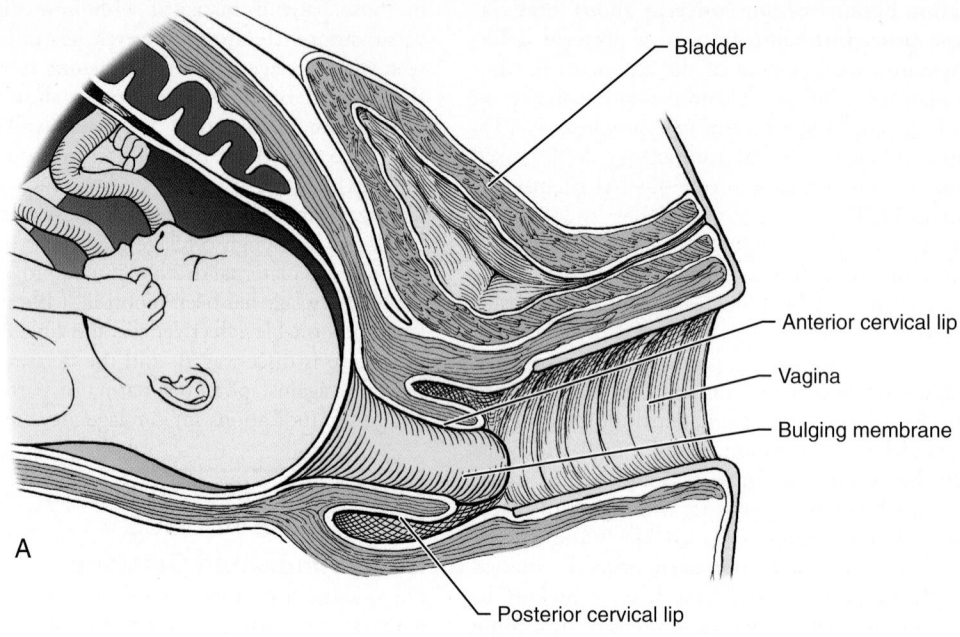

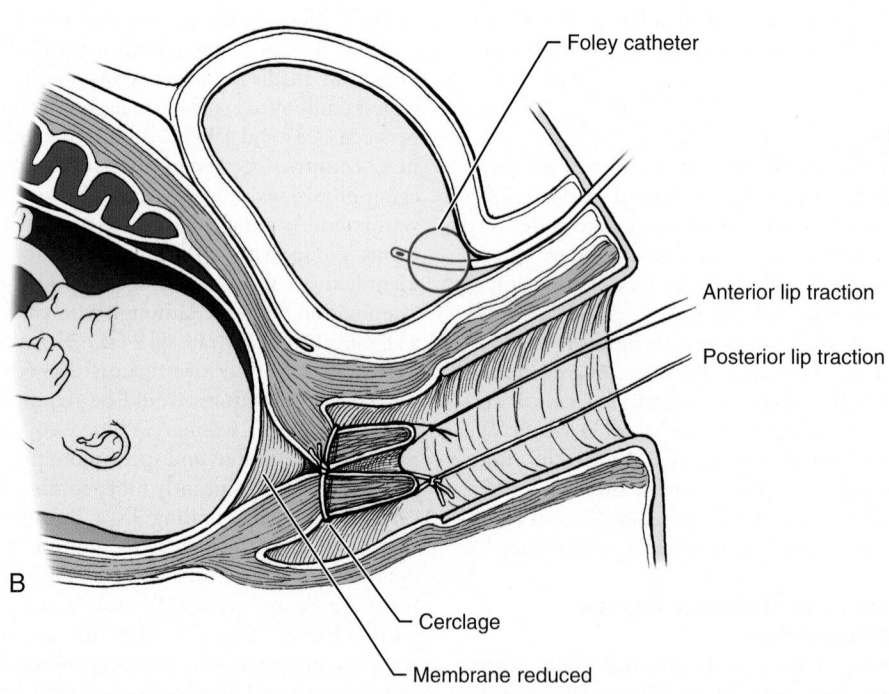

FIG 28-11 Emergent cerclage for bulging membranes at 23 weeks. **A,** Cervix dilated 3 cm with membranes protruding through the external cervical os into the vagina. **B,** Patient placed in Trendelenburg position and bladder filled with saline. Stay silk sutures are placed on anterior and posterior lip for traction while reducing membranes. McDonald cerclage is placed distal to reduced membranes.

compared a policy of history-indicated cerclage with a policy of TVU CL screening and cerclage only if CL shortened before 24 weeks in singleton gestations with prior PTBs showed similar maternal, perinatal, and PTB outcomes except that only 42% of women in the TVU CL group had a cerclage.[102] Despite the limited evidence to support history-indicated cerclage, one study performed by Fox and colleagues[103] reported that 75% of maternal-fetal medicine (MFM) specialists who responded to a

survey would place a cerclage in a patient with a history of a prior painless midgestation loss.

Branch and Cousins collectively tabulated over 25 case series of cerclage efficacy published between 1959 and 1981. Branch[104] estimated a precerclage survival range of 10% to 32% versus a perinatal survival range of 75% to 83% in the same cohorts of women managed with Shirodkar cerclage. Similarly, a case series that used McDonald cerclage reported a cohort perinatal

TABLE 28-1   RANDOMIZED TRIALS OF CERCLAGE FOR SONOGRAPHICALLY SUSPECTED CERVICAL INSUFFICIENCY

STUDY	POPULATION	N	SELECTION CRITERIA	GA FOR US EVALUATION (WK)	PRIMARY OUTCOME (WK)	CERCLAGE GROUP (%)	NO CERCLAGE GROUP (%)	BENEFIT?
Althuisius et al[101] (2001)	History or symptoms suggest CI	35	CL <25 mm	<27	PTB <34	0	44	Yes
Rust et al[102] (2001)	Many had risk factors	115	CL <25 mm or >25% funneling	16-24	PTB <34	35	36	No
To et al[65] (2004)	Unselected, generally low risk	253	CL ≤15 mm	22-24	PTB <33	22	26	No
Berghella et al[103] (2004)	Most had risk factors	61	CL <25 mm or >25% funneling	14-23	PTB <35	45	47	No
Owen et al[4] (2009)	Prior sPTB (17 to 33 wk)	301	CL <25 mm	16-21	PTB <35	32	42	Yes

CI, cervical insufficiency; *CL*, cervical length; *GA*, gestational age; *PTB*, preterm birth; *sPTB*, spontaneous preterm birth; *US*, ultrasound.

survival range of 7% to 50% before and 63% to 89% after cerclage. Cousins[105] estimated a "mean" survival before Shirodkar of 22% versus 82% post therapy and 27% and 74%, respectively, for investigators who used the McDonald technique. In total, more than 2000 patients have been reported in these historic cohort comparisons. As noted by Cousins, interpretation of these series is limited because (1) diagnostic criteria were inconsistent or were not always reported; (2) definitions of treatment success were inconsistent but were generally recorded as perinatal survival, as opposed to a gestational age-based end point; (3) treatment approaches were not always detailed and might involve multiple combinations of surgery, medication, bed rest, and other uncontrolled therapies; and (4) cases were not subcategorized according to etiology (e.g., anatomic defects versus a presumed functional cause). Nevertheless, based on compelling but potentially biased efficacy data, the surgical management of women with a history of clinically defined cervical insufficiency has become standard practice, and it has clearly shaped the way the average MFM provider practices. Although interpretation of efficacy based on historic control groups is always problematic, collectively these reports demonstrate that even women with typical histories may have successful pregnancies without cerclage and that cerclage as a treatment is not universally effective. Both of these observations support the multiple etiologies and interactive pathways characteristic of the spontaneous PTB syndrome.

Because of its unproven efficacy in randomized clinical trials and the attendant surgical risks, the recommendation for history-indicated cerclage should be limited to women with multiple midtrimester sPTBs when a careful history and physical examination suggest a dominant cervical component. Unless the physical examination confirms a significant cervical anatomic defect consistent with disruption of its circumferential integrity, the clinician should assess the history for other components of the PTB syndrome. Cervical insufficiency remains a diagnosis of exclusion.

Ultrasound-Indicated Cerclage

Under the presumption that shortened cervical length, with or without funneling at the internal os, is diagnostic of cervical insufficiency if it occurs in a singleton gestation and in a patient with a prior sPTB, several investigators have studied the effect of ultrasound-indicated cerclage on pregnancy outcomes. Retrospective analyses of uncontrolled use of cerclage in various

at-risk populations have given conflicting results, which suggests that cerclage was either effective[106] or ineffective.[56,107]

Later, five randomized trials of cerclage for sonographic indications were published (Table 28-1). Althuisius and colleagues in the Netherlands randomized high-risk patients, the majority of whom were believed to have cervical insufficiency based on their symptoms or obstetric history and midtrimester CL less than 25 mm. Both the cerclage and no-cerclage groups were instructed to use modified home rest. Of the 19 assigned to cerclage, no PTBs were reported before 34 weeks versus a 44% rate in the no cerclage–home rest group (*P* = .002). Rust and colleagues[109] enrolled 138 women who had various risk factors for PTB (including 12% with multiple gestations) and randomly assigned them to receive a McDonald cerclage or no cerclage after their CL shortened to less than 25 mm or they developed funneling of at least 25%. PTB before 34 weeks was observed in 35% of the cerclage group versus 36% of controls.

In a multinational trial, To and colleagues[65] screened 47,123 unselected women at 22 to 24 weeks' gestation with vaginal ultrasound to identify 470 with a shortened CL of 15 mm or less. Of these 470, 253 participated in a randomized trial whose primary outcome was the intergroup rates of delivery before 33 weeks' gestation. Women assigned to the cerclage group (*n* = 127) underwent a Shirodkar procedure. They had a similar rate of PTB as the control population (*n* = 126) 22% versus 26% (*P* = .44). The authors did not specifically comment on the proportion of women in the control group who were delivered in the midtrimester after a presentation consistent with clinically defined cervical insufficiency; however, they observed four stillbirths attributed to birth at 23 to 24 weeks and five neonatal deaths in deliveries at 23 to 26 weeks. In the cerclage group, the respective counts were three and four.

Berghella and colleagues[110] screened women with various risk factors for sPTB (e.g., prior PTB, curettages, cone biopsy, DES exposure) with vaginal scans every 2 weeks from 14 to 23 weeks' gestation and randomly assigned 61 with a cervical length less than 25 mm or funneling of at least 25% to a McDonald cerclage or to a no-cerclage control group. PTB before 35 weeks was observed in 45% of the cerclage group and in 47% of the control group.

The trial by Althuisius and colleagues[108] focused on women whom they believed had a clinical diagnosis of cervical insufficiency and who may have been candidates for history-indicated cerclage in the United States. Nevertheless, their study does suggest a potential role for cervical ultrasound in women with a clinical diagnosis of cervical insufficiency if the intent is to *avoid* cerclage when the CL is maintained at 25 mm or greater.

A meta-analysis[111] of the four randomized trials described earlier analyzed patient-level data to estimate whether certain subgroups of women with midtrimester cervical shortening might benefit from cerclage, where benefit was defined as a reduction in the relative risk of PTB before 35 weeks. They observed a marginal benefit from cerclage in women with singleton gestations and especially in those who had experienced a prior sPTB (RR, 0.6; 95% CI, 0.4 to 0.9). Paradoxically, they demonstrated a significant *detriment* in women with multiple gestations (RR, 2.15; 95% CI, 1.15 to 4.01). This harmful effect has never been confirmed in a randomized trial, nor have authors of cohort studies observed this relationship.[112-113]

Based on an earlier review of the utility of vaginal ultrasound for the diagnosis of cervical insufficiency,[114] a fifth randomized trial was performed by a consortium of 15 centers in the United States[4] and included only women who had had at least one prior sPTB at 17 to 34 weeks' gestation. They were followed with serial vaginal scans beginning at 16 weeks' gestation. As long as CL was at least 30 mm, scans were scheduled every 2 weeks, but the frequency was increased to weekly if the CL was 25 to 29 mm. Women who developed a short cervix (<25 mm) between 16 and 22 6/7 weeks were assigned to McDonald cerclage or no cerclage. These investigators observed a statistically significant decrease in previable births before 24 weeks (6% vs. 14%), perinatal mortality (9% vs. 16%), and birth before 37 weeks (45% vs. 60%), but a nonsignificant decrease was seen in the comparative rates of PTB before 35 weeks (32% vs. 42%). The number of patients with a short cervix that needed to be treated with cerclage to prevent one previable birth was 13. Of note was the observation that the benefit of cerclage was closely linked to cervical status. Women with a CL of less than 15 mm at randomization accrued a much greater benefit than those who were randomized with a CL of 15 to 24 mm. This finding suggested that shorter lengths are more likely to be associated with a primary cervical etiology and are thus more amenable to mechanical support, although the "optimal" CL (e.g., <25 mm, <15 mm) for recommending cerclage could not be established. Similarly, the finding of a U-shaped funnel (but not a V-shaped funnel) was also a significant additional risk factor for earlier birth, even considering CL; in these women, the beneficial effect of cerclage for prolonging gestation was also significantly pronounced.[115]

Considering the results of the multicenter trial mentioned above,[4] Berghella and colleagues performed a follow-up meta-analysis that included the findings of this trial with the original four studies.[116] **This patient-level analysis confirmed significant benefit of ultrasound-indicated cerclage for CLs less than 25 mm observed before 24 weeks' gestation in women with prior sPTB. Cerclage reduced PTB at cutoffs of less than 37, 35, 32, 28, and 24 weeks, and composite neonatal mortality and morbidity were also significantly lower (RR, 0.64; 95% CI, 0.45 to 0.91).**

Not uncommonly a patient presents with a prior midtrimester spontaneous birth that does not meet clinical criteria for cervical insufficiency. In these circumstances, she may have even undergone a history-indicated cerclage. Whether these women needed a history-indicated cerclage or if they should have had a repeat cerclage is controversial, and clinical judgment is important. However, accumulating evidence suggests that it is safe to follow

these women with CL measurements and avoid cerclage. A recent meta-analysis by Berghella and colleagues[102] of four randomized trials indicated that using sonographic CL to select women for cerclage, most women (58%) would avoid surgery yet have no greater risk of PTB than the cohorts who underwent history-indicated cerclage (RR, 0.97; 95% CI, 0.73 to 1.29).

In summary, collective results have established the utility of cervical length screening and ultrasound-indicated cerclage for a short cervix less than 25 mm in women with a prior sPTB (Box 28-4).

Physical Examination–Indicated Cerclage

Women who present with acute cervical insufficiency are often considered candidates for a physical examination–indicated cerclage. The limited data on the efficacy of this procedure reflect its rare presentation. Some investigators have reported fetal salvage rates in excess of 70%.[117] Aarts and colleagues[118] reviewed eight series published between 1980 and 1992 that comprised 249 patients who received a physical examination–indicated cerclage and estimated a mean neonatal survival rate of 64% (reported range, 22% to 100%). Novy and colleagues[106] published 35 cases of insufficiency in evolution (cervical dilation 2 to 5 cm); the two cohorts included 19 women who received physical examination–indicated cerclage and 16 who were managed with bed rest. Neonatal survival was 80% in the cerclage cohort versus 75% in the bed rest group. Two recent retrospective studies have supported the use of physical exam–indicated cerclage and reported a mean neonatal survival ("take-home-baby") rate of 50.7% and 64% and a mean pregnancy prolongation of 7.4 and 8.2 weeks, respectively.[119,120] Similar to previous reports,[118] Guducu and colleagues[119] further reported a diminished success rate (31%) in patients with membrane prolapsing into the vagina.

In a prospective, uncontrolled use of cerclage versus bed rest with cerclage utilized at the discretion of the attending physician, Olatunbosun and colleagues[121] studied women who presented with advanced cervical dilation greater than 4 cm. The cerclage group comprised 22 women, versus 15 in the bed-rest group. Although neonatal survival was not significantly different (17/22 with cerclage vs. 9/15 with bed rest, P = .3), gestational age at birth was a mean 4 weeks older in the cerclage group (33 vs. 29 weeks, P = .001). Rates of chorioamnionitis were similar between the two groups. A historic cohort study conducted by the Global Health Network for Perinatal and Reproductive Health examined outcomes in women between 14.0 and 25 6/7 weeks gestation when cervical dilation was identified.[122] Of 225 women, 152 received a physical examination–indicated cerclage, and 73 were managed expectantly. Although the groups were dissimilar because women with cervical dilation of 4 cm or more were more likely to be managed expectantly, cerclage was associated with a longer interval from presentation to delivery, improved neonatal outcome, and fewer births before 28 weeks compared with expectant management.

Althuisius and colleagues[123] performed a randomized clinical trial of physical examination–indicated cerclage plus bed rest versus bed rest alone in 23 women who presented with cervical dilation and membranes prolapsing to or beyond the external os before 27 weeks gestation. Both singleton and twin gestations were eligible; however, cervical dilation data were omitted, and so it is not known whether the groups were comparable. They observed a longer mean interval from presentation to delivery (54 days vs. 20 days; $P = .046$) in the cerclage group. Neonatal survival was 56% (9/16) with cerclage and 29% (4/14) in the bed-rest group. Although the survival differences were not statistically significant, composite neonatal morbidity, which included neonatal death, was significantly lower in the cerclage *and* bed-rest groups (63% [10/16] vs. 100% [14/14]) in the bed-rest alone group; $P = .02$).

Additional reports show that women who present with acute cervical insufficiency have an appreciable, approximately 50% incidence of bacterial colonization of their amniotic fluid or they demonstrate other markers of subclinical chorioamnionitis[124] or have proteomic markers of inflammation or bleeding.[125] Women with abnormal amniotic fluid markers have a much shorter presentation-to-delivery interval regardless of whether they receive a cerclage or are managed expectantly with bed rest. Mays and colleagues[124] performed amniocentesis in 18 women who presented with this syndrome and analyzed the amniotic fluid for glucose, lactate dehydrogenase, Gram stain, and culture; abnormal results suggested subclinical infection. Of 11 women who underwent cerclage with no evidence of subclinical infection, the neonatal survival was 100%, and the mean latent-phase duration from presentation to delivery was 93 days. Of the seven women with abnormal biochemistries in whom cerclage was withheld, no neonatal survivors were observed, and the mean latent phase was 4 days. In addition, seven women declined amniocentesis but did receive an emergent cerclage. Given that some of this group probably also had subclinical infection, it was predictable that the mean latent phase in this cohort was intermediate (17 days) as compared with the groups with amniotic fluid analyses. These investigators suggested that amniocentesis could aid in selecting candidates for emergent therapeutic cerclage. Diago-Almela and colleagues[126] have recently supported this finding in a prospective study of 31 patients presenting with bulging membranes who accepted amniocentesis. Of these, 20 amniotic fluid specimens revealed intraamniotic inflammation, or subclinical chorioamnionitis, defined as at least two of the following: interleukin 6 (IL-6) levels greater than 2.5 ng/mL, glucose levels below 15 mg/dL, leukocyte levels greater than 50/mm³, or positive leukocyte esterase. The remaining 11 had normal amniotic fluid markers, and nine of these patients accepted rescue cerclage. Four of nine delivered at term, and one patient who declined cerclage delivered at term. Those with intraamniotic inflammation/subclinical chorioamnionitis, in spite of being treated with antibiotics and bed rest, all delivered preterm, and 12 losses were seen in this group. Interestingly, of those with amniotic fluid that revealed inflammation, only seven had positive cultures at 5 days, and none had positive cultures in the normal-amniotic-fluid group. Receiver operating characteristic curve (ROC) analysis revealed that of the amniotic fluid markers, IL-6 had the highest diagnostic accuracy for survival using a cutoff of 2.90 ng/mL; all pregnancies with IL-6 above this level were lost. Their regression analysis further supported physical examination–indicated cerclage with low IL-6 and cervical length less than 30 mm as the best predictors of outcome. Interestingly, a sonographic marker of intrauterine subclinical infection, also known as "sludge," has been reported (see Fig. 28-2)[127] and is associated with suboptimal outcomes in several studies. Nevertheless, its clinical utility remains uncertain. **Although not currently standard practice, the evaluation of amniotic fluid for markers of infection and/or inflammation appears to have important prognostic value, but it is still unclear whether and to what extent the results should direct patient management.**

In summary, the optimal management of women who present with acute cervical insufficiency in evolution remains unclear. Although physical examination–indicated cerclage may benefit some, patient selection remains largely empiric. Although limited data exist on which to base firm management recommendations, collectively they demonstrate several important concepts: the earlier the gestational age at presentation, the more advanced the cervical dilation, and the presence of prolapsed membranes and IAI impart greater risk of poor neonatal outcome.

Cerclage in Multiple Gestations

Level 1 data are very limited on the effectiveness of cerclage in twin gestations with a short TVU CL. Cerclage is not beneficial and may in fact be harmful in these patients (215% increase in sPTB before 34 weeks) as per a meta-analysis of the only 49 twins with TVU CL less than 25 mm before 24 weeks, randomized to cerclage or no cerclage.[111] Larger RCTs are needed to determine whether cerclage in twins with a short TVU CL is beneficial. The subject of physically indicated cerclage in twins has not been studied in a proper RCT, and the data have been controversial. Until further studies in twins are properly evaluated, cerclage in twin gestations should be discouraged.

ALTERNATIVE TREATMENTS TO CERVICAL CERCLAGE

Nonsurgical interventions have been advocated for patients with presumed cervical insufficiency.

Activity Restriction

The rationale for the recommendation for bed rest alone or in conjunction with cerclage relies in the theoretic concept of putting less pressure on the cervix while in the recumbent position. **The validity of bed rest for treatment has not been scientifically proven, and some data suggest *worse* outcomes in patients placed on bed rest.**[74]

Pessary

Since the description by Vitsky in 1961 of the use of a vaginal pessary, instead of cerclage, for patients with cervical insufficiency,[128] several studies, mainly in Europe, suggest the same outcome for patients managed with this noninvasive modality compared with a surgical intervention. Arabin and colleagues[129] studied the use of a vaginal pessary in patients with a sonographically detected short cervix (Fig. 28-12). Patients managed with a pessary gained 99 days compared with 67 days for patients managed with bed rest alone ($P < .02$). In the last 2 years, several randomized studies have been done of asymptomatic pregnant patients with a short cervix detected by ultrasound in the

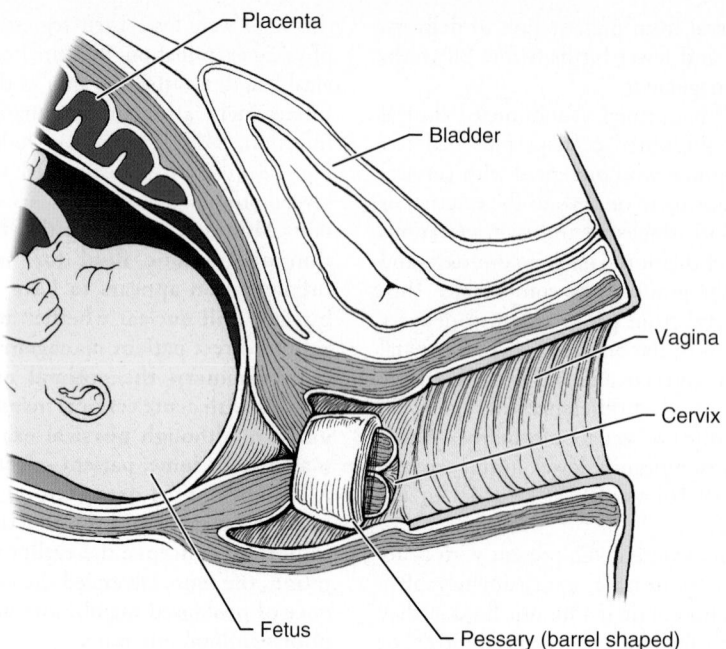

FIG 28-12 Vaginal pessary (Arabin type).

midtrimester, comparing an Arabin-type pessary to no intervention, and these have shown conflicting results. In the PECEP study (cervical pessary to prevent prematurity) conducted in Spain, patients with a singleton pregnancy with a cervical length less than 25 mm in the midtrimester were randomized to a pessary versus no intervention. The rates of preterm delivery before 34 weeks and 28 weeks were dramatically reduced in the patients managed with a pessary: 27% versus 6% ($P < .0001$) and 8% versus 2% ($P < .00058$). Furthermore, the pessary was not associated with maternal complications except for an increase in vaginal discharge.[130] In contrast, a similar study in China did not show differences in rates of preterm delivery before 37, 34, and 28 weeks in patients with a short cervix randomized to receive a pessary. Some of the criticisms of this study include the lack of adequate patient volume for adequate power and the low incidence of preterm delivery at less than 34 weeks (5.5%) in patients with a short cervix and no intervention.[131] In the only randomized study published to date of pessary use for prevention of prematurity in twin gestations (Pro TWIN study), the rate of prematurity was the same between control patients and the ones randomized to a pessary. However, benefit was found in patients whose cervical length was less than 38 mm (less than the tenth percentile).[132]

Several randomized studies of pessaries in singleton and multiple gestations with short CL are being conducted in both Europe and the United States (www.clinicaltrials.gov). **We must await the results of ongoing trials and assess the need for further prospective, randomized trials that compare pessary, cerclage, and progesterone before conclusions regarding the efficacy of any of these interventions can be established.**

Progesterone

RCTs[133,134] have shown that weekly 17-α-hydroxyprogesterone (17-OH-P) 250 mg intramuscularly (IM) started at about 16 weeks until about 36 weeks is associated with a significant, approximately 30% decrease in recurrent PTB. Based on these data, both the ACOG and SMFM have recommended that all

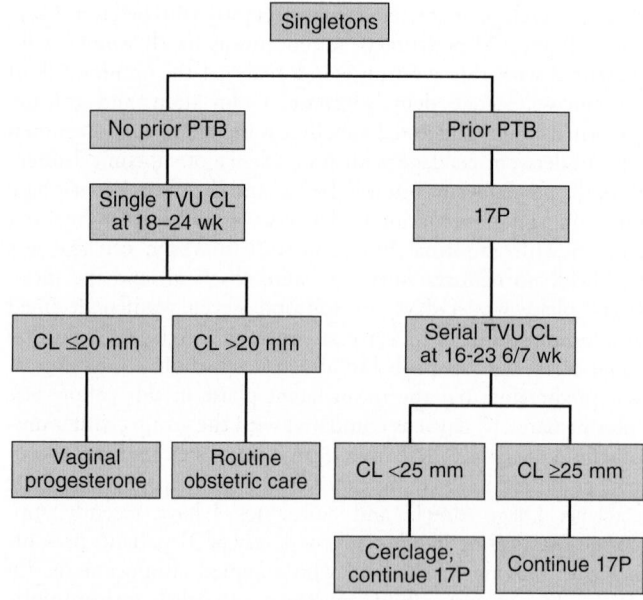

FIG 28-13 Use of progesterone for prevention of preterm birth. 17-P, 17-α hydroxyprogesterone; CL, cervical length; PTB, preterm birth; TVU, transvaginal ultrasound. (Modified from Society for Maternal-Fetal Medicine Publications Committee. Progesterone and preterm birth prevention: translating clinical trials data into clinical practice. *Am J Obstet Gynecol.* 2012;206[5]:376-386.)

women with a singleton pregnancy and a prior sPTB should receive this prophylactic therapy.[19,20] We agree that all women with an sPTB between 16 0/7 to 36 6/7 weeks should be eligible for this therapy. ACOG and SMFM use the algorithm seen in Figure 28-13 for management. At least two RCTs[136,137] have proposed that vaginal progesterone is also effective, and perhaps more effective, than 17-OH-P[137] in this clinical scenario. TVU CL is indicated in this population of singleton gestations with prior sPTB, even if the patient has already been given IM 17-OH-P or vaginal progesterone for prophylaxis. Although nonsignificant given their small numbers, studies have shown that cerclage for patients with TVU CL less than 25 mm before 24 weeks with a prior sPTB even on progesterone is associated with further cumulative prevention of sPTB.[138,139] **Further research is necessary to confirm the benefit of cerclage for women taking 17P and to evaluate the possible cumulative effects of other interventions for short TVU CL, including not only cerclage and progesterone but also perhaps nonsteroidal antiinflammatory agents, other tocolytics, and other pharmacologic agents.**

COMPARATIVE TRIALS OF TREATMENT OF CERVICAL INSUFFICIENCY

We have reviewed various approaches used to treat cervical insufficiency and their respective efficacies. Because randomized trial data are variously limited for each of the interventions compared with no-intervention controls, trials that compare the available treatment modalities are even less common. To date, nine systematic reviews to report on the above treatment modalities in the prevention or treatment of cervical insufficiency or PTB have been published in the Cochrane Database. Within these reviews, only one comparison trial between modalities has been included. In a study conducted by Keeler and colleagues,[140] 79 asymptomatic women with a short cervix (≤25 mm) detected on transvaginal CL screening between 16 and 24 weeks were randomized to either weekly IM injections of 17-OH-P caproate ($n = 37$) or McDonald cerclage ($n = 42$). No difference in spontaneous PTB prior to 35 weeks was observed (RR, 1.14; 95% CI, 0.67 to 1.93). A post hoc analysis conducted of women with a prior PTB again revealed no difference. However, secondary analysis of patients with a cervical length of 15 mm or less showed a 52% risk reduction in sPTB before 35 weeks with cerclage (RR, 0.48; 95% CI, 0.24 to 0.97).[141] In a retrospective cohort study conducted by Mackeen and colleagues of women who received a history-indicated cerclage, the authors compared 14 women who had received 17-OH-P with 80 women who had not. Once all outcomes were assessed, including PTB at various gestational age cutoffs, it was found that interval between cerclage placement and delivery, gestational age at delivery, and infant birthweight did not differ between groups.[142] A similar conclusion was reached by Szychowski and coworkers in a secondary analysis of the Vaginal Ultrasound Consortium Trial, where outcomes of women receiving 17-OH-P who had been randomized to cerclage or no cerclage in the setting of a short cervix (cervical length < 25 mm). Of the 99 women who received 17-OH-P, 47 received cerclage and 52 did not. Although a 36% decrease was noted in the odds of PTB < 35 weeks in those with a cerclage, this difference was not significant (aOR 0.64, 95% CI 0.27-1.52), possibly secondary to beta error.[139]

In a study conducted by Alfirevic and colleagues, the authors retrospectively and indirectly compared three management strategies for shortened cervical length in women with singletons and a prior spontaneous PTB before 34 weeks: ultrasound-indicated cerclage, vaginal progesterone, and cervical pessary. A total of 142 patients from the United States had undergone cerclage, 59 patients from the United Kingdom received vaginal progesterone, and 42 women from Spain received a cervical pessary.[143] The authors reported no difference in perinatal loss, neonatal morbidity, or PTB among the three groups, and concluded that cerclage, vaginal progesterone and pessary had similar efficacy in high risk patients with a short midtrimester cervical length.

Given the study design and different patient populations, definitive conclusions cannot be reached. Similarly, Conde-Agudelo and colleagues performed an adjusted, indirect meta-analysis of randomized controlled trials of different treatment strategies for midtrimester shortened cervical length in women with singleton pregnancies and a prior history of PTB. Within their analysis, they included four studies that compared vaginal progesterone to placebo (158 patients) and five studies evaluating cerclage versus no cerclage (504 patients). They concluded that either intervention was associated with a statistically significant reduction in both PTB <32 weeks and composite perinatal morbidity and mortality when compared to placebo/expectant management. Further, their adjusted indirect meta-analysis showed that both interventions had similar efficacy.[144] The recommendations from these indirect meta-analyses should be considered with caution because of the significant differences in baseline characteristics of the populations studied, making true comparisons difficult to interpret.

The above data highlight the need for quality randomized clinical trials comparing the various available interventions and, importantly, combinations of interventions (for example, progesterone plus cerclage). In the hopes of preventing adverse perinatal outcomes, providers might recommend dual or even triple intervention with the assumption that they will act synergistically (e.g. 17-OH-P for a history of PTB, ultrasound-indicated cerclage for cervical shortening and a supporting pessary when post-cerclage cervical changes are detected). A recent editorial by Griffin cautions against the use of combined strategies that have not been proven efficacious in combination.[145]

SUMMARY

Cervical insufficiency is rarely a distinct and well-defined clinical entity but only one part of a larger and more complex spontaneous preterm birth syndrome. The original paradigm of obstetric and gynecologic trauma as a common antecedent of cervical insufficiency has been replaced by the recognition of functional, as opposed to anatomic deficits as the more prevalent origin. Cervical competence functions along a continuum, influenced by both endogenous and exogenous factors that interact through various pathways with other recognized components of the PTB syndrome: uterine contractions and decidual/membrane activation. **The clinically convenient term, *cervical insufficiency,* probably represents an oversimplified, incomplete version of the broader, although poorly understood, pathophysiologic process.** Consequently, the continued use of traditional therapies, unsubstantiated by results of clinical trials, must be questioned. Effective, evidence-based management guidelines will stem from a more complete understanding of the PTB syndrome. This will improve patient selection and permit specifically tailored treatment regimens, confirmed by the results of well-designed intervention trials.

***Cervical insufficiency* remains primarily a clinical diagnosis. Cervical ultrasound demonstrating a short cervix has emerged as a proven, clinically useful screening and diagnostic tool in selected populations of asymptomatic high-risk women based on an obstetric**

history of a prior (early) spontaneous PTB. Women with history of preterm delivery who then develop shortened mid-trimester cervical length appear to have a treatable *component* of cervical insufficiency. Surgical intervention in the form of history-indicated cerclage, sonographically indicated cerclage, and physically indicated cerclage, may be beneficial in selective patients. The vast majority of women with prior sPTB can be followed with TVU CL screening, with ultrasound-indicated cerclage if the TVU CL becomes less than 25 mm before 24 weeks. Evidence continues to be developed for perioperative management strategies for cerclage placement. The use of abdominal/laparoscopic and/or robotic cerclage may be reasonable in rare, carefully selected patients. Additive and/or alternative interventions such as progesterone and vaginal pessary demonstrate promise but still require further evaluation to make final recommendations in the treatment of patients with a history consistent with cervical insufficiency or patients with a short cervical length in the midtrimester.

- Ultrasound indicated cerclage in twin gestation should not be performed because of the increase risk for preterm delivery with this intervention.
- There is a need for randomized studies to evaluate alternative treatments for cervical insufficiency such as pharmacologic therapy, and vaginal pessary.

KEY POINTS

- Cervical insufficiency is primarily a clinical diagnosis characterized by recurrent painless dilatation and spontaneous midtrimester loss.
- Cervical insufficiency is rarely a distinct and well-defined clinical entity, but only one component of the larger and more complex spontaneous preterm birth syndrome.
- Current evidence suggests that cervical competence functions along a continuum, influenced by both endogenous and exogenous factors, such as uterine contractions and decidual/membrane activation.
- The traditional nomenclature of cerclage type as prophylactic, therapeutic, and emergent should be replaced by history-indicated, ultrasound-indicated, and physical examination–indicated cerclage.
- There is no objective preconceptional diagnostic test for cervical insufficiency.
- History-indicated cerclage for patients with a clinical history of cervical insufficiency remains a reasonable approach.
- Cervical ultrasound for cervical insufficiency performs poorly as a screening test in low-risk women, but it has been proven to be a clinically useful screening and diagnostic tool in selected high-risk populations such as those with a prior sPTB who may have a treatable *component* of cervical insufficiency.
- In the vast majority of women with prior sPTBs, and even those with nonclassic clinical histories of cervical insufficiency, serial sonographic evaluations of the cervix may be an acceptable alternative approach to history-indicated cerclage.
- Physical examination–indicated cerclage may be beneficial in reducing PTB in a subgroup of patients without markers of infection.
- Abdominal cerclage may be considered for those rare patients with a history of failed vaginal cerclage.

REFERENCES

1. Culpepper N, Cole A, Rowland W, eds. *The Practice of Physick*. London: George Strawbridge; 1678:502.
2. Ludmir J, Sehdev HM. Anatomy and physiology of the cervix. *Clin Obstet Gynecol*. 2000;43:433.
3. Kuhn R, Pepperell R. Cervical ligation: a review of 242 pregnancies. *Aust N Z J Obstet Gynaecol*. 1977;17:79-83.
4. Owen J, Hankins G, Iams JD, et al. Multicenter randomized trial of cerclage for preterm birth prevention in high-risk women with shortened midtrimester cervical length. *Am J Obstet Gynecol*. 2009;201:375.e1-375.e8.
5. Danforth DN, Buckingham JC. Cervical incompetence: a reevaluation. *Postgrad Med*. 1962;32:345.
6. Danforth DN, Veis A, Breen M, et al. The effect of pregnancy and labor on the human cervix: changes in collagen, glycoproteins and gycosaminoglycans. *Am J Obstet Gynecol*. 1974;120:641.
7. Leppert PC, Yu SY, Keller S, et al. Decreased elastic fibers and desmosine content in incompetent cervix. *Am J Obstet Gynecol*. 1987;157:1134.
8. Dunn LJ, Dans P. Subsequent obstetrical performance of patients meeting the historical criteria for cervical incompetence. *Bull Sloan Hosp Women*. 1962;7:43.
9. Iams JD, Johnson FF, Sonek J, et al. Cervical competence as a continuum: a study of ultrasonography cervical length and obstetric performance. *Am J Obstet Gynecol*. 1995;172:1097.
10. Iams JD, Goldenberg RL, Meis PJ, et al. The length of the cervix and the risk of spontaneous premature delivery. *N Engl J Med*. 1996;334:567.
11. Craigo SD. Cervical incompetence and preterm delivery [editorial]. *N Engl J Med*. 1996;334:595.
12. Romero R, Gomez R, Sepulveda W. The uterine cervix, ultrasound and prematurity [editor comments]. *Ultrasound Obstet Gynecol*. 1992;2:385.
13. Larma JD, Iams JD. Is sonographic assessment of the cervix necessary and helpful? *Clin Obstet Gynecol*. 2012;55(1):324-335.
14. Iams JD. Identification of candidates for progesterone: why, who, how, and when? *Obstet Gynecol*. 2014;123(6):1317-1326.
15. Romero R, Espinoza J, Erez O, Hassam S. The role of cervical cerclage in obstetric practice: can the patient who could benefit from this procedure be identified? *Am J Obstet Gynecol*. 2006;194:1.
16. Hernandez-Andrade E1, Romero R, Ahn H, et al. Transabdominal evaluation of uterine cervical length during pregnancy fails to identify a substantial number of women with a short cervix. *J Matern Fetal Neonatal Med*. 2012;25(9):1682-1689.
17. Berghella V, Bega G. Ultrasound evaluation of the cervix. In: Callen PW, ed. *Ultrasonography in Obstetrics and Gynecology*. 5th ed. Philadelphia, PA: Saunders Elsevier; 2008:698-720.
18. Cahill AG, Odibo AO, Caughey AB, et al. Universal cervical length screening and treatment with vaginal progesterone to prevent preterm birth: a decision and economic analysis. *Am J Obstet Gynecol*. 2010;202(6):548.e1-548.e8.
19. Society for Maternal-Fetal Medicine Publications Committee, with assistance of Vincenzo Berghella. Progesterone and preterm birth prevention: translating clinical trials data into clinical practice. *Am J Obstet Gynecol*. 2012;206(5):376-386.
20. Committee on Practice Bulletins—Obstetrics, The American College of Obstetricians and Gynecologists. Practice bulletin no. 130: prediction and prevention of preterm birth. *Obstet Gynecol*. 2012;120(4):964-973.
21. Royal College of Obstetricians and Gynaecologists (RCOG). *Cervical cerclage*. London (UK): Royal College of Obstetricians and Gynaecologists (RCOG); 2011:21 (Green-top guideline; no. 60).
22. Berghella V, Tolosa JE, Kuhlman K, et al. Cervical ultrasonography compared with manual examination as a predictor of preterm delivery. *Am J Obstet Gynecol*. 1997;177:723-730.

23. *CLEAR guidelines.* Available at <https://clear.perinatalquality.org/>.
24. Berghella V. *Transvaginal ultrasound assessment of the cervix and prediction of spontaneous preterm birth.* <www.uptodate.com>.
25. Hassan SS, Romero R, Vidyadhari D, et al. PREGNANT Trial. Vaginal progesterone reduces the rate of preterm birth in women with a sonographic short cervix: a multicenter, randomized, double-blind, placebo-controlled trial. *Ultrasound Obstet Gynecol.* 2011;38(1):18-31.
26. Owen J, Yost N, Berghella V, et al. Mid-trimester endovaginal sonography in women at high risk for spontaneous preterm birth. *JAMA.* 2001;286:1340-1348.
27. Goldenberg RL, Iams JD, Miodovnik M, et al. The preterm prediction study: risk factors in twin gestations. National Institute of Child Health and Human Development Maternal-Fetal Medicine Units Network. *Am J Obstet Gynecol.* 1996;175:1047-1053.
28. Vendittelli F, Mamelle N. Transvaginal ultrasonography of the uterine cervix in hospitalized women with preterm labor. *Int J Gynaecol Obstet.* 2001;72:117-125.
29. Visintine J, Berghella V. Cervical length for prediction of preterm birth in women with multiple prior induced abortions. *Ultrasound Obstet Gynecol.* 2008;31:198-200.
30. Airoldi J, Berghella V. Transvaginal ultrasonography of the cervix to predict preterm birth in women with uterine anomalies. *Obstet Gynecol.* 2005;106:553-556.
31. Atrash HK, Hogue CJR. The effect of pregnancy termination on future reproduction. *Bailliere's Clin Obstet Gynaecol.* 1990;4:391-405.
32. Shah PS, Zao J, Knowledge Synthesis Group of Determinants of preterm/LBW births. Induced termination of pregnancy and low birthweight and preterm birth: a systematic review and meta-analyses. *Br J Obstet Gynaecol.* 2009;116:1425.
33. Kalish RB, Chasen ST. Impact of midtrimester dilation and evacuation on subsequent pregnancy outcome. *Am J Obstet Gynecol.* 2002;187:882-885.
34. Anonymous. Final report of of the Medical Research Council/Royal College of Obstetrics and Gynaecology multicenter randomized trial of cervical cerclage. *Br J Obstet Gynaecol.* 1993;100:516.
35. Bevis KS, Biggio JR. Cervical conization and the risk of preterm delivery. *Am J Obstet Gynecol.* 2011;205(1):19-27.
36. Ferenczy A, Choukroun D. The effect of cervical loop electrosurgical excision on subsequent pregnancy outcome: North American experience. *Am J Obstet Gynecol.* 1995;172:1246.
37. Althuisius SM, Shornagel GA. Loop electrosurgical excision procedure of the cervix and time of delivery in subsequent pregnancy. *Int J Gynecol Obstet.* 2001;72:31.
38. Kyrgiou M, Koliopoulos G. Obstetric outcomes after conservative treatment for intraepithelial or early invasive cervical lesions: systematic review and meta-analysis. *Lancet.* 2006;367(9509):489-498.
39. Heinonen A, Gissler M. Loop electrosurgical excision procedure and the risk for preterm delivery. *Obstet Gynecol.* 2013;121(5):1063-1068.
40. Jakobsson M, Gissler M. Preterm delivery after surgical treatment for cervical intraepithelial neoplasia. *Obstet Gynecol.* 2007;109(2 Pt 1):309-313.
41. Kyrgiou M, Mitra A, Arbyn M, et al. Fertility and early pregnancy outcomes after treatment for cervical intraepithelial neoplasia: systematic review and meta-analysis. *BMJ.* 2014;349:g6192.
42. Albrechtsen S, Rasmussen S. Pregnancy outcome before and after cervical conization: population based cohort study. *BMJ.* 2008;337:a1343.
43. Sadler L, Saftkas A, Wang W, et al. Treatment for cervical intraepithelial neoplasis and risk of preterm delivery. *JAMA.* 2004;29:2100.
44. Leiman G, Harrison NA. Pregnancy following conization of the cervix: complications related to cone size. *Am J Obstet Gynecol.* 1980;136:14.
45. Raio L, Ghezzi F, Di Naro E, et al. Duration of pregnancy after carbon dioxide laser conization of the cervix: influence of cone height. *Obstet Gynecol.* 1997;90:978.
46. Khalid S, Dimitriou E, Conroy R, et al. The thickness and volume of LLETZ specimens can predict the relative risk of pregnancy-related morbidity. *Br J Obstet Gynaecol.* 2012;119(6):685-691.
47. Conner SN, Frey HA, Cahill AG, Macones GA, Colditz GA, Tuuli MG. Loop electrosurgical excision procedure and risk of preterm birth: a systematic review and meta-analysis. *Obstet Gynecol.* 2014;123(4):752-761.
48. Poon LC, Savvas M, Zamblera D, Skyfta E, Nicolaides KH. Large loop excision of transformation zone and cervical length in the prediction of spontaneous preterm delivery. *BJOG.* 2012;119(6):692-698.
49. Kuoppala T, Saarikoski S. Pregnancy and delivery after cone biopsy of the cervix. *Arch Gynecol.* 1986;237:149.
50. Toaff R, Toaff ME. Diagnosis of impending late abortion. *Obstet Gynecol.* 1974;43:756.
51. Bergman P, Svenerund A. Traction test for demonstrating incompetence of internal os of the cervix. *Int J Fertil.* 1957;2:163.
52. Kiwi R, Neuman MR, Merkatz IR, et al. Determination of the elastic properties of the cervix. *Obstet Gynecol.* 1988;71:568.
53. Feltovich H, Hall TJ, Berghella V. Beyond cervical length: emerging technologies for assessing the pregnant cervix. *Am J Obstet Gynecol.* 2012;207(5):345-354.
54. Jones G. The weak cervix: failing to keep the baby in or infection out? *Br J Obstet Gynaecol.* 1998;105:1214-1215.
55. Owen J, Yost N, Berghella V, et al. Can shortened mid-trimester cervical length predict very early spontaneous preterm birth? *Am J Obstet Gynecol.* 2004;191:298.
56. Berghella V, Daly SF, Tolosa JE, et al. Prediction of preterm delivery with transvaginal ultrasonography of the cervix in patients with high-risk pregnancies: Does cerclage prevent prematurity? *Am J Obstet Gynecol.* 1999;181:809.
57. McMahon KS, Neerhof MC, Haney EI, et al. Prematurity in multiple gestations: identification of patients who are at low risk. *Am J Obstet Gynecol.* 2002;186:1137.
58. Honest H, Bachman LM, Coomarasamy A, et al. Accuracy of cervical transvaginal sonography in predicting preterm birth; a systematic review. *Ultrasound Obstet Gynecol.* 2003;22:305. 59.
59. Berghella V, Ludmir J, Simonazzi G, Owen J. Transvaginal cervical cerclage: evidence for perioperative management strategies. *Am J Obstet Gynecol.* 2013;209(3):181-192.
60. ACOG Practice Bulletin No.142: Cerclage for the management of cervical insufficiency. *Obstet Gynecol.* 2014;123(2 Pt 1):372-379.
61. Suhag A, Seligman NS, Bianchi I, Berghella V. What is the optimal gestational age for history-indicated cerclage placement? *Am J Perinatol.* 2010;27(6):469-474.
62. Lash AF, Lash SR. Habitual abortion: the incompetent internal os of the cervix. *Am J Obstet Gynecol.* 1950;59:68.
63. Shirodkar VN. A new method of operative treatment for habitual abortions in the second trimester of pregnancy. *Antiseptic.* 1955;52:299.
64. McDonald IA. Suture of the cervix for inevitable miscarriage. *J Obstet Gynecol Br Empire.* 1957;64:346.
65. To MS, Alfirevic Z, Heath VCF, et al. on behalf of the Fetal Medicine Foundation Second Trimester Screening Group: Cervical cerclage for prevention of preterm delivery in women with short cervix: randomized controlled trial. *Lancet.* 2004;363:1849.
66. Abdelhak YE, Sheen JJ, Kuczynski E, et al. Comparison of delayed absorbable suture v. non-absorbable suture for the treatment of incompetent cervix. *J Perinatal Med.* 1999;27:250.
67. Aarnoudse JG, Huisjes HJ. Complications of cerclage. *Acta Obstet Gynecol Scand.* 1979;58:225.
68. McDonald IA. Incompetence of the cervix. *Aust N Z J Obstet Gynaecol.* 1978;18:34.
69. Giraldo-Isaza MA, Fried GP, Hegarty SE, Suescum-Diaz MA, Cohen AW, Berghella V. Comparison of 2 stitches vs 1 stitch for transvaginal cervical cerclage for preterm birth prevention. *Am J Obstet Gynecol.* 2013;208(3):209.e1-209.e9.
70. Brix N, Secher NJ, McCormack CD, et al. Randomised trial of cervical cerclage, with and without occlusion, for the prevention of preterm birth in women suspected for cervical insufficiency. *Br J Obstet Gynaecol.* 2013;120(5):613-620.
71. Rust OA, Atlas RO, Jones KJ, Benham BN, Balducci J. A randomized trial of cerclage versus no cerclage among patients with ultrasonographically detected second-trimester preterm dilatation of the internal os. *Am J Obstet Gynecol.* 2000;183(4):830-835.
72. Steinberg ES, Santos AC. Surgical anesthesia during pregnancy. *Int Anesthesiol Clin.* 1980;28:58.
73. Chen L, Ludmir J, Miller FL, et al. Is regional better than general anesthesia for cervical cerclage? Nine years experience. *Anesth Analg.* 1990;70:Sl.
74. Grobman WA, Gilbert SA, Iams JD, et al. Activity restriction among women with a short cervix. *Obstet Gynecol.* 2013;121(6):1181-1186.
75. Bisulli M, Suhag A, Arvon R, Seibel-Seamon J, Visintine J, Berghella V. Interval to spontaneous delivery after elective removal of cerclage. *Am J Obstet Gynecol.* 2009;201(2):163.e1-163.e4.
76. Novy MJ. Transabdominal cervicoisthmic cerclage: a reappraisal 25 years after its introduction. *Am J Obstet Gynecol.* 1991;164:163.
77. Groom KN, Jones BA, Edmonds DK, Bennett PR. Preconception transabdominal cervicoisthmic cerclage. *Am J Obstet Gynecol.* 2004;191:230.

78. Debbs RH, DeLa Vega GA, Pearson S, Sehdev H, Marchiano D, Ludmir J. Transabdominal cerclage after comprehensive evaluation of women with previous unsuccessful transvaginal cerclage. *Am J Obstet Gynecol.* 2007;197(3):317.e1-317.e4.

79. Gallot D, Savary D, Laurichesse H, et al. Experience with three cases of laparoscopic transabdominal cervioisthmic cerclage and two subsequent pregnancies. *Br J Obstet Gynaecol.* 2003;110:696.

80. Cho CH, Kim TH, Kwon SH, et al. Laparoscopic transabdominal cervicoisthmid cerclage during pregnancy. *J Am Gynecol Laparosc.* 2003;10:363.

81. Burger NB, Brölmann HA, Einarsson JI, Langebrekke A, Huirne JA. Effectiveness of abdominal cerclage placed via laparotomy or laparoscopy: systematic review. *J Minim Invasive Gynecol.* 2011;18(6):696-704.

82. Wolfe L, DePasquale S, Adair D, Torres C, Stallings S, Briery C, et al. Robotic-assisted laparoscopic placement of transabdominal cerclage during pregnancy. *Am J Perinatol.* 2008;25:653-655.

83. Ludmir J, Jackson GM, Samuels P. Transvaginal cerclage under ultrasound guidance in cases of severe cervical hypoplasia. *Obstet Gynecol.* 1991;78:1067.

84. Guzman ER, Forster JK, Vintzileos AM, et al. Pregnancy outcomes in women treated with elective versus ultrasound-indicated cervical cerclage. *Ultrasound Obstet Gynecol.* 1998;12:323.

85. Berghella V, Daly SF, Tolosa JE, et al. Prediction of preterm delivery with transvaginal ultrasonography of the cervix in patients with high-risk pregnancies: does cerclage prevent prematurity? *Am J Obstet Gynecol.* 1999;181:809.

86. Aarts JM, Brons JT, Bruinse HW, et al. Emergency cerclage: a review. *Obstet Gynecol Surv.* 1995;50:459.

87. Locatelli A, Vergani P, Bellini P, Strobelt N, Arreghini A, Ghidini A. Amnioreduction in emergency cerclage with prolapsed membranes: comparison of two methods for reducing the membranes. *Am J Perinatol.* 1999;16(2):73-77.

88. Scheerer LJ, Lam F, Bartololucci L, et al. A new technique for reduction of prolapsed fetal membranes for emergency cervical cerclage. *Obstet Gynecol.* 1989;74:408.

89. Kurup M, Goldkrand JW. Cervical incompetence: elective, emergent, or urgent cerclage. *Am J Obstet Gynecol.* 1999;181:240.

90. Harger JH. Comparison of success and morbidity in cervical cerclage procedures. *Obstet Gynecol.* 1980;53:534.

91. Charles D, Edwards WR. Infectious complications of cerclage. *Am J Obstet Gynecol.* 1981;141:1065.

92. Baxter JK, Airoldi J, Berghella V. Short cervical length after history-indicated cerclage: is a reinforcing cerclage beneficial? *Am J Obstet Gynecol.* 2005;193(3 Pt 2):1204-1207.

93. Ludmir J, Bader T, Chen L, et al. Poor perinatal outcome associated with retained cerclage in patients with premature rupture of membranes. *Obstet Gynecol.* 1994;84:823.

94. Jenkins TM, Bergehlla V, Shlossman PA, et al. Timing of cerclage removal after preterm premature rupture of membranes: maternal and neonatal outcomes. *Am J Obstet Gynecol.* 2000;183:847.

95. McElrath TF, Norwitz ER, Lieberman ES, Heffner LJ. Management of cervical cerclage and preterm premature rupture of the membranes: should the stitch be removed? *Am J Obstet Gynecol.* 2000;183:840.

96. Galyean A, Garite TJ, Maurel K, Abril D, Adair CD, Browne P, et al. Removal versus retention of cerclage in preterm premature rupture of membranes: a randomized controlled trial. *Am J Obstet Gynecol.* 2014;211(4):399.e1-399.e7.

97. Dunn LE, Robinson JC, Steer CM. Maternal death following suture of incompetent cervix during pregnancy. *Am J Obstet Gynecol.* 1959;78:335.

98. Lazar P, Gueguen S, Dreyfus J, et al. Multicentred controlled trial of cervical cerclage in women at moderate risk of preterm delivery. *Br J Obstet Gynaecol.* 1984;91:731.

99. Dor J, Shalev J, Mashiach S, et al. Elective cervical suture of twin pregnancies diagnosed ultrasonically in the first trimester following induced ovulation. *Gynecol Obstet Invest.* 1982;13:55.

100. Rush RW, Isaacs S, McPherson K, et al. A randomized controlled trial of cervical cerclage in women at high risk for preterm delivery. *Br J Obstet Gynaecol.* 1984;91:724.

101. Althuisius SM, Dekker GA, Hummel P, et al. Final results of the cervical incompetence prevention randomized cerclage trial (CIPRACT): therapeutic cerclage with bed rest versus bed rest alone. *Am J Obstet Gynecol.* 2001;185:1106.

102. Rust OA, Atlas RO, Reed J, et al. Revisiting the short cervix detected by transvaginal ultrasound in the second trimester: why cerclage may not help. *Am J Obstet Gynecol.* 2001;185:1098.

103. Berghella V, Odibo AO, Tolosa JE. Cerclage for prevention of preterm birth in women with a short cervix found on transvaginal ultrasound: a randomized trial. *Am J Obstet Gynecol.* 2004;191:1311.

Additional references for this chapter are available at ExpertConsult.com.

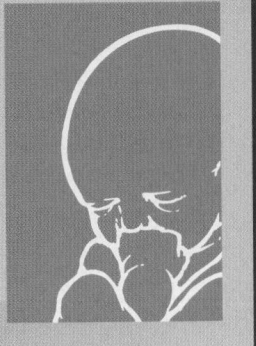

CHAPTER 29

Preterm Labor and Birth

HYAGRIV N. SIMHAN, JAY D. IAMS, and ROBERTO ROMERO

KEY ABBREVIATIONS

Adrenocorticotropic hormone	ACTH	Low birthweight	LBW
Assisted reproductive technology	ART	Matrix metalloproteinase	MMP
Bacterial vaginosis	BV	Messenger RNA	mRNA
Biophysical profile	BPP	Myosin light-chain kinase	MLCK
Bronchopulmonary dysplasia	BPD	National Institute of Child Health and Human Development	NICHD
Confidence interval	CI		
Corticotropin-releasing hormone	CRH	Necrotizing enterocolitis	NEC
Cyclic adenosine monophosphate	cAMP	Nitric oxide	NO
Cyclooxygenase	COX	Nonsteroidal antiinflammatory drugs	NSAIDs
Estrogen receptor	ER	Odds ratio	OR
Extremely low birthweight	ELBW	Omega-3 polyunsaturated fatty acid	PUFA
Ex utero intrapartum treatment	EXIT	Pathogen-associated molecular pattern	PAMP
Fetal inflammatory response syndrome	FIRS	Patent ductus arteriosus	PDA
Glycosaminoglycan	GAG	Polymerase chain reaction	PCR
Granulocyte-colony stimulating factor	G-CSF	Preterm premature rupture of membranes	PPROM
Group B *Streptococcus*	GBS		
In vitro fertilization	IVF	Progesterone receptor	PR
Interleukin-6	IL-6	Relative risk	RR
Intravenous	IV	Respiratory distress syndrome	RDS
Intraventricular hemorrhage	IVH	Retinopathy of prematurity	ROP

Thyrotropin-releasing hormone	TRH	Urokinase-type plasminogen activator	uPA
Tissue-type plasminogen activator	tPA	U.S. Food and Drug Administration	FDA
Tissue inhibitor of metalloproteinases	TIMP	Very low birthweight	VLBW
Tumor necrosis factor alpha	TNF-α	White blood cell	WBC

The average duration of a normal human pregnancy is 267 days, counted after conception, or 280 days (40 weeks) from the first day of the last normal menstrual period. Infants born at 39 and 40 weeks of gestation have the lowest rates of adverse outcomes. **Complications related to preterm birth (PTB) account for more newborn and infant deaths than any other cause.[1] Although advances in neonatal care have led to increased survival and reduced short- and long-term morbidity for infants born preterm, surviving infants have increased risks of visual and hearing impairment, chronic lung disease, cerebral palsy, and delayed development in childhood. The causes of PTB are diverse but can be usefully considered according to whether the parturitional process—which includes cervical remodeling, decidual membrane activation, and myometrial contractions—had begun before birth occurred. Preterm births that do not follow spontaneous initiation of parturition most often are iatrogenic, when the health of the mother or fetus is at risk** (e.g., with major hemorrhage, hypertension, or poor fetal growth).

DEFINITIONS

A *preterm birth* is commonly defined as one that occurs after 20 weeks' gestation and before the completion of 37 menstrual weeks of gestation regardless of birthweight. *Low birthweight* (LBW) is defined as birthweight below 2500 g regardless of gestational age; *very low birthweight* (VLBW) is birthweight below 1500 g, and *extremely low birth weight* (ELBW) is birthweight below 1000 g. Gestational age (GA) and birthweight (BW) are related by the terms *small for gestational age* (SGA; a BW less than the 10th percentile for GA), *average for gestational age* (AGA; BW between the 10th and 90th percentiles), *and large for gestational age* (LGA; BW above the 90th percentile). A *preterm* or *premature* infant is one born before 37 weeks of gestation—that is, 259 days from the first day of the mother's last normal menstrual period or 245 days after conception. The gestational boundaries of 20 and 37 weeks are historic, not scientific.[2] Infants born at 36, 37, and even 38 weeks of gestation may experience neonatal and even lifetime morbidity related to immaturity of one or more organs. The risk factors, etiologies, and recurrence risk for spontaneous births at 16 to 19 weeks do not differ from those of births at 20 to 25 weeks.[3,4] The American College of Obstetricians and Gynecologists (ACOG) and the Society for Maternal-Fetal Medicine (SMFM) have adopted the nomenclature *later preterm* ($34^{0/7}$ to $36^{6/7}$ weeks of gestation) and *early term* ($37^{0/7}$ to $38^{6/7}$ weeks of gestation) to acknowledge the contribution of gestational age in these ranges to neonatal risks.[5] **Recognition that some infants born after 37 weeks are not fully mature and that many births before 20 weeks arise from the same causes that lead to preterm births has led to reevaluation of these definitions and boundaries.**[6]

FREQUENCY OF PRETERM AND LOW-BIRTHWEIGHT DELIVERY

The World Health Organization (WHO) has estimated **that 9.6% of all births in 2005 were preterm—almost 13 million worldwide. Africa and Asia accounted for almost 11 million.**[7] Rates are lowest in Europe (6.2%), and the highest rates are seen in Africa (11.9%) and North America (10.6%). In the United States, the PTB rate rose from 10.6% in 1990 to 12.8% of all births in 2006. The rise resulted from improved pregnancy dating by ultrasound, which shifted the gestational age distribution to the left; increased use of assisted reproduction technology (ART); and, most importantly, from increased willingness to choose delivery when medical or obstetric complications occur after 34 weeks' gestation. The rate of PTB fell to its most recent nadir of 11.4% in 2013 (Fig. 29-1). The decline has been attributed to improved fertility practices that reduce the risk of higher-order multiple gestation; quality improvement programs that limit scheduled late-preterm and near-term births to only those with valid indications; and increased use of strategies to prevent recurrent PTB.

The rates of PTB vary substantially across the United States (Fig. 29-2). Reasons for the geographic variation are complex but are heavily influenced by the percentage of the population that is black. **Blacks have rates of PTB that are almost twofold higher than those of other racial/ethnic groups** (Fig. 29-3).

Outcomes for Infants Born Preterm

Gestational age at birth is strongly correlated with adverse pregnancy outcomes that include stillbirth (fetal death after 20 weeks' gestation), deaths of neonates (<28 days) and infants (<12 months), and long-term physical and intellectual morbidities.

PERINATAL MORTALITY

Perinatal mortality is defined as the sum of stillbirths after 20 weeks' gestation plus neonatal deaths through 28 days of life per 1000 total births (liveborn plus stillborn). Perinatal mortality increases markedly as gestational age and birthweight decline. Because this measure encompasses prenatal, intrapartum, and neonatal events, it reflects obstetric and neonatal care. Stillbirth and PTB have a similar epidemiologic profile, especially before 32 weeks. Rates of perinatal mortality declined between 1990 and 2003, mainly because of a decrease in fetal deaths after 27 weeks' gestation.[8]

Infant Mortality

The infant mortality rate is the number of deaths among liveborn infants before 1 year of age per 1000 *live* births. Although congenital malformations are often listed as the leading cause of infant mortality, this ranking is achieved by separating

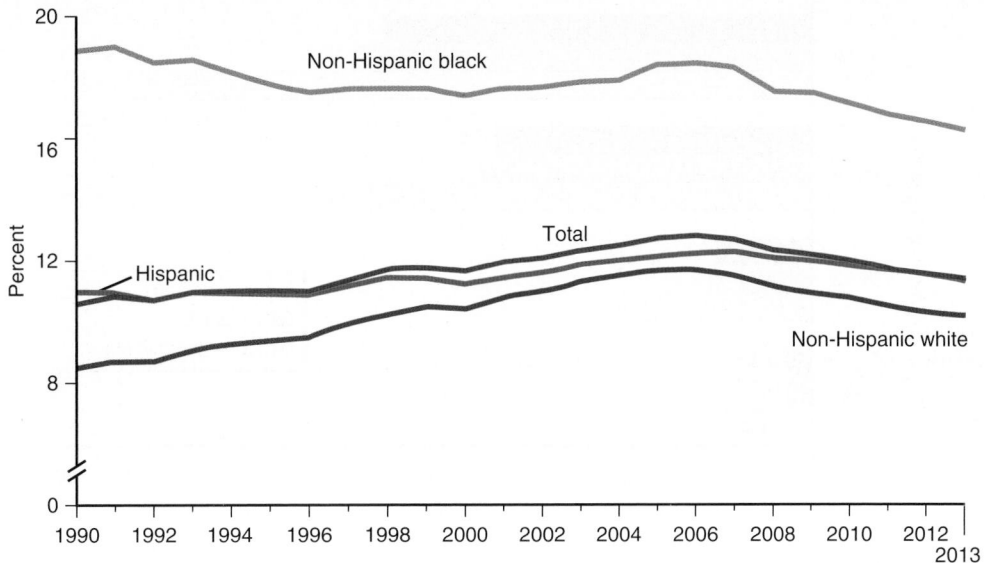

FIG 29-1 Preterm and low-birthweight rates: United States, final 1981 through 2009, preliminary 2009. (Modified from Hamilton BE, Martin JA, Ventura SJ. Births: preliminary data for 2009. *Natl Vital Stat Rep.* 2010;59[3].)

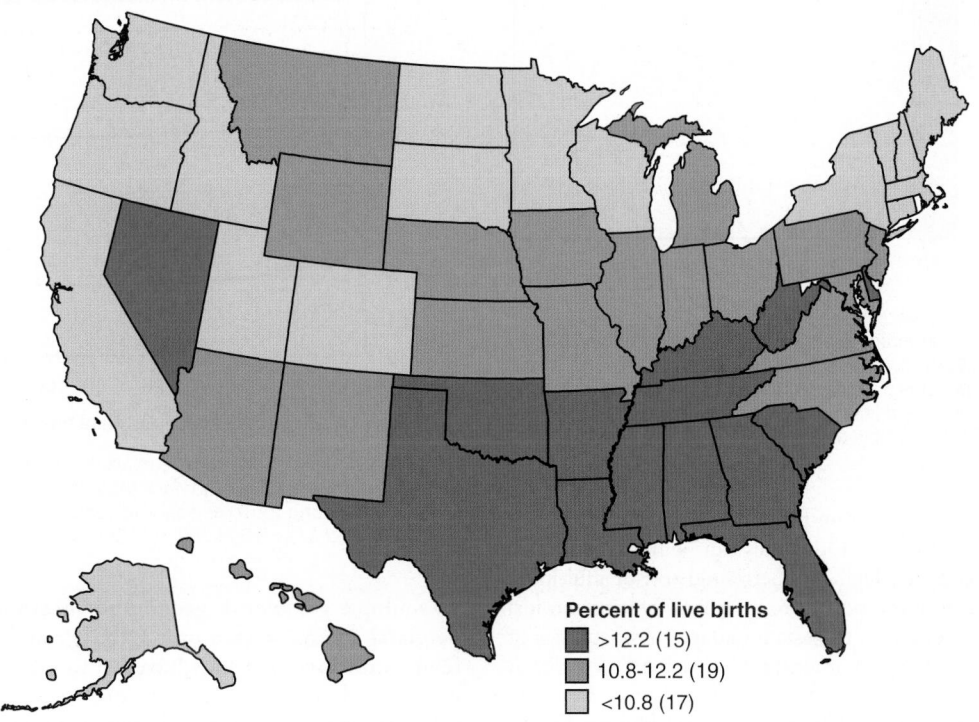

Percent of live births
- >12.2 (15)
- 10.8-12.2 (19)
- <10.8 (17)

FIG 29-2 Percentage of live preterm births in the United States by state, 2013. (From National Center for Health Statistics, final natality data. Available at www.marchofdimes.org/peristats.)

conditions related to PTB into several categories. The proportion of all infant deaths in the United States in 2008 by gestational age at birth is shown in Figure 29-4.

Infant and childhood mortality and morbidity in surviving preterm infants rise as gestational age at birth declines, and they vary with the level of neonatal care received. In 2008, the overall infant mortality rate was 6.6 infant deaths per 1000 live births; however, infant mortality rates varied widely by gestational age. For infants born at less than 32 weeks' gestation, the infant mortality rate was 175.5 infant deaths per 1000 live births, compared with a rate of 2.1 for infants born at 39

to 41 weeks' gestation, the age group with the lowest risk. Infant mortality rates generally decreased with increasing gestational age, and even infants born at 37 to 38 weeks had a mortality rate that was 50% higher than that for infants born at 39 to 41 weeks.

Regionalized care for high-risk mothers and preterm LBW infants, antenatal administration of corticosteroids, neonatal administration of exogenous pulmonary surfactant, and improved ventilator technology have improved outcomes for very preterm infants. Survival rates rise with gestational age at birth, from 6% for infants born at 22 weeks' gestation to more

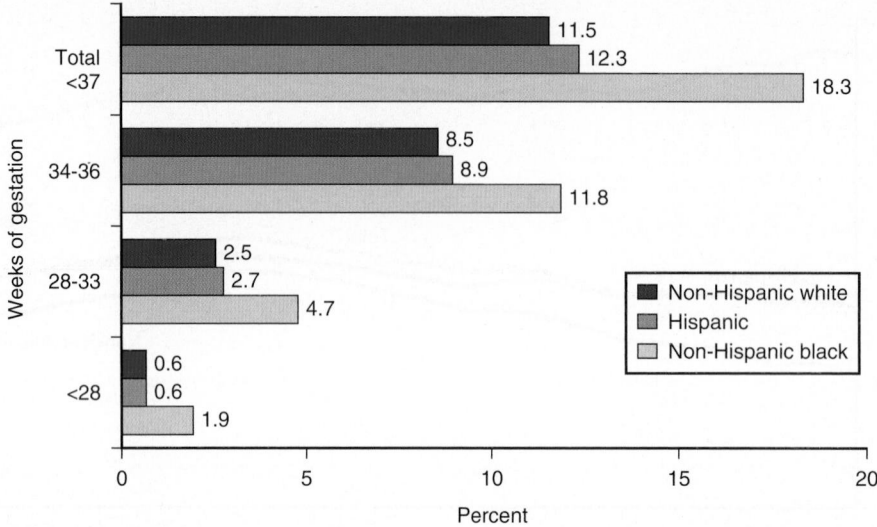

FIG 29-3 Percentage of live preterm births by racial group. (Data from Martin JA, Hamilton BE, Sutton PD, et al. Births: final data for 2008. *Natl Vital Stat Rep.* 2010;59[1]:1, 3-71.)

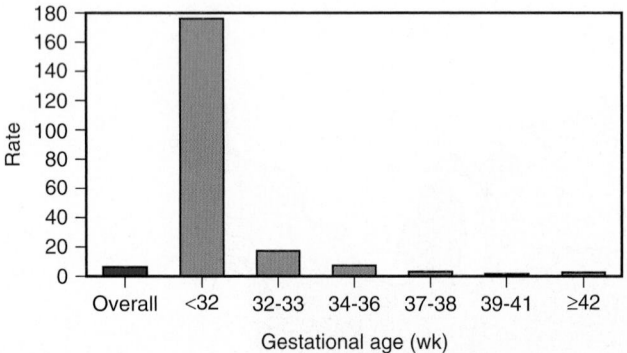

FIG 29-4 Proportion of all infant deaths in the United States in 2008 by gestational age at birth. (Modified from Centers for Disease Control and Prevention. Mathews TJ, MacDorman MF. Infant mortality statistics from the 2008 period linked birth/death data set. *Natl Vital Stat Rep.* 2012; 60[5]:1-27. Available at www.cdc.gov/nchs/vitalstats.htm.)

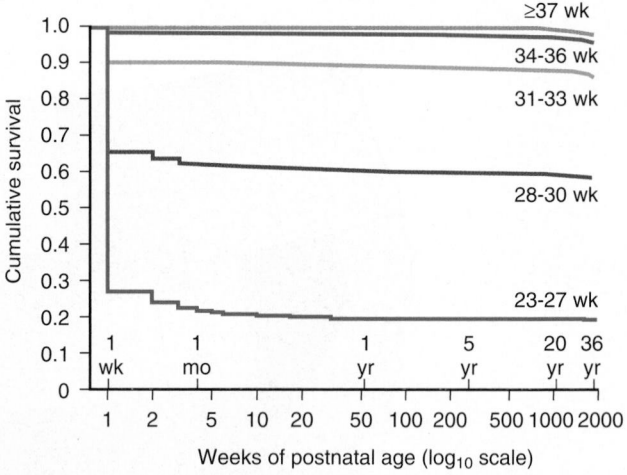

FIG 29-5 Cumulative long-term survival by gestational age at birth in 903,402 infants born in Norway. (Modified from Moster D, Lie RT, Markestad T. Long-term medical and social consequences of preterm birth. *N Engl J Med.* 2008;359[3]:262-273.)

than 90% at 28 weeks' gestation for infants cared for in tertiary intensive care units (ICUs).[9] Outcomes can be more accurately predicted by considering fetal number (singleton or multiple), gender, exposure or nonexposure to antenatal corticosteroids, and birthweight in addition to gestational age.[9] Probabilities of infant outcomes based upon antenatal factors can be estimated utilizing an online calculator available from the Eunice Kennedy Shriver National Institute of Child Health and Human Development (NICHD) Neonatal Research Network.[10] Long-term survival rates by gestational age at birth in 903,402 infants born in Norway[11] are shown in Figure 29-5.

Perinatal Morbidity

Preterm infants are at risk for specific diseases related to immaturity of various organ systems as well as to the causes and circumstances of PTB. **Common complications in premature infants include respiratory distress syndrome (RDS), intraventricular hemorrhage (IVH), bronchopulmonary dysplasia (BPD), patent ductus arteriosus (PDA), necrotizing enterocolitis (NEC), sepsis, apnea, and retinopathy of prematurity (ROP). Rates of morbidity vary primarily by gestational age but are also affected by birthweight, fetal number** (singleton

vs. multiple gestations), **geographic location, proximity to a neonatal intensive care unit (NICU), and any maternal or fetal conditions that may have led to PTB.** The frequency of major morbidity rises as gestational age decreases, especially before 30 weeks' gestation. Wide geographic variation is apparent in the frequency of neonatal morbidities, especially for VLBW infants. Reports of survival and morbidity also vary according to the denominator used. Obstetric datasets include all living fetuses at entry to the obstetric suite, whereas neonatal datasets exclude intrapartum and delivery room deaths and thus report rates based on newborns admitted to the nursery. Rates of survival and morbidity at the same gestational age and birthweight are thus somewhat higher in neonatal datasets.

Long-Term Outcomes

Major neonatal morbidities related to PTB that carry lifetime consequences include chronic lung disease, grades 3 and 4 intraventricular hemorrhage (associated with cerebral palsy), NEC, and vision and hearing impairment. Follow-up

BOX 29-1 DEMOGRAPHIC PROFILE OF WOMEN WITH SPONTANEOUS PRETERM BIRTH

- History of genital tract colonization, infection, or instrumentation
  - Urinary tract infection and bacteriuria
  - Sexually transmitted infections such as *Chlamydia*, gonorrhea, human papillomavirus, or *Trichomonas*
  - Bacterial vaginosis
  - Cervical dysplasia and treatment for this diagnosis
  - Spontaneous or induced abortion
- Black race
- Bleeding of uncertain origin in pregnancy
- History of a previous spontaneous preterm birth
- Uterine anomaly
- Use of assisted reproductive technology
- Multifetal gestation
- Cigarette smoking, substance abuse
- Prepregnancy underweight (body mass index <19.6) and prepregnancy obesity (body mass index >30)
- Periodontal disease
- Limited education, low income, and low social status
- Late registration for prenatal care
- High levels of personal stress in one or more domains of life

BOX 29-2 DEMOGRAPHIC AND MEDICAL PROFILE OF WOMEN WITH INDICATED PRETERM BIRTH

- Diabetes mellitus diagnosed before or during pregnancy
- Chronic or acute (preeclamptic) hypertension
- Obstetric disorders or risk conditions in the current or previous pregnancy
  - Preeclampsia
  - Previous uterine surgery (e.g., prior cesarean delivery via a vertical or T-shaped uterine incision)
  - Cholestasis
  - Placental disorders
    - Placenta previa
    - Premature separation (abruption) of the placenta
- Medical disorders
  - Seizures
  - Thromboembolism
  - Connective tissue disorders
  - Asthma and chronic bronchitis
  - Maternal human immunodeficiency virus or herpes simplex virus
  - Obesity
  - Smoking
- Advanced maternal age
- Fetal disorders
  - Fetal compromise
    - Chronic (poor fetal growth)
    - Acute (fetal distress; for example, abnormal fetal testing on a nonstress test or biophysical profile)
    - Excessive (polyhydramnios) or inadequate (oligohydramnios) amniotic fluid
    - Fetal hydrops, ascites, blood group alloimmunization
    - Birth defects
    - Fetal complications of multifetal gestation (e.g., growth deficiency, twin-to-twin transfusion syndrome)

studies of infants born preterm and of LBW infants reveal increased rates of cerebral palsy, neurosensory impairment, reduced cognition and motor performance, academic difficulties, and attention-deficit disorders.

The incidence of long-term morbidity in survivors is especially increased for those born before 26 weeks' gestation. In a study from the United Kingdom, 78% of 308 survivors born before 25 weeks' gestation were followed and compared with classmates of normal birthweight. Almost all had some disability at age 6 years: 22% had severe neurocognitive disabilities (cerebral palsy, IQ more than 3 standard deviations [SDs] below the mean, blindness, or deafness), 24% had moderate disability, 34% had mild disability, and 20% had no neurocognitive disability.

EPIDEMIOLOGY OF PRETERM BIRTH

The numerous maternal and fetal diagnoses that precede PTB may be considered according to whether parturition began spontaneously or not. **Spontaneous preterm parturition may first manifest as cervical softening and ripening, decidual activation, and/or uterine contractions. Cervical softening is the most common initial evidence that parturition has begun.** In women who later delivered spontaneously between 28 and 36 weeks' gestation, cervical length measurements at 22 to 24 weeks' gestation were significantly shorter than in women who delivered at term, indicating that cervical softening had begun before 24 weeks.[12] This same study found that more than half of women with evidence of very preterm cervical effacement delivered after 35 weeks' gestation, indicating that spontaneous preterm parturition does not always progress to PTB. Women with signs and symptoms of spontaneous preterm parturition often have one or more of the demographic characteristics shown in Box 29-1, but it is important to note that **approximately half of women who deliver preterm have no obvious risk factors.** Among 2521 women who received prenatal care at 10 collaborating university clinics, 323 (12.8%) delivered before 37 weeks' gestation. Of these, 234 (9.3% of the total and 72%

of those delivered preterm) were born after spontaneous initiation of parturition, and 89 (3.5% of the total and 27% of those delivered preterm) were born preterm because of medical or obstetric indications.[12]

As noted above, women whose PTB is not preceded by spontaneous parturition have medical and/or obstetric conditions that lead to the onset of parturition or to iatrogenic intervention to benefit the mother or fetus. Their demography reflects this (Box 29-2), and efforts to prolong pregnancy are primarily aimed at optimal management of their medical condition. This strategy is more successful in some—for example, those with diabetes mellitus, in whom maintenance of euglycemia often leads to birth at term—than in others, such as those with chronic hypertension, in whom effective blood pressure control does not prevent preeclampsia.

CLINICAL RISK FACTORS FOR SPONTANEOUS PRETERM BIRTH

Risk factors for spontaneous preterm birth (sPTB) arise from maternal factors, prior pregnancy history, and current pregnancy risks.

Maternal Factors

Many maternal factors impact PTB. These may be medical or dental, such as infection or disease; behavioral, related to maternal demographics or stress; or related to genetics and anatomy, including abnormalities of the genitourinary tract. Each of these factors will be discussed.

Medical
INFECTIONS

Systemic and genital tract infections are associated with PTB. In women in spontaneous preterm labor with intact membranes, lower genital tract flora are commonly found in the amniotic fluid, placenta, and membranes. The flora include *Ureaplasma urealyticum, Mycoplasma hominis, Fusobacterium* species, *Gardnerella vaginalis,* peptostreptococci, and *Bacteroides* species. Clinical and histologic evidence of intraamniotic inflammation and infection is more common as the gestational age at delivery decreases, especially before 30 to 32 weeks. **Bacteria in the amniotic fluid, whether detected by cultivation or by molecular methods, have been reported in 20% to 60% of women with preterm labor before 34 weeks' gestation.** The frequency of positive cultures increases as gestational age decreases, from 20% to 30% after 30 weeks to 60% at 23 to 24 weeks' gestation. Evidence of infection is less common after 34 weeks.

Bacterial vaginosis (BV) is a condition in which the ecosystem of the vagina is altered so that gram-negative anaerobic bacteria (e.g., *Gardnerella vaginalis, Bacteroides, Prevotella, Mobiluncus,* and *Mycoplasma* species) largely replace the normally predominant lactobacilli. **BV is associated with a twofold increased risk of sPTB. The association between BV and PTB is stronger when BV is detected early in pregnancy.** Despite the association, antibiotic eradication of BV does not consistently reduce the risk of PTB. Infections outside the genital tract have also been related to PTB, most commonly urinary tract and intraabdominal infections (e.g., pyelonephritis and appendicitis). The presumed mechanism of disease is inflammation of the nearby reproductive organs, but infections at remote sites—especially if they are chronic—have also been associated with increased risk of sPTB.

PERIODONTAL DISEASE
Women with periodontal disease have an increased risk of PTB that is not reduced by periodontal care, suggesting shared susceptibility rather than a cause-effect relation. The genitourinary and alimentary tracts are both major sites of microbial colonization where host immune factors defend the interior of the body, so shared risk factors are not surprising.

Genitourinary Tract Factors
CERVICAL LENGTH
Cervical length (CL) as measured by transvaginal ultrasound is inversely related to the risk of PTB in both singletons and twins. Women whose CL at 22 to 24 weeks' gestation was at or below the 10th percentile (25 mm by endovaginal ultrasound) had a 6.5-fold increased risk (95% confidence interval [CI], 4.5 to 9.3) of PTB before 35 weeks' gestation and a 7.7-fold increased risk (95% CI, 4.5 to 13.4) of PTB before 32 weeks' gestation when compared with women whose CL measurement was greater than the 75th percentile.[13] The explanation for the linkage between CL and PTB risk was once thought to reflect a "continuum of cervical competence" in which variable cervical resistance to uterine contractions explained the relationship. However, there is now substantial evidence that contractions do not herald the onset of PTB[14] and that progesterone supplementation slows the progression of cervical shortening and reduces the risk of PTB

when initiated before 24 weeks in women with and without a prior PTB.[15-19] These studies support the conclusion that **preterm cervical shortening (softening and ripening) is not the passive result of tissue weakness but instead is an active process indicating that pathologic preterm parturition has begun, regardless of its underlying cause.**[12]

CERVICAL PROCEDURES
A history of cervical surgery, including conization and the loop electrosurgical excision procedure (LEEP), has been suggested to be a risk factor for PTB. A recent meta-analysis supports the concept that when women with a history of LEEP are compared with women with prior dysplasia but no cervical excision, the risk of PTB is similar. This finding suggests that common factors for both PTB and dysplasia confound the association between LEEP and PTB.

CONGENITAL ABNORMALITIES OF THE UTERUS
Congenital structural abnormalities of the uterus, known as *müllerian fusion defects,* may affect the cervix, the uterine corpus, or both. **The risk of PTB in women with uterine malformations is 25% to 50% depending on the specific malformation and the obstetric history.** Implantation of the placenta on a uterine septum may lead to PTB by means of placental separation and hemorrhage. A T-shaped uterus in women exposed in utero to diethylstilbestrol (DES) has also been associated with an increased risk of preterm labor and birth.

Behavioral
In general, studies of behavioral influences on PTB have not found a consistent relationship between maternal activities and PTB, except with tobacco smoking.

SMOKING AND SUBSTANCE ABUSE
Smoking is associated with an increased risk of PTB, and unlike most other risks, it is amenable to intervention during pregnancy.

PHYSICAL ACTIVITY
Controversy exists as to whether excessive physical activity is associated with early delivery.

NUTRITIONAL FACTORS
Low maternal prepregnancy weight (body mass index [BMI] <19.8 kg/m^2) has been consistently found to be associated with an increased risk of PTB.[20,21] Prepregnancy overweight and obesity are also linked to an increased risk of PTB, especially extremely preterm birth.[22] Women who consume one or more servings of fish per month have lower rates of PTB than women who rarely or never eat fish.[23] Numerous studies of various nutritional deficiencies have been reported to be related to the risk of PTB, but there are few if any for which supplementation has been found to reduce the incidence of prematurity.

Demography, Stress, and Social Determinants of Health
Social disadvantage is persistently associated with increased risk of PTB: poverty; educational attainment; geographic residence in disadvantaged neighborhoods, states, and regions; and lack of access to prenatal care are all linked to significantly higher rates of PTB.[24] These associations were once deemed to be social, not medical, and thus beyond the reach of medical care. Stress[25] and depression[26] are consistently reported to have a moderate

TABLE 29-1 MAGNITUDE OF INCREASED RISK BASED ON EDUCATION AND RACE/ETHNICITY

YEARS OF EDUCATION	NON-HISPANIC BLACK	NON-HISPANIC WHITE	ASIAN/PACIFIC ISLANDER	NATIVE AMERICAN	HISPANIC
<8	19.6	11.0	11.5	14.8	10.7
8-12	16.8	9.9	10.5	11.8	10.4
13-15	14.5	8.3	9.1	9.9	9.3
≥16	12.8	7.0	7.5	9.4	8.4

From Behrman RE, Stith Butler A. Committee on understanding premature birth and assuring healthy outcomes: causes, consequences, and prevention. Washington, DC: National Academies Press; 2007.

TABLE 29-2 PRETERM BIRTH RATE PERCENTAGES BY MATERNAL RACE/ETHNICITY AND PRENATAL CARE ACCESS BY TRIMESTER OF INITIATION OF PRENATAL CARE, 1998-2000

TRIMESTER	NON-HISPANIC BLACK	NON-HISPANIC WHITE	ASIAN/PACIFIC ISLANDER	NATIVE AMERICAN	HISPANIC
First	14.7	8.3	8.6	10.4	9.7
Second	17.5	10.2	10.8	12.7	11.0
Third	16.0	10.0	9.5	12.3	10.0
No prenatal care	33.4	21.7	19.4	24.0	19.8

Data from National Committee on Health Statistics for U.S. birth cohorts from 1998 to 2000 and from Berhman RE, Butler AS. *Sociodemographic and Community Factors Contributing to Preterm Birth: Causes, Consequences, and Prevention.* Institute of Medicine (US) Committee on Understanding Premature Birth and Assuring Healthy Outcomes. Washington, DC: National Academies Press; 2007.

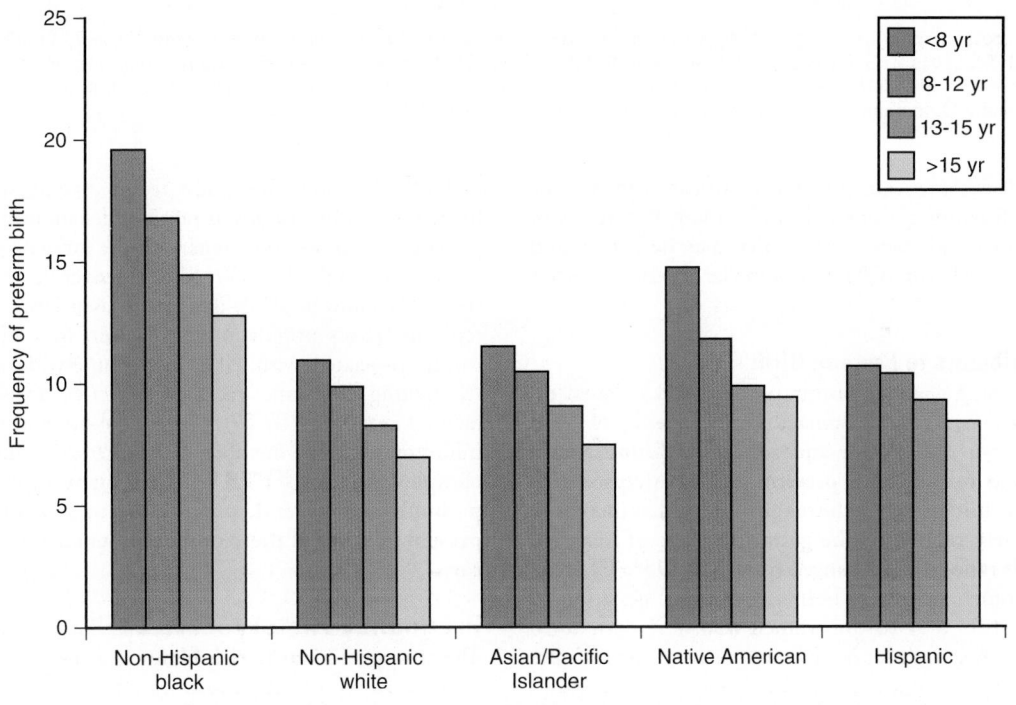

FIG 29-6 Risk of preterm birth according to educational level (years) by race/ethnicity (see Table 29-1). (Data from Behrman RE, Stith Butler A. *Committee on understanding premature birth and assuring healthy outcomes: causes, consequences, and prevention.* Washington, DC: National Academies Press; 2007.)

association with PTB, although the mechanisms again remain uncertain.

The effect of the social environment on reproduction has since been examined in greater detail and reveals evidence of a causative relationship. The magnitude of the increased risk of PTB according to educational level and race/ethnicity is shown in Table 29-1 and Figure 29-6.

A nearly twofold difference is seen in the rate of PTB for women of all racial and ethnic groups between those with the highest and lowest levels of education. Equally striking is the persistence of the disparity in rates of PTB in black women regardless of their educational level, and in Table 29-2 and as shown in Figure 29-7, their access to early prenatal care.

BLACK RACE

Black women have a uniquely increased risk for PTB when compared with women from any other racial or ethnic background.[27] In 2005 through 2007, the rate of PTB averaged 18.4% among black women, compared with 10.8% in Asian American, 11.6% in white, 12.6% in Hispanic, and 14.2% in Native American women. The disparity in the PTB rate persists after social and medical risk factors are accounted for[24,27,28] and

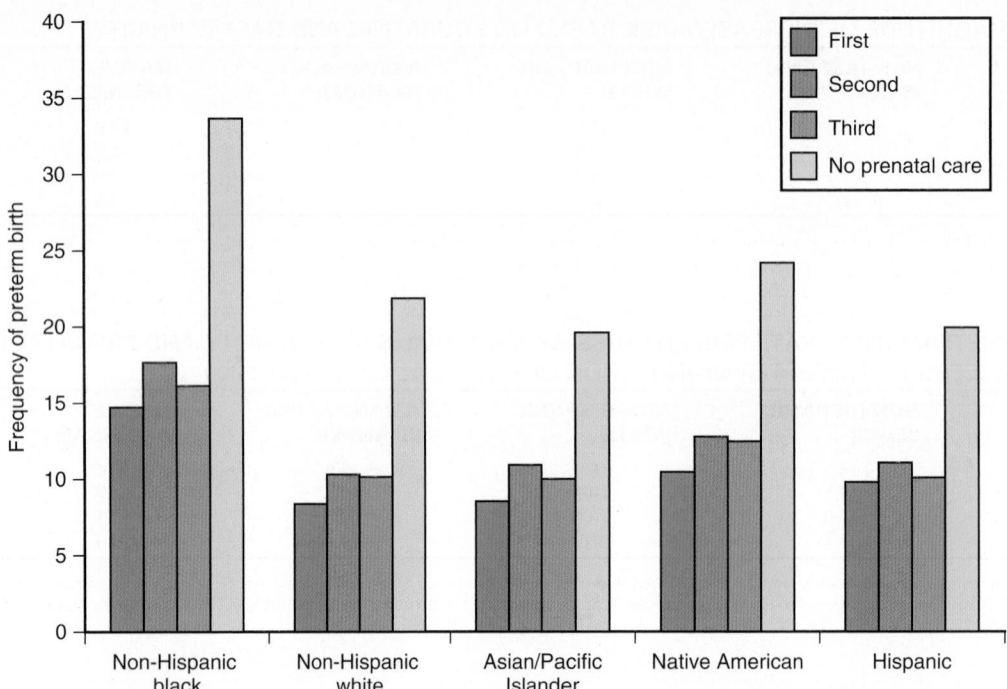

FIG 29-7 Risk of preterm birth according to access to early prenatal care by race/ethnicity and trimester (see Table 29-2). (Data from National Center for Health Statistics: U.S. Birth Cohorts From 1998 to 2000. From Berhman RE, Butler AS. *Sociodemographic and Community Factors Contributing to Preterm Birth: Causes, Consequences, and Prevention.* Institute of Medicine (US) Committee on Understanding Premature Birth and Assuring Healthy Outcomes. Washington, DC: National Academies Press; 2007.)

is evident in black Americans but not in African women. The origins of the disparity are not well understood. Regardless of the etiology, **all African American women may be considered to have an increased risk of PTB even in the absence of other risk factors.**

Genetic Contributors to Preterm Birth

The notion of some genetic contribution to PTB is based on several observations. First, a woman's family history of PTB influences her own risk. **Porter and colleagues found that a mother who was herself born preterm had an inceased risk for delivering a child preterm; the magnitude of that increased risk was inversely related to the gestational age of her own birth.** The odds ratio for PTB ranged from 1.18 (95% CI, 1.02 to 1.37) for women who were born at 36 weeks' gestation to 2.38 (95% CI, 1.37 to 4.16) for women who were born at 30 weeks' gestation. A second set of observations from twin studies supports a genetic contribution to PTB. Treloar and colleagues[29] studied 905 Australian female twin pairs to determine whether delivery had occurred more than 2 weeks before term. In this study, "all-cause" PTB was the outcome.[29,30] Twin-pair correlations were higher from monozygotic twin pairs than from dizygotic twin pairs ($r = 0.3 \pm 0.08$ vs. 0.03 ± 0.11 standard error [SE], respectively). Heritability was calculated at 17% for preterm delivery in the first pregnancy and 27% for preterm delivery in any pregnancy. A population-based twin study in Scandinavia investigated 868 monozygotic and 1141 dizygotic female twin pairs who delivered singletons between 1973 and 1993.[29,30] Correlation for gestational length was higher for monozygotic compared with dizygotic twins, and heritability estimates from model fitting were approximately 30% for gestational age and 36% for PTB. This heritability appears to be the result of maternal, rather than paternal, lineage. The pattern

of PTBs that occur in family pedigrees suggests that the most likely form of inheritance is nonmendelian; rather, the observed pedigrees are more consistent with the influence of many genes. Numerous studies have aimed at discovering variation in genes that contribute to PTB, and many associations have failed to replicate across populations. However, four genes are significantly associated with PTB in genome-wide studies: follicle-stimulating hormone receptor (*FSHR*), insulin-like growth factor 1 receptor (*IGF1R*), protein col-52, and serpin peptidase inhibitor, clade B, member 2 (*SERPINB2*). **Insights into the complex genetics of PTB hold promise for giving insight into pathophysiology and, potentially, to risk identification; at present, neither of these potential benefits influences clinical care.**

Pregnancy History

The strongest historic risk factor is a previous birth between 16 and 36 weeks' gestation. This history is often reported to confer a 1.5-fold to twofold increased risk but varies widely according to the number, sequence, and gestational age of prior PTBs (Fig. 29-8).

When the prior PTB occurs in a twin pregnancy, the risk of PTB in a subsequent singleton gestation rises as the gestational age at delivery of the twins falls below 34 weeks' gestation. There is minimal if any increased risk for women whose prior twin birth occurred after 34 weeks' gestation, but the risk of singleton PTB may be as much as 40% when the prior twin birth occurred before 30 weeks' gestation.

Prior stillbirth[31] and pregnancies ending between 16 and 20 weeks' gestation[3] are also associated with increased risk of PTB in subsequent pregnancies.

Pregnancy termination in the first and second trimesters is linked to an increased risk of subsequent PTB, especially when

PRIOR PRETERM DELIVERY STATUS BY ORDER AND GESTATIONAL AGE AT DELIVERY

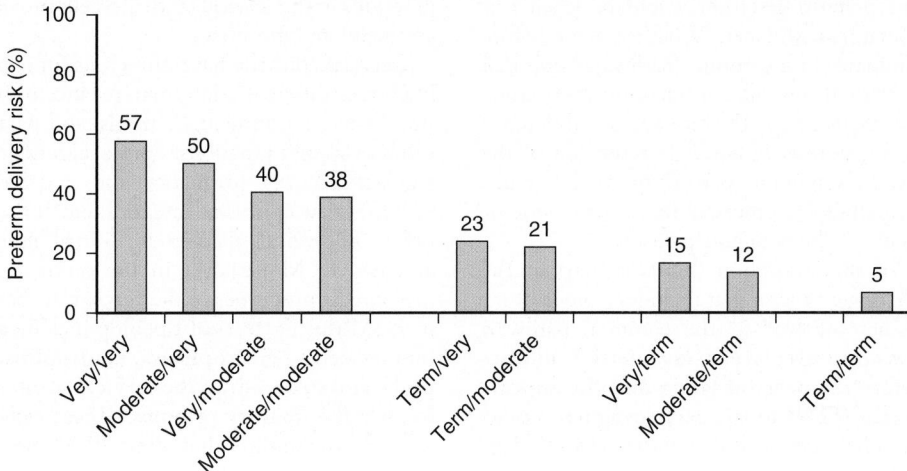

FIG 29-8 Risk of recurrent preterm birth in 19,025 women with two prior births according to the order and gestational age of the previous birth. Very preterm, 21 to 31 weeks' gestation; moderate preterm, 32 to 36 weeks' gestation. (Modified from McManemy J, Cooke E, Amon E, Leet T. Recurrence risk for preterm delivery. *Am J Obstet Gynecol.* 2007;196[6]:576.e1-e7.)

performed with mechanical dilation or curettage or when performed repeatedly.[32] Increased risk of PTB has been found after spontaneous, as well as induced, abortion.[33]

Current Pregnancy Risks

Mode of conception also affects the risk of PTB. The increased rate of PTB after assisted reproduction is due not only to the increased occurrence of multiple gestations but also to an increased rate of PTBs in singleton pregnancies as well. **A nearly twofold increased risk of PTB is observed in singleton pregnancies conceived with all methods of fertility care, including ovulation promotion.**[34] A meta-analysis of 15 studies that compared 12,283 pregnancies resulting from in vitro fertilization (IVF) with 1.9 million spontaneously conceived singleton births found approximately twofold increased rates of perinatal mortality, PTB, LBW and VLBW, and SGA infants born after IVF. Rates of PTB among multiple gestations do not appear to be increased after assisted conception relative to spontaneously conceived twins and triplets, so the explanation for the increased rates in singletons is unclear. Microbial colonization of the upper genital tract, increased stress among infertile couples, side effects of superovulation, and increased rates of birth defects have been proposed as possible causes.

Bleeding and Vanishing Twins

Women who experience unexplained vaginal bleeding after the first trimester have an increased risk of subsequent PTB that increases with the number of bleeding episodes. Perhaps reflecting similar causes, the risk of PTB is also increased in women whose pregnancies are complicated by a vanishing twin (see Chapter 32) or by an unexplained elevation in maternal serum alpha-fetoprotein.

Multifetal Gestation and Uterine Distension

Multifetal gestation is one of the strongest risk factors for PTB. Rates of preterm, very preterm, LBW, and VLBW births according to fetal number are described in Chapter 32. Slightly more than 50% of women with twins deliver before 37 weeks' gestation. The risk of early birth rises with the number of fetuses, which suggests uterine overdistension and fetal signaling as

potential pathways to the early initiation of labor. In addition to spontaneous preterm labor, multiple gestations are more commonly complicated by medical and obstetric disorders that lead to indicated preterm delivery. Poor fetal growth, fetal anomalies, hypertension, abruptio placentae, and fetal compromise are more common in multiple gestations and increase with the number of fetuses. The chorionicity of twin gestations is also an important factor in the risk for adverse pregnancy outcomes. **Monochorionic twin pregnancies are more likely than dichorionic twin gestations to be complicated by stillbirth and fetal growth restriction.** Newborn monochorionic twins are more likely than dichorionic twins to experience NEC and neurologic morbidity. It is unclear how much of the excess rate of PTB among monochorionic twins is due to indicated versus spontaneous PTB.

Risk-Scoring Systems

Attempts to develop scoring systems based on historic and epidemiologic data plus current pregnancy risk factors have had low sensitivity to identify women who will give birth preterm, but they have not included some of the historic risks listed here.

PATHOPHYSIOLOGY OF SPONTANEOUS PRETERM BIRTH

Term and preterm parturition share anatomic, physiologic, and biochemical features that are considered part of the common pathway of parturition. This pathway includes (1) cervical changes (*softening*, and *ripening*), (2) membrane/ decidual activation, and (3) increased uterine contractility. However, although spontaneous labor at term results from physiologic activation of the common pathway of parturition, preterm labor is the result of a *pathologic activation* of this pathway. The insult responsible for activation may lead to asynchronous recruitment of each pathway. **Asynchrony is recognized clinically as (1) cervical insufficiency when the process affects predominantly the cervix; (2) preterm uterine contractions when the process affects the myometrium; or (3) preterm premature rupture of membranes (PPROM) if**

the insult acts on the chorioamniotic membranes. Synchronous activation in the preterm gestation would be labeled as preterm labor with intact membranes. Whether at or before term, parturition culminates in a common pathway composed of cervical changes, persistent uterine contractions, and activation of the decidua and membranes. The fundamental difference is that labor at term is a normal physiologic activation of the common pathway, whereas preterm parturition is the result, entirely or in part, of pathologic processes that activate one or more of the components of the common pathway.

Although labor is of short duration (hours or days at the most), parturition is a longer process that includes a preparatory phase of the key tissues involved in the common pathway. Thus cervical changes occur over weeks, myometrial contractility is increased before the onset of labor, and the appearance of fetal fibronectin (FFN) in the cervicovaginal mucus can be considered to reflect extracellular matrix (ECM) degradation, which indicates activation of the decidua and membranes.

A fetal maturity–based signal for labor originates in the fetal hypothalamus and leads to increased secretion of corticotropin-releasing hormone (CRH), which in turn stimulates adrenocorticotropic hormone (ACTH) and cortisol production by the fetal adrenals, which ultimately leads to activation of the common pathway of parturition. The fetus may contribute to the onset of preterm labor in the context of the **fetal inflammatory response syndrome** (see below).

Spontaneous PTB may best be understood as a syndrome in which the clinical presentations of preterm labor, preterm ruptured membranes, and preterm cervical effacement and dilation without labor occur as the result of multiple etiologies that can occur alone or in combination. Some act to initiate preterm parturition acutely—for example, with acute posttraumatic placental abruption—but most follow a more subacute or indolent path over several weeks. It is helpful to remember that the normal process of parturition proceeds for several weeks before clinically evident labor begins. Thus pathologic stimuli of parturition may act in concert with the normal physiologic preparation for labor, especially after 32 weeks' gestation. Before 30 to 32 weeks, a greater proportion of preterm labor has a pathologic stimulus.

Cervical Changes: Softening and Ripening
The cervix is a critical structure in pregnancy and parturition; it must maintain structural integrity and act as a physical barrier during pregnancy and subsequently transition to allow passage of the fetus during delivery. This change is not acute; physiologic parturition occurs over the course of gestation and requires evolving biochemical and biomechanical changes in the cervix that manifest as cervical ripening.[35,36] Molecular processes that underlie cervical ripening are different between physiologic and pathologic parturition and may differ among etiologies of pathologic parturition.

Although collagen is the main contributor to the tensile strength of the cervix, glycosaminoglycans (GAGs) are critical to determining the viscoelastic properties of the tissue. GAGs are long, unbranched polysaccharides—vital components of the ECM—that serve many roles: they help to determine tissue hydration, which contributes to viscous tissue properties, and they stabilize the overall architecture of the ECM. In addition, small leucine-rich proteoglycans (GAGs linked to core proteins) such as decorin have been shown to interact with

soluble growth factors and mediators of inflammation. Tight junctions in the cervical epithelial cells provide structural support and regulate fluid fluxes.

Cervical epithelia have numerous functions that include proliferation, differentiation, maintenance of fluid balance, protection from environmental hazards, and paracellular transport of solutes via tight junctions. Epithelial functions must be carefully regulated during pregnancy and parturition, and molecules important in epithelial integrity and function are key components of cervical changes in animal models and in women at term. ECM turnover in the cervix is high, and thus the mechanical properties of the cervix can change rapidly. Changes in ECM during cervical ripening include **an influx of inflammatory cells—macrophages, neutrophils, mast cells, eosinophils, and so on—into the cervical stroma in a process similar to an inflammatory response. These cells produce cytokines and prostaglandins that affect ECM metabolism.** Prostaglandins effect cervical ripening physiologically and have been widely used as pharmacologic agents to ripen the cervix for induction of labor. Cervical ripening is influenced by estrogen, which induces ripening by stimulating collagen degradation, and by progesterone, which blocks these estrogenic effects. Furthermore, administration of a progesterone receptor antagonist can induce cervical ripening, and administration of progesterone has been reported to delay or even reverse ripening. Another mediator implicated in the mechanisms of cervical ripening is nitric oxide (NO), which can act as an inflammatory mediator.

Cervical changes normally precede the onset of labor, are gradual, and develop over several weeks. PTB is often preceded by cervical ripening over a period of weeks in the second and third trimesters, evidenced on clinical examination by softening and thinning of the cervix and on ultrasound examination of the cervix by cervical "funneling" and shortening of the length of the endocervical canal.

Increased Uterine Contractility
Labor is characterized by a change in uterine contractility from episodic uncoordinated myometrial contractures that last several minutes and produce little increase in intrauterine pressure to more coordinated contractions of short duration that produce marked increases in intrauterine pressure that ultimately effect delivery. **The change from the contracture to the contraction pattern typically begins at night, which suggests neural control.** The transition from contractures to contractions may progress to normal labor or may occur dyssynchronously as the result of inflammation (e.g., with maternal infection or abdominal surgery). Fasting may also induce the switch in humans. Oxytocin is produced by the decidua and the paraventricular nuclei of the hypothalamus, indicating both an endocrine and a paracrine role. **Plasma concentrations of oxytocin mirror uterine contractility, which suggests oxytocin may mediate the circadian rhythm in uterine contractility.**

Cellular communication is another feature of labor, promulgated by formation of gap junctions that develop in the myometrium before labor and disappear after delivery. Gap-junction formation and the expression of the gap-junction protein connexin 43 in the human myometrium is similar in term and preterm labor. These findings suggest that the **appearance of gap junctions and increased expression of connexin 43 may be part of the underlying molecular and cellular events responsible for the switch from contractures to**

contractions before the onset of parturition. Estrogen, progesterone, and prostaglandins have been implicated in the regulation of gap-junction formation and in influencing the expression of connexin 43. Lye and colleagues have proposed that changes in a set of distinct proteins called *contraction-associated proteins* are characteristic of this stage of parturition.

Decidual Membrane Activation

The maternal decidua and adjacent fetal membranes undergo anatomic and biochemical changes during the final weeks of gestation that ultimately result in a spontaneous rupture of the membranes. **Premature activation of this mechanism leads to PPROM, the clinical antecedent for up to 40% of all preterm deliveries.** Although rupture of the membranes normally occurs during the first stage of labor, histologic studies of prematurely ruptured membranes show decreased amounts of collagen types I, III, and V; increased expression of tenascin, expressed during tissue remodeling and wound healing; and disruption of the normal wavy collagen pattern, which suggests that preterm rupture is a process that precedes the onset of labor.

Structural ECM proteins such as collagens have been implicated in the tensile strength of the membranes, whereas the viscoelastic properties have been attributed to elastin. Dissolution of extracellular cements (e.g., fibronectins) is thought to be responsible for the process that allows the membranes to separate from the decidua after the birth of the infant. Degradation of the ECM, assessed by the detection of FFN, is part of the common pathway of parturition. The presence of FFN or pathogen-associated molecular patterns (PAMPs) in cervicovaginal secretions between 22 and 37 weeks' gestation is evidence of disruption of the decidual-chorionic interface and is associated with an increased risk of PTB.

The precise mechanism of membrane/decidua activation is uncertain, but matrix-degrading enzymes and apoptosis—programmed cell death—have been proposed. Increased levels of matrix metalloproteinases (MMPs) and their regulators (tissue inhibitors of metalloproteinases [TIMPs]) have been documented in the amniotic fluid of women with PPROM.

Apoptosis may also play a role in the mechanism of membrane rupture through increased expression of proapoptotic genes and decreased expression of antiapoptotic genes. MMP-9 may induce apoptosis in the amnion.

Fetal Participation in the Onset of Labor

A fetal signal contributes to the onset of labor in animals and humans. Destruction of the paraventricular nucleus of the fetal hypothalamus results in prolongation of pregnancy in sheep. The human counterpart to this animal experiment is anencephaly, which is also characterized by prolonged pregnancy when women with polyhydramnios are excluded. The current paradigm is that **once maturity has been reached, the fetal brain—specifically the hypothalamus—increases CRH secretion that, in turn, stimulates ACTH and cortisol production by the fetal adrenals. This increase of cortisol in sheep and of dehydroepiandrosterone sulfate (DHEAS) in primates eventually leads to activation of the common pathway of parturition.**

Preterm Parturition Syndrome

Obstetric taxonomy is largely based on clinical presentation, not the mechanism of disease. **Preterm labor may occur as the common clinical presentation of infection, vascular insult, uterine overdistension, abnormal allogeneic recognition, stress, or other pathologic processes. Often more than one of these factors is operative in the same patient. Thus preterm labor is a syndrome for which no single diagnostic test or treatment exists.** Obstetric syndromes share the following features:

- Multiple etiologies
- Chronicity
- Fetal involvement
- Clinical manifestations that are adaptive
- Variable susceptibility due to gene-environment interactions

Each of these features is true of PTB. As listed earlier, preterm labor clearly has *multiple etiologies*. Pathways to preterm labor are demonstrated to be *chronic,* as seen in the time interval between observation of a short cervix or increased concentrations of FFN in vaginal fluid in the midtrimester of pregnancy and subsequent preterm labor or delivery. *Fetal involvement* has been demonstrated in women with microbial invasion of the amniotic cavity, in which fetal bacteremia and cytokine production have been detected in 30% of women with PPROM and an amniotic fluid culture positive for microorganisms. Similarly, neonates born after spontaneous preterm labor or PPROM are more likely to be small for gestational age, which suggests chronically compromised fetal supply. Preterm labor may be seen as an *adaptive* mechanism of host defense against infection that allows the mother to eliminate infected tissue and allows the fetus to exit a hostile environment. If the clinical manifestations are adaptive, it is not surprising that treatments aimed at the common terminal pathway of parturition, such as tocolysis or cerclage, and not at the fundamental mechanism of disease-inducing activation of the pathway—myometrial contractility, cervical dilation, and effacement—would not be effective. Increasing evidence suggests gene-environment interaction in the steps leading to preterm labor complicated by the presence, and even perhaps the conflicting interests, of two genomes: maternal and fetal. This is most evident in studies of the relationship between maternal genital tract colonization and PTB. Finally, additional mechanisms may be at play that have not yet been identified.

Pathologic processes implicated in the preterm parturition syndrome include intrauterine inflammation/infection, vascular disorders, uterine overdistension, breakdown of maternal-fetal tolerance, allergy-induced causes, cervical insufficiency, and endocrine disorders.

Intrauterine Infection

Systemic maternal infections such as pyelonephritis and pneumonia are frequently associated with the onset of premature labor in humans. **Intrauterine infection is a frequent and important mechanism of disease leading to preterm delivery.** Intrauterine infection or systemic administration of microbial products to pregnant animals can result in preterm labor and delivery, and substantial evidence shows that subclinical intrauterine infections are associated with preterm labor and delivery. Moreover, fetal infection and inflammation have been implicated in the genesis of fetal or neonatal injury leading to cerebral palsy and chronic lung disease. **Microbiologic and histopathologic studies suggest that infection-related inflammation may account for 25% to 40% of cases of preterm delivery.**

Frequency of Intrauterine Infection in Spontaneous Preterm Birth

The prevalence of amniotic fluid cultures positive for microorganisms in women with preterm labor and intact membranes is approximately 13%, with additional instances of infection that are identifiable using polymerase chain reaction (PCR) techniques rather than culture. The earlier the gestational age at PTB, the more likely that microbial invasion of the amniotic cavity is present. **In PPROM, the prevalence of positive amniotic fluid cultures for microorganisms is approximately 32%.** Among women with a dilated cervix in the midtrimester, the prevalence of positive amniotic fluid cultures is 51%. Microbial invasion of the amniotic cavity occurs in 12% of twin gestations with preterm labor and when delivering a preterm neonate. The most common microorganisms found in the amniotic cavity are *Mycoplasma* and *U. urealyticum*.

Intrauterine Infection as a Chronic Process

Evidence in support of chronicity of intrauterine inflammation/infection is derived from studies of the microbiologic state of the amniotic fluid, as well as the concentration of inflammatory mediators, at the time of genetic amniocentesis. Genital mycoplasmas that include *M. hominis* and also *U. urealyticum* have been recovered from amniotic fluid samples obtained at second-trimester genetic amniocentesis, with subsequent preterm delivery and histologic chorioamnionitis, especially in those with *U. urealyticum*. **Increased levels of many inflammatory markers have been found in second-trimester amniotic fluid samples obtained from women who subsequently delivered preterm.** These observations suggest that infection and inflammation in the amniotic cavity in the midtrimester of pregnancy can lead to preterm delivery weeks later. The most advanced stage of intrauterine infection is fetal infection. Fetal bacteremia has been detected in blood obtained by cordocentesis in 33% of fetuses with positive amniotic fluid culture and in 4% of those with negative amniotic fluid culture.

Molecular mediators that trigger parturition (cytokines and other inflammatory mediators) are similar to those that protect the host against infection. **The onset of preterm labor in response to intrauterine infection is thus very likely a host defense mechanism with survival value for the mother and, after viability, for the fetus.**

Infection, Preterm Labor, and Neonatal Outcomes

The scenario postulated from the preceding evidence is that **microorganisms that reside in or ascend to reach the decidua may, depending on host defense and environmental influences, stimulate a local inflammatory reaction and the production of proinflammatory cytokines, chemokines, and inflammatory mediators.** This inflammatory process, which is initially extraamniotic, may produce cervical effacement, further inflammation of the choriodecidual interface, and uterine contractions, and it may progress to the amniotic fluid and ultimately to the fetus. Microorganisms are known to cross intact membranes into the amniotic cavity, where inflammatory mediators are produced by resident macrophages and other host cells within the amniotic cavity. Finally, microorganisms that gain access to the fetus may elicit a systemic inflammatory response, the fetal inflammatory response syndrome (FIRS), characterized by increased concentrations of interleukin-6 (IL-6) and other cytokines as well as cellular evidence of neutrophil and monocyte activation.

FIRS is a subclinical condition originally described in fetuses of mothers with preterm labor and intact membranes and PPROM. Fetuses with FIRS have a higher rate of neonatal complications and are frequently born to mothers with subclinical microbial invasion of the amniotic cavity. Evidence of multisystemic involvement in cases of FIRS includes increased concentrations of fetal plasma MMP-9, neutrophilia, a higher number of circulating nucleated red blood cells, and higher plasma concentrations of granulocyte-colony stimulating factor (G-CSF). The histologic hallmark of FIRS is inflammation in the umbilical cord (funisitis) or chorionic vasculitis. The systemic fetal inflammatory response may result in multiple organ dysfunction, septic shock, and death in the absence of timely delivery. Newborns with funisitis are at increased risk for neonatal sepsis and long-term handicaps that include BPD and cerebral palsy.

When the inflammatory process does not involve the chorioamniotic membranes and decidua, systemic fetal inflammation and injury may occur in the absence of labor with eventual delivery at term. An example of this is fetal alloimmunization (see Chapter 34), in which fetal plasma concentrations of IL-6 are elevated, but preterm labor does not occur.

Gene-Environment Interactions

Gene-environment interactions underlie many complex disorders such as atherosclerosis and cancer. **A gene-environment interaction is said to be present when the risk of a disease (occurrence or severity) among individuals exposed to both genotype and an environmental factor is greater or less than that predicted from the presence of either the genotype or the environmental exposure alone.** The inflammatory response to the presence of microorganisms is modulated by interactions between the host genotype and environment that determine the likelihood and course of some infectious diseases. An example of such an interaction has been reported for BV, an allele for tumor necrosis factor alpha (TNF-α) and preterm delivery. Maternal BV is a consistently reported risk factor for spontaneous preterm delivery, yet treatment of BV does not reliably prevent PTB in women with BV. One potential explanation has come from a study of PTB rates in women according to their carriage of BV and whether or not they had allele 2 of TNF-α, known to be associated with sPTB. Both BV (odds ratio [OR], 3.3; 95% CI, 1.8 to 5.9) and TNF-α allele 2 (OR, 2.7; 95% CI, 1.7 to 4.5) were associated with increased risk for preterm delivery, but the risk of sPTB was substantially increased (OR, 6; 95% CI, 1.9 to 21.0) in women with both BV and the TNF-α allele 2. It is reasonable to assume that other gene-environment interactions may contribute to PTB.

Uteroplacental Ischemia and Decidual Hemorrhage

After inflammation, the most common abnormalities seen in placental pathology specimens from sPTBs are vascular lesions of the maternal and fetal circulations. Maternal lesions include failure of physiologic transformation of the spiral arteries, atherosis, and thrombosis. Fetal abnormalities include a decreased number of villous arterioles and fetal arterial thrombosis.

One proposed mechanism linking vascular lesions and preterm labor/delivery is **uteroplacental ischemia**, evidenced in primate models and in studies that found failure of physiologic transformation in the myometrial segment of the spiral arteries—a phenomenon typical of preeclampsia and intrauterine growth restriction (IUGR)—in women with preterm labor and intact membranes and PPROM. Abnormal uterine artery Doppler velocimetry indicative of increased impedance to flow in the uterine circulation has been reported in women with apparently idiopathic preterm labor.

The mechanisms responsible for preterm parturition in cases of ischemia have not been determined, but uterine ischemia has been postulated to lead to increased production of uterine renin from the fetal membranes. Angiotensin II can induce myometrial contractility directly or through the release of prostaglandins.

Decidual necrosis and hemorrhage can activate parturition through production of thrombin, which stimulates myometrial contractility in a dose-dependent manner. Thrombin also stimulates production of MMP-1, urokinase-type plasminogen activator (uPA), and tissue-type plasminogen activator (tPA) by endometrial stromal cells in culture. Directly or indirectly, these factors can digest important components of the ECM in the chorioamniotic membranes. Thrombin/antithrombin complexes, a marker of in vivo generation of thrombin, are increased in plasma and amniotic fluid of women with preterm labor and PPROM. The decidua is a rich source of tissue factor, the primary initiator of coagulation and of thrombin activation. These observations are consistent with clinical associations among vaginal bleeding, retroplacental hematomas, and preterm delivery.

Uterine ischemia should not be equated with fetal hypoxemia. Studies of fetal cord blood do not support fetal hypoxemia as a cause or consequence of preterm parturition.

Uterine Overdistension

The mechanisms responsible for the increased frequency of PTB in multiple gestations and other disorders associated with uterine overdistension are unknown. Central questions are how the uterus senses stretch, and how these mechanical forces induce biochemical changes that lead to parturition. Increased expression of oxytocin receptor, connexin 43, and the *c-fos* messenger RNA (mRNA) have been consistently demonstrated in the rat myometrium near term. Progesterone blocks stretch-induced gene expression in the myometrium. Mitogen-activated protein kinases have been proposed to mediate stretch-induced *c-fos* mRNA expression in myometrial cells. Stretch can have effects on the membranes; for example, in vitro studies have demonstrated an increase in the production of collagenase, interleukin 8 (IL-8), and prostaglandin E_2 (PGE_2) as well as the cytokine pre–B-cell colony-enhancing factor. These observations provide a possible link between the mechanical forces that operate in an overdistended uterus and in the rupture of membranes.

Breakdown of Fetal-Maternal Tolerance

The fetoplacental unit is the most successful transplant. This is made possible by the development of a tolerogenic state, a state of immune tolerance during normal pregnancy that requires participation of the maternal and fetal immune systems as well as active suppression at the maternal-fetal interface. Recent evidence suggests that maternal antifetal rejection is a common mechanism of disease in premature labor. Chronic chorioamnionitis, a lesion in which maternal lymphocytes infiltrate the chorioamniotic membranes, is the most common pathologic finding in sPTB. Maternal lymphocytes can induce destruction of the

trophoblast in the chorion and can thus induce preterm labor. This lesion, as well as chronic villitis, is considered to represent evidence of maternal antifetal rejection.[37,38]

Allergy-Induced Preterm Labor

Case reports indicate that preterm labor has occurred after exposure to an allergen that generates an allergic-like mechanism (type I hypersensitivity reaction) and that some women with preterm labor have eosinophils as the predominant cells in amniotic fluid, suggesting a **form of uterine allergy.** Mast cells in the uterus produce histamine and prostaglandins, both of which can induce myometrial contractility. Premature birth can be induced by exposure to an allergen in sensitized animals, and it can be prevented by treatment with a histamine H_1 receptor antagonist.

Cervical Insufficiency

Prompted by knowledge of the relationship between a sonographic short cervix with and a subsequent PTB, the understanding of cervical function evolved from a categorical concept of cervical incompetence versus competence to one of "competence as a continuum."[13] However, subsequent analyses of these same data[12] were conducted in response to clinical trials that demonstrated that preterm cervical shortening (softening and ripening) is not the passive result of tissue weakness but instead is an active process that can be slowed or prevented by progesterone supplementation in some women.[15-19] These studies have led to the conclusion that a short cervix in the second trimester of pregnancy is evidence that parturition has begun, presumably triggered by decidual membrane activation in response to microbial colonization and/or decidual hemorrhage, perhaps aided by cervical factors and/or subclinical myometrial activity. Figure 29-9 shows the length of the cervix at 22 to 24 weeks' gestation and the subsequent rate of cervical

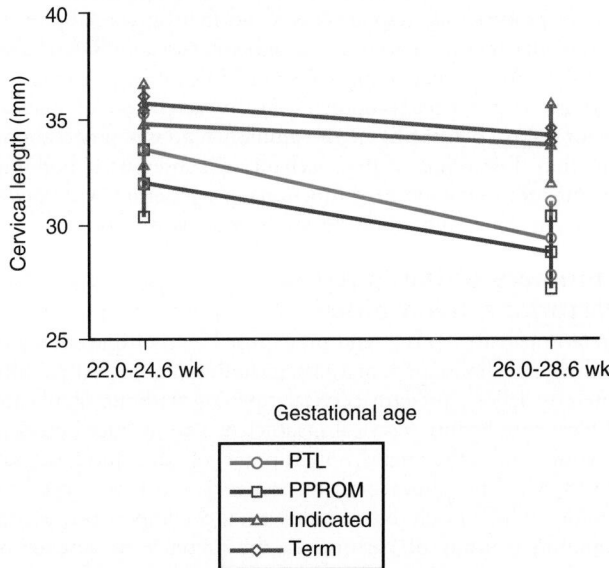

FIG 29-9 Length of the cervix at 22 to 24 weeks' gestation and the subsequent rate of cervical shortening in women who present after 28 weeks with preterm labor (PTL) or preterm premature rupture of membranes (PPROM) compared with women who delivered at term or preterm for medical indications.

shortening in women who later presented after 28 weeks' gestation with preterm labor or PPROM compared with women who delivered at term or preterm because of a medical indication. Significant differences in CL were already evident at 22 to 24 weeks, more than a month before clinical presentation, and accelerated for several weeks before clinical presentation.

Endocrine Disorders
Estrogen and progesterone play a central role in the endocrinology of pregnancy. **Progesterone is thought to maintain myometrial quiescence and inhibit cervical ripening. Estrogens have been implicated in increasing myometrial contractility and excitability as well as in the induction of cervical ripening before the onset of labor.** In many species, a fall in maternal serum progesterone concentration occurs before spontaneous parturition, but the mechanism for this progesterone withdrawal depends primarily on whether the placenta or the corpus luteum is the major source of progesterone.

A decrease in serum progesterone levels has not been demonstrated before parturition in humans. Nevertheless, inhibition of progesterone action could result in parturition. Alternative mechanisms posited to explain a suspension of progesterone action without a serum progesterone withdrawal include binding of progesterone to a high-affinity protein and thus a reduction in the functional active form; increased cortisol concentration that competes with progesterone for binding to the glucocorticoid receptors, resulting in functional progesterone withdrawal; and conversion of progesterone to an inactive form within the target cell before interaction with its receptor. None of these hypotheses are proven. Recent research has focused on alterations in the number and function of estrogen-progesterone receptors and progesterone binding.

The human progesterone receptor (PR) exists as two major subtypes, PR-A and PR-B. Another isoform, PR-C, has recently been described, but its function is not well understood. The human estrogen receptor (ER) also exists as two major subtypes, ERa and ERb. A functional progesterone withdrawal has been proposed in which expression of PR-A in the myometrium suppresses progesterone responsiveness and that functional progesterone withdrawal occurs by increased expression of PR-A relative to PR-B. An alternative mechanism of functional progesterone withdrawal has been proposed wherein activation of nuclear factor kappa B (NFκB) in the amnion represses progesterone function. Regardless of the mechanism, consensus is building for the idea that a localized functional progesterone withdrawal occurs in the myometrium during human parturition.

Summary of the Preterm Parturition Syndrome
Preterm parturition is a syndrome caused by multiple etiologies with several clinical presentations, including uterine contractility (preterm labor), preterm cervical ripening without significant clinical contractility (cervical insufficiency or advanced cervical dilation and effacement), or rupture of the amniotic sac (PPROM). The clinical presentation varies with the type and timing of the insult or stimulus to the components of the common pathway of parturition, the presence or absence of environmental cofactors, and individual variations of the host response by both mother and fetus. This conceptual framework has implications for the understanding of the mechanisms responsible for the initiation of preterm parturition as well as the diagnosis, treatment, and prevention of PTB.

CLINICAL CARE FOR WOMEN IN PRETERM LABOR
Clinical evaluation of preterm parturition begins with assessment of potential causes of labor, looking first for conditions that threaten the health of the mother and fetus. Acute maternal conditions—for example, pyelonephritis, pneumonia, asthma, peritonitis, trauma, and hypertension—or obstetric conditions that include preeclampsia, placental abruption, placenta previa, and chorioamnionitis, may mandate delivery. **Fetal compromise** may be acute, manifested by an abnormal fetal heart rate tracing, or it may be chronic, indicated by fetal growth restriction (FGR) or oligohydramnios; it may require delivery depending on the severity and potential for in utero versus ex utero treatment. **Fetal growth restriction** is more common in infants delivered after preterm labor or PPROM, even in apparently otherwise uncomplicated pregnancies. **Conditions that suggest specific therapy, such as preterm ruptured membranes or cervical insufficiency, should then be sought and treated accordingly.**

The next concerns are the accuracy of preterm labor diagnosis and the balance of risks and benefits that accompany active attempts to inhibit labor versus allowing delivery (Box 29-3).

DIAGNOSIS OF PRETERM LABOR
Given the pathways for preterm parturition described earlier, clinical recognition of preterm labor requires attention to the biochemical, as well as the biophysical, features of the onset of labor. Pathologic uterine contractility rarely occurs in isolation; cervical ripening and decidual membrane activation are almost always in progress as well, most often before uterine contractions are clinically evident. **Therefore preterm labor must be considered whenever a pregnant woman reports recurrent abdominal or pelvic symptoms that persist for several hours in the second half of pregnancy.** Symptoms of preterm labor such as pelvic pressure, increased vaginal discharge, backache, and menstrual-like cramps occur frequently in normal pregnancy and suggest preterm labor more by persistence than by severity. **Contractions may be painful or painless, depending**

BOX 29-3 DIAGNOSIS OF PRETERM LABOR AND INITIAL ASSESSMENT

- What is the gestational age, and what is the level of confidence about the accuracy of the gestational age?
- In the absence of advanced labor (cervical effacement >80% with dilation >2 cm) and a clear cause of preterm labor, what is the accuracy of the diagnosis of preterm labor?
- Are confirmatory diagnostic tests such as cervical sonography, fetal fibronectin, or amniocentesis for infection necessary?
- What is the anticipated neonatal morbidity and mortality at this gestational age in this clinical setting?
- Should labor be stopped?
- Is transfer to a more appropriate hospital required?
- Should fetal lung maturity be tested?
- What interventions can be applied that will reduce the risks of perinatal morbidity and mortality?
- Should drugs to arrest labor (tocolytics), glucocorticoids, or antibiotics be given?

on the resistance offered by the cervix. Contractions against a closed, uneffaced cervix are likely to be painful, but persistence of recurrent pressure or tightening may be the only symptoms when cervical effacement precedes the onset of contractions.

For decades, the clinical diagnosis of preterm labor has been based on the presence of regular, painful uterine contractions accompanied by cervical dilation and/or effacement. These criteria assume a crisp demarcation between preterm *parturition* and preterm *labor* that is increasingly understood as being more gradual than previously thought. If considered a screening criteria for the outcome "preterm birth," clinical signs and symptoms demonstrate poor sensitivity and specificity. Identifying women with preterm contractions who will actually deliver preterm is an inexact process. In like fashion, identifying those women who are at increased risk of not just PTB, but imminent PTB, remains elusive. A systematic review noted that approximately 30% of preterm labor cases resolved spontaneously. In subsequent studies, 50% of patients hospitalized for preterm labor actually delivered at term.

The inability to accurately distinguish women with an episode of preterm labor who will deliver preterm from those who deliver at term has greatly hampered the assessment of therapeutic interventions because as many as 50% of untreated (or placebo-treated) subjects do not actually deliver preterm. Optimal criteria for initiation of treatment are unclear. A contraction frequency of six or more per hour, cervical dilation of 3 cm, effacement of 80%, ruptured membranes, and bleeding are symptoms of preterm labor most often associated with preterm delivery. When lower thresholds for contraction frequency and cervical change are used, a *false-positive* diagnosis—defined in randomized controlled trials (RCTs) as delivery at term after treatment with placebo only—occurs in nearly 40% of women, but sensitivity does not rise. Difficulty in accurate diagnosis is the product of the high prevalence of the symptoms and signs of early preterm labor in normal pregnancy, the gradual onset of preterm labor discussed earlier, and the imprecision of digital examination of the cervix below 3 cm dilation and 80% effacement. The practice of initiating tocolytic drugs for contraction frequency without additional diagnostic criteria results in unnecessary treatment of women who are not at increased risk of imminent sPTB.[39]

Diagnostic Tests for Preterm Labor

Symptomatic women whose cervical dilation is less than 2 cm and whose effacement is less than 80% present a diagnostic challenge. **Diagnostic accuracy may be improved in these patients by testing other features of parturition such as cervical ripening; measurement of CL by transvaginal ultrasound; and decidual activation, tested by an assay for FFN in cervicovaginal fluid.**[40,41] Both tests aid diagnosis primarily by reducing false-positive results. Transabdominal ultrasound (TAU) has poor reproducibility for cervical measurement and should not be used clinically without confirmation by a transvaginal ultrasound (TVU). If the examination is properly performed, a CL of 30 mm or more by endovaginal sonography indicates that preterm labor is unlikely in symptomatic women.

Similarly, a negative FFN test in women with symptoms before 34 weeks' gestation with cervical dilation less than 3 cm can also reduce the rate of false-positive diagnosis if the result is returned promptly and the clinician is willing to act on a negative test result by not initiating treatment. When both tests were performed in a study of 206 women with possible preterm labor,

---

BOX 29-4   CLINICAL EVALUATION OF PATIENTS WITH POSSIBLE PRETERM LABOR

1. Patient presents with signs/symptoms of preterm labor
   - Persistent contractions, painful or painless
   - Intermittent abdominal cramping, pelvic pressure, or backache
   - Increase or change in vaginal discharge
   - Vaginal spotting or bleeding
2. General physical examination
   - Sitting pulse and blood pressure
   - Temperature
   - External fetal heart rate and contraction monitor
3. Sterile speculum examination
   - pH
   - Fern
   - Pooled fluid
   - Fibronectin swab (posterior fornix or external cervical os, avoiding areas with bleeding)
   - Cultures for *Chlamydia* (cervix), *Neisseria gonorrhoeae* (cervix), and group B *Streptococcus* (outer third of vagina and perineum)
4. Transabdominal ultrasound examination
   - Placental location
   - Amniotic fluid volume
   - Estimated fetal weight and presentation
   - Fetal well-being
5. Cervical examination (after ruptured membranes are excluded)
   a. Cervix >3 cm dilation, ≥80% effaced
      - Preterm labor diagnosis confirmed. Evaluate for tocolysis.
   b. Cervix 2 to 3 cm dilation, <80% effaced
      - Preterm labor likely but not established. Monitor contraction frequency and repeat digital examination in 30 to 60 minutes. Diagnose preterm labor if cervix changes. If not, send fibronectin or obtain transvaginal cervical ultrasound. Evaluate for tocolysis if any cervical change occurs, cervical length is <20 mm, or fibronectin is positive.
   c. Cervix <2 cm dilation and <80% effaced
      - Preterm labor diagnosis uncertain. Monitor contraction frequency, send fibronectin and/or obtain cervical sonography, and repeat digital examination in 1 to 2 hours. Evaluate for tocolysis if change in cervical dilation is 1 cm, effacement is >80%, cervical length is <20 mm, or fibronectin is positive.
6. Use of cervical ultrasound
   - Cervical length <20 mm *and* contraction criteria met: preterm labor
   - Cervical length 20 to 30 mm *and* contraction criteria met: probable preterm labor
   - Cervical length >30 mm: preterm labor *very unlikely* regardless of contraction frequency

---

the FFN test improved the performance of sonographic CL only when the sonographic CL was less than 30 mm (Box 29-4).

Amniocentesis for Women With Preterm Labor

The goal of care for women with preterm labor is to reduce perinatal morbidity and mortality, most of which is caused by immaturity of the respiratory, gastrointestinal, coagulation, and central nervous systems of the preterm infant. Fetal pulmonary immaturity is the most frequent cause of serious newborn illness, and the fetal pulmonary system is the only organ system whose function is directly testable before delivery. If the quality of obstetric dating is good and intrauterine fetal well-being is not compromised, the likelihood of neonatal RDS may be estimated from the gestational age.

Amniotic fluid studies may be useful in women with possible preterm labor in the following circumstances:

1. *Fetal pulmonary maturity testing.* Gestational age at birth is the best predictor of the frequency and severity of the consequences of prematurity to the newborn. Labor inhibition and antenatal glucocorticoid therapy are used when birth is anticipated to occur between 24 and 34 weeks' gestation. When dates are uncertain—such as with late prenatal care or fetal size larger than expected for dates, suggestive of a more advanced gestation—it may be reasonable in some circumstances to use amniotic fluid lung maturity studies to help guide management decisions.

2. *Testing for infection.* Among women with preterm labor and intact membranes, early gestational age, a short cervix, and progressive labor despite a tocolytic are all risk factors for occult amniotic fluid infection. In this setting, amniotic fluid studies for infection may guide the counseling of women and can influence management decisions in regard to antibiotics, inhibition of labor, and delivery. Amniotic fluid glucose (levels <20 mg/dL suggest intraamniotic infection) and Gram stain for bacteria, cell count, and culture may be used.

3. *Determining fetal karyotype.* The presence of polyhydramnios or a fetal anomaly suggests that preterm labor may have occurred because of uterine distension or placental insufficiency associated with fetal aneuploidy. Fluorescence in situ hybridization (FISH) studies for the most common aneuploid conditions can be available within 48 hours and do not require culture; chromosomal microarrays likewise do not require cell culture (see Chapter 10). In the absence of other fetal features suggestive of aneuploidy, the presence of preterm labor alone is an insufficient indication for the determination of a fetal karyotype.

TREATMENT FOR WOMEN IN PRETERM LABOR

Successful treatment with tocolytic drugs to inhibit labor after contractions have begun and cervical change has been documented is well established. However, treatment after membranes have ruptured does not prolong pregnancy sufficiently to allow further intrauterine growth and maturation, but therapy can often delay PTB long enough to permit **four interventions that have been shown to reduce neonatal morbidity and mortality:**

1. Antenatal transfer of the mother and fetus to the most appropriate hospital
2. Antibiotics in labor to prevent neonatal infection with group B *Streptococcus* (GBS)
3. Antenatal administration of glucocorticoids to the mother to reduce neonatal morbidity and mortality due to RDS, IVH, and other causes
4. Administration of maternal magnesium sulfate at the time of PTB before 32 weeks to reduce the incidence of cerebral palsy

Maternal Transfer
Many states have adopted systems of regionalized perinatal care in recognition of the advantages of concentrating care for preterm infants, especially those born before 32 weeks. Hospitals and birth centers that care for normal mothers and infants are designated as **level I.** Larger hospitals that care for the majority of maternal and infant complications are designated as **level II** centers; these hospitals have NICUs staffed and equipped to care for most infants with birthweights greater than 1500 g. **Level III** centers typically provide care for the sickest and smallest infants and for maternal complications that require intensive care. This three-tiered approach has been associated with improved outcomes for preterm infants.

Antibiotics
Women with preterm labor should be treated with antibiotics to prevent neonatal GBS infection (see Chapters 53 and 54). Because preterm infants have a greater risk of neonatal GBS infection than those born at term, intrapartum prophylaxis with penicillin is recommended.[42] This policy has successfully reduced the incidence of neonatal GBS infection to such a degree that most such infections now occur in full-term infants. Evidence also shows that infants born to women with PPROM have reduced perinatal morbidity when antepartum antibiotic prophylaxis has been administered for 3 to 7 days.

Antibiotic therapy in women with preterm labor and intact membranes is not effective in prolonging pregnancy or preventing preterm delivery. The failure of antibiotics to prolong pregnancy may be attributed to treatment of women whose preterm labor did not result from infection and to the timing of treatment relative to the infectious process. Rather than an acute infection due to the recent ascent of vaginal organisms into the uterus, the pathologic sequence in which infection-driven preterm labor occurs is often much more indolent. **Antimicrobial therapy for women in preterm labor should be limited to GBS prophylaxis, women with PPROM, or treatment of a specific pathogen** (e.g., urinary tract infection).

Antenatal Corticosteroids
Glucocorticoids act generally in the developing fetus to promote maturation over growth. In the lung, corticosteroids promote surfactant synthesis, increase lung compliance, reduce vascular permeability, and generate an enhanced response to postnatal surfactant treatment. Glucocorticoids have similar maturational effects on other organs including the brain, kidneys, and gut.

Studies by Liggins of mechanisms of parturition in sheep led to the discovery of the beneficial effect of antenatal glucocorticoids on the maturation and performance of the lung in prematurely born infants. Subsequent studies have shown conclusively that antepartum administration of the glucocorticoids betamethasone or dexamethasone to the mother reduces the risk of death, RDS, IVH, NEC, and PDA in the preterm neonate. Guidelines for appropriate clinical use of antenatal glucocorticoids have evolved from initial skepticism and selective use, through a period of broad and repeated treatment following the first NICHD panel report in 1994, to the practice of a single course of treatment for all women between 24 and 34 weeks' gestation who are at risk for preterm delivery within 7 days as recommended by the NICHD Consensus Panel in 2000. More recently, clinical trials support the notion that administration of a single rescue course of corticosteroids before 33 weeks' gestation improves neonatal outcome (e.g., it decreases RDS, ventilator support, and surfactant use) without apparent increased short-term risk.[43] **A single rescue course of antenatal** corticosteroids may be considered if the antecedent treatment was given more than 2 weeks prior, the gestational age is less than $32^{6/7}$ weeks, and the woman is judged by the clinician to be likely to give birth within the coming week. However, regularly scheduled repeat courses or multiple courses (i.e., more than two) are not recommended.[44] Betamethasone and dexamethasone, the only drugs found beneficial for this purpose, are potent glucocorticoids with limited if any mineralocorticoid effect. A course of treatment consists of two doses of 12 mg of betamethasone; the combination of 6 mg each of betamethasone acetate and betamethasone phosphate, administered intramuscularly twice, 24 hours apart; or four doses of 6 mg of dexamethasone given intramuscularly every 12 hours. Other corticosteroids (prednisolone, prednisone) and routes of administration (oral) are not suitable alternatives because of reduced placental transfer, lack of demonstrated benefit, and, in the case of oral dexamethasone, increased risk of adverse effects when compared with the intramuscular (IM) route.

Fetal Effects

Randomized placebo-controlled trials and meta-analyses confirm the beneficial effects of antenatal corticosteroids. Infants born to treated women were significantly less likely to experience RDS (OR, 0.53), IVH (OR, 0.38), or neonatal death (OR, 0.60). The beneficial effects on IVH are independent of the effects on respiratory function. Other morbidities of PTB are also reduced by antenatal glucocorticoids, including NEC, PDA, and BPD. Although both are considered effective, betamethasone may be superior to dexamethasone with respect to reduction of morbidity and mortality in the preterm newborn.

Other Fetal Effects of Glucocorticoids

Transient reduction in fetal breathing and body movements sufficient to affect the interpretation of the biophysical profile (BPP) have been described with both drugs but are more common after administration of betamethasone, typically lasting 48 to 72 hours after the second dose. Transient suppression of neonatal cortisol levels has been reported, but neonatal response to ACTH stimulation was unimpaired.

Maternal Effects

Antenatal glucocorticoids produce a transient rise in maternal platelet and white blood cell (WBC) counts that lasts 72 hours; a WBC count in excess of 20,000 is rarely due to steroids. Maternal glucose tolerance is also challenged, and treatment often requires insulin therapy to maintain euglycemia in those with previously well-controlled gestational or pregestational diabetes. Maternal blood pressure is unaffected by antenatal steroid treatment; neither betamethasone nor dexamethasone has a significant mineralocorticoid effect. Women treated with multiple courses of steroids during pregnancy had a blunted response to ACTH stimulation later in pregnancy and in the puerperium.

Duration of Benefit

The duration of the beneficial fetal effects after a single course of glucocorticoids is unclear. The issue is difficult to study because the interval between treatment and delivery in clinical trials is variable and because some effects may be transient, whereas others are permanent. Neonatal benefit has been most easily observed when the interval between the first dose and delivery exceeds 48 hours, but some benefit is evident after an incomplete course. One large multicenter trial found evidence of benefit for as long as 18 days after the initial course of treatment.

Risks of Antenatal Corticosteroid Treatment

The recommendation of the 1994 NICHD Consensus Conference to increase the use of antenatal steroids, coupled with uncertainty about the duration of neonatal protection from a single course of treatment and difficulty in predicting imminent preterm delivery, resulted in increased treatment of mothers at risk. Although more women received treatment, many did not deliver within 7 days but remained at risk and were treated weekly until delivery or 34 weeks' gestation. The safety and benefit of one course of steroids has never been questioned. Long-term follow-up studies of infants in the original cohorts of infants treated with a single course of antenatal steroids have displayed no differences in physical characteristics or mental function when compared with gestational age–matched controls. The increasing use of repeated courses prompted animal and human studies that have raised concerns about the effects of prolonged exposure to steroids on fetal growth and neurologic function. The animal studies may be summarized as showing reduced fetal growth and adverse brain and neurologic development in several species.

Human studies also observed reduced growth in fetuses exposed to multiple courses of antenatal steroids. An Australian study found a twofold increase in birthweights below the 10th percentile and significantly reduced head circumference in infants exposed to more than three antenatal courses of steroids. Others have also found reduced head circumference. Follow-up work from this Australian study noted that babies exposed to weekly doses of repeat antenatal corticosteroids demonstrate postnatal growth acceleration 3 to 5 weeks after birth.[45]

Sequelae of Antenatal Treatments to Reduce Fetal/Neonatal Morbidity
Respiratory Distress

The occurrence of RDS among infants born to women treated with steroid therapy has led to the investigation of alternative treatment approaches to further enhance pulmonary maturation. Neonatal treatment with surfactant is an effective adjunctive therapy that adds independently and synergistically to the benefit of corticosteroids in reducing RDS-related morbidity. More than 4600 women have been enrolled in 13 trials of maternal treatment with antenatal thyrotropin-releasing hormone (TRH) to reduce neonatal lung disease. No benefits to antenatal TRH have been found, compared with corticosteroids alone, for any neonatal outcome. Prenatal treatment with TRH actually increased the risk of adverse outcomes for infants in some trials.

Neurologic Morbidity

Antenatal maternal treatment with phenobarbital, vitamin K, and magnesium sulfate has been studied to reduce or prevent neonatal neurologic morbidity. Phenobarbital was not effective in reducing IVH when given alone or in combination with vitamin K.

Antenatal maternal treatment with magnesium has been inconsistently associated with reduced rates of IVH, cerebral palsy, and perinatal mortality in premature infants. A randomized placebo-controlled trial of antenatal magnesium conducted in 1062 women who delivered before 30 weeks' gestation found significantly lower rates of gross motor dysfunction and nonsignificant trends of reduced mortality and cerebral palsy in surviving infants in the treated group at 2 years of age. No significant adverse effects were noted in infants exposed to antenatal magnesium sulfate. In the 1990s, observational studies suggested an association between prenatal exposure to magnesium sulfate and less frequent subsequent neurologic morbidities. Subsequently, several large clinical studies have evaluated the evidence regarding magnesium sulfate, neuroprotection, and PTBs.[46-49] If tocolysis is indicated, the most effective agent with the most favorable side-effect profile should be given. None of the trials demonstrated significant pregnancy prolongation when magnesium sulfate was given for neuroprotection. **However, the available evidence suggests that magnesium sulfate given before anticipated early PTB reduces the risk of cerebral palsy in surviving infants.**[50]

The impact of gestational age on the neuroprotective effect of antenatally administered magnesium was assessed in a meta-analysis that included the five trials in the Cochrane review.[51] These trials were stratified by the gestational age at randomization: less than 32 to 34 weeks' gestation (5235 fetuses) or less than 30 weeks' gestation (3107 fetuses). Major findings were similar for both gestational age ranges[51]:

- No significant difference was found in the primary outcome of death or cerebral palsy at 18 to 24 months of corrected age or for the outcome of perinatal/infant death.
- The largest reduction in risk was for moderate to severe cerebral palsy.
- At less than 32 to 34 weeks' gestation, relative risk was 0.60 (95% CI, 0.43 to 0.84).
- At less than 30 weeks' gestation, relative risk was 0.54 (95% CI, 0.36 to 0.80).
- Statistically significant reductions were found in the risk of cerebral palsy (RR, 0.7 and 0.69 at less than 32 to 34 weeks' gestation and at less than 30 weeks' gestation, respectively) and for death or moderate to severe cerebral palsy (RR, 0.85 and 0.84 at less than 32 to 34 weeks' gestation and at less than 30 weeks' gestation, respectively).
- The numbers needed to treat to prevent one case of cerebral palsy in the less than 32 to 34 weeks' gestation group and in the less than 30 weeks' gestation group were 56 and 46, respectively.

A 4-g bolus of magnesium sulfate with a 1-g/hr maintenance dose is a regimen anticipated to have a more favorable side effect and safety profile than a higher-dose regimen. Neither the neuroprotective mechanism nor the dose response to magnesium sulfate is well understood. Although it seems likely that the neuroprotective effects of magnesium sulfate are secondary to residual concentrations of the drug in the neonate's circulation, data are insufficient regarding the maternal dose that confers neonatal benefit.

Administration of magnesium sulfate is appropriate for women with PPROM or preterm labor who have a high likelihood of imminent delivery (e.g., within 24 hours) **or before an indicated preterm delivery. If emergency delivery is necessary given maternal or fetal status, it should not be delayed to administer magnesium sulfate.** Therapy should be reserved for women who are at high risk of imminent delivery rather than for those who simply are diagnosed with preterm labor or PPROM. We do not recommend continuing the magnesium infusion for longer than 24 hours if delivery has not occurred.

TREATMENT PROTOCOL

We suggest limiting magnesium sulfate for neuroprotection to women who are at 24 to 32 weeks' gestation, given that the two largest trials of neuroprotective effects did not enroll women beyond this gestational age range.[49,52]

Magnesium sulfate must be given parenterally to achieve serum levels greater than the normal range. Therapeutic dosage regimens are similar to those used for intravenous (IV) seizure prophylaxis of preeclampsia. A loading dose of 4 g is given over 30 minutes, followed by an infusion of 1 g/hr.

If renal function is normal, magnesium is excreted rapidly in the urine. In patients with evidence of renal impairment—for example, oliguria or serum creatinine levels greater than 0.9 mg/dL—magnesium should be administered cautiously and should be followed with frequent vital signs, deep tendon reflexes, and magnesium serum levels, and doses should be adjusted accordingly. Magnesium sulfate should not be used in patients with myasthenia gravis because the magnesium ion competes with calcium. **Below is a clinical protocol for magnesium sulfate for fetal neuroprotection.**

1. Administer loading dose of 4 g magnesium sulfate in 10% to 20% solution over 30 minutes (60 mL of 10% magnesium sulfate in 1 L D_5 0.9 normal saline).
2. Maintenance dose of 1 g/hr (40 g of magnesium sulfate added to 1 L D_5 0.9 normal saline or Ringer's lactate at 50 mL/hr).
3. Limit IV fluid to 125 mL/hr. Follow fluid status closely; an indwelling urinary catheter is recommended.
4. Patients treated with magnesium sulfate should be assessed with the following examinations:
   a. Deep tendon reflexes and vital signs, including respiratory rate, should be recorded hourly.
   b. Intake and output should be measured every 2 to 4 hours.
   c. Magnesium levels should be monitored if any clinical concern about side effects exists.
5. Calcium gluconate should be readily available to reverse the respiratory depression that can be caused by magnesium.

Tocolysis in Preterm Labor

Because the contracting uterus is the most often recognized antecedent of PTB, stopping contractions has been the focus of therapeutic approaches. This strategy is based on the naïve assumption that clinically apparent contractions are commensurate with the initiation of the process of parturition; by logical extension, successfully inhibiting contractions should prevent delivery. The inhibition of myometrial contractions is called *tocolysis,* and an agent administered to that end is referred to as a *tocolytic.* **Although no medications have been approved for the indication of tocolysis by the U.S. Food and Drug Administration (FDA), a number of classes of drugs are used for this purpose.**

Efficacy

The efficacy of tocolytic drugs has been addressed through studies that compare one tocolytic drug with another, or less commonly, that compare a drug with a placebo in their ability to prolong pregnancy for 48 hours (the time sufficient to attain the benefit of antenatal corticosteroids), or 1 week (the time considered sufficient to gain significant additional in utero fetal maturation). **No studies have shown that any tocolytic can reduce the rate of PTB.** Most studies have been too small to allow firm conclusions, so reviews or meta-analyses wherein several studies of similar design are combined are the best available means to judge efficacy. The Cochrane Collaboration (www.cochrane.org) regularly produces meta-analyses of obstetric interventions that include tocolytic drugs. **Recent Cochrane meta-analyses of tocolytic agents indicate that calcium channel blockers and oxytocin antagonists can delay delivery by 2 to 7 days with the most favorable ratio of benefit to risk, that β-mimetic drugs delay delivery by 48 hours but carry greater side effects, that evidence is insufficient regarding cyclooxygenase (COX) inhibitors, and that magnesium sulfate is ineffective.**

Meta-analyses of studies of individual tocolytic drugs typically report limited prolongation of pregnancy but no decrease in PTB, and they rarely offer information about whether prolongation of pregnancy was accompanied by improved infant outcomes. Delayed delivery for 48 hours to allow antenatal transport and corticosteroids to reduce neonatal morbidity and mortality are thus the main rationale for use of these drugs.

Choosing a Tocolytic Agent
PHARMACOLOGY

Figure 29-10 depicts a myometrial cell and the sites of action of commonly used tocolytic agents. The key process in actin-myosin interaction, and thus contraction, is myosin light-chain phosphorylation. This reaction is controlled by myosin light-chain kinase (MLCK). **The activity of tocolytic agents can be explained by their effect on the factors that regulate the activity of this enzyme, notably calcium and cyclic adenosine monophosphate (cAMP).** For the myometrium to contract in a coordinated and effective manner (i.e., labor, whether term or preterm), individual smooth muscle cells must be functionally interconnected and able to communicate with adjacent cells. No agents used for tocolysis influence the function or expression of gap junctions.

CONTRAINDICATIONS TO TOCOLYSIS
Common maternal contraindications to tocolysis include preeclampsia or gestational hypertension with severe features, hemorrhage, and significant maternal cardiac disease. Although vaginal spotting may occur in women with preterm labor because of cervical effacement or dilation, any bleeding beyond light spotting is rarely due to labor alone. Placenta previa and placental abruption must be considered because both may be accompanied by uterine contractions. In general, both diagnoses place a woman at greater risk of hemodynamic compromise in the setting of tocolytic treatment. However, in rare instances, use of tocolysis in women with these dangerous diagnoses may be considered to achieve time for corticosteroids in the setting of extreme prematurity, when the bleeding is believed to occur in response to contractions. Such treatment is fraught with difficulty because even low doses of some tocolytic agents can be hazardous in a patient with bleeding. β-Mimetic agents and calcium channel blockers may hamper maternal cardiovascular response to hypotension, and cyclooxygenase inhibitors may impair platelet function. Cardiac disease is a contraindication because of the risks of tocolytic drug treatment in these patients. **Fetal contraindications to tocolysis include gestational age of greater than 37 weeks, fetal demise or lethal anomaly, chorioamnionitis, and evidence of acute or chronic fetal compromise.**

Tocolytic drugs may be safely used when standard protocols are followed. The choice of tocolytic requires consideration of the efficacy, risks, and side effects for each patient. Table 29-3 describes the side-effect profiles of commonly used tocolytic agents.

CALCIUM CHANNEL BLOCKERS
Calcium channel blockers are commonly used for treatment of hypertension, angina, and arrhythmias and are increasingly being used as tocolytic drugs. **Nifedipine** is the calcium channel blocker most studied as a tocolytic agent; it more selectively inhibits uterine contractions compared with other calcium blockers such as verapamil. Calcium channel blockers directly

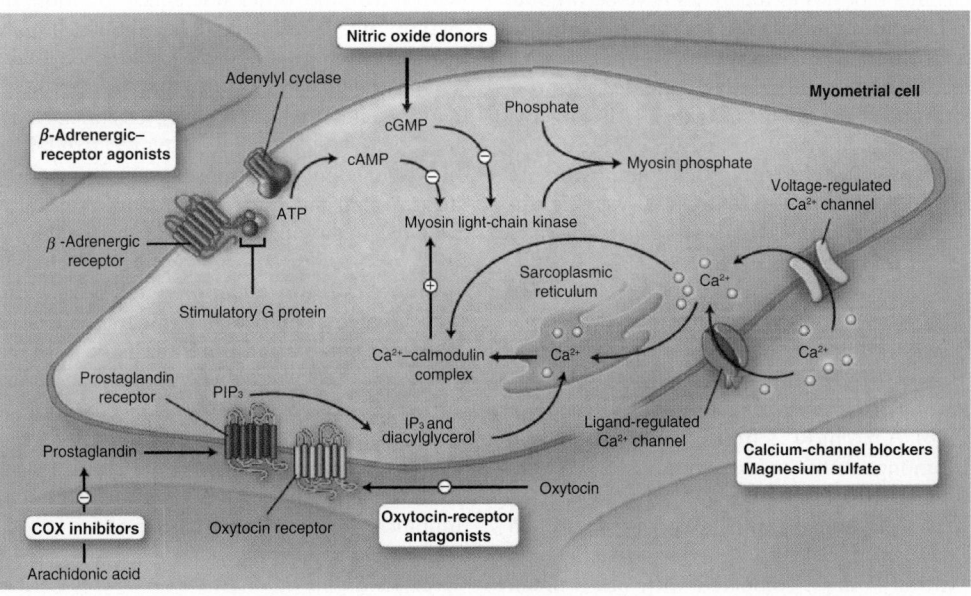

FIG 29-10 Site of action of commonly used tocolytics. ATP, adenosine triphosphate; cAMP, cyclic adenosine monophosphate; cGMP, cyclic guanosine monophosphate; COX, cyclooxygenase; IP, inositol triphosphate; PIP, phosphotidylinositol triphosphate.

TABLE 29-3   SIDE-EFFECT PROFILES OF TOCOLYTIC AGENTS

AGENT OR CLASS	SIDE EFFECTS MATERNAL	FETAL OR NEONATAL	CONTRAINDICATIONS
β-Adrenergic-receptor agonists	Tachycardia and hypotension, tremor (39% vs. 4% with placebo), shortness of breath (15% vs. 1% with placebo), chest discomfort (10% vs. 1% with placebo), pulmonary edema (0.3%), hypokalemia (39% vs. 6% with placebo), hyperglycemia (30% vs. 10% with placebo)	Tachycardia	Tachycardia-sensitive maternal cardiac disease, poorly controlled diabetes mellitus
Magnesium sulfate	Flushing, diaphoresis, nausea, loss of deep-tendon reflexes (serum levels of 9.6 to 12 mg/dL), respiratory paralysis (at serum levels of 12 to 18 mg/dL), cardiac arrest (at serum levels of 24 to 30 mg/dL); when used with calcium channel blockers, suppression of heart rate, contractility, and left ventricular systolic pressure and neuromuscular blockade	Data conflict with regard to effect on perinatal mortality	Myasthenia gravis
Calcium channel blockers	Dizziness, flushing, hypotension when used with magnesium sulfate; suppression of heart rate, contractility, and left ventricular systolic pressure and neuromuscular blockade; elevation of hepatic aminotransferase levels		Hypotension, preload-dependent cardiac lesions (e.g., aortic insufficiency)
COX inhibitors	Nausea, esophageal reflux, gastritis, and emesis; platelet dysfunction (rarely of clinical significance in patients without an underlying bleeding disorder)	In utero closure of ductus arteriosus (risk associated with use for >48 hr), PDA in neonate (conflicting data)	Platelet dysfunction or bleeding disorder, hepatic or renal dysfunction, gastrointestinal or ulcerative disease, asthma (in women with hypersensitivity to aspirin)
Oxytocin-receptor antagonists	Hypersensitivity injection-site reactions	For atosiban, an increased rate of fetal or infant death (may be attributable to the lower gestational age of infants in the atosiban group)	None
Nitric oxide donors	Dizziness, flushing, hypotension		Hypotension, preload-dependent cardiac lesions (e.g., aortic insufficiency)

COX, cyclooxygenase; *PDA,* patent ductus arteriosus.

block the influx of calcium ions through the cell membrane and also inhibit release of intracellular calcium from the sarcoplasmic reticulum, thus increasing calcium efflux from the cell. The ensuing decrease in intracellular free calcium leads to inhibition of calcium-dependent MLCK-mediated phosphorylation and results in myometrial relaxation. Calcium channel blockers are rapidly absorbed after oral administration. No placebo-controlled trials of calcium channel blockers as tocolytics have been done. **The Cochrane Collaboration meta-analyses support calcium channel blockers as short-term tocolytics, compared with other available agents, because of relatively greater suppression of contractions and fewer side effects than other agents in 12 reported trials.** Rates of birth within 7 days of treatment (relative risk [RR], 0.76; 95% CI, 0.60 to 0.97) and before 34 weeks' gestation (RR, 0.83; 95% CI, 0.69 to 0.99) were significantly reduced with calcium channel blockers, as were the rates of neonatal morbidities that included RDS (RR, 0.63; 95% CI, 0.46 to 0.88), NEC (RR, 0.21; 95% CI, 0.05 to 0.96), IVH (RR, 0.59; 95% CI, 0.36 to 0.98), and jaundice (RR, 0.73; 95% CI, 0.57 to 0.93) when compared with treatment with other tocolytics. Fewer women treated with calcium channel blockers ceased treatment owing to adverse drug reactions (RR, 0.14; 95% CI, 0.05 to 0.36). A recent RCT from Vis and colleagues[53] demonstrated that among women with symptoms of preterm labor and a CL between 10 and 30 mm with a negative FFN, nifedipine and placebo performed comparably with respect to delivery within 7 days. In the nifedipine group, three women (8.1%) delivered within 7 days, compared with one woman (2.8%) in the placebo group (difference −5.3%; one-sided 95% confidence limit, 4.5%). Median gestational ages at delivery

were for nifedipine 37 + 0 weeks' gestation (interquartile range [IQR], 34 + 6 to 38 + 5) and for the placebo 38 + 2 weeks' gestation (IQR, 37 + 0 to 39 + 6) weeks ($P = .008$).

MATERNAL EFFECTS
Nifedipine has fewer side effects when compared with β-mimetics and magnesium sulfate. Whereas hypotension occurs frequently with nifedipine, other side effects are more frequent with magnesium and β-mimetics. Nicardipine displayed similar advantages when compared in a randomized trial with magnesium. Pretreatment with IV fluids may reduce the frequency of maternal side effects related to hypotension such as headache (20%), flushing (8%), dizziness, and nausea (6%). Most effects are mild, but serious complications have been reported that include a documented myocardial infarction 45 minutes after the second dose of nifedipine given to a young, healthy woman. **Concomitant or sequential use of calcium channel blockers with β-mimetics is not recommended, nor is concurrent administration of magnesium, owing to reports of skeletal muscle blockade when nifedipine was given with magnesium sulfate.**

FETAL EFFECTS
Initial animal studies raised questions of fetal hypotension, but a study of women treated for preterm labor revealed no changes in the fetal middle cerebral artery, renal artery, ductus arteriosus, umbilical artery, or maternal vessels.

TREATMENT PROTOCOL
An optimal nifedipine dosing regimen has not been defined. A common approach is to administer an initial loading dose of

20 mg orally, followed by an additional 20 mg orally in 90 minutes. An alternative regimen is to administer 10 mg orally every 20 minutes for up to four doses. If contractions persist, 20 mg can be given orally every 3 to 8 hours for up to 72 hours, with a maximum dose of 180 mg/day. The half-life of nifedipine is approximately 2 to 3 hours, and the duration of action of a single orally administered dose is up to 6 hours. Plasma concentrations peak in 30 to 60 minutes. Nifedipine is almost completely metabolized in the liver and excreted by the kidney.

SUMMARY OF TREATMENT WITH CALCIUM CHANNEL BLOCKERS

Nifedipine has been used increasingly as a tocolytic because of its low incidence of significant maternal and fetal side effects and ease of administration. Nifedipine should not be combined with magnesium or β-mimetics, and it should be avoided in the presence of intrauterine infection, maternal hypertension, and cardiac disease. Use should follow published dosage schedules, and the cautions noted should be kept in mind.

MAGNESIUM SULFATE

The basis for the clinical use of magnesium sulfate as a labor-inhibiting agent is the observation from the 1960s of a reduction of human uterine myometrial contractility in vivo and in vitro. At a pharmacologic concentration (5 mmol/L), magnesium sulfate inhibits contractile response and decreases intracellular calcium concentration in pregnant human myometrial strips. Despite in vitro observations, the largest placebo-controlled randomized trial of magnesium as a tocolytic failed to demonstrate any benefit over a placebo in prolongation of pregnancy. **A meta-analysis that compared magnesium to controls observed no difference in the risk of birth within 48 hours of treatment for women given magnesium** (RR, 0.85; 95% CI, 0.58 to 1.25; 11 trials, 881 women). **Magnesium appeared to confer no benefit on the risk of preterm birth** (<37 weeks' gestation) **or very preterm birth** (<34 weeks' gestation). The risk of death (fetal and pediatric) was higher for infants exposed to magnesium (RR, 2.82; 95% CI, 1.20 to 6.62; 7 trials, 727 infants). The body of available literature fails to support efficacy of magnesium sulfate as a tocolytic agent. Thus in women at 24 to 32 weeks' gestation who are candidates for tocolysis, we recommend that another therapy be used for labor inhibition in women also receiving magnesium sulfate for fetal neuroprotection. Because of the increased risk of maternal complications with the concomitant use of nifedipine and magnesium sulfate, **an agent such as indomethacin may be a reasonable choice for tocolysis in the woman receiving magnesium sulfate for neuroprotection of the fetus.**

MATERNAL EFFECTS

Magnesium has a low rate of serious maternal side effects, but flushing, nausea, vomiting, headache, generalized muscle weakness, diplopia, and shortness of breath occur frequently. Chest pain and pulmonary edema have been reported with a frequency similar to that of β-mimetics.

NEONATAL EFFECTS

Magnesium crosses the placenta and achieves serum levels comparable to maternal levels, but serious short-term neonatal complications are uncommon. **Lethargy, hypotonia, and respiratory depression may occur.** Prolonged treatment for more than 7 days has been associated with neonatal bone abnormalities. One small trial suggested that magnesium sulfate may have adverse effects on neonatal and infant morbidity and mortality, but these observations were not confirmed by larger studies that enrolled more than 10 times as many subjects.

SUMMARY OF TREATMENT WITH MAGNESIUM SULFATE

Magnesium sulfate has historic familiarity, but tocolytic efficacy is not supported by data. However, magnesium may have a beneficial effect on the preterm newborn with respect to reducing the risk of cerebral palsy.

CYCLOOXYGENASE INHIBITORS

Prostaglandins are mediators of the final pathways of uterine muscle contraction. Prostaglandins cause an increase in free intracellular calcium levels in myometrial cells and an increased activation of MLCK, resulting in uterine contractions. Myometrial gap-junction formation, an important step in synchronized uterine activity, is enhanced by prostaglandins; given to pregnant women, prostaglandins can ripen the cervix or induce labor, depending on the dosage and route of administration. Prostaglandin synthase, also known as *cyclooxygenase* (COX), converts arachidonic acid to prostaglandin G_2. **Prostaglandin synthesis is increased when the COX-2 form of this enzyme is induced by cytokines, bacterial products such as phospholipases and endotoxins, and corticosteroids; it is reduced by the inhibition of COX with nonsteroidal antiinflammatory drugs** (NSAIDs). These agents vary in their activity, potency, and side-effect profile. Indomethacin is the NSAID most often used as a tocolytic, although it crosses the placenta. **Unlike aspirin, indomethacin binds reversibly to COX, so that inhibition lasts only until the drug is cleared metabolically.** Umbilical artery serum concentrations equal maternal levels within 6 hours of oral administration. The half-life in the mother is 4 to 5 hours, and in a full-term infant it is 15 hours, but it is significantly longer in preterm infants. The Cochrane review concluded that indomethacin administration was associated with a significant reduction in births before the 37th week of gestation, increased gestational age at birth, and increased birthweight.

MATERNAL EFFECTS

Prostaglandin inhibition has multiple side effects because of the abundance of prostaglandin-mediated physiologic functions. Nevertheless, **serious maternal side effects are uncommon when the agent is used in a brief course of tocolysis.** As with any NSAID, gastrointestinal side effects such as nausea, heartburn, and vomiting are common but usually mild. Less common but more serious complications include gastrointestinal bleeding, prolonged bleeding time, thrombocytopenia, and asthma in aspirin-sensitive patients. Prolonged treatment with NSAIDs can lead to renal injury, especially when other nephrotoxic drugs are used. Hypertensive women may rarely experience acute increased blood pressure after indomethacin treatment. The antipyretic effect of an NSAID may obscure a clinically significant fever. Maternal contraindications to indomethacin tocolysis include renal or hepatic disease, active peptic ulcer disease, poorly controlled hypertension, asthma, and platelet disorders.

FETAL AND NEONATAL EFFECTS

In actual practice, serious complications to the fetus/newborn with maternal administration of indomethacin have been rare, but risk of injury to the fetus is possible if treatment protocols are not followed carefully. **Three principal side effects raise concern: (1) in utero constriction of the ductus arteriosus, (2) oligohydramnios, and (3) neonatal pulmonary hypertension.** The ductal constriction occurs because formation of prostacyclin and PGE$_2$, which maintain ductal vasodilation, is inhibited by indomethacin. Doppler evidence of ductal constriction was found in 7 of 14 fetuses of women treated with indomethacin between 27 and 31 weeks' gestation, but it resolved within 24 hours after the medication was discontinued. The likelihood of ductal constriction increased from 5% to 10% before 32 weeks to 50% after 48 hours of treatment at 32 to 35 weeks. Ductal constriction is usually transient and responds to discontinuation of the drug, but persistent ductal constriction and irreversible right-sided heart failure have been reported. A review of fetal echocardiographs obtained from 61 women treated with indomethacin for preterm labor found evidence of ductal constriction in 50% of fetuses. A larger study of 124 women given indomethacin for labor inhibition for more than 48 hours revealed a 6.5% frequency of in utero ductal narrowing. **In both of these studies, the ductal narrowing reversed in all fetuses after cessation of medication.**

Oligohydramnios associated with indomethacin tocolysis is due to reduced fetal urine production, which is caused by **the indomethacin-induced reduction of normal prostaglandin inhibition of antidiuretic hormones and the direct effect on fetal renal blood flow.** Prolonged treatment with indomethacin incurs a 7% frequency of oligohydramnios. **These effects are reversible,** but neonatal renal insufficiency and death after several weeks of unmonitored antenatal maternal treatment has been reported.

Primary pulmonary hypertension in the neonate is a potentially fatal illness that has also been associated with prolonged (>48 hr) indomethacin therapy. **Primary neonatal pulmonary hypertension has not been reported within 24 to 48 hours of therapy,** but the incidence may be as high as 5% to 10% with long-term therapy, although a more modern series of longer-term use failed to identify an increased frequency of newborn pulmonary hypertension compared with untreated gestational age–matched controls.

Other complications—including NEC, small bowel perforation, PDA, jaundice, and IVH—have been observed when indomethacin administration was outside of standardized protocols that did not limit the duration of treatment or that used the drug after 32 weeks' gestation. No association with IVH was noted in studies in which standard protocols were used. A review of outcomes of 1621 fetuses treated in utero with indomethacin found no significant differences compared with 4387 infants not exposed.

Sulindac is an NSAID that has less placental transfer than indomethacin, but its tocolytic efficacy has not been studied in large numbers. Because of the effect on fetal urine production and amniotic fluid volume, **indomethacin may be an appropriate tocolytic when preterm labor is associated with polyhydramnios.** Indomethacin has been used to treat preterm labor in women with polyhydramnios and for polyhydramnios without labor. Uterine activity and pain associated with degenerating uterine fibroids in pregnancy also respond well to indomethacin.

TREATMENT PROTOCOL FOR INDOMETHACIN TOCOLYSIS
Indomethacin is well absorbed orally. The usual regimen is a 50-mg oral loading dose followed by 25 to 50 mg by mouth

every 6 hours. **Therapy is limited to 2 to 3 days** because of concern about side effects described earlier.

1. Limit use to preterm labor before 32 weeks' gestation in women with normal amniotic fluid volume and normal renal function.
2. Loading dose is 50 mg by mouth.
3. Give 25 mg orally every 6 hours for 48 hours.
4. If the drug is used beyond 48 to 72 hours, amniotic fluid volume should be monitored serially with ultrasound, and ductus arteriosus flow should be evaluated with Doppler echocardiography. If amniotic fluid is significantly reduced or the ductus is narrowed, the drug should be discontinued.
5. Discontinue therapy promptly if delivery seems imminent.
6. Fetal contraindications to the use of indomethacin include renal anomalies, chorioamnionitis, oligohydramnios, ductal-dependent cardiac defects, and twin-twin transfusion syndrome.

SUMMARY OF TREATMENT WITH INDOMETHACIN
Indomethacin is an effective tocolytic agent that is generally well tolerated by the mother. **Concern about fetal side effects has appropriately limited use of indomethacin to brief courses of therapy in patients with preterm labor before 32 weeks.**

β-MIMETIC TOCOLYTICS

β-Sympathomimetic drugs include terbutaline, ritodrine, and others that have been widely used as tocolytics for many years. Structurally related to epinephrine and norepinephrine, these agents act to relax smooth muscle; for example, in the bronchial tree, blood vessels, and myometrium through stimulation of the β-receptors, which are divided into β1 and β2 subtypes. The β1-receptors are largely responsible for the cardiac effects, whereas β2-receptors mediate smooth muscle relaxation, hepatic glycogen production, and islet cell release of insulin. Stimulation of β-receptors in the heart, vascular system, and liver accounts for the side effects of these drugs.

The most commonly used β-mimetic in the United States is terbutaline, marketed as a drug for asthma, but others that include albuterol, fenoterol, hexoprenaline, metaproterenol, nylidrin, orciprenaline, and salbutamol are used in other countries. Ritodrine was approved by the FDA as a parenteral tocolytic in 1980, but it did not achieve wide use because of frequent maternal side effects. Ritodrine is no longer marketed in the United States. Terbutaline has a rapid (3 to 5 minutes) effect when given subcutaneously. Published protocols often use subcutaneous administration, with a usual dose of 0.25 mg (250 μg) every 4 hours. A single subcutaneous dose of terbutaline to arrest contractions during the initial evaluation of preterm contractions may aid in the diagnosis of preterm labor. In one study, women whose contractions persisted or recurred after a single dose were more likely to have true preterm labor than those whose contractions ceased. **The Cochrane Database reported an analysis of 1332 women enrolled into 11 randomized placebo-controlled trials of β-mimetic drugs and found that treated subjects were less likely to deliver within 48 hours** (RR, 0.63; 95% CI, 0.53 to 0.75) **but not within 7 days.** Although a 48-hour delay in delivery allows sufficient time for in utero transfer and treatment with steroids, perinatal and neonatal death and perinatal morbidity were not reduced in this analysis. Side effects that required change or cessation of treatment were frequent.

SIDE EFFECTS AND COMPLICATIONS OF β-MIMETIC TOCOLYSIS

Maternal side effects of the β-mimetic drugs are common and diverse owing to the abundance of β-receptors in the body. Maternal tachycardia, chest discomfort, palpitation, tremor, headache, nasal congestion, nausea and vomiting, hyperkalemia, and hyperglycemia are significantly more common in women treated with β-mimetics. Most are mild and of limited duration, but serious maternal cardiopulmonary and metabolic complications have been reported.

Cardiopulmonary Complications of β-Mimetics. The β-mimetic agents produce a 5 to 10 mm Hg fall in diastolic blood pressure, and the extensive peripheral vasodilation makes it difficult to mount a normal response to hypovolemia. **Signs of excessive blood loss** (e.g., maternal and fetal tachycardia) **are masked by β-mimetics, so their use may be dangerous in women with antepartum hemorrhage. The most important steps to prevent cardiac complications are to (1) exclude patients with prior cardiac disease and (2) limit infusion rates so that maternal pulse does not exceed 130 beats/min.** Symptomatic cardiac arrhythmias and myocardial ischemia have occurred during β-agonist tocolytic therapy. **Tocolysis should be discontinued and oxygen administered whenever a patient develops chest pain during β-mimetic therapy.** Arrhythmias noted in association with β-mimetic therapy usually respond to discontinuation of the drug and oxygen administration. Baseline or routine electrocardiograms (ECGs) before or during treatment are not helpful. **An ECG is indicated if there is no response to oxygen and cessation of β-mimetic therapy. Pulmonary edema has been reported with β-mimetic therapy. Restricting the duration of treatment to less than 24 hours, careful attention to fluid status, and detection of complicating conditions such as intrauterine infection may reduce this risk.**

Metabolic Complications. **β-Mimetic agents induce transient hyperglycemia and hypokalemia during treatment.** Measurement of glucose and potassium before initiating therapy and, on occasion, during the first 24 hours of treatment, is appropriate to identify significant hyperglycemia (>180 mg/dL) or hypokalemia (<2.5 mEq/L). These metabolic changes are mild and transient, but prolonged treatment beyond 24 hours may induce significant alterations in maternal blood glucose, insulin levels, and energy expenditure. **The risk of abnormal glucose metabolism is further increased by simultaneous treatment with corticosteroids, a common combination for threatened preterm labor.** Other agents should be chosen for women with pregestational diabetes and usually for those with gestational diabetes as well. β-Mimetic treatment in these women requires frequent monitoring and insulin infusion to maintain euglycemia.

Neonatal Effects. **Neonatal hypoglycemia, hypocalcemia, and ileus may follow treatment with β-mimetics and can be clinically significant if the maternal infusion is not discontinued 2 hours or more before delivery.** Long-term data on neurodevelopmental outcomes in humans are lacking.

Protocols for continuous subcutaneous infusion of terbutaline have been reported to have fewer side effects than oral administration but did not improve rates of PTB or perinatal morbidity in randomized placebo-controlled trials. This drug has been the subject of an **FDA warning: "Terbutaline administered by injection or through an infusion pump should not be used in pregnant women for prevention or prolonged (beyond 48 to 72 hours) treatment of preterm labor due to the potential for serious maternal heart problems and death. In addition, oral terbutaline tablets should not be used for prevention or treatment of preterm labor."**[54] No placebo-controlled trials that demonstrate effectiveness have been reported since the FDA advisory was issued.

Given their potential for clinically significant side effects and the availability of alternatives, the **β-sympathomimetic agents should not be used in women with known or suspected heart disease, severe preeclampsia or eclampsia, pregestational gestational diabetes requiring insulin, or hyperthyroidism. These drugs are contraindicated when suspected preterm labor is complicated by maternal fever, fetal tachycardia, leukocytosis, or other signs of possible chorioamnionitis.**

SUMMARY OF TREATMENT WITH β-MIMETIC TOCOLYSIS

β-Mimetic drugs were once among the most commonly used tocolytics but have been replaced by agents with better safety and side-effect profiles. Terbutaline has relatively few serious side effects when used as a single subcutaneous injection of 0.25 mg to facilitate maternal transfer or to initiate tocolysis while another agent with a slower onset of action is being given. Long-term oral or subcutaneous treatment has not been shown in controlled trials to reduce prematurity or neonatal morbidity.

ATOSIBAN AND OTHER TOCOLYTIC AGENTS

Atosiban is a selective oxytocin-vasopressin receptor antagonist. Although commonly used in Europe, it is not available in the United States. In normal parturition, oxytocin stimulates contractions by inducing conversion of phosphatidylinositol to inositol triphosphate, which binds to a protein in the sarcoplasmic reticulum and causes release of calcium into the cytoplasm. A Cochrane review analyzed six randomized trials ($n = 1695$) that compared the oxytocin receptor antagonist atosiban to a placebo. Use of atosiban increased the risk of birth within 48 hours of initiation of treatment (RR, 2.50; 95% CI, 0.51 to 12.35), increased the risk of PTB at less than 28 weeks' gestation (RR, 2.25; 95% CI, 0.80 to 6.35), and increased the risk of PTB at less than 37 weeks' gestation (RR, 1.17; 95% CI, 0.99 to 1.37); however, none of these increases reached statistical significance. All neonatal morbidity and mortality outcomes evaluated were similar in both groups. There was, however, an imbalance in allocation of women with threatened preterm labor under 26 weeks' gestation such that significantly more women in this subgroup were allocated to the atosiban group. In addition, more women in the placebo group than in the atosiban group received rescue treatment, which may have confounded the estimate of the true effects of atosiban when compared with placebo. The use of rescue tocolytics complicated analysis of these trials because the criteria for switching therapies was not strictly defined. Finally, the trial protocol did not define how glucocorticoids should be used, which resulted in a great deal of variation in use among study sites. **The FDA declined to approve the use of atosiban for tocolysis because of concerns about the drug's safety when used in fetuses at less than 28 weeks' gestation.**[55]

Nitric oxide (NO) donors also promote myometrial relaxation. Meta-analysis of trials to compare NO donors to other agents support the notion that NO donors do not delay delivery or improve neonatal outcome when compared with placebo, no treatment, or alternative tocolytics such as ritodrine, albuterol, and magnesium sulfate. There was, however, a reduction in the number of deliveries prior to 37 weeks' gestation when compared with alternative tocolytics, but the number of deliveries before 32 and 34 weeks' gestation were not influenced. Side effects other than headache were reduced in women who received NO donors rather than other tocolytics. However, women were significantly more likely to experience headache when NO donors had been used.

Clinical Use of Tocolytic Drugs

Tocolytic therapy is used in several clinical circumstances. In a patient who is in active labor with advanced cervical effacement, the diagnosis is not in question, and the goal is prompt treatment to allow maternal transfer and time for corticosteroids and GBS prophylaxis. In this setting, initial treatment with oral indomethacin or oral nifedipine may be the best choice to stop contractions promptly. Treatment for preterm labor may be continued until contractions have stopped or occur less frequently than four times per hour without additional cervical change, or until a full course of corticosteroids therapy is completed after 48 hours.

PERSISTENT CONTRACTIONS

If contractions persist despite therapy, the wisdom of tocolytic treatment should be reevaluated. The cervix should be reexamined, and if dilation has progressed beyond 4 cm and imminent delivery is thought to be inevitable, tocolytic therapy in most cases should be discontinued. In the setting of progressive preterm labor despite labor inhibition, it is critical to acknowledge the higher probability of placental abruption and/or subclinical chorioamnionitis. Clinical evaluation with focused history, physical examination, and laboratory assessment should be used to address the probability of these conditions.

Some women will have persistent uterine contractions and may exhibit a "nonthreatening" cervical examination that does not change over serial examinations. If a fibronectin swab was collected before therapy was begun, it should be sent for analysis. A positive result is not confirmatory, but a negative fibronectin, if collected before performance of a digital examination, suggests that the risk of imminent delivery is low. Alternatively, a transvaginal cervical ultrasound examination may be performed. A CL of 30 mm or more substantially reduces the likelihood of imminent delivery.

Serum levels are not clinically helpful to adjust the dose of tocolytics. A change to a second agent, or combination therapy with multiple agents, may slow contractions but may also result in increased risks. Combined use of β-mimetics or magnesium sulfate with calcium channel blockers should also be avoided (Box 29-5).

Care After Acute Treatment for Preterm Labor
MAINTENANCE TOCOLYTIC TREATMENT

Continued suppression of contractions after acute tocolysis does not reduce the rate of PTB. Meta-analyses of these data also find no evidence of prolongation of pregnancy or decline in the frequency of PTB.

Posthospitalization surveillance with outpatient monitoring of uterine contractions did not improve the rate of delivery before 37 weeks' gestation, gestational age at delivery, or birthweight in any of three randomized trials or in a meta-analysis of these. A multicenter randomized trial in which uterine activity was monitored, but in which the data were masked from care

---

> **BOX 29-5 MANAGEMENT OF PERSISTENT CONTRACTIONS DESPITE 12 TO 24 HOURS OF TOCOLYSIS**
>
> 1. Is subclinical amniotic fluid infection present? Repeat clinical examination, white blood cell counts, and fetal assessment. Consider amniocentesis for glucose, Gram stain, leukocyte esterase, and culture.
> 2. Is the fetus compromised? Review the fetal heart tracings and, if needed, do a biophysical assessment.
> 3. Is there evidence of abruption? Is there a suspicion of uterine anomaly with implantation of the placenta on the septum? Evaluate vitals signs for evidence of hemodynamic response to blood loss and repeat hemoglobin, hematocrit, and fibrinogen and abdominal sonography for placental implantation site.
> 4. Is the diagnosis of preterm labor correct? Is the cervix changing? Perform a transvaginal cervical ultrasound to measure cervical length. Send a fibronectin swab.
> 5. If infection, fetal compromise and abruption can be excluded, stop parenteral tocolysis for 24 hours and observe. Contractions in most patients will stop spontaneously.

providers in one group, also found no improvement in the PTB rate when contraction data were used.

The duration of hospitalization for an episode of preterm labor varies according to several factors, including the examination of the cervix, ease of tocolysis, gestational age, obstetric history, distance from the hospital, and the availability of home and family support. Associated risk factors that may complicate or increase the risk of recurrent preterm labor—such as a positive genital culture for *Chlamydia* or gonorrhea, urinary tract infection, and anemia—should be addressed before discharge from hospital care. Social issues such as homelessness, availability of child care, or protection from an abusive partner are important determinants of a patient's ability to adhere to recommendations for medical care, and these issues must be considered before the patient is discharged from the hospital.

CONDUCT OF LABOR AND DELIVERY FOR THE PRETERM INFANT

Intrapartum care for women in labor before term is often complicated by conditions that increase the chance of intrapartum fetal compromise such as malpresentation, hypertension, amnionitis, abruption, oligohydramnios, or fetal growth restriction. When labor is induced preterm for maternal or fetal indications, the lower uterine segment and cervix may not be well prepared for labor, which leads to a prolonged latent phase.

Intrapartum Assessment of the Preterm Fetus

Intrapartum fetal surveillance has been associated with a significantly lower frequency of intrapartum death and neonatal seizures for preterm infants. **Ominous heart rate tracings in preterm fetuses have the same associations with fetal acidosis as they do later in gestation.** Mean fetal heart rate falls continuously, from 160 beats/min at 22 weeks' gestation to 140 beats/min at term, because of a gradual increase in parasympathetic tone. Fetal heart rate patterns should be considered as representative of well-being in the preterm fetus as they are at term.

Labor and Delivery

The duration of labor in preterm gestation may be shorter than that of term pregnancy. The active phase of the first stage and the second stage may be particularly brief. Care should be taken to ensure that the fetus does not have a precipitous delivery without control of the fetal head. Prophylactic forceps to "protect" the fetal head are of no benefit. The neonatal care team should be alerted to the circumstances of a PTB well in advance of the delivery so that appropriate personnel and equipment can be made available.

Cesarean Delivery

Routine cesarean delivery (CD) for all preterm or VLBW infants is not justified. Trends that favor CD disappear after adjustment for confounding factors. A review of studies of neonatal and maternal morbidities after vaginal versus CD for infants born between 24 and 36 weeks' gestation found increased maternal morbidity without clear benefit for the infant. Neonatal intracranial hemorrhage occurs as often before and after labor as it does during labor and delivery.

For infants in breech presentation, the reasons for CD are intuitive, particularly to avoid entrapment of the after-coming head and other manipulations that could lead to trauma or hypoxia (see Chapter 17). Older retrospective studies that suggested a benefit of CD led to the current custom of CD for preterm breech fetuses, but data in support of this practice are weak. It is illogical to perform a CD to avoid a traumatic vaginal delivery only to encounter a difficult CD because of an inadequate abdominal or uterine incision. The operation should be conducted to minimize the trauma of delivery through as roomy an incision as is necessary. In a study of delivery mode for high-risk (e.g., with preeclampsia, vaginal bleeding, abnormal heart rate tracing) versus low-risk (e.g., with preterm labor, incompetent cervix) pregnancies with VLBW infants, CD was found to be of no value in the low-risk group but was associated with significantly improved survival rates in the high-risk group. Considering these factors, optimal delivery of the VLBW fetus may at times appropriately lead to a decision to perform a CD without labor. Generally speaking, the appropriate mode of delivery for the preterm fetus ought to be based on similar standards of obstetric indications as at term.

Delayed Cord Clamping

In December of 2012, ACOG published a committee opinion recommending delayed umbilical cord clamping in preterm infants.[56] This opinion was endorsed by the American Academy of Pediatrics (AAP). The definitions of **early cord clamping and delayed cord clamping are quite varied in the literature. General consensus and review of numerous articles suggest that early cord clamping occurs within 30 seconds of delivery; late cord clamping occurs when the delay is greater than 30 seconds and up to 5 minutes, although most of the benefit occurs within the first 60 to 120 seconds.**[57] Delayed cord clamping (DCC) is associated with substantial benefits in hematologic characteristics. Following DCC, **preterm infants have higher initial hematocrits, higher circulating blood volumes, and higher diastolic blood pressures, and they require less resuscitation in the delivery room.**[58] In addition, DCC has been associated with lower transfusion rates in preterm infants.[59] Although polycythemia and higher bilirubin levels have been

linked to DCC, a statistically significant increased need for phototherapy has not been seen in the preterm population. A paucity of data exists to compare the alternative of umbilical cord milking to DCC. In the only direct comparison study[60] published to date (58 infants enrolled), no difference was noted between milking the cord four times and delaying clamping of the cord for 30 seconds. The published randomized studies on this topic have been relatively small (total of 173 infants randomized to cord milking and either immediate or delayed cord clamping) and thus *milking of the cord cannot be recommended as the standard of care for the preterm infant at this time.* The potential consequences of delaying resuscitation in preterm infants in order to provide DCC is a common concern among neonatal and obstetric providers. However, several studies have demonstrated that these concerns are unfounded. DCC of up to 60 seconds has no deleterious effect in regard to delivery room resuscitation as measured by Apgar scores at 1 and 5 minutes or the need for chest compressions and epinephrine. In fact, **in the VLBW population, DCC reduces the need for any delivery room resuscitation intervention, supplemental oxygen, or bag-mask ventilation.**[61] In addition, no increase in the rate of hypothermia has been noted in infants undergoing DCC.

PREVENTION OF PRETERM BIRTH

Care of PTB may be described according to the public health model as *tertiary* (treatment initiated *after* the parturitional process has begun to limit perinatal morbidity and mortality), *secondary* (identification and treatment for individuals with increased risk), or *primary* (prevention and reduction of risk in the population). Tertiary care described in the preceding section of this chapter has improved perinatal outcomes but has no effect on the incidence of PTB. Efforts to identify women likely to deliver preterm to reduce or eliminate their risk have not achieved high sensitivity, and, until recently, no effective interventions were available to reduce risk.

Prevention efforts aimed at risk factors have been undertaken with the expectation that PTB would decline in proportion to the contribution of that risk factor as a cause of PTB. The failure of this approach underlies the current understanding of PTB as a syndrome in which multiple factors, known and unknown, contribute to the initiation and progression of preterm parturition. Rather than a distinct entity for which there are specific tests, PTB is more appropriately considered as the result of various pathologic events that affect the timing and progress of parturition. Understanding maternal risk factors, symptoms, and tests as clues to steps in a parturitional sequence that may or may not progress to early delivery, rather than "tests for preterm labor," brings some clarity to the sometimes confusing literature on this subject.

Secondary Prevention of Preterm Birth

Identification and elimination or reduction of risk may be applied before and/or after conception.

Before Pregnancy

Prepregnancy medical risk factors occur in as many as 40% of PTBs, but preconceptional medical interventions to reduce PTB in these women have been disappointing. A history of second-trimester loss or PTB is most easily identified,[3,62] recalling that the risk increases as the gestational age of the previous PTB declines and as the number of PTBs increases. Preconceptional interventions include surgical correction of müllerian anomalies and preconceptional abdominal cerclage. A randomized trial in 1579 women of interconceptional home visits and counseling to reduce LBW and PTB reported no evidence of benefit. Another randomized placebo-controlled trial tested interconceptional antimicrobial treatment in women with a prior early PTB. Subjects were randomly assigned to receive metronidazole and azithromycin or placebo at 3-month intervals between pregnancies, but the recurrence risk of PTB was not improved.

During Pregnancy

Postconceptional prevention strategies have most often been studied in women with a prior PTB with a major risk factor such as multifetal gestation or bleeding and in women with a sign, symptom, or positive screening test indicative of increased risk. Previous editions of this text have noted the absence of any effective interventions, but recent studies have demonstrated reduced risk in selected populations; for example, in women with a prior PTB and with a short cervix.

Modification of Maternal Activity

Despite a lack of supporting evidence, bed rest, limited work, and reduced sexual activity are often recommended to reduce the risk of PTB in pregnancies at risk for indicated and spontaneous births. Yost and colleagues found no relationship between coitus and risk of recurrent PTB. **Grobman and coworkers[63] reported no relation between reduced activity and frequency of PTB in nulliparous women with CL less than 30 mm before 24 weeks.**

NUTRITIONAL SUPPLEMENTS

Supplemental use of omega-3 polyunsaturated fatty acids (PUFAs) has been recommended because populations with a high dietary intake have low rates of PTB, perhaps because omega-3 PUFAs reduce levels of proinflammatory cytokines. European trials of omega-3 supplements and supplemental fish oil found significant reductions in PTB, but a placebo-controlled U.S. trial of supplemental omega-3 PUFAs in women with a prior PTB found no benefit in women who were treated with 17-α-hydroxyprogesterone caproate.[64] Interestingly, women in both arms of this study who consumed more than one fish meal per month had a significantly lower rate of PTB than those who consumed fish once per month or less. **Trials of supplemental vitamins C and E and calcium have not demonstrated a reduction in PTB risk.[65]**

ENHANCED PRENATAL CARE

Although perhaps helpful in adolescents, programs of enhanced prenatal care that provide social support, home visits, and education have not reduced PTB. Frequent provider-initiated contact for women with a prior PTB also did not decrease recurrent PTB in randomized trials.

However, reduced rates of PTB have been reported for women receiving prenatal care in novel settings: group prenatal care in South Carolina,[66] a regional program to standardize care for an indigent population in Texas,[67] and specialized prematurity clinics in Utah and Ohio[68] for women with a prior PTB have all reported lower rates of premature birth, but all are retrospective and merit confirmation.

PERIODONTAL CARE

The association of periodontal disease with increased risk of prematurity prompted intensive study of the effects of periodontal care on the rate of PTB. Results have been negative, suggesting shared susceptibility rather than a causal linkage.

ANTIBIOTIC TREATMENT

Screening and antibiotic treatment of women with abnormal genital flora has been largely ineffective to prevent PTB. Antibiotic treatment for women with a prior PTB who have bacterial vaginosis was associated with reduced risk of recurrent PTB in secondary analyses. Reviews and meta-analyses have also been negative, and a U.S. Preventive Services Task Force review[69] cautioned that there may be "unintended potential for harm" from screening and treatment for bacterial vaginosis in pregnancy. Antibiotic prophylaxis has also been studied in women with positive fetal fibronectin test results. Rates of PTB were actually increased in fibronectin-positive women who received antibiotic treatment. Similar results were reported from a trial of antibiotics in women with *Trichomonas.*

PROGESTOGENS

Progestogen supplementation for women at risk for PTB has been investigated based on several plausible mechanisms of action, including reduced gap-junction formation and oxytocin antagonism leading to relaxation of smooth muscle, maintenance of cervical integrity, and antiinflammatory effects. Studies performed before 1990 in women with recurrent miscarriage and PTB were reviewed by Keirse,[70] who found "no support for the view that 17-α-hydroxyprogesterone caproate protects against miscarriage, but suggests that it does reduce the occurrence of PTB." **Subsequent randomized trials have demonstrated an approximately 40% decrease in the rate of PTB in women with a prior PTB and/or a short cervix (<15 to 20 mm before 24 weeks' gestation) who were treated with either intramuscular 17-α-hydroxyprogesterone caproate 250 mg weekly or with vaginal progesterone suppositories or cream daily between 16 and 36 weeks' gestation** (Table 29-4).[15-17,19,71,72]

Several randomized placebo-controlled trials have found that progestogen supplementation does not affect the rate of PTB in women with multifetal gestations, indicating that the

TABLE 29-4	STUDIES OF PROGESTOGENS TO REDUCE PRETERM BIRTH		
STUDY	**YEAR**	**POPULATION**	**EFFECT ON PTB RATE**
Keirse[70]*	1990	Meta-analysis	↓ 40%
da Fonseca[71]†	2003	History of PTB	↓ 40%
Meis[72]*	2003	History of PTB	↓ 35%
Fonseca[16]†	2007	Short cervix <15 mm	↓ 44%
O'Brien[17]†	2007	History of PTB without short cervix‡	No ↓
DeFranco[15]†	2007	History of PTB with short cervix§	↓
Hassan[19]†	2011	Short cervix 10 to 20 mm	↓ 45%

*17-α-hydroxyprogesterone caproate.
†Vaginal progesterone in various formulations.
‡Women likely to receive cerclage not enrolled. Mean cervical length at entry was 37 mm.
§Secondary analysis of O'Brien study subjects who later had a short cervix (<28 mm).
PTB, preterm birth variably defined.

mechanism of progesterone's action to reduce risk of PTB in singletons is not related to uterine stretch.[73-76]

Importantly, the effect of supplemental progesterone compounds is not universally observed in women with a prior PTB, indicating first that some pathways to recurrent PTB are not influenced by this therapy and also that many women with a prior PTB will deliver at term without treatment. The recurrence risk of sPTB without treatment is related to CL at 22 to 24 weeks' gestation and ranges from more than 35% in women whose CL is less than 25 mm to 15% in women with a CL of 25 to 35 mm and to less than 10% in those with a CL above 35 mm. In the only study of women with a previous PTB in which vaginal progesterone did not reduce the risk of recurrent PTB,[16] the mean CL at 18 to 22 weeks' gestation was 37 mm, which suggests that women with a prior PTB who also do not have a short cervix will not benefit from progesterone supplementation. Indeed, a secondary analysis of this study found a reduced risk of PTB in women who later had a short cervix.[15] **Taken together, these studies indicate that a *short cervix*, rather than *prior PTB*, is the most appropriate criterion for institution of vaginal progesterone therapy. However, a history of PTB will continue to be an indication for 17-α-hydroxyprogesterone caproate treatment until additional studies demonstrate that such treatment is unnecessary in women with a prior PTB who maintain a normal CL beyond 24 weeks' gestation.**

Trials of progestogens in women with other risk factors, such as a positive fetal fibronectin or bleeding, have not been reported. The mechanism of action is uncertain, but the absence of effect in multifetal gestation coupled with reductions in PTB in women with a short cervix suggest that the pathway may be related primarily to modulation of cervical softening, a conclusion also suggested by basic studies.

The optimal strategy to identify candidates for progesterone therapy has not been determined. Universal CL screening of all pregnant women at 18 to 24 weeks' gestation has been proposed based on two favorable cost-effectiveness studies[77,78] and expert opinion,[79] but universal application of any screening test in obstetric care is always accompanied by unanticipated costs and consequences, in this case likely related to reproducibility of cervical sonography and uncertain adherence to recommended treatment protocols.

An alternative list of indications for selective screening for a short cervix with transvaginal ultrasound is shown in Box 29-6. These women are candidates for screening with the expectation that progesterone supplementation will be considered if the CL measurement at 16 to 24 weeks' gestation is 20 mm or less. The value and timing of repeat cervical ultrasound in women with marginal CL measurements is uncertain. The schema suggested is likely to be modified by broader experience with cervical sonographic screening.

CERVICAL CERCLAGE

The relationship between a short cervix and the risk of PTB was initially interpreted as evidence of diminished cervical strength or competence, but subsequent clinical experience and interventional studies do not support that conclusion. Cerclage is an effective treatment for women with a history of PTB and a short cervix (see Chapter 28). Although beneficial for women with a prior PTB whose CL is very short (<15 to 25 mm),[80,81] cerclage treatment does not reduce PTB risk in women with an isolated short cervix (<15 mm) without a

> **BOX 29-6 INDICATIONS FOR CERVICAL ULTRASOUND SCREENING IN THE SECOND TRIMESTER**
>
> Any previous pregnancy delivered between 16 and 36 weeks' gestation
> All pregnancies conceived after fertility care
> All women with a history of cervical instrumentation
> - Cervical cone biopsy or loop electrosurgical excision procedure (LEEP)
> - Dilation and curettage for diagnosis or therapeutic indications, including first- and second-trimester pregnancy terminations
>
> All women with prior genital tract infections or persistently abnormal Papanicolaou smear
> All women with depression, low body mass index (BMI<19.6), or who smoke
> All women whose cervical length is <35 mm on a midtrimester transabdominal ultrasound examination
> - Women with signs or symptoms of preterm parturition in the current pregnancy
> - Vaginal bleeding or spotting without an obvious cause
> - Persistent symptoms of pelvic pressure, cramps, change in vaginal discharge after 16 weeks' gestation

history of PTB,[82] and it actually appears to increase the risk of PTB in women with a twin pregnancy and a short cervix.[82,83] In women with a prior PTB, cerclage is paradoxically most beneficial in those with the shortest CL (<15 mm),[80,81] which suggests that the benefit of cerclage may relate more to protection of exposed membranes than to bolstering cervical strength.

Clinical Use of Progesterone and Cerclage to Prevent Preterm Birth

The body of evidence that shows progesterone is effective in reducing the risk of PTB in women with a short cervix with or without a history of PTB has influenced the clinical care of women who would previously have been considered to be candidates for prophylactic history-indicated cervical cerclage. Similarly, results from the NICHD Vaginal Ultrasound Cerclage Trial[80] indicate that only 30% of the more than 1000 women with a history of a PTB between 17 and 34 weeks' gestation displayed a CL of 25 mm or less before 24 weeks' gestation when followed with cervical sonography. These observations led to development of the protocol displayed in Figure 29-11.[84] Cerclage is reserved for women with a history of cervical injury, uterine anomaly, and/or progressive cervical shortening to a length below 25 mm despite progesterone therapy. In these patients, cerclage is offered at 25 mm and is strongly urged if the CL is 15 mm or less or membranes are visible.

Late Preterm Birth

In 2008, 12.3% of births in the United States were preterm, and 71% of these (8.8%) were *late preterm*, occurring between $34^{0/7}$ and $36^{6/7}$ weeks' gestation (Fig. 29-12). Although these infants fare better than those born before 34 weeks' gestation, they experience substantially increased morbidity and mortality compared with infants born after 37 weeks' gestation, and they account for the overwhelming majority of admissions to the NICU. Approximately 70% of PTBs are spontaneous, but the relative percentage has declined in recent years because indicated PTBs have increased. **Other contributors to the decline in**

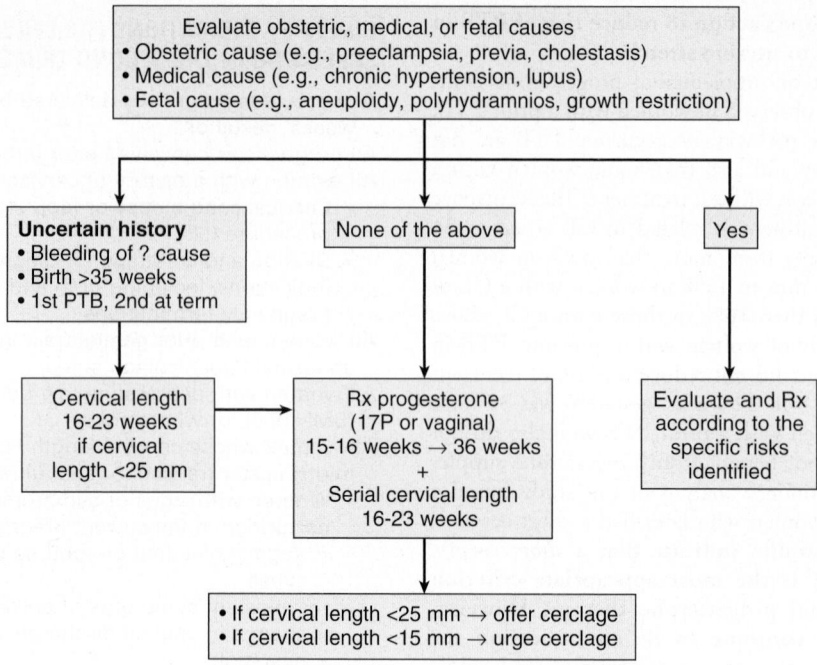

FIG 29-11 Care algorithm for women with a prior preterm birth (PTB) at 16 to 36 weeks' gestation. Rx, medical treatment. (Courtesy Ohio State University.)

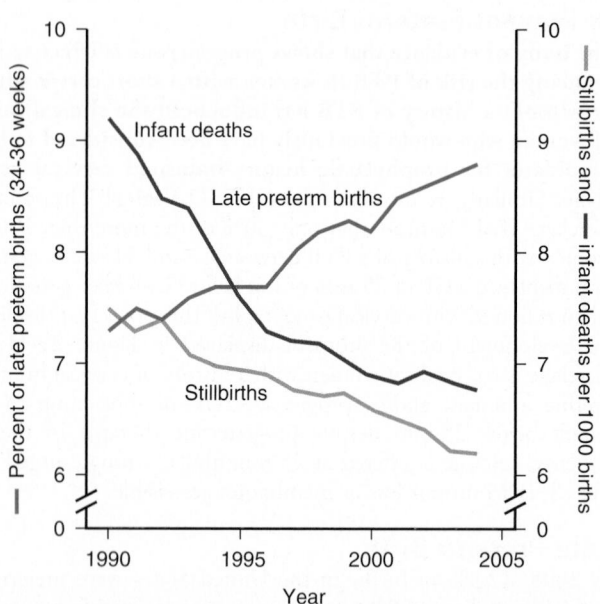

FIG 29-12 Trends in late-preterm birth, stillbirth, and infant mortality, United States, 1990-2004. (From Ananth CV, Gyamfi C, Jain L. Characterizing risk profiles of infants who are delivered at late preterm gestations: does it matter? *Am J Obstet Gynecol.* 2008;199[4]: 329-331.)

the proportion of late spontaneous PTBs that have occurred since 2006 include the decline in multifetal gestations related to fertility care and increased use of progesterone and cervical cerclage. The rise in PTBs between 1990 and 2006 in singletons was almost entirely explained by an increased rate of indicated PTBs between 34 and 36 weeks' gestation. The principal driver of this increase was an increased willingness to consider scheduled birth as a safer option than continuing the pregnancy in women with various pregnancy complications.

The decision to choose indicated PTB over continuation of the pregnancy at any gestational age carries great potential to create, as well as to prevent or reduce, perinatal morbidity and mortality. Unfortunately, the relative risks and benefits of delivery versus expectant management are difficult to weigh accurately, especially in the late preterm period. Before 34 weeks' gestation, clear benefit can be gained by daily increases in fetal maturity. At 34 weeks, the risks of immaturity have been considered to be acceptable in complicated pregnancies, but the morbidity and mortality rates for infants born between 34 and 37 weeks' gestation are higher than previously realized. Reddy and colleagues[85] examined the records of 292,627 late-preterm singleton births and found that 49% were associated with spontaneous labor. Remarkably, no reason was recorded in 23% of late PTBs. In another study,[86] 7.8% of all births and 65.7% of PTBs were late preterm. Of these, 29.8% followed spontaneous labor; 32.3% followed PPROM; 31.8% had an obstetric, maternal, or fetal condition that led to late PTB following induction of labor or cesarean delivery in the absence of labor; and 6.1%

were unknown. Specific guidelines for choosing late PTB in complicated pregnancies are lacking, but recent efforts to document the reasons and track the risks and benefits of these births are expected to help in the future (Table 29-5).[87]

Primary Prevention of Preterm Birth
Primary prevention strategies for PTB will require consistent efforts through education and public policy because the public and government currently underestimate the magnitude of the societal burden. Preconceptional interventions are needed because as many as 50% of PTBs occur in women without known risk factors.

Public Educational Interventions
Greater awareness of the increased risk of PTB in singleton gestations associated with assisted reproductive technology (ART) could affect attitudes and choices made in fertility care.

Similar strategies to reduce the prevalence of smoking, increase the use of condoms to prevent sexually transmitted infections, and promote recognition and early treatment of depression might all have an eventual effect on PTB rates. Promotion of long-acting reversible contraceptives for women at risk, especially after a preterm delivery, offers a chance to reduce the risk of recurrent PTB.

Public and Professional Policies
Policies promulgated by fertility specialists intended to reduce the risk of higher-order multiple gestation have been successful in Europe, Australia, and the United States. Rates of triplet and higher-order multiple pregnancies had been rising rapidly in the United States until 1998, when the increase was arrested by voluntary adoption of limitations on the number of ova transferred. The rate of higher-order multiples fell by 50% between 1996 and 2003. A societal approach to improve pregnancy

TABLE 29-5 GUIDANCE REGARDING TIMING OF DELIVERY WHEN CONDITIONS COMPLICATE PREGNANCY AT 34 WEEKS' GESTATION OR LATER

CONDITION	GESTATIONAL AGE* AT DELIVERY	GRADE OF RECOMMENDATION[†]
Placental and Uterine Issues		
Placenta previa[‡]	36-37 wk	B
Suspected placenta accreta, increta, or percreta with placenta previa[‡]	34-35 wk	B
Prior classical cesarean incision (upper segment uterine incision)[‡]	36-37 wk	B
Prior myomectomy necessitating cesarean delivery[‡]	37-38 wk (may require earlier delivery, similar to prior classical cesarean, in situations with more extensive or complicated myomectomy)	B
Fetal Issues		
Fetal growth restriction, singleton	*38-39 wk:* Otherwise uncomplicated, no concurrent findings	B
	34-37 wk: Concurrent conditions (oligohydramnios, abnormal Doppler studies, maternal risk factors, comorbidity)	B
	Expeditious delivery regardless of gestational age: Persistent abnormal fetal surveillance suggesting imminent fetal jeopardy	
Fetal growth restriction, twin gestation	*36-37 wk:* Dichorionic-diamniotic twins with isolated fetal growth restriction	B
	32-34 wk: Monochorionic-diamniotic twins with isolated fetal growth restriction	B
	Concurrent conditions (oligohydramnios, abnormal Doppler studies, maternal risk factors, comorbidity)	B
	Expeditious delivery regardless of gestational age: Persistent abnormal fetal surveillance suggesting imminent fetal jeopardy	
Fetal congenital malformations[‡]	*34-39 wk:* Suspected worsening of fetal organ damage	B
	Potential for fetal intracranial hemorrhage (e.g., vein of Galen aneurysm, neonatal alloimmune thrombocytopenia)	
	When delivery prior to labor is preferred (e.g., EXIT procedure)	
	Previous fetal intervention	
	Concurrent maternal disease (e.g., preeclampsia, chronic hypertension)	
	Potential for adverse maternal effect from fetal condition	
	Expeditious delivery regardless of gestational age:	B
	When intervention is expected to be beneficial	
	Fetal complications develop (abnormal fetal surveillance, new-onset hydrops fetalis, progressive or new-onset organ injury)	
	Maternal complications develop (mirror syndrome associated with fetal hydrops)	
Multiple gestations: dichorionic-diamniotic[‡]	38 wk	B
Multiple gestations (see Chapter 32): monochorionic-diamniotic[‡]	34-37 wk	B
Multiple gestations: dichorionic-diamniotic or monochorionic-diamniotic with single fetal death[‡]	At or after 34 wk, consider delivery (recommendation limited to pregnancies at or after 34 wk; if it occurs before 34 wk, individualize based on concurrent maternal or fetal conditions)	B
Multiple gestations: monochorionic-monoamniotic[‡]	32-34 wk	B
Multiple gestations: monochorionic-monoamniotic with single fetal death[‡]	Consider delivery; individualized according to gestational age and concurrent complications	B
Oligohydramnios, isolated and persistent[‡]	36-37 wk	B

Continued

TABLE 29-5 GUIDANCE REGARDING TIMING OF DELIVERY WHEN CONDITIONS COMPLICATE PREGNANCY AT 34 WEEKS' GESTATION OR LATER—cont'd

CONDITION	GESTATIONAL AGE* AT DELIVERY	GRADE OF RECOMMENDATION[†]
Maternal Issues		
Chronic hypertension, no medications[‡]	38-39 wk	B
Chronic hypertension, controlled on medication[‡]	37-39 wk	B
Chronic hypertension, difficult to control (requiring frequent medication adjustments)[‡]	36-37 wk	B
Gestational hypertension[§]	37-38 wk	B
Preeclampsia, severe[‡]	At diagnosis (recommendation limited to pregnancies at or after 34 wk)	C
Preeclampsia, mild[‡]	37 wk	B
Diabetes, pregestational, well controlled[‡]	LPTB or ETB not recommended	B
Diabetes, pregestational, with vascular disease[‡]	37-39 wk	B
Diabetes, pregestational, poorly controlled[‡]	34-39 wk (individualized to situation)	B
Diabetes, gestational, well controlled on diet[‡]	LPTB or ETB not recommended	B
Diabetes, gestational, well controlled on medication[‡]	LPTB or ETB not recommended	B
Diabetes, gestational, poorly controlled on medication[‡]	34-39 wk (individualized to situation)	B
Obstetric Issues		
Prior stillbirth, unexplained[‡]	LPTB or ETB not recommended	B
	Consider amniocentesis for fetal pulmonary maturity if delivery is planned at less than 39 wk	C
Spontaneous PTB: PPROM[‡]	34 wk (recommendation limited to pregnancies at or after 34 wk)	B
Spontaneous PTB: active preterm labor[‡]	Delivery if progressive labor or additional maternal or fetal indication	B

From Spong CY, Mercer BM, D'Alton M, et al. Timing of indicated late-preterm and early-term birth. *Obstet Gynecol.* 2011;118(2 Pt 1):323.
*Gestational age is in completed weeks; thus 34 weeks includes 340/7 weeks through 346/7 weeks.
[†]Grade of recommendation: recommendations or conclusions or both are based on good and consistent scientific evidence (A); based on limited or inconsistent scientific evidence (B); based primarily on consensus and expert opinion (C). The recommendations regarding expeditious delivery for imminent fetal jeopardy were not given a grade. The recommendation regarding severe preeclampsia is based largely on expert opinion; however, higher-level evidence is not likely to be forthcoming because this condition is believed to carry significant maternal risk with limited potential fetal benefit from expectant management after 34 weeks.
[‡]Uncomplicated, thus no fetal growth restriction, superimposed preeclampsia, and so on. If these are present, the complicating conditions take precedence, and earlier delivery may be indicated.
[§]Maintenance antihypertensive therapy should not be used to treat gestational hypertension.
ETB, early-term birth at 37$^{0/7}$ weeks through 38$^{6/7}$ weeks; *EXIT,* ex utero intrapartum treatment; *LPTB,* late-preterm birth at 34$^{0/7}$ weeks through 36$^{6/7}$ weeks; *PPROM,* preterm premature rupture of the membranes; *PTB,* preterm birth.

outcomes has been adopted in most European countries, where policies to protect pregnant women include minimum paid pregnancy leave, time off for prenatal visits, exemption from night shifts, and protection from workplace hazards. The European Programme of Occupational Risks and Pregnancy Outcome (EUROPOP) study of such policies found that **risk of PTB was increased among women who worked more than 42 hours per week** (OR, 1.33; CI, 1.1 to 1.6) **and who were required to stand for more than 6 hours per day** (OR, 1.26; CI, 1.1 to 1.5).

Social Determinants of Health

Racial disparities in health are not confined to perinatal medicine but rather are reflected throughout the life span. The increased rates of many illnesses in black and other disadvantaged groups are being addressed by the public health community through **the social determinants of health: (1) promotion of school attendance and completion, (2) food security, (3) neighborhood nutritional programs, (4) job fairs, and (5) an increasing role for hospital and health providers as local leaders.**[88]

SUMMARY

Preterm birth is a syndrome, the final result of several pathways that often overlap to initiate parturition. Obstetric interventions to reduce infant morbidity, such as antenatal glucocorticoids and antibiotics for group B streptococcal prophylaxis, are effective tertiary therapies but have no opportunity to reduce the incidence of PTB. Detection of pregnancies at risk through careful review of prior pregnancies, selective or universal use of cervical ultrasound screening to identify candidates for progesterone therapy, and selective use of cerclage are welcome advances. Adherence to protocols for timing of scheduled births and documentation of indications for iatrogenic PTB are needed to further reduce the rate of stillbirth while limiting the associated morbidity of late PTB.

KEY POINTS

- More than 70% of fetal, neonatal, and infant morbidity and mortality occurs in infants born preterm.
- The rate of PTB peaked in 2006 as the result of the increased use of assisted reproductive technology, ultrasound dating, and indicated preterm births. It has since declined largely because of the adoption of fertility practices to reduce the multifetal gestations associated with infertility treatment.
- Major risk factors for PTB are a history of previous preterm delivery, multifetal gestation, and bleeding after the first trimester of pregnancy; however, most women who deliver preterm have no apparent risk factors; therefore every pregnancy is potentially at risk.

◆ sPTB is a syndrome in which the parturition process may be initiated by one or more pathways that culminate in cervical ripening, decidual activation, uterine contractions, and ruptured membranes.

◆ Four interventions have been shown to reduce perinatal morbidity and mortality: (1) transfer of the mother and fetus to an appropriate hospital before PTB; (2) administration of maternal antibiotics to prevent neonatal Group B *Streptococcus* infection; (3) administration of maternal corticosteroids to reduce neonatal RDS, IVH, and neonatal mortality; and (4) administration of maternal magnesium sulfate at the preterm delivery at less than 32 weeks to reduce the incidence of cerebral palsy.

◆ The risk of recurrent PTB may be reduced in women with a prior PTB with 17-α-hydroxyprogesterone caproate and in women with a short cervix (<20 mm) by administration of prophylactic supplemental progesterone. Cervical cerclage should be reserved for women with a prior PTB and a short cervix.

REFERENCES

1. Callaghan WM, MacDorman MF, et al. The contribution of preterm birth to infant mortality rates in the United States. *Pediatrics.* 2006;118: 1566.
2. Fleischman AR, Oinuma M, et al. Rethinking the definition of term pregnancy. *Obstet Gynecol.* 2010;116:136.
3. Edlow AG, Srinivas SK, et al. Second-trimester loss and subsequent pregnancy outcomes: what is the real risk? *Am J Obstet Gynecol.* 2007;197 :581e1.
4. McManemy J, Cooke E, et al. Recurrence risk for preterm delivery. *Am J Obstet Gynecol.* 2007;196:576e1, discussion 576e6.
5. ACOG committee opinion no. 560: Medically indicated late-preterm and early-term deliveries. *Obstet Gynecol.* 2013;121(4):908-910.
6. Silver RM, Branch DW, Goldenberg RL, et al. Nomenclature for pregnancy outcomes: time for a change. *Obstet Gynecol.* 2011;118:1402.
7. Beck S, Wojdyla D, et al. The worldwide incidence of preterm birth: a systematic review of maternal mortality and morbidity. *Bull World Health Organ.* 2010;88:31.
8. MacDorman MF, Kirmeyer S. Fetal and perinatal mortality, United States, 2005. *Natl Vital Stat Rep.* 2009;57:1.
9. Stoll BJ, Hansen NI, et al. Neonatal outcomes of extremely preterm infants from the NICHD Neonatal Research Network. *Pediatrics.* 2010;126:443.
10. *Eunice Kennedy Shriver National Institute of Child Health and Human Development Neonatal Research Network. NICHD Neonatal Research Network (NRN): Extremely Preterm Birth Outcome Data.* <http://www.nichd.nih.gov/about/org/der/branches/ppb/programs/epbo/pages/epbo_case.aspx>.
11. Moster D, Lie RT, et al. Long-term medical and social consequences of preterm birth. *N Engl J Med.* 2008;359:262.
12. Iams JD, Cebrik D, Lynch C, et al. The rate of cervical change and the phenotype of spontaneous preterm birth. *Am J Obstet Gynecol.* 2011;205: 130.e1.
13. Iams JD, Goldenberg RL, et al. The length of the cervix and the risk of spontaneous premature delivery. National Institute of Child Health and Human Development Maternal Fetal Medicine Unit Network. *N Engl J Med.* 1996;334:567.
14. Iams JD, Newman RB, et al. Frequency of uterine contractions and the risk of spontaneous preterm delivery. *N Engl J Med.* 2002;346:250.
15. DeFranco EA, O'Brien JM, et al. Vaginal progesterone is associated with a decrease in risk for early preterm birth and improved neonatal outcome in women with a short cervix: a secondary analysis from a randomized, double-blind, placebo-controlled trial. *Ultrasound Obstet Gynecol.* 2007;30:697.
16. Fonseca EB, Celik E, et al. Progesterone and the risk of preterm birth among women with a short cervix. *N Engl J Med.* 2007;357:462.
17. O'Brien JM, Adair CD, et al. Progesterone vaginal gel for the reduction of recurrent preterm birth: primary results from a randomized, double-blind, placebo-controlled trial. *Ultrasound Obstet Gynecol.* 2007;30:687.
18. O'Brien JM, Defranco EA, et al. Effect of progesterone on cervical shortening in women at risk for preterm birth: secondary analysis from a multinational, randomized, double-blind, placebo-controlled trial. *Ultrasound Obstet Gynecol.* 2009;34:653.
19. Hassan SS, Romero R, et al. Vaginal progesterone reduces the rate of preterm birth in women with a sonographic short cervix: a multicenter, randomized, double-blind, placebo-controlled trial. *Ultrasound Obstet Gynecol.* 2011;38:18.
19b. Conner SN, Frey HA, Cahill AG, Macones GA, Colditz GA, Tuuli MG. Loop electrosurgical excision procedure and risk of preterm birth: a systematic review and meta-analysis. *Obstet Gynecol.* 2014;123(4):752-761.
20. Simhan HN, Bodnar LM. Prepregnancy body mass index, vaginal inflammation, and the racial disparity in preterm birth. *Am J Epidemiol.* 2006; 163:459.
21. Zhong Y, Cahill AG, et al. The association between prepregnancy maternal body mass index and preterm delivery. *Am J Perinatol.* 2010;27:293.
22. Cnattingius S, Villamor E, Johansson S, et al. Maternal overweight and obesity in early pregnancy and risk of infant mortality: a population based cohort study in Sweden. *JAMA.* 2013;309(22):2362-2370.
23. Klebanoff MA, Harper M, et al. Fish consumption, erythrocyte fatty acids, and preterm birth. *Obstet Gynecol.* 2011;117:1071.
24. Behrman R, Stith Butler A. *Preterm Birth: Causes, Consequences, and Prevention.* Report of the Committee on Understanding Premature Birth and Assuring Healthy Outcomes. Institute of Medicine. Washington, DC: National Academies Press; 2007.
25. Hobel CJ, Goldstein A, et al. Psychosocial stress and pregnancy outcome. *Clin Obstet Gynecol.* 2008;51:333.
26. Grote NK, Bridge JA, et al. A meta-analysis of depression during pregnancy and the risk of preterm birth, low birth weight, and intrauterine growth restriction. *Arch Gen Psychiatry.* 2010;67:1012.
27. Lu MC, Chen B. Racial and ethnic disparities in preterm birth: the role of stressful life events. *Am J Obstet Gynecol.* 2004;191:691.
28. Healy AJ, Malone FD, et al. Early access to prenatal care: implications for racial disparity in perinatal mortality. *Obstet Gynecol.* 2006;107:625.
29. Treloar SA, Macones GA, et al. Genetic influences on premature parturition in an Australian twin sample. *Twin Res.* 2000;3:80.
30. Clausson B, Lichtenstein P, et al. Genetic influence on birthweight and gestational length determined by studies in offspring of twins. *Br J Obstet Gynaecol.* 2000;107:375.
31. Getahun D, Lawrence JM, et al. The association between stillbirth in the first pregnancy and subsequent adverse perinatal outcomes. *Am J Obstet Gynecol.* 2009;201:378e1.
32. Watson LF, Rayner JA, et al. Modelling prior reproductive history to improve prediction of risk for very preterm birth. *Paediatr Perinat Epidemiol.* 2010;24:402.
33. Makhlouf M. Adverse pregnancy outcomes among women with prior spontaneous or induced abortions. *Am J Obstet Gynecol.* 2011;205: S204.
34. Reddy UM, Wapner RJ, et al. Infertility, assisted reproductive technology, and adverse pregnancy outcomes: executive summary of a National Institute of Child Health and Human Development workshop. *Obstet Gynecol.* 2007;109:967.
35. Word RA, Li XH, et al. Dynamics of cervical remodeling during pregnancy and parturition: mechanisms and current concepts. *Semin Reprod Med.* 2007;25:69.
36. Timmons B, Akins M, et al. Cervical remodeling during pregnancy and parturition. *Trends Endocrinol Metab.* 2010;21:353.
37. Kim CJ, Romero R, Kusanovic JP, et al. The frequency, clinical significance, and pathological features of chronic chorioamnionitis, a lesion associated with spontaneous preterm birth. *Mod Pathol.* 2010;23(7):1000-1011.
38. Lee J, Romero R, Xu Y, et al. A signature of maternal anti-fetal rejection in spontaneous preterm birth: chronic chorioamnionitis, anti-human leukocyte antigen antibodies, and C4d. *PLoS ONE.* 2011;6(2):e16806.
39. Swamy GK, Simhan HN, et al. Clinical utility of fetal fibronectin for predicting preterm birth. *J Reprod Med.* 2005;50:851.
40. Berghella V, Hayes E, et al. Fetal fibronectin testing for reducing the risk of preterm birth. *Cochrane Database Syst Rev.* 2008;CD006843.
41. Berghella V, Baxter JK, et al. Cervical assessment by ultrasound for preventing preterm delivery. *Cochrane Database Syst Rev.* 2009;CD007235.
42. Verani JR, McGee L, et al. Prevention of perinatal group B streptococcal disease—revised guidelines from CDC, 2010. *MMWR Recomm Rep.* 2010;59:1.

43. Garite TJ, Kurtzman J, et al. Impact of a "rescue course" of antenatal corticosteroids: a multicenter randomized placebo-controlled trial. *Am J Obstet Gynecol*. 2009;200:248e1.

44. ACOG Committee Opinion No. 475: Antenatal corticosteroid therapy for fetal maturation. *Obstet Gynecol*. 2011;117:422.

45. Battin M, Bevan C, Harding J. Growth in the neonatal period after repeat courses of antenatal corticosteroids: data from the ACTORDS randomised trial. *Arch Dis Child Fetal Neonatal Ed*. 2012;97(2):F99-F105.

46. Crowther CA, Hiller JE, et al. Effect of magnesium sulfate given for neuroprotection before preterm birth: a randomized controlled trial. *JAMA*. 2003;290:2669.

47. Marret S, Marpeau L, et al. Benefit of magnesium sulfate given before very preterm birth to protect infant brain. *Pediatrics*. 2008;121:225.

48. Marret S, Marpeau L, et al. Magnesium sulphate given before very-preterm birth to protect infant brain: the randomised controlled PREMAG trial. *Br J Obstet Gynaecol*. 2007;114:310.

49. Rouse DJ, Hirtz DG, et al. A randomized, controlled trial of magnesium sulfate for the prevention of cerebral palsy. *N Engl J Med*. 2008;359:895.

50. American College of Obstetricians and Gynecologists Committee on Obstetric Practice, Society for Maternal-Fetal Medicine. Committee Opinion No. 455: Magnesium sulfate before anticipated preterm birth for neuroprotection. *Obstet Gynecol*. 2010;115:669.

51. Costantine MM, Weiner SJ. Effects of antenatal exposure to magnesium sulfate on neuroprotection and mortality in preterm infants: a meta-analysis. *Obstet Gynecol*. 2009;114:354.

52. Crowther CA, Hiller JE, et al. Magnesium sulphate for preventing preterm birth in threatened preterm labour. *Cochrane Database Syst Rev*. 2002; CD001060.

53. Vis JY, et al. Randomized comparison of nifedipine and placebo in fibronectin-negative women with symptoms of preterm labor and a short cervix. *Am J Perinatol*. 2014 Dec 8.

54. *FDA Drug Safety Communication: New warnings against use of terbutaline to treat preterm labor*. <www.fda.gov/Drugs/DrugSafety/ucm243539.htm>.

55. *Food and Drug Administration, Center for Drug Evaluation and Research, Advisory Committee for Reproductive Health Drugs*. Available at <www.fda .gov/ohrms/dockets/ac/98/transcpt/3407t1.rtf>.

56. American College of Obstetricians and Gynecologists. Timing of umbilical cord clamping after birth. Committee Opinion No. 543. *Obstet Gynecol*. 2012;201:1522-1526.

57. Raju TN. Optimal timing for clamping the umbilical cord after birth. *Clin Perinatol*. 2012;39:889-900.

58. Rabe H, Reynolds G, Diaz-Rossello J. Early versus delayed umbilical cord clamping in preterm infants. *Cochrane Database Syst Rev*. 2004;(4):CD003248.

59. Oh W, Fanaroff AA, Carlo WA, et al. Effects of delayed cord clamping in very low birth weight infants. *J Perinatol*. 2011;31:S68-S71.

60. Rabe H, Jewison A, Alvarez RF, et al. Milking compared with delayed cord clamping to increase placental transfusion in preterm neonates. *Obstet Gynecol*. 2011;117:205-211.

61. Kaempf JW, Tomlinson MW, Kaempf AJ, et al. Delayed umbilical cord clamping in premature neonates. *Obstet Gynecol*. 2012;120:325-330.

62. Mazaki-Tovi S, Romero R, et al. Recurrent preterm birth. *Semin Perinatol*. 2007;31:142.

63. Grobman WA, Gilbert SA, Iams JD, et al. Activity restriction among women with a short cervix. *Obstet Gynecol*. 2013;121(6):1181-1186.

64. Harper M, Thom E, et al. Omega-3 fatty acid supplementation to prevent recurrent preterm birth: a randomized controlled trial. *Obstet Gynecol*. 2010;115:234.

65. Hauth JC, Clifton RG, et al. Vitamin C and E supplementation to prevent spontaneous preterm birth: a randomized controlled trial. *Obstet Gynecol*. 2010;116:653.

66. Picklesimer AH, Billings D, Hale N, et al. The effect of Centering Pregnancy: Group prenatal care on preterm birth in a low-income population. *Am J Obstet Gynecol*. 2012;206(5):415.e1-415.e7.

67. Leveno KJ, McIntire DD, Bloom SL, et al. Decreased preterm births in an inner-city public hospital. *Obstet Gynecol*. 2009;113:578.

68. Markham KB, Walker H, Lynch CD, et al. Preterm birth rates in a prematurity prevention clinic after adoption of progestin prophylaxis. *Obstet Gynecol*. 2014;123(1):34-39.

69. Nygren P, Fu R, Freeman M, et al. Evidence on the benefits and harms of screening and treating pregnant women who are asymptomatic for bacterial vaginosis: an update review for the U.S. Preventive Services Task Force. *Ann Intern Med*. 2008;148:220.

70. Keirse MJ. Progestogen administration in pregnancy may prevent preterm delivery. *Br J Obstet Gynaecol*. 1990;97:149.

71. da Fonseca EB, Bittar RE, Carvalho MH, et al. Prophylactic administration of progesterone by vaginal suppository to reduce the incidence of spontaneous preterm birth in women at increased risk: a randomized placebo-controlled double-blind study. *Am J Obstet Gynecol*. 2003;188:419.

72. Meis PJ, Klebanoff M, Thom E, et al. Prevention of recurrent preterm delivery by 17-alpha-hydroxyprogesterone caproate. *N Engl J Med*. 2003;348:2379.

73. Rouse DJ, Caritis SN, Peaceman AM, et al. A trial of 17 alpha-hydroxyprogesterone caproate to prevent prematurity in twins. *N Engl J Med*. 2007;357:454.

74. Combs CA, Garite T, Maurel K, et al. 17-hydroxyprogesterone caproate for twin pregnancy: a double-blind, randomized clinical trial. *Am J Obstet Gynecol*. 2011;204:e221.

75. Caritis SN, Rouse DJ, Peaceman AM, et al. Prevention of preterm birth in triplets using 17 alpha-hydroxyprogesterone caproate: a randomized controlled trial. *Obstet Gynecol*. 2009;113:285.

76. Combs CA, Garite T, Maurel K, et al. Failure of 17-hydroxyprogesterone to reduce neonatal morbidity or prolong triplet pregnancy: a double-blind, randomized clinical trial. *Am J Obstet Gynecol*. 2010;203:248.e1. Erratum in Am J Obstet Gynecol 204:166, 2011.

77. Cahill AG, Odibo AO, Caughey AB, et al. Universal cervical length screening and treatment with vaginal progesterone to prevent preterm birth: a decision and economic analysis. *Am J Obstet Gynecol*. 2010;202:548.e1.

78. Werner EF, Han CS, Pettker CM, et al. Universal cervical-length screening to prevent preterm birth: a cost-effectiveness analysis. *Ultrasound Obstet Gynecol*. 2011;38:32.

79. Campbell S. Universal cervical-length screening and vaginal progesterone prevents early preterm births, reduces neonatal morbidity and is cost saving: doing nothing is no longer an option. *Ultrasound Obstet Gynecol*. 2011;38:1.

80. Owen J, Hankins G, Iams JD, et al. Multicenter randomized trial of cerclage for preterm birth prevention in high-risk women with shortened midtrimester cervical length. *Am J Obstet Gynecol*. 2009;201:375.e1.

81. Berghella V, Rafael TJ, Szychowski JM, et al. Cerclage for short cervix on ultrasonography in women with singleton gestations and previous preterm birth: a meta-analysis. *Obstet Gynecol*. 2011;117:663.

82. Berghella V, Odibo AO, To MS, et al. Cerclage for short cervix on ultrasonography: meta-analysis of trials using individual patient-level data. *Obstet Gynecol*. 2005;106:181.

83. Jorgensen AL, Alfirevic Z, Tudur Smith C, et al. Cervical stitch (cerclage) for preventing pregnancy loss: individual patient data meta-analysis. *Br J Obstet Gynaecol*. 2007;114:1460.

84. Iams JD, Berghella V. Care for women with prior preterm birth. *Am J Obstet Gynecol*. 2010;203:89.

85. Reddy UM, Ko CW, Raju TN, Willinger M. Delivery indications at late-preterm gestations and infant mortality rates in the United States. *Pediatrics*. 2009;124:234.

86. Laughon SK, Reddy UM, Sun L, et al. Precursors for late preterm birth in singleton gestations. *Obstet Gynecol*. 2010;116:1047.

87. Spong CY, Mercer BM, D'Alton M, et al. Timing of indicated late-preterm and early-term birth. *Obstet Gynecol*. 2011;118:323.

88. Bryant AS, Worjoloh A, Caughey AB, Washington AE. Racial/ethnic disparities in obstetric outcomes and care: prevalence and determinants. *Am J Obstet Gynecol*. 2010;202:335.

Additional references for this chapter are available at ExpertConsult.com.

CHAPTER 30

Premature Rupture of the Membranes

BRIAN M. MERCER

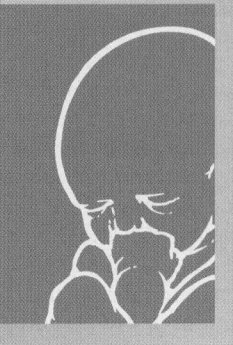

KEY ABBREVIATIONS

By mouth (per os)	PO
Confidence interval	CI
Fetal fibronectin	fFN
Group B *Streptococcus*	GBS
Herpes simplex virus	HSV
Human immunodeficiency virus	HIV
Insulin-like growth factor–binding protein 1	IGFBP-1
Intramuscular	IM
Intravenous	IV
Intraventricular hemorrhage	IVH
Lamellar body count	LBC
Maternal-Fetal Medicine Unit	MFMU
Matrix metalloproteinase	MMP
National Institute of Child Health and Human Development	NICHD
Neonatal intensive care unit	NICU
Odds ratio	OR
Periventricular leukomalacia	PVL
Phosphatidylglycerol	PG
Placental α-microglobulin 1	PAMG-1
Premature rupture of the membranes	PROM
Respiratory distress syndrome	RDS
Tissue inhibitors of matrix metalloproteinase	TIMP
U.S. Food and Drug Administration	FDA

Membrane rupture that occurs spontaneously before the onset of labor is described as premature rupture of the membranes (PROM) regardless of the gestational age at which it occurs. PROM complicates about 8% to 10% of pregnancies. Preterm PROM that occurs before 37 weeks' gestation affects about 1% of deliveries overall, and birth certificate data suggest that it is over twofold more common in blacks.[1] Like preterm labor and cervical insufficiency, PROM is considered a cause of spontaneous preterm birth. The relative contribution of PROM to prematurity appears to vary greatly among patient populations, affecting about 10% of preterm births in national databases but over 20% in certain high-risk populations. Its frequency appears to have declined during the past decade.[2-5]

PROM at any gestational age is associated with brief latency from membrane rupture to delivery and also increased risks for perinatal infection and umbilical cord compression due to oligohydramnios. Because of this, term and preterm PROM are significant causes of perinatal morbidity and mortality. When PROM occurs at term, the risk is low for severe neonatal complications with delivery of a noninfected and nonasphyxiated infant. Clinical management should be directed toward delivery. Although complications can occur, delivery at 32 to 36 weeks' gestation is generally associated with good infant outcomes, particularly if the fetus has documented pulmonary maturity. Given the risks of continued pregnancy and anticipated brief latency, delivery of the mature fetus is generally warranted, particularly at 34 weeks' gestation or later. At 32 to 33 weeks' gestation, the immature fetus may benefit from measures to accelerate fetal maturation and to prolong the pregnancy. With immediate delivery after preterm PROM at 23 to 31 weeks' gestation, the risk is significant for newborn complications that can be reduced through adequate delay of delivery. In the absence of contraindications, management is directed toward continuing the pregnancy with attention to potential complications that include umbilical cord compression, intrauterine infection, and abruptio placentae. When PROM occurs before the limit of viability, newborn death is inevitable with immediate delivery. Although conservative management may still result in a previable delivery, some women will benefit from extended latency with delivery of a potentially viable infant. **Regardless of the gestational age, the patient should be well informed regarding the potential maternal, fetal, and neonatal complications of PROM and preterm birth.** These issues are discussed in detail in this chapter.

FETAL MEMBRANE ANATOMY AND PHYSIOLOGY

The fetus develops within the amniotic sac, which is surrounded like a balloon by the fetal membranes. These membranes consist of a thin amnion layer that lines the amniotic cavity and a thicker outer chorion directly apposed to the maternal decidua. The amnion fuses to the chorion near the end of the first trimester of pregnancy, and these layers are subsequently attached by a collagen-rich connective tissue zone. For the remainder of the pregnancy, the fetal membranes include a single cuboidal amnion epithelium with subjacent compact and spongy connective tissue layers and a thicker chorion that consists of reticular and trophoblastic layers. Together, the amnion and chorion are stronger than either layer independently; individually, the amnion has greater tensile strength than the chorion.

As the pregnancy progresses, changes in collagen content and type, intercellular matrix, and cellular apoptosis result in structural weakening of the fetal membranes. Membrane remodeling is more evident near the internal cervical os and can be stimulated by thrombin-mediated increases in matrix metalloproteinases (e.g., MMP-1, MMP-2, MMP-9) and decreased levels of tissue inhibitors of matrix metalloproteinases (e.g., TIMP-1, TIMP-3) within the membranes, as well as increased poly (ADP-ribose) polymerase (PARP) cleavage.[6-8] Contractions subject the amniochorionic membranes to additional physical strain that can lead to membrane rupture. Should the fetal membranes not rupture before labor, advancing cervical dilation decreases the work needed to cause membrane rupture over the internal cervical os. **Preterm PROM likely results from a variety of factors that ultimately lead to accelerated membrane weakening through an increase in local cytokines and an imbalance in the interaction between MMPs and TIMPs, increased collagenase and protease activity, or other factors that cause increased intrauterine pressure** (e.g., polyhydramnios).[5-9]

ETIOLOGY OF PREMATURE RUPTURE OF THE MEMBRANES

A number of risk factors have been associated with the occurrence of preterm PROM. Among these are low socioeconomic status, uterine overdistension, second- and third-trimester bleeding, low body mass index (BMI), nutritional deficiencies of copper and ascorbic acid, maternal cigarette smoking, cervical conization or cerclage, pulmonary disease in pregnancy, connective tissue disorders (e.g., Ehlers-Danlos syndrome), and preterm labor or symptomatic contractions in the current gestation. Each risk factor, individually or in concert, could lead to PROM through the mechanisms outlined above. However, the ultimate

clinical cause of membrane rupture is often not apparent, and many at-risk patients will deliver at term without PROM.

Preterm PROM has also been linked to infections that involve the urogenital tract. *Neisseria gonorrhoeae, Chlamydia trachomatis,* and *Trichomonas vaginalis* have each been associated with preterm PROM.[10] Although *vaginal* group B β-hemolytic *Streptococcus* (GBS) colonization does not appear to be associated with preterm PROM, *cervical* colonization may be. **GBS bacteriuria is associated with preterm PROM and low-birth-weight infants.**[11,12] Although bacterial vaginosis has been linked to spontaneous preterm births, including preterm PROM, it is unclear whether bacterial vaginosis is the inciting condition that facilitates ascent of other bacteria to the upper genital tract, or whether it is simply a marker of maternal susceptibility to abnormal genital tract colonization.[13] Bacterial invasion can facilitate membrane rupture through direct release of proteases and also through stimulation of a host inflammatory response that results in the elaboration of local cytokines, MMPs, and prostaglandins. Histologic studies of the membranes after preterm PROM often demonstrate significant bacterial contamination along the choriodecidual interface with minimal involvement of the amnion.[14] Further evidence that links preterm PROM and genital tract infection is that these women have a high incidence of positive amniotic fluid cultures (25% to 35%) even in the absence of clinically suspected intrauterine infection.[15,16] Although some of these findings may reflect ascending infection subsequent to membrane rupture, it is probable that **ascending bacterial colonization and infection are integral to the pathogenesis of preterm PROM in many cases.**

Although the onset of vaginal fluid leakage is an acute event, evidence shows that the factors and events that lead to membrane rupture are sometimes subacute or even chronic. Women with a prior preterm birth (PTB), especially because of PROM, are at increased risk for PTB due to PROM in future pregnancies. Studies have also suggested associations exist between maternal inflammatory proteins, genotype, and spontaneous preterm birth (sPTB) due to preterm labor or PROM.[17,18] Further, asymptomatic women with a short cervical length in the second trimester are at increased risk for preterm PROM occurring many weeks later.[19]

PREDICTION AND PREVENTION OF PRETERM PREMATURE RUPTURE OF THE MEMBRANES

Once preterm PROM occurs, delivery is often required or inevitable. Optimally, prevention of PROM would offer the best opportunity to avoid its complications. **Prior PTB and especially prior preterm PROM (PPROM) have been associated with PPROM in a subsequent pregnancy.**[20] **The risk of recurrence increases with decreasing gestational age of the index PTB.** Those with a prior delivery near the limit of viability (23 to 27 weeks) have a 27.1% risk of subsequent PTB. Those with a prior history of PTB due to PROM have a 3.3-fold higher risk for PTB due to PROM (13.5% vs. 4.1%) and a 13.5-fold higher risk for PPROM before 28 weeks' gestation (1.8% vs. 0.13%) in a subsequent pregnancy (*P* < .01 for each). In an analysis from a prospective evaluation of PTB prediction, nulliparas and women with prior deliveries were evaluated separately because those without a prior birth lacked important historic information available to those with a prior term or preterm birth.[19] In that study, multivariable analysis revealed medical complications (including pulmonary disease in pregnancy), work during pregnancy, recent symptomatic uterine contractions, and bacterial vaginosis to be significant markers for subsequent PTB in nulliparas when assessed at 22 to 24 weeks' gestation (Table 30-1). **Among women with prior deliveries, prior PTB due to preterm labor or PROM and a positive cervicovaginal fetal fibronectin (fFN) screen were statistically significant clinical markers for subsequent PPROM after controlling for other factors.** Short cervical length (<25 mm) identified by transvaginal ultrasound and low maternal BMI (<19.8 kg/m^2) were associated with an increased risk for subsequent PROM in both nulliparas and multiparas. Nulliparas with a positive cervicovaginal fFN and a short cervix had a 16.7% risk for PTB due to PPROM. **Among multiparas, women with a prior PTB due to PROM, a short cervix on ultrasound, and positive cervicovaginal fFN screen had a 31-fold higher risk for PROM with delivery before 35 weeks' gestation (25% vs. 2.3%) than those without risk factors** (Table 30-2).

TABLE 30-1   MARKERS FOR PRETERM PREMATURE RUPTURE OF MEMBRANES BEFORE 37 WEEKS' GESTATION*

	NULLIPARAS (N = 1618)	MULTIPARAS (N = 1711)
Medical complications	3.7 (1.5-9.0)	—
Work in pregnancy	3.0 (1.5-6.1)	—
Symptomatic contractions within 2 weeks	2.2 (1.2-7.5)	—
Bacterial vaginosis	2.1 (1.1-4.1)	—
Low BMI (<19.8 kg/m^2)	2.0 (1.0-4.0)	1.8 (1.1-3.0)
Prior preterm birth due to PROM	—	3.1 (1.8-5.4)
Prior preterm birth due to preterm labor	—	1.8 (1.1-3.1)
Cervix <25 mm	3.7 (1.8-7.7)	2.5 (1.4-4.5)
Positive fetal fibronectin	—	2.1 (1.1-4.0)

Modified from Mercer BM, Goldenberg RL, Meis PJ, et al, for the NICHD-MFMU Network. The preterm prediction study: prediction of preterm premature rupture of the membranes using clinical findings and ancillary testing. *Am J Obstet Gynecol.* 2000;183:738.
*Results of multivariable analyses for nulliparas and multiparas (presented as odds ratios with 95% confidence intervals).
BMI, body mass index; *PROM,* premature rupture of the membranes.

TABLE 30-2   RISK FOR PRETERM BIRTH DUE TO PREMATURE RUPTURE OF THE MEMBRANES AMONG MULTIPARAS

	N	<37 WEEKS (%)	<35 WEEKS (%)
All multiparas	1711	5.0	2.3
No risk factors present	1351	3.2	0.8
Prior preterm birth due to PROM only	124	10.5	4.8
Prior preterm birth due to PROM and positive fFN*	13	15.4	15.4
Prior preterm birth due to PROM and short cervix†	26	23.1	15.4
All three risk factors present	8	25.0	25.0

Modified from Mercer BM, Goldenberg RL, Meis PJ, et al, for the NICHD-MFMU Network. The preterm prediction study: prediction of preterm premature rupture of the membranes using clinical findings and ancillary testing. *Am J Obstet Gynecol.* 2000;183:738.
*Positive fFN, cervicovaginal fFN screen positive (>50 ng/mL) at 22 to 24 weeks' gestation.
†Short cervix, cervix length <25 mm on transvaginal ultrasound at 22 to 24 weeks' gestation.
fFN, fetal fibronectin; *PROM,* premature rupture of the membranes.

Unfortunately, clinical risk-assessment systems identify only a small fraction of women who will ultimately deliver preterm. Although clinical and ancillary testing has increased our ability to identify women at increased risk because of potentially modifiable factors—such as cigarette smoking, poor nutrition, urinary tract and sexually transmitted infections, pulmonary disease, and severe polyhydramnios—it is unknown whether modification of these in a given patient will reduce the risk for PROM. Regardless, women at risk for PTB due to PROM based on clinical findings can be counseled regarding the symptoms of membrane rupture and contractions and can be encouraged to seek medical care should symptoms occur. Regarding ancillary testing, progesterone therapy has been recommended for prevention of PTB in asymptomatic women with a short cervix, and thus cervical length (CL) screening has potential value for both predictive and therapeutic reasons.[21] Alternatively, routine fFN screening has similar predictive value to CL measurement, but no effective intervention can be offered based on the results. Thus routine fFN testing after PTB due to PROM is not recommended. **Current evidence supports 17-α-hydroxyprogesterone caproate (17-P) treatment for women with a prior PTB due to PROM or preterm labor and also supports treatment with vaginal progesterone for asymptomatic women with a short cervical length.**[21-23] Data regarding the value of vitamin C supplementation in preventing PROM are conflicting and are not generally supportive. In one study, such treatment was associated with a lower risk (7.7% vs. 24.5%; $P = .02$).[24] Secondary analysis of another study suggested that treatment with vitamin C and E did not reduce sPTB or late preterm birth due to PROM but was associated with less frequent PTB due to PROM before 32 weeks' gestation.[25] However, a review of studies in which vitamin C was given alone or in combination with other supplements suggests a negative impact on membrane strength and an increased risk for PTB.[26,27] **Because of these findings, vitamin C supplementation to prevent PPROM is not currently recommended.**

CLINICAL COURSE AFTER PREMATURE RUPTURE OF THE MEMBRANES
Maternal Risks
Hallmarks of PROM include a brief latency from membrane rupture to delivery. On average, latency increases with decreasing gestational age at membrane rupture. At term, half of expectantly managed gravidas deliver within 5 hours and 95% deliver within 28 hours of membrane rupture.[28] **Of all women with PROM before 34 weeks, 93% deliver in less than 1 week.** After excluding those who require delivery soon after admission, 50% to 60% of those conservatively managed and treated with antibiotics for pregnancy prolongation will deliver within 1 week of membrane rupture.[29] Only a small proportion of women with membrane rupture (≤5%) can anticipate cessation of fluid leakage. About 86% of those with leakage after amniocentesis will reseal.[30,31]

RISKS OF PREMATURE RUPTURE OF THE MEMBRANES
Maternal Risks
Chorioamnionitis is the most common maternal complication after PPROM. This risk increases as the duration of membrane rupture becomes more prolonged and decreases with

advancing gestational age at PROM.[32] The risks of chorioamnionitis and endometritis increase with decreasing gestational age at PROM and also in different patient populations (13% to 60% for chorioamnionitis and 2% to 13%, for endometritis).[33,34] **Abruptio placentae can cause PROM or can occur subsequent to membrane rupture, and it affects 4% to 12% of these pregnancies.[35] Uncommon but serious complications of PROM managed conservatively near the limit of viability include retained placenta and hemorrhage, requiring dilation and curettage (12%); maternal sepsis (0.8%); and maternal death (0.14%).[36]**

Fetal and Neonatal Risks

Fetal complications after membrane rupture include infection and fetal distress due to umbilical cord compression or placental abruption. Umbilical cord compression due to oligohydramnios is not uncommon after PROM. Frank or occult umbilical cord prolapse can also occur, particularly with fetal malpresentation. Because of these factors, women with PROM have a higher risk for cesarean delivery for nonreassuring fetal heart rate (FHR) patterns than those with isolated preterm labor (7.9% vs. 1.5%). **Fetal death complicates 1% to 2% of cases of conservatively managed PROM.[29]**

The frequency and severity of neonatal complications after PROM vary inversely with gestational age at membrane rupture and at delivery. Respiratory distress syndrome (RDS) is the most common serious newborn complication after PPROM at any gestational age. Necrotizing enterocolitis (NEC), intraventricular hemorrhage (IVH), and sepsis are common with early PTB but are relatively uncommon when PPROM and delivery occur near term. Serious perinatal morbidities with delivery remote from term can lead to long-term sequelae such as chronic lung disease (CLD), visual or hearing difficulties, intellectual disabilities, developmental and motor delay, cerebral palsy, and death. Although specific data are not available for those who deliver after PPROM, general community-based survival and morbidity data suggest that long-term morbidities and death are uncommon with delivery after about 32 weeks' gestation.[37] It is controversial whether gestational age–specific mortality is increased for preterm infants who deliver after PPROM.[38,39]

PPROM increases the risk of neonatal sepsis twofold over that seen after PTB due to preterm labor with intact membranes.[40] Neonatal infection can result from the same organisms present in the amniotic fluid, or from others, and it can present as acute congenital pneumonia, sepsis, or meningitis. Late-onset bacterial or fungal infections can also occur. Accumulating evidence suggests that fetal and neonatal infection and inflammation are associated with an increased risk for long-term neurologic complications. Cerebral palsy and cystic periventricular leukomalacia (PVL), as well as cognitive impairment and death and neurodevelopmental impairment in extremely preterm infants, have been linked to chorioamnionitis, which is more commonly seen after PPROM and is more likely with conservative management after membrane rupture.[41,42] Elevated amniotic fluid cytokines and fetal systemic inflammation have also been associated with PPROM, PVL, and cerebral palsy.[43] **Although no data suggest that immediate delivery on admission with PROM will avert these sequelae, these findings highlight the importance of restricting conservative management after PROM to circumstances in which there is the potential to reduce neonatal morbidity through either antenatal corticosteroid** administration or extended pregnancy prolongation for fetal maturation.

Pulmonary hypoplasia is a severe complication of oligohydramnios in the second trimester that results from a lack of terminal bronchiole and alveolar development during the canalicular phase of pulmonary development.[44] It is most accurately diagnosed pathologically using radial alveolar counts and lung weights.[45] Clinical findings, such as a small chest circumference with severe respiratory distress and persistent pulmonary hypertension in the newborn, and radiographic findings—small, well-aerated lungs with a bell-shaped chest and elevation of the diaphragm—are also supportive of the diagnosis. Whether because of fluid efflux and tracheobronchial collapse after membrane rupture or through loss of intrinsic factors within the tracheobronchial fluid, pulmonary hypoplasia develops over weeks after membrane rupture. Pulmonary hypoplasia complicated an average of about 6% of cases in series of midtrimester PROM and carries a 70% mortality rate.[46] Its incidence is inversely correlated with gestational age at membrane rupture, and it complicates nearly 50% of cases with membrane rupture before 19 weeks and prolonged latency.[44,47] The frequency of pulmonary hypoplasia can be as high as 74% to 82% with PROM at 15 to 16 weeks, persistent oligohydramnios, and a latency of 28 days.[48] Lethal pulmonary hypoplasia rarely occurs with PROM after 26 weeks' gestation (0% to 1.4%).[49] However, other pulmonary complications such as pneumothorax and pneumomediastinum related to poor pulmonary compliance and high ventilatory pressures can occur with lesser degrees of this condition. Restriction deformities occur in about 1.5% of infants delivered after conservative management after midtrimester PROM but complicate up to 27% of fetuses with prolonged oligohydramnios.[36,50]

DIAGNOSIS OF PREMATURE RUPTURE OF THE MEMBRANES

The diagnosis of PROM involves clinical history and physical examination as well as laboratory evaluation in some cases. **The diagnosis of membrane rupture is confirmed by the presence of the following findings:**

- Visualization of amniotic fluid passing from the cervical canal *or*
- Vaginal sidewall or posterior fornix pH of more than 6.0 to 6.5 *and*
- Microscopic arborized crystals ("ferning"), owing to the interaction of amniotic fluid proteins and salts, from dried vaginal secretions obtained by swabbing the posterior fornix with a sterile swab.

False-positive pH results may occur with blood or semen contamination, alkaline antiseptics, or bacterial vaginosis. Cervical mucus can yield a false-positive ferning pattern; however, the crystals appear as more of a floral pattern. The fern pattern in samples heavily contaminated with blood is atypical and appears more "skeletonized." Prolonged leakage with minimal residual fluid can result in a false-negative result on visual inspection or pH or ferning testing. If the diagnosis is equivocal after initial testing, the patient can be placed in a Trendelenburg position and reexamined after a few hours. The diagnosis of membrane rupture can be made unequivocally by ultrasound-guided dye amnioinfusion (1 mL indigo carmine plus 9 mL sterile saline), followed by observation for passage of dye onto a perineal pad. **Although oligohydramnios without evident fetal urinary** tract malformations or fetal growth restriction may be suggestive of membrane rupture, ultrasound alone is not definitive.

Noninvasive cervicovaginal markers such as fFN, alpha-fetoprotein, prolactin, human chorionic gonadotropin (hCG), placental α-microglobulin 1 (PAMG-1), and insulin-like growth factor–binding protein 1 (IGFBP-1) have been studied for their ability to confirm or exclude membrane rupture, but most are unavailable for clinical use. Such testing is unneeded when the diagnosis is confirmed clinically. Further, although membrane rupture can be confirmed by the presence of PAMG-1 in cervicovaginal secretions, and the test's accuracy is relatively unaffected by the presence of blood,[51] it has also been found to be present in nearly one third of laboring women and in 1 of 20 nonlaboring women without suspected membrane rupture.[52]

MANAGEMENT OF PREMATURE RUPTURE OF THE MEMBRANES

General Considerations

Management of PROM is based primarily on an individual assessment of the estimated risk for fetal and neonatal complications should conservative management or delivery be pursued. The risks for maternal morbidity should also be considered, particularly when PROM occurs before the limit of potential viability (currently 23 weeks' gestational age). Regional factors may impact the potential risks and benefits of conservative management. In populations where the risk of intrauterine infection is high and the potential for extended latency without complications is low, the focus will tend to be on acceleration of fetal maturation, prevention of intrauterine infection, and delivery if fetal benefit from prolonged latency is not anticipated. Alternatively, in populations at low risk for intrauterine infection and with higher potential for prolonged latency, conservative management may be appropriate at a more advanced gestational age.

The diagnosis of membrane rupture is confirmed and the duration of membrane rupture is determined to assist the pediatric caregivers with subsequent management decisions. The patient is assessed for fetal presentation, contractions, findings suggestive of intrauterine infection, and evidence of fetal well-being. GBS carriage is ascertained, if available, from a recent anovaginal culture performed within the previous 5 weeks.

In general, digital cervical examinations should be avoided until it is determined that delivery is inevitable because such examination has been associated with a shortening of latency from membrane rupture to delivery.[53] Visualization of the cervix during a sterile speculum examination offers helpful information regarding cervical dilation and effacement. Brown and colleagues[54] found visual estimation to be within 1 cm of digitally determined cervical dilation in 64% and within 2 cm in 84% of examinations, whereas visually estimated cervical effacement was within 1 cm in 83% of cases. In addition to providing confirmatory evidence of membrane rupture, sterile speculum examination can provide the opportunity to inspect for cervicitis and to obtain appropriate cervical and vaginal cultures.

The benefit of narrow-spectrum intrapartum prophylaxis with intravenous (IV) penicillin G (5 million U and then 2.5 to 3 million U every 4 hr) or ampicillin (2 g IV, then 1 g IV every 4 hr) to prevent vertical transmission and early-onset neonatal

GBS sepsis from maternal GBS carriers has been well established, and the Centers for Disease Control and Prevention (CDC) published a revised guideline for the prevention of perinatal group B streptococcal disease in November 2010.[55,56] Current indications for intrapartum GBS prophylaxis and alternative antibiotic regimens for those with a penicillin allergy are discussed in Chapter 54. Known GBS carriers with PROM at any gestation and those with PPROM and unknown GBS status should receive intrapartum prophylaxis regardless of prior antibiotic treatment. GBS carriers with PROM and chorioamnionitis should receive broad-spectrum intrapartum antibiotic therapy, including agents effective against GBS. If chorioamnionitis is not suspected clinically and there is a recent negative anovaginal culture for GBS, intrapartum antibiotics should not be administered because of the potential for selection of resistant organisms should neonatal sepsis occur.[57]

Although practice varies regarding the management of PPROM, general consensus has been reached in regard to some issues. Gestational age should be established based on clinical history and earliest ultrasound assessment where available (Fig. 30-1). Ultrasound should be performed to assess fetal growth and position, residual amniotic fluid volume, and gross fetal abnormalities that might cause polyhydramnios and PROM. Those with advanced labor, intrauterine infection, significant vaginal bleeding, or nonreassuring fetal testing are best delivered. **If conservative management of PPROM is to be pursued, the patient should be admitted to a facility capable of providing emergent delivery for placental abruption, fetal malpresentation in labor, and fetal distress due to umbilical cord compression or in utero infection. The facility should also be capable of providing 24-hour neonatal resuscitation and intensive care because conservative management should generally be performed only when significant risk for neonatal morbidity and mortality is present.** If the need for transfer to a tertiary care facility is anticipated, this should occur early in the course of management to avoid emergent transfer once delivery is imminent or complications arise.

Management of Premature Rupture of the Membranes at Term

Despite some past controversy, studies have found that induction with oxytocin after PROM at term does not increase the risks for perinatal infection or cesarean delivery.[28,58-61] In fact, the largest prospective study to date has found that oxytocin induction after PROM at term reduces the duration of membrane rupture after PROM (median, 17.2 vs. 33.3 hr), and the frequencies of chorioamnionitis (4% vs. 8.6%) and postpartum fever (1.9% vs. 3.6%; $P \leq .008$ for each), without increasing cesarean deliveries (13.7% vs. 14.1%) or neonatal infections (2% vs. 2.8%).[28] An additional benefit of early oxytocin induction in this trial was a reduction in neonatal antibiotic therapy (7.5% vs. 13.7%; $P < .001$). Meta-analysis of 12 studies that comprised a total of 6814 women and studied early delivery versus expectant management for PROM at term confirmed less frequent chorioamnionitis and endometritis with planned delivery, with no increases in caesarean delivery or neonatal infection.[62] Fewer infants in the early delivery group required neonatal intensive care unit (NICU) or special care admission. Analysis of studies of prostaglandin versus oxytocin induction after PROM at or near term found increased chorioamnionitis (odds ratio [OR], 1.51; 95% confidence interval [CI], 1.07 to 2.12), neonatal infection (OR, 1.63; 95% CI, 1 to 2.66), and a

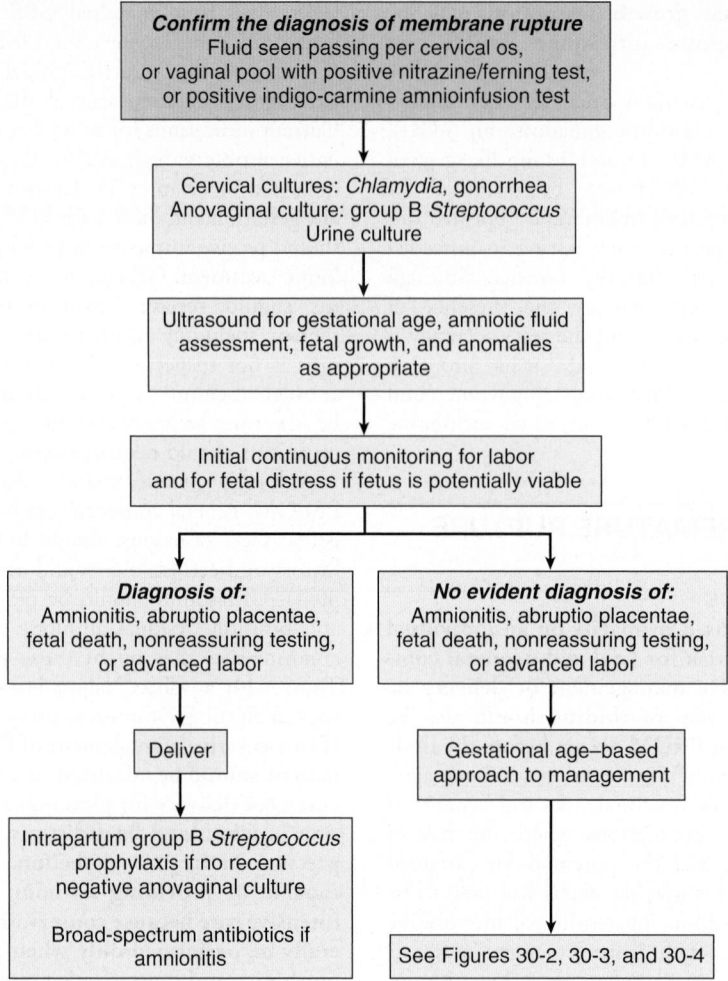

Confirm the diagnosis of membrane rupture
Fluid seen passing per cervical os,
or vaginal pool with positive nitrazine/ferning test,
or positive indigo-carmine amnioinfusion test

Cervical cultures: *Chlamydia*, gonorrhea
Anovaginal culture: group B *Streptococcus*
Urine culture

Ultrasound for gestational age, amniotic fluid
assessment, fetal growth, and anomalies
as appropriate

Initial continuous monitoring for labor
and for fetal distress if fetus is potentially viable

Diagnosis of:
Amnionitis, abruptio placentae,
fetal death, nonreassuring testing,
or advanced labor

No evident diagnosis of:
Amnionitis, abruptio placentae,
fetal death, nonreassuring testing,
or advanced labor

Deliver

Gestational age–based
approach to management

Intrapartum group B *Streptococcus*
prophylaxis if no recent
negative anovaginal culture

Broad-spectrum antibiotics if
amnionitis

See Figures 30-2, 30-3, and 30-4

FIG 30-1 Initial assessment and management of women with preterm premature rupture of the membranes. (From Mercer BM. Preterm premature rupture of the membranes: diagnosis and management. *Clin Perinatol.* 2004;31:765.)

prolonged NICU stay (OR, 1.43; 95% CI, 1.07 to 1.91) without improvement in cesarean delivery rates (OR, 0.92; 95% CI, 0.73 to 1.16) with prostaglandin treatment.[63] This meta-analysis was dominated by the TermPROM trial,[28] which found shorter latency from membrane rupture to delivery with oxytocin than with prostaglandin therapy (median, 17.2 vs. 23 hours; P <.001). Taken together, these data suggest that **women with PROM at term should be offered early delivery, generally with a continuous oxytocin infusion, to reduce the risk for maternal and neonatal complications.** Adequate time for latent phase of labor should be allowed. During labor, transcervical amnioinfusion of warm normal saline solution may prove useful if significant umbilical cord compression is suspected and immediate delivery is not required.[64,65]

Management of Preterm Premature Rupture of the Membranes Near Term (32 to 36 Weeks)

Severe acute newborn complications are uncommon when preterm birth occurs between 34 and 36 weeks' gestation. Antenatal corticosteroids for fetal maturation and magnesium sulfate for fetal/neonatal neuroprotection are not usually administered in this gestational age range.[37] Alternatively, **conservative**

management after PROM at 34 to 36 weeks' gestation only briefly prolongs pregnancy while increasing the likelihood of chorioamnionitis (16% vs. 2%; P = .001) without preventing neonatal complications.[66,67] A recent multicenter study regarding this issue suggested conservative management of women without GBS colonization to be preferable because newborn complications were not reduced with early delivery after PROM at 34 to 37 weeks' of gestation.[68,69] Whereas chorioamnionitis was twofold more common (5.6% vs. 2.3%, P = .045), conservative management was associated with less frequent newborn hypoglycemia and hyperbilirubinemia. **As such, conservative management of PROM that occurs at 34 to 37 weeks might be an option if the risk of intrauterine infection is considered to be low.**

Management of the woman with PROM at 32 to 33 weeks' gestation is more controversial because pulmonary and other gestational age–dependent complications can occur, but the likelihood of survival at this gestation is high and long-term complications are uncommon. Neerhoff and colleagues[67] found modest benefits in the duration of newborn hospital stay and the frequency of hyperbilirubinemia with conservative management at 32 to 33 weeks' gestation. Alternatively, two prospective trials that compared early delivery and conservative management of PROM near term have provided useful

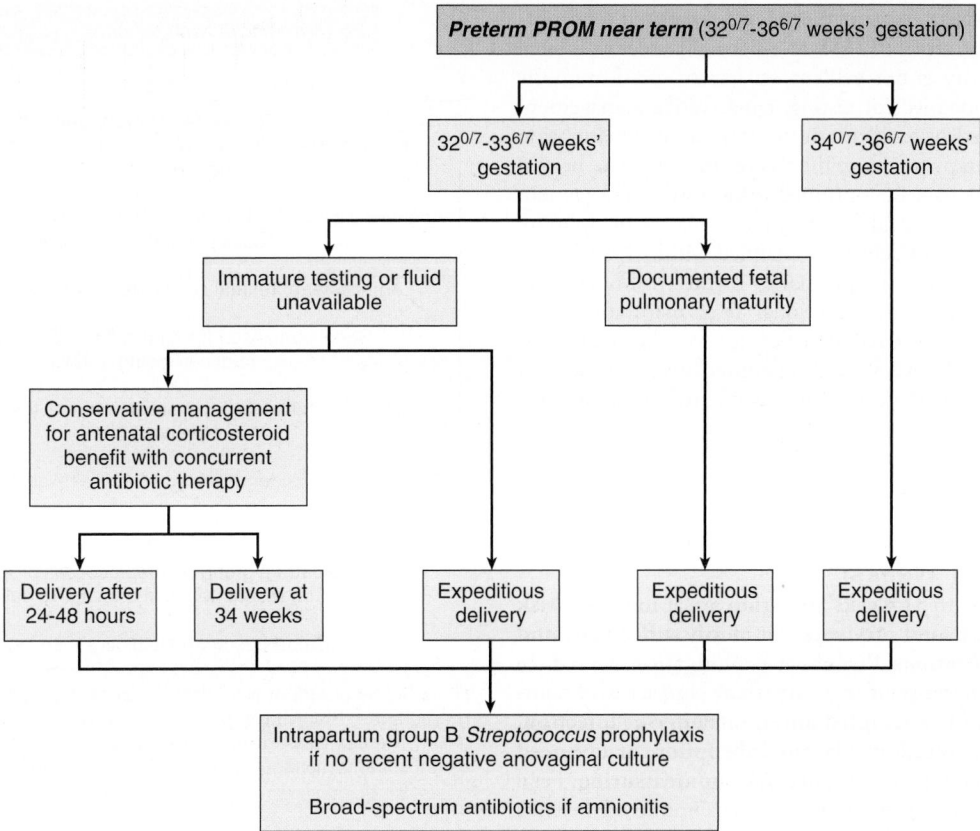

FIG 30-2 Management algorithm for preterm premature rupture of the membranes (PROM) near term (32 to 36 weeks' gestation). (From Mercer BM: Preterm premature rupture of the membranes: diagnosis and management. *Clin Perinatol.* 2004;31:765.)

insights. Cox and coworkers found conservative management of PROM at 30 to 33⁶ᐟ⁷ weeks' gestation to increase latency only briefly (59% vs. 100% delivered within 48 hr; $P < .001$).[70] In a study of PROM at 32 to 36⁶ᐟ⁷ weeks' gestation, Mercer and colleagues[71] observed only a 24-hour increase in latency with conservative management (36 vs. 14 hours; $P < .001$). However, both studies noted that conservative management increased the risk for chorioamnionitis (15% vs. 2%, $P = .009$ and 27.7% vs. 10.9%, $P = .06$, respectively) without evident reductions in newborn complications. Secondary analysis of those with PROM at 32 to 33⁶ᐟ⁷ weeks' gestation in the latter trial revealed similar trends regarding latency, infection, and infant morbidities.[72] The potential for umbilical cord compression during conservative management of PROM is highlighted by one stillbirth and the high incidence of nonreassuring FHR patterns found on intermittent monitoring in these studies.[70,71]

At 32 to 33 weeks' gestation, it can be helpful to assess fetal pulmonary maturity and to treat with antenatal corticosteroids those pregnancies without documented fetal maturity. Either vaginal pool or amniocentesis specimens can be used for testing. Because of the increased potential for inadvertent fetal or umbilical cord puncture during amniocentesis when the amniotic fluid volume is decreased, **vaginal pool specimen collection is preferable if an adequate specimen can be obtained.** If amniocentesis is required, color Doppler imaging can be helpful in differentiating umbilical cord loops from a small residual fluid pocket. Pulmonary phospholipids are not present in lavage fluid from the vagina when the membranes are intact.[73] Studies of women with ruptured membranes have found a high concordance rate (89% to 100%) between specimens collected vaginally and by amniocentesis for pulmonary phospholipids such as lecithin, phosphatidylglycerol (PG), phosphatidylinositol, phosphatidylethanolamine, and phosphatidylserine.[74] Lewis and associates[75] found no cases of RDS among infants delivered after a mature PG result from vaginal pool fluid. Similarly, in a study of vaginally collected samples, Russell and associates[76] found no cases of RDS after a mature lecithin-to-sphingomyelin (L/S) ratio or PG result. The presence of PG on perineal pad–collected fluid is predictive of fetal pulmonary maturity (97.8%), and its absence is predictive of pulmonary immaturity (33.7%).[77] The lamellar body count (LBC; ≥50,000 is considered mature) may be performed from vaginally collected amniotic fluid specimens and has been shown by some to have a high predictive value for fetal pulmonary maturity.[78] Amniotic fluid pulmonary maturity testing can be confounded by the presence of contaminants such as blood and meconium (see Chapter 11). Realistically, delivery should be considered if significant blood or meconium is present in a vaginal pool or an amniocentesis specimen after PROM.

Based on the available data, early delivery should be pursued when PROM occurs at 34 to 36 weeks' gestation (Fig. 30-2). The infant delivered after PROM at 30 to 33 weeks' gestation is at risk for infectious and other gestational age–dependent morbidities, but evidence of fetal pulmonary maturity at 32 to 33⁶ᐟ⁷ weeks' gestation suggests a low risk for complications with immediate delivery. Because of the increased risk for infectious morbidity and potential for occult umbilical cord compression with conservative management, **delivery should be initiated** before complications ensue if there is documented fetal pulmonary maturity after PROM at 32 to 33 weeks. If fetal pulmonary maturity is not evident on testing, or if amniotic fluid cannot be obtained for testing, conservative management with antenatal corticosteroid administration for fetal maturation and antibiotic therapy to reduce the risk for infection (see below) is appropriate. The issue of continued conservative management versus delivery after steroid treatment is a matter of opinion. Pragmatically, if elective delivery is planned within 1 week, it is unlikely that prolonging the pregnancy further will offer more opportunity for significant additional fetal maturation, and delivery should be considered after steroids have been administered. Alternatively, if several weeks of conservative management are to be attempted, there may be benefit to continuing the pregnancy.

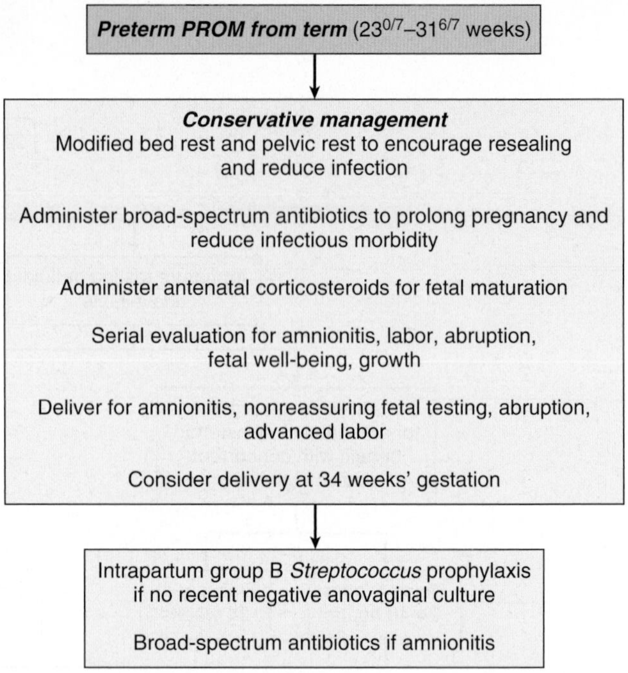

Management of Preterm Premature Rupture of the Membranes Remote From Term (23 to 31 Weeks)

Infants born at 23 to 31 weeks' gestation are at increased risk for perinatal death, and survivors commonly suffer acute and long-term complications. Pregnancy prolongation can reduce these risks, and because of this, inpatient conservative management is generally attempted unless intrauterine infection, significant vaginal bleeding, placental abruption, or advanced labor is evident or fetal testing becomes nonreassuring. Fetal malpresentation, funic presentation, human immunodeficiency virus (HIV), and primary herpes simplex virus (HSV) are examples of exceptions that might warrant expeditious delivery because of the increased potential for fetal death or infection with prolonged membrane rupture.

During conservative management, initial care generally consists of prolonged continuous FHR and maternal contraction monitoring for evidence of umbilical cord compression and occult contractions and to establish fetal well-being. If initial testing is reassuring, the patient can be transferred to an inpatient ward for modified bed rest (Fig. 30-3). Because the fetus with PPROM remote from term is at risk for heart rate abnormalities resulting from umbilical cord compression, fetal assessment should be performed at least daily. More frequent or continuous monitoring may be appropriate if intermittent FHR decelerations are present but findings are otherwise reassuring. Although both nonstress and biophysical profile testing have the ability to confirm fetal well-being in the setting of PPROM, FHR monitoring offers the opportunity to identify periodic heart rate changes and allows concurrent evaluation of uterine activity. Biophysical profile (BPP) testing may be confounded by the presence of oligohydramnios but can be helpful should the nonstress test (NST) result be equivocal (see Chapter 11). **Although a low initial amniotic fluid index is associated with shorter latency and an increased risk for chorioamnionitis, it does not accurately predict who will ultimately develop these complications and should not be used in isolation to make management decisions.** Prolonged bed rest in pregnancy may increase the risk for deep venous thrombosis (DVT).[79] Preventive measures such as leg exercises, antiembolic stockings, and/or prophylactic doses of subcutaneous heparin should be considered during conservative management of PROM (see Chapter 45).

Twofold to fourfold increases in perinatal mortality, IVH, and neonatal sepsis have been reported in infants born after

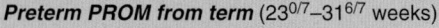

Preterm PROM from term (23^{0/7}–31^{6/7} weeks)

Conservative management
Modified bed rest and pelvic rest to encourage resealing and reduce infection

Administer broad-spectrum antibiotics to prolong pregnancy and reduce infectious morbidity

Administer antenatal corticosteroids for fetal maturation

Serial evaluation for amnionitis, labor, abruption, fetal well-being, growth

Deliver for amnionitis, nonreassuring fetal testing, abruption, advanced labor

Consider delivery at 34 weeks' gestation

Intrapartum group B *Streptococcus* prophylaxis if no recent negative anovaginal culture

Broad-spectrum antibiotics if amnionitis

FIG 30-3 Management algorithm for preterm premature rupture of the membranes (PROM) remote from term (23 to 31 weeks' gestation). (From Mercer BM. Preterm premature rupture of the membranes: diagnosis and management. *Clin Perinatol.* 2004;31:765.)

chorioamnionitis compared with gestational age–matched controls born to noninfected mothers.[33] **The clinical diagnosis is made when maternal fever** (temperature ≥38° C [100.4° F]) **with uterine tenderness and maternal or fetal tachycardia are identified in the absence of another evident source of infection. The maternal white blood cell (WBC) count can be helpful if clinical findings are equivocal.** An increase in the WBC count from a baseline level obtained on admission is suggestive of infection but may be artificially elevated if antenatal corticosteroids have been administered within 5 to 7 days. If additional confirmation of intrauterine infection is required, **amniocentesis may be helpful.**[15,80] A positive amniotic fluid culture is also supportive of a clinical suspicion of clinical chorioamnionitis (sensitivity, 65% to 85%; specificity, 85%), but the clinical diagnosis will likely become clear during the 48 hours needed to achieve a culture result. An **amniotic fluid glucose** concentration below 16 to 20 mg/dL (sensitivity and specificity, 80% to 90% for positive culture) or a **Gram stain positive for bacteria** are supportive of a clinically suspicious diagnosis of chorioamnionitis and can be rapidly obtained. However, the presence of WBCs only in amniotic fluid is not diagnostic of intrauterine infection after PROM. Elevated amniotic fluid interleukin levels have also been associated with an increased risk for early delivery and perinatal infectious morbidity, but cytokine analyses are not readily available in most clinical laboratories,[80] which limits their utility in clinical practice. **Once chorioamnionitis is diagnosed, broad-spectrum antibiotics should be initiated and delivery should be pursued.**

Corticosteroid Administration

A single course of antenatal corticosteroids, either betamethasone (12 mg intramuscularly [IM] every 24 hr for two doses) or dexamethasone (6 mg IM every 12 hours for four doses) before anticipated preterm birth has been shown to reduce the risks for RDS, IVH, NEC, perinatal death, and long-term neurologic morbidities. **Meta-analysis regarding antenatal corticosteroid administration after PPROM has confirmed steroid therapy to significantly reduce the risks for RDS** (20% vs. 35.4%), **IVH** (7.5% vs. 15.9%), **and NEC** (0.8% vs. 4.6%) **without increasing the risks for maternal** (9.2% vs. 5.1%) **or neonatal** (7.0% vs. 6.6%) **infection.**[81]

Repeated courses of antenatal corticosteroids after PPROM have been associated with increased newborn infection in some studies and have not been consistently associated with improvements in newborn outcomes.[82] Ghidini and colleagues[83] found less IVH and chorioamnionitis but no reduction in the risk for RDS with repeated antenatal corticosteroid doses. Alternatively, Abbasi and associates[82] observed a lower risk for RDS with more than one course of antenatal corticosteroids after PROM (34.9% vs. 45.2%). Given the potential risks and the lack of clear data supporting the benefit of repeated weekly antenatal corticosteroid administration, such treatment does not appear warranted. It remains to be determined whether a single repeat "rescue" course could benefit the woman who receives an initial course of antenatal corticosteroids after PROM near the limit of viability but then remains pregnant through 30 to 33 weeks' gestation.

Antibiotic Administration

The goal of antibiotic therapy during conservative management of PPROM remote from term is to treat or prevent ascending infection in order to prolong pregnancy and reduce perinatal infectious and gestational age–dependent morbidity. Meta-analyses have summarized a large number of randomized controlled clinical trials in this regard.[84,85] These evaluations suggest that **antibiotic treatment significantly prolongs latency after membrane rupture and reduces chorioamnionitis, and treatment also reduces the frequencies of newborn complications that include neonatal infection, the need for oxygen or surfactant therapy, and IVH.** Several published trials offer valuable insights regarding the potential role of adjunctive antibiotics in this setting. The National Institutes of Child Health and Human Development Maternal Fetal Medicine Units (NICHD-MFMU) Research Network studied women with PPROM remote from term (24 to 32 weeks, 0 days' gestation).[86,87] Participants received 48 hours of broad-spectrum IV therapy (ampicillin 2 g every 6 hours and erythromycin 250 mg every 6 hours), followed by 5 days of oral (PO) therapy (amoxicillin 250 mg every 8 hours and enteric-coated erythromycin base 333 mg every 8 hours) or a matching placebo. GBS carriers in both study arms received ampicillin for 1 week and then again in labor. Antibiotic treatment doubled the likelihood of remaining undelivered after 7 days, and this benefit persisted up to 3 weeks after randomization, suggesting that antibiotics successfully treat, rather than just suppress, subclinical infection. Antibiotics improved neonatal health by reducing the number of babies with one or more major infant complications from 53% to 44% (composite morbidity: death, RDS, early sepsis, severe IVH, severe NEC; $P < .05$) and also reduced individual newborn complications, including RDS (40.5% vs. 48.7%), stage 3 or 4 NEC (2.3% vs. 5.8%), patent ductus arteriosus (11.7% vs. 20.2%), and CLD (bronchopulmonary dysplasia: 20.5% vs. 13.0%; $P < .05$ for each). Regarding individual infectious morbidities, antibiotics reduced the frequencies of

chorioamnionitis overall (32.5% vs. 23%), and also neonatal sepsis (8.4% vs. 15.6%) and pneumonia (2.9% vs. 7%), among those who were not GBS carriers ($P \le .04$ for each). In a second multicenter placebo-controlled trial, Kenyon and colleagues[88] studied oral therapy with erythromycin, amoxicillin–clavulanic acid, or both for up to 10 days after PPROM before 37 weeks' gestation. In summary, erythromycin prolonged latency only briefly (not significant at 7 days) but did reduce the need for supplemental oxygen (31.1% vs. 35.6%) and the frequency of positive blood cultures (5.7% vs. 8.2%; $P = .02$ for both). Amoxicillin–clavulanic acid prolonged pregnancy (43.3% vs. 36.7% undelivered at 7 days) and reduced the need for supplemental oxygen (30.1% vs. 35.6%) but increased the risk for NEC (1.9% vs. 0.5%; $P \le .05$ for each). Long-term follow-up of infants delivered within this trial revealed no evident differences between antibiotic and control groups.[89] Subsequent studies have attempted to determine whether the duration of antibiotic therapy could be shortened but are of inadequate size and power to evaluate infant outcomes adequately.

In summary, **there is a role for a 7-day course of parenteral and oral antibiotic therapy with erythromycin and amoxicillin-ampicillin during conservative management of PROM remote from term, to prolong latency and to reduce infectious and gestational age–dependent neonatal complications. Extended-spectrum ampicillin–clavulanic acid treatment is not recommended because it may be harmful.**

Magnesium Sulfate for Neuroprotection

Administration of magnesium sulfate before early PTB will improve long-term infant outcomes and is recommended for anticipated deliveries before 32 weeks' gestation after PPROM regardless of attempts at conservative management.[90,91] In a large multicenter trial that studied this issue, 92% of participants had PROM before 32 weeks' gestation, and treatment was effective in preventing moderate/severe cerebral palsy (1.9% vs. 3.9%, $P = .03$) and cerebral palsy overall (4.2% vs. 7.3%, $P = .004$) by 2 years of age.[91] Magnesium sulfate was administered as a bolus of 6 g followed by an infusion of 2 g/hr for 12 hours if undelivered (or continued for imminent delivery). Retreatment was attempted for those initially undelivered and those who subsequently delivered before 34 weeks gestation.

Tocolysis

Limited evidence suggests that prophylactic tocolysis, administered after PPROM and before the onset of contractions, can prolong pregnancy briefly.[92] However, therapeutic tocolysis initiated only after the onset of contractions has not been shown to prolong latency after PPROM. A report from the National Institutes of Health (NIH) collaborative study on antenatal steroids suggested an association between tocolytic treatment after PPROM and subsequent neonatal RDS, but subsequent small prospective studies have found neither an increase nor a decrease in neonatal complications with such tocolytic treatment.[93] Although it is plausible that tocolysis could facilitate initial uterine quiescence to allow additional time for antibiotic and corticosteroid benefits, no studies have been done of therapy with traditional tocolytic agents after PPROM in which concurrent antenatal corticosteroid and antibiotic treatments were given. Further, weekly progesterone treatment failed to prolong latency after PROM in a recent small, randomized controlled trial.[94] Pending further study, **tocolysis and progesterone**

therapy are not recommended during conservative management of PPROM.

Cervical Cerclage

PPROM is a common complication after cervical cerclage placement, and it affects about one in four elective cerclages and half of emergent procedures.[95] Retrospective studies reveal that perinatal complications are similar to PROM without a cerclage if the stitch is removed on admission.[96] A single randomized controlled study of cerclage removal after PROM was discontinued when futility calculations determined that the power of the study would not be met. The investigation revealed no improvement in latency (56.3% vs. 45.8% delivered within 1 week, $P = .59$) and no improvement in newborn outcomes with cerclage retention. Despite being 1.7-fold more common in the study population, cerclage retention was not significantly associated with more frequent chorioamnionitis (41.7% vs. 25%, $P = .25$).[97] Retrospective studies that compared stitch removal and retention after PPROM have been small but have yielded consistent patterns.[98,99] Each has found insignificant trends toward increased maternal infections and only brief pregnancy prolongation; one study noted increased infant mortality and death due to sepsis when the cerclage was retained after PROM.[98] Because **no well-controlled study has found cerclage retention to improve newborn outcomes after PROM, early cerclage removal is recommended when PROM occurs.** The risks and benefits of short-term cerclage retention during antenatal corticosteroid are unknown.

Herpes Simplex Virus

Neonatal HSV infection most commonly results from direct maternal-fetal transmission during delivery, with newborn infection rates of 34% to 80% after primary and 1% to 5% after secondary maternal infection.[100] When neonatal HSV infection occurs, the infant mortality rate is 50% to 60%, and up to 50% of survivors will suffer serious sequelae.[101] Based on small case series of women with an active maternal genital HSV infection by Gibbs and colleagues[102] ($n = 9$) and Nahmias and colleagues ($n = 26$), both in 1971, the accepted belief has been that extended latency after membrane rupture (>4 to 6 hours) is associated with an increased risk for newborn infection. Major and coworkers[103] have reported on a case series of 29 gravidas managed expectantly with PROM before 32 weeks' gestation with active *recurrent* HSV lesions. Latency after membrane rupture ranged from 1 to 35 days, and cesarean delivery was performed if active lesions were present at the time of delivery. None of the infants delivered under this regimen developed neonatal herpes infection. **These data support conservative management of PROM complicated by recurrent maternal HSV infection when the likelihood of infant mortality and long-term complications with early delivery is high.** Prophylactic treatment with antiviral agents (e.g., acyclovir) to reduce viral shedding and the frequency of recurrences is prudent under this circumstance.

Management of Previable Premature Rupture of the Membranes

The cause of PROM before the limit of viability has implications for the anticipated pregnancy outcome and can be helpful in guiding counseling and management. Previable PROM subsequent to **second-trimester amniocentesis** is likely related to continued leakage of fluid through a small membrane defect without concurrent infection. Under this circumstance it is likely that the membranes will reseal, and extended pregnancy can be anticipated. Alternatively, previable PROM subsequent to **second-trimester bleeding,** oligohydramnios, or an elevated maternal serum alpha-fetoprotein level more likely reflects an abnormality of placentation and has a poorer prognosis. The patient with previable PROM and no indication for immediate delivery should be counseled regarding the potential risks and benefits of conservative management. Counseling should include a realistic appraisal of fetal and neonatal outcomes and the risks for maternal complications.

Most available data regarding women with PPROM near the limit of viability are derived from retrospective studies. **In a review of PPROM that occurred at or before 24 weeks' gestation, Waters and Mercer[36] found median latency to range from 6 to 13 days.** Another recent evaluation found that 38% delivered within 1 week and 69% delivered within 5 weeks after periviable PROM.[104] **Other maternal risks during conservative management of PROM at 24 weeks or less include chorioamnionitis (35%), abruptio placentae (19%), retained placenta (11%), and endometritis (14%).[37] Maternal sepsis (0.8%) and death (1 in 619 pregnancies overall) are rare but serious complications.** Conservative management can also lead to maternal muscle wasting, bone demineralization, and DVT due to prolonged bed rest. Overall, infant survival after conservatively managed periviable PROM occurs in 44% of cases, but this varies with gestational age at membrane rupture (14.4% before 22 weeks vs. 57.7% at 22 to 24 weeks). Stillbirth is common and complicates up to 23% to 53% of cases. Neonatal complications include pulmonary hypoplasia (19%), RDS (66%), grade III or IV intraventricular hemorrhage (5%), sepsis (19%), and NEC (4%) as well as long-term complications such as bronchopulmonary dysplasia (29%), stage III retinopathy of prematurity (5%), and contractures (3%). Prediction of individual outcomes is difficult because of the inability to predict the ultimate gestational age at delivery in any given case.

A potential management scheme for PROM before the limit of viability is presented in Figure 30-4. **Consensus has not yet been reached regarding the advantages of inpatient versus outpatient management for the patient who elects conservative management after previable PROM.** The benefits of an initial period of inpatient observation may include bed rest and pelvic rest to increase the opportunity for membrane resealing as well as early identification of infection, fetal demise, and abruption. A number of novel treatments, including amnioinfusion and fibrin-platelet-cryoprecipitate or Gelfoam sealing of the membranes, have been preliminarily investigated.[105-108] The risks and benefits of these aggressive interventions have not been adequately studied to suggest that such therapy be incorporated into routine clinical practice. **Typically, women with previable PROM who have been managed as outpatients are readmitted to the hospital once the pregnancy reaches the limit of viability.** Administration of antenatal corticosteroids for fetal maturation is appropriate at the limit of viability because early delivery is still anticipated.

During conservative management, serial ultrasound studies performed every 1 to 2 weeks can evaluate for reaccumulation of amniotic fluid and interval pulmonary growth. Although persistent severe oligohydramnios is a strong marker for subsequent development of lethal pulmonary hypoplasia, serial fetal biometric evaluation (e.g., lung length,

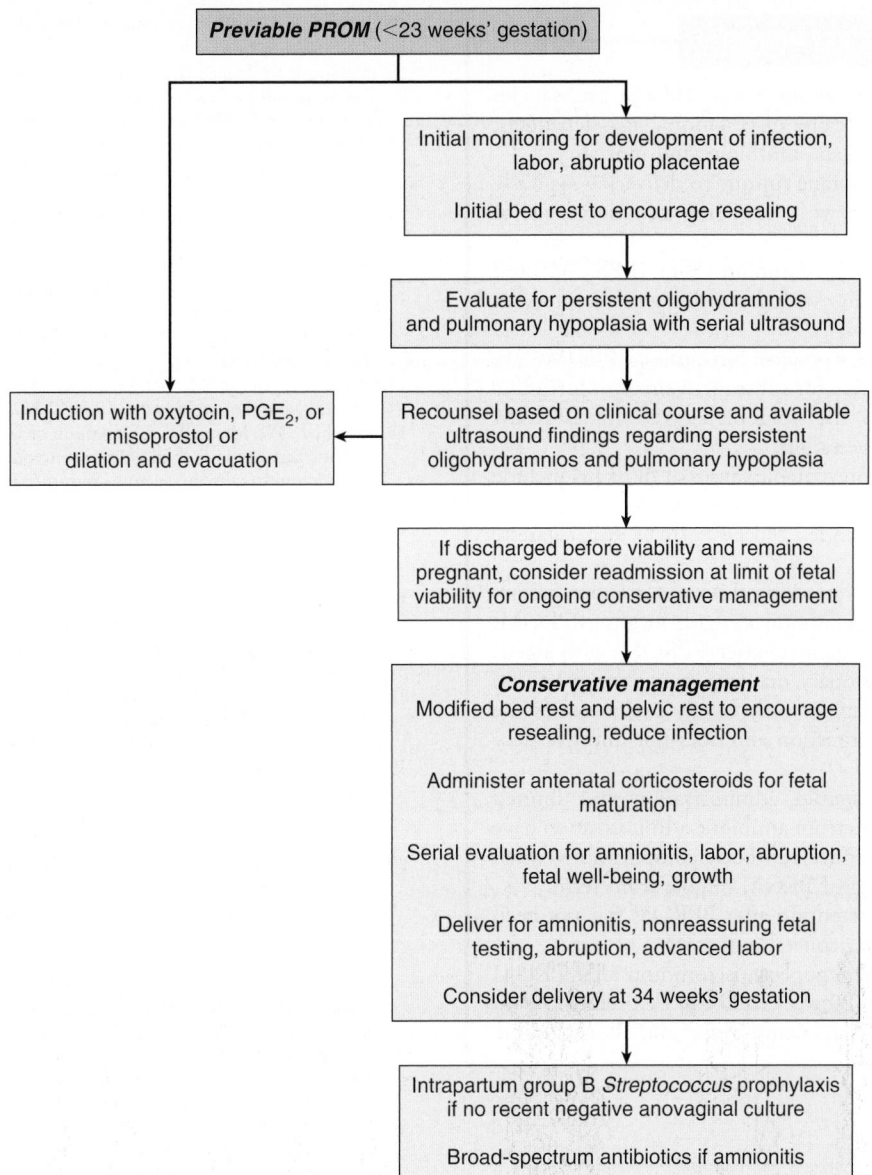

FIG 30-4 Management algorithm for previable premature rupture of the membranes (PROM) before the limit of potential viability (currently 23 weeks' gestation). PGE$_2$, prostaglandin E$_2$. (From Mercer BM. Preterm premature rupture of the membranes: diagnosis and management. *Clin Perinatol.* 2004;31:765.)

three-dimensional lung volume, chest circumference) and ratios that adjust for overall fetal size (thoracic-abdominal circumference, thoracic circumference–femur length) can demonstrate a lack of fetal pulmonary growth over time and have a high predictive value for lethal pulmonary hypoplasia.[44,47,109,110] Studies of pulmonary artery and ductus arteriosus waveform modulation with fetal breathing movements have shown some promise but can be technically difficult to perform.

Some women will choose to not undertake the potential risks for maternal complications after previable PROM either after initial counseling or with evidence of developing pulmonary hypoplasia. Delivery can be accomplished by labor induction with vaginal prostaglandin E$_2$, prostaglandin E$_1$ (misoprostol), high-dose IV oxytocin, or dilation and evacuation. The optimal approach depends on patient characteristics (e.g., gestational age, evident chorioamnionitis, prior cesarean delivery), available facilities, and physician experience.

SUMMARY

The potential for significant perinatal complications exists when PROM occurs at term or before term. Early delivery of the patient with PROM at or near term can reduce the risk for perinatal infections without increasing the likelihood of operative delivery. Careful conservative management of PROM remote from term offers the potential to reduce infectious and gestational age–dependent morbidities. Early transfer to a facility capable of providing urgent obstetric and neonatal intensive care is important should adequate facilities not be available locally. Regardless of the management approach, infants who deliver after PPROM and after PROM before the limit of potential viability are at high risk for perinatal complications, many of which cannot be avoided with current technology and management algorithms.

REFERENCES

1. Shen TT, DeFranco EA, Stamilio DM, Chang JJ, Muglia LJ. A population-based study of race-specific risk for preterm premature rupture of membranes. *Am J Obstet Gynecol.* 2008;199:373.
2. Ananth CV, Joseph KS, Oyelese Y, Demissie K, Vintzileos AM. Trends in preterm birth and perinatal mortality among singletons: United States, 1989 through 2000. *Obstet Gynecol.* 2005;105:1084.
3. Ananth CV, Joseph KS, Demissie K, Vintzileos AM. Trends in twin preterm birth subtypes in the United States, 1989 through 2000: impact on perinatal mortality. *Am J Obstet Gynecol.* 2005;193:1076.
4. Pakrashi T, Defranco EA. The relative proportion of preterm births complicated by premature rupture of membranes in multifetal gestations: a population-based study. *Am J Perinatol.* 2013;30:69.
5. Tucker JM, Goldenberg RL, Davis RO, et al. Etiologies of preterm birth in an indigent population: is prevention a logical expectation? *Obstet Gynecol.* 1991;77:343.
6. McParland PC, Taylor DJ, Bell SC. Mapping of zones of altered morphology and choriodeciduaic connective tissue cellular phenotype in human fetal membranes (amnion and decidua) overlying the lower uterine pole and cervix before labor at term. *Am J Obstet Gynecol.* 2003;189:1481.
7. McLaren J, Taylor DJ, Bell SC. Increased concentration of pro-matrix metalloproteinase 9 in term fetal membranes overlying the cervix before labor: implications for membrane remodeling and rupture. *Am J Obstet Gynecol.* 2000;182:409.
8. Kumar D, Schatz F, Moore RM, et al. The effects of thrombin and cytokines upon the biomechanics and remodeling of isolated amnion membrane, in vitro. *Placenta.* 2011;32:206.
9. Parry S, Strauss JF. Premature rupture of the fetal membranes. *N Engl J Med.* 1998;338:663.
10. McGregor JA, French JI, Parker R, et al. Prevention of premature birth by screening and treatment for common genital tract infections: results of a prospective controlled evaluation. *Am J Obstet Gynecol.* 1995;173:157.
11. Romero R, Mazor M, Oyarzun E, et al. Is there an association between colonization with group B Streptococcus and prematurity? *J Reprod Med.* 1989;34:797.
12. Regan JA, Klebanoff MA, Nugent RP, et al. Colonization with group B streptococci in pregnancy and adverse outcome. VIP Study Group. *Am J Obstet Gynecol.* 1996;174:1354.
13. Romero R, Chaiworapongsa T, Kuivaniemi H, Tromp G. Bacterial vaginosis, the inflammatory response and the risk of preterm birth: a role for genetic epidemiology in the prevention of preterm birth. *Am J Obstet Gynecol.* 2004;190:1509.
14. Romero R, Mazor M, Wu YK, et al. Infection in the pathogenesis of preterm labor. *Semin Perinatol.* 1988;12:262.
15. Gauthier DW, Meyer WJ. Comparison of Gram stain, leukocyte esterase activity, and amniotic fluid glucose concentration in predicting amniotic fluid culture results in preterm premature rupture of membranes. *Am J Obstet Gynecol.* 1992;167:1092.
16. Mercer BM, Moretti ML, Prevost RR, Sibai BM. Erythromycin therapy in preterm premature rupture of the membranes: a prospective, randomized trial of 220 patients. *Am J Obstet Gynecol.* 1992;166:794.
17. Macones GA, Parry S, Elkousy M, et al. A polymorphism in the promoter region of TNF and bacterial vaginosis: preliminary evidence of gene-environment interaction in the etiology of spontaneous preterm birth. *Am J Obstet Gynecol.* 2004;190:1504.
18. Romero R, Friel LA, Velez Edwards DR, et al. A genetic association study of maternal and fetal candidate genes that predispose to preterm prelabor rupture of membranes (PROM). *Am J Obstet Gynecol.* 2010;203:361.
19. Mercer BM, Goldenberg RL, Meis PJ, et al. for the NICHD-MFMU Network. The preterm prediction study: prediction of preterm premature rupture of the membranes using clinical findings and ancillary testing. *Am J Obstet Gynecol.* 2000;183:738.
20. Mercer BM, Goldenberg RL, Moawad AH, et al. for the NICHD-MFMU Network. The preterm prediction study: effect of gestational age and cause of preterm birth on subsequent obstetric outcome. *Am J Obstet Gynecol.* 1999;181:1216.
21. Hassan SS, Romero R, Vidyadhari D, et al. PREGNANT Trial. Vaginal progesterone reduces the rate of preterm birth in women with a sonographic short cervix: a multicenter, randomized, double-blind, placebo-controlled trial. *Ultrasound Obstet Gynecol.* 2011;38:18.
22. Meis PJ, Klebanoff M, Thom E, et al. for the NICHD-MFMU Network. Prevention of recurrent preterm delivery by 17 alpha-hydroxyprogesterone caproate. *N Engl J Med.* 2003;348:2379.
23. da Fonseca EB, Bittar RE, Carvalho MH, Zugaib M. Prophylactic administration of progesterone by vaginal suppository to reduce the incidence of spontaneous preterm birth in women at increased risk: a randomized placebo-controlled double-blind study. *Am J Obstet Gynecol.* 2003;188:419.
24. Casanueva E, Ripoll C, Tolentino M, et al. Vitamin C supplementation to prevent premature rupture of the chorioamniotic membranes: a randomized trial. *Am J Clin Nutr.* 2005;81:859.
25. Hauth JC, Clifton RG, Roberts JM, et al; Eunice Kennedy Shriver National Institute of Child Health and Human Development (NICHD) Maternal-Fetal Medicine Units Network (MFMU). Vitamin C and E supplementation to prevent spontaneous preterm birth: a randomized controlled trial. *Obstet Gynecol.* 2010;116:653.
26. Mercer BM, Abdelrahim A, Moore RM, et al. The impact of vitamin C supplementation in pregnancy and in vitro upon fetal membrane strength and remodeling. *Reprod Sci.* 2010;17:685.
27. Rumbold A, Crowther CA. Vitamin C supplementation in pregnancy. *Cochrane Database Syst Rev.* 2005;(2):CD004072.
28. Hannah ME, Ohlsson A, Farine D, et al. Induction of labor compared with expectant management for prelabor rupture of the membranes at term. *N Engl J Med.* 1996;334:1005.
29. Mercer B, Arheart K. Antimicrobial therapy in expectant management of preterm premature rupture of the membranes. *Lancet.* 1995;346:1271.
30. Gold RB, Goyer GL, Schwartz DB, et al. Conservative management of second trimester post-amniocentesis fluid leakage. *Obstet Gynecol.* 1989;74:745.
31. Johnson JW, Egerman RS, Moorhead J. Cases with ruptured membranes that "reseal.". *Am J Obstet Gynecol.* 1990;163:1024.
32. Hillier SL, Martius J, Krohn M, et al. A case-control study of chorioamnionic infection and histologic chorioamnionitis in prematurity. *N Engl J Med.* 1988;319:972.

33. Garite TJ, Freeman RK. Chorioamnionitis in the preterm gestation. *Obstet Gynecol.* 1982;59:539.

34. Simpson GF, Harbert GM Jr. Use of betamethasone in management of preterm gestation with premature rupture of membranes. *Obstet Gynecol.* 1985;66:168.

35. Gonen R, Hannah ME, Milligan JE. Does prolonged preterm premature rupture of the membranes predispose to abruptio placentae? *Obstet Gynecol.* 1989;74:347.

36. Waters TP, Mercer BM. The management of preterm premature rupture of the membranes near the limit of fetal viability. *Am J Obstet Gynecol.* 2009;201:230.

37. Mercer BM. Preterm premature rupture of the membranes. *Obstet Gynecol.* 2003;101:178.

38. Blumenfeld YJ, Lee HC, Gould JB, et al. The effect of preterm premature rupture of membranes on neonatal mortality rates. *Obstet Gynecol.* 2010;116:1381.

39. Chen A, Feresu SA, Barsoom MJ. Heterogeneity of preterm birth subtypes in relation to neonatal death. *Obstet Gynecol.* 2009;114:516.

40. Seo K, McGregor JA, French JI. Preterm birth is associated with increased risk of maternal and neonatal infection. *Obstet Gynecol.* 1992;79:75.

41. Wu YW, Colford JM Jr. Chorioamnionitis as a risk factor for cerebral palsy: a meta-analysis. *JAMA.* 2000;284:1417.

42. Pappas A, Kendrick DE, Shankaran S, et al; Eunice Kennedy Shriver National Institute of Child Health and Human Development Neonatal Research Network. Chorioamnionitis and early childhood outcomes among extremely low-gestational-age neonates. *JAMA Pediatr.* 2014; 168:137.

43. Yoon BH, Romero R, Kim CJ, et al. High expression of tumor necrosis factor-alpha and interleukin-6 in periventricular leukomalacia. *Am J Obstet Gynecol.* 1997;177:406.

44. Lauria MR, Gonik B, Romero R. Pulmonary hypoplasia: pathogenesis, diagnosis, and antenatal prediction. *Obstet Gynecol.* 1995;86:466.

45. Wigglesworth JS, Desai R. Use of DNA estimation for growth assessment in normal and hypoplastic fetal lungs. *Arch Dis Child.* 1981;56:601.

46. Moretti M, Sibai B. Maternal and perinatal outcome of expectant management of premature rupture of the membranes in midtrimester. *Am J Obstet Gynecol.* 1988;159:390.

47. Rizzo G, Capponi A, Angelini E, et al. Blood flow velocity waveforms from fetal peripheral pulmonary arteries in pregnancies with preterm premature rupture of membranes: relationship with pulmonary hypoplasia. *Ultrasound Obstet Gynecol.* 2000;15:98.

48. Winn HN, Chen M, Amon E, et al. Neonatal pulmonary hypoplasia and perinatal mortality in patients with midtrimester rupture of amniotic membranes: a critical analysis. *Am J Obstet Gynecol.* 2000;182:1638.

49. Nimrod C, Varela-Gittings F, Machin G, et al. The effect of very prolonged membrane rupture on fetal development. *Am J Obstet Gynecol.* 1984; 148:540.

50. Blott M, Greenough A. Neonatal outcome after prolonged rupture of the membranes starting in the second trimester. *Arch Dis Child.* 1988;63:1146.

51. Ramsauer B, Duwe W, Schlehe B, et al. Effect of blood on ROM diagnosis accuracy of PAMG-1 and IGFBP-1 detecting rapid tests. *J Perinat Med.* 2015;43(4):417-422.

52. Lee SE, Park JS, Norwitz ER, et al. Measurement of placental alpha-microglobulin-1 in cervicovaginal discharge to diagnose rupture of membranes. *Obstet Gynecol.* 2007;109:634.

53. Alexander JM, Mercer BM, Miodovnik M, et al. The impact of digital cervical examination on expectantly managed preterm rupture of membranes. *Am J Obstet Gynecol.* 2000;183:1003.

54. Brown CL, Ludwiczak MH, Blanco JD, Hirsch CE. Cervical dilation: accuracy of visual and digital examinations. *Obstet Gynecol.* 1993;81:215.

55. Verani JR, McGee L, Schrag SJ, for the Division of Bacterial Diseases, National Center for Immunization and Respiratory Diseases, Centers for Disease Control and Prevention (CDC). Prevention of perinatal group B streptococcal disease: revised guidelines from CDC, 2010. *MMWR Recomm Rep.* 2010;59:1.

56. Committee on Obstetric Practice. ACOG Committee Opinion No. 485: Prevention of early-onset group B streptococcal disease in newborns. *Obstet Gynecol.* 2011;117:1019.

57. Towers CV, Carr MH, Padilla G, Asrat T. Potential consequences of widespread antepartal use of ampicillin. *Am J Obstet Gynecol.* 1998;179:879.

58. Van der Walt D, Venter PF. Management of term pregnancy with premature rupture of the membranes and unfavourable cervix. *S Afr Med J.* 1989;75:54.

59. Grant JM, Serle E, Mahmood T, et al. Management of prelabour rupture of the membranes in term primigravidae: report of a randomized prospective trial. *Br J Obstet Gynaecol.* 1992;99:557.

60. Ladfors L, Mattsson LA, Eriksson M, Fall O. A randomised trial of two expectant managements of prelabour rupture of the membranes at 34 to 42 weeks. *Br J Obstet Gynaecol.* 1996;103:755.

61. Shalev E, Peleg D, Eliyahu S, Nahum Z. Comparison of 12- and 72-hour expectant management of premature rupture of membranes in term pregnancies. *Obstet Gynecol.* 1995;85:1.

62. Dare MR, Middleton P, Crowther CA, et al. Planned early birth versus expectant management (waiting) for prelabour rupture of membranes at term (37 weeks or more). *Cochrane Database Syst Rev.* 2006;(1):CD005302.

63. Tan BP, Hannah ME. Prostaglandins versus oxytocin for prelabour rupture of membranes at term. *Cochrane Database Syst Rev.* 2000;(2): CD000159.

64. Strong TH Jr, Hetzler G, Sarno AP, Paul RH. Prophylactic intrapartum amnioinfusion: a randomized clinical trial. *Am J Obstet Gynecol.* 1990; 162:1370.

65. Schrimmer DB, Macri CJ, Paul RH. Prophylactic amnioinfusion as a treatment for oligohydramnios in laboring patients: a prospective randomized trial. *Am J Obstet Gynecol.* 1991;165:972.

66. Naef RW 3rd, Allbert JR, Ross EL, et al. Premature rupture of membranes at 34 to 37 weeks' gestation: aggressive vs. conservative management. *Am J Obstet Gynecol.* 1998;178:126.

67. Neerhof MG, Cravello C, Haney EI, Silver RK. Timing of labor induction after premature rupture of membranes between 32 and 36 weeks gestation. *Am J Obstet Gynecol.* 1999;180:349.

68. Van der Ham DP, Vijgen SM, Nijhuis JG, et al; PPROMEXIL trial group. Induction of labor versus expectant management in women with preterm prelabor rupture of membranes between 34 and 37 weeks: a randomized controlled trial. *PLoS Med.* 2012;9:e1001208.

69. Tajik P, van der Ham DP, Zafarmand MH, et al. Using vaginal Group B Streptococcus colonisation in women with preterm premature rupture of membranes to guide the decision for immediate delivery: a secondary analysis of the PPROMEXIL trials. *BJOG.* 2014;121(10):1263-1272.

70. Cox SM, Leveno KJ. Intentional delivery vs. expectant management with preterm ruptured membranes at 30-34 weeks' gestation. *Obstet Gynecol.* 1995;86:875.

71. Mercer BM, Crocker L, Boe N, Sibai B. Induction vs. expectant management in PROM with mature amniotic fluid at 32-36 weeks: a randomized trial. *Am J Obstet Gynecol.* 1993;82:775.

72. Mercer BM in response to Repke JT, Berck DJ. Preterm premature rupture of membranes: a continuing dilemma. *Am J Obstet Gynecol.* 1994;170:1835.

73. Sbarra AJ, Blake G, Cetrulo CL, et al. The effect of cervical/vaginal secretions on measurements of lecithin/sphingomyelin ratio and optical density at 650 nm. *Am J Obstet Gynecol.* 1981;139:214.

74. Shaver DC, Spinnato JA, Whybrew D, et al. Comparison of phospholipids in vaginal and amniocentesis specimens of patients with premature rupture of membranes. *Am J Obstet Gynecol.* 1987;156:454.

75. Lewis DF, Towers CV, Major CA, et al. Use of Amniostat-FLM in detecting the presence of phosphatidylglycerol in vaginal pool samples in preterm premature rupture of membranes. *Am J Obstet Gynecol.* 1993;169:573.

76. Russell JC, Cooper CM, Ketchum CH, et al. Multicenter evaluation of TDx test for assessing fetal lung maturity. *Clin Chem.* 1989;35:1005.

77. Estol PC, Poseiro JJ, Schwarcz R. Phosphatidylglycerol determination in the amniotic fluid from a PAD placed over the vulva: a method for diagnosis of fetal lung maturity in cases of premature ruptured membranes. *J Perinat Med.* 1992;20:65.

78. Salim R, Zafran N, Nachum Z, et al. Predicting lung maturity in preterm rupture of membranes via lamellar bodies count from a vaginal pool: a cohort study. *Reprod Biol Endocrinol.* 2009;7:1.

79. Kovacevich GJ, Gaich SA, Lavin JP, et al. The prevalence of thromboembolic events among women with extended bed rest prescribed as part of the treatment for premature labor or preterm premature rupture of membranes. *Am J Obstet Gynecol.* 2000;182:1089.

80. Romero R, Yoon BH, Mazor M, et al. A comparative study of the diagnostic performance of amniotic fluid glucose, white blood cell count, interleukin-6, and Gram stain in the detection of microbial invasion in patients with preterm premature rupture of membranes. *Am J Obstet Gynecol.* 1993;169:839.

81. Harding JE, Pang J, Knight DB, Liggins GC. Do antenatal corticosteroids help in the setting of preterm rupture of membranes? *Am J Obstet Gynecol.* 2001;184:131.

82. Abbasi S, Hirsch D, Davis J, et al. Effect of single vs. multiple courses of antenatal corticosteroids on maternal and neonatal outcome. *Am J Obstet Gynecol.* 2000;182:1243.

83. Ghidini A, Salafia CM, Minior VK. Repeated courses of steroids in preterm membrane rupture do not increase the risk of histologic chorioamnionitis. *Am J Perinatol.* 1997;14:309.

84. Egarter C, Leitich H, Karas H, et al. Antibiotic treatment in premature rupture of membranes and neonatal morbidity: a meta-analysis. *Am J Obstet Gynecol*. 1996;174:589.

85. Kenyon S, Boulvain M, Neilson JP. Antibiotics for preterm rupture of membranes. *Cochrane Database Syst Rev*. 2013;(12):CD001058.

86. Mercer B, Miodovnik M, Thurnau G, et al. for the NICHD-MFMU Network. Antibiotic therapy for reduction of infant morbidity after preterm premature rupture of the membranes: a randomized controlled trial. *JAMA*. 1997;278:989.

87. Mercer BM, Goldenberg RL, Das AF, et al. for the NICHD-MFMU Network. What we have learned regarding antibiotic therapy for the reduction of infant morbidity. *Semin Perinatol*. 2003;27:217.

88. Kenyon SL, Taylor DJ, Tarnow-Mordi W; Oracle Collaborative Group. Broad spectrum antibiotics for preterm, prelabor rupture of fetal membranes: the ORACLE I Randomized trial. *Lancet*. 2001;357:979.

89. Kenyon S, Pike K, Jones DR, et al. Childhood outcomes after prescription of antibiotics to pregnant women with preterm rupture of the membranes: 7-year follow-up of the ORACLE I trial. *Lancet*. 2008;372:1310.

90. Doyle LW, Crowther CA, Middleton P, Marret S, Rouse D. Magnesium sulphate for women at risk of preterm birth for neuroprotection of the fetus. *Cochrane Database Syst Rev*. 2009;(1):CD004661.

91. Rouse DJ, Hirtz DG, Thom E, et al; Eunice Kennedy Shriver NICHD Maternal-Fetal Medicine Units Network. A randomized, controlled trial of magnesium sulfate for the prevention of cerebral palsy. *N Engl J Med*. 2008;359:895-905.

92. Weiner CP, Renk K, Klugman M. The therapeutic efficacy and cost-effectiveness of aggressive tocolysis for premature labor associated with premature rupture of the membranes. *Am J Obstet Gynecol*. 1988;159:216.

93. Curet LB, Rao AV, Zachman RD, et al. Association between ruptured membranes, tocolytic therapy, and respiratory distress syndrome. *Am J Obstet Gynecol*. 1984;148:263.

94. Briery CM, Veillon EW, Klauser CK, et al. Women with preterm premature rupture of the membranes do not benefit from weekly progesterone. *Am J Obstet Gynecol*. 2011;204:54.

95. Treadwell MC, Bronsteen RA, Bottoms SF. Prognostic factors and complication rates for cervical cerclage: a review of 482 cases. *Am J Obstet Gynecol*. 1991;165:555.

96. Yeast JD, Garite TR. The role of cervical cerclage in the management of preterm premature rupture of the membranes. *Am J Obstet Gynecol*. 1988;158:106.

97. Galyean A, Garite TJ, Maurel K, et al; Obstetrix Perinatal Collaborative Research Network. Removal versus retention of cerclage in preterm premature rupture of membranes: a randomized controlled trial. *Am J Obstet Gynecol*. 2014;211:399.

98. Ludmir J, Bader T, Chen L, et al. Poor perinatal outcome associated with retained cerclage in patients with premature rupture of membranes. *Obstet Gynecol*. 1994;84:823.

99. McElrath TF, Norwitz ER, Lieberman ES, Heffner LJ. Perinatal outcome after preterm premature rupture of membranes with in situ cervical cerclage. *Am J Obstet Gynecol*. 2002;187:1147.

100. Brown ZA, Vontver LA, Benedetti J, et al. Effects on infants of a first episode of genital herpes during pregnancy. *N Engl J Med*. 1987;317:1246.

101. Stagno S, Whitley RJ. Herpes virus infections of pregnancy. II. Herpes simplex virus and varicella zoster infections. *N Engl J Med*. 1985;313:1327.

102. Gibbs RS, Amstey MS, Lezotte DC. Role of cesarean delivery in preventing neonatal herpes virus infection. *JAMA*. 1993;270:94.

103. Major CA, Towers CV, Lewis DF, Garite TJ. Expectant management of preterm premature rupture of membranes complicated by active recurrent genital herpes. *Am J Obstet Gynecol*. 2003;188:1551.

104. Muris C, Girard B, Creveuil C, et al. Management of premature rupture of membranes before 25 weeks. *Eur J Obstet Gynecol Reprod Biol*. 2007;131:163.

105. Sciscione AC, Manley JS, Pollock M, et al. Intracervical fibrin sealants: a potential treatment for early preterm premature rupture of the membranes. *Am J Obstet Gynecol*. 2001;184:368.

106. Quintero RA, Morales WJ, Bornick PW, et al. Surgical treatment of spontaneous rupture of membranes: the amniograft-first experience. *Am J Obstet Gynecol*. 2002;186:155.

107. O'Brien JM, Barton JR, Milligan DA. An aggressive interventional protocol for early midtrimester premature rupture of the membranes using gelatin sponge for cervical plugging. *Am J Obstet Gynecol*. 2002;187:1143.

108. Roberts D, Vause S, Martin W, et al. Amnioinfusion in preterm premature rupture of membranes (AMIPROM): a randomised controlled trial of amnioinfusion versus expectant management in very early preterm premature rupture of membranes–a pilot study. *Health Technol Assess*. 2014;18:1.

109. Laudy JA, Tibboel D, Robben SG, et al. Prenatal prediction of pulmonary hypoplasia: clinical, biometric, and Doppler velocity correlates. *Pediatrics*. 2002;109:250.

110. Yoshimura S, Masuzaki H, Gotoh H, et al. Ultrasonographic prediction of lethal pulmonary hypoplasia: comparison of eight different ultrasonographic parameters. *Am J Obstet Gynecol*. 1996;175:477.

CHAPTER 31

Preeclampsia and Hypertensive Disorders

BAHA M. SIBAI

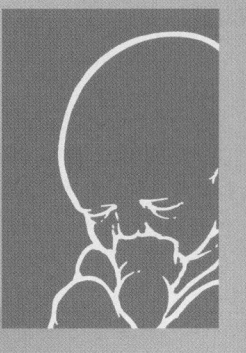

KEY ABBREVIATIONS

Acute fatty liver of pregnancy	AFLP	Glomerular filtration rate	GFR
Acute respiratory distress syndrome	ARDS	Hemolysis, elevated liver enzymes, and low platelets syndrome	HELLP
Alanine transaminase	ALT		
American College of Obstetricians and Gynecologists	ACOG	Hemolytic uremic syndrome	HUS
		Hypertensive disorders of pregnancy	HDP
Angiotensin-converting enzyme	ACE	Immune thrombocytopenic purpura	ITP
Aspartate transaminase	AST	Intrauterine growth restriction	IUGR
Biophysical profile	BPP	Lactate dehydrogenase	LDH
Blood pressure	BP	Low-dose aspirin	LDA
Body mass index	BMI	Magnetic resonance imaging	MRI
Central venous pressure	CVP	Mean arterial pressure	MAP
Computed tomography	CT	Nonstress test	NST
Confidence interval	CI	Placental-like growth factor	PLGF
Disseminated intravascular coagulation	DIC	Posterior reversible encephalopathy syndrome	PRES
Electrocardiogram	ECG		
Electroencephalography	EEG	Positive predictive value	PPV
False-positive rate	FPR	Preeclampsia	PE
Fetal growth restriction	FGR	Protein/creatinine ratio	P/C ratio
Gestational hypertension	GH	Pulmonary capillary wedge pressure	PCWP

Relative risk	RR	Thrombotic thrombocytopenic purpura	TTP
Respiratory distress syndrome	RDS	Thromboxane A$_2$	TXA$_2$
Small for gestational age	SGA	U. S. Preventive Services Task Force	USPSTF
Soluble fms-like tyrosine kinase 1	sFlt-1	Vascular endothelial growth factor	VEGF

Hypertensive disorders are among the most common medical complications of pregnancy; the reported incidence is between 5% and 10%,[1,2] although incidence varies among different hospitals, regions, and countries. These disorders are a major cause of maternal and perinatal mortality and morbidity worldwide.[3] The term *hypertension in pregnancy* is commonly used to describe a wide spectrum of patients who may have only mild elevations in blood pressure (BP) or severe hypertension with dysfunction of various organ systems. The clinical manifestations in these patients may be similar (e.g., hypertension, proteinuria); however, they may result from different underlying causes such as chronic hypertension, renal disease, or pure preeclampsia (PE). The three most common forms of hypertension that complicate pregnancy are (1) gestational hypertension, (2) preeclampsia, and (3) chronic essential hypertension.

DEFINITIONS

Gestational Hypertension

Hypertension may be present before pregnancy, or it may be diagnosed for the first time during pregnancy. In addition, in some women, hypertension may become evident only during labor or during the postpartum period. For clinical purposes, women with hypertension may be classified into one of the three categories listed above; these are described further in Table 31-1.[1,2] Recently, the diagnosis of PE and its subtypes have been expanded and revised by the members of the American College of Obstetricians and Gynecologists (ACOG) Task Force on Hypertension in Pregnancy[1]:

- Systolic BP greater than 140 mm Hg but less than 160 mm Hg *or*
- Diastolic BP greater than 90 mm Hg but less than 110 mm Hg *and*
- These pressures must be observed on at least two occasions 4 hours apart but no more than 7 days apart.[4]

Severe Hypertension

Severe hypertension refers to sustained elevations in systolic BP to at least 160 mm Hg and/or in diastolic BP to at least 110 mm Hg for at least 4 hours or once if the patient is receiving oral antihypertensive agents or received intravenous (IV) antihypertensive medications prior to the 4-hour period.

Proteinuria

Proteinuria may also be present before pregnancy, or it may be newly diagnosed during pregnancy. The definition of proteinuria is the same no matter when it occurs:

- Greater than 0.3 g in a 24-hour urine collection or protein/creatinine (P/C) ratio greater than 0.3. If it is not possible to measure 24-hour protein or P/C ratio, *proteinuria* can be defined as a dipstick measurement of at least 1+ on two occasions.
- Protein excretion in the urine increases in normal pregnancy from approximately 5 mg/dL in the first and second trimesters to 15 mg/dL in the third trimester. These low levels are not detected by dipstick. The concentration of urinary protein is influenced by contamination with vaginal secretions, blood, bacteria, or amniotic fluid. It also varies with urine specific gravity and pH, exercise, and posture.
- Proteinuria usually appears after hypertension in the course of the disease process, but in some women, it may appear before hypertension.

Edema

Edema is defined as excessive weight gain (>4 lb [1.8 kg] in 1 week) in the second or third trimester, and it may be the first sign of the potential development of PE. However, 39% of patients with eclampsia do not have edema.

Preeclampsia and Eclampsia

Preeclampsia is gestational hypertension (GH) plus proteinuria. Box 31-1 lists criteria for diagnosis of GH and PE. The ACOG Task Force on Hypertension in Pregnancy Group classifies PE based on whether it is has severe features. The term *mild preeclampsia* has been removed from the ACOG classification system and should not be used in clinical practice.

It is recognized that some women with GH may have undiagnosed chronic hypertension, whereas others will subsequently progress to develop the clinical syndrome of preeclampsia.[5] In general, the likelihood of progression to PE

TABLE 31-1   HYPERTENSIVE DISORDERS OF PREGNANCY

CLINICAL FINDINGS	CHRONIC HYPERTENSION	GESTATIONAL HYPERTENSION*	PREECLAMPSIA
Time of onset of hypertension	<20 wk	>20 wk	Usually in third trimester
Degree of hypertension	Mild or severe	Mild	Mild or severe
Proteinuria*	Absent	Absent	Usually present
Cerebral symptoms	May be present	Absent	Present in 30%
Hemoconcentration	Absent	Absent	Severe disease
Thrombocytopenia	Absent	Absent	Severe disease
Hepatic dysfunction	Absent	Absent	Severe disease

*Defined as 1+ or more (or protein/creatinine ratio >0.30) by dipstick testing on two occasions or 300 mg or more in a 24-hour urine collection or protein.

BOX 31-1   CRITERIA FOR MILD GESTATIONAL HYPERTENSION IN HEALTHY PREGNANT WOMEN

- Systolic blood pressure >140 mm Hg but <160 mm Hg and diastolic blood pressure >90 mm Hg but <110 mm Hg
- Proteinuria of <300 mg per 24-hr collection
- Platelet count of >100,000/mm³
- Normal liver enzymes
- Absent maternal symptoms
- Absent intrauterine growth restriction and oligohydramnios by ultrasound

TABLE 31-2	RECOMMENDED CRITERIA TO DIAGNOSE PREECLAMPSIA IN WOMEN WITH PREEXISTING MEDICAL CONDITIONS
CONDITION	**CRITERIA NEEDED**
Hypertension only	Proteinuria of ≥300 mg per 24 hr or thrombocytopenia
Hypertension plus proteinuria (renal disease or class F diabetes)	Worsening severe hypertension plus proteinuria and either new onset of symptoms, thrombocytopenia, or elevated liver enzymes

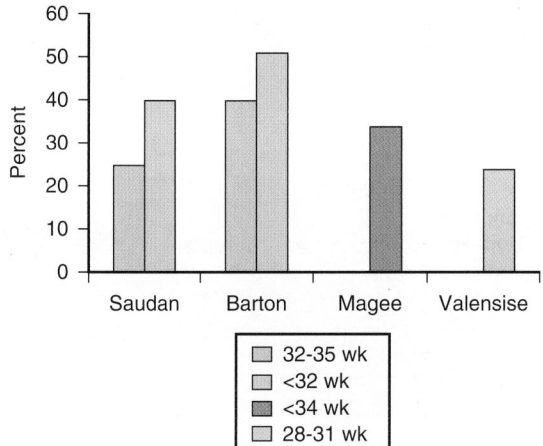

FIG 31-1 Rate of progression from gestational hypertension to pre-eclampsia by gestational age at diagnosis. (Data from references 5, 6, 7, and 8.)

depends on gestational age at time of diagnosis, with higher rates if the onset of hypertension is before 35 weeks' gestation (Fig. 31-1).[5-8]

Criteria for Preeclampsia or Gestational Hypertension With Severe Features

Preeclampsia, or *gestational hypertension with severe features,* is defined when either disorder is present in association with any of the following abnormalities:

- Systolic BP greater than 160 mm Hg or diastolic BP greater than 110 mm Hg on two occasions at least 4 hours apart while the patient is on bed rest or once if the patient has received prior antihypertensive therapy. Prompt treatment is recommended for severe BP values that are sustained for longer than 30 minutes.
- New-onset persistent cerebral symptoms (headaches) or visual disturbances
- Impaired liver function as indicated by abnormally elevated liver enzymes (at least twice the upper limit of normal [ULN]); severe, persistent right upper quadrant or epigastric pain that is unresponsive to medications and not accounted for by an alternative diagnosis; or both
- Pulmonary edema
- Thrombocytopenia (platelet count <100,000/μL)
- Progressive renal insufficiency (serum creatinine >1.1 mg/dL)

It is important to note that the amount of proteinuria, presence of oliguria, and presence of intrauterine growth restriction (IUGR) or fetal growth restriction (FGR) by ultrasound have been removed as criteria for the diagnosis of severe disease.

Eclampsia is defined as the occurrence of seizures after the second half of pregnancy not attributable to other causes.[9]

Chronic Hypertension

Chronic hypertension is defined as hypertension present prior to pregnancy or that is diagnosed before 20 weeks of gestation. Hypertension that persists for more than 3 months postpartum is also classified as chronic hypertension.[2,3]

Chronic Hypertension With Superimposed Preeclampsia

Women with chronic hypertension may develop superimposed preeclampsia, which increases morbidity for both the mother and fetus. The diagnosis of superimposed PE is based on one or both of the following findings: development of *new-onset proteinuria,* defined as the urinary excretion of 0.3 g or more of protein in a 24-hour specimen or a P/C ratio greater than 0.3 in women with hypertension and no proteinuria before 20 weeks' gestation; *or,* in women with hypertension and proteinuria before 20 weeks, severe exacerbation in hypertension plus development of symptoms *or* thrombocytopenia and abnormal liver enzymes (Table 31-2).[1,10,11]

The ACOG Task Force report on hypertension in pregnancy recommended that **superimposed preeclampsia** be stratified into two groups to guide management: (1) *superimposed preeclampsia,* defined as a sudden increase in blood pressure that was previously well controlled or escalation of antihypertensive medications to control BP, or (2) *new-onset proteinuria* (>300 mg/24-hour collection or a P/C ratio >0.3), or a sudden and sustained increase in proteinuria in a woman with known proteinuria before conception or early in pregnancy.

A diagnosis of **superimposed preeclampsia with severe features** should be made in the presence of any of the following: (1) severe-range BP (>160 mm Hg systolic or >110 mm Hg diastolic) despite escalation of antihypertensive therapy; (2) persistent cerebral symptoms such as headaches or visual disturbances; (3) significant increase in liver enzymes (at least two times the ULN concentration for a particular laboratory); (4) thrombocytopenia (platelet count <100,000/μL); or (5) new-onset and/or worsening renal insufficiency.

Gestational Hypertension

Gestational hypertension is the most frequent cause of hypertension during pregnancy. The incidence ranges between 6% and 29% in nulliparous women[2,4,12] and between 2% and 4% in multiparous women.[2] The incidence is markedly increased in patients with multiple gestations.[13-15] In general, most cases of GH develop at or beyond 37 weeks' gestation, and thus the overall pregnancy outcome is usually similar to that seen in women with normotensive pregnancies (Table 31-3).[4,5,12]

TABLE 31-3	PREGNANCY OUTCOME IN WOMEN WITH MILD GESTATIONAL HYPERTENSION			
	KNUIST ET AL[12] (*n* = 396)	HAUTH ET AL[4] (*n* = 715)	BARTON ET AL[5] (*n* = 405)	SIBAI[2] (*n* = 186)
Gestation at delivery (week)*	NR	39.7	37.4[†]	39.1
Before 37 weeks (%)	5.3	7.0	17.3	5.9
Before 34 weeks (%)	1.3	1.0	4.9	1.6
Birthweight (g)*	NR	3303	3038	3217
SGA (%)	1.5[‡]	6.9	13.8	7.0
<2500 g (%)	7.1	7.7	23.5	NR
Abruptio placentae (%)	0.5	0.3	0.5	0.5
Perinatal deaths (%)	0.8	0.5	0	0

Modified from Sibai BM. Diagnosis and management of gestational hypertension and preeclampsia. *Obstet Gynecol.* 2003;102:181.
*Mean values.
[†]Women who developed hypertension at 24 to 35 weeks.
[‡]Less than the third percentile.
NR, not reported; *SGA*, small for gestational age.

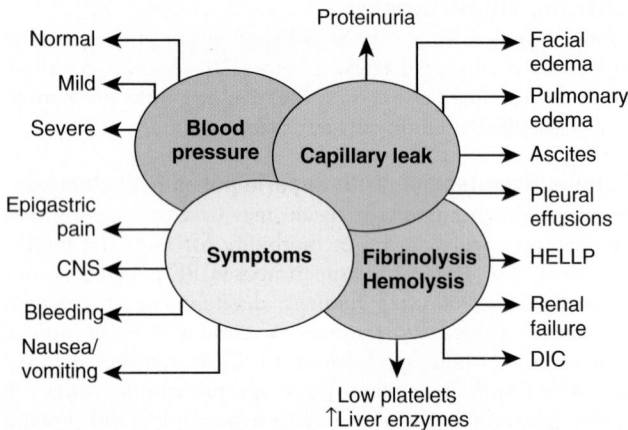

FIG 31-2 Maternal manifestations in preeclampsia. CNS, central nervous system; DIC, disseminated intravascular coagulation; HELLP, hemolysis, elevated liver enzymes, and low platelets.

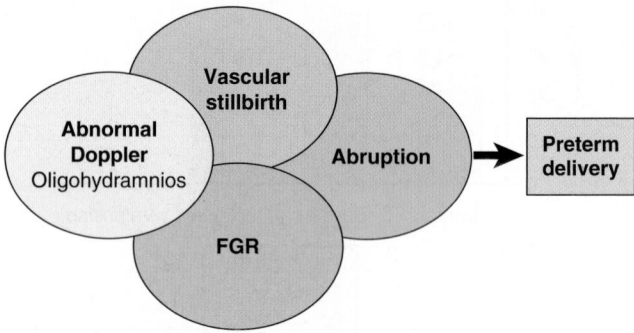

FIG 31-3 Fetal manifestations of preeclampsia. FGR, fetal growth restriction.

However, women with mild GH have higher rates of induction of labor.[4]

Maternal and perinatal morbidities are substantially increased in women with severe GH.[2,4] Indeed, these women have increased risk for morbidity compared with women with mild PE. The rates of abruptio placentae, preterm delivery (at <37 and 35 weeks), and small-for-gestational-age (SGA) infants in these women are similar to those seen in women with PE and severe features.[2,16] It remains unclear whether this increase in preterm delivery is secondary to scheduled early delivery according to physician preference or whether it occurs because of a disease process.

PREECLAMPSIA

Preeclampsia is a form of hypertension that is unique to human pregnancy. The clinical findings of PE can manifest as either a maternal syndrome (Fig. 31-2) **or a fetal syndrome** (Fig. 31-3).[17-19] In practice, the maternal syndrome of PE represents a clinical spectrum with major differences between near-term PE without demonstrable fetal effects and PE that is associated with low birthweight and preterm delivery.[17,20] PE is clearly a heterogeneous condition for which the pathogenesis may be different in women with various risk factors.[17,20,21] The pathogenesis of PE in nulliparous women may be different than that in women with preexisting vascular disease, multifetal gestations, diabetes mellitus, or previous PE. In addition, the

pathophysiology of early-onset PE may be different than that of PE that develops at term, during labor, or in the postpartum period.[17,20,21]

The incidence of preeclampsia ranges between 2% and 7% in healthy nulliparous women.[2,4,12] **In these women, PE is generally mild, with the onset near term or during labor** (75% of cases), **and the condition conveys only a minimally increased risk for adverse fetal outcome.**[2,4,12] In contrast, the incidence and severity of PE are substantially higher in women with multifetal gestation,[10,13,15,22] chronic hypertension,[10,11] previous PE,[23-28] pregestational diabetes mellitus,[10,29,30] or preexisting thrombophilias.[31]

Atypical Preeclampsia

The criteria for atypical preeclampsia include gestational proteinuria or FGR plus one or more of the following symptoms of preeclampsia: hemolysis, thrombocytopenia, elevated liver enzymes, early signs and symptoms of preeclampsia-eclampsia earlier than 20 weeks, and late postpartum preeclampsia-eclampsia (>48 hours postpartum).

Capillary Leak Syndrome: Facial Edema, Ascites and Pulmonary Edema, and Gestational Proteinuria

Hypertension is considered to be the hallmark for the diagnosis of preeclampsia. However, in some patients with PE, the disease may manifest as either a capillary leak (proteinuria, facial and vulvar edema, ascites, pulmonary edema); **excessive weight gain, particularly during the second and early third trimester; or a spectrum of abnormal hemostasis with multiple-organ dysfunction.** These women usually present

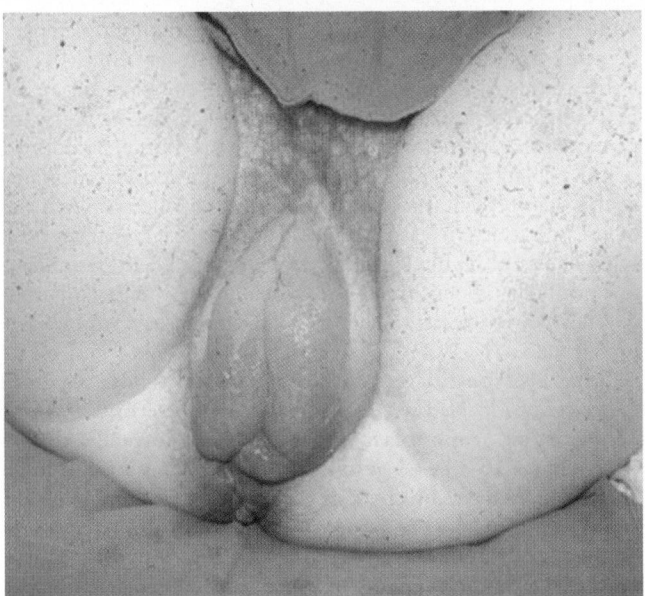

FIG 31-4 Vulvar edema in severe preeclampsia.

with clinical manifestations of atypical preeclampsia, such as proteinuria with or without facial edema, vulvar edema (Fig. 31-4), excessive weight gain (>4 lb/wk), ascites, or pulmonary edema in association with abnormalities in laboratory values or presence of symptoms but without hypertension.[32] Therefore we recommend that women with capillary leak syndrome with or without hypertension be evaluated for platelet, liver enzyme, and renal abnormalities. Those with symptoms such as new onset of unrelenting severe headache, severe visual disturbances, or abnormal blood tests should be considered to have PE.[32]

Gestational Proteinuria

It is generally agreed that urine dipstick protein measurements should be performed at each prenatal visit after 20 weeks' gestation. *Gestational proteinuria* is defined as urinary protein excretion of at least 300 mg per 24-hour timed collection, P/C ratio greater than 0.3, or persistent proteinuria (≥1+ on dipstick on at least two occasions at least 4 hr apart).[1,3] In addition, new-onset proteinuria greater than 2+ on one occasion is strongly associated with proteinuria of greater than 300 mg in 24 hours. The exact incidence of gestational proteinuria progressing to preeclampsia is unknown; however, isolated gestational proteinuria was identified in 4% of women enrolled in two multicenter trials.[33,34] In addition, these studies reported that 4.3% to 7% of patients had combined GH and gestational proteinuria. Thus it appears that at least one third of women with gestational proteinuria may progress to PE.[33,34] Indeed, some authors have suggested that gestational proteinuria alone may herald the early manifestations of impending preeclampsia.[33,35] **In the absence of other pathology, the patient should be treated as having potential PE and requires evaluation for the presence of symptoms; evaluation should include blood tests and frequent monitoring of BP** (at least twice per week or, alternatively, ambulatory home BP measurements), **and the patient should be educated about the signs and symptoms of PE. In addition, women in whom convulsions develop in association with hypertension and proteinuria during the first half of pregnancy should be considered to have eclampsia until proven otherwise.** These women should undergo ultrasound

examination of the uterus to rule out molar pregnancy or hydropic/cystic degeneration of the placenta. Measurement of uterine artery Doppler flow, which shows the classic "notching" characteristic of increased resistance in the placenta of patients with PE, is also recommended.[32]

Risk Factors for Preeclampsia

Several factors have been identified with increased risk for preeclampsia (Box 31-2). **Generally, PE is considered a disease of primigravid women.** The risk increases in those who have limited sperm exposure with the same partner before conception.[17,20,36] The protective effects of long-term sperm exposure with the same partner might provide an explanation for the high risk for PE in women younger than 20 years old. A previous abortion (spontaneous or induced) or a previous normal pregnancy with the same partner is associated with a lower risk for PE. However, this protective effect is lost with a change of partner or with prolonged interval between pregnancies.[37]

Both Scandinavian and U.S. studies have confirmed the importance of paternal factors as a contributor to PE as well as an interpregnancy interval greater than 7 years.[38,39] Using whole population data, Lie and colleagues[39] demonstrated that men who fathered one preeclamptic pregnancy were nearly twice as likely to father a preeclamptic pregnancy with a different woman (odds ratio [OR], 1.8; 95% confidence interval [CI], 1.2 to 2.6 after adjustment for parity), regardless of whether the new partner had a history of a preeclamptic pregnancy. Thus mothers had a substantially increased risk in their second pregnancy (2.9%) if their partner had fathered a preeclamptic first pregnancy with another woman. This risk was nearly as high as the average risk among primigravid women.[39]

Recent advances in assisted reproductive technology (ART) have been associated with an increased risk for preeclampsia.[14,15,40] Among the factors cited are a greater proportion of women older than 40 years, infertile women during their first gestation, multifetal gestation, obese women with polycystic ovary syndrome (PCOS), and women who become pregnant with donated gametes or embryos.[40] The use of donated gametes can influence the maternal-fetal immune interaction. In addition, infertile women with recurrent miscarriage are also reported to be at increased risk for PE.[41]

Obesity reflected as increased body mass index (BMI) heightens the risk for preeclampsia.[42] The worldwide increase in obesity is thus likely to lead to a rise in the frequency of PE.[43,44] Obesity has a strong link to insulin resistance, which is also a risk factor for PE. The exact mechanism by which obesity or insulin resistance is associated with PE is not well understood.

Earlier studies found an overall higher rate of thrombophilia in women with PE compared with controls.[31] Recently, a number of reports have failed to reproduce these findings.[45-46] The disparity in results may reflect the heterogeneity of the women being studied. In the largest series of preeclamptic women with thrombophilia, women had increasing risk for very early onset, severe disease (delivery before 28 weeks) compared with those who did not have thrombophilia.[31]

Pathophysiology

The etiology of preeclampsia remains unknown. Many theories have been suggested, but most of them have not withstood the test of time. Some of the theories still under consideration are listed in Box 31-3.[17, 47-50]

During normal pregnancy, impressive physiologic changes occur in the uteroplacental vasculature and in the cardiovascular system. These changes are most likely induced by the interaction of the fetal (parental) allograft with maternal tissue. The development of mutual immunologic tolerance in the first trimester is thought to lead to important morphologic and biochemical changes in the systemic and uteroplacental maternal circulation.

Uterine Vascular Changes

The human placenta receives its blood supply from numerous uteroplacental arteries that are developed by the action of migratory interstitial and endovascular trophoblasts into the walls *of the spiral arterioles*. This transforms the uteroplacental arterial bed into a low-resistance, low-pressure, high-flow system. The conversion of the spiral arterioles of the nonpregnant uterus into the uteroplacental arteries has been termed *physiologic changes*.[50,51] In a normal pregnancy, these trophoblast-induced vascular changes extend all the way from the intervillous space to the origin of the spiral arterioles that represent the radial arteries in the inner one third of the myometrium. **It is suggested that these vascular changes are effected in *two stages, "the conversion of the decidual segments of the spiral arterioles by a wave of endovascular trophoblast migration in the first trimester and the myometrial segments by a subsequent wave in the second trimester."*[52,53] *This process is reportedly associated with extensive fibrinoid formation and degeneration of the muscular layer in the arterial wall.*** These vascular changes result in the conversion of about 100 to 150 spiral arterioles into distended, tortuous, and funnel-shaped vessels that communicate through multiple openings into the intervillous space.

In contrast, pregnancies complicated by preeclampsia or by FGR demonstrate inadequate maternal vascular response to placentation. In these pregnancies, the previously mentioned vascular changes are usually found only in the decidual segments of the uteroplacental arteries. Hence the myometrial segments of the spiral arterioles continue to exhibit their characteristic musculoelastic architecture, thereby leaving them responsive to hormonal influences.[50,52] Additionally, the number of well-developed arterioles is smaller than that found in normotensive pregnancies.

It has been postulated that this defective vascular response to placentation is due to inhibition of the second wave of endovascular trophoblast migration that normally occurs from about 16 weeks' gestation onward. These pathologic changes may have the effect of curtailing the increased blood supply required by the fetoplacental unit in the later stages of pregnancy and may correlate with the decreased uteroplacental blood flow seen in most cases of preeclampsia.[50] Frusca and associates[52] studied placental bed biopsy specimens obtained during cesarean delivery from normal pregnancies ($n = 14$), preeclamptic pregnancies ($n = 24$), and chronic hypertensive pregnancies only ($n = 5$). Biopsy specimens from the preeclamptic group demonstrated abnormal vascular changes in every case, and 18 had acute atherosclerotic changes. In contrast, 13 of the 14 specimens from normotensive pregnancies had normal vascular physiologic changes. In addition, they found that the mean birthweight was significantly lower in the group with atherosclerosis than it was in the other group without such findings. It is important to note that these vascular changes may also be demonstrated in a significant proportion of normotensive pregnancies complicated by FGR. Meekins and associates[53] demonstrated that endovascular trophoblast invasion is not an all-or-none phenomenon in normal and preeclamptic pregnancies. These authors observed that morphologic features found in one spiral artery may not be representative of all vessels in a placental bed.

Vascular Endothelial Activation and Inflammation

The mechanism by which placental ischemia leads to the clinical syndrome of PE is thought to be related to the production of placental factors that enter the maternal circulation and result in endothelial cell dysfunction.[47-49,54] **Soluble fms-like tyrosine kinase 1 (sFlt-1) is a protein produced by the placenta. It acts by binding to the receptor-binding domains of vascular endothelial growth factor (VEGF), and it also binds to placental-like growth factor (PLGF). Increased levels of this protein in the maternal circulation results in reduced levels of free VEGF and free PLGF with resultant endothelial cell dysfunction.[54]**

Maternal serum and placental levels of sFlt-1 are increased in pregnancies complicated by preeclampsia values above seen during normal pregnancies. Maynard and coworkers[55] demonstrated that soluble placenta-derived VEGF receptor (sFlt-1)—an antagonist of VEGF and PLGF—is unregulated in PE, which leads to increased systemic levels of sFlt-1 that fall after delivery. Increased circulating sFlt-1 in PE is associated with decreased circulating levels of free VEGF and PLGF and results in endothelial dysfunction. The magnitude of increase in sFlt levels correlates with disease severity,[56] which lends further support to VEGF–soluble Flt balance and represents one of the final common pathophysiologic pathways.

First-trimester PLGF levels are decreased in future preeclamptic pregnancies and in pregnancies complicated by FGR, whereas sFlt levels do not differ from controls.[57] Again, these data are compatible with decidual angiogenic growth factors, in particular PLGF, as being essential for early placental development (PLGF is low in both FGR and preeclampsia), with a later involvement of sFlt as a fetal rescue signal steering the maternal response; that is, the degree of maternal systemic hypertension. This hypothesis is supported by Levine and colleagues,[56] who demonstrated that during the last 2 months of pregnancy in normotensive controls, the level of sFlt-1 increased and the level of PLGF decreased.

Levine and associates[58] investigated urinary PLGF levels in pregnant women with and without PE and found that among normotensive pregnant women, urinary PLGF increased during the first two trimesters, peaked at 29 to 32 weeks, and decreased thereafter. Among women who ultimately developed PE, the pattern of urinary PLGF was similar, but levels were significantly reduced beginning at 25 to 28 weeks. Particularly large differences were seen among those who subsequently developed early-onset PE and in those who delivered SGA infants.[58] A similar study suggested that urinary angiogenic factors can identify women with severe PE.[59]

During the past decade, our understanding of the molecular basis for the pathophysiologic abnormalities in preeclampsia has reached an unprecedented level. Clear appreciation now exists for the role of cell adhesion molecules (CAMs) and angiogenic proteins and for activation of the inflammatory system in the pathogenesis of microvascular dysfunction in women with PE.[47,48,56] Evidence also suggests an exaggerated inflammatory response (abnormal cytokine production and neutrophil activation) in women with the clinical findings of PE.[49] However, this enhanced inflammatory response is absent before the development of PE.[60]

Recent studies that have confirmed increased levels of asymmetric dimethylarginine at 23 to 25 weeks in pregnant women who develop PE have emphasized the importance of the nitric oxide–cyclic guanosine monophosphate (cGMP) pathway.[61,62] Endothelial dysfunction and inappropriate endothelial cell activation associated with alterations in nitric oxide levels in PE explains most typical clinical manifestations, including the increased endothelial cell permeability and increased platelet aggregation.[63]

Genetics and Genetic Imprinting

According to the genetic conflict theory, fetal genes are selected to increase the transfer of nutrients to the fetus, whereas maternal genes are selected to limit transfer in excess of some optimal level.[17,20] The phenomenon of genomic imprinting means that a similar conflict exists within fetal cells between genes that are maternally derived and those that are paternally derived. The conflict hypothesis suggests that placental factors (fetal genes) act to *increase* maternal BP, whereas maternal factors act to *reduce* BP.[20] Endothelial cell dysfunction may have evolved as a fetal rescue strategy to increase nonplacental resistance when the uteroplacental blood supply is inadequate.

Nilsson and associates[64] published a model that suggests a heritability estimate of 31% for PE and 20% for GH. It is unlikely that one major PE gene will be found because such a gene would be selected against through evolution, unless it also carried a major reproductive advantage. It is more likely that a rapidly growing number of susceptibility genes will be uncovered and that many of these will be found to interact with the maternal cardiovascular-hemostatic system or in the regulation of maternal inflammatory responses.[65] These loci segregate with different populations,[66] and it should be noted that these loci only explain a relatively small percentage of the overall cases of PE. In addition, although these linkage studies indicate maternal susceptibility, they do not exclude the additional involvement of fetal genes.[66] **Another important consideration regarding the genetics of PE is the confounding effect of the so-called fetal origins of adult disease hypothesis, which suggests that a hostile intrauterine environment for a female fetus would form the basis for the insulin resistance syndrome with its associated endothelial dysfunction and, as such, that it would lead to an increased risk for PE** (see Chapter 5).[20]

Epigenetic features and imprinting are also involved in the pathogenesis of PE.[66,67] Further evidence of the role of imprinting was recently suggested by Oudejans and van Dijk[66] and Nafee and associates.[67]

Changes in Prostanoids

Several investigators have described levels of the various prostaglandins and their metabolites throughout pregnancy. They have measured the concentrations of these substances in plasma, serum, amniotic fluid, placental tissues, urine, and cord blood. The data have been inconsistent, which reflects differences in methodology.[68,69] During pregnancy, prostanoid production increases in both maternal and fetoplacental tissues. Prostacyclin is produced by the vascular endothelium and in the renal cortex. It is a potent vasodilator and inhibitor of platelet aggregation. Thromboxane A_2 (TXA_2) is produced by the platelets and trophoblasts; it is a potent vasoconstrictor and platelet aggregator. Hence, these eicosanoids have opposite effects and play a major role in regulating vascular tone and vascular blood flow. **An imbalance in prostanoid production or catabolism has been suggested as being responsible for the pathophysiologic changes in preeclampsia.** However, the precise role by which prostaglandins are involved in the etiology of PE remains unclear.[20]

Lipid Peroxide, Free Radicals, and Antioxidants

Evidence is accumulating that lipid peroxides and free radicals may be important in the pathogenesis of preeclampsia.[40,50,70] Superoxide ions may be cytotoxic to the cell by changing the characteristics of the cellular membrane and producing membrane lipid peroxidation. Elevated plasma concentrations of free radical oxidation products precede the development of PE. In addition, some studies reported lower serum antioxidant activity in patients with PE than in those with normotensive pregnancies.[17,20]

Much of the controversy about oxidative stress is related to the nonspecificity of the markers. A recent study by Moretti and associates[71] measured oxidative stress "on line" in exhaled breath (not subjective to in vitro artifacts) and confirmed greater oxidative stress in women with PE compared with nonpregnant controls and those who had uncomplicated pregnancies.

Diagnosis of Preeclampsia

Preeclampsia is a clinical syndrome that embraces a wide spectrum of signs and symptoms that have been clinically

observed to develop alone or in combination. **Elevated BP is the traditional hallmark for diagnosis of the disease.** The diagnosis of PE and the severity of the disease process are generally based on maternal BP. Many factors may influence the measurement of BP, including the accuracy of the equipment used, the size of the sphygmomanometer cuff, duration of the rest period before recording, posture of the patient, and the Korotkoff phase used (phase IV or phase V for diastolic BP measurement). **It is recommended that all BP values be recorded with the woman in a sitting position for ambulatory patients or in a semireclining position for hospitalized patients.**[2,3,18,19] The right arm should be used consistently, and the arm should be in a roughly horizontal position at heart level. For diastolic BP measurements, both phases—muffling sound and disappearance sound—should be recorded. This is very important because the level measured at phase IV is about 5 to 10 mm Hg higher than that measured at phase V. A rise in BP has been used by several authors as a criterion for the diagnosis of hypertension in pregnancy. This definition is usually unreliable because a gradual increase in BP from the second to third trimester is seen in most normotensive pregnancies. Villar and Sibai[72] prospectively studied BP changes during the course of pregnancy in 700 young primigravidas and found that 137 patients (19.6%) had PE. The sensitivity and positive predictive values for PE of a threshold increase in diastolic BP of at least 15 mm Hg on two occasions were 39% and 32%, respectively. The respective values for a threshold increase in systolic pressures were 22% and 33%.

Three recent studies from New Zealand,[73] the United States,[74] and Turkey[75] investigated pregnancy outcomes in women with a rise in diastolic BP of more than 15 mm Hg but an absolute diastolic level below 90 mm Hg compared with gravidas who remained normotensive. The New Zealand report[73] and a Turkish study[75] included women with elevated BPs without proteinuria, whereas the American investigation[74] included women with an increased diastolic pressure by 15 mm Hg or more plus proteinuria (≥300 mg/24 hours). Overall, pregnancy outcomes were similar among women who remained normotensive and those who demonstrated a rise in diastolic pressure of 15 mm Hg or higher but did not reach 90 mm Hg. The use of a specific rise in BP over baseline as a diagnostic criterion is principally influenced by two factors: gestational age at time of first observation and frequency of BP measurements. Thus a 15 mm Hg rise in diastolic BP is unreliable to diagnose PE.

Prediction of Preeclampsia

A review of the world literature reveals that more than 100 clinical, biophysical, and biochemical tests have been recommended to predict or identify the patient at risk for future development of preeclampsia.[76-84] **The results of the pooled data for the various tests and the lack of agreement among serial tests suggest that none of these clinical tests is sufficiently reliable for use as a screening test in clinical practice.**[28]

Numerous biochemical markers have been proposed to predict which women are destined to develop PE. These biochemical markers were generally chosen on the basis of specific pathophysiologic abnormalities that have been reported in association with PE. Thus these markers have included markers of placental dysfunction, endothelial and coagulation activation, angiogenesis, and markers of systemic inflammation. However, the results of various studies to evaluate the reliability of these markers in predicting PE have been inconsistent, and many of

these markers suffer from poor specificity and predictive values that are too low for routine use in clinical practice.[80-88]

During the past decade, several prospective and nested case-control studies have found that certain maternal risk factors, biophysical clinical factors, and serum biomarkers obtained in the first trimester are associated with subsequent development of hypertensive disorders of pregnancy (HDP), GH, or PE.[79-83,89,90] These studies evaluated the use of these factors or markers alone or in combination, and they provided detection rates for various subtypes of hypertension and PE with a false-positive rate (FPR) of either 5% or 10%. Overall, neither the maternal factors nor the serum biomarkers, either alone or combined, had an adequate detection rate for either all HDPs or GH or PE developing at 37 weeks of gestation or later. In the same studies, using maternal factors and mean arterial pressure (MAP) in the first trimester, the detection rate for PE before 34 weeks was 73%, and for PE before 37 weeks, it was 60% with an FPR of 10%. Using data from the Maternal-Fetal Medicine Foundation, the use of combined maternal factors and biophysical and biochemical markers increased the detection rate to 95% for PE that required delivery before 34 weeks of gestation and 77% for PE that required delivery at before 37 weeks of gestation with an FPR of 10%.[90] However, the positive predictive value (PPV) for such a screen remained less than 10%. In addition, these studies were conducted in a heterogeneous group of women at various risks for HDP and PE. A recent study by Giguère and colleagues[91] evaluated combined maternal factors and serum markers measured in the first trimester in 7929 women who were at very low risk for GH (2.7%) and PE (1.8%). In those with PE, the incidence was 0.2% at less than 34 weeks and 1.2% at less than 37 weeks of gestation. They found that a clinical model that included maternal risk factors, BMI, and MAP had a detection rate of 54% and a PPV of 3% with an FPR of 10% for preeclampsia at less than 37 weeks of gestation, whereas a full model that also included serum biomarkers had a detection rate of 39% and a PPV of 2% for PE at less than 37 weeks of gestation.

Based on the results of this study and other reports in recent years, it is clear that evaluation of maternal clinical factors and other biophysical and biomarkers measured in the first trimester is useful only for the prediction of those who will ultimately progress to PE that will require delivery prior to 34 weeks of gestation. However, given the poor PPV for PE before 34 weeks and the poor detection rates for all cases of GH and PE, the clinical indications for a PE screening test in the first trimester remain unclear. **Currently, no prospective studies or randomized trials have evaluated the benefits and risks of first-trimester screening for prediction of PE. Until then, the use of such tests for screening should remain investigational.**[92]

Doppler ultrasound is a useful method to assess uterine artery blood flow velocity in the second trimester. An abnormal uterine artery velocity waveform is characterized by a high resistance index or by the presence of an early diastolic notch (unilateral or bilateral).[77,78,81] **Pregnancies complicated by abnormal uterine artery Doppler findings in the second trimester are associated with more than a sixfold increase in the rate of PE.**[77] However, the sensitivity of an abnormal uterine artery Doppler for predicting PE ranges from 20% to 60% with a PPV of 6% to 40%.[77,81] **Current data do not support Doppler studies for routine screening of pregnant women for PE, but uterine artery Doppler could be beneficial as a screening test**

BOX 31-4   INTERVENTIONS USED TO PREVENT PREECLAMPSIA

- High-protein and low-salt diet
- Nutritional supplementation (protein)
- Calcium
- Magnesium
- Zinc
- Fish and evening primrose oil
- Antihypertensive drugs, including diuretics
- Antithrombotic agents
- Low-dose aspirin
- Dipyridamole
- Heparin
- Vitamins E and C
- Sildenafil

in women at very high risk for PE if an effective preventive treatment should become available.

The ACOG task force report on hypertension in pregnancy recommends only using risk factors for identifying women considered at increased risk for PE.[1,3]

Prevention of Preeclampsia

Numerous clinical trials describe the use of various methods to prevent or reduce the incidence of preeclampsia.[28,92] Because the etiology of the disease is unknown, these interventions have been used in an attempt to correct theoretic abnormalities in PE. A detailed review of these trials is beyond the scope of this chapter; however, the results of these studies have been the subject of several recent systemic reviews.[92] **In short, randomized trials have evaluated protein or salt restriction; zinc, magnesium, fish oil, or vitamin C or E supplementation; the use of diuretics and other antihypertensive agents; and the use of heparin to prevent PE in women with various risk factors. These trials have had limited sample sizes, and results have revealed** *minimal to no benefit.* Some of the methods studied are summarized in Box 31-4.

Calcium Supplementation

The relationship between dietary calcium intake and hypertension has been the subject of several experimental and observational studies. Epidemiologic studies have documented an inverse association between calcium intake and maternal BP and the incidences of PE and eclampsia. The BP-lowering effect of calcium is thought to be mediated by alterations in plasma renin activity and parathyroid hormone.

Thirteen clinical studies (15,730 women) have compared the use of calcium with no treatment or with a placebo in pregnancy. These trials differ in the populations studied (low risk or high risk for hypertensive disorders of pregnancy), study design (randomization, double-blind, or use of a placebo), gestational age at enrollment (20 to 32 weeks' gestation), sample size in each group (range, 22 to 588), dose of elemental calcium used (156 to 2000 mg/day), and the definition of hypertensive disorders of pregnancy used.

In the Cochrane review, calcium supplementation was associated with reduced hypertension (relative risk [RR], 0.65; 95% CI, 0.53 to 0.81) and reduced PE (RR, 0.45; 95% CI, 0.31 to 0.65), particularly for those at high risk and with low baseline dietary calcium intake; for those with adequate calcium intake, the difference was not statistically significant. No side

effects of calcium supplementation have been recorded in the trials reviewed. **In contrast, a recent evidence-based review by the U.S. Food and Drug Administration (FDA) concluded that "the relationship between calcium and risk of hypertension in pregnancy is inconsistent and inconclusive, and the relationship between calcium and the risk of pregnancy-induced hypertension and preeclampsia is highly unlikely." At present, the benefit of calcium supplementation for PE prevention in women with low dietary calcium intake remains unclear.**[28] It is also important to note that none of the published randomized trials included women with high-risk factors such as previous PE, chronic hypertension, twins, or pregestational diabetes mellitus.[28] **Based on available data, the author does not recommend using calcium supplementation for the prevention of PE.**

Antiplatelet Agents Including Low-Dose Aspirin

Preeclampsia is associated with vasospasm and activation of the coagulation-hemostasis systems. Enhanced platelet activation plays a central role in the previously mentioned process and reflects abnormalities in the thromboxane-prostacyclin balance. Hence, several authors have used pharmacologic manipulation to alter the previously mentioned ratio in an attempt to prevent or ameliorate the course of PE.

Aspirin inhibits the synthesis of prostaglandins by irreversibly acetylating and inactivating cyclooxygenase (COX). In vitro, platelet COX is more sensitive to inhibition by low doses of aspirin (<80 mg) than vascular endothelial COX. This biochemical selectivity of low-dose aspirin appears to be related to its unusual kinetics, which result in presystemic acetylation of platelets exposed to higher concentrations of aspirin in the portal circulation.

Most randomized trials for the prevention of PE have used low-dose aspirin (LDA; 50 to 150 mg/dL). **The rationale for recommending LDA prophylaxis is the theory that the vasospasm and coagulation abnormalities in preeclampsia are caused partly by an imbalance in the TXA_2/prostacyclin ratio.**[20,28]

Recently, the Perinatal Antiplatelet Review of International Studies (PARIS) collaborative group performed a meta-analysis of the effectiveness and safety of antiplatelet agents, predominantly aspirin, for the prevention of PE. Thirty-one trials that involved 32,217 women are included in this review, and a 10% reduction was seen in the risk for PE associated with the use of antiplatelet agents (RR, 0.90; 95% CI, 0.84 to 0.96). For women with a previous history of hypertension or PE ($n = 6107$) who were assigned to antiplatelet agents, the relative risk for developing PE was 0.86 (95% CI, 0.77 to 0.97). No significant differences were found between treatment and control groups in any other measures of outcome. **The reviewers concluded that antiplatelet agents, largely LDA, have small to moderate benefits when used for prevention of PE.** LDA was also found to be safe. However, more information is clearly required to assess which women are most likely to benefit from this therapy, when treatment is optimally started, and what dose to use.[28]

Several studies have evaluated the efficacy of aspirin in the prevention of PE in high-risk pregnancies as determined by Doppler ultrasound or other risk factors when aspirin was used early in pregnancy. A meta-analysis suggested that LDA improves pregnancy outcome in these women when aspirin is started before 16 weeks' gestation. However, this review has numerous flaws in design and data analysis. A large multicenter study

TABLE 31-4 LOW-DOSE ASPIRIN IN HIGH-RISK WOMEN: NATIONAL INSTITUTE OF CHILD HEALTH AND HUMAN DEVELOPMENT TRIAL

| ENTRY CRITERIA | N | PREECLAMPSIA (%) | |
		ASPIRIN*	PLACEBO*
Normotensive and no proteinuria	1613	14.5	17.7
Proteinuria and hypertension	119	31.7	22.0
Proteinuria only	48	25.0	33.3
Hypertension only	723	24.8	25.0
Insulin-dependent diabetes	462	18.3	21.6
Chronic hypertension	763	26.0	24.6
Multifetal gestation	678	11.5	15.9
Previous preeclampsia	600	16.7	19.0

Data from Caritis SN, Sibai BM, Hauth J, et al, for the National Institute of Child Health and Human Development. Low-dose aspirin therapy to prevent preeclampsia in women at high risk. *N Engl J Med.* 1998;338:701.
*No difference was reported for any of the groups regarding the rate of preeclampsia.

sponsored by the National Institute of Child Health and Human Development (NICHD) included 2539 women with pregestational insulin-treated diabetes mellitus, chronic hypertension, multifetal gestation, or PE in a previous pregnancy and showed no beneficial effect from LDA in such high-risk women (Table 31-4).

During the past three decades, several randomized controlled trials (RCTs) and systematic reviews evaluated the benefits and risks of using LDA in pregnancy for the prevention of PE and its complications in women with one or more of the risk factors listed above. The results of the RCTs were conflicting, and the systematic reviews were inconclusive.[93] This is not surprising given that the published trials and those included in various reviews differed in regard to the enrolled study populations (minimal risk to extremely high risk for PE, preterm birth, FGR, and perinatal death), gestational age at enrollment (12 to 32 weeks), dose of aspirin utilized (50 to 150 mg/day), number of study subjects and number of centers in each trial, definition of PE and adverse perinatal outcomes, and whether the systemic review included unplanned subgroup analysis.[93]

The U.S. Preventive Services Task Force (USPSTF) recently published a report on LDA for the prevention of morbidity and mortality from preeclampsia.[94] The report contained an exhaustive review of published trials regarding the efficacy and safety of LDA in pregnancy for the prevention of PE and other adverse perinatal outcomes in women considered at high risk for PE. The review considered 15 randomized trials (8 quality) in women at increased risk for PE to evaluate maternal and perinatal benefits and 13 randomized trials (8 quality) to evaluate the incidence of PE. Preeclampsia incidence in women considered at increased risk ranged from 8% to 30%. In addition, two large observational studies were included to evaluate the safety of LDA use in pregnancy.

In women considered at increased risk for preeclampsia, the USPSTF members found that LDA administered after 12 weeks' gestation reduced the risk of PE by an average of 24% (pooled relative risk [PRR], 0.76; 95% CI, 0.62 to 0.95), **reduced the average risk of preterm birth by 14%** (PRR, 0.86; 95% CI, 0.76 to 0.98), **and reduced the risk of FGR by 20%** (PRR, 0.80; 95% CI, 0.65 to 0.99). In addition, they found that the magnitude of risk reduction with LDA for the above

complications was dependent on baseline risk for PE in the study population. Contrary to the results of other systematic reviews, they found that the beneficial effects of LDA were not dependent on the dose of LDA, and they were evident when LDA was used between 12 and 28 weeks' gestation. Moreover, they found that LDA did not increase the risk of bleeding complications (abruptio placentae, postpartum hemorrhage, neonatal intracerebral hemorrhage) or perinatal death. Based on results of this review, the **Task Force members recommended that women considered at increased risk for PE—that is, those with a history of PE, preexisting chronic hypertension or renal disease, pregestational diabetes, autoimmune disease, or multifetal gestation—should receive LDA** (81 mg/day) **starting at 12 to 28 weeks until delivery to reduce the likelihood of developing subsequent PE, preterm birth, or FGR.**

However, such recommendation is in contrast to that of the **ACOG Task Force on Hypertension in Pregnancy, which recommended LDA only to women with prior PE that resulted in delivery at less than 34 weeks or to those with prior recurrent PE.**

Heparin or Low-Molecular-Weight Heparin

Several observational studies and randomized trials have evaluated the prophylactic use of low-molecular-weight heparin (LMWH) for the prevention of PE and other adverse pregnancy outcomes. The results of these studies were the subject of several recent reviews. Two recent large randomized trials conducted in Italy[95] and in Canada[96] revealed that prophylactic LMWH does not reduce the rate of PE in women at high risk for this complication. In addition, a meta-analysis of published trials demonstrated no benefit from LMWH.[97] **Therefore it is the authors' opinion that LMWH should not be used for PE prevention.**

Vitamins C and E

Reduced antioxidant capacity, increased oxidative stress, or both in the maternal circulation and in the placenta have been proposed to play a major role in the pathogenesis of PE. Consequently, several trials were designed using vitamins C and E for the prevention of PE. The first trial suggested a beneficial effect from pharmacologic doses of vitamins E and C in women identified as being at risk for PE by means of abnormal uterine Doppler flow velocimetry. However, the study had limited sample size and must be confirmed in other populations. **In contrast, several randomized trials with large sample sizes in women at low risk and very high risk for PE found no reduction in the rate of PE with vitamin C and E supplementation** (Table 31-5).[29,98-103]

Laboratory Abnormalities in Preeclampsia

Women with preeclampsia may exhibit a symptom complex that ranges from minimal BP elevation to derangements of multiple-organ systems. The renal, hematologic, and hepatic systems are most likely to be involved.

Renal Function

Renal plasma flow and glomerular filtration rate (GFR) increase during normal pregnancy. These changes are responsible for a fall in serum creatinine, urea, and uric acid concentrations.[98] In PE, vasospasm and glomerular capillary endothelial swelling (glomerular endotheliosis) lead to an average reduction in GFR of 25% below the rate for normal pregnancy. Serum creatinine

TABLE 31-5 MULTICENTER TRIALS OF VITAMINS C AND E FOR THE PREVENTION OF PREECLAMPSIA

| STUDY GROUP | WOMEN | ENROLLMENT GESTATIONAL AGE (WEEKS) | PREECLAMPSIA | |
			VITAMINS C AND E (%)	PLACEBO (%)
ACTS[98]	Nulliparas	14 to 22	56/935 (6)	47/942 (5)
VIP[99]	High risk	14 to 22	181/1196 (15)	187/1199 (16)
Global Network[100]	High risk	12 to 20	49/355 (14)	55/352 (16)
WHO[101]	High risk	14 to 22	164/681 (24)	157/674 (23)
NICHD[102]	Nulliparas	9 to 16	358/4993 (7.2)	332/4976 (6.7)
INTAPP[103]	High risk	12 to 18	69/1167 (6)	68/1196 (5.7)
DAPIT[29]	Pregestational diabetes	8 to 22	57/375 (15)	70/3784 (19)

DAPIT, Diabetes and Preeclampsia Intervention Trial; *INTAPP,* International Trial of Antioxidants in the Prevention of Preeclampsia; *NICHD,* National Institute of Child Health and Development; *VIP,* Vitamins in Pregnancy; *WHO,* World Health Organization.

is rarely elevated in PE, but uric acid can be increased. In a study of 95 women with severe PE, Sibai and associates reported a mean serum creatinine of 0.91 mg/dL, a mean uric acid of 6.6 mg/dL, and a mean creatinine clearance of 100 mL/min.

The clinical significance of elevated uric acid levels in preeclampsia-eclampsia has been confusing. Hyperuricemia is associated with renal dysfunction, especially decreased renal tubular secretion, and has been consistently associated with glomerular endotheliosis. In addition, it has been linked with increased oxidative stress in PE. **Despite the fact that uric acid levels are elevated in women with PE, this test is not sensitive or specific for the diagnosis of PE or for predicting adverse perinatal outcome.**

Elevated uric acid levels above 6 mg/dL are often found in women with normotensive multifetal pregnancies. As a result, some authors have suggested that to secure a diagnosis of PE based on elevated uric acid values, the upper limit should be adjusted for those with multiple gestation. Elevated uric acid values are also found in women with acute fatty liver of pregnancy and underlying renal disease; therefore **it is suggested that uric acid values not be used for the diagnosis of PE or as an indication for delivery in women with PE.**

Hepatic Function

The liver is not primarily involved in preeclampsia, and hepatic involvement is observed in only 10% of women with severe PE. Fibrin deposition has been found along the walls of hepatic sinusoids in preeclamptic patients with no laboratory or histologic evidence of liver involvement. When liver dysfunction does occur in PE, mild elevation of serum transaminases is most common. Bilirubin is rarely increased in PE, but when elevated, the indirect fraction predominates. Elevated liver enzymes are a feature of the hemolysis, elevated liver enzymes, and low platelets (HELLP) syndrome, a variant of severe PE.

Hematologic Changes

Many studies have evaluated the hematologic abnormalities in women with preeclampsia. **Plasma fibrinopeptide A, D-dimer levels, and circulating thrombin-antithrombin complexes are higher in women with PE than in normotensive gravidas. In contrast, plasma antithrombin III activity is decreased.** These findings indicate enhanced thrombin generation.

Plasma fibrinogen rises progressively during normal pregnancy. In general, plasma fibrinogen levels are rarely reduced in women with PE in the absence of placental abruption.

Thrombocytopenia is the most common hematologic abnormality in women with severe PE. It is correlated with the severity of the disease process and the presence or absence of placental abruption. In a study of 1414 women with

hypertension during pregnancy, Burrows and Kelton found a platelet count of less than 150,000/mm³ in 15% of cases.

Leduc and associates studied the coagulation profile—the platelet count, fibrinogen, prothrombin time (PT), and partial thromboplastin time (PTT)—in 100 consecutive women with severe PE. A platelet count lower than 150,000/mm³ was found in 50% of the women, and a count lower than 100,000/mm³ was found in 36%. Thirteen women had a fibrinogen level of less than 300 mg/dL, and two had prolonged PT and PTT as well as thrombocytopenia on admission. These researchers found **the admission platelet count to be an excellent predictor of subsequent thrombocytopenia and concluded that fibrinogen levels, PT, and PTT should be obtained only in women with a platelet count of less than 100,000/mm³.** A recent study by Barron confirmed these observations in more than 800 women with hypertension in pregnancy.

Hemolysis, Elevated Liver Enzymes, and Low Platelets (HELLP) Syndrome

Considerable debate surrounds the definition, diagnosis, incidence, etiology, and management of HELLP syndrome.[104] Patients with such findings were previously described by many investigators. Weinstein considered it a unique variant of PE and coined the term *HELLP syndrome* for this entity. Barton and associates performed liver biopsies in patients with PE and HELLP syndrome, and periportal necrosis and hemorrhage were the most common histopathologic findings. In addition, they found that the extent of the laboratory abnormalities in HELLP syndrome, including the platelet count and liver enzymes, did not correlate with hepatic histopathologic findings.

LABORATORY CRITERIA FOR DIAGNOSIS

Various diagnostic criteria have been used for HELLP. *Hemolysis,* defined as the presence of microangiopathic hemolytic anemia, is the hallmark of the triad of HELLP syndrome.[104] The classic findings of microangiopathic hemolysis include an abnormal peripheral smear (schistocytes, burr cells, echinocytes), elevated serum bilirubin (indirect form), low serum haptoglobin levels, elevated lactate dehydrogenase (LDH) levels, and a significant drop in hemoglobin levels. A significant percentage of published reports included patients who had no evidence of hemolysis; hence, these patients will not fit the criteria for HELLP syndrome.[104] In some studies in which hemolysis is described, the diagnosis is suspect because it has been based on the presence of an abnormal peripheral smear (no description of type or degree of abnormalities) or elevated LDH levels (threshold of 180 to 600 U/L).

No consensus exists in the literature regarding the liver function test to be used or the degree of elevation in these tests to diagnose elevated liver enzymes. In his original report, Weinstein mentioned abnormal serum levels of aspartate transaminase (AST), abnormal alanine transaminase (ALT), and abnormal bilirubin values; however, specific levels were not suggested. In subsequent studies in which elevated liver enzymes were described, either AST or ALT, the values considered to be abnormal ranged from 17 to 72 U/L.[104] In clinical practice, many of these values are considered normal or slightly elevated.

Low platelet count is the third abnormality required to establish the diagnosis of HELLP syndrome; no consensus has been reached among various published reports regarding the diagnosis of thrombocytopenia. The reported cut-off values have ranged from 75,000/mm³ to 279,000/mm³, and a level of less than 100,000/mm³ is most often cited.[104]

Many authors have used elevated total LDH (usually >600 U/L) as a diagnostic criteria for hemolysis. Of the five isoforms of LDH, only two of them—LDH_1 and LDH_2—are released from ruptured red blood cells. In most women with severe preeclampsia-eclampsia, the elevation in total LDH is probably caused mostly by liver ischemia. Therefore many authors advocate that elevated bilirubin values (indirect form), abnormal peripheral smear, or a low serum haptoglobin level should be part of the diagnostic criteria for hemolysis.

Based on a retrospective review of 302 cases of HELLP syndrome, Martin and colleagues devised the following classification based on the nadir of the platelet count. **Class 1 HELLP syndrome was defined as a platelet nadir below 50,000/mm³, class 2 as a platelet nadir between 50,000 and 100,000/mm³, and class 3 as a platelet nadir between 100,000 and 150,000/mm³.** These classes have been used to predict the rapidity of recovery postpartum, maternal-perinatal outcome, and the need for plasmapheresis.

Hemolysis, defined as the presence of microangiopathic hemolytic anemia, is the hallmark of HELLP syndrome. The role of disseminated intravascular coagulation (DIC) in preeclampsia is controversial. **Most authors do not regard HELLP syndrome to be a variant of DIC because coagulation parameters such as PT, PTT, and serum fibrinogen are normal.**[85] However, the diagnosis of DIC can be difficult to establish in clinical practice. When sensitive determinants of this condition are used—such as antithrombin III, fibrinopeptide A, fibrin monomer, D-dimer, α_2-antiplasmin, plasminogen, prekallikrein, and fibronectin—many patients have laboratory values consistent with DIC. Unfortunately, these tests are time consuming and are not suitable for routine monitoring. Consequently, less sensitive parameters are often used. Sibai and associates defined DIC as the presence of thrombocytopenia, low fibrinogen levels (plasma fibrinogen <300 mg/dL), and fibrin split products above 40 mg/mL. These authors noted the presence of coagulopathy in 21% of 442 patients with HELLP syndrome. They

also found that most cases occurred in women who had antecedent placental abruption or peripartum hemorrhage, and it occurred in all four women in their study who had subcapsular liver hematomas. In the absence of these complications, the frequency of DIC was only 5%.

In view of the previously mentioned diagnostic problems, we recommended that uniform and standardized laboratory values be used to diagnose HELLP syndrome.[104] Plasma haptoglobin and bilirubin values should be included in the diagnosis of hemolysis. In addition, the degree of abnormality of liver enzymes should be defined as a certain number of standard deviations (SDs) from the normal value for each hospital population. Our laboratory criteria to establish the diagnosis are presented in Box 31-5.

CLINICAL FINDINGS

The reported incidence of HELLP syndrome in preeclampsia has been variable, which reflects the differences in diagnostic criteria. **The syndrome appears to be more common in white women and is also more common in preeclamptic women who have been managed conservatively.**[104]

Early detection of HELLP syndrome can be a challenge in that many women present with nonspecific symptoms or subtle signs of PE. The various signs and symptoms reported are not diagnostic of PE and may also be found in women with severe preeclampsia-eclampsia without HELLP syndrome.[104] Right upper quadrant or epigastric pain and nausea or vomiting have been reported with a frequency ranging from 30% to 90% (Table 31-6). Most women gave a history of malaise typical of a nonspecific viral-like syndrome for several days before presentation, which led one investigator to suggest performing laboratory investigations (complete blood count [CBC] and liver enzymes) in all pregnant women with suspected PE who have

---

BOX 31-5   CRITERIA TO ESTABLISH THE DIAGNOSIS OF HELLP SYNDROME

Hemolysis (as least two of these):
- Peripheral smear (schistocytes, burr cells)
- Serum bilirubin (≥1.2 mg/dL)
- Low serum haptoglobin

Severe anemia unrelated to blood loss

Elevated liver enzymes
- Aspartate transaminase or alanine transaminase at least twice the ULN
- Lactate dehydrogenase twice or more of the ULN

Low platelets (<100,000/mm³)

HELLP, hemolysis, elevated liver enzymes, and low platelets; *ULN,* upper limit of normal.

TABLE 31-6   SIGNS AND SYMPTOMS IN WOMEN WITH HELLP SYNDROME

	WEINSTEIN[108] (n = 57) (%)	SIBAI ET AL[107] (n = 509) (%)	MARTIN ET AL[106] (n = 501) (%)	RATH ET AL[109] (n = 50) (%)
Right upper quadrant epigastric pain	86	63	40	90
Nausea, vomiting	84	36	29	52
Headache	NR	33	61	NR
Hypertension	NR	85	82	88
Proteinuria	96	87	86	100

Modified from Sibai BM. Diagnosis, controversies, and management of HELLP syndrome. *Obstet Gynecol.* 2004;103:981.
HELLP, hemolysis, elevated liver enzymes, and low platelets; *NR,* not reported.

BOX 31-6 MEDICAL AND SURGICAL DISORDERS OFTEN CONFUSED WITH HELLP SYNDROME

- Acute fatty liver of pregnancy
- Appendicitis
- Gallbladder disease
- Glomerulonephritis
- Hemolytic uremic syndrome
- Hepatic encephalopathy
- Hyperemesis gravidarum
- Idiopathic thrombocytopenia
- Pyelonephritis
- Systemic lupus erythematosus
- Antiphospholipid antibody syndrome
- Thrombotic thrombocytopenic purpura
- Viral hepatitis

HELLP, hemolysis, elevated liver enzymes, and low platelets.

these symptoms during the third trimester.[104] Headaches are reported by 33% to 61% of the patients, whereas visual changes are reported in about 17%. A small subset of patients with HELLP syndrome may present with symptoms related to thrombocytopenia, such as bleeding from mucosal surfaces, hematuria, petechial hemorrhages, or ecchymosis.

Although most patients have hypertension (82% to 88%; see Table 31-6), it may be only mild in 15% to 50% of the cases and absent in 12% to 18%. Most of the patients (86% to 100%) have proteinuria by dipstick examination, although it has been reported to be absent in 13% of cases.

DIFFERENTIAL DIAGNOSIS

The presenting symptoms, clinical findings, and many of the laboratory findings in women with HELLP syndrome overlap with a number of medical syndromes, surgical conditions, and obstetric complications; therefore the differential diagnosis of HELLP syndrome should include any of the conditions listed in Box 31-6. Because some women with HELLP syndrome may present with gastrointestinal, respiratory, or hematologic symptoms in association with elevated liver enzymes or low platelets in the absence of hypertension or proteinuria, many initially are misdiagnosed as having other conditions such as upper respiratory infection, hepatitis, cholecystitis, pancreatitis, acute fatty liver of pregnancy (AFLP), or immune thrombocytopenic purpura (ITP).[104] Conversely, some women with other conditions—such as thrombotic thrombocytopenic purpura (TTP), hemolytic uremic syndrome (HUS), systemic lupus erythematosus (SLE), sepsis, or catastrophic antiphospholipid antibody syndrome—may be erroneously diagnosed as having HELLP syndrome. In addition, PE may occasionally be superimposed on one of these disorders, which further contributes to the diagnostic difficulty. Because of the remarkably similar clinical and laboratory findings of these disease processes, even the most experienced clinician can face a difficult diagnostic challenge. Therefore efforts should be made to attempt to identify an accurate diagnosis, given that management strategies may be different among these conditions. It is important to emphasize that affected women may have a variety of unusual signs and symptoms, none of which are diagnostic of severe PE. **Pregnant women with probable PE who present with atypical symptoms should have a CBC, a platelet count, and liver enzyme determinations irrespective of maternal BP findings.**

Occasionally, the presence of this syndrome is associated with hypoglycemia that leads to coma, severe hyponatremia, and cortical blindness. A rare but interesting complication of HELLP syndrome is transient nephrogenic diabetes insipidus. Unlike *central diabetes insipidus,* which results from the diminished or absent secretion of arginine vasopressin by the hypothalamus, *transient nephrogenic diabetes insipidus* is characterized by a resistance to arginine vasopressin mediated by excessive vasopressinase. It is postulated that elevated circulating vasopressinase may result from impaired hepatic metabolism of the enzyme.

MANAGEMENT OF HELLP SYNDROME

Management of preeclamptic women who present with HELLP syndrome is highly controversial.[104] Consequently, several therapeutic modalities have been described in the literature to treat or reverse HELLP syndrome. Most of these modalities are similar to those used in the management of severe PE remote from term (Box 31-7).

The clinical course of women with true HELLP syndrome is usually characterized by progressive and sometimes sudden deterioration in the maternal condition.[104] Because the presence of this syndrome has been associated with increased rates of maternal morbidity and mortality, many authors consider its presence to be an indication for immediate delivery. **There is also a consensus of opinion that prompt delivery is indicated if the syndrome develops beyond 34 weeks' gestation or earlier if obvious multiorgan dysfunction, DIC, liver infarction or hemorrhage, renal failure, suspected abruption, or nonreassuring fetal status are apparent.** Delivery is also indicated if the syndrome develops before 23 weeks' gestation.[1,104]

On the other hand, **considerable disagreement exists about the management of women with HELLP syndrome at or before 34 weeks of gestation when the maternal condition is stable, except for mild to moderate abnormalities in blood tests, and fetal condition is reassuring. In such patients, some authors recommend the administration of corticosteroids to accelerate fetal lung maturity followed by delivery after 24 hours,[104] whereas others recommend prolonging pregnancy until the development of maternal or fetal indications for delivery or until achievement of fetal lung maturity.** Some of the measures used in these latter cases have included one or more of the following: bed rest, antihypertensive agents, antithrombotic agents (LDA, dipyridamole), plasma volume expanders (crystalloids, albumin, fresh frozen plasma [FFP]), and corticosteroids (prednisone, prednisolone, dexamethasone, or betamethasone).[104]

EXPECTANT MANAGEMENT OF HELLP SYNDROME

Few large case series describe expectant management of women with true HELLP, partial HELLP, or severe PE with isolated liver enzyme elevation. In general, these reports suggest that transient improvement in laboratory values or pregnancy prolongation from a few days to a few weeks is possible in a select group of women with HELLP syndrome. It is important to note that most of the patients included in these studies were ultimately delivered within 1 week of expectant management.[104]

Investigators from the Netherlands have reported their experience with expectant management in women with HELLP syndrome before 34 weeks' gestation. Visser and Wallenburg reported the use of plasma volume expansion using invasive hemodynamic monitoring and vasodilators in 128 women with

HELLP syndrome before 34 weeks' gestation. Magnesium sulfate and steroids were not used in such women. Twenty-two of the 128 patients were delivered within 48 hours; the remaining 102 patients had pregnancy prolongation for a median of 15 days (range, 3 to 62 days). Fifty-five of these 102 women had antepartum resolution of HELLP syndrome, with a median pregnancy prolongation in these women of 21 days (range, 7 to 62 days). No maternal deaths or serious maternal morbidity was reported. However, 11 of the 128 pregnancies (8.6%) resulted in fetal death at 25 to 34.4 weeks, and 7 neonatal deaths (5.5%) at 27 to 32 weeks' gestation were reported.

Van Pampus and coworkers reported the use of bed rest, antihypertensive medication, and salt restriction in 41 women with HELLP syndrome before 35 weeks' gestation. Fourteen women (34%) were delivered within 24 hours; in the remaining 27 women, pregnancy was prolonged a median of 3 days (range, 0 to 59 days). Fifteen of these 27 women showed complete normalization of the laboratory values. No serious maternal morbidities were noted, but 10 fetal deaths were reported at 27 to 35.7 weeks' gestation.

The study by Ganzevoort and colleagues included 54 women with HELLP syndrome at the time of enrollment. In a subsequent publication, the same authors compared maternal and perinatal complications in these women to the respective outcomes in women without HELLP. They found that the median number of days of pregnancy prolongation and maternal and perinatal complications were similar between the two groups.

One randomized, double-blind trial compared prednisolone ($n = 15$) to placebo ($n = 16$) in patients with HELLP syndrome before 30 weeks' gestation. Prednisolone was given intravenously twice a day. The primary outcome measures were the entry-to-delivery interval and the number of "recurrent HELLP" exacerbations in the antepartum period. The mean entry-to-delivery interval was similar between the two groups (6.9 days for prednisolone and 8 days for placebo). Three cases of liver hematoma or rupture were reported, along with one maternal death in the placebo group. The perinatal mortality rate was similar between the two groups (20% in the prednisolone group and 25% in the placebo group).

The results of these studies suggest that expectant management is possible in a very select group of women with suspected HELLP syndrome before 34 weeks' gestation. However, despite pregnancy prolongation in some of these cases, the overall perinatal outcome was not improved compared with fetuses at a similar gestational age who were delivered within 48 hours after the diagnosis of HELLP syndrome.

Confounding variables make it difficult to evaluate any treatment modality proposed for this syndrome. Occasionally, some patients without true HELLP syndrome may demonstrate antepartum reversal of hematologic abnormalities following bed rest, use of corticosteroids, or plasma volume expansion. However, most of these patients experienced deterioration in either maternal or fetal condition within 1 to 10 days after conservative management. It is doubtful that such limited pregnancy prolongation will result in improved perinatal outcome, and maternal and fetal risks are substantial.[104]

In summary, the results of these studies suggest that expectant treatment is possible in a select group of women with HELLP syndrome before 34 weeks' gestation. However, the number of women who were studied in these reports is inadequate to evaluate maternal safety; therefore such treatment should be considered experimental. In addition, most experts—including members of the ACOG Task Force—recommend delivery of such patients after completion of a course of corticosteroids for fetal lung maturity or if the gestational age is less than 24 weeks.[1,3]

CORTICOSTEROIDS TO IMPROVE PREGNANCY OUTCOME IN WOMEN WITH HELLP SYNDROME

It is well established that antenatal glucocorticoid therapy reduces neonatal complications and neonatal mortality in women with severe PE at 34 weeks' gestation or less (see Chapter 29). The recommended regimens of corticosteroids for the enhancement of fetal maturity are betamethasone (12 mg intramuscularly every 24 hours, two doses) or dexamethasone (6 mg intramuscularly every 12 hours, four doses). These regimens have been identified as the most appropriate for this purpose because they readily cross the placenta and have minimal mineralocorticoid activity. However, it is unclear whether the same or different regimens are beneficial in women with HELLP syndrome.

Corticosteroids have been suggested as safe and effective drugs for improving maternal and neonatal outcome in women with HELLP or partial HELLP syndrome. A review of the literature reveals substantial differences in methodology, time of administration, and drug selection among investigators who advocate the use of corticosteroids in women with HELLP syndrome. Different regimens of steroids have been suggested for preventing respiratory distress syndrome (RDS) as well as to accelerate maternal recovery in the postpartum period.[104] The regimens of steroids used included intramuscular betamethasone (12 mg/12 hr or 24 hours apart on two occasions) or IV dexamethasone (various doses at various time intervals) or a combination of the two. Some studies used steroids only in the antepartum period (for 24 hours, 48 hours, repeat regimens, or chronically for weeks until delivery). In other studies, steroids were given for 48 hours before delivery and then were continued for 24 to 48 hours postpartum, whereas others recommend their administration only in the postpartum period.[104]

Some randomized trials have compared the use of high-dose dexamethasone to either no treatment or betamethasone in

TABLE 31-7   MATERNAL COMPLICATIONS WITH DEXAMETHASONE VERSUS PLACEBO IN HELLP SYNDROME

	NO. WITH PLACEBO (%)	NO. WITH DEXAMETHASONE (%)	CRUDE RELATIVE RISK (95% CI)
Acute renal failure*	8 (13)	6 (10)	0.8 (0.3-2.1)
Oliguria	4 (6)	5 (7.6)	1.3 (0.4-4.5)
Pulmonary edema*	1 (2)	3 (4.6)	3.1 (0.3-28)
Eclampsia	10 (15)	8 (14)	0.8 (0.3-1.9)
Infections	10 (15)	5(8)	0.5 (0.2-1.4)
Death	1 (2)	3 (5)	3.0 (0.3-28)
Platelet transfusion	10 (15)	12 (18)	1.2 (0.6-2.6)
Plasma transfusion	6 (9)	5 (8)	0.8 (0.3-2.6)

Modified from Fonseca JE, Mendez F, Catano C, Arias F. Dexamethasone treatment does not improve the outcome of women with HELLP syndrome: a double-blind, placebo-controlled, randomized clinical trial. *Am J Obstet Gynecol.* 2005;193:1591-1598.
*Only included patients without the event before randomization.
CI, confidence interval.

TABLE 31-8   MATERNAL COMPLICATIONS COMPARING DEXAMETHASONE VERSUS PLACEBO FOR POSTPARTUM HELLP SYNDROME

COMPLICATION*	DEXAMETHASONE (n = 56)		PLACEBO (n = 49)	
	n	%	n	%
Pulmonary edema	2	3.6	5	10.2
Hemorrhagic manifestation	20	35.7	16	32.7
Acute renal failure	9	16.1	12	24.5
Oliguria	27	48.2	22	44.9
Blood transfusion	16	28.6	19	38.6
Any complication	37	66.1	25	51
Death	2	3.6	2	4.1

Modified from Katz L, de Amorim MM, Figueiroa JN, Pinto e Silva JL. Postpartum dexamethasone for women with hemolysis, elevated liver enzymes, and low platelets (HELLP) syndrome: a double-blind, placebo-controlled, randomized clinical trial. *Am J Obstet Gynecol.* 2008;198:283.
*Each patient may have more than one complication.

TABLE 31-9   MATERNAL COMPLICATIONS IN 316 PREGNANCIES WITH HELLP SYNDROME, PARTIAL HELLP SYNDROME, OR SEVERE PREECLAMPSIA WITH NORMAL LABORATORY VALUES

	HELLP (n = 67)	PARTIAL HELLP (n = 71)	SEVERE HELLP (n = 178)
Blood products transfusion (%)	25*	4	3
Disseminated intravascular coagulation (%)	15*	0	0
Wound hematoma, infection (%)[†]	14[‡]	11[§]	2[§]
Pleural effusion (%)	6[‡]	0	1
Acute renal failure (%)	3[‡]	0	0
Eclampsia (%)	9	7	9
Abruptio placentae (%)	9	4	5
Pulmonary edema (%)	8	4	3
Subcapsular liver hematoma (%)	1.5	0	0
Intracerebral hemorrhage (%)	1.5	0	0
Death (%)	1.5	0	0

From Audibert F, Friedman SA, Frangieh AY, Sibai BM. Clinical utility of strict diagnostic criteria for the HELLP (hemolysis, elevated liver enzymes, and low platelets) syndrome. *Am J Obstet Gynecol.* 1996;175:460.
*P < .001, HELLP vs. partial and severe HELLP.
[†]Percentages of women who had cesarean delivery.
[‡]P < .05, HELLP vs. severe HELLP.
[§]P < .05, partial vs. severe HELLP.
HELLP, hemolysis, elevated liver enzymes, and low platelets.

women with presumed HELLP syndrome. These studies were summarized in a review by Sibai.[104] **The results of these studies demonstrated improved laboratory values and urine output in patients receiving dexamethasone but found no differences in serious maternal morbidity.** In addition, the number of patients studied was limited, and neither of these small studies used a placebo.

More recently, three randomized, double-blind placebo trials were conducted to evaluate dexamethasone versus placebo in women with antepartum and postpartum HELLP syndrome. Two of the trials were multicenter, and one was a single-center trial. The results of the two large, multicenter trials are summarized in Tables 31-7 and 31-8. Overall, these trials revealed no maternal benefit of using dexamethasone in women with HELLP syndrome.[105] **It is my opinion that corticosteroids should only be used for 48 hours to accelerate fetal lung maturity in women who have reached 24 to 34 weeks' gestation. In addition, it is recommended that dexamethasone not be used to treat maternal symptoms of HELLP syndrome either beyond 34 weeks or in the postpartum period.**[1,3]

MATERNAL AND PERINATAL OUTCOME

The presence of HELLP syndrome is associated with an increased risk for maternal death (1%) and increased rates of maternal morbidities such as pulmonary edema (8%), acute renal failure (3%), DIC (15%), abruptio placentae (9%), liver hemorrhage or failure (1%), acute respiratory distress syndrome (ARDS), sepsis, and stroke (<1%).[104] Pregnancies complicated by HELLP syndrome are also associated with

increased rates of wound hematomas and the need for transfusion of blood and blood products.[104] The rate of these complications depends on the population studied, the laboratory criteria used to establish the diagnosis, and the presence of associated preexisting medical conditions (chronic hypertension, lupus) or obstetric complications (abruptio placentae, peripartum hemorrhage, fetal demise, eclampsia).[104] The development of HELLP syndrome in the postpartum period also increases the risk for renal failure and pulmonary edema. The presence of placental abruption increases the risk for DIC, pulmonary edema, and renal failure and also increases the need for blood transfusions. Patients who have a large volume of ascites appear to have a high rate of cardiopulmonary complications. Finally, women who meet all the criteria suggested for diagnosis will have higher rates of maternal complications than those who have partial HELLP or elevated liver enzymes only (Table 31-9).

It is generally agreed that perinatal mortality and morbidity are substantially increased in pregnancies complicated by

the HELLP syndrome. The reported perinatal death rate in recent series ranged from 7.4% to 34%, and this high perinatal death rate is mainly experienced at a very early gestational age (<28 weeks) in association with severe FGR or placental abruption.[104] It is important to emphasize that neonatal morbidities in these pregnancies are dependent on gestational age at time of delivery, and they are similar when corrected for gestational age to those in preeclamptic pregnancies without the HELLP syndrome. The rate of preterm delivery is about 70%, and 15% occur before 28 weeks' gestation. As a result, these infants have a high rate of acute neonatal complications.

The HELLP syndrome may develop antepartum or postpartum. Analysis of 442 cases studied by Sibai and associates revealed that 309 (70%) had evidence of the syndrome antepartum, whereas 133 (30%) developed the condition postpartum. Four maternal deaths were reported, and morbidity was frequent (Table 31-10).

In the postpartum period, the time of onset of the manifestations can range from a few hours to 7 days, but most develop within 48 hours postpartum. Thus laboratory assessment for potential HELLP syndrome should be considered during the first 48 hours postpartum in women with significant hypertension or symptoms of severe PE. Eighty percent of the women who develop HELLP syndrome postpartum had PE before delivery, whereas 20% had no evidence of PE during either the antepartum or intrapartum periods. It is my experience that patients in this group are at increased risk for

the development of pulmonary edema and acute renal failure (Table 31-11). The differential diagnosis should include exacerbation of SLE, TTP, and HUS.

RECOMMENDED MANAGEMENT

The clinical course of women with HELLP syndrome is usually characterized by progressive and sometimes sudden deterioration in maternal and fetal condition. Therefore **patients with a suspected diagnosis of HELLP syndrome should be hospitalized immediately and observed in a labor and delivery unit (Fig. 31-5). Such patients should be managed as if they have PE with severe features and should initially receive IV magnesium sulfate as prophylaxis against convulsions and antihypertensive medications to maintain systolic BP below 160 mm Hg or diastolic BP below 105 mm Hg.**[104] This can be achieved with **a 5-mg bolus dose of hydralazine repeated as needed every 20 minutes for a maximal dose of 25 mg/hour. BP is recorded every 20 minutes during therapy and every hour once the desired values are achieved.** If hydralazine does not lower BP adequately, or if maternal side effects such as tachycardia or headaches develop, another agent such as labetalol or nifedipine can be used.

The **recommended dose of labetalol is 20 to 40 mg given intravenously every 10 minutes for a maximum of 300 mg, and the dose of nifedipine is 10 to 20 mg orally every 20 minutes for a maximum dose of 50 mg within an hour. During the observation period, maternal and fetal conditions should be followed carefully.**

The **recommended regimen of magnesium sulfate is a loading dose of 6 g given over 20 minutes, followed by a maintenance dose of 2 g/hr as a continuous IV solution.** Magnesium sulfate is initiated at the beginning of the observation period and is then continued during labor and for at least 24 hours postpartum. In those with abnormal renal function (oliguria or serum creatinine ≥1.2 mg/dL), the dose of magnesium sulfate should be reduced and perhaps even discontinued.

Once the diagnosis of HELLP syndrome is confirmed, a decision must be made regarding the need for delivery (see Fig. 31-5). Women with HELLP syndrome at less than 35 weeks' gestation should be referred to a tertiary care facility if their condition is stable. The first priority is to assess and stabilize the maternal condition, particularly BP and coagulation abnormalities. The next step is to evaluate fetal status with the use of fetal heart rate (FHR) monitoring, biophysical profile (BPP), or Doppler assessment of fetal vessels. Finally, a decision must be made as to whether delivery should be initiated or delayed for

TABLE 31-10 SERIOUS MATERNAL COMPLICATIONS IN 442 PATIENTS WITH HELLP SYNDROME

COMPLICATION	N (%)
Disseminated intravascular coagulation	92 (21)
Abruptio placentae	69 (16)
Acute renal failure	33 (8)
Severe ascites	32 (8)
Pulmonary edema	26 (6)
Pleural effusions	26 (6)
Cerebral edema	4 (1)
Retinal detachment	4 (1)
Laryngeal edema	4 (1)
Subcapsular liver hematoma	4 (1)
Adult respiratory distress syndrome	3 (1)
Death, maternal	4 (1)

From Sibai BM, Ramadan MK, Usta I, et al. Maternal morbidity and mortality in 442 pregnancies with hemolysis, elevated liver enzymes, and low platelets (HELLP syndrome). *Am J Obstet Gynecol.* 1993;169:1000.
HELLP, hemolysis, elevated liver enzymes, and low platelets.

TABLE 31-11 OUTCOME AND COMPLICATIONS OF HELLP SYNDROME IN RELATION TO TIME OF ONSET

	ANTEPARTUM ONSET (*n* = 309) (%)	POSTPARTUM ONSET (*n* = 133) (%)	RELATIVE RISK	95% CI
Delivery at <27 wk*	15	3	4.84	2.0-11.6
Delivery at 37-42 wk†	15	25	0.61	0.41-0.91
Pulmonary edema	5	9	0.50	0.24-1.05
Acute renal failure†	5	12	0.46	0.24-0.87
Eclampsia	7	10	0.73	0.38-1.40
Abruptio placentae	16	15	1.05	0.65-1.70
DIC	21	20	1.09	0.73-1.64

From Sibai BM, Ramadan MK, Usta I, et al. Maternal morbidity and mortality in 442 pregnancies with hemolysis, elevated liver enzymes, and low platelets (HELLP syndrome). *Am J Obstet Gynecol.* 1993;169:1000.
*P < .0007.
†P < .002.
CI, confidence interval; *DIC,* disseminated intravascular coagulation; *HELLP,* hemolysis, elevated liver enzymes, and low platelets.

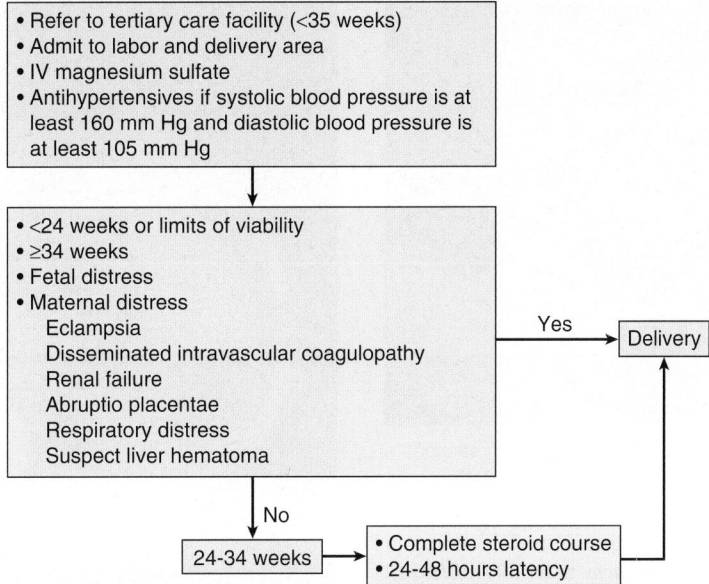

- Refer to tertiary care facility (<35 weeks)
- Admit to labor and delivery area
- IV magnesium sulfate
- Antihypertensives if systolic blood pressure is at least 160 mm Hg and diastolic blood pressure is at least 105 mm Hg

- <24 weeks or limits of viability
- ≥34 weeks
- Fetal distress
- Maternal distress
   - Eclampsia
   - Disseminated intravascular coagulopathy
   - Renal failure
   - Abruptio placentae
   - Respiratory distress
   - Suspect liver hematoma

Yes → Delivery

No

24-34 weeks

- Complete steroid course
- 24-48 hours latency

FIG 31-5 An algorithm for the management of hemolysis, elevated liver enzymes, and low platelets (HELLP) syndrome. IV, intravenous.

48 hours to allow the full benefit of corticosteroids. **Thus in practice, prompt delivery is undertaken in all patients with true HELLP syndrome except in those with a gestational age between 24 to 34 weeks with stable maternal and fetal conditions. These latter patients are given betamethasone and are generally then delivered within 24 hours after the last dose of corticosteroids. Maternal and fetal conditions are assessed continuously during this time. In some of these women, transient improvement in maternal laboratory values may be seen; however, delivery is still recommended despite such improvement.**[104]

INTRAPARTUM MANAGEMENT

The presence of HELLP syndrome is not an indication for immediate cesarean delivery, and such an approach might prove detrimental for both mother and fetus. The decision to perform a cesarean delivery should be based on gestational age, fetal condition, the presence of labor, and the cervical Bishop score. Elective cesarean delivery is recommended for all women with HELLP syndrome before 30 weeks' gestation who are not in labor and have a Bishop score of less than 5. Elective cesarean delivery is also undertaken for those with HELLP syndrome complicated by FGR or oligohydramnios, particularly if the gestational age is less than 32 weeks in the presence of an unfavorable cervical Bishop score (Box 31-8).

Women in labor and those whose membranes have ruptured are allowed to deliver vaginally in the absence of obstetric complications. When induction is indicated, labor is initiated with either oxytocin infusion or prostaglandins in patients with a gestational age of more than 30 weeks, irrespective of the amount of cervical dilation or effacement. A similar approach is used for those at 30 weeks' gestation or less if the cervical Bishop score is at least 5.

Maternal pain relief during labor and delivery can be provided by intermittent use of small doses of systemic opioids. Local infiltration anesthesia can be used for all vaginal deliveries if an episiotomy or repair of a laceration is necessary. The use of a pudendal block is contraindicated in these patients because of the risk for bleeding and hematoma formation into this area.

BOX 31-8 INDICATIONS AND MANAGEMENT DURING CESAREAN DELIVERY IN HELLP SYNDROME

Indications for Cesarean Delivery

- Nonreassuring fetal status
- Abnormal fetal presentation
- Gestation <30 weeks and Bishop score <5
- Gestation <32 weeks with IUGR or oligohydramnios and Bishop score <5
- Known subcapsular liver hematoma
- Suspected abruptio placentae

Management During Cesarean Delivery

- General anesthesia for platelet count <75,000/mm³
- Transfuse 6 U of platelets if count <40,000/mm³
- Insert subfascial drain
- Secondary skin closure or leave subcutaneous drain
- Observe for bleeding from upper abdomen before closure

HELLP, hemolysis, elevated liver enzymes, and low platelets; *IUGR*, intra-uterine growth restriction.

Epidural anesthesia is also contraindicated, particularly if the platelet count is less than 75,000/mm³. **Therefore general anesthesia is the method of choice for cesarean delivery in most thrombocytopenic women.** O'Brien and coworkers assessed the impact of glucocorticoid administration on the use of epidural anesthesia in 37 women with partial HELLP syndrome who had a platelet count of less than 90,000/mm³ before steroid administration. They found that administration of corticosteroids in these patients increased the use of epidural anesthesia, particularly in those who achieved a latency period of 24 hours before delivery (8 of 14 in the steroid group vs. 0 of 10 in the group that did not receive steroids; $P = .006$).

Platelet transfusions are indicated either before or after delivery in all patients with HELLP syndrome in the presence of significant bleeding—such as subcapsular hematoma of the liver, ecchymosis, bleeding from gums, oozing from

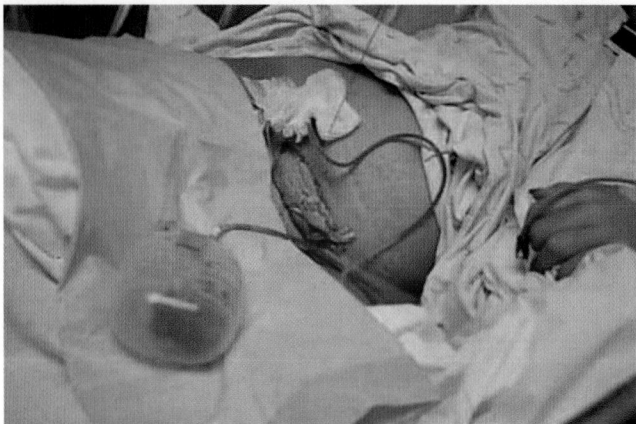

FIG 31-6 Subfascial drains used at the time of cesarean section.

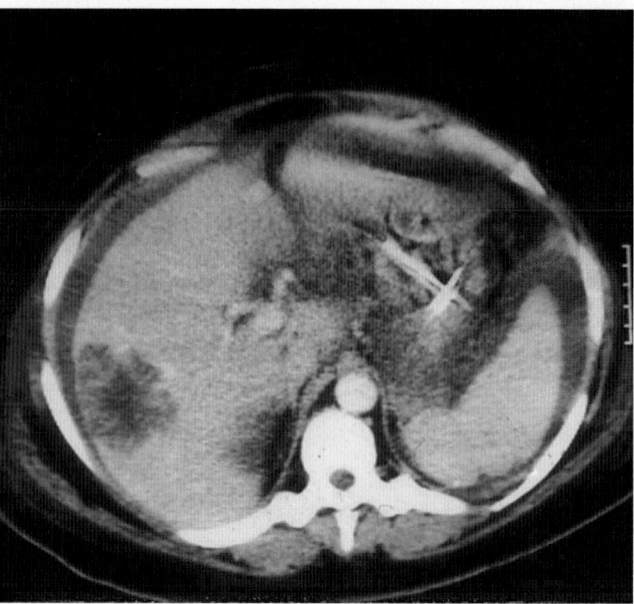

FIG 31-7 Computed tomographic scan of the liver demonstrates hepatic infarct.

puncture sites and wounds, or intraperitoneal bleeding—and in all those with a platelet count less than 20,000/mm³. However, repeated platelet transfusions are generally not necessary because of the short half-life of the transfused platelets in such patients. Correction of thrombocytopenia is also important before any surgery. Administration of 6 units of platelets is recommended in all patients with a platelet count less than 40,000 to 50,000/mm³ before intubation if cesarean delivery is needed. Generalized oozing from the incision site can occur during surgery or in the immediate postpartum period because of the continued drop in platelet count in some patients. The risk for hematoma formation at these sites is about 20%, and some prefer to use a vertical skin incision for this reason, whereas others use a subfascial drain and keep the skin incision open for at least 48 hours in women who require cesarean delivery (Fig. 31-6).[104]

POSTPARTUM MANAGEMENT

After delivery, patients with HELLP syndrome should receive close monitoring of vital signs, fluid intake and output, laboratory values, and pulse oximetry for at least 48 hours. IV magnesium sulfate prophylaxis is generally continued for 48 hours, and antihypertensive drugs are used if the systolic BP is at least 155 mm Hg or if the diastolic BP is at least 105 mm Hg. **In general, most women will show evidence of resolution of the disease process within 48 hours after delivery. However, some patients—especially those with placental abruption complicated by DIC, severe thrombocytopenia (platelet count <20,000/mm³), or severe ascites or those with significant renal dysfunction—may show delayed resolution or even deterioration in their clinical condition.** Such patients are at risk for the development of pulmonary edema from transfusion of blood and blood products, fluid mobilization, and compromised renal function. These patients are also at risk for acute tubular necrosis and may require dialysis and intensive monitoring for several days. Some authors have suggested that such patients might benefit from plasmapheresis or plasma transfusions. In practice, most of these women will recover with supportive therapy only. **If the patient continues to deteriorate for more than 72 hours after delivery, however, or shows improvement in laboratory values and then starts to show thrombocytopenia and abnormal liver enzymes again, a diagnosis of TTP/HUS should be considered. In such cases, plasmapheresis is indicated.**

The clinical and laboratory findings of HELLP syndrome may first appear during the postpartum period.[104] In these women, the time of onset of the manifestations ranges from a few hours to 7 days, although most develop within 48 hours postpartum.[104] Hence, all postpartum women and their health care providers should be educated to be aware of the signs and symptoms of HELLP syndrome. Management of patients with postpartum HELLP syndrome should be similar to that in the antepartum period, including the use of magnesium sulfate.

Hepatic Complications in HELLP Syndrome

Marked elevations in serum aminotransferases (>1000 to 2000 IU/L) are not typical of uncomplicated HELLP syndrome; however, when they do occur, the possibility of hepatic infarction and subcapsular hematoma of the liver must be considered. The differential diagnosis should also include AFLP, abruptio placentae with DIC, acute cholecystitis with sepsis, viral hepatitis, and TTP. In addition to the signs and symptoms of PE, physical examination findings consistent with peritoneal irritation and hepatomegaly may be present.

HEPATIC INFARCTION

Marked elevation in serum aminotransferases (usually 1000 to 2000 IU/L or higher) and LDH (usually 10,000 to 20,000 IU/L) associated with right upper quadrant pain and fever is characteristic of hepatic infarction; this diagnosis can be confirmed by hepatic imaging (Fig. 31-7). Follow-up imaging after delivery typically demonstrates resolution of the infarcts. These women may have underlying antiphospholipid antibody syndrome.[104]

HEPATIC HEMATOMA AND RUPTURE

HELLP syndrome may be complicated by hepatic rupture with the development of a hematoma beneath the Glisson capsule (Fig. 31-8). Histology of the liver adjacent to the rupture shows periportal hemorrhage and fibrin deposition along with a neutrophilic infiltrate suggestive of hepatic PE. The hematoma may remain contained or it may rupture, with resulting

Liver hematoma at 40 weeks
Pleural effusions, intubation

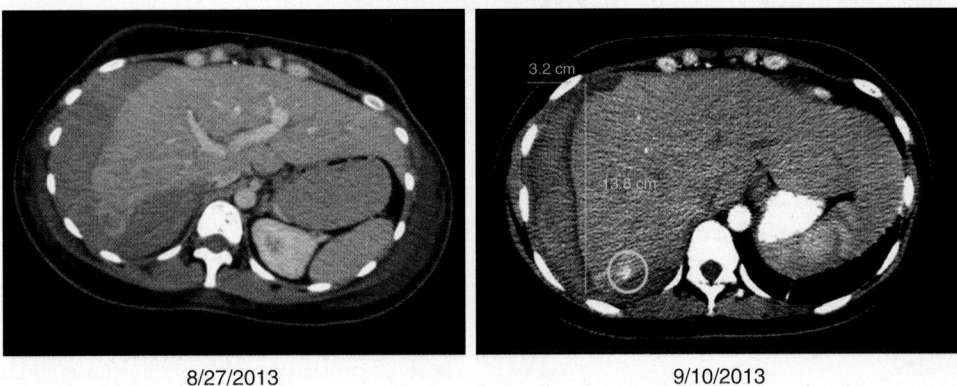

8/27/2013 9/10/2013

FIG 31-8 Computed tomographic scan of liver demonstrates subcapsular hematoma at presentation and 2 weeks postpartum.

hemorrhage into the peritoneal cavity. Women who develop a hepatic hematoma typically have abdominal pain, and many have severe thrombocytopenia, shoulder pain, nausea, and vomiting. The aminotransferases are usually modestly elevated, but values of 4000 to 5000 IU/L can occasionally be seen. If hepatic rupture occurs, swelling of the abdomen from hemoperitoneum and shock rapidly ensue.

The management of a contained hematoma is to support the patient with volume replacement and blood transfusion, as needed, with consideration for percutaneous embolization of the hepatic arteries. If the size of the hematoma remains stable and the laboratory abnormalities are resolving, the patient may be discharged home with outpatient follow-up. It may take months for the hematoma to resolve completely.

Surgical repair has been recommended for hepatic hemorrhage without liver rupture. This complication, however, can be managed conservatively in patients who remain hemodynamically stable. Management should include close monitoring of hemodynamics and coagulation status. Serial assessment of the subcapsular hematoma with ultrasound or computed tomography (CT) is necessary, as is immediate intervention for rupture or worsening of maternal status. It is important with conservative management to avoid exogenous sources of trauma to the liver—such as abdominal palpation, convulsions, or emesis—and to use care in transportation of the patient. Indeed, any sudden increase in intraabdominal pressure could potentially lead to rupture of the subcapsular hematoma (Fig. 31-9).

Rupture of a subcapsular hematoma of the liver is a life-threatening complication of HELLP syndrome. Profound hypovolemic shock in a previously hypertensive patient is the hallmark of hematoma rupture. In most instances, rupture involves the right lobe and is preceded by the development of a parenchymal hematoma. Patients frequently present with shoulder pain, shock, evidence of massive ascites, respiratory difficulty, pleural effusions, and often with a dead fetus. Ultrasound or CT of the liver should be performed to rule out the presence of subcapsular hematoma of the liver and to assess for the presence of intraperitoneal bleeding. Paracentesis can confirm intraperitoneal bleeding.

The presence of ruptured subcapsular liver hematoma that results in shock is a surgical emergency that requires acute multidisciplinary treatment (Box 31-9). Resuscitation should consist of massive transfusions of blood, correction of coagulopathy with FFP and platelets, and immediate laparotomy.

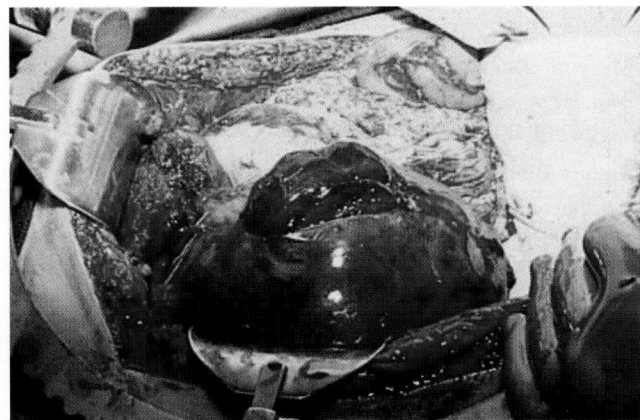

FIG 31-9 Subcapsular hematoma in a patient with hemolysis, elevated liver enzymes, and low platelets (HELLP) syndrome.

A team experienced in liver trauma surgery should be consulted. If hepatic rupture is suspected, an incision in the upper abdomen is necessary for adequate surgical exposure. A lower abdominal midline incision can be extended superiorly. If a Pfannenstiel incision was used for operative delivery, a separate upper abdominal midline incision should be made to maximize visualization of the upper abdomen and liver. Options at laparotomy include packing and drainage, surgical ligation of the hemorrhaging hepatic segments, embolization of the hepatic artery to the involved liver segment, and loose suturing of the omentum or surgical mesh to the liver to improve integrity. Shrivastava and associates in a case report described the successful use of an argon-beam coagulator to obtain hemostasis from a ruptured liver hematoma in a patient with HELLP syndrome, although previous experience with this modality was unsuccessful. **Even with appropriate treatment, maternal and fetal mortality is almost 50%. Mortality is most commonly associated with exsanguination with coagulopathy and sepsis.** Initial survivors are at increased risk for developing ARDS, pulmonary edema, liver failure, and acute renal failure in the postoperative period.

Reck and colleagues reviewed cases with HELLP syndrome–associated liver rupture (4 patients from their center in Germany and 49 identified from a MedLine literature search covering 1990 to 1999). Despite surgical interventions, HELLP syndrome–associated liver rupture carried a mortality rate of

39% (19 of 49) in their review. The main causes of death were hemorrhagic shock ($n = 11$) and multiorgan failure ($n = 7$). Based on their review, these authors suggested an interdisciplinary approach for patients with ruptured liver or hepatic failure that includes the use of temporary packing of the liver to control bleeding. In those patients with hepatic failure or uncontrollable hepatic hemorrhage, they noted that a liver transplantation as a last-resort measure must be considered.

LIVER TRANSPLANTATION FOR INTRACTABLE HEMORRHAGE
For women with intractable hemorrhage despite the previously described interventions, and for those with necrosis with subsequent liver failure, liver transplantation has been successful in case reports and case series. Shames and colleagues queried the Organ Procurement and Transplantation Network database regarding liver transplantations performed for complications from HELLP syndrome. Eight deceased donor liver transplantations were identified in the United States with this indication between October 1987 and November 2003. At the time of their review, six of the eight patients were alive, whereas two maternal deaths occurred within 1 month of transplantation. In addition, two patients required retransplantation. Based on the results of their review, these authors presented an algorithm in which liver transplantation is considered for patients with complicated HELLP syndrome, including ongoing, uncontrolled hemorrhage or liver necrosis and failure. **From our experience**

and review of the literature, we have developed a management plan of hepatic hematoma associated with HELLP syndrome. This plan emphasizes the potential for transfusion of large amounts of blood and blood products and the need for aggressive intervention if rupture of the hematoma is suspected (see Box 31-9). We recommend that 30 units of packed red blood cells, 20 U of FFP, 30 to 50 U of platelets, and 20 to 30 U of cryoprecipitate be available if rupture of a subcapsular hematoma is suspected.

We agree with the observations of others that a stable patient with an unruptured subcapsular hematoma should be conservatively managed. Constant monitoring must continue during this management, however, because patients can rapidly become unstable after rupture of the hematoma. Survival clearly is associated with rapid diagnosis and immediate medical or surgical stabilization, so these patients should be managed in an intensive care unit (ICU) with close monitoring of hemodynamic parameters and fluid status to avoid the potential for pulmonary edema or respiratory compromise.

Postpartum follow-up for patients with subcapsular hematoma of the liver should include serial CT, magnetic resonance imaging (MRI), or ultrasonography until the defect resolves. Although the data on subsequent pregnancy outcome after a subcapsular hematoma of the liver in pregnancy are limited, we have managed three such patients who have had subsequent normal maternal and fetal outcomes, and Wust and coworkers reported the successful outcome of four subsequent pregnancies in three women with a history of hepatic rupture and PE or HELLP syndrome.

Hemodynamic Monitoring in Preeclampsia
The cardiovascular hemodynamics of preeclampsia have been investigated over the years by many authors who have used various techniques for measurement of BP, cardiac output, pulmonary capillary wedge pressure (PCWP), and central venous pressure (CVP).

Hemodynamic findings in women with PE are variable. A review of the English literature demonstrates considerable disagreement regarding one or more of the hemodynamic parameters studied. This lack of agreement has been attributed to differences in the definition of PE, variable severity and duration of the disease process, presence of underlying cardiac or renal disease, techniques used to measure cardiac output and BP, and therapeutic interventions applied before obtaining the various measurements. In addition, the dynamic minute-to-minute fluctuation of the cardiovascular parameters studied makes it difficult to standardize the conditions under which these observations are made, which limits the value of a single measurement.

Invasive techniques have been used by many authors to study the hemodynamic findings in untreated women with severe PE. The reported cardiac index ranged from a low of 2.8 to a high of 4.8 L/m^2 per minute, and the reported PCWP ranged from a low of 3.3 to a high of 12 mm Hg. The findings suggest that cardiac index and PCWP are either low or normal in severe PE. The reported CVP values also ranged from 2 to 6 mm Hg. **The findings demonstrate that treated patients with PE have normal to high cardiac index, normal to high systemic vascular resistance index, and normal to high PCWP.**

In summary, variable hemodynamic findings accompany PE. Moreover, the clinical utility of invasive hemodynamic monitoring in PE is debatable. Most of the invasive monitoring data indicate that both cardiac output and systemic vascular resistance appear to be elevated in women with severe PE. This finding suggests that the problem in PE is a systemic vascular resistance that is inappropriately high for the level of cardiac output. Both the PCWP and the CVP appear to be in the low to normal range; however, no correlation is found between the two values.

Antepartum Management of Gestational Hypertension–Preeclampsia

GESTATIONAL HYPERTENSION

Women with gestational hypertension–preeclampsia (GH-PE) are at risk for progression to severe hypertension, PE with severe features, HELLP syndrome, or eclampsia.[1-8] The risks are increased with a lower gestational age at the time of diagnosis,[5-8] and therefore these patients require close observation of maternal and fetal conditions. Maternal evaluations require weekly prenatal visits; education about reporting preeclamptic symptoms; and evaluation of CBC, platelet count, liver enzymes, and serum creatinine.[1-3] Fetal evaluation includes ultrasound examination of fluid and estimated fetal weight at the time of diagnosis and weekly or twice weekly nonstress tests (NSTs) and evaluation of amniotic fluid volume (AFV).[1,3] Restriction of dietary salt and physical activity has not proved beneficial in the management of these patients.[1-3] Additionally, the results of several randomized trials reveal that control of maternal BP with antihypertensive drugs does not improve pregnancy outcome in these women.

In the absence of progression to severe disease, women with GH-PE can continue pregnancy until 37 weeks' gestation. During labor and immediately postpartum, they do not require seizure prophylaxis because the rate of eclampsia in these women is less than 1 in 500.[1,2]

The Hypertension and Preeclapmsia Intervention Trial At Term (HYPITAT) was a multicenter, open-label RCT conducted at 6 academic and 32 nonacademic hospitals in the Netherlands. It included 756 women with a singleton pregnancy at a gestational age between $36^{0/7}$ weeks and $41^{0/7}$ weeks who had mild GH ($n = 496$) or nonsevere GH ($n = 246$); 377 were randomized to induction, 379 to expectant monitoring. The primary outcome was a composite of adverse maternal outcomes: progression to severe disease or HELLP syndrome, eclampsia, pulmonary edema, placental abruption, postpartum hemorrhage, thromboembolic disease, or death. Secondary outcomes were a composite of adverse neonatal outcomes and rate of cesarean delivery. No cases of maternal, fetal, or neonatal death and no cases of eclampsia or abruption were reported in either group. However, women randomized to the induction group had a significant reduction in the primary outcome (31% vs. 44%; RR, 0.71; 95% CI, 0.59 to 0.86) mainly because of differences in the rates of severe hypertension. No differences were found in the overall secondary outcomes; however, subgroup analysis revealed significant differences in the primary outcomes in the group enrolled with mild PE (33% vs. 54%; RR, 0.61; 95% CI, 0.45 to 0.8) but not in those with mild GH (31% vs. 38%; RR, 0.81; 95% CI, 0.63 to 1.03). Unfortunately, the sample size was inadequate to answer the question in those with nonsevere GH only. Moreover, in the induction group, the rate of cesarean delivery was lower in nulliparous women and in those with a cervical Bishop score of less than 2, which refutes the belief that induction of labor in these women increases the rate of cesarean delivery. Results of this trial are summarized in Tables 31-12 and 31-13.

TABLE 31-12 MATERNAL OUTCOME IN RANDOMIZED TRIAL COMPARING INDUCTION AND EXPECTANT MONITORING IN MILD GESTATIONAL HYPERTENSION–PREECLAMPSIA

	INDUCTION ($n = 377$) (%)	EXPECTANT ($n = 379$) (%)	RELATIVE RISK (95% CI)
Composite adverse outcome	117 (31)	166 (44)	0.71 (0.59-0.86)
HELLP syndrome	4 (1)	11 (3)	0
Pulmonary edema	0	2 (1)	0
Abruptio placentae	0	0	0
Eclampsia	0	0	0
Maternal ICU admission	6 (2)	14 (4)	0
Cesarean delivery	54 (14)	72 (19)	0.75 (0.55-1.04)

Modified from Koopmans CM, Bijlenga D, Groen H, et al. Induction of labour versus expectant monitoring for gestational hypertension or mild pre-eclampsia after 36 weeks' gestation (HYPITAT): a multicentre, open-label randomize controlled trial. *Lancet.* 2009;374:979-988.
CI, confidence interval; *HELLP*, hemolysis, elevated liver enzymes, and low platelets; *ICU*, intensive care unit.

TABLE 31-13 NEONATAL OUTCOME IN RANDOMIZED TRIAL COMPARING INDUCTION VERSUS EXPECTANT MANAGEMENT IN MILD HYPERTENSION-PREECLAMPSIA

NEONATAL OUTCOME	NO. WITH INDUCTION (%)	NO. WITH EXPECTANT MONITORING (%)
Composite adverse outcome	24 (6)	32 (8)
Perinatal deaths	0	0
Apgar <7 at 5 min	7 (2)	9 (2)
Cord pH <7.05	9 (3)	19 (6)
Neonatal intensive care unit admission	10 (3)	8 (2)
Respiratory distress syndrome	1 (0.25)	1 (0.25)

Modified from Koopmans CM, Bijlenga D, Groen H, et al. Induction of labour versus expectant monitoring for gestational hypertension or mild pre-eclampsia after 36 weeks' gestation (HYPITAT): a multicentre, open-label randomized controlled trial. *Lancet.* 2009;374:979-988.

HOSPITALIZATION

In the past, management of these women has involved hospital bed rest for the duration of pregnancy with the belief that such management diminishes the frequency of progression to severe disease and allows rapid intervention in the event of sudden disease progression, including the development of placental abruption, eclampsia, or hypertensive crisis. However, these complications are extremely rare among compliant women with mild hypertension or nonsevere hypertension and absent symptoms. In addition, the results of two randomized trials in women with GH and several observational studies in women with mild hypertension and nonsevere PE suggest that most of these women can be safely managed at home or in a day care facility provided they undergo frequent maternal and fetal evaluation.[1-3]

BED REST

Complete or partial bed rest for the duration of pregnancy is often recommended for women with nonsevere hypertension–PE. No evidence to date suggests that this practice improves pregnancy outcome. In addition, no published randomized trials have compared complete bed rest and restricted activity in the management of women with PE. On the other hand, prolonged bed rest for the duration of pregnancy increases the risk for thromboembolism. The ACOG Task Force report recommends that bed rest not be used in management of GH-PE.[1]

BLOOD PRESSURE MEDICATIONS

Several randomized trials have described the use of antihypertensive drugs compared with no treatment or a placebo in the management of women with nonsevere hypertension or PE remote from term. Overall, these trials revealed lower rates of progression to severe disease with no improvement in perinatal outcome.[1-3] Of note, the sample size of these trials is inadequate to evaluate differences in FGR, abruptio placentae, perinatal death, or maternal outcome. It is recommended that antihypertensive medications not be used routinely to control mild levels of hypertension.

FETAL AND MATERNAL SURVEILLANCE

It is universally agreed that fetal testing is indicated during expectant management of women with GH or PE.[1-3] Most authorities in the United States recommend daily fetal movement counting (FMC) in association with either an NST or BPP to be performed at the time of diagnosis and serially thereafter until delivery (1 to 2 times per week).[1-3] Because uteroplacental blood flow may be reduced in some of these women, ultrasound estimation of fetal weight and amniotic fluid status is also recommended at the time of diagnosis and serially thereafter, with the frequency depending on findings. Doppler flow velocimetry is recommended in the presence of suspected IUGR.[1,3] The frequency of these tests is usually dependent on the severity of hypertension or PE, gestational age at the time of diagnosis, and fetal growth findings. Most clinical series suggest testing once weekly in women with GH or PE, twice weekly if fetal growth delay is suspected, and daily during expectant management of women with PE without severe features at less than 32 weeks' gestation. However, no large prospective studies have assessed outcomes of these monitoring techniques in women with GH or PE.

Maternal surveillance is indicated in all women with GH and PE. The goal of monitoring in women with GH is to observe progression of the condition to severe hypertension or to PE.[1-3] In women with PE, the goal is early detection of progression to PE with severe features. In those with severe features, the goal is to detect the development of organ dysfunction; therefore all such women should be evaluated for symptoms of organ dysfunction such as severe headaches, visual changes, altered mentation, right upper quadrant or epigastric pain, nausea or vomiting, and shortness of breath.[1-3] In addition, they should undergo laboratory testing for serum creatinine, platelet count, and liver enzymes. **Coagulation function tests are not necessary in the presence of a normal platelet count and liver enzymes. The frequency of laboratory testing will depend on the initial findings, the severity of the maternal condition, and the ensuing clinical progression.**

RECOMMENDED MANAGEMENT

The primary objective of management in women with GH-PE must always be safety of the mother and then delivery of a mature newborn that will not require intensive and prolonged neonatal care. This objective can be achieved by formulating a management plan that takes into consideration the severity of the disease process, gestational age, maternal and fetal status at the initial evaluation, presence of labor, and the wishes of the mother.

HYPERTENSION OR PREECLAMPSIA WITHOUT SEVERE FEATURES

Once the diagnosis of GH or PE is made, subsequent management will depend on the results of maternal and fetal evaluation (Fig. 31-10). **In general, women with disease that develops at 37 weeks' gestation or later should undergo induction of labor.**

In women who remain undelivered, close maternal and fetal evaluation are essential. These women are instructed to eat a regular diet with no salt restriction and to restrict their activity, but complete bed rest is not advised. Diuretics and antihypertensive medications are not used because of the potential to mask the diagnosis of severe disease.[1] At the time of initial and subsequent visits, women are educated and instructed about reporting symptoms of severe PE. **Those who are managed as outpatients are also advised to come to the hospital or outpatient facility immediately if they develop abdominal pain, significant headache, uterine contractions, vaginal spotting, or decreased fetal movement.**

In women with nonsevere GH, fetal evaluation should include an NST and an ultrasound examination of estimated fetal weight (EFW) and AFV using the amniotic fluid index (AFI). If the results are normal, repeat testing is performed every week as previously described.

Maternal evaluation includes weekly measurements of hematocrit, platelet count, serum creatinine, and liver function tests.

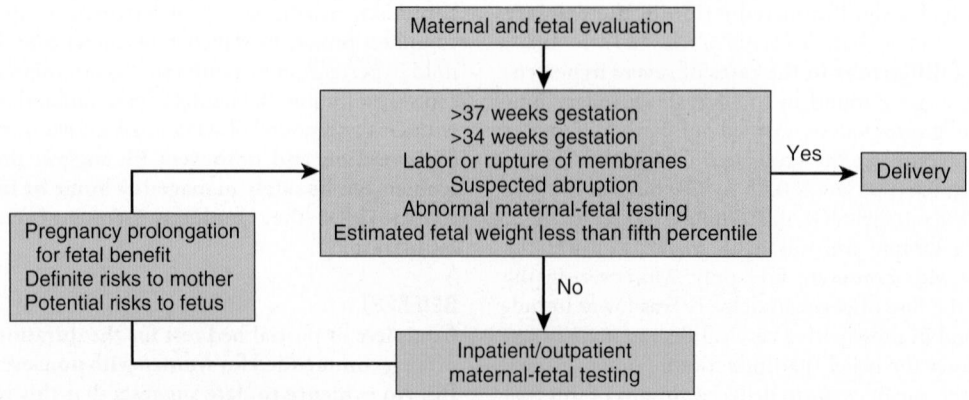

FIG 31-10 Management plan for patients with gestational hypertension–preeclampsia.

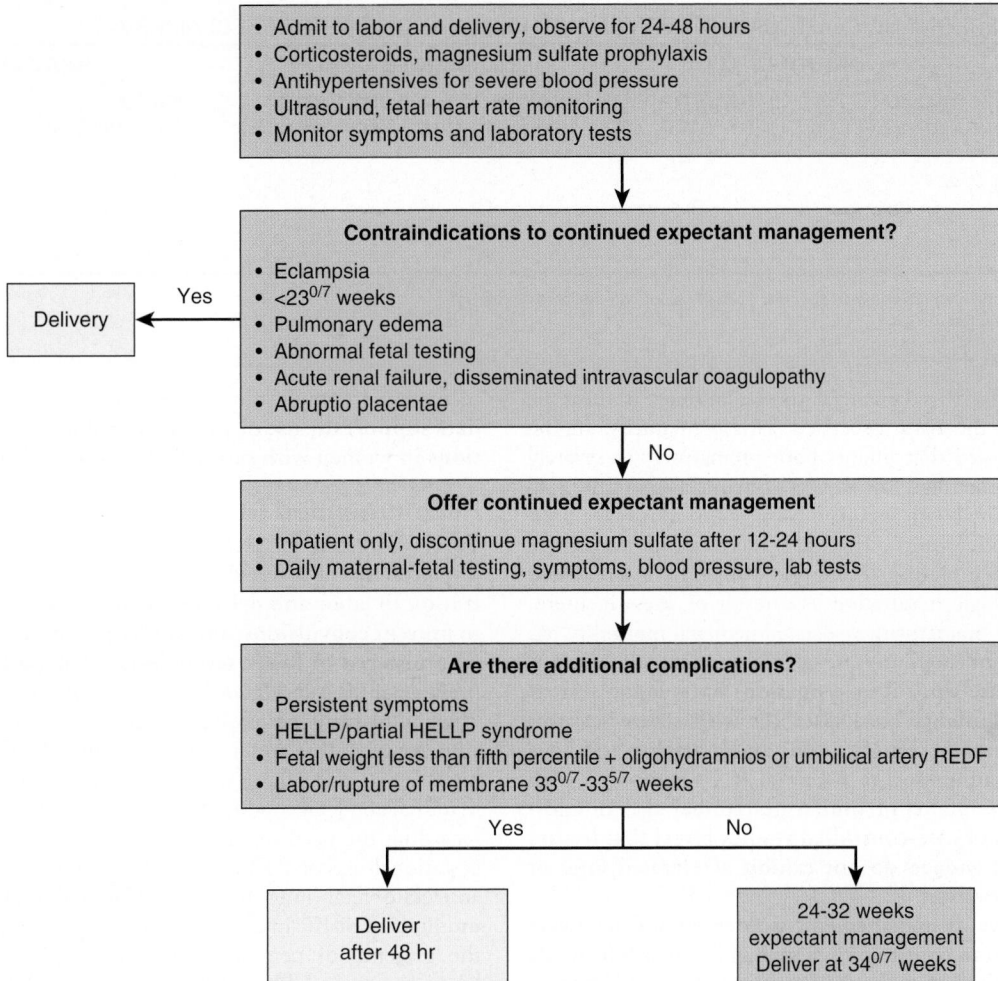

- Admit to labor and delivery, observe for 24-48 hours
- Corticosteroids, magnesium sulfate prophylaxis
- Antihypertensives for severe blood pressure
- Ultrasound, fetal heart rate monitoring
- Monitor symptoms and laboratory tests

Contraindications to continued expectant management?
- Eclampsia
- <23$^{0/7}$ weeks
- Pulmonary edema
- Abnormal fetal testing
- Acute renal failure, disseminated intravascular coagulopathy
- Abruptio placentae

Yes → Delivery

No

Offer continued expectant management
- Inpatient only, discontinue magnesium sulfate after 12-24 hours
- Daily maternal-fetal testing, symptoms, blood pressure, lab tests

Are there additional complications?
- Persistent symptoms
- HELLP/partial HELLP syndrome
- Fetal weight less than fifth percentile + oligohydramnios or umbilical artery REDF
- Labor/rupture of membrane 33$^{0/7}$-33$^{5/7}$ weeks

Yes → Deliver after 48 hr

No → 24-32 weeks expectant management Deliver at 34$^{0/7}$ weeks

FIG 31-11 Management plan for patients with preeclampsia with severe features before 34 weeks' gestation. HELLP, hemolysis, elevated liver enzymes, and low platelets; REDF, reversed end-diastolic flow.

The women are usually seen twice a week for evaluation of maternal BP, urine protein by dipstick or P/C ratio (GH only), and symptoms of impending eclampsia. This evaluation is extremely important for early detection of progression to severe disease. The onset of maternal symptoms and/or a sudden increase in BP to severe values requires prompt hospitalization for close evaluation.

In women with PE at less than 37 weeks' gestation but at more than 32 weeks, outpatient management can be considered for reliable patients with a systolic BP of 155 mm Hg or less or diastolic BP of 105 mm Hg or less and no symptoms. Women who do not satisfy these criteria are hospitalized, particularly those with PE before 32 weeks. During ambulatory management, women are instructed to have limited activity at home and are given instructions about prompt reporting of symptoms of severe disease; these women are then seen twice weekly. Fetal evaluation includes daily FMC, twice-weekly NST, and serial ultrasound evaluation of fetal growth and AFV. If disease progression is evident—that is, if a significant increase in BP to levels above the threshold mentioned previously, new onset of symptoms, evidence of abnormal blood tests, or abnormal fetal growth are apparent—these women are hospitalized for the duration of pregnancy. Women managed in the hospital receive similar maternal and fetal evaluations. Obstetric management is summarized in Figure 31-11.

PREECLAMPSIA WITH SEVERE FEATURES

The incidence of preeclampsia with severe features ranges from 0.6% to 1%.[105] Pregnancies complicated by PE with severe features are associated with serious maternal and perinatal complications, particularly preterm delivery, FGR, placental abruption, and perinatal death (Table 31-14). As a result, knowledge of the anticipated maternal, fetal, and neonatal risks is essential for appropriate counseling and management.

Expectant Management

The clinical course of PE with severe features may be characterized by progressive deterioration in both maternal and fetal conditions. **Because these pregnancies have been associated with increased rates of maternal morbidity and mortality and with significant risks for the fetus (growth restriction, hypoxemia, and death), it is generally agreed that all such patients should be delivered if the disease develops after 34 weeks' gestation.** Prompt delivery is also indicated when eclampsia is imminent—when persistent, severe symptoms do not respond to treatment—or in the presence of multiorgan dysfunction or severe IUGR (<5th percentile) in association with abnormal umbilical artery Doppler studies, such as reversed end-diastolic flow (REDF) or severe oligohydramnios (largest vertical pocket <2 cm), suspected placental abruption, nonreassuring fetal testing, gestational age less than 24 weeks, or fetal demise.[1-3,105]

TABLE 31-14   PREGNANCY OUTCOME IN WOMEN WITH MILD AND SEVERE PREECLAMPSIA

OUTCOME	HAUTH ET AL[4]		BUCHBINDER ET AL*[16]		HNAT ET AL[23]	
	MILD (n = 217) (%)	SEVERE (n = 109) (%)	MILD (n = 62) (%)	SEVERE (n = 45) (%)	MILD (n = 86) (%)	SEVERE (n = 70) (%)
Delivery at <37 wk	NR	NR	25.8	66.7	14.0	33.0
Delivery at <35 wk	1.9[†]	18.5[†]	9.7	35.6	2.3	18.6
SGA infant*	10.2	18.5	4.8	11.4	NR	NR
Abruptio placentae	0.5	3.7	3.2	6.7	0	1.4
Perinatal death	1.0	1.8	0	8.9	0	1.4

*Included women with previous preeclampsia. The other studies included only nulliparous women.
[†]Rates for delivery at <34 wk.
NR, not reported; SGA, small for gestational age.

Although delivery is beneficial to the mother, it must be weighed against the risks associated with prematurity. In the past, it was believed that infants born prematurely to severely preeclamptic women had lower rates of neonatal mortality and morbidity compared with infants of similar gestational age born to nonpreeclamptic women. This belief was based on the clinical impression that fetuses of preeclamptic women have accelerated lung and neurologic maturation as a result of stress in utero. Reduced risk for prematurity-associated neonatal morbidity has never been documented in case-control studies. In contrast, **several recent case-control investigations have demonstrated that premature infants born after PE with severe features have similar neonatal complications and mortality and have higher rates of admission to neonatal ICUs compared with other premature infants of similar gestational age. In addition, the results of case-controlled studies reveal that fetuses of preeclamptic women do not exhibit accelerated lung or neurologic maturation.**[104]

During expectant management, women should be aware that the decision to continue such management will be made on a daily basis and that the median time of pregnancy prolongation is *7 days with a range of 2 to 35 days.* Only three randomized trials have compared a policy of early elective delivery after corticosteroids with a policy of delayed delivery.[105] One trial was conducted in South Africa and included patients at a gestational age of 26 to 34 weeks, one United States trial included women at 28 to 32 weeks, and a recent trial from Latin American countries included patients with a gestational age of 28 to 34 weeks. The first two studies totaled 133 women and revealed improved neonatal outcome in those who had delivery delayed, whereas the multicenter Latin American study revealed no perinatal benefits and increased maternal morbidity. Nevertheless, the results of retrospective and observational studies of more than 2000 women suggest that **expectant management is associated with reduced short-term neonatal morbidity in a select group of women with a gestational age between 24 and 32 weeks.**[1,3,104]

In the past, uncertainty surrounded the efficacy and safety of corticosteroids administered to women with PE with severe features before 34 weeks' gestation. A prospective double-blind randomized trial of 218 women with severe PE with a gestational age between 26 and 34 weeks receiving either betamethasone (n = 110) or placebo (n = 108) reported a significant reduction in the rate of RDS (RR, 0.53; 95% CI, 0.35 to 0.82) in the steroid-treated group. Corticosteroid use also was associated with a reduction in the risks for neonatal intraventricular hemorrhage (RR, 0.35; 95% CI, 0.15 to 0.86), neonatal infection (RR, 0.39; 95% CI, 0.39 to 0.97), and neonatal death (RR, 0.5; 95% CI, 0.28 to 0.89). However, no differences were noted in maternal complications between the two groups. Thus **the data support the use of steroids to reduce neonatal complications in women with severe PE at 34 weeks' gestation or less.**

Recommended Management of Preeclampsia With Severe Features

The presence of severe disease mandates immediate hospitalization in labor and delivery. IV magnesium sulfate is begun to prevent convulsions, and antihypertensive medications are administered to lower severe levels of hypertension (systolic pressure ≥160 mm Hg *and/or* diastolic pressure ≥110 mm Hg). The aim of antihypertensive therapy is to keep the systolic pressure between 140 and 155 mm Hg and the diastolic pressure between 90 and 105 mm Hg. During the observation period, maternal and fetal conditions are assessed, and a decision is made regarding the need for delivery (see Fig. 31-11). Those with a gestational age of 24 to 34 weeks are given corticosteroids to accelerate fetal lung maturity. Maternal evaluation includes monitoring of BP, intake and urine output, cerebral status, and the presence of persistent severe epigastric pain, tenderness, labor, or vaginal bleeding. Laboratory evaluation includes a platelet count, liver enzymes, and serum creatinine. Fetal evaluation includes continuous fetal heart monitoring, a BPP, and ultrasound assessment of fetal growth and AFV. **Patients with resistant severe hypertension despite maximal doses of IV labetalol** (300 mg within an hour) **plus maximum doses of hydralazine** (25 mg) **or oral rapid-acting nifedipine** (50 mg) **or persistent cerebral symptoms while on magnesium sulfate are delivered irrespective of gestational age.**

After the initial evaluation, the need for immediate delivery versus the potential neonatal benefit and the relative maternal and fetal risks of expectant management should be determined.[33] Women who develop eclampsia, pulmonary edema, or documented or suspected placental abruption; those with DIC or moderate to severe renal dysfunction (serum creatinine ≥1.5 mg/dL); and those with gestational age less than $23^{0/7}$ weeks' gestation should be delivered after maternal stabilization. In addition, those with a nonreassuring FHR tracing (repetitive decelerations) and those with a persistent BPP of 4 or less should be delivered promptly.[33] Women with a fetus between $23^{0/7}$ and $23^{6/7}$ weeks should receive extensive counseling about the minimal neonatal benefit and high maternal complications from expectant management, and treatment should be individualized.

For pregnancies at $24^{0/7}$ weeks or greater without any indication for prompt delivery, corticosteroids are administered to accelerate fetal lung maturity.[33] **With a gestational age between $33^{0/7}$ to $33^{6/7}$ weeks, severe FGR with absent or reversed umbilical artery diastolic flow, largest amniotic fluid**

vertical pocket less than 2 cm, preterm labor or premature rupture of the membranes (PROM), HELLP syndrome or partial HELLP syndrome, or persistent symptoms—such as headaches, visual changes, epigastric or right upper quadrant pain, nausea, or vomiting—the fetus should be delivered no later than 24 hours after the last dose of corticosteroids. These gravidas should remain on magnesium sulfate with continuous monitoring of uterine contractions and FHR until delivery.

Women with a pregnancy between $24^{0/7}$ and $32^{6/7}$ weeks' gestation with stable maternal and fetal conditions during the initial 24-hour observation period are considered candidates for expectant management (see Fig. 31-11). In these women, magnesium sulfate is generally discontinued after 24 hours with transfer to a high-risk antepartum floor for close observation. Because of the potential for rapid deterioration in maternal and fetal conditions during expectant management, these women should generally be managed in a tertiary care hospital with adequate maternal and neonatal intensive care facilities. They should be cared for in consultation with a maternal-fetal medicine specialist, and the mother should receive counseling from a neonatologist.[33]

Oral antihypertensive medications are used as needed to keep systolic BP between 140 and 155 mm Hg and diastolic BP between 90 and 105 mm Hg.[33] Oral labetalol and oral calcium channel blockers (nifedipine or nicardipine) have been commonly used in reported studies. My regimen consists of an initial dose of labetalol of 200 mg every 8 hours to be increased up to 800 mg every 8 hours (600 to 2400 mg/day) as needed. If the maximal dose is inadequate to achieve the desired BP goal, short-acting oral nifedipine is added with an initial dose of 10 mg every 6 hours and is subsequently increased up to 20 mg every 4 hours (40 to 120 mg/day). An alternative regimen may include the long-acting (XL) version of nifedipine (30 to 60 mg) every 8 hours. During titration of oral antihypertensive agents, if the patient has persistent severe hypertensive episodes (systolic BP $\geq$160 mm Hg and/or diastolic BP $\geq$105 mm Hg), BP should be assessed every 15 minutes. If the BP remains in the severe range after 60 minutes, the patient should be transferred to the labor and delivery unit for more intensive monitoring and treatment with IV medications such as hydralazine or labetalol. Patients with resistant severe hypertension after maximal doses of IV hydralazine (25 mg) or labetalol (300 mg) should receive magnesium sulfate and be delivered. In addition, patients who develop persistent severe hypertension despite combined maximal doses of oral labetalol (2400 mg/day) plus short-acting nifedipine (120 mg/day) or nifedipine XL (180 mg/day) should also be considered for delivery.

Maternal assessment includes frequent evaluation of symptoms such as new onset of severe headaches that do not respond to repeated doses of analgesics, blurred or double vision or inability to see, confusion, persistent nausea, vomiting, epigastric or right upper quadrant pain, shortness of breath, uterine activity, and vaginal bleeding. In addition, intake and output should be closely monitored.[33]

Laboratory assessment includes daily testing of the CBC with platelet count, transaminases, LDH, and serum creatinine levels.[32] Coagulation studies are obtained only if thrombocytopenia or suspicion of abruption is present.

Fetal assessment includes daily fetal kick counts, at least daily NST with uterine activity monitoring with a BPP if the NST is nonreactive, and twice-weekly amniotic fluid assessment (see Chapter 11).[33] Ultrasound assessment of fetal growth is performed every 2 weeks.[33] Severe oligohydramnios (largest vertical pocket <2 cm) is considered an indication for delivery in women with a gestational age of more than 30 weeks irrespective of other fetal testing results. In those at 30 weeks or less of gestation, pregnancy may be continued with a reassuring NST, BPP, and umbilical artery Doppler studies. Umbilical artery Doppler studies are performed weekly, and they should be done more often when FGR is suspected or when testing reveals abnormal diastolic flow or severe oligohydramnios. If umbilical artery diastolic flow is absent, Doppler studies should be performed daily.

In general, most patients with preeclampsia without severe features managed expectantly will require delivery within 2 weeks, but some patients may continue their pregnancies for several weeks. It is important to emphasize that this therapy is appropriate only in a select group of patients and should be undertaken in a facility with adequate maternal and neonatal intensive care facilities. Once the decision is made for delivery, magnesium sulfate should be administered in labor and for at least 24 hours postpartum.[33]

Intrapartum Management

The goals of management of women with gestational hypertension-preeclampsia are early detection of FHR abnormalities and progression from mild to severe disease and prevention of maternal complications. Pregnancies complicated by PE, particularly those with severe disease or FGR, are at risk for reduced fetal reserve and placental abruption.[2] Therefore women with PE should receive continuous monitoring of FHR and uterine activity. The presence of uterine tachysystole or recurrent FHR decelerations may be the first sign of placental abruption in these women.

Some women with GH-PE progress to severe disease as a result of changes in cardiac output and stress hormones during labor. Therefore women with GH-PE should have BP recordings every hour and should be assessed for symptoms suggestive of severe disease. Those who develop severe hypertension or symptoms should be managed as patients with PE with severe features.

Maternal pain relief during labor and delivery can be provided by either systemic opioids or segmental epidural anesthesia. Epidural analgesia is considered to be the preferred method of pain relief in women whose GH and PE are nonsevere. Although no unanimity of opinion exists regarding the use of epidural anesthesia in women with PE with severe features, evidence suggests that epidural anesthesia is also safe in these women. A randomized trial of 116 women with severe PE who received either epidural analgesia or patient-controlled analgesia (PCA) reported no differences in cesarean delivery rates, and the group who received epidural had significantly better pain relief during labor.

The use of either epidural, spinal, or combined techniques of regional anesthesia is considered by most obstetric anesthesiologists to be the method of choice during cesarean delivery. In women with PE with severe features, general anesthesia carries the risk for aspiration and failed intubation owing to airway edema, and it is associated with marked increases in systemic and cerebral pressures during intubation and extubation.[1] Women with airway or laryngeal edema may require awake intubation under fiberoptic observation with the availability of immediate tracheostomy. Changes in systemic

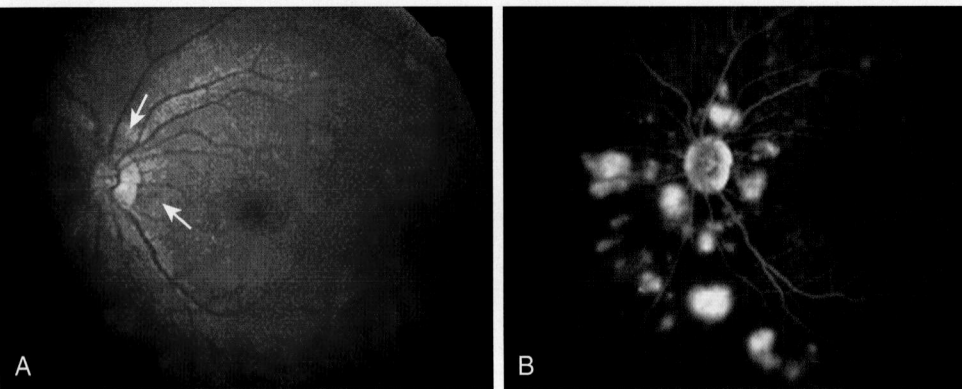

FIG 31-12 Retinal ischemia and injury in severe preeclampsia. **A,** Scattered, yellowish opaque lesions of the retinal pigment epithelium. **B,** Fluoroscein angiograms showing patchy delayed filling of the choriocapillaris.

and cerebral pressures may be attenuated by pretreatment with labetalol or nitroglycerine injections. It is important to recognize that regional anesthesia is contraindicated in the presence of coagulopathy or severe thrombocytopenia (platelet count <50,000/mm³).

Prevention of Eclamptic Seizures

Magnesium sulfate is the drug of choice to prevent convulsions in women with preeclampsia. The results of recent randomized trials revealed that magnesium sulfate is superior to placebo or no treatment for prevention of convulsions in women with PE with severe features. The overall results of these four trials demonstrate that magnesium sulfate prophylaxis, compared with placebo (two trials, 10,795 women), nimodipine (one trial, 1750 women), and no treatment (one trial, 228 women) in severe PE is associated with a significantly lower rate of eclampsia (RR, 0.39; 95% CI, 0.28 to 0.55). Results from one of the largest randomized trials to date, that of 10,141 women with PE in 33 nations (largely in the Third World), has been recently reported. Almost all the enrolled patients had severe disease by U.S. standards: 50% received antihypertensives before randomization, 75% received antihypertensives after randomization, and the remainder had severe PE or imminent eclampsia. Among all enrolled women, the rate of eclampsia was significantly lower in those assigned to magnesium sulfate (0.8% vs. 1.9%; RR, 0.42; 95% CI, 0.29 to 0.60). However, among the 1560 women enrolled in the western world, the rates of eclampsia were 0.5% in the magnesium group versus 0.8% with placebo, a difference that was not significant (RR, 0.67; 95% CI, 1.19 to 2.37).

Two randomized placebo-controlled trials evaluated the efficacy and safety of magnesium sulfate in women with mild PE. One of these trials included 135 women, and the other included only 222 women. No instances of eclampsia were reported in either group in both of these trials. In addition, **the findings of both studies revealed that magnesium sulfate does not affect either the duration of labor or the rate of cesarean delivery.** However, neither of these studies had an adequate sample size to address the efficacy of magnesium sulfate to prevent convulsions. Therefore **whether magnesium sulfate treatment benefits women with mild PE remains unclear.**

Control of Severe Hypertension

The objective of treating acute and sustained severe hypertension that lasts more than 60 minutes is to prevent cerebrovascular and cardiovascular complications such as encephalopathy, hemorrhage, and congestive heart failure (CHF) and to prevent retinal injury (Fig. 31-12).[1,2] For ethical reasons, no randomized trials have been done to determine the level of hypertension to treat in order to prevent these complications. Antihypertensive therapy is recommended by some for sustained systolic BP values of 160 mm Hg or more and for sustained diastolic values of 110 mm Hg or more. Some experts recommend treating diastolic levels of 105 mm Hg, and still others use a mean arterial BP of 130 mm Hg or more.[1,2] The definition of *sustained hypertension* is not clear and ranges from 30 minutes to 2 hours.

I recommend that antihypertensive medications are indicated with sustained elevations in systolic BP to levels of 160 mm Hg or greater and/or when diastolic BP is 105 mm Hg or higher for at least 60 minutes.[33] If the desired target of BP level is not achieved after maximum doses of IV medications are used, I recommend the insertion of an arterial line with the initiation of a continuous IV administration of medications such as nicardipine, nitroprusside, labetalol or nitroglycerine. This may require admitting the patient to an intensive care facility. Several antihypertensive medications can be used to treat severe hypertension in PE. The most commonly recommended medications include IV bolus doses of hydralazine, bolus doses of labetalol, or oral nifedipine (rapid-acting tablets or long-acting capsules). Other antihypertensive medications recommended for treatment of severe hypertension have included IV nicardipine and mini boluses of diazoxide.

Despite the extensive literature on the subject, it remains unclear which is the ideal antihypertensive medication to use in the acute control of hypertension in women with severe PE. The results of a recent meta-analysis of relevant randomized trials found that parenteral hydralazine was associated with more adverse effects compared with other antihypertensives; however, such a finding was not confirmed in a recent large randomized trial. **Based on the available evidence, hydralazine, labetalol, or nifedipine can be used to treat severe hypertension in PE.**[2,3,33] **The provider should be familiar with the dosage to be used, the expected response, and potential side effects of each of these drugs.** Both hydralazine and nifedipine are associated with tachycardia and headaches and thus are not the first drugs of choice in patients with a heart rate above 100 beats/min. In such case, labetalol is preferred. Labetalol, however, should be avoided in patients with moderate to severe asthma, bradycardia (heart rate <60 beats/min), and in those with CHF. Compared with other antihypertensive medications, nifedipine has the advantage of increased renal blood flow with an associated increase in urine output.[33] Thus it may be the drug of choice in those with decreased urine output and for treatment of severe hypertension in the postpartum period.[33] In the past, there has been a theoretic concern that the combined use of magnesium sulfate and nifedipine in patients with severe PE can result in excessive hypotension and neuromuscular blockade. However, a recent review on this subject found that therapy with both magnesium sulfate and nifedipine does not increase the risk for the previously described complications in women with PE. Nevertheless, if neuromuscular blockade develops in these patients, this can be easily reversed by the administration of 1 g of IV calcium gluconate.

For the treatment of severe hypertension in pregnancy, the recommended dosage is IV hydralazine given as bolus injections of 5 to 10 mg every 20 minutes for a maximal dose of 25 mg in 60 minutes. The recommended dose of labetalol is 20 to 80 mg intravenously every 10 minutes for a maximal dose of 300 mg; and the dosage of nifedipine is 10 to 20 mg orally every 20 minutes for a maximal dose of 50 mg within 60 minutes.[33] Sustained BP values of 160 mm Hg systolic or more or 105 to 110 mm Hg diastolic or more for at least 60 minutes require therapy intrapartum. It is important to emphasize that BP recordings during labor that utilize electronic equipment may not be reliable for lack of a standardized cuff position and for the effects of labor and pain. Therefore BP recordings should be accurately measured and then confirmed with a sphygmomanometer prior to the use of acute IV medications to treat severe sustained systolic hypertension. For women with severe thrombocytopenia and sustained systolic values greater than 150 mm Hg or diastolic readings greater than 100 mm Hg are the recommended thresholds for therapy.[33] **For this author, the first-line agent is IV labetalol, and if maximal doses are ineffective, hydralazine can be added. Oral nifedipine is my first choice in the postpartum period.**

Mode of Delivery

No randomized trials have compared the optimal method of delivery in women with GH-PE. A plan for vaginal delivery should be attempted in all women with disease without other indications for cesarean delivery and in most women with severe disease, particularly those beyond 30 weeks' gestation.[1,2,17] The decision to perform a cesarean delivery should be based on gestational age, fetal condition, presence of labor, and cervical Bishop score. In general, the presence of PE with severe features is not an indication for cesarean delivery per se.

No randomized trials have compared the optimal methods of delivery in patients with severe hypertension or severe PE. The method for delivery will depend on gestational age, cervical Bishop score, and fetal condition. The cesarean delivery rate among reported studies[33] in patients as less than 34 weeks' gestation ranged from 66% to 96% with the higher rates for patients with onset prior to 28 weeks' gestation. This high cesarean delivery rate is expected considering that a deterioration in either fetal or maternal condition is the indication for delivery during expectant management (high rates of severe FGR, oligohydramnios, nonreassuring fetal status, abnormal presentation, and maternal complications).[33] Thus, a very small percentage of these patients will be considered candidates for medical induction of labor.

Several retrospective studies have evaluated induction of labor in patients with PE before 34 weeks' gestation and absent any contraindication for induction. However, most of the women included in these studies had a gestational age beyond 32 weeks at the time of induction, and only two of these studies included data on patients earlier than 28 weeks undergoing induction of labor.[33] Both of these studies reported a cesarean delivery rate above 95% and thus recommended elective cesarean delivery in such patients.

In general, the decision to perform a cesarean delivery versus a trial of labor in such patients should be individualized and based on one or more of the following factors: fetal gestational age, fetal presentation, presence or absence of severe FGR, oligohydramnios, results of umbilical artery Doppler, BPP, FHR monitoring, presence of labor, and cervical Bishop score. On the basis of the available data, we recommend cesarean delivery for all women with a gestation of less than 28 weeks and for those with severe FGR, severe oligohydramnios, BPP of 4 or less, or reverse umbilical artery Doppler flow at less than 32 weeks of gestation.

Postpartum Management

During the immediate postpartum period, women with PE should receive close monitoring of BP and of symptoms consistent with severe disease, and accurate measurements of fluid intake and urinary output should be obtained.

These women often receive large amounts of IV fluids during labor as a result of prehydration before the administration of epidural analgesia, and IV fluids are given during the administration of oxytocin and magnesium sulfate in labor and postpartum. In addition, during the postpartum period, mobilization of extracellular fluid leads to increased intravascular volume. As a result, **women with severe PE—particularly those with abnormal renal function, capillary leak, or early-onset disease—are at increased risk for pulmonary edema and exacerbation of severe hypertension postpartum. Careful evaluation of the volume of IV fluids, oral intake, blood products, and urine output are advised in addition to monitoring by pulse oximetry and chest auscultation.**[2,33]

In general, most women with GH become normotensive during the first week postpartum.[1,2] In contrast, in women with PE, hypertension often takes longer to resolve. In addition, in some women with PE, an initial decrease in BP is seen immediately postpartum, followed by development of hypertension again between days 3 and 6. Moreover, a recent study found that resolution of hypertension and proteinuria may take up to 1 year postpartum. Oral antihypertensive drug treatment is recommended if the systolic BP is at least 150 mm Hg or if the diastolic BP is at least 100 mm Hg. Various agents may be used. A common regimen is to prescribe oral nifedipine, 10 mg every 6 hours, or long-acting nifedipine.[33] If the BP is well controlled and maternal symptoms are absent, the woman is discharged home with instructions for daily BP measurements by a home-visiting nurse for the first week postpartum or longer if necessary. Antihypertensive medications are discontinued if the BP remains below the hypertensive levels for at least 24 hours. Recently, some authors have suggested that 5 days of oral furosemide therapy (20 mg/dL) enhances recovery and reduces the need for antihypertensive therapy in women with severe disease.

Severe hypertension or PE with severe features may develop for the first time during the postpartum period. Hence, postpartum women should be educated about the signs and

symptoms of severe hypertension or PE. These women are at increased risk for eclampsia, pulmonary edema, stroke, and thromboembolism. **Therefore medical providers and personnel who respond to patient phone calls should be educated and instructed about symptoms of severe postpartum hypertension.** Women who have persistent new-onset severe headaches that do not respond to maximum doses of analgesics or who have persistent severe visual changes or new-onset epigastric pain with nausea or vomiting and those with sustained severe hypertension require evaluation and potential hospitalization. Some women may require magnesium sulfate for at least 24 hours and antihypertensive therapy. If neurologic symptoms exist or the symptoms do not respond to magnesium sulfate and lowering of maternal BP, brain imaging is undertaken to rule out the presence of cerebral pathology.

Maternal and Perinatal Outcomes With Preeclampsia

Maternal and perinatal morbidity is substantially increased in women with severe GH. Indeed, these women have higher morbidity rates than women with mild preeclampsia.[19] In addition, the rates of placental abruption, preterm delivery (at less than 37 and 35 weeks), and rates of SGA infants in these pregnancies are similar to those observed in women with PE with severe features. However, whether this increase in rate of preterm delivery is a result of early delivery chosen by the physician or because of the disease process itself remains unknown. Therefore these women should be managed as if they had severe PE.[33]

Maternal and perinatal outcomes in PE are usually dependent on one or more of the following four factors: (1) gestational age at onset of PE and at the time of delivery, (2) the severity of the disease process, (3) the presence of multifetal gestation, and (4) the presence of preexisting medical conditions such as pregestational diabetes, renal disease, or thrombophilias.

PE with severe features is also associated with an increased risk for maternal mortality (0.2%) and increased rates of maternal morbidity (5%), such as convulsions, pulmonary edema, retinal ischemia and injury (see Fig. 31-12), acute renal or liver failure, liver hemorrhage, DIC, and stroke. These complications are usually seen in women who develop PE before 32 weeks' gestation and in those with preexisting medical conditions.

Counseling Women Who Have Had Preeclampsia in Prior Pregnancies

We examined the pregnancy outcomes and incidences of PE in subsequent pregnancies and the frequency of chronic hypertension and diabetes mellitus in women who had severe PE (287 women) or eclampsia (119 women) in their first pregnancies (aged 11 to 25 yr) compared with 409 women (aged 12 to 25 yr) who remained normotensive during their first pregnancies. Each woman had at least one subsequent pregnancy (range, 1 to 11) and was followed for a minimum of 2 years (range, 2 to 24). **No significant difference was reported in the incidences of diabetes mellitus in the two groups** (1.3% vs. 1.5%), **but the incidence of chronic hypertension was significantly higher in the PE patients** (14.8% vs. 5.6%; $P < .001$). **This difference became even greater for women followed more than 10 years** (51% vs. 14%; $P < .001$). **The incidence of severe PE was also significantly higher in the second pregnancies** (25.9% to 4.6%) **and in the subsequent pregnancies** (12.2% to 5.0%) **of women with PE.**

In a later report, subsequent pregnancy outcome and long-term prognosis were studied in 108 women who had **severe PE in the second trimester.** These women were followed for a minimum of 2 years (range, 2 to 12 years) and had a total of 169 subsequent pregnancies. Fifty-nine subsequent pregnancies (35%) were normotensive, and 110 (65%) were complicated by PE. **Overall, 21% of all subsequent pregnancies were complicated by severe PE in the second trimester.** In addition, these women had a higher risk for developing chronic hypertension; the highest incidence was in those who had recurrent severe PE in the second trimester (55%).

Hnat and associates[23] reported subsequent pregnancy outcome in women with previous PE enrolled in a multicenter trial. The rate of recurrent PE was 17%. The authors also noted that these women had a high rate of severe PE and poor perinatal outcome. In addition, even in those who remained normotensive in their subsequent pregnancy, the likelihood of adverse pregnancy outcome (preterm delivery, SGA infants, and perinatal death) was greater.

Some women with PE remote from term may have placental abruption. The risk for this complication is increased significantly in those with PE before 34 weeks' gestation and particularly in those who have PE in the second trimester. **For women with PE complicated by placental abruption, the risk for abruption in subsequent pregnancies ranges from 5% to 20%.**

Pregnancy outcome and long-term prognosis were studied in 37 women with PE complicated by pulmonary edema, and 18 of these women had subsequent pregnancies. Ten of the 18 were normotensive, 4 were complicated by chronic hypertension, and 4 were had PE; 1 of the latter women also had pulmonary edema.

Pregnancy outcome and remote prognosis were also studied in 18 women with severe PE complicated by acute renal failure. All 18 had acute tubular necrosis, 9 of whom required dialysis, and 2 died within 8 weeks after birth. All women had serial evaluation of renal function, urine microscopic testing, and electrolyte studies at the onset of acute renal failure and during follow-up. All 16 surviving patients had normal renal function on long-term follow-up (average, 4 years). Four of the 16 women had seven subsequent pregnancies: one ended in miscarriage, one was complicated by PE at 35 weeks, and five were term pregnancies without complications.

Women with a history of HELLP syndrome are at increased risk for all forms of PE in subsequent pregnancies (Table 31-15). **In general, the rate of PE in subsequent pregnancies is about 20%, with significantly higher rates if the onset of HELLP syndrome is during the second trimester. The rate of recurrent HELLP syndrome ranges from 2% to 19%, and the most reliable data suggest a recurrence risk of less than 5%.** This lower rate of 5% has been recently confirmed by the results of a systemic review. Because of the previously mentioned risks, these women are informed that they are at increased risk for adverse pregnancy outcomes (preterm delivery, FGR, placental abruption, and fetal death) in subsequent pregnancies and therefore require close monitoring during subsequent gestations. At present, **no preventive therapy is available for recurrent HELLP syndrome.** Case series describe subsequent pregnancy outcomes in women with previous ruptured liver hematomas. We have followed three such women through four subsequent pregnancies without complications. Other authors have reviewed the literature and have reported on several such women, who

TABLE 31-15	PREGNANCY OUTCOME AFTER HELLP SYNDROME			
	NO. OF WOMEN	NO. OF PREGNANCIES	HELLP (%)	PREECLAMPSIA (%)
Sibai et al[110]	139	192	3	19
Sullivan et al[111]	122	161	19	23
Van Pampus et al[112]	77	92	2	16
Chames et al[113]*	40	42	6	52

Modified from Sibai BM. Diagnosis, controversies, and management of HELLP syndrome. *Obstet Gynecol.* 2004;103:981.
*HELLP (hemolysis, elevated liver enzymes, and low platelets) at 28 weeks' or less in a previous pregnancy.

had subsequent uneventful pregnancies under close maternal and fetal observation.

Liver function tests were studied in 54 women at a median of 31 months (range, 3 to 101 months) after pregnancies complicated by the HELLP syndrome. Serum levels of AST, LDH, and conjugated bilirubin were found to be normal. However, total bilirubin levels were elevated in 11 (20%) of the studied women. The authors of this report suggested the possibility that a dysfunction of the bilirubin-conjugating mechanism represents a risk factor for the development of this syndrome.

Two reports describe long-term renal function after HELLP syndrome. One of the reports included 23 patients whose pregnancies were complicated by HELLP syndrome and acute renal failure: 8 of these women had 11 subsequent pregnancies, 9 of which resulted in term gestation. All 23 women also had normal BP and renal function at an average follow-up of 4.6 years (range, 0.5 to 11 years). The other study compared renal function after at least 5 years after HELLP syndrome in 10 patients with the respective findings in 22 patients with previous normotensive gestation. No differences were reported in renal function tests between the two groups. These findings suggest that the development of HELLP syndrome with or without renal failure does not affect long-term renal function.

Remote Prognosis

Women with PE should also be counseled regarding future cardiovascular risks and risks for underlying renal disease. **Evidence suggests that women with PE remote from term are at particular increased risk for chronic hypertension later in life.** In addition, these patients—particularly those with recurrent PE—are more likely to have underlying renal disease. In a recent report, 86 Japanese women who had severe hypertension, severe proteinuria, or both during pregnancy had a postpartum renal biopsy. The authors found that women who had gestational proteinuria or PE before 30 weeks' gestation were more likely to have had underlying renal disease.

Several recent studies suggested that women who develop PE may be at increased risk for coronary artery disease later in life. Indeed, many of the risk factors and pathophysiologic abnormalities of PE are similar to those of coronary artery disease. Ramsey and associates demonstrated for the first time, using laser Doppler imaging in vivo, impaired microvascular function in women 15 to 25 years of age following a pregnancy complicated by PE. Thus microvascular dysfunction, which is associated with insulin resistance, may be a predisposing vascular mechanism for both coronary heart disease and PE. In addition, pregnancies complicated by PE are at increased risk for stroke later in life. **Therefore pregnancies complicated by PE may identify women at risk for vascular disease in later life and may provide the opportunity for lifestyle and risk-factor modification to alter their risk for complications.**

ECLAMPSIA

Eclampsia is the occurrence of convulsions or coma unrelated to other cerebral conditions with signs and symptoms of preeclampsia. Early writings of both the Egyptians and Chinese warned of the dangers of convulsions encountered during pregnancy. Hippocrates noted that headaches, convulsions, and drowsiness were ominous signs associated with pregnancy. The term *eclampsia* appeared in a treatise on gynecology written by Varandaeus in 1619. Clonic spasms in association with pregnancy were described by Pew in 1694. In 1772, De la Motte recognized that prompt delivery of pregnant women with convulsions favored their recovery.

Eclampsia **is defined as the development of convulsions or unexplained coma during pregnancy or postpartum in patients with signs and symptoms of PE.** In the western world, the reported incidence of eclampsia ranges from 1 in 2000 to 1 in 3448 pregnancies. The reported incidence is usually higher in tertiary referral centers, with multifetal gestation, and in those without prenatal care.[12]

Pathophysiology

The pathogenesis of eclamptic convulsions continues to be the subject of extensive investigation and speculation. Several theories and pathologic mechanisms have been implicated as possible etiologic factors, but none of these has been proved conclusively. It is not clear whether the pathologic features in eclampsia are a cause or an effect of the convulsions.[86]

Diagnosis

The diagnosis of eclampsia is secure in the presence of generalized edema, hypertension, proteinuria, and convulsions. However, women in whom eclampsia develops exhibit a wide spectrum of signs that range from severe hypertension, severe proteinuria, and generalized edema to absent or minimal hypertension, no proteinuria, and no edema.[86] Hypertension is considered the hallmark for the diagnosis of eclampsia. The hypertension can be severe (≥160 mm Hg systolic or ≥110 mm Hg diastolic), as in 20% to 54% of cases,[16,86] or it can be mild (systolic BP between 140 and 160 mm Hg or diastolic BP between 90 and 110 mm Hg), as in 30% to 60% of cases.[12,86] However, in 16% of cases, hypertension may be absent.[16] In addition, severe hypertension is more common in patients who develop antepartum eclampsia (58%) and in those who develop eclampsia at 32 weeks' gestation or later (71%).[16] Moreover, hypertension is absent in only 10% of women who develop eclampsia at or before 32 weeks' gestation.[16]

The diagnosis of eclampsia is usually associated with proteinuria (at least 1+ on a dipstick).[16,86] In a series of 399 women with eclampsia, substantial proteinuria (≥3+ on a dipstick) was present in only 48% of the cases, whereas proteinuria was absent in 14% of the cases.[16] Abnormal weight gain in excess of 2 lb/

wk (with or without clinical edema) during the third trimester might be the first sign before the onset of eclampsia. However, edema was absent in 26% of 399 eclamptic women studied.[16]

Several clinical symptoms are potentially helpful in establishing the diagnosis of eclampsia. These include persistent occipital or frontal headaches, blurred vision, photophobia, epigastric or right upper quadrant pain, and altered mental status. Women had at least one of these symptoms in 59% to 75% of the cases (Table 31-16). Headaches are reported by 50% to 75% of patients, whereas visual changes are reported in 19% to 32% of patients.[86] These symptoms may occur before or after the onset of convulsions.[86]

Time of Onset of Eclampsia

The onset of eclamptic convulsions can be during the antepartum, intrapartum, or postpartum period. The reported frequency of antepartum convulsions among recent series has ranged from 38% to 53% (Table 31-17),[16] whereas the frequency of postpartum eclampsia has ranged from 11% to 44%.[16] **Although most cases of postpartum eclampsia occur within the first 48 hours, some cases can develop beyond 48 hours postpartum and have been reported as late as 23 days postpartum.**[16] **In the latter cases, an extensive neurologic evaluation may be required to rule out the presence of other cerebral pathology.**[86]

Almost all cases of eclampsia (91%) develop in the third trimester (≥28 weeks).[16] The remaining cases occur between 21 and 27 weeks' gestation (7.5%) or at or before 20 weeks' gestation (1.5%).[16] **Eclampsia that occurs before the twentieth week of gestation is generally associated with molar or hydropic degeneration of the placenta with or without a coexistent fetus.**[32,86] Although rare, eclampsia can occur during the first half of pregnancy without molar degeneration of the placenta.[32,86] These women may be misdiagnosed as having hypertensive encephalopathy, a seizure disorder, or TTP. Women in whom convulsions develop in association with hypertension and proteinuria during the first half of pregnancy should be considered to have eclampsia until proved otherwise.[32] These women should have an ultrasound examination to rule out molar pregnancy or hydropic degeneration of the placenta, and they also should have an extensive neurologic and medical evaluation to rule out another pathologic process.

Late postpartum eclampsia is defined as eclampsia that occurs more than 48 hours but less than 4 weeks after delivery. **Historically, eclampsia was believed not to occur more than 48 hours after delivery. However, several recent reports have confirmed the existence of late postpartum eclampsia.**[86] These women have signs and symptoms consistent with PE in association with convulsions.[32,86] Some women demonstrate a clinical picture of PE during labor or immediately postpartum (56%), whereas others demonstrate these clinical findings for the first time more than 48 hours after delivery (44%). Of interest is the fact that late-postpartum eclampsia developed despite the use of prophylactic magnesium sulfate during labor and for at least 24 hours postpartum in previously diagnosed preeclamptic women.[86] Therefore women in whom convulsions develop in association with hypertension or proteinuria or with headaches or blurred vision after 48 hours of delivery should be considered to have eclampsia and initially treated as such.[32]

Cerebral Pathology

Autoregulation of the cerebral circulation is a mechanism for the maintenance of constant cerebral blood flow during changes in BP, and it may be altered in eclampsia. Through active changes in cerebrovascular resistance at the arteriolar level, cerebral blood flow normally remains relatively constant when cerebral perfusion pressure ranges between 60 and 120 mm Hg. In this normal range, vasoconstriction of cerebral vessels occurs in response to elevations in BP, whereas vasodilation occurs as BP is lowered. Once cerebral perfusion pressure exceeds 130 to 150 mm Hg, however, the autoregulatory mechanism fails. In extreme hypertension, the normal compensatory vasoconstriction may become defective, and cerebral blood flow increases. As a result, segments of the vessels become dilated, ischemic, and increasingly permeable. Thus exudation of plasma occurs and gives rise to focal cerebral edema and compression of the vessels, which results in a decreased cerebral blood flow.[86] Hypertensive encephalopathy, a possible model for eclampsia, is an acute clinical condition that results from abrupt severe hypertension and subsequent significant increases in intracranial pressure. Because this is an acute disturbance in the hemodynamics of cerebral arterioles, morphologic changes in anatomy may not be uniformly evident in pathologic material. Several autopsy findings that are relatively constant include cerebral swelling and fibrinoid necrosis of vessel walls.

The cause of eclampsia is unknown, and many questions regarding the pathogenesis of its cerebral manifestations remain unanswered. Cerebral pathology in cortical and subcortical

TABLE 31-16   SYMPTOMS IN WOMEN WITH ECLAMPSIA

	DOUGLAS & REDMAN[114] (*n* = 325) (%)	KATZ ET AL[115] (*n* = 53) (%)	CHAMES ET AL[116] (*n* = 89) (%)
Headache	50	64	70
Visual changes	19	32	30
Right upper quadrant epigastric pain	19	Not reported	12
At least one	59	Not reported	75

From Sibai BM. Diagnosis, differential diagnosis and management of eclampsia. *Obstet Gynecol.* 2005;105:402.

TABLE 31-17   TIME OF ONSET OF ECLAMPSIA IN RELATION TO DELIVERY

	DOUGLAS & REDMAN[114] (*n* = 383) (%)	KNIGHT[118] (*n* = 214) (%)	KATZ[115] (*n* = 53) (%)	TUFFNELL[117] (*n* = 82) (%)	MATTAR & SIBAI[15] (*n* = 399) (%)	CHAMES ET AL[116] (*n* = 89) (%)
Antepartum	38	96	53	45	53	67*
Intrapartum	18	41	36	12	19	—
Postpartum	44	75	11	26	28	33
<48 hr	39		5	24	11	7
>48 hr	5		6	2	17	26

*Includes antepartum and intrapartum cases.

white matter in the form of edema, infarction, and hemorrhage (microhemorrhage and intracerebral parenchymal hemorrhage) is a common autopsy finding in patients who die of eclampsia. However, although autopsy series provide information regarding the central nervous system (CNS) abnormality in patients who die of eclampsia, this information is not necessarily indicative of the CNS abnormality present in most patients who survive this condition.[86] The diagnosis of eclampsia is not dependent on any single clinical or diagnostic neurologic findings. Focal neurologic signs such as hemiparesis or an unconscious state are rare in cases of eclampsia reported from countries in the developed world.[86] **Although eclamptic patients may initially manifest a variety of neurologic abnormalities—including cortical blindness, focal motor deficits, and coma—fortunately, most have no permanent neurologic deficits.**[16,86] These neurologic abnormalities are probably due to a transient insult, such as hypoxia, ischemia, or edema.

Several neurodiagnostic tests—such as electroencephalography (EEG), CT, cerebral Doppler velocimetry, MRI, and cerebral angiography (both traditional and MRI angiography)—have been studied in women with eclampsia. In general, the EEG is acutely abnormal in most eclamptic patients; however, these abnormalities are not pathognomonic of eclampsia. In addition, the abnormal EEG findings are not affected by the use of magnesium sulfate. Moreover, lumbar puncture is not helpful in the diagnosis and management of eclamptic women. The results of CT and MRI studies reveal the presence of edema and infarction within the subcortical white matter and adjacent gray matter mostly in the parietooccipital lobes (Box 31-10). Cerebral angiography and Doppler velocimetry suggest the presence of vasospasm.

On the basis of cerebral imaging findings, attention has been directed to hypertensive encephalopathy as a model for the CNS abnormalities in eclampsia. The two conditions share many clinical, radiologic, and pathologic features. Normal cerebral blood flow autoregulation fails in patients with hypertensive encephalopathy and in some patients with eclampsia.[86] **Two theories have been proposed to explain these cerebral abnormalities, forced dilation and vasospasm,**[86] **and the forced dilation theory suggests that the lesions in eclampsia are caused by loss of cerebrovascular autoregulation.**

Recently, MRI and apparent diffusion coefficient mapping were used to characterize the relative frequency of vasogenic and cytotoxic edema in two small series of eclamptic women; cerebral edema (mostly vasogenic) was present in up to 93% to 100%. However, concurrent foci of infarction evidenced by reduced apparent diffusion coefficient (restricted diffusion) were present in 6 of 27 eclamptic women studied by Zeeman and colleagues and in 3 of 17 eclamptic and preeclamptic women studied by Loureiro and associates. In addition, 5 of the 6 women reported by Zeeman and colleagues had persistent abnormalities on repeat MRI testing 6 to 8 weeks later, which suggests these lesions might not be reversible. Moreover, 4 of the 17 women reported by Loureiro and associates had persistent MRI abnormalities at a median of 8 weeks of follow-up.

In summary, cerebral imaging findings in eclampsia are similar to those found in patients with hypertensive encephalopathy. The classic findings are referred to as *posterior reversible encephalopathy syndrome* (PRES); Figure 31-13 demonstrates such a lesion. This syndrome is also seen in patients with reversible cerebral vasoconstriction syndrome and is usually seen in patients who present in the postpartum period with signs and symptoms similar to eclampsia. The diagnosis is confirmed by angiogram (Fig. 31-14). **Cerebral imaging is not necessary for the diagnosis and management of most women with eclampsia; however, it is indicated for patients with focal neurologic deficits or prolonged coma. In these patients, hemorrhage and other serious abnormalities that require specific pharmacologic therapy or surgery must be excluded. Cerebral imaging may also be helpful in patients who have an atypical presentation for eclampsia** (onset before 20 weeks' gestation or more than 48 hours after delivery and eclampsia refractory to adequate magnesium sulfate therapy). Advances in MRI and magnetic resonance angiography (MRA), as well as in cerebral vascular Doppler velocimetry, may aid our understanding regarding the pathogenesis and may improve long-term outcome of this condition.[86]

Differential Diagnosis

The presenting symptoms, clinical findings, and many of the laboratory findings overlap with a number of medical and

---

BOX 31-10   REPORTED COMPUTED TOMOGRAPHY SCAN AND MAGNETIC RESONANCE IMAGING FINDINGS IN COMPLICATED ECLAMPSIA

Diffuse white matter low-density areas
Patchy areas of low density
Occipital white matter edema
Loss of normal cortical sulci
Reduced ventricular size
Acute hydrocephalus
Cerebral hemorrhage
- Intraventricular hemorrhage
- Parenchymal hemorrhage (high density)
Cerebral infarction
- Low-attenuation areas
- Basal ganglia infarctions

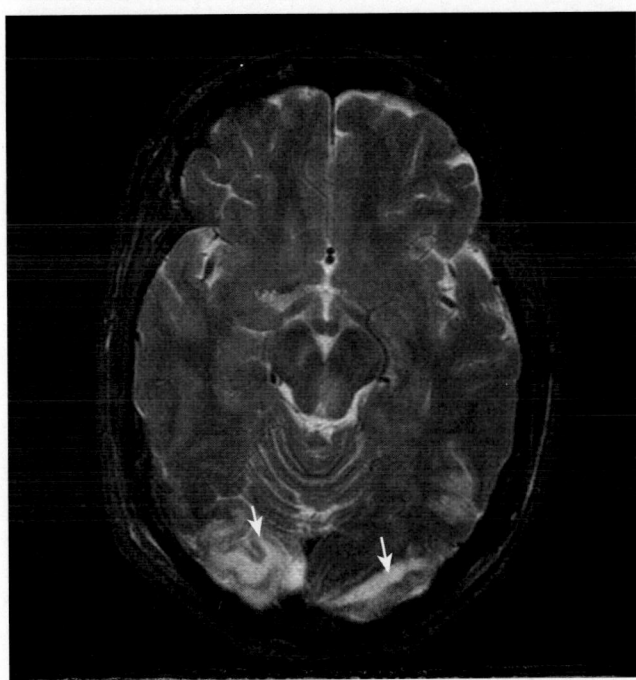

FIG 31-13 Magnetic resonance imaging of the brain reveals posterior reversible encephalopathy syndrome in a patient with eclampsia. *Arrows* point at vasogenic edema that is considered reversible.

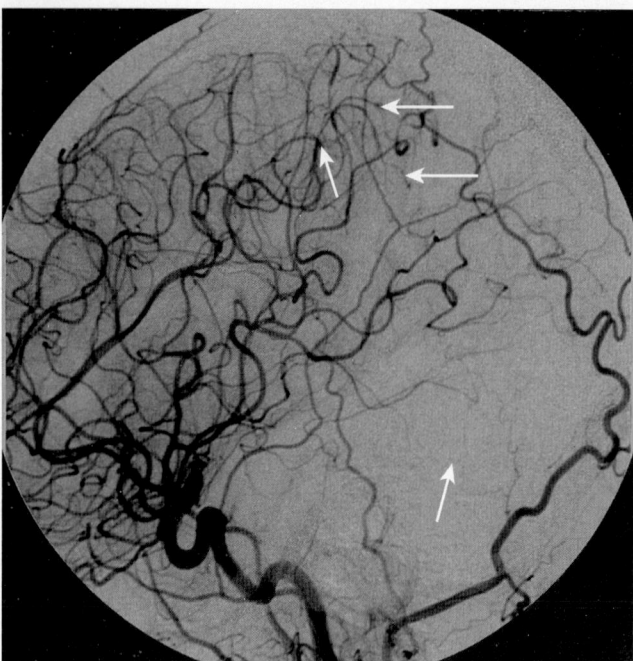

FIG 31-14 Cerebral arteriogram demonstrates cerebral vasoconstriction. *Arrows* show diffused vasoconstriction in small blood vessels.

BOX 31-11 DIFFERENTIAL DIAGNOSIS OF ECLAMPSIA

- Hypertensive encephalopathy
- Seizure disorder
- Hypoglycemia, hyponatremia
- Posterior reversible encephalopathy syndrome (PRES; see Fig. 31-13)
- Thrombotic thrombocytopenic purpura
- Postdural puncture syndrome
- Vasculitis, angiopathy
- Amniotic fluid embolism
- Cerebrovascular accident
- Hemorrhage
- Ruptured aneurysm or malformation
- Arterial embolism, thrombosis
- Cerebral venous thrombosis
- Hypoxic ischemic encephalopathy
- Angiomas

---

surgical conditions.[32] For convulsions that develop in association with hypertension or proteinuria during pregnancy or immediately postpartum, the most common cause is eclampsia. Rarely, other etiologies that produce convulsions in pregnancy or postpartum may mimic eclampsia.[86]

These diagnoses are particularly important in the presence of focal neurologic deficits, prolonged coma, or atypical eclampsia. In addition, in some patients, GH or PE may develop in association with disorders such as connective tissue disease, thrombophilias, seizure disorder, or hypertensive encephalopathy, which further contributes to the diagnostic difficulty. Therefore an effort should be made to identify an accurate diagnosis given that management strategies may differ among these conditions (Box 31-11).

Maternal and Perinatal Outcome

Eclampsia is associated with a slightly increased risk for maternal death in developed countries (0% to 1.8%),[86] but

the maternal mortality rate may be as high as 14% in developing countries. The high maternal mortality reported from developing countries occurs primarily among patients who have had multiple seizures outside the hospital and those without prenatal care. In addition, this high mortality rate could be attributed to the lack of resources and intensive care facilities needed to manage maternal complications from eclampsia. Of 4024 pregnancy-related deaths reported from 1979 to 1992, a total of 790 (19.6%) were considered to have been caused by PE-eclampsia, and 49% of these 790 were considered to have been related to eclampsia. In this series, the risk for death from PE or eclampsia was higher for women older than 30 years, those without prenatal care, and black women; the greatest risk for death was found among women with pregnancies at or before 28 weeks' gestation.

Pregnancies complicated by eclampsia are also associated with increased rates of maternal morbidities such as placental abruption (7% to 10%),[86] DIC (7% to 11%),[86] pulmonary edema (3% to 5%), acute renal failure (5% to 9%), aspiration pneumonia (2% to 3%), and cardiopulmonary arrest (2% to 5%).[86] ARDS and intracerebral hemorrhage are rare complications in series of eclamptic patients reported from the developed world. It is important to note that maternal complications are greatest among women who develop antepartum eclampsia, particularly among those who develop eclampsia remote from term.[86]

Perinatal mortality and morbidity remain high in eclamptic pregnancies. The reported perinatal death rate in recent series ranged from 5.6% to 11.8%.[86] This high perinatal death rate is related to prematurity, placental abruption, and severe FGR.[86] The rate of preterm delivery is about 50%, and about 25% of cases occur before 32 weeks' gestation.[86]

Is Eclampsia Preventable?

Prevention of eclampsia requires knowledge of its etiology and pathophysiology and of methods to predict patients at high risk for development of convulsions. However, as discussed earlier, the pathogenesis of eclampsia is largely unknown. Prevention of eclampsia can be *primary*, by preventing the development and/or progression of PE, or it can be *secondary*, by using pharmacologic agents that prevent convulsions in women with established PE. Prevention can also be *tertiary*, by preventing subsequent convulsions in women with established eclampsia.

Current management schemes designed to prevent eclampsia are based on early detection of GH or PE and subsequent use of preventive therapy in such women. Some of the recommended preventive therapies have included close monitoring (in-hospital or outpatient), use of antihypertensive therapy to keep maternal BP below a certain level (less than severe range or to normal values), timely delivery, and prophylactic use of magnesium sulfate during labor and immediately postpartum in those considered to have PE. These management schemes assume that the clinical course in the development of eclampsia is characterized by a gradual process that begins with progressive weight gain, followed by hypertension (mild to severe) and proteinuria, with the subsequent onset of premonitory symptoms, and ending with the onset of generalized convulsions or coma.[86] This clinical course may be present in some women who develop eclampsia in developed countries. However, recent data from large series of eclamptic women from the United States and Europe indicate that about 20% to 40% of eclamptic women do not have any premonitory signs or

symptoms before the onset of convulsions.[16] In many of these cases, the onset of convulsions is abrupt and does not follow an indolent progression from mild to severe disease before the onset of eclampsia.[86]

It is also assumed that appropriate and timely standard preventive therapy will prevent eclampsia in virtually all patients with GH-PE.[86] The efficacy of in-hospital management of patients with GH or PE for the prevention of eclampsia has not been evaluated in randomized trials. Moreover, data from retrospective studies from developed countries indicate that about 50% of eclamptic women develop their first convulsion while in the hospital under "close medical supervision."[86] Thus early and prolonged hospitalization of women with mild hypertension or PE may not prevent most cases of eclampsia.

Several randomized trials have described the use of antihypertensive drugs versus no treatment or a placebo in the treatment of women with mild hypertension or PE. Overall, these trials revealed lower rates of progression to severe disease. However, the study design and the sample size of these trials is inadequate to evaluate potential benefits regarding prevention of eclampsia.

Prophylactic magnesium sulfate is recommended only for women who are hospitalized with the established diagnosis of PE.[1-3] Its use is recommended only during labor and for 12 to 24 hours' postpartum[1-3]; therefore it can be expected to have a potential effect in preventing eclampsia that develops only during this time (40% of total).

Several randomized trials have compared the efficacy of magnesium sulfate with other anticonvulsive agents for the prevention of recurrent seizures in women with eclampsia. In these trials, **magnesium sulfate was compared with diazepam, phenytoin, and a lytic cocktail. Overall, these trials revealed that magnesium sulfate was associated with a significantly lower rate of recurrent seizures** (9.4% vs. 23.1%; RR, 0.41; 95% CI, 0.32 to 0.51) **and a lower rate of maternal death** (3% vs. 4.8%; RR, 0.62; 95% CI, 0.39 to 0.99) **than that observed with other agents.**

The low incidence of eclampsia in developed countries is probably related to prevention of cases of eclampsia in women with a classic presentation and with a classic progression from mild to severe PE.[86] As a result, most eclamptic cases described in reported series from the United States and Europe have an atypical presentation (abrupt onset, development of convulsions while receiving prophylactic magnesium sulfate, or onset of convulsions beyond 48 hours after delivery).[86] Indeed, most eclamptic convulsions in these series developed in hospitalized women, and in some of these women, the onset of convulsions was not preceded by warning signs or symptoms.[86] Overall, the percentage of eclampsia considered unpreventable in these series ranged from 31% to 87%.[86]

Transport of the Eclamptic Patient

During the past 20 years, a marked reduction has been seen in the incidence of eclampsia. Consequently, most obstetricians have little or no experience in the management of eclampsia. A recent survey of a random sample of obstetricians from all 50 states indicated that about 50% of obstetricians in private practice had not seen an eclamptic patient during the past year.

Because management of the eclamptic patient requires the availability of neonatal and obstetric ICUs and personnel with special expertise, it is recommended that eclamptic women at term be cared for only at level II or III hospitals with adequate facilities and with consultants from other specialties. For those eclamptic patients who are remote from term, referral should be made to a tertiary care center. The following steps should be taken before transfer of these critically ill patients:

1. The referring physician or nurse should consult with the physician at the perinatal center regarding the referral and appropriate treatment. All maternal records, including prenatal data and a detailed summary of the patient's condition, should be transmitted.
2. BP should be stabilized, and convulsions should be controlled.
3. Adequate prophylactic anticonvulsive medications should be given. An accepted regimen is 4 or 6 g IV magnesium sulfate as a loading dose over 20 minutes.
4. Maternal laboratory assessment (CBC with platelet count, liver enzymes) and fetal monitoring should be undertaken.

Patients should be sent in an ambulance with medical personnel in attendance for proper management in cases of subsequent convulsions.

Treatment of Eclamptic Convulsions

Eclamptic convulsions are a life-threatening emergency and require proper care to minimize morbidity and mortality. The development of an eclamptic convulsion is frightening to observe. Initially, the patient's face becomes distorted with protrusion of her eyes. This is followed by a congested facial expression. Foam often exudes from the mouth, and the woman usually bites her tongue unless it is protected. Respirations are absent throughout the seizure. The convulsion, which can be divided into two phases, typically continues for 60 to 75 seconds. The first phase, which lasts 15 to 20 seconds, begins with facial twitching and proceeds to the body becoming rigid with generalized muscular contractions. The second phase lasts about 60 seconds and consists of the muscles of the body alternately contracting and relaxing in rapid succession. This phase begins with the muscles of the jaw and rapidly involves the eyelids, other facial muscles, and then all the muscles of the body. Coma follows the convulsion, and the woman usually remembers nothing of the recent events. If she has repeated convulsions, some degree of consciousness returns after each convulsion. She may enter a combative state and may be agitated and difficult to control. Rapid and deep respirations usually begin as soon as the convulsions end. Maintenance of oxygenation is usually not a problem after a single convulsion; the risk for aspiration is low in the well-managed patient.

Because eclampsia is so frightening, the natural tendency is to attempt to abolish the convulsion. However, drugs such as diazepam should *not* be given in an attempt to stop or shorten the convulsion, especially if the patient does not have an IV line in place and someone skilled in intubation is not immediately available. If diazepam is used, no more than 5 mg should be given over 60 seconds. Rapid administration of diazepam may lead to apnea, cardiac arrest, or both.

Prevention of Maternal Injury During the Convulsions

The first priority in the management of eclampsia is to prevent maternal injury and to support cardiovascular function. During or immediately after the acute convulsive episode, supportive care should be given to prevent serious maternal injury and aspiration, assess and establish airway patency, and ensure maternal oxygenation. During this time, the bed's side rails should be elevated and padded; a padded tongue blade is inserted between the teeth (avoid inducing a gag reflex), and physical restraints may also be needed. To minimize the risk for aspiration, the patient should lie in the lateral decubitus position, and vomitus and oral secretions are suctioned as needed.[86] Aspiration may be caused by forcing the padded tongue blade to the back of the throat, stimulating the gag reflex with resultant vomiting.

Adequate oxygenation should be maintained during the convulsive episode because hypoventilation and respiratory acidosis often occur. Although the initial seizure lasts only a few minutes, it is important to maintain oxygenation by supplemental oxygen administration through a face mask with or without an oxygen reservoir at 8 to 10 L/min.[86] After the convulsion has ceased, the patient begins to breathe again, and oxygenation is rarely a problem. However, maternal hypoxemia and acidosis may develop in women who have had repetitive convulsions, in those with aspiration pneumonia or pulmonary edema, or as a result of a combination of these factors. **It is my policy to use transcutaneous pulse oximetry to monitor oxygenation in all eclamptic patients.** Arterial blood gas analysis is required if the pulse oximetry results are abnormal (oxygen saturation ≤92%). Sodium bicarbonate is not given unless the pH is below 7.10.

Prevention of Recurrent Convulsions

The next step in the management of eclampsia is to prevent recurrent convulsions. **Magnesium sulfate is the drug of choice to treat and prevent subsequent convulsions in women with eclampsia.[86] A loading dose of 6 g over 15 to 20 minutes is recommended, followed by a maintenance dose of 2 g per hour as a continuous IV solution.** About 10% of eclamptic women have a second convulsion after receiving magnesium sulfate.[86] In these women, another bolus of 2 g magnesium sulfate can be given intravenously over 3 to 5 minutes. An occasional patient will have recurrent convulsions while receiving adequate and therapeutic doses of magnesium sulfate. In this patient, recurrent seizures can be treated with Ativan 2 mg intravenously over 3 to 5 minutes.[86]

Rarely, a woman may experience an eclamptic seizure, lapse into a coma, and die. Magnesium toxicity should be considered in those women who do not regain consciousness. A case report of magnesium sulfate toxicity details the features of this serious complication. Within a few minutes of starting what was supposed to be a magnesium loading dose, 4 g magnesium sulfate in 250 mL saline, the patient went into cardiorespiratory arrest. Immediate resuscitation was performed, including intubation; about half of the loading dose had been given. A coma ensued that was believed to have been caused by an intracerebral accident or eclampsia; the loading dose was continued, and maintenance therapy was started. Initial blood gases were normal, and the electrocardiogram (ECG) was normal 15 minutes after the arrest. The patient's vital signs were stable; however, mechanical ventilatory support was required, and her pupils were nonreactive. Serum electrolytes, glucose, blood urea nitrogen, and creatinine were normal; CT scan of the head and cerebral angiograms were also normal. A magnesium level of 35 mg/dL was reported 3.5 hours later from a blood sample taken through femoral venipuncture at the time of arrest; the magnesium sulfate infusion was stopped immediately. During the first 5 hours after the cardiorespiratory arrest, 1344 mg of magnesium was excreted in the urine. Twelve hours after the arrest, an uncomplicated low vertical cesarean delivery was done for a

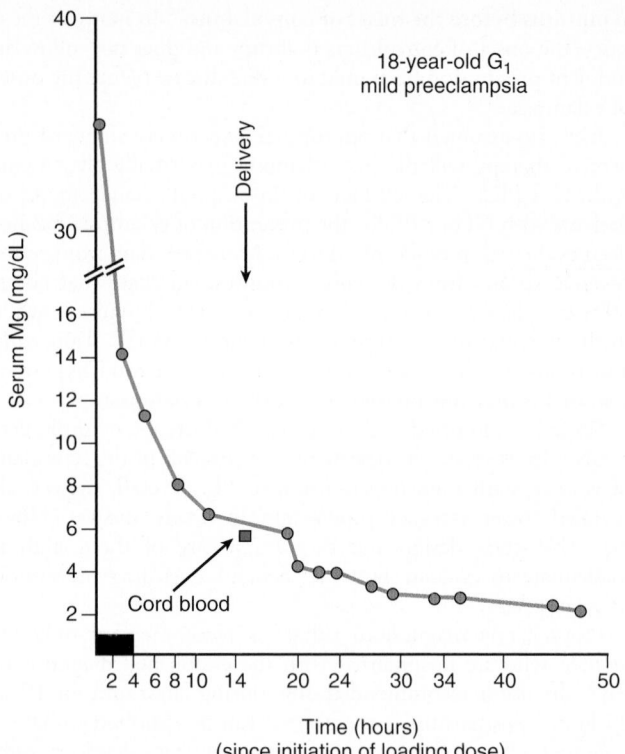

FIG 31-15 Magnesium levels over time in a patient with magnesium toxicity. (From McCubbin JH, Sibai BM, Abdella TN, et al. Cardiopulmonary arrest due to acute maternal hypermagnesemia [letter]. *Lancet.* 1981;1:1058.)

breech presentation. The 3160-g male infant had Apgar scores of 8 and 9 at 1 and 5 minutes, respectively. Maternal and cord blood magnesium levels at delivery were 5.8 mg/dL. Both mother and baby were discharged from the hospital with no apparent sequelae. Of interest, the patient reported she could hear and see what was occurring around her, but she could not make any movements while she was intubated. Figure 31-15 presents the maternal magnesium levels in this case.

Control of Severe Hypertension

The next step in the management of eclampsia is to reduce the BP to a safe range. The objectives of treating severe hypertension are to avoid loss of cerebral autoregulation and to prevent CHF without compromising cerebral perfusion or jeopardizing uteroplacental blood flow, which is already reduced in many women with eclampsia.[86] Thus **maintaining systolic BP between 140 and 160 mm Hg and diastolic BP between 90 and 105 mm Hg is a reasonable goal. This can be achieved with bolus 5 to 10 mg doses of hydralazine every 20 minutes or labetalol (20 to 40 mg intravenously) every 10 minutes as needed.**[86] Other potent antihypertensive medications, such as sodium nitroprusside or nitroglycerine, are rarely needed in eclampsia. Diuretics are not used except in the presence of pulmonary edema.

Intrapartum Management of Eclampsia

Maternal hypoxemia and hypercarbia cause FHR and uterine activity changes during and immediately after a convulsion. The FHR tracing may reveal bradycardia, transient late decelerations, decreased beat-to-beat variability, and compensatory tachycardia. Uterine contractions can increase in frequency and tone.[86] These changes usually resolve

spontaneously within 3 to 10 minutes after the termination of convulsions and correction of maternal hypoxemia. The patient should not be rushed to emergency cesarean delivery based on these findings, especially if the maternal condition remains stable.

In a review of 10 women who had undergone electronic internal fetal monitoring during an eclamptic convulsion, 6 had fetal bradycardia (FHR <120 beats/min) that varied in duration from 30 seconds to 9 minutes. The interval from onset of the seizure to the fall in FHR was 5 minutes. Transitory fetal tachycardia occurred frequently after the prolonged bradycardia. In addition, loss of beat-to-beat variability with transitory late decelerations occurred during the recovery phase. Uterine hyperactivity demonstrated by both increased uterine tone and increased frequency of uterine contractions occurs during an eclamptic seizure. The duration of the increased uterine activity varies from 2 to 14 minutes.

Fetal outcome is generally good after an eclamptic convulsion. The mechanism for the transitory fetal bradycardia may be a decrease in uterine blood flow caused by intense vasospasm and uterine hyperactivity. The absence of maternal respiration during the convulsion may also result in fetal hypoxia and heart rate changes. Because the FHR pattern usually returns to normal after a convulsion, other conditions should be considered if an abnormal pattern persists. It may take longer for the heart rate pattern to return to baseline in an eclamptic woman whose fetus is preterm with growth restriction. Placental abruption may occur after the convulsion and should be considered if uterine hyperactivity remains or the bradycardia persists.[86]

The presence of eclampsia is not an indication for cesarean delivery. The decision to perform a cesarean delivery should be based on gestational age, fetal condition, presence of labor, and cervical Bishop score.[86] Cesarean delivery is recommended for those with eclampsia before 30 weeks' gestation who are not in labor with an unfavorable cervix (Bishop score <5). Patients in labor or whose membranes have ruptured are allowed to deliver vaginally in the absence of obstetric complications. When labor is indicated, it is initiated with either oxytocin infusions or prostaglandins in all patients with a gestational age at or above 30 weeks, irrespective of the Bishop score. A similar approach is used for those before 30 weeks' gestation if the cervical Bishop score is at least 5.

Maternal pain relief during labor and delivery can be provided by either systemic opioids or epidural anesthesia as recommended for women with severe PE.[2] Either epidural, spinal, or combined techniques of regional anesthesia can be used for cesarean delivery. Regional anesthesia is contraindicated in the presence of coagulopathy or severe thrombocytopenia (platelet count <50,000/mm³). In women with eclampsia, general anesthesia increases the risk for aspiration and failed intubation due to airway edema and is associated with marked increases in

systemic and cerebral pressures during intubation and extubation.[86] Women with airway or laryngeal edema may require awake intubation under fiberoptic observation with the availability of immediate tracheostomy. Changes in systemic or cerebral pressures may be attenuated by pretreatment with labetalol or nitroglycerine injections.[86]

Postpartum Management of Eclampsia

After delivery, women with eclampsia should receive close monitoring of vital signs, fluid intake and output, and symptoms for at least 48 hours. These women usually receive large amounts of IV fluids during labor, delivery, and postpartum. In addition, during the postpartum period, mobilization of extracellular fluid leads to increased intravascular volume. As a result, women with eclampsia, particularly those with abnormal renal function; those with abruptio placentae; and those with preexisting chronic hypertension are at increased risk for pulmonary edema and exacerbation of severe hypertension postpartum.[86] Careful attention to fluid status is essential.

Parenteral magnesium sulfate should be continued for at least 24 hours after delivery or for at least 24 hours after the last convulsion. If oliguria is present (<100 mL/4 hr), both the rate of fluid administration and the dose of magnesium sulfate should be reduced. Once delivery has occurred, other oral antihypertensive agents such as labetalol or nifedipine can be used to keep systolic BP below 155 mm Hg and diastolic BP below 105 mm Hg. Nifedipine offers the benefit of improved diuresis in the postpartum period.

Subsequent Pregnancy Outcomes and Remote Prognosis

Women with a history of eclampsia are at increased risk for all forms of PE in subsequent pregnancies (Table 31-18). **In general, the rate of PE in subsequent pregnancies is about 25%, with substantially higher rates if the onset of eclampsia was in the second trimester. The rate of recurrent eclampsia is about 2%.** Because of these risks, these women should be informed that they are at increased risk for adverse pregnancy outcome in subsequent pregnancies. At present, no preventive therapy exists for recurrent antepartum eclampsia.

The long-term effects of eclampsia on maternal BP and neurologic outcome have been the subject of few reports. The findings of these studies revealed that eclampsia did not cause hypertension in women who were normotensive before the eclamptic pregnancy. Two of these studies found that the rate of chronic hypertension on follow-up was significantly higher in those who had eclampsia remote from term compared with those who had eclampsia at or beyond 37 weeks of gestation. In addition, one of these reports revealed that women who had eclampsia as multiparas were at increased risk for death from cardiovascular renal disease. Moreover, these investigations revealed no evidence of neurologic deficit during the follow-up period.

TABLE 31-18   RECURRENT PREECLAMPSIA-ECLAMPSIA IN WOMEN WITH ECLAMPSIA

	CHESLEY[119]	LOPEZ-LLERA & HORTA[120]	ADELUSI & OJENGBEDE[121]	SIBAI ET AL[122]
No. of women	171	110	64	182
No. of pregnancies	398	110	64	366
Eclampsia (%)	1.0	—	15.6	1.9
Preeclampsia (%)	23	35	27	22

From Sibai BM. Diagnosis, differential diagnosis and management of eclampsia. *Obstet Gynecol.* 2005;105:402.

CHRONIC HYPERTENSION

The frequency of chronic hypertension in pregnancy is estimated at 1% to 5%. It is more common in older obese women and in black women. Because of the current trend of childbearing at an older age and the obesity epidemic, it is expected that the incidence of chronic hypertension in pregnancy will continue to rise. During the new millennium, and estimating a prevalence of chronic hypertension during pregnancy of 3%, at least 120,000 pregnant women (3% of 4 million pregnancies) with chronic hypertension will be seen annually in the United States.

Definition and Diagnosis

In pregnancy, *chronic hypertension* is defined as elevated BP that is present and documented before conception. **In women whose prepregnancy BP is unknown, the diagnosis is based on the presence of *sustained hypertension* before 20 weeks of gestation, defined as either systolic BP of at least 140 mm Hg or diastolic BP of at least 90 mm Hg on at least two occasions measured at least 4 hours apart.**

The diagnosis may be difficult to establish in women with previously undiagnosed chronic hypertension who begin prenatal care after 16 weeks' gestation because physiologic decline in BP occurs at that time. An analysis of pregnancy outcome in 211 patients with mild chronic hypertension suggests that the use of antihypertensive drugs is not necessary to achieve a good pregnancy outcome (Table 31-19). The changes in average MAP throughout the course of pregnancy are summarized in Figure 31-16. This decrease may result in normal BP findings in the second trimester that will eventually increase again during the third trimester. These women are more likely to be erroneously diagnosed as having GH.

Women with chronic hypertension are at increased risk for superimposed PE. The development of superimposed PE is associated with high rates of adverse maternal and perinatal outcomes.[14] The diagnosis of superimposed PE should be made as described previously based on changes in BP, development of new-onset proteinuria, new-onset symptoms, or changes in laboratory tests.

Etiology and Classification

The etiology and severity of chronic hypertension are important considerations in the management of pregnancy. Chronic hypertension is subdivided into *primary* (essential) and *secondary* hypertension. Primary hypertension is by far the most common type of chronic hypertension seen during pregnancy (90%). In 10% of cases, chronic hypertension is secondary to one or more underlying disorders such as renal disease (glomerulonephritis, interstitial nephritis, polycystic kidneys, renal artery stenosis), collagen vascular disease (lupus, scleroderma), endocrine disorders (diabetes mellitus with vascular involvement, pheochromocytoma, thyrotoxicosis, Cushing disease, hyperaldosteronism), or coarctation of the aorta.

Chronic hypertension during pregnancy can be subclassified as either mild or severe, depending on the systolic and diastolic BP readings. Systolic and diastolic (Korotkoff phase V) BPs of at least 160 mm Hg or 110 mm Hg, respectively, constitute severe hypertension.

For management and counseling purposes, chronic hypertension in pregnancy is also categorized as either low risk or high risk, as described in Figure 31-17. **The patient is considered to**

TABLE 31-19	RATES OF ADVERSE PREGNANCY OUTCOME IN OBSERVATIONAL STUDIES DESCRIBING MILD CHRONIC HYPERTENSION IN PREGNANCY			
	PREECLAMPSIA (%)	**ABRUPTIO PLACENTAE (%)**	**DELIVERY <37 WK (%)**	**SGA (%)**
Rey & Couturier[124] (*n* = 337)	21	0.7	34.4	15.5
McCowan et al[123] (*n* = 142)	14	NR	16	11.0
Sibai et al[14] (*n* = 763)	25	1.5	33.3	11.1
Giannubilo et al[126] (*n* = 233)	28	0.5	NR	16.5
Chappell et al[125] (*n* = 822)	22	NR	22.7	27.2
Sibai et al[127] (*n* = 369)	17	2.4	29.3	15.0

NR, not reported; *SGA,* small for gestational age.

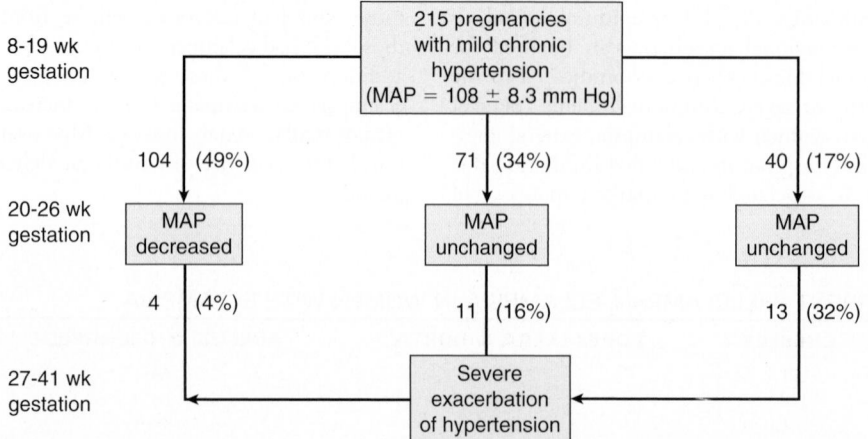

FIG 31-16 Mean arterial blood pressure (MAP) during pregnancy. (Modified from Sibai BM, Abdella TN, Anderson GD. Pregnancy outcome in 211 patients with mild chronic hypertension. *Obstet Gynecol.* 1983;61:571.)

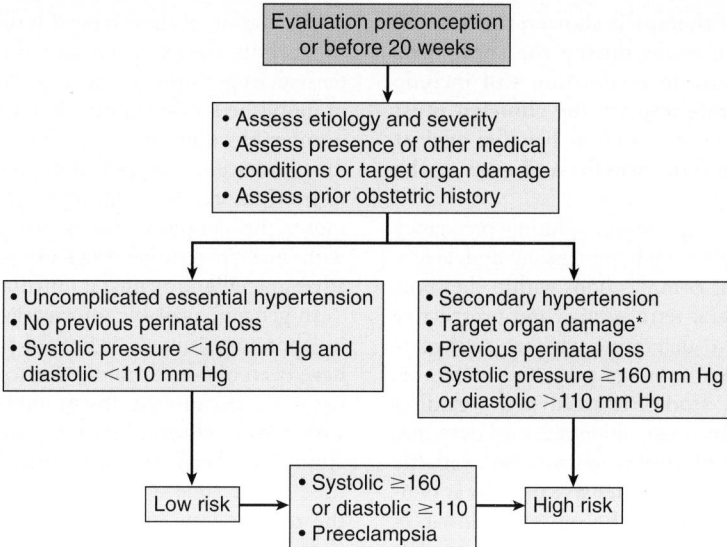

FIG 31-17 Initial evaluation of women with chronic hypertension. *Left ventricular dysfunction, retinopathy, dyslipidemia, maternal age >40 years, microvascular disease, stroke. (From Sibai BM. Chronic hypertension in pregnancy. *Obstet Gynecol.* 2002;100:369.)

be at low risk when she has mild essential hypertension without any organ involvement. The BP criteria are based on measurements at the initial visit irrespective of treatment with antihypertensive medications. For example, if the patient has a BP of 140/80 mm Hg on antihypertensive drugs, she is still classified as low risk. It is important to note that a patient initially classified as low risk early in pregnancy may become high risk if she later develops severe hypertension or PE.

Maternal and Perinatal Risks

Pregnancies complicated by chronic hypertension are at increased risk for the development of superimposed PE, placental abruption, and fetal growth restriction. The reported rates of PE in the literature in mild hypertension range from 14% to 28% (see Table 31-19).[14] The rate of PE in women with severe chronic hypertension ranges from 50% to 79%. Sibai and associates[14] studied the rate of superimposed PE among 763 women with chronic hypertension followed prospectively at several tertiary medical centers in the United States. The overall rate of superimposed PE was 25%. The rate was not affected by maternal age, race, or presence of proteinuria early in pregnancy; however, it was significantly greater in women who had hypertension for at least 4 years (31% vs. 22%), in those who had PE during a previous pregnancy (32% vs. 23%), and in those whose diastolic BP was 100 mm Hg or higher (42% vs. 24%).[14]

The reported rate of placental abruption in women with mild chronic hypertension has ranged from 0.7% to 2.7% (see Table 31-19). The rate in those with severe or high-risk hypertension may be 5% to 10%. In a recent multicenter study that included 763 women with chronic hypertension, the overall rate of abruption was reported at 1.5%, and the rate was significantly higher in those who developed superimposed PE than in those without this complication (3% vs. 1%, $P = .04$).[14] However, the rate was not influenced by maternal age, race, or duration of hypertension.[14] In addition, the results of a systematic review of nine observational studies revealed that in women with chronic hypertension, the rate of abruption is doubled

(OR, 2.1; 95% CI, 1.1 to 3.9) compared with normotensive patients.

In addition to PE and abruption, women with high-risk chronic hypertension are at increased risk for life-threatening maternal complications such as pulmonary edema, hypertensive encephalopathy, retinopathy, cerebral hemorrhage, and acute renal failure. These risks are particularly increased in women with uncontrolled severe hypertension, significant renal disease early in pregnancy, or left ventricular dysfunction before conception.

Fetal and neonatal complications are also increased in women with chronic hypertension. The risk for perinatal mortality is three to four times greater compared with that of the general obstetric population (OR, 3.4; 95% CI, 3.0 to 3.7). The likelihood of premature delivery and a growth-restricted infant is also increased in women with chronic hypertension. In women with severe chronic hypertension in the first trimester, the reported rates of preterm delivery were 62% to 70%, and the rates of an SGA infant were 31% to 40%. Recently, Sibai and associates[15] reported risk factors for adverse perinatal outcome in a secondary analysis of 763 women with mild chronic hypertension who were enrolled in a multicenter trial that compared low-dose aspirin with a placebo for the prevention of PE. They found that the development of superimposed PE was associated with higher rates of preterm delivery (OR, 3.9; 95% CI, 2.7 to 5.4), neonatal intraventricular hemorrhage (OR, 4.5; 95% CI, 1.5 to 14.2), and perinatal death (OR, 2.3; 95% CI, 1.4 to 4.8). In addition, the presence of proteinuria early in pregnancy was an independent risk factor associated with higher rates of preterm delivery (OR, 3.1; 95% CI, 1.8 to 5.3), an SGA infant (OR, 2.8; 95% CI, 1.6 to 5.0), and neonatal intraventricular hemorrhage (OR, 3.9; 95% CI, 1.3 to 11.6).[14]

Goals of Antihypertensive Therapy in Pregnancy

In nonpregnant individuals, long-term BP control can lead to significant reductions in the rates of stroke and cardiovascular morbidity and mortality. In contrast to hypertension in pregnancy, the duration of therapy is shorter, the benefits to the mother may not be obvious during the short time of treatment, and the exposure to medication will include both mother and fetus. In this respect, the clinician must balance the potential short-term maternal benefits against possible short-term and long-term benefits and risks to the fetus and infant.

Most women with chronic hypertension during pregnancy have mild, essential, uncomplicated hypertension and are at minimal risk for cardiovascular complications within the short time frame of pregnancy. Several retrospective and prospective studies have been conducted to determine whether antihypertensive therapy in these women improves pregnancy outcome. An overall summary of these studies revealed that regardless of the antihypertensive therapy used, maternal cardiovascular and renal complications were minimal or absent. **No available data suggest that short-term antihypertensive therapy is beneficial for the mother or the fetus in the setting of low-risk hypertension except for a reduction in the rate of exacerbation of hypertension. However, only three trials have had a sufficient sample size to evaluate the risks for superimposed PE and placental abruption.**

Recently, the benefits of tight blood pressure control versus less blood pressure control in women with chronic hypertension in pregnancy were studied in a large multicenter study, the Control of Hypertension in Pregnancy Study (CHIPS). The trial included 736 women with chronic hypertension; 361 were assigned to tight control and 371 were assigned to less tight control. The investigators found no difference between groups in primary outcome (pregnancy loss or high-level neonatal care) or in serious maternal complications. However, women in the less-tight control group had a higher rate of progression to severe hypertension. In contrast, the tight control group had a significantly higher rate of SGA infants (19.7% vs. 13.9%).

No placebo-controlled trials have examined the benefits of antihypertensive therapy in women with severe hypertension in pregnancy, and none are likely to be performed. **Antihypertensive therapy is necessary in women with severe hypertension to reduce the acute risks for stroke, CHF, and renal failure. In addition, control of severe hypertension can permit pregnancy prolongation and thereby improve perinatal outcome. However, no evidence suggests that control of severe hypertension reduces the rate of either superimposed PE or placental abruption.**

No trials have examined the treatment of women with chronic hypertension and other risk factors such as preexisting renal disease, diabetes mellitus, or cardiac disease. On the other hand, evidence from retrospective and observational studies suggests that uncontrolled mild to moderate hypertension may exacerbate target-organ damage during pregnancy in women with renal disease, diabetes mellitus with vascular disease, or left ventricular dysfunction. Therefore some authors recommend aggressive treatment of mild hypertension in these women because of the belief that such management may reduce both short- and long-term cardiovascular complications.

Safety of Antihypertensive Drugs in Pregnancy

The potential adverse effects of most commonly prescribed antihypertensive agents are either poorly established or unclearly quantified. Most of the evidence on harm associated with antihypertensives in pregnancy is limited to case reports. The interpretation of these reports is difficult because it is impossible to ascertain the exact number of women exposed to antihypertensive drugs during pregnancy. Also, it is likely that the number of published case reports is an underestimate of the actual number of women who experience the reported adverse reaction. This limitation is amplified by the fact that information related to previous exposure during pregnancy is nonexistent. Furthermore, the condition for which pregnant women are treated with antihypertensive drugs can be partially responsible for the adverse fetal and neonatal outcomes.

In general, available information about teratogenicity, except in laboratory animals, is limited and selective. All available data have been obtained from registries such as state Medicaid registry data. Because of absent multicenter randomized trials in women with chronic hypertension, no placebo-controlled evaluations have been done regarding the safety of these drugs when used at the time of conception and throughout pregnancy. At the present time, only minimal data are available to help the clinician evaluate the benefits or risks of most antihypertensive drugs when used in pregnancy. **Nevertheless, the limited data in the literature suggest potential adverse fetal effects, such as oligohydramnios and fetal-neonatal renal failure, when angiotensin-converting enzyme (ACE) inhibitors are used in the second or third trimester.** Similar effects are to be expected with the use of angiotensin II receptor blockers. Therefore these agents should be avoided once pregnancy is established (see Chapter 8).

The use of atenolol during the first and second trimesters has been associated with significantly reduced fetal growth along with decreased placental growth and weight. On the other hand, no such effects on fetal or placental growth have been reported with other β-blockers—such as metoprolol, pindolol, and oxprenolol—but data on the use of these agents in early pregnancy are very limited.

Prospective trials that have examined the effect of either methyldopa or labetalol in women with mild chronic hypertension revealed no adverse maternal or fetal outcomes with the use of these medications. In a large and unique trial in which methyldopa or labetalol was started between 6 and 13 weeks' gestation in patients with chronic hypertension, none of the exposed newborns had major congenital anomalies.

Clinical experience is extensive with the use of thiazide diuretics during pregnancy. The available data suggest that treatment with diuretics in the first trimester and throughout gestation is not associated with an increased risk for major fetal anomalies or adverse fetal-neonatal events. Information is sparse regarding the use of calcium channel blockers in women with mild chronic hypertension; however, **the available evidence suggests that the use of calcium channel blockers, particularly nifedipine, in the first trimester was not associated with increased rates of major birth defects.** The effects of nifedipine on fetal-neonatal outcome were evaluated in a prospective randomized trial of 283 women with mild to moderate hypertension in pregnancy in which 47% of the participants had chronic hypertension. Sixty-six of these women were enrolled between 12 and 20 weeks' gestation. In this study, the use of slow-release nifedipine was not associated with adverse fetal-neonatal outcomes.

The long-term effects on children of mothers exposed to antihypertensive drugs during pregnancy are lacking except for limited information concerning the use of methyldopa and nifedipine. A follow-up study of infants after 7.5 years showed no long-term adverse effects on development among those exposed to methyldopa in utero compared with infants not exposed to such treatment. A similar study that examined the effects of slow-release nifedipine after 1.5 years of follow-up demonstrated no adverse effects on development.

Recommended Management of Chronic Hypertension in Pregnancy

The primary objective in the management of pregnancies complicated by chronic hypertension is to reduce maternal risks and achieve optimal perinatal survival. This objective can be achieved by formulating a rational approach that includes preconception evaluation and counseling, early antenatal care, frequent antepartum visits to monitor both maternal and fetal well-being, timely delivery with intensive intrapartum monitoring, and proper postpartum management.

Evaluation and Classification

Women with chronic hypertension should ideally be counseled before pregnancy, when extensive evaluation and complete workup can be undertaken. Assessment of the etiology and severity of the hypertension, as well as the coexistence of other medical illnesses, and ruling out the presence of target-organ damage resulting from long-standing hypertension can be accomplished. An in-depth history should delineate in particular the duration of hypertension, the use of antihypertensive medications, their type, and the response to these medications. Also, attention should be given to the presence of cardiac or renal disease, diabetes mellitus, thyroid disease, and a history of cerebrovascular accident or CHF. A detailed obstetric history should include maternal and neonatal outcomes of previous pregnancies and should stress any history of the development of placental abruption, superimposed PE, preterm delivery, FGR, intrauterine fetal death, and neonatal morbidity and mortality.

Laboratory evaluation is obtained to assess the function of different organ systems likely to be affected by chronic hypertension and as a baseline for future assessments. **For all patients, these should include urinalysis, urine culture and sensitivity, 24-hour urine evaluations for protein, electrolytes, CBC, and screening for diabetes.**

Women with long-standing hypertension for several years, particularly those with a history of poor compliance or poor BP control, should be evaluated for target-organ damage that includes left ventricular hypertrophy, retinopathy, and renal injury. These women should undergo an ECG examination and echocardiography if the ECG is abnormal, ophthalmologic evaluation, and creatinine clearance.

Selectively, certain tests should be obtained to identify secondary causes of hypertension such as pheochromocytoma, primary hyperaldosteronism, or renal artery stenosis. These conditions require selective biochemical testing and are amenable to diagnosis with either CT or MRI. Pheochromocytoma should be suspected in women with paroxysmal severe hypertension, hyperglycemia, and sweating (see Chapter 43). Primary aldosteronism is extremely rare in pregnancy and should be considered in women with severe hypertension and marked hypokalemia (see Chapter 43). Based on this evaluation, the patient is then classified as having low-risk or high-risk chronic hypertension and is managed accordingly (Fig. 31-18).

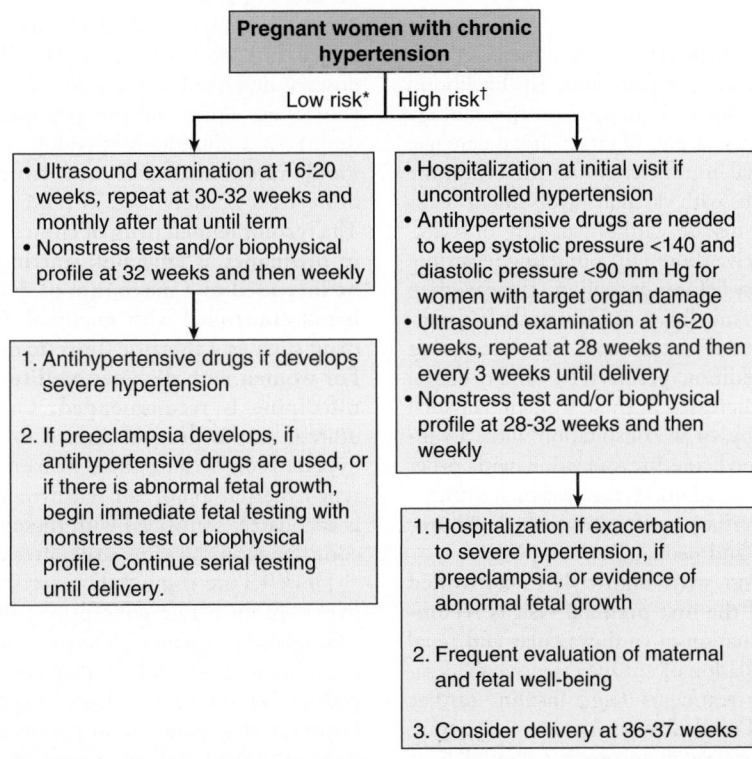

FIG 31-18 Antepartum management of chronic hypertension. *Low risk* (*) includes those with controlled hypertension on medication and those not receiving antihypertensive drugs; high risk (†) includes those with uncontrolled hypertension, left ventricular dysfunction, and/or coexisting medical diseases (renal, diabetes mellitus, systemic lupus erythematosus). (From Sibai BM. Chronic hypertension in pregnancy. *Obstet Gynecol.* 2002;100:369.)

LOW-RISK HYPERTENSION

Women with low-risk chronic hypertension without super-imposed PE usually have a pregnancy outcome similar to that of the general obstetric population. In addition, discontinuation of antihypertensive therapy early in pregnancy does not affect the rate of PE, abruptio placentae, or preterm delivery in these women. Many clinicians choose to discontinue antihypertensive treatment at the first prenatal visit because most of these women will experience a good pregnancy outcome without such therapy. Although many of these women will not require subsequent pharmacologic therapy, careful management is still essential (see Fig. 31-16). At the time of initial and subsequent visits, women are educated about nutritional requirements, weight gain, and sodium intake (maximum of 2.4 g/day). They are also counseled that consumption of alcohol and smoking during pregnancy can aggravate maternal hypertension and are associated with adverse effects on the fetus such as FGR and abruptio placentae. During each subsequent visit, they are observed closely for early signs of PE and FGR.

Fetal evaluation should include an ultrasound examination at 16 to 20 weeks' gestation, to be repeated at 30 to 32 weeks and monthly thereafter until term. **Antihypertensive treatment with either nifedipine or labetalol is initiated if the patient develops severe hypertension before term. The development of severe hypertension, PE, or abnormal fetal growth requires immediate fetal testing with NST or BPP. Women who develop severe hypertension require hospitalization, and those with documented FGR by ultrasound examination require intensive surveillance and often delivery.** If superimposed PE is diagnosed at or beyond 37 weeks, delivery is undertaken as well. In the absence of these complications, the pregnancy may be continued until 40 weeks' gestation.

HIGH-RISK HYPERTENSION

Women with high-risk chronic hypertension are at increased risk for adverse maternal and perinatal complications. The likelihood and impact of these complications will depend on the etiology of the hypertension as well as the degree of target-organ damage. Women with significant renal insufficiency (serum creatinine >1.4 mg/dL), diabetes mellitus with vascular involvement (class R/F), severe collagen vascular disease, cardiomyopathy, or coarctation of the aorta should receive thorough counseling regarding the adverse effects of pregnancy before conception. These women should be advised that pregnancy may exacerbate their condition, with the potential for CHF, acute renal failure requiring dialysis, and even death. In addition, perinatal loss and neonatal complications are markedly increased in these women. All such women should be managed by, or in consultation with, a subspecialist in maternal-fetal medicine in association with other medical specialists as needed. In addition, these women must be observed and delivered at a tertiary care center with the appropriate resources for maternal and neonatal care.

Hospitalization of women with high-risk uncontrolled hypertension at the time of the first prenatal visit is recommended. This facilitates evaluation of cardiovascular and renal status and also facilitates regulation of antihypertensive medications and other prescribed treatments (e.g., insulin, cardiac drugs, thyroid medications) if needed. Women who receive ACE inhibitors or angiotensin II receptor antagonists should have these medications discontinued under close observation. **Antihypertensive therapy with one or more of the drugs listed in Table 31-20 is subsequently used in all women with systolic**

TABLE 31-20	DRUGS USED TO TREAT HYPERTENSION IN PREGNANCY		
DRUG	**STARTING DOSE**	**MAXIMUM DOSE**	**COMMENTS**
Acute Treatment of Severe Hypertension			
Hydralazine	5-10 mg IV q20 min	20 mg*	Avoid in cases of tachycardia and persistent headaches
Labetalol	20-40 mg IV q10-15 min	220 mg*	Avoid in women with asthma or congestive heart failure
Nifedipine	10-20 mg oral q30 min	50 mg*	Avoid in case of tachycardia and palpitations
Long-Term Treatment of Hypertension			
Methyldopa	250 mg bid	4 g/day	
Labetalol	100 mg bid	2400 mg/day	
Nifedipine	10 mg bid	120 mg/day	
Thiazide diuretic	12.5 mg bid	50 mg/day	

*If desired blood pressure levels are not achieved, switch to another drug.

BP of 160 mm Hg or more or diastolic BP of 110 mm Hg or more. In women without target-organ damage, the aim of antihypertensive therapy is to keep systolic BP between 140 and 150 mm Hg and diastolic BP between 90 and 100 mm Hg. In addition, antihypertensive therapy is indicated in women with mild hypertension plus target-organ damage because of the short-term maternal benefits from lowering BP in such women. In these women, maintaining systolic BP below 140 mm Hg and diastolic BP below 90 mm Hg is advised. In some women, BP may be difficult to control initially, which demands the use of IV therapy with hydralazine or labetalol or oral short-acting nifedipine with doses as described in Table 31-20. For maintenance therapy, the choices are either oral methyldopa, labetalol, slow-release nifedipine, or a diuretic. Methyldopa remains the drug most commonly recommended to treat hypertension during pregnancy; however, it is rarely used in nonpregnant hypertensive women. **The recommended drug of choice for control of hypertension in pregnancy is labetalol, starting at 100 mg twice daily to be increased to a maximum of 2400 mg/day. If maternal BP is not controlled with maximal doses of labetalol, a second drug such as a thiazide diuretic or nifedipine may be added. For women with diabetes mellitus and vascular disease, oral nifedipine is recommended.** Oral nifedipine or a thiazide diuretic is the drug of choice for young black women with hypertension because these women often manifest a low-renin-type hypertension or salt-sensitive hypertension. If maternal BP is adequately controlled with these medications, the patient can continue with the same drug after delivery.

Diuretics are commonly prescribed in women with essential hypertension before conception, although the use of diuretics throughout pregnancy is controversial. Of concern, women who use diuretics from early in pregnancy do not have an increase in plasma volume to the degree expected in normal pregnancy. However, this reduction in plasma volume has not been shown to be associated with an adverse effect on fetal outcome. Therefore it is appropriate to start diuretics as a single agent during pregnancy or to use them in combination with other agents, particularly in women with excessive salt retention. However, diuretics should be discontinued immediately if superimposed PE develops or with evidence of suspected FGR because of the potential for reduced uteroplacental blood flow secondary to reduced plasma volume in women with these complications.

Early and frequent prenatal visits are the key for successful pregnancy outcome in women with high-risk chronic hypertension. These women need close observation throughout pregnancy and may require serial evaluation of 24-hour urine protein excretion and a CBC with a metabolic profile at least once every trimester. Further laboratory testing can be performed depending on the clinical progress of the pregnancy. During each visit, the woman should be advised about the adverse effects of smoking and alcohol abuse, and she should receive nutritional advice regarding diet and salt intake.

Fetal evaluation should include an ultrasound examination at 16 to 20 weeks' gestation, to be repeated at 28 weeks and subsequently every 3 weeks until delivery. NST or BPP testing is usually started at 28 to 32 weeks and then repeated weekly. **The development of uncontrolled severe hypertension or PE requires maternal hospitalization for more frequent evaluation of maternal and fetal well-being. The development of FGR also requires intensive surveillance, and the development of these complications at or beyond 34 weeks' gestation should be considered an indication for delivery.** In all other women, delivery should be considered at 36 to 37 weeks' gestation after documentation of fetal lung maturity.

Postpartum Management

Women with high-risk chronic hypertension are at risk for postpartum complications such as pulmonary edema, hypertensive encephalopathy, and renal failure. These risks are particularly increased in women with target-organ involvement, superimposed PE, or placental abruption. **In these patients, BP must be closely controlled for at least 24 hours after delivery.** IV labetalol or hydralazine can be used as needed, and diuretics may be appropriate in women with circulatory congestion and pulmonary edema. This therapy is usually required in those who develop exaggerated and sustained severe hypertension in the first week postpartum.

Oral therapy may be needed to control BP after delivery. In some women, it is often necessary to switch to a new agent such as an ACE inhibitor, particularly in those with pregestational diabetes mellitus and those with cardiomyopathy. Some patients may wish to breastfeed their infant, and all antihypertensive drugs are found in the breast milk, although the milk-to-plasma ratio of these drugs varies. Additionally, the long-term effect of maternal antihypertensive drugs on breastfeeding infants has not been specifically studied. Milk concentrations of methyldopa appear to be low and are considered to be safe. The β-blocking agents (atenolol and metoprolol) are concentrated in breast milk, whereas labetalol and propranolol have low concentrations. Concentrations of diuretic agents in breast milk are low; however, they may induce a decrease in milk production.

Little information is available about the transfer of calcium channel blockers to breast milk, but no side effects are apparent. ACE inhibitors and angiotensin II receptor antagonists should be avoided because of their effects on neonatal renal function, even though their concentrations appear to be low in breast milk (see Chapter 24).

Finally, in breastfeeding women, the use of methyldopa as a first-line oral therapy is a reasonable choice. If methyldopa is contraindicated, labetalol may be used.

HYPERTENSIVE EMERGENCIES IN CHRONIC HYPERTENSION

On rare occasions, pregnant women may present with life-threatening clinical conditions that require immediate control of BP, such as hypertensive encephalopathy, acute left ventricular failure, acute aortic dissection, or increased circulating catecholamines (pheochromocytoma, clonidine withdrawal, cocaine ingestion). Patients at highest risk for these complications include those using multiple drugs to control their hypertension and also women with underlying cardiac or chronic glomerular renal disease, superimposed PE in the second trimester, and placental abruption complicated by DIC. Although a diastolic BP of 115 mm Hg or greater is usually considered a hypertensive emergency, this level is actually arbitrary, and the rate of change of BP may be more important than its absolute level. The association of elevated BP with evidence of new or progressive end-organ damage determines the seriousness of the clinical situation.

Hypertensive Encephalopathy

Untreated essential hypertension progresses to a hypertensive crisis in up to 1% to 2% of cases for unknown reasons. **Hypertensive encephalopathy is usually seen in patients with a systolic BP above 220 mm Hg or a diastolic BP above 130 mm Hg.** Patients with an acute onset of hypertension may develop encephalopathy at pressure levels that are generally tolerated by those with chronic hypertension. Normally, cerebral blood flow is about 50 mL/min per 100 g tissue. When the BP falls, cerebral arterioles normally dilate, whereas when BP increases, they constrict to maintain constant cerebral blood flow. This mechanism usually remains operative between 60 and 120 mm Hg diastolic BP. **Hypertensive encephalopathy is currently considered to be a derangement of the autoregulation of cerebral arterioles, which occurs when the upper limit of autoregulation is exceeded.** With severe hypertension (130 to 150 mm Hg cerebral perfusion pressure), cerebral blood vessels constrict as much as possible and then reflex cerebral vasodilation occurs. This results in overperfusion, damage to small blood vessels, cerebral edema, and increased intracranial pressure (*breakthrough theory*). Others believe that hypertensive encephalopathy results from an exaggerated vasoconstrictive response of the arterioles that results in cerebral ischemia (*overregulation theory*). Patients who have impaired autoregulation that involves the cerebral arterioles may experience necrotizing arteriolitis, microinfarcts, petechial hemorrhages, multiple small thrombi, or cerebral edema. Typically, hypertensive encephalopathy has a subacute onset over 24 to 72 hours.

During a hypertensive crisis, other evidence for end-organ damage may be present: cardiac, renal, or retinal dysfunction secondary to impaired organ perfusion and loss of autoregulation of blood flow. Ischemia of the retina with flame-shaped retinal hemorrhages, retinal infarcts, or papilledema may occur and can cause decreased visual acuity. Impaired regulation of coronary blood flow and a marked increase in ventricular wall stress may result in angina, myocardial infarction (MI), CHF, malignant ventricular arrhythmia, pulmonary edema, or dissecting aortic aneurysm. Necrosis of the afferent arterioles of the glomerulus results in hemorrhages of the cortex and medulla, fibrinoid necrosis, and proliferative endarteritis that results in elevated serum creatinine (>3 mg/dL), proteinuria, oliguria, hematuria, hyaline or red blood cell casts, and progressive azotemia. Severe hypertension may result in placental abruption with resultant DIC. In addition, high levels of angiotensin II, norepinephrine, and vasopressin accompany ongoing vascular damage. These circulating hormones increase relative efferent arteriolar tone, which results in sodium diuresis and hypovolemia. Because levels of renin and angiotensin II are increased, the aldosterone level is also elevated. The impact of these endocrine changes may be important in maintaining the hypertensive crisis.

Treatment of Hypertensive Encephalopathy

The ultimate goal of therapy is to prevent the occurrence of a hypertensive emergency. Patients at risk for a hypertensive crisis should receive intensive management during labor and for a minimum of 48 hours after delivery. Although pregnancy may complicate the diagnosis, once the life-threatening conditions are recognized, pregnancy should not in any way slow or alter the mode of therapy. **The only reliable clinical criterion to confirm the diagnosis of hypertensive encephalopathy is prompt response of the patient to antihypertensive therapy. The headache and sensorium often clear dramatically, sometimes within 1 to 2 hours after the treatment.** The overall recovery may be somewhat slower in patients with uremia and when symptoms have been present for a prolonged period before the therapy is given. Sustained cerebrovascular deficits should suggest other diagnoses.

Patients with hypertensive encephalopathy or other hypertensive crisis should be hospitalized for bed rest. IV lines should be inserted for fluids and medications. Although the tendency is to restrict sodium intake in patients with a hypertensive emergency, volume contraction from sodium diuresis may be present. A marked drop in diastolic BP with a rise in heart rate on standing from the supine position is evidence of volume contraction. Infusion of normal saline solution during the first 24 to 48 hours to achieve volume expansion should be considered. Saline infusion can help decrease the activity of the renin-angiotensin-aldosterone axis and can result in better BP control. Simultaneous repletion of potassium losses and continuous monitoring of BP, volume status, urinary output, ECG readings, and mental status are mandatory. An intraarterial line provides the most accurate BP information. Laboratory studies include a CBC with differential, reticulocyte count, platelets, and blood chemistries. A urinalysis should be obtained for protein, glucose, blood, cells, casts, and bacteria. Assessment for end-organ damage in the CNS, retina, kidneys, and cardiovascular system should be done periodically. Antepartum patients should have continuous fetal monitoring.

LOWERING BLOOD PRESSURE IN HYPERTENSIVE ENCEPHALOPATHY

Certain risks are associated with an overly rapid or excessive reduction of elevated BP. The aim of therapy is to lower mean BP by no more than 15% to 25%. Small reductions in BP in the first 60 minutes, working toward a diastolic level of 100 to 110 mm Hg, have been recommended. Although cerebral blood flow is maintained constantly over a wide range of BPs, autoregulation has a lower and upper limit. In chronically hypertensive women who have a rightward shift of the cerebral autoregulation curve secondary to medial hypertrophy of the cerebral vasculature, lowering BP too rapidly may produce cerebral ischemia, stroke, or coma. Coronary blood flow, renal perfusion, and uteroplacental blood flow also may deteriorate, resulting in

acute renal failure, MI, fetal distress, or death. Hypertension that proves increasingly difficult to control is an indication to terminate the pregnancy. If the patient's outcome appears to be grave, consideration of perimortem cesarean delivery should be made.

The drug of choice in a hypertensive crisis is sodium nitroprusside. Other agents such as nitroglycerin, nifedipine, trimetaphan, labetalol, and hydralazine can also be used.

SODIUM NITROPRUSSIDE

Sodium nitroprusside causes arterial and venous relaxation by interfering with both influx and the intracellular activation of calcium. It is given as an IV infusion of 0.25 to 3 μg/kg/min. The onset of action is immediate, and its effect may last 3 to 5 minutes after discontinuing the infusion. Hypotension caused by nitroprusside should resolve within a few minutes of stopping the infusion because the drug's half-life is so short. If it does not resolve, other causes for hypotension should be suspected.

The effect of nitroprusside on uterine blood flow is controversial. Nitroprusside is metabolized into thiocyanate, which is excreted in the urine. Cyanide can accumulate if production is increased as a result of large doses (>10 μg/kg/min) or prolonged administration (>48 hours), or if there is renal insufficiency or decreased metabolism in the liver. Signs of toxicity include anorexia, disorientation, headache, fatigue, restlessness, tinnitus, delirium, hallucinations, nausea, vomiting, and metabolic acidosis. When it is infused at less than 2 μg/kg/min, cyanide toxicity is unlikely. At a maximal dose rate of 10 μg/kg/min, infusion should never last more than 10 minutes. Animal experiments and the few reported cases of nitroprusside use in pregnancy have revealed that **thiocyanate toxicity to mother and fetus rarely occur if it is used in a regular pharmacologic dose.** Tachyphylaxis to nitroprusside usually develops before toxicity occurs. Whenever toxicity is suspected, therapy should be initiated with 3% sodium nitrite at a rate not to exceed 5 mL/min up to a total dose of 15 mL. Then, infusion of 12.5 g of sodium thiosulfate in 50 mL of 5% dextrose in water over a 10 minute period should be started.

NITROGLYCERIN

Nitroglycerin is an arterial but mostly venous dilator. It is given as an IV infusion of 5 μg/min that is gradually increased every 3 to 5 minutes to titrate BP up to a maximal dose of 100 mg/min. **It is the drug of choice in PE associated with pulmonary edema and for control of hypertension associated with tracheal manipulation.** Side effects such as headache, tachycardia, and methemoglobinemia may develop. It is contraindicated in hypertensive encephalopathy because it increases cerebral blood flow and intracranial pressure.

KEY POINTS

- Hypertension is the most common medical complication during pregnancy.
- Preeclampsia is a leading cause of maternal mortality and morbidity worldwide.
- The pathophysiologic abnormalities of preeclampsia are numerous, but the etiology is unknown.
- At present, there is no proven method to prevent preeclampsia. However, low-dose aspirin may have a role in certain women.

- The HELLP syndrome may develop in the absence of maternal hypertension and proteinuria.
- Expectant management improves perinatal outcome in a select group of women with severe preeclampsia before 32 weeks' gestation.
- Magnesium sulfate is the preferred agent to prevent or treat eclamptic convulsions.
- Rare cases of eclampsia can develop before 20 weeks' gestation and beyond 48 hours postpartum.
- Antihypertensive agents do not improve pregnancy outcome in women with mild uncomplicated chronic hypertension.
- Labetalol is the drug of choice for the treatment of chronic hypertension during pregnancy; ACE inhibitors should not be used.

REFERENCES

1. American College of Obstetricians and Gynecologists. Task Force on Hypertension in Pregnancy. Hypertension in Pregnancy: Report of the American College of Obstetricians and Gynecologists' Task Force on Hypertension in Pregnancy. *Obstet Gynecol.* 2013;122:1122-1131.
2. Sibai BM. Diagnosis and management of gestational hypertension and preeclampsia. *Obstet Gynecol.* 2003;102:181.
3. Kuklina EV, Ayala C, Callaghan WM. Hypertensive disorders in pregnancy and severe obstetric morbidity in the United States. *Obstet Gynecol.* 2009;113:1299.
4. Hauth JC, Ewell MG, Levine RJ, et al. Pregnancy outcomes in healthy nulliparas who developed hypertension. Calcium for Preeclampsia Prevention Study Group. *Obstet Gynecol.* 2000;95:24.
5. Barton JR, O'Brien JM, Bergauer NK, et al. Mild gestational hypertension remote from term: progression and outcome. *Am J Obstet Gynecol.* 2001;184:979.
6. Saudan P, Brown MA, Buddle ML, Jones M. Does gestational hypertension become pre-eclampsia? *BJOG.* 1998;105:1177.
7. Magee LA, Von Dadelseen P, Bohun CM, et al. Serious perinatal complication of non-proteinuric hypertension: an international, multicenter, retrospective cohort study. *J Obstet Gynecol Can.* 2003;25:372.
8. Valensise H, Vasapelle B, Gagliardi G, Novelli GP. Early and late preeclampsia: two different maternal hemodynamic states in the latent phase of the disease. *Hypertension.* 2008;52:873.
9. Mattar F, Sibai BM. Eclampsia. VIII. Risk factors for maternal morbidity. *Am J Obstet Gynecol.* 2000;182:307.
10. Caritis S, Sibai B, Hauth J, et al. Low-dose aspirin to prevent preeclampsia in women at high risk. *N Engl J Med.* 1998;338:701.
11. Sibai BM, Lindheimer M, Hauth J, et al. Risk factors for preeclampsia, abruptio placentae, and adverse neonatal outcomes in women with chronic hypertension. National Institute of Child Health and Human Development Network of Maternal-Fetal Medicine Units. *N Engl J Med.* 1998;339:667.
12. Sibai BM, Hauth J, Caritis S, et al. Hypertensive disorders in twin versus singleton gestations. National Institute of Child Health and Human Development Network of Maternal-Fetal Medicine Units. *Am J Obstet Gynecol.* 2000;182:938.
13. Hernández-Díaz S, Werler MM, Mitchell AA. Gestational hypertension in pregnancies supported by infertility treatments: role of infertility, treatments, and multiple gestations. *Fertil Steril.* 2007;88:438.
14. Erez O, Vardi IS, Hallak M, et al. Preeclampsia in twin gestations: association with IVF treatments, parity and maternal age. *J Matern Fetal Neonatal Med.* 2006;19:141.
15. Sibai BM. Chronic hypertension in pregnancy. *Obstet Gynecol.* 2002;100:369.
16. Buchbinder A, Sibai BM, Caritis S, et al. Adverse perinatal outcomes are significantly higher in severe gestational hypertension than in mild preeclampsia. *Am J Obstet Gynecol.* 2002;186:66.
17. Steegers EA, von Dadelszen P, Duvekot JJ, Pijnenborg R. Pre-eclampsia. *Lancet.* 2010;376:631.
18. Canadian Hypertensive Disorders of Pregnancy (HDP) Working Group. Diagnosis, evaluation, and management of the hypertensive disorders of Pregnancy. *Pregnancy Hypertens.* 2014;4:105-145.
19. Tranquilli AL, Dekker G, Magee L, et al. The classification, diagnosis and management of the hypertensive disorders of pregnancy: A revised statement from the ISSHP. *Pregnancy Hypertens.* 2014;4(2):97-104.
20. Sibai B, Dekker G, Kupferminc M. Pre-eclampsia. *Lancet.* 2005;365:785.
21. Huppertz B. Placental origins of preeclampsia: challenging the current hypothesis. *Hypertension.* 2008;51:970.
22. Wen SW, Demissie K, Yang Q, Walker MC. Maternal morbidity and obstetric complications in triplet pregnancies and quadruplet and higher-order multiple pregnancies. *Am J Obstet Gynecol.* 2004;191:254.
23. Hnat MD, Sibai BM, Caritis S, et al. Perinatal outcome in women with recurrent preeclampsia compared with women who develop preeclampsia as nulliparas. *Am J Obstet Gynecol.* 2002;186:422.
24. Hernandez-Diaz S, Toh S, Cnattingius S. Risk of pre-eclampsia in first and subsequent pregnancies: prospective cohort study. *BMJ.* 2009;338:b2255.
25. Hjartardottir S, Leifsson B, Geirsson R, Steinthorsdottir V. Recurrence of hypertensive disorder in second pregnancy. *Am J Obstet Gynecol.* 2006;194:916.
26. Brown MA, Mackenzie C, Dunsmuir W, et al. Can we predict recurrence of pre-eclampsia or gestational hypertension? *BJOG.* 2007;114:984.
27. Van Rijn BB, Hoeks LB, Bots ML, et al. Outcomes of subsequent pregnancy after first pregnancy with early-onset preeclampsia. *Am J Obstet Gynecol.* 2006;194:723.
28. Barton JR, Sibai BM. Prediction and prevention of recurrent preeclampsia. *Obstet Gynecol.* 2008;112:359.
29. Diabetes and Pre-eclampsia Intervention Trial (DAPIT) Study Group. Vitamins C and E for prevention of pre-eclampsia in women with type 1 diabetes (DAPIT): a randomized placebo-controlled trial. *Lancet.* 2010;376:259.
30. Sibai BM. Vitamin C and E to prevent pre-eclampsia in diabetic women. *Lancet.* 2010;376:214.
31. Mello G, Parretti E, Marozio L. Thrombophilia is significantly associated with severe preeclampsia: results of a large scale case-controlled study. *Hypertension.* 2005;46:1270.
32. Sibai BM, Stella CL. Diagnosis and management of atypical preeclampsia-eclampsia. *Am J Obstet Gynecol.* 2009;200:481.
33. Holston A, Qian C, Karumanchi A, et al. Circulating angiogenic factors in gestational proteinuria without hypertension. *Am J Obstet Gynecol.* 2009;200:392.e1.
34. Villar A, Abdel-Aleem H, Merialdi M, et al. World Health Organization trial of calcium supplementation among low calcium intake pregnant women. *Am J Obstet Gynecol.* 2006;194:639.
35. Morikawa M, Yamada T, Cho K, et al. Pregnancy outcome of women who developed proteinuria in the absence of hypertension after mid-gestation. *J Perinat Med.* 2008;36:419.
36. Einarsson JI, Sangi-Haghpeykar H, Gardner NO. Sperm exposure and development of preeclampsia. *Am J Obstet Gynecol.* 2004;191:254.
37. Saftlas AF, Levine RJ, Klebanoff MA, et al. Abortion, changed paternity, and the risk of preeclampsia in nulliparous women. *Am J Epidemiol.* 2003;157:1108.
38. Esplin MS, Fausett MB, Fraser A, et al. Paternal and maternal components of the predisposition to preeclampsia. *N Engl J Med.* 2001;344:867.
39. Lie RT, Rasmussen S, Brunborg H, et al. Fetal and maternal contributions to risk of pre-eclampsia: a population based study. *Br Med J.* 1998;316:1343.
40. Wang JX, Knottnerus AM, Schuit G, et al. Surgically obtained sperm and risk of gestational hypertension and pre-eclampsia. *Lancet.* 2002;359:673.
41. Trogstad L, Magnus P, Moffett A, Stoltenberg C. The effect of recurrent miscarriage and infertility on the risk of pre-eclampsia. *BJOG.* 2009;116:108.
42. Catalano PM. Management of obesity in pregnancy. *Obstet Gynecol.* 2007;109:419.
43. Cedergren MI. Maternal morbid obesity and the risk of adverse pregnancy outcome. *Obstet Gynecol.* 2004;103:219.
44. Mbah AK, Kornosky JL, Kristensen S, et al. Super-obesity and risk of early and late pre-eclampsia. *BJOG.* 2010;117:997.
45. Said JM, Higgins JR, Moses EK, et al. Inherited thrombophilia polymorphisms and pregnancy outcomes in nulliparous women. *Obstet Gynecol.* 2010;115:5.
46. Silver RM, Zhao Y, Spong CY, Sibai B, et al. Prothrombin gene G20210A mutation and obstetric complications. *Obstet Gynecol.* 2010;115:14.
47. Myatt L, Webster RP. Vascular biology of preeclampsia. *J Thromb Haemost.* 2009;7:375.
48. Redman CW, Sargent IL. Immunology of pre-eclampsia. *Am J Reprod Immunol.* 2010;63:534.
49. Redman CS, Sargent IL. Placental stress and pre-eclampsia: a revised view. *Placenta.* 2009;30:38.

50. Pijnenborg R, Brosens I. Deep trophoblast invasion and spiral artery remodeling. In: Pijnenborg R, Brosens I, Romero R, eds. *Placental Bed Disorders: Basic Science and Its Translation to Obstetrics.* Cambridge, UK: Cambridge University Press; 2010:97.

51. Kong TY, DeWolf F, Robertson WB, Brosens I. Inadequate maternal vascular response to placentation in pregnancies complicated by preeclampsia and by small-for-gestational age infants. *BJOG.* 1986;93:1049.

52. Frusca T, Morassi L, Pecorell S, et al. Histological features of uteroplacental vessels in normal and hypertensive patients in relation to birthweight. *BJOG.* 1989;96:835.

53. Meekins JW, Pijnenborg R, Hanssens M, et al. A study of placental bed spiral arteries and trophoblast invasion in normal and severe preeclamptic pregnancies. *BJOG.* 1994;101:669.

54. Sibai BM. Discussion. Evidence supporting a role for blockade of the vascular endothelial growth factor system in the pathophysiology of preeclampsia. *Am J Obstet Gynecol.* 2004;190:1547.

55. Maynard SE, Min JY, Merchan J, et al. Excess placental soluble fms-like tyrosine kinase 1 (sFlt1) may contribute to endothelial dysfunction, hypertension, and proteinuria in preeclampsia. *Clin Invest.* 2003;111:649.

56. Levine RJ, Maynard SE, Qian C, et al. Circulating angiogenic factors and the risk of preeclampsia. *N Engl J Med.* 2004;350:672.

57. Thadhani R, Ecker JL, Mutter WP, et al. Insulin resistance and alterations in angiogenesis: additive insults that may lead to preeclampsia. *Hypertension.* 2004;43:988.

58. Levine RJ, Thadhani R, Qian C, et al. Urinary placental growth factor and risk of preeclampsia. *JAMA.* 2005;293:77.

59. Buhimschi CS, Norwitz ER, Funai E, et al. Urinary angiogenic factors cluster hypertensive disorders identify women with severe preeclampsia. *Am J Obstet Gynecol.* 2005;192:734.

60. Sibai BM. Preeclampsia: an inflammatory syndrome? *Am J Obstet Gynecol.* 2004;191:1061.

61. Savvidou MD, Hingorani AD, Tsikas D, et al. Endothelial dysfunction and raised plasma concentrations of asymmetric dimethylarginine in pregnant women who subsequently develop pre-eclampsia. *Lancet.* 2003; 361:1151.

62. Speer PD, Powers RW, Frank MP, et al. Elevated asymmetric dimethylarginine concentrations precede clinical preeclampsia, but not pregnancies with small-for-gestational-age infants. *Am J Obstet Gynecol.* 2008;198:112. e1.

63. Wang Y, Gu Y, Zhang Y, Lewis DF. Evidence of endothelial dysfunction in preeclampsia: decreased endothelial nitric oxide synthase expression is associated with increased cell permeability in endothelial cells from preeclampsia. *Am J Obstet Gynecol.* 2004;190:817.

64. Nilsson E, Salonen RH, Cnattingius S, Lichtenstein P. The importance of genetic and environmental effects for pre-eclampsia and gestational hypertension: a family study. *BJOG.* 2004;111:200.

65. Mutze S, Rudnik-Schoneborn S, Zerres K, Rath W. Genes and the preeclampsia syndrome. *J Perinat Med.* 2008;36:38.

66. Oudejans CB, van Dijk M. Placental gene expression and preeclampsia. *Placenta.* 2008;29:78.

67. Nafee TM, Farrell WE, Carroll WD, et al. Epigenetic control of fetal gene expression. *BJOG.* 2008;115:158.

68. Paarlberg KM, deJong CL, Van Geijn HP, et al. Vasoactive mediators in pregnancy-induced hypertensive disorders: a longitudinal study. *Am J Obstet Gynecol.* 1998;179:1559.

69. Mills JL, DerSimonian R, Raymond E, et al. Prostacyclin and thromboxane changes predating clinical onset of preeclampsia: a multicenter prospective study. *JAMA.* 1999;282:356.

70. Khankin EV, Royle C, Karumanchi A. Placental vasculature in health and disease. *Semin Thromb Hemost.* 2010;36:309.

71. Moretti M, Phillips M, Abouzeid A, et al. Increased breath markers of oxidative stress in normal pregnancy and in preeclampsia. *Am J Obstet Gynecol.* 2004;190:1184.

72. Villar MA, Sibai BM. Clinical significance of elevated mean arterial blood in second trimester and threshold increase in systolic or diastolic pressure during third trimester. *Am J Obstet Gynecol.* 1989;60:419.

73. North RA, Taylor RS, Schellenberg JC. Evaluation of a definition of preeclampsia. *BJOG.* 1999;106:767.

74. Levine RJ, Ewell MG, Hauth JC, et al. Should the definition of preeclampsia include a rise in diastolic blood pressure of ≥15 mmHg to a level <90 mmHg in association with proteinuria? *Am J Obstet Gynecol.* 2000;183:787.

75. Ohkuchi A, Iwasaki R, Ojima T, et al. Increase in systolic blood pressure of > or =30 mm Hg and/or diastolic blood pressure of > or =15 mm Hg during pregnancy: is it pathologic? *Hypertens Pregnancy.* 2003;22:275.

76. Wikstrom A-K, Wikstrom J, Larsson A, Olovsson M. Random albumin/creatinine ratio for quantitation of proteinuria in manifest pre-eclampsia. *BJOG.* 2006;113:930.

77. Gangaram R, Naicker M, Moodley J. Accuracy of the spot urinary microalbumin:creatinine ratio and visual dipsticks in hypertensive pregnant women. *Eur J Obstet Gynecol Reprod Biol.* 2009;144:146.

78. Lindheimer MD, Kanter D. Interpreting abnormal proteinuria in pregnancy: the need for a more pathophysiological approach. *Obstet Gynecol.* 2010;115:365.

79. Morris RK, Riley RD, Doug M, Deeks JJ, Kilby MD. Diagnostic accuracy of spot urinary protein and albumin to creatinine ratios for detection of significant proteinuria or adverse pregnancy outcome in suspected preeclampsia: systemic review and meta-analysis. *BMJ.* 2012;345:e4342.

80. De Paco C, Kametas N, Renceret G, Strobl I, Nicolaides KH. Maternal cardiac output between 11 and 13 weeks of gestation in the prediction of preeclampsia and small for gestational age. *Obstet Gynecol.* 2008; 111:292.

81. Cnossen JS, Vollebregt KC, de Vrieze N, et al. Accuracy of mean arterial pressure and blood pressure measurements in predicting preeclampsia: systematic review. *BMJ.* 2008;336:1117.

82. Cnossen JS, Morris RK, ter Riet G, et al. Use of uterine artery Doppler ultrasonography to predict pre-eclampsia and intrauterine growth restriction: a systemic review and bivariable meta-analysis. *CMAJ.* 2008;178:701.

83. Chaiworapongsa T, Romero R, Kusanovic JP, et al. Plasma soluble endoglin concentration in pre-eclampsia associated with an increased impedance to flow in the maternal and fetal circulations. *Ultrasound Obstet Gynecol.* 2010;35:155.

84. Espinoza J, Romero R, Nien JK, et al. Identification of patients at risk for early onset and/or severe preeclampsia with the use of uterine artery Doppler velocimetry and placental growth factor (published erratum appears in Am J Obstet Gynecol 2007;196:614). *Am J Obstet Gynecol.* 2007;196:326.e1.

85. Lapaire O, Shennan A, Stepan H. The preeclampsia biomarker soluble fms-like tyrosine kinase-1 and placental growth factor: current knowledge, clinical implications and future application. *Eur J Obstet Gynaecol Reprod Biol.* 2010;151:122.

86. Rana S, Karumanchi A, Levine FJ, et al. Sequential changes in antiangiogenic factors in early pregnancy and risk of developing preeclampsia. *Hypertension.* 2007;50:137.

87. Conde-Agudelo A, Romero R, Lindheimer MD. Tests to predict preeclampsia. In: Lindheimer MD, Roberts JM, Cunningham FG, eds. *Chesley's Hypertensive Disorders in Pregnancy.* Amsterdam: Academic Press, Elsevier; 2009:189.

88. Papageorghiou AT, Leslie K. Uterine artery Doppler in the prediction of adverse pregnancy outcome. *Curr Opin Obstet Gynecol.* 2007;19:103.

89. Kane SC, Da Silva Costa F, Brennecke SP. New directions in the prediction of pre-eclampsia. *Aust N Z J Obstet Gynaecol.* 2014;54:101.

90. Poon LC, Nicolaides KH. First-trimester maternal factors and biomarker screening for preeclampsia. *Prenat Diagn.* 2014;34:618.

91. Giguère Y1, Massé J, Thériault S, et al. Screening for pre-eclampsia early in pregnancy: performance of a multivariable model combining clinical characteristics and biochemical markers. *BJOG.* 2015;122:402.

92. Sibai BM. First trimester screening with combined maternal clinical factors, biophysical and biomarkers to predict preterm preeclampsia and hypertensive disorders: are they ready for clinical use? *BJOG.* 2015;122: 282-283.

93. Sibai BM. Therapy: Low-dose aspirin to reduce the risk of pre-eclampsia? *Nat Rev Endocrinol.* 2015;11(1):6-8.

94. Henderson JT, O'Connor E, Whitlock EP. Low-dose aspirin for prevention of morbidity and mortality from preeclampsia. *Ann Intern Med.* 2014;161:613-614.

95. Martinelli I, Ruggenenti P, Cetin I. Heparin in pregnant women with previous placenta-mediated pregnancy complications: a prospective, randomized, multicenter, controlled clinical trial. *Blood.* 2012;119: 3269-3275.

96. Rodger MA, Langlois NJ, de Vries JI, et al. Low-molecular-weight heparin for prevention of placenta-mediated pregnancy complications: protocol for a systematic review and individual patient data meta-analysis (AFFIRM). *Syst Rev.* 2014;3:69.

97. Rodger MA, Carrier M, Le Gal G, et al. Meta-analysis of low-molecular-weight heparin to prevent recurrent placenta-mediated pregnancy complications. *Blood.* 2014;123:822-828.

98. Rumbold AR, Cowther CA, Haslam RR, et al. Vitamins C and E and the risks of pre-eclampsia and perinatal complications. *N Engl J Med.* 2006; 354:1796.

99. Poston L, Briley AL, Seed PT, et al. Vitamin C and E in pregnant women at risk for pre-eclampsia (VIP trial): randomised placebo-controlled trial. *Lancet*. 2006;367:1145.

100. Spinnato JA, Freire S, Pinto E, Silva JL, et al. Antioxidant therapy to prevent pre-eclampsia: a randomised controlled trial. *Obstet Gynecol*. 2007;110:1311.

101. Villar J, Purwar M, Meraldi M, et al. World Health Organization multicenter randomised trial of supplementation with vitamins C and E among pregnant women at high-risk for pre-eclampsia in populations of low nutritional status from developing countries. *BJOG*. 2009;116:780.

102. Roberts JM, Myatt L, Spong CS, et al. Vitamins C and E to prevent complications of pregnancy-associated hypertension. *N Engl J Med*. 2010;362:1282.

103. Xu H, Perez-Cuevas R, Xiong X, et al. An international trial of antioxidants in the prevention of pre-eclampsia (INTAPP). *Am J Obstet Gynecol*. 2010;202:239.e1.

104. Sibai BM. Diagnosis, controversies, and management of the syndrome of hemolysis, elevated liver enzymes, and low platelets. *Obstet Gynecol*. 2004;103:981.

105. Woudstra DM, Chandra S, Hofmeyr GJ, Doswell T. Corticosteroids for HELLP (hemolysis, elevated liver enzymes, low platelets) syndrome in pregnancy. *Cochrane Database Syst Rev*. 2010;(9):CD008148.

106. Martin JN, Reinhart B, May WL, et al. The spectrum of severe preeclampsia: comparative analysis by HELLP syndrome classification. *Am J Obstet Gynecol*. 1999;108:1373.

107. Sibai BM, Ramadan MK, Usta I, et al. Maternal morbidity and mortality in 442 pregnancies with hemolysis, elevated liver enzymes, and low platelets (HELLP syndrome). *Am J Obstet Gynecol*. 1993;169:1000.

108. Weinstein L. Preeclampsia/eclampsia with hemolysis, elevated liver enzymes and thrombocytopenia. *Obstet Gynecol*. 1985;66:657.

109. Rath W, Loos W, Kuhn W, Graeff H. The importance of early laboratory screening methods for maternal and fetal outcome in cases of HELLP syndrome. *Eur J Obstet Gynecol Reprod Biol*. 1990;36:43.

110. Sibai BM, Ramadan MK. Acute renal failure in pregnancies complicated by hemolysis, elevated liver enzymes, and low platelets. *Am J Obstet Gynecol*. 1993;168:1682.

111. Sullivan CA, Magann EF, Perry KG, et al. The recurrence risk of the syndrome of hemolysis, elevated liver enzymes, and low platelets (HELLP) in subsequent gestations. *Am J Obstet Gynecol*. 1994;171:940.

112. Van Pampus MG, Wolf H, Mayruhu G, et al. Long-term follow up in patients with a history of (H)ELLP syndrome. *Hypertens Pregnancy*. 2001;20:15.

113. Chames MC, Haddad B, Barton JR, et al. Subsequent pregnancy outcome in women with a history of HELLP syndrome at < or =28 weeks of gestation. *Am J Obstet Gynecol*. 2003;188:1504.

114. Douglas KA, Redman CW. Eclampsia in the United Kingdom. *BMJ*. 1994;309:1395.

115. Katz VL, Farmer R, Kuller J. Preeclampsia into eclampsia: toward a new paradigm. *Am J Obstet Gynecol*. 2000;182:1389.

116. Chames MC, Livingston JC, Ivester TS, et al. Late postpartum eclampsia: a preventable disease? *Am J Obstet Gynecol*. 2002;186:1174.

117. Tuffnell DJ, Jankowicz D, Lindow SW, et al. Outcomes of severe pre-eclampsia/eclampsia in Yorkshire 1999/2003. *BJOG*. 2005;112:875.

118. Knight M. UKOSS. Eclampsia in the United Kingdom 2005. *BJOG*. 2007;114:1072.

119. Chesley LC. History. In: Chesley LC, ed. *Hypertensive Disorders in Pregnancy*. 2nd ed. New York: Appleton-Century-Crofts; 1978:17.

120. López-Llera M, Horta JLH. Pregnancy after eclampsia. *Am J Obstet Gynecol*. 1974;119:193.

121. Adelusi B, Ojengbede OA. Reproductive performance after eclampsia. *Int J Gynecol Obstet*. 1986;24:183.

122. Sibai BM, Sarinoglu C, Mercer BM. Eclampsia VII: pregnancy outcome after eclampsia and long-term prognosis. *Am J Obstet Gynecol*. 1992;166:1757.

123. McCowan LM, Buist RG, North RA, Gamble G. Perinatal morbidity in chronic hypertension. *BJOG*. 1996;103:123.

124. Rey E, Couturier A. The prognosis of pregnancy in women with chronic hypertension. *Am J Obstet Gynecol*. 1994;171:410.

125. Chappell LC, Enye S, Seed P, Driley AL, et al. Adverse perinatal outcomes and risk factors for preeclampsia in women with chronic hypertension: a prospective study. *Hypertension*. 2008;51:1002.

126. Giannubilo SR, Dell Uomo B, Tranquilli AL. Perinatal outcomes, blood pressure patterns and risk assessment of superimposed preeclampsia in mild chronic hypertensive pregnancy. *Eur J Obstet Gynecol Reprod Biol*. 2006;126:63.

127. Sibai BM, Koch M, Freire S, et al. The impact of a history of previous preeclampsia on the risk of superimposed preeclampsia and adverse pregnancy outcome in patients with chronic hypertension. *Am J Obstet Gynecol*. 2009;201:752.

Additional references for this chapter are available at ExpertConsult.com.

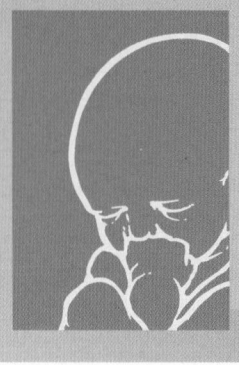

CHAPTER 32

Multiple Gestations

ROGER B. NEWMAN and ELIZABETH RAMSEY UNAL

KEY ABBREVIATIONS

17-Hydroxyprogesterone caproate	17-OH-P	Multiples of the median	MoM
American College of Obstetricians and Gynecologists	ACOG	National Institute of Child Health and Human Development	NICHD
Arterioarterial	AA	Necrotizing enterocolitis	NEC
Arteriovenous	AV	Neonatal intensive care unit	NICU
Body mass index	BMI	North American Fetal Therapy Network	NAFTNet
Deepest vertical pocket	DVP	Peak systolic velocity	PSV
Disseminated intravascular coagulation	DIC	Preterm birth	PTB
Dizygotic	DZ	Preterm premature rupture of the membranes	PPROM
Estimated fetal weight	EFW	Radiofrequency ablation	RFA
Fetal fibronectin	fFN	Respiratory distress syndrome	RDS
Follicle-stimulating hormone	FSH	Retinopathy of prematurity	ROP
Institute of Medicine	IOM	Selective termination	ST
Intrauterine fetal death	IUFD	Society for Maternal-Fetal Medicine	SMFM
Intrauterine growth restriction	IUGR	Transvaginal cervical length	TVCL
In vitro fertilization	IVF	Twin anemia-polycythemia sequence	TAPS
Low birthweight	LBW	Twin-twin transfusion syndrome	TTTS
Magnetic resonance imaging	MRI	Twin reversed arterial perfusion	TRAP
Middle cerebral artery	MCA	Very low birthweight	VLBW
Monochorionic	MC		
Multifetal pregnancy reduction	MPR		

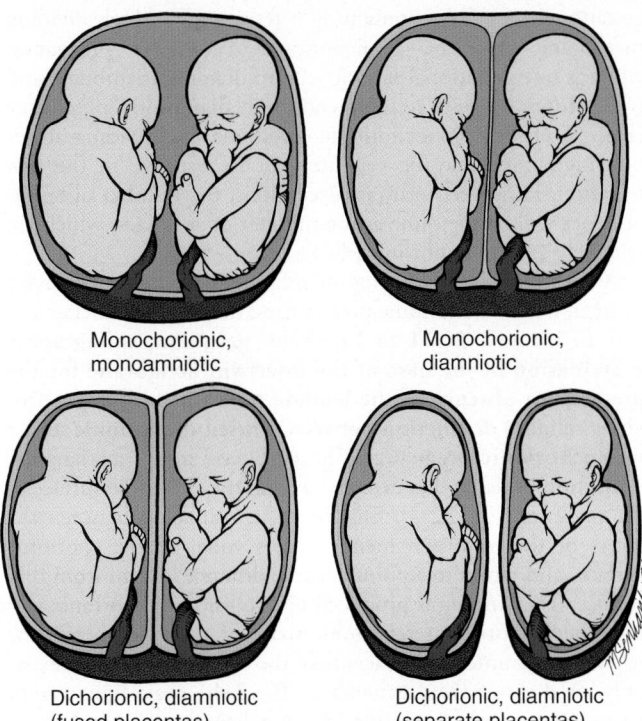

Monochorionic,
monoamniotic

Monochorionic,
diamniotic

Dichorionic, diamniotic
(fused placentas)

Dichorionic, diamniotic
(separate placentas)

FIG 32-1 Placentation in twin pregnancies.

TABLE 32-1	DETERMINATION OF MONOZYGOTIC TWIN PLACENTATION	
TIMING OF CLEAVAGE OF FERTILIZED OVUM	**RESULTING PLACENTATION**	**PERCENTAGE OF MONOZYGOTIC TWINS**
<72 hours	Diamniotic dichorionic	25-30
Days 4-7	Diamniotic monochorionic	70-75
Days 8-12	Monoamniotic monochorionic	1-2
≥Day 13	Conjoined	Very rare

Thus the type of placentation that develops is determined by the timing of this cleavage (Table 32-1).

MZ twins are at higher risk for adverse outcomes than are DZ twins. Not only do MZ twins have higher rates of anomalies than DZ twins, they also deliver earlier, have a lower birthweight, and have higher rates of intrauterine and neonatal death. However, several studies, including one that used DNA analysis to confirm zygosity, have shown that monochorionicity, rather than monozygosity per se, is the determining factor.

DISTRIBUTION AND CAUSES OF DIZYGOTIC VERSUS MONOZYGOTIC TWINNING

Among natural conceptions, DZ twins arise in about 1% to 1.5% of pregnancies, and MZ twins occur in 0.4% of pregnancies. Rates of spontaneous DZ twinning are greatly affected by maternal age, family history, and race. The risk for DZ twinning increases with maternal age and peaks at 37 years of age. Maternal family history, particularly in first-degree relatives, also increases the chance of spontaneous DZ twinning. Paternal family history contributes little or nothing to this risk. Finally, women of African descent have higher rates of DZ twinning than white women, who in turn have higher rates than women of Asian descent. For instance, in Japan, 1 in 250 newborns is a twin, whereas in Nigeria, 1 in 11 babies is a product of a twin gestation.

The causes of DZ twinning are much better understood than the causes of MZ twinning. **DZ twins result from multiple ovulation, which is associated with higher maternal follicle-stimulating hormone (FSH) levels.** FSH levels, and thus rates of DZ twinning, vary with season, geography, maternal age, and body habitus. Increases in DZ twins have been reported in summer months and in locations with more daylight hours and also in taller, heavier, and older mothers. Higher rates of DZ twinning have also been reported following discontinuation of birth control pills, presumably due to a rebound in FSH levels after discontinuation of hormonal suppression.

The causes of MZ twinning are less clear. No naturally occurring animal models for MZ twinning exist except for armadillos, which produce MZ quadruplets or octuplets. It has been proposed that MZ twinning in humans is a teratogenic event. Theories for MZ twinning in humans include fertilization of an "old" ovum with a more fragile zona pellucida or inadequate cytoplasm and with damage to the inner cell mass that leads to two separate points of regrowth and splitting of the fertilized ovum. MZ twinning rates are constant across all variables, with the exception of assisted reproduction. In vitro fertilization

The increase in multiple births during the past 30 years has been well documented, making multiple gestations one of the most common high-risk conditions encountered by obstetricians. The increase in multiples is due to assisted reproductive technology (ART), as well as older maternal age at childbirth, a known risk factor for spontaneous dizygotic twinning. Over the three decades between 1980 and 2009, the twin birth rate rose by 76%, from 18.9 per 1000 to 33.2 per 1000 births. Until 2004, the twin birth rate rose by approximately 2% each year. However, **since 2004, the twin birth rate has remained relatively stable, with a reported rate of 33.1 per 1000 births in 2012.**[1] Likewise, rates of triplets and higher-order multiples increased by more than 400% during the 1980s and 1990s, reaching an all-time high in 1998 at a rate of 193.5 per 100,000. Since then, the rate has generally trended downward. The 2012 rate of 124.4 per 100,000 births is the lowest since 1994.[1]

ZYGOSITY AND CHORIONICITY

Twins can be either monozygotic (MZ) or dizygotic (DZ). *Zygosity* refers to the genetic makeup of the twin pregnancy, and *chorionicity* indicates the pregnancy's placental composition (Fig. 32-1). **Chorionicity is determined by the mechanism of twinning and, in MZ twins, by the timing of embryo division. Early determination of chorionicity is vital because it is a major factor in determining obstetric risks, management, and outcomes.** Because they result from the fertilization of two different ova by two separate sperm, DZ twins always develop dichorionic diamniotic placentation because each blastocyst generates its own chorionic and amniotic sacs. An MZ twin pregnancy is created by the fertilization of one egg by one sperm and subsequent spontaneous cleavage of the fertilized ovum.

(IVF) and ovulation induction have been shown to produce higher rates of MZ twins. Against a spontaneous rate of 0.4% in the general population, studies have reported rates of MZ twinning more than tenfold higher in pregnancies conceived by assisted fertility. One theory to explain these increased rates of MZ twinning is that injury to the zona pellucida may be responsible for the increased tendency toward iatrogenic zygote splitting.

DIAGNOSIS OF MULTIPLE GESTATIONS

Prenatal ultrasound is invaluable to the early diagnosis of a multiple gestation. Before the advent of routine prenatal ultrasound, many twins were not diagnosed until late in gestation or at delivery. **Using transvaginal ultrasound, separate gestational sacs with individual yolk sacs can be identified as early as 5 weeks from the first day of the last menstrual period, and embryos with cardiac activity can usually be seen by 6 weeks.** Retromembranous collections of blood or fluid or a prominent fetal yolk sac should not be confused with a twin gestation. Another entity that could be confused with a multiple gestation would be a singleton pregnancy with a separate pseudosac in a bicornuate or didelphic uterus. The sonographer must be compulsive in examining the entire uterine cavity in order to avoid underdiagnosing or overdiagnosing a multiple gestation.

Determination of Chorionicity

Accurate determination of chorionicity and amnionicity early in pregnancy is vital to optimal obstetric care. A 2010 editorial argued that "there is no diagnosis of twins" but rather any twin gestation must be further classified at diagnosis as either monochorionic or dichorionic.[2] **Knowledge of chorionicity is essential in counseling patients on obstetric and neonatal risks because chorionicity is a major determinant of pregnancy outcome. Chorionicity is also crucial in making a surveillance and management plan because monochorionic twin gestations require closer surveillance for complications unique to monochorionic placentation, such as twin-twin transfusion syndrome (TTTS).**

Determination of chorionicity is easiest and most reliable when assessed in the first trimester. Between 6 and 10 weeks, counting the number of gestational sacs and evaluating the thickness of the dividing membrane is the most reliable method of determining chorionicity (Table 32-2). Two separate

TABLE 32-2	DETERMINATION OF CHORIONICITY AND AMNIONICITY IN FIRST-TRIMESTER PREGNANCIES		
PLACENTATION	**GESTATIONAL SACS**	**YOLK SACS**	**AMNIOTIC CAVITIES**
Dichorionic diamniotic	2	2	2 (thick dividing membrane)
Monochorionic diamniotic	1	2	2 (thin dividing membrane)
Monochorionic monoamniotic	1	1*	1

*Although this is nearly always true, there have been case reports of two yolk sacs in early pregnancy in twins later confirmed to be monoamniotic.

gestational sacs, each containing a fetus, and a thick dividing membrane represent a dichorionic diamniotic pregnancy, whereas one gestational sac with a thin dividing membrane and two fetuses suggests a monochorionic diamniotic pregnancy (Fig. 32-2). For monochorionic gestations, the dividing amniotic membrane may be very difficult to visualize in the first trimester. However, with rare exceptions, the number of amniotic sacs will be the same as the number of yolk sacs, which are relatively easy to count in early gestation.

After 9 weeks, the dividing membranes become progressively thinner, but in dichorionic pregnancies, they remain thicker and easy to identify. **At 11 to 14 weeks' gestation, sonographic examination of the base of the intertwin membrane for the presence or absence of the lambda, or twin peak, sign provides reliable distinction between a fused dichorionic and a monochorionic pregnancy.** The *twin peak sign* is a triangular projection of tissue that extends beyond the chorionic surface of the placenta (Fig. 32-3). This tissue is insinuated between the layers of the intertwin membrane, is wider at the chorionic surface, and tapers to a point at some distance inward from that surface. This finding is produced by extension of chorionic villi into the potential interchorionic space of the twin membrane where it encounters the placenta of the co-twin; this space exists only in dichorionic pregnancies. The twin peak sign cannot occur in monochorionic placentation because the single continuous chorion does not extend into the potential interamniotic space of the monochorionic diamniotic twin membrane.

After the early second trimester, determination of chorionicity and amnionicity becomes less accurate, and different techniques are used to assess placentation (Fig. 32-4). The sonographic prediction of chorionicity and amnionicity should be systematically approached by determining the number of placentae and the sex of each fetus and then by assessing the membranes that divide the sacs. In our own experience we found that using these criteria, **dichorionicity could be determined with 97.3% sensitivity and 91.7% specificity, and monochorionicity with 91.7% sensitivity and 97.3% specificity, in twin gestations first scanned at 22.6 ± 6.9 weeks.**[3] In some pregnancies with monochorionic diamniotic placentation, the dividing membranes may not be sonographically visualized because they are very thin. In other cases, they may not be seen because severe oligohydramnios causes them to be closely apposed to the fetus in that sac. This results in a "stuck twin" appearance, in which the trapped fetus remains firmly held against the uterine wall despite changes in maternal position. In many cases, a small portion of the dividing membrane can be seen extending from a fetal edge to the uterine wall (Fig. 32-5). Diagnosis of this condition confirms the presence of a monochorionic diamniotic gestation, which should be distinguished from a monoamniotic gestation, in which dividing amniotic membranes are absent. In the latter situation, free movement of both twins—and entanglement of their umbilical cords—can be demonstrated.

Determination of Zygosity

If a twin set is monochorionic, monozygosity can be inferred. If twins are different genders, with very rare anecdotal exceptions, they can be assumed to be DZ. It is estimated that based on these two findings, about 55% of all twins' zygosity can be determined by examination of the babies and placentae. Conversely, 45% of all twins (same-sex dichorionic twins) would need further genetic testing to determine zygosity.

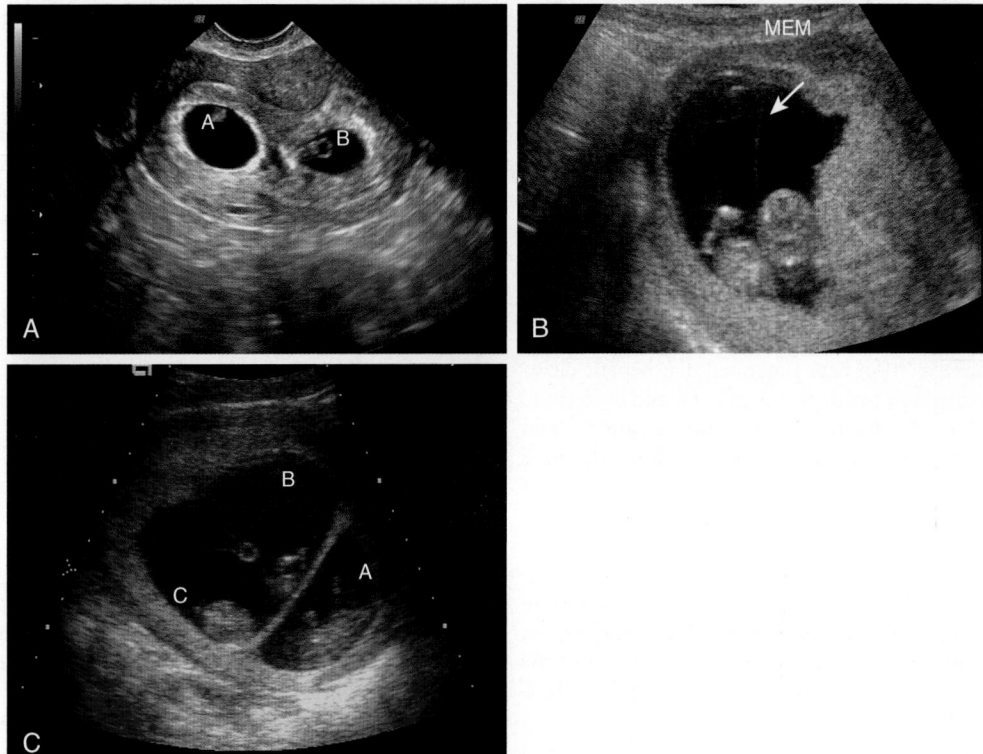

FIG 32-2 **A,** An early first-trimester dichorionic twin gestation. Note the clearly separate gestational sacs, each surrounded by a thick echogenic ring. **B,** A mid first-trimester monochorionic diamniotic twin pregnancy with a very thin, hairlike dividing membrane (MEM, *arrow*). **C,** An early first-trimester image of a dichorionic triamniotic triplet pregnancy. Note that monochorionic triplets B and C are separated by a very thin membrane, whereas triplet A—with its own placenta—is separated from B and C by a thick membrane.

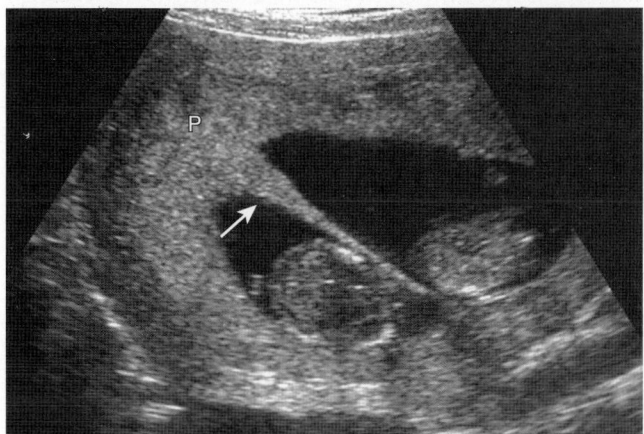

FIG 32-3 Twin peak sign in a dichorionic twin pregnancy. P, fused dichorionic placentae.

MATERNAL AND FETAL RISKS OF MULTIPLE GESTATION

Maternal Adaptation to Multifetal Gestation

The degree of maternal physiologic adaptation to pregnancy (see Chapter 3) **is exaggerated with a multiple gestation.** Levels of maternal progesterone, estriol, and human chorionic somatomammotropin (placental lactogen) are higher in multiple gestations than in singletons. This increase in human placental lactogen (hPL) modifies maternal metabolism and is thought to be the cause of the **increased risk for gestational diabetes** seen in multifetal pregnancies. Increased production of multiple placental proteins such as human chorionic gonadotropin (hCG)

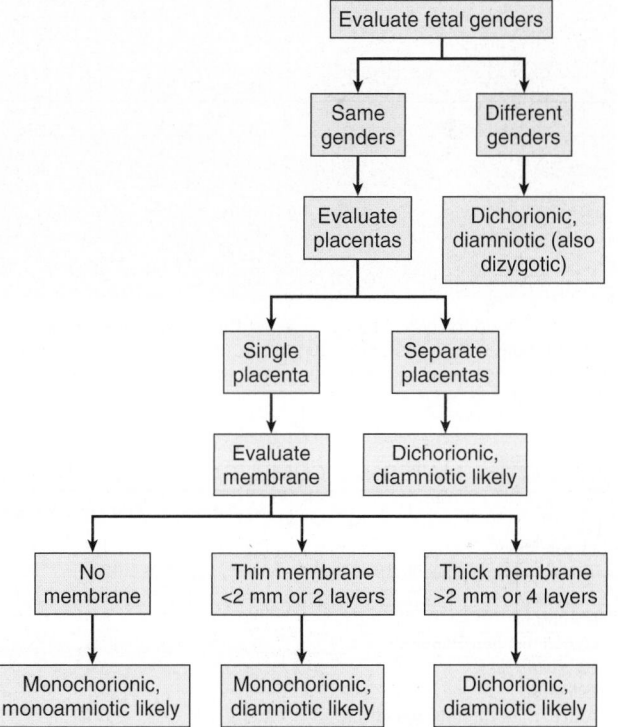

FIG 32-4 Algorithm for determination of chorionicity and amnionicity in the second and third trimesters.

may contribute to clinical conditions such as **a greater risk for hyperemesis,** and it complicates the interpretation of both first- and second-trimester maternal serum screening tests. Cardiovascular adaptations are also greater; both heart rate and stroke volume are increased compared with that of singleton gestations, thus increasing cardiac output. In addition to these cardiac changes, plasma volume expansion and total body water are remarkably increased in twin gestations. Partially as a consequence of increased total body water, colloid oncotic pressure is reduced. Clinical effects of the decreased colloid oncotic pressure are **increased dependent edema and a greater propensity for pulmonary edema.**

Studies using dye excretion have suggested that hepatic clearance capacity is reduced in pregnancy in general and even more so in twin gestation. As described previously, serum protein concentrations are decreased during pregnancy. Although this is partially due to increased total body water, likely some degree of reduced hepatic contribution of serum proteins is present that is again more exaggerated in multifetal gestation compared with singleton pregnancies. Most obvious to patients, marked uterine changes also occur. **By 25 weeks' gestation, the average twin gestation uterine size is equal to a term singleton pregnancy.** By term, the total uterine volume is often 10,000 mL, and the weight of the uterus and its contents can exceed 8 kg. These

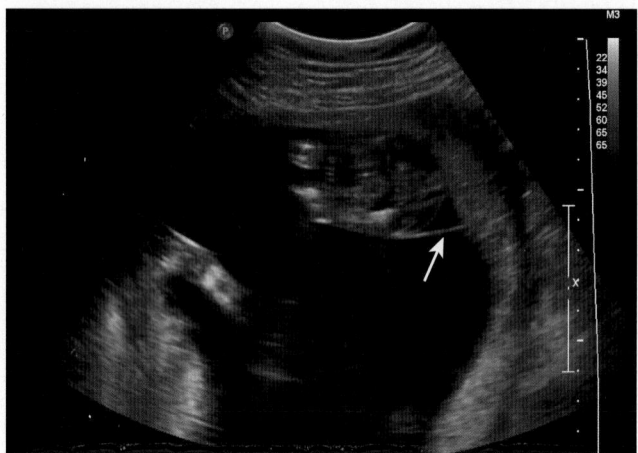

FIG 32-5 The donor twin "stuck" against the anterior uterine wall in a case of twin-twin transfusion syndrome. Note the small portion of membrane visible (*arrow*) extending from the edge of the fetus to the uterine wall.

changes are even more exaggerated with triplets and higher-order gestations.

Maternal Morbidity and Mortality

Virtually every obstetric complication, with the exception of macrosomia and postterm gestation, is more common with multiple gestations, and in general the risk rises proportionally to increasing plurality. Table 32-3 provides the relative risks for various obstetric complications in twin gestations compared with singletons.[4] In addition to the conditions listed in the table, multiples are associated with higher rates of gestational diabetes and rare but life-threatening conditions such as acute fatty liver and peripartum cardiomyopathy. **Additionally, women pregnant with multiples not only have higher risks for developing certain conditions but also are more likely to have more severe manifestations of those conditions.** For instance, Sibai and associates[5] showed that not only are mothers of twins more likely to develop preeclampsia (relative risk [RR], 2.62; 95% confidence interval [CI], 2.03 to 3.38), but twin mothers with preeclampsia also have higher rates of delivery before 37 weeks and before 35 weeks as well as higher rates of placental abruption and small-for-gestational-age (SGA) infants than singleton mothers with preeclampsia. A large retrospective analysis of 24,781 singleton, 6859 twin, 2545 triplet, and 189 quadruplet pregnancies found an incidence of pregnancy-related hypertensive conditions of 6.5% in singletons, 12.7% in twins, and 20% in triplets and quadruplets.[6] **Atypical presentations of preeclampsia are also more common in multifetal gestations, especially triplets and higher-order multiples.** One retrospective review of 21 triplet and 8 quadruplet pregnancies found that only half of the women who were delivered for preeclampsia had elevated blood pressures before delivery. Furthermore, proteinuria was present in only 3 of 16 women before delivery. Predominant presentations of preeclampsia in this series were laboratory abnormalities (chiefly elevated liver enzymes) and maternal symptoms.[7] One theory for the higher incidence of atypical preeclampsia in women with triplet and higher-order multiples is that the exaggerated hemodynamic changes found in higher-order multiples will mask the "typical" maternal manifestations of preeclampsia.

These increased maternal risks extend to life-threatening morbidity and even mortality. Multiple gestation has been found to be an independent risk factor for intensive care unit (ICU) admission.[8] Finally, **although fortunately still a very rare event, maternal death is also increased in multifetal gestations.** A

TABLE 32-3   MATERNAL COMPLICATIONS IN MULTIPLE GESTATIONS

	SINGLETON (*n* = 71,851) (%)	TWIN (*n* = 1694) (%)	RR	95% CI
Hyperemesis	1.7	5.1	3.0	2.1 to 4.1
Threatened spontaneous abortion	18.6	26.5	1.4	1.3 to 1.6
Anemia	16.2	27.5	1.7	1.5 to 1.9
Abruption	0.5	0.9	2.0	1.2 to 3.3
Gestational hypertension	17.8	23.8	1.3	1.2 to 1.5
Preeclampsia	3.4	12.5	3.7	3.3 to 4.3
Eclampsia	0.1	0.2	3.4	1.2 to 9.4
Antepartum thromboembolism	0.1	0.5	3.3	1.3 to 8.1
Manual placental extraction	2.5	6.7	2.7	2.2 to 3.2
Evacuation of retained products	0.6	2.0	3.1	2.0 to 4.8
Primary PPH (>1000 mL)	0.9	3.1	3.4	2.9 to 4.1
Secondary PPH	0.6	1.7	2.6	1.8 to 4.6
Postpartum thromboembolism	0.2	0.6	2.6	1.1 to 5.9

From Campbell DM, Templeton A. Maternal complications of twin pregnancy. *Int J Gynecol Obstet.* 2004;84:71-73.
CI, confidence interval; *PPH,* postpartum hemorrhage; *RR,* relative risk.

TABLE 32-4	BIRTH OUTCOMES FOR MULTIPLE GESTATIONS				
	MEAN BIRTHWEIGHT (g)	**MEAN GESTATIONAL AGE AT DELIVERY (WK)**	**DELIVERY <32 WK GESTATION (%)**	**LBW (%) (<2500 g)**	**VLBW (%) (<1500 g)**
Singleton	3296	38.7	1.6	6.4	1.1
Twins	2336	35.3	11.4	56.6	9.9
Triplets	1660	31.9	36.8	95.1	35.0
Quadruplets	1291	29.5	64.5	98.6	68.1
Quintuplet and higher-order	1002	26.6	95	94.6	86.5

Martin JA, Hamilton BE, Ventura SJ, et al. Births: Final data for 2009. National vital statistics reports; vol 60 no 1. Hyattsville, MD: National Center for Health Statistics, 2011.
LBW, low birthweight; *VLBW*, very low birthweight.

relative risk of 2.9 (95% CI, 1.4 to 6.1) for maternal death in women pregnant with multiples has been reported.[9]

Perinatal Morbidity and Mortality

Multifetal gestations carry significant perinatal risks. Babies who are products of multiple gestations have higher rates of low birthweight (LBW), very low birthweight (VLBW), earlier gestational age at delivery, and higher rates of neonatal and infant death and cerebral palsy (Table 32-4).[10] One in 8 twins and 1 in 3 triplets are born before 32 weeks' gestation compared with only 2 in 100 singletons. Additionally, the risk for infant death is dramatically higher than in singletons: twins are more than 4 times, triplets 10 times, and quadruplets more than 20 times as likely to die in infancy.[1] Rates of cerebral palsy have been estimated to be 4 to 8 times higher in twins than in singletons and as much as 47 times higher in triplets. Most of this increased risk is attributable to higher rates of early preterm delivery and VLBW in multiple gestations. Notably, although the overall rates of cerebral palsy are higher in twins than in singletons, LBW preterm twins do not have higher rates than similar-weight, gestational age–matched singletons. Interestingly, however, most studies have demonstrated higher rates of cerebral palsy for twins born at term weighing more than 2500 g than for comparable term singletons. This difference is mostly a reflection of the effect of monochorionicity on twin growth and development.

Fetal Anomalies

Fetuses in multiple gestations are known to be at increased risk for anatomic abnormalities, although the exact degree of risk is debated. The largest series[11] available, an international study of more than 260,000 twins, found an increased relative risk for major anomalies of 1.25 (95% CI, 1.21 to 1.28); anomalies were found in all organ systems. This study, however, was not informed on zygosity or chorionicity, and most experts believe that **much of the increased risk for structural anomalies in multiple gestation is associated with MZ twinning.**

A 2009 population-based study[12] from England found that rates of congenital anomalies were 1.7 times more frequent in twins compared with singletons (95% CI, 1.5 to 2.0) and that the relative risk for monochorionic twins was nearly twice that of dichorionic twins (RR, 1.8; 95% CI, 1.3 to 2.5). A Taiwanese series[13] of 844 twin sets compared with 4573 control singletons found a doubling of the relative risk of major congenital malformations in twins compared with singletons. When broken down by zygosity, the relative risks were 1.7 for DZ twins and 4.6 for MZ twins with an anomaly prevalence of 0.6% for singletons, 1% for DZ twins, and 2.7% for MZ twins. Anomalies were concordant in 18% of the MZ twins but in none of the DZ twins. Older studies have shown somewhat higher overall anomaly rates both for singletons and twins but found similar distributions. Thus **the overall evidence supports an approximately twofold increased risk for congenital anomalies in twins versus singletons, with most of this risk occurring in MZ twins.**

A strong association has been found between MZ twinning and midline structural defects. Nance[14] has presented evidence that a group of birth defects that involve midline structures—including symmelia, holoprosencephaly, exstrophy of the cloaca, and neural tube defects—may be associated with the MZ twinning process. Nance suggests that the MZ twinning process with its attendant opportunities for asymmetry, cytoplasmic deficiency, and competition in utero may favor the discordant expression of midline defects in these gestations.

ISSUES AND COMPLICATIONS UNIQUE TO MULTIPLE GESTATIONS

"Vanishing Twin"

The so-called vanishing twin is a well-known obstetric phenomenon, and this term refers to the **loss of one fetus of a multiple gestation early in pregnancy**. This is typically either asymptomatic or associated with spotting or mild bleeding. Landy and colleagues[15] reported on a series of 1000 first-trimester ultrasounds and found an incidence of twinning of just over 3%. After confirming a twin gestation (two embryos with heartbeats), 21.2% ultimately delivered singletons. In general, if two gestational sacs are confirmed by the first-trimester ultrasound, the chance of delivering twins is 63% for women younger than 30 years and 52% for women 30 years or older. If two embryos with cardiac activity are seen in the first trimester, the chance of a twin birth rises to 90% for women younger than 30 years and 84% for women 30 years or older.[16] Other investigators have shown that, not unexpectedly, the earlier the initial ultrasound, the greater the chance of a vanishing twin phenomenon. Additionally, monochorionic twin gestations are at higher risk for either a vanishing twin or a complete pregnancy loss than are dichorionic twins. A vanishing twin phenomenon is even more common in higher-order multiples. Dickey and colleagues[17] performed an ultrasound at 3.5 to 4.5 weeks postovulation and repeated the scan every 2 weeks until 12 weeks to assess the natural history of early pregnancy in higher-order gestations. Spontaneous loss of one or more sacs occurred in 53% of 132 triplets and in 65% of 23 quadruplets. Most of these losses were recognized earlier than 9 weeks' gestation.

First-Trimester Multifetal Pregnancy Reduction

The increasing use of ovulation induction and assisted reproduction has resulted in a growing number of multifetal pregnancies with three or more fetuses. **Because the risk for pregnancy loss,** preterm delivery, and long-term physical and neurodevelopmental morbidity for children who are products of multiple gestations is directly proportional to the number of fetuses being carried, first-trimester multifetal pregnancy reduction (MPR) has been advocated as a method to reduce the risks associated with prematurity. Currently, the method of choice is injection of potassium chloride into the thorax of one or more of the fetuses, most commonly performed transabdominally under real-time sonographic guidance. **Unless reduction of the entire monochorionic component is planned, the use of this technique is contraindicated in monochorionic pregnancies because of the vascular communications within the placenta.**

MPR is an outpatient procedure usually performed between 11 and 13 weeks, and chorionic villus sampling (CVS) can be performed on some or all of the fetuses before the procedure to confirm karyotype if desired. Ultrasound is used to map the location of each fetus, nuchal translucencies should be measured, and prophylactic antibiotics are often administered. Any fetus that appears small for gestational age, anatomically abnormal, abnormal in nuchal translucency measurement, or is known to have a karyotypic abnormality is included among those reduced. If a monochorionic twin component is present in a higher-order multiple gestation, the monochorionic set is generally targeted for reduction. If no abnormalities can be detected, the fetus or fetuses that are technically most accessible are chosen for reduction. In order to minimize the risk for premature rupture of the membranes whenever possible, the fetus whose sac overlies the internal cervical os is not electively reduced. Follow-up ultrasound examinations should be performed to confirm the success of the procedure and to monitor the growth of the remaining fetuses.

In deciding on the appropriateness of MPR for a multifetal pregnancy, the clinician must take into account not only the potential improvement in pregnancy outcome from reducing a higher-order multifetal pregnancy but also the risk of losing the entire desired pregnancy as a result of the procedure. Evans and colleagues[18] published a series of 3513 completed first-trimester MPR procedures from 11 centers in five countries. The overall loss rate was 9.6%, but each of the participating centers showed significant improvement in this parameter as the operators developed more experience. Additionally, loss rates increased steadily from 4.5% to 15.4% as the number of starting fetuses rose from three to six or more.

Stone and colleagues[19] also demonstrated a learning curve evidenced by fewer complications with increasing experience. A 2008 report of the most recent 1000 multifetal reductions (of >2000 procedures performed by their group at that time) found that the overall unintended pregnancy loss rate was 4.7%, a decrease from a 9.5% loss rate in the first 200 procedures at their institution. This 4.7% loss rate is unlikely to drop further because it approximates the baseline risk for pregnancy loss with twins in general. The rates of complete pregnancy loss by starting fetal number were 2.1%, 5.1%, 5.5%, and 11% for twins, triplets, quadruplets, and quintuplets or more, respectively. All patients except two reduced to twins or singletons; complete pregnancy loss rates by finishing fetal number were 3.8% for singletons and 5.3% for twins.

Although perinatal morbidity and mortality are clearly improved when pregnancies with quadruplets or greater are reduced to smaller numbers, the obstetric and perinatal advantages of reducing triplets to twins remain debatable. A 2006 meta-analysis attempted to answer this question.[20] The authors collected 893 pregnancies beginning as triplets, of which 411 were expectantly managed and 482 underwent MPR to twins. The rate of pregnancy loss before 24 weeks was higher in the MPR group (8.1% vs. 4.4%; $P = .036$). However, this risk was offset by a lower risk for delivery between 24 and 32 weeks in the MPR group (10.4% vs. 26.7%; $P < .0001$). The authors calculated that 7 reductions are needed to prevent one delivery before 32 weeks, and that 26 reductions would result in one loss before 24 weeks. Thus reducing triplets to twins may be associated with overall improvements in outcome. Since this meta-analysis, several other papers that reported outcomes in triplets reduced to twins have been published. A 2014 retrospective cohort study from the Netherlands compared 86 women with trichorionic triplets reduced to twins with 44 women with ongoing trichorionic triplet pregnancies and 824 women with conceived dichorionic twins. The study found that the median gestational age at delivery for reduced twins was 3 weeks longer than for triplets and 1 week shorter than for primarily conceived twins (36.1 weeks vs. 33.3 weeks vs. 37.1 weeks; $P < .001$). A significant difference was also found in birthweight (2217 g, 1700 g, and 2422 g in reduced twins, triplets, and primary twins, respectively; $P < .001$). However, no difference in survival was reported. In addition, no statistically significant reduction was noted in delivery prior to 24 weeks or prior to 32 weeks in the reduced twins compared with the triplets.[21] Another 2014 paper from Iran reported on 115 ART-conceived triplet pregnancies. Of those 115 triplet pregnancies, 57 were reduced to twins and 58 were not. The reduced pregnancies had a lower risk of preterm labor, higher birthweights, more advanced gestational age at delivery (35.1 vs. 32.4 weeks; $P = .002$), and lower rates of neonatal intensive care unit (NICU) admission. Additionally, they reported lower perinatal mortality in the reduced pregnancies (6% vs. 17.6%; $P = .007$).[22] Of course, it must be considered that inherent in a reduction procedure from triplets to twins is a one-third mortality rate. Offering the option of a multifetal reduction procedure to patients carrying triplets is medically reasonable, but whether this is perceived as a valuable option by the patient will depend on many factors, including the family's social, financial, ethical, and religious considerations.

Discordance for Anomalies

When an anomaly is detected in a twin gestation, even in an MZ set, the co-twin is usually normal. The diagnosis of discordance for a major anatomic abnormality places the parents in an extremely difficult position. Management choices include (1) expectant management of both fetuses, (2) termination of the entire pregnancy, or (3) selective termination of the anomalous fetus.

Several issues should be considered when counseling patients about the management of a multiple pregnancy complicated by discordant anomalies. These include (1) severity of the anomaly and certainty of diagnosis, (2) likelihood of survival or intact survival of the anomalous twin, (3) chorionicity, (4) effect of the anomalous fetus on the remaining fetus or fetuses, and (5) the parents' ethical beliefs. It is important to counsel patients if expectant management could result in adverse outcomes for the healthy twin. In dichorionic twins, the main issue is whether the presence of an anomalous co-twin is associated with a significantly increased risk of preterm delivery (e.g., an anomaly with polyhydramnios). For monochorionic twins, the issues are more complex. In addition to the possibility of preterm birth (PTB) associated with the presence of an anomalous co-twin, intrauterine fetal death (IUFD) of the anomalous fetus clearly has direct implications for the normal co-twin. As discussed elsewhere in this chapter, IUFD of one twin in a monochorionic pair is associated with a high rate of death or neurologic impairment of the co-twin.

Regarding the risk of PTB, the data are conflicting. Several papers have shown an increased risk of preterm delivery compared with twins in which neither fetus has a major structural anomaly.[23-25] A 2009 population-based study using the 1995 through 1997 United States Matched Multiple Births dataset compared more than 3000 normal co-twins of fetuses with nonchromosomal structural anomalies with more than 12,000 control twins unaffected by structural anomalies. They found higher rates of PTB (both <37 and <32 weeks), LBW, and perinatal mortality in the normal co-twins of affected fetuses. However, the differences in mean gestational age at delivery and mean birthweight, although statistically significant, were small (35.0 vs. 35.8 weeks, $P < .0001$, and 2265 vs. 2417 g, $P < .0001$, respectively).[26] A recent smaller paper did not find an increased risk of preterm delivery in twin pregnancies complicated by a major anomaly in one fetus. Harper and colleagues[27] compared 66 twin pregnancies discordant for anomalies with 1911 structurally normal twin pregnancies and found no difference in median gestational age at delivery (36.0 vs. 35.7 weeks for normal vs. anomalous pregnancies, respectively; $P = .43$).

Some papers have shown a small increased risk of perinatal mortality in normal co-twins of anomalous fetuses.[24,26] However, it should be noted that one of these papers did not have information on chorionicity, and several of the deaths in the other paper were in monochorionic sets. **Consequently, the evidence for an increased risk of perinatal mortality in dichorionic pregnancies discordant for major anomalies is inconclusive.** Other studies, even one of the papers that demonstrated a higher risk of preterm delivery, have not detected any differences in perinatal mortality or neonatal outcomes other than hospital length of stay.[23]

Selective Termination

Although multiple techniques have been used to effect selective termination (ST) of a single fetus in a multiple gestation, the most common approach in dichorionic gestations is intracardiac injection of potassium chloride.

Evans and collegues[28] reported the outcomes of 402 ST procedures in dichorionic twins from eight centers in four countries using ultrasound-guided intracardiac injection of potassium chloride. They reported successful ST in 100% of cases and delivery of one or more viable infants in more than 90% of cases. The complete pregnancy loss rate prior to 24 weeks was 7.1%, and no cases of disseminated intravascular coagulation (DIC) or serious maternal complications were reported.

In monochorionic twins, ST is far more challenging. Ablation of the umbilical cord of the anomalous fetus is needed to avoid back-bleeding through communicating vessels, which may precipitate death or neurologic injury in the remaining normal co-twin. Selective termination by cord occlusion can be considered in several circumstances involving monochorionic multiple gestations. These include:

1. Severely discordant anomalies
2. Severely discordant growth with high risk for IUFD at previable or periviable gestational ages

3. Twin reversed arterial perfusion (TRAP) sequence
4. Severe TTTS with associated discordant anomaly or in cases in which laser ablation was precluded by position of the fetus and placenta

Each of the above indications is discussed in more detail in the corresponding sections of this chapter.

Bipolar coagulation of the umbilical cord is probably the most commonly used technique, although radiofrequency ablation (RFA), laser coagulation, and ligation of the cord have also been successful. The site for port insertion is chosen according to the position of the placenta and the amniotic sac of the target fetus and its umbilical cord. Preferentially, the other sac is avoided. Sometimes amnioinfusion is necessary to expand the target sac.

Pregnancy outcomes for the surviving co-twin are relatively favorable after selective cord occlusion. Rossi and D'Addario[29] published a review of the literature regarding umbilical cord occlusion in complicated monochorionic twin pregnancies. They evaluated 12 studies that comprised 345 cases of cord occlusion at median gestational ages between 18 and 24 weeks. The overall survival rate for the remaining twin was 79% and was higher for cases after 18 weeks (89%) than for those undergoing the procedure earlier than 18 weeks (69%) regardless of the indication. Survival rates were 86% after RFA, 82% after bipolar cord coagulation, 72% after laser, and 70% after cord ligation. Long-term follow-up was not available for most studies. However, in one series, the incidence of developmental delay was 8% in 67 infants older than 1 year who underwent evaluation by a pediatrician.[30]

Intrauterine Fetal Demise of One Twin

Intrauterine fetal demise of one twin occurs most commonly during the first trimester. This phenomenon is known as a *vanishing twin* and was discussed earlier in this chapter. Although it can be associated with vaginal spotting, the loss of one conceptus early in the first trimester is often not clinically recognized, and the prognosis for the surviving twin is generally excellent. **IUFD of one fetus in a multiple gestation in the second or third trimester is much less common and complicates about 2.4% to 6.8% of twin pregnancies, but it can have more severe sequelae for the surviving fetus.** In triplet pregnancies, studies have reported single IUFD rates between 4.3% and 17%.

The etiology of IUFD in a multiple pregnancy may be similar to that for singletons or may be unique to the twinning process. Death in utero may be caused by conditions that affect only the demised twin, such as chromosomal or structural abnormalities, or by more global conditions such as maternal diseases, which put the entire pregnancy at risk. In diamniotic monochorionic pregnancies, IUFD may result from complications of TTTS or twin anemia-polycythemia sequence (TAPS), whereas cord entanglement is a major contributor to IUFD in monoamniotic monochorionic twins. Just as in singletons, however, the etiology of many IUFDs remains elusive.

Single IUFD in a twin gestation puts the surviving twin in jeopardy. In twin pregnancies complicated by demise of one twin, intrauterine death of the co-twin is reported in 12% to 15% of monochorionic gestations and in 3% to 4% of dichorionic gestations.[31,32] In a 2006 meta-analysis by Ong and associates[31] of twin pregnancies complicated by a single IUFD, preterm delivery occurred in 68% of monochorionic twins and in 57% of dichorionic twins, figures that include both spontaneous and iatrogenic preterm delivery. A more recent meta-analysis in 2011 by Hillman and colleagues[32] found strikingly similar rates of PTB: 68% for monochorionic and 54% for dichorionic twins. In the Hillman meta-analysis, overall PTB rates did not differ statistically by chorionicity except in the subgroup, in which IUFD occurred between 28 and 33 weeks. In this subgroup, preterm delivery was nearly 5 times more common in monochorionic compared with dichorionic twins (OR, 4.96; 95% CI, 1.6 to 15.8). The authors speculate that this difference may relate to iatrogenic delivery as a result of clinician concern for co-twin demise in monochorionic pregnancies. Neither of these meta-analyses had a control group of twins with two survivors. However, the reported percentages for PTB in the IUFD pregnancies are not markedly different than the 58.8% risk of preterm delivery reported by national vital statistics data for all twin pregnancies.[10] That said, some studies have shown an increased risk of PTB in twin pregnancies complicated by a single IUFD.[33]

Surviving co-twins of pregnancies complicated by a single IUFD are also at risk for brain injury. Pharoah and Adi[34] reported on a large cohort of all registered twin births in England and Wales between 1993 and 1995 and found a 20% risk of cerebral impairment in the surviving twins. That paper provided information on gender but not chorionicity or zygosity. The meta-analysis by Hillman and colleagues[32] reported the rate of abnormal postnatal (<4 weeks of delivery) cranial imaging and neurodevelopmental impairment after a single fetal death. Abnormal cranial imaging was found in 34% of monochorionic twins compared with 16% of dichorionic twins (not significant with OR 3.25; 95% CI, 0.66 to 16.10). Neurodevelopmental impairment followed single fetal death in 26% versus 2% for monochorionic and dichorionic twins, respectively (OR, 4.81; 95% CI, 1.4 to 16.6).

Multicystic encephalomalacia is believed to be a precursor to infant and childhood cerebral impairment in many cases; it results in **cystic lesions within the cerebral white matter distributed in areas supplied by the anterior and middle cerebral arteries, and it is associated with profound neurologic handicap** (Fig. 32-6). Patients with monochorionic placentation should thus be counseled about the risk of developing this condition and the resultant cerebral palsy or other serious neurodevelopmental handicap in the surviving twin. Ultrasound examination of the fetal brain may be suggestive of multicystic encephalomalacia but is not always definitive. Antenatal magnetic resonance imaging (MRI) of the fetal brain may also be useful in its detection. We currently offer fetal MRI to all patients with monochorionic placentae approximately 2 to 3 weeks after the demise of one fetus has been detected. If a normal MRI does not definitively rule out brain abnormalities, it is a very positive prognostic finding.

The most widely accepted hypothesis as to the cause of neurologic injury in surviving co-twins in a monochorionic pregnancy is that significant hypotension occurs at the time of the demise. After death of the first twin, the resulting low pressure in that twin's circulatory system causes blood from the survivor to rapidly back-bleed into the dead twin through placental anastomoses. If the resulting hypotension is severe, the surviving twin is at risk for both demise and ischemic damage to vital organs. The brain is at particular risk because of its high oxygen requirements. It should be stressed that, because the injury is coincident with the IUFD, rapid delivery of the co-twin following single IUFD in a monochorionic pregnancy will not improve the outcome.

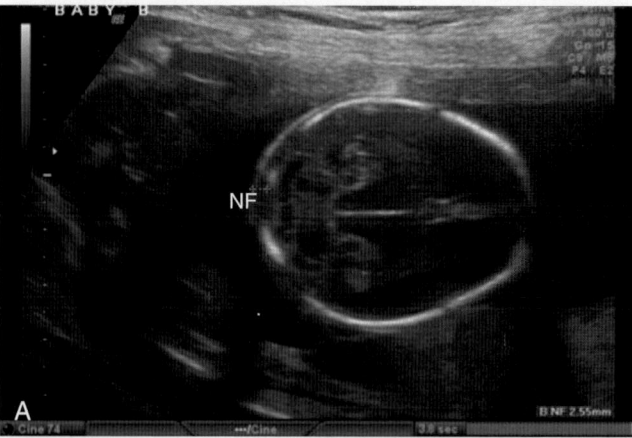

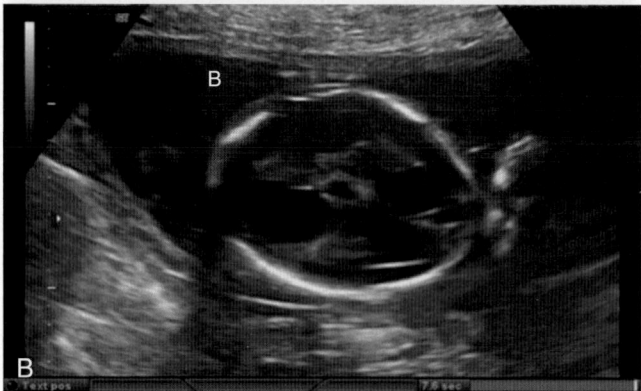

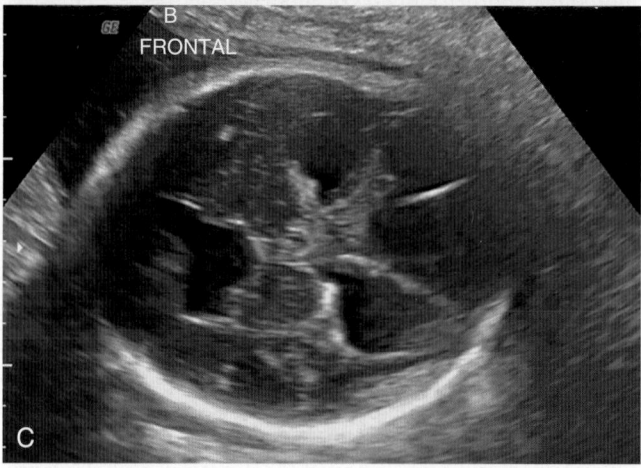

FIG 32-6 Ultrasound of the fetal brain of a monochorionic twin before **(A)** and after **(B, C)** intrauterine fetal death of the co-twin at 20 weeks' gestation. Note the normal brain anatomy in **A,** the dilation and cystic changes shortly after the co-twin's demise in **B,** and the residual irregular hydrocephalus and parenchymal loss 12 weeks later in **C.** B, twin B; NF, nuchal fold.

Until relatively recently, it was thought that intrauterine demise in a monochorionic twin gestation would not cause neurologic injury to its co-twin until at least the mid second trimester. However, in 2003, Weiss and coworkers[35] reported a case of injury to a fetus after IUFD of the co-twin at about 13 weeks. Multicystic encephalomalacia was diagnosed by ultrasound and MRI in the co-twin at 20 weeks. The patient was counseled regarding the likelihood of a poor prognosis and opted for termination. Multicystic encephalomalacia was confirmed pathologically, although the exact timing of the injury could not be determined.

Other maternal risks exist with single IUFD in a multifetal gestation. Cesarean delivery appears to be increased in these patients, often because of nonreassuring fetal status of the surviving twin. However, other adverse maternal outcomes such as hemorrhage, infection, and coagulopathy have *not* been found to be increased in twin mothers with a single IUFD.[33] It was originally estimated that the incidence of maternal DIC was 25% when a dead fetus was retained in a multiple gestation. However, only a few isolated cases of laboratory changes consistent with a subclinical coagulopathy have been reported under these circumstances. The estimated 25% incidence is certainly a gross overestimation. It is also reassuring to note that no cases of clinically significant coagulopathy have been reported in the extensive literature on selective termination and multifetal pregnancy reduction.

The optimal management for a single IUFD in multiple gestations is not well established, and recommendations are based mainly on expert opinion. **Clinical management depends on the gestational age, maternal status, or detection of in utero compromise of the surviving fetus or fetuses.** The goal is to optimize the outcome for the survivor while also avoiding unnecessary prematurity. Serial sonographic assessment of the surviving co-twin's growth is indicated, as is antenatal testing. However, when to initiate antenatal testing and the frequency of testing depends on clinical factors such as gestational age at the time of the IUFD.

The 2011 National Institute of Child Health and Human Development (NICHD) and Society for Maternal-Fetal Medicine (SMFM) workshop on timing of indicated late-preterm and early-term birth addressed the issue of a single IUFD in a twin pregnancy. If the IUFD occurs at 34 weeks or beyond, delivery should be considered.[36] In the 2014 Practice Bulletin on Multifetal Gestation, the American College of Obstetricians and Gynecologists (ACOG) gives a similar recommendation, stating that in the absence of other indications, a single IUFD in a twin pregnancy before 34 weeks should not prompt immediate delivery.[37] **In the authors' practices, a single IUFD in a monochorionic diamniotic pregnancy at or after 34 weeks would be an indication for delivery.** In a dichorionic pregnancy, delivery timing would be individualized based on the likely cause of the IUFD, the appropriateness of fetal growth, and fetal testing of the surviving co-twin.

Vaginal delivery is not contraindicated, and cesarean delivery is reserved for routine obstetric indications. Autopsy should be offered for the stillborn fetus but may not be helpful if the demise occurred several weeks earlier. Pathologic examination of the placenta is also recommended. In addition, the pregnancy history should be communicated to the pediatricians caring for the neonate.

Twin-Twin Transfusion Syndrome
Etiology
Twin-twin transfusion syndrome is exclusively a complication of monochorionic multifetal pregnancies. It occurs in 10% to 15% of monochorionic diamniotic gestations and is thus the most common life-threatening complication specific to this type of twinning. TTTS is characterized by an imbalance of fetal blood flow through communicating vessels across a shared placenta, which leads to **underperfusion of the donor twin and overperfusion of the recipient** (Fig. 32-7). **The donor twin develops oligohydramnios, and if it is chronic, intrauterine growth restriction (IUGR) ensues; the recipient**

twin experiences volume overload, which results in polyhydramnios that leads to uterine overdistension and increased intrauterine pressure, both of which may contribute to an increased risk for preterm labor and preterm premature rupture of the membranes (PPROM). On fetal echocardiography, the recipient demonstrates decreased ventricular function, tricuspid regurgitation, and cardiomegaly. Over time, recipient twins can develop functional right ventricular outflow tract obstruction and pulmonic stenosis. These cardiac abnormalities often progress during pregnancy and persist into the neonatal period.

TTTS can present at any gestational age, but earlier onset is associated with a poorer prognosis. If untreated, the reported mortality rates can range from 80% to 100%. Furthermore, if one fetus dies in utero, the surviving twin is at risk for death or multiorgan ischemia from acute exsanguination due to backbleeding into the circulation of the dead co-twin.

All monochorionic twins share vascular anastomoses and thus exist in a state of constant intertwin transfusion. As noted earlier, however, only a minority develop clinical TTTS. The following pathophysiology has been proposed to explain this observation. In monochorionic placentae, three types of vascular communication are possible: (1) arteriovenous (AV), (2) arterioarterial (AA), and (3) venovenous (VV). AA and VV anastomoses are usually superficial bidirectional anastomoses on the surface of the chorionic plate; however, **AV anastomoses—referred to as *deep anastomoses*—involve a shared cotyledon, which receives arterial supply from one twin and drains on the venous side to the other twin.** All these anastomoses are identifiable at the chorionic surface. Superficial anastomoses, especially those that are AA, are crucial for maintaining bidirectional flow. According to this hypothesis, an inadequacy of superficial AA and VV anastomoses, which help maintain balanced blood flow, allows TTTS to manifest due to an imbalance of deep AV anastomoses.

Diagnosis and Staging
The antenatal diagnosis of TTTS is made by ultrasound. The two classic criteria are monochorionic diamniotic twin gestation and oligohydramnios (deepest vertical pocket [DVP] <2 cm) in one amniotic sac and polyhydramnios (DVP >8 cm) in the other sac. A staging system for TTTS (Table 32-5) was developed in 1999 by Quintero and colleagues[38] to categorize disease severity and to standardize comparison of different treatment approaches. **Although the Quintero staging is widely used and has proved enormously useful in our understanding of TTTS, many experts have noted its limitations.** The stage does not always progress; and when patients worsen,

TABLE 32-5	QUINTERO STAGING FOR TWIN-TWIN TRANSFUSION SYNDROME
Stage I	Oligohydramnios, polyhydramnios sequence. Donor twin bladder visible.
Stage II	Oligohydramnios, polyhydramnios sequence. Donor twin bladder not visible. Doppler scan normal.
Stage III	Oligohydramnios, polyhydramnios sequence. Donor twin bladder not visible, and Doppler scans abnormal (absent or reversed end-diastolic velocity in the umbilical artery, reversed flow in the ductus venosus, or pulsatile flow in the umbilical vein).
Stage IV	One or both fetuses have hydrops.
Stage V	One or both fetuses have died.

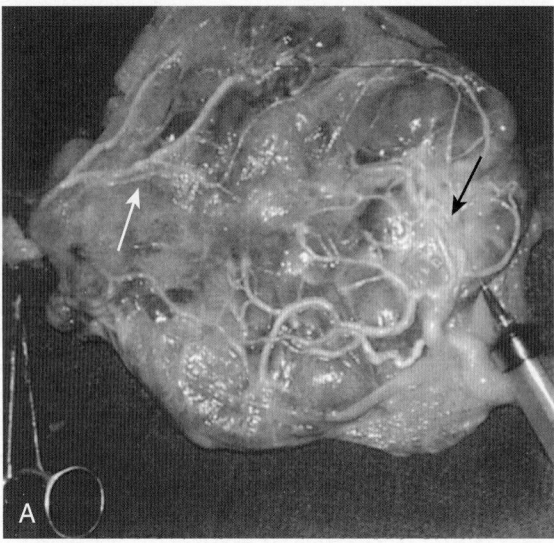

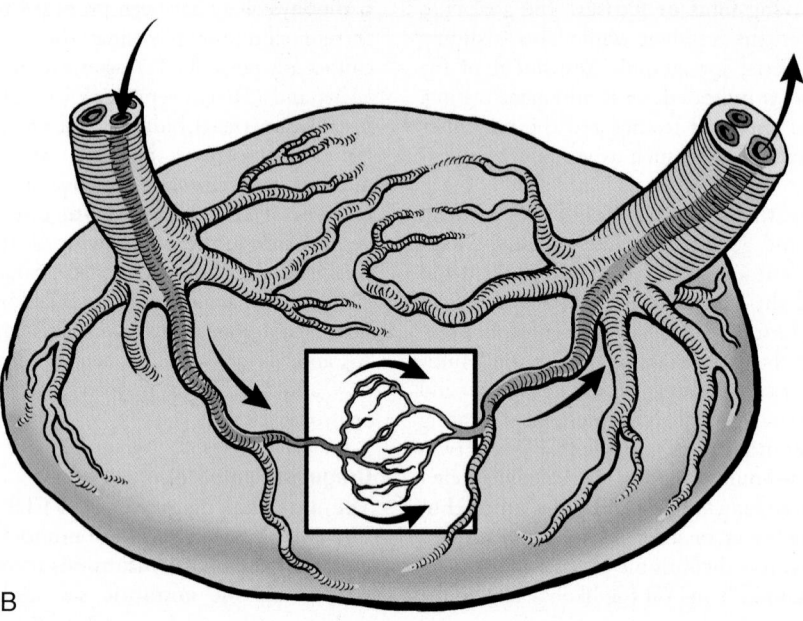

B

FIG 32-7 A, The placenta of a pregnancy complicated by twin-twin transfusion syndrome. Milk has been injected into an artery on the donor side of the placenta (*black arrow*). It can be seen returning through the venous circulation on that side but is also evident in the venous circulation of the recipient twin (*white arrow*). **B,** The arteriovenous shunt shown in A.

they do not always progress sequentially through the stages. For instance, a pregnancy can become stage 5 (fetal death) without progressing through stage 4 (hydrops); and an atypical stage III TTTS has been described with Doppler abnormalities but with a bladder still visible in the donor. Modifications of Quintero staging have been proposed that incorporate the differences in cardiovascular pathophysiology between donors and recipients. None of these proposed staging alternatives, however, has been validated in prospective studies.

TTTS most commonly presents between 15 and 26 weeks' gestation. Intensive ultrasound surveillance should be performed during this period to allow a timely diagnosis. Because an ultrasound interval of more than14 days has been associated with a higher stage of TTTS at diagnosis,[39] both ACOG and SMFM endorse an every-2-week ultrasound surveillance schedule for monochorionic diamniotic twins starting around 16 weeks.[37,40]

Management

When TTTS is diagnosed, five management options are available: (1) expectant management, (2) septostomy, (3) serial amnioreduction, (4) selective termination/cord occlusion, and (5) fetoscopic laser photocoagulation. Selective termination is only offered in extreme cases of advanced TTTS. Expectant management is generally not recommended in stage II or greater TTTS because of the poor perinatal outcomes associated with the disorder if untreated. **However, management depends on the gestational age at diagnosis and, despite the previously mentioned limitations of the Quintero staging system, on the severity of the clinical findings.**

SEPTOSTOMY

Septostomy involves intentional perforation of the dividing membrane, usually performed with a 20- or 22-gauge needle

under ultrasound guidance. This procedure can, in theory, equalize amniotic fluid volumes (AFVs) between amniotic sacs. The only randomized trial involving this technique compared septostomy with amnioreduction for the treatment of TTTS. The study was terminated early after enrollment of 73 women because the rate of survival of at least one infant was similar in both groups (78% vs. 80%; $P = .82$). The major advantage seen with septostomy was that women randomized to the septostomy group were more likely to require only a single procedure for treatment (64% vs. 46%; $P = .04$).[41] Because septostomy could functionally create an iatrogenic monoamniotic pregnancy with its own inherent risks, the procedure has been criticized and infrequently recommended as a therapeutic option for TTTS.

SERIAL AMNIOREDUCTION

In serial reduction amniocentesis, a needle is placed into the polyhydramniotic sac under ultrasound guidance. Amniotic fluid is withdrawn until the fluid volume normalizes (i.e., DVP <8 cm). Because of the large amount of fluid to be removed, attaching the needle to a closed-system vacuum container is more practical than withdrawing fluid manually. Amnioreduction is repeated as often as necessary to maintain a normal or near-normal AFV. The mechanism by which this procedure restores the amniotic fluid balance is unknown. Removing excessive fluid from the sac with polyhydramnios may result in decreased intraamniotic pressure that in turn may result in increased placental perfusion to the twin with oligohydramnios, especially through thin-walled superficial venous anastomoses with secondary improvement in its AFV. Additionally, normalizing the AFV may help prolong pregnancy by relieving uterine overdistension and pressure on the cervix.

Although no prospective studies are available with which to compare serial amnioreduction with conservative management, based on observational data, amnioreduction appears to offer a twofold to threefold increase in overall survival compared with no intervention. The exception may be late-onset (third-trimester) stage I TTTS that remains stable over a 1- to 2-week observation period. A large retrospective cohort study using the International Amnioreduction Registry to analyze 223 sets of twins with TTTS diagnosed prior to 28 weeks' gestation and treated with serial amnioreduction found a live birth rate of 78%, and 60% were alive 4 weeks after birth. IUFD of at least one twin occurred in 31% of the pregnancies. In 14% of cases, IUFD of both babies occurred. Of those babies alive 4 weeks after birth, 24% of the recipients and 25% of the donors had abnormal findings on cranial imaging. Poor prognostic factors for survival were earlier gestational age at diagnosis, no end-diastolic flow in the umbilical arteries, hydrops, LBW, and earlier gestational age at delivery. Complications within 48 hours of the procedure (spontaneous rupture of the membranes, spontaneous delivery, fetal distress, fetal death, and placental abruption) occurred in 15% of patients.[42]

LASER THERAPY

Laser ablation of placental anastomoses is the favored treatment option for early-onset TTTS (Fig. 32-8). In the United States, the use of laser photocoagulation to treat TTTS is restricted to gestations earlier than 26 weeks. Unlike both serial amnioreduction and septostomy, which are considered palliative procedures, laser ablation is the only therapeutic option that corrects the underlying pathophysiologic aberration that causes TTTS. Additionally, because laser ablation

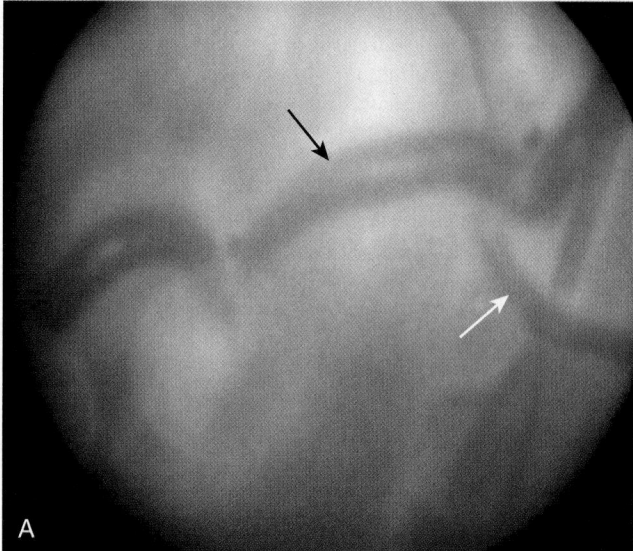
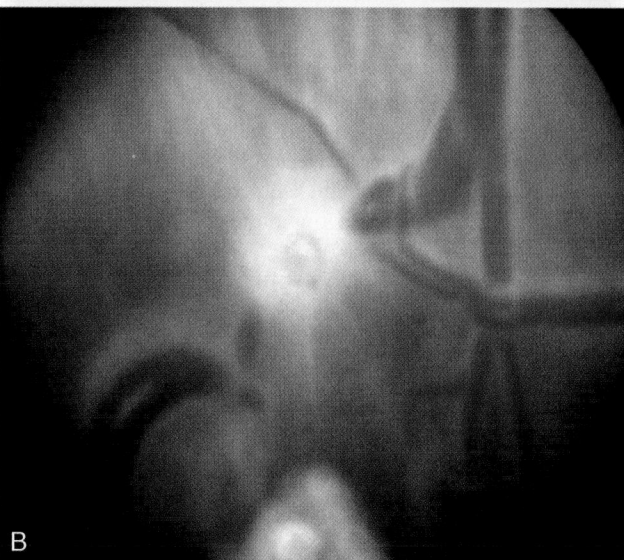

FIG 32-8 **A,** An artery from one twin going to a cotyledon, which is drained by a vein returning to the co-twin (*black arrow*). The cotyledon is also perfused by a small artery from the co-twin (*white arrow*) and is drained by a large vein going also to the co-twin. To preserve this cotyledon for the co-twin, the arterial perfusion to the cotyledon from the other twin is interrupted by laser photocoagulation of the other artery. **B,** The effect of photocoagulation. (Courtesy Timothy M Crombleholme, MD, University of Cincinnati College of Medicine.)

interrupts the vascular anastomoses between the fetuses, it has the advantage of being protective of the surviving twin should one twin succumb in utero.

In this procedure, first described by De Lia, the strategy is to ablate all anastomosing vessels that might connect the fetuses. The procedure is performed percutaneously under local or regional anesthesia. An endoscopic cannula is inserted into the amniotic cavity of the recipient fetus under ultrasound guidance at an angle perpendicular to the presumed vascular equator. The positions of the fetuses, umbilical cord insertions, and placenta are mapped. The operator visualizes the entire vascular equator and coagulates all visible anastomoses. Arteries are distinguishable from veins because they have a darker color and pass over the larger veins. Reduction amniocentesis is usually simultaneously performed. When the placenta is anterior, operative conditions are more difficult. Special instruments have been developed that include curved sheaths, flexible endoscopes, and a double-insertion technique. Most centers hospitalize patients for 1 or 2 postoperative days, and many experts use perioperative tocolytics and antibiotics.

OUTCOMES AFTER LASER THERAPY

In 2004, Senat and colleagues[43] published the results of the Eurofetus trial, a prospective multicenter randomized controlled trial (RCT) of endoscopic laser (semiselective technique) versus serial amnioreduction for the treatment of severe TTTS between 15 and 26 weeks' gestation. Following an interim analysis, the study was stopped after 142 patients had been treated. **Compared with the amnioreduction group, the laser group had a higher likelihood of survival for at least one twin to 28 days of life** (76% vs. 56%; $P = .009$) **and 6 months of age** (76% vs. 51%; $P = .002$). The median gestational age at delivery was significantly more advanced in the laser group (33.3 vs. 29.0 weeks; $P = .004$). Neonates from the laser group also had a lower incidence of periventricular leukomalacia (PVL) and were more likely to be free of neurologic deficits at 6 months of age (52% vs. 31%; $P = .003$). The authors concluded that **endoscopic laser coagulation of anastomoses is a more effective first-line treatment than serial amnioreduction for severe TTTS diagnosed before 26 weeks' gestation.** Although this study did include patients in all Quintero stages, most (90% of the laser group and 91% of the amnioreduction group) were stage II or III.

An NICHD-sponsored prospective multicenter trial is the only other randomized clinical trial to compare amnioreduction to fetoscopic laser photocoagulation.[44] That trial, in which all patients were Quintero stages II to IV, was stopped early after only 40 patients accrued, mainly because of recruitment difficulties but also because of concern about a trend toward more adverse fetal outcomes affecting the recipient twin in the laser arm. Analysis of the 40 patients showed no difference, either for donors or recipients, in the primary outcome of 30-day neonatal survival (55% in both arms for donors and 45% vs. 30% in the amnioreduction vs. laser arms for recipients; $P > .5$). The increased *fetal* mortality rate among recipients in the laser group was more pronounced in Quintero stage III and IV disease. The investigators concluded that the trial did not conclusively demonstrate the superiority of either treatment modality, although the results were severely limited by the small sample size.

Subsequently, both a Cochrane review and another meta-analysis that compared laser therapy with serial amnioreduction supported the use of endoscopic laser therapy in the treatment of severe TTTS. In the Cochrane review, at age 6 years, more children were alive without neurologic abnormality in the laser groups than in the amnioreduction groups (RR, 1.57; 95% CI, 1.05 to 2.34). However, no difference was apparent in overall death between amnioreduction and laser (RR, 0.87; 95% CI, 0.55 to 1.38).[45] The meta-analysis by Rossi and D'Addario[46] found improved overall survival (OR, 2.04; 95% CI, 1.52 to 2.76), decreased neonatal death (OR, 0.24; 95% CI, 0.15 to 0.4), and decreased neurologic morbidity (OR, 0.2; 95% CI, 0.12 to 0.33) with laser therapy compared with serial amnioreduction.

Short-term complications of laser ablation include placental abruption, PPROM, IUFD, and labor. In the Eurofetus trial, a 1% to 12% risk was reported for each of these complications in both the laser and amnioreduction groups. Rates of

IUFD, pregnancy loss, and PPROM within 7 days of the procedure were 1.5- to 5-fold higher in the laser group, although these differences did not reach statistical significance.[43] In the NICHD trial,[44] the incidence of PPROM before 28 weeks was 4.8% in the laser arm and 0% in the amnioreduction arm. Maternal complications are not consistently reported in the literature; however, no maternal deaths have been reported in all of the TTTS laser therapy literature, and serious complications such as pulmonary edema or blood transfusion appear to be very rare.

A few investigations have studied the long-term neurologic outcomes of babies treated in utero with laser ablation. Rossi and colleagues[47] performed a meta-analysis of 15 papers that described neurologic outcomes in children who underwent laser photocoagulation for TTTS. For those seven papers that reported neurologic morbidity at birth ($n = 895$ babies), the incidence was 6.1%. For the nine studies that reported follow-up at 6 to 48 months ($n = 1255$ babies), the incidence of neurologic impairment was 11.1%, and cerebral palsy was the most frequent neurologic diagnosis (39.7%). Neurologic impairment was identified equally between donors and recipients and between one survivor and two survivors for twin sets. Since publication of this meta-analysis, a long-term follow-up from the Eurofetus trial has been published.[48] This paper showed some improvement in neurologic outcome at age 6 years among 73 children who had undergone laser treatment compared with 47 children who had undergone amnioreduction. The survivors in the laser group had an 82% chance of a normal neurologic exam, compared with 72% in the amnioreduction group ($P = .12$). No difference was reported in neurologic outcomes between donors and recipients.

The current consensus is that laser ablation of vascular anastomoses is the optimal therapy for Quintero stage II to IV disease before 26 weeks' gestation. However, controversy exists as to the optimal management of stage I disease. This controversy is based on several observations. First, the prognosis for stage I patients can be quite good without laser surgery. In a series by Taylor and colleagues,[49] 70% of stage I patients treated with either expectant management, amnioreduction, or septostomy remained stable or regressed. O'Donoghue and colleagues[50] reviewed all cases of TTTS at their institution between 2000 and 2006 and identified 46 cases that presented with stage I TTTS, all of which were treated either expectantly or with amnioreduction. They found that 70% either remained stable or regressed. Rossi and D'Addario[51] published a review of the literature that included only stage I TTTS. They reported overall survival rates of 77% after amnioreduction, 85% after laser therapy, and 86% after expectant management. The progression to a more advanced stage was 15% for those pregnancies managed expectantly.

On the other hand, recent studies have shown that even in stage I and II TTTS, the recipient can suffer cardiac dysfunction, something not taken into account by the commonly used Quintero staging system. Michelfelder and associates[52] examined echocardiographic parameters of 42 TTTS patients, of whom 14 were stage I. Of the stage I patients, 57% had ventricular hypertrophy and 14% had atrioventricular valve dysfunction. Because it has been shown that cardiac dysfunction in the recipient improves after laser therapy but not after amnioreduction, this suggests that laser therapy may be the better choice in select patients who present with Quintero stage I TTTS. A single retrospective cohort study[53] published in 2009 directly compared outcomes in stage I patients treated with laser surgery versus expectant management. Of 50 women who presented with stage I TTTS, 40% underwent laser surgery and 60% were managed either expectantly, or, if maternal symptoms were present, with amnioreduction. Although short-term outcomes (gestational age at delivery and perinatal survival) were not significantly different between the two treatment groups, long-term neurodevelopmental impairment as determined by neurologic examination and neuropsychological developmental testing at a minimum of 2 years of age was decreased in the laser group (0/21 vs. 7/30; $P = .03$). This study raises the question as to whether ongoing neurologic injury is present from mild TTTS even if the disease does not progress and whether this damage could be prevented by interrupting the underlying pathophysiology of TTTS using laser ablation.

In summary, laser photocoagulation is considered optimal management of stage II and greater TTTS prior to 26 weeks' gestation. For stage I disease, pending further study, expectant management is reasonable; but some centers offer laser therapy to these women, especially when diagnosis is made in the early second trimester or when evidence of cardiac dysfunction is present. For women diagnosed with TTTS after 26 weeks, either expectant management or serial amnioreduction are recommended, and management decisions should be based on severity of disease. It is important to remember that even with optimal laser treatment of TTTS, it remains a serious disease with 20% to 50% overall perinatal mortality.[40]

SELECTIVE INTRAUTERINE GROWTH RESTRICTION IN MONOCHORIONIC TWIN PREGNANCIES

Selective IUGR (sIUGR) is defined as growth restriction, most commonly an estimated fetal weight below the 10th percentile of one twin with appropriate growth in the co-twin but without full criteria for TTTS. This condition has been reported in 10% to 15% of monochorionic diamniotic gestations and frequently presents at relatively early gestational ages, although sIUGR can also occur in dichorionic pregnancies. However, the course of early-onset sIUGR in a monochorionic pregnancy differs from early-onset IUGR in a singleton or dichorionic twin gestation. Umbilical artery (UA) Doppler findings cannot be interpreted in the same way as in singleton or dichorionic gestations because the waveforms represent not only the effects of placental insufficiency but also the influence of intertwin vascular communications. Usually the latency period is longer from abnormal Dopplers to delivery in monochorionic twins. Additionally, the initial UA Doppler findings (stage of sIUGR, see below) usually remain unchanged; that is, if Dopplers are initially normal, they rarely worsen, and a good prognosis is likely. In monochorionic compared with dichorionic twins, sIUGR is also associated with a higher frequency of abnormalities such as a two-vessel cord and marginal or velamentous cord insertions.

Gratacós and associates[54] have proposed a classification system for sIUGR based on UA Doppler findings. Type I is characterized by positive diastolic flow in the growth-restricted fetus, type II by persistently absent or reversed end-diastolic flow, and type III by intermittently absent or reversed end-diastolic flow. The cyclical pattern of intermittently abnormal Doppler flow is believed to be caused by transmitted waveforms from the larger to the smaller twin's cord due to the existence of large AA anastomoses. Pregnancies with type III sIUGR are reported to have both more frequent, as well as larger diameter, AA anastomoses than either uncomplicated monochorionic twin pregnancies or pregnancies with type I or II sIUGR.[54] Based on the type I through III classification system, Gratacós and associates[54] reported on 134 monochorionic diamniotic pregnancies complicated by sIUGR diagnosed before 26 weeks (39 type I, 30 type II, 65 type III). They reported unexpected IUFD of the smaller twin in 2.6%, 0%, and 15.4% of cases of type I, type II, and type III sIUGR, respectively. The corresponding numbers for IUFD of the normally grown twin were 2.6%, 0%, and 6.2%. Mean gestational ages at delivery for type I, type II, and type III sIUGR, were 35.4 weeks, 30.7 weeks, and 31.6 weeks, respectively. It should be noted that in 9 cases of type II and 4 cases of type III sIUGR, cord occlusion of the IUGR twin was performed for the benefit of the normally grown twin in the face of deterioration of the growth-restricted twin's status. Consequently, the above numbers do not necessarily represent the natural history of early-onset type II and III sIUGR in monochorionic twins. However, a study from Japan of expectantly managed sIUGR cases in monochorionic diamniotic gestations does provide some insight into the natural history of the disorder. Ishii and colleagues[55] reported on 23 type I, 27 type II, and 13 type III sIUGR pregnancies. Mean gestational age at delivery was 36 weeks, 28 weeks, and 31 weeks for types I through III, respectively. IUFD of the smaller twin occurred in 4.3%, 22.2%, and 15.4% of cases, respectively, and in the larger twin in 4.3%, 22.2%, and 0% of cases, respectively. In the Ishii study, the incidence of neurologic morbidity for the larger twin was 0%, 11.1%, and 38.5% for types I through III, respectively. For the smaller twin, the corresponding numbers were 4.3%, 14.8%, and 23.1%.

As evidenced by the above data, the prognosis for expectantly managed type I sIUGR is generally good, so close observation is preferred. The prognosis for type II and III sIUGR is much more guarded. Three management options are available for type II and III early-onset sIUGR in a monochorionic twin pregnancy:
1. Careful expectant management with an effort to maximize outcome for both twins
2. Cord occlusion of the IUGR twin, thus sacrificing the IUGR fetus to protect the larger twin from injury as a result of acute intertwin transfusion associated with smaller co-twin demise
3. Laser photocoagulation to physically separate the shared fetal circulations to help protect the larger co-twin from injury or death in the event of the smaller twin's demise

Detailed discussion of management options is beyond the scope of this chapter. The reader is referred to an excellent review article by Valsky and associates.[56]

TWIN ANEMIA-POLYCYTHEMIA SEQUENCE

Twin anemia-polycythemia sequence (TAPS) refers to the occurrence of a chronic and severe hemoglobin discordance in a monochorionic diamniotic twin pair in the absence of other criteria for TTTS. Prenatally, the diagnosis is made by middle cerebral artery (MCA) Doppler multiples of the median (MoM) of 1.5 or more in one twin and MoM of 0.8 or less in the other twin without amniotic fluid discordance that meets TTTS criteria. However, some experts have proposed an alternative criteria for the anemic twin; specifically, an MCA Doppler of MoM of 1.0 or less. Postnatally, criteria for anemia

TABLE 32-6	STAGING SYSTEM FOR TWIN ANEMIA-POLYCYTHEMIA SEQUENCE
STAGE	**FINDING**
1	Donor MCA-PSV >1.5 MoM and recipient MCA-PSV <1.0
2	Donor MCA-PSV >1.7 MoM and recipient MCA-PSV <0.8 MoM without other signs of fetal compromise
3	Stage 1 or 2, with critically abnormal Doppler ultrasound*
4	Hydrops of donor
5	IUFD of one or both fetuses

*Absent or reversed end-diastolic flow in umbilical artery, pulsatile flow in umbilical vein, increased pulsatility index or reversed flow in the ductus venosus.
IUFD, intrauterine fetal demise; *MCA,* middle cerebral artery; *MoM,* multiples of the median; *PSV,* peak systolic velocity.

and polycythemia are hemoglobin of 11 g/dL or less with reticulocytosis in the donor and hemoglobin of 20 g/dL or more in the recipient. A TAPS classification system has been proposed that is similar to the Quintero system for TTTS (Table 32-6).[57] Isolated TAPS can occur spontaneously in monochorionic pregnancies with an observed frequency of 3% to 5%, but it has been reported more commonly as a complication of laser photocoagulation for TTTS. Postlaser TAPS has been reported in up to 13% of laser-treated TTTS cases.

The cause of TAPS is thought to be the presence of only a few, very small AV anastomoses, which allow a slow transfusion of blood from the donor to the recipient. AA anastomoses are believed to be important in equilibrating the blood flow between twins and consequently are seen in 80% of uncomplicated monochorionic diamniotic gestations. In contrast, AA anastomoses are seen in only about 25% of TTTS pregnancies and are even more rare (11%) in pregnancies complicated by TAPS. Because of the possibility of TAPS, an MCA peak systolic flow velocity should be considered in the screening of all monochorionic multifetal pregnancies.

Ideal management of TAPS is not yet clear, but intrauterine transfusions—both intraperitoneal and intravenous (IV)—and laser treatment have been reported with good success. Expectant management is also a reasonable option. Regardless of management, survival rates for twins in a pregnancy complicated by TAPS have been reported to range from 75% to 100%. In utero intervention is not proven to be associated with clear differences in survival or long-term outcomes. The reader is also referred to two excellent reviews on TAPS by Slaghekke and coworkers[57] and by Baschat and Oepkes.[58]

Monoamniotic Twins

Monoamniotic twinning is an uncommon form of MZ twinning in which both fetuses occupy a single amniotic sac. Monoamniotic twins account for only 1% of all MZ pregnancies. Interestingly, as in conjoined twins, there is a female predominance: 55% to 74% of monoamniotic twin sets are reported to be female, although the reason for this difference is unclear.[59-63] **Historically, perinatal mortality rates for monoamniotic twins have been reported to approach 50%, attributed to premature delivery, growth restriction, and congenital anomalies** (seen in up to 25% of monoamniotic twin pregnancies) **but mostly to umbilical cord entanglement and cord accidents** (Fig. 32-9). Some degree of umbilical cord entanglement is present in virtually every monoamniotic twin pregnancy. More recent series of prenatally diagnosed cases suggest improved perinatal outcomes with mortality rates in the range of 7% to

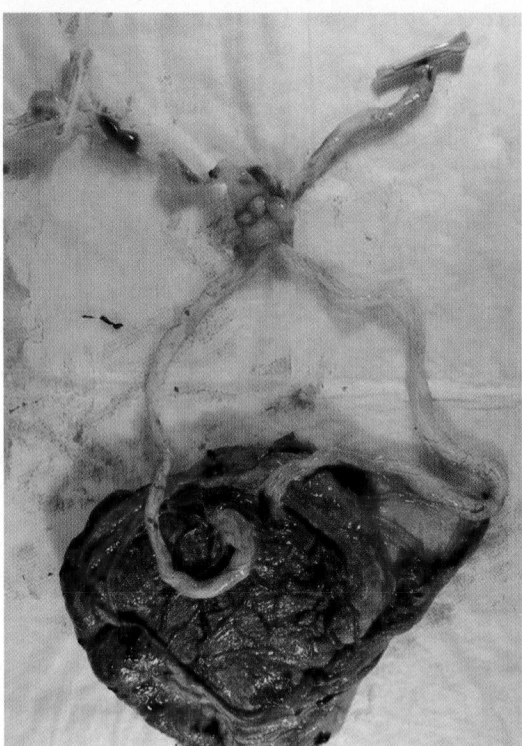

FIG 32-9 Entangled cords found during emergent cesarean delivery in a case of monochorionic monoamniotic twins at 32 weeks. Both babies did well.

20%[60-64] and as low as 2.4% to 2.8% when fetuses with anomalies are excluded.[65,66] **This improvement is likely due to prenatal diagnosis, use of antenatal corticosteroids, increased fetal surveillance, and elective early delivery.** Because cord accidents are the primary cause of fetal death, most management protocols emphasize intense fetal surveillance to identify significant umbilical cord constriction before fetal loss.

Rodis and coworkers[64] reviewed 13 cases of monoamnionicity at one tertiary care center over a 10-year period. All patients underwent serial ultrasound examinations and antenatal fetal surveillance two to seven times per week starting between 24 and 26 weeks' gestation, and 62% of the pregnancies were delivered for abnormal fetal testing. If undelivered earlier, all patients were delivered by cesarean delivery by 35 weeks' gestation. No fetal deaths were reported, and the mean gestational age at delivery was 32.9 weeks. Compared with 77 sets of monoamniotic twins from the literature that had not been diagnosed prenatally, these patients had a 71% reduction in the relative risk for perinatal mortality.

A more recent study evaluated the impact of routine hospitalization for fetal monitoring on perinatal survival and neonatal morbidity in a multicenter retrospective cohort study of 96 monoamniotic twin gestations.[61] Of 87 women with both twins surviving at 24 weeks, 43 patients were admitted electively at a median gestational age of 26.5 weeks for **inpatient surveillance and fetal testing two to three times daily.** The remaining 44 women were followed as outpatients with fetal testing one to three times weekly. None of the hospitalized patients experienced an IUFD, but 14.8% (13 of 88) of the fetuses of mothers followed as outpatients were stillborn. Statistically significant improvements in birthweight, gestational age at delivery, and neonatal morbidity were also noted among the electively hospitalized women. Two other smaller studies[67,68] have also compared inpatient with outpatient management and have found similar results. These studies suggest that **improved neonatal survival and decreased perinatal morbidity are achievable with monoamniotic twins admitted electively for daily fetal monitoring after viability, and we recommend offering hospital admission to all women with monoamniotic twins.**

The timing of admission should be the gestational age at which the mother would desire delivery for evidence of fetal compromise, generally 24 to 28 weeks. We obtain preadmission consultation with a neonatologist to discuss complications from prematurity at various gestational ages. After admission, we prophylactically administer antenatal corticosteroids because of the possibility of emergent delivery.

Some institutions perform continuous fetal monitoring in women electively admitted for monoamniotic twins. In actual practice, however, true continuous monitoring is never achievable. Quinn and colleagues[69] reviewed over 10,000 hours of fetal monitoring of monoamniotic twins and found that both fetuses were successfully monitored only 51.6% of the time. **We do not perform continuous monitoring, rather we recommend fetal heart rate (FHR) monitoring two or three times per day for 1 to 2 hours.** Although cord accidents cannot be predicted, FHR monitoring may reveal an increasing frequency of variable decelerations. If these are identified, continuous monitoring is recommended along with emergency delivery for worsening or nonreassuring fetal status. In the absence of nonreassuring fetal testing, the timing of elective delivery is not well established by prospective data. Multiple papers over the past 10 years have demonstrated a continued risk of sudden IUFD throughout gestation. Because of this continuing risk of unexpected fetal death, **most experts perform elective delivery following the administration of antenatal corticosteroid therapy between 32 and 34 weeks' gestation. Delivery at 32 to 34 weeks is associated with a low risk of serious neonatal morbidity counterbalanced against the unpredictable continuing IUFD risk.** Van Mieghem and colleagues[62] evaluated fetal and neonatal outcomes in 193 monoamniotic twin pairs managed

at eight European university hospitals between 2003 and 2012. In this study, the overall risk of fetal death was 18.1%, but of the 144 gestations with 2 live fetuses at 26 weeks' gestation, only 8 fetal deaths were reported. They compared the risk of IUFD to the risk of neonatal morbidity/mortality and calculated that the risk of IUFD exceeded the risk of a nonrespiratory neonatal complication at 32 weeks 4 days gestation. These researchers concluded that with close fetal surveillance instituted between 26 and 28 weeks of gestation and delivery at 33 weeks of gestation, the risk of stillbirth—as well as the risk of neonatal death or serious complication—is minimized.

The 2011 NICHD and SMFM workshop that addressed timing of indicated late-preterm and early-term birth recommended delivery of monoamniotic twins at 32 to 34 weeks.[36] The 2014 ACOG Practice Bulletin on multifetal gestation also acknowledges the limitations of the available evidence on management and delivery timing for monoamniotic twin gestations, but it states that delivery between 32 and 34 weeks is reasonable.[37]

Cesarean delivery has been recommended to eliminate the risk of intrapartum cord accidents, although vaginal delivery of these patients is not entirely contraindicated if careful fetal monitoring is performed. On the other hand, there have been case reports of a nuchal cord affecting the first twin being cut to facilitate delivery, only to discover that the cut cord actually belonged to the second twin. Given this issue and a high incidence of intrapartum nonreassuring fetal testing, **most experts recommend cesarean delivery for monoamniotic twin pregnancies.**

Twin Reversed Arterial Perfusion Sequence

The TRAP sequence, also known as *acardiac twinning*, is a malformation that occurs only in monochorionic pregnancies with a frequency of about 1 per 30,000 deliveries and 1 in 100 monochorionic twins. An acardiac twin is an extremely malformed fetus with either no heart at all or only rudimentary cardiac tissue in association with multiple other developmental abnormalities (Fig. 32-10). In about one third of acardiac twins,

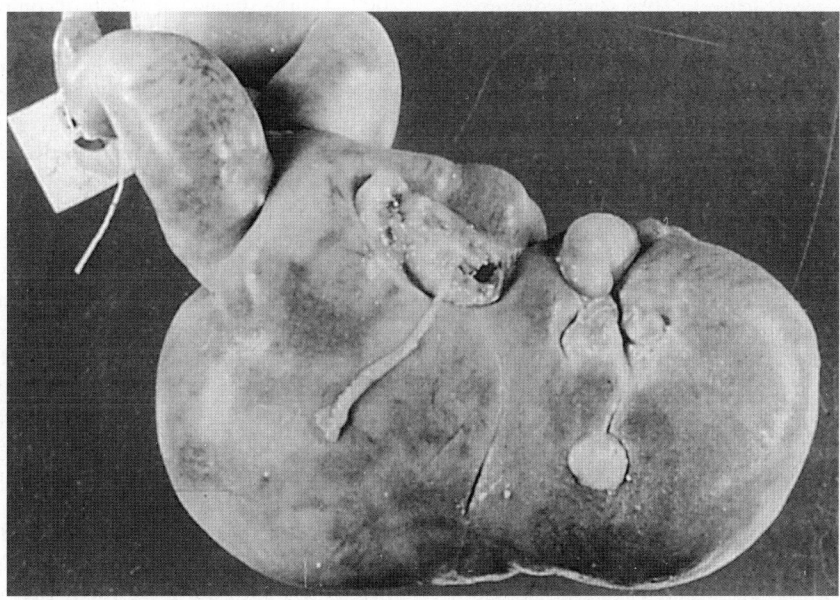

FIG 32-10 Acardiac twin. (Courtesy Dr. James Wheeler, Department of Surgical Pathology, Hospital of the University of Pennsylvania, Philadelphia.)

the karyotype has been found to be abnormal. A two-vessel cord is present in two thirds of acardiac twins, and polyhydramnios has been reported in around 70% of cases. The co-twin, referred to as the *pump twin,* is generally normal, although a 9% risk of aneuploidy has been reported.[70]

Patients with TRAP sequence have a monochorionic placenta with vascular anastomoses that sustain the life of the acardiac twin. The acardiac twin is perfused via direct UA-UA anastomosis at the placental surface. Blood flows from the normal pump twin's UAs back to the placenta. Then through this UA anastomosis, deoxygenated blood flows directly to the acardiac twin without passing through a placental capillary bed. In the acardiac twin's umbilical arteries, flow is thus retrograde, creating the TRAP sequence. **This poorly oxygenated blood preferentially perfuses the acardiac twin's lower body, contributing to the bizarre anomalies seen in acardiac fetuses.**

Antenatal diagnosis by ultrasound of an acardiac fetus coexisting with a normal co-twin is fairly straightforward, but **color Doppler is essential.** The only other entity in the differential diagnosis is an IUFD of one twin. However, continued growth of the abnormal, presumed dead twin rules this out, as does demonstration of umbilical blood flow in the presumed dead twin by color Doppler. Additionally, retrograde flow can be demonstrated to occur through the UAs.

The acardiac twin clearly has no chance of survival, but its presence is not innocuous for the normal pump twin. The pump twin is at increased risk for in utero cardiac failure and preterm delivery. In the absence of intervention, mortality rates of 50% or higher have been reported.[71] **The estimated weight of the acardiac twin** (calculated using the formula $1.2L^2 - 1.7L =$ weight in grams, where L is the longest dimension) **relative to the normal twin is an important prognostic factor.** Moore and colleagues[71] reported on a series of 49 pregnancies complicated by TRAP sequence. Other than four therapeutic amniocenteses, none of the pregnancies underwent invasive therapies. They reported 90% preterm delivery, 40% polyhydramnios, and 30% cardiac failure of the normal pump twin when the weight ratio of the acardiac to normal pump twin was more than 70%, compared with 75% preterm delivery, 30% polyhydramnios, and 10% cardiac failure for the normal pump twin when the weight ratio was less than 70%. In that same series, no pump twins had cardiac failure when the weight ratio was less than 50%. Among all 49 cases in the series, the mean gestational age at delivery was 29 weeks, and the mean birthweight of the pump twin was 1378 g.

When faced with a monochorionic pregnancy complicated by TRAP sequence, three options are available: (1) expectant management, (2) delivery, or (3) interruption of the vascular communication between the twins. Many experts use a ratio of weight of acardiac twin to weight of pump twin of 0.5 (50%) as a criterion for invasive intervention. Other factors that suggest a need for intervention are hydrops, polyhydramnios, and abdominal circumference of the acardiac twin greater than or equal to that of the pump twin.

Expectant management is reasonable in the absence of poor prognostic features, and good survival rates have been reported (88% in one series) when the weight ratio of the acardiac to pump twin is 50% or less.[72] If expectant management is undertaken, weekly surveillance that includes fetal echocardiography is recommended. Delivery may be indicated if signs of cardiac decompensation are noted at a viable gestational age. In the face

of poor prognostic features remote from term, interruption of the vascular communication between the twins should be considered. This intervention is most commonly performed between 16 and 26 weeks. Current treatment modalities include occlusion of the acardiac twin's umbilical cord by bipolar cord coagulation, laser ablation, or RFA. The optimal treatment approach has not yet been definitively determined.

A recent meta-analysis of intrafetal laser treatment for TRAP sequence found an 82% survival rate for the pump twin. The median gestational age at delivery was 37 weeks and 1 day.[73] A report by the North American Fetal Therapy Network (NAFTNet)[74] on outcomes for all patients ($n = 98$) who underwent RFA for TRAP at NAFTNet institutions between 1998 and 2008 found an 80% overall survival to 30 days of life for pump twins with a median gestational age at delivery of 37 weeks 0 days.

Conjoined Twins

Conjoined twins are another rare complication of MZ twinning. They are believed to occur when a single embryo incompletely divides between 13 and 15 days after fertilization instead of splitting earlier. This event gives rise to monochorionic monoamniotic placentation with conjoined fetuses, and it occurs with a frequency of about 1 in 50,000 pregnancies. Most conjoined twins are female, with a reported female/male ratio of 2:1 or 3:1.

Conjoined twins are classified according to their site of union. The most common location is the chest (thoracopagus), followed by the anterior abdominal wall (omphalopagus), the buttocks (pygopagus), the ischium (ischiopagus), and the head (cephalopagus; Fig. 32-11 and Videos 32-1 and 32-2). Organs are shared to varying degrees. Major congenital anomalies of one or both twins are common, and polyhydramnios is present in almost half of the reported cases of conjoined twins.

The mortality rate is high, as evidenced by a retrospective case series from the Children's Hospital of Philadelphia.[75] That series identified an incidence of 28% intrauterine death, 54% early neonatal death, and 18% overall survival among 14 sets of conjoined twins managed at their institution between 1996 and 2002. Another series[76] of 36 sets of conjoined twins from a single center in Brazil between 1998 and 2010 reported similar results: after excluding the nearly 40% who underwent termination of pregnancy, the survival rate was 13.6%.

Ultrasound can establish this diagnosis in utero as early as the first trimester based on visualization of monoamnionicity and a bifid fetal pole. Three-dimensional ultrasound, color Doppler, fetal echocardiography, and MRI can be used to complement two-dimensional ultrasound imaging to confirm the diagnosis, determine the extent of organ sharing, and definitively classify the type of conjoined twinning. If the diagnosis is confirmed before viability, pregnancy termination should be offered. **If the patient desires expectant management, she should be counseled that the prognosis for survival and successful separation depends on the degree of organ and vascular sharing between the two fetuses, especially the heart.** Multimodality fetal evaluation as previously described should be used prenatally to survey fetal anatomy. **To optimize postnatal management, patients with conjoined twins should be cared for by a multidisciplinary team during the antenatal period, including maternal-fetal medicine specialists, neonatologists, pediatric anesthesiologists, pediatric surgeons, and appropriate pediatric subspecialists.**

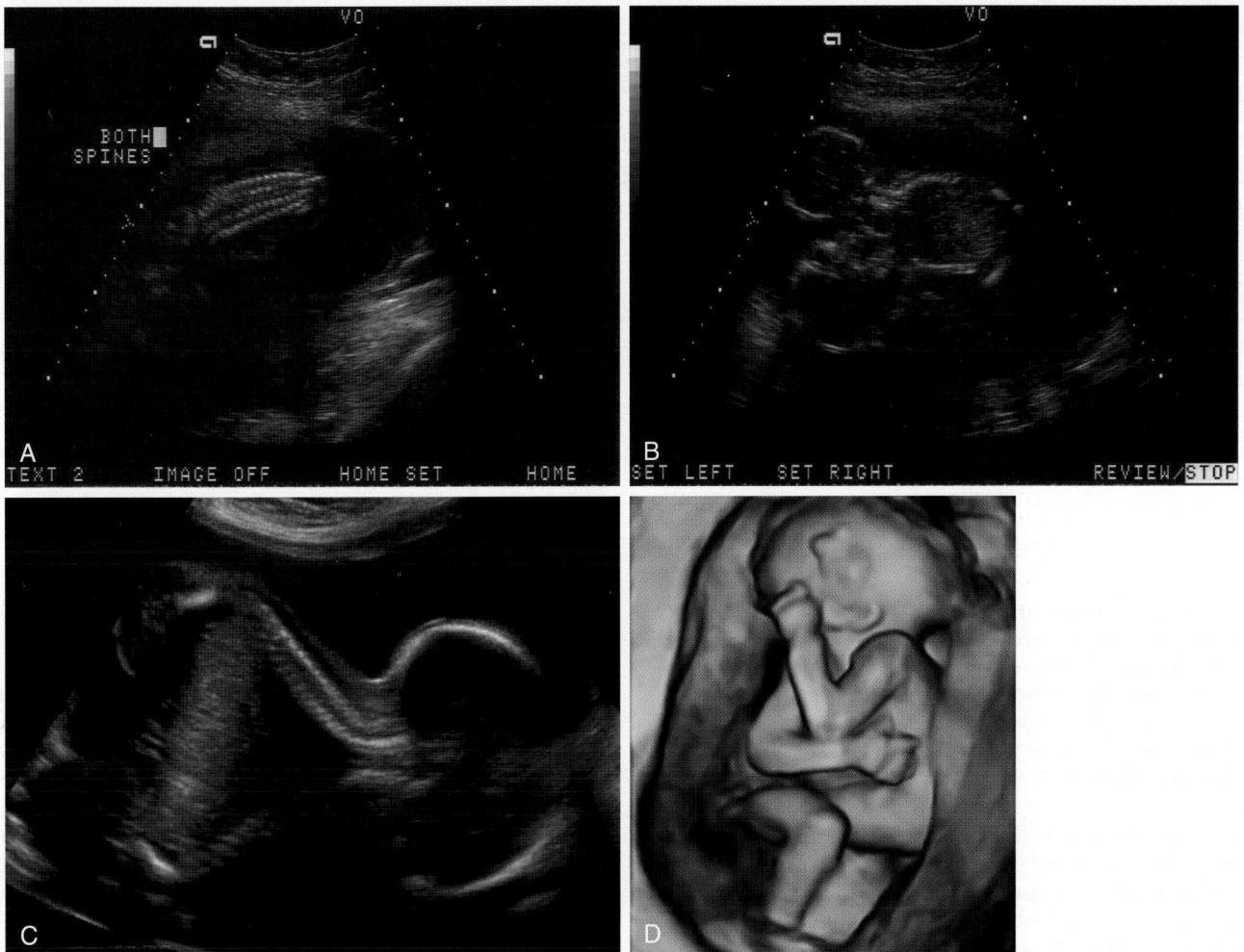

FIG 32-11 A and **B,** Late first-trimester images of thoracopagus conjoined twins. This twin set had one trunk with two parallel spinal columns (**A**) leading to two separate necks and heads (**B**). **C** and **D,** Cephalopagus conjoined twins with a single cranium but two separate spines, conjoined to the level just above the pelvis. (This case is depicted in Videos 32-1 and 32-2.)

If any evaluation and treatment beyond palliation is planned, patients with conjoined twins should deliver at a tertiary care facility where neonatal and pediatric specialists with experience in the care of conjoined twins are available. Cesarean delivery near term will be necessary to minimize maternal and fetal injury. For conjoined twins, a mean gestational age at delivery of 34 to 35 weeks has been reported.[75,76] If the twins are believed to be nonviable and are believed to be small enough to pass through the birth canal without traumatizing the mother, vaginal delivery can be considered. In the above mentioned series from Brazil, all conjoined twins at less than 27 weeks' gestation were delivered vaginally.

Of conjoined twins who are deemed appropriate for and survive to undergo elective separation, survival rates approach 80%. If conjoined twins require emergent separation, however, survival rates are much lower, around 25% to 30%.[77] Although the long-term follow-up of conjoined twins who have undergone successful surgical separation is limited, the data seem favorable. Survivors frequently require additional surgeries following the initial separation, but many achieve educational levels similar to their singleton peers.

ANTEPARTUM MANAGEMENT OF MULTIFETAL PREGNANCY
Maternal Nutrition and Weight Gain

The two factors that most influence pregnancy outcome are gestational age at delivery and the adequacy of fetal growth. Nutritional status during gestation is closely linked to both these outcomes. The increased physiologic stress of a multifetal pregnancy demands **a 10% higher maternal resting energy expenditure.** To meet this heightened metabolic expenditure, multiple gestations require modification of the caloric intake and weight gain recommendations established for singleton pregnancies. **The higher risks of LBW, PTB, and neonatal complications in twin pregnancies create a situation in which enhancement of maternal nutrition has the potential to provide tremendous positive impact.**

Both total maternal weight gain and the timing of that weight gain are critical to optimizing twin birthweight and perinatal outcomes. Luke and colleagues[78] have shown **that weight gain before 28 weeks accounts for 80% of the effects of maternal weight gain on infant birthweights.** Underscoring this point,

TABLE 32-7 RECOMMENDED RATES OF MATERNAL WEIGHT GAIN IN TWIN PREGNANCIES

GESTATIONAL AGE PERIOD	UNDERWEIGHT (BMI <19.8)	NORMAL WEIGHT (BMI 19.8-26)	OVERWEIGHT (BMI 26.1-29)	OBESE (BMI >29)
Early (<20 wk)	1.25-1.75 lb/wk	1-1.5 lb/wk	1-1.25 lb/wk	0.75-1 lb/wk
Mid (21-28 wk)	1.5-1.75 lb/wk	1.25-1.75 lb/wk	1-1.5 lb/wk	0.75-1.25 lb/wk
Late (≥29 wk)	1.25 lb/wk	1 lb/wk	1 lb/wk	0.75 lb/wk

From Luke B, Hediger ML, Nugent C, et al. Body mass index–specific weight gains associated with optimal birth weights in twin pregnancies. *J Reprod Med.* 2003;48:217-224.
BMI, body mass index.

TABLE 32-8 2009 INSTITUTE OF MEDICINE RECOMMENDATIONS FOR WEIGHT GAIN IN PREGNANCY

PREPREGNANCY BMI	BMI (kg/m²) WHO CRITERIA	TOTAL WEIGHT GAIN SINGLETON (lb)	TOTAL WEIGHT GAIN TWINS (lb)
Underweight	<18.5	28-40	No recommendations made
Normal weight	18.5-24.9	25-35	37-54
Overweight	25.0-29.9	15-25	31-50
Obese	≥30.0	11-20	25-42

From Rasmussen KM, Yaktine AL, editors. *Institute of Medicine (Committee to Reexamine IOM Pregnancy Weight Guidelines, Food and Nutrition Board and Board on Children, Youth, and Families). Weight Gain During Pregnancy: Reexamining the Guidelines.* Washington, DC: National Academies Press; 2009.
BMI, body mass index; *WHO,* World Health Organization.

these researchers demonstrated that even when weight gain is appropriate after 24 weeks, suboptimal gain before 24 weeks is still associated with earlier delivery and poor intrauterine growth. Body mass index (BMI)–specific weight gain patterns associated with ideal twin pregnancy outcomes, defined as a birthweight of 2850 to 2950 g at 36 weeks or later, are summarized in Table 32-7. Although the BMI categories used are slightly different from current BMI definitions, the differences in recommended weight gain by BMI category can easily be appreciated. Compared with singleton gestations, **these recommended rates of weight gain are more than double early in pregnancy** (0 to 20 weeks), **about 50% higher during mid-pregnancy** (20 to 28 weeks), **and about 25% higher late in gestation** (28 to 38 weeks).[79]

The crucial role of early weight gain and the pronounced benefits of appropriate weight gain in underweight women suggest that **early weight gain provides improved maternal nutrient stores for use later in pregnancy when fetal demands increase. Additionally, optimal maternal nutrition and weight gain early in pregnancy may enhance placental growth,** thus providing a better ongoing nutrient supply to the babies. Both of these mechanisms may explain why adequate weight gain in late pregnancy after inadequate gain in early pregnancy does not provide complete recovery in either fetal growth or outcomes. The implementation of these nutritional principles as part of an enhanced nutritional clinical program for twins at the University of Michigan was associated with improvements in virtually all important obstetric and neonatal outcomes in a prospective cohort trial.[80]

Using the data published by Luke and colleagues but with slight changes in the BMI categories, the Institute of Medicine (IOM) issued new BMI-specific weight-gain recommendations for twin pregnancy in 2009; these recommendations are summarized in Table 32-8. Several studies have examined perinatal outcomes using the IOM recommendations for maternal weight gain and have found improved outcomes among women who meet the IOM weight-gain goals. For instance, Fox and coworkers[81] retrospectively studied a cohort of 297 twin pregnancies from a private maternal-fetal medicine practice, applying the 2009 IOM guidelines to compare pregnancy outcomes between those women who achieved or failed to achieve these

recommendations. They found that women with a prepregnancy BMI in the normal or overweight categories who met the weight-gain recommendations demonstrated significantly better outcomes. **Normal-weight women who achieved the IOM weight-gain recommendations had significantly larger babies and a greater likelihood of babies weighing more than 2500 g.** Overweight women who met the weight-gain recommendations had more advanced gestational ages at delivery and a heavier weight of the larger twin. Both normal-weight and overweight women who met weight-gain goals had reductions in both overall and spontaneous PTB. Notably, the IOM guidelines do not provide a specific weight-gain recommendation for women with an underweight prepregnancy BMI who are pregnant with twins. However, because the singleton literature clearly demonstrates that underweight women benefit the most from optimal gestational weight gain, special attention should be given to nutritional counseling and achievement of weight-gain goals in this population.

Although increased maternal weight gain during pregnancy is associated with improved outcomes, maternal weight retention and its long-term health effects are also a concern. Therefore in the setting of multiple gestation, emphasis should be placed on appropriate weight gain, while avoiding gains that exceed the IOM recommendations.

Spontaneous Preterm Birth

Patients with a multiple gestation are at significant risk for preterm labor and delivery. **Refining the risk for PTB in each individual patient improves pregnancy management by selecting those patients who may benefit most from increased surveillance and interventions while simultaneously minimizing unnecessary interventions in lower-risk women.**

The use of ultrasound transvaginal cervical length (TVCL) measurements and fetal fibronectin (fFN) sampling can help stratify PTB risk in multiple gestations. A 2010 meta-analysis that included 21 studies with a total of 3523 women pregnant with twins found that in asymptomatic women, a **TVCL of 20 mm or less between 20 and 24 weeks' gestation was the best predictor of PTB before 32 and before 34 weeks.** A TVCL of 20 mm or less increased the probability of birth before 32 weeks from 6.8% to 42.4% and increased the risk of birth before

34 weeks from 15.3% to 61.9%. At a gestational age of 20 to 24 weeks, a TVCL of 25 mm or less increased the risk of delivery before 32 weeks from 3.5% to 25.8%, and it increased the risk of delivery before 37 weeks from 41.2% to 75.5%. A TVCL of 25 mm or more reduced the risk of delivery before 28 weeks to 1.4% and the risk of delivery before 37 weeks to 36.8%.[82]

In addition to the absolute cervical length (CL), **the degree of change in the cervical length over time may also be an important predictor of PTB in twins**. Fox and coworkers[83] studied a historical cohort of 121 asymptomatic twin pregnancies who had two TVCL measurements taken 2 to 6 weeks apart between 18 and 24 weeks' gestation. They found that CL shortening of 20% or more over this interval was associated with a greater risk for PTB before 28, 30, 32, and 34 weeks compared with women whose CL remained stable (15.8% vs. 1% at <28 weeks, 15.8% vs. 2% at <30 weeks, 31.6% vs. 5% at <32 weeks, and 36.8% vs. 12.9% at <34 weeks; all P values $\leq$ .03). Most striking was the fact that this association with PTB remained significant even when patients with a CL less than 25 mm were excluded.

Fetal fibronectin has also been studied as a predictor of spontaneous PTB risk in multifetal pregnancies. A 2010 meta-analysis[84] that included 15 studies with a total of 1221 women found that **in symptomatic mothers of twins, fFN had good predictive value**. A positive fFN in this setting increased the risk of delivery within 7 days of testing from 7.7% to 24.5%, and a negative result decreased the risk of delivery within 7 days to 1.6%.

The use of these tests can help guide management decisions, such as frequency of office visits or whether work or activity restriction is prudent. Identification of a patient at particularly high risk for preterm delivery based on her CL, fFN, or a combination of the two can allow for heightened surveillance and may permit timely interventions such as tocolysis or steroid administration. On the other hand, documentation of an above-average (>35 mm) or stable CL in midgestation can allow both patient and physician to feel comfortable with a patient continuing with her normal activities, avoiding the temptation to implement unnecessary restrictions or interventions.

Unfortunately, although studies such as those mentioned above allow us to determine which multiple gestations are at greatest risk for spontaneous PTB, limited options are available to prevent PTB. Of note, however, few PTB prevention studies have been carried out in the highest-risk multiple gestations based on transvaginal CLs or a positive fFN. The following section discusses the relative merits of proposed interventions to prevent spontaneous PTB in multiple gestations.

Bed Rest and Hospitalization

A Cochrane review[85] analyzed seven randomized trials that included 713 women and 1426 babies and concluded that **routine hospitalized bed rest was not associated with a decrease in PTB in multifetal pregnancies**. A trend toward fewer LBW babies was noted (RR, 0.92; 95% CI, 0.85 to 1.00), although this trend did not extend to VLBW infants. Because no evidence suggests that routine hospitalization is beneficial for patients with multiples, these women should be hospitalized only for the same obstetric indications as singletons. **For asymptomatic twin pregnancies in women with a reassuring CL and no prior history of PTB, we do not recommend either cessation of work or rest at home.**

Tocolysis

Prophylactic tocolysis has been evaluated in multiple gestations and was not found to be effective. In contrast, short-term use of agents for acute tocolysis in preterm labor is helpful to gain time for administration of corticosteroids to enhance fetal lung maturity and allow transport to a tertiary care facility. Tocolytic use in multiple gestations, however, must be accompanied by careful monitoring of the maternal condition. Because of the exaggerated maternal cardiovascular adaptations to a multiple gestation, women pregnant with multiples are predisposed to cardiopulmonary complications, most notably pulmonary edema. This risk is heightened with β-adrenergic agents and when tocolytics are used in combination with corticosteroids and intravenous fluids. **In 2011, the U.S. Food and Drug Administration (FDA) issued a boxed warning on terbutaline, stating that it should not be used in an injectable form beyond 48 to 72 hours to treat preterm labor—and that it should not be used *at all* in an oral form—because of the potential for serious maternal cardiovascular problems and death.** Because of the FDA warning and known higher risks of tocolysis in multifetal pregnancies, use of terbutaline in multiple gestations should be discouraged. **At our institution, intravenous magnesium sulfate is used as a first-line acute tocolytic.** When needed in patients before 32 weeks' gestation, we add oral indomethacin for 48 hours. After 32 weeks, we have also used short-acting nifedipine for tocolysis, assuming the maternal blood pressure tolerates its use.

Progesterone

INTRAMUSCULAR 17-HYDROXYPROGESTERONE CAPROATE

After 17-hydroxyprogesterone caproate (17-OH-P) was shown to be effective in reducing recurrent PTB in singletons, there was interest in using it in populations with other risk factors for spontaneous preterm delivery, such as multiple gestations. Numerous RCTs have been done using 17-OH-P in doses that range from 250 mg weekly, the dose proven effective in singleton gestations, to 500 mg twice weekly in multifetal gestations. Most of the twin populations were unselected, but one study[86] enrolled only women with a TVCL of 25 mm or less. **None of these studies have shown any benefit associated with the use of 17-OH-P in multiple gestation.**[86-90] An interesting dilemma arises when caring for a woman pregnant with multiples who has had a prior singleton spontaneous PTB. Unfortunately, no data exist to inform decision making on whether to offer weekly 17-OH-P in this scenario.

VAGINAL PROGESTERONE

Vaginally administered progesterone has been shown in multiple studies to be beneficial in prolonging gestation in singleton pregnancies with a short cervix. Vaginal progesterone is recommended by ACOG as a management option in asymptomatic women with a singleton gestation and incidentally identified CL of 20 mm or less prior to 24 weeks of gestation. The 2007 trial by Fonseca and associates[91] examined the effect of nightly vaginal progesterone in women with a short midgestation CL and included twin gestations, although twins made up only 10.4% ($n = 13$) of the placebo group and 8.8% ($n = 11$) of the treatment group. This study randomized women with a transvaginal CL of 15 mm or less at a median of 22 weeks' gestation to either 200 mg of vaginal progesterone or placebo. They found that administration of nightly vaginal progesterone decreased spontaneous delivery before 34 weeks from 34.3% to 19.2%

($P < .05$). In the subgroup of twin gestations, vaginal progesterone was associated with a similar reduction in preterm delivery, although the difference did not reach statistical significance because of the small sample size. Since publication of that paper, multiple RCTs have examined the use of vaginal progesterone gel 90 mg daily or vaginal micronized progesterone suppositories in doses that ranged from 100 to 400 mg daily in women pregnant with multiples.[92-97] **None of the studies that enrolled only multiple gestations showed an improvement in the primary outcome, but the study by Cetingoz and colleagues[93] that enrolled women at high risk for PTB** (of whom 40% in the placebo group and 48.7% in the daily 100-mg micronized vaginal progesterone group had twins) **found a statistically significant increase in the risk of delivery before 37 weeks** (3.48; 95% CI, 1.16 to 10.46)**, but not before 34 weeks, in twin gestations in which the mother received placebo compared with those who received progesterone.**[93] None of these studies enrolled the highest-risk multiple gestations based on TVCL or other factors such as prior spontaneous PTB.

Two meta-analyses have been published that help distill the results of these various studies that have examined the use of intramuscular and vaginal progesterone in multifetal gestations. The first is a 2012 meta-analysis of individual patient data by Romero and colleagues[98] that included five trials of vaginal progesterone in women with an asymptomatic short cervix in the midtrimester. Overall, the five trials included 775 women and 827 infants. **In the subgroup of women with a twin gestation, the investigators found a nonsignificant 30% reduction in the rate of PTB before 33 weeks in women given progesterone compared with those who received placebo** (RR, 0.70; 95% CI, 0.34 to 1.44), **and a statistically significant reduction in composite adverse neonatal outcomes** (RR, 0.52; 95% CI, 0.29 to 0.93).

The more recent individual patient data meta-analysis evaluated the effectiveness of progesterone in improving twin pregnancy outcomes and included 13 trials with 3768 women and 7536 babies.[99] The primary outcome was a composite of perinatal mortality and severe neonatal morbidity. The results demonstrated no reduction in adverse outcome with either 17-OH-P or vaginal progesterone in the overall analysis. However, in a subgroup analysis of women with twins and a TVCL of 25 mm or less who received vaginal progesterone, a statistically significant reduction was seen in adverse perinatal outcome (RR, 0.56; 95% CI, 0.42 to 0.75) when TVCL was measured prior to 24 weeks.

The authors' interpretation of the available literature on progesterone to prevent PTB in twins is that no evidence is available to support the use of intramuscular 17-OH-P in any multifetal gestation, nor should any form of progesterone be used in unselected multiple pregnancies. However, although more study is needed to confirm this finding, because of the evidence of neonatal benefit in twin pregnancies with a TVCL of 25 mm or less, vaginal progesterone should be offered to these women. Evidence is insufficient to support a specific dose or to support gel versus a micronized progesterone suppository.

Cerclage

Results of studies using cervical cerclage to prolong pregnancy in multiple gestations have been disappointing. **Prophylactic cerclage has been studied and was found to be ineffective in both twins and triplets.** Even in the presence of cervical shortening, no clear benefit of cerclage placement in patients with twins has been demonstrated. Newman and coworkers[100] prospectively followed 147 twin pregnancies in women who underwent transvaginal ultrasonographic CL measurements between 18 and 26 weeks' gestation. Cerclage was offered to all 33 women with a transvaginal cervical length of 25 mm or less, and a cerclage was placed in 21 women. No differences were reported between the cerclage and no-cerclage groups with regard to length of gestation, birthweight, delivery before 34 weeks, PPROM, or VLBW. A 2005 meta-analysis of ultrasound-indicated cerclage found that in the subgroup with twins, cerclage placement was actually associated with a statistically significant increase in birth before 35 weeks (75% vs. 36%).[101] Because cerclage is a surgical procedure that may be associated with adverse sequelae for both the mother and her fetuses, it is recommended that **cerclage placement in multiple gestations be restricted to women with either a strongly suggestive history of cervical insufficiency or objectively documented cervical insufficiency based on physical examination. Neither prophylactic nor ultrasound-indicated cerclage are of benefit in multifetal gestations.**

Pessary

In the last few years, there has been renewed interest in pessary placement for prevention of spontaneous PTB. The Cervical Pessary in Pregnant Women with a Short Cervix (PECEP) study, an RCT of pessary versus expectant management in singleton pregnancies with a TVCL less than 25 mm at a mean gestational age of 22 weeks, showed a reduction in birth before 34 weeks as well as an improvement in neonatal outcomes in the pessary group.[102] Pessary use has also been studied in a prospective RCT of multifetal gestations conducted in 40 centers in the Netherlands. The ProTWIN trial[103] randomized 813 women pregnant with multiple gestations, of which 98% were twins, to either expectant management or pessary placement. Fifty-five percent of women in both groups were nulliparous, and only 7% in the pessary group and 6% in the control group had a prior spontaneous PTB. TVCL was measured between 16 and 22 weeks. Only 1% of women in both groups had funneling, and the median TVCL was 43.6 mm in the pessary group and 44.2 mm in the control group. **In the overall analysis, no difference was seen in neonatal outcomes; gestational age at delivery; or delivery before 28 weeks, 32 weeks, or 37 weeks between women randomized to pessary and those randomized to expectant management.** The study had originally included a planned a priori analysis of all women with TVCL less than 25 mm, but because very few women met this criterion, that analysis was changed to TVCL below the 25th percentile. When the analysis was restricted to women with TVCL below the 25th percentile, which corresponded to 38 mm, median gestational age at delivery was longer in the pessary group than in the control group (36.4 vs. 35.0 weeks, $P < .05$). Pessary use was associated with a reduced risk of delivery before 28 weeks (OR, 0.23; 95% CI, 0.06 to 0.87) and before 32 weeks (OR, 0.49; 95% CI, 0.24 to 0.97) but not before 37 weeks (OR, 0.82; 95% CI, 0.54 to 1.24) in the group of women with TVCL below the 25th percentile. Additionally, among women with a shorter cervix at enrollment, the risk of a composite adverse neonatal outcome was decreased in the pessary group (OR, 0.40; 95% CI, 0.19 to 0.83). The results of this study show that pessary placement is not effective in prolonging gestation or improving outcomes when used routinely in twin pregnancies, but **the subgroup analysis of women** with TVCL below the 25th percentile suggests that pessary could be effective in women pregnant with twins who also have a short cervix. In the 2014 Practice Bulletin on Multifetal Gestation, ACOG cites the ProTWIN study and concludes that "based on available evidence, the use of prophylactic cervical pessary is not recommended in multifetal pregnancies."[37] Further study is needed to determine whether pessary use could be of value in multifetal pregnancies with a short cervix, a population in which evidence-based interventions are lacking.

Antenatal Testing

Multiple gestations are at increased risk for uteroplacental insufficiency, IUGR, and stillbirth; for this reason, antenatal surveillance in the form of nonstress tests (NSTs) or biophysical profiles (BPPs) is often performed. Retrospective data show that both NSTs and BPPs can effectively detect compromised twin gestations and can be interpreted the same as in singletons. However, any recommendations on specific surveillance protocols are based on expert opinion, because no prospective data are available upon which to base a recommendation. **ACOG does not recommend antenatal testing for uncomplicated dichorionic twins, but the 2014 ACOG practice bulletin on antenatal testing does list monochorionicity as an indication, although no specific testing schedule is suggested.**[104] In the United States, most institutions perform weekly or twice weekly antenatal testing on monochorionic twins starting at around 32 to 34 weeks. Although ACOG does not list dichorionic twins as an indication for routine antenatal testing, **the authors feel it is reasonable to perform routine weekly NSTs or BPPs in this population, in part because of the limitations in detection of IUGR.** The 2009 NICHD reevaluation of antenatal testing does not specify by chorionicity, but they list weekly testing at 32 weeks as a reasonable strategy for twins with normal fetal growth.[105] **At the authors' institutions, weekly NST or BPP is initiated at 32 weeks for monochorionic diamniotic twins and at 34 weeks for dichorionic twins.** More frequent or earlier onset of testing is initiated for twins with additional complications such as IUGR, discordant growth, or underlying maternal medical disorders such as diabetes or hypertension.

Even fewer data are available for triplet and higher-order multiple gestations. However, because the stillbirth risk increases with increasing plurality, it is reasonable to begin antenatal testing earlier for triplets than for twins. **The 2009 NICHD document lists initiation of antenatal testing at 28 weeks as a reasonable strategy for triplets.**[105] **We preferentially perform BPPs instead of NSTs in triplets or higher plurality because of the difficulty in consistently and efficiently obtaining and interpreting NSTs with more than two fetuses.**

Fetal Growth Surveillance

Although ultrasound is an imperfect predictor of fetal weight, it is the only method available for assessing individual fetal growth in multiple gestations. Data indicate that **twins grow at the same rate as singletons until 30 to 32 weeks gestation, after which their growth velocity slows compared with singletons.**[106-108] A study that used 1991 to 1995 National Center for Health Statistics data found that singleton, twin, and triplet birthweights prior to 28 weeks gestation were similar regardless of plurality. However, by 30 weeks gestation, differences in birthweights began to be identified. By 32 weeks, the median birthweight in twins and triplets was reduced by 300 g and 450 g, respectively, compared with singletons.[106] A retrospective study in Scotland studied all twins ($n = 131$) delivered at a single institution between 1994 and 1996. Each pregnancy had ultrasounds every 2 to 3 weeks after 24 weeks to assess fetal growth, and growth velocities were calculated. The study found that biparietal diameter (BPD) and abdominal area growth velocities slowed significantly after 30 weeks. This slowing of growth was present regardless of whether the pregnancy subsequently delivered preterm.[107] A prospective longitudinal study of 162 twin pregnancies that underwent ultrasound assessment of fetal growth every 2 weeks starting at 16 weeks gestation reported slowing of growth velocities for BPD, femur length (FL), and abdominal circumference (AC) after 32 weeks.[108]

Formulas developed specifically for ultrasound estimation of twin fetal weights have been studied, but these twin formulas have not proven to be superior to standard singleton formulas typically used. **It is recommended that twin fetal weights should be estimated using singleton formulas, taking into account multiple biometric parameters. Additionally, because growth is a dynamic process, patients with multifetal gestations should be followed throughout pregnancy. It is recommended that all patients with twins undergo ultrasound evaluation of fetal growth at least every 4 weeks after 20 weeks and more frequently if IUGR or growth discordance is suspected. Additionally, ultrasounds should be performed every 2 weeks in monochorionic twins beginning at 16 weeks to screen for TTTS.**

Discordant Growth

Significant discordance in weight between twins is most commonly defined as a greater than 20% difference in actual or estimated twin weights (the difference between the weights divided by the weight of the larger twin). In a cohort of 293 twin pregnancies, birthweight discordance of 10%, 15%, 20%, and 25% was reported in 48.8%, 34.5%, 23.5%, and 18.8% of twin pregnancies, respectively.[109] Because DZ twins are genetically distinct, they might easily be programmed to have obviously different weights at birth. There are, however, several pathologic situations in which either monochorionic or dichorionic twins may develop substantial weight differences. These include TTTS, the combination of an anomalous fetus with a normal co-twin, umbilical cord abnormalities that affect a single twin, and selective IUGR that affects only one twin. Although it has been argued that twin weight discordance is not concerning if both babies' estimated weights remain appropriate for gestational age, discordance, especially when severe, suggests the possibility of clinically significant growth restriction.

Although it is generally agreed that weight discordance in twins should be calculated, the degree of discordance that confers an increased risk of adverse outcomes is subject to debate. The ESPRiT trial prospectively followed twin pregnancies with serial sonography, including growth assessments every 2 weeks. Analyzing data for 977 twin pregnancies, they found that perinatal morbidity and mortality increased with birthweight discordance above 18%. This threshold remained the same regardless of chorionicity after cases of TTTS were excluded.[110] Adverse perinatal outcome was roughly twofold higher (hazard ratio [HR], 2.1; 95% CI, 1.6 to 2.8) in twins with discordance of 18% or more, even when both twin weights were appropriate for gestational age. The hazard ratio for adverse perinatal outcome rose more than fourfold (HR, 4.5; 95% CI,

1.8 to 10.8) if one twin in a discordant pair was growth restricted, defined as below the 5th percentile in birthweight.

Another recent retrospective cohort study that involved 895 dichorionic and 250 monochorionic pregnancies reported different results. All pregnancies were cared for at a single tertiary care center between 1990 and 2008. Exclusion criteria were monoamnionicity, TTTS, structural anomalies and, importantly, growth-restricted twins (birthweight below the 10th percentile). The study found that a birthweight discordance of 20% or more did not affect outcome in appropriately grown dichorionic gestations. However, in monochorionic twins, a birthweight discordance of 20% or more was associated with an increased risk of delivery before 34 weeks and before 28 weeks and with a higher risk of admission to the NICU. The paper concluded that when neither twin was growth restricted, growth discordance was a risk factor for adverse perinatal outcomes only in monochorionic twin gestations.[111]

Most of the available literature on twin weight discordance and associated outcomes has used birthweight, rather than discordance, in estimated fetal weight (EFW). Of course, ultrasound estimation of fetal weight is the only information available to guide antenatal management. Khalil and associates[109] compared sonographically estimated fetal weights and fetal growth discordance to actual birthweights that occurred within 48 hours of the ultrasound. Ultrasound correctly identified growth discordance ($\geq$10%, $\geq$15%, $\geq$20%, and $\geq$25%) in 69% to 86% of cases, with greater accuracy at the extremes of growth discordance. **Because ultrasound diagnosis of fetal growth discordance and IUGR is imperfect, we recommend using the presence of EFW discordance of 20% or more as an indication for heightened surveillance even when neither fetus meets criteria for IUGR. This recommendation applies to both dichorionic and monochorionic twins, but more caution should be used in monochorionic gestations with the same degree of estimated growth discordance compared with a dichorionic pregnancy.** Based on the ESPRiT study data, using a cutoff of 18% or more discordance would also be reasonable.

SPECIALIZED TWIN CLINICS

The value of specialized twin clinics has been described. **In these clinics, where women carrying twins are seen at regular intervals by the same obstetric team, several advantages accrue. Patients are followed by a small group of focused caregivers and benefit from the accumulated experience of a specialized service.** Two studies have examined the effects of such clinics and have found improvements in outcomes. One study demonstrated reduced rates of VLBW babies, NICU admissions, and perinatal mortality,[112] whereas the other showed improvements in gestational age and birthweight and reduced rates of PPROM, preterm labor and delivery, preeclampsia, and LBW and VLBW infants as well as reductions in NICU admissions and individual complications such as respiratory distress syndrome (RDS), necrotizing enterocolitis (NEC), and retinopathy of prematurity (ROP).[113] Although they lack a prospective randomized design, these studies suggest that intensive education, multidisciplinary care, and surveillance combined with careful attention to maternal nutrition and weight gain can improve outcomes in twin pregnancies. Figure 32-12 outlines a reasonable management algorithm for antepartum care unique to twin gestations.

TIMING OF DELIVERY IN MULTIPLE GESTATIONS

Concern over preterm delivery in twin pregnancies sometimes overshadows decision making regarding the appropriate timing of delivery for mothers with a multiple gestation who remain pregnant at or near term. **Numerous population-based studies suggest that the nadir of perinatal complications occurs at earlier gestational ages in multiple gestations compared with singletons.**

Unfortunately, the hypothesis that elective early delivery of twins leads to better outcomes has not been subjected to rigorous prospective study. Until recently the only randomized study of elective early delivery of twins was an underpowered Japanese study, with only 17 women in the induction group and 19 in the expectant management group. Women with both uncomplicated dichorionic and monochorionic pregnancies and a cephalic first twin were randomized at 37 weeks to either labor induction or expectant management. No differences were apparent in birthweight, Apgar score, or cesarean delivery rate, and no fetal deaths occurred in either group.[114] More recently, Dodd and associates[115] performed a randomized trial of delivery timing at term for uncomplicated twin pregnancies. Two hundred thirty-five women with uncomplicated dichorionic or monochorionic diamniotic twins were randomized to delivery at 37 weeks ($n = 116$) versus at or after 38 weeks ($n = 119$). Recruitment was stopped well short of the sample-size goal of 460 women due to insufficient funding. The study found a decreased rate of the primary outcome, which was a composite of adverse neonatal outcomes, in the 37-week delivery group (4.7% vs. 12.2%; RR, 0.39; 95% CI, 0.20 to 0.75; $P = .005$). However, this apparent improvement in overall outcome was solely a result of a decrease in birthweight below the 3rd percentile (3.0% vs. 10.1%; $P = .004$). No difference was reported in any other individual infant outcome, nor were differences found in maternal outcomes or mode of delivery. The difference in mean birthweight between groups was statistically significant (2.74 kg vs. 2.83 kg in the 37-week vs. the greater than 38-week groups, respectively; $P = .01$) but arguably clinically insignificant. For this reason, as well as the fact that the study was significantly underpowered, the question of optimal delivery timing for uncomplicated twins remains unanswered. Furthermore, it is unlikely that a trial to definitively answer this question would ever be feasible to perform.

As mentioned previously, numerous population-based studies suggest a perinatal benefit associated with the early delivery of twins. Kahn and colleagues[116] reviewed nearly 300,000 twin pairs and found 39 weeks to be the point of intersection that minimized both the fetal and neonatal death rates. They found that the prospective risk for stillbirth in twins equaled that of postterm singletons by 36 to 37 weeks' gestation. Another analysis by Sairam and associates[117] evaluated more than 4000 multiple pregnancies, of which more than 99% were twins, and found that the fetal death rate at 39 weeks' gestation in a twin pregnancy exceeded that of a postterm singleton pregnancy. Twins at 37 to 38 weeks' gestation had stillbirth rates equivalent to those of postterm singletons.

Given consistent evidence of increased risk in twin pregnancies that extend past 38 to 39 weeks' gestation (analogous to a postdate singleton gestation), **a rational delivery approach would be elective delivery at 38 weeks in well-dated, uncomplicated dichorionic twin pregnancies** (Fig. 32-13). Allowing

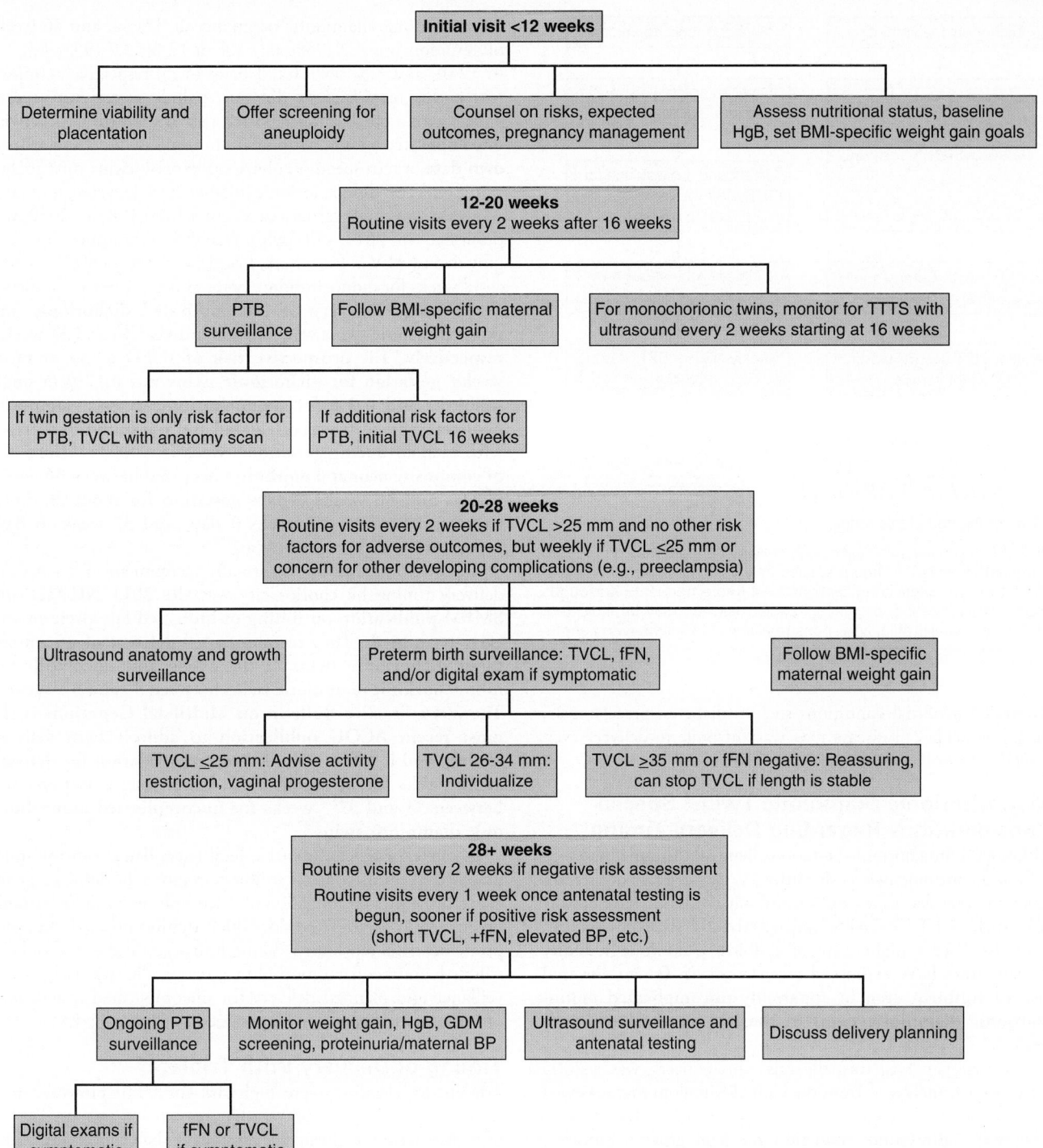

FIG 32-12 Suggested algorithm for antepartum management of twin gestations. BMI, body mass index; BP, blood pressure; fFN, fetal fibronectin; GDM, gestational diabetes mellitus; Hct, hematocrit; HgB, hemoglobin; PTB, preterm birth; TVCL, transvaginal cervical length; TTTS, twin-twin transfusion syndrome.

a dichorionic twin gestation to go past 38 weeks requires convincing evidence of normal fetal growth, amniotic fluid volume, and fetal testing as well as a patient desire to extend the pregnancy. **Prolongation of a twin pregnancy past 39 weeks is not advisable because of clear risk without any known benefit.** Unfortunately, few of these population-based studies differentiated between dichorionic and monochorionic pregnancies, and further studies were needed to define the optimal

delivery timing for monochorionic twins; this evidence will be discussed below.

Of course, the timing of delivery in the face of either maternal or fetal complications is influenced by severity and clinical judgment and will require modification of the guidelines outlined in Figure 32-13. For instance, an IUGR twin or a pregnancy with significant discordance in EFWs may be an indication for earlier delivery even if all other testing is normal. Likewise, poorly

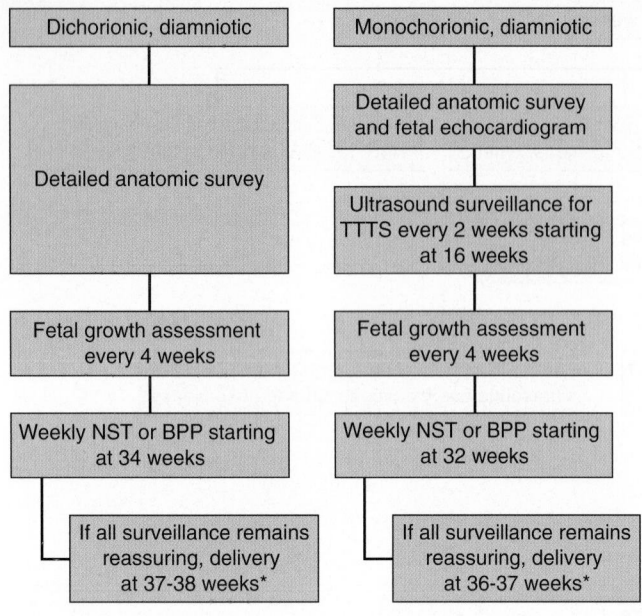

*Aim for the end of this range

FIG 32-13 Antenatal surveillance and delivery timing for uncomplicated diamniotic twins. This figure applies only to uncomplicated twins. If any fetal or maternal complications exist, more frequent ultrasounds and antenatal testing, as well as earlier delivery, may be indicated. BPP, biophysical profile; NST, nonstress test; TTTS, twin-twin transfusion syndrome.

controlled maternal conditions such as diabetes, preeclampsia, lupus, or sickle cell disease may warrant preterm delivery even if fetal growth is appropriate.

Monochorionic Diamniotic Twins: Special Considerations Regarding Delivery Timing

Although monochorionic gestations share all the same increased risks as dichorionic twins—for instance, elevated risk of preterm labor and preeclampsia—monochorionic twins also have unique risks such as TTTS, TAPS, and selective IUGR; consequently, they also have a higher risk of stillbirth. Additionally, **many investigators have expressed recent concern for an elevated risk of stillbirth even in apparently uncomplicated monochorionic diamniotic twins in the late-preterm/early-term period.**

The first paper to formally raise this concern was a 2005 retrospective analysis[118] from the United Kingdom that reviewed 151 uncomplicated monochorionic pregnancies. The patients underwent ultrasound evaluation for fetal growth, amniotic fluid, and UA Dopplers every 2 weeks. The study reported a prospective risk of stillbirth after 32 weeks of 4.3% (1 in 23). Since publication of that paper, over a dozen studies on stillbirth risk and optimal delivery timing for monochorionic diamniotic twins have been published. Most show a lower stillbirth risk than reported in the Barigye paper. The results of these studies are conflicting, and differences in antenatal surveillance regimens, as well as inclusion or exclusion of certain complications, make synthesis of the information difficult. A 2013 meta-analysis[119] of nine studies reported the risk of stillbirth per monochorionic diamniotic pregnancy at 32, 34, and 36 weeks of gestation to be 1.6%, 1.3%, and 0.9%, respectively. Four of the nine studies had a dichorionic control group. Compared with the uncomplicated dichorionic pregnancies, the odds ratio for stillbirth per

monochorionic diamniotic pregnancy at 32, 34, and 36 weeks of gestation was 4.2 (95% CI, 1.4 to 12.6), 3.7 (95% CI, 1.1 to 12.0), and 8.5 (95% CI, 1.6 to 44.7), respectively. Importantly, this meta-analysis did not include several very recent papers with a much lower reported risk of stillbirth in otherwise uncomplicated monochorionic diamniotic twins. The authors' own data, a retrospective cohort study of all twins (601 dichorionic and 167 monochorionic pregnancies) delivered at or after 34 weeks at a single tertiary care center from 1987 to 2010, was published in 2014. All twins received ultrasounds for fetal growth and AFV at least every 4 weeks and weekly NSTs starting at 32 weeks for monochorionic twins and at 34 weeks for dichorionic twins. **Delivery of uncomplicated dichorionic and monochorionic twins was recommended at 38 and 37 weeks, respectively. The prospective risk of IUFD at 34 or more weeks' gestation for dichorionic twins was 0.17%** (a single stillbirth) **and 0.0% for monochorionic twins. Composite neonatal morbidity was calculated and was found to decrease with each advancing gestational week** ($P < .0001$). **The nadir of composite neonatal morbidity occurred between 36 weeks 0 days and 36 weeks 6 days gestation for monochorionic twins and between 37 weeks 0 days and 37 weeks 6 days gestation for dichorionic twins.**[120]

The first organization to formally recommend differences in delivery timing by chorionicity was **the 2011 NICHD and SMFM publication on timing of indicated late-preterm and early-term birth. They recommended delivery of uncomplicated dichorionic twins at 38 weeks and uncomplicated monochorionic diamniotic twins between 34 and 37 weeks.**[36] **The 2014 Practice Bulletin on Multifetal Gestations is the most recent ACOG publication to address twin delivery timing, and it offers a similar recommendation for delivery at 38 weeks for uncomplicated dichorionic gestations and between 34 and 37$^{6/7}$ weeks for uncomplicated monochorionic diamniotic twins.**[37]

In our experience, intensive fetal surveillance can minimize unexpected third-trimester stillbirth in monochorionic pregnancies. This allows prolongation of uncomplicated monochorionic pregnancy to 36 to 37 weeks, which significantly reduces composite neonatal morbidity. Taking into account the risks of both stillbirth and neonatal morbidity, a reasonable approach to surveillance and planned delivery for uncomplicated monochorionic diamniotic gestations is outlined in Figure 32-13.

Timing of Delivery With Triplets

Triplets are clearly at very high risk for PTB. However, in a review of more than 15,000 triplet pregnancies, as many as 15% of triplets were undelivered at 36 weeks. That same study found that the point of intersection between a falling neonatal death rate and a rising stillbirth rate occurred at 36 weeks' gestation.[116] **Most experts agree that it is reasonable to offer delivery of uncomplicated triplets anytime between 35 and 36 weeks.**

MODE OF DELIVERY IN MULTIPLE GESTATIONS

A number of factors must be considered when determining the mode of delivery for patients with multifetal gestations. These variables include the gestational age, estimated weights of the fetuses, their positions relative to each other, the availability of real-time ultrasound on the labor floor and in the delivery room, and the ability to monitor each twin independently during the

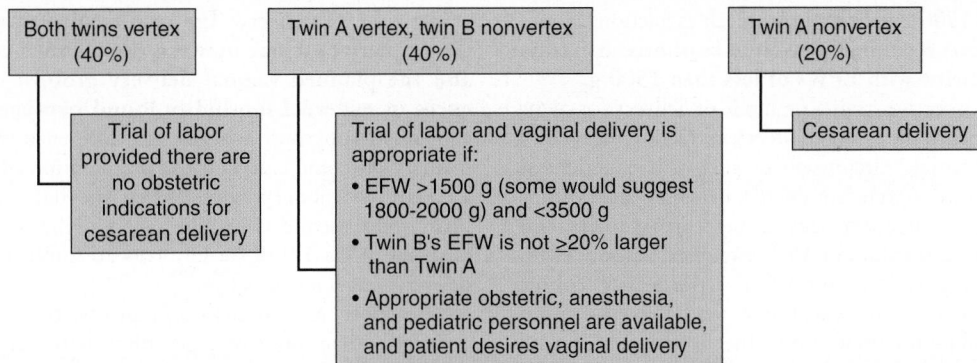

FIG 32-14 Algorithm for mode of delivery in diamniotic twins. (Monoamniotic twins should have cesarean delivery.) EFW, estimated fetal weight.

entire intrapartum period. Carefully considering all these variables is essential because multiple gestations are inherently at higher risk during the intrapartum period. The recent available literature on mode of delivery in twin gestations is summarized below.

All combinations of intrapartum twin presentations can be classified into three groups: (1) twin A vertex, twin B vertex; (2) twin A nonvertex, twin B either vertex or nonvertex; and (3) twin A vertex, twin B nonvertex. In a series of 362 twin deliveries presented by Chervenak and associates,[121] these presentations were found in 42.5%, 19.1%, and 38.4% of cases, respectively. Each scenario is discussed in turn, and recommendations are summarized in Figure 32-14.

Vertex-Vertex Twins

A trial of labor and vaginal delivery is appropriate for all vertex-vertex twin gestations, regardless of gestational age or estimated fetal weight. No clear benefit to routine cesarean delivery of vertex-vertex twins has been found in the literature, including VLBW deliveries. However, it is important to note that the presentation of the second twin may change in 5% to 10% of cases after delivery of the presenting twin. The obstetrician should always discuss this possibility with the patient before delivery, and the obstetric team should always have a clear plan for the management of an unexpected nonvertex second twin.

Nonvertex Presenting Twin

Twin pregnancies with a nonvertex presenting twin are nearly always managed by cesarean delivery. Historically, this was because of a fear of interlocking fetal heads during delivery of breech-vertex twins. However, interlocking fetuses are exceedingly rare. More concerning is extension of the fetal head of the presenting breech twin, which predisposes to a more difficult breech extraction and risk of cervical spine injury. Currently, in an era in which nearly all singleton breech fetuses are delivered by elective cesarean delivery (see Chapter 17), cesarean delivery is also the optimal mode of delivery for twin pregnancies with a nonvertex-presenting fetus.

Vertex-Nonvertex Twins

Although the route of delivery for the previous two scenarios is noncontroversial, the management of patients whose twins are in a vertex-breech or vertex-transverse lie is subject to significant debate. When the second twin is nonvertex after delivery of the first twin, the two options for vaginal delivery are breech extraction or external cephalic version (ECV). Although ECV is an acceptable strategy, it has been shown to be associated with more delivery complications and higher rates of cesarean delivery than breech extraction.[122] **Thus, provided the obstetrician is sufficiently trained in breech extraction and the fetus is of appropriate size, breech extraction is the preferable option for achievement of vaginal delivery with a nonvertex second twin** (see Chapter 17).

Some obstetricians have voiced concerns regarding the safety of breech extraction and have questioned whether outcomes are equivalent to cesarean delivery. Chervenak and colleagues[121] cite several older references in which depressed Apgar scores and increased perinatal mortality rates were associated with vaginal breech delivery of the second twin. However, in the same report, the authors analyze their own extensive experience, along with a review of the published literature, and conclude that breech extraction of a second twin is a safe and appropriate option if the EFW is more than 2000 g. Although the data supported the safety of breech extraction for babies who weigh more than 1500 g, the investigators chose 2000 g—rather than 1500 g—to allow for the margin of error of an ultrasound-estimated fetal weight.

The safety of breech extraction for second twins is supported by what was until recently the only randomized trial of cesarean delivery versus breech extraction. Rabinovici and associates[123] randomized 66 women with vertex-nonvertex twins of more than 35 weeks' gestation to vaginal delivery with breech extraction or cesarean delivery. They found no differences in neonatal outcomes and no cases of birth trauma or neonatal death. Not surprisingly, maternal febrile morbidity was greater in the cesarean delivery group.

Several other large case series and cohort studies have also supported the safety of breech extraction of second twins. Gocke and colleagues[122] retrospectively analyzed 136 sets of vertex-nonvertex twins with a birthweight higher than 1500 g in whom delivery of the second twin was managed by primary cesarean delivery, ECV, or primary breech extraction. No differences were noted in the incidence of neonatal mortality or morbidity among the three delivery modes, although ECV was associated with a higher failure rate than breech extraction along with a higher rate of nonreassuring FHR patterns, cord prolapse, and compound presentation. The authors concluded that primary breech extraction of a second nonvertex twin weighing more than 1500 g is a reasonable alternative to either cesarean delivery or ECV. Fishman and coworkers[124] and Greig and colleagues[125] examined the records of more than 1200 twin gestations and concluded that no evidence supported cesarean delivery for nonvertex second twins who weighed more than 1500 g. In fact, Greig's data did not show poorer outcomes even for babies who weighed less than 1500 g delivered by breech extraction. Nonetheless, **most experts recommend avoidance of breech extractions on second twins with EFWs of less than 1500 g.**

Two recent retrospective studies on mode of delivery for twins lend further support to the safety of breech extraction for second twins under appropriate circumstances and with experienced operators. Both studies were conducted in single institutions with strict protocols for active second-stage management and immediate breech extraction of the nonvertex second twin. Schmitz and colleagues[126] performed a retrospective cohort study of 758 consecutive twin sets at more than 35 weeks' gestation with a cephalic-presenting twin. The investigators found that the neonatal composite morbidity for the second twin did not differ between planned cesarean and planned vaginal delivery. The second, more recent study by Fox and coworkers[127] examined a retrospective cohort of 287 twin pregnancies from a single tertiary care academic medical center. Once again, following a strict second-stage management protocol, all nonvertex second twins underwent immediate breech extraction, and all nonengaged vertex second twins were delivered by immediate internal podalic version and subsequent breech vaginal delivery. The study found no difference in the rates of 5-minute Apgar scores lower than 7 or a cord pH lower than 7.2 between the planned vaginal delivery ($n = 130$) and planned cesarean delivery groups ($n = 157$). Both of these studies were retrospective and were conducted in a single center by experienced obstetricians using a strict protocol for second-stage management.

Another recent multicenter prospective study revealed similar results. In a prespecified secondary analysis of the ESPRiT study, Breathnach and colleagues[128] analyzed perinatal outcomes by mode of delivery in 971 diamniotic twin pregnancies delivered at eight centers in Ireland. Decisions on timing and mode of delivery were deferred to the lead clinician managing each case and were not prespecified by the study protocol. Of those 971 pregnancies, 441 (45%) were deemed to be appropriate for trial of labor. Of those 441 women, 338 (77%) had a successful vaginal delivery of both twins. The most common indication for cesarean delivery during a trial of labor was arrest of the first stage of labor. Breech extraction of the second twin was performed in 29% of those 338 successful vaginal deliveries, and no differences were found in perinatal outcomes by planned mode of delivery. When they analyzed predictors of successful vaginal delivery for both babies, only multiparity and spontaneous conception were independently associated with successful vaginal birth. Four percent of women who underwent a trial of labor had vaginal delivery of the first twin and cesarean delivery of the second twin.

In 2013, a large randomized trial of delivery mode in twin pregnancies was published. This multicenter, multinational study randomized 2804 women pregnant with diamniotic twins and a cephalic-presenting first twin between 32 weeks 0 days and 38 weeks 6 days gestation to either planned cesarean or planned vaginal delivery. **The primary outcome was a composite of fetal or neonatal death or serious morbidity.** In the planned cesarean delivery group, 89.9% of women underwent cesarean delivery of both babies, and in the planned vaginal delivery group, 56.2% had successful vaginal delivery of both twins. In the planned vaginal group, 4.2% of women underwent vaginal delivery of the first twin and cesarean delivery of the second twin. The paper does not state how many women had vaginal breech delivery of the second twin, but 36.4% of the planned vaginal delivery group had twins in cephalic/noncephalic presentation

at the time of delivery. **The results showed no difference in the primary outcome between the planned cesarean delivery and the planned vaginal delivery groups, nor were differences in maternal morbidity found between the groups.** In a planned subgroup analysis, no difference was found in the primary outcome based on the presentation of the second twin (cephalic vs. noncephalic). When the data were analyzed by birth order, second twins did have a higher risk of the primary outcome (OR, 1.9; 95% CI, 1.34 to 2.69); however, cesarean delivery was not protective.[129]

The above retrospective and prospective data on mode of delivery in diamniotic twin gestations with a cephalic-presenting first twin, including two randomized trials, show that **in selected women under appropriate conditions and with experienced obstetricians and supporting staff, no benefit to routine cesarean delivery is evident.** However, the importance of operator training and experience for safe vaginal delivery of twins cannot be underestimated, particularly when the second twin is in a nonvertex presentation. During the past decade, concerns about outcomes associated with singleton breech deliveries have led to virtual abandonment of vaginal delivery of breech-presenting singletons. As a consequence, **fewer obstetricians are acquiring or maintaining the skills needed to safely perform vaginal breech deliveries.**

Triplets

Although vaginal delivery is an option for patients with triplets, no large prospective studies have established its safety. Adequate monitoring of three fetuses throughout labor and delivery is challenging. **As a result, elective cesarean delivery of patients with three or more live fetuses of viable gestational age is in most cases the optimal management strategy.** Vaginal delivery of triplets should probably be restricted to those cases with EFWs greater than 1800 g, at least the first two triplets in a cephalic presentation, and obstetricians experienced in such deliveries.

INTRAPARTUM MANAGEMENT OF TWIN VAGINAL DELIVERY

Safe vaginal delivery of multiples requires careful preparation and multidisciplinary cooperation among obstetrics, anesthesia, nursing, and neonatology or pediatrics. On admission to labor and delivery, both fetal presentations should be confirmed by ultrasound. If a recent (<1 to 2 weeks) ultrasound-estimated fetal weight for both babies is not available, this should be obtained and documented. As discussed earlier, knowledge of the presentation, gestational age, and estimated weight of each twin permits the establishment of a plan regarding the anticipated route of delivery. Additionally, the discussion between obstetric providers and the patient regarding mode of delivery should be thoroughly documented in the medical record.

If a trial of labor is elected, both fetuses should be continuously monitored. Although the woman may labor in a standard room, the delivery itself is best performed in an operating room (OR) in the event that general anesthesia or cesarean delivery is emergently needed. **We typically transfer the patient to the OR bed for delivery. Epidural anesthesia for labor and delivery is also advisable and is advocated by ACOG.**[37] The pain control afforded by an epidural enhances maternal cooperation, allows a wider range of obstetric procedures to be performed

Personnel and Location
- Availability of a fully staffed operating room for the delivery with staff capable of performing an emergency cesarean delivery
- Skilled obstetric attendants present
- Anesthesiologist present at delivery
- Sufficient neonatal personnel for resuscitation of two infants

Supplies
- Equipment to continuously monitor both fetuses throughout labor and delivery
- Portable ultrasound for intrapartum use
- Premixed oxytocin
- Methergine, 15-methyl $PGF_{2\alpha}$, and misoprostol for postpartum hemorrhage
- Nitroglycerin and terbutaline for uterine relaxation
- Obstetric forceps and vacuum (including Piper forceps for aftercoming head)
- Blood products

quickly, and is available for anesthesia if emergent cesarean delivery becomes necessary. Box 32-1 provides a list of personnel and equipment that should be prepared for each planned vaginal delivery of a multiple gestation.

Time Interval Between Deliveries

Historically, many investigators have considered the time interval between delivery of the first and second babies to be an important intrapartum variable that affects the outcome of twin pregnancies. After delivery of the first twin, uterine inertia may develop, the umbilical cord of the second twin can prolapse, and placental abruption may occur; each of these poses a risk to the undelivered second twin. In addition, the cervix can constrict, making rapid delivery of the second twin extremely difficult if nonreassuring fetal status develops. **Many reports have suggested that the interval between deliveries should ideally be 15 minutes or less and certainly not more than 30 minutes.** Most of the data in support of this view, however, were obtained before the advent of continuous and dual intrapartum fetal monitoring capability.

Rayburn and associates[130] reported the outcome of 115 second twins delivered vaginally at or beyond 34 weeks' gestation after the vertex delivery of their co-twin. Continuous monitoring of the FHR was performed in all cases. Oxytocin was used if uterine contractions subsided within 10 minutes after delivery of the first twin. In this series, 70 second twins were delivered within 15 minutes of the first twin, 28 within 16 to 30 minutes, and 17 more than 30 minutes later. The longest interval between deliveries was 134 minutes. All of these infants survived, and none had a traumatic delivery. All 17 of the neonates delivered beyond 30 minutes had 5-minute Apgar scores between 8 and 10. In another series reported by Chervenak and colleagues,[131] when the FHR of the second twin was monitored with ultrasound visualization throughout the period between twin deliveries, no relationship was found between the length of the interdelivery interval and low 5-minute Apgar scores.

Although some second twins may require rapid delivery, most can be safely followed with FHR surveillance and can remain undelivered for substantial periods of time. This less hurried approach when the second twin is not demonstrating signs of nonreassuring fetal status may reduce the incidence of both maternal and fetal trauma associated with difficult deliveries performed to meet arbitrary deadlines.

SUMMARY

The patient who carries more than one fetus presents a formidable challenge to the obstetrician. The elevated maternal risk and perinatal morbidity and mortality seen in multiple gestations, compared with singletons, are due to a variety of factors, many of which cannot currently be altered. However, extraordinary technologic advances during the past 25 years have given us new insights into problems peculiar to multifetal pregnancies and has provided tools with which to detect and treat those problems. Early diagnosis of multiple gestations, determination of chorionicity, and serial surveillance with ultrasound and antenatal testing offer the potential for administering specialized regimens to selected patients, which we believe will lead to a beneficial impact on the outcome of those pregnancies.

KEY POINTS

- Twinning is one of the most common high-risk conditions in all of obstetrics. Both maternal and perinatal morbidity and mortality are significantly higher in multifetal gestations than in singleton pregnancies.
- Chorionicity is a critical determinant of pregnancy outcome and management, and as such it should be ascertained by ultrasound as early in gestation as possible.
- Monochorionic pregnancies are at higher risk than dichorionic pregnancies and have increased rates of spontaneous abortion, congenital anomalies, IUGR, and IUFD in addition to a 10% to 15% risk for TTTS, a complication unique to monochorionic pregnancies.
- Multiple gestations benefit from specialized care, which includes attention to maternal nutrition and weight gain, serial assessment of fetal growth by ultrasound, and careful surveillance for signs of preterm labor.
- Routine bed rest, prophylactic tocolytics, prophylactic cerclage, prophylactic progesterone, and prophylactic pessary have not been shown to be effective in prolonging multiple gestations. However, none of these interventions has been adequately studied in the highest-risk women based on prior obstetric history or current short cervical lengths.
- The nadir of perinatal complications and an increase in stillbirth risk occurs earlier in twin gestations than in singletons. Uncomplicated dichorionic twins appear to have the best outcomes between 37 and 38 weeks, and uncomplicated monochorionic diamniotic twin outcomes are best when delivery occurs between 36 and 37 weeks. We recommend scheduled delivery at the later end of this range.
- Monoamniotic twin outcomes are best when managed with a combination of prophylactic antenatal corticosteroids, hospitalization for daily fetal assessment, and elective cesarean delivery between 32 and 34 weeks.

◆ Mode of delivery should take into account gestational age, fetal presentations, estimated weights, and the experience and skill of the obstetrician; a trial of labor is appropriate when both twins are vertex.

◆ Mode of delivery should be individualized for vertex-nonvertex twins, and cesarean delivery is optimal when the presenting twin is nonvertex.

REFERENCES

1. Martin JA, Hamilton BE, Osterman JK, et al. *Births: Final data for 2012. National vital statistics reports; vol 62 no 9.* Hyattsville, MD: National Center for Health Statistics.; 2013.
2. Moise K, Johnson A. There is NO diagnosis of twins. *Am J Obstet Gynecol.* 2010;203:1-2.
3. Scardo JA, Ellings JM, Newman RB. Prospective determination of chorionicity, amnionicity and zygosity in twin gestations. *Am J Obstet Gynecol.* 1995;173:1376-1380.
4. Campbell DM, Templeton A. Maternal complications of twin pregnancy. *Int J Gynecol Obstet.* 2004;84:71-73.
5. Sibai BM, Hauth J, Caritis S, et al. Hypertensive disorders in twin versus singleton gestations. *Am J Obstet Gynecol.* 2000;182:938-942.
6. Day MC, Barton JR, O'Brien JM, et al. The effect of fetal number on the development of hypertensive conditions of pregnancy. *Obstet Gynecol.* 2005;106:927-931.
7. Hardardottir H, Kelly K, Bork MD, et al. Atypical presentation of preeclampsia in high-order multifetal gestations. *Obstet Gynecol.* 1996;87:370-374.
8. Bouvier-Colle MH, Varnoux N, Salanave B, et al. Case control study of risk factors for obstetric patients' admission to intensive care units. *Eur J Obstet Gynec and Reprod Biol.* 1997;79:173-177.
9. Senat MV, Ancel PY, Bouvier-Colle MH, et al. How does multiple pregnancy affect maternal mortality and morbidity? *Clin Obstet Gynecol.* 1998;41:79-83.
10. Martin JA, Hamilton BE, Ventura SJ, et al. *Births: Final data for 2009. National vital statistics reports; vol 60 no 1.* Hyattsville, MD: National Center for Health Statistics.; 2011.
11. Mastroiacovo P, Castilla EE, Arpino C, et al. Congenital malformations in twins: an international study. *Am J Med Genet.* 1999;83:117-124.
12. Glinianaia SV, Rankin J, Wright C. Congenital anomalies in twins: a register-based study. *Hum Reprod.* 2008;23:1306-1311.
13. Chen CJ, Wang CJ, Yu MW, et al. Perinatal mortality and prevalence of major congenital malformations of twins in taipei city. *Acta Genet Med Gemellol.* 1992;41(2–3):197-203.
14. Nance WE. Malformations unique to the twinning process. *Prog Clin Biol Res.* 1981;69A:123-133.
15. Landy HJ, Weiner S, Corson SL, et al. The "vanishing twin:" ultrasonographic assessment of fetal disappearance in the first trimester. *Am J Obstet Gynecol.* 1986;155(1):14-19.
16. Dickey RP, Olar TT, Curole SN, et al. The probability of multiple births when multiple gestational sacs or viable embryos are diagnosed at first trimester ultrasound. *Hum Reprod.* 1990;5(7):880-882.
17. Dickey RP, Taylor SN, Lu PY, et al. Spontaneous reduction of multiple pregnancy: incidence and effect on outcome. *Am J Obstet Gynecol.* 2002;186(1):77-83.
18. Evans MI, Berkowitz RL, Wapner RJ, et al. Improvement in outcomes of multifetal pregnancy reduction with increased experience. *Am J Obstet Gynecol.* 2001;184(2):97-103.
19. Stone J, Ferrara L, Kamrath J, et al. Contemporary outcomes with the latest 1000 cases of multifetal pregnancy reduction. *Am J Obstet Gynecol.* 2008;199:406.e1-406.e4.
20. Papageorghiou AT, Avgidou K, Bakoulas V, et al. Risks of miscarriage and early preterm birth in trichorionic triplet pregnancies with embryo reduction versus expectant management: new data and systematic review. *Hum Reprod.* 2006;21(7):1912-1917.
21. van de Mheen L, Everwijn SM, Knapen MF, et al. The effectiveness of multifetal pregnancy reduction in trichorionic triplet gestation. *Am J Obstet Gynecol.* 2014;210:e1-e6.
22. Shiva M, Mohammadi Yeganeh L, Mirzaagha E. Comparison of the outcomes between reduced and nonreduced triplet pregnancies achieved by assisted reproductive technology. *Aust N Z J Obstet Gynaecol.* 2014;54:424-427.
23. Alexander JM, Ramus R, Cox SM, et al. Outcome of twin gestations with a single anomalous fetus. *Am J Obstet Gynecol.* 1997;177(4):849-852.
24. Gul A, Cebeci A, Aslan H, et al. Perinatal outcomes of twin pregnancies discordant for major fetal anomalies. *Fetal Diagn Ther.* 2005;20(4):244-248.
25. Nassar AH, Adra AM, Gómez-Marín O, et al. Perinatal outcome of twin pregnancies with one structurally affected fetus: a case-control study. *J Perinatol.* 2000;20(2):82-86.
26. Sun LM, Chen XK, Wen SW, et al. Perinatal outcomes of normal cotwins in twin pregnancies with one structurally anomalous fetus: a population-based retrospective study. *Am J Perinatol.* 2009;26:51-56.
27. Harper LM, Odibo AO, Rehl KA, et al. Risk of preterm delivery and growth restriction in twins discordant for structural anomalies. *Am J Obstet Gynecol.* 2012;206(1):70.e1-e5.
28. Evans MI, Goldberg JD, Horenstein J, et al. Selective termination for structural, chromosomal, and mendelian anomalies: international experience. *Am J Obstet Gynecol.* 1999;181:893-897.
29. Rossi AC, D'Addario V. Umbilical cord occlusion for selective feticide in complicated monochorionic twins: a systematic review of the literature. *Am J Obstet Gynecol.* 2009;200:123-129.
30. Lewi L, Gratacós E, Ortibus E, et al. Pregnancy and infant outcome of 80 consecutive cord coagulations in complicated monochorionic multiple pregnancies. *Am J Obstet Gynecol.* 2006;194(3):782-789.
31. Ong S, Zamora J, Khan K, et al. Prognosis for the co-twin following single-twin death: a systematic review. *BJOG.* 2006;113:992-998.
32. Hillman SC, Morris RK, Kilby MD. Co-Twin prognosis after single fetal death: a systematic review and meta-analysis. *Obstet Gynecol.* 2011;118:928-940.
33. Kaufman HK, Hume RF, Calhoun BC, et al. Natural history of twin gestation complicated by in utero fetal demise: associations of chorionicity, prematurity, and maternal morbidity. *Fetal Diagn Ther.* 2003;18:442-446.
34. Pharoah PO, Adi Y. Consequences of in-utero death in a twin pregnancy. *Lancet.* 2000;355:1597-1602.
35. Weiss JL, Cleary-Goldman J, Budorick N, et al. Multicystic encephalomalacia after first trimester intrauterine fetal demise in monochorionic twins. *Am J Obstet Gynecol.* 2004;190(2):563-565.
36. Spong CY, Mercer BM, D'Alton M, et al. Timing of indicated late-preterm and early-term birth. *Obstet Gynecol.* 2011;118:323-333.
37. Multifetal gestations: twin, triplet, and higher-order multifetal pregnancies. Practice Bulletin No. 144. American College of Obstetricians and Gynecologists. *Obstet Gynecol.* 2014;123:1118-1132.
38. Quintero RA, Morales WJ, Allen MH, et al. Staging of Twin-Twin Transfusion Syndrome. *J Perinatology.* 1999;19(8):550-555.
39. Thorson HL, Ramaeker DM, Emery SP. Optimal interval for ultrasound surveillance in monochorionic twin gestations. *Obstet Gynecol.* 2011;117:131-135.
40. Society for Maternal-Fetal Medicine, Simpson LL. Twin-twin transfusion syndrome. *Am J Obstet Gynecol.* 2013;208(1):3-18.
41. Moise KJ, Dorman K, Lamvu G, et al. A randomized trial of amnioreduction versus septostomy in the treatment of twin-twin transfusion syndrome. *Am J Obstet Gynecol.* 2005;193(3 Pt 1):701-707.
42. Mari G, Roberts A, Detti L. Perinatal morbidity and mortality rates in severe twin-twin transfusion syndrome: results of the international amnioreduction registry. *Am J Obstet Gynecol.* 2001;185(3):708-715.
43. Senat MV, Deprest J, Boulvain M, et al. Endoscopic laser surgery versus serial amnioreduction for severe twin-to-twin transfusion syndrome. *NEJM.* 2004;351(2):136-144.
44. Crombleholme TM, Shera D, Lee H, et al. A prospective randomized multicenter trial of amnioreduction vs. selective fetoscopic laser photocoagulation for the treatment of severe twin-twin transfusion syndrome. *Am J Obstet Gynecol.* 2007;197(4):396.e1-e9.
45. Roberts D, Neilson JP, Kilby MD, et al. Interventions for the treatment of twin-twin transfusion syndrome. *Cochrane Database Syst Rev.* 2014;(1):Art. No.: CD002073.
46. Rossi AC, D'Addario V. Laser therapy and serial amnioreduction as treatment for twin-twin transfusion syndrome: a meta-analysis and review of the literature. *Am J Obstet Gynecol.* 2008;198(2):147-152.
47. Rossi AC, Vanderbilt D, Chmait RH. Neurodevelopmental outcomes after laser therapy for twin-twin transfusion syndrome: a systematic review and meta-analysis. *Obstet Gynecol.* 2011;118:1145-1150.

48. Salomon LJ, Örtqvist L, Aegerter P, et al. Long-term developmental follow-up of infants who participated in a randomized clinical trial of amniocentesis vs laser photocoagulation for the treatment of twin-to-twin transfusion syndrome. *Am J Obstet Gynecol*. 2010;203:444.e1-e7.

49. Taylor MJ, Govender L, Jolly M, Wee L, Fisk NM. Validation of the Quintero staging system for twin-twin transfusion syndrome. *Obstet Gynecol*. 2002;100(6):1257-1265.

50. O'Donoghue K, Cartwright E, Galea P, et al. Stage 1 twin-to-twin transfusion syndrome: rates of progression and regression in relation to outcome. *Ultrasound Obstet Gynecol*. 2007;30(7):958-964.

51. Rossi AC, D'Addario V. Survival outcomes of twin-twin transfusion syndrome stage I: a systematic review of literature. *Am J Perinatol*. 2013; 30(1):5-10.

52. Michelfelder E, Gottliebson W, Border W. Early manifestations and spectrum of recipient twin cardiomyopathy in twin-twin transfusion syndrome: relation to Quintero stage. *Ultrasound Obstet Gynecol*. 2007; 30(7):965-971.

53. Wagner MM, Lopriore E, Klumper FJ. Short and long-term outcomes in stage 1 twin-to-twin transfusion syndrome treated with laser surgery compared with conservative management. *Am J Obstet Gynecol*. 2009; 201(3):286.e1-e6.

54. Gratacós E, Lewi L, Muñoz B, et al. A classification system for selective intrauterine growth restriction in monochorionic pregnancies according to umbilical artery Doppler flow in the smaller twin. *Ultrasound Obstet Gynecol*. 2007;30:28-34.

55. Ishii K, Murakoshi T, Takahashi Y, et al. Perinatal outcome of monochorionic twins with selective intrauterine growth restriction and different types of umbilical artery Doppler under expectant management. *Fetal Diagn Ther*. 2009;26:157-161.

56. Valsky DV, Eixarch E, Martinez JM, et al. Selective intrauterine growth restriction in monochorionic twins: pathophysiology, diagnostic approach and management dilemmas. *Sem Fetal Neonatal Med*. 2010;15:342-348.

57. Slaghekke F, Kist WJ, Oepkes D, et al. Twin anemia-polycythemia sequence: diagnostic criteria, classification, perinatal management and outcome. *Fetal Diagn Ther*. 2010;27:181-190.

58. Baschat AA, Oepkes D. Twin anemia-polycythemia sequence in monochorionic twins: implications for diagnosis and treatment. *Am J Perinatol*. 2014;31:525-530.

59. Hack KE, Derks JB, Schaap AH, et al. Perinatal outcomes of monoamniotic twin pregnancies. *Obstet Gynecol*. 2009;113:353-360.

60. Roque H, Gillen-Goldstein J, Funai E, et al. Perinatal outcomes in monoamniotic gestations. *J Matern Fetal Neonatal Med*. 2003;13:414-421.

61. Heyborne KD, Porreco RP, Garite TJ, et al. Improved perinatal survival of monoamniotic twins with intensive inpatient monitoring. *Am J Obstet Gynecol*. 2005;192(1):96-101.

62. Van Mieghem T, De Heus R, Lewi L, et al. Prenatal management of monoamniotic twin pregnancies. *Obstet Gynecol*. 2014;124:498-506.

63. Morikawa M, Yamada T, Yamada T, et al. Prospective risk of intrauterine fetal death in monoamniotic twin pregnancies. *Twin Res Hum Genet*. 2012;15(4):522-526.

64. Rodis JF, McIlveen PF, Egan JF, et al. Monoamniotic twins: improved perinatal survival with accurate prenatal diagnosis and antenatal fetal surveillance. *Am J Obstet Gynecol*. 1997;177:1046-1049.

65. Allen VM, Windrim R, Barrett J, et al. Management of monoamniotic twin pregnancies: a case series and systematic review of the literature. *BJOG*. 2001;108:931-936.

66. Baxi LV, Walsh C. Monoamniotic twins in contemporary practice: a single-center study of perinatal outcomes. *J Mat Fet Neonatal Med*. 2010;23(6):506-510.

67. Ezra Y, Shveiky D, Ophir E, et al. Intensive management and early delivery reduce antenatal mortality in monoamniotic twin pregnancies. *Acta Obstet Gynecol Scand*. 2005;84:432-435.

68. DeFalco LM, Sciscione AC, Megerian G, et al. Inpatient versus outpatient management of monoamniotic twins and outcomes. *Am J Perinatol*. 2006;23:205-212.

69. Quinn KH, Cao CT, Lacoursiere DY, et al. Monoamniotic twin pregnancy: continuous electronic fetal monitoring – an impossible goal? *Am J Obstet Gynecol*. 2011;204:161.e1-e6.

70. Healey MG. Acardia: Predictive Risk Factors for the Cotwin's Survival. *Teratology*. 1994;50:205-213.

71. Moore TR, Gale S, Benirschke K. Perinatal outcome of forty-nine pregnancies complicated by acardiac twinning. *Am J Obstet Gynecol*. 1990; 163:907-912.

72. Jelin E, Hirose S, Rand L, et al. Perinatal outcome of conservative management versus fetal intervention for twin reversed arterial perfusion sequence with a small acardiac twin. *Fetal Diagn Ther*. 2010;27: 138-141.

73. Pagani G, D'Antonio F, Khalil A, et al. Intrafetal laser treatment for twin reversed arterial perfusion sequence: cohort study and meta-analysis. *Ultrasound Obstet Gynecol*. 2013;42:6-14.

74. Lee H, Bebbington M, Crombleholme T. The North American Fetal Therapy Network Registry Data on Outcomes of Radiofrequency Ablation for Twin-Reversed Arterial Perfusion Sequence. *Fetal Diagn Ther*. 2013;33: 224-229.

75. MacKenzie TC, Crombleholme TM, Johnson MP, et al. The natural history of prenatally diagnosed conjoined twins. *J Pediatr Surg*. 2002;37: 303-309.

76. Brizot ML, Liao AW, Lopes LM, et al. Conjoined twins pregnancies: experience with 36 cases from a single center. *Prenat Diagn*. 2011;31: 1120-1125.

77. Spitz L. Conjoined Twins. *Prenat Diagn*. 2005;25:814-819.

78. Luke B, Min SJ, Gillespie B, et al. The importance of early weight gain in the intrauterine growth and birth weight of twins. *Am J Obstet Gynecol*. 1998;179:1155-1161.

79. Luke B, Hediger ML, Nugent C, et al. Body mass index-specific weight gains associated with optimal birth weights in twin pregnancies. *J Reprod Med*. 2003;48:217-224.

80. Luke B, Brown MB, Misiunas R, et al. Specialized prenatal care and maternal and infant outcomes in twin pregnancy. *Am J Obstet Gynecol*. 2003;189(4):934-938.

81. Fox NS, Rebarber A, Roman AS, et al. Weight gain in twin pregnancies and adverse outcomes: examining the 2009 Institute of Medicine Guidelines. *Obstet Gynecol*. 2010;116:100-106.

82. Conde-Agudelo A, Romero R, Hassan SS, et al. Transvaginal sonographic cervical length for the prediction of spontaneous preterm birth in twin pregnancies: a systematic review and meta-analysis. *Am J Obstet Gynecol*. 2010;203:128.e1-e12.

83. Fox NS, Rebarber A, Klauser CK, et al. Prediction of spontaneous preterm birth in asymptomatic twin pregnancies using the change in cervical length over time. *Am J Obstet Gynecol*. 2010;202:155.e1-e4.

84. Conde-Agudelo A, Romero R. Cervicovaginal fetal fibronectin for the prediction of spontaneous preterm birth in multiple pregnancies: a systematic review and meta-analysis. *J Mat Fet Neonatal Med*. 2010;23(12): 1365-1376.

85. Crowther CA, Han S. Hospitalisation and bed rest for multiple pregnancy. *Cochrane Database Syst Rev*. 2010;(7):CD000110.

86. Senat MV, Porcher R, Winer N, et al. Prevention of preterm delivery by 17 alpha-hydroxyprogesterone caproate in asymptomatic twin pregnancies with a short cervix: a randomized controlled trial. *Am J Obstet Gynecol*. 2013;208:194.e1-e8.

87. Lim AC, Schuit E, Bloemenkamp K, et al. 17-Hydroxyprogesterone Caproate for the Prevention of Adverse Neonatal Outcome in Multiple Pregnancies: A Randomized Controlled Trial. *Obstet Gynecol*. 2011;118: 513-520.

88. Combs CA, Garite T, Maurel K, et al. 17-hydroxyprogesterone caproate for twin pregnancy: a double-blind, randomized clinical trial. *Am J Obstet Gynecol*. 2011;204:221.e1-e8.

89. Caritis SN, Rouse DJ, Peaceman AM, et al. Prevention of preterm birth in triplets using 17 alpha-hydroxyprogesterone caproate: a randomized controlled trial. *Obstet Gynecol*. 2009;113:285-292.

90. Rouse DJ, Caritis SN, Peaceman AM, et al. A trial of 17 alpha-hydroxyprogesterone caproate to prevent prematurity in twins. *N Engl J Med*. 2007;357:454-461.

91. Fonseca EB, Celik E, Parra M, et al. Progesterone and the risk of preterm birth among women with a short cervix. *N Engl J Med*. 2007;357: 462-469.

92. Norman JE, Owen P, Mactier H, et al. Progesterone for the Prevention of Preterm Birth in Twin Pregnancy (STOPPIT): a randomized, double-blind, placebo-controlled study and meta-analysis. *Lancet*. 2009;373: 2034-2040.

93. Cetingoz E, Cam C, Sakallı M, et al. Progesterone effects on preterm birth in high-risk pregnancies: a randomized placebo-controlled trial. *Arch Gynecol Obstet*. 2011;283:423-429.

94. Serra V, Perales A, Meseguer J, et al. Increased doses of vaginal progesterone for the prevention of preterm birth in twin pregnancies: a randomised controlled double-blind multicentre trial. *BJOG*. 2013;120: 50-57.

95. Wood S, Ross S, Tang S, et al. Vaginal progesterone to prevent preterm birth in multiple pregnancy: a randomized controlled trial. *J Perinat Med*. 2012;40:593-599.

96. Aboulghar MM, Aboulghar MA, Amin YM, et al. The use of vaginal natural progesterone for prevention of preterm birth in IVF/ICSI pregnancies. *Reprod Biomed Online.* 2012;25:133-138.

97. Rode L, Klein K, Nicolaides KH, et al. Prevention of preterm delivery in twin gestations (PREDICT): a multicenter, randomized, placebo-controlled trial on the effect of vaginal micronized progesterone. *Ultrasound Obstet Gynecol.* 2011;38:272-280.

98. Romero R, Nicolaides K, Conde-Agudelo A, et al. Vaginal progesterone in women with an asymptomatic sonographic short cervix in the midtrimester decreases preterm delivery and neonatal morbidity: a systematic review and meta-analysis of individual patient data. *Am J Obstet Gynecol.* 2012;206:124.e1-e19.

99. Schuit E, Stock S, Rode L, et al. Effectiveness of progestogens to improve perinatal outcome in twin pregnancies: an individual participant data meta-analysis. *BJOG.* 2015;122(1):27-37.

100. Newman RB, Krombach S, Myers MC, et al. Effect of cerclage on obstetrical outcome in twin gestations with a shortened cervical length. *Am J Obstet Gynecol.* 2002;186(4):634-640.

101. Berghella V, Odibo AO, To MS, et al. Cerclage for short cervix on ultrasonography. *Obstet Gynecol.* 2005;106(1):181-189.

102. Goya M, Pratcorona L, Merced C, et al. Cervical pessary in pregnant women with a short cervix (PECEP): an open-label randomised controlled trial. *Lancet.* 2012;379(9828):1800-1806.

103. Liem S, Schuit E, Hegeman M, et al. Cervical pessaries for prevention of preterm birth in women with a multiple pregnancy (ProTWIN): a multicentre, open-label randomised controlled trial. *Lancet.* 2013;382(9901):1341-1349.

104. Antepartum fetal surveillance. Practice Bulletin No. 145. American College of Obstetricians and Gynecologists. *Obstet Gynecol.* 2014;124:182-192.

105. Signore C, Freeman RK, Spong CY. Antenatal testing—a reevaluation. *Obstet Gynecol.* 2009;113:687-701.

106. Alexander GR, Kogan M, Martin J, et al. What are the fetal growth patterns of singletons, twins, and triplets in the United States? *Clin Obstet Gynecol.* 1998;41(1):114-125.

107. Taylor GM, Owen P, Mires GJ. Foetal growth velocities in twin pregnancies. *Twin Res.* 1998;1:9-14.

108. Smith AP, Ong S, Smith NC, Campbell D. A Prospective longitudinal study of growth velocity in twin pregnancy. *Ultrasound Obstet Gynecol.* 2001;18:485-487.

109. Khalil A, D'Antonio F, Dias T, et al. Ultrasound estimation of birth weight in twin pregnancy: comparison of biometry algorithms in the STORK multiple pregnancy cohort. *Ultrasound Obstet Gynecol.* 2014;44(2):210-220.

110. Breathnach FM, McAuliffe FM, Geary M, et al. Definition of intertwin birth weight discordance. *Obstet Gynecol.* 2011;118(1):94-103.

111. Harper LM, Weis MA, Odibo AO, et al. Significance of growth discordance in appropriately grown twins. *Am J Obstet Gynecol.* 2013;208(5):393.e1-e5.

112. Ellings JM, Newman RB, Hulsey TC, et al. Reduction in very low birth weight deliveries and perinatal mortality in a specialized, multidisciplinary twin clinic. *Obstet Gynecol.* 1993;81(3):387-391.

113. Luke B, Brown MB, Misiunas R, et al. Specialized prenatal care and maternal and infant outcomes in twin pregnancy. *Am J Obstet Gynecol.* 2003;189(4):934-938.

114. Suzuki S, Otsubo Y, Sawa R, et al. Clinical trial of induction of labor versus expectant management in twin pregnancy. *Gynecol Obstet Invest.* 2000;49:24-27.

115. Dodd JM, Crowther CA, Haslam RR, et al. Elective birth at 37 weeks of gestation versus standard care for women with an uncomplicated twin pregnancy at term: the Twins Timing of Birth Randomised Trial. *BJOG.* 2012;119(8):964-973.

116. Kahn B, Lumey LH, Zybert PA, et al. Prospective risk of fetal death in singleton, twin, and triplet gestations: implications for practice. *Obstet Gynecol.* 2003;102:685-692.

117. Sairam S, Costeloe K, Thilaganathan B. Prospective risk of stillbirth in multiple gestation pregnancies: a population-based analysis. *Obstet Gynecol.* 2002;100:638-641.

118. Barigye O, Pasquini L, Galea P, et al. High risk of unexpected late fetal death in monochorionic twins despite intensive ultrasound surveillance: a cohort study. *PLoS Med.* 2005;2:e172.

119. Danon D, Sekar R, Hack KE, Fisk NM. Increased stillbirth in uncomplicated monochorionic twin pregnancies: a systematic review and meta-analysis. *Obstet Gynecol.* 2013;121:1318-1326.

120. Burgess JL, Unal ER, Nietert PJ, et al. Risk of late-preterm stillbirth and neonatal morbidity for monochorionic and dichorionic twins. *Am J Obstet Gynecol.* 2014;210:578e1-578e9.

121. Chervenak FA, Johnson RE, Youcha S, et al. Intrapartum management of twin gestation. *Obstet Gynecol.* 1985;65:119-124.

122. Gocke SE, Nageotte MP, Garite T, et al. Management of the nonvertex second twin: primary cesarean section, external version or primary breech extraction. *Am J Obstet Gynecol.* 1989;161(1):111-114.

123. Rabinovici J, Barkai G, Reichman B, et al. Randomized management of the second nonvertex twin: vaginal delivery or cesarean section. *Am J Obstet Gynecol.* 1987;156:52-56.

124. Fishman A, Grubb DK, Kovacs BW, et al. Vaginal delivery of the nonvertex second twin. *Am J Obstet Gynecol.* 1993;168:861-864.

125. Greig PC, Veille JC, Morgan T, Henderson L. The effect of presentation and mode of delivery on neonatal outcome in the second twin. *Am J Obstet Gynecol.* 1992;167:901-906.

126. Schmitz T, Carnavalet Cde C, Azria E, et al. Neonatal outcomes of twin pregnancy according to the planned mode of delivery. *Obstet Gynecol.* 2008;111:695-703.

127. Fox NS, Silverstein M, Bender S, et al. Active second-stage management in twin pregnancies undergoing planned vaginal delivery in a U.S. population. *Obstet Gynecol.* 2010;115:229-233.

128. Breathnach FM, McAuliffe FM, Geary M, et al. Prediction of safe and successful vaginal twin birth. *Am J Obstet Gynecol.* 2011;205:237.e1-e7.

129. Barrett JF, Hannah ME, Hutton EK, et al. A randomized trial of planned cesarean or vaginal delivery for twin pregnancy. *N Engl J Med.* 2013;369:1295-1305.

130. Rayburn WF, Lavin JP, Miodovnik M, et al. Multiple gestation: Time interval between delivery of the first and second twins. *Obstet Gynecol.* 1984;63:502-506.

131. Chervenak FA, Johnson RE, Berkowitz RL, et al. Intrapartum external version of the second twin. *Obstet Gynecol.* 1983;62:160-165.

CHAPTER 33

Intrauterine Growth Restriction

AHMET ALEXANDER BASCHAT and HENRY L. GALAN

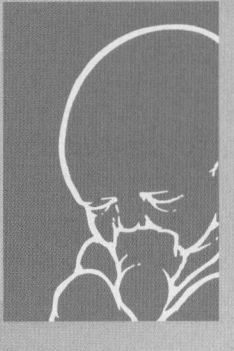

KEY ABBREVIATIONS

Abdominal circumference	AC	Intrauterine growth restriction	IUGR
Absent end-diastolic velocity	AEDV	Intraventricular hemorrhage	IVH
Alpha-fetoprotein	AFP	Low birthweight	LBW
Amniotic fluid index	AFI	Multiples of the median	MoM
Amniotic fluid volume	AFV	Necrotizing enterocolitis	NEC
Average for gestational age	AGA	Neonatal intensive care unit	NICU
Biophysical profile	BPP	Nonstress test	NST
Biparietal diameter	BPD	Nucleated red blood cell	NRBC
Cerebroplacental Doppler ratio	CPR	Placental growth factor	PIGF
Computerized cardiotocography	cCTG	Polymerase chain reaction	PCR
Contraction stress test	CST	Pregnancy-associated plasma protein A	PAPP-A
Ductus venosus	DV	Respiratory distress syndrome	RDS
Estimated date of confinement	EDC	Reversed end-diastolic velocity	REDV
Femur length	FL	Selective intrauterine growth restriction	sIUGR
Fetal activity count	FAC	Small for gestational age	SGA
Fetal growth restriction	FGR	Sonographically estimated fetal weight	SEFW
Fetal heart rate	FHR	Systolic/diastolic ratio	S/D
Head circumference	HC	Transcerebellar diameter	TCD
Human chorionic gonadotropin	hCG		

The identification of pregnancies at risk for preventable perinatal handicap is a primary goal of the obstetric care provider. Pregnancies in which adverse intrauterine conditions result in failure of the fetus to reach its growth potential constitute such a high-risk group. Next to prematurity, intrauterine growth restriction (IUGR) is the second leading cause of perinatal mortality.

Compared with appropriately grown counterparts, perinatal mortality rates in growth-restricted neonates are 6 to 10 times greater; perinatal mortality rates as high as 120 per 1000 for all cases of IUGR and 80 per 1000 after exclusion of anomalous infants have been reported. As many as 53% of preterm stillbirths and 26% of term stillbirths are growth

restricted. In survivors, the incidence of intrapartum asphyxia may be as high as 50%.[1] Prevention of some perinatal complications that lead to adverse outcomes in growth-restricted fetuses is possible with appropriate prenatal identification and management. This chapter reviews normal and disturbed fetal growth, the definition of abnormal fetal growth, the impact of fetal growth restriction, and the incorporation of this knowledge into screening, diagnosis, and management of these high-risk pregnancies. *Intrauterine growth restriction* (IUGR), *fetal growth restriction* (FGR), and *small for gestational age* (SGA) are terms frequently used interchangeably when describing the small fetus.

REGULATION OF FETAL GROWTH

Fetal growth is regulated at multiple levels and requires successful development of the placental interface between maternal and fetal compartments. In the early first trimester, anchoring villi that originate from the cytotrophoblast connect the decidua to the uterus and thereby establish placental adherence. This allows formation of vascular connections between the maternal circulation and the intervillous space so that increasing quantities of placental secretory products can reach the maternal circulation (see Chapter 1).

The villous trophoblast becomes the primary placental site of maternal-fetal exchange. By 16 weeks' gestation, the maternal microvillous and fetal basal layer are only 4 microns apart, posing little resistance to passive diffusion. Elaboration of active transport mechanisms for three major nutrient classes—glucose, amino acids, and free fatty acids—and an increase in the villous surface area raise the capacity and efficiency of active transplacental transport. Vascular throughput across the placenta also increases in the maternal and fetal compartments. Extravillous cytotrophoblast invasion of the maternal spiral arteries results in progressive loss of the musculoelastic media, a process paralleled on the fetal side by continuous villous vascular branching. **This results in significant reduction of blood flow resistance in the uterine and umbilical vessels, which converts both circulations into low-resistance, high-capacitance vascular beds.** Owing to these developments, as much as 600 mL/min of maternal cardiac output reaches a placental exchange area of up to 12 m[2] at term. In the fetal compartment this is matched with a blood flow volume of 200 to 300 mL/kg/min throughout gestation. This magnitude of maternal blood flow is necessary to ensure maintenance of placental function that is energy intensive and consumes as much as 40% of the oxygen and 70% of the glucose supplied. Optimal fetal growth and development depends on a magnitude of maternal nutrient and oxygen delivery to the uterus that leaves sufficient surplus for fetal substrate utilization.

Of the actively transported primary nutrients, glucose is the predominant oxidative fuel, whereas amino acids are major contributors to protein synthesis and muscle bulk. Glucose and, to a lesser extent, amino acids drive the insulin-like growth factors axis and therefore stimulate longitudinal fetal growth.

Concurrent development and maturation of the fetal circulation as a conduit for nutrient and waste delivery allows preferential partitioning of nutrients in the fetus. Nutrient- and oxygen-rich blood from the primitive villous circulation enters the fetus via the umbilical vein. The ductus venosus (DV) is the first vascular partitioning shunt encountered. Through modulation in DV shunting, the proportion of umbilical venous blood distributed to the liver and heart changes with advancing gestation. **Near term, 18% to 25% of umbilical venous flow shunts through the DV to reach the right atrium in this high-velocity stream; 55% reaches the dominant left hepatic lobe, and 20% reaches the right liver lobes** (Fig. 33-1). The differences in direction and velocity of blood entering the right atrium ensures that nutrient-rich blood is distributed to the left ventricle, myocardium, and brain while low-nutrient venous return is distributed to the placenta for reoxygenation and waste exchange. **This process of blood distribution is referred to as *preferential streaming.*** [2] In addition to this overall distribution of left- and right-sided cardiac output, several organs can modify local blood flow to meet oxygen and nutrient demands by autoregulation.

When the milestones in maternal, placental, and fetal development are met, placental and fetal growth progress normally. The metabolic and vascular maternal adaptations promote a steady and enhanced nutrient delivery to the uterus, and placental transport mechanisms allow for efficient bidirectional exchange of nutrients and waste. **Placental and fetal growth across the three trimesters are characterized by sequential cellular hyperplasia, hyperplasia plus hypertrophy, and lastly, by hypertrophy alone.** Placental growth follows a sigmoid curve that plateaus in midgestation preceding exponential third-trimester growth of the fetus. During this exponential fetal growth phase of 1.5% per day, initial weight gain is due to longitudinal growth and muscle bulk and therefore correlates with glucose and amino acid transport. **Eighty percent of fetal fat gain is accrued after 28 weeks' gestation, providing essential body stores in preparation for extrauterine life.** From 32 weeks onward, fat stores increase from 3.2% of fetal body weight to 16%, which accounts for the significant reduction in body water content.[3]

Several possible mechanisms may challenge compensatory capacity of the maternal-placental-fetal unit to such an extent that failure to reach the growth potential may be the end result.

DEFINITION AND PATTERNS OF FETAL GROWTH RESTRICTION

Normal fetal growth involves hyperplasia and hypertrophy on a cellular level. Disturbance of fetal growth dynamics can lead to a reduced cell number, cell size, or both, ultimately resulting in abnormal weight, body mass, or body proportion at birth. The classification of abnormal growth has evolved significantly over the last century. From its modern origins in 1919 when Yippo was the first to label neonates with a birthweight below 2500 g as "premature" to the description of individualized growth potential, the recognition of the SGA neonate has advanced significantly. With the advent of ultrasound, the recognition and study of fetal growth abnormalities extended into the prenatal period. It is important to note that several definitions that describe abnormal growth are used interchangeably in the obstetric and pediatric literature, but they do not necessarily describe the same population.

The terminology for classifying fetal growth disorders has specifically expanded over the last four decades, which has led to confusion among the various terms used. **From the 1960s, growth has been classified by the absolute birthweight value as *low birthweight*** (LBW; <2500 g), ***very low birthweight*** (VLBW; <1500 g), ***extremely low birth weight*** (ELBW; <1000 g), **or *macrosomia*** (>4000 g). Subsequently, studies by

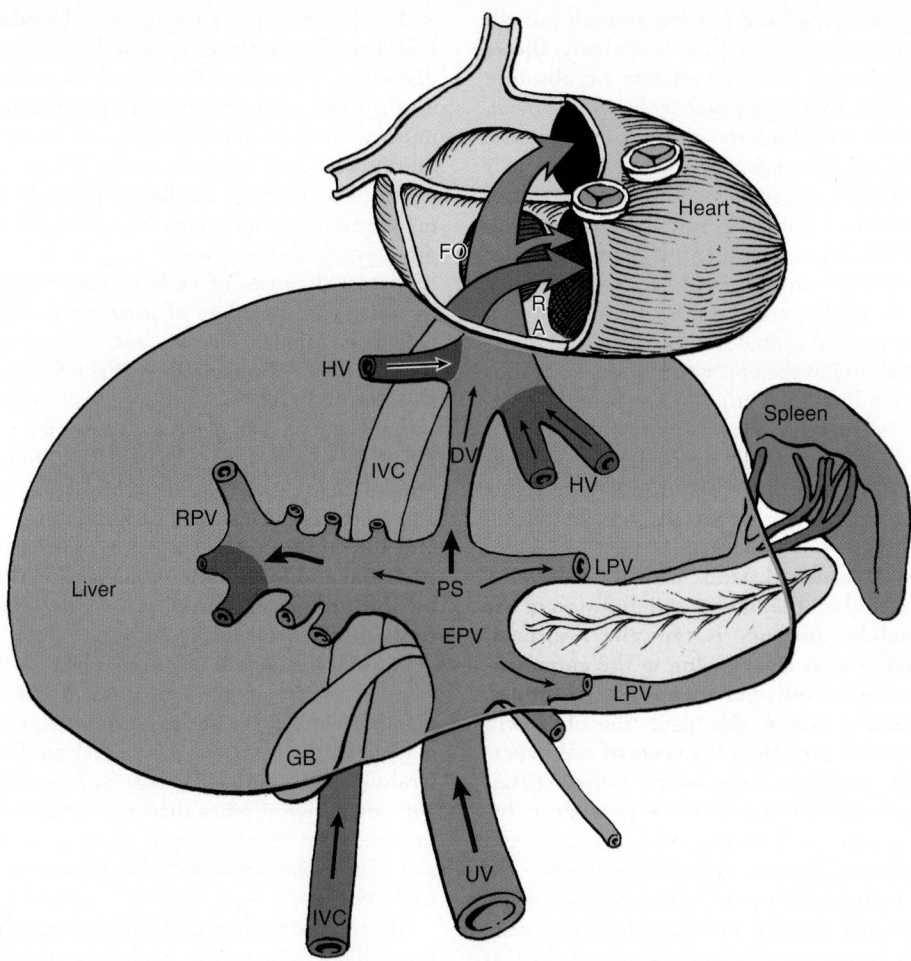

FIG 33-1 Fetal umbilical and hepatic venous circulation. The *arrows* indicate the direction of blood flow, and the color shows the oxygen content (*red* = high, *purple* = medium, *blue* = low). DV, ductus venosus; EPV, extrahepatic portal vein; FO, foramen ovale; GB, gallbladder; HV, hepatic vein; IVC, inferior vena cava; LPV, left portal vein; PS, portal sinus; RA, right atrium; RPV, right portal vein; UV, umbilical vein. (From Mavrides E, Moscoso G, Carvalho JS, et al. The anatomy of the umbilical, portal and hepatic venous systems in the human fetus at 14-19 weeks of gestation. *Ultrasound Obstet Gynecol.* 2001;18:598.)

Lubchenco, Usher, Battaglia, and others demonstrated that only the comparison of the actual birthweight to the expected weight in a population at the same gestational age identified small neonates at risk for adverse outcome. Adopting this concept of "light" and "heavy" for gestational age served as an introduction of population-based reference ranges for birthweight in the 1970s and allowed classification of growth by the birthweight percentile. **This resulted in the currently accepted classification of birthweight as *very small for gestational age*** (VSGA; <3rd percentile), *small for gestational age* (SGA; <10th percentile), *average for gestational age* (AGA; 10th to 90th percentile), **or** *large for gestational age* (LGA; >90th percentile). Although birthweight percentiles are superior in identifying the small neonate, they fail to account for proportionality of growth and the growth potential of the individual. Therefore neonates with a normal birthweight percentile but abnormal body proportion as a result of differential growth delay may be missed. Similarly, birthweight percentiles do not distinguish between the small neonate normally grown given his or her genetic potential and the neonate that is growth restricted because of a disease process.

The detection of abnormal body mass or proportions is based on anthropometric measurements and ratios that are relatively

independent of sex and race and, to a certain extent, gestational age and therefore also the traditional birthweight percentiles. **The ponderal index** ([birthweight in grams/crown heel length]^3 × 100) **has a high accuracy for the identification of SGA** and macrosomia. The ponderal index correlates more closely with perinatal morbidity and mortality than traditional birthweight percentiles, but it may miss the proportionally small and lean growth-restricted neonate. Several studies are currently underway to determine the most appropriate statistical methods to calculate the personalized growth potential across ethnicities. It is anticipated that these will improve the accurate prenatal identification of the SGA fetus.

The classification of abnormal growth during fetal life marks a significant advance because it opens the possibility of prenatal detection that leads to preventive or therapeutic management. The concept of percentiles has been adapted to the ultrasound biometry of the fetus. Accordingly, parameters of head, abdominal, and skeletal growth are related to population-based reference ranges. The prenatal diagnosis of FGR based on ultrasound biometry is described in detail below.

In addition to the detection of smaller individual measurements and lower weight, **two principal patterns of disturbed fetal growth have been described: asymmetric and** symmetric. In the *asymmetric growth pattern,* somatic growth (e.g., the abdominal circumference [AC] and lower body) **shows a significant delay, whereas there is relative or absolute sparing of head growth. In the *symmetric growth pattern,* body and head growth are similarly affected.** Asymmetric growth patterns result from two processes. First, liver volume is reduced because of depletion of glycogen stores as the result of limited nutrient supply, which leads to a decrease in AC. Second, elevations in placental blood flow resistance increase right cardiac afterload and promote diversion of the cardiac output toward the left ventricle because of the parallel arrangement of the fetal circulation and the presence of central shunts. Blood and nutrient supply to vital structures in the upper part of the body thus increase, presumably resulting in relative "head sparing." Symmetrically restricted fetal growth typically results when interference with the growth process results in decreased cell numbers and cell size, typically resulting from a first-trimester insult. As a result, all parts of the body are equally affected, which produces uniformly small growth.

The pattern of fetal growth depends on the underlying cause of growth delay and on the timing and duration of the insult. Uteroplacental insufficiency is typically associated with asymmetric fetal growth delay owing to the aforementioned mechanisms. Aneuploidy, nonaneuploid syndromes, and viral infections either disrupt the regulation of growth processes or interfere with growth at the stage of cell hyperplasia. This typically results in a symmetric growth delay. Specific conditions such as skeletal dysplasia may produce distinct growth patterns by their differential impacts on axial and peripheral skeletal growth. Because growth is dynamic, the pattern of growth restriction may evolve in the course of gestation. Placental disease may initially present with relative head sparing but eventually progresses to symmetric growth delay as placental insufficiency worsens. Alternatively, the acute course of a fetal viral illness may temporarily result in arrested growth with subsequent resumption of a normal growth pattern.

Although the definition and classification of FGR has significantly evolved, research is still ongoing. Small fetal and neonatal sizes have to be considered as a physical sign rather than a specific disease that warrants further investigation of underlying causes. Given that the term *small for gestational age* simply identifies a fetus below a specific weight cutoff without identifying any underlying cause, the SGA designation will be used for this chapter when no underlying cause is evident. The terms *intrauterine growth restriction* and *fetal growth restriction* imply that some pathologic process has prohibited attainment of genetic growth potential, and these terms will be used accordingly in this chapter with a focus on underlying placental pathology. From the perspective of the managing obstetrician, prenatal identification of IUGR is most relevant because it allows appropriate prospective fetal management. Conversely, prenatal identification of the constitutionally small fetus will allow the obstetrician to reassure the patient. To formulate a uniform approach to prenatal detection and perinatal management, an understanding of the maternal and fetal impact of placental insufficiency is essential.

ETIOLOGIES OF INTRAUTERINE GROWTH RESTRICTION

The precise mechanisms by which various conditions interfere with normal placentation and culminate in either pregnancy loss or IUGR are of great importance. **Conditions that result in FGR broadly consist of maternal, uterine, placental, and fetal disorders.** These conditions result in growth delay by affecting nutrient and oxygen delivery to the placenta (maternal causes), nutrient and oxygen transfer across the placenta (placental causes), and fetal nutrient uptake or regulation of growth processes (fetal causes). In clinical practice, considerable overlap may occur between the conditions that determine manifestation, progression, and outcome.

Maternal causes of FGR include vascular disease such as hypertensive disorders of pregnancy, diabetic vasculopathy, collagen vascular disease, and thrombophilia and chronic renal disease. Abnormalities of the fetus and/or placenta can also result in FGR. Chromosomal abnormalities, congenital malformations, and genetic syndromes have been associated with less than 10% of cases of IUGR.[4] Similarly, although long recognized as a cause of growth restriction, intrauterine infection also accounts for less than 10% of all cases. **However, genetic and infectious etiologies are of special importance because perinatal and long-term outcomes are ultimately determined by the underlying condition, with little potential impact through perinatal interventions.**

Growth restriction has been observed in 53% of cases of trisomy 13 and in 64% of cases of trisomy 18 and may be manifest as early as the first trimester. Other conditions that may present with FGR include skeletal dysplasia and de Lange syndrome. The online database of inheritance in man lists over 100 genetic syndromes that may be associated with FGR. Of the infectious agents, herpes, cytomegalovirus (CMV), rubella, and *Toxoplasma gondii* are well-documented causes of symmetric IUGR.

The common causes of IUGR are listed in Box 33-1. Recognition of these is important in planning the diagnostic workup for specific underlying conditions.

Although it is beyond the scope of this chapter to discuss the spectrum of clinical consequences, it needs to be

---

BOX 33-1   ETIOLOGIES AND RISK FACTORS FOR INTRAUTERINE GROWTH RESTRICTION

Maternal
- Hypertensive disease
- Pregestational diabetes
- Cyanotic cardiac disease
- Autoimmune disease
- Restrictive pulmonary disease
- High altitude (>10,000 feet)
- Tobacco/substance abuse
- Malabsorptive disease/malnutrition
- Multiple gestation

Fetal
- Teratogenic exposure
- Fetal infection
- Genetic disorders
- Structural abnormalities

Placental
- Primary placental disease
- Placental abruption and infarction
- Placenta previa
- Placental mosaicism

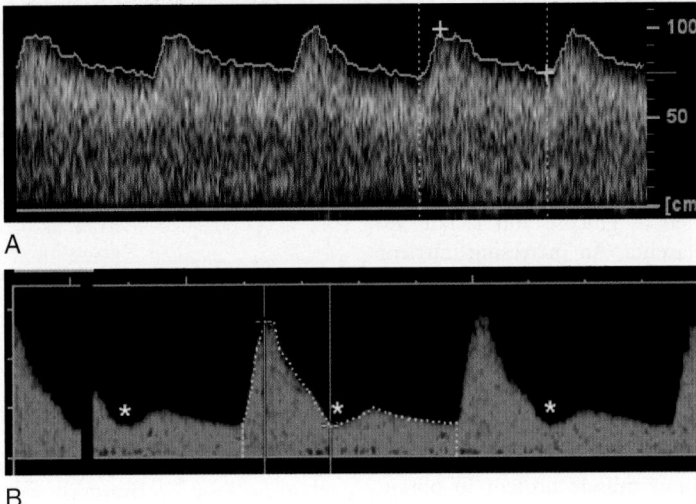

FIG 33-2 A, Uterine artery flow-velocity waveforms. Normal trophoblast invasion results in a low-resistance, high-capacitance placental vascular circulation that can be documented with uterine artery Doppler velocimetry. The flow-velocity waveform in **A** was obtained at 24 weeks' gestation and shows high diastolic flow velocities. Such a flow pattern indicates successful trophoblast invasion. **B,** The second waveform shows lower diastolic velocities and an early diastolic notch (*asterisks*). This flow pattern is reflective of increased blood flow resistance in the spiral arteries and downstream placental vascular bed. Persistence of notching beyond 24 weeks' gestation is associated with an increased risk of fetal growth restriction and/or hypertensive disorders of pregnancy.

recognized that the diagnosis and prognosis of FGR in twin pregnancies is critically determined by the chorionicity (see Chapter 32). *Selective intrauterine growth restriction (sIUGR) is a specific term applied to FGR that occurs in monochorionic twins. The prognosis and risk profile can be determined based on the umbilical artery flow pattern.*[5]

MATERNAL AND FETAL MANIFESTATIONS OF INTRAUTERINE GROWTH RESTRICTION

The impact and clinical manifestations of placental insufficiency depend on the gestational age at onset and the severity and type of the placental disease. Early interference with normal placentation affects all levels of placental and fetal development and culminates in the most severe clinical picture, which may result in miscarriage or early stillbirth. If sufficient supply to the placental mass can be established, further placental differentiation may be possible, but suboptimal maternal adaptation to pregnancy and deficient nutrient delivery pose limitations. If adaptive mechanisms permit ongoing fetal survival, early-onset growth restriction with its many fetal manifestations develops. If placental disease is mild or successful compensation has occurred, the consequences of nutrient shortage may remain largely subclinical, only to be unmasked through their restrictive effect on exponential fetal growth in the second to third trimester. In these cases, late-onset growth delay, a decrease in adipose tissue, or abnormal body proportions at birth may be the consequence.

Maternal Impacts

Placental dysfunction affects several aspects of maternal adaptation to pregnancy. Associations between poor placentation with suboptimal maternal volume expansion, increased vascular reactivity, and a "flat" curve on the glucose tolerance test have been described. Abnormalities of placental vascular development are of special interest because they can be detected by Doppler ultrasound of the uterine arteries and frequently predate clinical disease (Fig. 33-2). When trophoblast invasion remains confined to the decidual portion of the myometrium, maternal spiral and radial arteries fail to undergo the physiologic transformation into low-resistance vessels, which is generally expected by 22 to 24 weeks. **Maternal placental floor infarcts, fetal villous obliteration, and fibrosis each increase placental blood flow resistance, producing a maternal-fetal placental perfusion mismatch that decreases the effective exchange area.** With progressive vascular occlusion, fetoplacental flow resistance is increased throughout the vascular bed, and eventually, metabolically active placental mass is reduced. The diagnostic and screening utility of ultrasound findings suggestive of such pathology are discussed below.

Fetal Impacts

When placental dysfunction compromises nutrient delivery and triggers fetal mobilization of hepatic glycogen stores, physical manifestation of growth delay becomes clinically apparent. In addition to the cardinal sign of FGR, metabolic, endocrine, hematologic, cardiovascular, and behavioral manifestations of placental insufficiency have been described that relate to the severity and duration of placental dysfunction. Of these, cardiovascular and central nervous system (CNS) responses are best studied because their noninvasive assessment is readily achieved by multivessel Doppler, gray-scale ultrasonography, and fetal heart rate (FHR) analysis and can therefore be utilized for fetal surveillance. Appreciating the variety of fetal manifestations helps to understand the potential limitations of antenatal surveillance and provides a basis on which to appreciate the possible short- and long-term impacts of placental insufficiency.

Metabolic manifestations occur early in growth-restricted fetuses. This is because with mild to moderate decline in uterine nutrient delivery, fetal supply is compromised first, whereas placental nutrition is preferentially maintained. With progression of placental insufficiency, nutrient deficits become universal and result in decreased fetal and placental size. Accordingly, with mild restrictions in oxygen and glucose supply, fetal demands are still met by increased fractional extraction. **When uterine oxygen delivery falls below a critical value** (0.6 mmol/min/kg fetal body weight in sheep), **fetal oxygenation begins to fall and is eventually accompanied by fetal hypoglycemia.** The initially mild hypoglycemia results in a blunted fetal pancreatic insulin response that allows gluconeogenesis from hepatic glycogen stores. The minimal hepatic glycogen stores in the fetus are quickly depleted as glucose and lactate are preferentially diverted to the placenta. An increasing nutrient deficit leads to worsening fetal hypoglycemia, which decreases the maintenance of fetal oxidative metabolism and placental nutrition. With a more significant limitation of oxidative metabolism associated with downregulation of placental transport mechanisms and intensifying hypoglycemia, the use of other fetal energy sources becomes necessary, and more widespread metabolic consequences ensue. Limitation of amino acid transfer and breakdown of endogenous muscle protein to obtain gluconeogenic amino acids depletes branched-chain and other essential amino acids.[6] Simultaneously, lactate accumulates because of the limited capacity for oxidative metabolism. Placental transfer of fatty acids loses its selectivity, particularly for essential fatty acids. Reduced utilization leads to increased fetal free fatty acid and triglyceride levels with a subsequent failure to accumulate adipose stores. In this setting of advancing malnutrition, cerebral and cardiac metabolism of lactate and ketones is upregulated to remove these accumulating products of anaerobic metabolism. Acid-base balance can be maintained as long as acid production is met by sufficient buffering capacity of fetal hemoglobin and an equal disposition by the various organs. **Thus metabolic compromise progresses from simple hypoglycemia, hypoxemia, and decreased levels of essential amino acids to overt hypoaminoacidemia, hypercapnia, hypertriglyceridemia, and hyperlacticemia. The lactate production is exponentially correlated to the degree of acidemia that generally results from this metabolic state.[7] A summary of metabolic responses is provided in** Table 33-1.

Fetal endocrine manifestations of placental insufficiency are relevant because they are responsible for the downregulation of growth and developmental processes. Decreases in fetal glucose and amino acids indirectly downregulate insulin and insulin-like growth factors (IGFs) I and II as the principal endocrine regulators of longitudinal growth. Leptin-coordinated deposition of fat stores is similarly affected. In addition, pancreatic cellular dysfunction becomes evident through a decreased insulin/glucose ratio and impaired fetal glucose tolerance. Significant elevations of corticotropin-releasing hormone (CRH), adrenocorticotropic hormone (ACTH), and cortisol and a decline in active vitamin D and osteocalcin all correlate with the severity of placental dysfunction. **These hormonal imbalances are believed to have additional negative impacts on linear and growth, bone mineralization, and the potential for postpartum catch-up growth.**

In growth-restricted fetuses, declining function at all levels of the thyroid axis correlates to the degree of hypoxemia. Thyroid gland dysfunction may develop as indicated by low levels of thyroxine and triiodothyronine despite elevated thyroid-stimulating hormone (TSH) levels. In other instances, central production of TSH may be responsible for fetal hypothyroidism. Finally, downregulation of thyroid hormone receptors may limit the biologic activity of circulating thyroid hormones in specific target tissues such as the developing brain.[8]

TABLE 33-1	SUMMARY OF METABOLIC RESPONSES TO PLACENTAL INSUFFICIENCY
SUBSTRATE	**CHANGE**
Glucose	Decreased proportional to the degree of fetal hypoxemia
Amino acids	Significant decrease in branched-chain amino acids (valine, leucine, isoleucine) as well as lysine and serine; in contrast, hydroxyproline is elevated. The decrease in essential amino acids is proportional to the degree of hypoxemia.
	Elevated amniotic fluid glycine to valine ratio
	Elevations in amniotic fluid ammonia with a significant positive correlation with the fetal ponderal index
Fatty acids and triglycerides	Decrease in long-chain polyunsaturated fatty acids (docosahexaenoic and arachidonic acids), decrease in overall fatty acid transfer only with significant loss of placental substance
	Hypertriglyceridemia due to decreased utilization
	Lower cholesterol esters
Oxygen and carbon dioxide	Degree of hypoxemia proportional to villous damage; correlates significantly with hypercapnia, acidemia and hypoglycemia, and hyperlacticemia

Elevations in serum glucagon, adrenaline, and noradrenaline and stimulation of the fetal glucocorticoid axis have immediate effects that promote the mobilization of hepatic glycogen stores and peripheral gluconeogenesis. However, persistent alterations of these hormones may have a causative relationship with the development of diabetes and vascular complications in adult life.

Fetal hematologic responses to placental insufficiency are important because they initially provide a compensatory mechanism for hypoxemia and acidemia but eventually become contributory to the escalation of placental vascular dysfunction. Fetal hypoxemia is a trigger for erythropoietin release and stimulation of red blood cell (RBC) production through both medullary and extramedullary sites, which results in polycythemia.[9] Oxygen-carrying capacity and the buffering capacity are thus increased through the elevation in hemoglobin count. If extramedullary hematopoiesis is increasingly induced by prolonged tissue hypoxemia and/or acidosis, the nucleated red blood cell (NRBC) count rises owing to the escape of these cells from these sites. **Thus elevated NRBC counts correlate with metabolic and cardiovascular status and are independent markers for poor perinatal outcome.** In advanced placental insufficiency, more complex hematologic abnormalities supervene that may result from dysfunctional erythropoiesis, placental consumption of platelets, and vitamin and iron deficiency. Subsequently, fetal anemia and thrombocytopenia are observed, particularly in fetuses with marked elevation of placental blood flow resistance and evidence of intraplacental thrombosis, which suggests a causative relationship. **Increase in whole blood viscosity, decrease in RBC membrane fluidity, and platelet aggregation may be important precursors in the acceleration of placental vascular occlusion and dysfunction.**[10]

Growth-restricted fetuses also show evidence of immune dysfunction at the cellular and humoral level. Decreases in immunoglobulin, absolute B-cell counts, total white blood cell (WBC) counts, and neutrophil, monocyte, and lymphocyte subpopulations—as well as selective suppression of T-helper and cytotoxic T cells—are all related to the degree of acidemia. These immune deficiencies explain the higher susceptibility of growth-restricted neonates to infection after delivery.

Fetal cardiovascular responses to placental insufficiency can be subdivided into early and late based on the degree of deterioration of cardiovascular status and the associated derangement of fetal acid-base balance (see below).[11] *Early responses* are typically adaptive in nature and result in preferential nutrient streaming to essential organs. The combination of elevated placental blood flow resistance and impaired transplacental gas transfer has several effects on the fetal circulation. Normally, nutrient-rich oxygenated blood enters the fetus via the umbilical vein and reaches the liver as the first major organ. One of the earliest cardiovascular signs of placental insufficiency is a decrease in the magnitude of umbilical venous flow volume. In response to these changes in umbilical venous nutrition content and blood flow volume, the proportion of umbilical venous blood diverted through the ductus venosus toward the fetal heart increases.[12] This change in venous shunting across the DV increases the proportion of nutrient-rich umbilical venous blood that bypasses the liver and reaches the left side of the heart through the foramen ovale.[13] Because of the presence of central shunts at the level of the foramen ovale and ductus arteriosus, differential changes in downstream blood flow resistance can affect the proportion of cardiac output delivered through each ventricle (Fig. 33-3). Elevation of blood flow resistance in the pulmonary vascular bed and subdiaphragmatic circulation (lower body and placenta) increase right ventricular afterload. A drop in cerebral blood flow resistance decreases left ventricular afterload. As a consequence, **shunting of nutrient-rich blood from the DV through the foramen ovale to the left side of the heart increases, and left ventricular output rises in relation to the right cardiac output.**[14] At the aortic isthmus, blood coming from the right ventricle through the ductus arteriosus is diverted toward the aortic arch, thereby supplementing this central shift in cardiac output from right to left. **This relative shift in cardiac output toward the left ventricle that results in increased blood flow to the myocardium and brachiocephalic circulation has been termed** *redistribution,* **which indicates a compensatory mechanism in response to placental insufficiency.**

Late circulatory responses are associated with deterioration of cardiovascular status and are predominantly observed in early-onset growth delay, which requires delivery prior to 34 weeks.[15] Redistribution is only effective as long as adequate forward cardiac function is maintained. Marked elevations in placental blood flow resistance and progressive placental insufficiency can lead to an impairment of cardiac function. When this occurs, several aspects of cardiovascular homeostasis can be affected. **Ineffective preload handling and elevation in central venous pressure may result from ineffective redistribution, a measurable decline in cardiac output, and a decline in cardiac forward function.** The hallmark of this advancing deterioration in cardiovascular state is loss of diastolic forward flow in the umbilical circulation and a marked decline of forward flow in the venous system.[16] **Finally, myocardial dysfunction and cardiac dilatation may result in holosystolic tricuspid insufficiency and spontaneous FHR decelerations, followed by fetal demise.**[17]

Fetal organs also have the ability to regulate their individual blood flow through autoregulation. Such autoregulatory mechanisms have been identified in the myocardium, adrenal glands, spleen, liver, celiac axis, mesenteric vessels, and kidneys. These autoregulatory mechanisms are evoked at different levels of compromise and their effect is

TABLE 33-2	ARTERIAL AND VENOUS DOPPLER INDICES
INDEX	**CALCULATION**
Arterial Doppler Indices	
Systolic/diastolic (S/D) ratio	$\dfrac{\text{Systolic peak velocity}}{\text{Diastolic peak velocity}}$
Resistance index (RI)	$\dfrac{\text{Systolic} - \text{End-diastolic peak velocity}}{\text{Systolic peak velocity}}$
Pulsatility index (PI)	$\dfrac{\text{Systolic} - \text{End-diastolic peak velocity}}{\text{Time averaged maximum velocity}}$
Venous Doppler Indices	
Inferior vena cava preload index	$\dfrac{\text{Peak velocity during atrial contraction}}{\text{Systolic peak velocity}}$
Ductus venosus preload index	$\dfrac{\text{Systolic} - \text{Diastolic peak velocity}}{\text{Systolic peak velocity}}$
Inferior vena cava and ductus venosus pulsatility index for veins (PIV)	$\dfrac{\text{Systolic} - \text{Diastolic peak velocity}}{\text{Time averaged maximum velocity}}$
Inferior vena cava and ductus venosus peak velocity index for veins (PVIV)	$\dfrac{\text{Systolic} - \text{Atrial contraction peak velocity}}{\text{Diastolic peak velocity}}$
Percentage reverse flow	$\dfrac{\text{Systolic time averaged velocity}}{\text{Diastolic time averaged velocity}} \times 100$

typically complementary to central blood flow redistribution by enhancing perfusion of vital organs as long as cardiovascular homeostasis is maintained. A summary of Doppler findings and their physiologic significance in the context of placental insufficiency is provided in Table 33-2.

Fetal behavioral responses to placental insufficiency and characteristics of the FHR reflect developmental status and undergo significant changes with advancing gestation. Progressive sophistication of fetal behavior and increasing variation of the FHR reflect differentiation of central regulatory centers and expansion of central processing capability. **Normally, behavioral milestones progress from the initiation of gross body movements and fetal breathing in the first trimester to coupling of fetal behavior** (e.g., heart rate reactivity) **and integration of rest-activity cycles into stable behavioral states** (states 1 through 4 F) **by 28 to 32 weeks' gestation** (see Chapter 11). A steady decrease in baseline heart rate that reflects increasing vagal tone accompanies these developments. In addition, short- and long-term variability and variation, as well as the amplitude of accelerations, increase with advancing gestation, which reflects increased central processing. **With the completion of these milestones, heart rate reactivity by traditional criteria is present in 80% of fetuses by 32 weeks' gestation.** Differences in maturational state and behavioral state, disruption of neural pathways, and declining oxygen tension may all modulate or even abolish fetal behavior or heart rate characteristics.

Because variations of fetal behavior and the FHR may be due to several factors, observation of several variables over a sufficient length of time is necessary to separate physiologic from pathologic variation. Biophysical profile (BPP) scoring quantifies fetal behavior by assessing tone, movement, breathing activity, and

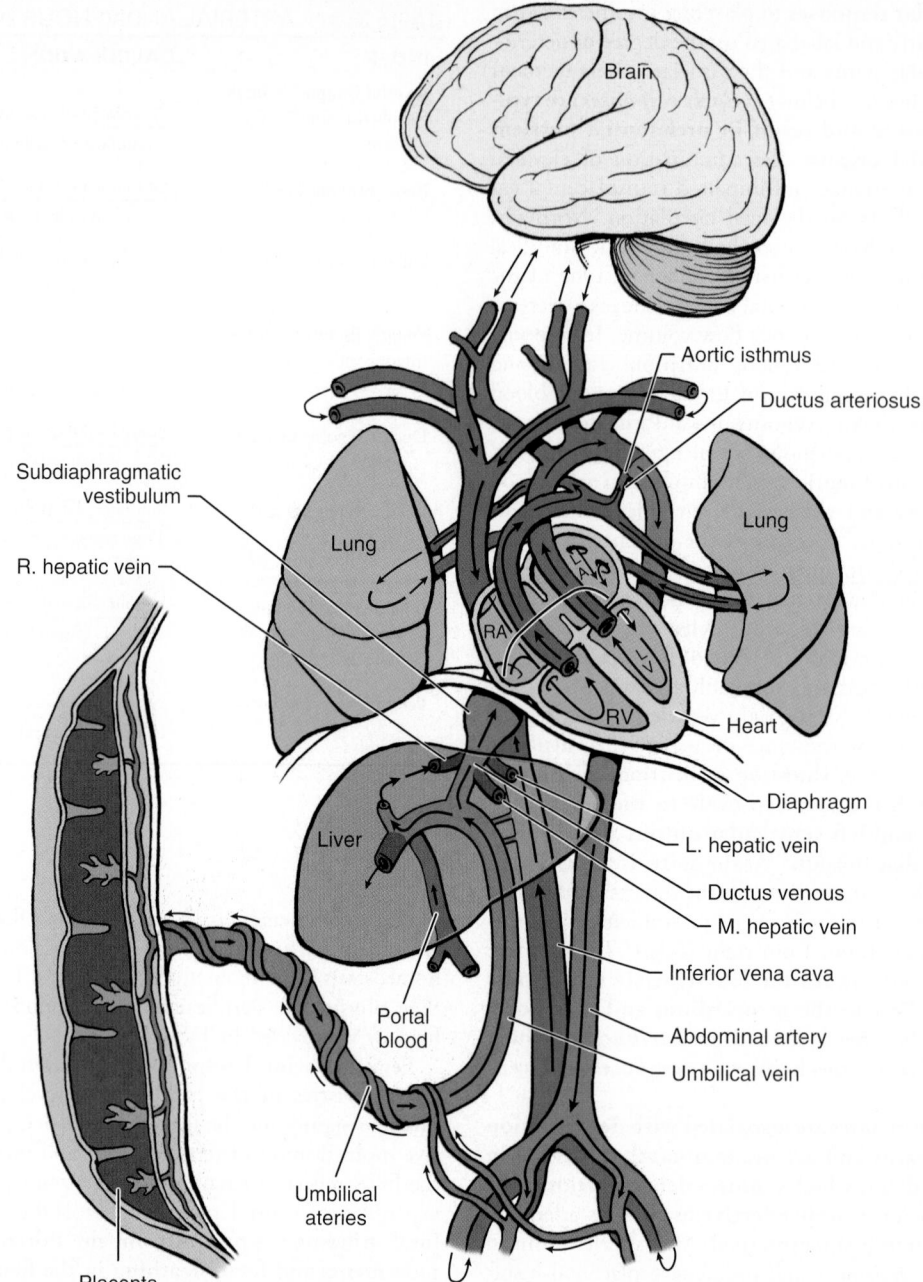

FIG 33-3 Schematic presentation of the fetal circulation. This figure illustrates the serial partitioning of nutrient- and oxygen-rich blood reaching the fetus via the umbilical vein. The first partition at the level of the ductus venosus distributes the majority of umbilical venous blood to the liver. Umbilical venous blood that continues toward the heart is partitioned toward the left ventricle (LV) at the foramen ovale. This blood supplies the brain and upper part of the body via the brachiocephalic circulation and the myocardium via the coronary circulation. A minor proportion of blood from the right ventricle (RV) supplies the lungs, and the remainder continues through the ductus arteriosus toward the aorta. At the aortic isthmus bloodstreams coming from the aorta are partitioned based on the relationship of blood flow resistance in the brachiocephalic and subdiaphragmatic circulations. Whereas net forward flow is maintained under physiologic conditions, diastolic flow reversal occurs when brachiocephalic resistance falls and/or subdiaphragmatic (placental) resistance rises. Finally, the major proportion of descending aortic blood is partitioned at the umbilical arteries to return to the placenta for respiratory and nutrient exchange. LA, left atrium; RA, right atrium. (From Baschat AA. The fetal circulation and essential organs—a new twist to an old tale. *Ultrasound Obstet Gynecol.* 2006;27:349.)

FHR reactivity in an observation period of at least 30 minutes (see Chapter 11). Amniotic fluid volume (AFV) assessment has traditionally been a part of the BPP. From the second trimester onward, AFV is primarily related to fetal urine production and therefore renal perfusion (see Chapter 35). **Thus AFV assessment provides an indirect assessment of renal/vascular status and constitutes the main longitudinal monitoring component of the BPP** (see below). **Visual FHR analysis is associated with interobserver and intraobserver variability.** These are circumvented by computerized cardiotocography (cCTG) analysis of the fetal heart rate. The cCTG assesses short-term, long-term, and mean minute variation and periods of high variation in addition to traditional FHR parameters that also allow longitudinal observations.

In growth-restricted fetuses with chronic hypoxemia and mild placental dysfunction, the primary CNS response is a delay in all aspects of CNS maturation.[18] With the help of computerized research tools, a delay in behavioral development has been documented under such circumstances. The combination of delayed central integration of FHR control, decreased fetal activity, and chronic hypoxemia results in a higher baseline heart rate with lower short- and long-term variation (on computerized analysis) and delayed development of heart rate reactivity.[19] These maturational differences in FHR parameters are particularly evident between 28 and 32 weeks.

Despite the maturational delay of some aspects of CNS function, several centrally regulated responses to acid-base status are still preserved. Therefore the growth-restricted fetus still maintains behavioral responses to a decline in acid-base status independently of the cardiovascular status. **In contrast, the declining AFV that commonly accompanies the sequential loss of biophysical variables appears to be related to renal blood flow and the degree of vascular redistribution.**[20]

With worsening fetal hypoxemia, a decline in global fetal activity initiates the cascade of late behavioral responses characteristic of placental insufficiency.[21] With further deepening hypoxemia, fetal breathing movement ceases.

Gross body movements and tone decrease further until they are no longer observed in the traditional examination period.[22,23] **Traditional FHR variables are frequently abnormal by this time. Reduction of global fetal activity and loss of fetal coupling** (absence of heart rate reactivity and fetal breathing movements) **are typically observed at a mean pH between 7.10 and 7.20.** Loss of tone and movement is characteristic as the pH drops further. Late decelerations of the FHR may develop because of a relative drop in oxygen tension that exceeds 8 torr (see Chapter 15). Spontaneous decelerations as a result of direct depression of cardiac contractility or "cardiac" late decelerations typically herald fetal demise.

DIAGNOSTIC TOOLS IN FETAL GROWTH RESTRICTION

Fetal growth restriction is a syndrome marked by failure of the fetus to reach its growth potential with consequences related to the underlying disorder as well as the severity of fetal disease. Because IUGR may be the consequence of many underlying etiologies, the differential diagnosis always includes maternal disease, placental insufficiency, aneuploidy, nonaneuploid syndromes, and viral infection. For appropriate patient counseling and choice of management options, comprehensive prenatal evaluation must go beyond the assessment of fetal size, utilizing a diagnostic approach aimed at identifying the underlying causes. **After confirming small fetal size, stratification into three patient groups is of particular importance. The first group consists of constitutionally small but otherwise normal fetuses.** These will not usually require any intervention and therefore do not need antenatal surveillance. **The second group consists of fetuses with aneuploidy, nonaneuploid syndromes, or viral infection.** In these conditions, prognosis is largely determined by the underlying disease, with little potential for impact by perinatal interventions. Sensitive and knowledgeable counseling of the parents about the likely prognosis in these conditions is especially important in such cases. **The third group consists of fetuses with placental disease in which progressive deterioration of the fetal condition worsens the**

prognosis. This subset of patients is most likely to benefit from fetal surveillance and subsequent intervention. Although grayscale ultrasonography provides important clues to the presence of IUGR, the liability of preterm delivery and iatrogenic complications is great if the diagnosis is based solely on biometry. Although maternal disease is readily apparent through a history and physical examination, the accurate evaluation of a possible fetal disorder and stratification of risk requires the integration of several diagnostic modalities that evaluate fetal, placental, and amniotic fluid characteristics.[24-26]

Fetal Biometry

Ultrasound criteria have emerged as the diagnostic standard used in the identification of FGR. For this purpose, sonographic measurements of fetal bony and soft structures are related to reference ranges for gestation. The primary measurements utilized to evaluate fetal growth include those of the fetal head, abdominal circumference, and long bones. The most important calculated ultrasound variable of fetal growth is the sonographically estimated fetal weight (SEFW), and numerous investigators have identified distinct fetal ultrasound parameters that are useful in the calculation of the SEFW.[27] All of the techniques incorporate an index of abdominal size as a variable contributing to the estimation of fetal weight. **Population-specific formulae have been derived to generate reference limits that generally have 95% confidence limits that deviate approximately 15% around the actual value.**

Accurate estimation of fetal growth from these fetal measurements requires knowledge of the gestational age as a reference point to calculate percentile ranks. **An estimated date of confinement (EDC) should be based on the last menstrual period when the sonographic estimate of gestational age is within the predictive error** (7 days in the first, 14 days in the second, and 21 days in the third trimester). **Once the EDC is set by this method or by a first-trimester ultrasound, it should not be changed because such practice interferes with the ability to diagnose IUGR.**

Measurement of the biparietal diameter (BPD) alone is a poor tool for the detection of IUGR. The physiologic variation in size inherent with advancing gestation is high. The majority of growth-restricted fetuses who present with asymmetric growth restriction and delayed flattening of the cranial growth curve would be detected relatively late. Factors that interfere with a technically adequate measurement of the BPD include alterations of the cranial shape by external forces (oligohydramnios, breech presentation) and direct anteroposterior position of the fetal head.

The head circumference (HC) is not subject to the same extrinsic variability as the BPD. The measurement technique is important because calculated HC measurements are systematically smaller than those directly measured, thus the nomogram selected should be based on measurements obtained using the same methodology. As a screening tool for IUGR, the HC poses a similar problem as the BPD in that two thirds of IUGR fetuses with asymmetric growth pattern would be detected late.

The transcerebellar diameter (TCD) is one of the few soft tissue measurements that correlate well with gestational age, being relatively spared from the effects of mild to moderate uteroplacental dysfunction.[28] Whether its measurement offers any advantage over bony measurements in the assessment of compromised fetal growth is controversial.

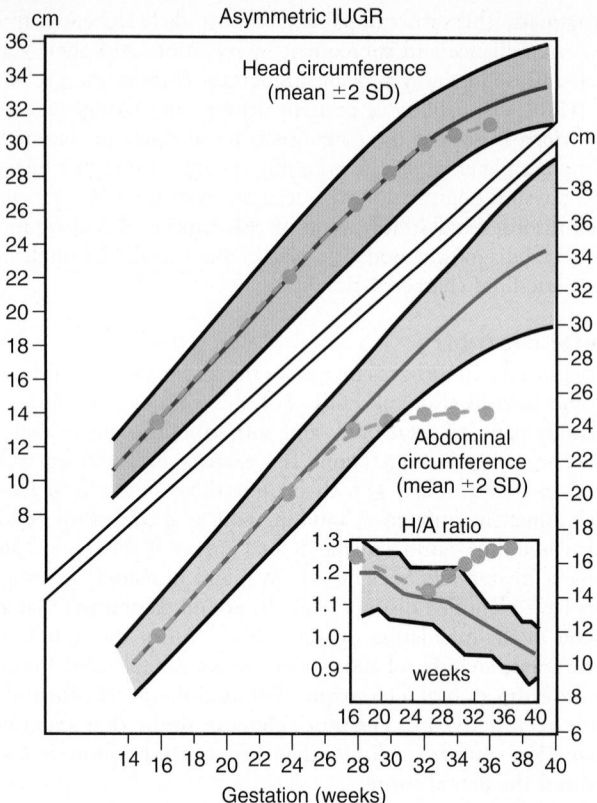

FIG 33-4 Growth chart in a case of asymmetric intrauterine growth restriction (IUGR). Although head circumference is preserved, abdominal circumference growth falls off early in the third trimester. For this reason, the head/abdomen (H/A) ratio shown in the lower right corner of the graph becomes elevated. SD, standard deviation. (From Chudleigh P, Pearce JM. *Obstetric Ultrasound.* Edinburgh: Churchill Livingstone; 1986.)

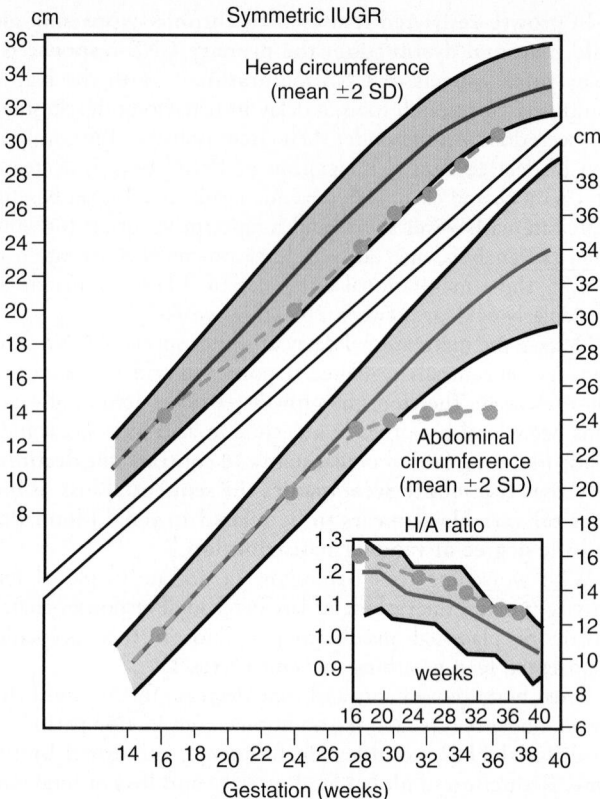

FIG 33-5 Growth chart in a case of symmetric intrauterine growth restriction (IUGR). Note the early onset of both head circumference and abdominal circumference growth restriction. For this reason, the head/abdomen (H/A) ratio shown in the lower right corner remains normal. SD, standard deviation. (From Chudleigh P, Pearce JM. *Obstetric Ultrasound.* Edinburgh: Churchill Livingstone; 1986.)

The AC is the single best measurement for the detection of IUGR.[29] The most accurate AC is the smallest directly measured circumference obtained in a perpendicular plane of the upper abdomen at the level of the hepatic vein between fetal respirations. The AC percentile has both the highest sensitivity and negative predictive value for the sonographic diagnosis of IUGR whether defined postnatally by birthweight percentile or ponderal index. **Using the 10th percentiles as cutoffs, the AC has a higher sensitivity** (98% vs. 85%) **but lower positive predictive value (PPV) than the SEFW** (36% vs. 51%). **Its sensitivity is further enhanced by serial measurements at least 14 days apart.**[30] Because of its high sensitivity, some type of abdominal measurement should be part of every sonographic growth evaluation. However, because the AC reflects fetal nutrition, it should be excluded from the calculation of the composite gestational age after the early second trimester.

Calculation of the ratio between the head and abdominal circumference (HC/AC ratio) has been proposed as a tool to increase detection of the fetus with asymmetric growth restriction (Figs. 33-4 and 33-5). In the normally growing fetus, the HC/AC ratio exceeds 1.0 before 32 weeks' gestation, is approximately 1.0 at 32 to 34 weeks' gestation, and falls below 1.0 after 34 weeks' gestation. In fetuses with asymmetric growth restriction, the HC remains larger than that of the body and results in an elevated HC/AC ratio,[31] whereas the ratio remains normal in symmetric IUGR, in which both direct measurements are equally affected (see Figs. 33-4 and 33-5). Using the HC/AC

ratio, 70% to 85% of growth-restricted fetuses are detected, with a reduction in false-negative diagnoses. Thus even when determined in the latter part of pregnancy, a single set of measurements can be very helpful in evaluating the status of fetal growth. **However, both the sensitivity and the PPV of the HC/AC ratio for growth restriction does not equal either the AC percentile or the SEFW.**[32]

When measurement of the HC is difficult because of fetal position, comparisons can be made of the femur length (FL)—which is relatively spared in asymmetric IUGR—to the AC. **The FL/AC ratio is 22 at all gestational ages from 21 weeks to term; therefore this ratio can be applied without knowledge of the gestational age. An FL/AC ratio greater than 23.5 suggests IUGR.**

Several formulae have been devised to calculate the SEFW. Using a multifactorial equation and a measurement of abdominal size, a weight can be predicted and related to gestational age. Formulae that incorporate the FL may increase the accuracy of in utero weight estimation for the fetus with IUGR. Because the SEFW cannot be measured directly but is calculated from a combination of directly measured parameters, the error in the estimate is increased. **The accuracy of most formulae (±2 standard deviations [SDs]) is ± 10%, and none has proven superior to the first devised by Warsof and reported by Sheppard.** As noted earlier, the SEFW has a lower sensitivity but higher PPV than the AC and does not add to the AC percentile for the diagnosis of IUGR. However, an SEFW below the 10th percentile provides a graphic image that makes it easy for both patient and referring physician to conceptualize. **Therefore use of the estimated fetal weight (EFW) has become the most common method for characterizing fetal size and thereby growth abnormalities.**

Reference Ranges That Define Fetal Growth

An absolute threshold to define IUGR can be applied to any of the fetal biometric parameters. These criteria have been statistically defined, rather than outcome based, and use either a threshold percentile ranking (nonnormative data) or a number of standard deviations below the mean (normative data) as cutoffs. *Small for gestational age* **is defined as a birthweight below the population 10th percentile corrected for gestational age. However, this cutoff has also been the most widely used criterion for defining growth restriction at birth.** This definition has also been adopted for the prenatal period by using an SEFW below the 10th percentile as an indicator of IUGR. Because such an approach is purely based on a weight threshold, it can only serve as a screen for the identification of the small fetus at risk for adverse outcomes. **Approximately 70% of infants with a birthweight below the 10th percentile are normally grown** (i.e., constitutionally small) **and are not at risk for adverse outcomes because they present one end of the normal spectrum for neonatal size.**[33] **The remaining 30% consist of infants who are truly growth restricted and are at risk for increased perinatal morbidity and mortality.** When the cutoff for an abnormal birthweight is adjusted to the 3rd percentile, the proportion of true growth-restricted infants identified increases, whereas some with milder forms of IUGR will be missed. The principal advantage of a lower percentile cutoff is the identification of fetuses at greatest need for antenatal surveillance. This is further emphasized by the increased mortality for birthweights through the 15th percentile with an odds ratio of 1.9 for mortality in newborns with birthweights between the 10th and 15th percentiles. Because the percentile cutoffs to define abnormal growth continue to be a matter of debate, risk assessment based on weight alone is further hampered by discrepancies between the SEFW and the actual birthweight. Live birthweight criteria do not appropriately describe SEFWs, and **a significant association of preterm birth with FGR is apparent.**[34] The weights of preterm infants are not normally distributed as they are at term, which produces a significant discrepancy between birthweight-defined growth curves and SEFW-defined growth curves in preterm gestation.[35] **SEFW growth curves are generated from patient samples that represent the entire obstetric population at any gestational age. In contrast, preterm live birth normative data tables reflect only those individuals who have delivered under abnormal circumstances.** Thus the SEFW growth curves consistently demonstrate higher fetal weights over the range of preterm gestation than do birthweight-generated growth curves. **Therefore use of an SEFW cutoff below the 10th percentile is more appropriate to define abnormal fetal growth because the ability to identify fetuses at greater perinatal risk is increased.**[36] For the AC, a cutoff of the 2.5 percentile is appropriate because reference ranges are based on a cross section of small, appropriately grown preterm and term newborns. However, because reference limits are based on healthy women delivering appropriately nourished neonates at term, less than the 10th percentile cutoff is consistent with IUGR.

Because of the limitation of population-based reference ranges to assess fetal growth, **individualized growth models have been proposed by several investigators.**[1,37] The obvious advantage is the lack of dependency on population-based normative data and the ability to detect a true, singularly defined growth restriction even with EFWs above the 10th percentile for the population. Some of these models require three sequential sonograms. This includes baseline biometry in the second trimester, a second sonogram to establish growth potential for an individual morphometric parameter, and a third scan to identify a growth abnormality. Because this approach is cumbersome in clinical practice, other models have been developed that account for variables that contribute the majority of the variance to newborn size. These include early pregnancy weight, maternal height, ethnic group, parity, and sex.[1] Using these variables and fetal growth patterns, the estimated size of a fetus of a given mother can be projected at term and estimated at any specific point in gestation. Deviations from this projected growth pattern can then be recognized. Overall, the diagnostic advantages of these individualized growth models has been questioned when compared with the sequential comparison of the percentile ranking of individual or composite growth parameters to population-based growth curves.

Fetal growth, as opposed to fetal size, is a dynamic process that requires more than a single evaluation for its estimation. The appropriate observation interval for the evaluation of fetal growth has been based on the assumptions that growth is continuous, rather than sporadic, and that the identification of growth is limited by the technical capability of the ultrasound equipment used to measure the fetus. **The recommended interval between ultrasound evaluations of fetal growth is 3 weeks because shorter intervals increase the likelihood of a false-positive diagnosis.**

In summary, the ability to correctly identify growth-restricted fetuses at risk for adverse outcome by weight estimates alone is limited. Individualized or sequential growth assessment performs better than a single measurement of fetal size. Improved stratification of risk requires the integration of additional diagnostic tests.

Fetal Anatomic Survey

The sonographic survey of fetal anatomy may provide a clue to the underlying etiology of IUGR. The anatomic survey should focus on markers of aneuploidy, nonaneuploid syndromes, and fetal infection as well as structural malformations. The relationship between aneuploidy and fetal anomalies such as omphalocele, diaphragmatic hernia, congenital heart defects, and sonographic markers such as echogenic bowel, nuchal thickening, and abnormal hand positioning are discussed in Chapter 9. Abnormalities of skull contour, thoracic shape, or disproportional shortening of the long bones may be suggestive of a skeletal dysplasia. Markers for viral infection may be nonspecific but include echogenicity and calcification in organs such as the brain and liver.[38] Identification of any of these abnormalities on ultrasound may help to establish a differential diagnosis and can impact the prognosis.

Amniotic Fluid Assessment

From the second trimester onward, regulation of AFV is primarily dependent on fetal urine output, production of pulmonary fluid, and fetal swallowing (see Chapter 35). **Placental dysfunction and fetal hypoxemia both may result in decreased** perfusion of the fetal kidneys with subsequent oliguria and decreasing AFV.[39] Although the accuracy of ultrasound in the assessment of actual AFV is poor, two techniques are used that can provide important diagnostic and prognostic information.[40] A vertical pocket of amniotic fluid measuring 1 cm or more was historically considered indicative of an adequate fluid volume. Criteria for AFV assessment were subsequently broadened. A 2-cm vertical pocket was considered *normal,* 1 to 2 cm was *marginal,* and less than 1 cm was *decreased.* Alternatively, AFV may be assessed by the sum of vertical pockets from the four quadrants of the uterine cavity. This four-quadrant amniotic fluid index (AFI) nomogram (see Fig. 33-3) is compared with gestational reference ranges. **Despite the availability of these numerical methods for estimating the AFV, an overall clinical impression of reduced amniotic fluid may be most important.** Ultrasound criteria for a subjectively reduced AFV include a maximum vertical pocket less than 3 cm, the fetus in a flexion attitude with limited room for movement, a small or empty bladder and stomach, and molding of the uterus around the fetal body. In addition, movement of the transducer frequently generates uterine contractions, which may be associated with variable decelerations.

Overall, estimation of AFV in itself is a poor screening method for IUGR or fetal acidemia. However, in clinical practice, it is an important diagnostic and prognostic tool. Oligohydramnios may be the first sign of FGR detected on ultrasonography preceding an assessment for lagging fetal growth. If gestational age is known, ultrasound assessment of fetal growth based on the HC, AC, FL, and SEFW can be performed. **If gestational age is unknown, measurements of the FL/AC ratio and a single amniotic fluid pocket have to be used because they are independent of gestational age. Up to 96% of fetuses with fluid pockets less than 1 cm may be growth restricted.**[41] When growth delay is already suspected, assessments of AFV can help with a differential diagnosis. In the setting of small fetal size, abundant AFV suggests aneuploidy or fetal infection, whereas normal or decreased amniotic fluid is compatible with placental insufficiency. **The volume of amniotic fluid also has prognostic significance for the course of labor.** Groome and colleagues[42] demonstrated that oligohydramnios associated with fetal oliguria is associated with a higher rate of intrapartum complications that may be attributed to reduced placental reserve.

Doppler Velocimetry

Similar to the assessment of AFV, the role of Doppler velocimetry in the management of FGR is unique because it serves as a diagnostic, as well as a monitoring, tool. Doppler flow-velocity waveforms may be obtained from arterial and venous vascular beds in the fetus. **Arterial Doppler waveforms provide information on downstream vascular resistance, which may be altered because of structural changes in the vasculature or regulatory changes in vascular tone. The systolic/diastolic (S/D) ratio, the resistance index (RI), and the pulsatility index (PI) are the three Doppler indices most widely used to analyze arterial blood flow resistance** (see Table 33-2). An increase in blood flow resistance manifests with a relative decrease in end-diastolic velocity that results in an increase in all three Doppler indices. Of these, the pulsatility index has the smallest measurement error and narrower reference limits. With extreme increases in blood flow resistance, end-diastolic forward flow velocity may be absent or reversed, referred

to as *absent end-diastolic velocity* (AEDV) or *reversed end-diastolic velocity* (REDV; Fig. 33-6).

Venous Doppler parameters complement evaluation of fetal cardiovascular status by providing an assessment of cardiac forward function. Forward blood flow in the venous system is determined by cardiac compliance, contractility, and afterload and is characterized by a triphasic flow pattern that reflects pressure volume changes in the atria throughout the cardiac cycle.[43] The descent of the AV ring during ventricular systole and passive diastolic ventricular filling generates the systolic and diastolic peaks respectively (the S-wave and the D-wave). The sudden increase in right atrial pressure with atrial contraction in late diastole causes a variable amount of reverse flow that produces a second trough after the D-wave (the a-wave; Fig. 33-7). The magnitude of forward flow during the atrial systole varies considerably in individual veins, and reversal may be physiologic in the inferior vena cava and hepatic veins but is always abnormal in the ductus venosus. **Multiple venous Doppler indices have been described to characterize this complex waveform without any clear advantages of individual indices** (see Table 33-2).

The vessels that are of primary importance in the differential diagnosis of placental dysfunction are the umbilical artery (UA) and the middle cerebral artery (MCA). Randomized trials and meta-analyses confirm that the combined use of fetal biometry and UA Doppler significantly reduces perinatal mortality and iatrogenic intervention because documentation of placental vascular insufficiency effectively separates growth-restricted fetuses that require surveillance and possible intervention from constitutionally small fetuses.[44,45]

A free umbilical cord loop is examined with continuous or pulsed Doppler ultrasound far from the fetal and placental insertions. Most current ultrasound equipment allows concurrent use of color and pulsed Doppler with improved reproducibility of measurements. **Vascular damage that affects approximately 30% of the placenta produces elevations in the Doppler index.** More marked abnormalities result in umbilical artery AEDV or REDV. **Milder forms of placental vascular dysfunction, especially near term, may not produce elevation of UA blood flow resistance sufficient to be detectable by traditional Doppler methods.**[46] If placental gas exchange is significantly impaired, resulting in fetal hypoxemia, a decrease in MCA Doppler resistance may occur (Fig. 33-8). Another Doppler index frequently used clinically to detect this condition is the ratio between UA pulsatility as an index of vasoconstriction in the placenta and MCA pulsatility as an index of vasodilation in the fetal brain. In milder forms of placental disease with near minimal increase in UA blood flow resistance, the cerebroplacental Doppler ratio (CPR) may decrease. Grammellini and coworkers demonstrated that a value below 1.08 identified small fetuses at risk for adverse outcome. **Subsequently, Bahado-Singh and coworkers**[47] **indicated that the predictive accuracy of the CPR decreased after 34 weeks' gestation. This is presumably attributable to an increasing number of growth-restricted fetuses who may have normal UA blood flow resistance near term but demonstrate isolated "brain sparing" as the only sign of placental insufficiency of oxygen transfer. These fetuses are at risk for adverse outcomes.**

Because of the variable presentation of IUGR across gestation, comprehensive Doppler assessment of placental function should include the umbilical and middle cerebral arteries. For the UA,

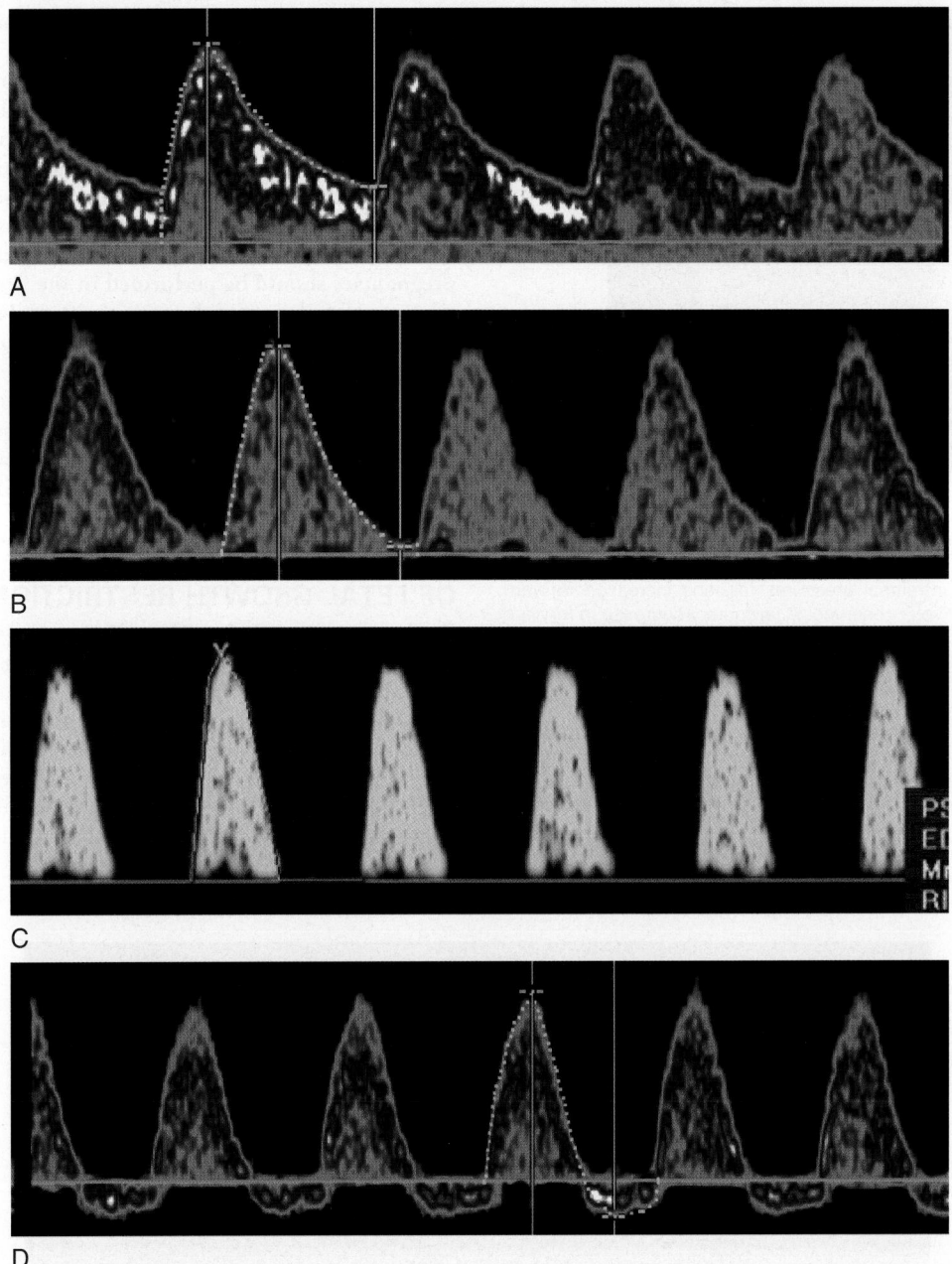

FIG 33-6 Umbilical artery flow-velocity waveforms. **A,** The normal umbilical artery flow-velocity waveform has positive end-diastolic velocities that increase toward term, reflecting a falling blood flow resistance in the villous vascular tree. **B,** Moderate abnormalities in the villous vascular structure raise the blood flow resistance and are associated with a decline in end-diastolic velocities. When a significant proportion of the villous vascular tree is abnormal, end-diastolic velocities may be absent **(C)** or even reversed **(D).**

an abnormal test result is defined as a Doppler index measurement of greater than 2 SDs above the gestational age mean and/or a loss of end-diastolic velocity. As with growth curves, it is best to use nomograms developed from a local or comparable population. For the CPR and also for the MCA, a greater than 2-SD decrease of the index is considered abnormal. In a setting of small fetal size, these findings identify those fetuses at greatest risk for adverse outcome (Figs. 33-9 to 33-12).

Invasive Testing

Several invasive tests for the evaluation of the fetus with suspected growth restriction have been described. From a clinical standpoint, only a few studies are of critical importance. These include maternal toxoplasmosis, other infections, rubella, CMV, and herpes infection (TORCH) serology and invasive fetal testing to obtain amniotic fluid and/or fetal blood for karyotyping or microarray analysis to rule out a chromosomal abnormality such as trisomies 13, 18, or 21 or a submicroscopic deletion or duplication (Table 33-3). Trisomy 18 may present with the unusual combination of growth restriction and polyhydramnios (see Chapter 10). If the diagnosis of a lethal anomaly can be made with certainty, cesarean delivery for fetal distress is unnecessary and may be prevented. Viral polymerase chain reaction (PCR) studies can be performed if clinical

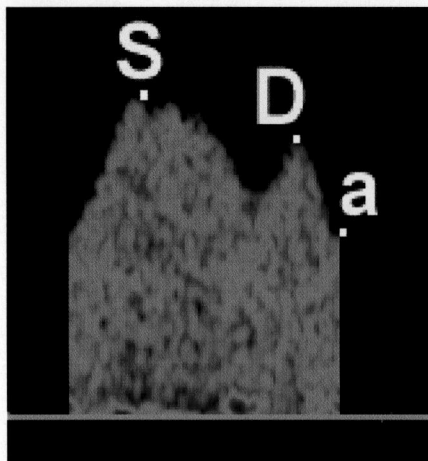

FIG 33-7 Venous flow-velocity waveform. A typical venous flow-velocity waveform is shown. The triphasic waveform (systole [S], diastole [D], atrial contraction [a]) reflects volume flow changes during the cardiac cycle. With descent of the atrioventricular valves during ventricular systole, intraatrial pressures fall, and increased forward flow during the S-wave is observed. A temporary decrease in forward flow occurs when the atrioventricular valve ring ascends at the end of ventricular systole, producing the first trough in the flow-velocity waveform. When atrial pressures exceed intraventricular pressures, the atrioventricular valves open, resulting in the rapid influx of blood into the ventricles. The associated increase in venous flow results in the D-wave. With initiation of a new cardiac cycle, atrial contraction results in a sharp rise in intraatrial pressure and a decline in venous forward flow. This second trough is called the *a-wave* because it is produced by atrial contraction.

suspicion is based on the ultrasound examination or the maternal history.

In summary, ultrasound examination is the primary diagnostic tool for the evaluation of fetal growth. In the presence of risk factors and clinical conditions associated with IUGR, a comprehensive gray-scale ultrasound examination of fetal anatomy along with biometry and an assessment of amniotic fluid characteristics is required. In the absence of routine clinical indications, ultrasound screening of these high-risk pregnancies should be performed in the first or early second trimester for dating and again at 32 to 34 weeks. If small fetal size is documented, Doppler ultrasound of the umbilical and middle cerebral arteries and invasive tests when indicated are of critical importance to identify fetuses most likely to benefit from antenatal surveillance and perinatal interventions. A diagnostic algorithm that utilizes this combination of test parameters is depicted in Figure 33-13.[48]

SCREENING AND PREVENTION OF FETAL GROWTH RESTRICTION

Fetal growth restriction as a disease entity fulfills several criteria that potentially justify a screening program. It is a common clinical problem with an identifiable predisease state that leaves enough time for potential interventions. Although treatment options in utero are limited (see below), interventions that improve outcome exist. The various screening methods that have been proposed include identification of risk factors in addition to serum and ultrasound tests.

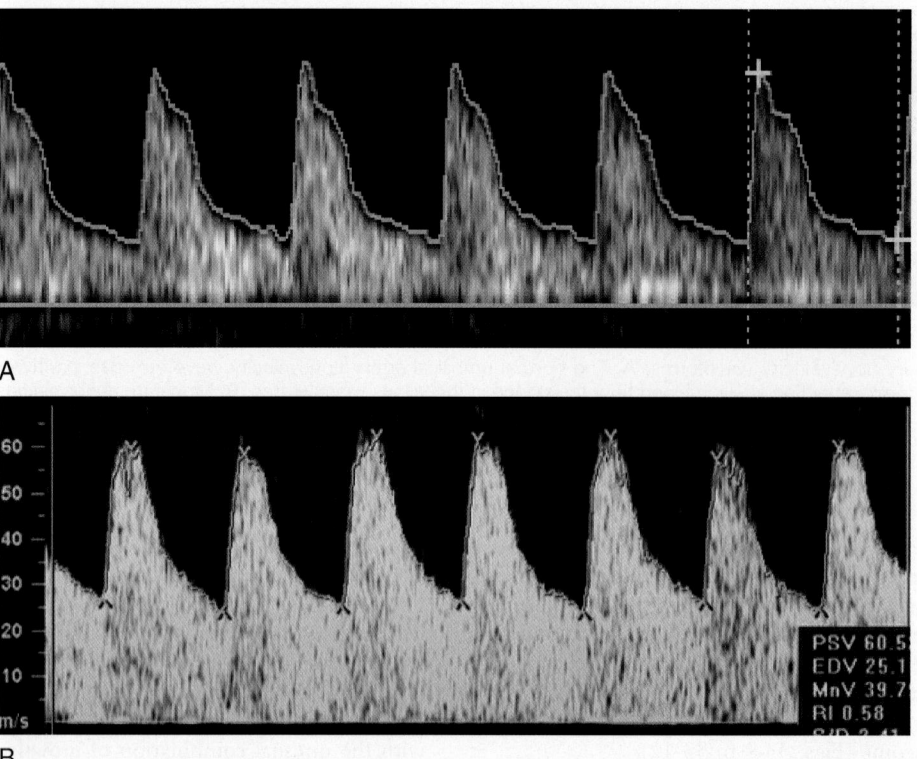

FIG 33-8 Middle cerebral artery flow-velocity waveform. **A,** The normal middle cerebral artery flow pattern has relatively little diastolic flow. With progressive placental dysfunction, an increase in the diastolic velocity results in a decrease in the Doppler index (brain sparing). **B,** With brain sparing, the systolic downslope of the waveform becomes smoother so that the waveform almost resembles that of the umbilical artery. The associated rise in the mean velocity results in a marked decline in the Doppler index.

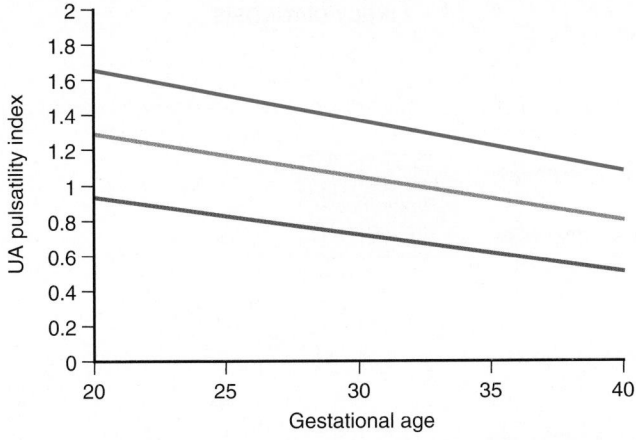

FIG 33-9 Umbilical artery (UA) pulsatility index with advancing gestational age. Displayed are the reference ranges (mean and 95% confidence interval).

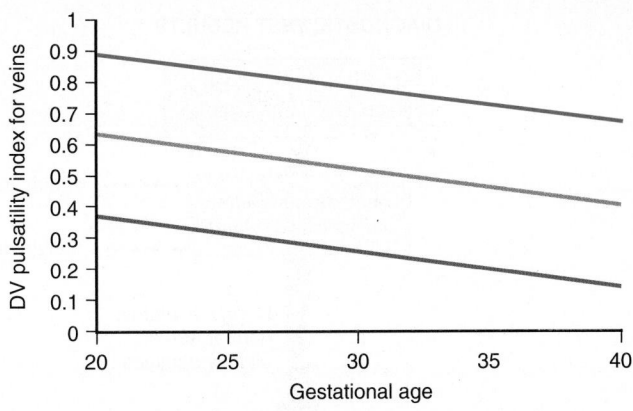

FIG 33-12 Ductus venosus (DV) pulsatility index for veins with advancing gestational age. This graph displays the gestational reference range (mean and 95% confidence interval) of the ductus venosus pulsatility index for veins calculated from cross-sectional data in 232 normal singleton fetuses.

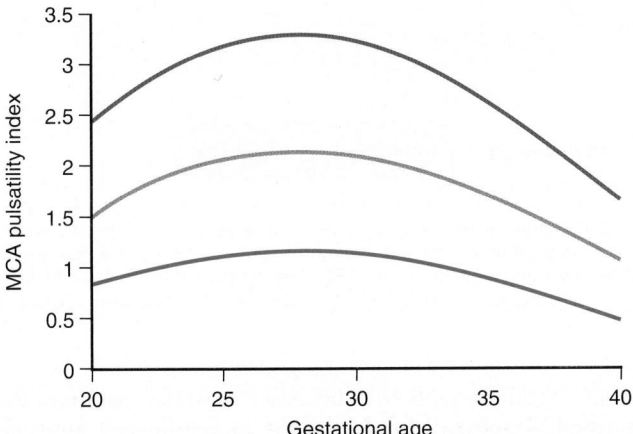

FIG 33-10 Middle cerebral artery (MCA) pulsatility index with advancing gestational age. The graph shows the mean and 95% confidence intervals.

TABLE 33-3	CHROMOSOMAL ABNORMALITIES AND INTRAUTERINE GROWTH RESTRICTION		
ULTRASOUND FINDINGS PRESENT			**ABNORMAL KARYOTYPE**
IUGR	**ANOMALY**	**HYDRAMNIOS**	
X			12/180 (7%)
X	X		18/57 (32%)
X		X	6/22 (27%)
X	X	X	7/15 (47%)

From Eydoux P, Choiset, A, LePorrier, N, et al. Chromosomal prenatal diagnosis: study of 936 cases of intrauterine abnormalities after ultrasound assessment. *Prenat Diagn.* 1989;9:255.
IUGR, intrauterine growth restriction.

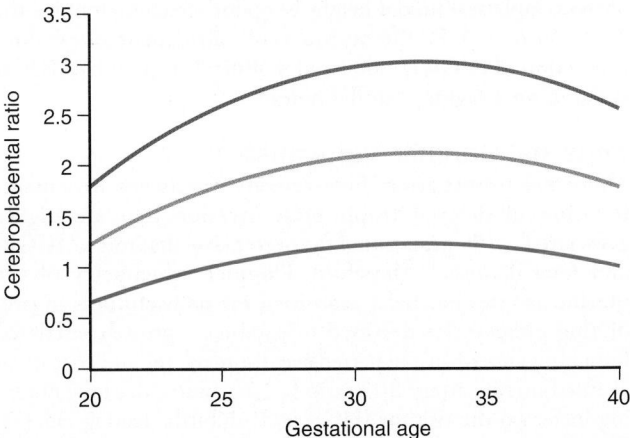

FIG 33-11 Cerebroplacental Doppler ratio with advancing gestational age. This graph displays the gestational reference range (mean and 95% confidence interval) of the cerebroplacental ratio based on paired measurements of the middle cerebral and umbilical artery pulsatility indices.

Maternal History

A history of poor pregnancy outcome is clearly correlated with the subsequent delivery of a growth-restricted infant. **A prior birth of a growth-restricted infant is the obstetric factor most often associated with the subsequent birth of a growth-restricted infant.** These study populations did include women with underlying medical problems. A retrospective study of 83 multigravidas who had delivered growth-restricted infants noted that the perinatal wastage from their 200 prior pregnancies was 41%. This striking figure, which includes spontaneous abortions as well as neonatal and intrauterine deaths, points to the significance of poor obstetric history as a risk factor for IUGR. **The history of delivery of a growth-restricted infant in the first pregnancy is associated with a 25% risk of delivering a second infant below the 10th percentile.** After two pregnancies complicated by IUGR, the risk is increased fourfold for birth of a subsequent growth-restricted infant. When all indices of risk have been applied, the one third of patients considered at highest risk for delivering a growth-restricted infant actually deliver over 60% of infants identified as growth restricted. The two thirds of women not considered at risk for delivering a growth-restricted infant contribute to one third of deliveries with a birthweight below the 10th percentile. The majority of these babies are considered constitutionally small.

DIAGNOSTIC TEST RESULTS   LIKELY DIAGNOSIS

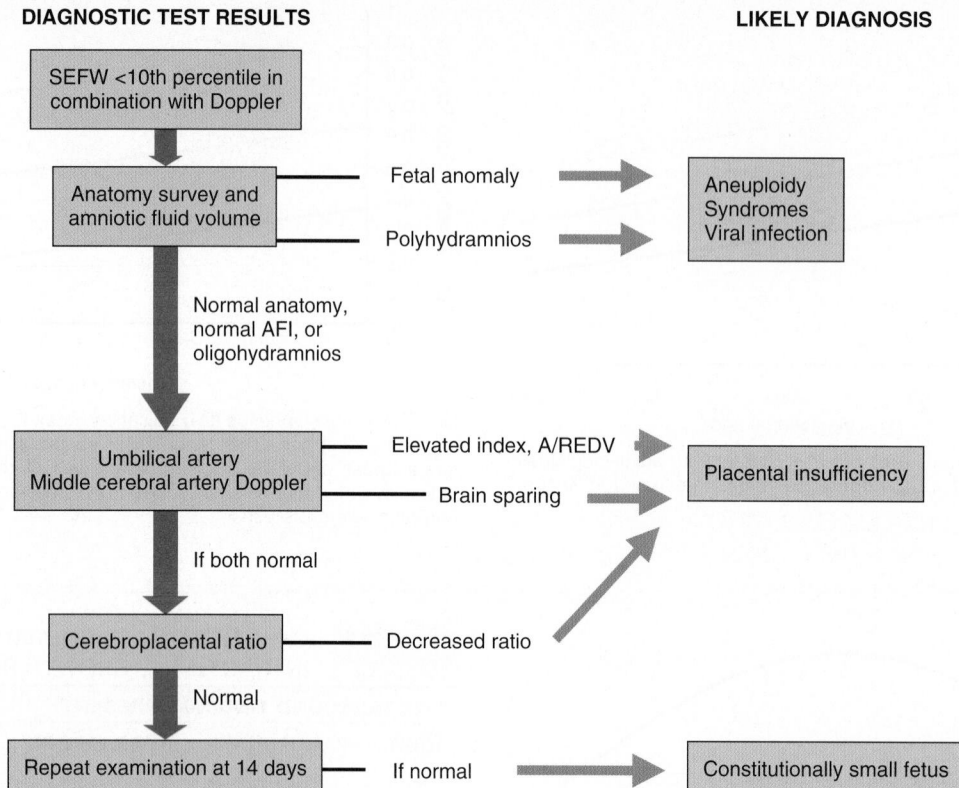

FIG 33-13 An integrated diagnostic approach to the fetus with suspected fetal growth restriction. This figure displays a decision tree following the evaluation of fetal anatomy, amniotic fluid volume, and umbilical and middle cerebral artery Doppler. The most likely clinical diagnosis based on the test results is presented on the right-hand side. A high index of suspicion for aneuploidy and viral and nonaneuploid syndromes needs to be maintained at all times. AFI, amniotic fluid index; A/REDV, absent/reversed end-diastolic flow; SEFW, sonographically estimated fetal weight. (Data from Unterscheider J, Daly S, Geary MP, et al. Optimizing the definition of intrauterine growth restriction: the multicenter prospective PORTO Study. *Am J Obstet Gynecol.* 2013;208:290.e1-e6.)

Maternal Serum Analytes

At least four hormone/protein markers measured in the maternal sera during the early second trimester are associated with subsequent IUGR. These include serum estriol, human placental lactogen (hPL), human chorionic gonadotrophin (hCG), and alpha-fetoprotein (AFP). Elevated maternal serum alpha-fetoprotein (MSAFP) and elevated hCG levels in the second trimester are considered markers of abnormal placentation and have been associated with an increased risk for IUGR.[49] Most studies conclude that **a single, unexplained elevated value of 2 to 2.5 multiples of the median (MoM) raises the risk of growth restriction fivefold to tenfold.**

Several first-trimester serum analytes associated with early abnormalities in placenta angiogenesis and development have been identified. These show significant differences in their distribution among pregnancies at risk of developing early-onset preeclampsia or FGR prior to 34 weeks' gestation. Of these markers, **a decrease in the pregnancy-associated plasma protein A (PAPP-A) or the placental growth factor (PlGF) have shown the most consistent predictive performance.** The advantage of PAPP-A is the current commercial availability as part of the first-trimester screen for aneuploidy. In this setting, a decrease in the PAPP-A below 0.8 MoM is associated with an increased risk for subsequent placental dysfunction.

Clinical Examination

From the early second trimester on, each antenatal visit includes the measurement of the distance between the maternal uterine fundus and the symphysis pubis. **After 20 weeks' gestation, the normal symphyseal-fundal height in centimeters approximates the weeks' gestation after allowances for maternal height and fetal station. After 20 weeks' gestation, a lag of the symphyseal-fundal height of 4 cm or more suggests growth restriction.** The reported sensitivities of symphyseal fundal height screening for IUGR range from 27% to 85%, and the PPVs range from 18% to 50%. Although the measurement of the symphyseal fundal height is a poor screening tool for the detection of IUGR, **the accuracy of subsequent ultrasound prediction of IUGR is enhanced if clinical suspicion of IUGR is based on a lagging fundal height.**

Maternal Doppler Velocimetry

Abnormal uterine artery flow-velocity waveforms are a manifestation of delayed trophoblast invasion that are highly associated with gestational hypertensive disorders, IUGR, and fetal demise.[50] Therefore, Doppler velocimetry of the uterine arteries has been examined for its usefulness in predicting pregnancies destined to produce a growth-restricted fetus. In women with hypertensive disorders, the presence of an elevated uterine artery S/D ratio (>2.6) and/or diastolic notching increased the risk for IUGR and stillbirth (see Fig. 33-17). **The changes in uterine artery flow patterns precede those observed in the umbilical artery and antedate FGR.** Subsequent studies used various cutoffs to define an abnormal test result. These include S/D ratios above 2.18 at 18 weeks, RI above 0.58 at 18 to 24 weeks, PI above the 95th percentile

(1.45) at 22 to 24 weeks, or the presence of notches. The screen positive rate ranges between 5% and 13% according to the gestational age and the criterion used to define an abnormal test result. In low-risk patients, a uterine artery Doppler resistance profile that is high, persistently notched, or both identifies women at high risk for preeclampsia and IUGR, with sensitivities and PPVs as high as 72% and 35%, respectively, when performed between 22 and 23 weeks' gestation. Uterine artery Doppler is better at predicting severe, rather than mild, disease. The likelihood ratio of abnormal uterine artery impedance for the development of IUGR was 3.7 with higher sensitivity for severe early-onset forms. Meta-analysis of the utility of uterine artery Doppler in the prediction of intrauterine death yields a likelihood ratio of 2.4 for patients with an abnormal result. Combining uterine artery Doppler velocimetry with other tests can improve screening sensitivities. The combination of abnormal second-trimester maternal uterine artery Doppler velocimetry and maternal glucose tolerance testing that demonstrate a "flat" response results in a PPV of 94% and a sensitivity of 54% for FGR. The presence of a normal uterine artery flow-velocity waveform bears a high negative predictive value, with a likelihood ratio of 0.5 and 0.8 for the development of preeclampsia and IUGR, respectively.

Integrated Approach to Screening

Several markers reflect early failure of normal placental development in the first trimester. One marker is abnormal maternal cardiovascular adaptation to pregnancy, which results in a delay in the physiologic drop of mean arterial blood pressure (BP). Deficient trophoblast invasion is associated with a slower than anticipated drop in uterine artery blood flow resistance, and placental expression of analytes that relate to normal development is altered. When these markers are considered in isolation, their prediction of subsequent placental dysfunction is inaccurate. Therefore **an integrated screening algorithm has been developed that uses multiple independent risk factors that include a prior history of preeclampsia, maternal first-trimester body mass index (BMI), BP, uterine artery pulsatility index, and the PAPP-A MoM.** This combined model is capable of predicting early-onset preeclampsia or FGR with 80% to 90% sensitivity and a 5% to 10% false-positive rate. Although the predictive accuracy of this algorithm needs to be confirmed in a variety of population settings, this approach offers the important advantage of early stratification of risk with potential for intervention.

Preventive Strategies

Efforts to prevent FGR have been disappointing. Low-dose aspirin has been extensively evaluated as a possible preventive agent for improving placental vascular development by virtue of its inhibitory action on platelet aggregation. However, whereas the use of aspirin in the second trimester has been found to be safe, initiation of therapy in the second trimester improves neither placental function nor long-term outcome. Because subsets of patients with a poor obstetric history appear to derive a benefit from aspirin, the utility of first-trimester uterine artery screening with subsequent aspirin therapy has been investigated. The choice of target population profoundly affects the utility of this approach. Although low-risk patients derive little benefit, high-risk patients—those with thrombophilia, hypertension, or a past history of either preeclampsia or IUGR—given low-dose aspirin because of bilateral uterine artery notching at 12 to 14 weeks experience an 80% reduction of placental disease compared with placebo-matched controls. However, only women who were initiated on aspirin before 16 weeks' gestation derive a 50% to 60% reduction in the relative risk for development of preeclampsia or FGR.[51]

It appears prudent to regard poor obstetric history, unexplained elevations in second-trimester MSAFP, flat oral glucose tolerance curves, and abnormal second-trimester uterine artery Doppler velocimetry as important risk factors for IUGR that warrant further investigation when the clinical suspicion of IUGR arises and/or maternal preeclampsia develops. Such patients should undergo ultrasound estimation of fetal size and a full diagnostic workup if these factors are confirmed.

MANAGEMENT IN CLINICAL PRACTICE

Before developing a management plan, it is important that the major underlying etiologies have been addressed by a comprehensive diagnostic workup as described above. **It is worth stressing that the majority of fetuses thought to be growth restricted are constitutionally small and require no intervention. Approximately 15% exhibit symmetric growth restriction attributable to an early fetal insult for which there is no effective therapy. Here, an accurate diagnosis is essential. Finally, approximately 15% of small fetuses have growth restriction as a result of placental disease or reduced uteroplacental blood flow.** Once the diagnosis of placental insufficiency has been made, appropriate therapeutic options may be explored. However, ongoing assessment of fetal growth and parameters of fetal well-being is a more critical component of clinical management in defining the intervention thresholds when the balance of fetal versus neonatal risks favors delivery.

Therapeutic Options

Elimination of contributors such as stress, smoking, and alcohol and drug use is advocated. Tobacco smoke contains a number of substances that are vasoactive and can cause vasoconstriction. Anecdotally, the authors have observed cases of IUGR with absent end-diastolic flow in the umbilical artery in which diastolic flow returned upon cessation of maternal smoking. Nonspecific therapies include bed rest in the left lateral decubitus position to increase placental blood flow. Although an inadequate diet has not been clearly established as a cause of growth restriction in the United States, dietary supplementation may be helpful in those with poor weight gain or low prepregnancy weight. In patients with chronic malnutrition, improved fetal growth has been reported with total parenteral nutrition. Consideration should be given to hospitalized bed rest, which has the advantages of positive enforcement of rest and facilitation of daily fetal testing. The decision for inpatient versus outpatient management is based on the severity of the maternal and/or fetal condition and the local standard of care.

Maternal hyperoxygenation has been examined in several studies for potential benefits in the treatment of the compromised growth-restricted fetus. Studies by several groups confirm that maternal hyperoxygenation can raise the fetal cord blood pO_2.[52] Techniques used included administration of 55% oxygen by face mask or 2.5 L/min by nasal prong. Prolongation of pregnancy from the first recognition of the compromised fetal condition ranged from 9 days to 5 weeks. However, fetal growth velocity was not improved. In addition, fetuses subjected to oxygen therapy had more hypoglycemia, thrombocytopenia, and disseminated intravascular coagulation (DIC) compared with controls. The primary role of maternal hyperoxygenation may reside in the safe short-term prolongation of pregnancy to allow the administration of corticosteroids to reduce the risk of neonatal respiratory distress syndrome (RDS) and intraventricular hemorrhage (IVH) in anticipation of a preterm delivery. There may also be benefit by gaining additional time in utero for improved survival and fetal maturity.

Maternal hyperalimentation as a means of intrauterine feeding of the growth-restricted fetus is an attractive therapeutic concept. Increasing the maternal concentration of amino acids leads to an increased umbilical uptake of some amino acids to the fetus, but no change is seen in the three essential amino acids: lysine, histidine, and threonine. These data further support that total parenteral nutrition can reverse abnormal fetal growth secondary to maternal nutritional deprivation. However, it does not overcome abnormal placental function. Outcomes are neither improved in animal models nor in human pregnancies. Therefore maternal hyperalimentation only plays a role in patients in whom malnutrition has been established as the underlying cause of growth delay.

Maternal volume expansion as a therapeutic concept is based on the observation that poor maternal blood volume status is associated with adverse pregnancy outcome.[53] In a small group of centrally monitored women with abnormal placental Doppler studies, volume expansion was associated with reappearance of umbilical artery end-diastolic velocities and a significant improvement of neonatal survival.

Low-dose aspirin in combination with dipyridamole administered from 16 weeks' gestation was first reported in 1987 by Wallenburg and Rotmans to significantly reduce the incidence of FGR in women with a history of recurrent IUGR. Women receiving therapy had a rate of FGR of 13%, compared with 61% in an untreated control group. No treated woman had a child with severe growth restriction (birthweight <2.3 percentile) compared with 27% in the untreated group. **In 1997, a meta-analysis of the efficacy of low-dose aspirin** (50 to 100 mg/day) **demonstrated a significant reduction in the frequency of IUGR when low-dose aspirin was used. A dose-dependent relationship is apparent: higher doses** (100 to 150 mg/day) **were significantly more effective in preventing IUGR than were lower doses** (50 to 80 mg/day).

Two recent randomized trials illustrate important considerations regarding the use of aspirin to prevent preeclampsia and IUGR. In a study of patients randomized at 24 weeks' gestation based on the uterine artery flow-velocity waveform, low-dose aspirin was not associated with any improvement in placental function or perinatal outcome. Conversely, in patients with a poor obstetric history (thrombophilia, hypertension, history of either preeclampsia or IUGR) randomized at 12 to 14 weeks based on the uterine artery flow-velocity waveforms, those who received aspirin experienced an 80% reduction in placental disease compared with placebo-matched controls. Therefore **it appears that aspirin works best in patients with significant risk factors for IUGR and that the therapeutic optimal window to commence aspirin therapy lies between 12 and 16 weeks' gestation when branching angiogenesis of the placenta is ongoing.**

Although the overall safety of aspirin has been documented in a large patient population, concerns about a possible association with abdominal wall defects have been raised with

administration in the early first trimester. Therefore, **we suggest deferral of indicated therapy until completion of organogenesis at 12 weeks' gestation.** Selected patients who present in the second trimester may still derive benefit from aspirin, and patients should be counseled on an individualized basis. Aspirin prophylaxis can be discontinued at any point after 34 weeks' gestation because bleeding risks at delivery and during regional anesthesia outweigh the benefits of prolonging gestation.

Corticosteroids are a universally available antenatal therapeutic option that positively affects outcome by enhancing lung maturation and preventing IVH. The impact of prenatal glucocorticoid administration on the neonatal complication rate in the growth-restricted newborn has recently been examined by Bernstein and coworkers[35] in a study of 19,759 newborns between 500 and 1500 g. After controlling for a different set of confounding variables, **this study demonstrated a significant reduction in neonatal RDS, IVH, and death when prenatal glucocorticoids were administered.** These benefits were not qualitatively different from those observed in appropriately sized newborns. **Other studies have also refuted that the "stress" of the intrauterine condition enhances maturation and protects against prematurity.** In contrast, a smaller study demonstrated no benefit to neonatal outcome when perinatal glucocorticoids were used. Although these studies indicate the need for randomized comparison of management, they also clearly show no benefit from the omission of antenatal corticosteroids. **We recommend administration of a complete 48-hour course of antenatal steroids to any growth-restricted fetus when delivery is anticipated before 34 weeks' gestation, if this can be safely accomplished.**

When corticosteroids are administered, it is important to account for their effect on fetal testing parameters when interpreting antenatal surveillance results. Betamethasone, for example, temporarily reduces FHR variation on days 2 and 3 after the first injection, together with a 50% decrease in fetal body movements and a near cessation of fetal breathing movements. Subsequently, the number of fetuses with abnormal BPP scores increases significantly by 48 hours after steroid administration, with a return to the preadministration state at 72 hours.[54] In contrast, maternal and fetal Doppler findings are not affected to the same degree during this period. A transient decrease in the MCA blood flow resistance has been reported 48 hours after betamethasone administration.

ASSESSMENT OF FETAL WELL-BEING

Once the diagnosis of FGR has been made and the differential diagnostic options have been explored, fetal assessment is instituted (see Chapter 11). **Serial ultrasound evaluations of fetal growth are continued every 3 to 4 weeks and should include determinations of the BPD, HC/AC ratio, fetal weight, and AFV.** The institution of antenatal surveillance is a critical component in the management of the growth-restricted fetus. The goal is to avoid stillbirth and optimize the timing of delivery, which requires consideration of the appropriate intervention threshold and the choice of the appropriate surveillance intervals. Relationships between fetal testing parameters and subsequent outcome determine the balance between fetal and neonatal risks and therefore define intervention thresholds. In contrast, changes in the rate of clinical progression determine the surveillance interval for patients where delivery is not yet indicated. Growth-restricted fetuses are at risk for worsening placental function, subsequent deterioration of acid-base status, decompensation, stillbirth, and long-term adverse health outcomes into adulthood. Although prevention of long-term morbidity is an attractive goal, information is insufficient on its relationships with prenatal variables to direct management with long-term outcomes in mind. Of the many short-term outcomes that have been related to fetal status, only a few are presently of clinical relevance. Fetal acidemia and major neonatal complications have a significant impact on subsequent neurodevelopment, whereas the combination of fetal and neonatal deaths determines the overall perinatal mortality.[55] **The likelihood of fetal acidemia and stillbirth is therefore the strongest fetal criterion for intervention. In contrast, gestational age–specific expectations for neonatal complications and survival force conservative management.** Whereas neonatal complications are typically multifactorial and not accurately predicted prenatally, anticipation of fetal risks remains as the primary goal. Therefore antenatal surveillance tests need to predict fetal acid-base status, rate of anticipated progression, and the resulting risk for deterioration and stillbirth. The monitoring tools available to achieve this include the traditional nonstress test (NST), contraction stress test, (CST), BPP scoring, and Doppler sonography.

Maternal Monitoring of Fetal Activity

Maternal monitoring of fetal activity has been used extensively in Great Britain, Scandinavia, and Israel for the assessment of pregnancies complicated by IUGR. **Fetal activity charting in pregnancies complicated by FGR predicts subsequent distress in labor.**[56] A simple technique for monitoring fetal movement is the minimum requirement of 10 movements in a 2-hour period. If this criterion is not met, additional testing is warranted. In an outpatient setting, maternal kick counts or fetal activity counts (FAC) supplement medically administered antenatal surveillance. In compliant patients with an appropriate level of awareness of fetal movements, it may also be helpful in modifying monitoring intervals as fetal deterioration occurs.

Fetal Heart Rate Analysis

The traditional NST is a visually analyzed record of the FHR baseline, variability, and episodic changes. Normal FHR characteristics are determined by gestational age, maturational and functional status of central regulatory centers, and oxygen tension. A "reactive" NST exhibits two 15-beat accelerations above the baseline maintained for 15 seconds in a 30-minute monitoring period. When the NST is analyzed as part of the five-component BPP score, reactivity criteria that account for gestational age are applied (see below). **Irrespective of the context, a "reactive" NST indicates absence of fetal acidemia at the moment of the FHR recording. Many growth-restricted fetuses with a normal heart rate tracing can have low-normal pO_2 values, but acidemia is virtually excluded by a reactive NST. Heart rate reactivity also correlates highly with a fetus not in immediate danger of intrauterine demise. Nonreactive NST results, on the other hand, are often falsely positive and require further evaluation. The development of repetitive decelerations may reflect fetal hypoxemia or cord compression as a result of the development of oligohydramnios and has been associated with a high perinatal mortality rate.**[57]

The CST is an additional option for testing placental respiratory reserve.[58] Positive CST results have been reported in 30% of pregnancies complicated by proven growth restriction. **In one study, 30% of growth-restricted infants had nonreactive NST results, and 40% had positive CST results.**[59] **Ninety-two percent of IUGR infants with a nonreactive positive pattern exhibited perinatal morbidity. However, a 25% to 50% false-positive rate has been associated with the CST by some investigators. A possible role for the CST may be evaluation of placental reserve prior to induction in IUGR fetuses in whom vaginal delivery is attempted.**

Marked intraobserver and interobserver variability of visual FHR analysis has been identified as a potential factor affecting the prediction of fetal status. Currently, traditional FHR parameters and short- and long-term variation of the heart rate in milliseconds, length of episodes with low and high variation, and the rate of signal loss can be assessed by computerized analysis. The objective assessment of these variables circumvents the issue of observer variability, and a direct correlation between FHR variation and pO_2 in the umbilical vein as assessed at cordocentesis prior to the onset of labor has been documented. **A computerized documentation of a mean minute variation below 3.5 msec has been reported to predict an umbilical artery cord pH less than 7.20 with over 90% sensitivity. In addition, FHR variation usually decreases gradually in the weeks that precede the appearance of late decelerations and fetal hypoxemia and is therefore the most useful computerized FHR parameter for longitudinal assessment in IUGR.** As with the traditional NST, gestational age, time of day, and the presence of fetal rest-activity cycles also need to be taken into account in the interpretation of computerized results. Wide normal ranges are apparent for FHR patterns and their variations, but the individual fetus shows a certain intrafetal consistency throughout gestation. For monitoring of trends, each fetus should therefore serve as its own control, using recordings of standardized duration and appropriate reference ranges.

In summary, **a visually reactive FHR provides assurance of fetal well-being at the time of analysis.** Whereas the traditional NST is most sensitive in the prediction of fetal normoxemia, computerized analysis appears to be superior in the prediction of hypoxemia and acidemia. Once traditional reactivity is lost, computerized analysis of heart rate variation is a potential tool available for ongoing longitudinal analysis. Computerized FHR analysis is more widely used in Europe. FHR analysis itself does not assess the severity of disease and most importantly does not anticipate the rate of deterioration; therefore frequency of surveillance cannot be based on FHR testing. To address these issues, additional fetal tests are available.

Amniotic Fluid Volume

In the context of fetal surveillance, assessment of AFV provides an indirect measure of vascular status. **A relationship between oligohydramnios and progressive deterioration of arterial and venous Doppler studies has been documented in growth-restricted fetuses and prolonged pregnancies.**

Therefore declining AFV is suggestive of ineffective downstream delivery of cardiac output and allows some form of longitudinal monitoring even in the absence of Doppler studies. **If the NST is reactive, a concurrent assessment of the AFV constitutes the *modified biophysical profile* (MBPP) and provides assurance of fetal well-being if both parameters are normal.** Interventions based on twice-weekly MBPP scores result in similar perinatal outcomes as with weekly contraction stress testing and therefore have largely replaced the latter. **When the FHR is nonreactive, relying on a normal AFV assessment** alone is inadequate, and a full BPP that incorporates multiple parameters of fetal well-being should be done because of its superior performance in identifying jeopardized fetuses.

Biophysical Parameters

The five-component fetal BPP was developed by Manning and colleagues and has been widely used in the surveillance of growth-restricted fetuses. A graded system is applied to categorize fetal tone, movement, breathing movement, heart rate reactivity, and a maximum amniotic fluid pocket as *normal* (2 points) or *abnormal* (0 points). If used in the context of the BPP, fetal heart rate reactivity criteria that account for gestational age are used. *Reactivity* **has been defined prior to 32 weeks' gestation as accelerations greater than 10 beats/min sustained for more than 10 seconds; between 32 to 36 weeks' gestation, accelerations greater than 15 beats/min sustained for more than 15 seconds; and after 36 weeks' gestation, accelerations greater than 20 beats/min sustained for more than 20 seconds.** In anatomically normal fetuses, the presence of the dynamic variables is related to physiologic variations in maturation and behavioral state as well as acid-base status. Vintzileos and coworkers have demonstrated that four components of the BPP are affected at different levels of hypoxemia and acidemia. The earliest manifestations of abnormal fetal biophysical activity consist of the loss of heart rate reactivity along with the absence of fetal breathing. This is followed by decreased fetal tone and movement in association with more advanced acidemia, hypoxemia, and hypercapnia. **Because of the relationship between AFV and vascular status, amniotic fluid assessment provides the only marker of chronic hypoxemia and is the only longitudinal monitoring component of the BPP.**

Growth-restricted fetuses preserve acute central responses to acid-base status despite their maturational delay and are at risk for oligohydramnios. **The five-component BPP accounts best for physiologic and individual variations in behavior and therefore remains closely related to arterial pH in fetuses with IUGR without anomalies from 20 weeks onward.**[60] **An abnormal score of 4 or less is associated with a mean pH of less than 7.20, and sensitivity in the prediction of acidemia is 100% for a score of 2 or less. A normal score and normal AFV indicate the absence of fetal acidemia at the time of testing.** Longitudinal observations in growth-restricted fetuses have shown that the BPP deteriorates late and often rapidly.[20] Whereas an abnormal BPP is associated with escalating risks for stillbirth and perinatal mortality, a normal score allows no anticipation of fetal deterioration and stillbirth.

In summary, assessment of fetal biophysical variables provides an accurate measure of fetal status at the time of testing. In the patient with a nonreactive NST, a full five-component BPP must be performed. As a back-up test for a nonreactive FHR test, the BPP leads to lower rates of intervention, when compared with the CST, without jeopardizing perinatal outcome. In the presence of normal AFV, a normal BPP of 8 (−2 for a nonreactive NST) or 10 is reassuring of fetal well-being. Nevertheless, in the absence of knowledge about placental vascular status, the rate of progression cannot be anticipated and may require even daily testing in severe IUGR. The development of oligohydramnios is concerning and frequently requires modification of management or delivery. The knowledge of fetal Doppler status is complementary to BPP because it improves the anticipation of fetal deterioration and provides an additional means to assess fetal state.[61]

Doppler Ultrasound

Doppler parameters are influenced by several variables that include vascular histology and tone and fetal blood pressure. Placental respiratory function is related to the integrity of the villous vasculature, and a decrease in arterial pO_2 can trigger autoregulatory adjustments of vascular smooth muscle tone. As diagnostic tools, elevated umbilical artery blood flow resistance and/or MCA brain sparing provide evidence of placental dysfunction. The utility of Doppler ultrasound in the assessment of fetal well-being is based on the relationship between Doppler parameters with metabolic status, rate of disease progression, and the risk for stillbirth. **This utility is greatest for early-onset growth restriction, which is associated with more marked Doppler abnormalities than late-onset disease that requires delivery after 34 weeks, especially in early-onset placental dysfunction.**[18,62] Distinction between early and late fetal vascular responses to placental insufficiency provides a useful framework within which to estimate these risks.

Early responses to placental insufficiency are observed in mild placental vascular disease when umbilical artery end-diastolic velocity is still present. A decrease in the CPR provides an early and sensitive marker of redistribution of cardiac output that often precedes overt growth delay by up to 2 weeks. The reduction of fetal growth velocity generally mirrors the elevation in umbilical artery blood flow resistance and is followed by decreasing MCA impedance (brain sparing). The nadir of cerebral blood flow resistance is typically reached after a median of 2 weeks and is followed by an increase in aortic blood flow impedance.[63] **Early cardiovascular responses are considered compensatory because they occur at a time when cardiac function is normal, and they are typically accompanied by preferential perfusion of vital organs and the placenta. Although the fetus may be hypoxemic, the risk for acidemia is low.**

Late responses to placental insufficiency are observed when accelerating placental disease results in loss or reversal of umbilical artery end-diastolic velocity, and when fetal deterioration becomes evident through parallel elevations in placental blood flow resistance and venous Doppler indices. **Although the development of abnormal venous blood flows has been documented in many veins, the precordial veins—including the ductus venosus, the inferior vena cava, and the umbilical vein—are typically utilized in clinical practice** (Figs. 33-14 and 33-15). When fetal compromise accelerates, a further steady rise is seen in umbilical blood flow resistance; venous Doppler indices escalate over a wide range, and the development of oligohydramnios and metabolic academia is characteristic of ineffective downstream delivery of cardiac output.[64] In the final stages of compromise, cardiac dilatation with holosystolic tricuspid insufficiency, complete fetal inactivity, short-term heart rate variation below 3.5 ms, and spontaneous "cardiac" late decelerations of the FHR can be observed as preterminal events (Fig. 33-16).[65]

In the past, the major focus of Doppler studies for the assessment of fetal health has been the umbilical circulation. The association between an elevation in Doppler blood flow indices in the UA, increased disturbance of placental perfusion, and the deterioration of fetal acid-base status proportional to the degree of the Doppler abnormality has been demonstrated by several

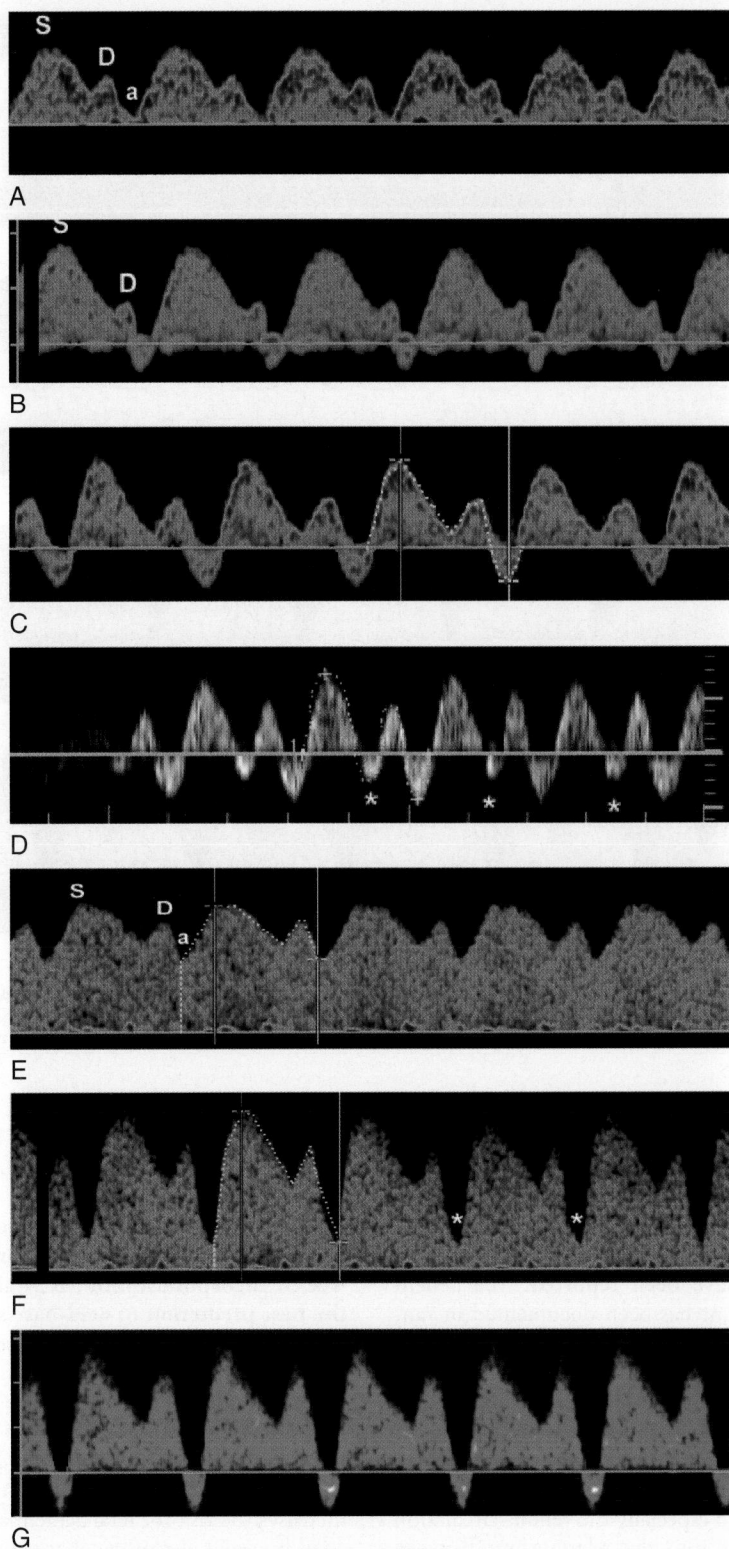

FIG 33-14 Normal and abnormal precordial venous flow-velocity waveforms. The inferior vena cava and ductus venosus are the most commonly evaluated precordial veins, whereas the umbilical venous flow-velocity waveform is predominantly assessed qualitatively. **A,** The inferior vena cava shows the typical triphasic pattern with systolic and diastolic peaks (*S, D,* respectively). **B,** The a-wave may be reversed under physiologic conditions. **C,** An abnormal inferior vena cava flow-velocity waveform shows a relative decrease in forward flow during the first trough, the D-wave, and the a-wave. **D,** Under extreme circumstances, flow may be reversed during the first trough (*asterisks*). **E,** In contrast to the inferior vena cava, the ductus venous has antegrade blood flow throughout the cardiac cycle with forward velocities during the S-, D-, and a-waves. **F,** A decrease in atrial systolic forward velocities (*asterisks*) is the first sign of abnormality and results in an increased Doppler index. **G,** With marked elevation of central venous pressure, blood flow may reverse during atrial systole.

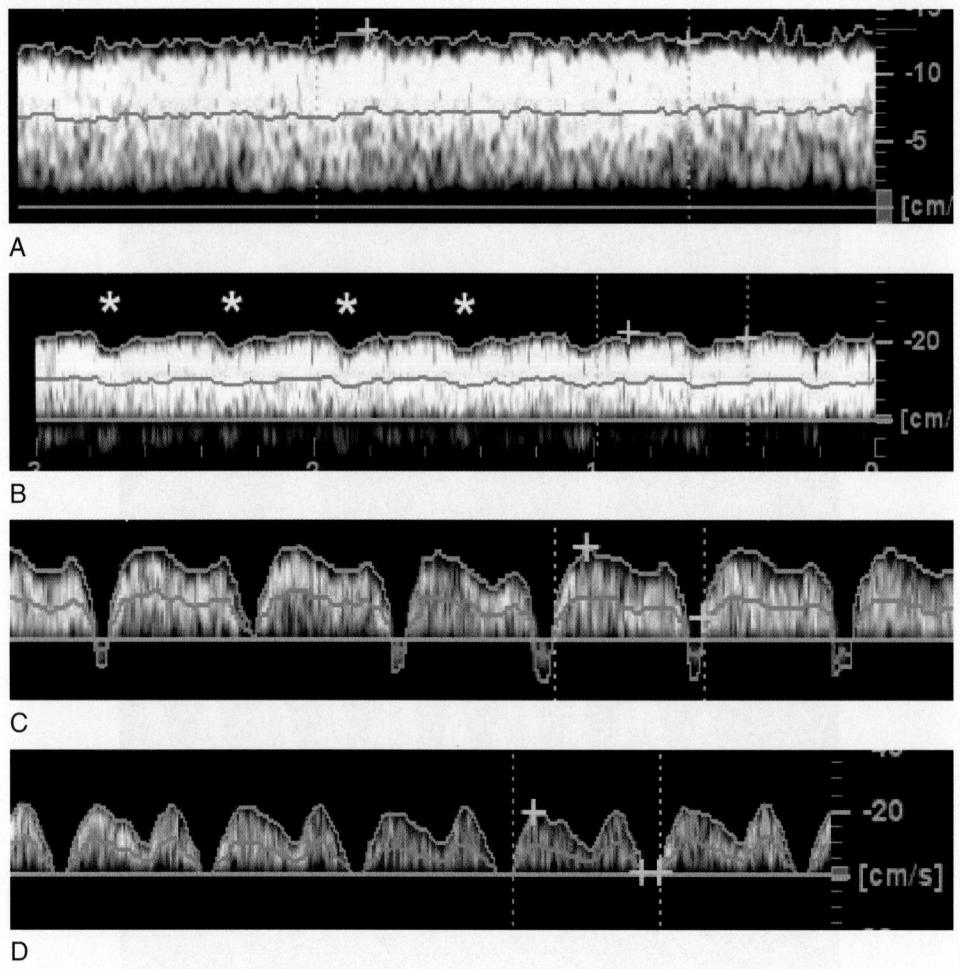

A

B

C

D

FIG 33-15 Normal and abnormal umbilical venous flow velocity. Umbilical venous blood flow is usually constant **(A)**. Monophasic umbilical venous pulsations (*asterisks*) may be observed with moderate elevations of placental blood flow resistance and/or oligohydramnios **(B)**. Retrograde propagation of increased central venous pressure first results in biphasic and then triphasic pulsations (**C** and **D**, respectively).

investigators. In the fetal compartment, elevation of the UA **Doppler index is observed when approximately 30% of the fetal villous vessels are abnormal. Absence or even reversal of UA end-diastolic velocity can occur when 60% to 70% of the villous vascular tree is damaged.**[66] **Incidences of intra-uterine hypoxia that range from 50% to 80% in fetuses with absent end-diastolic flow have been reported.** The benefit of UA Doppler in management has been documented in randomized controlled trials and meta-analyses. **In these studies, when used in conjunction with standard antepartum testing, UA Doppler was associated with a decrease of up to 38% in perinatal mortality, antenatal admissions, inductions of labor, and cesarean deliveries for fetal distress in labor in women considered at high risk.** However, several studies that have examined the cerebral and especially the venous circulation have provided greater insight into the relationships between Doppler abnormality and outcome. Previous work has reported that development of umbilical venous pulsations in fetuses with absent end-diastolic velocities in the UA was associated with a fivefold increase in mortality. Arduini and colleagues[67] demonstrated that gestational age at onset, maternal hypertension, and the development of pulsations in the umbilical venous velocities were significantly correlated with the interval of time between diagnosis and delivery for late decelerations of the FHR. Subsequently, several studies have confirmed that fetuses

with abnormal arterial velocities who also developed abnormal precordial venous velocities had a higher morbidity and mortality than fetuses without abnormal venous flow.[68] These studies and subsequent analyses confirm that **fetal Doppler assessment based on the UA alone is no longer appropriate, particularly in the setting of early-onset IUGR prior to 34 weeks. Incorporation of MCA and venous Doppler provide the best prediction of acid-base status, risk of stillbirth, and the anticipated rate of progression.**

In growth-restricted fetuses with an elevated Doppler index in the UA, brain sparing in the presence of normal venous Doppler parameters is typically associated with hypoxemia but a normal pH.** Elevation of venous Doppler indices, either alone or in combination with umbilical venous pulsations, increases the risk for fetal acidemia. This association is strengthened by serial elevations of the ductus venosus Doppler index. Depending on the cutoff (2 vs. 3 SD) and the combinations of veins examined, sensitivity for prediction of acidemia ranges from 70% to 90%, and specificity from 70% to 80%. **Abnormal venous Doppler parameters are the strongest Doppler predictors of stillbirth. Even among fetuses with severe arterial Doppler abnormalities (e.g., AEDV or REDV), the risk of stillbirth is largely confined to those fetuses with abnormal venous Dopplers.**[68] The likelihood of stillbirth increases with the degree of venous Doppler abnormality. Particularly ominous

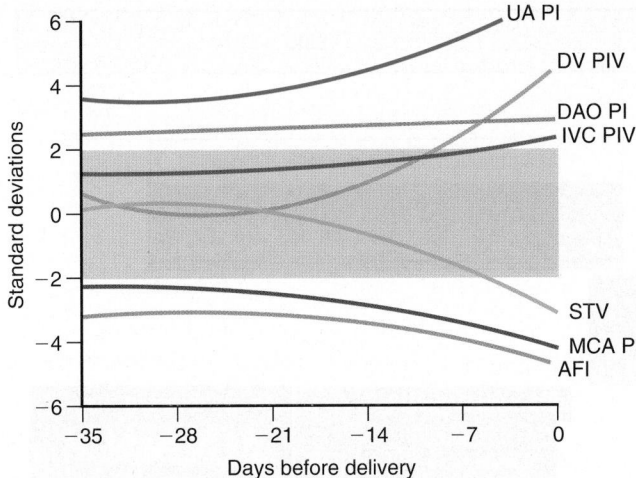

FIG 33-16 Longitudinal progression of antenatal testing variables. This figure displays trends in arterial and venous Doppler parameters (DAO, descending aorta; DV, ductus venosus; IVC, inferior vena cava; MCA, middle cerebral artery; PI, pulsatility index; PIV, pulsatility index for veins; UA, umbilical artery), amniotic fluid index (AFI), and computerized fetal heart rate short-term variation (STV) in relation to delivery expressed as standard deviation for growth-restricted fetuses delivered before 32 weeks' gestation. The graph demonstrates that arterial Doppler parameters may be abnormal for more than 5 weeks prior to delivery, whereas venous Doppler parameters and the short-term variation deteriorate in the week prior to delivery for fetal indications. (From Hecher K, Bilardo CM, Stigter RH, et al. Monitoring of fetuses with intrauterine growth restriction: a longitudinal study. *Ultrasound Obstet Gynecol.* 2001;18:564.)

venous Doppler findings are absence or reversal of the ductus venous a-wave and biphasic/triphasic umbilical venous pulsations. In the setting of a 25% stillbirth rate in a population with preterm severe IUGR, these Doppler findings have a 65% predictive sensitivity and 95% specificity.[69]

Although neonatal morbidity is primarily determined by gestational age at delivery, and neonatal mortality is the product of several factors, both of these outcomes are also related to fetal Doppler studies. Arterial redistribution and brain sparing are not associated with a significant rise in major neonatal complications. In contrast, a 2-SD elevation of the DV Doppler index is associated with a threefold increase in neonatal complications, and further escalation of DV Doppler indices leads to an elevenfold increase in this relative risk. **The neonatal mortality rate in fetuses with absent or reversed UA end-diastolic velocity ranges from 5% to 18% when the venous Doppler indices are normal. Elevation of the DV Doppler index greater than 2 SDs doubles this mortality rate, although predictive sensitivity is only 38% with a specificity of 98%.**

In summary, Doppler evaluation of the umbilical, cerebral, and precordial vessels of the growth-restricted fetus provides important diagnostic and prognostic information. Fetal acidemia and the risk of stillbirth are high with progressive elevation of venous Doppler indices. **Advancing Doppler abnormalities indicate acceleration of disease and require increased frequency of fetal monitoring. In growth-restricted fetuses, Doppler evaluation is complementary to all other surveillance modalities.**

Invasive Fetal Testing

In the past, direct determination of fetal acid-base status by cordocentesis was often performed with fetal karyotyping.

Nicolini and colleagues examined 58 growth-restricted fetuses using cordocentesis for acid-base evaluation in addition to karyotyping. They found significant differences in pH, partial pressure of carbon dioxide (pCO_2), pO_2, and the base equivalent in fetuses with no evidence of end-diastolic flow by UA Doppler velocimetry. However, they observed no relationship between acid-base determination and perinatal outcome. Pardi and colleagues[70] examined umbilical blood acid-base status in 56 growth-restricted fetuses and demonstrated an association between acid-base status and the results of cardiotocographic and UA Doppler waveform analysis. If both FHR and Doppler studies were normal, neither hypoxemia nor acidemia was noted. When both tests were abnormal, 64% of the growth-restricted fetuses demonstrated abnormal acid-base analysis. The prognostic significance of these abnormalities remains unclear. Lack of benefit, the complication rate, accuracy of noninvasive assessment of fetal acid-base status, and finally the availability for rapid karyotyping techniques from amniocytes all mean that **cordocentesis is rarely necessary today.**

Anticipating the Progression to Fetal Compromise

The anticipation of clinical progression is a critical component in the management of the fetus with IUGR because it determines fetal surveillance intervals as well as the timing for intervention. Although deterioration of fetal status is manifested in all surveillance modalities, accelerating disease is best anticipated by AFV status and arterial and venous Doppler parameters (Fig. 33-17). **However, the gestational age at onset has an important impact on the clinical presentation and, accordingly, on the diagnosis and management of FGR. In early-onset growth delay** (prior to 34 weeks' gestation), **the significantly decreased survival rates—as well as the higher mortality following immediate delivery—places special emphasis on safe pregnancy prolongation in these situations.[71,72] Late-onset FGR** (presenting after 34 weeks' gestation) **does not typically pose a dilemma for delivery timing because delivery thresholds can be low given the lower neonatal risks. However, late-onset FGR is a significant clinical problem that contributes to over 50% of unanticipated stillbirths at term.[73]** Therefore a more pressing issue in term pregnancies is the recognition of growth-restricted fetuses, rather than the timing of their delivery (see earlier sections on diagnostic tools and clinical examination). Once the fetus with IUGR has been identified, recognizing the important differences in management helps to clarify the nature of decisions that need to be based on the results of the surveillance examination. The principal choices that need to be made at each monitoring visit are whether intervention is needed and the interval to the next visit. The intervention threshold is based on the balance of fetal and neonatal risks, and it is high at early gestation given the high neonatal morbidity but successively decreases as gestation advances. The monitoring interval is often empirically defined but needs to be shortened if fetal signs of deterioration are present that indicate an acceleration of the disease. This in turn requires an appreciation of the typical pattern of progression in early- and late-onset FGR.[11,74]

Umbilical artery Doppler alone provides inaccurate prediction because progression to abnormal FHR parameters is highly variable and may range from 0 to 49 days, as reported in a study by Farine and coworkers. In general, early-onset IUGR that presents prior to 28 weeks' gestation is associated with more

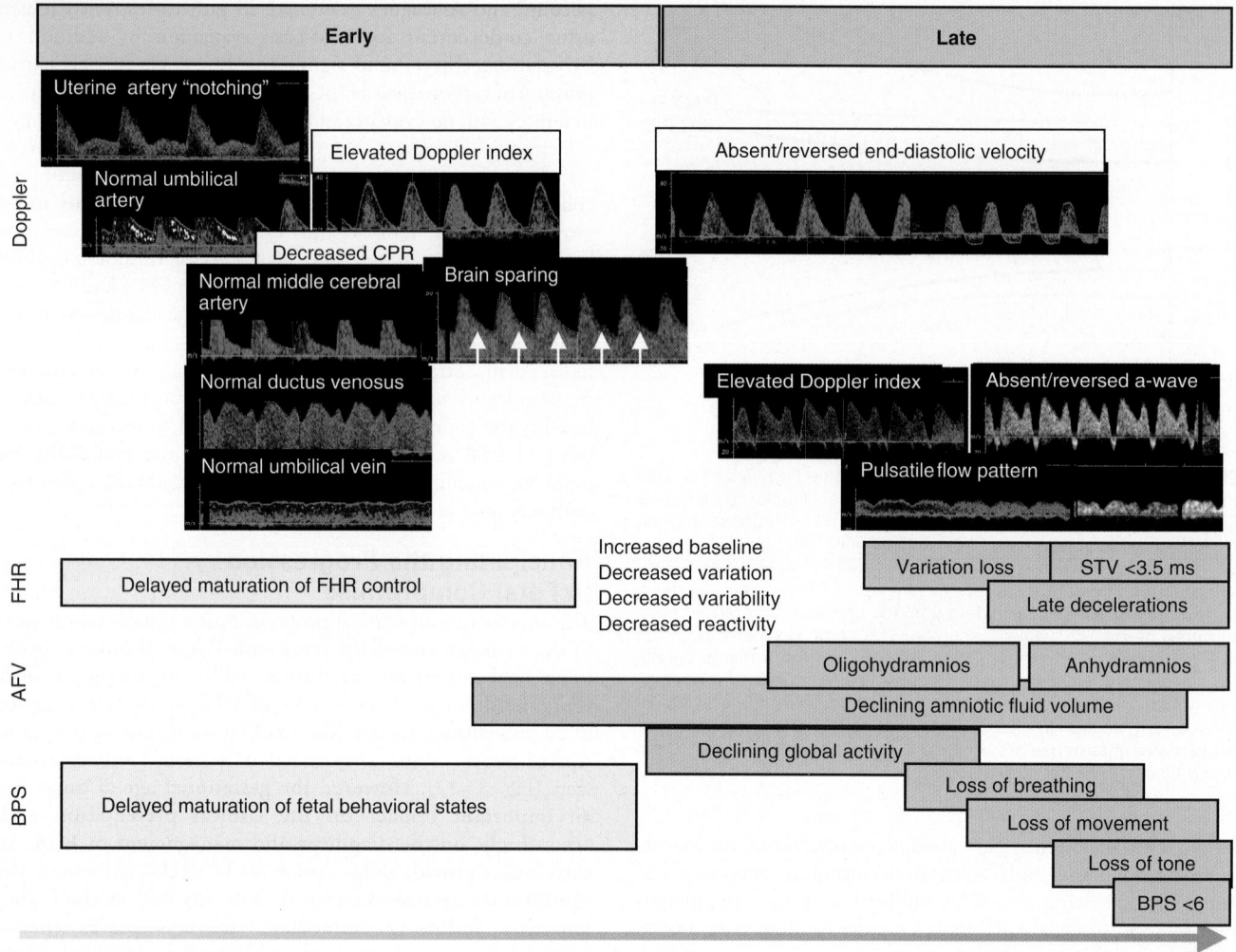

FIG 33-17 Progression of compromise in various monitoring systems. This figure summarizes the early and late responses to placental insufficiency. Doppler variables in the placental circulation precede abnormalities in the cerebral circulation. Fetal heart rate (FHR), amniotic fluid volume (AFV), and biophysical profile score (BPS) are still normal at this time, and computerized analysis of fetal behavioral patterns is necessary to document a developmental delay. With progression to late responses, venous Doppler abnormality in the fetal circulation is characteristic and often precedes the sequential loss of fetal dynamic variables and frequently accompanies the decline in AFV. The decline in biophysical variables shows a reproducible relationship with acid-base status. Because the BPS is a composite score of five variables, an abnormal BPS less than 6 often develops late and may be sudden. Absence or reversal of the ductus venous a-wave, decrease of the short-term variation (STV) of the computerized FHR analysis, spontaneous late decelerations, and an abnormal BPS are the most advanced testing abnormalities. If adaptation mechanisms fail and the fetus remains undelivered, stillbirth ensues. CPR, cerebroplacental ratio.

significant placental vascular problems that produce marked Doppler changes. In contrast, IUGR that presents near term is typically associated with milder placental disease and therefore more subtle Doppler findings. Decreasing AFV and behavioral responses are preserved throughout gestation irrespective of Doppler status. Accordingly, longitudinal progression and clinical findings may vary based on gestational age and may be further modulated by maternal disease.[75] Beyond 34 weeks, when the UA waveform may be normal or near normal, assessment of the MCA flow-velocity waveform and/or the CPR may be necessary to provide an estimate of placental disease and direct the frequency of testing.[47] In fetuses with elevated placental blood flow resistance, onset of MCA brain sparing or a decline in the AFI indicate accelerating disease. Once brain sparing is established, the next level of deterioration occurs when UA end-diastolic velocity is lost and parallel elevations in placental blood flow resistance and precordial venous Doppler

indices are observed. Although this may happen after several weeks, the anticipation of such deterioration may require twice-weekly, rather than weekly, testing. When accelerating fetal compromise occurs, it is associated with a further rise in umbilical blood flow resistance (leading to REDV), whereas venous Doppler indices escalate over a wide range of distribution (see Fig. 33-15). **Studies by Baschat, Ferrazzi, Hecher, and Bilardo indicate that 40% of preterm growth-restricted fetuses that deteriorate in utero have an increased DV Doppler index the week prior to delivery** (Figs. 33-18 and 33-19; see also Fig. 33-16). On the day of delivery, an additional 20% deteriorated further. Elevations of precordial venous Doppler indices also precede sudden deterioration of the BPP by a median of 1 week in fetuses with elevated UA blood flow resistance. These findings have an important impact on testing frequency. For example, in a preterm growth-restricted fetus where venous Doppler indices are elevated, a BPP of 10 does not provide assurance that fetal

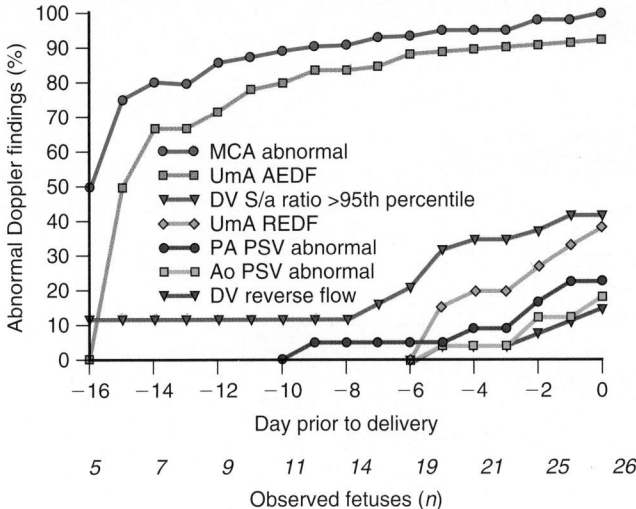

FIG 33-18 Early and late Doppler findings in growth-restricted fetuses. This figure displays cumulative onset time curves of Doppler abnormalities for each fetal vessel examined. Middle cerebral artery (MCA) brain sparing and umbilical artery (UmA) absent end-diastolic flow (AEDF) are observed up to 16 days before delivery. Ao PSV, aortic peak systolic velocity; DV, ductus venosus; PA PSV, pulmonary artery peak systolic velocity; REDF, reverse end-diastolic flow; S/a, ratio of maximum forward velocity during ventricular systole and atrial systole. (Modified from Ferrazzi E, Bozzo M, Rigano S, et al. Temporal sequence of abnormal Doppler changes in the peripheral and central circulatory systems of the severely growth-restricted fetus. *Ultrasound Obstet Gynecol.* 2002;19:140.)

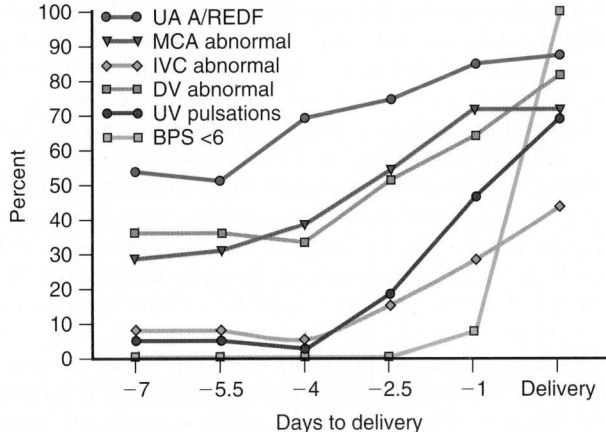

FIG 33-19 Sequential deterioration of Doppler and biophysical parameters. This figure shows the percentage of abnormal Doppler findings in individual vessels and the incidence of a biophysical profile score (BPS) below 6 in the last week prior to delivery represented by the lines. A/REDF, absent or reversed end-diastolic flow; DV, ductus venosus; IVC, inferior vena cava; MCA, middle cerebral artery; UA, umbilical artery; UV, umbilical vein. Deterioration of Doppler findings precedes decline in biophysical profile score. (From Baschat AA, Gembruch U, Harman CR. The sequence of changes in Doppler and biophysical parameters as severe fetal growth restriction worsens. *Ultrasound Obstet Gynecol.* 2001;18:571.)

status will remain stable for the following week. In fact, a sizeable proportion of these fetuses may have a BPP score of less than 6 after a median time of just 1 day.[20] Therefore, thrice-weekly or even daily testing may be necessary in such fetuses. This is illustrated in a study by Divon and coworkers in which the authors performed a daily BPP in fetuses with absent UA end-diastolic velocity. Delivery was indicated for maternal reasons, a BPP

below 6, oligohydramnios, documented lung maturity, or a gestational age beyond 36 weeks' gestation. No stillbirths and no cord artery pH below 7.20 were reported using this intensive monitoring approach.

More recent work reported through the Prospective Observational Trial to Optimize Pediatric Health in IUGR (PORTO) study identifies one of the challenges in Doppler evaluation of the severely growth-restricted fetus prior to 34 weeks' gestation.[48] **Pregnancies at increased risk of adverse outcome were those with an abnormal UA Doppler study and, in particular, those with an EFW below the third percentile with or without oligohydramnios.** However, after approximately 31 weeks, it appears that these growth-restricted fetuses do not follow a dominant pattern or sequence of Doppler abnormalities as seen earlier in gestation, and it cannot be predicted what Doppler abnormality pattern a given fetus will follow prior to an abnormal biophysical test. However, it remains clear that by the time severe venous Doppler changes are detected, the fetus is frequently acidemic.[76] Of note, a substantial number of fetuses with absent UA flow were managed as inpatients and were not included in the PORTO trial after 30 weeks' gestation.

The clinical progression in Doppler and biophysical abnormalities is observed in approximately 70% to 80% of growth-restricted fetuses prior to 34 weeks' gestation.[11,20] Two rates of progression have been described that can be anticipated based on the UA end-diastolic velocity (EDV). In pregnancies in which UA EDV is lost within the first 2 weeks of diagnosis, deterioration to venous Doppler and biophysical abnormalities within 4 weeks is common (Fig. 33-20). If UA EDV is maintained for longer periods, deterioration may not occur for 6 weeks after diagnosis. In late-onset growth restriction that presents beyond 34 weeks' gestation, several other presentations are possible. UA blood flow resistance may be normal, and brain sparing may be observed as the only Doppler sign of perceived hypoxemia that requires an increase in surveillance frequency to twice weekly.[15] Alternatively, Doppler findings may be normal, and oligohydramnios and/or a decline of biophysical variables may be the only signs of placental insufficiency. On a similar note, the speed of progression may vary significantly in these different clinical scenarios, and persistence of normal umbilical Doppler parameters for up to 9 weeks before new-onset brain sparing is observed is not unusual. In recognition of these variable time scales and patterns of deterioration, it is evident that **the combination of several testing modalities is more likely to provide evidence of deterioration. If BPP scoring is used, particular attention needs to be placed on the amniotic fluid, because this is the only component that reflects longitudinal progression. The most comprehensive approach that addresses cardiovascular and behavioral responses in IUGR fetuses across all gestational ages has been described as "integrated fetal testing."**

Integrated fetal testing utilizes a surveillance approach to pregnancies with IUGR that requires familiarity with the combined assessment of the five-component BPP and arterial and venous Doppler studies.[77] Doppler examination includes evaluation of the UA, MCA, DV, and free umbilical vein flow-velocity waveform. The testing is always supplemented with maternal assessment of fetal movement ("kick counts"). Surveillance is initiated no earlier than 24 weeks' gestation. In fetuses with elevated UA pulsatility, positive end-diastolic flow, and absence of any additional abnormality, weekly BPP is performed along with multivessel Doppler

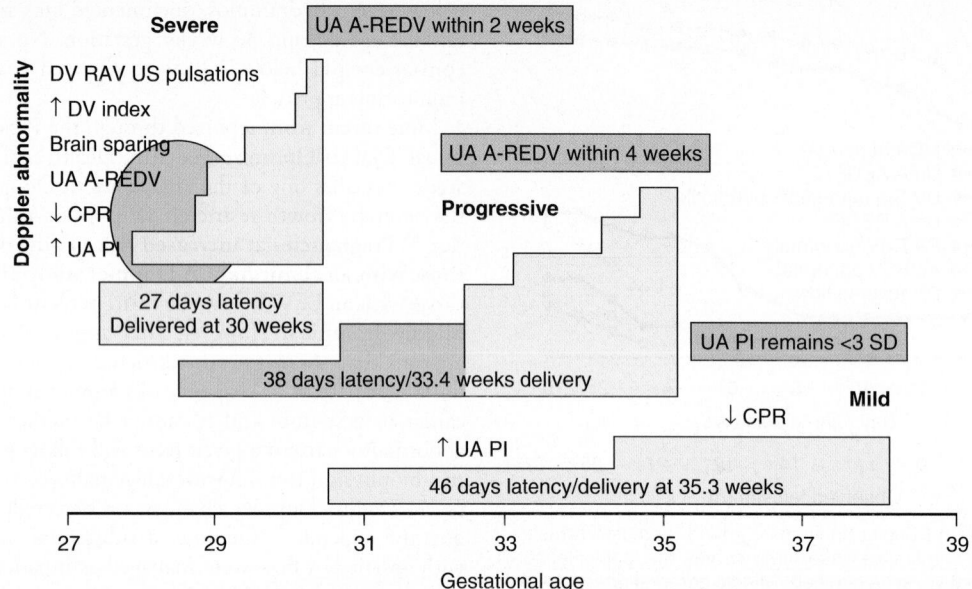

FIG 33-20 Two rates of progression can be anticipated based on the umbilical artery (UA) end-diastolic velocity (EDV). Losing UA EDV within the first 2 weeks of diagnosis commonly leads to deterioration to venous Doppler and biophysical abnormalities within 4 weeks (middle section of the figure). However, UA EDV can be maintained for longer periods, and deterioration may not occur for 6 weeks after diagnosis (bottom section of figure). A-REDV, absent/reversed end-diastolic velocity; CPR, cerebroplacental ratio; DV, ductus venosus; PI, pulsatility index; RAV, reverse atrial systolic velocity; US, ultrasound.

monitoring studies every 2 weeks. With the onset of brain sparing, Doppler monitoring intervals are shortened to weekly visits. In fetuses with an AFI of less than 5 cm or AEDV in the umbilical artery, surveillance intervals are shortened to every 3 to 4 days. With elevation of the DV Doppler index to less than 2 SD, testing frequency is increased to every 2 to 3 days. Further escalation of the DV Doppler index may require daily testing, and inpatient admission may be prudent based on local practice. Any change in maternal condition, especially the development of preeclampsia, calls for reassessment of fetal status irrespective of the last examination result (Fig. 33-21).

TIMING OF DELIVERY

In the absence of definitive fetal therapy, proper timing of delivery is often the critical management issue when dealing with the growth-restricted fetus. **In principle, the decision for delivery always weighs fetal risks against risks that can be anticipated as a result of delivery.** The risks of prematurity are of primary concern and make management of the preterm growth-restricted fetus particularly challenging. Typically, the decline in neonatal mortality is greatest between 24 and 28 weeks, whereas morbidity declines progressively thereafter toward 32 weeks. Although surprisingly few randomized management studies address the issue of delivery timing in IUGR, the Growth Restriction Intervention Trial (GRIT) clarified several important points.[78] This prospective multicenter study randomized more than 500 women with complicating FGR into immediate versus delayed delivery when their managing physicians were unsure about the timing of delivery. In the conservatively managed group, delivery was delayed until a point when their managing obstetricians were no longer unsure about the need to deliver or when fetal testing became overtly normal. With a median delay of 4.5 days, no significant differences in short-term outcome were identified

between the two groups (Table 33-4). **The perinatal mortality with early delivery was associated with a higher rate of neonatal deaths, whereas delaying delivery increased the risk for stillbirth.** Delivery timing also had little effect on neurodevelopment at 2 years of age. However, in the subset of fetuses delivered before 32 weeks, a trend toward poor neurodevelopment was primarily attributable to neonatal complications that occurred as a result of prematurity. In 2010, Walker and colleagues[79] reported on the 6- to 13-year GRIT study outcomes and found the two groups to be similar for cognitive, language, behavior, and motor ability (half of original cohort). This suggests that neurologic impairment may already be set by the time the fetus with IUGR reaches the point of delivery. Other observational studies have also addressed the impact of gestational age on perinatal morbidity. In prenatally identified growth-restricted fetuses, the effect of gestational age overshadows all other perinatal variables. **After 27.0 weeks, when survival and intact survival first exceed 50%, a birthweight below 550 g is associated with a high risk for neonatal death.**[80,81] **It appears that fetal deterioration of venous Doppler parameters begins to have an independent impact on neonatal survival from 28 weeks onward as postpartum morbidities become less frequent with advancing gestation.**[72] **Gestational age is also an important factor affecting perinatal mortality in patients who remain undelivered. More recent data from the Trial of Randomized Umbilical and Fetal Flow in Europe (TRUFFLE) study**[82] **confirm the trend of improved outcome with advancing gestational age. This was a randomized clinical trial of delivery of severely growth-restricted fetuses based on either FHR monitoring, early DV changes, or late DV changes** (absent or reversed a-wave; see Fig. 33-14). **In contrast to prior studies, the neonatal outcomes are significantly better, which has been attributed to a standardized management approach and improvement of neonatal care in the last decade.**[83] **A recently published 2-year follow-up study showed that**

IUGR UNLIKELY		
Normal AC, AC growth rate and HC/AC ratio UA, MCA Doppler, BPS, and AFV normal	Asphyxia extremely rare low risk for intrapartum distress	Deliver for obstetric or maternal factors only, follow growth

IUGR		
AC <5th, low AC growth rate, high HC/AC ratio, abnormal UA and/or CPR, normal MCA and veins, BPS ≥8/10, AFV normal	Asphyxia extremely rare Increased risk for intrapartum distress	Deliver for obstetric or maternal factors only, Every 2 weeks Doppler Weekly BPS

With blood flow redistribution

IUGR diagnosed based on above criteria Low MCA, normal veins BPS ≥8/10, AFV normal	Hypoxemia possible, asphyxia rare Increased risk for intrapartum distress	Deliver for obstetric or maternal factors only, weekly Doppler BPS 2 times/week

With significant blood flow redistribution

UA A/REDV normal veins BPS ≥6/10, oligohydramnios	Hypoxemia common, acidemia or asphyxia possible Onset of fetal compromise	>34 weeks: deliver <32 weeks: antenatal steroids Repeat all testing daily

With proven fetal compromise

Significant redistribution present Increased DV pulsatility BPS ≥6/10, oligohydramnios	Hypoxemia common, acidemia or asphyxia likely	>32 weeks: deliver <32 weeks: admit, Steroids, individualize testing daily vs. tid

With fetal decompensation

Compromise by above criteria Absent or reversed DV a-wave, pulsatile UV BPS <6/10, oligohydramnios	Cardiovascular instability, metabolic compromise, stillbirth imminent, high perinatal mortality irrespective of intervention	Deliver at tertiary care center with the highest level of NICU care

FIG 33-21 Integrated fetal testing and management protocol. The management algorithm for pregnancies complicated by intrauterine growth restriction (IUGR) is based on the ability to perform arterial and venous Doppler as well as a full five-component biophysical profile score (BPS). AC, abdominal circumference; AFV, amniotic fluid volume; A/REDV, absent/reversed end-diastolic velocity; CPR, cerebroplacental ratio; DV, ductus venosus; HC, head circumference; MCA, middle cerebral artery; NST, nonstress test; NICU, neonatal intensive care unit; tid, three times daily; UA, umbilical artery. (From Baschat AA, Hecher K. Fetal growth restriction due to placental disease. *Semin Perinatol.* 2004;28:67.)

liveborn fetuses delivered on the basis of late DV changes (absent or reversed a-wave) **demonstrated a reduction in neuroimpairment.**[84]

Frigoletto has previously emphasized that the majority of fetal deaths in IUGR occur after the 36th week of gestation and before the onset of labor. The Disproportionate Intrauterine Growth Intervention Trial at Term (DIGITAT) randomized trial[85] **illustrates that neonatal morbidity is still a concern until 38 weeks' gestation. For these reasons, a definite delivery indication other than the presence of suspected growth delay is required prior to 38 weeks' gestation.**[85] **One limitation of the DIGITAT trial was a lack of UA and MCA Doppler assessment or integration in the study.**

These investigations illustrate several points that are of critical importance in the management of pregnancies complicated by IUGR today. Patients need to be aware that growth-restricted fetuses have different viability thresholds and neonatal risk

statistics than their appropriately grown counterparts. The major risk for the undelivered growth-restricted fetus is progression of hypoxemia to acidemia and stillbirth. Delivery is therefore typically indicated when the risk for these complications is high or there is no added benefit from prolongation of pregnancy. In the preterm growth-restricted fetus, **the risk for acidemia and stillbirth is highest when repetitive late decelerations are observed in association with oligohydramnios and/or anhydramnios, when the BPP is below 6, when the DV Doppler index elevation escalates beyond 3 SDs, or when reversal of the DV a-wave is observed with accompanying umbilical venous pulsations.** In the growth-restricted fetus beyond 37 weeks, risks of unanticipated stillbirth increase when brain sparing, loss of heart rate reactivity, or a decrease in the AFV are observed.[15] A recent study from the Washington University group[86] demonstrated that although the overall risk of stillbirth is low in fetuses beyond 37 weeks, an increase in stillbirth risk

TABLE 33-4   OUTCOMES IN THE GROWTH RESTRICTION INTERVENTION TRIAL (GRIT)

	IMMEDIATE (N = 296)	DELAYED (N = 291)
Gestational age at entry (weeks)	32 (30-34)	32 (29-34)
Steroids already given	191 (70%)	189 (69%)
Days gained in utero	0.9 (0.4-1.2)	4.9 (2-10.8)
Birth weight (g)	1200 (875-1705)	1400 (930-1940)
Apgar <7 at 5 min	25 (9%)	17 (6%)
Cord pH <7.0	2 (1%)	4 (2%)
Death prior to discharge	29 (10%)	27 (9%)
Stillbirth	2	9
Neonatal death	23	12
Death >28 days	4	6
Survivors after 2 yr	256	251
Developmental delay at age 2 yr for patients delivered at 24 to 31 wk	14 (13%)	5 (5%)

Data from The GRIT study group. A randomised trial of timed delivery for the compromised preterm fetus: short term outcomes and Bayesian interpretation. *BJOG.* 2003;110:27; and Thornton JG, Hornbuckle J, Vail A, et al; The GRIT study group: Infant well-being at 2 years of age in the Growth Restriction Intervention Trial (GRIT): multicentred randomized trial. *Lancet.* 2004;364:513.

occurs with each advancing week for ongoing pregnancies. Thus they recommend delivery of the IUGR fetus at 37 to 38 weeks. The study is limited by its retrospective nature and that the growth-restricted fetuses that died in utero may not have been identified and followed with Doppler or antenatal testing.

General Considerations

Surveillance and management considerations are most challenging in preterm pregnancies, which places the highest demand on the accuracy of fetal testing before 34 weeks' gestation. Once FGR is suspected or anticipated, appropriate fetal testing and daily maternal assessment of fetal activity should be instituted. Ultrasound examinations to assess fetal growth should be scheduled every 2 to 4 weeks. As long as studies show continued fetal head growth and testing results remain reassuring, no intervention is required. An understanding of the strengths and limitations of individual surveillance tests in this context is important. The NST and fetal dynamic variables (fetal breathing, movement, and tone) provide assurance of fetal well-being at the time of testing. Because the traditional NST is frequently nonreactive in preterm fetuses, it is often inadequate as a stand-alone test of fetal well-being. A combination of UA Doppler and a five-component BPP are the surveillance tests of choice in preterm growth-restricted fetuses that circumvent this limitation of the NST alone. In the presence of UA end-diastolic velocity, normal AFV, and a normal BPP, weekly testing is sufficient. Testing frequency is adjusted according to fetal status with strict criteria for delivery as indicated above. In preterm growth-restricted fetuses in which timing of delivery is most critical, the combination of multiple modalities, including arterial and venous Doppler, offers the most comprehensive approach to assess fetal well-being.[61,87] Such integrated fetal testing is suggested for centers experienced with the performance of these studies. In the preterm growth-restricted fetus who presents before 34 weeks' gestation, consideration should always be given to administration of steroids if necessary, with continuous FHR monitoring and oxygen supplementation. Beyond 34 weeks' gestation, an amniocentesis to access lung maturity to direct timing of

delivery should be considered. Delivery at 38 weeks is an option that should be discussed in all pregnancies complicated by SGA because of the difficulties in accurately identifying fetal deterioration at this gestational age. Even with optimal management, there may be a yet undefined background morbidity that is predetermined by the condition and not amenable to treatment.

The following recommendations regarding the timing of delivery of the SGA fetus are made with the understanding that these guidelines are primarily based on retrospective studies, registries, and expert opinion; definitive randomized clinical studies are otherwise lacking or inconclusive. These guidelines are consistent with those produced by the American College of Obstetricians and Gynecologists (AGOG).

Between 24 and 29 Weeks' Gestation

Between 24 and 27 weeks' gestation, a growth-restricted fetus is periviable, and interventions are typically undertaken for maternal conditions such as severe preeclampsia. Thresholds for fetal indications should be high, which requires strong evidence of fetal compromise and risk of stillbirth. Management is frequently individualized, and a multidisciplinary approach is helpful in stressing that outcome may be poor even with maximal support in the neonatal intensive care unit (NICU). Parents need to be aware that despite maximum management and effort, perinatal mortality exceeds of 50%.[80,81] Based on retrospective studies, 29 weeks' gestation may be an important milestone to reach. Gestational age appears to be the strongest predictor of intact survival until 29 weeks, and 94% of perinatal morality has been reported to occur prior to 29 weeks' gestation.[80,88] Delivery triggers can be considered to be any one or a combination of FHR tracing with decelerations, BPP of 4 or less, or reverse a-wave in the ductus venosus, a marker of fetal acidemia.

Between 29 and 34 Weeks' Gestation

Fetal indications for delivery should be based on firm evidence of fetal compromise with an attempt to complete a course of antenatal corticosteroids whenever possible. Indications may include any one or combination of FHR tracing with decelerations, BPP of 4 or less, or absent or reverse a-wave in the ductus venosus.

Between 34 and 37 Weeks' Gestation

Between 34 and 37 weeks' gestation, lower delivery thresholds are acceptable and may include absent fetal growth (in particular arrested head growth), oligohydramnios, documented lung maturity on amniocentesis, Doppler evidence of accelerating disease, and maternal comorbidity.

Beyond 37 Weeks

If an SGA fetus has continued appropriate interval growth, normal Doppler studies, normal AFV, normal antepartum testing, and no maternal comorbidities, this may represent a normal or constitutionally small fetus. Delivery may be accomplished between 38 to 39 weeks' gestation.

DELIVERY

The premature growth-restricted fetus requires the highest level of NICU care; therefore predelivery transport to an appropriate institution is recommended in all cases of early-onset IUGR.

Because many growth-restricted infants suffer intrapartum asphyxia, intrapartum management demands continuous FHR monitoring. In principle the route of delivery is determined by the severity of the fetal and maternal condition, along with other obstetric factors. Cesarean delivery without a trial of labor is indicated when the risks of vaginal delivery are unacceptable to the mother and fetus. These circumstances include prelabor evidence of fetal acidemia, spontaneous late decelerations, or late decelerations with minimal uterine activity. In addition, absent and reversed end-diastolic flow in the UA is associated with a high incidence of fetal intolerance of labor. Thus cesarean delivery is often required and should be considered for these severely growth-restricted fetuses. In the instance of less abnormal fetal test results, typically in the setting of a more advanced gestational age, selection of the route of delivery is based on the Bishop score, AFV, and difficulty anticipated in inducing labor. The presence of IUGR has been considered a relative contraindication to the use of prostaglandin for cervical preparation by some authors. If cervical ripening is considered, preinduction oxytocin challenge testing may be helpful in determining the likelihood and safety of vaginal delivery. Pharmacologic or mechanical ripening of the cervix, coupled with labor in the left lateral decubitus position with supplemental oxygen, increases the likelihood of a successful vaginal delivery. During labor, a tracing without late decelerations is predictive of a good outcome in cases complicated by IUGR. However, with late decelerations, the incidence of asphyxia in growth-restricted infants is far greater than in normally grown infants.

OUTCOME

IUGR can transiently and/or permanently impair neonatal well-being. The potential effects of this condition at birth and from complications that occur in the neonatal period have been most extensively studied. However, additional effects of this perinatal period on intermediate and long-term health are starting to emerge. Recently, a new area of research into the fetal origin of maternal diseases has also pointed out how exposure to a hostile intrauterine environment can be a predisposing factor for the development in adulthood of cardiovascular diseases and endocrine disturbances (see Chapter 5). An understanding of these outcomes will become important when the focus of management strategies shifts from the prevention of fetal and neonatal morbidity to the improvement of intermediate- and long-term development. Studies that examine the relationship between FGR and postdelivery outcomes are therefore best separated into those that focus on short-term outcomes and those that focus on long-term outcomes.

Short-Term Outcomes

Initial reports that evaluated the association between FGR and neonatal morbidity suggested the possibility of a protective effect of IUGR, with reduced occurrence of RDS and IVH. Subsequent studies do not support these early assumptions. No differences were found in indices of fetal lung maturity and the frequency of the need for ventilator support comparing gestational age-matched SGA and AGA fetuses. Most recently, several large trials suggest that RDS, necrotizing enterocolitis (NEC), IVH, clotting disorders, and multiorgan failure are significantly more likely to occur in growth-restricted neonates.[89,90] Mortality rates are uniformly higher when IUGR is present. These data

should put to rest the notion that FGR is associated with any reduction in newborn illness. Additional neonatal morbidities that must be anticipated include meconium aspiration, hypoglycemia, and electrolyte abnormalities.

Meconium aspiration occurs more frequently in IUGR than in appropriately grown infants and is largely observed after 34 weeks. Gasping in utero in response to asphyxia appears to contribute to this problem. Historically, careful suctioning of the nasopharynx and oropharynx with the DeLee catheter at delivery was used to decrease the incidence of this complication; however, more recent data show that this is not the case. Clearing of the airway can be accomplished at delivery by direct laryngoscopy and aspiration by an experienced pediatrician. To effect immediate attention to the many potential neonatal problems, appropriate pediatric support should be present in the delivery room when an infant suspected of being growth restricted is to be delivered.

Hypoglycemia is frequently observed in growth-restricted infants owing to their inadequate glycogen reserves and a gluconeogenic pathway that is less sensitive to hypoglycemia than that of the normally grown infant.[89] In anticipation of this risk for hypoglycemia, frequent blood glucose monitoring should be instituted in all growth-restricted infants. **Hypocalcemia**, another well-recognized problem in IUGR, may be the result of relative hypoparathyroidism, a result of intrauterine acidosis.

Hyperphosphatemia secondary to tissue breakdown may also contribute. Frequent calcium monitoring is essential because symptoms are nonspecific and are similar to those associated with hypoglycemia.

Hyponatremia that results from impaired renal function is also frequently reported in growth-restricted infants. The renal complications associated with IUGR may be attributed to asphyxia, which can produce central nervous system injury and can lead to inappropriate antidiuretic hormone (ADH) secretion.[89]

Neonates with growth restriction are at risk for polycythemia, anemia, thrombocytopenia, and complex hematologic derangements that may be problematic well beyond delivery.[10] **Polycythemia** is observed three to four times more frequently in the growth-restricted infant than in weight-matched controls. Polycythemia results from hypoxia-stimulated production of red blood cells (RBCs) and from transfer of blood volume from the placental to the fetal circulation in the face of intrauterine asphyxia. Thus these infants produce more RBCs that are shunted to them if hypoxia occurs during labor. Polycythemia leads to increased RBC breakdown, accounting in part for the high incidence of **hyperbilirubinemia** in these infants. Polycythemia is a criterion for, but does not necessarily lead to, hyperviscosity, which can result in capillary bed sludging and thrombosis. Multiple organ systems can be affected and can lead to pulmonary hypertension, cerebral infarction, and NEC. Anemia can be observed in preterm fetuses with growth restriction with markedly abnormal placental blood flow studies, and thrombocytopenia frequently accompanies the anemia. The risk for thrombocytopenia is increased more than tenfold if UA end-diastolic velocity is absent. The cause for these abnormalities could involve a combination of dysfunctional erythropoiesis coupled with placental consumption of platelets and RBCs. Neonates with such complex hematologic abnormalities are frequently unable to sustain their blood cell counts despite repeated substitution of blood products.

Hypothermia is another common problem for the growth-restricted infant and results from decreased body fat stores secondary to intrauterine malnourishment.[89] If unrecognized and untreated, hypothermia can contribute to the metabolic deterioration of an already unstable growth-restricted infant.

Finally, growth-restricted neonates are at increased risk for perinatal death in light of the multiple complications that may arise in the fetal and neonatal periods. The range of reported perinatal mortality is variable but depends clearly on the level of perinatal management received: infants who received optimal intrapartum and neonatal management have a lower perinatal mortality than age-matched controls who did not have such intensive care.[90]

Long-Term Outcomes

Following delivery, the ultimate growth potential for growth-restricted infants appears to be good. The degree of catch-up growth observed in several longitudinal studies suggests that **these infants can be expected to have normal growth curves and a normal, albeit slightly reduced size as adults.** In an 8-year follow-up study of children who weighed less than 1500 g at birth,[91] 75% of growth-restricted infants achieved a height and weight above the 10th percentile. Of infants whose birthweight fell below the 3rd percentile, 60% had reached the 25th percentile for weight at 8 years. However, 50% of the children with small HCs still had HCs below the 10th percentile at the 8-year follow-up visit in spite of their growth in height and weight.[91] Others observed that growth-restricted infants experienced a period of catch-up growth in early infancy but remained near the 25th percentile through age 47 months, and infants with birthweights less than 1250 g remained below the third percentile for height and weight at 1 year in 38% to 46% of cases, respectively.[92] In general, those infants who suffered growth restriction near the time of delivery do tend to catch up. However, those neonates with earlier onset and more longstanding growth restriction in utero continue to lag behind.

The issue of long-term neurologic sequelae remains unresolved. In 1972, Fitzhardinge and Steven[93] evaluated a group of 96 growth-restricted infants and noted that 50% of males and 36% of females had poor school performance and, overall, 25% had minimal cerebral dysfunction. Major neurologic deficits were much less frequent. Other studies have shown low birthweight and short gestation to be risk factors for cerebral palsy. However, **the vast majority of children with cerebral palsy were not growth restricted.**

The positive effect of intrapartum surveillance for the growth-restricted fetus is reflected in the data of Low and colleagues.[94] In a study of 88 growth-restricted infants, they reported no severe neurologic sequelae. They did detect a lag in mental development that was significant in the growth-restricted babies when compared with appropriately grown controls, especially in the group with birthweights less than 2300 g. This study correlates well with other data on LBW babies, showing that **growth-restricted infants with HCs below the 10th percentile have two to three times the number of serious neurologic sequelae of their normocephalic counterparts.** Others have found that term infants with IUGR and HCs less than 2 SD below the mean had significantly poorer performance on intelligence and visual motor development testing at age 7 when compared with their control siblings.[95] In an examination of 7-year-olds who suffered no perinatal complications despite IUGR and who were matched for social class with a control

group, Walther showed an increase in teacher-identified hyperactivity, poor concentration, and clumsiness. In a study of school performance in 8-year-olds matched for socioeconomic status, Robertson and colleagues demonstrated a tendency toward hyperactivity in preterm growth-restricted children compared with control groups. Low and colleagues[96] have shown that in 9- to 11-year-olds, only FGR and socioeconomic status contributed independently to the presence of learning deficits. Intrapartum fetal asphyxia assessed by UA base deficit was not associated with learning deficits in this group of children.

Few studies have related neurodevelopment to a full complement of antenatal surveillance parameters. A study of predominantly preterm growth-restricted infants that evaluated 2-year developmental outcomes reported **gestational age at delivery, birthweight, and reversal of UA end-diastolic velocity as the main determinants of motor and neurosensory morbidity.** Interestingly, fetal deterioration of venous Doppler or biophysical parameters did not have a statistical impact on neurodevelopment.[97]

The pattern that emerges from evaluation of these data emphasizes that **neurologic outcome depends on the degree of growth restriction, especially the impact on head growth, its time of onset, the gestational age of the infant at birth, and the postnatal environment.** An early intrauterine insult between 10 and 17 weeks' gestation could limit neuronal cellular multiplication and would obviously have a profound effect on neurologic function. In the third trimester, brain development is characterized by glial multiplication, dendritic arborization, establishment of synaptic connections, and myelinization—all of which continue during the first 2 years of life. Recovery after a period of impaired growth in the third trimester is therefore more likely to occur. Thus **the preterm appropriately grown infant has more normal neurologic development and fewer severe neurologic deficits than its preterm growth-restricted counterpart.** Developmental milestones and neurologic development of mature infants with IUGR and mature infants of normal birthweight are similar. Presumably, this also reflects heightened physician awareness of the growth-restricted infant that allows detection, appropriate antepartum management, intrapartum therapy, and early pediatric intervention. The premature growth-restricted infant suffers from increased susceptibility to intrauterine asphyxia and all of the neonatal complications of the premature infant in addition to those of the infant with IUGR. **If growth restriction is associated with lagging head growth before 26 weeks, even mature infants have significant developmental delay at 4 years of age.**

The long-term impacts at age 6 to 13 years of age were reported for the GRIT study. In the absence of any specific delivery triggers, the cognitive development was identical in both groups. In summary, these findings are concerning, which emphasizes the fact that the intrauterine environment has significant impact on neurodevelopment *before* management issues at delivery arise and, accordingly, it is unlikely that intervention trials will demonstrate a large impact of delivery timing on neurodevelopment.[97]

Gestational programming of growth-restricted fetuses has received considerable attention over the past 10 to 15 years. Infants born growth restricted have an increased risk of metabolic syndrome, obesity, hypertension, diabetes, and stroke from coronary artery disease. For a more in-depth review of fetal programming and long-term adult outcomes from IUGR, the reader is referred to Chapter 5.

REFERENCES

1. Savchev Wolfe HM, Gross TL, Sokol RJ. Recurrent small for gestational age birth: perinatal risks and outcomes. *Am J Obstet Gynecol*. 1987;157:288.
2. Mavrides E, Moscoso G, Carvalho JS, et al. The anatomy of the umbilical, portal and hepatic venous systems in the human fetus at 14-19 weeks of gestation. *Ultrasound Obstet Gynecol*. 2001;18:598.
3. Sparks JW, Girard JR, Battaglia FC. An estimate of the caloric requirements of the human fetus. *Biol Neonate*. 1980;38:113.
4. Khoury MJ, Erickson D, Cordero JE, et al. Congenital malformations and intrauterine growth retardation: a population study. *Pediatrics*. 1988;82:83.
5. Cowles T, Tatlor S, Zneimer S, et al. Association of confined placental mosaicism with intrauterine growth restriction [abstract]. *Am J Obstet Gynecol*. 1994;170:273.
6. Paolini CL, Marconi AM, Ronzoni S, et al. Placental transport of leucine, phenylalanine, glycine, and proline in intrauterine growth-restricted pregnancies. *J Clin Endocrinol Metab*. 2001;86:5427.
7. Soothill PW, Nicolaides KH, Campbell S. Prenatal asphyxia, hyperlacticaemia, hypoglycaemia, and erythroblastosis in growth retarded fetuses. *Br Med J*. 1987;294:1051.
8. Kilby MD, Gittoes N, McCabe C, et al. Expression of thyroid receptor isoforms in the human fetal central nervous system and the effects of intrauterine growth restriction. *Clin Endocrinol (Oxf)*. 2000;53:469.
9. Thilaganathan B, Athanasiou S, Ozmen S, et al. Umbilical cord blood erythroblast count as an index of intrauterine hypoxia. *Arch Dis Child Fetal Neonatal Ed*. 1994;70:F192.
10. Baschat AA, Kush M, Berg C, et al. The hematologic profile of neonates with growth restriction is associated with the rate and degree of prenatal Doppler deterioration. *Ultrasound Obstet Gynecol*. 2013;41:66-72.
11. Ferrazzi E, Bozzo M, Rigano S, et al. Temporal sequence of abnormal Doppler changes in the peripheral and central circulatory systems of the severely growth-restricted fetus. *Ultrasound Obstet Gynecol*. 2002;19:140.
12. Bellotti M, Pennati G, De Gasperi C, et al. Simultaneous measurements of umbilical venous, fetal hepatic, and ductus venosus blood flow in growth-restricted human fetuses. *Am J Obstet Gynecol*. 2004;190:1347.
13. Kiserud T. The ductus venosus. *Semin Perinatol*. 2001;25:11.
14. Reed KL, Anderson CF, Shenker L. Changes in intracardiac Doppler flow velocities in fetuses with absent umbilical artery diastolic flow. *Am J Obstet Gynecol*. 1987;157:774.
15. Crimmins S, Desai A, Block-Abraham D, Berg C, Gembruch U, Baschat AA. A comparison of Doppler and biophysical findings between liveborn and stillborn growth-restricted fetuses. *Am J Obstet Gynecol*. 2014;211(6):669.e1-669.e10.
16. Hecher K, Campbell S, Doyle P, et al. Assessment of fetal compromise by Doppler ultrasound investigation of the fetal circulation. Arterial, intracardiac, and venous blood flow velocity studies. *Circulation*. 1995;91:129.
17. Rizzo G, Capponi A, Pietropolli A, et al. Fetal cardiac and extracardiac flows preceding intrauterine death. *Ultrasound Obstet Gynecol*. 1994;4:139.
18. Arduini D, Rizzo G, Caforio L, et al. Behavioural state transitions in healthy and growth retarded fetuses. *Early Hum Dev*. 1989;19:155.
19. Henson G, Dawes GS, Redman CW. Characterization of the reduced heart rate variation in growth-retarded fetuses. *Br J Obstet Gynaecol*. 1984;91:751.
20. Baschat AA, Gembruch U, Harman CR. The sequence of changes in Doppler and biophysical parameters as severe fetal growth restriction worsens. *Ultrasound Obstet Gynecol*. 2001;18:571.
21. Ribbert LS, Nicolaides KH, Visser GH. Prediction of fetal acidaemia in intrauterine growth retardation: comparison of quantified fetal activity with biophysical profile score. *Br J Obstet Gynaecol*. 1993;100:653.
22. Vintzileos AM, Fleming AD, Scorza WE, et al. Relationship between fetal biophysical activities and umbilical cord blood gas values. *Am J Obstet Gynecol*. 1991;165:707.
23. Manning FA, Snijders R, Harman CR, et al. Fetal biophysical profile score. VI. Correlation with antepartum umbilical venous fetal pH. *Am J Obstet Gynecol*. 1993;169:755.
24. Ott WJ. Intrauterine growth restriction and Doppler ultrasonography. *J Ultrasound Med*. 2000;19:661.
25. Hecher K, Spernol R, Stettner H, et al. Potential for diagnosing imminent risk for appropriate- and small for gestational fetuses by Doppler examination of umbilical and cerebral arterial blood flow. *Ultrasound Obstet Gynecol*. 1995;5:247.
26. Baschat AA. Pathophysiology of fetal growth restriction: implications for diagnosis and surveillance. *Obstet Gynecol Surv*. 2004;59:617.
27. Hadlock FP, Harrist RB, Sharman RS, et al. Estimation of fetal weight with the use of head, body, and femur measurements—a prospective study. *Am J Obstet Gynecol*. 1985;151:333.
28. Smith PA, Johansson D, Tzannatos C, et al. Prenatal measurement of the fetal cerebellum and cisterna cerebellomedullaris by ultrasound. *Prenat Diagn*. 1986;6:133.
29. Baschat AA, Weiner CP. Umbilical artery Doppler screening for detection of the small fetus in need of antepartum surveillance. *Am J Obstet Gynecol*. 2000;182:154.
30. Divon MY, Chamberlain PF, Sipos L, et al. Identification of the small for gestational age fetus with the use of gestational age-independent indices of fetal growth. *Am J Obstet Gynecol*. 1986;155:1197.
31. Campbell S, Thoms A. Ultrasound measurement of the fetal head to abdomen circumference ratio in the assessment of growth retardation. *Br J Obstet Gynaecol*. 1977;84:165.
32. Warsof SL, Cooper DJ, Little D, et al. Routine ultrasound screening for antenatal detection of intrauterine growth retardation. *Obstet Gynecol*. 1986;67:33.
33. Ott WJ. The diagnosis of altered fetal growth. *Obstet Gynecol Clin North Am*. 1988;15:237.
34. Weiner CP, Sabbagha RE, Vaisrub N, et al. A hypothetical model suggesting suboptimal intra-uterine growth in infants delivered preterm. *Obstet Gynecol*. 1985;65:323.
35. Bernstein IM, Meyer MC, Capeless EL. "Fetal growth charts": comparison of cross-sectional ultrasound examinations with birthweight. *Maternal Fetal Med*. 1994;3:182.

36. Lackman F, Capewell V, Richardson B, et al. Fetal or neonatal growth curve: which is more appropriate in predicting the impact of fetal growth on the risk of perinatal mortality? *Am J Obstet Gynecol.* 1999;180:S145.

37. Rossavik IK, Deter RL. Mathematical modeling of fetal growth. I. Basic principles. *J Clin Ultrasound.* 1984;12:529.

38. Baschat AA, Towbin J, Bowles NE, et al. Is adenovirus a fetal pathogen? *Am J Obstet Gynecol.* 2003;189:758.

39. Veille JC, Kanaan C. Duplex Doppler ultrasonographic evaluation of the fetal renal artery in normal and abnormal fetuses. *Am J Obstet Gynecol.* 1989;161:1502.

40. Magann EF, Chauhan SP, Barrilleaux PS, et al. Amniotic fluid index and single deepest pocket: weak indicators of abnormal amniotic volumes. *Obstet Gynecol.* 2000;96:737.

41. Manning FA, Hill LM, Platt LD. Qualitative amniotic fluid volume determination by ultrasound: antepartum detection of intrauterine growth retardation. *Am J Obstet Gynecol.* 1981;193:254.

42. Groome LJ, Owen J, Neely CL, et al. Oligohydramios: antepartum fetal urine production and intrapartum fetal distress. *Am J Obstet Gynecol.* 1991;165:1077.

43. Hecher K, Campbell S. Characteristics of fetal venous blood flow under normal circumstances and during fetal disease. *Ultrasound Obstet Gynecol.* 1996;7:68.

44. Neilson JP, Alfirevic Z. Doppler ultrasound for fetal assessment in high risk pregnancies. *Cochrane Database Sys Rev.* 2000;(2):CD000073.

45. Westergaard HB, Langhoff-Roos J, Lingman G, et al. A critical appraisal of the use of umbilical artery Doppler ultrasound in high-risk pregnancies: use of meta-analyses in evidence-based obstetrics. *Ultrasound Obstet Gynecol.* 2001;17:466.

46. Yagel S, Anteby EY, Shen O, et al. Simultaneous multigate spectral Doppler imaging of the umbilical artery and placental vessels: novel ultrasound technology. *Ultrasound Obstet Gynecol.* 1999;14:256.

47. Bahado-Singh RO, Kovanci E, Jeffres A, et al. The Doppler cerebroplacental ratio and perinatal outcome in intrauterine growth restriction. *Am J Obstet Gynecol.* 1999;180:750.

48. Unterscheider J, Daly S, Geary MP, et al. Optimizing the definition of intrauterine growth restriction: the multicenter prospective PORTO Study. *Am J Obstet Gynecol.* 2013;208(4):290.e1-e6.

49. Yaron Y, Cherry M, Kramer RL, et al. Second-trimester maternal serum marker screening: maternal serum alpha-fetoprotein, beta-human chorionic gonadotropin, estriol, and their various combinations as predictors for pregnancy outcome. *Am J Obstet Gynecol.* 1999;181:968.

50. Bower S, Kingdom J, Campbell S. Objective and subjective assessment of abnormal uterine artery Doppler flow velocity waveforms. *Ultrasound Obstet Gynecol.* 1998;12:260.

51. Bujold E, Roberge S, Lacasse Y, et al. Prevention of preeclampsia and intrauterine growth restriction with aspirin therapy started early in pregnancy—a meta analysis. *Obstet Gynecol.* 2010;116:402.

52. Battaglia C, Artini PG, D'Ambrogio G, et al. Maternal hyperoxygenation in the treatment of intrauterine growth retardation. *Am J Obstet Gynecol.* 1992;167:430.

53. Karsdorp VH, van Vugt JM, Dekker GA, et al. Reappearance of end-diastolic velocities in the umbilical artery following maternal volume expansion: a preliminary study. *Obstet Gynecol.* 1992;80:679.

54. Deren O, Karaer C, Onderoglu L, et al. The effect of steroids on the biophysical profile and Doppler indices of umbilical and middle cerebral arteries in healthy preterm fetuses. *Eur J Obstet Gynecol Reprod Biol.* 2001;99:72.

55. Soothill PW, Ajayi RA, Campbell S, et al. Relationship between fetal acidemia at cordocentesis and subsequent neurodevelopment. *Ultrasound Obstet Gynecol.* 1992;2:80.

56. Matthews DD. Maternal assessment of fetal activity in small-for-dates infants. *Obstet Gynecol.* 1975;45:488.

57. Pazos R, Vuolo K, Aladjem S, et al. Association of spontaneous fetal heart rate decelerations during antepartum nonstress testing and intrauterine growth retardation. *Am J Obstet Gynecol.* 1982;144:574.

58. Gabbe SG, Freeman RD, Goebelsmann U. Evaluation of the contraction stress test before 33 weeks ' gestation. *Obstet Gynecol.* 1978;52:649.

59. Lin CC, Devoe LD, River P, et al. Oxytocin challenge test and intrauterine growth retardation. *Am J Obstet Gynecol.* 1981;140:282.

60. Ribbert LS, Snijders RJ, Nicolaides KH, et al. Relationship of fetal biophysical profile and blood gas values at cordocentesis in severely growth-retarded fetuses. *Am J Obstet Gynecol.* 1990;163:569.

61. Baschat AA, Galan HL, Bhide A, et al. Doppler and biophysical assessment in growth restricted fetuses: distribution of test results. *Ultrasound Obstet Gynecol.* 2006;27:41.

62. Savchev S, Figueras F, Sanz-Cortes M, et al. Evaluation of an optimal gestational age cut-off for the definition of early- and late-onset fetal growth restriction. *Fetal Diagn Ther.* 2014;36(2):99-105.

63. Harrington K, Thompson MO, Carpenter RG, et al. Doppler fetal circulation in pregnancies complicated by pre-eclampsia or delivery of a small for gestational age baby: 2. Longitudinal analysis. *Br J Obstet Gynaecol.* 1999;106:453.

64. Bilardo CM, Wolf H, Stigter RH, et al. Relationship between monitoring parameters and perinatal outcome in severe, early intrauterine growth restriction. *Ultrasound Obstet Gynecol.* 2004;23:119.

65. Guzman ER, Vintzileos AM, Martins M, et al. The efficacy of individual computer heart rate indices in detecting acidemia at birth in growth-restricted fetuses. *Obstet Gynecol.* 1996;87:969.

66. Morrow RJ, Adamson SL, Bull SB, et al. Effect of placental embolization on the umbilical artery velocity waveform in fetal sheep. *Am J Obstet Gynecol.* 1989;161:1055.

67. Arduini D, Rizzo G, Romanini C. The development of abnormal heart rate patterns after absent end-diastolic velocity in umbilical artery: analysis of risk factors. *Am J Obstet Gynecol.* 1993;168:50.

68. Baschat AA. Doppler application in the delivery timing of the preterm growth-restricted fetus: another step in the right direction. *Ultrasound Obstet Gynecol.* 2004;23:111.

69. Baschat AA, Gembruch U, Weiner CP, et al. Qualitative venous Doppler waveform analysis improves prediction of critical perinatal outcomes in premature growth-restricted fetuses. *Ultrasound Obstet Gynecol.* 2003;22:240.

70. Pardi G, Cetin I, Marconi AM, et al. Diagnostic value of blood sampling in fetuses with growth retardation. *N Engl J Med.* 1993;328:692.

71. The GRIT study group. A randomised trial of timed delivery for the compromised preterm fetus: short term outcomes and Bayesian interpretation. *BJOG.* 2003;110:27.

72. Baschat AA, Cosmi E, Bilardo CM, et al. Predictors of neonatal outcome in early-onset placental dysfunction. *Obstet Gynecol.* 2007;109:253.

73. Froen JF, Gardosi JO, Thurmann A, et al. Restricted fetal growth in sudden intrauterine unexplained death. *Acta Obstet Gynecol Scand.* 2004;83:801.

74. Hecher K, Bilardo CM, Stigter RH, et al. Monitoring of fetuses with intrauterine growth restriction: a longitudinal study. *Ultrasound Obstet Gynecol.* 2001;18:564.

75. Hershkovitz R, Kingdom JC, Geary M, et al. Fetal cerebral blood flow redistribution in late gestation: identification of compromise in small fetuses with normal umbilical artery Doppler. *Ultrasound Obstet Gynecol.* 2000;15:209.

76. Unterscheider J, Daly S, Geary MP, et al. Predictable progressive Doppler deterioration in IUGR: does it really exist? *AJOG.* 2014;209:539e1-e7.

77. Baschat AA. Integrated fetal testing in growth restriction: combining multivessel Doppler and biophysical parameters. *Ultrasound Obstet Gynecol.* 2003;21:1.

78. Thornton JG, Hornbuckle J, Vail A, et al., The GRIT study group. Infant well-being at 2 years of age in the Growth Restriction Intervention Trial (GRIT): multicentred randomized trial. *Lancet.* 2004;364:513.

79. Walker DM, Marlow N, Upstone L, et al. Long term outcomes in a randomized trial of timing of delivery in fetal growth restriction. *Am J Obstet Gynecol.* 2011;204:34.e1.

80. Baschat AA, Bilardo CM, Germer U, et al. Thresholds for intervention in severe early onset growth restriction. *Am J Obstet Gynecol.* 2004;191:S143.

81. Garite TJ, Clark R, Thorp JA. Intrauterine growth restriction increases morbidity and mortality among premature neonates. *Am J Obstet Gynecol.* 2004;191:481.

82. Lees C, Marlow N, Arabin B, et al. Perinatal morbidity and mortality in early-onset fetal growth restriction: cohort outcomes of the trial of randomized umbilical and fetal flow in Europe (TRUFFLE). *Ultrasound Obstet Gynecol.* 2013;42:400-408.

83. Lees CC, Marlow N, van Wassenaer-Leemhuis A, et al. 2 year neurodevelopmental and intermediate perinatal outcomes in infants with very preterm fetal growth restriction (TRUFFLE): a randomized trial. *Lancet.* 2015 (E pub ahead of print).

84. Boers KE, van Wyk L, van der Post JA, et al. DIGITAT Study Group. Neonatal morbidity after induction vs expectant monitoring in intrauterine growth restriction at term: a subanalysis of the DIGITAT RCT. *Am J Obstet Gynecol.* 2012;206(4).

85. Trudell AS, Cahill AG, Tuuli MG, et al. Risk of stillbirth after 37 weeks in pregnancies complicated by small-for-gestational-age fetuses. *Am J Obstet Gynecol.* 2013;208:376.e1-e7.

86. Baschat AA, Gembruch U, Weiner CP, et al. Combining Doppler and biophysical assessment improves prediction of critical perinatal outcomes. *Am J Obstet Gynecol.* 2002;187:S147.

87. Mariari G, Hanif F, Treadwell MC, Kruger M. Gestational age at delivery and Doppler waveforms in very preterm intrauterine growth-restricted fetuses as predictors of perinatal mortality. *J Ultrasound Med.* 2007;26: 555-559.

88. McIntire DD, Bloom SL, Casey BM, et al. Birth weight in relation to morbidity and mortality among newborn infants. *N Engl J Med.* 1999; 340:1234.

89. Ley D, Wide-Swensson D, Lindroth M, et al. Respiratory distress syndrome in infants with impaired intrauterine growth. *Acta Paediatr.* 1997;10:1090.

90. Kitchen WH, Richards A, Ryan MM, et al. A longitudinal study of very low-birthweight infants. II: Results of controlled trial of intensive care and incidence of handicaps. *Dev Med Child Neurol.* 1979;21:582.

91. Kitchen WH, McDougall AB, Naylor FD. A longitudinal study of very low-birthweight infants. III: Distance growth at eight years of age. *Dev Med Child Neurol.* 1980;22:1633.

92. Kumar SP, Anday EK, Sacks LM, et al. Follow-up studies of very low birthweight infants (1,250 grams or less) born and treated within a perinatal center. *Pediatrics.* 1980;66:438.

93. Fitzhardinge PM, Steven EM. The small-for-dates infant. II: Neurological and intellectual sequelae. *Pediatrics.* 1972;50:50.

94. Low JA, Galbraith RS, Muir D, et al. Intrauterine growth retardation: a preliminary report of long-term morbidity. *Am J Obstet Gynecol.* 1978; 130:534.

95. Strauss R, Dietz WH. Growth and development of term children born with low birth weight: effects of genetic and environmental factors. *J Pediatr.* 1998;133:67.

96. Low JA, Handley-Derry MH, Burke SO, et al. Association of intrauterine fetal growth retardation and learning deficits at age 9 to 11 years. *Am J Obstet Gynecol.* 1992;167:1499.

97. Baschat AA, Viscardi RM, Hussey-Gardner B, Hashmi N, Harman C. Infant neurodevelopment following fetal growth restriction: relationship with antepartum surveillance parameters. *Ultrasound Obstet Gynecol.* 2009; 33:44-50.

Additional references for this chapter are available at ExpertConsult.com.

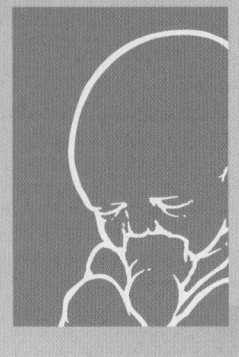

Red Cell Alloimmunization

KENNETH J. MOISE JR

KEY ABBREVIATIONS

American Association of Blood Banks	AABB
American College of Obstetricians and Gynecologists	ACOG
Cytomegalovirus	CMV
Circulating cell-free fetal DNA	ccffDNA
Deoxyribonucleic acid	DNA
Diphosphatidylglycerol	DPG
Fetal blood sampling	FBS
Fetomaternal hemorrhage	FMH
Grams per deciliter	g/dL
Hemolytic disease of the fetus and newborn	HDFN
Hemolytic disease of the newborn	HDN
Intraperitoneal transfusion	IPT
International unit(s)	IU
Intrauterine transfusion	IUT
Intravascular transfusion	IVT
Intravenous immune globulin	IVIG
Kleihauer-Betke	KB
Middle cerebral artery	MCA
Microgram	μg
Rhesus immune globulin	RhIG
Single nucleotide polymorphisms	SNPs

NOMENCLATURE

Exposure to foreign red cell antigens invariably results in the production of anti–red cell antibodies in a process known as *red cell alloimmunization*, formerly termed *isoimmunization*. The expression *sensitization* can be used interchangeably with *Rhesus alloimmunization*. The active transport of these antibodies across the placenta during pregnancy results in fetal anemia, hyperbilirubinemia, and ultimately hydrops fetalis. Before the advent of obstetric ultrasound, the perinatal effects of maternal red cell alloimmunization could be recognized only after birth in the affected neonate. Thus the neonatal consequences of maternal red cell alloimmunization came to be known as *hemolytic disease of the newborn* (HDN). Because the peripheral blood smear of these infants demonstrated a large percentage of circulating immature red cells known as *erythroblasts,* the newborn entity was also known as *erythroblastosis fetalis.* Today, ultrasound and fetal blood sampling (FBS) make the detection of the severely anemic fetus a reality. For this reason, **the term *hemolytic disease of the fetus and newborn* (HDFN) would appear more appropriate to describe this disorder.**

HISTORIC PERSPECTIVES

The first case of HDFN was probably described by a midwife in 1609 in the French literature: a twin gestation in which the first fetus was stillborn and the second twin developed jaundice and died soon after birth.[1] In 1932, Diamond[2] proposed that the clinical entities of erythroblastosis fetalis, icterus gravis neonatorum, and hydrops fetalis represented different manifestations of the same disease. Seven years later, Levine and Stetson[3] described an antibody in a woman who gave birth to a stillborn fetus. The patient experienced a severe hemolytic transfusion reaction after later receiving her husband's blood. In 1940, Landsteiner and Weiner[4] injected red blood cells from rhesus monkeys into rabbits. The antibody isolated from these rabbits was used to test human blood samples from whites, and agglutination was noted in 85% of individuals. The following year Levine and colleagues[5] were able to demonstrate a causal relationship between Rhesus D (RhD) antibodies in RhD-negative women and HDFN in their offspring.

The advent of therapy for HDFN began in 1945 with the description by Wallerstein[6] of the technique of neonatal exchange transfusion. Later Liley[7] proposed the use of amniotic fluid bilirubin assessment as an indirect measure of the degree of fetal hemolysis. Sir William Liley's major contribution to the story of rhesus disease was the introduction of the fetal intraperitoneal transfusion (IPT).[8] He learned from a visiting fellow who had returned from Africa that the infusion of red blood cells into the peritoneal cavity of children with sickle-cell disease produced normal-appearing red blood cells on peripheral blood smear. Liley realized that he had previously inadvertently entered the peritoneal cavity of fetuses at the time of amniocentesis, based on the marked contrast in the yellow hue of the ascitic fluid as compared with amniotic fluid. He postulated that purposeful entry into the fetal peritoneal cavity could be accomplished. After three unsuccessful attempts that resulted in fetal demises, the fourth fetus was delivered at 34[1/7] weeks' gestation after undergoing two successful IPTs. Early attempts at IPT used fluoroscopy for needle guidance. With the introduction of real-time ultrasound in the early 1980s, IPT became a safer procedure as fluoroscopy was abandoned. Charles Rodeck[9] is credited with the first intravascular fetal transfusion (IVT) using a fetoscope to guide the transfusion needle into a placental plate vessel. Just 1 year later, investigators in Denmark performed the first ultrasound-guided IVT using the intrahepatic portion of the umbilical vein.[10]

The 1990s saw the introduction of genetic techniques using amniocentesis to determine fetal red cell typing.[11] The turn of the century brought the noninvasive detection of fetal anemia through Doppler ultrasound of the fetal middle cerebral artery (MCA) and the use of fetal typing through cell-free DNA in maternal plasma.[12,13]

INCIDENCE

The advent of the routine administration of antenatal and postpartum rhesus immune globulin (RhIG) has resulted in a marked reduction in cases of red cell alloimmunization secondary to the RhD antigen. The Centers for Disease Control and Prevention (CDC) last required the reporting of rhesus alloimmunization as a medical complication of pregnancy on U.S. birth certificates in the year 2002.[14] In that year, the most recent for which epidemiologic data are available, the incidence was reported to be 6.7 cases of rhesus alloimmunization per 1000 live births.

Clearly, a shift to other red cell antibodies associated with HDFN has occurred as a result of the decreasing incidence of RhD alloimmunization. In a series of over 8000 pregnant patients between 2007 and 2011, a positive screen for an antibody associated with HDFN was found in 1.2% of samples.[15] Anti-E was the most common antibody encountered; RhD antibody accounted for only 19% of the significant antibodies (Fig. 34-1).

PATHOPHYSIOLOGY

Although the placenta was once thought to be an absolute barrier to the transfer of cells between the maternal and fetal compartments, we now appreciate that the placental interface allows for the bidirectional movement of both intact cells and free DNA. The putative "grandmother theory" of rhesus red cell alloimmunization probably occurs more commonly than first

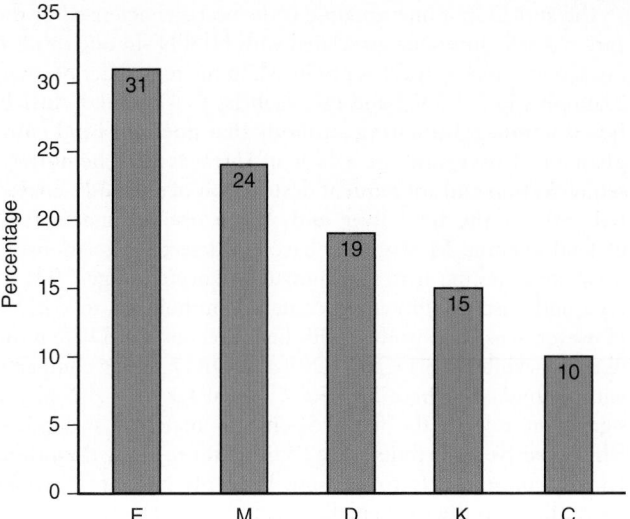

FIG 34-1 Incidence of maternal anti–red cell antibodies associated with hemolytic disease of the fetus and newborn (HDFN) at a tertiary care institution between 2007 and 2011. E, M, D, K, and C are antibodies. (Modified from Smith HM, Shirey RS, Thoman SK, Jackson JB. Prevalence of clinically significant red blood cell alloantibodies in pregnant women at a large tertiary care facility. *Immunohematology.* 2013;29: 127-130.)

thought. In this paradigm, maternal RhD-positive red cells gain access to the circulation of the RhD-negative fetus at the time of delivery. **As many as one fourth of RhD-negative babies have been shown to be immunized in early life as a result of their delivery.**[16,17] The immune response of an Rh-negative individual to RhD-positive red cells has been characterized into one of three groups: (1) responders, (2) hyporesponders, and (3) nonresponders. About 60% to 70% of individuals are *responders* who develop an antibody to relatively small volumes of red cells; in these individuals, the probability of immunization increases with escalating volumes of cells. A small percentage of responders can be called *hyperresponders* in that they will be immunized by very small quantities of red cells. The second group of individuals (10% to 20%), *hyporesponders,* can be immunized only by exposure to very large volumes of cells. Finally, the 10% to 20% of individuals who remain appear to be *nonresponders.*

In most cases of red cell alloimmunization, a fetomaternal hemorrhage (FMH) occurs in the antenatal period or, more commonly, at the time of delivery. If a maternal ABO blood type incompatibility exists between the mother and her fetus, anti-A and/or anti-B antibodies lyse the fetal cells in the maternal circulation and destroy the RhD antigen.[18,19] Even if this protective effect is not present, **only 13% of deliveries of RhD-positive fetuses result in RhD alloimmunization in RhD-negative women who do not receive RhIG.** The vast majority of RhD-alloimmunized women produce an immunoglobulin G (IgG) response as their initial antibody. *Responders* may represent a group of individuals who had their initial exposure to the RhD antigen at birth because of FMH.[17] After a sensitizing event, the human antiglobulin anti-D titer can usually be detected after 5 to 16 weeks. However, approximately half of alloimmunized patients are *sensibilized.* In this scenario, an antibody screen will be negative, but memory B lymphocytes are present that can create an anti-D antibody response. When faced with the challenge of a subsequent pregnancy involving an RhD-positive fetus, the anti-D titer becomes detectable.

The anti-D immune response is the best characterized of the anti–red cell antibodies associated with HDFN. In one third of cases, only subclass IgG1 is produced; in the remainder of cases, a combination of IgG1 and IgG3 subclasses is found.[20] **Anti-D IgG is a nonagglutinating antibody that does not bind complement. This results in a lack of intravascular hemolysis; sequestration and subsequent destruction of antibody-coated red cells in the fetal liver and spleen are the mechanism of fetal anemia.** Most studies have not detected a relationship between a specific maternal human leukocyte antigen (HLA) type and susceptibility to become alloimmunized to RhD.[21] However, sensitized women with high titers of anti-D are more likely to exhibit the DQB1*0201 and DR17 alleles compared with women who have low titers.[22] Fetal sex may also play a significant role in the fetal response to maternal antibodies. **RhD-positive male fetuses are 13 times more likely than their female counterparts to become hydropic and are 3 times more likely to die of their disease.**[23]

Anemia results in several important physiologic changes in the fetus. Reticulocytosis from the bone marrow can be detected by FBS once the hemoglobin deficit exceeds 2 g/dL compared with norms for gestational age; erythroblasts are released from the fetal liver once the hemoglobin deficit reaches 7 g/dL or greater.[24] In an effort to increase oxygen delivery to peripheral tissues, fetal cardiac output increases and 2-3 diphosphatidyl-glycerol (DPG) levels are enhanced.[25,26] Tissue hypoxia appears as anemia progresses despite these physiologic changes. An increased umbilical artery lactate level is noted when the fetal hemoglobin falls below 8 g/dL, and increased venous lactate can be detected when the hemoglobin level falls below 4 g/dL.[27] **Hydrops fetalis, the accumulation of extracellular fluid in at least two body compartments, is a late finding in cases of fetal anemia. Its exact pathophysiology is unknown.** Enhanced hepatic erythropoietic function with subsequent depressed synthesis of serum proteins has been proposed as the explanation for the lower serum albumin levels that have been detected.[28] Colloid osmotic pressure appears decreased.[29] However, experimental animal models in which fetal plasma proteins have been replaced with saline did not produce hydrops.[30] An alternative hypothesis is that tissue hypoxia due to anemia enhances capillary permeability. In addition, iron overload due to ongoing hemolysis may contribute to free radical formation and endothelial cell dysfunction.[31] Central venous pressures do appear elevated in the hydropic fetus with HDFN. This may cause a functional blockage of the lymphatic system at the level of the thoracic duct as it empties into the left brachiocephalic vein.[29] This theory is supported by reports of poor absorption of donor red cells infused into the intraperitoneal cavity in cases of hydrops.[32]

RHESUS ALLOIMMUNIZATION AND FETAL/NEONATAL HEMOLYTIC DISEASE OF THE NEWBORN

Genetics

Initial concepts on the genetics of the Rh antigens proposed the presence of three distinct genes.[33] Newer DNA techniques have allowed for the localization of the Rh locus to the short arm of chromosome 1.[34] **Only two genes were identified, an *RHD* gene and an *RHCE* gene.** Each gene is 10 exons in length with 96% homology. These genes presumably represent a duplication of a common ancestral gene. Production of two distinct proteins

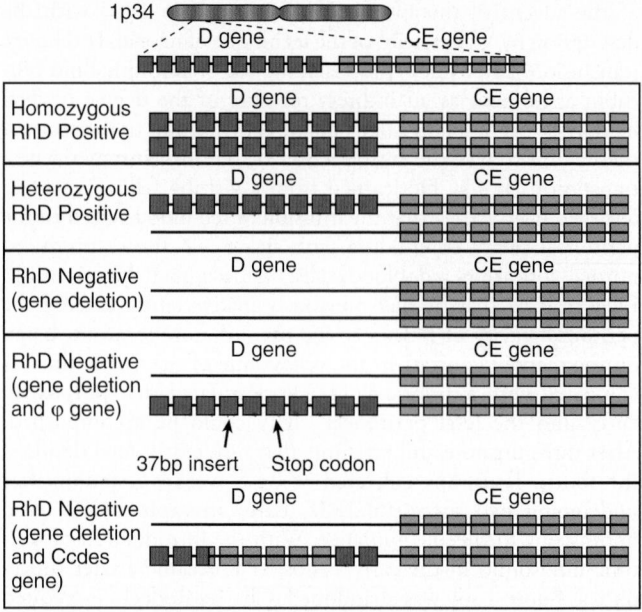

FIG 34-2 Schematic of Rh gene locus on chromosome 1. The homozygous RhD-positive state, heterozygous RhD-positive state, RhD-negative with heterozygosity for the *RhD* pseudogene, and RhD-negative with heterozygosity for the *RHCcdes* gene are demonstrated. (Modified from Moise KJ. Hemolytic disease of the fetus and newborn. In Creasy RK, Resnik R, Iams J, eds. *Maternal-Fetal Medicine: Principles and Practice*, ed 5. Philadelphia: Elsevier; 2004.)

from the *RHCE* gene probably occurs as a result of alternative splicing of messenger RNA.[35] One nucleotide difference, cytosine to thymine, in exon 2 of the *RHCE* gene results in a single amino acid change of a serine to proline. This causes the expression of the *C* antigen as opposed to the *c* antigen.[36] A single cytosine-to-guanine change in exon 5 of the *RHCE* gene, producing a single amino acid change of a proline to alanine, results in formation of the *e* antigen instead of the *E* antigen.

The gene frequency found in different ethnic groups can be traced to the Spanish colonization in the fifteenth and sixteenth centuries. Populations native to certain land masses have a less than 1% incidence of RhD negativity—Eskimos, Native Americans, Japanese, and Chinese individuals. The Basque tribe in Spain is noted to have a 30% incidence of Rh negativity. This may well be the origin of the *RHD* gene deletion that is the most common genetic basis of the RhD-negative state in whites (Fig. 34-2). Whites of European descent exhibit a 15% incidence of RhD negativity, whereas an 8% incidence is found in blacks and Hispanics of Mexico and Central America. This latter incidence probably reflects ethnic diversity secondary to Spanish colonization of the New World.

Further study of the *RHD* gene has revealed significant heterogeneity. Several of these genetic modifications result in a lack of expression of the RhD phenotype. Although these individuals may have an aberrant RhD gene present, serologic methods do not detect the RhD antigen on the surface of the red cells. One such example is the *RHD* pseudogene, which has been found in 69% of South African blacks and 24% of American blacks (see Fig. 34-2).[37] In this situation, all 10 exons of the *RHD* gene are present. However, translation of the gene into a messenger RNA (mRNA) product does not occur owing to the presence of a stop codon in the intron between exons 3 and 4. Thus, no RhD protein is synthesized, and the patient is serologically RhD negative. Similarly, the *RHCcdes* gene has been detected in 22% of American blacks. It appears to contain exons 1, 2, 9, and 10 as well as a portion of exon 3 of the original *RHD* gene, with other exons being duplicated from the *RHCE* gene. In the Taiwanese population of RhD-negative individuals, five different exons of the *RHD* gene were evaluated.[38] Seventeen percent of individuals had all five exons detected, and an additional 135 demonstrated the presence of at least one of the five exons tested.

PREVENTION OF RhD HEMOLYTIC DISEASE IN THE FETUS AND NEWBORN

History

The history of rhesus prophylaxis can be traced to three unique individuals. Vincent Freda was an obstetric resident who developed an interest in HDFN.[39] He was allowed to spend part of the fourth year of his residency at Columbia Presbyterian Medical Center in the laboratory of Alexander Weiner, one of the first investigators to identify the "Rh factor." When Freda returned to Columbia, he went on to establish a serology laboratory and later organized the Rh Antepartum Clinic in 1960. A seat on the hospital transfusion committee became vacant, and in an unprecedented move based on his interest, the chairman of obstetrics and gynecology, Howard C. Taylor, Jr., appointed Freda to this position even though he had not completed his residency. The chairman of pathology responded with the appointment of John Gorman to the committee, a resident in pathology with an interest in blood banking. It is here that these two individuals met and developed the collaboration that would one day end in the introduction of RhIG. In 1906, Theobald Smith[40] found that guinea pigs given excess passive antibody failed to become immunized to diphtheria toxin. Freda and Gorman proposed that anti-D could be used in a similar fashion to prevent alloimmunization after delivery. They enlisted the aid of William Pollack, a senior protein chemist at Ortho Diagnostics, who developed an IgG globulin fraction from high-titered donor plasma. An initial grant application to the National Institutes of Health was rejected; however, funding was secured from the New York City Health Research Council on a second attempt. This was followed by a year's negotiations with lawyers in the state capital to allow the investigators to perform their clinical trials at the Sing Sing prison in New York beginning in 1961 (John Gorman; personal communication, 2009). Nine RhD-negative male volunteers were injected monthly with RhD-positive cells for five successive months.[41] Four of the men were immunized with intramuscular RhIG 24 hours before the injection of the red cells. Four of the five controls became alloimmunized to RhD, whereas none of the treated individuals developed anti-RhD antibodies. Their second experiment involved 27 inmates at Sing Sing, 13 controls and 14 treated. Red cells were given intravenously. However, the warden of Sing Sing would not allow the investigators to return on any fixed schedule that would enable the prisoners to know the time and day of their revisit. He was concerned that this exact foreknowledge could involve the prisoners in an escape plan. The investigators gladly accepted this limitation as they reasoned that pregnant women who delivered over a weekend would probably not receive RhIG until Monday, up to 72 hours after delivery, owing to the closure of blood banks on weekends, as was commonly practiced at the time. None of the men who received RhIG were alloimmunized, whereas 8 of 13 controls developed anti-RhD antibodies. After two additional experiments at Sing Sing in this second group of individuals, Freda and Gorman[41] went on to conduct a clinical trial in postpartum women at Columbia Presbyterian Medical Center starting in March of 1964. Of the 100 patients that received RhIG, none became sensitized, as compared with a rate of 12% sensitization to RhD in the control group. In a follow-up study in these patients in their next pregnancy, none of the treated patients developed antibodies; 5 of 10 controls were alloimmunized and delivered infants affected by HDFN.

A parallel track of investigation was being undertaken by a group of British researchers in Liverpool. This group reasoned that the natural protective effect of ABO incompatibility between a mother and her fetus in preventing the formation of anti-D antibody could be used as a preventative strategy. A preparation of plasma that contained anti-D IgM was formulated and was administered intravenously to male volunteers.[42] Although initial short-term antibody studies were promising, eventually 8 of 13 treated men became immunized to RhD, compared with only 1 of 11 controls. After the publication of the initial work of Freda and colleagues[43] describing the use of a gamma globulin fraction of the plasma, the British group visited the New York investigators and obtained a sample of their gamma globulin preparation. The Liverpool group[44] began their clinical trial in postpartum women with evidence of FMH by Kleihauer-Betke (KB) stain in April 1964, and they were subsequently credited with the first publication of a successful clinical trial in women.

An observational trial in Canada was initiated and determined that the baseline rate of antenatal sensitization to RhD was 1.8%.[45] Between 1968 and 1974, a trial of antenatal prophylaxis using injections of 300 µg of RhIG at 28 and 34 weeks' gestation followed. As compared with the previous observational study, none of the women demonstrated the development of anti-D antibodies. In a subsequent investigation that involved RhIG administered only at 28 weeks' gestation, only 0.18% of women became sensitized.

In 1968, RhIG was approved by the Division of Biologics Standards of the National Institutes of Health for general clinical use in the United States as RhoGAM (Ortho-Clinical Diagnostics, Inc.). **Recommendations for use during the immediate postpartum period were set forth by the American College of Obstetricians and Gynecologists (ACOG)[46] in 1970. The Food and Drug Administration (FDA) approved the use of antenatal RhIG in 1981. Routine antenatal prophylaxis at 28 to 29 weeks' gestation was proposed by ACOG later that same year.[47]**

Preparations

Four polyclonal products derived from human plasma are currently available in the United States for the prevention of RhD alloimmunization. Two of the products (RhoGAM [Kedrion Biopharma] and HyperRho S/D [Grifols USA]) can only be given intramuscularly because they are derived from human plasma through Cohn cold ethanol fractionation, a process that results in contamination with IgA and other plasma proteins. The remaining two products (WinRho-SDF, [Cangene Corporation] and Rhophlac [CSL Behring]) are prepared through sepharose column and ion-exchange chromatography, respectively. At present, all available products are subject to solvent detergent treatment to inactivate enveloped viruses; many manufacturers also use an additional micropore filtration step to further reduce the chance for viral contamination.

Additionally, thimerosal, a mercury preservative used to prevent bacterial and fungal contamination, has been removed from all RhIG products used in the United States.

The dwindling resource of plasma donors for RhIG manufacture has led to the search for a synthetic product. Several monoclonal anti-D antibodies and a synthetic polyclonal immune globulin consisting of 25 recombinant anti-D antibodies have been developed but are still being studied in human clinical trials. In the future, one of these products may replace the current polyclonal products derived from human plasma.

Indications

All pregnant patients should undergo determination of blood type and an antibody screen at the first prenatal visit. In the past, all Rh negative patients underwent additional testing to see if they were *Du positive*. This terminology was later changed to classify these patients as *weak Rh positive* individuals. In one series of 500 pregnant patients, this occurred in 1% of whites, 2.6% of blacks, and 2.7% of Hispanics.[48] The recommendation in the past was that these individuals should be considered Rh positive, and RhIG was not indicated.[48] Subsequent research found that the *weak D* individuals can belong to one of two groups; some of these patients have intact D antigens that are expressed in reduced numbers on the surface of the red cells (Fig. 34-3). These individuals are *not* at risk for rhesus alloimmunization. **In others with a weak D phenotype, the individual has inherited a gene that results in a variant expression of the D antigen. In these cases, one or more of the D antigen epitopes are missing, and the patient can become alloimmunized to these missing portions of the D antigen. Severe HDFN has been reported in these cases when a maternal antibody develops to the missing epitope.[49] Although clinical trials have not been undertaken, the current recommendation is that these patients should receive RhIG.**

Confusion can arise depending on when and where the patient undergoes red cell typing. Standards from the American Association of Blood Banks (AABB) recommend that reagents that detect weak D should *not* be used for prenatal typing.[50] This guideline results in all weak D patients being called Rh negative and subsequently receiving antenatal RhIG. Newer monoclonal reagents used in an indirect antiglobulin test that can detect weak D are used at blood donor centers. These reagents are used to be sure that weak D blood is not administered to an Rh-negative recipient, resulting in a potential for alloimmunization. This will result in the same individual, now a blood donor, being called *RhD positive*—very confusing to the patient and to the clinician.

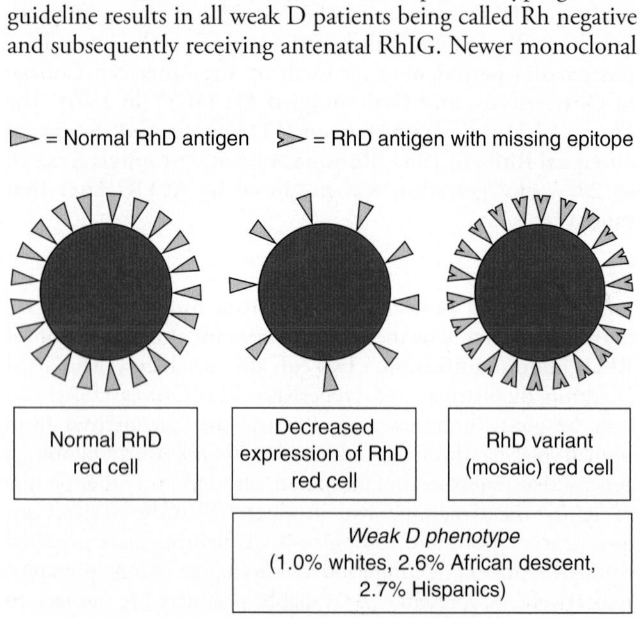

More recently, a work group of the AABB and the College of American Pathologists has suggested that weak D types 1, 2, and 3 can be managed as if they are RhD positive with no need for RhIG.[51] *RHD* genotyping would be required in all pregnant patients to identify this subgroup with weak D. This proposal has not yet been adopted by ACOG.

If there is no evidence of anti-D alloimmunization in the RhD-negative woman, the patient should receive 300 µg of RhIG at 28 weeks of gestation.[48] The 2% background incidence of RhD alloimmunization in the antenatal period can be expected to decline to 0.1%. In the United Kingdom, an antenatal protocol of administering 100 µg (500 IU) of RhIG at 28 and 34 weeks is used in primigravida women.[52] Limited resources have not allowed for extension of this protocol to all subsequent pregnancies. The issue of repeating an antibody screen at 28 weeks before the administration of RhIG is controversial. A recent study of over 2000 women found an incidence of sensitization prior to 28 weeks' gestation to occur in only 0.099% of pregnancies.[53] In addition, the authors of this study did not find the practice to be cost-effective. Although ACOG leaves the decision to repeat the antibody screen up to the obstetric provider, the AABB and the U.S. Preventative Services Task Force recommend that a repeat screen be obtained before antenatal RhIG.[50,54] If a repeat antibody screen is to be undertaken, a maternal blood sample can be drawn at the same office visit as the RhIG injection. Although the administration of the exogenous anti-D will eventually result in a weakly positive titer, this will not occur in the short interval of several hours due to the slow absorption from the intramuscular site.

A new paradigm is developing in antenatal prophylaxis. Early studies in pregnant women carrying a male fetus indicated that 3% of the circulating cell-free fetal DNA (ccffDNA) in the maternal circulation in the first trimester is fetal in origin; this increases to 6% by the third trimester.[55] The source of this DNA appears to be apoptosis of placental villi. Fetal DNA is rapidly cleared from the maternal circulation with a mean half-life of 16 minutes after cesarean delivery; after vaginal delivery, fetal free DNA is cleared by 100 hours.[56,57] The presence of fetal *RHD* DNA sequences in the maternal circulation was first reported by Lo and colleagues.[13] Clinical assays for the determination of the fetal RhD status were subsequently developed. Approximately 40% of Rh-negative pregnant women will carry an Rh-negative fetus; thus rhesus immune globulin would not be indicated in the antepartum period if this can be accurately determined.

Screening of RhD-negative pregnant patients to determine whether antepartum RhIG should be undertaken is routinely now practiced in Denmark and the Netherlands as well as in regions of Sweden, France, and England.[58] In some of these situations, ccffDNA screening was implemented as part of a new antepartum prophylaxis program because of the limited availability of RhIG. However, in the United States, plasma collected from sensitized male volunteer donors is used to manufacture RhIG. Therefore the availability of RhIG is unrestricted. Others

▷ = Normal RhD antigen   ▷ = RhD antigen with missing epitope

| Normal RhD red cell | Decreased expression of RhD red cell | RhD variant (mosaic) red cell |

Weak D phenotype
(1.0% whites, 2.6% African descent, 2.7% Hispanics)

FIG 34-3 Depiction of a normal RhD-positive red cell as well as red cells noted in individuals with weak D variants.

TABLE 34-1	INDICATIONS FOR RHESUS IMMUNE GLOBULIN	
INDICATION	**LEVEL OF EVIDENCE***	
Spontaneous miscarriage	A	
Elective abortion	A	
Threatened miscarriage	C	
Ectopic pregnancy	A	
Hydatidiform mole	B	
Genetic amniocentesis	A	
Chorion villus biopsy	A	
Fetal blood sampling	A	
Placenta previa with bleeding	C	
Suspected abruption	C	
Intrauterine fetal demise	C	
Blunt trauma to the abdomen	C	
At 28 weeks' gestation unless father of fetus is RhD negative	A	
Amniocentesis for fetal lung maturity	A	
External cephalic version	C	
Within 72 hours of delivery of an RhD-positive infant	A	
After administration of RhD-positive blood component	C	

Modified from Prevention of RhD alloimmunization. American College of Obstetricians and Gynecologists Practice Bulletin 1999;4.
*A = high, B = moderate, C = low.

have argued that the potential for infection with prions and other viruses supports an ethical approach to limiting antenatal RhIG to only those patients who need it.[59] A cost-neutral strategy would appear to be the optimal approach to the implementation of ccffDNA. Several studies have determined that the break-even costs of ccffDNA testing would range from $29 to $119 for the saved doses of RhIG to offset the costs of evaluating all RhD-negative pregnant women.[60,61] In addition, even at an accuracy of 99%, as many 3000 patients in the United States would be misdiagnosed with an RhD-negative fetus, when the fetus is actually RhD positive. These cases would result in missed opportunities for the prevention of antenatal alloimmunization and an estimated 21 new cases of Rh alloimmunization annually. Continuation of the practice of obtaining cord serology at birth would allow these "misses" to be correctly diagnosed at the time of delivery when postpartum RhIG is indicated. Currently, the use of ccffDNA to guide antenatal RhIG use is not a guideline from any major U.S. organization, although this may change in the near future.

Although not well studied, level A scientific evidence has been cited by ACOG to address additional indications for the antepartum administration of RhIG.[48] **These include spontaneous miscarriage, elective abortion, ectopic pregnancy, genetic amniocentesis, chorionic villus sampling, and FBS** (Table 34-1). A dose of 50 μg of RhIG is effective until 13 weeks' gestation owing to the small volume of red cells in the fetoplacental circulation. However, most hospitals and offices do not stock this dose of RhIG because the cost is equivalent to that of the standard dose of 300 μg.

The use of RhIG in other scenarios that involve the possibility of FMH are lacking. However, most experts agree that such events as hydatidiform mole, threatened miscarriage, fetal death in the second or third trimester, blunt trauma to the abdomen, and external cephalic version warrant strong consideration for the use of RhIG.[48]

The practice of evaluating a persistent maternal anti-D titer as an indication that additional RhIG is not required after an antenatal event is to be discouraged. Although the precise mechanism for the protective effect of RhIG is unknown, an excess amount of exogenous antibody in relation to the volume of RhD-positive red cells in the maternal circulation is essential for effective prophylaxis. Both animal and human studies have demonstrated that a low level of RhIG can actually enhance the chance for alloimmunization.[18] In the words of Vincent Freda, "The rule of thumb should be to administer Rh immune globulin when in doubt, rather than to withhold it."

Because the half-life of RhIG is approximately 16 days, 15% to 20% of patients receiving it at 28 weeks' gestation have a very low anti-D titer (usually 2 or 4) at the time of admission for labor at term.[62] In North America, the current recommendation is to administer 300 μg of RhIG within 72 hours of delivery if umbilical cord blood typing reveals an RhD-positive infant.[50] This is sufficient for protection from sensitization due to an FMH of 30 mL of fetal whole blood. In the United Kingdom, 100 μg is given at delivery. Approximately 1 in 1000 deliveries will be associated with an excessive FMH; risk factors identify only 50% of these cases.[63] **Both ACOG and AABB now recommend routine screening of all women at the time of delivery for excessive FMH.** A qualitative yet sensitive test for FMH, the *rosette test*, is first performed. Results return as positive or negative; a negative result warrants administration of a standard 300 μg dose of RhIG. If the rosette is positive, a KB stain or fetal cell stain using flow cytometry is undertaken to quantitate the amount of the FMH. The AABB then recommends that the percentage of fetal blood cells be multiplied by a factor of 50 (to account for an estimated maternal blood volume of 5000 mL) to calculate the volume of the FMH. This volume is divided by 30 to determine the number of vials of RhIG to be administered. A decimal point is rounded up or down for values greater than 0.5 or less than 0.5, respectively. Because this calculation includes an inaccurate estimation of the maternal blood volume, one additional vial of RhIG is added to the calculation. As an example, a 3% KB stain is calculated to indicate a 150-mL FMH. Dividing this number by 30 yields five vials of RhIG with one additional vial added; therefore the blood bank would prescribe 6 vials of RhIG (a total of 1800 μg) for this patient. However, a recent survey by the American College of Pathologists of its member blood banks noted that even following these guidelines, an inadequate dose of RhIG was recommended in 9% of cases and an excessive dose was recommended in 12% of cases.[64]

No more than 5 mL RhIG should be administered by the intramuscular route in one 24-hour period. Should a large dose of RhIG be necessary, an alternative method would be to give the calculated dose using one of the intravenous (IV) preparations of RhIG now available. Doses of up to 600 μg (3000 IU) can be administered every 8 hours until the total dose has been achieved. **Should RhIG be inadvertently omitted after delivery, some protection has been proven with administration within 13 days; recommendations have been made to administer it as late as 28 days after delivery.**[63] If delivery is planned within 48 hours of amniocentesis for fetal lung maturity, RhIG can be deferred until after delivery. **If delivery occurs less than 3 weeks from the administration of RhIG used for antenatal indications such as external cephalic version, a repeat dose is unnecessary unless a large FMH is detected at the time of delivery.**[50]

Failed prophylaxis after the appropriate dose of RhIG is administered is rare. However, once postpartum administration is undertaken, the anti-D antibody screen may remain positive for up to 6 months. Anti-D that persists after this time is likely to be the result of sensitization.

Administration of RhIG after a postpartum tubal ligation is controversial. The possibility of a new partner in conjunction with the availability of in vitro fertilization would seem to make the use of RhIG in these situations prudent. In some cases, RhD-negative red cells may be in short supply if the patient presents after major trauma such as a motor vehicle accident with the need for massive transfusion. In these cases, RhD-positive blood could not be used as a life-saving alternative if the patient is alloimmunized to RhD through her previous delivery. RhIG is not effective once alloimmunization to the RhD antigen has occurred. At present, prophylactic immune globulin preparations to prevent other forms of red cell alloimmunization such as anti-K1 do not exist.

Diagnostic Methods

Maternal Antibody Determination

Once a maternal antibody screen reveals the presence of an anti-D antibody, a titer is the first step in the evaluation of the RhD-sensitized patient during the first affected pregnancy. Previous titer methodologies using albumin or saline should no longer be used because they detect varying levels of IgM antibody. The pentamer structure of this class of antibody does not allow for transplacental passage; therefore, the contribution of IgM to the titer quantitation has no clinical relevance. **The human antiglobulin titer** (indirect Coombs test) **is used to determine the degree of alloimmunization because it measures the maternal IgG response.** Most titer values in the obstetric literature are reported as dilutions (e.g., 1:32). By blood-banking convention, however, titer values should be reported as the reciprocal of the last tube dilution that demonstrates a positive agglutination reaction, that is, a final dilution of 1:16 is equivalent to a titer of 16.

Variation in results between laboratories is not uncommon because many commercial laboratories use enzymatic treatment of red cells to prevent failed detection of low titer samples. This method causes a marked elevation in titer as compared with the use of nonenzymatic treated cells. Because standard tube methodology uses red cell agglutination as the indicator reaction, subjective interpretation of end points by the laboratory technologist accounts for the variation in results. In addition, inherent subtle differences in the indicator red cell preparations may play a role because their shelf life is only 1 month, and serial titers may require the use of different reagent lots. For these reasons, serial titers should be run in tandem using stored sera from the previous draw.

In the same laboratory, the titer should not vary by more than one dilution if the two samples are run in tandem. Thus an initial titer of 8 that returns at 16 does not represent a true increase in the amount of antibody in the maternal circulation. In addition, the clinician should be aware that newer gel microcolumn assays will result in higher titers than conventional tube testing. In one study, the mean titer was 3.4-fold increased with gel technology.[65] **A critical titer is defined as the anti–red cell titer associated with a significant risk for hydrops fetalis.** When this is present, further fetal surveillance is warranted. This value will vary with institution and methodology; however, **in most centers, a critical titer for anti-D between 8 and 32 is usually used.**

In the United Kingdom, quantitation of anti-D is undertaken through the use of an automated technique using a device known as the *AutoAnalyzer*. Red cell samples are mixed with agents to enhance agglutination by the anti-D antibodies. Agglutinated cells are separated from nonagglutinated cells and are then lysed. The amount of released hemoglobin is then compared with an international standard; results are reported as international units per milliliter. Levels of less than 4 IU/mL are rarely associated with HDFN; a maternal anti-D level of less than 15 IU/mL has been associated with only mild fetal anemia.[66]

Fetal Blood Typing

Several techniques have been used to determine the fetal blood type if the patient's partner is determined to be heterozygous for the involved red cell antigen. In 50% of cases in which the fetus is found to be antigen negative, further maternal and fetal testing is unnecessary. Historically, initial attempts at fetal testing in these cases used serology on blood obtained by ultrasound-directed cordocentesis. Unfortunately, this technique placed half of the antigen-negative fetuses at a 1% to 2% chance of procedure-related loss (see Chapter 10). Investigators went on to use chorionic villus sampling to obtain genetic material for detection of the *RHD* gene. However, the major disadvantage of this method is that disruption of the chorion villi during the procedure can result in FMH and a rise in maternal titer, thereby worsening the fetal disease.[67] Therefore this procedure should be discouraged unless the patient plans to terminate all antigen-positive fetuses detected. In 1990, amniocentesis was described as a reliable method for assessing the fetal blood type through DNA testing.[11] **This method has now been replaced in almost all countries, including the United States, by the use of fetal *RHD* determination using ccffDNA.** In addition, the test can be performed with reliable results at as early as 10 weeks' gestation.[68]

The initial step in determining the fetal RhD type involves an assessment of paternity and paternal zygosity. Once undertaken using serologic testing and population statistics, molecular techniques can now be used to accurately determine the paternal genotype at the *RHD* locus.[69] However, some authorities have argued that issues with paternity can be averted by omitting this step and testing every pregnancy with ccffDNA for fetal *RHD* determination.

In a recent series of more than 1000 patients, ccffDNA testing for *RHD* was found to be accurate in 99% of cases.[70] An *RHD* positive result on free DNA testing can be considered reliable because *RHD* positive genetic material cannot be from a maternal source. An RhD-negative result with ccffDNA is more problematic. If fetal DNA fails to amplify in a background of overwhelming maternal DNA in the plasma, an *RHD* negative result will be obtained. One internal control that can be used is the detection of the *SRY* gene found in male fetuses. The presence of this gene in free DNA indicates that fetal DNA is present, and an *RHD* negative result is reliable.[62] In the case of a female fetus, the presence of single nucleotide polymorphisms (SNPs) not found in the maternal white cells can be used as an internal control.[71] If different polymorphisms than those found in the mother are noted in the plasma sample, these are of paternal origin; thus fetal DNA is present. In this situation, the finding of an *RHD* negative fetus can be considered reliable. **In the cases with an inconclusive result, a repeat maternal**

sample can be submitted or amniocentesis can be undertaken to determine the fetal *RHD* status.

Amniocentesis to Follow the Severity of Hemolytic Disease of the Fetus and Newborn

Historically, amniocentesis was routinely used in the alloimmunized pregnancy to measure the amount of bilirubin (ΔOD_{450}) as an indirect indication of the degree of fetal hemolysis. Results were plotted on specialized curves first introduced by William Liley[7] and later modified by John Queenan.[72] **The advent of noninvasive testing for fetal anemia with middle cerebral artery MCA Doppler (see below) has now replaced serial amniocenteses for ΔOD_{450}.**

Fetal Blood Sampling

Ultrasound-directed FBS—also known as *percutaneous umbilical blood sampling, cordocentesis,* and *funipuncture*—allows direct access to the fetal circulation to obtain important laboratory values such as fetal blood type, hematocrit, direct Coombs test, reticulocyte count, and total bilirubin. Although serial FBS was once proposed as a primary method of fetal surveillance after a maternal critical titer is reached, it has been associated with a 1% to 2% rate of fetal loss and up to a 50% risk for FMH with subsequent worsening of the alloimmunization.[73] For these reasons, **FBS is reserved for patients with elevated peak systolic MCA Doppler velocities.**

Ultrasound

Perhaps the greatest advance in the management of the alloimmunized pregnancy has been the use of ultrasound. Gestational age can be accurately established to evaluate fetal parameters that vary with gestational age such as the peak systolic MCA Doppler velocities. *Hydrops fetalis* is defined as the presence of extracellular fluid in at least two fetal compartments. Often, ascites is the first sign of impending hydrops, with scalp edema and pleural effusions noted with worsening anemia. **When hydrops is present, fetal hemoglobin deficits of 7 to 10 g/dL from the mean hemoglobin value for the corresponding gestational age can be expected.**[74] Unfortunately, this represents the end-stage state of fetal anemia. Survival with intrauterine transfusion (IUT) is markedly reduced in these cases. In addition, **the early second-trimester fetus can be severely anemic without signs of hydrops.**[75] Therefore many investigators have sought alternative ultrasound parameters that could predict the early onset of anemia. In one large series, fetal abdominal circumference (AC), head/abdomen circumference (HC/AC) ratio, intraperitoneal volume, intrahepatic and extrahepatic umbilical venous diameter, and placental thickness failed to accurately predict a fetal hemoglobin deficit of greater than 5 g/dL from the mean.[76] Because the fetal liver and spleen represent sites of extramedullary hematopoiesis and the destruction and sequestration of sensitized red cells in cases of severe HDFN, enlargement of these organs has been evaluated. Both splenic perimeter and hepatic length correlate with the degree of fetal anemia. However, neither has gained widespread acceptance for noninvasive fetal surveillance in red cell alloimmunization.

The severely anemic fetus exhibits an increased cardiac output in an effort to enhance oxygen delivery to peripheral tissues.[26] In addition, fetal anemia is associated with a lower blood viscosity that produces fewer shearing forces in blood vessels; this results in increased blood velocities. Using these principles, **Doppler ultrasound has been used to study the**

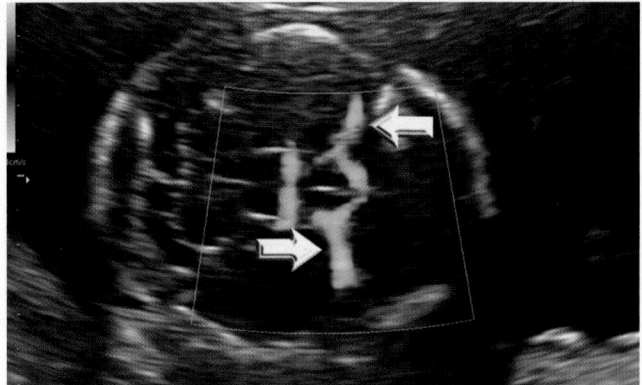

FIG 34-4 Power Doppler image of the fetal circle of Willis. *Arrows* point to locations where the pulsed Doppler gate should be placed for obtaining the fetal peak middle cerebral artery Doppler velocity.

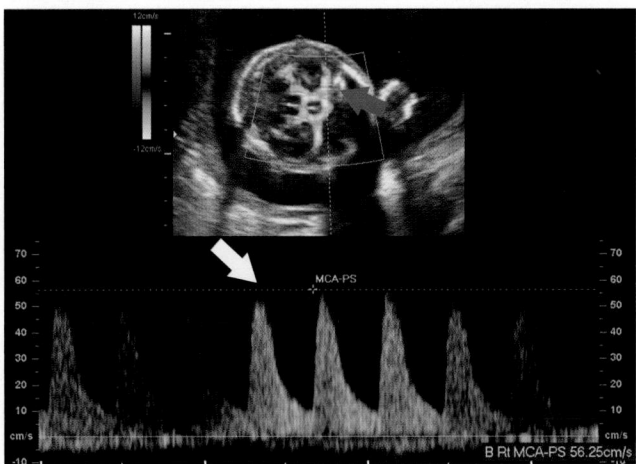

FIG 34-5 Pulsed Doppler of the peak systolic velocity. The *blue arrow* at the top of figure indicates the location of the pulsed Doppler gate; the *white arrow* indicates the measurement using on-board software of a peak velocity of 56.25 cm/sec.

peak systolic velocity (PSV) in the fetal MCA to predict fetal anemia. A value of greater than 1.5 multiples of the median (MoM) for the corresponding gestational age predicts moderate to severe fetal anemia with a sensitivity of 88% and a negative predictive rate of 89%.[12]

Serial MCA Doppler studies are now the mainstay of surveillance for fetal anemia in the red cell alloimmunized pregnancy. Careful attention to technique is paramount in using this method of surveillance. Because the anteroposterior axis of the fetal head typically lies in a transverse plane, the examiner can use either fetal MCA vessel for interrogation. First, the anterior wing of the sphenoid bone at the base of the skull is located. Color or power Doppler is then used to locate the MCA (Fig. 34-4). The angle of insonation is maintained as close to zero as possible by positioning the ultrasound transducer on the maternal abdomen (Figs. 34-5 and 34-6). The MCA vessel closer to the maternal abdominal wall is usually studied, although the posterior vessel will give equivalent results.[77] Angle-correction software is not typically used, although studies have demonstrated that its use can still result in an accurate determination of the MCA velocity.[78] The Doppler gate is then placed in the proximal MCA where the vessel arises from the carotid siphon. Measurements in the more distal aspect of the vessel will be

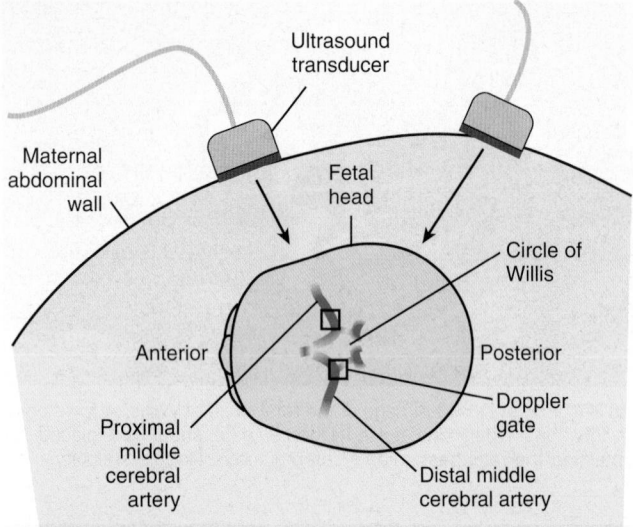

FIG 34-6 Correct determination of the fetal peak middle cerebral artery Doppler velocity.

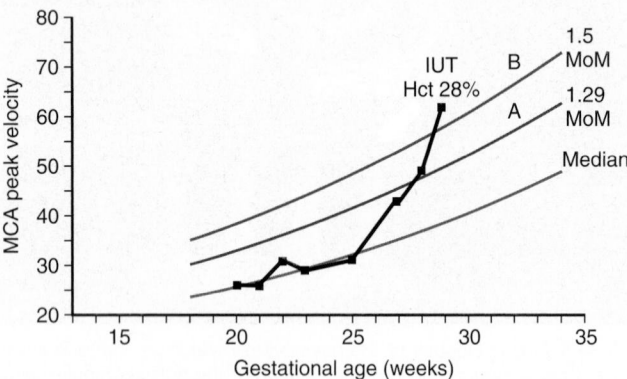

FIG 34-7 Serial middle cerebral artery (MCA) Doppler studies in one patient who required intrauterine transfusion (IUT). Hct, hematocrit; MoM, multiples of the median.

inaccurate because reduced peak velocities will be obtained. The fetus should be in a quiescent state during the Doppler examination because accelerations of the fetal heart rate can result in a decrease in the PSV, especially late in the third trimester.[79] Several authorities have reported transient decreases in the peak MCA velocity after the administration of antenatal steroids to enhance fetal lung maturity. This effect usually lasts for 24 to 48 hours after the last dose.

MCA measurements can be obtained reliably as early as 18 weeks' gestation. Studies are repeated every 1 to 2 weeks depending on the trend (Fig. 34-7). Values should be converted to MoM using Internet-based calculators (e.g., www.perinatology.com).

CLINICAL MANAGEMENT

The approach using the available diagnostic tools is based on the patient's history of fetal or neonatal manifestations of HDFN. **As a general rule, the patient's first RhD-sensitized pregnancy involves minimal fetal/neonatal disease; but subsequent gestations are associated with worsening degrees of anemia.**

First Affected Pregnancy

Once sensitization to the RhD antigen is detected, maternal titers are repeated every month until approximately 24 weeks; titers are repeated every 2 weeks thereafter (Fig. 34-8). If paternity is assured, blood is drawn from the patient's partner to determine his *RHD* status and zygosity (DNA testing). Once a critical maternal titer is reached (usually 32), serial MCA Doppler studies are initiated at approximately 24 weeks' gestation. These are then repeated every 1 to 2 weeks depending on their trend. In cases of a heterozygous paternal phenotype or questionable paternity, ccffDNA testing should be sent to a DNA reference laboratory to determine the fetal RhD status. In the case of an RhD-negative paternal blood type or a fetal *RHD* negative genotype, further maternal and fetal monitoring is unwarranted as long as paternity is assured.

If presence of an *RHD* positive fetus is evident (homozygous paternal phenotype or *RHD* positive fetus by DNA testing), serial fetal surveillance is indicated. If an MCA Doppler returns at greater than 1.5 MoM, cordocentesis should be undertaken at an experienced referral center, with blood readied for IUT if the fetal hematocrit is less than 30%.

Previously Affected Fetus or Infant

If the patient has a history of a previous perinatal loss related to HDFN, a previous need for IUT, or a previous need for neonatal exchange transfusion, she should be referred to a tertiary care center with experience in the management of the severely alloimmunized pregnancy. In these cases, maternal titers are *not* predictive of the degree of fetal anemia. In the case of a heterozygous paternal phenotype or questionable paternity, ccffDNA analysis to determine the fetal *RHD* status is indicated. **Amniocentesis can be used after 15 weeks' gestation to determine the status of the fetal red cell antigen in cases of other maternal antibodies such as anti-Kell.** Serial MCA Doppler measurements should begin at 18 weeks' gestation and should be repeated every 1 to 2 weeks.

INTRAUTERINE TRANSFUSION
Technique

IUTs today are performed under continuous ultrasound guidance with direct infusions of red blood cells into the umbilical cord vessels or into the intrahepatic portion of the umbilical vein of the fetus.[80] Some centers continue to use the intraperitoneal approach as part of a combined technique with an intravascular transfusion (IVT) in an effort to create a reservoir of red cells between procedures.[81]

Typically, a freshly donated, cytomegalovirus (CMV)-negative unit of type O, RhD-negative red blood cells is cross-matched to a maternal blood sample. Extended cross-matching to the mother can decrease the chance of new antibody formation. The unit is leukoreduced and irradiated with 25 Gy to prevent graft-versus-host reaction. It is then washed and packed to a final hematocrit of approximately 75% to 80% to prevent volume overload in the fetus.

The patient is admitted to the labor and delivery unit as an outpatient. The procedure is typically performed in the operating room, especially when a viable gestational age has been reached should an emergency delivery be necessary. The skin is prepped with hexachlorophene, and sterile drapes are applied. A long-acting local anesthetic is administered, and conscious sedation may help alleviate the patient's anxiety. A 20-gauge

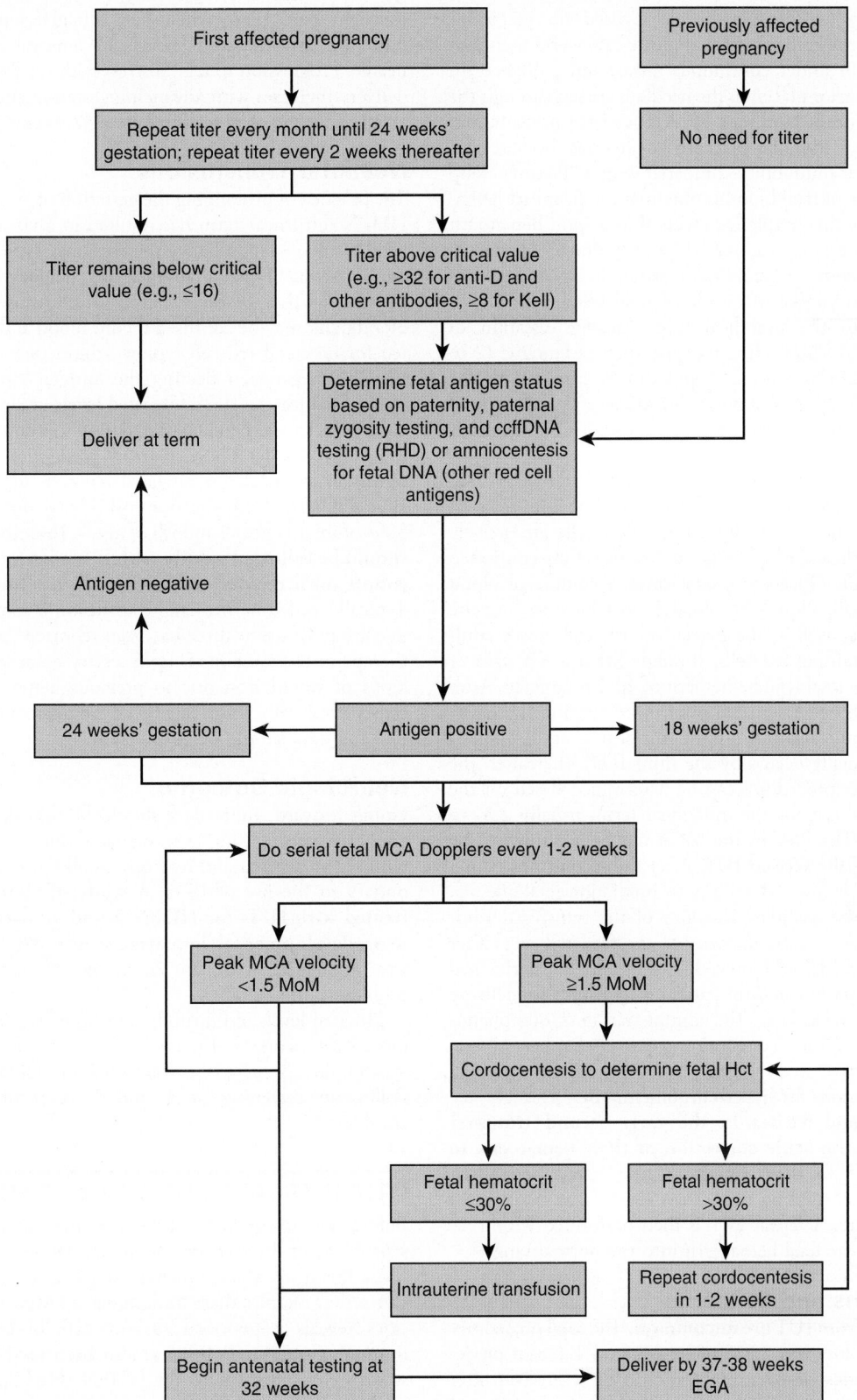

FIG 34-8 Algorithm for clinical management of a patient with red cell alloimmunization. EGA, estimated gestational age; Hct, hematocrit; MCA, middle cerebral artery; MoM, multiples of the median.

procedure needle (a 22-gauge needle is used for gestations <22 weeks) is introduced into the amniotic cavity and then into the umbilical vein under continuous ultrasound guidance. In the case of an anterior placenta, the needle is passed through the placental mass into the cord root. With a posterior placentation, the cord insertion into the placenta is preferred because this represents a site of immobility compared with a "floating" loop of cord. A sample of fetal blood is obtained for an initial hematocrit. Optimally, the sample is processed as a spun hematocrit or through the use of an automated hemocytometer located in the operating room. A short-term paralytic agent such as vecuronium (0.01 mg/kg of estimated fetal weight [EFW]) is administered into the umbilical vein, causing cessation of fetal movement. A short-acting narcotic such as fentanyl (2 to 3 µg/kg EFW) can also be used and can be mixed with the vecuronium.[82] Paralysis is almost immediate and lasts 2 to 3 hours. The amount of packed red blood cells to be infused is based on the EFW determined by ultrasound. Using a donor unit hematocrit of 78%, a factor of 0.02 multiplied by the EFW in grams will calculate the dose of red cells to be administered to raise the fetal hematocrit by 10%.[83] Red cells are actively infused through the use of a syringe and sterile tubing connected to the donor unit. Once the predetermined volume of blood is infused, a small aliquot of blood is obtained to measure the hematocrit, as well as the percentage of fetal versus adult hemoglobin-containing red cells, through either a KB stain or flow cytometry. A final fetal hematocrit of 40% is targeted. After the first IUT, subsequent procedures can be empirically scheduled at 14-day intervals until suppression of fetal erythropoiesis is noted. This usually occurs by the third IUT. Thereafter, the interval for repeat procedures can be determined based on the decline in hematocrit for the individual fetus, usually a 3- to 4-week interval. **The PSV in the MCA has been shown to be useful in timing the second IUT.** After the second procedure, the MCA Doppler loses its validity in predicting fetal anemia, perhaps due to the changing rheology of the transfused adult red cells that make up the majority of the fetal red mass after serial IUTs.[84] The final IUT procedure is usually not performed past 35 weeks' gestation, and the patient is scheduled for delivery approximately 3 weeks later. The administration of oral phenobarbital (30 mg tid) for 10 days prior to delivery has been shown in one retrospective study to decrease the need for neonatal exchange transfusions for hyperbilirubinemia by 75%.[85]

Severely anemic fetuses in the early second trimester do not tolerate the acute correction of their hematocrit to normal values.[86] In these situations, the initial hematocrit should not be increased by more than fourfold at the time of the first procedure. A repeat IVT is then performed within 48 hours to correct the fetal hematocrit into the normal range.[87]

Complications and Outcome

Complications from IUT are uncommon. The total procedure-related perinatal loss was 3.8% of fetuses and 1.2% of procedures in one series of over 300 procedures.[88] Survival after IUT varies with the center, its experience, and the presence of hydrops fetalis. **An overall survival rate of 91% has been reported in one series of over 1400 procedures.**[89] The presence of fetal hydrops, particularly if this does not resolve after several IUTs, has been associated with a lower rate of perinatal survival.[90] Preterm premature rupture of the membranes (PPROM) and chorioamnionitis occur rarely. Fetal bradycardia is usually

transient, particularly when there is inadvertent puncture of the umbilical artery, and responds to removal of the procedure needle. Progression to fetal distress with the need for emergency delivery increases with advancing gestation and may complicate as many as 5% of procedures after 32 weeks' gestation.[91]

Neonatal Transfusions

The practice of prolonging the gestation of the treated fetus with HDFN until near term has resulted in a virtual absence of the need for neonatal exchange transfusions. Typically, these infants are born with a virtual absence of reticulocytes with a red cell population that consists mainly of transfused red cells. The blood bank may be confused if cord blood at delivery is submitted for neonatal red cell typing—the neonate will be typed as O, RhD-negative, reflecting the antigen status of the donor blood used for the IUTs. Elevated levels of circulating maternal antibodies in the neonatal circulation in conjunction with suppression of the fetal bone marrow production of red cells often results in the need for neonatal red cell "top-up" transfusions after discharge from the nursery; this occurs in approximately 50% of infants near 1 month of age.[92] **Therefore these children should be followed weekly with hematocrits and reticulocyte counts until recovery of hematopoietic function is evident.** Typically, only one neonatal transfusion is required, although a maximum of up to three has been reported. Supplemental iron therapy in these infants is unnecessary because they have excess levels of stored iron due to previous hemolysis in utero and lysis of red cells from the IUTs. Supplemental folate therapy (0.5 mg/day) should be considered.

Neurologic Outcome

Going forward, more data should be available to counsel the patient regarding long-term neonatal outcomes because fetuses with severe anemia and hydrops are likely to survive today secondary to the use of IVTs. **A study of almost 300 children treated with IUTs for HDFN found an overall incidence of neurodevelopmental impairment of 4.8%.**[93] Severe hydrops was associated with an elevenfold increase in neurologic problems.

Elevated levels of bilirubin have been associated with hearing loss in the neonate. Therefore, newborn screening for hearing loss would appear to be warranted in children with HDFN. Follow-up screening at 1 and 2 years of age should be considered.

OTHER TREATMENT MODALITIES

Before the advent of the IUT, maternal plasmapheresis represented one of the few therapeutic modalities for severe HDFN. Most literature reports include single cases or relatively small case series. Despite these limitations, a review[94] of the published cases reveals a perinatal survival rate of 69%. Intravenous immune globulin (IVIG) has also been used effectively as the sole antenatal treatment for HDFN. Hydrops fetalis was less likely to occur, and the onset of anemia occurred later in pregnancies treated with IVIG. **Some experts have proposed a combined approach in patients with a previous perinatal loss in the early second trimester when technical limitations make the success of IUT unlikely.**[95] Plasmapheresis is started at 12 weeks' gestation and repeated three times in that week. The maternal titer should be expected to be reduced by 50%.

IVIG is then given to replace the globulin fraction removed by plasmapheresis in the form of a 2 g/kg loading dose after the third plasmapheresis; this is followed by 1 g/kg/week of IVIG until 20 weeks' gestation.

FUTURE THERAPEUTIC OPTIONS

Patients with high anti–red cell titers and recurrent perinatal loss in the second trimester have few options other than artificial insemination with red cell antigen–negative donor semen, surrogate pregnancy, or preimplantation diagnosis (if the father is heterozygous). **Peptides associated with the proliferation of T-helper cells in the development of antibody to the RhD antigen and monoclonal anti-D blocking antibodies are currently being investigated to ameliorate an established anti-D response, thereby preventing severe HDFN in a subsequent pregnancy.**[96,97] Proteasome inhibitors used in in the suppression of antibodies in transplant rejection and in cases of multiple myeloma may prove useful for suppression of RhD alloimmunization prior to pregnancy.[98]

HEMOLYTIC DISEASE OF THE FETUS AND NEWBORN DUE TO NON-RhD ANTIBODIES

Antibodies to the red cell antigens Lewis, I, M, and P are often encountered through antibody screening during prenatal care. Because these antibodies are typically of the IgM class, they are not associated with HDFN.[99]

However, antibodies to more than 50 other red cell antigens have been reported to be associated with HDFN (Table 34-2). **More important, only three antibodies—anti-RhD, anti-Rhc, and anti-Kell (K1)—cause significant enough fetal hemolysis that treatment with IUT is considered necessary.** In one series from a tertiary care center for IUT in the Netherlands, 85% of cases involved anti-D; 10%, anti-K1; and 3.5%, anti-c. In addition, one case each of anti-E, anti-e, and anti-Fy^a was also reported.[100]

Rhc

Anti-c antibody should be considered equivalent to anti-D regarding its potential to cause HDFN. In one report, 25% of

TABLE 34-2 NON-RhD ANTIBODIES AND ASSOCIATED HEMOLYTIC DISEASE OF THE FETUS AND NEWBORN

ANTIGEN SYSTEM	SPECIFIC ANTIGEN	ANTIGEN SYSTEM	SPECIFIC ANTIGEN	ANTIGEN SYSTEM	SPECIFIC ANTIGEN
Frequently Associated With Severe Disease					
Kell	-K (K1)				
Rhesus	-c				
Infrequently Associated With Severe Disease					
Colton	-Co^a	MNS	-Mur	Scianna	-Sc2
	-Co3		-M^V		-Rd
Diego	-ELO		-s	Other Ags	-Bi
	-Di^a		-s^D		-Good
	-Di^b		-S		-
Heibel					
	-Wr^a		-U		-HJK
	-Wr^b		-Vw		-Ht^a
Duffy	-Fy^a	Rhesus	-Be^a		-Jones
Kell	-Js^b		-C		-Joslin
	-k (K2)		-Ce		-Kg
	-Kp^a		-C^w		-Kuhn
	-Kp^b		-ce		-Li^a
	-K11		-E		-MAM
	-K22		-E^w		-
Niemetz					
	-Ku		-Evans		-REIT
	-Ul^a		-G		-Reiter
Kidd	-Jk^a		-Go^a		-Rd
MNS	-En^a		-Hr		-Sharp
	-Far		-Hr$_o$		-Vel
	-Hil		-JAL		-Zd
	-Hut		-Rh32		
	-M		-Rh42		
	-Mi^a		-Rh46		
	-Mt^a		-STEM		
	-MUT		-Tar		
Associated With Mild Disease					
Duffy	-Fy^b	Kidd	-Jk^b	Rhesus	-Riv
	-Fy^3		-Jk^3		-RH29
Gerbich	-Ge^2	MNS	-Mit	Other	-At^a
	-Ge^3	Rhesus	-C^X		-JFV
	-Ge^4		-D^w		-Jr^a
	-Ls^a		-e		-Lan
Kell	-Js^a		-HOFM		
			-LOCR		

From Moise KJ. Hemolytic disease of the fetus and newborn. In Creasy RK, Resnik R, Iams J, eds. *Maternal-Fetal Medicine, Principles and Practice,* ed 5. Philadelphia: Elsevier; 2004.
Ag, antigen; *HDFN,* hemolytic disease of the fetus and newborn.

TABLE 34-3   GENE FREQUENCIES (%) AND ZYGOSITY (%) FOR OTHER RED CELL ANTIGENS ASSOCIATED WITH HEMOLYTIC DISEASE OF THE NEONATE

	WHITE		BLACK		HISPANIC	
	Antigen + Heterozygous		**Antigen + Heterozygous**		**Antigen + Heterozygous**	
C	70	50	30	32	81	51
c	80	50	96	32	76	51
E	32	29	23	21	41	36
e	97	29	98	21	95	36
K (K1)	9	97.8	2	100		
k (K2)	99.8	8.8	100	2		
M	78	64	70	63		
N	77	65	74	60		
S	55	80	31	90		
s	89	50	97	29		
U	100	—	99	—		
Fy^a	66	26	10	90		
Fy^b	83	41	23	96		
Jk^a	77	36	91	63		
Jk^b	72	32	43	21		

Modified from Moise KJ. Hemolytic disease of the fetus and newborn. In Creasy RK, Resnik R, Iams J, eds. *Maternal-Fetal Medicine: Principles and Practice*, ed 5. Philadelphia: Elsevier; 2004.

antigen-positive fetuses were noted to have severe HDFN, 7% were hydropic, and 17% required IUTs for therapy.[101]

RhC, RhE, and Rhe
RhC, RhE, and Rhe antibodies are often found in low titer in the alloimmunized patient with anti-D. Their presence may be additive to the fetal hemolytic effect of anti-D.[102] When they occur alone, mild HDFN is usually the clinical course. Only a handful of case reports have indicated the need for treatment with IUT with each of these antibodies.[100,103]

Duffy
The Duffy antigen system consists of two antigens, Fy^a and Fy^b. Only anti-Fy^a has been associated with mild HDFN.[104]

Kidd
The Kidd antigen system consists of two antigens, Jk^a and Jk^b. Rare cases of mild HDFN have been reported.

Kell
The Kell antigen system includes 23 different members. Antibodies to at least nine of the Kell antigens have been associated with HDFN. The most common of these is Kell (also designated *K, K1*) and cellano (*k, K2*). Additional antibodies that have been reported to be causative for HDFN include -Penny (*Kp^a, K3*), -Rautenberg (*Kp^b, K4*), -Peltz (*Ku, K5*), -Sutter (*Js^a, K6*), -Matthews (*Js^b, K7*), -Karhula (*Ul^a, K10*) and -K22.[95] Unlike the case of other hemolytic antibodies, fetal anemia due to Kell (anti-K1) sensitization is thought to be secondary to not only hemolysis but also to suppression of fetal erythropoiesis.[105]

The majority of cases of K1 sensitization are secondary to previous maternal blood transfusion, usually as a result of postpartum hemorrhage in a previous pregnancy. Because 92% of individuals are Kell negative, the initial management of the K1-sensitized pregnancy should entail paternal red cell typing and genotype testing. If the paternal typing returns K1-negative (kk) and paternity is assured, no further maternal testing is undertaken. The majority of Kell-positive individuals will be heterozygous (Table 34-3). Amniocentesis can be used to determine the fetal genotype in these cases because ccffDNA for fetal Kell typing is currently only available in Europe. A **lower maternal critical antibody value of 8 has been proposed to begin fetal surveillance.**[106] **Serial MCA Doppler studies have proven effective in detecting fetal anemia.**[107]

KEY POINTS

◆ Alloimmunization to the RhD, Kell (K1), and Rhc red cell antigens is the main cause for severe HDFN.

◆ Despite the widespread use of RhIG, approximately six cases of RhD alloimmunization occur annually per 1000 live births in the United States.

◆ *Hydrops fetalis* is defined as extracellular fluid in two fetal compartments; it represents the end-stage of fetal anemia in HDFN.

◆ The rhesus D, C, c, E, and e antigens are coded by two genes located on the short arm of chromosome 1.

◆ The rule of thumb should be to administer RhIG when in doubt, rather than to withhold it.

◆ A critical maternal antibody titer can be used in the first affected pregnancy to decide when to begin further fetal testing.

◆ The fetal peak systolic MCA Doppler velocity can be used to determine the onset of fetal anemia.

◆ In the case of a heterozygous paternal phenotype for a particular red cell antigen, fetal typing can be undertaken through ccffDNA in maternal plasma for the *RHD* gene; fetal DNA typing for other red cell antigens can be obtained through amniocentesis.

◆ Intravascular fetal intrauterine transfusions are the mainstay of fetal therapy with an overall perinatal survival of greater than 90%.

◆ Except in cases of alloimmunization to Kell antigens, irregular red cell antibodies in pregnancy should be managed in a similar fashion to RhD.

REFERENCES
1. Bowman JM. RhD hemolytic disease of the newborn. *N Engl J Med*. 1998;339(24):1775-1777.

2. Diamond LE, Baty JM. Erythroblastosis fetalis and its association with universal edema of the fetus, icterus gravis neonatorium and anemia of the newborn. *J Pediatr.* 1932;1:269.
3. Levine P, Stetson R. An usual case of intragroup agglutination. *JAMA.* 1939;113:126-127.
4. Landsteiner K, Weiner AS. An agglutinable factor in human blood recognized by immune sera for rhesus blood. *Proc Soc Exper Biol Med.* 1940;43:223.
5. Levine P, Katzin EM, Burham L. Isoimmunization in pregnancy: its possible bearing on etiology of erythroblastosis foetalis. *JAMA.* 1941;116:825-827.
6. Wallerstein H. Treatment of severe erythroblastosis by simultaneous removal and replacement of blood of the newborn infant. *Science.* 1946;103:583-584.
7. Liley AW. Liquor amnii analysis in the management of pregnancy complicated by rhesus sensitization. *Am J Obstet Gynecol.* 1961;82:1359-1370.
8. Liley AW. Intrauterine transfusion of foetus in haemolytic disease. *BMJ.* 1963;2:1107-1109.
9. Rodeck CH, Kemp JR, Holman CA, Whitmore DN, Karnicki J, Austin MA. Direct intravascular fetal blood transfusion by fetoscopy in severe Rhesus isoimmunisation. *Lancet.* 1981;1(8221):625-627.
10. Bang J, Bock JE, Trolle D. Ultrasound-guided fetal intravenous transfusion for severe rhesus haemolytic disease. *Br Med J (Clin Res Ed).* 1982;284(6313):373-374.
11. Bennett PR, Le Van Kim C, Colin Y, et al. Prenatal determination of fetal RhD type by DNA amplification. *N Engl J Med.* 1993;329(9):607-610.
12. Mari G. for the Collaborative Group for Doppler Assessment of the Blood Velocity in Anemic Fetuses. Noninvasive diagnosis by Doppler ultrasonography of fetal anemia due to maternal red-cell alloimmunization. *N Engl J Med.* 2000;342:9-14.
13. Lo YM, Bowell PJ, Selinger M, et al. Prenatal determination of fetal RhD status by analysis of peripheral blood of rhesus negative mothers. *Lancet.* 1993;341(8853):1147-1148.
14. Martin JA, Hamilton BE, Sutton PD, Ventura SJ, Menacker F, Munson ML. Births: final data for 2003. *National Vital Statistics Reports.* 2003;54(2):1-116.
15. Smith HM, Shirey RS, Thoman SK, Jackson JB. Prevalence of clinically significant red blood cell alloantibodies in pregnant women at a large tertiary-care facility. *Immunohematol.* 2013;29(4):127-130.
16. Carapella-de Luca E, Casadei AM, Pascone R, Tardi C, Pacioni C. Maternofetal transfusion during delivery and sensitization of the newborn against the rhesus D-antigen. *Vox Sang.* 1978;34(4):241-243.
17. Pollack W. Rh hemolytic disease of the newborn: its cause and prevention. *Prog Clin Biol Res.* 1981;70:185-302.
18. Pollack W, Gorman JG, Hager HJ, Freda VJ, Tripodi D. Antibody-mediated immune suppression to the Rh factor: animal models suggesting mechanism of action. *Transfusion.* 1968;8(3):134-145.
19. Pollack W, Gorman JG, Freda VJ, Ascari WQ, Allen AE, Baker WJ. Results of clinical trials of RhoGAM in women. *Transfusion.* 1968;8(3):151-153.
20. Pollock JM, Bowman JM. Anti-Rh(D) IgG subclasses and severity of Rh hemolytic disease of the newborn. *Vox Sang.* 1990;59(3):176-179.
21. Kumpel BM. Monoclonal anti-D development programme. *Transpl Immunol.* 2002;10(2–3):199-204.
22. Hilden JO, Gottvall T, Lindblom B. HLA phenotypes and severe Rh(D) immunization. *Tissue Antigens.* 1995;46(4):313-315.
23. Ulm B, Svolba G, Ulm MR, Bernaschek G, Panzer S. Male fetuses are particularly affected by maternal alloimmunization to D antigen. *Transfusion.* 1999;39(2):169-173.
24. Nicolaides KH, Thilaganathan B, Rodeck CH, Mibashan RS. Erythroblastosis and reticulocytosis in anemic fetuses. *Am J Obstet Gynecol.* 1988;159(5):1063-1065.
25. Lestas AN, Bellingham AJ, Nicolaides KH. Red cell glycolytic intermediates in normal, anaemic and transfused human fetuses. *Br J Haematol.* 1989;73(3):387-391.
26. Copel JA, Grannum PA, Green JJ, et al. Fetal cardiac output in the isoimmunized pregnancy: a pulsed Doppler-echocardiographic study of patients undergoing intravascular intrauterine transfusion. *Am J Obstet Gynecol.* 1989;161(2):361-365.
27. Soothill PW, Nicolaides KH, Rodeck CH, Clewell WH, Lindridge J. Relationship of fetal hemoglobin and oxygen content to lactate concentration in Rh isoimmunized pregnancies. *Obstet Gynecol.* 1987;69(2):268-271.
28. Nicolaides KH, Warenski JC, Rodeck CH. The relationship of fetal plasma protein concentration and hemoglobin level to the development of

hydrops in rhesus isoimmunization. *Am J Obstet Gynecol.* 1985;152(3):341-344.
29. Moise KJ Jr, Carpenter RJ Jr, Hesketh DE. Do abnormal Starling forces cause fetal hydrops in red blood cell alloimmunization? *Am J Obstet Gynecol.* 1992;167(4 Pt 1):907-912.
30. Moise AA, Gest AL, Weickmann PH, McMicken HW. Reduction in plasma protein does not affect body water content in fetal sheep. *Pediatr Res.* 1991;29(6):623-626.
31. Berger HM, Lindeman JH, van Zoeren-Grobben D, Houdkamp E, Schrijver J, Kanhai HH. Iron overload, free radical damage, and rhesus haemolytic disease. *Lancet.* 1990;335(8695):933-936.
32. Lewis M, Bowman JM, Pollock J, Lowen B. Absorption of red cells from the peritoneal cavity of an hydropic twin. *Transfusion.* 1973;13(1):37-40.
33. Fischer RA, Race RR. Rh gene frequencies in Britain. *Nature.* 1946;157:48-49.
34. Cherif-Zahar B, Mattei MG, Le Van Kim C, Bailly P, Cartron JP, Colin Y. Localization of the human Rh blood group gene structure to chromosome region 1p34.3-1p36.1 by in situ hybridization. *Hum Genet.* 1991;86(4):398-400.
35. Le Van Kim C, Cherif-Zahar B, Raynal V, et al. Multiple Rh messenger RNA isoforms are produced by alternative splicing. *Blood.* 1992;80(4):1074-1078.
36. Carritt B, Kemp TJ, Poulter M. Evolution of the human RH (rhesus) blood group genes: a 50 year old prediction (partially) fulfilled. *Hum Mol Genet.* 1997;6(6):843-850.
37. Singleton BK, Green CA, Avent ND, et al. The presence of an RHD pseudogene containing a 37 base pair duplication and a nonsense mutation in Africans with the Rh D-negative blood group phenotype. *Blood.* 2000;95(1):12-18.
38. Lee YL, Chiou HL, Hu SN, Wang L. Analysis of RHD genes in Taiwanese RhD-negative donors by the multiplex PCR method. *J Clin Lab Anal.* 2003;17(3):80-84.
39. Dunn LJ. Prevention of isoimmunization in pregnancy developed by Freda and Gorman. *Obstet Gynecol Surv.* 1999;54(suppl 12):S1-S6.
40. Smith T. Active immunity produced by so-called balanced or neutral mixtures of diptheria toxin and anti-toxin. *J Exp Med.* 1909;11:241.
41. Freda VJ, Gorman JG, Pollack W, Robertson JG, Jennings ER, Sullivan JF. Prevention of Rh isoimmunization. Progress report of the clinical trial in mothers. *JAMA.* 1967;199(6):390-394.
42. Finn R, Clarke CA, Donohoe WT, et al. Experimental studies on the prevention of Rh haemolytic disease. *Br Med J.* 1961;5238:1486-1490.
43. Freda VJ, Gorman JG, Pollack W. Successful prevention of experimental Rh sensitization in man with anti-Rh gamma2-globulin antibody: A preliminary report. *Transfusion.* 1964;4:26-32.
44. Clarke CA, Sheppard PM. Prevention of rhesus haemolytic disease. *Lancet.* 1965;19:343.
45. Bowman JM, Chown B, Lewis M, Pollock JM. Rh isoimmunization during pregnancy: antenatal prophylaxis. *Can Med Assoc J.* 1978;118(6):623-627.
46. *Prenatal antibody screening and use of Rho (D) immune globulin (human).* American College of Obstetricians and Gynecologists Technical Bulletin 1970;13.
47. *The selective use of Rho(D) immune globulin (RhIG).* American College of Obstetricians and Gynecologists Technical Bulletin Update 1981;61.
48. *Prevention of RhD alloimmunization.* American College of Obstetricians and Gynecologists Practice Bulletin 1999;4.
49. Cannon M, Pierce R, Taber EB, Schucker J. Fatal hydrops fetalis caused by anti-D in a mother with partial D. *Obstet Gynecol.* 2003;102(5 Pt 2):1143-1145.
50. Levitt J. *Standards for Blood Banks and Transfusion Services.* 29th ed. Bethesda, MD: American Association of Blood Banks; 2014.
51. Sandler SG, Roseff SD, Domen RE, Shaz B, Gottschall JL. Policies and procedures related to testing for weak D phenotypes and administration of Rh immune globulin: results and recommendations related to supplemental questions in the Comprehensive Transfusion Medicine survey of the College of American Pathologists. *Arch Pathol Lab Med.* 2014;138(5):620-625.
52. Urbaniak SJ. Consensus conference on anti-D prophylaxis, April 7 & 8, 1997: final consensus statement. Royal College of Physicians of Edinburgh/Royal College of Obstetricians and Gynaecologists. *Transfusion.* 1998;38(1):97-99.
53. Abbey R, Dunsmoor-Su R. Cost-benefit analysis of indirect antiglobulin screening in rh(d)-negative women at 28 weeks of gestation. *Obstet Gynecol.* 2014;123(5):938-945.

54. U.S. Preventive Service Task Force. Recommendation statement: Screening for Rh(D) incompatibility. Rockville. *MD.* 2004.

55. Lo YM, Tein MS, Lau TK, et al. Quantitative analysis of fetal DNA in maternal plasma and serum: implications for noninvasive prenatal diagnosis. *Am J Hum Genet.* 1998;62(4):768-775.

56. Lo YM, Zhang J, Leung TN, Lau TK, Chang AM, Hjelm NM. Rapid clearance of fetal DNA from maternal plasma. *Am J Hum Genet.* 1999;64(1):218-224.

57. Nelson M, Eagle C, Langshaw M, Popp H, Kronenberg H. Genotyping fetal DNA by non-invasive means: extraction from maternal plasma. *Vox Sang.* 2001;80(2):112-116.

58. Moise KJ. Selected use of antenatal Rhesus-immune globulin based on free fetal DNA. *BJOG.* 2015;122(12):1687.

59. Kent J, Farrell AM, Soothill P. Routine administration of Anti-D: the ethical case for offering pregnant women fetal RHD genotyping and a review of policy and practice. *BMC Pregnancy Childbirth.* 2014;14:87.

60. Teitelbaum L, Metcalfe A, Clarke G, Parboosingh JS, Wilson R, Johnson JM. Costs and benefits of non-invasive fetal RhD determination. *Ultrasound Obstet Gynecol.* 2015;45(1):84-88.

61. Hawk AF, Chang EY, Shields SM, Simpson KN. Costs and Clinical Outcomes of Noninvasive Fetal RhD Typing for Targeted Prophylaxis. *Obstet Gynecol.* 2013;122(3):579-585.

62. Goodrick J, Kumpel B, Pamphilon D, et al. Plasma half-lives and bioavailability of human monoclonal Rh D antibodies BRAD-3 and BRAD-5 following intramuscular injection into Rh D-negative volunteers. *Clin Exp Immunol.* 1994;98(1):17-20.

63. Bowman JM. Controversies in Rh prophylaxis. Who needs Rh immune globulin and when should it be given? *Am J Obstet Gynecol.* 1985; 151(3):289-294.

64. Ramsey G. Inaccurate doses of R immune globulin after Rh-incompatible fetomaternal hemorrhage: survey of laboratory practice. *Arch Pathol Lab Med.* 2009;133(3):465-469.

65. Novaretti MC, Jens E, Pagliarini T, Bonifacio SL, Dorlhiac-Llacer PE, Chamone DA. Comparison of conventional tube test with diamed gel microcolumn assay for anti-D titration. *Clin Lab Haematol.* 2003;25(5): 311-315.

66. Nicolaides KH, Rodeck CH. Maternal serum anti-D antibody concentration and assessment of rhesus isoimmunisation. *BMJ.* 1992;304(6835): 1155-1156.

67. Moise KJ Jr, Carpenter RJ Jr. Chorionic villus sampling for Rh typing: clinical implications [letter; comment]. *Am J Obstet Gynecol.* 1993; 168(3 Pt 1):1002-1003.

68. Moise KJ Jr, Boring NH, O'Shaughnessy R, et al. Circulating cell-free fetal DNA for the detection of RHD status and sex using reflex fetal identifiers. *Prenat Diagn.* 2013;33(1):95-101.

69. Pirelli KJ, Pietz BC, Johnson ST, Pinder HL, Bellissimo DB. Molecular determination of RHD zygosity: predicting risk of hemolytic disease of the fetus and newborn related to anti-D. *Prenat Diagn.* 2010;30(12–13): 1207-1212.

70. Chitty LS, Finning K, Wade A, et al. Diagnostic accuracy of routine antenatal determination of fetal RHD status across gestation: population based cohort study. *BMJ.* 2014;349:g5243.

71. Tynan JA, Angkachatchai V, Ehrich M, Paladino T, van den Boom D, Oeth P. Multiplexed analysis of circulating cell-free fetal nucleic acids for noninvasive prenatal diagnostic RHD testing. *Am J Obstet Gynecol.* 2010; 204:251.e1-e6.

72. Queenan JT, Tomai TP, Ural SH, King JC. Deviation in amniotic fluid optical density at a wavelength of 450 nm in Rh-immunized pregnancies from 14 to 40 weeks' gestation: a proposal for clinical management. *Am J Obstet Gynecol.* 1993;168(5):1370-1376.

73. Weiner CP, Williamson RA, Wenstrom KD, et al. Management of fetal hemolytic disease by cordocentesis. II. Outcome of treatment. *Am J Obstet Gynecol.* 1991;165(5 Pt 1):1302-1307.

74. Nicolaides KH, Soothill PW, Clewell WH, Rodeck CH, Mibashan RS, Campbell S. Fetal haemoglobin measurement in the assessment of red cell isoimmunisation. *Lancet.* 1988;1(8594):1073-1075.

75. Yinon Y, Visser J, Kelly EN, et al. Early intrauterine transfusion in severe red blood cell alloimmunization. *Ultrasound Obstet Gynecol.* 2010;36(5): 601-606.

76. Nicolaides KH, Fontanarosa M, Gabbe SG, Rodeck CH. Failure of ultrasonographic parameters to predict the severity of fetal anemia in rhesus isoimmunization. *Am J Obstet Gynecol.* 1988;158(4):920-926.

77. Abel DE, Grambow SC, Brancazio LR, Hertzberg BS. Ultrasound assessment of the fetal middle cerebral artery peak systolic velocity: A comparison of the near-field versus far-field vessel. *Am J Obstet Gynecol.* 2003;189(4):986-989.

78. Ruma MS, Swartz AE, Kim E, Herring AH, Menard MK, Moise KJ Jr. Angle correction can be used to measure peak systolic velocity in the fetal middle cerebral artery. *Am J Obstet Gynecol.* 2009;200(4):397 e1-e3.

79. Swartz AE, Ruma MS, Kim E, Herring AH, Menard MK, Moise KJ Jr. The effect of fetal heart rate on the peak systolic velocity of the fetal middle cerebral artery. *Obstet Gynecol.* 2009;113(6):1225-1229.

80. Nicolini U, Santolaya J, Ojo OE, et al. The fetal intrahepatic umbilical vein as an alternative to cord needling for prenatal diagnosis and therapy. *Prenat Diagn.* 1988;8(9):665-671.

81. Moise KJ Jr, Carpenter RJ Jr, Kirshon B, Deter RL, Sala JD, Cano LE. Comparison of four types of intrauterine transfusion: effect on fetal hematocrit. *Fetal Ther.* 1989;4(2–3):126-137.

82. Moise KJ Jr, Deter RL, Kirshon B, Adam K, Patton DE, Carpenter RJ Jr. Intravenous pancuronium bromide for fetal neuromuscular blockade during intrauterine transfusion for red-cell alloimmunization. *Obstet Gynecol.* 1989;74(6):905-908.

83. Giannina G, Moise KJ Jr, Dorman K. A simple method to estimate the volume for fetal intravascular transfusion. *Fetal Diagn Ther.* 1998;13: 94-97.

84. Scheier M, Hernandez-Andrade E, Fonseca EB, Nicolaides KH. Prediction of severe fetal anemia in red blood cell alloimmunization after previous intrauterine transfusions. *Am J Obstet Gynecol.* 2006;195(6): 1550-1556.

85. Trevett TN Jr, Dorman K, Lamvu G, Moise KJ Jr. Antenatal maternal administration of phenobarbital for the prevention of exchange transfusion in neonates with hemolytic disease of the fetus and newborn. *Am J Obstet Gynecol.* 2005;192(2):478-482.

86. Moise KJ Jr, Mari G, Fisher DJ, Huhta JC, Cano LE, Carpenter RJ Jr. Acute fetal hemodynamic alterations after intrauterine transfusion for treatment of severe red blood cell alloimmunization. *Am J Obstet Gynecol.* 1990;163(3):776-784.

87. Radunovic N, Lockwood CJ, Alvarez M, Plecas D, Chitkara U, Berkowitz RL. The severely anemic and hydropic isoimmune fetus: changes in fetal hematocrit associated with intrauterine death. *Obstet Gynecol.* 1992;79(3): 390-393.

88. Sainio S, Nupponen I, Kuosmanen M, et al. Diagnosis and treatment of severe hemolytic disease of the fetus and newborn: a 10-year nationwide retrospective study. *Acta Obstet Gynecol Scand.* 2015;94(4):383-390.

89. Lindenburg IT, van Kamp IL, van Zwet EW, Middeldorp JM, Klumper FJ, Oepkes D. Increased perinatal loss after intrauterine transfusion for alloimmune anaemia before 20 weeks of gestation. *BJOG.* 2013;120(7): 847-852.

90. van Kamp IL, Klumper FJ, Bakkum RS, et al. The severity of immune fetal hydrops is predictive of fetal outcome after intrauterine treatment. *Am J Obstet Gynecol.* 2001;185(3):668-673.

91. Klumper FJ, van Kamp IL, Vandenbussche FP, et al. Benefits and risks of fetal red-cell transfusion after 32 weeks gestation. *Eur J Obstet Gynecol Reprod Biol.* 2000;92(1):91-96.

92. Saade GR, Moise KJ, Belfort MA, Hesketh DE, Carpenter RJ. Fetal and neonatal hematologic parameters in red cell alloimmunization: predicting the need for late neonatal transfusions. *Fetal Diagn Ther.* 1993;8(3): 161-164.

93. Lindenburg IT, Smits-Wintjens VE, van Klink JM, et al. Long-term neurodevelopmental outcome after intrauterine transfusion for hemolytic disease of the fetus/newborn: the LOTUS study. *Am J Obstet Gynecol.* 2012;206(2):141 e1-e8.

94. Moise KJ, Whitecar PW. Antenatal therapy for haemolytic disease of the fetus and newborn. In: Hadley A, Soothill P, eds. *Alloimmune disorders in pregnancy. Anaemia, thrombocytopenia and neutropenia in the fetus and newborn,* Vol. 1. 1st ed. Cambridge, U.K.: Cambridge University Press; 2002:173-202.

95. Ruma MS, Moise KJ Jr, Kim E, et al. Combined plasmapheresis and intravenous immune globulin for the treatment of severe maternal red cell alloimmunization. *Am J Obstet Gynecol.* 2007;196(2):138 e1-e6.

96. Hall AM, Cairns LS, Altmann DM, Barker RN, Urbaniak SJ. Immune responses and tolerance to the RhD blood group protein in HLA-transgenic mice. *Blood.* 2005;105(5):2175-2179.

97. Nielsen LK, Green TH, Sandlie I, Michaelsen TE, Dziegiel MH. In vitro assessment of recombinant, mutant immunoglobulin G anti-D devoid of hemolytic activity for treatment of ongoing hemolytic disease of the fetus and newborn. *Transfusion.* 2008;48(1):12-19.

98. Kubiczkova L, Pour L, Sedlarikova L, Hajek R, Sevcikova S. Proteasome inhibitors - molecular basis and current perspectives in multiple myeloma. *J Cell Mol Med*. 2014;18(6):947-961.

99. Brecher ME. *Technical Manual of the American Association of Blood Banks*. 15th ed. Bethesda, MD: American Association of Blood Banks; 2005.

100. van Kamp IL, Klumper FJ, Oepkes D, et al. Complications of intrauterine intravascular transfusion for fetal anemia due to maternal red-cell alloimmunization. *Am J Obstet Gynecol*. 2005;192(1):171-177.

101. Hackney DN, Knudtson EJ, Rossi KQ, Krugh D, O'Shaughnessy RW. Management of pregnancies complicated by anti-c isoimmunization. *Obstet Gynecol*. 2004;103(1):24-30.

102. Spong CY, Porter AE, Queenan JT. Management of isoimmunization in the presence of multiple maternal antibodies. *Am J Obstet Gynecol*. 2001;185(2):481-484.

103. Joy SD, Rossi KQ, Krugh D, O'Shaughnessy RW. Management of pregnancies complicated by anti-E alloimmunization. *Obstet Gynecol*. 2005; 105(1):24-28.

104. Hughes L, Rossi K, Krugh D, O'Shaughnessy R. Management of pregnancies complicated by anti-Fya alloimmunization. *Am J Obstet Gynecol*. 2004;191:S164.

105. Vaughan JI, Manning M, Warwick RM, Letsky EA, Murray NA, Roberts IA. Inhibition of erythroid progenitor cells by anti-Kell antibodies in fetal alloimmune anemia. *N Engl J Med*. 1998;338(12):798-803.

106. Bowman JM, Pollock JM, Manning FA, Harman CR, Menticoglou S. Maternal Kell blood group alloimmunization. *Obstet Gynecol*. 1992; 79(2):239-244.

107. van Dongen H, Klumper FJ, Sikkel E, Vandenbussche FP, Oepkes D. Non-invasive tests to predict fetal anemia in Kell-alloimmunized pregnancies. *Ultrasound Obstet Gynecol*. 2005;25(4):341-345.

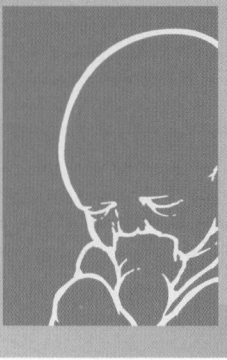

Amniotic Fluid Disorders

WILLIAM M. GILBERT

KEY ABBREVIATIONS

Amniotic fluid	AF
Amniotic fluid index	AFI
Amniotic fluid volume	AFV
Antiphospholipid syndrome	APS
Intrauterine fetal death	IUFD
Intrauterine growth restriction	IUGR
Maximum vertical pocket	MVP
Neonatal intensive care unit	NICU
Odds ratio	OR
Perinatal mortality rate	PMR
Premature rupture of the membranes	PROM
Twin-to-twin transfusion syndrome	TTTS

OVERVIEW

Abnormalities of amniotic fluid volume (AFV) raise the concern for an underlying fetal or maternal complication during pregnancy or fetal/neonatal compromise. The perinatal mortality rate (PMR) approaches 90% to 100% with severe oligohydramnios in the second trimester and can exceed 50% with significant polyhydramnios in midpregnancy.[1-5] Although these two extreme conditions are rare, other less drastic examples are more common and can impact pregnancy outcome. Efforts to study abnormalities of amniotic fluid (AF) are complicated by the fact that despite over 30 years of research in various human and animal models, little is known about the processes involved in normal AFV regulation. Many of the disease states associated with the extremes of AFV are better understood than the physiologic processes that maintain the normal state.

This chapter explores what is known about the normal mechanisms that effect the production and removal of AF, including fetal urination, swallowing, lung liquid, and intramembranous absorption. The normal changes in AFV and composition across

gestation are reviewed, as well as AFV abnormalities that include oligohydramnios and polyhydramnios, along with the possible underlying causes and treatment modalities.

AMNIOTIC FLUID VOLUME

Attempts to measure true AFV are difficult because of obvious limitations. To measure the actual volume of AF, an inert dye must be injected into the amniotic cavity via amniocentesis, and samples of amniotic fluid must be obtained to determine a dilution curve. Although the dye injection technique is considered the gold standard for determining actual AFV and is compared with other methods of estimating AFV, such as ultrasound, it is impractical to utilize an invasive test to assess AFV in clinical practice.

Despite these limitations, Brace and Wolf[6] identified all published measurements of AFV in 12 studies with 705 individual AFV measurements; for each week of gestation, wide variation was seen in AFV (Fig. 35-1). The greatest variation occurred at 32 to 33 weeks of gestation, when the normal range was 400 to 2100 mL (5th to 95th percentile); this represents a wide normal range. One of the most interesting findings of the Brace and Wolf study is that **from 22 through 39 weeks of gestation, the average volume of AF** (black dots on Fig. 35-1) **remained unchanged despite an increase in fetal weight from about 500 g to 3500 g, a sevenfold increase.**[6] Using the dye dilution technique, others found that the normal range was less and the peak AFV occurred at 40 weeks of gestation, instead of 30 to 38 weeks.[7] These studies suggest **the AFV is closely regulated throughout pregnancy.**

Ultrasound Assessment of Amniotic Fluid Volume

Ultrasound has largely replaced clinical assessment of AFV based on the Leopold maneuver or fundal height measurements. However, AF disorders should be suspected when the uterus measures too large or too small for the gestational age. **Polyhydramnios may be present if the maternal uterus is large for gestational age (LGA) or if the fetus cannot be easily palpated**

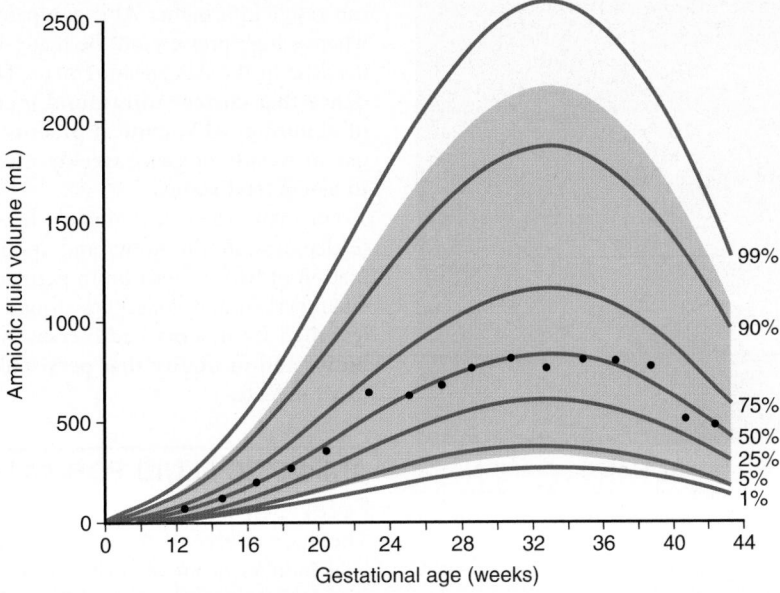

FIG 35-1 Nomogram showing amniotic fluid volume as a function of gestational age. The black dots are the mean for each 2-week interval. Percentiles are calculated from a polynomial regression equation and standard deviation of residuals. (From Brace RA, Wolf EJ. Normal amniotic fluid volume throughout pregnancy. *Am J Obstet Gynecol.* 1989;161:382.)

or is ballotable. The diagnosis of oligohydramnios is a consideration when the fundal height is small for gestational age (SGA) or the fetus is easily palpated.

Early ultrasound estimations of AFV were made by measuring the maximum vertical pocket (MVP) of AF.[8] Chamberlain and colleagues[9] and Mercer and colleagues[10] found that perinatal morbidity and mortality rates were increased with an MVP of less than 1 cm and 0.5 cm, respectively. These lower values of the MVP identified at-risk fetuses, but the low sensitivity for identifying the majority of pregnancy complications associated with oligohydramnios was unacceptable and prompted other investigators to select higher cut-off values.

Subsequently, Phelan and others[11-13] proposed a four quadrant assessment of AF referred to as the *amniotic fluid index* (AFI). After 20 weeks, the uterus is divided into four equal quadrants, as shown in Figure 35-2. The deepest pocket of AF is measured in each quadrant, making sure that the ultrasound transducer is perpendicular to the floor and that fetal body parts and umbilical cord do not interfere with the vertical measurement (Fig. 35-3). The sum of the MVP in each quadrant equals the AFI.[13] Moore and Cayle[13] performed a cross-sectional study of 791 normal pregnancies; the 5th and 95th percentile of the AFI varied for each gestational age. At the 95th percentile, the AFI at 35 to 36 weeks' gestation was 24.9 cm, and it was 19.4 cm at 41 weeks' gestation. The variation in the AFI at the 5th percentile was less than that of the 95th percentile, but it still varied by as much as 2.5 cm. Finally, the investigators reported the interobserver and intraobserver variation to be 3.1% and 6.7%, respectively, which is acceptable for this commonly performed procedure. Comparing the ultrasound estimation of the AFV by the AFI (Fig. 35-4) with the actual measured volume (see Fig. 35-1) demonstrates very similar appearing curves.

Studies that have compared estimates of AFV by ultrasound (MVP and AFI) with actual measurements taken by the dye-dilution technique demonstrate that MVP and AFI

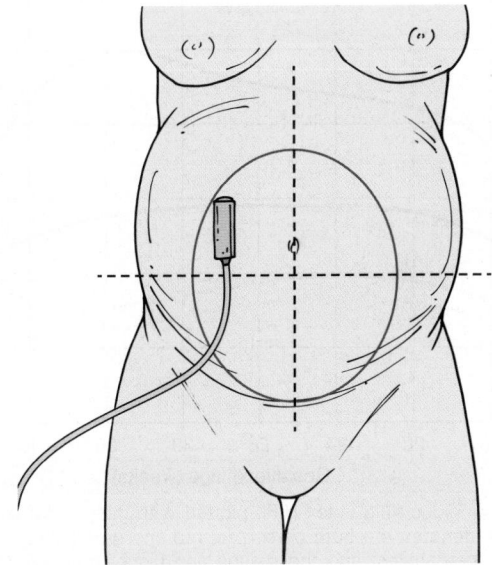

FIG 35-2 Schematic diagram of the technique for measuring the four-quadrant amniotic fluid index.

measurements are poor predictors of actual AFV. Dildy and colleagues[14] found that the AFI overestimated the actual volume in 88% of cases at lower volumes, and it underestimated the actual volume in 54% of cases at higher volumes. However, this difference should not alter clinical practice. Magann and colleagues[15] reported a sensitivity of 10% (specificity 96%) for an AFI measurement of less than 5 cm (oligohydramnios), and the sensitivity was 5% (specificity 98%) for MVP up to 2 cm. For cases of suspected polyhydramnios, an AFI greater than 20 cm had a sensitivity of 29% (specificity 97%), as did an MVP of greater than 8 cm (specificity 94%). The MVP method had fewer false-positive tests compared with the AFI.[15] Based on these findings, the authors concluded that the MVP is superior

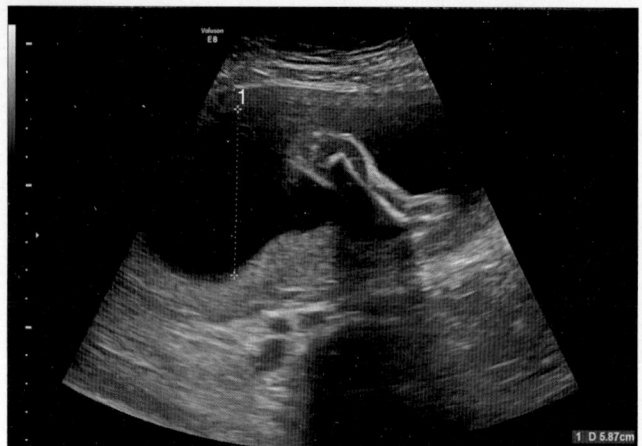

FIG 35-3 Ultrasound image demonstrates measurement of the maximum vertical pocket (MVP) within the uterus by holding the transducer perpendicular to the floor and determining the MVP of amniotic fluid in centimeters.

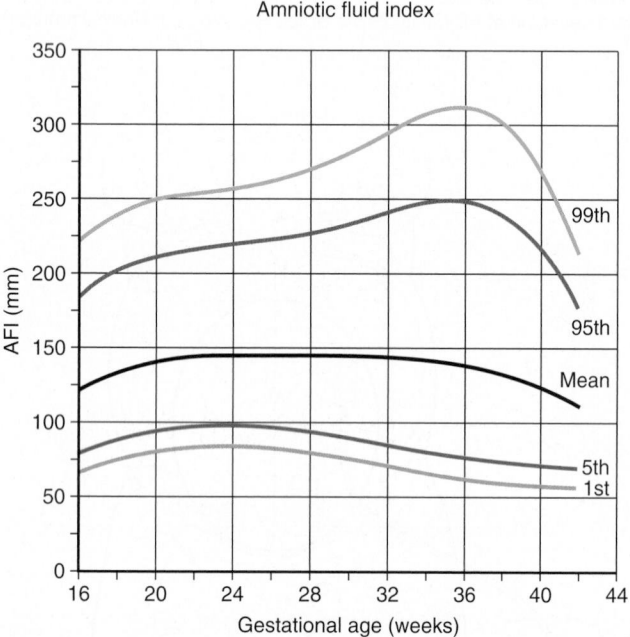

FIG 35-4 Amniotic fluid index (AFI) plotted with gestational age. The black line denotes the 50th percentile; red and green lines, the 5th and 95th percentiles; and the orange and black lines, +2 standard deviations (2.5th and 97.5th percentiles). (From Moore TR, Cayle JE. The amniotic fluid index in normal human pregnancy. *Am J Obstet Gynecol.* 1990;162:1168.)

to the AFI.[16] In contrast, Moore[17] found the AFI superior to the MVP for identifying cases of oligohydramnios but found the two methods similar at predicting polyhydramnios. In a recent review, Moise[18] found that the MVP was superior to the AFI in diagnosing oligohydramnios using an MVP less than 2 cm. **Although the MVP appears to be the preferred method to diagnose oligohydramnios near term, the vast majority of research on ultrasound measurement of AFV utilizes the AFI.**

Differences in ultrasound technique, specifically the pressure of the transducer on the maternal abdomen, can affect the accuracy of the ultrasound measurement of AF. Low pressure can result in a higher AFI, compared with moderate pressure, whereas high pressure on the maternal abdomen can result in a decrease in the AFI measurement. **Despite overwhelming evidence that current ultrasound methods are poor predictors of abnormal AFV, clinical practice continues to include the use of weekly or twice-weekly ultrasound estimates of AFV to assess fetal status.**

For many years, investigators have tried with mixed success to demonstrate the utility and applicability of ultrasound estimation of AFV in relation to perinatal outcome. Early work by Chamberlain and colleagues[9] found that **when the MVP was less than 1 cm, a marked increase was seen in perinatal morbidity and mortality that persisted even after correcting for birth defects.**

AMNIOTIC FLUID FORMATION
Fetal Urine
The main source of AF is fetal urination. In the human, the fetal kidneys begin to make urine before the end of the first trimester, and production of urine increases until term. Many different animal models have been used to study fetal urine production. The fetal sheep provides an excellent model for comparative human study owing to its similar fetal weight at term, its sufficient size to allow catheter placement, and the fact that the sheep fetus has a low risk of premature labor after catheter placement. In the fetal sheep, urine production has been reported to be approximately 200 to 1200 mL/day in the last third of pregnancy.[19-21] Efforts to measure human fetal urine production have been accomplished by ultrasound measurements of the change in fetal bladder volume over time. Wladimiroff and Campbell[22] initially measured three dimensions of the fetal bladder every 15 minutes and reported a human fetal urine production rate of 230 mL/day at 36 weeks of gestation, which increased to 655 mL/day at term. Others found similar volumes using the same technique. Interestingly, using the same technique but measuring the change in volume every 2 to 5 minutes, Rabinowitz and colleagues[23] found fetal urine production to be much greater than previously predicted (1224 mL/day). This was confirmed by three-dimensional (3-D) ultrasound and computer modeling.[24] Fetal urine-production rates from several studies are shown in Figure 35-5.[22,23,25-28] **Human fetal urine-production rate appears to be approximately 1000 to 1200 mL/day at term, which suggests that the entire AFV is replaced more frequently than every 24 hours.**

Lung Liquid
Fetal lung liquid also plays an important role in AF formation. For years, it was presumed that actual movement of AF into the fetal lungs occurred; however, recent data offer no support for this concept.[29,30] In fact, throughout gestation, the fetal lungs produce fluid that exits the trachea and is either swallowed or leaves the mouth and enters the amniotic compartment. In fetal sheep experiments, the lungs have been reported to produce volumes of up to 400 mL/day, with 50% being swallowed and 50% exiting via the mouth.[31-35] Although we do not have direct measurements in humans, the presence of surfactant in the AF near term provides evidence for the outward flow of lung liquid. During normal fetal life, fetal breathing movements provide a "to-and-fro" movement of AF into and out of the trachea, upper lungs, and mouth with a net outward movement of fetal lung liquid into the AF.[36]

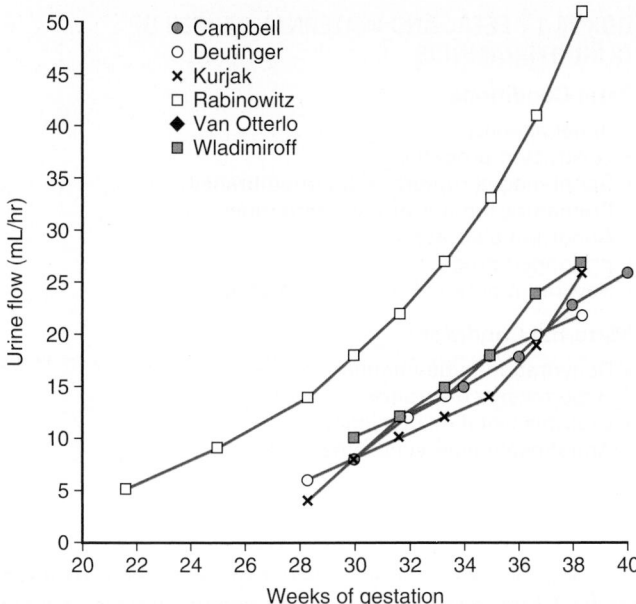

FIG 35-5 Normal changes in fetal urine flow rates across gestation. Lines represent mean values for six studies in the literature,[35-40] whose first authors are shown. The highest line is data from Rabinowitz and colleagues and represents bladder volume measurements every 5 minutes, instead of every 15 minutes, as is the case for the other five studies. (Studies referenced from Gilbert WM, Brace RA: Amniotic fluid volume and normal flows to and from the amniotic cavity. *Semin Perinatol.* 1993;7:150.)

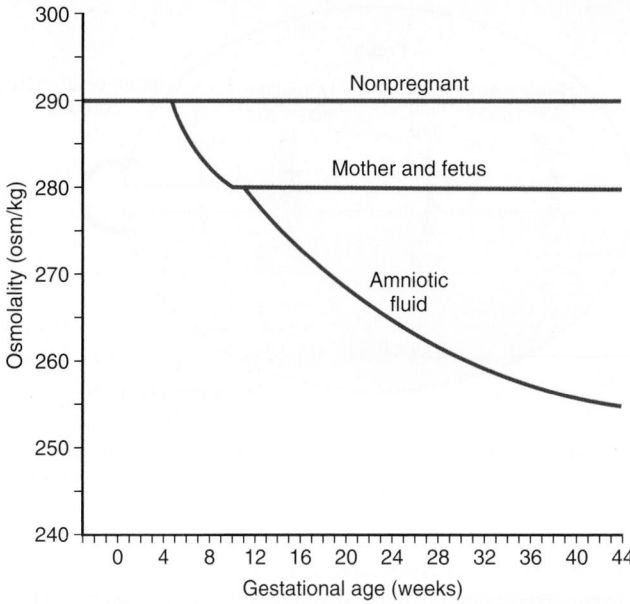

FIG 35-6 Change in maternal and fetal plasma and in amniotic fluid osmolality across gestation. (From Gilbert WM, Moore TR, Brace RA. Amniotic fluid volume dynamics. *Fetal Med Review.* 1991;3:89.)

AMNIOTIC FLUID REMOVAL
Fetal Swallowing

In the human, fetal swallowing begins early in gestation and contributes to the removal of AF. In the fetal sheep, swallowing has mostly been measured in the latter half of pregnancy and appears to increase with increasing gestational age. Sherman and colleagues[37] reported that the ovine fetus swallows volumes of 100 to 300 mL/kg/day in episodes that last 2 minutes. In the term ovine fetus, that volume represents a daily swallowing rate of 350 to 1000 mL/day for a 3.5-kg fetus. This is obviously more than the adult sheep, which drinks 40 to 60 mL/kg daily.

Many different techniques have been used to determine swallowing rates in the animal model, including repetitive sampling of injected dye and actual flow probe measurements.[19,37] For obvious reasons, actual measurement of human fetal swallowing is much more difficult. Human fetal swallowing was studied in the distant past by injecting radioactive chromium–labeled erythrocytes and Hypaque (Amersham Health, Princeton, NJ) into the amniotic compartment, and swallowing rates of 72 to 262 mL/kg/day were found in studies in the 1960s.[29,38] Abramovich[39] injected colloidal gold into the human amniotic compartment and found that fetal swallowing increased with advancing gestational age. He also found similar swallowing rates to those previously reported.[38] Obviously, similar studies could not be performed today, but this information is helpful in our understanding of human fetal swallowing. **Fetal swallowing does not remove the entire volume of fluid that enters the amniotic compartment from fetal urine production and lung liquid; therefore other mechanisms of AF removal such as intramembranous absorption must occur.**

Intramembranous Absorption

One major stumbling block to the understanding of AFV regulation was the discrepancy in volume between fetal urine and lung-liquid production and its removal by swallowing. If the measurements and estimates of AF production and removal were accurate, at least 500 to 750 mL/day of excess fluid would enter the amniotic compartment, which should have resulted in acute polyhydramnios. This does not occur under normal conditions (see Fig. 35-1); therefore a second route for AF removal has been suggested, namely the intramembranous pathway.[24,40-43] This process describes the movement of water and solutes between the amniotic compartment and the fetal blood, which circulates through the fetal surface of the placenta. The large osmotic gradient (Fig. 35-6) between AF and fetal blood provides a substantial driving force for the movement of AF into the fetal blood. Intramembranous absorption has been described in detail in the fetal sheep and has also been demonstrated in the rhesus monkey fetus.[43] Several anecdotal studies suggest that intramembranous absorption also occurs in humans. Heller[44] and Renaud and colleagues[45] each injected labeled amino acids into the amniotic compartments of women, who were shortly thereafter delivered by cesarean section. Both groups found high levels of the amino acids concentrated in the placenta within 45 minutes of injection. They concluded that the amino acids had to have been absorbed by some route other than swallowing in order to explain the rapid absorption into the fetal circulation within the placenta. **Intramembranous absorption could easily explain this movement. This route of absorption is now being actively investigated, and researchers have noted that 200 to 500 mL/ day leaves the amniotic compartment under normal physiologic conditions.**[40,41,46] In addition, it has been reported that absorption through the intramembranous pathway can increase almost tenfold under experimental conditions in sheep.[47] Figure 35-7 summarizes all currently identified avenues for fluid entry and exit from the amniotic compartment and measured or estimated volumes. The flow of fluid into and out of the amniotic

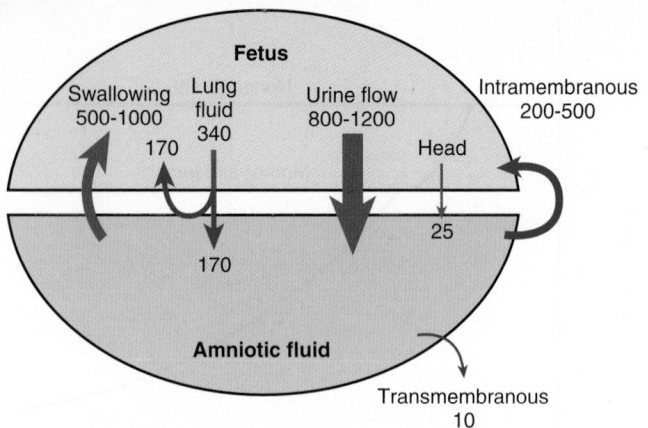

FIG 35-7 All known pathways for fluid and solute entry and exit from the amniotic fluid in the fetus near term. Arrow size is relative to associated flow rate. Solid red arrows represent directly measured flows, whereas the blue arrows represent estimated flows. The numbers represent volume flow in milliliters per day. The curved portion of the double arrow represents lung fluid that is directly swallowed after leaving the trachea, whereas the straight portion represents lung fluid that enters the amniotic cavity from the mouth and nose. (From Gilbert WM, Moore TR, Brace RA. Amniotic fluid volume dynamics. *Fetal Med Review.* 1991;3:89.)

cavity appears to be in a state of balance. Recent work on the mechanisms associated with intramembranous absorption suggests that four intramembranous transport mechanisms act in concert and include (1) a unidirectional bulk transport of AF and solutes out of the AF into the fetal circulation, (2) passive bidirectional diffusion of solutes, (3) passive bidirectional water movement, and (4) unidirectional transport of lactate into the AF.[46] In spite of these new findings, overall AFV regulation still needs further investigation.

OLIGOHYDRAMNIOS

The incidence of oligohydramnios varies depending on which definition is used; reported rates vary between 1% and 3%.[48] The incidence of oligohydramnios is much higher (19% to 20%) among women undergoing antepartum testing for an underlying maternal or fetal indication.[16] Three studies reported actual measurements of AFV for oligohydramnios from less than 200 mL to 500 mL.[6,49,50] With the advent of ultrasound estimation of AFV, multiple thresholds have been reported.[3,8] **In clinical practice, an MVP less than 1 to 2 cm or an AFI less than 5 cm are commonly used as criteria for the diagnosis of oligohydramnios.**

Chamberlain and colleagues[9] reported a fiftyfold increase in PMR for pregnancies with an MVP of less than 1 cm. This report was instrumental in raising concern about the risk of stillbirth and neonatal mortality in the presence of oligohydramnios. A second, less often reported finding of that study was that 40% of the cases with oligohydramnios also had other confounding factors such as intrauterine growth restriction (IUGR), maternal hypertensive disorders, and congenital malformations. Other investigators have reported that oligohydramnios in the prolonged pregnancy has an increased risk of meconium staining of the AF, fetal distress in labor, and low 1-minute Apgar scores.[48]

The PMR approaches 100% when the AFV is greatly decreased early in pregnancy, especially in midpregnancy.[1-3] The cause of the decrease or absence of AF largely determines the perinatal

outcome (Box 35-1). With renal agenesis, virtually 100% of newborns die because of pulmonary hypoplasia. **AF is required for fetal lung development during certain periods of early and mid gestation.** If premature rupture of the membranes (PROM) results in a loss of all AF, neonatal survival will vary based on the gestational age when the membranes ruptured and whether intraamniotic infection was the cause of the membrane rupture.[51] Oligohydramnios can also occur with maternal conditions such as hypertensive disorders or the antiphospholipid syndrome (APS). In these cases, if the fetus is large enough to survive outside of the uterus, there may be little impact on perinatal outcome other than the consequences of prematurity.[51]

A common incidental finding is the existence of a low AFI in an otherwise normal pregnancy. Because the diagnosis of oligohydramnios has been associated with poor perinatal outcomes, many women who are at or near term are sent to labor and delivery to be considered for induction solely because of a low AFI. Frequently, their cervical examination is unfavorable for induction, and an induction is attempted in spite of this; often this ends in a cesarean delivery for failed induction. **Although the evidence for induction in the prolonged pregnancy is solid** (see Chapter 36), **the term or preterm patient with isolated oligohydramnios may not need immediate delivery.** Having said this, borderline oligohydramnios has been found to be a predictor of SGA newborns with an increase in admissions to the neonatal intensive care unit (NICU) but no other significant morbidities.[52] Lagrew and colleagues[53] reported that 41% of women with oligohydramnios, as determined by the AFI, had a normal AFI 3 to 4 days later. They also found that a normal AFI measurement was valid for 1 week, which suggests that the test need not be repeated more often except in certain high-risk situations. Magann and colleagues[16] examined 1001 high-risk women who underwent antepartum testing. They found that those with an AFI of less than 5 cm (19% of cases) had similar outcomes to those whose AFI was in the normal range, and these researchers concluded that an AFI of less than 5 cm was not an indication for delivery.[16] Rainford and colleagues[54] examined 232 women at more than 37 weeks of gestation who had an AFI of less than 5 cm (19%). They found outcomes to be no worse when compared with those whose AFI was in the normal range. In fact, the risk of meconium staining of the AF was found to be increased (35% vs. 16%) in the normal group.[54] Finally, Casey and colleagues[48] examined 6423 women at more than 34 weeks' gestation with an AFI of less than 5 cm and found an increase in intrauterine fetal death (IUFD), admissions to the NICU, neonatal death, low birthweight (LBW), and meconium aspiration syndrome (MAS) compared with women with an AFI of greater than 5 cm. If the birth defects and IUGR were removed, no difference was seen in admissions to the NICU, neonatal death, or respiratory distress syndrome (RDS).[48] This suggests that IUGR and birth defects contributed to the increased morbidity and mortality, not the oligohydramnios. **All cases with oligohydramnios should be evaluated for evidence of IUGR and should be followed with antepartum testing.**

Evaluation and Treatment of Oligohydramnios

When the diagnosis of oligohydramnios is made in the second trimester, it is vitally important to obtain a complete history and physical exam and to perform a targeted ultrasound to help identify a cause (see Box 35-1). The patient should be questioned for any history consistent with rupture of the membranes, leakage of clear or bloody fluid, or wetness of her underwear. If there is a question of possible rupture of the membranes (ROM), a sterile speculum examination should be performed in an attempt to obtain fluid that can be examined for evidence of rupture. Specific tests include evidence of ferning on microscopy examination, a neutral pH on nitrazine paper, and pooling of fluid in the posterior vagina. Commercial tests are also available that screen for ROM: these include AmniSure (Qiagen, Hilden, Germany) and ROM Plus (Clinical Innovations, Murray, Utah), which check for certain proteins from the AF in the vagina. These tests reportedly have a higher sensitivity and specificity than either the fern or nitrazine tests. Next, a targeted ultrasound should be performed to assess the amount of AF present; evaluate fetal anatomy, including the kidneys and bladder; and determine appropriate interval growth. If the fetus is normally grown with kidneys and bladder visualized, more often than not, the amniotic membrane has ruptured prematurely (PROM). If kidneys and bladder cannot be seen, the diagnosis is most likely renal agenesis. Renal agenesis is uniformly fatal, whereas PROM can have a reasonable prognosis if it occurs after fetal viability and if infection is not present.

Although severe oligohydramnios has an increased PMR later in the third trimester, it is still not as high as earlier in pregnancy.[3,48,55] Other studies have reported similar increases in perinatal mortality associated with oligohydramnios, but most have not corrected for other underlying medical conditions.[8] Because of the increase in perinatal morbidity and mortality associated with oligohydramnios in prolonged pregnancy, delivery is recommended (see Chapter 36). As discussed earlier, the patient who presents with isolated oligohydramnios in the third trimester may be a candidate for expectant management.[16,48,54]

Several investigators have attempted to treat oligohydramnios with the oral administration of water in the hope of "hydrating" the fetus through the mother. Animal studies have demonstrated that a close relationship exists between the hydration status of the mother and the fetus.[56,57] Attempts to dehydrate the mother have resulted in dehydration of the fetus, and in some cases vice versa. In human pregnancies, Goodlin and colleagues[58] found that the maternal intravascular volume was low in cases of idiopathic oligohydramnios, and that by increasing the maternal intravascular volume, the oligohydramnios resolved. In a randomized study, the oral administration of water increased the AFI in women with oligohydramnios.[59] The treatment group that drank 2 L of water within 4 hours of a repeat AFI measurement had a significantly greater increase in

TABLE 35-1	CHANGE IN AMNIOTIC FLUID INDEX 4-6 HOURS AFTER ORAL WATER HYDRATION	
	CONTROL (*N* = 20)	**HYDRATION** (*N* = 20)
Before Treatment		
AFI (cm)	17.7 ± 5.0	18.4 ± 4.7
USG	1.013 + 0.007	1.015 + 0.008
After Treatment		
AFI (cm)	16.2 ± 4.5*	21.4 ± 4.5[†]
USG	1.019 ± 0.009[†]	1.006±0.006[†]
Delta AFI (cm)	−1.5 ± 2.7	3.0 ± 2.4
Intake (mL)	1576 + 607	1596 + 465

From Kilpatrick SJ, Safford KL. Maternal hydration increases amniotic fluid index in women with normal amniotic fluid. *Obstet Gynecol.* 1993;81:50.
*P < .02, paired *t* test before vs. after treatment.
[†]P < .0001, paired *t* test before vs. after treatment.
AFI, amniotic fluid index; *Intake,* amount of fluid intake over the previous 24 hours other than the 2 L; *USG,* urine specific gravity; *Delta AFI,* change in AFI from before to after treatment.

AFI on repeat testing (6.3 cm) than the control group (5.1 cm).[59] A follow-up study of women with a normal AFI demonstrated that the amount of water ingested could increase or decrease their AFI.[60] As illustrated in Table 35-1, the AFI significantly increased in the oral hydration group compared with the control group. The control group was given what was thought to be a "normal" volume of water to drink, but the AFI actually decreased and urine osmolality increased. This suggests that the mothers were actually dehydrated during the control portion of the study. **Both groups demonstrated that the AFI can be influenced by increasing or decreasing water intake orally.**

Many other studies have shown a similar improvement in AFV with either oral or intravenous administration of water and/or crystalloids.[61-63] In a prospective randomized trial of women with an AFI between 6 and 24 cm, the patients were either hydrated with 1 L of water over 1 hour and placed in the left lateral recumbent position or were not orally hydrated but were placed in the left lateral recumbent position. AFIs were measured every 15 minutes for 90 minutes. Both groups saw a similar increase in the AFI at 15 and 30 minutes, but the hydration group saw a further increase at 45 minutes, which suggests that oral hydration—and simple bed rest alone, but to a lesser extent—can improve the AFI.[63] Several researchers have reported success in improving AFV in women with oligohydramnios by the injection of a crystalloid solution into the amniotic compartment during an amniocentesis.[64] Most of these studies, however, have been case reports; because no large prospective studies have been performed, the routine use of this approach for cases of severe oligohydramnios in mid gestation cannot be justified.

Oligohydramnios in Labor

Almost 30 years ago, Gabbe and colleagues[65] worked with fetal monkeys and noted that when AF was removed from the amniotic compartment, variable decelerations in the fetal heart rate developed. These decelerations resolved when the AF was replaced, suggesting that cord compression was the cause of the decelerations. Since that time, multiple investigators have studied amnioinfusion as a technique by which to treat variable decelerations in labor. **Although most report a decrease in the frequency of variable decelerations, few have demonstrated any decrease in perinatal morbidity or mortality or in the cesarean delivery rate.**[66-69] Amnioinfusion has been studied as a possible therapy in the case of thick meconium. In several small prospective studies, it has been shown to improve neonatal outcomes, including meconium visualized below the newborn vocal cords and meconium aspiration syndrome.[70-73] Sadovsky and colleagues[74] found that with the randomization of women with greater than light meconium to a control or amnioinfusion treatment group, 29% of control newborns had meconium below the umbilical cords, whereas none of the treated newborns did. A meta-analysis of the therapeutic use of amnioinfusion for thick meconium demonstrated a reduction (odds ratio [OR] 0.3; 95% confidence interval [CI], 0.19 to 0.46) in meconium below the vocal cords at delivery.[75] A more recent, multicenter, randomized trial of 1998 women in labor at 36 weeks' gestation or later with thick meconium did not find that amnioinfusion reduced the risk of moderate or severe meconium aspiration syndrome or perinatal death.[76] **Based on this large multicenter trial, ACOG recommends against routine prophylactic amnioinfusion for the dilution of meconium–stained amniotic fluid.**[77]

POLYHYDRAMNIOS

The incidence of polyhydramnios is 1% to 2%. The earlier in gestation polyhydramnios occurs and the greater the amount of fluid, the higher the perinatal morbidity and mortality.[4] Ultrasound assessment of the MVP or AFI is used to confirm the diagnosis of polyhydramnios.

Many authors define *polyhydramnios* as an MVP of greater than 8 cm, whereas others use an AFI of 25 cm or greater. Hill and colleagues[78] divided their patients with polyhydramnios into three groups: *mild* (MVP 8 to 11 cm, 79% of cases), *moderate* (MVP 12 to 15 cm, 16.5%), and *severe* (MVP ≥16 cm, 5%). Overall, the perinatal mortality rate was 127.5/1000, which corrected to 58.8/1000 when lethal malformations were excluded. This value is markedly increased over the background rate. A specific cause was identified in only 16% of the pregnancies with mild, 90% with moderate, and 100% with severe polyhydramnios. Fetal and maternal conditions associated with polyhydramnios are shown in Box 35-2. In a follow-up study, Many and colleagues[79] examined 275 women with polyhydramnios to determine whether its degree had any influence on the rate of prematurity. Although excessive AF did not impact the rate of prematurity, the presence of anomalies or diabetes mellitus was associated with an increased risk of preterm delivery.[80] **Severe polyhydramnios in the second trimester has a significant PMR due to prematurity or aneuploidy.**[81,82] Pregnancy complications associated with polyhydramnios have been reported to increase the risk for placental abruption and postpartum hemorrhage as a result of overdistension or rapid deflation of the uterus, and this should be taken into consideration in the plan of care.

Evaluation and Treatment of Polyhydramnios

The pregnant woman who presents with a rapidly enlarging uterus in mid pregnancy, with or without preterm labor, needs to be evaluated by an ultrasound examination to measure the AFV and assess fetal anatomy. Esophageal atresia with or without tracheoesophageal fistula can present with early-onset severe polyhydramnios due to an obstruction of swallowing. Other gastrointestinal obstructions such as duodenal atresia may result in polyhydramnios.[78] When a structural defect is seen in a fetus with polyhydramnios, consideration should be given to performing an amniocentesis for microarray analysis (see Chapter 10).

BOX 35-2   FETAL AND MATERNAL CAUSES OF POLYHYDRAMNIOS

Fetal Conditions

Congenital anomalies
- Gastrointestinal obstruction, central nervous system abnormalities, cystic hygroma, nonimmune hydrops, sacrococcygeal teratoma, cystic adenoid malformations of lung

Aneuploidy

Genetic disorders
- Achondrogenesis type 1-B
- Muscular dystrophies
- Bartter syndrome

Twin-to-twin transfusion syndrome

Infections
- Parvovirus B-19

Placental abnormalities
- Chorioangioma

Maternal Conditions

Idiopathic

Poorly controlled diabetes mellitus

Fetomaternal hemorrhage

Another common cause of acute, severe polyhydramnios in the second trimester is the twin-to-twin transfusion syndrome (TTTS; see Chapter 32). The ultrasound findings associated with TTTS are marked polyhydramnios of the receiving twin and absent AFV or marked oligohydramnios of the donor twin. **When polyhydramnios occurs in the third trimester of pregnancy, it is usually mild and is not associated with a structural defect.**[78] Although the vast majority of cases in the third trimester are idiopathic, the other causes of polyhydramnios must be excluded (see Box 35-2).

In many cases, polyhydramnios may be transient. Mild or transient polyhydramnios is usually idiopathic and has a favorable prognosis.[83] However, complications of pregnancy are greater when the AFV remains markedly elevated during pregnancy, including preterm delivery (2.7-fold increase), preeclampsia (2.7-fold increase), IUFD (7.7-fold increase), and neonatal demise (7.7-fold increase). In such cases, antenatal and maternal surveillance is warranted.

A meta-analysis of 43 studies found that polyhydramnios (AFI >24 cm or MVP >8 cm) was predictive of macrosomia with an OR of 11.5 (95% CI, 4.1 to 32.9), which suggests that this should be taken into account when considering delivery options.[84] Treatment options for patients with polyhydramnios are usually tailored to the underlying cause. With mild idiopathic polyhydramnios—in which the workup is negative, and follow-up ultrasound demonstrates persistent polyhydramnios—antepartum testing with fetal kick counts or nonstress tests may be prudent. Antepartum surveillance is recommended for women with polyhydramnios and poorly controlled diabetes mellitus.

With severe polyhydramnios associated with preterm labor, one medical treatment option involves the administration of a prostaglandin inhibitor such as indomethacin, which decreases fetal urine production.[85-87] This effect occurs within 5 hours of starting the medication and decreases the AFV within 24 hours.[85,86,88] Although indomethacin has been shown to be relatively safe when given over a short period of time, such as 72 hours, prolonged use may be associated with risks to the fetus such as premature closure, narrowing of the ductus arteriosus within the fetal heart, and renal abnormalities in the newborn period.[86,87] Complications related to indomethacin use worsen with advancing gestational age, and such treatment beyond 31 to 32 weeks of gestation should be avoided.[88] The use of repetitive amnioreductions, in which amniocentesis is performed and large volumes (1 to 5 L) of AF are removed through plastic tubing into a vacuum bottle, does prolong pregnancies in a number of cases but may need to be repeated on a regular basis.[5,88]

KEY POINTS

- Amniotic fluid is dynamic, with large volume flows into and out of the amniotic compartment each day.
- Clinical estimates of actual AFV based on ultrasound measurements of the AFI or MVP are not accurate in predicting true volume.
- In the presence of IUGR or a prolonged gestation, oligohydramnios is associated with significant increases in perinatal morbidity and mortality.
- Preterm or term isolated oligohydramnios is not associated with an increase in perinatal morbidity or mortality with an otherwise normal fetus.
- Early-onset or severe polyhydramnios is associated with aneuploidy, congenital malformations, preterm delivery, and an increased perinatal mortality rate.
- The cause of mild polyhydramnios, especially in the latter part of the third trimester, is usually idiopathic or related to diabetes mellitus and has little impact on perinatal survival.
- AFV as estimated by the AFI may be expanded with increased maternal oral ingestion of water and/or bed rest in the left lateral recumbent position.
- Short-term use of indomethacin decreases fetal urine production and can reduce AFV within 24 hours of administration; prolonged use should be avoided because of the risk of premature closure of the ductus arteriosus and renal abnormalities in the newborn.

REFERENCES

1. Hackett GA, Nicolaides KH, Campbell S. The value of Doppler ultrasound assessment of fetal and uteroplacental circulations when severe oligohydramnios complicates the second trimester of pregnancy. *Br J Obstet Gynaecol.* 1987;94:1074.
2. Barss VA, Benacerraf BR, Frigoletto FD. Second trimester oligohydramnios, a predictor of poor fetal outcome. *Obstet Gynecol.* 1984;64:608.
3. Mercer LJ, Brown LG. Fetal outcome with oligohydramnios in the second trimester. *Obstet Gynecol.* 1986;67:840.
4. Wier PE, Raten G, Beisher N. Acute polyhydramnios–a complication of monozygous twin pregnancy. *Br J Obstet Gynaecol.* 1979;86:849.
5. Reisner DP, Mahony BS, Petty CN, et al. Stuck twin syndrome: outcome in thirty-seven consecutive cases. *Am J Obstet Gynecol.* 1993;169:991.
6. Brace RA, Wolf EJ. Characterization of normal gestational changes amniotic fluid volume. *Am J Obstet Gynecol.* 1989;161:382.
7. Magann EF, Sandlin AT, Ounpraseuth ST. Amniotic fluid and the clinical relevance of the sonographically estimated amniotic fluid volume: oligohydramnios. *J Ultrasound Med.* 2011;30(11):1573.
8. Manning FA, Hill LM, Platt LD. Qualitative amniotic fluid volume determination by ultrasound: antepartum detection of intrauterine growth retardation. *Am J Obstet Gynecol.* 1981;139:254.
9. Chamberlain PF, Manning FA, Morrison I, et al. Ultrasound evaluation of amniotic fluid volume. I: The relationship of marginal and decreased amniotic fluid volumes to perinatal outcome. *Am J Obstet Gynecol.* 1984;150:245.
10. Mercer LJ, Brown LG, Petres RE, et al. A survey of pregnancies complicated by decreased amniotic fluid. *Am J Obstet Gynecol.* 1984;149:355.
11. Phelan JP, Ohn MO, Smith CV, et al. Amniotic fluid index measurements during pregnancy. *J Reprod Med.* 1987;32:603.
12. Rutherford SE, Phelan JP, Smith CV, et al. The four quadrant assessment of amniotic fluid volume: an adjunct to antepartum fetal heart rate testing. *Obstet Gynecol.* 1987;70:353.
13. Moore TR, Cayle JE. The amniotic fluid index in normal human pregnancy. *Am J Obstet Gynecol.* 1990;162:1168.
14. Dildy GA 3rd, Lira N, Moise KJ, et al. Amniotic fluid volume assessment: comparison of ultrasonographic estimates versus direct measurements with a dye-dilution technique in human pregnancies. *Am J Obstet Gynecol.* 1992;167:986.
15. Magann EF, Chauhan SP, Barrilleaux PS, et al. Amniotic fluid index and single deepest pocket: Weak indicators of abnormal amniotic volumes. *Obstet Gynecol.* 2000;96:737.
16. Magann EF, Chauhan SP, Doherty DA, et al. The evidence for abandoning the amniotic fluid index in favor of the single deepest pocket. *Am J Perinatol.* 2007;24(9):549-555.
17. Moore TR. Superiority of the four-quadrant sum over the single-deepest-pocket technique in ultrasonographic identification of abnormal amniotic fluid volumes. *Am J Obstet Gynecol.* 1990;163:762.
18. Moise KJ Jr. Toward consistent terminology: assessment and reporting of amniotic fluid volume. *Semin Perinatol.* 2013;37:370.
19. Tomoda S, Brace RA, Longo L. Amniotic fluid volume and fetal swallowing rate in sheep. *Am J Physiol.* 1985;249:R133.
20. Gresham EL, Rankin JH, Makowski EL, Meschia G, Battaglia FC. An evaluation of fetal renal function in a chronic sheep preparation. *J Clin Invest.* 1972;51:149.
21. Wintour EM, Barnes A, Brown EH, et al. Regulation of amniotic fluid volume and composition on the ovine fetus. *Obstet Gynecol.* 1978;52:689.
22. Wladimiroff JW, Campbell S. Fetal urine-production rates in normal and complicated pregnancy. *Lancet.* 1974;1:151.
23. Rabinowitz R, Peters MT, Vyas S, et al. Measurement of fetal urine production in normal pregnancy by real-time ultrasonography. *Am J Obstet Gynecol.* 1989;161:1264.
24. Gilbert WM, Cheung CY, Brace RA. Rapid intramembranous absorption into the fetal circulation of arginine vasopressin injected intraamniotically. *Am J Obstet Gynecol.* 1991;164:1013.
25. Lee SM, Park SK, Shim SS, et al. Measurement of fetal urine production by three-dimensional ultrasonography in normal pregnancy. *Ultrasound Obstet Gynecol.* 2007;30(3):281.
26. van Otterlo LC, Wladimiroff JW, Wallenburg HC. Relationship between fetal urine production and amniotic fluid volume in normal pregnancy and pregnancy complicated by diabetes. *Br J Obstet Gynaecol.* 1977;84:205.
27. Kurjak A, Kirkinsen P, Latin V, et al. Ultrasonic assessment of fetal kidney function in normal and complicated pregnancies. *Am J Obstet Gynecol.* 1981;141:266.
28. Deutinger J, Bartl W, Pfersmann C, et al. Fetal kidney volume and urine production in cases of fetal growth retardation. *J Perinat Med.* 1987;15:307.
29. Duenhoelter JH, Pritchard JA. Fetal respiration: quantitative measurements of amniotic fluid inspired near term by human and rhesus fetuses. *Am J Obstet Gynecol.* 1976;125:306.
30. Seeds AE. Current concepts of amniotic fluid dynamics. *Am J Obstet Gynecol.* 1980;138:575.
31. Adamson TM, Brodecky V, Lambert TF, et al. The production and composition of lung liquids in the in-utero foetal lamb. In: Comline RS, Cross KW, Dawes GS, Nathaniel PW, eds. *Foetal and Neonatal Physiology.* Cambridge, UK: Cambridge University Press; 1973:208.
32. Mescher EJ, Platzker A, Ballard PL, et al. Ontogeny of tracheal fluid, pulmonary surfactant, and plasma corticoids in the fetal lamb. *J Appl Physiol.* 1975;39:1017.
33. Olver RE, Strang LB. Ion fluxes across the pulmonary epithelium and the secretion of lung liquid in the foetal lamb. *J Physiol.* 1974;241:327.
34. Lawson EE, Brown ER, Torday JS, et al. The effect of epinephrine on tracheal fluid flow and surfactant efflux in fetal sheep. *Am Rev Respir Dis.* 1978;118:1023.
35. Brace RA, Wlodek ME, Cook ML, et al. Swallowing of lung liquid and amniotic fluid by the ovine fetus under normoxic and hypoxic conditions. *Am J Obstet Gynecol.* 1994;171:764.
36. Patrick J, Campbell K, Carmichael L, et al. Patterns of human fetal breathing at 30–31 and 38–39 weeks' gestational age. *Obstet Gynecol.* 1980;56:24.

37. Sherman DJ, Ross MG, Day L, et al. Fetal swallowing: correlation of electromyography and esophageal fluid flow. *Am J Physiol.* 1990;258:R1386.
38. Prichard JA. Deglutition by normal and anencephalic fetuses. *Obstet Gynecol.* 1965;25:289.
39. Abramovich DR. Fetal factors influencing the volume and composition of liquor amnii. *J Obstet Gynaecol Br Commonw.* 1970;77:865.
40. Gilbert WM, Brace RA. The missing link in amniotic fluid volume regulation: Intramembranous absorption. *Obstet Gynecol.* 1989;74:748.
41. Gilbert WM, Brace RA. Novel determination of filtration coefficient of ovine placenta and intramembranous pathway. *Am J Physiol.* 1990;259:R1281.
42. Gilbert WM, Moore TR, Brace RA. Amniotic fluid volume dynamics. *Fet Med Rev.* 1991;3:89.
43. Gilbert WM, Eby-Wilkens EM, Tarantal AF. The missing-link in Rhesus monkey amniotic fluid volume regulation: Intramembranous absorption. *Obstet Gynecol.* 1997;892:462.
44. Heller L. Intrauterine amino acid feeding of the fetus. In: Bode H, Warshaw J, eds. *Parenteral Nutrition in Infancy and Childhood.* New York, NY: Plenum Press; 1974:206.
45. Renaud R, Kirschtetter L, Koehl D, et al. Amino-acid intraamniotic injections. In: Persianinov LS, Chervakova TV, Presl J, eds. *Recent Progress in Obstetrics and Gynaecology.* Amsterdam: Excerpta Medica; 1974:234.
46. Brace RA, Anderson DF, Cheung CY. Regulation of amniotic fluid volume: Mathematical model based on intramembranous transport mechanisms. *Am J Physiol Regul Integr Comp Physiol.* 2014;307(10):R1260-R1273.
47. Faber JJ, Anderson DF. Absorption of amniotic fluid by amniochorion in sheep. *Am J Physiol.* 2002;282:H850.
48. Casey BM, McIntire DD, Bloom SL, et al. Pregnancy outcomes after antepartum diagnosis of oligohydramnios at or beyond 34 weeks' gestation. *Am J Obstet Gynecol.* 2000;182:909.
49. Magann EF, Nolan TE, Hess LW, et al. Measurement of amniotic fluid volume: accuracy of ultrasonography techniques. *Am J Obstet Gynecol.* 1992;167:1533.
50. Horsager R, Nathan L, Leveno KJ. Correlation of measured amniotic fluid volume and sonographic predictions of oligohydramnios. *Obstet Gynecol.* 1994;83:955.
51. Hill MH. Oligohydramnios: Sonographic diagnosis and clinical implications. *Clin Obstet Gynecol.* 1997;40:314.
52. Hashimoto K, Kasdaglis T, Jain S, et al. Isolated low-normal amniotic fluid volume in the early third trimester: association with adverse perinatal outcomes. *J Perinat Med.* 2013;41(4):349.
53. Lagrew DC, Pircon RA, Nageotte M, et al. How frequently should the amniotic fluid index be repeated? *Am J Obstet Gynecol.* 1992;167:1129.
54. Rainford M, Adair R, Scialli AR, et al. Amniotic fluid index in the uncomplicated term pregnancy. Prediction of outcome. *J Reprod Med.* 2001;46:589.
55. Jeng CJ, Lee JF, Wang KG, et al. Decreased amniotic fluid index in term pregnancy. Clinical significance. *J Reprod Med.* 1992;37:789.
56. Ross MG, Ervin MG, Leake RD, et al. Bulk flow of amniotic fluid water in response to maternal osmotic challenge. *Am J Obstet Gynecol.* 1983;147:697.
57. Woods LL. Fetal renal contribution to amniotic fluid osmolality during maternal hypertonicity. *Am J Physiol.* 1986;250:R235.
58. Goodlin RC, Anderson JC, Gallagher TF. Relationship between amniotic fluid volume and maternal plasma volume expansion. *Am J Obstet Gynecol.* 1983;146:505.
59. Kilpatrick SJ, Safford K, Pomeroy T, et al. Maternal hydration affects amniotic fluid index (AFI). *Am J Obstet Gynecol.* 1991;164:361.
60. Kilpatrick SJ, Safford KL. Maternal hydration increases amniotic fluid index in women with normal amniotic fluid volumes. *Obstet Gynecol.* 1993;81:49.
61. Flack NJ, Sepulveda W, Bower S, Fisk NM. Acute maternal hydration in third-trimester oligohydramnios: effects on amniotic fluid volume, uteroplacental perfusion, and fetal blood flow and urine output. *Am J Obstet Gynecol.* 1995;173:1186-1191.
62. Doi S, Osada H, Seki K, et al. Effect of maternal hydration on oligohydramnios: a comparison of three volume expansion methods. *Obstet Gynecol.* 1998;92:525.
63. Ulker K, Melek C. Effect of maternal hydration on the amniotic fluid volume during maternal rest in the left lateral decubitus position. *J Ultrasound Med.* 2013;32:955.
64. Sepulveda W, Flack NJ, Fisk NM. Direct volume measurement at midtrimester amnioinfusion in relation to ultrasonographic indexes of amniotic fluid volume. *Am J Obstet Gynecol.* 1994;170:1160.
65. Gabbe SG, Ettinger BB, Freeman RK, et al. Umbilical cord compression associated with amniotomy: laboratory observations. *Am J Obstet Gynecol.* 1976;126:353.
66. Nageotte MP, Bertucci L, Towers CV, et al. Prophylactic amnioinfusion in pregnancies complicated by oligohydramnios: a prospective study. *Obstet Gynecol.* 1991;77:677.
67. Ogundipe OA, Spong CY, Ross MG. Prophylactic amnioinfusion for oligohydramnios: A reevaluation. *Obstet Gynecol.* 1994;84:544.
68. Schrimmer DB, Macri CJ, Paul RH. Prophylactic amnioinfusion as a treatment for oligohydramnios I laboring patients: a prospective randomized trial. *Am J Obstet Gynecol.* 1991;165:972.
69. Miyazaki FS, Taylor NA. Saline amnioinfusion for relief of variable or prolonged decelerations. *Am J Obstet Gynecol.* 1983;146:670.
70. Chanhan SP, Rutherford SE, Hess LW, et al. Prophylactic intrapartum amnioinfusion for patients with oligohydramnios. *J Reprod Med.* 1992;37:817.
71. Wenstrom KD, Parsons MT. The prevention of meconium aspiration in labor using amnioinfusion. *Obstet Gynecol.* 1989;73:647.
72. Eriksen NL, Hostetter M, Parisi VM. Prophylactic amnioinfusion in pregnancies complicated by thick meconium. *Am J Obstet Gynecol.* 1994;171:1026.
73. Macri CJ, Schrimmer DB, Leung A, et al. Prophylactic amnioinfusion improves outcome of pregnancy complicated by thick meconium and oligohydramnios. *Am J Obstet Gynecol.* 1992;167:117.
74. Sadovsky Y, Amon E, Bade ME, et al. Prophylactic amnioinfusion during labor complicated by meconium: a preliminary report. *Am J Obstet Gynecol.* 1989;161:613.
75. Pierce J, Gaudier FL, Sanchez-Ramos L. Intrapartum amnioinfusion for meconium-stained fluid: meta-analysis of prospective trials. *Obstet Gynecol.* 2000;95:1051.
76. Fraser WD, Hofmeyr J, Lede R, et al. Amnioinfusion for the prevention of the meconium aspiration syndrome. *N Engl J Med.* 2005;353:909.
77. ACOG Committee on Obstetric Practice. *Committee Opinion No. 346: Amnioinfusion does not prevent meconium aspiration syndrome,* 2014.
78. Hill LM, Breckle R, Thomas ML, et al. Polyhydramnios: ultrasonically detected prevalence and neonatal outcome. *Obstet Gynecol.* 1987;69:21.
79. Many A, Hill LM, Lazebnik N, et al. The association between polyhydramnios and preterm delivery. *Obstet Gynecol.* 1995;86:389.
80. Chamberlain PF, Manning FA, Morrison I, et al. Ultrasound evaluation of amniotic fluid volume II: the relationship of increased amniotic fluid volume to perinatal outcome. *Am J Obstet Gynecol.* 1984;150:250.
81. Pauer HU, Viereck V, Krauss V, et al. Incidence of fetal malformations in pregnancies complicated by oligo- and polyhydramnios. *Arch Gynecol Obstet.* 2003;268:52.
82. Desmedt EJ, Henry OA, Beischer NA. Polyhydramnios and associated maternal and fetal complications in singleton pregnancies. *Br J Obstet Gynaecol.* 1990;97:1115.
83. Golan A, Wolman I, Sagi J, et al. Persistence of polyhydramnios during pregnancy-its significance and correlation with maternal and fetal complications. *Gynecol Obstet Invest.* 1994;37:18.
84. Morris RK, Meller CH, Tamblyn J, et al. Association and prediction of amniotic fluid measurements for adverse pregnancy outcome: systematic review and meta-analysis. *BJOG.* 2014;121(6):686.
85. Stevenson KM, Lumbers ER. Effects of indomethacin on fetal renal function, renal and umbilicoplacental blood flow and lung liquid production. *J Dev Physiol.* 1992;17:257.
86. Kirshon B, Moise KJ, Wasserstrum N, et al. Influence of short-term indomethacin therapy on fetal urine output. *Obstet Gynecol.* 1988;72:51.
87. Mamopoulos M, Assimakopoulos E, Reece EA, et al. Maternal indomethacin therapy in the treatment of polyhydramnios. *Am J Obstet Gynecol.* 1990;162:1225.
88. Moise KJ. Polyhydramnios. *Clin Obstet Gynecol.* 1997;40:266.

Additional references for this chapter are available at ExpertConsult.com.

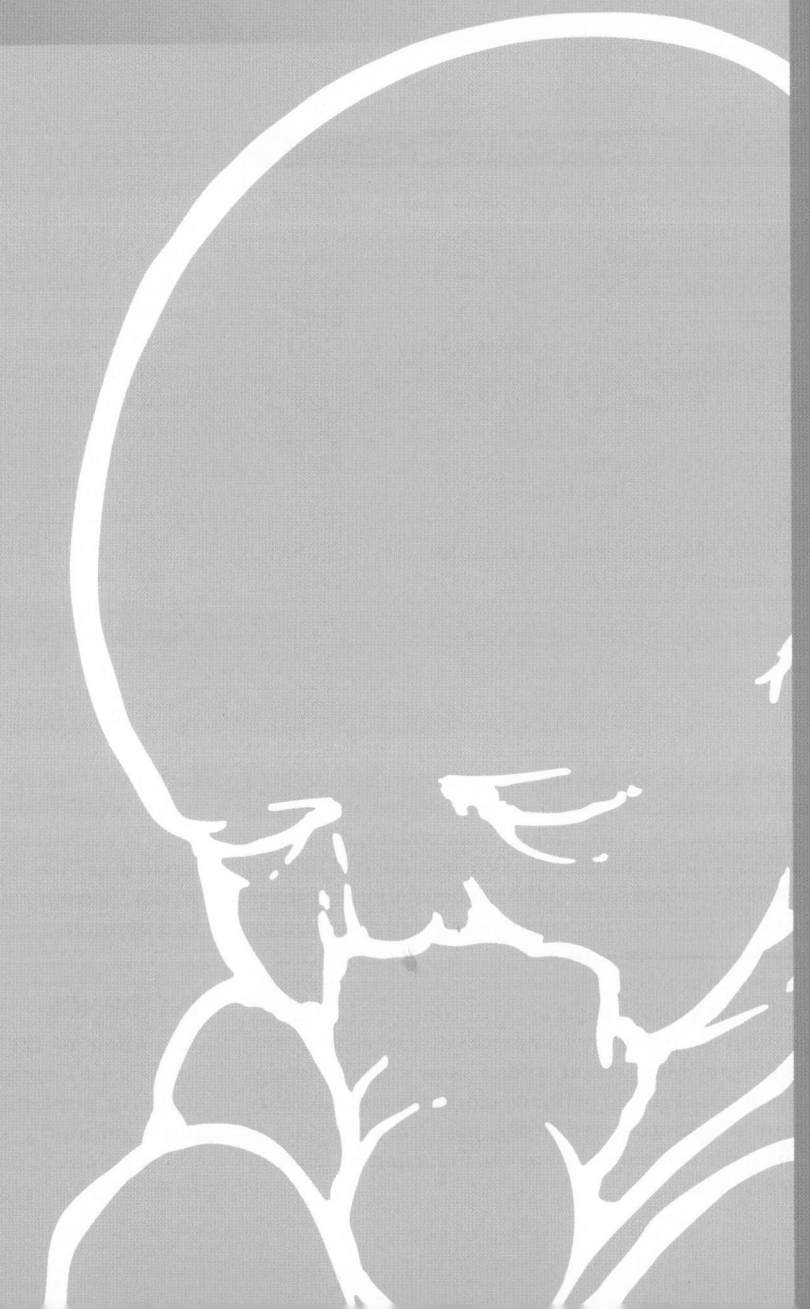

Pregnancy and Coexisting Disease

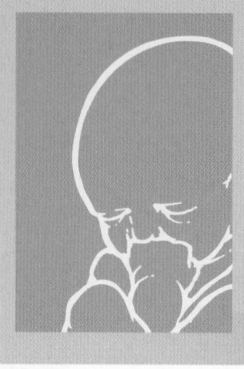

CHAPTER 36

Prolonged and Postterm Pregnancy

ROXANE RAMPERSAD and GEORGE A. MACONES

KEY ABBREVIATIONS

American College of Obstetricians and Gynecologists	ACOG
Amniotic fluid index	AFI
Confidence interval	CI
Estimated date of delivery	EDD
International Federation of Gynecology and Obstetrics	FIGO
Last menstrual period	LMP
Odds ratio	OR
Perinatal mortality rate	PMR
Randomized controlled trial	RCT
Relative risk	RR
Society for Maternal-Fetal Medicine	SMFM
World Health Organization	WHO

Obstetricians have long recognized the detrimental effects of preterm delivery, but for the last century, there has also been concern for pregnancies that have gone beyond the normal period of gestation. Early descriptions from prolonged pregnancies described a large fetus and resulted in a difficult delivery with an increased risk of stillbirth.[1] Later descriptions suggested that a posterm fetus not only could be large but also small for gestational age.[2] These concerns led some to adopt a practice of inducing labor to avoid complications in prolonged pregnancies. This practice was variable, and somewhat controversial, because the upper limit of pregnancy was not well defined and the risks were inconsistent. **More recent studies show a small but significantly increased risk in perinatal morbidity and mortality in posterm pregnancies, and hence, posterm pregnancy is one of the most common reasons for induction of labor in the United States.**

DEFINITION

The American College of Obstetricians and Gynecologists (ACOG), International Federation of Gynecology and Obstetrics (FIGO), and the World Health Organization (WHO) have defined a *posterm pregnancy* as a **gestation that has completed or gone beyond 42, weeks or 294 days, from the first day of the last menstrual period** (LMP).[3-5] This gestational age cutoff has been used for several decades and was first suggested based on early studies that reported an increased risk of fetal death at 42 weeks and beyond.[6] However, in view of more recent perinatal mortality data derived from accurately dated pregnancies, **it would be reasonable to conclude that the gestational age that warrants clinical concern should be 41 weeks.**

Many terms have been used in the literature, including *postmature, postdates, prolonged,* and *posterm.* These terms have been used with varying definitions, which has led to some confusion regarding proper terminology. Recently ACOG and the Society for Maternal-Fetal Medicine (SMFM) has endorsed the use of new terminology recommended by the Defining Term Pregnancy Workgroup to decrease confusion among physicians, patients, and researchers and to designate gestational ages at higher risk.[7-8] Pregnancies are now designated to be "early term" if they are $37^{0/7}$ weeks through $38^{6/7}$ weeks. Full term is defined at $39^{0/7}$ weeks through $40^{6/7}$ weeks. **Pregnancies are to be designated as "late term" if they are $41^{0/7}$ weeks through $41^{6/7}$ weeks. Posterm will continue to be defined as $42^{0/7}$ weeks and beyond.**

INCIDENCE

According to the vital statistics reported by the Centers for Disease Control and Prevention (CDC), the overall incidence of posterm pregnancies was 5.6% in 2012 and has not significantly changed compared with previous years.[9] Other published studies have shown varying frequency of posterm pregnancies depending on the population studied. The incidence of prolonged pregnancies in European countries also varies widely, with rates as low as 0.4% in Austria and as high as 7% in Denmark and Sweden.[10] These differences are most likely explained by different approaches for managing pregnancies beyond the estimated date of delivery (EDD) and different criteria for gestational age dating.

ETIOLOGY

The etiology of the majority of pregnancies that are late term or postterm is unknown, but some pregnancies may be defined as late term or postterm as the result of an error in dating. It is common practice to assign an EDD based on the LMP. This practice has been proven by several studies to be unreliable and may have led to the incorrect classification of a pregnancy as late term or postterm.[11]

Understanding the events that lead to parturition in human gestation may help to provide clues to the pathophysiology in prolonged pregnancies. **Parturition is the result of a complex interplay among the mother, fetus, and placenta.**[12] The mechanism in human gestation is unknown but may be similar to that of other mammals. In sheep, the hypothalamic-pituitary-adrenal (HPA) axis is important in the timing of birth. The release of corticotropin-releasing hormone (CRH) from the fetal brain results in the secretion of adrenocorticotropic hormone (ACTH) from the pituitary gland and cortisol from the adrenal gland.[13] The increase in cortisol parallels an increase in the secretion of prostaglandin and estrogens and a fall in progesterone.[13] Decreases in progesterone and increases in prostaglandins are known triggers of uterine myometrium. Further support for the role of the HPA axis in the initiation of labor is seen in studies with hypophysectomized sheep; disruption of the HPA axis results in prolonged pregnancy.[14] More recent studies have proposed a similar involvement of the HPA axis in human gestation, and its dysregulation may play a role in prolonged pregnancies.

Early studies likened anencephaly to the hypophysectomized sheep. It is hypothesized that the absence of the fetal brain in the anencephalic fetus may result in a similar dysfunction of the HPA axis and may lead to prolonged gestation. Epidemiologic studies of anencephalic pregnancies have observed prolongation of pregnancy.[15] These findings support current thinking that the interaction between the fetal brain and placenta plays an important role in triggering labor.

Pregnancies complicated by placental sulfatase deficiency, an X-linked recessive disorder characterized by the absence of the enzyme steroid sulfatase, are marked by abnormally low estriol levels and, in general, fail to go into spontaneous labor.[16] This is an example of a genetic etiology for prolonged pregnancy and lends further support to the important role of the placenta in the initiation of labor.

A number of observational studies have identified risk factors for postterm pregnancy including primigravidity, prior postterm pregnancy, male fetus, obesity, and a genetic predisposition.[17-23] A 10-year cohort study of births in Norway failed to find a strong association of risk factors with postterm pregnancy but may have had a bias toward nondetection.[17] Intergenerational studies suggest a genetic predisposition for postterm pregnancy. Mothers who themselves were postterm also have an increased risk of prolonged pregnancy. Twin studies have found higher rates of concordance for postterm pregnancy among female twins, compared with male twins, implicating a maternal influence on the risk for prolonged pregnancy.[22]

DIAGNOSIS

The diagnosis of truly late term and postterm pregnancy is based on accurate gestational dating. The three most commonly used methods to determine the EDD are (1) knowledge of the date of the LMP, (2) knowledge of the timing of intercourse, and (3) early ultrasound assessment. Other methods have been described but are rarely used in contemporary practice, including the determination of uterine size, quickening, ability to detect fetal heart tones by Doppler auscultation, and fundal height measurement. In most cases, the date of conception is rarely known and therefore is infrequently used to determine gestational age. The EDD is most commonly assigned based on the first day of the LMP, but this assumes that conception occurs on the fourteenth day of the menstrual cycle. This method can be very inaccurate because the timing of ovulation is variable among an individual's menstrual cycles and between individuals.[24,25] Basing gestational age solely on the LMP generally results in an overestimation of gestational age and may result in a higher frequency of induction of labor for presumed postterm pregnancy.

The use of ultrasound to determine the accuracy of gestational dating based on the LMP is superior to the use of the LMP alone. The EDD is most accurately determined if the crown-rump length is measured in the first trimester with an error of ± 5 to 7 days. Boyd and colleagues[26] showed that the incidence of patients whose pregnancy exceeded 293 days was 7.5% based on menstrual dating and declined to 2.6% when dates were determined by early sonographic examination. A similar conclusion was reached by Gardosi and associates,[27] who evaluated 24,675 spontaneous, normal singleton deliveries and showed a decline in the postterm (>294 days) pregnancy rate from 9.5% when pregnancies were dated by LMP to 1.5% when ultrasound dating was used. These authors also reported that about 72% of routine labor inductions at 42 weeks' gestation were not indicated because they were performed before the patients reached 42 weeks based on ultrasound assessment of gestational age. Similarly, Nguyen and coworkers[28] evaluated 14,805 spontaneous deliveries with a reliable LMP and showed that ultrasound dating reduced the proportion of deliveries beyond 294 days of gestation by 39% (from 7.9% to 5.2%). Bennett and colleagues[29] confirmed these findings in a prospective, randomized study of 218 women and found fewer postterm inductions of labor in women dated by a first-trimester sonogram when compared with women whose dates were established by second-trimester sonography.

PERINATAL MORBIDITY AND MORTALITY

Numerous studies have evaluated the risk to the fetus in late-term and postterm pregnancies. Early descriptive studies found that pregnancies that continued past their EDD had an increased risk of fetal death. In 1963, McClure[6] found a twofold increase in "fetal distress" at 42 weeks with an increase in operative deliveries and surmised that 42 weeks constituted a significant risk to the fetus and proposed intervening with induction of labor or cesarean delivery to avoid the risk of fetal death. Early studies were likely fraught with inaccurate dating and inconsistent definitions of postterm pregnancy. Lastly, it is important to note that these studies included pregnancies complicated by fetal anomalies, intrauterine growth restriction (IUGR), and mothers with coexisting medical conditions, all of which increase the risk of fetal demise.

More recent observational studies that have evaluated the risk of perinatal mortality at each gestational week show an increased risk as gestational age advances beyond the EDD.[30-32] Divon and associates[33] evaluated fetal and neonatal mortality rates in 181,524 accurately dated full-term, late-term, and postterm pregnancies. A significant increase in fetal mortality was detected from 41 weeks' gestation onward (odds ratios [ORs] of 1.5, 1.8, and 2.9 at 41, 42, and 43 weeks, respectively). Campbell and colleagues[17] performed a multivariate analysis of factors associated with perinatal death among 65,796 singleton postterm births (≥294 days). Three variables were identified as independent predictors of perinatal mortality: (1) birthweight lower than the 10th percentile for gestational age had a relative risk (RR) of 5.7 and a 95% confidence interval (CI) of 4.4 to 7.4; (2) maternal age 35 years or greater had an RR of 1.88 and a 95% CI of 1.2 to 2.9; and (3) birthweight at the 90th percentile for gestational age or above was associated with a modest protective effect for perinatal death (RR, 0.51; 95% CI, 0.26 to 1.0).

Many of these studies have used perinatal mortality rate (PMR), which has been suggested by Smith[34] and others to be an inappropriate assessment of risk to the fetus. The denominator in the calculation of the PMR is the number of deliveries.[34-37] As stated by Smith,[34] "Estimating the probability of an event requires that the number of events (numerator) be divided by the number of subjects at risk for that event (denominator)." Therefore it seems logical to calculate fetal mortality as fetal deaths per 1000 ongoing pregnancies, rather than per 1000 deliveries. When Hilder and colleagues[35] used ongoing pregnancies in a large retrospective study that included 171,527 births, higher rates of stillbirth were found. A nadir was seen at 41 weeks, but compared with 37 weeks' gestation, an eightfold increase in stillbirths at 43 weeks was reported (Fig. 36-1). Using the Scottish birth registry, Smith[37a] also found a significant increase in the risk of stillbirth from 37 weeks (0.4/1000) to 43 weeks (11.5/1000).

Several studies have examined the association of perinatal morbidity with postterm pregnancy. **Clausson and colleagues[38] evaluated a large Swedish database of term and postterm** (defined as ≥294 days) **singleton, normal neonates and showed that postterm pregnancies were associated with an increased frequency of neonatal convulsions, meconium aspiration syndrome, and Apgar scores of less than 4 at 5 minutes** (Table 36-1). Tunon and associates[39] compared neonatal intensive care unit (NICU) admission rates among 10,048 term pregnancies and 246 postterm pregnancies (≥296 days by both scan and LMP dates). Postterm pregnancy was associated with a significant increase in NICU admissions (OR, 2.05; 95% CI, 1.35 to 3.12).

Guidetti and colleagues[40] reported an increased incidence of perinatal morbidity at 41 weeks' gestation or greater. Maternal and fetal complications were evaluated in a large (n = 45,673) retrospective cohort study by Caughey and Musci.[41] These authors documented a significant increase in the rate of intrauterine fetal death (IUFD) beyond 41 weeks. They concluded that risks to both the mother and the infant increase as pregnancy progresses beyond 40 weeks' gestation.

Oligohydramnios

Oligohydramnios is a common finding in postterm pregnancies; it is presumably the result of fetal hypoxemia, which may result in altered renal perfusion and decreased urine production.[42]

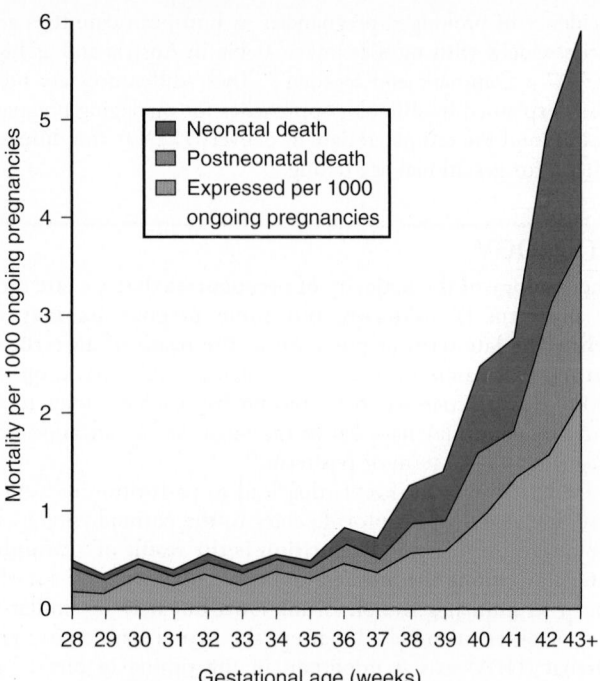

FIG 36-1 The summed mortality at each gestation for the rate of stillbirth (*red*), neonatal death (*blue*), and postneonatal death (*green*) expressed per 1000 ongoing pregnancies. (Modified from Hilder L, Costeloe K, Thilaganathan B. Prolonged pregnancy: evaluating gestation specific risks of fetal and infant mortality. *BJOG.* 1998;105:169.)

TABLE 36-1	NEONATAL MORBIDITY IN POSTTERM AVERAGE AND SGA INFANTS	
COMPLICATIONS	**TERM AGA NEONATES***
Convulsions	
Term SGA	2.3 (1.6-3.4)
Postterm AGA	1.5 (1.2-2.0)
Postterm SGA	3.4 (1.5-7.6)
Meconium Aspiration	
Term SGA	2.4 (1.6-3.4)
Postterm AGA	3.0 (2.6-3.7)
Postterm SGA	1.6 (0.5-5.0)
Apgar Score <4 at 5 min	
Term SGA	2.2 (1.4-3.4)
Postterm AGA	2.0 (1.5-2.5)
Postterm SGA	3.6 (1.5-8.7)

Modified from Clausson B, Cnattinguis S, Axelsson O. Outcomes of post-term births: the role of fetal growth restriction and malformations. *Obstet Gynecol.* 1999;94:758.
*Values are presented as odds ratios (confidence interval).
AGA, average for gestational age; *SGA,* small for gestational age.

Doppler studies of renal blood flow are conflicting.[43,44] Thus the etiology of oligohydramnios in postterm pregnancies is still debated.

Regardless of the pathophysiology of oligohydramnios in postterm pregnancies, in a setting of oligohydramnios, the risk of perinatal morbidity and mortality is increased.[45] The importance of oligohydramnios was identified by Leveno and coworkers,[46] who used its presence to explain the increased incidence of abnormal antepartum and intrapartum fetal heart rate (FHR) abnormalities seen in prolonged pregnancies. These authors suggested that prolonged FHR decelerations that represented cord compression preceded 75% of cesarean deliveries for fetal jeopardy. The association between a reduced amniotic fluid index (AFI) and variable decelerations is well documented and is likely related to cord compression.[47,48] Meconium passage in amniotic fluid has also been associated with oligohydramnios, and it is postulated that the hypoxemia may result in rectal sphincter relaxation. Some studies have shown meconium-stained fluid as high as 29% in postterm pregnancies complicated by oligohydramnios.[49] See Chapter 35 for further discussion of oligohydramnios.

A prospective, blinded observational study of 1584 pregnancies was performed by Morris and colleagues[50] to assess the usefulness of ultrasound assessment of amniotic fluid in the prediction of adverse outcome in prolonged pregnancies. The authors demonstrated that an AFI of less than 5 cm, but not a single deepest vertical pocket less than 2 cm, was significantly associated with birth asphyxia or meconium aspiration. In addition, a significant association was found between an AFI of less than 5 cm and fetal distress in labor, cord arterial pH less than 7.0, and low Apgar scores.

The presence of oligohydramnios is often cited as an indication for delivery of pregnancies that reach term gestation or beyond. Importantly, no large, prospective, randomized studies have documented the benefits of delivery in this setting. **Still, given the well-described association between oligohydramnios and adverse pregnancy outcome at or beyond term, delivery is a reasonable choice for patients with oligohydramnios.**

Fetal Growth

The risk of macrosomia has been shown to increase with advancing gestational age, although the majority of prolonged pregnancies are appropriately grown. In a sample of 7000 pregnancies between 39 and 42 weeks, McLean and coworkers[51] found an increase in both fetal weight and head circumference. Eden and associates[52] observed that, compared with term pregnancies, postterm pregnancies have a twofold increase in the risk for macrosomia; and in these pregnancies, macrosomia was associated with a greater risk of operative delivery and shoulder dystocia leading to fetal injury.

Chervenak and colleagues[54] investigated the use of ultrasound to evaluate the estimated fetal weight (EFW) in pregnancies greater than 41 weeks and also found an increased incidence of fetal weight greater than 4000 g. They also showed an increase in the risk of cesarean delivery (22%) because of protracted and arrested labors when compared with nonmacrosomic infants (10%; $P < .01$). The positive and negative predictive values were 70% and 87%, respectively. However, a similar study of pregnancies at 41 weeks or greater found an absolute error of approximately 8% and a positive predictive value of 64% when ultrasound was used to estimate fetal weight within 1 week of delivery.[54] **ACOG[53] has warned that the diagnosis of fetal macrosomia by ultrasound is not precise and that early induction of labor or cesarean delivery has not been shown to reduce the morbidity associated with fetal macrosomia.**

Postmaturity

Postmaturity, another complication of prolonged pregnancies, occurs in approximately 10% to 20% of such pregnancies.[55-57] The "postmature" infant has decreased subcutaneous fat and lacks lanugo and vernix. The features are similar to those of IUGR, and some authors believe that postmaturity is really another manifestation of IUGR. Postmaturity is also associated with an increased incidence of meconium-stained fluid.

Meconium

Meconium-stained fluid can be seen at any gestational age, although several studies have documented a significantly increased risk of meconium-stained fluid in postterm pregnancies. Meconium aspiration is a serious neonatal condition that results in decreased lung compliance, abnormal production of surfactant, and a chemical pneumonitis (see Chapter 22).

MATERNAL COMPLICATIONS

Prolonged pregnancies are also associated with significant risk to the mother. Not only is anxiety significant as the pregnancy advances beyond the EDD but the risk of maternal morbidity during the intrapartum period is also increased. Caughey and colleagues[58] studied 119,254 women who delivered at 37 weeks and beyond and found an increased risk in significant perineal laceration (OR, 1.19; 95% CI, 1.09 to 1.22), chorioamnionitis (OR, 1.32; 95% CI, 1.21 to 1.44), endomyometritis (OR, 1.46; 95% CI, 1.14 to 1.87), postpartum hemorrhage (OR, 1.21; 95% CI, 1.10 to 1.32), and cesarean delivery (OR, 1.28; 95% CI, 1.20 to 1.36). The indications for cesarean delivery in this study were nonreassuring FHR and cephalopelvic disproportion.

MANAGEMENT

Accurate assessment of gestational age is paramount in the management of late-term and postterm pregnancies. When ultrasound is used to confirm menstrual dating, the incidence of late-term and postterm pregnancies and unnecessary interventions are decreased.[59] Because late-term and postterm pregnancies have an increased risk of fetal mortality, modern management includes the use of antenatal fetal surveillance and carefully timed intervention.

Antenatal Surveillance

Given the increased risk of stillbirth, antenatal surveillance is recommended in the management of prolonged and postterm pregnancies. Testing options for fetal surveillance include monitoring of fetal kick counts, nonstress test (NST), contraction stress test (CST), biophysical profile (BPP), and modified biophysical profile (NST and AFI). Few data are available with adequate power to assess the timing of initiation or frequency of fetal testing in prolonged pregnancies. **However, based on the studies on perinatal morbidity and mortality discussed above, it would seem prudent to initiate fetal testing no later than 41 weeks of gestation.** A number of small studies suggest that twice-weekly antepartum testing is superior to once a week in prolonged pregnancies. Johnson and associates[60] reported results on twice-weekly testing with BPP in 293 patients followed beyond 42 weeks. No stillbirths were observed in this small series.

No large randomized controlled trials (RCTs) have compared different modalities of fetal surveillance in prolonged pregnancies. One RCT of 145 pregnancies beyond 42 weeks compared BPP with modified BPP (mBPP).[61] This study found a significant increase in abnormal testing in the mBPP group (42% vs. 20.5%, OR, 3.5; 99% CI, 1.3 to 9.1) but no difference in cord blood gases and neonatal outcome between the two groups. Studies have not shown one modality of antepartum surveillance to be superior to another.[61]

ACOG proposed that amniotic fluid volume (AFV) should be assessed when surveillance is initiated for late-term

pregnancies because oligohydramnios has been associated with abnormal fetal heart tracings, umbilical cord compression, and meconium-stained fluid. Chamberlain and coworkers[62] studied 7582 complicated pregnancies and found an increase in the risk of fetal demise with decreased amniotic fluid.

A paucity of data are available to demonstrate improved neonatal outcomes in postterm pregnancies when testing is used. Still, given the well-described increase in stillbirth in postterm pregnancies, **ACOG currently recommends the initiation of fetal surveillance at 41 weeks or beyond with assessment of AFV.**[3]

Umbilical artery Doppler measurements are sometimes used in cases of suspected placental insufficiency, and hence it might be imagined that this modality could be useful in postterm pregnancies. However, umbilical artery Doppler measurements have not been shown to be useful in the management of prolonged pregnancies.[63]

Expectant Management Versus Induction of Labor

Until the recent ACOG guidelines, expectant management was acceptable when the cervix was unfavorable. **New evidence, as discussed below, supports the induction of labor after $42^{0/7}$ weeks and by $42^{6/7}$ weeks to decrease the risk of perinatal morbidity and mortality,** and it may be considered for pregnancies between $41^{0/7}$ weeks and $41^{6/7}$ weeks.

Several clinical trials have compared induction of labor to expectant management in pregnancies that have progressed beyond their EDD. Hannah and associates[64] performed one of the largest clinical trials, wherein 3407 pregnant women were randomized at 41 weeks to induction or expectant management with fetal surveillance. Delivery was indicated if the pregnancy reached 44 weeks or if fetal compromise was evident. No difference was reported in the perinatal mortality and neonatal morbidity, although the rate of cesarean delivery was increased in the expectantly managed group. No cases of fetal demise were reported in the induction group, and two were reported in the expectantly managed group.

Another RCT of 440 uncomplicated pregnancies performed by the National Institute of Child Health and Human Development (NICHD) Network of Maternal-Fetal Medicine Units compared induction at 42 weeks versus expectant management until cervical effacement, dilation, or evidence of fetal compromise was apparent.[65] The primary outcome was perinatal or maternal death or a composite of variables for perinatal morbidity. Secondary outcomes for this trial included cesarean delivery, maternal infection, blood transfusion, severe variable or late decelerations, and a 5-minute Apgar score less than 4. No differences were detected in primary outcome or rates of cesarean delivery. The study concluded that either induction or expectant management at 42 weeks was deemed acceptable practice.

More recently, Sanchez-Ramos and colleagues[66] published a meta-analysis that included 16 RCTs and 6588 patients and found a 20% rate of cesarean delivery in uncomplicated pregnancies induced at 41 weeks compared with 22% in the expectantly managed group. A nonsignificant but numerically lower perinatal mortality rate was reported for the induction group (0.09% vs. 0.33%, OR, 0.41; 95% CI, 0.14 to 1.18). They also found no differences in NICU admission and meconium aspiration.

The most recent Cochrane review,[67] updated in 2012, is a meta-analysis of 22 RCTs. The review included 9383 patients and looked at the potential benefits or harms of labor induction

at or beyond 40 weeks' gestation versus expectant management. The primary outcome was perinatal mortality, which included IUFD and neonatal death in the first week of life. Labor induction was associated with a small but significant reduction in perinatal death (RR, 0.31; 95% CI, 0.12 to 0.88) with no impact on the rate of cesarean delivery (RR, 0.89; 95% CI, 0.81 to 0.97). **This Cochrane meta-analysis suggests that induction may yield slightly improved perinatal outcomes.**

Labor Induction

Several studies have addressed membrane sweeping as a method for labor induction in an attempt to reduce the occurrence of postterm pregnancies (see Chapter 13). Membrane sweeping is the digital separation of the membranes from the lower uterine segment during a cervical examination. This practice is thought to increase the levels of endogenous prostaglandin, which results in uterine contractions. An RCT conducted by de Miranda and colleagues[68] enrolled 742 patients at 41 weeks' gestation and randomized them to serial sweeping of membranes every 48 hours until 42 weeks, or until labor was initiated, or to no intervention. They found a decrease in the risk of postterm pregnancy in the first group; 23% were postterm (RR, 0.57; 95% CI, 0.46 to 0.71) compared with 41% in the no-intervention group. The number needed to treat (NNT) for this trial was six patients. Previously published trials have not shown a significant difference, but these studies limited membrane sweeping to a single episode.[69,70] The most recent Cochrane review of trials that enrolled pregnant patients from 38 to 41 weeks to membrane sweeping found a reduced rate of pregnancies that continued past 41 weeks' gestation, with an NNT of eight patients.[71] Although this practice may be effective in some pregnant patients, the procedure is known to cause maternal discomfort and bleeding. Also, evidence is limited regarding membrane sweeping in women colonized with group B *Streptococcus*. **Thus patients who can consider this option should be selected carefully and counseled appropriately.**

Some have attempted to predict the likelihood of successful induction using transvaginal ultrasound of the cervix and fetal fibronectin. Pandis and colleagues[72] compared Bishop score with ultrasound cervical assessment and found cervical length to be more predictive of a successful labor induction than Bishop score (with a sensitivity and specificity of 87% and 71% vs. 58% and 27%, respectively). Although the results of this study are promising, transvaginal ultrasound assessment of the cervix to predict induction success is not commonly used. Attempts to evaluate the role of a fetal fibronectin in cervical secretions as a predictor of the onset of spontaneous labor have been inconclusive. In fact, Rozenberg and associates[73] have shown that the spontaneous onset of labor within 7 days of evaluation is predicted by a Bishop score greater than 7 and a cervical length less than 25 mm but not with a positive fetal fibronectin (fFN).

Prostaglandins are most commonly used for labor induction in patients with an unfavorable cervix or a Bishop score less than 6. Studies have shown both misoprostol (prostaglandin E1 [PGE$_1$]) and dinoprostone (prostaglandin E2 [PGE$_2$]) to be efficacious in postterm pregnancy, and either preparation is acceptable.[64,65,74]

LONG-TERM NEONATAL OUTCOMES

A paucity of information exists on neonates born at 42 weeks and later. Ting and coworkers[75] evaluated a population enrolled in the Collaborative Perinatal Study in Philadelphia and found that surviving children could not be differentiated from their matched controls either physically or mentally. Shime and colleagues[76] found similar results in children followed at 1 and 2 years of age. They assessed intelligence by the Griffiths Mental Development Scale and found no difference when these children were compared with those from term births. **Based on these small and older studies, no difference in long-term neonatal outcome is apparent.**

MULTIPLE GESTATION

No defined gestational age cutoff has been established to define a prolonged pregnancy in twin, triplet, or higher-order multiples. The average gestation lengths for twin, triplet, and quadruplet pregnancies are 36, 33, and 29 weeks, respectively. The nadir of stillbirth occurs at 38 weeks for twins and at 35 weeks for triplets, and it is unknown for quadruplets and higher-order multiples.[77] Intuitively, because we use rates of perinatal mortality to define these cutoffs for singletons, we should do the same for multiple gestations. No current strategies have been recommended as these pregnancies approach the above gestational ages, although **it would seem reasonable to utilize antenatal testing as these gestational ages approach and to accomplish delivery at the nadir of stillbirth risk** (see Chapter 32).

KEY POINTS

- Ultrasonography, preferably done in the first trimester, is the most accurate method with which to establish the EDD.

- No gestational cutoff has been established by which to define a prolonged pregnancy in multiple gestations. The risk for stillbirth increases after 38 weeks in twins and after 35 weeks in triplets.

- Late-term and postterm pregnancies are associated with an increased risk for perinatal morbidity and mortality, oligohydramnios, macrosomia, postmaturity, and maternal morbidity.

- It seems prudent to initiate antenatal fetal surveillance at 41 weeks in a normal, uncomplicated pregnancy in the absence of IUGR.

- Antenatal fetal surveillance at 41 weeks should include an mBPP at least once a week.

- If the cervix is favorable at 41 weeks, induction of labor can be considered.

- Delivery after $42^{0/7}$ weeks and by $42^{6/7}$ weeks is recommended based on the small but increased risk of perinatal morbidity and mortality.

- Either prostaglandin preparation, PGE_1 or PGE_2, can be used for induction of the postterm pregnancy.

REFERENCES

1. Ballantyne JW. The problem of the postmature infant. *J Obstet Gynaecol Br Emp*. 1902;2:521.
2. Clifford SH. Postmaturity with placental dysfunction, clinical syndrome and pathologic findings. *J Pediatr*. 1954;44:1.
3. American College of Obstetricians and Gynecologists. Practice bulletin no. 146: Management of late-term and postterm pregnancies. *Obstet Gynecol*. 2014;124(2 Pt 1):390-396.
4. World Health Organization (WHO). Recommended definition terminology and format for statistical tables related to the perinatal period and rise of a new certification for cause of perinatal deaths. Modifications recommended by FIGO as amended, October 14, 1976. *Acta Obstet Gynecol Scand*. 1977;56:347.
5. Federation of Gynecology and Obstetrics (FIGO). *Report of the FIGO Subcommittee on Perinatal Epidemiology and Health Statistics Following a Workshop in Cairo, November 11-18, 1984*. London: International Federation of Gynecology and Obstetrics; 1986:54.
6. McClure-Brown JC. Postmaturity. *JAMA*. 1963;186(12):81.
7. ACOG Committee Opinion No 579. Definition of term pregnancy. *Obstet Gynecol*. 2013;122:1139-1140.
8. Spong CY. Defining "Term" Pregnancy Recommendations From the Defining Term Pregnancy Workgroup. *JAMA*. 2013;309(23):2445.
9. Martin JA, Hamilton BE, Osterman MJ, et al. *Births: Final data for 2012. National vital statistics reports*. Vol. 62 no 9. Hyattsville, MD: National Center for Health Statistics; 2013.
10. Zeitlin J, Blondel B, Alexander S, Bréart G, PERISTAT Group. Variation in rates of postterm birth in Europe: reality or artefact? *BJOG*. 2007; 114(9):1097.
11. Gardosi J. Dating of pregnancy: time to forget the last menstrual period. *Ultrasound Obstet Gynecol*. 1997;9:367.
12. Norwitz ER, Robinson JN, Challis JR. The control of labor. *N Engl J Med*. 1999;341:660.
13. Challis JR, Sloboda D, Matthews SG, et al. The fetal placental hypothalamic-pituitary-adrenal (HPA) axis, parturition and postnatal health. *Mol Cell Endocrinol*. 2001;185(1–2):135.
14. Nathanielsz PW. Endocrine mechanisms of parturition. *Annu Rev Physiol*. 1978;40:411.
15. Naeye RL, Blanc WA. Organ and body growth in anencephaly: A quantitative, morphological study. *Arch Pathol*. 1971;91(2):140.
16. Rabe T, Hösch R, Runnebaum B. Sulfatase deficiency in the human placenta: clinical findings. *Biol Res Pregnancy Perinatol*. 1983;4(3):95.
17. Campbell MK, Ostbye T, Irgens LM. Post-term birth: risk factors and outcomes in a 10-year cohort of Norwegian births. *Obstet Gynecol*. 1997; 89:543.
18. Mogren I, Stenlund H, Högberg U. Recurrence of prolonged pregnancy. *Int J Epidemiol*. 1999;28:253.
19. Olesen AW, Basso O, Olsen J. Risk of recurrence of prolonged pregnancy. *BMJ*. 2003;326:476.
20. Kistka ZA, Palomar L, Boslaugh SE, et al. Risk for postterm delivery after previous postterm delivery. *Am J Obstet Gynecol*. 2007;196:241.
21. Divon MY, Ferber A, Nisell H, Westgren M. Male gender predisposes to prolongation of pregnancy. *Am J Obstet Gynecol*. 2002;187:1081.
22. Laursen M, Billie C, Olesen AW, et al. Genetic influence on prolonged gestation: a population-based Danish twin study. *Am J Obstet Gynecol*. 2004;190:489.
23. Stotland NE, Washington AE, Caughey AB. Prepregnancy body mass index and the length of gestation at term. *Am J Obstet Gynecol*. 2007;197:378.
24. Munster K, Schmidt L, Helm P. Length and variation in the menstrual cycle: a cross-sectional study from a Danish county. *Br J Obstet Gynaecol*. 1992;99(5):422.
25. Creinin MD, Keverline S, Meyn LA. How regular is regular? An analysis of menstrual cycle regularity. *Contraception*. 2004;70(4):289.
26. Boyd ME, Usher RH, McLean FH, Kramer MS. Obstetric consequences of postmaturity. *Am J Obstet Gynecol*. 1988;158:334.
27. Gardosi J, Vanner T, Francis A. Gestational age and induction of labor for prolonged pregnancy. *Br J Obstet Gynaecol*. 1997;104:792.
28. Nguyen TH, Larsen T, Engholm G, Møller H. Evaluation of ultrasound-estimated date of delivery in 17,450 spontaneous singleton births: do we need to modify Naegele's rule? *Ultrasound Obstet Gynecol*. 1999;14:23.
29. Bennett KA, Crane JM, O'Shea P, et al. First trimester ultrasound screening is effective in reducing postterm labor induction rates: a randomized controlled trial. *Am J Obstet Gynecol*. 2004;190:1077.
30. Ingemarsson I, Kallen K. Stillbirths and rate of neonatal deaths in 76,761 postterm pregnancies in Sweden, 1982-1991: a register study. *Acta Obstet Gynecol Scand*. 1997;76:658.
31. Yudkin PL, Wood L, Redman CW. Risk of unexplained stillbirth at different gestational ages. *Lancet*. 1987;1:1192.
32. Feldman GB. Prospective risk of stillbirth. *Obstet Gynecol*. 1992;79:547.
33. Divon MY, Haglund B, Nisell H, et al. Fetal and neonatal mortality in the post-term pregnancy: the impact of gestational age and fetal growth restriction. *Am J Obstet Gynecol*. 1998;178:726.

34. Smith GC. Estimating risks of perinatal death. *Am J Obstet Gynecol.* 2005;192:17.

35. Hilder L, Costeloe K, Thilaganathan B. Prolonged pregnancy: evaluating gestation-specific risks of fetal and infant mortality. *Br J Obstet Gynaecol.* 1998;105:169.

36. Cotzias CS, Paterson-Brown S, Fisk NM. Prospective risk of unexplained stillbirth in singleton pregnancies at term: population based analysis. *BMJ.* 1999;319:287.

37. Huang DY, Usher RH, Kramer MS, et al. Determinants of unexplained antepartum fetal deaths. *Obstet Gynecol.* 2000;95:215.

37a. Smith GC. Life-table analysis of the risk of perinatal death at term and post term in singleton pregnancies. *Am J Obstet Gynecol.* 2001;184: 489-496.

38. Clausson B, Cnattingius S, Axelsson O. Outcomes of post-term births: the role of fetal growth restriction and malformations. *Obstet Gynecol.* 1999; 94:758.

39. Tunon K, Eik-Nes SH, Grottum P. Fetal outcome in pregnancies defined as post-term according to the last menstrual period estimate, but not according to the ultrasound estimate. *Ultrasound Obstet Gynecol.* 1999;14:12.

40. Guidetti DA, Divon MY, Langer O. Postdate fetal surveillance: is 41 weeks too early? *Am J Obstet Gynecol.* 1989;161:91.

41. Caughey AB, Musci TJ. Complications of term pregnancies beyond 37 weeks of gestation. *Obstet Gynecol.* 2004;103:57.

42. Nicolaides KH, Peters MT, Vyas S, et al. Relation of rate of urine production to oxygen tension in small for gestational age fetuses. *Am J Obstet Gynecol.* 1990;162:387.

43. Gresham EL, Rankin JH, Makowski EL, Meschia G, Battaglia FC. An evaluation of fetal renal function in chronic sheep preparation. *J Clin Invest.* 1972;51:149.

44. Bar-Hava I, Divon MY, Sardo M, Barnhard Y. Is oligohydramnios in post-term pregnancy associated with redistribution of fetal blood flow? *Am J Obstet Gynecol.* 1995;173:519.

45. Phelan JP, Ahn MO, Smith CV, et al. Amniotic fluid index measurements during pregnancy. *J Reprod Med.* 1987;32:601.

46. Leveno KJ, Quirk JG Jr, Cunningham FG, et al. Prolonged pregnancy. I. Observations concerning the causes of fetal distress. *Am J Obstet Gynecol.* 1984;150:465.

47. Gabbe SG, Ettinger BB, Freeman RK, Martin CB. Umbilical cord compression associated with amniotomy: laboratory observations. *Am J Obstet Gynecol.* 1976;126:353.

48. Miyazaki FS, Taylor NA. Saline amnioinfusion for relief of variable or prolonged decelerations. A preliminary report. *Am J Obstet Gynecol.* 1983; 146:670.

49. Crowley P, O'Herlihy C, Boylan P. The value of ultrasound measurement of amniotic fluid volume in management of prolonged pregnancies. *Br J Obstet Gynaecol.* 1984;91:444.

50. Morris JM, Thompson K, Smithey J, et al. The usefulness of ultrasound assessment of amniotic fluid in predicting adverse outcome in prolonged pregnancy: a prospective blinded observational study. *Br J Obstet Gynecol.* 2003;110:989.

51. McLean FH, Boyd ME, Usher RH, Kramer MS. Post-term infants: too big or too small? *Am J Obstet Gynecol.* 1991;164:619.

52. Eden RD, Seifert LS, Winegar A, Spellacy WN. Perinatal characteristics of uncomplicated postdate pregnancies. *Obstet Gynecol.* 1987;69(3 Pt 1):296.

53. ACOG Practice Bulletin. *Fetal macrosomia, No. 22,* 2000.

54. Chervenak LJ, Divon MY, Hirsch J, et al. Macrosomia in the post-date pregnancy: is routine sonography screening indicated? *Am J Obstet Gynecol.* 1989;161:753.

55. Shime J, Librach CL, Gare DJ, Cook CJ. The influence of prolonged pregnancy on infant development at one and two years of age: a prospective controlled study. *Am J Obstet Gynecol.* 1986;154:341.

56. Vorherr H. Placental insufficiency in relation to postterm pregnancy and fetal postmaturity. Evaluation of fetoplacental function; management of postterm gravida. *Am J Obstet Gynecol.* 1975;123:67.

57. Mannino F. Neonatal complications of postterm gestation. *J Reprod Med.* 1988;33:271.

58. Caughey AB, Stotland NE, Washington AE, Escobar GJ. Maternal and obstetric complications of pregnancy are associated with increasing gestational age at term. *Am J Obstet Gynecol.* 2007;196:155.

59. Whitworth M, Bricker L, Neilson JP, Dowswell T. Ultrasound for fetal assessment in early pregnancy. *Cochrane Database Syst Rev.* 2010;(4): CD007058.

60. Johnson JM, Harman CR, Lange IR, Manning FA. Biophysical profile scoring in the management of the post term pregnancy: an analysis of 307 patients. *Am J Obstet Gynecol.* 1986;154:269.

61. Alfirevic Z, Walkinshaw SA. A randomized controlled trial of simple compared with complex antenatal fetal monitoring after 42 weeks gestation. *Br J Obstet Gynaecol.* 1995;102(8):638.

62. Chamberlain PF, Manning FA, Morrison I, et al. Ultrasound evaluation of amniotic fluid volume. I. The relationship of marginal and decreased amniotic fluid volumes to perinatal outcome. *Am J Obstet Gynecol.* 1984;150: 245.

63. Zimmermann P, Alback T, Koskinen J, et al. Doppler flow velocimetry of the umbilical artery, uteroplacental arteries and fetal middle cerebral artery in prolonged pregnancy. *Ultrasound Obstet Gynecol.* 1995;5:189.

64. Hannah ME, Hannah WJ, Hellman J, et al. Induction of labor as compared with serial antenatal monitoring in post-term pregnancies. A randomized controlled trial. The Canadian Multicenter Post-term Pregnancy Trial Group. *N Engl J Med.* 1992;327:1587.

65. The National Institute of Child Health and Human Development Network of Maternal Fetal Medicine Units. A clinical trial of induction of labor versus expectant management in post term pregnancy. *Am J Obstet Gynecol.* 1994;170:716.

66. Sanchez-Ramos L, Olivier F, Delke I, Kaunitz AM. Labor induction versus expectant management for postterm pregnancies: a systematic review with meta-analysis. *Obstet Gynecol.* 2003;101:1312.

67. Gülmezoglu AM, Crowther CA, Middleton P. Induction of labour for improving birth outcomes for women at or beyond term. *Cochrane Database Syst Rev.* 2012;(4):CD004945.

68. de Miranda E, van der Bom JG, Bonsel GJ, et al. Membrane sweeping and prevention of post-term pregnancy in low-risk pregnancies: a randomised controlled trial. *BJOG.* 2006;113(4):402.

69. Crane J, Bennett K, Young D, et al. The effectiveness of sweeping membranes at term: a randomized trial. *Obstet Gynecol.* 1997;89(4):586.

70. Wong SF, Hui SK, Choi H, Ho LC. Does sweeping of membranes beyond 40 weeks reduce the need for formal induction of labour? *BJOG.* 2002; 109(6):632.

71. Boulvain M, Stan CM, Irion O. Membrane sweeping for induction of labour. *Cochrane Database Syst Rev.* 2005;(1):CD000451.

72. Pandis GK, Papageorghiou AT, Ramanathan VG, et al. Preinduction sonographic measurement of cervical length in the prediction of successful induction. *Ultrasound Obstet Gynecol.* 2001;18:623.

73. Rozenberg P, Goffinet F, Hessabi M. Comparison of the Bishop score ultrasonographically measured cervical length, and fetal fibronectin assay in predicating time until delivery and type of delivery at term. *Am J Obstet Gynecol.* 2000;182:108.

74. Meydanli MM, Caliskan E, Burak F, et al. Labor induction post-term with 25 micrograms vs. 50 micrograms of intravaginal misoprostol. *Int J Gynaecol Obstet.* 2003;81(3):249.

75. Ting RV, Wang MH, Scott TF. The dysmature infant: associated factors and outcome at 7 years of age. *J Pediatr.* 1977;90:943.

76. Shime J, Librach CL, Gare DJ, Cook CJ. The influence of prolonged pregnancy on infant development at one and two years of age: a prospective controlled study. *Am J Obstet Gynecol.* 1986;154:341.

77. Luke B. Reducing fetal deaths in multiple births: optimal birthweights and gestational ages for infants of twin and triplet births. *Acta Genet Med Gemellol (Roma).* 1996;45:333.

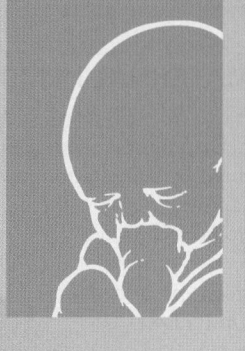

CHAPTER 37

Heart Disease in Pregnancy

JASON DEEN, SUCHITRA CHANDRASEKARAN, KAREN STOUT, and THOMAS EASTERLING

KEY ABBREVIATIONS

Activated partial thromboplastin time	aPTT	Myocardial infarction	MI
Acute respiratory distress syndrome	ARDS	New York Heart Association	NYHA
American College of Cardiology	ACC	Patent ductus arteriosus	PDA
Aortic diameter	AD	Peripartum cardiomyopathy	PPCM
Atrial septal defect	ASD	Positive end-expiratory pressure	PEEP
Body surface area	BSA	Pulmonary artery wedge pressure	PAWP
β-type natriuretic peptide	BNP	Pulmonary flow	Q_P
Cardiac index	CI	Pulmonary vascular resistance	PVR
Cardiac output	CO	Relative risk	RR
Central venous pressure	CVP	Right ventricle	RV
Congenital heart disease	CHD	Stroke volume	SV
Ejection fraction	EF	Systemic flow	Q_S
Electrocardiogram	ECG	Systemic vascular resistance	SVR
Heart rate	HR	Total peripheral resistance	TPR
International normalized ratio	INR	Transposition of the great arteries	TGA
Left ventricular outflow tract	LVOT	Unfractionated heparin	UFH
Low-molecular-weight heparin	LMWH	Ventricular septal defect	VSD
Mean arterial pressure	MAP		

Cardiovascular adaptations to pregnancy are well tolerated by healthy young women. However, these adaptations are of such magnitude that they can significantly compromise women with abnormal or damaged hearts. Without accurate diagnosis and appropriate care, heart disease in pregnancy can be a significant cause of maternal mortality and morbidity. Under more optimal conditions, many women with significant disease can experience good outcomes and should not necessarily be discouraged from becoming pregnant. This chapter develops an understanding of cardiovascular physiology as a basis for care of the pregnant woman with heart disease. Although published experience with more common conditions can be used to support these principles, information regarding many other conditions is limited to case reports. Data from case reports may, however, be biased toward more complicated cases with more adverse outcomes. The best care for women with heart disease is usually achieved from a thorough understanding of maternal cardiovascular physiology, knowledge of existing literature, and extensive clinical experience brought by a multidisciplinary team of clinicians.

MATERNAL HEMODYNAMICS

Hemodynamics refers to the relationship between blood pressure, cardiac output, and vascular resistance. Blood pressure is measured by auscultation, use of an automated cuff, or directly with an intraarterial catheter. Cardiac output is measured by dilutional techniques that require central venous access, by Doppler or two-dimensional (2-D) echocardiographic techniques, or by electrical impedance. Peripheral resistance is calculated using Ohm's law:

$$TPR = (MAP \times 80)/CO$$

where *TPR* is total peripheral resistance (in dyne · sec · cm^{-5}), *MAP* is mean arterial pressure (in millimeters of mercury [mm Hg]), and *CO* is cardiac output (in liters per minute).

Pregnancy and events unique to pregnancy, such as labor and delivery, are associated with significant and frequently predictable changes in these parameters. The hemodynamic changes of pregnancy, although well tolerated by an otherwise healthy woman, may be tolerated poorly by a woman with significant cardiac disease. Therefore the importance of understanding these changes and placing them in the context of a specific cardiac lesion cannot be overstated.

The maternal hemodynamics of 89 nulliparous women who remained normotensive throughout pregnancy are described in Figure 37-1.[1] MAP falls sharply in the first trimester and reaches a nadir by midpregnancy. Thereafter blood pressure increases slowly and reaches near nonpregnant levels by term. Cardiac output rises throughout the first and second trimesters and reaches a maximum by the middle of the third trimester. **In the supine position, a pregnant woman in the third trimester may experience significant hypotension as a result of venocaval occlusion by the gravid uterus.** In normal pregnancy, venocaval occlusion may produce symptoms such as diaphoresis, tachycardia, or nausea but will rarely result in significant complications. Fetal heart rate (FHR) decelerations may be observed but usually resolve when the mother, often spontaneously, shifts to a more comfortable position. Women with significant right or left ventricular outflow obstruction, such as aortic stenosis, may seriously decompensate in the supine position as a result of poor ventricular filling. Cardiac output (CO) is the product of heart rate (HR) and stroke volume (SV):

$$CO = HR \times SV$$

HR and SV increase as pregnancy progresses to the third trimester. After 32 weeks, SV falls, with the maintenance of CO becoming more and more dependent on HR. Vascular resistance falls in the first and early second trimesters. The magnitude of the fall is sufficient to offset the rise in CO, which results in a net decrease in blood pressure.

Labor, delivery, and the postpartum period are times of acute hemodynamic changes that may result in maternal decompensation. Labor itself is associated with pain and anxiety, and tachycardia is a normal response. Significant catecholamine release increases afterload. Each uterine contraction acutely redistributes 400 to 500 mL of blood from the uterus to the central circulation. In Figure 37-2, Robson and colleagues[2] describe the hemodynamic changes associated with unmedicated labor. **HR, blood pressure, and CO all increase with uterine contractions, and the magnitude of the change increases as labor advances.** Obstructive cardiac lesions impede the flow of blood through the heart, blunting the expected rise

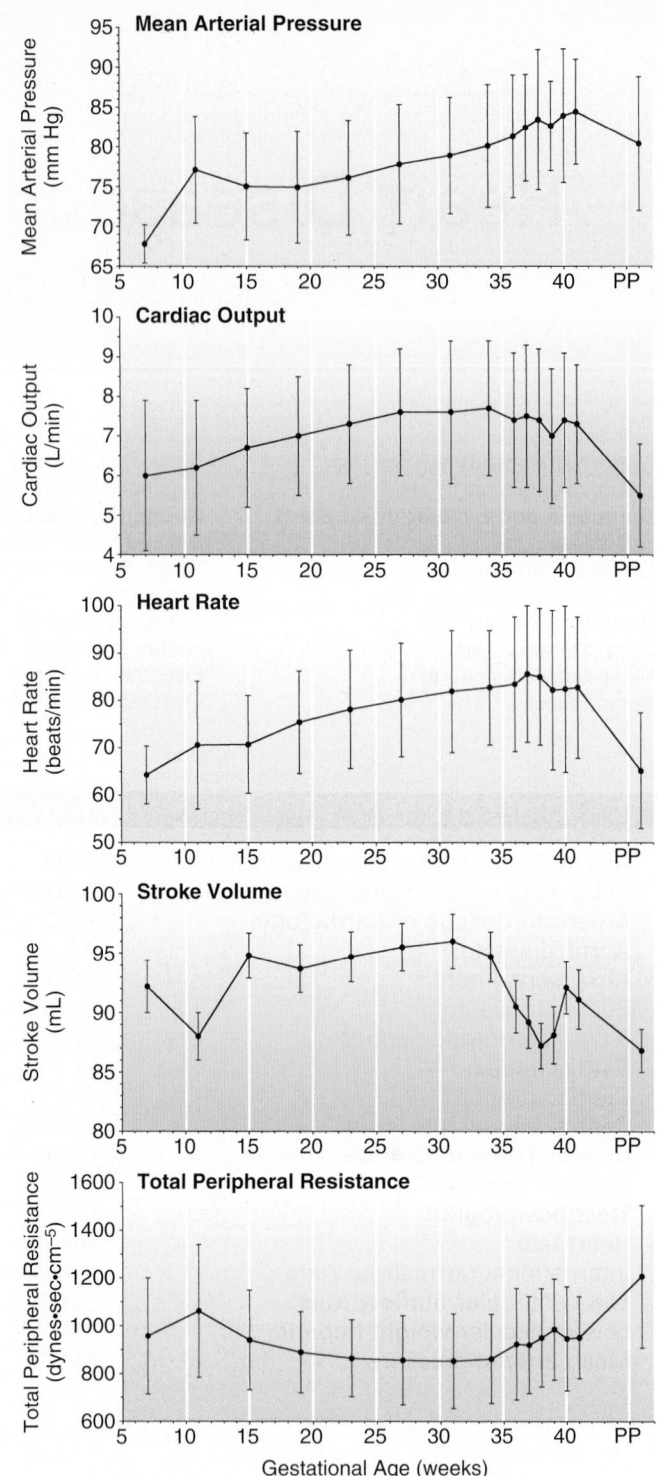

FIG 37-1 Changes in hemodynamic parameters throughout pregnancy (mean ± standard deviation). PP, postpartum.

in CO at the expense of increasing pulmonary pressures and pulmonary congestion. In Figure 37-3, intrapartum hemodynamic changes of a patient with aortic stenosis and a peak gradient of 160 mm Hg are shown.[3] In this individual, pulmonary pressures rise in parallel with uterine contractions.

Immediately after delivery, blood from the uterus is returned to the central circulation. In normal pregnancy, this compensatory mechanism protects against the hemodynamic effects that

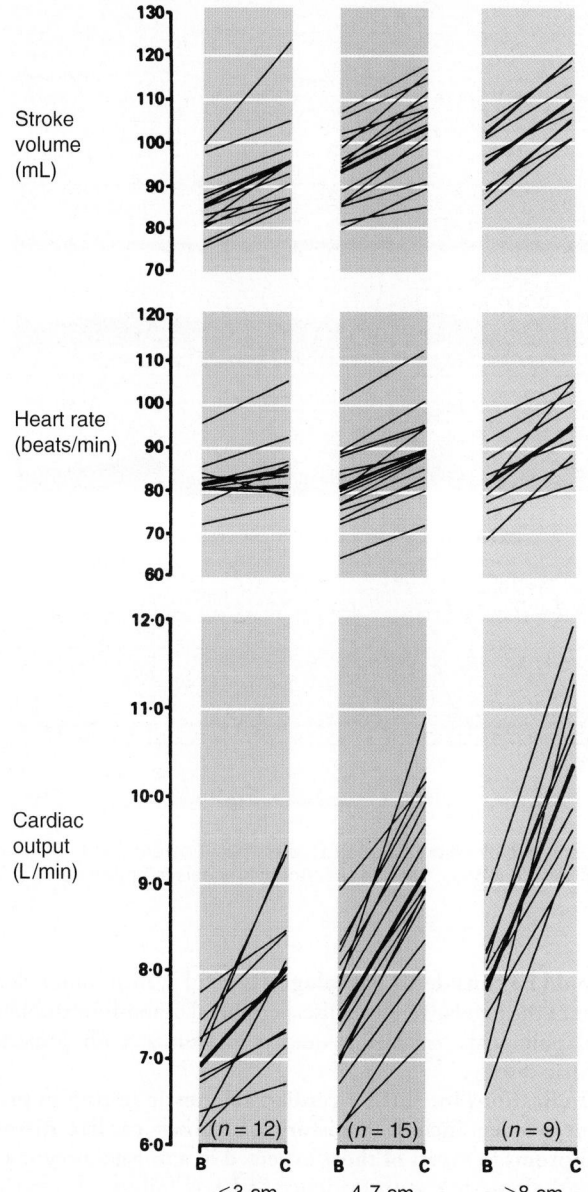

FIG 37-2 Changes in hemodynamic parameters at three different points during labor (≤3 cm, 4-7 cm, and ≥8 cm). Each line represents the change in an individual subject. B, before contraction; C, during contraction. (From Robson S, Dunlop W, Boys R, Hunter S. Cardiac output during labour. *BMJ*. 1987;295:1169.)

may accompany postpartum hemorrhage. **In the context of cardiac disease, this acute centralization of blood may increase pulmonary pressures and pulmonary congestion.**[4] During the first 2 postpartum weeks, extravascular fluid is mobilized, diuresis ensues, and vascular resistance increases, returning to nonpregnant norms. Decompensation during postpartum fluid mobilization is common in women with mitral stenosis. Volume loading coupled with vasoconstriction may also unmask maternal cardiomyopathy. Unsuspected cardiac disease may be diagnosed when a woman returns to the emergency department several days postpartum with dyspnea and oxygen desaturation. Maternal CO usually normalizes by 2 weeks postpartum.

Three key features of the maternal hemodynamic changes in pregnancy are particularly relevant to the management of

women with cardiac disease: **(1) increased CO, (2) increased HR, and (3) reduced vascular resistance.** In conditions such as mitral stenosis, in which CO is relatively fixed, the drive to achieve an elevated CO may result in pulmonary congestion. If a patient has an atrial septal defect (ASD), the incremental increase in systemic flow associated with pregnancy will be magnified in the pulmonary circulation to the extent that pulmonary flow exceeds systemic flow. If, for example, a shunt ratio of 3:1 is maintained in pregnancy, pulmonary flow may be as high as 20 L/min and may be associated with increasing dyspnea and potential desaturation.

Many cardiac conditions are HR dependent. Flow across a stenotic mitral valve is dependent on the proportion of time in diastole. Tachycardia reduces left ventricular (LV) filling and CO. Coronary blood flow is also dependent on the length of diastole. Patients with aortic stenosis have increased wall tension and therefore increased myocardial oxygen requirements. Tachycardia reduces coronary perfusion time in diastole while simultaneously further increasing myocardial oxygen requirements, and the resulting imbalance between oxygen demand and supply may precipitate myocardial ischemia. Patients with complex congenital heart disease (CHD) can experience significant tachyarrhythmias. The increasing HR in pregnancy may be associated with a worsening of tachyarrhythmias.

Reduction in vascular resistance may be beneficial to some patients, and afterload reduction reduces cardiac work. Cardiomyopathy, aortic regurgitation, and mitral regurgitation all benefit from reduced afterload. Alternatively, patients with intracardiac shunts, in which right and LV pressures are nearly equal when the patient is not pregnant, may reverse their shunt during pregnancy and may desaturate because of right-to-left shunting.

Blood Volume

Very early in the first trimester, pregnant women experience an expansion of renal blood flow and glomerular filtration rate (GFR). Filtered sodium increases by about 50%. Despite physiologic changes that would promote loss of salt and water and contraction of blood volume, **the pregnant woman will expand her blood volume by 40% to 50%.** In part, the stimulation to retain fluid may be a response to the fall in vascular resistance and reduction in blood pressure. The renin-angiotensin system is activated, and the plasma concentration of aldosterone is elevated. Although the simplicity of this explanation is attractive, the actual process is probably much more complicated.

As plasma volume expands, the hematocrit falls, and hematopoiesis is stimulated. Red cell mass will expand from 18% to 25% depending on the status of individual iron stores. Physiologic anemia with a maternal hematocrit between 30% and 35% does not usually complicate pregnancy in the context of maternal heart disease. More significant anemia, however, may increase cardiac work and induce tachycardia. Microcytosis due to iron deficiency may impair perfusion of the microcirculation of patients who are polycythemic because of cyanotic heart disease; this is because microcytic red blood cells are less deformable. Iron and folate supplementation may be appropriate.

In a similar fashion, serum albumin concentration falls by 22% despite an expansion of intravascular albumin mass by 20%. **As a result, serum oncotic pressure falls in parallel by 20% to about 19 mm Hg.**[5] In normal pregnancy, intravascular fluid balance is maintained by a fall in interstitial oncotic pressure. However, if LV filling pressure becomes elevated or if pulmonary vascular integrity is disrupted, pulmonary edema

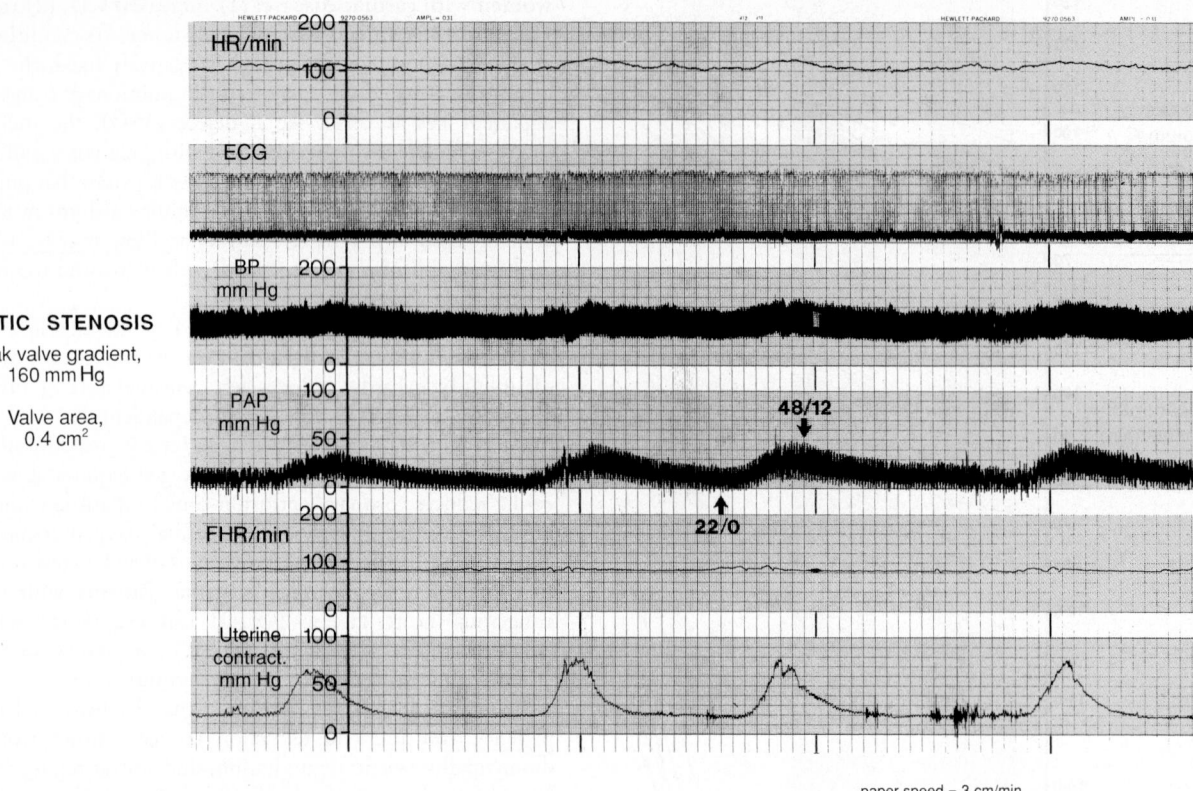

FIG 37-3 Hemodynamic monitoring of a patient with severe aortic stenosis in labor. BP, blood pressure; ECG, electrocardiogram; FHR, fetal heart rate; HR, heart rate; PAP, pulmonary artery pressure. (From Easterling T, Chadwick H, Otto C, Benedetti T. Aortic stenosis in pregnancy. *Obstet Gynecol.* 1988;72:113.)

will develop earlier in the disease process than in nonpregnant women.

DIAGNOSIS AND EVALUATION OF HEART DISEASE

Many women with heart disease have been diagnosed and treated before pregnancy. For example, in women with prior surgery for CHD, detailed historic information may be available. Others report only that they have a murmur or "a hole in their heart." Alternatively, heart disease may be diagnosed for the first time during pregnancy owing to symptoms precipitated by increased cardiac demands.

The classic symptoms of cardiac disease are palpitations, shortness of breath with exertion, and chest pain. Because these symptoms also may accompany normal pregnancy, a careful history is needed to determine whether the symptoms are out of proportion to the stage of pregnancy. Symptoms are of particular concern in a patient with other reasons to suspect underlying cardiac disease, such as being native to an area where rheumatic heart disease is prevalent.

A systolic flow murmur is present in 80% of pregnant women, most likely because of the increased flow volume in the aorta and pulmonary artery. Typically, a flow murmur is grade 1 or 2, midsystolic, loudest at the cardiac base, and not associated with any other abnormal physical examination findings. A normal physiologic split second heart sound is heard in patients with a flow murmur. **Any diastolic murmur and any systolic murmur that is loud** (grade 3/6 or higher) **or radiates to the carotids should be considered pathologic.** Careful evaluation for elevation of the jugular venous pulse, peripheral cyanosis or clubbing, and pulmonary crackles is needed in women with suspected cardiac disease.

Indications for further cardiac diagnostic testing in pregnant women include a history of known cardiac disease, symptoms in excess of those expected in a normal pregnancy, a pathologic murmur, evidence of heart failure on physical examination, or arterial oxygen desaturation in the absence of known pulmonary disease. The preferred next step in evaluation of pregnant women with suspected heart disease is transthoracic echocardiography. A chest radiograph is helpful only if congestive heart failure (CHF) is suspected. An electrocardiogram (ECG) may be nonspecific but could show changes suggestive of the underlying heart disease, such as right ventricular (RV) hypertrophy and biatrial enlargement, seen in patients with significant mitral stenosis. If symptoms are consistent with a cardiac arrhythmia, an event monitor or 24-hour ECG monitor may be indicated. Rarely, cardiac catheterization is needed for full diagnosis of valvular disease or CHD. The exception is an acute coronary syndrome during pregnancy, in which the risk for radiation exposure with cardiac catheterization is small compared with the benefit of early diagnosis and early revascularization to prevent myocardial infarction (MI).

Echocardiography provides detailed information on cardiac anatomy and physiology that allows optimal management of women with heart disease. Basic data obtained on echocardiography include left ventricular ejection fraction, pulmonary artery systolic pressure, qualitative evaluation of RV systolic function,

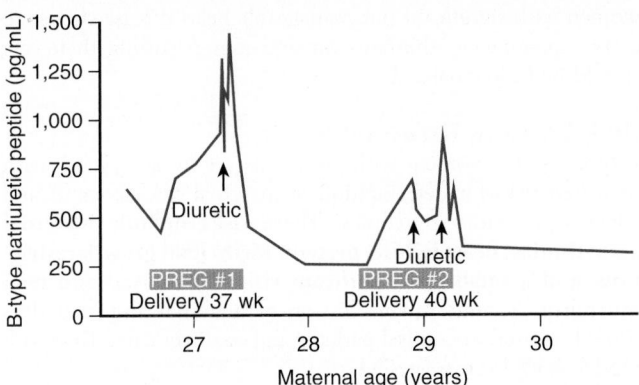

FIG 37-4 Changes in B-type natriuretic protein in a patient across two pregnancies.

and evaluation of valve anatomy and function. When valvular stenosis is present, the pressure gradient (ΔP) across the valve is calculated from the **Doppler-derived velocity (v) of flow across the valve ($\Delta P = 4v^2$).** Similarly, pulmonary artery systolic pressure can be calculated from the maximal Doppler velocity obtained across a tricuspid regurgitant jet.

Aortic valve area is calculated using the continuity equation. Stroke volume (SV) is calculated from the product of the cross-sectional area of the left ventricular outflow tract (LVOT) and the time-velocity integral derived from Doppler evaluation of the outflow tract. A time-velocity integral is then derived from the stenotic valve. Because the LVOT and the aortic valve are in continuity, SVs across each are equal. Therefore valve area can be derived by dividing the SV by the aortic valve time-velocity integral. Mitral valve area is measured directly by 2-D planimetry or by the Doppler pressure half-time method. In patients with congenital disease, detailed evaluation of anatomy and previous surgical repair is possible. When complex CHD is present or when image quality is suboptimal, transesophageal imaging provides improved image quality. Cardiac magnetic resonance imaging (MRI) may be used to define complex anatomy that is not well evaluated by echocardiography, but caution must be taken with magnetic resonance contrast agents such as gadolinium.

Serum levels of B-type (β) natriuretic peptide (BNP) and N-terminal pro-BNP (NT-proBNP) rise in response to volume loading conditions and have been used outside pregnancy as predictors of adverse outcomes in patients with cardiac disease. Serum levels of BNP of 100 pg/mL or less and NT-proBNP of 125 pg/mL or less have been demonstrated to have strong negative predictive values for adverse cardiac outcomes in pregnant women with heart disease.[6,7] In our practice, we use BNP to identify potentially adverse effects of volume loading in pregnancy and to guide therapy. Figure 37-4 describes the course of serum BNP levels across two pregnancies in a woman with hypertrophic cardiomyopathy. The time frame of each of the pregnancies is easily identifiable by a marked rise in BNP, and the impact of the initiation and dose adjustments in diuretic therapy with furosemide can be identified by sharp reductions in BNP.

GENERAL CARE

Management of cardiac disease in pregnancy is frequently complicated by unique social and psychological concerns. Women who had CHD as children may have experienced multiple hospitalizations and may be fearful of the medical environment. Some have been cautioned against pregnancy and therefore never expected to bear children. Women with rheumatic heart disease have frequently lived outside the traditional medical care system owing to conditions of poverty, immigration, and cultural differences. Care must be exercised to facilitate their access to care and their comfort with the environment of care. Their practitioner must be patient but persistent in the face of deviations from more traditional standards of compliance and medical care.

Deterioration in cardiac status during pregnancy is frequently insidious. Continuity of care with a single provider facilitates early intervention before overt decompensation. Regular visits should include particular attention to heart rate, weight gain, and oxygen saturation. An unexpected increase in weight may indicate the need for more aggressive outpatient therapy. A fall in oxygen saturation often precedes a clearly abnormal chest examination or radiograph. Regular use of a structured history of symptoms (Box 37-1) alerts the physician to a change in condition. A regular review of symptoms also educates patients and reinforces their collaborative roles as "partners in care."

The physiologic changes of pregnancy are usually continuous; therefore they offer adequate time for maternal compensation despite cardiac disease. **Intercurrent events superimposed on pregnancy in the context of maternal heart disease are usually responsible for acute decompensation.** During the antepartum period, the most common of these are febrile episodes. Screens for bacteriuria and vaccination against influenza and pneumococcus (*Streptococcus pneumoniae*) are appropriate. Patients should be instructed to report symptoms of upper respiratory infection, particularly fever. Many women with heart disease—but especially adolescents, recent immigrants, and those living in poverty—are also at risk for iron deficiency. Prophylaxis against anemia with iron and folate supplementation may decrease cardiac work.

One strategy is described in Box 37-2; these general principles for care are similar for most cardiac diagnoses. **Physiologically, the ideal labor for a woman with heart disease is short and pain free.** Although induction of labor facilitates organization of care and early pain control, shortening the duration of pregnancy by 1 or 2 weeks at the cost of a 2- or 3-day induction of labor is not worthwhile. Induction of labor with a favorable cervix is therefore preferred. Some patients with severe cardiac disease benefit from invasive hemodynamic monitoring with an arterial catheter and a pulmonary artery catheter. These methods are discussed in detail later. Cesarean delivery is usually reserved for obstetric indications. The American Heart Association (AHA) does not recommend routine antibiotic prophylaxis for the prevention of endocarditis, although it is optional in

BOX 37-2 STANDARD CARDIAC CARE FOR LABOR AND DELIVERY

1. Accurate diagnosis
2. Mode of delivery based on obstetric indications
3. Medical management initiated early in labor
   - Prolonged labor avoided
   - Induction with a favorable cervix
4. Maintenance of hemodynamic stability
   - Invasive hemodynamic monitoring when required
   - Initial, compensated hemodynamic reference point
   - Specific emphasis based on particular cardiac condition
5. Avoidance of pain and hemodynamic responses
   - Epidural analgesia with narcotic/low-dose local technique
6. Consideration for prophylactic antibiotics when at risk for endocarditis
7. Avoidance of maternal pushing
   - Caudal block for dense perineal anesthesia
   - Low forceps or vacuum delivery
8. Avoidance of maternal blood loss
   - Proactive management of the third stage
   - Early but appropriate fluid replacement
9. Early volume management postpartum
   - Often careful but aggressive diuresis

high-risk patients having a vaginal delivery. Because bacteremia is common at the time of vaginal delivery and cesarean delivery,[8] many practitioners will provide antibiotic prophylaxis in all patients at risk. In contrast to AHA recommendations, compelling arguments in support of broad use of antibiotic prophylaxis have been made, citing limited large-scale studies that support the recommendations and the high cost and risk associated with endocarditis.[9]

Women with significant heart disease should be counseled before pregnancy regarding the risk of pregnancy, interventions that may be required, and potential risks to the fetus. However, women with significant uncorrected disease often present with an ongoing established pregnancy. In this situation, the risks and benefits of termination of pregnancy versus those of continuing a pregnancy should be addressed. **The decision to become pregnant or carry a pregnancy in the context of maternal disease is a balance of two forces: the objective medical risk, including the uncertainty of that estimate, and the value of the birth of a child to an individual woman and her partner.** The first goal of counseling is to educate the patient. Only a few cardiac diseases represent an overwhelming risk for maternal mortality: Eisenmenger syndrome, pulmonary hypertension with RV dysfunction, and Marfan syndrome with significant aortic dilation and severe LV dysfunction. Most other conditions require aggressive management and significant disruption in lifestyle. Intercurrent events such as antepartum pneumonia or obstetric hemorrhage pose the greatest risk for initiating life-threatening events; fastidious care can reduce, but does not eliminate, the risk for these events. Maternal CHD increases the risk for CHD in the fetus from 1% to about 4% to 6%.[9,10] Marfan syndrome and some forms of hypertrophic cardiomyopathy are inherited as autosomal-dominant conditions, and offspring of these women carry a 50% chance of inheriting the disease. The second goal of counseling is to help each woman integrate the medical information into her individual value system and her individual desire to become a mother. Many

women with significant but manageable heart disease choose to carry a pregnancy. The basis for decisions regarding their care should be individualized.

Risk-Scoring Strategies

Pregnancy in women with heart disease is associated with increased risks for deterioration of maternal cardiac status and adverse pregnancy outcomes. **These risks include maternal arrhythmias, heart failure, preterm birth, fetal growth restriction, and a small but significant risk of maternal and fetal mortality.** Accurate quantification of maternal and fetal risks should be used to counsel patients and to direct care. Three risk models have been suggested.

The Cardiac Disease in Pregnancy (CARPREG) score was derived from a prospective descriptive study of 562 pregnant women with cardiac disease that included congenital or acquired lesions and arrhythmias.[11] The scoring system was created to estimate the risk of experiencing a primary cardiac event. The predictors in this scoring system include (1) a prior cardiac event—heart failure, transient ischemic attack, or stroke before pregnancy; (2) baseline New York Heart Association (NYHA) class greater than II or cyanosis; (3) mitral valve area less than 2 cm^2, aortic valve area less than 1.5 cm^3, or peak LVOT gradient greater than 30 mm Hg by echocardiography; and (4) reduced systemic ventricular systolic function with an ejection fraction (EF) of less than 40%.

The ZAHARA (*Zwangerschap bij Aangeboren Hartafwijkingen* [Pregnancy In Congenital Heart Disease]) score was derived from a nationwide database of 1302 pregnant women with CHD.[12] Predictors identified to be associated with maternal cardiac complications included (1) prior arrhythmia, (2) NYHA class III or IV, (3) LVOT gradient greater than 50 mm Hg or aortic valve area less than 1.0 cm^2, (4) mechanical valve prosthesis, (5) systemic atrioventricular (AV) valve regurgitation (moderate/severe), (6) pulmonary AV valve regurgitation (moderate to severe), (7) cardiac medication prior to pregnancy, and (8) cyanotic heart disease, both corrected and uncorrected. This study also externally validated the prior CARPREG study and noted that the CARPREG score overestimated the risk.

The modified World Health Organization (WHO) classification uses four categories determined largely by diagnosis: *class I* includes uncomplicated, mild pulmonary stenosis; *class II* comprises unoperated ASD, ventricular septal defect (VSD), and repaired tetralogy of Fallot; *class III* includes mechanical valves, systemic right ventricle, Fontan circulation, unrepaired cyanotic heart disease, other complex CHD, Marfan syndrome with an aorta 40 to 45 mm in width or bicuspid aortic valve with an aorta 45 to 50 mm; and *class IV* describes pulmonary hypertension/Eisenmenger syndrome, systemic EF less than 30%, systemic dysfunction of NYHA class III or IV, severe mitral stenosis, severe symptomatic aortic stenosis, Marfan syndrome with aorta greater than 45 mm, bicuspid valve with aorta greater than 50 mm, or severe coarctation.[13]

The ZAHARA II study was performed to validate and compare CARPREG, ZAHARA I, and the modified WHO risk models for pregnant women with CHD.[14] ZAHARA II enrolled 213 women and included patients only with congenital structural heart disease. Overall, primary cardiovascular events were observed in 22 of the pregnancies (10.3%). The most frequent events included clinically significant arrhythmias, followed by heart failure and thrombotic events. It was noted that the ZAHARA I and CARPREG scores overestimated risk. The modified WHO classification performed as the best available risk-assessment model for estimating cardiovascular risk.

From the scoring systems, common features can be identified that individually or collectively may predict adverse outcome. For patients with several risk factors, the impact on outcome may be more than additive, as suggested by the structures of the scoring systems: (1) prior cardiac event, (2) NYHA class III or IV, (3) LVOT obstruction, (4) reduced systemic EF, (5) mechanical prosthesis, (6) moderate to severe AV valve regurgitation, (7) cardiac medications prior to pregnancy, and (8) cyanotic heart disease. The WHO system based on diagnoses incorporates risk associated with pulmonary hypertension and RV dysfunction, severe mitral stenosis, dilated aortas, and single-ventricle repairs not specifically captured by CARPREG or ZAHARA.

Although it seems optimal to be able to assign a direct risk score to a woman when counseling her during pregnancy, all of the studies above highlight the challenge in being able to create the ideal scoring system. Each category of CHD carries varied risks based on maternal hemodynamic and cardiovascular function findings. It is therefore important to understand the different risk scores; although ultimately, the individual cardiovascular functional parameters and overall hemodynamic stability of each patient must be understood to provide the most individualized care for each woman.

VALVULAR DISEASE

The American College of Cardiology (ACC) and the AHA have published guidelines for the management of valvular heart disease, including some guidelines for management during pregnancy.[15] These guidelines create a general framework for preconceptional care and care during pregnancy, realizing that treatment of a specific patient must be individualized.

Mitral Stenosis

Mitral stenosis is most commonly caused by rheumatic heart disease and is the most common acquired valvular lesion in pregnant women. Valvular dysfunction progresses continuously throughout life. Deterioration may be accelerated by recurrent episodes of rheumatic fever, an immunologic response to group A β-hemolytic Streptococcus (GBS) infections. The incidence of rheumatic fever in a population is heavily influenced by conditions of poverty and crowding. These same individuals are at risk for having reduced access and use of health care resources and may present undiagnosed or untreated.

Patients with asymptomatic mitral stenosis have a 10-year survival rate of greater than 80%. Once a patient is significantly symptomatic, the 10-year survival rate without treatment is less than 15%. In the presence of pulmonary hypertension, mean survival falls to less than 3 years. Death is due to progressive pulmonary edema, right-sided heart failure, systemic embolization, or pulmonary embolism.[15]

Stenosis of the mitral valve impedes the flow of blood from the left atrium to the left ventricle during diastole. The normal mitral valve area is 4 to 5 cm². Symptoms with exercise can be expected with valve areas less than or equal to 2.5 cm². Symptoms at rest are expected at less than or equal to 1.5 cm². The left ventricle responds with Starling mechanisms to increased venous return with increased performance, elevating CO in response to demand. The left atrium is limited in its capacity to respond, and therefore **CO is limited by the relatively passive flow of blood through the valve during diastole; increased venous return results in pulmonary congestion rather than increased CO.** Thus the drive for increased CO in pregnancy cannot be achieved, resulting in increased pulmonary congestion. The relative tachycardia experienced in pregnancy shortens diastole, decreases LV filling, and therefore further compromises CO and increases pulmonary congestion.

The diagnosis of mitral stenosis in pregnancy before maternal decompensation is uncommon. Fatigue and dyspnea on exertion are characteristic symptoms of mitral stenosis but are also ubiquitous among pregnant women. Although the presence of a diastolic rumble may suggest mitral stenosis, this finding is subtle and may be overlooked or not appreciated. Not uncommonly, an intercurrent event such as a febrile episode will result in exaggerated symptoms and the diagnosis of pulmonary edema or oxygen desaturation. Under these circumstances, particularly in the context of a patient from an at-risk group, an echocardiogram should be performed to rule out mitral valvular disease.

Echocardiographic diagnosis of mitral stenosis is based on the characteristic appearance of the stenotic, frequently calcified valve. Calculation of valve area from the Doppler pressure half-time method or by 2-D planimetry provides an objective measure of severity. Valve areas of 1 cm² or less usually require pharmacologic management during pregnancy and invasive hemodynamic monitoring during labor, whereas those 1.4 cm² or less usually require careful expectant management. Left atrial enlargement identifies a patient at risk for atrial fibrillation, subsequent atrial thrombus, and the potential for systemic embolization. Embolic complications have been reported in pregnant women with atrial enlargement without atrial fibrillation. Pulmonary hypertension, a complication of worsening mitral disease, can be diagnosed and quantified with Doppler evaluation of the regurgitant jet across the tricuspid valve. **Elevated pulmonary pressures may be due to hydrostatic forces associated with elevated left atrial pressures or, in more advanced disease, may result from pathologic elevations of pulmonary vascular resistance (PVR).** Hydrostatic pulmonary hypertension may respond to therapy that lowers left atrial pressure. Pulmonary hypertension due to elevated PVR is life threatening in pregnancy and may precipitate right-sided heart failure in the postpartum period.

Pregnancy does not negatively affect the natural history of mitral stenosis. Chesley[16] reviewed the medical histories of 134 women with functionally severe mitral stenosis who survived pregnancies between 1931 and 1943. These women lived before modern management of mitral stenosis and therefore represent the natural history of the disease. By 1974, only nine of the cohort remained alive. Their death rate was exponential; during each year of follow-up, the rate for the remaining cohort was 6.3%. Women with subsequent pregnancies had comparable survival to those who did not become pregnant again, allowing the authors to conclude that pregnancy did not negatively affect long-term outcome.

The goal of antepartum care in the context of mitral stenosis is to achieve a balance between the drive to increase CO and the limitations of flow across the stenotic valve. Most women with significant disease require diuresis with a drug such as furosemide. In addition, β-blockade reduces heart rate, improves diastolic flow across the valve, and relieves pulmonary congestion. Al Kasab and associates[17] evaluated the impact of β-blockade on 25 pregnant women with significant mitral stenosis. Figure 37-5 describes the functional status of women before pregnancy and during pregnancy before and after β-blockade. The deterioration associated with pregnancy and the subsequent improvement with treatment is evident. Fastidious antepartum care as described earlier should supplement pharmacologic management.

Women with a history of rheumatic valvular disease who are at risk for contact with populations with a high prevalence of streptococcal infection should receive prophylaxis with daily oral penicillin G or monthly benzathine penicillin. Most pregnant women live in close contact with groups of children and usually are considered at risk.

Atrial fibrillation (AF) is a complication associated with mitral stenosis due to left atrial enlargement. Rapid ventricular response to AF may result in sudden decompensation. Digoxin, β-blockers, or calcium channel blockers can be used to control ventricular response. In the context of hemodynamic decompensation, electrical cardioversion may be necessary. Anticoagulation with heparin should be used before and after cardioversion to prevent systemic embolization. Patients with chronic AF and a history of an embolic event should also undergo anticoagulation. Anticoagulation may be considered in women with a left atrial dimension of 55 mm or greater.

Labor and delivery can frequently precipitate decompensation in patients with critical mitral stenosis. Pain induces tachycardia, and uterine contractions increase venous return and thereby increase pulmonary congestion. Women with critical mitral stenosis frequently cannot tolerate the work of pushing in the second stage. Clark and coworkers[4] described the abrupt elevation in pulmonary artery pressures in the immediate postpartum period associated with return of uterine blood to the general circulation (Fig. 37-6). **Aggressive, anticipatory diuresis will reduce pulmonary congestion and the potential for oxygen desaturation.**

The hemodynamics of women with symptomatic stenosis or a valve area of 1 cm^2 or less may benefit from management with the aid of a pulmonary artery catheter. Ideally, hemodynamic parameters are assessed when the patient is well compensated, early in labor. These findings serve as a reference point to guide subsequent therapy. Pain control is best achieved with an epidural, and heart rate control is maintained through pain control and β-blockade. To avoid pushing, the second stage is shortened with low forceps or vacuum delivery; cesarean delivery is reserved for obstetric indications. Aggressive diuresis is initiated immediately postpartum. In a series of 80 pregnancies managed with a range of severity, the most common complications were pulmonary edema (31%) and arrhythmia (11%). When valve area was 1 cm^2 or less, the rate of pulmonary edema was higher (56%), as was the rate of arrhythmia (33%).[18] These rates will be dependent on the effectiveness of medical management and the timing of presentation and diagnosis.

Aggressive medical management, including hospital bed rest in selected cases, is sufficient to manage most women with mitral stenosis. The woman with uncommonly severe disease may require surgical intervention. Although successful valve replacement and open commissurotomy have been reported in pregnancy, they are now rarely needed. Two reports detail successful balloon valvotomy in a series of 40 and 71 women with minimal complications.[19,20] Complications of balloon valvuloplasty outside of pregnancy occur at the following rates:

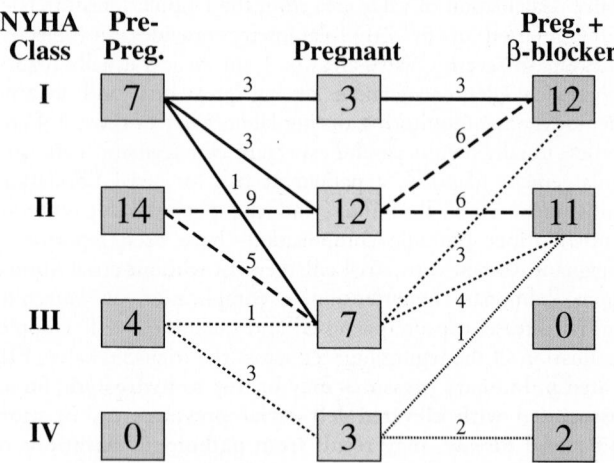

FIG 37-5 The effects of β-blockade on functional status of women with mitral stenosis. NYHA, New York Heart Association. (From Al Kasab S, Sabag T, Al Zaibag M, et al. Beta-adrenergic receptor blockade in the management of pregnant women with mitral stenosis. *Am J Obstet Gynecol.* 1990;163:37.)

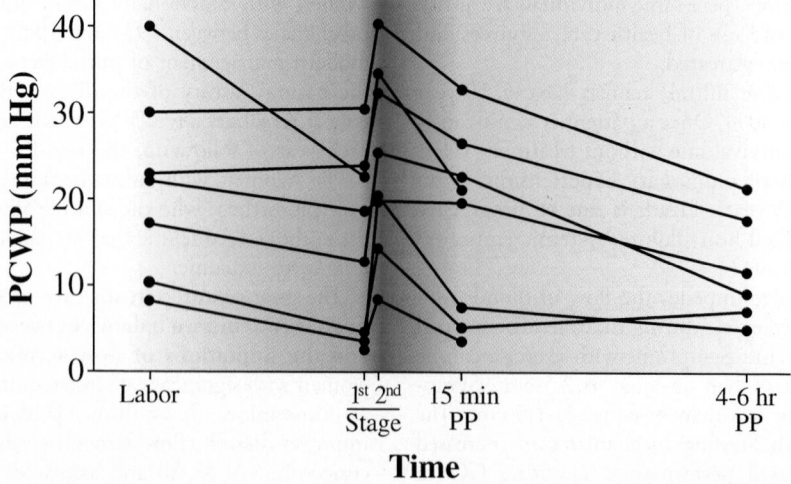

FIG 37-6 The changes in pulmonary capillary wedge pressure (PCWP) associated with delivery and subsequent diuresis in women with mitral stenosis. PP, postpartum. (From Clark S, Phelan J, Greenspoon J, et al. Labor and delivery in the presence of mitral stenosis: central hemodynamic observations. *Am J Obstet Gynecol.* 1985;152:384.)

mortality (0.5%), cerebrovascular accident (1%), and mitral regurgitation that requires surgery (2%). Mitral valvuloplasty in pregnancy has been reported with success rates of 95% or greater. The incidence of severe mitral regurgitation that required surgery was 4.6% in the larger series at long-term follow-up; no women required surgery for acute mitral regurgitation during pregnancy. The rate of fetal loss was between 1% and 2%. **Medical management should be clearly exhausted before assuming these risks during pregnancy, when emergent intervention such as valve replacement is more complicated and carries a significant risk to the fetus.**

Rheumatic disease can also affect the aortic valve. In the context of aortic stenosis that is critically dependent on ventricular filling, management of significant mitral stenosis that limits ventricular filling is particularly complicated.

Mitral Regurgitation

Mitral regurgitation may be due to a chronic progressive process such as rheumatic valve disease or myxomatous mitral valve disease, frequently associated with mitral valve prolapse. As regurgitation increases over time, forward flow is maintained at the expense of LV dilation with eventual impaired contractility. Left atrial enlargement may be associated with AF that should be managed with ventricular rate control and anticoagulation. The patient with chronic mitral regurgitation may remain asymptomatic even with exercise. Preconceptional counseling should include consideration of valve replacement in consultation with a cardiologist. In general, valve replacement is recommended for (1) symptomatic patients, (2) AF, (3) EF less than 60%, (4) LV end-diastolic dimension greater than 40 mm, or (5) pulmonary systolic pressure greater than 50 mm Hg.[15] As discussed later, the benefits of valve replacement before pregnancy must be balanced against the risks associated with a prosthetic valve in pregnancy and the potential for prosthetic valve deterioration in pregnancy. If surgery is required, valve repair—rather than replacement—is preferred when possible to avoid the need for anticoagulation.

Acute mitral regurgitation in young patients is uncommon and may be associated with ruptured chordae tendineae as a result of endocarditis or myxomatous valve disease. Without time for LV compensation, forward flow may be severely compromised; urgent valve surgery is usually required. Inotropic LV support and systemic afterload reduction can be used to stabilize the patient.

The hemodynamic changes associated with pregnancy can be expected to have mixed effects. A reduction in systemic vascular resistance (SVR) tends to promote forward flow. The drive to increase CO will exacerbate LV volume overload, and increased atrial dilation may initiate AF. Pulmonary congestion can be managed by careful diuresis with the knowledge that adequate forward flow is usually dependent on a high preload to achieve adequate LV filling. AF should be managed as in the nonpregnant state. An increase in SVR due to progressive hypertension secondary to advancing preeclampsia may significantly impair forward flow and should be treated. Labor and delivery should be managed with standard cardiac care. Catecholamine release that occurs as a result of pain or stress impairs forward flow; therefore particular attention should be paid to LV filling. **Excessive preload results in pulmonary congestion, and insufficient preload will not fill the enlarged left ventricle and will result in insufficient forward flow.** A pulmonary artery catheter can be used to determine appropriate filling pressure in

early labor or before induction. Although a large v-wave may complicate the interpretation of pulmonary artery wedge pressure, the pulmonary artery diastolic pressure can be used as a reference point. Diuresis in the early postpartum period may be required.

Myxomatous mitral valve disease or mitral valve prolapse is a common condition that affects as many as 12% of young women. **In the absence of conditions of abnormal connective tissue such as Marfan or Ehlers-Danlos syndrome and clinically significant mitral regurgitation, women with mitral prolapse can be expected to have uncomplicated pregnancies.** They may experience an increase in tachyarrhythmias that can be treated with β-blockers, and the use of prophylactic antibiotics may be considered at the time of delivery.

Aortic Stenosis

Most patients who develop calcific stenotic trileaflet aortic valves do so outside their childbearing years (age 70 to 80 years). Patients with bicuspid valves develop significant stenosis after the age of 50 to 60 years. Rheumatic disease can also affect the aortic valve, usually after the development of significant mitral disease. Most pregnant women with significant aortic stenosis have congenitally stenotic valves: bicuspid valves with congenitally fused leaflets, unicuspid valves, or tricuspid valves with fused leaflets.

The natural history of aortic stenosis is characterized by a long, asymptomatic period. With increasing outflow obstruction, patients develop angina, syncope, and LV failure. Without valve replacement, only 50% of patients will survive 5 years after the development of angina; 3 years after the development of syncope; and 2 years after the development of LV failure. Although valve replacement is the only definitive treatment for calcific aortic stenosis, valvuloplasty may prove beneficial in some young adults whose valves are not calcified. Medical management of symptomatic patients is not generally efficacious. Mechanical valve replacement requires anticoagulation, which complicates subsequent pregnancies.

Young women with aortic stenosis are usually asymptomatic. Although they may develop increasing exercise intolerance in pregnancy, the progression is insidious and not easily distinguished from the effects of normal pregnancy. The diagnosis is usually made by the auscultation of a harsh systolic murmur. **The murmur can easily be distinguished from a physiologic murmur of pregnancy by its harshness and radiation into the carotid arteries.** Diagnosis is confirmed by echocardiography whereby the pressure gradient across the valve can be measured by Doppler, and the valve area can be calculated with the continuity equation. Many women with significant aortic stenosis experience the expected increase in CO associated with pregnancy.[3] Increased flow across the fixed, stenotic valve results in a proportionately increased gradient across the valve. Although the pressure gradient during pregnancy may be higher than that observed postpartum, these differences are not significant.

Four series of patients with aortic stenosis in pregnancy have been reported.[3,21-23] The reports summarize experiences with wide ranges in severity of disease and management ranging from the 1960s and 1970s to the present. Arias and Pineda[21] described a series of 23 cases managed before 1978 with a maternal mortality rate of 17%. More recent series, however, do not demonstrate this high level of maternal risk.[3,22,23] The potential for serious adverse outcomes reported by Arias should, however, serve as an indication for intensive management. The rate of mortality should not necessarily be used as an indication for termination or surgical intervention. Pregnant patients have been successfully managed with aortic gradients in excess of 160 mm Hg.[3] In general, patients with a peak aortic gradient of 60 mm Hg or less have had uncomplicated courses. Those with higher gradients require increasingly intensive management.

Aortic valve replacement and balloon valvotomy have been reported during pregnancy. Balloon valvotomy in a young patient without valve calcification can provide significant long-term palliation. Valvotomy before pregnancy may provide an interval of hemodynamic stability sufficient to complete a pregnancy without the complications associated with a mechanical prosthetic valve. **Consideration for valve replacement or valvotomy during pregnancy should be reserved for patients who remain clinically symptomatic despite hospital care.** In general, intervention should not be based solely on a pressure gradient or valve area.

Aortic stenosis is a condition of excess LV afterload. Ventricular hypertrophy increases cardiac oxygen requirements, whereas increased diastolic ventricular pressure impairs coronary perfusion. **Each increases the potential for myocardial ischemia.** The left ventricle requires adequate filling to generate sufficient systolic pressure to produce flow across the stenotic valve. **Given a hypertrophied ventricle and some degree of diastolic dysfunction, the volume-pressure relationship is very steep. A small loss of LV filling results in a proportionately large fall in LV pressure and, therefore, a large fall in forward flow and CO.** The pregnant patient with significant aortic stenosis is very sensitive to loss of preload associated with hemorrhage or epidural-induced hypotension. The window of appropriate filling pressure is narrow. Excess fluid may result in pulmonary edema; insufficient fluid may result in hypotension and coronary ischemia. **In general, pulmonary edema associated with excess preload is much easier to manage than hypotension due to hypovolemia.**

Appropriate antepartum care is described earlier. Given that most aortic stenosis in young women is congenital in origin, fetal echocardiography is indicated. Although some controversy persists, cesarean delivery is generally reserved for obstetric indications. Pain during labor and delivery can be safely managed with regional analgesia using a low-dose bupivacaine and narcotic technique. Dense anesthesia during the second stage can be obtained with minimal hemodynamic complications using a caudal catheter. Patients with gradients above 60 to 80 mm Hg may benefit from the use of a pulmonary artery and arterial catheter during labor. Hospital admission one day before planned induction of labor with a favorable cervix is preferred, and a prolonged induction should be avoided. Pulmonary artery and radial artery catheters, as well as epidural and caudal catheters, are placed. The patient should be gently hydrated overnight to achieve a pulmonary artery wedge pressure (PAWP) of 12 to 15 mm Hg. Some patients with milder disease spontaneously diurese in the face of a volume load such that an elevation in PAWP cannot be achieved. An elevated PAWP serves as a buffer against a loss of preload. If PAWP falls with bleeding or the onset of anesthesia, volume can be administered before a reduction in forward flow occurs. In general, pushing is minimized, and the second stage is shortened with operative vaginal delivery. Antibiotics may be considered for the prevention of endocarditis.

Postpartum patients should be monitored hemodynamically for 24 to 48 hours. Diuresis is usually spontaneous, and the patient can be allowed to find her predelivery compensated state. When diuresis must be induced to treat pulmonary edema, it should be done gently and carefully. Predelivery hemodynamic parameters should be used as an end point. Some have found that a significant delay in valve replacement in women with quite severe disease is associated with maternal complications.[3] In a larger cohort of women with less severe disease followed for 6 years and compared with a matched cohort who had not been pregnant, women who experienced a pregnancy had a reduction in event-free survival.[24] These observations may be the result of accelerated valve deterioration due to pregnancy. For this reason, valve replacement within weeks of delivery may be indicated.

Aortic Regurgitation

Aortic regurgitation is most often due to a congenitally abnormal valve. Other causes include Marfan syndrome, endocarditis, and rheumatic disease. As with mitral regurgitation, the left ventricle compensates for decreased forward flow with an increase in LV end-diastolic volume. Afterload reduction prevents progressive LV dilation and is recommended for patients with LV dysfunction or dilation. Valve replacement is generally recommended for (1) NYHA functional class III and class IV symptoms, (2) an EF less than 50%, or (3) an LV end-systolic dimension greater than 50 mm.[12] Acute regurgitation may be due to aortic root dissection or endocarditis and usually represents a medical emergency that requires urgent valve replacement.

The reduction in vascular resistance associated with pregnancy tends to improve cardiac performance. If afterload reduction has been achieved with an angiotensin-converting enzyme (ACE) inhibitor or an angiotensin receptor blocker (ARB) before pregnancy, hydralazine or a calcium channel blocker such as nifedipine should be substituted. Modest heart rate elevations should be tolerated, and bradycardia may be associated with increased regurgitation due to prolongation of diastole. Labor and delivery are managed with standard cardiac care, and pulmonary artery catheterization is not usually required. As the hemodynamic changes associated with pregnancy resolve, a rise in vascular resistance should be anticipated and afterload reduction maintained.

Prosthetic Valves

Definitive therapy for significant valvular disease requires surgical repair or, more commonly, replacement. Mechanical valves are durable but require anticoagulation. When used in a young woman, bioprosthetic valves usually require replacement during her lifetime. Reports of pregnancies associated with prosthetic valves suggest significant variability in outcomes, and these have been reviewed in detail by Elkayam and Bitar[25] and within the 2014 AHA/ACC Valvular Heart Disease Guidelines.[15] Reported outcomes must be interpreted in the context of the cohorts of patients reported and the circumstances of clinical care.

Decisions that surround the timing and choice of valve replacement for a woman of reproductive age are complex. Managing a pregnancy with moderate valve disease may be less complicated than managing a pregnancy with a prosthetic valve. The durability of a mechanical valve has considerable advantages for a young person, but it is associated with more adverse outcomes in pregnancy. **Delay in valve replacement until childbearing is completed is appropriate when the severity of heart disease is believed to be manageable in pregnancy.**

Bioprosthetic valves have relatively low rates of complications in pregnancy. Some women, particularly those with CHD, will have residual hemodynamic issues associated with their primary condition that are not addressed with valve replacement. The impact of pregnancy on the life of a bioprosthetic valve has been studied.[26] Ten-year graft survival following two pregnancies was 16.7%, compared with 54.8% following a single pregnancy, which suggests that pregnancy may adversely affect the life of a bioprosthetic valve. **Accelerated deterioration of bioprosthetic valves in the setting of pregnancy has been confirmed by several studies.**[25,28-30]

Anticoagulation is required with a mechanical valve. Management of anticoagulation in pregnant women with mechanical prosthetic valves remains very controversial because commonly used anticoagulants have significant maternal and fetal adverse effects, and no single agent is safe throughout all stages of pregnancy. Interpretation of reported outcomes must be made in the context of valve location, thrombogenicity of the particular valve, strategies for anticoagulation and monitoring of effectiveness, and social context including compliance. Mechanical valves in the mitral position will be expected to have more thrombotic complications than those in the aortic position. Older-generation valves, such as Björk-Shiley or Starr-Edwards, may be in place in a pregnant woman and will be more likely to have thrombotic complications. **When strategies for anticoagulation without dose adjustment are used in pregnancy, particularly in the case of heparin therapy, increased thrombotic complications are to be expected. Outcomes are better when clinical care teams are experienced with monitoring and dosing anticoagulation and work to achieve compliance.**

Recommendations regarding anticoagulation in pregnancy for women with mechanical valves have been published by the ACC and AHA,[15] the American College of Chest Physicians,[31] and by Elkayam and Bitar.[25] Each have largely drawn information from the same sources but in doing so have made substantially different recommendations regarding the use of warfarin or heparin. Physicians who care for pregnant women with mechanical heart valves should be familiar with each set of recommendations and should use them for guidance in counseling patients and establishing a plan.

Ideally, patients are evaluated and counseled preconceptionally. An effective plan of birth control is used until a pregnancy is planned; therefore long-acting reversible contraceptives should be considered. Progestin-based systems may reduce menstrual bleeding for women on warfarin. Once a pregnancy is desired, a clear plan for anticoagulation in the first trimester should be in place, with clinical systems available to immediately implement the plan once a pregnancy is identified. Early surveillance for a potential pregnancy is essential.

First Trimester

Warfarin is clearly teratogenic when used in the first trimester, and its use in pregnancy has been extensively reviewed.[32] A teratogenic window between 6 and 9 gestational weeks has been suggested. Exposure in this timeframe results in an incidence of warfarin embryopathy of approximately 6%. Exposure to less than 5 mg/day has been suggested to decrease the incidence to as low as 3%. If adequate anticoagulation can be maintained with less than 5 mg/day of warfarin, oral anticoagulation could be considered after appropriate counseling. An increase in dosing should be expected in pregnancy and may limit use of this strategy. Many women will choose therapy with low-molecular-weight heparin (LMWH). Conversion can be accomplished

shortly after the first missed period and with confirmation of pregnancy.

Second and Third Trimester

Management during the second and third trimesters (prior to labor) remains controversial. Treatment with warfarin offers superior anticoagulation compared with heparin therapy. The magnitude of maternal risk assumed with heparin therapy will be dependent on valve type and location and on the quality of anticoagulation achieved. Weight-based dosing, treatment without aggressive monitoring, and noncompliance are associated with unacceptably high rates of thromboembolic complications. Three studies[33-35] have reported a total 35 pregnancies with therapeutic factor Xa levels without thrombotic complications. Three patients experienced complications with subtherapeutic factor Xa levels.

The magnitude of risk to the fetus in the second and third trimesters associated with warfarin exposure is also unclear. Minor levels of dose-dependent neurologic dysfunction with exposure after the first trimester have been reported as have trends for an increased risk for intelligence quotient (IQ score) below 80 (odds ratio [OR], 3.1; 95% confidence interval (CI), 0.8 to 11.6).[32] Preterm labor in the context of anticoagulation with warfarin will be associated with risks for fetal bleeding as well as the potential need for urgent operative delivery, which places the mother at risk for hemorrhage.

The AHA/ACC guidelines recommend treatment with warfarin in the second and third trimesters but suggest that dose-adjusted LMWH is a reasonable option for women who choose not to be on an oral anticoagulant.[15] The American College of Chest Surgeons (ACCS) supports use of dose-adjusted LMWH, dose-adjusted unfractionated heparin (UFH), or warfarin in the second and third trimesters.[31] The review recognizes that "the choice of anticoagulant regimen is so value and preference dependent (risk of thrombosis vs. risk of fetal abnormalities) that we consider the decision to be completely individualized."

Labor and Delivery

Prior to delivery, conversion to heparin-based therapy is uniformly recommended. Continuous intravenous (IV) management with UFH or LMWH has been suggested. IV therapy will usually require chronic vascular access and comes with an associated risk for line infection and endocarditis. Treatment is stopped such that delivery can be accomplished without anticoagulation.

Postpartum

IV heparin is consistently recommended after delivery. Initiating intravenous UFH without a bolus may decrease the risk for bleeding complications, and conversion to warfarin once the risk for bleeding is low is recommended. Avoiding the use of LMWH while bridging to warfarin may also reduce the incidence of bleeding. Oral anticoagulation is not contraindicated with breastfeeding.

Treatment with warfarin to achieve an international normalized ratio (INR) of 2.5 to 3.5 has been recommended.[25] Treatment with LMWH requires careful monitoring and dose adjustment, and the total dose should be expected to increase substantially throughout pregnancy. Substantial variability in anti–factor Xa levels should be expected over a dosing interval and may result in subtherapeutic trough levels.[36] Peak levels of 1.5 IU/mL or less, midinterval levels of approximately 1.0 IU/

mL, and trough levels of 0.6 IU/mL have been recommended.[25] Twice-daily dosing will be required at a minimum, and thrice-daily dosing may be required to achieve an appropriate trough without an excessively high peak concentration. Treatment with intravenous UFH to achieve an activated partial thromboplastin time (aPTT) greater than 2.0 has been recommended[25] in addition to simultaneous treatment with low-dose aspirin.[15]

If valve thrombosis is encountered, thrombolysis should be considered because successful thrombolytic therapy of a clotted valve in pregnancy has been reported. Although thrombolysis is safe and effective for many patients, embolic complications, bleeding, and death have been reported in pregnancy. Surgery such as cesarean delivery cannot be performed in proximity to thrombolytic therapy.

Management of pregnant women with mechanical heart valves is complex. Counseling balances risks of alternative therapies that rely on less than optimal data and the values and risk willingness of individual patients. Management of anticoagulation, whether it be with warfarin or LMWH, is nuanced and relies heavily on clinical experience in monitoring and dose adjustment.

CONGENITAL HEART DISEASE

Congenital heart disease is present in 0.7% to 1% of live births and accounts for as many as 30% of infants with birth anomalies. Before the development of corrective surgery, many children died shortly after birth or in childhood. In 1939, the first patent ductus arteriosus (PDA) was ligated. In 1945, the first Blalock-Thomas-Taussig shunt was performed for palliation of cyanotic heart disease. In 1953, cardiac bypass was introduced. Introduction of surgery under hypothermia in the late 1960s permitted longer and more complex repairs. Of children who survived surgery to correct tetralogy of Fallot between 1955 and 1960, the 23-year survival was 86%, approaching the expected survival rate of 96% for normal children. Before the 1960s, rheumatic heart disease was more common in pregnancy than CHD by a ratio of 4 : 1. By the 1980s, the ratio was 1 : 1. Currently, congenital disease is now estimated to exceed rheumatic disease by 4 : 1. Although most enter pregnancy with known heart disease, some women have their disease first recognized because of the hemodynamic demands of pregnancy.

Increased survival of children with congenital disease has created a population of young women with complex medical and psychosocial conditions entering their childbearing years. Those whose CHD was diagnosed in infancy have frequently experienced multiple cardiothoracic surgeries and extended hospitalizations. They have lived with continued concerns from parents and health care professionals regarding their ongoing health problem. Their childhood has been described as "growing up heart sick."[37] Some describe a lack of information regarding childbearing and contraception. They "seemed to believe that someone else could and would decide whether they should become pregnant." Kovacs and coworkers[38] describe the contraception and pregnancy advice women with CHD recall receiving from their health care providers, and in many cases, women received either no information or the information they did receive was inaccurate. **Health care providers should strive to (1) objectively share information regarding reproductive health care; (2) direct decision making toward the patient, rather than toward parents and health care professionals; and (3) improve self-esteem and body image.** When treating CHD

TABLE 37-1 INCIDENCE OF CONGENITAL HEART DEFECTS IN CHILDHOOD AND IN PREGNANCY

DEFECT	CHILDHOOD (%)	PREGNANCY (%)
Ventricular septal defect	35	13
Atrial septal defect	9	9
Patent ductus arteriosus	8	2.7
Pulmonary stenosis	8	8
Aortic stenosis	6	20
Coarctation of the aorta	6	8
Tetralogy of Fallot	5	12
Transposition of the great vessels	4	5.4

Data from Shime J, Mocarski E, Hastings D, et al. Congenital heart disease in pregnancy: short- and long-term implications. *Am J Obstet Gynecol.* 1987;156:313; and Findlow D, Doyle E. Congenital heart disease in adults. *Br J Anaesth.* 1997;78:416.

TABLE 37-2 NEONATAL OUTCOME WITH CONGENITAL HEART DISEASE: LIVEBORN VERSUS TERMINATION

	LIVEBORN INFANT (%)	TERMINATION (%)
Noncyanotic	86	5
Cyanotic	85	26
Corrected	95	17
Palliative	87	17
Uncorrected	71	42

Data from Whittemore R, Hobbins J, Engle M. Pregnancy and its outcome in women with and without surgical treatment of congenital heart disease. *Am J Cardiol.* 1982;50:641.

during pregnancy, there must be a willingness to acknowledge and address the impact of the patient's disease on her life.

Table 37-1 summarizes the distribution of CHD in childhood and in pregnancy.[23,39] The spontaneous closure of lesions such as VSD and correction of a patent ductus are reflected by reduced reporting in pregnancy. The increased reporting of aortic stenosis in pregnancy is probably due to a worsening of disease with age and the ease of recognition during pregnancy. The complexity and diversity of CHD confounds our ability to describe the prognosis or a management plan for the breadth of conditions. **Major risks in pregnancy include (1) cyanosis; (2) left (or systemic) ventricular dysfunction and poor functional status; (3) pulmonary hypertension and Eisenmenger syndrome, particularly with RV dysfunction; and (4) severe left (or systemic) outflow tract obstruction.**

Neonatal complications are more likely when pregnant women have heart disease, particularly if one or more of the major risk factors listed above is present.[9,11,23,39] Neonatal outcomes have been most clearly described based on the presence or absence of maternal cyanosis. Table 37-2 is derived from a report[9] of 482 pregnancies from 233 women with CHD who delivered between 1968 and 1982. The rate of terminations was higher in the group of women with cyanotic heart disease and was particularly high (42%) in those with uncorrected lesions. This reflects the anticipated poor neonatal outcome and maternal risks associated with uncorrected cyanotic disease. It is likely that patients with more severe disease are overly represented in the group of women who chose to terminate, which would bias the group who continued pregnancy toward a better outcome: 86% to 90% of pregnancies without cyanosis ended in a live birth, and 71% with an uncorrected lesion also delivered successfully. Given an expected baseline rate of miscarriage, these outcomes are good. Corrected cyanotic disease was associated with outcomes comparable to noncyanotic disease. Other adverse neonatal outcomes, including low birthweight, are concentrated among women with uncorrected cyanotic heart disease. In a report of 96 pregnancies among 44 women with cyanotic CHD, 43% resulted in a live birth and spontaneous abortion and stillbirth occurred in 51% and 6%, respectively.[40] Among the live births, 37% were premature. The mean birthweight among those born full term was 2575 g (2100 to 3600 g). A report[23] of 144 pregnancies from women with CHD delivered between 1976 and 1986 details a similar rate of prematurity (35%) with 53% born small for gestational age (SGA, mean birthweight 2400 g ± 800).

Common maternal complications include CHF and pulmonary edema (4%), arrhythmia (4%), and hypertension (6%). CHF and hypertension were often associated with uncorrected LV outflow obstruction.[9,23] Arrhythmias were observed after surgery in and around atrial or ventricular septa. Maternal death was uncommon, 0 per 482 pregnancies in one series[9] and 1 per 144 pregnancies in a second.[23] Maternal deaths are most commonly reported in association with Eisenmenger syndrome, which is discussed more fully later.

Men and women with CHD are at increased risk for having children with CHD. In a prospective study with aggressive pediatric evaluation, Whittemore and associates[9] estimated the incidence to be as high as 14.2%. In a retrospective study, Rose and coworkers[41] found the risk to be 8.8%. The rate of CHD associated with an affected mother is 2 to 3.5 times that observed with an affected father. **Specific parental defects are not generally associated with the same defect in the child; the risk for cardiac maldevelopment is inherited rather than the risk for a specific defect.** The risk for CHD and the character of the risk should be discussed with an affected mother. In Whittemore's[9] report, 58 of 60 affected infants were diagnosed with relatively benign correctable lesions (ASD, VSD, pulmonary stenosis, aortic stenosis, PDA, or mitral valve prolapse). Only two infants from 372 pregnancies (0.5%) were diagnosed with complex CHD. Gill and colleagues[10] examined the recurrence pattern of CHD in 6640 pregnancies for whom fetal echocardiography was obtained because of a family history of CHD. The recurrence rate was 2.9% (95% CI, 2% to 4%) for mothers with CHD, a rate lower than that reported by others. However, the study is limited to diagnoses established by fetal echocardiography and therefore may underrepresent the true incidence of abnormalities. The type and severity of the cardiac defect seen in the mother did not predict the type or severity of the cardiac defect in the offspring, with a few exceptions. Atrioventricular canal defects, especially those associated with situs abnormalities, had a highly concordant recurrence rate.[10] CHD-associated 22q11.2 deletion (DiGeorge syndrome, velocardiofacial syndrome) will be inherited as an autosomal-dominant condition. Many parents with CHD will not have been previously screened for genetic syndromes; therefore referral for genetic counseling and possible screening should be considered, particularly in the context of conotruncal abnormalities and other associated anomalies. **All women who have CHD should undergo fetal echocardiographic examination at approximately 18 to 22 weeks' gestation.**

Contraceptive counseling should be offered to all women with CHD. **Given the problems experienced growing up with heart disease, contraceptive education should probably be initiated as part of general health care education before the overt need for birth control.** In the context of CHD, complications associated with pregnancy are usually greater than those associated with any form of birth control. Cyanosis, pulmonary hypertension, low CO, dilated cardiac chambers, passive-flow venous conduits (e.g., Fontan), and atrial fibrillation place patients at risk for thrombosis. This small group of women should probably avoid combined estrogen-progestin oral contraceptives. Progestin-only pills are not associated with risk for thrombosis but require regular dosing to achieve optimal efficacy. Parenteral progestins are safe for women with cardiac disease and are extremely effective. They do cause irregular bleeding, which may be significant if the patient is anticoagulated. The intrauterine device (IUD) may also be a suitable choice for women with congenital heart lesions.

Isolated Septal Defects

VSDs and ASDs represent greater than 40% of CHD identified in childhood. In adulthood, 50% of large VSDs (>1.5 cm) lead to the development of Eisenmenger syndrome, and 10% of patients with uncorrected ASDs develop pulmonary hypertension. The management of Eisenmenger syndrome in pregnancy is discussed later.

A harsh S1-coincident systolic murmur that radiates to the left sternal border but not to the carotids suggests the presence of a VSD. The diagnosis can be confirmed by 2-D echocardiography with color-flow Doppler that demonstrates shunting across the ventricular septum. The peak velocity of the jet across the septum can be used to assess the pressure gradient between the ventricles. A high velocity between ventricles indicates a large pressure gradient between the right and left ventricles and the absence of pulmonary hypertension. In the absence of associated cardiac lesions and pulmonary hypertension, the presence of a VSD does not usually complicate pregnancy. Small defects create loud murmurs but are not usually hemodynamically significant, although the high-velocity jet of a small lesion does create a risk for endocarditis.

ASDs are more difficult to diagnose by auscultation. The characteristic finding, a split S_2 that is fixed with respiration, is subtle and usually not appreciated without specific attention. Increased right-sided blood flow secondary to shunting across the defect may create a pulmonary flow murmur that will be augmented in pregnancy. In the absence of other anomalies, the significance of the ASD is related to its size. Hemodynamically significant defects result in left-to-right shunting from the systemic circulation to the pulmonary circulation that causes right atrial and ventricular enlargement. Atrial arrhythmias are commonly associated with atrial enlargement. Increased pulmonary blood flow may result in dyspnea on exertion and restriction of activity. As with VSDs, Eisenmenger syndrome may develop, but this usually occurs at an older age.

Piesiewicz and colleagues[42] reported 54 pregnancies in women with secundum ASDs. **Impaired functional status (NHYA class III or IV) increased from 5.5% in the second trimester to 11.1% in the third trimester.** Although left-to-right shunting was present in all patients in the second trimester, three patients (5.5%) developed bidirectional shunting in the third trimester. One additional patient reversed her shunt. RV diameter and systolic pulmonary artery pressure increased from the second to third trimester (34.1 ± 8.4 mm Hg to 39.1 ± 12.2 mm Hg). Over the same time frame, the pulmonary flow (Q_p)/ systemic flow (Q_s) ratio decreased. Increased flow associated with pregnancy appears to adversely affect RV function and pulmonary pressures. The fall in Q_p/Q_s suggests that the rise in pulmonary pressure is due to increased PVR. The authors also reported supraventricular arrhythmias in 50% of women in the third trimester.

The patient with a significant VSD or ASD shunt can be expected to normally expand her CO during pregnancy. However, the price of a normal systemic CO is a high pulmonary flow. The pregnant patient may begin to experience symptoms at rest that she previously noted with exercise. She may also experience an increase in tachyarrhythmias. Heart rate control with a β-blocker may provide symptomatic relief, and early diuresis may benefit the patient postpartum. Elevated pulmonary blood flow associated with pregnancy could accelerate the progression of pulmonary vascular disease. In the absence of associated anomalies, arrhythmias, and pulmonary hypertension, the presence of an ASD does not usually complicate pregnancy.

Patent Ductus Arteriosus

The diagnosis of a PDA is suggested by the characteristic continuous murmur at the upper left sternal border. Most cases are identified in childhood and are treated with surgical or transcatheter procedures. Of patients with an uncorrected patent ductus, as many as 50% develop Eisenmenger syndrome, usually in childhood. In adults with a small patent ductus, the major risk is endocarditis. **In the absence of Eisenmenger syndrome, pregnancy is not usually complicated.** As with the ASD, the increase in pulmonary blood flow associated with the increase in CO in pregnancy may result in increased dyspnea with exertion and at rest. Early diuresis may benefit the patient postpartum.

Tetralogy of Fallot

Tetralogy of Fallot is a syndrome of abnormalities that results from malalignment of the conoventricular septum. It is characterized by (1) RV outflow tract (RVOT) obstruction, (2) VSD, (3) overriding aorta, and (4) RV hypertrophy. **Tetralogy of Fallot is the most common cyanotic CHD,** and it was among the first to be successfully surgically palliated by Blalock, Thomas, and Taussig in 1945 and subsequently physiologically repaired. Therefore a significant number of adults with CHD have repaired tetralogy of Fallot. The severity of the clinical presentation in infancy is dependent on the degree of RVOT obstruction. More severe obstruction leads to more significant cyanosis from right-to-left shunting. Surgical repair generally includes closure of a VSD and relief of RVOT obstruction. Some patients with repaired tetralogy of Fallot have near-normal cardiac physiology, but many have residual lesions that may complicate pregnancy.

Some patients had palliative classic Blalock-Thomas-Taussig shunts in infancy using the subclavian artery to connect the systemic circulation with the pulmonary circulation, thus increasing pulmonary blood flow and reducing cyanosis. As a consequence, blood pressures in the arm supplied by the transected artery may not be reflective of aortic pressure. Patients should be asked if one arm is unreliable for blood pressure measurements, or they should be examined to look for evidence of a thoracotomy scar that indicates an affected ipsilateral arm, which should not be used for blood pressure measurements.

Efforts to relieve the RVOT obstruction may be incomplete and may result in persistent pulmonary stenosis. More often, significant pulmonary insufficiency is a consequence of the transannular patch approach used to enlarge the outflow tract and valve annulus. Several studies have demonstrated that women with severe pulmonary insufficiency and RV dysfunction are more likely to have complications with pregnancy. Balci and colleagues[43] reported a series of 74 women with tetralogy of Fallot who had 157 pregnancies. Eight percent experienced cardiac complications that included supraventricular tachycardia ($n = 8$), heart failure ($n = 2$), and thromboembolism ($n = 1$). The use of cardiac medications prior to pregnancy was identified as an important predictor of cardiovascular events.

Tetralogy of Fallot is often well tolerated during pregnancy. Preconceptional evaluation should include assessment of right and left ventricular size and function along with the severity of the pulmonary insufficiency or stenosis, with consideration given to repair of severe pulmonary insufficiency before pregnancy if appropriate.

Transposition of the Great Arteries

Transposition of the great arteries (TGA) is present in only 5% of pregnant women with CHD but is overrepresented in the publication of case reports and case series. **In complete TGA, systemic venous blood returns to the right atrium and passes through the tricuspid valve, into the RV, and directly into the transposed aorta. Although this is an adequate circulation for fetal life, infants decompensate at birth owing to ineffective systemic circulation.** Some will have an ASD sufficiently large to achieve adequate systemic blood flow and oxygenation; others will require an immediate palliative procedure to open the atrial septum (balloon atrial septostomy).

TGA was first definitively corrected in 1957 with the Senning procedure, then it was standardized in 1964 with the Mustard operation. In both procedures, a baffle is constructed through the left and right atria so that systemic venous return is channeled through the mitral valve into the left ventricle, and pulmonary venous return is directed through the tricuspid valve into the right ventricle (atrial switch operation). With a modest surgical intervention, the right and left pumps are placed in series with physiologic flow of systemic venous return through the pulmonary circulation. **The right ventricle (RV), as the systemic ventricle, must work against systemic resistance, and the tricuspid valve is exposed to systemic pressures. Long-term complications are associated with failure of the systemic RV and arrhythmia.** Of patients who survive the first 30 days after repair, 90% will be alive in 10 years and 87% will be alive in 20 years. After 13 years, only 5% suffer significant disability (NYHA classes II through IV).[44] A more physiologic repair can be achieved when transposition is accompanied by a VSD. The ventricular septum is reconstructed so that the aortic outflow tract lies within the left ventricle, and a conduit is constructed to connect the RV to the pulmonary artery (Rastelli repair). The pulmonary conduit is prone to stenosis with deterioration of the transplanted valve. More recently, a direct surgical switch between the pulmonary artery and the aorta has been performed (arterial switch operation). Given the time when these operations were introduced, fewer young women entering pregnancy will have an atrial repair; however, increasing numbers will have an arterial repair.

The hemodynamic changes of pregnancy will have a mixed impact on a patient with an atrial repair. Increased CO *increases* the volume load on the right heart, and decreased vascular resistance *reduces* afterload on the right heart. Table 37-3 summarizes nine papers that reported a total of 49 pregnancies in 36

TABLE 37-3	PREGNANCY OUTCOMES WITH TRANSPOSITION OF THE GREAT ARTERIES

	N (%)
Women	36
Pregnancies	49
Live births	41 (84%)
Miscarriages	5
Terminations	2
Fetal deaths	1
Premature birth (<35 wk)	5 (12%)
Congenital heart disease	0 (0%)
Congestive heart failure	6 (15%)
Arrhythmia	8 (20%)

Data from references 23, 45-52.

TABLE 37-4	PREGNANCY OUTCOMES WITH CONGENITALLY CORRECTED TRANSPOSITION OF THE GREAT ARTERIES

	N (%)
Women	54
Cyanotic	4 (10%)
Pregnancies	125
Cyanotic	13 (12%)
Live births	96 (77%)
Miscarriages*	23
Terminations	6
Fetal deaths	1
Premature birth (<35 wk*)	9 (9%)
Congenital heart disease	1 (1%)
Congestive heart failure	6 (6%)
Arrhythmia	2 (2%)
Cerebrovascular accident	1 (1%)

Data from Therrien J, Barnes I, Somerville J. Outcome of pregnancy in patients with congenitally corrected transposition of the great arteries. Am J Cardiol. 1999;84:820; Connolly H, Grogan M, Warnes C. Pregnancy among women with congenitally corrected transposition of great arteries. J Am Coll Cardiol. 1999;33:1692; Kowalik E, Klisiewicz A, Biernacka E, et al. Pregnancy and long-term cardiovascular outcomes in women with congenitally corrected transposition of the great arteries. Int J Gynaecol Obstet. 2014;125:154-157.
*Miscarriages and premature births were concentrated among cyanotic mothers.

women.[23,44-51] No maternal mortality was reported, and neonatal outcomes were generally good. Two women entered pregnancy with disability due to their heart disease (NYHA classes III and IV), and one delivered at 26 weeks as a result of preterm labor; the other developed severe CHF near term and died 19 months postpartum. CHF was frequently associated with uncontrolled tachyarrhythmias.

Zentner and colleagues[52] compared long-term outcomes after atrial repair in 19 women who completed 42 pregnancies with 15 women who never became pregnant. The group without pregnancies had greater numbers of women with *complex TGA*, defined as the presence of a VSD with or without pulmonary stenosis: 74% of pregnancies resulted in full-term infants (median gestational age, 39 [37.2 to 40] weeks; median birthweight, 3.0 [2.4 to 3.5] kg), and 26% of the infants were born premature (median gestational age 35 [31 to 40] weeks; median birthweight, 2.3 [1.3 to 2.4] kg). Within 12 months of pregnancy, three women had hospital admissions for heart failure, two had clinically significant arrhythmias, and one experienced sudden cardiac death. After a median follow-up of 5 (2 to 15) years, more women in the pregnancy group experienced a decline in their RV systolic function that necessitated medications (13 vs. 3), and two women required implantable cardioverter-defibrillator (ICD) placement. Canobbio and coworkers[53] reported a series derived from a registry. Of significance, this report is based on diverse practices rather than from centers with considerable experience managing CHD. Forty women carried 54 pregnancies that resulted in live births: 36 had Mustard repairs, and four had Senning repairs. In six pregnancies, heart failure developed in the second or third trimesters. In five, heart failure developed postpartum. One woman required transplantation postpartum, one died of heart failure 1 month after delivery, and another died 4 years later. This report clearly documents the potential for adverse outcome.

Tobler and associates[54] reported on 17 pregnancies in nine women with arterial repairs. One developed nonsustained ventricular tachycardia, and one developed a valve thrombosis.

Congenitally corrected TGA (ventricular inversion) is characterized by the passage of systemic venous blood into the right atrium, directly into the morphologic LV, and out through the transposed pulmonary artery. Pulmonary venous return passes directly from the left atrium into the morphologic RV and out through the aorta. The RV again serves as the systemic ventricle. Congenitally corrected TGA may be an isolated anomaly but may also be associated with other anomalies that result in cyanosis. See Table 37-4 for a summary of three series

of pregnancies with congenitally corrected TGA.[55-57] Again, maternal and neonatal outcomes are good and are consistent with outcomes associated with other acyanotic forms of CHD. Miscarriage and premature birth are concentrated among those with cyanotic lesions.

Young women with surgically or congenitally corrected TGA can successfully complete pregnancy. Nevertheless, they require aggressive management by an experienced team. Women who are functionally impaired or who are cyanotic before pregnancy can expect more adverse outcomes and may deteriorate postpartum. Evaluation before pregnancy should include assessment of functional status, evaluation of right systemic heart function, and confirmation of normal oxygenation. When the right side of the heart is the systemic heart, pharmacologic afterload reduction should be maintained until pregnancy is confirmed. ACE inhibitors should be discontinued early in the first trimester. Postpartum, the systemic RV should be considered "at risk" to fail and should be managed with rate control (β-blocker), afterload reduction (ACE inhibitor), and appropriate management of preload (diuresis; see Tables 37-3 and 37-4).

The reported experience with TGA is to date the most extensive for any complex defect. The conclusions drawn from this experience are probably applicable to other, less common conditions with a systemic RV. **Functional status and cyanosis are the most reliable predictors of complicated pregnancies.** Arrhythmia is common and is frequently the cause of cardiac decompensation.

Fontan Procedure

The Fontan procedure was initially performed to achieve a physiologic palliation of tricuspid atresia by connecting the right atrium directly to the pulmonary artery. **The Fontan procedure and subsequent modifications are currently used to correct a variety of complex congenital heart conditions characterized by a single functional ventricle.** The operation achieves a noncyanotic state, with passive flow of systemic venous return

TABLE 37-5	PREGNANCY OUTCOMES AFTER FONTAN PALLIATION

	N (%)
Women	27
Pregnancies	43
Live births	19 (44%)
Miscarriages	19
Terminations	6
Fetal deaths	0
Premature birth (<35 wk)	3 (15%)
Congenital heart disease	1 (5%)
Congestive heart failure	3 (15%)
Arrhythmia	3 (16%)

Data from Canobbio M, Mair D, Van der Velde M, et al. Pregnancy outcomes after the Fontan repair. *J Am Coll Cardiol.* 1996;28:763; and Drenthen W, Pieper PG, Roos-Hesselink JW, et al, on behalf of the ZAHARA investigators. Pregnancy and delivery in women after Fontan palliation. *Heart.* 2006;92:1290.

through the lungs and a functionally systemic ventricle. Without a pulmonary pump, the cardiac price for this result is intolerance of increased intrathoracic pressure and elevated central venous pressure (CVP).

Experience with pregnancy in women after Fontan palliation is limited. In a survey of 76 women of reproductive age, Canobbio and associates[58] reported that 66% were counseled not to become pregnant despite a stable surgical outcome and a strong desire to have children. The remaining 34% were not counseled regarding pregnancy. Despite counseling against pregnancy, contraceptive use was inconsistent. Although the miscarriage rate was higher than in the general population, the preterm birth rate was low. Maternal complications were limited to arrhythmia, usually atrial, and CHF in the postpartum period. Although not reported in these small series, sluggish flow through the pulmonary circulation may increase the risk for thrombosis. The incidence of pulmonary emboli in nonpregnant patients with Fontan circulation may be as high as 17%. Another series reported 10 pregnancies in 6 women.[59] Of the 10 pregnancies, 5 ended in miscarriage before 12 weeks, and 1 was ectopic. Of the 4 completed pregnancies, 1 woman had a decline of NYHA class with both of her pregnancies, and the second pregnancy was complicated by atrial flutter. The other two women did not have maternal complications. These series remain small, and thus the ability to extrapolate to the individual with Fontan physiology is difficult, **but the uniqueness of the Fontan physiology warrants care in institutions with expertise in adult CHD.** Table 37-5 summarizes the outcomes with Fontan palliation of 43 pregnancies from 27 women reported by these groups.[58,59]

Eisenmenger Syndrome

Eisenmenger syndrome describes pulmonary-systemic shunting associated with cyanosis and increased pulmonary pressures secondary to pulmonary vascular disease. **Eisenmenger syndrome may develop from any intracardiac shunt that results in blood from the high-pressure systemic circulation being directed into the pulmonary circulation.** Systemic pressure and excessive flow lead to microvascular injury, obliteration of pulmonary arterioles and capillaries, and in the end, elevated PVR. The time to onset of shunt reversal is variable, but most patients who have a large VSD or large PDA develop shunt reversal in infancy. Shunt reversal in those with an ASD is delayed until early adulthood. Survival at 10 years from diagnosis is 80%; at 25 years, it is 42%.[60]

Patients with Eisenmenger syndrome are at risk for CHF, hemoptysis due to pulmonary hemorrhage, sudden death due to arrhythmia, cerebrovascular accident (CVA), and hyperviscosity syndrome. The diagnosis should be considered in any cyanotic patient and is confirmed by echocardiography with the demonstration of increased pulmonary pressure and an intracardiac shunt. If the shunt is due to an ASD or a PDA, cardiac MRI may be necessary to establish the diagnosis. Treatment is nonspecific and includes supportive care and avoidance of destabilizing events such as surgery and unnecessary medications. Symptomatic hyperviscosity syndrome due to an elevated hematocrit can be treated with hydration and, if necessary, phlebotomy. Iron deficiency, preexisting or secondary to phlebotomy, can exacerbate hyperviscosity; microcytic cells are less deformable and are therefore more prone to occlude the microcirculation. Definitive therapy can be achieved only with heart-lung or lung transplantation. However, the 4-year survival with lung transplantation is less than 50%, a less favorable prognosis than that for many patients with Eisenmenger syndrome.

VSD, ASD, and PDA are responsible for 89% of reported cases of Eisenmenger syndrome in pregnancy.[61] Each lesion is initially associated with shunting from the systemic circulation to the pulmonary circulation. As PVR and pulmonary pressures increase over time and approach systemic pressures, the characteristic murmurs of a VSD or PDA may diminish. **Reversal of flow from the pulmonary to the systemic circulation and the development of hypoxemia with increasing hematocrit herald the development of Eisenmenger syndrome. The fall in SVR associated with pregnancy may initiate right-to-left shunting in a patient not previously cyanotic.**

In 1979, Gleicher and colleagues[62] reviewed published cases of Eisenmenger syndrome in pregnancy. Seventy pregnancies from 44 women were evaluated; 52% of the women died during pregnancy, and 30% of the pregnancies resulted in maternal death. The risks for death associated with first, second, and third pregnancies were 36%, 27%, and 33%, respectively. A first successful pregnancy did not confirm the safety of subsequent pregnancies. Most deaths (70%) occurred at the time of delivery or within 1 week postpartum. Excessive blood loss was associated with 35% of deaths, whereas thromboembolic conditions were responsible for 44%. Maternal mortality associated with cesarean delivery (80%) exceeded that associated with vaginal delivery (34%). Maternal death was not reported with first-trimester termination of pregnancy. Only 26% of pregnancies resulted in a term birth. Fifty-five percent of newborns were delivered preterm, and 32% were small for gestational age.

A more modern review[63] of cases in the United Kingdom between 1991 and 1995 confirms the poor prognosis for pregnant women with Eisenmenger syndrome despite considerable advancement in the management of cardiac disease in pregnancy. Mortality remains extremely high: 40% of the women died, and most deaths (96%) occurred within the first 35 days postpartum. Late diagnosis (relative risk [RR], 5.4) and delayed hospitalization significantly increased maternal mortality.

Although the risks associated with Eisenmenger syndrome in pregnancy are clear, appropriate management is controversial. Decreased activity, hospitalization, and oxygen supplementation are usually used. Reduction of pulmonary pressures and improved systemic oxygen saturation after oxygen supplementation indicate that PVR is not fixed and suggest a better prognosis. Intercurrent antepartum events such as pneumonia or a urinary tract infection are poorly tolerated. Preventing microcytosis with iron supplementation may decrease the risk for microvascular slugging.

Cesarean delivery is reserved for obstetric indications and is avoided whenever possible. Hemodynamic stability must be maintained during labor and postpartum. When PVR is not fixed, oxygen supplementation may decrease pulmonary pressures. Systemic hypotension from hemorrhage or sympathectomy from epidural analgesia results in increased right-to-left shunting, increased hypoxemia, increased PVR, and worsening of the shunt. Volume overload or excessive systemic resistance, particularly postpartum, may further tax the failing right side of the heart. A pulmonary artery catheter and a peripheral arterial catheter are usually used to guide hemodynamic management. Narcotic-based regional analgesia provides adequate pain relief without excessive hemodynamic instability. Anticoagulation remains controversial. If patients are anticoagulated, caution should be exercised to avoid excessive treatment and associated hemorrhage.

Although use of a selective pulmonary vasodilator, inhaled nitric oxide (NO), has been reported to reduce pulmonary pressures, increase CO, and improve systemic oxygenation, maternal death was not averted. Use of sildenafil and L-arginine has been reported with apparent hemodynamic benefit and the survival of a single patient. Other case reports used pulmonary vasodilators with improved pregnancy outcomes, but nonetheless, maternal risk remains high. **Unlike many cardiac conditions in pregnancy, meticulous care frequently fails to prevent maternal death.**

Coarctation of the Aorta

Coarctation of the aorta results from a constriction of the aorta at or about the level of the ductus arteriosus or left subclavian artery. Patients have a characteristic discrepancy in blood pressure between their right arm and lower extremities. Complications include dissection at the site of coarctation, rupture of associated cranial berry aneurysms, heart failure, and ischemic heart disease associated with cephalic hypertension.

Modern reports of uncorrected coarctation in pregnancy are limited. Historically, pregnancy was associated with a maternal mortality rate of 9% owing to aortic rupture, CHF, CVAs, and endocarditis. β-Blockade may serve to protect against dissection and may promote diastolic flow through the aortic narrowing.

Pediatric screening identifies most significant coarctations, which leads to repair. After repair, systemic hypertension may persist and may require treatment. In two reports of 216 pregnancies in 104 women, 41 were complicated by hypertension and one suffered a lethal dissection at 36 weeks.[64,65]

SUMMARY

An increasing cohort of young women with corrected CHD will be presenting to their obstetricians pregnant and desiring to bear children. Some basic conclusions can be drawn from our experience with CHD to date. **First, Eisenmenger syndrome and pregnancy remain a lethal combination. New, effective strategies for therapy are not anticipated. Second, cyanotic heart disease in the absence of pulmonary hypertension is associated with increased rates of miscarriage and preterm birth. Third, mothers with cardiac disability (NYHA classes III and IV) or with evidence of right heart dilation have** a more complicated course in pregnancy. **Fourth, arrhythmias may become worse in pregnancy and may precipitate cardiac decompensation.** Aggressive pharmacologic treatment is appropriate. Finally, many young women who are initially without cardiac disability and are acyanotic can have successful pregnancies.

CARDIOMYOPATHY

Dilated cardiomyopathy is characterized by the development of pulmonary edema in the context of LV dysfunction and dilation. Patients usually present with signs and symptoms of pulmonary edema: dyspnea, cough, orthopnea, tachycardia, and occasionally, hemoptysis. Although characteristic of heart failure, these symptoms of pulmonary edema may also be due to previously undiagnosed congenital or rheumatic heart disease, preeclampsia, embolic disease, intrinsic pulmonary disease, or sepsis or from tocolysis. The diagnosis of cardiomyopathy is made in the clinical circumstances of characteristic signs and symptoms and findings of LV dysfunction and dilation on echocardiographic examination. The finding of an elevated B-type natriuretic peptide (BNP) can be used to help discriminate patients who need more definitive testing such as an echocardiogram. An elevated level may also be found with women with diastolic dysfunction or other conditions in which cardiac volume loading and stretch are increased. Ventricular dysfunction may be due to conditions extrinsic to the heart, such as thyrotoxicosis or hypertension, or to intrinsic myocardial dysfunction. Accurate diagnosis directs appropriate therapy and permits assessment of long-term prognosis.

Peripartum cardiomyopathy is a rare syndrome of heart failure that presents in late pregnancy or postpartum. The diagnosis is made after excluding other causes of pulmonary edema and heart failure. Failure to adhere to a rigorous definition of disease in the literature confounds conclusions regarding etiology and prognosis. A definition based on criteria for idiopathic dilated cardiomyopathy has been suggested (Box 37-3).[66] The incidence is estimated to be between 1 in 1300 and 1 in 15,000.[67] Although some of the variability in reported incidence is due to regional and ethnic differences, much is due to the imprecise definition of the disease. The cause of peripartum cardiomyopathy is unknown. Nutritional and immunologic mechanisms have been proposed. The prevalence of antibodies to echovirus and Coxsackie virus is not higher among women with cardiomyopathy compared with controls.

The mortality rate for peripartum cardiomyopathy (PPCM) is reported to be 25% to 50%. Death is usually due to progressive CHF, arrhythmia, or thromboembolism. Within 6 months, half of patients demonstrate resolution of LV dilation;

BOX 37-3 DIAGNOSTIC CRITERIA FOR PERIPARTUM CARDIOMYOPATHY

1. Heart failure within the last month of pregnancy or within 5 months postpartum
2. Absence of prior heart disease
3. No determinable cause
4. Echocardiographic indication of left ventricle dysfunction
   - Ejection fraction of <45% or fractional shortening of <30%
   - Left ventricle end-diastolic dimension of >2.7 cm/m²

their prognosis is very good. Of those who do not show resolution, an 85% mortality rate can be expected within the next 4 to 5 years.[68] The magnitude of risk for subsequent pregnancies after PPCM is unclear. A recent survey of 67 pregnancies in 63 women suggests a mortality rate of 8% when LV dysfunction has not resolved and 2% in patients with normal function.[69]

Women with established dilated cardiomyopathy who enter pregnancy with known disease are reported to have less severe outcomes. As might be expected, moderate to severe LV dysfunction and NYHA class III and IV symptoms are associated with worse outcomes. In a series of 36 pregnancies in 32 women, no deaths were reported. Three women developed pulmonary edema, and arrhythmia complicated six pregnancies. Pregnant women were much less likely to be treated with diuretics and β-blockers than were nonpregnant women.[70]

Women with a diagnosis of PPCM in a previous pregnancy are at risk for heart failure in a subsequent pregnancy. If LV ejection fraction (LVEF) has not normalized, the mortality rate may be as high as 19%.[71] In those in whom LVEF has normalized, a worsening of function and an increased incidence of symptoms of heart failure can be expected. Aggressive, appropriate pharmacologic management is frequently required.

Acute treatment of cardiomyopathy is directed at improving cardiac function and treating the inciting event. Diuretics are used to decrease preload and relieve pulmonary congestion, and digoxin may improve myocardial contractility and facilitate rate control when AF is present. Afterload reduction is achieved with ACE inhibitors postpartum or hydralazine before delivery. β-Blockade in stable, euvolemic patients has been clearly demonstrated to improve cardiac function and survival outside of pregnancy and should not be withheld from pregnant women. Significantly dilated and hypokinetic cardiac chambers pose a risk for clot formation and systemic embolization. Anticoagulation with heparin antepartum or warfarin postpartum should be considered. Implanted defibrillators have been used in pregnancy without significant complications. Arrhythmia is a common cause of death associated with cardiomyopathy outside pregnancy. Hemodynamic management during labor and delivery is frequently directed by a pulmonary artery catheter. Pain control decreases cardiac work and reduces tachycardia. A carefully dosed epidural is appropriate. Cesarean delivery is reserved for obstetric indications.

The postpartum period represents a time of particular risk. Women have received exogenous volume loading from IV fluids during labor; blood volume is centralized with uterine contractions, extravascular fluid is mobilized, tachycardia persists, and SVR increases. Each physiologic change will work toward LV decompensation, therefore preemptive HR control, diuresis, and afterload reduction should be used.

MYOCARDIAL INFARCTION

Myocardial infarction is a rare event among women of reproductive age. Recent studies suggest a rate between 2.8 and 6.2 per 100,000 deliveries.[71,72] **An increased risk for MI in pregnancy is consistently associated with maternal age greater than 40 years, chronic hypertension, diabetes, smoking, migraine headache, transfusion, and postpartum infection.**[72]

Owing to the rarity of the event, information regarding MI in pregnancy is derived from case reports and is therefore subject to considerable reporting bias. Elkayam and associates[73] summarized 150 cases between 2006 and 2011 (Table 37-6).

TABLE 37-6	MYOCARDIAL INFARCTION IN PREGNANCY

	N (%)
Pregnancies	150
Mean age ± SD	34 ± 6 yr
Age range	17 to 52 yr
Anterior infarction	69%
Multiparous	47%
Hypertension	15%
Diabetes mellitus	9%
Smoking	25%
Family history of MI	9%
Hyperlipidemia	20%
Preeclampsia	7%
CHF after MI	38%
Coronary anatomy	
Stenosis	27%
Thrombus	17%
Dissection	43%
Spasm	2%
Normal	9%
Death	
Maternal	7%
Infant	5%

Data from Elkayam U, Jalnapurkar S, Barakkat MN, et al. Pregnancy-associated acute myocardial infarction: a review o contemporary experience in 150 cases between 2006 and 2011. *Circulation.* 2014;129:1695-1702.
CHF, congestive heart failure; *MI,* myocardial infarction; *SD,* standard deviation.

Coronary dissection and normal coronary arteries are observed in almost 50% of cases. Delivery within 2 weeks of infarction may be associated with a maternal mortality rate as high as 50%. MI has been reported in association with cigarette smoking, hyperlipidemia, hypertension, diabetes mellitus, and family history of coronary artery disease as well as pheochromocytoma, Ehlers-Danlos type IV, antiphospholipid syndrome, multiple gestation, and sickle cell anemia. Medications such as ergot alkaloids given for bleeding, bromocriptine for lactation suppression, ritodrine and nifedipine for tocolysis, and prostaglandin E_2 in conjunction with severe hypertension have also been associated with MI (see Table 37-6).

The diagnosis of MI in pregnancy is often delayed because of the rarity of the event and common symptoms of pregnancy. During normal pregnancy, most women experience some increase in exercise intolerance and dyspnea. Chest pain due to reflux is common. **However, ST-segment elevation is not a normal finding, and in the context of ongoing chest pain, it should markedly increase the suspicion of acute MI.** The MB fraction of creatinine kinase isoenzymes may be elevated at cesarean delivery as well. Troponin I levels are not elevated during labor and delivery. If confusion regarding the appropriate diagnosis exists in the context of a constellation of findings suggestive of MI, an echocardiogram can be used to confirm abnormal wall motion in the ischemic region.

Acute therapy is based on rapid coronary reperfusion. Coronary angioplasty and stenting have been reported in pregnancy and should not be withheld when appropriate for the mother's condition. Thrombolytic therapy has also been used in pregnancy.[73] Although effective, there may be a small but real incidence of associated maternal bleeding, preterm delivery, or fetal loss. Furthermore, thrombolytic drugs are contraindicated in patients with coronary dissection,[74] and given the high incidence of coronary dissection in pregnant patients with acute MI, the use of thrombolytic drugs likely should be avoided. Surgery after thrombolytic therapy is associated with significant risk for hemorrhage.

Medications commonly used in the management of MI—such as morphine, organic nitrates, lidocaine, β-blockers, aspirin, magnesium sulfate, and calcium antagonists—may be used in appropriate doses in pregnancy. Clopidogrel should be strictly reserved for use after stenting procedures, whereas other glycoprotein IIb/IIIa inhibitors (bivalirudin, prasugrel, and ticagrelor) should be avoided. Use of clopidogrel at the time of cesarean delivery or other surgical procedures can lead to significant bleeding complications. Care should be taken to avoid the supine position and maternal hypotension during procedures, and a viable fetus should be monitored.

Elective delivery within 2 weeks of infarction should be avoided because it is associated with an increased risk for maternal death. Cesarean delivery is reserved for obstetric indications. Labor and delivery are managed with standard cardiac care, and pain is controlled, usually with carefully administered regional analgesia; tachycardia is prevented with pain control and is treated with β-blockers as needed. Hemodynamic stability is maintained, frequently using information from pulmonary and peripheral arterial catheters. Maternal pushing is avoided, and the second stage of labor is shortened with low forceps or vacuum. Diuresis is gently initiated postpartum with diuretics.

The experience with pregnancy after a remote MI is limited. Of 33 reported cases, recurrent infarction and significant complications have not been reported.[75]

MARFAN SYNDROME

Marfan syndrome is an autosomal-dominant genetic disorder caused by an abnormal gene for fibrillin on chromosome 15. Disease prevalence is estimated to be four to six per 10,000. Sporadic cases represent 15% of those diagnosed. The production of abnormal connective tissue results in the characteristic feature of the disease: aortic root dilation, dislocation of the optic lens, deformity of the anterior thorax, scoliosis, long limbs, joint laxity, and arachnodactyly. Diagnosis is usually based on family history and physical examination that includes ocular, cardiovascular, and skeletal features.

When Marfan syndrome is untreated, life expectancy is reduced by one third, and most deaths are due to aortic dissection and rupture. Elective aortic repair is associated with a low mortality rate (1.5%), whereas emergent repair results in a much higher mortality rate (11.7%). Therefore elective repair has been recommended when the aortic root diameter measures 5.0 cm.[76] Using an absolute aortic diameter (AD) as an indication for surgery ignores relevant differences in aortic size associated with patients of different stature. These considerations are particularly important when caring for young women. An aortic ratio between measured and predicted AD can be calculated. A ratio of less than 1.3 with a dilation rate of less than 5% per year suggests a low risk for a cardiovascular event. The predicted diameter for young adults can be calculated as follows:

$$AD_{predicted} = 1.02 + (0.98 \times body\ surface\ area)$$

The risk for aortic dissection is associated with the rate of change of blood pressure in the aorta over time in systole. Although simple reduction in blood pressure does not reduce the risk for dissection, β-blockade lowers the risk for reaching a critical cardiac end point at 10 years, from about 20% to 10%.

TABLE 37-7   MARFAN SYNDROME IN PREGNANCY

	N (%)
Women	113
Pregnancies	291
Live births	234 (80%)
Miscarriages	15 (5%)
Terminations	10 (3%)
Fetal deaths	1 (0.3%)
Aortic events	6 (2%)
Dissection	3 (1%)
Rapid dilation	2 (0.7%)
Valve dysfunction	1 (0.3%)
Death	0

Data from Meijboom LJ, Vos FE, Timmermans J, Boers GH, Zwinderman AH, Mulder BJ. Pregnancy and aortic root growth in the Marfan syndrome: a prospective study. *Eur Heart J.* 2005;26:914-920; Donnelly RT, Pinto NM, Kocolas I, Yetman AT. The immediate and long-term impact of pregnancy on aortic growth rate and mortality in women with Marfan syndrome. *J Am Coll Cardiol.* 2012;60:224-229; and Rossiter J, Repke J, Morales A, et al. A prospective longitudinal evaluation of pregnancy in the Marfan syndrome. *Am J Obstet Gynecol.* 1995;173:1599.

Literature surveys[77] **of case reports suggest a maternal mortality rate associated with Marfan syndrome in pregnancy in excess of 50%.** These case reports likely represent a bias of reporting more severely affected pregnancies. Three prospective population-based studies[78-80] are summarized in Table 37-7. Aortic events—dissection, rapid dilation, or aortic valve dysfunction—occurred in 2% of cases (*n* = 6). Of the three patients who experienced aortic dissection, two had prior dissections and the remaining had a prepregnancy AD of 4.2 cm. Two patients experienced rapid progressive dilation of the aorta, defined as greater than 5 mm from baseline. The final patient with a 4.9 cm aortic root had progression of aortic insufficiency from mild to severe by 38 weeks of gestation.

These studies suggest that women with mild disease, defined as an AD less than 4 cm, can attempt pregnancy with only modest risk. The risk associated with more advanced disease is certainly greater. **Given the data available, a precise risk for death from aortic dissection or rupture cannot be quantified, although patients with a prior aortic dissection or an AD greater than 4.5 cm likely are at higher risk. For women with ADs greater than 4 cm, prophylactic aortic graft and valve replacement is recommended before pregnancy.**[76] They will then assume the risk associated with an artificial valve and the risk associated with the remaining aorta. These risks may be significant; however, adequate data do not exist to quantify the risks. Fifty percent of the offspring of women with Marfan syndrome can be expected to have the disease.

Management of pregnancies affected by Marfan syndrome should begin with an accurate assessment of the aortic root. An absolute diameter, or preferably an aortic ratio, can be used to assess specific risk. The aortic root should be protected from hemodynamic forces with β-blockade. A resting HR of about 70 beats/min can usually be achieved. Although β-blockade may potentially contribute to impaired fetal growth, this risk is outweighed by the maternal risk without such treatment.

Labor and delivery are managed with standard cardiac care, with particular emphasis on the prevention of tachycardia. Patients with aortic roots less than 4 cm can be delivered vaginally, reserving cesarean delivery for obstetric indications. Some authors have recommended cesarean delivery for women with larger roots based on concerns about increased pressure in the aorta during labor, although data do not exist to make this a firm recommendation.

PULMONARY HYPERTENSION

Although pulmonary hypertension is fundamentally a pulmonary disease, the major pathologic impact is on the right side of the heart. The incidence of primary pulmonary hypertension is 1 to 2 per 1 million, and women are affected more commonly than men. Secondary pulmonary hypertension may develop as a complication of cardiac disease such as mitral stenosis or secondary to intrinsic pulmonary disease. Drugs such as cocaine or appetite suppressants may also be associated with pulmonary hypertension. If left untreated, the median survival after diagnosis is 2.5 years.[81] More recently, survival has been reported to be 68% to 77% at 1 year, 40% to 56% at 3 years, and 22% to 38% at 5 years.[82] As might be expected, right heart failure and NYHA class III and IV symptoms predict adverse outcome. General therapy may include limitation of extreme exercise, supplemental oxygen, diuresis, and in some cases, anticoagulation.

Pulmonary vasodilator therapy generally improves symptoms, and lifestyle changes may improve survival. About 10% of patients will respond to high-dose calcium channel blockers. Of those who initially respond to nifedipine, the 5-year survival rate is 95%. IV prostacyclin is associated with a higher response rate but is also associated with side effects such as headache, jaw pain, diarrhea, flushing, and leg pain. A long-term IV line is required, and the dose must be increased on a regular basis. The 5-year survival rate for those who require treatment with prostacyclin is 54%. Subcutaneous, oral, and inhaled prostacyclin are also available, although each has limitations because of the route and timing of delivery.

Sildenafil, a cyclic guanosine monophosphate phosphodiesterase inhibitor, increases the endogenous production of nitric oxide and therefore operates as a potent vasodilator. Treatment with sildenafil improves functional status and hemodynamic profile, and ease of administration is a significant advantage.

The maternal mortality with severe pulmonary hypertension is reported to be as high as 50%.[83] Although a review of reported cases suggests an improvement in mortality from 30% between 1978 and 1996 to 17% between 1997 and 2007, the risk remains high. The improvement may be associated with the advent of vasodilator therapy, which highlights the value of a team with considerable experience in pharmacologic management of pulmonary hypertension. **Sudden, irreversible deterioration in the postpartum period is common, and as many as 75% of deaths will occur postpartum.**[84]

The symptoms of pulmonary hypertension are nonspecific. Increasing fatigue and shortness of breath are associated with progressive right-sided heart failure but are also ubiquitous in pregnancy. They can easily be attributed to a presumed upper respiratory infection. Hoarseness may be a result of impingement on the laryngeal nerve by an enlarged pulmonary artery. Patients may exhibit disproportionate lower extremity edema or oxygen desaturation out of proportion for a presumed illness. The diagnosis can be confirmed with echocardiography, in which the velocity of the regurgitant jet across the tricuspid valve can estimate pulmonary systolic pressure. A dilated, hypokinetic RV with displacement of the intraventricular septum into the LV suggests right-sided heart failure.

Pulmonary hypertension with RV dysfunction is poorly tolerated in pregnancy. A mortality rate between 17% and 30% should be expected. Antepartum management often requires hospitalization, and oxygen therapy may reduce PVR and may improve RV performance. Pharmacologic treatment with pulmonary vasodilators may also be effective,[82,85] and anticoagulation with heparin should be considered. Worsening disease will usually be manifest by falling CO rather than rising RV pressure. Labor and delivery should be managed with standard cardiac care, with particular attention to RV filling as assessed by measurement of CVP. **Although the RV requires adequate filling to generate forward flow against an elevated PVR, modest elevations in CVP may precipitate increasing RV dysfunction.** Given fluid mobilization postpartum and the potential need to treat volume loss associated with delivery, appropriate filling may be difficult to achieve; in these cases, aggressive diuresis may be required. Modest underloading or overloading of the RV can result in rapid decompensation and death.

Women with pulmonary hypertension and RV dysfunction should be strongly discouraged from becoming pregnant. Because pulmonary artery pressures fall as the RV fails, the condition of the RV may be a more important consideration than an absolute systolic pulmonary pressure. Some women may consider pregnancy after a favorable response to treatment with pulmonary vasodilators. In a small series, two women whose pulmonary pressures and RV function had normalized carried three pregnancies successfully while being treated with nifedipine or prostacyclin. Neither experienced deterioration in their condition during the first year postpartum.

OTHER CONDITIONS

Young women may experience **malignant ventricular arrhythmias** due to idiopathic ventricular fibrillation, cardiomyopathy, long-QT syndrome, CHD, or hypertrophic cardiomyopathy. An ICD can effectively protect these patients from sudden death. In a report of 44 pregnancies, no women experienced generator erosion or lead fractures due to the expanding pregnancy. Twenty-five percent experienced electrical discharges during pregnancy without complication.[86]

Hypertrophic cardiomyopathy is a genetic condition usually inherited in an autosomal-dominant pattern with variable penetrance. Although the condition can be subclassified, the physiologic impact of different forms is similar. Patients are at risk for malignant arrhythmia, diastolic dysfunction, and outflow tract obstruction. A risk for sudden death is suggested by a family history of sudden death, extreme hypertrophy (LV wall ≥30 mm), a history of syncope, nonsustained ventricular tachycardia, and hypotension with exercise. Arrhythmia risk is managed with an ICD and β-blockade. Volume loading during pregnancy in the face of diastolic dysfunction may result in pulmonary edema. Serum BNP can be used to direct volume management with diuretics. LV outflow tract obstruction is uncommon in young women. Reduced ventricular filling associated with blood loss, dehydration, or tachycardia will increase the functional obstruction. Management of hypertrophic cardiomyopathy has been recently reviewed.[87]

Reviews of case reports suggest a maternal mortality rate of 1% to 2% in these cases.[88-90] Given the biases associated with case report–derived data, this estimate probably sets an upper limit of expected mortality. Thaman and colleagues[90] reported 271 pregnancies in 127 women with hypertrophic cardiomyopathy, complicated by only two cases of pulmonary edema postpartum that resolved with appropriate therapy. In pregnancy, increased blood volume and LV dimension will tend to benefit the patient. Increased heart rate will not benefit the patient;

therefore β-blockers are generally used to manage tachycardia and some arrhythmias, and ICDs may also be used. Labor and delivery are managed with standard cardiac care with particular emphasis given to ensuring generous LV filling. **Excessive volume loading may reveal a stiff ventricle and diastolic dysfunction. In some patients, a relatively small increase in vascular volume results in a substantial increase in pulmonary pressure, pulmonary congestion, and desaturation.** Although diastolic dysfunction may be difficult to diagnose by echocardiography, careful attention to an O_2 saturation monitor during labor and postpartum can reveal the need for augmented diuresis. Supine hypotension must be carefully avoided, and obstetric bleeding should be treated early and aggressively with volume replacement.

CRITICAL CARE: HEMODYNAMIC MONITORING AND MANAGEMENT

Diseases unique to pregnancy, the physiologic stresses of pregnancy, and the special conditions that surround labor and delivery operate to create circumstances in which intensive care may be necessary more frequently than would be required among young nonpregnant individuals. Specialists in intensive care may not be familiar with the physiology of pregnancy and associated unique conditions such as preeclampsia or amniotic fluid embolus. They may also be unfamiliar with maternal-fetal physiologic relationships and decision making that must balance the needs of the mother and the fetus. **Therefore obstetricians must be familiar with basic principles and techniques of critical care medicine in order to primarily manage critically ill pregnant women or to serve as valuable consultants to a critical care team.**

Acute indications for invasive hemodynamic monitoring can be broadly categorized based on questions of physiology (Box 37-4). Severe preeclampsia, sepsis, acute respiratory distress syndrome (ARDS), pneumonia, previously undiagnosed heart disease, and fluid management after resuscitation from obstetric hemorrhage are the most common conditions that require hemodynamic monitoring. Certain conditions, particularly maternal heart disease as discussed earlier, require a planned prospective decision for invasive monitoring. In these cases, the therapeutic window for hemodynamic management is narrow, and knowledge of the patient's baseline compensated hemodynamic status can serve as a goal for intrapartum management.

In many cases, initial therapy can and should be based empirically on an understanding of the patient's pathophysiology. If subsequent interventions are needed, specific data obtained from hemodynamic monitoring may be required. Physicians with abundant experience treating a particular disease may rely less on invasive monitoring because an improved understanding makes the clinical course more predictable. In contrast, physicians with less experience may have a lower threshold for using invasive hemodynamic monitoring. Therefore understanding principles of management is particularly important for obstetricians who do not necessarily anticipate critically ill patients in their practice.

Hemodynamic Monitoring

The objective of hemodynamic monitoring is to provide continuous assessment of systemic and intracardiac pressures and to provide the means to determine CO and therefore to calculate systemic and pulmonary resistances. An arterial catheter is usually placed in the radial artery to measure systemic pressure, and the diastolic pressure obtained usually correlates well with noninvasive measurements. Systolic pressure may be significantly higher than noninvasive measurements because of a very brief peak in pressure in early systole. The spike in pressure contributes little to MAP. The noninvasive measurement is usually more clinically relevant to the patient's condition. The arterial catheter permits easy access to arterial blood sampling and relieves the patient from the discomfort of frequent blood draws.

Measurement of intracardiac pressures and CO are obtained through the insertion of a catheter into the central venous circulation and advancement into and through the right side of the heart. Venous access is most commonly obtained through the right internal jugular vein; a subclavian approach may also be used. Traditionally, insertion is guided by using the sternocleidomastoid muscle and the clavicle as landmarks. The higher-frequency ultrasound transducer found on a vaginal probe can also be used to facilitate insertion under direct visualization. Once central venous access has been obtained and confirmed, a pulmonary artery catheter can be "floated" into the right side of the heart and pulmonary artery. Figure 37-7 demonstrates the waveforms and normal pressure values found as the catheter passes through the heart. Success in floating the catheter is initially confirmed by observation of characteristic waveforms in the RV, pulmonary artery, and wedged position and subsequently with a radiograph. In experienced hands, complications from pulmonary artery catheterization are uncommon and include pneumothorax (<0.1%), pulmonary infarction (0 to 1.3%), pulmonary artery rupture (<0.1%), and septicemia (0.5% to 2.0%). Arrhythmias are usually transient and are associated with passage of the catheter through the RV. If the patient has significant pulmonary hypertension, difficulty may be encountered maintaining placement in the pulmonary artery.

Once the catheter has been successfully placed, continuous readings of CVP and pulmonary artery pressures can be

---

BOX 37-4   INDICATIONS FOR HEMODYNAMIC MONITORING

1. Why is the patient hypoxic?
   - Are pulmonary capillary pressures high because of relative volume overload (e.g., mitral stenosis postpartum)?
   - Are pulmonary capillary pressures high because of depressed cardiac function (e.g., cardiomyopathy)?
   - Is capillary membrane integrity intact (e.g., acute respiratory distress syndrome, pneumonia)?
2. Why is the patient persistently hypertensive?
   - Is vascular resistance elevated?
   - Is cardiac output elevated?
3. Why is the patient hypotensive?
   - Is left ventricle filling pressure low (e.g., after hemorrhage)?
   - Is vascular resistance low (e.g., as with septic shock)?
4. Why is the patient's urine output low?
   - Is left ventricle filling pressure low, resulting in low cardiac output?
5. Is the patient expected to be unstable in labor?
   - Is the window of left ventricle filling narrow (e.g., aortic stenosis)?
   - Will normal physiologic changes associated with delivery be tolerated poorly (e.g., volume loading postpartum, mitral stenosis, pulmonary hypertension)?

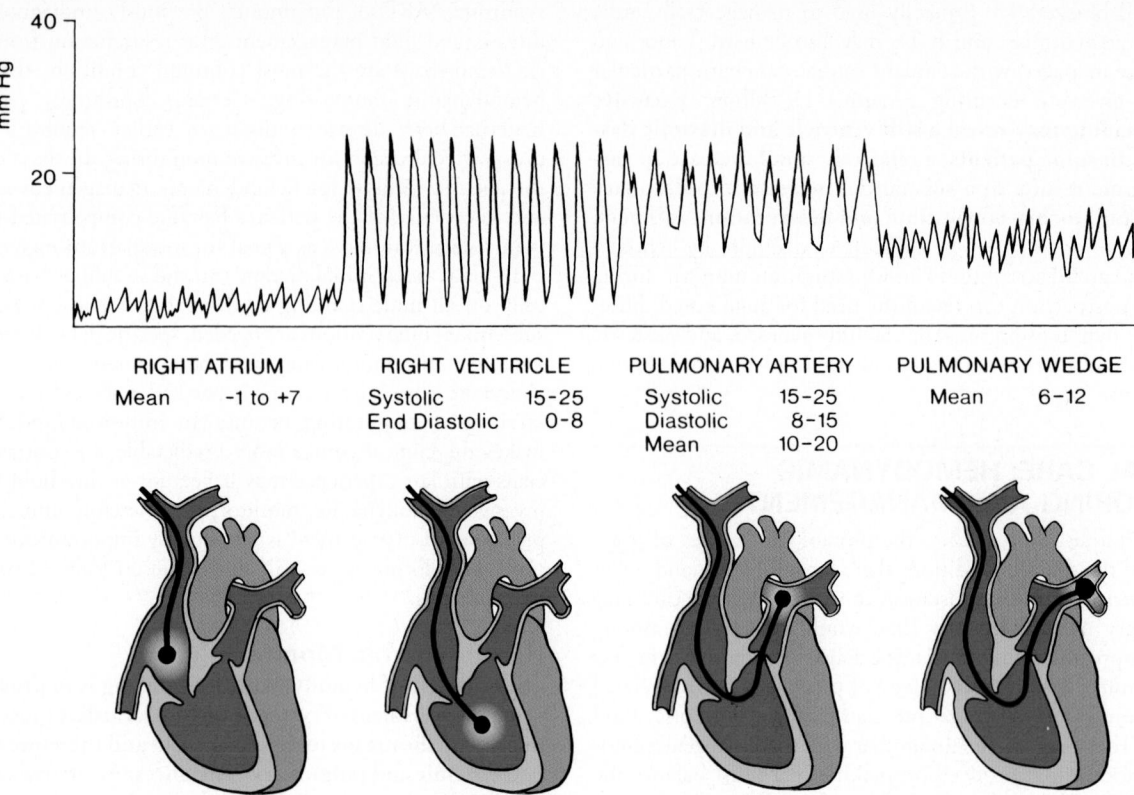

FIG 37-7 Hemodynamic waveforms and normal pressure values associated with catheter positions during advancement of a pulmonary artery catheter.

obtained. By inflating the balloon at the catheter tip, the catheter can be wedged in the pulmonary artery to obtain a PAWP, which reflects the filling pressure—preload—in the left ventricle. CVP measured in the right atrium is a measure of RV filling pressure. In pregnant women, CVP cannot be assumed to accurately reflect LV filling. Right atrial pressures and systolic pulmonary pressures can be measured noninvasively by echocardiography.

CO is measured by thermodilution. A bolus of cold fluid is injected into the right atrium, and a curve of temperature change over time is recorded as the bolus passes through the pulmonary artery. From the shape of the curve, CO can be calculated; when the CO is higher, the dilutional curve is shorter in time and greater in maximal temperature change. More recently, catheters have been equipped with a heating element in the right atrial segment so that continuous measurement of CO can be performed. CO can be measured noninvasively with Doppler and impedance techniques. Doppler technique has been validated under a wide range of clinical circumstances.[91-94] The impedance technique tends to underestimate CO in pregnancy but accurately reflects changes in hemodynamics in many conditions. In conditions of pathologically high flow, impedance may significantly underestimate CO.[95-97] Cardiac index can be derived from CO in order to adjust for maternal size and equals CO divided by body surface area (BSA). However, BSA does not seem to be related to CO in pregnancy, therefore CO is usually preferred.[94] When CO is measured noninvasively and CVP is not available, resistance is expressed as total peripheral resistance (TPR) rather than SVR. In most clinical conditions, the differences between the two are not important.

Table 37-8 summarizes the formulae used to calculate hemodynamic parameters not directly measured. Normal values for

TABLE 37-8   CALCULATED HEMODYNAMIC VARIABLES

	CALCULATION	UNITS
Mean arterial pressure (MAP)	$\dfrac{sBP + 2(dBP)}{3}$	mm Hg
Stroke volume (SV)	$\dfrac{CO \cdot 1000}{HR}$	mL
Systemic vascular resistance (SVR)	$\dfrac{(MAP - CVO) \cdot 80}{CO}$	dyne $\cdot$ sec $\cdot$ cm^{-5}
Total peripheral resistance (TPR)	$\dfrac{MAP \cdot 80}{CO}$	dyne $\cdot$ sec $\cdot$ cm^{-5}
Pulmonary vascular resistance (PVR)	$\dfrac{80(mPAP - PAWP)}{CO}$	dyne $\cdot$ sec $\cdot$ cm^{-5}

CO, cardiac output; *CVO*, central venous oxygen; *dBP*, diastolic blood pressure; *mPAP*, mean pulmonary artery pressure; *PAWP*, pulmonary artery wedge pressure; *sBP*, systolic blood pressure.

CO, MAP, HR, SV, and TPR are summarized in Figure 37-1. In a study of 10 normal pregnant women at term, Clark and coworkers[98] determined that CVP, pulmonary artery pressure, PAWP, and LV work index were not different from nonpregnant measurements made about 3 months postpartum. The relationship between PAWP and LV work index fell within the normal range for nonpregnant individuals, suggesting normal contractility in pregnancy. PVR was 34% lower, and colloid osmotic pressure was reduced by 14%.

Hemodynamic Management

Strategies of hemodynamic therapy that may be applicable to a variety of clinical circumstances are discussed in this section. As outlined earlier, the use of hemodynamic monitoring should be directed at answering specific questions of maternal pathophysiology. To achieve a particular goal, a number of physiologic interventions are possible. Each of these interventions will precipitate a secondary or compensatory response. The secondary response, if excessive, may adversely affect the patient. The choice of intervention from available options will often be determined by the potential for and magnitude of adverse effect. **Hemodynamic monitoring permits the physician to choose an intervention and subsequently assess the positive and negative effects.**

Disruption of alveolar capillary fluid dynamics is frequently associated with acute oxygen desaturation due to excess alveolar fluid. Pulmonary edema is usually due to excess hydrostatic capillary pressure (e.g., cardiomyopathy, mitral stenosis) or to a disruption of alveolar capillary membrane integrity (e.g., pneumonia, ARDS). **Although a reduction in serum oncotic pressure is rarely a primary cause of pulmonary edema, the reduced serum albumin level in normal pregnancy can act in synergy with other forces and result in earlier or more severe pulmonary edema than would normally occur.**

The use of pulse oximetry facilitates the early detection of maternal desaturation. Oxygen supplementation improves maternal saturation but does not correct the underlying cause. If desaturation is progressive, further intervention will be required. In the normal heart, diuresis to reduce preload works to decrease alveolar water in patients with elevated PAWP and in patients with capillary leak. A reduction in capillary pressure from high normal to low normal will reduce the egress of water across damaged membranes. In many circumstances, these interventions are made empirically based on a diagnosis and an understanding of maternal physiology. For example, tocolysis with β-mimetic agents can induce pulmonary edema. Timely diagnosis, discontinuation of the offending agent, oxygen supplementation, and a single diuretic dose will usually be sufficient therapy. When initial interventions do not achieve an adequate effect, invasive monitoring may be required to direct subsequent care. Maternal diuresis to improve oxygen saturation, when excessive, may lead to a reduction in CO. **Fetal decompensation is usually encountered before a significant reduction in maternal perfusion and hypotension.** The maternal PAWP and CO can be used to direct maternal diuresis. If desaturation continues despite hemodynamic management, intubation may be required. Positive end-expiratory pressure (PEEP) can be used to increase intraalveolar pressure to impede the forces that drive water into alveolar spaces. PEEP may impede venous return and decrease CO as a result of the effects of the associated increase in extracardiac intrathoracic pressure. A PAWP in excess of PEEP is required for adequate ventricular filling. Only in the sickest of pregnant women will PEEP have a clinically significant impact on CO.

Disorders of blood pressure and perfusion can be managed with the knowledge of maternal hemodynamics. Figure 37-8 describes the relationships between MAP, CO, and vascular resistance. CO and MAP are represented on the x-axis and y-axis, respectively. Resistance is represented by diagonal isometric lines. Vasodilators or vasopressors that act on resistance produce vectors of change that run perpendicular to lines of resistance. Interventions that decrease (β-blockers, diuresis) or increase (dopamine, volume) CO produce vectors of change that run roughly parallel to lines of resistance. The region labeled "normal" represents the goal of therapy. Plotting patient data on

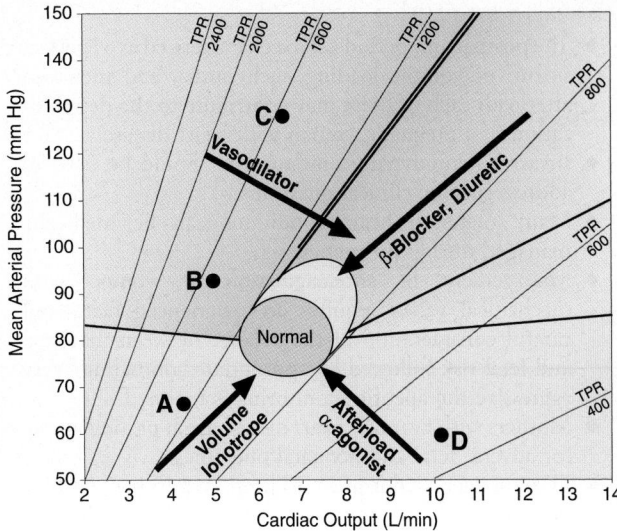

FIG 37-8 Hemodynamic flow chart. Cardiac output and mean arterial pressure are plotted on the x-axis and y-axis, respectively. Diagonal lines are isometric lines of vascular resistance. Anticipated vectors of change can be used to predict patient response to intervention. TPR, total peripheral resistance.

the chart allows the clinician to visually determine the vector or combination of vectors that could return hemodynamics to normal.

Patient A represents a patient who is hypotensive with a low CO, as might be expected after hemorrhage or in heart failure. Given a low PAWP associated with hemorrhage, volume administration would be expected to create a vector that would return hemodynamics to normal. Alternatively, the patient could have a normal or high PAWP associated with heart failure and would need an inotropic agent such as dopamine. Patient B has a normal blood pressure but a high vascular resistance and low CO such as might be expected with a cardiomyopathy. Afterload reduction with a medication such as hydralazine will produce a vector of vasodilation and will return hemodynamics to normal. Patient C is hypertensive with a mixed hemodynamic pattern. She will need a combination of vectors to approach normal hemodynamics (e.g., hydralazine and β-blocker). Patient D is hypotensive and hyperdynamic with a low vascular resistance, hemodynamics that might be found in a patient with early sepsis. Treatment with volume could increase pressure but at the expense of high filling pressures and a potentially negative impact on developing ARDS. Alternatively, a small dose of an α-adrenergic agent such as phenylephrine would create a vector perpendicular to lines of resistance and would return hemodynamics to normal.

KEY POINTS

- ◆ Hemodynamic changes in pregnancy may adversely affect maternal cardiac performance.
- ◆ Intercurrent events such as infection during pregnancy are usually the cause of decompensation.
- ◆ Women with heart disease in pregnancy frequently have unique psychosocial needs.
- ◆ Labor, delivery, and postpartum are periods of hemodynamic instability.

◆ The postpartum period can be characterized as a "perfect storm" of volume loading, tachycardia, and increased afterload; each of these may contribute to the destabilization of a pregnant woman with heart disease.

◆ Invasive hemodynamic monitoring should be used to address specific clinical questions.

◆ Many maternal heart conditions can be medically managed during pregnancy.

◆ Management of anticoagulation in women with mechanical valves requires an experienced team and careful consideration of the balance between maternal and fetal risk followed by appropriate counseling. Very aggressive therapeutic monitoring is required.

◆ Mothers with cyanotic heart disease are at particular risk for adverse fetal and neonatal outcomes.

◆ Eisenmenger syndrome, Marfan syndrome with a dilated aorta, and pulmonary hypertension with right heart dysfunction are associated with a very high risk for maternal mortality.

◆ Many women with congenital heart disease can successfully complete a pregnancy.

◆ Preconceptual counseling is based on achieving a balance between medical information and the patient's value system.

REFERENCES

1. Easterling T, Benedetti T, Schmucker B, et al. Maternal hemodynamics in normal and preeclamptic pregnancies: a longitudinal study. *Obstet Gynecol.* 1990;76:1061.
2. Robson S, Dunlop W, Boys R, et al. Cardiac output during labour. *BMJ.* 1987;295:1169.
3. Easterling T, Chadwick H, Otto C, et al. Aortic stenosis in pregnancy. *Obstet Gynecol.* 1988;72:113.
4. Clark S, Phelan J, Greenspoon J, et al. Labor and delivery in the presence of mitral stenosis: central hemodynamic observations. *Am J Obstet Gynecol.* 1985;152:384.
5. Whittaker P, Lind T. The intravascular mass of albumin during pregnancy: a serial study in normal and diabetic women. *BJOG.* 1993;100:587.
6. Tanous D, Siu S, Jennifer Mason J, et al. B-type natriuretic peptide in pregnant women with heart disease. *J Am Coll Cardiol.* 2010;56:1247-1253.
7. Kampman M, Balci1 A, van Veldhuisen D, et al. N-terminal pro-B-type natriuretic peptide predicts cardiovascular complications in pregnant women with congenital heart disease. *Eur Heart J.* 2014;35:708-715.
8. Boggess K, Watts D, Hillier S, et al. Bacteremia shortly after placental separation during cesarean section. *Obstet Gynecol.* 1996;87:779.
9. Whittemore R, Hobbins J, Engle M. Pregnancy and its outcome in women with and without surgical treatment of congenital heart disease. *Am J Cardiol.* 1982;50:641.
10. Gill H, Splitt M, Sharland G, et al. Patterns of recurrence of congenital heart disease: an analysis of 6,640 consecutive pregnancies evaluated by detailed fetal echocardiography. *J Am Coll Cardiol.* 2003;42:923.
11. Siu S, Sermer M, Colman J, et al. Prospective multicenter study of pregnancy outcomes in women with heart disease. *Circulation.* 2001;104:515-521.
12. Drenthen W, Boersma E, Balci A, et al. Predictors of pregnancy complications in women with congenital heart disease. *Eur Heart J.* 2010;31:2124-2132.
13. Regitz-Zagrosek V, Blomstrom LC, Borghi C, et al. ESC Guidelines on the management of cardiovascular diseases during pregnancy: the Task Force on the Management of Cardiovascular Diseases during Pregnancy of the European Society of Cardiology (ESC). *Eur Heart J.* 2011;32:3147-3197.
14. Balci A, Sollie-Szarynska K, van der Bijl A, et al. Prospective validation and assessment of cardiovascular and offspring risk models for pregnant women with congenital heart disease. *Heart.* 2014;100:1373-1381.
15. Nishimura R, Otto C, Bonow R, et al. 2014 AHA/ACC Guideline for the Management of Patients With Valvular Heart Disease: A Report of the American College of Cardiology/American Heart Association Task Force on Practice Guidelines. *J Am Coll Cardiol.* 2014;63:e57-e185.
16. Chesley L. Severe rheumatic cardiac disease and pregnancy: the ultimate prognosis. *Am J Obstet Gynecol.* 1980;136:552.
17. Al Kasab S, Sabag T, Al Zaibag M, et al. Beta-adrenergic receptor blockade in the management of pregnant women with mitral stenosis. *Am J Obstet Gynecol.* 1990;163:37.
18. Silversides CK, Colman JM, Sermer M, et al. Cardiac risk in pregnant women with rheumatic mitral stenosis. *Am J Cardiol.* 2003;91:1382.
19. Routray SN, Mishra TK, Swain S, et al. Balloon mitral valvuloplasty during pregnancy. *Int J Gynaecol Obstet.* 2004;85:18-23.
20. Esteves CA, Munoz JS, Braga S, et al. Immediate and long-term follow-up of percutaneous balloon mitral valvuloplasty in pregnant patients with rheumatic mitral stenosis. *Am J Cardiol.* 2006;98:812-816.
21. Arias F, Pineda J. Aortic stenosis and pregnancy. *J Reprod Med.* 1978;20:229.
22. Lao T, Sermer M, MaGee L, et al. Congenital aortic stenosis and pregnancy: a reappraisal. *Am J Obstet Gynecol.* 1993;169:540.
23. Shime J, Mocarski E, Hastings D, et al. Congenital heart disease in pregnancy: short- and long-term implications. *Am J Obstet Gynecol.* 1987;156:313.
24. Tzemos N, Silversides CK, Colman JM, et al. Late cardiac outcomes after pregnancy in women with congenital aortic stenosis. *Am Heart J.* 2009;157:474.
25. Elkayam U, Bitar F. Valvular heart disease and pregnancy part II: prosthetic valves. *J Am Coll Cardio.* 2005;46:403-410.
26. Lee C, Wu C, Lin P, et al. Pregnancy following cardiac prosthetic valve replacement. *Obstet Gynecol.* 1994;83:353.
27. Deleted in review.
28. Jamieson W, Miller D, Atkins C, et al. Pregnancy and bioprostheses: influence on structural valve deterioration. *Ann Thorac Surg.* 1995;60:S282-S287.
29. Crawford M. Cardiovascular disease in pregnancy. Foreword. *Cardiol Clin.* 2012;30:ix.
30. Regitz-Zagrosek V, Blomstrom Lundqvist C, Borghi C, et al. ESC Guidelines on the management of cardiovascular diseases during pregnancy: the task force on the management of cardiovascular diseases during pregnancy of the European Society of Cardiology (ESC). *Eur Heart J.* 2011;32:3147-3197.
31. Bates S, Greer I, Middeldorp S, et al. American College of Chest Physicians. VTE, thrombophilia, antithrombotic therapy, and pregnancy: antithrombotic therapy and prevention of thrombosis, 9th ed.: American College of Chest Physicians Evidence-Based Clinical Practice Guidelines. *Chest.* 2012;141(2 suppl):e691S-736S.
32. Van Driel D, Wesseling J, Sauer P, et al. Teratogen update: fetal effects after in utero exposure to coumarins overview of cases, follow-up findings, and pathogenesis. *Teratology.* 2002;66:127-140.
33. Quinn J, Klemperer K, Ruth Brooks R, et al. Use of high intensity adjusted dose low molecular weight heparin in women with mechanical heart valves during pregnancy: a single-center experience. *Haematologica.* 2009;94:1608-1612.
34. Abildgaard U, Sandset P, Hammerstrøm J, et al. Management of pregnant women with mechanical heart valve prosthesis: Thromboprophylaxis with low molecular weight heparin. *Thromb Res.* 2009;124:262-267.
35. Saeed C, Frank J, Pravin M, et al. A Prospective Trial Showing the Safety of Adjusted-Dose Enoxaparin for Thromboprophylaxis of Pregnant Women With Mechanical Prosthetic Heart Valves. *Clin Appl Thromb Hemost.* 2011;7:313-319.
36. Barbour LA, Oja JL, Schultz LK. A prospective trial that demonstrates that dalteparin requirements increase in pregnancy to maintain therapeutic levels of anticoagulation. *Am J Obstet Gynecol.* 2004;191:1024.
37. Gantt L. Growing up heartsick: the experiences of young women with congenital heart disease. *Health Care Women Int.* 1992;13:241.
38. Kovacs AH, Harrison JL, Colman JM, et al. Pregnancy and contraception in congenital heart disease: what women are not told. *J Am Coll Cardiol.* 2008;12:577.
39. Findlay D, Doyle E. Congenital heart disease in adults. *Br J Anaesth.* 1997;78:416.
40. Presbitero P, Somerville J, Stone S, et al. Pregnancy in cyanotic congenital heart disease: outcome of mother and fetus. *Circulation.* 1994;89:2673-2676.
41. Rose V, Gold R, Lindsay G, et al. A possible increase in the incidence of congenital heart defects among the offspring of affected patients. *J Am Coll Cardiol.* 1985;6:376.

42. Piesiewicz W, Goch A, Binokowski Z, et al. Changes in the cardiovascular system during pregnancy in females with secundum atrial septal defect. *Polish Heart J.* 2004;60:218.

43. Balci A, Drenthen W, Mulder BJ, et al. Pregnancy in women with corrected tetralogy of Fallot: occurrence and predictors of adverse events. *Am Heart J.* 2011;161:307-313.

44. Genoni M, Jenni R, Hoerstrup S, et al. Pregnancy after atrial repair for transposition of the great arteries. *Heart.* 1999;81:276.

45. Nwosu U. Pregnancy following Mustard operation for transposition of great arteries. *J Tenn Med Assoc.* 1992;85:509.

46. Neukermans K, Sullivan T, Pitlick D. Successful pregnancy after the Mustard operation for transposition of the great arteries. *Am J Cardiol.* 1988;57:838.

47. Megerian G, Bell E, Huhta J, et al. Pregnancy outcome following Mustard procedure for transposition of the great arteries: a report of five cases and review of the literature. *Obstet Gynecol.* 1994;83:512.

48. Lynch-Salomond D, Maze S, Combs C. Pregnancy after Mustard repair for transposition of the great arteries. *Obstet Gynecol.* 1993;82:676.

49. Lao T, Sermer M, Colman J. Pregnancy following surgical correction for transposition of the great arteries. *Obstet Gynecol.* 1994;83:665.

50. Dellinger E, Hadi H. Maternal transposition of the great arteries in pregnancy: a case report. *J Reprod Med.* 1994;39:324.

51. Clarkson P, Wilson N, Neutze J, et al. Outcome of pregnancy after the Mustard operation for transposition of the great arteries with intact ventricular septum. *Am Coll Cardiol.* 1994;24:190.

52. Zentner D, Wheeker M, Grigg L. Does pregnancy contribute to systemic right ventricular dysfunction in adults with an atrial switch operation? *Heart Lung Circ.* 2012;21:433.

53. Canobbio MM, Morris CD, Graham TP, Landzberg MJ. Pregnancy outcomes after atrial repair for transposition of the great arteries. *Am J Cardiol.* 2006;98:668.

54. Tobler D, Fernandes SM, Wald RM, et al. Pregnancy outcomes in women with transposition of the great arteries and arterial switch operation. *Am J Cardiol.* 2010;106:417.

55. Therrien J, Barnes I, Somerville J. Outcome of pregnancy in patients with congenitally corrected transposition of the great arteries. *Am J Cardiol.* 1999;84:820.

56. Connolly H, Grogan M, Warnes C. Pregnancy among women with congenitally corrected transposition of great arteries. *J Am Coll Cardiol.* 1999;33:1692.

57. Kowalik E, Klisiewicz A, Biernacka E, et al. Pregnancy and long-term cardiovascular outcomes in women with congenitally corrected transposition of the great arteries. *Int J Gynaecol Obstet.* 2014;125:154-157.

58. Canobbio M, Mair D, Van der Velde M, et al. Pregnancy outcomes after the Fontan repair. *J Am Coll Cardiol.* 1996;28:763.

59. Drenthen W, Pieper PG, Roos-Hesselink JW, on behalf of the ZAHARA investigators, et al. Pregnancy and delivery in women after Fontan palliation. *Heart.* 2006;92:1290.

60. Vongpatanasin W, Brickner E, Hillis L, et al. The Eisenmenger syndrome in adults. *Ann Intern Med.* 1998;128:745.

61. Weiss B, Zemp L, Burkhardt S, et al. Outcome of pulmonary vascular disease in pregnancy: a systematic overview from 1978 through 1996. *J Am Coll Cardiol.* 1998;31:1650.

62. Gleicher N, Midwall J, Hochberger D, et al. Eisenmenger's syndrome and pregnancy. *Obstet Gynecol Surv.* 1979;34:721.

63. Yentis S, Steer P, Plaat F. Eisenmenger's syndrome in pregnancy: maternal and fetal mortality in the 1990's. *BJOG.* 1998;105:921.

64. Vriend JW, Drenthen W, Pieper PG, et al. Outcome of pregnancy in patients after repair of aortic coarctation. *Eur Heart J.* 2005;26:2173.

65. Beauchesne LM, Connolly HM, Ammash NM, et al. Coarctation of the aorta: outcome of pregnancy. *J Am Coll Cardiol.* 2001;38:1728.

66. Hibbard J, Lindheimer M, Lang R. A modified definition for peripartum cardiomyopathy and prognosis based on echocardiography. *Obstet Gynecol.* 1999;94:311.

67. Lampert M, Lang R. Peripartum cardiomyopathy. *Am Heart J.* 1995;130:860.

68. Ostrzega E, Elkayam U. Risk of subsequent pregnancy in women with a history of peripartum cardiomyopathy: results of a survey. *Circulation.* 1995;92:1.

69. Elkayam U, Tummala PP, Rao K, et al. Maternal and fetal outcomes of subsequent pregnancies in women with peripartum cardiomyopathy. *N Engl J Med.* 2001;344:1567.

70. Sliwa K, Hilfiker-Kleiner D, Petrie MC, et al. Current state of knowledge on aetiology, diagnosis, management, and therapy of peripartum cardiomyopathy: a position statement from the Heart Failure Association of the European Society of Cardiology Working Group on peripartum cardiomyopathy. *Eur J Heart Fail.* 2010;12:767.

71. Ladner HE, Danielsen B, Gilbert WM. Acute myocardial infarction in pregnancy and the puerperium: a population-based study. *Obstet Gynecol.* 2005;105:480.

72. James AH, Jamison MG, Biswas MS, et al. Acute myocardial infarction in pregnancy: a United States population-based study. *Circulation.* 2006; 113:1564.

73. Elkayam U, Jalnapurkar S, Barakkat MN, et al. Pregnancy-associated acute myocardial infarction: a review of contemporary experience in 150 cases between 2006 and 2011. *Circulation.* 2014;129:1695-1702.

74. Alfonso F. Spontaneous coronary artery dissection: new insights from the tip of the iceberg? *Circulation.* 2012;126:667-670.

75. Dufour P, Occelli B, Puech F. Brief communication: pregnancy after myocardial infarction. *Int J Obstet Gynecol.* 1997;59:251.

76. Hiratzka L, Bakris G, Beckman J, et al. ACCF/AHA/AATS/ACR/ASA/SCA/SCAI/SIR/STS/SVM guidelines for the diagnosis and management of patients with thoracic aortic disease. *J Am Coll Cardiol.* 2010;55: e27-e129.

77. Elkayam U, Ostrzega E, Shotan A, et al. Cardiovascular problems in pregnant women with the Marfan syndrome. *Ann Intern Med.* 1995;123:117.

78. Meijboom LJ, Vos FE, Timmermans J, Boers GH, Zwinderman AH, Mulder BJ. Pregnancy and aortic root growth in the Marfan syndrome: a prospective study. *Eur Heart J.* 2005;26:914-920.

79. Donnelly RT, Pinto NM, Kocolas I, Yetman AT. The immediate and long-term impact of pregnancy on aortic growth rate and mortality in women with Marfan syndrome. *J Am Coll Cardiol.* 2012;60:224-229.

80. Rossiter J, Repke J, Morales A, et al. A prospective longitudinal evaluation of pregnancy in the Marfan syndrome. *Am J Obstet Gynecol.* 1995;173:1599.

81. D'Alonzo GE, Barst R, Ayres S, et al. Survival in patients with primary pulmonary hypertension. *Ann Intern Med.* 1991;115:343.

82. Humbert M, Sitbon O, Simonneau G. Treatment of pulmonary arterial hypertension. *N Engl J Med.* 2004;351:1425.

83. Martinez J, Comas C, Sala X, et al. Maternal primary pulmonary hypertension associated with pregnancy. *Eur J Obstet Gynaecol Reprod Biol.* 1994;54:143.

84. Branko M, Weiss MD, Lea Z, et al. Outcome of pulmonary vascular disease in pregnancy: a systematic overview from 1978 through 1996. *JACC.* 1998;31:1650.

85. Easterling T, Ralph D, Schmucker B. Pulmonary hypertension in pregnancy: treatment with pulmonary vasodilators. *Obstet Gynecol.* 1999;93:494.

86. Natale A, Davidson T, Geiger M, et al. Implantable cardioverter-defibrillators and pregnancy. *Circulation.* 1997;96:2808.

87. Maron BJ. Hypertrophic cardiomyopathy: a systematic review. *JAMA.* 2002;287:1308.

88. Shah D, Sunderji S. Hypertrophic cardiomyopathy and pregnancy: report of a maternal mortality and review of the literature. *Obstet Gynecol Surv.* 1985;40:444.

89. Piacenza J, Kirkorian G, Audra P, et al. Hypertrophic cardiomyopathy and pregnancy. *Eur J Obstet Gynaecol Reprod Biol.* 1998;80:17.

90. Thaman R, Varnava A, Hamid MS, et al. Pregnancy related complications in women with hypertrophic cardiomyopathy. *Heart.* 2003;89:752.

91. Robson S, Dunlop W, Moore M, et al. Combined Doppler and echocardiographic measurement of cardiac output: theory and application in pregnancy. *BJOG.* 1987;94:1014.

92. Lee W, Rokey R, Cotton D. Noninvasive maternal stroke volume and cardiac output determinations by pulsed Doppler echocardiography. *Am J Obstet Gynecol.* 1988;158:505.

93. Easterling T, Carlson K, Schmucker B, et al. Measurement of cardiac output in pregnancy by Doppler technique. *Am J Perinatol.* 1990;7:220.

94. Easterling T, Watts D, Schmucker B, et al. Measurement of cardiac output during pregnancy: validation of Doppler technique and clinical observations in preeclampsia. *Obstet Gynecol.* 1987;69:845.

95. de Swiet M, Talbert D. The measurement of cardiac output by electrical impedance plethysmography in pregnancy: are the assumptions valid? *BJOG.* 1986;93:721.

96. Easterling T, Benedetti T, Carlson K, et al. Measurement of cardiac output in pregnancy: impedance versus thermodilution techniques. *BJOG.* 1989;96:67.

97. Masaki D, Greenspoon J, Ouzounian J. Measurement of cardiac output in pregnancy by thoracic electrical bioimpedance and thermodilution. *Am J Obstet Gynecol.* 1989;161:680.

98. Clark S, Cotton D, Lee W, et al. Central hemodynamic assessment of normal pregnancy. *Am J Obstet Gynecol.* 1989;161:1439.

Additional references for this chapter are available at ExpertConsult.com.

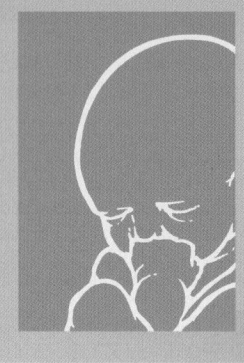

CHAPTER 38

Respiratory Disease in Pregnancy

JANICE E. WHITTY and MITCHELL P. DOMBROWSKI

KEY ABBREVIATIONS

Acquired immunodeficiency syndrome	AIDS	Latent tuberculosis infection	LTBI
Amniotic fluid index	AFI	Leukotriene-receptor agonist	LTRA
Bacille Calmette-Guérin	BCG	Metered-dose inhaler	MDI
Community-acquired methicillin-resistant *Staphylococcus aureus*	CA-MRSA	National Asthma Education and Prevention Program	NAEPP
Confidence interval	CI	Odds ratio	OR
Direct amplification test	DAT	Peak expiratory flow rate	PEFR
Dry-powder inhaler	DPI	Percutaneous transthoracic needle aspiration	PTNA
Forced expiratory volume in 1 second	FEV_1		
Forced vital capacity	FVC	*Pneumocystis jiroveci* pneumonia	PJP
Highly active antiretroviral therapy	HAART	Positive end-expiratory pressure	PEEP
Human immunodeficiency virus	HIV	Purified protein derivative	PPD
Interferon-γ release assay	IGRA	Rifampin	RIF
Intrauterine growth restriction	IUGR	Tuberculosis	TB
Isoniazid	INH	Tuberculin skin testing	TST
Long-acting β-agonist	LABA	U.S. Food and Drug Administration	FDA

Pulmonary diseases are among the most common medical complications of pregnancy. The occurrence of pulmonary disease during gestation may result in increased morbidity or mortality for both the mother and her fetus. Pregnancy may have an adverse or positive impact on the pulmonary function of the gravida depending on the particular complication that is being encountered. The cardiorespiratory changes that occur in pregnancy are reviewed in Chapter 3, and the obstetrician and medical consultants should have a thorough understanding of these changes and their potential effects on the respiratory disease in question. It is also extremely important to realize that most diagnostic tests used to evaluate pulmonary function are not harmful to the fetus and, if indicated, should be performed during gestation. In this section, we discuss some of the respiratory complications that may be encountered during gestation,

the impact of pregnancy on the disease, and the potential impact of the disease on pregnancy.

PNEUMONIA IN PREGNANCY

Pneumonia is an uncommon complication of pregnancy, observed in 0.78 to 2.7 per 1000 deliveries.[1,2] However, **pneumonia contributes to considerable maternal mortality and is reportedly the most common nonobstetric infection to cause maternal mortality in the peripartum period.**[3] Before the introduction of antibiotic therapy, maternal mortality was as high as 24%.[2] However, **with modern management and antibiotic therapy, the maternal mortality rate currently ranges from 0% to 4%.**[1,3,4] **Preterm delivery is a significant complication of pneumonia; even with antibiotic therapy and**

modern management, it continues to occur in 4% to 43% of affected pregnancies.[1,3,4]

The incidence of pneumonia in pregnancy may be increasing primarily as a reflection of the declining health status of certain segments of the childbearing population.[1] In addition, the epidemic of human immunodeficiency virus (HIV) infection has increased the number of potential mothers at risk for opportunistic lung infections. HIV infection further predisposes the pregnant woman to the infectious complications of the acquired immunodeficiency syndrome (AIDS).[5] Reported incidence rates range from 97 to 290 cases per 1000 HIV-infected people per year.[6] **HIV-infected people are 7.8 times more likely to develop pneumonia** than non–HIV-infected individuals with similar risk factors.[6] Women with medical conditions that increase the risk for pulmonary infection, such as cystic fibrosis, are now living to childbearing age more often than in the past. This disorder also contributes to the increased incidence of pneumonia in pregnancy.

Pneumonia can complicate pregnancy at any time during gestation and may be associated with preterm birth, poor fetal growth, and perinatal loss. Benedetti and colleagues[3] described 39 cases of pneumonia in pregnancy. Sixteen gravidae presented before 24 weeks' gestation, 15 between 25 and 36 weeks' gestation, and eight presented after 36 weeks' gestation. Twenty-seven patients in this series were followed to completion of pregnancy, and only two required delivery during the acute phase of pneumonia. Of these 27 patients, three suffered a fetal loss, and 24 delivered live fetuses; one neonatal death was due to prematurity.[1] Madinger and associates[4] reported 25 cases of pneumonia that occurred among 32,179 deliveries and observed that fetal and obstetric complications were much more common than in earlier studies. **Preterm labor occurred in 11 of 21 patients who had complete follow-up data, and pneumonia was present at the time of delivery in 11 patients. Preterm labor was more likely in those women who experienced bacteremia, required mechanical ventilation, or had a serious underlying maternal disease.** In addition to the complication of preterm labor, three perinatal deaths occurred in this series. In Berkowitz and La Sala's report[1] of 25 patients with pneumonia that complicated pregnancy, full-term delivery of normally grown infants occurred in 14 women, one delivered preterm, three had a voluntary termination of pregnancy, three had term deliveries of growth-restricted babies, and four were lost to follow-up. Birthweight was significantly lower in the study group (2770 ± 224 g vs. 3173 ± 99 g in the control group; $P < .01$). In this series, pneumonia complicated 1 in 367 deliveries, and the authors attributed the increase in the incidence of pneumonia in this population to a decline in general health status that included anemia and a significant incidence of cocaine use in the study group (52% vs. 10% in the general population) as well as HIV positivity in the study group (24% vs. 2% in controls). **Madinger and associates[4] reported preterm labor in 44% of cases with antepartum pneumonia, with a preterm birth rate of 36%. Maternal complications of pneumonia include respiratory failure and mechanical ventilation in 10% to 20%, bacteremia in 16%, and empyema in 8%.**[1,4] Respiratory failure due to pneumonia accounts for 12% of intubations during pregnancy.[7] A recent report by Chen and colleagues[8] documents that women with pneumonia during pregnancy have a significantly higher risk of low-birthweight (LBW) infants, preterm birth, small-for-gestational-age (SGA) infants, infants with low Apgar scores,

cesarean delivery, and preeclampsia/eclampsia compared with unaffected women.

BACTERIOLOGY

Most series that have described pneumonia complicating pregnancy have used incomplete methodologies to diagnose the etiologic pathogens involved, relying primarily on cultures of blood and sputum. In most cases, no identifiable pathogen is reported; however, ***Streptococcus pneumoniae* and *Haemophilus influenzae* remain the most common identifiable causes of pneumonia in pregnancy.**[1,3] Because comprehensive serologic testing has rarely been undertaken, the true incidence of viral pneumonia, *Legionella,* and *Mycoplasma* pneumonia in pregnancy is difficult to estimate. In Berkowitz and LaSala's series,[1] one patient had *Legionella* species. **Several unusual pathogens have been reported to cause pneumonia in pregnancy, including mumps, infectious mononucleosis, swine flu, influenza A, varicella, coccidioidomycosis, and other fungi.**[9] **Varicella pneumonia complicates primary varicella infections in 9% of infections in pregnancy, compared with 0.3% to 1.8% in the nonpregnant population.**[10] Influenza A has a higher mortality in pregnant than in nonpregnant patients. **The increase in virulence of viral infections reported in pregnancy may be secondary to the alterations in maternal immune status that characterize pregnancy, including reduced lymphocyte proliferative response, reduced cell-mediated cytotoxicity, and a decrease in the number of helper T lymphocytes** (see Chapter 4).[11,12] Viral pneumoniae can also be complicated by superimposed bacterial infection, particularly with pneumococcus (*S. pneumoniae*). **Recent reports have been made of community-acquired methicillin-resistant *Staphylococcus aureus* (CA-MRSA) causing necrotizing pneumonia in pregnancy and postpartum.**[11-13]

Chemical pneumonitis results after the aspiration of gastric contents, and it can be superinfected with pathogens present in the oropharynx and gastric juices, primarily anaerobes and gram-negative bacteria.[9]

Heterosexual transmission of HIV has become an increasingly important mode of transmission. Many women infected with HIV are of childbearing age, and they are at risk for developing *Pneumocystis jiroveci* pneumonia (PJP) during pregnancy. The reported maternal mortality rate from PJP is as high as 50%.[14] Although the risk for maternal mortality is high with PJP infection, most HIV-infected pregnant women in the United States today receive PJP prophylaxis. This practice may actually lead to a decrease in the incidence and mortality from PJP pneumonia in pregnancy.

BACTERIAL PNEUMONIA

***Streptococcus pneumoniae* (*pneumococcus*) is the most common bacterial pathogen to cause pneumonia in pregnancy, and *H. influenzae* is the next most common.** These pneumoniae typically present as acute illness accompanied by fever, chills, purulent productive cough, and a lobar pattern on chest radiograph (Fig. 38-1). **Streptococcal pneumonia produces a "rusty" sputum, and gram-positive diplococci appear on Gram stain with asymmetric consolidation and air bronchograms on chest radiograph. *H. influenzae* is a gram-negative coccobacillus that produces consolidation and air bronchograms, often in the upper lobes.** Less frequent

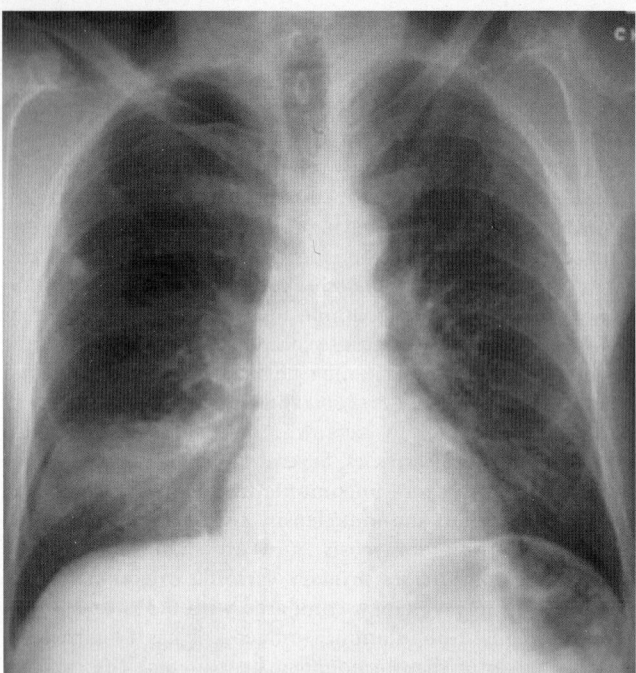

FIG 38-1 Right lower lobe pneumonia.

bacterial pathogens include *Klebsiella pneumoniae,* a gram-negative rod that causes extensive tissue destruction with air bronchograms, pleural effusion, and cavitation noted on chest radiograph. Patients with *Staphylococcus aureus* pneumonia present with pleuritis, chest pain, purulent sputum, and consolidation without air bronchograms noted on chest radiograph. Community-acquired methicillin-resistant *Staphylococcus aureus* (CA-MRSA) can present with a viral-like prodrome that progresses to severe pneumonia with high fever, hypotension, and hemoptysis followed by septic shock and need for ventilator support.[11] Severe cases of CA-MRSA have been reported during influenza seasons or associated with a preceding influenza illness in 33% to 71% patients.[11] Leukopenia can be observed and has been found to be a predictor of poor outcome.[11] Patients can present with multilobar infiltrates and cavitation. Mortality from CA-MRSA pneumonia in the United States and Europe is reportedly greater than 50%.

Patients with atypical pneumonia pathogens—such as *M. pneumoniae, L. pneumophila,* and *Chlamydia pneumoniae* (Taiwan acute respiratory [TWAR] agent)—present with gradual onset and a lower fever, appear less ill, and have a mucoid sputum and a patchy or interstitial infiltrate on chest radiograph. The severity of the findings on chest radiograph is usually out of proportion to the mild clinical symptoms. *M. pneumoniae* is the most common organism responsible for atypical pneumonia and is best detected by the presence of cold agglutinins, which are present in 70% of cases.

The normal physiologic changes in the respiratory system associated with pregnancy result in a loss of ventilatory reserve. This, coupled with the relative immunosuppression that accompanies pregnancy, puts the mother and fetus at great risk from respiratory infection. **Therefore any gravida suspected of having pneumonia should be managed aggressively. Hospital admission is generally recommended**, and an investigation should be undertaken to determine the pathologic etiology. In a study of 133 women admitted with pneumonia during

pregnancy and managed using protocols based on the British and American Thoracic Societies' admission guidelines for management in nonpregnant individuals,[15] the authors reported that if the American Thoracic Society (ATS) guidelines had been used, 25% of the pregnant women with pneumonia could have avoided admission.[15,16] None of the gravidae who would have been managed as outpatients using the American criteria had any complications.[17] If the British Thoracic Society guidelines had been used, 66% of the pregnant women in this group would have been assigned to outpatient therapy. However, of those, 14% would have required readmission for complications. Of note, most of the 133 women who were hospitalized with pneumonia in this study did not receive a chest radiograph for confirmation of diagnosis. This limits the value of the study for use in guiding admission criteria for pneumonia in pregnancy. **Therefore until additional information is available, admission for all pregnant women with pneumonia is prudent.**

Workup should include physical examination, arterial blood gases, chest radiograph, sputum for Gram stain and culture, and blood cultures. Several recently published studies have called into question the use of cultures to identify the microbiology of community-acquired pneumonia. **The successful identification of the bacterial etiology with cultures has been found to range from 2.1% to about 50%.**[18,19] Review of available clinical data reflects an overall reliance on clinical judgment and the patient response to treatment to guide therapy. Other tests are available to identify the etiology of pneumonia that do not require culture and are more sensitive and specific. **An assay approved by the U.S. Food and Drug Administration (FDA) for pneumococcal urinary antigen has been assessed in several studies.**[20] **The sensitivity for identifying pneumococcal disease in adults is reportedly 60% to 90% with specificity close to 100%.**[20] In one study, the pneumococcal antigen was detected in 26% of patients in whom no pathogen had been identified.[21] This suggests that cases undiagnosed by standard testing can be identified with the assay. In this study, **10% of samples from patients with pneumonia caused by other agents were positive for the pneumococcal assay, which indicates a potential problem with specificity.**[21] Therefore if the response to therapy directed at pneumococcus (*Streptococcus pneumoniae*) is inadequate, coverage for other potential pathogens should be added. A test is available for *Legionella* urinary antigen as well, with a sensitivity of 70% and specificity of 90% for serogroup 1.[22] This is especially useful in the United States and Europe because about 85% of *Legionella* isolates are serogroup 1.[22] *Legionella* is a common cause of severe community-acquired pneumonia; therefore the urinary antigen for serogroup 1 should be considered for any patient who requires admission to an intensive care unit (ICU) for pneumonia.[22]

Percutaneous transthoracic needle aspiration (PTNA) has been advocated as a valuable and safe method to increase the chance of establishing a causative agent in pneumonia.[23] This test should be reserved for use in compromised individuals, when tuberculosis (TB) is suspected in the absence of a productive cough, and in selected cases of chronic pneumonia, pneumonia associated with neoplasm or foreign body, suspected PJP pneumonia, and suspected conditions that necessitate lung biopsy.[17]

When admission for pneumonia is required, evidence suggests that inpatient and 30-day mortality have been reduced when antibiotics are administered within 8 hours. **Therefore current U.S. federal standards require that the first dose of antibiotics be administered within 4 hours of arrival to the hospital.**[24] **Empiric antibiotic coverage should be started, usually with a macrolide for mild illness with addition of a β-lactam for severe illness.** Yost and colleagues[15] demonstrated that monotherapy with erythromycin was adequate in 118 of 119 women with pneumonia in pregnancy. **A macrolide combined with a β-lactam is safe and will provide adequate coverage for most community-acquired bacterial pneumoniae, including *Legionella*.** Dual coverage has been demonstrated to improve response to therapy even for abbreviated macrolide regimens.[17] This is theoretically because of an added antiinflammatory effect of the macrolides.[19] Azithromycin administration has been shown to be an independent predictor of positive outcome and reduced length of hospital stay in mild to moderate community-acquired pneumonia.[17] However, **the use of macrolides to treat community-acquired pneumonia should be limited when possible because their use has also been associated with increased penicillin resistance among patients with *S. pneumoniae*.**[25]

Once the results of the antigen, sputum culture, blood cultures, Gram stain, and serum studies are obtained and a pathogen has been identified, antibiotic therapy should be directed toward the identifiable pathogen. **The quinolones as a class should be avoided in pregnancy because they may damage developing fetal cartilage. However, with the emergence of highly resistant bacterial pneumonia, their use may be lifesaving and therefore justified in specific circumstances.** The respiratory quinolones are not only effective against highly penicillin-resistant *S. pneumoniae* strains, their use reportedly does not increase resistance.[25-27] **The respiratory quinolones include levofloxacin, gatifloxacin, and moxifloxacin. These are ideal agents for community-acquired pneumonia because they are highly active against penicillin-resistant strains of *S. pneumoniae*. They are also active against *Legionella* and the other atypical pulmonary pathogens.** Another advantage is a favorable pharmacokinetic profile such that blood/lung levels are the same whether the drug is administered orally or intravenously.[28] Arguments against more extensive respiratory quinolone use are based on concerns about the potential for developing resistance, the variable incidence of *Legionella*, and cost. An additional caveat is that the respiratory quinolones are partially effective against mycobacterial TB. Therefore evaluation for this infection should be done when considering the use of quinolones for pneumonia. **If CA-MRSA pneumonia is suspected, vancomycin or linezolid should be added to empiric therapy.**[11] Additional therapy with clindamycin can be considered in difficult-to-treat cases because it has been shown to reduce production of staphylococcal exotoxins.[26] **CA-MRSA is susceptible to fluoroquinolones and trimethoprim-sulfamethoxazole and often are only resistant to β-lactams.**[11]

In addition to antibiotic therapy, oxygen supplementation should be given, and frequent arterial blood gas measurements should be obtained. **Arterial saturation should be monitored with pulse oximetry with a goal of maintaining the PO_2 at 70 mm Hg, a level necessary to ensure adequate fetal oxygenation. When the gravida is afebrile for 48 hours and has signs of clinical improvement, an oral cephalosporin or macrolide, or both, can be initiated and intravenous (IV) therapy discontinued. A total of 10 to 14 days of treatment should be completed.**

Pneumococcal polysaccharide vaccination prevents pneumococcal pneumonia in otherwise healthy populations with an efficacy of 65% to 84%.[17] **The vaccine is safe in pregnancy and should be administered to high-risk gravidae.** Those at high risk include individuals with sickle cell disease secondary to autosplenectomy, patients who have had a surgical splenectomy, and individuals who are immunosuppressed. **An additional advantage to maternal immunization with the pneumococcal vaccine is that several studies have demonstrated a significant transplacental transmission of vaccine-specific antibodies.**[27] **After in utero exposure to the vaccine, significantly high concentrations of pneumococcal antibodies are present in infants at birth and at 2 months of age.**[27] **In addition, colostrum and breast milk antibodies are significantly increased in women who have received the pneumococcal vaccine.**[28]

Pneumonia in pregnancy can be complicated by respiratory failure that requires mechanical ventilation. In such cases, team management should include the obstetrician, a maternal-fetal medicine specialist, and an intensivist. In addition to meticulous management of the gravida's respiratory status, maintenance of the left lateral recumbent position is advocated to improve uteroplacental perfusion. **The potentially viable fetus should be monitored with continuous fetal monitoring. Serial ultrasound examinations for amniotic fluid index (AFI) and growth will help to guide clinical management. If positive end-expiratory pressure (PEEP) greater than 10 cm H_2O is required to maintain oxygenation, central venous monitoring should be instituted to adequately monitor volume status** and maintain maternal and uteroplacental perfusion. **No evidence suggests that elective delivery results in an overall improvement in respiratory function**[29]; therefore elective delivery should be undertaken with caution. **However, if clear evidence of fetal compromise or profound maternal compromise and impending demise is apparent, delivery should be accomplished.**

VIRAL PNEUMONIA
Influenza Virus
Every year in the United States, an estimated 4 million cases of pneumonia occur that complicate influenza; this represents the sixth leading cause of death in this country.[30] Although three types of influenza virus—types A, B, and C—can cause human disease, **most epidemic infections are due to influenza A,**[9] **which typically has an acute onset after a 1- to 4-day incubation period and first manifests as high fever, coryza, headache, malaise, and cough. In uncomplicated cases, the chest examination and chest radiograph remain clear.**[9] **If symptoms persist longer than 5 days, especially in a pregnancy, complications should be suspected.** Pneumonia may complicate influenza as the result of either secondary bacterial infection or primary viral infection of the lung parenchyma. **In the epidemic of 1957, autopsies demonstrated that pregnant women most commonly died of fulminant viral pneumonia, whereas nonpregnant patients died most often of secondary bacterial infection.**[31] A large nested case-control study evaluated the rate of influenza-related complications over 17 influenza seasons in women enrolled in the Tennessee Medicaid system.[32] This study demonstrated a high risk for hospitalization for influenza-related reasons in low-risk pregnant women during the last trimester of pregnancy. The authors predicted that 25 of 10,000 women in the third trimester during the influenza season

will be hospitalized with influenza-related complications.[32] **A more recent matched cohort study using the administrative database of pregnant women enrolled in the Tennessee Medicaid population examined pregnant women aged 25 to 44 years with respiratory hospitalization during influenza seasons in 1985 to 1993.**[33] **In this population of pregnant women, those with asthma accounted for half of all respiratory hospitalizations during influenza season. Of pregnant women with the diagnosis of asthma, 6% required respiratory hospitalization during the influenza season** (odds ratio [OR], 10.63; 95% confidence interval [CI], 8.61 to 13.83) compared with women without a medical comorbidity. This study detected no significant increases in adverse perinatal outcome associated with respiratory hospitalization during flu season.[33]

Early data on pandemic 2009 influenza A (H1N1) suggest pregnant women had an increased risk for hospitalization and death. Siston and associates[34] identified 788 pregnant women in the United States with H1N1. Thirty died (5% of all reported H1N1 deaths in this period). Among 509 hospitalized women, 115 (22.5%) were admitted to an ICU. **Pregnant women who began treatment more than 4 days after symptom onset were more likely to be admitted to an ICU** (56.9% vs. 9.4%; relative risk [RR], 6.0; 95% CI, 3.5 to 10.6) **than those treated within 2 days after symptom onset.**[34]

Primary influenza pneumonia is characterized by rapid progression from a unilateral infiltrate to diffuse bilateral disease. The gravida may develop fulminant respiratory failure that requires mechanical ventilation and PEEP. **When pneumonia complicates influenza in pregnancy, antibiotics should be started, directed at the likely pathogens that can cause secondary infection:** *Staphylococcus aureus, Streptococcus pneumoniae* (pneumococcus), *H. influenzae,* **and certain enteric gram-negative bacteria. Antiviral agents, such as amantadine and ribavirin, can be considered. It has been recommended that the influenza vaccine be given routinely to gravidae during the flu season** (October to March) regardless of the trimester to prevent the occurrence of influenza and to prevent the development of secondary pneumonia. In addition to maternal protection, **prospective studies have demonstrated higher cord blood antibody levels to influenza in babies born to mothers immunized during pregnancy.** Disease onset is delayed and severity of the influenza is decreased in infants who have higher antibody levels.[35]

Varicella Virus

Varicella zoster is a DNA virus that usually causes a benign self-limited illness in children but may infect up to 2% of all adults.[36] **Varicella infection occurs in 0.7 of every 1000 pregnancies.**[37] Pregnancy may increase the likelihood of varicella pneumonia complicating the primary infection.[37,38] **Varicella pneumonia occurs most often in the third trimester, and the infection is likely to be severe.**[37,38] **The maternal mortality from varicella pneumonia is reportedly as high as 35% to 40%, compared with 11% to 17% in nonpregnant individuals. With modern management, mortality has decreased dramatically. One review reported three deaths in 28 women with varicella pneumonia.**[37] **Another described 347 pregnant women with Varicella zoster infection. Of these, 18 (5.2%) had pneumonia treated with acyclovir. None died.** The authors noted that women with varicella pneumonia were significantly more likely to be current smokers (OR, 5.1; 95% CI, 1.6 to 16) and to have 100 or more skin lesions.[39] A more recent study

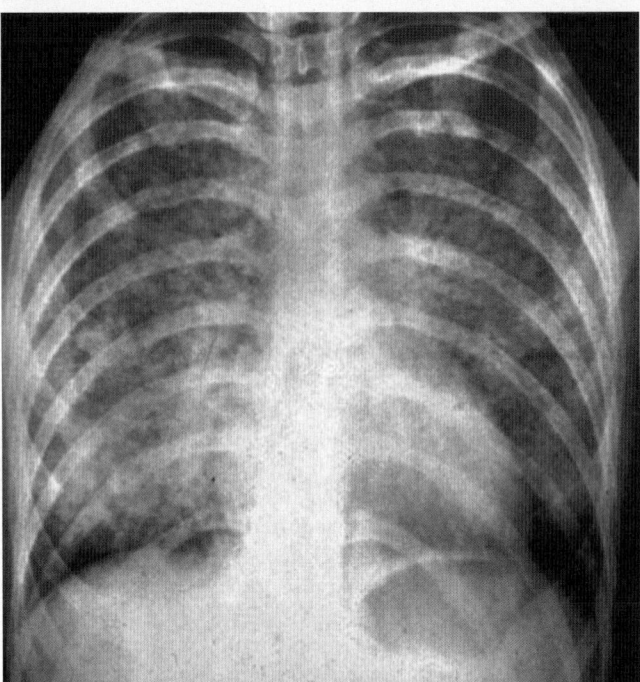

FIG 38-2 This chest radiograph demonstrates bilateral nodular and interstitial pneumonia characteristic of varicella pneumonia. The patient—a 27-year-old gravida 6, para 2, abortus 3—was exposed to varicella infection in her two children. Characteristic skin vesicles of varicella occurred several days before the development of pulmonary symptoms. She required endotracheal intubation and mechanical ventilation for 6 days and was treated with intravenous acyclovir and ceftazidime for possible superimposed infection. The patient recovered fully and delivered a healthy infant at term.

by Zhang and colleagues[38] reported 935 cases of varicella pneumonia in pregnancy in the United States and no maternal deaths.

Varicella pneumonia usually presents 2 to 5 days after the onset of fever, rash, and malaise and is heralded by the onset of pulmonary symptoms that include cough, dyspnea, pruritic chest pain, and hemoptysis. The severity of the illness may vary from asymptomatic radiographic abnormalities to fulminant pneumonitis and respiratory failure (Fig. 38-2). **All gravidae with varicella pneumonia should be aggressively treated with antiviral therapy and admitted to the ICU for close observation.** Acyclovir, a DNA polymerase inhibitor, should be started. **The early use of acyclovir has been associated with an improved hospital course after the fifth day and a lower mean temperature, lower respiratory rate, and improved oxygenation and survival.**[40] **Treatment with acyclovir is safe in pregnancy.** Among 312 exposed pregnancies, no increase was seen in the number of birth defects, and no consistent pattern of congenital abnormalities was apparent.[41] **A dose of 7.5 mg/kg intravenously every 8 hours has been recommended.** The use of varicella immune globulin to prevent infection in individuals exposed to varicella is not possible because it is no longer available in the United States.

Varicella vaccine is a live attenuated vaccine, and it is the first vaccine against the herpesvirus. Extensive prelicensure studies have demonstrated that the **vaccine is safe and efficacious against varicella; therefore varicella vaccine was added to the universal childhood immunization schedule in the United States in 1995.** The program of universal childhood vaccination against varicella in the United States **has resulted in a sharp decline in the rate of death from varicella.**[42] **This vaccine is not recommended for use in pregnancy.** However, the overall decline in the incidence of varicella secondary to vaccination will likely result in a decreased incidence of varicella infection and varicella pneumonia in pregnancy.

A recent study assessed the risk for congenital varicella syndrome and other birth defects in offspring of women who inadvertently received the varicella vaccine during pregnancy or within 3 months of conception.[43] **Fifty-eight women received their first dose of varicella vaccine during the first or second trimester, and no cases of congenital varicella syndrome were identified among 56 live births** (rate, 0%; 95% CI, 0 to 15.6). Among the prospective reports of live births, five congenital anomalies were reported. No specific pattern of anomalies was identified in either the susceptible cohort or the sample population as a whole. Although the numbers in the study are small, the results should provide some reassurance to health care providers and women with inadvertent exposure before or during pregnancy.[43]

Pneumocystis jiroveci Pneumonia

Pneumocystis jiroveci **(PJP), formerly *Pneumocystis carinii* pneumonia (PCP) remains the most prevalent opportunistic infection in patients infected with HIV.**[44] **It is an AIDS-defining illness that occurs more frequently when the helper T-cell count (CD4⁺) is less than 200 cells/mm³.**[44] **When AIDS is complicated by PJP, the mortality rate is 10% to 20% during the initial infection, but this rate can increase substantially with the need for mechanical ventilation.** The transmission of *Pneumocystis* is not fully understood, although some evidence suggests person-to-person transmission as the most likely mode; however, acquisition from environmental sources may also occur.[44]

The symptoms of PJP are nonspecific; therefore it may be difficult to diagnose. **Typical radiographic features of PJP are bilateral perihilar interstitial infiltrates that become increasingly homogeneous and diffuse as the disease progresses** (Fig. 38-3). **The diagnosis of PJP requires microscopic examination to identify *Pneumocystis* from a clinical source such as sputum, bronchoalveolar fluid, or lung tissue** (Fig. 38-4). *Pneumocystis* cannot be propagated in culture. The fungus has trophic forms as well as a cyst state, which can be detected with a modified Papanicolaou, Wright-Giemsa, or Gram-Weigert stain.[44] **Monoclonal antibodies are useful for detecting *Pneumocystis* as well.** The application of polymerase chain reaction (PCR) to detect *Pneumocystis* has been an area of active research and may be valuable for detection in sputum and bronchoalveolar lavage fluid.[43] **Trimethoprim-sulfamethoxazole is the preferred treatment for PJP. Thus far, resistance to this therapeutic agent has not been identified.**[44]

A significant number of new infections with HIV are occurring in women of childbearing age. **As of 1995, more than 80% of women with AIDS were of reproductive age. PJP pneumonia is the most common cause of AIDS-related death in the United States.** Literature on PJP in pregnancy is scarce, but one report describes five cases of PJP in pregnancy and also reviews the literature.[45] **In this series of 22 pregnant women with PJP, 11 patients (50%) died of pneumonia. The incidence of respiratory failure in this series was 59%.** In individuals who required mechanical ventilation, the survival rate was 31%. The average gestational age was 25 weeks, with a range

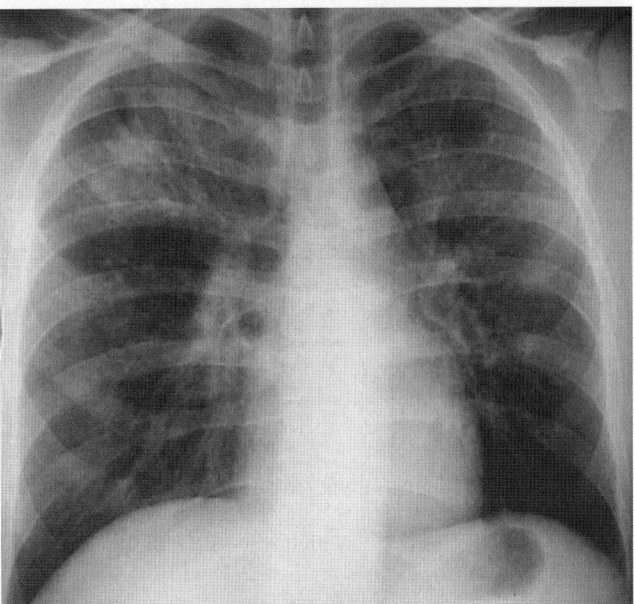

FIG 38-3 *Pneumocystis jiroveci* (formerly *P. carinii*) pneumonia with mixed interstitial and alveolar opacities, a ground-glass appearance.

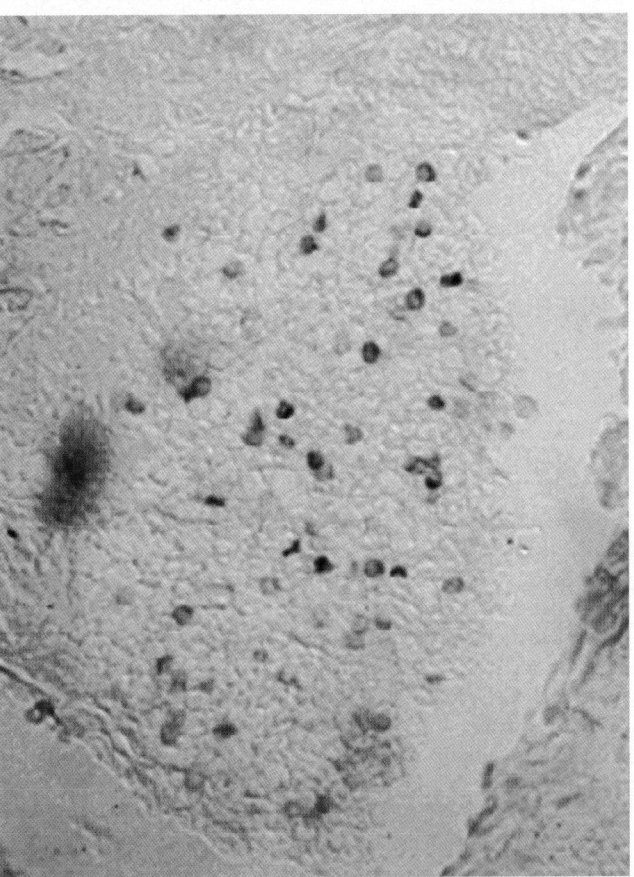

FIG 38-4 Wright-Giemsa stain of *Pneumocystis jiroveci* (formerly *P. carinii*) pneumonia.

of 6 weeks' gestation up to 1 week postpartum. Fifteen of the 22 patients had CD4⁺ counts performed, and the mean was 93 cells/mm³. The patients in this series were treated with a variety of regimens, including trimethoprim-sulfamethoxazole alone, trimethoprim-sulfamethoxazole and steroids, and pentamidine isethionate. Six patients received trimethoprim-sulfamethoxazole alone, and six were given trimethoprim-sulfamethoxazole and steroids; four patients (66%) survived in each group. Only 12 babies survived; five stillbirths were reported, and four neonates died shortly after birth. In this series, **PJP pneumonia complicating pregnancy in the third trimester had a better maternal and fetal outcome compared with disease in the first or second trimester. Evidence also suggested that treatment with trimethoprim-sulfamethoxazole with or without steroids was associated with an increased survival rate.**[45]

The high mortality rate in this series may be skewed by the fact that this is a retrospective review, and severe cases are more likely to be reported than mild ones. In addition, all the women in this series were unaware of their HIV infection until the diagnosis of PJP was made; therefore none had received PJP prophylaxis.[45]

In summary, PJP pneumonia remains a dreaded complication of HIV infection and an AIDS-defining illness. The maternal and fetal mortality rate is very high when PJP complicates pregnancy. **Primary prophylaxis against PJP with trimethoprim-sulfamethoxazole in HIV-infected adults, including pregnant women and patients receiving highly active antiretroviral therapy (HAART), should begin when the CD4$^+$ count is less than 200 cells/mm^3 or when the patient has a history of oropharyngeal candidiasis** (see Chapter 53).[46] Prophylaxis should be discontinued when the CD4$^+$ cell count increases to more than 200 cells/mm^3 for a period of 3 months.[44] The use of HAART, as well as prophylaxis with trimethoprim-sulfamethoxazole, may decrease the incidence of PJP pneumonia in developed countries. However, many countries worldwide do not have the resources for HAART and therefore remain a reservoir for infection with PJP.

TUBERCULOSIS IN PREGNANCY

The incidence of TB in the United States began to decline in the early part of the twentieth century and fell steadily until 1953, when the introduction of isoniazid led to a dramatic decrease, from 84,000 cases in 1953 to 22,255 cases in 1984.[47] However, since 1984, there have been significant changes in TB morbidity trends. **From 1985 through 1991, reported cases of TB increased by 18%, representing about 39,000 more cases than expected had the previous downward trend continued. This increase is due to many factors, including the HIV epidemic, deterioration in the health care infrastructure, and significantly more cases among immigrants.**[47] The emergence of drug-resistant TB has also become a serious concern. In New York City, in 1991, 33% of TB cases were resistant to at least one drug, and 19% were resistant to both isoniazid (INH) and rifampin (RIF).[48] Between 1985 and 1992, the number of TB cases in women of childbearing age increased by 40%.[49] One report noted TB-complicated pregnancies in 94.8 cases per 100,000 deliveries between 1991 and 1992.[49,50]

Diagnosis

Most gravidae diagnosed with TB in pregnancy are asymptomatic. The ATS and the Centers for Disease Control and Prevention (CDC) issued a statement on targeted tuberculin testing for latent tuberculosis infection (LTBI).[51,52] This is a strategic component of TB control that identifies people at high risk for developing TB who would benefit from treatment of LTBI if detected. **Those at risk include people who have had recent**

BOX 38-1 HIGH-RISK FACTORS FOR TUBERCULOSIS

- Close contact with people known or suspected to have tuberculosis
- Medical risk factors known to increase risk for disease if infected
- Birth in a country with a high tuberculosis prevalence
- Medically underserved status
- Low income
- Alcohol addiction
- Intravenous drug use
- Residency in a long-term care facility (e.g., correctional institution, mental institution, nursing home or facility)
- Health professionals working in high-risk health care facilities

---

BOX 38-2 CLINICAL RISK FACTORS FOR DEVELOPING ACTIVE TUBERCULOSIS

- Human immunodeficiency virus infection
- Recent tuberculosis infection
- Injection drug use
- Silicosis
- Solid organ transplantation
- Chronic renal failure
- Jejunoileal bypass
- Diabetes mellitus
- Carcinoma of the head or neck
- Underweight by >15%

---

infection with TB and those who have clinical conditions associated with an increased risk for progression of LTBI to active TB (Boxes 38-1 and 38-2).

All gravidae at high risk for TB should be screened with tuberculin skin testing (TST) This is usually done with subcutaneous administration of intermediate-strength purified protein derivative (PPD).[51] If anergy is suspected, control antigens such as *Candida,* mumps, or tetanus toxoids should also be placed. **The sensitivity of the PPD is 90% to 99% for exposure to TB. The tine test is not recommended for screening because of its low sensitivity.**

The PPD remains the most commonly used screening test for TB. **Three cut-off levels have been recommended for defining a positive tuberculin reaction: greater than 5 mm, greater than 10 mm, and 15 mm or more induration (Fig. 38-5). Induration of greater than 5 mm is a positive reaction in individuals with highest risk for conversion to active TB (see Box 38-2). Interferon-γ release assays (IGRAs), an alternative diagnostic tool for LTBI, have specificity of greater than 95% for diagnosis of latent TB infection.**[53] **The sensitivity for T-SPOT.*TB* (Oxford Immunotec) appears to be higher than that of the QuantiFERON TB Gold in-Tube (QFT-GIT) test** (Cellestis Ltd., Melbourne, Australia) or TST, **approximately 90%, 80%, and 80%, respectively. CDC 2012 guidelines indicate that IGRAs can be used in place of, but not in addition to, TST in all situations—including pregnancy—in which the CDC recommends TST as an aid in diagnosing *Mycobacterium tuberculosis* infection. IGRA results can be available in 24 to 48 hours, and no follow-up visit is required for diagnosis. Because IGRAs are not affected by Bacille**

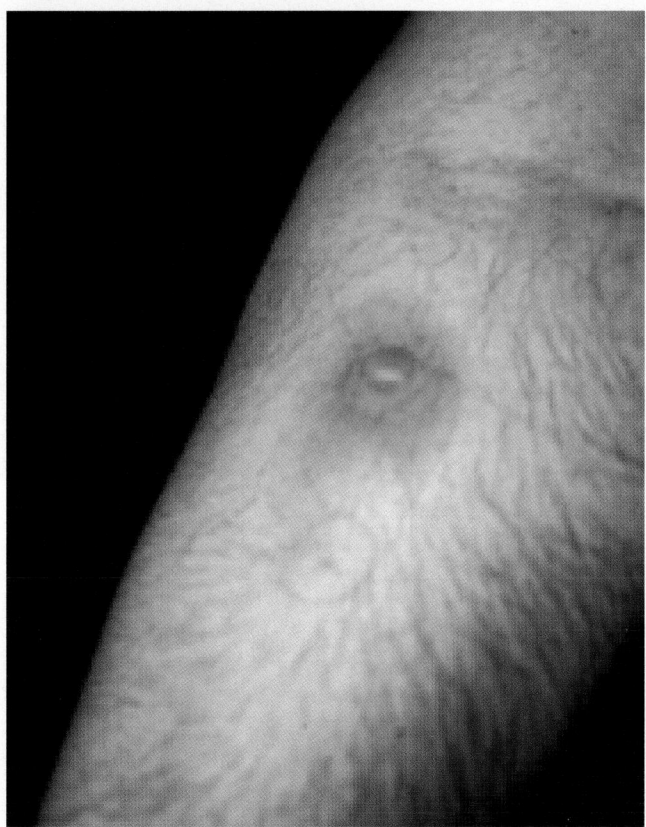

FIG 38-5 Positive purified protein derivative: induration >10 mm.

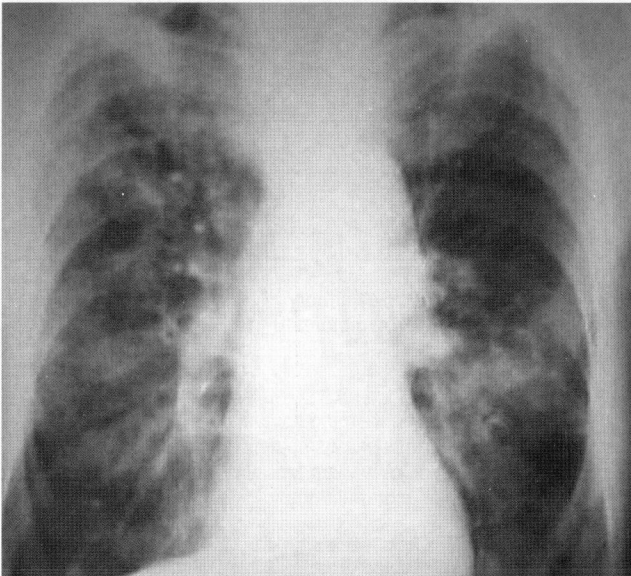

FIG 38-6 Pulmonary tuberculosis.

Calmette-Guérin (BCG) vaccination status, they are useful for evaluation of LTBI in BCG-vaccinated individuals.

Immigrants from areas where TB is endemic may have received the BCG vaccine. Such individuals likely have a positive response to the PPD.[54] However, this reactivity should wane over time. Therefore the PPD can be used to screen these patients for TB unless their skin tests are known to be positive. If the BCG vaccine was given 10 years earlier and the PPD is positive with a skin test reaction of 10 mm or more, that individual should be considered infected with TB and should be managed accordingly.[54]

Women with a positive PPD skin test must be evaluated for active TB with a thorough physical examination for extrapulmonary disease and a chest radiograph once they are beyond the first trimester. Symptoms of active TB include cough (74%), weight loss (41%), fever (30%), malaise and fatigue (30%), and hemoptysis (19%).[55] Individuals with active pulmonary TB may have radiographic findings that include adenopathy, multinodular infiltrates, cavitation, loss of volume in the upper lobes, and upper medial retraction of hilar markings (Fig. 38-6). The finding of acid-fast bacilli in early-morning sputum specimens confirms the diagnosis of pulmonary TB. Two direct amplification tests (DATs) have been approved by the FDA, the *Mycobacterium tuberculosis* Direct test (MTD; Gen-Probe, San Diego, CA) and the Amplicor *Mycobacterium tuberculosis* (Amplicor MTB) test (Roche Diagnostic Systems, Branchburg, NJ).[56,57] Both tests amplify and detect *M. tuberculosis* 16S ribosomal DNA. When testing acid-fast stain smear-negative respiratory specimens, the specificity remains greater than 95%, but the sensitivity ranges from 40% to 77%.[56,57] To date, these tests are FDA approved only for

testing acid-fast stain smear-positive respiratory specimens obtained from untreated patients or those who have received no more than 7 days of anti-TB therapy.

Extrapulmonary TB occurs in up to 16% of cases in the United States; however, in patients with AIDS, the pattern may occur in 60% to 70%.[58] Extrapulmonary sites include lymph nodes, bone, kidneys, and breasts. Extrapulmonary TB appears to be rare in pregnancy. Extrapulmonary TB that is confined to the lymph nodes has no effect on obstetric outcome, but TB at other extrapulmonary sites does adversely affect the outcome of pregnancy.[59] Rarely, mycobacteria invade the uteroplacental circulation, and congenital TB results.[49] The diagnosis of congenital TB is based on one of the following factors: (1) demonstration of primary hepatic complex or cavitating hepatic granuloma by percutaneous liver biopsy at birth; (2) infection of the maternal genital tract or placenta; (3) lesions noted in the first week of life; or (4) exclusion of the possibility of postnatal transmission by a thorough investigation of all contacts, including attendants.[49]

Prevention

Most gravidae with a positive PPD in pregnancy are asymptomatic with no evidence of active disease and are therefore classified as having LTBI. The risk for progression to active disease is highest in the first 2 years of conversion. It is important to prevent the onset of active disease while minimizing maternal and fetal risk. An algorithm for management of the positive PPD is presented in Figure 38-7. In women with a known recent conversion (2 years) to a positive PPD and no evidence of active disease, the recommended prophylaxis is INH, 300 mg/day, starting after the first trimester and continuing for 6 to 9 months. INH should be accompanied by pyridoxine (vitamin B_6) supplementation, 50 mg/day, to prevent the peripheral neuropathy associated with INH treatment. Women with an unknown or prolonged duration of PPD positivity (>2 years) should receive INH, 300 mg/day, for 6 to 9 months after delivery. INH prophylaxis is not recommended for women older than 35 years who have an unknown or prolonged PPD positivity in the absence of active disease.

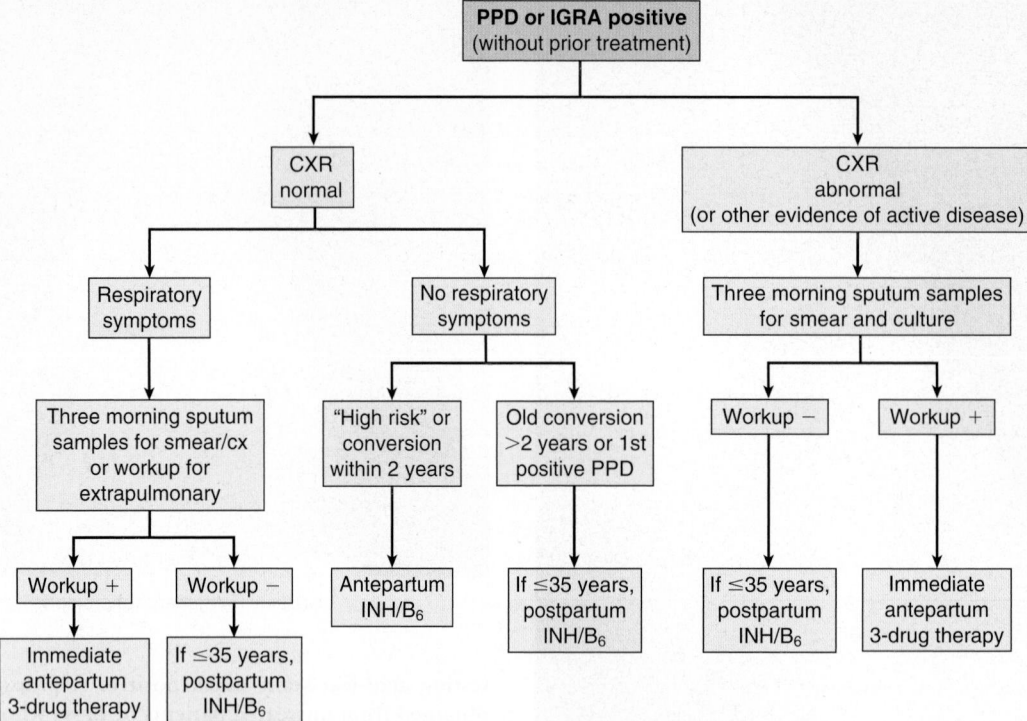

FIG 38-7 Algorithm for the management of positive purified protein derivative (PPD). CX, culture; CXR, chest x-ray; IGRA, interferon-γ release assay; INH, isoniazid.

The use of INH is discouraged in this group because of an **increased risk for hepatotoxicity. INH is associated with hepatitis in both pregnant and nonpregnant adults. The risk for liver inflammation in pregnancy from INH use is rare, and therefore this therapy should be instituted when the risk for conversion to active disease is high.**[54] Monthly monitoring of liver function tests may prevent this adverse outcome. Among individuals receiving INH, 10% to 20% develop mildly elevated liver function tests. These changes resolve once the drug is discontinued.

Treatment

The gravida with active TB should be treated initially with INH, 300 mg/day, combined with RIF, 600 mg/day (Table 38-1).[60] Resistant disease results from initial infection with resistant strains (33%), or it can develop during therapy. **If resistance to INH is identified or anticipated, ethambutol should be added, 2.5 g/day, and the treatment period should be extended to 18 months.**[60] Ethambutol is teratogenic in animals; however, this has not been demonstrated in humans. The most common side effect of ethambutol therapy is optic neuritis. Streptomycin should be avoided during pregnancy because it is associated with eighth nerve damage in neonates.[61] **Antituberculous agents not recommended for use in pregnancy include ethionamide, streptomycin, capreomycin, kanamycin, cycloserine, and pyrazinamide.** However, recent case reports that document use of the above-mentioned antituberculous agents in pregnancy have revealed no adverse fetal or neonatal effects. No congenital abnormalities were reported, and pregnancy outcome in the individuals treated was good.[60,61] **Untreated TB has been associated with higher morbidity and mortality among pregnant women;** therefore the management of the gravida with multidrug-resistant TB should

be individualized. The patient should be counseled about the small risk for teratogenicity and the increased risk for maternal and fetal morbidity and mortality from progression of disease when treatment is delayed. **The risk for postpartum transmission of TB to the baby may be higher among infants born to mothers with drug-resistant TB.**[62,63] **Therefore in patients with active disease at the time of delivery, separation of the mother and newborn should be accomplished to prevent infection of the newborn.**

Women who are being treated with antituberculous drugs may breastfeed. Only 0.75% to 2.3% of INH and 0.05% of RIF is excreted into breast milk. Ethambutol excretion into breast milk is also minimal. However, if the infant is concurrently taking oral antituberculous therapy, excessive drug levels may be reached in the neonate, and breastfeeding should be avoided. **Breastfed infants of women receiving INH therapy should receive a multivitamin supplement that includes pyridoxine.**[52] **Neonates of women on antituberculous therapy should have a PPD skin test at birth and again at 3 months of age. Infants born to women with active TB at the time of delivery should receive INH prophylaxis (10 mg/kg/day) until maternal disease has been inactive for 3 months** as evidenced by negative maternal sputum cultures. Active TB in the neonate should be treated appropriately with INH and RIF immediately upon diagnosis or with multiagent therapy should drug-resistant organisms be identified. **Infants and children at high risk for intimate and prolonged exposure to untreated or ineffectively treated individuals should receive the BCG vaccine.**

Summary

In summary, high-risk gravidae should be screened for TB and treated appropriately with INH prophylaxis for infection

TABLE 38-1 ANTITUBERCULOSIS DRUGS

DRUG	FORM	DAILY DOSE	WEEKLY DOSE	MAJOR ADVERSE REACTIONS
First-Line Drugs (for Initial Treatment)				
Isoniazid	PO or IM	10 mg/kg up to 300 mg	15 mg/kg up to 900 mg	Hepatic enzyme elevation, peripheral neuropathy hepatitis, hypersensitivity
Rifampin	PO	10 mg/kg up to 600 mg	10 mg/kg up to 600 mg	Orange discoloration of secretions and urine, nausea, vomiting, hepatitis, febrile reaction, purpura (rare)
Pyrazinamide	PO	15 to 30 mg/kg up to 2 g	50 to 70 mg/kg	Hepatotoxicity, hyperuricemia, arthralgias, skin rash, GI upset
Ethambutol	PO	15 mg/kg up to 2.5 g	50 mg/kg	Optic neuritis (decreased red-green color discrimination, decreased visual acuity), skin rash
Streptomycin	IM	15 mg/kg up to 1 g	25 to 30 mg/kg up to 1 g	Ototoxicity, nephrotoxicity
Second-Line Drugs (Daily Therapy)				
Capreomycin	IM	15 to 30 mg/kg up to 1 g		Auditory, vestibular, and renal toxicity
Kanamycin	IM	15 to 30 mg/kg up to 1 g		Auditory and renal toxicity, rare vestibular toxicity
Ethionamide	PO	15 to 20 mg/kg up to 1 g		GI disturbance, hepatotoxicity, hypersensitivity
Para-aminosalicylic acid	PO	150 mg/kg up to 1 g		GI disturbance, hypersensitivity, hepatotoxicity, sodium load
Cycloserine	PO	15 to 20 mg/kg up to 1 g		Psychosis, convulsions, rash

GI, gastrointestinal; *IM*, intramuscular; *PO*, by mouth.

without overt disease and with dual antituberculous therapy for active disease, and the newborn should also be screened for evidence of TB. Proper screening and therapy will result in a good outcome for mother and fetus in most cases.

ASTHMA IN PREGNANCY

Up to 8% of pregnancies are complicated by asthma, which may be the most common potentially serious medical condition to complicate pregnancy.[64] In general, the prevalence of and morbidity from asthma are increasing; however, asthma mortality has decreased in recent years. Asthma is characterized by chronic airway inflammation with increased airway responsiveness to a variety of stimuli and airway obstruction that is partially or completely reversible. Insight into the pathogenesis of asthma has changed with the recognition that airway inflammation is present in nearly all cases. **Current medical management for asthma emphasizes treatment of airway inflammation to decrease airway responsiveness and prevent asthma symptoms. The National Asthma Education and Prevention Program (NAEPP) Working Group has found that "it is safer for pregnant women with asthma to be treated with asthma medications than it is for them to have asthma symptoms and exacerbations."**[64]

Diagnosis

The enlarging uterus elevates the diaphragm about 4 cm with a reduction of the functional residual capacity (FRC). However, no clinically significant alterations occur in forced vital capacity (FVC), peak expiratory flow rate (PEFR), or forced expiratory volume in 1 second (FEV_1) in normal pregnancy.

Diagnosis of asthma in pregnancy is no different than for a nonpregnant patient. Asthma typically includes characteristic symptoms (wheezing, chest cough, shortness of breath, chest tightness), **temporal relationships** (fluctuating intensity, worse at night), **and triggers** (e.g., allergens, exercise, infections). Wheezing on auscultation would support the diagnosis, but its absence does not rule it out. Ideally, such a diagnosis would be confirmed by demonstrating airway obstruction on spirometry that is at least partially reversible and greater than a 12% increase in FEV_1 after inhalation of albuterol.[65,66] However, reversible airway obstruction may not be demonstrable in some patients with asthma. In patients with a clinical picture

consistent with asthma in whom reversible airway obstruction cannot be demonstrated, a trial of asthma therapy is reasonable. In such patients, a positive response to asthma therapy can establish the presumptive diagnosis during pregnancy. If methacholine testing is deemed necessary to confirm asthma, it should be delayed until postpartum.[64]

In patients who present with new respiratory symptoms during pregnancy, the most common differential diagnosis would be dyspnea (breathlessness) of pregnancy, which can usually be differentiated from asthma by its lack of cough, wheezing, chest tightness, or airway obstruction. Other differential diagnosis considerations include gastroesophageal reflux, chronic cough from postnasal drip, and bronchitis.

The NAEPP defined *mild intermittent, mild persistent, moderate persistent,* and *severe persistent asthma* according to daytime and nighttime symptoms—wheezing, cough, or dyspnea—and objective tests of pulmonary function.[64] The most commonly used pulmonary function parameters are the PEFR and FEV_1. Current NAEPP guidelines suggest classifying degree of asthma *severity* in patients not on controller medication and degree of asthma *control* in patients on controller medication (Table 38-2).[65,66] In another study,[67] pregnant patients who had mild asthma by symptoms and pulmonary function but who required regular medications to control their asthma were found to be similar to those with moderate asthma with respect to asthma exacerbations; those who required regular systemic corticosteroids to control asthma symptoms were similar to patients with severe asthma with respect to exacerbations. Using the Juniper Quality of Life Questionnaire, asthma-specific quality of life in early pregnancy was found to be related to subsequent asthma morbidity but not to perinatal outcomes.[68]

Effects of Pregnancy on Asthma

Asthma during pregnancy has been associated with considerable maternal morbidity. In a large prospective study, the effects of pregnancy on asthma were found to be variable: 23% improved and 30% become worse during pregnancy.[67] Women with *mild asthma* had an exacerbation rate of 12.6% and a hospitalization rate of 2.3%; those with *moderate asthma* had an exacerbation rate of 25.7% and a hospitalization rate of 6.8%; and those with *severe asthma* had an exacerbation rate of 51.9% and a hospitalization rate of 26.9%.[67]

TABLE 38-2   CLASSIFICATION OF ASTHMA SEVERITY AND CONTROL IN PREGNANT PATIENTS

ASTHMA CONTROL*	WELL CONTROLLED	NOT WELL CONTROLLED		VERY POORLY CONTROLLED
Asthma severity[†]	Mild intermittent	Mild persistent	Moderate persistent	Severe persistent
Symptom frequency, albuterol use	≤2 days/week	>2 days/week but not daily	Daily symptoms	Throughout the day
Nighttime awakening	≤2 times/month	>2 times/month	>1 time/week	≥4 times/week
Interference with normal activity	None	Minor limitation	Some limitation	Extremely limited
FEV$_1$ or peak flow (% predicted/personal best)	>80%	>80%	60% to 80%	<60%

Modified from Quick Reference NAEPP Expert Panel Report: Managing asthma during pregnancy: Recommendations for pharmacologic treatment—2004 update. *J Allergy Clin Immunol.* 2005;115:34-36.
*Assess in patients on long-term-control medications to determine whether step-up, step-down, or no change in therapy is indicated.
†Assess severity in patients who are not on long-term-control medications; see Table 38-5 to determine starting controller therapy based on severity.
FEV$_1$, forced expiratory volume in 1 second.

Effects of Asthma on Pregnancy

Compared with women without a history of asthma, women with asthma have been reported to have higher risks for complications of pregnancy even after adjustment for potential confounders.[69]

In a 2013 retrospective cohort study based on medical record data from 12 clinical centers in the United States from 2002 to 2008, Mendola and colleagues[70] found that the 17,404 gravidae with asthma had increased risks for nearly all outcomes studied. Women with asthma had significantly higher adjusted odds ratios for preeclampsia (1.14; 95% CI, 1.06 to 1.22), superimposed preeclampsia (1.34; CI, 1.15 to 1.56), gestational diabetes (1.11; CI, 1.03 to 1.19), placental abruption (1.22; CI, 1.09 to 1.36), placenta previa (1.30; CI, 1.08 to 1.56), and maternal seizures (1.79; CI, 1.21 to 2.63). Asthmatic women had higher odds of preterm birth (1.17; CI, 1.12 to 1.23), preterm premature rupture of the membranes (PPROM; OR, 1.18; CI, 1.07 to 1.30), medically indicated preterm delivery (1.14; CI, 1.01 to 1.29), breech presentation (1.13; CI, 1.05 to 1.22), hemorrhage (1.09; CI, 1.03 to 1.16), pulmonary embolism (1.71; CI, 1.05 to 2.79), and maternal ICU admission (1.34; CI, 1.04 to 1.72). Patients with asthma were less likely to have spontaneous labor (0.87; CI, 0.84 to 0.90) and vaginal delivery (0.84; CI, 0.80 to 0.87).

A significant increase in congenital malformations (adjusted OR, 1.48; CI, 1.04 to 2.09) has also been associated with exacerbations during the first trimester.[71] Although residual confounding or common pathogenic factors may explain some of these associations, observational data that show strong associations between poor asthma control (based on symptoms, pulmonary function, or exacerbations) and these increased risks suggest potential benefits of active asthma management in pregnancy in terms of improved pregnancy outcomes.[69,72,73] **Prospective studies that actively managed asthma during pregnancy have generally had excellent perinatal outcomes.**[73-79] Significantly increased adverse outcomes included preterm birth before 37 weeks' gestation among those who had severe disease or required oral corticosteroids, increased preeclampsia and growth restriction among those with daily symptoms, and an increased rate of cesarean delivery among those with moderate or severe asthma.[73,78] Although these studies show that the gravida with mild or moderate asthma can have excellent maternal and perinatal outcomes, important caveats apply when interpreting them. Prospective studies have tended to find fewer significant adverse associations, possibly because of better asthma surveillance and treatment. In addition, women who enroll in research studies tend to be more compliant and better motivated than the general public. The lack of finding more adverse outcomes among women with severe persistent asthma may also be a function of the relatively small numbers and the resulting lack of statistical power. Nonetheless, these prospective studies are reassuring in their consensus of good pregnancy outcomes, and they do not contradict that suboptimal control of asthma during pregnancy is associated with increased risk to the mother and baby.[65,78] In fact, a significant relationship has been reported between lower FEV$_1$ during pregnancy and increased risk for low birthweight and prematurity.[80]

Asthma Management

The ultimate goal of asthma therapy during pregnancy is to maintain adequate oxygenation of the fetus by prevention of hypoxic episodes in the mother. Other goals include achievement of minimal or no maternal symptoms day or night, minimal or no exacerbations, no limitations of activities, maintenance of normal or near-normal pulmonary function, minimal use of albuterol, and minimal or no adverse effects from medications. Consultation or comanagement with an asthma specialist may aid in the evaluation of the role of allergy and irritants, completion pulmonary function tests, or reevaluation of the medication plan should difficulties arise in achieving the goals of therapy or if the patient has severe asthma. **Effective management of asthma during pregnancy relies on four integral components: (1) objective measures for assessment and monitoring, (2) patient education, (3) avoidance or control of asthma triggers, and (4) pharmacologic therapy.**

Objective Measures for Assessment and Monitoring

Subjective measures of lung function by either the patient or physician can be an insensitive and inaccurate assessment of airway hyperresponsiveness, airway obstruction, and asthma severity. **The FEV$_1$ is the single best measure of pulmonary function.** When adjusted for confounders, a mean FEV$_1$ lower than 80% predicted has been found to be significantly associated with increased preterm delivery before 32 weeks and before 37 weeks and birthweight less than 2500 g.[80] However, measurement of FEV$_1$ requires a spirometer. **The PEFR correlates well with the FEV$_1$ and has the advantage that it can be measured reliably with inexpensive, disposable, portable peak flowmeters.** Self-monitoring of PEFR provides valuable insight into the course of asthma and helps detect early signs of deterioration so that timely therapy can be instituted. Because many pregnant women have increased symptoms, even those with mild or well-controlled disease need to be monitored with PEFR and FEV$_1$

testing as well as by observing their symptoms during pregnancy.[65] The typical PEFR in pregnancy is 380 to 550 L/min. The patient should establish her "personal best" PEFR then calculate her individualized PEFR zones: green greater than 80%, yellow 50% to 80%, and red zone less than 50% of personal best PEFR.

Patient Education

The patient should be made aware that controlling asthma during pregnancy is especially important for the well-being of the fetus. She should have a basic understanding of the medical management of asthma during pregnancy, including self-monitoring of PEFRs and the correct use of inhalers. She should be instructed on proper PEFR technique: make the measurement while standing, take a maximal inspiration, and note the reading on the peak flowmeter. Women who smoke should be encouraged to quit. Active smoking, but not passive smoking, has been associated with increased asthma symptoms and fetal growth abnormalities.[81] Women should also be instructed to avoid and control other asthma triggers.

All patients should be educated regarding the relationship between asthma and pregnancy: instruction about self-treatment should include inhaler techniques, the importance of adherence to medication, and control of potential environmental triggers. The patient should know that discontinuation of medications during pregnancy is associated with more severe asthma for all categories of asthma severity.[82] Caregivers should discuss self-reported adherence to treatment with controller medication, and they should address any barriers to optimal adherence (e.g., cost, convenience, concern about side effects). **The importance of adherence to treatment should be stressed.** Advice on environmental control measures for reducing exposure to allergens can be provided on the basis of the results of allergy testing.

Patients should be provided with a schedule for maintenance medications and doses of rescue therapy for increased symptoms. It is important to explain when and how to increase controller medications, when and how to use prednisone, how to recognize a severe exacerbation, and when and how to seek urgent or emergency care. A written asthma action plan is optimal, an example of which is available at http://www.nhlbi.nih.gov/files/docs/public/lung/asthma_actplan.pdf.

Avoidance or Control of Asthma Triggers

Limiting adverse environmental exposures during pregnancy is important for controlling asthma. Irritants and allergens that provoke acute symptoms also increase airway inflammation and hyperresponsiveness. Avoiding or controlling such triggers can reduce asthma symptoms, airway hyperresponsiveness, and the need for medical therapy.[66] Association of asthma with allergies is common; 75% to 85% of patients with asthma have positive skin tests to common allergens that include animal dander, house dust mites, cockroach antigens, pollens, and molds. Other common nonimmunologic triggers include tobacco smoke, strong odors, air pollutants, food additives such as sulfites, and certain drugs including aspirin and β-blockers. Another trigger can be strenuous physical activity. For some patients, exercise-induced asthma can be avoided with inhalation of albuterol 10 to 30 minutes before exercise.

Specific measures for avoiding asthma triggers include using allergen-impermeable mattress and pillow covers, removing carpeting, weekly washing of bedding in hot water, avoiding tobacco smoke, inhibiting mite and mold growth by reducing

TABLE 38-3	STEP THERAPY MEDICAL MANAGEMENT OF ASTHMA DURING PREGNANCY	
STEP		**ASTHMA SEVERITY**
1. No daily medications; albuterol as needed		Mild intermittent
2. Low-dose inhaled corticosteroid (alternatives: LTRA or theophylline*)		Mild persistent
3. Medium-dose inhaled corticosteroid† (alternatives: low-dose inhaled corticosteroid and LABA, LTRA, or theophylline*)		Moderate persistent
4. Medium-dose inhaled corticosteroid and LABA (alternatives: medium-dose inhaled corticosteroid plus LTRA or theophylline*)		Moderate persistent
5. High-dose inhaled corticosteroid and LABA		Severe persistent
6. High-dose inhaled corticosteroid and LABA and oral prednisone		Severe persistent

Modified from Quick Reference NAEPP Expert Panel Report: Managing asthma during pregnancy: Recommendations for pharmacologic treatment—2004 update. *J Allergy Clin Immunol.* 2005;115:34-36.
*Theophylline (serum level, 5-12 μg/mL).
†We have modified step 3 to reflect the choice of a medium-dose inhaled corticosteroid over a low-dose inhaled corticosteroid plus a LABA because of the lack of safety data on the use of a LABA during pregnancy.
LABA, long-acting β-agonist; *LTRA,* leukotriene-receptor agonist.

humidity, and leaving the house when it is vacuumed. Stuffed animals in the bed can also be a trigger. Ideal animal dander control involves removing the pet from the home; allergic women should at least keep furry pets out of the bedroom. Cockroaches can be controlled by poison baits or traps and eliminating exposed food or garbage.

The use of allergen immunotherapy, or "allergy shots," has been shown to be effective in improving asthma in allergic patients.[66] However, anaphylaxis is a risk for allergy injections—especially early in the course of immunotherapy, when the dose is being escalated—and anaphylaxis during pregnancy has been associated with fetal and maternal death. In a patient who is receiving a maintenance or near-maintenance dose, not experiencing adverse reactions to the injections, and apparently deriving clinical benefit, continuation of immunotherapy is recommended.[69] In such patients, a dose reduction may be considered to further decrease the chance of anaphylaxis. Risk-benefit considerations do not usually favor *beginning* allergy shots during pregnancy.

Pharmacologic Therapy

Medications for asthma are divided into *long-term controllers* that prevent asthma manifestations—inhaled corticosteroids, long-acting β-agonists, leukotriene modifiers, and theophylline—and *rescue therapy,* such as with albuterol, to provide quick relief of symptoms.

Women who have previously been prescribed asthma medications should be asked about their use to classify their current level of therapy according to a step-care approach (Table 38-3) and to assess potential adherence problems and barriers. **Asthma medication has been reported to significantly decline in the first trimester according to the number of prescriptions filled; a 23% decrease in inhaled corticosteroids, a 13% decrease in β-agonist, and a 54% decrease in rescue corticosteroids was noted.**[83] Moreover, a substantial proportion of asthma exacerbations during pregnancy have been associated with nonadherence to inhaled corticosteroids. In addition to assessing adherence, asking about past medications and their effectiveness and any side effects can help guide subsequent management decisions.

It is safer for pregnant women with asthma to be treated with asthma medications than it is for them to have asthma symptoms and exacerbations.[64] Typical dosages of commonly used asthma medications are listed in Table 38-4. Low, medium, and high doses of inhaled corticosteroid are presented in Table 38-5. The step-care therapeutic approach uses the least amount of drug intervention necessary to control a patient's severity of asthma.

Step Therapy

The step-care therapeutic approach increases the number and frequency of medications with increasing asthma severity.[64,66] Based on clinical trials in patients with varying degrees of disease severity, medications (see Table 38-3) are considered to be "preferred" or "alternative" at each step of therapy. Patients who do not respond optimally to treatment should be stepped up to more intensive medical therapy. Patients with poorly controlled asthma should generally be stepped up one step, and those with very poorly controlled asthma (see Table 38-2) should be increased by two steps.[69] Once control is achieved and sustained for several months, a step-down approach can be considered but should be undertaken cautiously and gradually to avoid compromising the stability of the asthma control. For some patients, it may be prudent to postpone attempts to reduce therapy that is effectively controlling the patient's asthma until after delivery.[64] In the case of a patient who had a favorable response to an alternative drug before becoming pregnant, it would be appropriate to maintain the therapy that successfully controlled the patient's asthma before pregnancy. However, when initiating new treatment for asthma during pregnancy, preferred medications should be considered first rather than alternative treatment options.[64]

Inhaled Corticosteroids

Inhaled corticosteroids are the preferred treatment for the management of all levels of persistent asthma during pregnancy.[64] Airway inflammation is present in nearly all cases; therefore inhaled corticosteroids have been advocated as first-line therapy even for patients with mild persistent asthma. In a prospective observational study of 504 pregnant women, those who were not initially treated with inhaled budesonide or beclomethasone had a 17% acute exacerbation rate, compared with only a 4% rate among those treated with inhaled corticosteroids from the start of pregnancy.[77] Randomized controlled trials with pregnant patients have shown that inhaled beclomethasone is more effective than theophylline in improving pulmonary function[79] and that prescribing inhaled beclomethasone in addition to oral corticosteroids and inhaled β-agonists at the time of discharge after hospitalization for asthma reduces subsequent asthma readmissions compared with oral corticosteroids and inhaled β-agonists alone.[84]

No consistent evidence links inhaled corticosteroid use to increases in congenital malformations or adverse perinatal outcomes.[64,85] Because more data are available on budesonide use during pregnancy, it is the preferred inhaled corticosteroid,[86] and it is the only inhaled corticosteroid with an FDA pregnancy category B rating. However, if asthma is well controlled by a different inhaled corticosteroid, it may be continued during pregnancy. No human pregnancy data are available for the glucocorticoid ciclesonide.[85]

Inhaled β₂-Agonists

As-needed use of inhaled β₂-agonists is currently recommended for all levels of asthma during pregnancy.[64] Albuterol has a rapid onset of effect in the relief of acute bronchospasm through smooth muscle relaxation and is an excellent bronchoprotective agent for pretreatment before exercise; however, β₂-agonists are associated with tremor, tachycardia, and palpitations. They do not block the development of airway hyperresponsiveness. An increased frequency of bronchodilator use could be an indicator of the need for additional antiinflammatory therapy. Appropriate β₂-agonist use appears to be safe during pregnancy.[64,87]

TABLE 38-4	TYPICAL DOSAGES OF ASTHMA MEDICATIONS
Albuterol MDI	2 to 4 puffs every 4-6 hours as needed
Salmeterol DPI	1 blister 2 times/day
Formoterol	1 capsule 2 times/day
Fluticasone/ salmeterol (Advair) DPI	1 inhalation 2 times/day; strength (100, 250, 500) depends on severity of asthma
Montelukast	10-mg tablet at night
Zafirlukast	20-mg tablet twice daily
Prednisone	7.5 to 60 mg/day for active symptoms or maintenance therapy for severe persistent asthma
Theophylline	Start 200 mg 2 times/day orally, target serum levels of 5 to 12 μg/mL (decrease dosage by half if treated with erythromycin or cimetidine)
Ipratropium MDI	2 to 3 puffs every 6 hours

Modified from Quick Reference NAEPP Expert Panel Report: Managing asthma during pregnancy: Recommendations for pharmacologic treatment—2004 update. *J Allergy Clin Immunol.* 2005;115:34-36.
DPI, dry-powder inhaler; *MDI,* metered-dose inhaler.

TABLE 38-5	COMPARATIVE DAILY DOSES FOR INHALED CORTICOSTEROIDS			
	DAILY DOSE*	**LOW DOSE**	**MEDIUM DOSE**	**HIGH DOSE**
Beclomethasone MDI	40 to 80 μg/puff	80 to 240 μg	240 to 480 μg	>480 μg
Budesonide DPI	90 or 180 μg/inhalation	180 to 540 μg	540 to 1080 μg	>1080 μg
Flunisolide MDI	80 μg/puff	320 μg	320 to 640 μg	>640 μg
Fluticasone MDI	44, 110, or 220 μg/puff	88 to 264 μg	264 to 440 μg	>440 μg
Fluticasone DPI	50, 100, or 250 μg/inhalation	100 to 300 μg	300 to 500 μg	>500 μg
Mometasone DPI	110 or 220 μg/inhalation	110 to 220 μg	220 to 440 μg	>440 μg
Ciclesonide MDI	80 or 160μg/puff	160 to 320 μg	320 to 640 μg	>640 μg

Modified from Asthma Care Quick Reference 2012. National Institutes of Health publication No. 12-5075. Available at http://www.nhlbi.nih.gov/files/docs/guidelines/asthma_qrg.pdf.
*Note that total daily puffs are usually divided as a twice-a-day regimen.
DPI, dry-powder inhaler; *MDI,* metered-dose inhaler.

Salmeterol and formoterol are long-acting β-agonist (LABA) preparations. Although human data are limited, the safety of LABAs during human pregnancy is considered likely based on the inhalational route and the generally reassuring data for short-acting β-agonists in addition to animal data.[64,85] LABAs should only be used in combination with inhaled corticosteroids during pregnancy, and they have been shown to be more effective than leukotriene-receptor antagonists (LTRAs) and theophylline as add-on therapy to inhaled corticosteroids.[66] The efficacy of these drugs during pregnancy is largely extrapolated from studies performed in nonpregnant patients.

Omalizumab

Omalizumab is a humanized monoclonal antibody to immuno-globulin (Ig) E and is an FDA category B drug. An observational registry (the Xolair Pregnancy Registry [EXPECT]) to evaluate exposure to omalizumab had 128 outcomes as of July of 2011. The number of miscarriages (8), fetal deaths (1), preterm deliveries (19), and major birth defects (5) were not inconsistent with expectations for women with moderate to severe asthma.[88] Because of the paucity of safety data and the potential risk of anaphylaxis, omalizumab should not be initiated during pregnancy; a possible exception may be the patient who has allergies and remains uncontrolled despite medical management presented in Table 38-3. However, it would seem reasonable to continue omalizumab among women with severe asthma who become pregnant.

Theophylline

Theophylline is an alternative treatment for mild and moderate persistent asthma during pregnancy (see Table 38-3).[64] Subjective symptoms of adverse theophylline effects include insomnia, heartburn, palpitations, and nausea; high doses have been observed to cause jitteriness, tachycardia, and vomiting in neonates. **Dosing guidelines have recommended that serum theophylline concentrations be maintained at 5 to 12 μg/mL during pregnancy.**[64] Treatment with cimetidine, erythromycin, or azithromycin can decrease clearance with resultant toxicity; in such cases it may be appropriate to decrease the dosage of theophylline by half.[79] Theophylline is only indicated for chronic therapy and is not effective for the treatment of acute exacerbations during pregnancy.

Theophylline has not been shown to be associated with congenital anomalies.[64,85] In one randomized controlled trial, no differences were found in asthma exacerbations or perinatal outcomes in a cohort that received theophylline compared with the cohort that received inhaled beclomethasone.[79] However, the theophylline cohort had significantly more reported side effects and discontinuation of study medication, and they had an increased proportion of those with an FEV_1 lower than 80% predicted.

Leukotriene Moderators

Leukotrienes are arachidonic acid metabolites that have been implicated in causing bronchospasm, mucous secretion, and increased vascular permeability. Bronchoconstriction associated with aspirin ingestion can be blocked by LTRAs. Montelukast and zafirlukast are both designated pregnancy category B. Although human data are limited for LTRA use in pregnancy, their use has not been associated with an increase in congenital anomalies.[85,89] **Leukotriene modifiers are less effective as single agents than inhaled corticosteroids and are less effective than LABAs as add-on therapy.**[66]

Oral Corticosteroids

Prednisone is indicated for the maintenance therapy of severe persistent asthma (see Tables 38-3 and 38-4). For outpatient treatment of acute exacerbations, prednisone may be given 40 to 60 mg per day in one or two divided doses for 3 to 10 days.[64] In a retrospective study, pregnant asthmatic women were found to be undertreated with systemic corticosteroids when compared with nonpregnant patients in an emergency department (ED); they were also nearly 4 times more likely to return to the same ED within 2 weeks for asthma symptoms.[90]

Oral corticosteroid use during the first trimester of pregnancy was associated with a threefold increased risk for isolated cleft lip (background incidence is about 0.1%) with or without cleft palate.[64,85] Oral corticosteroid use has also been associated with an increased incidence of preeclampsia, preterm delivery, and low birthweight.[73,75,85,87] However, it is difficult to separate the effects of the oral corticosteroids on these outcomes from the effects of severe or uncontrolled asthma. Because of the uncertainties in these data and the definite risks of severe uncontrolled asthma to the mother and fetus, **the NAEPP recommends the use of oral corticosteroids when indicated for the long-term management of severe persistent asthma or for exacerbations during pregnancy.**[64]

Management of Allergic Rhinitis and Gastroesophageal Reflux

Rhinitis, sinusitis, and gastroesophageal reflux may exacerbate asthma symptoms, and their management should be considered an integral aspect of asthma care. Intranasal corticosteroids are the most effective medications for control of allergic rhinitis. Loratadine and cetirizine are recommended second-generation antihistamines. Oral decongestant ingestion during the first trimester has been associated with gastroschisis; therefore short-term (≤3 days) intranasal decongestants or intranasal corticosteroids should be considered before use of oral decongestants.[64] Controlling gastroesophageal reflux with acid reducers may improve asthma control.

Antenatal Asthma Management

In general, data are lacking to guide the optimal obstetric management of the woman with asthma, and recommendations are based on extrapolation of data from other clinical settings and expert opinion.[69] Women with asthma should be offered influenza vaccination as appropriate. Patients with persistent asthma should be considered to be at risk for pregnancy complications. Adverse outcomes can be increased by underestimation of asthma severity and undertreatment of asthma. The first prenatal visit should include a detailed medical history with attention to coexisting medical conditions that could complicate the management of asthma, including rhinitis, sinusitis, reflux, or depression. The patient should be questioned about smoking history and the presence and severity of symptoms, episodes of nocturnal asthma, the number of days of work missed, and emergency care visits associated with asthma. Asthma severity or control should be determined (see Table 38-2). The type and amount of asthma medications, including the number of puffs of albuterol used per week, should be noted.

Those with moderate or severe asthma should have scheduling of prenatal visits based on clinical judgment. In addition to routine care, monthly or more frequent evaluations of asthma history (emergency visits, hospital admissions, symptom frequency, symptom interference with sleep or activity, medications, dosages, and compliance) and pulmonary function (FEV₁ or PEFR) are recommended. Patients should be instructed on proper dosing and administration of their asthma medications.

Daily PEFR monitoring should be considered for patients with moderate or severe asthma and especially for patients who have difficulty perceiving signs of worsening asthma. It may be helpful to maintain an asthma diary that contains daily assessment of asthma status and includes PEFR measurements, symptoms and activity limitations, doctor visits, and a record of regular and as-needed medications taken. Identifying and avoiding asthma triggers, especially smoking, can lead to improved maternal well-being with less need for medications. Specific recommendations can be made for appropriate environmental controls based on the patient's history of exposure and, when available, results of blood or skin testing for IgE–mediated sensitivity to inhalant allergen asthma triggers.

Women with asthma that is not well controlled, or those who have an exacerbation, may benefit from additional fetal surveillance in the form of ultrasound examinations and antenatal fetal testing.[64] Because asthma has been associated with intrauterine growth restriction (IUGR) and preterm birth, it is useful to establish pregnancy dating accurately by first-trimester ultrasound. The intensity of antenatal surveillance of fetal well-being should be considered on the basis of the severity of the asthma as well as any other high-risk features of the pregnancy that may be present.

Home Management of Asthma Exacerbations

An asthma exacerbation that causes minimal problems for the mother may have severe sequelae for the fetus. Patients should be instructed on rescue management and should be educated to recognize signs and symptoms of early asthma exacerbations such as coughing, chest tightness, dyspnea, or wheezing or by a 20% decrease in their PEFR. This is important so that prompt home rescue treatment may be instituted to avoid maternal and fetal hypoxia. In general, patients should use inhaled albuterol, 2 to 4 puffs every 20 minutes for up to 1 hour (Box 38-3). **The**

BOX 38-3   HOME MANAGEMENT OF ACUTE ASTHMA EXACERBATIONS

Use albuterol MDI 2 to 4 puffs and measure PEFR.
Poor response:
- If PEFR is <50% predicted and severe wheezing and shortness of breath occur or decreased fetal movement is apparent, repeat albuterol 2 to 4 puffs by MDI and seek emergency care.

Incomplete response:
- If PEFR is 50% to 80% predicted or if persistent wheezing and shortness of breath occur, repeat albuterol treatment 2 to 4 puffs by MDI at 20-minute intervals up to two more times. If repeat PEFR is 50% to 80% predicted or if decreased fetal movement is noted, contact caregiver or seek emergency care.

Good response:
- If PEFR is >80% predicted, no wheezing or shortness of breath occur, and the fetus is moving normally, the patient can continue inhaled albuterol, 2 to 4 puffs by MDI, every 3 to 4 hours as needed.

Modified from Quick Reference NAEPP Expert Panel Report: Managing asthma during pregnancy: Recommendations for pharmacologic treatment—2004 update. *J Allergy Clin Immunol.* 2005;115:34-36.
MDI, metered-dose inhaler; *PEFR,* peak expiratory flow rate.

---

response is considered good if symptoms are resolved or if they become subjectively mild, normal activities can be resumed, and the PEFR is more than 80% of the personal best. For asthma exacerbations that can be managed at home, a course of oral prednisone is recommended, 40 to 60 mg per day in a single dose or in two divided doses for 3 to 10 days.[64] The patient should seek further medical attention if the response is incomplete or if fetal activity is decreased.

Hospital and Emergency Department Management of Asthma Exacerbations

The principal goal should be the prevention of hypoxia. Measurement of oxygenation through pulse oximetry is essential, and arterial blood gases may be obtained if oxygen saturation remains less than 95%. Chest radiographs are not commonly needed. **Continuous electronic fetal monitoring should be initiated if gestation has advanced to the point of potential fetal viability. Albuterol** (2.5 to 5 mg every 20 minutes for three doses, then 2.5 to 10 mg every 1 to 4 hours as needed, or 10 to 15 mg/hour continuously) **should be delivered by a nebulizer driven with oxygen.**[64] Occasionally, nebulized treatment is not effective because the patient is moving air poorly; in such cases, 0.25 mg terbutaline can be administered subcutaneously every 20 minutes for three doses. Guidelines for the management of asthma exacerbations are presented in Box 38-4.

Systemic glucocorticoids are indicated for those with a poor response to treatment after 1 hour or as initial therapy for those who were taking prednisone. Methylprednisolone, prednisolone, or prednisone should be given 40 to 80 mg/day in a single or divided dose until peak flow reaches 70% of predicted or personal best, and then the dosage is tapered as the patient improves.[64] For patients who have a severe exacerbation, a higher initial dose of 120 to 180 mg/day given over 3 to 4 divided doses should be continued for 48 hours and then tapered as above.[64,66] In severe exacerbations if the patient is unresponsive to the initial regimen, consider treatment with magnesium sulfate, a bronchodilator.

Labor and Delivery Management of Asthma

Asthma medications should not be discontinued during labor and delivery. Although asthma is usually quiescent during labor, consideration should be given to assessing PEFR. The patient should be kept hydrated and should receive adequate analgesia to decrease the risk for bronchospasm. It is commonly recommended that women who are currently taking systemic corticosteroids or who have received several short courses of systemic corticosteroids during pregnancy receive IV corticosteroids (e.g., hydrocortisone at a dose of 100 mg every 8 hours) during labor and for 24 hours after delivery to prevent adrenal crisis.[69] An elective delivery should be postponed if the patient is having an exacerbation. It is rarely necessary to perform a cesarean delivery for an acute asthma exacerbation; maternal and fetal compromise usually respond to aggressive medical management.

Prostaglandin E₂ (PGE₂) or PGE₁ can be used for cervical ripening, management of spontaneous or induced abortions, or postpartum hemorrhage, although the patient's respiratory status should be monitored.[65] **Methylergonovine and especially carboprost (15-methyl PGF₂ₐ) can cause bronchospasm.**[65] If tocolysis is needed, magnesium sulfate and terbutaline are preferable because they are bronchodilators; in contrast,

BOX 38-4   EMERGENCY DEPARTMENT AND HOSPITAL-BASED MANAGEMENT OF ASTHMA EXACERBATION

Initial Assessment and Treatment

History and examination (auscultation, use of accessory muscles, heart rate, respiratory rate), PEFR or FEV_1, oxygen saturation, and other tests as indicated:

- If severe exacerbation (FEV_1 or PEFR is <50% with severe symptoms at rest), high-dose albuterol by nebulization every 20 minutes or continuously for 1 hour, inhaled ipratropium bromide, and systemic corticosteroids
- Initiate fetal assessment (consider fetal monitoring and/or BPP if fetus is potentially viable)
- Albuterol by MDI or nebulizer, up to three doses in the first hour
- Oral corticosteroid if no immediate response is seen or if the patient was recently treated with a systemic corticosteroid
- Oxygen to maintain pulse oximetry saturation >95%
- Repeat assessment: symptoms, physical examination, PEFR, oxygen saturation
- Continue albuterol every 60 minutes for 1 to 3 hours provided improvement is evident

Repeat Assessment

- Symptoms, physical examination, PEFR, oxygen saturation, other tests as needed
- Continue fetal assessment

Good Response

- FEV_1 or PEFR ≥70%
- Response sustained 60 minutes after last treatment
- No distress
- Physical examination: normal
- Reassuring fetal status
- Discharge home

Incomplete Response

- FEV_1 or PEFR ≥50% but <70%
- Mild or moderate symptoms
- Continue fetal assessment until patient has stabilized

- Monitor FEV_1 or PEFR, oxygen saturation, pulse
- Continue inhaled albuterol and oxygen
- Inhaled ipratropium bromide
- Systemic (oral or intravenous) corticosteroid
- Individualize decision for hospitalization

Poor Response

- FEV_1 or PEFR <50%
- PCO_2 >42 mm Hg
- Physical examination: symptoms severe, drowsiness, confusion
- Continue fetal assessment
- Admit to ICU

Impending or Actual Respiratory Arrest

- Admit to ICU
- Intubation and mechanical ventilation with 100% oxygen
- Nebulized albuterol plus inhaled ipratropium bromide
- Intravenous corticosteroid

Intensive Care Unit

- Inhaled albuterol hourly or continuously plus inhaled ipratropium bromide
- Intravenous corticosteroid
- Oxygen
- Possible intubation and mechanical ventilation
- Continue fetal assessment until patient has stabilized

Discharge Home

- Continue treatment with albuterol
- Oral systemic corticosteroid if indicated
- Initiate or continue inhaled corticosteroid until review at medical follow-up
- Patient education:
  - Review medicine use
  - Review/initiate action plan
  - Recommend close medical follow-up

Modified from Quick Reference NAEPP Expert Panel Report: Managing asthma during pregnancy: Recommendations for pharmacologic treatment—2004 update. *J Allergy Clin Immunol.* 2005;115:34-36.
BPP, biophysical profile; *FEV_1,* forced expiratory volume in 1 second; *ICU,* intensive care unit; *MDI,* Metered-dose inhaler; *PCO_2,* partial pressure of carbon dioxide; *PEFR,* peak expiratory flow rate.

indomethacin might induce bronchospasm in the aspirin-sensitive patient.[65] Use of calcium channel blockers for tocolysis among patients with asthma has not been reported, although an association with bronchospasm has not been observed with wide clinical use. Nonselective β-blockers may trigger bronchospasm.

Lumbar anesthesia has the benefit of reducing oxygen consumption and minute ventilation during labor. Fentanyl or butorphanol may be safer than morphine or meperidine, which can cause histamine release, but evidence of bronchospasm during labor is lacking. Communication among the obstetric, anesthetic, and pediatric caregivers is important for optimal care.

Breastfeeding

In general, only small amounts of asthma medications enter breast milk. Prednisone, theophylline, antihistamines, inhaled corticosteroids, LTRAs, and β2-agonists are not considered to be contraindications for breastfeeding.[64,65] However, among sensitive neonates, theophylline may cause vomiting, feeding difficulties, jitteriness, and cardiac arrhythmias.

Summary

Asthma is an increasingly common problem during pregnancy. Mild and moderate asthma can be associated with excellent maternal and perinatal pregnancy outcomes, especially if patients are managed according to contemporary NAEPP recommendations. Severe and poorly controlled asthma may be associated with increased prematurity, preeclampsia, growth restriction, and a need for cesarean delivery. Severe asthma exacerbations can result in maternal morbidity and mortality and can have commensurate adverse pregnancy outcomes. The management of asthma during pregnancy should be based on objective assessment, trigger avoidance, patient education, and step therapy. Asthma medications should be continued during pregnancy and while breastfeeding.

RESTRICTIVE LUNG DISEASE

Restrictive ventilatory defects occur when lung expansion is limited because of alterations in the lung parenchyma or

because of abnormalities in the pleura, chest wall, or the neuromuscular apparatus. These conditions are characterized by a reduction in lung volumes and an increase in the ratio of FEV_1 to FVC.[91] The interstitial lung diseases include idiopathic pulmonary fibrosis, sarcoidosis, hypersensitivity pneumonitis, pneumoconiosis, drug-induced lung disease, and connective tissue disease. **Additional conditions that cause a restrictive ventilatory defect include pleural and chest wall diseases and extrathoracic conditions such as obesity, peritonitis, and ascites.**[91] Restrictive lung disease in pregnancy has not been well studied. Consequently, little is known about the effects of restrictive lung disease on the outcome of pregnancy or the effects of pregnancy on the disease process itself. Boggess and colleagues[92] presented data on nine pregnant women with interstitial and restrictive lung disease who were prospectively managed. Diagnoses included idiopathic pulmonary fibrosis, hypersensitivity pneumonitis, sarcoidosis, kyphoscoliosis, and multiple pulmonary emboli. Three of the gravidae described in this paper had severe disease characterized by a vital capacity of 1.5 L or less (50% predicted) or a diffusing capacity less than or equal to 50% predicted. Five of the patients had exercise-induced oxygen desaturation, and four patients required supplemental oxygen. One patient in the group had an adverse outcome and was delivered at 31 weeks; she subsequently required mechanical ventilation for 72 hours. All other patients were delivered at or beyond 36 weeks with no adverse intrapartum or postpartum complications. All infants were at or above the 30th percentile for growth. The authors concluded that restrictive lung disease was well tolerated in pregnancy. However, exercise intolerance was common; therefore early oxygen supplementation may be required.

Sarcoidosis

Sarcoidosis is a systemic granulomatosis disease of undetermined etiology that often affects young adults. **Pregnancy outcome for most women with sarcoidosis is good.**[93,94] In a study of 35 pregnancies in 18 patients with sarcoidosis, disease activity remained stable in nine patients. During pregnancy, improvement was demonstrated in six patients, and in three, a worsening of the disease was reported.[93] During the postpartum period, 15 patients remained stable; however, in three women, a progression of the disease continued. Another retrospective study presented 15 pregnancies complicated by maternal sarcoidosis over a 10-year period.[94] **Eleven of these patients remained stable, two experienced disease progression, and two died as a result of severe complications of severe sarcoidosis. In this group, factors indicative of a poor prognosis reportedly included parenchymal lesions on chest radiograph, advanced radiographic staging, advanced maternal age, low inflammatory activity, requirement for drugs other than steroids, and the presence of extrapulmonary sarcoidosis.**[94] **Both of the patients who succumbed during gestation had severe disease at the onset of pregnancy. The overall cesarean delivery rate was 40%; in addition, 27% of infants (4 of 15) weighed less than 2500 g.** None of the patients developed preeclampsia. One possible explanation for the commonly observed improvement in sarcoidosis may be the increased concentration of cortisol during pregnancy. However, because sarcoidosis improves spontaneously in many nonpregnant patients, the improvement may be coincident with, but not due to, pregnancy.

One study examined 17 pregnancies in 10 patients and concluded that pregnancy had no consistent effect on the course of the disease.[95] Scadding[96] separated patients into three categories based on characteristic patterns of their chest radiographs. When the chest radiograph had resolved before pregnancy, the normal radiograph persisted throughout gestation. In women with resolving radiographic changes before pregnancy, resolution continued throughout the prenatal period. Patients with inactive fibrotic residual disease had stable chest radiographs, and those with active disease tended to have partial or complete resolution of those changes during pregnancy. Most patients in this latter group, however, experienced exacerbation of the disease within 3 to 6 months after delivery.[96]

Patients with pulmonary hypertension complicating restrictive lung disease may suffer a mortality rate as high as 50% during gestation. These patients need close monitoring during labor and delivery and postpartum. Invasive monitoring with a pulmonary artery catheter may be indicated to optimize cardiorespiratory function. **Gravidae with restrictive lung disease, including pulmonary sarcoidosis, may benefit from early institution of steroid therapy for evidence of worsening pulmonary status.** Individuals with evidence of severe disease need close monitoring and may require supplemental oxygen therapy during gestation.

During labor, consideration should be given to early use of epidural anesthesia, if it is not contraindicated. The proactive institution of pain management in this population will minimize pain, decrease sympathetic response, and therefore decrease oxygen consumption during labor and delivery. **The use of general anesthesia should be avoided, if possible,** because these patients may develop pulmonary complications after general anesthesia, including pneumonia and difficulty weaning from the ventilator. **In addition, close fetal surveillance throughout gestation is warranted because impaired oxygenation may compromise fetal growth.**

An additional consideration is the need to counsel all women with restrictive lung disease about the potential for continued impairment of their respiratory status during pregnancy, particularly if their respiratory disease is deteriorating at the time of conception. The individual with clinical signs consistent with pulmonary hypertension or severe restrictive disease should be cautioned about the possibility of maternal mortality due to worsening pulmonary function during gestation.

In summary, although the literature on restrictive lung disease in pregnancy is limited, it supports the conclusion that most patients with restrictive lung disease complicating pregnancy—which includes those with pulmonary sarcoidosis—will have a favorable pregnancy outcome. However, the clinician should keep in mind that a subgroup of women with restrictive lung disease can have significant worsening of their clinical condition during gestation.

Cystic Fibrosis

Cystic fibrosis (CF) involves the exocrine glands and epithelial tissues of the pancreas, sweat glands, and mucous glands in the respiratory, digestive, and reproductive tracts. **Chronic obstructive pulmonary disease (COPD), pancreatic exocrine insufficiency, and elevated sweat electrolytes are present in most patients with CF.** The disease is **genetically transmitted with an autosomal-recessive pattern of inheritance.** The CF gene was identified and cloned in 1989; the gene is localized to chromosome 7, and the molecular defect that accounts for the majority of cases has been identified. **In the United States, about 4% of the white population are heterozygous carriers of the CF gene, and the disease occurs in 1 in 3000 live white births.** Morbidity and mortality in CF is usually secondary to progressive chronic bronchial pulmonary disease. Pregnancy and the attendant physiologic changes can stress the pulmonary, cardiovascular, and nutritional status of women with CF. The purpose of this section is to familiarize the obstetrician with the physiologic effects of this complex disease and the impact of the disease on pregnancy and the impact of pregnancy on the disease. Additional factors that need to be addressed are the genetics of this disorder (see Chapter 10) and the implications for the newborn, as well as social issues, including who will raise the child should the mother succumb to her disease.

Survival for patients with CF has increased dramatically since 1940. According to the Cystic Fibrosis Foundation's patient registry, mean survival in 2008 had increased to 39.6 years. Women had a slightly lower median age of survival (27.3 years) compared with men (29.6 years). The reasons for sex differences in mortality are unclear. **Today, more than 45% of individuals with CF in the United States are older than 18 years.** This increase in survival of patients with CF is likely secondary to earlier diagnosis and intervention and to advances in antibiotic therapy and nutritional support. **Therefore, more women with CF are now entering reproductive age. In contrast to men with CF, who for the most part are infertile, women with CF are more often fertile. Infertility in women with CF may occasionally be due to anovulatory cycles and secondary amenorrhea, which result from significant malnutrition associated with advanced disease. A more common reason for infertility appears to result from alteration in the physiologic properties of cervical mucus.**

The first case of CF complicating pregnancy was reported in 1960. The annual number of CF pregnancies reported to the Cystic Fibrosis Foundation's patient registry doubled between 1986 and 1990, with 52 pregnancies reported in 1986 and 111 pregnancies reported in 1990. This same registry more recently reported on a total of 680 pregnancies in 8136 women between 1985 and 1997. This documents a dramatic increase in pregnancy complicated by CF, and increasing numbers are reported in other countries as well. **Because the number of women with CF who achieve pregnancy is steadily increasing, it is important that the obstetrician be familiar with the disease. Liberal consultation with a CF specialist should be obtained because a team effort will increase the chance for an improved pregnancy outcome.**

Effect of Pregnancy on Cystic Fibrosis

The physiologic changes associated with pregnancy (see Chapter 3) are well tolerated by healthy gravidae; however, those with CF may adapt poorly. During pregnancy, an increase in resting minute ventilation at term may approach 150% of control values due to the increased oxygen consumption and increased carbon dioxide burden that occur during pregnancy. In addition, increased levels of circulating progesterone stimulates the respiratory drive. Enlargement of the abdominal contents and upward displacement of the diaphragm lead to a decrease in functional residual volume and a decrease in residual volume. Pregnancy is also accompanied by subtle alterations in gas exchange with widening of the alveolar-arterial oxygen gradient

that is most pronounced in the supine position. These alterations in pulmonary function are of little consequence to the normal pregnant woman. However, in the gravida with CF, these changes may contribute to respiratory decompensation that can lead to an increase in morbidity and mortality for the mother and the fetus.

During normal pregnancy, blood volume increases by an average of 50%. Cardiac output increases as well and reaches a plateau in midpregnancy. During labor, blood volume rises acutely, in large part because of the release of blood from the contracting uterus, and it is additionally increased after delivery secondary to augmented venous return with the release of caval obstruction.

Women with CF and advanced lung disease may suffer from pulmonary hypertension with high pulmonary artery pressures. Regardless of the etiology, pulmonary hypertension is associated with unacceptable maternal risk during pregnancy and is considered to be a contraindication to pregnancy. Women with significant pulmonary hypertension may develop cardiovascular collapse at the time of labor and delivery, with a maternal mortality rate that exceeds 25%. Additionally, **women with pulmonary hypertension may not be able to adequately increase cardiac output during pregnancy; therefore they suffer uteroplacental insufficiency that leads to intrauterine growth restriction and stillbirth.**

Nutritional requirements are increased during pregnancy, and about 300 kcal/day in additional fuel is needed to meet the requirements of mother and fetus. **Most patients with CF have pancreatic exocrine insufficiency. As a result, digestive enzymes and bicarbonate ions are diminished, which results in maldigestion, malabsorption, and malnutrition.**

Several reports suggest that **patients who have mild CF, good prepregnancy nutritional status, and less impairment of lung function tolerate pregnancy well. However, those with poor clinical status, malnutrition, hepatic dysfunction, or advanced lung disease are at increased risk from pregnancy.**[97,98] Kent and Farquharson[98] reviewed the literature and reported 217 pregnancies. In this series, the frequency of preterm delivery was 24.3%, and the perinatal death rate was 7.9%. **Poor outcomes were associated with a maternal weight gain of less than 4.5 kg and an FVC of less than 50% of predicted. A series of pregnancies in women with CF described by Edenborough and colleagues**[99] **reported 18 live births (81.8%), one third of which were preterm deliveries, and 18.2% of patients had abortions. Four maternal deaths occurred within 3.2 years after delivery.** In this series, lung function was available before delivery, immediately after delivery, and after pregnancy. Although the patients demonstrated a decline of 13% in FEV_1 and 11% in FVC during pregnancy, most returned to baseline pulmonary function after pregnancy. Although most of the women tolerated pregnancy well, **those with moderate to severe lung disease—an FEV_1 less than 60% of predicted—more often had preterm infants and had increased loss of lung function compared with those with milder disease.**[99] **In two series, prepregnancy FEV_1 was found to be the most useful predictor of outcome in pregnant women with CF.**[99,100] **In addition, a positive correlation was found between prepregnancy FEV_1 and maternal survival.**

Another report examined survival in 8136 women enrolled in the U.S. Cystic Fibrosis Foundation National Patient Registry from 1985 to 1997,[101] and 680 of these became pregnant. The authors matched the 680 women in an index year to 3327 control women with CF. Women who reported a pregnancy were more likely to have had a higher percentage of predicted FEV_1 (67.5% predicted vs. 67.1% predicted, respectively; $P > .001$) and a higher weight (52.9 vs. 46.4 kg, respectively; $P > .001$). The 10-year survival rate in pregnant women (77%; 95% CI, 71% to 82%) was higher than in those women who did not become pregnant. A separate analysis that matched the pregnant patient's FEV_1 percent of predicted, age, *Pseudomonas aeruginosa* colonization, and pancreatic function obtained similar results. In this cohort, pregnancy was not harmful in any subgroup, which included patients with an FEV_1 40% of predicted or diabetes mellitus.[101] **The authors concluded that women with CF who became pregnant were initially healthier and had better 10-year survival rates than women with CF who did not become pregnant.**

A 2014 report by Patel and colleagues[102] describes 1119 deliveries in women with CF in the United States, compared with 12,627,627 women without the disease, and documents an increased risk of death, mechanical ventilation, pneumonia, acute renal failure, preterm labor, diabetes, asthma, and an adverse composite CF outcome; however, the absolute risks were low. **Pulmonary involvement in CF includes chronic infection of the airways and bronchiectasis. Selective infection with certain microorganisms occurs, such as *S. aureus*, *H. influenzae*, *P. aeruginosa*, and *Burkholderia cepacia*, although *P. aeruginosa* is the most frequent pathogen.** Parenteral antibiotics are the mainstays of treatment for these acute infections. However, pregnancy- and CF–associated alterations in pharmacokinetics can have grave consequences for these patients. It is well known that pregnant subjects have lower serum levels and higher urine levels of antibiotics than nonpregnant subjects. The lower levels in plasma are attributed to the increase in volume of distribution and an increase in glomerular filtration and renal clearance of the drugs, therefore monitoring drug levels is indicated when therapeutic response is less than optimal.

Counseling Patients with Cystic Fibrosis in Pregnancy

Several factors must be considered when counseling a woman with CF who is considering pregnancy, including the possibility that her fetus will have CF (see Chapter 10). **When the mother has CF and the proposed father is a white individual of unknown genotype, the risk for the fetus having CF is 1 in 50, compared with 1 in 3000 in the general white population. If the prospective father is a known carrier of a CF mutation, the risk to the fetus increases to 1 in 2.** If, however, DNA testing does not identify a CF mutation in the prospective father, it is still possible that the father is a carrier of an unidentified CF mutation, making the risk for CF to the offspring 1 in 492.[103]

It is important that the woman with CF be advised about the potential adverse effects of pregnancy on maternal health status. Factors that may predict poor outcome include prepregnancy evidence of poor nutritional status, significant pulmonary disease with hypoxemia, and pulmonary hypertension. Liver disease and diabetes mellitus are also poor prognostic factors. **Gravidae with poor nutritional status, pulmonary hypertension (cor pulmonale), and deteriorating pulmonary function early in gestation should consider therapeutic abortion because the risk for maternal mortality may be unacceptably high.**

The woman with CF who is considering pregnancy should also give consideration to the need for strong psychosocial and physical support after delivery. The rigors of child rearing may add to the risk for maternal deterioration during this period. Family members should also be willing to provide physical and emotional support and should be aware of the potential for deterioration in the mother's health and the potential for maternal mortality. **In addition, the need for care of a potentially preterm growth-restricted neonate with all of its attendant morbidities and potential mortality should be discussed.** Over the long term, the woman and her family should also consider the fact that her life expectancy may be shortened by CF. **Overall, 20% of mothers with CF succumb to the disease before the child's tenth birthday, and this number increases to 40% if the FEV_1 is less than 40% of predicted.**[104] Plans should be made for rearing of the child in the event of maternal death.

Management of the Pregnancy Complicated by Cystic Fibrosis

Care of the gravida with CF should be a coordinated team effort. Physicians familiar with CF, its complications, and management should be included as well as a maternal-fetal medicine specialist and neonatal team. The gravida should be assessed for potential risk factors such as severe lung disease, pulmonary hypertension, poor nutritional status, pancreatic failure, and liver disease—preferably before attempting gestation, but certainly during the early months of pregnancy. **Gravidae should be advised to be 90% of ideal body weight before conception if possible. A weight gain in pregnancy of 11 to 12 kg is recommended.**[105] **Frequent monitoring of weight, blood glucose, hemoglobin, total protein, serum albumin, prothrombin time, and fat-soluble vitamins A and E is suggested.**[105] At each visit, the history of caloric intake and symptoms of maldigestion and malabsorption should be taken, and pancreatic enzymes should be adjusted if needed. **Patients who are unable to achieve adequate weight gain through oral nutritional supplements may be given nocturnal enteral nasogastric tube feedings. In this situation, the risk for aspiration should be considered, especially in patients with a history of gastroesophageal reflux, which is common in CF. If malnutrition is severe, parenteral hyperalimentation may be necessary for successful completion of the pregnancy. Baseline pulmonary function should be assessed, preferably before conception. Assessment should include FVC, FEV_1, lung volumes, pulse oximetry, and arterial blood gases,** if indicated. **These values should be serially monitored during gestation, and deterioration in pulmonary function should be addressed immediately. An echocardiogram can assess the patient for pulmonary hypertension and cor pulmonale,** and if this is diagnosed, the gravida should be advised of the high maternal risk.

Early recognition and prompt treatment of pulmonary infections are important in the management of the pregnant woman with CF. **Treatment includes IV antibiotics in the appropriate dose, keeping in mind the increased clearance of these drugs secondary to pregnancy and CF.** Plasma levels of aminoglycosides should be monitored and adjusted as indicated. **Chest physical therapy and bronchial drainage are also important components of the management of pulmonary infections in CF. Because *P. aeruginosa* is the most frequently isolated bacterium associated with chronic endobronchitis**

and bronchiectasis, antibiotic regimens should include coverage for this organism.

If the patient with CF has pancreatic insufficiency and diabetes mellitus, careful monitoring of blood glucose and insulin therapy are indicated. As previously mentioned, pancreatic enzymes may need to be replaced to optimize the patient's nutritional status. **Because of malabsorption of fats and frequent use of antibiotics, the patient with CF is prone to vitamin K deficiency; therefore prothrombin time should be checked regularly, and parenteral vitamin K should be administered if the prothrombin time is elevated.**

When managing pregnancy in a woman with CF, it is imperative to recognize that the fetus is at risk for uteroplacental insufficiency and IUGR. The maternal nutritional status and weight gain during pregnancy will likewise affect fetal growth; therefore **fundal height should be measured routinely, and serial ultrasound evaluations of fetal growth and amniotic fluid volume should be made.** Fetal kick counts may be useful for monitoring fetal status starting at 28 weeks. **If fetal compromise is evident, nonstress testing should be started at 32 weeks or sooner;** if fetal compromise is severe—such as no interval fetal growth, persistent decelerations, or poor biophysical profile scoring—delivery should be accomplished. Likewise, **evidence of profound maternal deterioration such as a marked and sustained decline in pulmonary function, development of right-sided heart failure, refractory hypoxemia, and progressive hypercapnia and respiratory acidosis may be indications for early delivery.** If the fetus is potentially viable, the administration of betamethasone may be beneficial. Vaginal delivery should be attempted when possible.

Labor, delivery, and the postpartum period can be particularly dangerous for the patient with CF. The augmentation in cardiac output stresses the cardiovascular system and can lead to cardiopulmonary failure in the patient with pulmonary hypertension and cor pulmonale. These patients are also more likely to develop right-sided heart failure. **Heart failure should be treated with aggressive diuresis and supplemental oxygen, and management can be optimized by insertion of a pulmonary artery catheter to monitor right- and left-sided filling pressures. Pain control will reduce the sympathetic response to labor and tachycardia. This will benefit the patient who demonstrates pulmonary or cardiac compromise.** In the patient with a normal partial thromboplastin time, insertion of an epidural catheter for continuous epidural analgesia may be beneficial. This is also useful in the event a cesarean delivery is indicated because general anesthesia and its possible effects on pulmonary function can be avoided. **If general anesthesia is needed, preoperative anticholinergic agents should be avoided because they tend to promote drying and inspissation of airway secretions.** Close fetal surveillance is also extremely important because the fetus who may have been suffering from uteroplacental insufficiency during gestation is more prone to develop evidence of fetal compromise during labor. **Cesarean delivery should be reserved for the usual obstetric indications.**

In summary, more women with CF are living to childbearing age and are capable of conceiving. Clinical experience thus far has demonstrated that **pregnancy in women with CF and mild disease is well tolerated, but women with severe disease have an associated increase in maternal and fetal morbidity and mortality.** The potential risk to any individual with CF desirous of pregnancy should be assessed and discussed with the patient and her family in detail.

KEY POINTS

- Pneumonia is the most common nonobstetric infection that causes maternal mortality, and preterm delivery complicates pneumonia in up to 43% of cases. *Streptococcus pneumoniae* is the most common bacterial pathogen to cause pneumonia.

- To treat pneumonia, empiric antibiotic coverage should be started that includes a third-generation cephalosporin and a macrolide, such as azithromycin, to cover atypical pathogens. If CA-MRSA is suspected, add vancomycin or linezolid.

- The HIV-infected gravida with a CD4+ count of less than 200 cells per cubic millimeter should receive prophylaxis with trimethoprim-sulfamethoxazole, as well as HAART, to prevent PJP pneumonia.

- High-risk gravidae should be screened for TB and treated appropriately with isoniazid prophylaxis for infection without overt disease and with dual anti-TB therapy for active disease. If resistant TB is identified, ethambutol, 2.5 g/day, should be added to therapy, and the treatment period should be extended to 18 months.

- IGRAs can be used for screening for TB and are helpful in cases where BCG vaccine has been given.

- Inhaled corticosteroids are the preferred treatment for persistent asthma in pregnancy.

- It is safer for pregnant women with asthma to be treated with asthma medications than it is for them to have asthma symptoms and exacerbations.

- Inhaled albuterol is recommended for rescue therapy during pregnancy.

- Step-care therapy uses the principle of tailoring medical therapy according to asthma severity.

- The interstitial lung diseases include idiopathic pulmonary fibrosis, sarcoidosis, hypersensitivity pneumonitis, drug-induced lung disease, and connective tissue disease. Restrictive lung disease is generally well tolerated in pregnancy; however, exercise intolerance and need for oxygen supplementation may develop.

- Gravidae with pulmonary hypertension complicating restrictive lung disease may suffer a high mortality rate.

- An increasing number of women with cystic fibrosis are surviving to the reproductive years and usually maintain their fertility with meticulous management of pulmonary function, including pulmonary toilet and aggressive surveillance for signs of pulmonary infection and treatment with antibiotics in adequate doses. Close attention to nutrition is required secondary to maldigestion, malabsorption, and malnutrition, which can complicate cystic fibrosis. Gravidae with reassuring pulmonary function studies, good nutritional status, near-normal chest radiographs, and only mild obstructive lung disease will tolerate pregnancy well. Fetal growth should be monitored closely.

REFERENCES

1. Berkowitz K, LaSala A. Risk factors associated with the increasing prevalence of pneumonia during pregnancy. *Am J Obstet Gynecol*. 1990;163:981.
2. Munn MB, Groome LJ, Atterbury JL, et al. Pneumonia as a complication of pregnancy. *J Matern Fetal Med*. 1999;8:151.

3. Benedetti TJ, Valle R, Ledger W. Antepartum pneumonia in pregnancy. *Am J Obstet Gynecol.* 1982;144:413.

4. Madinger NE, Greenspoon JS, Ellrodt AG. Pneumonia during pregnancy: has modern technology improved maternal and fetal outcome? *Am J Obstet Gynecol.* 1989;161:657.

5. Koonin LM, Ellerbrock TV, Atrash HK, et al. Pregnancy-associated deaths due to AIDS in the United States. *JAMA.* 1989;261:1306.

6. Dinsmoor MJ. HIV infection and pregnancy. *Med Clin North Am.* 1989;73:701.

7. Jenkins TM, Troiano NH, Graves CR, et al. Mechanical ventilation in an obstetric population: characteristics and delivery rates. *Am J Obstet Gynecol.* 2003;188:549.

8. Chen YH, Keller J, Wang IT, Lin CC, Lin HC. Pneumonia and pregnancy outcomes: a nationwide population-based study. *Am J Obstet Gynecol.* 2012;e1-e7.

9. Rodrigues J, Niederman MS. Pneumonia complicating pregnancy. *Clin Chest Med.* 1992;13:679.

10. Haake DA, Zakowski PC, Haake DL, et al. Early treatment with acyclovir for varicella pneumonia in otherwise healthy adults: retrospective controlled study and review. *Rev Infect Dis.* 1990;12:788.

11. Mercieri M, Di Rosa R, Pantosti A, et al. Critical pneumonia complicating early-stage pregnancy. *Anesth Analg.* 2010;110:852.

12. Rotas M, McCalla S, Liu C, Minkoff H. Methicillin-resistant Staphylococcus aureus necrotizing pneumonia arising from an infected episiotomy site. *Obstet Gynecol.* 2007;109:108.

13. Asnis D, Haralambou G, Tawiah P. Methicillin-resistant Staphylococcus aureus necrotizing pneumonia arising from an infected episiotomy site [letter to the editor]. *Obstet Gynecol.* 2007;110:188.

14. Ahmad H, Mehta NJ, Manikal VM, et al. Pneumocystis carinii pneumonia in pregnancy: division of infectious disease. *Chest.* 2001;120:666.

15. Yost P, Bloom S, Richey S, et al. Appraisal of treatment guidelines of antepartum community acquired pneumonia. *Am J Obstet Gynecol.* 2000;183:131.

16. American Thoracic Society. Guidelines for the initial management of adults with community-acquired pneumonia: diagnosis assessment of severity, and initial antimicrobial therapy. *Am Rev Respir Dis.* 1993;148:1418.

17. Harrison BD, Farr BM, Connolly CK, et al. The hospital management of community-acquired pneumonia: recommendation of the British Thoracic Society. *J R Coll Physicians Lond.* 1987;21:267.

18. Campbell SG, Marrie TJ, Anstey R, et al. Utility of blood cultures in management of adults with community acquired pneumonia discharged from the emergency department. *Emerg Med J.* 2003;20:521.

19. Pimentel LP, McPherson SJ. Community-acquired pneumonia in the emergency department: a practical approach to diagnosis and management. *Emerg Med Clin North Am.* 2003;21:395.

20. Murdoch DR, Laing RT, Mills GD, et al. Evaluation of a rapid immunochromatographic test for detection of Streptococcus pneumoniae antigen in urine samples from adults with community-acquired pneumonia. *J Clin Microbiol.* 2001;39:3495.

21. Gutierrez F, Rodriequez JC, Ayelo A, et al. Evaluation of the immunochromatographic Binax NOW assay for detection of Streptococcus pneumoniae urinary antigen in a prospective study of community-acquired pneumonia in Spain. *Clin Infect Dis.* 1996;36:286.

22. Waterer GW, Baselski VS, Wunderink RG. Legionella and community-acquired pneumonia: a review of current diagnostic test from a clinician's viewpoint. *Am J Med.* 2001;110:41.

23. Niederman MS, Ahmed OA. Community-acquired pneumonia in elderly patients. *Clin Geriatr Med.* 2003;19:101.

24. Golden WE, Brown P, Godsey N. CMS release new standards for community acquired pneumonia. *J Ark Med Soc.* 2003;99:288.

25. Cunha BA. Empiric therapy of community-acquired pneumonia. *Chest.* 2004;125:1913.

26. Hidron A, Low C, Hoing E, Blumberg H. Emergence of community-acquired methicillin-resistant Staphylococcus aureus strain USA300 as a cause of necrotizing community-onset pneumonia. *Lancet Infect Dis.* 2009;9:384.

27. Muñoz FM, Englund JA, Cheesman CC, et al. Maternal immunization with pneumococcal polysaccharide vaccine in the third trimester of gestation. *Vaccine.* 2001;20:826.

28. Shahid NS, Steinhoff MC, Hoque SS, et al. Serum, breast milk, and infant antibody after maternal immunization with pneumococcal vaccine. *Lancet.* 1995;346:1252.

29. Tomlinson MW, Caruthers TJ, Whitty JE, Gonik B. Does delivery improve maternal condition in the respiratory-compromised gravida? *Obstet Gynecol.* 1998;91:108.

30. National Center for Health Statistics. National hospital discharge survey: annual summary 1990. *Vital Health Stat.* 1992;13:1.

31. Hollingsworth HM, Pratter MR, Irwin RS. Acute respiratory failure in pregnancy. *J Intensive Care Med.* 1989;4:11.

32. Neuzil KM, Reed GW, Mitchel EF, et al. Impact of influenza on acute cardiopulmonary hospitalizations in pregnant women. *Am J Epidemiol.* 1998;148:1094.

33. Hartert TV, Neuzil KM, Shintani AK, et al. Maternal morbidity and perinatal outcome among pregnant women with respiratory hospitalizations during influenza season. *Am J Obstet Gynecol.* 2003;189:1705.

34. Siston AM, Rasussen SA, Honein MA, et al. Pandemic 2009 Influenza A (H1N1) virus illness among pregnant women in the United States. *JAMA.* 2010;303:1517.

35. Harper SA, Fukuda K, Uyeka TM, et al. Prevention and control of influenza: recommendations of the Advisory Committee on Immunization Practice (ACIP). *MMWR Recomm Rep.* 2003;52:1.

36. Cox SM, Cunningham FG, Luby J. Management of varicella pneumonia complicating pregnancy. *Am J Perinatol.* 1990;7:300.

37. Esmonde TG, Herdman G, Anderson G. Chickenpox pneumonia: an association with pregnancy. *Thorax.* 1989;44:812.

38. Zhang HJ, Patenaude V, Abenhaim H. Maternal outcomes in pregnancies affected by varicella zoster virus infections. *Obstet Gynecol Suppl.* 2014;1:86S-87S.

39. Smego RA, Asperilla MO. Use of acyclovir for varicella pneumonia during pregnancy. *Obstet Gynecol.* 1991;78:1112.

40. Jones AM, Thomas N, Wilkins EG. Outcome of varicella pneumonitis in immunocompetent adults requiring treatment in a high dependency unit. *J Infect.* 2001;43:135.

41. Andrews EB, Yankaskas BC, Cordero JF, et al. Acyclovir in pregnancy registry: six years' experience. *Obstet Gynecol.* 1992;79:7.

42. Nguyen HQ, Jumaan AO, Seward JF. Decline in mortality due to varicella after implementation of varicella vaccination in the United States. *N Engl J Med.* 2005;352:450.

43. Shields KE, Galil K, Seward J, et al. Varicella vaccine exposure during pregnancy: data from the first 5 years of the pregnancy registry. *Obstet Gynecol.* 2001;98:14.

44. Thomas CF Jr, Limper AH. Pneumocystis pneumonia. *N Engl J Med.* 2004;350:2487.

45. Ahmad H, Mehta NJ, Manikal VM, et al. Pneumocystis carinii pneumonia in pregnancy. *Chest.* 2001;120:666.

46. Masur H, Kaplan JE, Holmes KK. Guidelines for preventing opportunistic infections among HIV-infected persons-2002: recommendations of the U.S. Public Health Service and the Infectious Disease Society of America. *Ann Intern Med.* 2002;137:435.

47. Centers for Disease Control and Prevention. Initial therapy for tuberculosis in the era of multidrug resistance–recommendations of the advisory council for the elimination of tuberculosis. *MMWR Recomm Rep.* 1993;42:1.

48. Frieden TR, Sterling T, Pablos-Mendez A, et al. The emergence of drug-resistant tuberculosis in New York City. *N Engl J Med.* 1993;328:521.

49. Cantwell MF, Shehab AM, Costello AM. Brief report: congenital tuberculosis. *N Engl J Med.* 1994;330:1051.

50. Margono F, Mroveh J, Garely A, et al. Resurgence of active tuberculosis among pregnant women. *Obstet Gynecol.* 1994;83:911.

51. Centers for Disease Control and Prevention. The use of preventive therapy for tuberculosis infection in the United States. *MMWR Recomm Rep.* 1990;39:9.

52. Griffith DE. Mycobacteria as pathogens of respiratory infection. *Infect Dis Clin North Am.* 1998;12:593.

53. Pai M, Denkinger CM, Kik SV, et al. Gamma interferon release assays for detection of Mycobacterium tuberculosis infection. *Clin Microbiol Rev.* 2014;27:3.

54. Centers for Disease Control and Prevention. The role of BCG vaccine in the prevention and control of tuberculosis in the United States: a joint statement by the Advisory Council for the Elimination of Tuberculosis and the Advisory Committee on Immunization Practices. *MMWR Recomm Rep.* 1996;45:1.

55. Good JT, Iseman MD, Davidson PT, et al. Tuberculosis in association with pregnancy. *Am J Obstet Gynecol.* 1981;140:492.

56. American Thoracic Society Workshop. Rapid diagnostic tests for tuberculosis—what is the appropriate use? *Am J Respir Crit Care Med.* 1997;155:1804.

57. Barnes PF. Rapid diagnostic tests for tuberculosis, progress but no gold standard. *Am J Respir Crit Care Med.* 1997;155:1497.

58. American Thoracic Society. Mycobacteriosis and the acquired immunodeficiency syndrome. *Am Rev Respir Dis.* 1987;136:492.

59. Jana N, Vasishta K, Saha SC, Ghosh K. Obstetrical outcomes among women with extrapulmonary tuberculosis. *N Engl J Med*. 1999;341:645.

60. Fox CW, George RB. Current concepts in the management and prevention of tuberculosis in adults. *J la State Med Soc*. 1992;144:363.

61. Robinson GC, Cambion K. Hearing loss in infants of tuberculosis mothers treated with streptomycin during pregnancy. *N Engl J Med*. 1964;271:949.

62. Lessnau KL, Qarah S. Multidrug-resistant tuberculosis in pregnancy: case report and review of the literature. *Chest*. 2003;123:953.

63. Shin S, Guerra D, Rich M, et al. Treatment of multidrug-resistant tuberculosis during pregnancy: a report of 7 cases. *Clin Infect Dis*. 2003;36:996.

64. Quick Reference NAEPP Expert Panel Report: Managing asthma during pregnancy: Recommendations for pharmacologic treatment—2004 update. *J Allergy Clin Immunol*. 2005;115:34-36.

65. ACOG Practice Bulletin number 90. Asthma in pregnancy. *Obstet Gynecol*. 2008;111:457-464.

66. *National Asthma Education and Prevention Program Expert Panel Report 3.* Guidelines for the diagnosis and management of asthma–Full Report 2007. <http://www.nhlbi.nih.gov/guidelines/asthma/asthgdln.pdf>.

67. Schatz M, Dombrowski M, Wise R, et al., for The NICHD Maternal-Fetal Medicine Units Network, and NHLBI. Asthma morbidity during pregnancy can be predicted by severity classification. *J Allergy Clin Immunol*. 2003;112:283-288.

68. Schatz M, Dombrowski M, Wise R, et al. The relationship of asthma-specific quality of life during pregnancy to subsequent asthma and perinatal morbidity. *J Asthma*. 2010;47:46-50.

69. Schatz M, Dombrowski M. Asthma in pregnancy. *N Engl J Med*. 2009;360(18):62-68.

70. Mendola P, Laughon K, Männistö T, et al. Obstetric complications among US women with asthma. *Am J Obstet Gynecol*. 2013;208:127, e1-e8.

71. Blais L, Forget A. Asthma exacerbations during the first trimester of pregnancy and the risk of congenital malformations among asthmatic women. *J Allergy Clin Immunol*. 2008;121:1379-1384.

72. Murphy V, Namazy J, Powell H, et al. A meta-analysis of adverse perinatal outcomes in women with asthma. *BJOG*. 2011;118:1314-1323.

73. Bracken M, Triche E, Belanger K, et al. Asthma symptoms, severity, and drug therapy: A prospective study of effects on 2205 pregnancies. *Obstet Gynecol*. 2003;1024:739-752.

74. Mihrshani S, Belousov E, Marks G, Peat J. Pregnancy and birth outcomes in families with asthma. *J Asthma*. 2003;40:181-187.

75. Schatz M, Zeiger R, Hoffman C, et al. Perinatal outcomes in the pregnancies of asthmatic women: a prospective controlled analysis. *Am J Respir Crit Care Med*. 1995;151:1170-1174.

76. Minerbi-Codish I, Fraser D, Avnun L, et al. Influence of asthma in pregnancy on labor and the newborn. *Respiration*. 1998;65:130-135.

77. Stenius-Aarniala B, Hedman J, Teramo K. Acute asthma during pregnancy. *Thorax*. 1996;51:411-414.

78. Dombrowski M, Schatz M, Wise R, et al. for the NICHD Maternal-Fetal Medicine Units Network, and the NHLBI: Asthma during pregnancy. *Obstet Gynecol*. 2004;103:5-12.

79. Dombrowski M, Schatz M, Wise R, et al., for the NICHD Maternal-Fetal Medicine Units Network, and the NHLBI. Randomized trial of inhaled beclomethasone dipropionate versus theophylline for moderate asthma during pregnancy. *Am J Obstet Gynecol*. 2004;190:737-744.

80. Schatz M, Dombrowski M, Wise R, et al., for the NICHD Maternal-Fetal Medicine Units Network, and the NHLBI. Spirometry is related to perinatal outcomes in pregnant women with asthma. *Am J Obstet Gynecol*. 2006;194:120-126.

81. Newman RB, Momirova V, Dombrowski M, et al., for the Eunice Kennedy Shriver National Institute of Child Health and Human Development Maternal-Fetal Medicine Units (MFMU) Network. The effect of active and passive household cigarette smoke exposure on pregnant women with asthma. *Chest*. 2010;137:601-608.

82. Belanger K, Hellenbrand M, Holford T, Bracken M. Effect of pregnancy on maternal asthma symptoms and medication use. *Obstet Gynecol*. 2010;3:559-567.

83. Enriquez R, Wu P, Griffin M, et al. Cessation of asthma medication in early pregnancy. *Am J Obstet Gynecol*. 2006;195:149-153.

84. Wendel P, Ramin S, Barnett-Hamm C, et al. Asthma treatment in pregnancy: A randomized controlled trial. *Am J Obstet Gynecol*. 1996;175:150-154.

85. Briggs G, Freeman R, eds. *Drugs in Pregnancy and Lactation*. 10th ed. Philadelphia: Wolters Kluwer; 2015.

86. Kallen B, Rydhstroem H, Aberg A. Congenital malformations after use of inhaled budesonide in early pregnancy. *Obstet Gynecol*. 1999;93:392-395.

87. Schatz M, Dombrowski M, Wise R, et al., for the NICHD Maternal-Fetal Medicine Units Network, and the NHLBI. The relationship of asthma medication use to perinatal outcomes. *J Allergy Clin Immunol*. 2004;113:1040-1045.

88. Namazy J, Cabana M, Scheuerle A, et al. The Xolair pregnancy registry (expect): An observational study of the safety of omalizumab during pregnancy in women with asthma. *Am J Respir Crit Care Med*. 2012;185:A4221.

89. Sarkar M, Koren G, Kalra S, et al. Montelukast use during pregnancy: a multicentre, prospective, comparative study of infant outcomes. *Eur J Clin Pharmacol*. 2009;65:1259-1264.

90. McCallister J, Benninger C, Frey H, et al. Pregnancy related treatment disparities of acute asthma exacerbations in the emergency department. *Respir Med*. 2011;105:1434-1440.

91. King TE Jr. Restrictive lung disease in pregnancy. *Clin Chest Med*. 1992;13:607.

92. Boggess KA, Easterling TR, Raghu G. Management and outcome of pregnant women with interstitial and restrictive lung disease. *Am J Obstet Gynecol*. 1995;173:1007.

93. Agha FP, Vade A, Amendola MA, Cooper RF. Effects of pregnancy on sarcoidosis. *Surg Gynecol Obstet*. 1982;155:817.

94. Haynes de Regt R. Sarcoidosis and pregnancy. *Obstet Gynecol*. 1987;70:369.

95. Reisfield DR. Boeck's sarcoid and pregnancy. *Am J Obstet Gynecol*. 1958;75:795.

96. Scadding JG. *Sarcoidosis*. London: Eyre & Spottiswoode; 1967:519.

97. Canny GJ, Corey M, Livingstone RA, et al. Pregnancy and cystic fibrosis. *Obstet Gynecol*. 1991;77:850.

98. Kent NE, Farquharson DF. Cystic fibrosis in pregnancy. *Can Med Assoc J*. 1993;149:809.

99. Edenborough FP, Stableforth DE, Webb AK, et al. Outcome of pregnancy in women with cystic fibrosis. *Thorax*. 1995;50:170.

100. Olson GL. Cystic fibrosis in pregnancy. *Semin Perinatol*. 1997;21:307.

101. Goss CH, Rubenfel GD, Otto K, Aitken ML. The effect of pregnancy on survival in women with cystic fibrosis. *Chest*. 2003;124:1460.

102. Patel EM, Swamy GK, Heine RP, Kuller JA, James AH, Grotegut CA. Medical and obstetric complications among pregnant women with cystic fibrosis. *Am J Obstet Gynecol*. 2014;212:98, e1-9.

103. Lemna WK, Feldman GL, Kerem B, et al. Mutation analysis for heterozygote detection and the prenatal diagnosis of cystic fibrosis. *N Engl J Med*. 1990;322:291.

104. Edonborough FP, Mackenzie WE, Stableforth DE. The outcome of 72 pregnancies in 55 women with cystic fibrosis in the United Kingdom 1977-1996. *BJOG*. 2000;107:254.

105. Cole BN, Seltzer MH, Kassabian J, et al. Parenteral nutrition in a pregnant cystic fibrosis patient. *JPEN J Parenter Enteral Nutr*. 1987;11:205.

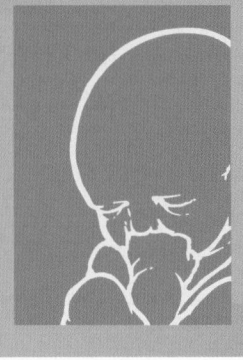

Renal Disease in Pregnancy

DAVID F. COLOMBO

KEY ABREVIATIONS	
American College of Obstetricians and Gynecologists	ACOG
Adult respiratory distress syndrome	ARDS
Acute renal failure	ARF
Arginine vasopressin	AVP
Asymptomatic bacteriuria	ASB
Blood urea nitrogen	BUN
Disseminated intravascular coagulation	DIC
End-stage renal disease	ESRD
Erythropoietin	EPO
Glomerular filtration rate	GFR
Glucose-6-phosphate dehydrogenase	G6PD
Hemolytic uremic syndrome	HUS
Intrauterine growth restriction	IUGR
Immunoglobulin	Ig
Intravenous pyelogram	IVP
Mycophenolate mofetil	MMF
Positive end-expiratory pressure	PEEP
Red blood cell	RBC
Urinary tract infection	UTI
White blood cell	WBC

OVERVIEW

Prior to just decades ago, women with preexisting renal disease were strongly discouraged from attempting pregnancy because of the expectation of poor perinatal outcome and the likelihood of renal disease progression. Currently, through better understanding of the prognosis and treatment of kidney disease during pregnancy, women with most renal conditions are no longer discouraged from attempting conception. This even holds true for women who have undergone renal transplantation.

This chapter first reviews the normal changes in the kidney and urinary collecting system in pregnancy and then it follows with the basic evaluation of maternal renal status, acute and chronic renal disorders in pregnancy, and the treatment of the post–renal transplant patient.

ALTERED RENAL PHYSIOLOGY IN PREGNANCY

Pregnancy is associated with significant anatomic changes in the kidney and its collecting system (see Chapter 3). These changes begin to occur shortly after conception and may persist for several months postpartum.[1,2] The kidney is noted to increase in size and weight during the course of a pregnancy. **Of more clinical significance is the marked dilation of the collecting system, including both the renal pelvis and ureters. This dilation is most pronounced on the right side and is most likely due to hormonal changes** (i.e., from progesterone, endothelin, relaxin) **and mechanical obstruction by the gravid uterus** (Fig. 39-1).[3-5]

Renal plasma flow increases greatly during pregnancy.[6] It peaks by the end of the first trimester, and although it decreases near term, it remains higher than in the nonpregnant woman. This change is due in part to increased cardiac output and decreased renal vascular resistance. **The glomerular filtration rate (GFR) increases by 50% during a normal gestation.**[7] It rises early in pregnancy and remains elevated throughout gestation, and the percentage increase in GFR is greater than the percentage increase in renal plasma flow. This leads to an elevation of the filtration fraction, which results in a fall in serum blood urea nitrogen (BUN) and serum creatinine values.

Because GFR increases to such a great degree, electrolytes, glucose, and other filtered substances reach the renal tubules in greater amounts. The kidney handles sodium efficiently, reabsorbing most of the filtered load in the proximal convoluted tubule. Glucose reabsorption, however, does not increase proportionately during pregnancy. The average renal threshold for

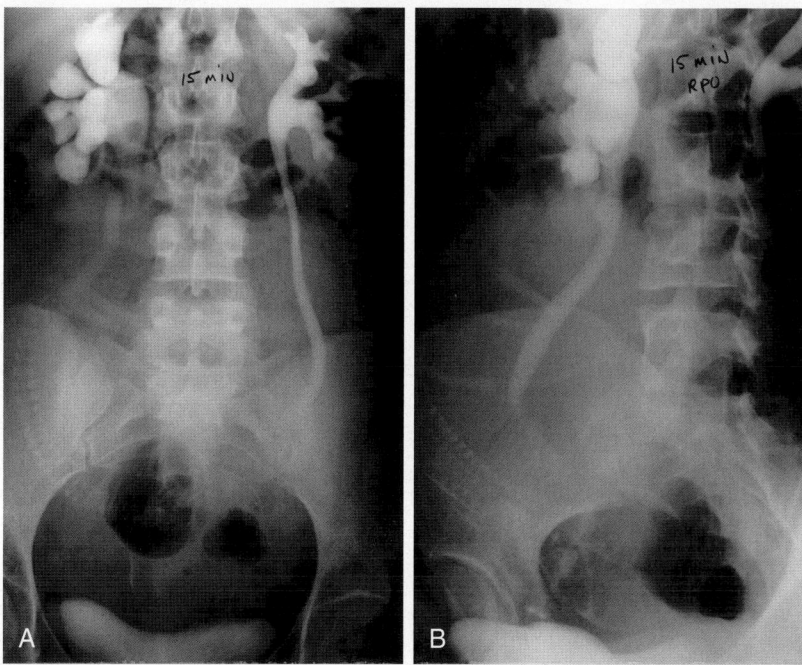

FIG 39-1 A, An intravenous pyelogram of a gravid patient in the late second trimester with flank pain. The image was taken in the anteroposterior view 15 minutes after the instillation of contrast dye. Note the dilation of the renal pelves bilaterally, with the right side more dilated than the left. The fetus is seen in the vertex position. **B,** The same patient in the right lateral view.

glucose is reduced to 155 mg/dL from 194 mg/dL in the non-pregnant individual.[8] Therefore **glycosuria can be a feature of normal pregnancy.**

Urate is handled by filtration and secretion. Its clearance increases early in pregnancy and leads to lower serum levels of uric acid. In late pregnancy, urate clearance and serum urate levels return to their prepregnancy values. **Serum urate levels are elevated in women with preeclampsia.** Whether this is due to decreased renal plasma flow, hemoconcentration, renal tubular dysfunction, or other renal circulatory changes remains unclear. A summary of the renal changes in normal pregnancy is shown in Table 39-1.

ASYMPTOMATIC BACTERIURIA

The prevalence of asymptomatic bacteriuria (ASB) in sexually active women has been reported to be as high as 5% to 6%.[9,10] The diagnosis of ASB is based on a clean-catch voided urine specimen. **To secure a diagnosis, the urine culture should reveal greater than 100,000 colonies/mL of a single organism.**[11] Some investigators have suggested that two consecutively voided specimens should contain the same organism prior to establishing the diagnosis of bacteriuria.[12,13] Bacteriuria occurs in 2% to 7% of pregnancies, particularly in multiparous women, a similar prevalence as seen in nonpregnant women. The pathogenic organisms are also similar in species and virulence factors to those observed in nonpregnant women (see Chapter 53); thus the basic mechanism of entry of bacteria into the urinary tract is likely to be the same for both groups. Bacteriuria often develops in the first month of pregnancy and is frequently associated with a reduction in urine concentrating ability, which suggests involvement of the kidney.[7] **The smooth muscle relaxation and subsequent ureteral dilation that accompany pregnancy are believed to facilitate the ascent of bacteria from the bladder to the kidney. As a result, untreated bacteriuria during**

TABLE 39-1	SUMMARY OF RENAL CHANGES IN NORMAL PREGNANCY	
ALTERATION	**MANIFESTATION**	**CLINICAL RELEVANCE**
Increased renal size	Renal length is about 1 cm greater on radiographs.	Postpartum decreases in size should not be mistaken for parenchymal loss.
Dilation of pelves, calyces, and ureters	Dilation resembles hydronephrosis on ultrasound or IVP and is usually more prominent on the right side.	Should not be mistaken for obstructive uropathy. Upper urinary tract infections can be more virulent.
Changes in acid-base metabolism	The renal bicarbonate reabsorption threshold decreases.	Serum bicarbonate is 4 to 5 mM/L lower in pregnancy. PCO_2 is 10 mm Hg lower in normal pregnancy. PCO_2 of 40 mm Hg represents retention in pregnancy.
Renal water osmoregulation	The osmotic threshold for AVP release decreases.	Serum osmolarity is decreased by approximately 10 mOsm/L.

Modified from Lindheimer M, Grünfeld JP, Davison JM. Renal disorders. In Barron WM, Lindheimer M, editors. *Medical Disorders During Pregnancy*, 3rd ed. St. Louis: Mosby; 2000:39-70.
AVP, vasopressin; *IVP,* intravenous pyelography; PCO_2, carbon dioxide tension.

pregnancy has a greater propensity to progress to pyelone-phritis (up to 40%) than in nonpregnant women.[14] If a urine culture is negative for bacteria at the first prenatal visit, the risk of developing acute cystitis is less than 1%.[10,15]

It is important to diagnose and treat ASB in pregnancy. If left untreated, a symptomatic urinary tract infection (UTI) will

BOX 39-1   ANTIMICROBIAL TREATMENT REGIMENS FOR PREGNANT WOMEN WITH BACTERIURIA*

- Amoxicillin 500 mg 3 times a day
- Ampicillin 500 mg 4 times a day
- Cephalexin 500 mg 4 times a day
- Nitrofurantoin 100 mg 4 times a day
- Sustained release nitrofurantoin 100 mg 2 times a day
- Trimethoprim 160 mg with sulfamethoxazole 800 mg 2 times a day

*The agent of choice should be given for a 7-day course. A repeat urine culture is recommended 2 weeks after the treatment has been completed.

develop in up to 40% of these patients.[6,10,16] **Recognition and therapy for ASB can eliminate 70% of acute UTIs in pregnancy.** Nonetheless, 2% of pregnant women with negative first-trimester urine cultures develop symptomatic cystitis or pyelonephritis. This group accounts for 30% of the cases of acute UTI that develop during gestation. **The American College of Obstetricians and Gynecologists (ACOG) recommends routine screening of all women for ASB at their first prenatal visit.[17] Some debate has surrounded whether the patient should collect a first void sample or simply a clean-catch sample.** In pregnant women, the contamination rate of midstream samples is comparable for morning and clean-catch samples.[18] Other than progression to more serious infection, however, little evidence suggests that ASB has an effect on pregnancy outcome.[9,19]

Escherichia coli **is the organism responsible for most cases of ASB and UTI during pregnancy.** Women can therefore be safely treated with nitrofurantoin, ampicillin, cephalosporins, and short-acting sulfa drugs (Box 39-1). Sulfa compounds should be avoided near term because they compete for bilirubin-binding sites on albumin in the fetus and newborn and therefore pose a risk for kernicterus. Nitrofurantoin should not be used in patients with glucose-6-phosphate dehydrogenase (G6PD) deficiency because of the risk for hemolytic crisis; if the fetus has a G6PD deficiency, it may also experience hemolysis. **Therapy for ASB is recommended for 7 days, and a follow-up culture should be performed 1 to 2 weeks after discontinuing therapy.** Approximately 15% of women will experience a reinfection or will not respond to initial therapy. Therapy in these cases should be reinstituted after careful microbial sensitivity testing. Women with a recurrent UTI during pregnancy and those with a history of pyelonephritis should eventually undergo imaging of the upper urinary tract. This procedure may be delayed until 3 months postpartum so that the anatomic changes of pregnancy can regress.

Occasionally it can be difficult to distinguish severe cystitis from pyelonephritis, although the presence of fever suggests upper tract infection. Although the drugs used for treatment are similar, pyelonephritis during pregnancy generally requires intravenous (IV) antibiotics. Sandberg and coinvestigators[20] studied symptomatic UTI in 174 women and found that C-reactive protein was elevated in 91% of pregnant women with acute pyelonephritis and in only 5% of women with cystitis. They also noted that the urine-concentrating ability was lower in women with acute pyelonephritis. Because the erythrocyte sedimentation rate is normally elevated in pregnancy, they found that this was not a useful parameter for distinguishing pyelonephritis from cystitis.

PYELONEPHRITIS

Pyelonephritis complicates 1% to 2% of all pregnancies and can result in significant maternal morbidity, and it is among the most common nonobstetric causes for hospitalization during pregnancy.[21] A recent 18-year retrospective analysis showed "the incidence of acute antepartum pyelonephritis during pregnancy was 0.5% (2894/543,430). Women with pyelonephritis in pregnancy were more likely to be black or Hispanic, young, less educated, and nulliparous; they initiate prenatal care late in gestation and use tobacco during pregnancy. Pregnancies of women with pyelonephritis, compared with those without, were more likely to be complicated by anemia (26.3% vs. 11.4%; odds ratio [OR], 2.6; 95% confidence interval [CI], 2.4 to 2.9), septicemia (1.9% vs. 0.03%; OR, 56.5; 95% CI, 41.3 to 77.4), acute pulmonary insufficiency (0.5% vs. 0.04%; OR, 12.5; 95% CI, 7.2 to 21.6), acute renal dysfunction (0.4% vs. 0.03%; OR, 16.5; 95% CI, 8.8 to 30.7), and spontaneous preterm birth (10.3% vs. 7.9%; OR, 1.3; 95% CI, 1.2 to 1.5). Most of the preterm births in this series occurred between 33 and 36 weeks.[22] **Recurrent pyelonephritis** has been implicated as a cause of fetal death and intrauterine growth restriction (IUGR). As noted above, an association between acute pyelonephritis and preterm labor is apparent.[23,24] Fan and coworkers,[25] however, have shown that if pyelonephritis is aggressively treated, it does not increase the likelihood of premature delivery or low birthweight. Hill and colleagues[26] reported 440 cases of acute pyelonephritis over a 2-year period and noted the disease to be more common in younger primigravid women without racial predilection. The majority of cases (53%) presented during the second trimester. The most common pathogen was *E. coli*, which accounted for 83% of cases; gram-positive organisms accounted for another 11.6%.[26]

Acute pyelonephritis during pregnancy is most often treated on an inpatient basis with IV antibiotics. Empiric therapy should be begun as soon as the presumptive diagnosis is established. Therapy can be tailored to the specific organism after antibiotic sensitivities have been determined, and because septicemia may occasionally result from pyelonephritis, blood cultures should be obtained if patients do not respond rapidly to initial antibiotic therapy. **Generally, a broad-spectrum first-generation cephalosporin is the initial therapy of choice.** Fan and coinvestigators[25] reviewed 107 cases of pyelonephritis and noted that 33% of the cases were resistant to ampicillin and 13% were resistant to first-generation cephalosporins; current rates of resistance to ampicillin and first-generation cephalosporins are likely higher. If resistance to more common therapies is encountered, a later-generation cephalosporin or an aminoglycoside can be safely administered. Peak and trough aminoglycoside levels should be measured whenever these are used, and serum creatinine and BUN level should be followed as well. During the febrile period, acetaminophen treatment is advised to keep the maternal temperature below 38° C.

IV antibiotic therapy should be continued for 24 to 48 hours after the patient becomes afebrile and costovertebral angle tenderness subsides. After the cessation of IV therapy, treatment with appropriate oral antibiotics is recommended for 10 to 14 days. Upon termination of therapy, urine cultures should be obtained each trimester for the remainder of gestation. **After an episode of acute pyelonephritis, antibiotic suppression should also be implemented and should be continued for the remainder of the pregnancy.** Nitrofurantoin 100 mg once or twice daily is an acceptable regimen for suppression. In a study by Van Dorsten and colleagues,[27] nitrofurantoin suppression reduced the rate of subsequent positive cultures from 38% to 8%. However, nitrofurantoin did not lower the rate of positive cultures if inpatient antibiotic selection was inappropriate or if the urine culture was positive at the time of discharge.

The most common maternal complications associated with pyelonephritis are anemia, septicemia, transient renal dysfunction, and pulmonary insufficiency.[26] **Pulmonary injury that resembles adult respiratory distress syndrome (ARDS) can occur in pregnant women with acute pyelonephritis.[26] Clinical manifestations of this complication usually occur 24 to 48 hours after the patient is admitted for pyelonephritis.[28,29] Some of these women will require intubation, mechanical ventilation,[6] and positive end-expiratory pressure (PEEP). ARDS is believed to result from endotoxin-induced alveolar capillary membrane injury.** Towers and colleagues[30] found evidence of pulmonary injury in 11 of 130 patients with pyelonephritis. A fever of greater than 39.4°C, a maternal heart rate above 110 beats/min, and gestation beyond 20 weeks were factors associated with increased risk for pulmonary injury. The most predictive factors were fluid overload and tocolytic therapy.

Women with prior urinary tract surgery are at increased risk for pyelonephritis. Austenfeld and Snow[31] reported 64 pregnancies in 30 women who had previously undergone ureteral reimplantation for vesicoureteral reflux. During pregnancy, 57% of these women experienced one or more UTIs, and 17% had more than one UTI or an episode of pyelonephritis.[31] More frequent urine cultures and aggressive therapy during pregnancy are recommended for this group of high-risk parturients.

ACUTE RENAL DISEASE IN PREGNANCY
Urolithiasis

Urolithiasis affects 0.03% of all pregnancies, a frequency similar to that of the general population.[32] Colicky abdominal pain, recurrent UTI, and hematuria suggest urolithiasis.[33] If the diagnosis is suspected, IV pyelogram (IVP) should be considered, which limits this study to the minimum number of exposures necessary to make the diagnosis. Ultrasound can also be used to establish the diagnosis without radiation exposure. However, ultrasound alone may be limited in securing a diagnosis of urolithiasis. In a recent multicenter, longitudinal study the authors noted, "Of the group treated surgically after imaging with ultrasound alone, 23% had no evidence of a ureteral stone, resulting in the lowest positive predictive value of the modalities used. Alternative imaging techniques, particularly low-dose computerized tomography, offer improved diagnostic information that can optimize management and avoid unnecessary intervention."[34] Newer ultrasound flow studies can actually follow flow from the ureter to the bladder, and they can detect obstruction without the use of ionizing radiation. If transabdominal ultrasound is limited, transvaginal ultrasound can also be used to visualize the distal ureter.[35] Urine microscopy may detect crystals and can help distinguish the type of stone before it is passed. Serum calcium, phosphorous, and urate levels should be assayed for any woman with renal calculi to assist in the evaluation for possible hyperparathyroidism and gout.

Because of the physiologic hydroureter of pregnancy, 75% to 85% of women with symptomatic urolithiasis will spontaneously pass their stones.[33] Treatment should therefore be conservative and should consist of hydration and narcotic analgesia.[36]** Epidural anesthesia has been advocated to establish a segmental block from T11 to L2, although it is unknown whether this promotes passage of the stone. **Ureteral stenting to relieve obstruction is an option for managing pregnant women with renal stones. For refractory cases, nephrostomy tubes can also be used.** It should be noted that pregnancy increases the risk of stent encrustation, which requires frequent stent exchange every 4 to 6 weeks until delivery.[37] **Lithotripsy is contraindicated during pregnancy.[38]**

Recurrent UTI with urease-containing organisms causes precipitation of calcium phosphate in the kidney that may lead to the development of staghorn calculi. Surgery is rarely indicated in women with this condition during gestation. Individuals with staghorn calculi should have frequent urine cultures, and bacteriuria should be treated aggressively. Recurrent infections pose a risk for chronic pyelonephritis with resultant loss of kidney function.

Glomerular Disease

Acute glomerulonephritis is an uncommon complication of pregnancy, with a reported incidence of 1 per 40,000 pregnancies.[39] Poststreptococcal glomerulonephritis is rarely observed in the adult population. In this disorder, renal function tends to deteriorate during the acute phase of the disease but usually recovers in time.[40] **Acute glomerulonephritis can be difficult to distinguish from preeclampsia. Periorbital edema, a striking clinical feature of acute glomerulonephritis, is often seen in preeclampsia. However, hematuria, red blood cell (RBC) casts in the urine sediment, and depressed serum complement levels support the diagnosis of glomerulonephritis.** A rise in antistreptolysin O titers may secure the diagnosis of poststreptococcal glomerulonephritis.

Treatment of acute glomerulonephritis in pregnancy is similar to that for the nonpregnant individual. Blood pressure control is essential, and careful attention to fluid balance is advised. Sodium intake should be restricted to 500 mg/day during the acute disease, and serum potassium levels must also be carefully monitored.

Packham and coworkers[41] extensively reviewed 395 pregnancies in 238 women with primary glomerulonephritis. Remarkably, only 51% of the infants were born after 36 weeks' gestation. Excluding therapeutic abortion, the fetal loss rate was 20%, with 15% occurring after 20 weeks' gestation. IUGR was noted in 15% of the cases, and maternal renal function deteriorated in 15% of pregnancies and failed to resolve following delivery in 5% of the study population. Hypertension was recorded in 52% of the pregnancies and developed prior to 32 weeks' gestation in 26%. In most cases, this blood pressure elevation was not an exacerbation of chronic hypertension. Eighteen percent of the women who developed de novo hypertension in pregnancy remained hypertensive postpartum, and increased proteinuria was recorded in 59% of these pregnancies and was irreversible in 15%. **The highest incidence of fetal and maternal complications in women with glomerular disease occurred in those with primary focal and segmental hyalinosis and sclerosis, whereas the lowest incidence was observed in non–immunoglobulin A (IgA) diffuse mesangial proliferative glomerulonephritis.[41]** The presence of severe vessel lesions on renal biopsy was associated with a significantly higher rate of fetal loss after 20 weeks' gestation. Packham and coworkers[42] also studied 33 pregnancies in 24 patients with biopsy-proven membranous glomerulonephritis. Fetal loss occurred in 24% of pregnancies, preterm delivery was reported in 43%, and a term liveborn infant was delivered in only 33% of patients. Hypertension was noted in 46% of these pregnant women, and 30% had proteinuria in the nephrotic range during the first trimester. The presence of significant proteinuria during the first trimester correlated with poor fetal and maternal outcome.

Jungers and associates[43] described 69 pregnancies in 34 patients with IgA glomerulonephritis. The fetal loss rate in this group was 15%. Preexisting hypertension was statistically associated with poor fetal outcome. Hypertension at the time of conception also correlated with a deterioration of maternal renal function during pregnancy. Hypertension in the first pregnancy was highly predictive of recurrence of hypertension in a subsequent pregnancy. Kincaid-Smith and Fairley[44] analyzed 102 pregnancies in 65 women with IgA glomerulonephritis and noted that hypertension occurred in 63% of pregnancies, and it was severe in 18%. In this subset of women, a decline in renal function was observed in 22%. Abe[45] reported 240 pregnancies in 166 women with preexisting glomerular disease and found that 8% of the pregnancies resulted in a spontaneous abortion, 6% in a stillbirth, and 86% in a liveborn infant. Most losses occurred in women with a GFR less than 70 mL/min and preexisting hypertension. Even though the majority of women with significant renal insufficiency had good pregnancy outcomes, the long-term prognosis for these cases was worse if the GFR was less than 50 mL/min and the serum creatinine was more than 1.5 mg/dL.[45] The histopathogenic diagnosis of membranoproliferative glomerulonephritis seemed to carry the worst prognosis: 29% developed hypertension and 33% demonstrated a long-term decrease in renal function.

Imbasciati and Ponticelli[46] summarized six studies that comprised a total of 906 pregnancies in 558 women with preexisting glomerular disease. The overall perinatal mortality was 13%. Hypertension, azotemia, and nephrotic-range proteinuria were the strongest predictive factors for a poor pregnancy outcome. In this report, the histologic type of glomerulonephritis had little correlation with pregnancy outcome. Hypertension persisted in 3% to 12% of patients who developed hypertension for the first time during pregnancy. In 25% of patients, hypertension worsened during pregnancy and normalized postpartum.[46] Some of these cases represented superimposed preeclampsia. However, this diagnosis can be difficult to establish in women with baseline hypertension and proteinuria. Remarkably, only 3% of these 166 women experienced an acceleration of their glomerular disease after pregnancy.

Acute Renal Failure in Pregnancy

Acute renal failure (ARF) is defined as a urine output of less than 400 mL in 24 hours. To establish the diagnosis, ureteral and urethral obstruction must be excluded. The incidence of ARF during pregnancy is approximately 1 per 10,000. It is most frequently observed following sepsis or in cases of sudden severe volume depletion as a result of hemorrhage.[47] ARF may also be observed with marked volume contraction associated with severe preeclampsia,[48,49] dehydration from hyperemesis gravidarum, and with acute fatty liver of pregnancy.[48,51]

The incidence of ARF in pregnancy has decreased over the years. Stratta and colleagues[52] reported 81 cases of pregnancy-related ARF between 1958 and 1987, which accounted for 9% of the total number of ARF cases that required dialysis during that time. In three successive 10-year periods (1958–1967,

1968–1977, and 1978–1987), the incidence of pregnancy-related ARF fell from 43% to 2.8% of the total number of cases of ARF. The incidence declined from 1 in 3000 to 1 in 15,000 pregnancies over the study period.[52] In these 81 cases of ARF, 11.6% experienced irreversible renal damage, the majority of which occurred in the setting of severe preeclampsia-eclampsia.[52]

Renal ischemia is a common phenomenon in cases of ARF. With mild ischemia, quickly reversible prerenal failure results; with more prolonged ischemia, acute tubular necrosis occurs. This process is also reversible because glomeruli are not affected. Severe ischemia, however, may produce acute cortical necrosis. This pathology is irreversible, although on occasion, a small amount of renal function is preserved.[53] Stratta and colleagues[54] have reported 17 cases of ARF complicating pregnancies over 15 years, and all were observed in the setting of preeclampsia-eclampsia; cortical necrosis occurred in 29.5% of the cases, and progression of ARF to cortical necrosis did not appear to be related to maternal age, parity, gestational age, duration of preeclampsia prior to delivery, or eclamptic seizures. **The only significant risk factor associated with cortical necrosis was placental abruption.** In another study, Turney and coworkers[16] demonstrated that acute cortical necrosis, which occurred in 12.7% of their patients with ARF, was associated with a 100% mortality within 6 years.

Sibai and colleagues[55] studied the remote prognosis in 31 consecutive cases of ARF in patients with hypertensive disorders of pregnancy. Eighteen of the 31 patients had "pure" preeclampsia, whereas 13 pregnancies had other hypertensive disorders and renal disease; of the 18 patients with pure preeclampsia, 5% required dialysis during hospitalization, and all 18 patients had acute tubular necrosis. Of the other 13 women, 42% required dialysis, and three patients had bilateral cortical necrosis. **The majority of pregnancies in both groups were complicated by placental abruption and hemorrhage.**[55] All 16 surviving patients in the pure preeclampsia group recovered normal renal function on long-term follow-up. Conversely, 9 of the 11 surviving patients in the nonpreeclamptic group required long-term dialysis, and four ultimately died of end-stage renal disease.[55] In a follow-up study, Turney and colleagues[16] found that maternal survival was adversely affected by increasing age. Their 1-year maternal survival rate was 78.6%, and follow-up of survivors showed normal renal function up to 31 years after ARF.

Individuals with reversible ARF experience a period of oliguria of variable duration followed by polyuria, or a high-output phase. It is important to recognize that BUN and serum creatinine levels continue to rise early in the polyuric phase. During the recovery phase, urine output approaches normal. In these patients, it is important to monitor electrolytes frequently and to carefully treat any imbalance. The urine to plasma osmolality ratio should be determined early in the course of the disease. If the ratio is 1.5 or greater, prerenal pathology is likely, and the disorder tends to be of shorter duration and of less severity. A ratio near 1.0 suggests acute tubular necrosis.

The main goal of treatment is the elimination of the underlying cause. Volume and electrolyte balance must be evaluated frequently. To assess volume requirements, invasive hemodynamic monitoring may be useful. This is especially true during the polyuric phase. Central hyperalimentation may also be required if renal failure is prolonged.

Acidosis frequently occurs in cases of ARF. Therefore, arterial blood gases should be followed regularly. **Acidosis must be**

treated promptly because it can exacerbate hyperkalemia, which can be fatal. If hyperkalemia develops, potassium restriction should be instituted immediately. Sodium bicarbonate, used to treat acidosis, may overload the patient with sodium and water. In such cases, peritoneal dialysis or hemodialysis may be necessary. **The main indications for dialysis in ARF of pregnancy are hypernatremia, hyperkalemia, severe acidosis, volume overload, and worsening uremia.**

Hemolytic Uremic Syndrome

The hemolytic uremic syndrome (HUS) is a rare idiopathic disorder that must be considered when a patient exhibits signs of hemolysis and decreasing renal function, particularly during the third trimester and in the postpartum period. This idiopathic syndrome may occur as early as the first trimester and as late as 2 months postpartum, and it is part of a spectrum of disease that may also include thrombotic thrombocytopenic purpura (TTP; see Chapter 44).[16,56-59] Most individuals have no predisposing factors. Prodromal symptoms include vomiting, diarrhea, and a flulike illness. A review of 49 cases documented a 61% mortality rate, although with improved intensive care monitoring and treatment, the prognosis is now much improved.

Disseminated intravascular coagulation (DIC) with hemolysis usually accompanies HUS. However, DIC is not the cause of the syndrome. Microscopically, the kidney shows thrombotic microangiopathy. The glomerular capillary wall is thick, and biopsy specimens taken later in the course of the disease show severe nephrosclerosis and deposition of the third component of complement (C_3).

Some investigators believe that this syndrome is due to decreased renal production of prostacyclin,[60,61] infusions of which have been used to treat these patients, although such therapy remains experimental. One observer noted a decrease in antithrombin III in a woman with postpartum HUS. This patient was successfully treated with an infusion of antithrombin III concentrate.[62]

Coratelli and coworkers[56] reported a case of HUS diagnosed at 13 weeks' gestation and confirmed by renal biopsy. Circulating endotoxin was detected and was progressively reduced by hemodialysis performed daily from the third to the ninth day of the disease. Complete normalization of renal function occurred by day 34. These investigators propose that initiation of early dialysis may play an important role in supporting patients through the disease process. They also propose that endotoxins are key pathogenic factors in the disorder.[56] In contrast, Li and coworkers[63] failed to measure any endotoxin in a patient's serum who developed HUS after an uncomplicated cesarean delivery; this patient eventually underwent dialysis and recovered. **Plasma exchange in cases of ARF caused by postpartum HUS can be vital to the treatment of this condition.**[61]

Polycystic Kidney Disease

Adult polycystic kidney disease is an autosomal-dominant disorder that usually begins to manifest during the fifth decade of life. Reproductive-age women may occasionally display symptoms, and hypertension is a key component of this disorder. If a woman with adult polycystic kidney disease becomes pregnant, hypertension may be greatly exacerbated and may not improve following delivery.[46] However, the overall prognosis for the disorder does not appear to worsen with an increasing number of pregnancies.

Vesicoureteral Reflux

Although vesicoureteral reflux may be exacerbated with pregnancy, it usually does not result in morbidity unless reflux becomes severe. If reflux is significant enough to warrant surgery, this should ideally be undertaken prior to pregnancy. Even with surgical correction, women with ureterovesical reflux remain at increased risk for pyelonephritis and should have urine cultures performed frequently.[46] If indicated prior to pregnancy, antibiotic suppression should be continued.

Brandes and Fritsche[64] have reported a case of ARF that resulted from ureteral obstruction by a gravid uterus. This case was complicated by a twin gestation with polyhydramnios at 34 weeks' gestation. The serum creatinine level peaked at 12.2 mg/dL but resolved immediately after amniotomy.[64] In cases remote from term, ureteral stenting or dialysis may be necessary if significant obstruction and/or reflux is present.

Renal Artery Stenosis

Renal artery stenosis is rarely discovered during pregnancy.[65] This disorder may present as chronic hypertension with superimposed preeclampsia or as recurrent isolated preeclampsia. Although Doppler flow studies may be suggestive, renal angiography is the most specific and sensitive diagnostic test. Percutaneous transluminal angioplasty can be carried out at the time of angiography.[65]

Nephrotic Syndrome

The nephrotic syndrome was initially described as a 24-hour urine protein excretion equal to or in excess of 3.5 g, reduced serum albumin, edema, and hyperlipidemia.[66] **Currently, the syndrome is defined by proteinuria alone, which is often the result of glomerular damage.**[66] The most common etiology of nephrotic syndrome in pregnancy, especially in the third trimester, is preeclampsia. Other etiologies include membranous and membranoproliferative glomerulopathy, minimal change glomerulopathy, lupus nephropathy, hereditary nephritis, diabetic nephropathy, renal vein thrombosis, and amyloidosis.[67]

Women with a newly diagnosed or persistent nephrotic syndrome need close monitoring during pregnancy. Whenever possible, the etiology of the proteinuria should be determined. In some cases, steroid therapy may be used to treat this condition; however, depending on the etiology, its use can actually aggravate the underlying disease process.[67] One common complication of nephrotic syndrome in pregnancy is profound edema secondary to protein excretion, which is further complicated by the normal decline in serum albumin associated with pregnancy.[67] Another complication is the development of a hypercoagulable state precipitated by urinary losses of antithrombin III, reduced levels of proteins C and S, hyperfibrinogenemia, and enhanced platelet aggregation.[68] For this reason, prophylactic anticoagulation may be considered for affected pregnant women.

CHRONIC RENAL DISEASE IN PREGNANCY

Chronic renal disease can be silent until its advanced stages. Because obstetricians routinely test women's urine for the presence of protein, glucose, and ketones, they may be the first to detect chronic renal disease.

Any gravida with more than trace proteinuria should collect a 24-hour urine specimen for creatinine clearance and total protein excretion. Prior to pregnancy, 24-hour urinary protein excretion should not exceed 0.2 g. During gestation, quantities up to 0.3 g per day may be considered normal (see Chapter 3). Moderate proteinuria (<2 g/day) is often seen with glomerular disease.

Microscopic examination of the urine can reveal much about renal status. If renal disease is suspected, a catheterized specimen should be obtained. More RBCs than one to two per high-power field (hpf) or RBC casts are indicative of glomerular disease. Less frequently, they suggest trauma or malignant hypertension. Increased numbers of white blood cells (WBCs)—that is, more than one to two per high-power field— or the appearance of WBC casts is usually indicative of acute or chronic infection. Cellular casts are found in the presence of renal tubular dysfunction, and hyaline casts are associated with significant proteinuria.

The obstetrician can easily be misled when relying solely on BUN and serum creatinine levels to assess renal function. A 70% decline in creatinine clearance, an indirect measure of GFR, can be seen before a significant rise in serum BUN or serum creatinine occurs. Little change in serum creatinine or in the BUN may be observed until the creatinine clearance falls below 50 mL/min. Below that level, small decrements in creatinine clearance can lead to marked azotemia as reflected by significant increases in serum BUN and creatinine. **A single creatinine clearance value less than 100 mL/min is therefore not diagnostic of renal disease. An incomplete 24-hour urine collection is the most frequent cause of this finding. An abnormal clearance rate should prompt a repeat assay.**

Serum urate is an often overlooked but helpful parameter in detecting renal dysfunction. **Excretion of uric acid is dependent not only on glomerular filtration but also on tubular secretion.** Therefore an elevated serum urate in the presence of a normal BUN and serum creatinine may implicate tubular disease, and a solitary increase in uric acid may also signify impending or early preeclampsia.

Effect of Pregnancy on Renal Function

Although baseline creatinine clearance is decreased in women with chronic renal insufficiency, a physiologic rise will often occur in pregnancy. A moderate fall in creatinine clearance may then be observed during late gestation in patients with renal disease. This decline is typically more severe in women with diffuse glomerular disease and typically reverses after delivery.

The long-term effect of pregnancy on renal disease remains controversial. If the serum creatinine is less than 1.5 mg/dL, pregnancy appears to have little effect on the long-term prognosis. However, pregnancy is associated with an increased incidence of pyelonephritis in patients with chronic renal disease. Few data are available concerning the long-term effect of pregnancy on renal disease in women with significant azotemia. **Occasionally, some women with a baseline serum creatinine of more than 1.5 mg/dL will experience a significant decrease in renal function during gestation that does not improve during the postpartum period.**[46,69] This deterioration occurs more frequently in women with diffuse glomerulonephritis; however, it is not possible to predict which women with renal insufficiency will have a permanent decline in renal function. Moreover, if renal function significantly deteriorates during gestation, termination of pregnancy may not reverse the process. Therefore termination cannot be routinely recommended for patients who become pregnant and whose baseline serum creatinine level exceeds 1.5 mg/dL solely based on the consideration of preserving maternal renal function. Ideally, women with chronic renal disease should be counseled prior to conception about the potential decline in renal function.

Severe hypertension remains the greatest threat to a pregnant patient with chronic renal disease. Left uncontrolled, hypertension can lead to cerebral hemorrhage and deteriorating renal function. Most pregnant women with chronic renal dysfunction also have preexisting hypertension.[11,70] Approximately 50% of these women will have worsening hypertension as pregnancy progresses, and diastolic blood pressures of 110 mm Hg or greater will develop in about 20% of cases.[71] Those women with diffuse proliferative glomerulonephritis and nephrosclerosis appear to be at the greatest risk for the development of severe hypertension.

Worsening proteinuria is common during pregnancy complicated by chronic renal disease and often reaches the nephrotic range.[71] In general, massive proteinuria alone does not carry an increased risk for mother or fetus.[72] Low serum albumin, however, has been correlated with low birthweight.[73] The development of massive proteinuria is not necessarily a harbinger of preeclampsia, although women with proteinuria are clearly at increased risk for this complication. **In late pregnancy, it can be particularly difficult to differentiate preeclampsia from worsening chronic renal disease. For this reason, an evaluation in the first trimester to establish a baseline for creatinine clearance and total protein is essential.**

Effect of Chronic Renal Disease on Pregnancy

More than 85% of women with chronic renal disease will have a surviving infant if renal function is well preserved. Earlier reports were more pessimistic and cited a 6% incidence of stillbirth, a 5% incidence of neonatal death, and an increased risk for second-trimester loss.[71] If hypertension is uncontrolled and if renal function deteriorates, the likelihood of pregnancy loss is still high.[41] Antepartum fetal surveillance and advances in neonatal care have contributed to an improved perinatal outcome in these patients. One study reported a total fetal loss rate of 14% that included miscarriage, stillbirths, and neonatal deaths.[70]

The outlook for pregnancies complicated by severe renal insufficiency with a baseline serum creatinine level more than 1.5 mg/dL is less certain. This is due in part to the limited number of pregnancies reported in these women. One study reported no surviving infants when the maternal BUN was greater than 60 mg/dL.[72] Other investigations, however, have found that about 80% of such pregnancies resulted in surviving infants.[70,74] **Preterm birth and IUGR remain important complications, with the reported incidence of preterm birth ranging from 20% to 50%.**[71,75]

Imbasciati and Ponticelli[46] summarized three studies that comprised 81 pregnancies in 78 women with serum creatinine concentrations greater than 1.4 mg/dL. The perinatal loss rate was only 9%. However, 33% of the infants were growth restricted, and 50% were born preterm secondary to either maternal or fetal indications. Of concern, 33% of the women showed acceleration of their renal disease after delivery. Some individuals believe that growth restriction may be due to the lack of normal plasma volume increase as the pregnancy progresses. Cunningham and colleagues[76] demonstrated that women with moderate renal dysfunction exhibit increased creatinine clearance and plasma volume expansion during gestation, whereas women with severe renal dysfunction generally do not.[76]

Management of Chronic Renal Disease in Pregnancy

A 24-hour urine collection for creatinine clearance and total protein excretion should be obtained in women with known renal disease as soon as the pregnancy is confirmed. These parameters should be monitored periodically. A general guideline is to see patients every 2 weeks until 32 weeks' gestation and weekly thereafter.

Control of hypertension is critical in managing patients with chronic renal disease. Home blood pressure monitoring is advised for women with underlying hypertension, and β-blockers, calcium channel blockers, and hydralazine can be used to treat blood pressure effectively as long as the dosages are monitored carefully. Clonidine is occasionally useful in refractory patients. Doxazosin and prazosin may also be used if necessary. Angiotensin-converting enzyme (ACE) inhibitors are contraindicated because these drugs have been associated with fetal and neonatal oliguria/anuria[77,78] as well as anomalies.[79] In one study, 1 of 19 exposed infants had anuria and required dialysis.[77,76] Congenital anomalies, including microcephaly and encephalocele,[77] have been associated with the use of ACE inhibitors (see Chapter 8).[75]

The use of diuretics in pregnancy is controversial.[80,81] For massive debilitating edema, a short course of diuretics can be helpful, although electrolytes must be monitored carefully. Salt restriction does not appear to be beneficial once edema has developed; however, it should be instituted without hesitation in pregnant women with true renal insufficiency.

Fetal growth should be assessed with serial ultrasonography, because growth restriction is common in women with chronic renal disease. Antepartum fetal heart rate testing is often initiated at 28 to 32 weeks' gestation.[11]

If the patient manifests anemia in the presence of chronic renal disease, use of erythropoietin (EPO) may be considered. Because of the molecule's large size, recombinant EPO does not appear to cross the placenta. No cases of fetal morbidity or mortality were noted in a literature review[82] that spanned from 2002 through 2012. Use of EPO may be especially important for women who decline blood products.[82] One area of concern when using EPO in these patients is the possible exacerbation of hypertension.[83,84]

The timing of delivery should be individualized. Maternal indications for delivery include uncontrollable hypertension, the development of superimposed preeclampsia, and decreasing renal function after fetal viability has been reached. Fetal indications are dictated by assessment of fetal growth and biophysical testing.

Renal biopsy is rarely indicated during pregnancy, and it is not advised after 34 weeks' gestation, when delivery of the fetus and subsequent biopsy would prove a safer alternative. Excessive bleeding secondary to the greatly increased renal blood flow has been reported by some but not all observers.[80,85] If coagulation indices are normal and blood pressure is well controlled, morbidity should be no greater than that observed in the nonpregnant individual.[86] Packham and Fairley[87] reported a series of 111 renal biopsies performed in 104 pregnant women over 20 years. The complication rate was 4.5%. The most likely clinical dilemma necessitating renal biopsy in a pregnant woman would be the development of nephrotic syndrome and increasing hypertension between 22 and 32 weeks' gestation. In this case, renal biopsy can distinguish chronic renal disease from preeclampsia and could significantly impact management.

Hemodialysis in Pregnancy

Women with chronic hemodialysis can have successful pregnancies.[88-94] However, many women with chronic renal failure experience oligomenorrhea, and their fertility is often impaired.[95] These women commonly fail to use contraception; therefore it is important that testing be undertaken if a pregnancy is suspected.

As in all patients with impaired renal function, the most important aspect of care is meticulous control of blood pressure. During dialysis, wide fluctuations in blood pressure can occur.[96] Sudden volume shifts should be avoided because they may compromise fetal well-being.[91,92] In late pregnancy, continuous fetal heart rate monitoring should be carried out during dialysis.[97] If possible, positioning on the left side with uterine displacement away from the vena cava is preferred. During dialysis, careful attention to electrolyte balance is advised. Because pregnant women are in a state of chronic compensated respiratory alkalosis, a large reduction in serum bicarbonate should be avoided. Dialysates that contain glucose and bicarbonate are preferred, and those containing citrates should be avoided.[94]

Women should be counseled that a successful pregnancy will often require longer and more frequent periods of dialysis,[89,94,96,98] and a dose response to dialysis and pregnancy outcome is apparent. A recent study that compared outcomes in patients with end-stage renal disease (ESRD) found "a dose response between dialysis intensity and pregnancy outcomes emerged, with live birth rates of 48% in women dialyzed ≤20 hours per week and 85% in women dialyzed >36 hours per week ($P = .02$), with a longer gestational age and greater infant birthweight for women dialyzed more intensively. Pregnancy complications were few and manageable. We conclude that pregnancy may be safe and feasible in women with ESRD receiving intensive hemodialysis."[99] A diet that includes at least 70 g of protein and 1.5 g of calcium daily is recommended. Weight gain should be limited to 0.5 kg between dialysis sessions. Chronic anemia is often a problem in patients on hemodialysis. The hematocrit should be kept above 25%, and transfusion with packed RBCs or EPO therapy may be necessary to accomplish this objective.[89]

Criteria for initiating hemodialysis during pregnancy is controversial.[100] Some investigators believe that beginning regular hemodialysis in patients with moderate renal insufficiency may improve pregnancy outcome.[91] Redrow and coworkers[92] reported 14 pregnancies in 13 women undergoing dialysis, 10 of which were successful. Five of eight pregnancies managed with chronic ambulatory peritoneal dialysis or chronic cycling peritoneal dialysis utilizing an automatic cycler for short exchanges were successful. The investigators hypothesize several advantages for peritoneal dialysis that include a more constant chemical and extracellular environment for the fetus, higher hematocrit levels, infrequent episodes of hypotension, and no need for heparin. They also postulate that intraperitoneal insulin facilitates the management of blood glucose in patients with diabetes and that intraperitoneal magnesium used in the dialysate reduces the likelihood of preterm labor.

Preterm birth occurs more frequently in women undergoing dialysis.[101] Progesterone is removed during dialysis, and at least one group has advocated that parenteral progesterone therapy should be administered to the patient undergoing dialysis.[102] In their review, Yasin and Bey Doun[94] report a 40.7% incidence of premature labor.

Renal Transplant

Pregnancy following renal transplantation has become increasingly common.[103] Many previously anovulatory patients begin ovulating postoperatively and regain fertility as renal function normalizes.[104] As with women who receive hemodialysis, many transplant recipients do not recognize that they are pregnant until well into the second trimester. A recent report of all women in the United Kingdom who became pregnant after a renal transplant included 105 pregnancies identified in 101 recipients. The median prepregnancy creatinine was 1.3 mg/dL. Preeclampsia developed in 24% compared with 4% of the comparison group. Median gestation at delivery was 36 weeks, and 52% of these women delivered before 37 weeks. Twenty-four infants (24%) were small for gestational age (SGA; <10th centile). Two cases of acute rejection were reported (2%). Potential predictive factors for poor pregnancy outcome included more than one previous kidney transplant ($P = .03$), first-trimester serum creatinine greater than 1.4 mg/dL ($P = .001$), and diastolic blood pressure over 90 mm Hg in the second ($P = .002$) and third trimesters ($P = .05$).[105] Similar studies have provided consistent results and have demonstrated an overall lower rate of morbidity and adverse pregnancy complications when compared with patients with ESRD on dialysis.[106] These outcomes hold true even for women who received a renal transplant during childhood. Wyld and colleagues[107] found that pregnancy outcomes for these women are similar to those for more recent transplant recipients, with no difference in the rates of live births, SGA infants, or gestational age at delivery.

Many transplant recipients will discontinue all medications after discovering they are pregnant. The importance of continuing immunosuppressive therapy cannot be emphasized strongly enough to renal allograft recipients. Glucocorticoids, especially prednisone, are metabolized in the placenta by 11β-hydroxysteroid dehydrogenase type 1 (11β-HSD1), and only limited amounts reach the fetus.[108] Azathioprine cannot be activated in the fetus because of its lack of inosinate pyrophosphorylase.[109] Azathioprine has been shown to cause decreased levels of IgG and IgM as well as a smaller thymic shadow on chest x-ray in these neonates.[110] Chromosomal aberrations, which cleared within 20 to 32 months, have also been demonstrated in lymphocytes of infants exposed to azathioprine in utero.[111] The long-term implications of this treatment are not yet known, and IUGR has also been reported in infants born to mothers receiving this medication.[112] These risks are clearly outweighed by the benefits, including reducing the risk of allograft rejection that may occur if medication is discontinued. Of note, a single report describes a successful kidney transplant during pregnancy in the first trimester. The patient received a kidney from her father at approximately 13 weeks' gestation, and she went on to experience a successful pregnancy.[113]

Cyclosporine A appears to be relatively safe for use during gestation but does hold some risks. Women may develop arterial hypertension secondary to its interference with the normal hemodynamic adaptation to pregnancy.[114] Cyclosporine metabolism appears to be increased during pregnancy and, as such, the dose may need to be increased to maintain therapeutic levels.[115] Cyclosporine crosses the placenta, and although no evidence of teratogenesis exists, its safety in pregnancy has not been established.[116,117] In the absence of maternal hypertension, IUGR has been reported with use of cyclosporine A.[118] However, most women who receive cyclosporine have had no complications attributable to the drug, and the risk of allograft rejection certainly outweighs the risk to the fetus from the medication.

Mycophenolate mofetil (MMF) has been shown to cause adverse effects on fetal development and is associated with first-trimester loss and congenital defects. These anomalies include cleft lip and palate, limb anomalies, heart defects, and renal anomalies.[119] **This drug is contraindicated in pregnancy.**

Sirolimus is also contraindicated in pregnancy. This medication has been shown to be embryotoxic and is associated with increased fetal mortality.[119] It is recommended that women who wish to conceive be switched from this medication prior to becoming pregnant.[119]

Tacrolimus has been poorly studied in pregnancy. In 100 pregnancies in patients who were taking tacrolimus, 68 live births were reported, 60% of which were premature. Four infants had malformations, but no consistent pattern of anomalies was reported.[120] Patients taking tacrolimus require frequent monitoring of renal function and their drug levels.

Davison[121] reviewed 1569 renal transplants in 1009 women and found that 22% of the women elected to abort their pregnancies, 16% had a spontaneous abortion, and 8% experienced perinatal deaths. Furthermore, he observed that 45% of the surviving pregnancies were delivered preterm, and 22% were complicated by IUGR. In addition, 3% of the infants were born with major malformations, a rate no different from that expected in the background population. Preeclampsia complicated 30% of the pregnancies, but as previously noted, the diagnosis is difficult to make in a patient who may already have hypertension and proteinuria. The allograft rejection rate in these women was 9%, a rate no different from that expected in a nonpregnant population.[121] The long-term rejection rate was also the same as for women who had not experienced a pregnancy.

During pregnancy, renal allograft recipients must be carefully watched for signs of rejection. As previously mentioned, significant episodes of rejection may occur in as many as 9% of transplant recipients during gestation. Unfortunately, **the clinical hallmarks of rejection—fever, oliguria, tenderness, and decreasing renal function—are not always exhibited by the pregnant patient. Occasionally, rejection may mimic pyelonephritis or preeclampsia, which occurs in approximately one-third of renal transplant patients. In these cases, renal biopsy is indicated to distinguish rejection from preeclampsia.** Rejection has been known to occur during the puerperium, when maternal immune competence returns to its prepregnancy level.[122] Therefore it may be advisable to increase the dose of immunosuppressive medications in the immediate postpartum period.

Infection can be disastrous for the renal allograft; therefore urine cultures should be obtained at least monthly during pregnancy, and any bacteriuria should be aggressively treated. It is crucial to recognize that the allograft is denervated, and pain may not accompany pyelonephritis; the only symptoms may be fever and nausea.

Renal function, as determined by 24-hour creatinine clearance and protein excretion, should be assessed monthly. Approximately 15% of transplant recipients will exhibit a significant

BOX 39-2 GUIDELINES FOR RENAL ALLOGRAFT RECIPIENTS CONSIDERING PREGNANCY

- Wait 2 years after cadaver transplant or 1 year after a graft from a living donor.
- Immunosuppression should be at maintenance levels.
- Plasma creatinine should be <1.5 mg/dL.
- Hypertension should be absent or easily controlled.
- Minimal to no proteinuria should be present.
- Active graft rejection should not be evident.
- No pelvicalyceal distension should be apparent on a recent ultrasound or intravenous pyelogram.
- Prednisone dose should be 15 mg/day.
- Azathioprine dose should be 2 mg/kg/day.
- Cyclosporine A dose should be 2-4 mg/kg (available data on the use of this drug in pregnancy includes <150 patients).

Modified from Lindheimer M, Katz A. Pregnancy in the renal transplant patient. *Am J Kidney Dis.* 2000;19:173.

decrease in renal function in late pregnancy.[67] This condition usually, but not always, reverses after pregnancy. Proteinuria develops in about 40% of patients near term but most often disappears soon after delivery unless significant hypertension is present.

Similar to women with chronic renal disease, serial ultrasonography should be used to assess fetal growth, and antepartum fetal heart rate testing should be considered at 28 to 32 weeks' gestation. Approximately 50% of renal allograft recipients will deliver preterm. Preterm labor, preterm rupture of membranes, and IUGR are commonly observed. Cesarean delivery is reserved for obstetric indications. Allograft recipients may have an increased frequency of cephalopelvic disproportion from pelvic osteodystrophy as a result of prolonged renal disease with hypercalcemia or extended steroid use.[123] The transplanted kidney, however, rarely obstructs vaginal delivery despite its pelvic location.

Although many successful pregnancies have been reported in renal allograft recipients, no consensus has been reached as to when it is safe to attempt pregnancy after transplantation. Lindheimer and Katz[124] have suggested some guidelines, which are summarized in Box 39-2.

KEY POINTS

- Asymptomatic bacteriuria complicates 5% to 7% of pregnancies. If left untreated, it will result in symptomatic urinary tract infections in 40% of women.
- Pyelonephritis complicates 1% to 2% of pregnancies and generally requires inpatient treatment.
- Women with glomerular disease can have successful pregnancies, but pregnancy loss rates increase greatly if the patient has preexisting hypertension.
- Creatinine clearance can decline 70% before significant increases are seen in the BUN or serum creatinine level. Therefore a 24-hour urine specimen for creatinine clearance should be collected from any pregnant woman with underlying renal disease.
- The chance of a successful pregnancy outcome is reduced if the creatinine clearance is less than 50 mL/min or if the serum creatinine level is more than 1.5 mg/dL.

- Severe hypertension poses the greatest threat to the pregnant woman with chronic renal disease.
- Growth restriction and preeclampsia are common complications in women with chronic renal disease. Frequent sonograms and antepartum fetal surveillance at 28 weeks' gestation are recommended in affected pregnancies.
- Women with chronic renal disease are often anovulatory. Following transplantation, ovulation may resume, which can result in an unplanned pregnancy.
- Women should wait 2 years after receiving a cadaver renal allograft and 1 year after receiving a living allograft before attempting conception. Furthermore, no signs of allograft rejection should be apparent.
- Renal transplant patients may remain on cyclosporine or azathioprine throughout gestation, although levels may need to be adjusted during pregnancy. Other immunosuppressive medications such as mycophenolate mofetil and sirolimus are contraindicated.
- Renal function may decline as a result of pregnancy among patients with renal disease. An increased risk for this decline is observed in women with an elevated serum creatinine level (above 1.5mg/dL) and hypertension.

REFERENCES

1. Cietak KA, Newton JR. Serial quantitative maternal nephrosonography in pregnancy. *Br J Radiol.* 1985;58:405-413.
2. Cietak KA, Newton JR. Serial qualitative maternal nephrosonography in pregnancy. *Br J Radiol.* 1985;58:399-404.
3. Rassmussen PE, Nielson FR. Hydronephrosis during pregnancy: a literature survey. *Eur J Obstet Gynecol Reprod Biol.* 1988;27:249-259.
4. Danielson LA, Sherwood OD, Conrad KP. Relaxin is a potent vasodilator in conscious rats. *J Clin Invest.* 1999;103(4):525-533.
5. Conrad KP, Gandley RE, Ogawa T, Nakanishi S, Danielson LA. Endothelin mediates renal vasodilation and hyperfiltration during pregnancy in chronically instrumented conscious rats. *Am J Physiol.* 1999;276(5):767-776.
6. Davison JM, Sprott MS, Selkon JB. The effect of covert bacteriuria in schoolgirls on renal function at 18 years and during pregnancy. *Lancet.* 1984;2(8404):651-655.
7. Davidson J. Changes in renal function and other aspects of homeostasis in earily pregnancy. *J Obstet Gynaecol Br Commonw.* 1974;81:1003.
8. Christensen P. Tubular reabsorbtion of glucose during pregnancy. *Scand J Clin Lab Invest.* 1958;10:364.
9. Sheffield JS, Cunningham FG. Urinary tract infection in women. *Obstet Gynecol.* 2005;106(5 Pt 1):1085-1092.
10. Hooton TM, Scholes D, Stapleton AE, et al. A prospective study of asymptomatic bacteriuria in sexually active young women. *N Engl J Med.* 2000;343(14):992-997.
11. Bear R. Pregnancy in patients with renal disease: a study of 44 cases. *Obstet Gynecol.* 1976;48:13.
12. Norden C, Kass E. Bacteriuria of pregnancy—a critical reappraisal. *Annu Rev Med.* 1968;19:431.
13. McFadyen I, Eykryn S, Gardner N. Bacteriuria of pregnancy. *J Obstet Gynaecol Br Commonw.* 1973;80:385.
14. Smaill F, Vazquez JC. Antibiotics for asymptomatic bacteriuria in pregnancy. *Cochrane Database Syst Rev.* 2015;(8):CD000490.
15. Whalley P. Bacteriuria of pregnancy. *Am J Obstet Gynecol.* 1967;97:723-738.
16. Turney JH, Ellis CM, Parsons FM. Obstetric acute renal failure 1956-1987. *Br J Obstet Gynaecol.* 1989;96:679.
17. American Acadamy of Pediatrics and American College of Obstetricans and Gynecologists. *Guidlines for Prenatal Care.* 5th ed. Elk Grove Village,

IL: American Acadamy of Pediatrics and American College of Obstetricans and Gynecologists; 2002.

18. Schneeberger C, van den Heuvel ER, Erwich JJ, Stolk RP, Visser CE, Geerlings SE. Contamination rates of three urine-sampling methods to assess bacteriuria in pregnant women. *Obstet Gynecol.* 2013;121(2 Pt 1): 299-305.

19. Smaill F. Antibiotics for asymptomatic bacteriuria in pregnancy. *Cochrane Database Syst Rev.* 2001;(2):CD000490.

20. Sandberg T, Likin-Janson G, Eden CS. Host response in women with symptomatic urinary tract infection. *Scand J Infect Dis.* 1989;21:67.

21. Plattner MS. Pylonephritis in pregnancy. *J Perinatol Neonat Nurs.* 1994;8:20.

22. Wing DA, Fassett MJ, Getahun D. Acute pyelonephritis in pregnancy: an 18-year retrospective analysis. *Am J Obstet Gynecol.* 2014;210(3): 216-219.

23. Brumfitt W. The significance of symptomatic and asymptomatic infection in pregnancy. *Contrib Nephrol.* 1981;25:23.

24. Gilstrap L, Leveno K, Cunningham F, et al. Renal infections and pregnancy outcome. *Am J Obstet Gynecol.* 1981;141:709.

25. Fan YD, Pastorek JG 2nd, Miller JM, Mulvey J. Acute pyelonephritis in pregnancy. *Am J Perinatol.* 1987;4:324.

26. Hill JB, Sheffield JS, McIntire DD, Wendel GD Jr. Acute Pyelonephritis in Pregnancy. *Obstet Gynecol.* 2005;105(1):18-23.

27. Van Dorstan JP, Lenke RR, Schifrin BS. Pylonephritis in pregnancy: the role of in-hospital management and nitrofurantoin suppression. *J Reprod Med.* 1987;32:895.

28. Cunningham FG, Lucas MJ, Hankins GD. Pulmonary injury complicating antepartum pyelonephritis. *Am J Obstet Gynecol.* 1987;156:797.

29. Pruett K, Faro S. Pylonephritis associated with respiratory distress. *Obstet Gynecol.* 1987;69:444.

30. Towers CV, Kaminskas CM, Garite CM, et al. Pulmonary injury associated with antepartum pyelonephritis: Can at risk patients be identified? *Am J Obstet Gynecol.* 1991;164:974.

31. Austenfeld MS, Snow BW. Complications of pregnancy in women after reimplantation for vesicoureteral reflux. *J Urol.* 1988;140:1103.

32. Harris R, Dunnihoo D. The incidence and significance of urinary calculi in pregnancy. *Am J Obstet Gynecol.* 1967;99:237.

33. Butler EL, Cox SM, Eberts EG, Cunningham FG. Symptomatic nephrolithiasis complicating pregnancy. *Obstet Gynecol.* 2000;96(5 Pt 1): 753-756.

34. White WM, Johnson EB, Zite NB, et al. Predictive value of current imaging modalities for the detection of urolithiasis during pregnancy: a multicenter, longitudinal study. *J Urol.* 2013;189(3):931-934.

35. Laing FC, Benson CB, DiSalvo DN. Distal uretral calculi: detection with vaginal ultrasound. *Radiology.* 1994;192:545.

36. Strong D, Murchison R, Lynch D. The management of ureteral calculi during pregnancy. *Obstet Gynecol Surv.* 1978;146:604.

37. Parulkar BG, Hopkins TB, Wollin MR. Renal colic during pregnancy. *J Urol.* 1998;159:365.

38. Deliveliotis CH, Argyropoulos B, Chrisofos M, Dimopoulos CA. Shockwave lithotripsy in unrecognised pregnancy: interruption or continuation? *J Endourol.* 2001;15:787.

39. Nadler N, Salinas-Madrigal L, Charles A, Pollack V. Acute glomerulonephritis during late pregnancy. *Obstet Gynecol.* 1969;34:277.

40. Wilson C. Changes in renal function. In: Morris N, Browne J, eds. *Nontoxemic Hypertension in Pregnancy*. Boston: Little Brown; 1958:177.

41. Packham DK, North RA, Fairly KF, et al. Primary glomerulonephritis and pregnancy. *Q J Med.* 1989;71:537.

42. Packham DK, North RA, Fairly KF, et al. Membranous glomerulonephritis and pregnancy. *Clin Nephrol.* 1988;30:487.

43. Jungers P, Forget D, Houillier P, et al. Pregnancy in IgA nephropathy, reflux nephropathy, and focal glomerular sclerosis. *Am J Kidney Dis.* 1987;9:334.

44. Kincaid-Smith P, Fairley KF. Renal disease in pregnancy. Three controversial areas: mesangial IgA nephropathy, focal glomerular sclerosis (focal and segmental hyalinosis and sclerosis), and reflux nephropathy. *Am J Kidney Dis.* 1987;9:328.

45. Abe S. An overview of pregnancy in women with underlying renal disease. *Am J Kidney Dis.* 1991;17:112.

46. Imbasciati E, Ponticelli C. Pregnancy and renal disease: predictors for fetal and maternal outcome. *Am J Nephrol.* 1991;11:353.

47. Davison J. Renal Disease. In: deSwiet M, ed. *Medical Disorders in Obstetric Practice*. Oxford: Blackwell; 1984:236.

48. Pertuiset N, Grunfeld JP. Acute renal failure in pregnancy. *Baillieres Clin Obstet Gynaecol.* 1987;1:873.

49. McDonald SD, Han Z, Walsh MW. Kidney disease after preeclampsia: a systematic review and meta-analysis. *Am J Kidney Dis.* 2010;55:1026.

50. Krane NK. Acute renal failure in pregnancy. *Arch Intern Med.* 1988; 148:2347.

51. Grunfeld JP, Pertuiset N. Acute renal failure in pregnancy. *Am J Kidney Dis.* 1987;9:359.

52. Stratta P, Canavese C, Dogliani M, et al. Pregnancy related acute renal failure. *Clin Nephrol.* 1989;32:14.

53. Grunfeld JP, Ganeval D, Bournerias F. Acute renal failure in pregnancy. *Kidney Int.* 1980;18:179.

54. Stratta P, Canavese C, Colla L, et al. Acute renal failure in preeclampsia-eclampsia. *Gynecol Obstet Invest.* 1987;27:225.

55. Sibai B, Villar MA, Mabie BC. Acute renal failure in hypertensive disorders of pregnancy: pregnancy outcome and remote prognosis in thirty-one consecutive cases. *Am J Obstet Gynecol.* 1990;162:777.

56. Coratelli P, Buongiorno E, Passavanti G. Endotoxemia in hemolytic uremic syndrome. *Nephron.* 1988;50:365.

57. Robson J, Martin A, Burkley V. Irreversible postpartum renal failure: a new syndrome. *Q J Med.* 1968;37:423.

58. Seconds A, Louradour N, Suc J, Orfila C. Postpartum hemolytic uremic syndrome: a study of three cases with a review of the literature. *Clin Nephrol.* 1979;12:229.

59. Creasey GW, Morgan J. Hemolytic uremic syndrome after ectopic pregnancy: postectopic nephrosclerosis. *Obstet Gynecol.* 1987;69:448.

60. Remuzzi G, Misiani R, Marchesi D, et al. Treatment of hemolytic uremic syndrome with plasma. *Clin Nephrol.* 1979;12:279.

61. Webster J, Rees A, Lewis P, Hensby C. Prostacyclin deficiency in haemolytic uraemic syndrome. *BMJ.* 1980;281:271.

62. Brandt P, Jesperson J, Gregerson G. Post-partum haemolytc-uremic syndrome successfully treated with antithrombin III. *BMJ.* 1980;281:449.

63. Li PK, Lai FM, Tam JS, Lai KN. Acute renal failure due to postpartum haemoltic uremic syndrome. *Aust N Z J Obstet Gynaecol.* 1988;28:228.

64. Brandes JC, Fritsche C. Obstructive acute renal failure by a gravid uterus: a case report and review. *Am J Kidney Dis.* 1991;18:398.

65. Hayborn KD, Schultz MF, Goodlin RC, Durham JD. Renal artery stenosis during pregnancy: a review. *Obstet Gynecol Surv.* 1991;46:509.

66. Coe FL, Brenner BM. Approach to the patient with diseases of the kidney and urinary tract. In: Fauci AS, Braunwald E, Isselbacher KJ, et al., eds. *Principles of Internal Medicine.* 14th ed. New York: McGraw-Hill; 1998: 1495-1498.

67. Davison J, Lindheimer M. Pregnancy in women with renal allografts. *Semin Nephrol.* 1984;4:240.

68. Denker BM, Brenner BM. Cardinal manifestations of renal disease. In: Fauci AS, Braunwald E, Isselbacher KJ, et al., eds. *Principles of Internal Medicine.* 14th ed. New York: McGraw-Hill; 1998:258-262.

69. Hou S. Pregnancy in women with chronic renal disease. *N Engl J Med.* 1985;312:839.

70. Hou S, Grossman S, Madias N. Pregnancy in women with renal disease and moderate renal insufficiency. *Am J Med.* 1985;78:185.

71. Katz A, Davison J, Hayslett J, et al. Pregnancy in women with kidney disease. *Kidney Int.* 1980;18:192.

72. Mackay E. Pregnancy and renal disease: a ten-year study. *Aust N Z J Obstet Gynaecol.* 1963;3:21.

73. Studd J, Blainey J. Pregnancy and the nephrotic syndrome. *BMJ.* 1969;1:276.

74. Kincaid-Smith P, Fairley K, Bullen M. Kidney disease and pregnancy. *Med J Aust.* 1967;11:1155.

75. Surian M, Imbasciati E, Banfi G, et al. Glomerular disease and pregnancy. *Nephron.* 1984;36:101.

76. Cunningham FG, Cox SG, Harstad TW, et al. Chronic renal disease and pregnancy outcome. *Am J Obstet Gynecol.* 1990;163:453.

77. Piper JM, Ray WA, Rosa FW. Pregnancy outcome following exposure to angiotensin-converting enzyme inhibitors. *Obstet Gynecol.* 1992;80:429.

78. Hulton SA, Thompson PD, Cooper PA, Rothberg AD. Angiotensin-converting enzyme inhibitors in pregnancy may result in neonatal renal failure. *S Afr Med J.* 1990;78:673.

79. Cooper WO, Hernandez-Diaz S, Arbogast PG, et al. Major congenital malformations after first-trimester exposure to ACE inhibitors. *N Engl J Med.* 2006;354(23):2443-2451.

80. Sibai B, Grossman R, Grossman H. Effects of diuretics on plasma volume in pregnancy with long term hypertension. *Am J Obstet Gynecol.* 1984; 150:831.

81. Rodriquez S, Leikin S, Hillar M. Neonatal thrombocytopenia associated with antepartum administration of thiazide drugs. *N Engl J Med.* 1964; 270:881.

82. Sienas L, Wong T, Collins R, Smith J. Contemporary uses of erythropoietin in pregnancy: a literature review. *Obstet Gynecol Surv.* 2013;68(8):594-602.

83. Lundby C, Olsen NV. Effects of recombinant human erythropoietin in normal humans. *J Physiol.* 2011;589(Pt 6):1265-1271.

84. Berglund B, Ekblom B. Effect of recombinant human erythropoietin treatment on blood pressure and some haematological parameters in healthy men. *J Intern Med.* 1991;229(2):125-130.

85. Lindheimer M, Spargo B, Katz A. Renal biopsy in pregnancy-induced hypertension. *J Reprod Med.* 1975;15:189.

86. Lindheimer M, Fisher K, Spargo B, Katz A. Hypertension in pregnancy: a biopsy with long term follow-up. *Contrib Nephrol.* 1981;25:71.

87. Packham DK, Fairley K. Renal biopsy: indications and complications in pregnancy. *Br J Obstet Gynaecol.* 1987;94:935.

88. Ackrill P, Goodwin F, Marsh F, et al. Successful pregnancy in patient on regular dialysis. *BMJ.* 1975;2:172.

89. Kobayashi H, Matsumoto Y, Otsubo O, et al. Successful pregnancy in a patient undergoing chronic hemodialysis. *Obstet Gynecol.* 1981;57:382.

90. Savdie E, Caterson R, Mahony J, Clifton-Bligh P. Successful pregnancies treated by haemodialysis. *Med J Aust.* 1982;2:9.

91. Cohen D, Frenkel Y, Maschiach S, Eliahou HE. Dialysis during pregnancy in advanced chronic renal failure patients: outcome and progression. *Clin Nephrol.* 1988;29:144.

92. Redrow M, Cherem L, Elliott J, et al. Dialysis in the management of pregnant patients with renal insufficiency. *Medicine.* 1988;67:199.

93. Hou S. Pregnancy in women requiring dialysis for renal failure. *Am J Kidney Dis.* 1987;9:368.

94. Yasin SY, Bey Doun SW. Hemodialysis in pregnancy. *Obstet Gynecol Surv.* 1988;43:655.

95. Lim V, Henriquez C, Sievertsen G, Prohman L. Ovarian function in chronic renal failure: evidence suggesting hypothalamic anovulation. *Ann Intern Med.* 1980;57:7.

96. Nageotte MP, Grundy HO. Pregnancy outcome in women requiring chronic hemodialysis. *Obstet Gynecol.* 1988;72:456.

97. Luders C, Castro MC, Titan SM. Obstetric outcomes in pregnant women on long-term dialysis: a case series. *Am J Kidney Dis.* 2010;56:77.

98. EDTA Registration Committee. Successful pregnancies in women treated by dialysis and kidney transplantation. *Br J Obstet Gynaecol.* 1980;87:839.

99. Hladunewich MA, Hou S, Odutayo A, et al. Intensive hemodialysis associates with improved pregnancy outcomes: a Canadian and United States cohort comparison. *J Am Soc Nephrol.* 2014;25(5):1103-1109.

100. Asamiya Y, Otsubo S, Matsuda Y. The importance of low blood urea nitrogen levels in pregnant patients undergoing hemodialysis to optimize birth weight and gestational age. *Kidney Int.* 2009;75:1217.

101. Fine L, Barnett E, Danovitch G, et al. Systemic lupus erythematosus in pregnancy. *Ann Intern Med.* 1981;94:667.

102. Johnson T, Lorenz R, Menon K, Nolan G. Successful outcome of a pregnancy requiring dialysis: effects on serum progesterone and estrogens. *J Reprod Med.* 1979;22:217.

103. Gill JS, Zalunardo N, Rose C, Tonelli M. The pregnancy rate and live birth rate in kidney transplant recipients. *Am J Transplant.* 2009;9:1541.

104. Merkatz I, Schwartz G, David D, et al. Resumption of female reproductive function following renal transplantation. *JAMA.* 1971;216:1749.

105. Bramham K, Nelson-Piercy C, Gao H, et al. Pregnancy in renal transplant recipients: a UK national cohort study. *Clin J Am Soc Nephrol.* 2013;8(2):290-298.

106. Saliem S, Patenaude V, Abenhaim HA. Pregnancy outcomes among renal transplant recipients and patients with end-stage renal disease on dialysis. *J Perinat Med.* 2015. Epub ahead of print.

107. Wyld ML, Clayton PA, Kennedy SE, Alexander SI, Chadban SJ. Pregnancy outcomes for kidney transplant recipients with transplantation as a child. *JAMA Pediatr.* 2015;169(2):e143626.

108. Penn I, Markowski E, Harris P. Parenthood following renal transplantation. *Kidney Int.* 1980;18:221.

109. Saarikoski S, Sappala M. Immunosuppression during pregnancy: transmission of azathioprine and its metabolites from mother to fetus. *Am J Obstet Gynecol.* 1973;115:1100.

110. Cote C, Meuwissen H, Pickering R. Effects on the neonate of prednisone and azathioprine administered to the mother during pregnancy. *J Pediatr.* 1974;85:324.

111. Price H, Salaman J, Laurence K, Langmaid H. Immunosuppressive drugs and the fetus. *Transplantation.* 1976;21:294.

112. Scott J. Fetal growth retardation associated with maternal administration of immunosuppressive drugs. *Am J Obstet Gynecol.* 1977;128:668.

113. Hold P, Wong C, Dhanda R, Walkinshaw S, Bakran A. Successful renal transplantation during pregnancy. *Am J Transplant.* 2005;5(9):2315-2317.

114. Ponticelli C, Montagnino G. Causes of arterial hypertension in kidney transplantation. *Contrib Nephrol.* 1987;54:226.

115. McKay DB, Josephson MA. Pregnancy in recipients of solid organs—effects on the mother and child. *N Engl J Med.* 2006;354:1281.

116. Derfler K, Schuller A, Herold C, et al. Successful outcome of a complicated pregnancy in a renal transplant recipient taking cyclosporin A. *Clin Nephrol.* 1988;29:96.

117. Salamalekis EE, Mortakis AE, Phocas I, et al. Successful pregnancy in a renal transplant recipient taking cyclosporin A: hormonal and immunological studies. *Int J Gynaecol Obstet.* 1989;30:267.

118. Pickerell MD, Sawers R, Michael J. Pregnancy after renal transplantation: severe intrauterine growth retardation during treatment with cyclosporin A. *BMJ.* 1988;1:825.

119. Sifontis MN, Coscia LA, Constantinescu S. Pregnancy outcomes in solid organ transplant recipients with exposure to mycophenolate mofetil or sirolimus. *Transplantation.* 2006;82:1698.

120. Kainz A, Harabacz I, Cowlrick IS. Review of the course and outcome of 100 pregnancies in 84 women treated with tacrolimus. *Transplantation.* 2000;70:1718.

121. Davison J. Renal transplantation and pregnancy. *Am J Kidney Dis.* 1987;9:374.

122. Parsons V, Bewick M, Elias J, et al. Pregnancy following renal transplantation. *J R Soc Med.* 1979;72:815.

123. Huffer W, Kuzela D, Popovtzer M. Metabolic bone disease in chronic renal failure in renal transplant patients. *Am J Pathol.* 1975;78:385.

124. Lindheimer M, Katz A. Pregnancy in the renal transplant patient. *Am J Kidney Dis.* 2000;19:173.

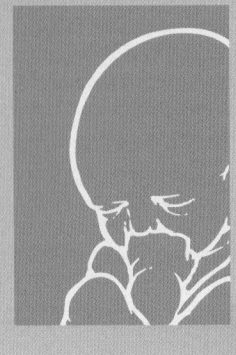

CHAPTER 40

Diabetes Mellitus Complicating Pregnancy

MARK B. LANDON, PATRICK M. CATALANO, and STEVEN G. GABBE

KEY ABBREVIATIONS

American College of Obstetricians and Gynecologists	ACOG	Infant of a diabetic mother	IDM
		Insulin-dependent diabetes mellitus	IDDM
American Diabetes Association	ADA	Low-density lipoprotein	LDL
Australian Carbohydrate Intolerance Study in Pregnant Women	ACHOIS	Maternal-Fetal Medicine Unit	MFMU
		Maternal serum alpha-fetoprotein	MSAFP
Biophysical profile	BPP	Maturity-onset diabetes of youth	MODY
Continuous subcutaneous insulin infusion	CSII	National Institute of Child Health and Human Development	NICHD
Depot medroxyprogesterone acetate	DMPA	Nonstress test	NST
Diabetic ketoacidosis	DKA	Oral contraceptive	OC
Disposition index	DI	Phosphatidylglycerol	PG
Free fatty acid	FFA	Randomized controlled trial	RCT
Gestational diabetes mellitus	GDM	Respiratory distress syndrome	RDS
Glucose tolerance test	GTT	Total urinary protein excretion	TPE
Glucose transporter	GLUT	Tumor necrosis factor alpha	TNF-α
Hemoglobin A1c	HbA1c	Urinary albumin excretion	UAE
High-density lipoprotein	HDL	Very-low-density lipoprotein	VLDL
Hyaline membrane disease	HMD		

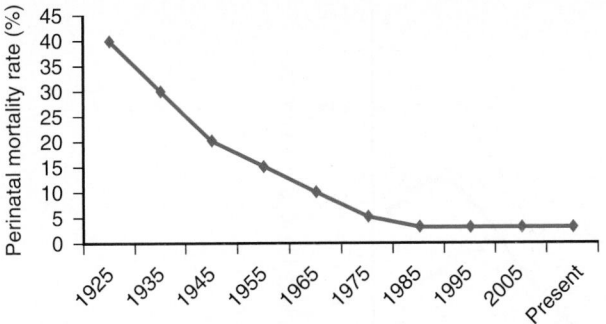

FIG 40-1 Perinatal mortality rate in pregnancy complicated by insulin-dependent diabetes mellitus.

Insulin therapy was introduced nearly 100 years ago and remains perhaps the most important landmark in the care of pregnancy for the diabetic woman. Before insulin became available, pregnancy was not advised because it was likely to be accompanied by fetal mortality and also came with a substantial risk for maternal death. Over the past 30 years, however, management techniques have been developed that can prevent many complications associated with the diabetic pregnancy. These advances, based on our understanding of the pathophysiology, have resulted in perinatal mortality rates in optimally managed cases that approach those of the normal population. This dramatic improvement in perinatal outcome can be largely attributed to clinical efforts to establish improved maternal glycemic control both before conception and during gestation (Fig. 40-1). Excluding major congenital malformations, which continue to plague pregnancies in women with preexisting (type 1 and type 2) diabetes mellitus (DM), perinatal loss for the woman with diabetes has fortunately become an uncommon event.

Although the benefit of careful regulation of maternal glucose levels is well accepted, failure to establish optimal glycemic control—as well as other factors—continues to result in significant perinatal morbidity. Clinical experience has also resulted in recognition of the impact that vascular complications can have on pregnancy and the manner in which pregnancy can affect these disease processes. With current management techniques and a skilled, organized team approach, successful pregnancies have become the norm even for women with significant complications of DM.

Gestational diabetes mellitus (GDM), the most common type of diabetes found in pregnancy, is increasing in frequency worldwide. GDM continues to represent a significant challenge for both clinicians and investigators. After nearly 60 years since the concept of GDM was introduced, and as a recent result of large-scale observational studies and treatment trials, the clinical significance of this disorder is now accepted. However, controversy still remains concerning screening techniques, diagnostic criteria, thresholds for insulin initiation, and whether oral hypoglycemic agents are a suitable treatment.

Before considering these clinical issues, it is important to review the metabolic effects of pregnancy in relation to the pathophysiology of DM.

PATHOPHYSIOLOGY
Normal Glucose Tolerance
Significant alterations occur in maternal metabolism during pregnancy, which provide for adequate maternal nutritional

stores in early gestation to meet the increased maternal and fetal metabolic demands of late gestation and lactation. Although we are apt to think of DM as a disorder exclusively of maternal glucose metabolism, in fact **DM affects all aspects of nutrient metabolism.** In this section we consider maternal glucose metabolism as it relates to pancreatic β-cell production of insulin and insulin clearance, endogenous (i.e., primarily hepatic) glucose production, and suppression with insulin and peripheral glucose insulin sensitivity. We also address maternal protein and lipid insulin metabolism. Lastly, the effects of these alternations on maternal metabolism are examined as they relate to maternal energy expenditure and fetal growth.

Glucose Metabolism
Normal pregnancy has been characterized as a "diabetogenic state" because of the progressive increase in postprandial glucose levels and increased insulin response in late gestation. **However, early gestation can be viewed as an anabolic state because of the increases in maternal fat stores and decreases in free fatty acid (FFA) concentration, particularly in normal weight and obese women.** Garcia-Patterson and colleagues[1] have described significant decreases in maternal insulin requirements in early gestation in women with type 1 diabetes (Fig. 40-2). The mechanism for the decrease in insulin requirements has been ascribed to various factors that include increased insulin sensitivity and decreased substrate availability secondary to factors such as nausea, the fetus acting as a glucose sink, and enhanced maternal insulin secretion; however, the exact mechanism is not known. Longitudinal studies in women with normal glucose tolerance have shown significant alterations in all aspects of glucose metabolism as early as the end of the first trimester.[2]

Progressive increases are seen in insulin secretion in response to an intravenous (IV) glucose challenge with advancing gestation (Fig. 40-3). The increases in insulin concentration are more pronounced in lean women, compared with obese women, most probably as a response to the greater decreases in insulin sensitivity in lean women, as will be described later. Data regarding insulin clearance in pregnancy are limited. In separate studies, Bellman, Lind, and colleagues and Burt and Davidson reported no difference in insulin disappearance rate when insulin was infused intravenously in late gestation compared with nongravid subjects. In contrast, using a radiolabeled insulin, Goodner and Freinkel described a 25% increase in insulin turnover in a pregnant compared with a nonpregnant rat model. Using the euglycemic clamp, Catalano and associates[3] reported a 20% increase in insulin clearance in lean women and a 30% increase in insulin clearance in obese women by late pregnancy (Fig. 40-4). Although the placenta is rich in insulinase, the exact mechanism for the increased insulin clearance in pregnancy remains speculative.

Although there is a progressive decrease in fasting glucose with advancing gestation, this decrease is most probably a result of the increase in plasma volume in early gestation and the increase in fetoplacental glucose utilization in late gestation. Using various stable isotope methodologies in cross-sectional study designs, Kalhan and Cowett were the first to describe increased fasting hepatic glucose production in late pregnancy. Additionally, using a stable isotope of glucose in a prospective longitudinal study design, Catalano and coworkers[4] reported a **30% increase in maternal fasting hepatic glucose production with advancing gestation** (Fig. 40-5), which remained significant even after adjusting for maternal weight gain. Tissue

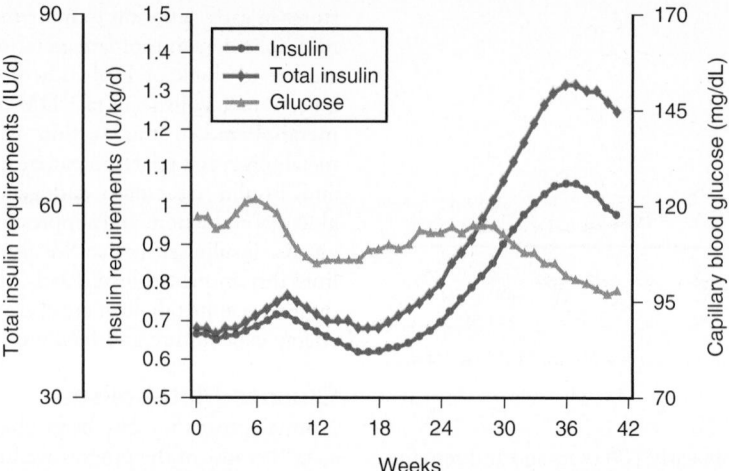

FIG 40-2 Mean insulin requirements and self-monitored blood glucose in women with type 1 diabetes. (Modified from Garcia-Patterson A, Gich I, Amini SB, et al. Insulin requirements throughout pregnancy in women with type 1 diabetes mellitus: three changes of direction. *Diabetologia*. 2010;53:446.)

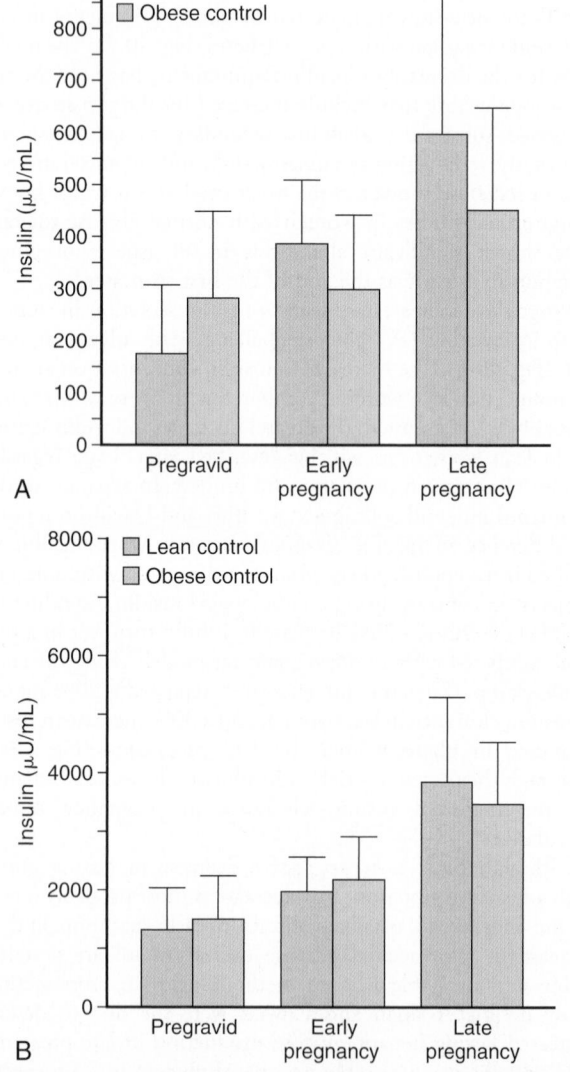

FIG 40-3 Longitudinal increase in insulin response to an intravenous glucose challenge in lean and obese women with normal glucose tolerance: pregravid and early and late pregnancy. **A,** First phase: area under the curve from 0 to 5 minutes. **B,** Second phase: area under the curve from 5 to 60 minutes.

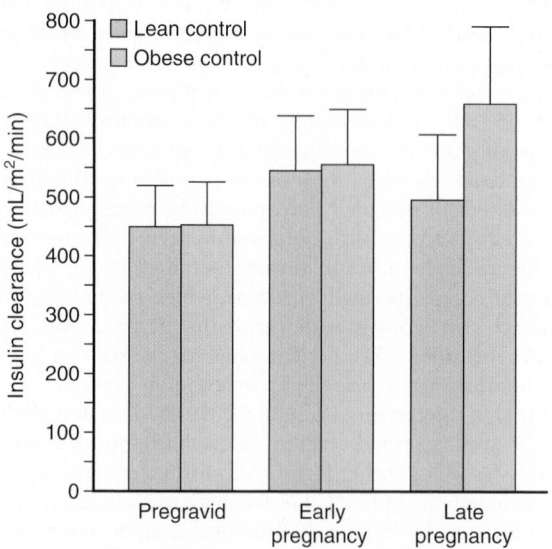

FIG 40-4 Longitudinal increases in metabolic clearance rate of insulin (mL/m²/min) in lean and obese women with normal glucose tolerance: pregravid and early and late pregnancy.

sensitivity to insulin involves both liver and peripheral tissues, primarily skeletal muscle. The increase in fasting maternal hepatic glucose production occurs despite a significant increase in fasting insulin concentration, which indicates a decrease in maternal hepatic glucose sensitivity in women with normal glucose tolerance in late pregnancy. In obese women, a further decrease of insulin to suppress hepatic glucose production was seen in late gestation, thereby indicating a further decrease in hepatic insulin sensitivity in obese women.

Estimates of peripheral insulin sensitivity in pregnancy have included measurements of insulin response to a fixed oral or IV glucose challenge or the ratio of insulin to glucose under a variety of experimental conditions. Methodologies such as the minimal model and the euglycemic-hyperinsulinemic clamp have improved our ability to quantify peripheral insulin sensitivity. In lean women in early gestation, Catalano and colleagues[5] reported a 40% decrease in maternal peripheral insulin sensitivity using the euglycemic-hyperinsulinemic clamp. However, when adjusted for changes in insulin concentrations during the

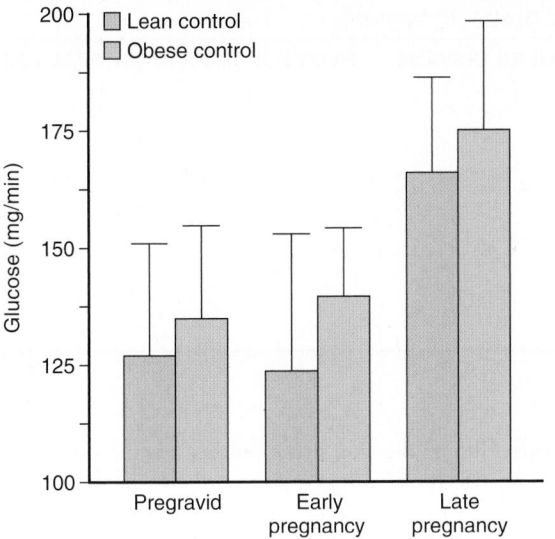

FIG 40-5 Longitudinal increase in basal endogenous (primarily hepatic) glucose production (mg/min) in lean and obese women with normal glucose tolerance: pregravid and early and late pregnancy.

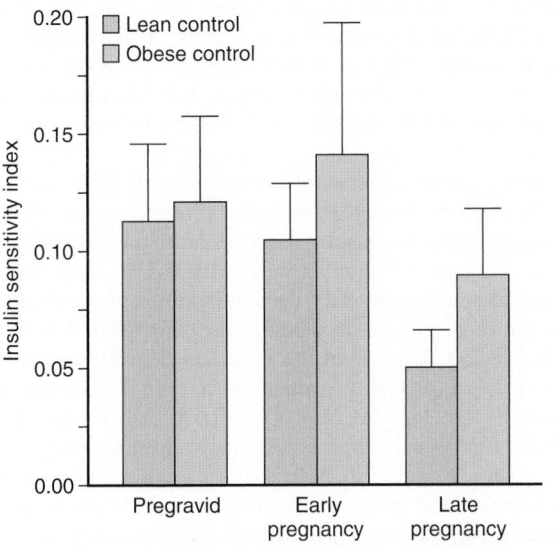

FIG 40-6 Longitudinal changes in the insulin sensitivity index (glucose infusion rate adjusted for residual endogenous glucose production and insulin concentrations achieved during the glucose clamp) in lean and obese women with normal glucose tolerance: pregravid and early and late gestation.

clamp and residual hepatic glucose production (i.e., the insulin sensitivity index), insulin sensitivity *decreased* only 10% (Fig. 40-6). In contrast, a 15% *increase* was seen in the insulin sensitivity index in obese women in early pregnancy compared with pregravid estimates.[6] Hence, the decrease in insulin requirements in early gestation observed in some women may be a consequence of an increase in insulin sensitivity, particularly in women with decreased insulin sensitivity before conception.

Compared with the varied metabolic alterations in early pregnancy, consensus has been reached regarding the decrease in peripheral insulin sensitivity in late gestation. Spellacy and Goetz were among the first investigators to report an increase in insulin response to a glucose challenge in late gestation. Additionally, Burt demonstrated that pregnant women experienced

less hypoglycemia in response to exogenous insulin in comparison with nonpregnant subjects. **Later research by Fisher and associates (using a high-dose glucose infusion test), by Buchanan and colleagues (using the Bergman minimal model), and by Ryan and coworkers[7] and Catalano and associates[2] (using the euglycemic-hyperinsulinemic clamp) all demonstrated a decrease in insulin sensitivity ranging from 33% to 78% in late gestation.** However, all these quantitative estimates of insulin sensitivity are overestimates because of non–insulin-mediated glucose disposal by the fetus and placenta. Hay and colleagues reported that in the pregnant ewe model, about one third of maternal glucose use was accounted for by uterine, placental, and fetal tissue. Additionally, Marconi and coworkers reported that based on human fetal blood sampling, fetal glucose concentration was a function of fetal size and gestational age in addition to maternal glucose concentration.

The decrease in insulin sensitivity during pregnancy has been ascribed to an increased production of various placental and maternal hormones, such as human placental lactogen (hPL), progesterone, estrogen, cortisol, and prolactin. However, recent evidence has focused on the role of several new mediators of insulin resistance such as leptin, tumor necrosis factor alpha (TNF-α), and resistin. Kirwan and coworkers[8] reported that TNF-α was inversely correlated with the changes in insulin sensitivity from the time before conception through late gestation. In combination with other placental hormones, multivariate stepwise regression analysis revealed that **TNF-α was the strongest independent predictor of insulin sensitivity in pregnancy, accounting for about half of the variance in the decrease in insulin sensitivity during gestation.**

Pregnancy has been characterized as a chronic low-grade inflammatory condition because of the increase in activation of circulating blood leukocytes.[9] The inflammation of pregnancy is further enhanced by maternal prepregnancy obesity. This increase in low-grade inflammation, particularly observed in obese women, has been related to increases in macrophage infiltration in both maternal white adipose tissue and the placenta. The increase in inflammation has been associated with increased circulating C-reactive protein (CRP) and interleukin-6 (IL-6). Both of these factors may exacerbate the increased insulin resistance previously noted in obese women with normal glucose tolerance because of effects on the postreceptor insulin-signaling cascade. These inflammatory cytokines may then relate to increased substrate availability for the developing fetus and resultant macrosomia.

Placental glucose transport is a process that takes place through facilitated diffusion. Glucose transport is dependent on a family of glucose transporters referred to as the *GLUT glucose transporter family*. **The principal glucose transporter in the placenta is GLUT1, which is located in the syncytiotrophoblast.[10] GLUT1 is located on both the microvillus and basal membranes.** Basal membrane GLUT1 may be the rate-limiting step in placental glucose transport. A twofold to threefold increase is seen in the expression of syncytiotrophoblast glucose transporters with advancing gestation. Although GLUT3 and GLUT4 expression have been identified in placental endothelial cells and intervillous nontrophoblastic cells, respectively, the role they may play in placental glucose transport remains speculative.

Debate has been ongoing regarding the location and/or function of insulin receptors in the placenta. In early pregnancy, insulin receptors are abundant on the syncytiotrophoblast, the

TABLE 40-1   MODIFIED WHITE CLASSIFICATION OF PREGNANT DIABETIC WOMEN

CLASS	DIABETES ONSET AGE (yr)	DURATION (yr)	VASCULAR DISEASE	NEED FOR INSULIN OR ORAL AGENT
Gestational Diabetes				
A₁	Any	Any	−	−
A₂	Any	Any	−	+
Pregestational Diabetes				
B	>20	<10	−	+
C	10 to 19	or 10 to 19	−	+
D	<10	or >20	+	+
F	Any	Any	+	+
R	Any	Any	+	+
T	Any	Any	+	+
H	Any	Any	+	+

Modified from White P. Pregnancy complicating diabetes. *Am J Med.* 1949;7:609.

cellular layer in contact with maternal blood. In late gestation, insulin receptors are increased on the placental vascular endothelium (i.e., in contact with fetal blood). Maternal insulin response in early pregnancy, as is often seen in women who are obese or who have diabetes, was strongly related to placental weight at birth.[11] Placental weight at birth has the strongest correlation with birthweight, that is, fat and lean body mass.[11] The implication of these data is that early maternal pregnancy metabolism, insulin resistance and response, may affect placental growth and gene expression, which only becomes clinically manifest as fetal overgrowth in late gestation.

DIABETES MELLITUS

Diabetes mellitus is a chronic metabolic disorder characterized by either absolute or relative insulin deficiency that results in increased glucose concentrations. Although glucose intolerance is the common outcome of DM, the pathophysiology remains heterogeneous. The two major classifications of DM are *type 1,* formerly referred to as *insulin-dependent* or *juvenile-onset diabetes,* and *type 2,* formerly referred to as *non–insulin-dependent* or *adult-onset diabetes.* During pregnancy, classification of women with diabetes has often relied on the White classification,[12] first proposed in the 1940s. This classification is based on factors such as the age of onset of diabetes and duration as well as end-organ involvement, primarily retinal and renal (Table 40-1).

All forms of diabetes can occur during pregnancy. However, in addition to types 1 and 2 diabetes, genetic causes of diabetes exist, the most common of which is maturity-onset diabetes of youth (MODY), characterized by β-cell dysfunction; it has an autosomal-dominant mode of inheritance and usually becomes manifest in young adulthood. Mutations in the glucokinase gene are a frequent cause of MODY. Various mutations have been described, and each mutation is associated with varying degrees of disease severity. The most common of these mutations, MODY2, occurs in the European population and involves the glucokinase gene. Because the age of onset of diabetes in women with MODY coincides with the reproductive years, it may be difficult to distinguish between type 1 DM and MODY. The glucokinase gene acts as a sensor in the β-cell, which leads to a secretory defect in insulin response. **Ellard and colleagues reported that 2.5% of women with GDM in the United Kingdom have the glucokinase mutation,** whereas Stoffel, in a small population in the United States, reported that 5% of patients had a glucokinase in mutation. In another U.S. population, Sewell and colleagues[13] reported no cases in 72 pregnant women with GDM or recently diagnosed pregestational

diabetes. The implication if the mother has the mutation is an increased risk for fetal macrosomia, whereas if the mutation is inherited from the father, the implication for the fetus is a significant decrease in growth secondary to relative insulinopenia.

Type 1 Diabetes Mellitus

Type 1 diabetes mellitus is usually characterized by an abrupt onset at a young age and absolute insulinopenia with lifelong requirements for insulin replacement. Although depending on the population, the onset of type 1 diabetes may occur in individuals in their third or fourth decades of life. Although the phenotype of the individual with type 1 diabetes has often been conceptualized as being thin, in an 18-year follow-up study, the prevalence of overweight increased by 47%, and the prevalence of obesity increased sevenfold. Patients with DM may have a genetic predisposition for antibodies directed against their pancreatic islet cells. The degree of concordance for the development of type 1 diabetes in monozygotic twins is 33%, suggesting that the events subsequent to the development of autoantibodies and appearance of glucose intolerance are also related to environmental factors. Because of the complete dependence on exogenous insulin, pregnant women with type 1 diabetes are at increased risk for the development of diabetic ketoacidosis (DKA). Additionally, because intensive insulin therapy is used in women with type 1 diabetes to decrease the risk for spontaneous abortion and congenital anomalies in early gestation, these women are at increased risk for hypoglycemic reactions. Studies by Diamond and Rosenn have shown that women with type 1 diabetes are more likely to experience hypoglycemic reactions during pregnancy because of diminished counterregulatory epinephrine and glucagon response to hypoglycemia. The deficiency in this counterregulatory response may be in part due to an independent effect of pregnancy.

The alterations in glucose metabolism in women with type 1 diabetes are not well characterized. Because of maternal insulinopenia, insulin response during gestation can only be estimated relative to pregravid requirements. Estimates of the change in insulin requirements are complicated by the degree of preconceptional glucose control and potential presence of insulin antibodies. Garcia-Patterson[1] reported on the change in insulin requirements in women with type 1 diabetes and strict glucose control prior to conception. In early pregnancy, both insulin requirements and total insulin peak at 9 weeks' gestation and reach a nadir at 16 weeks to baseline prepregnancy levels. After 16 weeks, insulin requirements gradually increase through 37 weeks. This represents a total increase in insulin requirements of 5.19% per week and about a twofold increase relative to prepregnancy requirements. A 5% decrease in insulin requirements after 36 weeks' gestation was also noted by McManus and Ryan. The decrease in insulin requirements was associated with a longer duration of DM but not with adverse perinatal outcome. The fall in insulin requirements in early pregnancy in women with type 1 diabetes may be a reflection of increased insulin sensitivity as was previously described.

Schmitz and associates have evaluated the longitudinal changes in insulin sensitivity in women with type 1 diabetes in early and late pregnancy, as well as postpartum, in comparison with nonpregnant women with type 1 diabetes. **In the pregnant women with type 1 diabetes, a 50% decrease in insulin sensitivity was observed only in late gestation.** No significant difference was found in insulin sensitivity in pregnant women with type 1 diabetes in early pregnancy or within 1 week of delivery compared with nonpregnant women with type 1 diabetes. Therefore based on the available data, women with type 1 diabetes appear to have a similar decrease in insulin sensitivity compared with women with normal glucose tolerance. Relative to the issue of placental transporters (GLUT1), a report by Jansson and Powell describes an increase in both basal GLUT1 expression and glucose transport activity from placental tissue in women with White class D pregnancies.

Type 2 Diabetes and Gestational Diabetes

The pathophysiology of type 2 diabetes involves abnormalities of both insulin-sensitive tissue (i.e., both a decrease in skeletal muscle and hepatic sensitivity to insulin) and β-cell response as manifested by an inadequate insulin response for a given degree of glycemia. Initially in the course of the development of type 2 diabetes, the insulin response to a glucose challenge may be increased relative to that of individuals with normal glucose tolerance but is inadequate to maintain normoglycemia. Whether decreased insulin sensitivity precedes β-cell dysfunction in the development of type 2 diabetes continues to be debated. Arguments and experimental data support both hypotheses.

Despite the limitations of any classification system, certain generalizations can be made regarding women with type 2 diabetes or GDM. These individuals are typically older and more often are heavier compared with individuals with normal glucose tolerance. The onset of the disorder is usually insidious, with few patients complaining of the classic triad of polydipsia, polyphagia, and polyuria. Individuals with type 2 diabetes are often initially recommended to lose weight, increase their activity (i.e., exercise), and follow a diet low in saturated fats and high in complex carbohydrates. Oral agents are often used to increase insulin response, enhance insulin sensitivity, or increase renal excretion of glucose. Individuals with type 2 diabetes may eventually require insulin therapy to maintain euglycemia but are at significantly less risk for DKA. **Data from monozygotic twin studies have reported a lifetime risk for both twins developing type 2 diabetes that ranges between 58% and almost 100%, suggesting that the disorder has a strong genetic component.**

Type 2 pregestational diabetes is usually classified as class B diabetes according to the White classification system. Women who develop GDM—that is, glucose intolerance first recognized during pregnancy—share many of the metabolic characteristics of women with type 2 diabetes. Although earlier studies reported a 10% to 35% incidence of islet cell antibodies in women with GDM as measured by immunofluorescence techniques, research using specific monoclonal antibodies has described a much lower incidence, on the order of 1% to 2%,[14] which suggests a low risk for type 1 diabetes in women with GDM. Furthermore, postpartum studies of women with GDM have demonstrated defects in insulin secretory response and decreased insulin sensitivity, indicating that typical type 2 abnormalities in glucose metabolism are present in women with GDM. The alterations in insulin secretory response and insulin resistance in women with a previous history of GDM compared with a weight-matched control group may differ depending on whether the women with previous GDM are lean or obese.[15] Thus in women with GDM, the hormonal events of pregnancy may represent an unmasking of a genetic susceptibility to type 2 diabetes.

Significant alterations in glucose metabolism are found in women who develop GDM relative to women with normal glucose tolerance. Decreased insulin response to a glucose challenge has been demonstrated by Yen, Fisher, and Buchanan and their colleagues in women with GDM in late gestation. In prospective longitudinal studies of both lean and obese women with GDM, Catalano and associates[5] also showed a progressive decrease in first-phase insulin response in late gestation in lean women who develop GDM compared with a weight-matched control group (Fig. 40-7). In contrast, in obese women who develop GDM, no difference in first-phase insulin response was reported, but rather a significant increase was seen in second-phase insulin response to an IV glucose challenge compared with that of a weight-matched control group (see Fig. 40-7). These differences in insulin response may be related to the ethnicity of the various study groups. Although the metabolic clearance rate of insulin is increased with advancing gestation, no evidence suggests that a significant difference exists between women with normal glucose tolerance and those with GDM.[6]

Fasting glucose concentrations decrease with advancing gestation in women who develop mild GDM. In late pregnancy, however, hepatic glucose production increases in women with GDM in comparison with a matched control group.[5,6] In late gestation, women with GDM have increased fasting insulin concentrations (Fig. 40-8) and less suppression of hepatic glucose production during insulin infusion, thereby indicating decreased hepatic glucose insulin sensitivity in women with GDM compared with a weight-matched control group.[5,6,16] In the studies of Xiang and associates,[16] a significant correlation was found between fasting FFA concentrations and hepatic glucose production, which suggests that increased FFA concentrations may contribute to hepatic insulin resistance.

Women with GDM have decreased insulin sensitivity in comparison with weight-matched control groups. Ryan and colleagues[7] were the first to report a 40% decrease in insulin sensitivity in women with GDM compared with a pregnant control group in late pregnancy using a hyperinsulinemic-euglycemic clamp. Xiang and associates[16] found that women with GDM who had normal glucose tolerance within 6 months of delivery had significantly decreased insulin sensitivity as estimated by the glucose clearance rate during a hyperinsulinemic-euglycemic clamp compared with that of a matched control group. Using similar techniques, Catalano and coworkers[5,6] described the longitudinal changes in insulin sensitivity in both lean and obese women who developed GDM in comparison with a matched control group. Women who developed GDM had decreased insulin sensitivity compared with that of the matched control group (Fig. 40-9). The differences in insulin sensitivity were greatest before and during early gestation; by late gestation, the differences in insulin sensitivity between the

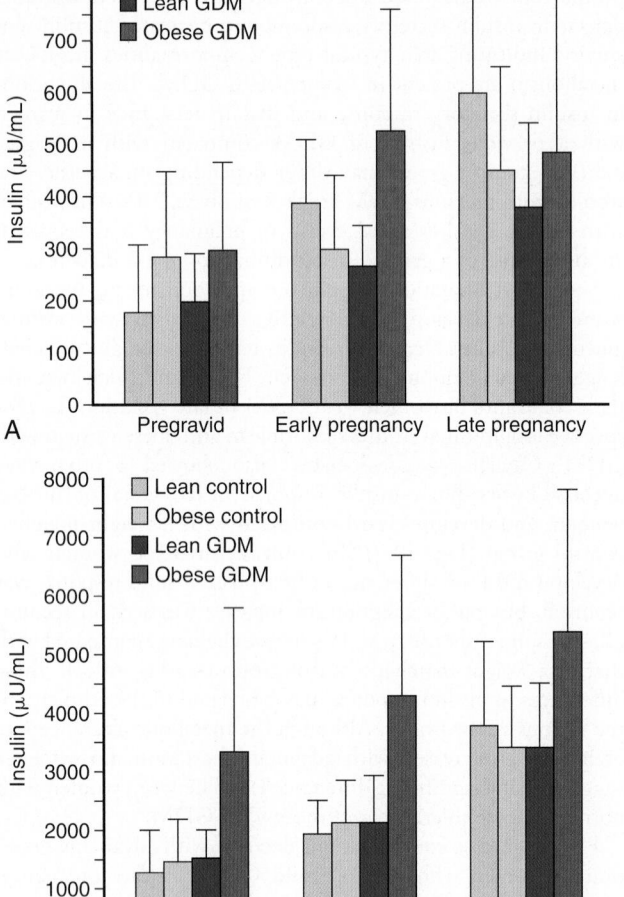

FIG 40-7 Longitudinal increase in insulin response to an intravenous glucose challenge in lean and obese women with normal glucose tolerance and gestational diabetes mellitus (GDM): pregravid and early and late pregnancy. **A,** First phase: area under the curve from 0 to 5 minutes. **B,** Second phase: area under the curve from 5 to 60 minutes.

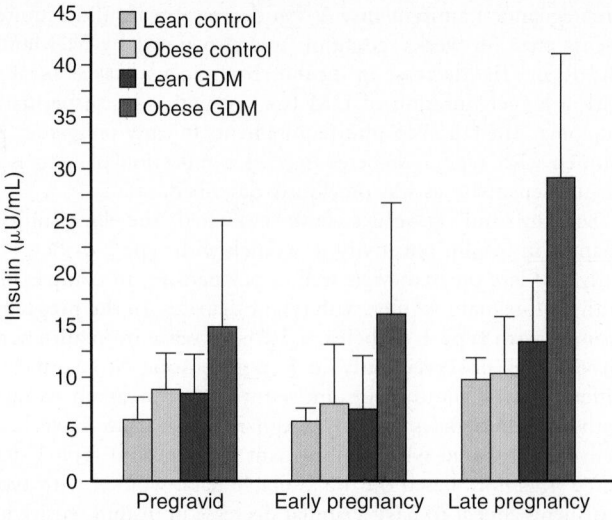

FIG 40-8 Longitudinal increase in basal or fasting insulin (μg/mL) in lean and obese women with normal glucose tolerance and gestational diabetes mellitus (GDM): pregravid and early and late pregnancy.

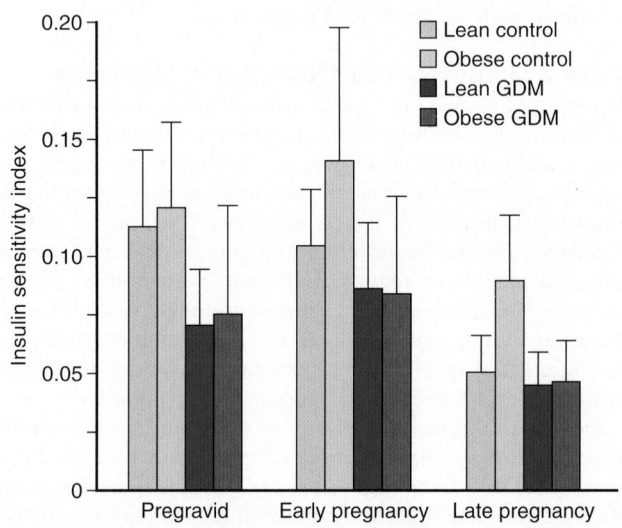

FIG 40-9 Longitudinal changes in the insulin sensitivity index (glucose infusion rate adjusted for residual endogenous glucose production and insulin concentrations achieved during the glucose clamp) in lean and obese women with normal glucose tolerance and gestational diabetes mellitus (GDM): pregravid and early and late pregnancy.

groups were less pronounced but still significant. Of interest, an increase in insulin sensitivity was noted from the time before conception through early pregnancy (12 to 14 weeks), particularly in those women with the greatest decreases in insulin sensitivity before conception. **The changes in insulin sensitivity from the time before conception through early pregnancy were significantly correlated with changes in maternal weight gain and energy expenditure.** The relationship between these alterations in maternal glucose insulin sensitivity and weight gain and energy expenditure may help explain the decrease in maternal weight gain and insulin requirements in women with diabetes in early gestation.[1] In summary, the various degrees of decreased insulin sensitivity observed in late pregnancy in women with normal glucose tolerance or gestational diabetes are but a reflection of their individual prepregnancy insulin sensitivity. Unless unforeseen severe metabolic events occur during pregnancy, relatively uniform decreases are apparent in insulin sensitivity with advancing gestation in all women.

The interactions of β-cell response and insulin sensitivity are hallmarks of the metabolic adaptations of pregnancy. As described by Bergman, the relationship between insulin response and insulin resistance is fixed in nonpregnant individuals and follows a hyperbolic curve (i.e., the disposition index [DI]; Fig. 40-10). Buchanan described a similar relationship between insulin response and insulin action during pregnancy. Indeed, when the DI has been compared between women with normal glucose tolerance and GDM both during and after pregnancy, the failure of the β-cell to compensate for insulin resistance in GDM has been similar to the hyperbolic changes in the control group (see Fig. 40-10). This relationship between insulin sensitivity and insulin resistance, however, may not hold in early pregnancy, when both an increase in insulin sensitivity and insulin response may be evident.

Studies in human skeletal muscle and adipose tissue have demonstrated that postreceptor defects in the insulin-signaling cascade are related to decreased insulin sensitivity in pregnancy.

Garvey and colleagues were the first to demonstrate that there were no significant differences in the glucose transporter (GLUT4) responsible for insulin action and skeletal muscle in pregnant compared with nonpregnant women. Based on the studies of Friedman and colleagues[17] in pregnant women with normal glucose tolerance and GDM, as well as in weight-matched nonpregnant control subjects, defects were apparent in the insulin-signaling cascade relating to pregnancy and to what may be additional abnormalities in women with gestational diabetes. **All pregnant women appeared to have a decrease in expression of insulin receptor substrate 1 (IRS1).** The down-regulation of the IRS1 protein closely parallels the decreased ability of insulin to induce additional steps in the insulin-signaling cascade, which results in movement of the GLUT4 to the cell surface membrane to facilitate glucose transport into the cell. The downregulation of IRS1 protein closely parallels the ability of insulin to stimulate 2-deoxyglucose uptake in vitro. In addition to the previous mechanisms, **women with GDM demonstrate a distinct decrease in the ability of insulin**

receptor-β, **that component of the insulin receptor not on the cell surface, to undergo tyrosine phosphorylation. The additional defect in the insulin-signaling cascade results in a 25% lower glucose transport activity** (Fig. 40-11).

Amino Acid Metabolism

Although glucose is the primary source of energy for the fetus and placenta, no appreciable amounts of glucose are stored as glycogen in the fetus or placenta. However, accretion of protein is essential for growth of fetoplacental tissue. Nitrogen retention is increased in pregnancy in both maternal and fetal compartments, and this increase results in about 0.9 kg of maternal fat-free mass by 27 weeks.[18] A significant decrease is apparent in most basal maternal amino acid concentrations in early pregnancy before the accretion of significant maternal or fetal tissue. These anticipatory changes in amino acid metabolism occur after a shorter period of fasting in comparison with nonpregnant women and may be another example of the accelerated starvation of pregnancy described by Freinkel and coworkers.[19] Furthermore, amino acid concentrations, such as of serine, correlate significantly with fetal growth in both early and late gestation.[20] Maternal amino acid concentrations were significantly decreased in mothers of small-for-gestational-age (SGA) neonates in comparison with maternal amino acid concentrations in appropriately grown neonates.

Based on a review of various studies, Duggleby and Jackson have estimated that during pregnancy, protein synthesis is similar to that in nonpregnant women in the first trimester. **However, a 15% increase in protein synthesis occurs during the second trimester, and a further increase is seen in the third trimester, by about 25%.** Additionally, interindividual differences at each time point are marked, and these differences have a strong relationship with fetal growth: mothers who had increased protein turnover in midpregnancy had babies who had increased lean body mass after adjustment for important covariables.

Amino acids can be used for protein accrual or they can be oxidized as an energy source. Estimation of urea synthesis using stable isotopes has been performed in a number of studies. In general, a modest shift in oxidation occurs in early pregnancy with an accrual of amino acids for protein synthesis in late

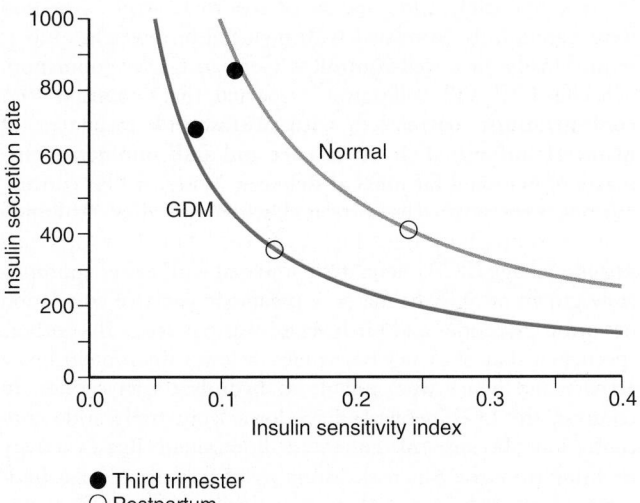

● Third trimester
○ Postpartum

FIG 40-10 Insulin sensitivity index. GDM, gestational diabetes mellitus.

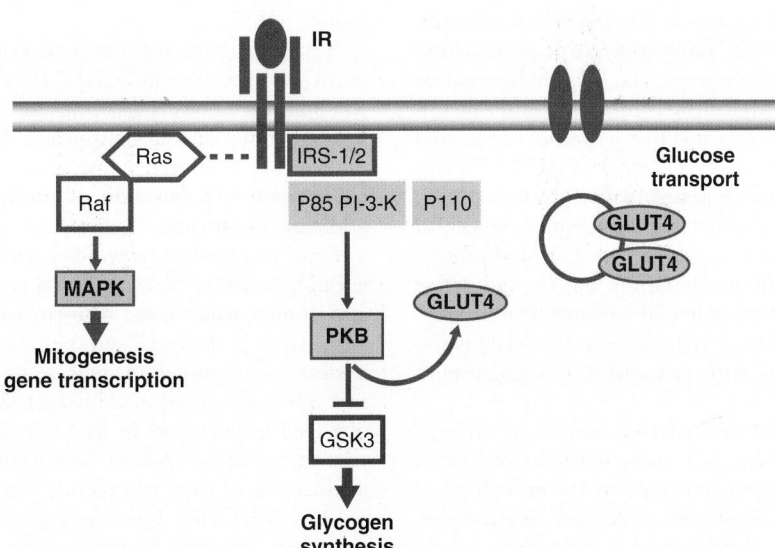

FIG 40-11 Schematic model of insulin-signaling cascade in skeletal muscle. GLUT, glucose transporter; IR, insulin receptor; IRS, insulin receptor substrate.

gestation. Kalhan and colleagues reported significant pregnancy-related adaptations in maternal protein metabolism early in gestation before any significant increase in fetal protein accretion. Catalano and associates have also reported decreased amino acid insulin sensitivity based on a decreased suppression of leucine turnover during insulin infusion in late gestation. Some evidence suggests an increase in basal leucine turnover in women with GDM compared with that of a matched control group. Whether these decreases in amino acid insulin sensitivity are related to decreased whole-body and liver protein synthesis or increased breakdown are not known at this time.

Cetin and associates reported that placental amino acid exchange is altered in pregnancies complicated by GDM. Ornithine concentrations were significantly increased in women with GDM compared with controls, and in the cord blood of infants of women with GDM, significant increases were observed in multiple amino acids, including phenylalanine and leucine, but decreases in glutamate were also found. The investigators speculate that in infants of women with GDM, the altered in utero fetal milieu affects fetal growth through multiple mechanisms that affect various nutrient compartments.

Amino acids are actively transported across the placenta from mother to fetus through energy-requiring amino acid transporters. These transporters are highly stereospecific, but they have low substrate specificity. Additionally, they may vary in location between the microvillus and basal membranes. Decreased amino acid concentrations have been reported in growth-restricted neonates in comparison with appropriately grown neonates, and decreased amino acid transporter activity has been implicated as a possible mechanism. However, the potential role, if any, of placental amino acid transporters in the development of fetal macrosomia in women with diabetes is currently unknown.

Lipid Metabolism

Although ample literature supports the changes in glucose metabolism during gestation, the data regarding the alterations in lipid metabolism are meager by comparison. Darmady and Postle[21] measured serum cholesterol and triglyceride before, during, and after pregnancy in 34 normal women and observed a decrease in both cholesterol and triglyceride at about 7 weeks' gestation. Both of the levels increased progressively until term, and then a decrease was seen in serum triglyceride postpartum. The decrease was more rapid in women who breastfed compared with those women who bottle-fed their infants.[21] Additionally, Knopp and coworkers[22] have reported that a twofold to fourfold increase occurs in total triglyceride concentration and a 25% to 50% increase is seen in total cholesterol concentration during gestation. A 50% increase in low-density lipoprotein (LDL) cholesterol and a 30% increase in high-density lipoprotein (HDL) cholesterol is seen by midgestation, but these decrease slightly in the third trimester. Maternal triglyceride and very-low-density lipoprotein (VLDL) triglyceride levels in late gestation are positively correlated with maternal estriol and insulin concentrations.

A study by Vahratian and associates examined the changes in lipid levels during pregnancy in normal-weight compared with overweight and obese women from 6 to 10 through 32 to 36 weeks' gestation. The levels of total cholesterol, triglycerides, and LDL and HDL cholesterol increased throughout gestation. Although the concentrations in the overweight and obese women were generally higher in early pregnancy, the rate of change of LDL cholesterol and total cholesterol was lower in later gestation.

FFAs have been associated with fetal overgrowth, particularly of fetal adipose tissue. A significant difference in the arteriovenous FFA concentration is seen at birth, much the same as with arteriovenous glucose concentration. Multiple clinical studies suggest the contribution of maternal lipids to fetal growth and in particular to adiposity. Knopp and coworkers[22] reported that neonatal birthweight was positively correlated with triglyceride and FFA concentrations in late pregnancy. Similar conclusions were reached by Ogburn and colleagues, who showed that insulin concentrations decrease FFA concentrations, inhibit lipolysis, and result in increased fat deposition. Kleigman reported that infants of obese women had an increased birthweight and skinfold thickness and higher FFA levels compared with infants of lean women. DiCianni and associates[23] reported that in women with a positive glucose screen but normal glucose tolerance, their serum triglycerides and prepregnancy body mass index (BMI) had a significant correlation with birthweight at term. In Australia, Nolan and coworkers showed that nonfasting maternal triglycerides measured at 9 to 12 weeks' gestation were significantly correlated with neonatal birthweight ratio at term. Finally, in a well-controlled German GDM population, Schaeffer-Graf and colleagues[24] reported that **maternal FFA concentrations correlated with ultrasound estimates of neonatal abdominal circumference and anthropometric estimates of neonatal fat mass at delivery.** Maternal FFA concentrations were positively correlated with cord FFA. Although FFA concentrations were higher in cord blood of large-for-gestational-age (LGA) neonates compared with either appropriately grown or SGA neonates, a paradoxic negative correlation of cord triglycerides and birthweight was reported. The authors speculated that SGA newborns have a lower lipoprotein lipase activity and hence were unable to hydrolyze triglycerides. In contrast, the LGA neonates have lower cord triglyceride concentrations because of enhanced lipoprotein lipase activity resulting from their increased number of fat cells. Similar findings were noted by Merzouk and coworkers in growth-restricted infants. Lastly, the placentae of women with GDM have increased expression of genes related to inflammation and lipid metabolism in comparison with those of a BMI-matched control group.

In summary, in women with evidence of decreased insulin sensitivity (obesity and/or GDM) in addition to glucose, maternal lipid metabolism accounts for a significant proportion of fetal growth, particularly adiposity. These data support the original work by **Freinkel,[25] which proposed that fetal growth or overgrowth is a function of multiple nutritional factors in addition to glucose.**

Lipid metabolism in women with diabetes mellitus is influenced by whether the woman has type 1 or type 2 diabetes. This also applies when these women become pregnant. In women with type 2 diabetes and gestational diabetes, Knopp and coworkers[22] reported an increase in triglyceride and a decrease in HDL concentration. However, Montelongo and colleagues observed little change in FFA concentrations through all three trimesters after a 12-hour fast. Koukkou and coworkers noted an increase in total triglyceride but lower LDL cholesterol in women with GDM. Increased triglyceride concentrations during pregnancy have also been reported to be related to the development of GDM and preeclampsia in women with normal pregravid glucose tolerance, both of which are related to increased insulin resistance. In women with type 1 diabetes, no change was observed in total triglycerides, but a lower cholesterol concentration was reported secondary to a decrease in HDL. This is of interest because HDL acts as a plasma antioxidant, and thus a lower HDL level may be related to the increase in congenital malformations in women with type 1 diabetes. Oxidative stress has been implicated as a potential factor in the incidence of anomalies in women with type 1 diabetes.

Hyperinsulinemic-euglycemic clamp studies in pregnant women with normal glucose tolerance and GDM revealed a decreased ability of insulin to suppress plasma FFAs with advancing gestation. Insulin's ability to suppress plasma FFAs was lower in women with GDM compared with women with normal glucose tolerance.

Taken together, these studies demonstrate decreased nutrient insulin sensitivity in all women with advancing gestation. These decreases in insulin sensitivity are further exacerbated by the presence of decreased pregravid maternal insulin sensitivity, which manifests in later pregnancy as GDM and results in greater nutrient availability and higher ambient insulin concentrations for the developing fetoplacental unit, which may eventually result in fetal overgrowth.

Maternal Weight Gain and Energy Expenditure

Estimates of the energy cost of pregnancy range from a cost of 80,000 kcal to a net savings of up to 10,000 kcal.[26] As a result, the recommendations for nutritional intake in pregnancy differ and depend on the population being evaluated. Furthermore, recommendations for individuals within a population may be more diverse than previously believed, making general guidelines for nutritional intake difficult.

The theoretic energy cost of pregnancy was originally estimated by Hytten and Leitch[18] using a factorial method. The additional cost of pregnancy consisted of (1) the additional maternal and fetoplacental tissue accrued during pregnancy and (2) the additional "running cost" of pregnancy (e.g., the work of increased cardiac output). In Hytten's model, the greatest increases in maternal energy expenditure occur between 10 and 30 weeks' gestation, primarily because of maternal accretion of adipose tissue. However, the mean increases in maternal adipose tissue vary considerably among various ethnic groups. Forsum and associates reported a mean increase of more than 5 kg of adipose tissue in Swedish women, whereas Lawrence and colleagues found no increase in adipose tissue stores in women from the Gambia.

Basal metabolic rate accounts for 60% to 70% of total energy expenditure in individuals not engaged in competitive physical activity, and this correlates well with total energy expenditure. As with the changes in maternal accretion of adipose tissue, wide variations are seen in the change in maternal basal metabolic rate during gestation, not only in different populations but again within relatively homogeneous groups. The cumulative energy changes in basal metabolic rate range from a high of 52,000 kcal in Swedish women to a net savings of 10,700 kcal in women from the Gambia without nutritional supplementation. **The mean increase in basal metabolic rate in Western women relative to a nonpregnant, nonlactating control group averages about 20% to 25%.** However, the coefficient of variation of basal metabolic rate ranges from 93% in women in the United Kingdom to more than 200% in Swedish women.[27] When assessing energy intake in relation to energy expenditure,

however, estimated energy intake remains lower than the estimates of total energy expenditure. These discrepancies have usually been explained by factors such as increased metabolic efficiency during gestation, decreased maternal activity, and unreliable assessment of food intake.[26]

Data in nonpregnant subjects may help explain some of the wide variations in metabolic parameters during human gestation, even with homogeneous populations. Swinburn and colleagues reported that in the Pima Indian population, subjects with decreased insulin sensitivity gained less weight compared with more insulin-sensitive subjects (3.1 vs. 7.6 kg) over a period of 4 years. Furthermore, the percentage weight change per year was highly correlated with glucose disposal as estimated from clamp studies. Catalano and coworkers[28] evaluated the changes in maternal accretion of body fat and basal metabolic rate in lean and obese women with normal GDM. Women who developed GDM had decreased insulin sensitivity in early gestation compared with a matched control group and had significantly smaller increases in body fat than women with normal glucose tolerance. A significant inverse correlation was found between the changes in fat accretion and insulin sensitivity (i.e., women with decreased pregravid insulin sensitivity had less accretion of body fat compared with women with increased pregravid insulin sensitivity).

In the basal state, lean women increase the use of carbohydrate as a metabolic fuel, whereas in obese women, there is an increased use of lipids for oxidative needs. However, with the decrease in insulin sensitivity in late gestation, all women have an increase in fat oxidation and decrease in nonoxidative glucose metabolism (storage). These increases in lipid oxidation are positively correlated with the increases in maternal leptin concentrations, possibly accounting for a role of leptin in human pregnancy. The result of these studies emphasize that an inverse relationship exists between the changes in maternal insulin sensitivity and accretion of adipose tissue in early gestation. The ability of women with decreased pregravid glucose insulin sensitivity (obese women and women with GDM) to conserve energy, not significantly increase body fat, and make sufficient nutrients available to produce a healthy fetus supports the hypothesis that decreased maternal insulin sensitivity may have a reproductive metabolic advantage in women when food availability is marginal (i.e., the thrifty gene hypothesis). In contrast, decreased maternal insulin sensitivity before conception in areas where food is plentiful and a sedentary lifestyle is more common and may manifest as GDM, and this increases the long-term risk for both diabetes and obesity in the woman and her offspring.[28]

PERINATAL MORBIDITY AND MORTALITY
Fetal Death

In the past, sudden and unexplained stillbirth occurred in 10% to 30% of pregnancies complicated by type 1 DM, also called *insulin-dependent diabetes mellitus* (IDDM). Although relatively uncommon today, such losses still plague the pregnancies of patients who do not receive optimal care. Mathiesen and colleagues[29] reported 25 stillbirths among 1361 singleton births of women with type 1 diabetes. In this series, the offspring of women with type 1 or type 2 diabetes were five times more likely to be stillborn compared with those of mothers without diabetes. Stillbirths have been observed most often after the 36th week of pregnancy in patients with poor glycemic control, hydramnios, fetal macrosomia, vascular disease, or preeclampsia. Women with vascular complications may develop fetal growth restriction (FGR) and intrauterine fetal demise (IUFD) as early as the second trimester.

Excessive stillbirth rates in pregnancies complicated by diabetes have been linked to chronic intrauterine hypoxia.[30] Extramedullary hematopoiesis, frequently observed in stillborn infants of diabetic mothers (IDMs), supports chronic intrauterine hypoxia as a likely cause of these intrauterine fetal deaths. Studies of fetal umbilical cord blood samples in pregnant women with type 1 diabetes have demonstrated relative fetal erythremia and lactic acidemia. Maternal diabetes may also produce alterations in red blood cell (RBC) oxygen release and placental blood flow. Reduced uterine blood flow is thought to contribute to the increased incidence of intrauterine growth restriction (IUGR) observed in pregnancies complicated by diabetic vasculopathy. Ketoacidosis and preeclampsia, two factors known to be associated with an increased incidence of intrauterine deaths, may further decrease uterine blood flow.

Alterations in fetal carbohydrate metabolism also may contribute to intrauterine asphyxia. Considerable evidence links hyperinsulinemia and fetal hypoxia. Hyperinsulinemia induced in fetal lambs by an infusion of exogenous insulin produces an increase in oxygen consumption and a decrease in arterial oxygen content.[30] Persistent maternal-fetal hyperglycemia occurs independent of maternal uterine blood flow, which may not be increased enough to allow for enhanced oxygen delivery in the face of increased metabolic demands. Thus hyperinsulinemia in the fetus of the diabetic mother appears to increase the metabolic rate and oxygen requirement in the fetus. Other factors such as hyperglycemia, ketoacidosis, preeclampsia, and maternal vasculopathy can also reduce placental blood flow and fetal oxygenation.

Congenital Malformations

Congenital malformations are the most important cause of perinatal loss in pregnancies complicated by type 1 and type 2 DM. In the past, these anomalies were responsible for only 10% of all perinatal deaths. Malformations now account for 30% to 50% of perinatal mortality. Neonatal deaths exceed stillbirths in pregnancies complicated by pregestational DM, and fatal congenital malformations are responsible for this pattern.

Most studies have documented a two to sixfold increase in major malformations in infants of type 1 and type 2 diabetic mothers. A large population-based cohort study of Canadian women revealed a 23% decline in congenital malformations in diabetic pregnancies from 1996 through 2010; however, the relative risk (RR) for malformations remained elevated in women with preexisting diabetes (RR, 2.33; 95% confidence interval [CI], 1.59 to 3.43). In a prospective analysis, Simpson and associates observed an 8.5% incidence of major anomalies in the diabetic population, whereas the malformation rate in a small group of concurrently gathered control subjects was 2.4%. Similar figures were obtained in the Diabetes in Early Pregnancy Study in the United States. The incidence of major anomalies was 2.1% in 389 control patients and 9% in 279 diabetic women. A recent case-control study of 13,030 infants with congenital anomalies and 4895 controls revealed a prevalence in type 1 diabetes of 2.2% versus 0.5% and in type 2 diabetes of 5.1% versus 3.7% in controls. In general, the incidence of major malformations in worldwide

TABLE 40-2	FREQUENCY OF CONGENITAL MALFORMATIONS IN INFANTS OF DIABETIC MOTHERS	
STUDY (YEAR)	***N***	**%**
Mills et al[97] (1988)	25/279	9.0
Greene[98] (1993)	35/451	7.7
Steel[99] (1982)	12/239	7.8
Fuhrmann et al[100] (1983)	22/292	7.5
Simpson et al[101] (1983)	9/106	8.5
Albert et al[102] (1996)	29/289	10.0

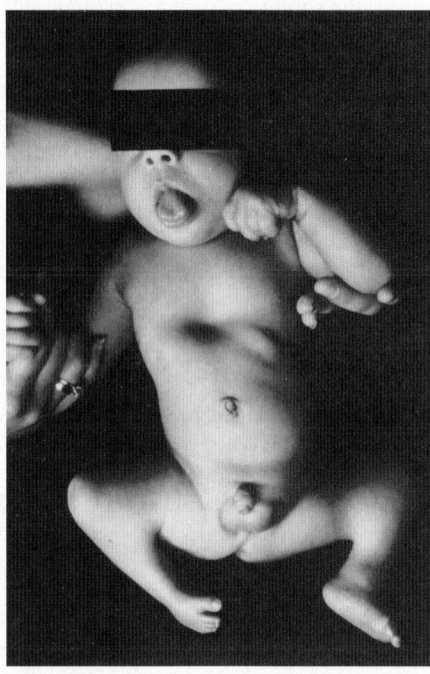

FIG 40-12 Infant of a diabetic mother with sacral agenesis and hypoplastic lower extremities.

studies of offspring of diabetic women has ranged from 7.5% to 10% (Table 40-2).

The insult that causes malformations in IDMs affects most organ systems and must act before the seventh week of gestation. Central nervous system malformations—particularly anencephaly, open spina bifida, and holoprosencephaly—are increased tenfold. Cardiac anomalies are the most common malformations seen in IDMs, with ventricular septal defects and complex lesions such as transposition of the great vessels increased fivefold. The congenital defect thought to be most characteristic of diabetic embryopathy is sacral agenesis or caudal dysplasia, an anomaly found 200 to 400 times more often in offspring of diabetic women (Fig. 40-12). However, this defect is not pathognomonic for diabetes because it also occurs in nondiabetic pregnancies.

Impaired glycemic control and associated derangements in maternal metabolism appear to contribute to abnormal embryogenesis. Maternal hyperglycemia has been proposed by most investigators as the primary teratogenic factor, but hyperketonemia, hypoglycemia, somatomedin inhibitor excess, and excess free oxygen radicals have also been suggested (Box 40-1). The profile of a woman most likely to produce an anomalous infant would include a patient with poor periconceptional glucose control, long-standing diabetes, and vascular disease.

BOX 40-1 PROPOSED FACTORS ASSOCIATED WITH TERATOGENESIS IN PREGNANCY COMPLICATED BY DIABETES MELLITUS

- Hyperglycemia
- Ketone body excess
- Somatomedin inhibition
- Arachidonic acid deficiency
- Free oxygen radical excess

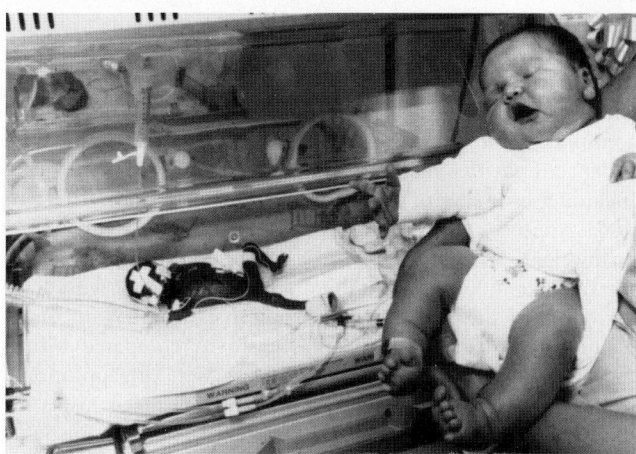

FIG 40-13 Two extremes of growth abnormalities in pregnancies complicated by diabetes mellitus. On the left is a severely growth-restricted infant, and on the right is a macrosomic infant.

Genetic susceptibility to the teratogenic influence of diabetes may also be a factor.

Several mechanisms have been proposed by which the previously mentioned teratogenic factors produce malformations. Freinkel and colleagues first suggested that anomalies might arise from inhibition of glycolysis, the key energy-producing process during embryogenesis. They found that the addition of D-mannose to the culture medium of rat embryos inhibited glycolysis and produced growth restriction and derangement of neural tube closure. Freinkel and colleagues stressed the sensitivity of normal embryogenesis to alterations in these key energy-producing pathways, a process he labeled "fuel-mediated" teratogenesis. Goldman and Baker suggested that the mechanism responsible for the increased incidence of neural tube defects (NTDs) in embryos cultured in a hyperglycemic medium may involve a functional deficiency of arachidonic acid, because supplementation with arachidonic acid or myo-inositol will reduce the frequency of NTDs in this experimental model. Pinter and Reece, along with Pinter and associates, confirmed these studies and demonstrated that hyperglycemia-induced alterations in neural tube closure include disordered cells, decreased mitoses, and changes indicative of premature maturation. Pinter and colleagues further demonstrated that hyperglycemia during organogenesis has a primary deleterious effect on yolk sac function with resultant embryopathy.

Altered oxidative metabolism from maternal diabetes may cause increased production of free oxygen radicals in the developing embryo, which are likely teratogenic. Supplementation of oxygen radical–scavenging enzymes, such as superoxide dismutase, to the culture medium of rat embryos protects against growth delay and excess malformations. It has been suggested that excess free oxygen radicals may have a direct effect on embryonic prostaglandin biosynthesis. Free oxygen radical excess may enhance lipid peroxidation, and in turn, generated hydroperoxides might stimulate thromboxane biosynthesis and might inhibit prostacyclin production, an imbalance that could have profound effects on embryonic development. Finally, oxidative stress in diabetic rats is associated with the accumulation of glycation products and altered vascular endothelial growth factor (VEGF) expression in cardiovascular regions of the developing heart associated with endocardial cushion defects.

Fetal Macrosomia

Macrosomia **has been variously defined as birthweight greater than 4000 to 4500 g, as well as LGA, in which birthweight is above the 90th percentile for population and sex-specific growth curves. Fetal macrosomia complicates as many as 50% of pregnancies in women with GDM and 40% of pregnancies complicated by type 1 and type 2 diabetes, which includes some women treated with intensive glycemic control** (Fig. 40-13). Delivery of an infant weighing greater than 4500 g occurs 10 times more often in women with diabetes compared with a population of women with normal glucose tolerance.

According to the Pedersen hypothesis, maternal hyperglycemia results in fetal hyperglycemia and hyperinsulinemia, which results in excessive fetal growth. Increased fetal β-cell mass may be identified as early as the second trimester. Evidence in support of the Pedersen hypothesis has come from the studies of amniotic fluid and cord blood insulin and C-peptide concentrations. Both are increased in the amniotic fluid of insulin-treated women with diabetes at term and correlate with neonatal fat mass. Lipids and amino acids, which are elevated in pregnancies complicated by GDM, may also play a role in excessive fetal growth by either stimulating the release of insulin and other growth factors from the fetal pancreatic β-cells and placenta or by providing the necessary nutrients for excessive fetal growth. **Infants of mothers with GDM have an increase in fat mass, compared with fat-free mass, in comparison with infants of women with normal glucose tolerance. Additionally, the growth is disproportionate, with chest-to-head and shoulder-to-head ratios larger than those of infants of women with normal glucose tolerance.** These anthropometric differences may contribute to the higher rate of shoulder dystocia and birth trauma observed in these infants.

The results of several clinical series have validated the Pedersen hypothesis inasmuch as tight maternal glycemic control has been associated with a reduction in macrosomia and, in particular, with a reduction in fat mass. Using daily capillary glucose values obtained during the second and third trimesters in women who required insulin, Landon and colleagues reported a rate of 9% for macrosomia when mean values were below 110 mg/dL compared with 34% when less optimal control was achieved. Jovanovic and associates have suggested that 1-hour postprandial glucose measurements correlate best with the frequency of macrosomia. After controlling for other factors, these authors noted that the strongest prediction for birthweight was third-trimester nonfasting glucose measurements.

In a series of metabolic studies, Catalano and associates[31] estimated body composition in 186 neonates using anthropometry. Fat-free mass, which represented 86% of mean birthweight, accounted for 83% of the variance in birthweight; and fat mass, which made up only 14% of birthweight, accounted for 46% of the variance in birthweight. In addition, significantly greater fat-free mass was observed in male compared with female infants. Using independent variables such as maternal height, pregravid weight, weight gain during pregnancy, parity, paternal height and weight, neonatal sex, and gestational age, the authors accounted for 29% of the variance in birthweight, 30% of the variance in fat-free mass, and 17% of the variance in fat mass. Including estimates of maternal insulin sensitivity in 16 additional subjects, they were able to explain 48% of the variance in birthweight, 53% of the variance in fat-free mass, and 46% of the variance in fat mass. Studies by Caruso and colleagues have corroborated these findings, reporting that women with unexplained FGR had greater insulin sensitivity compared with a control group of women whose infants were an appropriate weight for their gestational age. The potential mechanisms for this relate to the possibility that maternal circulating nutrients for glucose, FFAs, and amino acids available for placental transport to the fetus are decreased because of the relative increase in maternal insulin sensitivity. A positive correlation between birthweight and weight gain has been observed in women with normal glucose tolerance. The correlation was strongest in women who were lean before conception, and it became progressively weaker as pregravid weight for height increased. In women with GDM, no significant correlations were found between maternal weight gain and birthweight irrespective of pregravid weight for height. Although these studies emphasize the role of the maternal metabolic environment and fetal growth, Kim and colleagues[32] have reported that GDM actually contributed the least (2.0% to 8.0%) to the development of LGA infants in a general obstetric population, whereas excessive gestational weight gain contributed the most (33.3% to 37.7%).

Normalization of birthweight in infants of women with GDM, however, may in itself not help those infants achieve optimal growth. In a study of approximately 400 infants of women with normal glucose tolerance and GDM, Catalano and coworkers[31] showed that the infants of women with GDM had increased fat mass, but not lean body mass or weight, compared with a control group even after adjustment for potential confounding variables (Table 40-3). Similarly, when only infants who were an appropriate size for their gestational age (i.e., between the 10th and 90th percentiles) were examined, the infants of the women with GDM had significantly greater fat mass and percentage of body fat but had less lean mass compared with the control group, and no difference was observed in birthweight. Of note, in the infants of the women with GDM, the strongest correlations with fat mass were fasting glucose and gestational age; this accounted for 17% of the variance in infant fat mass.

Hypoglycemia

Neonatal hypoglycemia, a blood glucose level less than 35 to 40 mg/dL during the first 12 hours of life, results from a rapid drop in plasma glucose concentrations following clamping of the umbilical cord. Hypoglycemia, a byproduct of hyperinsulinemia, is particularly common in macrosomic newborns, in whom rates exceed 50%. We have observed an overall rate of 27% in offspring of diabetic women delivered at our institution. The degree of hypoglycemia may be influenced by at least two factors: maternal glucose control during the latter half of pregnancy during labor and delivery. Prior poor maternal glucose control can result in fetal β-cell hyperplasia, which leads to exaggerated insulin release following delivery. IDMs who exhibit hypoglycemia have elevated cord C-peptide and free insulin levels at birth and show an exaggerated pancreatic response to glucose loading. The hyperinsulinemia and resultant hypoglycemia typically lasts for several days following birth.

Respiratory Distress Syndrome

Experimental animal studies have provided evidence that hyperglycemia and hyperinsulinemia can affect pulmonary surfactant biosynthesis, and in vitro studies have documented that insulin can interfere with substrate availability for surfactant biosynthesis. Insulin excess may interfere with the normal timing of glucocorticoid-induced pulmonary maturation in the fetus. Cortisol apparently acts on pulmonary fibroblasts to induce synthesis of fibroblast-pneumocyte factor, which then acts on type II cells to stimulate phospholipid synthesis. Carlson and coworkers demonstrated that insulin blocks cortisol action at the level of the fibroblast by reducing the production of fibroblast-pneumocyte factor.

Clinical studies to investigate the effect of maternal diabetes on fetal lung maturation have produced conflicting data. The role of amniocentesis in determining fetal lung maturity is discussed with timing and mode of delivery. Several studies suggest that in women with well-controlled diabetes whose fetus is delivered at 38 to 39 weeks' gestation, the risk for respiratory distress syndrome (RDS) is no higher than that observed in the general population. Kjos and Walther[33] studied the outcome of 526 diabetic gestations delivered within 5 days of amniotic fluid fetal lung maturation testing and reported hyaline membrane disease (HMD) in five neonates (0.95%), all of whom were delivered before 34 weeks' gestation. Mimouni and associates compared outcomes of 127 IDMs with matched controls and concluded that well-controlled diabetes in pregnancy is not a direct risk factor for the development of RDS. Yet cesarean delivery not preceded by labor and prematurity, both of which are increased in diabetic pregnancies, clearly increases the likelihood of neonatal respiratory disease. With cesarean delivery, many of these cases represent retained lung fluid or transient tachypnea of the newborn, which usually resolves within the first days of life.

Calcium and Magnesium Metabolism

Neonatal hypocalcemia, with serum levels below 7 mg/dL or an ionized level less than 4 mg/dL, occurs at an increased rate in IDMs when controlling for predisposing factors such as prematurity and birth asphyxia. With modern management, the frequency of neonatal hypocalcemia is less than 5% in IDMs. Hypocalcemia in IDMs has been associated with a failure to increase parathyroid hormone synthesis following birth. Decreased serum magnesium levels have also been documented in pregnant diabetic women as well as in their infants. Mimouni and associates described reduced amniotic fluid magnesium

TABLE 40-3	NEONATAL BODY COMPOSITION		
	GDM (N = 195)	**NGT (N = 220)**	**P VALUE**
Weight (g)	3398 ± 550	3337 ± 549	.26
FFM (g)	2962 ± 405	2975 ± 408	.74
Fat mass (g)	436 ± 206	362 ± 198	.0002
Body fat	12.4 ± 4.6	10.4 ± 4.6	.0001

Modified from Catalano PM, Tyzbir ED, Allen SR, et al. Evaluation of fetal growth by estimation of body composition. *Obstet Gynecol.* 1987;156:1089.
FFM, fat-free mass; *GDM,* gestational diabetes mellitus; *NGT,* normal glucose tolerance.

concentrations in women with type 1 DM. These findings may be explained by a drop in fetal urinary magnesium excretion, which would accompany a relative magnesium-deficient state. Paradoxically, magnesium deficiency may then inhibit fetal parathyroid hormone secretion.

Hyperbilirubinemia and Polycythemia

Hyperbilirubinemia is frequently observed in the IDM. Neonatal jaundice has been reported in as many as 25% to 53% of pregnancies complicated by pregestational DM and 38% of pregnancies in women with GDM. Jaundice observed in IDMs can be attributed largely to prematurity. However, jaundice is also increased in macrosomic IDMs.

Although severe hyperbilirubinemia may be observed independent of polycythemia, a common pathway for these complications most likely involves increased RBC production, which is stimulated by increased erythropoietin (EPO) in the IDM. Presumably, the major stimulus for red cell production is a state of relative hypoxia in utero. Cord EPO levels generally are normal in IDMs whose mothers demonstrate good glycemic control during gestation; however, hemoglobin A1c (HbA1c) values in late pregnancy are significantly elevated in mothers of hyperbilirubinemic infants.

Cardiomyopathy

A transient form of cardiomyopathy may occur in IDMs. Among symptomatic infants, septal hypertrophy may cause left ventricular outflow obstruction. Although most infants are asymptomatic, respiratory distress or signs of cardiac failure may arise. Cardiac hypertrophy likely results from fetal hyperinsulinemia, which leads to fat and glycogen deposition in the myocardium. Thus cardiomyopathy generally occurs in pregnancies complicated by macrosomia in which glucose levels are poorly controlled. Elevated levels of B-type natriuretic peptide (BNP) produced during cardiac stress have been reported in umbilical blood of IDMs and have been correlated with maternal glycemic control. In most cases, symptoms of cardiomyopathy improve over several weeks with supportive care, and echocardiographic changes resolve as well.

MATERNAL CLASSIFICATION AND RISK ASSESSMENT

Priscilla White first noted that the patient's age at onset of diabetes, the duration of the disease, and the presence of vasculopathy significantly influenced perinatal outcome. Her classification system has been widely applied to pregnant women with diabetes, and a modification of this scheme is presented in Table 40-1. Counseling a patient and formulating a plan of management requires assessment of both maternal and fetal risk. The White classification may facilitate this evaluation, yet consideration of glycemic control in early pregnancy is also vital to risk assessment.

Class A₁ DM includes those women who have demonstrated carbohydrate intolerance during an oral glucose tolerance test (GTT); however, their fasting and postprandial glucose levels are maintained within physiologic range by dietary regulation alone. Class A₂ includes women with GDM who require medical management that consists of insulin or oral hypoglycemic therapy in response to repetitive elevations of fasting or postpartum glucose levels following dietary intervention.

Two international workshop conferences on gestational diabetes sponsored by the American Diabetes Association (ADA) in cooperation with the American College of Obstetricians and Gynecologists (ACOG) recommended that the term *gestational diabetes,* rather than *class A diabetes,* be used to describe women with carbohydrate intolerance of variable severity with onset or recognition during the present pregnancy. The definition applies whether insulin or only diet modification is used for treatment and whether the condition persists after pregnancy. It does not exclude the possibility that unrecognized glucose intolerance may have antedated the pregnancy or may have begun with pregnancy. **The increasing frequency of type 2 diabetes has drawn attention to the need to distinguish diabetes first identified in early pregnancy as most likely representing cases of "overt diabetes."** The term *gestational diabetes* fails to specify whether the patient requires dietary adjustment alone or treatment with diet and insulin. This distinction is important because those women who are normoglycemic while fasting appear to have a significantly lower perinatal mortality rate. Women with GDM who require medical management are at greater risk for a poor perinatal outcome than those whose diabetes is controlled by diet alone.

Women who require insulin are designated by the letters B, C, D, R, F, and T. Class B patients are those whose onset of disease occurs after age 20 years. They have had diabetes for less than 10 years and have no vascular complications. Included in this subgroup of patients are those who have been previously treated with oral hypoglycemic agents.

Class C diabetes includes patients whose onset of disease was between the ages of 10 and 19 years and those who have had the disease for 10 to 19 years. Vascular disease is not present.

Class D represents women whose disease is of 20 years' duration or more, those whose disease onset occurred before the age of 10 years, and those who have benign retinopathy. The latter includes microaneurysms, exudates, and venous dilation.

Nephropathy

Renal disease develops in 25% to 30% of women with IDDM, with a peak incidence after 16 years of diabetes. **Overt diabetic nephropathy is diagnosed in women with type 1 or type 2 DM when persistent proteinuria exists in the absence of infection or other urinary tract disease. Damm and colleagues[34] have reported the prevalence of diabetic nephropathy during pregnancy to be 2.3% (5/220) in women with type 2 diabetes and 2.5% (11/445) in women with type 1 diabetes.** The criteria for diagnosis in the nonpregnant state includes a total urinary protein excretion (TPE) of greater than 500 mg in 24 hours or greater than 300 mg in 24 hours of urinary albumin excretion (UAE).

Before the development of overt diabetic nephropathy, some individuals develop incipient diabetic nephropathy defined by repetitive increases in UAE known as *microalbuminuria.* The diagnosis is established from a 24-hour urine collection exhibiting UAE of 20 to 199 μg/min or 30 to 299 mg in 24 hours. It is important to note that women who exhibit microalbuminuria in early pregnancy have a 35% to 60% risk for superimposed preeclampsia.[35] Without specific interventions, about 80% of individuals with type 1 diabetes who develop sustained microalbuminuria experience an increase in UAE of 10% to 20% per year, leading to overt nephropathy. In the nonpregnant individual, improvement of glycemic and blood pressure control has been demonstrated to reduce the risk for, or slow the progression

TABLE 40-4 COMPARATIVE STUDIES OF OUTCOMES IN CLASS F DIABETES MELLITUS

	KITZMILLER ET AL[103]	GRENFEL ET AL[104]	REECE ET AL[105]	ULLMO ET AL[106]	ROSENN ET AL[107]
No. of subjects	26	20	31	45	61
Chronic hypertension	31%	27%	22%	26%	47%
Initial creatinine >1.9 mg/dL	38%	10%	22%	11%	—
Initial proteinuria >3 g/24 hr	8.3%	—	22%	13%	—
Preeclampsia	15%	55%	35%	53%	51%
Cesarean delivery	—	72%	70%	80%	82%
Perinatal survival (%)	88.9	100	93.5	100	94%
Major anomalies	3 (11.1%)	1 (4.3%)	3 (9.7%)	2 (4%)	4 (6%)
Intrauterine growth restriction (%)	20.8	—	19.4	11.0	11%
Delivery					
<34 wk (%)	30.8	27	22.5	15.5	25%
34-36 wk (%)	40.7	23	32.3	35.5	28%
>36 wk (%)	28.5	50	45.2	49	47%

of, diabetic nephropathy. Renoprotective or antihypertensive therapy consisting of either angiotensin-converting enzyme (ACE) inhibitors or angiotensin II receptor blockers (ARBs) is indicated in nonpregnant women with diabetes who exhibit microalbuminuria or overt nephropathy. **In contrast, both ACE inhibitors and ARBs are contraindicated during pregnancy because they may result in fetal proximal tubal dysgenesis and oligohydramnios.** A population-based study by Cooper and colleagues[36] has indicated potential teratogenesis in women who received ACE inhibitors in early pregnancy and thus calls into question whether such agents are advised in women attempting conception. These researchers studied a cohort of 29,507 infants enrolled in Tennessee Medicaid born between 1985 and 2000 for whom there was no evidence of maternal diabetes. A total of 209 infants with exposure to ACE inhibitors during the first trimester alone were compared with 202 infants exposed to other antihypertensives during the first trimester and with 29,096 infants with no exposure to any antihypertensive agents during pregnancy. Major congenital malformations were identified from linked vital records and hospitalization claims during the first year of life. Infants with only first-trimester exposure to ACE inhibitors had an increased risk for major congenital malformations (RR, 2.71; 95% CI, 1.72 to 4.27) compared with infants who had no fetal exposure to other antihypertensive medications during only the first trimester. The increased risk conferred by ACE inhibitor exposure manifested as primarily anomalies of the cardiovascular and central nervous systems. Clearly, given this information, the risk and benefits of use of ACE inhibitors in diabetic women planning pregnancy must be considered.

Women with diabetic nephropathy have a significantly reduced life expectancy. Disease progression is characterized by hypertension, declining glomerular filtration rate (GFR), and eventual end-stage renal disease (ESRD) that requires dialysis or transplantation. In women with overt nephropathy, ESRD occurs in 50% by 10 years and in greater than 75% by 20 years.

Class F describes pregnant women with underlying renal disease. This includes those with reduced creatinine clearance or proteinuria of at least 500 mg in 24 hours measured during the first 20 weeks of gestation. Two factors present before 20 weeks' gestation appear to be predictive of adverse perinatal outcome in these women (e.g., preterm delivery, low birthweight, or preeclampsia): proteinuria greater than 3 g per 24 hours and serum creatinine greater than 1.5 mg/dL.

In a series of 45 class F women, 12 women had such risk factors.[37] Preeclampsia developed in 92%, with a mean

gestational age at delivery of 34 weeks, compared with an incidence of preeclampsia of 36% in 33 women without these risk factors who reached an average gestational age of 36 weeks. Remarkably, perinatal survival was 100% in this series, and no deliveries occurred before 30 weeks' gestation. Comparable series' detailing perinatal outcomes in class F patients are presented in Table 40-4.

The management of the diabetic woman with nephropathy requires great expertise. Limitation of dietary protein, which may reduce protein excretion in nonpregnant patients, has not been adequately studied during pregnancy. Although controversial, some nephrologists recommend a modified reduction in protein intake for pregnant women with nephropathy. **Control of hypertension in pregnant women with diabetic nephropathy is crucial to prevent further deterioration of kidney function and to optimize pregnancy outcome. Suboptimal control of blood pressure has been associated with a significantly increased risk for preterm delivery in this population. Thus in contrast to higher suggested thresholds for treatment in nondiabetic individuals, some have recommended instituting antihypertensive therapy to maintain blood pressure less than 135/85 mm Hg in pregnant women with nephropathy.[38] Prospective studies to evaluate blood pressure targets in pregnant women with diabetic nephropathy have not been conducted.** Because calcium channel blockers have renoprotective effects similar to those of ACE inhibitors and do not appear to be teratogenic, these agents are our first choice for treatment of hypertension in pregnant women with diabetic nephropathy. Whether such agents benefit normotensive pregnant women with microalbuminuria or nephropathy has not been determined. Other options for treatment include labetalol or hydralazine.

Studies are limited and conflict as to whether a permanent worsening of diabetic renal disease in women with mild to moderate renal insufficiency occurs as a result of pregnancy. Several small studies of women with serum creatinine greater than 1.5 mg/dL suggest that pregnancy may be associated with a more rapid decline in postpartum renal function. The increased risk of ESRD in nondiabetic women with previous preeclampsia also raises the question as to whether preeclampsia has an independent effect on the incidence and progression of diabetic nephropathy. **In summary, no deleterious effect on the progression of diabetic nephropathy is apparent provided that serum creatinine is in the normal range and significant proteinuria is absent in early pregnancy.**[39] In a review of 35 pregnancies complicated by diabetic nephropathy, proteinuria increased in 69%, and hypertension developed in 73%. After delivery, proteinuria declined in 65% of cases. In only two patients did protein excretion increase after gestation. In Gordon's series, 26 women (58%) had more than a 1-g increase in proteinuria, and by the third trimester, 25 (56%) excreted more than 3 g in 24 hours. In most cases, protein excretion returned to baseline levels after gestation.

Normal pregnancy is marked by an approximate 50% increase in GFR, and thus a rise in creatinine clearance, accompanied by a modest decline in serum creatinine. Most women with diabetic nephropathy, however, do not exhibit a rise in creatinine clearance during gestation. In a study of 46 class F pregnancies, Gordon and colleagues reported a mean decrease in creatinine clearance of 7.9%. When evaluated according to initial creatinine clearance, no difference in the degree of change was noted when subjects were classified according to first-trimester renal function. Whereas few patients exhibited a rise in creatinine clearance, other smaller studies have demonstrated an increase in creatinine clearance in about one third of women. Given the importance of blood pressure control in reducing cardiovascular and renal complications in the nonpregnant state, Carr and colleagues[40] studied the effect of poorly controlled hypertension in early pregnancy on renal function in 43 women with type 1 diabetes with nephropathy. Those women with mean arterial pressure in excess of 100 mm Hg demonstrated higher serum creatinine levels (1.23 vs. 0.895 mg/dL) compared with women with controlled hypertension.

With overt diabetic nephropathy, both albumin and total protein excretion may rise significantly during gestation. Importantly, a rise in total protein excretion to levels exceeding 300 mg in 24 hours may also be observed in women both with and without microalbuminuria in early pregnancy. Biesenbach and Zazgornik reported an average increase by the third trimester in total protein excretion to 478 mg in 24 hours in seven women with microalbuminuria in early pregnancy. This observation underscores the importance of obtaining baseline 24-hour urine measurements for total protein in all diabetic women because confusion arises as to the significance when new-onset macroalbuminuria or proteinuria is detected during the third trimester. Despite this recommendation, it may be challenging to distinguish preeclampsia from the natural progression of diabetic nephropathy, which often manifests as progressive proteinuria during pregnancy.

Gordon and colleagues[37] have detailed the progressive rise in proteinuria during pregnancy in 46 class F pregnancies. The mean increase in proteinuria between initial values and third-trimester values was 3.08 (± 4 g) in 24 hours. Twenty-six women (58%) had more than a 1-g increase in proteinuria, and by the third trimester, 25 (56%) excreted more than 3 g in 24 hours, including three women who exceeded 10 g in 24 hours. The mean change in proteinuria was not correlated with alterations in creatinine clearance, and a similar increase in proteinuria was observed during pregnancy regardless of the initial level present.

In summary, changes in creatinine clearance are variable during pregnancy in women with diabetic nephropathy. Most women with nephropathy will not exhibit a normal rise in creatinine clearance. Protein excretion will frequently rise during gestation to levels that can reach the nephrotic range.

With improved survival of diabetic patients after renal transplantation, a growing number of kidney recipients have now achieved pregnancy (class T). Attempting pregnancy is not advised until 2 years after transplantation. Mycophenolate is contraindicated during pregnancy, and a decision as to whether to discontinue this drug prior to conception should be individualized. Most diabetic renal transplant patients have underlying hypertension, although in one series of 28 women, preeclampsia was diagnosed in only 17% of cases. Allograft rejection occurred in one case. Overall, despite an increase in deliveries before 37 weeks, perinatal survival was 100%. These excellent results have come from improvements in both perinatal management and newer immunosuppressive regimens.

Many transplantation centers strive to perform combined kidney-pancreas transplantations in diabetic individuals with ESRD. Gilbert-Hayn and McGrory reviewed pregnancy outcomes in 43 pancreas-kidney recipients, of whom 66% developed hypertension and 77% had pregnancies that resulted in preterm birth. In this series, 6% of women experienced a rejection episode during pregnancy.

Retinopathy

Class R diabetes designates women with proliferative retinopathy, which represents neovascularization or growth of new retinal capillaries. These vessels may cause vitreous hemorrhage with scarring and retinal detachment, which results in vision loss. As with nephropathy, prevalence of retinal disease is highly related to the duration of diabetes. At 20 years, nearly 80% of diabetic individuals have some element of diabetic retinopathy. Background changes are generally apparent, whereas proliferative diabetic retinopathy fortunately complicates only 3% of pregnancies. Excellent glycemic control prevents retinopathy and may slow its progression. Parity is not associated with a risk for subsequent retinopathy; however, pregnancy does convey more than a twofold independent risk for progression of existing retinopathy. **Progression of diabetic retinopathy during pregnancy is associated with (1) retinal status at inception, (2) duration and early onset of diabetes, (3) elevated first-trimester HbA1c and persistent poor glycemic control or rapid normalization of blood glucose, and (4) hypertension.**[41] Retinopathy may worsen significantly during pregnancy despite the major advances that have been made in diagnosis and treatment of existing retinopathy. Ideally, women planning a pregnancy should have a comprehensive eye examination and treatment before conception. For those discovered to have proliferative changes during pregnancy, laser photocoagulation therapy with careful follow-up has helped maintain many pregnancies to a gestational age at which neonatal survival is likely.

In a large series of 172 patients, including 40 cases with background retinopathy and 11 with proliferative changes, only one patient developed new-onset proliferative retinopathy during pregnancy. A review of the literature by Kitzmiller and colleagues[42] confirms the observation that progression to proliferative retinopathy during pregnancy rarely occurs in women with background retinopathy or in those without any eyeground changes. Of the 561 women in these two categories, only 17 (3%) developed neovascularization during gestation. In contrast, 23 of 26 (88.5%) with untreated proliferative disease experienced worsening retinopathy during pregnancy.

Pregnancy may increase the prevalence of some background retinal changes. Characteristic streak-blob hemorrhages and soft exudates have been noted, and such retinopathy may progress despite strict metabolic control. At least two studies have related worsening retinal disease to plasma glucose at the first prenatal visit as well as the magnitude of improvement in glycemia during early pregnancy. In a subset of 140 women without proliferative retinopathy at baseline followed in the Diabetes in Early Pregnancy Study, progression of retinopathy was seen in 10.3%, 21.1%, 18.8%, and 54.8% of patients with no retinopathy, microaneurysms only, mild nonproliferative retinopathy, and moderate to severe nonproliferative retinopathy at baseline, respectively. Elevated glycosylated hemoglobin at baseline and the magnitude of improvement of glucose control through week 14 were associated with a higher risk for progression of retinopathy. Women with an initial glycohemoglobin greater than 6 standard deviations (SDs) above the control mean were nearly three times as likely to experience worsening retinopathy compared with those within 2 SDs of the mean. Whether improving control or simply suboptimal control contributes to a deterioration of background retinopathy remains uncertain. Hypertension may also be a significant risk factor for the progression of retinopathy during pregnancy. **For women with proliferative changes, laser photocoagulation is indicated, and most will respond to this therapy. However, women who demonstrate severe florid disc neovascularization that is unresponsive to laser therapy during early pregnancy may be at great risk for deterioration of their vision.** Termination of pregnancy may need to be considered in this group of patients.

In labor, women with proliferative retinopathy are generally advised to avoid the Valsalva maneuver to reduce the risk for retinal hemorrhage. Shortening of the second stage of labor or cesarean delivery has been advocated; however, studies are lacking that address this issue.

In addition to background and proliferative eye disease, vasoocclusive lesions associated with the development of macular edema have been described during pregnancy. Cystic macular edema is most often found in patients with proteinuric nephropathy and hypertensive disease, leading to retinal edema; macular capillary permeability is a feature of this process, and the degree of macular edema is directly related to the fall in plasma oncotic pressure present in these women. In one series, seven women with minimal or no retinopathy before becoming pregnant developed severe macular edema associated with preproliferative or proliferative retinopathy during the course of their pregnancies. Although proliferation was controlled with photocoagulation, the macular edema worsened until delivery in all cases and was often aggravated by photocoagulation. Although both macular edema and retinopathy regressed after delivery in some patients, in others, these pathologic processes persisted and resulted in significant visual loss.

Coronary Artery Disease

Class H diabetes refers to the presence of diabetes of any duration associated with ischemic myocardial disease. Symptomatic coronary artery disease is rare in type 1 diabetic women who are younger than 35 years. It is unknown whether the small number of women who have coronary artery disease are at an increased risk for infarction during gestation. The maternal mortality rate exceeded 50% for cases of infarction during pregnancy reported before 1980; however, all but 1 of 23 cases reported from 1980 to 2005 survived. A high index of suspicion for ischemic heart disease should be maintained in women with long-standing diabetes because anginal symptoms may be minimal in women, and infarction may present as congestive heart failure. Although more than a dozen reports have described successful pregnancies following myocardial infarction (MI) in diabetic women, cardiac status should be carefully assessed early in gestation or, preferably, before pregnancy. If

electrocardiographic (ECG) abnormalities are encountered, echocardiography may be used to assess ventricular function, or modified stress testing may be performed. The decision to undertake a pregnancy in a woman with type 1 or type 2 DM and coronary artery disease needs to be made only after serious consideration. The potential for morbidity and mortality must be thoroughly reviewed with the patient and her family. The management of MI during pregnancy is discussed in Chapter 37.

EARLY SCREENING FOR OVERT DIABETES AND DETECTION OF GESTATIONAL DIABETES MELLITUS

The frequency of diabetes complicating pregnancy has generally been estimated to be as high as 6% to 7% with approximately 90% of these cases representing women with GDM.[43] Utilizing a pregnancy risk-assessment monitoring system between 2007 and 2010, DeSisto and colleagues[43] confirmed that the prevalence of GDM is rising in the United States and may now be as high as 9.2%. The increasing frequency of GDM can be attributed to the worldwide obesity epidemic as well the introduction of less stringent criteria for the diagnosis now being adapted by some institutions. An increased prevalence of GDM is found in women of ethnic groups that have high frequencies of type 2 diabetes. These include women of Hispanic, African, Native American, Asian, and Pacific Island ancestry. Women with GDM represent a group with significant risk for developing glucose intolerance later in life. O'Sullivan projected that 50% of women with GDM would become diabetic in follow-up at 22 to 28 years. Kjos and colleagues reported that 60% of Latina women will develop type 2 diabetes, and this level of risk may actually be manifest by 5 years after the GDM index pregnancy. The likelihood for subsequent diabetes increases when GDM is diagnosed in early pregnancy and when maternal fasting glucose levels are elevated. Presumably, some of these women with impaired β-cell function may represent cases of unidentified preexisting type 2 diabetes.

As noted earlier, GDM is a state restricted to pregnant women whose impaired glucose tolerance (IGT) is discovered during pregnancy. Because in most cases, patients with GDM have normal fasting glucose levels, some challenge of glucose tolerance must be undertaken. Traditionally, obstetricians relied on historic and clinical risk factors to select those patients most likely to develop GDM. This group included patients with a family history of diabetes and those whose past pregnancies were marked by an unexplained stillbirth or the delivery of a malformed or macrosomic infant. Obesity, hypertension, glycosuria, and maternal age older than 25 years were other indications for screening. Although multiple risk factors may increase the likelihood of GDM, more than half of all women who exhibit an abnormal GTT lack any of these risk factors.

The ACOG suggests that all pregnant women be screened for GDM, whether by the patient's medical history, clinical risk factors, or laboratory screening tests to determine blood glucose levels (Box 40-2). Screening is generally performed at 24 to 28 weeks' gestation, when the "diabetogenic state" of pregnancy has been established. ACOG also recommends early pregnancy screening for undiagnosed type 2 diabetes in women with a previous history of GDM, a history of impaired glucose metabolism, or those who are obese. Studies validating various approaches to early pregnancy screening for both type 2 diabetes and GDM are, however, lacking. A simple approach to early screening for diabetes is to obtain an HbA1c level in women believed to be at greatest risk. A diagnosis of overt diabetes is made if the level is greater than or equal to 6.5%. If the level is between 5.7% and 6.4%, suggesting impaired glucose tolerance, a diagnostic oral GTT is performed. For those women with normal results or those with an HbA1c level less than 5.7%, screening for GDM is then undertaken at 24 to 28 weeks. Recently, Hughes and colleagues[44] suggested that an early HbA1c level greater than or equal to 5.9% is optimal for detecting overt diabetes in women at less than 20 weeks' gestation and also identifies women at increased risk of adverse pregnancy outcomes.

Despite the widespread acceptance of screening for and treating GDM in the United States, expert panels have only recently recognized the benefit of GDM screening programs altogether.[45,46] The criteria for the diagnosis of GDM originally designated a population at increased risk for the development of type 2 diabetes in later life. The fact that O'Sullivan's original work that established the criteria used for the diagnosis of GDM failed to evaluate an association between mild carbohydrate tolerance and perinatal outcome led many to question the overall significance of this diagnosis.

The Hyperglycemia and Adverse Pregnancy Outcome (HAPO) study was designed to aid in the development of internationally agreed-upon diagnostic criteria for GDM based on their predictive value for pregnancy outcome.[47] This landmark multicenter international study allowed for analysis of blinded, 75-g, 2-hour oral GTT data in more than 25,000

gravidas without pregestational diabetes. Glycemia was evaluated in relation to various perinatal and maternal outcomes. **Increases in each of the three values on the 75-g, 2-hour oral GTT were associated with graded increases in the likelihood of outcomes such as an LGA infant, cesarean delivery, fetal C-peptide levels, and neonatal adiposity** (Fig. 40-14). The HAPO study investigators did not offer specific recommendations for the diagnostic criteria of GDM. Because a continuous association was found between glucose values and perinatal outcome, it was apparent that any new recommended diagnostic criteria would need to be arrived at by consensus. To meet this challenge, the International Association of Diabetes and Pregnancy Study Groups (IADPSG) convened a workshop conference in 2008.[48] An odds ratio of 1.75 greater than the mean was selected for the outcomes of increased neonatal body fat, LGA, and cord serum C-peptide greater than the 90th percentile, which yielded the recommended diagnostic criteria for GDM (Table 40-5).

Importantly, the IADPSG task force recommended that a 75-g, 2-hour oral GTT be performed universally during pregnancy and that the diagnosis of GDM be made when any single value on the oral GTT was met or exceeded.[48] Using the proposed criteria, 17.8% of the HAPO study population would be identified as having GDM. A recent retrospective cohort study confirmed a greater than twofold increased risk of LGA infants among the offspring of untreated women who met only the IADPSG criteria for diagnosis of GDM (and not the ACOG accepted Carpenter and Coustan criteria) when compared with a control population.[46] There are, however, no data from randomized treatment trials regarding therapeutic interventions for the expanded group of women identified as having GDM using IADPSG criteria for the diagnosis. This important consideration was paramount to the conclusions of the 2013 Eunice Kennedy Shriver National Institute of Child Health and Human Development (NICHD) Consensus Development Conference on diagnosing GDM.[49] The conferees recommended that health care providers continue to use a two-step approach to the screening and diagnosis of GDM because no evidence suggests that using the 2-hour oral GTT criteria to diagnose GDM would lead to clinically significant improvements in maternal or newborn outcomes and that a significant increase in health care costs would accompany adoption of the IADPSG criteria. Another major concern with the IADPSG approach is the reliance on a single oral GTT value to confer the diagnosis of GDM.[49] Theoretic cost-benefit analyses have suggested a benefit to using the IADPSG criteria; however, one such study recognized the benefit to hinge on follow-up and potential prevention of type 2 diabetes in the additional group of women identified as having GDM using IADPSG criteria. Proponents of the IADPSG approach to diagnosis cite (1) the fact that the two-step approach may miss approximately 25% of GDM in those who pass the 50-g screen yet demonstrate an abnormal oral GTT, and (2) the rate of prediabetes in women in the United States is approximately 26%, and this figure is not very different from the rate of GDM using the IADPSG criteria. A recent systematic review of diagnostic thresholds for GDM concluded that a pragmatic approach to the diagnosis of GDM utilizing a HAPO study odds ratio (OR) of 2.0 as a threshold, in contrast to the IADPSG criteria (OR, 1.75), warrants further consideration, until additional analysis of the data comparing mutually exclusive groups of women is provided and large randomized controlled trials (RCTs) to investigate different diagnostic thresholds

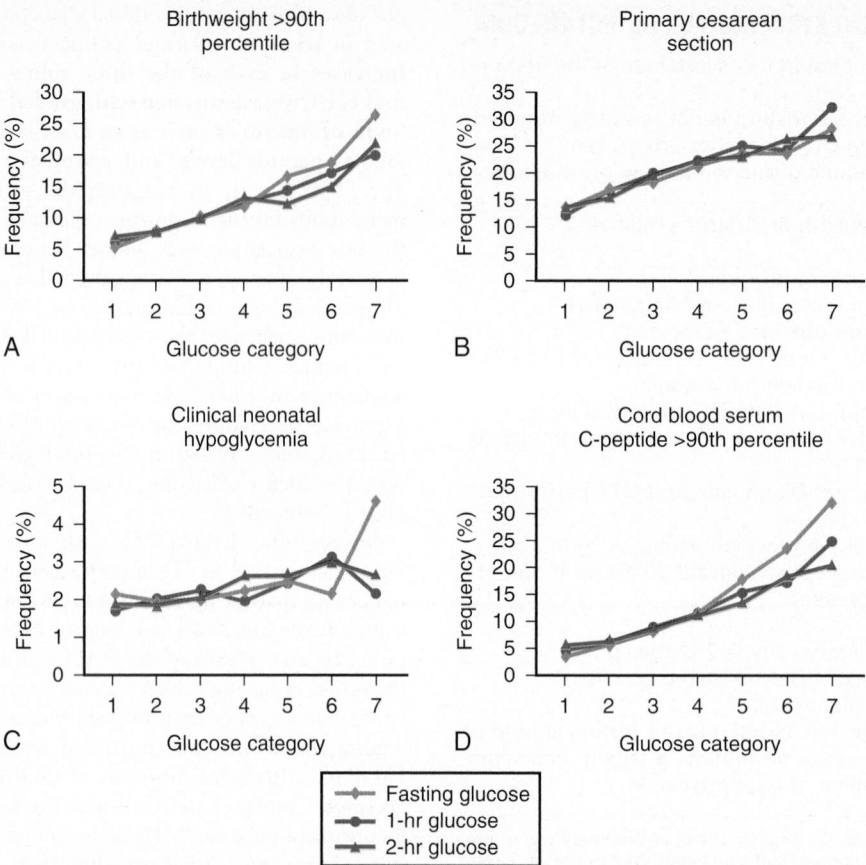

FIG 40-14 Frequency of perinatal and maternal outcomes in relation to maternal glycemia. (Modified from Metzger BE, Lowe LP, Dyer AR, for the HAPO Study Cooperative Research Group: Hyperglycemia and adverse pregnancy outcomes. *N Engl J Med.* 2008;358:1991.)

TABLE 40-5	INTERNATIONAL ASSOCIATION OF DIABETES AND PREGNANCY STUDY GROUPS' DEFINITION OF GDM*		
	GLUCOSE		**FREQUENCY OF GDM (%)**
Fasting glucose	92 mg/dL	Alone	8.3
1-hr glucose	180 mg/dL	Plus	5.7 = 14
2-hr glucose	153 mg/dL	Plus	2.1 = 16.1†

From Metzger BE, Gabbe SG, Persson B, for the International Association of Diabetes and Pregnancy Study Groups Consensus Panel. Recommendations on the diagnosis and classification of hyperglycemia in pregnancy. *Diabetes Care.* 2010;33:676.
*Based on a universal, 75-g, 2-hr glucose tolerance test. Diagnosis of GDM is made if one value is met or exceeded.
†Approximately 1.7% of the HAPO study population were unblinded because of fasting glucose ≥105 mg/dL and/or at 2 hr, ≥200 mg/dL. As a result, the frequency of GDM in this population would be 17.8%.
GDM, gestational diabetes mellitus.

are completed.[50,51] Utilizing an OR of 2.0 with HAPO-derived data would result in a frequency of GDM of approximately 10%, in contrast to the 18% when using the proposed IADPSG thresholds.[52] To date, two observational and one cross-sectional study have confirmed a markedly increased frequency of GDM utilizing the IADPSG criteria for diagnosis without a reduction in LGA infants.[53,54] The ADA recently summarized the dilemma concerning the two strategies—the IADPSG one-step approach using a 2-hour, 75-g oral GTT versus the traditional two-step method using a diagnostic 3-hour oral GTT—with the following key points:

1. Data are insufficient to strongly demonstrate the superiority of one strategy over the other.
2. The decision of which strategy to implement must therefore be made based on relative values placed on currently unmeasured factors (e.g., cost-benefit estimation; willingness to change practice based on correlation studies, rather than on clinical intervention trial results; relative role of cost considerations; and available infrastructure).
3. Further research is needed to resolve these uncertainties.

At the present time, most practitioners in the United States continue to perform glucose-challenge screening followed by a diagnostic 100-g oral GTT (two-step approach). The 50-g glucose challenge may be performed in the fasting or fed state. Sensitivity is improved if the test is performed in the fasting state. **A plasma value between 130 and 140 mg/dL is commonly used as a threshold for performing a 3-hour oral GTT** (Table 40-6). Coustan and coworkers have demonstrated that 10% of women with GDM have screening test values between 130 and 139 mg/dL. This study indicated that the sensitivity of screening would be increased from 90% to nearly 100% if universal screening were used with a threshold of 130 mg/dL. The prevalence of positive screening tests that require further diagnostic testing increases from 14% (140 mg/dL) to 23% (130 mg/dL), which is accompanied by about a 12% increase in the overall cost to diagnose each case of GDM.

Using the plasma cutoff of 135 to 140 mg/dL, approximately 15% to 20% of patients with an abnormal screening value can be expected to have an abnormal 3-hour oral GTT. Patients

TABLE 40-6	DETECTION OF GDM		
SCREENING TEST (50 g, 1 hr)		**PLASMA (mg/dL, 130-140)**	
Oral GTT*	**NDDG**	**Carpenter & Coustan**	
Fasting glucose	105	95	
1-hr glucose	190	180	
2-hr glucose	165	155	
3-hr glucose	145	110	

*Diagnosis of gestational diabetes is made when any two values are met or exceeded in a 100-g, 3-hour test.
GDM, gestational diabetes mellitus; *GTT*, glucose tolerance test; *NDDG*, National Diabetes Data Group.

TABLE 40-7	TARGET PLASMA GLUCOSE LEVELS IN PREGNANCY
TIME	**GLUCOSE LEVEL (mg/dL)**
Before breakfast	60-90
Before lunch, supper, bedtime snack	60-105
One hour after meals	≤140
Two hours after meals	≤120
2 AM to 6 AM	>60

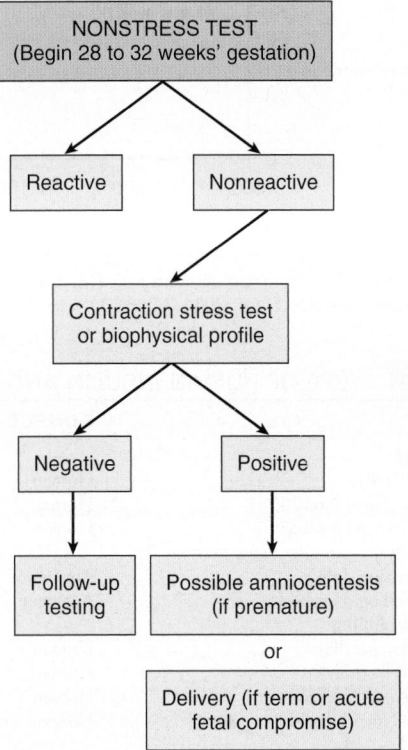

FIG 40-15 Algorithm for antepartum fetal testing.

whose 1-hour screening value exceeds 190 mg/dL (10.5 mmol/L) will exhibit an abnormal oral GTT in 90% of cases. In women with a screening value between 190 and 215 mg/dL, it is preferable to check a fasting blood glucose level before administering a 100-g carbohydrate load. If the fasting glucose is greater than 95 mg/dL, the patient is treated for GDM.

The criteria for establishing the diagnosis of gestational diabetes based on a 100-g, 3-hour oral GTT are listed in Table 40-6. Both sets of diagnostic criteria are endorsed by ACOG. The U.S. National Diabetes Data Group (NDDG) criteria represent a theoretic conversion of O'Sullivan's thresholds in whole blood. Carpenter and Coustan prefer to use another modification of these data, which is supported by a comparison of the old Somogyi-Nelson method and current plasma glucose oxidase assays. Several studies have confirmed that patients diagnosed using the less stringent Carpenter and Coustan criteria experience as much perinatal morbidity (macrosomia and cesarean delivery) as subjects diagnosed by the NDDG criteria. In one study of 26,000 women that compared the two sets of criteria using cross-sectional data, the diagnosis of GDM increased approximately 50% utilizing the Carpenter-Coustan criteria. A recent secondary analysis of the NICHD Maternal-Fetal Medicine Units (MFMU) Network RCT for mild GDM demonstrated that the beneficial treatment effect was seen in subjects diagnosed by both NDDG and Carpenter-Coustan criteria. Using either of the two 100-g, 3-hour oral GTT criteria, the patient must have at least two abnormal glucose determinations to be diagnosed with GDM.

TREATMENT OF THE PATIENT WITH TYPE 1 OR TYPE 2 DIABETES MELLITUS

Clinical efforts aimed at optimizing maternal control are considered the key component responsible for the decline in perinatal deaths in pregnancies complicated by DM over the past few decades. Self-monitoring of blood glucose, combined with intensive insulin therapy, has resulted in improved glycemia for many pregnant diabetic women. Women with pregestational diabetes should monitor their glucose control six to eight times daily using glucose-oxidase-impregnated reagent strips and a glucose reflectance meter. Target glucose levels for control of diabetes during pregnancy have been established largely based on expert opinion (Table 40-7). A recent review of twelve studies concerning patterns of glycemia in normal pregnancy suggested that glucose concentrations are significantly lower than suggested normal therapeutic targets (Fig. 40-16).[55]

The technology of continuous glucose monitoring (CGM) has been studied in pregnant diabetic women. By providing a total of 288 measurements daily, compared with six to eight blood glucose measurements using self-monitoring of blood glucose, CGM can provide a more complete glycemic profile and can presumably detect unrecognized postprandial hyperglycemia as well as symptomatic hypoglycemia. A randomized trial of 71 women with pregestational diabetes confirmed a lower third-trimester HbA1c level and reduced birthweight and macrosomia in women who underwent CGM.

Insulin therapy is recommended by the ADA as the primary medication to achieve optimal glycemic control in pregnant women with both type 1 and type 2 diabetes. Women with type 2 diabetes may present in early pregnancy on an oral agent for treatment of their diabetes. Our approach is to continue metformin therapy in well-controlled type 2 diabetic women, whereas those receiving other agents are generally switched to insulin therapy. Many type 2 diabetic women who enter pregnancy with their disease controlled with metformin will eventually require the addition of insulin to their regimen. To achieve the best glycemic control possible for each patient, conventional insulin therapy is abandoned during pregnancy in favor of intensive therapy. Insulin regimens have classically included multiple injections of

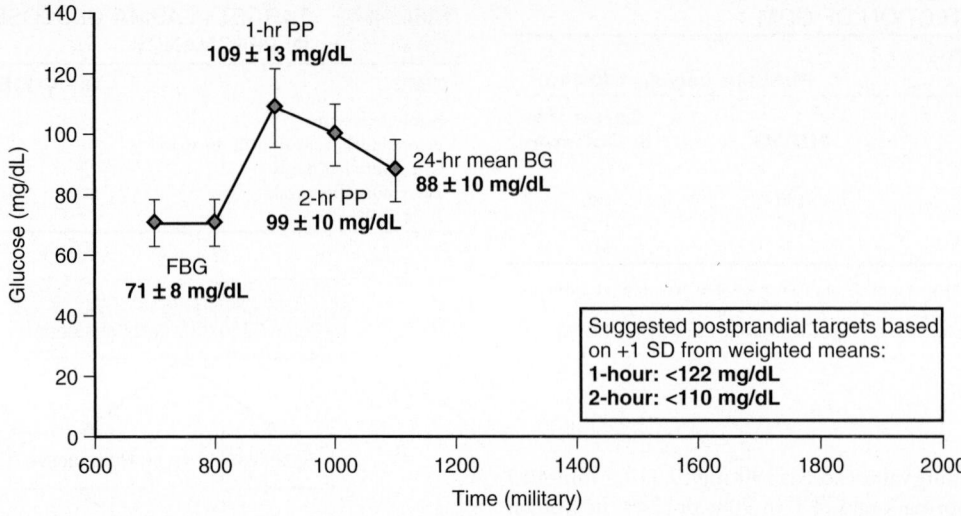

FIG 40-16 Patterns of glycemia in normal pregnancy. BG, blood glucose; FBG, fasting blood glucose; PP, postpartum; SD, standard deviation. (From Hernandez TL, Friedman JE, Van Pelt RE, Barbour LA. Patterns of glycemia in normal pregnancy: should the current therapeutic targets be challenged? *Diabetes Care.* 2011;34:1660.)

TABLE 40-8	TYPE OF HUMAN INSULIN AND INSULIN ANALOGUES			
	SOURCE	ONSET (HR)	PEAK (HR)	DURATION (HR)
Short Acting				
Humulin R (Lilly)	Human	0.5	2-4	5-7
Velosulin H (Novo Nordisk)	Human	0.5	1-3	8
Novolin R (Novo Nordisk)	Human	0.5	2.5-5	6-8
Rapid Acting				
Lispro (Humalog, Lilly)	Analogue	0.25	0.5-1.5	4-5
Aspart (NovoLog, Nordisk)	Analogue	0.25	1-3	3-5
Intermediate Acting				
Humulin Lente (Lilly)	Human	1-3	6-12	18-24
Humulin NPH (Lilly)	Human	1-2	6-12	18-24
Novolin l (Novo Nordisk)	Human	2.5	7-15	22
Novolin N (Novo Nordisk)	Human	1.5	4-20	24
Long Acting				
Glargine (Lantus, Sanofi)	Analogue	1	—	24
Detemir (Levemir, Novo Nordisk)	Analogue	1-2	—	24

insulin—usually before breakfast, lunch, the evening meal, and often at bedtime—complemented by self-monitoring of blood glucose and adjustment of insulin dose according to glucose profiles. Patients are instructed on dietary composition, insulin action, recognition and treatment of hypoglycemia, adjusting insulin dosage for exercise and sick days, as well as monitoring for hyperglycemia and potential ketosis. **These principles form the foundation for intensive insulin therapy in which an attempt is made to simulate physiologic insulin requirements. Insulin administration is provided for both basal needs and meals, and rapid adjustments are made in response to glucose measurements. The treatment regimen generally involves three to four daily injections or the use of continuous subcutaneous insulin infusion (CSII) devices.** With either approach, frequent self-monitoring of blood glucose is fundamental to achieve the therapeutic objective of physiologic glucose control. Glucose determinations are made in the fasting state and before lunch, dinner, and at bedtime. Postprandial and nocturnal values are also advised. Patients are instructed on an insulin dose for each meal and at bedtime, if necessary. Mealtime insulin needs are determined by the composition of the meal, the premeal glucose measurement, and the level of activity anticipated following the meal. Basal or intermediate-acting insulin

requirements are determined by periodic 2:00 AM to 4:00 AM glucose measurements, as well as late afternoon values, which reflect morning intermediate-acting insulin action.

In patients whose diabetes is not well controlled, a brief period of hospitalization may be necessary for the initiation of therapy. Patients are encouraged to contact their physician at any time if questions should arise concerning the management of their diabetes. **During pregnancy, we advise women to report their glucose values by telephone, fax, or e-mail on at least a weekly basis.**

Insulin therapy must be individualized with dosage determinations tailored to diet and exercise. Insulin requirements during pregnancy have been reported to average 0.7 U/kg in the first trimester, increasing to 1.1 U/kg by term, although the variation in requirements is considerable. Garcia-Patterson and colleagues have noted a steady increase in insulin requirements from 16 to 37 weeks, and unstable requirements are common before 16 weeks. **Semisynthetic human insulin preparations and newer insulin analogues** (Table 40-8) **are preferred for use during pregnancy. Insulin lispro and insulin aspart are rapid-acting insulin preparations that have replaced regular insulin.** Insulin lispro features reversal of proline and lysine at positions B28 and B29, and because it remains in monomeric form, it is rapidly absorbed. Its duration of action is shorter than that of regular insulin, so unexpected hypoglycemia hours after injection is avoided. Insulin lispro appears to be safe for use during pregnancy and is a category B drug. Insulin aspart has also been compared with human insulin in women with type 1 diabetes during pregnancy, and comparable fetal outcomes have been observed among both groups; however, limited information exists concerning glycemia in treated women (see Table 40-8).

The long-acting insulin analogues glargine and detemir have been designed to more accurately mimic basal insulin secretion. Observational data would suggest that use of insulin glargine is safe during pregnancy; it has a flat profile, compared with neutral protamine Hagedorn (NPH), so that when administered with rapid-acting insulin, unpredictable spikes in insulin levels and resultant hypoglycemia appear to be less common. **However, the flat profile of glargine may be undesirable during pregnancy when variation in basal insulin needs are likely. For this reason, we frequently suggest that women who receive glargine change to a twice-daily regimen of NPH insulin. A multicenter trial that compared insulin detemir with NPH insulin in 310 type 1 diabetic pregnant women demonstrated equivalent efficacy of insulin detemir with respect to hypoglycemic episodes and HbA1c levels.[56] The U.S. Food and Drug Administration (FDA) has now designated insulin detemir as a class B medication. Our approach is to maintain patients on insulin detemir if their blood glucose is well controlled.**

Insulin is generally administered in three to five injections. We prefer a four-injection regimen, although most patients present taking a combination of intermediate-acting (NPH) and short-acting (lispro or aspart) insulin before dinner and breakfast. As a general rule, the amount of intermediate-acting insulin will exceed the short-acting component by a 2:1 ratio. Patients usually receive two thirds of their total dose with breakfast and the remaining third in the evening as a combined dose at dinner or split into components with short-acting or rapid-acting insulin at dinner and intermediate-acting insulin at bedtime in an effort to minimize periods of nocturnal hypoglycemia. These episodes frequently occur when the mother is in a relative fasting state, whereas placental and fetal glucose consumption continue. Finally, some women may require a small dose of short-acting insulin before lunch, thus constituting a four-injection regimen.

Open-loop CSII pump therapy is preferred by many women with type 1 diabetes during pregnancy. The pump is a battery-powered unit that may be worn like a beeper during most daily activities. These systems provide continuous short-acting insulin therapy through a subcutaneous infusion. The basal infusion rate and bolus doses to cover meals are determined by frequent self-monitoring of blood glucose.

Pregnant women may need to be hospitalized before initiation of pump therapy. Women must be educated regarding the strategy of continuous infusion and should have their glucose stabilized over several days. This requires that multiple blood glucose determinations be made for the prevention of periods of hyperglycemia and hypoglycemia. Most recently, pump therapy has been linked with a CGM system to provide this information. Glucose values may become normalized with minimal amplitude of daily excursions in most patients.

Episodes of hypoglycemia are often reduced with pump therapy. When they do occur, they are usually secondary to errors in dose selection or failure to adhere to the required diet. The risk for nocturnal hypoglycemia, which is increased in the pregnant state, necessitates that great care be undertaken in selecting patients for CSII. Patients using the pump who fail to exhibit normal counterregulatory responses to hypoglycemia should probably check their glucose values at 2:00 AM to 3:00 AM to detect nocturnal hypoglycemia.

The mechanics of the CSII systems are relatively simple. A fine-gauge infusion cannula is attached by connecting tubing to the pump. This cannula is reimplanted every 2 to 3 days at a different site, usually in the anterior abdominal wall. Rapid-acting insulin (usually insulin lispro) is stored in the pump syringe. Infusion occurs at a basal rate, which can be fixed or altered for a specific time of day by a computer program. For example, the basal rate can be programmed for a lower dose at night. Preprandial boluses can be adjusted manually before each meal and snack. Half of the total daily insulin is usually given as the basal rate with the remainder given as boluses infused before each meal. The largest bolus (30% to 35%) is administered with breakfast, followed by 25% before dinner and 15% to 20% before snacks.

Patients without any pancreatic reserve may have rapid elevations of blood glucose if the pump fails or if intercurrent infection is present. Since the advent of buffered insulin, insulin aggregation leading to occlusion of the Silastic infusion tubing is uncommon. Failure of the pump is associated with a steady rise in ketonemia in the nonpregnant patient.

It is unclear whether CSII is superior to multiple-injection regimens. Coustan and colleagues randomized 22 patients to intensive conventional therapy with multiple injections versus pump therapy. No differences were found between the two treatment groups with respect to outpatient mean glucose levels, glycosylated hemoglobin levels, or glycemic excursions. Gabbe and colleagues reported a large retrospective cohort study of women who began pump therapy during gestation compared with a group treated with multiple-injection regimens. Women using pumps, most with insulin lispro, had fewer hypoglycemic reactions and comparable glucose control and pregnancy outcomes. Notably, **a systematic review that compared randomized trials of CSII versus multiple-injection regimens revealed no difference in measures of glycemic control or pregnancy outcome.[57]**

Diet therapy is critical to successful regulation of maternal diabetes. A program that consists of three meals and several snacks is used for most patients. Dietary composition should be 40% to 60% complex high-fiber carbohydrates, 20% protein, and 30% to 40% fat with less than 10% saturated fats, up to 10% polyunsaturated fatty acids, and the remainder derived from monosaturated sources. Caloric intake is established based on prepregnancy weight and weight gain during gestation. Weight reduction is not advised. Patients with a BMI of 22 to 27 should consume about 35 kcal/kg ideal body weight. Obese women (BMI > 30) may be managed with an intake as low as 15 kcal/kg actual weight. Any further caloric restriction that results in ketonuria requires an increase in caloric consumption. In general, caloric distribution is as follows: 10% to 20% with breakfast, 20% to 30% with lunch, 30% to 40% percent with dinner, and up to 30% as snacks. Snacks may be necessary to minimize episodes of hypoglycemia, especially at bedtime (Box 40-3).

The presence of maternal vasculopathy should be thoroughly assessed early in pregnancy by an ophthalmologist familiar with diabetic retinopathy. Ophthalmologic examinations are performed during each trimester and are repeated

more often if retinopathy is detected. Baseline renal function is established by assaying a 24-hour urine collection for creatinine clearance and protein. An ECG and urine culture are also obtained.

Most patients with type 1 and type 2 DM are followed with outpatient visits at 1- to 2-week intervals. At each visit, control is assessed and adjustments in insulin dosage are made; however, patients should be instructed to call at any time if periods of hypoglycemia (<60 mg/dL) or hyperglycemia (>200 mg/dL) occur. Ketone testing is advised for persistent glucose levels that exceed 200 mg/dL. **The increased risk for hypoglycemia in pregnant individuals may be related to defective glucose counterregulatory hormone mechanisms, and both epinephrine and glucagon appear to be suppressed in pregnant diabetic women during hypoglycemia.** For these reasons, patients should test glucose levels frequently, and family members should be instructed on the technique of glucagon injection for the treatment of severe reactions. Box 40-4 provides some important lessons we have learned over the years in caring for our patients.

Ketoacidosis

With the implementation of antenatal care programs that stress strict metabolic control of blood glucose levels for women who require insulin, diabetic ketoacidosis (DKA) has fortunately become a less common occurrence. DKA has been reported to complicate between 0.5% and 3.0% of diabetic pregnancies.[58] Kilvert and colleagues reported 11 cases of ketoacidosis in 635 insulin-treated pregnancies over a 20-year period. One fetal loss and one spontaneous miscarriage complicated the affected pregnancies.

DKA can occur in the newly diagnosed diabetic patient, and the hormonal milieu of pregnancy may become the background for this phenomenon. Because pregnancy is a state of insulin resistance marked by enhanced lipolysis and ketogenesis, DKA may develop in a pregnant woman with glucose levels that barely exceed 200 mg/dL (11.1 mmol/L). This phenomenon has been referred to as *euglycemic ketoacidosis*. DKA occurs in a background of impaired insulin action with an increase in counterregulatory hormones such as glucagon, cortisol, and catecholamines. Thus, because of the contrainsulin state of pregnancy with a predisposition to lipolysis, DKA may be diagnosed during pregnancy with minimal hyperglycemia accompanied by a fall in plasma bicarbonate (anion gap acidosis), a pH value less than 7.30, and ketonemia.

Early recognition of signs and symptoms of DKA improves both maternal and fetal outcome. As in the nonpregnant state, clinical signs of volume depletion follow the symptoms of hyperglycemia, which include polydipsia and polyuria. Malaise, headache, nausea, and vomiting are common complaints. **A pregnant diabetic woman with poor fluid intake and persistent vomiting over 8 to 12 hours should be evaluated for potential DKA.** A low serum bicarbonate level prompts an arterial blood gas determination to rule out this diagnosis. Occasionally, DKA presents in a woman with undiagnosed diabetes who receives β-mimetic agents such as terbutaline to arrest preterm labor.

Once the diagnosis of DKA is established and the patient is stabilized, she should be transported to a facility where tertiary care in both perinatology and neonatology is available. Therapy hinges on the meticulous correction of metabolic and fluid abnormalities. An attempt at treatment of any underlying cause for DKA, such as infection, should be initiated as well. The general management of DKA in pregnancy is outlined in Box 40-5. **Fluid resuscitation and insulin infusion should be maintained even in the face of normoglycemia until bicarbonate levels return to normal, indicating that acidemia has cleared.** DKA does represent a substantial risk for fetal compromise, and the combined effects of maternal acidosis, hyperglycemia-induced hyperinsulinemia, dehydration, and electrolyte abnormalities may result in stillbirth. Not surprisingly, fetal heart rate monitoring may reveal late decelerations (Fig. 40-17). Fortunately, **successful fetal resuscitation often accompanies correction of maternal acidosis.** However, this process may take several hours. Therefore every effort should be made to correct and stabilize the mother's condition before intervening and delivering a preterm infant.

ANTEPARTUM FETAL EVALUATION

Maternal diabetes can result in fetal hyperglycemia and hyperinsulinemia and can thereby increase the risk for fetal hypoxia. Thus protocols for antepartum fetal assessment in pregnancies complicated by DM have been incorporated into the care plan for outpatient monitoring. A program of fetal surveillance is initiated during the third trimester, when the risk for sudden intrauterine death increases (Tables 40-9 and 40-10). To date, no randomized trials of fetal monitoring have been done in pregnancies complicated by diabetes to provide clinical evidence, so decisions regarding the timing of initiation of testing, as well as the frequency, often follow local custom. **Because improvement in maternal glucose control has played a major**

BOX 40-5 MANAGEMENT OF DIABETIC KETOACIDOSIS DURING PREGNANCY

Intravenous Fluids

Isotonic sodium chloride is used, with total replacement of 4-6 L in the first 12 hr.

- Insert intravenous catheters: Maintain hourly flow sheet for fluids and electrolytes, potassium, insulin, and laboratory results.
- Administer normal saline (0.9% NaCl) at 1-2 L/hr for the first hour.
- Infuse normal saline at 250 to 500 mL/hr depending on hydration state (8 hr). If serum sodium is elevated, use half-normal saline (0.45% NaCl).
- When plasma or serum glucose reaches 200 mg/dL, change to 5% dextrose with 0.45% NaCl at 150-250 mL/hr.
- After 8 hr, use half-normal saline at 125 mL/hr.

Potassium

Establish adequate renal function (urine output ~50 mL/hr).

- If serum potassium is <3.3 mEq/L, hold insulin and give 20-30 mEq K^+/hr until K^+ is >3.3 mEq/L or is being corrected.
- If serum K^+ is >3.3 mEq/L but <5.3 mEq/L, give 20-30 mEq K^+ in each liter of IV fluid to keep serum K^+ between 4 and 5 mEq/L.
- If serum K^+ is >5.3 mEq/L, do not give K^+ but check serum K^+ every 2 hr.

Insulin

Use regular insulin intravenously.

- Consider a loading dose of 0.1-0.2 U/kg as an IV bolus depending on plasma glucose.
- Begin continuous insulin infusion at 0.1 U/kg/hr.
- If plasma or serum glucose does not fall by 50-70 mg/dL in the first hour, double the insulin infusion every hour until a steady glucose decline is achieved.
- When plasma or serum glucose reaches 200 mg/dL, reduce insulin infusion to 0.05-0.1 U/kg/hr.
- Keep plasma or serum glucose between 100 and 150 mg/dL until resolution of diabetic ketoacidosis.

Bicarbonate

Assess need, and provide based on pH.

- pH >7.0: No HCO_3 is needed.
- pH is 6.9-7.0: Dilute $NaHCO_3$ (50 mmol) in 200 mL H_2O with 10 mEq KCl and infuse over 1 hr. Repeat $NaHCO_3$ administration every 2 hr until pH is 7.0. Monitor serum K^+.
- pH <6.9-7.0: Dilute $NaHCO_3$ (100 mmol) in 400 mL H_2O with 20 mEq KCl and infuse for 2 hr. Repeat $NaHCO_3$ administration every 2 hr until pH is 7.0. Monitor serum K^+.

TABLE 40-9 ANTEPARTUM FETAL SURVEILLANCE IN LOW-RISK INSULIN-DEPENDENT DIABETES MELLITUS*

STUDY	INDICATED
Ultrasonography at 4- to 6-wk intervals	Yes
Maternal assessment of fetal activity, daily at 28 wk	Yes
NST at 32 wk; BPP or CST if NST is nonreactive	Yes
Amniocentesis for lung profile	Yes, if elective delivery is planned before 39 wk

*Excellent control, no vasculopathy (classes B, C), no stillbirth.
BPP, biophysical profile; CST, contraction stress test; NST, nonstress test.

TABLE 40-10 ANTEPARTUM FETAL SURVEILLANCE IN HIGH-RISK INSULIN-DEPENDENT DIABETES MELLITUS*

STUDY	INDICATED
Ultrasonography at 4- to 6-wk intervals	Yes
Maternal assessment of fetal activity daily at 28 wk	Yes
NST; BPP or CST if NST is nonreactive	Initiate at 28-30 wk
Consider amniocentesis for lung profile prior to 38 wk	

*Poor control (macrosomia, hydramnios), vasculopathy (classes D, F, R), prior stillbirth.
BPP, biophysical profile; CST, contraction stress test; NST, nonstress test.

women with preexisting diabetes, 25% of women had greater than a 15% fall in insulin requirements, which was associated with an increased risk of preeclampsia and SGA infants.[59] Prospective studies are needed to confirm these findings in order to guide clinical management when insulin requirements decline in late pregnancy.

Maternal assessment of fetal activity serves as a simple screening technique in a program of fetal surveillance. During the third trimester, women are instructed to perform daily fetal movement counts. Women with a variety of high-risk antepartum conditions, including diabetes, appear to have an increased incidence of alarming fetal activity patterns. Although the false-negative rate with maternal monitoring of fetal activity is low (~1%), the false-positive rate may be as high as 60%. Although generally believed to be associated with decreased fetal movement, maternal hypoglycemia may actually stimulate fetal activity.

The nonstress test (NST) remains the preferred primary method to assess antepartum fetal well-being in the patient with DM. If the NST is nonreactive, a biophysical profile (BPP) or contraction stress test (CST) is then performed (see Fig. 40-15). We generally begin heart rate monitoring by 32 weeks' gestation. Two studies have also demonstrated an increased fetal death rate within 1 week of a reactive NST in pregnancies complicated by IDDM compared with other high-risk gestations. **If the NST is to be used as the primary method of antepartum heart rate testing, we prefer that it be done at least twice weekly after the patient reaches 32 weeks' gestation. In some centers, twice-weekly testing includes an NST followed several days later by a BPP. In patients with vascular disease, poor glucose control, or suspected FGR in whom the incidence of abnormal tests and intrauterine deaths is greater, testing is often initiated between 28 and 32 weeks' gestation.**

Doppler umbilical artery velocimetry has been proposed as a clinical tool for antepartum fetal surveillance in pregnancies at risk for placental vascular disease (see Chapter 33). Because Doppler studies of the umbilical artery may be predictive of fetal

role in reducing perinatal mortality in diabetic pregnancies, antepartum fetal monitoring tests are now used primarily to reassure the obstetrician and to avoid unnecessary premature intervention. These techniques have few false-negatives results, and in a woman with well-controlled diabetes and no vasculopathy or significant hypertension, reassuring antepartum testing allows the fetus to benefit from further maturation in utero. A subset of women who had diabetes prior to gestation will have falling insulin requirements in late pregnancy, which in limited cohort studies have not been associated with adverse outcomes. However, in a recent retrospective review of 139 pregnancies of

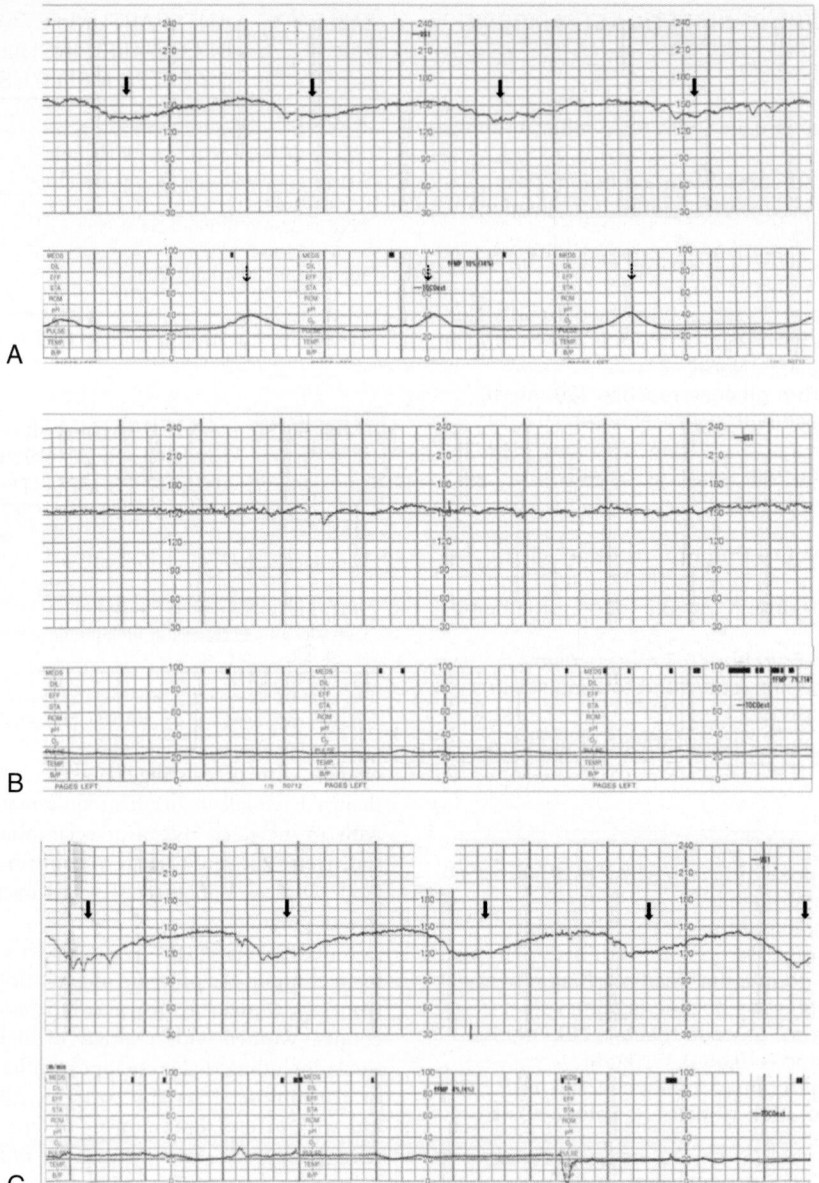

FIG 40-17 Fetal heart rate monitoring during an acute episode of diabetic ketoacidosis. **A,** Recurrent late decelerations are observed. **B,** Following hydration and correction of acidosis, the tracing improves. **C,** Fetal tracing in a patient with acute diabetic ketoacidosis at 34 weeks' gestation demonstrating repetitive late decelerations (solid arrows) and minimal variability. An emergency cesarean delivery was performed. The arterial cord pH was 6.85. (From Sibai B. Diabetic ketoacidosis in pregnancy. *Obstet Gynecol.* 2014;123:167.)

outcome in diabetic pregnancies complicated by vascular disease, we reserve the use of screening Doppler measurements for women with nephropathy or hypertensive disease. Elevated placental resistance, as evidenced by an increased systolic-to-diastolic ratio, is associated with FGR and preeclampsia in these high-risk patients. In contrast, patients with well-controlled diabetes without vascular disease rarely demonstrate abnormal fetal umbilical artery waveforms.

It is important not only to include the results of antepartum fetal testing but also to weigh all of the clinical features that involve the mother and fetus before deciding to intervene for suspected fetal compromise, especially if this decision may result in a preterm delivery (see Tables 40-9 and 40-10). Our review of studies that comprised 993 diabetic women revealed that in 5% of cases, an abnormal test of fetal condition led to delivery. It appears that outpatient testing pro-

tocols work well in diabetic patients who require insulin. Abnormal fetal testing is more common in women whose diabetes is poorly controlled and in those who have hypertension or significant vasculopathy that may be associated with FGR. It follows that these subgroups probably benefit most from a program of antepartum fetal surveillance.

Ultrasound can be a valuable tool in evaluating fetal growth, estimating fetal weight, and detecting hydramnios and malformations. Maternal serum alpha-fetoprotein (MSAFP) determination at 16 weeks' gestation is often used in association with a detailed ultrasound study during the midtrimester in an attempt to detect NTDs and other anomalies (see Chapter 10). Levels of MSAFP, unconjugated estriol (uE$_3$), and inhibin A in diabetic women are lower than those in the nondiabetic population. A lower threshold for the upper limit of normal (ULN) for MSAFP, 1.5 multiples of the median (MoM), may thus be preferable in pregnancies complicated by DM in order to help detect spina bifida and other major malformations that are increased in this population. **A comprehensive ultrasound examination at 18 to 20 weeks, as well as fetal echocardiography performed at 20 to 22 weeks, is undertaken to diagnose fetal anomalies. Whereas the risk for defects, including cardiac anomalies, is increased with markedly elevated maternal HbA1c levels, the frequency in women with moderate control remains elevated compared with that of nondiabetic pregnancies. Thus we prefer to utilize fetal echocardiography as a screening tool in all type 1 and type 2 diabetic pregnancies.** Greene and Benacerraf performed detailed sonography in the midtrimester and detected 18 of 32 malformations in a series of 432 diabetic pregnancies. The specificity was in excess of 99%, and the negative predictive value was 97%. Spina bifida was identified in all cases; however, ventricular septal defects, limb abnormalities, and facial clefts were missed. A review of the prenatal diagnosis experience in 289 women with IDDM in the Ohio State University Diabetes in Pregnancy Program revealed 29 anomalies, of which 12 were cardiac, 14 were noncardiac, and 3 were combined. Twelve of 15 cardiac (80%) and 10 of 17 noncardiac lesions (59%) were identified prenatally. When considering cardiac defects alone, we could not identify a glycosylated hemoglobin cutoff for these anomalies. Starikov and colleagues[60] identified 30 fetal cardiac defects in a series of 535 diabetic women and noted the risk to be 8.3% in women with an HbA1c greater than 8.5%, compared with 3.9% in those below this cutoff.

Ultrasound examinations should be performed during the third trimester to assess fetal growth. The detection of fetal macrosomia, the leading risk factor for shoulder dystocia, is important in the selection of patients who are best delivered by cesarean section. **An increased rate of cephalopelvic disproportion and shoulder dystocia, accompanied by significant risk for traumatic birth injury and asphyxia, has been consistently associated with vaginal delivery of large infants. The risk for such complications rises exponentially when birthweight exceeds 4 kg, and it is greater for the fetus of a diabetic mother when compared with a fetus with similar weight whose mother does not have diabetes** (Fig. 40-18).[61]

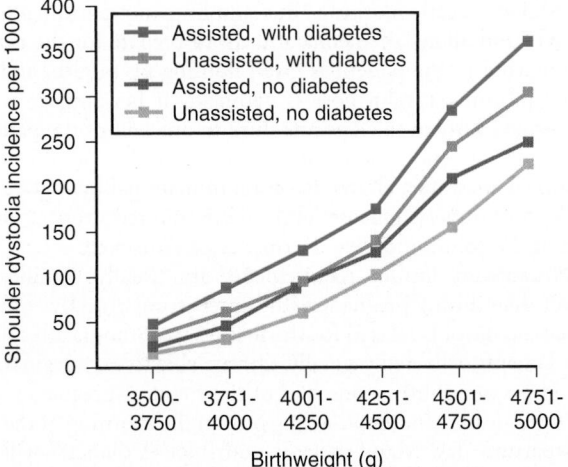

FIG 40-18 Frequency of shoulder dystocia for increasing birthweight by maternal diabetes status and method of vaginal delivery, spontaneous or assisted. (Modified from Nesbitt TS, Gilbert WM, Herrchen B. Shoulder dystocia and associated risk factors with macrosomic infants born in California. *Am J Obstet Gynecol.* 1998;17:476.)

Sonographic measurements of the fetal abdominal circumference have proved most helpful in predicting fetal macrosomia. The abdomen is likely to be large because of increased subcutaneous fat deposition. However, it is critical to recognize that a single ultrasound examination may have limited accuracy in predicting macrosomia at term in women with diabetes. Using serial sonographic examinations, accelerated abdominal growth may be identified between 28 and 32 weeks' gestation in pregnancies complicated by diabetes.[62]

TIMING AND MODE OF DELIVERY

Delivery should be delayed until fetal maturation has taken place, provided diabetes is well controlled and antepartum surveillance remains normal. The ACOG suggests delivery be delayed until 39 weeks in women without vascular disease whose diabetes is well controlled. In our practice, induction of labor is often planned at 39 to 40 weeks' gestation in such patients. For diabetic women with vascular disease, it has been suggested that delivery may be undertaken at 37 to 39 weeks. Women with vascular disease are delivered prior to 37 weeks only if hypertension worsens, if significant FGR is present, or if biophysical testing mandates early delivery. Depending on clinical circumstances, antenatal corticosteroids may be administered to accelerate fetal lung maturity. This must be done with caution because significant maternal hyperglycemia may be observed for several days after antenatal corticosteriods are given. In women with poor glycemic control, an individualized approach to the timing of delivery is recommended. Options may include late preterm or early term delivery or amniocentesis to assess lung maturity prior to delivery. **Tests of fetal lung maturity appear to have the same predictive value in diabetic pregnancies as in the normal population.**

The presence of the acidic phospholipid phosphatidylglycerol (PG) is the final marker of fetal pulmonary maturation. Several authors have suggested that fetal hyperinsulinemia may be associated with delayed appearance of PG and an increased incidence of RDS. Landon and coworkers have correlated the appearance of PG in amniotic fluid with maternal glycemic control during gestation. RDS may occur in the IDM with a mature lecithin-to-sphingomyelin (L/S) ratio or fetal lung maturity index but absent PG. Moore[63] compared PG production in amniotic fluid specimens from 295 diabetic women and 590 matched controls and reported that the onset of PG production was delayed in GDM from 35.9 ± 1.1 weeks to 37.3 ± 1 weeks and to 38.7 ± 0.9 weeks in pregestational diabetic pregnancies. In this study, delayed appearance of PG was not associated with the level of glycemic control. In addition, the lamellar body count may be used to assess amniotic fluid for lung maturity; cut-off values in diabetic patients are similar to those in the nondiabetic population (see Chapter 11).

When antepartum testing suggests fetal compromise, delivery must be considered. If amniotic fluid analysis yields a test result that indicates lung maturity, delivery should be accomplished promptly. In the presence of presumed lung immaturity, the decision to proceed with delivery should be based on confirmation of deteriorating fetal condition by several tests that show abnormal values. For example, if the NST and the BPP indicate fetal compromise, delivery is indicated. Finally, several maternal indications exist for delivery that include significant preeclampsia, worsening renal function, and deteriorating vision secondary to proliferative retinopathy.

Choosing the route of delivery for the diabetic patient remains controversial. **Cesarean delivery rates as high as 50% are common in series of pregestational diabetic women.** This figure is likely to represent the practice trends of most obstetricians and perinatologists in the United States. A trial of labor following previous cesarean delivery may be undertaken in select cases and has a reported success rate of 64%.

The increased rate of shoulder dystocia and brachial plexus injury in the offspring of diabetic women has prompted adoption of early induction strategies, as well as selection of patients for cesarean delivery, based on ultrasound estimation of fetal size. Such approaches are limited by the relative inaccuracy of ultrasound prediction of birthweight. Despite the limitations, Kjos and colleagues demonstrated that induction at 38 weeks in a population of women with GDM was associated with a lower frequency of LGA infants and shoulder dystocia without an increased rate of cesarean delivery. This is in contrast to studies of induction in nondiabetic women, in which suspected macrosomia is apparently associated with an increased rate of cesarean delivery. In a decision tree analysis of cost-effectiveness, Rouse and colleagues found that whereas elective cesarean delivery for macrosomia to prevent permanent brachial plexus injury was prohibitively expensive in the nondiabetic woman, at a cost of several million dollars per permanent brachial plexus injury prevented, 489 cesarean deliveries—at a cost per avoided birth injury of $880,000 per case—for those diabetic pregnancies with an estimated fetal size greater than 4000 g seemed to be at least tenable.

The overall risk for shoulder dystocia in the macrosomic fetus of an IDM is greater than in large infants of normal pregnancy. The risk for shoulder dystocia with a fetal weight greater than 4000 g in diabetic gravidae is about 30%. Somewhat less impressive yet significantly greater frequencies of shoulder dystocia for delivery of a macrosomic fetus of IDMs, compared with non-IDMs, have been reported by Nesbitt and colleagues (see Fig. 40-18).[61] At present, the ACOG recommends consideration of cesarean delivery in diabetic women when estimated fetal weight exceeds 4500 g. Our approach continues to be to consider cesarean delivery when the estimated weight is 4000 to 4500 g after evaluating obstetric history and clinical pelvimetry. Despite attempts to select patients with obvious fetal macrosomia for elective cesarean delivery, arrest of dilation or descent despite adequate labor should alert the physician to the possibility of cephalopelvic disproportion. Approximately 25% of deliveries of macrosomic infants (>4000 g) following a prolonged second stage are complicated by shoulder dystocia; therefore it follows that cesarean delivery should be considered in a diabetic woman who demonstrates significant protracted labor or failure of descent.

GLUCOREGULATION DURING LABOR AND DELIVERY

Because neonatal hypoglycemia is in part related to maternal glucose levels during labor, it is important to maintain maternal plasma glucose levels within the physiologic normal range. The patient is given nothing by mouth after midnight of the evening before induction or elective cesarean delivery. The usual bedtime dose of insulin is administered, or for women receiving pump therapy, the infusion is continued overnight. Upon arrival to labor and delivery, early in the morning, the patient's capillary glucose level is assessed with a bedside

BOX 40-6   INSULIN MANAGEMENT DURING LABOR AND DELIVERY

- Usual dose of intermediate-acting insulin is given at bedtime.
- Morning dose of insulin is withheld.
- Intravenous infusion of normal saline is begun.
- Once active labor begins or glucose levels fall to <70 mg/dL, the infusion is changed from saline to 5% dextrose and is delivered at a rate of 2.5 mg/kg/min.
- Glucose levels are checked hourly using a portable reflectance meter allowing for adjustment in the infusion rate.
- Regular (short-acting) insulin is administered by intravenous infusion if glucose levels exceed 140 mg/dL.

From Jovanovic L, Peterson CM. Management of the pregnant, insulin-dependent diabetic woman. *Diabetes Care.* 1980;3:63.

reflectance meter. In women who use continuous insulin infusion pumps, this therapy may be used during the latent phase of labor or early in the induction process. Basal infusion rates are generally reduced, and boluses may be given based on carbohydrate consumption and to correct hyperglycemia. Once active labor begins, IV infusion of both insulin and glucose is then begun based on maternal glucose levels (Box 40-6). Also, 10 U of short-acting insulin may be added to 1000 mL of solution containing 5% dextrose. An infusion rate of 100 to 125 mL/hr (1 U/hr) will result in good glucose control in most cases. Insulin may also be infused from a syringe pump at a dose of 0.25 to 2 U/hr and adjusted to maintain normal glucose values. Glucose levels are recorded hourly during the active phase of labor, and the infusion rate is adjusted accordingly. Patients with well-controlled diabetes are often euglycemic once active labor begins and then require increased glucose infusion at a rate of 2.5 mg/kg/min, which mimics strenuous exercise requirements. During the second stage of labor, in response to hyperglycemia associated with increased catecholamine secretion, it may be necessary to increase the insulin infusion.

When cesarean delivery is to be performed, it should be scheduled for early morning. This simplifies intrapartum glucose control and allows the neonatal team to prepare for the care of the newborn. The patient is given nothing by mouth, and her usual morning insulin dose is withheld. If her surgery is not performed early in the day, one third to one half of the patient's intermediate-acting dose of insulin may be administered. Regional anesthesia allows detection of maternal hypoglycemia. Following surgery, glucose levels are monitored every 2 hours, and an IV solution of 5% dextrose is administered.

Postpartum insulin requirements are usually significantly lower than during pregnancy. The antepartum objective of tight glucose control is relaxed for the first 24 to 48 hours after delivery. Patients delivered vaginally who are able to eat a regular diet are given one third to one half of their end-of-pregnancy dose of NPH insulin and rapid-acting insulin the morning of the first postpartum day. Many patients with type 2 diabetes will not require insulin for 24 to 48 hours postpartum, and these women can be managed with insulin or oral agents as preferred; frequent glucose determinations are used to guide insulin dosage. Most patients are stabilized on this regimen within a few days after delivery.

Whether they receive insulin or oral agents, women with diabetes are encouraged to breastfeed. The additional 500 kcal required daily are given as approximately 100 g of carbohydrate and 20 g of protein. The insulin dose may be somewhat lower in lactating diabetic women. Hypoglycemia appears to be common in the first week after delivery and immediately after nursing.

MANAGEMENT OF THE WOMAN WITH GESTATIONAL DIABETES

Is There a Benefit to the Treatment of Gestational Diabetes Mellitus?

The frequency of GDM has increased worldwide, and up to 14% of pregnancies are affected.[64] With both an increased incidence and the proposed lowering of the threshold for diagnosis, the health care costs of GDM can be expected to rise proportionally. It follows that whether a benefit exists to the treatment of GDM has assumed even greater importance now than in the past.

The 2013 guidelines of the U.S. Preventive Services Task Force (USPSTF)[45] acknowledged a treatment benefit for GDM for the first time. Their systematic review and meta-analysis concluded that treatment of GDM results in less preeclampsia, shoulder dystocia, and macrosomia.

Randomized Treatment Trials for Gestational Diabetes Mellitus

Two important RCTs conducted over the last decade have provided high-level evidence that treatment of GDM confers both maternal and perinatal benefits. The Australian Carbohydrate Intolerance Study in Pregnant Women (ACHOIS) was a multicenter, 10-year randomized treatment trial of 1000 women conducted at 14 sites in Australia.[65]

Treatment was associated with a significant reduction in the rate of the primary outcome, a composite of serious perinatal complications (perinatal death, shoulder dystocia, birth trauma that included fracture or nerve palsy; adjusted RR, 0.33; 95% CI, 0.14 to 0.75). Overall, seven infants in the treatment group had a serious complication (all shoulder dystocia) compared with 23 infants in the untreated group, of whom five experienced perinatal death, four had birth trauma, and 16 had shoulder dystocia.

Among secondary neonatal outcomes, no significant differences were found in the rates of neonatal hypoglycemia that required IV therapy, jaundice that required phototherapy, or respiratory disease that required supplemental oxygen. Neonatal intensive care unit (NICU) admissions were remarkably high in both groups: 71% in treated versus 61% in untreated patients ($P = .01$). Importantly, treatment did reduce the frequency of LGA infants from 22% to 13% and birthweight greater than 4000 g from 21% to 10%. Among maternal outcomes, preeclampsia was significantly reduced with treatment (12% vs. 18%).

The ACHOIS study was followed by the NICHD MFMU Network RCT of 958 cases of mild GDM.[66] In this study, mild GDM was defined as a fasting glucose less than 95 mg/dL with two of the three postglucose values exceeding established thresholds.

These investigators found no significant difference in the frequency of the primary composite perinatal outcome—perinatal death, neonatal hypoglycemia, elevated cord C-peptide level, or

TABLE 40-11	RESULTS OF RANDOMIZED CONTROLLED TRIALS FOR TREATMENT OF GESTATIONAL DIABETES MELLITUS	
	LANDON ET AL[66] **(2009)**	**CROWTHER ET AL**[65] **(2005)**
Preeclampsia	↓	↓
Weight gain	↓	↓
LGA infant	↓	↓
Neonatal fat mass	↓	—
Shoulder dystocia	↓	Not studied

LGA, large for gestational age.

birth trauma—in the treatment group (32.4%) compared with the usual care group (37%; $P = .14$). Several key differences in secondary outcomes, however, were observed with treatment, including a lower frequency of LGA infants with birthweight exceeding 4000 g and decreased neonatal fat mass.

Among maternal outcomes, rates of labor induction were similar between groups; however, cesarean delivery was performed less often in treated women (26.9% vs. 33.8). This rate remained lower after excluding cases of abnormal presentation, prior cesarean delivery, placenta previa, and oligohydramnios (13% vs. 19.7%; $P = .011$). A lower rate of shoulder dystocia (1.5% vs. 4%) and preeclampsia or gestational hypertension (8.6% vs. 13.6%) was also found in the treatment group.

In summary, the NICHD MFMU trial demonstrated that although treatment of mild GDM did not reduce the frequency of several neonatal morbidities characteristic of diabetic pregnancy, it did lower the risk for fetal overgrowth, neonatal fat mass, shoulder dystocia, cesarean delivery, and hypertensive disorders of pregnancy.[66] **These findings, along with those reported in the ACHOIS study, have confirmed a benefit to treatment of even mild carbohydrate intolerance of pregnancy** (Table 40-11).

Treatment of the Woman with Gestational Diabetes Mellitus

The mainstay of treatment of GDM remains nutritional counseling and dietary intervention. The optimal diet should provide caloric and nutrient needs to sustain pregnancy without resulting in significant postprandial hyperglycemia. Women with GDM generally do not need hospitalization for dietary instruction and management. Once the diagnosis is established, women are begun on a dietary program of 2000 to 2500 kcal daily. This represents approximately 35 kcal/kg of present pregnancy weight. For women who are overweight and obese, a reduction in caloric intake to 25 kcal/kg/day and 15 kcal/kg/day (present pregnancy weight), respectively, may be advised. Jovanovic-Peterson and Peterson have noted that the usually prescribed diet composed of 50% to 60% carbohydrate will cause excessive weight gain and postprandial hyperglycemia and will require insulin therapy in 50% of patients. For this reason, these authors have suggested limiting carbohydrates to 33% to 40% of calories. Barbour[67] has noted that with carbohydrate restriction, many women will substitute fat and thereby potentially transfer excess FFAs, which are associated with fetal fat accretion.

Complex carbohydrates are preferred to simple carbohydrates because they are less likely to produce significant postprandial hyperglycemia. A randomized crossover study found that liberalizing complex carbohydrate intake in GDM women resulted in achievement of glycemia below current targets and also lowered postprandial FFA concentrations.[68] In spite of the widespread prevalence of GDM, Hernandez and colleagues[69] have noted that only six RCTs of 250 women have provided the evidence that a diet higher in complex carbohydrate and lower in simple sugar and saturated fat may be effective in blunting postprandial hyperglycemia and thereby preventing worsened insulin resistance and promoting excess fetal growth. Clearly, additional clinical trials are needed to help define the optimal diet for women with GDM. In light of the 2009 Institute of Medicine (IOM) recommendations concerning weight gain during pregnancy, the question arises as to their applicability to women with GDM. These guidelines did not specify recommendations for women with diabetes, yet limited weight gain may be advisable in obese diabetic women. The IOM recommends a weight gain of 11 to 20 lb for obese women (BMI 30 or greater). A specified carbohydrate-limited diet in obese women with GDM both improves glycemic control and reduces weight gain. An independent effect of maternal obesity, weight gain, and diabetes on birthweight is also apparent.

Once the patient with GDM is placed on an appropriate diet, surveillance of blood glucose levels is necessary to be certain that glycemic control has been established. We prefer to have patients perform daily self-monitoring of blood glucose that consists of a fasting glucose level and three postprandial determinations. We provide women with GDM with a reflectance meter and carefully review values following the initial week of diet intervention. In women with good control on diet therapy alone, the frequency of testing can be reduced and tailored accordingly. We do not use CGM in women with GDM, although reports exist of improved glycemic control and pregnancy outcomes in women with GDM utilizing this technology.[70]

Glycemic target thresholds of fasting glucose less than 95 mg/dL, 1-hour postprandial glucose less than 140 mg/dL, and 2-hour postprandial glucose less than 120 mg/dL have been suggested by the Fifth International Workshop Conference on GDM. If a patient repetitively exceeds established thresholds, pharmacologic therapy is recommended. In our experience, if the majority of values at a particular time point are elevated, pharmacologic therapy should be initiated. Approximately 25% to 50% of women with GDM require insulin or oral agents. Some cases are managed with a single dose of bedtime NPH insulin to treat isolated fasting hyperglycemia, whereas others require treatment of postprandial hyperglycemia with insulin lispro or aspart at appropriate mealtimes. Up to four injections daily may be necessary to achieve adequate control. Whereas some have recommended calculating starting insulin dosage based on body weight, we have typically prescribed 15 to 20 U of NPH insulin in the morning and at bedtime (if fasting glucose is elevated) along with 5 to 10 U of rapid-acting insulin to cover specific mealtime elevations. Continued monitoring of glucose levels with feedback allows the practitioner to make frequent adjustments in the insulin regimen. It is important to recognize that use of the previously mentioned cutoffs for initiating insulin are based on data regarding increased perinatal morbidity when such values are exceeded in women with preexisting diabetes. Data have yet to be gathered from controlled trials to identify ideal glycemic targets for prevention of fetal morbidity associated with GDM.

An observational study conducted by Langer and colleagues found that women with a fasting glucose between 96 and 105 mg/dL have a greater incidence of LGA infants (28.6%) when receiving diet therapy alone compared with those receiving both diet therapy and insulin. In women with an initial fasting glucose between 95 and 104 mg/dL, 70% required insulin therapy to achieve optimal control.

During the past 15 years, oral hypoglycemic therapy has become a suitable alternative to insulin treatment in women with GDM. At present, glyburide is the most commonly prescribed medication in the United States for the treatment of GDM.[71] **Nicholson and colleagues[72] performed a systematic review of the evidence from randomized trials and observational studies and concluded that glycemia was equivalent in women who received oral hypoglycemic agents compared with those who received insulin.** Moreover, no evidence suggested increased adverse neonatal outcomes with the use of oral hypoglycemic agents. ACOG recognizes that either insulin or oral agents may be appropriate first-line therapy for GDM. At present, data are insufficient to recommend treatment with any oral agent other than glyburide or metformin. In a landmark study, Langer and colleagues[73] reported results from a randomized trial of 404 women who received insulin versus glyburide and noted similar improvement in glycemia with both regimens. The frequency of macrosomia and neonatal hypoglycemia was similar in the two study groups. Only 4% of women failed glyburide therapy and required a change to insulin. Cord blood analysis revealed no detectable glyburide in exposed pregnancies. Subsequently, Hebert and colleagues reported that glyburide appears to cross the placenta in significant amounts; this observation has raised concerns regarding the safety of this agent. Importantly, clinical studies have revealed increased rates of neonatal hypoglycemia with glyburide use in GDM. It is, however, unknown whether glyburide can affect progression to type 2 diabetes in treated women or whether glucose homeostasis is altered later in life in their offspring.

Following Langer's randomized trial, several smaller studies reported success in achieving good glycemic control with glyburide but with slightly higher failure rates (15% to 20%). Jacobson and colleagues recently reported on the implementation of glyburide as an alternative to insulin in a large managed-care organization. These authors noted a similar frequency of LGA infants and macrosomia among 268 women treated with insulin compared with 236 who received glyburide. In this nonrandomized study, more women in the glyburide group achieved lower mean fasting and postprandial glucose levels compared with insulin-treated subjects. Importantly, the authors noted an increased rate of preeclampsia, need for neonatal phototherapy, and birth injury in the glyburide group, all of which point to the need for further study concerning safety.

Lain and colleagues performed a randomized trial of 99 women with GDM that compared glyburide with insulin treatment. These authors reported no increase in neonatal fat mass, BMI, ponderal index, or anthropometric measures in glyburide-treated offspring, although a significantly greater rate of infant birthweights higher than 4000 g was observed in the glyburide-treated group (22% vs. 2.4%). Similar to insulin therapy, glyburide action must be carefully balanced with meals and snacks to prevent maternal hyperglycemia. **Observational data suggest that glyburide may be less successful in obese women and in those with marked hyperglycemia discovered early in gestation.** In our experience, most women with fasting glucose levels of 115 mg/dL or higher will fail to achieve adequate glucose control with glyburide and will require insulin therapy

BOX 40-7 SUMMARY OF GLYBURIDE VERSUS INSULIN TREATMENT IN GESTATIONAL DIABETES MELLITUS

- Maternal fasting and postprandial glycemia comparable to that with insulin treatment
- Glyburide failure rate of 15%-20%
- Glyburide failures associated with earlier diagnosis of gestational diabetes and fasting glucose levels >110-115 mg/dL
- Comparable neonatal outcomes
- Significant cost savings

(Box 40-7). The usual dose of glyburide is 2.5 to 20 mg daily in divided doses, usually before breakfast and dinner, although pharmacokinetic studies during pregnancy indicate that a daily dose as great as 30 mg may be necessary to achieve adequate control. Caritis and Hebert have suggested that glyburide is optimally administered 30 to 60 minutes prior to a meal.

Metformin has also been used for treatment of GDM. Although metformin clearly crosses the placenta, it does not appear to be teratogenic. Rowan and colleagues[74] randomized 761 women with GDM at 20 to 33 weeks to metformin and insulin as needed versus insulin therapy alone. No differences in perinatal outcomes were reported, and a composite of perinatal morbidity—neonatal hypoglycemia, respiratory distress, birth trauma, prematurity, and need for phototherapy in the infant—was observed in about one third of women in each group. Metformin use was well tolerated, and treated women gained less weight than those who received insulin; however, 46% of these women required supplemental insulin to achieve glycemic control. A 2-year follow-up study of the offspring from this trial reported no significant difference in total body fat or central adiposity between infants of metformin-treated mothers versus those of insulin-treated mothers; however, an increase in subcutaneous adiposity was reported. Carlsen and colleagues[75] reported that in offspring of women who were continued on with metformin treatment for polycystic ovary syndrome, no difference was reported at birth in infant weight or length; however, at 1 year of age, the offspring of the women who used metformin in pregnancy were heavier than in the placebo group (10.2 ± 1.2 vs. 9.7 ± 1.1 kg, $P = .003$). Further follow-up of these children is necessary to determine the significance of this finding. Another, smaller follow-up study[76] at 18 months of children exposed to metformin in utero found these offspring to be taller and heavier than insulin-exposed children. Body composition did not differ between the two groups.

It appears that glyburide may be superior to metformin in achieving satisfactory glucose control in women with GDM. A randomized trial[77] of 149 women compared metformin with glyburide for the treatment of GDM and found that 35% of women randomized to metformin, compared with 16% who received glyburide, required insulin to achieve adequate control.

Exercise may serve as a useful adjunctive treatment for women with GDM. Physical exercise may improve glycemic control because increased insulin sensitivity accompanies cardiovascular conditioning. A randomized study of 41 women with GDM who manifested elevated fasting glucose levels and would normally require insulin therapy utilized a supervised bicycle ergometry training program. No statistical differences were observed in weekly blood glucose determinations between the study groups. Another study that used arm ergometry three times per week resulted in a significant reduction in mean fasting glucose in the exercise group as well as a reduction in glucose concentration following a 1-hour, 50-g challenge. Because the total number of women with GDM studied in randomized trials is limited, the role of exercise as a primary therapy in GDM remains unknown. Nonetheless, a program of moderate exercise has been advocated by the ADA as part of the treatment of GDM.

Women with GDM that is well controlled are at low risk for an IUFD. For this reason, we do not routinely institute antepartum fetal heart rate testing in uncomplicated diet-controlled GDM. Women with a hypertensive disorder, a history of a prior stillbirth, or suspected macrosomia do undergo fetal testing.[78] Additionally, those who require insulin or oral agents for treatment of GDM undergo twice-weekly heart rate testing at 32 weeks' gestation. Using such a protocol at the Ohio State University Hospital Diabetes in Pregnancy Program, we observed only six intrauterine deaths in more than 3500 women with uncomplicated GDM in the past 25 years. Thus it appears that the third-trimester stillbirth rate in these patients is no higher than that of the general obstetric population. A study of 389 women with GDM documented an antepartum stillbirth rate of 7.7 per 10,000, which was not significantly different from the rate of 4.8 per 1000 observed in nondiabetic low-risk patients. In this study, because only 7% of fetuses were delivered on the basis of a low BPP score, the benefit of testing all GDM pregnancies remains in question. At present, without prospective studies to compare outcomes in monitored and unmonitored women with GDM without other risk factors, it is not possible to determine whether any benefits exist to antepartum fetal surveillance in this population.

Because many obstetricians have extrapolated the increased risk for stillbirth in women with type 1 or type 2 diabetes to those with GDM, a remarkable number of GDM pregnancies are subject to scheduled delivery at term. At present, the ACOG suggests that if GDM is well controlled on diet or medication, delivery should not be undertaken prior to 39 weeks' gestation. If glycemic control is suboptimum, ACOG recommends that the decision to schedule late-preterm or early-term birth in such cases should be individualized. As with antepartum fetal testing, in the otherwise uncomplicated group, should scheduled induction be the standard approach for these pregnancies complicated by GDM? Available observational and retrospective data do not permit an evidence-based recommendation. Rosenstein and colleagues[78] have recommended that women with class A2 GDM routinely undergo induction at 39 weeks based on a large retrospective cohort that indicated that infant mortality at 39 weeks (8.7/1000) was statistically lower than the risk of stillbirth plus infant mortality with expectant management over an additional week (15.2/1000). A secondary analysis[79] of the MFMU trial of treatment of mild GDM revealed that induction of labor prior to 40 weeks' gestation does not increase the rate of cesarean delivery.

Kjos and colleagues conducted a prospective randomized trial of active induction of labor at 38 weeks' gestation versus expectant management in a series that included 187 women with GDM who required insulin. The cesarean delivery rate was not significantly different in the expectant-management group (31%) compared with the active-induction group (25%); however, an increased prevalence of LGA infants (23% vs. 10%) was observed in the expectant-management group. Moreover, the frequency of shoulder dystocia was 3% in this group, with

TABLE 40-12	DIAGNOSTIC CRITERIA FOR DIABETES MELLITUS, IMPAIRED FASTING GLUCOSE, AND IMPAIRED GLUCOSE TOLERANCE		
TEST	DIABETES	IMPAIRED FASTING GLUCOSE	IMPAIRED GLUCOSE TOLERANCE
Fasting plasma glucose	Fasting plasma glucose ≥126 mg/dL	Fasting plasma glucose 100-125 mg/dL	Not applicable
75-g 2-hr oral glucose tolerance test	Fasting plasma glucose ≥126 mg/dL *or* 2-hr plasma glucose ≥200 mg/dL	Fasting plasma glucose 100-125 mg/dL	2-hr plasma glucose 140-199 mg/dL

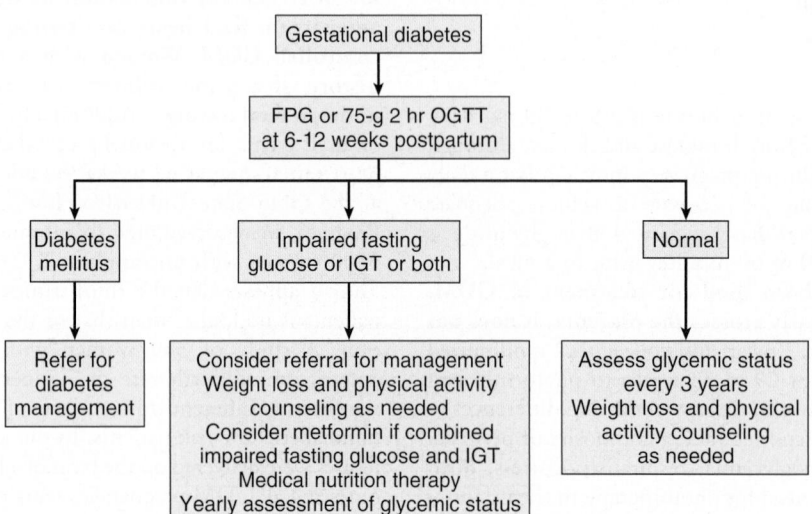

FIG 40-19 Management of postpartum glucose screening results. FPG, fasting plasma glucose; IGT, impaired glucose tolerance; OGTT, oral glucose tolerance test. (Modified from American College of Obstetricians and Gynecologists Committee Opinion No. 435, June 2009.)

no cases reported in those undergoing induction at 38 weeks' gestation. These data led the authors to conclude that scheduled elective induction should be considered in insulin-requiring patients with GDM because it does not increase the risk for cesarean delivery and it lowers the risk for shoulder dystocia. In women managed expectantly, monitoring of fetal growth should be considered because of an apparent increasing risk for macrosomia with advancing gestational age. As with women with preexisting diabetes, scheduled cesarean delivery to prevent birth trauma is offered to women with suspected macrosomia or a history of prior shoulder dystocia. A range of 58 to 588 cesarean deliveries with an estimated fetal weight of 4500 g and 148 to 962 cesarean deliveries with an estimated fetal weight of 4000 g have been suggested as needed to prevent a single case of permanent brachial plexus injury.[80] We use the same estimated weight cutoffs in considering the mode of delivery in pregnancies complicated by GDM as previously discussed with regard to pregnancies complicated by preexisting diabetes.

POSTPARTUM FOLLOW-UP OF WOMEN WITH GESTATIONAL DIABETES MELLITUS

Women with GDM have a sevenfold increased risk for developing type 2 diabetes compared with women who do not have diabetes during pregnancy.[81] Follow-up studies for up to 28 years of O'Sullivan's original cohort of women indicated a prevalence of diabetes in 50% to 60% of women with previous GDM. A follow-up study of up to 10 years in 11,270 women with GDM compared with 174,146 women without GDM revealed a 15.7% frequency of diabetes in patients with a history

of GDM compared with 1% in the non-GDM population.[82] Findings of abnormal carbohydrate intolerance may manifest early in the postpartum period depending on the population studied and its risk factors. As many as one third of women with GDM will have overt diabetes, impaired fasting glucose, or IGT identified during postpartum testing conducted within 6 to 12 weeks of delivery (Table 40-12). Thus both the ADA and the ACOG (Fig. 40-19) recommend postpartum glucose testing following a diagnosis of GDM. Nevertheless, the prevalence of postpartum glucose screening with either a fasting plasma glucose or a 2-hour oral GTT has ranged from only 23% to 58% in seven reported studies.[82] Most recently, a retrospective cohort study of 2016 GDM women in the United Kingdom found that only 18.5% underwent follow-up screening at 6 months and that annual screening remained constant at approximately 20%. A report of 11,825 women with GDM from a large health maintenance organization indicated that postpartum testing was performed in only 50% (n = 5939) of eligible women. In this series, of 5857 women with test results, 16.3% (n = 956) had impaired fasting glucose or IGT, whereas 1.1% (n = 66) were found to have overt diabetes. After adjustment for demographic and clinical factors, abnormal postpartum test results were associated with having required insulin or oral agents during pregnancy and with a longer period from delivery to postpartum testing.

Some debate surrounds whether postpartum glucose testing can be limited to fasting glucose versus a 75-g 2-hour oral GTT. Whereas some have reported sufficiently high sensitivity using a fasting glucose alone (cutoff of 6 mmol/L or 108 mg/dL) to detect diabetes in women with prior GDM, more recent reports indicate the need for a complete 75-g 2-hour oral GTT to achieve satisfactory sensitivity. McClean and colleagues reported 272 abnormal postpartum oral GTTs (27.6%), with 109 women identified as having frank diabetes. Eleven of these (10%) had fasting plasma glucose less than or equal to 6 mmol/L (≤108 mg/dL), as did 62% of 114 cases of IGT. These authors concluded that a postpartum fasting plasma glucose is not sensitive enough in a high-risk population to classify glucose tolerance status accurately. However, only 5 of 109 women with overt diabetes did not require insulin during pregnancy, and of these, three had a postpartum fasting plasma glucose of less than or equal to 6 mmol/L. **Currently, the ACOG recommends using either a fasting plasma glucose or a 75-g 2-hour oral GTT at 6 to 12 weeks' postpartum** (see Fig. 40-19). **The optimal frequency of subsequent testing has not been established; however, the ADA recommends repeat testing at least every 3 years for women with prior GDM and normal results of postpartum screening.**

Given the high risk for subsequent diabetes in women with prior GDM, this population is ideally suited for preventive strategies to lower their risk for deteriorating carbohydrate tolerance.[84-86] Ample evidence shows that breastfeeding improves immediate postpartum glucose tolerance, yet much less is known about whether lactation prevents progression to type 2 diabetes. However, substantial evidence shows that both lifestyle changes and pharmacotherapy can prevent or delay the progression of IGT to type 2 diabetes following GDM.[84,85] In the Diabetes Prevention Program, which compared lifestyle changes to metformin therapy, intensive lifestyle changes of diet and exercise resulted in an average weight loss of 15 lb, most of which was sustained throughout the study. Fewer individuals randomized to lifestyle intervention developed diabetes (14%) compared with the metformin group (22%) and placebo-treated subjects (29%). When women with a history of GDM in this population were studied, Ratner and colleagues[86] found that metformin and lifestyle intervention were similarly effective in reducing the incidence of diabetes in women with a history of GDM. In women with a history of GDM and IGT, the incidence of subsequent diabetes was reduced by 50% and 53% in subjects who received metformin and lifestyle intervention, respectively, compared with placebo. It follows that women with GDM found to have IGT on postpartum glucose tolerance testing should be referred for preventive therapy.

Women with GDM are at high risk for recurrence in future pregnancies. Getahum and colleagues found a 41.3% incidence in second pregnancies in this group. These authors also documented that the risk for GDM is significantly increased in the third pregnancy if the first pregnancy was complicated with GDM compared with a first affected pregnancy followed by an unaffected pregnancy. **Because of the high recurrence risk with previous GDM, we recommend early pregnancy screening or testing, followed by screening at 24 to 28 weeks, or testing in those not found to have GDM earlier in pregnancy.**

Long-Term Effects of Glucose Intolerance on Mother and Fetus

The metabolic syndrome encompasses a myriad metabolic disturbances that include core metabolic problems such as obesity, insulin resistance, and hyperinsulinemia. Related metabolic dysfunctions include hyperlipidemia, hypertension, inflammation, and atherosclerotic vascular disease. The metabolic alterations in pregnancy provide a useful paradigm for the long-term risks of both mother and fetus relative to metabolic dysfunction.

Based on the original work of O'Sullivan and colleagues, GDM is a significant risk factor for the later development of type 2 diabetes. These findings have been replicated in a number of studies. **In a review of the incidence of type 2 diabetes in women with a previous history of GDM, Kim and associates[87] reported that the cumulative incidence of type 2 diabetes increased markedly in the first 5 years after delivery and plateaued after 10 years to about 50%. Elevated fasting glucose during pregnancy was the most common risk factor.**

During pregnancy, women with GDM have an increased risk for hypertensive disorders such as preeclampsia. Carr and coworkers reported that women with a family history of type 2 diabetes and a history of prior GDM are at a threefold higher risk for developing the metabolic syndrome. Additionally, such women were at increased risk for cardiovascular dysfunction such as coronary artery disease and stroke. Hence, not only is the diagnosis of GDM in pregnancy a harbinger of chronic metabolic disease, it also offers an opportunity to initiate efforts to prevent cardiovascular disease in this at-risk population.

The developmental origins of health and disease (DOHAD), or a perinatal programming concept, has recently gained wider acceptance because of the increase in childhood and adult obesity. However, the effect of a hyperglycemic environment on long-term fetal development has been recognized for decades. On the basis of the Pima Indian studies of Pettitt and associates,[88] children of Pima women are at increased risk for both diabetes and obesity. This risk persisted when the offspring of the women with diabetes were compared with that of their siblings born before the mother developed glucose intolerance. These studies were later confirmed and expanded on by Dabelea and colleagues,[89] also in a Pima Indian population. **In fact, the strongest risk factor for diabetes in Pima Indian children is being exposed to maternal diabetes while in utero, independent of maternal obesity and birthweight.** In a white population, Boney reported not only that the LGA children of the women with GDM had an increased risk for diabetes and obesity but also that 50% had evidence of the metabolic syndrome; however, this risk was no longer significant after adjustment for maternal obesity. In a recent multiethnic study, Hillier and coworkers observed that increasing levels of hyperglycemia, particularly fasting hyperglycemia less than the level diagnostic for GDM, were associated with an increased risk for childhood obesity. More recently, **Clausen and associates reported that the risk for being overweight was twofold greater in the young adults of mothers with GDM or type 1 diabetes. The risk for the metabolic syndrome was also increased fourfold in comparison with a matched cohort from the same background population.[90] In contrast to these findings, two systematic reviews and meta-analyses have concluded that childhood obesity associations with GDM may be attenuated with adjustment for maternal obesity or BMI.** In summary, observations are inconsistent with respect to the risk for childhood obesity in the offspring of GDM women. The potential improvement in long-term childhood outcomes with treatment of GDM has been addressed in follow-up studies of the two large randomized treatment trials for GDM.[91,92] In a 4- to 5-year follow-up of children from the ACHOIS study, Gillman and colleagues[91] reported that treatment did not result in a change in offspring BMI. Similarly, Landon and colleagues[92] followed

500 children at ages 5 to 10 years from the MFMU study of mild GDM and found no overall reduction in childhood obesity or metabolic dysfunction in the offspring of treated women. These authors did note an association between neonatal and childhood obesity with a treatment effect suggested in female offspring with the highest neonatal fat mass. Importantly, both the ACHOIS and MFMU RCTs included women with mild GDM, and thus it remains open to question whether fetal programming of metabolic function in GDM can have an intergenerational effect that may be modified by treatment.

PREPREGNANCY COUNSELING OF WOMEN WITH PREEXISTING DIABETES MELLITUS

Anomalies of the cardiac, renal, and central nervous systems arise during the first 7 weeks of gestation, a time when it is most unusual for patients to seek prenatal care. Therefore the management and counseling of women with diabetes in the reproductive age group should begin before conception. Additionally, preconception care for women with diabetes can reduce the occurrence of other adverse birth outcomes. A cost-benefit analysis that estimated a frequency of 2.2% of U.S. births annually to women with preexisting diabetes suggested that universal preconception care might avert 8397 preterm deliveries, 3725 birth defects, and 1872 perinatal deaths with discounted lifetime costs averted as high as $4.3 billion for the affected cohort of children.[93] In the United Kingdom, about 50% of diabetic women receive preconception counseling, whereas estimates as low as 20% have been reported in the United States. Prepregnancy counseling includes an assessment of vascular status and glycemic control. Physicians who care for young women with diabetes must be aware of the importance of such counseling. At this time, the nonpregnant patient can learn techniques for self-monitoring of blood glucose as well as the need for proper dietary management. Folic acid dietary supplementation at a dose of at least 0.4 mg daily should be prescribed to reduce the frequency of NTDs, although it has not specifically been studied in the diabetic population. During counseling, questions may be answered regarding risk factors for complications and the plan for general management of diabetes in pregnancy. Planning for pregnancy should optimally be accomplished over several months, and glycosylated hemoglobin measurements are performed to aid in the timing of conception (Box 40-8).

A reduced rate of major congenital malformations in patients optimally managed before conception has been consistently observed with special diabetes clinics. Mills and associates reported that diabetic women registered before pregnancy had fewer infants with anomalies compared with late registrants (4.9% vs. 9%). Although the incidence of 4.9% remains higher than that in a normal control population (2%), normalization of glycemia was not established in the early-entry group. Kitzmiller and colleagues studied 84 women with pregestational DM who were recruited for preconception education and management during a 7-year period. A group of 110 pregnancies in women with IDDM who presented in the first trimester without preconceptional counseling served as controls in this study. One anomaly (1.2%) occurred in the preconception group compared with 12 malformations (10.9%) in the control population.

Glycosylated hemoglobin levels obtained during the first trimester may be used to counsel diabetic women regarding

---

BOX 40-8   PREPREGNANCY CARE FOR DIABETIC WOMEN

- Multidisciplinary care team: Obstetrician, endocrinologist, diabetes educator, nutritionist
- Evaluation for vascular complications
  - Retinal examination
  - Assess renal function: Serum creatinine and evaluation for proteinuria
- Evaluation for cardiovascular status
  - Hypertension
  - Ischemic cardiac disease: Electrocardiogram if longstanding diabetes, hypertension, or symptoms
- Review medications
  - Angiotensin-converting enzyme inhibitors, angiotensin II receptor blockers, and statins are best avoided if planning conception.
  - Folate supplementation is recommended.
- Assessment of glycemic control
  - Measure HbA1c every 2 months.
  - Target HbA1c should be ≤7.0%.
  - Contraception is not advised until glucose is well controlled.
- Promote healthy lifestyle
  - Regular exercise
  - Nutrition counseling and weight loss for obese women
  - Smoking cessation

---

the risk for an anomalous infant. Miller and colleagues first observed that elevated HbA1c concentrations early in pregnancy correlated with an increased incidence of malformations. In a series of 58 patients with elevated glycosylated hemoglobin levels, 13 malformed infants (22%) were noted. This is in contrast to a 3.4% incidence of major malformations in 58 women whose glycosylated hemoglobin levels were in the normal range. Overall, the risk for a major fetal anomaly may be as high as 25% when the glycosylated hemoglobin level is several percent above normal values. Greene reported that 14 of 35 pregnancies with a glycosylated hemoglobin that exceeded 12.8% were complicated by major malformations. In his series from the Joslin Diabetes Clinic, the risk for major anomalies did not become evident until glycosylated hemoglobin values exceeded 6 SD above the mean. The risk for spontaneous abortion also appears to be increased with marked elevations in glycosylated hemoglobin. However, for diabetic women with good glucose control, there appears to be no greater likelihood of miscarriage. In summary, women with type 1 or type 2 DM should be advised to achieve an HbA1c level close to the upper limit of the normal range before conceiving in order to reduce the risk for a major fetal malformation or miscarriage.

CONTRACEPTION

No evidence suggests that DM impairs fertility; thus family planning is an important consideration for the diabetic woman. A careful history and complete gynecologic examination and counseling are required before selecting a method of contraception. Barrier methods of birth control continue to be safe and inexpensive. When used correctly with a spermicide, the diaphragm has a failure rate of less than 10%. **Because no risks are inherent to the diaphragm and other barrier methods, and because these methods do not affect carbohydrate** metabolism, they have become the preferred interim method of contraception for women with DM. The intrauterine device (IUD) may also be used by diabetic women without concerns about an increased risk for infection.

Combined oral contraceptives (OCs) are the most effective reversible method of contraception with failure rates generally less than 1%. The low-dose preparations are not associated with an increased risk of developing diabetes in women with prior GDM; however, controversy continues in regard to their use in women with overt diabetes. The serious side effects of OC use, including thromboembolic disease and MI, may be increased in diabetic women who use combined OCs.[95] A retrospective study of 136 diabetic women found five cardiovascular complications in those who primarily used low-dose pills. Three patients had cerebrovascular accidents, one had an MI, and one had an axillary vein thrombosis. Despite diabetes increasing the risk for cerebral thromboembolism fivefold compared with controls, this risk was not enhanced by use of combined OCs in a retrospective case-control study.

In one report, several diabetic women exhibited rapid progression of retinopathy with OC use. Klein and colleagues[95] studied the impact of OCs in a cross-sectional study of 384 insulin-dependent women and reported no association between OCs and progression of vascular complications. For physicians who prescribe low-dose OCs to diabetic women, their use should probably be restricted to patients without serious vascular complications or additional risk factors such as a strong family history of myocardial disease or smoking. In these women, a monophasic preparation (progestin only) may be considered. In women taking OCs, the lowest dose of estrogen and progesterone should be used. Patients should have blood pressure monitoring after the first cycle and quarterly, with baseline and follow-up lipid levels obtained as well.

Women who use OCs may demonstrate increased resistance to insulin as a result of a diminished concentration of insulin receptors. Despite the fact that carbohydrate metabolism may be affected by the progestin component of the pill, disturbances in diabetic control are actually uncommon with its use. Triphasic OCs may also be used safely in women with a history of GDM without other risk factors. Kjos and colleagues[96] performed a prospective randomized study of 230 women with recent GDM. OC users were randomized to low-dose norethindrone or levonorgestrel preparations in combination with ethinyl estradiol. The rate of subsequent diabetes in OC users was 15% to 20% after 1 year of follow-up. This rate was not significantly different from that in non-OC users (17%). Importantly, no adverse effects on total cholesterol, low-density lipoprotein (LDL), high-density lipoprotein (HDL), or triglycerides were found with OC use. In a separate study, Kjos and colleagues found that progestin-only preparations were associated with an increased risk for diabetes during breastfeeding.

At present, little information is available concerning long-acting progestins in women with diabetes or previous GDM. A statistically significant yet clinically limited deterioration in carbohydrate tolerance has been reported in healthy depot medroxyprogesterone acetate (DMPA) users. As observed with other progestins, DMPA may lower serum triglyceride and HDL cholesterol levels but not LDL or total cholesterol. For this reason, DMPA is not recommended as a first-line method of contraception for women with diabetes. The progestin-only OC would be preferred because it does not produce significant metabolic effects in diabetic women.

KEY POINTS

- Pregnancy has been characterized as a diabetogenic state because of increased postprandial glucose levels in late gestation.
- Both hepatic and peripheral (tissue) insulin sensitivity are reduced in normal pregnancy. As a result, a progressive increase in insulin secretion follows a glucose challenge.
- In women with GDM, the hormonal milieu of pregnancy may represent an unmasking of a susceptibility to the development of type 2 DM.
- According to the Pedersen hypothesis, maternal hyperglycemia results in fetal hyperglycemia and hyperinsulinemia, which results in excessive fetal growth and perinatal morbidities. Tight maternal glycemic control is associated with a reduced risk for fetal macrosomia.
- Congenital malformations occur with a twofold to sixfold increased rate in offspring of women with pregestational diabetes compared with that of the normal population. Impaired glycemic control and associated derangement in maternal metabolism appear to contribute to abnormal embryogenesis.
- Women with class F (nephropathic) diabetes have an increased risk for preeclampsia and preterm delivery that correlates with their degree of renal impairment.
- Diabetic retinopathy may worsen during pregnancy, yet for women optimally treated with laser photocoagulation before pregnancy, significant deterioration of vision is uncommon.
- Screening for GDM is generally performed between 24 and 28 weeks' gestation. A two-step method that consists of a 50-g screen and a diagnostic 100-g oral glucose tolerance test is commonly performed in the United States.
- Treatment of women with type 1 and type 2 DM during pregnancy requires intensive therapy that consists of frequent self-monitoring of blood glucose and aggressive insulin dosing by multiple injections or continuous subcutaneous insulin infusion (insulin pump).
- The cornerstone of treatment for GDM is dietary therapy. Insulin and oral agents are reserved for individuals who manifest significant fasting hyperglycemia or postprandial glucose elevations despite dietary intervention.
- Antepartum fetal assessment for women with both pregestational diabetes or GDM is based on the degree of risk believed to be present in each case. Glycemic control, prior obstetric history, and the presence of vascular disease or hypertension are important considerations.
- Delivery should generally be delayed in patients whose glucose is well controlled until 39 weeks' gestation. The mode of delivery for the suspected large fetus remains controversial. In cases of suspected macrosomia, cesarean delivery has been recommended to prevent a traumatic birth.
- Women with type 1 and type 2 DM should seek prepregnancy consultation. Efforts to improve glycemic control before conception have been associated with a significant reduction in the rate of congenital malformations in the offspring of such women.

REFERENCES

1. Garcia-Patterson A, Gich I, Amini SB, et al. Insulin requirements throughout pregnancy in women with type 1 diabetes mellitus: three changes of direction. *Diabetologia*. 2010;53:446.
2. Catalano PM, Tyzbir ED, Roman NM, et al. Longitudinal changes in insulin release and insulin resistance in non-obese pregnant women. *Am J Obstet Gynecol*. 1991;165:1667.
3. Catalano PM, Drago NM, Amini SB. Longitudinal changes in pancreatic B cell function and metabolic clearance rate of insulin in pregnant women with normal and abnormal glucose tolerance. *Diabetes Care*. 1998; 21:403.
4. Catalano PM, Tyzbir ED, Wolfe RR, et al. Longitudinal changes in basal hepatic glucose production and suppression during insulin infusion in normal pregnant women. *Am J Obstet Gynecol*. 1992;167:913.
5. Catalano PM, Tyzbir ED, Wolfe RR, et al. Carbohydrate metabolism during pregnancy in control subjects and women with gestational diabetes. *Am J Physiol*. 1993;264:E60.
6. Catalano PM, Huston L, Amini SB, Kalhan SC. Longitudinal changes in glucose metabolism during pregnancy in obese women with normal glucose tolerance and gestational diabetes. *Am J Obstet Gynecol*. 1999; 180:903.
7. Ryan EA, O'Sullivan MJ, Skyler JS. Insulin action during pregnancy: studies with the euglycemic clamp technique. *Diabetes*. 1985;34:380.
8. Kirwan JP, Hauguel-de Mouzon S, Lepercq J, et al. TNFα is a predictor of insulin resistance in human pregnancy. *Diabetes*. 2002;51:2207.
9. Sacks GP, Studena K, Sargent K, et al. Normal pregnancy and preeclampsia both produce inflammatory changes in peripheral blood leukocytes akin to those of sepsis. *Am J Obstet Gynecol*. 1999;180:1310.
10. Barros LF, Yudilevich DL, Jarvis SM, et al. Quantitation and immunolocalization of glucose transporters in the human placenta. *Placenta*. 1995; 16:623.
11. O'Tierney-Ginn P, Presley L, Minium J, Hauguel deMouzon S, Catalano PM. Sex-specific effects of maternal anthropometrics on body composition at birth. *Am J Obstet Gynecol*. 2014;211:292, e1-e9.
12. White P. Pregnancy complicating diabetes. *Am J Med*. 1949;7:609.
13. Sewell MF, Presley LH, Holland SH, Catalano PM. Genetic causes of maturity onset diabetes of the young may be less prevalent in American pregnant women recently diagnosed with diabetes mellitus than in previously studied European populations. *J Matern Fetal Neonatal Med*. 2015;28:1113-1115. [Epub 2014 Jul 30].
14. Catalano PM, Tyzbir ED, Sims EA. Incidence and significance of islet cell antibodies in women with previous gestational diabetes mellitus. *Diabetes Care*. 1990;13:478.
15. Ryan EA, Imes S, Liu D, et al. Defects in insulin secretion and action in women with a history of gestational diabetes. *Diabetes*. 1995;44:506.
16. Xiang AH, Peters RH, Trigo E, et al. Multiple metabolic defects during late pregnancy in women at high risk for type 2 diabetes. *Diabetes*. 1999;48:848.
17. Friedman JE, Ishizuka T, Shao J, et al. Impaired glucose transport and insulin receptor tyrosine phosphorylation in skeletal muscle from obese women with gestational diabetes. *Diabetes*. 1999;48:1807.
18. Hytten FE, Leitch I. The gross composition of the components of weight gain. In: *The Physiology of Human Pregnancy*. 2nd ed. London: Blackwell Scientific; 1971:371.
19. Freinkel N, Metzger BE, Nitzan M, et al. "Accelerated starvation" and mechanisms for the conservation of maternal nitrogen during pregnancy. *Isr J Med Sci*. 1972;8:426.
20. Kalkhoff RK, Kandaraki E, Morrow PG, et al. Relationship between neonatal birth weight and maternal plasma amino acids profiles in lean and obese nondiabetic women with type 1 diabetic pregnant women. *Metabolism*. 1988;37:234.
21. Darmady JM, Postle AD. Lipid metabolism in pregnancy. *BJOG*. 1982;82:211.
22. Knopp RH, Chapman M, Bergeline RO, et al. Relationship of lipoprotein lipids to mild fasting hyperglycemia and diabetes in pregnancy. *Diabetes Care*. 1980;3:416.
23. DiCianni G, Miccoli R, Volpe L, et al. Maternal triglyceride levels and newborn weight in pregnant women with normal glucose tolerance. *Diabet Med*. 2005;22:21.
24. Schaefer-Graf UM, Graf K, Kulbacka I, et al. Maternal lipids as strong determinants of fetal environment and growth in pregnancies with gestational diabetes mellitus. *Diabetes Care*. 2008;31:1858.
25. Freinkel N. Banting Lecture of 1980: of pregnancy and progeny. *Diabetes*. 1980;29:1023.
26. Prentice AM, Poppitt SD, Goldberg CR, et al. Energy balance in pregnancy and lactation. In: Allen L, King J, Lonnerdal B, eds. *Nutrient Regulation During Pregnancy, Lactation and Infant Growth*. New York: Plenum; 1994:11.
27. Forsum E, Kabir N, Sadurskis A, Westerp K. Total energy expenditure of healthy Swedish women during pregnancy and lactation. *Am J Clin Nutr*. 1992;56:334.
28. Catalano PM, Thomas A, Huston-Presley L, Amini SB. Increased fetal adiposity: a very sensitive marker of abnormal in utero development. *Am J Obstet Gynecol*. 2003;189:1698.
29. Mathieson ER, Ringholm I, Damm P. Stillbirth in diabetic pregnancies. *Best Pract Res Clin Obstet Gynaecol*. 2011;25:105.
30. Philips AF, Dubin JW, Matty PJ, Raye JR. Arterial hypoxemia and hyperinsulinemia in the chronically hyperglycemic fetal lamb. *Pediatr Res*. 1982;16:653.
31. Catalano PM, Tyzbir ED, Allen SR, et al. Evaluation of fetal growth by estimation of body composition. *Obstet Gynecol*. 1992;79:46.
32. Kim SY, Sharma AJ, Sappenfield W, Wilson HG, Salihu HM. Association of maternal body mass index, excessive weight gain, and gestational diabetes mellitus with large-for-gestational-age births. *Obstet Gynecol*. 2014;123:737.
33. Kjos SL, Walther F. Prevalence and etiology of respiratory distress in infants of diabetic mothers: predictive value of lung maturation tests. *Am J Obstet Gynecol*. 1990;163:898.
34. Damm JA, Asbjörnsdóttir B, Callesen NF, et al. Diabetic nephropathy and microalbuminuria in pregnant women with type 1 and type 2 diabetes: prevalence, antihypertensive strategy, and pregnancy outcome. *Diabetes Care*. 2013;36:3489.
35. Ekbom P, Damm P, Feldt-Rasmussen B, Feldt-Rasmussen U, Mølvig J, Matheisen ER. Pregnancy outcome in type 1 diabetic women with microalbuminuria. *Diabetes Care*. 2001;24:1739.
36. Cooper WO, Hernandez-Diaz S, Arbogast PG, et al. Major congenital malformations after first-trimester exposure to ACE inhibitors. *N Engl J Med*. 2006;354:2443.
37. Gordon M, Landon MB, Samuels P, et al. Perinatal outcome and long-term follow-up associated with modern management of diabetic nephropathy (class F). *Obstet Gynecol*. 1996;87:401.
38. Nielsen LR, Müller C, Damm P, Mathiesen ER. Reduced prevalence of early preterm delivery in women with type 1 diabetes and microalbuminuria–possible effect of early antihypertensive treatment during pregnancy. *Diabet Med*. 2006;23:426.
39. Powe CE, Thadhani R. Diabetes and the kidney in pregnancy. *Semin Nephrol*. 2011;31:59.
40. Carr DB, Koontz GL, Gardell A, et al. Diabetic nephropathy I pregnancy: suboptimal hypertensive control associated with preterm delivery. *Am J Hypertens*. 2006;19:513.
41. Kitzmiller JL, Brown ER, Phillippe M, et al. Diabetic nephropathy and perinatal outcome. *Am J Obstet Gynecol*. 1981;141:741.
42. Kitzmiller JL, Jovanovic L, Brown F, et al., eds. *Managing preexisting diabetes and pregnancy. Technical reviews and consensus. Recommendations for Care*. American Diabetes Association; 2008.
43. DeSisto CL, Kim SY, Sharma AJ. Prevalence estimates of gestational diabetes mellitus in the United States, Pregnancy Risk Assessment Monitoring System (PRAMS), 2007-2010. *Prev Chronic Dis*. 2014;11:E104.
44. Hughes RC, Moore MP, Gullam JE, Mohamed K, Rowan J. An early pregnancy HbA1c ≥5.9% (41 mmol/mol) is optimal for detecting diabetes and identifies women at increased risk of adverse pregnancy outcomes. *Diab Care*. 2014;37:2953-2959.
45. Hartling L, Dryden DM, Guthrie A, et al. Benefits and harms of treating gestational diabetes mellitus: a systematic review and meta-analysis for the U.S. Preventive Services Task Force and the National Institutes of Health Office of Medical Applications of Research. *Ann Intern Med*. 2013;159(2): 123-129.
46. U.S. Preventive Services Task Force Recommendation Statement. Screening for gestational diabetes mellitus. *Ann Intern Med*. 2008;148:759.
47. The HAPO Study Cooperative Research Group. Hyperglycemia and adverse pregnancy outcome (HAPO) study: associations with neonatal anthropometrics. *Diabetes*. 2009;58:453.
48. Ethridge JK Jr, Catalano PM, Waters TP. Perinatal outcomes associated with the diagnosis of gestational diabetes made by the international association of the diabetes and pregnancy study groups criteria. *Obstet Gynecol*. 2014;124:571.
49. National Institutes of Health consensus development conference statement: diagnosing gestational diabetes mellitus, March 4-6, 2013. *Obstet Gynecol*. 2013;122:358.

50. Cundy T, Ackermann E, Ryan EA. Gestational diabetes: new criteria may triple the prevalence but effect on outcomes is unclear. *BMJ.* 2014;348:1567.

51. McIntyre HD. Diagnosing gestational diabetes mellitus: rationed or rationally related to risk? *Diabetes Care.* 2013;36:2879.

52. Hartling L, Dryden DM, Guthrie A, et al. Diagnostic thresholds for gestational diabetes and their impact on pregnancy outcomes: a systematic review. *Diabet Med.* 2014;31:319.

53. Ryan EA. Clinical diagnosis of gestational diabetes. *Clin Obstet Gynecol.* 2013;56:774.

54. Oriot P, Selvais P, Radikov J, et al. Assessing the incidence of gestational diabetes and neonatal outcomes using the IADPSG guidelines in comparison with the Carpenter and Coustan criteria in a Belgian general hospital. *Acta Clin Belg.* 2014;69:8.

55. Hernandez TL, Friedman JE, Van Pelt RE, Barbour LA. Patterns of glycemia in normal pregnancy: should the current therapeutic targets be challenged? *Diabetes Care.* 2011;34:1660.

56. Mathiesen ER, Hod M, Ivanisevic M, et al. Maternal efficacy and safety outcomes in a randomized, controlled trial comparing insulin detemir with NPH insulin in 310 pregnant women with type 1 diabetes. *Diabetes Care.* 2012;35:2012.

57. Mukhopadhyay A, Farrell T, Fraser RB, Ola B. Continuous subcutaneous insulin infusion vs. intensive conventional insulin therapy in pregnant diabetic women: a systematic review of metaanalysis of randomized, controlled trials. *Am J Obstet Gynecol.* 2007;197:447.

58. Sibai BM, Viteri OA. Diabetic ketoacidosis in pregnancy. *Obstet Gynecol.* 2014;123:167.

59. Padmanabhan S, McLean M, Cheung NW. Falling insulin requirements are associated with adverse obstetric outcomes in women with preexisting diabetes. *Diabetes Care.* 2014;37:2685-2692.

60. Starikov R, Bohrer J, Goh W, et al. Hemoglobin A1c in pregestational diabetic gravidas and the risk of congenital heart disease in the fetus. *Pediatr Cardiol.* 2013;34:1716.

61. Nesbitt TS, Gilbert WM, Herrchen B. Shoulder dystocia and associated risk factors with macrosomic infants born in California. *Am J Obstet Gynecol.* 1998;179:476.

62. Landon MB, Mintz MG, Gabbe SG. Sonographic evaluation of fetal abdominal growth: predictor of the large-for-gestational age infant in pregnancies. *Am J Obstet Gynecol.* 1989;160:115.

63. Moore TR. A comparison of amniotic fluid pulmonary phospholipids in normal and diabetic pregnancy. *Am J Obstet Gynecol.* 2002;186:641.

64. Metzger BE, Buchanan TA, Coustan DR, et al. Summary and recommendations of the Fifth International Workshop-Conference on Gestational Diabetes Mellitus. *Diabetes Care.* 2010;30:3154.

65. Crowther CA, Hiller JE, Moss JR, et al. Effect of treatment of gestational diabetes mellitus on pregnancy outcomes. *N Engl J Med.* 2005;352:2477.

66. Landon MB, Spong CY, Thom E, et al. A multicenter, randomized trial of treatment for mild gestational diabetes. *N Engl J Med.* 2009;361:1339.

67. Barbour LA. Unresolved controversies in gestational diabetes: implications on maternal and infant health. *Curr Opin Endocrinol Diabetes Obes.* 2014;21:264.

68. Hernandez TL, Van Pelt RE, Anderson MA, et al. A higher-complex carbohydrate diet in gestational diabetes mellitus achieves glucose targets and lowers postprandial lipids: a randomized crossover study. *Diabetes Care.* 2014;37:1254.

69. Hernandez TL, Anderson MA, Chartier-Logan C, Friedman JE, Barbour LA. Strategies in the nutritional management of gestational diabetes. *Clin Obstet Gynecol.* 2013;56:803.

70. Yu F, Lv L, Liang Z, et al. Continuous glucose monitoring effects on maternal glycemic control and pregnancy outcomes in patients with gestational diabetes mellitus: a prospective cohort study. *J Clin Endocrinol Metab.* 2014;99:4674-4682.

71. Camelo Castilo W, Boggess K, Stürmer T, et al. Trends in glyburide compared with insulin use for gestational diabetes treatment in the United States, 2000-2011. *Obstet Gynecol.* 2014;123:1177.

72. Nicholson W, Bolen S, Witkop CT, et al. Benefits and risk of oral agents compared with insulin in women with gestational diabetes: a systematic review. *Obstet Gynecol.* 2009;113:193.

73. Langer O, Conway DL, Berkus MD, et al. A comparison of glyburide and insulin in women with gestational diabetes mellitus. *N Engl J Med.* 2000;343:1134.

74. Rowan JA, Hague WM, Wanzhen G, et al. Metformin versus insulin for treatment of gestational diabetes. *N Engl J Med.* 2008;358:208.

75. Carlsen SM, Martinussen MP, Vanky E. Metformin's effect on first-year weight gain: a follow-up study. *Pediatrics.* 2012;13:1222.

76. Ijäs H, Vääräsmäki M, Saarela T, Keravuo R, Raudaskoski T. A follow-up of a randomized study of metformin and insulin in gestational diabetes mellitus: growth and development of the children at the age of 18 months. *BJOG.* 2015;122:994.

77. Moore LE, Clokey D, Rappaport VJ, Curet LB. Metformin compared with glyburide in gestational diabetes: a randomized trial. *Obstet Gynecol.* 2010;115:55.

78. Rosenstein MG, Cheng YW, Snowden JM, et al. The risk of stillbirth and infant death stratified by gestational age in women with gestational diabetes. *Am J Obstet Gynecol.* 2012;206:1.

79. Sutton AL, Mele L, Landon MB, et al., Eunice Kennedy Shriver National Institute of Child Health and Human Development Maternal-Fetal Medicine Units Network. Delivery timing and cesarean delivery risk in women with mild gestational diabetes mellitus. *Am J Obstet Gynecol.* 2014;211:244.

80. Garabedian C, Deruelle P. Delivery (timing, mode, glycemic control) in women with gestational diabetes. *J Gynecol Obstet Bio Reprod.* 2010;39:S274.

81. Bellamy L, Casas JP, Hingorani AD, Williams D. Type 2 diabetes mellitus after gestational diabetes: a systemic review and meta-analysis. *Lancet.* 2009;373:1773.

82. Chodick G, Elchalal U, Sella T, et al. Epidemiology. The risk of overt diabetes mellitus among women with gestational diabetes: a population-based study. *Diabet Med.* 2010;27:852.

83. Hunt KJ, Logan SL, Conway DL, Korte JE. Postpartum screening following GDM: how well are we doing? *Curr Diab Rep.* 2010;10:235.

84. McGovern A, Butler L, Jones S, et al. Diabetes screening after gestational diabetes in England: a quantitative retrospective cohort study. *Br J Gen Pract.* 2014;64(618):e17-e23.

85. Knowler WC, Barrett-Conner E, Fowler SE, et al. Reduction in the incidence of type 2 diabetes with lifestyle intervention or metformin. *N Engl J Med.* 2002;346:393.

86. Ratner RE, Christophi CA, Metzer BE, et al. Prevention of diabetes in women with a history of gestational diabetes: effects of metformin and lifestyle interventions. *J Clin Endocrinol Metab.* 2008;93:4774.

87. Kim C, Newton KM, Knopp RH. Gestational diabetes and the incidence of type 2 diabetes: a systemic review. *Diabetes Care.* 2002;25:1862.

88. Pettitt DJ, Knowler WC, Baird HR, et al. Gestational diabetes: Infant and maternal complications of pregnancy in relation to third-trimester glucose tolerance in the Pima Indians. *Diabetes Care.* 1980;3:458.

89. Dabelea D, Pettitt DJ. Intrauterine diabetic environment confers risks for type 2 diabetes mellitus and obesity in the offspring, in addition to genetic susceptibility. *J Pediatr Endocrinol Metab.* 2001;14:1085.

90. Clausen TD, Mathiesen ER, Hansen T, et al. High prevalence of type 2 diabetes and pre-diabetes in adult offspring of women with gestational diabetes mellitus or type 1 diabetes: the role of intrauterine hyperglycemia. *Diabetes Care.* 2008;31:340.

91. Gillman MW, Oakey H, Baghurst PA, et al. Effect of treatment of gestational diabetes mellitus on obesity in the next generation. *Diabetes Care.* 2010;33:964.

92. Landon MB, Rice MM, Varner MW, et al., the Eunice Kennedy Shriver National Institute of Child Health and Human Development Maternal-Fetal Medicine Units (MFMU) Network. Mild gestational diabetes and long-term child health. *Diabetes Care.* 2015;38:445.

93. Peterson C, Grosse SD, Li R, et al. Preventable health and cost burden of adverse birth outcomes associated with pregestational diabetes in the United States. *Am J Obstet Gynecol.* 2015;212:74, e1-e9.

94. Lidegard O. Oral contraceptives, pregnancy, and the risk of cerebral thromboembolism: the influence of diabetes, hypertension, migraine, and previous thrombotic disease. *Br J Obstet Gynecol.* 1995;102:153.

95. Klein BE, Moss SE, Klein R. Oral contraceptives in women with diabetes. *Diabetes Care.* 1990;13:895.

96. Kjos SL, Shoupe D, Douyan S, et al. Effect of low-dose oral contraceptives on carbohydrate and lipid metabolism in women with recent gestational diabetes: results of a controlled, randomized, prospective study. *Am J Obstet Gynecol.* 1990;163:182.

97. Mills JL, Knopp RH, Simpson JP, et al. Lack of relation of increased malformation rates in infants of diabetic mothers to glycemic control during organogenesis. *N Engl J Med.* 1988;318:671.

98. Greene MF. Prevention and diagnosis of congenital anomalies in diabetic pregnancies. *Clin Perinatol.* 1993;20:533.

99. Steel JM, Johnstone FD, Smith AF, et al. Five years' experience of a pre-pregnancy clinic for insulin-dependent diabetics. *Br Med J.* 1982;285:353.

100. Fuhrmann K, Reiher H, Semmler K, et al. Prevention of congenital malformations in infants of insulin-dependent diabetic mothers. *Diabetes Care.* 1983;6:219.

101. Simpson JL, Elias S, Martin O, et al. Diabetes in pregnancy, Northwestern University Series (1977-1981). I. Prospective study of anomalies in offspring of mothers with diabetes mellitus. *Am J Obstet Gynecol*. 1983;146:263.

102. Albert TJ, Landon MB, Wheller JJ, et al. Prenatal detection of fetal anomalies in pregnancies complicated by insulin-dependent diabetes mellitus. *Am J Obstet Gynecol*. 1996;174:1424.

103. Kitzmiller JL. Diabetic nephropathy. In: Reece EA, Coustan DR, Gabbe SG, eds. *Diabetes in pregnancy*. Philadelphia: Lippincott Williams & Wilkins; 2004:383.

104. Grenfel A, Brudnell JM, Doddridge MC, Watkins PJ. Pregnancy in diabetic women who have proteinuria. *Q J Med*. 1986;59:379.

105. Reece EA, Coustan DR, Hayslett JP, et al. Diabetic nephropathy: pregnancy performance and fetomaternal outcome. *Am J Obstet Gynecol*. 1988;159:56.

106. Ullmo S, Vial Y, Di Bernardo S, et al. Pathologic ventricular hypertrophy in the offspring of diabetic mothers: a retrospective study. *Eur Heart J*. 2007;28:1319.

107. Rosenn BM, Miodovnik M, Khoury JC, et al. Outcome of pregnancy in women with diabetic nephropathy. *Am J Obstet Gynecol*. 1997;176:S631.

Additional references for this chapter are available at ExpertConsult.com.

Obesity in Pregnancy

PATRICK M. CATALANO

KEY ABBREVIATIONS

Body mass index	BMI
Cell-free DNA	cfDNA
Centers for Disease Control and Prevention	CDC
Centre for Maternal and Child Enquiries	CMACE
First-and Second-Trimester Evaluation of Risk Research Consortium	FASTER
Gestational diabetes mellitus	GDM
Hemolysis, elevated liver enzymes, low platelets syndrome	HELLP
High-density lipoprotein	HDL
Institute of Medicine	IOM
Insulin sensitivity index	ISI
Large for gestational age	LGA
Low-molecular-weight heparin	LMWH
Magnetic resonance imaging	MRI
Maternal-Fetal Medicine Unit	MFMU
National Health and Nutrition Examination Survey	NHANES
Nonalcoholic fatty liver disease	NAFLD
Negative pressure wound therapy	NPWT
Randomized controlled trial	RCT
Royal College of Obstetricians and Gynaecologists	RCOG
Single nucleotide polymorphism	SNP
Surgical site infection	SSI
Trial of labor after cesarean	TOLAC
United States Department of Agriculture	USDA
Venous thromboembolism	VTE
Very-low-density lipoprotein	VLDL
World Health Organization	WHO

OVERVIEW

Obesity in women is such a common problem that the implications relative to pregnancy often are overlooked, or possibly ignored, because of the lack of specific treatments. For example, medical treatment of hypertension or diabetes mellitus involves medications that have relatively rapid onset, and the effects of treatment can be quantitatively monitored. In contrast, the management of obesity—in addition to medical and surgical treatments—requires long-term approaches that include public health and economic initiatives, nutrition, and behavioral modifications. Therefore an understanding of the management of obesity during pregnancy begins prior to conception and continues through the postpartum period; that is, it must be seen from a life-course perspective. Although the care of the obese women during pregnancy requires the involvement of the obstetrician/gynecologist, depending on the comfort level of the provider, other health care professionals can offer specific expertise relative to management.

PREVALENCE OF OBESITY IN WOMEN OF REPRODUCTIVE AGE

Obesity is commonly classified by the body mass index (BMI), which is weight in kilograms divided by height in meters squared (kg/m^2) using the World Health Organization (WHO) criteria. Underweight is less than 18.5, normal weight is 18.5 to 24.9, overweight is 25.0 to 29.9; obese class I, is 30.0 to 34.9, obese class II is 35.0 to 39.9, and obese class III is 40 or more.[1] **Based on the 2011 to 2012 National Health and Nutrition Examination Survey (NHANES), the prevalence of obesity in women of reproductive age** (20 to 39 years) **in the United States was 31.8%** (95% confidence interval [CI], 28.5 to 35.5), **whereas overweight plus obesity was 58.5%** (95% CI, 51.4 to 65.2) **of that population.**[2] The prevalence of overweight and obesity is higher in non-Hispanic black and Mexican women in the United States (Table 41-1). BMI is often used as a measure that correlates with fat mass. In nonpregnant women of reproductive age, BMI explains about 50%

TABLE 41-1   PREVALENCE OF OBESITY AND OVERWEIGHT IN WOMEN OF REPRODUCTIVE AGE*

ALL RACE/ ETHNICITY GROUPS	NON-HISPANIC WHITE	NON-HISPANIC BLACK	HISPANIC	MEXICAN AMERICAN
31.9 (28.6-35.5)	26.9 (23.0-31.3)	56.2 (44.3-67.5)	34.4 (30.9-38.2)	37.8 (33.2-42.7)
55.8 (49.6-61.9)	50.7 (43.1-58.2)	74.2 (65.9-81.1)	65.4 (59.9-70.5)	68.8 (62.1-74.8)

Data from National Health and Nutrition Examination Survey 2009–2010. Values are mean ± standard deviation.
*Reproductive age is 20 to 39 years old.

to 70% of the variance in fat mass. However, because of the increase in total body water that occurs with advancing gestation, the correlation becomes progressively less robust.[3] Because of racial differences in body composition, the WHO has discussed different cutoff criteria for the classification of obesity in Asian women.[4]

Based on Centers for Disease Control and Prevention (CDC) data, no significant change occurred in the prevalence of obesity in women of reproductive age from 2003 through 2004 to 2011 through 2012.[2] From 1999 through 2010, however, obesity (BMI ≥30) in women aged 20 to 39 years appeared to increase, from 28.4% (95% CI, 24.4 to 32.4) to 34.0% (95% CI, 29.0 to 39.1), again with a higher prevalence in non-Hispanic black and Mexican American women.[5] Of greater concern is the increasing prevalence of grade II obesity (17.2%; 95% CI, 14.2 to 20.7) and grade III obesity (7.5%; 95% CI, 5.8 to 9.7) in women aged 20 to 39 years from 2009 through 2010.[6]

Multiple social, environmental, behavioral, and biologic determinants lead to the development of obesity. Major single-gene defects (homozygosity for recessive alleles) account for about 5% of early-onset severe obesity.[7,8] About 60 single nucleotide polymorphisms (SNPs) have been associated with obesity based on genome-wide significance levels.[7,9] Although when taken individually, each of these factors may only account for a small proportion of the variance in obesity, when taken together, their combination and interactions explain a far greater proportion of the variance.[7]

Multiple commonly held beliefs are associated with the development of obesity, and many more are associated with prescriptions to achieve weight loss.[10] In the simplest terms, weight loss or gain is related to the balance between energy intake and energy expenditure, although the relationships are not linear. For example, if a person increases energy expenditure by walking an extra mile per day and maintains caloric intake constant, the weight loss over time will be only approximately 20% of expected.[11] This is because the physiologic compensation for changes in energy expenditure or requirements to maintain the decreased weight are less than would be expected if the relationships were linear.[12]

As obstetrician/gynecologists, we encourage our patients to breastfeed. Although many maternal and neonatal benefits accompany breastfeeding, the concept that infants who are breastfed are less likely to be obese in later life did not hold true in a randomized controlled trial (RCT) of more than 13,000 children followed for more than 6 years.[13] The previous reports may have been affected by confounding and selection bias.

METABOLISM IN OBESE PREGNANT WOMEN

Large epidemiologic studies have reported that obese women gain less weight during pregnancy compared with nonobese women.[14] Based on small longitudinal metabolic studies in healthy lean and obese women before and during early and late

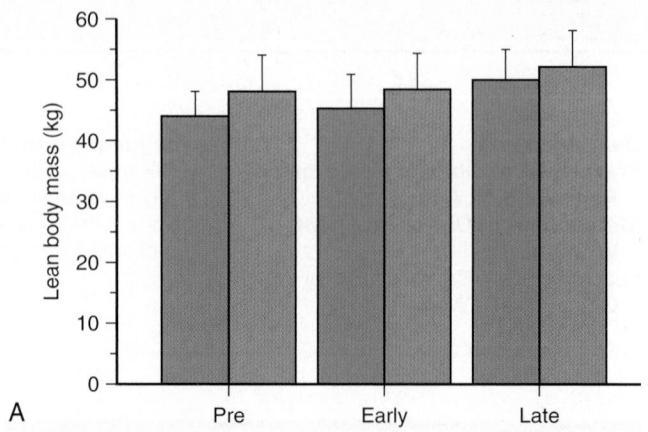

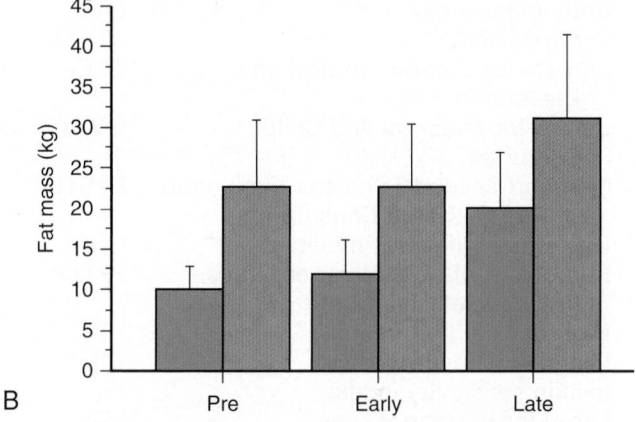

FIG 41-1 A, Longitudinal changes (mean ± standard deviation [SD]) in lean body mass in lean (*blue bars, n* = 5) and obese women (*red bars, n* = 6) before pregnancy *(Pre)* and in early (12-14 weeks) and late pregnancy (34-36 weeks). Change over time, *P* = .0001, and group, *P* = .34. **B,** Longitudinal changes (mean ± SD) in fat mass in lean (*blue bars, n* = 5) and obese women (*red bars, n* = 6) before pregnancy and in early (12-14 weeks) and late pregnancy (34-36 weeks). Change over time, *P* = .0001 and group, *P* = .02. (From Catalano P, Resi V, Presley L, Hauguel-deMouzon. Changes in maternal lipid metabolism in lean and obese pregnancy are related to fetal adiposity. Reproductive Sciences 22, number 1 [supplement], March 25-28, 2015, 62nd Annual Meeting, San Francisco CA. Abstract F-137.)

gestation, significant changes were observed over time and between groups. **A significant increase in lean and fat mass was reported in both lean and obese women, but a greater increase in fat mass was seen in lean women** (Fig. 41-1). A significant 23% increase in resting energy expenditure over time was not different between groups (Fig. 41-2, *A*). Basal carbohydrate oxidation increased 68% over time and was greater in obese women (see Fig. 41-2, *B*). A 40% decrease in insulin sensitivity was reported as estimated by the glucose infusion rate during the hyperinsulinemic-euglycemic clamp divided by the

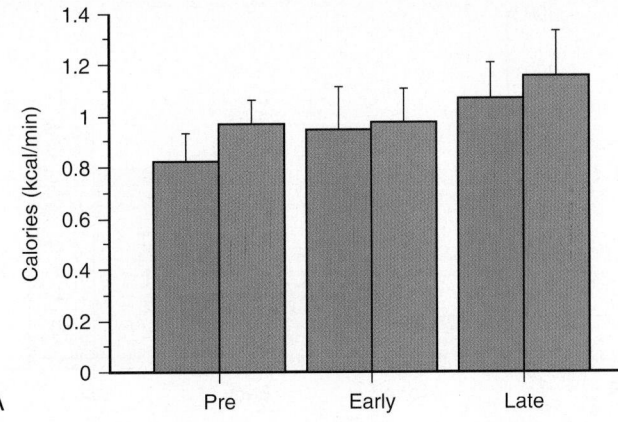

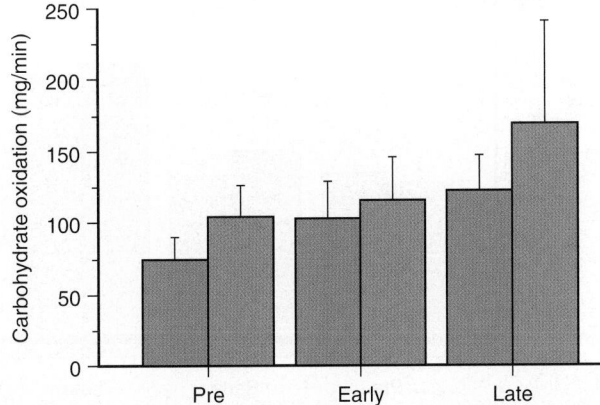

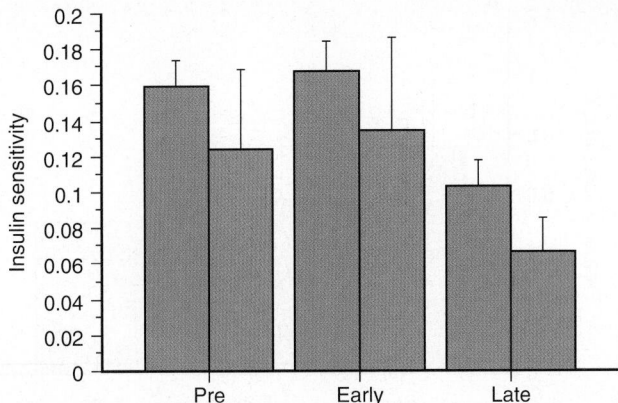

FIG 41-3 Longitudinal changes in insulin sensitivity index (mean ± standard deviation [SD]) as estimated by the hyperinsulinemic-euglycemic clamp (mg/kg/min) in lean (*blue bars, n = 5*) and obese women (*red bars, n = 6*) before pregnancy (*Pre*) and in early (12-14 weeks) and late pregnancy (34-36 weeks). Change over time, $P = .0001$, and group, $P = .07$. (From Catalano P, Resi V, Presley L, Hauguel-deMouzon. Changes in maternal lipid metabolism in lean and obese pregnancy are related to fetal adiposity. Reproductive Sciences 22, number 1 [supplement], March 25-28, 2015, 62nd Annual Meeting, San Francisco CA. Abstract F-137.)

FIG 41-2 **A,** Longitudinal changes (mean ± standard deviation [SD]) in resting metabolic rate in lean (*blue bars, n = 5*) and obese women (*red bars, n = 6*) before pregnancy (*Pre*) and in early (12-14 weeks) and late pregnancy (34-36 weeks). Change over time, $P = .0002$, and group, $P = .22$. **B,** Longitudinal changes (mean ± SD) in carbohydrate oxidation in lean (*blue bars, n = 5*) and obese women (*red bars, n = 6*) before pregnancy and in early (12-14 weeks) and late pregnancy (34-36 weeks). Change over time, $P = .008$, and group, $P = .04$. (From Catalano P, Resi V, Presley L, Hauguel-deMouzon. Changes in maternal lipid metabolism in lean and obese pregnancy are related to fetal adiposity. Reproductive Sciences 22, number 1 [supplement], March 25-28, 2015, 62nd Annual Meeting, San Francisco CA. Abstract F-137.)

mean insulin concentrations (i.e., the insulin sensitivity index [ISI]) in lean and obese women over time, with a trend ($P = .07$) for a greater decrease in obese compared with lean women (Fig. 41-3). As a result of the significant decrease in insulin sensitivity, fat oxidation increased 220% during the clamp in both lean and obese women ($P = .003$) because of the decreased ability to suppress lipolysis. Basal free fatty acids decreased 16% over time ($P = .02$), and a 62% increase was seen in free fatty acids with insulin infusion during the clamp ($P = .0004$), but no significant difference was noted between groups (Fig. 41-4). Although a 61% increase in fasting cholesterol and a 260% increase in triglycerides ($P = .0001$) were observed over time, no significant difference was found between lean and obese women (Fig. 41-5). Others have reported that in late pregnancy, obese women have increases in circulating triglycerides, very-low-density lipoprotein (VLDL) cholesterol, and lower high-density lipoprotein (HDL) as compared with that of lean women.[15-18] In summary, **significant increases in many lipid components are seen during pregnancy, some of which are increased to a greater degree in obese, compared with lean, women.**

Recommendations for Gestational Weight Gain in Obese Women

Weight gain recommendations for pregnancy were first published by the Institute of Medicine (IOM) in 1990.[19] At that time, prior to the increased prevalence of obesity in the population, the purpose was to establish recommendations for a healthy gestational weight gain for both the mother and her fetus primarily because of concerns for low birthweight and nutritional status. The recommendation for weight gain for women who were *obese*—defined as a prepregnancy BMI greater than 29—was at least 15 lb. Since that time, a significant increase has been seen in the number of women of childbearing age who are overweight or obese. Women also are becoming pregnant at an older age and with an increasing number of chronic medical conditions such as hypertension and diabetes. Hence, in 2009, the IOM revised the gestational weight guidelines taking into account more recent literature and the increased proportion of overweight and obesity in women of reproductive age (Table 41-2).[20]

Although the 2009 IOM recommendations for gestational weight gain are not dramatically different from the 1990 guidelines except in regard to obese women, other substantive differences were apparent. These include using the WHO criteria for defining pregravid BMI[1] and eliminating specific recommendations for certain populations that included women of short stature, pregnant adolescents, and different racial or ethnic groups.[20] **Based on these more recent definitions, excessive gestational weight gain occurs in 38% of normal-weight women, 63% of overweight women, and 46% of obese women. Excessive gestational weight gain is a significant factor for postpartum weight retention and hence is a significant contributor to the obesity epidemic.**[21]

Some authors have suggested that weight gain for obese women less than that specified in the current IOM recommendations may improve some perinatal outcomes.[22] However, potential fetal risks relate to inadequate gestational weight gain in obese women.[23] Although the issue of gestational weight gain

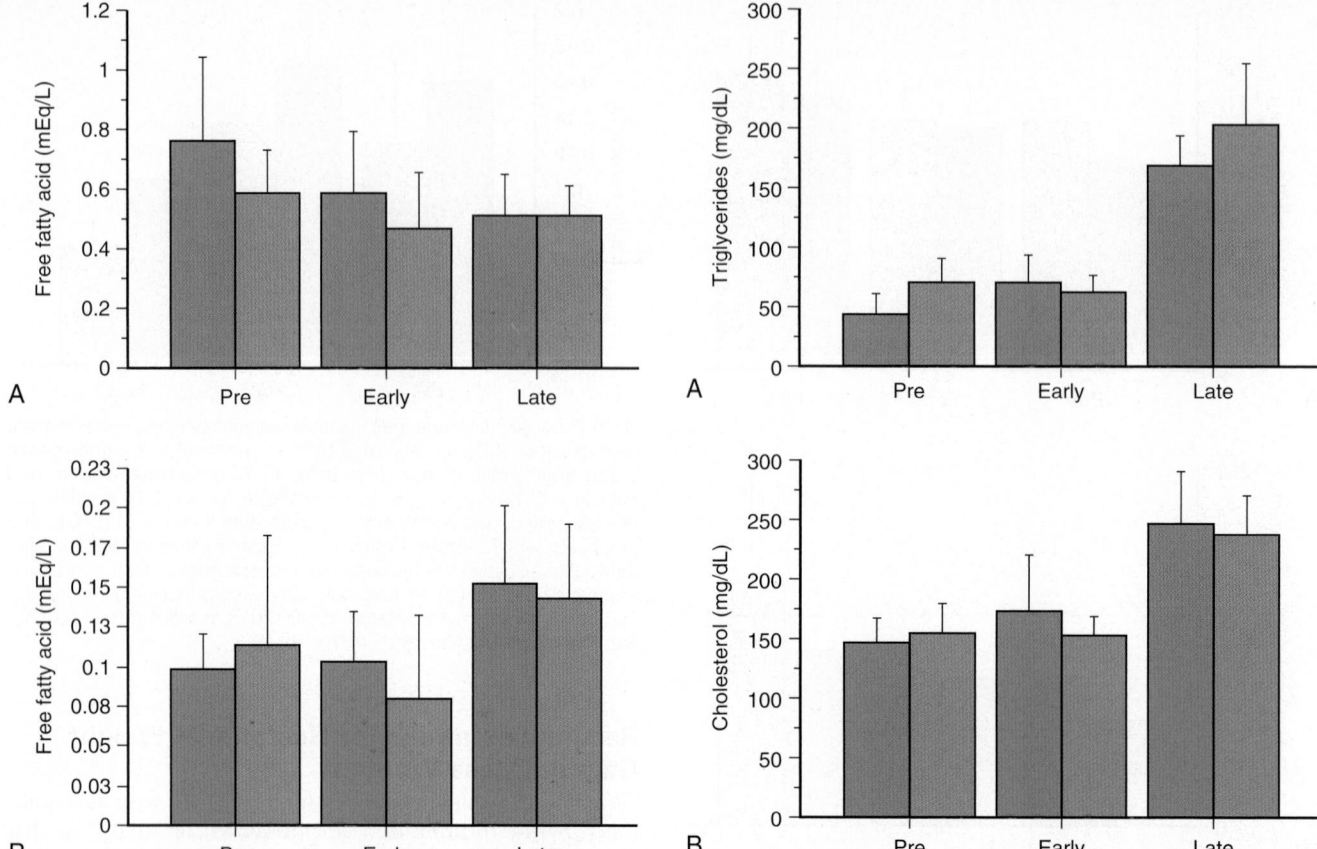

FIG 41-4 **A,** Longitudinal changes in basal free fatty acid concentration (mean ± standard deviation [SD]) in lean (*blue bars, n* = 5) and obese women (*red bars, n* = 6) before pregnancy *(Pre)* and in early (12-14 weeks) and late pregnancy (34-36 weeks). Change over time, *P* = .02, and group, *P* = .30. **B,** Longitudinal changes in free fatty acid concentration during the hyperinsulinemic-euglycemic clamp in lean (*blue bars, n* = 5) and obese women (*red bars, n* = 6) before pregnancy and in early (12-14 weeks) and late pregnancy (34-36 weeks). Change over time, *P* = .0004, and group, *P* = .82. (From Catalano P, Resi V, Presley L, Hauguel-deMouzon. Changes in maternal lipid metabolism in lean and obese pregnancy are related to fetal adiposity. Reproductive Sciences 22, number 1 [supplement], March 25-28, 2015, 62nd Annual Meeting, San Francisco CA. Abstract F-137.)

FIG 41-5 **A,** Longitudinal changes in basal triglyceride concentration in lean (*blue bars, n* = 5) and obese women (*red bars, n* = 6) before pregnancy *(Pre)* and in early (12-14 weeks) and late pregnancy (34-36 weeks). Change over time, *P* = .0001, and group, *P* = .22. **B,** Longitudinal changes in basal cholesterol concentrations in lean (*blue bars, n* = 5) and obese women (*red bars, n* = 6) before pregnancy and in early (12-14 weeks) and late pregnancy (34-36 weeks). Change over time, *P* = .0001, and group, *P* = .67. (From Catalano P, Resi V, Presley L, Hauguel-deMouzon. Changes in maternal lipid metabolism in lean and obese pregnancy are related to fetal adiposity. Reproductive Sciences 22, number 1 [supplement], March 25-28, 2015, 62nd Annual Meeting, San Francisco CA. Abstract F-137.)

| TABLE 41-2 | RECOMMENDATIONS FOR TOTAL AND RATE OF WEIGHT GAIN DURING PREGNANCY BY PREPREGNANCY BMI | | |

PREPREGNANCY BMI	BMI (kg/m²)	TOTAL WEIGHT GAIN (RANGE) (lb)	RATES OF WEIGHT GAIN* IN TRIMESTERS 2 AND 3 (MEAN AND RANGE) (lb/wk)
Underweight	<18.5	28-40	1 (1-1.3)
Normal weight	18.5-24.9	25-35	1 (0.8-1)
Overweight	25.0-29.9	15-25	0.6 (0.5-0.7)
Obese (includes all classes)	≥30.0	11-20	0.5 (0.4-0.6)

From Rasmussin KM, Abrams B, Bodnar LM, et al. Weight gain during pregnancy: re-examining the guidelines. Institute of Medicine, 2009.
*Calculations assume a 0.5-2 kg (1.1-4.4 lb) weight gain in the first trimester.
BMI, body mass index.

is much debated in the United States, it is noteworthy that recommendations in other countries are not uniform. The Society of Obstetricians and Gynecologists of Canada[24] have adopted the 2009 IOM recommendations,[20] whereas recommendations from Sweden[25] and China[26] are unique to their own populations. Finally, the Centre for Maternal and Child Enquiries (CMACE) and Royal College of Obstetricians and

Gynaecologists (RCOG) have no clinical recommendations or clinical guidelines for weight gain during pregnancy.[27]

During pregnancy, medications for weight management are not recommended because of safety concerns and side effects.[28] The classical anorexiants, such as phentermine, alter the release and reuptake of neurotransmitters that impact appetite. Other drugs such as orlistat reduce intestinal fat absorption by inhibiting pancreatic lipase. Metformin, which decreases hepatic glucose production, has been associated with decreased gestational weight gain in some studies when used to treat mild gestational diabetes mellitus (GDM).[29] Metformin has not been used solely to manage gestational weight gain, and it crosses the placenta in significant amounts.[29]

The primary weight-management strategies during pregnancy are dietary control, exercise, and behavior modification. These strategies have been used either alone[30,31] or in combination[32,33] to avoid excessive gestational weight gain. None of these strategies is uniform. For example, with diet, some studies have examined the role of food having a low glycemic index,[30] whereas others have used probiotic interventions.[34] Unfortunately, the authors of a recent Cochrane review concluded that **there is not enough evidence to recommend any specific intervention for preventing excessive weight gain in pregnancy,** because studies have suffered from methodologic limitations, small sample sizes, and insufficient power to detect clinically meaningful effect size.[35] In general, **nutritional strategies, rather than exercise, appear to be more useful in avoiding excessive gestational weight gain in pregnancy.**[36]

PREGNANCY COMPLICATIONS IN OBESE WOMEN

Early Pregnancy

A number of pregnancy complications are associated with obesity. **The risk of spontaneous abortion** (odds ratio [OR], 1.2; 95% CI, 1.01 to 1.46) **and recurrent miscarriage** (OR, 3.5; 95% CI, 1.03 to 12.01) **is increased in obese women** as compared with age-matched controls.[37] **The risk of congenital anomalies is also increased in obese mothers, who are at increased risk for pregnancies affected by neural tube, cardiovascular, orofacial, and limb-reduction anomalies.**[38]

Based on the Northern Congenital Abnormality Survey, routine ultrasound detected **46.2%** (1146 of 2483) **of structural anomalies in fetuses with a normal karyotype.**[39] Detection rates decreased significantly with increasing maternal BMI (P = .0007, test for trend), **and the odds of detection of any anomaly were significantly lower in obese women than in those with a normal BMI** (adjusted OR [aOR], 0.77; 95% CI, 0.60 to 0.99).[39] Factors associated with the decreased ability to detect congenital anomalies in obese women include the distance from the skin surface to the fetus, resolution/penetration of sonographic equipment, prolonged time to complete the examination, and the experience of the sonographer.[40] Potential means to optimize image quality in obese pregnant women include a vaginal approach in the first trimester, using the maternal umbilicus as an acoustic window, and tissue harmonic imaging.[40] Fetal magnetic resonance imaging (MRI) obviates many of these technical problems, but because its use is limited by cost and availability, the use of MRI for routine screening of anomalies is not recommended.[41]

In the First- And Second-Trimester Evaluation of Risk (FASTER) Research Consortium trial, the detection rate for cardiac anomalies among women with a BMI less than 25 was higher (21.6%) at a significantly lower false-positive rate (FPR, 78.4%; 95% CI, 77.3 to 79.5) compared with obese women (8.3% detection rate with an FPR of 91.7%; 95% CI, 90.1 to 92.2). In a logistic regression model, maternal obesity significantly decreased the likelihood of sonographic detection of common anomalies (aOR, 0.7; 95% CI, 0.6 to 0.9).[42]

Maternal obesity also affects measures of serum analytes because of the increased plasma volume in obese pregnant women. Although weight adjustment for analytes related to neural tube defects (NTDs) and trisomy 18 improves detection rates, this adjustment does not increase detection rates for trisomy 21.[41] In prenatal testing for trisomies 21 and 18 using cell-free DNA (cfDNA), the false-positive rates were significantly lower (P = .03) than with standard screening (serum biochemical assays with or without nuchal translucency measurement). The positive predictive value for cfDNA was also better for trisomy 21 (45.5% vs. 4.2%) and trisomy 18 (40.0% vs. 8.3%). The median BMI in this study was 27.4 (range, 15.5 to 59).[43] It should be noted, however, that these test characteristics were for "positive" results and did not take into account results from women who were unable to have results obtained from the assay, an occurrence that is more common as BMI increases. Also, maternal obesity is associated with an increase in total, but not fetal, cfDNA. In a small study, total cfDNA increased 1.7% per BMI unit, and when adjusted for blood volume, it increased 3.2% per BMI unit. Therefore in the future, cfDNA values may need to be adjusted for maternal BMI for better interpretation of clinical data.[44]

Mid to Late Pregnancy

The risk of metabolic problems is increased, which includes GDM[45] and preeclampsia,[46] as is the risk of cardiac dysfunction, proteinuria, sleep apnea, and nonalcoholic fatty liver disease (NAFLD)[47,48] in obese as compared with normal-weight pregnant women. Because of the increased insulin resistance often observed in obese women before pregnancy, preexisting subclinical metabolic dysfunction may become manifest as obstetric conditions such as preeclampsia, gestational diabetes, and obstructive sleep apnea (OSA)[49] and are associated with adverse pregnancy outcomes.[50-52] These disorders may have a higher prevalence in certain racial or ethnic groups including black Africans and Southern Asians.[53] In early gestation, hypertension, suspected glucose intolerance, or OSA should be screened for at the first antenatal visit with a history, physical examination, and laboratory and clinical studies as needed. Women with suspected OSA—those with symptoms of snoring, excessive daytime sleepiness, witnessed apneas, or unexplained hypoxia—should be referred to a sleep medicine specialist for evaluation and possible treatment.[54] Although universal screening for gestational diabetes is recommended at 24 to 28 weeks gestation, screening for glucose intolerance in early gestation (gestational diabetes or overt diabetes) should be based on risk factors that include maternal obesity, known impaired fasting or 2-hour glucose levels based on a 75-g glucose tolerance test, or previous gestational diabetes (see Chapter 40).[55] It has not been determined, however, whether universal testing early in pregnancy to detect overt diabetes is of clinical value or is cost-effective.[56] In addition, NAFLD—the most common liver disease in developed countries—usually presents with elevated liver function tests.[57] NAFLD is related to increased insulin resistance and is often confused with other disorders of liver function during pregnancy such as the hemolysis, elevated liver enzymes, low platelets (HELLP) syndrome.

Is there any treatment to prevent metabolic complications such as gestational diabetes in obese women once they are pregnant? Lifestyle interventions in studies of small numbers of obese women to prevent the development of GDM have not been successful.[58,59] A Cochrane review reported that no conclusive evidence for exercise in pregnancy to prevent GDM was available to guide practice.[60] Supplementation with a probiotic and myo-inositol in two European studies has been reported to reduce the frequency of gestational diabetes.[61,62] However, these trials were conducted in nonobese populations. Although prevention of preeclampsia with calcium supplementation and vitamin C and E have not been successful,[63,64] optimizing glucose control in women with GDM may decrease the rate of preeclampsia.[65] The administration of low-dose aspirin (60 to 80 mg/day) in the late first trimester is suggested in women with a medical history of early-onset preeclampsia and preterm delivery at less than $34^{0/7}$ weeks or preeclampsia in more than one prior pregnancy.[66]

Not only is the risk of indicated preterm deliveries increased[67] **because of the aforementioned antepartum complications, the risk of idiopathic preterm birth is also increased**[68] **in overweight and obese pregnant women. The risk of stillbirth also increases** (test for trend, $P < .01$) **with progressive degrees of maternal obesity:** BMI class I (adjusted hazard ratio [aHR], 1.3; 95% CI, 1.2 to 1.4), BMI class II (aHR, 1.4; 95% CI, 1.3 to 1.6), and extreme obesity (aHR, 1.9; 95% CI, 1.6 to 2.1). A further increased risk of stillbirth was seen in obese black, compared with obese white, mothers.[69] The underlying etiology for intrauterine fetal death in obese women is unknown, and as such, no specific recommendations exist regarding prevention other than optimizing general obstetric care relative to medical or obstetric conditions. **Although obese women are at increased risk for adverse perinatal outcomes, data are insufficient to recommend antenatal surveillance in this population without additional clinical indications.**[70] As a noninvasive option, fetal movement counts, such as kick counts, are suggested (see Chapter 11).

Intrapartum Complications

At delivery, obese women are at increased risk of cesarean delivery, endometritis, wound rupture/dehiscence, and venous thrombosis, and they have an almost twofold increased risk of composite maternal morbidity and a fivefold risk of neonatal injury.[71] The unadjusted ORs of cesarean delivery are 1.46 (95% CI, 1.34 to 1.60), 2.05 (95% CI, 1.86 to 2.27), and 2.89 (95% CI, 2.28 to 3.79) for overweight, obese, and severely obese women, respectively, compared with normal-weight women.[72] Maternal obesity alone is not an indication for induction of labor.[73] However, obese women are at increased risk of a prolonged pregnancy and have an increased rate of induction of labor.[74] Although compared with spontaneous labor, induction of labor is associated with an increased risk of cesarean delivery in obese women,[75] no specific recommendations have been made to decrease the risk of primary cesarean delivery in this population.[76]

The length of labor in nulliparous women is proportional to maternal BMI.[77] In a study that adjusted for maternal height, labor induction, membrane rupture, oxytocin use, epidural anesthesia, net maternal weight gain, and fetal size, the median duration of labor from 0 to 10 cm was significantly longer in overweight and obese women. In overweight women, the prolongation was between 4 and 6 cm, and for obese women, labor was slower before 7 cm.[78] **In a mixed nulliparous and multiparous cohort, the second stage of labor was not significantly different among normal, overweight, and obese women.** The intrauterine pressure generated during a standardized Valsalva maneuver also was not significantly different among the various weight groups.[79]

The rate of trial of labor after cesarean (TOLAC) has been decreasing since the mid-1990s and is now less than 10% (see Chapter 20).[76] TOLAC success rates are inversely related to BMI: for a BMI less than 19.8, the rate is 83.1%; when BMI is between 19.8 and 26, the rate is 79.9%; between 26.1 and 29, the rate is 69.3%; and when BMI exceeds 29, the rate is 68.2% ($P < .001$). Similarly, gaining over 40 lb during pregnancy is associated with a decreased TOLAC success rate (66.8% vs. 79.1%, $P < .001$).[80] Class III women undergoing a TOLAC had greater composite morbidity—which included prolonged hospital stay, endometritis, rupture/dehiscence, and neonatal injury (fractures, brachial plexus injuries, and lacerations)—compared with class III women having an elective cesarean delivery, although absolute morbidities were small.[71] The risk is increased significantly for postpartum atonic hemorrhage (>1000 mL) for class III obese women after a vaginal delivery (5.2%) and instrumental delivery (13.6%), compared with normal-weight women (4.4%), but not after cesarean delivery.[81]

Maternal obesity significantly increases the risk of anesthetic complications. The CMACE/RCOG recommendations state that women with a pregravid BMI greater than 40 should have an antenatal consultation with an obstetric anesthesiologist to discuss and document anesthetic management plans for labor and delivery (see Chapter 16).[27] For all other obese women, early consultation with an obstetric anesthesiologist at the time of admission to labor and delivery should be considered to obtain proper equipment to monitor blood pressure, establish venous access, and screen for relevant comorbid conditions.[82] The risk of epidural failure is greater in obese women, compared with normal weight and overweight women[83]; therefore early labor epidural placement should be considered. This may mitigate increased time in the obese patient from decision for an emergency cesarean to delivery. Compared with normal-weight women, severely obese women at term have significantly greater hypotension and prolonged fetal heart rate decelerations after controlling for epidural bolus dose and hypertensive disorders.[84] The combination of spinal anesthesia and obesity significantly impairs respiratory function for up to 2 hours after the procedure.[85] General anesthesia also poses a risk for the obese pregnant women because of potential difficulties with endotracheal intubation (see Chapter 16).[86] However, general anesthesia is not a contraindication in obese women, but consideration should be given to the need for preoxygenation, proper positioning of the patient, and fiberoptic equipment intubation availability.[87]

Broad-spectrum antimicrobial prophylaxis is recommended for all cesarean deliveries unless the patient is already receiving antibiotics for conditions such as chorioamnionitis.[88] In a study of normal weight, overweight, and obese women, after 2-g dosing 30 to 60 minutes before skin incision, cefazolin concentrations in adipose tissue were inversely proportional to BMI. In obese and extremely obese patients, adipose tissue concentrations of cefazolin at the time of skin incision were less than the minimally inhibitory concentration for gram-negative rods (<4 μg/g of tissue) in 20% and 33% of obese and severely obese patients, respectively.[89] However, differences in clinical outcomes have not been established, and a proper dosing based on BMI has not been recommended.

The optimal type of skin incision for primary cesarean delivery in order to decrease morbidity in obese class II and III patients has not been resolved. Using data from a perinatal

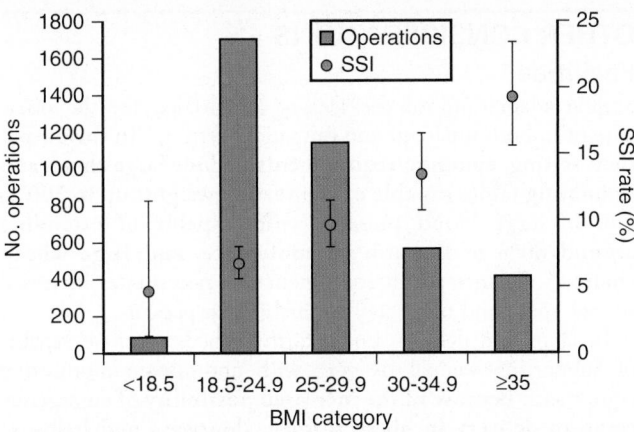

FIG 41-6 Frequency of surgical site infection (SSI) following cesarean delivery in women stratified by maternal body mass index (BMI). (From Wloch C, Wilson J, Lamagni T, et al. Risk factors for surgical site infection following cesarean section in England: results from a multicenter cohort study. *BJOG.* 2012;119:1324-1333.)

database, it was reported that a vertical skin incision was associated with a higher rate of wound complications than a transverse incision.[90] More recent data from a secondary analysis of the Maternal-Fetal Medicine Unit's (MFMU) cesarean registry, which used a composite of wound complications (infection, seroma, hematoma, wound evisceration, and fascial dehiscence) as the primary outcome, reported that in a univariate analysis, patients with a vertical skin incision had a significantly higher rate of wound complications; however, after adjustment for confounding factors, a vertical incision was associated with a significantly lower risk for wound complications.[91] The discrepancy was most likely explained by selection bias. Others have reported that in obese women with a voluminous panniculus, a supraumbilical incision was associated with favorable outcomes.[92]

Closure with suture of subcutaneous tissue greater than 2 cm in depth can significantly decrease the incidence of wound disruption.[93] The additional use of a subcutaneous drain with bulb suction in obese women with at least 4 cm of subcutaneous fat was not effective in preventing wound complications and may have potentiated postcesarean wound complications.[94] Compared with normal-weight women, the risk of surgical site infections (SSIs) is increased following a cesarean delivery in overweight women (OR, 1.6; 95% CI, 1.2 to 2.2), obese class I women (OR, 2.4; 95% CI, 1.7 to 3.4), and obese class II and III women (OR, 3.7; 95% CI, 2.6 to 5.2; Fig. 41-6).[95] Subcutaneous skin thickness greater than 3 cm is a significant risk factor (OR, 2.8; 95% CI, 1.3 to 5.9) for postcesarean wound infection after adjusting for maternal BMI.[96] Types of skin preparation, skin-closure techniques, and supplemental oxygen have not proved useful in decreasing the rate of postcesarean infectious morbidity.[97-99]

POSTPARTUM CONSIDERATIONS
Maternal
Obesity is a risk factor for venous thromboembolism (VTE) in the general population (see Chapter 45).[100] In a case-control study[101] of over 71,000 women in Denmark, the relative risk of VTE in obese women during pregnancy was 9.7 (95% CI, 3.1 to 30.8), and during the postpartum period, it was 2.8 (95% CI, 0.8 to 9.8) after adjustment for age, parity, clomiphene citrate stimulation, and diabetes. Obesity also was associated

with a higher risk of pulmonary embolism (aOR, 14.9; 95% CI, 3.0 to 74.8). However, these data are associated with very wide confidence intervals that limit confidence in the precision of the estimate. The Pregnancy and Thrombosis Working Group[100] in the United States recommends consideration of thromboprophylaxis only in selected patients and notes that data are insufficient to recommend routine pharmacologic prophylaxis in patients having a cesarean delivery.[101] **Because cesarean delivery increases the risk of VTE, placement of pneumatic compression devices has been recommended for all patients before and after cesarean delivery by the American College of Obstetricians and Gynecologists** (ACOG).[102] In contrast, the RCOG in the United Kingdom recommends obese women who have two or more additional risk factors such as smoking should be considered for prophylactic low-molecular-weight heparin (LMWH) as early in pregnancy as practical and should continue this therapy until 6 weeks postpartum. Additionally, the RCOG recommends that obese women who have one or more additional risk factors for VTE should be considered for LMWH for 7 days after delivery.[27]

Few randomized trials have addressed management of wound complications following cesarean delivery.[103] Risk factors for wound complications in addition to maternal obesity include diabetes, chorioamnionitis, corticosteroids, stress, and poor nutrition.[104] In a retrospective study of 2492 cesarean deliveries, the risk of postcesarean infection was 18.4%, and risk was highest among obese women (OR, 1.43; 95% CI, 1.09 to 1.88) after adjustment for diabetes and emergent/elective cesarean deliveries. Among women with diabetes, obesity increased the risk of postcesarean infection to an even greater extent (OR, 2.06; 95% CI, 1.13 to 3.75).[105] Management of the infected postcesarean wound includes antibiotics and evacuation of any hematoma/seroma. **An open wound can be managed in any of three ways: with secondary closure, closure by secondary intention with dressings, and closure by secondary intention using negative pressure wound therapy** (NPWT). Secondary closure and NPWT are associated with improved healing times compared with closure by secondary intention with dressings in nonpregnant patients.[104]

Excessive gestational weight gain is associated with short- and long-term postpartum weight retention.[106] In the Danish birth cohort (*n* = 60,892), underweight women retained an average of 2.3 kg and obese women lost 1.7 kg by 6 months postpartum. However, the variation of weight loss was great in the overweight and obese women, and the crude risks for postpartum weight retention showed only moderate associations with pregravid BMI. The greatest contribution to retention of over 5 kg at 6 months postdelivery was the degree of excessive weight gain during pregnancy. For example, women who gained in excess of 20 kg had a risk of postpartum weight retention that was sixfold greater than women who gained 10 to 15 kg.[107] Similar findings were reported among Asian populations.[108]

In the Fit for Delivery study, although behavioral intervention did not result in a significant decrease in gestational weight gain in overweight/obese women, a significant increase was reported among those who received the intervention in the proportion of overweight/obese women (30.7% vs. 18.7%) who returned to or were below their pregravid weight by 6 months postpartum.[109] Traditional means to decrease postpartum weight reduction have used behavioral intervention that involves diet and physical activity.[110] In a small study, use of the Internet-based program from the United States Department of Agriculture

(USDA), MyPyramid Menu Planner for Moms—which computes energy needs to achieve a defined weight loss based on demographic, anthropometric, and lactation status—resulted in significantly increased weight loss compared with a control group.[111] In a larger study in breastfeeding women that compared a Mediterranean-style diet with the MyPyramid menu planner for pregnancy and breastfeeding, both groups achieved a similar degree of moderate weight loss (−2.3 ± 3.4 kg vs. −3.1 ± 3.4 kg, respectively) over 4 months.[112] In an RCT in which women were followed over 10 months, family-based behavioral intervention did not result in a significant increase in postpartum weight loss compared with a control group. In a multivariate analysis, only baseline energy intake, work status, and breastfeeding were significant predictors of weight change.[113] Finally, in a Cochrane analysis, diet alone or diet plus exercise, but not exercise alone, helped women lose weight postpartum. Pregravid obesity, but not gestational weight gain, has been associated with early termination of breastfeeding[114] and also with postpartum anemia.[115] For breastfeeding women, more evidence is required to discern whether diet or exercise or both are detrimental for either mother or infant.[116]

The optimal treatment of obesity in pregnancy is prevention of obesity *before* pregnancy occurs. As discussed previously, the obstetrician/gynecologist, either in conjunction with other health care providers or individually, may consider using prepregnancy behavioral modification such as motivational interviewing to achieve behavioral change in areas such as weight control.[117] **Although achieving a normal BMI is the ideal, based on the results of the Look Ahead trial, a weight loss of even 5% to 7% significantly improved metabolic health.**[118]

Weight loss between pregnancies in obese women has been shown to decrease the risk of a large for gestational age (LGA) infant (aOR, 0.61; 95% CI, 0.52 to 0.73), **whereas an interpregnancy weight gain was associated with an increased risk of delivering an LGA infant** (aOR, 1.37; 95% CI, 1.21 to 1.54). Risk of a small-for-gestational-age (SGA) infant was not increased unless there was a loss of more than 8 kg/m².[119] The interpregnancy interval in women who lost weight in this study was longer than that seen in the women who gained weight between pregnancies, which underscores the importance of contraceptive counseling in this population.[120]

Neonate/Child
The infants of obese women are at increased risk for fetal macrosomia and, more specifically, for increased body fat compared with infants of normal-weight women.[121,122] Long-term risks for the offspring include an increased risk of the metabolic syndrome[123] and childhood obesity.[124] The risk of childhood obesity in offspring of obese women persists even after adjustment for complications such as GDM.[125] In a large Scandinavian study, higher maternal BMI was associated with an increased risk of asthma.[126] Maternal obesity has also been linked to altered behavior in the offspring, including an increased risk of autism spectrum disorders, childhood developmental delay, and attention-deficit/hyperactivity disorder.[127] However, as compelling as these data may seem, it is impossible in these observational studies to separate other prenatal and postnatal influences from obesity on outcomes in the offspring. Socioeconomic issues, behavior, activity, and diet within families often are not adjusted for the analysis of metabolic outcomes in the offspring of obese women, and thus the potential for confounding remains.[128]

OTHER CONSIDERATIONS
Facilities
Several adaptations of the facility are needed for the obese patient in both inpatient and outpatient settings. **In the outpatient setting, common requirements include large chairs and examining tables capable of supporting weights up to 500 to 750 lb, large blood pressure cuffs capable of extending around 80% of the arm circumference, and large wheelchairs.**[129] An increase in equipment size necessitates increased storage space and more staff to safely assist patients.

In labor and delivery units, birthing beds must be capable of supporting vaginal delivery with appropriate monitoring equipment. **Because of the increased possibility of emergency cesarean delivery in obese women, doorways and hallways require enough space to accommodate large beds and additional staff moving patients safely.** In the operating room, motorized lifts to assist obese patient onto the operating table[130] and sufficient space to allow staff to move safely and efficiently are necessary.[27] **Operating tables need to be strong enough to safely support patients with weights up to 500 to 750 lb and should have attachments to increase the width of tables.** Although no consensus has been reached in regard to the optimal positioning of the obese patient at the time of cesarean delivery,[131] operating tables should be able to accommodate various positions to the satisfaction of anesthesia and obstetric staff. **Long instruments are also necessary to facilitate the surgeon's access to the proper tissue planes.** Finally, consideration should be given to practice drills for staff to safely prepare for emergency cesarean delivery of the obese patient, particularly for those with a BMI greater than 40.

KEY POINTS

- Behavioral modification of diet or diet plus exercise can decrease excessive gestational weight gain in obese women.
- Weight gain in pregnancy should be based on pregravid BMI and should follow the IOM recommendations.
- Obese women should be counseled as to the limitation of ultrasound in identifying structural anomalies.
- At the first prenatal visit, obese women should be screened for glucose intolerance.
- Antenatal fetal surveillance is not recommended for obese women without other maternal or fetal indications.
- Obese women should be counseled about the increased risk of cesarean delivery for obese, compared with normal-weight, women.
- Closure of subcutaneous tissue greater than 2 cm, but not placement of subcutaneous drains, decreases the risk of postpartum cesarean wound complications.
- Excessive gestational weight gain is a significant risk factor for postpartum weight retention.
- Behavioral interventions that use diet and/or diet and exercise can improve postpartum weight reduction but not exercise alone.
- Because of the increase in plasma volume in obese women, consideration should be given to increase the bolus of preepidural intravenous fluid and dosage of prophylactic antibiotics for cesarean delivery.

REFERENCES

1. World Health Organization. *Obesity: Preventing and managing the global epidemic.* Geneva: World Health Organization; 2000.
2. Ogden CL, Carroll MD, Kit BK, et al. Prevalence of childhood and adult obesity in the United States, 2011-2012. *JAMA.* 2014;311:806-814.
3. Lindsay CA, Huston L, Amini SB, et al. Longitudinal changes in the relationship between body mass index and percent body fat in pregnancy. *Obstet Gynecol.* 1997;39:337-382.
4. Nishida C, WHO Expert Consultation. Appropriate body-mass index for Asian populations and its implications for policy and intervention strategies. *Lancet.* 2004;363:157-163.
5. Flegal KM, Carroll MD, Ogden CL, et al. Prevalence and trends in obesity among US adults, 1999-2008. *JAMA.* 2010;303:235-241.
6. Flegal KM, Carroll MD, Kit BK, et al. Prevalence of obesity and trends in the distribution of body mass index among US adults, 1999-2010. *JAMA.* 2012;307:491-497.
7. Katzmarzyk PT, Barlow S, Bouchard C, et al. An evolving scientific basis for the prevention and treatment of pediatric obesity. *Int J Obes.* 2014;38(7):887-905.
8. Ramachandrappa S, Farooqi IS. Genetic approaches to understanding human obesity. *J Clin Invest.* 2011;121:2080-2086.
9. Speliotes EK, Willer CJ, Berndt S, et al. Association analyses of 249,796 individuals reveal eighteen new loci associated with body mass index. *Nat Genet.* 2010;42:937-948.
10. Casazza K, Fontaine KR, Astrup A, et al. Myths, Presumptions, and facts about obesity. *N Engl J Med.* 2013;368:446-454.
11. Thomas DM, Schoeller DA, Redman LA, et al. A computational model to determine energy intake during weight loss. *Am J Clin Nutr.* 2010;92:1326-1331.
12. Hall KD, Heymsfield SB, Kemnitz JW, Klein S, Schoeller DA, Speakman JR. Energy balance and its components: implications for body weight regulation. *Am J Clin Nutr.* 2012;95:989-994.
13. Kramer MS, Matush L, Vanilovich I, et al. A randomized breast-feeding promotion intervention did not reduce child obesity in Belarus. *J Nutr.* 2009;139:417S-421S.
14. Chu SY, Callaghan WM, Bish CL, et al. Gestational weight gain by body mass index among US women delivering live births, 2004-2005: fueling future obesity. *Am J Obstet Gynecol.* 2009;200:271, e1-e7.
15. Fahraeus L, Larsson-Cohn U, Wallentin L. Plasma lipoproteins including high density lipoprotein subfractions during normal pregnancy. *Obstet Gynecol.* 1985;66:468-472.
16. Alvarez JJ, Montelongo A, Iglesias A, et al. Longitudinal study on lipoprotein profile, high density lipoprotein subclass, and postheparin lipases during gestation in women. *J Lipid Res.* 1996;37:299-308.
17. Sattar N, Tan CE, Han TS, et al. Association of indices of adiposity with atherogenic lipoprotein subfractions. *Int J Obes.* 1998;22:432-439.
18. Ramsay JE, Ferrell WR, Crawford L, et al. Maternal obesity is associated with dysregulation of metabolic, vascular, and inflammatory pathways. *J Clin Endocrinol Metab.* 2002;87:4231-4237.
19. Committee on Nutritional Status During Pregnancy and Lactation, Institute of Medicine. *Nutrition During Pregnancy: Part I: Weight Gain, Part II: Nutrient Supplements.* The National Academies Press; 1990:1-480.
20. Rasmussen KM, Abrams B, Bodnar LM, et al. *Weight gain during pregnancy: reexamining the guidelines.* Institute of Medicine; 2009.
21. Rasmussen KM, Abrams B, Bodnar LM, et al. Recommendations for weight gain during pregnancy in the context of the obesity epidemic. *Obstet Gynecol.* 2010;116:1191-1195.
22. Artal R, Lockwood CJ, Brown HL. Weight gain recommendations in pregnancy and the obesity epidemic. *Obstet Gynecol.* 2010;115:152-155.
23. Catalano PM, Mele L, Landon MB, et al., for the Eunice Kennedy Shriver National Institute of Child Health and Human Development Maternal-Fetal Medicine Units Network. Inadequate weight gain in overweight and obese pregnant women: what is the effect on fetal growth? *Am J Obstet Gynecol.* 2014;211:137, e1-7.
24. Society of Obstetricians and Gynecologists of Canada. Obesity in Pregnancy: SOGC Clinical Practice Guideline. *JOGC.* 2010;239:165-173.
25. Cedergren MI. Optimal gestational weight gain for body mass index categories. *Obstet Gynecol.* 2007;110:759-764.
26. Wong W, Tang NLS, Lau TK, Wong W. A new recommendation for maternal weight gain in Chinese women. *J Am Diet Assoc.* 2000;100:791-796.
27. CMACE/RCOG Guidelines Committee. *Management of women with obesity in pregnancy.* Royal College of Obstetricians and Gynaecologists; 2010:1-29.
28. WIN Weight-Control Information Network. Prescription medications for the treatment of obesity. *NIDDK.* 2013;1-8.
29. Rowan JA, Hague WM, Gao W, et al. for the MiG Trial Investigators. Metformin versus insulin for the treatment of gestational diabetes. *N Engl J Med.* 2008;358:2003-2015.
30. Moses RG, Casey SA, Quinn EG, et al. Pregnancy and glycemic index outcomes study: effects of low glycemic index compared with conventional dietary advice on selected pregnancy outcomes. *Am J Clin Nutr.* 2014;99:517-523.
31. Santos IA, Stein R, Fuchs SC, et al. Aerobic exercise and submaximal functional capacity in overweight pregnant women: a randomized trial. *Obstet Gynecol.* 2005;106:243-249.
32. Vinter CA, Jensen DM, Ovesen P, Beck-Nielsen H, Jørgensen JS. The LiP (Lifestyle in Pregnancy) study: a randomized controlled trial of lifestyle intervention in 360 obese pregnant women. *Diabetes Care.* 2011;34:2502-2507.
33. Dodd JM, Turnbull D, McPhee A, et al., for the LIMIT Randomised Trial group. Antenatal lifestyle advice for women who are overweight or obese: LIMIT randomised trial. *BMJ.* 2014;348:g1285.
34. Ilmonen J, Isolauri E, Poussa T, Laitinen K. Impact of dietary counselling and probiotic intervention on maternal anthropometric measurements during and after pregnancy: a randomized placebo-controlled trial. *Clin Nutr.* 2011;30:156-164.
35. Muktabhant B, Lumbiganon P, Ngamjarus C, Dowswell T. Interventions for preventing excessive weight gain during pregnancy. *Cochrane Database Syst Rev.* 2012;(4):CD007145.
36. Thangaratinam S, Rogozinska E, Jolly K, et al. Effects of interventions in pregnancy on maternal weight and obstetric outcomes: meta-analysis of randomised evidence. *BMJ.* 2012;344:e2088.
37. Lashen H, Fear K, Sturdee DW. Obesity is associated with increased risk of first trimester and recurrent miscarriage: matched case-control study. *Hum Reprod.* 2004;19:1644-1646.
38. Stothard KJ, Tennant PW, Bell R, Rankin J. Maternal overweight and obesity and the risk of congenital anomalies: a systemic review and meta-analysis. *JAMA.* 2009;301:636-650.
39. Best KE, Tennant PW, Bell R, Rankin J. Impact of maternal body mass index on the antenatal detection of congenital anomalies. *BJOG.* 2012;119:1503-1511.
40. Weichert J, Hartge DR. Obstetrical sonography in obese women: a review. *J Clin Ultrasound.* 2011;39:209-216.
41. Racusin D, Stevens B, Campbell G, et al. Obesity and the risk and detection of fetal malformations. *Semin Perinatol.* 2012;36:213-221.
42. Aagaard-Tillery KM, Flint Porter T, Maline FD, et al. Influence of maternal BMI on genetic sonography in the FaSTER trial. *Prenat Diagn.* 2010;30:14-22.
43. Bianchi DW, Parker RL, Wentworth J, et al., for the CARE Study Group. DNA sequencing versus standard prenatal aneuploidy screening. *N Engl J Med.* 2014;370:799-808.
44. Vora NL, Johnson KL, Basu S, et al. A multi-factorial relationship exists between total circulating cell-free DNA levels and maternal BMI. *Prenat Diagn.* 2012;32:912-914.
45. Weiss JL, Malone FD, Emig D, et al., for the FASTER Research Consortium. Obesity, obstetric complications and cesarean delivery rate: a population-based screening study. *Am J Obstet Gynecol.* 2004;190:1091-1097.
46. Anderson NH, McCowan LM, Fyfe EM, et al., on behalf of the SCOPE Consortium. The impact of maternal body mass index on the phenotype of pre-eclampsia: a prospective cohort study. *BJOG.* 2012;119:589-595.
47. Catalano PM. Management of obesity in pregnancy. *Obstet Gynecol.* 2007;109:419-433.
48. Facco FL. Sleep-disordered breathing and pregnancy. *Semin Perinatol.* 2011;35:335-339.
49. Pien GW, Pack AI, Jackson N, et al. Risk factors for sleep-disordered breathing in pregnancy. *Thorax.* 2014;69:371-377.
50. Sohlberg S, Stephansson O, Cnattingius S, Wikström AK. Maternal body mass index, height, and risks of preeclampsia. *Am J Hypertens.* 2012;25:120-125.
51. Chu SY, Callaghan WM, Kim SY, et al. Maternal obesity and risk of gestational diabetes mellitus. *Diabetes Care.* 2007;30:2070-2076.
52. Chen YH, Kang JH, Lin CC, et al. Obstructive sleep apnea and the risk of adverse pregnancy outcomes. *Am J Obstet Gynecol.* 2012;206:136, e1-e5.
53. Makgoba M, Savvidou MD, Steer PJ. An analysis of the interrelationship between maternal age, body mass index and racial origin in the development of gestational diabetes mellitus. *BJOG.* 2012;119:276-282.

54. Louis J, Auckley D, Bolden N. Management of obstructive sleep apnea in pregnant women. *Obstet Gynecol.* 2012;119:864-868.

55. ACOG Practice Bulletin. Clinical management guidelines for obstetrician-gynecologists. Gestational diabetes mellitus. *Obstet Gynecol.* 2013; 122(Pt 1):406-416.

56. International Association of Diabetes and Pregnancy Study Groups Consensus Panel. International Association of Diabetes and Pregnancy Study Groups recommendations on the diagnosis and classification of hyperglycemia in pregnancy. *Diabetes Care.* 2010;33:676-682.

57. Page LM, Girling JC. A novel cause for abnormal liver function tests in pregnancy and the puerperium: non-alcoholic fatty liver disease. *BJOG.* 2011;118:1532-1535.

58. Callaway LK, Colditz PB, Byrne NM, et al., Bambino Group. Prevention of gestational diabetes. Feasibility issues for an exercise intervention in obese pregnant women. *Diabetes Care.* 2010;33:1457-1459.

59. Oostdam N, van Poppel MN, Wouters MG, et al. No effect of the FitFor2 exercise programme on blood glucose, insulin sensitivity, and birthweight in pregnant women who were overweight and at risk for gestational diabetes: results of a randomised controlled trial. *BJOG.* 2012;119:1098-1107.

60. Han S, Middleton P, Crowther CA. Exercise for pregnant women for preventing gestational diabetes mellitus. *Cochrane Database Syst Rev.* 2012;(7):CD009021.

61. Luoto R, Laitinen K, Nermes M, et al. Impact of maternal probiotic-supplemented dietary counselling on pregnancy outcome and prenatal and postnatal growth: a double-blind, placebo-controlled study. *Br J Nutr.* 2010;103:1792-1799.

62. D'Anna R, Scilipoti A, Giordano D, et al. Myo-Inositol supplementation and onset of gestational diabetes mellitus in pregnancy women with a family history of type 2 diabetes. A prospective, randomized, placebo-controlled study. *Diabetes Care.* 2013;36:854-857.

63. Levine RJ, Hauth JC, Curet LB, et al. Trail of calcium to prevent pre-eclampsia. *N Engl J Med.* 1997;337:69-76.

64. Roberts JM, Myatt L, Spong CY, et al. Vitamins C and E to prevent complications of pregnancy-associated hypertension. *N Engl J Med.* 2010;362:1282-1291.

65. Yogev Y, Xenakis EM, Langer O. The association between preeclampsia and the severity of gestational diabetes: the impact of glycemic control. *Am J Obstet Gynecol.* 2004;191:1655-1660.

66. Executive Summary: Hypertension in pregnancy. American College of Obstetricians and Gynecologists. *Obstet Gynecol.* 2013;122:1122-1131.

67. McDonald SD, Han Z, Mulla S, Beyene J, Knowledge Synthesis Group. Overweight and obesity in mothers and risk of preterm birth and low birth weight infants: systematic review and meta-analyses. *BMJ.* 2010;341:c3428.

68. Cnattiangius S, Villamor E, Johansson S, et al. Maternal obesity and risk of preterm delivery. *JAMA.* 2013;309:2362-2370.

69. Salihu HM, Dunlop AL, Hedayatzadeh M, et al. Extreme obesity and risk of stillbirth among black and white gravidas. *Obstet Gynecol.* 2007;110:552-557.

70. Signore C, Freeman RK, Spong CY. Antenatal testing – a reevaluation: Executive summary of a Eunice Kennedy Shriver NICHD workshop. *Obstet Gynecol.* 2009;113:687-701.

71. Hibbard JU, Gilbert S, Landon MB, et al., for the NICHD Maternal-Fetal medicine Units Network. Trial of labor or repeat cesarean delivery in women with morbid obesity and previous cesarean delivery. *Obstet Gynecol.* 2006;108:125-133.

72. Chu SY, Kim SY, Schmid CH, et al. Diagnostic in Obesity Comorbidities. Maternal obesity and risk of cesarean delivery: a meta-analysis. *Obes Rev.* 2007;8:385-394.

73. ACOG Practice Bulletin. Clinical management guidelines for obstetrician-gynecologists. Induction of Labor. *Obstet Gynecol.* 2009;114(Pt 1):386-397.

74. Arrowsmith S, Wray S, Quenby S. Maternal obesity and labor complications following induction of labour in prolonged pregnancy. *BJOG.* 2011;118:578-588.

75. Wolfe KB, Rossi RA, Warshak CR. The effect of maternal obesity on the rate of failed induction of labor. *Am J Obstet Gynecol.* 2011;205:128, e1-123.e7.

76. Safe prevention of the primary cesarean delivery. Obstetric Care Consensus No. 1. American College of Obstetricians and Gynecologists. *Obstet Gynecol.* 2014;123:693-711.

77. Nuthalapaty FS, Rouse DJ, Owen J. The association of maternal weight with cesarean risk, labor duration, and cervical dilation rate during labor induction. *Obstet Gynecol.* 2004;103:452-456.

78. Vahratian A, Zhang J, Troendle JF, et al. Maternal prepregnancy overweight and obesity and the pattern of labor progression in term nulliparous women. *Obstet Gynecol.* 2004;104:943-951.

79. Buhimschi CA, Buhimschi IA, Malinow AM, et al. Intrauterine pressure during the second stage of labor in obese women. *Obstet Gynecol.* 2004;103:225-230.

80. Juhasz G, Gyamfi C, Gyamfi P, et al. Effect of body mass index and excessive weight gain on success of vaginal birth after cesarean delivery. *Obstet Gynecol.* 2005;106:741-746.

81. Bloomberg M. Maternal obesity and risk of postpartum hemorrhage. *Obstet Gynecol.* 2011;118:561-568.

82. Tan T, Sia AT. Anesthesia considerations in the obese gravida. *Semin Perinatol.* 2011;35:350-355.

83. Dresner M, Brocklesby J, Bamber J. Audit of the influence of body mass index on the performance of epidural analgesia in labour and the subsequent mode of delivery. *BJOG.* 2006;113:1178-1181.

84. Vricella LK, Louis JM, Mercer BM, et al. Impact of morbid obesity on epidural anesthesia complications in labor. *Am J Obstet Gynecol.* 2011;205:370, e1-e6.

85. Von Ungern-Sternberg BS, Regli A, Bucher E, et al. Impact of spinal anesthesia and obesity on maternal respiratory function during elective caesarean section. *Anesthesia.* 2004;59:743-749.

86. Mhyre JM. Anesthetic management for the morbidly obese pregnant woman. *Int Anesthesiol Clin.* 2007;45:51-70.

87. Dresner M. The 30 min decision to delivery time is unrealistic in morbidly obese women. *Int J Obstet Anesth.* 2010;19:435-437.

88. Use of prophylactic antibiotics in labor and delivery. Practice Bulletin No. 120. American College of Obstetricians and Gynecologists. *Obstet Gynecol.* 2011;117:1473-1483.

89. Pevzner L, Swank M, Krepel C, et al. Effects of maternal obesity on tissue concentrations of prophylactic cefazolin during cesarean delivery. *Obstet Gynecol.* 2011;117:877-882.

90. Wall PD, Deucy EE, Glantz JC, et al. Vertical skin incisions and wound complications in the obese parturient. *Obstet Gynecol.* 2003;102:952-956.

91. Marrs CC, Houssa HN, Sibai BM, et al. The relationship between primary cesarean delivery skin incision type and wound complications is women with morbid obesity. *Am J Obstet Gynecol.* 2014;201:319, e1-4.

92. Tixier H, Thouvenot S, Coulange L, et al. Cesarean section in morbidly obese women: supra or subumbilical transverse incision? *Acta Obstet Gynecol Scand.* 2009;88:1049-1052.

93. Naumann RW, Hauth JC, Woen J, et al. Subcutaneous tissue approximation in relation to wound disruption after cesarean delivery in obese women. *Obstet Gynecol.* 1995;85:412-416.

94. Ramsey PS, White AM, Guinn DA, et al. Subcutaneous tissue reapproximation, along in combination with drain, in obese women undergoing cesarean delivery. *Obstet Gynecol.* 2005;105:967-973.

95. Wloch C, Wilson J, Lamagni T, Harrington P, Charlett A, Sheridan E. Risk factors for surgical site infection following caesarean section in England: results from a multicentre cohort study. *BJOG.* 2012;119:1324-1333.

96. Vermillion ST, Lamoutte C, Soper DE. Wound infection after cesarean: effect of subcutaneous tissue thickness. *Obstet Gynecol.* 2000;95:923-926.

97. Hadiati DR, Hakimi M, Nurdiati DS. Skin preparation for preventing infection following caesarean section. *Cochrane Database Syst Rev.* 2012;(9):CD007462.

98. Mackeen AD, Berghella V, Larsen ML. Techniques and materials for skin closure in caesarean section. *Cochrane Database Syst Rev.* 2012;(11):CD003577.

99. Scifres CM, Leighton BL, Fogertey PJ, et al. Supplemental oxygen for the prevention of postcesarean infectious morbidity: a randomized controlled trial. *Am J Obstet Gynecol.* 2011;205:267, e1-9.

100. Duhl AJ, Paidas MJ, Ural SH, et al., for the Pregnancy and Thrombosis Working Group. Antithrombotic therapy and pregnancy: consensus report and recommendations for prevention and treatment of venous thromboembolism and adverse pregnancy outcomes. *Am J Obstet Gynecol.* 2007;197:457, e1-21.

101. Larsen TB, Sørensen HT, Gislum M, et al. Maternal smoking, obesity, and risk of venous thromboembolism during pregnancy and the puerperium: A population-based nested case-control study. *Thromb Res.* 2007;120:505-509.

102. Obesity in pregnancy. Committee Opinion No. 549. American College of Obstetrics and Gynecologists. *Obstet Gynecol.* 2013;121:213-217.

103. Thromboembolism in pregnancy. Practice Bulletin No. 123. American College of Obstetricians and Gynecologists. *Obstet Gynecol*. 2011;118:718-729.

104. Tipton AM, Cohen SA, Chelmow D. Wound infection in the obese pregnant woman. *Semin Perinatol*. 2011;35:345-349.

105. Sarsam SE, Elliott JP, Lam GK. Management of wound complications from cesarean delivery. *Obstet Gynecol Surv*. 2005;60:462-473.

106. Leth RA, Uldbjerg N, Nørgaard M, et al. Obesity, diabetes, and the risk of infections diagnosed in hospital and post-discharge infections after cesarean section: a prospective cohort study. *Acta Obstet Gynecol Scand*. 2011;90:510-519.

107. Nehring I, Schmoll S, Beyerlein A, et al. Gestational weight gain and long-term postpartum weight retention: a meta-analysis. *Am J Clin Nutr*. 2011;94:1225-1231.

108. Nohr EA, Vaeth M, Baker JL, et al. Combined associations of prepregnancy body mass index and gestational weight gain with the outcome of pregnancy. *Am J Clin Nutr*. 2008;87:1750-1759.

109. Cheng HR, Walker LO, Tseng YF, Lin PC. Post-partum weight retention in women in Asia: a systematic review. *Obes Rev*. 2011;12:770-780.

110. Phelan S, Phipps MG, Abrams B, et al. Randomized trial of a behavioral intervention to prevent excessive gestational weight gain: the Fit for delivery study. *Am J Clin Nutr*. 2011;93:772-779.

111. Choi J, Fukuoka Y, Lee JH. The effects of physical activity and physical activity plus diet interventions on body weight in overweight or obese women who are pregnant or in postpartum: A systematic review and meta-analysis of randomized controlled trials. *Prev Med*. 2013;56:351-364.

112. Colleran HL, Lovelady CA. Use of MyPyramid menu planner for moms in a weight-loss intervention during lactation. *J Acad Nutr Diet*. 2012;112:553-558.

113. Stendell-Hollis NR, Thompson PA, West JL, et al. A comparison of Mediterranean-style and MyPyramid diets on weight loss and inflammatory biomarkers in postpartum breastfeeding women. *J Womens Health*. 2013;22:48-57.

114. Wiltheiss GA, Lovelady CA, West DG, Brouwer RJ, Krause KM, Østbye T. Diet quality and weight change among overweight and obese postpartum women enrolled in a behavioral intervention program. *J Acad Nutr Diet*. 2013;113:54-62.

115. Baker JL, Michaelsen KF, Sørensen TI, Rasmussen KM. High prepregnant body mass index is associated with early termination of full and any breastfeeding in Danish women. *Am J Clin Nutr*. 2007;86:404-411.

116. Bodnar LM, Siega-Riz AM, Cogswell ME. High prepregnancy BMI increases the risk of postpartum anemia. *Obes Res*. 2004;12:941-948.

117. Amorim Adegboye AR, Linne YM. Diet or exercise, or both, for weight reduction in women after childbirth. *Cochrane Database Syst Rev*. 2013;(7):CD005627.

118. ACOG Committee Opinion No 423. Motivational interviewing: A tool for behavior change. *Obstet Gynecol*. 2009;113:243-246.

119. The Look AHEAD Research Group. Long-term effects of a lifestyle intervention on weight and cardiovascular risk factors in individuals with type 2 diabetes: four-year results of the Look AHEAD trial. *Arch Intern Med*. 2010;170:1566-1575.

120. Jain AP, Gavard JA, Rice JJ, et al. The impact of interpregnancy weight change on birthweight in obese women. *Am J Obstet Gynecol*. 2013;208:205, e1-7.

121. de Bocanegra HT, Chang R, Howell M, et al. Interpregnancy intervals: impact of postpartum contraceptive effectiveness and coverage. *Am J Obstet Gynecol*. 2014;201:311, e1-8.

122. Sewell MF, Huston-Presley L, Super DM, Catalano P. Increased neonatal fat mass, not lean body mass, is associated with maternal obesity. *Am J Obstet Gynecol*. 2006;195:1100-1103.

123. Hull HR, Kinger MK, Knehans AW, et al. Impact of maternal body mass index on neonate birthweight and body composition. *Am J Obstet Gynecol*. 2008;198:416, e1-6.

124. Boney CM, Verma A, Tucker R, et al. Metabolic syndrome in childhood: association with birth weight, maternal obesity, and gestational diabetes mellitus. *Pediatrics*. 2005;115:e290-e296.

125. Catalano PM, Farrell K, Thomas A, et al. Perinatal risk factors for childhood obesity and metabolic dysregulation. *Am J Clin Nutr*. 2009;90:1303-1313.

126. Philipps LH, Santhakumaran S, Gale C, et al. The diabetic pregnancy and offspring BMI in childhood: a systematic review and meta-analysis. *Diabetologia*. 2011;54:1957-1966.

127. Patel SP, Rodriguez A, Little MP, et al. Associations between pre-pregnancy obesity and asthma symptoms in adolescents. *J Epidemiol Community Health*. 2012;66:809-814.

128. Krakowiak P, Walker CK, Bremer AA, et al. Maternal metabolic conditions and risk for autism and other neurodevelopmental disorders. *Pediatrics*. 2012;129:e1121-e1128.

129. O'Reilly JR, Reynolds RM. The risk of maternal obesity to the long-term health of the offspring. *Clin Endocrinol*. 2013;78:9-16.

130. Kriebs JM. Obesity as a complication of pregnancy and labor. *J Perinat Neonatal Nurs*. 2009;23:15-22.

131. James DC, Mahner MA. Caring for the extremely obese. *MCN*. 2009;34:24-30.

132. Cluver C, Novikova N, Hofmeyr GJ, Hall DR. Maternal position during caesarean section for preventing maternal and neonatal complications. *Cochrane Database Syst Rev*. 2010;(6):CD00723.

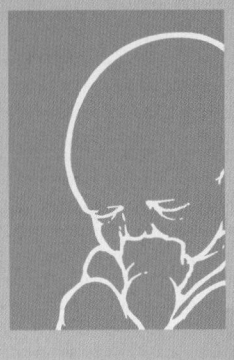

CHAPTER 42

Thyroid and Parathyroid Diseases in Pregnancy

JORGE H. MESTMAN

KEY ABBREVIATIONS

1,25-dihydroxyvitamin D	$1,25[OH]_2D_3$	Parathyroid hormone–related protein	PTHrP
American Association of Clinical Endocrinologists	AACE	Postpartum thyroiditis	PPT
American College of Obstetricians and Gynecologists	ACOG	Pregnancy and lactation–associated osteoporosis	PLO
American Thyroid Association	ATA	Primary hyperparathyroidism	PHPT
Antithyroglobulin antibody	TgAb	Propylthiouracil	PTU
Antithyroid drug	ATD	Subclinical hypothyroidism	SCH
Carbimazole	CMZ	Thyroid-binding inhibitor	TBI
Endocrine Society	ES	Thyroid-binding inhibitor immunoglobulin	TBII
Familial hypocalciuric hypercalcemia	FHH	Thyroid-receptor antibody	TRAb
Familial isolated primary hyperparathyroidism	FIHPT	Thyroid function test	TFT
		Thyroid peroxidase	TPO
Fine-needle aspiration biopsy	FNAB	Thyroid peroxidase antibody	TPOAb
Free thyroxine	FT_4	Thyroid-stimulating hormone	TSH
Free thyroxine index	FT_4I	Thyroid-stimulating immunoglobulin	TSI
Free triiodothyronine	FT_3		
Free triiodothyronine index	FT_3I	Thyroid stimulation–blocking antibody	TSBA
Human chorionic gonadotropin	hCG		
Hyperemesis gravidarum	HG	Thyrotropin-releasing hormone	TRH
Immunoglobulin G	IgG	Thyroxine	T_4
Intelligence quotient	IQ	Thyroxine-binding globulin	TBG
Intrauterine growth restriction	IUGR	Total triiodothyronine	TT_3
Levothyroxine	L-thyroxine	Total thyroxine	TT_4
Methimazole	MMI	Triiodothyronine	T_3
Neonatal severe primary hyperparathyroidism	NSPHPT	Thyroid-stimulating hormone receptor antibody	TRAb, TSHRAb
Parathyroid hormone	PTH		

Along with diabetes mellitus, thyroid diseases are the most frequent endocrine pathology seen in pregnancy; parathyroid diseases, on the other hand, are rare but may present a diagnostic and therapeutic challenge to the obstetrician. The obstetrician should be aware of the symptoms and signs of the particular disease, the effect of pregnancy on the interpretation of endocrine tests, and the transfer of hormones and medications across the placenta with potential complications for the fetus and neonate. It is imperative that a team approach be used in the management of these conditions; **the close cooperation of the obstetrician, endocrinologist, neonatologist, pediatric endocrinologist, and anesthesiologist** *well in advance of the delivery time* **will offer the patient the best maternal and perinatal outcomes.**

PARATHYROID DISEASES

Although uncommon in pregnancy, parathyroid diseases may produce significant perinatal and maternal morbidity and mortality if not diagnosed and properly managed.

Calcium Homeostasis During Pregnancy

Parathyroid hormone (PTH) and 1,25-dihydroxyvitamin D $(1,25[OH]_2D_3)$ are responsible for maintaining calcium homeostasis. **About 50% of serum calcium is protein bound, mostly to albumin; 10% is complexed to anions; and 40% circulates free as ionized calcium. During pregnancy, active transfer of maternal calcium to the fetus occurs.** A full-term infant requires 25 to 30 g of calcium during the course of pregnancy for new bone mineralization, most of it in the third trimester.

Total serum calcium during gestation is 8% below postpartum levels.[1] **Ionized calcium levels, however, remain unchanged throughout gestation.** Serum phosphate and renal tubular reabsorption of phosphorus also remain normal throughout pregnancy. Maternal serum PTH levels are slightly decreased in the first half of pregnancy (about 20% of the mean nonpregnant values) but return to normal by midgestation.[2]

Blood levels of $1,25(OH)_2D_3$ (calcitriol), the active metabolite of vitamin D, increase early in gestation to twice the nonpregnancy level in the third trimester. This increase comes as a result of stimulation of maternal renal 1α-hydroxylase activity by estrogen, placental lactogen, and PTH as well as synthesis of calcitriol by the placenta. Also, 24-hour urinary calcium excretion increases with each trimester of gestation and decreases in the postpartum period,[2] which reflects the increased intestinal calcium absorption induced by higher levels of 1,25-hydroxyvitamin D during gestation.

Parathyroid hormone–related protein (PTHrP), a peptide responsible for the hypercalcemia found in many malignant tumors, increases in early pregnancy. The source of maternal serum PTHrP is multiple, and both fetal and maternal sites have been postulated (placenta, myometrium, amnion, decidua, fetal parathyroid glands, breast, umbilical cord). PTHrP increases 1α-hydroxylase activity with an increase in $1,25(OH_2)D_3$; in addition, PTHrP plays a role in placental calcium transport and may also help protect the maternal skeleton during pregnancy.

Serum calcitonin levels are higher during pregnancy and in the postpartum period compared with nonpregnant controls.

Osteocalcin is a bone-specific protein released by osteoblasts into the circulation proportional to the rate of new bone formation. **Markers of bone resorption increase during pregnancy and reach values in the last trimester of pregnancy up to twice the normal level.** These changes are consistent with the increase in bone turnover at the time of maximal transfer of maternal calcium to the fetus.

After delivery, urinary calcium excretion is reduced; ionized serum calcium remains within normal limits; and total calcium, 1,25-hydroxyvitamin D, and serum PTH return to prepregnancy levels. Intestinal absorption of calcium decreases to the nonpregnant rate as a result of the previously mentioned return to normal levels of $1,25(OH)_2D_3$.[1] Early concern for calcium loss in lactating mothers, with the development of osteopenia, has not been confirmed, and **extra calcium supplementation during breastfeeding appears to be unnecessary** because calcium supplementation above normal does not significantly reduce the amount of lost bone during gestation.[5] The alteration in calcium and bone metabolism that accompanies human lactation represents a physiologic response that is independent of calcium intake.

Hyperparathyroidism

The prevalence of primary hyperparathyroidism (PHPT) is 0.5%. The incidence of the disease in pregnancy is unknown, but it is definitely rare, and most of the reported cases have been single ones complemented with a review of the literature. With the introduction of routine, automated techniques in clinical medicine and with early diagnosis, most patients with PHPT are symptom free, and their serum calcium elevation is mild. In nonpregnant PHPT patients, indications for surgery include (1) serum calcium greater than 1 mg/dL (>0.25 mmol/L) above the upper limit of normal; (2) bone densitometry with a T score of −2.5 or greater at the lumbar spine, total hip, femoral neck, or distal third of the radius; (3) vertebral fracture; (4) creatinine clearance below 60 mL/min; or (5) clinical signs and symptoms of a stone or visualization of a stone on imaging. It is estimated that 10% of PHPT patients have a mutation in one of 11 genes. They may occur as part of complex disorders, such as multiple endocrine neoplasia (MEN) syndromes 1 through 4; as a familial disorder, familial isolated primary hyperparathyroidism (FIHPT); in the syndrome of familial hypocalciuric hypercalcemia (FHH); and in the syndrome of neonatal severe primary hyperparathyroidism (NSPHPT). In practice, genetic testing is indicated in cases of primary hyperparathyroidism (1) in the presence of multigland disease, (2) in the very young (before pregnancy), (3) with parathyroid carcinoma or atypical adenoma, and (4) with a family history of hypercalcemia in first-degree relatives. Genetic testing is expensive; therefore patients should be referred to genetic counselors, and appropriate tests should be performed by accredited centers.

The first case of PHPT during pregnancy was reported in 1931. Shortly thereafter, the first case of neonatal hypocalcemia to cause tetany in a mother with undiagnosed hypercalcemia due to hyperparathyroidism was described by Friderichsen. **The most common cause of PHPT in pregnancy is a single parathyroid adenoma, which is present in about 80% of all cases.** Primary hyperplasia of the four parathyroid glands accounts for about 15% of the cases reported, 3% are due to multiple adenomas, and only a few cases due to parathyroid carcinoma have been reported in the English literature. In 1962, Ludwig reviewed the literature on the subject and described 21 women with 40 pregnancies: the incidence of fetal wastage was 27.5%; and neonatal tetany as a result of hypocalcemia, representing the first indication of maternal hyperparathyroidism, occurred in 19% of these cases. In contrast to the previous high neonatal morbidity and mortality, reviewing the literature from 1976 to 1990, Kelly[3] found only two perinatal deaths (5%) among 37 infants born of hyperparathyroid mothers. Two additional cases of perinatal deaths were reported in mothers with hypercalcemic crisis.

In the nonpregnant state, almost 70% of patients are symptom free, and the diagnosis is made through the routine use of biochemical screening. In pregnancy, because routine calcium determinations are not routinely performed, manifestations of the disease are present in almost 70% of the diagnosed patients. In a review of 70 pregnant women, gastrointestinal symptoms such as nausea, vomiting, and anorexia were present in 36% of patients, whereas 34% presented with weakness and fatigue. In 26%, mental symptoms that included headaches, lethargy, agitation, emotional lability, confusion, and inappropriate behavior were reported. Nephrolithiasis was detected in 36%, bone disease in 19%, acute pancreatitis in 13%, and hypertension in 10%. Only 24% of these patients were symptom free.

Parathyroid cancer is a rare cause of hyperparathyroidism, with very few cases documented in pregnancy. Serum calcium levels are significantly higher than in other cases of PHPT, and perinatal mortality and morbidity are significant. Hypercalcemia with values above 13 mg/dL in the presence of a palpable neck mass should raise a strong suspicion of parathyroid carcinoma. On the contrary, in the presence of mild hypercalcemia and a neck mass, the most common cause of the neck lesion is a thyroid nodule. One other clinical feature of parathyroid carcinoma is poor response to the usual clinical therapeutic measures such as intensive hydration and loop diuretics. Surgery is the only effective therapy.

Hyperparathyroidism should be considered in the differential diagnosis of acute pancreatitis during pregnancy, which has been reported in 13% of women with primary hyperparathyroidism. The incidence of *acute pancreatitis* in nonpregnant hyperparathyroid women is about 1.5% and is less than 1% in normal pregnancy. It is mostly likely to occur during the last trimester of pregnancy or the postpartum period but has also been reported in the first trimester of pregnancy, mimicking hyperemesis gravidarum (HG). **Serum calcium should be obtained in any pregnant woman with persistent significant nausea, vomiting, and abdominal pain.**

Hyperparathyroid crisis, a serious complication of PHPT, has been reported during gestation and the postpartum period and is characterized by severe nausea and vomiting, generalized weakness, changes in mental status, and severe dehydration. Hypertension may be present and should be differentiated from preeclampsia. The serum calcium level is frequently higher than 14 mg/dL; hypokalemia and elevation in serum creatinine are routinely seen. If not recognized and treated promptly, hyperparathyroid crisis may progress to uremia, coma, and death. Of the 12 cases reported in the literature, four occurred in the postpartum period. Patients presented with severe nausea, vomiting, and elevation in serum creatinine due to dehydration. Serum calcium levels higher than 20 mg/dL were reported in three cases, and three patients died. In addition, six cases have been associated with pancreatitis, and four fetal deaths have also been reported.

Bone disease in patients with PHPT is now unusual, but in early series, it was a common complication. Radiologic evaluation of the bones showed diffuse demineralization, subperiosteal resorption of the phalanges, and in severe cases, single or multiple cystic lesions and generalized osteoporosis.

Shani and associates reported[4] five cases of excessive amniotic fluid in mothers with PHPT and serum calcium levels between 11.3 and 14 mg/dL. The authors suggested that the fetal polyuria was, similar to adult polyuria, a common finding in patients with hyperparathyroidism.

The two most common causes of neonatal morbidity are prematurity and neonatal hypocalcemia, and the latter is related to levels of maternal hypercalcemia. In early reports, it was often the only clue of maternal hyperparathyroidism. Neonatal hypocalcemia develops between the second and fourteenth day of life and lasts for a few days.

Preeclampsia has been reported in some cases of PHPT. Hultin and coworkers examined whether parathyroid adenoma, the main cause of hyperparathyroidism, diagnosed and treated before pregnancy is associated with preeclampsia. They reviewed the records of 52 women, between 1973 and 1997 with the diagnosis of parathyroid adenoma confirmed by surgery and compared them with 519 women without the disease, all of whom had a subsequent singleton pregnancy. They concluded that PHPT due to a single adenoma diagnosed and treated before delivery is significantly associated with preeclampsia (adjusted odds ratio [aOR], 6.89; 95% confidence interval [CI], 2.30 to 20.58; $P < .0001$). Therefore treated PHPT should be considered a risk factor for preeclampsia in future pregnancies.

The clinical manifestations of PHPT and pregnancy complications—maternal, fetal, and neonatal—are directly related to the serum calcium level. Dochez and Ducarme reviewed 34 published articles in English and French on the characteristics of PHPT, clinical presentations, pregnancy complications, birth outcomes, and management of PHPT during pregnancy. They emphasized the need to rule out FHH and hereditary syndromes such as multiple endocrine neoplasia syndrome (MEN-1 or MEN-2) and familial parathyroid hyperplasia. Nephrolithiasis was the most common finding in symptomatic patients during pregnancy; other maternal complications include depression, constipation, bone fracture, maternal heart rhythm disorders, pancreatitis, parathyroid crisis, and HG. Maternal hypertension and preeclampsia were observed in 25% of these patients.

The diagnosis of PHPT is based on persistent hypercalcemia in the presence of increased PTH or a PTH level inappropriate for the level of serum calcium.[5] In pregnancy, because of the presence of hypoalbuminemia, a persistent total serum calcium value higher than 9.5 mg/dL is suspicious for hypercalcemia. A determination of 24-hour urinary calcium excretion is helpful in the diagnosis, because most women with PHPT have an increase in urinary calcium excretion above the usual hypercalciuria of normal pregnancy. Urinary calcium excretion is low or low normal in the syndrome of familial hypocalciuric hypercalcemia (FHH), another cause of hypercalcemia that must be included in the differential diagnosis. The serum alkaline phosphatase level may be increased in PHPT. However, it is also increased in normal pregnancy. **Ultrasonography of the neck is the current first-line investigation during pregnancy for localization of parathyroid diseases, with a sensitivity of 69% and a specificity of 94% in experienced hands. Parathyroid contrast imaging studies are contraindicated in pregnancy.**

Hypercalcemia

Differential Diagnosis

Although most young women with hypercalcemia have PHPT, other unusual causes should be ruled out, mainly

BOX 42-1 CAUSES OF HYPERCALCEMIA IN PREGNANCY AND THE PUERPERIUM

Hyperparathyroidism (most common)
Rare causes related to pregnancy
    Familial hypocalciuric hypercalcemia*
    Postpartum hypercalcemia in hypoparathyroidism
    Parathyroid hormone–related protein induced
      hypercalcemia
Other causes not related to pregnancy
  Malignancy
  Endocrine
    • Thyrotoxicosis
    • Adrenal insufficiency
  Vitamin overdose
    • Vitamin D
    • Vitamin A
  Drugs
    • Thiazide diuretics
    • Lithium
  Granulomatous disease
    • Sarcoidosis
    • Tuberculosis
    • Histoplasmosis
    • Coccidioidomycosis
Milk alkali syndrome
Acute and chronic renal failure
Total parenteral nutrition

From Mestman JH. Endocrine diseases in pregnancy. In Sciarra JJ, editor. *Gynecology and Obstetrics.* Philadelphia: Lippincott-Raven; 1997:11.
*Different expression with significant neonatal manifestations.

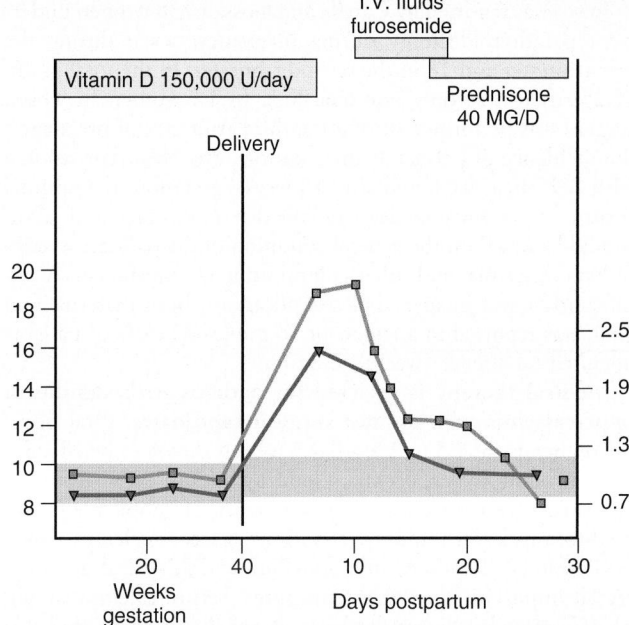

FIG 42-1 Serum calcium (triangles) and creatinine (squares) levels during pregnancy and 1 month after delivery in a woman with hypoparathyroidism who was treated with vitamin D and calcium. Normal range indicated by green shading.

endocrine disorders, vitamin D or A overdose, the use of thiazide diuretics, or granulomatous diseases (Box 42-1). A brief discussion of three uncommon syndromes associated with hypercalcemia during pregnancy follows.

FHH is an autosomal-dominant condition with a high penetrance for hypercalcemia. The disorder is associated with an inactivating mutation in the gene for the calcium-sensing receptor. Mild hypercalcemia, a slight elevation in serum PTH, mild hypermagnesemia, and low urinary calcium excretion are the typical findings. Infants born to mothers with FHH may present with different clinical manifestations: (1) asymptomatic hypercalcemia can develop in an affected offspring if the mother is a carrier for FHH, (2) severe neonatal hypocalcemia can return to normal a few weeks after delivery, or (3) severe neonatal hypercalcemia can occur in infants homozygous for the FHH gene defect.

Postpartum hypercalcemia can occur in women with treated hypoparathyroidism, and the mechanism for hypercalcemia is not well understood. Nausea and vomiting develop a few days after delivery; therefore patients with treated hypoparathyroidism should be followed postpartum with serum calcium determinations, and vitamin D should be discontinued if hypercalcemia occurs. In severe cases, intravenous fluids and glucocorticoid therapy are required (Fig. 42-1).

A few cases of hypercalcemia mediated by PTHrP during pregnancy and postpartum have been reported. In one case, hypercalcemia developed in two successive pregnancies. In the second pregnancy, serum PTHrP levels were elevated to three times normal, and the infant was born with mild hypercalcemia that returned to normal within 24 hours after delivery. In a second case, a 25-year-old woman had massive bilateral breast enlargement at 24 weeks' gestation. Her serum calcium level was 14.3 mg/dL, but her serum PTH level was undetectable. She underwent bilateral mastectomy during pregnancy. The immunohistochemical studies demonstrated PTHrP antigenic activity in breast tissue.

Therapy

Surgery is the only effective treatment for PHPT, and the procedure is safe when performed by a surgeon with extensive experience in neck surgery.[6] The cure rate is excellent, and complications due to surgery are low, particularly in the presence of a single lesion. Improvements in the outcome of surgery and avoidance of intraoperative and postoperative complications include (1) preoperative parathyroid adenoma localization by ultrasonography, (2) minimally invasive parathyroidectomy techniques, (3) intraoperative PHPT monitoring to confirm successful surgery, and (4) detection and management of postpartum hypocalcemia.

Although guidelines for the management of PHPT in nonpregnant individuals have been suggested, the proper medical management of PHPT in pregnancy has not been uniformly agreed on. For asymptomatic pregnant women in whom serum calcium is not greater than 1 mg above normal range, close follow-up with proper hydration and avoidance of medications that could elevate calcium, such as thiazide diuretics, is reasonable. Because most of the neonatal complications have been reported in patients with symptomatic disease, a surgical approach is indicated in such patients and in those with complications such as nephrolithiasis, bone disease, and persistent hypercalcemia (>1 mg above the normal range). **It is preferable to perform the surgery in the second trimester of pregnancy.**

In a series reported by Carella and Gossain, 38 women underwent parathyroidectomy during pregnancy, seven during the first trimester and 18 in the second trimester. In the total group of 25, there was only one fetal loss. In 12 women in whom surgery was performed during the third trimester of pregnancy, the incidence of perinatal complications was 58%. For women with PHP first diagnosed after 28 weeks' gestation, the optimal treatment strategy is unclear, and the decision in such a situation should be based on the general condition of the patient, severity of hypercalcemia, and other complicating circumstances. A significantly lower incidence of complications, both maternal and fetal, was reported in a review of 16 published cases of patients operated on after 27 weeks' gestation.

Medical therapy is reserved for patients with significant hypercalcemia who are not surgical candidates. Oral phosphate therapy of 1.5 to 2.5 g/day has been shown to be effective in controlling hypercalcemia. Good hydration, early treatment of urinary tract infections, and avoidance of supplements and medications known to cause elevations in serum calcium—such as vitamin D, vitamin A, aminophylline, and thiazide diuretics—are all important therapeutic measures. Serum calcium should be determined on a regular basis. A novel oral agent that acts directly on the calcium sensor, cinacalcet hydrochloride, has been used in isolated cases. It reduces serum calcium in combination with calcitonin.[7]

In patients undergoing surgical treatment, hypocalcemia—albeit transient—may occur after surgery in some cases. Therefore serum calcium should be checked every 6 hours, and if the patient develops hypocalcemic symptoms, intravenous (IV) calcium in the form of calcium gluconate (1 to 2 g of calcium-gluconate, equivalent to 90 to 180 mg elemental calcium, in 50 mL of 5% dextrose) can be infused over 10 to 20 minutes. Oral calcitriol 0.5 mg every 8 to 12 hours and oral calcium should be started when oral feeding is tolerated. In patients with bone disease, postsurgical hypocalcemia may be profound; therefore aggressive treatment is needed. These patients may benefit from vitamin D supplementation in the form of calcitriol, 0.25 to 0.5 μg/day, for a few days before operative intervention.

Hypoparathyroidism

The most common etiology of hypoparathyroidism is damage to or removal of the parathyroid glands in the course of surgery for thyroid gland pathology. The incidence of permanent hypoparathyroidism after thyroid surgery has been estimated to be between 0.2% and 3.5%. In many cases, hypocalcemia in the immediate postoperative period is only transitory. Idiopathic hypoparathyroidism is much less common and is frequently associated with other autoimmune endocrinopathies as part of the polyglandular autoimmune syndrome type 1.

The requirement for calcium supplementation and vitamin D may decrease in some women with hypoparathyroidism during the second half of pregnancy and lactation. In a few cases, hypocalcemic symptoms ameliorate with progression of pregnancy. The explanation for these findings is not clear but may be related to the increased intestinal absorption of calcium and/or the production of vitamin D by the placenta.

Clinical clues for the diagnosis of hypoparathyroidism include a previous history of thyroid surgery and clinical, radiologic, and laboratory information. **Typical symptoms of hypocalcemia are numbness and tingling of the fingers and toes and around the lips.** Patients may complain of carpopedal spasm, laryngeal stridor, and dyspnea. Convulsions may be a manifestation of severe hypocalcemia. On physical examination, patients with idiopathic hypoparathyroidism demonstrate changes in the teeth, skin, nails, and hair as well as papilledema and cataracts. Chvostek sign, a twitch of the facial muscles—notably those of the upper lip—when a sharp tap is given over the facial nerve, is seen in many patients with hypocalcemia. Chvostek sign has also been described in 10% of normal adults. Trousseau sign is another manifestation of hypocalcemia. It is the induction of spasm of the hand and forearm by reducing the circulation in the arm with a blood pressure cuff. The constriction should be maintained above the systolic blood pressure for 2 minutes before the test is considered negative.

The diagnosis of hypoparathyroidism is confirmed by the presence of persistent low serum calcium and high serum phosphate levels. Serum PTH is low in primary hypoparathyroidism. The differential diagnosis of hypocalcemia includes rickets and osteomalacia.

Radiologic bone changes characterized by generalized skeletal demineralization, subperiosteal bone resorption, bowing of the long bones, osteitis fibrosa cystica, and rib and limb deformities may be present in the newborn as a consequence of intrauterine hyperparathyroidism. Loughead and colleagues[8] described 16 infants of hypoparathyroid mothers, and secondary hyperparathyroidism in the infants resolved by 1 month of age.

Treatment of hypoparathyroidism in pregnancy does not differ from that in the nonpregnant state, including a normal high-calcium diet and vitamin D supplementation. Normal calcium supplementation during pregnancy is about 1.2 g/day. Calcitriol, 1 to 3 μg/day, is used almost routinely in most patients affected with hypoparathyroidism. Calcitriol must be given in divided doses because its half-life is much shorter than that of vitamin D. If vitamin D is used, the dose is in the range of 50,000 to 150,000 IU/wk. Vitamin D requirements may decrease in some patients by the second half of gestation. The importance of compliance with medications should be strongly emphasized, particularly when calcitriol is prescribed, in view of its short half-life. The major problem in the treatment of hypoparathyroidism is the recurrence of hypercalcemia and hypocalcemia; therefore serum calcium determinations should be performed at regular intervals.

Lactation in mothers taking vitamin D may be contraindicated because a metabolite of vitamin D, 25-hydroxyvitamin D, has been detected in breast milk in high concentration in a mother taking 50,000 IU of vitamin D daily. Regardless of the form of vitamin D prescribed, serum calcium determinations should be done in the postpartum period, particularly in breast-feeding mothers.

Pseudohypoparathyroidism

Pseudohypoparathyroidism encompasses several different disorders, having as a common feature varying degrees of target-organ resistance to PTH. In some forms of the syndrome, somatic changes are present that include short stature, obesity, a round face, brachydactyly, and mental retardation with brain calcifications. This variant is known as *Albright syndrome type 1a.* Most patients suffer from hypocalcemia due to a derangement of renal 1α-hydroxylase and production of calcitriol, and a few cases have been reported during pregnancy. Infants are at risk for intrauterine fetal hyperparathyroidism, perhaps because of the relative maternal hypocalcemia during pregnancy.

Vitamin D Deficiency

Classically, vitamin D deficiency was related to the development of rickets, with its subsequent impact on obstetric care. Deformities of weight-bearing bones, including the pelvis, prevented vaginal delivery in mothers affected by the disease.[9] In recent years, however, conflicting results have been published on the potential deleterious effect of vitamin D deficiency in a variety of medical problems from autoimmune disease to cancer. Several reviews on obstetric, fetal, and neonatal outcomes have been reported.[9] The normal reference range values for serum vitamin D (25[OH]D), the active metabolite of vitamin D, are controversial, with values varying between 20 and 40 ng/mL, equivalent to 50 to 100 nmol/L.

Many studies in the past few years had linked low maternal 25(OH)D levels with maternal, fetal, and neonatal complications. In a report from Amsterdam, mothers with singleton pregnancies and serum 25(OH)D levels below 29.9 nmol/L (12 ng/mL) had infants with a lower birthweight and a higher incidence of growth restriction than mothers with values of over 50 nmol/L (20 ng/mL). Hart and colleagues examined the relationship between maternal vitamin D deficiency at 18 weeks' gestation and long-term health outcomes in 901 mother-offspring pairs in Perth, Western Australia. The incidence of serum 25(OH)D deficiency (<50 nmol/L [<20 ng/mL]) was present in 36% of the pregnant women. After adjusting for relevant covariates, women with vitamin D deficiency had children with impaired lung development at age 6, neurocognitive deficiencies at age 10, increased risk of eating disorders in adolescence, and lower peak bone mass at age 20.

Recent systemic reviews and meta-analyses of observational studies and randomized controlled trials (RCTs) have failed to corroborate earlier observations. Theodoratou and colleagues[10] concluded that despite a few hundred systematic reviews and meta-analyses, highly convincing evidence for a clear role of vitamin D does not exist for any outcome, but associations with a selection of outcomes are probable. De-Regil and colleagues[11] reviewed six small trials with a total of 1023 women and compared five studies with vitamin D supplementation versus no treatment or placebo. The authors concluded that the use of vitamin D supplements during pregnancy improves vitamin concentrations as measured by 25-hydroxyvitamin D at term. However, the clinical significance of this finding has yet to be determined because quality evidence related to the clinical benefits of vitamin supplementation during pregnancy is insufficient. It is apparent that more studies are needed, preferably an RCT to understand the interrelationship with other factors such as age, ethnicity, seasonal variation, BMI, medical diseases, gestational age, and so on. Further studies on serum PTH and its relationship to serum vitamin D may be warranted. In the meantime, the practicing obstetrician will have to decide for each individual patient whether determination of 25(OH)D levels is indicated, what the normal values for pregnancy are, whether they are trimester specific, what the proper treatment should be, and how often the test needs to be repeated in pregnancy; this must be done also taking into consideration the cost of the tests and the possible implications for the fetus and newborn.

In 2010, the Institute of Medicine (IOM)[12] reviewed nearly 1000 published studies that included reports of protection from cancer, autoimmune disease, heart disease, and diabetes with vitamin D supplementation. In brief, they recommended that the lower normal limit for serum 25(OH)D should be "about" 20 ng/mL or 50 nmol/L. **For women who are not pregnant, the authors of the report recommend a daily vitamin D dietary allowance of 600 IU with an upper limit intake of 4000 IU; for calcium, they recommended a 1000-mg dietary allowance and an upper limit intake of 2500 mg a day. In the presence of vitamin D insufficiency/deficiency, it is reasonable to normalize serum levels as early as possible, preferably starting early in pregnancy. Detection of women at risk for vitamin D deficiency by proper history seems reasonable until the results of an RCT become available.** Recent evidence suggests that vitamin D deficiency is common during pregnancy, especially among high-risk groups that include vegetarians, women with limited sun exposure (e.g., those who live in cold climates, reside in northern latitudes, or wear sun and winter protective clothing), and ethnic minorities, especially those with darker skin. For pregnant women thought to be at increased risk of vitamin D deficiency, maternal serum 25(OH)D levels can be considered and should be interpreted in the context of the individual clinical circumstance.

The American College of Obstetricians and Gynecologists (ACOG) has stated, "At this time there is insufficient evidence to support a recommendation for screening all pregnant women for vitamin D deficiency. For pregnant women thought to be at increased risk of vitamin D deficiency, maternal serum 25(OH)D levels can be considered and should be interpreted in the context of the individual clinical circumstance. When vitamin D deficiency is identified during pregnancy, most experts agree that 1000 to 2000 IU/day of vitamin D is safe."

Osteoporosis

The condition of idiopathic osteoporosis related to pregnancy, *pregnancy and lactation–associated osteoporosis* (PLO), was recognized in the 1950s. In the past few years, interest has increased in several clinical aspects of osteoporosis in pregnancy and lactation.[13] Although the prevalence is unknown, approximately 120 cases have been reported. Another form of rare pregnancy-associated osteoporosis is called *transient osteoporosis of pregnancy*. It usually presents in the third trimester of pregnancy—sometimes with very severe pain while walking or standing, usually localized in the hip—and it sometimes leads to hip fracture, with complete recovery a few months postpartum. Preexisting secondary causes of osteoporosis such as vitamin D deficiency, celiac disease, anorexia nervosa, mastocytosis, and hyperparathyroidism or hyperthyroidism should always be considered. Severe PLO may prompt screening for an underlying monogenetic bone disorder when associated with one of the following three features: (1) severely reduced bone density; (2) family history of osteoporosis or multiple fractures, joint hypermobility, blue sclerae, congenital blindness, or severely reduced vision; or (3) a history of fractures before pregnancy.

Although osteoporosis has been diagnosed during pregnancy, pregnancy unmasks low bone mass, it does not cause it. Postural changes during pregnancy, including increased lordosis, when superimposed on a small and transient decrease in bone mass may lead to pain and even fractures. In a study of 24 women with symptoms of bone pain for many years, 18 complained of back pain, 5 complained of hip pain, and 1 complained of ankle pain in late pregnancy and up to 8 months after delivery; radiologic examination of the spine showed vertebral deformities in 17, bone mass was measured in 21, evidence of osteoporosis was found in 7, and 13 were osteopenic. The authors concluded that bone mass was probably low before pregnancy and that a transient and slight decrease in bone mass during pregnancy could have weakened the bone further.

A recent study identified 78 cases with exposure to bisphosphonates before conception or during pregnancy. Although it did not demonstrate serious adverse effects, cases of increased spontaneous abortions, shortened gestational age, low neonatal birthweight, and transient hypocalcemia of the newborn were reported. Etidronate appears to be the agent to use in women with severe disease who are planning pregnancy, although the drug should be stopped a few months before conception.

The impact of lactation on the progression of osteoporosis is controversial. It has been suggested that lactation by itself is not a determinant of bone mineral density. Although one investigation reported that lactation for more than 8 months was associated with greater bone mineral density at both the femoral neck and shaft, another study found that nursing for longer than 9 months produced a greater decrease in bone mass than observed during the first 6- to 9-month period of nursing. Given this controversy, the health care provider must decide whether cessation of lactation is advisable in the management of osteoporosis. Bolzetta and colleagues studied 752 women (mean age, 64.5 ± 9.3 years) of whom 23% reported vertebral osteoporotic fractures. The women with vertebral fractures had breastfed their infants for longer periods (11.8 ± 12.9 vs. 9.3 ± 11.2 months, $P = .03$) and had more pregnancies (2.6 ± 2.2 vs. 2.2 ± 1.3, $P = .002$). Breastfeeding for more than 18 months was associated with a twofold risk of developing vertebral fractures (OR, 2.12; 95% CI, 1.14 to 5.38; $P = .04$), particularly in those without current or past use of drugs that positively affect bone. The authors concluded that an association exists between long periods of breastfeeding and vertebral fractures, which supports a role for lengthy lactation as a risk factor for osteoporotic fractures after menopause.

Heparin-associated osteoporosis has been reported during pregnancy that may be related to the total dose of heparin.[14] **The authors concluded that heparin adversely affected bone density in about one third of exposed patients.**

THYROID DISEASES

Thyroid disorders in pregnancy present a unique opportunity for health care professionals to use a similar "team approach" that has successfully improved the care of women with diabetes mellitus. Because of changes in thyroid economy that occur early in pregnancy, it is imperative to advise women with chronic thyroid diseases to plan their pregnancies and contact their health care professionals before or as soon as the diagnosis of pregnancy is confirmed. Autoimmune thyroid disease occurs five to eight times more often in women than in men, and its course could be affected by the immunologic changes that occur in pregnancy and in the postpartum period.[15,16]

In early pregnancy, the maternal thyroid gland is challenged with an increased demand for thyroid hormone secretion, due mainly to (1) the increase in thyroxine-binding globulin (TBG) secondary to the effect of estrogens on the liver; (2) the stimulatory effect of human chorionic gonadotropin (hCG) on the thyroid-stimulating hormone (TSH) receptor; (3) high concentrations of type 3 iodothyronine deiodinase (D3), which degrades thyroxine and triiodothyronine to inactive compounds; and (4) the supply of iodine available to the thyroid gland. In the United States, the iodine content in the diet—although decreased in past decades—appears to be insufficient in only about 10% of pregnancies. **The suggested total daily iodine ingestion for pregnant women is 229 µg/day, and for lactating women, it is 289 µg/day; prenatal vitamins should contain 150 µg of iodine in the form of potassium iodine.[17]**

The normal thyroid gland is able to compensate for the increase in thyroid hormone demands by increasing its secretion of thyroid hormones and maintaining them within normal limits throughout gestation. However, in those situations in which there is a subtle pathologic abnormality of the thyroid gland, such as chronic autoimmune thyroiditis, or in women on thyroid hormone replacement therapy, the normal increase in the production of thyroid hormones is not met. As a consequence, the pregnant woman could develop biochemical markers of hypothyroidism (i.e., an elevation in serum TSH).

Active secretion of thyroid hormones by the fetal thyroid gland commences at about 18 weeks' gestation, although iodine uptake by the fetal gland occurs between 10 and 14 weeks.[18] Transfer of thyroxine (T_4) from mother to embryo occurs from early pregnancy. Maternal T_4 has been demonstrated in coelomic fluid at 6 weeks and in the fetal brain at 9 weeks. Maternal transfer continues until delivery but only in significant amounts in the presence of fetal hypothyroidism. Thyroid hormone receptor gene expression has been shown in human fetal brain by 8 weeks' gestation, which supports the important role of maternal thyroid hormone during the first trimester of human pregnancy in fetal brain development.

The levels of maternal thyroid hormone concentrations, both total thyroxine (TT_4) and total triiodothyronine (TT_3), increase from early pregnancy as the result of an elevation in TBG and a reduced peripheral TBG degradation rate. TBG reaches a plateau by 20 weeks' gestation and remains unchanged until delivery. Despite these acute changes in total hormone concentration, **the serum free fractions of both T_4 and T_3 remain within normal limits,** unless supply of iodine to the mother is decreased or abnormalities of the thyroid gland are present.

Human chorionic gonadotropin (hCG) is a weak thyroid stimulator that acts on the maternal thyroid gland TSH receptor; peak hCG values are reached by 9 to 12 weeks' gestation. In situations in which there is a high production of hCG—such as in cases of multiple pregnancies, hydatidiform mole, and HG—serum free T_4 (FT_4) concentrations rise to levels seen in thyrotoxicosis, with a transient suppression in serum TSH values.

Goiter is commonly seen in pregnancy in areas of iodine deficiency. However, in the United States and other areas of the world with sufficient iodine intake, the thyroid gland does not clinically increase in size during pregnancy. **Therefore the detection of a goiter in pregnancy is an abnormal finding that needs careful evaluation.** The most common cause of diffuse goiter is chronic autoimmune thyroiditis or Hashimoto thyroiditis. Most patients are euthyroid, and the diagnosis is made by the determination of thyroid antibodies, mainly thyroid peroxidase (TPO). Antibody concentration decreases during pregnancy and increases in the postpartum period. High values in the first trimester of pregnancy are predictors of the syndrome of postpartum thyroid dysfunction.

Thyroid Function Tests

Measurement of serum TSH is the most practical, simple, and economic screening test for thyroid dysfunction.[19] Normal TSH concentrations, as well as serum FT_4 and TT4 determinations,

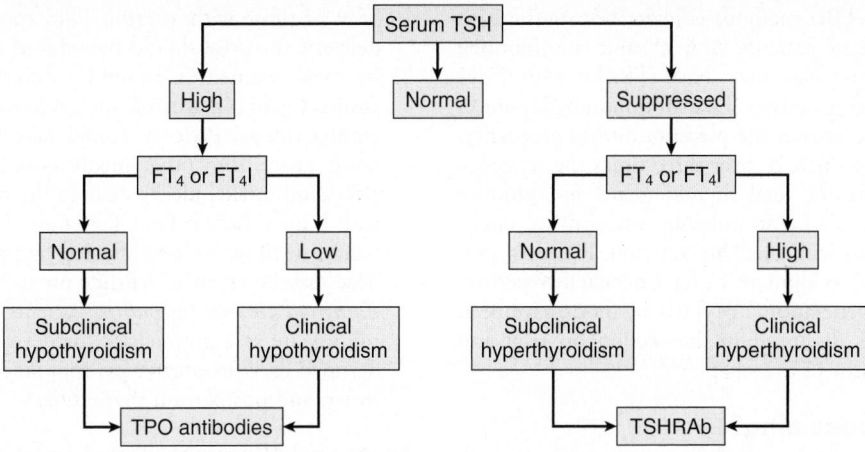

FIG 42-2 Algorithm for the interpretation of thyroid function tests in pregnancy. Serum thyroid-stimulating hormone (TSH) upper limit of normal in the first trimester of pregnancy is 2.5 mIU/L; in the second and third trimesters, it is 3 mIU/L. The serum TSH lower limit of normal in the first trimester of pregnancy may be as low as 0.1 mIU/L or may even be undetectable. Subclinical hyperthyroidism in the absence of TSH receptor antibodies (TSHRAbs) is a normal first-trimester physiologic finding. Presence of serum thyroid peroxidase (TPO) antibodies is consistent with a diagnosis of chronic thyroiditis. Presence of TSHRAb is consistent with the diagnosis of Graves disease. FT_4, free thyroxine; FT_4I, free thyroxine index.

are trimester specific and depend on iodine intake in a given population, ethnicity, and assay performance; serum TSH is lower in the first trimester compared with prepregnancy values and with the second and third trimester of pregnancy. An elevated serum TSH value is consistent with the diagnosis of primary hypothyroidism, whereas a low one, with few exceptions, is a normal finding in the first trimester (Fig. 42-2) secondary to the stimulatory effect of hCG on the thyroid gland TSH receptor. Significant clinical data[19] support a serum TSH below 2.5 mIU/L in the first trimester, and less than 3.0 mIU/L in the second and third trimesters, as the upper limit of normal.[20] However, studies from China, the United Kingdom, and India that have used a specific reference range for their populations reported TSH reference ranges in the first trimester up to 4.5 mIU/L.[21-23] Guidelines from the American Thyroid Association (ATA) and the Endocrine Society (ES) recommend the use of trimester-specific reference ranges for serum TSH and FT_4 in a given population, and when not available, they recommend a serum TSH upper limit of normal of 2.5 mIU/L in the first trimester and up to 3.0 mIU/L in the second and third trimesters, as noted above. **Because most pregnant women present for their first obstetric visit after 6 weeks gestation, the upper serum TSH limit of 2.5 mIU/L is reasonable for detection of hypothyroidism.**

A word of caution is required regarding the determination of FT_4 levels in the different trimesters of pregnancy. A significant inconsistency is found in FT_4 values in the second half of pregnancy among the different immunoassays, as reported by commercial laboratories, because of both the methodology used and the variation in dietary iodine intake among the different populations studied. FT_4 values in the lower limits of normal, and even in the hypothyroid range, are not uncommonly seen in daily clinical practice, particularly in the third trimester of pregnancy. Lee and colleagues[24] compared the diagnostic performances of two different immunoassays to traditional approaches for estimating FT_4 (total T_4 and FT_4 index [FT_4I]) relative to the physiologic TSH changes known to occur throughout pregnancy. They studied euthyroid women who were negative for TPO antibody in the first, second, and third trimesters of gestation. Control women were premenopausal nonpregnant women

matched for ethnicity. Serum TT_4, as expected, was elevated in all three trimesters, and serum FT_4I was elevated in the first trimester compared with controls ($P < .05$) and returned to the nonpregnant range in the second and third trimesters. In contrast, FT_4 values were either comparable or lower than controls as measured by two different immunoassays, and by the second and third trimesters, they were about 65% of controls. The authors concluded that TT_4 and FT_4I retained an appropriate inverse relationship with serum TSH throughout pregnancy and appeared to provide a more reliable FT_4 estimate than the FT_4 test. Because the determination of FT_4 by the dialysis method—the gold standard for FT_4 assessment—or the use of tandem mass spectrometry are not routinely available, the determination of TT_4 adjusted by a factor of 1.5 for pregnant patients has been suggested.[24] Therefore it is imperative for the practicing physician to be familiar with the interpretation and significance of the thyroid tests as reported by a given commercial laboratory.

A suppressed serum TSH value and high concentrations of FT_4 or FT_4I is diagnostic of hyperthyroidism. However, in rare situations, hyperthyroidism may be diagnosed in the presence of suppressed TSH and normal concentrations of FT_4, such as in the case of an autonomous thyroid nodule. In such cases, a serum TT_3 or free triiodothyronine index (FT_3I) determination should be obtained.

Thyroid-Stimulating Hormone Receptor Antibodies

Graves disease is caused by direct stimulation of the thyroid epithelial cells by TSH receptor-stimulating antibodies (TSHRAbs, or TRAbs). Highly sensitive and specific assays for detection of TRAbs are now commercially available that are very valuable in assessing fetal and neonatal risk in pregnancy, not only in women with active disease but also in those with a previous history of Graves hyperthyroidism, both in spontaneous remission and after ablation therapy. TRAbs are also used in the differential diagnosis of hyperthyroidism, when the etiology is not clinically evident. Two methods are used for measuring TRAbs, *competition-based assays* (thyroid-binding inhibitor [TBI]–thyroid-binding inhibitor immunoglobulin [TBII] assays) or *bioassays* that detect cyclic adenosine monophosphate (cAMP) production (thyroid-stimulating immunoglobulin [TSI] assays).

The specificity of TBI-TBII methods is lower because positive tests may be obtained in patients with chronic autoimmune (Hashimoto) thyroiditis who may have TRAbs with TSH receptor (TSHR)-blocking activity. Like all immunoglobulin G (IgG) molecules, TRAb crosses the placenta during pregnancy, and in significant titers—that is, over three times the reference range—it can stimulate the fetal thyroid gland and produce hyperthyroidism (TRAbs with stimulating function) or, rarely, hypothyroidism (TRAbs with blocking activity). Recently, predictable levels for the development of fetal/neonatal hyperthyroidism using second-generation TBI-TBII methods have been reported. This topic is discussed in the section on fetal and neonatal hyperthyroidism in this chapter.

Prepregnancy Counseling

The physician may be faced with different clinical situations when counseling a woman suffering from thyroid disease who is contemplating pregnancy:

1. *Hyperthyroidism diagnosed "de novo" or under antithyroid drug (ATD) treatment.* A choice of the three classic therapeutic options for hyperthyroidism treatment should be given: (1) long-term ATD therapy, (2) radioactive iodine-131 (^{131}I) ablation, or (3) near-total thyroidectomy. Potential side effects of ATDs on the fetus should be discussed with the future parents. ^{131}I ablation therapy should be avoided in patients with positive TRAb titers because serum levels increase following ^{131}I therapy, and the effect persists for several years; fetuses whose mothers have titers above three times the normal level in the second half of pregnancy are at risk of fetal and neonatal hyperthyroidism. Surgery is another option selected by some physicians and patients concerned about the potential side effects of ATDs or radioactive treatment. **Regardless of the form of therapy chosen, it is important for the patient to be euthyroid at the time of conception.** In a large series of untreated hyperthyroid pregnant women, a doubling in the incidence of congenital malformations was reported in the first trimester compared with euthyroid women.

2. *Previous treatment with ^{131}I for thyroid carcinoma.* It is reasonable for patients treated with ablative doses of ^{131}I to wait 6 months to 1 year after completion of treatment before conception. Data obtained from 2673 pregnancies in patients treated for thyroid carcinoma but without significant external radiation to the ovaries were analyzed by Garsi and colleagues, who found no evidence that exposure to radioiodine affects the outcome of subsequent pregnancies and offspring.

3. *Treated hypothyroidism.* **Women under treatment with thyroid hormone usually require an increase in L-thyroxine dose soon after conception.**[25,26] The increase in requirements is observed as early as the first 6 to 8 weeks after the last menstrual period. As soon as the diagnosis of pregnancy is made, thyroid function tests should be performed, and thyroid doses should be adjusted accordingly. It has been recommended to add two extra doses of L-thyroxine per week to the customary doses as soon as the diagnosis of pregnancy is confirmed until the results of thyroid function tests become available.[26] Recently it was reported that in hypothyroid women (excluding those who underwent thyroidectomy because of thyroid cancer) on L-thyroixine replacement therapy, if the serum TSH was below 1.3 mIU/L before conception, only 17% of women needed an increase in L-thyroxine in the first trimester of pregnancy compared with 58% of those with a serum TSH above 1.3 mIU/L.[81] After delivery, the dose should be reduced to prepregnancy levels in most women. Common medications may affect the absorption of L-thyroxine, such as ferrous sulfate and calcium, among others. Patients should take L-thyroxine at least 2 hours apart from other medications and 1 hour before or after food intake, ideally early in the morning on awakening and 1 hour before food ingestion. However, during pregnancy, in those women affected by nausea or vomiting, the dose may be taken at bedtime on an empty stomach.

4. *Euthyroid chronic thyroiditis.* Patients with Hashimoto thyroiditis are at a greater risk for developing hypothyroidism de novo early in pregnancy, spontaneous abortions, prematurity, and postpartum thyroiditis.[27]

Maternal-Placental-Fetal Interactions

Studies over the past few decades have shown an important role of maternal thyroid hormones in embryogenesis.[18,28] Maternal T_4 crosses the placenta in the first half of pregnancy at a time when the fetal thyroid gland is not functional, and maternal TSH does not cross the placenta. Thyrotropin-releasing hormone (TRH) does cross the placental barrier, but its physiologic significance is unknown.

Methimazole (MMI), propylthiouracil (PTU), and carbimazole (CMZ)—a drug that is metabolized to methimazole—do cross the placenta, may induce congenital malformations if given early in pregnancy, and if given in inappropriately high doses may produce fetal goiter and hypothyroidism. Preparations that contain iodine given in large doses or for prolonged periods are contraindicated in pregnancy because accumulation by the fetal thyroid may induce goiter and hypothyroidism.

As mentioned above, TRAb crosses the placenta, and serum concentrations decrease with progression of pregnancy. However, its titers increase significantly in Graves hyperthyroidism after therapy with ^{131}I.

Hyperthyroidism

Autoimmune hyperthyroidism affects pregnancy in about 0.1% to 0.4% of patients.[29] Classically, it has been stated that Graves disease is the most common cause of hyperthyroxinemia in pregnancy; other etiologies are uncommon (Box 42-2). As will be discussed subsequently, hyperthyroidism due to inappropriate secretion or action of hCG is recognized as the most common cause of transient hyperthyroidism in pregnancy.[30] In our experience, single toxic adenoma and multinodular toxic goiter are found in less than 10% of cases. Subacute thyroiditis is rarely seen during gestation.

Gestational Hyperthyroidism

Also known as *gestational thyrotoxicosis, transient hyperthyroidism of hyperemesis gravidarum,* and *transient nonautoimmune hyperthyroidism of early pregnancy,* this condition is defined as transient hyperthyroidism in the first trimester of pregnancy due, with few exceptions, to high titers of hCG secretion that stimulate the TSH receptor. The most common causes of gestational hyperthyroidism are HG, multiple gestation, and hydatidiform mole. Other isolated reports included hyperplacentosis.

Transient Hyperthyroidism of Hyperemesis Gravidarum

Hyperemesis gravidarum (HG) is characterized by severe nausea and vomiting with onset between 4 and 8 weeks' gestation that requires frequent visits to the emergency department and sometimes repeated hospitalizations for IV hydration.[31] Weight loss of at least 5 kg, ketonuria, abnormal liver function tests, and hypokalemia are common findings, depending on the severity of vomiting and dehydration. FT_4 and TT_4 levels are elevated, sometimes up to four to six times the normal values, whereas TT_3 and FT_3 values are elevated in up to 40% of affected women, although FT_3 values are not as high as those of serum FT_4.[30] The TT_3/TT_4 ratio is less than 20, compared with Graves hyperthyroidism, in which the ratio is more than 20. Serum TSH measured by a sensitive assay is consistently undetected or suppressed. **Despite the significant biochemical hyperthyroidism, signs and symptoms of hypermetabolism are mild or absent.** Patients may complain of mild palpitations and heat intolerance, but perspiration, proximal muscle weakness, and frequent bowel movements are rare. On physical examination, ophthalmopathy and goiter are absent, a mild tremor of the outstretched fingers is occasionally seen, and tachycardia may be present due in part to dehydration. Significant in the medical history is the lack of hyperthyroid symptoms before conception because most patients with Graves disease diagnosed for the first time during gestation give a history of hypermetabolic symptoms that antedate conception. Spontaneous normalization of hyperthyroxinemia parallels the improvement in vomiting and weight gain, and most cases resolve spontaneously between 14 and 20 weeks' gestation, although persistence of hyperthyroidism beyond 20 weeks' gestation has been reported in 15% to 25% of cases. Suppressed serum TSH may lag for a few more weeks after normalization of free thyroid hormone levels (Fig. 42-3). **Antithyroid medications are not needed.** In one series in which antithyroid medication was used, pregnancy outcome was not significantly different from that of a similar group of patients who received no therapy. Occasionally, severe vomiting and hyperthyroidism may require parenteral nutrition.

The degree of thyroid abnormalities is directly related to the severity of vomiting and weight loss. In 67 patients studied by Goodwin and colleagues,[30] liver and electrolyte abnormalities were routinely found in women with worse symptoms, including severe vomiting, weight loss of at least 5 kg, and significant dehydration. They also presented with more significant elevations in FT_4 levels and suppression of serum TSH values; indeed, in 30% of their patients, serum TSH was undetectable (<0.04 mIU/L). Those with a lesser degree of hyperemesis had a less severe disorder of thyroid function.

BOX 42-2   CAUSES OF HYPERTHYROIDISM IN PREGNANCY

Immune Thyroid Disease

Graves disease
Chronic thyroiditis
Sporadic silent thyroiditis

Nonautoimmune Thyroid Disease

Multinodular goiter
Toxic adenoma
Subacute thyroiditis

Gestational Thyrotoxicosis

Multiple gestations
Nausea and vomiting
Hyperemesis gravidarum
• Trophoblastic tumor
• Hydatidiform mole
• Choriocarcinoma

Iatrogenic

Excessive levothyroxine intake
• Overtreatment
• Factitious
Iodine induced

From Patil-Sisodia K, Mestman JH. Graves hyperthyroidism and pregnancy: a clinical update. *Endocr Pract.* 2010;16:118-129.

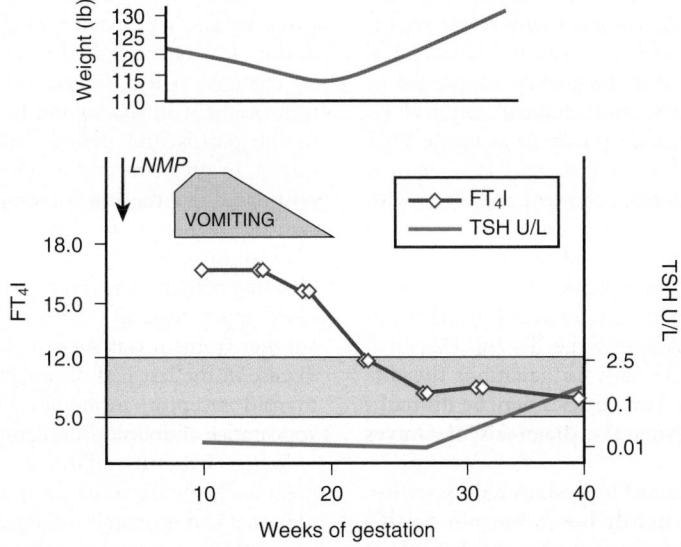

FIG 42-3 A representative example of transient hyperthyroidism of hyperemesis gravidarum. By week 6, vomiting begins; it becomes severe by week 10. Serum free thyroxine index (FT_4I) is elevated, and thyrotropin is suppressed. By weeks 16 to 18, vomiting subsides with marked improvement of the FT_4I value. During this period, the patient loses 3.6 kg. By week 18, the serum FT_4I returns to normal, but the serum thyrotropin remains suppressed until week 26. The patient improves and gains weight and delivers a healthy infant at term. The orange band indicates the reference range. LNMP, last normal menstrual period; TSH, thyroid-stimulating hormone.

TABLE 42-1   DIAGNOSIS OF GRAVES HYPERTHYROIDISM VERSUS GESTATIONAL THYROTOXICOSIS

	GRAVES HYPERTHYROIDISM	GESTATIONAL THYROTOXICOSIS
Symptoms before pregnancy	++	–
Symptoms during pregnancy	+/++	–/+
Nausea, vomiting	–/+	+++
Goiter, ophthalmopathy	+	–
Thyroid receptor antibodies	+	–
Thyroid ultrasound	Vascularity	Normal

From Patil-Sisodia K, Mestman JH. Graves hyperthyroidism and pregnancy: a clinical update. *Endocr Pract.* 2010;16:118-129.
–, None; +, mild; ++, severe.

Transient hyperthyroidism due to HG should be suspected in women who present in the first few weeks after conception with sudden onset of severe nausea and vomiting and thyroid tests in the hyperthyroid range. These patients do not complain of hypermetabolic symptoms that antedate pregnancy, goiter is not detected by palpation, and symptoms or signs of tissue thyrotoxicosis are mild or absent. In addition, screens for thyroid anti-TPO antibodies and TRAbs, markers of autoimmune thyroid disease, are negative. The differential diagnosis may also be difficult because vomiting can also be a presenting symptom of the hyperthyroidism of Graves disease (Table 42-1).

The cause of the elevations of thyroid hormones in patients with HG is the endocrine effect of hCG.[32] Most likely, high levels of hCG—a known stimulator of the TSH receptor—play an important role, as does the prolongation in its biologic activity seen in twin pregnancies. A significant, albeit weak, correlation has been found between the degree of thyroid stimulation and total hCG levels in normal women and in those with hyperemesis.[32] Titers of more than 200,000 mIU/mL of hCG consistently bring serum TSH to undetectable values. A case has been reported in a mother and daughter with recurrent hyperemesis, in whom hCG levels were not elevated. Both were heterozygous for a missense mutation in the extracellular domain of the thyrotropin receptor. The mutant receptor was more sensitive than the wild-type receptor to hCG, which accounted for the occurrence of hyperthyroidism despite the presence of normal hCG levels.

As noted previously, the diagnosis of transient hyperthyroidism of HG should be considered in women with severe vomiting, no clinical manifestations of Graves disease, biochemical evidence of hyperthyroidism in early pregnancy, suppressed or undetectable serum TSH values, and elevated serum FT_4. Normal serum TSH in early pregnancy may be as low as 0.01 mIU/L; therefore the presence of elevated serum FT_4 is required for the diagnosis. Vomiting should be persistent and severe with a significant weight loss because most women with morning sickness of pregnancy have normal thyroid function tests. The syndrome may repeat in future pregnancies.

HG may also occur in women with Graves hyperthyroidism. It may occur during remission of the disease, explained by the additional action of hCG early in gestation; **the differential diagnosis between the two entities may be difficult, but the presence of TRAb favors the diagnosis of Graves hyperthyroidism.**[33]

Obstetric outcome is not affected by gestational hyperthyroidism. Birthweight may be slightly lower, but not significantly different, compared with fetuses of control mothers and is related to maternal weight loss.

Gestational trophoblastic diseases, partial and complete hydatidiform moles, and choriocarcinoma are other causes of hyperthyroidism early in pregnancy.

BOX 42-3   POTENTIAL MATERNAL AND FETAL COMPLICATIONS OF GRAVES HYPERTHYROIDISM

MATERNAL	FETAL
Miscarriage	Low birthweight
Pregnancy-induced hypertension	• Prematurity
Preterm delivery	• Small for gestational age
Congestive heart failure	• Intrauterine growth
Thyroid storm	restriction
Placental abruption	Stillbirth
Infection	Thyroid dysfunction
	• Fetal hyperthyroidism
	• Fetal hypothyroidism
	• Neonatal hyperthyroidism
	• Neonatal goiter
	• Neonatal central hypothyroidism

From Patil-Sisodia K, Mestman JH. Graves hyperthyroidism and pregnancy: a clinical update. *Endocr Pract.* 2010;16:118-129.

Graves Disease

The natural course of hyperthyroidism due to Graves disease in pregnancy is characterized by an exacerbation of symptoms in the first trimester and during the postpartum period and an amelioration of symptoms in the second half of pregnancy. Stimulation of the thyroid gland by hCG in the first trimester and an elevation in TRAb values have been suggested as the cause of the exacerbation. Immunologic responses caused by changes in lymphocyte subsets could explain spontaneous improvement in the second half of pregnancy and recurrences in the postpartum period. In a study that compared Graves disease in pregnant and nonpregnant women, Kung and Jones postulated that the amelioration of symptoms seen with progression of pregnancy was due to a decrease in the titers of TRAbs with stimulating activity and an increase in TRAbs with thyroid-blocking activity. The reverse was true in the postpartum period, when aggravation of Graves hyperthyroidism usually occurs. In another study, it was suggested that the amelioration of Graves disease in the last half of pregnancy is induced by a decrease of thyroid receptor antibodies (TRAbs, TSIs) but not by the appearance of thyroid stimulation–blocking antibodies (TSBAs).

When hyperthyroidism is properly managed throughout pregnancy, the outcome for mother and fetus is good; however, maternal and neonatal complications for mothers with untreated or poorly controlled hyperthyroidism are significantly increased (Box 42-3).[34]

In most patients in whom the diagnosis is made for the first time during pregnancy, hyperthyroid symptoms antedate conception. The clinical diagnosis of thyrotoxicosis may present difficulties during gestation because many symptoms and signs are commonly seen in normal pregnancy, such as mild palpitations, heart rate between 90 and 100 beats/min, mild heat intolerance, shortness of breath on exercise, and warm skin. However, some clinical clues increase the likelihood of the diagnosis of hyperthyroidism: presence of goiter, ophthalmopathy, proximal muscle weakness, tachycardia with a pulse rate of more than 100 beats/min, and weight loss or inability to gain weight despite a good appetite. Occasionally, the patient may be seen for the first time in congestive heart failure, and the etiologic diagnosis is difficult because many of the physical findings are suggestive of cardiac valvular disease, particularly mitral insufficiency or stenosis. Hyperthyroidism under poor control is frequently complicated by preeclampsia, small-for-gestational-age (SGA) infants, and preterm delivery. The physician should suspect hyperthyroidism in the presence of systolic hypertension with an inappropriately low diastolic blood pressure and a wide pulse pressure, which is also seen in other conditions such as aortic insufficiency.

Classic symptoms of hyperthyroidism include nervousness, increased sweating, increased appetite, heat intolerance, insomnia, proximal muscle weakness, irritability, changes in personality, frequent bowel movements, decreased tolerance to exercise (sometimes manifested as shortness of breath), eye irritation, frequent lacrimation, pruritus, and weight loss. Not all symptoms are present in a given patient; therefore the physician should be aware of subtle complaints, particularly in the presence of weight loss or inability to gain weight. As mentioned previously, in the first trimester of pregnancy, differentiating the diagnosis from transient hyperthyroidism of HG presents a real challenge for the health care professional.

On physical examination, the thyroid gland is enlarged in almost every pregnant woman with Graves disease. Indeed, the absence of a goiter makes the diagnosis unlikely in young people. The gland is diffusely enlarged, between two and six times the normal size, and varies from soft to firm; sometimes it is irregular to palpation, with one lobe being more prominent than the other. A thrill may be felt or a bruit may be heard, indications of a hyperdynamic circulation. Examination of the eyes may reveal obvious ophthalmopathy, but in most cases, exophthalmos is absent or mild, with one eye slightly more prominent than the other with retraction of the upper lid. Extraocular movements may be impaired on careful eye examination. Stare is common, as is injection or edema of the conjunctiva. Severe ophthalmopathy is rare in pregnancy; glucocorticoid therapy and surgical orbital wall decompression may be required to restore visual acuity. Pretibial myxedema is rare, seen in less than 10% of women. A hyperdynamic heart with a loud systolic murmur is a common finding. Proximal muscle weakness, fine tremor of the outstretched fingers, and hyperkinetic symptoms are seen frequently. The skin is warm and moist, and palmar erythema is accentuated.

As discussed previously (see Thyroid Function Tests), almost every patient with Graves disease will have an elevated FT_4 concentration. **An undetected TSH value in the presence of a high FT_4, or FT4I or TT_4 adjusted for pregnancy confirms the diagnosis of hyperthyroidism.**[29] In some unusual situations, the serum FT_4 may be at the upper limit of normal or slightly elevated, in which case the determination of TT_3 or adjusted TT_3 will confirm the diagnosis of hyperthyroidism. Thyroid peroxidase antibodies (TPOAbs) or thyroid antimicrosomal antibodies, markers of thyroid autoimmune disease, are elevated in most patients with Graves disease, although it is of no clinical relevance for the diagnosis; the titers of TRAb, both TBII and TSI, are elevated, which confirms the clinical diagnosis of Graves hyperthyroidism, and their actual titers have a prognostic importance for fetal and neonatal hyperthyroidism (see later discussion).

Significant maternal and perinatal morbidity and mortality were reported in early studies of pregnancies complicated by hyperthyroidism. In the past 25 years, however, there has been a significant decrease in the incidence of maternal and fetal complications directly related to improved control of maternal hyperthyroidism (see Box 42-3).[34-36] In patients whose hyperthyroidism is poorly controlled, one of the most common maternal complications is pregnancy-induced hypertension (PIH). In women with uncontrolled hyperthyroidism, the risk for severe preeclampsia was five times greater than that in patients with controlled disease.[34] Other complications include preterm delivery, placental abruption, birthweight less than 2500 g, stillbirth, and miscarriage. Congestive heart failure may occur in women untreated or treated for a short period in the presence of PIH or operative delivery. Left ventricular dysfunction is usually detected by echocardiography in women with cardiovascular manifestations. Although these changes are reversible, they may persist for several weeks or months after achieving a euthyroid state. In one study, reduction in peripheral vascular resistance and higher cardiac output were still present despite normalization of T_4 levels. This is an important finding with significant clinical implications. **Left ventricular decompensation in hyperthyroid pregnant women may develop in the presence of superimposed preeclampsia, at the time of delivery, or with undercurrent complications such as anemia or infection.** We have seen congestive heart failure in the first half of pregnancy in women with long-standing hyperthyroidism. It is likely that the aggravation of hyperthyroidism seen in the first part of pregnancy played an important role in the development of this complication. Careful monitoring of fluid administration is imperative in these situations. Thyroid storm has been observed in pregnancy and was reported 2 weeks postpartum in a woman whose hyperthyroidism was uncontrolled during pregnancy in association with multiorgan failure.

Fetal and neonatal complications are also related to maternal control of hyperthyroidism. Intrauterine growth restriction (IUGR), prematurity, stillbirth, and neonatal morbidity are the most common complications. Millar and coworkers[34] demonstrated that uncontrolled hyperthyroidism during the entire gestation was associated with a ninefold greater incidence of low-birthweight (LBW) infants compared with the control population. The incidence of LBW infants was almost 2.5 times greater in those whose hyperthyroidism was treated during pregnancy but who became euthyroid at some time during gestation. In mothers who achieved a euthyroid state before or early in pregnancy, the incidence of LBW infants was no different from that in the control population. Delivery of an SGA infant is correlated with the presence of maternal thyrotoxicosis lasting more than 30 weeks of pregnancy, a duration of Graves disease of approximately 10 years, and the onset of Graves disease before age 20 years. The reported incidences of spontaneous abortions (25.7%) and premature delivery (14.9%) in mothers who were hyperthyroid at the time of conception are higher than those in euthyroid mothers, 12.8% and 9.5%, respectively. Neonatal central hypothyroidism has been reported in infants whose mothers remained hyperthyroid throughout their pregnancies.

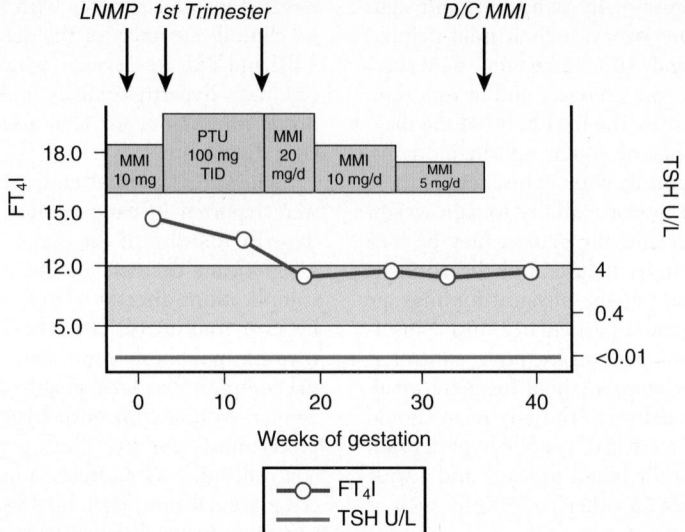

FIG 42-4 A representative example of management of hyperthyroidism in pregnancy. The patient is hyperthyroid at time of conception on methimazole (MMI) 10 mg daily. When pregnancy is diagnosed, MMI is discontinued, and propylthiouracil (PTU) is added at a dosage of 150 mg three times daily. By the end of the first trimester, PTU is discontinued and MMI is given at a dosage of 20 mg daily. By week 20, the free thyroxine index (FT_4I) is almost normal, and the MMI dosage is reduced to 10 mg. By week 26, the FT_4I is in the upper reference range and thyrotropin remains suppressed; the MMI dosage is reduced to 5 mg daily. The FT_4I remains in the upper reference range, and by week 34 MMI is discontinued (D/C), and the patient remains euthyroid until delivery. The orange band indicates the reference range. LNMP, last normal menstrual period; TSH, thyroid-stimulating hormone.

Many of these infants recovered normal thyroid function in a few weeks, whereas another group had long-standing hypopituitary dysfunction.[37]

The use of ultrasonography for monitoring the size of the fetal thyroid gland as an indicator of thyroid dysfunction and possible need for therapeutic intervention was evaluated by Luton and associates in France.[38] In a group of hyperthyroid women considered to be at high risk (presence of TRAbs) and on antithyroid therapy, fetal goiter was detected in 11 of 41 patients. Four fetuses were hyperthyroid, and seven were hypothyroid secondary to high doses of maternal antithyroid drug treatment; all of them benefited from adjusting drug therapy. The authors concluded that ultrasonography of the fetal thyroid gland by an experienced ultrasonographer is an excellent diagnostic tool, in conjunction with close teamwork, to ensure normal fetal thyroid function.

Treatment of hyperthyroidism is essential to prevent maternal, fetal, and neonatal complications (Fig. 42-4). **The goal of treatment is normalization of thyroid tests as soon as possible and maintenance of euthyroidism with the minimal amount of antithyroid medication.** Excessive amounts of ATDs crossing the placenta may affect the fetal thyroid, with the development of fetal hypothyroidism with or without goiter. Patients should be monitored at regular intervals, and the dose of their medications should be adjusted to keep the FT_4 or FT_4I or TT_4 very close to the upper limit of the reference range for pregnancy, or just above it. Momotani and associates[35] showed that fetal serum TSH was elevated even in mothers with FT_4 within the normal range; furthermore, they demonstrated that normalization of *maternal* serum TT_3 is a risk factor for the development of fetal hypothyroidism, which supports the recommendations that serum TT_3 determination should rarely be used to assess maternal thyroid function during gestation.

To achieve a euthyroid state, and with the aim to keep the FT_4 in the upper limit of the nonpregnant reference range and even slightly above normal, thyroid tests should be performed every 2 weeks at the beginning of treatment and every 2 to 4 weeks when euthyroidism is achieved. Because of the immunologic changes that occur with the progression of pregnancy, the requirement for antithyroid medications decreases after the second half of gestation. Some women with small goiters, a short duration of symptoms, low serum TRAb titers, and taking minimal amounts of antithyroid medication are able to discontinue ATDs by 34 weeks' gestation or beyond. It is estimated that 30% to 40% are able to remain euthyroid without antithyroid therapy in the last few weeks of pregnancy.[34,36]

In a study of 44 women in 46 pregnancies, the correlation among TRAb activity, the dose of antithyroid therapy, and neonatal outcome was studied.[36] Medication was discontinued in 30 pregnancies 3 to 18 weeks before delivery. Neonatal thyrotoxicosis was seen in four infants whose mothers' TBII levels exceeded 70% (normal, <15%). Interestingly, of the infants born with elevated serum TSH, maternal TBII was less than 30% in most, suggesting that in Graves disease–associated hyperthyroid pregnancies, a low TBII titer is an indication to use the minimal amount of antithyroid therapy to avoid the development of fetal hypothyroidism with or without goiter.

In the United States, the two available ATDs are PTU and MMI. Both drugs are effective in controlling symptoms. Recently, the risk for hepatic toxicity with PTU was revisited. An alarming number of deaths and cases requiring liver transplantation were noted (Box 42-4). MMI can also induce liver toxicity, but these effects are milder, confined to cholestasis, not associated with liver failure, and seen more frequently in patients older than 61 years. It is estimated that about 4000 pregnant women per year in the United States would be expected to be treated with ATDs, most of them with PTU, as recommended per previous practice guidelines. Taylor and Vaidya[40] found six reported cases of PTU-induced liver failure; it has been estimated that four women per year will have severe PTU-related hepatic complications.[39] **Although the incidence of both liver toxicity with PTU and embryopathy from MMI are very low,**

BOX 42-4 SIDE-EFFECT PROFILES OF METHIMAZOLE VERSUS PROPYLTHIOURACIL

METHIMAZOLE	PROPYLTHIOURACIL
Skin rash	Skin rash
Pruritus	Pruritus
Migratory polyarthritis	Migratory polyarthritis
Lupus-like syndrome	Lupus-like syndrome
Cholestatic jaundice	Propylthiouracil hepatotoxicity
Agranulocytosis	• Hepatitis
Methimazole embryopathy	• Fulminant liver failure
• Choanal atresia ± esophageal atresia	Propylthiouracil embryopathy
• Aplasia cutis	• Neck
• Hearing loss	• Urinary tract
• Dysmorphic facial features	
• Developmental delay	
• Congenital cardiac malformations	

From Patil-Sisodia K, Mestman JH. Graves hyperthyroidism and pregnancy: a clinical update. *Endocr Pract.* 2010;16:118-129.

a panel convened by the U.S. Food and Drug Administration (FDA) and the ATA recommended the use of PTU only in the first trimester of pregnancy with a change to MMI in the second trimester (see Fig. 42-4).[41] Other indications for the preferential use of PTU over MMI are drug allergy to MMI and in thyroid storm, because of the ability of PTU to inhibit peripheral conversion of T_4 to T_3.

To our knowledge, no studies have shown PTU to be superior to MMI in the management of hyperthyroidism in pregnancy; both drugs have similar placental transfer kinetics. Furthermore, when the efficacies of both drugs were compared, euthyroidism was achieved equally with equivalent amounts of drugs and at the same weeks of treatment. Neonatal outcomes were no different in both groups.

Aplasia cutis congenita, a localized lesion in the parietal area of the scalp characterized by congenital absence of the skin and a punched-out ulcer-like lesion, has occurred in a small group of infants born to mothers on MMI therapy. Only one case has been reported with the use of PTU. However, the incidence in the general population is 0.03% of newborns.

Several studies have described a specific embryopathy in infants born to mothers treated with MMI in the first trimester of pregnancy.[42] This has been named *methimazole embryopathy*, and it includes choanal atresia (failure of the nasal passages to develop), tracheoesophageal fistula, esophageal atresia, omphalocele, hypothelia and athelia (failure of the nipples to develop), minor dysmorphic features, and developmental delay. Very few cases have been described, and none with the use of PTU. The prevalence of these malformations in the general population is 1 in 2500 for esophageal atresia and 1 in 1000 for choanal atresia. The doses of MMI were 5 to 50 mg/day in one study; in the second study, both affected mothers took more than 20 mg/day. In an epidemiologic report, Barbero and associates[42] described an OR of 18 (95% CI, 3 to 121) for choanal atresia among infants whose mothers received MMI in the first trimester compared with the general population; however, the authors could not exclude the possibility that hyperthyroidism itself may be associated with this and other abnormalities. Recently, congenital heart defects were reported in children whose mothers

were exposed to MMI with carbimazole (MMI-CMZ) early in pregnancy. In one study, echocardiography was performed in 60 of the 68 neonates born of mothers with Graves disease, and four cases of congenital heart defects were diagnosed (two atrial septal defects, one ventricular septal defect, and one tetralogy of Fallot).[43] In the Danish Civil Registration System study,[44-46] 1097 children exposed to MMI-CMZ and 564 children exposed to PTU in early pregnancy were followed after birth for a median of 8.3 years and were compared with 881,730 unexposed children. They reported a series of congenital malformations in neonates exposed to PTU in early pregnancy; they tended to be less severe than the ones observed with MMI and affected mainly the face and neck area and the urinary system. Some of these malformations were detected within 2 years after birth and needed surgery. The adjusted risk for face and neck region defects (preauricular and branchial sinus fistula/cyst) was 4.92, and for the urinary system (single cyst of the kidney and hydronephrosis) it was 2.73. Previous studies did not show PTU-associated congenital malformations of any statistical significance. Yoshihara and colleagues in Japan studied the pregnancy outcomes of 6744 women with 5967 live births that included 1426 women treated with MMI and 1578 with PTU. The overall rate of major anomalies in the MMI group was 4.1% (most of them part of the MMI embryopathy syndrome), a rate significantly higher than the 2.1% in the control group. The incidence of congenital malformations in the PTU group was not different from that of the control group. The contrast between the PTU anomalies in the Danish and Japanese studies could be due to the follow-up of the newborns in the Danish study 2 years after birth.

The reports of congenital malformations in children exposed to PTU opens a new dilemma in the management of hyperthyroidism in women planning pregnancy, and in all women of reproductive age, because unplanned pregnancy is reported to be over 50% in our population. The ATA and ES both recommend either prescribing PTU in women with active hyperthyroidism who are planning a pregnancy or switching from MMI to PTU as soon as the diagnosis of pregnancy is confirmed. Laurberg and Andersen reviewed the literature on the association between the periods of exposure in early pregnancy and the development of birth defects. They concluded that high risk was confined to gestational weeks 6 through 10, the major period of organogenesis. PTU-associated defects might occur if PTU is given later than gestational week 5, which suggests that the risk of birth defects could be minimized if pregnant women stop ATD intake before gestational week 6. Their recommendation for fertile women on drug therapy is to receive written instructions (1) to perform a pregnancy test within a few days after a missed menstrual period; (2) if the test is positive, to contact their physician; (3) if feasible, to discontinue ATD therapy and follow thyroid tests weekly for the remaining of the first trimester; and (4) if drug therapy is needed, PTU should be used because birth defects seem to be less severe with PTU.

The initial recommended dose of PTU is 100 to 450 mg/day, given every 8 hours, and for MMI, 10 to 20 mg/day given in a single daily dose; very seldom is a larger initial dose required. MMI is given once or twice daily, which allows for improvement in patient compliance. Because of its shorter half-life, PTU should be given every 8 hours. **In our experience, 20 mg/day of MMI or 100 to 150 mg of PTU three times a day is an effective initial dose in most patients.** Drug side effects are related to the ATD dose. Those with large goiters and longer duration of the disease may need higher doses at the initiation of therapy. In patients with minimal symptoms, an initial dose of 10 mg of MMI daily or PTU 50 mg two or three times a day may be initiated. In the majority of patients, clinical improvement is seen in 2 to 6 weeks, and improvement in thyroid tests occurs within the first 2 weeks of therapy, with normalization to chemical euthyroidism in 3 to 7 weeks. Resistance to drug therapy is unusual, most likely a result of poor patient compliance. **Once clinical improvement occurs, mainly weight gain and reduction in tachycardia, the dose of antithyroid medication may be reduced by half of the initial dose.** The daily dose is adjusted every few weeks according to the clinical response and the results of thyroid tests, and serum TSH remains suppressed despite the normalization of thyroid hormone levels; normalization of serum TSH is an indicator to reduce the dose of medication. If an exacerbation of symptoms or worsening of the thyroid tests occurs, the amount of antithyroid medication is doubled.

The main concerns of maternal drug therapy are the potential side effects in the fetus, mainly goiter and hypothyroidism, as well as birth defects—hence the importance of using the minimal drug dose to keep FT_4 in the upper limit of the reference range or just above the normal nonpregnant range. However, small elevations in serum TSH in the neonate have been reported even with lower doses of antithyroid medication. Furthermore, in one study, cord blood FT_4 values were not correlated with the antithyroid medication dose at term. As mentioned previously,[36] in the presence of maternal TBII values less than 30%, the dose of MMI required to control hyperthyroidism may be lower than in women with elevated TBII titers, and such a dose may protect the fetus from hypothyroidism. **We do not recommend adding T_4 to ATD therapy** (block-replace regimen) **in the management of Graves disease in pregnancy. It is difficult to interpret the serum T_4 level, and this may lead to more unnecessary antithyroid medications.**

In addition to PTU-induced liver failure, side effects of ATDs occur in 3% to 5% of treated patients (see Box 42-4). **The most common complications of both drugs are pruritus and skin rash,** which usually resolve after switching to the other antithyroid medication. However, allergies to both antithyroid medications have been reported in a pregnant woman with type 1 diabetes mellitus. In general, the rash occurs 2 to 6 weeks after initiation of therapy. Because pruritus may be an initial symptom of hyperthyroidism, it is customary to ask the patient during the first visit whether she is bothered by this. Other complications that are much less common are migratory polyarthritis, a lupus-like syndrome, and cholestatic jaundice. Agranulocytosis, a serious but unusual complication, has been reported in 1 in 300 patients receiving PTU or MMI. It manifests as fever, malaise, gingivitis, and sore throat. Agranulocytosis occurs in the first 12 weeks of therapy and appears to be related to the dose of medication. Patients should be made aware of the potential adverse effects of these drugs at the time the prescription is given and should be advised to discontinue the medication at once if these effects appear. In this setting, a leukocyte count should be obtained immediately. Although some have recommended routine white blood cell counts in patients on antithyroid therapy, such testing is not indicated because granulocytopenia or agranulocytosis may appear without warning symptoms.

β-Adrenergic blocking agents (propranolol 20 to 40 mg every 6 hours or atenolol 25 to 50 mg/day) **are very effective in controlling hyperdynamic symptoms and are indicated for the first few weeks in patients who have symptoms.** One situation in which β-adrenergic blocking agents may be very effective is in the treatment of severe hyperthyroidism during labor. In a case reported in which both mother and fetus were affected, labetalol was infused at a rate of 2 mg/min and controlled maternal and fetal tachycardia within 45 minutes.

Subtotal thyroidectomy in pregnancy is effective in managing severe hyperthyroidism. However, indications for surgical treatment are few and include allergy to ATDs, requirements of large doses of medication, patient preference, and the exceptional case of resistance to drug therapy. Two issues are significant when advising surgical therapy: first, the mother should be prepared with β-adrenergic blocking agents to render her hemodynamically stable and with Lugol's solution for at least 10 days to reduce thyroid gland vascularity (use of potassium iodide for a short time is not contraindicated); and second, a determination of TRAb is of the utmost importance because a value three times greater than normal places the fetus at risk for fetal hyperthyroidism.[47]

[131]I therapy is contraindicated in pregnancy because when given after 12 weeks' gestation, it could produce fetal hypothyroidism.[48] A pregnancy test is mandatory in any woman of childbearing age before a therapeutic or diagnostic dose of ^{131}I is administered.

Iodine crosses the placenta. If given in large amounts and for prolonged periods, it may produce a fetal goiter and hypothyroidism. Therefore its therapeutic use is not recommended in pregnancy. However, iodine was used in small amounts (6 to 40 mg/day) in a group of pregnant Japanese women with mild hyperthyroidism. Elevation in serum TSH was observed in 2 of 35 newborns, and the mothers were slightly hyperthyroid at the time of delivery. Despite this observation, iodine therapy is not routinely indicated in the treatment of hyperthyroidism in pregnancy.

Breastfeeding should be permitted if the daily dose of PTU or MMI is less than 300 mg/day or 20 mg/day, respectively. It is prudent to give the total dose in divided doses after each feeding. Occasionally, thyroid function tests may be done in the baby.[49] In a very provocative study, PTU was given to lactating hyperthyroid mothers whose infants were born with elevated serum TSH levels. Infant TSH levels normalized even with continuation of PTU therapy by the mothers. In another study, thyroid tests were done at regular intervals in breastfed infants of mothers taking up to 20 mg of MM daily and showed no evidence of hypothyroidism. The authors followed the children up to 74 months of age and found no evidence of physical or intellectual developmental deficits compared with 176 controls.

Fetal surveillance with serial ultrasounds, nonstress tests (NSTs), and biophysical profiles (BPPs) is indicated for patients with uncontrolled hyperthyroidism, in the presence of fetal tachycardia or IUGR, in pregnancies complicated by preeclampsia, or when indicated for other obstetric or medical complications.

Treatment of Thyroid Storm

Thyroid storm is a clinical diagnosis based on severe signs of thyrotoxicosis with significant hyperpyrexia (>103° F) and neuropsychiatric symptoms essential for the clinical diagnosis. Tachycardia with a pulse rate that exceeds 140 beats/min is not uncommon, and congestive heart failure is a frequent complication. Gastrointestinal symptoms such as nausea and vomiting accompanied by liver compromise have been reported. Burch and Wartofsky have derived a scoring system based on clinical symptoms to predict the likelihood of thyroid storm. Laboratory tests show the classic hyperthyroid changes, although the actual elevation in FT$_4$ values does not help in the diagnosis.

Management includes the following:

1. Admission to the intensive care unit is initiated for supportive therapy such as fluids and correction of electrolyte abnormalities, oxygen therapy as needed, and control of hyperpyrexia. Acetaminophen is the drug of choice because aspirin may increase free thyroid hormones.
2. Management of congestive heart failure is undertaken, which may require large doses of digoxin.
3. Proper antibiotic therapy is instituted in case of infection.
4. To control hyperadrenergic symptoms, β-adrenergic blocker therapy can be used, such as propranolol 60 to 80 mg every 4 hours orally or 1 mg/min intravenously. Esmolol, a short-acting β-acting antagonist, can be given intravenously with a loading dose of 250 to 500 µg/kg of body weight followed by continuous infusion at 50 to 100 µg/kg/min.
5. MMI 30 mg or PTU 300 mg every 6 hours can also be used. If the patient is unable to take oral medications, a nasogastric tube may be needed; thioamides block the synthesis of thyroid hormones in a few hours.
6. One hour after the administration of thioamides, iodine is administered in the form of Lugol's solution, 10 drops three times a day, or sodium iodide is given intravenously 1 g every 12 hours.
7. Glucocorticoids are also helpful because they reduce the peripheral conversion of serum T$_4$ to T$_3$. They are administered in the form of hydrocortisone every 8 hours or equivalent amounts of other glucocorticoids.

In summary, thyroid storm is a life-threatening condition with a mortality rate of 20% to 30%,[50] and it requires early recognition and aggressive therapy in an intensive unit care setting.

Fetal Hyperthyroidism

In mothers with hyperthyroidism due to Graves disease, either active or past, high concentrations of TRAb that cross the placental barrier stimulate fetal production of thyroid hormones and may cause fetal hyperthyroidism. However, in mothers with active disease who are under drug treatment, the hyperactive fetal thyroid is controlled by maternal therapy, and the fetus remains euthyroid during fetal life. Within a few days after birth, when the beneficial effect of antithyroid therapy ceases, the neonate may develop neonatal hyperthyroidism (see the section, "Neonatal Hyperthyroidism"). **Women at risk for an infant with fetal hyperthyroidism are those with a history of Graves disease previously treated with ablation therapy, either by surgery or with ^{131}I, with elevated TRAb titers despite maternal euthyroidism.** The fetuses of women with Graves disease–associated hyperthyroidism who undergo therapeutic thyroidectomy in the second trimester of pregnancy are also at risk for hyperthyroidism if the mother carries high titers of TRAb.[47] The fetal thyroid TSH receptor starts responding to TSI stimulation during the second trimester, and the placental transfer of IgG from mother to fetus increases by the end of the second trimester, reaching a level in the fetus similar to that of the mother at about 30 weeks' gestation.

Fetal hyperthyroidism is diagnosed in the presence of persistent fetal tachycardia (>160 beats/min), **IUGR,** oligohydramnios, hydrops, and occasionally a goiter identified on ultrasonography, sometimes manifested as hyperextension of the fetal neck.[51] The diagnosis may be confirmed by measuring thyroid hormone levels in cord blood obtained by cordocentesis. Serial cordocentesis for monitoring drug therapy has been proposed, but its value has been questioned.[52,53] A fetal heart monitor tracing that demonstrated a sustained baseline of 170 to 180 beats/min with moderate variability that exhibited accelerations without decelerations was present in two fetuses of hyperthyroid mothers. The authors stated that "this pattern is unique to fetal thyrotoxicosis." Heckel and associates reviewed nine cases of fetal hyperthyroidism treated with antithyroid medications. Fetal tachycardia was the most frequent sign, whereas oligohydramnios and IUGR were reported in only two cases. Fetal goiter was detected by ultrasonography in three cases. Treatment consisted of antithyroid medication given to the mother (MMI, 10 to 20 mg/day),[54] and the dose is guided by the improvement and resolution of fetal tachycardia, a decrease in the goiter size, and normalization of fetal growth—all are indicators of good therapeutic response.

Luton and associates performed clinical fetal evaluation in 72 mothers with a past or present history of Graves hyperthyroidism. The main tools were the determination of maternal TRAb and fetal ultrasonography; cordocentesis was rarely indicated. In 31 mothers, TRAb titers were undetectable, and none of the patients received antithyroid medications. All infants were born euthyroid. Of 30 women positive for TRAb and on antithyroid drug therapy, neonatal function was normal. Eleven fetuses were diagnosed with goiter by ultrasonography, and seven of them were hypothyroid at birth. Their mothers had low TRAb titers and had received antithyroid therapy, probably in higher doses than needed. In the four hyperthyroid newborns, maternal TRAb titers were very high, and their mothers may not have received enough medication. The authors recommended monthly fetal ultrasonography after 20 weeks' gestation with determination of TRAb early in gestation and again by 24 to 28 weeks' gestation.

In summary, the diagnosis of fetal hyperthyroidism should be suspected in the presence of fetal tachycardia, IUGR, oligohydramnios or polyhydramnios, and accelerated bone maturation (the presence of the distal femoral ossification center before 31 weeks' gestation) with or without fetal goiter in mothers with active hyperthyroidism or in women with a history of Graves disease treated previously by ablation therapy in the presence of high titers of serum TRAb. The indications for ordering a determination of TRAbs are described in Box 42-5. This should

---

BOX 42-5   INDICATIONS FOR MATERNAL DETERMINATION OF THYROID-BLOCKING ANTIBODIES

Fetal or neonatal hyperthyroidism in previous pregnancies
Active disease or treatment with antithyroid drugs
Thyroidectomy during pregnancy
Euthyroid, postablation (surgery, Iodine-131)
Presence of:
- Fetal tachycardia
- Intrauterine growth restriction
- Incidental fetal goiter on ultrasound
- Accelerated bone maturation

From Mestman JH. Endocrine diseases in pregnancy. In Sciarra JJ, editor. *Gynecology and Obstetrics*. Philadelphia: Lippincott-Raven; 1997:27.

be done in patients at risk between 22 and 28 weeks' gestation, although some investigators recommended this test early in pregnancy and late in the second trimester.[51] The diagnosis may be confirmed by the determination of fetal thyroid hormones by cordocentesis in those centers with expertise in this technique.

Neonatal Hyperthyroidism

Neonatal hyperthyroidism is infrequent, with an incidence of 1% to 5% of infants born to mothers with Graves disease; therefore it affects 1 in 50,000 neonates. **In most cases, the disease is caused by the transfer of maternal immunoglobulin antibodies with stimulating activity to the fetus.** When present in high concentrations in maternal serum, these TSH receptor antibodies with stimulating activity (TRAbs) cross the placental barrier, stimulate the TSH receptor of the fetal thyroid gland, and may produce fetal or neonatal hyperthyroidism. Thyroid-stimulating receptor (TSHR) responsiveness to TSH develops early in the second trimester. When the mother is treated with antithyroid medications, the fetus benefits from maternal therapy and remains euthyroid during pregnancy despite the high circulating antibody titer. However, the protective effect of the ATD is lost after delivery, and neonatal hyperthyroidism may develop within a few days after birth. High titers of TRAb, a threefold increase over baseline, in the third trimester of pregnancy are a predictor of neonatal hyperthyroidism. If neonatal hyperthyroidism is not recognized and treated properly, neonatal mortality could be as high as 30%. Because the half-life of the antibodies is only a few weeks, complete resolution of neonatal hyperthyroidism is the rule.

Sporadic cases of neonatal hyperthyroidism without evidence of the presence of circulating TSI in the mother or infant have been published. Activation of mutations in the TSH receptor molecule is the cause of this entity. It is inherited as an autosomal-dominant trait and, in contrast to Graves neonatal hyperthyroidism, the condition persists indefinitely. Treatment with antithyroid medications followed by thyroid ablation therapy will eventually be needed.

As described previously, two methods are currently available for the determination of TRAb: receptor assays that measure thyroid-binding inhibitory immunoglobulins (TBII) and bioassays that measure the ability of TRAb to stimulate the production of cAMP (TSI). Abeillon-du Payrat and colleagues reported their experience with a second-generation TBII assay in 47 neonates born to 42 mothers with history of Graves disease. The assay result was considered positive above a cutoff value of 1.5 IU/L. A value over 5 IU/L measured in the second trimester indicated a risk of neonatal hyperthyroidism (sensitivity 100%, specificity 43%). Nine infants were born with hyperthyroidism: four who were asymptomatic resolved spontaneously within 3 to 45 days; in the other five infants, ATD treatment was needed, and two infants were admitted to the neonatal intensive care unit. The TBII value normalized after a median of 3 months. Interestingly, four of the nine mothers were on thyroid replacement therapy following thyroid ablation therapy, three with surgery and one with [131]I. No mother with a TSI (bioassay) below 400% gave birth to a hyperthyroid neonate. Besançon and associates evaluated the course of thyroid function and clinical outcome during the first postnatal month in babies born to mothers with Graves disease. Of the 68 babies, 33 of their mothers were on drug therapy during pregnancy, and their TRAb assay was positive. They recommend measuring TRAb in cord blood because a positive value indicates a high risk of neonatal hyperthyroidism. Of note, serum FT_4 should be repeated in the neonate between 3 and 5 days because a rapid FT_4 elevation during the first postnatal week is predictive of hyperthyroidism. Levy-Shraga and colleagues retrospectively studied the outcome of 96 neonates of mothers with Graves disease. Four infants were diagnosed with overt neonatal hyperthyroidism. In a subgroup of 77 newborns with subclinical hyperthyroidism, serum FT_4 levels peaked at day 5 and returned to normal by day 14 postpartum. Elevated FT_4 was associated with poor weight gain in the first 2 weeks of life. Serum TSH may remain suppressed for up to 3 months. These authors also advised thyroid tests between days 3 and 5 after birth to ensure early detection of neonatal hyperthyroidism.

Neonatal Central Hypothyroidism

Infants of untreated hyperthyroid mothers may be born with transient central hypothyroidism of pituitary or hypothalamic origin. High levels of T_4 cross the placental barrier and feed back to the fetal pituitary with suppression of fetal pituitary TSH. The diagnosis is made in the presence of a low FT_4 and a normal or low TSH level in cord blood. This complication should be avoidable with proper management of maternal hyperthyroidism.[37] Prolonged suppression of pituitary TSH production in some infants may produce a chronic state of hypothalamic-pituitary-thyroid axis dysfunction.

Resistance to Thyroid Hormone Syndrome

Described by Weiss and Refetoff and colleagues, resistance to thyroid hormone (RTH) is a syndrome of reduced end-organ responsiveness to thyroid hormone caused primarily by mutations in the thyroid hormone receptor β-gene, characterized by elevated free thyroid hormones with nonsuppressed TSH and with signs of hyperthyroidism in some tissues and hypothyroidism in others. The clinical manifestations include goiter and tachycardia, and the prevalence is about 1/40,000 live births. Unaffected fetuses of mothers with RTH syndrome and affected fetuses from normal mothers are at risk for poor obstetric outcome. Anselmo and associates reported 36 couples with 9 mothers and 9 fathers affected by the disease and with 18 unaffected relatives. The rates of miscarriage were 23.7% when the mother was affected, 6.7% when the father was affected, and 8.8% with unaffected first-degree relatives, with a rate of 8.1% in the general population. The birthweights of unaffected infants born to affected mothers were lower than those of affected newborns, who in addition had a lower serum TSH at birth. This finding suggests that high maternal thyroid hormone levels produced fetal thyrotoxicosis and had a direct toxic effect on the fetus. The approach to a pregnant patient with the RTH syndrome would depend on the genotype of the fetus. This requires obtaining the genotype of the fetus from DNA through amniocentesis or chorionic villus sampling, a history of the course and outcome of previous pregnancies, and information about other family members with RTH syndrome.

Hypothyroidism

Until 1980, few cases of pregnancy in women with myxedema were published because it was believed that most hypothyroid women were infertile. Soon after the determination of serum TSH became commercially available to confirm the diagnosis of primary hypothyroidism, a few series of hypothyroidism in pregnancy were described.[55,56] The incidence of hypothyroidism, defined at the time of these original publications as an elevation in serum TSH above 5 mIU/L, was reported to be between 2% and 4%.[57,58]

Etiology and Classification of Hypothyroidism

The two most common etiologies of primary hypothyroidism in countries with sufficient dietary iodine supply are autoimmune (Hashimoto) thyroiditis and post–thyroid ablation therapy, either surgical or ^{131}I induced. Others include congenital disease (about 1 in 3000 births in the United States), drug-induced hypothyroidism (with lithium, amiodarone, iodine excess, and ATDs), and prior head and neck radiation for nonthyroid malignant disease. Earlier studies in women with "hypothyroxinemia," diagnosed as a low serum protein-bound iodine (serum TSH was not available for the diagnosis of hypothyroidism), reported a high incidence of congenital malformations, perinatal mortality, and impaired mental and somatic development in infants of hypothyroid women. In contrast, recent reports have shown no increase in the incidence of congenital malformations. Secondary hypothyroidism includes diseases of the pituitary gland or hypothalamus. Autoimmune hypophysitis as a cause of secondary hypothyroidism is of interest to the obstetrician for its relationship to Sheehan syndrome.[59]

Regardless of the etiology, primary hypothyroidism is classified as either *subclinical hypothyroidism* (normal serum FT$_4$ and elevated serum TSH) or *overt clinical hypothyroidism* (low serum T$_4$ and elevated TSH or normal FT$_4$ with serum TSH values >10 mIU/L). The spectrum of pregnant women diagnosed with hypothyroidism includes (1) women with subclinical and overt hypothyroidism diagnosed for the first time during pregnancy; (2) hypothyroid women who are not consistent in taking their medication or those who discontinue thyroid therapy before or at the time of conception because of poor medical advice or because of the misconception that thyroid medications may affect the fetus; (3) women on thyroid replacement therapy who require larger doses in pregnancy (30% to 40% on prepregnancy levothyroxine therapy); (4) hyperthyroid patients on excessive amounts of ATD therapy; (5) rarely in the United States, those with severe iodine deficiency; and (6) some patients on lithium or amiodarone therapy.

SUBCLINICAL HYPOTHYROIDISM

Subclinical hypothyroidism (SCH) diagnosed in the first trimester of pregnancy has been associated with maternal, fetal, and neonatal complications in some but not all studies. The most commonly reported complications are miscarriage, preterm delivery, and preeclampsia.[57-62] Others include gestational diabetes, gestational hypertension, placental abruption, and low birthweight. Lower intelligence quotients (IQs) in these infants and other neurocognitive deficits have been described in the past,[63,64] but this has not been confirmed recently.

Most patients with subclinical hypothyroidism do not have overt clinical symptoms. Thyroid tests may be requested by the physician because of vague symptoms that resemble hypothyroidism, a patient or family history of thyroid disease, or findings in the physical examination such as the presence of a goiter. As will be discussed later (in the section on screening), in women who present for preconception counseling or at the time of the first obstetric visit, a selective list of potential risk factors should be evaluated, and if any are positive, thyroid tests should be obtained. **One laboratory test diagnostic of subclinical hypothyroidism is an elevated serum TSH in the presence of normal trimester-specific FT$_4$ levels.** A determination of TPOAbs is helpful to determine the etiology of hypothyroidism because they are present in 70% to 80% of hypothyroid patients of childbearing age. As mentioned earlier in the section "Thyroid Function Tests," **the recommended serum TSH upper limit of normal, if gestation-specific reference ranges are not available, is 2.5 mIU/L in the first trimester and up to 3 mIU/L in the second and third trimesters.**[65,66] A significant number of women on thyroid replacement therapy have become hypothyroid, most of them subclinical, by the time of the first obstetric visit because of the physiologic increase in the need for thyroid hormones in the first trimester of pregnancy.[25,26] Taylor and colleagues reported that in the United Kingdom, 46% of levothyroxine-treated women aged 18 to 45 years had a serum TSH level greater than 2.5 mIU/L; among pregnant women who had their TSH measured in the first trimester, 62.8% had a TSH level greater than 2.5 mU/L, with 7.4% greater than 10 mU/L.

Casey and associates[61] undertook a prospective thyroid screening study to evaluate pregnancy outcomes in women with subclinical hypothyroidism diagnosed before 20 weeks' gestation. Compared with euthyroid women, pregnancies of women with subclinical hypothyroidism were three times more likely to be complicated by placental abruption, a very preterm birth (before 34 weeks' gestation), and admission of their newborns to the neonatal intensive care nursery. Respiratory distress syndrome was twice as likely. In contrast, Cleary-Goldman and colleagues[62] reported no adverse outcomes in a group of 247 women with subclinical hypothyroidism diagnosed on the basis of a serum TSH more than the 97.5th percentile (TSH >4.29 mIU/L) and FT$_4$ between the 2.5th and 97.5th percentiles (0.3 and 0.71 ng/dL).

In a randomized study by Negro and colleagues[67] in southern Italy, 4657 women were screened for serum TSH and TPOAbs within the first 11 weeks of gestation. Of this group, 642 women presented with a serum TSH between 2.5 and 5 mIU/L and negative TPOAbs. The pregnancy loss (miscarriage) rate was 6.1%, compared with 3.6% in women with a serum TSH below 2.5 mIU/L ($P = .006$). Liu and associates performed thyroid function tests in 3315 women at low risk for thyroid dysfunction at 4 to 8 weeks' gestation from iodine-sufficient areas of China. The pregnancy-specific reference range for TSH in their population was 0.29 to 5.22 mIU/L. They also determined thyroid antibodies, TPOAb and antithyroglobulin antibody (TgAb). The risk of miscarriage was not significantly increased in women with serum TSH greater than 2.5 and less than 5.22 mIU/L, compared with women with TSH less than 2.5 mIU/L (3.5% vs. 2.2%) with exception of those women with positive thyroid antibodies (10.0% vs. 3.5%). In a prospective study from Australia of 152 women in the first trimester, Schneuer and associates[68] reported a significant increase in miscarriages in those women with a serum TSH greater than 2.9 mIU/L. In a review of five studies that evaluated SCH and miscarriages, only two of them showed a significant association of SCH and miscarriage. Taylor and colleagues[69] found no increased in miscarriage in first-trimester women on levothyroxine replacement therapy with serum TSH greater than 2.5 and less than 4.5 mIU/L compared with those with a serum TSH below 2.51 mIU/L. Of interest, the adjusted odds of miscarriage in women with serum TSH greater than 10 mIU/L was 3.95 versus 1.0 in women with a serum TSH between 0.2 and 2.5 mIU/L. The above studies emphasize the importance of the serum TSH–specific reference range for different populations, which may be affected by ethnicity, geographic region, and iodine intake.

NEUROLOGIC DEVELOPMENT AND SUBCLINICAL HYPOTHYROIDISM

In 1999, a retrospective study reported neuropsychological development in young children of mothers diagnosed early in pregnancy with hypothyroidism, a group of them with slight elevations in serum TSH. In a recent study from the United Kingdom, Lazarus and colleagues conducted a randomized trial of pregnant women at a median gestational age of 12.3 weeks. A serum TSH above the 97.5th percentile, FT_4 levels below 2.5th percentile, or both were considered diagnostic of thyroid deficiency. Two groups of patients were studied: 390 in the screening group and 404 in the control group; 150 µg of levothyroxine were prescribed to women in the screening group at a median of 13.3 weeks. The dose was adjusted to achieve serum TSH values of 0.1 to 1.0 mIU/L, and the primary outcome was the infant's IQ at 3 years of age. **The authors concluded that no benefit was found with routine screening for maternal hypothyroidism at about 12 to 13 weeks' gestation in the prevention of impaired childhood cognitive function.** In contrast, two recent studies suggested that normalization of thyroid function in hypothyroid women by midgestation avoids neurodevelopmental defects in the children.[70,71] A recently completed study organized by the National Institute of Child Health and Human Development (NICHD)[71a,71b] included a total of 97,226 pregnant women from 14 institutions in the United States. In this randomized trial, women with subclinical hypothyroidism or hypothyroxinemia received L-thyroxine or placebo. The obstetric outcomes and the neurocognitive function of the offspring at 5 years were not significantly different.

CLINICAL HYPOTHYROIDISM

The diagnosis of clinical or overt hypothyroidism in pregnancy is confirmed by the presence of an elevated serum TSH and an FT_4 below the trimester-specific reference range or a serum TSH greater than 10 mIU/L irrespective of the serum thyroxine level. Patients with overt hypothyroidism may complain of tiredness, cold intolerance, fatigue, muscle cramps, constipation, irregular menstrual periods, infertility, and deepening of the voice. On physical examination, the skin may be dry and cold, deep tendon reflexes may be delayed, and bradycardia may be detected as well as periorbital edema. A goiter is present in almost 80% of patients in whom the etiology is chronic thyroiditis. In the other 20% of women with chronic thyroiditis, no goiter is found; this is called *atrophic thyroiditis*, also known as *primary myxedema* or *chronic thyroiditis without goiter*. Of course, a well-healed scar in the neck suggests that the patient has had a prior surgical thyroidectomy. The degree of severity of the clinical symptoms varies with the thyroid abnormalities on testing, although correlation is not always good between clinical and chemical parameters. It is important to emphasize that many patients with frank hypothyroidism by laboratory tests offer no specific complaints. Spontaneous pregnancies have been reported in newly diagnosed women with a serum TSH higher than 150 mIU/L at the time of the first obstetric visit.[56] The mean TSH value at the time of diagnosis of overt hypothyroidism was 89.7 ± 86.2 mIU/mL (normal, 0.4 to 5.0) with a mean FT_4I of 2.1 ± 1.5 (normal, 4.5 to 12).[57] **Serum thyroid antibodies—TPOAbs, also known as** *antimicrosomal antibodies*—**are elevated in almost 95% of patients with autoimmune hypothyroidism.**

As in the case of hyperthyroidism, untreated overt hypothyroidism is associated with adverse neonatal outcomes that include premature birth, SGA infants, and in one study, an increased prevalence of fetal death. **One of the most common obstetric complications is preeclampsia, with an incidence of 21% in a combined study of 60 patients with overt hypothyroidism.**[56,57] Preeclampsia has not been reported in all series, although some of them were retrospective analyses. Low birthweight was detected in 16.6% of births, mostly related to preterm delivery. Hirsh and coworkers retrospectively compared outcomes of 101 pregnant women with serum TSH greater than 20 mIU/L at diagnosis of pregnancy with a control group of 205 euthyroid pregnant women identified from the 2009–2010 computerized database of a health maintenance organization in Israel. The mean duration of clinical hypothyroidism during pregnancy was 21.2 ±13.2 weeks, and in 36 cases (34.9%), all TSH levels during pregnancy remained elevated. The incidence of severe hypothyroidism (TSH >20 mIU/L) was 1.1% of all hypothyroid mothers. Surprisingly, the incidence of miscarriages, prematurity, and other pregnancy complications was not different between the control and study groups. The authors speculated that the low incidence of complications could be due to the normal median FT_4 level at the time of maximal serum TSH measurement and intensive levothyroxine therapy in addition to the thorough obstetric management provided in their country.

ISOLATED HYPOTHYROXINEMIA

The term *isolated hypothyroxinemia* is reserved for those patients in areas of sufficient dietary iodine intake with values less than the trimester-specific FT_4 reference range in the presence of normal serum TSH values. Although the pathophysiologic explanation for such an entity is not clear, maternal hypothyroxinemia is extremely frequent in endemic areas of iodine deficiency and is associated with increased perinatal morbidity and mortality and an increased incidence of hypothyroidism in neonates.[72] Recently, a study from China found that isolated hypothyroxinemia was associated with iron deficiency, both before pregnancy and in the first trimester.

Two reports from iodine-sufficient countries confirmed previous reports of the adverse role of maternal hypothyroxinemia in the neuropsychological development of children. Li and colleagues collected serum from 1268 women at 16 to 20 weeks' gestation at Shenyang Maternal and Neonatal Health Clinic in an area described as "iodine sufficient." Intellectual and motor development scores were evaluated in the children at 25 to 30 months of age using the Bayley Scales of Infant Development. Eighteen women (1.8%) were diagnosed as having subclinical hypothyroidism; 19 women were hypothyroxinemic (1.5%); and 34 (2.6%) were euthyroid with an elevated level of TPOAbs. The authors concluded that maternal subclinical hypothyroidism, hypothyroxinemia, and euthyroidism with elevated serum TPOAb titers are all statistically significant predictors of lower motor and intellectual development at 25 to 30 months. In a population-based cohort study in the Netherlands, Henrichs and colleagues[64] observed that mild and severe hypothyroxinemia were associated with a higher risk for expressive language delay across all ages. categorized as either mild (OR, 1.44; 95% CI, 1.09 to 1.91; $P = .010$) or severe (OR, 1.8; 95% CI, 1.24 to 2.61; $P = .002$).

BOX 42-6   INDICATIONS FOR THYROID TESTING IN PREGNANCY

History of thyroid dysfunction or prior thyroid surgery
Age greater than 30 years
Symptoms of thyroid dysfunction or the presence of goiter
Thyroid peroxidase antibody positive
Type 1 diabetes or other autoimmune disorders
History of head/neck radiation
Family history of thyroid dysfunction
Morbid obesity (body mass index ≥ 40 kg/m^2)
Use of amiodarone or lithium or recent administration of iodinated radiologic contrast
Unexplained infertility
Residing in an area of known moderate to severe iodine sufficiency

From Stagnaro-Green A et al. Guidelines of the American Thyroid Association for the Diagnosis and Management of Thyroid Disease During Pregnancy and Postpartum. *Thyroid.* 2011;21:1081.

No adverse obstetric outcomes were reported by Casey and associates[73] in evaluating 17,289 women before 20 weeks' gestation: the prevalence of hypothyroxinemia was 1%, subclinical hypothyroidism was 3%. A study by Lazarus and colleagues[74] included patients with hypothyroxinemia along with women with hypothyroidism who were treated with levothyroxine, and no difference was found in the IQs of children of treated mothers compared with the children of untreated mothers.

It is important to recognize that the assay technique used to determine FT$_4$, particularly in the second half of pregnancy, may be more difficult to perform.[24]

Universal Versus Selective Screening for Thyroid Disease

Despite the potential obstetric and pediatric complications from maternal thyroid dysfunction reported in the past 50 years, the consistency of reports on the incidence of maternal subclinical and clinical hypothyroidism in the first trimester, and our recognized difficulty in diagnosing the disease both by medical history and physical examination, **when and how to screen for thyroid disease in pregnant and nonpregnant individuals remains a very controversial issue, and different positions have been adopted by several medical organizations.** A consensus development conference on subclinical thyroid disease was sponsored by the American Association of Clinical Endocrinologists (AACE), the ATA, and the ES. Their recommendation was based on an extensive review of the published literature available at that time, and it limited thyroid tests to women at high risk for thyroid disease.[75] In 2007, the Committee on Obstetric Practice of the American College of Obstetricians and Gynecologists (ACOG) stated, "Without evidence that identification and treatment of pregnant women with subclinical hypothyroidism improves maternal or infant outcomes, routine screening for subclinical hypothyroidism currently is not recommended." **It is reasonable to perform a determination of serum TSH at the first obstetric visit in those women at higher risk for thyroid dysfunction** (Box 42-6). In the second version of the ES guidelines and the ATA Clinical Guidelines for Thyroid and Pregnancy,[76] universal screening is not recommended, but it is strongly suggested that health care professionals personally ask during preconception counseling or in the first obstetric visit about risk factors for thyroid disease. **The main**

barrier to universal screening is the lack of RCTs that demonstrate a reversal of both obstetric and intellectual abnormalities in the offspring after normalization of thyroid deficiency by maternal L-thyroxine replacement therapy.

Several studies have consistently demonstrated the failure to recognize women at risk for thyroid dysfunction when using a case-finding strategy, based on actual thyroid dysfunction symptoms, a personal or family history of thyroid disease, and obstetric history.

Vaidya and coworkers[77] offered thyroid function tests early in pregnancy to 1560 women to evaluate the effectiveness of universal screening versus case finding. They showed that targeted screening would still have missed about one third of all pregnant women with an elevated serum TSH. They divided women early in pregnancy into two groups, a low-risk group that included 75% of the women and a high-risk group that comprised the remaining 25%. The high-risk group included those with a personal and family history of thyroid disorders or other autoimmune disease and current and past treatment with ATDs, L-thyroxine, radioiodine, or thyroid surgery. Forty women, 2.6% of the total group, had an elevated serum TSH, and 70% of them were in the high-risk group.

Similar conclusions have been reported in other studies. Wang and coworkers performed thyroid tests in the first trimester of pregnancy and classified 367 women (12.7%) out of 2899 as high risk, following the recommendations of the ES guidelines.[20] Of the 2899, 294 had thyroid dysfunction: hypothyroidism was reported in 7.5%, most of which was subclinical hypothyroidism; 1% had hyperthyroidism; and 0.9% had hypothyroxinemia. Positive antibodies were detected in 279 (9.6%), and 196 of them were euthyroid. The prevalence of thyroid dysfunction in the high-risk group was higher than in the low-risk group (15% vs. 9.4%; $P = .001$). However, of the 217 women with an elevated serum TSH, 171 (78.8%) belonged to the low-risk group. The authors concluded that a case-finding strategy for screening thyroid function in the high-risk group would miss about 81.6% of women with an elevated serum TSH and 80.4% women with hyperthyroidism. In a study from the Czech Republic, Horacek and colleagues concluded that more than 55% of pregnant women at risk would be missed if only those with high-risk criteria were examined. The authors stated that a more extensive screening of thyroid autoimmunity and dysfunction seems warranted.

Ong and colleagues performed thyroid tests and evaluated levels of β-hCG and pregnancy-associated plasma protein A (PAPP-A) in 2411 women, mostly white, in Western Australia between 9 and 14 weeks' gestation. Their objective was to determine whether thyroid function tests performed with first-trimester screening predicts adverse pregnancy outcomes. One hundred thirty-three women (5.5%) had serum TSH greater than 2.15 mIU/L (above the 97.5th percentile for the first trimester), five of whom (0.2%) had a serum TSH greater than 10 mIU/L. On multivariate analysis, neither maternal serum TSH greater than 2.15 mIU/L nor TSH as a continuous variable predicted primary or secondary outcomes. **Their conclusions were that testing TSH as part of first-trimester screening does not predict adverse pregnancy outcomes.** The authors question whether screening is justified to detect these cases.

Negro and colleagues[78] reported on a prospective randomized study of 4562 women in southern Italy. Thyroid tests were done very early in pregnancy. Their conclusion was that universal screening did not affect the rate of adverse events in comparison to targeted high-risk case finding, implying a negative outcome. As discussed in the section on subclinical hypothyroidism, in the same article by Negro and associates, a subgroup of low-risk patients detected to be hypothyroid were treated with L-thyroxine and were compared with a nontreated group. The rate of pregnancy-related adverse events was reduced by nearly 40% after detection and treatment.

A cost-effectiveness approach to compare universal screening with case finding was reported in two studies, and both concluded that universal screening is cost-effective compared with a case-finding strategy.[79] However, Thung and colleagues added in their conclusions that a wide range of circumstances should be considered before universal screening is adopted. The same position was voiced by Stagnaro-Green and Schwartz.

A number of barriers must be considered before universal routine thyroid function screening can be recommended in pregnancy.[80] They include the selection of thyroid tests to be used (TSH, FT$_4$, TPOAb), the threshold applied to characterize an abnormality, weeks of gestation, appropriate intervention, and monitoring. **The second issue still in dispute is the management of hypothyroid women in the preconceptional period.** It is accepted that most of these women will need an increase in the L-thyroxine dose soon after conception.[25,26] It could be argued whether the target of serum TSH between 0.3 and 2.5 mIU/L before pregnancy is reasonable in anticipation of the increase in T$_4$ requirements. Abalovich and associates[81] reported that when the serum TSH is below 1.3 mIU/L before conception, only 17% of women need an increase in L-thyroxine in the first trimester. It has also been recommended that women on L-thyroxine therapy be advised at the time of confirmation of pregnancy to increase their dose empirically by two doses a week until the results of the thyroid tests are available.[26]

The Controlled Antenatal Thyroid Screening trial[74] failed to show any benefit of levothyroxine therapy on the cognitive function of children of mothers with hypothyroidism or hypothyroxinemia. An argument about the study is that mothers did not receive thyroxine therapy until a median gestational age of 13.4 weeks. As mentioned above, a small number of children whose hypothyroid mothers started levothyroxine therapy after the first trimester of pregnancy had no neurocognitive deficits when evaluated after 5 years of age.[70,71] As previously mentioned, the NICHD Maternal-Fetal Medicine Units Network study of universal screening and L-thyroxine treatment for women with subclinical hypothyroidism or euthyroid chronic thyroiditis diagnosed during pregnancy showed no differences in the obstetric outcomes or neurocognitive development of the offspring at 5 years of age. **The practicing physician should consider this new information when deciding whether universal screening versus case finding is warranted and which women may benefit from thyroxine therapy.**

Euthyroid Chronic or Hashimoto Thyroiditis

Chronic or Hashimoto thyroiditis[83] is a benign inflammatory disorder of the thyroid gland with a prevalence in women of childbearing age of 5% to 20%. **Chronic autoimmune thyroid disease is more common in women with other autoimmune diseases, particularly type 1 diabetes.**

In the United States, the incidence is greater in the white than in the black population. The classic clinical picture is characterized by the presence of a goiter with a firm, rubbery consistency that moves freely on swallowing. Absence of a goiter (atrophic thyroiditis) may be present in 20% to 30% of patients.

On presentation, patients have no symptoms of thyroid dysfunction. A goiter is discovered on routine physical examination, by neck ultrasonography, or by the patient or a family member or acquaintance. The diagnosis may be suggested by a hyperechoic pattern on an ultrasound of the thyroid gland, and **diagnosis is confirmed by the presence of thyroid autoantibodies (TPOAb or TgAb).** The actual antibody titer is not correlated with the size of the goiter, symptoms, or severity of the disease. From a practical point of view, determination of TgAb is unnecessary if TPOAbs are positive. It is estimated that 5% of women with chronic thyroiditis have an isolated positive TgAb and a significantly higher serum TSH compared with women who do not have autoimmune thyroiditis. Patients with euthyroid chronic thyroiditis may develop hypothyroidism over time. The odds ratio was 8 over 20 years in those women with a normal serum TSH and positive antibodies.[27]

The importance of diagnosing chronic thyroiditis in women of childbearing age relates to the potential consequences in pregnancy and in the postpartum period. Women with chronic thyroiditis who are known to be euthyroid should be evaluated early in pregnancy because they are at risk for developing hypothyroidism de novo, with an increased risk of miscarriages, prematurity (according to some studies), and breech presentation.[84]

In rare situations, women with chronic thyroiditis—particularly those without a goiter, the atrophic form—may have high titers of serum TRAb-blocking antibodies compared with the stimulating antibodies present in women with Graves hyperthyroidism. These antibodies cross the placenta, and at high titers, they block the fetal TSH receptor and cause transient congenital hypothyroidism.[85] The neonatal disease resolves spontaneously over 3 to 6 months, but these infants should receive levothyroxine and should be closely followed for several years. **Therefore in mothers who have given birth to infants with congenital hypothyroidism, TRAb should be determined.**

In 1990, Stagnaro-Green and colleagues[84] reported a twofold to threefold increased risk for spontaneous abortion in euthyroid women with positive thyroid autoantibodies, studies confirmed by later publications. Preterm delivery was associated with the presence of thyroid antibodies in three out of four reports from Belgium, Italy, Japan, and Pakistan. A significant increase in preterm premature rupture of the membranes in TPOAb-positive euthyroid mothers was also reported.

Regarding the therapeutic use of L-thyroxine in women with euthyroid chronic thyroiditis (normal serum TSH and positive TPO antibodies), there is only one published study.[86] The authors performed thyroid tests that included TPOAbs in a group of 984 women early in pregnancy; 113 (11.7%) of them were TPOAb positive, with normal serum TSH values (reference range, 0.27 to 4.2 mIU/L). Their first obstetric visit was at 10.3 ± 3.1 weeks. Fifty-seven TPOAb-positive women were treated with L-thyroxine, with a dose between 0.5 and 1 µg/kg per day according to TSH values and TPOAb titers. They were compared with 58 untreated TPOAb-positive women and a control group of TPOAb-negative women. Two end points were evaluated: the incidences of miscarriage and preterm delivery. **The L-thyroxine–treated group had an incidence of complications similar to that of the control group, whereas the untreated chronic thyroiditis group had a threefold increase in miscarriages and preterm deliveries and in addition developed impaired thyroid function in the second half of pregnancy.**

A higher incidence of thyroid autoimmunity has been reported in women with polycystic ovary syndrome (PCOS) and idiopathic infertility. Of 992 women who attended a fertility clinic in Belgium, 16% had evidence of thyroid autoimmunity. Both antibodies were present in 74, only TPOAb was present in 41, and 48 had isolated TgAb detected.[87] In a Dutch study, in a selected group of women between 25 and 30 years of age, the prevalence of TgAb and TPOAb was 14% and 12%, respectively. Based on these and other studies, **it appears reasonable, in an infertility workup, to determine serum TgAb in the presence of a negative serum TPOAb.**

Infertile women seeking treatment should have serum TSH measured before treatment is started and every 2 weeks after the initiation of treatment because the risk of developing hypothyroidism is significant. Furthermore, the early diagnosis of hypothyroidism and prompt levothyroxine therapy may improve pregnancy outcome.

There is also agreement in the literature that the presence of TPOAb in the first trimester of pregnancy is a risk factor for the development of postpartum thyroiditis (see the later section, "Postpartum Thyroid Dysfunction").

Treatment of Hypothyroidism

L-Thyroxine is the drug of choice for the treatment of hypothyroidism. **In view of the complications mentioned previously, it is important to normalize thyroid tests as early as possible before conception or soon after the diagnosis of pregnancy.** In women on L-thyroxine replacement therapy, how much the dose will need to be increased from prepregnancy levels depends on the etiology of the hypothyroidism.[88] Loh and colleagues reported an increase in L-thyroxine dose of 16% by the second trimester in patients with primary hypothyroidism and reported a 51% increase following ablation therapy for Graves disease by surgery or ^{131}I therapy. For patients with a history of thyroid cancer, the increase was 21% by the second trimester, depending on the level of TSH suppression recommended for cancer patients. In newly diagnosed pregnant women, the levothyroxine dose may be calculated according to body weight (2 to 2.4 µg/kg/day), a dose higher than recommended in nonpregnant patients (1.7 to 2 µg/kg/day). In patients with severe hypothyroidism, the normalization of serum TSH is delayed, but normal serum FT_4 or FT_4I values are achieved in the first 2 weeks of therapy if sufficient L-thyroxine is administered. Abalovich and colleagues retrospectively analyzed seventy-seven patients with newly diagnosed hypothyroidism in pregnancy. The objective was to normalize the serum TSH to a value less than 2.5 mIU/L in the first trimester and less than 3.0 mIU/L in the second and third trimesters. The authors suggested that if the serum TSH is less than 4.2 mIU/L, the levothyroxine starting dose should be 1.2 µg/kg/day; with TSH greater than 4.2 and less than 10 mIU/L, 1.42 µg/kg/day is appropriate; and for women with overt hypothyroidism, 2.33 µg/kg/day is required. Only 11% and 23% of SCH and chronic hypothyroidism, respectively, required dose adjustment. The time at which a euthyroid state was achieved was 6.06 ± 3.3 days in SCH and 5.3 ± 1.8 days in overt hypothyroidism.

Women planning their pregnancies should have a serum TSH below 2.5 mIU/L, ideally closer to 1 mIU/L, given the greater requirements expected early in gestation. The serum TSH should be repeated every 2 to 6 weeks during the first 20 weeks' gestation and at 24 to 28 weeks and at 32 to 34 weeks. The aim is to keep serum TSH, as well as serum FT_4 or FT_4I, within normal trimester-specific reference ranges. The T_4 dose should be adjusted. Increased thyroid requirements are seen in about 20% to 30% of patients in the second half of pregnancy. Immediately after delivery, patients should return to their prepregnancy dose. Interference in the absorption of T_4 was discussed previously.[20]

Hypothyroid treated women who require in vitro fertilization (IVF) should have their thyroid tests measured before the initiation of controlled ovarian hyperstimulation. In a group of 72 selected hypothyroid women on replacement therapy and with a serum TSH below 2.5 mIU/L, determination of serum TSH was obtained at three points: (1) before treatment, (2) at the time of hCG administration, and (3) at 16 days after hCG administration. Serum TSH levels were 1.7 ± 0.7 at baseline, 2.9 ± 1.3 at the time of hCG administration, and 3.2 ± 1.7 mIU/L after 16 days. Serum TSH exceeded 2.5 mIU/L in 46 women (63.8%) and in 49 (68%) 16 days after hCG administration. The authors suggested strictly monitoring serum TSH in hypothyroid-treated women during IVF cycles, adjusting therapy if necessary. Karmon and colleagues[89] evaluated differences in intrauterine insemination (IUI) outcomes among euthyroid women with preconceptional serum TSH values in the normal (0.4 to 2.4 mIU/L) and high-normal (2.5 to 4.9 mIU/L) ranges. No autoimmunity tests were available. Data were obtained from a single family center and comprised a total of 1477 women who underwent 4064 IUI cycles. No difference in adverse outcomes was reported between the groups. The above studies[89,90] should remind us that as health professionals who take care of women planning a pregnancy, the lack of uniformity in the results of well-planned medical protocols and discrepancies in their observations complicate our ability to counsel these patients.

Single Nodule of the Thyroid Gland

The incidence of thyroid nodularity in pregnancy has been studied by several groups using ultrasonography. The three studies were done in Belgium, Germany, and China—areas of mild iodine deficiency, where the incidence of thyroid nodules is increased. They examined the frequency of nodules, the effect of progression of pregnancy on nodule size, and new nodule formation. Together they showed a prevalence of 3% to 23%, the incidence being higher with increasing parity.

It is estimated that nodular thyroid disease is clinically detectable in 10% of pregnant women. The size of the thyroid nodule clinically detectable is 1.0 to 1.5 cm. In most cases, it is discovered during the first routine clinical examination or is detected by the patient. The probability for a single or solitary thyroid nodule to be malignant is between 5% and 10%, depending on risk factors such as previous radiation therapy to the head, neck, or chest; rapid growth of a painless nodule; patient age; and family history of thyroid cancer. Papillary carcinoma accounts for almost 75% to 80% of malignant tumors, and follicular neoplasms account for 15% to 20%; a few percent are represented by medullary thyroid carcinoma. Undifferentiated thyroid carcinoma is extremely rare in patients younger than 50 years.

The incidence of thyroid carcinoma in the general population has risen significantly in recent decades, perhaps because of the increased detection of small papillary cancers, from 3.6 per 100,000 in 1973 to 8.7 per 100,000 in 2002—a 2.4-fold increase (95% CI, 2.2 to 2.6; $P <.001$ for trend). In part, this increase could be explained by the routine use of thyroid ultrasonography.

EVALUATION OF A PALPABLE THYROID NODULE
IN PREGNANCY: THERAPEUTIC OPTIONS

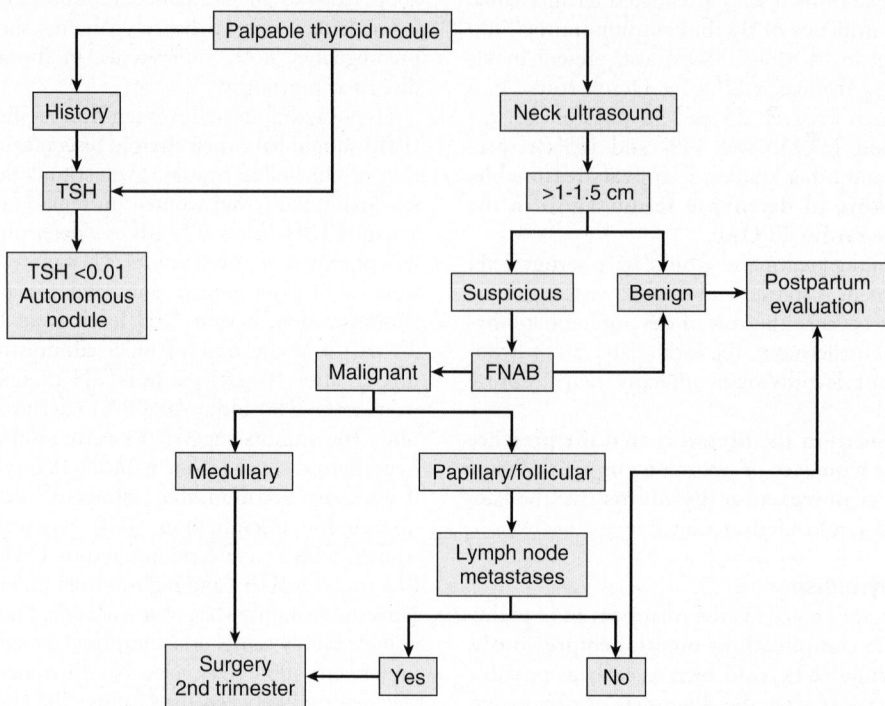

FIG 42-5 American Thyroid Association clinical guidelines for thyroid and pregnancy. FNAB, fine-needle aspiration biopsy; TSH, thyroid-stimulating hormone.

It is estimated that as many as 14 of every 100,000 pregnancies in the United States are complicated by a new diagnosis of thyroid cancer. In a retrospective study from the California Cancer Registry from 1991 to 1999, 129 cases of thyroid cancer were diagnosed during pregnancy; 3.3 per 100,000 were diagnosed before pregnancy; 0.3 per 100,000 were diagnosed at the time of delivery; and 10.8 per 100,000 were diagnosed within 1 year after delivery.

There is a paucity of information in the literature regarding the management and timing of the workup in the presence of thyroid nodularity. The ATA management guidelines for patients with thyroid nodules and differentiated thyroid carcinoma[91] recommended a similar evaluation of thyroid nodules in pregnancy as for the nonpregnant patient, with the exception, of course, that a radionuclide scan is contraindicated. In the presence of a thyroid nodule, they stressed the importance of a careful medical history, including a family history of malignant thyroid disease. If the family history is positive for familial medullary thyroid carcinoma or multiple endocrine neoplasia type 2, the evaluation of the nodule and management requires a more aggressive approach.

Careful examination of the neck enables the physician to define and characterize the thyroid lesion (Fig. 42-5). In addition to the size of the nodule, the consistency, tenderness, fixation to the skin, and presence of metastasis in the thyroid bed should be noted. A hard, painless nodule that measures more than 2 cm in diameter is suspicious of malignancy. Serum TSH and FT_4 need to be assessed. A suppressed or undetectable TSH value in the presence of a single or dominant thyroid nodule is consistent with an autonomous or "hot" thyroid nodule, in which case a fine-needle aspiration biopsy (FNAB) is not

indicated; these are rarely malignant. Interpretation of TSH values requires caution because a low or suppressed value may be present in a number of pregnancies in the first trimester. Serum calcitonin determination is reserved for patients with a family history of medullary thyroid carcinoma.[91] In expert hands, high-resolution real-time ultrasound is very helpful in defining the size of the lesion, characterizing the dominant nodule in a multinodular gland, and identifying characteristics of the lesion suspicious for malignancy: microcalcifications, a hypoechoic pattern, or irregular margins among other findings, such as whether the lesion is solid, cystic, or mixed. If FNAB of the nodule is indicated, pregnancy is not a contraindication, and FNAB may be performed at any time during gestation irrespective of gestational age. The importance of a competent cytopathologist in the interpretation and diagnosis of the specimens cannot be overemphasized.

In the presence of a single thyroid nodule detected on physical examination or a dominant nodule in a multinodular gland, the following approach is recommended by the ATA Clinical Guidelines for Thyroid and Pregnancy[76] (see Fig. 42-5):

1. In the presence of a solid lesion smaller than 1 to 1.5 cm, follow-up in the postpartum period is indicated.
2. Nodules larger than 1 to 1.5 cm should be considered for FNAB if ultrasound findings are suspicious.
3. In the presence of tracheal obstruction, immediate surgery is indicated.
4. If the FNAB is diagnostic of malignancy or it is a suspicious lesion, surgery may be postponed until after delivery except with lymph node metastases, if the diagnosis is a large primary lesion, or if extensive lymph node involvement is apparent in a medullary cancer.

5. Surgery can be postponed until after delivery during the last weeks of pregnancy, and FNAB could be safely postponed until after delivery.

6. A woman with a malignant lesion or a rapidly growing lesion should be offered surgery in the second trimester of gestation.

7. Women with follicular lesions or early-stage papillary carcinoma may postpone surgery until after delivery because these lesions are not expected to progress rapidly.

When advising pregnant women on the evaluation of a thyroid nodule, it must be kept in mind that the incidence of malignancy is between 5% and 10%, and in most cases, the tumors are slow growing.

It is generally agreed that elective surgery should be avoided in the first trimester and after 24 weeks' gestation because of the potential risks for spontaneous abortion and premature delivery, respectively. Based on clinical experience, the recommendations for total thyroidectomy in the second trimester are to avoid unnecessary exposure of the embryo to anesthetic drugs and to avoid potential prematurity due to surgery. However, no well-controlled study is available to support such recommendations.[92] One report showed a higher risk for complications from thyroid and parathyroid surgery during pregnancy. Thyroidectomy during pregnancy was associated with a complication rate of 21%, compared with 8%, for malignant lesions and 27%, compared with 14%, for benign lesions. This was a retrospective, cross-sectional analysis of hospital discharge data. Complications included suspected fetal compromise, abortion, and cesarean delivery and hysterectomy. A skilled surgeon with ample experience in thyroid surgery should perform the procedure.

In one retrospective study, a conservative approach to the management of a single thyroid nodule was recommended.[93] In this report, 61 women were pregnant at the time of the diagnosis of differentiated thyroid carcinoma. Fourteen women were operated on during pregnancy, whereas the other 47 women underwent surgical treatment 1 to 84 months after delivery. The authors concluded that both diagnostic studies and initial therapy might be delayed until after delivery in most patients. Yasmeen and associates reviewed cancer registry data and compared disease-related survival in 6505 women diagnosed with thyroid cancer during pregnancy or 1 year after delivery. No significant difference in outcome was apparent up to 11 years later compared with an age-matched nonpregnant cohort.

Recently, 15 women diagnosed with thyroid cancer during pregnancy or within 1 year postpartum were compared with 61 women matched for age whose cancer was treated before pregnancy. The authors reported that women diagnosed in pregnancy or in the first year postpartum were more likely to have persistent or recurrent disease and suggested that estrogen may play a role in these poorer outcomes.[94] Messuti and colleagues studied retrospectively 340 women younger than 45 years with differentiated thyroid cancer and compared persistence/recurrence of thyroid tumor in three groups: (1) those diagnosed at least 2 years after delivery, (2) those diagnosed during pregnancy and within 2 years after delivery, and (3) women who were nulliparous at the time of diagnosis. These researchers concluded that persistence/recurrence of disease was significantly higher in the group diagnosed during or within 2 years of delivery than in the control group ($P = .023$), which is consistent with the study by Moosa and colleagues.[94] Further studies are needed before a firm recommendation can be offered to patients diagnosed with thyroid cancer in pregnancy or postpartum.

Patients With Known Thyroid Cancer Before Pregnancy

Pregnancy does not appear to be a risk factor for recurrences in women with a previous history of treated thyroid cancer and no evidence of residual disease. Leboeuf and colleagues[95] published a retrospective analysis of 36 women who became pregnant a median of 4.3 years after initial therapy for differentiated thyroid carcinoma. They were evaluated a median of 4 months after delivery (0.1 to 1.7 years), and serum thyroglobulin values were available before and after pregnancy. Two women treated with thyroidectomy and radioactive iodine and one treated with thyroidectomy alone, whose serum thyroglobulin values were elevated before pregnancy, had new evidence of disease with an increase in thyroglobulin values and cervical nodes detected by ultrasonography. The authors concluded that pregnancy "is probably a mild stimulus to cancer growth as evidenced by minor disease progression in some patients with known structural disease before pregnancy."

Hirsch and associates[96] evaluated 63 consecutive women, for a total of 90 births, who were followed at their institution from 1992 to 2009 and who had given birth at least once after total thyroidectomy, and they evaluated 58 who received ^{131}I for papillary thyroid cancer. Serum thyroglobulin values and neck ultrasound were compared before and after pregnancy. In this study, levels of serum TSH during pregnancy were correlated with disease persistence before pregnancy and disease progression during pregnancy. They concluded that pregnancy does not cause thyroid cancer recurrence in survivors who have no structural or biochemical evidence of disease persistence at the time of conception. The conclusions from both studies indicate no progression of the disease in women free of disease before pregnancy. However, the possibility of progression exists in those patients who have evidence of residual cancer at the time of conception.

Women on suppressive T_4 therapy for thyroid cancer before pregnancy must continue with therapy, adjusting the levothyroxine dose to keep serum TSH at the same level as before pregnancy and serum TFT_4 within the normal reference range.[97,98] In women treated with ^{131}I therapy after thyroidectomy for thyroid cancer, a potential concern exists for future fertility and a risk for complications, mainly birth defects. Miscarriages, preterm delivery, stillbirth, and congenital abnormalities were not reported in a systemic review of the literature by Sawka and coworkers.[99] Irregular menses in the first year after treatment occurred in 27% of women following radioactive iodine treatment, and early menopause occurred in some women. Garsi and colleagues[100] described 483 patients exposed to ^{131}I treatment for thyroid carcinoma and concluded that **no evidence suggests that exposure to radioiodine affects the outcome of subsequent pregnancies and offspring.**

Postpartum Thyroid Dysfunction

Postpartum thyroiditis (PPT) **is defined as transient thyroid dysfunction in the first year after delivery in women who were euthyroid before pregnancy on no thyroid therapy.**[101,102] PPT also occurs following spontaneous or medically induced abortions.[103] **The etiology in most cases is autoimmune chronic (Hashimoto) thyroiditis, with a few cases due to hypothalamic or pituitary lesions** (Box 42-7).[104]

PPT, a variant of Hashimoto or chronic thyroiditis, is the most common cause of thyroid dysfunction in the postpartum period. Women with type 1 diabetes mellitus and other

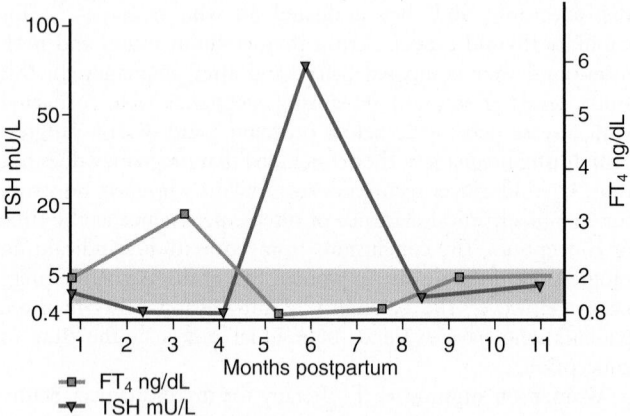

FIG 42-6 Clinical course of postpartum thyroiditis. The green band indicates the reference range. FT$_4$, free thyroxine; TSH, thyroid-stimulating hormone.

autoimmune diseases are at higher risk for developing PPT.[105] The clinical diagnosis is not always obvious, and the clinician should be concerned about nonspecific symptoms such as tiredness, fatigue, depression, palpitations, and irritability in women following the birth of a child or after a miscarriage or abortion. Fatigue is the most common complaint.[106] Predictors for the development of PPT include high titers of TPOAb in the first trimester of gestation, family or personal history of thyroid disease, presence of goiter, and smoking. Patients at risk should be evaluated in the first year postpartum at 3, 6, and 12 months after delivery.

Postpartum thyroiditis may also develop in women with negative antibodies. In a study from the Netherlands, the authors suggested two forms of PPT: an autoimmune form, which is most common and eventually will develop into chronic hypothyroidism, and a nonautoimmune form without antibodies that appears to be transient without progressing to permanent hypothyroidism. This has recently been confirmed.[102] The incidence of PTT in women with negative TPOAb was 1.7%.

The clinical course of PPT is not uniform (Fig. 42-6). In about one third of cases, mild symptoms of hyperthyroidism may develop between 1 and 4 months postpartum. On physical examination, a goiter is felt in most cases and is firm and non-tender to palpation. Tachycardia may be detected. Thyroid tests are in the hyperthyroid range, and thyroid antibodies (TPOAbs) are elevated in the vast majority of cases. Titers of TRAb, a marker of Graves disease, are negative. In one third of the patients, the hyperthyroid phase is followed by hypothyroidism (3 to 7 months) and return to a euthyroid state by 7 to 12 months after delivery. Antibody titers have a tendency to increase during this process, and a change in the size of the goiter is usually noted. In one third of patients, the course of PPT is different, characterized by an initial episode of hypothyroidism between 3 and 7 months postpartum without the initial hyperthyroid phase. The permanent incidence of hypothyroidism 12 months after delivery ranges from 2% to 21%. By 5 years after the diagnosis of PPT, most studies report an incidence of permanent hypothyroidism of 50%. In summary, presentation of PPT is characterized by (1) an episode of hyperthyroidism (1 to 3 months), followed by hypothyroidism (3 to 7 months) and reverting to euthyroidism (after the seventh month); (2) an episode of hyperthyroidism (1 to 4 months) reverting to euthyroidism; (3) an episode of hypothyroidism (3 to 7 months) reverting to a euthyroid state; and (4) permanent hypothyroidism after the hypothyroid phase (see Fig. 42-6). **It is recommended that a diagnosis of PPT be considered for any thyroid abnormality that occurs within 1 year after a delivery or miscarriage.**

Graves hyperthyroidism may recur after delivery with an exacerbation in the first 3 months or between 6 and 12 months postpartum. The symptoms of hyperthyroidism are more severe than those in patients with PPT, and patients with Graves disease benefit from antithyroid medications. On physical examination, women with Graves hyperthyroidism may present with ophthalmopathy, a visible goiter, and in many situations a bruit. Titers of TRAb are positive. If not contraindicated, as in breastfeeding mothers, a 4- or 24-hour thyroid radioactive iodine uptake (RAIU) is helpful in establishing the etiology. It will be very low in patients with PPT, whereas it is high normal or elevated in patients with recurrent hyperthyroidism due to Graves disease. Ide and colleagues studied 42 women with newly developed hyperthyroidism after delivery. Eighteen patients had Graves disease and 24 had thyroiditis. Twelve of 14 patients who developed thyrotoxicosis in the first 3 months postpartum had postpartum thyroiditis; all patients who developed thyrotoxicosis after 6.5 months postpartum had Graves disease. TRAbs were positive in all women with Graves hyperthyroidism and were negative in those with PPT. **The late postpartum period (8 to 12 months)** is associated with the risk of developing **Graves disease** de novo. Whether hyperthyroidism is due to a recurrence or new onset of Graves disease, treatment with antithyroid medications is indicated, or the physician may advise ablation therapy.

Although most patients with PPT recover spontaneously, treatment is indicated for symptomatic patients. In the presence of hyperthyroid symptoms, β-adrenergic blocking drugs (propranolol 10 to 40 mg every 6 hr or atenolol 25 to 50 mg every 24 hr) are effective in controlling the symptoms. Antithyroid medications are not effective because the hyperthyroxinemia is secondary to the release of thyroid hormones due to the acute injury to the gland (destructive hyperthyroidism). For hypothyroid symptoms, small amounts of L-thyroxine (50 μg/day) will control symptoms and allow for spontaneous recovery of thyroid function after discontinuation of the drug. However, in women who desire future pregnancies, it has been recommended that L-thyroxine therapy be continued because these patients are at high risk for developing hypothyroidism in a future pregnancy.[107]

Preventing PPT with the administration of selenium during pregnancy in women with chronic thyroiditis was evaluated by Negro and associates. They studied two groups of pregnant women: 77 received 200 μg/day of selenium during pregnancy and postpartum, and 74 were given a placebo. A significant reduction was seen in the incidence of PPT between both groups: 28.6% of women receiving selenium developed PPT compared with 48.6% of those taking placebo ($P < .01$). Future studies will be needed to confirm these findings.

KEY POINTS

◆ Hyperthyroidism due to Graves disease needs to be differentiated in the first trimester of pregnancy from the syndrome of gestational thyrotoxicosis.

◆ Recent reports indicate increased risk for liver failure with the use of propylthiouracil (PTU); it is recommended that PTU be used in the first trimester of pregnancy and methimazole (MMI) after 13 weeks' gestation. MMI is not indicated in the first trimester because of the potential risk for the syndrome of MMI embryopathy. PTU may also be teratogenic, but the risk is much less than that associated with MMI.

◆ Women with Graves disease planning a pregnancy should be informed of the teratogenicity of antithyroid drugs.

◆ The dose of antithyroid medications should be adjusted frequently, aiming to use the minimal amount of drug that will keep the FT_4 at the upper limit of normal.

◆ Breastfeeding is not contraindicated in women on antithyroid therapy, provided that the maximal daily dose is 300 mg of PTU and 20 mg of MMI.

◆ Hypothyroid women on thyroid replacement therapy should have their thyroid tests checked at the time of planning their pregnancy, and they should have their serum TSH adjusted to close to 1 mIU/L.

◆ Women on suppressive T_4 therapy for thyroid cancer before pregnancy must continue with therapy. The levothyroxine dose should be adjusted to keep serum TSH at the same level before pregnancy and to keep FT_4 within the normal reference range.

◆ In hypothyroid women, thyroid tests should be performed at the time pregnancy is diagnosed and should be checked every 2 to 4 weeks in the first trimester. An increase in levothyroxine dose is needed in more than 50% of patients on thyroid replacement therapy.

◆ Women with risk factors for thyroid disease—such as a family history of thyroid disease, the presence of a goiter, or a history of PPT—should be studied before or early in pregnancy. Determinations of serum TSH and TPOAb are recommended in these women.

◆ Postpartum thyroiditis affects up to 16.7% of all women in the postpartum period. Women with chronic thyroiditis are at higher risk for developing the syndrome. Long-term follow-up is strongly advised because up to 50% of these patients will develop permanent hypothyroidism in 5 to 10 years.

REFERENCES

1. Kovacs CS, Kronenberg HM. Maternal fetal calcium and bone metabolism during pregnancy, puerperium and lactation. *Endocr Rev.* 1997;18:832.
2. Dahlman T, Sjoberg HE, Bucht E. Calcium homeostasis in normal pregnancy and puerperium: a longitudinal study. *Acta Obstet Gynecol Scant.* 1994;73:393.
3. Kelly T. Primary hyperparathyroidism during pregnancy. *Surgery.* 1991;110:1028.
4. Shani H, Sivan E, Cassif E, et al. Maternal hypercalcemia as a possible cause of unexplained fetal polyhydramnios: a case series. *Am J Obstet Gynecol.* 2008;199:410.e1.
5. Ficinski M, Mestman JH. Primary hyperparathyroidism during pregnancy. *Endocr Pract.* 1996;2:362.
6. Pothiwala P, Levine SN. Parathyroid surgery in pregnancy: review of the literature and localization by aspiration for parathyroid hormone levels. *J Perinatol.* 2009;29:779.
7. Horjus C, Groot I, Telting D, et al. Cinacalcet for hyperparathyroidism in pregnancy and puerperium. *J Pediatr Endocrinol Metab.* 2009;22:741.
8. Loughead JL, Mughal Z, Mimouni F, et al. Spectrum and natural history of congenital hyperparathyroidism secondary to maternal hypocalcemia. *Am J Perinatol.* 1990;7:350.
9. Barrett H, McEleduff A. Vitamin D and pregnancy: an old problem revisited. *Best Pract Res Clin Endocrinol Metab.* 2010;24:527.
10. Theodoratou E, Tzoulaki I, Zgaga L, Ioaannidis JPA. Vitamin D and multiple health outcomes: umbrella review of systematic reviews and meta-analysis of observational studies and randomized trials. *BMJ.* 2014;348:2035.
11. De-Regil LM, Palacios C, Ansary A, Kulier R, Peña-Rosas JP. Vitamin D supplementation for women during pregnancy. *Cochrane Database Syst Rev.* 2012;(2):CD008873.
12. Ross CA, Abrams SA, Aloia JF, et al: Dietary reference intake for calcium and vitamin D: report at a glance. Institute of Medicine of the National Academies, released date: 11/20/2010.
13. Wiser J, Florio I, Neff M, et al. Changes in bone density and metabolism in pregnancy. *Acta Obstet Gynecol Scand.* 2005;94:349.
14. Barbour LA, Kick SD, Steiner JF, et al. A prospective study of heparin induced osteoporosis in pregnancy using bone densitometry. *Am J Obstet Gynecol.* 1994;170:862.
15. Glinoer D. The regulation of thyroid function in pregnancy: pathways of endocrine adaptation from physiology to pathology. *Endocr Rev.* 1997;18:404.
16. Krassas GE, Poppe K, Glineor D. Thyroid function and human reproductive health. *Endocr Rev.* 2010;31:702.
17. Pearce EN. Iodine in pregnancy: is salt iodization enough? *J Clin Endocrinol Metab.* 2008;93:2466.
18. Kratzsch J, Pulzer F. Thyroid gland development and defects. *Best Pract Res Clin Endocrinol Metab.* 2008;22:57.
19. Glinoer D, Spencer CA. Serum TSH determinations in pregnancy: how, when and why? *Nat Rev Endocrinol.* 2010;6:526.
20. Abalovich M, Amino N, Barbour LA, et al. Management of thyroid dysfunction during pregnancy and postpartum: an Endocrine Society clinical practice guideline. *J Clin Endocrinol Metab.* 2007;92:S1.
21. Li C, Shan A, Mao J, et al. Assessment of thyroid function during first trimester pregnancy: what is the rational upper limit of serum TSH during the first trimester in Chinese pregnant women? *J Clin Endocr Metab.* 2014;99:73-79.
22. Tyler PN, Minassian C, Rehman A, et al. TSH levels and risk of miscarriage in women on long-term levothyroxine: a community-based study. *J Clin Endocrinol Metab.* 2014;9:3895-3902.
23. Marwaha RK, Chopra S, Gopalakrishnan S, et al. Establishment of reference range for thyroid hormones in normal pregnant Indian women. *Br J Obstet Gynaecol.* 2008;115:602-660.
24. Lee RH, Spencer CA, Mestman JH, et al. Free T4 immunoassays are flawed during pregnancy. *Am J Obstet Gynecol.* 2009;200:260.e1.
25. Mandel SL, Larsen PR, Seely EW, et al. Increased need for thyroxine during pregnancy in women with primary hypothyroidism. *N Engl J Med.* 1990;323:91.
26. Yassa L, Marqusee E, Fawcett R, et al. Thyroid hormone early adjustment in pregnancy: the THERAPY trial. *J Clin Endocrinol Metab.* 2010;95:3234.
27. Lazarus JH, Hall R, Othman S, et al. The clinical spectrum of postpartum thyroid disease. *QJM.* 1996;89:429.
28. de Escobar GM, Obregon MJ, del Rey FE. Is neuropsychological development related to maternal hypothyroidism or to maternal hypothyroxinemia? *J Clin Endocrinol Metab.* 2000;85:3975.

29. Patil-Sisodia K, Mestman JH. Graves hyperthyroidism and pregnancy: a clinical update. *Endocr Pract.* 2010;16:118.

30. Goodwin TM, Montoro MN, Mestman JH. Transient hyperthyroidism and hyperemesis gravidarum: clinical aspects. *Am J Obstet Gynecol.* 1992; 167:648.

31. Niebyl JR. Nausea and vomiting in pregnancy. *N Engl J Med.* 2010; 363:1544.

32. Goodwin TM, Hershman JM. Hyperthyroidism due to inappropriate production of human chorionic gonadotropin. *Clin Obstet Gynceol.* 1997; 40:32.

33. Tagami T, Hagiwara H, Kimura T, et al. The incidence of gestational hyperthyroidism and postpartum thyroiditis in treated patients with Graves' disease. *Thyroid.* 2007;17:767.

34. Millar LK, Wing DA, Leung AS, et al. Low birth weight and preeclampsia in pregnancies complicated by hyperthyroidism. *Obstet Gynecol.* 1994; 84:946.

35. Momotani N, Noh J, Oyangi H, et al. Antithyroid drug therapy for Graves' disease during pregnancy: optimal regimen for fetal thyroid status. *N Engl J Med.* 1986;315:24.

36. Mortimer RH, Tyack SA, Galligan JP, et al. Graves' disease in pregnancy: TSH receptor binding inhibiting immunoglobulins and maternal and neonatal thyroid function. *Clin Endocrinol (Oxf).* 1990;32:141.

37. Kempers MJE, van Trotsenburg ASP, van Tijn DA. Disturbance of the fetal thyroid hormone state has long-term consequences for treatment of thyroidal and central congenital hypothyroidism. *J Clin Endocrinol Metab.* 2005;90:4094.

38. Luton D, LeGac I, Vuillard E. Management of Graves' disease during pregnancy: the key role of fetal thyroid gland monitoring. *J Clin Endocrinol Metab.* 2005;90:6093.

39. Copoper DS, Rivkees SA. Putting propylthiouracil in perspective. *J Clin Endocriol Metab.* 2009;94:1881.

40. Taylor PN, Vaidya B. Side effects of anti-thyroid drugs and their impact on the choice of treatment for thyrotoxicosis in pregnancy. *Eur Thyroid J.* 2012;1(3):176-185.

41. Bahn RS, Burch HS, Cooper DS, et al. The role of propylthiouracil in the management of Graves' disease in adults: report of a meeting jointly sponsored by the American Thyroid Association and the Food and Drug Administration. *Thyroid.* 2009;19:673-674.

42. Barbero P, Valdez R, Rodriguez H, et al. Choanal atresia associated with maternal hyperthyroidism treated with methimazole: a case control study. *Am J Med Genet.* 2008;146A:2390.

43. Besancon A, Beltrand J, Le Gac I, et al. Management of neonates born to women with Graves' disease: a cohort study. *Eur J Endocrinol.* 2014;170: 855f-862f.

44. Andersen SL, Olsen J, Wu CS, Laurberg P. Birth defects after early pregnancy use of antithyroid drugs: A Danish nationwide study. *J Clin Endocrinol Metab.* 2013;98:4373-4381.

45. Andersen SL, Olsen J, Wu CS, Laurberg P. Severity of birth defects after propylthiouracil exposure in early pregnancy. *Thyroid.* 2014;24: 1530-1540.

46. Laurberg P, Andersen SL. Antithyroid drug use in early pregnancy and birth defects: time windows of relative safety and high risk? *Eur J Endocrinol.* 2014;171:R13-R20.

47. Laurberg P, Bournaud C, Karmisholt J, et al. Management of Graves' hyperthyroidism in pregnancy: focus on both maternal and foetal thyroid function, and caution against surgical thyroidectomy in pregnancy. *Eur J Endocrinol.* 2009;160:1.

48. Stoffer SS, Hamburger JI. Inadvertent 131I therapy for hyperthyroidism in the first trimester of pregnancy. *J Nucl Med.* 1976;17:146.

49. Azizi F, Khoshmiat M, Bahrainian M, et al. Thyroid function and intellectual development of infants nursed by mothers taking methimazole. *J Clin Endocrinol Metab.* 2000;85:3233.

50. Nayakk B, Burman K. Thyrotoxicosis and thyroid storm. *Endocrinol Metab Clin North Am.* 2006;35:663.

51. Polak M, Luton D. Fetal thyroidology. Best practice and research. *Clin Endocrinol Metab.* 2014;28:161-173.

52. Polak M, Leger J, Oury JF, et al. Fetal cord blood sampling in the diagnosis and the treatment of fetal hyperthyroidism in the offspring of a euthyroid mother producing thyroid stimulating immunoglobulins. *Ann Endocrinol (Paris).* 1997;58:338.

53. Kilpatrick S. Umbilical blood sampling in women with thyroid disease in pregnancy: is it necessary? *Obstet Gynecol.* 2003;189:1.

54. Van Vliet G, Polak M, Ritzen EM. Treating fetal thyroid and adrenal disorders through the mother. *Nat Clin Pract.* 2008;4:675.

55. Davis LE, Leveno KJ, Cunningham FG. Hypothyroidism complicating pregnancy. *Obstet Gynecol.* 1988;72:108.

56. Leung AS, Millar LK, Koonings PP, et al. Perinatal outcome in hypothyroid pregnancies. *Obstet Gynecol.* 1993;81:349.

57. Klein RZ, Haddow JE, Faix JD, et al. Prevalence of thyroid deficiency in pregnant women. *Clin Endocrinol (Oxf).* 1991;35:41.

58. McClain M, Lambert-Messerlian G, Haddow JE. Sequential first- and second-trimester TSH, free thyroxine, and thyroid antibody measurements in women with known hypothyroidism: FaSTER trial study. *Am J Obstet Gynecol.* 2008;199:129.e1.

59. Gutenberg A, Hans V, Puchner M, et al. Primary hypophysitis: clinical-pathological correlations. *Eur J Endocrinol.* 2006;155:101.

60. Burman KD. Controversies surrounding pregnancy, maternal thyroid status and fetal outcome. *Thyroid.* 2009;19:323.

61. Casey BM, Dashe JS, Wells CE, et al. Subclinical hypothyroidism and pregnancy outcome. *Obstet Gynecol.* 2005;105:239.

62. Cleary-Goldman J, Malone FD, Lambert-Messerlian G, et al. Maternal thyroid hypofunction and pregnancy outcome. *Obstet Gynecol.* 2008; 112:85.

63. Haddow JE, Palomaki GE, Allan WC, et al. Maternal thyroid deficiency during pregnancy and subsequent neuropsychological development of the child. *N Engl J Med.* 1999;341:549.

64. Henrichs J, Bongers-Schokking JJ, Schenk JJ, et al. Maternal thyroid function during early pregnancy and cognitive functioning in early childhood: the generation R study. *J Clin Endocrinol Meetab.* 2010;95:4227.

65. De Groot L, Abalovich M, Alexander EK, et al. Management of thyroid dysfunction during pregnancy and postpartum: an Endocrine Society clinical practice guideline. *J Clin Endocrinol Metab.* 2012;97:2543-2565.

66. Stagnaro-Green A, Abalovich M, Alexander E, et al. American Thyroid Association Taskforce on Thyroid Disease During Pregnancy and Postpartum. Guidelines of the American Thyroid Association for the diagnosis and management of thyroid disease in pregnancy and postpartum. *Thyroid.* 2011;21:1081-1125.

67. Negro R, Schwartz A, Gismondi R, et al. Increased pregnancy loss rate in thyroid antibody negative women with TSH levels between 2.5 and 5.0 in the first trimester of pregnancy. *J Clin Endocrinol Metab.* 2010;95:E44.

68. Schneuer FJ, Nassar N, Tasevski V, et al. Association and predictive accuracy of high TSH serum levels in first trimester and adverse pregnancy outcomes. *J Clin Endoc Metab.* 2012;97:3115-3122.

69. Tyler PN, Minassian C, Rehman A, et al. TSH levels and risk of miscarriage in women on long-term levothyroxine: a community-based study. *J Clin Endocrinol Metab.* 2014;9:3895-3902.

70. Downing S, Halpern L, Carswell J, Brown RS. Severe maternal hypothyroidism corrected prior to the third trimester associated with normal cognitive outcome in the offspring. *Thyroid.* 2012;22:625-630.

71. Momotani N, Iwana S, Momotani K. Neurodevelopment in children born to hypothyroid mothers restored to normal thyroxine (T4) concentration by late pregnancy in Japan: no apparent influence of maternal T4 deficiency. *J Clin Endocrinol Metab.* 2012;97:1104-1108.

71a. Casey B. Effect of treatment of maternal subclinical hypothyroidism or hypothyroxinemia on IQ in offspring. *Am J Obstet Gynecol.* 2016;214:S2.

71b. Peaceman A. Effect of treatment of maternal subclinical hypothyroidism and hypothyroxinemia on pregnancy outcomes. *Am J Obstet Gynecol.* 2016;214:S200.

72. Glinoer D. Maternal and fetal impact of chronic iodine deficiency. *Clin Obstet Gynecol.* 1997;40:102.

73. Casey BM, Dashe JS, Spong CY, et al. Perinatal significance of isolated maternal hypothyroxinemia identified in the first half of pregnancy. *Obstet Gynecol.* 2007;109:1129.

74. Lazarus JH, Bestwick JP, Channon S, et al. Antenatal thyroid screening and childhood cognitive function. *N Engl J Med.* 2013;36:493-501.

75. American Thyroid Association. Statement on early maternal thyroid insufficiency: recognition, clinical management and research direction. *Thyroid.* 2005;15:77.

76. Stagnaro-Green A, et al. Guidelines of the American Throid Association for the Diagnosis and Management of Thyroid Disease During Pregnancy and Postpartum. *Thyroid.* 2011;21:1081.

77. Vaidya B, Anthony S, Biklous M, et al. Detection of thyroid dysfunction in early pregnancy: universal screening or targeted high-risk case finding? *J Clin Endocrinol Metab.* 2007;92:203.

78. Negro R, Schwartz A, Gismondi R, et al. Universal screening versus case finding for detection and treatment of thyroid hormone dysfunction during pregnancy. *J Clin Endocrinol Metab.* 2010;95:1699.

79. Thung S, Funai EF, Grobman WA. The cost-effectiveness of universal screening in pregnancy for subclinical hypothyroidism. *Am J Obstet Gynecol.* 2009;200:267.

80. Brent GA. Diagnosing thyroid dysfunction in pregnant women: is case finding enough? *[Editorial] J Clin Endocrinol Metab.* 2007;92:39.

81. Abalovich M, Alcaraz G, Kleiman-Rubinsztein J, et al. The relationship of preconception thyrotropin levels to requirements for increasing the levothyroxine dose during pregnancy in women with primary hypothyroidism. *Thyroid*. 2010;20:1175.

82. Deleted in review.

83. Pearce EN, Farwell AP, Braverman LE. Thyroiditis. *N Engl J Med*. 2003; 348:2646.

84. Stagnaro-Green A, Roman SH, Cobin RH, et al. Detection of at-risk pregnancy by means of highly sensitive assays for thyroid autoantibodies. *JAMA*. 1990;264:1422.

85. Matsuura N, Yamada Y, Nohara Y, et al. Familial neonatal transient hypothyroidism due to maternal TSH binding inhibitor immunoglobulins. *N Engl J Med*. 1980;303:738.

86. Negro R, Formoso G, Mangieri T, et al. Levothyroxine treatment in euthyroid pregnant women with autoimmune thyroid disease: effects on obstetrical complications. *J Clin Endocrinol Metab*. 2006;91:2587.

87. Unuane D, Velkeniers B, Anckaert E, et al. Thyroglobulin autoantibodies: is there any added value in the detection of thyroid autoimmunity in women consulting for fertility treatment? *Thyroid*. 2013;23:1022-1028.

88. Loh JA, Wartofsky L, Jonklaas J, et al. The magnitude of increased levothyroxine requirements in hypothyroid pregnant women depends upon the etiology of the hypothyroidism. *Thyroid*. 2009;19:269.

89. Busnelli A, Somigliana E, Benaglia L, et al. Thyroid axis dysregulation during *in vitro* fertilization in hypothyroid-treated patients. *Thyroid*. 2014;24(11):1650-1655.

90. Karmon AE, Batsis M, Chavarro JE, Souter I. Preconceptional thyroid-stimulating hormone levels and outcomes of intrauterine insemination among euthyroid infertile women. *Fertil Steril*. 2015;103(1):258-263.

91. Cooper DS, Doherty GM, Haugen BR, et al. Revised American Thyroid Association Management Guidelines for patients with thyroid nodules and differentiated thyroid cancer. *Thyroid*. 2009;19:1167.

92. Sam S, Molitch ME. Timing and special concerns regarding endocrine surgery during pregnancy. *Endocrinol Metab Clin North Am*. 2003;32:337.

93. Moosa M, Mazzaferri EL. Outcome of differentiated thyroid cancer diagnosed in pregnant women. *J Clin Endocrinol Metab*. 1997;82:2862.

94. Vannucchi G, Perrino M, Rossi S, et al. Clinical and molecular features of differentiated thyroid cancer diagnosed during pregnancy. *Euro J Endocrinol*. 2010;162:145.

95. Mannisto T, Vaarasmaki M, Pouta A, et al. Antithyroperoxidase antibody and antithyroglobulin antibody positivity during the first trimester of pregnancy is a major risk for perinatal death. *J Clin Endocrinol Metab*. 2009;94:772.

96. Hrisch D, Levy S, Tsvetov G, et al. Impact of pregnancy on outcome and prognosis of survivors of papillary thyroid cancer. *Thyroid*. 2010;20:1179.

97. Mazzaferri E. Approach to the pregnant patient with thyroid cancer. *J Clin Endoc Metab*. 2011;96:265-272.

98. Imran SA, Rajaraman M. Managemet of differentiated thyroid cancer in pregnancy. *J Thyroid Res*. 2011;2011:549609.

99. Sawka AM, Lakra DC, Lea J, et al. A systematic review examining the effects of therapeutic radioactive iodine on ovarian function and future pregnancy in female thyroid cancer survivors. *Clin Endocrinol (Oxf)*. 2008;69:479.

100. Garsi JP, Schlumberger M, Rubino C, et al. Therapeutic administration of I131 for differentiated thyroid cancer: Radiation dose to ovaries and outcome of pregnancy. *J Nucl Med*. 2008;49:845.

101. Nicholson WK, Robinson KA, Smallridge RC, et al. Prevalence of postpartum thyroid dysfunction: a quantitative review. *Thyroid*. 2006;16:573.

102. Stagnaro-Green A, Schwartz A, Gismondi R, et al. High rate of persistent hypothyroidism in a large scale prospective study in postpartum thyroiditis in Southern Italy. *J Clin Endocrinol Metab*. 2011;96:652-657.

103. Marquesee E, Hill JA, Mandel SJ. Thyroiditis after pregnancy loss. *J Clin Endocrinol Metab*. 1997;82:2455.

104. Landek-Salgado MA, Gutenberg A, Lupi I, et al. Pregnancy, postpartum autoimmune thyroiditis and autoimmune hypophysitis: intimate relationships. *Autoimmun Rev*. 2010;9:153.

105. Alvarez-Marfany M, Roman SH, Drexler AJ, et al. Long term prospective study of postpartum thyroid dysfunction in women with insulin dependent diabetes mellitus. *J Clin Endocrinol Metab*. 1994;79:10.

106. Amino N, Mori H, Iwatani O, et al. High prevalence of transient postpartum thyrotoxicosis and hypothyroidism. *N Engl J Med*. 1982;306:849.

107. Stagnaro-Green A. Postpartum thyroiditis. *Best Pract Res Clin Endocrinol Metab*. 2004;18:303.

Additional references for this chapter are available at ExpertConsult.com.

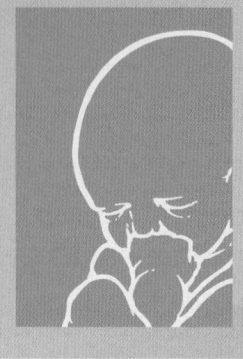

CHAPTER 43

Pituitary and Adrenal Disorders in Pregnancy

MARK E. MOLITCH

KEY ABBREVIATIONS	
Adrenocorticotropic hormone	ACTH
Arginine vasopressin	AVP
Clinically nonfunctioning adenoma	CNFA
Desmopressin	dDAVP
Diabetes insipidus	DI
Follicle-stimulating hormone	FSH
Growth hormone	GH
Human chorionic gonadotropin	hCG
Insulin-like growth factor I	IGF-1
Luteinizing hormone	LH
Magnetic resonance imaging	MRI
Prolactin	PRL
Thyroid-stimulating hormone	TSH

ANTERIOR PITUITARY

Anterior Pituitary Hormone Changes in Pregnancy

During pregnancy, the normal pituitary gland enlarges considerably as a result of estrogen-stimulated lactotroph hyperplasia.[1,2] Prolactin (PRL) levels rise gradually throughout gestation to prepare the breast for lactation.[3] Beginning in the second half of pregnancy, circulating levels of a growth hormone (GH) variant made by the syncytiotrophoblastic epithelium of the placenta increase, and pituitary GH secretion decreases as a result of the negative feedback effects of insulin-like growth factor I (IGF-1).[4,5] Pregnant patients with acromegaly have autonomous GH secretion; both forms of GH therefore persist in the blood.[6]

Cortisol levels rise progressively over the course of a normal gestation and result in a twofold to threefold increase by term due both to the estrogen-induced increase in corticosteroid-binding globulin (CBG) levels and an increase in cortisol production, so that the bioactive "free" fraction, urinary free cortisol levels, and salivary cortisol levels are also increased.[7,8]

Pituitary Tumors

Pituitary adenomas cause problems because of hormone hypersecretion and by causing hypopituitarism, and pregnancy-induced alterations in hormone secretion complicate the evaluation of patients with pituitary neoplasms. The influence of various types of therapy on the developing fetus also affects therapeutic decision making.

Prolactinoma

Hyperprolactinemia commonly causes symptoms of galactorrhea, amenorrhea, and infertility.[9] The differential diagnosis of hyperprolactinemia is extensive,[9] but this discussion will focus on the patient with prolactinoma. The choice of therapy has important consequences for decisions regarding pregnancy. **Transsphenoidal surgery for *microadenomas* is curative in 50% to 60% of prolactinomas after accounting for recurrences, and it rarely causes hypopituitarism when it is performed by experienced neurosurgeons on women with tumors less than 10 mm in diameter.**[10] For patients with *macroadenomas*, tumors 10 mm in diameter or larger, surgical cure rates are lower, and the risk of causing hypopituitarism is considerably greater.[10]

The dopamine agonists bromocriptine and cabergoline are the primary mode of medical therapy, restoring ovulatory menses in about 80% and 90% of cases, respectively,[9,10] **and reducing *macroadenoma* size.** A reduction in size of 50% or more occurs in 50% to 75% of patients with bromocriptine and in more than 90% of patients with cabergoline.[10]

The stimulatory effect of the hormonal milieu of pregnancy and the withdrawal of the dopamine agonist may result in significant prolactinoma enlargement (Fig. 43-1). Tumor enlargement that required intervention during pregnancy has been reported in 18 of 764 (2.4%) women with microadenomas, 50 of 238 (21%) with macroadenomas that had not undergone prior surgery or radiotherapy, and 7/148 (4.7%) with macroadenomas that had undergone prior surgery or radiotherapy.[11-14] In almost all cases, such enlargement was successfully treated with reinstitution of a dopamine agonist.[14] If the pregnancy is sufficiently advanced, another approach is to deliver the baby electively.[14] Surgical decompression is only resorted to if these other approaches fail.[14]

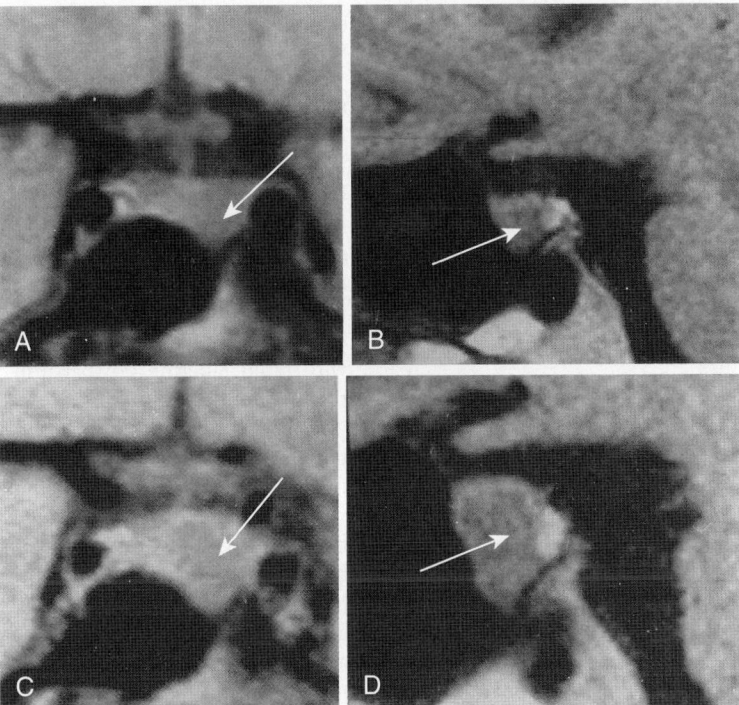

FIG 43-1 Coronal and sagittal magnetic resonance imaging scans of an intrasellar prolactin- secreting macroadenoma in a woman before conception (**A** and **B**) and at 7 months of gestation (**C** and **D**). Note the marked tumor enlargement at the latter point, at which time the patient was complaining of headaches. (From Molitch ME. Medical treatment of prolactinomas. *Endocrinol Metab Clin North Am.* 1999;28:143-170.)

When a dopamine agonist is stopped once a woman has missed her menstrual period and pregnancy is diagnosed, no increase in spontaneous abortions, ectopic pregnancies, trophoblastic disease, multiple pregnancies, or malformations were found in over 6000 pregnancies in which bromocriptine was used and in 822 pregnancies in which cabergoline was used.[11-15] Although data on safety of continuous dopamine agonist therapy during pregnancy are limited, treatment is probably not harmful.[14]

Patients with large macroadenomas should be assessed monthly for symptoms of tumor enlargement, and visual fields should be tested each trimester. PRL levels may rise without tumor enlargement and may not rise with tumor enlargement; therefore such tests are often misleading[16] and should not be done. In some patients, postpartum PRL levels and tumor sizes are actually reduced compared with values before pregnancy.[17] Therefore many women may be ovulatory postpartum and would not need resumption of a dopamine agonist. Nursing does not cause an increase of PRL levels nor does it increase headaches or visual disturbances suggestive of tumor enlargement.[18]

Acromegaly

Acromegaly is associated with infertility in about two thirds of cases because of associated hyperprolactinemia, hypopituitarism due to tumor mass effects, and even increased GH/IGF-1 levels (menses are restored with lowering of GH/IGF-1 levels); two or more of these causes occur in about one quarter of cases.[19] **Most patients with acromegaly are treated with surgery as primary therapy; those not cured by surgery are usually treated medically with the somatostatin analogues octreotide and lanreotide.**[20] Cabergoline may also be helpful in some cases.[20]

Conventional assays cannot distinguish between normal pituitary GH and the placental GH variant.[4] If it is critical to make a diagnosis of acromegaly during pregnancy, it may be possible by demonstrating GH pulsatility with frequent sampling, given that GH secretion in acromegaly is highly pulsatile but that of the placental variant is not.[6,21]

Only four patients with GH-secreting tumors have been reported to have enlargement of their tumors with a resultant visual field defect, in one case during pregnancy.[22-25] However, in one of these cases tumor enlargement was more likely due to octreotide withdrawal, and in another, it was due to hemorrhage into the tumor. Therefore as with prolactinomas, patients with acromegaly with macroadenomas should be monitored for symptoms of tumor enlargement and visual field testing.

Because of GH-induced insulin resistance, the risk of gestational diabetes is increased in acromegalic patients along with salt retention and gestational hypertension.[26,27] Cardiac disease has not proved to be an issue in pregnant women with acromegaly.[26,27]

The considerations regarding the use of bromocriptine and cabergoline in women with prolactinomas also apply to those with acromegaly. Fewer than 50 pregnant patients treated with somatostatin analogues have been reported, and no malformations were found in their children.[26-28] However, a decrease in uterine artery blood flow has been reported with short-acting octreotide,[28] and one fetus appeared to have intrauterine growth restriction (IUGR) that responded positively to a lower dose of long-acting release octreotide.[25] Octreotide binds to somatostatin receptors in the placenta and crosses the placenta,[28] and it can therefore affect developing fetal tissues in which somatostatin receptors are widespread. I recommend that octreotide and other somatostatin analogues be discontinued if pregnancy is considered and that contraception be used when these drugs are administered, and most[25,29] but not all[28] others concur. A reasonable option could be to switch to short-acting somatostatin analogues so that these can be continued until pregnancy is diagnosed and then stopped; their short half-life would then prevent fetal exposure. On the other hand, these drugs can control tumor growth, and for enlarging tumors, their reintroduction during pregnancy may be warranted rather than operating. Pegvisomant, a GH receptor antagonist, has been given to a patient with acromegaly during pregnancy without harm,[30] but its safety has not been established.

Thyrotropin-Secreting Tumors

Only three cases of pregnancy occurring in women with thyrotropin (thyroid-stimulating hormone [TSH])-secreting tumors have been reported.[31-33] In one of these cases, octreotide was stopped but had to be reinstituted to control tumor size.[31] In a second, octreotide was continued during pregnancy for tumor size control.[32] The most pressing issue with such tumors is the need to control hyperthyroidism during pregnancy, which can usually be done with standard antithyroid drugs (Chapter 43).[33] However, with growing macroadenomas, octreotide may be necessary for tumor size control,[31,32] and it is possible that it may be necessary to control the hyperthyroidism if thionamides are ineffective.

Clinically Nonfunctioning Adenomas

Pregnancy would not be expected to influence tumor size in patients with clinically nonfunctioning adenomas (CNFAs). Indeed, only two cases have been reported in which tumor enlargement during pregnancy resulted in a visual field defect.[22,34] In the second case, the patient responded rapidly to bromocriptine treatment, probably due to shrinkage of the lactotroph hyperplasia with decompression of the chiasm and probably with little or no direct effect on the tumor itself.[34]

Most CNFAs are actually gonadotroph adenomas. Two patients have been reported who had gonadotroph adenomas that secreted intact follicle-stimulating hormone (FSH) with a resultant ovarian hyperstimulation syndrome[35,36]; both became pregnant, one after having the FSH hypersecretion controlled by bromocriptine[35] and the second following surgical removal of the tumor.[36]

Hypopituitarism

Hypopituitarism may be partial or complete, and loss of gonadotropin secretion is common. Induction of ovulation may be difficult, and a variety of techniques have been used by reproductive endocrinologists, including administration of hCG and FSH,[37,38] pulsatile gonadotropin-releasing hormone,[37,38] and in vitro fertilization.[39,40] The malformation rate is normal in such pregnancies, but there seems to be an increased frequency of cesarean deliveries, miscarriages, and small-for-gestational-age (SGA) babies.[34,38,40]

Because of increased thyroxine turnover and volume of distribution in pregnancy, thyroxine (T_4) levels usually fall and TSH levels rise with a fixed thyroxine dose over the course of gestation.[41] The average increase in thyroxine needed in these patients is about 0.05 mg/day. Because patients with hypothalamic/pituitary dysfunction may not elevate their TSH levels normally in the face of the increased need for thyroxine, it is reasonable to increase the thyroxine supplementation by 0.025 mg after the first 4 to 6 weeks and by an additional 0.025 mg after the second trimester, also following total T_4 levels.

The dose of chronic glucocorticoid replacement does not usually need to be increased during pregnancy.[8] **Hydrocortisone is metabolized by the placental enzyme 11β-hydroxysteroid dehydrogenase 2 (11β-HSD2); thus the fetus is generally protected from any overdose of hydrocortisone. The usual dose is in the range of 12 to 15 mg/m²** given in two or three divided doses; 10 mg in the morning and 5 mg in the afternoon is a common regimen.[8] Additional glucocorticoids are needed for the stress of labor and delivery, such as 75 mg of intravenous (IV) hydrocortisone every 8 hours with rapid tapering postpartum.[8] Prednisolone does not cross the placenta, and prednisone crosses only minimally.[42] Suppression of neonatal adrenal function in offspring of women taking prednisone during pregnancy is very uncommon,[43] and the amounts passed in breast milk are negligible.[44]

Few data are available on the use of GH during pregnancy in hypopituitary individuals, and in most series, GH therapy has been stopped at conception.[45] Because the GH variant, which is biologically active, is produced by the placenta in substantial amounts beginning in the second half of pregnancy, and it can access the maternal circulation (see above), then at most the mother would be GH deficient only in the first half of pregnancy. When Curran and colleagues[45] analyzed 25 pregnancies that occurred in 16 patients with GH deficiency during which GH therapy was not continued, they found no adverse outcome for either the fetus or the mother from omitting GH therapy and concluded that GH replacement therapy during pregnancy is not essential for GH-deficient women.

Sheehan Syndrome

Sheehan syndrome consists of pituitary necrosis secondary to ischemia that occurs within hours of delivery,[46] usually secondary to hypotension and shock from an obstetric hemorrhage. The degree of ischemia and necrosis dictates the subsequent patient course (Table 43-1). This syndrome rarely occurs in current obstetric practice.[47]

Acute necrosis is suspected in the setting of an obstetric hemorrhage in which hypotension and tachycardia persist following adequate replacement of blood products. Failure to lactate and hypoglycemia may also occur.[46] Investigation should include obtaining blood samples for adrenocorticotropic hormone (ACTH), cortisol, prolactin, and free thyroxine. The ACTH stimulation test would be normal because the adrenal cortex would not be atrophied. Free thyroxine levels may prove normal initially because the hormone has a half-life of 7 days, and an additional sample should be sent after 1 week. Prolactin levels

TABLE 43-1	SYMPTOMS AND SIGNS OF SHEEHAN SYNDROME	
ACUTE FORM	**CHRONIC FORM**
Hypotension	Light headedness
Tachycardia	Fatigue
Failure to lactate	Failure to lactate
Hypoglycemia	Persistent amenorrhea
Extreme fatigue	Decreased body hair
Nausea and vomiting	Dry skin
	Loss of libido
	Nausea and vomiting
	Cold intolerance

are usually low in this setting. Diabetes insipidus (DI) may also occur and would be revealed with dehydration testing.[48]

If acute necrosis is suspected, treatment with saline and stress doses of corticosteroids should be instituted immediately after drawing the blood for testing. If later free thyroxine levels become low, therapy with levothyroxine is indicated. Additional pituitary testing with subsequent therapy should be delayed until recovery.

When milder forms of infarction occur, diagnosis may be delayed for months or years.[46] These women generally have a history of amenorrhea, decreased libido, failure to lactate, breast atrophy, loss of pubic and axillary hair, fatigue, and symptoms of secondary adrenal insufficiency with nausea, vomiting, diarrhea, and abdominal pain.[46] Rarely, some women retain gonadotropin secretion and may have normal menses and fertility.[43]

Lymphocytic Hypophysitis

Lymphocytic hypophysitis is thought to be autoimmune, with infiltration and destruction of the parenchyma of the pituitary and infundibulum by lymphocytes and plasma cells.[49-51] Generally occurring during pregnancy or in the postpartum period,[49-51] this condition is associated with symptoms of hypopituitarism or an enlarging mass lesion with headaches and visual field defects, and it is suspected based on its timing and lack of association with an obstetric hemorrhage or prior history of menstrual difficulties or infertility.[49-51] DI may also occur.[49-51] On magnetic resonance imaging (MRI) scans, diffuse enhancement is usually seen rather than a focal lesion that might indicate a tumor.[49-51] The clinical picture often allows a clinical diagnosis to be made without invasive procedures.

Treatment of lymphocytic hypophysitis is generally conservative and involves identification and correction of any pituitary deficits, especially of ACTH secretion, which is particularly common in this condition.[49-51] Data regarding the beneficial effects of high-dose corticosteroid treatment are inconclusive.[50] Surgery to debulk but not remove the gland is indicated in the presence of uncontrolled headaches, visual field defects, and progressive enlargement on scan. Spontaneous regression and resumption of partial or normal pituitary function may occur, although most patients progress to chronic panhypopituitarism.[49-51]

POSTERIOR PITUITARY

The set point for plasma osmolality at which arginine vasopressin (AVP) is secreted and thirst is stimulated is reduced approximately 5 to 10 mOsm/kg in pregnancy.[52] The placenta produces vasopressinase, an enzyme that rapidly inactivates AVP, thereby greatly increasing its clearance.[53,54]

Standard water deprivation tests, which require 5% weight loss, should be avoided during pregnancy because they can cause uterine irritability and can alter placental perfusion. Instead, desmopressin (dDAVP) is used to assess urinary concentrating ability.[53] Urinary concentrating ability in the pregnant patient should be determined in the seated position, because the lateral recumbent position inhibits maximal urinary concentration.[52]

Diabetes Insipidus

Central DI may develop in pregnancy because of an enlarging pituitary lesion, lymphocytic hypophysitis, or hypothalamic disease. Because of the increased clearance of AVP by placental vasopressinase, DI usually worsens during gestation, and subclinical DI may become manifest.[53-55] Desmopressin is resistant to vasopressinase and provides satisfactory, safe treatment during gestation, although a higher dose may be required.[56] During monitoring of the clinical response, clinicians should remember that the normal sodium concentration is 5 mEq/L lower during pregnancy,[52] and dDAVP transfers minimally into breast milk.[56]

Transient AVP-resistant forms of DI secondary to placental production of vasopressinase may occur spontaneously in one pregnancy but not in a subsequent one.[57] Some of these patients may respond to dDAVP therapy. Another rare cause of transient DI of pregnancy is placental abruption, in which the abruption causes a rise in vasopressinase.[58]

Acute fatty liver of pregnancy and other disturbances of hepatic function such as hepatitis may be associated with late-onset transient DI of pregnancy in some patients.[59] In some cases, this has been associated with the hemolysis, elevated liver enzymes, low platelets (HELLP) syndrome.[60] It is presumed the hepatic dysfunction is associated with reduced degradation of vasopressinase, which further increases vasopressinase levels and the clearance of AVP. Polyuria may develop either prior to delivery or postpartum.

DI that develops postpartum may be a result of Sheehan syndrome. Transient DI of unknown etiology has been described postpartum, lasting only days to weeks.[61]

Congenital nephrogenic DI is a rare X-linked disorder caused by a mutation in the vasopressin V2 receptor gene, which predominantly affects males.[53] Female carriers of this disease may have significant polyuria during pregnancy. Treatment is with thiazide diuretics,[54] which should be used with caution in pregnant women.

ADRENALS

In addition to the changes during pregnancy in cortisol outlined previously, plasma renin activity, angiotensin II, and aldosterone increase threefold to sevenfold during pregnancy, and blood volume is also increased.[62]

Cushing Syndrome

Fewer than 150 cases of Cushing syndrome in pregnancy have been reported.[63-69] Less than 50% of the pregnant patients described had pituitary adenomas, a similar number had adrenal adenomas, and more than 10% had adrenal carcinomas.[63-68] Pregnancies associated with the ectopic ACTH syndrome have been reported only rarely.[65,67,68] In many cases, the hypercortisolism first became apparent during pregnancy, with improvement and even remission after parturition.[65,66,68] Recently, cases have been reported of pregnancy-induced Cushing syndrome from human chorionic gonadotropin (hCG)-induced stimulation of ectopic luteinizing hormone (LH)/hCG receptors on the adrenal.[69]

Diagnosing Cushing syndrome during pregnancy may be difficult. Both conditions may be associated with weight gain in a central distribution, fatigue, edema, emotional upset, glucose intolerance, and hypertension. The striae associated with normal pregnancy are usually pale, but they are red or purple in Cushing syndrome. Hirsutism and acne may point to excessive androgen production, and proximal myopathy and bone fractures point to Cushing syndrome.

The laboratory evaluation is difficult. Elevated total and free serum cortisol and ACTH levels and urinary free cortisol excretion are compatible with that of normal pregnancy. The overnight dexamethasone test usually demonstrates inadequate suppression during normal pregnancy.[8,67] ACTH levels are normal to elevated even with adrenal adenomas,[8,63-65] perhaps because of the production of ACTH by the placenta or from the nonsuppressible stimulation of pituitary ACTH by placental corticotropin-releasing hormone (CRH).

A persistent circadian variation in the elevated levels of total and free serum cortisol during normal pregnancy may be most helpful in distinguishing Cushing syndrome from the hypercortisolism of pregnancy, because this finding is characteristically absent in all forms of Cushing syndrome.[7,8] Midnight levels of salivary cortisol during pregnancy have not yet been standardized.[66] In some cases, MRI scanning of the pituitary (without contrast) or ultrasound of the adrenal may be helpful, but the high frequencies of "incidentalomas" in both glands makes interpretation of imaging difficult.[70,71] Little experience has been reported with CRH stimulation testing or petrosal venous sinus sampling during pregnancy.[65,67,68]

Cushing syndrome is associated with a pregnancy loss rate of 25% due to spontaneous abortion, stillbirth, and early neonatal death because of extreme prematurity.[63,66-68] The passage of cortisol across the placenta may rarely result in suppression of the fetal adrenals.[72] Hypertension develops in most mothers with Cushing syndrome, and diabetes and myopathy are frequent. Postoperative wound infection and dehiscence are common after cesarean delivery.

In a review of 136 pregnancies collected from the literature, Lindsay and colleagues[67] found that the frequency of live births increased from 76% to 89% when active treatment was instituted by a gestational age of 20 weeks. Therefore treatment during pregnancy has been advocated.[63,67,68]

Medical therapy for Cushing syndrome during pregnancy with metyrapone and ketoconazole is not very effective,[66-68] and IUGR has been reported with ketoconazole.[67] **The FDA has issued a black-box warning for ketoconazole with respect to severe liver toxicity; therefore its use cannot be recommended.** Mitotane should be avoided because of fetal toxicity. Two new medications have recently been approved for the treatment of Cushing disease. Mifepristone, a cortisol receptor blocker, is highly effective, but because it is also a progesterone receptor blocker and an abortifacient, it cannot be used during pregnancy.[73] **Pasireotide is a new somatostatin analogue with modest efficacy in patients with Cushing disease.**[74] **It has the adverse effect of hyperglycemia, and there is no experience with its use during pregnancy.** However, the same cautions discussed above for somatostatin analogues should also hold true for the use of pasireotide in a patient with Cushing disease.

Transsphenoidal resection of a pituitary ACTH-secreting adenoma and laparoscopic resection of adrenal adenomas have been carried out successfully in several patients during the second trimester.[66-68] The live birth rate is approximately 87% after unilateral or bilateral adrenalectomy.[67] **Although any surgery poses risks for the mother and fetus,**[75] **it appears that with Cushing syndrome, the risks of not operating are considerably higher than those of proceeding with surgery.**

Adrenal Insufficiency

In developed countries, the most common etiology for primary adrenal insufficiency is autoimmune adrenalitis. Primary adrenal insufficiency from infections (**tuberculosis** or fungal), bilateral metastatic disease, hemorrhage, or infarctions is uncommon. Secondary adrenal insufficiency from pituitary neoplasms or glucocorticoid suppression of the hypothalamic-pituitary-adrenal axis may also occur.

Recognition of adrenal insufficiency may be difficult because many of the clinical features are found in normal pregnancies, including weakness, lightheadedness, syncope, nausea, vomiting, hyponatremia, and increased pigmentation. Addisonian hyperpigmentation may be distinguished from chloasma of pregnancy by its presence on the mucous membranes, on extensor surfaces, and on unexposed areas. Weight loss, hypoglycemia, salt craving, and excessive hyponatremia should prompt a clinical evaluation. **If unrecognized, maternal adrenal crisis may ensue at times of stress, such as a urinary tract infection or labor.**[76-78] **The fetoplacental unit largely controls its own steroid milieu, so maternal adrenal insufficiency generally causes no problems with fetal development.** Women with Addison disease are relatively infertile, and babies born to mothers with Addison disease have increased risks of preterm birth, low birthweight, and an increased rate of cesarean delivery.[79] Severe maternal hyponatremia or metabolic acidosis and poor maternal compliance with therapy may cause a poor fetal outcome.[76-78] Association with other autoimmune conditions such as anticardiolipin antibodies may lead to additional risks such as miscarriage.[80]

Adrenal insufficiency may be associated with laboratory findings of hyponatremia, hyperkalemia, hypoglycemia, eosinophilia, and lymphocytosis. Early morning plasma cortisol levels of 3.0 μg/dL (83 nmol/L) or less confirm adrenal insufficiency, whereas a cortisol level greater than 19 μg/dL (525 nmol/L) in the first or early second trimester excludes the diagnosis in a clinically stable patient.[81] However, plasma cortisol levels may fall in the normal "nonpregnant" range due to the increase in CBG concentrations in the second and third trimesters, but they will not be appropriately elevated for the stage of pregnancy.[82] Normal basal and cosyntropin (250 μg)-stimulated cortisol values have been established for pregnant women; for the first, second, and third trimesters, basal morning values (mean ± standard deviation [SD]) were 9.3 ± 2.2 μg/dL (257 ± 61 nmol/L), 14.5 ± 4.3 μg/dL (401 ± 119 nmol/L), and 16.6 ± 4.2 μg/dL (459 ± 116 nmol/L). Stimulated values were 29.5 ± 16.1 μg/dL (815 ± 445 nmol/L), 37.9 ± 9.0 μg/dL (1047 ± 249 nmol/L), and 34.7 ± 7.5 μg/dL (959 ± 207 nmol/L).[83] The 1-μg low-dose cosyntropin test has been reported to be accurate at 24 to 34 weeks' gestation using a cutoff of 30 μg/dL (828 nmol/L).[81] With primary adrenal insufficiency, ACTH levels will be elevated, and a level above 100 pg/mL (22 pmol/L) is consistent with the diagnosis.[84] However, ACTH will not be low with secondary forms because of placental production of this hormone, albeit insufficient to maintain normal maternal adrenal function.

In the unstable patient, empiric glucocorticoid therapy of hydrocortisone 50 to 75 mg IV should be administered pending the results of diagnostic testing. Thereafter, doses of 50 to 75 mg every 6 to 8 hours should be given in the face of severe stress and during labor.[78] Despite the normal increase in plasma cortisol during pregnancy, baseline maternal replacement doses of corticosteroids usually are not different from those required in the nonpregnant state.[78] Mineralocorticoid replacement requirements usually do not change during gestation, although some clinicians have reduced doses of fludrocortisone in the third trimester in an attempt to treat Addisonian patients who develop edema, exacerbation of hypertension, and preeclampsia.[78]

Patients who have received glucocorticoids as antiinflammatory therapy are presumed to have adrenal axis suppression for at least 1 year following cessation of such therapy.[85] These patients should be treated with stress doses of glucocorticoids during labor and delivery. They are at risk for postoperative wound infection and dehiscence, as are patients with endogenous Cushing syndrome, and their offspring are at risk for transient adrenal insufficiency.

Primary Hyperaldosteronism

Primary hyperaldosteronism rarely has been reported in pregnancy and is most often caused by an adrenal adenoma.[86-89] Reports of glucocorticoid-remediable hyperaldosteronism in pregnancy are rare.[90] The elevated aldosterone levels found in affected patients during pregnancy are similar to those in normal pregnant women, but the plasma renin activity is suppressed.[88] Moderate to severe hypertension develops in 85%, proteinuria in 52%, and hypokalemia in 55% of patients; symptoms may include headache, malaise, and muscle cramps.[86-89] Placental abruption and preterm delivery are also risks.[86,87] Interestingly, the very high progesterone levels of pregnancy may have an antimineralocorticoid effect at the renal tubules, and thus the hypertension and hypokalemia may ameliorate during pregnancy in some women.[89]

Spironolactone, the usual nonpregnant therapy for hyperaldosteronism, is contraindicated in pregnancy because it crosses the placenta and is a potent antiandrogen, which can cause ambiguous genitalia in a male fetus.[86] Eplerenone, a more selective aldosterone receptor blocker without antiandrogen activity, has been used successfully in one case during pregnancy without any untoward consequences for the fetus.[91] Surgical therapy may be delayed until after delivery if hypertension can be controlled with agents safe in pregnancy, such as amiloride, methyldopa, labetalol, and calcium channel blockers.[86,87] On the other hand, laparoscopic removal of an aldosterone-producing adenoma during pregnancy has been reported.[88] Potassium supplementation may be required, but the hypokalemia may ameliorate in pregnancy because of the antikaliuretic effect of progesterone. Both hypertension and hypokalemia may exacerbate postpartum because of removal of the progesterone effect.[89]

Pheochromocytoma

Exacerbation of hypertension is the typical presentation of pheochromocytoma, which can often be mistaken for pregnancy-induced hypertension or preeclampsia.[92-95] As the uterus enlarges and an actively moving fetus compresses the neoplasm, maternal complications such as severe hypertension, hemorrhage into the neoplasm, hemodynamic collapse, myocardial infarction, cardiac arrhythmias, congestive heart failure, and cerebral hemorrhage may occur. In 10% of patients, tumors may be outside of the adrenal, such as at the aortic bifurcation, and are particularly prone to hypertensive episodes with changes in position, uterine contractions, fetal movement, and Valsalva maneuvers.[92-95] Unrecognized pheochromocytoma has been associated with a maternal mortality rate of 50%.[92-95]

Placental transfer of catecholamines is minimal,[96] likely because of high placental concentrations of catechol O-methyltransferase and monoamine oxidase.[96] Adverse fetal effects such as hypoxia are a result of catecholamine-induced uteroplacental vasoconstriction and placental insufficiency[92,93] and of maternal hypertension, hypotension, or vascular collapse. Placental abruption may also occur.[92]

Diagnosis requires a high index of suspicion. Preconception screening of families known to have multiple endocrine neoplasia (MEN) type 2, von Hippel-Lindau disease, and neurofibromatosis is important.[97] The diagnosis should be considered in pregnant women with severe or paroxysmal hypertension, particularly in the first half of pregnancy or in association with orthostatic hypotension or episodic symptoms of pallor, anxiety, headaches, palpitations, chest pain, or diaphoresis.

Laboratory diagnosis of pheochromocytoma relies on measuring urine metanephrines and catecholamines and plasma metanephrines.[92-95] This is unchanged from the nonpregnant state because catecholamine metabolism is not altered by pregnancy per se. If possible, methyldopa and labetalol should be discontinued because these agents may interfere with the quantification of the catecholamines.[98] Tumor localization with MRI, with high-intensity signals noted on T_2-weighted images, provides the best sensitivity without fetal exposure to ionizing radiation.[92,93]

Differentiation from preeclampsia is generally simple. Edema, proteinuria, and hyperuricemia found in women with preeclampsia are absent in those with pheochromocytomas. Plasma and urinary catecholamines may be modestly elevated in severe preeclampsia and other serious pregnancy complications that require hospitalization, although they remain normal in mild preeclampsia or in pregnancy-induced hypertension.[99] Catecholamine levels are two to four times normal after an eclamptic seizure, however.[100]

Initial medical management involves α-blockade with phenoxybenzamine, phentolamine, prazosin, or labetalol. All of these agents are well-tolerated by the fetus, but phenoxybenzamine is considered the preferred agent because it provides long-acting, stable, noncompetitive blockade.[92-95] Phenoxybenzamine is started at a dose of 10 mg twice daily, with titration until the hypertension is controlled. Placental transfer of phenoxybenzamine occurs[101] but is generally considered safe.[92-95] However, two neonates of mothers treated with phenoxybenzamine have been reported with respiratory distress and hypotension that required ventilatory and inotropic support.[102] Beta-blockade is reserved for treating maternal tachycardia or arrhythmias that persist after full α-blockade and volume repletion.[92-95] β-Blockers may be associated with fetal bradycardia and with IUGR but are generally safe, with wide experience concerning their use.[93] All of these potential fetal risks are small compared with the risk of fetal wastage from unblocked high maternal levels of catecholamines. Hypertensive emergencies should be treated with phentolamine (1 to 5 mg) or nitroprusside, although the latter should be limited because of potential fetal cyanide toxicity.

Timing of surgical excision of the neoplasm is controversial and may depend on the success of the medical management and the location of the tumor. Pressure from the uterus, motion of the fetus, and labor contractions are all stimuli that may cause an acute crisis. In the first half of pregnancy, surgical excision may proceed once adequate α-blockade is established, although the risk of fetal loss may be higher with first-trimester surgery. In the early second trimester, fetal loss is less likely with surgery compared with the first trimester, and the size of the uterus will not make excision difficult. If a pheochromocytoma is not recognized until the second half of gestation, increasing uterine size makes surgical exploration challenging. Successful laparoscopic excision of pheochromocytomas has been described in the second trimester.[92-95] Other options include combined cesarean delivery and tumor resection or delivery followed by tumor resection at a later date.

Although successful vaginal delivery has been reported,[103] rates of maternal mortality have been higher than with cesarean delivery. Labor may result in uncontrolled release of catecholamines secondary to pain and uterine contractions. Severe maternal hypertension may lead to placental ischemia and fetal hypoxia. Cesarean delivery is most common, but in the well-blocked patient, vaginal delivery may be possible with pain management with epidural anesthesia and use of techniques of passive descent and instrumented delivery.

KEY POINTS

- About 30% of prolactin-secreting macroadenomas enlarge significantly during pregnancy.
- Dopamine agonists can be used safely for the treatment of prolactinomas if stopped when pregnancy is diagnosed.
- In patients with acromegaly, the risks of gestational diabetes and hypertension are increased.
- Gonadotropins, gonadotropin-releasing hormone, and assisted reproductive technology have been used successfully to achieve pregnancy in women with hypopituitarism.
- Sheehan syndrome is very uncommon with modern obstetric practice but still must be thought of in the postpartum unstable patient following hemorrhage.
- Lymphocytic hypophysitis that occurs during pregnancy is often associated with ACTH deficiency and may be fatal.
- Subclinical diabetes insipidus may become manifest during pregnancy because of placental vasopressinase.
- Cushing syndrome is associated with adverse outcomes for mother and fetus and should be treated aggressively during pregnancy.
- Although maintenance glucocorticoid replacement does not need to be increased in pregnant women with either hypopituitarism or primary adrenal insufficiency, stress doses of hydrocortisone are needed during labor and delivery and other stressful situations.
- Pheochromocytomas must be treated aggressively and usually require surgical resection during the pregnancy.

REFERENCES

1. Scheithauer BW, Sano T, Kovacs KT, et al. The pituitary gland in pregnancy. A clinicopathologic and immunohistochemical study of 69 cases. *Mayo Clin Proc.* 1990;65:461.
2. Elster AD, Sanders TG, Vines FS, et al. Size and shape of the pituitary gland during pregnancy and post-partum: Measurement with MR imaging. *Radiology.* 1991;181:531.
3. Rigg LA, Lein A, Yen SS. Pattern of increase in circulating prolactin levels during human gestation. *Am J Obstet Gynecol.* 1977;129:454.
4. Frankenne F, Closset J, Gomez F, et al. The physiology of growth hormones (GHs) in pregnant women and partial characterization of the placental GH variant. *J Clin Endocrinol Metab.* 1988;66:1171.
5. Eriksson L, Frankenne F, Edèn S, Hennen G, Von Schoultz B. Growth hormone 24-h serum profiles during pregnancy–lack of pulsatility for the secretion of the placental variant. *Br J Obstet Gynaecol.* 1989;96:949.
6. Beckers A, Stevenaert A, Foidart JM, Hennen G, Frankenne F. Placental and pituitary growth hormone secretion during pregnancy in acromegalic women. *J Clin Endocrinol Metab.* 1990;71:725.
7. Nolten WE, Lindheimer MD, Rueckert PA, et al. Diurnal patterns and regulation of cortisol secretion in pregnancy. *J Clin Endocrinol Metab.* 1980;51:466.
8. Lindsay JR, Nieman LK. The hypothalamic-pituitary-adrenal axis in pregnancy: challenges in disease detection and treatment. *Endocr Rev.* 2005;26:775.
9. Melmed S, Casanueva FF, Hoffman AR, et al. Diagnosis and treatment of hyperprolactinemia: an Endocrine Society Clinical Practice Guideline. *J Clin Endocrinol Metab.* 2011;96:273-288.
10. Gillam MP, Molitch ME, Lombardi G, et al. Advances in the treatment of prolactinomas. *Endocr Rev.* 2006;27:485.
11. Lebbe M, Hubinont C, Bernard P, et al. Outcome of 100 pregnancies initiated under treatment with cabergoline in hyperprolactinaemic women. *Clin Endocrinol.* 2010;73:230.
12. Ono M, Miki N, Amano K, et al. Individualized high-dose cabergoline therapy for hyperprolactinemic infertility in women with micro- and macroprolactinomas. *J Clin Endocrinol Metab.* 2010;95:2672.
13. Colao A, Abs R, Bárcena DG, et al. Pregnancy outcomes following cabergoline treatment: extended results from a 12-year observational study. *Clin Endocrinol.* 2008;68:66.
14. Molitch ME. Endocrinology in pregnancy: management of the pregnant patient with a prolactinoma. *Eur J Endocrinol.* 2015;172:R205-R213.
15. Stalldecker G, Mallea-Gil MS, Guitelman M, et al. Effects of cabergoline on pregnancy and embryo-fetal development: retrospective study on 103 pregnancies and a review of the literature. *Pituitary.* 2010;13:345.
16. Divers WA, Yen SS. Prolactin-producing microadenomas in pregnancy. *Obstet Gynecol.* 1983;62:425.
17. Domingue ME, Devuyst F, Alexopoulou O, Corvilain B, Maiter D. Outcome of prolactinoma after pregnancy and lactation: a study on 73 patients. *Clin Endocrinol (Oxf).* 2014;80:642.
18. Ikegami H, Aono T, Koizumi K, et al. Relationship between the methods of treatment for prolactinomas and the puerperal lactation. *Fertil Steril.* 1987;47:867.
19. Grynberg M, Salenave S, Young J, et al. Female gonadal function before and after treatment of acromegaly. *J Clin Endocrinol Metab.* 2010;95:4518.
20. Katznelson L, Laws ER Jr, Melmed S, et al. Acromegaly: an Endocrine Society Clinical Practice Guideline. *J Clin Endocrinol Metab.* 2014;99:3933.
21. Barkan AL, Stred SE, Reno K, et al. Increased growth hormone pulse frequency in acromegaly. *J Clin Endocrinol Metab.* 1989;69:1225.
22. Kupersmith MJ, Rosenberg C, Kleinberg D. Visual loss in pregnant women with pituitary adenomas. *Ann Intern Med.* 1994;121:473.
23. Okada Y, Morimoto I, Ejima K, et al. A case of active acromegalic woman with a marked increase in serum insulin-like growth factor-1 levels after delivery. *Endocr J.* 1997;44:117.
24. Cozzi R, Attanasio R, Barausee M. Pregnancy in acromegaly: a one-center experience. *Eur J Endocrinol.* 2006;155:279.
25. Caron P, Broussaud S, Bertherat J, et al. Acromegaly and pregnancy: a retrospective multicenter study of 59 pregnancies in 46 women. *J Clin Endocrinol Metab.* 2010;95:4680.
26. Cheng V, Faiman C, Kennedy L, et al. Pregnancy and acromegaly: a review. *Pituitary.* 2012;15:59.
27. Cheng S, Grasso L, Martinez-Grozco JA, et al. Pregnancy in acromegaly: experience from two referral centers and systematic review of the literature. *Clin Endocrinol.* 2012;76:264.
28. Maffei P, Tamagno G, Nardelli GB, et al. Effects of octreotide exposure during pregnancy in acromegaly. *Clin Endocrinol.* 2010;72:668.
29. Karaca Z, Tanriverdi F, Unluhizarci K, et al. Pregnancy and pituitary disorders. *Eur J Endocrinol.* 2010;162:453.
30. Brian SR, Bidlingmaier M, Wajnrajch MP, Weinzimer SA, Inzucchi SE. Treatment of acromegaly with pegvisomant during pregnancy: maternal and fetal effects. *J Clin Endocrinol Metab.* 2007;92:3374.
31. Caron P, Gerbeau C, Pradayrol L, et al. Successful pregnancy in an infertile woman with a thyrotropin-secreting macroadenoma treated with the somatostatin analog (octreotide). *J Clin Endocrinol Metab.* 1996;81:1164.
32. Blackhurst G, Strachan MW, Collie D, et al. The treatment of a thyrotropin-secreting pituitary macroadenoma with octreotide in twin pregnancy. *Clin Endocrinol.* 2002;56:401.

33. Chaiamnuay S, Moster M, Katz MR, Kim YN. Successful management of a pregnant woman with a TSH secreting pituitary adenoma with surgical and medical therapy. *Pituitary*. 2003;6:109.

34. Masding MG, Lees PD, Gawne-Cain ML, et al. Visual field compression by a non-secreting pituitary tumour during pregnancy. *J Roy Soc Med*. 2003;96:27.

35. Murata Y, Ando H, Nagasaka T, et al. Successful pregnancy after bromocriptine therapy in an anovulatory woman complicated with ovarian hyperstimulation caused by follicle-stimulating hormone-producing plurihormonal pituitary microadenoma. *J Clin Endocrinol Metab*. 2003;88:1988.

36. Sugita T, Seki K, Nagai Y, et al. Successful pregnancy and delivery after removal of gonadotrope adenoma secreting follicle-stimulating hormone in a 29-year-old amenorrheic woman. *Gynecol Obstet Invest*. 2005;59:138.

37. Hall R, Manski-Nankervis J, Goni N, et al. Fertility outcomes in women with hypopituitarism. *Clin Endocrinol*. 2006;65:71.

38. Overton CE, Davis CJ, West C, et al. High-risk pregnancies in hypopituitary women. *Human Reprod*. 2002;17:1464.

39. Esfandiari N, Gotlieb L, Casper RF. Live birth of healthy triplets after in vitro fertilization and embryo transfer in an acromegalic woman with elevated growth hormone. *Fertil Steril*. 2005;83:1041.

40. Kübler K, Klingmüller D, Gembruch U, et al. High-risk pregnancy management in women with hypopituitarism. *J Perinatol*. 2009;29:89.

41. Mandel SJ, Larsen PR, Seely EW, et al. Increased need for thyroxine during pregnancy in women with primary hypothyroidism. *N Engl J Med*. 1990;323:91.

42. Beitins IZ, Bayard F, Ances IG, et al. The transplacental passage of prednisone and prednisolone in pregnancy near term. *J Pediatr*. 1972;81:936.

43. Kenny FM, Preeyasombat C, Spaulding JS, et al. Cortisol production rate: IV. Infants born of steroid-treated mothers and of diabetic mothers. Infants with trisomy syndrome and with anencephaly. *Pediatrics*. 1966; 137:960.

44. McKenzie SA, Selley JA, Agnew JE. Secretion of prednisolone into breast milk. *Arch Dis Child*. 1975;50:894.

45. Curran AJ, Peacey SR, Shalet SM. Is maternal growth hormone essential for a normal pregnancy? *Eur J Endocrinol*. 1998;139:54.

46. Kelestimur F. Sheehan's syndrome. *Pituitary*. 2003;6:181.

47. Feinberg E, Molitch M, Endres L, et al. The incidence of Sheehan's syndrome after obstetric hemorrhage. *Fertil Steril*. 2005;84:975.

48. Iwasaki Y, Oiso Y, Yamauchi K, et al. Neurohypophyseal function in postpartum hypopituitarism: impaired plasma vasopressin response to osmotic stimuli. *J Clin Endocrinol Metab*. 1989;68:560.

49. Caturegli P, Newschaffer C, Olivi A, et al. Autoimmune hypophysitis. *Endocr Rev*. 2005;26:599.

50. Carmichael JD. Update on the diagnosis and management of hypophysitis. *Curr Opin Endocrinol Diabetes Obes*. 2012;19:314.

51. Glezer A, Bronstein MD. Pituitary autoimmune disease: nuances in clinical presentation. *Endocrine*. 2012;42:74.

52. Lindheimer MD, Davison JM. Osmoregulation, the secretion of arginine vasopressin and its metabolism during pregnancy. *Eur J Endocrinol*. 1995; 132:133.

53. Ananthakrishnan S. Diabetes insipidus in pregnancy: etiology, evaluation, and management. *Endocr Pract*. 2009;15:377.

54. Aleksandrov N, Audibert F, Bedard MJ, et al. Gestational diabetes insipidus: a review of an underdiagnosed condition. *J Obstet Gynaecol Can*. 2010;32:225.

55. Iwasaki Y, Oiso Y, Kondo K, et al. Aggravation of subclinical diabetes insipidus during pregnancy. *N Engl J Med*. 1991;324:522.

56. Ray JG. DDAVP use during pregnancy: an analysis of its safety for mother and child. *Obstet Gynecol Survey*. 1998;53:450.

57. Brewster UC, Hayslett JP. Diabetes insipidus in the third trimester of pregnancy. *Obstet Gynecol*. 2005;105:1173.

58. Wallia A, Bizhanova A, Huang W, et al. Acute diabetes insipidus mediated by vasopressinase after placental abruption. *J Clin Endocrinol Metab*. 2013;98:881.

59. Kennedy S, Hall PM, Seymour AE, et al. Transient diabetes insipidus and acute fatty liver of pregnancy. *Br J Obstet Gynaecol*. 1994;101:387.

60. Ellidokuz E, Uslan I, Demir S, et al. Transient postpartum diabetes insipidus associated with HELLP syndrome. *J Obstet Gynaecol Res*. 2006;32:602.

61. Raziel A, Rosenberg T, Schreyer P, et al. Transient postpartum diabetes insipidus. *Am J Obstet Gynecol*. 1991;164:616.

62. Wilson M, Morganti AA, Zervoudakis I, et al. Blood pressure, the renin-aldosterone system and sex steroids throughout normal pregnancy. *Am J Med*. 1980;8:97.

63. Bevan JS, Gough MH, Gillmer MD, Burke CW. Cushing's syndrome in pregnancy: the timing of definitive treatment. *Clin Endocrinol (Oxf)*. 1987;27:225.

64. Chico A, Manzanares JM, Halperin I, et al. Cushing's disease and pregnancy. *Eur J Obstet Gynecol Reprod Biol*. 1996;64:143.

65. Guilhaume B, Sanson ML, Billaud L, et al. Cushing's syndrome and pregnancy: aetiologies and prognosis in twenty-two patients. *Eur J Med*. 1992;1:83.

66. Madhun ZT, Aron DC. Cushing's disease in pregnancy. In: Bronstein MD, ed. *Pituitary Tumors and Pregnancy*. Norwell, MA: Kluwer Academic Publishers; 2001:149.

67. Lindsay JR, Jonklaas J, Oldfield EH, et al. Cushing's syndrome during pregnancy: personal experience and review of the literature. *J Clin Endocrinol Metab*. 2005;90:3077.

68. Vilar L, Freitas Mda C, Lima LH, Lyra R, Kater CE. Cushing's syndrome in pregnancy: an overview. *Arq Bras Endocrinol Metabol*. 2007;51: 1293.

69. Chui MH, Ozbey NC, Ezzat S, et al. Case report: Adrenal LH/hCG receptor overexpression and gene amplification causing pregnancy-induced Cushing's syndrome. *Endocr Pathol*. 2009;20:256.

70. Molitch ME. Management of incidentally found nonfunctional pituitary tumors. *Neurosurg Clin N Amer*. 2012;23:543.

71. Kannan S, Remer EM, Hamrahian AH. Evaluation of patients with adrenal incidentalomas. *Curr Opin Endocrinol Diabetes Obes*. 2013; 20:161.

72. Kreines K, DeVaux WD. Neonatal adrenal insufficiency associated with maternal Cushings syndrome. *Pediatrics*. 1971;47:516.

73. Fleseriu M, Molitch ME, Gross C, et al. on behalf of the SEISMIC study investigators. A new therapeutic approach in the medical treatment of Cushing's syndrome: glucocorticoid receptor blockade with mifepristone. *Endocr Pract*. 2013;19:313.

74. Colao A, Petersenn S, Newell-Price J, et al. for the Pasireotide B2305 Study Group. A 12-month phase 3 study of pasireotide in Cushing's disease. *N Engl J Med*. 2012;366:914.

75. Cohen-Kerem R, Railton C, Orfen D, et al. Pregnancy outcome following non-obstetric surgical intervention. *Am J Surgery*. 2005;190:467.

76. Albert E, Dalaker K, Jorde R, et al. Addison's disease and pregnancy. *Acta Obstet Gynecol Scand*. 1989;68:185.

77. Otta CF, de Meresian PS, Iraci GS, et al. Pregnancies associated with primary adrenal insufficiency. *Fertil Steril*. 2008;90:1199.

78. Ambrosi B, Barbetta L, Morricone L. Diagnosis and management of Addison's disease during pregnancy. *J Endocrinol Invest*. 2003;26:698.

79. Björnsdottir S, Cnattingius S, Brandt L, et al. Addison's disease in women is a risk factor for an adverse pregnancy outcome. *J Clin Endocrinol Metab*. 2010;95:5249.

80. Grottolo A, Ferrari V, Mariano M, et al. Primary adrenal insufficiency, circulating lupus anticoagulant and anticardiolipin antibodies in a patient with multiple abortions and recurrent thrombotic episodes. *Haematologica*. 1988;73:517.

81. McKenna DS, Wittber GM, Nagaraja HN, et al. The effects of repeat doses of antenatal corticosteroids on maternal adrenal function. *Am J Obstet Gynecol*. 2000;183:669.

82. Nolten WE, Lindheimer MD, Oparil S, et al. Desoxycorticosterone in normal pregnancy: I. sequential studies of the secretory patterns of desoxycorticosterone, aldosterone, and cortisol. *Am J Obstet Gynecol*. 1978; 132:414.

83. Suri D, Moran J, Hibbard JU, et al. Assessment of adrenal reserve in pregnancy: defining the normal response to the adrenocorticotropin stimulation test. *J Clin Endocrinol Metab*. 2006;91:3866.

84. Grinspoon SK, Biller BM. Clinical review 62: laboratory assessment of adrenal insufficiency. *J Clin Endocrinol Metab*. 1994;79:79.

85. Schlaghecke R, Kornely E, Santen RT, et al. The effect of long-term glucocorticoid therapy on pituitary-adrenal responses to exogenous corticotropin-releasing hormone. *N Engl J Med*. 1992;326:226.

86. Robar CA, Poremba JA, Pelton JJ, et al. Current diagnosis and management of aldosterone-producing adenomas during pregnancy. *Endocrinologist*. 1998;8:403.

87. Okawa T, Asano K, Hashimoto T, et al. Diagnosis and management of primary aldosteronism in pregnancy: case report and review of the literature. *Am J Perinatol*. 2002;19:31.

88. Nursal TZ, Caliskan K, Ertorer E, et al. Laparoscopic treatment of primary hyperaldosteronism in a pregnant patient. *Can J Chir*. 2009;52:E188.

89. Krysiak R, Samborek M, Stojko R. Primary aldosteronism in pregnancy. *Acta Clin Belg*. 2012;67:130.

90. Wyckoff JA, Seely EW, Hurwitz S, et al. Glucocorticoid-remediable aldosteronism and pregnancy. *Hypertension*. 2000;35:668.

91. Cabassi A, Rocco R, Berretta R, Regolisti G, Bacchi-Modena A. Eplerenone use in primary aldosteronism during pregnancy. *Hypertension*. 2012;59:e18.

92. Oliva R, Angelos P, Kaplan E, et al. Pheochromocytoma in pregnancy. A case series and review. *Hypertension*. 2010;55:600.

93. Sarathi V, Lila AR, Bandgar TR, et al. Pheochromocytoma and pregnancy: a rare but dangerous combination. *Endocr Pract*. 2010;16:300.

94. Lenders JW. Pheochromocytoma and pregnancy: a deceptive connection. *Eur J Endocrinol*. 2012;166:143.

95. Biggar MA, Lennard TW. Systematic review of phaeochromocytoma in pregnancy. *Br J Surg*. 2013;100:182.

96. Saarikoski S. Fate of noradrenaline in the human fetoplacental unit. *Acta Physiol Scand*. 1984;421(suppl):1.

97. Fishbein L, Orlowski R, Cohen D. Pheochromocytoma/paraganglioma: review of perioperative management of blood pressure and update on genetic mutations associated with pheochromocytoma. *J Clin Hypertens*. 2013;15:428.

98. Sheps SG, Jiang NS, Klee GC. Diagnostic evaluation of pheochromocytoma. *Endocrinol Metab Clin North Am*. 1988;17:397.

99. Pederson EB, Rasmussen AB, Christensen NJ, et al. Plasma noradrenaline and adrenaline in pre-eclampsia, essential hypertension in pregnancy and normotensive pregnant control subjects. *Acta Endocrinol*. 1982;99:594.

100. Khatun S, Kanayama N, Hossain B, et al. Increased concentrations of plasma epinephrine and norepinephrine in patients with eclampsia. *Eur J Obstet Gynecol Reprod Biol*. 1997;74:103.

101. Santeiro ML, Stromquist C, Wyble L. Phenoxybenzamine placental transfer during the third trimester. *Ann Pharmacother*. 1996;30:1249.

102. Aplin SC, Yee KF, Cole MJ. Neonatal effects of long-term maternal phenoxybenzamine therapy. *Anesthesiology*. 2004;100:1608.

103. Schenker JG, Granat M. Phaeochromocytoma and pregnancy—An updated appraisal. *Aust NZ J Obstet Gynaecol*. 1982;22:1.

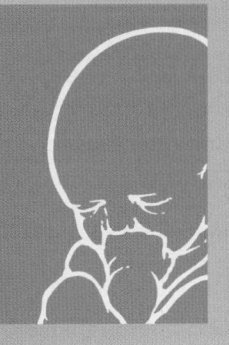

CHAPTER 44

Hematologic Complications of Pregnancy

PHILIP SAMUELS

KEY ABBREVIATIONS

Chorionic villus sampling	CVS
Hemolysis, elevated liver enzymes, low platelets	HELLP
Hemolytic uremic syndrome	HUS
Human immunodeficiency virus	HIV
Immune thrombocytopenic purpura	ITP
Immunoglobulin G	IgG
Intravenous immunoglobulin	IVIG
Mean corpuscular volume	MCV
Polymerase chain reaction	PCR
Red blood cell	RBC
Thrombotic thrombocytopenic purpura	TTP
Unusually large multimers of von Willebrand factor	ULVWf
Urinary tract infection	UTI
von Willebrand cleaving enzyme	ADAMTS13
von Willebrand disease	vWD
von Willebrand factor	vWF

PREGNANCY-ASSOCIATED THROMBOCYTOPENIA

Affecting approximately 4% of pregnancies, thrombocytopenia is the most frequent hematologic complication of pregnancy that results in consultation. As gestation progresses, platelet counts generally fall slightly owing to hemodilution and increased destruction.[1] Commonly, platelet counts will reach a nadir of 120,000/mm[3] during pregnancy; however, they should not fall below the normal range. **In pregnancy, the vast majority of cases of mild to moderate thrombocytopenia are caused by gestational thrombocytopenia.[2] This form of thrombocytopenia has little likelihood of causing maternal or neonatal complications.[3]** The obstetrician, however, should rule out other etiologies of thrombocytopenia that are associated with severe maternal or perinatal morbidity. The common and rare causes of thrombocytopenia in the gravida at term are shown in the Box 44-1.

Gestational Thrombocytopenia

Most patients with gestational thrombocytopenia generally have a platelet count of 120,000 to 149,000/mm[3]. However, about 1% of patients with gestational thrombocytopenia will have a platelet count of 50,000 to 99,000/mm[3]. **These patients require no therapy, and the fetus appears to be at negligible risk of being born with clinically significant thrombocytopenia or a bleeding diathesis.** This distinct entity was first suggested but not specifically defined in a study published in 1986 by Hart and colleagues.[4] In this report, 28 of 116 pregnant women (24%) who were evaluated prospectively during an 8-month period had platelet counts less than 150,000/mm[3] at least once during pregnancy. In all 17 patients who were followed after delivery, platelet counts returned to normal. These researchers were actually describing gestational thrombocytopenia before the condition had been recognized as a distinct entity. Samuels and colleagues[5] also investigated 74 mothers with gestational thrombocytopenia. Regardless of platelet antibody status, none of the infants born to these mothers demonstrated thrombocytopenia. Burrows and Kelton[6] have further shown that **there is little risk to the mother or neonate in cases of gestational thrombocytopenia.** In their study of 1357 healthy, pregnant women, 112 (8.3%) had platelet counts less than 150,000/mm[3]. The lowest platelet count was 97,000/mm[3]. The incidence of thrombocytopenia (platelet count < 150,000/mm[3]) in the infants of these 112 women was 4.3%, not statistically different from infants born to healthy pregnant women without thrombocytopenia (1.5%).[5] None of these infants had platelet counts less than 100,000/mm[3]. Indeed, the reports by Samuels and colleagues[5] and Burrows and Kelton[6] have convincingly demonstrated that gestational thrombocytopenia is a distinct and common entity that requires no treatment. However, **the obstetrician must use judgment in giving this diagnosis because no test exists**

BOX 44-1 CAUSES OF THROMBOCYTOPENIA DURING PREGNANCY

Common Causes

Gestational thrombocytopenia
Severe preeclampsia
Hemolysis, elevated liver enzymes, low platelets (HELLP) syndrome
Disseminated intravascular coagulation

Uncommon Causes

Immune thrombocytopenic purpura
Antiphospholipid antibody syndrome
Systemic lupus erythematosus
Human immunodeficiency virus (HIV) infection

Rare Causes

Thrombotic thrombocytopenic purpura
Hemolytic uremic syndrome
Type 2b von Willebrand syndrome
Hemoglobin SC crisis with splenic sequestration
Folic acid deficiency
Hematologic malignancies
May-Hegglin anomaly (congenital thrombocytopenia)
Wiskott-Aldrich syndrome

BOX 44-2 PENTAD OF FINDINGS IN THROMBOTIC THROMBOCYTOPENIC PURPURA*

Microangiopathic hemolytic anemia[†]
Thrombocytopenia[†]
Neurologic abnormalities[†] that include confusion, headache, paresis, visual hallucinations, seizures
Fever
Renal dysfunction

---

*The classic pentad is found in only 40% of patients.
[†]These three findings are present in 74% of patients.

---

for this disorder. **If platelet counts continue to fall to levels below 50,000/mm³, other diagnoses should be entertained.**

The decrease in platelet count that occurs in gestational thrombocytopenia is not merely the result of dilution of platelets with increasing blood volume; it also appears to be due to an acceleration of the normal increase in platelet destruction that occurs during pregnancy. This is demonstrated by the fact that the mean platelet volume (MPV) is increased in patients with gestational thrombocytopenia. However, if the platelet counts fall below 20,000/mm³ or if clinical bleeding is present, further investigation and intervention are warranted. This scenario, however, is rare, and it is difficult to determine whether these patients with profound thrombocytopenia have gestational thrombocytopenia or thrombocytopenia from another cause. Platelet antibody testing should only be utilized if suspicion is high for immune thrombocytopenic purpura (ITP). This would include a platelet count less than 50,000/mm³.

Immune Thrombocytopenic Purpura

Immune thrombocytopenic purpura affects 1 to 3 per 1000 pregnancies and rarely causes neonatal complications. Although rare cases of neonatal thrombocytopenia have been reported, fetal complications are almost nonexistent.[5] Therefore the focus should be on maternal disease and well-being.

In general, **pregnancy has not been determined to cause ITP or to change its severity**, but rare exceptions do exist. Harrington and associates[7] were the first to demonstrate that ITP was humorally mediated, and Shulman and colleagues[8] showed that the mediator of this disorder was immunoglobulin G (IgG). These findings were confirmed when Cines and Schreiber[9] developed the first platelet antiglobulin test, a radioimmunoassay, in 1979. Today, this test is usually performed using an enzyme-linked immunosorbent assay (ELISA) or flow cytometry. Newer assays have shown that these autoantibodies may be directed against specific platelet surface glycoproteins, including the IIb/IIIa and Ib/IX complexes.[10] In vivo, after the platelets are coated with antibody, they are removed from circulation by binding to the Fc receptors of macrophages in the reticuloendothelial system, especially the spleen. **Approximately 90% of women with ITP have platelet-associated IgG.[9] Unfortunately, this is not specific for ITP, because studies have shown that these tests are also positive in women with gestational thrombocytopenia and preeclampsia.**

To make the issue more confusing, the pathogenesis of ITP in children and adults usually differs. Childhood ITP most often follows a viral infection and clinically presents with petechiae and bleeding. This form of ITP is generally self-limited and disappears over time. Conversely, adults have milder bleeding and easy bruisability and are often diagnosed after a prolonged period of subtle symptoms. Adult ITP usually runs a chronic course, and long-term therapy is often eventually needed. Many pregnancies occur in women in their late teens and early twenties. In these women with a history of ITP, it may be difficult to ascertain whether the patient has childhood ITP or adult ITP. The distinction is important for counseling concerning long-term prognosis.

ITP has a predisposition for women aged 18 to 40 years, with an overall female-male ratio of 1.7.[11] It is a diagnosis of exclusion. The patient must have isolated thrombocytopenia with an unremarkable peripheral smear. She must have only bleeding clinically consistent with a depressed platelet count, such as petechiae. She must not be taking any medication, herbal compound, or illicit drug that may cause thrombocytopenia. Finally, the patient must have no other disease process than can cause thrombocytopenia, such as those listed in the box earlier in this chapter.[11,12] The American Society of Hematology has published a review of ITP that details the diagnostic and therapeutic guidelines.[13]

Thrombotic Thrombocytopenic Purpura and Hemolytic Uremic Syndrome

These two conditions are characterized by microangiopathic hemolytic anemia and severe thrombocytopenia. Pregnancy does not predispose a patient to these conditions, but they should be considered when evaluating the gravida with severe thrombocytopenia. Thrombotic thrombocytopenic purpura (TTP) is characterized by a pentad of findings, which are shown in Box 44-2.[14,15] **The complete pentad occurs only in approximately 40% of patients, but approximately 75% have a triad of microangiopathic hemolytic anemia, thrombocytopenia, and neurologic changes.[16]** Pathologically, these patients have thrombotic occlusions of arterioles and capillaries.[14] These occur in multiple organs, and no specific clinical manifestation for the disease is recognized. The clinical picture reflects the organs that are involved.

TTP/hemolytic uremic syndrome (HUS) may mimic preeclampsia. Because preeclampsia is much more common than this disorder, it should be considered first. However, **delay in diagnosing TTP/HUS can have fatal consequences**.

To diagnose the hemolytic anemia associated with TTP, the indirect antiglobulin (Coombs) test must be negative. This rules out an immune-mediated cause for the hemolytic anemia. Lactate dehydrogenase (LDH) should be elevated, the indirect bilirubin should be increased, and haptoglobin should be decreased, indicating ongoing hemolysis. Schistocytes are usually seen on the peripheral smear, if it is carefully reviewed. These tests all signify hemolysis, but specificities and sensitivities differ. For instance, LDH can be elevated in liver disease. Schistocytes are very specific but manifest themselves once the hemolysis is severe. The clinician should use the clinical picture, as well as some of these tests, to make the diagnosis of hemolysis. To be classified as TTP, the platelet count should be less than 100,000/mm^3. In renal insufficiency associated with TTP, the urine sediment is usually normal with an occasional red blood cell (RBC). This finding helps distinguish this disorder from a lupus flare, which more often has associated hematuria and casts. The serum creatinine is usually greater than 2 mg/dL. This degree of renal dysfunction is unusual, but not rare, in preeclampsia. Proteinuria, more than a trace amount, is usually seen on urine dipstick.

The neurologic findings in TTP are usually nonspecific. They include headache, confusion, and lethargy. Infrequently, generalized tonic-clonic seizures occur. Terrell and coworkers[17] examined the epidemiology of TTP/HUS occurring in Oklahoma between 1996 and 2004. In 206 reported cases, they found that 37% were idiopathic. However, 13% were associated with an autoimmune disease, and 7% occurred in pregnancy and postpartum. These researchers were able to project that the annual incidence of suspected TTP/HUS is 11 cases per million population, whereas the annual incidence of proven cases is 4.5 cases per million.[17] **If this disease is so rare, why include it in a text on obstetrics? Because if untreated, TTP carries a 90% mortality rate, whereas treatment with plasma exchange decreases the mortality rate to 20%.** Therefore obstetricians must be aware of this disease process so it can be quickly and aggressively treated.

Tsai and colleagues[18,19] **have found that a decrease of ADAMTS13 (the von Willebrand cleaving enzyme) activity is strongly associated with TTP.** This metalloprotease, also known as *von Willebrand cleaving enzyme*, cleaves unusually large multimers of von Willebrand factor (ULVWf). Activity can be decreased from a decrease in the metalloprotease or antibodies against it. If a deficiency in the activity and/or concentration of ADAMTS13 is apparent, ULVWf circulates in increased amounts, leading to increased platelet aggregation and the initiation of TTP. ADAMTS13 can be readily assayed in clinical laboratories. Ferrari and colleagues[20] have shown that **all four immunoglobulin subclasses of anti-ADAMTS13 antibodies are associated with TTP, but the IgG4 subclass is most common.** Congenital TTP is usually associated with a mutation of *ADAMTS13* that leads to a profound decrease in its activity.[21] Moatti-Cohen and colleagues[21] queried the French registry of thrombotic microangiopathies and found that 24% of women who developed TTP during pregnancy had the congenital type (Upshaw-Schulman syndrome) compared with less than 5% of total adult cases. Weiner[22] has published the most extensive literature review concerning TTP.

In this series of 45 patients, **40 developed the disease antepartum, and 50% occurred before 24 weeks' gestation. The mean gestational age at onset of symptoms was 23.4 weeks.** This finding may be helpful when trying to distinguish TTP from other causes of thrombocytopenia and microangiopathic hemolytic anemia that occur during gestation. In Weiner's review, the fetal and maternal mortality rates were 84% and 44%, respectively. These mortality rates are overly pessimistic, because this series included many patients who contracted the disease before plasma infusion/exchange therapy was utilized to treat TTP.

However, TTP may be confused with rarely occurring early-onset severe preeclampsia. **In preeclampsia, antithrombin III levels are frequently low, and this is not the case with TTP. This test, therefore, may be a useful discriminator between these two disorders.**

Although HUS has many features in common with TTP, it usually has its onset in the postpartum period. Patients with HUS display a triad of microangiopathic hemolytic anemia, acute nephropathy, and thrombocytopenia. HUS is rare in adults, and the thrombocytopenia is usually milder than that seen in TTP, with only 50% of patients having a platelet count less than 100,000/mm^3 at the time of diagnosis. The thrombocytopenia worsens as the disease progresses. A major difference between TTP and HUS is that 15% to 25% of patients with HUS develop chronic renal disease. HUS often follows infections with verotoxin-producing enteric bacteria. Cyclosporine therapy, cytotoxic drugs, and oral contraceptives may predispose adults to develop HUS. **The majority of cases of HUS that occur in pregnancy develop at least 2 days after delivery.** In fact, in one series, only 9 of 62 cases (14.5%) of pregnancy-associated HUS occurred antepartum. Four of these nine patients developed symptoms on the day of delivery. The mean time from delivery to development of HUS in patients in this series was 26.6 days. The maternal mortality rate may exceed 50% in postpartum HUS; however, this mortality rate is based on historic data. With plasmapheresis and dialysis, the likelihood of maternal death is probably much less. **It is not important to make the distinction between TTP and HUS, because the initial therapy for both disorders is plasmapheresis.**

EVALUATION OF THROMBOCYTOPENIA DURING PREGANCY AND THE PUERPERIUM

Before deciding on a course to follow in treating the patient with thrombocytopenia, the obstetrician must evaluate the patient and attempt to ascertain the etiology of her low platelet count, realizing that gestational thrombocytopenia will be the most likely diagnosis. Important management decisions are dependent on arriving at an accurate diagnosis; therefore a complete medical history is critically important. It is essential to learn whether the patient has previously had a depressed platelet count or bleeding diathesis. It is also important to know whether these clinical conditions occur coincidentally with pregnancy. A complete medication history should be elicited, because certain medications—such as heparin, many antibiotics, and histamine-2 blockers—can result in profound maternal thrombocytopenia. The obstetric history should focus on whether any maternal or neonatal bleeding problems occurred in the past. **Excessive bleeding from an episiotomy site or cesarean delivery incision site or bleeding from intravenous (IV) sites during labor should alert the physician to the possibility of thrombocytopenia in the previous pregnancy.** The obstetrician should also question whether the infant had any bleeding diathesis or any problem occurred following a circumcision. The obstetrician should also ask pertinent questions to determine whether severe preeclampsia or hemolysis, elevated liver enzymes, and low platelets (HELLP) syndrome is the cause of her thrombocytopenia. The treatment of preeclampsia and HELLP are discussed in Chapter 31. All thrombocytopenic pregnant women should be carefully evaluated for the presence of risk factors for human immunodeficiency virus (HIV) infection, because this infection can cause an ITP-like syndrome. Also, a family history should be elicited because familial forms of thrombocytopenia exist.

An accurate assessment of gestational age should also be carried out. This is important not only in helping to determine the etiology of the thrombocytopenia but also in the timing of delivery. A thorough physical examination of the patient should be performed, and the physician should look for the presence of ecchymoses or petechiae. The conjunctivae and nail beds often reveal petechiae when they are not readily apparent elsewhere on the body. Blood pressure should be determined to ascertain whether the patient has impending preeclampsia. If the patient is developing HELLP syndrome, scleral icterus may be present, and an eye exam should be performed to look for evidence of arteriolar spasm or hemorrhage.

It is imperative that a peripheral blood smear be examined by an experienced physician or technologist whenever a case of pregnancy-associated thrombocytopenia is diagnosed. The presence or absence of evidence of microangiopathic hemolysis on the smear will help establish a diagnosis. This specialist can also rule out platelet clumping, which will result in a factitious thrombocytopenia. Platelet clumping in ethylenediaminetetraacetic acid (EDTA, a lavender-top tube) occurs in about 3 per 1000 individuals and may lead to a spurious diagnosis of thrombocytopenia. If platelet clumping is suspected, the physician should ask the laboratory to perform a platelet count on citrate-collected blood (a blue-top tube). If the count is normal, platelet clumping is likely, and the patient is not thrombocytopenic. Other laboratory evaluations should be performed as necessary to rule out preeclampsia and HELLP syndrome as well as disseminated intravascular coagulation (DIC). If a diagnosis of ITP is entertained, appropriate platelet antibody testing may aid in the diagnosis but is of limited utility during pregnancy.

After determining the etiology of thrombocytopenia, the physician can better determine whether imminent delivery is necessary, if the thrombocytopenia should be treated before initiating delivery, or if the low platelet count should be monitored during an ongoing pregnancy.

THERAPY OF THROMBOCYTOPENIA DURING PREGNANCY

Gestational Thrombocytopenia

Gestational thrombocytopenia, the most common form of thrombocytopenia encountered in the third trimester, requires no special intervention or therapy. The most important therapeutic issue is to refrain from treatment and testing that may lead to unnecessary intervention or iatrogenic preterm delivery. In patients with mild to moderate thrombocytopenia and no antenatal or antecedent history of thrombocytopenia, the patient should be treated as a normal pregnant patient. If the maternal platelet count drops below 50,000/mm^3, the patient may still have gestational thrombocytopenia, but not enough data are available on mothers with counts this low to

determine whether any maternal or fetal risks exist. These patients, therefore, should be treated as if they have de novo ITP. Although approximately 4% of patients have gestational thrombocytopenia, less than 1% of alternate uncomplicated pregnant women will have gestational thrombocytopenia with platelet counts less than 100,000/mm^3.[6]

Immune Thrombocytopenic Purpura

Treatment of the gravida with ITP during pregnancy and the puerperium requires special attention to the mother, because platelet counts can drop to very low numbers during gestation. As in other cases of thrombocytopenia, maternal therapy needs to be instituted only if a bleeding diathesis is evident or to prevent a bleeding complication if surgery is anticipated. Usually no spontaneous bleeding is present unless the platelet count falls below 20,000/mm^3.[23] In a meta-analysis of 17 studies, the risk of fatal hemorrhage in an individual younger than 40 years of age with a platelet count less than 30,000/mm^3 was 0.4%. The predicted 5-year mortality rate in this setting was 2.2%.[23] **Surgical bleeding does not usually occur until the platelet count is less than 50,000/mm^3. The American Society of Hematology presently recommends that hospital admission is not necessary unless the platelet count falls to below 20,000/mm^3 or if clinical bleeding is present.**[21]

The conventional forms of raising the platelet count in the patient with ITP include glucocorticoid therapy, IV gamma globulins, platelet transfusions, and splenectomy. If the patient has clinical bleeding or if the platelet count is below 20,000/mm^3, there is usually a need to raise the platelet count in a relatively short period of time. Although oral glucocorticoids can be used, IV glucocorticoids may work more rapidly. Any steroid with a glucocorticoid effect can be used. However, **hematologists have had the most experience with methylprednisolone. This medication can be given intravenously and has very little mineralocorticoid effect.** It is important to avoid steroids with strong mineralocorticoid effects because these agents can disturb electrolyte balance, cause fluid retention, and result in hypertension. The usual dose of methylprednisolone is 1.0 to 1.5 mg/kg of *total body weight* intravenously daily in divided doses. It usually takes approximately 2 days for a response, but it may take up to 10 days for a maximum response. Even though methylprednisolone has very little mineralocorticoid effect, some may be observed because of the large dose being administered. Therefore **it is important to follow the patient's electrolytes.** The likelihood is low that methylprednisolone will cause neonatal adrenal suppression because little crosses the placenta. It is metabolized by placental 11β-dehydrogenase type 1 to an inactive 11-keto metabolite. Park-Wyllie and colleagues[24] performed a meta-analysis, which confirmed the general safety of glucocorticoids during pregnancy. They did, however, find a 3.4-fold increased risk of cleft lip and palate with first-trimester exposure. The risk/benefit ratio should be discussed with the patient before initiation of therapy (see Chapter 8).

After the platelet count has risen satisfactorily using IV methylprednisolone, the patient can be switched to oral prednisone. The usual dose is 60 to 100 mg/day. Prednisone can be given in a single dose, but less gastrointestinal upset occurs with divided doses. The physician can rapidly taper the dose to 30 to 40 mg/day and decrease it slowly thereafter. The dose should be titrated to keep the platelet count at approximately 100,000/mm^3. If therapy is initiated with oral prednisone, the usual daily dose is 1 mg/kg total body weight.

The likelihood of a favorable response to glucocorticoids is about 70%. It is important to realize that **if the patient has been taking glucocorticoids for a period of at least 2 to 3 weeks, she may have adrenal suppression and should undergo increased doses of steroids during labor and delivery to avoid an adrenal crisis. Tapering should be done slowly thereafter.** Also, if the patient has been taking glucocorticoids for some time, she may experience significant side effects, including fluid retention, hirsutism, acne, striae, poor wound healing, and monilia vaginitis. In rare circumstances, patients on long-term steroids during gestation can develop osteopenia or cataract formation. The chance of any fetal or neonatal side effects from the glucocorticoids, however, is remote.

Although glucocorticoids are the mainstays of treating maternal thrombocytopenia, up to 30% of patients do not respond to these medications. In such cases, IV immunoglobulin (IVIG) is used. This agent probably works by binding to the IgG Fc receptors on reticuloendothelial cells and preventing destruction of platelets. It may also adhere to receptors on platelets and prevent antiplatelet antibodies from binding to these sites. The usual dose is 0.4 g/kg/day for 3 to 5 days. However, it may be necessary to use as much as 1 g/kg/day. The response usually begins in 2 to 3 days and peaks in 5 days. An alternative regimen is to give 1 g/kg once and observe the patient. Often this single dose will result in an adequate increase in platelets. The length of this response is variable, and the timing of the dose is extremely important. If the obstetrician wants a peak platelet count for delivery, therapy should be instituted about 5 to 8 days before the planned delivery. The most frequent adverse reaction is postinfusion headache, which may be lessened by slowing the infusion rate.

IVIG is a blood product from many pooled donors. Early in its use, concerns were raised about hepatitis C transmission. No recent cases of viral infection from IVIG use have been reported. This is due to careful donor screening as well as an intensive purification process. IVIG should be used before seriously contemplating splenectomy, because some patients experience long-term remission with IVIG, and others have a spontaneous increase in platelet counts postpartum. In severe life-threatening hemorrhage, recombinant factor VIIa can be used in conjunction with other therapies. This is a very expensive and complicated therapy that should only be undertaken with the assistance of a physician familiar with its use.

IV anti-D has been used in emergent settings in Rh-positive, direct antiglobulin–negative patients. In life-threatening situations, when other methods fail, this could be considered an option. The usual dose is 50 to 75 µg/kg.[25] Anti-D binds to IgG Fc receptors different than those bound by IVIG.

The **American Society of Hematology** (ASH) has made specific recommendations for treating ITP in pregnancy.[21] They state that virtually no indication exists for cordocentesis to determine the fetal platelet count. This group recommends **no pharmacologic treatment in the first or second trimesters unless the platelet count is less than 30,000/mm³ or if clinically significant bleeding is evident. If the count is between 10,000/mm³ and 30,000/mm³ in the second or third trimester, IVIG is recommended. The ASH does not recommend platelet transfusion unless the platelet count falls below 10,000/mm³.**

In the midtrimester, splenectomy can also be used to raise the maternal platelet count. This procedure is reserved for those who do not respond to medical management, with the platelet count remaining below 20,000/mm³ and with clinical bleeding. It can also be performed postpartum if the patient does not respond to medical management. In extremely emergent cases of life-threatening bleeding or unresponsiveness to other therapies, splenectomy can be performed at the time of cesarean delivery after extending a midline incision cephalad.

In an emergent situation, platelets can be transfused during cesarean delivery if significant clinical bleeding is evident. Platelets can be transfused before a vaginal delivery if the mother's platelet count is less than 10,000/mm³ or at any count if clinically significant bleeding is present. **Each "pack" of platelets increases the platelet count by approximately 10,000/mm³. The half-life of these platelets is extremely short because the same antibodies and reticuloendothelial cell clearance rates that affect the mother's endogenous platelets also affect the transfused platelets. However, if platelets are transfused at the beginning of surgery, hemostasis adequate to carry out the surgical procedure should be provided.**

If the patient with profound thrombocytopenia undergoes cesarean delivery, certain surgical precautions should be taken. Needless to say, the key is adequate surgical hemostasis. The bladder flap may be left open to avoid hematoma formation. If the parietal peritoneum is closed, subfascial drains are helpful if hemostasis is imperfect. If the peritoneum is not closed, the peritoneal edges should be carefully inspected to make certain no bleeding vessels are present. Small "bleeders" may not be apparent if the patient is hypotensive; therefore the operator must watch for bleeding as the blood pressure rises toward the end of the surgical case. If severe, life-threatening hemorrhage occurs, recombinant factor VIIa and platelet transfusion can be used.

In summary, the treatment of thrombocytopenia during gestation is dependent on its etiology. The obstetrician need not act on the mother's platelet count unless it is below 30,000/mm³, if it is below 50,000/mm³ with evidence of clinical bleeding, or if surgery is anticipated.[9] In these cases, the treatment depends on the diagnosis. Furthermore, whether delivery needs to be expedited or can be delayed is also dependent on the etiology of thrombocytopenia, the patient's physical health, fetal well-being, and gestational age.

MANAGEMENT OF THROMBOTIC THROMBOCYTOPENIC PURPURA AND HEMOLYTIC UREMIC SYNDROME

Before the use of plasma exchange, maternal and fetal outcomes in pregnancies complicated by TTP were uniformly poor.[17] The first cases treated with plasma exchange for TTP during pregnancy were reported in 1984, and no large series of patients with TTP in pregnancy have been undertaken. A review of 11 patients described in case reports reveals that **the prognosis has improved greatly with plasma infusion and plasma exchange.**[25] These researchers also demonstrated that cyclosporin may increase the duration of remission. In one case report, TTP relapses were prevented by using prophylactic monthly plasma exchange throughout gestation.[26] If TTP is suspected, plasma exchange should be initiated immediately.

HUS has been more difficult to treat, and only a few case reports have appeared. **Supportive therapy remains the mainstay in cases of HUS,** although dialysis is often necessary with close attention to fluid management. Platelet function inhibitors were used in two cases during pregnancy. Plasma infusion and plasma exchange can be attempted, but the results have not been as good as those observed in cases of TTP. Vincristine has been administered with some success in nonpregnant patients but has not been tried in pregnancy, and prostacyclin infusion has been effective in children but has not been used during pregnancy.

FETAL/NEONATAL ALLOIMMUNE THROMBOCYTOPENIA

In neonatal alloimmune thrombocytopenia, a rare disorder, the mother lacks a specific platelet antigen and develops antibodies to this antigen. The disease is somewhat analogous to Rh isoimmunization but involves platelets. If the fetus inherits an antigen from its father and the mother lacks the antigen, maternal antibody can develop and can cross the placenta. This results in severe neonatal thrombocytopenia and possibly fetal intracranial hemorrhage. The mother, however, will have a normal platelet count. **The most common antibodies noted in these patients is anti–HPA-1a antibodies, although several other antibodies have been identified.** If this disorder is suspected, the mother's blood should be sent to a reference laboratory with experience in diagnosing neonatal alloimmune thrombocytopenia. **These patients should be managed in a tertiary care center with experience caring for mothers and infants with this rare disorder.** Transfusion of maternal platelets into the neonate has improved outcome in these cases. After birth or in utero, the child can be transfused with the mother's platelets (because she lacks the antigen) or with donor platelets known to lack the antigen. Bussel and colleagues[27] demonstrated that neonates who had an older sibling that was affected, especially with an antenatal intracranial hemorrhage, had lower platelet counts than the index pregnancy.[28] Pacheco and colleagues[29] have described an excellent algorithm based on risk stratification for evaluating mothers at risk of having a neonate with alloimmune thrombocytopenia. It describes all of the testing that should be performed. McQuilten and colleagues[30] reviewed the experience in Australia and showed that cordocentesis with transfusion, IVIG administration, and corticosteroids have all been used with good results. Kamphuis and Oepkes[31] reviewed the experience in the Netherlands and demonstrated that weekly IVIG alone can virtually prevent fetal/neonatal intracranial hemorrhage in neonatal alloimmune thrombocytopenia; therefore they believe that fetal blood sampling should be abandoned because of its risks. Rayment and coworkers[32] searched the Cochrane database and the Childbirth Group's trial register to ascertain whether they could discern the optimal management of alloimmune thrombocytopenia. They reviewed four trials that involved 206 patients. Because of incomplete data and differences in interventions, they could not conclude the best treatment plan for these patients.[32] They convincingly show that more randomized studies to look at medication doses and timing need to be performed.[31]

IRON DEFICIENCY ANEMIA

During a singleton pregnancy, maternal plasma volume gradually expands by approximately 50% (1000 mL). The total RBC mass also increases but only by approximately 300 mg (25%), and this starts later in pregnancy. It is not surprising, therefore, that **hemoglobin and hematocrit levels usually fall during gestation. These changes are not necessarily pathologic but usually represent a physiologic alteration of pregnancy.** By 6

BOX 44-3   CAUSES OF ANEMIA DURING PREGNANCY

Common Causes: 85% of Anemia
Physiologic anemia
Iron deficiency

Uncommon Causes
Folic acid deficiency
Vitamin B_{12} deficiency
Hemoglobinopathies
- Sickle cell disease
- Hemoglobin SC
- β-Thalassemia minor
Bariatric surgery
Gastrointestinal bleeding

Rare Causes
Hemoglobinopathies
- β-Thalassemia major
- α-Thalassemia
Syndromes of chronic hemolysis
- Hereditary spherocytosis
- Paroxysmal nocturnal hemoglobinuria
Hematologic malignancy

weeks postpartum, in the absence of excessive blood loss during the puerperium, hemoglobin and hematocrit levels have returned to normal if the mother has adequate iron stores.

Most clinicians diagnose anemia when the hemoglobin concentration is less than 11 g/dL or the hematocrit is less than 32%.[33] **Using these criteria, 50% of pregnant women are anemic.** Many women have hemoglobin concentrations as low as 10 gm/dL and recover. The incidence of anemia changes depending on the population studied. It is unfortunate that this problem is often ignored; in developing nations, iron deficiency is an overwhelming problem, and worldwide, many maternal deaths occur because of excessive blood loss in those who were already anemic. Causes of anemia are shown in Box 44-3.

Approximately 75% of anemia that occurs during pregnancy is secondary to iron deficiency. Ho and colleagues[34] performed elaborate hematologic evaluations of 221 gravidas at term in Taiwan. None of the studied patients received an added iron preparation during gestation. Of the previously nonanemic patients, 10.4% developed clinical anemia after a full-term delivery. Of these 23 patients, 11 (47.8%) developed florid iron deficiency anemia, and another 11 demonstrated moderate iron depletion. The other anemic patient in the group had folate deficiency. Of the 198 nonanemic gravidas at term, 46.5% showed evidence of iron depletion stores even though they had a normal hematocrit.[34]

To distinguish the normal physiologic changes of pregnancy from those of pathologic iron deficiency, the normal iron requirements of pregnancy (Table 44-1) and the proper use of hematologic laboratory parameters must be understood. In adult women, iron stores are located in the bone marrow, liver, and spleen in the form of ferritin, which constitutes approximately 25% (500 mg) of the 2 g of iron stores found in the normal woman. Approximately 65% of stored iron is located in the circulating RBCs. **If the dietary iron intake is poor, the interval between pregnancies is short, or the delivery is complicated by hemorrhage, iron deficiency anemia readily and rapidly develops.**

TABLE 44-1	IRON REQUIREMENTS FOR PREGNANCY AND THE PUERPERIUM	
FUNCTION		**REQUIREMENT**
Increased red blood cell mass		450 mg
Fetus and placenta		360 mg
Vaginal delivery		190 mg
Lactation		1 mg/day

TABLE 44-2	ELEMENTAL IRON AVAILABLE FROM COMMON GENERIC IRON PREPARATIONS	
PREPARATION		**ELEMENTAL IRON (mg)**
Ferrous gluconate 325 mg		37-39
Ferrous sulfate 325 mg		60-65
Ferrous fumarate 325 mg		107

The first pathologic change to occur in iron deficiency anemia is the depletion of bone marrow, liver, and spleen iron stores. This may take a few weeks to a few months depending on the level of the woman's iron stores. Over a period of a few weeks, the serum iron level falls, as does the percentage saturation of transferrin. The total iron-binding capacity rises simultaneously with the fall of iron, because this is a reflection of unbound transferrin. A falling hemoglobin and hematocrit follow within 2 weeks. Microcytic hypochromic RBCs are released into the circulation. If this is a pure iron deficiency, a reticulocytosis will occur within 3 days of initiating therapy, and the hemoglobin concentration will increase within a week. However, it may take more than a month to completely replete iron stores. A patient who has a very low hemoglobin as a result of iron deficiency immediately postpartum should return to normal by her 6-week postpartum visit. If iron deficiency is combined with folate or vitamin B12 deficiency, normocytic and normochromic RBCs are observed on the peripheral blood smear.

Care must be taken when using laboratory parameters to establish the diagnosis of iron deficiency anemia during gestation. A serum iron concentration less than 60 mg/dL with a less than 16% saturation of transferrin is suggestive of iron deficiency. Conversely, a single normal serum iron concentration does not rule out iron deficiency. For example, a patient may take iron for several days, and this may result in a transiently normal serum iron concentration while iron stores are still negligible. An increase in iron-binding capacity is not reliable, however, because 15% of pregnant women without iron deficiency show an increase in this parameter.[35] If a patient has been iron deficient for an extended period of time, her serum iron level can rise before she has depleted her iron stores. **The ferritin level indicates the total status of her iron stores.** Serum ferritin levels normally decrease minimally during pregnancy. However, a significantly reduced ferritin concentration is indicative of iron deficiency anemia and is the best parameter to judge the degree of iron deficiency. However, ferritin levels are variable and can change 25% from one day to the next.[36] Tran and colleagues[37] have demonstrated that iron deficiency is the only possible diagnosis for a low ferritin. If a ferritin of 41 ng/mL is used as a cutoff, serum ferritin has 98% sensitivity and 98% specificity in diagnosing iron deficiency.[38] This is true if there is no concomitant infectious or inflammatory process.

Ahluwalia[39] compared iron status in normal and obese pregnant women and found by comparing ferritin that obese women had decreased iron stores. It was also found that obese pregnant women had higher concentrations of the inflammatory marker hepcidin, the concentration of which correlated directly with iron status; it was therefore surmised that chronic inflammation in obese pregnant women may impede their ability to absorb iron.

As part of a large study that included 1171 pregnant women between 1999 and 2006, Mei and colleagues,[40] working through the National Centers for Chronic Disease Prevention and Health

Promotion, assessed total body iron using ferritin and soluble transferrin receptor concentrations. They found that iron deficiency increased during pregnancy from 6.9% ± 2.2% in the first trimester to 29.5% ± 2.7% in the third trimester. The prevalence of iron deficiency was highest in women with a parity of at least two. Iron deficiency was significantly higher in Mexican-American and non-Hispanic black women. Statistical analysis showed that this difference was not due to educational level or family income.[40]

Bone marrow aspiration is rarely necessary for the diagnosis of iron deficiency. It is reserved for persistent anemia with confusing hematologic parameters and can be safely performed during pregnancy.

Whether all women should receive prophylactic iron in addition to that contained in prenatal vitamins during pregnancy remains controversial. In reviewing the Cochrane database, Milman and colleagues[41] found that 20% of fertile women have iron stores greater than 500 mg, which is the required minimum for pregnancy. They also noted that 40% of women have iron stores between 100 and 500 mg, and 40% have virtually no iron stores. Based on these data, **most women do need some iron supplementation.** No consensus was reached, however, on how much iron supplementation may be needed in patients with iron deficiency.

In pregnancy, iron absorption from the duodenum increases, providing 1.3 to 2.6 mg of elemental iron daily. An acid environment in the duodenum helps this absorption; therefore the frequent ingestion of antacid medications commonly used by many patients decreases the absorption of iron. Chronic use of H_2 blockers and proton pump inhibitors also diminishes iron absorption. Vitamin C, in addition to the iron, may increase the acidic environment of the stomach and increase absorption. In patients who do not show clear signs of iron deficiency, it is uncertain whether prophylactic iron, in addition to what is in prenatal vitamins, leads to an increased hemoglobin concentration at term. Iron prophylaxis, however, is safe because only amounts that can be used are absorbed. With the exception of dyspepsia and constipation, side effects are few. **One 325 mg tablet of ferrous sulfate daily provides adequate prophylaxis. It contains 60 mg of elemental iron, 10% of which is absorbed.** If the iron is not needed, it will not be absorbed and will be excreted in the feces. The standard generic iron tablets and the amount of elemental iron they provide are listed in Table 44-2.

In iron-deficient patients, one iron tablet three times daily has been recommended, although the evidence-based source of this recommendation is difficult to ascertain. Most individuals can absorb as much iron as they need taking iron twice daily. Iron should be taken 30 minutes before meals to allow maximum absorption. However, when taken in this manner, dyspepsia and nausea are more common. Therapy, therefore, must be individualized to maximize patient compliance. Reveiz and colleagues[33] examined the Cochrane database to see whether an optimal treatment for iron deficiency during pregnancy could be discerned. They identified 23 trials that comprised 3198 women. Many of the trials were from low-income countries, were generally small, and had poor methodology. Although oral iron supplementation led to a reduction in the incidence of anemia, it was not possible to assess the effects of treatment by severity of anemia. The authors concluded that despite a high incidence and significant ramifications of this disease, a paucity of good-quality trials exists. Whereas these trials could be relatively easy to design and would be relatively inexpensive compared with so many other investigations being carried out, a lack of interest among researchers and funding institutions in the United States is apparent.

Young and colleagues[42] studied the effectiveness of weekly iron supplementation and found it to be almost as effective as daily supplementation in raising the hemoglobin concentration in iron-deficient patients. This approach can be used in patients with less than optimal compliance. Yakoob and Bhutta[43] systematically reviewed 31 studies in the Cochrane database to determine whether routine iron supplementation affects the incidence of anemia in pregnancy. They included studies that used iron alone and iron with folic acid and found a 73% reduction in anemia with routine supplementation. However, no difference was found in rates of anemia at term with intermittent iron-folate when compared with daily supplementation (relative risk [RR], 1.61; 95% confidence interval [CI], 0.82 to 3.14).

For those patients who are noncompliant or unable to take oral iron and are severely anemic, IV iron can be given. Singh and colleagues[44] found that parenteral iron can be safely given and significantly raises the hematocrit in patients. It also raises the serum ferritin. Hallak and coworkers[45] examined the safety and efficacy of parenteral iron administration. Of 26 patients receiving parenteral iron, only one developed signs of mild allergy during the test dose and was excluded from the study. The remaining 21 pregnant patients completed the course of therapy and received a mean of 1000 mg of elemental iron. Their hemoglobin increased an average of 1.6 g/dL from the beginning to the end of therapy and rose another 0.8 g/dL during the following 2 weeks. Ferritin levels increased from 2.9 ng/mL at the beginning of therapy to 122.8 ng/dL by the end of treatment. Ferritin levels decreased to a mean of 109.4 ng/mL 2 weeks later, demonstrating that the iron was being utilized. Only mild transient side effects were noted; therefore the authors concluded that parenteral iron therapy can be used safely during pregnancy.

Parenteral iron is indicated in those who cannot or will not take oral iron therapy and are not anemic enough to require transfusion. In fact, by building iron stores in the patients before delivery, we may be able to prevent a need for transfusion postpartum in the severely anemic patient. Iron dextran comes in a concentration of 50 mg/mL. It can be given intramuscularly or intravenously, although intramuscular injection is very painful. **Iron dextran can result in anaphylaxis caused by dissociation of the iron and carbohydrate components.** The reaction may be immediate or delayed; therefore a 0.5 mL test dose should be given, and epinephrine should be readily available. Anaphylaxis usually occurs within several minutes but may take 2 days to develop. **In the past 3 years, our group has given iron dextran to 14 patients. Two developed a severe reaction within minutes of the test dose. Although neither patient developed shortness of breath, both exhibited severe bone pain and myalgias.** The dosage for iron

TABLE 44-3 PARENTERAL IRON ADMINISTRATION

MEDICATION	DOSE	PREPARATION
Iron dextran	Total dose (mL) = 0.0442 (desired Hb − observed Hb) × LBW + (0.26 × LBW), 100 mg/dose maximum	50 mg elemental iron/mL
Iron sucrose	100 mg/dose, usually 1 dose/day, usually 10 doses needed	20 mg elemental iron/mL
Sodium ferric gluconate complex	125 mg/dose, usually 1 dose/day, usually 8 doses needed	12.5 mg of elemental iron/mL

Hb, hemoglobin; *LBW,* lean body weight.

dextran therapy is shown in Table 44-3. Although iron dextran is rarely used in the United States and Canada, in developing nations, this compound is the only parenteral iron readily available, and therefore its discussion is included in this chapter.

Today, two other agents with excellent safety records are available for parenteral iron therapy. Both of these compounds have the disadvantage of requiring multiple doses to accomplish what can be done with one dose of iron dextran; however, they have the advantage of less likelihood of a severe adverse reaction. Iron sucrose complex is given intravenously, usually daily, with a maximum dose of 100 mg. Patients generally require 10 doses (1 g) to obtain the desired rise in ferritin and subsequent rise in hemoglobin concentration. Sodium ferric gluconate complex can be used similarly, and the maximum dose is 125 mg. It is usually given daily, and eight doses (1 g) are most often required to obtain the desired results. Sodium ferric gluconate appears to have the least risk of adverse side effects. If the patient has concomitant renal insufficiency, subcutaneous erythropoietin can be given to help raise the hemoglobin concentration if iron stores have already been increased. These agents should be used only in patients with severe iron deficiency who cannot absorb iron or who will not or cannot take oral iron. A parenteral iron overdose can lead to hemosiderosis.

It is still uncertain whether anemia results in an increased risk for poor pregnancy outcome. In their literature review, Scholl and Hediger[46] concluded that anemia diagnosed in early pregnancy is associated with preterm delivery and low birthweight (LBW). In this study, women with iron deficiency anemia had twice the risk of preterm delivery and three times the risk of delivering an LBW infant. Preterm labor, however, is a multifactorial problem, and many other confounders were present in this study. Yip[47] reviewed the literature concerning pregnancy outcome with anemia and found through epidemiologic studies an association between moderate anemia and poor perinatal outcome, yet he was unable to determine whether this relationship was causal. Sifakis and Pharmakides[48] observed that hemoglobin concentrations below 6 g/dL are associated with preterm birth, spontaneous abortion, LBW, and fetal deaths. Nevertheless, a mild to moderate anemia did not appear to have any significant effect on fetal outcomes. Hemminki and Starfield[49] reviewed controlled trials and concluded that routine iron administration did not decrease preterm labor or raise birthweight. Conversely, Stephansson and colleagues[50] found an increased risk of stillbirth and growth-restricted infants in women with hemoglobin concentrations greater than 14.6 g/dL at their prenatal visit. Demmouche and colleagues[51] found that nearly 50% of 207 women were anemic, and 14.43% were severely anemic with a hemoglobin less than 9 g/dL. No difference in birthweight was reported between anemic and nonanemic pregnant women.

In summary, iron deficiency is very prevalent in the general pregnant population. **In developing nations, severe anemia is alarmingly common and is a major cause of maternal morbidity and mortality.** Routine iron administration as formulated in prenatal vitamins should be used unless it is certain that the patient is iron replete. Iron prophylaxis can be taken as one iron tablet daily, or as one study showed, it can be given on a weekly basis. An association between adverse pregnancy outcome and maternal anemia, especially severe anemia, may exist; however, it is uncertain whether this is a causal relationship.

MEGALOBLASTIC ANEMIA

Folic acid, a water-soluble vitamin, is found in strawberries, green vegetables, peanuts, and liver. Folate stores are located primarily in the liver and are usually sufficient for 6 weeks. After 3 weeks of a diet deficient in folate, the serum folate level falls. Two weeks later, hypersegmentation of neutrophils occurs. After 17 weeks without folic acid ingestion, RBC folate levels drop. In the next week, a megaloblastic bone marrow develops. **During pregnancy, folate deficiency is the most common cause of megaloblastic anemia. The daily folate requirement in the nonpregnant state is approximately 50 μg, but this rises at least fourfold during gestation. Fetal demands increase the requirement, as does the decrease in the gastrointestinal absorption of folate during pregnancy.**

Clinical megaloblastic anemia seldom occurs before the third trimester of pregnancy. If the patient is at risk for folate deficiency or has mild anemia, an attempt should be made to detect this disorder before megaloblastosis occurs. Serum folate and RBC folate levels are the best tests for folate deficiency. Whereas serum folate reflects recently ingested folate, **RBC folate levels give a better idea of folate status at the tissue level.**

Folate deficiency rarely occurs in the fetus and is not a cause of significant perinatal morbidity. However, some evidence shows that fetuses homozygous for the C677T variant of the gene that encodes for 5,10-methylene tetrahydrofolate reductase have a 20% lower folate level and may be at risk for a neural tube defect (NTD). Because infants born to mothers with type 1 and type 2 diabetes mellitus have an increased incidence of NTDs, Kaplan and colleagues[52] studied 31 pregnant women with diabetes and 54 controls to determine whether aberrations in folate metabolism are apparent in patients with diabetes. They found no differences in how ingested folate is processed in the pregnant patient with diabetes. **Prenatal vitamins that require physician prescription contain 1 mg of folic acid, and most nonprescription prenatal vitamins contain 0.8 mg of folic acid. These amounts are more than adequate to prevent and treat folate deficiency. Women with significant hemoglobinopathies, patients taking anticonvulsant medications, women carrying a multiple gestation, and women with frequent conception may require more than 1 mg of supplemental folate daily. Often, 4 mg of folic acid is recommended daily because this is the dose that has been shown to reduce the risk of recurrent NTDs.** However, no studies have demonstrated the optimal dose of folic acid in women with the conditions listed above. If the patient is folic acid deficient, her reticulocyte count will be depressed. Within 3 days after the administration of

sufficient folic acid, reticulocytosis usually occurs. In fact, **folic acid deficiency should be considered when a patient has unexplained thrombocytopenia.** The leukopenia and thrombocytopenia that accompany megaloblastosis are rapidly reversed, and **the hematocrit level may rise as much as 1% per day after 1 week of folate replacement.**

Vollsett and colleagues[53] performed a retrospective analysis of 14,492 pregnancies in 5883 women in Norway to determine whether elevated homocysteine levels are associated with pregnancy complications. An elevated homocysteine level is often found with depressed folate levels, so they compared those in the upper quartile of homocysteine levels with those in the lower quartile. They noted a 32% higher risk for preeclampsia (odds ratio [OR], 1.32), a 38% greater risk for prematurity (OR, 1.38), and a 10% increased risk for very low birthweight (OR, 2.01). All trends were statistically significant, but the limitations inherent in retrospective epidemiologic studies apply here.[53] Munger and associates[54] investigated serum folate, RBC folate, active pyridoxine, and homocysteine concentrations in 347 pregnancies complicated by facial clefting and in 469 controls. Low RBC and serum folate levels were significantly associated with an increased risk of clefting, whereas pyridoxine and homocysteine levels were not. Therefore homocysteine does not appear to have an etiologic role in clefting.

Iron deficiency is frequently observed in association with folic acid deficiency. If a patient with folate deficiency does not develop a significant reticulocytosis within 1 week after administration of sufficient replacement therapy, appropriate tests for iron deficiency should be performed.

Until recently, the prevalence of vitamin B_{12} deficiency in pregnancy was unusual. However, bariatric surgery has become increasingly common. Individuals who were morbidly obese and not ovulating suddenly ovulate and become pregnant, and now **we regularly encounter individuals with vitamin B_{12} deficiency following bariatric surgery.** Cobalamin is found only in animal products, and the daily minimum required intake is 6 to 9 μg. Total body stores are 2 to 5 mg, and one half of this is stored in the liver. For cobalamin to be absorbed, an individual needs (1) acid-pepsin in the stomach, (2) intrinsic factor secreted by parietal cells in the stomach, (3) pancreatic proteases, and (4) an intact ileum with receptors to bind the cobalamin–intrinsic factor complex. **Because of the abundant vitamin B_{12} stores in the body, it takes several years for a clinical vitamin B_{12} deficiency to develop.**[55] Prolonged vitamin B_{12} deficiency can result in subacute combined degeneration, which involves the dorsal horns and lateral columns of the spinal cord. This can result in sensory and proprioception deficits, which can progress and cause serious disabilities. Fortunately, these changes are reversible when detected early.

In addition to bariatric surgery, gastrointestinal diseases such as Crohn disease may lead to an inability to absorb vitamin B_{12}. Because of advances in medical care, more individuals with these chronic disorders are becoming pregnant. As primary care physicians for women, we must be prepared to diagnose and coordinate care in these complex patients. Furthermore, we are encountering more patients taking metformin, which is being prescribed for polycystic ovarian syndrome (PCOS) and other disorders in addition to type 2 diabetes mellitus and gestational diabetes. It is important to note that this medication can also result in vitamin B_{12} deficiency, because approximately 10% to 30% of patients taking metformin may have depressed vitamin B_{12} levels, which can be reversed with increased calcium intake.[56] The major causes of vitamin B_{12} deficiency are listed in Box 44-4.

Megaloblastic anemia usually leads to a suspicion of folate or vitamin B_{12} deficiency. As noted earlier, if an associated iron deficiency is present, the RBC indices may portray a normocytic, normochromic picture. Therefore it is important to look at more specific tests for vitamin B_{12} and folate deficiencies. Vitamin B_{12} levels may fall during pregnancy, but this finding may not represent a pathologic process. Also, serum vitamin B_{12} levels may be normal in up to 5% of individuals with a true deficiency.[57]

Evaluation of methylmalonate and homocysteine levels can be used to distinguish folate deficiency from vitamin B_{12} deficiency. Vitamin B_{12} is a cofactor in the metabolism of both methylmalonic acid and homocysteine. A deficiency in vitamin B_{12} will therefore lead to an increased concentration of both of these compounds. Folic acid is a cofactor in the metabolism of homocysteine, therefore a folate deficiency will lead to an elevated homocysteine level. Savage and colleagues[57] found elevated methylmalonic acid levels in 98% of individuals with a vitamin B_{12} deficiency but in only 12% of individuals with a folate deficiency; he also found elevated homocysteine levels in 96% of individuals with a vitamin B_{12} deficiency and in 91% of individuals with a folate deficiency. Figure 44-1 schematically shows how to incorporate methylmalonic acid and homocysteine testing into the evaluation of megaloblastic anemia.

HEMOGLOBINOPATHIES

Hemoglobin is a tetrameric protein composed of two pairs of polypeptide chains with a heme group attached to each chain. The normal adult hemoglobin A1 (HbA1) comprises 95% of hemoglobin. It consists of two α-chains and two β-chains. The remaining 5% of hemoglobin usually consists of HbA2, which contains two α- and two δ-chains, and HbF, with two α- and two γ-chains. In the fetus, HbF (fetal hemoglobin) declines during the third trimester of pregnancy, reaching its permanent nadir several months after birth. Hemoglobinopathies arise when a change occurs in the structure of a peptide chain or a defect compromises the ability to synthesize a specific polypeptide chain. The patterns of inheritance are often straightforward, and the prevalences of the most common hemoglobinopathies in black adults are listed in Table 44-4.

Hemoglobin S

Hemoglobin S, a variant form of hemoglobin, is present in patients with sickle cell disease (HbSS) and sickle cell trait (HbAS). A single substitution of valine for glutamic acid at the sixth position in the β-polypeptide chain causes a significant change in the physical characteristics of this hemoglobin. At low oxygen tensions, RBCs that contain HbS assume a sickle shape. Sludging in small vessels occurs and results in microinfarction of the affected organs. Sickle cells have a life span of 5 to 10 days, compared with 120 days for a normal RBC. Sickling is triggered by dehydration, hypoxia, or acidosis. Infants with sickle cell anemia show no signs of the disease until the concentration of HbF falls to adult levels. Some patients do not experience symptoms until adolescence.

Approximately 1 in 12 black adults in the United States is heterozygous for HbS and therefore has sickle cell trait (HbAS) and carries the affected gene. **These individuals generally have 35% to 45% HbS and are asymptomatic. The child of two individuals with sickle cell trait has a 50% probability of inheriting the trait and a 25% probability of actually having**

BOX 44-4   CAUSES OF VITAMIN B_{12} DEFICIENCY THAT MAY BE ENCOUNTERED IN PREGNANCY

- Strict vegetarian diet
- Use of proton pump inhibitors
- Metformin
- Gastritis
- Gastrectomy
- Ileal bypass
- Crohn disease
- Sprue
- *Helicobacter pylori* infection

TABLE 44-4   FREQUENCY OF COMMON HEMOGLOBINOPATHIES IN BLACK ADULTS IN THE UNITED STATES

HEMOGLOBIN TYPE	FREQUENCY
Hemoglobin AS	1 in 12
Hemoglobin SS	1 in 708
Hemoglobin AC	1 in 41
Hemoglobin CC	1 in 4790
Hemoglobin SC	1 in 757
Hemoglobin S/β-thalassemia	1 in 1672

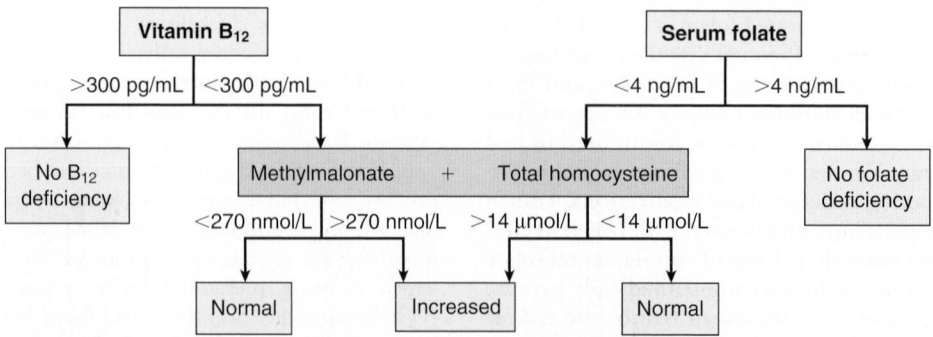

Increased methylmalonate and folate levels indicate vitamin B_{12} deficiency.
Normal methylmalonate and increased homocysteine levels indicate folate deficiency.

FIG 44-1 Use of methylmalonate and homocysteine levels in the workup of megaloblastic anemia.

sickle cell disease. One of every 625 black children born in the United States is homozygous for HbS, and the frequency of sickle cell disease among blacks is 1 in 708. **All at-risk patients should undergo hemoglobin electrophoresis.** Although it is more expensive, it will identify all patients with aberrant hemoglobin types.

The traditional teaching is that women with sickle cell trait are not at increased risk for maternal and perinatal morbidity. A report by Larrabee and Monga[58] questions this. In their study, 162 women with HbAS had a 24.7% incidence of preeclampsia compared with 10.3% of controls. Furthermore, the mean birthweight of infants born to women with HbAS was 3082 g compared with 3369 g for controls ($P < .0001$). The rate of postpartum endometritis was 12.3% for sickle trait patients, compared with 5.1% for controls ($P < .001$), despite similar rates of cesarean delivery. This study indicates that **we should increase our surveillance in patients with HbAS.**

If a patient has HbAS, the spouse/partner should be tested, and if both are carriers of a hemoglobinopathy, prenatal diagnosis should be offered. This can be done rapidly by DNA analysis with polymerase chain reaction (PCR) amplification of DNA fragments. Testing can be performed on amniocytes, and the diagnosis can also be made by chorionic villus sampling (CVS).

A study conducted on patients from Michigan highlights the possibility that adolescents with sickle cell disease may not receive adequate contraceptive counseling.[59] These researchers at Nationwide Children's Hospital found that of 250 women with sickle cell disease, only 20 had filled prescriptions for contraception. Among the 195 adolescents, 49 underwent 59 pregnancies during the study period. The authors suggest that significant gaps may exist in family planning care for young women with sickle cell disease.

Painful vasoocclusive episodes that involve multiple organs are the clinical hallmark of sickle cell disease. The most common sites for these episodes are the extremities, joints, and abdomen. Vasoocclusive episodes can also occur in the lung and can result in pulmonary infarction. **Analgesia, oxygen, and hydration are the clinical foundations for treating these painful crises, and physicians often underestimate the associated pain.** Patients have often received many narcotics and may have a tolerance to the usual dosage of these medications. **It is very important to treat this pain, no matter how much narcotic pain medication is needed. If the obstetrician is uncomfortable with these large doses, he or she should consult with a pain specialist with experience in this area.**

Sickle cell disease can affect virtually all organ systems. **Osteomyelitis** is common, and osteomyelitis caused by *Salmonella* is found almost exclusively in these patients. The risk of **pyelonephritis** is increased, especially during pregnancy. Sickling may also occur in the renal medulla, in which oxygen tension is reduced, resulting in papillary necrosis. These patients also exhibit renal tubular dysfunction and hyposthenuria. Because of chronic hemolysis and decreased RBC survival, patients with sickle cell anemia often demonstrate some degree of jaundice. Biliary stasis commonly occurs during crises, and **cholelithiasis** is seen in about 30% of cases. Because of chronic anemia, **high-output cardiac failure** can occur. Left ventricular hypertrophy and cardiomegaly are common.

Pregnancies complicated by sickle cell disease are at risk for poor perinatal outcomes. The rate of spontaneous abortion may be as high as 25%, and the perinatal mortality rate is approximately 15%. Powars and coworkers[60] studied 156 pregnancies in 79 women with sickle cell anemia. In this group, the perinatal mortality rate was 52.7% before 1972 and 22.7% after that time. In a report by Seoud and coworkers,[61] the perinatal mortality rate was 10.5%. Much of this poor perinatal outcome is related to preterm birth. **Approximately 30% of infants born to mothers with sickle cell disease have birthweights less than 2500 g.** In the report by Seoud and coworkers,[61] the mean birthweight was 2443 g. In a multicenter study, Smith and colleagues[62] reported that 21% of infants born to mothers with sickle cell disease were small for gestational age (SGA). It has been hypothesized that sickling in the uterine vessels may lead to decreased fetal oxygenation and intrauterine growth restriction (IUGR).

Persistent HbF in the mother decreases episodes of painful crises during pregnancy and may also have a protective effect on the neonate. Morris and colleagues[63] studied 270 singleton pregnancies in 175 women with sickle cell disease and found an overall rate of fetal wastage of 32.2%. **Mothers with high HbF levels had a significantly lower perinatal mortality rate.** Hydroxyurea reduces the incidence of painful crises and increases HbF concentration and is especially useful in children, although its safety in pregnancy has not been established. If an individual becomes pregnant while using hydroxyurea, it should be discontinued, but pregnancy termination is not justified. Parvovirus B19 infection is usually asymptomatic in pregnant women but can cause fetal hydrops. In women with AS or SS hemoglobin, parvovirus B19 can result in an acute hemolytic anemia.[64]

Stillbirth rates of 8% to 10% have been described in patients with sickle cell disease, although these rates include studies that took place many years ago. Whereas the widespread use of antenatal fetal testing has reduced the number of stillbirths significantly, the rates of preterm delivery are higher. These fetal deaths happen not only during crises but also unexpectedly; therefore **careful antepartum fetal testing must be used that includes serial ultrasonography to assess fetal growth.** Anyaegbunam and coworkers[65] examined Doppler flow velocimetry in patients with hemoglobinopathies and showed abnormal systolic/diastolic ratios for the uterine or umbilical arteries in 88% of patients with HbSS compared with 7% with HbAS and 4% with HbAA. Howard and colleagues[66] observed that maternal exchange transfusions did not change uteroplacental Doppler blood flow velocimetry in these patients, which suggests that although maternal well-being may be improved, no change in uteroplacental pathology occurs.

Although maternal mortality is rare in patients with sickle cell anemia, maternal morbidity is significant. Infections are common and occur in 50% to 67% of women with HbSS. Most are urinary tract infections (UTIs), which can be detected by frequent urine cultures. Common infecting organisms for the bladder, kidneys, lungs, and other sites include *Streptococcus pneumoniae*, *Haemophilis influenzae* type B, *Escherichia coli*, *Salmonella*, and *Klebsiella*. Patients with HbAS are at greater risk for a UTI and should be screened. Pulmonary infection and infarction are also common, and **patients with sickle cell anemia should receive pneumococcal vaccine before pregnancy.** Maternal deaths have been reported in association with pulmonary complications in sickle cell disease. **Any infection demands prompt attention, because fever, dehydration, and acidosis results in further sickling and painful crises.** The incidence of **pregnancy-induced hypertension** is increased in patients with sickle cell anemia and may complicate almost one third of pregnancies in these patients.[62] A study by Villers and colleagues[67] delineated maternal risks and pregnancy complications in 17,952 deliveries in women with sickle cell disease between 2000 and 2003. **They observed that cerebral vein thrombosis, pneumonia, pyelonephritis, deep venous thrombosis, transfusion, postpartum infections, sepsis, and systemic inflammatory response syndrome (SIRS) were statistically more common in women with sickle cell disease. Furthermore, they found that pregnancy-related complications including hypertensive disorders, antepartum bleeding, abruption, preterm labor, growth restriction, and urinary tract infections were much more common in parturients with sickle cell disease. Seaman and colleagues[68] reviewed the Pennsylvania Health Care Cost Containment Council database to investigate maternal morbidity in 212 women with HbSS. They found that thromboembolic phenomena were 1 to 1.5 times greater in these individuals than in the general population, especially in patients with sickle cell crisis and pneumonia.**

The care of the pregnant patient with sickle cell anemia must be individualized and meticulous. These patients benefit from care in a medical center experienced in treating the multitude of problems that can complicate such pregnancies. From early gestation, good dietary habits should be promoted, and a folic acid supplement of at least 1 mg/day should be administered as soon as pregnancy is confirmed. This is because these patients are in a state of chronic hemolysis, and folic acid is needed for their increased hematopoiesis. Although hemoglobin and hematocrit levels are decreased, iron supplements should not be routinely given. Serum iron and ferritin levels should be checked monthly, and iron supplementation should be started only when these levels are diminished. Often, because of ongoing hemolysis, serum ferritin values are significantly higher in pregnant women with HbSS disease than in those with HbAA disease. Routine iron supplementation, even with prenatal vitamins, should not be given, because iron overload can lead to hemosiderosis and even hemochromatosis. Patients with sickle cell anemia may benefit from an echocardiogram in the first trimester because they are at increased risk for hypertensive and other cardiovascular complications during pregnancy.

No role exists for prophylactic transfusions in these patients. Although a few studies showed decreased maternal and neonatal morbidity with exchange transfusion,[69,70] Koshy and colleagues[71] followed 72 pregnant patients with sickle cell anemia: half received prophylactic transfusions and half received transfusions only for medical or obstetric emergencies. **No significant difference was seen in perinatal outcome between the offspring of mothers who received prophylactic transfusions and those who did not. Two risk factors were identified as harbingers of an unfavorable outcome: the occurrence of a perinatal death in a previous pregnancy and twins in the current pregnancy. Even though no difference in perinatal morbidity and mortality was reported, prophylactic transfusion did appear to decrease significantly the incidence of painful crises.**

Mahomed[72] reviewed the Cochrane database and found that evidence was insufficient to make any conclusions about the use of prophylactic RBC transfusion in patients with sickle cell disease. Many of the cited studies did not show evidence of benefit to the fetus from exchange transfusion. A review by Hassell[73] summarized the various small studies and concluded

that prophylactic transfusion does not improve fetal and neonatal outcome. He did not, however, attempt to quantify changes in maternal well-being.

In a study of 128 patients, Ngo and colleagues[74] attempted to delineate whether prophylactic partial exchange transfusion improved fetal/neonatal outcomes. Although their control group comprised patients with HbAA, they demonstrated significant perinatal/neonatal complications in patients with sickle cell disease who received prophylactic exchange transfusions. The study would have been much stronger had they used a control group of patients with HbSS who had not received exchange transfusions.

Transfusion should be reserved for the same indications that would be used if the patient were not pregnant. However, in the postpartum period, the obstetrician should realize that the patient with HbSS will not increase her hemoglobin/hematocrit as quickly as would the patient with HbAA.

Vaginal delivery is preferred for patients with sickle cell disease, and cesarean delivery should be reserved for obstetric indications. Patients should labor in the left lateral recumbent position and should receive supplemental oxygen. Although adequate hydration should be maintained, fluid overload must be avoided. Conduction anesthesia is recommended because it provides excellent pain relief and can be used for cesarean delivery if necessary. Winder and colleagues[75] reported a case in which epidural anesthesia was used antepartum to relieve a painful crisis, and the patient's hospital stay was significantly shortened. Figure 44-2 provides a schematic presentation of the care of patients with sickle cell anemia. It can also be adapted to patients with other hemoglobinopathies.

Hemoglobin SC Disease

Hemoglobin C is another β-chain variant. It results from a G to A point mutation in the first nucleotide of codon 6. The gene is present is 2% of blacks. Clinically significant HbSC disease occurs in 1 in 833 black adults in the United States. **Women with both S and C hemoglobin suffer less morbidity in pregnancy than do patients with only HbS.** As in sickle cell disease, however, the incidence of early spontaneous pregnancy loss and pregnancy-induced hypertension are increased. Because patients with SC disease can have only mild symptoms, this hemoglobinopathy may remain undiagnosed until a crisis occurs during pregnancy.

Whereas patients with HbSS often undergo "autosplenectomy" as a result of splenic infarction, patients with HbSC may have an enlarged, tender spleen. **Crises in patients with HbSC may be marked by sequestration of a large volume of RBCs in the spleen accompanied by a dramatic fall in hematocrit.[76] Because these patients have increased splenic activity, they may be mildly thrombocytopenic throughout pregnancy and may become profoundly thrombocytopenic during a crisis.** During gestation, patients with HbSC should receive the same program of prenatal care outlined for women with HbSS (see Fig. 44-2).

Thalassemia

Thalassemia is due to a defect in the rate of globin chain synthesis. Any of the polypeptide chains can be affected. As a result, production and accumulation of abnormal globin subunits occurs and leads to ineffective erythropoiesis and a decreased life span of RBCs. The disease may range from minimal suppression of synthesis of the affected chain to its

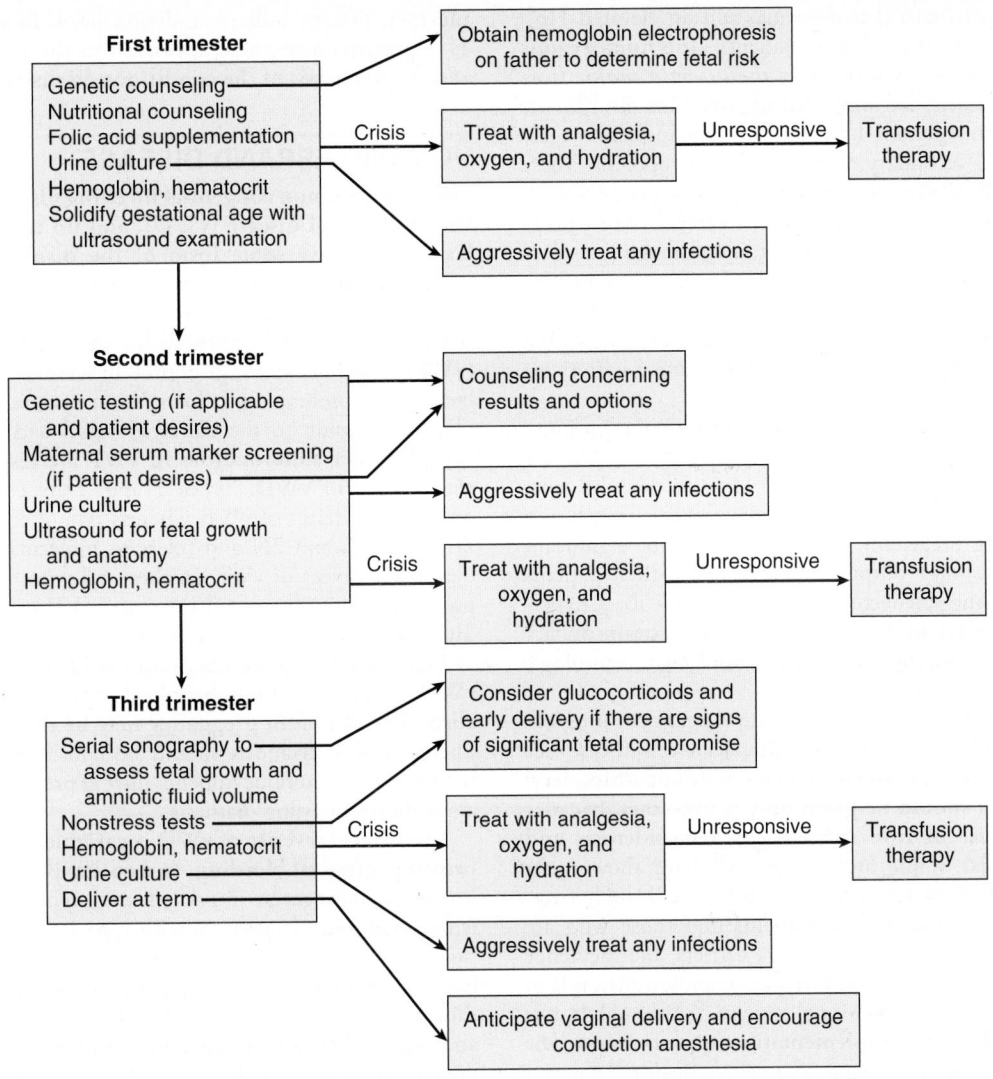

First trimester

Genetic counseling
Nutritional counseling
Folic acid supplementation
Urine culture
Hemoglobin, hematocrit
Solidify gestational age with
ultrasound examination

Obtain hemoglobin electrophoresis
on father to determine fetal risk

Crisis → Treat with analgesia,
oxygen, and hydration *Unresponsive* → Transfusion
therapy

Aggressively treat any infections

Second trimester

Genetic testing (if applicable
and patient desires)
Maternal serum marker screening
(if patient desires)
Urine culture
Ultrasound for fetal growth
and anatomy
Hemoglobin, hematocrit

Counseling concerning
results and options

Aggressively treat any infections

Crisis → Treat with analgesia,
oxygen, and
hydration *Unresponsive* → Transfusion
therapy

Third trimester

Serial sonography to
assess fetal growth and
amniotic fluid volume
Nonstress tests
Hemoglobin, hematocrit
Urine culture
Deliver at term

Consider glucocorticoids and
early delivery if there are signs
of significant fetal compromise

Crisis → Treat with analgesia,
oxygen, and
hydration *Unresponsive* → Transfusion
therapy

Aggressively treat any infections

Anticipate vaginal delivery and encourage
conduction anesthesia

FIG 44-2 Schematic presentation of the care of patients with sickle cell anemia.

complete absence. Either α- or β-thalassemia can occur, and heterozygous patients are often asymptomatic.

Thalassemia can be detected by prenatal diagnosis. Prenatal diagnosis of β-thalassemia can be accomplished by DNA from villi or amniocytes. Because there are many β-globin mutations, it is important to report the patient's ethnicity and the geographic region of the family when submitting specimens. The laboratory can then test for specific mutations based on this information and will be able to identify β-thalassemia in 90% of cases. α-Thalassemia is also amenable to prenatal diagnosis using quantitative PCR or Southern blot analysis. **The American College of Obstetricians and Gynecologists (ACOG) recommends thalassemia screening for pregnant women with a low mean corpuscular volume (MCV) and no evidence of iron deficiency.**[77]

Homozygous α-thalassemia results in the formation of tetramers of β-chains known as *hemoglobin Bart*. This hemoglobinopathy can result in hydrops fetalis. Ghosh and coinvestigators[78] reported their experience caring for 26 Chinese women who were at risk to deliver a fetus with homozygous α-thalassemia. Six of the 26 fetuses were affected. In two of the six cases, progressive fetal ascites appeared before 24 weeks'

gestation. These pregnancies were terminated, and the diagnoses were confirmed. The remaining four patients had evidence of IUGR by 28 weeks' gestation. At later gestational ages, an increase in the transverse cardiac diameter was seen in the affected fetuses. Woo and colleagues[79] reported that umbilical artery velocimetry revealed **a hyperdynamic circulatory state in fetuses that were hydropic because of α-thalassemia.** In a study from Taiwan, Hsieh and colleagues[80] demonstrated that umbilical vein blood flow measurements can help to distinguish hydrops fetalis caused by hemoglobin Bart from hydrops fetalis from other causes. The umbilical vein diameter, blood velocity, and blood flow in fetuses with hemoglobin Bart were usually higher than those in fetuses with hydrops fetalis due to other etiologies.

β-Thalassemia is the most common form of thalassemia, although patients with the heterozygous state are usually asymptomatic; they are detected by an increase in their level of both HbA2 and HbF. HbE is another β-chain variant found generally in patients from Southeast Asia. The clinical course is variable and is similar to that described for β-thalassemia. In the homozygous state of β-thalassemia, synthesis of HbA1 may be completely suppressed. HbA2 levels of greater than 50% are found in 40% of patients with β-thalassemia, and an elevated HbF level is observed in 50% of these patients. **The homozygous state of β-thalassemia is known as** *thalassemia major* (formerly known as *Cooley anemia*). Patients with this disorder are transfusion dependent and have marked hepatosplenomegaly and bone changes secondary to increased hematopoiesis. These individuals usually die of infectious or cardiovascular complications, have a decreased life expectancy, and **rarely become pregnant.** They also have a high rate of infertility, although successful full-term pregnancies have been reported. The few patients who do become pregnant generally exhibit severe anemia and congestive heart failure.[81] Prenatal care is dependent on transfusion therapy similar to that used in the care of the patient with sickle cell disease.

Heterozygous β-thalassemia has different forms of expression. Patients with *thalassemia minima* have microcytosis but are asymptomatic. Those with *thalassemia intermedia* exhibit splenomegaly and significant anemia and may become transfusion dependent during pregnancy. Their anemia can be significant enough to produce high-output cardiac failure. If these patients have not undergone splenectomy, they are at risk for a hypersplenic crisis as seen in HbSC disease. Also, extramedullary hematopoiesis may impinge on the spine, resulting in neurologic symptoms.

These patients should be managed with a treatment program similar to that followed for patients with sickle cell disease (see Fig. 44-2). **As in the case of sickle hemoglobinopathies, iron supplementation should be given only if necessary, because indiscriminate use of iron can lead to hemosiderosis and hemochromatosis.** White and coworkers[82] have shown that patients with a β-thalassemia usually have a much higher ferritin concentration than normal patients and those who are α-thalassemia carriers. In β-thalassemia carriers, the incidence of iron deficiency anemia is four times less common than it is in α-thalassemia carriers and in normal patients.[82] Although iron is not necessary, **folic acid supplementation appears important in β-thalassemia carriers.** Leung and coinvestigators[83] showed that the daily administration of folate significantly increased the predelivery hemoglobin concentration in both nulliparous and multiparous patients.

Patients who are transfusion dependent can develop iron overload, but few data are available on the safety of iron chelating agents during pregnancy. Ricchi and colleagues[84] report a case of successful pregnancy while using deferasirox in the first trimester. The pregnancy went to term, and no fetal malformations were reported. This therapy has not been reported in other pregnancies; therefore chelating agents should only be used in emergent situations.

As in the case of sickle cell disease, antepartum fetal evaluation is essential in patients with thalassemia who are anemic. Patients with clinically significant thalassemia should undergo serial ultrasonography to track fetal growth as well as nonstress testing to evaluate fetal well-being. Asymptomatic thalassemia carriers need no special testing.

Occasionally, individuals will inherit two hemoglobinopathies, such as sickle cell thalassemia (HbS thalassemia). The prevalence of this disorder among adult blacks in the United States is 1 in 1672.[85] The clinical course is variable: if minimal suppression of β-chains occurs, patients may be free of symptoms; however, with total suppression of β-chain synthesis, a clinical picture similar to that of sickle cell disease will develop. The course of these patients during pregnancy is quite variable,

and their therapy must be individualized. **In summary,** Figure 44-3 **presents a stepwise approach to the workup of anemia and the diagnosis of the conditions discussed in this chapter.**

VON WILLEBRAND DISEASE

The most common congenital bleeding disorder in humans is von Willebrand disease (vWD), and up to 1% of the population may have some form of the disorder. Type 1 is an autosomal-dominant disorder, whereas type 3 and occasionally type 2 are autosomal recessive.[86] vWD is related to **quantitative or qualitative abnormalities of von Willebrand factor (vWF).** This multimeric glycoprotein serves as carrier protein of factor VIII, prolonging its life span in plasma. It also promotes platelet adhesion to the damaged vessel and platelet aggregation. **Distinct abnormalities of vWF are responsible for the three types of vWD.** Types 1 and 3 are characterized by a quantitative defect of vWF, whereas type 2 comprises subtypes 2A, 2B, 2M, and 2N and refers to molecular variants with a qualitative defect of vWF. In these subtypes, there are various problems in binding of vWF to factor VII or platelet surface.[87] The knowledge of the structure of the vWF gene and the use of PCR have led to the identification of the molecular basis of vWD in a significant number of patients.[88] **In type 2B, the only clinical symptom in pregnancy may be thrombocytopenia.**[89] Therefore this diagnosis should be considered in the gravida with isolated thrombocytopenia during pregnancy who exhibits a significant bleeding diathesis.

The clinical severity of vWD is variable. Menorrhagia, easy bruising, gingival bleeding, and epistaxis are common. Menorrhagia is most severe in patients with types 2 and 3 vWD but is most common in patients with type 1 disease. In a compilation of two studies, 17% of women with severe menorrhagia had a form of vWD.[90] Some patients may be entirely asymptomatic until they have severe bleeding after surgery or trauma, and **von Willebrand disease does not appear to affect fetal growth or development.**

Classically, the bleeding time is prolonged in patients with vWD as a result of diminished platelet aggregation. Occasionally, the activated partial thromboplastin time (aPTT) is also abnormal. This is only seen when the factor VIII activity is extremely low.[91] **In pregnancy, clotting factors that include the factor VIII complex increase, and the patient's bleeding time may improve as gestation progresses.**[90] This is especially true for type 1A vWD. In type 1B, the patient may not correct her bleeding time.[90] In type 2B, the platelet count decreases, which may be exacerbated in pregnancy.[91] There will, however, be an improvement in the vWF multimeric pattern.[92]

Heavy bleeding may be encountered in patients with vWD undergoing elective or spontaneous first-trimester pregnancy loss because the levels of factor VIII have not yet risen.[93] **Most important, postpartum hemorrhage may be a serious problem. The concentration of factor VIII appears to determine the risk of hemorrhage.** If the level is greater than 50% of normal and the patient has a normal bleeding time, excessive bleeding should not occur at vaginal delivery.[87] In a study by Kadir and colleagues,[93] 18.5% of patients with vWD experienced a significant postpartum hemorrhage, and 6 of 31 patients required transfusion. The clinical course during labor is variable. In a study by Chediak and colleagues,[94] bleeding complications were seen in six of eight (75%) pregnancies. Five of the newborns had vWD, one of whom was born with a scalp hematoma.

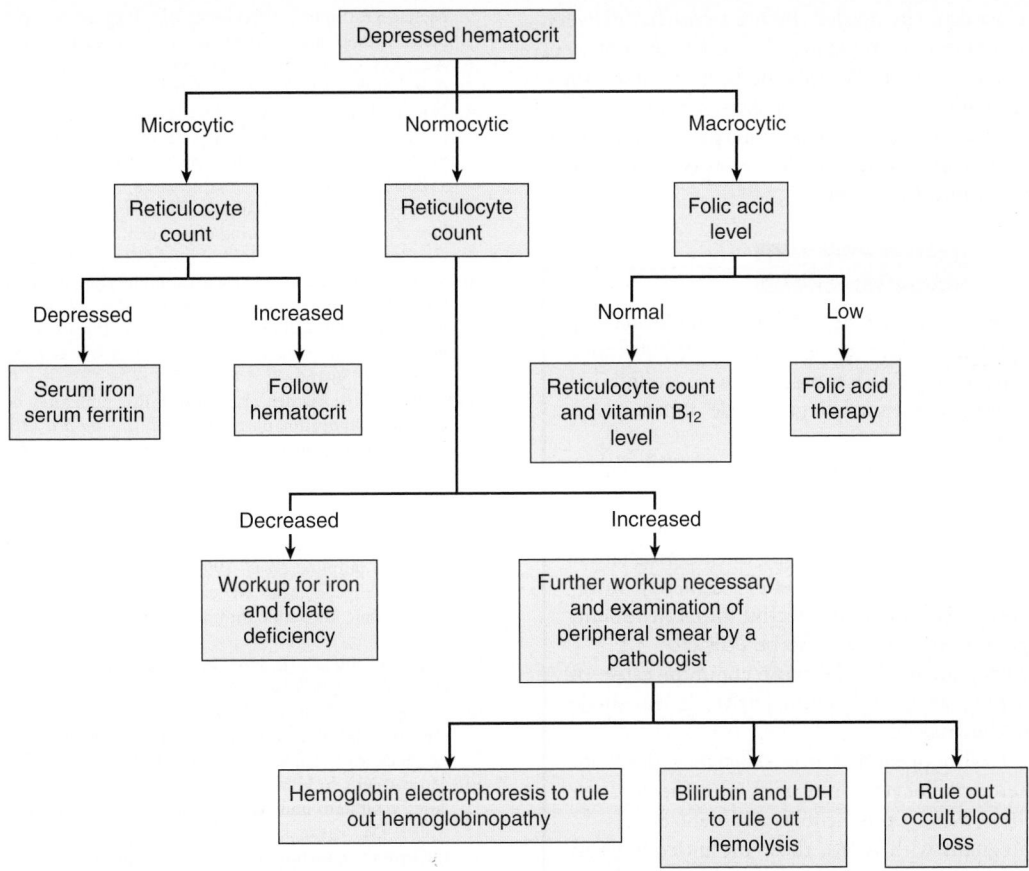

FIG 44-3 Evaluation of anemia. LDH, lactate dehydrogenase.

Conversely, Conti and associates[95] reported no bleeding complications during the puerperium in five women with vWD. Ieko and colleagues[96] demonstrated that factor VIII concentrate could raise the platelet levels in patients with type 2B vWD. Ito and coinvestigators[55] followed six women with type 1 vWD in 10 term pregnancies, three induced abortions, and one spontaneous abortion. Bleeding complications occurred within 1 week after term delivery and immediately after both spontaneous and induced abortions. Pacheco and coworkers[97] published a comprehensive review of vWD coexisting with pregnancy. This study confirmed that most type I patients do not need treatment as long as the factor VIII concentration is greater than 50%. They also stressed the need for close postpartum follow-up because levels of vWF can plummet a few days postpartum. It was recommended that pudendal anesthesia and operative vaginal delivery be avoided if possible.[97]

As noted earlier, **bleeding during pregnancy is rare because levels of factor VIII and vWF increase during pregnancy. However, shortly after delivery, they drop. If the factor VIII level is less than 50%, treatment during labor and delivery should be initiated. Hemorrhage can also occur several days postpartum.** Therefore factor VIII levels should be checked before the patient goes home after delivery.

Desmopressin is the treatment of choice for type 1 vWD.[98] It elicits the release of vWF from endothelial cells. Intranasal preparations of 300 μg are usually used, although the half-life of desmopressin is about 8 hours, so the dose should be repeated every 12 hours. In emergent or preoperative situations, 0.3 μg/kg of desmopressin can be given intravenously over 30 minutes.[97] Desmopressin can rarely cause hyponatremia and fluid retention.[98] Patients can develop tachyphylaxis with desmopressin, so it should not be used for prolonged periods. Also, desmopressin can initiate uterine contractions and should be used with caution in patients in the second or early third trimesters of pregnancy.

For those women who do not respond to desmopressin or for those with vWD types other than 1A, Humate-P or Alphanate should be used. These commercially available concentrates of **antihemophiliac factor** have been tested extensively in clinical studies. They contain two to three times more vWF than they do factor VIII concentrate.[99] The usual dose of Humate-P or Alphanate is 20 to 50 U/kg. During labor, this can be given every 12 hours. For labor and delivery, usually the lower end of the dosage range will suffice. If a cesarean delivery is needed, the upper end of the dosage range should be used. These compounds have been heated at high temperature and treated with solvents and detergents to inactivate blood-borne viruses. It is important to note that products that contain highly purified factor VIII obtained by recombinant DNA should not be used. They contain very little vWF and are ineffective in vWD. Therefore the infused factor VIII has a very short half-life because vWF is essential to prevent the degradation of factor VIII. **Bleeding during pregnancy is rare.** Patients with classic type 1 vWD usually need no treatment owing to the increase in factor VIII levels during pregnancy. Those with a history of postpartum hemorrhage should be given an IV dose of desmopressin immediately after delivery, and the dose should be repeated 24 hours later. For those with types 2 and 3 disease, factor VIII/vWF concentrates are occasionally needed. Before a cesarean delivery, factor VIII activity should be measured. If it is less than 50% of expected, patients with type 1 vWD should be given desmopressin, and patients with vWD type 2 or type 3 should receive factor VIII/vWF concentrate.[100] **In an emergent situation, if the type of vWD is not known with certainty, factor VIII/vWF concentrate should be used.**

KEY POINTS

◆ Four percent of pregnancies will be complicated by maternal platelet counts of less than 150,000/mm³. The vast majority of these patients have gestational thrombocytopenia with a benign course and need no intervention.

◆ Surgical bleeding occurs if the platelet count falls below 50,000/mm,³ and spontaneous bleeding occurs if the platelet count falls below 20,000/mm³. Platelet counts below 30,000/mm³ warrant therapy during pregnancy.

◆ In the second and third trimesters of pregnancy, intravenous immunoglobulin is an effective initial treatment, although glucocorticoids can also be utilized.

◆ Iron deficiency anemia is the most common cause of anemia in pregnancy, and serum ferritin is the single best test to diagnose it.

◆ If a patient with presumed iron deficiency does not increase her reticulocyte count with iron therapy, she may also have a concomitant folic acid deficiency.

◆ Patients pregnant with twins, those on anticonvulsant therapy, those with a hemoglobinopathy, and those who conceive frequently need supplemental folic acid during gestation.

◆ Most hereditary hemoglobinopathies can be detected in utero, and prenatal diagnosis should be offered to the patient early in pregnancy. Early testing can be done using DNA analysis from the chorionic villus sampling specimen.

◆ As in the nonpregnant patient, analgesia, hydration, and oxygen are the key factors in treating pregnant women with sickle cell crisis.

◆ Women with sickle cell disease are at high risk for maternal complications during the puerperium and should be closely monitored.

◆ Patients with sickle cell disease are at increased risk for a fetus with growth restriction and adverse fetal outcomes; therefore they warrant frequent sonography and antepartum fetal evaluation.

◆ Any woman with a low mean corpuscular volume without evidence of iron deficiency should be screened for thalassemia.

◆ In the pregnant patient with von Willebrand disease, the normal increase in the factor VIII clotting complex reduces the risk of bleeding, but levels can fall postpartum and can place the patient at risk for delayed postpartum hemorrhage.

REFERENCES

1. Jensen JD, Wiedmeier SE, Henry E, et al. Linking maternal platelet counts with neonatal platelet counts and outcomes using the data repositories of a multihospital health care system. *Am J Perinatol.* 2011;28:597.
2. McRae KR, Samuels P, Schreiber AD. Pregnancy-associated thrombocytopenia: pathogenesis and management. *Blood.* 1992;80:2697.
3. Aster RH. Gestational thrombocytopenia. A plea for conservative management. *N Engl J Med.* 1990;323:264.
4. Hart D, Dunetz C, Nardi M, et al. An epidemic of maternal thrombocytopenia associated with elevated antiplatelet antibody in 116 consecutive pregnancies: relationship to neonatal platelet count. *Am J Obstet Gynecol.* 1986;154:878.
5. Samuels P, Bussel JB, Braitman LE, et al. Estimation of the risk of thrombocytopenia in the offspring of pregnant women with presumed immune thrombocytopenia purpura. *N Engl J Med.* 1990;323:229.
6. Burrows RF, Kelton JG. Fetal thrombocytopenia and its relationship to maternal thrombocytopenia. *N Engl J Med.* 1993;329:1463.
7. Harrington WI, Minnich V, Arimura G. The autoimmune thrombocytopenias. In: Tascantins LM, ed. *Progress in Hematology.* New York: Grune Stratton; 1956:166.
8. Shulman MR, Marder VJ, Weinrach RS. Similarities between thrombocytopenia in idiopathic purpura. *Ann N Y Acad Sci.* 1965;124:449.
9. Cines DB, Schreiber AD. Immune thrombocytopenia: use of a Coombs antiglobulin test to detect IgG and C3 on platelets. *N Engl J Med.* 1979;300:106.
10. He R, Reid DM, Jones CE, Shulman NR. Spectrum of Ig classes, specificities, and titers of serum anti glycoproteins in chronic idiopathic thrombocytopenia purpura. *Blood.* 1994;83:1024.
11. Stasi R, Stipa E, Masi M, et al. Long-term observation of 208 adults with chronic idiopathic thrombocytopenic purpura. *Am J Med.* 1995;98:4536.
12. Cines DB, Bussell JB. How I treat idiopathic thrombocytopenic purpura (ITP). *Blood.* 2005;106:2244.
13. George JN, Woolf SH, Raskob GE, et al. Idiopathic thrombocytopenic purpura: a practice guideline developed by explicit methods for the American Society of Hematology. *Blood.* 1996;88(1):3-40.
14. Moschcowitz E. Hyaline thrombosis of the terminal arterioles and capillaries: a hitherto undescribed disease. *Proc N Y Pathol Soc.* 1924;24:21.
15. Miller JM, Pastorek JG. Thrombotic thrombocytopenic purpura and the hemolytic uremic syndrome in pregnancy. *Clin Obstet Gynecol.* 1991;34:64.
16. Ridolfi RL, Bell WR. Thrombotic thrombocytopenic purpura: report of 25 cases and a review of the literature. *Medicine.* 1981;60:413.
17. Terrell DR, Williams LA, Vesely SK, et al. The incidence of thrombotic thrombocytopenic purpura-hemolytic uremic syndrome: all patients, idiopathic patients, and patients with severe ADAMTS-13 deficiency. *J Thrombo Haemost.* 2005;3:1432.
18. Tsai HM, Rice L, Sarode R, et al. Antibody inhibitors to von Willebrand factor metalloproteinase and increased binding of von Willebrand factor to platelets in ticlopidine-associated thrombotic thrombocytopenic purpura. *Ann Intern Med.* 2000;132:794.
19. Tsai HM. Advances in the pathogenesis, diagnosis and treatment of thrombotic thrombocytopenic purpura. *J Am Soc Nephrol.* 2003;14:1072.
20. Ferrari S, Mudde GC, Rieger M, et al. IgG subclass distribution of anti-ADAMTS13 antibodies in patients with acquired thrombotic thrombocytopenic purpura. *J Thromb Hemost.* 2009;7:1703.
21. Moatti-Cohen M, Garrec C, Wolf M, et al. Unexpected frequency of Upshaw-Schulman syndrome in pregnancy-onset thrombotic thrombocytopenic purpura. *Blood.* 2012;119(24):5888-5897.
22. Weiner CP. Thrombotic microangiopathy in pregnancy and the postpartum period. *Semin Hematol.* 1987;24:119.
23. Cohen YC, Dbulbegovic B, Shamai-Lubovitz O, Mozes B. The bleeding risk and natural history of idiopathic thrombocytopenic purpura in patients with persistent low platelet counts. *Arch Intern Med.* 2000;160:1630.
24. Park-Wyllie L, Mazzotta P, Pastuszak A, et al. Birth defects after maternal exposure to corticosteroids: prospective cohort study and meta-analysis of epidemiological studies. *Teratology.* 2000;62:385.
25. Egerman RS, Witlin AG, Friedman SA, Sibai BM. Thrombotic thrombocytopenic purpura and hemolytic uremic syndrome in pregnancy: review of 11 cases. *Am J Obstet Gynecol.* 1996;175:950.
26. Abou-Nassar K, Karsh J, Giulivi A, Allan D. Successful prevention of thrombotic thrombocytopenic purpura (TTP) relapse using monthly prophylactic plasma exchanges throughout pregnancy in a patient with systematic lupus erythematosus and a prior history of refractory TTP and recurrent fetal loss. *Transfus Apher Sci.* 2010;43:29.
27. Bussel JB, Zabusky MR, Berkowitz RL, McFarland JG. Fetal alloimmune thrombocytopenia. *N Engl J Med.* 1997;337(1):22.
28. Menell JS, Bussel JB. Antenatal management of thrombocytopenias. *Clin Perinatol.* 1994;21:591.

29. Pacheco LD, Berkowitz RL, Moise KJ Jr, et al. fetal and neonatal alloimmune thrombocytopenia: a management algorithm based on risk stratification. *Obstet Gynecol.* 2011;118:1157.

30. McQuilten ZK, Wood EM, Savoia H, Cole S. A review of pathophysiology and current treatment for neonatal alloimmune thrombocytopenia (NAIT) and introducing the Australian NAIT registry. *Aust N Z J Obstet Gynecol.* 2011;51:191.

31. Kamphuis MM, Oepkes D. Fetal and neonatal alloimmune thrombocytopenia: prenatal interventions. *Prenat Diagn.* 2011;31:712.

32. Rayment R, Brunskill SJ, Soothill PW, et al. Antenatal interventions for fetomaternal alloimmune thrombocytopenia. *Cochrane Database Syst Rev.* 2011;(5):CD004226.

33. Reveiz L, Gyte GM, Cuervo LG, Casasbuenas A. Treatments for iron-deficiency anaemia in pregnancy. *Cochrane Database Syst Rev.* 2011;(10):CD003094.

34. Ho CH, Yuan CC, Yeh SH. Serum ferritin, folate and cobalamin levels and their correlation with anemia in normal full-term pregnant women. *Eur J Obstet Gynecol Reprod Biol.* 1987;26:7.

35. Carr MC. Serum iron-TIBC in the diagnosis of iron deficiency anemia during pregnancy. *Obstet Gynecol.* 1971;38:602.

36. Boued JL. Iron deficiency: assessment during pregnancy and its importance in pregnant adolescents. *Am J Clin Nutr.* 1994;59:5025.

37. Tran TN, Eubanks SK, Schaffer KJ, Zhou CY, Linder MC. Secretion of ferritin by rat hepatoma cells and its regulation by inflammatory cytokines and iron. *Blood.* 1997;90:4979.

38. van den Broek NR, Letsky EA, White SA, Shenkin A. Iron status in pregnant women; which measurements are valid? *Br J Haematol.* 1998;103:817.

39. Ahluwalia N. Diagnostic utility of serum transferrin receptors measurement in assessing iron status. *Nutr Rev.* 1998;56:133.

40. Mei Z, Cogswell ME, Looker AC, et al. Assessment of iron status in US pregnant women from the National Health and Nutrition Examination Survey (MHANES), 1999-2006. *Am J Clin Nutr.* 2011;93:1312.

41. Milman N, Bergholt T, Byg KE, et al. Iron status and iron balance during pregnancy. A critical reappraisal of iron supplementation. *Acta Obstet Gynecol Scand.* 1999;78:749.

42. Young MW, Lupafya E, Kapenda E, Bobrow EA. The effectiveness of weekly iron supplementation in pregnant women of rural northern Malawi. *Trop Doct.* 2000;30:84.

43. Yakoob MY, Bhutta ZA. Effect of routine iron supplementation with or without folic acid on anemia during pregnancy. *BMC Public Health.* 2011;11:S21.

44. Singh K, Fong YF, Kuperan P. A comparison between intravenous iron polymaltose complex (Ferrum Hausmann) and oral ferrous fumarate in the treatment of iron deficiency anaemia in pregnancy. *Eur J Haematol.* 1998;60:119.

45. Hallak M, Sharon AS, Diukman R, et al. Supplementing iron intravenously in pregnancy: a way to avoid blood transfusions. *J Reprod Med.* 1997;42:99.

46. Scholl TO, Hediger ML. Anemia and iron-deficiency anemia: compilation of data on pregnancy outcome. *Am J Clin Nutr.* 1994;59:4925.

47. Yip R. Significance of abnormally low or high hemoglobin concentration during pregnancy: special consideration of iron nutrition. *Am J Clin Nutr.* 2000;72:272S.

48. Sifakis S, Pharmakides G. Anemia in pregnancy. *Ann N Y Acad Sci.* 2000;900:125.

49. Hemminki E, Starfield B. Routine administration of iron and vitamins during pregnancy: review of controlled clinical trials. *Br J Obstet Gynaecol.* 1978;85:404.

50. Stephansson O, Dickman PW, Johansson A, Cnattingius S. Maternal hemoglobin concentration during pregnancy and risk of stillbirth. *JAMA.* 2000;284:2611.

51. Demmouche A, Lazrag A, Moulessehoul S. Prevalence of anaemia in pregnant women during the last trimester: consequence for birth weight. *Rev Med Pharmacol Sci.* 2011;15:436.

52. Kaplan JS, Iqbal S, England BG, et al. Is pregnancy in diabetic women associated with folate deficiency? *Diabetes Care.* 1999;22:1017.

53. Vollsett SE, Refsum H, Irgens LM, et al. Plasma total homocysteine, pregnancy complications, and adverse pregnancy outcomes: the Hordaland homocysteine study. *Am J Clin Nutr.* 2000;71:962.

54. Munger RG, Tamura T, Johnston KE, et al. Oral clefts and maternal biomarkers of folate-dependent one-carbon metabolism in Utah. *Birth Defects Res.* 2011;91:153.

55. Ito M, Yoshimura K, Toyoda N, Wada H. Pregnancy and delivery in patient with von Willebrand's disease. *J Obstet Gynaecol Res.* 1997;23:37.

56. Bauman WA, Shaw S, Jayatilleke E, et al. Increased intake of calcium reverses vitamin B-12 malabsorption induced by metformin. *Diabetes Care.* 2000;23:1227.

57. Savage DG, Lindenbaum J, Stabler SP, Allen RH. Sensitivity of serum methylmalonic acid and total homocysteine determinations for diagnosing cobalamin and folate deficiencies. *Am J Med.* 1994;96:238.

58. Larrabee KD, Monga M. Women with sickle cell trait are at increased risk for preeclampsia. *Am J Obstet Gynecol.* 1997;177:425.

59. O'Brien SH, Klima J, Reed S, et al. Hormonal contraception use and pregnancy in adolescents with sickle cell disease: analysis of Michigan Medicaid claims. *Contraception.* 2011;83:134.

60. Powars DR, Sandhu M, Niland-Weiss J, et al. Pregnancy in sickle cell disease. *Obstet Gynecol.* 1986;67:217.

61. Seoud MA, Cantwell C, Nobles G, Levy OL. Outcome of pregnancies complicated by sickle cell disease and sickle-C hemoglobinopathies. *Am J Perinatol.* 1994;11:187.

62. Smith JA, England M, Bellevue R, et al. Pregnancy in sickle cell disease: experience of the cooperative study of sickle cell disease. *Obstet Gynecol.* 1996;87:199.

63. Morris JS, Dunn DT, Poddorr D, Serjeant GR. Hematological risk factors for pregnancy outcome in Jamaican women with homozygous sickle cell disease. *Br J Obstet Gynaecol.* 1994;101:770.

64. Miller ST, Sleeper LA, Pegelow CH, et al. Prediction of adverse outcomes in children with sickle cell disease. *N Engl J Med.* 2000;342:8.

65. Anyaegbunam A, Langer O, Brustman L, et al. The application of uterine and umbilical artery velocimetry to the antenatal supervision of pregnancies complicated by maternal sickle hemoglobinopathies. *Am J Obstet Gynecol.* 1988;159:544.

66. Howard RJ, Tuck SM, Pearson TC. Blood transfusion in pregnancy complicated by sickle cell disease: effects on blood rheology and uteroplacental Doppler velocimetry. *Clin Lab Haematol.* 1994;16:253.

67. Villers MA, Mamison MG, DeCastro LM, James AH. Morbidity associated with sickle cell disease in pregnancy. *Am J Obstet Gynecol.* 2008;199:125.

68. Seaman CD, Yabes J, Li J, Moore CG, Ragni MV. Venous thromboembolism in pregnant women with sickle cell disease: a retrospective database analysis. *Thromb Res.* 2014;134:1249.

69. Cunningham FG, Pritchard JA, Mason R. Pregnancy and sickle cell hemoglobinopathies: results with and without prophylactic transfusions. *Obstet Gynecol.* 1983;62:419.

70. Morrison JC, Schneider JM, Whybrew WD, et al. Prophylactic transfusions in pregnant patients with sickle hemoglobinopathies: benefit versus risk. *Obstet Gynecol.* 1980;56:274.

71. Koshy M, Burd L, Wallace D, et al. Prophylactic red-cell transfusions in pregnant patients with sickle cell disease: a randomized cooperative study. *N Engl J Med.* 1988;319:1447.

72. Mahomed K. Prophylactic versus selective blood transfusion for sickle cell anaemia during pregnancy. *Cochrane Database Syst Rev.* 2000;(2):CD000040.

73. Hassell K. Pregnancy and sickle cell disease. *Hematol Oncol Clin North Am.* 2005;19:903.

74. Ngo C, Kayem G, Habibi A, et al. Pregnancy in sickle cell disease: maternal and fetal outcomes in a population receiving prophylactic partial exchange transfusions. *Eur J Obstet Gynecol Reprod Biol.* 2010;153:138.

75. Winder AD, Johnson S, Murphy J, Ehsanipoor R. Epidural analgesia for treatment of a sickle cell crisis during pregnancy. *Obstet Gynecol.* 2011;118:495.

76. Solanki DL, Kletter GG, Castro O. Acute splenic sequestration crises in adults with sickle cell disease. *Am J Med.* 1986;80:985.

77. ACOG Practice Bulletin 78. Hemoglobinopathies in pregnancy. *Obstet Gynecol.* 2007;109:229.

78. Ghosh A, Tan MH, Liang ST, et al. Ultrasound evaluation of pregnancies at risk for homozygous alpha-thalassaemia-1. *Prenat Diagn.* 1987;7:307.

79. Woo JS, Liang ST, Lo RL, Chan FY. Doppler blood flow velocity waveforms in alpha-thalassemia hydrops fetalis. *J Ultrasound Med.* 1987;6:679.

80. Hsieh FJ, Chang FM, Huang HC, et al. Umbilical vein blood flow measurement in nonimmune hydrops fetalis. *Obstet Gynecol.* 1988;71:188.

81. Mordel N, Birkenfeld A, Goldfarb AN, Rachmilewitz EA. Successful full-term pregnancy in homozygous beta-thalassemia major: case report and review of the literature. *Obstet Gynecol.* 1989;73:837.

82. White JM, Richards R, Jelenski G, et al. Iron state in alpha and beta thalassaemia trait. *J Clin Pathol.* 1986;39:256.

83. Leung CF, Lao TT, Chang AM. Effect of folate supplement on pregnant women with beta-thalassaemia minor. *Eur J Obstet Gynecol Reprod Biol.* 1989;33:209.

84. Ricchi P, Costantini S, Spasiano A, et al. A case of well-tolerated and safe deferasirox administration during the first trimester of a spontaneous

pregnancy in an advanced maternal age thalassemic patient. *Acta Haematol.* 2011;125:222.

85. Schmidt RM. Laboratory diagnosis of hemoglobinopathies. *JAMA.* 1973;224:1276.

86. Castaman G, Rodeghiero F. Current management of von Willebrand's disease. *Drugs.* 1995;50:602.

87. Pacheco LD, Constantine MM, Saade GR, et al. Von Willebrand disease and pregnancy: a practical approach for the diagnosis and treatment. *Am J Obstet Gynecol.* 2010;203:194.

88. Mazurier C, Ribba AS, Gaucher C, Meyer D. Molecular genetics of von Willebrand disease. *Ann Genet.* 1998;41:34.

89. Giles AR, Hoogendoorn H, Benford K. Type IIB von Willebrand's disease presenting as thrombocytopenia during pregnancy. *Br J Haematol.* 1987;67:349.

90. Kouides PA. Females with von Willebrand disease: 72 years as the silent majority. *Haemophilia.* 1998;4:665.

91. Casonato A, Sarrori MT, Bertomoro A, et al. Pregnancy-induced worsening of thrombocytopenia in a patient with type IIB von Willebrand's disease. *Blood Coagul Fibrinolysis.* 1991;2:33.

92. Nichols WL, Hutlin MB, James AH, et al. Von Willebrand disease: evidence-based diagnosis and management guidelines. The National Heart, Lung and Blood Institute (NHLBI) Expert Panel report. *Haemophilia.* 2008;14:171.

93. Kadir RA, Lee CA, Sabin CA, et al. Pregnancy in women with von Willebrand's disease or factor XI deficiency. *Br J Obstet Gynaecol.* 1998;105:314.

94. Chediak JR, Alban GM, Maxey B. Von Willebrand's disease and pregnancy: management during delivery and outcome of offspring. *Am J Obstet Gynecol.* 1986;155:618.

95. Conti M, Mari D, Conti E, et al. Pregnancy in women with different types of von Willebrand disease. *Obstet Gynecol.* 1986;68:282.

96. Ieko M, Sakurama S, Sagan A, et al. Effect of factor VIII concentrate on type IIB von Willebrand's disease-associated thrombocytopenia presenting during pregnancy in identical twin mothers. *Am J Hematol.* 1990;35:26.

97. Pacheco LD, Constantine MM, Saade GR, et al. von Willebrand disease and pregnancy: a practical approach for diagnosis and treatment. *Am J Obstet Gynecol.* 2010;203:194.

98. Mannucci PM. Treatment of von Willebrand's disease. *N Engl J Med.* 2004;351:683.

99. Bertolini DM, Butler CS. Severe hyponatremia secondary to desmopressin therapy in von Willebrand's disease. *Anesth Intensive Care.* 2000;28:199.

100. Nitu-Whalley IC, Griffloen A, Harrington C, Lee CA. Retrospective review of the management of elective surgery with desmopressin and clotting factor concentrates in patients with von Willebrand disease. *Am J Hematol.* 2001;66:280.

Additional references for this chapter are available at ExpertConsult.com.

CHAPTER 45

Thromboembolic Disorders in Pregnancy

CHRISTIAN M. PETTKER and CHARLES J. LOCKWOOD

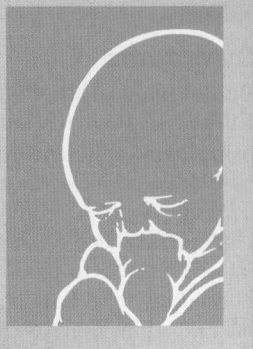

KEY ABBREVIATIONS

Activated partial thromboplastin time	aPTT
American College of Obstetricians and Gynecologists	ACOG
Activated protein C	APC
Adenosine diphosphate	ADP
Antiphospholipid antibody	APA
Antiphospholipid syndrome	APS
Computed tomography	CT
Computed tomographic pulmonary angiography	CTPA
Deep venous thrombosis	DVT
Disseminated intravascular coagulation	DIC
Enzyme-linked immunosorbent assay	ELISA
Factor V Leiden	FVL
Heparin-induced thrombocytopenia	HIT
Inferior vena cava	IVC
International normalized ratio	INR
Low-molecular-weight heparin	LMWH
Magnetic resonance angiography	MRA
Magnetic resonance imaging	MRI
Protein Z–dependent protease inhibitor	ZPI
Pulmonary embolus	PE
Systemic lupus erythematosus	SLE
Thrombin-activatable fibrinolysis inhibitor	TAFI
Thromboxane A_2	TXA_2
Tissue factor	TF
Tissue factor pathway inhibitor	TFPI
Type 1 plasminogen activator inhibitor	PAI-1
Unfractionated heparin	UFH
Urokinase-type plasminogen activator	uPA
Venous thromboembolism	VTE
Venous ultrasonography	VUS
Ventilation-perfusion scan	V/Q scan

BACKGROUND AND HISTORIC NOTES

Pregnancy, childbirth, and the puerperium pose serious challenges to a woman's hemostatic system. Whereas implantation, placentation, and uterine spiral artery remodeling lead to the development of the high-volume, high-flow, low-resistance uteroplacental circulation required for human fetal development, they require enhanced hemostatic responsiveness to avoid potentially fatal hemorrhage. **The price paid for this essential hemostatic adaptation to human hemochorial placentation is an increased risk of superficial and deep venous thrombosis (DVT) and pulmonary embolus (PE).** Acquired or inherited thrombophilias, obesity, advanced maternal age, advanced parity, antepartum hospitalizations, surgery, and infection are major risk factors for DVT and PE in pregnancy and the puerperium. The expeditious identification and prompt treatment of thrombotic events is critical to avoiding death and serious postphlebitic sequelae.

DIAGNOSES AND DEFINITIONS

Thrombosis is the obstruction or occlusion of a vessel by a blood clot. Venous thromboembolism (VTE) includes venous thrombosis of the deep venous system of the lower (common) or upper (uncommon) extremity (DVT). Thrombosis or inflammation of the *superficial* venous system is generally not associated with morbidity, although in some cases it can develop into or be associated with DVT or PE. In fact, 10% to 20% of superficial thrombosis cases in nonpregnant patients are associated with DVT. **Pulmonary embolus is the obstruction of the pulmonary artery or one of its branches, arising from a clot from a DVT in approximately 90% of cases.** A majority of PE cases are due to deportment of thrombus from the lower extremities; for the purposes of this chapter, *pulmonary embolus* will refer to VTE of the pulmonary vasculature (rather than air, fat, or amniotic fluid embolism).

Symptoms

Deep Venous Thrombosis

Clinical findings typical of DVT include erythema, warmth, pain, edema, and tenderness localized to the area of the thrombosis. Occasionally, a palpable cord may be present that corresponds to a thrombosed vein. **Homans sign** is pain and tenderness elicited on compression of the calf muscles by squeezing the muscles or by dorsiflexion of the foot. These are rather nonspecific signs and symptoms that involve a broad differential diagnosis, including cellulitis, ruptured or strained muscle or tendon, trauma, ruptured popliteal (Baker) cyst, cutaneous vasculitis, superficial thrombophlebitis, and lymphedema. The specificity of these manifestations is less than 50%, and among patients with these signs and symptoms, the diagnosis of DVT is confirmed by objective testing in only approximately one third of the group.[1,2]

Pulmonary Embolism

Tachypnea (>20 breaths/min) and tachycardia (>100 beats/min) are present in 90% of patients with acute PE, but these findings lack specificity and generate a broad differential diagnosis.[3] Presyncope and syncope are rarer symptoms and indicate a massive embolus.[4]

EPIDEMIOLOGY AND INCIDENCE

Occurring in approximately in 1 in 1500 pregnancies, VTE is a relatively uncommon disorder but is a leading cause of mortality and serious morbidity in pregnant women.[5-12] This rate represents a nearly tenfold increase compared with nonpregnant women of comparable childbearing age. According to the most recent U.S. vital statistics, from 2006 through 2010, VTE was a leading cause of maternal mortality that contributed to 9% of pregnancy-related deaths.[13] Classic teaching viewed the postpartum period as the period of maximal thrombotic occurrence. However, management styles of prior eras that included prolonged puerperal bed rest and estrogen to suppress lactation likely inflated this risk.[10] More recent studies have shown that a majority of thromboembolic events happen in the antepartum period.[5,7,14-16] Given its shorter duration, and after adjusting for duration of exposure, the day-to-day relative risk of VTE is about threefold to eightfold higher in the puerperium.[12] New evidence suggests that the risk for a thrombotic event extends out to 12 weeks postpartum, although the absolute increase in risk is quite low after 6 weeks.[17]

GENETICS

It is well known that inherited mutations in various components of the coagulation cascade, the so-called inherited thrombophilias, contribute to significant risk for thrombosis, especially in the presence of other risk factors such as pregnancy, surgery (e.g., cesarean delivery), trauma, infection, or immobility. **Factor V Leiden is the most common mutation and accounts for over 40% of inherited thrombophilias in most studies.** Most of these genetic mutations act in an autosomal-dominant manner, thus one mutation will incur an elevated risk for VTE; individuals with two mutations will have higher risks for thrombotic events than those with one. Patients with a strong family history of thrombotic events who have screened negative for the panel of known thrombophilia mutations likely have an as yet unrecognized gene defect in a specific component of the coagulation

cascade. The details of the known inherited thrombophilias are discussed later in this chapter.

PHYSIOLOGY OF HEMOSTASIS

Vasoconstriction and Platelet Action

Vasoconstriction and platelet activity play a primary initial role in limiting blood loss following vascular disruption and endothelial damage. Vasoconstriction limits blood flow and also limits the size of thrombus necessary to repair the defect. Platelet adherence to damaged vessels is mediated by the formation of von Willebrand factor (vWF) "bridges" anchored at one end to subendothelial collagen and at the other to the platelet glycoprotein Ib (GP Ib)/factor IX/V receptor.[18] Platelet adhesion stimulates release of α-granules that contain vWF, thrombospondin, platelet factor 4, fibrinogen, β-thromboglobulin, and platelet-derived growth factor as well as dense granules that contain adenosine diphosphate (ADP) and serotonin. These latter molecules, when combined with the release of thromboxane A_2 (TXA_2), contribute to further vasoconstriction and platelet activation. In addition, ADP causes a conformational change in the platelet GP IIb/IIIa receptor that promotes aggregation by forming interplatelet fibrinogen, fibronectin, and vitronectin bridges.[19]

Coagulation Cascade

Platelet action alone is insufficient to provide adequate hemostasis in the face of a substantial vascular insult; in this setting, the coagulation cascade—with resultant fibrin plug formation—is required to restore hemostasis. Tissue factor (TF), a cell membrane-bound glycoprotein, is the primary initiator of the coagulation cascade.[20] It is expressed constitutively by epithelial, stromal, and perivascular cells throughout the body and in abundance by endometrial stromal cells and the pregnant uterine decidua.[20,21] TF is also present in low concentrations in blood, on activated platelets, and in high levels in amniotic fluid, which accounts for the coagulopathy seen in amniotic fluid embolism.[22] It is interesting to note that although intrauterine survival is possible in the absence of platelets or fibrinogen, it is not possible in the absence of TF.[23] Clotting is initiated by the binding of TF to factor VII, the only clotting factor with intrinsic coagulation activity in its zymogenic form (Fig. 45-1).

Following endothelial injury and in the presence of ionized calcium, perivascular cell- or platelet-bound TF comes into contact with factor VII on anionic cell membrane phospholipids. Factor VII has low intrinsic clotting activity but can be autoactivated after binding to TF, or it can be activated by thrombin or activated factors such as IXa, Xa, or XIIa.[20,24] The TF–activated factor VII (VIIa) complex initiates the elements of the coagulation cascade by activating both factors IX and X. Activated factor IX (IXa) complexes with its cofactor VIIIa to indirectly activate X. Once generated, Xa binds with its cofactor Va to convert prothrombin (factor II) to thrombin (factor IIa). Cofactors V and VIII can each be activated by either thrombin or Xa, and XIIa activates XI on the surface of activated platelets, which provides an alternative route to IX activation. Factor XII can be activated by kallikrein/kininogen as well as by plasmin. **The key event of hemostasis occurs when thrombin cleaves fibrinogen to produce fibrin.** Fibrin monomers self-polymerize and are cross-linked by thrombin-activated factor XIIIa. Although TF is the initiator of hemostasis, thrombin is the ultimate arbiter of clotting; it not only activates platelets

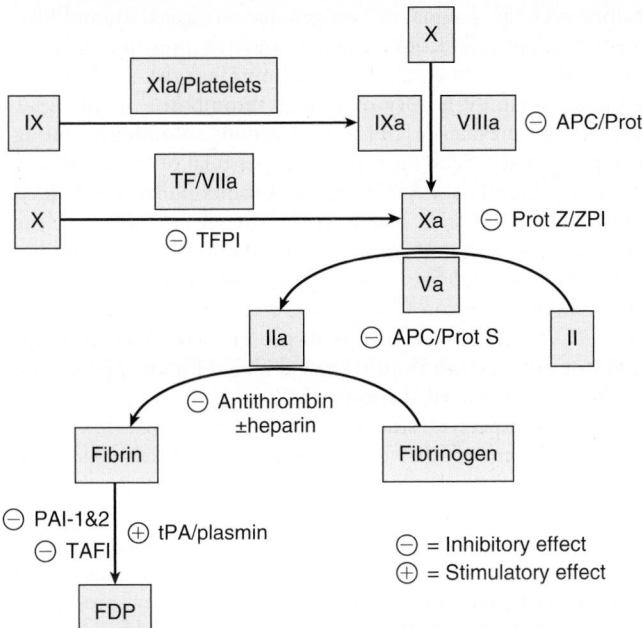

FIG 45-1 Hemostatic, thrombotic, and fibrinolytic pathways. APC, activated protein C; FDP, fibrin degradation product; PAI, plasminogen activator inhibitor; PROT, protein; TAFI, thrombin-activatable fibrinolysis inhibitor; TFPI, tissue factor pathway inhibitor; tPA, tissue-type plasminogen activator; ZPI, protein Z–dependent protease inhibitor.

and generates fibrin, it also activates critical clotting factors and cofactors (V, VII, VIII, XI, and XIII). Figure 45-1 provides a diagram of the interaction of the various components of the coagulation cascade.

Anticoagulant System

The risk of thrombosis, the inappropriate and excessive activation of the clotting cascade, is restrained by the anticoagulant system (see Fig. 45-1). Evidence shows that the coagulation system "idles" like a car engine to quickly respond to vascular injury, and thus **the anticoagulant system performs the critical role of preventing inappropriate acceleration of clotting.**[24] Tissue factor pathway inhibitor (TFPI) binds to the prothrombinase complex (factor Xa/TF/factor VIIa) to stop TF-mediated clotting.[25] However, as noted, factor XIa generation can bypass this block. Moreover, in the 10 to 15 seconds before TFPI-mediated prothrombinase inhibition, sufficient quantities of factors Va, VIIIa, IXa, and Xa and thrombin are generated to sustain clotting for some time. As a result, additional physiologic anticoagulant molecules are required to maintain blood fluidity.

Paradoxically, thrombin also plays a pivotal role in the anticoagulant system by binding to thrombomodulin, which causes a conformation change that allows it to activate protein C. The activated protein C (APC) molecule binds to anionic endothelial cell membrane phospholipids on damaged vessels or to the endothelial cell protein-C receptor (EPCR) to inactivate factors Va and VIIIa.[26] Protein S is an important cofactor in this process because it enhances APC activity. Factor Va is also a cofactor in APC-mediated factor VIIIa inactivation.

Factor Xa can also be inhibited by the protein Z–dependent protease inhibitor (ZPI). When ZPI forms a complex with its cofactor, protein Z, its inhibitory activity is enhanced a thousandfold, although ZPI can also inhibit factor XIa independent

of protein Z.[27] Deficiencies of protein Z can promote both bleeding and thrombosis, although the latter predominates particularly in the presence of other thrombophilias.

Thrombin activity is modulated by a number of serine protease inhibitors—such as heparin cofactor II, α-2 macroglobulin, and antithrombin—which serve to inactivate thrombin and Xa. The most active inhibitor within this group is antithrombin, which binds to either thrombin or factor Xa and then to heparin or other glycosaminoglycans, augmenting antithrombin's rate of thrombin inactivation more than a thousandfold.[28,29] The other two inhibitors work in a similar fashion to inhibit thrombin.

Clot Lysis and Fibrinolysis

Fibrinolysis is a further critical element in preventing overwhelming thrombosis (see Fig. 45-1). Tissue-type plasminogen activator (tPA), an endothelial enzyme metabolized by the liver, becomes embedded in fibrin and cleaves plasminogen to generate plasmin, which in turn cleaves fibrin into fibrin degradation products; the latter are indirect measures of fibrinolysis. These fibrin degradation products can also inhibit thrombin action, a favorable effect when production is limited, but a contributor to disseminated intravascular coagulation (DIC) when production is excessive. A second plasminogen activator, urokinase-type plasminogen activator (uPA), is produced by endothelial cells. A series of fibrinolysis inhibitors also prevent hemorrhage from premature clot lysis. The α-2 plasmin inhibitor is bound to the fibrin clot, where it prevents premature fibrinolysis. Platelets and endothelial cells release type 1 plasminogen activator inhibitor (PAI-1), an inactivator of tPA. In pregnancy, the decidua is also a rich source of PAI-1,[30] whereas the placenta produces mostly type 2 (PAI-2). The thrombin-activatable fibrinolysis inhibitor (TAFI) is another fibrinolytic inhibitor that is also activated by the thrombin-thrombomodulin complex.[31] TAFI modifies fibrin and renders it resistant to inactivation by plasmin.

PATHOPHYSIOLOGY OF THROMBOSIS IN PREGNANCY

Characteristic physiologic changes in decidual and systemic hemostatic systems occur in pregnancy in preparation for the hemostatic challenges of implantation, placentation, and childbirth. Decidual TF and PAI-1 expression are greatly increased in response to progesterone, and levels of placental-derived PAI-2, which are negligible prior to pregnancy, increase until term.[30,31] Pregnancy is associated with systemic changes that enhance hemostatic capability and promote thrombosis. For example, **a doubling occurs in circulating concentrations of fibrinogen, and 20% to 1000% increases are seen in factors VII, VIII, IX, X, and XII, all of which peak at term in preparation for delivery.**[32] Levels of vWF also increase up to 400% at term.[32] In contrast, levels of prothrombin and factor V remain unchanged, and levels of factor XIII and XI decline modestly. **Concomitantly, there is a 40% to 60% decrease in the levels of free protein S, conferring an overall resistance to activated protein C.**[32,33] Further reductions in free protein-S concentrations are caused by stress, cesarean delivery, and infection; this accounts for the high rate of PE following cesarean deliveries, particularly in association with prolonged labor and endomyometritis. **Coagulation parameters** may normalize as early as 3 weeks postpartum, but **they generally return to baseline at 6 to 12 weeks.**

The risk of thrombosis in pregnancy is also related to physical changes in the gravid woman. **Venous stasis in the lower extremities results from compression of the inferior vena cava (IVC) and pelvic veins by the enlarging uterus.**[34,35] Despite the presence of the sigmoid colon promoting uterine dextrorotation, ultrasound findings indicate lower flow velocities in the left leg veins throughout pregnancy.[36] This would explain why multiple studies have confirmed that **the incidence of thrombosis is far greater in the left leg than in the right.**[5,15] Hormone mediated increases in deep vein capacitance secondary to increased circulating levels of estrogen and local production of prostacyclin and nitric oxide also contribute to the increased risk of thrombosis.

Antiphospholipid Syndrome

Overall, antiphospholipid syndrome (APS) is responsible for approximately 14% of thromboembolic events in pregnancy.[37,38] The diagnosis of APS requires the presence of prior or current vascular thrombosis or characteristic obstetric complications together with at least one laboratory criterion, such as anticardiolipin antibodies (immunoglobulin G [IgG] or IgM greater than 40 GPL [1 GPL unit is 1 μg of IgG antibody] or 40 MPL [1 MPL unit is 1 μg of IgM antibody] or greater than the 99th percentile), anti–β-2 glycoprotein-I (IgG or IgM greater than the 99th percentile), or lupus anticoagulant.[39] Refer to Chapter 46 for details of diagnosis and treatment of APS.

The antiphospholipid antibodies (APAs) are a class of self-recognition immunoglobulins whose epitopes are proteins bound to negatively charged phospholipids. These antibodies must be present on two or more occasions at least 12 weeks apart for diagnosis[39] and are present in 2.2% of the general obstetric population, and most affected patients have uncomplicated pregnancies.[40] **Thus providers should use caution when ordering and interpreting tests in the absence of APS-qualifying clinical criteria.**

APS has been associated with both venous (DVT, PE) and arterial vascular events (stroke). A meta-analysis of 18 studies has shown elevated risk of DVT, PE, and recurrent VTE among patients with systemic lupus erythematous (SLE) who test positive for APA. Overall, when compared with those SLE patients who do not test positive for either test, those with lupus anticoagulants and anticardiolipin antibodies have a respective sixfold and twofold increased risk of venous thrombosis.[41] These antibodies also pose a risk to patients without SLE. The lifetime prevalence of arterial or venous thrombosis in affected non-SLE patients is approximately 30%, with an event rate of 1% per year.[42,43] The risks of thromboembolic events are highly dependent on the presence of other predisposing factors that include pregnancy, estrogen exposure, immobility, surgery, and infection. As noted above, APS has also been associated with adverse pregnancy outcome and accounts for 14% of VTE in pregnancy.[37,38] In fact, the risk of a thrombotic event in pregnancy is 5% even with prophylaxis.[44] All patients who present with VTE in pregnancy or in the postpartum period should have an appropriate APS workup.

Inherited Thrombophilias

The inherited thrombophilias are a heterogeneous group of genetic disorders associated with arterial and venous thrombosis as well as fetal loss. As with APAs, the occurrence of a thromboembolic event is highly dependent on other predisposing factors such as pregnancy, exogenous estrogens, immobility, obesity, surgery, infection, trauma, and the presence of other thrombophilias. However, the most important risk modifier is a personal or family history of venous thrombosis.[45] Table 45-1 presents the prevalence and risk of venous thrombosis among pregnant patients with and without a personal or family history of venous thrombosis. As noted, the thrombophilias are divided into high and low risk based on the overall risk of VTE. The screening for and management of inherited thrombophilias during and around the time of pregnancy has been recently addressed by American College of Obstetricians and Gynecologists (ACOG).[46] **All patients who present with VTE in pregnancy or postpartum should be considered for an appropriate workup for inherited thrombophilias.**

Recent prospective studies have suggested that lower-risk inherited thrombophilias may have an even weaker association with maternal thrombosis than that reported by the retrospective studies cited in Table 45-1. For example, a prospective study of 4885 low-risk women screened in the first trimester of pregnancy noted that 134 (2.7%) carried the factor V Leiden mutation, but none had a thromboembolic event during pregnancy or the in puerperium (95% confidence interval [CI], 0% to 2.7%).[47] In two other prospective studies[48,49] that involved 584 Irish and 4250 British pregnant women again screened for factor V Leiden early in pregnancy, no thrombotic episodes were noted among carriers. Said and associates[50] tested 1707 Australian nulliparous women blindly for factor V Leiden, the prothrombin gene G20210A mutation, and a thrombomodulin polymorphism prior to 22 weeks and reported an expected prevalence of heterozygosity for the factor V Leiden and prothrombin G20210A gene mutations and homozygosity for the thrombomodulin polymorphism of 5.39%, 2.38%, and 3.51%, respectively; again, none of the patients developed VTEs. However, one prospective study[51] of 2480 women tested for activated protein-C resistance/factor V Leiden early in pregnancy observed that affected patients had an eightfold increase in VTE. Thus the true risk of thrombosis in patients with low-risk inherited thrombophilias is probably lower than that suggested by retrospective case-control and cohort studies and is also likely dependent on the presence of concomitant risk factors such as a strong family history, obesity, and surgery.

Risk Factors and Associations

Virchow triad—vascular stasis, hypercoagulability, and vascular trauma—describes the three classic antecedents to thrombosis, and many of the physiologic changes of pregnancy contribute to these criteria. Other pregnancy-specific risk factors for thrombosis include increased parity, postpartum endomyometritis, operative vaginal delivery, and cesarean delivery. The latter is associated with a substantial ninefold increase in VTE risk compared with vaginal delivery.[14] Risk factors not unique to pregnancy include age greater than 35 years, obesity, trauma, immobility, infection, smoking, nephrotic syndrome, hyperviscosity syndromes, cancer, surgery (particularly orthopedic procedures), and a history of DVT or PE (Table 45-2). **Admission to the hospital in pregnancy may be associated with a seventeenfold increased risk for VTE compared with a nonhospitalized cohort, with this risk remaining high (sixfold) for the 28 days after admission.**[52] In vitro fertilization (IVF) has been shown to increase the risk for VTE in the first trimester in a cross-sectional study in Sweden, although the overall absolute risk is still rather low.[53]

TABLE 45-1 INHERITED THROMBOPHILIAS AND ASSOCIATION WITH VENOUS THROMBOEMBOLISM IN PREGNANCY

RISK	THROMBOPHILIA TYPE	PREVALENCE IN THE EUROPEAN POPULATION	PREVALENCE IN PATIENTS WITH VTE IN PREGNANCY	RR/OR OF VTE IN PREGNANCY (95% CI)	PROBABILITY OF VTE IN PREGNANT PATIENTS WITH PERSONAL OR FAMILY HX	PROBABILITY OF VTE IN PREGNANT PATIENTS WITHOUT PERSONAL OR FAMILY HX	STUDY
High risk	FVL homozygous	0.07%*	<1%*	25.4 (8.8-66)	≫10%	1.5%	45, 124-127
	Prothrombin gene G20210A mutation homozygous	0.02%*	<1%*	N/A	≫10%	2.8%	128, 129
	Antithrombin III deficiency	0.02%-1.1%	1%-8%	119	11%-40%	3.0%-7.2%	124, 127, 128
	Compound heterozygous (FVL/ prothrombin G20210A)	0.17%+	<1%+	84 (19-369)	4.7% (overall probability of VTE in pregnancy)		45, 124, 130
Low risk	FVL heterozygous	5.3%	44%	6.9 (3.3-15.2)	>10%	0.26%	45, 124-126, 131
	Prothrombin G20210A mutation heterozygous	2.9%	17%	9.5 (2.1-66.7)	>10%	0.37%-0.5%	45, 124, 129, 130
	Protein C deficiency	0.2%-0.3%	<14%	13.0 (1.4-123)	NA	0.8%-1.7%	124, 127, 128, 132
	Protein S deficiency	0.03%-0.13%	12.4%	NA	NA	<1%-6.6%	45, 124, 128, 133

*Calculated based on a Hardy-Weinberg equilibrium.
CI, confidence interval; *FVL*, factor V Leiden; *HX*, history; *NA*, Data not available; *OR*, odds ratio; *PREG*, pregnant; *PROB*, probability; *PTS*, patients; *RR*, relative risk; *VTE*, venous thromboembolism.

Complications

Thromboembolism is associated with serious complications that include arrhythmia, hypoxia, pulmonary hypertension, heart failure, and postthrombotic syndrome of the extremities. Thromboembolism is a major cause of death worldwide; thus prompt diagnosis and treatment is a priority. When confronted with the signs and symptoms suggestive of VTE, rapid initiation of the workup and treatment is essential to avoid complications. Complications of anticoagulation, such as bleeding or thrombocytopenia, are also a reality and should be avoided.

Considerations in Management of Pregnant Women

Pregnancy and the postpartum period are considered a high-risk period for thromboembolism. Key considerations in the workup and management of pregnant women are the selection of appropriate diagnostic tools and anticoagulation regimens with special concern regarding pregnancy-related changes and fetal exposures.

Diagnosis of Venous Thromboembolism
DEEP VENOUS THROMBOSIS
CLINICAL SIGNS AND SYMPTOMS

The clinical findings typical of DVT include erythema, warmth, pain, edema, and tenderness localized to the area of the thrombosis. Occasionally, a palpable cord may correspond to a thrombosed vein. Homans sign is the pain and tenderness elicited on compression of the calf muscles by squeezing the muscles or by dorsiflexion of the foot. These are rather nonspecific signs and symptoms that involve a broad differential diagnosis that includes cellulitis, ruptured or strained muscle or tendon, trauma, ruptured popliteal (Baker) cyst, cutaneous vasculitis, superficial thrombophlebitis, and lymphedema. In fact, as noted above, evidence suggests that the specificities of these manifestations are less than 50%, and among patients with these signs and symptoms, the diagnosis of DVT is confirmed by objective testing in only approximately one third of the group.[1,2]

RISK-SCORING SYSTEM

Work by Chan and colleagues[54] demonstrated that subjective assessment by "thrombosis experts" of clinical risk of DVT in symptomatic pregnant patients can categorize patients prior to diagnostic testing into two groups, one *low risk* (1.5% prevalence, 98.5% negative predictive value) and the other *non-low risk* (25% prevalence). **Three factors—symptoms in the left leg, a leg circumference discrepancy of 2 cm or more, or first-trimester presentation—were highly predictive of DVT.** Furthermore, this study and one additional validation study demonstrated that patients who lack all three criteria were at no risk for VTE.[55] Thus determination of prediagnostic study risk can be helpful before proceeding to the selection and interpretation of diagnostic tests.

IMAGING

Contrast venography, an invasive technique that involves the injection of dye into a vein distal to the site of suspected thrombosis, followed by radiographic imaging is now rarely used for diagnosis of DVT. The risks of radiation and contrast allergy, as well as its technical difficulty, particularly preclude its use in pregnancy.[56]

The most common diagnostic modality used in the evaluation of patients with suspected DVT is venous ultrasonography (VUS) with or without color Doppler. This modality has virtually replaced the cumbersome and less accurate impedance

TABLE 45-2	RISK FACTORS FOR VENOUS THROMBOEMBOLISM	
GENERAL	**PREGNANCY RELATED**	
Age >35 years	Increased parity	
Obesity	Postpartum endomyometritis	
Trauma	Operative vaginal delivery	
Immobility	Cesarean delivery	
Infection		
Smoking		
Nephrotic syndrome		
Hyperviscosity syndromes		
Cancer		
Surgery, especially orthopedic		
Prior deep venous thromboembolism or pulmonary embolism		
Hospital admission		

plethysmography technique. The ultrasound transducer is placed over the common femoral vein beginning at the inguinal ligament and is then sequentially moved to image the greater saphenous vein, the superficial femoral vein, and the popliteal vein to its trifurcation with the deep veins of the calf. Compression VUS involves the application of pressure with the probe to determine whether the vein under investigation is compressible. **The most accurate ultrasonic criterion for diagnosing venous thrombosis is noncompressibility of the venous lumen in a transverse plane under gentle probe pressure using duplex and color flow Doppler imaging.**[1] The overall sensitivity and specificity of VUS has been reported at 90% to 100% for proximal vein thromboses, but traditionally it has been considered lower for the detection of calf vein thromboses.[57] This is confirmed by a more recent meta-analysis, which demonstrated that in nonpregnant patients, duplex ultrasound has a pooled sensitivity of 96.4% for proximal (knee or thigh) DVT and 75.2% for distal (calf) DVT, and total specificity is 94.3%.[58]

Magnetic resonance imaging (MRI) appears to have equivalent test performance characteristics to VUS. One meta-analysis demonstrated a sensitivity of 91.5% and specificity of 94.8% for diagnosis of DVT in nonpregnant patients with suspected DVT or PE.[59] Similar to VUS, sensitivity is also improved for distal, compared with proximal, thrombi (93.9% vs. 62.1%). The advantage of MRI may be in the ability to detect more centralized DVT, like those in the pelvic, iliac, or femoral veins.

D-DIMER ASSAYS

Laboratory evaluation of serum concentrations of D-dimer, a product of the degradation of fibrin by plasmin, has been increasingly advocated as a helpful test in the diagnosis of DVT in the nonpregnant population. Testing relies on the use of monoclonal antibodies to D-dimer fragments. The most accurate and reliable tests for D-dimer appears to be two rapid enzyme-linked immunosorbent assays (ELISAs; Instant-IA D-dimer [Stago] and Vidas DD [bioMérieux]) and a rapid whole blood assay (SimpliRED D-dimer [Agen Biomedical]). The test is limited by factors that may contribute to false-positive testing, including pregnancy, postpartum and postoperative periods, and superficial thrombophlebitis.[60,61] In particular, **normal pregnancy causes a physiologic increase in D-dimer, with levels that exceed the threshold for normal in 78% and 100% of patients in the second and third trimesters, respectively.**[62] The performance of the SimpliRED D-dimer test was evaluated by Chan and colleagues[54] in a prospective cohort of pregnant patients at risk for

DVT. In this population, who had a DVT prevalence of 8.7%, sensitivity of D-dimer testing was 100% and specificity was 60%. Utility in particular appeared to be stratified across gestation; false-positive rates were 0%, 24%, and 51% for the first, second, and third trimesters, respectively. The value of D-dimer testing in pregnancy may lie in its ability to rule out disease because this same study showed a negative predictive value of 100% with a 95% confidence interval of 95% to 100%. The value of D-dimer testing in the late second and third trimesters is likely to be lower than in the first half of pregnancy because patients in the late second and third trimester will likely have levels above the threshold. Thus at this time, although D-dimer appears useful as a test to rule out a DVT, its routine use in pregnancy cannot be endorsed.

WORKUP OF PATIENTS WITH SUSPECTED DEEP VENOUS THROMBOSIS

The diagnostic paradigm outlined in Figure 45-2 can be used to diagnose DVT in pregnant patients with maximal sensitivity and specificity. Risk may be stratified as in the section above (see "Risk-Scoring System").

PULMONARY EMBOLUS

CLINICAL SIGNS AND SYMPTOMS

Tachypnea (>20 breaths/min) and tachycardia (>100 beats/min) are present in 90% of patients with acute PE, but these findings lack specificity and generate a broad differential diagnosis.[3] Presyncope and syncope are rarer symptoms and indicate a massive embolus.[4]

NONSPECIFIC STUDIES

The classic electrocardiography (ECG) changes associated with PE are the S1, Q3, and inverted T3. Other findings include nonspecific ST changes, right bundle branch block, or right axis deviation. These findings are usually associated with cor pulmonale and right-sided heart strain or overload, reflective of more serious cardiopulmonary compromise. About 26% to 32% of patients with massive PE had the above-mentioned ECG changes.[63] These findings are why the Royal College of Obstetricians and Gynaecologists (RCOG)[64] have recommended that an ECG be performed in women who present with signs and symptoms of an acute PE. **Arterial blood gases and oxygen saturation have limited value in the assessment of acute PE, particularly in a pregnant population.** Measurements of PO_2 are greater than 80 mm Hg in 29% of PE patients younger than 40 years of age.[65] In another study, up to 18% of patients with PE had PO_2 measurements of more than 85 mm Hg.

The chest radiograph may be abnormal in up to 84% of affected patients.[3] The common findings on radiography are pleural effusion, pulmonary infiltrates, atelectasis, and elevated hemidiaphragm. The eponymous findings of pulmonary infarction such as a wedge-shaped infiltrate (Hampton hump) or decreased vascularity (Westermark sign) are rare.[66] Although a normal chest radiograph in the setting of dyspnea, tachypnea, and hypoxemia in a patient without known preexistent pulmonary or cardiovascular disease is suggestive of PE, a chest radiograph cannot be used to confirm the diagnosis.[66] It is useful, however, in the workup for PE as a tool for selecting the correct diagnostic modality (ventilation-perfusion [V/Q] scan vs. computed tomography [CT] scan; see below).

A large PE can create changes consistent with cor pulmonale and right-sided heart strain. Large emboli in the main

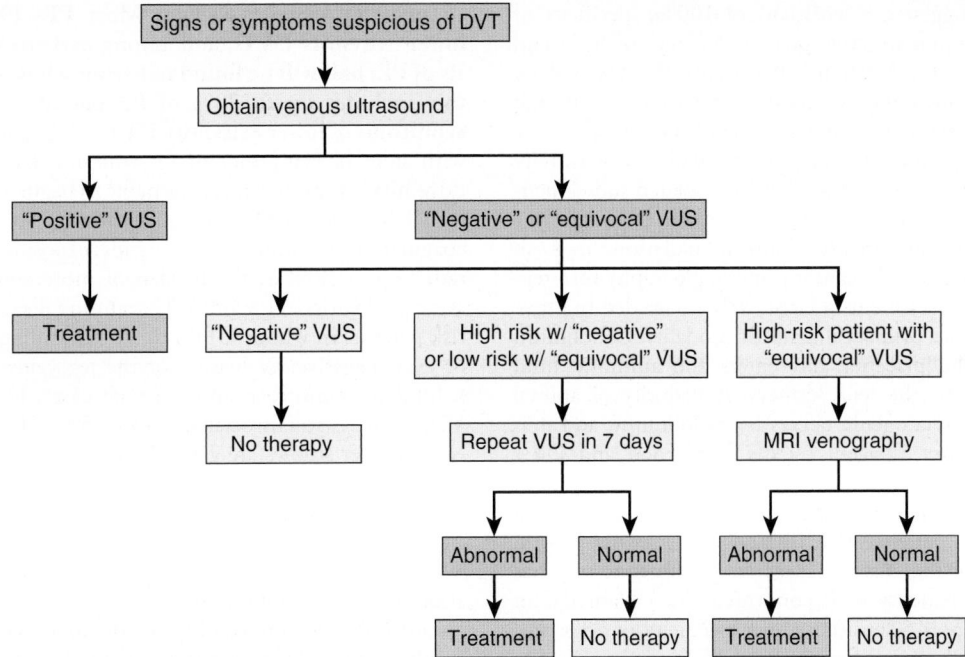

FIG 45-2 Diagnostic algorithm for suspected deep venous thrombosis. MRI, magnetic resonance imaging; VUS, venous ultrasonography.

pulmonary artery and its primary branches can result in acute right-sided heart failure, which is the ultimate cause of death in most patients with PE. Between 30% and 80% of patients with PE display echocardiographic abnormalities in right ventricular size or function.[67-69] Typical findings include a dilated and hypokinetic right ventricle, tricuspid regurgitation, and absence of preexisting pulmonary arterial or left-sided heart pathology. Transesophageal echocardiography with or without contrast appears to improve the imaging of main or right pulmonary artery emboli and, occasionally, of left pulmonary artery clots.[70] For these reasons, **bedside echocardiography can be very useful for the unstable patient or the patient unable to travel for other imaging studies.**

Ventilation-Perfusion Scanning. Perfusion scanning uses intravenously injected radioisotope-labeled albumin macroaggregates that deposit in the pulmonary capillary bed. Ventilation scanning involves the inhalation of radiolabeled aerosols, whose distribution is evaluated by gamma camera. The comparison of these two images allows for interpretation of characteristic patterns that are then used to assign diagnostic probabilities (high, intermediate, or low). More than 90% of high-risk patients with high probability ventilation-perfusion (V/Q) scans have a PE, whereas less than 6% of low-risk patients with low-probability scans have a PE. **Given that most young, healthy women have little underlying lung pulmonary pathology, the diagnostic efficacy of V/Q scanning in pregnancy is substantially higher than that in older, nonpregnant patients.**

Spiral Computed Tomographic Pulmonary Angiography. Spiral CT scanning (computed tomographic pulmonary angiography [CTPA]) requires injection of intravenous (IV) contrast while simultaneously imaging the distribution of contrast in the pulmonary vasculature with a CT scanner.[66] Although this can be an effective judge of large, segmental, and central emboli, CT is of limited value with small subsegmental vessels and horizontally oriented vessels in the right middle lobe. One strength of CTPA is its utility in diagnosing nonembolic pulmonary phenomena such as pneumonia or pulmonary edema.

In nonpregnant patients, CTPA is often the modality of choice; however, this is not likely the case in pregnancy. Several studies have shown that **CTPA performs less well in pregnant compared with nonpregnant cohorts.** Andreou and associates[71] demonstrated in a small study of 32 patients with suspected PE that contrast enhancement of the pulmonary arteries is reduced in pregnant women compared with nonpregnant women, likely due to the increased cardiac output of pregnancy. Another reason may be the more frequent dilution or interruption of contrast by nonopacified blood from the lower vena cava in pregnancy.[72] Comparing CTPA imaging in 40 pregnant patients with that in 40 nonpregnant patients, U-King-Im and colleagues[73] also demonstrated a threefold higher rate of suboptimal studies in the pregnant population (27.5% vs. 7.5%).

Ventilation-Perfusion Scanning Versus Computed Tomographic Pulmonary Angiography. V/Q scanning and CTPA have been directly compared in pregnant patients by Cahill and colleagues,[74] who retrospectively evaluated a cohort of 304 pregnant or postpartum women evaluated for pulmonary embolism. CTPA was performed in 108 women, and a V/Q scan was done in 196. In women with a normal chest radiograph, CTPA yielded nondiagnostic results 5.4 times more often than V/Q scanning (30.0% vs. 5.4%). As would be expected, in those patients with an abnormal chest radiograph, V/Q scanning was more often nondiagnostic. Ridge and colleagues[72] evaluated these two techniques prospectively in a total of 50 patients. Again, they found that CTPA more often gave a nondiagnostic result (35.7% vs. 2.1%), and V/Q scanning was adequate for diagnosis more frequently (35.7% vs. 4%). For these reasons, as well as considerations of radiation exposure (see below), **V/Q scanning is the modality of choice for pregnant patients with suspected PE and a normal chest radiograph.**

Magnetic Resonance Angiography. Magnetic resonance angiography (MRA) may be performed using MRI during IV injection of gadolinium. Faster image-acquisition rates and improved image timing to respiratory and cardiac motion have allowed this technique to be utilized. Preliminary experience by Meaney and colleagues[75] suggested a sensitivity of 100%, specificity of 95%, and positive and negative predictive values of 87% and 100%, respectively, for MRA in 30 patients also assessed by classic pulmonary angiography. Another prospective study that involved 141 patients showed an overall sensitivity of only 77% in comparison to pulmonary angiography, with the sensitivity broken down to 40%, 84%, and 100% for isolated subsegmental, segmental, and central pulmonary emboli, respectively.[76] Because MRA does not involve ionizing radiation, it is an appealing alternative to CT scanning and angiography for pregnancy, and further assessment in large trials are needed to prove its ultimate utility as a primary diagnostic modality. Gadolinium contrast crosses the placenta and enters the amniotic fluid through excretion by the fetal kidneys. A majority of animal studies suggest no teratogenic effects by gadolinium, and it is considered a category C agent by the U.S. Food and Drug Administration (FDA), although it should be used with caution.

D-Dimer Assays. The D-dimer assay appears to have much lower sensitivity in patients with PE and thus it is not helpful as a test for ruling out disease. Negative D-dimer testing has been observed in patients with confirmed PE.[77] Damodaram and associates[78] report a sensitivity and specificity of 73% and 15% for D-dimer in testing for suspected PE in pregnancy. The difference in D-dimer test performance for PE in pregnancy may be due to the smaller clot burden compared with DVT coupled with the increase in intravascular plasma volume of pregnancy. This unacceptably high false-negative rate indicated **no role for D-dimer testing in the workup of pregnant patients with suspected PE.**

Lower Extremity Evaluation. **Most PEs (90%) arise from lower extremity DVTs, and among patients with the diagnosis of PE, half will be found to harbor a lower extremity DVT; this includes up to 20% of PE patients without signs or symptoms of lower extremity DVT.**[79-81] In patients who present with signs or symptoms of PE who also have left-sided lower extremity symptoms, it is reasonable to begin with lower extremity VUS to detect DVT because the need for therapeutic anticoagulation is similar. This avoids exposure to the ionizing radiation, as well as the burden of more complicated testing, associated with CTPA and V/Q scanning. Furthermore, in high-risk patients in whom CTPA or V/Q scanning is nondiagnostic or even negative, evaluation of the leg veins for DVT can be helpful to reinforce results. In such cases, however, a negative VUS study is still associated with a 25% risk of PE, which suggests further studies are generally needed.[82]

WORKUP OF PATIENTS WITH SUSPECTED PULMONARY EMBOLUS

Workup of patients with suspected PE should begin with evaluation of their cardiorespiratory status to determine whether they are critically ill; this would include an ECG and chest radiograph. Patients who are stable hemodynamically with favorable oxygenation status (oxygen saturation >80%) should be evaluated in a carefully ordered fashion, taking into account the possibility of lower extremity DVT and the results of the chest radiograph (Fig. 45-3), according to an algorithm advocated by a panel of experts from the American Thoracic Society, the Society of Thoracic Radiology, and ACOG.[83] If lower extremity

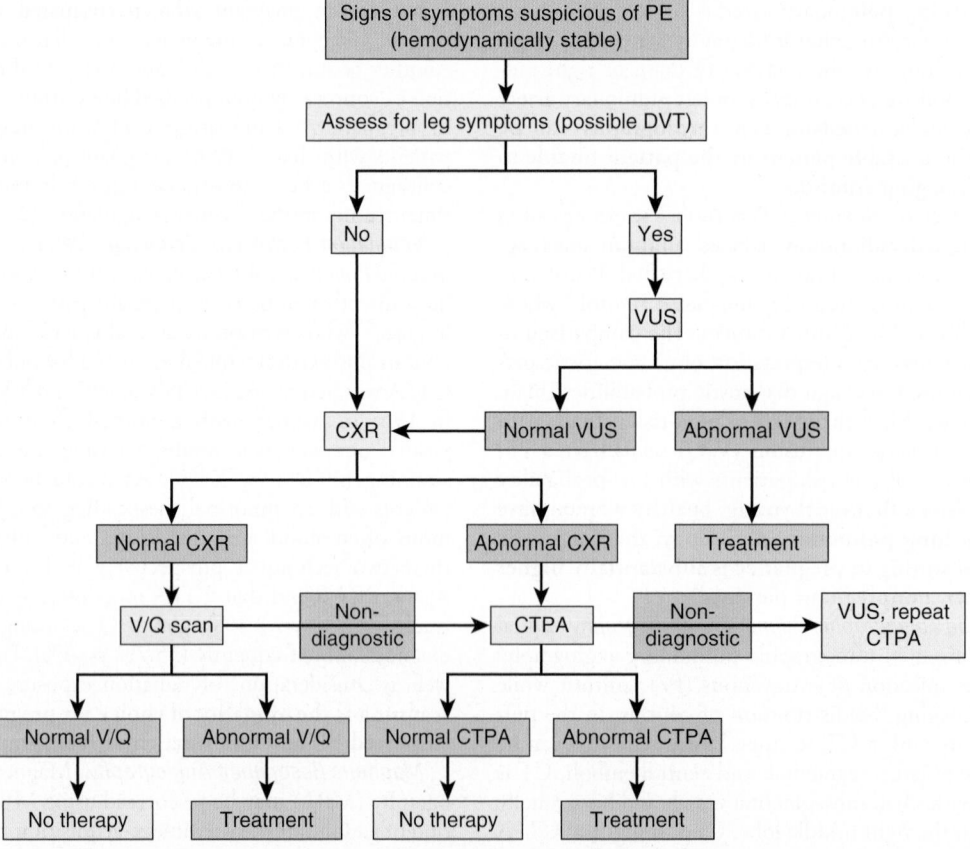

FIG 45-3 Diagnostic algorithm for suspected pulmonary embolus (PE) in a hemodynamically stable patient. CTPA, computed tomographic pulmonary angiography; CXR, chest radiograph; DVT, deep venous thrombosis; V/Q, ventilation-perfusion; VUS, venous ultrasound.

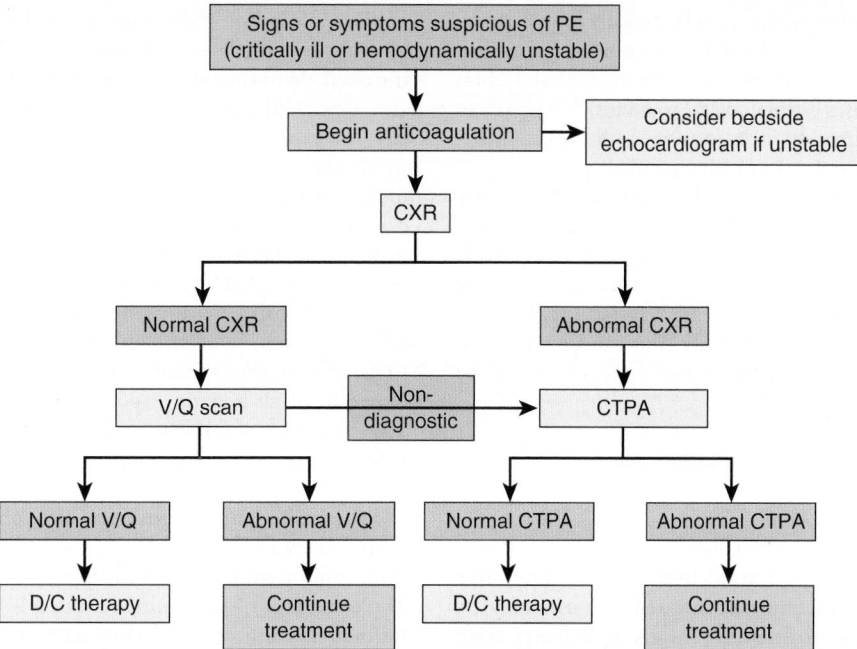

FIG 45-4 Diagnostic algorithm for suspected pulmonary embolism (PE) in a critically ill or hemodynamically unstable patient. CTPA, computed tomographic pulmonary angiography; CXR, chest radiograph; D/C, discontinue; V/Q, ventilation-perfusion.

symptoms are present, particularly if left sided, VUS can be performed; if results are positive, therapeutic anticoagulation should begin. **Chest radiography should definitely be performed when VUS is negative or when no lower extremity signs or symptoms are apparent. Although the chest radiograph is not typically used in the actual diagnosis, it allows for proper selection of the next diagnostic test. V/Q scan is performed if the chest radiograph is normal.** A positive (high or moderate probability) V/Q scan should prompt therapeutic anticoagulation. A negative test should exclude the diagnosis. A nondiagnostic result—such as intermediate probability/equivocal test in any patient and a low-probability result in a high-risk patient (one with prior VTE, known thrombophilia, family history of thrombosis in a first-degree relative under 50 years of age, or other clinical risk factors)—should trigger performance of CTPA.

For such patients, and for those with an abnormal chest radiograph, CTPA is the diagnostic modality of choice. Positive tests will prompt initiation of anticoagulation. In the patient with an abnormal chest radiograph who has a negative CTPA, the true etiology of the chest pathology is often seen on CT. Alternatively, if the CTPA is nondiagnostic, further testing is performed, such as MRA or serial lower extremity VUS studies.

In the critically ill patient, anticoagulation should be started—in the absence of contraindications—and a similar protocol is followed (Fig. 45-4). Very unstable patients who cannot be transported safely can be evaluated with a bedside echocardiogram, which may have more test accuracy in this setting.

Radiation Exposure from Diagnostic Procedures
FETAL EXPOSURE
The diagnosis of DVT and PE in pregnant patients poses unique challenges because of concerns in regard to fetal radiation exposure. ACOG advises that exposure to less than 5 rads has not been associated with increases in pregnancy loss or fetal

TABLE 45-3	FETAL RADIATION EXPOSURE OF VARIOUS IONIZING MODALITIES
RADIOLOGIC MODALITY	**FETAL RADIATION EXPOSURE (RADS)**
Chest radiograph	<0.01
Venography	
Limited, shielded	<0.05
Full (unilateral), unshielded	0.31
Pulmonary angiography	
Brachial vein	0.05
Femoral vein	0.22-0.37
Ventilation-perfusion scan	0.007-0.031
Ventilation scan	0.001-0.019
Perfusion scan	0.006-0.012
Spiral computed tomography	0.013

Modified from Toglia M, Weg J. Venous thromboembolism during pregnancy. *N Engl J Med.* 1996;335(2):108-114.

anomalies.[84] Exposure to ionizing radiation doses above 1 rad, however, may create a marginally increased risk of childhood leukemia (from 1/3000 baseline to 1/2000).[85,86] Table 45-3 outlines the *fetal* radiation exposure of different radiation modalities. **A combination of chest x-ray, V/Q scan, and pulmonary angiography exposes the fetus to less than 0.5 rads.**[10] CTPA is associated with only slightly lower radiation levels for the fetus compared with V/Q scanning. Although the concern for possible adverse effects should not prevent a medically important test from being performed, judicious use and selection of tests is advised.

MATERNAL EXPOSURE
Radiation exposure to the maternal breast is also an important consideration when choosing tests because the increased glandularity and proliferative state of the pregnant breast presumably make it more radiosensitive. This is an important concern with respect to cumulative radiation exposure and

cancer risk.[87] V/Q scanning results in substantially lower maternal breast radiation exposure. CTPA is estimated to expose maternal breast tissue to 150 times more ionizing radiation than V/Q scanning[88] with doses estimated at 2 to 6 rads.[89,90] This dose can be reduced approximately 50% to 60% with breast shielding, without significant reduction in image quality.[91]

MRI and ultrasonography have not been associated with any adverse fetal effects, and teratogenic effects have not been described after administration of gadolinium contrast media.[92] Concerns about fetal goiter following maternal radiographic contrast exposure suggest that fetal heart rate monitoring may be used to detect the reduced variability that can be seen with fetal hypothyroidism, and neonatal thyroid function should be tested during the first week of life.[92]

Management of Venous Thromboembolism
PREVENTION
PERIOPERATIVE PREVENTION
Evidence is very limited regarding the value of perioperative thromboprophylaxis with cesarean delivery.[93,94] **Perioperative administration of low-dose unfractionated heparin may be appropriate in patients undergoing cesarean delivery with clear risk factors such as obesity, malignancy, immobility, or a high-risk chronic medical disease.** As noted, patients with low-risk thrombogenic thrombophilias require postoperative prophylaxis. Nonpharmacologic interventions aimed at preventing VTE include graduated elastic compression stockings and pneumatic compression devices. In pregnancy, a cohort study suggested that the use of graduated compression stockings reduced the prevalence of postpartum VTE from 4.3% to 0.9%.[95] **Because these stockings and pneumatic compression devices pose no hemorrhagic risk and do little harm, they should be strongly considered for thromboprophylaxis in all patients with risk factors, such as those patients who are hospitalized or immobilized, including pregnant or postoperative cesarean patients.** The left lateral decubitus position in the third trimester may also reduce the risk of VTE.

PRECONCEPTION COUNSELING
Preconception counseling is particularly important for patients at high-risk for recurrent VTE in pregnancy and for patients with a recent VTE. Patients on long-term anticoagulation before pregnancy, for example, should be advised of the risks of pregnancy. In particular, patients on warfarin can be counseled that they would be advised to switch from warfarin to a heparin-based regimen upon finding out about pregnancy. In particular, it would be helpful for the woman to know that the risks of warfarin embryopathy are highest between the sixth and twelfth weeks of pregnancy, so vigilance on tracking the last menstrual period is important.

THERAPY
UNFRACTIONATED HEPARIN
Unfractionated heparin (UFH) affects anticoagulation by enhancing antithrombin activity, increasing factor Xa inhibitor activity, and inhibiting platelet aggregation.[96] UFH, an FDA category C agent, does not cross the placenta and is not teratogenic.[97] The chief side effects of heparin include hemorrhage, osteoporosis, and thrombocytopenia. The former is more common with treatment coinciding with surgery or liver disease or with concomitant aspirin use. Heparin-associated bone loss is usually reversible and correlates more with therapy that exceeds

15,000 U/day for more than 6 months and can be opposed by supplemental calcium use (1500 mg/day).[98,99] **Heparin-induced thrombocytopenia (HIT) occurs in 3% of patients,** and type 1 HIT is the most common form; it occurs within days of exposure, is self-limited, and is not associated with a significant risk of hemorrhage or thrombosis. Immunoglobulin-mediated type 2 HIT, on the other hand, is rare and usually occurs 5 to 14 days following initiation of therapy; paradoxically, it increases the risk of thrombosis. Monitoring for HIT should include serial platelet counts every 2 to 3 days from day 4 until day 14 or until heparin is stopped, whichever occurs first.[100] A 50% decline in platelet count from its pretreatment maximum suggests immune-mediated HIT type 2 and should prompt cessation of all heparin exposure, including that in IV flushes. The diagnosis of HIT type 2 can be confirmed by serotonin release assays, heparin-induced platelet aggregation assays, flow cytometry, or solid-phase immunoassays.[101]

Protamine sulfate reverses the effect of intravenously administered UFH. It is given by slow IV infusion of less than 20 mg/min, with no more than 50 mg given over 10 minutes. The total dose of protamine required is calculated based on the residual amount of circulating heparin, with a ratio of 1 mg of protamine sulfate necessary for every 100 U of residual circulating heparin. Residual heparin is calculated by assuming a half-life of 30 to 60 minutes of IV heparin. However, repeated serial administrations of lower doses of protamine, coinciding with serial measurements of the activated partial thromboplastin time (aPTT), are required when the heparin is dosed subcutaneously.

LOW-MOLECULAR-WEIGHT HEPARIN
The low-molecular-weight heparins (LMWHs)—dalteparin, enoxaparin, and tinzaparin—are reliable and safe alternatives to UFH and have fewer side effects. Enzymatic manipulation of standard heparin produces lower molecular weight molecules with equivalent anti–factor Xa but little or no antithrombin effects. The LMWHs have longer half-lives, and a closer correlation exists between anti–factor Xa activity and body weight than subcutaneously administered UFH. We suggest following anti–factor Xa levels in pregnant patients, although this is not universal practice, because the variability in binding, distribution, metabolism, and excretion is far greater. However, this approach may be justified in pregnancy because of an increased rate of subprophylactic levels in pregnancy in patients on standard 40-mg once-daily enoxaparin dosing, which may be due to enhanced renal clearance.[102,103] The LMWHs (pregnancy category B) do not cross the placenta and do not enter breast milk, and the risk of hemorrhage associated with LMWH is lower. **However, regional anesthesia is contraindicated within 18 to 24 hours of therapeutic LMWH administration.** Accordingly, we recommend switching to UFH at 36 weeks or earlier if preterm delivery is expected. Protamine is not as effective in fully reversing the anti–factor Xa activity of LMWH, although it may reduce bleeding. Dosing of 1 mg of protamine for every 100 antifactor Xa units of LMWH can normalize aPTT values, but antifactor Xa levels can only be reversed by 80%.[104,105] Whereas the risk of HIT type 2 is lower in patients who receive LMWH, platelet counts should still be checked every 2 to 3 days from day 4 to day 14.[100,106,107]

FONDAPARINUX
Fondaparinux is a synthetic heparin pentasaccharide that complexes with the antithrombin binding site for heparin to permit

the selective inactivation of factor Xa but not thrombin. A major advantage of this medication is that there does not appear to be a risk of HIT type 2. It has comparable efficacy to both LMWH and UFH in nonpregnant patients.[108,109] Although fondaparinux has been used in a small number of pregnant patients without complication,[110-113] umbilical cord plasma concentrations at 10% of those of maternal plasma have been demonstrated, which suggests limited transplacental passage.[114] Use of fondaparinux should be limited to women without other therapeutic alternatives, such as those with a history of HIT type 2 or heparin allergies and those who have failed other anticoagulants.

COUMARIN

The coumarins are vitamin K antagonists that block the vitamin K–dependent, function-enhancing posttranslational modifications of prothrombin and factors VII, IX, and X as well as the anticlotting agents protein C and S. Coumadin (warfarin) has been shown to be effective for both the primary and secondary prevention of VTE, stroke, myocardial infarction, and systemic embolism due to artificial valves and atrial fibrillation.[115] **Warfarin is a pregnancy category X medication because fetal exposure can cause nasal and midface hypoplasia, microphthalmia, mental retardation, and other ocular, skeletal, and central nervous system malformations** (see Chapter 8). Teratogenic potential is greatest between the 6th and 12th weeks of pregnancy, and the risk of warfarin also includes fetal hemorrhage. As a result, warfarin is rarely used during gestation, although the exceptional case of a patient requiring therapeutic anticoagulation who cannot be sufficiently treated with the heparins may require its use (e.g., certain patients with artificial heart valves). Warfarin is also favored in the postpartum period because it is safe to use during lactation.

Therapy is started at a dose of 5 to 10 mg for 2 days, with subsequent doses titrated to achieve an international normalized ratio (INR) of 2.0 to 3.0. Peak effects occur within 72 hours, and its half-life is from 36 to 42 hours.[115] **Warfarin metabolism is greatly affected by genetic polymorphisms, making the response to particular dosing regimens unpredictable.** A pharmacogenetic approach to warfarin dosing includes testing for particular variations in vitamin K and warfarin metabolic enzymes and using this information to formulate a dosing regimen that expeditiously achieves a proper maintenance dose.[116] A criticism of this approach is that pharmacogenetics only account for 30% to 50% of the variability in response because environment, diet, and comorbidities often have a significant influence as well. A nomogram for predicting warfarin dosing, based on patient-specific responses to warfarin doses as assessed by day 3 and day 5 INRs, has been proposed by Lazo-Langner and associates.[117] Avoiding the need for costly genetic testing, this protocol accounts for individual variation of warfarin metabolism.

Because of protein C's shorter half-life relative to the other vitamin K–dependent clotting factors, warfarin may initially create a prothrombotic state, particularly in pregnancy. Thus patients who are started on warfarin postpartum should be on therapeutic doses of UFH or LMWH for 5 days and until the INR is therapeutic for 48 hours. Coumadin effects can be reversed by vitamin K.[118] The INR generally normalizes within 6 hours of a 5 mg dose of vitamin K and within 4 days with cessation of warfarin therapy. Fresh-frozen plasma can be used to achieve immediate reversal of effects. RCOG recommends avoiding warfarin until at least the fifth postpartum day and

TABLE 45-4	WEIGHT-BASED NOMOGRAM FOR UNFRACTIONATED HEPARIN

Give a bolus of 80 U/kg, followed by a maintenance dosage of 18 U/kg/hr following aPTT values every 6 hr and with the following adjustments for aPTT values obtained:

aPTT VALUE	ADJUSTMENT
<35 sec (<1.2× control value)	Repeat full bolus (80 U/kg) then increase infusion rate by 4 U/kg/hr
35-45 sec (1.2-1.5× control)	Repeat half bolus (40 U/kg) then increase infusion rate by 2 U/kg/hr
46-70 sec (1.6-2.3× control)	No change in infusion rate
71-90 sec (2.4-3× control)	Decrease infusion rate by 2 U/kg/hr
>90 sec (>3× control)	Stop infusion for 1 hour then decrease to 3 U/kg/hr

Modified from Raschke R, Reilly B, Guidry J, Fontana J, Srinivas S. The weight-based heparin dosing nomogram compared with a "standard care" nomogram. A randomized controlled trial. *Ann Intern Med.* 1993;119:874-881.
aPTT, activated partial thromboplastin time.

even longer in patients at increased risk for postpartum hemorrhage.[64]

TREATMENT OF ACUTE DEEP VENOUS THROMBOSIS OR PULMONARY EMBOLUS

Women with new-onset VTE diagnosed during pregnancy should receive therapeutic anticoagulation, and this treatment should be continued for at least 20 weeks. If this period of time expires before the end of the postpartum period, prophylactic anticoagulation should be initiated in patients without highly thrombogenic thrombophilias and should be continued for 6 weeks to 6 months postpartum, depending on the severity of the thrombotic event and the underlying risk factors. During pregnancy, UFH and the LMWHs are the drugs of choice given their efficacy and safety profile. **Therapeutic doses of the LMWH enoxaparin may start at 1 mg/kg subcutaneously twice daily.** Dosing should be titrated to achieve anti–factor Xa levels of 0.6 to 1.0 U/mL when tested 4 hours after injection because of inconsistent efficacy of this weight-based regimen in pregnant patients.[119] UFH for acute DVT or PE is initially given intravenously and is titrated to keep the aPTT at 1.5 to 2.5 times control (checked every 4 to 6 hours during the titration period), usually according to weight-based protocols (Table 45-4).[120] IV heparin should be continued for 5 to 10 days or until clinical improvement is noted. This regimen can be changed to subcutaneous injections every 8 to 12 hours to keep the aPTT at 1.5 to 2.0 times control when tested 6 hours after injection.

Prophylactic Anticoagulation Recommendations for Low-, Moderate-, and High-Risk Groups. Risk stratification based on the likelihoods of recurrence, such as in Table 45-1, is the essential foundation of the recommendations for antepartum and postpartum anticoagulation in patients without recent or active VTE. This issue has recently been addressed by ACOG[121] and is summarized in Table 45-5. The first principle is that **the postpartum period represents a time of elevated risk, particularly in patients with risk factors.** For this reason, anticoagulation recommendations in the postpartum period are typically a maintenance of antepartum recommendations or an increase. The second principle is that **the various thrombophilias can be classified into high- and low-risk types, and anticoagulation recommendations for each type will be different depending on whether the patient has a personal history of VTE.** Third, **patients with recurrent VTE who have tested negative**

TABLE 45-5	ANTICOAGULATION IN PREGNANCY: INDICATIONS, TYPES, AND TIMING		
INDICATION	**DESCRIPTION**	**ANTEPARTUM**	**POSTPARTUM**
VTE in current pregnancy		Therapeutic LMWH/UFH to complete 20-week course, then therapeutic or prophylactic LMWH/UFH regimen as appropriate based on thrombophilia or risk factors	Therapeutic LMWH/UFH regimen to complete 20-week course, followed by prophylactic LMWH or postpartum warfarin
High-risk thrombophilia • FVL homozygous • Prothrombin G20210A mutation homozygous	History of one prior VTE	Therapeutic or prophylactic LMWH/UFH	Therapeutic or prophylactic LMWH regimen or postpartum warfarin; dosing/level to match antepartum regimen
• FVL/prothrombin G20210A mutation double heterozygous • Antithrombin III deficiency	No history of VTE	Prophylactic LMWH/UFH	Prophylactic LMWH or postpartum warfarin
Low-risk thrombophilia • FVL heterozygous	History of one prior VTE	Prophylactic LMWH/UFH or surveillance without anticoagulation	Prophylactic LMWH/UFH or postpartum warfarin
• Prothrombin G20210A mutation heterozygous • Protein C deficiency • Protein S deficiency	No history of VTE	Surveillance without anticoagulation or prophylactic LMWH/UFH	Surveillance without anticoagulation or prophylactic LMWH/UFH or postpartum warfarin if patient has additional risk factors
No thrombophilia	History of one prior VTE (pregnancy or estrogen related)	Prophylactic LMWH/UFH or surveillance without anticoagulation	Prophylactic LMWH or postpartum warfarin
	History of one prior VTE (idiopathic)	Prophylactic LMWH/UFH or surveillance without anticoagulation	Prophylactic LMWH or postpartum warfarin
Two or more prior VTE episodes (thrombophilia or no thrombophilia)	On long-term anticoagulation	Therapeutic LMWH/UFH	Resumption of long-term anticoagulation therapy
	Not on long-term anticoagulation	Therapeutic or prophylactic LMWH/UFH	Therapeutic or prophylactic LMWH/UFH

Modified from American College of Obstetricians and Gynecologists. Practice Bulletin no. 123: Thromboembolism in pregnancy. *Obstet Gynecol.* 2011;118(3):718-729.
FVL, factor V Leiden; *LMWH,* low-molecular-weight heparin; *UFH,* unfractionated heparin; *VTE,* venous thromboembolism.

for the known inherited thrombophilias likely have an underlying pathology (e.g., an undiagnosed genetic malformation in a step in the coagulation cascade) and should be cared for cautiously.

After this stratification, appropriate dosing is chosen (Table 45-6). Dosing regimens are categorized into prophylactic and therapeutic types. Prophylactic therapy is warranted in all patients with low to moderate risk during pregnancy and the postpartum period. **Typical prophylactic doses of the LMWH enoxaparin may start at 40 mg subcutaneously daily.** Weight-based dosing in pregnant patients may be unreliable, and some investigators, but not all, recommend titrating doses to achieve anti–factor Xa levels of 0.1 to 0.2 U/mL 4 hours after injection. UFH prophylaxis may range from 5000 to 10,000 units subcutaneously every 12 hours, with dosing adjusted by trimester and based on weight. Because of inconsistent efficacy in pregnant patients, and because the aPTT cannot be followed in prophylactic dosing, this dosing may be titrated to achieve heparin levels (by protamine titration assay) of 0.1 to 0.2 U/mL.[122] Therapeutic dosing of LMWH and UFH should be followed with anti–factor Xa levels or aPTT, respectively, as in Table 45-6. Postpartum anticoagulation is typically done with LMWH (prophylactic or therapeutic dosing), warfarin, or a newer agent if the patient is on long-term anticoagulation.

INFERIOR VENA CAVA FILTERS

The use of IVC filters is primarily restricted to patients with absolute contraindications to medical anticoagulation or those who have failed therapeutic anticoagulation. Pregnant patients in need of prophylaxis with a history of HIT type 2 or with true heparin or LMWH allergies are potential candidates for IVC filters. However, the introduction of fondaparinux may eliminate this need. The use of IVC filters is discouraged in younger patients, but newer retrievable filters may be appropriate.[123]

TABLE 45-6	EXAMPLE ANTICOAGULATION REGIMENS	
TYPE	**DRUG AND DOSING**	**SURVEILLANCE**
Prophylactic LMWH	Enoxaparin 40 mg SC once daily	*Consider* target anti-Xa levels of 0.1-0.2 U/mL 4 hours after injection
Therapeutic LMWH	Enoxaparin 1 mg/kg/12 hr	Target anti-Xa levels of 0.6-1.0 U/mL tested 4 hours after injection
Prophylactic UFH	First trimester: UFH 5000-7500 units SC/12 hr Second trimester: UFH 7500-10,000 units SC/12 hr Third trimester: UFH 10,000 units SC/12 hr	aPTT should be in the normal range *Consider* target heparin levels of 0.1-0.2 U/mL
Therapeutic UFH	UFH 10,000 U (or more)/12 hr	Target aPTT in 1.5-2.5× control range tested 6 hours after injection
Warfarin (postpartum, therapeutic)	Begin 5-10 mg oral daily and titrate to INR target	Overlap UFH or LMWH therapy until INR is >2.0 for more than 2 days; target INR, 2.0-3.0

Modified from American College of Obstetricians and Gynecologists Practice Bulletin no. 123: Thromboembolism in Pregnancy. *Obstet Gynecol.* 2011;118(3):718-729.
aPTT, activated partial thromboplastin time; *INR,* international normalized ratio; *LMWH,* low-molecular-weight heparin; *SC,* subcutaneously; *UFH,* unfractionated heparin; *Xa,* activated factor X.

DELIVERY AND ANESTHESIA CONCERNS

As noted earlier, the major concerns of therapeutic anticoagulation in pregnancy are regional anesthesia use and the risk of hemorrhage. Regional anesthesia is contraindicated within 18 to 24 hours of therapeutic LMWH use, thus LMWH should be converted to UFH at 36 weeks or earlier if clinically indicated.

Vaginal or cesarean delivery more than 24 hours after therapeutic LMWH dosing should not pose a risk of hemorrhage, although protamine sulfate may be necessary to partially reverse anticoagulation. Protamine sulfate may also be used to normalize completely an elevated aPTT in patients on therapeutic UFH near the time of delivery. Heparin anticoagulation may be restarted 3 to 6 hours after vaginal delivery and 6 to 8 hours after cesarean delivery. Coumadin anticoagulation may be started on the first postpartum or postoperative day, although it should be recognized that RCOG recommends waiting until at least the fifth day postpartum. As noted earlier, because of the paradoxic increase in APC resistance and factor VIII after starting coumadin, therapeutic doses of the heparins should be continued for 5 days and until the INR reaches therapeutic range (2.0 to 3.0) for 2 successive days.

The risk of hemorrhage or complication from regional anesthesia is minimal when administered more than 12 hours after a prophylactic dose of LMWH. Again, given the difficulty of timing administration with the onset of labor, we recommend converting from LMWH to UFH at 36 weeks or earlier as clinically indicated. As with therapeutic use, anticoagulation may be restarted 3 to 6 hours after vaginal delivery and 6 to 8 hours after cesarean delivery.

POSTPARTUM BREASTFEEDING
UFH does not cross into breast milk and is therefore considered safe during breastfeeding. Warfarin is also considered safe for breastfeeding because it does not accumulate in breast milk and has no effect on the coagulation of breastfeeding neonates. Long-term use of UFH is associated with bone loss, typically in doses higher than 15,000 U/day and for use longer than 6 months. Bone density typically recovers over time after discontinuing heparin.

KEY POINTS
- Pregnancy, childbirth, and the puerperium pose serious hemorrhagic challenges that are met by increased decidual and systemic clotting potential.
- VTE is a leading cause of mortality and serious morbidity in pregnant women, with a prevalence of 1 per 1000 to 1 per 2000 pregnancies; the greatest risk of fatal PE occurs following caesarean deliveries.
- Inherited and acquired thrombophilias account for most VTEs in pregnancy.
- VUS is the most common diagnostic modality used in the evaluation of patients with suspected DVT, with an overall sensitivity and specificity of 90% to 100% for proximal vein thromboses.
- In stable patients with suspected PE and leg signs or symptoms, VUS should be performed because it may avoid the risks of radiation exposure and may detect a DVT, the cause of the PE.
- Stable patients with suspected PE should have a chest radiograph to determine the diagnostic test to be used. A nondiagnostic chest radiograph should therefore prompt performance of a V/Q scan. A patient with abnormal chest radiography should be evaluated with spiral CTPA.
- Heparin remains the mainstay of therapy for VTE, with its most serious but rare complication being immunoglobulin-mediated HIT type 2, which usually occurs 5 to 14 days following initiation of therapy and paradoxically increases the risk of thrombosis.
- Thromboprophylaxis is warranted in high- and moderate-risk groups based on a history of VTE and the presence of thrombophilia and should be selected according to overall risk for recurrence.
- Protamine sulfate can entirely reverse the anticoagulant effect of UFH and can partially (80%) reverse the effect of LMWH.
- Graduated elastic compression stockings and pneumatic compression devices appear to reduce the likelihood of VTE in pregnancy and, at a minimum, should be used in all high-risk patients and should be strongly considered for all patients undergoing cesarean delivery. (We follow this recommendation in our own practice).

REFERENCES
1. Hirsh J, Hoak J. Management of Deep Vein Thrombosis and Pulmonary Embolism: A Statement for Healthcare Professionals from the Council on Thrombosis (in Consultation with the Council on Cardiovascular Radiology), American Heart Association. *Circulation.* 1996;93:2212-2245.
2. Sandler D, Martin J, Duncan J, et al. Diagnosis of deep-vein thrombosis: comparison of clinical evaluation, ultrasound, plethysmography, and venoscan with x-ray venogram. *Lancet.* 1984;8405:716-719.
3. Stein P, Terrin M, Hales C, et al. Clinical, laboratory, roentgenographic, and electrocardiographic findings in patients with acute pulmonary embolism and no pre-existing cardiac or pulmonary disease. *Chest.* 1991;100:598-603.
4. Fedullo P, Tapson V. The evaluation of suspected pulmonary embolism. *N Engl J Med.* 2003;349:1247-1256.
5. Ginsberg J, Brill-Edwards P, Burrows R, et al. Venous thrombosis during pregnancy: leg and trimester of presentation. *Thromb Haemost.* 1992;67:519-520.
6. Kierkegaard A. Incidence and diagnosis of deep vein thrombosis associated with pregnancy. *Acta Obstet Gynecol Scand.* 1983;62:239-243.
7. Rutherford S, Montoro M, McGehee W, Strong T. Thromboembolic disease associated with pregnancy: an 11-year review (SPO Abstract). *Obstet Gynecol.* 1991;164:286.
8. Simpson E, Lawrenson R, Nightingale A, Farmer R. Venous thromboembolism in pregnancy and the puerperium: incidence and additional risk factors from a London perinatal database. *BJOG.* 2001;108:56-60.
9. Stein P, Hull R, Jayali F, et al. Venous thromboembolism in pregnancy: 21-year trends. *Am J Med.* 2004;117:121-125.
10. Toglia M, Weg J. Venous thromboembolism during pregnancy. *N Engl J Med.* 1996;335(2):108-114.
11. Treffers P, Huidekoper B, Weenink G, Kloosterman G. Epidemiological observations of thrombo-embolic disease during pregnancy and the puerperium, in 56,022 women. *Int J Gynaecol Obstet.* 1983;21(4):327-331.
12. McColl M, Ramsay J, Tait R, et al. Risk factors for pregnancy associated venous thromboembolism. *Thromb Haemost.* 1997;78:1183-1188.
13. Creanga AA, Berg CJ, Syverson C, Seed K, Bruce C, Callaghan WM. Pregnancy-related mortality in the United States. *Obstet Gynecol.* 2015;125:5-12.
14. Macklon N, Greer I. Venous thromboembolic disease in obstetrics and gynecology: the Scottish experience. *Scott Med J.* 1996;41:83-86.
15. Bergqvist A, Bergqvist D, Hallbook T. Deep vein thrombosis during pregnancy: a prospective study. *Acta Obstet Gynecol Scand.* 1983;62:443-448.
16. Bergqvist D, Hedner U. Pregnancy and venous thrombo-embolism. *Acta Obstet Gynecol Scand.* 1983;62:449-453.
17. Kamel H, Navi BB, Sriram N, Hovsepian DA, Devereux RB, Elkind MS. Risk of a thrombotic event after the 6-week postpartum period. *N Engl J Med.* 2014;370(14):1307-1315.
18. Ruggeri Z, Dent J, Saldivar E. Contribution of distinct adhesive interactions to platelet aggregation in flowing blood. *Blood.* 1999;94:172-178.

19. Pytela R, Pierschbacher M, Ginsberg M, Plow E, Ruoslahti E. Platelet membrane glycoprotein IIb/IIIa: member of a family of Arg-Gly-Asp-specific adhesion receptors. *Science*. 1986;231:1559-1562.

20. Nemerson Y. Tissue factor and hemostasis. *Blood*. 1988;71:1-8.

21. Preissner K, de Boer H, Pannekoek H, de Groot P. Thrombin regulation by physiological inhibitors: the role of vitronectin. *Semin Thromb Hemost*. 1996;165:1335-1341.

22. Lockwood C, Bach R, Guha A, Zhou X, Miller W, Nemerson Y. Amniotic fluid contains tissue factor, a potent initiator of coagulation. *Am J Obstet Gynecol*. 1991;165:1335-1341.

23. Mackman N. Role of tissue factor in hemostasis, thrombosis, and vascular development. *Arterioscler Thromb Vasc Biol*. 2004;24:1015-1022.

24. Mackman N. The role of tissue factor and factor VIIa in hemostasis. *Anesth Analg*. 2009;108(5):1447-1452.

25. Broze GJ Jr. The rediscovery and isolation of TFPI. *J Thromb Haemost*. 2003;1:1671-1675.

26. Dahlback B. Progress in the understanding of the protein C anticoagulant pathway. *Int J Hematol*. 2004;79:109-116.

27. Broze GJ Jr. Protein Z-dependent regulation of coagulation. *Thromb Haemost*. 2001;86:8-13.

28. Preissner K, Zwicker L, Muller-Berghaus G. Formation, characterization and detection of a ternary complex between protein S, thrombin and antithrombin III in serum. *Biochem J*. 1987;243:105-111.

29. Bouma B, Meijers J. New insights into factors affecting clot stability: a role for thrombin activatable fibrinolysis inhibitor. *Semin Hematol*. 2004;41:13-19.

30. Schatz F, Lockwood C. Progestin regulation of plasminogen activator inhibitor type-1 in primary cultures of endometrial stromal and decidual cells. *JCEM*. 1993;77:621-625.

31. Lockwood C, Krikun G, Schatz F. The decidua regulates hemostasis in the human endometrium. *Semin Reprod Endocrinol*. 1999;17:45-51.

32. Bremme K. Haemostatic changes in pregnancy. *Best Pract Res Clin Haematol*. 2003;16:153-168.

33. Paidas MJ, Ku DH, Lee MJ, et al. Protein Z, protein S levels are lower in patients with thrombophilia and subsequent pregnancy complications. *J Thromb Haemost*. 2005;3(3):497-501.

34. Wright H, Osborn S, Edmunds D. Changes in the rate of flow of venous blood in the leg during pregnancy, measured with radioactive sodium. *Surg Gynecol Obstet*. 1950;90:481.

35. Goodrich S, Wood J. Peripheral venous distensibility and velocity of venous blood flow during pregnancy or during oral contraceptive therapy. *Am J Obstet Gynecol*. 1964;90:740.

36. Macklon N, Greer I, Bowman A. An ultrasound study of gestational and postural changes in the deep venous system of the leg in pregnancy. *BJOG*. 1997;104:191-197.

37. Girling J, de Swiet M. Inherited thrombophilia and pregnancy. *Curr Opin Obstet Gynecol*. 1998;10:135-144.

38. Ginsberg J, Wells P, Brill-Edwards P, et al. Antiphospholipid antibodies and venous thromboembolism. *Blood*. 1995;86(10):3685-3691.

39. Miyakis S, Lockshin MD, Atsumi T, et al. International consensus statement on an update of the classification criteria for definite antiphospholipid syndrome (APS). *J Thromb Haemost*. 2006;4(2):295-306.

40. Lockwood C, Romero R, Feinberg R, Clyne L, Coster B, Hobbins J. The prevalence and biologic significance of lupus anticoagulant and anticardiolipin antibodies in the general obstetric population. *Am J Obstet Gynecol*. 1989;161:369-373.

41. Wahl D, Guillemin F, de Maistre E, Perret C, Lecompte T, Thibaut G. Risk for venous thrombosis related to antiphospholipid antibodies in systemic lupus erythematous–a meta-analysis. *Lupus*. 1997;6:646-673.

42. Galli M, Barbui T. Antiphospholipid antibodies and thrombosis: strength of association. *Hematol J*. 2003;4:180-186.

43. Garcia-Fuster M, Fernandez C, Forner M, Vaya A. Risk factors and clinical characteristics of thromboembolic venous disease in young patients: a prospective study. *Med Clin (Barc)*. 2004;123:217-219.

44. Branch D, Silver R, Blackwell J, Reading J, Scott J. Outcome of treated pregnancies in women with antiphospholipid syndrome: an update of the Utah experience. *Obstet Gynecol*. 1992;80:612-620.

45. Zotz R, Gerhardt A, Scharf R. Inherited thrombophilia and gestational venous thromboembolism. *Best Pract Res Clin Haematol*. 2003;16:243-259.

46. ACOG Practice Bulletin No. 138: Inherited Thrombophilias in Pregnancy. *Obstet Gynecol*. 2013;122(3):706-717.

47. Dizon-Townson D, Miller C, Sibai B, et al. The relationship of the factor V Leiden mutation and pregnancy outcomes for mother and fetus. *Obstet Gynecol*. 2005;106(3):517-524.

48. Clark P, Walker ID, Govan L, Wu O, Greer IA. The GOAL study: a prospective examination of the impact of factor V Leiden and ABO(H) blood groups on haemorrhagic and thrombotic pregnancy outcomes. *Br J Haematol*. 2008;140(2):236-240.

49. Murphy RP, Donoghue C, Nallen RJ, et al. Prospective evaluation of the risk conferred by factor V Leiden and thermolabile methylenetetrahydrofolate reductase polymorphisms in pregnancy. *Arterioscler Thromb Vasc Biol*. 2000;20(1):266-270.

50. Said JM, Higgins JR, Moses EK, et al. Inherited thrombophilia polymorphisms and pregnancy outcomes in nulliparous women. *Obstet Gynecol*. 2010;115(1):5-13.

51. Lindqvist PG, Svensson PJ, Marsaal K, Grennert L, Luterkort M, Dahlback B. Activated protein C resistance (FV:Q506) and pregnancy. *Thromb Haemost*. 1999;81(4):532-537.

52. Abdul Sultan A, West J, Tata LJ, Fleming KM, Nelson-Piercy C, Grainge MJ. Risk of first venous thromboembolism in pregnant women in hospital: population based cohort study from England. *BMJ*. 2013;347:f6099.

53. Henriksson P, Westerlund E, Wallen H, Brandt L, Hovatta O, Ekbom A. Incidence of pulmonary and venous thromboembolism in pregnancies after in vitro fertilisation: cross sectional study. *BMJ*. 2013;346:e8632.

54. Chan WS, Lee A, Spencer FA, et al. Predicting deep venous thrombosis in pregnancy: out in "LEFt" field? *Ann Intern Med*. 2009;151(2):85-92.

55. Righini M, Jobic C, Boehlen F, et al. Predicting deep venous thrombosis in pregnancy: external validation of the LEFT clinical prediction rule. *Haematologica*. 2013;98(4):545-548.

56. Heijboer H, Cogo A, Buller H, Prandoni P, ten Cate J. Detection of deep vein thrombosis with impedance plethysmography and real-time compression ultrasonography in hospitalized patients. *Arch Intern Med*. 1992;152: 1901-1903.

57. Kassai B, Boissel J, Cucherat M, Sonie S, Shah N, Leizorovicz A. A systematic review of the accuracy of ultrasound in the diagnosis of deep venous thrombosis in asymptomatic patients. *Thromb Haemost*. 2004;91: 655-666.

58. Goodacre S, Sampson F, Thomas S, van Beek E, Sutton A. Systematic review and meta-analysis of the diagnostic accuracy of ultrasonography for deep vein thrombosis. *BMC Med Imaging*. 2005;5:6.

59. Sampson FC, Goodacre SW, Thomas SM, van Beek EJ. The accuracy of MRI in diagnosis of suspected deep vein thrombosis: systematic review and meta-analysis. *Eur Radiol*. 2007;17(1):175-181.

60. Epiney M, Boehlen F, Boulvain M, et al. D-dimer levels during delivery and the postpartum. *J Thromb Haemost*. 2005;3:268-271.

61. Koh S, Pua H, Tay D, Ratnam S. The effects of gynaecological surgery on coagulation activation, fibrinolysis, and fibrinolytic inhibitor in patients with and without ketorolac infusion. *Thromb Res*. 1995;79:501-514.

62. Kline JA, Williams GW, Hernandez-Nino J. D-dimer concentrations in normal pregnancy: new diagnostic thresholds are needed. *Clin Chem*. 2005;51(5):825-829.

63. Junker R, Nabavi D, Wolff E, et al. Plasminogen activator inhibitor-1 4G/4G genotype is associated with cerebral sinus thrombosis in factor V Leiden carriers. *Thromb Haemost*. 1998;80:706-707.

64. Royal College of Obstetricians and Gynaecologists. Thromboembolic Disease in Pregnancy and the Puerperium: Acute Management. *Green-top Guideline No. 37b*. April 2015, Available at <https://www.rcog.org.uk/globalassets/documents/guidelines/gtg-37b.pdf>.

65. Green R, Meyer T, Dunn M, Glassroth J. Pulmonary embolism in younger adults. *Chest*. 1992;101:1507-1511.

66. Tapson V, Carroll B, Davidson B, et al. The diagnostic approach to acute venous thromboembolism. Clinical practice guideline. American Thoracic Society. *Am J Respir Crit Care Med*. 1999;160:1043-1066.

67. Come P. Echocardiographic evaluation of pulmonary embolism and its response to therapeutic interventions. *Chest*. 1992;101:151S-162S.

68. Kasper W, Meinertz T, Kersting F, Lollgen H, Limbourg P, Just H. Echocardiography in assessing acute pulmonary hypertension due to pulmonary embolism. *Am J Cardiol*. 1980;45:567-572.

69. Gibson N, Sohne M, Buller H. Prognostic value of echocardiography and spiral computed tomography in patients with pulmonary embolism. *Curr Opin Pulm Med*. 2005;11:380-384.

70. Pruszczyk P, Torbicki A, Pacho R, et al. Noninvasive diagnosis of suspected severe pulmonary embolism: transesophageal echocardiography vs spiral CT. *Chest*. 1997;112:722-728.

71. Andreou AK, Curtin JJ, Wilde S, Clark A. Does pregnancy affect vascular enhancement in patients undergoing CT pulmonary angiography? *Eur Radiol*. 2008;18(12):2716-2722.

72. Ridge CA, McDermott S, Freyne BJ, Brennan DJ, Collins CD, Skehan SJ. Pulmonary embolism in pregnancy: comparison of pulmonary CT

angiography and lung scintigraphy. *AJR Am J Roentegenol.* 2009;193(5): 1223-1227.

73. U-King-Im J, Freeman S, Boylan T, Cheow H. Quality of CT pulmonary angiography for suspected pulmonary embolus in pregnancy. *Eur Radiol.* 2008;18(12):2709-2715.

74. Cahill AG, Stout MJ, Macones GA, Bhalla S. Diagnosing pulmonary embolism in pregnancy using computed-tomographic angiography or ventilation-perfusion. *Obstet Gynecol.* 2009;114(1):124-129.

75. Meaney J, Weg J, Chenevert T, Stafford-Johnson D, Hamilton B, Prince M. Diagnosis of pulmonary embolism with magnetic resonance angiography. *N Engl J Med.* 1997;336:1422-1427.

76. Oudkerk M, van Beek EJ, Wielopolski P, van Ooijen PM, Brouwers-Kuyper EM, Bongaerts AH, et al. Comparison of contrast-enhanced magnetic resonance angiography and conventional pulmonary angiography for the diagnosis of pulmonary embolism: a prospective study. *Lancet.* 2002;359(9318):1643-1647.

77. To MS, Hunt BJ, Nelson-Piercy C. A negative D-dimer does not exclude venous thromboembolism (VTE) in pregnancy. *J Obstet Gynaecol.* 2008; 28(2):222-223.

78. Damodaram M, Kaladindi M, Luckit J, Yoong W. D-dimers as a screening test for venous thromboembolism in pregnancy: is it of any use? *J Obstet Gynaecol.* 2009;29(2):101-103.

79. Girard P, Musset D, Parent F, Maitre S, Phlippoteau C, Simonneau G. High prevalence of detectable deep venous thrombosis in patients with acute pulmonary embolism. *Chest.* 1999;116(4):903-908.

80. Girard P, Sanchez O, Leroyer C, et al. Deep venous thrombosis in patients with acute pulmonary embolism: prevalence, risk factors, and clinical significance. *Chest.* 2005;128(3):1593-1600.

81. Yamaki T, Nozaki M, Sakurai H, Takeuchi M, Soejima K, Kono T. Presence of lower limb deep vein thrombosis and prognosis in patients with symptomatic pulmonary embolism: preliminary report. *Eur J Vasc Endovasc Surg.* 2009;37(2):225-231.

82. Stein P, Hull R, Saltzman H, Pineo G. Strategy for diagnosis of patients with suspected pulmonary embolism. *Chest.* 1993;103:1553-1559.

83. Leung AN, Bull TM, Jaeschke R, et al. American Thoracic Society documents: an official American Thoracic Society/Society of Thoracic Radiology Clinical Practice Guideline–Evaluation of Suspected Pulmonary Embolism in Pregnancy. *Radiology.* 2012;262(2):635-646.

84. ACOG Committee Opinion. Number 299, September 2004 (replaces No. 158, September 1995). Guidelines for diagnostic imaging during pregnancy. *Obstet Gynecol.* 2004;104(3):647-651.

85. Brent R. The effect of embryonic and fetal exposure to x-ray, microwaves, and ultrasound: counseling the pregnant and nonpregnant patient about these risks. *Semin Oncol.* 1989;16:347-368.

86. Stewart A, Kneale G. Radiation dose effects in relation to obstetric x-rays and childhood cancers. *Lancet.* 1970;1(7658):1185-1188.

87. Einstein AJ, Henzlova MJ, Rajagopalan S. Estimating risk of cancer associated with radiation exposure from 64-slice computed tomography coronary angiography. *JAMA.* 2007;298(3):317-323.

88. Bourjeily G, Paidas M, Khalil H, Rosene-Montella K, Rodger M. Pulmonary embolism in pregnancy. *Lancet.* 2010;375(9713):500-512.

89. Hopper KD, King SH, Lobell ME, TenHave TR, Weaver JS. The breast: in-plane x-ray protection during diagnostic thoracic CT–shielding with bismuth radioprotective garments. *Radiology.* 1997;205(3):853-858.

90. Hurwitz LM, Yoshizumi TT, Reiman RE, et al. Radiation dose to the female breast from 16-MDCT body protocols. *AJR Am J Roentgenol.* 2006;186(6):1718-1722.

91. Parker MS, Kelleher NM, Hoots JA, Chung JK, Fatouros PP, Benedict SH. Absorbed radiation dose of the female breast during diagnostic multidetector chest CT and dose reduction with a tungsten-antimony composite breast shield: preliminary results. *Clin Radiol.* 2008;63(3):278-288.

92. Webb J, Thomson H, Morcos SK, Members of the Contrast Media Safety Committee of European Society of Urogenital Radiology (ESUR). The use of iodinated and gadolinium contrast media during pregnancy and lactation. *Eur Radiol.* 2005;15:1234-1240.

93. Burrows R, Gan E, Gallus A, Wallace E, Burrows E. A randomised double-blind placebo controlled trial of low molecular weight heparin as prophylaxis in preventing venous thrombolic events after caesarean section: a pilot study. *BJOG.* 2001;108(8):835-839.

94. Gates S, Brocklehurst P, Ayers S, Bowler U. Thromboprophylaxis in Pregnancy Advisory Group. Thromboprophylaxis and pregnancy: two randomized controlled pilot trials that used low-molecular-weight heparin. *Am J Obstet Gynecol.* 2004;191:1296-1303.

95. Zaccoletti R, Zardini E. Efficacy of elastic compression stockings and administration of calcium heparin in the prevention of puerperal thromboembolic complications. *Minerva Ginecol.* 1992;44:263-266.

96. Hirsh J. Heparin. *N Engl J Med.* 1991;324:1565-1574.

97. Ginsberg J, Hirsh J, Turner D, Levine M, Burrows R. Risks to the fetus of anticoagulant therapy during pregnancy. *Thromb Haemost.* 1989;61:197-203.

98. Griffith G, Nichols GJ, Asher J, Flanagan B. Heparin Osteoporosis. *JAMA.* 1965;193:85-88.

99. Dahlman T. Osteoporotic fractures and the recurrence of thromboembolism during pregnancy and the puerperium in 184 women undergoing thromboprophylaxis with heparin. *Am J Obstet Gynecol.* 1993;168:1265-1270.

100. Warkentin T, Greinacher A. Heparin-induced thrombocytopenia: recognition, treatment, and prevention. The Seventh ACCP Conference on Antithrombotic and Thrombolytic Therapy. *Chest.* 2004;126:311S-337S.

101. Walenga J, Jeske W, Fasanella A, Wood J, Ahmad S, Bakhos M. Laboratory diagnosis of heparin-induced thrombocytopenia. *Clin Appl Thromb Hemost.* 1999;5(suppl 1):S21-S27.

102. Casele HL, Laifer SA, Woelkers DA, Venkataramanan R. Changes in the pharmacokinetics of the low-molecular-weight heparin enoxaparin sodium during pregnancy. *Am J Obstet Gynecol.* 1999;181(5 Pt 1):1113-1117.

103. Fox NS, Laughon SK, Bender SD, Saltzman DH, Rebarber A. Anti-factor Xa plasma levels in pregnant women receiving low molecular weight heparin thromboprophylaxis. *Obstet Gynecol.* 2008;112(4):884-889.

104. Hirsh J, Raschke R. Heparin and low-molecular-weight heparin: the Seventh ACCP Conference on Antithrombotic and Thrombolytic Therapy. *Chest.* 2004;126(3 suppl):188S-203S.

105. Holst J, Lindblad B, Bergqvist D, et al. Protamine neutralization of intravenous and subcutaneous low-molecular-weight heparin (tinzaparin, Logiparin). An experimental investigation in healthy volunteers. *Blood Coagul Fibrinolysis.* 1994;5:795-803.

106. Fausett M, Vogtlander M, Lee R, et al. Heparin-induced thrombocytopenia is rare in pregnancy. *Am J Obstet Gynecol.* 2001;185:148-152.

107. Lepercq J, Conard J, Borel-Derlon A, et al. Venous thromboembolism during pregnancy: a retrospective study of enoxaparin safety in 624 pregnancies. *BJOG.* 2001;108:1134-1140.

108. Buller H, Davidson B, Decousus H, et al. Fondaparinux or enoxaparin for the initial treatment of symptomatic deep venous thrombosis: a randomized trial. *Ann Intern Med.* 2004;140:867-873.

109. Buller H, Davidson B, Decousus H, et al. Subcutaneous fondaparinux versus intravenous unfractionated heparin in the initial treatment of pulmonary embolism. *N Engl J Med.* 2003;349:1695-1702.

110. Harenberg J. Treatment of a woman with lupus and thromboembolism and cutaneous intolerance to heparins using fondaparinux during pregnancy. *Thromb Res.* 2007;119(3):385-388.

111. Knol HM, Schultinge L, Erwich JJ, Meijer K. Fondaparinux as an alternative anticoagulant therapy during pregnancy. *J Thromb Haemost.* 2010;8:1876-1879.

112. Mazzolai L, Hohlfeld P, Spertini F, Hayoz D, Schapira M, Duchosal MA. Fondaparinux is a safe alternative in case of heparin intolerance during pregnancy. *Blood.* 2006;108(5):1569-1570.

113. Winger EE, Reed JL. A retrospective analysis of fondaparinux versus enoxaparin treatment in women with infertility or pregnancy loss. *Am J Reprod Immunol.* 2009;62(4):253-260.

114. Dempfle C. Minor transplacental passage of fondaparinux in vivo. *N Engl J Med.* 2004;350:1914-1915.

115. Hirsh J, Dalen J, Anderson D, et al. Oral anticoagulants: mechanism of action, clinical effectiveness, and optimal therapeutic range. *Chest.* 2001; 119(1 suppl):8S-21S.

116. Lazo-Langner A, Kovacs MJ. Predicting warfarin dose. *Curr Opin Pulm Med.* 2010;16(5):426-431.

117. Lazo-Langner A, Monkman K, Kovacs MJ. Predicting warfarin maintenance dose in patients with venous thromboembolism based on the response to a standardized warfarin initiation nomogram. *J Thromb Haemost.* 2009;7(8):1276-1283.

118. Ansell J, Hirsh J, Poller L, Bussey H, Jacobson A, Hylek E. The Pharmacology and Management of the Vitamin K Antagonists. The Seventh ACCP Conference on Antithrombotic and Thrombolytic Therapy. *Chest.* 2004; 126:204S-233S.

119. Barbour L, Oja J, Schultz L. A prospective trial that demonstrates that dalteparin requirements increase in pregnancy to maintain therapeutic levels of anticoagulation. *Am J Obstet Gynecol.* 2004;191:1024-1029.

120. Raschke R, Reilly B, Guidry J, Fontana J, Srinivas S. The weight-based heparin dosing nomogram compared with a "standard care" nomogram. A randomized controlled trial. *Ann Intern Med*. 1993;119:874-881.

121. ACOG Practice Bulletin no. 123: Thromboembolism in Pregnancy. *Obstet Gynecol*. 2011;118(3):718-729.

122. Barbour LA, Smith JM, Marlar RA. Heparin levels to guide thromboembolism prophylaxis during pregnancy. *Am J Obstet Gynecol*. 1995;173(6): 1869-1873.

123. Ferraro F, D'Ignazio N, Matarazzo A, Rusciano G, Iannuzzi M, Belluomo Anello C. Thromboembolism in pregnancy: a new temporary caval filter. *Minerva Anestesiol*. 2001;67:381-385.

124. Gerhardt A, Scharf R, Beckmann M, Struve S, Bender H, Pillny M, et al. Prothrombin and factor V mutations in women with a history of thrombosis during pregnancy and the puerperium. *N Engl J Med*. 2000;342: 374-380.

125. Juul K, Tybjaerg-Hansen A, Steffensen R, Kofoed S, Jensen G, Nordestgaard B. Factor V Leiden: The Copenhagen City Heart Study and 2 meta-analyses. *Blood*. 2002;100:3-10.

126. Price D, Ridker P, Factor V. Leiden mutation and the risks for thromboembolic disease: a clinical perspective. *Ann Intern Med*. 1997;127: 895-903.

127. Franco R, Reitsma P. Genetic risk factors of venous thrombosis. *Hum Genet*. 2001;109:369-384.

128. Friedrich P, Sanson B, Simioni P, Zanardi S, Huisman M, Kindt I, et al. Frequency of pregnancy-related venous thromboembolism in anticoagulant factor-deficient women: implications for prophylaxis. *Ann Intern Med*. 1996;125:955-960.

129. Aznar J, Vaya A, Estelles A, Mira Y, Segui R, Villa P, et al. Risk of venous thrombosis in carriers of the prothrombin G20210A variant and factor V Leiden and their interaction with oral contraceptives. *Haematologica*. 2000;85:1271-1276.

130. Emmerich J, Rosendaal F, Cattaneo M, Margaglione M, De Stefano V, Cumming T, et al. Combined effect of factor V Leiden and prothrombin 20210A on the risk of venous thromboembolism—pooled analysis of 8 case-control studies including 2310 cases and 3204 controls. Study Group for Pooled-Analysis in Venous Thromboembolism. *Thromb Haemost*. 2001;86:809-816.

131. Ridker P, Miletich J, Hennekins C, Buring J. Ethnic distribution of factor V Leiden in 4047 men and women. Implications for venous thromboembolism screening. *JAMA*. 1997;277:1305-1307.

132. Vossen C, Conard J, Fontcuberta J, Makris M, Van Der Meer F, Pabinger I, et al. Familial thrombophilia and lifetime risk of venous thrombosis. *J Thromb Haemost*. 2004;2:1526-1532.

133. Goodwin A, Rosendaal F, Kottke-Marchant K, Bovill E. A review of the technical, diagnostic, and epidemiologic considerations for protein S assays. *Arch Pathol Lab Med*. 2002;126:1349-1366.

CHAPTER 46

Collagen Vascular Diseases in Pregnancy

JEANETTE R. CARPENTER and D. WARE BRANCH

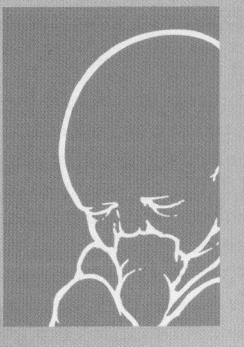

KEY ABBREVIATIONS

Anti-β2–glycoprotein I antibody	aβ2-GP-I	Low-molecular-weight heparin	LMWH
Anticardiolipin antibody	aCL	Lupus nephritis	LN
American College of Obstetricians and Gynecologists	ACOG	Major histocompatibility complex	MHC
		Mycophenolate mofetil	MMF
American College of Rheumatology	ACR	Methotrexate	MTX
Antinuclear antibody	ANA	Neonatal lupus erythematosus	NLE
Antiphospholipid antibody	aPL	Nonsteroidal antiinflammatory drug	NSAID
Antiphospholipid syndrome	APS	Normal sinus rhythm	NSR
Azathioprine	AZA	Preterm birth	PTB
Catastrophic antiphospholipid syndrome	CAPS	Rheumatoid arthritis	RA
Congenital heart block	CHB	Recurrent early miscarriage	REM
C-reactive protein	CRP	Rheumatoid factor	RF
Deep venous thrombosis	DVT	Small for gestational age	SGA
Erythrocyte sedimentation rate	ESR	Systemic lupus erythematosus	SLE
Estimated glomerular filtration rate	EGFR	Sjögren syndrome	SS
Hydroxychloroquine	HCQ	Systemic sclerosis	SSc
Intrauterine growth restriction	IUGR	Tumor necrosis factor alpha	TNF-α
Intravenous immunoglobulin	IVIG	Regulatory T cell	T$_{REG}$
Lupus anticoagulant	LAC	Unfractionated heparin	UFH

SYSTEMIC LUPUS ERYTHEMATOSUS

Epidemiology and Etiology

Systemic lupus erythematosus (SLE) is a chronic inflammatory and autoimmune disorder that can affect multiple organ systems, including the skin, joints, kidneys, central nervous system, heart, lungs, and liver.

SLE is more prevalent among women than men, and most women who are affected by the disease manifest it at some point during their reproductive years. Not infrequently, an initial diagnosis is made during the course of an evaluation for pregnancy complications or during pregnancy or the postpartum period. Significant racial differences are apparent in disease prevalence: black women have a prevalence of 405 per 100,000 compared with a prevalence of 164 per 100,000 among white women.[1]

Genetic predisposition appears to be an important contributing factor to the development of SLE in that 5% to 12%

of relatives of SLE patients also have the disease. The concordance for SLE is high (~25%) among monozygotic twins. Rare genetic factors such as deficiencies in complement components and mutations in the *TREX1* gene, which encodes a DNA-degrading enzyme—as well as more common single nucleotide polymorphisms (SNPs) in the major histocompatibility complex (MHC)—are associated with the development of SLE.[2] Although an individual may be genetically predisposed to develop SLE, the cause appears to be multifactorial. Studies have identified various exposures—such as to the Epstein-Barr virus, ultraviolet (UV) light, and silica dust—as having associations with SLE.[3] Emerging research suggests that such exposures may mediate the development of SLE through epigenetic changes that cause sustained alterations in gene expression.[3]

Consistent with the higher prevalence of SLE among women, **hormonal factors appear to play an important role. Early menarche, oral contraceptives, and postmenopausal hormone replacement have all been associated with an increased risk for SLE.**[4]

Clinical Manifestations

The clinical course of SLE is characterized by periods of disease "flares" interspersed with periods of remission. The most common presenting symptoms of SLE include arthralgias, fatigue, malaise, weight change, Raynaud phenomenon, fever, photosensitive rash, and alopecia. Constitutional symptoms will be present in nearly all women at some point in their disease course. **More than 90% of individuals with SLE will experience arthralgias,** which are typically migratory and most commonly involve the proximal interphalangeal and metacarpophalangeal joints, wrists, and knees. The arthralgias of SLE typically improve as the day progresses. **Most patients also have skin manifestations at some point in the course of the disease, and the classic presentation is a malar "butterfly" rash that worsens with sun exposure.** For women who present in the postpartum period, some SLE symptoms—such as fatigue and hair loss—may be easily overlooked. More severe but less common manifestations include discoid lupus (inflammatory skin lesions that result in scarring), lupus nephritis (LN), pleurisy, pericarditis, and seizures or psychosis.

Diagnosis

The American College of Rheumatology (ACR) has devised a set of diagnostic criteria for SLE. These criteria were most recently revised in 1997 (Table 46-1) and are highly sensitive and specific for SLE. To be diagnosed with SLE, **a patient must have at least four of the 11 clinical and laboratory criteria, either serially or simultaneously. It should be emphasized, however, that some women with features of SLE might not meet the strict diagnostic criteria but can still be at risk for pregnancy complications. These women may benefit from increased surveillance and even treatment.**

Because nearly all individuals with SLE will have a positive antinuclear antibody (ANA) titer, this is a reasonable initial screening test for women with suggestive symptoms. If the ANA test is negative, a diagnosis of SLE is highly unlikely. However, an elevated ANA titer is not specific for SLE because it can also be seen in other autoimmune conditions such as Sjögren syndrome, scleroderma, and rheumatoid arthritis (RA). **Anti–double-stranded DNA (anti-dsDNA) and anti-Smith (anti-Sm) antibodies are more highly specific for SLE, albeit less sensitive.** Anti-dsDNA titers are frequently elevated in

TABLE 46-1	REVISED AMERICAN COLLEGE OF RHEUMATOLOGY CRITERIA FOR CLASSIFICATION OF SYSTEMIC LUPUS ERYTHEMATOSUS (1982 AND 1997)
Malar rash	Fixed erythema, flat or raised, over the malar eminences that tends to spare the nasolabial folds
Discoid rash	Erythematous raised patches with adherent keratotic scaling and follicular plugging; atrophic scarring may occur in older lesions
Oral ulcers	Oral or nasopharyngeal ulceration, usually painless
Arthritis	Nonerosive arthritis involving two or more peripheral joints, characterized by tenderness, swelling, or effusion
Serositis	Pleuritis (convincing history of pleuritic pain, rubbing heard by a physician, or evidence of pleural effusion) Pericarditis documented by ECG or rub or evidence of effusion
Renal	Persistent proteinuria greater than 0.5 g/day or greater than 3+ if quantitation is not performed Cellular casts: Red cell, hemoglobin, granular, tubular, or mixed
Neurologic	Seizures in the absence of offending drugs or known metabolic derangements (e.g., uremia, ketoacidosis, or electrolyte imbalance) Psychosis in the absence of drugs or metabolic derangements
Hematologic	Hemolytic anemia with reticulocytosis Leukopenia <4000/mm^3 on two or more occasions Lymphopenia <1500/mm^3 on two or more occasions Thrombocytopenia <100,000/mm^3 in the absence of drugs
Immunologic	Anti-DNA: Antibody to native DNA in abnormal titer Anti-Sm: Presence of antibody to Sm nuclear antigen Positive finding of antiphospholipid antibodies based on* (1) an abnormal serum level of IgG or IgM anticardiolipin antibodies, (2) a positive test result for lupus anticoagulant using a standard method, or (3) a false-positive serologic test for syphilis for 6 months
Antinuclear antibody	An abnormal titer of ANA by immunofluorescence or an equivalent assay at any point in time and in the absence of drugs known to be associated with drug-induced lupus syndrome

For the purposes of enrollment in clinical studies, a person is defined as having systemic lupus erythematosus (SLE) if four or more of the 11 criteria are present, serially or simultaneously.
*Testing for antiphospholipid antibodies should also include IgG and IgM anti-β2–glycoprotein I antibodies.
ANA, antinuclear antibody; *ECG,* electrocardiograph; *Ig,* immunoglobulin.

the setting of a disease flare, whereas Anti-Sm antibodies are detected in 30% to 40% of individuals with SLE and are associated with LN. Antiribonucleoprotein (anti-RNP) antibodies are associated with myositis and Raynaud phenomenon. **Patients with either SLE or Sjögren syndrome may also have anti-Ro/SSA and anti-La/SSB antibodies, which are particularly relevant to the obstetric patient because of the association with neonatal lupus erythematosus (NLE) and congenital heart block (CHB).**

Lupus Flare in Pregnancy

Studies on the risk of SLE flare in pregnancy have yielded inconsistent results. In the 1960s and 1970s, studies suggested a significant risk for disease flare in pregnancy with accompanying high rates of adverse maternal and fetal/neonatal outcomes. However, more recent studies indicate that pregnancy may not significantly increase the risk of an SLE flare.[5,6] If flares do occur in pregnancy, they are generally not severe and are relatively easily treated.[7] **The best predictor of the course of SLE during** gestation is the state of disease activity at the onset of pregnancy. In one study, approximately one third of women who were in remission for at least 6 months prior to pregnancy suffered an SLE flare compared with two thirds of women with active disease at the beginning of pregnancy.[8] Thus **women with SLE should be counseled to delay pregnancy until their disease has been in remission for at least 6 months.**

The detection of SLE flare in pregnancy requires frequent clinical assessment and astute clinical judgment. **Flares in pregnancy most commonly manifest as fatigue, joint pain, rash, and proteinuria. Assessing anti-dsDNA titers and complement (C3 and C4) levels may provide additional evidence of disease flares in women with clinical symptoms.** The routine assessment of anti-dsDNA and complement levels in *asymptomatic* women is of doubtful clinical utility.[9]

Lupus Nephritis in Pregnancy

Renal manifestations are present in approximately half of all patients with SLE. Although LN may be suspected based on hematuria, proteinuria, and casts on urinalysis, confirmation of the diagnosis requires a renal biopsy. According to the International Society of Nephrology and the Renal Pathology Society, six classes of LN have been defined, with the most common and severe form being class IV, or diffuse LN.[10] All patients with active diffuse LN have proteinuria and hematuria, and a significant subset of patients will progress to nephrotic syndrome, hypertension, and renal insufficiency. **Women with LN, particularly active disease, are at especially increased risk for adverse pregnancy outcomes that include hypertensive disorders of pregnancy, disease flares, low birthweight infants, and indicated preterm delivery.**[11] Similar to SLE in general, the activity of LN during pregnancy is related to disease status at conception. In one study, an LN flare was seen in only 9% of cases in which the disease was in remission for at least 5 months prior to pregnancy, compared with 66% of cases in which disease was clinically active at conception.[12] Women with baseline renal insufficiency are at greatest risk. Ideally, assessment of baseline renal status—serum creatinine and urine protein excretion—is done prior to planning a pregnancy. If the patient is already pregnant, assessment as early as feasible in the pregnancy is recommended. **As a general rule, a serum creatinine of 1.4 to 1.9 mg/dL** (estimated glomerular filtration rate [EGFR] ~30 to 59 mL/min/1.73 m^2) **is a relative contraindication to pregnancy given the substantial risk of midterm pregnancy complications that might require preterm delivery. Most experts consider a serum creatinine of 2.0 mg/dL or greater** (EGFR ~15 to 29 mL/min/1.73 m^2) **to be an absolute contraindication to pregnancy, again because of the substantial risk of pregnancy complications requiring extreme preterm birth (PTB) and the threat to long-term renal function.** Women with moderate and especially severe baseline renal insufficiency should be counseled regarding the small (5% to 10%) but real risk of an irreversible decline in renal function during pregnancy.[13]

Women with LN often have increasing proteinuria across gestation, related in part to increased glomerular filtration. However, an isolated increase in proteinuria without new-onset or worsening hypertension or a significant rise in serum creatinine should not be an indication for preterm delivery. Furthermore, the American College of Obstetricians and Gynecologists (ACOG) no longer considers proteinuria a necessary diagnostic criterion for preeclampsia.

Distinguishing between a flare in SLE (and LN) and preeclampsia can pose a clinical dilemma. Both entities can present with hypertension and proteinuria. If the pregnancy is at or near term, delivery may be the most prudent strategy. Preeclampsia should resolve after delivery. However, if the pregnancy is still very preterm, distinguishing between a disease flare and preeclampsia is more critical. A SLE flare can usually be treated, such as with corticosteroids, to prolong the pregnancy and optimize neonatal outcomes. Because elevated anti-dsDNA titers and low complement levels are often seen in active SLE, assessing them may aid in distinguishing between a disease flare and preeclampsia. However, it should be emphasized that hypocomplementemia can also be seen in preeclampsia.[14] **Examination of the urine sediment** may also provide useful information because hematuria and cellular casts often accompany an LN flare but are not characteristic of preeclampsia. Renal biopsy may be considered in difficult cases but is usually avoided during pregnancy unless management of the pregnancy is incumbent upon the results.

Women with severe LN are often treated with mycophenolate mofetil (MMF), a significant teratogen that is contraindicated in pregnancy. MMF is typically replaced by azathioprine (AZA) when a pregnancy is planned or soon after conception in an unplanned pregnancy. In one study, preconceptional replacement of MMF with AZA among women with inactive disease did not lead to an increase in LN flares in the 3 to 6 months prior to a confirmed pregnancy.[15]

Pregnancy Complications

Women with SLE do not appear to be less fertile than women without SLE, but they are at increased risk for multiple adverse pregnancy outcomes that include pregnancy loss, PTB, preeclampsia, and intrauterine growth restriction (IUGR).

Pregnancy Loss

Studies from the 1960s and 1970s reported pregnancy loss rates as high as 50% among women with SLE. Although rates of pregnancy loss appear to have declined over the decades, probably related to improved treatment and surveillance, women with SLE are still at greater risk for pregnancy loss compared with women who do not have SLE. One study found that even women with disease remission at the onset of pregnancy had a risk of miscarriage or fetal death of 17% compared with 5% for women without SLE.[16] A meta-analysis reported a spontaneous abortion rate of 16% and a stillbirth rate of 3.6% among women with SLE.[11] The National Institutes of Health (NIH) sponsored Predictors of Pregnancy Outcome: Biomarker In Antiphospholipid Antibody Syndrome and Systemic Lupus Erythematosus (PROMISSE), a study that followed a cohort of women with inactive or mild-to-moderate SLE activity at conception. Because patients were enrolled in the late first or early second trimesters, early pregnancy loss was not assessed. However, **the overall fetal death rate among these women was 4%, and the neonatal death rate was 1%.**[17]

Active disease at the onset of pregnancy confers an increased risk for pregnancy loss. Among a cohort of 267 pregnancies followed between 1987 and 2002, 77% resulted in a live birth among women with high-activity SLE compared with 88% among those with low-activity disease.[18] In addition to disease activity, LN, hypertension, and antiphospholipid antibodies (aPLs) are all associated with an increased risk for pregnancy loss (see Chapter 27).[19]

Intrauterine Growth Restriction

The increased risk for stillbirth among women with SLE is likely related to higher rates of placental insufficiency and IUGR (see Chapter 33), particularly among pregnancies complicated by active disease, hypertension, LN, and/or antiphospholipid syndrome (APS). **Although the rate of IUGR among pregnancies complicated by SLE has been reported to be as high as 40%,**[20] **modern treatments and improved pregnancy surveillance have probably decreased this rate**. A study from the National Inpatient Sample analyzed over 16 million hospital admissions for childbirth and found that 5.6% of women with SLE carried a diagnosis of IUGR, compared with 1.5% among women without SLE (this difference was not statistically significant).[21] In the PROMISSE study, 8% of infants of women with mild to moderate SLE were small for gestational age (SGA).[17] **Chronic, high-dose glucocorticoid treatment is also a risk factor for IUGR.** Because of the increased risk for IUGR and stillbirth, it is standard practice to assess fetal growth intermittently with ultrasound after 20 weeks and to perform antenatal testing (nonstress tests or biophysical profiles) in the third trimester.

Preterm Birth

Women with SLE have an approximately threefold increased risk for PTB.[22] In the PROMISSE study, 9% of pregnancies delivered before 36 weeks.[17] Most of these PTBs are not spontaneous but are rather iatrogenic, the result of fetal or maternal indications (IUGR, preeclampsia, disease flare, deteriorating renal function, etc.). Women with active disease, aPLs, LN, and hypertension are at particular risk for PTB. In one study, a full-term delivery was achieved in only 26% of women with high-activity SLE compared with 61% of women with low-activity disease or remission.[23] High-dose glucocorticoids have also been associated with an increased risk for preterm premature rupture of membranes.

Hypertensive Disorders of Pregnancy

Hypertensive disorders (gestational hypertension or preeclampsia) **occur in 10% to 30% of pregnancies with SLE.**[5,21] The risk for preeclampsia is particularly increased in women with LN and/or chronic hypertension. Preeclampsia may develop in as many as two thirds of women with LN[23] and is a frequent indication for iatrogenic PTB. It appears that preeclampsia is also more likely to develop at an earlier gestational age among women with a history of LN compared with those without such a history (37.5 weeks vs. 34.5 weeks in one study[24]). **Daily low-dose aspirin** (typically 81 mg in the United States) **beginning early in pregnancy is recommended for women with SLE, particularly those with renal manifestations, because evidence suggests this may modestly decrease the risk of developing preeclampsia.**[25]

As mentioned previously, it may be difficult in some cases to distinguish between an SLE flare and preeclampsia, and astute clinical judgment is required. Hospitalization for maternal and fetal monitoring, administration of antenatal steroids, and thoughtful determination of the need for delivery is frequently indicated in these cases.

Neonatal Lupus Erythematosus

Neonatal lupus erythematosus is an acquired autoimmune condition related to the transplacental transfer of anti-Ro/SSA and anti-La/SSB antibodies. NLE most commonly presents as an erythematous, scaling, plaquelike rash that begins in the early neonatal period and may persist for 1 to 2 months. Less common manifestations of NLE include hematologic abnormalities (leukopenia, hemolytic anemia, thrombocytopenia) and hepatosplenomegaly. Fortunately, the incidence of NLE is low. **Among all pregnant women with SLE, the risk of NLE is less than 5%.** Of those women with SLE who test positive for anti-Ro/SSA and anti-La/SSB antibodies, at most 15% to 20% will have an affected newborn. Many mothers of newborns with NLE will not carry a current diagnosis of SLE. However, a significant number of these women will develop symptomatic autoimmune disease, often Sjögren syndrome, in the future. They should therefore be counseled to seek medical evaluation if symptoms of SLE or Sjögren syndrome develop.

The most serious manifestation of NLE is complete heart block. It is most frequently diagnosed at a routine prenatal visit when a fixed fetal bradycardia of 50 to 80 beats/min is detected. CHB is most commonly diagnosed between 16 and 24 weeks' gestation, and it is rarely diagnosed in the third trimester. It is caused by the binding of antibodies to antigens in fetal cardiac tissue with subsequent damage to the cardiac conduction system and, ultimately, complete atrioventricular (AV) dissociation. Some cases progress to endocardial fibroelastosis, which can result in cardiac failure that leads to fetal hydrops and fetal death. Among women with anti-Ro/SSA and anti-La/SSB antibodies, the risk for CHB in the fetus is only 1% to 2%. However, women with a prior affected child have a recurrence risk for CHB of 15% to 20% in subsequent pregnancies.[26] Fetal genetic factors, such as certain human leukocyte antigen (HLA) polymorphisms, may modify susceptibility to the development of CHB.[27] **Although many clinicians routinely test pregnant women with SLE for anti-Ro/SSA and anti-La/SSB antibodies, this practice is not without controversy given that CHB is infrequent, antenatal treatment to alter outcome is of uncertain efficacy, and a positive test result may cause unnecessary maternal anxiety.**

Complete CHB is irreversible and is associated with an overall mortality rate of at least 20% (5% stillborn).[28] **The majority of survivors require a pacemaker.** In one series of 102 cases, a prenatal diagnosis of CHB was associated with a 43% risk of mortality in the first two decades of life.[29] Among a registry of 325 offspring with cardiac manifestations of NLE, predictors of a stillbirth or postnatal death included hydrops, endocardial fibroelastosis, earlier diagnosis, and a lower ventricular rate.[30] In addition, the case fatality rate was significantly higher among minorities (32.1% for blacks compared with 14.3% for whites).[30]

Management of Pregnancies Complicated by Systemic Lupus Erythematosus

Because SLE commonly affects women at some point during their reproductive years, the clinician should be familiar with the high-risk nature of these pregnancies and the altered management and increased surveillance required. **Ideally, women with SLE would present for a preconceptional visit such that disease remission could be ensured, medications reviewed, and counseling performed.**

Table 46-2 outlines recommendations for the management of pregnancies complicated by SLE. **Key components include the assessment of disease activity and renal manifestations, surveillance for preeclampsia, surveillance of fetal growth, and antenatal testing. Co-management with a rheumatologist is particularly important for women with severe manifestations**

TABLE 46-2	RECOMMENDATIONS FOR MANAGEMENT OF PREGNANCIES COMPLICATED BY SYSTEMIC LUPUS ERYTHEMATOSUS
Baseline assessment	• Antiphospholipid antibodies: Lupus anticoagulant, anticardiolipin IgG/IgM, and anti-β2–glycoprotein I IgG/IgM • Review current medications and risks • Consider testing for anti-Ro/SSA and anti-La/SSB antibodies (controversial)
Lupus nephritis	• Serum creatinine every 4 to 6 weeks • Baseline urine protein assessment (24-hour urine collection or spot protein/creatinine ratio) • Urine culture each trimester* • Increased surveillance for signs and symptoms of preeclampsia
Intrauterine growth restriction (IUGR)	• Monthly ultrasonographic assessment of fetal growth after 24 to 28 weeks
Stillbirth	• NST/AFI or BPP beginning at 32 weeks unless indicated earlier (e.g., due to IUGR) • Delivery by 39 weeks unless indicated earlier (e.g., due to IUGR, preeclampsia, worsening renal function)
Chronic steroid therapy	• Early and repeated screening for gestational diabetes • Stress-dose steroids at delivery, particularly for women on more than 20 mg/day of prednisone for more than 3 weeks†
Antiphospholipid antibodies	• Daily low-dose aspirin • Consideration of prophylactic or therapeutic heparin, depending on laboratory results and clinical history (see section on antiphospholipid syndrome)
Lupus flare	• Continuation, or possibly initiation, of hydroxychloroquine • Postpartum monitoring for increased disease activity

*Sulfa antibiotics may exacerbate lupus symptoms in some patients. Consider other antibiotics for the treatment of urinary tract infections.
†Intravenous hydrocortisone 100 mg every 8 hours for 2 to 3 doses is one regimen.
AFI, amniotic fluid index; BPP, biophysical profile; IG, immunoglobulin; IUGR, intrauterine growth restriction; NST, nonstress test.

or active disease. Furthermore, some women experience a disease flare in the postpartum period; therefore the obstetrician should carefully assess disease activity at postpartum visits, and follow-up with rheumatology in the 1 to 3 months following delivery is usually recommended.

Management of Congenital Heart Block

Given that complete CHB is irreversible and that the prognosis is grave, efforts have focused on trying to predict and prevent the development of CHB. Some experts have proposed serial fetal echocardiograms with Doppler monitoring of the PR interval or kinetocardiography in women with anti-Ro/SSA and anti-La/SSB antibodies, particularly in those with a prior fetus affected by CHB. However, these practices are controversial, and no formal guidelines for the type and frequency of monitoring have been established. Neither fetal Doppler PR interval monitoring nor kinetocardiography have been associated with proven benefit, in part because progression to CHB can occur rapidly and without discernable progression through first- and second-degree block. In spite of this, many experts—including expert rheumatologists and pediatric cardiologists—recommend serial PR interval monitoring of the fetus in a woman with anti-SSA/Ro and anti-SSB/La antibodies. In our experience, the inclinations of the local pediatric cardiology team play a dominant

role in deciding upon the nature and frequency of such monitoring.

Even with early detection of cardiac conduction abnormalities or new-onset CHB, no credible evidence suggests that medical interventions alter outcomes. Current treatment recommendations are based on expert opinion and relatively small studies, all nonrandomized. Several case series have described use of fluorinated steroids such as dexamethasone for the treatment of either cardiac conduction abnormalities or new-onset CHB.[31-33] The PR Interval and Dexamethasone Evaluation (PRIDE) study enrolled 40 women with anti-Ro/SSA antibodies and a fetus with any degree of heart block diagnosed echocardiographically.[31] Thirty women were treated with dexamethasone and 10 declined treatment. No cases of CHB reverted, treated or untreated. Among six treated fetuses with second-degree block, three remained in second-degree block, two reverted to normal sinus rhythm (NSR), and one progressed to complete block. Two treated fetuses had first-degree block, and both reverted to NSR after initiation of dexamethasone. However, the one untreated fetus with first-degree block was in NSR at birth. Although case selection in this nonrandomized study likely played a role, no perinatal deaths were reported in the nontreated group compared with deaths (20%) in the dexamethasone group. Treatment with steroids was associated with more preterm and SGA infants; the potential adverse effects of steroids must thus be weighed against the limited data that support a benefit in cases of early cardiac conduction abnormalities.

Although experts generally agree that steroid treatment should not be expected to reverse CHB, at least one group of investigators has concluded that steroid treatment might reverse or improve hydrops, reduce morbidity, and improve 1-year survival.[32] Others disagree.[30,34] In addition to steroid treatment, β-stimulation—such as with terbutaline, ritodrine, or salbutamol—has been administered in some cases of a very low fetal heart rate (<55 beats/min) in an attempt to increase the heart rate and prevent hydrops. Once again, data to support this treatment strategy are very limited.[32] Table 46-3 outlines management strategies for CHB.

Strategies to prevent conduction abnormalities altogether would certainly seem attractive, and three preventive treatments have been considered. Glucocorticoids are not recommended as preventative treatment for women at high risk of CHB due to lack of proven benefit and because most fetuses will not develop CHB. Furthermore, chronic glucocorticoid therapy is associated with some maternal and fetal risks, including potential programming effects on offsprings' hypothalamic-pituitary-adrenal axis and neurodevelopment (see Chapter 5).

Two multicenter prospective observational studies have evaluated intravenous immunoglobulin (IVIG) as a preventative agent.[35,36] The two studies enrolled a total of 44 women at high risk for CHB. The results do not indicate that IVIG is effective at preventing the development of CHB, and it should not be used for this purpose outside of approved research protocols.

More recent data suggest a potential benefit of hydroxychloroquine (HCQ) in decreasing the risk of NLE cardiac complications among high-risk women.[37-40] In a historic cohort of 257 pregnancies in women with anti-Ro/SSA antibodies and a previous child affected with CHB, HCQ use beginning in the first trimester was associated with significantly decreased odds of cardiac NLE (0.23; 95% confidence interval [CI], 0.06 to 0.92), defined as second- or third-degree block or

TABLE 46-3	MANAGEMENT APPROACHES FOR CONGENITAL HEART BLOCK
Anti-Ro/SSA, anti-La/SSB antibodies, no previously affected child	• Risk of CHB is 1%-2%, routine monitoring of the fetal PR interval is usually not recommended (controversial)
Anti-Ro/SSA, anti-La/SSB antibodies, previously affected child	• Risk of CHB is 15%-20% • Give hydroxychloroquine beginning in the first trimester (400 mg/day) • Consider serial monitoring of the fetal PR interval (controversial) with weekly pulsed Doppler echocardiography*
First-degree heart block[†]	• Patient may revert to normal sinus rhythm; monitor for progression • Consider dexamethasone treatment at 4 mg/day (controversial)
Second-degree heart block[†]	• Monitor for progression • Consider dexamethasone treatment at 4 mg/day upon diagnosis • Discontinue dexamethasone if condition progresses to complete block except with evidence of hydrops • Given potential adverse effects, consider discontinuation of dexamethasone if heart block reverts
First-degree (complete) heart block[†]	• Monitor for hydrops • Give dexamethasone if hydrops develops • Consider oral terbutaline (2.5-7.5 mg every 4-6 hr) for an FHR <55 beats/min[‡]

*Highest risk period for development of CHB is between 18 and 24 weeks' gestation.
[†]Fetal echocardiography is recommended to rule out structural heart disease.
[‡]Caution is warranted with chronic terbutaline therapy because of reported serious maternal adverse events. Terbutaline should especially be avoided in women with diabetes, hypertension, hyperthyroidism, seizures, or a history of arrhythmias.
CHB, congenital heart block; *FHR,* fetal heart rate.

isolated cardiomyopathy.[38] Given the low risk for fetal harm (see the section on medications) and potential benefit, initiation of HCQ in the first trimester should be considered among women positive for anti-Ro/SSA antibodies who have had a prior affected child.

Drug Used to Treat Systemic Lupus Erythematosus and Pregnancy Considerations

It should be noted that as of June of 2015, the U.S. Food and Drug Administration (FDA) Pregnancy and Lactation Labeling Final Rule requires that the pregnancy safety letter categories of A, B, C, D, and X be removed from drug labels and replaced by a risk summary, clinical considerations, and available data. The goal of this change is to better assist health care providers in assessing the benefits versus risks of medications in pregnancy. This rule also requires that labels be updated when the information is outdated.

Drugs with Acceptable Risk Profiles in Pregnancy (See Chapter 8)

HYDROXYCHLOROQUINE

Past concerns regarding HCQ being associated with fetal ocular toxicity and ototoxicity (FDA category C) have not been confirmed by studies published within the past 15 years.[39,41] One study of 114 HCQ-exposed pregnancies, most in the first trimester, compared with 455 unexposed pregnancies found no significant difference in the rate of congenital anomalies.[41] Moreover, the continuation of HCQ during pregnancy may be beneficial; one retrospective analysis[42] showed that women who remained on HCQ had less severe SLE flares and

thus required lower doses of glucocorticoids. Evidence also suggests that HCQ may prevent CHB in at-risk fetuses.[37,38,40] Given the possible benefits and the apparent lack of harm, many experts now recommend that women on HCQ who become pregnant continue the medication during pregnancy. It is also a favored agent for the treatment of SLE flares in pregnancy, and **HCQ is compatible with breastfeeding.**

GLUCOCORTICOIDS

SLE flares in pregnancy are most commonly treated with glucocorticoids. Nonfluorinated steroids, such as prednisone and methylprednisolone (both FDA category C) **are preferred in pregnancy** because the placenta metabolizes these agents to an inactive metabolite, which results in limited fetal exposure. Some studies have reported a small increased risk of cleft lip and palate with first-trimester glucocorticoid use,[43] but other studies have not confirmed these findings.[44] If the risk for orofacial clefts is increased, this increase appears to be small. **Prolonged use of glucocorticoids is associated with an increased risk for maternal bone loss, gestational diabetes, hypertension and preeclampsia, and adrenal suppression.** The use of prednisone in moderate to high doses may be associated with preterm rupture of membranes (PROM) and fetal growth restriction.[45] Women taking glucocorticoids should be screened early for gestational diabetes, and the test should be repeated at the usual 24 to 28 weeks if normal. Those on 20 mg/day or more of prednisone for at least 3 weeks are at greatest risk of adrenal suppression and should receive **stress-dose steroids during labor and delivery.** One stress-dose regimen is 100 mg of intravenous (IV) hydrocortisone every 8 to 12 hours for two to three doses. The risk of adrenal suppression for women taking 5 mg or less per day of prednisone is very small, and stress-dose steroids are not indicated. For women who take more than 5 mg and less than 20 mg per day, many clinicians still administer stress-dose steroids, although simply continuing women on their daily steroid dose is probably adequate. In general, **prednisone is compatible with breastfeeding, although for women who take more than 20 mg per day, it may be prudent to delay feeding for 4 hours after the dose.**

NONSTEROIDAL ANTIINFLAMMATORY DRUGS

Nonsteroidal antiinflammatory drugs (NSAIDs) are considered first-line treatment for autoimmune disease symptoms such as arthralgias or arthritis. First trimester NSAID exposure was not associated with an increase in the rate of congenital malformations or a decrease in infant survival in several large population-based studies.[46,47] It is controversial as to whether first- and early second-trimester use of NSAIDs is associated with an increased risk of spontaneous abortion. **Third-trimester NSAID use may cause premature closure of the fetal ductus arteriosus, particularly after 30 weeks' gestation, and oligohydramnios. For these reasons, NSAIDs are FDA category C before 30 weeks and category D thereafter.** NSAIDs should be used judiciously in the late first and second trimesters of pregnancy and should be generally avoided after 28 to 30 weeks. The single exception **is low-dose aspirin, which can be taken safely throughout pregnancy. Daily low-dose aspirin may provide modest risk reduction for the development of preeclampsia among high-risk women.**[48] Data are limited regarding cyclooxygenase 2 (COX-2) inhibitors such as celecoxib in pregnancy, and it is recommended that these agents be avoided. **NSAIDs are compatible with breastfeeding.**

AZATHIOPRINE

Azathioprine (FDA category D) is used in the prevention of transplant rejection and in the treatment of SLE and LN. Although teratogenicity has been documented in animal studies, the human placenta lacks the enzyme that metabolizes AZA to its active metabolite, 6-mercaptopurine. As a result, very little active drug reaches the fetal circulation. Human studies have not found an increased risk for teratogenicity. Some studies have found increased rates of IUGR, PTB, and impaired neonatal immunity with AZA use in pregnancy. However, it is difficult to determine whether these outcomes are related to AZA use or the underlying disease.[49] **AZA, often in combination with glucocorticoids, is thus the preferred treatment for severe or active SLE in pregnancy. Most experts consider AZA to be compatible with breastfeeding, although long-term follow-up of exposed infants is limited.** Avoiding feeding for 4 to 6 hours after a dose will markedly decrease the amount of drug in breastmilk.

CYCLOSPORINE A

Cyclosporine A (FDA category C) is a calcineurin inhibitor sometimes used in the treatment of LN or severe arthritis. The drug is an immunosuppressive that inhibits the production and release of interleukin 2 (IL-2). Animal studies have demonstrated very low transplacental transfer of cyclosporine. Human studies are conflicting, but probably very little drug enters the fetal circulation. **Data obtained primarily from organ transplant patients indicate a very low risk of teratogenicity, but the risk for PTB and SGA infants may be increased.**[45] The drug may also cause a rise in maternal creatinine. **Women on cyclosporine are generally discouraged from breastfeeding, although data are limited regarding adverse outcomes.**

Drugs with Uncertain or Higher Risk Profiles in Pregnancy
CYCLOPHOSPHAMIDE

Cyclophosphamide (FDA category D) is an alkylating agent used in the treatment of LN and vasculitis. **This drug is teratogenic and should not be used at all in the first trimester.** Use of cyclophosphamide may be considered in the second and third trimesters in the rare patient with very severe and progressive disease manifestations. *Cyclophosphamide is not compatible with breastfeeding.*

Drugs Contraindicated in Pregnancy
MYCOPHENOLATE MOFETIL

Mycophenolate mofetil (FDA category D) is an inhibitor of purine biosynthesis and is used in the treatment of LN. *MMF is absolutely contraindicated in pregnancy due its abortifacient and teratogenic properties.* MMF is associated with an increased risk for cleft lip and palate, micrognathia, microtia, and abnormalities of the ear canals. Women should avoid pregnancy until they have been off MMF for at least 6 weeks. **No data are available regarding MMF use and breastfeeding, and it is considered contraindicated.**

ANTIPHOSPHOLIPID SYNDROME

Antiphospholipid syndrome (APS) is an autoimmune condition associated with venous and arterial thrombosis, and adverse pregnancy outcomes that include recurrent early miscarriage (REM), fetal death, early preeclampsia, and placental insufficiency. Diagnosis of APS is confirmed by persistently positive aPLs, a heterogeneous group of autoantibodies directed against either negatively charged phospholipids or glycoproteins bound to these phospholipids. **The diagnosis of APS is confirmed by the detection of one or more of three aPLs: lupus anticoagulant (LAC), anticardiolipin antibodies (aCL), and anti-β2–glycoprotein I (aβ2-GP-I) antibodies.** The classification criteria for APS were most recently revised in 2006 (Box 46-1).[50]

BOX 46-1 REVISED CLASSIFICATION CRITERIA FOR THE ANTIPHOSPHOLIPID ANTIBODY SYNDROME*

Clinical Criteria

Vascular Thrombosis†
1. One or more clinical episodes of arterial, venous, or small-vessel thrombosis in any tissue or organ *and*
2. Thrombosis confirmed by objective, validated criteria (i.e., unequivocal findings of appropriate imaging studies or histopathology) *and*
3. For histopathologic confirmation, thrombosis should be present without significant evidence of inflammation in the vessel wall

PREGNANCY MORBIDITY
1. One or more unexplained deaths of a morphologically normal fetus at or beyond the 10th week of gestation, with normal fetal morphology documented by ultrasound or by direct examination of the fetus *or*
2. One or more premature births of a morphologically normal neonate at or before the 34th week of gestation because of eclampsia or severe preeclampsia or placental insufficiency‡ *or*
3. Three or more unexplained consecutive spontaneous abortions before the 10th week of gestation with maternal anatomic or hormonal abnormalities and paternal and maternal chromosomal causes excluded

Laboratory Criteria
1. Lupus anticoagulant present in plasma on two or more occasions at least 12 weeks apart, detected according to the guidelines of the International Society on Thrombosis and Hemostasis
2. Anticardiolipin antibody of IgG and/or IgM isotype in blood present in medium or high titer (i.e., >40 GPL or MPL or >99th percentile) on at least two occasions at least 12 weeks apart, measured by standardized ELISA
3. Anti-β2–glycoprotein I antibody of IgG and/or IgM isotype in serum or plasma (in titer >99th percentile) present in medium or high titer on at least two occasions at least 12 weeks apart, measured by standardized ELISA

Modified from Miyakis S, Lockshin MD, Atsumi T, et al. International consensus statement on an update of the classification criteria for definite antiphospholipid syndrome (APS). *J Thromb Haemost.* 2006;4: 295-306.
*Must meet at least one clinical and one laboratory criterion for diagnosis of "definite" APS.
†Superficial venous thrombosis is not included in the clinical criteria.
‡Features of placental insufficiency may include: (1) abnormal or nonreassuring fetal surveillance, such as a nonreactive nonstress test; (2) abnormal Doppler flow in the umbilical artery (e.g. absent end-diastolic flow); (3) oligohydramnios; or (4) infant birthweight below the 10th percentile for gestational age.
ELISA, enzyme-linked immunosorbent assay; *GPL,* IgG phospholipid units; *Ig,* immunoglobulin; *MPL,* IgM phospholipid units.

Clinical Presentation

APS may occur as a primary condition or in association with another autoimmune disease, most commonly SLE. **Prevalence and incidence are uncertain**, although definite APS in the absence of other autoimmune conditions is probably no more common than SLE. If low-titer positive tests for one or more of the three aPLs (usually aCL or aβ2-GP-I) are included, aPLs are found in a small percentage (<5%) of healthy women[51] and in up to 40% of patients with SLE.[52] **In the absence of a history of thrombosis or pregnancy morbidity, the risks associated with an incidentally identified positive test for aPL among otherwise healthy women are not well understood, and these women should not be diagnosed with APS.**

The most common thrombotic presentation of APS is deep venous thrombosis (DVT) of the lower extremity, which represents about two thirds of thrombotic APS cases.[53] The most common arterial presentation is stroke; positive aPL results are found in up to 20% of ischemic stroke patients younger than 50 years of age.[54] Small vessel thrombosis may present as nephropathy. Compared with heritable thrombophilias, APS is more likely to manifest with thromboses in diverse or unusual locations such as the intracranial (stroke), hepatic, and intraabdominal venous or arterial circulations.

APS should be considered in the differential diagnosis of venous or arterial thrombosis and also with any of the following adverse pregnancy outcomes:

- Three or more otherwise unexplained *recurrent early miscarriages,* defined as preembryonic or embryonic losses at less than 10 weeks' gestation
- One or more otherwise unexplained fetal deaths (≥10 weeks' gestation)
- A history of PTB occurring at less than 34 weeks' gestation secondary to severe preeclampsia or placental insufficiency

Recurrent Early Miscarriage

Although studies have found that up to 15% of women with REM have positive aPL results,[55] the data are flawed by poor standardization of aPL assays, inclusion of women with other causes of REM, inconsistent selection of controls, variability in the type of aPLs or isotypes tested, and variable definitions of aPL positivity and REM.[56] As a result, women with REM should only be diagnosed with APS if they meet accepted international criteria.[57] This topic is discussed in greater detail in Chapter 27.

Stillbirth

In a recent analysis from the Stillbirth Collaborative Research Network's multicenter, population-based case-control study of stillbirths and live births, **9.6% of fetal death cases at 20 or more weeks' gestation were associated with a positive test for aPLs** (aCL or aβ2-GP-I antibodies) **compared with 6% of live birth cases—a statistically significant difference.**[58] Among otherwise unexplained cases, immunoglobulin G (IgG) aCL and IgM aCL antibodies were associated with fivefold and twofold increased odds of fetal death, respectively. Positive IgG aβ2-GP-I antibodies were associated with a threefold increased odds of fetal death. **The authors concluded that 14% of otherwise unexplained fetal deaths were attributable to APS.** In the recently published prospective Nimes Obstetricians and Hematologists Antiphospholipid Syndrome (NOH-APS) study,[59] women with well-characterized APS who had either REM or a prior fetal death suffered an 8.3% and 15.9% rate of fetal loss,

respectively, in their next observed pregnancy in spite of treatment with enoxaparin and low-dose aspirin.

Placental Insufficiency

The association between aPL and PTB before 34 weeks due to severe preeclampsia or placental insufficiency (manifested as IUGR) is somewhat uncertain because studies are flawed by poor standardization of laboratory tests, concerns related to cases and controls selection, and the variable definitions of preeclampsia and placental insufficiency. These issues notwithstanding, several studies suggest **that a median of 7.9% of women with severe preeclampsia have positive tests for aPL, compared with 0.5% for controls.**[60,61] In the NOH-APS study, 10% of women with well-characterized APS developed severe preeclampsia in spite of enoxaparin and low-dose aspirin treatment.[59] So although PTB before 34 weeks' gestation due to severe preeclampsia or placental insufficiency is included in the clinical criteria for APS, experts agree that further study is warranted.[57]

The most serious but rare thrombotic presentation of APS is catastrophic APS (CAPS). This condition is characterized by rapid-onset, often small vessel thrombosis, multiorgan dysfunction, a systemic inflammatory response, involvement of unusual organ systems (e.g., renal or hepatic), and a high mortality rate.

Although not included in the international diagnostic criteria, aPLs are associated with other clinical features that include immune thrombocytopenia, hemolytic anemia, cardiac valvular disease, chronic skin ulcers, myelopathy, chorea, migraine, epilepsy, and cognitive impairment, particularly among patients with SLE.

Diagnosis

Definite Antiphospholipid Syndrome

As defined by the international criteria, at least one clinical criterion and positive aPL are required for the diagnosis of definite APS (see Box 46-1).[50] Clinicians should recognize that the clinical criteria are relatively common and nonspecific for APS, such that the final diagnosis of APS ultimately rests on positive aPL. Specifically, the laboratory criteria require that a patient have medium to high titers of aCL IgG or IgM antibodies, aβ2-GP-I IgG or IgM antibodies, or LAC. Because other conditions can result in transiently positive aPL, persistently positive results on two or more occasions at least 12 weeks apart are needed. Laboratories are required to delineate medium or high titer results for aCL and greater than 99% results for aβ2-GP-I antibodies. The development of standard calibrators and international "units" for the aCL assay has established greater than 40 IgG units ("GPL") or IgM units ("MPL") as being a medium or high titer. The status of IgA isotypes is a matter of ongoing investigation, but currently IgA aCL or aβ2-GP-I antibodies are not recognized as diagnostic of APS.

It should also be emphasized that LAC is a better predictor of pregnancy morbidity or thrombosis than aCL or aβ2-GP-I antibodies.[62,63] False-positive LAC results may occur in the setting of anticoagulant drugs. Higher titers and the IgG isotype of aCL and aβ2-GP-I antibodies are more specific for APS-related clinical manifestations. Finally, some experts hold that triple aPL positivity (LAC, aCL, and aβ2-GP-I) is of greater clinical significance than double or single aPL positivity.

Catastrophic Antiphospholipid Syndrome

Catastrophic antiphospholipid syndrome (CAPS) can occur in pregnancy and should be considered in the differential

diagnosis that includes hemolytic uremic syndrome (HUS) and thrombotic thrombocytopenic purpura (TTP). According to international criteria, the diagnosis of CAPS is based on thromboses in three or more organs in less than a week, microthrombosis in at least one organ, and persistent aPL positivity.[64] In practice, features of microthrombosis vary from biopsy-proven thrombosis in small vessels to clinical ischemia resulting from occlusion of arterioles and capillaries. Given the often vague features of microthromboses and the substantial mortality rate associated with CAPS, a high index of suspicion is warranted in patients who present with fewer than three organ systems involved.

Possible or Probable Antiphospholipid Syndrome and Equivocal Cases

In certain scenarios, it may not be prudent to wait 12 weeks to confirm initially positive aPL results before considering treatment. For example, after weighing the risks and potential benefits, thromboprophylaxis might be considered in a woman with a history of fetal death who is newly pregnant and initially tests positive for aPL. In the case of CAPS, the high mortality rate should prompt consideration of aggressive treatment without waiting for confirmation of persistently positive aPL.

At the other end of the clinical spectrum are patients who meet the clinical criteria for APS but have "equivocal" aPL results. One frequent scenario is the woman with REM and persistently low-positive aCL or aβ2-GP-I antibody results (i.e., aCL result of 20 to 39 GPL or MPL units). In such cases, clinicians are often faced with the difficult decision as to whether low-dose heparin "treatment" in the next pregnancy is reasonable, in spite of the lack of evidence of efficacy in such cases.

Management of Antiphospholipid Syndrome in Pregnancy

Treatment during Pregnancy

Management of APS during pregnancy is aimed at minimizing or eliminating the risks of thrombosis, miscarriage, fetal death, preeclampsia, placental insufficiency, and iatrogenic preterm birth. With currently recommended management strategies, the likelihood of a successful pregnancy (delivery of a viable infant) in a woman diagnosed with APS exceeds 70%.

The combination of a heparin agent and low-dose aspirin is the current recommended treatment for APS in pregnancy because it serves to provide thromboprophylaxis and may improve pregnancy outcomes. Ideally aspirin is started preconceptionally because of its possible beneficial effects on implantation. Because some patients with APS have immune thrombocytopenia, the platelet count should be assessed prior to starting treatment. Heparin is usually begun in the early first trimester after demonstrating either an appropriately rising serum human chorionic gonadotropin (hCG) or the presence of a live embryo on ultrasonography. Most APS patients with a history of thrombosis are maintained on long-term anticoagulation, frequently warfarin. To minimize the risk of warfarin embryopathy, these patients should be transitioned from warfarin to a heparin agent either prior to or very early in pregnancy.

Women with APS diagnosed on the basis of obstetric criteria who do *not* have a history of thrombosis may be classified into one of two groups: (1) those with REM or (2) those with one or more previous fetal deaths (≥10 weeks gestation) or previous early delivery (<34 weeks' gestation) because of severe preeclampsia or placental insufficiency. Most experts recommend prophylactic-dose heparin and low-dose aspirin for these patients.

Heparin treatment to improve obstetric outcomes in women with APS is not without controversy. Four heparin treatment trials have been conducted in women diagnosed with APS predominantly based on REM.[65-68] In two of these, the proportion of successful pregnancies substantially improved with the addition of unfractionated heparin (UFH) to low-dose aspirin.[65,66] The other two trials used low-molecular-weight heparin (LMWH) and did not find a significant benefit when combined with low-dose aspirin,[67,68] primarily because the live birth rates in the patients treated with aspirin only were quite good (70% to 75%). Two studies have compared UFH with LMWH, each paired with low-dose aspirin, in women with predominant REM and found no differences in outcomes.[69,70] Furthermore, several studies have reported successful pregnancy outcomes in excess of 70% among women with predominant REM who were treated with low-dose aspirin alone.[71,72] A Cochrane systematic review concluded that although the quality of available studies was not high, "combined UFH and aspirin may reduce pregnancy loss by 54%" in women with APS based on REM.[73] The American College of Chest Physicians recommends antepartum administration of prophylactic or intermediate-dose UFH or prophylactic LMWH in women who fulfill the laboratory criteria for APS and meet the clinical criteria for REM.[74] In contrast, a recent ACOG practice bulletin states that for women with APS without a preceding thrombotic event, either clinical surveillance or prophylactic heparin may be used in the antepartum period but that "prophylactic doses of heparin and low-dose aspirin during pregnancy...should be considered."[75]

Treatment to prevent adverse pregnancy outcomes in women with APS and fetal death (≥10 weeks' gestation) or previous early delivery (<34 weeks' gestation) due to severe preeclampsia or placental insufficiency has not been established by well-designed trials. So although heparin treatment is frequently initiated in such patients, professional guidelines have avoided making unequivocal recommendations for its use in the prevention of these later adverse pregnancy outcomes.[74,75]

Box 46-2 summarizes the recommended treatment regimens for APS in pregnancy. Three important clinical points are relevant with regard to treatment aimed at preventing adverse outcomes in pregnant women with APS. First, women with APS and prior thrombosis represent a high-risk population that should be treated with appropriate anticoagulant agents during pregnancy and the postpartum period.[74,75] Second, even in the absence of a prior thrombosis, women with repeatedly positive tests for LAC or medium to high titers of aCL or aβ2-GP-I antibodies are at increased risk for pregnancy-associated thrombosis, which favors at least prophylactic UFH or LMWH during pregnancy and the postpartum period. Finally, even in the absence of prior thrombosis, most women with a history of REM, fetal death, or early PTB due to severe preeclampsia or placental insufficiency will opt for "treatment" if it is felt to be relatively safe. Considering that prophylactic UFH or LMWH regimens are rarely associated with serious adverse effects such as clinically significant osteopenia, significant bleeding, or heparin-induced thrombocytopenia, most clinicians are agreeable to treatment in these patients.

Postpartum thromboprophylaxis with UFH, LMWH, or warfarin (international normalized ratio [INR] 2 to 3) **should be strongly considered in all women with APS and is absolutely indicated in women with prior thrombosis,** most of whom will restart their long-term anticoagulation regimen.[75] In patients with no previous thrombosis, treatment is usually continued for 6 weeks following delivery. **Both heparin and warfarin are safe for breastfeeding mothers.** In patients with obstetric APS and without prior thrombosis, recent data suggest that long-term low-dose aspirin may decrease the risk of an initial thrombosis event.[76]

In the past, case series and small trials indicated that glucocorticoid treatment of APS in pregnancy results in outcomes comparable to those achieved with heparin.[77,78] However, glucocorticoids are associated with adverse effects that include gestational diabetes, weight gain, and premature rupture of membranes. Randomized trials have not demonstrated a benefit from the use of IVIG, when either added to heparin or used alone.[56,79,80]

Refractory Obstetric Antiphospholipid Syndrome

Experienced clinicians are likely to encounter patients with recurrent fetal death or extreme PTB due to severe preeclampsia or placental insufficiency despite treatment with low-dose aspirin and heparin. Such "refractory obstetric APS" cases are extremely challenging because little evidence is available to guide treatment. These women should be counseled regarding the potential

for grave maternal risks and the need for extremely premature delivery in subsequent pregnancies. One group reported a 60% rate of successful pregnancies in 18 women with refractory obstetric APS when prednisolone was added to standard low-dose aspirin and heparin treatment in the first trimester.[81] **Because inflammation appears to be a key component of aPL-related adverse pregnancy outcomes, modulators of excessive inflammation may be beneficial.** The authors are familiar with a handful of anecdotal reports of successful pregnancies using such agents as IVIG, HCQ, and etanercept (a tumor necrosis factor [TNF] inhibitor) in addition to low-dose aspirin and a heparin agent. Statin agents are being investigated for the prevention of recurrent preeclampsia, and therapy trials are currently underway (e.g., NCT01717586). Fluvastatin treatment reduces proinflammatory and prothrombotic biomarkers in persistently positive aPL patients.[82] Complement inhibitors such as eculizumab or pexelizumab may hold promise, but data are extremely limited, potential adverse effects exist, and such agents are costly.

Catastrophic Antiphospholipid Syndrome

The management of suspected or proven CAPS requires a multidisciplinary approach with hematologic and rheumatologic expertise. The optimal management of CAPS is not well defined. However, because the mortality rate is so high, aggressive empiric treatments are typically pursued that include anticoagulation with IV heparin, high-dose steroids, and plasma exchange. A full discussion of the management of CAPS is beyond the scope of this chapter.

Pregnancy Complications and Surveillance

In addition to the risk of fetal loss, women with definite APS are at significantly increased risk of developing preeclampsia and placental insufficiency. Case series of highly selected patients, many of whom had prior thrombosis or SLE, indicate that hypertensive disorders or placental insufficiency complicate 20% of pregnancies with APS and lead to a high rate of iatrogenic PTB.[77] In the prospective, observational PROMISSE study, 144 women with aPL, APS, or SLE and confirmed, repeatedly positive aPL were identified.[62] Despite contemporary management, usually with UFH or LMWH and low-dose aspirin, 19.4% of these women suffered an adverse obstetric outcome; among these, 8% suffered a fetal death after 12 weeks, and 8% required delivery prior to 34 weeks because of hypertensive disorders. Risks of adverse obstetric outcome were particularly elevated among women with repeatedly positive LAC, a history of SLE, or prior thrombosis. The NOH-APS study included 500 women with obstetric APS and excluded women with a history of thrombosis.[59] All were treated with low-dose aspirin and prophylactic LMWH. Overall, including miscarriages at less than 10 weeks' gestation, the live birth rate was just under 70%, similar to controls, but PTBs were observed in nearly 25% of APS cases (12% at less than 34 weeks' gestation). PTBs were largely the result of severe preeclampsia with or without IUGR. Among women with ongoing pregnancies at 20 weeks, 25% went on to suffer preeclampsia, IUGR, abruption, or a combination of these, compared with a rate of 17.5% in the controls.

The risk of APS-related pregnancy complications is dependent on the population in which the diagnosis of APS is made. Women who meet criteria for APS because of REM but who are otherwise healthy are not at high

risk of thrombosis, fetal death, preeclampsia, or placental insufficiency.[65-67] In the NOH-APS study, severe preeclampsia occurred in less than 3% of women with a diagnosis of APS based on REM.[59]

Serial ultrasounds to assess fetal growth and amniotic fluid volume are recommended in pregnancies complicated by APS. In pregnancies without evidence of maternal hypertension or fetal compromise, surveillance with nonstress tests or biophysical profiles should begin at 32 weeks. In the setting of suspected IUGR, hypertension, or thrombocytopenia, earlier institution of fetal surveillance is warranted.

RHEUMATOID ARTHRITIS

Rheumatoid arthritis (RA) is an autoimmune disease characterized by chronic, symmetric inflammatory arthritis of the synovial joints. RA affects 1% to 2% of U.S. adults, and as with SLE, RA is more common among females than males. Although the incidence of RA increases with age, it is still occasionally encountered among reproductive-aged women. A genetic susceptibility to RA is evidenced by the higher disease concordance among monozygotic twins compared with dizygotic twins (15% vs. 3.6%).[83] Also, relatives of individuals with RA are at increased risk for RA as well as for other connective tissue diseases. Several variant alleles of the *HLA-DRB1* gene appear to play primary roles in disease susceptibility.[84]

Clinical Manifestations

The onset of RA is often insidious, with the gradual development of symmetric peripheral polyarthritis and morning stiffness. Involvement of the metacarpophalangeal and proximal interphalangeal joints is characteristic, and significant deformity of these joints may become apparent as the disease progresses. Systemic symptoms occur commonly and include fatigue, weakness, weight loss, and malaise. Rheumatoid nodules develop in 20% to 30% of patients. These local proliferations of small vessels, fibroblasts, and histiocytes within the subcutaneous tissue occur most commonly on pressure points such as the extensor surfaces of the forearms; they may be painful and may interfere with joint and nerve function. Treatment involves local injections of glucocorticoids and an anesthetic and, in rare cases, surgical excision. A minority of patients with RA develop extraarticular manifestations that include pleuritis, pericarditis, neuropathy, vasculitis, scleritis, and renal disease.

Diagnosis

In 2010, the ACR, in collaboration with the European League Against Rheumatism, released revised classification criteria for RA (Table 46-4).[85] These new diagnostic criteria represent a shift in focus to the early features of RA that are most predictive of later erosive disease. **"Definite" RA is based on confirmed synovitis in at least one joint, absence of another cause for the synovitis, and a score of at least 6 out of 10 on a standardized assessment in four clinical domains: (1) degree of joint involvement; (2) serologic testing; (3) response from acute phase reactants; and (4) duration of symptoms.**

Seventy to eighty percent of patients with RA test positive for rheumatoid factor (RF) antibodies. RF immunoglobulins are produced from B cells stimulated by CD4+ T-cell cytokines. These CD4+ T cells are activated by unknown antigens and play a key role in the inflammatory damage seen in RA. **However, RF antibodies are somewhat nonspecific because 5% to 10%**

TABLE 46-4	2010 AMERICAN COLLEGE OF RHEUMATOLOGY/EUROPEAN LEAGUE AGAINST RHEUMATISM CLASSIFICATION CRITERIA FOR RHEUMATOID ARTHRITIS

TARGET POPULATION	SCORE
1. Patients with at least one joint with definite clinical synovitis (swelling)	
2. Patients with synovitis not better explained by another disease	

CLASSIFICATION CRITERIA

(Score-based algorithm: Add score of categories A through D; a score of 6 out of 10 or greater is needed for classification of definite RA)

A. **Joint involvement**	
1 large joint	0
2 to 10 large joints	1
1 to 3 small joints (with or without involvement of large joints)	2
4 to 10 small joints (with or without involvement of large joints)	3
More than 10 joints (at least one small joint)	5
B. **Serology** (at least one test result is needed for classification)	
Negative RF *and* negative ACPA	0
Low-positive RF *or* low-positive ACPA	2
High-positive RF *or* high-positive ACPA	3
C. **Acute-phase reactants** (at least one test result is needed for classification)	
Normal CRP *and* normal ESR 0	0
Abnormal CRP *or* normal ESR 1	1
D. **Duration of symptoms**	
Less than 6 weeks	0
At least 6 weeks	1

Modified from Aletaha D, Neogi T, Silman AJ, et al. 2010 Rheumatoid arthritis classification criteria: an American College of Rheumatology/European League Against Rheumatism collaborative initiative. *Arthritis Rheum.* 2010;62:2569-2581.
ACPA, anticitrullinated protein antibody; *CRP,* C-reactive protein; *ESR,* erythrocyte sedimentation rate; *RA,* rheumatoid arthritis; *RF,* rheumatoid factor.

of the general, healthy population will test positive for RF. Furthermore, RF may be detected in the setting of certain viral infections and in other autoimmune conditions such as SLE and Sjögren syndrome. Antibodies to citrullinated peptides/proteins (ACPAs) have better specificity for RA and sensitivity similar to that of RF. The laboratory evaluation for RA also includes testing of acute phase reactants such as C-reactive protein (CRP) and erythrocyte sedimentation rate (ESR). Elevations in CRP and ESR suggest an aberrant inflammatory response. Patients with RA frequently also have anemia, thrombocytosis, leukocytosis, and a positive antinuclear antibody (ANA).

Pregnancy Considerations

The majority of women, perhaps as many as 80% to 90%, experience some improvement in their RA symptoms during pregnancy, although only approximately 50% have more than moderate improvement. Improvements in joint pain and stiffness generally begin in the first trimester and persist through several weeks postpartum. Women who experience symptom improvement in one pregnancy will usually observe similar improvements in subsequent pregnancies. **Most women who experience an improvement in symptoms during pregnancy will relapse postpartum, typically in the first 3 months. It does not appear that pregnancy has any significant effects on the long-term course of RA.**

RA patients have been shown to have functionally defective regulatory T cells (T$_{REGS}$), critical inhibitors of autoimmunity that suppress CD4+ and CD8+ T-cell cytokine production and B-cell immunoglobulin production. The generally favorable course of RA in pregnancy may be related to the normal increase in circulating T_{REGS} that occurs during pregnancy. Hormonal changes may also modulate RA disease activity. Many women experience improvement in RA symptoms during the luteal phase of the menstrual cycle, when progesterone levels are highest.

Not only do RA symptoms usually improve during pregnancy, but RA disease activity does not appear to significantly impact pregnancy outcomes. Women with RA typically have uneventful pregnancies without increased risks for PTB, preeclampsia, or IUGR. Certain antirheumatic medications, however, are associated with increased pregnancy risks. **Disease activity and medication use should ideally be assessed during a preconceptional visit.**

Antirheumatic Drugs
Drugs With Acceptable Risk Profiles in Pregnancy
The use of NSAIDs, glucocorticoids, and HCQ in pregnancy were discussed in the section on SLE.

SULFASALAZINE
Sulfasalazine (FDA category B) is a combination of a sulfa antibiotic and salicylate. Most of the data regarding safety in pregnancy come from women with inflammatory bowel disease. Although sulfasalazine and its metabolite sulfapyridine cross the placenta, large studies have not found an increase in congenital malformations with use in pregnancy.[86] Because sulfasalazine acts as a dihydrofolate reductase inhibitor, it is recommended that women considering pregnancy take at least 0.4 mg of folic acid daily. **Sulfasalazine is compatible with breastfeeding.**

Drugs with Uncertain or Higher Risk Profiles in Pregnancy
TUMOR NECROSIS FACTOR-α INHIBITORS
Several TNF inhibitors (all FDA category B) are used for the long-term control of RA. These include infliximab, etanercept, adalimumab, certolizumab, and golimumab. Inhibition of TNF-α increases circulating T_{REG} cells and restores their capacity to inhibit cytokine production. All of the TNF inhibitors except certolizumab are transferred across the placenta. Animal studies of infliximab, adalimumab, and certolizumab have not demonstrated an increase in congenital anomalies. An association between TNF inhibitors and fetal vertebral anomalies, anal atresia, cardiac defects, tracheoesophageal fistula, esophageal atresia, renal anomalies, and limb dysplasia (VACTERL) syndrome has been reported,[87] but a subsequent study from a European congenital malformation database did not confirm these findings.[88] Indeed, published experience with hundreds of pregnancies exposed to TNF inhibitors suggests that these agents are not teratogenic and are not associated with adverse pregnancy outcomes. Proceedings of the ACR Reproductive Health Summit stated that **although human data are somewhat limited, "TNF inhibitors are considered to be compatible with pregnancy."** Some providers recommend avoiding TNF inhibitors in the third trimester in order to limit early postnatal exposure, but this should be weighed against the risk of an increase in disease activity without treatment. Small amounts of etanercept, infliximab, and adalimumab have been reported in breast milk, although it is uncertain whether this poses a risk to the neonate. **The choice to breastfeed while taking TNF inhibitors should be made after a thorough discussion of potential risks and benefits.**

BIOLOGIC AGENTS
This continually expanding class of agents includes anakinra (interleukin-1 receptor antagonist, FDA category B), rituximab (chimeric monoclonal antibody leading to B-cell depletion, FDA category C), abatacept (inhibitor of T-cell co-stimulation, FDA category C), and tocilizumab (interleukin-6 receptor inhibitor, FDA category C). **These drugs may be used to treat autoimmune disease not sufficiently controlled with traditional therapies, but data regarding the use of these medications in pregnancy are extremely limited.** Case reports in humans generally suggest little fetal risk.[89-91] According to the manufacturer, when given to monkeys during organogenesis, tocilizumab caused abortion (embryo or fetal death) at doses just above those used in humans. Rituximab treatment later in pregnancy can cause B-cell lymphocytopenia in the neonate that persists for several months.[92] Given the overall relatively limited experience with these medications in pregnancy, **it is prudent to avoid their use unless the woman is refractory to other therapies and the severity of disease warrants continuation.** Likewise, the safety of breastfeeding while taking these medications is unknown. **Patients who choose to breastfeed should do so only after a thorough discussion of potential risks and benefits.**

Drugs Contraindicated in Pregnancy
METHOTREXATE
Methotrexate (MTX, FDA category X) is a folate antagonist used for long-term, maintenance immunosuppression in patients with autoimmune conditions, including SLE and RA. **MTX is an abortifacient in early pregnancy and a potent teratogen** associated with craniofacial anomalies, neural tube defects, abnormal facies, and neurodevelopmental delay. The greatest risks are with exposure prior to 10 weeks, with one study reporting a 9% rate of congenital anomalies and a 25% risk of miscarriage.[45] The drug is widely distributed in maternal tissues and may persist for up to 4 months in the liver. **All reproductive-aged women taking MTX should be warned of its teratogenic risks and advised to remain on effective contraception.** For those considering pregnancy, conception should be delayed for at least three menstrual cycles after discontinuation of MTX. *MTX is found in low levels in breastmilk and is considered contraindicated in breastfeeding.*

LEFLUNOMIDE
Some patients with RA are treated with leflunomide, an FDA category X disease-modifying antirheumatic drug (DMARD). Leflunomide is sometimes also used to treat lupus-related skin manifestations. The drug's mechanism of action is inhibition of dihydroorotate dehydrogenase, an enzyme necessary for pyrimidine biosynthesis. *Leflunomide is teratogenic in humans and is absolutely contraindicated in pregnancy.* In a recent report, 2 of 16 exposed offspring had major anomalies and 3 had minor anomalies.[93] The major metabolite (teriflunomide) is detectable in the serum of patients for up to 2 years after discontinuation of the drug. Patients on leflunomide should be counseled to avoid pregnancy until serum drug levels are less than 0.02 mg/L on two tests performed 2 weeks apart. This may take up to 2 years. Drug elimination can be hastened by administering cholestyramine (8 g orally three times daily for 11 days) with follow-up of serum drug levels to assure elimination. **No data are available regarding leflunomide and breastfeeding, and it is considered contraindicated.**

Management of Pregnancies Complicated by Rheumatoid Arthritis

Because the majority of women with RA have improvement in their disease during pregnancy, many can discontinue their antirheumatic drugs. **Mild to moderate joint pain can usually be managed with acetaminophen or low-dose glucocorticoids.** Physical therapy may be helpful in some cases. **No alterations to routine prenatal care are necessary for women with mild, uncomplicated RA.** Routine serial ultrasounds to assess fetal growth and antenatal testing are unnecessary. **Because the risk of postpartum disease exacerbation is high, it is important to assess symptoms at postpartum visits and to arrange appropriate follow-up with rheumatology.** Some experts recommend reinitiating antirheumatic drug treatment after delivery in all women with RA, regardless of disease activity.

SYSTEMIC SCLEROSIS

Systemic sclerosis (SSc), or systemic scleroderma, is a heterogeneous autoimmune disorder characterized by small vessel vasculopathy, the presence of characteristic autoantibodies, and fibroblast dysfunction that leads to increased extracellular matrix deposition and progressive fibrosis of the skin and visceral tissues. The small vessel vasculopathy manifests most commonly as Raynaud phenomenon and in severe cases as renal crisis. SSc is rare and occurs in only 1 to 2 per 100,000 individuals in the United States annually. Similar to other autoimmune disorders, it is more common in women than in men. But in contrast to SLE, **SSc is infrequently encountered in pregnancy because the peak age of onset is in the fifth decade.**

Clinical Manifestations

Early symptoms of SSc include subcutaneous swelling with muscle and joint pain, and more than 90% of patients will experience Raynaud phenomenon. When combined with skin thickening, Raynaud phenomenon is specific for SSc; however, the phenomenon also occurs in 5% of the general population, and thus will frequently be seen by obstetricians.

Two main subsets of SSc have been recognized: *diffuse cutaneous SSc* usually involves cutaneous fibrosis of the forearms and is associated with a greater risk for serious internal organ manifestations such as renal crisis, pulmonary fibrosis, and myocardial fibrosis; *limited cutaneous SSc* involves fibrosis of the distal extremities and face and is associated with digital ulcerations. CREST syndrome—calcinosis of the skin, Raynaud phenomenon, esophageal dysmotility, sclerodactyly, and telangiectasias— falls under this latter category.

The most frequent visceral symptoms of SSc are heartburn and dysphagia related to esophageal dysmotility. Involvement of the lower gastrointestinal tract can lead to malabsorption, diarrhea, and constipation. Cardiopulmonary manifestations (i.e., pulmonary hypertension, cardiac arrhythmias) are of particular concern in pregnancy.

Renal involvement is usually mild, but 10% to 20% of patients with diffuse disease will develop renal crisis, which manifests as acute onset of severe hypertension, progressive renal insufficiency, and hemolytic anemia. Renal crisis results in progression to end-stage renal disease in a significant proportion of affected individuals and is a major cause of mortality in SSc patients.

Diagnosis

The ACR and European League Against Rheumatism released classification criteria for SSc in 2013.[94] These criteria were primarily designed to identify SSc patients for inclusion in studies. Because significant clinical heterogeneity exists among SSc patients, it should be noted that some individuals might not meet these strict diagnostic criteria. According to these criteria, **the presence of skin thickening of the fingers extending proximal to the metacarpophalangeal joints is sufficient for the diagnosis of SSc.** The diagnosis is supported by visceral organ involvement and the presence of certain autoantibodies. **Most patients with SSc have a positive ANA.** Antitopoisomerase I, anticentromere, and anti-RNA polymerase III antibodies are highly specific for SSc but have only moderate sensitivity.[95] Individuals with SSc may also be positive for aPL.

Pregnancy Considerations

Because pregnancy in women with SSc is uncommon, relatively few data are available regarding the impact of pregnancy on the disease and the risk of pregnancy complications. **If SSc is clinically stable at the onset of pregnancy and the woman is without obvious renal, cardiac, or pulmonary disease, maternal outcomes are generally good.** Raynaud phenomenon may improve in pregnancy related to greater vasodilation, although gastrointestinal manifestations related to esophageal dysmotility may become more prominent. The risk for renal crisis during pregnancy is probably not increased for women without preexisting kidney disease, but distinguishing this complication from preeclampsia may be challenging. In the case of renal crisis, the urine sediment is either normal or shows only mild proteinuria with few cells or casts. **Hemolytic-uremic syndrome** can also have a similar presentation to SSc renal crisis and should be part of the differential diagnosis, particularly in postpartum patients. Some authors have reported that women with SSc have an increased risk of spontaneous abortion both before and after their diagnosis.[96,97] Other studies have not confirmed these findings,[98] although women with late, diffuse SSc probably do have a higher rate of miscarriage.[98]

PTB is more common among women with SSc, particularly those with diffuse disease.[98] The risks for preeclampsia and IUGR are threefold higher among women with SSc when compared with the general population, likely related to the vascular pathology of the disease and frequent renal involvement.[99] One of the largest published series found that pregnancies in women with SSc, compared with the general obstetric population, were significantly more likely to complicated by PTB (25% vs. 12%) and IUGR (6% vs. 1%).[100] Indeed, PTBs among women with SSc are usually indicated, rather than spontaneous, due to hypertensive complications and IUGR.

Management of Pregnancies Complicated by Systemic Sclerosis

Preconceptional counseling is critical for women with SSc. Those with diffuse, progressive disease and significant cardiac, pulmonary, or renal involvement are at particularly high risk for adverse maternal and fetal outcomes. **Women should be evaluated for pulmonary hypertension, which is a contraindication to pregnancy.** Active renal disease increases the risk for crisis during pregnancy with the accompanying risks of end-stage renal disease and mortality.

Even among nonpregnant individuals, the treatment of SSc is challenging and noncurative. Treatment of diffuse disease is typically organ specific. Symptomatic relief of arthralgias and myalgias should be limited to acetaminophen or low-dose glucocorticoids if possible. Ultraviolet light therapy, topical glucocorticoids, and vitamin D analogues may be used to treat cutaneous manifestations. Many women take proton pump inhibitors (FDA category C) for upper gastrointestinal symptoms, and they can be continued in pregnancy because data do not suggest significant fetal risks. Raynaud phenomenon is often treated with oral vasodilators, in particular calcium channel blockers (CCBs). Although definitive proof of fetal safety is lacking, CCBs are FDA category C drugs and are probably safe to continue in pregnancy. Avoidance of cold, stress, nicotine, caffeine, and sympathomimetic decongestants may also improve Raynaud symptoms.

Renal crisis is specifically treated with angiotensin-converting enzyme (ACE) inhibitors. Although these agents are usually contraindicated in pregnancy because of risks of teratogenicity and effects on fetal renal function, **SSc renal crisis carries such a high risk of morbidity and mortality that the use of an ACE inhibitor in pregnancy may be justified in this specific circumstance.** In patients with renal crisis, intensive care admission with continuous fetal monitoring may be indicated. Many patients will also require dialysis. Decisions regarding delivery should be guided by maternal stability and prognosis, gestational age, and results of fetal monitoring.

No evidence-based guidelines have been established for prenatal care in women with SSc. Clinicians should have a low threshold to investigate any new and unusual symptoms, especially as they might relate to visceral organ involvement. **Particular attention should be paid to those women with diffuse disease, and an increase in the frequency of prenatal visits to every 1 to 2 weeks is prudent.** Women should be closely monitored for preeclampsia because SSc appears to increase this risk. Serial ultrasounds after 18 to 20 weeks to assess fetal growth and antenatal testing at 30 to 32 weeks are also reasonable.

Delivery among women with advanced skin disease may be complicated by poor wound healing. Some women will be at increased anesthetic risk because of problems with IV access, difficult intubation, and increased risk for aspiration. **Among those with diffuse and severe disease, a multidisciplinary approach with rheumatology, anesthesiology, and even nephrology, cardiology, or pulmonology** (depending on the specific organs involved) **is recommended. Intensive care management may even be necessary in some cases.**

SJÖGREN SYNDROME

Sjögren syndrome (SS) is a chronic autoimmune disorder characterized by decreased lacrimal and salivary gland function, which leads to dry eyes and dry mouth. Extraglandular manifestations commonly include fatigue, arthralgias, myalgias, and Raynaud phenomenon. Less common extraglandular manifestations include interstitial lung disease, dysphagia, liver function abnormalities, nephritis, central and/or peripheral nervous system manifestations, and an increased risk for lymphoma in the long term. SS occurs in a primary form and in a secondary form associated with other autoimmune conditions, primarily SLE and RA. **Pregnancy outcomes among women with SS are similar to those without the disease. However, women with SS may be positive for anti-Ro/SSA antibodies, with the accompanying risks for NLE and CHB.**

KEY POINTS

- ◆ SLE is the most common serious autoimmune disease that affects women of reproductive age.
- ◆ SLE disease activity at the onset of pregnancy is the most important determinant of the course of the disease in pregnancy.
- ◆ Women with SLE should be counseled to postpone pregnancy until a sustained remission for at least 6 months has been achieved.
- ◆ For women with lupus nephritis, moderate renal insufficiency (serum creatinine 1.5 to 2 mg/dL) is a relative contraindication to pregnancy, and advanced renal insufficiency (creatinine >2 mg/dL) should be considered an absolute contraindication to pregnancy.
- ◆ The risk for NLE, and in particular CHB, in fetuses or neonates of women with SLE is low. The highest-risk group for CHB is seen in women with anti-Ro/SSA or anti-La/SSB antibodies and a prior affected child (15% to 20% recurrence).
- ◆ Women with SLE who become pregnant on hydroxychloroquine should generally continue this medication because it may decrease the risk of disease flares.
- ◆ The diagnosis of APS is incumbent upon either arterial or venous thrombosis or obstetric morbidity and repeatedly positive testing for lupus anticoagulant and/or medium to high titers of anticardiolipin or anti-B2–glycoprotein I IgG or IgM antibodies.
- ◆ All women with APS and prior thrombosis should receive full anticoagulation during pregnancy and postpartum.
- ◆ Pregnant women with an APS diagnosis based upon recurrent early miscarriage without prior thrombosis should receive either low-dose aspirin alone or combined with a prophylactic dose of heparin.
- ◆ Pregnant women with an APS diagnosis based upon fetal death, early preeclampsia, or placental insufficiency and without prior thrombosis should generally receive low-dose aspirin combined with prophylactic heparin.
- ◆ Most women with rheumatoid arthritis will experience an improvement in symptoms during pregnancy, but the risk for postpartum relapse is high.
- ◆ Women with systemic sclerosis generally have favorable pregnancy outcomes but should be carefully assessed for visceral organ (i.e., renal, cardiac, or pulmonary) involvement.

REFERENCES

1. Chakravarty EF, Bush TM, Manzi S, Clarke AE, Ward MM. Prevalence of adult systemic lupus erythematosus in California and Pennsylvania in 2000: estimates obtained using hospitalization data. *Arthritis Rheum.* 2007;56:2092-2094.
2. Moser KL, Kelly JA, Lessard CJ, Harley JB. Recent insights into the genetic basis of systemic lupus erythematosus. *Genes Immun.* 2009;10:373-379.
3. Costenbader KH, Gay S, Alarcon-Riquelme ME, Iaccarino L, Doria A. Genes, epigenetic regulation and environmental factors: which is the most relevant in developing autoimmune diseases? *Autoimmun Rev.* 2012;11:604-609.

4. Costenbader KH, Feskanich D, Stampfer MJ, Karlson EW. Reproductive and menopausal factors and risk of systemic lupus erythematosus in women. *Arthritis Rheum.* 2007;56:1251-1262.

5. Lockshin MD. Pregnancy does not cause systemic lupus erythematosus to worsen. *Arthritis Rheum.* 1989;32:665-670.

6. Urowitz MB, Gladman DD, Farewell VT, Stewart J, McDonald J. Lupus and pregnancy studies. *Arthritis Rheum.* 1993;36:1392-1397.

7. Petri M, Howard D, Repke J. Frequency of lupus flare in pregnancy. The Hopkins Lupus Pregnancy Center experience. *Arthritis Rheum.* 1991;34:1538-1545.

8. Hayslett JP. Maternal and fetal complications in pregnant women with systemic lupus erythematosus. *Am J Kidney Dis.* 1991;17:123-126.

9. Clowse ME, Magder LS, Petri M. The clinical utility of measuring complement and anti-dsDNA antibodies during pregnancy in patients with systemic lupus erythematosus. *J Rheumatol.* 2011;38:1012-1016.

10. Weening JJ, D'Agati VD, Schwartz MM, et al. The classification of glomerulonephritis in systemic lupus erythematosus revisited. *J Am Soc Nephrol.* 2004;15:241-250.

11. Smyth A, Oliveira GH, Lahr BD, Bailey KR, Norby SM, Garovic VD. A systematic review and meta-analysis of pregnancy outcomes in patients with systemic lupus erythematosus and lupus nephritis. *Clin J Am Soc Nephrol.* 2010;5:2060-2068.

12. Jungers P, Dougados M, Pelissier C, et al. Lupus nephropathy and pregnancy: report of 104 cases in 36 patients. *Arch Intern Med.* 1982;142:771-776.

13. Moroni G, Quaglini S, Banfi G, et al. Pregnancy in lupus nephritis. *Am J Kidney Dis.* 2002;40:713-720.

14. Mellembakken JR, Hogasen K, Mollnes TE, Hack CE, Abyholm T, Videm V. Increased systemic activation of neutrophils but not complement in preeclampsia. *Obstet Gynecol.* 2001;97:371-374.

15. Fischer-Betz R, Specker C, Brinks R, Aringer M, Schneider M. Low risk of renal flares and negative outcomes in women with lupus nephritis conceiving after switching from mycophenolate mofetil to azathioprine. *Rheumatology.* 2013;52(6):1070-1076.

16. Georgiou PE, Politi EN, Katsimbri P, Sakka V, Drosos AA. Outcome of lupus pregnancy: a controlled study. *Rheumatology.* 2000;39:1014-1019.

17. Buyon JP, Kim M, Guerra M, et al. Predictors of pregnancy outcome in a prospective, multiethnic cohort of lupus patients. *Ann Intern Med.* 2015;163:153-163.

18. Clowse ME, Magder LS, Witter F, Petri M. The impact of increased lupus activity on obstetric outcomes. *Arthritis Rheum.* 2005;52:514-521.

19. Clowse ME, Magder LS, Witter F, Petri M. Early risk factors for pregnancy loss in lupus. *Obstet Gynecol.* 2006;107:293-299.

20. Agaarwal N, Sawhney H, Vasishta K, et al. Pregnancy in patients with systemic lupus erythematosus. *Aust N Z J Obstet Gynaecol.* 1999;39:28-30.

21. Clowse ME, Jamison M, Myers E, James AH. A national study of the complications of lupus in pregnancy. *Am J Obstet Gynecol.* 2008;199:127 e121-127 e126.

22. Clark CA, Spitzer KA, Laskin CA. Decrease in pregnancy loss rates in patients with systemic lupus erythematosus over a 40-year period. *J Rheumatol.* 2005;32:1709-1712.

23. Nossent HC, Swaak TJ. Systemic lupus erythematosus. VI. Analysis of the interrelationship with pregnancy. *J Rheumatol.* 1990;17:771-776.

24. Bramham K, Hunt BJ, Bewley S, et al. Pregnancy outcomes in systemic lupus erythematosus with and without previous nephritis. *J Rheumatol.* 2011;38:1906-1913.

25. Schramm AM, Clowse ME. Aspirin for prevention of preeclampsia in lupus pregnancy. *Autoimmune Dis.* 2014;2014:920467.

26. Buyon JP, Clancy RM, Friedman DM. Autoimmune associated congenital heart block: integration of clinical and research clues in the management of the maternal / foetal dyad at risk. *J Intern Med.* 2009;265:653-662.

27. Meisgen S, Ostberg T, Salomonsson S, et al. The HLA locus contains novel foetal susceptibility alleles for congenital heart block with significant paternal influence. *J Intern Med.* 2014;275(6):640-651.

28. Buyon JP, Hiebert R, Copel J, et al. Autoimmune-associated congenital heart block: demographics, mortality, morbidity and recurrence rates obtained from a national neonatal lupus registry. *J Am Coll Cardiol.* 1998;31:1658-1666.

29. Jaeggi ET, Hamilton RM, Silverman ED, Zamora SA, Hornberger LK. Outcome of children with fetal, neonatal or childhood diagnosis of isolated congenital atrioventricular block. A single institution's experience of 30 years. *J Am Coll Cardiol.* 2002;39:130-137.

30. Izmirly PM, Saxena A, Kim MY, et al. Maternal and fetal factors associated with mortality and morbidity in a multi-racial/ethnic registry of anti-SSA/Ro-associated cardiac neonatal lupus. *Circulation.* 2011;124(18):1927-1935.

31. Friedman DM, Kim MY, Copel JA, Llanos C, Davis C, Buyon JP. Prospective evaluation of fetuses with autoimmune-associated congenital heart block followed in the PR Interval and Dexamethasone Evaluation (PRIDE) Study. *Am J Cardiol.* 2009;103:1102-1106.

32. Jaeggi ET, Fouron JC, Silverman ED, Ryan G, Smallhorn J, Hornberger LK. Transplacental fetal treatment improves the outcome of prenatally diagnosed complete atrioventricular block without structural heart disease. *Circulation.* 2004;110:1542-1548.

33. Saleeb S, Copel J, Friedman D, Buyon JP. Comparison of treatment with fluorinated glucocorticoids to the natural history of autoantibody-associated congenital heart block: retrospective review of the research registry for neonatal lupus. *Arthritis Rheum.* 1999;42:2335-2345.

34. Eliasson H, Sonesson SE, Sharland G, et al. Isolated atrioventricular block in the fetus: a retrospective, multinational, multicenter study of 175 patients. *Circulation.* 2011;124:1919-1926.

35. Pisoni CN, Brucato A, Ruffatti A, et al. Failure of intravenous immunoglobulin to prevent congenital heart block: Findings of a multicenter, prospective, observational study. *Arthritis Rheum.* 2010;62:1147-1152.

36. Friedman DM, Llanos C, Izmirly PM, et al. Evaluation of fetuses in a study of intravenous immunoglobulin as preventive therapy for congenital heart block: Results of a multicenter, prospective, open-label clinical trial. *Arthritis Rheum.* 2010;62:1138-1146.

37. Izmirly PM, Kim MY, Llanos C, et al. Evaluation of the risk of anti-SSA/Ro-SSB/La antibody-associated cardiac manifestations of neonatal lupus in fetuses of mothers with systemic lupus erythematosus exposed to hydroxychloroquine. *Ann Rheum Dis.* 2010;69:1827-1830.

38. Izmirly PM, Costedoat-Chalumeau N, Pisoni CN, et al. Maternal use of hydroxychloroquine is associated with a reduced risk of recurrent anti-SSA/Ro-antibody-associated cardiac manifestations of neonatal lupus. *Circulation.* 2012;126:76-82.

39. Costedoat-Chalumeau N, Amoura Z, Duhaut P, et al. Safety of hydroxychloroquine in pregnant patients with connective tissue diseases: a study of one hundred thirty-three cases compared with a control group. *Arthritis Rheum.* 2003;48:3207-3211.

40. Tunks RD, Clowse ME, Miller SG, Brancazio LR, Barker PC. Maternal autoantibody levels in congenital heart block and potential prophylaxis with anti-inflammatory agents. *Am J Obstet Gynecol.* 2013;208(1):64e1-64e7.

41. Diav-Citrin O, Blyakhman S, Shechtman S, Ornoy A. Pregnancy outcome following in utero exposure to hydroxychloroquine: a prospective comparative observational study. *Reprod Toxicol.* 2013;39:58-62.

42. Clowse ME, Magder L, Witter F, Petri M. Hydroxychloroquine in lupus pregnancy. *Arthritis Rheum.* 2006;54:3640-3647.

43. Carmichael SL, Shaw GM, Ma C, et al. Maternal corticosteroid use and orofacial clefts. *Am J Obstet Gynecol.* 2007;197:585e1-585e7.

44. Bay Bjørn AM, Ehrenstein V, Hundborg HH, Nohr EA, Sørenson HT, Nørgaard M. Use of corticosteroids in early pregnancy is not associated with risk of oral clefts and other congenital malformations in offspring. *Am J Ther.* 2014;21:73-80.

45. Ostensen M, Khamashta M, Lockshin M, et al. Anti-inflammatory and immunosuppressive drugs and reproduction. *Arthritis Res Ther.* 2006;8:209.

46. Kozer E, Nikfar S, Costei A, Boskovic R, Nulman I, Koren G. Aspirin consumption during the first trimester of pregnancy and congenital anomalies: a meta-analysis. *Am J Obstet Gynecol.* 2002;187:1623-1630.

47. Nezvalova-Henriksen K, Spigset O, Nordeng H. Effects of ibuprofen, diclofenac, naproxen, and piroxicam on the course of pregnancy and pregnancy outcome: a prospective cohort study. *Br J Obstet Gynaecol.* 2013;120:948-959.

48. Askie LM, Duley L, Henderson-Smart DJ, Stewart LA, PARIS Collaborative Group. Antiplatelet agents for prevention of pre-eclampsia: a meta-analysis of individual patient data. *Lancet.* 2007;369:1791-1798.

49. Goldstein LH, Dolinsky G, Greenberg R, et al. Pregnancy outcome of women exposed to azathioprine during pregnancy. *Birth Defects Res A Clin Mol Teratol.* 2007;79:696-701.

50. Miyakis S, Lockshin MD, Atsumi T, et al. International consensus statement on an update of the classification criteria for definite antiphospholipid syndrome (APS). *J Thromb Haemost.* 2006;4:295-306.

51. Lockwood CJ, Romero R, Feinberg RF, Clyne LP, Coster B, Hobbins JC. The prevalence and biologic significance of lupus anticoagulant and

anticardiolipin antibodies in a general obstetric population. *Am J Obstet Gynecol.* 1989;161:369-373.

52. Branch DW, Gibson M, Silver RM. Clinical practice. Recurrent miscarriage. *N Engl J Med.* 2010;28(363):1740-1747.

53. Andreoli L, Chighizola CB, Banzato A, Pons-Estel GJ, Ramire de Jesus G, Erkan D. Estimated frequency of antiphospholipid antibodies in patients with pregnancy morbidity, stroke, myocardial infarction, and deep vein thrombosis: a critical review of the literature. *Arthritis Care Res (Hoboken).* 2013;65:1869-1873.

54. Bushnell CD, Goldstein LB. Diagnostic testing for coagulopathies in patients with ischemic stroke. *Stroke.* 2000;31:3067-3078.

55. Clark CA, Laskin CA, Spitzer KA. Anticardiolipin antibodies and recurrent early pregnancy loss: a century of equivocal evidence. *Hum Reprod Update.* 2012;18:474-484.

56. Triolo G, Ferrante A, Ciccia F, et al. Randomized study of subcutaneous low molecular weight heparin plus aspirin versus intravenous immunoglobulin in the treatment of recurrent fetal loss associated with antiphospholipid antibodies. *Arthritis Rheum.* 2003;48:728-731.

57. de Jesus GR, Agmon-Levin N, Andrade CA, et al. 14th International Congress on Antiphospholipid Antibodies: Task Force Report on Obstetric Antiphospholipid Syndrome. *Autoimmun Rev.* 2014;13(8):795-813.

58. Silver RM, Parker CB, Reddy UM, et al. Antiphospholipid antibodies in stillbirth. *Obstet Gynecol.* 2013;122:1-18.

59. Bouvier S, Cochery-Nouvellon E, Lavigne-Lissalde G, et al. Comparative incidence of pregnancy outcomes in treated obstetric antiphospholipid syndrome: the NOH-APS observational study. *Blood.* 2014;123:404-413.

60. Lee RM, Brown MA, Branch DW, Ward K, Silver RM. Anticardiolipin and antibeta2-glycoprotein-I antibodies in preeclampsia. *Obstet Gynecol.* 2003;102(2):294-300.

61. Cerevera R, Piette UC, Font J, et al. Antiphospholipid syndrome. Clinical and immunologic manifestations and patterns of disease expression in a cohort of 1,000 patients. *Arthritis Rheum.* 2002;46:1019-1027.

62. Lockshin MD, Kim M, Laskin CA, et al. Prediction of adverse pregnancy outcome by the presence of lupus anticoagulant, but not anticardiolipin antibody, in patients with antiphospholipid antibodies. *Arthritis Rheum.* 2012;64:2311-2318.

63. Pengo V, Ruffatti A, Legnani C, et al. Incidence of a first thromboembolic event in asymptomatic carriers of high-risk antiphospholipid antibody profile: a multicenter prospective study. *Blood.* 2001;118:4714-4718.

64. Asherson R, Cervera R, de Groot P, et al. Catastrophic antiphospholipid syndrome: international consensus statement on classification criteria and treatment guidelines. *Lupus.* 2003;12:530-534.

65. Kutteh WH. Antiphospholipid antibody-associated recurrent pregnancy loss: treatment with heparin and low-dose aspirin is superior to low-dose aspirin alone. *Am J Obstet Gynecol.* 1996;174:1584-1589.

66. Rai R, Cohen H, Dave M, et al. Randomised controlled trial of aspirin and aspirin plus heparin in pregnant women with recurrent miscarriage associated with phospholipid antibodies (or antiphospholipid antibodies). *Br Med J.* 1997;314:253-257.

67. Farquharson RG, Quenby S, Greaves M. Antiphospholipid syndrome in pregnancy: a randomized, controlled trial of treatment. *Obstet Gynecol.* 2002;100:408-413.

68. Laskin CA, Spitzer KA, Clark CA, et al. Low molecular weight heparin and aspirin for recurrent pregnancy loss: results from the randomized, controlled Hep/ASA trial. *J Rheumatol.* 2009;36:279-287.

69. Stephenson MD, Ballem PJ, Tsang P, et al. Treatment of antiphospholipid antibody syndrome (APS) in pregnancy: a randomized pilot trial comparing low molecular weight heparin to unfractionated heparin. *J Obstet Gynaecol Can.* 2004;26:729-734.

70. Noble LS, Kutteh WH, Lashey N, et al. Antiphospholipid antibodies associated with recurrent pregnancy loss: prospective, multicenter, controlled pilot study comparing treatment with low-molecular-weight heparin versus unfractionated heparin. *Fertil Steril.* 2005;83:684-690.

71. Silver R, MacGregor SN, Sholl JS, Hobart JM, Neerhof MG, Ragin A. Comparative trial of prednisone plus aspirin versus aspirin alone in the treatment of anticardiolipin antibody-positive obstetric patients. *Am J Obstet Gynecol.* 1993;169:1411-1417.

72. Pattison NS, Chamley LW, Birdsall M, Zanderigo AM, Liddel HS, McDougall J. Does aspirin have a role in improving pregnancy outcome for women with the antiphospholipid syndrome? A randomized controlled trial. *Am J Obstet Gynecol.* 2000;183:1008-1012.

73. Empson MB, Lassere M, Craig JC, Scott JR. Prevention of recurrent miscarriage for women with antiphospholipid antibody or lupus anticoagulant. *Cochrane Database Syst Rev.* 2005;(2):Art. No.CD002859.

74. Bates SM, Greer IA, Middeldorp S, Veenstra DL, Prabulos AM, Vandvik PO, et al. VTE, thrombophilia, antithrombotic therapy, and pregnancy. Antithrombotic Therapy and Prevention of Thrombosis, 9th ed: American College of Chest Physicians Evidence-Based Clinical Practice Guidelines. *Chest.* 2012;141(2 suppl):e691S-e736S.

75. Antiphospholipid syndrome. Practice Bulletin No. 132. American College of Obstetricians and Gynecologists. *Obstet Gynecol.* 2012;120:1514-1521.

76. Arnaud L, Mathian A, Ruffatti A, et al. Efficacy of aspirin for the primary prevention of thrombosis in patients with antiphospholipid antibodies: An international and collaborative meta-analysis. *Autoimmun Rev.* 2014;13:281-291.

77. Branch DW, Silver RM, Blackwell JL, Reading JC, Scott JR. Outcome of treated pregnancies in women with antiphospholipid syndrome: an update of the Utah experience. *Obstet Gynecol.* 1992;80:614-620.

78. Cowchock FS, Reece EA, Balaban D, Branch DW, Plouffe L. Repeated fetal losses associated with antiphospholipid antibodies: a collaborative randomized trial comparing prednisone with low-dose heparin treatment. *Am J Obstet Gynecol.* 1992;166:1318-1323.

79. Branch DW, Peaceman AM, Druzin M, et al. A multicenter, placebo-controlled pilot study of intravenous immune globulin treatment of antiphospholipid syndrome during pregnancy. The Pregnancy Loss Study Group. *Am J Obstet Gynecol.* 2000;182:122-127.

80. Vaquero E, Lazzarin N, Valensise H, et al. Pregnancy outcome in recurrent spontaneous abortion associated with antiphospholipid antibodies: a comparative study of intravenous immunoglobulin versus prednisone plus low-dose aspirin. *Am J Reprod Immunol.* 2001;45:174-179.

81. Bramham K, Thomas M, Nelson-Piercy C, Khamashta M, Hunt B. First-trimester low-dose prednisolone in refractory antiphospholipid antibody-related pregnancy loss. *Blood.* 2011;117:6948-6951.

82. Erkan D, Willis R, Murthy VL, et al. A prospective open-label pilot study of fluvastatin on proinflammatory and prothrombotic biomarkers in antiphospholipid antibody positive patients. *Ann Rheum Dis.* 2014;73:1176-1180.

83. Silman AJ, MacGregor AJ, Thomson W, et al. Twin concordance rates for rheumatoid arthritis: results from a nationwide study. *Br J Rheumatol.* 1993;32(10):903-907.

84. De Vries N, Tijssen H, van Riel PL, van de Putte LB. Reshaping the shared epitope hypothesis: HLA-associated risk for rheumatoid arthritis is encoded by amino acid substitutions at positions 67-74 of the HLA-DRB1 molecule. *Arthritis Rheum.* 2002;46(4):921-928.

85. Aletaha D, Neogi T, Silman AJ, et al. 2010 Rheumatoid arthritis classification criteria: an American College of Rheumatology/European League Against Rheumatism collaborative initiative. *Arthritis Rheum.* 2010;62:2569-2581.

86. Viktil KK, Engeland A, Furu K. Outcomes after anti-rheumatic drug use before and during pregnancy: a cohort study among 150,000 pregnant women and expectant fathers. *Scand J Rheumatol.* 2010;41:196-201.

87. Carter JD, Ladhani A, Ricca LR, Valeriano J, Vasey FB. A safety assessment of tumor necrosis factor antagonists during pregnancy: a review of the Food and Drug Administration database. *J Rheumatol.* 2009;36:635-641.

88. Crijns HJ, Jentink J, Garne E, et al. The distribution of congenital anomalies within the VACTERL association among tumor necrosis factor antagonist-exposed pregnancies is similar to the general population. *J Rheumatol.* 2011;38:1871-1874.

89. Chakravarty EF, Murray ER, Kelman A, Farmer P. Pregnancy outcomes after maternal exposure to rituximab. *Blood.* 2011;117:1499-1506.

90. Ostensen M, Brucato A, Carp H, et al. Pregnancy and reproduction in autoimmune rheumatic diseases. *Rheumatology.* 2011;50:657-664.

91. Ojeda-Uribe M, Afif N, Dahan E, et al. Exposure to abatacept or rituximab in the first trimester of pregnancy in three women with autoimmune diseases. *Clin Rheumatol.* 2013;32:695-700.

92. Friedrichs B, Tiemann M, Salwende H, Verpoort K, Wenger MK, Schmitz N. The effects of rituximab treatment during pregnancy on a neonate. *Haematologica.* 2006;91:1426-1427.

93. Cassina M, Johnson DL, Robinson LK, et al. Pregnancy outcome in women exposed to leflunomide before or during pregnancy. *Arthritis Rheum.* 2012;64:2085-2094.

94. Van den Hoogen F, Khanna D, Fransen J, et al. 2013 Classification criteria for systemic sclerosis: An American College of Rheumatology/European League Against Rheumatism Collaborative initiative. *Arthritis Rheum.* 2013;65:2737-2747.

95. LeRoy EC, Black C, Fleischmajer R, et al. Scleroderma (systemic sclerosis): classification, subsets and pathogenesis. *J Rheumatol.* 1988;15:202-205.

96. Silman AJ, Black C. Increased incidence of spontaneous abortion and infertility in women with scleroderma before disease onset: a controlled study. *Ann Rheum Dis.* 1988;47:441-444.

97. Giordano M, Valentini G, Lupoli S, et al. Pregnancy and systemic sclerosis. *Arthritis Rheum.* 1985;28:237-238.

98. Steen VD. Pregnancy in women with systemic sclerosis. *Obstet Gynecol.* 1999;94:15-20.

99. Chakravarty EF, Khanna D, Chung L. Pregnancy outcomes in systemic sclerosis, primary pulmonary hypertension, and sickle cell disease. *Obstet Gynecol.* 2008;111:927-934.

100. Taraborelli M, Ramoni V, Brucato A, et al. Brief report: successful pregnancies but a higher risk of preterm births in patients with systemic sclerosis: an Italian multicenter study. *Arthritis Rheum.* 2012;64(6): 1970-1977.

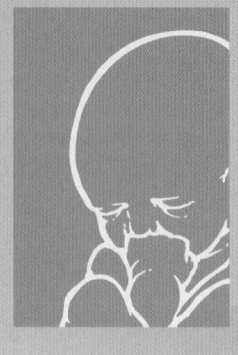

CHAPTER 47

Hepatic Disorders During Pregnancy

MITCHELL S. CAPPELL

KEY ABBREVIATIONS

Acute fatty liver of pregnancy	AFLP
Acute intermittent porphyria	AIP
Computed tomography	CT
Disseminated intravascular coagulation	DIC
Endoscopic retrograde cholangiopancreatography	ERCP
Esophagogastroduodenoscopy	EGD
γ-Glutamyl transpeptidase	GGTP
Gastroesophageal reflux disease	GERD
Hepatobiliary iminodiacetic acid scan	HIDA
Hepatocellular cancer	HCC
Hyperemesis gravidarum	HG
Intrahepatic cholestasis of pregnancy	ICP
Long-chain 3-hydroxyacyl coenzyme A dehydrogenase	LCHAD
Magnetic resonance cholangiopancreatography	MRCP
Magnetic resonance imaging	MRI
Nausea and vomiting of pregnancy	NVP
Right upper quadrant	RUQ
Total parenteral nutrition	TPN
Transjugular intrahepatic portosystemic shunt	TIPS

Hepatic, biliary, and pancreatic disorders are relatively uncommon but are not rare during pregnancy. For example, during pregnancy about 3% of women develop serum liver function test abnormalities,[1] and about 1 in 500 develop potentially life-threatening hepatic diseases that endanger fetal viability.[2,3]

Hepatic, biliary, and pancreatic disorders are often complex and clinically challenging problems during pregnancy. First, the differential diagnosis during pregnancy is extensive and includes both disorders related and unrelated to pregnancy. Second, the clinical presentation and natural history of these disorders may be altered during gestation. Indeed, some disorders—such as intrahepatic cholestasis of pregnancy—are unique to gestation. Third, the diagnostic evaluation may need to be slightly altered because of pregnancy. Nonetheless, almost all radiologic tests can be done judiciously to maintain fetal safety. Fourth, **the interests of both the mother and the fetus must be considered in therapeutic decisions. Usually these interests do not conflict, because generally, what is good for the mother is good for the fetus.** Sometimes, however, maternal therapy must be modified to substitute alternative but safer therapy because of concerns about drug teratogenicity.[4] Rarely, maternal and fetal interests are diametrically opposed, as in the use of chemotherapy for maternal cancer, a therapy that is potentially life-saving to the mother but dangerous to the fetus.[5] These conflicts raise significant medical, legal, and ethical issues.

Obstetricians, hepatologists, surgeons, and internists should be familiar with hepatic, biliary, and pancreatic disorders that can present in pregnancy and how these conditions affect and are affected by pregnancy. This chapter reviews these conditions with a focus on features unique to pregnancy.

PHYSIOLOGIC EFFECTS OF PREGNANCY AND ASSESSMENT OF LIVER DISEASE

Abdominal assessment is modified during pregnancy. The expanding gravid uterus can displace abdominal viscera and may conceal an abdominal mass on physical examination.[5] During the first and second trimesters of pregnancy, blood pressure normally declines modestly. A rise in blood pressure during pregnancy may, therefore, portend preeclampsia or eclampsia. Physiologic alterations of laboratory values during pregnancy include mild leukocytosis, physiologic anemia of pregnancy, and electrolyte changes, particularly mild hyponatremia[6] (see Chapter 3). The risk of thromboembolic phenomena is increased during pregnancy because of mild hypercoagulopathy from hyperestrogenemia and vascular stasis from vascular compression by the enlarged gravid uterus.[7] The changes in serum glucose levels during pregnancy are complex. Normal pregnancy is characterized by fasting hypoglycemia, postprandial hyperglycemia, and hyperinsulinemia.[8] Meticulous control of the serum glucose level is important in diabetic patients for proper fetal development.

Pregnancy does not affect the liver span. The liver may be pushed cephalad by the gravid uterus, but a liver span greater than 12 cm, when appreciated, remains a valid indicator of hepatomegaly. **Spider angiomata and palmar erythema, cutaneous lesions often associated with chronic liver disease, may appear transiently during normal pregnancy without underlying liver disease, presumably because of hyperestrogenemia during pregnancy.**[9] During pregnancy, the serum alkaline phosphatase level normally increases mildly as a result of placental synthesis; the serum albumin level also declines, primarily from hemodilution and secondarily from decreased hepatic synthesis. Serum bilirubin levels tend to change little during pregnancy because of the effect of mildly impaired hepatic excretion balanced by the opposing effects of hemodilution and hypoalbuminemia.[10] Serum bile acids tend to mildly increase during gestation because of impaired hepatic transport and biliary secretion. Serum levels of cholesterol, triglycerides, and phospholipids increase moderately during pregnancy as a result of increased hepatic synthesis.[11] The serum aminotransferase levels are largely unaffected by pregnancy. Changes of serum levels of common blood tests during pregnancy are summarized in Box 47-1 (see Appendix I, "Normal Values in Pregnancy").

DIFFERENTIAL DIAGNOSIS OF HEPATOBILIARY SYMPTOMS AND CONDITIONS DURING PREGNANCY

Maternal Jaundice

As in the general population, acute viral hepatitis is the most common cause of jaundice during pregnancy.[2,3] The differential diagnosis of jaundice during the first and second trimesters of pregnancy also includes drug hepatotoxicity and gallstone disease such as acute cholecystitis, choledocholithiasis, ascending cholangitis, or gallstone pancreatitis. In addition to these disorders, the differential of jaundice during the third trimester includes pregnancy-related causes such as

---

BOX 47-1   CHANGES IN ROUTINE LABORATORY TESTS AND LIVER FUNCTION TESTS DURING PREGNANCY

Mildly Decreased Serum Levels
- Sodium
- Albumin

Moderately Decreased Blood Level
- Hematocrit: physiologic anemia of pregnancy

Mildly Increased Blood or Serum Levels
- Leukocyte count
- Alkaline phosphatase
- Amylase

Moderately Increased Serum Levels
- Serum bile acids
- Cholesterol
- Triglycerides

Other
- Glucose level: fasting hypoglycemia, postprandial hyperglycemia

---

intrahepatic cholestasis of pregnancy; acute fatty liver of pregnancy (AFLP); and hemolysis, elevated liver enzymes, and low platelets (HELLP) syndrome. Moderate direct hyperbilirubinemia without jaundice during the third trimester may also be due to preeclampsia, eclampsia, and Budd-Chiari syndrome. Predominantly indirect hyperbilirubinemia during pregnancy is usually due to hemolysis (including the HELLP syndrome) or Gilbert syndrome.

Right Upper Quadrant Abdominal Pain

The differential diagnosis of right upper quadrant (RUQ) abdominal pain is extensive during pregnancy (Box 47-2). In addition to hepatic, biliary, gastrointestinal (GI), and renal disorders that can occur in nonpregnant patients, the differential includes diseases related to pregnancy. In the medical history, the pain intensity, nature, temporal pattern, radiation pattern, exacerbating factors, and alleviating factors help narrow the differential diagnosis. **Biliary colic** produces a waxing and waning intensity of pain. **Acute cholecystitis** is associated with RUQ pain and pain referred to the right shoulder. The pain of **acute pancreatitis** is often boring in quality, located in the abdominal midline, and radiating to the back. Careful physical examination of the abdomen that includes inspection, palpation, and auscultation can further pinpoint the cause of the pain. **Laboratory evaluation of significant abdominal pain routinely includes a complete blood count (CBC), serum electrolytes, and liver function tests (LFTs) as well as a leukocyte differential, coagulation profile, and serum lipase determination.** In evaluating the laboratory results, gestational changes in normative values, as mentioned earlier, must be considered. Radiologic tests may be extremely helpful diagnostically, but the choice of radiologic imaging is constrained by the pregnancy, as discussed below. **RUQ pain and abnormal LFTs in the setting of new-onset hypertension should strongly suggest preeclampsia with hepatic involvement.** RUQ pain and abnormal LFTs in the setting of thrombocytopenia and microangiopathic hemolysis, as demonstrated by the presence of schistocytes in a peripheral blood smear, should strongly suggest the HELLP syndrome.

BOX 47-2   DIFFERENTIAL DIAGNOSIS OF RIGHT UPPER QUADRANT ABDOMINAL PAIN DURING PREGNANCY

Hepatic Disorders
- Hepatitis
- Hepatic vascular engorgement
- Hepatic hematoma
- Hepatic malignancy

Biliary Tract Disease
- Biliary colic
- Choledocholithiasis
- Cholangitis
- Cholecystitis

Diseases Related to Pregnancy
- Preeclampsia or eclampsia
- Hemolysis, elevated liver enzymes, and low platelets (HELLP) syndrome
- Acute fatty liver of pregnancy
- Hepatic hemorrhage or rupture

Renal Disorders
- Pyelonephritis
- Nephrolithiasis

Gastrointestinal Disorders
- Peptic ulcer disease
- Perforated duodenal ulcer

Other Conditions
- Rib fracture
- Shingles

Referred Pain From Another Disease
- Pneumonia
- Pulmonary embolus or infarct
- Pleural effusion
- Radiculopathy
- Inferior wall myocardial infarction
- Colon cancer

Occasionally, the pregnancy is not known by the patient or is not revealed to the physician, particularly in early pregnancy, when physical findings are absent. The physician should be vigilant for possible pregnancy in a fertile woman with abdominal pain, particularly in the setting of missed menses, because pregnancy affects the differential diagnosis, clinical evaluation, and mode of therapy. Pregnancy tests should be performed early in the evaluation of acute abdominal pain in a fertile woman.

Nausea and Vomiting

Nausea and vomiting may be ubiquitous during pregnancy, and nausea and vomiting of pregnancy (NVP) is the most common cause (see Chapter 6). It typically begins at about 6 weeks and abates at about 18 weeks[12] and is caused by the physiologic effects of the pregnancy without demonstrable mucosal or mural disease. **Hyperemesis gravidarum (HG) is a serious and potentially life-threatening form of NVP associated with loss of more than 5% of the pregravid weight.** HG is a diagnosis of exclusion, based on nausea and vomiting that occur early in pregnancy and that gradually resolve during the middle second trimester and unassociated with other symptoms. **The differential diagnosis of nausea and vomiting during pregnancy also includes hepatic and pancreatobiliary diseases such as**

pancreatitis, viral hepatitis, symptomatic cholelithiasis, acute cholecystitis, AFLP, and occasionally intrahepatic cholestasis of pregnancy. GI causes include gastroesophageal reflux disease (GERD), peptic ulcer disease, viral gastroenteritis, appendicitis, gastroparesis diabeticorum, and GI obstruction. Other causes include adnexal torsion, pyelonephritis, urolithiasis, and Addison disease (glucocorticoid deficiency).

Pruritus

The differential diagnosis of pruritus during pregnancy includes intrahepatic cholestasis of pregnancy, cholestatic viral hepatitis, primary sclerosing cholangitis, primary biliary cirrhosis, and mechanical choledochal obstruction from benign or malignant strictures. Pruritus sometimes occurs physiologically during pregnancy; this pruritus is typically mild, localized, unassociated with other symptoms, and unassociated with abnormal liver function tests (see Chapter 50). **Important clues that pruritus may be due to the intrahepatic cholestasis of pregnancy include pruritus that begins during the third trimester of pregnancy with no history of chronic liver disease, absence of abdominal pain, pruritus that affects mostly the hands and feet, and only mild to moderately elevated serum transaminase and bilirubin levels.**

Hepatic Lesions

Hepatic lesions identified on abdominal imaging studies are classified as cystic or solid. The differential of cystic hepatic lesions includes simple hepatic cysts, hepatic cysts associated with polycystic kidney disease, Caroli disease (a rare inherited disorder characterized by dilation of the intrahepatic bile ducts), bacterial abscesses, amebic abscesses, intraparenchymal hemorrhage, hemangiomas, echinococcal cysts, and rarely hepatic malignancies. The differential of a solid hepatic mass includes hepatic adenoma, focal nodular hyperplasia, hepatocellular carcinoma, and hepatic metastases.

Ascites

Hepatic causes of ascites during pregnancy include cirrhosis, AFLP, Budd-Chiari syndrome, portal vein thrombosis, hepatic fibrosis, and hepatocellular carcinoma. Other causes of ascites during pregnancy include ovarian cancer, abdominal tuberculosis, cardiac failure, protein-losing nephropathy, and severe protein malnutrition (kwashiorkor).

Neonatal Cholestasis

Neonatal cholestasis is characterized by conjugated hyperbilirubinemia, pale stools, and dark urine. The differential includes neonatal prematurity; anatomic anomalies such as biliary atresia; infections such as cytomegalovirus or toxoplasmosis; and metabolic defects such as cystic fibrosis, alpha 1antitrypsin deficiency, or bile acid synthetic defects. Neonates frequently have unconjugated (indirect) hyperbilirubinemia or physiologic jaundice due to increased production and decreased clearance of bilirubin. The bilirubin may peak at 7 mg/dL several days after birth but rapidly normalizes within about 1 week thereafter. Unconjugated neonatal hyperbilirubinemia may also be due to hemolysis, sepsis, or Gilbert syndrome.

ABDOMINAL IMAGING DURING PREGNANCY

Fetal safety during diagnostic imaging is a concern for pregnant patients. Ultrasonography is considered safe and is the preferred abdominal imaging modality during pregnancy.[13] Unfortunately, the test sensitivity depends on operator technique, patient cooperation, and patient anatomy. For example, test sensitivity is decreased by abdominal fat and intestinal gas.[13] **No reported harmful effects result from magnetic resonance imaging (MRI) during pregnancy**, but few data are available on safety during the first trimester or with use of gadolinium.[14] However, **gadolinium has not been associated with adverse fetal outcomes in a number of individual case reports or in limited case series**. MRI is preferable to computed tomography (CT) scanning during pregnancy to avoid ionizing radiation, but gadolinium administration should be avoided during MRI in the first trimester.[15] Rapid-sequence MRI is preferable to conventional MRI because of briefer exposures.

Radiation can cause fetal mortality, growth restriction, chromosomal mutations, and neurologic abnormalities that include mental retardation, and they increase the risk of childhood leukemia (see Chapter 8).[16] Radiation dosage is the most important risk factor, but fetal age at exposure is also important. Fetal mortality is greatest from radiation exposure during the first 2 weeks after conception, and the risk of neurologic malformations is greatest during the first trimester, when organogenesis occurs.[16] The patient should undergo counseling before diagnostic roentgenography. Exposure to more than 15 rads during the second and third trimesters or more than 5 rads during the first trimester should prompt consideration of termination of pregnancy.[16] **Diagnostic studies with high radiation exposure, such as abdominal CT, typically expose the fetus to less than 1 rad and should therefore be considered when indicated.**[15] The physician ordering a roentgenographic study can consult with a medical physicist to estimate the fetal exposure. Fetal radiation exposure should be minimized by shielding the abdomen above the uterus and using narrow collimation and rapid-sequence studies. When performing abdominal CT scans with contrast, precontrast films can be reduced or eliminated to reduce radiation exposure.

THERAPEUTIC ENDOSCOPY DURING PREGNANCY
Therapeutic Endoscopic Retrograde Cholangiopancreatography

Choledocholithiasis usually requires urgent therapy because of potentially life-threatening ascending cholangitis or gallstone pancreatitis. Symptomatic choledocholithiasis is best managed by therapeutic endoscopic retrograde cholangiopancreatography (ERCP) in the nonpregnant patient to avoid complex biliary surgery during cholecystectomy. In experienced hands, therapeutic ERCP in the general population has acceptable morbidity of about 5% and low mortality of about 0.5%.[17] Therapeutic ERCP is theoretically more attractive than biliary surgery for choledocholithiasis during pregnancy because surgery entails a significant risk of fetal loss.[18] Aside from maternal risks, therapeutic ERCP during pregnancy entails theoretic risks to the fetus from induction of premature labor, medication and radiation teratogenicity, placental abruption or fetal trauma during endoscopic intubation, cardiac arrhythmias, systemic hypotension, and transient hypoxia.[17]

A literature review of about 350 cases of ERCP during pregnancy noted three larger studies that encompassed over 100 patients in total and numerous small case series or individual case reports.[19] Almost all pregnant patients in all these studies

required therapeutic intervention, mostly for choledocholithiasis. The outcome after ERCP was favorable in the three larger studies in terms of maternal health, maintenance of pregnancy, and eventual fetal outcome.[19] Complications included maternal pancreatitis in 5% to 16%, one spontaneous abortion 3 months after ERCP, one neonatal demise 26 hours after delivery, and a prematurity rate of 8%.[19] These relatively favorable results were confirmed in the review of the rest of the approximately 350 cases. Although the individual studies were generally flawed because of small study size, retrospective design, and limited follow-up after delivery, the consistency of the favorable results across so many studies argues forcefully that **ERCP is justifiable during pregnancy for appropriate indications and contemplated therapeutic intervention**. These results have been further confirmed in additional individual studies[20,21] and literature reviews.[22] In particular, **therapeutic ERCP can be performed during pregnancy to help avoid complex biliary surgery or to postpone cholecystectomy until after parturition**. Special precautions to minimize fetal risks from ERCP during pregnancy include consideration for consultation with a neonatologist, radiation physicist, and anesthesiologist before ERCP; referral to a tertiary medical center for management by a team of experts; lead shielding of the mother's abdomen except for the region of the proximal pancreas and biliary tree; use of a modern fluoroscope to minimize radiation leakage; avoidance of spot radiographs for documentation because they require considerable radiation energy; and, if possible, delay ERCP until the second trimester to reduce radiation teratogenicity.[17]

Endoscopic Variceal Sclerotherapy or Banding

Pregnancy appears to increase the risk of variceal bleeding from portal hypertension because of the gestational increase in plasma volume.[23] Endoscopic ligation (banding) or sclerotherapy are particularly attractive therapies for variceal bleeding during pregnancy because the alternative of transjugular intrahepatic portosystemic shunt (TIPS) requires radiation, and the surgical alternatives can cause fetal loss.** Esophagogastroduodenoscopy (EGD) can be performed during pregnancy with relatively low fetal risks and should certainly be considered when strongly indicated, such as for acute upper GI hemorrhage.[17,24] **Endoscopic banding and sclerotherapy** raise concerns beyond that of diagnostic EGD from the additional procedure time, the typically severe underlying maternal illness, and the therapy itself. **Variceal banding** is preferred over sclerotherapy in the general (nonpregnant) population. Scant clinical data exist on variceal banding during pregnancy and comprise one small case series and individual case reports. These data suggest relatively favorable maternal and fetal outcomes after variceal banding compared with the poor prognosis in untreated patients.[19] More clinical data exist on **sclerotherapy** during pregnancy. In one clinical series, 10 patients underwent a mean of three endoscopic sclerotherapy sessions during pregnancy, five for active variceal bleeding and five for prophylaxis.[25] Hemostasis was achieved in all actively bleeding patients. One patient suffered a complication from sclerotherapy of an esophageal stricture, which was successfully treated using perioral esophageal dilators. All patients had a normal vaginal delivery at term.[25] Nine other patients successfully underwent endoscopic sclerotherapy for actively or recently bleeding esophageal varices with delivery of healthy infants in all cases.[17] One study reported less favorable pregnancy outcomes after endoscopic sclerotherapy, attributable to the underlying maternal disease.

TABLE 47-1	CLINICAL PRESENTATION AND TREATMENT DURING PREGNANCY OF COMMON PANCREATIC DISORDERS MINIMALLY AFFECTED BY PREGNANCY			
DISEASE OR DISORDER	**SYMPTOMS AND SIGNS**	**LABORATORY FINDINGS**	**TREATMENT**
Acute pancreatitis	Epigastric pain radiating to back, nausea and vomiting, pyrexia; abdominal tenderness, guarding, distension	Increased serum lipase, leukocytosis; abdominal ultrasound can reveal pancreatomegaly, peripancreatic inflammation, inhomogeneous pancreas	Discontinue oral intake; provide aggressive IV hydration, analgesia, and nasojejunal feeding or TPN for a prolonged bout of pancreatitis
Acute cholecystitis	Epigastric or RUQ pain, nausea and vomiting, tachycardia, Murphy sign	Leukocytosis, variably, mildly elevated LFTs; abdominal ultrasound shows a thickened gallbladder wall, pericholecystic fluid, gallstones in gallbladder	Discontinue oral intake; provide IV hydration, analgesia, and antibiotics; cholecystectomy can be performed during pregnancy, most safely during the second trimester
Choledocholithiasis with ascending cholangitis	RUQ pain, pyrexia, jaundice (Charcot triad); epigastric tenderness	Leukocytosis, jaundice, variably elevated other LFTs; abdominal ultrasound shows dilated choledochus, possible gallstones in gallbladder; ERCP reveals dilated choledochus, choledocholithiasis	Discontinue oral intake; provide IV hydration, antibiotics; ERCP with sphincterotomy may be performed during pregnancy to address choledocholithiasis

ERCP, endoscopic retrograde cholangiopancreatography; IV, intravenous; LFTs, liver function tests; RUQ, right upper quadrant; TPN, total parenteral nutrition.

Four of seventeen pregnant patients undergoing endoscopic sclerotherapy for variceal bleeding due to noncirrhotic portal hypertension had adverse pregnancy outcomes of stillbirth or neonatal death.[26] Still, **the available data should justify endoscopic therapy during pregnancy for actively bleeding esophageal varices, after informed consent, because of poor outcomes with the alternative available therapies.**

Team Approach and Informed Consent

A team approach with consultation and referral helps optimize the management of complex diseases during pregnancy that affect both the mother and the fetus and that require disparate areas of expertise. The obstetrician may consult with the hepatologist regarding timing of delivery in patients with obstetric-related hepatic disease. The gastroenterologist contemplating therapeutic ERCP for symptomatic choledocholithiasis may consult with the obstetrician about the optimal procedure timing and with the anesthesiologist about analgesia during endoscopy. The internist may discuss with the radiologist the benefits versus risks of radiologic tests, and the radiologist may in turn consult with a physicist about methods to monitor and reduce fetal radiation exposure. **Complex hepatic problems during pregnancy are best handled at a tertiary hospital with the requisite experience and expertise.**

The patient should be informed about the consequences to both herself and her fetus of diagnostic tests and therapy and should be actively involved in medical decisions. The patient makes the decision under the vigilant guidance of the experts and with input from her partner, family, and friends. When an intervention, such as roentgenographic tests, entails significant potential fetal risk, a signed, witnessed, and informed consent is recommended even though this intervention would be routine and would not require consent in a nonpregnant patient.

PANCREATOBILIARY DISEASE

Acute Pancreatitis

Acute pancreatitis occurs in about 1 per 3000 pregnancies, most commonly during the third trimester.[27,28] Gallstones cause about 70% of cases because alcoholism is relatively uncommon during pregnancy.[29,30] The risk of cholesterol stones is increased during pregnancy because of increased cholesterol secretion into bile.[28] Other causes include drugs, abdominal surgery, trauma, hyperlipidemia, hyperparathyroidism,

vasculitis, and infections such as mumps or mononucleosis.[29] The risk of pancreatitis from hyperlipidemia is increased during pregnancy because of the significant elevation of triglyceride levels during late pregnancy.[31] Some cases are idiopathic.

The clinical presentation, diagnostic tests, and treatment of pancreatobiliary disorders during pregnancy are summarized in Table 47-1. **Pregnancy does not significantly alter the clinical presentation of acute pancreatitis.**[29,30] **Epigastric pain is the most common symptom.** The pain commonly radiates to the back, and nausea, emesis, and pyrexia frequently occur. Signs include midabdominal tenderness, abdominal guarding, hypoactive bowel sounds, abdominal distension, and increased tympany. Severe cases are associated with shock and pancreatic ascites. Turner sign, bruising of the flanks, or Cullen sign, superficial edema and bruising around the umbilicus, suggest retroperitoneal bleeding.[29,30]

Acute pancreatitis is diagnosed by finding typical abnormalities in two of the following three parameters: (1) clinical presentation, (2) laboratory tests, or (3) radiologic examinations. Typical symptoms of pancreatitis include epigastric or RUQ pain and nausea and vomiting. Serum lipase is a reliable marker of acute pancreatitis during pregnancy because the lipase level is unchanged during normal pregnancy. The serum amylase level is a less specific marker of pancreatitis because it mildly rises during late pregnancy,[32] and it can rise due to diabetic ketoacidosis, renal failure, bowel perforation, or bowel obstruction. Hypertriglyceridemia can falsely lower the serum amylase level in pancreatitis, but the lipase level remains elevated.[4] A serum alanine aminotransferase level more than three times the upper limit of normal strongly suggests biliary pancreatitis. Abdominal ultrasonography is useful in gauging pancreatic inflammation in thin patients with mild to moderate acute pancreatitis, but CT scanning is better at delineating areas of pancreatic necrosis in patients with severe pancreatitis.[30] Abdominal CT is, however, generally discouraged during pregnancy because of potential teratogenicity. Abdominal ultrasonography is also useful to detect cholelithiasis and bile duct dilatation, but endoscopic ultrasonography is required to reliably detect choledocholithiasis. Because of fetal risks from ionizing radiation with ERCP,[28] magnetic resonance cholangiopancreatography (MRCP) is preferable to ERCP as a diagnostic study to visualize the common bile duct during pregnancy, unless endoscopic therapy is contemplated. **Acute pancreatitis during pregnancy is often mild and usually responds to medical**

therapy that includes intravenous (IV) fluid administration, gastric acid suppression, analgesia, sometimes nasogastric suction, and discontinuation of oral intake. Meperidine is the traditional choice for analgesia because it does not cause contraction of the sphincter of Oddi. Short-term administration of meperidine appears to be relatively safe during pregnancy.[33] Pancreatitis complicated by a pancreatic phlegmon, abscess, sepsis, or hemorrhage necessitates antibiotic therapy, total parenteral nutrition (TPN), and possible radiologic aspiration or surgical debridement with patient monitoring in an intensive care unit (ICU).[30,34] Large and persistent pancreatic pseudocysts require endoscopic or radiologic drainage or surgery.[30] Endoscopic sphincterotomy can be performed for gallstone pancreatitis during pregnancy with minimal fetal radiation exposure.[35] Pregnancy should not delay these therapies. **Laparoscopic cholecystectomy can be utilized during pregnancy and is best performed during the second trimester after organogenesis has occurred and before the growing gravid uterus interferes with visualization of the laparoscopic field.** Maternal mortality is low in uncomplicated pancreatitis but exceeds 10% in complicated pancreatitis.[30] Fetal outcome is generally good for mild to moderate pancreatitis but can be poor with severe pancreatitis. However, moderately severe pancreatitis is occasionally associated with fetal death during the first trimester and is associated with premature labor in the third trimester.[36] Nutritional requirements for TPN for severe pancreatitis should include the extra nutritional requirements of the gravida.[37]

Cholelithiasis and Cholecystitis

Pregnancy promotes bile lithogenicity and sludge formation because estrogen increases cholesterol synthesis, and progesterone impairs gallbladder motility.[38] In large population surveys using abdominal ultrasonography, 12% of pregnant women in Chile had cholelithiasis,[39] and 8% of pregnant women in the United States[40] had cholelithiasis or biliary sludge detected by abdominal ultrasonography. **Most gallstones are asymptomatic during pregnancy,[41] although symptoms of gallstone disease during pregnancy are the same as those in other patients.[39,41]** The usual initial symptom is biliary colic, pain located in the epigastrium or RUQ that may radiate to the back or shoulders. The pain typically increases over several hours then plateaus and subsides over several hours. It can occur spontaneously or can be induced by eating a fatty meal. Diaphoresis, nausea, and emesis are common. Physical examination is unremarkable, other than occasional RUQ tenderness. About two thirds of patients with biliary colic will experience recurrent attacks during the ensuing 2 years.[4]

More severe complications of cholelithiasis include **cholecystitis, choledocholithiasis, jaundice, ascending cholangitis, hepatic abscess, and gallstone pancreatitis. Pregnancy does not increase the frequency or severity of these complications.**[41] **Acute cholecystitis** is a chemical inflammation usually caused by cystic duct obstruction by a gallstone. It is **the third most common nonobstetric surgical emergency during pregnancy with an incidence of about 4 cases per 10,000 pregnancies.**[30] As in biliary colic, the pain is located in the epigastrium and RUQ, but the pain is usually more severe, prolonged, and associated with other clinical findings that include nausea, emesis, pyrexia, tachycardia, right-sided subcostal tenderness, Murphy sign, and leukocytosis.[42] A positive Murphy sign is increased discomfort or inspiratory arrest (a catching of the breath) during deep inspiration when the examiner palpates the gallbladder

fossa just beneath the liver edge. Serum biochemical parameters of liver function and serum levels of amylase may be mildly abnormal. **Ultrasound is very helpful in diagnosing acute cholecystitis during pregnancy,** and it may demonstrate cholelithiasis. Findings compatible with acute cholecystitis include gallbladder wall thickening, pericholecystic fluid, and a positive sonographic Murphy sign in which inspiratory arrest is elicited by pressing the ultrasound transducer probe against the gallbladder fossa during inspiration. Cholescintigraphy with 99mTc hepatobiliary iminodiacetic acid (HIDA) scan is sometimes used to confirm acute cholecystitis in nonpregnant patients, but it is rarely required during pregnancy even though it is believed to be relatively safe to the fetus when strongly indicated. Jaundice suggests choledocholithiasis, and pronounced hyperamylasemia suggests gallstone pancreatitis.

Most cases of biliary colic and some cases of very mild acute cholecystitis can be managed conservatively with close observation, expectant management, and deferral of surgery to the immediate postpartum period.[34,43] However, **most patients with recurrent biliary colic or acute cholecystitis undergo cholecystectomy.**[39,42,44] Preoperative management includes discontinuing oral intake and then administering IV fluids, analgesia, and usually antibiotics.[38] Ampicillin, cephalosporins, and clindamycin are relatively safe antibiotics during pregnancy.[42,45] **Cholecystectomy is best performed during the second trimester; cholecystectomy during the first trimester is occasionally associated with fetal loss, and cholecystectomy during the third trimester may be associated with premature labor.**[42,44] Cholecystectomy has become increasingly accepted during the first and third trimesters because of improved surgical outcomes,[44] although tocolysis may be necessary during cholecystectomy performed in the third trimester. Intraoperative cholangiography is only performed during pregnancy for strong indications to avoid radiation teratogenicity. Laparoscopic cholecystectomy is safe during pregnancy and is best performed during the second trimester.[4,43] Both maternal and fetal mortality from acute cholecystitis is less than 2.5% during pregnancy.[41]

Choledocholithiasis

Symptomatic choledocholithiasis is uncommon during pregnancy. Choledocholithiasis can produce gallstone pancreatitis manifested by pyrexia, nausea, and severe abdominal pain or ascending cholangitis manifested by pyrexia, RUQ pain, and jaundice (Charcot triad).[30] Endoscopic ultrasound is relatively safe in pregnancy and is sensitive in detecting choledocholithiasis.[46] Patients with choledocholithiasis and gallstone pancreatitis should undergo ERCP and sphincterotomy with stone extraction, as previously described. Pancreatography can be avoided to minimize fetal radiation exposure.[35] These patients then usually undergo cholecystectomy postpartum but can, if necessary, undergo cholecystectomy antepartum, especially during the second trimester, with acceptable maternal and fetal risks.[30] Cholecystectomy can be performed by laparoscopic, rather than open, techniques during the first or second trimester of pregnancy.[47]

Choledochal Cysts

Choledochal cysts are rare. They typically produce a diagnostic triad of abdominal pain, jaundice, and a palpable abdominal mass in nonpregnant patients. Choledochal cysts are classified into types 1 through 4, depending upon which segment of the biliary tree is dilated.[48] Choledochal cysts can initially present during pregnancy, which can exacerbate the abdominal pain and increase the jaundice because of choledochal compression by the enlarged gravid uterus. However, pregnancy can mask the palpable abdominal mass because of the size of the uterus.[49,50] Severe pain suggests cyst rupture or concomitant pancreatitis.[49] A choledochal cyst is often diagnosed by abdominal ultrasound, although cholangiography is sometimes required. MRI is preferred over abdominal CT or diagnostic ERCP for determining the anatomy. Surgical management is generally recommended for symptomatic choledocholithiasis because of the risk of recurrent cholangitis and malignant degeneration. The standard surgery is cystectomy, cholecystectomy, and reconstitution of biliary-intestinal flow by either a Roux-en-Y hepaticojejunostomy or choledochojejunostomy.[50] Medical management, including antibiotics and temporary percutaneous or endoscopic drainage, may sometimes suffice until delivery.[49,50]

COMMON LIVER DISEASES INCIDENTAL TO PREGNANCY
Acute Viral Hepatitis A, B, and C
Acute viral hepatitis A, B, and C present similarly in pregnancy as in the nonpregnant state (see Chapter 52). In a review of 13 cases of **hepatitis A** that occurred during the second or third trimesters of pregnancy, many of the mothers had mild to moderate gestational complications such as premature contractions or transient vaginal bleeding, but all pregnancies had favorable outcomes.[51] **Acute hepatitis B** is usually self-limited and mild during pregnancy. Patients with very severe or prolonged acute hepatitis B may be considered as candidates for lamivudine therapy.[52] Typical symptoms of acute viral hepatitis include anorexia, nausea, malaise, and RUQ discomfort. Patients with acute hepatitis A or hepatitis B typically have highly elevated serum aminotransferase levels, and jaundice may also be apparent. **Acute hepatitis C** is frequently subclinical and typically causes only mild serum aminotransferase level elevations. Maternal mortality is rare from acute hepatitis A, B, or C during pregnancy. Fetal mortality and neonatal morbidity is increased by acute hepatitis A or B but is still relatively low.

Hepatitis E
Hepatitis E, while rare and sporadic in industrialized countries, is the most common epidemic waterborne form of hepatitis in middle- to low-income countries. It usually spreads by fecal-oral transmission through a contaminated water supply. Infected patients typically have a prodrome with malaise and pyrexia, followed by an acute illness with anorexia, nausea, vomiting, abdominal pain, and jaundice. Patients often have hepatomegaly and usually have significant elevations of the serum aminotransferase levels. The infection is typically mild and self-limited without chronicity or clinical sequelae.

Pregnant patients have a more severe illness, with frequent fulminant hepatitis. The mortality rate rises progressively with increasing gestational age, up to about 20% for acute infection in the third trimester.[53] Maternal infection is likewise associated with a high risk of fetal or neonatal mortality. Medical management is supportive, and fulminant hepatitis should be managed in an ICU and may require liver transplantation. The cause of the increased severity of hepatitis E during pregnancy is unknown but may relate to attenuated cellular immunity during pregnancy.[54]

In the United States, hepatitis E infection is rare and is not routinely tested for in the evaluation of acute hepatitis. However, patients with acute hepatitis should be evaluated for hepatitis E if they have recently traveled to an endemic area and have had hepatitis A, B, and C excluded by serologic tests. Hepatitis E testing should also be considered in patients who present with fulminant hepatitis of unclear etiology who lack a travel history to endemic regions. The infection is generally diagnosed by detecting hepatitis E antibodies in the serum. Acute infection is indicated by the presence of immunoglobulin M (IgM) antibodies, whereas prior infection is characterized by detecting IgG antibodies. Detection of the virus in blood by polymerase chain reaction (PCR) is more accurate than serologic tests. Tests for hepatitis E are not commercially available in the United States but may be obtained via the Centers for Disease Control and Prevention (CDC). The infection is largely prevented by public health measures, such as a clean water supply. Pregnant women should avoid travel to endemic areas, should not drink water from the municipal water supply in endemic areas, should not consume uncooked shellfish or vegetables from endemic areas, and should wash all fruit from endemic areas using uncontaminated water. Table 47-2 summarizes the clinical presentation, diagnostic tests, and treatment during pregnancy complicated by hepatitis E as well as other hepatic disorders significantly affected by pregnancy.

TABLE 47-2	CLINICAL PRESENTATION AND TREATMENT DURING PREGNANCY OF HEPATIC DISORDERS SIGNIFICANTLY AFFECTED BY PREGNANCY		
DISEASE OR DISORDER	**SYMPTOMS AND SIGNS**	**LABORATORY FINDINGS**	**TREATMENT**
Hepatitis E	Anorexia, nausea and vomiting, RUQ abdominal pain, jaundice, hepatomegaly	Significantly elevated aminotransferase levels, mild jaundice; IgM antibodies to hepatitis E; PCR positive for hepatitis E virus	Supportive care and prevention by public health measures; avoid drinking municipal water in endemic areas
Acute intermittent porphyria	Diffuse abdominal pain, vomiting, constipation, neuropsychiatric abnormalities	Increased porphobilinogen and δ-aminolevulinic acid levels in urine	Hematin, parenteral glucose; avoid precipitating drugs and fasting; narcotics or phenothiazines relieve symptoms
Budd-Chiari syndrome	Abdominal pain, hepatomegaly, and ascites	Moderately elevated bilirubin and alkaline phosphatase, relatively normal aminotransferase levels; Doppler ultrasound, hepatic venography, or MRA will show no flow in the hepatic vein	Low-sodium diet and diuretics manage ascites and fluid retention; consider anticoagulation, balancing benefits against risks, and thrombolytic therapy or angioplasty for an acute clot; data are limited on this therapy during pregnancy

IgM, immunoglobulin M; *PCR,* polymerase chain reaction; *MRA,* magnetic resonance angiography; *RUQ,* right upper quadrant.

Chronic Hepatitis B

Pregnancy does not appear to significantly affect the progression of chronic hepatitis B.[55] Despite immunotolerance during pregnancy, acute flares are relatively uncommon in patients with chronic hepatitis B. **Maternal chronic hepatitis B infection may, however, be transmitted to the neonate, usually during delivery.**[56] **The risk of vertical transmission is about 90% in mothers who are positive for the hepatitis B e antigen (HBeAg), but it is about 25% in mothers who are HBeAg negative.**[57] Perinatal infection is clinically important because infected neonates tend to become chronic carriers and then have a markedly increased risk of developing hepatocellular carcinoma in adulthood. All pregnant women are tested for hepatitis B surface antigen (HBsAg) in the United States.[55] **Infants born to mothers with acute or chronic hepatitis B infection should be passively immunized with hepatitis B hyperimmune globulin and should be actively immunized with hepatitis B vaccine immediately after birth** to prevent neonatal infection from intrapartum exposure.[58] Recent data suggest that treatment of chronic hepatitis B in pregnancy with lamivudine or tenofovir is feasible, safe, and effective in reducing maternal viral load. This therapy is currently an area of active research.[59,60]

Chronic Hepatitis C

Women with chronic hepatitis C may exhibit transient normalization of their serum aminotransferase levels associated with an increase in the serum viral load during pregnancy, possibly because of mildly attenuated immunity.[61] The clinical significance of this phenomenon in terms of progression of the liver disease is unclear, but chronically infected patients may develop mild progression of their liver disease, as evidenced by increased hepatic fibrosis during pregnancy.

The risk of vertical transmission of hepatitis C from a chronically infected mother with viremia to the neonate is about 5%.[62] This rate of vertical transmission is much lower than that for hepatitis B. Viral transmission to the neonate is unlikely (<2%) in mothers who have an undetectable viral load. In contrast, women positive for the human immunodeficiency virus (HIV) can have hepatitis C transmission rates as high as 20% to 40%. Infants born to mothers with hepatitis C infection should undergo periodic testing for hepatitis C during the first 18 months of life to detect persistent infection. Directly acting antiviral drugs are now able to achieve a sustained undetectable hepatitis C viral load and should be considered in pregnancy as more safety data become available.[63]

Wilson Disease

Noncirrhotic women treated for early Wilson disease have relatively intact fertility and may therefore become pregnant. Their serum levels of copper and ceruloplasmin increase during pregnancy,[64] and therefore they require maintenance therapy to prevent a flare of disease that can increase maternal morbidity and fetal mortality. Although the data are limited, trientine (triethylene tetramine dihydrochloride) or zinc therapy for Wilson disease may be continued during pregnancy without significant fetal toxicity.[65] D-penicillamine is potentially teratogenic; therefore its use during pregnancy should be limited when alternatives are available. Women with cirrhosis from Wilson disease have increased risks of complications during pregnancy that include intrauterine growth restriction (IUGR) and preeclampsia.

Autoimmune Hepatitis

Women with autoimmune hepatitis should be maintained on immunosuppressive therapy during pregnancy. Glucocorticoids appear to be relatively safe during pregnancy,[66] and the U.S. Food and Drug Administration (FDA) rates prednisone as a category B drug during gestation. Patients with well-compensated and well-controlled autoimmune hepatitis tolerate pregnancy well while maintained on this therapy and have only a moderately increased rate of perinatal complications.[66,67] These patients typically have a reversible mild deterioration of serum parameters of liver function during pregnancy, particularly of serum bilirubin and alkaline phosphatase, attributed to the cholestatic effects of gestation. Patients who discontinue their immunosuppressive therapy can develop severe acute flares.

Hepatic Hemangiomas, Cysts, and Abscesses

Hepatic hemangiomas are the most common benign tumors of the liver in the general population. The vast majority of hepatic hemangiomas smaller than 5 cm are asymptomatic in the general population. **Hepatic hemangiomas appear to behave similarly during pregnancy.** Rare symptoms attributable to hemangiomas include RUQ pain, abdominal distension, or symptoms such as nausea that are attributable to impingement of adjacent viscera. Serious complications during pregnancy include consumptive coagulopathy with hemolysis, thrombocytopenia, and hypofibrinogenemia (Kasabach-Merritt syndrome); intrahepatic hemorrhage; and spontaneous hepatic rupture. Patients with large hemangiomas are at greater risk for these complications. Warning signs include progressively increasing symptoms and rapid lesion growth, although these complications are rare during pregnancy. Among 20 patients with very large hemangiomas, only one case of hepatic rupture and one case of intrahepatic hemorrhage occurred in 27 pregnancies.[68] Nearly all hemangiomas, including moderately large lesions, appear to be indolent during pregnancy and can therefore be observed without interventional therapy. MRI is the imaging modality of choice to follow hemangioma size during gestation because of high sensitivity, high specificity, and reduced fetal risks compared with CT.

Focal nodular hyperplasia is the second most common cause of a benign hepatic mass. It is usually asymptomatic during pregnancy and is often detected incidentally during obstetric ultrasonography.[13,46] This lesion occasionally grows during gestation, possibly because of estrogen stimulation. Most cases can be observed without intervention. It rarely causes hepatic hemorrhage or biliary obstruction as a result of compression by the enlarged gravid uterus.[68-70] Clinical findings may include abdominal pain, jaundice, or hypotension. Surgical intervention is occasionally necessary for these complications.[69,70]

Hepatic cysts may be isolated or associated with polycystic kidney disease, malignancy, or amebic or echinococcal infection.[69,71] Pyogenic liver abscesses during pregnancy arise from ascending cholangitis, appendicitis, or diverticulitis.[69,70] Both antibiotics and percutaneous drainage are usually indicated.

Hepatocellular Carcinoma and Hepatic Metastases

Hepatocellular carcinoma (HCC) usually occurs in the setting of cirrhosis secondary to chronic viral hepatitis, hemochromatosis, or alcoholism. It is rarely diagnosed during pregnancy.[69,70] The poor prognosis during pregnancy may result from delayed diagnosis or mild immunosuppression during pregnancy.

Screening high-risk patients with abdominal ultrasonography can detect HCC earlier.[69,72] The fibrolamellar variant of HCC, typically found in younger women, has a better prognosis. In addition, hepatic metastases from colon cancer can also occur during pregnancy.[5]

LIVER DISEASES SIGNIFICANTLY AFFECTED BY PREGNANCY

Hepatic Adenomas

Hepatic adenomas are benign hepatic tumors promoted by hyperestrogenemia. They are composed of large plates of adenoma cells, which are typically larger than ordinary hepatocytes. Pregnancy is associated with accelerated adenoma growth and consequent development of symptoms such as nausea, vomiting, and RUQ pain. Risks during pregnancy include adenoma hemorrhage or intraperitoneal rupture. On MRI, adenomas are typically well demarcated, hyperintense on T2-weighted images, and enhance further with gadolinium administration. **Hepatic adenomas that are symptomatic, larger than 5 cm in diameter, or exhibit evidence of hemorrhage should be considered for surgical excision before conception in women contemplating pregnancy, and they should be evaluated for possible excision if first diagnosed during pregnancy.**[73]

Acute Intermittent Porphyria

The porphyrias are rare diseases caused by deficiency of various heme biosynthetic enzymes that result in accumulation of toxic porphyrin precursors. Acute intermittent porphyria (AIP), the result of a porphobilinogen deaminase deficiency, is the most common hepatic porphyria and has a frequency of about 1 per 10,000 people. It is transmitted as an autosomal trait with incomplete penetrance[74] and is strongly affected by environmental factors, including female sex hormone levels. Women have more severe symptoms than men, and their symptoms are exacerbated by oral contraceptive administration, menstruation, and pregnancy.[74,75] About one third of female patients present initially during pregnancy or immediately postpartum. Hyperemesis gravidarum is a common precipitant. Diffuse abdominal pain is frequently seen, and other symptoms include vomiting, constipation, and neuropsychiatric abnormalities.[74] Autonomic abnormalities can cause tachycardia, hypertension, or ileus. Unlike other porphyrias, AIP lacks dermatologic manifestations. Attacks can recur during pregnancy.

AIP should be considered in any pregnant patient with abdominal pain and a puzzling diagnostic evaluation. Increased urinary levels of porphobilinogen and δ-aminolevulinic acid are diagnostic.[74] Management includes avoidance of precipitating drugs, avoidance of fasting, and possible administration of hematin or parenteral glucose.[74] Also, abdominal pain and nausea and vomiting should be treated with narcotic analgesics or phenothiazines. The maternal mortality is less than 10%, with a fetal mortality of 13% and frequent delivery of low-birthweight infants.[74,75] Genetic counseling is recommended.

Sickle Cell Hemoglobinopathies

The sickle cell hemoglobinopathies—including hemoglobin SS, hemoglobin SC, and hemoglobin S/β-thalassemia—are the most common hematologic disorders during pregnancy (see Chapter 44). They primarily occur in blacks. Patients with these hemoglobinopathies are prone to develop preeclampsia, eclampsia, or sickle cell crisis during pregnancy.[76,77] They can also exhibit ischemia and microinfarction of multiple organs including extremities, joints, and abdominal viscera,[77] and abdominal pain during a sickle cell crisis can be excruciating. Hemoglobin SS patients have an increased risk of acute cholecystitis during pregnancy.[41,77] Maternal mortality during pregnancy in patients with SS disease is almost 0.1% and comprises nearly six times the general maternal mortality.[77] These maternal hemoglobinopathies significantly increase fetal mortality.[76] Fetal complications related to compromised placental perfusion include IUGR, low birthweight, and preterm delivery.

Portal Hypertension

Pregnancy is uncommon in cirrhotic women because they frequently experience anovulation and amenorrhea secondary to abnormal estrogen and endocrine hormone metabolism.[78] However, patients with well-compensated early cirrhosis occasionally become pregnant. The plasma volume gradually increases during pregnancy to a maximum of about 40% above baseline.[79] The primary contributing factor is sodium retention mediated by increased serum aldosterone, estrogen, and renin levels, but water retention is a secondary factor.[79] Maternal cardiac output increases in proportion with the plasma volume. Portal pressure appears to physiologically increase during pregnancy as a result of these increases in plasma volume and cardiac output as well as from the increased vascular resistance due to external compression of the inferior vena cava by the gravid uterus. Pregnancy can, therefore, exacerbate preexisting portal hypertension with shunting of blood into portosystemic collaterals, particularly esophageal varices, which leads to increased intravariceal pressure and an associated increased risk of variceal hemorrhage. About 30% of pregnant patients with portal hypertension develop variceal hemorrhage, as do about 75% of pregnant patients with preexisting esophageal varices.[79] **The risk of variceal hemorrhage is highest during the second trimester, when portal hypertension peaks, and during labor, when venous collateral resistance abruptly increases from use of the Valsalva maneuver during pushing.**

Pregnancy has variable effects on the progression of cirrhosis. **About 25% of cirrhotics experience hepatic failure during pregnancy, whereas others have relatively stable hepatic function during pregnancy.**[80] Some treatments for specific liver diseases must be modified during pregnancy to avoid fetal toxicity. Maternal mortality in patients with cirrhosis may be as high as 10%.[78] Pregnant women with cirrhosis have worse pregnancy outcomes than other patients, with only about a 60% live birth rate.[81] Pregnant patients with more advanced cirrhosis have worse fetal outcomes.[81]

Portal hypertension without cirrhosis is usually due to portal vein obstruction or hepatic fibrosis. Fertility is much better preserved in portal hypertension without cirrhosis than with cirrhosis. Pregnant patients, therefore, more frequently have portal hypertension without cirrhosis than with cirrhosis. **Noncirrhotic patients with portal hypertension** have a much lower mortality from each episode of variceal hemorrhage than cirrhotic patients because of better preserved liver function, a lower incidence of coagulopathy or thrombocytopenia, and a much lower risk of hepatic failure precipitated by variceal hemorrhage.

Women with prior variceal hemorrhage or with borderline liver function who are contemplating pregnancy should be advised of the high risks of maternal hepatic

decompensation or variceal hemorrhage during pregnancy and of the relatively poor fetal prognosis. They should also be advised of the risk of transmitting genetic hepatic diseases, such as alpha-1 antitrypsin deficiency, or of transmitting hepatotropic viral infections, such as hepatitis B, to their offspring. **Women with well-compensated chronic liver disease without prior variceal hemorrhage should undergo EGD before conception for risk stratification.** Patients with silent esophageal varices are at high risk of variceal hemorrhage during pregnancy, whereas patients without esophageal varices are at low risk of this complication during pregnancy. Patients with esophageal varices should be informed of the benefits of β-adrenergic receptor antagonists during pregnancy to reduce portal pressure; however, they should also be advised of the fetal risks of these medications, which may include fetal bradycardia and growth restriction.

About 2.5% of cirrhotic patients experience splenic artery rupture during pregnancy. Pregnant patients with portal hypertension should undergo an ultrasound examination with Doppler studies of the upper abdomen to screen for splenic artery aneurysms at the time of their routine antenatal pelvic ultrasound. **Administration of iron is contraindicated in pregnant patients with hemochromatosis and is inadvisable in pregnant patients with several other types of chronic liver disease, such as chronic hepatitis C.** Routine serum parameters of liver function, including a coagulation profile, should be serially monitored during pregnancy. Variceal hemorrhage in pregnancy is managed the same as it would be in a nonpregnant patient: initial treatment includes endoscopic variceal banding or sclerotherapy, as described earlier; octreotide therapy is normally administered before the endoscopic therapy and is maintained for several days after endoscopic treatment in nonpregnant patients. Several cases of prolonged administration of octreotide for pituitary tumors have been reported in pregnant patients with good pregnancy outcomes.[82] Propranolol has been safely used during pregnancy to treat portal hypertension but may cause fetal problems as noted above. During parturition, the second stage of labor should be shortened to minimize portal hypertension. IV fluids should be administered cautiously to avoid volume overload, and any coagulopathy should be corrected to minimize the risk of intrapartum variceal hemorrhage.[79]

Budd-Chiari Syndrome

The *Budd-Chiari syndrome* **refers to hepatic vein thrombosis or occlusion that increases the hepatic sinusoidal pressure, and it can lead to portal hypertension or hepatic necrosis.**[83] Many cases are secondary to congenital vascular anomalies or hypercoagulopathies. This syndrome is rare in general and is consequently rare in pregnancy, although pregnancy tends to promote this disorder owing to a hypercoagulable state.[84,85] This syndrome usually presents in the last trimester or in the puerperium. The characteristic clinical triad is abdominal pain, hepatomegaly, and ascites.[84,85] Acute and chronic presentations occur. The serum bilirubin and alkaline phosphatase levels are typically moderately elevated with normal to mildly elevated serum aminotransferase levels. **This syndrome is diagnosed by pulsed Doppler ultrasound, hepatic venography, or magnetic resonance angiography** (MRA).[84-86] Without therapy, death usually occurs within a decade of diagnosis, and the **definitive therapy is liver transplantation.** Selective thrombolytic therapy and surgical or radiologic relief of portal hypertension for intractable

ascites or variceal bleeding have also been described.[84,85] Anticoagulant therapy is often administered long term during pregnancy to prevent further thrombotic events but is associated with a moderate risk of bleeding events, especially during delivery.[87] Maternal outcome is generally good, but about 30% of pregnancies result in fetal demise.[87] Patients have had subsequent successful pregnancies after undergoing liver transplantation for Budd-Chiari syndrome that presented during the puerperium.[86]

Pregnancy After Liver Transplantation

Although cirrhotic women are often infertile, women often regain fertility after successful liver transplantation for cirrhosis with restoration of liver function. **Immunosuppressive therapy should be maintained during pregnancy after liver transplantation.** Tacrolimus and azathioprine appear to be safe in pregnancy. Mycophenolate mofetil (MMF) should be stopped if possible before pregnancy (see Chapter 39). Pregnancy appears to be relatively well tolerated after liver transplantation provided the transplanted liver functions well before conception. Maternal complications during pregnancy include hypertension, preeclampsia, infections associated with immunosuppression, and occasionally acute hepatic rejection.[88] Chronic immunosuppression with prednisone may result in gestational diabetes. The fetal outcome is variable, with a large increase in fetal or neonatal mortality and a moderate increase in neonatal complications, particularly prematurity and low birthweight. However, about 70% of liveborn babies do well.[88]

LIVER DISEASE STRONGLY RELATED TO OR UNIQUE TO PREGNANCY

Alcoholism During Pregnancy

About 10% of woman drink heavily or binge drink during pregnancy.[89] Alcohol is a teratogen that causes central nervous system defects (see Chapter 8), and alcoholism during pregnancy can result in the fetal alcohol syndrome (FAS), characterized by facial abnormalities such as a smooth philtrum, growth restriction, and neurodevelopmental deficits. Heavy drinking of alcohol during the first trimester can cause major anatomic brain abnormalities, including reduced brain volume. Affected infants occasionally develop hepatic dysfunction manifested by hepatomegaly, fatty liver, or elevations of serum aminotransferase or alkaline phosphatase levels.[90]

Hepatic Involvement in Hyperemesis Gravidarum

About 15% of patients with hyperemesis gravidarum experience liver dysfunction. The most prominent abnormality is manifold elevations of the serum aminotransferase levels, but jaundice or pruritus may also occur.[91] The hepatic dysfunction may be related to dehydration, malnutrition, and electrolyte abnormalities. This dysfunction is typically mild and resolves with cessation of the vomiting and reversal of the underlying metabolic abnormalities (see Chapter 6).

Herpes Simplex Hepatitis

Herpes simplex hepatitis is uncommon during pregnancy. However, about half of all cases of this hepatitis in immunocompetent adults occur during pregnancy, possibly because of attenuated immunity. This hepatitis has a high mortality during

TABLE 47-3 CLINICAL PRESENTATION AND TREATMENT DURING PREGNANCY OF COMMON HEPATIC DISORDERS STRONGLY RELATED OR UNIQUE TO PREGNANCY

DISEASE OR DISORDER	SYMPTOMS AND SIGNS	LABORATORY FINDINGS	TREATMENT
Herpes simplex hepatitis	RUQ abdominal pain after prodrome of upper respiratory tract symptoms and pyrexia; oral or genital cutaneous vesicular eruptions	Highly elevated serum aminotransferase levels, moderately increased serum bilirubin; viral culture or histologic analysis of infected tissue is diagnostic	Acyclovir or similar antiviral drugs
Intrahepatic cholestasis of pregnancy	Intense pruritus, occasional anorexia and nausea	Modestly elevated serum bilirubin and alkaline phosphatase levels; moderately elevated serum aminotransferase levels; elevated total bile acid level is diagnostic	Ursodeoxycholic acid (also antihistamines, phenobarbitol, or cholestyramine); delivery rapidly and completely relieves cholestasis
Acute fatty liver of pregnancy	Anorexia, nausea and vomiting, malaise, fatigue, RUQ abdominal pain	Variable, mildly elevated LFTs; hepatic imaging excludes other disorders; test for LCHAD mutation; long-chain 3-hydroxyacyl metabolites accumulate; liver biopsy (usually unnecessary) shows microsteatosis in hepatocytes; DIC may occur in severely ill patients	Specific treatments for specific complications (e.g., blood products for DIC); prompt delivery should occur after maternal stabilization; patients rapidly improve after delivery

AST, aspartate aminotransferase; *CT,* computed tomography; *DIC,* disseminated intravascular coagulation; *LCHAD,* long-chain 3-hydroxyacyl coenzyme A dehydrogenase; *LFTs,* liver function tests; *RUQ,* right upper quadrant.

pregnancy due to a propensity for viral dissemination and delayed diagnosis.[92] Patients typically present with RUQ pain, very high serum aminotransferase levels, and mild to moderate hyperbilirubinemia after a brief viral prodrome with fever and upper respiratory tract symptoms. An oral or genital cutaneous vesicular eruption in association with highly elevated serum aminotransferase levels should suggest the diagnosis. The diagnosis may be confirmed by viral culture or histologic analysis of infected tissue. Unlike hepatic diseases such as AFLP or preeclampsia with liver disease, for which early delivery is often curative, early delivery is not recommended for herpes simplex hepatitis; rather acyclovir therapy is the treatment of choice. Table 47-3 summarizes the clinical presentation and treatment during pregnancy of herpes simplex hepatitis and other hepatic disorders strongly related to or unique to pregnancy.

Intrahepatic Cholestasis of Pregnancy

The incidence of intrahepatic cholestasis of pregnancy (ICP) ranges from about 2 per 10,000 in the United States to about 20 per 10,000 in Europe.[93] The cardinal symptom is pruritus due to cholestasis and accumulated bile salts in the dermis. The pruritus typically most severely affects the palms and soles of the feet, becomes worse at night, and begins in the third trimester. The pruritus can be intense and can cause psychologic distress. Patients occasionally experience anorexia, nausea, and vomiting. Proposed etiologic factors include genetic predisposition, as illustrated by the extremely high rate in the indigenous Araucanian people of Chile and by familial clustering; gestational hyperestrogenemia, as supported by the known cholestatic effect of estrogen; and abnormal progesterone metabolism, as supported by the cholestatic effects of sulfated progesterone metabolites.[79] This syndrome is sometimes related to defects in the multidrug resistance type 3 (MDR-3) gene that encodes for the canalicular phospholipid pump protein.[94] Aside from family history, risk factors include multiple gestations and occurrence of this syndrome during previous pregnancies. Patients have elevated fasting serum levels of total bile acids, particularly conjugated bile acids and especially cholic acid.[79,94,95] Patients typically exhibit hyperbilirubinemia that is mild and predominantly

conjugated; about 10% of patients develop jaundice. The serum level of alkaline phosphatase is modestly elevated, and the level of γ-glutamyl transpeptidase (GGTP) is normal. The serum aminotransferase levels are generally severalfold higher than normal,[94] but hepatic imaging studies reveal normal hepatic parenchyma and anatomy. Liver biopsy demonstrates bile staining of hepatocytes and bile plugs in biliary cannaliculi without necroinflammatory activity, findings consistent with cholestasis. The risk of gestational diabetes mellitus is also increased.

Ursodeoxycholic acid is the generally recommended therapy.[96] It tends to normalize the serum bile acid profile and decreases the pruritus by stimulating bile acid excretion.[97] Other treatments designed to ameliorate the pruritus and/or lower the serum bile acid concentration include hydroxyzine, an antihistamine, phenobarbitol, cholestyramine, and S-adenosyl methionine.[79]

Delivery results in rapid and complete relief of the cholestasis, and maternal outcome is usually good without long-term sequelae. However, the gestational cholestasis increases the risk of postpartum cholesterol cholelithiasis. **Vitamin K deficiency that results from mild steatorrhea, associated with the cholestasis itself or the cholestyramine therapy for the cholestasis, increases the risk of postpartum hemorrhage. The prothrombin time may be monitored during pregnancy, especially near parturition, and vitamin K can be administered as necessary.** ICP results in a significantly increased incidence of poor fetal outcomes such as meconium ileus, premature delivery, or stillbirth. Antepartum fetal testing with twice-weekly nonstress tests is a reasonable plan. In the absence of nonreassuring testing, consideration should be given for delivery at about 37 weeks' gestation.[98] Cholestasis recurs in approximately two thirds of subsequent pregnancies.

Acute Fatty Liver of Pregnancy

Acute fatty liver of pregnancy (AFLP) is a rare but severe disease characterized by hepatic microvesicular steatosis associated with mitochondrial dysfunction. It is related to an autosomally inherited mutation that causes deficiency of the long-chain 3-hydroxyacyl coenzyme A dehydrogenase (LCHAD), a fatty acid β-oxidation enzyme.[4] The most common mutation that leads to AFLP is the G1528C mutation.[99] This mutation leads to accumulation of hepatotoxic long-chain 3-hydroxyacyl metabolites produced by the fetus and placenta. It usually manifests in the third trimester and is rarely observed immediately postpartum.[83,100] AFLP occurs in about 1 per 10,000 pregnancies[2,3] and is more common in primiparas and twin pregnancies. About half of these patients exhibit signs of preeclampsia.[100-102]

The initial symptoms—including anorexia, nausea, emesis, malaise, fatigue, and headache—are nonspecific.[83,100] About half of the patients have epigastric or RUQ pain and about half have hypertension.[101,102] Physical examination may reveal hepatic tenderness, usually without hepatomegaly. Serum aminotransferase and bilirubin levels are variably elevated, and jaundice usually manifests later in the course of the illness or after delivery. **Characteristic laboratory findings in severely affected patients include a prolonged prothrombin time, hypofibrinogenemia, and increased serum levels of fibrin split products from DIC and/or hepatic decompensation. Other laboratory abnormalities include increased serum levels of ammonia, uric acid, blood urea nitrogen (BUN), and creatinine.**[83,101,102] Hepatic imaging studies primarily help to exclude other disorders or detect hepatic hemorrhage.[101]

Liver biopsy is usually diagnostic but is *not* indicated for suspected AFLP unless the presentation is atypical or postpartum jaundice is prolonged.[2,101] Hepatic pathology reveals intracytoplasmic microsteatosis in hepatocytes, preservation of hepatic architecture, and isolated foci of inflammatory and necrotic cells.[101,102] Sinusoidal deposition of fibrin is usually not present in AFLP but is usually observed in preeclampsia and eclampsia. **AFLP differs from severe acute viral hepatitis in that the serum aminotransferase levels in AFLP rarely exceed 1000 U/L, the viral serologic tests are negative, and hepatic pathologic analysis reveals much less inflammatory infiltration and hepatocytic necrosis.**[83,99,101,102] **AFLP may be difficult to distinguish from HELLP syndrome and preeclampsia or eclampsia with DIC.**

Fortunately, the definitive treatment for all these disorders is prompt delivery after maternal stabilization that may include a glucose infusion to treat hypoglycemia related to hepatic dysfunction, transfusion of fresh-frozen plasma or platelets as necessary to reverse coagulopathies, transfusion of packed erythrocytes to correct anemia from bleeding related to DIC, and administration of albumin to address the hypoalbuminemia from liver dysfunction. Other complications include pulmonary edema, pancreatitis, diabetes insipidus, seizures, coma, and hepatic failure manifested by jaundice, encephalopathy, ascites, or variceal bleeding.[101,102] The complications may require specific therapy: lactulose for hepatic encephalopathy, hemodialysis for renal failure, blood transfusions and endoscopic therapy for GI bleeding, and desmopressin for diabetes insipidus.

Most patients improve clinically within several days after delivery, and their liver function tests normalize. The maternal mortality is low with early diagnosis, appropriate supportive therapy, and early delivery. The fetal mortality of AFLP is 10% to 15%.[3,101,103] The mother, her partner, and the neonate should be tested for LCHAD mutations. Genetic testing is available for the G1528C mutation, but it is unavailable for the other, less common mutations.[104] **AFLP rarely recurs in subsequent pregnancies.**[101]

SUMMARY

Although relatively uncommon, hepatic, biliary, and pancreatic disorders during pregnancy are clinically important because of their potentially severe effects on the mother and fetus. These disorders are often complex, and such problems during pregnancy are clinically challenging. The differential diagnosis is particularly extensive during pregnancy because it includes pregnancy-related as well as unrelated conditions. The patient history, physical examination, laboratory data, and radiologic findings will usually provide the diagnosis. Abdominal ultrasound is generally the recommended radiologic imaging modality. Maternal and fetal survival have recently improved in many of these life-threatening conditions, such as liver disease during pregnancy, because of enhanced diagnostic technology, better maternal and fetal monitoring, earlier diagnosis, and more refined therapies.

KEY POINTS

- The differential of hepatobiliary conditions is extensive in pregnancy and includes pregnancy-related disorders in addition to disorders unrelated to pregnancy. Indeed, several clinical syndromes are unique to pregnancy, such as intrahepatic cholestasis of pregnancy and acute fatty liver of pregnancy.
- Pregnancy affects the normative values of serum parameters of liver function and pancreatic injury. During pregnancy, the serum level of albumin declines, and the serum levels of amylase, alkaline phosphatase, bile acids, cholesterol, and triglycerides rise. Yet these serum parameters are still clinically important measures of liver function and pancreatic injury during pregnancy, provided the changes in normative values are appreciated.
- Many causes of significant to severe liver dysfunction during pregnancy—including preeclampsia, eclampsia, HELLP syndrome, and AFLP—are rapidly relieved and completely reversed by delivery of the baby. Delivery is generally the definitive therapy for these disorders.
- Pregnancy aggravates preexisting portal hypertension and increases the risk of variceal hemorrhage. As in nonpregnant patients, endoscopic banding and sclerotherapy appear to be first-line therapies for esophageal variceal bleeding in pregnant patients.
- Pregnancy greatly aggravates acute hepatitis E infection, hepatocellular adenomas, acute intermittent porphyria, and herpes simplex hepatitis.
- Neonates born to mothers who have acute or chronic hepatitis B are at high risk of vertical transmission of infection during delivery. Such infants should be passively immunized with hepatitis B hyperimmune globulin and actively immunized with hepatitis B vaccine at birth to prevent this infection.

REFERENCES

1. Ch'ng CL, Morgan M, Hainsworth I, Kingham JG. Prospective study of liver dysfunction in pregnancy in Southwest Wales. *Gut.* 2002;51:876-880.
2. Knox TA, Olans LB. Liver disease in pregnancy. *N Engl J Med.* 1996;335:569-576.
3. Riely CA. Liver disease in the pregnant patient; American College of Gastroenterology. *Am J Gastroenterol.* 1999;94:1728-1732.
4. Cappell MS, Friedel D. Abdominal pain during pregnancy. *Gastroenterol Clin North Am.* 2003;32:1-58.
5. Cappell MS. Colon cancer during pregnancy. *Gastroenterol Clin North Am.* 2003;32:341-383.
6. Delgado I, Neubert R, Dudenhauseu JW. Changes in white blood cells during parturition in mothers and newborns. *Gynecol Obstet Invest.* 1994;38:227-235.
7. Stirling Y, Woolf L, North WR, et al. Haemostasis in normal pregnancy. *Thromb Haemost.* 1984;52:176-182.
8. Phelps RL, Metzger BE, Freinkel N. Carbohydrate metabolism in pregnancy. XVII. Diurnal profiles of plasma glucose, insulin, free fatty acids, triglycerides, cholesterol, and individual amino acids in late normal pregnancy. *Am J Obstet Gynecol.* 1981;140:730-736.
9. Bean WB, Cogswell R, Dexter M. Vascular changes of the skin in pregnancy: vascular spiders and palmar erythema. *Surg Obstet Gynecol.* 1949;88:739-752.
10. Bacq Y, Zarka O, Brechot JF, et al. Liver function tests in normal pregnancy: a prospective study of 103 pregnant women and 103 matched controls. *Hepatology.* 1996;23:1030-1034.
11. Knopp RH, Warth MR, Carrol CJ. Lipid metabolism in pregnancy. I. Changes in lipoprotein triglyceride and cholesterol in normal pregnancy and the effects of diabetes mellitus. *J Reprod Med.* 1973;10:95-101.
12. Goodwin TM. Hyperemesis gravidarum. *Clin Obstet Gynecol.* 1998;41(3):597-605.
13. Derchi LE, Serafini G, Gandolfo N, Gandolfo NG, Martinoli C. Ultrasound in gynecology. *Eur Radiol.* 2001;11:2137-2155.
14. Shellock FG, Crues JV. MR procedures: biologic effects, safety, and patient care. *Radiology.* 2004;232:635-652.
15. Osei EK, Faulkner K. Fetal doses from radiological examinations. *Br J Radiol.* 1999;72:773-780.
16. Toppenberg KS, Hill DA, Miller DP. Safety of radiographic imaging during pregnancy. *Am Fam Physician.* 1999;59:1813-1820.
17. Cappell MS. The fetal safety and clinical efficacy of GI endoscopy during pregnancy. *Gastroenterol Clin North Am.* 2003;32:123-179.
18. Dixon NP, Faddis DM, Silberman H. Aggressive management of cholecystitis during pregnancy. *Am J Surg.* 1987;154:292-294.
19. Friedel D, Stavropoulos S, Iqbal S, Cappell MS. Gastrointestinal endoscopy in the pregnant woman. *World J Gastrointest Endosc.* 2014;6(5):156-167.
20. Tang SJ, Mayo MJ, Rodriguez-Frias E, et al. Safety and utility of ERCP during pregnancy. *Gastrointest Endosc.* 2009;69(3):453-461.
21. Jamidar PA, Beck GJ, Hoffman BJ, et al. Endoscopic retrograde cholangiopancreatography in pregnancy. *Am J Gastroenterol.* 1995;90:1263-1267.
22. Date RS, Kaushal M, Ramesh A. A review of the management of gallstone disease and its complications in pregnancy. *Am J Surg.* 2008;196:599-608.
23. Pritchard JA. Changes in the blood volume during pregnancy and delivery. *Anesthesiology.* 1965;26:393-399.
24. Cappell MS, Colon VJ, Sidhom OA. A study of eight medical centers of the safety and clinical efficacy of esophagogastroduodenoscopy in 83 pregnant females with follow-up of fetal outcome with comparison control groups. *Am J Gastroenterol.* 1996;91:348-354.
25. Kochhar R, Kumar S, Goel RC, Sriram PV, Goenka MK, Singh K. Pregnancy and its outcome in patients with noncirrhotic portal hypertension. *Dig Dis Sci.* 1999;44:1356-1361.
26. Aggarwal N, Sawhney H, Vasishta K, Dhiman RK, Chawla Y. Noncirrhotic portal hypertension in pregnancy. *Int J Gynaecol Obstet.* 2001;72:1-7.
27. Eddy JJ, Gideonsen MD, Song JY, et al. Pancreatitis in pregnancy. *Obstet Gynecol.* 2008;112(5):1075-1081.
28. Pitchumoni CS, Yegneswaran B. Acute pancreatitis in pregnancy. *World J Gastroenterol.* 2009;15(45):5641-5646.
29. Laraki M, Harti A, Bouderka MA, Barrou H, Matar N, Benaguida M. Acute pancreatitis and pregnancy. *Rev Fr Gynecol Obstet.* 1993;88:514-516.
30. Ramin KD, Ramsey PS. Disease of the gallbladder and pancreas in pregnancy. *Obstet Gynecol Clin North Am.* 2001;28:571-580.
31. Lippi G, Albiero A, Salvagno GL, Scevarolli S, Franchi M, Guidi CC. Lipid and lipoprotein profile in physiologic pregnancy. *Clin Lab.* 2007;53:173-177.
32. Karsenti D, Bacq Y, Brechot JF, Mariotte N, Vol S, Tichet J. Serum amylase and lipase activities in normal pregnancy: a prospective case-control study. *Am J Gastroenterol.* 2001;96:697-699.
33. Briggs GG, Freeman RK, Yaffe SJ. Meperidine. In: *Drugs in pregnancy and lactation: a reference guide to fetal and neonatal risk.* Philadelphia: Lippincott Williams & Wilkins; 2005:999-1000.
34. Swisher SG, Schmit PJ, Hunt KK, et al. Biliary disease during pregnancy. *Am J Surg.* 1994;168(6):576-579.
35. Barthel JS, Chowdhury T, Miedema BW. Endoscopic sphincterotomy for the treatment of gallstone pancreatitis during pregnancy. *Surg Endosc.* 1998;12:394-399.
36. Legro RS, Laifer SA. First-trimester pancreatitis: maternal and neonatal outcome. *J Reprod Med.* 1995;40:689-695.
37. Badgett T, Feingold M. Total parenteral nutrition in pregnancy: case review and guidelines for calculating requirements. *J Matern Fetal Med.* 1997;6(4):215-217.
38. Van Bodegraven AA, Bohmer CJ, Manoliu RA, et al. Gallbladder contents and fasting gallbladder volumes during and after pregnancy. *Scand J Gastroenterol.* 1998;33:993-997.
39. Valdivieso V, Covarrubias C, Siegel F, Cruz F. Pregnancy and cholelithiasis: pathogenesis and natural course of gallstones diagnosed in early puerperium. *Hepatology.* 1993;17:1-4.
40. Ko CW, Beresford SA, Schulte SJ, Matsumoto AM, Lee SP. Incidence, natural history, and risk factors for biliary sludge and stones during pregnancy. *Hepatology.* 2005;41(2):359-365.
41. Davis A, Katz VL, Cox R. Gallbladder disease in pregnancy. *J Reprod Med.* 1995;40:759-762.
42. Ghumman E, Barry M, Grace PA. Management of gallstones in pregnancy. *Br J Surg.* 1997;84:1645-1650.
43. Date RS, Kaushai M, Ramesh A. A review of the management of gallstone disease and its complications in pregnancy. *Am J Surg.* 2008;196(4):599-608.
44. Glasgow RE, Visser BC, Harris HW, et al. Changing management of gallstone disease during pregnancy. *Surg Endosc.* 1998;12:241-246.
45. Dashe JS, Gilstrap LC 3rd. Antibiotic use in pregnancy. *Obstet Gynecol Clin North Am.* 1997;24:617-629.
46. Snady H. Endoscopic ultrasonography in benign pancreatic disease. *Surg Clin North Am.* 2001;81:329-344.
47. Jelin EB, Smink DS, Vernon AH, Brooks DC. Management of biliary tract disease during pregnancy: a decision analysis. *Surg Endosc.* 2008;22(1):54-60.
48. Wu DQ, Zhang LX, Wang QS, Tan WH, Hu SJ, Li PL. Choledochal cysts in pregnancy: case management and literature review. *World J Gastroenterol.* 2004;10(20):3065-3069.
49. Hewitt PM, Krige JE, Bornman PC, Terblanche J. Choledochal cyst in pregnancy: a therapeutic dilemma. *J Am Coll Surg.* 1995;181:237-240.
50. Nassar AH, Chakhtoura N, Martin D, Parra-Davila E, Sleeman D. Choledochal cysts diagnosed in pregnancy: a case report and review of treatment options. *J Matern Fetal Med.* 2001;10:363-365.
51. Elinav E, Ben-Dov IZ, Shapira Y, et al. Acute hepatitis A infection in pregnancy is associated with high rates of gestational complications and preterm labor. *Gastroenterology.* 2006;130:1129-1134.
52. Potthoff A, Rifai K, Wedemeyer H, Deterding K, Manns M, Strassburg C. Successful treatment of fulminant hepatitis B during pregnancy. *Z Gastroenterol.* 2009;47:667-670.
53. Kumar A, Beniwal M, Kar P, Sharma JB, Murthy NS. Hepatitis E: In pregnancy. *Int J Gynecol Obstet Surv.* 2005;60:7-8.
54. Kar P, Jilani N, Husain SA, et al. Does hepatitis E viral load and genotypes influence the final outcome of acute liver failure during pregnancy? *Am J Gastroenterol.* 2008;103(10):2495-2501.
55. Jonas MM. Hepatitis B and pregnancy: an underestimated issue. *Liver Int.* 2009;29(suppl 1):133-139.
56. Arevalo JA. Hepatitis B in pregnancy. *West J Med.* 1989;150:668-674.
57. Tong MJ, Thursby M, Rakela J, McPeak C, Edwards VM, Mosley JW. Studies on the maternal-infant transmission of the viruses which cause acute hepatitis. *Gastroenterology.* 1981;80:999-1004.
58. Vranckx R, Alisjahbana A, Meheus A. Hepatitis B virus vaccination and antenatal transmission of HBV markers to neonates. *J Viral Hepat.* 1999;6:135-139.

59. Shi Z, Yang Y, Li X, Schreiber A. Lamivudine in late pregnancy to interrupt in utero transmission of hepatitis B. *Obstet Gynecol.* 2010;116:147-159.

60. Trepo C, Chan HL, Lok A. Hepatitis B virus infection. *NEJM.* 2014;384:2053-2063.

61. Conte D, Fraquelli M, Prati D, Colucci A, Minola E. Prevalence and clinical course of chronic hepatitis C virus (HCV) infection and rate of HCV vertical transmission in a cohort of 15,250 pregnant women. *Hepatology.* 2000;31:751-755.

62. Su GL. Hepatitis C in pregnancy. *Curr Gastroenterol Rep.* 2005;7:45-49.

63. Webster DP, Klenerman P, Dusheiko GM. Hepatitis C. *Lancet.* 2015;385:1124-1135.

64. Walshe JM. The management of pregnancy in Wilson's disease treated with trientine. *Q J Med.* 1986;58:81-87.

65. Brewer GJ, Johnson VD, Dick RD, Hedera P, Fink JK, Kluin KJ. Treatment of Wilson's disease with zinc. XVII: treatment during pregnancy. *Hepatology.* 2000;31:364-370.

66. Aggarwal N, Chopra S, Sun V, Sikka P, Dhiman RK, Chawla Y. Pregnancy outcome in women with autoimmune hepatitis. *Arch Gynecol Obstet.* 2011;284(1):19-23.

67. Heneghan MA, Norris SM, O'Grady JG, Harrison PM, McFarlane IG. Management and outcome of pregnancy in autoimmune hepatitis. *Gut.* 2001;48:97-102.

68. Cobey FC, Salem RR. A review of liver masses in pregnancy and proposed algorithm for their diagnosis and management. *Am J Surg.* 2004;187:181-191.

69. Athanassiou AM, Craigo SD. Liver masses in pregnancy. *Semin Perinatol.* 1998;22:166-177.

70. Maged DA, Keating HJ 3rd. Noncystic liver mass in the pregnant patient. *South Med J.* 1990;83:51-53.

71. Kesby GJ. Pregnancy complicated by symptomatic adult polycystic liver disease. *Am J Obstet Gynecol.* 1998;179:266-267.

72. Entezami M, Hardt W, Ebert A, Runkel S, Becker R. Hepatocellular carcinoma as a rare cause of excessive rise in alpha-fetoprotein in pregnancy. *Zentralbl Gynakol.* 1999;121:503-505.

73. Wilson CH, Manas DM, French JJ. Laparoscopic liver resection for hepatic adenoma in pregnancy. *J Clin Gastroenterol.* 2011;45(9):828-833.

74. Jeans JB, Savik K, Gross CR, et al. Mortality in patients with acute intermittent porphyria requiring hospitalization: a United States case series. *Am J Med Genet.* 1996;65:269-273.

75. Milo R, Neuman M, Klein C, Caspi E, Arlazoroff A. Acute intermittent porphyria in pregnancy. *Obstet Gynecol.* 1989;73:450-452.

76. Smith JA, Espeland M, Bellevue R, Bonds D, Brown AK, Koshy M. Pregnancy in sickle cell disease: experience of the Cooperative Study of Sickle Cell Disease. *Obstet Gynecol.* 1996;87:199-204.

77. Villers MS, Jamison MG, de Castro LM, James AH. Morbidity associated with sickle cell disease in pregnancy. *Am J Obstet Gynecol.* 2008;199(2):125 e1-125 e5.

78. Joshi D, James A, Quaglia A, Westbrook RH, Heneghan MA. Liver disease in pregnancy. *Lancet.* 2010;375(9714):594-605.

79. Sandhu BS, Sanyal AJ. Pregnancy and liver disease. *Gastroenterol Clin North Am.* 2003;32:407-436.

80. Tan J, Surti B, Saab S. Pregnancy and cirrhosis. *Liver Transpl.* 2008;14(8):1081-1091.

81. Westbrook RH, Yeoman AD, O'Grady JG, Harrison PM, Devlin J, Heneghan MA. Model for end-stage liver disease score predicts outcome in cirrhotic patients during pregnancy. *Clin Gastroenterol Hepatol.* 2011;9:694-699.

82. Chandraharan E, Arulkumaran S. Pituitary and adrenal disorders complicating pregnancy. *Curr Opin Obstet Gynecol.* 2003;15:101-106.

83. Wolf JL. Liver disease in pregnancy. *Med Clin North Am.* 1996;80:1167-1187.

84. Singh V, Sinha SK, Nain CK, et al. Budd-Chiari syndrome: our experience of 71 patients. *J Gastroenterol Hepatol.* 2000;15:550-554.

85. Slakey DP, Klein AS, Venbrux AC, Cameron JL. Budd-Chiari syndrome: current management options. *Ann Surg.* 2001;233:522-527.

86. Salha O, Campbell DJ, Pollard S. Budd-Chiari syndrome in pregnancy treated by caesarean section and liver transplant. *Br J Obstet Gynaecol.* 1996;103:1254-1256.

87. Rautou PE, Angermayr B, Garcia-Pagan JC, et al. Pregnancy in women with known and treated Budd-Chiari syndrome: maternal and fetal outcomes. *J Hepatol.* 2009;51:47-54.

88. Nagy S, Bush MC, Berkowitz R, Fishbein TM, Gomez-Lubo V. Pregnancy outcome in liver transplant recipients. *Obstet Gynecol.* 2003;102(1):121-128.

89. *Morbidity and Mortality Weekly Report.* Alcohol Use and Binge Drinking Among Women of Childbearing Age: United States, 2006–2010. Available at <http://www.cdc.gov/mmwr/preview/mmwrhtml/mm6128a4.htm?s_cid=mm6128a4_e>.

90. Lefkowitch JH, Rushton AR, Feng-Chen KC. Hepatic fibrosis in fetal alcohol syndrome: pathologic similarities to adult alcoholic liver disease. *Gastroenterology.* 1983;85:951-957.

91. Abell TL, Riely CA. Hyperemesis gravidarum. *Gastroenterol Clin North Am.* 1992;21(4):835-849.

92. Kang AH, Graves CR. Herpes simplex hepatitis in pregnancy: a case report and review of the literature. *Obstet Gynecol Surv.* 1999;54:463-468.

93. Davidson KM. Intrahepatic cholestasis of pregnancy. *Semin Perinatol.* 1998;22:104-111.

94. Bacq Y, Sapey T, Brechot MC, Pierre F, Fignon A, Dubois F. Intrahepatic cholestasis of pregnancy: a French prospective study. *Hepatology.* 1997;26(2):358-364.

95. Heikkinen J. Serum bile acids in the early diagnosis of intrahepatic cholestasis of pregnancy. *Obstet Gynecol.* 1983;61:581-587.

96. Pathak B, Shaibani L, Lee RH. Cholestasis of pregnancy. *Obstet Gynecol Clin North Am.* 2010;37:269-282.

97. Kondrackiene J, Beurs U, Kupcinkas L. Efficacy and safety of ursodeoxycholic acid versus cholestyramine in intrahepatic cholestasis of pregnancy. *Gastroenterology.* 2005;129(3):894-901.

98. Rioseco AJ, Ivankovic MB, Manzur A, et al. Intrahepatic cholestasis of pregnancy: a retrospective case-control study of perinatal outcome. *Am J Obstet Gynecol.* 1994;170:890-895.

99. Rajasri AG, Srestha R, Mitchell J. Acute fatty liver of pregnancy (AFLP): an overview. *J Obstet Gynaecol.* 2007;27(3):237-240.

100. Monga M, Katz AR. Acute fatty liver in the second trimester. *Obstet Gynecol.* 1999;93:811-813.

101. Castro MA, Fassett MJ, Reynolds TB, et al. Reversible peripartum liver failure: a new perspective on the diagnosis, treatment, and cause of acute fatty liver of pregnancy, based on 28 consecutive cases. *Am J Obstet Gynecol.* 1999;181:389-395.

102. Mabie WC. Acute fatty liver of pregnancy. *Gastroenterol Clin North Am.* 1992;21:951-960.

103. Pereira SP, O'Donohue J, Wendon J, Williams R. Maternal and perinatal outcome in severe pregnancy-related liver disease. *Hepatology.* 1997;26:1258-1262.

104. Bellig LL. Maternal acute fatty liver of pregnancy and the associated risk for long-chain 3-hydroxyacyl-coenzyme a dehydrogenase (LCHAD) deficiency in infants. *Adv Neonatal Care.* 2004;4(1):26-32.

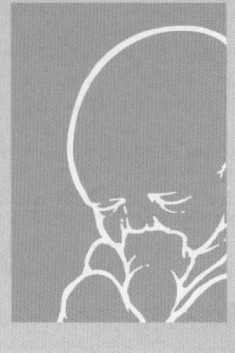

CHAPTER 48

Gastrointestinal Disorders During Pregnancy

MITCHELL S. CAPPELL

KEY ABBREVIATIONS

Carcinoembryonic antigen	CEA
Computed tomography	CT
Crohn disease	CD
Ectopic pregnancy	EP
Esophagogastroduodenoscopy	EGD
Gastroesophageal	GE
Gastroesophageal reflux disease	GERD
Human chorionic gonadotropin	hCG
Hyperemesis gravidarum	HG
Inflammatory bowel disease	IBD
Irritable bowel syndrome	IBS
Lower esophageal sphincter	LES
Magnetic resonance imaging	MRI
Nausea and vomiting of pregnancy	NVP
Nonsteroidal antiinflammatory drug	NSAID
Pelvic inflammatory disease	PID
Peptic ulcer disease	PUD
Small bowel obstruction	SBO
Ulcerative colitis	UC

Gastrointestinal (GI) complaints and disorders are common in women,[1] including in their childbearing years, and thus often occur during pregnancy. These complaints and disorders present unique clinical challenges during pregnancy. First, the differential diagnosis during pregnancy is extensive. Aside from GI disorders unrelated to pregnancy, their complaints may be caused by obstetric or gynecologic disorders related to pregnancy or other intraabdominal diseases incidental to pregnancy. Moreover, some GI conditions—such as hyperemesis gravidarum (HG)—are unique to pregnancy. Second, the clinical presentation and natural history of GI disorders can be altered during pregnancy, as described below for appendicitis. Third, the diagnostic evaluation may need to be altered because of pregnancy. For example, radiologic tests and invasive

examinations may raise concerns about their fetal safety during pregnancy. Fourth, the interests of both the mother and the fetus must be considered in therapeutic decisions during pregnancy. Usually, these interests do not conflict because what is good for the mother is generally good for the fetus. Sometimes, however, maternal therapy must be modified to substitute alternative but safer therapy because of concerns about drug teratogenicity (e.g., substituting a histamine 2 [H2]-receptor antagonist for misoprostol, an abortifacient that is contraindicated during pregnancy).[2,3] Rarely, the maternal and fetal interests are diametrically opposed, as in the use of chemotherapy for maternal cancer, a therapy that can be life-saving to the mother but life-threatening to the fetus.[4] These conflicts raise significant medical, legal, and ethical issues.

The obstetrician and gynecologist, as well as the gastroenterologist and surgeon, should be familiar with the medical and surgical GI conditions that can present in pregnancy and how these conditions affect and are affected by pregnancy. This chapter reviews GI symptoms and disorders during pregnancy with a focus on aspects of these disorders unique to pregnancy.

PHYSIOLOGIC EFFECTS OF PREGNANCY ON ABDOMINAL DISORDERS

Abdominal assessment during pregnancy is modified by displacement of abdominal viscera by the expanding gravid uterus. For example, the location of maximal abdominal pain and tenderness from acute appendicitis migrates superiorly and laterally as the appendix is displaced by the growing gravid uterus.[5] A rigid abdomen with rebound tenderness remains a valid indicator of peritonitis during pregnancy, but abdominal wall laxity and the interposition of the gravid uterus between the appendix and the anterior abdominal wall in late pregnancy may mask the classical signs of peritonitis.[6] An abdominal mass may be missed on physical examination because of an enlarged, gravid uterus.[4]

Many extraintestinal abdominal conditions or disorders are promoted by pregnancy. Mild hydronephrosis and hydroureter are common during pregnancy, particularly during the early third trimester, because of diminished muscle tone in the urinary tract from elevated progesterone levels and mechanical obstruction from uterine compression. Hydronephrosis in pregnancy is usually asymptomatic but can cause positional abdominal discomfort.[7] Mucosal immunity may be attenuated during pregnancy as part of the physiologic immunologic tolerance for the foreign fetal antigens.[8] This phenomenon, as well as urinary stasis during pregnancy, contributes to an increased rate of cystitis and pyelonephritis. Pregnancy also promotes cholelithiasis because of increased cholesterol synthesis and gallbladder hypomotility related to gestational hormones.

Pregnancy modifies GI physiology. Gastroesophageal reflux is promoted by gastric compression by the enlarged gravid uterus and by decreased lower esophageal sphincter tone due to increased serum progesterone and motilin levels during pregnancy. Pregnancy also increases the risk of aspiration of gastric contents for the same reasons, and gastric acid secretion may decrease as a result of increased progesterone levels. In addition, small bowel motility decreases during pregnancy.[9] Constipation is promoted by decreased intestinal motility, mild intestinal compression by the enlarged gravid uterus, and increased recumbence from bed rest during pregnancy. Physiologic nausea and vomiting of pregnancy (NVP) is described below.

Physiologic alterations of laboratory values during pregnancy include, among others, mild leukocytosis, physiologic anemia of pregnancy, mild dilutional hypoalbuminemia, mildly increased alkaline phosphatase level, and electrolyte changes, particularly mild hyponatremia (see Appendix 1, "Normal Values in Pregnancy").[5,10] The erythrocyte sedimentation rate is physiologically elevated and is a less reliable monitor of inflammatory activity during pregnancy.[11] Gestational hormones, particularly estrogen, contribute to a mild hypercoagulopathy by increasing the synthesis of clotting factors. Thromboembolic phenomena are also promoted by intraabdominal vascular stasis from vascular compression by the enlarged gravid uterus.

The fetus poorly tolerates maternal hypotension, hypovolemia, anemia, and hypoxia. This intolerance affects the type and timing of therapy for abdominal disorders during pregnancy. The gravid uterus can compress the inferior vena cava in the supine position and thereby compromise venous return, aggravating systemic hypoperfusion from hypovolemia or GI bleeding. Simply turning the patient to the left side to displace the uterus may relieve this compression, improve venous return, and normalize the blood pressure.[10] The heart rate increases by 10 to 15 beats/min during pregnancy, but the blood pressure normally declines modestly; therefore a rise in blood pressure during pregnancy may portend preeclampsia or eclampsia. Drugs that are normally safe and indicated in nonpregnant women must be evaluated in terms of fetal safety before administration during pregnancy.

DIFFERENTIAL DIAGNOSIS AND EVALUATION OF GASTROINTESTINAL SYMPTOMS DURING PREGNANCY

Physiologic changes during pregnancy may cause abdominal symptoms that include nausea, emesis, early satiety, bloating, pyrosis, and abdominal discomfort. Serious disorders that produce these symptoms may, therefore, be difficult to distinguish from physiologic changes during pregnancy. **Significant symptoms should not be dismissed as normal during**

BOX 48-1 DIFFERENTIAL DIAGNOSIS OF RIGHT LOWER QUADRANT ABDOMINAL PAIN

Gastrointestinal Disorders

Appendicitis
Crohn disease
Ruptured Meckel diverticulum
Intestinal intussusception
Cecal perforation
Colon cancer
Ischemic colitis
Irritable bowel syndrome

Renal Diseases

Nephrolithiasis
Cystitis
Pyelonephritis

Obstetric and Gynecologic Diseases

Ruptured ectopic pregnancy
Ovarian tumors
Ovarian cyst rupture
Ovarian torsion
Endometriosis
Uterine leiomyomas

Other

Trochanteric bursitis

---

pregnancy without a careful history, physical examination, and appropriate evaluation.

Occasionally, the pregnancy is not known by the patient or is not revealed to the physician, particularly in early pregnancy, when physical findings are absent. The physician should be vigilant for possible pregnancy in a fertile woman with abdominal symptoms, particularly in the setting of missed menses, because pregnancy affects the differential diagnosis, clinical evaluation, and mode of therapy. Pregnancy tests should be performed early in the evaluation of significant abdominal symptoms in this situation.

Abdominal Pain

The differential diagnosis of abdominal pain during pregnancy is extensive in that it includes obstetric conditions in addition to the usual GI and other intraabdominal conditions in the general population.[5] Abdominal discomfort without other symptoms or signs can be due to an enlarging uterus, fetal pressure against adjacent organs, and Braxton-Hicks uterine contractions associated with normal pregnancy. **The abdominal pain is typically localized to the abdominal quadrant in which the afflicted organ is located, as illustrated for pain in the right lower quadrant in** Box 48-1. This general rule has occasional exceptions in nonpregnant patients because of referred pain from nearby regions, but it has more frequent exceptions during pregnancy because of displacement of viscera by the growing gravid uterus and referred or poorly localized pain from obstetric conditions.

In the medical history, the pain intensity, nature, temporal pattern, radiation, exacerbating factors, and alleviating factors help narrow the differential diagnosis. Abdominal pain increases progressively in appendicitis but is nonprogressive in viral gastroenteritis. The pain from obstruction of the small

TABLE 48-1 COMMON CAUSES OF ACUTE, SEVERE ABDOMINAL PAIN DURING PREGNANCY: PAIN CHARACTERISTICS AND DIAGNOSTIC TESTS

CONDITION	LOCATION	CHARACTER	RADIATION	DIAGNOSTIC TESTS
Ruptured ectopic pregnancy	Lower abdomen or pelvis	Localized, severe	None	Serum β-hCG, abdominal ultrasound
Pelvic inflammatory disease	Lower abdomen or pelvis	Gradual in onset, localized	Flanks and thighs	Abdominal ultrasound
Appendicitis	First periumbilical, later RLQ (RUQ in late pregnancy)	Gradual in onset, becomes focal	Back or flank	Abdominal ultrasound in appropriate clinical setting
Acute cholecystitis	RUQ	Focal	Right scapula, shoulder or back	Abdominal ultrasound, serum liver function tests
Pancreatitis	Epigastric	Localized, boring	Middle of back	Serum lipase and amylase, abdominal ultrasound
Perforated peptic ulcer	Epigastric or RUQ	Burning, boring	Right back	Abdominal ultrasound, laparotomy
Urolithiasis	Abdomen or flanks	Varies from intermittent and aching to severe and unremitting	Groin	Urinalysis, abdominal ultrasound, and occasionally fluoroscopy with contrast urography

hCG, human chorionic gonadotropin *RLQ,* right lower quadrant; *RUQ,* right upper quadrant.

intestine may be intermittent but is severe, and renal and biliary colic also produce a waxing and waning intensity of pain. Acute cholecystitis is associated with RUQ pain as well as pain referred to the right shoulder. The pain of acute pancreatitis is often boring in quality, located in the abdominal midline, and radiates to the back. Careful physical examination of the abdomen that includes inspection, palpation, and auscultation can further pinpoint the etiology. Laboratory evaluation of significant abdominal pain routinely includes a complete blood count, serum electrolytes, and liver function tests and often includes a leukocyte differential, coagulation profile, and serum lipase determination. In evaluating the laboratory results, gestational changes in normative values, as mentioned earlier, must be considered. Radiologic tests may be extremely helpful diagnostically.

When the diagnosis is uncertain, close and vigilant monitoring by a surgical team with frequent abdominal examination and regular laboratory tests can often clarify the diagnosis. The character, severity, localization, or instigating factors of abdominal pain often change with time. For example, acute appendicitis typically changes from a dull, poorly localized, moderate pain to an intense and focal pain as the inflammation extends from the appendiceal wall to the surrounding peritoneum. The differential diagnosis of severe abdominal pain is described in Table 48-1.

GI causes of abdominal pain are discussed below under their individual headings in this chapter, and hepatobiliary causes are discussed in the prior chapter on hepatic disorders. Obstetric causes of abdominal pain are also prominent during pregnancy. **Ectopic pregnancy** (EP) classically presents with abdominopelvic pain and vaginal bleeding after a period of amenorrhea. The pain may initially be diffuse and vague but later becomes focal and severe. Physical signs include mild uteromegaly, cervical tenderness, and an adnexal mass. EP is often differentiated from a viable intrauterine pregnancy by serial beta–human chorionic gonadotropin (β-hCG) determinations,[12] but it is better differentiated from intrauterine pregnancy by transabdominal or transvaginal pelvic ultrasonography with simultaneous β-hCG determination.[13] Rupture of an ectopic pregnancy often presents with abdominal pain, rebound tenderness, and hypotension.[12]

In an **abdominal (heterotopic) pregnancy,** the abdominal pain is associated with signs of abdominal tenderness; a closed, noneffaced cervix; and a palpable mass distinct from the uterus.[5] Sonography and other radiologic modalities, as well as serial β-hCG determinations, are used to detect and localize the pregnancy. Abdominal pain is the most common symptom of heterotopic pregnancy. Abdominal ultrasound is sometimes diagnostic, but laparotomy may be required for the diagnosis.

The lower abdominal pain associated with **preterm labor** is characteristically associated with vaginal discharge or spotting. Back pain and vaginal pressure commonly occur. The diagnosis is made by cervical examination, either by transvaginal ultrasound or digitally. The abdominal pain from **spontaneous abortion**—whether threatened, incomplete, or complete—tends to be mild to moderate, crampy, and diffuse and is typically associated with vaginal bleeding. **Placenta previa** sometimes presents with abdominal pain or painful uterine contractions in late pregnancy. Vaginal hemorrhage is, however, the predominant symptom. Sonography is usually diagnostic.[13] Although **placental abruption** commonly causes abdominal pain, it is typically distinguished from GI disorders by the presence of vaginal bleeding. Patients typically exhibit uterine tenderness and frequent uterine contractions. **Uterine rupture** usually presents in laboring women with abnormal fetal heart rate recordings or fetal death, uterine tenderness, peritoneal irritation, hypotension, and vaginal bleeding.

Severe preeclampsia can present with right upper quadrant (RUQ) pain and elevated serum transaminase levels. Patients exhibit hypertension and proteinuria that starts after 20 weeks' gestation. Patients with **hemolysis, elevated liver enzymes, and low platelets (HELLP) syndrome** often have epigastric or RUQ pain. Patients have hemolysis with a microangiopathic peripheral blood smear, elevated liver transaminase levels, and thrombocytopenia. **Acute fatty liver of pregnancy (AFLP)** often presents with abdominal pain, nausea and vomiting, anorexia, and jaundice. Liver biopsy demonstrates intracytoplasmic microsteatosis in hepatocytes. The definitive treatment for these three pregnancy-related conditions of preeclampsia, HELLP syndrome, and AFLP is prompt delivery after maternal stabilization, provided that the fetus is sufficiently mature (see Chapters 31 and 47).

Choriocarcinoma, a malignant trophoblastic proliferation, typically presents with an abdominal mass and vaginal bleeding but may cause abdominal pain. The symptoms usually occur after term pregnancy, abortion, or incomplete evacuation of a hydatidiform mole. The diagnosis is suggested by persistently elevated β-hCG levels in the absence of pregnancy.

Gynecologic disorders are also in the differential of abdominal pain during pregnancy. The lower abdominal pain from pelvic inflammatory disease (PID) is typically associated with pyrexia and vaginal discharge.[14] Hemorrhagic infarction of large uterine leiomyomas (fibroids), called the *painful myoma syndrome,* is characterized by severe abdominal pain, nausea, emesis, pyrexia, and uterine bleeding. Ultrasonography or magnetic resonance imaging (MRI) is usually diagnostic. The abdominal pain of a tuboovarian abscess is frequently associated with a palpable lower abdominal mass, pyrexia, and leukocytosis. Patients often have risk factors such as prior pelvic surgery, assisted reproduction, or PID.[15] MRI or sonography is helpful in the diagnosis, but laparoscopy is often required for confirmation.

Adnexal torsion typically causes lower abdominal pain that is sharp and sudden in onset. Signs include unilateral lower quadrant tenderness, a palpable adnexal mass, cervical tenderness, or rebound tenderness from peritonitis. Ultrasonography, including duplex scanning, is valuable in the detection of adnexal masses, particularly cysts. The abdominal pain from early ovarian cancer tends to be vague and diffuse. Patients may also complain of abdominal distension and urinary frequency. Abdominal sonography is highly sensitive at mass detection but is insufficiently accurate at distinguishing malignant from benign ovarian lesions.[13] Surgery may be required to confirm the diagnosis and for definitive therapy.

The differential of abdominal pain during pregnancy also includes renal disorders. Symptoms from **cystitis** may include suprapubic discomfort without frank abdominal pain, but patients usually have urinary frequency, urgency, or dysuria.[16] The diagnosis is made by urinalysis and urine culture in the appropriate clinical setting. Symptoms from **acute pyelonephritis** include pyrexia, chills, nausea, emesis, and flank pain. The pain may radiate to the abdomen or pelvis and may cause costovertebral tenderness. Patients often have risk factors such as nephrolithiasis, recurrent lower urinary tract infections, diabetes mellitus, or congenital ureteral abnormalities.[8] The diagnosis is usually made by urine and blood cultures in the appropriate clinical setting. Renal ultrasound is performed in patients who fail to respond clinically within 3 days of instituting therapy or who have recurrent infection. The abdominal pain from **urolithiasis** typically radiates from the back or abdomen to the groin. Other symptoms include gross hematuria, nausea, emesis, urinary urgency, and urinary frequency.[17] Ultrasonography is the standard initial diagnostic test during pregnancy.[17]

Patients with **sickle cell hemoglobinopathies** that include hemoglobin SS, hemoglobin SC, and hemoglobin S/β-thalassemia are prone to sickle cell crises during pregnancy. Patients are usually black, and the abdominal pain in sickle cell crisis can be excruciating.

Upper Gastrointestinal Symptoms
Nausea and Vomiting
Nausea and vomiting during pregnancy is most commonly because of NVP or HG, idiopathic disorders without demonstrable mucosal or mural disease. The differential diagnosis of nausea and vomiting includes many other conditions (Box 48-2). NVP should be diagnosed only after exclusion of organic disorders by the history, physical findings, blood tests, and appropriate diagnostic studies. Misdiagnosis of nausea and vomiting as NVP, rather than more severe diseases, can be catastrophic. However, the great majority of nausea and vomiting during the first half of pregnancy is from NVP.

Dyspepsia or Pyrosis
The differential diagnosis of dyspepsia or pyrosis (heartburn) during pregnancy is listed in Box 48-3. **During pregnancy,**

BOX 48-2 DIFFERENTIAL DIAGNOSIS OF NAUSEA AND VOMITING DURING PREGNANCY

- Nausea and vomiting of pregnancy
- Hyperemesis gravidarum
- Pancreatitis
- Symptomatic cholelithiasis
- Viral hepatitis
- Peptic ulcer disease
- Gastric cancer
- Intestinal obstruction
- Intestinal pseudoobstruction
- Gastroparesis diabeticorum
- Gastritis
- Gastroesophageal reflux disease
- Acute pyelonephritis
- Drug toxicity
- Vagotomy
- Preeclampsia/eclampsia
- Acute fatty liver of pregnancy
- Hemolysis, elevated liver enzymes, and low platelets (HELLP syndrome)
- Anorexia nervosa/bulimia
- Other neuropsychiatric disorders

BOX 48-3 DIFFERENTIAL DIAGNOSIS OF DYSPEPSIA OR PYROSIS DURING PREGNANCY

- Gastroesophageal reflux disease
- Peptic ulcer disease
- Nausea and vomiting of pregnancy
- Hyperemesis gravidarum
- Pancreatitis
- Biliary colic
- Acute cholecystitis
- Viral hepatitis
- Appendicitis
- Acute fatty liver of pregnancy (in late pregnancy)
- Irritable bowel syndrome/nonulcer dyspepsia

---

gastroesophageal reflux disease (GERD) is extremely common,[18] **whereas peptic ulcer disease (PUD) is relatively uncommon.** The diagnosis of GERD, rather than PUD, is suggested by pain that radiates substernally, or pain exacerbated by drinking acidic citrus drinks, or recumbency. Symptoms include water brash or regurgitation of an excessive amount of acidic saliva and the presence of extraintestinal manifestations, including nocturnal asthma, hoarseness, laryngitis, or periodontal disease. Patients with dyspepsia or pyrosis during pregnancy can usually be managed symptomatically without undergoing diagnostic esophagogastroduodenoscopy (EGD), as discussed below.

Hematemesis
Upper GI bleeding is uncommon, but not rare, during pregnancy because pregnant patients are generally relatively young adults. NVP increases the risk of hemorrhage from a Mallory-Weiss tear, and decreased lower esophageal sphincter (LES) pressure and increased intragastric pressure during pregnancy promote gastroesophageal reflux that can cause hemorrhage. **The most common causes of GI hemorrhage during pregnancy are GERD, gastritis, Mallory-Weiss tears, and ulcers.**[19,20] Unusual causes include esophageal varices and gastric cancer. Patients with upper GI bleeding that causes hemodynamic instability are approached much the same as nonpregnant patients

but with a few exceptions. In the general population, the hematocrit is not a reliable indicator of the severity of bleeding because of the lag between blood loss and the decline in the hematocrit. **The hematocrit is an even less reliable indicator of bleeding severity during pregnancy because of the conflicting effects of intravascular fluid accumulation and increased erythrocyte mass during normal pregnancy.** Maternal blood pressure is not a reliable indicator of fetal well-being. Fluid, including transfusions of packed erythrocytes when indicated, should be aggressively administered to pregnant patients with acute GI bleeding because of the extraordinary fetal sensitivity to hypoperfusion, the difficulty in assessing volume status during pregnancy, and the usually satisfactory cardiac function of pregnant patients.

Dysphagia

The differential of dysphagia during pregnancy is similar to that in the general adult population, except that esophageal cancers are uncommon in these relatively young adults. Pregnant patients with acquired immunodeficiency syndrome (AIDS) can have dysphagia or painful swallowing, odynophagia, from esophageal candidiasis or esophageal lymphoma. Dysphagia from a peptic stricture is uncommon in pregnant patients, despite their high frequency of GERD, because their GERD is typically short term and moderate. Achalasia is a motility disorder that typically presents with a high resting LES pressure, failure of the LES to relax with swallowing, nonperistaltic esophageal muscle contractions, dysphagia, and weight loss.

Definitive therapy for severe dysphagia is best performed before, rather than during, pregnancy to assure adequate nutrition during gestation, a paramount concern for normal fetal development. Thus surgery for severe achalasia or other benign esophageal diseases should be performed before pregnancy.

Lower Gastrointestinal Symptoms

Diarrhea

The pathogenesis and differential diagnosis of diarrhea in pregnant women is similar to that in the nonpregnant population.[21] Acute diarrhea is usually caused by viral, bacterial, or parasitic enteropathogens. Viral agents, such as rotavirus and Norwalk virus, typically cause an acute self-limited diarrhea with upper GI symptoms and rare long-term sequelae. Bacterial causes of diarrhea include *Campylobacter, Shigella,* pathogenic *Escherichia coli,* and *Salmonella.* Pseudomembranous colitis from *Clostridium difficile* infection must be considered in the differential diagnosis when the diarrhea starts after antibiotic administration. Bacterial pathogens tend to produce frequent, small-volume stools, abdominal pain, and pyrexia. Inflammation of intestinal mucosa may produce fecal blood or leukocytes. Bacterial colitis is usually diagnosed by stool analysis and stool cultures. Pregnant patients with advanced human immunodeficiency virus (HIV) infection are prone to opportunistic enteric bacterial, fungal, parasitic, and viral infections, which often cause diarrhea. Noninfectious causes of diarrhea include medications, functional causes, food intolerances, and inflammatory bowel disease (IBD); in addition, hyperthyroidism can cause hyperdefecation. The initial management of severe acute diarrhea includes intravenous (IV) hydration, correction of electrolyte disorders, and consideration of discontinuing oral feedings. Stool studies include bacterial culture and sensitivity, ova and parasites, *C. difficile* toxin, and fecal leukocytes. Flexible sigmoidoscopy can be considered despite pregnancy for persistent refractory diarrhea if the stool studies are unrevealing. Reversal of nutritional deficiencies from profound acute or chronic diarrhea is especially important during pregnancy to maintain fetal well-being.

Constipation

Constipation is very common in pregnant women and affects up to one-fourth of this population.[22] Pregnancy tends to promote constipation from poor fluid intake due to nausea and vomiting, iron supplementation, decreased patient mobility, slowed GI transit predominantly from the effects of progesterone,[9] and GI compression by the enlarged gravid uterus.[21]

General measures can reverse these constipating factors during pregnancy. Adequate fluid intake and moderate exercise are important. Increased fiber intake—either by increasing dietary fiber, such as with wheat bran or psyllium husks, or by administering medications such as methylcellulose—is recommended to promote stool bulk and softness. Patients should be advised to defecate in the morning or after meals when colonic motor activity is stimulated via the gastrocolonic reflex. Sorbitol and lactulose, poorly absorbed sugars that cause an osmotic diarrhea, may be effective for constipation during pregnancy; however, they may cause abdominal bloating and flatulence. They should be used with caution in patients with diabetes, and they should be avoided in pregnant patients with nausea because they can exacerbate this symptom. Stimulant laxatives such as senna or bisacodyl may be considered in patients with severe constipation who fail to respond to conservative measures, bulk laxatives, or osmotic laxatives. **Laxatives to be avoided during pregnancy include castor oil, because it may initiate premature uterine contractions, and hypertonic saline laxatives such as phospho soda, because they promote sodium and water retention, which is inadvisable during pregnancy; in addition, they may cause renal failure in patients who are dehydrated or have preexisting renal insufficiency.**[21,23] Rarely, constipation is the first manifestation of severe GI disease during pregnancy.

Red Blood Per Rectum

Hemorrhoids are the most common cause of rectal bleeding during pregnancy. Other causes in the differential diagnosis include ulcerative colitis (UC), Crohn disease (CD), a rectal fissure, and infectious colitis as well as unusual diagnoses during pregnancy such as diverticular bleeding, bowel ischemia, or colon cancer.

DIAGNOSTIC TESTING DURING PREGNANCY

Radiologic Imaging

Fetal safety during diagnostic imaging is a concern for pregnant patients and pregnant medical personnel. **Ultrasonography is considered safe during pregnancy and is the preferred imaging modality for abdominal pain during pregnancy.**[13] Unfortunately, test sensitivity depends on operator technique, patient cooperation, and the patient's anatomy in that sensitivity is decreased by abdominal fat and intestinal gas (see Chapter 9).[13] MRI is preferable to computed tomography (CT) during pregnancy to avoid ionizing radiation, and gadolinium administration should be avoided if feasible during MRI in the first trimester.[24] Rapid-sequence MRI is preferable to conventional MRI because of briefer exposure. The patient should undergo counseling before diagnostic roentgenography.

Data concerning fetal malformations, growth restriction, and mortality from ionizing radiation are derived from past

TABLE 48-2	GENERAL PRINCIPLES REGARDING ABDOMINAL IMAGING TESTS DURING PREGNANCY
TEST	**SAFETY DURING PREGNANCY**
Abdominal ultrasound	Considered safe and is the preferred imaging modality during pregnancy; unfortunately, this test is less sensitive and less specific than other imaging modalities for many abdominal disorders
Magnetic resonance imaging	Considered safe; some avoid administering gadolinium, but no firm evidence of teratogenicity or other harm exists
Radiographs	Single radiographs entail a small but acceptable fetal risk; limit fetal radiation exposure by shielding, collimation, rapid-sequence studies, and modern x-ray equipment
Computed tomography	Consider magnetic resonance imaging as alternative when abdominal ultrasound is nondiagnostic. Computed tomography may be required in rare circumstances (e.g., to avoid surgery for possible but unproven appendicitis) and is safe if not repeated several times. Consult with a radiation physicist to minimize fetal radiation exposure

experience, particularly from survivors of the atomic bombs in Japan and the nuclear accident in Chernobyl. Radiation can cause chromosomal mutations and neurologic abnormalities, including mental retardation, and it moderately increases the risk of childhood leukemia.[25] Radiation dosage is the most important risk factor, but fetal age at exposure and proximity to the radiation source are also important factors (see Chapter 8). Diagnostic studies with the most radiation exposure, such as IV pyelography or barium enema, typically expose the fetus to less than 1 rad.[24] Thus one diagnostic fluoroscopic procedure is safe in pregnancy. In decisions regarding roentgenographic tests, the risks from radiation exposure must be weighed against the benefits of diagnosing a severe condition. Fetal radiation exposure should be minimized by fetal shielding, collimation, and rapid-sequence studies. Consultation with a radiation physicist may help reduce radiation exposure. Adverse fetal effects from iodinated contrast have not been reported, and these contrast materials can be used when indicated. The safety of radiologic abdominal imaging during pregnancy is briefly summarized in Table 48-2.

Endoscopy During Pregnancy

Endoscopy is often performed in the evaluation of abdominal symptoms in nonpregnant patients. Flexible sigmoidoscopy is used to evaluate minor lower GI complaints including rectal symptoms, whereas EGD is performed to evaluate epigastric pain, dyspepsia, or pyrosis. Although endoscopy is extremely safe in the general population, endoscopy during pregnancy raises the unique issue of fetal safety. Endoscopy could potentially cause fetal complications from the medications used, placental abruption or fetal trauma during endoscopic intubation, cardiac arrhythmias, systemic hypotension or hypertension, and transient hypoxia. The teratogenicity of medications is of particular concern in the first trimester during organogenesis.

Sigmoidoscopy seems to be relatively safe during pregnancy. No woman suffered endoscopic complications in a study of 46 patients undergoing sigmoidoscopy during pregnancy.[26] Excluding one unknown pregnancy outcome and four voluntary abortions, 38 of 41 pregnant women delivered healthy infants, including 27 at full term. Study patients did not have a worse outcome than pregnant controls matched for sigmoidoscopy

indications who did not undergo sigmoidoscopy in terms of mean infant Apgar scores at birth, the rates of fetal or neonatal demise, premature delivery, low birthweight, and delivery by cesarean section. Additionally, no endoscopic complications were reported in 13 flexible sigmoidoscopies during pregnancy analyzed by a mailed survey of 3300 gastroenterologists.[20] All pregnancies resulted in delivery of healthy infants at term.

These studies, in addition to scattered case reports, strongly suggest that sigmoidoscopy during pregnancy does not induce labor or cause congenital malformations and should be strongly considered in medically stable patients with clear indications. Sigmoidoscopy is not recommended during pregnancy for questionable indications, such as routine cancer screening or surveillance, which can be deferred until at least 6 weeks postpartum. Sigmoidoscopy should be performed with careful maternal monitoring that includes electrocardiography (ECG), blood pressure, and pulse oximetry after obstetric consultation and medical stabilization. Analgesic medication should be minimized during sigmoidoscopy, especially during the first trimester.

Data are currently limited on colonoscopy during pregnancy. The two largest studies comprised 20 and 8 pregnant patients.[26,27] In the study of 20 pregnant patients, 16 colonoscopies were performed during the second trimester. Excluding one successful therapeutic colonoscopy to decompress a severely dilated colon from colonic pseudoobstruction, colonoscopy was diagnostic in 10 of 19 cases, which included diagnoses of ulcerative, ischemic, Crohn, and lymphocytic colitis. Colonoscopy led to therapeutic changes in the management of seven patients, and two minor maternal procedural complications of mild transient hypotension occurred without clinical sequelae. Fetal outcomes were generally favorable: all infants were born healthy except for one spontaneous abortion and one infant born with congenital defects.

Colonoscopy should be considered, particularly during the second trimester, for very strong indications—such as suspected colon cancer—after obtaining informed consent that includes the theoretic but unsubstantiated fetal risks of colonoscopy. Colonoscopy should be considered questionable during the first trimester, even though at times it can be justified for extremely clear indications. A polyethylene glycol (PEG) balanced electrolyte solution is generally preferred over a sodium phosphate (Fleet phospho soda) solution to cleanse the colon for colonoscopy because sodium phosphate is associated with renal failure or electrolyte abnormalities in dehydrated or otherwise at-risk patients.[28] Colonoscopic tattooing of colonic lesions is performed using India ink or methylene blue in the nonpregnant population, but methylene blue should not be used during pregnancy because of potential fetotoxicity.

EGD is relatively safe for the fetus and the pregnant mother. In a case-controlled study[19] of 83 EGDs performed during pregnancy at a mean gestational age of 20 weeks, the indications for EGD included GI bleeding in 37, abdominal pain in 28, vomiting in 14, and other indications in 4. EGD did not cause any maternal complications and did not lead to labor. Excluding 6 voluntary abortions and 3 unknown pregnancy outcomes, 70 of 74 patients (95%) delivered healthy infants. In this study, the four adverse pregnancy outcomes—three stillbirths or deaths from severe prematurity and one involuntary abortion—occurred in high-risk pregnancies and were unrelated to EGD temporally or etiologically. No liveborn infant had any congenital malformation noted in the neonatal nursery. The pregnancy outcome in study patients included the mean Apgar scores at

1 and 5 minutes and the frequency of low birthweight, infant deaths, congenital defects, and delivery by cesarean section and was not statistically significantly different from the mean scores or rates in a group of 48 pregnant controls matched for EGD indications who did not undergo EGD because of their pregnancy. The two patient groups had similar pregnancy outcomes even though the study patients generally were sicker and had a stronger indication for EGD than the controls. This study and two other studies of 60 pregnant patients undergoing EGD during the first trimester[29] and of 30 pregnant patients undergoing EGD during pregnancy[30] suggest that EGD is at least as safe as not performing the procedure in pregnant patients with a strong indication for EGD. Similar results were noted in a report of 73 pregnant patients who underwent EGD, analyzed by a mailed survey of 3300 gastroenterologists.[20]

EGD is recommended during pregnancy for hemodynamically significant upper GI bleeding. It is rarely helpful, and rarely necessary, for nausea and vomiting or even HG during pregnancy. EGD is reserved for atypical situations, such as severe and refractory nausea and vomiting accompanied by significant abdominal pain, hematemesis, or signs of gastroduodenal obstruction. EGD is neither necessary nor indicated to evaluate typical symptoms of GERD during pregnancy and **should be reserved for cases when the presentation is atypical and severe, when the condition is refractory to intense pharmacologic therapy, when esophageal surgery is contemplated, and when complications such as GI bleeding or dysphagia supervene.** EGD is useful in diagnosing complicated PUD, including gastric outlet obstruction, malignant gastric ulcer, refractory ulcer, and persistently bleeding ulcer. EGD should be performed in relatively stable patients with ECG monitoring after obstetric consultation and after normalization of vital signs, which may require transfusion of packed erythrocytes and supplemental oxygenation. Fetal monitoring should be performed at a gestational age when intervention for nonreassuring fetal status would be considered. Informed consent is particularly important during pregnancy. The patient should be informed of the benefits and apparent safety of endoscopy, but she should also be cautioned that the potential fetal risks are incompletely characterized. **General measures to increase the risk/benefit ratio of endoscopy during pregnancy are listed in** Table 48-3.[31-34]

Video capsule endoscopy (VCE) is routinely used for recurrent GI bleeding after nondiagnostic EGD and colonoscopy. The most common serious complication of VCE in the general population is capsule retention.[35] Pregnancy may theoretically promote capsule retention because of displacement and impingement of bowel loops by the enlarged gravid uterus. Few data exist on VCE safety during pregnancy.[36] A review of the literature revealed only one case performed during pregnancy, in which VCE identified the bleeding site and "the patient and the fetus did well."[37] VCE is currently considered experimental during pregnancy but may be considered for recurrent, life-threatening GI hemorrhage after excluding upper GI and colonic etiologies.

Team Approach and Informed Consent

A team approach with consultation and referral helps optimize the management of complex diseases during pregnancy that affect both the mother and the fetus and that require disparate areas of expertise. The gastroenterologist contemplating endoscopy may consult with the obstetrician about the optimal timing for the procedure and with the anesthesiologist about analgesia during endoscopy. The internist may discuss with the radiologist the benefits versus risks of radiologic tests, and the radiologist may in turn consult with a physicist about methods to monitor and reduce fetal radiation exposure. The surgeon may consult with the obstetrician about the timing of abdominal surgery in relation to the pregnancy and about performing simultaneous cesarean delivery and abdominal surgery. These complex problems during pregnancy are best handled at a tertiary hospital, where the requisite experience and expertise is available. Pregnancy complicated by significant GI disease is best managed by an obstetrician who specializes in high-risk pregnancies.

The patient should be informed about the consequences to both herself and her fetus of diagnostic tests and therapy and should be actively involved in these medical decisions. Under the vigilant guidance of medical experts, the patient makes the decision with advice provided by her partner, family, and friends. When an intervention entails significant potential fetal risk, such as roentgenographic tests, a signed, witnessed, and informed consent is recommended even though this intervention would

TABLE 48-3	GENERAL PRINCIPLES TO IMPROVE THE RISK/BENEFIT RATIO OF GASTROINTESTINAL ENDOSCOPY DURING PREGNANCY
PRINCIPLE	**EXAMPLE**
Perform endoscopy only for strong indications	Colonoscopy for suspected colon cancer
Avoid endoscopy or defer it until delivery for weak or elective indications	Colonoscopy for routine colon cancer screening
Use the safest drugs (Food and Drug Administration category B preferable or at most category C) in the lowest possible dosages for sedation and analgesia	Propofol (category B) or fentanyl (category C) but not diazepam (category D) because of possible, albeit unlikely, association with congenital cleft palate
Consult an anesthesiologist regarding drug safety during pregnancy	Monitored anesthesia care (MAC) with anesthesiologist present during endoscopy
It is preferable to perform endoscopy in the second trimester, if possible, to avoid potential teratogenicity during fetal organogenesis in the first trimester and to avoid premature labor or adverse effects on the neonate after delivery in the third trimester	If possible, defer endoscopy during the first trimester until the second trimester, and defer endoscopy during the third trimester until after delivery.
Minimize procedure time	Performed by an experienced, expert endoscopist
Obstetric support should be available for a pregnancy-related procedure complication	Performed in an in-hospital endoscopy suite rather than a physician's office or ambulatory surgical center

Modified from Cappell MS. Endoscopy in pregnancy: risks versus benefits. *Nature Clin Pract Gastroenterol Hepatol.* 2005;2(9):376-377; Cappell MS. The fetal safety and clinical efficacy of gastrointestinal endoscopy during pregnancy. *Gastroenterol Clin North Am.* 2003;32:123-79; Cappell MS. Sedation and analgesia for gastrointestinal endoscopy during pregnancy. *Gastrointest Endosc Clin North Am.* 2006;16(1):1-31; and American Society for Gastrointestinal Endoscopy. ASGE guideline: guidelines for endoscopy in pregnant and lactating women. *Gastrointest Endosc.* 2005;61(3):357-362.

be routine and would not require consent in a nonpregnant patient.

GASTROINTESTINAL DISORDERS

Key differences during pregnancy in the clinical presentation, diagnosis, and therapy of GI disorders are summarized in Box 48-4.

Predominantly Upper Gastrointestinal Disorders

Nausea and Vomiting of Pregnancy and Hyperemesis Gravidarum

Nausea and vomiting occurs in more than 50% of pregnancies. It typically begins at about 5 weeks' gestation and abates by about 18 weeks. It has been called "morning sickness" but is more accurately called *nausea and vomiting of pregnancy* (NVP) or *emesis gravidarum* because it occurs throughout the day.[38] This condition should be viewed as a physiologic, rather than pathologic, process during early pregnancy because it is generally associated with favorable maternal and fetal outcomes (see Chapter 6). **Hyperemesis gravidarum (HG) is a severe, pathologic form of NVP characterized by a greater than 5% loss of prepregnancy weight and otherwise unexplained ketonuria.** The weight loss is paradoxic because patients normally gain weight during pregnancy.[39] HG occurs in only about 0.5% of pregnancies.[40]

The pathophysiology of HG is unknown but is believed to be multifactorial. Human chorionic gonadotropin (hCG) has been proposed as an etiologic factor because the serum hCG level peaks when HG is most severe, and the serum hCG level is higher in patients with HG than it is in other pregnant patients.[41] Other postulated etiologic factors include gestational hyperestrogenemia, gastric dysrhythmias, and hyperthyroidism.[40]

Patients with NVP have only mild to moderate symptoms, no weight loss, and lack evidence of dehydration, vitamin deficiencies, and other nutritional deficiencies. Aside from severe nausea and vomiting, symptoms of HG may include xerostomia, sialorrhea or ptyalism, and dysgeusia. Physical findings reflective of hypovolemia include dry mucous membranes, poor skin turgor, and orthostatic hypotension or hypotension. Serum electrolyte abnormalities include hyponatremia, hypocalcemia, and hypokalemia. Patients may demonstrate prerenal azotemia, and chronic vomiting of gastric contents may cause hypochloremic metabolic alkalosis. An increased hematocrit reflects hemoconcentration from hypovolemia. Patients with severe vomiting may develop abnormal liver function tests, particularly elevations of the serum aminotransferases. Patients may exhibit mild, transient hyperthyroidism that manifests as low thyroid-stimulating hormone (TSH) levels as a result of elevated serum hCG levels,[42] and inadequate nutrition may lead to vitamin or micronutrient deficiencies.

NVP and HG are diagnoses of exclusion arrived at only after excluding other conditions by appropriate tests. An abdominopelvic ultrasound is performed to exclude other causes of nausea and vomiting, as well as gestational trophoblastic disease and multiple gestation, conditions associated with HG. Patients with epigastric or RUQ pain should have determinations of serum liver function tests and serum lipase levels to rule out hepatobiliary and pancreatic disease. Patients with nausea and vomiting complicated by dysphagia or hematemesis may require EGD.

Risk factors for HG include a first pregnancy, multiple gestation, molar pregnancy, prior unsuccessful pregnancy, and prior HG.[39] Like NVP, HG typically begins early in pregnancy; severe vomiting that begins after the first trimester is unlikely from HG. In other pregnancy-related conditions that cause nausea and vomiting—including AFLP, preeclampsia, and HELLP syndrome—the nausea and vomiting typically begins in the second half of pregnancy.

Patients with mild nausea during pregnancy typically require counseling and reassurance without pharmacologic therapy. Patients with NVP often benefit from eating small, frequent meals to avoid gastric distension that may trigger nausea and from eating a bland diet that emphasizes salty crackers, soups, starches, and chicken while avoiding spicy, fatty, or fibrous foods.[40] Avoiding strenuous work and taking frequent naps may also be helpful. Patients with NVP associated with heartburn and regurgitation should be instructed about antireflux measures and diet and lifestyle modifications and should receive mild antireflux medications.

Patients with more severe NVP may benefit from drug therapy. Bendectin—which contains vitamin B_6 and doxylamine, an antihistamine—was once commonly administered for NVP but was withdrawn in 1983 due to unproven allegations of teratogenicity.[40] A subsequent meta-analysis reported no increase in the incidence of birth defects after in utero exposure to Bendectin.[43] **Vitamin B_6 (pyridoxine), a component of Bendectin, has been used by itself to treat mild-to-moderate NVP with some success.**[44] A delayed-release form of doxylamine-pyridoxine (Diclectin) is currently approved in the United States and Canada to treat NVP and should be the first-line pharmacotherapy. Dopamine antagonists, such as promethazine, or selective serotonin antagonists, such as ondansetron, have been used successfully and safely as antiemetics for these conditions.[45] Other therapies for HG include ginger, metoclopramide, and methylprednisone.

Therapy for HG is initially focused on aggressive IV rehydration and restoration of electrolyte deficiencies. Vitamins should be replaced, and thiamine should be administered before dextrose to prevent Wernicke encephalopathy. After IV repletion, the diet is gradually advanced as tolerated, initially to salty fluids and then to a bland diet. Nutritional consultation is recommended. Nasoenteral or nasogastric feedings are useful alternatives in patients who cannot tolerate oral feedings. Total parenteral nutrition (TPN) is rarely necessary. Patients should avoid environmental stimuli that trigger their nausea and vomiting. Patients should eat as soon as they feel hungry to avoid eating on an empty stomach, which can exacerbate nausea.

NVP is classically associated with a favorable pregnancy outcome, but in addition to the psychological stress in the expectant mother, it has been linked to possible physical and psychosocial disorders later in childhood.[46] The maternal and fetal prognosis of HG is relatively favorable provided that the nausea and vomiting are reversed, and the mother gains adequate weight during the remainder of the pregnancy.[47]

Gastroesophageal Reflux and Peptic Ulcer Disease

The incidence of pyrosis approaches 80% during pregnancy.[5] **The incidence of GERD is likewise high during pregnancy**[48] **and may relate to a hypotonic LES and delayed GI transit attributed to gestational hormones, especially progesterone, and gastric compression by the gravid uterus.** GERD manifests in pregnancy, as in nonpregnant patients, by pyrosis,

BOX 48-4 KEY DIFFERENCES DURING PREGNANCY IN THE CLINICAL PRESENTATION AND DIAGNOSIS OF GASTROINTESTINAL DISORDERS

Mallory-Weiss Tear

Much more common cause of upper GI bleeding during pregnancy due to mechanical trauma at the GE junction from nausea and vomiting of pregnancy or HG.

Nausea and Vomiting

Extremely common during pregnancy. Nausea begins at about 5 weeks' gestation and abates between 12 and 18 weeks and is related to elevated serum hCG levels during early pregnancy.

Hyperemesis Gravidarum

Severe form of nausea and vomiting during pregnancy characterized by a more than 5% loss of prepregnancy weight, serum electrolyte disorders, and ketonuria. This condition requires aggressive therapy.

Gastroesophageal Reflux

GE reflux is extremely common during pregnancy due to reduced LES tone due to gestational elevation of serum progesterone level and gastric compression by the enlarged gravid uterus. Although it may produce bothersome symptoms during pregnancy, serious complications of GE reflux are unusual during pregnancy.

Acute Appendicitis

Displacement of appendix by the enlarged gravid uterus during late pregnancy may cause the point of maximal abdominal pain and tenderness to migrate several centimeters superiorly and laterally from the McBurney point. Rate of appendiceal perforation from appendicitis is increased during pregnancy attributed to delayed diagnosis. Ultrasound is the imaging test of choice during pregnancy to diagnose appendicitis to avoid fetal exposure to ionizing radiation. Appendectomy may be performed during pregnancy but is safest during the second trimester.

Intestinal Obstruction

More common in third trimester because of mechanical effects of the enlarged gravid uterus, IO can occur during parturition because of mechanical effects of descent of the fetal head and abrupt decrease in uterine size. Despite pregnancy, supine and upright radiographs are necessary to diagnose and monitor IO. Unremitting, complete IO generally requires surgery despite pregnancy.

Intestinal Pseudoobstruction

Although risk of intestinal pseudoobstruction or adynamic ileus is increased after cesarean or vaginal delivery, this complication is still uncommon. It is generally managed medically without surgical intervention as in nonpregnant patients.

Colonic Pseudoobstruction

Despite limited clinical data, colonoscopy can be considered for colonic decompression when the only alternative is surgery, provided that colonic necrosis is not suspected. Parenteral neostigmine is often administered therapeutically in nonpregnant patients but may be contraindicated during pregnancy.

Colon Cancer

Uncommon during pregnancy because of younger age of pregnant patients, iron deficiency anemia is common during pregnancy due to increased gestational demands and is much less often associated with colon cancer in pregnant patients than it is in the elderly. Colon cancer diagnosed during pregnancy is often located in the rectum or sigmoid colon and frequently presents at an advanced pathologic stage, attributed to delayed diagnosis. Pregnant patients have a high incidence (25%) of ovarian metastases from colon cancer. Colonoscopy may be necessary during pregnancy before surgery for colon cancer to obtain a pathologic diagnosis and to exclude synchronous lesions. When cancer is diagnosed during the first half of pregnancy, cancer surgery should be promptly performed to minimize risk of metastases. Bilateral salpingo-oophorectomy is indicated for ovarian metastases.

Inflammatory Bowel Disease

Ulcerative colitis does not generally affect fertility, whereas Crohn disease mildly decreases fertility. Patients with inactive or mild inflammatory bowel disease at conception tend to have the same disease activity during pregnancy. Patients with active disease at conception can have active disease during pregnancy with an increased risk of poor fetal outcomes, especially for Crohn disease. Flexible sigmoidoscopy is generally well tolerated during pregnancy and can be used to help diagnose a disease flare. Corticosteroids, sulfasalazine, and 5-aminosalicylates can be administered during pregnancy. Azathioprine is classified as FDA class D during pregnancy, but gastroenterologists sometimes continue this medication during pregnancy to maintain remission. However, the TNF inhibitors infliximab, adalimumab, and certolizumab are apparently safer alternatives and are rated as FDA category B during pregnancy. Methotrexate is contraindicated during pregnancy.

Hemorrhoids

Hemorrhoids are extremely common during pregnancy due to vascular engorgement, vascular compression from the enlarging gravid uterus, and increased straining at defecation because of constipation. Medical therapy is generally recommended because hemorrhoidal symptoms usually resolve spontaneously soon after delivery.

Mesenteric Ischemia and Infarction

Risk of mesenteric ischemia is mildly increased during pregnancy due to mild hypercoagulability from hyperestrogenemia, but risk is still relatively low because mesenteric ischemia is predominantly a disease of the elderly.

Splenic Artery Rupture

Risk of splenic artery aneurysm rupture markedly increases during pregnancy due to estrogen weakening the elasticity of the arterial wall, but overall risk is still relatively low.

FDA, Food and Drug Administration; *GE,* gastroesophageal; *GI,* gastrointestinal; *hCG,* human chorionic gonadotropin; *HG,* hyperemesis gravidarum; *IO,* intestinal obstruction; *LES,* lower esophageal sphincter; *TNF,* tumor necrosis factor.

regurgitation, water brash, dyspepsia, hypersalivation, or, rarely, pulmonary symptoms. Symptoms may be exacerbated by ingesting certain foods, such as acidic drinks, or by recumbency. Complications of GERD include hemorrhagic esophagitis, dysphagia from reflux-induced esophageal stricture, and Barrett esophagus or adenocarcinoma. These complications generally relate to severe, long-standing, poorly controlled GERD. During pregnancy, GERD tends to be mild and of short duration, coincident with the pregnancy, so these complications are rare. EGD is the best test to diagnose reflux esophagitis. Characteristic findings are erosions, exudates, erythema, or ulcers just above the gastroesophageal (GE) junction. EGD can be performed during pregnancy if necessary but is generally reserved for complications from GERD such as GI hemorrhage or dysphagia.

Symptomatic peptic ulcer disease is uncommon during pregnancy, and antecedent PUD often improves during pregnancy.[49] **Nausea, emesis, dyspepsia, and anorexia are so frequent during pregnancy that PUD cannot be diagnosed solely by symptomatology during pregnancy.**[50] The most common cause of a duodenal ulcer is *Helicobacter pylori* infection. Nonsteroidal antiinflammatory drugs (NSAIDs), including aspirin, can cause gastric or duodenal ulcers. These ulcers more commonly present with GI bleeding than abdominal pain, possibly because of the analgesic properties of NSAIDs.[51]

Although the efficacy of modern acid-suppressive drugs has rendered lifestyle modifications less important in the nonpregnant patient with GERD or PUD, lifestyle modifications remain important in the pregnant patient because of concern about drug teratogenicity.[50,52] **Pregnant patients with GERD or PUD should avoid caffeine, alcohol, smoking cigarettes, and NSAID use, although acetaminophen is safe and the cyclooxygenase 2 (COX-2) inhibitors are less gastrotoxic than the nonselective NSAIDs.**[51] **Patients with GERD should elevate the head of their bed and avoid wearing tight belts. They should avoid recumbency after eating and discontinue oral intake 3 hours before bedtime.**

Antacids are generally safe for the fetus, although those that contain sodium bicarbonate should be used with caution throughout pregnancy because such antacids may cause fluid overload or metabolic alkalosis.[53] Antacids and dietary measures often suffice during the first trimester for minimally symptomatic disease.[2] Antacids must be administered frequently because of low potency, and frequent administration can cause diarrhea or constipation and electrolyte or mineral abnormalities. Orally administered sucralfate has minimal systemic absorption and is generally believed to be safe during pregnancy, but its aluminum content is of concern to the fetus in mothers with renal insufficiency.[54] Misoprostol can cause labor and cervical ripening.[3] H2-receptor antagonists are useful in treating GERD and PUD when symptoms are more severe or occur later in pregnancy.[2,54] Ranitidine and famotidine are preferable because nizatidine is possibly toxic to the fetus,[55] and cimetidine has antiandrogenic effects.[56] **Proton pump inhibitors were initially reserved for refractory, severe, or complicated GERD or PUD during pregnancy but have recently been increasingly used for moderate disease because of accumulating evidence of relative fetal safety.** Lansoprazole, rabeprazole, and pantoprazole (Food and Drug Administration [FDA] pregnancy category B) appear to be relatively safe and are therefore the recommended agents in this class during pregnancy.[57,58] Omeprazole is rated only as FDA category C during pregnancy, but a study

in 2001 that involved 863 infants exposed to omeprazole during the first trimester revealed rates of stillbirth and congenital malformations comparable to those of unexposed controls.[59] Metoclopramide is probably not teratogenic, but it can cause maternal side effects. **Drug therapy for *H. pylori* eradication should be deferred until after parturition and lactation because of concern about the fetal safety of antibiotics, such as clarithromycin and metronidazole.**[60]

Surgery for GERD is best performed either before or after pregnancy.[2,54] Endoscopic therapy is the initial intervention for bleeding from GERD or PUD,[32,49] but a hemodynamically unstable patient refractory to endoscopic therapy requires expeditious surgery, because the fetus poorly tolerates maternal hypotension.[61,62] Patients in advanced pregnancy should undergo cesarean delivery just before gastric surgery for GI bleeding.[61,62] Pregnant patients with PUD may also require surgery for gastric outlet obstruction, refractory ulcer, or a malignant ulcer.[63]

Diaphragmatic Rupture

In diaphragmatic rupture, abdominal contents herniate through a diaphragm weakened by congenital defects or abdominal or chest trauma. The risk of rupture is increased during pregnancy because of increased pressure on the diaphragm from recurrent vomiting during the first half of pregnancy, rapid growth of the gravid uterus during the second trimester, or the Valsalva (breath holding) and Kristeller (fundal pressure) maneuvers during labor. Even during pregnancy, diaphragmatic rupture is rare, but it is potentially catastrophic when it occurs during pregnancy, and both maternal and fetal mortality from bowel strangulation exceed 40%.[64] Increased intraabdominal pressure from the enlarged gravid uterus increases the risk. Herniorrhaphy is recommended during the first two trimesters for eventrated diaphragmatic hernia, even if asymptomatic, because of the high mortality without surgery.[64,65] Early recognition of eventrated or strangulated viscera is crucial to reduce mortality. Expectant management is advised for asymptomatic patients during the third trimester, followed by cesarean delivery and herniorrhaphy when the fetus is sufficiently mature. Cesarean delivery is the preferred route of delivery and avoids the increased abdominal pressure during active labor, which can cause bowel strangulation.[65]

Predominantly Lower Gastrointestinal Disorders

Acute Appendicitis

Acute appendicitis is the most common nonobstetric surgical emergency during pregnancy with an incidence of about 1 per 1000 pregnancies.[6,66] **Appendiceal obstruction, usually from an appendicolith, is the primary etiologic event, although stasis and other factors are also implicated. As the appendiceal lumen distends secondary to appendiceal obstruction, the patient initially experiences poorly localized periumbilical pain. Severe luminal distension, mural inflammation and edema, and bacterial translocation produce somatic pain that becomes severe and well localized at the McBurney point, which is located in the right lower quadrant one third of the way from the anterior superior iliac spine to the umbilicus. Displacement of the appendix by the gravid uterus during late pregnancy may cause the point of maximal abdominal pain and tenderness to migrate superiorly and laterally from the McBurney point, but this migration typically extends only a few centimeters away from the McBurney**

point during late pregnancy.[5] Rectal or pelvic tenderness may occur in early pregnancy but is unusual in late pregnancy as the appendix migrates from its pelvic location. Other clinical findings include anorexia, nausea, emesis, pyrexia, tachycardia, and abdominal tenderness.[67] Periappendiceal inflammation or peritonitis causes involuntary guarding and rebound tenderness. Involuntary guarding and rebound tenderness are less reliable signs of peritonitis in late pregnancy because of abdominal wall laxity and elevation of the anterior abdominal wall away from the inflamed appendix by the growing gravid uterus.[6] Patients may have significant leukocytosis and neutrophilia in the leukocyte differential.[68]

Radiologic imaging is indicated to reduce the incidence of negative appendectomy when the diagnosis is suspected but remains ambiguous after routine laboratory studies. Although CT is the preferred imaging test in nonpregnant patients because of its high diagnostic accuracy, **sonography is the initial imaging test of choice during pregnancy** to avoid fetal exposure to radiation from CT. In a comprehensive review, ultrasound was 86% sensitive and 81% specific in the diagnosis of appendicitis in adults or adolescents.[69] Diagnostic findings include appendiceal mural thickening, periappendiceal fluid, and a noncompressible tubular structure 6 mm or more in diameter that is closed at one end and open at the other. **Appendicitis cannot be excluded if the appendix is not visualized on ultrasound.** Ultrasound can also help exclude other pathology, such as an adnexal mass.[13] Factors associated with diminished test sensitivity include maternal obesity, the third trimester of pregnancy, and an inexperienced radiologist.

MRI is the appropriate next test in the pregnant patient if the abdominal ultrasound is inconclusive. In a study of 148 pregnant women with suspected appendicitis during pregnancy, MRI was 100% sensitive and 93% specific for the diagnosis of acute appendicitis.[70] CT can be performed with modifications to limit fetal radiation exposure to less than 300 mrad if MRI is unavailable. Abnormal CT findings with appendicitis include right lower quadrant inflammation; a nonfilling, enlarged tubular structure; and an appendicolith.

Up to one quarter of pregnant women with appendicitis develop an appendiceal perforation.[5] This high rate is attributed to delayed diagnosis during pregnancy. The diagnosis may be missed in pregnant patients for a number of reasons: (1) leukocytosis, a classic sign of acute appendicitis, occurs physiologically during pregnancy; (2) nausea and emesis, common symptoms of acute appendicitis, are also common during pregnancy; and (3) the abdominal pain is sometimes atypically located.[68] Other diseases are often confused with appendicitis. The differential diagnosis of appendicitis in pregnancy is shown in Box 48-5. Appendiceal displacement predisposes to rapid development of generalized peritonitis after perforation because the omentum is not nearby to contain the infection.

Appendicitis during pregnancy mandates prompt appendectomy after IV hydration and correction of electrolyte abnormalities. Appendectomy is safer for the fetus during the second trimester than during the first trimester.[71] Antibiotics are generally administered for uncomplicated appendicitis and are absolutely required for appendicitis complicated by perforation, abscess, or peritonitis.[5] Cephalosporins, clindamycin, gentamicin, and penicillins including ampicillin/sulbactam are considered safe during gestation.[5] Clindamycin is preferred over metronidazole for anaerobic coverage, even though both are category B drugs in pregnancy.[60] Clindamycin/gentamicin is a

relatively inexpensive, effective, and safe antibiotic combination; quinolones are not recommended. **Laparoscopy should be considered during the first two trimesters or even later by experienced operators for nonperforated appendicitis or when the diagnosis is uncertain.[72]** Appendectomy is recommended even if appendicitis is not evident at surgery.[67,68] Maternal mortality from appendicitis is about 0.1% without appendiceal perforation, but with perforation, mortality exceeds 4%.[66] Fetal mortality is about 2% without perforation but exceeds 30% with appendiceal perforation.[66]

Intestinal Obstruction

Acute intestinal obstruction is the second most common nonobstetric abdominal emergency with an incidence of 1 per 2500 pregnancies.[73-75] It may be incidental or secondary to pregnancy, and obstruction more commonly occurs in the third trimester because of the mechanical effects of the enlarged gravid uterus.[76] In particular, some cases occur at term because of the mechanical effects from descent of the fetal head and the abrupt decrease in uterine size at delivery.[73,74] Adhesions, particularly from prior gynecologic surgery or appendectomy, cause 60% to 70% of small bowel obstruction (SBO) during pregnancy.[74,77] Other causes of SBO include neoplasms, particularly ovarian, endometrial, or cervical malignancies; CD; external or internal

---

BOX 48-5 DIFFERENTIAL DIAGNOSIS OF APPENDICITIS DURING PREGNANCY

Gynecologic Conditions

Ruptured ovarian cyst
Adnexal torsion
Pelvic inflammatory disease or salpingitis
Endometriosis
Ovarian cancer

Obstetric Causes

Placental abruption
Chorioamnionitis
Endometritis
Uterine fibroid degeneration
Labor (preterm or term)
Viscus perforation after abortion
Ruptured ectopic pregnancy

Gastrointestinal Causes

Crohn disease
Colonic diverticulitis (right side)
Cholecystitis
Pancreatitis
Mesenteric lymphadenitis
Gastroenteritis
Colon cancer
Intestinal obstruction
Hernia (incarcerated inguinal or internal)
Colonic intussusception
Ruptured Meckel diverticulum
Colonic perforation
Acute mesenteric ischemia

Other Causes

Pyelonephritis
Urolithiasis

hernias; volvulus; and intussusception.[73,74] Rare causes of SBO include ectopic pregnancy; prior radiotherapy; and intraluminal gallstones, fecoliths, or other concretions. Colonic obstruction can be caused by adhesions, colon cancer, other neoplasms, diverticulitis, and volvulus.[73,74]

Intestinal obstruction classically presents with a symptomatic triad of abdominal pain, emesis, and obstipation.[73,74] The pain may be constant or periodic. SBO is more painful than colonic obstruction, and the pain with SBO may be diffuse and poorly localized and may radiate to the back, flanks, or perineum.[78] Abdominal pain is milder with volvulus and intussusception. Intestinal malrotation may produce nonspecific symptoms of mild, crampy abdominal pain and nonbilious emesis.[79] Intestinal strangulation with compromised bowel perfusion may be heralded by abdominal guarding and rebound tenderness. Emesis occurs more frequently and earlier in SBO than in colonic obstruction.[73,74] Constipation from complete intestinal obstruction is usually severe and unremitting and is associated with abdominal pain.[74] The abdomen is typically distended and tympanitic to percussion because of an inability to defecate or pass flatus. Bowel sounds are high-pitched, hypoactive, and tinkling in early intestinal obstruction and become absent in late obstruction.

The approach to intestinal obstruction is the same in pregnancy as in the general population except that decisions are more urgently required because both the fetus and the mother are at risk. Fetal exposure to radiation is a concern, but supine and upright abdominal radiographs are needed to diagnose and monitor intestinal obstruction.[74] The diagnosis is strongly suggested by radiographic findings of distended bowel loops that contain air-fluid levels, particularly with differential air-fluid levels. An abrupt transition between distended and nondistended bowel favors the diagnosis of intestinal obstruction over intestinal pseudoobstruction. Volvulus is suspected when a single bowel loop is grossly dilated.

Surgery is recommended for unremitting and complete intestinal obstruction, whereas medical management is recommended for intermittent or partial obstruction.[73] Parenteral fluids are aggressively administered in all patients with intestinal obstruction to reverse the fluid and electrolyte deficits caused by emesis and fluid sequestration but are particularly important during pregnancy to sustain uterine perfusion. Nasogastric suction helps decompress the bowel. Maternal mortality is about 5%, and fetal mortality ranges from 20% to 30%.[73,77] Morbidity and mortality from intestinal obstruction are increased by delayed diagnosis.

Intestinal Pseudoobstruction

Intestinal pseudoobstruction, adynamic ileus, is characterized by severe abdominal distension detected on physical examination and diffuse intestinal dilatation noted on abdominal roentgenogram. Patients may also present with diffuse abdominal pain and hypoperistalsis on abdominal auscultation. Intestinal pseudoobstruction is diagnosed only after exclusion of mechanical intestinal obstruction by the clinical presentation, laboratory studies, and early clinical evolution. Patients with mechanical obstruction tend to be much sicker than those with pseudoobstruction for the same degree of intestinal dilatation as detected by abdominal imaging and tend to progress more rapidly. **Intestinal pseudoobstruction is a well-described but uncommon complication of cesarean or vaginal delivery.**[80,81] **Patients with pseudoobstruction have**

nausea, emesis, obstipation, and diffuse abdominal pain that typically evolves over several days.**[80] Patients often have hypoperistalsis, whereas pyrexia, leukocytosis, and increasing abdominal tenderness may herald GI ischemia. **Treatment includes nasogastric aspiration, parenteral fluid administration, repletion of electrolytes, and rectal tube decompression. The pseudoobstruction usually spontaneously resolves.**[80]

Therapeutic options for severe colonic pseudoobstruction (Ogilvie syndrome), manifested by a cecal diameter greater than 10 cm on abdominal roentgenogram, include colonoscopic decompression or surgical therapies such as cecostomy, cecectomy with diverting ileostomy, or colonic resection when intestinal necrosis supervenes.[82] Colonoscopy can be considered for colonic pseudoobstruction during the second trimester of pregnancy when the only alternative is surgery.[27] Parenteral neostigmine is often administered for colonic pseudoobstruction in nonpregnant patients but may be contraindicated during pregnancy.[80] Mortality approaches 10% with impending perforation but reaches 70% after cecal perforation.[82]

Colon Cancer

Colon cancer is uncommon during pregnancy with an estimated incidence of 1 per 13,000 to 1 per 50,000 pregnancies (see Chapter 49).[4,83] With approximately 4 million pregnancies annually in the United States, these incidence estimates translate into 80 to 300 colon cancers during pregnancy each year.

The clinical presentation and evaluation of colon cancer in pregnant patients is similar to that in other patients, with notable exceptions. **Common symptoms of colon cancer in pregnant patients include abdominal pain, rectal bleeding, nausea and vomiting, and abdominal distension.**[4,84] **However, colon cancer tends not to produce signs until it has advanced.** About one fifth of colon cancers occur in the rectum in the general population, whereas about two thirds of colon cancers occur in the rectum during pregnancy.[85] This shift during pregnancy may be an artifact due to increased self-referral resulting from increased patient attention to rectal symptoms because of rectal compression by the gravid uterus or from increased physician detection due to frequent pelvic and rectal examinations during pregnancy.[4] Rectal examination is essential in the evaluation of suspected colon cancer during pregnancy because this cancer often arises in the rectum during pregnancy and may then be palpable by digital rectal exam. Stool should be tested for the presence of occult blood. The finding of occult blood has a low positive predictive value for colon cancer or adenomas during pregnancy because of the low disease prevalence in this rather young patient population. Iron deficiency anemia is common during pregnancy due to increased gestational demands. Iron deficiency anemia, therefore, is not nearly as strongly associated with colon cancer in the pregnant patient as it is in the elderly patient.[4] Patients who present with colon cancer during pregnancy are relatively young and may therefore have predisposing factors, including hereditary nonpolyposis colon cancer (HNPCC), familial polyposis coli, Peutz-Jeghers syndrome, and longstanding IBD.[86]

During pregnancy, colon cancer often presents at an advanced pathologic stage attributed to delayed diagnosis.[85] Advanced pathologic stage is highly correlated with a poor prognosis. The incidence of ovarian metastases from colon cancer in women is only about 5% but increases to about 25% in women younger than 40 years.[87] Pregnant patients are typically younger than 40 years and seem to have a similarly high incidence of ovarian metastases.[4] Although abdominal CT is the imaging modality of choice for detection of hepatic metastases from colon cancer in the general population, CT is relatively contraindicated during pregnancy, and abdominal ultrasound is substituted for hepatic evaluation. This test is highly sensitive for metastatic lesions over 2 cm in diameter but is poorly sensitive for metastatic lesions less than 1 cm in diameter. Hepatic metastases typically produce discrete echogenic masses, and MRI may be required to detect small hepatic metastases.[88] Complete colonoscopy is indicated preoperatively in nonpregnant patients for pathologic diagnosis and for excluding synchronous colonic lesions. Colonoscopy may, therefore, be necessary during pregnancy before colon cancer surgery for the same reasons. Colonoscopy may be technically difficult during late pregnancy because of colonic compression by the uterus. If the gestation is advanced, and the fetus is viable, it may be preferable to induce labor and then perform colonoscopy and cancer surgery.

Surgery is the primary curative therapy for colon cancer. In the absence of distant metastases, the primary tumor is resected with wide surgical margins at least 5 cm beyond the edge of gross tumor together with resection of regional mesenteric lymph nodes. In the presence of widespread distant metastases, only palliative surgery is considered. The timing and type of surgery during pregnancy depends on gestational age, maternal prognosis, and intraoperative findings as well as maternal desires. **When the cancer is diagnosed during the first half of pregnancy, cancer surgery should be promptly performed to minimize the risk of metastases.**[4] Such surgery can often be performed without removing the gravid uterus and disturbing the pregnancy.[85] Total abdominal hysterectomy is recommended to facilitate access to the rectum when needed for intraoperative exposure, when the mother's life expectancy is less than the time needed for the fetus to become viable, or when the cancer extends into the uterus. Otherwise, when the cancer appears resectable, curative surgery should be performed leaving the pregnancy intact.[4] **When the cancer is diagnosed during the second half of pregnancy, cancer surgery should ideally be delayed until but not beyond the time that good neonatal outcome is normally expected—at about 32 weeks' gestation—because further delay permits cancer growth and metastasis.**[84] Bilateral salpingo-oophorectomy is indicated for ovarian metastases. Colon cancer surgery is associated with a moderately increased, but still acceptable, rate of fetal death but is associated with a high risk of preterm delivery and low birthweight.[89] Serum carcinoembryonic antigen (CEA) levels obtained before surgery provide a baseline to monitor response to surgery and chemotherapy. Pregnancy does not significantly alter the serum CEA level.[90]

Pregnant patients considering adjuvant chemotherapy should be counseled about the potential fetal risks as well as the potential maternal benefits. Chemotherapy is generally contraindicated during the first trimester and should be restricted during this trimester to patients with Dukes stage C cancer who accept a significant teratogenic risk after informed and written consent. Chemotherapy is much less teratogenic during the second and third trimesters, after organogenesis is completed. Patients who refused preoperative chemotherapy during the first trimester because of fetal teratogenicity should consider receiving postoperative chemotherapy during the second trimester when the risk is reduced. Although pelvic radiotherapy is often performed for rectal cancer with local extramural extension, this therapy is perilous to the fetus and is contraindicated during pregnancy. Radiotherapy is possible only after delivery or termination of pregnancy.

Patients younger than 40 years generally have a poor prognosis from colon cancer, attributed to delayed diagnosis and advanced pathologic stage at diagnosis.[91] Likewise, when diagnosed during pregnancy, the maternal prognosis from colon cancer—whether colonic or rectal—is poor. Fetal prognosis depends on the pathologic stage of the maternal cancer, gestational age at diagnosis, and type and timing of therapy. Fetal viability is endangered by severe maternal debility and malnourishment from advanced cancer because the fetus depends upon maternal homeostasis and nutrition for normal development. A few healthy infants have been born after colorectal cancer surgery, including abdominoperineal resection, early in pregnancy.[4] When the cancer is diagnosed late in pregnancy, the fetus is less affected by maternal illness because of improved fetal viability after delivery. The overall fetal prognosis from maternal colon cancer is generally relatively favorable because the diagnosis is usually made near term. Infant survival is about 80%.[4] However, liveborn infants are often born prematurely and often have a low birthweight, factors associated with an increased risk of pulmonary complications and subsequent neurodevelopmental handicaps.

Novel diagnostic modalities for colon cancer diagnosis with promising applications in pregnancy include VCE, in which the colon may be imaged by a microcamera placed within a pill-sized device swallowed by the patient,[92] and a large array of genetic markers that detect genetic abnormalities associated with colon cancer in minute quantities of DNA in stool shed from colonic mucosa.[93]

Inflammatory Bowel Disease

The inflammatory bowel diseases, UC and DC, are immunologically mediated disorders that peak in incidence during a woman's reproductive life. In women younger than 40 years of age, the incidence of UC is 40 to 100 per 100,000, and the incidence of CD is 5 to 10 per 100,000.[5] **UC is a colonic mucosal disease manifested by bloody diarrhea, crampy abdominal pain, and pyrexia. CD can involve any part of the GI tract but most commonly involves the terminal ileum or colon. It is characterized by diarrhea, abdominal pain, anorexia, pyrexia, and malnutrition. Patients with CD may have fistulae and anorectal disease. Extraintestinal manifestations of IBD include arthritis, uveitis, sclerosing cholangitis, and cutaneous lesions.**

UC does not significantly affect fertility, although fertility decreases after colonic resection for UC.[94,95] CD, however, mildly decreases fertility because of extension of ileal inflammation to the nearby fallopian tubes or ovaries, scarring after surgery of the nearby reproductive organs, and the systemic effects of malnutrition.[96] IBD activity is mostly independent of pregnancy. **Patients with inactive or mild disease before conception tend to have the same disease activity during pregnancy. Active disease at conception increases the likelihood of active disease during pregnancy and of a poor pregnancy outcome that includes spontaneous abortion, miscarriage, stillbirth, or premature delivery.**[97,98] During pregnancy, the onset of CD—and to a lesser extent UC—is associated with increased fetal loss.[98]

Differentiating the signs and symptoms of IBD from physiologic changes related to pregnancy or from other obstetric, gynecologic, or surgical conditions may be difficult. Nausea,

TABLE 48-4 PHARMACOLOGIC THERAPY FOR INFLAMMATORY BOWEL DISEASE DURING PREGNANCY

DRUG	FDA CATEGORY DURING PREGNANCY	RECOMMENDATION DURING PREGNANCY
Sulfasalazine	B	Relatively safe, but concern exists about sulfa moiety causing neonatal jaundice
Mesalamine	B	Mesalamine is relatively safe
Infliximab (anti-TNF)	B	Not teratogenic in mice exposed to an analogous antibody, but clinical data are insufficient
Adalimumab (anti-TNF)	B	Believed to be relatively safe drug during pregnancy based on animal data, little clinical data; drug manufacturer is placing patients receiving this drug during pregnancy on a national registry
Certolizumab (anti-TNF)	B	Animal studies have not revealed fetal toxicity, and clinical data are sparse
Loperamide	B	Loperamide is relatively safe
Metronidazole	B	Avoid during first trimester (carcinogenic in rodents)
Corticosteroids	C	Relatively safe, concern regarding fetal adrenal function and maternal hyperglycemia; monitor the neonates of mothers who received substantial doses of corticosteroids during pregnancy
Ciprofloxacin	C	Use with caution, small studies show no significant risk during pregnancy
Diphenoxylate	C	Avoid; a possible teratogen
Cyclosporine	C	Cyclosporine is embryotoxic and fetotoxic at very high doses in rats and rabbits
6-Mercaptopurine	D	Avoid starting after conception, might cause IUGR
Azathioprine	D	Avoid starting after conception, might cause IUGR, teratogenic in laboratory animals
Methotrexate	X	Methotrexate is a contraindicated teratogen and abortifacient

FDA, Food and Drug Administration; *IUGR,* intrauterine growth restriction; *TNF,* tumor necrosis factor.

emesis, abdominal discomfort, and constipation may be noted during any pregnancy but may also signal a flare of IBD. The differential diagnosis of acute right lower quadrant abdominal pain in a pregnant woman with CD includes an exacerbation of CD, ectopic pregnancy, appendicitis, or adnexal disease. Pyrexia, bloody diarrhea, and weight loss suggest an exacerbation of CD.

The diagnostic evaluation is influenced by the pregnancy, but indicated tests should be performed. Laboratory evaluation includes a complete blood count, serum chemistry profile, and electrolyte determinations and takes into account the physiologic alterations of late pregnancy to include anemia, leukocytosis, and hypoalbuminemia. Flexible sigmoidoscopy is well tolerated during pregnancy without maternal complications or fetal toxicity.[32] Colonoscopy has been safely performed during pregnancy, especially during the second trimester, but the experience in the first and third trimesters is relatively limited.[27] Diagnostic roentgenographic tests that involve ionizing radiation, such as abdominopelvic CT, are best deferred until after delivery.[97]

The beneficial effects of IBD therapy on the mother and fetus must be weighed against the potential of fetal toxicity and teratogenicity (Table 48-4; see Chapter 8). However, **active disease poses greater risk to the fetus than most therapies.**[99] Corticosteroids are generally safe during pregnancy except that they may modestly increase the risk of cleft lip or palate, exacerbate gestational diabetes, and aggravate preeclampsia.[100] Corticosteroids should be administered at the lowest possible dose during pregnancy and should be avoided during the first trimester, when the hard palate is forming. **Sulfasalazine and 5-aminosalicylates are safe and should be used when required during pregnancy.**[95,97] Methotrexate is not safe, rather it is an abortifacient associated with congenital skeletal malformations.[101] **The FDA categorizes azathioprine and 6-mercaptopurine (6-MP) as class D drugs during pregnancy, but many gastroenterologists continue these medications during pregnancy if required to maintain remission.**[97,102] Anti–tumor necrosis factor (TNF) biologic therapies appear to be safer alternatives during pregnancy (see Table 48-4), although their safety during pregnancy is somewhat controversial because of limited data. One study found a high rate of congenital malformations reported to the FDA associated

with this drug class,[103] but another study noted a low rate.[104] One large investigation showed no increase in birth defects. This class of drugs should generally be discontinued before a contemplated pregnancy but may be used during pregnancy to control active current disease. Metronidazole is safe during pregnancy, but some advise avoidance during the first trimester.[105] The antidiarrheal agent diphenoxylate should be avoided during pregnancy because of case reports of teratogenicity when administered during the first trimester.[5]

Emergency surgery for toxic megacolon, intestinal obstruction, or massive bleeding should be done expeditiously, whereas elective surgery such as fistulectomy should be performed during the second trimester or postpartum.[98,106] Severe perianal CD may necessitate cesarean delivery because an episiotomy during vaginal delivery can exacerbate perianal disease.[107]

Hemorrhoids

Hemorrhoids are common in adults and are particularly common during pregnancy, especially during the third trimester or immediately postpartum, with an estimated incidence of 25% during pregnancy.[108] Contributing factors during pregnancy include increased constipation, resulting in increased straining at defecation; expansion of the circulating blood volume, resulting in venous dilatation and engorgement; and vascular compression from the enlarging gravid uterus, resulting in venous stasis.[21] Hemorrhoids above the dentate line are *internal,* whereas those below the dentate line are *external.*

Hemorrhoids characteristically produce a clinical triad of bright red blood per rectum that resembles the color of arterial blood; blood coating, rather than blood admixed with stool; and postdefecatory bleeding, most commonly noted on the toilet paper.[109] Other clinical manifestations include anorectal discomfort, pruritus, or pain associated with prolapse, thrombosis, or incarceration of hemorrhoids.

When the pain from external hemorrhoids is mild to moderate, recommended conservative treatment includes stool softeners, a high-fiber diet, increased liquid intake, topical analgesics, and warm sitz baths.[21] Therapy for hemorrhoids is primarily directed at treating the constipation. Hemorrhoidectomy can be safely performed during pregnancy using local anesthesia for severely painful or acutely thrombosed external hemorrhoids. General measures for internal hemorrhoids similarly include fiber supplements, fluids, and a high-fiber diet to decrease constipation; switching to a slow-release iron supplement to mitigate the constipating effects of iron; topical local anesthetics for anorectal discomfort; skin protectants applied after defecation to reduce anal pruritus; and avoidance of straining during bowel movements.[21] Therapies for severe or refractory symptoms from internal hemorrhoids include band ligation, injection, sclerotherapy, and coagulation. These therapies are generally safe and effective during pregnancy.[110] Invasive therapy, however, is rarely necessary for external or internal hemorrhoids because the symptoms spontaneously resolve soon after delivery.[108]

Mesenteric Ischemia and Infarction

Bowel infarction can occur during pregnancy secondary to intestinal obstruction or mesenteric venous thrombosis.[111] Digoxin, ergot alkaloids, cocaine, and other vasoconstrictors are also associated with mesenteric ischemia.[112] Mild hypercoagulability from hyperestrogenemia during pregnancy may contribute to a mildly increased risk of mesenteric ischemia compared with other middle-aged patients, but this risk is not high because mesenteric ischemia is predominantly a disease of the elderly. Patients with mesenteric venous thrombosis typically have an insidious onset of poorly localized abdominal pain with a relatively unremarkable physical examination.[113] The thrombosis is diagnosed by the noninvasive modalities of MRI or CT scanning and by the invasive modality of the venous phase of angiography. Hematologic evaluation for hypercoagulopathy is recommended.[111]

Irritable Bowel Syndrome

The irritable bowel syndrome (IBS) is most common in younger women, and the pathogenesis is poorly defined. Both intestinal motor and sensory abnormalities, particularly hyperalgesia, have been described.[114] **IBS is diagnosed, according to the Rome III criteria, by the presence of both abdominal pain and disordered defecation for at least 6 months with at least two of the following: (1) pain relief by a bowel movement, (2) onset of pain related to a change in stool frequency, and (3) onset of pain related to a change in stool appearance.**[115] **Endoscopic, radiologic, and histologic intestinal studies reveal no evident organic disease. Young women typically have diarrhea-predominant IBS but sometimes have primarily constipation or alternating diarrhea and constipation. Abdominal bloating and distension are common symptoms.**

Few data exist concerning the effect of pregnancy on IBS.[116] The onset of IBS typically predates the pregnancy and rarely begins during pregnancy. **IBS is believed to be generally mild during pregnancy,**[117] **and gestational hormones—particularly progesterone—may exacerbate the symptoms of IBS.**[118] Presumed IBS in the absence of warning signs or symptoms such as rectal bleeding, pyrexia, or weight loss should not require invasive tests such as sigmoidoscopy. However, signs and symptoms of organic disease such as rectal bleeding or involuntary weight loss should not be attributed to IBS without proper evaluation. In particular, sigmoidoscopy is indicated for significant nonhemorrhoidal rectal bleeding during pregnancy.[26]

Symptoms of IBS are best treated during pregnancy by dietary modification or behavioral therapy rather than with systemic drugs.[119] Patients with diarrhea-predominant IBS may benefit from elimination of foods from the diet that precipitate diarrhea, such as alcohol, caffeinated beverages, poorly digestible sugars, and fatty foods. Pregnant patients usually consume large amounts of dairy products in their diet to ensure adequate calcium intake, and some may benefit from lactase supplements when ingesting dairy products. Dietary fiber and fluid ingestion may improve constipation-predominant IBS. Polysaccharide bulking agents, such as methylcellulose, appear to be safe because of a lack of systemic absorption.[75] IBS is not believed to affect fertility and pregnancy outcome in the absence of nutritional deficiencies or concomitant disorders.[116]

Splenic Artery Aneurysm Rupture

Splenic artery aneurysm rupture is associated with pregnancy, possibly because of the effects of gestational hormones on the elastic properties of the arterial wall. Rupture most commonly occurs in the third trimester. Patients typically present suddenly in hemorrhagic shock with left upper quadrant abdominal pain and free intraperitoneal fluid. The diagnosis is suggested by demonstration of a calcified rim from the aneurysm on plain abdominal roentgenogram and is confirmed by abdominal CT scanning or angiography. Treatment consists of fluid resuscitation and prompt surgery, with ligation of the splenic artery and splenectomy. The maternal mortality exceeds 75%, and the fetal mortality exceeds 90%.[120] Splenic artery aneurysms should therefore be surgically corrected even if asymptomatic.[120,121] Abdominal aortic and renal aneurysms can also rupture during pregnancy.

SUMMARY

The differential diagnosis of abdominal symptoms and signs is particularly extensive in pregnancy. The differential includes GI, obstetric, gynecologic, and other disorders that are related or unrelated to the pregnancy. The patient history, physical examination, laboratory data, and radiologic findings usually provide the diagnosis of abdominal disorders during pregnancy. The pregnant woman has physiologic alterations that affect the clinical presentation, including atypical normative laboratory values. Abdominal ultrasound is generally the recommended radiologic imaging modality. MRI may be performed as indicated, and gadolinium administration should be avoided during the first trimester. Flexible sigmoidoscopy and EGD can be performed during gestation when indicated. Concerns about the fetus may occasionally limit the pharmacotherapy during pregnancy. Early diagnosis is critical to improve maternal and fetal survival, which have recently improved for many life-threatening GI conditions—such as appendicitis—because of improved diagnostic modalities, better maternal and fetal monitoring, improved laparoscopic technology, and earlier and better therapy.

KEY POINTS

◆ The differential diagnosis of GI symptoms and signs such as abdominal pain is particularly extensive during pregnancy. Aside from GI and other intraabdominal disorders incidental to pregnancy, the differential includes obstetric, gynecologic, and GI disorders related to pregnancy.

◆ Pregnancy can affect the clinical presentation, frequency, or severity of GI diseases. For example, gastroesophageal reflux disease markedly increases in frequency, and peptic ulcer disease decreases in frequency or may become inactive during pregnancy.

◆ Abdominal ultrasound is the safest and most commonly used abdominal imaging modality to evaluate GI conditions during pregnancy. Other common abdominal imaging modalities, particularly computed tomography, raise serious concerns about fetal safety.

◆ Esophagogastroduodenoscopy and flexible sigmoidoscopy can be performed when strongly indicated during pregnancy, such as for significant acute upper and lower GI bleeding, respectively.

◆ Most GI drugs appear to be relatively safe for the fetus (FDA categories B and C) and can be used with caution when clearly indicated during pregnancy, especially during the second and third trimesters after organogenesis has occurred. Drugs to be avoided during pregnancy include methotrexate (category X), some chemotherapeutic agents, and a few antibiotics.

REFERENCES

1. Powers RD, Guertter AT. Abdominal pain in the ED (emergency department): stability and change over 20 years. *Am J Emerg Med.* 1995;13: 301-303.
2. Broussard CN, Richter JE. Treating gastro-esophageal reflux disease during pregnancy and lactation: what are the safest therapy options. *Drug Saf.* 1998;19:325-337.
3. Costa SH, Vessey MP. Misoprostol and illegal abortion in Rio de Janeiro, Brazil. *Lancet.* 1993;341:1258-1261.
4. Cappell MS. Colon cancer during pregnancy. *Gastroenterol Clin North Am.* 2003;32:341-383.
5. Cappell MS, Friedel D. Abdominal pain during pregnancy. *Gastroenterol Clin North Am.* 2003;32:1-58.
6. Tracey M, Fletcher HS. Appendicitis in pregnancy. *Am Surg.* 2000;66: 555-559.
7. Puskar D, Balagovic I, Filipovic A, et al. Symptomatic physiologic hydronephrosis in pregnancy: incidence, complications and treatment. *Eur Urol.* 2001;39:260-263.
8. Petersson C, Hedges S, Stenqvist K, et al. Suppressed antibody and interleukin-6 responses to acute pyelonephritis in pregnancy. *Kidney Int.* 1994;45:571-577.
9. Lawson M, Kern F Jr, Everson GT. Gastrointestinal transit time in human pregnancy: prolongation in the second and third trimesters followed by postpartum normalization. *Gastroenterology.* 1985;89:996-999.
10. Martin C, Varner MW. Physiologic changes in pregnancy: surgical implications. *Clin Obstet Gynecol.* 1994;37:241-255.
11. Van den Broe NR, Letsky EA. Pregnancy and the erythrocyte sedimentation rate. *Br J Obstet Gynaecol.* 2001;108:1164-1167.
12. Wong E, Suat SO. Ectopic pregnancy: a diagnostic challenge in the emergency department. *Eur J Emerg Med.* 2000;7:189-194.
13. Derchi LE, Serafini G, Gandolfo N, et al. Ultrasound in gynecology. *Eur Radiol.* 2001;11:2137-2155.
14. Blanchard AC, Pastorek JG 2nd, Weeks T. Pelvic inflammatory disease during pregnancy. *South Med J.* 1987;80:1363-1365.
15. Friedler S, Ben-Shachar I, Abramov Y, et al. Ruptured tubo-ovarian abscess complicating transcervical cryopreserved embryo transfer. *Fertil Steril.* 1996;65:1065-1066.
16. Millar LK, Cox SM. Urinary tract infections complicating pregnancy. *Infect Dis Clin North Am.* 1997;11:13-26.
17. Evans HJ, Wollin TA. The management of urinary calculi in pregnancy. *Curr Opin Urol.* 2001;11:379-384.
18. Marrero JM, Goggin PM, de Caestecker JS, Pearce JM, Maxwell JD. Determinants of pregnancy heartburn. *Br J Obstet Gynaecol.* 1992;99: 731-734.
19. Cappell MS, Colon VJ, Sidhom OA. A study at eight medical centers of the safety and clinical efficacy of esophagogastroduodenoscopy in 83 pregnant females with follow-up of fetal outcome and with comparison to control groups. *Am J Gastroenterol.* 1996;91:348-354.
20. Frank B. Endoscopy in pregnancy. In: Karlstadt RG, Surawicz CM, Croitoru R, eds. *Gastrointestinal disorders during pregnancy.* Arlington, VA: American College of Gastroenterology; 1994:24-29.
21. Wald A. Constipation, diarrhea, and symptomatic hemorrhoids during pregnancy. *Gastroenterol Clin North Am.* 2003;32:309-322.
22. Bradley CS, Kennedy CM, Turcea AM, Rao SS, Nygaard IE. Constipation in pregnancy: prevalence, symptoms, and risk factors. *Obstet Gynecol.* 2007;110(6):1351-1357.
23. Russman S, Lamerato L, Motsko SP, Pezzullo JC, Faber MD, Jones JK. Risk of further decline in renal function after the use of oral sodium phosphate or polyethylene glycol in patients with a preexisting glomerular filtration rate below 60 mL/min. *Am J Gastroenterol.* 2008;103(11): 2707-2716.
24. Karam PA. Determining and reporting fetal radiation exposure from diagnostic radiation. *Health Phys.* 2000;79(suppl 5):S85-S90.
25. Toppenberg KS, Hill DA, Miller DP. Safety of radiographic imaging during pregnancy. *Am Fam Physician.* 1999;59:1813-1820.
26. Cappell MS, Colon VJ, Sidhom OA. A study at 10 medical centers of the safety and efficacy of 48 flexible sigmoidoscopies and 8 colonoscopies during pregnancy with follow-up of fetal outcome and with comparison to control groups. *Dig Dis Sci.* 1996;41:2353-2361.
27. Cappell MS, Fox SR, Gorrepati N. Safety and efficacy of colonoscopy during pregnancy: an analysis of pregnancy outcome in 20 patients. *J Reprod Med.* 2010;55(3–4):115-123.
28. Vinod J, Bonheur J, Korelitz BI, Panagopoulos G. Choice of laxatives and colonoscopic preparation in pregnant patients from the viewpoint of obstetricians and gastroenterologists. *World J Gastroenterol.* 2007;13(48): 6549-6552.
29. Debby A, Golan A, Sadan O, Glezerman M, Shirin H. Clinical utility of esophagogastroduodenoscopy in the management of recurrent and intractable vomiting in pregnancy. *J Reprod Med.* 2008;53(5):347-351.
30. Bagis T, Gumurdulu Y, Kayaselcuk F, Yilmaz ES, Killicadag E, Tarim E. Endoscopy in hyperemesis gravidarum and Helicobacter pylori infection. *Int J Gynaecol Obstet.* 2002;79(2):105-109.
31. Cappell MS. Endoscopy in pregnancy: risks versus benefits. *Nat Clin Pract Gastroenterol Hepatol.* 2005;2(9):376-377.
32. Cappell MS. The fetal safety and clinical efficacy of gastrointestinal endoscopy during pregnancy. *Gastroenterol Clin North Am.* 2003;32: 123-179.
33. Cappell MS. Sedation and analgesia for gastrointestinal endoscopy during pregnancy. *Gastrointest Endosc Clin N Am.* 2006;16(1):1-31.
34. Qureshi WA, Rajan E, Adler DG, et al. ASGE guideline: guidelines for endoscopy in pregnant and lactating women. *Gastrointest Endosc.* 2005; 61(3):357-362.
35. Figueiredo P, Almeida N, Lopes S, et al. Small-bowel capsule endoscopy in patients with suspected Crohn's disease: diagnostic value and complications. *Diagn Ther Endosc.* 2010;2010:pii: 101284. E pub 2010 Aug 5.
36. Storch I, Barkin JS. Contraindications to capsule endoscopy: do any still exist? *Gastrointest Endosc Clin N Am.* 2006;16(2):329-336.
37. Hogan RB, Ahmad N, Hogan RB 3rd, et al. Video capsule endoscopy detection of jejunal carcinoid in life-threatening hemorrhage, first trimester pregnancy. *Gastrointest Endosc.* 2007;66(1):205-207.
38. Lacroix R, Eason E, Melzack R. Nausea and vomiting during pregnancy: A prospective study of its frequency, intensity, and patterns of change. *Am J Obstet Gynecol.* 2000;182:931-937.
39. Hamaoui E, Hamaoui M. Nutritional assessment and support during pregnancy. *Gastroenterol Clin North Am.* 2003;32:59-121.
40. Koch KL, Frissora CL. Nausea and vomiting during pregnancy. *Gastroenterol Clin North Am.* 2003;32:201-234.
41. Tan PC, Tan NC, Omar SZ. Effect of high levels of human chorionic gonadotropin and estradiol on the severity of hyperemesis gravidarum. *Clin Chem Lab Med.* 2009;47(2):165-171.
42. Lockwood CM, Grenache DG, Gronowski AM. Serum human chorionic gonadotropin concentrations greater than 400,000 IU/L are invariably associated with suppressed serum thyrotropin concentrations. *Thyroid.* 2009;19(8):863-868.
43. McKeigue PM, Lamm SH, Linn S, Kutcher JS. Bendectin and birth defects: 1. A meta-analysis of the epidemiologic studies. *Teratology.* 1994;50(1):27-37.
44. Sahakian V, Rouse D, Sipes S, Rose N, Niebyl J. Vitamin B6 is effective therapy for nausea and vomiting of pregnancy: a randomized, double-blind placebo-controlled study. *Obstet Gynecol.* 1991;78:33-36.

45. Tan PC, Khine PP, Vallikannu N, Omar SZ. Promethazine compared with metoclopramide for hyperemesis gravidarum: a randomized controlled trial. *Obstet Gynecol.* 2010;115(5):975-981.

46. Martin RP, Wisenbaker J, Huttunen MO. Nausea during pregnancy: relation to early childhood temperament and behavior problems at twelve years. *J Abnorm Child Psychol.* 1999;27:323-329.

47. Dodds L, Fell DB, Joseph KS, Allen VM, Butler B. Outcomes of pregnancies complicated by hyperemesis gravidarum. *Obstet Gynecol.* 2006; 107(2 Pt 1):285-292.

48. Castro Lde P. Reflux esophagitis as the cause of heartburn in pregnancy. *Am J Obstet Gynecol.* 1967;98:1-10.

49. Cappell MS. Gastric and duodenal ulcers during pregnancy. *Gastroenterol Clin North Am.* 2003;32:263-308.

50. Winbery SL, Blaho KE. Dyspepsia in pregnancy. *Obstet Gynecol Clin North Am.* 2001;28:333-350.

51. Cappell MS, Schein JR. Diagnosis and treatment of nonsteroidal anti-inflammatory drug-associated upper gastrointestinal toxicity. *Gastroenterol Clin North Am.* 2000;29:97-124.

52. Lalkin A, Magee L, Addis A, et al. Acid-suppressing drugs during pregnancy. *Can Fam Physician.* 1997;43:1923-1926.

53. Nakatsuka T, Fujikake N, Hasebe M, et al. Effects of sodium bicarbonate and ammonium chloride on the incidence of furosemide-induced fetal skeletal anomaly, wavy rib, in rats. *Teratology.* 1993;48:139-147.

54. Charan M, Katz PO. Gastroesophageal reflux disease in pregnancy. *Curr Treat Options Gastroenterol.* 2001;4:73-81.

55. Morton DM. Pharmacology and toxicity of nizatidine. *Scand J Gastroenterol.* 1987;22(suppl l36):1-8.

56. Koren G, Zemlickis DM. Outcome of pregnancy after first trimester exposure to H-2 receptor antagonists. *Am J Perinatol.* 1991;8:37-38.

57. *Physicians Desk Reference.* 70th ed. 2010. Montvale, NJ: PDR Network; 2016.

58. Briggs GG, Freeman RK, Yaffe SJ. *Drugs in Pregnancy and Lactation.* 9th ed. Philadelphia: Lippincott Williams & Wilkins; 2011.

59. Kallen BA. Use of omeprazole during pregnancy: no hazard demonstrated in 955 infants exposed during pregnancy. *Eur J Obstet Gynecol Reprod Biol.* 2001;96(1):63-68.

60. Dashe JS, Gilstrap LC 3rd. Antibiotic use in pregnancy. *Obstet Gynecol Clin North Am.* 1997;24:617-629.

61. Aston NO, Kalaichandran S, Carr JV. Duodenal ulcer hemorrhage in the puerperium. *Can J Surg.* 1991;34:482-483.

62. Schein M. Choice of emergency operative procedure for bleeding duodenal ulcer. *Br J Surg.* 1991;78:633-634.

63. Chan YM, Ngai SW, Lao TT. Gastric adenocarcinoma presenting with persistent, mild gastrointestinal symptoms in pregnancy: a case report. *J Reprod Med.* 1999;44:986-988.

64. Dumont M. Diaphragmatic hernia and pregnancy. *J Gynecol Obstet Biol Reprod.* 1990;19:395-399.

65. Kurzel RE, Naunheim KS, Schwartz RA. Repair of symptomatic diaphragmatic hernia during pregnancy. *Obstet Gynecol.* 1988;71:869-871.

66. Mazze RI, Kallen B. Appendectomy during pregnancy: a Swedish registry of 778 cases. *Obstet Gynecol.* 1991;77:835-840.

67. Tamir IL, Bongard FS, Klein SR. Acute appendicitis in the pregnant patient. *Am J Surg.* 1990;160:571-575.

68. Mourad J, Elliott JP, Erickson L, et al. Appendicitis in pregnancy: new information that contradicts long-held clinical beliefs. *Am J Obstet Gynecol.* 2000;182:1027-1029.

69. Terasawa T, Blackmore CC, Bent S, Kohlwes RJ. Systematic review: computed tomography and ultrasonography to detect acute appendicitis in adults and adolescents. *Ann Intern Med.* 2004;141(7):537-546.

70. Pedrosa I, Lafornara M, Pandharipande PV, Goldsmith JD, Rofsky NM. Pregnant patients suspected of having acute appendicitis: effect of MR imaging on negative laparotomy rate and appendiceal perforation rate. *Radiology.* 2009;250(3):749-757.

71. Andersen B, Nielsen TF. Appendicitis in pregnancy: diagnosis, management and complications. *Acta Obstet Gynecol Scand.* 1999;78(9): 758-762.

72. De Perrot M, Jenny A, Morales M, et al. Laparoscopic appendectomy during pregnancy. *Surg Laparosc Endosc Percutan Tech.* 2000;l0:368-371.

73. Connolly MM, Unti JA, Nom PF. Bowel obstruction in pregnancy. *Surg Clin North Am.* 1995;75:101-113.

74. Perdue PW, Johnson HW Jr, Stafford PW. Intestinal obstruction complicating pregnancy. *Am J Surg.* 1992;164:384-388.

75. Pandolfino J, Vanagunas A. Gastrointestinal complications of pregnancy. In: Sciarra JJ, ed. *Gynecology and Obstetrics, revised edition.* Vol. 3. Philadelphia: Lippincott Williams & Wilkins; 2003:1-14 [Chapter 30].

76. Davis MR, Bohon CJ. Intestinal obstruction in pregnancy. *Clin Obstet Gynecol.* 1983;26:832-842.

77. Meyerson S, Holtz T, Ehrinpreis M, et al. Small bowel obstruction in pregnancy. *Am J Gastroenterol.* 1995;90:299-302.

78. Dufour P, Haentjens-Verbeke K, Vinatier D, et al. Intestinal obstruction and pregnancy. *J Gynecol Obstet Biol Reprod.* 1996;25:297-300.

79. Rothstein RD, Rombeau JL. Intestinal malrotation during pregnancy. *Obstet Gynecol.* 1993;81:817-819.

80. Fielding LP, Schultz SM. Treatment of acute colonic pseudo-obstruction. *J Am Coll Surg.* 2001;192:422-423.

81. Roberts CA. Ogilvie's syndrome after cesarean delivery. *J Obstet Gynecol Neonatal Nurs.* 2000;29:239-246.

82. Sharp HT. Gastrointestinal surgical conditions during pregnancy. *Clin Obstet Gynecol.* 1994;37:306-315.

83. Woods JB, Martin JN Jr, Ingram FH, Odom CD, Scott-Conner CE, Rhodes RS. Pregnancy complicated by carcinoma of the colon above the rectum. *Am J Perinatol.* 1992;9:102-110.

84. Nesbitt JC, Moise KJ, Sawyers JL. Colorectal carcinoma in pregnancy. *Arch Surg.* 1985;120(5):636-640.

85. Bernstein MA, Madoff RD, Caushaj PF. Colon and rectal cancer in pregnancy. *Dis Colon Rectum.* 1993;36:172-178.

86. Minter A, Malik R, Ledbetter L, Winokur TS, Hawn MT, Saif MW. Colon cancer in pregnancy. *Cancer Control.* 2005;12(3): 196-202.

87. Tsukamoto N, Uchino H, Matsukuma K, Kamura T. Carcinoma of the colon presenting as bilateral ovarian tumors during pregnancy. *Gynecol Oncol.* 1986;24:386-391.

88. Chen MM, Coakley FV, Kaimel D, Laros RK Jr. Guidelines for computed tomography and magnetic resonance imaging use during pregnancy and lactation. *Obstet Gynecol.* 2008;112(2 Pt 1):333-340.

89. Kort B, Katz VL, Watson WJ. The effect of nonobstetric operation during pregnancy. *Surg Gynecol Obstet.* 1993;177:371-376.

90. Lamerz R, Ruider H. Significance of CEA determinations in patients with cancer of the colon-rectum and the mammary gland in comparison to physiological states in connection with pregnancy. *Bull Cancer.* 1976;63: 573-586.

91. Smith C, Butler JA. Colorectal cancer in patients younger than 40 years of age. *Dis Colon Rectum.* 1989;32:843-846.

92. Rokkas T, Papaxoinis K, Triantafyllou K, Ladas SD. A meta-analysis evaluating the accuracy of colon capsule endoscopy in detecting colon polyps. *Gastrointest Endosc.* 2010;71(4):792-798.

93. Imperiale TF, Ransohoff DF, Itzkowitz SH, Turnbull BA, Ross ME, the Colorectal Cancer Study Group. Fecal DNA versus fecal occult blood for colorectal-cancer screening in an average-risk population. *N Engl J Med.* 2004;351:2704-2714.

94. Ording Olsen K, Juul S, Berndtsson I, Oresland T, Laurberg S. Ulcerative colitis: female fecundity before diagnosis, during disease, and after surgery compared with a population sample. *Gastroenterology.* 2002;122(1): 15-19.

95. Jospe ES, Peppercorn MA. Inflammatory bowel disease and pregnancy: a review. *Dig Dis.* 1999;17:201-207.

96. Woolfson K, Cohen Z, McLeod RS. Crohn's disease and pregnancy. *Dis Colon Rectum.* 1990;33:869-873.

97. Friedman S. Management of inflammatory bowel disease during pregnancy and nursing. *Semin Gastrointest Dis.* 2001;12:245-252.

98. Rajapakse R, Korelitz BI. Inflammatory bowel disease during pregnancy. *Curr Treat Options Gastroenterol.* 2001;4:245-251.

99. Sachar D. Exposure to mesalamine during pregnancy increased preterm deliveries (but not birth defects) and decreased birth weight. *Gut.* 1998;43:316.

100. Park-Wyllie L, Mazzotta P, Pastuszak A, et al. Birth defects after maternal exposure to corticosteroids: prospective cohort study and meta-analysis of epidemiological studies. *Teratology.* 2000;62(6):385-392.

101. Hausknecht RU. Methotrexate and misoprostol to terminate early pregnancy. *N Engl J Med.* 1995;333:537-540.

102. Alstead EM, Ritchie JK, Lennard-Jones JE, Farthing MJ, Clark ML. Safety of azathioprine in pregnancy in inflammatory bowel disease. *Gastroenterology.* 1990;99:443-446.

103. Carter JD, Ladhani A, Ricca LR, Valeriano J, Vasey FB. A safety assessment of tumor necrosis factor antagonists during pregnancy: a review of the Food and Drug Administration database. *J Rheumatol.* 2009;36(3): 635-641.

104. Ali YM, Kuriya B, Orozco C, Cush JJ, Keystone EC. Can tumor necrosis factor inhibitors be safely used in pregnancy? *J Rheumatol.* 2010;37(1): 9-17.

105. *Antimicrobial therapy for obstetric patients*. Education Bulletin No. 245. American College of Obstetricians and Gynecologists, March 1998.

106. Hill J, Clark A, Scott NA. Surgical treatment of acute manifestations of Crohn's disease during pregnancy. *J R Soc Med*. 1997;90:64-66.

107. Ilnyckyji A, Blanchard JF, Rawsthorne P, Bernstein CN. Perianal Crohn's disease and pregnancy: role of the mode of delivery. *Am J Gastroenterol*. 1999;94:3274-3278.

108. Staroselsky A, Nava-Ocampo A, Vohra S, Koren G. Hemorrhoids in pregnancy. *Can Fam Physician*. 2008;54:189-190.

109. Cappell MS, Friedel D. The role of sigmoidoscopy and colonoscopy in the diagnosis and management of lower gastrointestinal disorders: endoscopic findings, therapy, and complications. *Med Clin North Am*. 2002;86: 1253-1288.

110. Medich DS, Fazio VW. Hemorrhoids, anal fissure, and carcinoma of the colon, rectum, and anus during pregnancy. *Surg Clin North Am*. 1995;75: 77-88.

111. Engelhardt TC, Kerstein MD. Pregnancy and mesenteric venous thrombosis. *South J Med*. 1989;82:1441-1443.

112. Cappell MS. Colonic toxicity of administered drugs and chemicals. *Am J Gastroenterol*. 2004;99:1175-1190.

113. Cappell MS. Intestinal (mesenteric) vasculopathy: I. Acute superior mesenteric arteriopathy and venopathy. *Gastroenterol Clin North Am*. 1998;27:783-825.

114. Verne GN, Robinson ME, Price DD. Hypersensitivity to visceral and cutaneous pain in the irritable bowel syndrome. *Pain*. 2001;93:7-14.

115. Longstreth GF, Thompson WG, Chey WD, Houghton CA, Mearin F, Spiller RC. Functional bowel disorders. *Gastroenterology*. 2006;130: 1480-1491.

116. Kane SV, Sable K, Hanauer SB. The menstrual cycle and its effect on inflammatory bowel disease and irritable bowel syndrome: a prevalence study. *Am J Gastroenterol*. 1998;93:1867-1872.

117. Johnson P, Mount K, Graziano S. Functional bowel disorders in pregnancy: effect on quality of life, evaluation and management. *Acta Obstet Gynecol Scand*. 2014;93(9):874-879.

118. Mathias JR, Clench MH. Relationship of reproductive hormones and neuromuscular disease of the gastrointestinal tract. *Dig Dis*. 1998;16: 3-13.

119. West L, Warren J, Cutts T. Diagnosis and management of irritable bowel syndrome, constipation, and diarrhea in pregnancy. *Gastroenterol Clin North Am*. 1992;21:793-802.

120. Stanley JC, Wakefield TW, Graham LM, et al. Clinical importance and management of splanchnic artery aneurysms. *J Vasc Surg*. 1986;3: 836-840.

121. Hallet JW Jr. Splenic artery aneurysms. *Semin Vasc Surg*. 1995;8: 321-326.

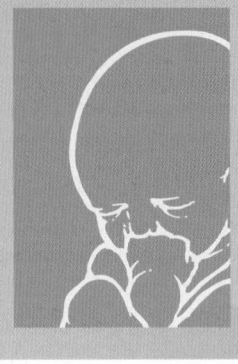

CHAPTER 49

Neurologic Disorders in Pregnancy

ELIZABETH E. GERARD and PHILIP SAMUELS

KEY ABBREVIATIONS

American Academy of Neurology	AAN	Intramuscular	IM
American Heart Association	AHA	Intrauterine device	IUD
Antiepileptic drug	AED	Intrauterine growth restriction	IUGR
Arteriovenous	AV	Liverpool and Manchester	LMNG
Arteriovenous malformation	AVM	Neurodevelopmental Group	
Australian Register of Antiepileptic Drugs	APR	Magnetic resonance imaging	MRI
in Pregnancy		Magnetic resonance angiography	MRA
Attention-deficit/hyperactivity disorder	ADHD	Magnetic resonance venogram	MRV
Autism spectrum disorder	ASD	Multiple sclerosis	MS
Autosomal-dominant frontal lobe epilepsy	ADFLE	Neural tube defect	NTD
Autosomal-dominant temporal lobe	ADTLE	Neurodevelopmental disorder	NDD
epilepsy		Neurodevelopmental Effects of	NEAD
Centers for Disease Control and	CDC	Antiepileptic Drugs	
Prevention		North American AED Pregnancy Registry	NAAPR
Central nervous system	CNS	Periventricular nodular heterotopia	PVNH
Cerebral venous thrombosis	CVT	Posterior reversible encephalopathy	PRES
Cerebrospinal fluid	CSF	syndrome	
Computed tomography angiography	CTA	Pregnancy and Multiple Sclerosis study	PRIMS
Computed tomography	CT	Reversible cerebral vasoconstriction	RCVS
Disease-modifying agent	DMA	syndrome	
Electroencephalogram	EEG	Small for gestational age	SGA
Electromyography	EMG	Sodium channel, voltage-gated type 1	SCN1A
Enzyme-inducing antiepileptic drug	EIAED	alpha subunit	
European Medicine Agency	EMA	Subarachnoid hemorrhage	SAH
Expanded Disability Status Scale	EDSS	Sudden unexpected death in epilepsy	SUDEP
U.S. Food and Drug Administration	FDA	Thymus helper	Th
Idiopathic intracranial hypertension	IICH	Tissue plasminogen activator	tPA
Intelligence quotient	IQ	World Health Organization	WHO

EPILEPSY AND SEIZURES

Epilepsy affects approximately 1% of the general population and is the most frequent major neurologic complication encountered in pregnancy. It is important that the practicing obstetrician becomes familiar with the basic treatment of epilepsy and the implications for the patient and fetus. Many of the antiepileptic drugs (AEDs) used to treat epilepsy are also used to treat psychiatric and pain disorders and are commonly prescribed to women of childbearing age; this makes an understanding of their implications for pregnancy imperative for any clinician managing these patients.

A diagnosis of epilepsy is made in the setting of two unprovoked seizures or one seizure in a patient with clinical features that make a second seizure likely, such as findings on brain magnetic resonance imaging (MRI) or electroencephalogram (EEG) that are consistent with a diagnosis of epilepsy or a family history of epilepsy. Epilepsy syndromes can be divided into *generalized* and *focal* epilepsies. An epilepsy syndrome is defined by the constellation of clinical features of a patient's seizures as well as their imaging and EEG findings. It is important to note that both types of epilepsy syndromes can present with a wide spectrum of seizure types. Convulsions or tonic-clonic seizures, colloquially referred to as "generalized" seizures, can occur in patients with either generalized or focal epilepsies. It is important to work with a patient's neurologist to have an understanding of the patient's epilepsy syndrome because this has significant implications for treatment and also sometimes gives insight into the etiology of the patient's seizure disorder. It may also have a role in predicting the course of the seizure disorder during pregnancy.

Genetic generalized epilepsies, also known as *idiopathic generalized epilepsies,* are presumed to be genetic in origin, although most cases do not exhibit a mendelian inheritance pattern or have varying degrees of penetrance; first-degree relatives are often not affected. Patients with genetic generalized epilepsy can have myoclonic, absence, or tonic-clonic seizures. They may have only one or a combination of those seizure types. These patients are typically treated with "broad-spectrum" AEDs that include lamotrigine, levetiracetam, topiramate, valproate, and zonisamide. The majority of other AEDs—including, but not limited to, carbamazepine, gabapentin, oxcarbazepine, phenytoin, and pregabalin—are considered "narrow spectrum" and can provoke myoclonic or absence seizures in patients with genetic generalized epilepsies, even if the patient does not have a history of these seizure types. The newest AEDs, such as lacosamide and perampanel, are approved for treatment of focal epilepsies but are being studied for use in generalized epilepsies.

Focal epilepsy is the most common type of epilepsy in adult patients. Whereas the etiology of most focal epilepsies often remains unknown, an underlying cause must be ruled out because **they may occur secondary to an acquired abnormality such as a tumor, vascular malformation, brain injury, or infectious or autoimmune disorder that affects the brain.** An increasing number of genetic causes of focal epilepsies have also been identified recently, including some with autosomal-dominant inheritance patterns. Patients with focal epilepsy may present with focal seizures with or without loss of consciousness, previously known as *simple partial* and *complex partial seizures,* and/or focal seizures that progress to a tonic-clonic seizure, previously known as a *secondarily generalized seizure.*

The manifestations of focal seizures depend on where in the brain the seizure begins. The most commonly encountered focal epilepsy is temporal lobe epilepsy, which frequently presents with focal seizures with loss of awareness. These seizures are characterized by alteration of awareness that typically lasts 30 seconds to 2 minutes and may be accompanied by semipurposeful movements of the face and hands. The break in awareness is often underreported by patients and even their family members because patients do not remember this part of the seizure, and they may seem to observers to be interacting with their environment. These seizures can be preceded by an aura, such as a feeling of fear or an "epigastric rising," a sensation that begins in the stomach and that may rise to the chest and head, but an aura also may not be present or remembered. These seizures have the potential to progress to tonic-clonic seizures. Patients with focal epilepsy can be treated with broad- or narrow-spectrum AEDs; however, if the diagnosis is uncertain, it is best to begin with broad-spectrum drugs. The choice of the first AED usually depends on characteristics of the patient and the side effects of the drug. In women of childbearing age, the teratogenic potential of the AEDs should be a strong consideration; this will be discussed below.

Most women with epilepsy will need to remain on AEDs during their childbearing years and throughout pregnancy. Exceptions include patients with childhood epilepsy, which can remit in adulthood. In select cases of adult-onset epilepsy, patients who have been seizure free for 2 to 4 years may attempt to wean from seizure medications under a neurologist's supervision. Several factors that include the patient's seizure pattern and MRI and EEG findings affect this decision. Seizure freedom in the 9 months prior to pregnancy predicts a good chance of seizure control during pregnancy.[1] Thus in an appropriate patient who wanted to stop AED therapy before pregnancy, weaning her off seizure medication should be started at least 1 year before becoming pregnant. **Unfortunately, women with epilepsy may abruptly stop all medications as soon as they find out that they are pregnant,[2] which puts both the mother and fetus at risk.**

Uncontrolled seizures increase the risk of maternal injury and death and potentially expose the infant to transient anoxia.[3] The direct fetal effects of seizures during pregnancy have only been studied in a few case reports. Tonic-clonic seizures during delivery were associated with fetal bradycardia followed by tachycardia in two cases, although the infants were reportedly unaffected on delivery.[4] Fetal death at 33 weeks' gestation was associated with intraventricular hemorrhage in one patient following a tonic-clonic seizure; the patient had had three tonic-clonic seizures in pregnancy.[5] Focal seizures with loss of consciousness were associated with prolonged uterine contraction in one patient reported by Nei and colleagues.[6] The fetal heart rate also fell from 140 to 78 beats/min. In a population-based study from Taiwan, Chen and colleagues[7] studied 1016 pregnant women with epilepsy. Women with seizures during pregnancy had increased risks of preterm delivery (odds ratio [OR], 1.63), small-for-gestational-age (SGA) infants (OR, 1.37), and low-birthweight infants (OR, 1.36) compared with women without epilepsy. When compared with women with epilepsy but without tonic-clonic seizures during pregnancy, patients with seizures had an increased risk of SGA infants (OR, 1.34).

Two studies have raised significant alarm about the risk of epilepsy in pregnancy. The U.K. confidential inquiry into maternal deaths found that **women with epilepsy were 10 times** more likely to die during pregnancy or during the postpartum period.[8] Similarly, a recent study by MacDonald and associates[9] evaluated delivery hospitalization records in the United States and also reported a more than tenfold increase in deaths during delivery in women with epilepsy. In the U.K. study, 3 of 14 maternal deaths appeared to be directly related to complications of seizures (drowning, hypoxia, trauma), and the other 11 were attributed to **sudden unexpected death in epilepsy (SUDEP),[10] defined as the sudden and unexpected, nontraumatic, and nondrowning death of a person with epilepsy without a detected toxicologic or anatomic cause of death.** Mechanisms of SUDEP are uncertain, but risk factors include refractory and tonic-clonic seizures and noncompliance with medications. The U.K. inquiry pointed out that 8 of the 14 women with epilepsy who died in their cohort had not been referred to a provider with knowledge of epilepsy and had not received prepregnancy counseling. Additionally, they noted that one third of the women had difficult social circumstances that may have limited their access to care. Domestic abuse was present in at least two cases, and one patient had schizophrenia.[8] The causes of maternal mortality in the U.S. population study are not known, but it was observed that these patients had an increased risk of major comorbidities that included diabetes, hypertension, psychiatric conditions, and alcohol and substance abuse.[11] They were also at increased risk of preeclampsia, preterm labor, stillbirth, and cesarean delivery.[9]

Whereas these two studies that describe increased mortality in women with epilepsy point to the importance of further research into the optimal management of pregnant women with epilepsy and their comorbidities, they should be put into context for women with epilepsy so as not to deter them from pursuing pregnancy. Although the relative risk was significantly increased, the absolute risk of maternal death in women with epilepsy in the study by MacDonald and colleagues[9] was 80 per 100,000 births (0.08%). Similarly, Edey and colleagues[10] analyzed the U.K. inquiry and estimated the rate of deaths during pregnancy and the postpartum period among women with epilepsy to be 100 per 100,000 births (0.1%). These studies do point to the need for close medical supervision of pregnancies in women with epilepsy and the importance of prepregnancy counseling and planning. **The obstetrician and neurologist must work closely together to guide the patient through her pregnancy. Through this cooperation, the majority of pregnant women with seizure disorders can have a successful pregnancy with minimal risk to mother and fetus.**

EPILEPSY AND FERTILITY

Epilepsy and epilepsy treatment may adversely affect fertility in some women. Several population studies have demonstrated that birth rates are lower in both men and women with epilepsy compared with unaffected individuals.[12-15] In many studies these decreased birth rates were not explained by lower marriage rates in patients with epilepsy. However, these epidemiologic studies are unable to control for nonbiologic factors that may affect reproduction rates, such as decreased libido, which has been reported in patients with epilepsy, or patients' concerns about having a child because of fears about the implications of the condition or their medications. Sukumaran and colleagues[16] prospectively followed 375 Indian women trying to conceive and found that 38.4% were infertile after at least 1 year of trying to conceive. Risk factors for infertility

include taking AEDs, particularly multiple AEDs. However, age and lower educational level also played a role in the study.

Many lines of evidence suggest that potentially, both epilepsy and AEDs may have adverse effects on reproductive function. Seizures, particularly temporal lobe seizures, are known to disrupt the hypothalamic-pituitary-gonadal axis, and certain AEDs can affect sex steroid metabolism and sex hormone binding globulin concentrations. Increased risks of polycystic ovarian syndrome, premature ovarian insufficiency, and hypogonadotropic hypogonadism have been reported in women with epilepsy.[17,18] **Miscarriage rates, however, do not seem to be increased in women with epilepsy.**[19]

EPILEPSY AND PREGNANCY
Teratogenic Effects of Antiepileptic Drugs
Women with epilepsy are at increased risk of having pregnancies complicated by major congenital malformations. This risk appears to be related to exposure to AEDs during pregnancy rather than the epilepsy.[20] Not all AEDs are the same in terms of their teratogenic potential or the patterns of malformations with which they are associated (see Chapter 8). Over the past 15 years, prospective studies of the effects of AEDs on teratogenesis have largely replaced older retrospective case series. A few prospective studies of the cognitive effects of AED exposure during pregnancy have also been pivotal in our understanding of AED-associated risks. The most well-studied AEDs in pregnancy are valproate, carbamazepine, and lamotrigine. Of these drugs, **valproate has been consistently demonstrated to carry a risk of major congenital malformations significantly greater than that of other AEDs and baseline population rates, typically 1% to 3% depending on the study population. It has also been clearly associated with adverse cognitive and behavioral developmental outcomes.**

Lamotrigine has been associated with relatively low rates of teratogenesis, and although cognitive data are mostly reassuring, this still needs further clarification. Levetiracetam is less well studied, but promising early data have led to a dramatic increase in its use in pregnant women and those planning pregnancy. **Lamotrigine and levetiracetam are now the most commonly prescribed AEDs for women of childbearing age.**[21] Carbamazepine also appears to be a reasonable choice for women who plan to conceive, although its use has been declining in this population.[21]

The section below summarizes the available information on the best-studied and most prescribed AEDs. The majority of the information we have on structural teratogenesis is derived from several international pregnancy registries (Table 49-1). It is important to note that each of these registries uses slightly different methodologies in regard to means of recruitment, infant assessment control groups, and duration of follow-up.[22] These differences account for some of the variability in results; however, when the findings are looked at in aggregate, clear patterns emerge regarding the relative teratogenic risk of individual AEDs.

Valproate
Rates of major congenital malformations with first-trimester exposure to valproate monotherapy range from 4.7% to 13.8%.[23-27] In the two largest prospective cohorts from the United Kingdom and Ireland (1290 valproate exposures)[28] and the European Registry of Antiepileptic Drugs and Pregnancy

TABLE 49-1 RATE OF MAJOR CONGENITAL MALFORMATIONS WITH INDIVIDUAL ANTIEPILEPTIC DRUGS WHEN USED AS MONOTHERAPY

REGISTRY	STUDY	RATE OF MAJOR CONGENITAL MALFORMATIONS WITH INDIVIDUAL ANTIEPILEPTIC DRUGS AS MONOTHERAPY*								
		CBZ	GBP	LTG	LEV	OXC	PHB	PHT	TPM	VPA
Australian Pregnancy Registry	Vajda, 2014	5.5% (346)	0% (14)	4.6% (307)	2.4% (82)	5.9% (17)	0% (4)	2.4% (41)	2.4% (42)	13.8% (253)
Danish Registry	Mølgaard, 2011		1.7% (59)	3.7% (1019)	0 % (58)	2.8% (393)			4.6% (108)	
EURAP	Tomson, 2011	5.6% (1402)		2.9% (1280)	1.6% (126)	3.3% (184)	7.4% (217)	5.8% (103)	6.8% (73)	9.7% (1010)
Finland National Birth Registry	Artama, 2005	2.7% (805)								10.7% (263)
GSK Lamotrigine Registry	Cunnington, 2011			2.2% (1558)						
North American AED Pregnancy Registry	Hernandez, 2012	3.0% (1033)	0.7% (145)	2.0% (1562)	2.4% (450)	2.2% (182)	5.5% (199)	2.9% (416)	4.2% (359)	9.3% (323)
Norwegian Medical Birth Registry	Veiby, 2014	2.9% (685)		3.4% (833)	1.7% (118)	1.8% (57)	7.4% (27)		4.2% (48)	6.3% (333)
Swedish Medical Birth Registry	Tomson, 2012	2.7% (1430)	0% (18)	2.9% (1100)	0% (61)	3.7% (27)	14% (7)	6.7% (119)	7.7% (52)	4.7% (619)
U.K./Ireland pregnancy registry	Campbell, 2014 Mawhinney, 2013 Morrow, 2006 Hunt, 2008	2.6% (1657)	3.2% (32)	2.3% (2098)	0.7% (304)			3.7% (82)	9% (203)	6.7% (1290)

Data from Gerard E, Pack AM. Pregnancy registries: what do they mean to clinical practice? *Curr Neurol Neurosci Rep*. 2008;8(4):325-332.
*Numbers in parentheses indicate number of pregnancies enrolled.
AED, antiepileptic drug; *CBZ*, carbamazepine; *GBP*, gabapentin; *LEV*, levetiracetam; *LTG*, lamotrigine; *OXC*, oxcarbazepine; *PHB*, phenobarbital; *PHT*, phenytoin; *TPM*, topiramate; *VPA*, valproic acid.

(EURAP, 1010 valproate exposures),[29] the malformation rates were 6.7% and 9.7%, respectively.

In the European Surveillance of Congenital Anomalies (EUROCAT) database, a population-based database of 14 European countries, valproate exposure was associated with an increased risk of several specific defects.[30] Compared with control pregnancies, those exposed to valproate monotherapy were at statistically increased risk for spina bifida (OR, 12.7), craniosynostosis (OR, 6.8), cleft palate (OR, 5.2), hypospadias (OR, 4.8), atrial septal defects (OR, 2.5), and polydactyly (OR, 2.2). These numbers, however, describe only relative risk and can be hard for a patient to understand. **Tomson and Battino**[24] **compiled the data of 22 prospective studies that reported on specific AED-associated malformations and reported the absolute risks of neural tube defects (NTDs, 1.8%), cardiac malformations (1.7%), hypospadias (1.4%), and oral clefts (0.9%).**

In addition to significantly increasing the risk of birth defects, **valproate exposure during pregnancy has also been associated with cognitive and behavioral teratogenesis.** Two prospective studies of children exposed to AEDs in utero have recently been published, the Neurodevelopmental Effects of Antiepileptic Drugs (NEAD) study[31] and a study by the Liverpool and Manchester Neurodevelopmental Group (LMNG).[32] Both recruited women with epilepsy in the first trimester of pregnancy and followed the development of their children until age 6. In contrast to many earlier studies of the cognitive effects of AEDs, both of these investigations controlled for several important confounding variables, including maternal intelligence quotient (IQ)—an important predictor of a child's cognitive performance. Of note, the two studies did overlap: 92 children from the LMNG study were also enrolled in the NEAD study. The NEAD study ultimately evaluated 224 children at age 6 who had been exposed to carbamazepine, lamotrigine, phenytoin, or valproate monotherapy. The LMNG study

assessed 198 six-year-old children born to women with epilepsy who took AED monotherapy ($n = 143$) or polytherapy ($n = 30$) or no medication ($n = 25$) during pregnancy and a control group of 210 children of the same age. In the NEAD study, exposure to valproate monotherapy was associated with a significant decrease in mean full-scale IQ (FSIQ) by 7 to 10 points compared with children exposed to carbamazepine, lamotrigine, or phenytoin. The LMNG found that exposure to first-trimester doses of valproate greater than 800 mg/day was associated with a significant decrease in FSIQ by 9.7 points when compared with a control group.[32] The mean FSIQ of children exposed to low valproate doses (≤800 mg/day) was also lower than that of controls, but this did not meet statistical significance. The low-dose group, did, however, have significantly lower verbal IQ scores and an increased need for educational intervention.[32]

A population study that utilized the National Psychiatric Registry and birth registries in Denmark found that school-age children whose mothers were prescribed valproate monotherapy during pregnancy had a significantly increased risk of receiving a formal diagnosis of autism or autism spectrum disorder (ASD).[33] In the valproate-exposed cohort, the absolute risk of autism was 2.5%, whereas the rate in the general population was 0.48%, and the risk of ASD was 4.42%, with a baseline risk of ASD of 1.53%. The rates of autism and ASD in children born to mothers with epilepsy who did not take valproate during pregnancy did not differ from baseline population rates. A recent nested study[34] from the Australian Pregnancy Registry also found that of 26 children between 6 and 8 years of age who were exposed to valproate monotherapy, one tested in the "autistic range" and one tested in the "concern for autistic range" on a standardized assessment. The overall risk of autistic traits was 7.7% in the monotherapy group. In this study, the risk of autistic traits was greatest in the valproate polytherapy group (7/15; 46.7%) and was dose related in the valproate monotherapy group.

The LMNG also found an increased risk of behavioral abnormalities in their antenatally recruited cohort at 6 years of age. Because of the relatively smaller numbers in this cohort, the study examined the aggregate risk of several different neurodevelopmental disorders (NDDs) in exposed children, including autism and ASD, attention-deficit/hyperactivity disorder (ADHD), and dyspraxia as based on diagnoses received from professionals outside of the study. An NDD was diagnosed in 12% of 50 children exposed to valproate monotherapy and in 15% of 20 children exposed to valproate in polytherapy.[35] These rates were significantly elevated compared with an NDD rate of 1.87% in the 214 control children.

Carbamazepine

In its 2009 guidelines, the American Academy of Neurology (AAN) stated, "Carbamazepine probably does not substantially increase the risk of major congenital malformations in the offspring of women with epilepsy."[36] This conclusion was based on one class I study[37] from the United Kingdom and the Ireland Pregnancy Registry that did not find a difference between the rate of malformations in carbamazepine-exposed pregnancies and those of an internal control group. At the time, carbamazepine was the only medication that the AAN felt had strong enough evidence to support this conclusion. Across seven pregnancy registries, rates of major malformations in pregnancies exposed to carbamazepine monotherapy have ranged from 2.6% to 5.5%.[23-29] The two largest studies, the United Kingdom and Ireland Pregnancy Registries ($n = 1657$) and the EURAP registry ($n = 1402$) reported rates of 2.6% and 5.6%, respectively. Of note, the two registries that reported higher rates of major anomalies with carbamazepine exposure—the Australian and EURAP registries—both follow the exposed infants to 1 year and beyond, whereas the other registries performed the last assessment for malformations at birth or 3 months.[22] In the EURAP registry, malformations that were most likely to be picked up between 2 and 12 months were cardiac, hip, and renal malformations.[24] The rates of anomalies increased for several drugs at the later assessment, but rates with carbamazepine were most affected.

In the EUROCAT database, carbamazepine exposure was specifically associated with an increased risk of NTDs compared with unexposed controls (OR, 2.6; 95% confidence interval [CI], 1.2 to 5.3).[38] However, the risk of spina bifida with carbamazepine exposure was still significantly lower than the risk with valproate (OR, 0.2; 95% CI, 0.1 to 0.6) and was not different from the risk of exposure to other AEDs when valproic acid was excluded. The EUROCAT study did not find a specific association between carbamazepine exposure and other major malformations that included oral clefts, diaphragmatic hernia, hypospadias, and total anomalous venous return.[38] In the compiled registry data prepared by Tomson and Battino,[24] the absolute risks of certain anomalies with exposure to carbamazepine monotherapy were reported for NTDs (0.8%), cardiac malformations (0.3%), hypospadias (0.4%), and oral clefts (0.36%).

Early studies of carbamazepine's effect on cognitive development were conflicting, and many were limited by retrospective design or did not control for important confounders. A Cochrane review[39] of prospective studies published prior to 2014 concluded that the reported effects of carbamazepine on developmental scores were largely accounted for by variability between studies and identified no clear risk of delayed development in infants and toddlers exposed to carbamazepine. The

meta-analysis also reported no evident adverse effect of carbamazepine exposure on the IQ of school-age children.[39] In the NEAD study, no specific effects of carbamazepine exposure on IQ were identified when this group of children was compared with the lamotrigine- and phenytoin-exposed cohorts at age 6.[31] The recent LMNG study also found no difference in the adjusted mean IQ scores between the 6-year-old carbamazepine-exposed children and controls, but verbal IQ was 4.2 points lower in the exposed children. Additionally, the relative risk of having an IQ below 85 was significantly increased in the carbamazepine cohort.[32] Both the NEAD and LMNG studies demonstrated that, compared with valproate exposure, prenatal carbamazepine exposure was less likely to be associated with adverse cognitive effects.[31,32]

The LMNG found no increased risk for formally diagnosed NDDs at 6 years in the carbamazepine-exposed children when compared with controls.[35] The large Danish population study by Christensen and colleagues[33] also found no increased risk of autism or ASD in teenagers and children with prenatal carbamazepine exposure. An earlier study in Aberdeen, Scotland reported that two of 80 (2.5%) of carbamazepine-exposed children had an ASD, which is above the population rate (0.25%) but lower than that of the valproate group (8.9%).[40] These findings are limited by the small number of cases, the absence of a control group, and retrospective recruitment of only 41% of the original AED-exposed cohort, which potentially introduced a selection bias. The more recent study[34] of autistic traits from the Australian Registry also recruited mothers retrospectively from the prospectively identified cohort (63% enrollment). This study reported scores consistent with autism in one of 34 children exposed to carbamazepine and scores that raised "concern for autism" in another child based on a standardized assessment. The overall rate of autistic traits was 5.9%. The authors advise that this increase should be interpreted with caution because no discernable dose-effect of carbamazepine and no increased risk were seen in pregnancies exposed to polytherapy regimens that excluded valproate. The majority of these polytherapy regimens did include carbamazepine.[34]

Lamotrigine

Rates of major malformations with lamotrigine exposure have been consistently low and range from 2% to 4.6%, across eight prospective registries.[24-29,41,42] Initially, the North American AED Pregnancy Registry (NAAPR) reported a tenfold increased risk in oral clefts with lamotrigine monotherapy exposure. However, with a larger sample size, this risk was reevaluated and reported as a fourfold increased risk (absolute risk with lamotrigine, 0.45%).[26] A case-control study,[43] however, found no specific increased risk of oral clefting with lamotrigine, and other registries have reported much lower rates of clefting with lamotrigine exposure (0.1% to 0.25%).[37,41,44] The absolute risks of clefting reported by Tomson and Battino[24] was 0.15%. The composite risk of other specific malformations in this review were 0.6% for cardiac defects, 0.12% for NTDs, and 0.36% for hypospadias.[24]

In two independent cohorts from the United Kingdom, developmental scores of infants prenatally exposed to lamotrigine did not differ from those of controls.[45,46] In the LMNG cohort, at 6 years of age, the IQ scores of the lamotrigine-exposed children did not differ from those of controls.[32] Additionally, in the NEAD study, FSIQ scores in children exposed to lamotrigine were significantly higher than those of valproate-exposed children and did not differ from those of carbamazepine- or phenytoin-exposed children.[31] However, both valproate and lamotrigine exposure were associated with decreased verbal IQ relative to nonverbal IQ.[31] In a Norwegian population-based mail survey, parents of lamotrigine-exposed infants also reported impaired language functioning and an increase in autistic traits observed in their children.[47] Parental ratings of the 6-year-old children prenatally exposed to lamotrigine in the NEAD study suggested that they may be at increased risk for ADHD, but the teacher ratings in a subgroup of these children did not substantiate this finding, and no tendency toward social impairment was detected.[48] In contrast to these parental observations, the LMNG found no increased risk of formally diagnosed NDDs in lamotrigine-exposed children,[35] and the population study by Christensen and colleagues[33] found no increased risk of autism or ASD.

Levetiracetam

Levetiracetam is a relatively new AED, and to date, just over 1000 pregnancies have been reported across eight prospective registries, which have each recruited relatively small cohorts. The major malformation rates across these registries range from 0% to 2.4%.[24-27,29,41,49] Developmental effects of levetiracetam have been assessed in one study of 51 levetiracetam-exposed children recruited from pregnancies identified in the U.K. Epilepsy and Pregnancy Register.[50] At 36 to 54 months, the developmental scores of the exposed children did not differ from those of controls but were better than a group exposed to valproate. Because this is the only investigation of developmental outcomes with levetiracetam exposure, it will need to be replicated in future studies.

Phenytoin

Despite the fact that phenytoin is one of the oldest AEDs still in use, little certainty exists in regard to its teratogenic implications. **In 1975, Hanson and Smith[51] described a specific fetal hydantoin syndrome associated with in utero phenytoin exposure.** They noted growth and performance delays and craniofacial abnormalities that included clefting and limb anomalies, including hypoplasia of nails and distal phalanges. They later reported that this was present in 11% of 35 exposed infants and that 31% of exposed infants had some aspects of the syndrome.[52] Yet other studies have not substantiated this. In 1988, Gaily and colleagues[53] reported no evidence of the hydantoin syndrome in 82 women exposed in utero to phenytoin. Some of the patients had hypertelorism and hypoplasia of the distal phalanges, but none had the full hydantoin syndrome. The true prevalence of this syndrome and contributing factors has not been established, and it has largely fallen out of current literature.

The more recent pregnancy registries have not focused on the description of syndromes. Of note, the major malformations studied in these registries do not include many of the skeletal abnormalities included in the fetal hydantoin syndrome. Rates of anomalies in these registries have ranged from 2.4% to 6.7% across five registries,[24,26,27,29,37] but only 761 pregnancies have been enrolled in these studies, and the individual cohorts are small. The largest cohort studied in the NAAPR published a major malformation rate of 2.9% among 416 phenytoin-exposed pregnancies.[26] Tomson and Battino[24] reported the **rates of specific malformations with phenytoin exposure: 0.4% for cardiac malformations, 0% for NTDs, 0.2% for oral clefts, and 0.5% for hypospadias.**

The cognitive implications of phenytoin exposure have only been evaluated in a few prospective studies. The 2014 Cochrane review[39] found that the methodologies of these studies were too disparate to perform a meta-analysis. The review concluded that **phenytoin exposure was associated with better developmental and cognitive outcomes than valproate exposure and that no discernable differences between phenytoin and carbamazepine exposure were present in terms of development and IQ.** In the NEAD study, average FSIQ and verbal IQ scores of the phenytoin-exposed children were significantly higher than those of the valproate-exposed cohort and were not different from those of children exposed to carbamazepine or lamotrigine. Because the study did not include an unexposed control group, it is unknown whether the phenytoin group would differ from unexposed children.[31] In terms of behavioral effects, Vinten and associates[54] reported no difference between parentally assessed adaptive behaviors in the phenytoin-exposed Norwegian children when compared with unexposed controls born to mothers with epilepsy.

Phenobarbital

Phenobarbital is rarely used as a first-line AED in developed countries given its adverse cognitive and metabolic side effects and the availability of alternative medications with fewer adverse effects. It is very difficult to wean patients from phenobarbital, however, and this process often leads to worsened seizure control. Thus, unless pregnancy is planned well in advance, many women previously taking phenobarbital may remain on it. In the NAAPR, phenobarbital was associated with a risk of major malformations of 5.5% in 199 pregnancies, and cardiac malformations were the most frequent malformation reported. In a pooled analysis of 765 barbiturate-exposed pregnancies, Tomson and Battino[24] reported a rate of 3.5% for cardiac malformations and a 1% risk or oral clefts. The absolute risk of NTDs and hypospadias in this analysis was 0.2% for each.

Retrospective studies of the effect of phenobarbital on cognitive and educational outcomes of exposed children have reported mixed results.[55-58] The largest prospective study[59] of phenobarbital and cognitive outcomes evaluated a cohort of 114 Danish men who had been exposed to phenobarbital in utero between 1959 and 1961. The most common indication for phenobarbital was pregnancy-related hypertension, and mothers with epilepsy were not evaluated. Thus the exposure to phenobarbital was likely shorter in duration than in the children of mothers with epilepsy. The phenobarbital-exposed group had significantly lower IQ scores compared with controls, and children exposed in the third trimester were most affected. In a subset of 33 subjects, this effect was driven by lower verbal IQ compared with children exposed to other AEDs in monotherapy. In a prospective study, Thomas and colleagues[60] also found lower IQs in a group of 12 phenobarbital-exposed children. None of the studies to evaluate the cognitive effects of phenobarbital have accounted for the maternal IQ, which is an important predictor of the child's IQ.

Other Antiepileptic Drugs

A paucity of data is available to describe the teratogenic risks of other AEDs commonly used to treat epilepsy. The rate of major malformations with oxcarbazepine exposure among 393 prospective cases in the Danish birth registry was 2.8%. Other cohorts are smaller.[41] In the NAAPR study,[61] no major anomalies were reported in a cohort of 98 pregnancies exposed to zonisamide monotherapy, but this was interpreted with caution given the small sample size. The study did demonstrate an increased risk of low birthweight with both zonisamide and topiramate exposure. Recently, concern has been raised that topiramate is a significant teratogen, although sample sizes are still small. In the NAAPR study, the risk of major anomalies was 4.2% in 359 pregnancies.[26] **The registry also reported a tenfold increased risk of oral clefts in the topiramate cohort compared with that of an external control group; this corresponded to an absolute risk of 1.4%,[26]** which resulted in the **U.S. Food and Drug Administration (FDA) reclassification of topiramate from class C to class D for pregnancy. This concern has been corroborated by subsequent cohorts and meta-analyses.**[62,63] Studies of the effect of oxcarbazepine, zonisamide, and topiramate on cognitive and behavioral development are limited.

Little useful information is available on the effect of human in utero exposure to other AEDs that include benzodiazepines, eslicarbazepine, ethosuximide ezogabine, felbamate, gabapentin, lacosamide, perampanel, pregabalin, rufinamide, and vigabatrin. The manufacturers of lacosamide, a recently introduced AED, caution that it is known to antagonize the collapsin response mediator protein 2, which is involved in axonal growth and neuronal differentiation and appears to have adverse effects on brain development in rodents.[64]

Effect of Antiepileptic Drug Dose
The risk of major malformations has been shown to be dose related for several AEDs. In the EURAP registry, for example, valproate monotherapy was associated with a malformation risk of 5.6% with preconception doses of less than 750 mg/day and a risk of 24.6% with doses greater than 1500 mg/day.[29] Similar correlations between the risk of birth defects and preconception AED dose were also noted for carbamazepine, lamotrigine, and phenobarbital. Additionally, dose effects on cognitive and behavioral development have been noted for valproate,[32,34,65] although more data on the relationship between cognitive teratogenesis and dose of both valproate and other AEDs are needed. Further research is also required on the relevance of serum concentrations, instead of dose, because of the substantial differences in AED metabolism among individuals. For now, preparing a woman with epilepsy for pregnancy involves trying to identify the minimum therapeutic dose and corresponding drug level to control her seizures.

Polytherapy
It was previously thought that AED polytherapy always posed more of a teratogenic risk than monotherapy and that polytherapy should be avoided whenever possible. This conclusion was based on several prior studies that demonstrated a higher rate of major malformations with polytherapy. However, a recent study from the NAAPR suggested that the results of these prior studies were largely driven by polytherapy combinations that included valproate. Within the NAAPR, Holmes and colleagues[66] reported that the risk of major anomalies with lamotrigine and valproate therapy was 9.1%, whereas it was 2.9% for the combination of lamotrigine and any other AED. Similarly, they reported that carbamazepine and valproate polytherapy was associated with a major malformation risk of 15.4%, which was much higher than the 2.5% risk seen with the combination of carbamazepine and any other AED. The authors also

highlighted similar findings that had been reported in the United Kingdom Epilepsy and Pregnancy Registry[37] and the International Lamotrigine Pregnancy Registry.[42] Studies on cognitive development have suggested the same trend. In an Australian cohort, Nadebaum and colleagues[65] found that in utero exposure to valproate polytherapy was associated with significantly lower FSIQ and verbal comprehension scores than exposure to valproate monotherapy or polytherapy combinations without valproate. The LMNG also reported that only polytherapies that included valproate were linked to decreased mean FSIQ and verbal IQ in school-age children.[32]

The mainstay of epilepsy therapy, especially in women of childbearing age, is still to try to find the one AED that best controls a patient's seizures at the minimum therapeutic dose or level. However, in certain cases, polytherapy may be preferable to monotherapy. For example, women with idiopathic generalized epilepsies have a limited number of AEDs that are appropriate for their condition. Valproate is an effective option for this type of epilepsy but is a poor choice for these women. When one AED—such as levetiracetam or lamotrigine—is ineffective for these patients, the combination of the two may sometimes be effective and likely carries a reduced risk of teratogenesis when compared with valproate monotherapy. Given the emerging information on the relationship between AED dose and malformation risk for most AEDs, more research is needed to determine whether polytherapy combinations that involve low doses of two AEDs are ever preferable to a single non-valproate AED at a high dose.

Effects of Pregnancy on Anticonvulsant Medications
Although most pregnancy studies to date have focused on AED dose, AED levels are probably far more important and should be studied in the future. Although drug manufacturers and laboratories publish standard therapeutic windows for individual AEDs, these large ranges have little relevance for a given patient with epilepsy. **AED metabolism varies greatly by individual, and each patient has her own therapeutic drug level at which seizures are best controlled. This is typically within the standard window but may be above or below it. Therefore it is important to understand and establish this drug level prior to pregnancy whenever possible, because levels of anticonvulsant medications can change dramatically during pregnancy, and in many cases, decreasing AED levels have been associated with loss of seizure control.** When prepregnancy levels have not been obtained, they should be drawn as early as possible in the first trimester. Whereas a trough level is ideal, it is usually not practical or safe for women to hold medications for a blood draw. It is more important that they have levels drawn at a convenient and roughly standard time relative to their AED dose. For certain AEDs, including phenytoin and sometimes carbamazepine and valproate, free (unbound) drug levels are available and preferable.

Many factors—including altered protein binding, delayed gastric emptying, nausea and vomiting, changes in plasma volume, changes in the volume of distribution, and even folic acid supplementation—can affect the levels of anticonvulsant medications. Additionally, changes in AED metabolism can be dramatically altered by the pregnant state.

Lamotrigine is the most common AED prescribed in pregnancy, and it is utilized to treat both epilepsy and bipolar disorder. It is also the best example of the substantial effects of pregnancy on AED metabolism. Lamotrigine clearance depends heavily on glucuronidation, a process induced by the increases in estrogen during pregnancy. **Over the course of a pregnancy, lamotrigine clearance increases by over 200% in the majority of women with epilepsy.**[67] **Lamotrigine doses need to be increased substantially over the course of a pregnancy in order to maintain prepregnancy levels and seizure control.** Doses of 600 to 900 mg/day are not uncommon by the end of pregnancy. Lamotrigine metabolism decreases rapidly after delivery and returns to baseline within 3 weeks of delivery. To avoid toxicity, it is important to give patients a postpartum dosing plan to taper their dose starting immediately after delivery and then decrease back toward the baseline dose. Leaving a patient on slightly more than her prepregnancy dose is also common, especially in patients with brittle seizure control who may be especially susceptible to the effects of sleep deprivation.

Although less well studied, oxcarbazepine clearance is also dependent on glucuronidation.[68] In the EURAP registry, patients taking oxcarbazepine or lamotrigine during pregnancy were noted to have poorer seizure control than those taking other AEDs.[69,70] Less than half of those using lamotrigine or oxcarbazepine had their doses adjusted, which suggests therapeutic drug monitoring may not have been regularly performed. In contrast, levels of free and total carbamazepine—as well as a metabolite of carbamazepine—are relatively stable throughout pregnancy,[71] and seizure control appears to be better in patients taking carbamazepine.[72,73] **Given the interindividual variation in AED metabolism and susceptibility to changes during pregnancy, checking AED drug levels monthly is recommended for all AEDs.**

Pregnancy and Seizure Frequency

For the majority of women with epilepsy (54% to 80%), seizure frequency will remain similar to their baseline seizure frequency. Across several studies, seizure frequency increased in 15.8% to 32% of women and decreased in 3% to 24%.[1,69,74,75] **Seizure freedom for 9 months prior to pregnancy is associated with an 84% to 92% chance of remaining seizure free during pregnancy.**[1] Genetic generalized epilepsies seem to be associated with less of a risk of seizures during pregnancy than focal epilepsies, although both groups of patients are at increased risk of seizures in the peripartum and postpartum periods.[1,69,76]

A recent study from the Australian Register of Antiepileptic Drugs in Pregnancy (APR) suggested that the AEDs taken during pregnancy might predict seizure control.[73] The authors reported that the risk of seizures was lowest with valproate (27%), levetiracetam (31.8%), and carbamazepine (37.8%), whereas an increased risk of seizures was seen with lamotrigine (51.3%). Phenytoin (51.2%) and topiramate (54.8%) were also associated with a relatively higher risk of seizures, but the sample sizes of these groups were small. As mentioned above, the EURAP registry has also reported a higher risk of seizures in patients taking lamotrigine or oxcarbazepine.[69,70] In contrast to the APR, a small study by Reisinger and colleagues[72] found a relatively high risk of seizure deterioration in patients treated with levetiracetam monotherapy (47%) when they compared seizures during pregnancy to each patient's baseline. The NAAPR also notes that rates of seizures during pregnancies managed with levetiracetam were similar to the rates in patients treated with lamotrigine.[26] The increasing metabolism and falling AED levels

of many of the newer AEDs including lamotrigine likely play an important role in the variable seizure control reported. Both the APR and EURAP registries reported that lamotrigine dosing had been increased in fewer than 50% of cases analyzed.[69,73] Future prospective studies, during which therapeutic drug monitoring and appropriate dose adjustments are made, will be necessary to understand whether AED metabolism is the principal reason for worsening seizure control with certain AEDs or if other factors play a role.

Obstetric and Neonatal Outcomes

Women with epilepsy may be at increased risk for obstetric complications. Historically, studies on obstetric complications had yielded mixed results. A 2009 evidence-based review from the AAN reported that insufficient evidence was available to support or refute an increased risk of preeclampsia or gestational hypertension in women with epilepsy. They also stated that preterm labor was probably not increased, at least not to moderate levels (1.5 times the baseline risk) except in women with epilepsy who smoked.[1] Since then, population studies from the United States and Norway have associated epilepsy with a mild to moderate risk of preeclampsia (OR, 1.59 to 1.7) and preterm labor (OR, 1.54 to 1.6) when compared with that of women without epilepsy.[9,77] *Preterm labor* was defined as labor before 34 weeks in the Norwegian study and before 37 weeks in the U.S. study. In the Norwegian study by Borthen and colleagues,[78] the risk of these complications in women with epilepsy who did not take AEDs was not increased. However, the possibility that these patients may have had milder epilepsy must be considered. Borthen and colleagues[78] also studied 205 epileptic women from a single Norwegian hospital and found an increased risk of severe preeclampsia in these patients compared with unaffected women.

Epilepsy and AED use are typically not indications for cesarean delivery (CD); however, CD may be more common in women with epilepsy. The reasons for this association are unclear and has not been seen consistently across all studies.[9,77-79] In their hospital-based study, Borthen and colleagues[78] found no significant increased risk of CD if preterm labor was accounted for. Induction of labor may also be more common in women with epilepsy.[9,78] Prospective studies are needed to determine the reasons for labor induction and CD in women with epilepsy. It is unclear if this is related to other complications in these women or physician or patient concern about seizures during late pregnancy or delivery.

Bleeding complications at delivery may also be increased in women with epilepsy, although again studies have been conflicting on this point.[79] Population studies from Norway and the United States both suggest a small but significantly increased risk of postpartum hemorrhage.[9,80]

According to the 2009 AAN literature review and recommendations, evidence was sufficient to suggest a near twofold **increased risk of SGA infants born to epileptic women taking AEDs,** but the group felt data were inadequate on the risk of intrauterine growth restriction (IUGR).[36] A recent study from a prospective registry in Norway studied 287 children born to women with epilepsy and found that they had an increased risk of being SGA and having a ponderal index below the tenth percentile.[81] AED exposure was the strongest predictor of a low ponderal index, but seizure frequency was not controlled for. In yet another Norwegian study,[25] topiramate was specifically associated with SGA infants, and in an investigation from the NAAPR, both topiramate and zonisamide were associated with lower birthweights in exposed infants.[61] A Taiwanese study by Chen and colleagues found that seizures during pregnancy were associated with an increased risk of SGA.

The recent U.S. population study found a mild but significantly increased risk of stillbirth in women with epilepsy (OR, 1.27; 95% CI, 1.17 to 1.38).[9] Two other population studies from Denmark and Norway found a trend toward an increased stillbirth risk of similar magnitude, but the effect was not statistically significant.[82,83] Little else about fetal outcomes of infants born to women with epilepsy is known. The AAN did conclude that the offspring of women using AEDs were at greater risk for a low 1-minute Apgar score.[84]

Preconception Counseling for Women With Epilepsy

Ideally, preconception counseling for a woman with epilepsy should begin at the time of diagnosis and with prescription of the first AED. Unfortunately, this is not always possible. For most patients, the obstetrician must stress that the patient has a greater than 90% chance of having a successful pregnancy that results in a normal newborn. A detailed history of medication use, seizure types, and seizure frequency should be obtained. The patient must be informed that if she has frequent seizures before conception, this pattern will probably continue. Furthermore, if she has frequent seizures, in most cases, she should be encouraged to delay conception until control is optimized. The obstetrician must stress that controlling seizures is of primary importance. For patients with seizures that have been refractory to one to two medications, inpatient video EEG monitoring is often indicated to determine whether the patient is a surgical candidate. Inpatient video EEG monitoring is also recommended in intractable cases or in any patient with atypical features to rule out a diagnosis of nonepileptic seizures. It can be very difficult to diagnose nonepileptic seizures based on clinical history, but some features that should raise suspicion of this diagnosis are closed eyes during a seizure, long duration of seizure activity that waxes and wanes, and a history of abuse.

Valproate is a poor first choice as an AED for any woman of childbearing age. In addition to the adverse effects on pregnancy, valproate is associated with weight gain, hirsutism, and signs of polycystic ovarian syndrome (PCOS). **Lamotrigine and levetiracetam are better choices and are quickly becoming the most commonly prescribed drugs for women of childbearing age.** They are often used in both focal and generalized epilepsies. Carbamazepine is also a reasonable option for women with focal epilepsy. If these medications are not effective, however, a woman may need to be switched to an AED with higher teratogenic risk or undefined risk. In these cases the patient should be counseled on the available information and unknowns, but again, the importance of seizure control should be stressed. In some women with genetic generalized epilepsies, valproate is the only drug that effectively controls their seizures. Valproate therapy is not a reason to terminate pregnancy, and despite the relatively increased risks of teratogenesis, the majority of women taking valproate will have healthy children. For all AEDs, pre-pregnancy counseling should include trying to find the minimum therapeutic dose/level needed. This is of utmost importance in women taking valproate.

As discussed above, it is important to establish baseline AED levels prior to pregnancy in order to set a target for dose adjustment during pregnancy. A minimum of two levels taken at a similar time of day is advisable to establish a given individual's therapeutic range.

Unfortunately, the majority of pregnancies in women with epilepsy are unplanned,[85] which emphasizes the need for appropriate selection of an AED for women of childbearing age and the need for early preconception counseling. **Changing AEDs once a woman is already pregnant is usually not recommended.** Structural teratogenesis occurs early in the first trimester, and the potential effects of exposure are likely already underway by the time a woman learns she is pregnant. Additionally, switching drugs during the first trimester exposes the fetus to polytherapy and potentially breakthrough seizures during this critical time. Given the increasing knowledge of the adverse cognitive effects of valproate, which are mostly thought to occur in the third trimester, some specialists have switched women off valproate typically to levetiracetam. No available evidence supports or refutes this approach, but it should only be considered in select patients whose history suggests that they may have a good chance of responding to a different drug and are in the care of an epilepsy specialist who can monitor them closely.

If the patient has had no seizures during the past 2 to 4 years, an attempt may be made to withdraw her from anticonvulsant medications. This is usually done over a 1- to 3-month period, slowly reducing the medication, and should not be done close to or during pregnancy. Up to 50% of patients relapse and need to start their medications again. This withdrawal should be attempted only if the patient is completely seizure free and has a normal EEG, and it should only be done with the help of a neurologist. Based on a patient's history, many neurologists will recommend that the patient refrain from driving for a period of time during and after the wean.

Genetic Counseling

A detailed family history should be taken in the process of counseling women with epilepsy. A history of congenital malformations in the family increases the chances of having an affected child. In particular, in women taking valproate, those who have had prior pregnancies complicated by a malformation have a significantly increased risk of having a second child with a malformation, regardless of whether they were taking valproate at the time of the prior pregnancy.[86]

It is also important to take a family history that includes seizure disorders, including febrile seizures, and intellectual disability. Many patients are concerned about the risk of passing epilepsy on to their child. Only a few epidemiologic studies have looked at the inheritance patterns of epilepsy. **For most patients with epilepsy, the risk of passing it on to their children is higher than the approximate 1% to 2% risk in the general population; however, the absolute risk remains low.** Factors associated with a low risk are late onset of epilepsy in the parent and a known acquired cause of epilepsy such as a vascular malformation, stroke, or trauma. Patients with an early onset of epilepsy, epilepsy of unknown cause, and a family history of epilepsy—particularly in a first-degree relative—have a higher risk. Epilepsy associated with intellectual disability may also be more likely to be genetic. Across many studies, the "genetic" generalized epilepsies or idiopathic generalized epilepsies have a higher risk of inheritance than focal epilepsy. Interestingly, a consistent finding in several epidemiologic studies is that mothers with epilepsy have a much higher chance of having a child with epilepsy than do fathers with epilepsy. The most recent large population study from Rochester, Minnesota reviewed the medical records of all 660 probands with epilepsy born between 1935 and 1994 and all their first-degree relatives.[87] This study also found that epilepsy was more likely to be inherited from the mother, although when analyzed separately, this effect was only true for focal epilepsies, not generalized epilepsies. When all types of epilepsy were considered, the cumulative incidence to age 40 of epilepsy in a child of a woman with epilepsy was 5.39%, which correlates to a fivefold increased risk from the baseline population. The authors recommended taking the standard error into account and counseling women that **on average, the risk of passing on epilepsy is 2.69% to 8%**. In children of women with generalized epilepsy, the incidence was 8.34% (1.36% to 15.36% risk, considering standard error), and if the mother had focal epilepsy, the incidence was 4.43% (1.43% to 7.43%).

This type of epidemiologic data can be useful for patients with epilepsy of unknown cause, but they should not be used to counsel all patients indiscriminately. It is critical that the neurologist and obstetrician take a patient's individual clinical and family history into account before advising on the risks of passing on epilepsy.

An increasing number of epilepsy genes and familial syndromes have been discovered that can substantially alter the risk of inheriting an epileptic disorder.[88] Autosomal-dominant forms of epilepsy, such as autosomal-dominant frontal lobe epilepsy (ADFLE) and autosomal-dominant temporal lobe epilepsy (ADTLE), are highly penetrant familial epilepsies that should be considered in a patient with one or more first-degree relatives with a similar epilepsy syndrome. Mutations in the sodium channel, voltage gated, type 1 alpha subunit (*SCN1A*) gene have variable penetrance and expressivity, and they can present with a range of manifestations. Even within one family, some individuals with the mutation will be unaffected, some will have simple febrile seizures or a mild epilepsy syndrome that persists into adulthood, whereas others can have Dravet syndrome, a severe epileptic encephalopathy. Preimplantation genetic testing for these disorders is available only for some syndromes and is controversial. However, recognizing these family syndromes definitely changes the counseling on the risk of inheriting epilepsy. Other genetic syndromes associated with epilepsy have more serious complications. For example, bilateral periventricular nodular heterotopia (PVNH; Fig. 49-1) is an uncommon cause of focal epilepsy. Approximately 50% of female patients with PVNH will have a mutation in the filamin A gene.[89] This is an X-linked–dominant mutation that is typically lethal in males in the third trimester or in the immediate postnatal period. Female patients may have no manifestations other than the periventricular nodules, which represent aberrant neuronal migration, and epilepsy. An echocardiogram is recommended in these women, because they can have cardiac anomalies. Other examples of critical genetic diagnoses are mitochondrial disorders that can present with epilepsy. Whereas a comprehensive review of the genetics of epilepsy is beyond the scope of this chapter, **genetic counseling is an important option for many prospective parents with epilepsy, and certain clinical findings or key features in a family history, such as other affected relatives or frequent miscarriages, make specialized counseling essential.**

Folic Acid Supplementation

The 2009 AAN practice guidelines recommend folic acid supplementation of 0.4 to 4 mg/day for all women of

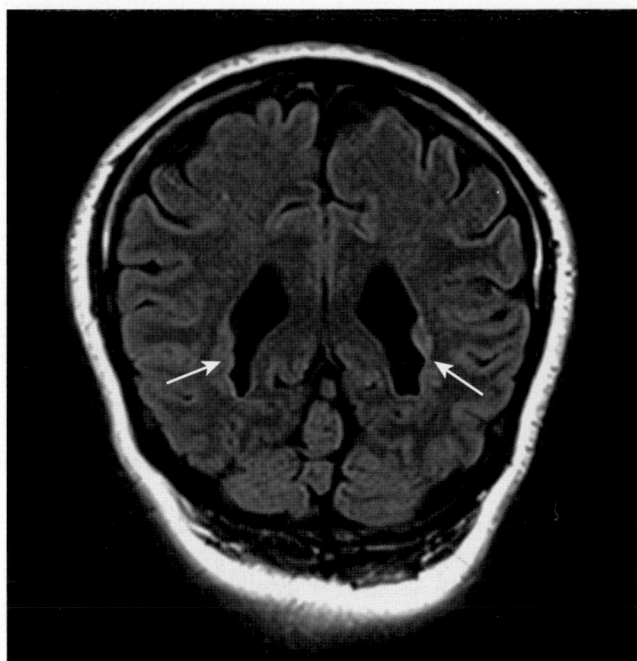

FIG 49-1 Bilateral periventricular nodular heterotopia (PVNH). Magnetic resonance imaging (MRI) of a 28-year-old primigravida with intractable focal epilepsy who presented for neurologic evaluation at 24 weeks' gestation. Her prior MRI demonstrated bilateral PNVH (*white arrows* point to abnormal cortical tissue lining the ventricles bilaterally). In up to 50% of women, this syndrome is associated with an X-linked dominant mutation in the filamin A gene that is often lethal in male fetuses in the third trimester or the first few postnatal days. In females, this mutation is associated with the above migrational abnormalities and focal seizures. Female patients may have normal or slightly low intelligence quotients (IQs). This case illustrates the importance of early prepregnancy neurologic evaluation and genetic counseling.

childbearing age who take AEDs.[90] These recommendations are largely extrapolated from studies that have demonstrated that folic acid supplementation reduces the risk for NTDs in the general population.[91] Additionally, low first-trimester serum folic acid levels have been correlated with an increased risk for congenital malformations in the offspring of women with epilepsy, and several AEDs are known to lower folic acid levels.[92,93] Little direct evidence is available to suggest that folic acid reduces the risk of major anomalies in women taking AEDs, although the AAN practice guidelines state that prior studies might have been underpowered to detect a benefit.[90] One study by Pittschieler and colleagues[94] suggested that folic acid may reduce the risks of miscarriage in women with epilepsy. The NEAD study[31] also found an association between higher IQs in children of mothers with epilepsy who took periconceptional folic acid supplementation (≥0.4 mg). It is unclear whether this effect was specific to AED use because similar beneficial effects on cognitive development have been noted in the general population. The optimal dose of folic acid for women taking AEDs is not known. A recent study of women without epilepsy found delayed psychomotor development in children of women exposed to doses greater than 5 mg compared with women who took doses of 0.4 to 1 mg, which raises concerns about the practice of high-dose supplementation.[95] More research is needed to determine the optimal dose of folic acid in women with epilepsy. In the meantime, **supplementation with 0.4 to 1 mg in all women**

of childbearing age taking AEDs should be recommended. Many clinicians increase the dose to 4 mg of folic acid when a patient is trying to conceive or is pregnant.

Vitamin D deficiency is also common in women with epilepsy. This occurs because anticonvulsants may interfere with the conversion of 25-hydroxycholecalciferol to 1,25-dihydroxycholecalciferol, the active form of vitamin D. **Ideally, 25-hydroxyvitamin D levels should be checked and optimized prior to pregnancy.** A supplemental dose of 1000 to 2000 IU of vitamin D_3 in addition to a prenatal vitamin is reasonable during pregnancy. Additionally, because folic acid supplementation can mask the hematologic effects of vitamin B_{12} deficiency, B_{12} levels should also be checked in women with epilepsy.

Care of the Patient During Pregnancy

Once the patient becomes pregnant, it is of the utmost importance to establish accurate gestational dating. This will prevent any confusion over fetal growth in later gestation. **AED levels should be checked as soon as possible and then monthly. Adjustments should be made to keep the patient's AED level around her prepregnancy or early pregnancy level.**

An early anatomic ultrasound at 14 to 15 weeks' gestation can identify signs suggestive of NTDs in women at high risk (see Chapter 9). At approximately 16 weeks' gestation, the patient should undergo blood testing with maternal serum alpha-fetoprotein screening in an attempt to detect any NTD. Coupled with ultrasonography, these data result in a detection rate of more than 90% for open NTDs (see Chapter 10). **At 18 to 22 weeks, the patient should undergo a specialized, detailed anatomic ultrasound to determine whether congenital malformations, including NTDs, are present. If adequate views of the fetal heart are not obtained, a fetal echocardiogram can be performed at 20 to 22 weeks' gestation to detect cardiac malformations, which are among the more common malformations in women taking any antiepileptic medications.** In the United States, no official recommendations have been made on the use of fetal cardiac echo studies in women with epilepsy, but the 2009 Italian guidelines do advise this examination for all women taking AEDs.[96]

As previously noted, there appears to be an increased risk for IUGR in fetuses exposed in utero to anticonvulsant medications. If the patient's weight gain and fundal growth appear appropriate, regular ultrasound examinations to assess fetal weight are probably unnecessary. If, however, if poor fundal growth is suspected or if the patient's habitus precludes adequate assessment of this clinical parameter, serial ultrasonography for fetal weight discernment can be performed.

Antepartum fetal evaluation with nonstress testing is not necessary in all mothers with seizure disorders, but it should be considered for patients who have active seizures in the third trimester.

Vitamin K Supplementation

Third-trimester vitamin K supplementation in women taking certain enzyme-inducing AEDs (EIAEDs) is a historic practice based on a concern for an increased risk of intracranial neonatal hemorrhage and clotting factor deficiencies associated with EIAED exposure reported in early case studies.[97,98] EIAEDs include phenobarbital, phenytoin, carbamazepine, and oxcarbazepine. **A more recent study of 662 women with epilepsy taking EIAEDs did not find any increased risk of bleeding**

in the neonate if the infant received 1 mg of vitamin K intramuscularly at birth.[99] This problem is rare today because most neonates are given vitamin K at birth. The 2009 AAN guidelines state that evidence is insufficient to recommend for or against the practice of peripartum vitamin K supplementation.[90] Another recent study evaluated the risk of maternal postpartum hemorrhage in women with epilepsy and also found no significant difference in the risk of bleeding in women taking EIAEDs versus controls.[100] There was also no difference in the risk of bleeding in women taking EIAEDs who supplemented with vitamin K and those who did not.

Labor and Delivery

Although epidemiologically there may be an increased risk of induction of labor and CD in women with epilepsy, these interventions should not be recommended to women with epilepsy without specific additional obstetric, medical, or neurologic indications. Most women with epilepsy have successful vaginal deliveries. Although no evidence exists to support or challenge epidural analgesia in patients with epilepsy, it is typically utilized to decrease stress and allow the mother to rest during a long labor.

The risk of seizures during labor in women with epilepsy is 3.5% or less, and seizures are most common in patients who have had seizures during pregnancy.[69,70] Whenever a seizure occurs, acute seizure management involves assessing the patient's clinical stability, including respiratory and circulatory function. Nothing should be put in the mouth of a seizing patient, but supplemental oxygen should be provided, and suctioning of secretions can be performed if possible. Ideally, the patient should be turned on her left side to increase blood supply to the fetus. Short-acting benzodiazepines, typically lorazepam 0.1 mg/kg to 0.2 mg/kg with a maximum of 10 mg, are the mainstay of acute seizure treatment. If the seizure does not resolve within 2 minutes, lorazepam should be given. In most cases this is followed by intravenous (IV) fosphenytoin or phenytoin if seizures persist. *Status epilepticus* is defined by seizures that last more than 5 minutes. In the rare case of tonic-clonic status in pregnancy, intubation and stabilization with anesthesia may be required. Fetal monitoring should begin as soon as possible after a seizure, if it is not already in place. Transient fetal heart rate changes may be seen and can be tolerated temporarily, but if fetal bradycardia persists, the clinician must assume fetal compromise or placental abruption and must proceed with CD.

New Onset of Seizures in Pregnancy and in the Puerperium

Occasionally, seizures are diagnosed for the first time during pregnancy, which may present a diagnostic dilemma. **If the seizures occur in the third trimester, they are eclampsia until proven otherwise and should be treated as such until the physician can perform a proper evaluation.** The treatment of eclampsia is delivery, but the patient must first be stabilized (see Chapter 31). Magnesium sulfate, instead of AEDs, is the treatment of choice for eclamptic seizures. It is often difficult, however, to distinguish eclampsia from an epileptic seizure. The patient may be hypertensive initially after an epileptic seizure and may exhibit some myoglobinuria secondary to muscle breakdown, which will test as proteinuria on a routine urinalysis. The diagnosis becomes clearer over time, but in either case, rapid thoughtful action must be undertaken. The first physician to attend a patient after a seizure may not be an obstetrician/

gynecologist, and magnesium sulfate may not be started acutely; this should be remedied as soon as possible.

If the patient develops seizures for the first time at an earlier gestational age, she should be evaluated and started on the proper medication. The physician must look for acquired causes of seizures that include trauma, infection, metabolic disorders, space-occupying lesions, central nervous system (CNS) bleeding, and ingestion of drugs such as cocaine and amphetamines. Blood samples should be obtained for electrolytes, glucose, ionized calcium, magnesium, renal function studies, and toxicologic studies while IV access is being established. If the patient experienced a tonic-clonic seizure and the attending physician believes, based on clinical history, that this is probably new-onset epilepsy with a high likelihood of recurrence, she should be started on the appropriate anticonvulsant medication while awaiting the results of any laboratory studies. **Although lamotrigine is one of the most commonly prescribed drugs for women planning pregnancy, it is typically not practical to start it when epilepsy presents in pregnancy.** The lamotrigine titration schedule is at least 6 weeks because of an increased risk of a Stevens-Johnson reaction in patients taking this drug, especially if it is titrated quickly. In addition, accelerated lamotrigine metabolism in pregnancy makes it virtually impossible to achieve a therapeutic level in a pregnant woman over a reasonable time period. Similar considerations apply to oxcarbazepine. **For new-onset epilepsy, levetiracetam is often used first because it can be started quickly and does not carry a high risk of rash.** An unfortunate side effect of levetiracetam, however, is an increase in depressed mood or irritability; this should be assessed in women starting this drug.

Any patient who experiences seizures for the first time during pregnancy without a known cause should undergo an EEG and intracranial imaging. In studying only eclamptic patients, Sibai and colleagues[101] found that EEGs were initially abnormal in 75% of patients but normalized within 6 months in all women studied. Although this group found no uniform abnormalities on computed tomography (CT) in this series of eclamptic patients, they did find that 46% and 33% had some abnormal findings on EEG and CT, respectively. Most of the findings were nonspecific and were not helpful in diagnosis or treatment. An MRI is indicated in most cases of new-onset seizures and may be helpful if eclampsia is suspected.

Breastfeeding and the Postpartum Period

The levels of anticonvulsant medications must be monitored frequently during the first few weeks postpartum (see Chapter 23) because they can rise rapidly. **If the patient's medication dosages were increased during pregnancy, they will need to be decreased over the 3 weeks after delivery to levels at or slightly higher than that of the prepregnancy period.** As discussed above, this is especially important for lamotrigine.

The benefits of breastfeeding have been well established and include the promotion of mother-infant bonding (see Chapter 24).[102] **Whereas AEDs taken by the mother are present in breast milk to varying degrees, few data suggest neonatal harm from exposure through breast milk.** The NEAD study[103] found that infants exposed to carbamazepine, lamotrigine, phenytoin, and valproate in breast milk had higher IQs and language scores at 6 years than those infants whose mothers did not breastfeed. An improvement in parent-reported developmental abilities of children was also noted in breastfed infants in a Norwegian cohort of AED-exposed children at 6 and 18 months,

although the effect was not sustained at 36 months.[104] Neither study found adverse effects on developmental outcomes related to breast milk exposure for the studied drugs (carbamazepine, lamotrigine, phenytoin, and valproate). Although further prospective studies of AED exposure via breast milk are necessary, for most AEDs, the theoretic concern of prolonged infant exposure likely does not outweigh the known benefits of breastfeeding. Some experts advise caution with AEDs with longer half-lives, such as phenobarbital and zonisamide, although again the concern is largely theoretic.

Postpartum Safety

Breastfeeding should be supported and encouraged for most women with epilepsy; however the sleep deprivation associated with trying to feed a newborn may put her at risk for seizures. **A key part of managing a pregnancy in women with epilepsy is discussing seizure safety with her and her family.** Partners or other members of a patient's support system should assist with night feedings with either pumped milk or formula so that the patient can get a stretch of uninterrupted sleep, typically 6 to 8 hours depending on the patient. The patient may have to pump milk additional times during the day to maintain this supply. Other safety recommendations include giving baths only in the presence of another adult and changing diapers on a pad on the floor instead of on a changing table. Avoiding stairs when possible and using a stroller, rather than an infant carrier strapped to the mother, should also be considered. The importance of not allowing infants to sleep in the parents' bed should also be emphasized. Lastly, women with epilepsy are at increased risk for postpartum depression, a topic that should be discussed with the patient and her family prior to delivery and after.

Contraception

Contraceptive counseling is an important part of preconception and postpartum planning in women with epilepsy, and drug-drug interactions are numerous between AEDs and hormonal contraception. Both the Centers for Disease Control and Prevention (CDC) and the World Health Organization (WHO) have released evidence-based reviews on the use of specific types of contraception in women taking AEDs.[105,106] The most reliable form of reversible contraception is the intrauterine device (IUD), and this is considered the contraceptive method of choice for most women with epilepsy. Both the copper and levonorgestrel IUD are appropriate. If hormonal methods are considered, the physician should review the considerations laid out by the CDC and WHO before initiating treatment.

MULTIPLE SCLEROSIS

Multiple sclerosis (MS) is a chronic autoimmune demyelinating disease that affects women more often than men, and the ratio of affected females to males has been increasing over time.[107] **The onset of symptoms usually occurs between the ages of 20 and 40 years, and thus it commonly affects women of childbearing age.** The diagnosis of MS is often made years after the initial onset of symptoms. Common presenting symptoms include weakness, paresthesias or numbness of one or both lower extremities, visual complaints that include optic neuritis, and loss of coordination. MS primarily affects the white matter of the CNS, and lesions may involve the spinal cord, brainstem, cerebral hemispheres, and optic tracts. The hallmark of diagnosis is that it causes lesions "disseminated over space and time." **The**

most common form of the disease, relapsing remitting MS, is characterized by periodic exacerbations with complete or partial remissions. Only 10% to 15% of patients show steady progression at the time of onset, but over time, the majority of patients with MS will develop secondary progressive MS with continuing accumulation of neurologic deficits and disability.

Because symptoms of an MS attack can be subtle, it is often easy to attribute them to pregnancy. Many pregnant women complain of being more awkward or having some weakness. If these symptoms are persistent or progressive, they should not be ignored, and the patient should be referred for neurologic consultation. An MRI of the brain and sometimes an MRI of the spinal cord are necessary to make the diagnosis of MS. Gadolinium contrast is helpful to identify acute demyelinating lesions, but it should *not* be administered to pregnant women. Even without contrast, an MRI can be valuable in evaluating a patient with suspected MS or new symptoms in the setting of a prior diagnosis of MS.

Multiple Sclerosis and Fertility

The relationship between MS and fertility is unclear. Similar to women with epilepsy, women with MS are less likely to have children than are unaffected women.[108,109] However, it is not completely clear whether this is due to biologic reasons or to the reproductive decisions of women with MS. Other factors may play a role, such as sexual dysfunction, which is common in MS patients. Translational studies have suggested that women with MS may have reduced ovarian reserve based on elevated follicle-stimulating hormone (FSH) and decreased anti-Müllerian hormone (AMH) levels; AMH is a marker of ovarian reserve.[110,111] Additionally, women with MS are also more likely to utilize assisted reproductive technology (ART).[112] It should be noted, however, that in vitro fertilization (IVF) procedures that utilize gonadotropin-releasing hormone (GnRH) agonists have been shown to increase MS disease activity, particularly if the cycle is not successful.[113-115]

Effect of Pregnancy on Multiple Sclerosis

The risk of MS relapses is reduced during gestation but may increase transiently in the postpartum period. Convincing evidence shows that the risk of MS attacks is decreased during the course of pregnancy. It is hypothesized that the lower rate of disease activity during gestation may be attributable to a pregnancy-induced shift from thymus helper 1 (Th 1) cytokines to Th 2 cytokines to facilitate immune tolerance (see Chapter 4). The Pregnancy and Multiple Sclerosis (PRIMS) study prospectively followed 269 pregnancies in 254 women with MS across 12 European countries.[116,117] They found that the annual rate of relapse declined during pregnancy, especially in the third trimester. A rebound of disease activity was noted in the first 3 months postpartum, but subsequently the relapse frequency returned to baseline. Of note, the rate of relapse over the entire pregnancy year—9 months gestation plus 3 months postpartum—did not differ from the baseline rate, and only 28% of patients experienced a postpartum relapse. **Most importantly, no change in disability progression was noted over the duration of the study.**[117,118] A meta-analysis of 13 studies published prior to 2011 found that the annualized relapse rate significantly decreased from a baseline of 0.43 per year to 0.26 per year during pregnancy.[119] In the year following delivery, the average annualized rate of relapse increased to 0.7 per year.

Despite the transient increase in postpartum relapses seen in women with MS, pregnancy likely has a neutral effect on long-term disease progression. Weinshenker and colleagues[120] showed no association between long-term disability and (1) total number of term pregnancies, (2) the timing of pregnancy relative to the onset of MS, or (3) the worsening of MS in relation to a pregnancy. Verdru and associates[121] studied 200 women with MS and found that pregnancy delays the onset of long-term disability. As an index of progression, they used the length of time from onset of disease until wheelchair dependence. In patients with at least one pregnancy after diagnosis, the mean time to wheelchair dependence was 18.6 years compared with 12.5 years for other women. Similarly, Runmarker and Andersen[122] observed a decreased risk of MS onset in parous women compared with nulliparous women and reported that women who were pregnant after the onset of MS had a decreased risk of developing progressive disease. A recent retrospective study of 1317 Canadian women with MS also found that pregnancy slowed the rate of conversion to irreversible disability based on the Expanded Disability Status Scale (EDSS).[123] However, in terms of long-term risk of conversion to secondary progressive MS—as judged by an EDSS of 6, when a walking aid is required—women who had been pregnant had a lower risk, at trend levels, of converting to this form of the disease at 5 years but an increased risk at 10 years postpartum. These longer-term effects were not statistically significant and require further study. The apparent slowed progression of disability may also be influenced by the fact that women with more severe disease are less likely to conceive after the onset of MS. A population-based study of 2105 women, also from Canada, found that when confounding variables such as age at disease onset were considered, pregnancy had no effect on the time to progress to an EDSS score of 6.[124]

Effect of Multiple Sclerosis on Pregnancy Outcomes

Although more data are needed, **MS does not seem to have any significant effect on the course of pregnancy or fetal outcomes.** Some early studies had suggested that MS may affect fetal birthweight, but important confounders were not assessed. The largest study to date by van der Kop and colleagues[125] also controlled for important confounders such as parity and prior preterm births but found **no association between MS and preterm birth or newborn birthweight.**

Disease-Modifying Agents and Pregnancy

The field of MS therapy is rapidly evolving, and unfortunately, information on the risks related to MS therapies during pregnancy and lactation is sorely lacking. **The mainstay of treatment for acute MS relapses is corticosteroids or, rarely, other immunomodulatory treatments.** Corticosteroids are used symptomatically to lessen the severity and hasten recovery from acute neurologic symptoms, but they do not seem to alter the course of the disease. In 1993, the first disease-modifying agent (DMA), interferon-β, was introduced. Since then, a steady increase has occurred in available DMAs. **These therapies are utilized to reduce relapse rates; decrease MRI progression, one marker of MS disease activity; and lessen cumulative disability in patients with MS. They are not used to treat acute MS relapses.** DMAs are divided into *first-line* and *second-line* agents (Table 49-2). Second-line therapies are usually

TABLE 49-2 DISEASE-MODIFYING AGENTS FOR MULTIPLE SCLEROSIS: TERATOGENIC RISK AND RECOMMENDED WASHOUT PERIOD

DISEASE MODIFYING AGENT	ANIMAL STUDIES	HUMAN STUDIES	RECOMMENDED WASHOUT
First-Line Disease-Modifying Agents			
Glatiramer acetate	No concerns raised	No concerns, although studies were small	1 month
Interferon-β	Increased spontaneous abortion	No changes in rates of conception, spontaneous abortion, or MCM; may be associated with preterm birth and decreased birthweight and length	1 month
BG-12/dimethyl fumarate	Embryo toxicity, spontaneous abortion, neurobehavioral issues	No increased risk of MCM or spontaneous abortion in 69 pregnancies	1 month
Fingolimod	Embryolethality and fetal malformations (ventricular septal defect, persistent truncus arteriosus)	In humans, spontaneous abortion rate 24% (slightly increased from baseline) in 89 pregnancies; "abnormal fetal development" also noted in 7.6%	2 months
Teriflunomide	Embryotoxic and teratogenic effects	No increased risk of spontaneous abortion or MCM in 83 pregnancies where mother was exposed	24 months; "washout protocol" recommended to achieve plasma concentrations less than 0.02 mg/mL
Second-Line Disease-Modifying Agents			
Natalizumab	Increased risk of spontaneous abortion	No increased risk of MCM in 101 pregnancies; hematologic issues in infants exposed in third trimester	2 to 3 months, although some advise continuation to conception
Alemtuzumab	Increased risk of fetal death	Limited data, no increased risk of spontaneous abortion in 134 pregnancies	4 months
Mitoxantrone	Limited data	Decreased weight, increased prematurity	6 months; consider fertility preservation (may cause amenorrhea)

MCM, major congenital malformation; *MS*, multiple sclerosis.

reserved for patients who have failed a first-line agent and those who have very active disease.

Given that few data are available on the safety of DMAs in pregnancy and the fact that MS attacks are usually less frequent in pregnancy, most experts recommend stopping DMAs prior to conception. Highly effective contraception is also recommended for women who utilize these therapies. It is worth noting that many of the observational reports of MS, including the prospective PRIMS study, took place before DMAs were available. Since then, a few studies have suggested that use of DMAs prior to conception or during gestation decreases the risk for postpartum relapses.[118,126,127] Postpartum relapse rates are also lower in patients whose MS activity had been well controlled in the year prior to pregnancy.[126,128] Deciding which DMA is best for a woman with MS who is of reproductive age, as well as the appropriate time to stop the drug and contraception when trying to conceive, is a complex decision based on the patient's disease burden, the specific drug she is taking, and her personal concerns. These decisions should be made in consultation with her treating neurologist. Available information on the various DMAs available are summarized below and in Table 49-2.

First-Line Agents

First-line DMAs include interferon-β, glatiramer acetate, dimethyl fumarate, and teriflunomide. The Food and Drug Administration (FDA) also considers fingolimod a first-line drug for the treatment of MS, although the European Medicine Agency (EMA) does not. **Of the first-line therapies, experts agree that interferon-β and glatiramer acetate can be continued up to the time that contraception is stopped. Some have suggested that they can even be continued until a pregnancy is confirmed.**[118] In some rare cases, glatiramer acetate is continued during pregnancy.

Interferon-β formulations (interferon beta-1a and interferon beta-1b) are subcutaneous or intramuscular (IM) injections used at intervals that range from daily to every other week based on the formulation. These were among the first DMAs introduced for the treatment of MS, yet a relative paucity of information remains concerning the use of interferon-β therapy in pregnancy. However, lately, the number of available studies on this topic has increased.

Of note, interferons are large molecules that must be transferred across the placenta by active transport, and this process likely does not occur until after the first trimester.[129] Animal studies had suggested an increased risk of spontaneous abortions with interferon-β exposure; however, this has not held up in observational human studies. Sandberg-Wollheim and colleagues[130] dissected data on 1022 cases of interferon beta-1a exposure during pregnancy. To avoid bias, they only included outcomes for prospective data (n = 425) and found 324 normal infants were delivered at term (76.2%), 4 infants were born with malformations (0.9%), 4 third-trimester stillbirths occurred (0.9%, 1 with anomalies), along with 5 ectopic pregnancies (1.2%), 49 (11.5%) first-trimester spontaneous abortions, and 39 (9.2%) elective abortions. The authors reported that these results are not dissimilar to the general population, but no control group was included. Amato and colleagues[131] investigated first-trimester exposure to interferon β-1a or -1b. They compared these patients with those who were never treated or who discontinued treatment at least 4 weeks before conception. Of the 88 exposed fetuses, no increase was found in spontaneous abortion, malformations, or developmental abnormalities over a median follow-up of 2.1 years, although the incidence of low birthweight was increased and infants were shorter at birth. **In a systematic review of reports of DMA exposure in pregnancy, Lu and colleagues[132] summarized that prospective cohort studies of fair to good quality have found that**

interferon-β exposure may be associated with preterm delivery (before 37 weeks), **as well as lower weight and length at birth, but did not find an association between interferon exposure and birthweight below 2500 g, major malformations, or spontaneous abortion.** Recently, the manufacturers of interferon β-1b released information on the largest prospective cohort of pregnancies exposed to this interferon from their international pharmacovigilance database.[133] Among 1045 pregnancies, no increased risk of spontaneous abortions or major anomalies was reported compared with expected population rates. They also detected no change in preterm birth or SGA infants. It should be noted that the majority of patients in these studies had limited exposure to interferon-β (average of 4 to 8 weeks), and no conclusions can be reached about exposure throughout pregnancy or long-term effects.

Glatiramer acetate is also used to treat frequent relapses in those with relapsing remitting MS. It is a large macromolecule that likely does not pass the placenta.[129] Preclinical studies did not demonstrate adverse effects of glatiramer acetate on offspring of exposed animals, and thus it received a class B designation from the FDA. Studies of glatiramer acetate in pregnancy are based on small cohorts, but two studies have evaluated women exposed to the drug throughout pregnancy. Salminen and coworkers[134] prospectively followed 13 women exposed to glatiramer from preconception through pregnancy and the postpartum period and found no congenital anomalies, and the treatment was well tolerated. Fragoso and colleagues[135] retrospectively evaluated 11 women who used glatiramer continuously for at least 7 months during pregnancy. Children were followed for at least 1 year after birth. No congenital anomalies, neonatal complications, or developmental abnormalities were seen in the children. Postnatal MS relapse rates remained significantly lower than antenatal rates in these women.[135] Although data are significantly limited by the small sample sizes, most experts feel that **glatiramer acetate is the DMA of choice if one must be used during pregnancy, although the patient's history of response to this drug must also be considered.**

Dimethyl fumarate, teriflunomide, and **fingolimod** are oral agents that have been recently introduced and have been shown to reduce relapse rates, as well as disability scores, in patients with MS. They are popular given that they are oral formulations. Animal studies have raised concern for embryolethality and teratogenicity of these medications, and clinical experience with these drugs in human pregnancy is limited to accidental exposures in clinical trials and postmarketing surveillance. It is recommended that effective contraception be used with each of these drugs and that they *not* be continued in pregnancy. In addition, given the long-term effects and half-lives of some of these oral agents, it is recommended that they be stopped prior to discontinuation of contraception (see Table 49-2). A special "washout" protocol is advised for teriflunomide.

In animal studies of **dimethyl fumarate,** an increased risk of spontaneous abortion and adverse fetal outcome (decreased fetal weight and delayed ossification) were seen at supratherapeutic doses and were thought to be due to maternal toxicity.[136] Neurodevelopmental effects were observed in animals at all doses tested. No increased risk of spontaneous abortion or fetal abnormalities was noted in 69 reports of human pregnancies exposed to dimethyl fumarate in clinical trials or postmarketing surveillance.[137]

Teriflunomide has been associated with embryotoxicity and teratogenicity in animals.[138] In 83 pregnancies of women with MS and 22 pregnancies of partners of men with MS taking teriflunomide, the risks of spontaneous abortions or fetal abnormalities were not increased.[139] Because of the concern of teratogenesis, as well as the long half-life of teriflunomide, contraception is recommended during and after treatment. A "washout" protocol with activated charcoal or cholestyramine is recommended for women who plan to conceive and for those who become pregnant while taking the drug. In a systematic review, an international multidisciplinary consortium recommended that for teriflunomide, **"Conception should be tied to plasma concentration levels less than 0.02 mg/mL rather than to the 5 maximal half-lives algorithm for exponential decay."**[140] Because teriflunomide is also present in the sperm of men who take the drug, a similar protocol is recommended for men planning to conceive.

Animal studies of **fingolimod** have demonstrated embryolethality and teratogenic effects with doses lower than those recommended in humans.[141] In a report of 89 pregnancies that occurred during the clinical studies of the drug, the rate of spontaneous abortions was 24% (slightly higher than the expected baseline rate of 15% to 20% according to the authors), and five cases of "abnormal fetal development" were reported that included one case of each of acrania, bowing of the tibia, tetralogy of Fallot, intrauterine death, and failure of fetal development.[142]

Second-Line Agents

Natalizumab is a humanized monoclonal immunoglobulin (Ig) G4 antibody to human α4 integrin that works against many processes involved in human development. However, it is a large molecule that should not cross the placenta. Wehner and colleagues[143] set out to examine postnatal development in monkeys exposed to this medication. In the first cohort of monkeys, an increase in spontaneous abortions occurred. However, the rate in the control group was low (7%). In the second cohort studied, the spontaneous abortion rates were equivalent in both groups. These researchers found no adverse effects on the general health, survival, development, or immunologic structure or function of the newborn monkeys whose mothers were treated with natalizumab. Ebrahimi and colleagues[144] reported on 101 pregnancies in patients who received natalizumab during pregnancy or up to 8 weeks before the last menstrual period. The patients were ascertained from a prospective registry of MS patients and were paired with disease-matched controls. The authors found no significant difference in the presence of malformations, low birthweight, or preterm birth between the two groups. In a case series of 13 pregnancies in 12 women with highly active MS who were treated with natalizumab in the third trimester, Haghikia and colleagues[145] reported mild to moderate hematologic abnormalities, including thrombocytopenia and anemia, in 10 of 13 infants. In most children, the abnormalities resolved without consequence within 4 months of delivery. One child had subclinical bleeding and another was born with a cystic abnormality in the thalamic region thought to be due to prior hemorrhage, although no developmental consequences were obvious at 2 years of age. No consensus has been reached on when to stop natalizumab prior to conception. Some experts recommend, based on the above data, that the drug can be continued up to the time of conception, checking pregnancy tests before each infusion.[118] Others believe waiting 1 to 3 months before conceiving is appropriate.[129] The antibody can be removed from the blood with a series of plasma exchanges, but this is rarely thought to be necessary.

Alemtuzumab is another humanized monoclonal antibody approved as a second-line drug for MS in 2013. It is directed against CD52 and causes a long-lasting depletion of lymphocytes. It is given as a yearly infusion and can be complicated by immune-mediated thyroid disease in one third of patients. Animal exposure to alemtuzumab during gestation increased the risk of fetal death in rodents.[138] Limited data are available in humans. In the only clinical abstract,[146] 139 pregnancies in 104 patients were reported. The rate of spontaneous abortion was 17%, which the authors stated was comparable to that of the general population. Eleven adverse events without a clear pattern were also reported, along with one case of thyrotoxic crisis. Contraception is therefore recommended for 4 months after discontinuing alemtuzumab.[138]

Mitoxantrone is a second-line agent for the treatment of MS, and cyclophosphamide is occasionally used for severe cases. Both treatments can cause amenorrhea in one third of patients, and cyclophosphamide is associated with ovarian toxicity.[138] In animals, cyclophosphamide has been shown to cause genetic abnormalities in female germ cells; however, very little is known about the effects of mitoxantrone and cyclophosphamide during pregnancy. The risks of both are felt to outweigh potential benefits of both in pregnancy. It is recommended that contraception be continued for 6 months after mitoxantrone and 3 months after cyclophosphamide have been stopped.

Prepregnancy Counseling for Patients With Multiple Sclerosis

Women with MS should be counseled about reproductive choices at the time of diagnosis and before starting a DMA. The topic should also be revisited regularly. **Patients should be reassured that the vast majority of women with MS can have healthy pregnancies and that MS in the mother does not pose an adverse risk to the fetus.** Additionally, they should be told that pregnancy will likely reduce the risk of MS flares temporarily, and although they may worsen in some women in the postpartum period, pregnancy likely does not have any adverse effect on long-term disease course. The decision of whether to start a DMA and which DMA to start depends on the patient's disease burden and timeline for conception.

Timing of conception is very important for a woman with MS, given that disease burden prior to conception may affect the course of the pregnancy. For a woman with very active disease, a neurologist might recommend treatment with a DMA for 1 year to obtain better disease control before conception. Of course, given uncertainties around ovarian function in women with MS, the patient's age and an assessment of fertility may also be considered. Women who require treatment with drugs such as cyclophosphamide or mitoxantrone may want to consider fertility preservation prior to beginning treatment. Women should be counseled on the recommended timeline to continue contraception following discontinuation of a DMA (see Table 49-2).

Some women with MS may be concerned about the risk of passing the disease on to their children. MS is a polygenic disorder and combined effects of genetic susceptibility and environment determines an individual's risk. **The risk of developing MS in a child with a single parent with MS is 2% to 2.5%.**[147] Whereas this is a twentyfold increase from the baseline population risk, the absolute likelihood that a mother will pass MS on to her child is still very low and usually is not a reason to avoid pregnancy.[118]

Women with MS should also receive general prenatal counseling that includes stressing the importance of supplementation with a prenatal vitamin. **Vitamin D deficiency** is gaining more attention as an environmental factor that affects susceptibility to MS and MS relapses. Vitamin D deficiency in a mother may also affect her child's subsequent risk of developing MS. In a small open-label trial, pregnant women with MS and low vitamin D levels were randomized to 50,000 IU of vitamin D_3 a week, starting at weeks 12 to 16 of gestation, or routine care.[148] The group of six who received "high-dose" vitamin D had normal postpartum levels of vitamin D, whereas the nine patients who received routine care did not. No adverse effects of supplementation were reported during pregnancy or 6 months postpartum, although no conclusions can be made about long-term fetal effects. Patients who received the high-dose vitamin D appeared to do better in terms of EDSS and relapse rate, but these data are limited by the small sample size and open-label methodology. The optimal dose of vitamin D in pregnancy is not known, but a consortium of experts recommended that 1000 to 2000 IU daily should be safe.[140] Ideally, the vitamin D level should be checked and optimized before pregnancy, and a dose of 1000 to 2000 IU can be continued in pregnancy.

Management of Multiple Sclerosis During Pregnancy

No specific changes in routine obstetric care are recommended for women with MS. Women with disturbances in bladder function may be more prone to urinary tract infections and need to be monitored more frequently. Urinalysis and culture should be checked in the setting of new or worsening symptoms because infections can often exacerbate the presentation of MS.

If an acute and severe MS relapse occurs during pregnancy, treatment with corticosteroids may hasten recovery. The typical regimen is 1 g of methylprednisolone daily for 3 to 7 days, which can be given intravenously or orally; no oral taper is used. Methylprednisolone or the equivalent dose of prednisolone and prednisone are recommended if steroids are needed because less than 10% of these steroids pass across the placenta. When possible, it is recommended that steroid use be minimized in pregnancy, and ideally, it should be avoided in the first trimester. Safety information on the fetal effects of steroids is limited but some older studies associated steroid exposure with an increased risk of cleft lip and palate (see Chapter 8).[140] Questions were also raised by studies that suggested low birthweight and premature delivery as a result of steroid use. IV immunoglobulin (IVIG) can be used as an alternative to steroids or when steroids fail, but safety data on IVIG is also limited.[140] Monthly IVIG or steroids can also be considered for women with active disease during pregnancy to decrease the risk of relapses.

Labor and Delivery

In the past, anesthesiologists had been concerned that epidural analgesia might somehow worsen the disease or promote relapses. In both the PRIMS study[116,117] and a large Italian cohort,[149] only 18% to 19% of women with MS received epidural analgesia. In the PRIMS study, a trend was seen toward a higher relapse rate in the first 3 months postpartum in women who received epidurals, but this effect did not reach statistical significance. **In the Italian study by Pastò and colleagues,[149] no increase was seen in relapse rate or EDSS score 1 year after delivery in women with MS who had received epidural anesthesia.**

Perceptions of the risk of anesthesia may have changed. A more recent population-based study performed in Canada found that nulliparous women with MS received epidural or spinal anesthesia at a rate similar to that of the general population. However, multiparous women with MS were more likely to receive epidural analgesia.[150]

Cesarean delivery is usually not indicated in women with MS. Only in rare cases of severe or active disease that affects the spinal cord may MS affect a patient's ability to labor safely. Across five studies assessed in a recent meta-analysis, cesarean delivery rates varied from 9.6% to 42%,[119] which likely reflects the variability of practice among different cultures and practitioners. Pastò and colleagues[149] found no association between cesarean delivery and relapse rate or disability scores in Italian women with MS.

Breastfeeding and the Postpartum Period

Breastfeeding in women with MS is a controversial and actively debated topic. Some studies have suggested that breastfeeding has a protective effect on MS relapses, whereas others report no effect on disease activity. **The PRIMS study found that breastfeeding had no effect on the rate of MS relapses in the first 3 months postpartum.**[116,117] A more recent study of 302 pregnant women with MS treated at Italian MS centers also found no effect of breastfeeding on disease activity. The authors noted that breastfeeding may not be possible for women with high disease burden.[128] Other studies have suggested, however, that breastfeeding—particularly exclusive breastfeeding—may reduce the likelihood of MS relapses in the postpartum period.[151,152] A 2012 meta-analysis of 12 studies of MS and breastfeeding found that women who did not breastfeed were nearly twice as likely to have at least one relapse in the postpartum period.[153] This result was significant but was limited by the variability of the studies available. The authors cautioned that it is not possible to completely control for the possibility that women with more benign disease may also be more likely to breastfeed.

The decision to breastfeed is made more complicated by a woman or her doctor's desire for her to resume DMAs. **Most experts state that DMAs should not be resumed while a woman is breastfeeding.**[118,129,138] However, **this recommendation is based on a lack of evidence about the safety of these drugs in breastfeeding rather than evidence of harm.** Unfortunately, this conservative approach will likely prevent the ability to gather important data on the safety of some of these therapies during breastfeeding, as has been done with AEDs, and may make patients more reluctant to breastfeed.

Both interferons and glatiramer acetate are large molecules that are not orally bioavailable. It is unlikely that they pass into breastmilk, although this has not been studied systematically. Interferon β-1a transfer into breastmilk was assessed in six women, and the relative infant dose was estimated at 0.006%. No adverse effects were noted in the infants who were exposed through breastmilk.[154] In another small study of glatiramer acetate and breastfeeding, no problems were noted in nine infants exposed through breastmilk for an average of 3.6 months.[135] Nevertheless, official recommendations continue to state that all DMAs should be held in women who plan to breastfeed, and thus most women must make a choice between breastfeeding and resuming a DMA. A minority of physicians are comfortable with patients breastfeeding while taking glatiramer acetate.[129] It is important to note, however, that the

onset of action of these first-line therapies is delayed, typically by 2 months, and even if they are started immediately postpartum, they may not provide protection from relapses in the immediate postpartum period. Pulse doses of IVIG[155-157] or methylprednisolone[158] have been tried to prevent relapses in the postpartum period, but differing results and methodologic limitations make it difficult to draw firm conclusions about the benefit of this approach.[118]

Postpartum, women with MS will often need help with their own care and the care of their infant. This depends greatly on the patient's level of disability and whether she experiences a relapse. For all patients who are pregnant or considering pregnancy, it is helpful to discuss the need for support from friends and family members in the postpartum period as well as to prepare a contingency plan for infant care in the event of a disabling MS relapse.

HEADACHE

Headache disorders can be divided into two classes, primary and secondary. *Primary headache disorders* include migraine and tension-type headaches as well as cluster headaches, although the latter are rare in women. Both migraine and tension-type headaches improve in pregnancy, although some may persist. The biggest challenge in evaluating headache is to rule out *secondary headache disorders* (Fig. 49-2), which are symptomatic of underlying and potentially deleterious pathologies. Most patients with primary headaches such as migraine have a prior history of a similar headache pattern. Any new symptoms or headache pattern and all new-onset headaches, even if they have a migrainous quality, should prompt evaluation for underlying causes. It is also important to be aware of the appropriate treatments for these conditions.

Migraine

Headaches are extremely common in women, and the majority of migraine headaches occur in women of childbearing age. Migraines are associated with vasodilation of the cerebral

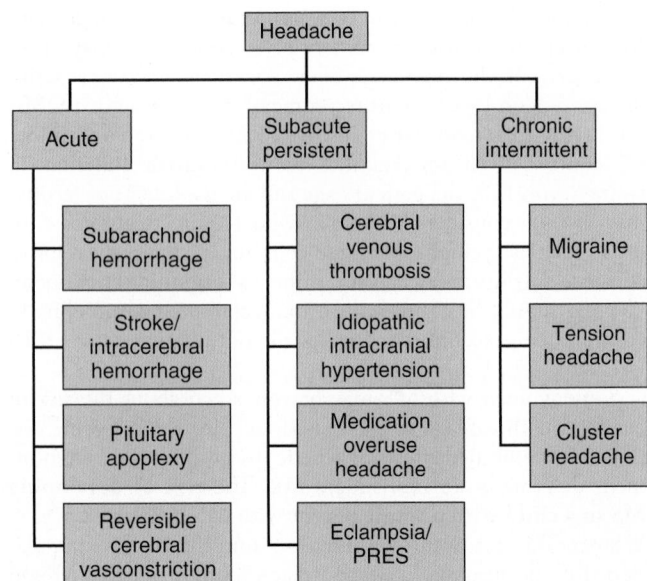

FIG 49-2 Differential diagnosis of headaches in pregnancy. PRES, posterior reversible encephalopathy syndrome.

vasculature and typically last several hours. Onset is usually subacute and the headache is often unilateral and pounding and is often accompanied by photosensitivity and/or phonosensitivity and nausea. Migraines can be classified as those with aura and those without. *Migraines with aura* are characterized by reversible focal neurologic symptoms that occur before the headache. Visual auras are common, but aphasia or unilateral numbness or weakness may also occur, which sometimes makes such headaches difficult to distinguish from transient ischemic attacks. The migraine aura should be fully reversible in 5 to 60 minutes, and sometimes the aura can occur without a headache.

Migraine symptoms tend to improve during pregnancy. Maggioni and colleagues[159] found that 80% of patients experienced either complete remission or a 50% reduction in headaches during pregnancy. Improvement was more common after the first trimester. Migraine type does not seem to be a prognostic factor. Those with menstrual (catamenial) migraines had the most improvement. However, 4% to 8% show significant worsening during pregnancy. In a study by Ertresvåg and colleagues,[160] 58% of subjects with migraine reported having no headache during pregnancy. Transient neurologic symptoms were more common in patients with a history of migraine. Chen

and Leviton[161] examined data from the large, prospective Collaborative Perinatal Project of 55,000 pregnancies. They found that less than 2% of women in the sample were considered to have migraines at their initial prenatal visit. Of the 484 (of 508) women with a complete data set, 17% experienced complete cessation of headache throughout pregnancy, and an additional 62% had two or fewer headaches in the third trimester. Only 21% of these women had no improvement in their headache. The authors examined all available demographic and pregnancy factors and could find none that could be used to predict headache improvement during pregnancy.

Using a nationwide population-based database in Taiwan, Chen and colleagues[162] identified 4911 women with migraines who delivered from 2001 to 2003. After adjusting for confounders, they found an increased risk for low birthweight (OR, 1.16), preterm birth (OR, 1.24), cesarean delivery (OR, 1.16), and preeclampsia (OR, 1.34). Although these increases were not large, they were all statistically significant.[162] More research needs to be undertaken to determine whether these increases apply to different populations and if they are clinically significant.

Migraine treatment is divided into abortive and prophylactic treatments (Tables 49-3 and 49-4). Given the anticipated improvement of migraines during pregnancy, most women do

---

TABLE 49-3 ABORTIVE TREATMENTS FOR PRIMARY HEADACHES IN PREGNANCY

	BEST STUDIED/ RECOMMENDED	MALFORMATION RISK	OTHER COMMENTS	BREASTFEEDING COMPATIBLE
Preferred				
Nonpharmacologic measures	Hydration, sleep, caffeine	NA		Yes
Acetaminophen	Acetaminophen	No known associations with MCMs have been reported.	Recent concerns over associations with behavioral abnormalities[*] and asthma[†] have been raised, but more research is needed.	Yes
NSAIDs	Ibuprofen	Possible associations were found with cardiac anomalies and oral clefts, but studies vary.	NSAIDs must be avoided in the third trimester because of increased risk of premature PDA closure and oligohydramnios; an association with asthma in children was recently reported, but more research is needed.[†]	Yes
Antiemetics	Metoclopramide	No association was found with MCMs in limited studies.	A risk of tardive dyskinesia is present for the mother.	Yes
Less Preferred				
Triptans	Sumatriptan	Data from case series suggest no increased risk of MCMs, but these were usually cases of inadvertent first-trimester use.	Effects on later pregnancy have not been well studied.	Yes
Opiates	Oxycodone	Recent study links first-trimester opiates to increased risk of certain MCMs, including heart defects and spina bifida.[‡]	Typically ineffective for migraine, these agents can create dependence; neonatal withdrawal has also been noted with use near term.	Yes, but monitor infant for sedation
Avoid if Possible				
Barbiturates	Butalbital	No data are available on butalbital in animals or humans, but extrapolating from phenobarbital data, an increased risk of MCMs is likely.	Based on phenobarbital data, concern exists for cognitive effects of butalbital exposure; risk of neonatal withdrawal is present with use near term.	Not recommended because of the long half-life and potential for sedation
Ergots	Dihydroergotamine Erogtamine	Data are limited.	Ergots cause vasoconstriction of uterine vessels and are potentially abortifacient; therefore use is contraindicated in pregnancy.	Not recommended because of nausea, vomiting, and weakness in the infant and suppression of prolactin in the mother.

[*]Sordillo JE, Scirica CV, Rifas-Shiman SL, et al. Prenatal and infant exposure to acetaminophen and ibuprofen and the risk for wheeze and asthma in children. *J Allergy Clin Immunol.* 2015;135(2):441-448.
[†]Broussard CS, Rasmussen SA, Reefhuis J, et al. Maternal treatment with opioid analgesics and risk for birth defects. *Am J Obstet Gynecol.* 2011;204(4):314.e1.
[‡]Liew Z, Ritz B, Rebordosa C, Lee PC, Olsen J. Acetaminophen use during pregnancy, behavioral problems, and hyperkinetic disorders. *JAMA Pediatr.* 2014;168(4):313-320.
MCM, major congenital malformation; *N/A,* not applicable; *NSAID,* nonsteroidal antiinflammatory drug; *PDA,* patent ductus arteriosus.

TABLE 49-4   PROPHYLACTIC TREATMENTS FOR PRIMARY HEADACHE DISORDERS IN PREGNANCY

	BEST STUDIED/ RECOMMENDED	MALFORMATION RISK	OTHER COMMENTS	BREASTFEEDING COMPATIBLE
Preferred				
Nonpharmacologic measures	Stress reduction Acupuncture Physical therapy	No known association	Many chronic migraneurs will not need any prophylactic migraine medications in pregnancy	Yes
Magnesium	Magnesium sulfate	Limited data	The FDA recommends upper limit of 350 mg/day; may decrease risk of eclampsia, but may have GI side effects	Yes
Coenzyme Q10	Coenzyme Q10	Limited data Not recommended for use prior to 20 weeks' gestation	May decrease risk of preeclampsia in migraneurs when given after 20 weeks	Probably
Less Preferred				
β-Blockers	Propranolol Metoprolol	Limited data Possible intrauterine growth restriction	Possible fetal bradycardia, hypoglycemia, respiratory depression; stop 2 to 3 days before delivery to avoid fetal bradycardia and impairment of uterine contractions	Yes Propranolol seems to pose low risk
Tricyclic antidepressants	Amitriptyline	Limited data; possible limb deformities, CNS effects with higher doses, but none noted in range of 10 to 50 mg/day	Drug of choice for tension-type headache prophylaxis in pregnancy, if needed	Probably Low levels are found in breast milk
Calcium channel blockers	Verapamil	Limited data on high doses in pregnancy	Drug of choice for cluster headache prophylaxis in pregnancy if needed; monitor maternal ECG for heart block every 6 months or with dose changes; consider increased fetal monitoring	Probably Maternal doses up to 360 mg/day are used without adverse effect
Avoid if Possible				
Topiramate	Topiramate	Increased risk of MCM, especially oral clefts	Increased risk for SGA infants, possible cognitive effects on infant though not well studied	Possibly compatible but not well studied If used, monitor infant for metabolic acidosis, lethargy, and overheating
Valproic acid	Valproic acid	Substantially increased risk of MCMs including spina bifida	Increased risk of adverse cognitive outcomes such as lower IQ and autism; contraindicated in pregnancy for treatment of migraine	Yes
Lithium	Lithium	Associated with fetal cardiac anomalies as well as polyhydramnios, cardiac arrhythmias, hypoglycemia, diabetes insipidus, and thyroid abnormalities	Not indicated for the treatment of migraine; used for cluster headache; contraindicated for headache treatment in pregnancy; associated with neonatal withdrawal	Possibly compatible, but caution is advised because of hypotonia and ECG changes in infant; lithium can be considered in closely monitored patients

CNS, central nervous system; *ECG,* electrocardiogram; *FDA,* U.S. Food and Drug Administration; *GI,* gastrointestinal; *IQ,* intelligence quotient; *MCM,* major congenital malformation; *SGA,* small for gestational age.

not need to take prophylactic treatment, and such treatment is usually weaned prior to conception. Nonpharmacologic measures such as sleep, hydration, and relaxation techniques are the first-line treatment for migraines during gestation. For drug therapy, acetaminophen is initially recommended. Ibuprofen can be used in the first and second trimester, but the use of nonsteroidal antiinflammatory drugs (NSAIDs) should be avoided if possible after 24 weeks' gestation. When used for more than 48 hours, these agents can cause oligohydramnios and premature closure of the ductus arteriosus. Although opiates are often prescribed during pregnancy, these are actually not preferred for migraine treatment because they are typically ineffective, increase nausea, and decrease gastric motility. Antiemetic therapy may be helpful, but barbiturates should be avoided if possible.

Sumatriptan, a serotonin receptor agonist, is very successful in treating migraines acutely. In a review by O'Quinn and colleagues,[163] no untoward effects were reported in 76 first-trimester exposures to sumatriptan. Using logistic regression, Olesen and colleagues[164] compared 34 pregnancies with sumatriptan exposures with 89 migraine controls and 15,995 healthy women. They found that the risk of preterm birth was elevated with exposure (OR, 6.3) as was the risk of IUGR.[164] They do state that they did not control for disease severity. A larger study by Källén and Lygner[165] did not confirm these findings. **In 658 infants whose mothers used sumatriptan during pregnancy, no significant difference in prematurity or low birthweight was noted.**[165] Hilaire and colleagues[166] found birth defects in 3% to 5% of infants exposed to sumatriptan in the first trimester, a rate not greater than expected.

Recent studies have demonstrated that sumatriptan can be used during pregnancy. In a large Norwegian database, no increase in congenital anomalies or other adverse pregnancy outcomes was reported. However, increases were seen in intrapartum bleeding (OR, 1.5) and uterine atony (OR, 1.4). Ephross and Sinclair[167] reviewed 528 first-trimester exposures to sumatriptan and 57 to naratriptan and observed an anomaly rate similar to that of the background population; however, this study had no control group. Evans and Lorber described all available studies from 1990 through 2007 and also contacted the manufacturers of seven triptan medications; **they concluded that data are sufficient to recommend the use of sumatriptan for treatment of migraine in the first trimester** and also feel that naratriptan and rizatriptan are probably safe. Although these medications are acceptable for use in the second and third trimesters, little information is available regarding their use in late pregnancy. **Soldin and colleagues[168] confirm these findings and also stress that sumatriptan should be the triptan of choice because more data are available concerning its use in pregnancy.**

Ergotamine should be avoided during pregnancy. Previous reports have suggested that it may cause birth defects that have a vascular disruptive etiology. In addition, ergots are uterotonic and have an abortifacient potential.

Dietary factors may precipitate migraine attacks. Therefore careful history may uncover foods that should be avoided, including foods that contain monosodium glutamate (MSG), red wine, cured meats, and strong cheeses that contain tyramine. Relative hypoglycemia and alcohol can also trigger migraine attacks. Many individuals have recommended, without supporting evidence, dietary supplements and vitamins for migraine prevention. In a small study, Maizels and colleagues[169] demonstrated a possible role for riboflavin and magnesium in the prevention of migraines.

Secondary Headache in Pregnancy

Headaches during pregnancy can be a symptom of underlying intracranial pathology. Concerning causes of secondary headache in pregnancy include idiopathic intracranial hypertension, cerebral venous thrombosis (CVT), subarachnoid hemorrhage, and stroke. **Symptoms that should prompt further evaluation include abrupt onset of symptoms, persistent headache, and positional component. Any associated focal neurologic signs or vision changes should also prompt additional investigation unless they are a typical part of a patient's migraine aura. Patients with primary headache disorders can get secondary headaches, so any change in pattern or new symptoms should also be considered evidence of a possible underlying problem.**

Idiopathic Intracranial Hypertension (Pseudotumor Cerebri)

Idiopathic intracranial hypertension (IIH) may complicate 2% to 12% of pregnancies.[170] It had been thought to occur more frequently in pregnant women, particularly those who are obese. However, in a study by Ireland and colleagues,[171] the incidence in pregnant women and in oral contraceptive users was no higher than that in control groups. The headache of IIH is usually subacute in onset and is present daily. It may be aggravated by lying down and may be worse in the morning. However, the positional component is not always typical. **More than 90% of patients with IIH have headaches, and 40% have horizontal diplopia.[170]** Patients with IIH may also report transient visual obscurations that last less than one minute and may also report pulsatile tinnitus. **Papilledema is a characteristic feature of the condition and is present in the majority of cases. If left untreated, IIH can progress to permanent visual loss.** To establish the diagnosis, other causes of intracranial

hypertension must be excluded, such as an intracranial mass or CVT, and elevated cerebrospinal fluid (CSF) pressure (>250 mm H20) with normal CSF composition must be demonstrated.[172] MRI and magnetic resonance venogram (MRV) of the brain without contrast are the imaging modalities of choice and must be performed before a lumbar puncture to avoid herniation in the setting of a mass lesion. The pathogenesis of this disorder is unknown, but CSF prolactin is markedly elevated. Prolactin appears to have an affinity for receptors in the choroid plexus, where CSF is produced. Prolactin has osmoregulatory functions and therefore may have a role in the increased CSF production found in IIH, although some believe that reduced CSF reabsorption is the etiology. **Pregnancy outcome appears to be unaffected by IIH,[172] and no increase in fetal wastage or congenital anomalies are reported.**

The main objectives of treatment for IIH are relief of pain and preservation of vision. The patient should be followed closely with visual acuity and visual field determinations at intervals indicated by the clinical condition. In patients with mild disease, analgesics and close follow-up may be adequate. Moderate weight loss is recommended. For patients without improvement or those at risk for visual deterioration, acetazolamide—a carbonic anhydrase inhibitor that reduces CSF production—is the first-line treatment. Lee and colleagues[173] treated 12 patients with acetazolamide during pregnancy and reported no adverse fetal outcomes. They reviewed the English language literature and found nothing to contradict this assertion. The usual dose of acetazolamide is 500 mg twice daily. Steroids are rarely used for IIH; they are reserved for cases with impending vision loss in patients awaiting a surgical intervention. Serial lumbar punctures to reduce CSF pressure are rarely necessary but can effectively lower intracranial pressure transiently. Surgical approaches are reserved for refractory patients in whom rapid visual deterioration occurs. The two most common procedures are optic nerve sheath fenestration and lumboperitoneal or ventriculoperitoneal shunt.

IIH is not usually an indication for cesarean delivery. A review of the literature reveals that 73% of the reported patients delivered vaginally. Although no data are available to confirm this, the Valsalva maneuver—which can increase CSF pressure—should be minimized when possible. Therefore the second stage of labor should be shortened by operative vaginal delivery if possible. **Both epidural and spinal anesthesia, when expertly administered, can be safely used in patients with IIH.** However, in patients with lumboperitoneal shunts, the anesthetic should be directed away from the spinal canal. Month and Vaida[174] reported a successful spinal epidural technique during which 5 to 6 mL of CSF withdrawn at the time of analgesia provided additional relief.

Cerebral Vein Thrombosis

In patients with cerebral venous thrombosis (CVT), the chief symptoms are similar to those of IIH because the initial manifestations are due to increased intracranial pressure. **Patients typically present with a subacute, progressive, unremitting headache that may be worse when lying down.** As in IIH, patients may have diplopia and pulsatile tinnitus. Patients with CVT may also demonstrate papilledema. CVT can be complicated by a venous infarction with or without bleeding, which often leads to focal neurologic deficits and seizures. Severe headache with vomiting can be seen and should raise concern for acute worsening, such as associated stroke or hemorrhage. CVT occurs most frequently during the immediate postpartum period but can occur at any stage of pregnancy. It is often attributed to a hypercoagulable state. An incidence of 1 in 10,000 pregnancies was suggested in one study.[175] Vora and colleagues[176] reviewed 37,420 pregnancies in a Mumbai, India hospital between 2002 and 2006 and found a 0.1% incidence of thrombotic phenomena. Of these, 10% were documented cortical vein thromboses, confirming the incidence of 1 in 10,000 pregnancies.[176] CVT can be misdiagnosed as a postepidural headache, and this should be considered in the differential diagnosis. When CVT has a positional component, it should be worse lying and better standing, whereas a low-pressure headache often exhibits the reverse. These patterns are not always observed in individual patients, however; therefore CVT should be considered in the differential of all postpartum headaches.

MRI and MRV of the brain are the diagnostic tests of choice, and IV contrast is not needed to make the diagnosis. Anticoagulation, typically with low-molecular-weight heparin (LMWH), is the mainstay of treatment during pregnancy and breastfeeding. Workup for underlying thrombophilias is indicated to determine the duration of treatment. Prothrombin and factor V Leiden mutations can be performed during pregnancy, but other tests of hypercoagulability should be assessed 6 weeks or more after delivery (see Chapter 45). Seizures can be treated symptomatically with anticonvulsants, although little evidence is available to suggest the appropriate duration of AED treatment. Many neurologists and neurosurgeons advocate expectant management and do not routinely use AEDs for these symptomatic seizures. **Women who have had a CVT during pregnancy should avoid hormonal contraception, and women with a history of clotting while on hormonal contraception should use prophylactic anticoagulation during pregnancy.**

Subarachnoid Hemorrhage
Subarachnoid hemorrhage (SAH) usually manifests with a sudden "thunderclap" headache that is often associated with vomiting, stiff neck, and fluctuations of consciousness. Patients often refer to it as the "worst headache of their life." This presentation is a medical emergency that necessitates an emergency head CT scan, which is better than an MRI for visualizing bleeding. Even if the CT scan is negative, a lumbar puncture is indicated in patients with a suspicious history to exclude intrathecal blood. Up to 50% of aneurysmal SAHs are preceded by a "sentinel" bleed and a headache that should not go undiagnosed. The rate of SAH complicating pregnancy is approximately 1 per 10,400.[177] Robinson and coworkers[178] evaluated 26 patients with spontaneous SAH during pregnancy and found that approximately half were caused by aneurysms and half by arteriovenous (AV) malformations. They observed that AV malformations are more common in patients younger than 25 years of age and usually bleed before 20 weeks' gestation. Conversely, aneurysms occurred in patients older than 30 years of age and usually bled in the third trimester.

Cerebral angiography can be used to pinpoint the origin of cerebral bleeding. SAH due to aneurysms should be treated surgically whenever possible. In one study, SAH without early surgery resulted in a maternal mortality of 63% and a fetal mortality of 27%. With early surgery, the risk of mortality was lowered to 11% and 5%, respectively.[179] Surgery under hypothermia or hypotension appears to cause no adverse fetal effects. At an appropriate gestational age, the fetal heart rate should be monitored during the procedure. If fetal bradycardia occurs, the patient's blood pressure should be raised sufficiently to normalize the fetal heart rate.

Reversible Cerebral Vasoconstriction
Reversible cerebral vasoconstriction syndrome (RCVS) can present with a similar "thunderclap" headache. It may also present with focal neurologic deficits, seizures, and fluctuating levels of consciousness. RCVS can be complicated by stroke, nonaneurysmal SAH, and cerebral edema. Postpartum angiopathy is a type of RCVS often seen in the immediate postpartum period and is characterized by severe headaches with reversible narrowing of the intracranial vessels. Diagnosis can often be made by MRI and magnetic resonance angiography (MRA) of the brain. Alternatively, computed tomographic angiography (CTA) may be used for imaging or, rarely, an angiogram is needed. Treatment with nimodipine appears to help the headaches.[180] In a review of cerebrovascular disorders of pregnancy, however, Feske and Singhal[183] point out that postpartum angiopathy is on the same spectrum as eclampsia and posterior reversible encephalopathy syndrome (PRES; see Chapter 31, Figs. 31-13 and 31-14). Despite the lack of proteinuria in postpartum angiopathy/RCVS, the similarities of imaging findings suggest that they are likely mediated by the same pathologic process. Thus the authors argue that magnesium sulfate infusions similar to those used in eclampsia should be given to women with postpartum angiopathy to control blood pressure and seizures.

STROKE
Strokes can be divided into ischemic and hemorrhagic strokes. **Ischemic strokes** are usually the result of an arterial occlusion from cardioembolism and can also occur secondary to a CVT. Arterial dissection is also a common cause of stroke in young people and may be seen in pregnancy. **Hemorrhagic strokes** can be secondary to a variety of causes and may occur from severe hypertension alone or may be secondary to an underlying aneurysm or vascular malformation. Ischemic strokes can also exhibit hemorrhagic conversion. **Preeclampsia and eclampsia are risk factors for both ischemic and hemorrhagic strokes.**

Ischemic Stroke
Ischemic stroke is diagnosed in 34 per 100,000 deliveries, with 1.4 deaths per 100,000. The risk of stroke is increased in patients older than 35 years and in black women. Del Zotto and colleagues[181] reviewed multiple worldwide databases and showed that varied incidences between 4 and 41 per 100,000 deliveries. The highest risk was in patients with preeclampsia. Predisposing factors such as preeclampsia, chronic hypertension, or hypotensive episodes can be demonstrated in about one third of these patients. Brown and colleagues[182] investigated ischemic stroke in women recruited between 1992 and 1996 and again between 2001 and 2003. They found that preeclampsia was statistically associated with an increased risk of ischemic stroke (OR, 1.59; 95% CI, 1.00 to 2.52). Of note, women with a history of preeclampsia were more likely to eventually experience a non–pregnancy-related ischemic stroke. Half of the pregnancy-related cases occurred during the immediate postpartum period, and the remainder occurred during the second and third trimesters.

Ischemic stroke typically presents with acute focal neurologic symptoms. Headache can be present in 17% to 34% of cases. The workup should be done swiftly and starts with a noncontrast CT of the head. Acute treatment of disabling stroke due to arterial occlusion in nonpregnant patients is with IV or intraarterial recombinant tissue plasminogen activator (tPA). Little is known about the efficacy and safety of tPA in pregnant women because they were excluded from the clinical trials for tPA therapy. However, in acute ischemic strokes due to arterial thrombosis, the benefits of tPA likely outweigh the risks, even in pregnant women. Feske and Singhal[183] reviewed the case reports of 11 women who received IV or intraarterial thrombolysis. They concluded that 10 of the patients had no major complications from the thrombolysis and mentioned that the one patient who died had a major complicating illness. Seven of the exposed fetuses were delivered without complications. One fetus died along with the mother, two pregnancies were terminated, and one spontaneous abortion occurred in a fetus whose mother had bacterial endocarditis. The authors point out that **although tPA can be considered for pregnant women with arterial occlusion, it should probably be avoided in patients with preeclampsia/eclampsia given the increased risk of intracranial hemorrhage in these cases.**

Patients with acute strokes should typically be monitored in an intensive care setting, especially if tPA was given. Tight blood pressure control is required, and for major strokes, aggressive management of intracranial pressure may be needed. Further workup of ischemic stroke includes an MRI of the brain along with MRA of the head and neck. In some cases, CTA or angiography is needed. All patients with possible embolic stroke should have a transthoracic echo with agitated saline to exclude a patent foramen ovale. Blood tests should include a lipid panel, hemoglobin A1C level, erythrocyte sedimentation rate, and C-reactive protein level.

Hemorrhagic Stroke and Vascular Malformations

Based on a review of prior epidemiologic studies, Feske and Singhal[183] estimated the incidence of hemorrhagic stroke in pregnancy to be between 5 and 35 per 100,000 patients. The likelihood of a hemorrhagic stroke increases more dramatically in pregnancy than the risk for an ischemic stroke.

Evidence conflicts in regard to the effect of pregnancy on the behavior of arteriovenous malformations (AVMs).[178,185,186] Although it is uncertain whether incidental AVMs are at greater risk of bleeding during pregnancy, one study found that in 27 women who presented with hemorrhage due to AVMs in pregnancy, 26% had recurrent bleeding during or immediately after pregnancy. This is higher than the annual 6% risk expected in nonpregnant patients.[187] There also appears to be a significantly heightened risk of bleeding from an AVM on the day of delivery.[186]

In considering the above information, a 2001 consensus statement from the American Heart Association (AHA) recommended that **a woman with a known AVM should consider treatment prior to conceiving, and when an AVM is discovered during pregnancy, risks of treatment should be weighed against the risk of hemorrhage.** The committee felt that in most cases, such a risk-benefit analysis will not support elective treatment of AVMs during pregnancy.[187] Typically, AVMs found incidentally without hemorrhage are managed expectantly, but surgical intervention is considered in a woman with an AVM that has hemorrhaged.[183]

If the patient has undergone corrective surgery for an aneurysm or an AVM, she should be allowed to deliver vaginally. Moderate increases in blood pressure do not cause spontaneous hemorrhage in nonpregnant patients with intracranial AVMs. If the aneurysm or AVM has not been surgically corrected, a cesarean delivery is often recommended because of concern about the effects of increased blood pressure and intracranial pressure during delivery and prior observations of increased bleeding on the day of delivery.[178,183] However, in truth, no direct evidence is available to show that cesarean delivery is more protective against bleeding from an AVM than vaginal delivery.[187]

CARPAL TUNNEL SYNDROME

The medial border of the carpal tunnel consists of the pisiform and hamate bones, and its lateral border consists of the scaphoid and trapezium bones. They are covered on the palmar surface by the flexor retinaculum. **The median nerve and flexor tendons pass through this carpal tunnel, which has little room for expansion. If the wrist is extremely flexed or extended, the volume of the carpal tunnel is reduced. In pregnancy, weight gain and edema can produce a carpal tunnel syndrome that results from compression of the median nerve.** The association between carpal tunnel syndrome and pregnancy was first reported in 1957. Although many pregnant women complain of pain on the palmar surface of the hand, few actually have the true carpal tunnel syndrome. Stolp-Smith and colleagues[188] found that 50 of 14,579 pregnant patients (0.34%) who presented between 1987 and 1992 actually met criteria for carpal tunnel syndrome. **Commonly, the syndrome consists of pain, numbness, and tingling in the distribution of the median nerve in the hand and wrist. This includes the thumb, index finger, long finger, and radial side of the ring finger on the palmar aspect.** These symptoms/signs can be accompanied by dysesthetic wrist pain, loss of grip strength, and problems with dexterity. Compressing the median nerve and percussing the wrist and forearm with a reflex hammer, the Tinel maneuver, often exacerbates the pain. In severe cases, weakness and decreased motor function can occur. The definitive diagnosis is made by electromyography, but this test is often unnecessary.

McLennan and coworkers[189] studied 1216 consecutive pregnancies. Of these patients, 427 (35%) reported hand symptoms. Fewer than 20% of these 427 affected women described the classic carpal tunnel syndrome. No patient required operative intervention. Most symptoms were bilateral and commenced in the third trimester of pregnancy. **Ekman-Ordeberg and colleagues[190] found a 2.3% incidence of carpal tunnel syndrome in a prospective study of 2358 pregnancies. The syndrome appeared to be more common in primigravidae with generalized edema.** Increased weight gain during pregnancy also raises the risk.[189] A recent prospective study of 639 Dutch pregnant women found a 34% prevalence of carpal tunnel syndrome based on a standardized questionnaire.[191] Symptoms were more likely to occur after 32 weeks' gestation and were associated with symptoms of fluid retention when adjusting for body mass index (BMI), age, parity, and depression scores.

Padua and colleagues[192] conducted a systematic literature review concerning carpal tunnel syndrome in pregnancy. Of the 214 studies reviewed, only six fulfilled their criteria for inclusion. Neurophysiologically confirmed carpal tunnel syndrome ranged from 7% to 43% of those who presented with symptoms. Clinically diagnosed carpal tunnel syndrome ranged from 31% to 62%. Of note in 50% of cases, symptoms persisted for more than a year, and in 30%, symptoms were still present 3 years postpartum.

Supportive and conservative therapies are usually adequate for the treatment of carpal tunnel syndrome. Symptoms often subside in the postpartum period as total body water returns to normal.[193] Pain scores fall by half during the first week after delivery and by half again during the next week. The reduction in score is strongly correlated with loss of the weight gained during pregnancy. However, about half of the women with carpal tunnel syndrome during pregnancy still have some symptoms 1 year later. This occurs more commonly in those whose symptoms started early in pregnancy. Carpal tunnel syndrome that develops during breastfeeding may also last longer.[193]

Splints placed on the dorsum of the hand, which keep the wrist in a neutral position and maximize the capacity of the carpal tunnel, often provide dramatic relief. Local injections of glucocorticoids may also be used in severe cases. Although diuretics may help to control the symptoms of carpal tunnel syndrome over a short period of time, their use is not recommended because the symptoms return rather rapidly after the cessation of treatment.

Surgical correction of this syndrome should not be delayed in patients with deteriorating muscle tone and/or motor function. Even small changes can be documented by electromyography (EMG), which can be performed without harm during pregnancy. Decompression surgery for carpal tunnel syndrome is a simple procedure that can be safely carried out during pregnancy using local anesthesia, an axillary block, or a Bier block. With new endoscopic approaches, the procedure is even less invasive. Assmus and Hashemi[194] describe the outcomes for 314 hands surgically treated during pregnancy or in the puerperium for carpal tunnel syndrome. One hundred thirty-three cases were performed during pregnancy, most in the last trimester, and included four who had both hands treated simultaneously; 98% of patients reported good or excellent results. Local anesthesia was used in all cases, and no complications were reported. These authors recommend surgery if sensory loss is present or if motor latency is more than 5 msec on nerve conduction studies. **It is important to warn patients that carpal tunnel syndrome can persist for several years postpartum and can recur in future pregnancies.**[192]

KEY POINTS

♦ Epilepsy affects approximately 1% of the general population and is the most frequent neurologic complication of pregnancy.

♦ Prepregnancy counseling is imperative in the patient with epilepsy.

♦ Valproic acid has been associated with a significantly increased risk of major congenital malformations and adverse cognitive outcomes, including lower IQs and an increased risk of autism, when compared with other AEDs and with the general population.

♦ AEDs known to have a low risk of structural teratogenesis—such as lamotrigine, levetiracetam, or carbamazepine—should be tried as first-line agents in

women with epilepsy over AEDs that have been less well studied or valproic acid.

♦ Ultimately, the AED that best controls the patient's seizures should be used during pregnancy. Efforts to reach the minimum therapeutic dose should be attempted well in advance of pregnancy.

♦ Because of the changes in plasma volume, drug distribution, and metabolism that occur during pregnancy, anticonvulsant levels should be checked prior to conception and monthly during pregnancy. Dose adjustments to maintain prepregnancy levels are an important part of seizure control for many AEDs, especially lamotrigine.

♦ Women using AEDs should take folic acid 0.4 mg to 4 mg daily prior to and throughout pregnancy. They should also be offered a specialized ultrasound for careful assessment of major congenital malformations.

♦ Understanding a patient's epilepsy syndrome is necessary to give appropriate counseling on the risk of inheritance of epilepsy in offspring.

♦ Assisted reproductive techniques can precipitate MS relapses.

♦ Pregnancy does not hasten the onset or progression of MS. In fact, exacerbations are decreased during pregnancy.

♦ DMAs used to decrease the rate of relapses and disability in MS are typically not recommended during pregnancy because MS relapses tend to be less frequent during gestation, and data on exposure risk are still limited. A washout period is recommended for many DMAs.

♦ Increasing data on DMA use in pregnancy is available; for some patients, certain DMAs—such as glatiramer acetate and interferon-β—can be used in pregnancy.

♦ Breastfeeding in MS is controversial. Exclusive breastfeeding may reduce the risk of MS relapses, but treatment with DMAs is typically not recommended for women who are breastfeeding.

♦ Any new headache or new headache type that presents in pregnancy requires workup for an underlying potentially deleterious cause.

♦ Nonpharmacologic treatments are considered first-line therapies for migraine in pregnancy, which typically improves without treatment.

♦ Although opiates are commonly prescribed for migraine in pregnancy, they are actually not very effective migraine medications.

♦ Carpal tunnel syndrome is common in pregnancy and usually responds to conservative splinting, glucocorticoid injection, or both. Surgery can be safely undertaken if indicated during pregnancy.

REFERENCES

1. Harden CL, Hopp J, Ting TY, et al. Practice parameter update: management issues for women with epilepsy–focus on pregnancy (an evidence-based review): obstetrical complications and change in seizure frequency: report of the Quality Standards Subcommittee and Therapeutics and Technology Assessment Subcommittee of the American Adacemy of Neurology and American Epilepsy Society. *Neurology.* 2009;73(2):126-132.
2. Williams J, Myson V, Steward S, et al. Self-discontinuation of antiepileptic medication in pregnancy: Detection by hair analysis. *Epilepsia.* 2002; 43(8):824-831.

3. Sveberg L, Svalheim S, Taubøll E. The impact of seizures on pregnancy and delivery. *Seizure*. 2015;4-7.
4. Teramo K, Hiilesmaa V, Bardy A, Saarikoski S. Fetal Heart Rate during a Maternal Grand Mal Epileptic Seizure. *J Perinat Med*. 1979;7:3-6.
5. Minkoff H, Schaffer RM, Delke I, Grunebaum AN. Diagnosis of Intracranial Hemorrhage in Utero after a Maternal Seizure. *Obstet Gynecol*. 1985;65:22S-24S.
6. Nei M, Daly S, Liporace J. A maternal complex partial seizure in labor can affect fetal heart rate. *Neurology*. 1998;51(3):904-906.
7. Chen YH, Chiou HY, Lin HC, Lin HL. Affect of seizures during gestation on pregnancy outcomes in women with epilepsy. *Arch Neurol*. 2009;66(8):979-984.
8. Cantwell R, Clutton-Brock T, Cooper G, et al. Saving Mothers' Lives: Reviewing maternal deaths to make motherhood safer: 2006-2008. The Eighth Report of the Confidential Enquiries into Maternal Deaths in the United Kingdom. *BJOG*. 2011;118(suppl 1):1-203.
9. MacDonald SC, Bateman BT, McElrath TF, Hernández-Díaz S. Mortality and morbidity during delivery hospitalization among pregnant women with epilepsy in the United States. *JAMA Neurol*. 2015;02115:1-8.
10. Edey S, Moran N, Nashef L. SUDEP and epilepsy-related mortality in pregnancy. *Epilepsia*. 2014;55(7):e72-e74.
11. French JA, Meador K. Risks of epilepsy during pregnancy: how much do we really know? *JAMA Neurol*. 2015;6-7.
12. Artama M, Isojärvi JIT, Auvinen A. Antiepileptic drug use and birth rate in patients with epilepsy: a population-based cohort study in Finland. *Hum Reprod*. 2006;21(9):2290-2295.
13. Dansky LV, Andermann E, Andermann F. Marriage and fertility in epileptic patients. *Epilepsia*. 1980;21(3):261-271.
14. Webber MP, Hauser WA, Ottman R, Annegers JF. Fertility in persons with epilepsy: 1935-1974. *Epilepsia*. 1986;27(6):746-752.
15. Viinikainen K, Heinonen S, Eriksson K, Kälviäinen R. Fertility in women with active epilepsy. *Neurology*. 2007;69(22):2107-2108.
16. Sukumaran SC, Sarma PS, Thomas SV. Polytherapy increases the risk of infertility in women with epilepsy. *Neurology*. 2010;75(15):1351-1355.
17. Klein P, Serje A, Pezzullo JC. Premature ovarian failure in women with epilepsy. *Epilepsia*. 2001;42(12):1584-1589.
18. Harden CL, Pennell PB. Neuroendocrine considerations in the treatment of men and women with epilepsy. *Lancet Neurol*. 2013;12(1):72-83.
19. Bech BH, Kjaersgaard MI, Pedersen HS, et al. Use of antiepileptic drugs during pregnancy and risk of spontaneous abortion and stillbirth: population based cohort study. *BMJ*. 2014;349:g5159.
20. Holmes LB, Harvey EA, Coull BA, et al. The teratogenicity of anticonvulsant drugs. *N Engl J Med*. 2001;344(15):1132-1138.
21. Wen X, Meador KJ, Hartzema A. Antiepileptic drug use by pregnant women enrolled in Florida Medicaid. *Neurology*. 2015;84(9):944-950.
22. Gerard E, Pack AM. Pregnancy registries: What do they mean to clinical practice? *Curr Neurol Neurosci Rep*. 2008;8(4):325-332.
23. Artama M, Auvinen A, Raudaskoski T, Isojärvi I, Isojärvi J. Antiepileptic drug use of women with epilepsy and congenital malformations in offspring. *Neurology*. 2005;64(11):1874-1878.
24. Tomson T, Battino D. Teratogenic effects of antiepileptic drugs. *Lancet Neurol*. 2012;11(9):803-813.
25. Veiby G, Daltveit AK, Engelsen BA, Gilhus NE. Fetal growth restriction and birth defects with newer and older antiepileptic drugs during pregnancy. *J Neurol*. 2014;261(3):579-588.
26. Hernández-Díaz S, Smith CR, Shen A, et al. Comparative safety of antiepileptic drugs during pregnancy. *Neurology*. 2012;78(21):1692-1699.
27. Vajda FJ, Graham J, Roten A, Lander CM, O'Brien TJ, Eadie M. Teratogenicity of the newer antiepileptic drugs–the Australian experience. *J Clin Neurosci*. 2012;19(1):57-59.
28. Campbell E, Kennedy F, Russell A, et al. Malformation risks of antiepileptic drug monotherapies in pregnancy: updated results from the UK and Ireland Epilepsy and Pregnancy Registers. *J Neurol Neurosurg Psychiatry*. 2014;2013-2015.
29. Tomson T, Battino D, Bonizzoni E, et al. Dose-dependent risk of malformations with antiepileptic drugs: an analysis of data from the EURAP epilepsy and pregnancy registry. *Lancet Neurol*. 2011;10(7):609-617.
30. Jentink J, Loane MA, Dolk H, et al. Valproic acid monotherapy in pregnancy and major congenital malformations. *N Engl J Med*. 2010;362(23):2185-2193.
31. Meador KJ, Baker GA, Browning N, et al. Fetal antiepileptic drug exposure and cognitive outcomes at age 6 years (NEAD study): a prospective observational study. *Lancet Neurol*. 2013;12(3):244-252.
32. Baker G, Bromley RL, Briggs M, et al. IQ at 6 years following in utero exposure to antiepileptic drugs: a controlled cohort study. *Neurology*. 2015;84:382-390.
33. Christensen J, Grønborg TK, Sørensen MJ, et al. Prenatal valproate exposure and risk of autism spectrum disorders and childhood autism. *JAMA*. 2013;309(16):1696-1703.
34. Wood AG, Nadebaum C, Anderson V, et al. Prospective assessment of autism traits in children exposed to antiepileptic drugs during pregnancy. *Epilepsia*. 2015;56:1047-1055.
35. Bromley RL, Mawer GE, Briggs M, et al. The prevalence of neurodevelopmental disorders in children prenatally exposed to antiepileptic drugs. *J Neurol Neurosurg Psychiatry*. 2013;84(6):637-643.
36. Harden CL, Meador KJ, Pennell PB, et al. Practice parameter update: management issues for women with epilepsy–focus on pregnancy (an evidence-based review): teratogenesis and perinatal outcomes: report of the Quality Standards Subcommittee and Therapeutics and Technology Assessment Subcommittee. *Neurology*. 2009;73(2):133-141.
37. Morrow J. Malformation risks of antiepileptic drugs in pregnancy: a prospective study from the UK Epilepsy and Pregnancy Register. *J Neurol Neurosurg Psychiatry*. 2006;77(2):193-198.
38. Jentink J, Dolk H, Loane MA, et al. Intrauterine exposure to carbamazepine and specific congenital malformations: systematic review and case-control study. *BMJ*. 2010;341:c6581.
39. Bromley R, Weston J, Adab N, et al. Treatment for epilepsy in pregnancy: neurodevelopmental outcomes in the child. In: Bromley R, ed. *Cochrane Database of Systematic Reviews*. Chichester, UK: John Wiley & Sons, Ltd; 2014.
40. Rasalam AD, Hailey H, Williams JH, et al. Characteristics of fetal anticonvulsant syndrome associated autistic disorder. *Dev Med Child Neurol*. 2005;47(8):551-555.
41. Mølgaard-Nielsen D, Hviid A. Newer-generation antiepileptic drugs and the risk of major birth defects. *JAMA*. 2011;305(19):1996-2002.
42. Cunnington MC, Weil JG, Messenheimer JA, Ferber S, Yerby M, Tennis P. Final results from 18 years of the International Lamotrigine Pregnancy Registry. *Neurology*. 2011;76(21):1817-1823.
43. Dolk H, Jentink J, Loane M, Morris J, De Jong-van den Berg LT, EUROCAT Antiepileptic Drug Working Group. Does lamotrigine use in pregnancy increase orofacial cleft risk relative to other malformations? *Neurology*. 2008;71(10):714-722.
44. Cunnington M, Ferber S, Quartey G, et al. Effect of dose on the frequency of major birth defects following fetal exposure to lamotrigine monotherapy in an international observational study. *Epilepsia*. 2007;48(6):1207-1210.
45. Bromley RL, Mawer G, Love J, et al. Early cognitive development in children born to women with epilepsy: a prospective report. *Epilepsia*. 2010;51(10):2058-2065.
46. Cummings C, Stewart M, Stevenson M, Morrow J, Nelson J. Neurodevelopment of children exposed in utero to lamotrigine, sodium valproate and carbamazepine. *Arch Dis Child*. 2011;96(7):643-647.
47. Veiby G, Daltveit AK, Schjølberg S, et al. Exposure to antiepileptic drugs in utero and child development: a prospective population-based study. *Epilepsia*. 2013;54(8):1462-1472.
48. Cohen MJ, Meador KJ, Browning N, et al. Fetal antiepileptic drug exposure: Adaptive and emotional/behavioral functioning at age 6 years. *Epilepsy Behav*. 2013;29(2):308-315.
49. Mawhinney E, Craig J, Morrow J, et al. Levetiracetam in pregnancy: results from the UK and Ireland epilepsy and pregnancy registers. *Neurology*. 2013;80(4):400-405.
50. Shallcross R, Bromley RL, Cheyne CP, et al. In utero exposure to levetiracetam vs valproate: development and language at 3 years of age. *Neurology*. 2014;82(3):213-221.
51. Hanson W, Smith DW. The fetal hydantoin syndrome. *J Pediatr*. 1975;87(2):285-290.
52. Hanson JW, Myrianthopoulos NC, Harvey MA, Smith DW. Risks to the offspring of women treated with hydantoin anticonvulsants, with emphasis on the fetal hydantoin syndrome. *J Pediatr*. 1976;89(4):662-668.
53. Gaily E, Granström ML, Hiilesmaa V, Bardy A. Minor anomalies in offspring of epileptic mothers. *J Pediatr*. 1988;112(4):520-529.
54. Vinten J, Bromley RL, Taylor J, Adab N, Kini U, Baker GA. The behavioral consequences of exposure to antiepileptic drugs in utero. *Epilepsy Behav*. 2009;14(1):197-201.
55. Dessens AB, Cohen-Kettenis PT, Mellenbergh GJ, Koppe JG, van De Poll NE, Boer K. Association of prenatal phenobarbital and phenytoin exposure with small head size at birth and with learning problems. *Acta Paediatr*. 2000;89(5):533-541.
56. van der Pol MC, Hadders-Algra M, Huisjes HJ, Touwen BC. Antiepileptic medication in pregnancy: late effects on the children's central nervous system development. *Am J Obstet Gynecol*. 1991;164:121-128.

57. Dean JC, Hailey H, Moore SJ, Lloyd DJ, Turnpenny PD, Little J. Long term health and neurodevelopment in children exposed to antiepileptic drugs before birth. *J Med Genet.* 2002;39(4):251-259.

58. Hill RM, Verniaud WM, Rettig GM, Tennyson LM, Craig JP. Relation between antiepileptic drug exposure of the infant and developmental potential. In: Janz D, Dam M, Richens A, Bossi L, Helge H, Schmidt D, eds. *Epilepsy, Pregnancy and the Child.* New York, NY: Raven Press; 1982: 409-417.

59. Reinisch JM, Sanders SA, Mortensen EL, Rubin DB. In utero exposure to phenobarbital and intelligence deficits in adult men. *JAMA.* 1995;274(19):1518-1525.

60. Thomas SV, Sukumaran S, Lukose N, George A, Sarma PS. Intellectual and language functions in children of mothers with epilepsy. *Epilepsia.* 2007;48(12):2234-2240.

61. Hernández-Díaz S, Mittendorf R, Smith CR, Hauser WA, Yerby M, Holmes LB. Association between topiramate and zonisamide use during pregnancy and low birth weight. *Obstet Gynecol.* 2014;123(1):21-28.

62. Margulis AV, Mitchell AA, Gilboa SM, et al. Use of topiramate in pregnancy and risk of oral clefts. *Am J Obstet Gynecol.* 2012;207(5):405.e1-405.e7.

63. Alsaad AM, Chaudhry SA, Koren G. First trimester exposure to topiramate and the risk of oral clefts in the offspring: A systematic review and meta-analysis. *Reprod Toxicol.* 2015;53:45-50.

64. *Lacosamide (Vimpat) prescribing information.* <http://www.vimpat.com/pdf/vimpat_PI.pdf>.

65. Nadebaum C, Anderson VA, Vajda F, Reutens DC, Barton S, Wood AG. Language skills of school-aged children prenatally exposed to antiepileptic drugs. *Neurology.* 2011;76(8):719-726.

66. Holmes LB, Mittendorf R, Shen A, Smith CR, Hernández-Díaz S. Fetal effects of anticonvulsant polytherapies: different risks from different drug combinations. *Arch Neurol.* 2011;68(10):1275-1281.

67. Polepally AR, Pennell PB, Brundage RC, et al. Model-based lamotrigine clearance changes during pregnancy: clinical implication. *Ann Clin Transl Neurol.* 2014;1(2):99-106.

68. Petrenaite V, Sabers A, Hansen-Schwartz J. Seizure deterioration in women treated with oxcarbazepine during pregnancy. *Epilepsy Res.* 2009;84(2-3):245-249.

69. Battino D, Tomson T, Bonizzoni E, et al. Seizure control and treatment changes in pregnancy: Observations from the EURAP epilepsy pregnancy registry. *Epilepsia.* 2013;54(9):1621-1627.

70. EURAP Study Group. Seizure control and treatment in pregnancy: observations from the EURAP epilepsy pregnancy registry. *Neurology.* 2006;66: 354-360.

71. Johnson EL, Stowe ZN, Ritchie JC, et al. Carbamazepine clearance and seizure stability during pregnancy. *Epilepsy Behav.* 2014;33(6):49-53.

72. Reisinger TL, Newman M, Loring DW, Pennell PB, Meador KJ. Antiepileptic drug clearance and seizure frequency during pregnancy in women with epilepsy. *Epilepsy Behav.* 2013;29(1):13-18.

73. Vajda FJ, O'Brien T, Lander C, Graham J, Eadie M. The efficacy of the newer antiepileptic drugs in controlling seizures in pregnancy. *Epilepsia.* 2014;55(8):1229-1234.

74. Cagnetti C, Lattanzi S, Foschi N, Provinciali L, Silvestrini M. Seizure course during pregnancy in catamenial epilepsy. *Neurology.* 2014;83(4):339-344.

75. La Neve A, Boero G, Francavilla T, Plantamura M, De Agazio G, Specchio LM. Prospective, case-control study on the effect of pregnancy on seizure frequency in women with epilepsy. *Neurol Sci.* 2014;36(1):79-83.

76. Thomas SV, Syam U, Devi JS. Predictors of seizures during pregnancy in women with epilepsy. *Epilepsia.* 2012;53(5):2010-2013.

77. Borthen I, Eide MG, Veiby G, Daltveit AK, Gilhus NE. Complications during pregnancy in women with epilepsy: Population-based cohort study. *BJOG.* 2009;116(13):1736-1742.

78. Borthen I, Eide MG, Daltveit AK, Gilhus NE. Obstetric outcome in women with epilepsy: A hospital-based, retrospective study. *BJOG.* 2011;118(8):956-965.

79. Borthen I. Obstetrical complications in women with epilepsy. *Seizure.* 2015;28:32-34.

80. Borthen I, Eide MG, Daltveit AK, Gilhus NE. Delivery outcome of women with epilepsy: A population-based cohort study. *BJOG.* 2010; 117(12):1537-1543.

81. Farmen AH, Grundt J, Tomson T, et al. Intrauterine growth retardation in foetuses of women with epilepsy. *Seizure.* 2015;28:76-80.

82. Veiby G, Daltveit AK, Engelsen BA, Gilhus NE. Pregnancy, delivery, and outcome for the child in maternal epilepsy. *Epilepsia.* 2009;50(9): 2130-2139.

83. Bech BH, Kjaersgaard MI, Pedersen HS, et al. Use of antiepileptic drugs during pregnancy and risk of spontaneous abortion and stillbirth: population based cohort study. *BMJ.* 2014;349:g5159.

84. Harden CL, Meador KJ, Pennell PB, et al. Practice parameter update: management issues for women with epilepsy—focus on pregnancy (an evidence-based review): teratogenesis and perinatal outcomes: report of the Quality Standards Subcommittee and Therapeutics and Technology Assessment Subcommittee. *Neurology.* 2009;73(2):133-141.

85. Davis AR, Pack AM, Kritzer J, Yoon A, Camus A. Reproductive history, sexual behavior and use of contraception in women with epilepsy. *Contraception.* 2008;77(6):405-409.

86. Vajda FJ, O'Brien TJ, Graham J, Lander CM, Eadie MJ. Prediction of the hazard of foetal malformation in pregnant women with epilepsy. *Epilepsy Res.* 2014;108(6):1013-1017.

87. Peljto AL, Barker-Cummings C, Vasoli VM, et al. Familial risk of epilepsy: A population-based study. *Brain.* 2014;137(3):795-805.

88. Poduri A, Sheidley BR, Shostak S, Ottman R. Genetic testing in the epilepsies—developments and dilemmas. *Nat Rev Neurol.* 2014;10(5): 293-299.

89. Sheen V, Walsh C. X-Linked Periventricular Heterotopia Clinical Diagnosis Genetically Related (Allelic) Disorders. In: Pagon R, Adam M, Ardinger H, eds. *GeneReviews(R).* Seattle: University of Washington; 2009.

90. Harden CL, Pennell PB, Koppel BS, et al. Practice parameter update: management issues for women with epilepsy—focus on pregnancy (an evidence-based review): vitamin K, folic acid, blood levels, and breastfeeding: report of the Quality Standards Subcommittee and Therapeutics and Technology Assessment Subcommittee of the American Academy of Neurology and American Epilepsy Society. *Neurology.* 2009;73(2):142-149.

91. Blencowe H, Cousens S, Modell B, Lawn J. Folic acid to reduce neonatal mortality from neural tube disorders. *Int J Epidemiol.* 2010;39(suppl 1): i110-i121.

92. Kjaer D, Horvath-Puhó E, Christensen J, et al. Antiepileptic drug use, folic acid supplementation, and congenital abnormalities: a population-based case-control study. *BJOG.* 2008;115(1):98-103.

93. Linnebank M, Moskau S, Semmler A, et al. Antiepileptic drugs interact with folate and vitamin B12 serum levels. *Ann Neurol.* 2011;69(2): 352-359.

94. Pittschieler S, Brezinka C, Jahn B, et al. Spontaneous abortion and the prophylactic effect of folic acid supplementation in epileptic women undergoing antiepileptic therapy. *J Neurol.* 2008;255(12):1926-1931.

95. Valera-Gran D, García de la Hera M, Navarrete-Muñoz EM, et al. Folic Acid Supplemnts During Pregnancy and Child Psychomotor Development After the First Year of Life. *JAMA Pediatr.* 2014;168(11):e142611.

96. Aguglia U, Barboni G, Battino D, et al. Italian consensus conference on epilepsy and pregnancy, labor and puerperium. In. *Epilepsia.* 2009;50: 7-23.

97. Milunsky A, Jick H, Jick SS, et al. Multivitamin/folic acid supplementation in early pregnancy reduces the prevalence of neural tube defects. *JAMA.* 1989;262(20):2847-2852.

98. Bleyer WA, Skinner AL. Fatal Neonatal Hemorrhage After Maternal Anticonvulsant Therapy. *JAMA.* 1976;235(6):626-627.

99. Kaaja E, Kaaja R, Matila R, Hiilesmaa V. Enzyme-inducing antiepileptic drugs in pregnancy and the risk of bleeding in the neonate. *Neurology.* 2002;58(4):549-553.

100. Sveberg L, Vik K, Henriksen T, Taubøll E. Women with epilepsy and post partum bleeding—Is there a role for vitamin K supplementation? *Seizure.* 2015;28:85-87.

101. Sibai BM, Spinnato JA, Watson DL, Lewis JA, Anderson GD. Eclampsia. IV. Neurological findings and future outcome. *Am J Obstet Gynecol.* 1985;152(2):184-192.

102. Ip S, Chung M, Raman G, Trikalinos TA, Lau J. A summary of the Agency for Healthcare Research and Quality's evidence report on breastfeeding in developed countries. *Breastfeed Med.* 2009;4(suppl 1):S17-S30.

103. Meador KJ. Breastfeeding and antiepileptic drugs. *JAMA.* 2014;311(17): 1797-1798.

104. Veiby G, Engelsen BA, Gilhus NE. Early child development and exposure to antiepileptic drugs prenatally and through breastfeeding: a prospective cohort study on children of women with epilepsy. *JAMA Neurol.* 2013; 70(11):1367-1374.

105. Gaffield ME, Culwell KR, Lee CR. The use of hormonal contraception among women taking anticonvulsant therapy. *Contraception.* 2011;83(1): 16-29.

106. Stephens JW, Thacker SB, Casey CG, et al. U.S. Medical Eligibility Criteria for Contraceptive Use, 2010. *MMWR Recomm Rep.* 2010;59(RR–4): 1-86.

107. Trojano M, Lucchese G, Graziano G, et al. Geographical Variations in Sex Ratio Trends over Time in Multiple Sclerosis. *PLoS ONE.* 2012;7(10).

108. Cavalla P, Rovei V, Masera S, et al. Fertility in patients with multiple sclerosis: Current knowledge and future perspectives. *Neurol Sci.* 2006; 27(4):231-239.

109. Roux T, Courtillot C, Debs R, Touraine P, Lubetzki C, Papeix C. Fecundity in women with multiple sclerosis: an observational mono-centric study. *J Neurol.* 2015;262(4):957-960.

110. Thöne J, Kollar S, Nousome D, et al. Serum anti-Müllerian hormone levels in reproductive-age women with relapsing-remitting multiple sclerosis. *Mult Scler.* 2015;21(1):41-47.

111. Grinsted L, Heltberg A, Hagen C, Djursing H. Serum sex hormone and gonadotropin concentrations in premenopausal women with multiple sclerosis. *J Intern Med.* 1989;226(4):241-244.

112. Jalkanen A, Alanen A, Airas L. Pregnancy outcome in women with multiple sclerosis: results from a prospective nationwide study in Finland. *Mult Scler.* 2010;16(8):950-955.

113. Michel L, Foucher Y, Vukusic S, et al. Increased risk of multiple sclerosis relapse after in vitro fertilisation. *J Neurol Neurosurg Psychiatry.* 2012; 83(8):796-802.

114. Correale J, Farez MF, Ysrraelit MC. Increase in multiple sclerosis activity after assisted reproduction technology. *Ann Neurol.* 2012;72(5): 682-694.

115. Hellwig K, Schimrigk S, Beste C, Müller T, Gold R. Increase in relapse rate during assisted reproduction technique in patients with multiple sclerosis. *Eur Neurol.* 2009;61(2):65-68.

116. Confavreux C, Hutchinson M, Hours MM, Cortinovis-Tourniaire P, Moreau T. Rate of pregnancy-related relapse in multiple sclerosis. Pregnancy in Multiple Sclerosis Group. *N Engl J Med.* 1998;339(5): 285-291.

117. Vukusic S, Hutchinson M, Hours M, et al. Pregnancy and multiple sclerosis (the PRIMS study): Clinical predictors of post-partum relapse. *Brain.* 2004;127(6):1353-1360.

118. Vukusic S, Marignier R. Multiple sclerosis and pregnancy in the "treatment era". *Nat Rev Neurol.* 2015;11(5):280-289.

119. Finkelsztejn A, Brooks JB, Paschoal FM, Fragoso YD. What can we really tell women with multiple sclerosis regarding pregnancy? A systematic review and meta-analysis of the literature. *BJOG.* 2011;118(7):790-797.

120. Weinshenker BG, Hader W, Carriere W, Baskerville J, Ebers GC. The influence of pregnancy on disability from multiple sclerosis: a population-based study in Middlesex County, Ontario. *Neurology.* 1989;39(11): 1438-1440.

121. Verdru P, Theys P, D'Hooghe MB, Carton H. Pregnancy and multiple sclerosis: the influence on long term disability. *Clin Neurol Neurosurg.* 1994;96(1):38-41.

122. Runmarker B, Andersen O. Pregnancy is associated with a lower risk of onset and a better prognosis in multiple sclerosis. *Brain.* 1995;118(Pt 1): 253-261.

123. Karp I, Manganas A, Sylvestre MP, Ho A, Roger E, Duquette P. Does pregnancy alter the long-term course of multiple sclerosis? *Ann Epidemiol.* 2014;24(7):504-508.e2.

124. Ramagopalan S, Yee I, Byrnes J, Guimond C, Ebers G, Sadovnick D. Term pregnancies and the clinical characteristics of multiple sclerosis: a population based study. *J Neurol Neurosurg Psychiatry.* 2012;83(8): 793-795.

125. van der Kop ML, Pearce MS, Dahlgren L, et al. Neonatal and delivery outcomes in women with multiple sclerosis. *Ann Neurol.* 2011;70(1): 41-50.

126. Hughes SE, Spelman T, Gray OM, et al. Predictors and dynamics of postpartum relapses in women with multiple sclerosis. *Mult Scler.* 2014; 20(6):739-746.

127. Fragoso YD, Boggild M, MacIas-Islas MA, et al. The effects of long-term exposure to disease-modifying drugs during pregnancy in multiple sclerosis. *Clin Neurol Neurosurg.* 2013;115(2):154-159.

128. Portaccio E, Ghezzi A, Hakiki B, et al. Breastfeeding is not related to postpartum relapses in multiple sclerosis. *Neurology.* 2011;77(2): 145-150.

129. Coyle PK. Multiple Sclerosis in Pregnancy. *Continuum (Minneap Minn).* 2014;20:42-59.

130. Sandberg-Wollheim M, Alteri E, Moraga MS, Kornmann G. Pregnancy outcomes in multiple sclerosis following subcutaneous interferon beta-1a therapy. *Mult Scler.* 2011;17(4):423-430.

131. Amato MP, Portaccio E, Ghezzi A, et al. Pregnancy and fetal outcomes after interferon-β exposure in multiple sclerosis. *Neurology.* 2010;75(20): 1794-1802.

132. Lu E, Wang BW, Guimond C, Synnes A, Sadovnick D, Tremlett H. Disease-modifying drugs for multiple sclerosis in pregnancy: a systematic review. *Neurology.* 2012;79(11):1130-1135.

133. Romero RS, Lünzmann C, Bugge JP. Pregnancy outcomes in patients exposed to interferon beta-1b. Table 1. *J Neurol Neurosurg Psychiatry.* 2015;86(5):587-589.

134. Salminen HJ, Leggett H, Boggild M. Glatiramer acetate exposure in pregnancy: Preliminary safety and birth outcomes. *J Neurol.* 2010;257(12): 2020-2023.

135. Fragoso YD, Finkelsztejn A, Kaimen-Maciel DR, et al. Long-term use of glatiramer acetate by 11 pregnant women with multiple sclerosis: A retrospective, multicentre case series. *CNS Drugs.* 2010;24(11):969-976.

136. *Tecfidera (dimethyl fumarate) highlights of prescribing information.* 2015. Patient information approved by the FDA. <http://www.tecfiderahcp.com/pdfs/full-prescribing-information.pdf?utm_source=bing&utm_medium=cpc&utm_term=Tecfidera+Prescribing+Information&utm_campaign=Branded_Sitelink>.

137. Gold R, Phillips JT, Havrdova E, et al. Delayed-release dimethyl fumarate and pregnancy: preclinical studies and pregnancy outcomes from clinical trials and postmarketing experience. *Neurol Ther.* 2015;4(2):93-104.

138. Amato MP, Portaccio E. Fertility, Pregnancy and Childbirth in Patients with Multiple Sclerosis: Impact of Disease-Modifying Drugs. *CNS Drugs.* 2015;29(3):207-220.

139. Henson L, Benamor M, Truffinet P, Kieseier B. Updated pregnancy outcomes in patients and partners of patients in the teriflunomide clinical trial program [abstract]. *Neurology.* 2014;82(10 suppl):4-161.

140. Bove R, Alwan S, Friedman JM, et al. Management of Multiple Sclerosis During Pregnancy and the Reproductive Years. *Obstet Gynecol.* 2014; 124(6):1157-1168.

141. *Gilenya (fingolimod) highlights of prescribing information. Patient information approved by the FDA.* Novartis, revised August 2015. <http://www.fda.gov/Safety/MedWatch/SafetyInformation/ucm266123.htm>.

142. Karlsson G, Francis G, Koren G, et al. Pregnancy outcomes in the clinical development program of fingolimod in multiple sclerosis. *Neurology.* 2014;82(8):674-680.

143. Wehner NG, Shopp G, Osterburg I, Fuchs A, Buse E, Clarke J. Postnatal development in cynomolgus monkeys following prenatal exposure to natalizumab, an alpha4 integrin inhibitor. *Birth Defects Res B Dev Reprod Toxicol.* 2009;86(2):144-156.

144. Ebrahimi N, Herbstritt S, Gold R, Amezcua L, Koren G, Hellwig K. Pregnancy and fetal outcomes following natalizumab exposure in pregnancy. A prospective, controlled observational study. *Mult Scler.* 2015;21: 198-205.

145. Haghikia A, Langer-Gould A, Rellensmann G, et al. Natalizumab use during the third trimester of pregnancy. *JAMA Neurol.* 2014;71(7): 891-895.

146. Mccomb P, Achiron A, Giovanni G, Brinar V, Margolin D, Palmer J. Pregnancy outcomes in the alemtuzumab multiple sclerosis clinical development program [Abstract]. In: *Joint ACTRIMS-ECTRIMS Congress.* Boston: 2014.

147. Compston A, Coles A. Multiple sclerosis. *Lancet.* 2002;359(9313): 1221-1231.

148. Etemadifar M, Janghorbani M. Efficacy of high-dose vitamin D3 supplementation in vitamin D deficient pregnant women with multiple sclerosis: Preliminary findings of a randomized-controlled trial. *Iran J Neurol.* 2015;14(2):67-73.

149. Pastò L, Portaccio E, Ghezzi A, et al. Epidural analgesia and cesarean delivery in multiple sclerosis post-partum relapses: the Italian cohort study. *BMC Neurol.* 2012;12:165.

150. Lu E, Zhao Y, Dahlgren L, et al. Obstetrical epidural and spinal anesthesia in multiple sclerosis. *J Neurol.* 2013;260(10):2620-2628.

151. Hellwig K, Haghikia A, Rockhoff M, Gold R. Multiple sclerosis and pregnancy: experience from a nationwide database in Germany. *Ther Adv Neurol Disord.* 2012;5(5):247-253.

152. Langer-Gould A, Huang SM, Gupta R, et al. Exclusive breastfeeding and the risk of postpartum relapses in women with multiple sclerosis. *Arch Neurol.* 2009;66(8):958-963.

153. Pakpoor J, Disanto G, Lacey MV, Hellwig K, Giovannoni G, Ramagopalan SV. Breastfeeding and multiple sclerosis relapses: A meta-analysis. *J Neurol.* 2012;259(10):2246-2248.

154. Hale TW, Siddiqui AA, Baker TE. Transfer of Interferon β-1a into Human Breastmilk. *Breastfeed Med.* 2012;7(2):123-125.

155. Achiron A, Kishner I, Dolev M, et al. Effect of intravenous immunoglobulin treatment on pregnancy and postpartum-related relapses in multiple sclerosis. *J Neurol.* 2004;251(9):1133-1137.

156. Confavreux C. Intravenous immunoglobulins, pregnancy and multiple sclerosis. *J Neurol.* 2004;251(9):1138-1139.

157. Haas J, Hommes OR. A dose comparison study of IVIG in postpartum relapsing-remitting multiple sclerosis. *Mult Scler.* 2007;13(7):900-908.

158. de Seze J, Chapelotte M, Delalande S, Ferriby D, Stojkovic T, Vermersch P. Intravenous corticosteroids in the postpartum period for reduction of acute exacerbations in multiple sclerosis. *Mult Scler.* 2004;10(5):596-597.

159. Maggioni F, Alessi C, Maggino T, Zanchin G. Headache during pregnancy. *Cephalalgia.* 1997;17(7):765-769.

160. Ertresvåg JM, Zwart JA, Helde G, Johnsen HJ, Bovim G. Headache and transient focal neurological symptoms during pregnancy, a prospective cohort. *Acta Neurol Scand.* 2005;111(4):233-237.

161. Chen TC, Leviton A. Headache recurrence in pregnant women with migraine. *Headache.* 1994;34(2):107-110.

162. Chen HM, Chen SF, Chen YH, Lin HC. Increased risk of adverse pregnancy outcomes for women with migraines: A nationwide population-based study. *Cephalalgia.* 2010;30(4):433-438.

163. O'Quinn S, Ephross SA, Williams V, Davis RL, Gutterman DL, Fox AW. Pregnancy and perinatal outcomes in migraineurs using sumatriptan: A prospective study. *Arch Gynecol Obstet.* 1999;263(1-2):7-12.

164. Olesen C, Steffensen FH, Sørensen HT, Nielsen GL, Olsen J. Pregnancy outcome following prescription for sumatriptan. *Headache.* 2000;40(1):20-24.

165. Källén B, Lygner PE. Delivery outcome in women who used drugs for migraine during pregnancy with special reference to sumatriptan. *Headache.* 2001;41(4):351-356.

166. Hilaire ML, Cross LB, Eichner SF. Treatment of migraine headaches with sumatriptan in pregnancy. *Ann Pharmacother.* 2004;38(10):1726-1730.

167. Ephross SA, Sinclair SM. Final Results From the 16-Year Sumatriptan, Naratriptan, and Treximet Pregnancy Registry. *Headache.* 2014;54(7):1158-1172.

168. Soldin OP, Dahlin J, O'Mara DM. Triptans in pregnancy. *Ther Drug Monit.* 2008;30(1):5-9.

169. Maizels M, Blumenfeld A, Burchette R. A combination of riboflavin, magnesium, and feverfew for migraine prophylaxis: A randomized trial. *Headache.* 2004;44(9):885-890.

170. Kesler A, Kupferminc M. Idiopathic intracranial hypertension and pregnancy. *Clin Obstet Gynecol.* 2013;56(2):389-396.

171. Ireland B, Corbett JJ, Wallace RB. The search for causes of idiopathic intracranial hypertension. A preliminary case-control study. *Arch Neurol.* 1990;47(3):315-320.

172. Koontz WL, Herbert WN, Cefalo RC. Pseudotumor cerebri in pregnancy. *Obstet Gynecol.* 1983;62(3):324-327.

173. Lee AG, Pless M, Falardeau J, Capozzoli T, Wall M, Kardon RH. The use of acetazolamide in idiopathic intracranial hypertension during pregnancy. *Am J Ophthalmol.* 2005;139(5):855-859.

174. Month RC, Vaida SJ. A combined spinal-epidural technique for labor analgesia and symptomatic relief in two parturients with idiopathic intracranial hypertension. *Int J Obstet Anesth.* 2012;21(2):192-194.

175. Abraham J, Rao PS, Inbaraj SG, Shetty G, Jose CJ. An epidemiological study of hemiplegia due to stroke in South India. *Stroke.* 1970;1(6):477-481.

176. Vora S, Ghosh K, Shetty S, Salvi V, Satoskar P. Deep venous thrombosis in the antenatal period in a large cohort of pregnancies from western India. *Thromb J.* 2007;5:9.

177. Miller HJ, Hinkley CM. Berry aneurysms in pregnancy: a 10 year report. *South Med J.* 1970;63(3):279.

178. Robinson JL, Hall CS, Sedzimir CB. Arteriovenous malformations, aneurysms, and pregnancy. *J Neurosurg.* 1974;41(1):63-70.

179. Dias MS, Sekhar LN. Intracranial hemorrhage from aneurysms and arteriovenous malformations during pregnancy and the puerperium. *Neurosurgery.* 1990;27(6):855-866.

180. Ducros A, Boukobza M, Porcher R, Sarov M, Valade D, Bousser MG. The clinical and radiological spectrum of reversible cerebral vasoconstriction syndrome. A prospective series of 67 patients. *Brain.* 2007;130(12):3091-3101.

181. Del Zotto E, Giossi A, Volonghi I, Costa P, Padovani A, Pezzini A. Ischemic Stroke during Pregnancy and Puerperium. *Stroke Res Treat.* 2011;2011(Table 1):606780.

182. Brown DW, Dueker N, Jamieson DJ, et al. Preeclampsia and the risk of ischemic stroke among young women: results from the Stroke Prevention in Young Women Study. *Stroke.* 2006;37(4):1055-1059.

183. Feske SK, Singhal AB. Cerebrovascular disorders complicating pregnancy. *Continuum (Minneap Minn).* 2014;20(1 Neurology of Pregnancy):80-99.

184. Kittner SJ, Stern BJ, Feeser BR, et al. Pregnancy and the risk of stroke. *N Engl J Med.* 1996;335(11):768-774.

185. Horton JC, Chambers WA, Lyons SL, Adams RD, Kjellberg RN. Pregnancy and the risk of hemorrhage from cerebral arteriovenous malformations. *Neurosurgery.* 1990;27(6):867-872.

186. Parkinson D, Bachers G. Arteriovenous malformations. Summary of 100 consecutive supratentorial cases. *J Neurosurg.* 1980;53(3):285-299.

187. Ogilvy CS, Stieg PE, Awad I, et al. AHA Scientific Statement: Recommendations for the management of intracranial arteriovenous malformations: a statement for healthcare professionals from a special writing group of the Stroke Council, American Stroke Association. *Stroke.* 2001;32(6):1458-1471.

188. Stolp-Smith KA, Pascoe MK, Ogburn PL. Carpal tunnel syndrome in pregnancy: Frequency, severity, and prognosis. *Arch Phys Med Rehabil.* 1998;79(10):1285-1287.

189. McLennan HG, Oats JN, Walstab JE. Survey of hand symptoms in pregnancy. *Med J Aust.* 1987;147(11-12):542-544.

190. Ekman-Ordeberg G, Sälgeback S, Ordeberg G. Carpal tunnel syndrome in pregnancy. A prospective study. *Acta Obstet Gynecol Scand.* 1987;66(3):233-235.

191. Meems M, Truijens S, Spek V, Visser L, Pop V. Prevalence, course and determinants of carpal tunnel syndrome symptoms during pregnancy: a prospective study. *BJOG.* 2015;122(8):1112-1118.

192. Padua L, Di Pasquale A, Pazzaglia C, Liotta GA, Librante A, Mondelli M. Systematic review of pregnancy-related carpal tunnel syndrome. *Muscle Nerve.* 2010;42(5):697-702.

193. Wand JS. Carpal tunnel syndrome in pregnancy and lactation. *J Hand Surg [Br].* 1990;15(1):93-95.

194. Assmus H, Hashemi B. Surgical treatment of carpal tunnel syndrome in pregnancy: results from 314 cases. *Nervenarzt.* 2000;71(6):470-473.

CHAPTER 50

Malignant Diseases and Pregnancy

RITU SALANI and LARRY J. COPELAND

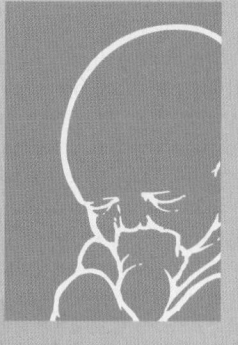

KEY ABBREVIATIONS

Acute lymphoblastic leukemia	ALL
Acute myeloid leukemia	AML
Acute nonlymphocytic leukemia	ANLL
Alpha-fetoprotein	AFP
Beta human chorionic gonadotropin	β-hCG
Carcinoembryonic antigen	CEA
Central nervous system	CNS
Chronic myelocytic leukemia	CML
Computed tomography	CT
Fine-needle aspiration	FNA
Food and Drug Administration	FDA
Gestational trophoblastic disease	GTD
Gray	Gy
Hodgkin lymphoma	HL
Magnetic resonance imaging	MRI
Non-Hodgkin lymphoma	NHL

The juxtaposition of life and death can present numerous emotional and ethical conflicts to the patient, her family, and her physicians. The diagnosis of cancer for anyone is understandably frightening. To deal with cancer in the context of pregnancy is particularly burdensome, because the patient may have to balance competing maternal and fetal interests. On occasion, a pregnant woman may be required to make decisions that affect her life or longevity versus the life or the well-being of her unborn child. Cancer in pregnancy complicates the management of both the cancer and the pregnancy. Diagnostic and therapeutic interventions must carefully address the associated risks to both the patient and the fetus. Informed decisions require evaluation of a number of factors, and with counseling, these considerations are the foundation on which treatment decisions are made. An evolution has taken place in the philosophy of care, from one of total disregard of the pregnancy with frequent immediate termination to a more thoughtful approach in which management decisions consider both maternal and fetal outcomes so as to limit risk of death or morbidity to both.

It is estimated that approximately 20% to 30% of malignancies occur in women younger than age 45 years.[1] **Although cancer is the second most common cause of death for women in their reproductive years, only about 1 in 1000 pregnancies is complicated by cancer.**[2] Because no large prospective studies have addressed cancer treatment in pregnancy, physicians tend to base treatment strategies on small retrospective studies or anecdotal reports that occasionally present conflicting information.[1,2] **A successful outcome is dependent on a cooperative multidisciplinary approach.** The management plan must be formulated within a medical, moral, ethical, legal, and religious framework that is acceptable to the patient and guided by communication and educational resources of the health care team.

Delays in diagnosis of cancer during pregnancy are common for various reasons: (1) many of the presenting symptoms of cancer are often attributed to the pregnancy; (2) many of the physiologic and anatomic alterations of pregnancy can compromise physical examination; (3) serum tumor markers such as β-human chorionic gonadotropin (β-hCG), alpha-fetoprotein (AFP), and cancer antigen 125 (CA 125) are increased during pregnancy; and (4) the ability to optimally perform either imaging studies or invasive diagnostic procedures may be altered during pregnancy. Because the gestational age is significant when evaluating the risks of treatments, it is important to determine gestational age accurately. An early ultrasound evaluation may be useful to ensure accurate dating.

The malignancies most commonly encountered in the pregnant patient are breast cancer, cervical cancer, and melanoma—cancers that most commonly occur in this age group—but also ovarian, thyroid, and colorectal cancer as well as leukemia and lymphoma.[2,3] The frequencies of these diseases complicating pregnancy may increase secondary to the trend to delay childbearing, and age is the most potent predictor of cancer. Before specific malignancies are discussed below, some general principles are reviewed.

CHEMOTHERAPY DURING PREGNANCY
Pharmacology of Chemotherapy During Pregnancy

Because pregnancy profoundly changes maternal physiology (see Chapter 3), the potential exists for altered pharmacokinetics associated with chemotherapy. Orally administered medications are subject to changes in gastrointestinal (GI) motility. Peak drug concentrations are decreased owing to the 50% expansion in plasma volume, which produces a longer drug half-life unless a concurrent increase occurs in metabolism or excretion. The increase in plasma proteins and fall in albumin may alter drug availability, and amniotic fluid may act as a pharmacologic third space that potentially increases toxicity because of delayed metabolism and excretion. Hepatic oxidation and renal blood flow are both elevated during pregnancy and may influence the metabolism and excretion of most drugs.[4] However, because pharmacologic studies in pregnant women are lacking, we currently assume that initial drug dosages are similar to those given to the nonpregnant woman, and adjustments to dose are based on toxicity on a course-by-course basis. **Because most antineoplastic agents can be found in breast milk, breastfeeding is contraindicated** (see Chapter 24).[4]

Drug Effects on the Fetus

All drugs undergo animal teratogenicity testing, and based on these results, the drugs are assigned risk categories (Table 50-1) by the U.S. Food and Drug Administration (FDA).[5] Based on this system, most chemotherapeutic agents are rated as C, D, or X. However, animal teratogenicity testing cannot always be reliably extrapolated to humans. For example, a drug (e.g., aspirin) may show teratogenic effects in animals but will not affect humans. The opposite is also true and, as such, has serious potential to do harm; for example, a drug may demonstrate no animal teratogenicity (e.g., thalidomide), but it can cause serious human anomalies (see Chapter 8). Because detailed ultrasonography may fail to identify subtle anatomic but serious functional abnormalities before 20 weeks' gestation, patients should be appropriately counseled and may want to consider the option of pregnancy termination if first-trimester chemotherapy is planned or administered. **The risk of teratogenicity during the second and third trimesters is significantly reduced and is likely no different from that for pregnant women who are not exposed to chemotherapy.**[4]

Although the literature that addresses chemotherapy administration during pregnancy is somewhat limited and dated, literature reviews provide us with some information regarding the frequency of affected offspring.[4,6] Because antineoplastic agents target the rapidly dividing malignant cell, it could be expected that the exposed fetus would be particularly susceptible to serious toxicity. Clear documentation of such is not the case. Excluding the intentional use of abortifacients, it is difficult to

TABLE 50-1 FOOD AND DRUG ADMINISTRATION RISK CATEGORIES FOR DRUG USE DURING PREGNANCY

CATEGORY	DEFINITION
A	Controlled studies have demonstrated no risk in the first trimester, and the possibility of fetal harm appears remote.
B	*Either* animal studies have failed to identify a risk but no controlled studies have been done in women *or* animal studies have shown an unconfirmed adverse effect.
C	*Either* animal studies have revealed adverse effects and no controlled studies have been done in women *or* studies in women and animals are not available. Use the drugs only if the potential benefit justifies the potential risks.
D	Evidence of fetal risk exists, but the benefits may be acceptable despite the risk in either a life-threatening situation or a serious disease for which safer drugs are ineffective.
X	Studies in animals or humans have demonstrated fetal abnormalities, and the risk of the drug clearly outweighs any possible benefit.

From Amant F, Han SN, Gziri MM, Dekrem J, Van Calsteren K. Chemotherapy during pregnancy. *Curr Opin Oncol.* 2012;24:580-586.

clearly demonstrate that the use of chemotherapy results in an increase in the clinically recognized spontaneous abortion rate over the expected 15% to 20%. However, **if continuation of the pregnancy is desired, chemotherapy is not advised in the first trimester because of an increased rate of major malformations that ranges from 10% to 17% with single-agent therapy and up to 25% with combination chemotherapy.**[6] **Administration in the second and third trimester has been associated with intrauterine growth restriction (IUGR), stillbirth, and low birthweight.**[6,7] Maternal effects such as chemotherapy-induced nausea and vomiting may also affect fetal growth and birthweight.[8] Because early induction of labor or surgical delivery is often a component of the overall treatment plan, it has been difficult to identify premature birth as a specific result of the chemotherapy. Preterm delivery has been reported to occur in more than half of pregnancies associated with malignancies, with a majority being iatrogenically induced and associated with increased neonatal morbidity.[6] Therefore the timing of delivery and consideration of delay of therapy in the case of early-stage disease should be part of the treatment planning.

When chemotherapy is administered during the latter half of gestation, fetal organ toxicity has not been reported as a major problem, although neonatal myelosuppression and hearing loss have been reported.[6,9] Although second malignancies, impaired growth and development, intellectual impairment, and infertility have been reported after chemotherapy administration to children, the delayed effects of in utero exposure are less well documented.[6,9] Although few data are available, concerns regarding cognitive development have been evaluated, and the outcomes are comparable to those of individuals not exposed to chemotherapy in utero. Growth and fertility in these children have also been shown to be similar to those not exposed.[9]

Classification of Chemotherapy Agents
Antimetabolites

Historically, the antimetabolite aminopterin was used as an abortifacient, and in cases of failed abortion, the risk of fetal malformation was about 50%. Methotrexate has replaced aminopterin for chemotherapeutic purposes, and although similar types of anomalies occur, a lower overall frequency (<10%) has been reported.[8] **In the first trimester, methotrexate has been associated with skeletal and central nervous system (CNS) defects.** Although no anomalies were reported in the second and third trimesters, methotrexate was associated with low birthweight and neonatal myelosuppresion.[9] The use of low-dose methotrexate for systemic diseases (e.g., rheumatic disease and psoriasis) does not appear to produce teratogenicity.[10] In a prospective study, 5-fluorouracil, in combination with other agents, was well tolerated and resulted in no perinatal deaths.[8]

Alkylating Agents

Alkylating agents such as **cyclophosphamide and chlorambucil** are commonly used for the management of malignancies. Unfortunately, most of these agents have demonstrated some teratogenic potential when administered in the first trimester, with defects that include renal agenesis, ocular abnormalities, and cleft palate.[8] In the second and third trimesters, alkylating agents have been shown to be acceptably safe.[1,9]

Antitumor Antibiotics

Even when administered in early pregnancy, antitumor antibiotics—such as doxorubicin, idarubicin, bleomycin, and daunorubicin—appear to demonstrate a low risk of teratogenicity. Doxorubicin has been associated with one case of multiple anomalies; however, the patient was receiving combination chemotherapy.[9] One potential reason for the low rate of anthracycline-associated teratogenicity is its questionable ability to cross the placenta.[4]

Vinca Alkaloids

Although potent teratogens in animals, vincristine and vinblastine do not appear to be as teratogenic in humans.[8] In limited studies, vinca alkaloids were well tolerated in both early and later stages of pregnancy.[9]

Platinum Agents

Platinum agents have been used with relatively acceptable risks, and normal outcomes have been reported along with cases of IUGR. In addition, case studies have reported hearing loss and ventriculomegaly in 2.7% of patients exposed to cisplatin.[1] One case of bilateral hearing loss was noted in the offspring of a woman treated with carboplatin in the second trimester of pregnancy. However, the cause cannot be fully attributed to the platinum agent because other causes of hearing loss were also present, including prematurity and administration of gentamycin in the neonatal period.[8]

Miscellaneous

Taxane chemotherapy is used in the treatment of malignant tumors of multiple sites, and experience with this class of drugs remains limited, although a few reports to date are favorable.[8,9]

Targeted Therapies

Despite the emerging role of targeted agents in cancer treatment, they have been used only inadvertently in pregnancy. Trastuzumab has been linked to oligohydramnios, and its use is not recommended in pregnancy.[1] Rituximab has been associated with transient neonatal lymphopenia, and further studies are necessary to determine an accurate safety profile. Imatinib has been associated with low birthweight and premature delivery, whereas erlotinib showed no adverse effects in one case. The antiangiogenic agents (bevacizumab, sunitinib, and sorafenib) are not recommended for use in pregnant women.[1]

RADIATION THERAPY

Ionizing radiation is a known teratogen, and the developing embryo is particularly sensitive to its effects. Doses higher than 0.20 Gray (Gy) are considered teratogenic. Effects during early pregnancy are typically lethal or result in congenital malformations. During late gestation, radiation may cause specific organ damage in addition to mental retardation, skeletal anomalies, and ophthalmologic abnormalities. Reports have indicated that radiation exposure in utero increases the risk of malignancies such as leukemia and other childhood tumors, particularly when exposure occurred in the first trimester.[1,9] It is important to remember that these data are conflicting and are extrapolated from data derived from atomic catastrosphes.[9] Regardless, recommendations for radiation exposure in pregnancy should be less than 0.05 Gy.[1,9] **Radiation therapy should be postponed until the postpartum period, and consideration should be given to suitable alternative therapies such as surgery or chemotherapy. If delay of therapy is not possible, termination of the pregnancy may be required.**

SURGERY AND ANESTHESIA

Aspects of surgery are addressed later in the sections on specific cancers, but some general principles should be considered first. Although complications of surgery can threaten the fetus, extraperitoneal surgery is not related to spontaneous abortion or preterm labor. Surgery can be performed safely in all three trimesters.[11] **If flexibility in timing exists, abdominal or pelvic surgery is best performed in the second trimester to limit the risk of first-trimester spontaneous abortion or preterm labor.** In the first trimester, progesterone therapy is indicated (weeks 7 to 12) following resection of the corpus luteum. When laparoscopy is selected for abdominal surgery, the open technique is recommended to avoid injury to the uterus.[11] Perioperative cautions include attention to the relative safety of all drugs administered. When appropriate, antibiotic prophylaxis can be safely administered.[11] Fever secondary to either infection or atelectasis should be treated promptly because it may be associated with fetal abnormalities.

No evidence suggests that significant risks of anesthesia exist independent of coexisting disease (see Chapter 16).[12] Preoxygenation is critical due to the increase in oxygen consumption, which can lead to desaturation.[11] In the second and third trimesters, careful attention to positioning is required so as to avoid compression of the vena cava from the enlarged uterus. Use of local or regional anesthesia should be considered. Finally, continuous or intermittent fetal monitoring should be used when extrauterine survival is possible.

PREGNANCY FOLLOWING CANCER TREATMENT

With improved survival rates for many childhood and adolescent malignancies, the clinician must be prepared to offer prenatal counseling to the young woman who presents with a cancer history. Issues worthy of review and in need of clarification for the obstetrician and the patient are listed in Box 50-1.

Previous abdominal irradiation for a Wilms tumor appears to adversely affect the risk of pregnancy complications, including increased perinatal mortality, low birthweight, and abnormal pregnancy. In contrast, a review of pregnancies following treatment for Hodgkin lymphoma revealed no increase in poor pregnancy outcome.[13] However, the rate of ovarian failure following the multiple drug combinations is greater than 50% in some reports.[13] Also, a combination of pelvic irradiation and chemotherapy for Hodgkin disease results in an even higher rate of ovarian failure. Over recent years, a number of women with early cervical cancer have received fertility preservation surgery with radical trachelectomy and regional lymphadenectomy. The preliminary fertility and pregnancy outcomes have been favorable.[14]

Will pregnancy increase the risk of recurrence or accelerate recurrence? Even in women with estrogen receptor–positive breast cancer, there is no evidence that subsequent pregnancy adversely affects survival. In addition to the altered hormonal milieu, concern is also directed toward the potential for accelerated tumor activity associated with alterations in the pregnant patient's immune system. No available data support this concern; however, **it has been recommended that after a cancer diagnosis, pregnancy should be delayed for at least 2 years, during which recurrence risk is highest.**

CANCER DURING PREGNANCY
Breast Cancer
The estimated number of breast cancer cases in women in the United States exceeds 230,000 cases with approximately 40,000 deaths each year.[15] Although the lifetime risk of developing breast cancer is 1 in 8, the risk is 1 in 206 for women 40 years or younger. Each year, this results in approximately 7% to 15% of premenopausal breast cancers being diagnosed in women who are pregnant or lactating or within 1 year after delivery.[16-18] Although an increase in the frequency of breast cancer complicating pregnancy has been predicted because of delayed childbearing, **recent publications are consistent with a frequency of breast cancer concurrent with pregnancy of 1 per 3000 to 10,000 live births.**[17]

In general, the risk of breast cancer is directly related to the duration of ovarian function. Therefore both early menarche and late menopause appear to increase the likelihood of developing breast cancer. However, interruption of the normal cyclic ovarian

function by pregnancy appears to be protective. This apparent protective effect may be secondary to the normal hormonal milieu of pregnancy that produces epithelial proliferation, followed by marked differentiation and mitotic rest. Multiparous women, particularly those who breastfeed, have a lower risk of developing breast cancer than do nulliparous women. However, based on one study of almost 90,000 women, breastfeeding may not be an independent protective factor.[19] Paradoxically, carriers of *BRCA1* and *BRCA2* mutations may have an increased risk of developing breast cancer by having children.[20]

Diagnosis and Staging
Breast abnormalities should be evaluated in the same manner as in a nonpregnant patient. The most common presentation of breast cancer in pregnancy is a painless lump discovered by the patient. Because the breast changes become more pronounced in later pregnancy, it is important to perform a thorough breast examination at the initial visit (see Chapter 24). Despite the striking physiologic breast changes of pregnancy, including nipple enlargement and increases in glandular tissue that result in engorgement and tenderness, a newly found or persistent breast mass should be evaluated promptly. Diagnostic delays may increase the risk of nodal involvement and are often attributed to physician reluctance to evaluate breast complaints or abnormal findings in pregnancy.[21] **The lengths of delays in diagnosis of breast cancer in pregnancy are commonly 3 to 7 months or longer and may result in more advanced stages of diagnosis compared with the general population.**[18,21]

Although bilateral serosanguinous discharge may be normal in late pregnancy, less common presentations such as **bloody nipple discharge should be evaluated with mammography and ultrasound.**[16] In cases of mastitis or breast abscesses or for evaluation of breast edema or inflammation, a skin biopsy should be considered to evaluate for inflammatory breast cancer.

Mammography in pregnancy is controversial. Although the radiation exposure to the fetus is negligible, the hyperproliferative changes in the breast during pregnancy are characterized by increased tissue density, which makes interpretation more difficult.[9,16] **Breast ultrasound has a high sensitivity and specificity and can distinguish between solid and cystic masses, which makes it the preferred imaging modality for pregnant women.** Magnetic resonance imaging (MRI) without gadolinium has also been used; however, data are limited in regard to its accuracy in this population. Percutaneous biopsy is recommended for any lesion that does not meet criteria for a simple cyst.[18] Fine-needle aspiration (FNA) of a mass for cytologic study may be used, but it is often misleading because of changes in the breast during pregnancy. **For breast masses, a core needle biopsy is the preferred method for histologic diagnosis.**[18]

Before proceeding with treatment, staging should be undertaken. All draining lymph nodes should be evaluated. Recent studies have evaluated the role of sentinel lymph node dissection in pregnant women with breast cancer. Although blue dye is associated with a risk of anaphylaxis and should not be used, several reports have demonstrated the safety of sentinel lymph node biopsy using a low-dose lymphoscintigraphy with 99m-Technetium–labeled sulfur colloid. This technique may be considered in select cases at an experienced center.[18,22,23] **The contralateral breast must be carefully assessed. Laboratory tests should include baseline liver function tests and serum tumor markers, carcinoembryonic antigen (CEA), and also cancer antigen 15-3 (CA 15-3), which appears to be a useful**

tumor marker for monitoring breast cancer in pregnancy.[24] A chest radiograph is indicated, and if the liver function tests are abnormal, the liver can be evaluated by ultrasound. If bone metastases are suspected, a bone scan can be performed in pregnancy. In a symptomatic patient, radiographs of the specific symptomatic bones are advised. However, in an asymptomatic patient with normal blood tests, because the yield is low, bone scanning is usually not performed.

Treatment

The treatment of breast carcinoma at any time is often overshadowed by psychological and emotional factors. Because of potential risks to the developing fetus, treatment decisions carry an additional burden. **Therapy must be individualized in accordance with present knowledge and with the specific desires of the patient, gestational age, and tumor stage and biology; at all times, maternal treatment should adhere to standard recommendations.** At the time of diagnosis, it is important to have a baseline assessment of fetal growth and development by ultrasound as well as routine fetal monitoring throughout the pregnancy and treatment.[11]

LOCAL THERAPY

The usual criteria for breast-preserving therapy versus modified radical mastectomy pertain to the patient with breast cancer in stages I to III.[2,16] Although breast surgery can be safely performed in all trimesters with minimal fetal risks, the use of radiation is complicated by the presence of the pregnancy.[18,21] **Consideration should be given to the delay of irradiation until after delivery.** Experimental calculations suggest that when the fetus is within the true pelvis, a tumor dose of 5 Gy will expose the fetus to 0.010 to 0.015 Gy. Later in pregnancy, parts of the fetus may receive as much as 0.200 Gy.[21] Because these levels exceed the upper limit of safety, alternative approaches should be considered, and reports have shown that in the late second or third trimester, delaying treatment without impacting maternal outcome may be reasonable.

PREGNANCY TERMINATION

Because early studies suggested more unfavorable outcomes in pregnant women, it was assumed that the hormonal changes of pregnancy contributed to rapid tumor growth; therefore therapeutic abortion was frequently advised. At present, a harmful effect of continuing pregnancy has *not* been demonstrated in most published series.[2] Although data are limited, **studies have shown similar survival outcome if the patient had a spontaneous pregnancy loss, chose to terminate, or continued the pregnancy.**[8,25] However, it is difficult to evaluate potential selection bias toward performing an abortion in patients with advanced disease. Because young women tend to have hormone receptor–negative tumors, it is difficult to make an argument, based on hormonal concerns, for either termination of pregnancy or oophorectomy as an adjunct to therapy.[16]

CHEMOTHERAPY

In general, **women who present with either metastatic breast carcinoma or rapidly progressive inflammatory carcinoma should avoid any delays in therapy.** Immediate initiation of chemotherapy is critical to providing the patient with inflammatory carcinoma with any chance for long-term survival. **If the patient has a clinical indication for adjuvant chemotherapy other than inflammatory carcinoma, the delay of instituting chemotherapy and awaiting fetal pulmonary maturity should be considered in select third-trimester situations.** Current literature shows that the use of cytotoxic agents for breast cancer in pregnancy is relatively safe; and anthracycline-based regimens, which are the most widely used, are associated with a favorable safety profile.[22] Additional agents such as 5-fluorouracil, cyclophosphamide, and taxanes have also been used, but data on these agents are limited.[21,22] Others concur with the use of chemotherapy in the second and third trimesters in the management of breast cancer.[16,18] Pregnancy is a contraindication to the use of tamoxifen because of the risk of adverse fetal outcomes, including craniofacial malformations and ambiguous genitalia. Data regarding the safety of trastuzumab in pregnancy are limited, and currently it is not recommended because of reports of oligohydramnios and neonatal deaths as a result of respiratory and renal failure.[18,21]

Prognosis

As with any malignant disease, prognosis best correlates with the anatomic extent of disease at the time of diagnosis. **Outcomes in stage I and II disease are favorable, and survival rates approach 86% to 100%; however, the presence and extent of nodal involvement is especially predictive of prognosis in both nonpregnant and pregnant patients.**[8] Although nodal status is of prognostic significance, the number of positive nodes is also important. In the pregnant patient, the 5-year survival rate is 82% for patients with three or fewer positive nodes and 27% if greater than three nodes contain tumor.[26] **Probably because of the associated delays in diagnosis, pregnancy appears to increase the frequency of nodal disease, with 53% to 71% of patients exhibiting nodal involvement at diagnosis.**[26,27]

Reports have demonstrated that up to 60% to 80% of breast cancer cases in the pregnant population are estrogen receptor negative and have a rate of *ERBB2* positivity between 25% and 58%.[20,25] In addition to a higher incidence of lymph node metastases, breast tumors in pregnant women are more frequently reported to be larger and to be of a higher grade that those of their nonpregnant counterparts.[16,27] However, these rates are histologically identical to the nonpregnant patient of similar age, and when controlled for age and stage, pregnancy does not seem to affect prognosis adversely.[25,27] Of note, pregnant women with early-stage disease who had a delay in therapy did not experience a negative effect on disease-free survival.[28] However, breast cancer therapy during pregnancy is feasible, and patients should be counseled thoroughly.[21] Although infants exposed to chemotherapy for breast cancer in utero had a lower birthweight and more complications, this was not clinically significant, and most adverse outcomes were associated with preterm delivery; thus full-term delivery should be planned when possible.[28]

SUBSEQUENT PREGNANCY

Although the consensus is that subsequent pregnancies do not adversely affect survival, recommendations have been made regarding the timing of a subsequent pregnancy.[29] **It is generally advised that women with node-negative disease wait 2 to 3 years, and this interval should be extended to 5 years for patients with positive nodes.** Others have advised that no delay is indicated for the patient with a good prognosis who does not receive postoperative adjuvant chemotherapy.[29] It has been advised that patients should undergo a complete metastatic workup before a subsequent pregnancy.

Lactation and Breast Reconstruction

Lactation is possible in a small percentage of patients after breast-conserving therapy for early-stage breast cancer.[30] Lumpectomy using a radial incision, rather than the cosmetically preferred circumareolar incision, is less likely to disrupt ductal anatomy (see Chapter 24). Disruption of the ductal system may increase the rate of mastitis. Breastfeeding is contraindicated in women receiving chemotherapy, because significant levels of the drug can be found in breast milk.

Breast reconstruction with the use of autologous tissue has increased secondary to questions about the use of silicone-filled implants. The transverse rectus abdominis myocutaneous (TRAM) flap is one popular method of breast reconstruction. Because the donor site is a portion of the anterior abdominal wall, there is potential concern when the patient develops abdominal distension from pregnancy. In one case report and review of the literature, nine women who became pregnant following breast reconstruction experienced no problem with anterior abdominal wall integrity.[31] However, because data are limited, it may be best to address reconstruction in the postpartum period.

Lymphoma

Hodgkin Lymphoma

Approximately 36,000 cases of lymphoma were expected to be diagnosed in women in the United States in the year 2015, and only about 11% of these would have been Hodgkin lymphoma (HL).[15] **HL is the second most commonly diagnosed cancer in women aged 15 to 29 years, and it presents at a mean age of 32 years.** Lymphomas complicate approximately 1 in 6000 pregnancies, and few large series have evaluated the many issues that affect these women.[17,32] However, spontaneous abortion, stillbirth rates, preterm births, and adverse pregnancy outcomes do not appear to be increased or affected by the course of the disease, and **termination of pregnancy should not be routinely advised.**[32,33] Although some advocate therapeutic abortion for the patient with a first-trimester pregnancy and HL to allow complete staging, others limit therapeutic abortion to those women who require infradiaphragmatic radiation or those with extensive systemic symptoms or visceral disease.

Women with HL frequently present with enlarged cervical or axillary lymph nodes, and the diagnosis is established by biopsy of the suspicious nodes. The presence of systemic symptoms such as night sweats, pruritus, or weight loss suggests more extensive disease. In a series of 17 women diagnosed with HL during pregnancy, the average time of diagnosis was 22 weeks' gestation, and systemic symptoms were uncommon.[33] Clinical staging for lymphoma requires systemic evaluation by history, laboratory findings, bone marrow, and radiographic imaging. Clinical treatment and staging are individualized. Although pathologic staging for HL in the nonpregnant patient may involve laparotomy and splenectomy, these are not generally performed in pregnancy. **The routine evaluation for HL during pregnancy includes a single anterior/posterior view chest radiograph, liver function tests, serum creatinine clearance, complete blood count, erythrocyte sedimentation rate, and lymph node and bone marrow biopsy.** Evaluation of the abdomen is compromised by the gravid uterus, and MRI is preferred because it can accurately assess nodes, liver, and spleen. Chest tomography or computed tomographic (CT) scan of the mediastinum may be necessary to evaluate nodal enlargement in the chest. Isotope scans of the liver and bone are best avoided

STAGE	DESCRIPTION
TABLE 50-2	**STAGING CLASSIFICATION OF HODGKIN DISEASE**
I	Involvement of a single lymph node region (I) or of a single extralymphatic organ site (I_E)
II	Involvement of two or more lymph node regions on the same side of the diaphragm (II) or localized involvement of an extralymphatic organ site and of one or more lymph node regions on the same side of the diaphragm (II_E)
III	Involvement of lymph node regions on both sides of the diaphragm (III), which also may be accompanied by localized involvement of an extralymphatic organ or site (III_E), the spleen (III_S), or both (III_{SE})
IV	Diffuse or disseminated involvement of an extralymphatic organ with or without localized lymph node involvement (liver, bone marrow, lung, skin)

Symptoms of unexplained fever, night sweats, and unexplained weight loss of 10% of normal body weight results in classification of patients as B; absence of these symptoms is denoted as A.

during pregnancy, but ultrasonography is safe and may provide useful information.

Disease stage is the most important factor in treatment planning and prognosis (Table 50-2). The survival rate for early-stage HL exceeds 90%, whereas patients with disseminated nodal disease have a 5-year survival rate of about 50%. As expected, patients with stage IV disease have poor survival rates. Radiation therapy is the mainstay of treatment for early-stage HL, and combination chemotherapy is used for the treatment of advanced-stage disease with organ involvement. **Most investigators agree that treatment should not be withheld during pregnancy except in early-stage disease, particularly if the diagnosis is made in late gestation.**

Radiotherapy to the supradiaphragmatic regions may be performed with abdominal shielding after the first trimester. When this approach is chosen, irradiation should be delayed until after the first trimester, total fetal dose should be limited to 0.1 Gy or less, and the goal is partial therapy with completion therapy after delivery. Spontaneous abortion has been reported with an estimated first-trimester fetal dose of 0.09 Gy secondary to scatter from delivering 44 Gy to the chest of a patient receiving treatment for a recurrence.[34] In general, if the estimated exposure to a first-trimester fetus is expected to exceed 0.1 Gy or if combination chemotherapy is planned for the first trimester, therapeutic abortion should be considered because of an increased risk of fetal malformations.[35] Asymptomatic early-stage disease that presents in the second half of pregnancy may be followed closely while preparations are made for early delivery.[34] The use of corticosteroids and single-agent chemotherapy have been proposed for the patient with systemic symptoms.

Subdiaphragmatic or advanced disease requires chemotherapy, and commonly used regimens include doxorubicin, bleomycin, vinblastine, and dacarbazine (ABVD) and mechlorethamine, vincristine, procarbazine, and prednisone (MOPP).[32,34] Because many of these chemotherapeutic agents are known teratogens, such treatment is best avoided in the first trimester. A systematic review found 42 pregnancies in which HL was treated with chemotherapy, and 17 were exposed to chemotherapy in the first trimester, which resulted in six congenital anomalies and three spontaneous abortions.[36] Similar treatments should also be approached with caution later in pregnancy, although most case reports have documented only IUGR and neonatal

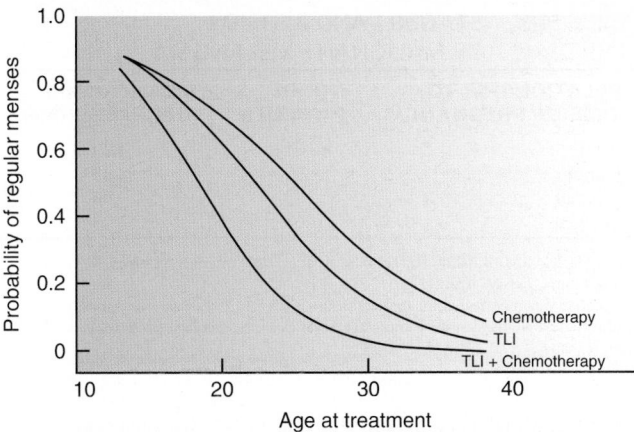

FIG 50-1 Probability of regular menses after chemotherapy, total lymphoid irradiation (TLI), and TLI and chemotherapy in patients with Hodgkin disease. The synergistic effect is more apparent in younger women. (From Horning SJ, Hoppe RT, Kaplan HS. Female reproduction after treatment for Hodgkin disease. *N Engl J Med.* 1981;304:1377.)

neutropenia as complications. Long-term follow-up toxicity studies are lacking.

Following therapy for HL, it has been suggested that pregnancy planning should take into consideration that about 80% of recurrences manifest within 2 years. Treatments for HL may compromise the reproductive potential of young patients.[13,37] As reflected in Figure 50-1, ovarian failure is more likely to occur in older patients even if treated with fewer courses of chemotherapy.[37] Early studies reported normal ovarian function in only 12% of women following therapy for HL, and combined treatment with radiation and chemotherapy have been found to lead to the highest risk of ovarian failure. **More recent series have shown the pregnancy rate among reproductive-age HL survivors to be similar to that of the normal female population.** Regimen changes that have occurred since the earlier reports include improved pelvic shielding during primary irradiation, ovarian transposition when pelvic radiation is required, and more frequent use of the ABVD regimen instead of MOPP. Depending on their availability, new reproductive technologies that include oocyte donation and embryo cryopreservation can be considered in select situations.

Patients who become pregnant after treatment for HL do not demonstrate increased adverse perinatal outcomes such as fetal wastage, preterm birth, and birth defects when compared with sibling controls.[32] Although fetal anomalies have occurred after treatment for HL, chromosomal abnormalities or a new gene mutation have not been diagnosed.[37] The absence of a repetitive pattern of malformations makes it difficult to imply a causal relationship between any birth defects observed and previous therapy for Hodgkin disease.

General recommendations, therefore, include delaying therapy until at least the second trimester due to the increased first-trimester fetal risk. After the first trimester, therapy should not be delayed for patients with symptomatic, subdiaphragmatic, or progressive HL. Treatment options include supradiaphragmatic radiation therapy for early-stage disease and combination chemotherapy for bulky, subdiaphragmatic, progressive, or advanced disease. Radiation fields should be tailored to limit fetal dose, and a maximal fetal dose calculation should be performed prior to treatment. Pregnant women with HL should be managed by a maternal-fetal medicine specialist, and

whether pregnancy termination should be pursued will depend on the clinical situation.

Non-Hodgkin Lymphoma

Non-Hodgkin lymphoma (NHL) occurs at a mean age of 42 years and is therefore observed less frequently than Hodgkin lymphoma with approximately 100 cases reported in pregnancy. **In general, NHL is more likely to complicate pregnancy because more patients have an aggressive histology and advanced-stage disease.** Indolent lymphomas are less common in younger patients and are rarely described in pregnancy. Up to 70% of NHL in pregnancy is diffuse large B-cell lymphoma.[38] Interestingly, reproductive organs—particularly the breasts and ovaries—are commonly involved in pregnancy-associated lymphoma compared with aged-matched counterparts.[32]

With the exception of aggressive histologic types, the management of lymphoma may be deferred in the first trimester because of the typical indolent nature of the disease. When initiated, treatment often includes chemotherapy and targeted therapy. If required, radiotherapy can be considered in local fields away from the pelvis in late gestational stages; however, it is typically postponed until after delivery.[32]

Treatment regimens evaluated in pregnancy include cyclophosphamide, doxorubicin, vincristine, and prednisone (CHOP) with or without bleomycin, which did not have an adverse effect on pregnancy outcomes.[36] Non-CHOP regimens were associated with several unfavorable outcomes that included miscarriage, intrauterine fetal demise, and transient neonatal leukopenia. The anti-CD20 antibody rituximab has been evaluated in limited cases with acceptable toxicities; however, further studies are warranted.[32]

Acute Leukemia

Although the incidence of leukemia in pregnancy is not specifically known, it is estimated to occur in fewer than 1 in 75,000 to 100,000 pregnancies.[17] **Acute leukemia represents about 90% of leukemias that coexist with pregnancy. Acute myeloid leukemia (AML) accounts for about 60% and acute lymphoblastic leukemia (ALL) for about 30% of cases. More than three fourths of the cases are diagnosed after the first trimester.**[32,39] **The prognosis for acute leukemia in pregnancy is guarded.**[39] Although no evidence suggests that pregnancy adversely affects the prognosis of acute leukemia, optimal and immediate care of the pregnant patient with acute leukemia necessitates a team effort and is best achieved in a cancer referral center.[40,41]

The diagnosis of acute leukemia is rarely difficult. The signs and symptoms of anemia, granulocytopenia, and thrombocytopenia include fatigue, fever, infection, and easy bleeding or petechiae, which usually prompts a complete blood count. A normal or elevated white blood cell count (WBC) is present in up to 90% of patients with ALL, although a WBC in excess of 50,000 is found in only one fourth of patients. In contrast, patients with acute nonlymphocytic leukemia (ANLL) may present with a markedly elevated WBC, although one third may exhibit leukopenia. The diagnosis of leukemia should be confirmed by bone marrow biopsy and aspirate. The biopsy material is usually hypercellular with leukemic cells. The smear of the aspirate reveals decreased erythrocyte and granulocytic precursors as well as megakaryocytes. Leukemic cells comprise greater than half of the marrow's cellular elements in most patients. The morphology of the marrow and the peripheral leukemic cells help to distinguish between lymphocytic and nonlymphocytic leukemias. This latter group includes acute myelocytic (granulocytic), promyelocytic, monocytic, and myelomonocytic leukemias and erythroleukemia. Acute myelocytic leukemia is the most common form of ANLL. Patients who develop ANLL as a result of previous chemotherapy have a particularly poor response to treatment.

Acute leukemia requires immediate treatment regardless of gestational age because delay may result in poorer maternal outcomes. When ALL is diagnosed in the first trimester, termination is recommended due to the effect on both the fetus and the mother. This is in part due to the need for intensive treatment that includes stem cell transplantation, which is contraindicated in gestation.[42] **However, numerous reports have documented successful pregnancies in patients with acute leukemia who were aggressively treated with leukapheresis and combination chemotherapy in the second and third trimesters.**[32] Although reports have shown no serious long-term effects of in utero exposure to chemotherapy, it is important to counsel patients that acute leukemia and its therapy are associated with a high rates of spontaneous abortion, stillbirth, preterm delivery, and fetal growth restriction.[40,42,43] **If the mother is exposed to cytotoxic drugs within 1 month of delivery, the newborn should be monitored closely for evidence of granulocytopenia or thrombocytopenia.**

Chronic Leukemia

Chronic leukemia accounts for approximately 10% of cases of leukemia during pregnancy. A majority of cases are chronic myelocytic leukemia (CML) because the median age is 35 years, compared with chronic lymphocytic leukemia (CLL), which has a median age of 60 years and makes cases during pregnancy rare.[40]

CML is characterized by excessive production of mature myeloid cell elements, with granulocyte counts that average 200,000/dL. Most patients have thrombocytosis and a mild normochromic normocytic anemia. Platelet function is often abnormal, although hemorrhage is usually limited to patients with marked thrombocytopenia. CML tends to be indolent, and normal hematopoiesis is only mildly affected in the early stages of disease. Therefore delay of aggressive treatment is more feasible than with acute leukemia. Unless complications such as severe systemic symptoms, autoimmune hemolytic anemia, recurrent infection, or symptomatic lymphatic enlargement occur, treatment for chronic leukemia should be withheld until after delivery. When necessary, therapy may consist of interferon-alfa, steroids, and chemotherapy agents or more recently, tyrosine kinase inhibitors such as imatinib. However, whereas the data are limited, **it does appear that early exposure to imatinib is associated with a high rate of congenital anomalies and miscarriage.**[44,45] Imatinib therapy initiated in the second and third trimesters may not add significant additional risk, but better outcome data are necessary before this can be ensured.[44]

Melanoma

The incidence of malignant melanoma is increasing in the childbearing years, with reported ranges from 1% to 3.3% in pregnant or lactating women; it accounts for 8% of malignancies diagnosed in gestation.[1,2,46] A topic of continued debate is whether pregnancy exerts a negative effect on the course of malignant melanoma. Prognostic features of the primary tumor include tumor thickness, ulceration, and location.[46,47] Reports

TABLE 50-3	STAGES I AND II STUDY OF MALIGNANT MELANOMA	
RELATIONSHIP TO TIME OF PREGNANCY	**NO. OF PATIENTS**	**MEAN TUMOR THICKNESS (mm)**
Before	85	1.29
During	92	2.38*
After all	143	1.96
Between	68	1.78

From MacKie RM, Bufalino R, Morabito A, et al. Lack of effect on pregnancy outcome of melanoma. *Lancet.* 1991;337:653.
*P = .004. When corrected for tumor thickness, survival rates were not different. Multivariate analysis identified tumor thickness as an independent prognostic variable, not pregnancy.

have suggested that melanoma that arises during pregnancy is associated with an aggressive clinical course; it is more likely to be diagnosed at an advanced stage, to have an increased tumor thickness, to be found in locations associated with a poor prognosis and therefore to have a shorter disease-free interval.[9,48-51] A meta-analysis of melanoma suggested that pregnancy-associated melanomas did appear to have poorer outcomes.[52] **However, after correcting for tumor thickness, survival rates were similar, and other studies show no increase in poor prognostic location of lesions in the pregnant patient and comparable survival outcomes to nonpregnant cohorts (Table 50-3).**[46,47] A large population-based study found no data to support the notion of advanced stage, thicker tumors, increased rate of lymph node metastases, or worsened survival in women with melanoma diagnosed during pregnancy when compared with nonpregnant women.[53] This series also noted that maternal and neonatal outcomes were equivalent to those of pregnant women without melanoma.[53]

Once the diagnosis is suspected, biopsy is recommended. **The methods used to describe the depth of invasion for melanoma are depicted in** Figure 50-2. **Wide surgical excision with appropriate margins remains the most effective modality for the treatment of melanoma.** Sentinel or complete lymph node dissection has been used successfully.[9] Because adjuvant chemotherapy has not demonstrated improved survival, it is not recommended for the pregnant patient because of the potential risk to the fetus. However, it may be appropriate to plan for early delivery to allow initiation of therapy.

Despite rare reports of regression after delivery, no studies support any benefit associated with therapeutic abortion.[51] Given the aggressive nature of the current therapies available for metastatic disease, it is appropriate to consider termination of pregnancy when managing advanced disease that presents in the first trimester.[51]

The patient who has undergone apparent successful treatment for a malignant melanoma may express concern about the safety of a future pregnancy. No adverse impact on recurrence or survival has been identified in most studies that have addressed this issue.[48] However, the timing of subsequent pregnancy deserves some consideration. The probability for survival of a specific cancer should be evaluated based on the known prognostic variables. The 5-year survival rate for the patient with a melanoma less than 1.5 mm thick is 90%. For a tumor of intermediate thickness (1.5 to 4 mm), the 5-year survival rate is 50% to 75%, and for a more deeply invasive tumor, survival is less than 50%. Some studies report that approximately 60% to 70% of patients develop their recurrence within 2 years, and 80% to 90% within 5 years.[51] Based on this information, **it is generally**

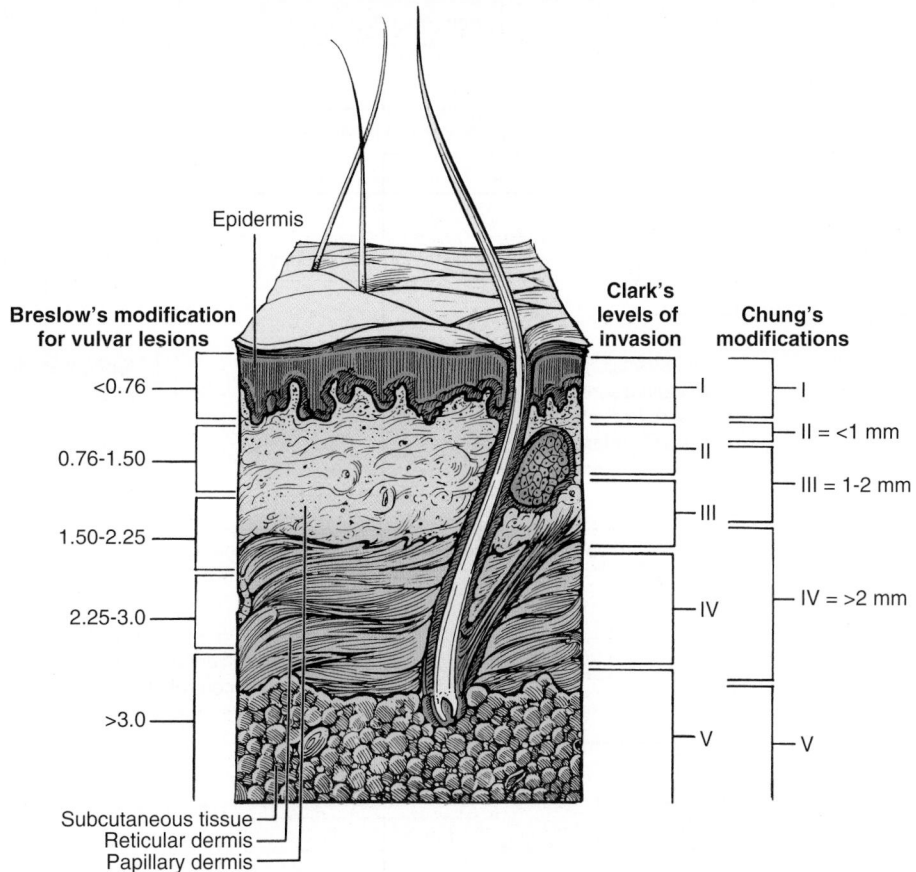

Epidermis

Breslow's modification
for vulvar lesions

Clark's
levels of
invasion

Chung's
modifications

<0.76 —— I —— I

0.76-1.50 —— II —— II = <1 mm

1.50-2.25 —— III —— III = 1-2 mm

2.25-3.0 —— IV —— IV = >2 mm

>3.0 —— V —— V

Subcutaneous tissue
Reticular dermis
Papillary dermis

FIG 50-2 Schematic comparison of the different levels of invasion for melanoma. (From Gordon AN. Vulvar tumors. In Copeland LJ [ed]: *Textbook of Gynecology,* ed 2. Philadelphia: WB Saunders; 2000:1202.)

recommended that patients wait 2 to 3 years before attempting another pregnancy, especially with nodal disease.[48]

Cervical Cancer

Cervical cancer is the most common gynecologic malignancy associated with pregnancy. It occurs in approximately 1 to 2 per 2000 to 10,000 pregnancies, and approximately 3% (1 in 34 cases) of all invasive cervical cancers occur during pregnancy.[1,2,17] Although it is the only cancer whose screening is part of the prenatal evaluation, the true incidence is difficult to ascertain because of the reporting biases associated with the reports that originate from large referral centers. Also, various reports may include patients who have preinvasive lesions as well as those diagnosed in the postpartum period.

The initial obstetric visit should include visualization of the cervix and cervical cytology, if indicated. If the cervix appears friable, cervical cytology alone may not be sufficient to alert the physician to the presence of a malignant tumor. **False-negative cervical cytology is at increased risk in pregnancy owing to excess mucus and bleeding from cervical eversion; therefore it is necessary to obtain a biopsy to ensure that tissue friability or a lesion is not secondary to tumor.** The most common symptoms for cervical cancer are vaginal bleeding or discharge, although approximately one third of pregnant patients with cervical cancer are asymptomatic at the time of diagnosis.

Cervical cytology suggestive of a squamous intraepithelial lesion or a report of atypical glandular cells during pregnancy requires appropriate clinical evaluation (Fig. 50-3). Colposcopy during pregnancy is usually enhanced by the physiologic eversion of the lower endocervical canal. However, vascular changes and redundant vagina may alter or obscure normal visualization and may make interpretation difficult, and referral to a gynecologic oncologist may be appropriate. During pregnancy, failure to visualize the entire transformation zone and squamocolumnar junction is uncommon. **Although endocervical curettage is not recommended during pregnancy, lesions that involve the lower endocervical canal can often be directly visualized and biopsied. Whereas the pregnant cervix is hypervascular, serious hemorrhage from an outpatient biopsy is uncommon, and the risk of bleeding is offset by the risk of missing an early invasive cancer.** Following a colposcopy evaluation with appropriate tissue sampling, most patients with preinvasive lesions can be followed with repeat colposcopy at 6- to 8-week intervals to delivery and postpartum.[17]

When necessary during pregnancy, cone biopsy should ideally be performed during the second trimester because of increased risks of abortion in the first trimester and rupture of membranes or premature labor in the third trimester.[54] Because complications from conization of the pregnant cervix are common, **therapeutic conization for intraepithelial squamous lesions is contraindicated during pregnancy. Diagnostic cone biopsy in pregnancy is reserved for patients whose colposcopic-directed biopsy has shown superficial invasion (suspected microinvasion) or in other situations in which an invasive lesion is suspected but cannot be confirmed by biopsy.** When a cone biopsy is necessary during pregnancy, the clinician should

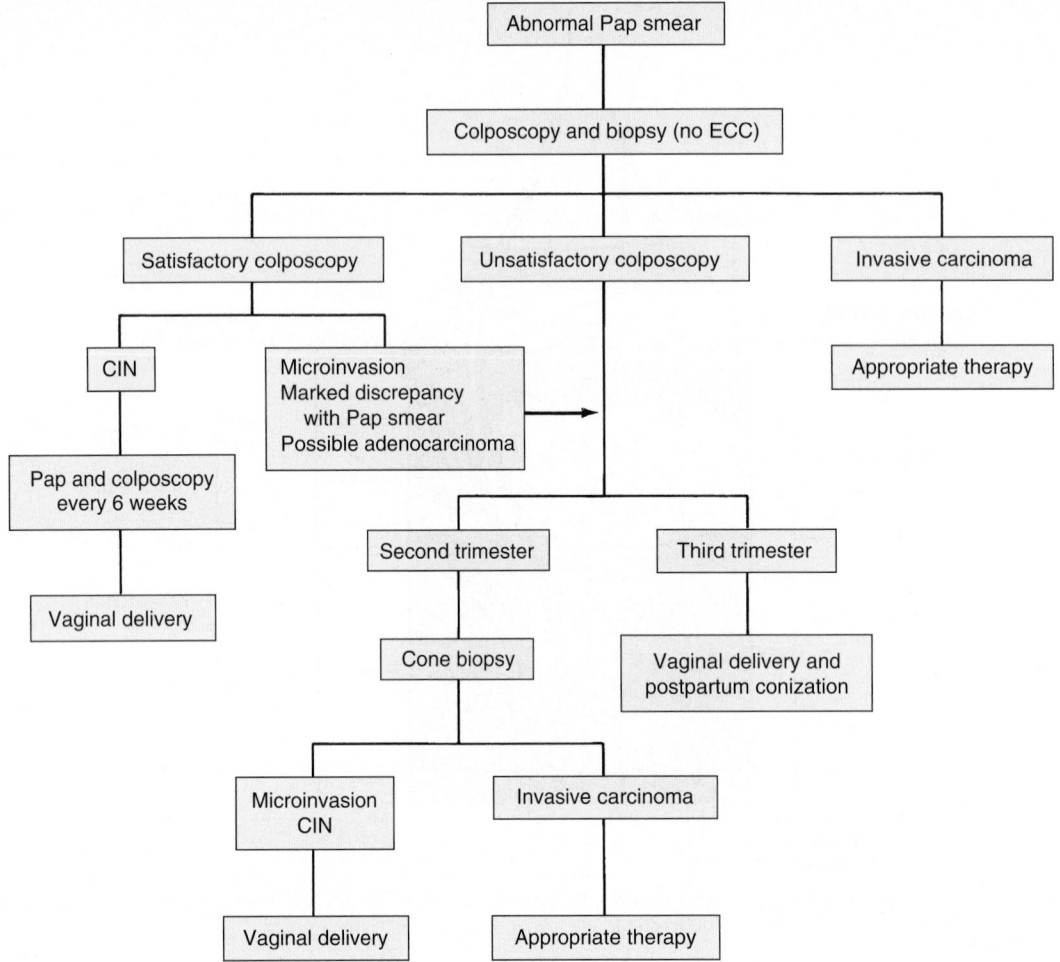

FIG 50-3 Suggested protocol for evaluation of abnormal cervical cytology in pregnancy. ECC, endocervical curettage; CIN, cervical intraepithelial neoplasia. (From Hacker NF, Berek JS, Lagasse LD, et al. Carcinoma of the cervix associated with pregnancy. *Obstet Gynecol*. 1982;59:735.)

keep in mind the anatomic alteration of the cervix secondary to pregnancy. A shallow disklike cone is usually satisfactory to clarify the diagnosis with a minimum of morbidity. Of importance, patients who have had a conization during pregnancy are at higher risk for residual disease, therefore close follow-up is essential.

Considering the routine practice of cervical evaluation in early pregnancy, a preponderance of early-stage disease diagnosed in the first trimester would be expected. Surprisingly, this is not the case, **and the diagnosis of cervical cancer is commonly made postpartum rather than during pregnancy. Furthermore, although stage IB disease is the most common stage found, all stages are represented in significant numbers.** Both patient and physician factors contribute to the delays in diagnosis, and these include lack of prenatal care, failure to obtain cervical cytology or biopsy of gross cervical abnormalities, false-negative cytology, and failure to evaluate abnormal cytology or vaginal bleeding properly.

Following the diagnosis of invasive cervical cancer, a staging evaluation is indicated. The standard cervical staging is clinical and is usually based on the results of physical examination and modification of routine testing, such as chest radiograph with abdominal shielding and sonography to detect hydronephrosis. If additional retroperitoneal imaging is desired for the evaluation

of lymphadenopathy, consideration should be given to using MRI because it does not involve ionizing radiation.

Microinvasion
In patients with a microinvasive squamous carcinoma with negative margins on cone biopsy, consideration can be given to conservative management until delivery. The risk of occult metastatic disease is predominantly dependent on two pathologic features: (1) the depth of invasion and (2) the presence or absence of lymph–vascular space involvement.[55] Whether the cone biopsy can be considered sufficient long-term therapy or whether a postpartum hysterectomy with or without lymphadenectomy should be performed is also based on the detailed analysis of the pathologic features of the cone biopsy. In these cases, consultation with a gynecologic oncologist is appropriate.

Invasive, Early-Stage Disease
Because the definitive treatment of invasive cervical cancer is not compatible with continuation of pregnancy, the clinical question that must be addressed is when to proceed with delivery so that therapy can be completed. Considering this requirement, treatment options will be influenced by gestational age, tumor stage and metastatic evaluation, and maternal desires and expectations regarding the pregnancy. The

management of early invasive cervical cancer (stages IA2, IB, and IIA) in the young patient usually includes radical hysterectomy, pelvic lymphadenectomy, and aortic lymph node sampling.[56] The primary advantage of this treatment approach over radiation therapy for these patients is preservation of ovarian function. For the woman with a high probability of having a poor prognostic lesion that would require postoperative irradiation, consideration can be given to performing a unilateral or bilateral oophoropexy at the time of the hysterectomy. The ovarian suspension should be intraperitoneal, because retroperitoneal placement seems to predispose to subsequent ovarian cyst formation. In the first trimester, this surgery is usually carried out with the fetus in utero. In the third trimester, the radical hysterectomy and lymphadenectomy are performed after completion of a high classical cesarean delivery. Delays in therapeutic intervention have not been reported to increase recurrence rates for patients with small-volume stage I disease.[56] Although the pelvic vessels are large, the dissection is enhanced by more easily defined tissue planes.[56]

Second-trimester presentations are more problematic. Studies have supported delay in management of early-stage disease until after fetal viability in women diagnosed after 20 weeks' gestation.[17,57] Other reports have suggested the administration of one to three cycles of platinum-based chemotherapy, allowing an additional 7 to 15 weeks of fetal maturation. This neoadjuvant approach, chemotherapy before either surgery or irradiation, has been reported in nine cases of cervical cancer diagnosed during pregnancy; three patients, all with advanced disease, ultimately died of disease, but all neonatal outcomes were normal.[57] In terms of general fetal salvage and outcome, the risk of extreme prematurity would far outweigh the risk of the chemotherapy exposure. Although this management of second-trimester cervical cancer presentations seems logical, little information is available about this treatment approach. In cases diagnosed remote from fetal maturity, between 20 and 30 weeks' gestation, assessment of nodal involvement should be considered and will dictate further recommendations for management.[57]

Invasive, Locally Advanced Disease

The management of the patient with more advanced local disease is based on treatment with chemotherapy and irradiation, both external beam to treat the regional nodes and shrink the central tumor and brachytherapy to complete the delivery of a tumoricidal dose to the cervix and adjacent tissues.[57] Coordinating a chemoradiation treatment plan for pregnant patients with stage IIB, stage III, and stage IVA disease is challenging. **The patient with a first-trimester pregnancy can usually be treated in the standard fashion with initiation of chemotherapy and external radiation therapy to the pelvis or an extended field, as dictated by standard treatment guidelines. Most of these patients proceed to abort spontaneously within 2 to 5 weeks of initiating the radiation.** Patients in the late first trimester are least likely to abort spontaneously, and it may be necessary to perform a uterine evacuation on the completion of external therapy in some patients. Following either spontaneous abortion or uterine evacuation, the brachytherapy component of the radiation therapy can proceed in the standard fashion. Second- or third-trimester patients should have a high classic cesarean delivery before starting standard chemotherapy and irradiation. Again, it would seem appropriate to strongly consider neoadjuvant chemotherapy for this group of patients, especially the patient with a second-trimester or early third-trimester

presentation, when the opportunity for further fetal maturation can be provided.

Invasive, Distant Metastasis

Metastatic disease to extrapelvic sites carries a poor prognosis. Although a select few patients with aortic node metastasis may receive curative therapy, it is unlikely for the patient with either pulmonary, bone, or supraclavicular lymph node metastases to be cured. Personal patient choices and ethical considerations are the major factors guiding treatment in these situations.

Small cell neuroendocrine tumors of the cervix associated with pregnancy are rare. Neoadjuvant or adjuvant chemotherapy may be used, and long-term survivors have been reported.[58] These tumors are considered to be histologically aggressive, and pregnancy preservation is not recommended. However, each case should be individualized.[47,48]

Method of Delivery

Controversy continues to surround the issue of the method of delivery for the term patient with cervical cancer. It seems unjustifiably risky to encourage vaginal delivery of a patient with a large, firm, barrel-shaped tumor or a large, friable, hemorrhagic exophytic tumor. However, many patients with small-volume stage IB, IIA, and early IIB tumors are potential candidates for vaginal delivery. **Whether vaginal delivery promotes systemic dissemination of tumor cells is unknown, although the general opinion is that survival rates are not influenced by the mode of delivery.**

Although systemic tumor dissemination secondary to vaginal delivery has not been documented, there are reports of episiotomy implants for both squamous carcinoma and adenocarcinoma following vaginal delivery.[59] Episiotomy implants are sufficiently rare that the risk should not be a determining factor for a given patient. However, **the episiotomy should be carefully followed in a cervical cancer patient who delivers vaginally.** Episiotomy nodules in these patients must be promptly evaluated by biopsy, because an early diagnosis may permit curative therapy.[59] Diagnostic delays secondary to suspicion of the nodules representing a stitch abscess should be avoided.

Survival

Although some authors have suggested that the survival of patients with cervical cancer associated with pregnancy is compromised, most reports indicate that the prognosis is not altered.[57]

Ovarian Cancer

Although adnexal masses are often observed in pregnancy, only 2% to 5% are malignant ovarian tumors.[60] **Ovarian cancer occurs in approximately 1 in 10,000 to 1 in 56,000 pregnancies.**[17,60] With the increased use of diagnostic ultrasound, ovarian cysts and neoplasms are more frequently encountered in early pregnancy.[60,61] Ultrasonic features associated with an increased risk of malignancy include the presence of excrescences/papillary structures, irregular borders, septations/complex appearance, and presence of ascites; any of these features should prompt further evaluation.[61]

Whereas the three major categories of ovarian tumors—epithelial, including borderline tumors; germ cell; and sex-cord stromal—occur during pregnancy, the majority are diagnosed in early stages and result in favorable outcomes.[60] Germ cell tumors account for 30% to 50%, followed by sex-cord

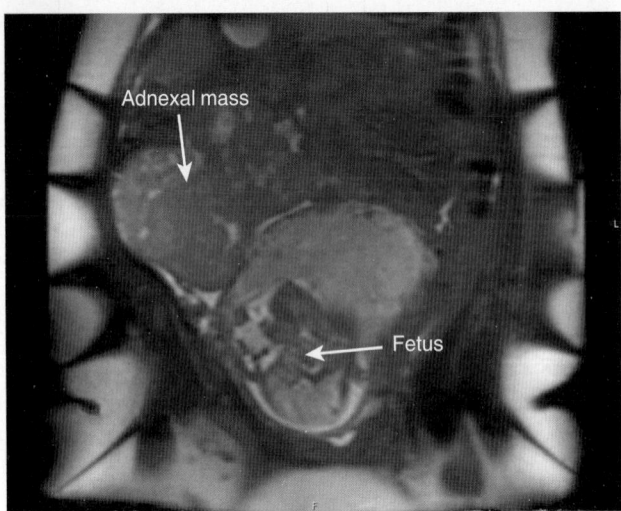

FIG 50-4 Magnetic resonance imaging of an ovarian malignancy diagnosed during pregnancy.

stromal tumors and epithelial tumors; the remainder are metastatic tumors to the ovary.[60] This distribution is undoubtedly skewed by the reporting bias associated with rare tumors. Of note, **the majority of epithelial ovarian tumors that complicate pregnancy are grade 1, or low malignant potential, or early stage; and not uncommonly, these tumors are both low grade and stage I.**

Management of the adnexal mass in pregnancy is controversial. The risks of surgical intervention may favor a conservative approach.[60,61] Serial sonograms may be of some value in determining the nature and biologic potential of the tumor. A number of opposing risks require consideration before following a conservative approach. The risk of greatest concern is that a delay of surgical intervention could permit a malignant ovarian tumor to spread, resulting in a decreased opportunity for cure. However, considering the rarity of advanced-stage poorly differentiated epithelial tumors in this age group, this risk is relatively small. Although ovarian tumors may be the cause of obstructed labor, this is uncommon.[61] **Skilled sonographic examination or MRI (Fig. 50-4) is essential to determining the potential for malignancy based on size and imaging characteristics.** Serial sonographic evaluations will also identify the rare tumor that remains in the pelvis as the gestation progresses. Because most ovarian masses relocate to the abdomen as the pregnancy advances, other explanations should be considered for persistent pelvic masses, including pelvic kidney, uterine fibroids, and colorectal or bladder tumors.

There does appear to be an increased probability that an adnexal mass during pregnancy will undergo torsion or rupture, and surgical intervention for these events is associated with higher fetal loss than with an elective procedure.[60] **Prompt surgical exploration is also performed for the mass associated with ascites or when metastatic disease is evident.** Because surgical exploration during pregnancy is associated with an increase in pregnancy loss and neonatal morbidity, it is ideal to delay surgical intervention until term or after delivery. However, if intervention is required during pregnancy, surgery should be performed after 16 weeks of gestation to reduce the risk of spontaneous abortion and allow the resolution of functional cysts.[60,61]

When a malignant ovarian tumor is encountered at laparotomy, surgical intervention should be similar to that for the nonpregnant patient. If the gestation is preterm, and the tumor appears confined to one ovary, consideration should be given to limiting the staging to removal of the involved ovary, cytologic washings, omentectomy, pelvic and paraaortic lymph node dissection, and a thorough manual exploration of the abdomen and pelvis.[62] The potential benefit of more extensive staging may be offset by higher pregnancy loss or neonatal morbidity. Before surgery, a comprehensive discussion with the patient should guide the extent of surgery if metastatic disease, especially a high-grade epithelial lesion, is encountered. Depending on the gestational age and the patient's desires, limited surgery followed by chemotherapy and additional extirpative surgery following delivery may be offered in select cases.[62]

Preoperative serum tumor markers are of limited value during pregnancy secondary to the physiologic increases in β-hCG, AFP, and CA 125. The mean CA 125 level increases slightly during the first trimester and then normalizes during the second trimester.[63] However, following diagnostic confirmation of a malignant ovarian tumor, the appropriate serum markers may be useful to monitor the course of the disease.

Virilizing ovarian tumors during pregnancy are most commonly secondary to theca-lutein cysts, and their evaluation and management should be conservative. These benign exaggerated physiologic "tumors" may redevelop with subsequent pregnancies.[60,61]

Postoperative Adjuvant Therapy

Postoperative adjuvant therapy should follow the treatment guidelines for the nonpregnant patient. Although it may be reasonable for patients with low-risk, low-stage tumors to have adjuvant therapy delayed until after delivery, **patients with advanced epithelial tumors should receive combination chemotherapy. The standard therapy is the combination of a platinum agent and paclitaxel, and tolerability of this regimen in pregnancy has been demonstrated.**[62] A number of favorable treatment outcomes has also been reported in pregnant patients who have malignant germ cell and sex cord stromal tumors, and consultation with a gynecologic oncologist is warranted.[64]

Vulvar and Vaginal Cancer

Because vulvar and vaginal cancers usually occur after age 40, the diagnosis of either disease concurrent with pregnancy is rare. Fewer than 30 cases of vulvar carcinoma diagnosed and treated during pregnancy have been reported.[62,65] Vulvar carcinoma in pregnancy is typically diagnosed in early stages. The diagnosis is based on biopsy, and neither pregnancy nor the young age of a patient should discourage the biopsy of a vulvar mass. Because verrucous squamous carcinoma tends to be misdiagnosed as condyloma, it is important to inform the pathologist of the clinical characteristics of unusually large or aggressive condyloma-like lesions. Surgical management is similar to that used in the nonpregnant patient, with the preference being to perform surgery in the second trimester to avoid the fetal risks of exposure to anesthesia in the first trimester and the maternal risks associated with operating on the hypervascular vulva in the third trimester. If vulvar carcinoma is diagnosed after 36 weeks' gestation, treatment is generally deferred until the postpartum period.[57,62] Vaginal delivery has been reported following surgical resection of vulvar cancers during pregnancy.[62]

Vaginal carcinoma is less common than vulvar carcinoma. The same limitations apply to vaginal cancer as apply to locally advanced cervical cancer in pregnancy. The cornerstone of treatment is irradiation therapy. Clear cell adenocarcinoma of the vagina has been reported in 16 pregnant patients, and 13 were long-term survivors.[66]

Endometrial Cancer

Approximately 35 cases of endometrial cancer associated with pregnancy have been reported in the literature, and only 30% of cases are associated with a viable fetus.[67] Although more than half of these cases were diagnosed in the first trimester, abnormal bleeding later in pregnancy or postpartum may be the presenting symptom of this tumor. Fortunately, a majority of cases of endometrial cancer in pregnancy are diagnosed with stage I disease (88%) and grade 1 tumors (80%). With extensive counseling and a thorough evaluation to exclude metastatic disease, these patients may be candidates for conservative treatment with hormonal manipulation, repeat endometrial evaluation, and modifications of risk factors to preserve fertility.[67]

Gastrointestinal Cancers
Upper Gastrointestinal Cancers

The diagnostic delay in detecting pregnancy-related upper GI cancers is often attributable to the frequency and duration of GI symptoms in pregnancy. In the United States, stomach cancer is rarely diagnosed in women during the reproductive years. During pregnancy, persistent severe upper GI symptoms are best evaluated by gastroduodenoscopy rather than radiologic studies.[17] Because curative resection of localized stomach cancer is possible in only approximately 30% of patients, it is imperative that treatment not be delayed.

Malignant hepatic tumors are rare during the reproductive years. Hepatocellular tumors detected during pregnancy should be resected, because the maternal and fetal mortality associated with subcapsular hemorrhage and liver rupture during pregnancy is high. In patients with unresectable hepatomas, therapeutic abortion can be considered to decrease the risk of subsequent rupture and bleeding.

Colon and Rectal Cancer

The incidence of colon cancer during pregnancy is about 1 in 13,000 liveborn deliveries.[68] Because pregnancy is often accompanied by constipation and exacerbations of hemorrhoids and anal fissures, the symptoms of colorectal carcinoma—namely, rectal bleeding, anemia, altered bowel movements, abdominal pain, and backache—tend to be attributed to the pregnancy, and diagnostic delay is common. **The majority of colorectal carcinomas during pregnancy are rectal and palpable on rectal examination, in contrast to more proximal lesions found in the nonpregnant patient.**[68] Patients with unexplained hypochromic microcytic anemia should be evaluated with stool guaiac testing. If a colorectal lesion is suspected, endoscopic methods of evaluation are preferred to radiologic imaging studies. Unfortunately, most cases of colorectal cancer are not diagnosed until late pregnancy or at the time of delivery. Delays in diagnosis are probably responsible for a higher likelihood of advanced-stage colorectal cancer in pregnancy and an associated poor prognosis.[68]

Management of colon cancer is determined by gestational age at diagnosis and tumor stage. During the first half of pregnancy, colon resection with anastomosis is indicated for colon or appendiceal cancers.[69] Abdominoperineal resection or low anterior resection has been accomplished up to 20 weeks' gestation without disturbing the gravid uterus. In some cases, access to the rectum may not be possible without a hysterectomy or uterine evacuation.

In late pregnancy, a diverting colostomy may be necessary to relieve a colonic obstruction and allow the development of fetal maturity before instituting definitive therapy. Some patients with a diagnosis after 20 weeks may opt to continue the pregnancy to fetal viability. Vaginal delivery is planned unless the tumor is obstructing the pelvis or is located on the anterior rectum. If cesarean delivery is performed, tumor resection can be accomplished immediately. Although reports are limited in regard to chemotherapy with oxaliplatin, 5-fluorouracil (FU), and leucovorin in pregnancy, neoadjuvant chemotherapy or radiation therapy for colorectal carcinoma in the pregnant patient has not demonstrated sufficient response to risk fetal exposure.[70]

Urinary Tract Cancers

Just over 100 cases of renal cell carcinoma have been reported during pregnancy.[71] Diagnosis is typically made by a combination of symptoms that include the presence of a palpable mass, flank pain, refractory urinary tract symptoms, or hematuria. Initial evaluation consists of ultrasound followed by MRI. Although each case should be individualized based on stage, symptoms, and risks to pregnancy, surgery is the mainstay of treatment. Cases of successful nephrectomy during pregnancy have been reported.

Bladder cancer during pregnancy is rare with fewer than 30 cases reported.[71,72] The most common symptoms are painless hematuria and abdominal pain. Diagnostic evaluation consists of urethrocystoscopy, urinary cytology, and renal ultrasonography, which can all be performed safely in pregnancy.[72] **Bladder cancer has even been diagnosed on routine obstetric ultrasound examination,** and it can be managed by local fulguration or resection if it is well differentiated and superficial. Less differentiated, deeply invasive, and recurrent tumors may require a partial or complete cystectomy. Treatment of urethral carcinoma varies with the size and location and may include surgical excision or interstitial brachytherapy implants.

CENTRAL NERVOUS SYSTEM TUMORS

The spectrum of CNS tumors found in pregnant patients is similar to those found in nonpregnant patients.[73] In pregnancy, 32% of brain tumors are gliomas, 29% are meningiomas, 15% are acoustic neuromas, and the other 24% are divided among other, more rare subtypes. Spinal tumors account for only one eighth of the CNS tumors and are most often vertebral hemangiomas (61%) and meningiomas (18%). Unfortunately, the presenting symptoms of headache, nausea, and vomiting are often attributed to normal complaints of pregnancy, which results in a delay of diagnosis. Meningiomas, pituitary adenomas (see Chapter 43), acoustic neuromas, and vertebral hemangiomas may demonstrate rapid enlargement during pregnancy. This may be secondary to fluid retention, increase in blood volume, or hormonal stimulation. MRI is the preferred imaging technique used to diagnose intracranial neoplasms.[73]

Whereas high-grade glial tumors should undergo prompt diagnosis and treatment, low-grade glial tumors such as astrocytomas and oligodendrogliomas do not usually require

immediate intervention. Adjuvant cranial radiotherapy with abdominal shielding should be considered for patients with high-grade tumors. Successful surgical removal of a variety of CNS tumors has been reported.[74,75] Corticosteroids are recommended to reduce the surrounding edema of intracranial masses. The role of adjuvant chemotherapy should be individualized.[73] Although rare, if a prolactin-secreting adenoma enlarges or is symptomatic, bromocriptine may be used with a favorable safety profile (see Chapter 43). Because painful contractions and pushing increase intracranial pressure, it is recommended that labor be as pain free as possible, and the second stage of labor should be assisted with forceps to reduce the risk of herniation.

NEONATAL OUTCOMES

In addition to maternal outcomes, the impact of cancer and its therapy on the fetus/neonate needs to be considered. Consultation with maternal-fetal medicine and a neonatology team as soon as possible is recommended.[17] In a series of 180 pregnancies affected by cancer, the mean gestational age at delivery was 36.2 (± 2.9) weeks' gestation.[6] Over 45% of all deliveries occurred before 37 weeks, and 8% occurred before 32 weeks. Induction was performed in 89.7% of the preterm deliveries for maternal cancer (88%) and obstetric indications (12%).[6]

Over 50% of the neonates were admitted to the neonatal intensive care unit (NICU) with prematurity as the most common indication.[6] Of note, neonates exposed to chemotherapy for ALL near the time of delivery may experience hematologic toxicity.[6,76] When assessing neonatal outcomes, the rates of major and minor malformations were comparable to those of the general population.[6,76]

FETAL-PLACENTAL METASTASIS

Metastatic spread of a maternal primary tumor to the placenta or fetus is rare, with approximately 100 cases reported. In general, the biologically aggressive spectrum of malignancies seem to carry the highest risk for fetal metastases. **Malignant melanoma is the most frequently reported tumor metastatic to the placenta, and it also has a high rate of fetal metastases.**[77,78] Other cancers that have been reported to metastasize to the products of conception include hematologic malignancies, breast cancer, lung cancer, sarcoma, and gynecologic cancers.[77] When the diagnosis of cancer in pregnancy is present, recommendations include a thorough macroscopic and microscopic evaluation of the placenta and cytologic examination of maternal and umbilical cord blood. Neonates should be examined every 6 months for 2 years with a physical examination, chest radiograph, and liver function tests.[77]

FERTILITY PRESERVATION

It is estimated that every year, approximately 55,000 cases of cancer will be diagnosed in Americans under the age of 35 years.[79] Because of better treatments, survival rates among young patients has improved, which highlights the need to address the impact of cancer and its treatment on fertility. **The risk of infertility may be a direct result of the disease, surgery, chemotherapy agents and dose, radiation, and age.**[79] Although based on limited studies and selection bias, the use of fertility preservation techniques in appropriately selected patients has

not been shown to have inferior oncologic outcomes when compared with standard therapy. Surgical options for fertility preservation include radical trachelectomy and ovarian transposition for cervical cancer and retention of the contralateral ovary and uterus in ovarian cancer. Additional options include the use of medical management for endometrial cancer and pelvic shielding for radiation therapy.

Infertility is associated with psychosocial distress, and options for fertility preservation should be addressed as soon as possible.

When treatment renders a high risk of resultant infertility, consultation with a reproductive specialist may be warranted. Options for fertility preservation vary depending on the age and potential impact of the treatment on fertility.[17] Embryo cryopreservation is the most established method, and in those women who do not have a partner, oocyte cryopreservation can be performed. However, these options require hormonal stimulation and a possible delay in cancer treatment. Although less well studied, other options include the use of oocyte collection and ovarian tissue cryopreservation.[79,80] Once thought to be beneficial, the use of gonadotropin-releasing hormone (GnRH) agonists in women receiving chemotherapy for breast cancer was not associated with a higher rate of ovarian function preservation.[81] When fertility cannot be preserved, patients should be advised on options such as gestational surrogacy and adoption.

Cancer survivors should be counseled on contraception options to reduce the risk of unintended pregnancy. Selection of contraception is based on status and type of malignancy and compliance. Additionally, hormonal contraception may be contraindicated because of a negative impact on cancer outcomes (e.g., breast cancer) or an increase in the risk of adverse side effects, such as thrombosis.[17]

GESTATIONAL TROPHOBLASTIC DISEASE AND PREGNANCY-RELATED ISSUES

It is uncommon for a normal viable pregnancy to be complicated by gestational trophoblastic disease (GTD). A comprehensive summary of the evaluation and management of the complete spectrum of GTD is beyond the scope of this chapter. However, the aspects of GTD related to general obstetric and postpartum care are reviewed.

Hydatidiform Mole (Complete Mole)

The incidence of hydatidiform mole has great geographic variability. In the United States, it occurs in approximately 1 in 1000 to 1 in 1500 pregnancies. The two clinical risk factors that carry the highest risk of a molar pregnancy are (1) the extremes of the reproductive years (age 50 or older is associated with a relative risk of over 500) and (2) the history of a prior hydatidiform mole (the risk for development of a second molar pregnancy is 1% to 2%, and the risk of a third after two is approximately 25%).[82,83] Patients with these risk factors should have an ultrasound evaluation of uterine contents in the first trimester. Although historically, approximately 50% of patients were not diagnosed with a molar pregnancy before vaginal expulsion of molar tissue, currently, in developed countries, most patients are diagnosed either by ultrasound while asymptomatic or by ultrasound for the evaluation of vaginal spotting or cramping symptoms. Approximately 95% of complete hydatidiform moles have a 46,XX paternal homologous chromosomal pattern.

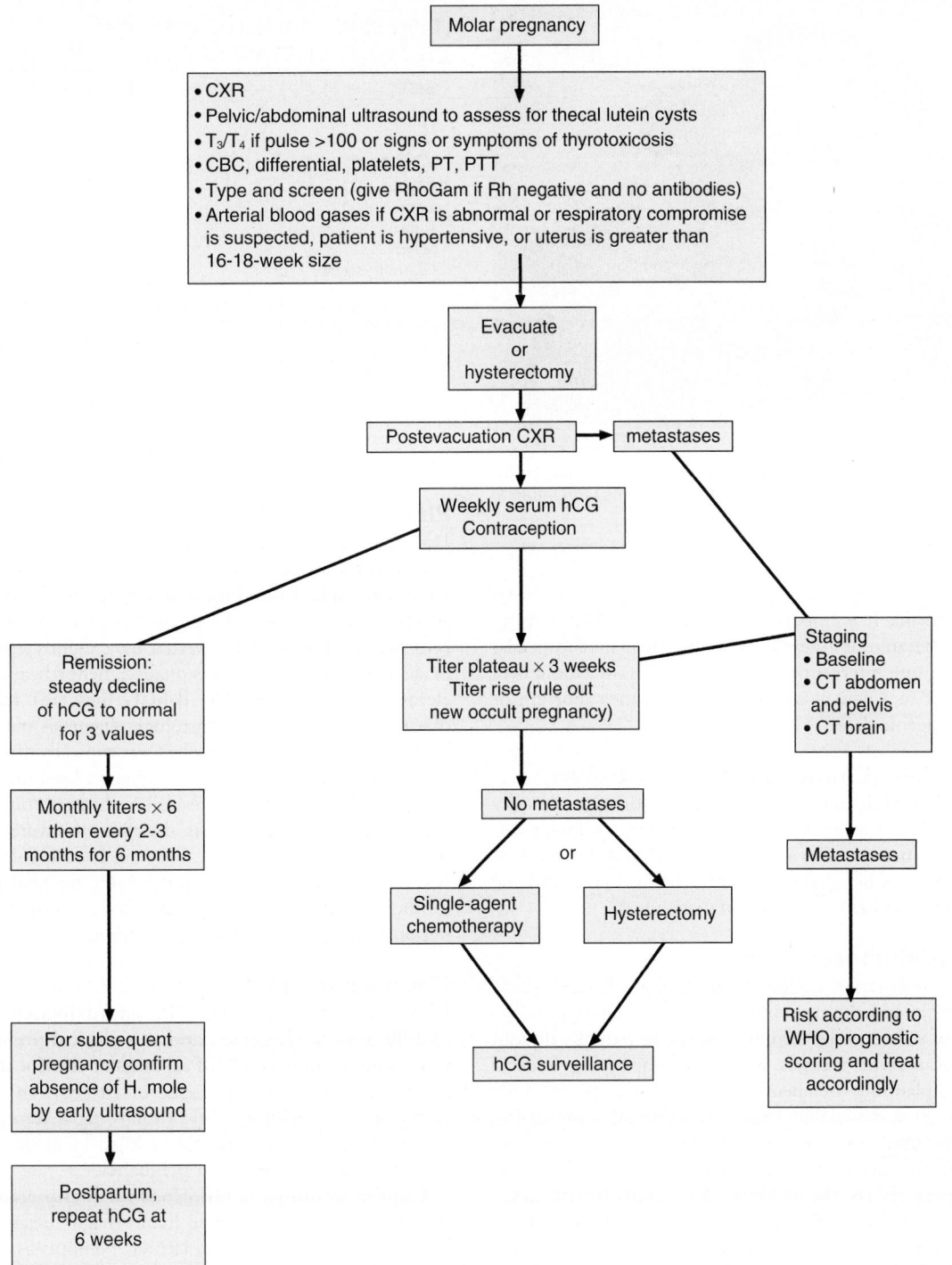

FIG 50-5 Algorithm for the management of molar pregnancy. CBC, complete blood count; CT, computed tomography; CXR, chest x-ray; hCG, human chorionic gonadotropin; H. mole, hydatidiform mole; PT, prothrombin time; PTT, partial thromboplastin time; WHO, World Health Organization. (From Finfer SR: Management of labor and delivery in patients with intracranial neoplasms. *Br J Anaesth* 1991;67:784.)

The safest technique for evacuating a hydatidiform mole is with the suction aspiration technique. Oxytocin should not be initiated until the patient is in the operating room and evacuation is imminent in order to minimize the risk of embolization of trophoblastic tissue. The alternative management for the older patient who requests concurrent sterilization is hysterectomy. Following either evacuation or hysterectomy, weekly β-hCG levels are drawn until the hCG titer is within

normal limits for 3 weeks. The titers are then observed at monthly intervals for 6 to 12 months. Figure 50-5 illustrates an algorithm for molar pregnancy management.

For the patient with a complete molar pregnancy, the risk of requiring chemotherapy for persistent GTD is approximately 20%. Clinical features that increase this risk include delayed hemorrhage, excessive uterine enlargement, theca-lutein cysts, serum hCG greater than 100,000 mIU/mL, and maternal

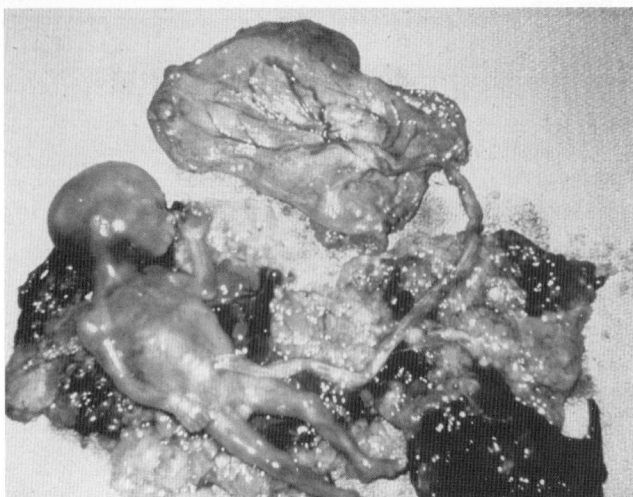

FIG 50-6 Partial mole with dead fetus of abnormal karyotype. (From Finfer SR. Management of labor and delivery in patients with intracranial neoplasms. *Br J Anaesth.* 1991;67:784.)

TABLE 50-4	COMMON SITES FOR METASTATIC CHORIOCARCINOMA	
SITE	**PERCENT**	
Lung	60-95	
Vagina	40-50	
Vulva/cervix	10-15	
Brain	5-15	
Liver	5-15	
Kidney	0-5	
Spleen	0-5	
Gastrointestinal	0-5	

From Finfer SR. Management of labor and delivery in patients with intracranial neoplasms. *Br J Anaesth.* 1991;67:784.
Frequencies vary depending on whether data are based on autopsy studies or obtained from pretreatment imaging.

age older than 40. It is important not to misinterpret a rising β-hCG level because of a new intervening pregnancy as persistent GTD because intervention with chemotherapy would be a significant risk to a new gestation, inducing either abortion or possible teratogenic defects.

Invasive Mole (Chorioadenoma Destruens)
Because invasion of the myometrium by molar tissue is clinically occult, it is difficult to assess the true incidence, although it is estimated to be between 5% and 10%. The clinical hallmark of an invasive mole is hemorrhage, which can be severe, and the bleeding may be either vaginal or intraperitoneal.

Partial Hydatidiform Mole
Most partial moles have a triploid (paternally inherited, diandric) karyotype, and the next most common are tetraploidies. A minority of partial moles exhibit a mosaic or partially diploid karyotype. Karyotype analysis of the accompanying fetus is important in planning therapeutic intervention. A partial mole associated with a nonviable fetal chromosomal abnormality requires either mechanical or medically induced uterine evacuation (Fig. 50-6).[84] In the presence of an abundance of hydropic tissue, there is always the concern that trophoblastic tissue embolization may occur during uterine contractions induced to evacuate molar tissue. **The management of a patient with sonographic findings suggestive of a diagnosis of a partial mole is particularly challenging if the karyotype analysis of the fetus is diploid, especially if the diagnosis is made in the second or third trimester.** When a normal karyotype exists, it is appropriate to consider diagnostic possibilities other than partial mole, such as a twin gestation—one normal developing fetus and one molar pregnancy. Also, degenerative changes (hydropic villi), retroplacental hematomas, placental abnormalities (chorioangiomas), degenerative uterine myomas, and aborted tissue—sometimes referred to as a "transitional mole"—may lead to imaging abnormalities that are difficult to interpret.

Approximately 2% to 6% of patients develop persistent GTD after a partial molar pregnancy.[85] Therefore because choriocarcinoma can follow a true partial mole, these patients require the same postevacuation surveillance and management as the patient with a complete mole, with a follow-up of at least 6 months.[86]

Placental Site Trophoblastic Tumor
Less than 1% of all patients with GTD have placental site trophoblastic tumor. Although this tumor usually presents with abnormal vaginal bleeding following a term pregnancy, it can also be a sequela to a molar pregnancy or abortion. The postpartum presentation is characterized by a slightly enlarged uterus; persistent bleeding, or occasionally amenorrhea; and a slightly elevated β-hCG level. **The β-hCG may not reliably reflect disease progression.** The histologic diagnosis may be obtained by uterine curettage, possibly hysteroscopically directed. Because this disease tends to metastasize late and be somewhat resistant to chemotherapy, surgical excision (hysterectomy) should be considered. If the patient is desirous of future childbearing, management considerations that have been reported with some success include systemic chemotherapy, regional infusion chemotherapy, uterine curettage, and local excision of tumor by hysterotomy and uterine reconstruction.[87]

Choriocarcinoma
Choriocarcinoma develops in approximately 1 in every 40,000 term pregnancies, and this clinical presentation represents about one fourth of all cases of choriocarcinoma. The other cases follow molar disease or an abortion (spontaneous, therapeutic, or ectopic). GTD following a term pregnancy is always either choriocarcinoma or a placental site trophoblastic tumor, assuming a singleton pregnancy.

Choriocarcinoma is notorious for masquerading as other diseases. This is secondary to hemorrhagic metastases that produce symptoms such as hematuria, hemoptysis, hematemesis, hematochezia, stroke, or vaginal bleeding. The common sites for metastatic disease are listed in Table 50-4. The diagnosis of choriocarcinoma is based on history, imaging studies, and a serum β-hCG level. Histologic confirmation is neither necessary for the diagnosis nor as a prerequisite to initiate therapy. Again, it is essential to exclude the presence of a new gestation as the source of a rising β-hCG level before extensive diagnostic imaging or therapeutic intervention. **It is also important to rule out phantom β-hCG production if the clinical scenario warrants, such as situations with low titers and no histologic or convincing imaging evidence of GTD.**

The complexities of the general treatment approach or treatment for special situations is beyond the scope of this chapter. It is recommended that the reader refer to a gynecology or gynecologic oncology resource for discussions of the therapeutic subtleties and pitfalls. Choriocarcinoma should be managed by a gynecologic oncologist, preferably one with a special interest in the disease.

KEY POINTS

- Because many of the common complaints of pregnancy are also early symptoms of metastatic cancer, pregnant women with cancer are at risk for delays in diagnosis and therapeutic intervention.

- The safest time for most cancer therapies in pregnancy is in the second and third trimesters, thereby avoiding induction of teratogenic risks or miscarriage in the first trimester. For most malignancies diagnosed during the second trimester, chemotherapy should be undertaken as indicated because fetal risk is generally lower than the risk of delaying treatment or proceeding with preterm delivery.

- Antimetabolites and alkylating agents present the greatest hazard to the developing fetus.

- Diagnostic delays for breast cancer in pregnancy are often attributed to physician reluctance to properly evaluate breast complaints or abnormal findings in pregnancy.

- Treatment for Hodgkin disease may compromise the reproductive potential, and combined treatment with irradiation and chemotherapy are associated with the highest risk of ovarian failure.

- If a mother is exposed to cytotoxic drugs within 1 month of delivery, the newborn should be monitored closely for evidence of granulocytopenia or thrombocytopenia.

- The effect of pregnancy on the clinical course of melanoma has been the subject of debate. When corrected for tumor thickness, pregnancy does not appear to be an independent prognostic variable for survival.

- After stratifying for stage and age, patients with pregnancy-associated cervical carcinoma have survival rates similar to those of the nonpregnant patient.

- Because most malignant ovarian tumors found in pregnancy are either germ cell tumors or low-grade, early-stage epithelial tumors, the therapeutic plan will usually permit continuation of the pregnancy and preservation of fertility.

- Although rare, most colorectal carcinomas in pregnancy are detectable on rectal examination, underscoring the need for a rectal examination at the patient's first prenatal visit.

- Phantom β-hCG should be ruled out in patients suspected of having gestational trophoblastic disease when not documented by other clear clinical evidence (histology, imaging, and clinical history), especially when β-hCG titers are low.

REFERENCES

1. Pentheroudakis G, Orecchia R, Hoekstra HJ, Pavlidis N. Cancer, fertility and pregnancy: ESMO clinical practice guidelines for diagnosis, treatment and follow-up. *Ann Oncol.* 2010;21:V226.
2. Pavlidis NA. Coexistence of pregnancy and malignancy. *Oncologist.* 2002;7:279.
3. Andersson TM, Johansson AL, Fredriksson I, Lambe M. Cancer during pregnancy and the postpartum period: a population based study. *Cancer.* 2015.
4. Amant F, Han SN, Gziri MM, Dekrem J, Van Calsteren K. Chemotherapy during pregnancy. *Curr Opin Oncol.* 2012;24:580-586.
5. Briggs GG, Freeman RK, Yaffe SJ. *Drugs in Pregnancy and Lactation: A Reference Guide to Fetal and Neonatal Risk.* 8th ed. Philadelphia: Lippincott, Williams & Wilkins; 2008.
6. Van Calsteren K, Hyens L, De Smet F, et al. Cancer during pregnancy: an analysis of 215 patients emphasizing the obstetrical and the neonatal outcomes. *J Clin Oncol.* 2009;28:683.
7. Zemlickis D, Lishner M, Degendorfer P, et al. Fetal outcome after in utero exposure to cancer chemotherapy. *Arch Intern Med.* 1992;152:573.
8. Cardonick E, Iacobucci A. Use of chemotherapy during human pregnancy. *Lancet Oncol.* 2004;5:283.
9. Weisz B, Meirow D, Schiff E, Lishner M. Impact and treatment of cancer during pregnancy. *Exper Rev Anticancer Ther.* 2004;4:889.
10. Schardein JL. Cancer chemotherapeutic agents. In: Schardein JL, ed. *Chemically Induced Birth Defects.* 2nd ed. New York: Marcel Dekker; 1993.
11. Amant F, Han SN, Gziri MM, Vandenbroucke T, Verheecke M, Van Calsteren K. Management of cancer in pregnancy. *Best Pract Res Clin Obstet Gynaecol.* 2015;29:741.
12. Mazze RI, Kallen B. Reproductive outcome after anesthesia and operation during pregnancy: a registry study of 5405 cases. *Am J Obstet Gynecol.* 1989;161:1178.
13. Clark ST, Radford JA, Crowther D, et al. Gonadal function following chemotherapy for Hodgkin disease: a comparative study of MVPP and a seven-drug hybrid regimen. *J Clin Oncol.* 1995;13:134.
14. Plante M, Renaud MC, François H, Roy M. Vaginal radical trachelectomy: an oncologically safe fertility-preserving surgery. An updated series of 72 cases and review of the literature. *Gynecol Oncol.* 2004;94:614.
15. Siegel RL, Miller KD, Jemal A. Cancer statistics, 2015. *Cancer.* 2015; 65(1):5-29.
16. Ring A. Breast cancer and pregnancy. *Breast.* 2007;16:S155.
17. Salani R, Billingsley CC, Crafton SM. Cancer and pregnancy: an overview for obstetricians and gynecologists. *Am J Obstet Gynecol.* 2014;211(1): 7-14.
18. Amant F, Loibl S, Neven P, Van Calsteren K. Breast cancer in pregnancy. *Lancet.* 2012;379:570-579.
19. Michels KB, Willett WC, Rosner BA, et al. Prospective assessment of breastfeeding and breast cancer incidence among 89,877 women. *Lancet.* 1996;347:431.
20. Jernstrom H, Lerman C, Ghadirian P, et al. Pregnancy and risk of early breast cancer in carriers of BRCA1 and BRCA2. *Lancet.* 1999;354:1846.
21. Amant F, Deckers S, Van Calsteren K, et al. Breast cancer in pregnancy: recommendations of an international consensus meeting. *Eur J Cancer.* 2010;4:3158.
22. Zagouri F, Psaltopoulou T, Dimitrakakis C, Bartsch R, Dimopoulos MA. Challenges in managing breast cancer during pregnancy. *J Thorac Dis.* 2013;5(suppl 1):S62-S67.
23. Gentilini O, Cremonesi M, Trifiro G, et al. Safety of sentinel node biopsy in pregnant patients with breast cancer. *Ann Oncol.* 2004;15:1348.
24. Botsis D, Sarandakou A, Kassanos D, et al. Breast cancer markers during normal pregnancy. *Anticancer Res.* 1999;19:3539.
25. Cardonick E, Dougherty R, Grana G, Gilmandyar D, Ghaffar S, Usmani A. Breast cancer during pregnancy: Maternal and fetal outcomes. *Cancer J.* 2010;16:76-82.
26. King RM, Welch JS, Martin JK Jr, Coul CB. Carcinoma of the breast associated with pregnancy. *Surg Gynecol Obstet.* 1985;160:228.
27. Amant F, von Minckwitz G, Han SN, et al. Prognosis of women with primary breast cancer diagnosed during pregnancy: results from an international collaborative study. *J Clin Oncol.* 2013;31:2532-2539.
28. Loibl S, Han SN, Minckwitz GV, et al. Treatment of breast cancer during pregnancy: an observation study. *Lancet Oncol.* 2012;13:887-896.
29. Blakely LJ, Buzdar AU, Lozada JA, et al. Effects of pregnancy after treatment for breast carcinoma on survival and risk of recurrence. *Cancer.* 2004;100:465.
30. Higgins S, Haffty B. Pregnancy and lactation after breast-conserving therapy for early-stage breast cancer. *Cancer.* 1994;73:2175.
31. Miller MJ, Ross ME. Case report: pregnancy following breast reconstruction with autologous tissue. *Cancer Bull.* 1993;45:546.
32. Brenner B, Avivi I, Lishner M. Haematological cancers in pregnancy. *Lancet.* 2012;379:580-587.

33. Gelb AB, van de Rijn M, Warnke RA. Pregnancy-associated lymphomas. A clinicopathologic study. *Cancer.* 1996;78:304.

34. Jacobs C, Donaldson SS, Rosenberg SA, Kaplan HS. Management of the pregnant patient with Hodgkin's disease. *Ann Intern Med.* 1981;95:649.

35. Friedman E, Jones GW. Fetal outcome after maternal radiation treatment of supradiaphragmatic Hodgkin's disease. *Can Med Assoc J.* 1993;149:1281.

36. Azim HA, Pavlidis N, Peccatori FA. Treatment of the pregnant mother with cancer: a systematic review on the use of cytotoxic, endocrine, targeted agents and immunotherapy during pregnancy. Part II: Hematological tumors. *Cancer Treat Rev.* 2010;36:110.

37. Dein RA, Mennuti MT, Kovach P, Gabbe SG. The reproductive potential of young men and women with Hodgkin's disease. *Obstet Gynecol Surv.* 1984;39:474.

38. Aviles A, Neri N. Hematological malignancies and pregnancy: a final report of 84 children who received chemotherapy in utero. *Clin Lymphoma.* 2001;2:173.

39. Caligiuri MA, Mayer RJ. Pregnancy and leukemia. *Semin Oncol.* 1989; 16:338.

40. Antonelli NM, Dotters DJ, Katz VL, Kuller JA. Cancer in pregnancy: a review of the literature. Part II. *Obstet Gynecol Surv.* 1996;51:135.

41. Chang A, Patel S. Treatment of acute myeloid leukemia during pregnancy. *Ann Pharmacother.* 2014;49(1):48-68.

42. Avivi I, Brenner B. Management of acute myeloid leukemia during pregnancy. *Future Oncol.* 2014;10(8):1407-1415.

43. Aviles A, Niz J. Long-term follow-up of children born to mothers with acute leukemia during pregnancy. *Med Pediatr Oncol.* 1988;16:3.

44. Pye SM, Cortes J, Ault P, et al. The effects of imatinib on pregnancy outcome. *Blood.* 2008;111:5505.

45. Bhandari A, Rolen K, Sha BK. Management of chronic myelogenous leukemia in pregnancy. *Anticancer Res.* 2015;35:1-12.

46. Stensheim H, Møller B, van Dijk T, et al. Cause-specific survival for women diagnosed with cancer during pregnancy or lactation: a registry-based cohort study. *J Clin Oncol.* 2009;27:45.

47. Houghton AN, Flannery J, Viola MV. Malignant melanoma of the skin occurring during pregnancy. *Cancer.* 1981;48:407.

48. MacKie RM, Bufalino R, Morabito A, et al. Lack of effect on pregnancy outcome of melanoma. *Lancet.* 1991;337:653.

49. Slingluff CL Jr, Reintgen D, Vollmer RT, et al. Malignant melanoma arising during pregnancy: a study of 100 patients. *Ann Surg.* 1990;211:552-557.

50. Travers R, Sober A, Barnhill R, et al. Increased thickness of pregnancy-associated melanoma: a study of the MGH pigmented lesion clinic. *Melanoma Res.* 1993;3:44.

51. Ross MI. Melanoma and pregnancy: prognostic and therapeutic considerations. *Cancer Bull.* 1994;46:412.

52. Byrom L, Olsen C, Knight L, Khosrotehrani K, Green AC. Increased mortality for pregnancy-associated melanoma: systematic review and meta-analysis. *J Eur Acad Dermatol Venereol.* 2015;29:1457.

53. O'Meara AT, Cress R, Xing G, Danielsen B, Smith LH. Malignant melanoma in pregnancy: a population based evaluation. *Cancer.* 2005;103:1217-1226.

54. Hannigan EV. Cervical cancer in pregnancy. *Clin Obstet Gynecol.* 1990;33:837.

55. Copeland LJ, Silva EG, Gershenson DM, et al. Superficially invasive squamous cell carcinoma of the cervix. *Gynecol Oncol.* 1992;45:307.

56. Sood AK, Sorosky JI, Krogman S, et al. Surgical management of cervical cancer complicating pregnancy: a case-control study. *Gynecol Oncol.* 1996;63:294.

57. Amant F, Van Calsteren K, Halaska M, et al. Gynecologic cancers in pregnancy: guidelines of an international consensus meeting. *Int J Gynecol Cancer.* 2009;19:S1.

58. Balderston KD, Tewari K, Gregory WT, et al. Neuroendocrine small cell cervix cancer in pregnancy: long-term survivor following combined therapy. *Gynecol Oncol.* 1998;71:128.

59. Cliby WA, Dodson WA, Podratz KC. Cervical cancer complicated by pregnancy: episiotomy site recurrences following vaginal delivery. *Obstet Gynecol.* 1994;84:179.

60. Leiserowitz GS, Xing G, Cress R, et al. Adnexal masses in pregnancy: how often are they malignant? *Gynecol Oncol.* 2006;101:315.

61. Schwartz N, Timor-Tritsch IE, Wang E. Adnexal masses in pregnancy. *Clin Obstet and Gynecol.* 2009;52:570.

62. Latimer J. Gynaecological malignancies in pregnancy. *Curr Opin Obstet Gynecol.* 2007;19:140.

63. Kobayashi F, Sagawa N, Nakamura K, et al. Mechanism and clinical significance of elevated CA 125 levels in the sera of pregnant women. *Am J Obstet Gynecol.* 1989;160:563.

64. Young RH, Dudley AG, Scully RE. Granulosa cell, Sertoli-Leydig cell and unclassified sex-cord stromal tumors associated with pregnancy: a clinical pathological analysis of 36 cases. *Gynecol Oncol.* 1984;18:181.

65. Bakour SH, Jaleel H, Weaver JB, et al. Vulvar carcinoma presenting during pregnancy, associated with recurrent bone marrow hypoplasia: a case report and literature review. *Gynecol Oncol.* 2002;87:207.

66. Senekjian EK, Hubby M, Bell DA, et al. Clear cell adenocarcinoma of the vagina and cervix in association with pregnancy. *Gynecol Oncol.* 1986;24:207.

67. Yael HK, Lorenza P, Evelina S, et al. Incidental endometrial adenocarcinoma in early pregnancy: a case report and review of the literature. *Int J Gynecol Cancer.* 2009;19:1580.

68. Woods JB, Martin JN Jr, Ingram FH, et al. Pregnancy complicated by carcinoma of the colon above the rectum. *Am J Perinatol.* 1992;9:102.

69. Nesbitt JC, Moise KJ, Sawyers JL. Colorectal carcinoma in pregnancy. *Arch Surg.* 1985;120:636.

70. Gensheimer M, Jones CA, Graves CR, et al. Administration of oxaliplatin to pregnant patients with rectal cancer. *Cancer Chemother Pharmacol.* 2009;63:371.

71. Boussios S, Pavlidis N. Renal cell carcinoma in pregnancy: a rare coexistence. *Clin Transl Oncol.* 2014;16:122-127.

72. Yeaton-Massey A, Brookfield KF, Aziz N, Mrazek-Pugh B, Chueh J. Maternal bladder cancer diagnosed at routine first-trimester obstetric ultrasound examination. *Obstet Gynecol.* 2013;122:464-466.

73. Verheecke M, Halaska M, Lok CA, et al. Primary brain tumours, meningiomas and brain metastases in pregnancy: report on 27 cases and review of literature. *Eur J Cancer.* 2014;59:1462-1471.

74. Finfer SR. Management of labor and delivery in patients with intracranial neoplasms. *Br J Anaesth.* 1991;67:784.

75. Blumenthal DT, Parreno MG, Batten J, et al. Management of malignant gliomas during pregnancy: a case series. *Cancer.* 2008;113:3349.

76. Backes CH, Moorehead PA, Nelin LD. Cancer in pregnancy: fetal and neonatal outcomes. *Clin Obstet Gynecol.* 2011;54(4):574-590.

77. Pavlidis N, Pentheroudakis G. Metastatic involvement of placenta and foetus in pregnant women with cancer. *Recent Results Cancer Res.* 2008;178:183-194.

78. Alexander A, Samlowski WE, Grossman D, et al. Metastatic melanoma in pregnancy: risk of transplacental metastases in the infant. *J Clin Oncol.* 2003;21:2179-2186.

79. Lee SJ, Schover LR, Partridge AH, et al. American Society of Clinical Oncology recommendations on fertility preservation in cancer patients. *J Clin Oncol.* 2006;24:2917-2931.

80. Jeruss JS, Woodruff TK. Preservation of fertility in patients with cancer. *N Engl J Med.* 2009;360:902-911.

81. Munster PN, Moore AP, Ismail-Khan R, et al. Randomized trial using gonadotropin-releasing hormone agonist triptorelin for the preservation of ovarian function during (neo)adjuvant chemotherapy for breast cancer. *J Clin Oncol.* 2012;30(5):533-538.

82. Bandy LC, Clarke-Pearson DL, Hammond CB. Malignant potential of gestational trophoblastic disease at the extreme ages of reproductive life. *Obstet Gynecol.* 1984;64:395.

83. Berkowitz RS, Goldstein DP, Bernstein MR, Sablinska B. Subsequent pregnancy outcomes in patients with molar pregnancies and gestational trophoblastic tumors. *J Reprod Med.* 1987;32:680.

84. Copeland LJ. Gestational trophoblastic neoplasia. In: Copeland LJ, ed. *Textbook of Gynecology.* 2nd ed. Philadelphia: WB Saunders; 2000:1414.

85. Rice LW, Berkowitz RS, Lage JM, Goldstein DP. Persistent gestational trophoblastic tumor after partial molar pregnancy. *Gynecol Oncol.* 1993;48:165.

86. Seckl MH, Fisher RA, Salerno G, et al. Choriocarcinoma and partial hydatidiform moles. *Lancet.* 2000;356:36.

87. Leiserowitz GS, Webb MJ. Treatment of placental site trophoblastic tumor with hysterotomy and uterine reconstruction. *Obstet Gynecol.* 1996;88:696.

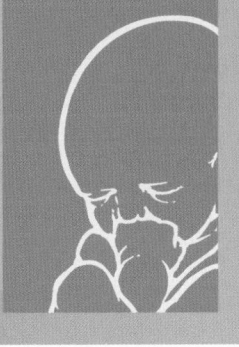

CHAPTER 51

Skin Disease and Pregnancy

ANNIE R. WANG and GEORGE KROUMPOUZOS

KEY ABBREVIATIONS	
Atopic dermatitis	AD
Atopic eruption of pregnancy	AEP
Estrogen receptor	ER
Intrahepatic cholestasis of pregnancy	ICP
Malignant melanoma	MM
Pemphigoid gestationis	PG
Polymorphic eruption of pregnancy	PEP
Prurigo of pregnancy	PP
Pruritic folliculitis of pregnancy	PFP
Psoralen with ultraviolet light A	PUVA
Ultraviolet light B	UVB

This chapter reviews the physiologic skin changes induced by pregnancy, along with preexisting skin diseases and tumors, and also outlines the diagnosis and treatment of melanoma, pruritis, and specific dermatoses of pregnancy. Common skin conditions discussed in the text are defined in Table 51-1.

PHYSIOLOGIC SKIN CHANGES INDUCED BY PREGNANCY

The human skin undergoes substantial changes during pregnancy, induced by the combined effect of endocrine, metabolic, mechanical, and blood flow alterations. **Although they may prompt cosmetic complaints, such physiologic changes are not associated with risks to the mother or fetus and can be expected to resolve or improve postpartum** (Box 51-1).[1,2] However, some changes such as melasma, varicosities, and pregnancy-associated hyperkeratosis of the nipple[3] may persist postpartum.

Pigmentary Changes

Mild forms of localized or generalized hyperpigmentation occur to some extent in up to 90% of pregnant women and are most noticeable in the areolae, nipples, genital skin, axillae, and inner thighs. Familiar examples include the darkening of the *linea alba* (*linea nigra*) and periareolar skin. Melasma, also termed *chloasma* or *mask of pregnancy,* refers to the facial hyperpigmentation reported in up to 70% of pregnant women.[2] Hyperpigmented, symmetric, poorly demarcated patches are commonly seen on the malar areas (*malar pattern*) and are often distributed over the entire central face (*centrofacial pattern*; Fig. 51-1). In 16% of cases, hyperpigmentation occurs on the ramus of the mandible (mandibular pattern).[4,5] Melasma results from melanin deposition in the epidermis (70%), dermal macrophages (10% to 15%), or both (20%). It is likely secondary to the hormonal changes of gestation with increased expression of α-melanocyte–stimulating hormone. Melasma typically is exacerbated by exposure to ultraviolet and visible light.[5,6] Hyperpigmentation is often more pronounced in brunettes and women with more melanocytes than in women with lighter baseline skin tone; the use of a broad-spectrum sunscreen with a high sun protection factor (SPF) during pregnancy may decrease the severity of hyperpigmentation.

Melasma usually resolves postpartum but may recur in subsequent pregnancies or with the use of oral contraceptives.[4] Troublesome persistent melasma can be treated postpartum with topical hydroquinone 2% to 4% and sunscreen, with or without a topical retinoid and mild topical steroid.[7] Despite treatment postpartum, melasma persists in approximately 30% of patients, especially in women with the dermal or mixed subtypes in which the deeper level of pigmentation results in decreased efficacy of topical agents. Combination therapies including laser treatment[8,9] and chemical peels[10] may be effective in resistant cases. There have been no reports of adverse fetal effects from laser skin treatment during pregnancy. Most laser

TABLE 51-1   COMMON SKIN CHANGES AND DISEASES

CONDITION	DESCRIPTION
Pseudoacanthosis nigricans	Hyperpigmentation of the skin folds and neck that mimic acanthosis nigricans
Dermal melanocytosis	Clusters of melanocytes abnormally located in the dermis that result in ill-defined bluish-gray patches
Vulvar melanosis	Irregularly distributed patches of pigmentation on the vulva
Pregnancy-associated hyperkeratosis of the nipple	Focal hyperkeratosis, at times with wartlike papules, of the apex of the nipple
Miliaria	Sweat retention that reflects obstruction of eccrine sweat ducts
Hyperhidrosis	Skin disorder characterized by increased sweat secretion
Dyshidrosis	Recurrent vesicular eruption of palms and soles
Fox-Fordyce disease	Chronic pruritic disorder of the apocrine glands characterized by blockage of the apocrine duct and sweat retention
Onycholysis	Detachment of the nail plate from the nail bed
Subungual hyperkeratosis	Deposition of keratinous material on the distal nail beds
Palmoplantar pompholyx eczema	See *dyshidrosis* above (former name for *pompholyx*)
Acne conglobata	Variant of acne vulgaris characterized by severe eruptive nodulocystic lesions without systemic manifestations
Pemphigus vulgaris	Autoimmune bullous disorder of the skin and oral mucosa produced by antidesmoglein-3 antibodies that cause intraepidermal acantholysis
Pemphigus vegetans	Variant of pemphigus vulgaris characterized by pustules that form fungoid vegetations or papillomatous proliferations
Pemphigus foliaceus	Autoimmune bullous skin disorder produced by antidesmoglein-3 antibodies that cause subcorneal acantholysis
Spitz nevi	Seen predominantly in children or young adults and characterized by prominent epithelioid and/or spindled melanocytes that can have atypical features

BOX 51-1   PHYSIOLOGIC SKIN CHANGES IN PREGNANCY

Pigmentary

COMMON
Hyperpigmentation
Melasma

UNCOMMON
Jaundice
Pseudoacanthotic changes
Dermal melanocytosis
Hyperkeratosis of the nipple
Vulvar melanosis

Hair Cycle and Growth
Hirsutism
Postpartum telogen effluvium
Postpartum male-pattern alopecia
Diffuse hair thinning (late pregnancy)

Nail
Subungual hyperkeratosis
Distal onycholysis
Transverse grooving
Brittleness and softening

Glandular
Increased eccrine function
Increased sebaceous function
Decreased apocrine function

Connective Tissue
Striae
Skin tags (*molluscum fibrosum gravidarum*)

Vascular
Spider telangiectasias
Pyogenic granuloma (*granuloma gravidarum*)
Palmar erythema
Nonpitting edema
Severe labial edema
Varicosities
Vasomotor instability
Gingival hyperemia
Hemorrhoids

Mucous Membrane
Gingivitis
Chadwick sign
Goodell sign

experts agree that laser radiation does not penetrate through the skin into deeper soft tissues; therefore it should not affect the fetus or the placenta. Still, because of potential liability issues, most dermatologists and plastic surgeons prefer not to perform laser procedures during gestation.

Uncommon pigmentary patterns such as pseudoacanthosis nigricans,[11] dermal melanocytosis, vulvar melanosis, and verrucous areolar hyperpigmentation can also be seen in pregnancy (see Box 51-1).[12] Postinflammatory hyperpigmentation secondary to specific dermatoses of pregnancy (see the section "Specific Dermatoses of Pregnancy") is also common in women with more highly pigmented skin types.

Vascular Changes

As a result of the combination of rising estrogen levels and increased blood volume in pregnancy, blood flow to the skin increases 4 to 16 times in the first 2 months of pregnancy and doubles again during the third month; this results in significant vascular sequelae (see Box 51-1). Spider nevi (spider angiomata) and telangiectasias develop in approximately two thirds of white women and 10% of black women between the second and fifth months of pregnancy and usually resolve within 3 months postpartum (Fig. 51-2, *A*).[1,4] Approximately 10% of women have persistent spider nevi; treatment with electrodessication or pulsed dye laser is effective in women who find these cosmetically troubling.

Palmar erythema, likely secondary to capillary engorgement, is also very common and occurs in up to 70% of white and 30% of black women. Whereas varicosities of the distal leg veins and hemorrhoidal veins develop in more than 40% of women, thrombosis within these superficial varicosities occurs infrequently (<10%). Nonpitting edema can be seen on the ankles (70%) and face (50%) and is most pronounced in the early months of gestation. Varicosities may regress postpartum but usually not completely and are likely to recur in subsequent pregnancies.

Gum hyperemia and gingivitis are common and frequently result in mild bleeding from the gums during routine oral hygiene. This is most prominent during the third trimester and resolves postpartum. Good dental hygiene will minimize symptoms. Periodontal disease has been associated with adverse pregnancy outcomes, so women without a recent dental examination should be referred.[13]

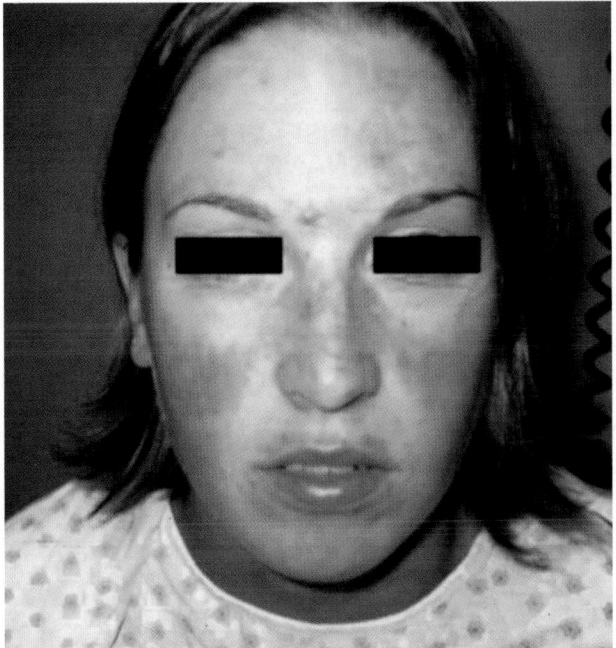

FIG 51-1 Centrofacial type of melasma involving the cheeks, nose, upper lip, and forehead.

The pyogenic granuloma of pregnancy, known as *granuloma gravidarum* or *pregnancy epulis*, is a benign proliferation of capillaries that usually occurs in the gingiva but can occasionally be identified on the lip or extramucosal sites (see Fig. 51-2, *B*). Pyogenic granulomas commonly appear between the second and fifth months of pregnancy and affect up to 2% of pregnancies.[4] Presenting as a vascular, deep red or purple, exuberant, often pedunculated nodule between the teeth or on the buccal or lingual surface of the marginal gingiva, a pyogenic granuloma may be more likely after mucosal trauma. Spontaneous shrinkage of the tumor usually occurs postpartum, and most cases do not require treatment. Surgical excision or electrosurgical destruction should be reserved for cases complicated by excessive bleeding or severe discomfort.

Connective Tissue Changes

Striae gravidarum, also called *striae distensae* or "stretch marks," **develop in up to 90% of white women between the sixth and seventh months of gestation.**[4] Risk factors include younger maternal age, excessive pregnancy weight gain, and concomitant use of corticosteroids; however, genetic susceptibility plays a key role. Striae are most prominent on the abdomen, breasts, buttocks, groin, and axillae; whereas usually asymptomatic, a proportion of patients complain of mild to moderate pruritus. The treatment of striae gravidarum is a challenge; at present, no optimal treatment is available. The erythema (red color) of early striae responds well to various pulsed-dye lasers or intense pulsed light. The red color tends to become pale over time, with or without treatment, but the atrophic lines never disappear completely and do not respond to laser treatment. Topical tretinoin 0.1% cream has been shown to improve the appearance of the striae, decreasing the length by 20%, and is occasionally used in combination with topical glycolic acid (up

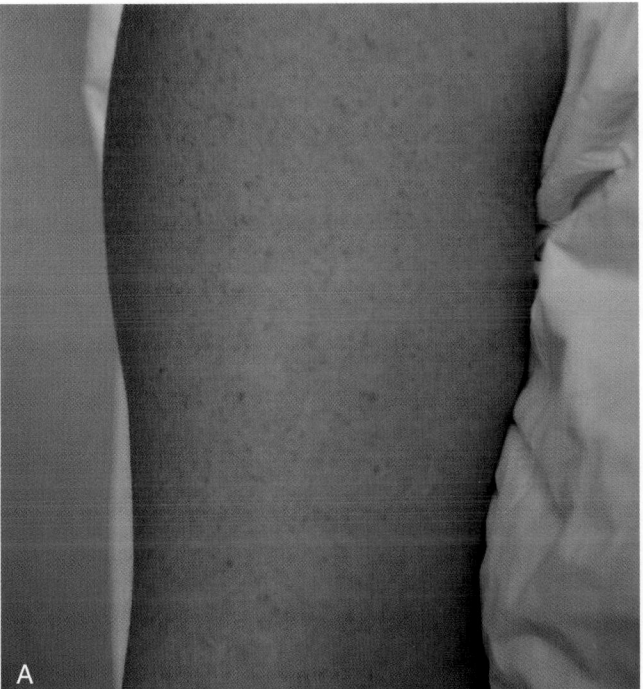 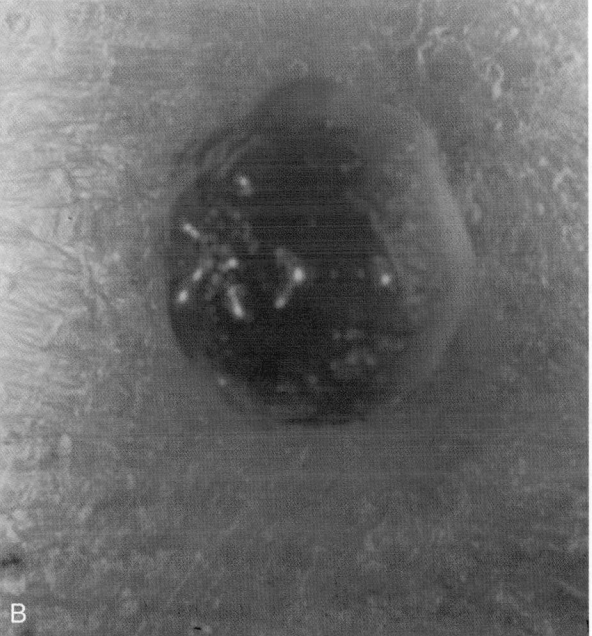

FIG 51-2 **A,** Numerous telangiectasias and spider angiomata on the arm of a pregnant woman. **B,** Pyogenic granuloma of pregnancy (*granuloma gravidarum*), a benign vascular proliferation, is typically seen as a nodule on the gingivae and is shown here at a less common extramucosal site.

to 20%) in an effort to increase elastin content of the affected areas.[14] Nevertheless, tretinoin can be very irritating to the skin and does not make striae completely disappear. No topical therapy prevents or affects the course of striae; they become less apparent postpartum but may never disappear.

Skin tags *(molluscum fibrosum gravidarum)* present as 1- to 5-mm fleshy, pedunculated, exophytic growths on the neck, axillae, inframammary region, or groin and usually appear during the later months of gestation. Treatment can be postponed until completion of the pregnancy because lesions may regress postpartum. Cryotherapy with liquid nitrogen or shave removal is effective for persistent or enlarging lesions. Skin tags do not have malignant potential, and treatment is unnecessary unless inflammation or ulceration develops.

Glandular Changes

Increased eccrine function has been reported during pregnancy and may account for the increased prevalence of miliaria, hyperhidrosis, and dyshidrosis.[4,12] **Conversely, apocrine activity may decrease** during gestation, which contributes to the decreased prevalence of Fox-Fordyce disease and possibly hidradenitis suppurativa in pregnancy.[2] Changes in sebaceous function are variable, and the effects of pregnancy on acne vulgaris are unpredictable. Treatment for acne vulgaris during pregnancy is discussed below. During pregnancy, the sebaceous glands on the areolae enlarge *(Montgomery's glands or tubercles)*.

Hair and Nail Changes

Most pregnant women develop mild hirsutism that affects their face, trunk, and extremities that commonly regresses within 6 months postpartum. In addition, **postpartum hair shedding *(telogen effluvium)* may be noted as a greater proportion of hairs enter the telogen phase** (Fig. 51-3). The severity of *telogen effluvium* varies considerably, and the hair loss becomes noticeable when more than 40% to 50% of the hair is affected. Recovery is spontaneous, and no effective treatment is available. Patients can be counseled that hair thinning usually resolves

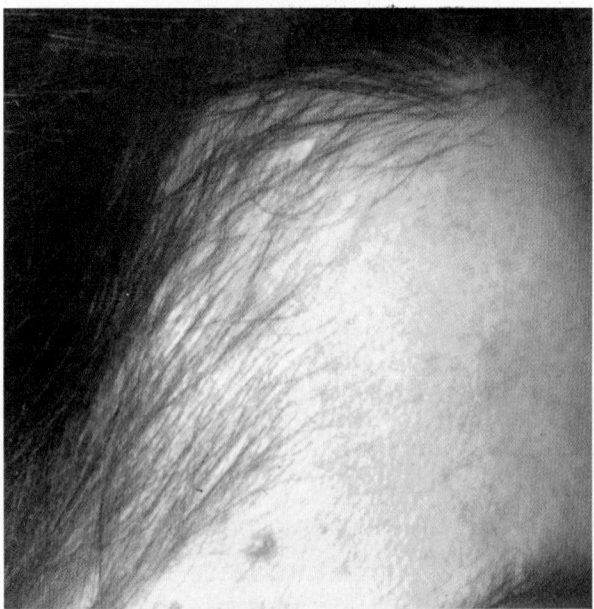

FIG 51-3 *Telogen effluvium* that develops within 5 months postpartum typically presents with temporal recession and hair thinning.

within 1 to 5 months but that complete resolution may occasionally take up to 15 months.[1,4] Frontoparietal hair recession and diffuse hair thinning in the later months of pregnancy have been noted in some women. Nail changes can be seen as early as the first trimester of gestation that include brittleness, onycholysis, subungual hyperkeratosis, and transverse grooving. No specific treatment is available for nail changes during pregnancy, and most are expected to resolve postpartum. An attempt should be made to eliminate external sensitizers, such as nail polish removers, and infections. The nails should be kept short if they are brittle or prone to onycholysis.[6]

PREEXISTING SKIN DISEASES AND TUMORS AFFECTED BY PREGNANCY

Pregnancy can aggravate or, less often, improve many skin conditions and primary skin tumors (see Video 51-1).[15] Diseases that may improve during pregnancy include atopic dermatitis, acne, chronic plaque psoriasis, Fox-Fordyce disease, hidradenitis suppurativa, linear immunoglobulin A (IgA) dermatosis, sarcoidosis, Behçet disease, urticaria, and autoimmune progesterone dermatitis (see Table 51-1).

Atopic Eczema and Dermatitis

Atopic dermatitis (AD), also known as *atopic eczema,* is a very common skin condition and is often exacerbated by pregnancy, although remission has been noted in up to 24% of cases.[16] Two large studies that used diagnostic criteria established in pediatric populations indicated a high prevalence of AD in pregnancy, including "new AD" (AD presenting for the first time in pregnancy); however, the true prevalence may be revised as the criteria for gestational AD are refined.[16-20] Risk factors include a history of prior atopy (27%), family history of atopy (50%), and offspring with infantile AD (19%). Other risk factors for AD include black or Asian race and tobacco use.[21,22] The prevalence of intrinsic ("nonallergic") versus extrinsic (IgE associated) AD[23] during gestation is unknown, although a small study showed that intrinsic AD is more affected by pregnancy.[24]

Most patients present with lesions in the flexural surfaces of the extremities, occasionally with concomitant lesions on the trunk. Less common presentations are palmoplantar pompholyx eczema and follicular and facial eczema. In pregnancy, eczematous lesions can develop bacterial or viral superinfection (i.e., *eczema herpeticum* secondary to herpes simplex virus); treatment with dicloxacillin or a first-generation cephalosporin should be used as necessary in these cases. *Eczema herpeticum* and disseminated herpetic infection, the latter of which may lead to fetal risk, should be promptly treated with intravenous (IV) acyclovir to minimize maternal and fetal risks.

AD is not associated with an increased risk of adverse fetal outcomes. The effects of breastfeeding and maternal food antigen avoidance during pregnancy on AD in the offspring are controversial. **Treatment for gestational exacerbations of AD is primarily symptomatic. A moisturizer and low potency to midpotent topical steroid is the first-line treatment.** Systemic antihistamines, such as chlorpheniramine or diphenhydramine, can also be used as necessary for relief of pruritus. A short course of oral steroids may be required for severe AD. Ultraviolet light B (UVB) is a safe second-line treatment for eczema in pregnancy. There is less experience with the newer topical immunomodulators (pimecrolimus, tacrolimus).[25] Although their bioavailability is limited (<5%) and no pattern of anomalies has been reported after exposure to these drugs in utero, several infants have had neonatal hyperkalemia.[26] Therefore these immunomodulators should be used as third-line treatment for refractory AD that has not responded to UVB. If systemic agents are needed for refractory AD, cyclosporine is the safest option.

The course of gestational AD in the postpartum period has not been studied. Irritant hand dermatitis and nipple eczema are often seen postpartum.[1] Irritant hand dermatitis is treated with emollients and hand protection. Nipple eczema can evolve into painful fissures and can be complicated with bacterial superinfection, most commonly with *Staphylococcus aureus*. Superinfected nipple eczema should be treated with a topical steroid combined with a topical or systemic antibiotic.

Acne Vulgaris

The effects of pregnancy on acne vulgaris are unpredictable. **In one study, pregnancy affected acne in approximately 70% of women, with 41% reporting improvement and 29% reporting a worsening with pregnancy.**[27] Two patients had improvement in one pregnancy and exacerbation in another. Some patients may develop acne for the first time during pregnancy or in the postpartum period (*postgestational acne*). Comedonal acne should be treated with topical keratolytic agents, such as benzoyl peroxide, whereas inflammatory acne should be treated with azelaic acid, topical erythromycin, topical clindamycin, or oral erythromycin base. Although first-trimester use of topical tretinoin has not been associated with an increased rate of congenital malformations in controlled studies, the number of reported exposures is too small to exclude a small increased risk. A theoretic concern remains, and the use of tretinoin during pregnancy is therefore not recommended (see Chapter 8).

Other Inflammatory Skin Diseases

Recurrent flares of urticaria may worsen in pregnancy. Of interest, these flares show common features with hereditary angioedema and may have been exacerbated in the past by oral contraceptive use or prior to menses. Chronic plaque psoriasis may develop for the first time during pregnancy. **Women with existing chronic psoriasis can be counseled that between 40% and 63% of women have symptomatic improvement, compared with only 14% of women who have symptomatic deterioration**; postpartum flares are common (80%).[28] Topical steroids and topical calcipotriene are relatively safe treatment options for localized psoriasis in pregnancy.[29] For severe psoriasis that has not responded to topical medications, UVB or a short course of cyclosporine are considered second-line treatment options.

Autoimmune Progesterone Dermatitis

Autoimmune progesterone dermatitis is caused by hypersensitivity to progesterone through autoimmune or nonimmune mechanisms. Although this rare dermatosis can take various forms (urticarial, papular, vesicular, or pustular), the hallmark is recurrent cyclic lesions that usually appear during the luteal phase of the menstrual cycle. Limited information is available regarding the effects of pregnancy on autoimmune progesterone dermatitis. Case series report instances of both improvement and exacerbation.[30] Increased cortisol levels and/or the gradual increase in the sex hormone levels during pregnancy with subsequent hormonal desensitization in some patients are both possible mechanisms for observed improvement. Diagnosis is based on either an immediate local urticarial reaction or, more

frequently, a delayed hypersensitivity reaction following intradermal challenge with synthetic progesterone. Intramuscular administration of progesterone should be avoided in these patients because it has been associated with angioedema. Circulating antibodies to progesterone or the corpus luteum have been detected by indirect immunofluorescence in several patients. The sensitivity of this test seems to be lower than that of the intradermal progesterone challenge, therefore these antibodies are not widely used to confirm this diagnosis. No specific therapy for the condition during pregnancy has been proposed. Autoimmune estrogen dermatitis has also been reported in a patient who presented with urticaria in early pregnancy.[31]

Impetigo Herpetiformis

Impetigo herpetiformis is a rare variant of generalized pustular psoriasis that develops primarily during pregnancy, often in association with hypocalcemia[32] **or low serum levels of vitamin D.**[33] Although familial occurrence has been reported, more commonly a personal or family history of psoriasis is absent. The eruption usually develops in the third trimester but can also start in earlier trimesters and postpartum. Whereas the overwhelming majority of cases resolve postpartum, persistent cases have been reported and can be associated with oral contraceptive use.[34] Various infections during pregnancy may also trigger a flare of pustular psoriasis in a genetically predisposed individual.[35]

Impetigo herpetiformis is characterized by numerous grouped, discrete, sterile pustules at the periphery of erythematous patches (Fig. 51-4, *A*). Lesions typically originate in the major flexures (axillae, inframammary areas, groin, and gluteal fold) and progress onto the trunk, usually sparing the face, hands, and feet. Painful mucosal erosions may also develop. Onycholysis, or complete nail shedding secondary to subungual lesions, has been reported. Constitutional symptoms are common and include fever, malaise, diarrhea, and vomiting with resultant dehydration. Rarely, patients develop complications secondary to hypocalcemia that include tetany, convulsions, and delirium. Common laboratory findings are leukocytosis and elevated erythrocyte sedimentation rate; rarer perturbations include hypocalcemia, decreased serum vitamin D levels, and signs of hypoparathyroidism. Historically reported maternal risks such as tetany, seizures, delirium, and death from cardiac or renal failure or septicemia are uncommon. Fetal risks such as stillbirth and fetal abnormalities secondary to placental insufficiency[33] have been reported even when the condition was well controlled.[36] **Whereas maternal prognosis is excellent with early diagnosis, aggressive treatment, and supportive care, an increased risk of perinatal mortality may persist despite maternal treatment.**[37] The risk is difficult to quantify because it is based on sparse case reports that span decades. Intensive fetal monitoring should be considered until the mother is stabilized. After acute treatment, the appropriate degree of fetal surveillance is not known; however, periodic assessment of fetal well-being is prudent after viability.

Definite diagnosis of impetigo herpetiformis is based on histopathology that shows typical features of pustular psoriasis (see Fig. 51-4, *B*). Direct and indirect skin immunofluorescence is negative. Systemic steroids are first-line therapy for impetigo herpetiformis, and 20 to 40 mg/day of prednisone is usually effective. Cases of pustular psoriasis exacerbated by pregnancy have been treated with cyclosporine.[37] Calcium and vitamin D replacement therapy should be undertaken if necessary and can

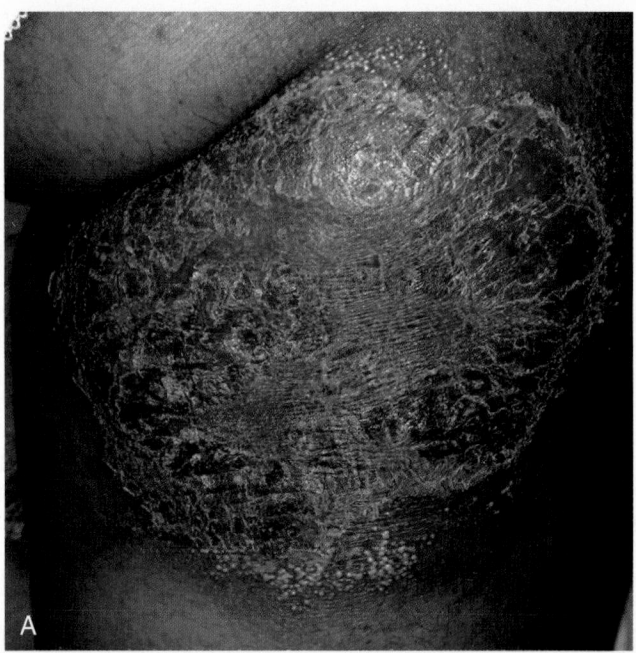

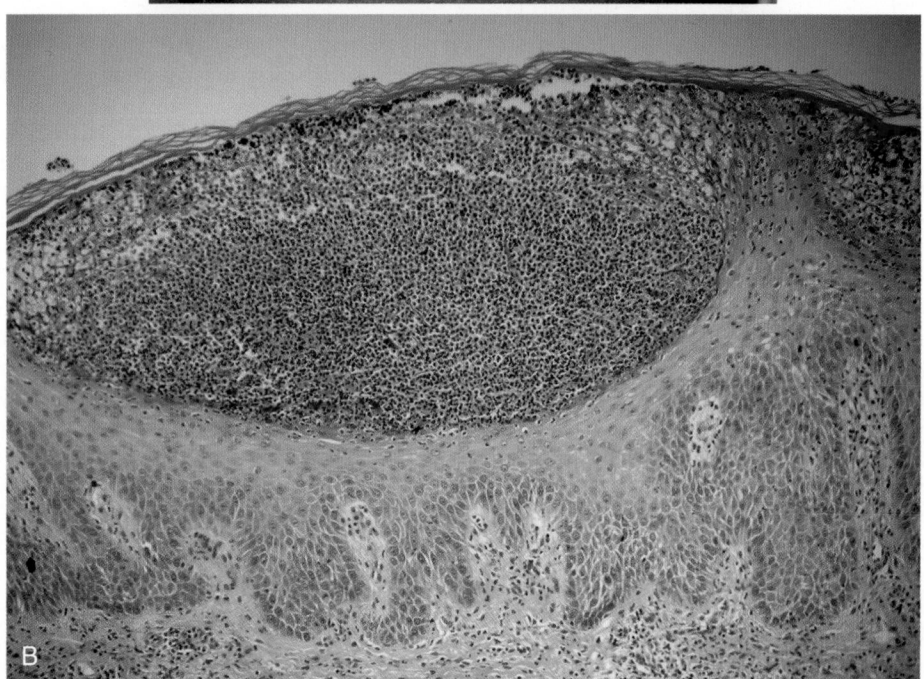

FIG 51-4 A, Impetigo herpetiformis: discrete, grouped, sterile pustules at the periphery of an erythematous crusted plaque. **B,** Histopathology of impetigo herpetiformis shows the characteristic Kogoj spongiform pustule, formed of neutrophils in the uppermost portion of the spinous layer (hematoxylin-eosin stain). (Courtesy Aleksandr Itkin, MD.)

lead to remission of the eruption.[25] Systemic antibiotics should be administered if bacterial superinfection is suspected. Post-inflammatory hyperpigmentation may develop, but scarring is usually absent. Impetigo herpetiformis has been treated postpartum with oral steroids, oral retinoids,[38] and photochemotherapy (psoralen with ultraviolet light A [PUVA])[39] as single agents or in combination. Resistant cases can be treated with a combination of PUVA and clofazimine or methotrexate postpartum (methotrexate is contraindicated during pregnancy [category X], and both methotrexate and clofazimine are contraindicated during breastfeeding).

Cutaneous Manifestations of Autoimmune Disorders

Cutaneous lesions may be prominent in some individuals affected by autoimmune disorders, and these patients often have questions regarding how pregnancy will affect the appearance of these lesions. The cutaneous manifestations of chronic discoid lupus are not affected by pregnancy. Cutaneous flares of systemic lupus erythematosus can usually be managed with oral steroid treatment. Dermatomyositis/polymyositis may show exacerbation of the characteristic heliotrope rash in approximately half of affected individuals.[40] The cutaneous progression of scleroderma is not significantly altered by pregnancy, and symptoms of Raynaud phenomenon may improve. Pregnant women with limited skin disease do significantly better than those with diffuse scleroderma.[41] The medical and obstetric management of pregnancies complicated by collagen vascular disease is discussed in detail in Chapter 46.

Bullous Disorders

Bullous dermatologic disorders develop secondary to autoantibodies that target constituents of the skin and oral mucosa. **Pemphigus vulgaris,[42] vegetans, or foliaceus may develop or worsen during pregnancy,** whereas linear IgA disease may improve.[43] In more than 50% of cases of pemphigus vulgaris, lesions may initially appear within the oral cavity. Diffuse skin involvement with multiple flaccid vesicles follows with confluence of vesicles forming large eroded areas. Skin biopsy with immunofluorescence studies are needed for a definitive diagnosis. Biopsy for routine histopathology and immunofluorescence is indicated in patients with new-onset lesions, most critically to differentiate pemphigus from herpes (*pemphigoid*) gestationis (see that section below). In cases of pemphigus, fetal and neonatal skin lesions can occur secondary to transplacental transfer of IgG antibodies, but these resolve spontaneously within 2 to 3 weeks after birth. Pemphigus should be treated with oral corticosteroids, and high doses may be required. A recent study of 49 pregnancies complicated by pemphigus vulgaris showed a 12% perinatal mortality. Forty-five percent of live neonates had pemphigus lesions at birth.[44] Increased fetal surveillance is prudent in pregnancies affected by active pemphigus, although the effectiveness of this surveillance in preventing morbidity and fetal loss is not known.

Acrodermatitis enteropathica is a rare autosomal-recessive disorder of zinc deficiency characterized by dermatitis, diarrhea, and alopecia. Vesiculobullous and/or eczematous skin lesions can develop on the extremities and at periorificial sites such as the mouth and perianal and genital areas. The disease usually flares early in gestation[45] as serum zinc levels decrease, but it may also flare with oral contraceptive use.

Skin Tumors

Most skin neoplasms that present or enlarge during pregnancy are benign, and this includes pyogenic granuloma, hemangioma, hemangioendothelioma, glomus tumor, glomangioma, dermatofibroma, dermatofibrosarcoma protuberans, leiomyoma, keloid, desmoid tumor, and neurofibroma. **Melanocytic nevi may develop, enlarge, or darken during pregnancy, but these changes are less dramatic than previously thought.** A mild degree of histopathologic atypia has been reported in a few studies. Pennoyer and colleagues[46] compared photographs of moles taken during the first trimester and again in the third trimester. Only 3% of nevi enlarged during pregnancy, and another 3% regressed. In contrast, dysplastic nevi in women with familial dysplastic nevus syndrome do have a tendency to increase in size and undergo color change during pregnancy.[47] Spitz nevi, another class of common pigmented benign neoplasms, may also increase in size or erupt during pregnancy.[48] Studies that used dermoscopy showed that the pigment network of nevi becomes thicker and more prominent, and the globules darken during pregnancy; these features, however, return to their original state within 1 year after delivery.[49] Any suspicious pigmented skin lesion should prompt a dermatologic referral. The "ABCDE" clinical criteria for pigmented lesions—*asymmetry, border* irregularity, *color* variegation, *diameter* greater than 6 mm, and *evolution* (i.e., an enlarging or otherwise changing lesion)—are helpful in determining which lesions are of higher malignant potential.[50] Seborrheic keratoses are also common and may enlarge or darken during gestation. None of these benign lesions requires treatment during pregnancy; the pregnant patient should be reassured that these changes are benign and may improve postpartum.

Malignant Melanoma

Malignant melanoma (MM; see Chapter 50) is the most common malignancy in pregnancy and accounts for 31% of all malignant tumors diagnosed in pregnancy[51] with an overall incidence that ranges between 2.8 and 8.5 cases per 100,000 women.[52,53] Some studies have shown that melanomas that develop during pregnancy are thicker than those in nonpregnant women,[54] possibly because of a delayed diagnosis due to a shared misconception by the patient and/or her physician that darkening and changing of a nevus is normal in pregnancy. However, after correcting for tumor thickness, no effect on prognosis was apparent. Despite initial concerns, **several epidemiologic studies to evaluate the effect of pregnancy status at diagnosis suggest that the 5-year survival rate is not affected after controlling for confounding factors.**[53,55-57] However, data are insufficient for stage III and IV disease.[58] The major prognostic determinants of survival in patients with localized melanoma are tumor (Breslow) thickness and ulceration status,[59] and level of invasion is only significant in women with tumors more than 1 mm in thickness.

Inconclusive evidence supports the role of estrogen receptors (ERs) in melanoma. Most studies did not show an increased risk of melanoma recurrence with oral contraceptives or hormone replacement therapy (HRT) use.[60,61] Some studies have found melanoma cell lines that lack type I ERs,[62,63] but others have demonstrated an inhibitory effect of estrogens on melanoma cell lines through type II ERs.[61] In fact, decreased levels of ERβ expression, which antagonizes the proliferative behaviors of ERα, have been seen in more invasive MM with increased Breslow thickness.[64] Higher levels of ERβ have been demonstrated in melanoma cells of pregnant women compared with melanoma cells in men, thus potentially implicating ERβ and female sex as a protective and prognostic factor in MM.[65,66] **Wide local excision of the primary melanoma should be performed in stages I through III, and conservative excision should be undertaken in stage IV.**[58,67] Sentinel lymph node biopsy (SLNB) is indicated for a tumor stage of T1b or greater if thickness is greater than 0.75 mm. **SLNB is the most powerful prognostic factor in clinically localized melanoma.** However, because allergic reactions to the isosulfan blue dye used in the procedure have been reported, Schwartz and colleagues[67] proposed the use of radiocolloid alone for SLNB in the first trimester. The authors also proposed that wide local excision and SLNB with blue dye can be delayed until after delivery in women who are in the second half of pregnancy and have already undergone narrow excision of their MM with negative margins. Regarding other staging procedures, chest radiography with appropriate shielding and ultrasound of the abdomen and liver should be performed in stage IIB/IIIA.[58] In stages greater than IIIA, magnetic resonance imaging (MRI) of the head and positron emission tomography (PET)/computed tomography (CT) scans should be performed; MRI carries a risk for tissue overheating and should not be used in the first trimester.[58]

Complete lymph node dissection is warranted in stages I and II if SLNB is positive, and therapeutic lymph node dissection should be undertaken in stage III.[58] As far as management of stage IV patients, elective termination and tailored treatment should be considered in the first trimester, whereas tailored treatment and induction when the fetus is viable should be considered in the second and third trimesters.[58] However, termination of pregnancy in stage IV patients does not affect the outcome of MM in the mother,[68] and the risk of fetal metastasis remains remote.

Melanoma is the most common type of malignancy to metastasize to the placenta and fetus, and it represents 31% of such metastases.[69] However, it should be emphasized that placental and/or fetal metastases are extraordinarily rare (27 cases) and that even in the setting of placental metastasis, fetal metastasis only occurs in 17% of cases. Histologic evaluation of the placenta should be performed because of potentially microscopic placental metastasis with known association to fetal melanoma. The presence of placental metastases is associated with widespread disease and dismal maternal survival. The role of systemic therapy in preventing metastases to the placenta and fetus has not been adequately studied.

No standard guidelines are available for patients who desire to become pregnant after the diagnosis and treatment of melanoma. A nonsignificant decrease in mortality in pregnancy subsequent to a melanoma diagnosis has been reported.[53] The primary reason to delay pregnancy following a recent diagnosis of melanoma is the time-dependent risk of tumor recurrence and subsequent maternal mortality. One study showed that 83% of stage II MM recurrences were within 2 years of initial treatment.[55] Schwartz and colleagues[67] suggested waiting 2 years in patients with thin melanomas and 3 to 5 years in thicker lesions before becoming pregnant again. Patients should be counseled on a case-by-case basis depending primarily on risk of recurrence, taking into account the thickness of their original tumor and other prognostic factors. Women with a significant risk of recurrence may want to delay pregnancy until they can be assured of a low recurrence risk. In women with a thin tumor with a low risk of recurrence, no delay may be necessary.

PRURITUS IN PREGNANCY

Itching is the most common dermatologic symptom of pregnancy. Mild pruritus attributed to pregnancy (*pruritus gravidarum*) is common and occurs most frequently over the abdomen. Pruritus has been reported in up to 17% of pregnancies,[70] but a more recent report suggests that significant pruritus that requires a more thorough evaluation occurs in only 1.6% of patients.[71] **A broad differential diagnosis needs to be considered; the constellation of clinical and laboratory findings will help establish a diagnosis and guide management decisions.** Pruritic skin diseases not specifically related to pregnancy, such as AD and scabies, should be considered. In cases of pruritus without eruption, systemic diseases are more likely. Intrahepatic cholestasis of pregnancy (ICP) is a common etiology (see Chapter 47 for diagnosis and management); however, other conditions—such as lymphoma and liver, renal, and thyroid disease—should also be considered.[12] In the patient with pruritus and skin lesions other than excoriations, referral to a dermatologist for evaluation of a specific dermatosis of pregnancy (see

below) is appropriate, unless a clear etiologic agent for a systemic or topical allergic reaction can be elucidated.

SPECIFIC DERMATOSES OF PREGNANCY

The term *specific dermatoses of pregnancy* refers to a group of skin diseases encountered predominantly during or immediately following pregnancy and includes **only those skin diseases that result directly from the state of gestation or the products of conception** (see Video 51-2).[16] Included in this definition are pemphigoid (herpes) gestationis (PG); polymorphic eruption of pregnancy (PEP), also called *pruritic urticarial papules and plaques of pregnancy* (PUPPP); prurigo of pregnancy (PP); and pruritic folliculitis of pregnancy (PFP; Table 51-2). A recent reclassification[17] included ICP in the specific dermatoses of pregnancy and grouped AD, PP, and PFP under "atopic eruption of pregnancy" (AEP). However, some studies have not confirmed the association of PP and PFP with atopy, and some features of AEP need to be further clarified.[18]

Pemphigoid (Herpes) Gestationis

Pemphigoid gestationis (PG) is a rare autoimmune skin disease that affects between 1 in 7000 and 1 in 50,000 pregnancies.[20] Although PG and bullous pemphigoid recognize the same antigen[72] and share certain features, PG is confined to pregnant women and those affected by gestational trophoblastic disease (GTD). Some authors[73] have suggested that exposure to paternal antigens may play a critical role in disease initiation, but "skip pregnancies" with the same partner have been reported and would argue against this association. Of interest, expression of the PG antigen in the placenta begins in the midtrimester, which correlates with the timing of clinical symptoms. The antibody that incites the pathology in PG belongs to the IgG1 subclass and recognizes the NC16A2 (MCW-1) epitope in the noncollagenous domain (NC16A) of the transmembrane 180-kd antigen (bullous pemphigoid antigen 2).[74] PG primarily affects whites with only scattered case reports in blacks[75]; this observation is consistent with the association between PG and the human leukocyte antigens (HLAs) DR3 (61% to 80%), DR4 (52%), or both (43% to 50%), which are less frequent in the black population.

Clinically, **PG usually presents in the second or third trimester of pregnancy with extremely pruritic urticarial lesions that typically begin on the abdomen and trunk and commonly involve the umbilicus** (Fig. 51-5, *A*). These urticarial plaques rapidly progress to widespread bullous lesions (see Fig. 51-5, *B*) that may affect the palms and soles but rarely the face and mucous membranes. Tense bullous lesions arise in both inflamed and clinically normal skin and usually heal without scarring. Up to 25% of cases can present in the postpartum period, although these may represent recrudescences of previously undiagnosed mild PG. The most important clinical and laboratory features of PG are summarized in Table 51-2.

Although the differential diagnosis of PG includes drug eruption, erythema multiforme, and allergic contact dermatitis, the most common diagnosis to exclude is the far more common PEP (see below). **PEP can manifest with urticarial and/or vesicular lesions almost indistinguishable from those of PG, although PEP classically begins in the abdominal striae and spares the umbilicus.** Definitive diagnosis should be based on immunofluorescence of perilesional skin that demonstrates the hallmark finding of PG: linear C3 deposition along

TABLE 51-2   OVERVIEW OF SPECIFIC DERMATOSES OF PREGNANCY

	U.S. RATES	CLINICAL DATA	LESION MORPHOLOGY AND DISTRIBUTION	IMPORTANT LABORATORY FINDINGS	FETAL RISKS
Pemphigoid gestationis (PG)	1:50,000	Second or third trimester or postpartum Flare at delivery (75%) Resolution postpartum with a good chance of recurrence in future pregnancies	Abdominal urticarial lesions progress into a generalized bullous eruption.	Skin immunofluorescence shows linear deposition of C3 along basement membrane.	Neonatal PG SGA infants Preterm delivery
Polymorphic eruption of pregnancy (PEP)	1:130 to 1:300	Third trimester or postpartum *Primigravidae* Resolution postpartum Association with multiple gestation No recurrence in future pregnancies	Polymorphous eruption starts in the abdominal striae and shows periumbilical sparing.	None	None
Atopic eruption of pregnancy (AEP)	>50% of pruritic dermatoses	First or second trimester Resolution postpartum with possible recurrence in future pregnancies	Flexural surfaces, neck, chest, trunk	Serum IgE elevations (20% to 70%)	None
Prurigo of pregnancy (PP)	1:300 to 1:450	Second or third trimester Resolution postpartum with recurrence in future pregnancies	Grouped excoriated papules over the extensor extremities and occasionally the abdomen	None	None
Pruritic folliculitis of pregnancy (PFP)	>30 cases	Second or third trimester Resolution postpartum with possible recurrence in future pregnancies	Follicular papules and pustules	Biopsy: sterile folliculitis	None

Modified from Kroumpouzos, G, Cohen LM. Specific dermatoses of pregnancy: an evidence-based systematic review. *Am J Obstet Gynecol.* 2003;18:1083.
Ig, immunoglobulin; *SGA,* small for gestational age.

the basement membrane zone, which is absent in PEP.[1] Interestingly, a small recent study showed C4d positivity at the basement membrane zone on paraffin sections in PG but not in PEP; this may eliminate the second biopsy for immunofluorescence but needs confirmation.[76] Skin histopathology shows a spongiotic epidermis, marked papillary dermal edema, and an eosinophilic infiltrate. Serum antibody titers with conventional indirect immunofluorescence do not correlate with the course of disease but parallel disease activity when BP-180 NC16A enzyme-linked immunosorbent assay (ELISA) was used.[77]

Oral corticosteroids remain the cornerstone of treatment in PG. The majority of patients will respond rapidly to treatment with relatively low-dose prednisone (20 to 40 mg/day). In resistant cases, doses as high as 180 mg/day have been tried. Once new blister formation has been suppressed, prednisone should be tapered to 5 to 10 mg/day. Typically, up to 75% of patients will experience spontaneous resolution or improvement in the late third trimester, and steroid treatment can often be discontinued. However, because PG typically flares at delivery or within the days following delivery, steroid doses can be increased in anticipation. A subset of patients will have persistent PG or recurrent flares that last weeks or months. Patients at risk for prolonged or chronic PG tend to be older with higher parity, with more widespread lesions and a history of PG in prior pregnancies.[78] Oral contraceptive use has been implicated in postpartum flares; 20% to 50% of patients who use oral contraceptives within 6 months of delivery have associated flares. This association should be considered when counseling patients on their contraceptive options. Breastfeeding was associated with a significantly shorter duration of active lesions in one study,[79] but this has been debated. PG recurs in 95% of future pregnancies, and lesions may be more severe, appear earlier in gestation, and persist longer postpartum. Treatment for chronic, recalcitrant PG is generally unsatisfactory, although case reports

have described success with plasmapheresis; immunoapheresis; chemical oophorectomy with goserelin; ritodrine; rituximab; and high-dose intravenous immune globulin (IVIG) combined with cyclosporine or other immunosuppressant medications. Minocycline or doxycycline combined with nicotinamide and immunosuppressive and antiinflammatory agents such as cyclophosphamide, azathioprine, rituximab, pyridoxine, sulfapyridine, gold, methotrexate, or dapsone have been used postpartum in refractory cases with some success, but their use is limited to nonlactating patients.[20]

The maternal effects of PG are largely limited to symptomatic pruritus and a small risk of lesion superinfection. An association between PG and Graves disease has been reported, and PG[80] is an indication for performing both immediate and periodic screening tests of thyroid function. **An association with small-for-gestational-age (SGA) infants and preterm delivery has been reported,** but the effect of PG on the fetus remains difficult to estimate from the small study cohorts due to the rarity of the disease. The largest cohort to date compared fetal outcome between the affected and unaffected pregnancies of 74 women; 16% of pregnancies with active PG delivered prior to 32 weeks, compared with 2% of the unaffected pregnancies.[81] Mild placental insufficiency has been postulated as a mechanism, therefore sonographic evaluation of fetal interval growth and third-trimester fetal surveillance is appropriate. Finally, **approximately 5% to 10% of neonates will manifest bullous skin lesions** (neonatal PG) **secondary to passive transplacental transfer of PG antibody.**[82] Parents should be reassured that these lesions will resolve spontaneously without scarring over a period of a few weeks as the maternal antibodies clear from the infant's blood. However, parents should be counseled about the signs and symptoms of bacterial superinfection so that timely treatment can prevent progression to systemic infection.

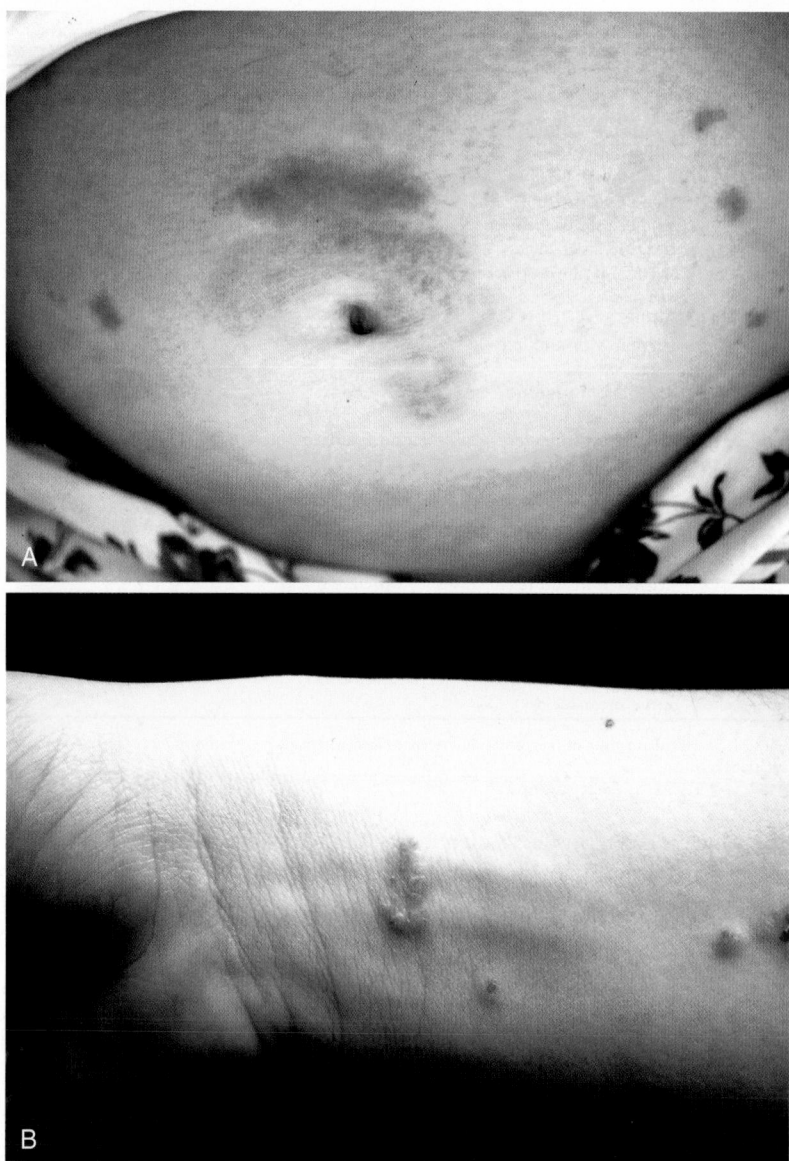

FIG 51-5 A, Pruritic abdominal urticarial plaques develop in the early phase of pemphigoid (herpes) gestationis and typically involve the umbilicus. **B,** Characteristic tense vesicles on an erythematous base on the forearm in a patient with PG. (From Kroumpouzos G: Skin disease. In James DK, Steer PJ, Weiner CP, Gonik B, Crowther CA, Robson SC: *High-Risk Pregnancy: Management Options,* 4th ed, Philadelphia: Elsevier Saunders; 2011, p. 929.)

Polymorphic Eruption of Pregnancy

Polymorphic eruption of pregnancy (PEP), also known as *pruritic urticarial papules and plaques of pregnancy* **(PUPPP), is the most common specific dermatosis of pregnancy and affects between 1 in 130 and 1 in 300 pregnancies.** It occurs classically in primigravidae in the mid to late third trimester and has been associated with a slight predominance of male babies (55%).[20,83,84] **Lesions typically begin in the abdominal striae and spare the periumbilical region in up to two thirds of cases** (Fig. 51-6, *A*).[1,85] PEP can be difficult to characterize because the eruption is polymorphous and can include urticarial and occasionally vesicular, purpuric, polycyclic, or targetoid lesions reminiscent of erythema multiforme or herpes gestationis (see Fig. 51-6, *B*).[84] Although lesions can spread over the trunk and extremities, they usually spare the palms and soles, and involvement of the face is very unusual.

Generalized PEP may resemble a toxic erythema or atopic dermatitis (see Fig. 51-6, *C*).

Skin histopathology is often nonspecific and shows spongiotic dermatitis with variable numbers of eosinophils. In contrast to PG, immunofluorescence studies and serologic tests are typically negative. IgE elevation (uncontrolled) was reported in 28% of PEP cases in a recent study,[86] but the significance and specificity of IgE elevations in pregnancy remain unclear.[18] The high prevalence (55%) of a personal or family history of atopy[86] has not been confirmed by other studies. The pathogenesis of PEP has not been established, but the immunohistologic profile of skin lesions[87] suggests a delayed hypersensitivity reaction to an unknown antigen. Some authors have proposed that rapid abdominal wall distension in primigravidae may trigger an inflammatory process; this has been supported by the association between PEP and multiple-gestation pregnancy, excess

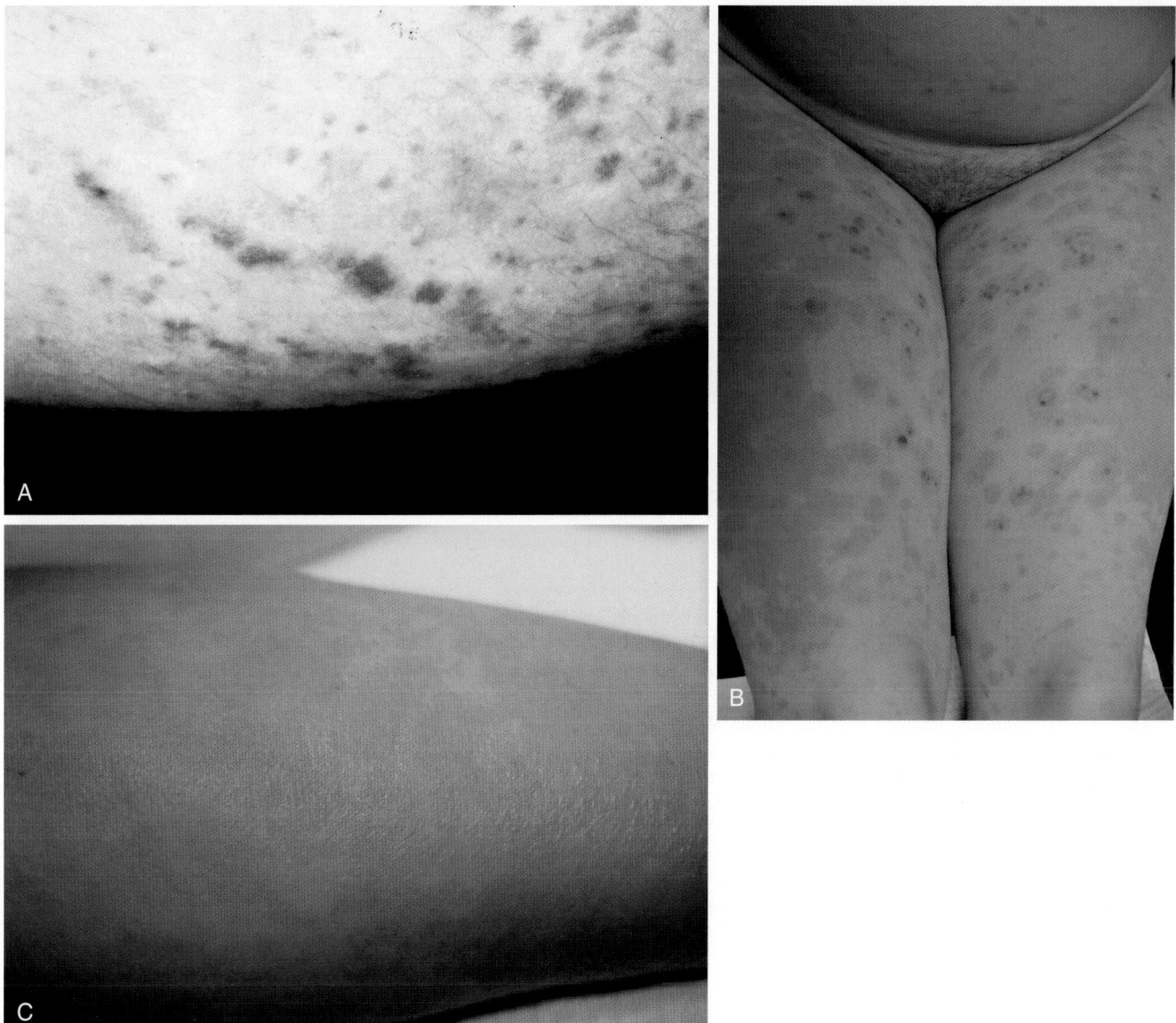

FIG 51-6 A, Pruritic urticarial papules and plaques of pregnancy (PUPPP) include urticarial lesions that typically start in the abdominal striae. **B,** Vesicular lesions superimposed on urticarial plaques and targetoid lesions reminiscent of erythema multiforme or pemphigoid (herpes) gestationis. **C,** Widespread PUPPP may resemble a toxic erythema or atopic dermatitis. (Courtesy Helen Raynham, MD.)

maternal weight gain, and fetal macrosomia.[88,89] **A meta-analysis revealed a tenfold higher prevalence of multiple gestation in pregnancies affected by PEP.**[85] Multiple-gestation pregnancy is associated with higher estrogen and progesterone levels, and progesterone has been shown to aggravate the inflammatory process at the tissue level. Interestingly, increased progesterone receptor levels have been detected in skin lesions of PEP.[90] Finally, fetal DNA has been detected in PEP lesions.[91] Still, the importance of microchimerism in the pathogenesis of PEP remains uncertain.

PEP is not associated with adverse maternal or fetal outcomes. The association with cesarean delivery in two recent studies needs to be clarified.[92] The goal of therapy is the relief of maternal discomfort. Mild PEP can be treated with antipruritic topical medications, topical steroids, and oral antihistamines. In cases of severe itching, a short course of oral prednisone may be necessary. UVB has been used anecdotally.[85]

Atopic Eruption of Pregnancy

AEP is a clinical entity that encompasses prurigo of pregnancy (PP), pruritic folliculitis of pregnancy (PFP), and atopic dermatitis (AD); this includes *new* AD, defined as AD that develops for the first time in gestation.[17,93,94] This reclassification was suggested given the clinical overlap of an atopic diathesis—that is, a personal or family history of atopy or elevated IgE levels—seen in 79% of all affected patients. Further, AEP patients had an earlier eczematous onset, and 75% of patients developed symptoms prior to the third trimester.[17] Features of patchy eczema (*E-type* AEP, seen in 67%) and papular/prurigo (*P-type* AEP, seen in 33%) can coexist.[17,93,94] In addition, up to 34% of patients with AEP had a history of AEP in prior pregnancies.[17] Atopic sites—flexural surfaces; face and neck, including the vee of the neck and upper chest; and the trunk (68%)—were the most frequently involved areas.[16,17] Hand and

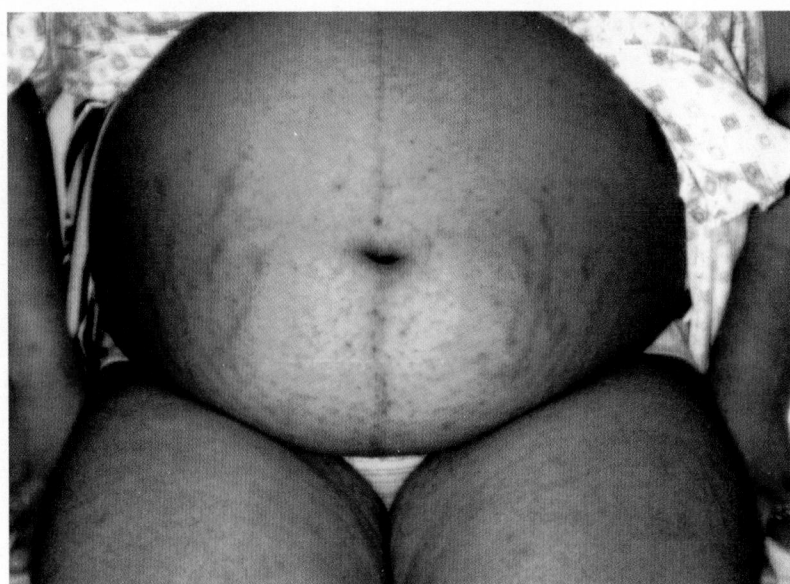

FIG 51-7 Pruritic folliculitis of pregnancy appears as discrete follicular erythematous or pigmented papules on the abdomen.

foot eczema and, less commonly, eczema of the nipple/areola, dyshidrosis, and follicular eczema have been reported. The likelihood for eczematous flares in nonpregnant and postpartum states has not been elucidated.

Differential diagnoses include obstetric cholestasis, contact dermatitis, drug eruptions, and infestations such as scabies. **The earlier onset, prior to the third trimester, may help distinguish AEP from other pregnancy dermatoses such as pemphigoid gestationis and PEP.** No histopathologic distinction exists between AEP and PEP. Maternal and fetal prognosis is unaffected in the absence of superinfection. As with all AD, the risk of bacterial or viral infection is increased. Management is as discussed in the AD section.

Prurigo of Pregnancy

Prurigo of pregnancy (PP) affects between 1 in 300 and 1 in 450 pregnancies. It manifests itself with grouped excoriated or crusted pruritic papules over the extensor surfaces of the extremities and occasionally on the trunk and elsewhere (see Table 51-2).[1] The condition lacks pathognomonic histopathologic features, and skin immunofluorescence is negative. Serologic tests may show elevated IgE levels.[16] Early reports[95] of a dismal fetal outcome in patients with PP have not been confirmed by subsequent studies, and **PP has not been associated with increased maternal risk.** PP should be differentiated from pruritic dermatoses unrelated to pregnancy, other specific dermatoses of pregnancy, drug eruptions, arthropod bites, and infestations such as scabies. PP is treated with moderately potent topical steroids, if necessary intralesional or under occlusion, and oral antihistamines.[85] A short course of oral steroids is rarely required.

PP has been associated with a family history of intrahepatic cholestasis of pregnancy (ICP; see Chapter 47). **It has been proposed that PP and ICP are closely related conditions, distinguished only by the absence of primary lesions in ICP.**[16] These authors reported an association with a personal or family history of AD and elevation of serum IgE (uncontrolled) and suggested that PP may be the result of ICP in women with an atopic predisposition. A reclassification of PP under AEP by the same group[17] has been debated[18] because some PP patients have no history of AD and no established atopic background, and several PP patients fulfill only minor criteria of atopy.[17] Furthermore, the association with atopy has not been confirmed by other groups, and the importance of mild serum IgE elevations in pregnancy has been controversial.[18,20]

Pruritic Folliculitis of Pregnancy

Pruritic folliculitis of pregnancy (PFP) is a rare specific dermatosis of pregnancy, the exact prevalence of which remains unknown (see Table 51-2). Approximately 30 cases have been reported.[20] **PFP presents with pruritic follicular erythematous papules and pustules that affect primarily the trunk** (Fig. 51-7).[96] PFP resolves spontaneously at delivery or postpartum but may recur in subsequent pregnancies.[71] The histopathology is that of folliculitis, and special stains for microorganisms are negative. Skin immunofluorescence studies and serology are negative. The differential diagnosis of PFP includes an infectious folliculitis and specific dermatoses of pregnancy. An infectious folliculitis can be ruled out with stains for microorganisms and cultures from the pustular lesions. PFP was associated with decreased birthweight and a male to female ratio of 2:1 in one study.[16] Preterm delivery was reported in one case, but no other maternal or fetal risks have been noted.

The pregnant patient should be reassured that **PFP resolves postpartum and has not been associated with substantial risks for the fetus.** PFP has been treated with low potency or midpotent topical steroids, benzoyl peroxide, and UVB.[97] The etiology of PFP remains unknown. Increased serum androgen levels in PFP or association with ICP have been reported but were probably coincidental. It has been postulated that PFP may be a form of hormonally induced acne, based on clinical similarities with the acne that develops after the administration of systemic steroids or progestogens.[98] Other authors[71] have considered PFP to be a variant of PEP based on reports of follicular lesions in some PEP patients. Nevertheless, the clinical presentation and histopathology of PFP differs overall from those of PEP. An association with *Pityrosporum* has been debated.[99] A reclassification[17] of PFP under AEP on the basis of personal and family history of eczema in a patient with PFP has been debated[18] because history of atopy has not been reported in other PFP cases. Further studies are required to define whether PFP is a distinct specific dermatosis of pregnancy.

KEY POINTS

- With the physiologic skin changes of pregnancy, no risks are incurred for the mother or fetus. The changes should be expected to resolve postpartum.
- Preexisting melanocytic nevi may show mild changes in pregnancy, but no increased risk for malignant transformation exists.
- Preexisting skin disorders are more likely to worsen than improve in pregnancy; atopic dermatitis (eczema) is the most common dermatosis in pregnancy.
- Prognosis of melanoma is not adversely affected by pregnancy.
- Pruritus occurs in up to 3% to 14% of pregnancies. A constellation of clinical and laboratory findings is crucial to establishing etiology.
- Impetigo herpetiformis (pustular psoriasis of pregnancy) is often associated with reduced calcium or vitamin D. Serious maternal and fetal risks are associated with this disease.
- PG typically flares at delivery, and treatment is with oral steroids. Mild fetal risks—such as small-for-gestational-age infants, preterm delivery, and neonatal PG—have been associated with this disease.
- PEP commonly starts in the abdominal striae and spares the periumbilical area. It is associated with multiple gestation pregnancy, but no maternal or fetal risks are apparent.
- PP and PFP carry no maternal or fetal risks.

REFERENCES

1. Kroumpouzos G, Cohen LM. Dermatoses of pregnancy. *J Am Acad Dermatol.* 2001;45:1.
2. Winton GB, Lewis CW. Dermatoses of pregnancy. *J Am Acad Dermatol.* 1982;6:977.
3. Higgins WM, Jenkins J, Horn T, et al. Pregnancy-associated hyperkeratosis of the nipple: a report of 25 patients. *JAMA Dermatol.* 2013;149:722.
4. Wong RC, Ellis CN. Physiologic skin changes in pregnancy. *J Am Acad Dermatol.* 1984;10:929.
5. Sanchez NP, Pathak MA, Sato S, et al. Melasma: a clinical, light microscopic, ultrastructural, and immunofluorescence study. *J Am Acad Dermatol.* 1981;4:698.
6. Snell RS, Bischitz PG. The effects of large doses of estrogen and progesterone on melanin pigmentation. *J Invest Dermatol.* 1960;35:73.
7. Kligman AM, Willis I. A new formula for depigmenting human skin. *Arch Dermatol.* 1975;111:40.
8. Angsuwarangsee S, Polnikorn N. Combined ultrapulse CO2 laser and Q-switched alexandrite laser compared with Q-switched alexandrite laser alone for refractory melasma: split-face design. *Dermatol Surg.* 2003;29:59.
9. Tse Y, Levine VJ, McClain SA, et al. The removal of cutaneous pigmented lesions with the Q-switched ruby laser and the Q-switched neodymium: yttrium-aluminum-garnet laser: a comparative study. *J Dermatol Surgery Oncol.* 1994;20:795.
10. Lee GY, Kim HJ, Whang KK. The effect of combination treatment of the recalcitrant pigmentary disorders with pigmented laser and chemical peeling. *Dermatol Surg.* 2002;28:1120.
11. Kroumpouzos G, Avgerinou G, Granter S. Acanthosis nigricans without diabetes during pregnancy. *Br J Dermatol.* 2002;146:925.
12. Kroumpouzos G. Skin disease. In: James DK, Steer PJ, Weiner CP, Gonik B, Crowther CA, Robson SC, eds. *High-Risk Pregnancy: Management Options.* 4th ed. Philadelphia: Elsevier Saunders; 2011:929.
13. Khader YS, Ta'ani Q. Periodontal diseases and the risk of preterm birth and low birth weight: a meta-analysis. *J Periodontol.* 2005;76:161.
14. Rangel O, Arias I, Garcia E, Lopez-Padilla S. Topical tretinoin 0.1% for pregnancy-related abdominal striae: an open-label, multicenter, prospective study. *Adv Ther.* 2001;18:181.
15. Winton GB. Skin diseases aggravated by pregnancy. *J Am Acad Dermatol.* 1989;20:1.
16. Vaughan Jones SA, Hern S, Nelson-Piercy C, et al. A prospective study of 200 women with dermatoses of pregnancy correlating the clinical findings with hormonal and immunopathological profiles. *Br J Dermatol.* 1999;141:71.
17. Ambros-Rudolph CM, Müllegger RR, Vaughan-Jones SA, et al. The specific dermatoses of pregnancy revisited and reclassified: results of a retrospective two-center study on 505 pregnant patients. *J Am Acad Dermatol.* 2006;54:395.
18. Cohen LM, Kroumpouzos G. Pruritic dermatoses of pregnancy: to lump or to split? *J Am Acad Dermatol.* 2007;56:708.
19. Hanifin JM, Rajka G. Diagnostic features of atopic eczema. *Acta Derm Venereol.* 1980;92(suppl):44.
20. Kroumpouzos G. Specific dermatoses of pregnancy: advances and controversies. *Expert Rev Dermatol.* 2010;5:633.
21. Moore MM, Rifas-Shiman SL, Rich-Edwards JW, et al. Perinatal predictors of atopic dermatitis occurring in the first six months of life. *Pediatrics.* 2004;113:468.
22. Schafer T, Dirschedl P, Kunz B. Maternal smoking during pregnancy and lactation increases the risk for atopic eczema in the offspring. *J Am Acad Dermatol.* 1997;36:550.
23. Wuthrich B, Schmid-Grendelmeier P. The atopic eczema/dermatitis syndrome. Epidemiology, natural course, and immunology of the IgE-associated ("extrinsic") and the nonallergic ("intrinsic") AEDS. *J Investig Allergol Clin Immunol.* 2003;13:1.
24. Cho S, Kim HJ, Oh SH, et al. The influence of pregnancy and menstruation on the deterioration of atopic dermatitis symptoms. *Ann Dermatol.* 2010;22:180.
25. Hale EK, Pomeranz MK. Dermatologic agents during pregnancy and lactation: an update and clinical review. *Int J Dermatol.* 2002;41:197.
26. Kainz A, Harabacz I, Cowlrick IS, et al. Review of the course and outcome of 100 pregnancies in 84 women treated with tacrolimus. *Transplantation.* 2000;70:1718.
27. Shaw JC, White LE. Persistent acne in adult women. *Arch Dermatol.* 2001;137:1252.
28. Boyd AS, Morris LF, Phillips CM, et al. Psoriasis and pregnancy: hormone and immune system interaction. *Int J Dermatol.* 1996;35:169.
29. Tauscher AE, Fleischer AB Jr, Phelps KC, et al. Psoriasis and pregnancy. *J Cutan Med Surg.* 2002;6:561.
30. Bierman SM. Autoimmune progesterone dermatitis of pregnancy. *Arch Dermatol.* 1973;107:896.
31. Lee AY, Lee KH, Lim YG. Oestrogen urticaria associated with pregnancy. *Br J Dermatol.* 1999;141:774.
32. Bajaj AK, Swarup V, Gupta OP, et al. Impetigo herpetiformis. *Dermatologica.* 1977;155:292.
33. Ott F, Krakowski A, Tur E, et al. Impetigo herpetiformis with lowered serum level of vitamin D and its diminished intestinal absorption. *Dermatologica.* 1982;164:360.
34. Oumeish OY, Farraj SE, Bataineh AS. Some aspects of impetigo herpetiformis. *Arch Dermatol.* 1982;118:103.
35. Rackett SC, Baughman RD. Impetigo herpetiformis and Staphylococcus aureus lymphadenitis in a pregnant adolescent. *Pediatric Dermatol.* 1997;14:387.
36. Beveridge GW, Harkness RA, Livingston JR. Impetigo herpetiformis in two successive pregnancies. *Br J Dermatol.* 1966;78:106.
37. Finch TM, Tan CY. Pustular psoriasis exacerbated by pregnancy and controlled by cyclosporin A [Letter]. *Br J Dermatol.* 2000;142:582.
38. Gimenez-Garcia R, Gimenez Garcia MC, Llorente de la Fuente A. Impetigo herpetiformis: response to steroids and etretinate. *Int J Dermatol.* 1989;28:551.
39. Breier-Maly J, Ortel B, Breier F, et al. Generalized pustular psoriasis of pregnancy (impetigo herpetiformis). *Dermatology.* 1999;198:61.
40. Gutierrez G, Dagnino R, Mintz G. Polymyositis/dermatomyositis and pregnancy. *Arthritis Rheum.* 1984;27:291.
41. Steen VD. Scleroderma and pregnancy. *Rheum Dis Clin North Am.* 1997;23:133.

42. Yair D, Shenhav M, Botchan A, et al. Pregnancy associated with pemphigus. *Br J Obstet Gynecol*. 1995;102:667.

43. Collier PM, Kelly SE, Wojnarowska FW. Linear IgA disease and pregnancy. *J Am Acad Dermatol*. 1994;30:407.

44. Kardos M, Levine D, Gürkan HM, et al. Pemphigus vulgaris in pregnancy: analysis of current data on the management and outcomes. *Obstet Gynecol Surv*. 2009;64:739.

45. Bronson DM, Barsky R, Barsky S. Acrodermatitis enteropathica: recognition at long last during a recurrence in pregnancy. *J Am Acad Dermatol*. 1983;9:140.

46. Pennoyer JM, Grin CM, Driscoll MS. Changes in size of melanocytic nevi during pregnancy. *J Am Acad Dermatol*. 1997;36:378.

47. Ellis DL. Pregnancy and sex steroid hormone effects on nevi of patients with dysplastic nevus syndrome. *J Am Acad Dermatol*. 1991;25:467.

48. Onsun N, Saracoglu S, Demirkesen C, et al. Eruptive widespread Spitz nevi: can pregnancy be a stimulating factor? *J Am Acad Dermatol*. 1999; 40:866.

49. Rubegni P, Sbano P, Burroni M, et al. Melanocytic skin lesions and pregnancy: digital dermoscopy analysis. *Skin Res Technol*. 2007;13:143.

50. Brodell RT, Helms SE. The changing mole: additional warning signs of malignant melanoma. *Postgrad Med*. 1998;104:145.

51. Steinheim H, Moller B, van Dijk T, Fossa SD. Cause-specific survival for women diagnosed with cancer during pregnancy or lactation: a registry-based cohort study. *J Clin Onc*. 2009;27:45.

52. O'Meara AT, Cress R, Xing G, Danielsen B, Smith LH. Malignant melanoma in pregnancy. A population-based evaluation. *Cancer*. 2005;103:1217.

53. Lens MB, Rosdahl I, Ahlbom A, et al. Effect of pregnancy on survival in women with cutaneous malignant melanoma. *J Clin Oncol*. 2004;22:4369.

54. Travers RL, Sober AJ, Berwick M, et al. Increased thickness of pregnancy-associated melanoma. *Br J Dermatol*. 1995;132:876.

55. Mackie RM, Bufalino R, Morabito A, et al. Lack of effect of pregnancy on outcome of melanoma. *Lancet*. 1991;337:653.

56. Wong JH, Sterns EE, Kopald KH, et al. Prognostic significance of pregnancy in stage I melanoma. *Arch Surg*. 1989;124:1227.

57. Johansson AL, Andersson TM, Plym A, et al. Mortality in women with pregnancy-associated malignant melanoma. *J Am Acad Dermatol*. 2014;71: 1093.

58. Tierney E, Kroumpouzos G, Rogers G. Skin Tumors. In: Kroumpouzos G, ed. *Text Atlas of Obstetric Dermatology*. Philadelphia, PA: Lippincott Williams & Wilkins; 2014:141-151.

59. Balch CM. Prognostic factors analysis of 17,600 melanoma patients: validation of the American Joint Committee on Cancer melanoma staging system. *J Clin Oncol*. 2001;19:3622.

60. Smith M, Fine JA, Barnhill RL, Berwick M. Hormonal and reproductive influences and risk of melanoma in women. *Int J Epidemiol*. 1998;27:751.

61. Lama G, Angelucci C, Bruzzese N, et al. Sensitivity of human melanoma cells to oestrogens, tamoxifen and quercetin: is there any relationship with type I and II oestrogen binding site expression? *Melanoma Res*. 1999;9:530.

62. Flowers JL, Seigler HF, McCarty KS, et al. Absence of estrogen receptors in human melanoma as evaluated by monoclonal antiestrogen receptor antibody. *Arch Dermatol*. 1987;123:764.

63. Lecavalier MA, From L, Gaid N. Absence of estrogen receptors in dysplastic nevi and malignant melanoma. *J Am Acad Dermatol*. 1990;23:242.

64. Di Giorgi V, Gori A, Grazzini M, et al. Estrogens, estrogen receptors and melanoma. *Expert Rev Anticancer Ther*. 2011;11:739-747.

65. Thorn M, Adam HO, Ringborg U, et al. Long-term survival in malignant melanoma with special reference to age and sex as prognostic factors. *J Natl Cancer Inst*. 1987;79:969.

66. Ries LG, Pollack ES, Young JL. Cancer patient survival: surveillance, epidemiology and end results program, 1973-79. *J Natl Cancer Inst*. 1983; 70:693.

67. Schwartz JL, Mozurkewich EL, Johnson TM. Current management of patients with melanoma who are pregnant, want to get pregnant, or do not want to get pregnant [editorial]. *Cancer*. 2003;97:2130.

68. Leachman SA, Jackson R, Eliason MJ, et al. Management of melanoma during pregnancy. *Dermatol Nurs*. 2007;19:145.

69. Alexander A, Samlowski WE, Grossman D, et al. Metastatic melanoma in pregnancy: risk of transplacental metastases in the infant. *J Clin Oncol*. 2003;21:2179.

70. Furhoff A. Itching in pregnancy. *Acta Med Scand*. 1974;196:403.

71. Roger D, Vaillant L, Fignon A, et al. Specific pruritic diseases of pregnancy. A prospective study of 3192 pregnant women. *Arch Dermatol*. 1994;130: 734.

72. Morrison LH, Labib RS, Zone JJ, et al. Herpes gestationis autoantibodies recognize a 180-kd human epidermal antigen. *J Clin Invest*. 1988;81:2023.

73. Kelly SE, Black MM. Pemphigoid gestationis: placental interactions. *Semin Dermatol*. 1989;8:12.

74. Engineer L, Bhol K, Ahmed AR. Pemphigoid gestationis: a review. *Am J Obstet Gynecol*. 2000;183:483.

75. Shornick JK, Meek TJ, Nesbitt LT, Gilliam JN. Herpes gestationis in blacks. *Arch Dermatol*. 1984;120:511.

76. Kwon EJ, Ntiamoah P, Shulman KJ. The utility of C4d immunohistochemistry on formalin-fixed paraffin-embedded tissue in the distinction of polymorphic eruption of pregnancy from pemphigoid gestationis. *Am J Dermatopathol*. 2013;35:787.

77. Sitaru C, Powell J, Messer G, et al. Immunoblotting and enzyme-linked immunosorbent assay for the diagnosis of pemphigoid gestationis. *Obstet Gynecol*. 2004;103:757.

78. Boulinguez S, Bedane C, Prost C, et al. Chronic pemphigoid gestationis: comparative clinical and immunopathological study of 10 patients. *Dermatology*. 2003;206:113.

79. Holmes RC, Black MM, Jurecka W, et al. Clues to the etiology and pathogenesis of herpes gestationis. *Br J Dermatol*. 1983;109:131.

80. Shornick JK, Black MM. Secondary autoimmune diseases in herpes gestationis (pemphigoid gestationis). *J Am Acad Dermatol*. 1992;26:563.

81. Shornick JK, Black MM. Fetal risks in herpes gestationis. *J Am Acad Dermatol*. 1992;26:63.

82. Karna P, Broecker AH. Neonatal herpes gestationis. *J Pediatr*. 1991;119:299.

83. Lawley TJ, Hertz KC, Wade TR, et al. Pruritic urticarial papules and plaques of pregnancy. *JAMA*. 1979;241:1696.

84. Aronson IK, Bond S, Fiedler VC, et al. Pruritic urticarial papules and plaques of pregnancy: clinical and immunopathologic observations in 57 patients. *J Am Acad Dermatol*. 1998;39:933.

85. Kroumpouzos G, Cohen LM. Specific dermatoses of pregnancy: an evidence-based systematic review. *Am J Obstet Gynecol*. 2003;188:1083.

86. Rudolph CM, Al-Fares S, Vaughan-Jones SA, et al. Polymorphic eruption of pregnancy: clinicopathology and potential risk factors in 181 patients. *Br J Dermatol*. 2006;154:54.

87. Carli P, Tarocchi S, Mello G, et al. Skin immune system activation in pruritic urticarial papules and plaques of pregnancy. *Int J Dermatol*. 1994; 33:884.

88. Cohen LM, Capeless EL, Krusinski PA, et al. Pruritic urticarial papules and plaques of pregnancy and its relationship to maternal-fetal weight gain and twin pregnancy. *Arch Dermatol*. 1989;125:1534.

89. Elling SV, McKenna P, Powell FC. Pruritic urticarial papules and plaques of pregnancy in twin and triplet pregnancies. *J Eur Acad Dermatol Venereol*. 2000;14:378.

90. Im S, Lee ES, Kim W, et al. Expression of progesterone receptor in human keratinocytes. *J Korean Med Sci*. 2000;15:647.

91. Aractingi S, Bertheau P, Le Goue C, et al. Fetal DNA in skin of polymorphic eruptions of pregnancy. *Lancet*. 1998;352:1898.

92. Regnier S, Fermand V, Levy P, et al. A case-control study of polymorphic eruption of pregnancy. *J Am Acad Dermatol*. 2008;58:63.

93. Koutroulis I, Papoutsis J, Kroumpouzos G. Atopic dermatitis in pregnancy: current status and challenges. *Obst Gynecol Surv*. 2011;66:654.

94. Kroumpouzos G, Cohen LM. Prurigo, Pruritic Folliculitis, and Atopic Eruption of Pregnancy. In: Kroumpouzos G, ed. *Text Atlas of Obstetric Dermatology*. Philadelphia, PA: Lippincott Williams & Wilkins; 2014: 205-216.

95. Spangler AS, Reddy W, Bardawil WA, et al. Papular dermatitis of pregnancy: a new clinical entity? *JAMA*. 1962;181:577.

96. Zoberman E, Farmer ER. Pruritic folliculitis of pregnancy. *Arch Dermatol*. 1981;117:20.

97. Kroumpouzos G, Cohen LM. Pruritic folliculitis of pregnancy. *J Am Acad Dermatol*. 2000;43:132.

98. Kroumpouzos G, Cohen LM. Diseases of pregnancy and their treatment. In: Krieg T, Bickers D, Miyachi Y, eds. *Therapy of Skin Diseases*. Berlin: Springer Verlag; 2010:677.

99. Kroumpouzos G. Pityrosporum folliculitis during pregnancy is not pruritic folliculitis of pregnancy. *J Am Acad Dermatol*. 2005;53:1098.

Maternal and Perinatal Infection: Chlamydia, Gonorrhea, and Syphilis in Pregnancy

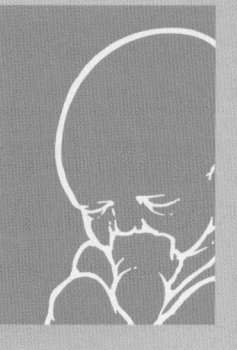

CHAPTER 52

JESSICA L. NYHOLM, KIRK D. RAMIN, and DANIEL V. LANDERS

KEY ABBREVIATIONS

By mouth (per os)	PO
Centers for Disease Control and Prevention	CDC
Central nervous system	CNS
Cerebrospinal fluid	CSF
Direct fluorescence assay	DFA
Elementary body	EB
Enzyme immunoassay	EIA
Human immunodeficiency virus	HIV
Human papillomavirus	HPV
Institute of Medicine	IOM
Intramuscularly	IM
Intravenously	IV
Lipopolysaccharide	LPS
Major outer membrane protein	MOMP
Morbidity and Mortality Weekly Report	MMWR
Nucleic acid amplification test	NAAT
Polymerase chain reaction	PCR
Rapid plasma reagin	RPR
Reticulate body	RB
Ribonucleic acid	RNA
Sexually transmitted disease	STD
Venereal disease research laboratory	VDRL
World Health Organization	WHO

Maternal and perinatal infections represent common complications of the peripartum interval. In many industrialized nations, the role of sexually transmitted pathogens is declining in its relative contribution to infections in women; however, in the United States and developing nations, the epidemic persists. Many of these pathogens are either proved or presumed to play an integral role in infectious morbidities of pregnancy and the neonatal period, and thus understanding the social, economic, and pathophysiologic burden is essential. Indeed, as our ability to readily screen the population as a whole has improved for the most prevalent or serious of these infectious agents—*Chlamydia trachomatis, Neisseria gonorrhoeae,* and *Treponema pallidum*—epidemiologic statistics have provided evidence for their implied role in preterm labor, preterm premature rupture of the membranes, intrauterine growth restriction, neonatal conjunctivitis, neonatal pneumonia, and congenital syphilis. Thus a greater understanding of the role of these prevalent pathogens in mediating disease pathogenesis has mandated that the obstetrician be well versed in the identification and management of these organisms. In this chapter, we review current trends in epidemiology, diagnosis, treatment, and prevention of common sexually transmitted infections.

CHLAMYDIA

Epidemiology

The two most valuable sources of incidence and prevalence data on sexually transmitted pathogens are provided by the Centers for Disease Control and Prevention (CDC) and the World Health Organization (WHO). The CDC reports sexually transmitted disease (STD) estimates for the United States using reported cases and estimates after accounting for underreporting. The Institute of Medicine (IOM) provides WHO estimates on worldwide incidences and prevalence of the four curable sexually transmitted infections: *Chlamydia,* gonorrhea, syphilis, and *Trichomonas.* **Overall, the WHO 2008 global estimate places the incidence at 105.7 million new cases of chlamydia infection, 106.1 million new cases of gonorrhea, and 10.6 million new cases of syphilis among people aged 15 to 49 years.** In addition, epidemiologic studies have revealed a number of basic principles regarding STDs: (1) sexually active adolescents have the highest rates of STDs of any age group[1]; (2) sex differences are observed in the transmission of the most prevalent STDs, with more efficient transmission from men to women; (3) curable STDs (i.e., not human immunodeficiency virus [HIV], human papillomavirus [HPV], or chronic recurrent herpes simplex virus [HSV]) are associated with more serious long-term consequences in women than in men; (4) having one or more STDs predisposes an individual to acquisition and transmission of other STDs; (5) STDs in developing nations are often constantly prevalent at a high rate and affect all age groups; and (6) marked racial disparity is apparent.

Genital tract chlamydial infections are generally ascribed to *C. trachomatis* and account for the most prevalent reported infectious disease in the United States. In 2013, more than 1.4 million cases were reported to the CDC.[2] However, the actual presumed number of new cases in the United States, accounting for estimates of underreporting, is estimated at 3 million annually.[1] **These infections present unique problems for public health control programs because 50% to 70% of these infections are clinically silent in women.** Unrecognized and untreated, the bacteria may remain infectious in the host for months and is readily transmitted to sex partners. Furthermore, **most reported infections occur in the 15- to 24-year-old age group,** individuals who often do not participate in preventive health care programs. Estimates on worldwide exposure approximate that 90 million new cases of *C. trachomatis* infection occur on an annual basis, which accounts for a rising majority of perinatal and neonatal complications.[3-6] Of note, a primary goal of the Healthy People 2010 U.S. health promotion initiative is the elimination of racial disparities among multiple sexually transmitted pathogens. An assessment of the racial disparities of nationally notifiable disease for the year 2002 revealed a nearly tenfold increased rate for *Chlamydia* in blacks compared with whites (805.9 vs. 90.2 per 100,000).[7] In 2013, the rate of *Chlamydia* remained 6.4 times higher among blacks compared with whites, although the rate in whites doubled in that same span of time (1147.2 vs. 180.3 per 100,000).[2]

The cost of treatment, prevention, and management of complications of chlamydial infections is estimated at $2.4 billion annually.[4-6] Taken together, these factors have resulted in **the endorsement of a nationwide broad-based screening program by both the CDC and IOM.**

Pathogenesis

Chlamydia is a sexually transmitted pathogen generally associated with endocervical infection.[8,9] Species of *Chlamydia* were initially serotyped according to their biologic and biochemical properties, and a greater than 95% homology in their 16s ribosomal ribonucleic acid (RNA) sequences was observed. Subsequent molecular analyses led to the reclassification of some *C. psittaci* strains as *C. pneumoniae,* a human pathogen, and *C. pecorum,* a pathogen of ruminants. Nevertheless, of the four species mentioned here, **only *C. trachomatis* and *C. pneumoniae* claim primates as their endogenous hosts.** Each of the species bears multiple strains based on serotype, which in turn are associated with distinct clinical entities. These are summarized in Table 52-1.

Chlamydiae are obligate intracellular bacteria that grow in eukaryotic epithelial cells, and they have a unique growth cycle, distinct from all other pathogens. During the 1970s, the infectivity and growth cycle of chlamydiae was initially characterized.[10-14] Known to specifically infect the cuboidal or nonciliated columnar epithelial cells common to the endocervix, urethra, and conjunctiva, this growth cycle involves infection of a susceptible host cell through a receptor-specific phagocytic process. This phagocytic process involves chlamydiae *elementary bodies* (EBs) that bind to the host cell through a heparin sulfate–like molecule to glycosaminoglycan receptors, and these subsequently are phagocytosed into cytoplasmic vacuoles termed *phagosomes.*[15] In this fashion, chlamydiae may be considered to

TABLE 52-1	SPECTRUM OF HUMAN AND MAMMALIAN DISEASES CAUSED BY CHLAMYDIAE SEROTYPES	
SPECIES SEROTYPE	**ACUTE DISEASES**	**CLINICAL SEQUELAE**
Chlamydia trachomatis A, B, Ba, C D-K	Conjunctivitis, acute urethral syndrome, cervicitis, endometritis, salpingitis, inclusion conjunctivitis, neonatal pneumonia	Trachoma, proctitis, epididymitis, Reiter syndrome, pelvic inflammatory disease, ectopic pregnancy, tubal infertility, Fitz-Hugh–Curtis syndrome
L1, L2, L3	Lymphogranuloma venereum	Reactive airway disease
Chlamydia pneumoniae	Pharyngitis, sinusitis, bronchitis, community-acquired pneumonia	Infection is often asymptomatic or mild with only rare life-threatening infection
Chlamydia psittaci Parrots, cats, ewes	Atypical pneumonia, conjunctivitis	Spontaneous abortion

have a unique biphasic life cycle with dimorphic forms that are functionally and morphologically distinct. Once endocytosed, the EB differentiates into a larger pleomorphic form called the *reticulate body* (RB), which replicates by binary fission. The chlamydiae remain in the phagosome throughout their growth cycle, presumptively as an acquired means of escaping host lysosomes.[12-13] The endosome is transported to the distal region of the Golgi apparatus and incorporates host-derived sphingolipids into the inclusion membrane. Thus it appears that chlamydiae are able to intercept host vesicular traffic bound for the plasma membrane to sequester lipids and possibly other host substances synthesized in the Golgi. Subversion of host vesicular traffic may represent a dual advantage for chlamydiae in obtaining materials from the host for its metabolism as well as in modifying the inclusion membrane to evade lysosomal fusion and immune detection.

Because chlamydiae depend on their host cell for the generation of adenosine triphosphate (ATP), they require viable cells for survival.[16] Chlamydiae are incapable of de novo nucleotide biosynthesis and thus are dependent on host nucleotide pools. In this manner, this unique pathogen may be considered to be viruslike. On the other hand, chlamydiae resemble a bacterial pathogen in that they contain both DNA and RNA; have a modified rigid cell wall with a lipopolysaccharide (LPS) similar to that in the outer membrane of gram-negative bacteria, albeit lacking the intervening peptidoglycan layer; and multiply by binary fission.[12-16]

Some interesting insights into the interaction of chlamydiae and the host immune system have emerged in the past decade. These new observations include the extensive but unexpected polymorphism of the major outer membrane protein (MOMP), the evidence for genetic susceptibility to disease, and the association of antibody response to the 60-kDa heat shock protein CHSP60 with the development of adverse sequelae following ocular and genital infections. By way of summary, **MOMP is a major target for protective host immune responses, such as neutralizing antibodies and possibly protective T-cell responses.**[17,18] The basis for MOMP antigenic variation is allelic polymorphism at the omp-1 locus, and immune selection appears to be occurring in host populations frequently exposed to *C. trachomatis.*[19] Combined with the observations that clear genetic susceptibility to disease is apparent, because only a subset of infected individuals appear to have long-term complications after acute or repeated chlamydial infections, it is now believed that **chronic immune activation plays a role in propagating clinical disease.**[20] Thus susceptibility to chlamydial pelvic inflammatory disease (PID) in a study of sex workers in Nairobi, Kenya has been associated with a human leukocyte antigen (HLA) class I allele, HLA-A31.[21-23] Similarly, allelic variation in the class II allele (DQ) have been shown to be positively associated with *C. trachomatis* tubal infertility.[23,24]

In addition to host genotype playing a role in determining the severity of *Chlamydia*-mediated disease, **aberrations in humoral immunity also appear to modulate clinical disease.** Antibody response to a 57-kDa chlamydial protein was initially observed more frequently in women with tubal infertility than in controls.[9,20] This protein was subsequently identified as a heat shock protein (HSP) of the GroEL family of stress proteins. The association between antibody response to CHSP60 and PID, ectopic pregnancy, tubal infertility, and trachoma has been subsequently observed in a number of population-based serotype studies.[9,10] Suffice it to say that although it remains unclear whether antibody to CHSP60 is causally involved in chlamydial immunopathogenesis or is merely a marker of persistent chlamydial infection, in cells that remain infected with *C. trachomatis,* the constitutive expression of CHSP60 may provide continued antigenic stimulation for the CHSP60 antibody response observed in persons with long-term sequelae. Moreover, observed immunopathology may also result from aberrations in self-tolerance mediated by shared and similar epitopes between CHSP60 and endogenous HSP60, which in turn results in a classic immune cascade that leads to tissue damage.

Diagnosis

Because curative antibiotic therapies for chlamydial infections are available and inexpensive, early diagnosis is an essential component of management and prevention. Historically, isolation of *Chlamydia* in cell culture was the traditional method for laboratory diagnosis, and it has remained the gold standard because of its specificity. However, culture requires expensive equipment, technical expertise, and stringent transport conditions to preserve specimen viability. Thus **chlamydial culture has been replaced by nucleic acid amplification tests (NAATs), which are currently recommended for screening for urogenital *C. trachomatis* in men and women, regardless of symptoms.**[25] The common characteristic among NAATs is that they are designed to amplify nucleic acid sequences that are specific for the organism being detected and thus do not require viable organisms. The increased sensitivity of NAATs is attributable to their ability to produce a positive signal from as little as a single copy of the target DNA or RNA. **NAATs can be utilized to test for *C. trachomatis* in endocervical swabs from women, urethral swabs from men, first-catch urine from both men and women, and vaginal swabs from women.**[25] **The ability of NAATs to detect *C. trachomatis* without a pelvic examination is a key advantage of NAATs, and this ability facilitates screening men and women in nontraditional screening venues.** Although false-positive and false-negative results can occur, the performance of NAATs for testing for *C. trachomatis* is superior to both culture and other nonculture tests. The sensitivity of NAATs is generally greater than 90%, and specificity is greater than 99%.[25] Given the performance of the NAATs,

TABLE 52-2 SCREENING FOR *CHLAMYDIA TRACHOMATIS* INFECTIONS IN PREGNANCY

When to screen	• All pregnant women <25 years and older women at increased risk. • Retest in the third trimester for women <25 years or at increased risk. • Women treated during pregnancy should be retested 3-4 weeks after treatment and be retested within 3 months.
How to screen	• Nucleic acid amplification tests (NAATs) of urine, endocervix, or vagina are preferred.*
Diagnostic criteria	• Positive NAATs are diagnostic.

Modified from Workowski KA, Bolan GA; Centers for Disease Control and Prevention. Sexually transmitted diseases treatment guidelines, 2015. *MMWR Morb Mortal Wkly Rep.* 2015;64(RR-03):1-137.
*Cell culture, direct immunofluorescence, enzyme immunosorbent assay, and nucleic acid hybridization of endocervical specimens are also available.

supplemental testing of NAAT-positive specimens is no longer recommended by the CDC. An additional consideration when using NAATs for detection of *C. trachomatis* is that they are not approved by the Food and Drug Administration (FDA) for test of cure because nucleic acid may remain from noninfective bacteria following treatment for up to 3 weeks after infection with *C. trachomatis.*

Other antigen-detection methods—such as enzyme immunoassay (EIA), direct fluorescence assay (DFA), nucleic acid hybridization/probe tests, and nucleic acid genetic transformation tests—are also available but are generally not recommended for routine testing for genital tract specimens. Additionally, serology screening has limited or no value in testing for uncomplicated genital *C. trachomatis* infection and should not be used for screening because previous chlamydial infection frequently elicits long-lasting antibodies that cannot be easily distinguished from the antibodies produced in a current infection. Table 52-2 summarizes the screening recommendations for *C. trachomatis* in pregnancy.

Treatment

The recommended treatment regimen for uncomplicated genital *Chlamydia* infection has remained largely unchanged since 1998, with the exception of amoxicillin now being considered an alternative regimen due to treatment failures in response to penicillin-class antibiotics in vitro and in animal studies. **In pregnancy, the CDC recommends azithromycin in a single 1-g oral dose** (Box 52-1). Amoxicillin 500 mg orally three times daily for 7 days and various erythromycin formulations are also available with dosing that can be utilized as an alternative regimen (see Box 52-1). **Doxycycline, ofloxacin, and levofloxacin are part of the treatment options in a nonpregnant patient; however, they are contraindicated in pregnancy and should not be used in this population.** To minimize transmission and reinfection, patients should be instructed to abstain from sexual intercourse for 7 days after single-dose therapy or until completion of a 7-day regimen and should also be instructed to abstain from sexual intercourse until all of their sex partners have been treated for the same duration. **A repeat chlamydial test should be performed 3 to 4 weeks after treatment is completed.** Longitudinal studies of *Chlamydia*-infected adolescent female patients have demonstrated a high risk for *Chlamydia* reinfection and for other STD infections within a few months of initial diagnosis. Because of the high incidence of

Chlamydia infection that can occur in the months following a treated infection, CDC guidelines recommend that health care providers repeat testing 3 months after infection.[26] Additionally, **women under the age of 25 and patients at high risk for *Chlamydia* infection should be retested in the third trimester of pregnancy.** In addition to treating the pregnant woman, any sex partners within the preceding 60 days of diagnosis—or the most recent sex partner, if that has been longer than 60 days—should be evaluated and treated to help reduce the rate of reinfection as well as infection of others.[26]

GONORRHEA

Epidemiology

The reported incidence of *Neisseria gonorrhoeae* infection was 333,004 cases in the United States in 2013 (106.1 cases per 100,000).[2] However, the actual number of reported cases may be underrepresented by as much as 40%, yielding a U.S. estimate of 700,000 cases annually.[27] In contrast to *Chlamydia*, the worldwide prevalence of gonorrhea may be significantly less than that observed in the United States, as supported by epidemiologic data from Canada and Western Europe.[28]

Historically, a review of trends in the incidence of reported gonorrhea in the United States from 1941 to 1997 reveals peak increases among both men and women in the interval around World War II and again in 1975, peaking at 473 cases per 100,000.[27] The steady decline since 1975 has been accompanied by three interesting observations. First, the male-to-female ratio of reported cases not only declined from a high of 3:1, it changed to a female prevalence in 2013, by a ratio of 1:2.[2,8] Second, racial disparity is noted, with a 12.4-fold higher rate among blacks compared with whites (426.6 vs. 34.5 per 100,000).[2] **Third, the single greatest determinant of** gonorrhea incidence since 1975 has so far been age: annual reported cases are highest in adolescents aged 15 to 19 years (459.2 per 100,000) **and in young adults aged 20 to 24 years** (541.6 per 100,000).[2]

Pathogenesis

In contrast to chlamydiae species, the pathogenesis of *N. gonorrhoeae* and human disease is more straightforward and reflects classic bacterial pathogenesis. ***N. gonorrhoeae* is a gram-negative diplococcus for which humans are the only natural host.** Like the other endocervical infectious pathogens, gonorrhea also bears a predilection for the columnar epithelium, which lines the mucous membranes of the anogenital tract.[27,29] Gonococcal pathogens adhere to these mucosal cells through attachment of pili and other surface proteins, which results in the release of lipopolysaccharide and likely instigates mucosal damage. Following adherence, *N. gonorrhoeae* is pinocytosed and is thereby transported into epithelial cells. Unlike chlamydiae, the gonococcus does not replicate in the phagosome, and hence it evades lysosomal degradation. **Rather gonococci persist in the host by virtue of their ability to alter the host environment.** In sum, multiple structures of *N. gonorrhoeae* enable pathogenesis by a variety of immune-evasive mechanisms that include immunoglobulin A (IgA) protease, iron repression, and cell-adherence mechanisms.[27,29]

Diagnosis

The gold standard for diagnosis of gonorrhea infection was previously isolation of the organism by culture. Traditionally, specimens are streaked on a selective (Thayer-Martin or Martin-Lewis) or nonselective (chocolate agar) medium. Inoculated media are incubated at 35° to 36.5°C in an atmosphere supplemented with 5% CO_2 and are evaluated at 24 and 48 hours. Subsequent diagnosis is made by identification of the organism with growth on the medium, with a Gram stain and oxidase test on colonies identifying Gram-negative, oxidase-positive diplococci morphology. A confirmed laboratory diagnosis of *N. gonorrhoeae* cannot be made on the basis of these tests alone. However, **antimicrobial therapy should be initiated following an initial presumptive test result, but additional tests must be performed to confirm the identity of an isolate as *N. gonorrhoeae*.** Whereas culture isolation is also suitable for non–genital tract specimens, using selective media is necessary if the anatomic source of the specimen normally contains other bacterial species.

The advantages of gonorrheal culture are high sensitivity and specificity, low cost, suitability for use with different types of specimens, and the ability to retain the isolate for additional testing. The major disadvantage of culture for *N. gonorrhoeae* is that specimens must be transported under conditions adequate to maintain the viability of organisms. Another disadvantage is that a minimum of 24 to 48 hours is required from specimen collection to the report of a presumptive culture result.[25] Due to the technical difficulties with culture, other nonculture tests were developed. However, the importance of maintaining the option of culture remains important for *N. gonorrhoeae*. **Indications for culture for *N. gonorrhoeae* include testing in suspected cases of treatment failure, monitoring antibiotic resistance, and testing in cases of suspected extragenital infection and exposure due to sexual abuse.**

As with *C. trachomatis*, the **current recommended test for routine screening for *N. gonorrhoeae* is NAATs** regardless of

TABLE 52-3	SCREENING FOR *NEISSERIA GONORRHOEAE* INFECTIONS IN PREGNANCY
When to screen	• Women <25 years and older women at increased risk. • Women treated during pregnancy should be retested 3 months after infection.
How to screen	• Nucleic acid amplification tests (NAATs) of urine, endocervix, or vagina are preferred.*
Diagnostic criteria	• A positive NAAT is diagnostic.

Modified from Workowski KA, Bolan GA; Centers for Disease Control and Prevention. Sexually transmitted diseases treatment guidelines, 2015. *MMWR Morb Mortal Wkly Rep.* 2015;64(RR-03):1-137.
*Cell culture and nucleic acid hybridization of endocervical specimens are also available.

BOX 52-2 RECOMMENDED TREATMENT REGIMEN* FOR UNCOMPLICATED GENITAL *NEISSERIA GONORRHOEAE* INFECTIONS IN PREGNANCY[†]

Standard Regimen

Ceftriaxone, 250 mg intramuscularly in a single dose
Plus azithromycin, 1g orally in a single dose

Modified from Workowski KA, Bolan GA; Centers for Disease Control and Prevention. Sexually transmitted diseases treatment guidelines, 2015. *MMWR Morb Mortal Wkly Rep.* 2015;64(RR-03):1-137.
*The Centers for Disease Control and Prevention recommends treating individuals with a positive gonorrhea test result for both gonorrhea and *Chlamydia*. Consult with an infectious disease specialist if the patient has cephalosporin allergy and spectinomycin is not available.
[†]Sex partners within the preceding 60 days of diagnosis, or most recent sex partner if that has been longer than 60 days, should be evaluated and treated for *Neisseria Gonorrhoeae*.

symptoms.[25] **NAATs can be utilized to test for *N. gonorrhoeae* in endocervical swabs from women, urethral swabs from men, first-catch urine from both men and women, and vaginal swabs from women.**[25] **The ability of NAATs to detect *N. gonorrhoeae* without a pelvic examination is a key advantage of NAATs, and this ability facilitates screening men and women in nontraditional screening venues.** Whereas false-positive and false-negative results can occur, the performance of NAATs for testing for *N. gonorrhoeae* is superior to both culture and other nonculture tests. The sensitivity of NAATs is generally greater than 90%, and specificity is greater than 99%.[25] **Given the performance of NAATs, supplemental testing of NAAT-positive specimens is no longer recommended by the CDC.** An additional consideration when using NAATs for detection of *N. gonorrhoeae* is that they are not FDA approved for test of cure because nucleic acid may remain from noninfective bacteria following treatment for up to 2 weeks.

Additional tests have been studied for *N. gonorrhoeae* testing. Nucleic acid hybridization assays are available to detect *N. gonorrhoeae*, although they are not recommended for routine use and are no longer routinely available. A large number of EIA tests for detecting *N. gonorrhoeae* infection have been studied, but their performance and cost characteristics for *N. gonorrhoeae* infection have not made them competitive with other available tests.[25] Similar to EIAs, DFA is also not appropriate as a diagnostic test for the direct detection of *N. gonorrhoeae* in clinical specimens.[25] A serologic screening or diagnostic assay is not available for *N. gonorrhoeae*. Table 52-3 reviews the recommended screening for *N. gonorrhoeae* in infections in pregnancy.

Treatment

Although uncomplicated genital gonorrhea infections can be treated with single-dose therapy, fewer oral treatment options are available compared with the efficacious therapies available for chlamydial infections (Box 52-2). Moreover, recent emergence of quinolone-resistant *N. gonorrhoeae* in California, Hawaii, Asia, and the Pacific Islands has led to the generalized recommendation that these agents should not be used to treat gonorrhea infections acquired in these areas or in areas with an increased prevalence of quinolone resistance.[25] The CDC recommendations became somewhat complicated in July 2002, when Wyeth Pharmaceuticals discontinued cefixime. However, in April of 2008, Lupin Pharmaceuticals began manufacturing and providing cefixime tablets. Currently, cefixime is only recommended for the treatment of uncomplicated genital *N. gonorrhoeae* infections if ceftriaxone is not available. In addition, **because of the risk for coinfectivity with *N. gonorrhoeae* and**

C. trachomatis, the CDC recommends empirically treating patients with positive gonorrhea test results for both gonorrhea and *Chlamydia*.[25]

In 2007, the Gonococcal Isolate Surveillance Project (GISP) found 27% of *N. gonorrhoeae* infections were resistant to penicillin, tetracycline, ciprofloxacin, or a combination of these antibiotics. In 2009, the CDC Working Group for Cephalosporin-Resistant Gonorrhea Outbreak Response Plan was convened to address the growing resistance to these antibiotics by *N. gonorrhoeae*.[30] In their *Morbidity and Mortality Weekly Report* from May of 2011, the CDC reviewed five cases of urethral gonorrhea with high mean inhibitory capacities (9.1%) of azithromycin, which represented 10% of those treated for *N. gonorrhoeae* in San Diego County from August to October of 2009.[31] In this monograph, the CDC reinforced the 2010 STD Treatment Guidelines that recommend dual therapy with 250 mg ceftriaxone and 1 g of azithromycin orally for uncomplicated urogenital, rectal, and pharyngeal gonorrhea. The CDC does not recommend azithromycin as monotherapy in the treatment of gonorrhea due to the concern over development of resistance and reported treatment failures. Spectinomycin can be used to treat uncomplicated urogenital infections with good success; however, it is expensive and not produced in the United States. As with chlamydial infections, any sex partners within the preceding 60 days of diagnosis—or the most recent sex partner, if the interval has been longer than 60 days—should be evaluated and treated for gonorrhea to help reduce the rate of reinfection as well as the infection of others. These guidelines are also consistent with the 2015 CDC recommendations (see Box 52-2).

SYPHILIS
Epidemiology

Historically, syphilis has long been recognized as a chronic systemic infectious process secondary to infection with the spirochete *Treponema pallidum*. Throughout the centuries, epidemics of syphilis have been periodically reported. In the United States, the observed incidence of primary and secondary syphilis initially mirrored that of gonorrhea (reflecting the principle that epidemiologic synergy among the STDs occurs), with a rising peak during and shortly after World War II to 76 per 100,000 population to its reported nadir of 4 per 100,000 from 1955 through 1957.[32] Since the mid-1950s, recurrent epidemics have occurred, the most recent in 1985 to 1990, with a peak incidence of 23.5 cases per 100,000.[33] Beginning in 2001, syphilis increased each year to 13,997 cases in 2009.[1] In 2010 there was a decline in the rate of syphilis, with a subsequent increase of 22% between 2011 and 2013.[2] The increased rate of syphilis during this period was seen for men only; the rates for women remained the same.[2]

Of concern are observations from both the WHO and CDC that the prevalence of syphilis in both the United States and developing nations has fluctuated over the past two decades. Noted again are elements of racial disparity, with a disproportionate number of cases in blacks compared with whites (16.8 vs. 3.0 per 100,000), and sex and age disparity, with a predilection for women aged 20 to 24 years.[2,27]

Pathogenesis

Syphilis is a chronic disease caused by the spirochete *Treponema pallidum*. *T. pallidum* belongs to the order Spirochaetales, characterized by slender, nonflagellated, flexuous, tightly spiraled protozoa-like organisms. It is an anaerobic and obligate human parasite. Motility is attained by the flexuous bending of its long slender body. **This motility is responsible for the attainment of access through disrupted integument, mostly mucous membranous, primarily during sexual contact.** *T. pallidum* invades the host and evades the host defense mechanisms while **being completely dependent on the host for survival.** It lacks the fundamental biosynthetic machinery to create complex molecules and fatty acids.[34,35] The ability to evade the host defense mechanisms stems from its basic construct of an inner membrane with few integral membrane proteins that protrude through the surface to gain exposure through the outer membrane.[36] Berman[37] concluded that this construct "may provide some understanding of how the organism elicits such a vigorous inflammatory and immunological response but manages to evade immunological clearance, although a paucity of surface proteins means that its surface presents few targets for a host immune response."

Following mucosal invasion, an incubation period of about 1 week to 3 months ensues until the chancre appears to herald the primary infection. The chancre arises at the point of entry by the spirochetes and is a broad-based, typically nontender ulcerated lesion that gives a characteristic "woody" or "rubbery" feel on palpation. It is seldom secondarily infected, and it resolves without medical treatment in 3 to 6 weeks. The organism then hematogenously spreads through the body during the period in which the immune system has responded, usually about 4 to 10 weeks.[27] Secondary syphilis is characterized by a generalized maculopapular eruption, constitutional symptoms, major organ involvement, and lymphadenopathy. Like the other major organ systems, the central nervous system (CNS) is invaded in about 40% of individuals during this hematogenous phase.[38,39] Secondary syphilis resolves over 2 to 6 weeks as the patient enters the latent phase of the disease.[27] The latent phase is divided into *early latent* (<1 year) and *late latent* (>1 year) disease, during which no symptoms or signs of clinical disease are noted. If left untreated, progression to tertiary disease with cardiovascular system, CNS, and musculoskeletal system involvement occurs. The organism has an affinity for the arterioles, and the inflammatory response that follows results in obliterative endarteritis and subsequent end-organ destruction.[40] In immunocompromised individuals (e.g., those on immune-suppressive medications, those with HIV infection), the progression to tertiary disease, especially of the CNS, is known to occur early after the onset of disease.

Diagnosis

The ability to diagnose infection with *T. pallidum* has been problematic for two primary reasons. The first is the failure of the organism, as of yet, to be cultured on an artificial medium. The second lies in the long-recognized tendency of the clinical manifestations to mimic a variety of other diseases. Reports continue to surface touting the difficulty with which syphilis is recognized at any stage.[41] Primary syphilis often goes unrecognized by the infected individual. Although the primary genital lesion of syphilis, the chancre, is commonly recognized by affected males, women more often than not fail to identify this lesion because it typically occurs without associated constitutional symptoms. **If primary syphilis is suspected, examination of the serous exudates from the chancre under darkfield microscopy can definitively diagnose the condition by identification of the flexuous-bodied (spiral) organism.** Unfortunately, darkfield microscopy lacks sensitivity, owing in part to specimen collection technique. The lesion must be abraded with a gauze sponge or cotton-tipped applicator until bleeding ensues; the clinician must then squeeze the lesion to express clear serum, which is pressed onto a microscope slide. DFAs have the advantage that they can be performed on slides that are air dried as well as on stored paraffin-embedded tissue.[42] Polymerase chain reaction (PCR) has increased the sensitivity for detection in samples obtained from genital lesions, cerebrospinal fluid (CSF), amniotic fluid, serum, and paraffin-embedded tissue.[43]

Because most individuals infected with *T. pallidum* are in the asymptomatic latent phase of the disease, serologic testing is the primary means of diagnosis. Two types of serologic tests are currently available, nontreponemal tests and treponemal tests. The *nontreponemal tests* include the rapid plasma reagin (RPR) and the Venereal Disease Research Laboratories (VDRL) tests. False-positive reactions occur with nontreponemal tests secondary to viral infections or autoimmune disease.[26] If a nontreponemal test is positive, a *treponemal test* is subsequently performed to confirm the diagnosis of syphilis. The treponemal tests include the fluorescent treponemal antibody absorbed (FTA-ABS) tests, the *T. pallidum* passive particle agglutination assay (TP-PA), as well as other EIAs and chemiluminescence immunoassays.[26] Once appropriately treated, most individuals—pregnant or not—lose reactivity to these nontreponemal serologic tests. **For most individuals, the treponemal tests remain positive lifelong.**[44] Table 52-4 reviews the recommended screening for syphilis infections in pregnancy.

Although in most HIV-infected individuals serologic testing is accurate and reliable, occasionally a clinician will encounter patients with expressed lesion exudates or biopsy-proven disease, and serologic testing is negative.[44] **The following recommendations for diagnosing syphilis in HIV-infected individuals have been made by the CDC.**[45] First, individuals with HIV should be screened for syphilis, and all sexually active individuals with syphilis should be screened for HIV. If clinical examination and findings suggest syphilis in the presence of negative serologic testing, DFA for *T. pallidum* staining of lesion exudates and biopsy or darkfield microscopic examination should be performed. In these individuals, all laboratories should titrate the nontreponemal tests (RPR, VDRL) to the exact final end point

TABLE 52-4	SCREENING SYPHILIS INFECTIONS IN PREGNANCY
When to screen	• All women should be screened at their first prenatal visit. • Repeat screening should be performed in all pregnancies early in the third trimester. • Patients should be screened at delivery if not screened previously or if at high risk.
How to screen*	• Treponemal and nontreponemal test
Diagnostic criteria	• Positive treponemal *and* nontreponemal test

Modified from Workowski KA, Bolan GA; Centers for Disease Control and Prevention. Sexually transmitted diseases treatment guidelines, 2015. *MMWR Morb Mortal Wkly Rep.* 2015;64(RR-03):1-137.
Cell culture and nucleic acid hybridization of endocervical specimens are also available.

to better guide response to therapy. Finally, neurosyphilis must be entertained as a diagnosis in HIV-infected individuals, and appropriate consultations should be obtained to better interpret serologic results.

Neurosyphilis is diagnosed in non–HIV-infected and in HIV-infected patients by examination of CSF obtained by a spinal tap. Individuals in whom CSF testing should be considered include those with neurologic or ophthalmologic symptoms, active tertiary disease, or treatment failure and HIV-positive individuals.[26] Spinal tap and examination of CSF is not currently recommended in non–HIV-infected individuals who have early asymptomatic syphilis.[26]

Treatment

It was not long after the introduction of penicillin, about the time of World War II, that it became recognized as the primary antimicrobial for the treatment of syphilis. **Penicillin has been effective in the treatment of disease and in the prevention of disease progression in both nonpregnant and pregnant women, and it has also been used in the prevention and treatment of congenital syphilis** (Box 52-3).[26,46] CDC 2015 treatment guidelines recommend benzathine penicillin G—2.4 miU intramuscularly (IM) as a single dose—for primary, secondary, and early latent syphilis in both pregnant and nonpregnant women.[26] Late latent syphilis and latent syphilis of unknown duration are treated with benzathine penicillin G, 2.4 miU IM weekly for three doses (7.2 miU total).[26] If a dose is missed during pregnancy it is recommended that a full treatment course be repeated. Treatment can precipitate a Jarish-Herxheimer reaction, which can lead to preterm labor and or fetal distress. Women being treated for syphilis in pregnancy should be counseled to seek evaluation if they develop fever, contractions, or decreased fetal movement.

Individuals with documented allergies to penicillin present a particular treatment problem. Treatment recommendations differ depending on whether the penicillin-allergic individual is pregnant. Due to the increased risk for treatment failure with alternative therapies, close follow-up is crucial to determine treatment response. Penicillin is the only therapy that has been proven to be effective in the treatment of congenital syphilis, syphilis in pregnant women, and neurosyphilis, and the alternative therapies should not be considered for these.[26] These aforementioned patients should be managed in conjunction with an infectious disease specialist and should undergo penicillin desensitization and penicillin therapy. **The initial evaluation of patients with a penicillin allergy should begin with skin testing with both major and minor determinants.**[26]

BOX 52-3   RECOMMENDED TREATMENT REGIMENS* FOR *TREPONEMA PALLIDUM* INFECTIONS

Primary, Secondary, Early Latent Disease

Benzathine penicillin G, 2.4 million U IM as a single dose

Late Latent and Latent Disease of Unknown Duration

Benzathine penicillin G, 2.4 miU IM weekly for three doses (7.2 miU total)

Tertiary Disease

NEUROSYPHILIS

Aqueous crystalline penicillin G, 18 to 24 miU/day IV (3 to 4 miU every 4 hours or continuous infusion) for 10 to 14 days *or*

Procaine penicillin G, 2.4 miU IM once daily with probenecid 500 mg PO four times a day for 10 to 14 days if compliance can be ensured

WITHOUT NEUROSYPHILIS

Benzathine penicillin G, 2.4 miU IM weekly for 3 weeks (7.2 miU total)

Penicillin Allergy (Documented)

IN PREGNANCY

Desensitization and penicillin therapy as above

Modified from Workowski KA, Bolan GA; Centers for Disease Control and Prevention (CDC): Sexually transmitted diseases treatment guidelines, 2015. *MMWR Morb Mortal Wkly Rep.* 2015;64(RR-03):1-137.
*The CDC recommends penicillin as the treatment of choice in individuals with syphilis.
IM, intramuscularly; *IV,* intravenously; *miU,* million units; *PO,* per os.

Those with a reported penicillin allergy and negative skin testing may receive penicillin therapy. However, patients who have had a positive skin test should undergo penicillin desensitization with subsequent administration of penicillin therapy.[26,47]

Therapy for tertiary syphilis is dependent on the presence or absence of neurosyphilis. Provided CSF examination is negative, individuals are treated with benzathine penicillin G, 2.4 miU IM weekly for 3 weeks (7.2 miU total).[26] If neurosyphilis has been diagnosed, aqueous crystalline penicillin G, 18 to 24 miU IV daily (3 to 4 miU every 4 hours or continuous infusion) is given for 10 to 14 days. An alternative therapy in compliant individuals is procaine penicillin, 2.4 miU IM once daily, along with probenecid, 500 mg orally four times a day for 10 to 14 days.[26] A follow-up CSF evaluation is recommended to assess response to therapy.

CONGENITAL SYPHILIS

Congenital syphilis continues to be a problem worldwide, and as such, the WHO has established elimination of congenital syphilis as one of the millennium goals.[48] **In 2008, it was estimated that approximately 1.86 million cases of syphilis occurred in pregnant women around the world. In their most recent report, the CDC summarized congenital syphilis surveillance data for 2013**, which indicated that congenital syphilis rates decreased among all racial and ethnic minority populations from 2009 to 2013, with the exception of Native Americans and Alaska Natives.[2] However, the rates of congenital syphilis remain disproportionately high in blacks and Hispanics.[2] The rates of congenital syphilis per 100,000 liveborn infants were determined from U.S. natality data and demonstrated a decrease from 10.4 to 8.4 cases per 100,000 live births between 2009 and 2012, respectively. **This reflects a decrease in primary and secondary syphilis rates among reproductive-aged women, a decline from 1.5 to 0.9 cases per 100,000.**[2]

Congenital syphilis infection results from transplacental migration of the organism to the fetus. Congenital disease can occur at any stage of maternal infection and at any gestational age.[49] Past theories of a placental impasse during the first half of gestation were disproved by pathologic examination of infected first-trimester abortuses and by the demonstration of living organisms in amniotic fluid obtained by amniocentesis in the early second trimester.[49,50] It is now believed that **transplacental infection must be close to 100% during the early stages of maternal disease because of the known hematogenous spread, with rates of transmission falling to 10% as bacteremia abates with the subsequent mounting of the maternal immunologic response during late latent disease.**[51-53] Also of importance in the pathogenesis of fetal disease is knowledge of fetal immunologic development. Disease early in gestation incites little response because the fetal immune system functions little until midgestation. Following this period, the fetus is able to mount a vigorous response with marked endarteritis and end-organ involvement. **The risk for adverse pregnancy outcome in pregnant women with syphilis that was untreated is approximately 52%.**[54] **The specific risks include a higher risk for miscarriage or stillbirth (21%), neonatal death (9.3%), premature birth or low birthweight (5.8%), and clinical evidence of congenital infection (15%) when compared with the risks in women without syphilis.**[54]

Nonimmune fetal hydrops, polyhydramnios, and intrauterine fetal demise have long been associated with congenital syphilis. Recent reports confirm the constellation of nonimmune hydrops (ascites, pleural effusion, scalp or skin edema), hepatomegaly, polyhydramnios, and placentomegaly as markers for congenital syphilis.[55,56] **Hollier and colleagues**[57] **prospectively identified and followed 24 women with untreated syphilis to better define the pathophysiology of fetal disease.** Ultrasound examination with amniocentesis and funipuncture was performed. The infected pregnant women were treated with benzathine penicillin G given IM per the CDC guidelines (see Box 52-3). Six women had primary, 12 had secondary, and 6 had early latent syphilis disease. Sixteen of these fetuses (67%) had either congenital syphilis or *T. pallidum* identified in the amniotic fluid specimens. **Maternal stage of disease—primary, secondary, and early latent—correlated with fetal infection rates of 50%, 67%, and 83%, respectively. Ultrasound examination was abnormal in 16 of the 24 fetuses (67%).** Thirteen of these fetuses had hepatomegaly, three had hepatomegaly and ascites, and one had nonimmune hydrops. Increased placental thickness was seen in 17 (71%), and hydramnios was observed in only one fetus with an abnormal ultrasound. **This study demonstrates the utility of ultrasound examination in the diagnosis and management of the syphilis-infected gravida and her unborn child. This is supported by the CDC, which recommends sonographic evaluation of the fetus for evidence of congenital infection if syphilis is diagnosed after 20 weeks' gestation.**

In an effort to reduce the incidence of congenital syphilis, the CDC recommends screening all pregnant women at the time of their first prenatal visit, and again early in the third trimester. In addition, women should be screened at delivery if not previously screened, or if they are at high risk.[26] If prenatal screening is not available, patients should be screened at delivery.[42]

The implementation of appropriate screening and treatment of pregnant women should theoretically result in the elimination of congenital syphilis.[37,51] Despite these screening recommendations, attempts at targeted mass treatment for syphilis in populations at risk in order to reduce outbreaks and ultimately wipe out congenital syphilis have met with failure.[58] **It was estimated by the WHO that approximately one third of women who received prenatal care were not tested for syphilis.**[48] Children continue to be born with increased prematurity, low birthweight, hepatomegaly, and cutaneous and bone lesions in both developing and developed nations.[59] **Almost 90% of stillbirths attributed to congenital syphilis occur among women who are never treated or who are treated inappropriately.**[60] Alexander and colleagues[61] examined the CDC guidelines for the treatment of maternal syphilis among 340 gravidae and found better than 95% success for all stages of clinical disease in preventing congenital disease. Sheffield and associates[62] evaluated 43 women who received antepartum therapy with treatment failure and revealed that preterm delivery (<36 weeks), a short interval between treatment and delivery, a higher VDRL titer at the time of treatment and delivery, and early stage of maternal disease were associated with treatment failure. The optimal management (transplacental through maternal therapy vs. neonatal) of the fetus with severe or advanced clinical disease remains unknown and requires consultation with experienced clinicians.[63]

KEY POINTS

- All pregnant women younger than 25 years or those at increased risk should be screened for *Chlamydia* and gonorrhea during pregnancy.
- Women younger than 25 and those at high risk for sexually transmitted infections should be rescreened for *Chlamydia* during the third trimester.
- Syphilis screening should be performed at the first prenatal visit as well as early in the third trimester. Repeat testing should be performed at the time of delivery in patients at high risk for syphilis.
- If syphilis testing was not done during pregnancy, it should be performed postpartum prior to the patient's discharge from the hospital.
- NAATs of urine, the endocervix, or the vagina is the preferred screening test for both *Chlamydia* and gonorrhea.
- Screening for syphilis can be performed using either a treponemal or nontreponemal test.
- Penicillin is the antimicrobial of choice in treating syphilis among pregnant women and for reducing the incidence of congenital syphilis.
- Pregnant women with a penicillin allergy and syphilis infection should undergo penicillin desensitization with subsequent penicillin therapy.

REFERENCES

1. Wall KM, Khosropour CM, Sullivan PS. *Centers for Disease Control and Prevention. Sexually Transmitted Disease Surveillance 2009.* Atlanta: U.S. Department of Health and Human Services; 2010.

2. Centers for Disease Control and Prevention. *Sexually Transmitted Disease Surveillance 2013.* Atlanta: U.S. Department of Health and Human Services; 2014.

3. Hammerschlag MR, Anderka M, Semine DZ, et al. Prospective study of maternal and infantile infection with *Chlamydia trachomatis. Pediatrics.* 1979;64:142.

4. Mangione-Smith R, O'Leary J, McGlynn EA. Health and cost-benefits of Chlamydia screening in young women. *Sex Transm Dis.* 1999;26:309.

5. Sweet RL, Landers DV, Walker C, et al. *Chlamydia trachomatis* infection and pregnancy outcome. *Am J Obstet Gynecol.* 1987;156:824.

6. Schachter J, Grossman M, Sweet RL, et al. Prospective study of perinatal transmission of *Chlamydia trachomatis. JAMA.* 1986;255:3374.

7. Centers for Disease Control and Prevention. Racial Disparities in Nationally Notifiable Diseases-United States, 2002. *MMWR Morb Mortal Wkly Rep.* 2005;54(9).

8. Stamm WE. *Chlamydia trachomatis* infections of the adult. In: Holmes KK, Sparling PF, Mardh P-A, et al., eds. *Sexually Transmitted Diseases.* New York: McGraw-Hill; 1999:407.

9. Sweet RS, Gibbs R. Chlamydial Infections. In: Sweet R, Gibbs R, eds. *Infectious Diseases of the Female Reproductive Tract.* 4th ed. Philadelphia: Lippincott Williams & Wilkins; 2002:57.

10. Schachter J. Chlamydial infections. *N Engl J Med.* 1978;298:428.

11. Sweet RS, Schachter J, Landers DV. Chlamydial infections in obstetrics and gynecology. *Clin Obstet Gynecol.* 1983;26:143.

12. Friis RR. Interaction of L cells and *Chlamydia psittaci:* entry of the parasite and host responses to its development. *J Bacteriol.* 1972;110:706.

13. Kuo CC, Wang SP, Grayson JT. Effect of polycations, polyanions, and neuraminidase on the infectivity of trachoma-inclusion conjunctivitis and LGV organisms in HeLa cells: sialic acid residues as possible receptors for trachoma-inclusion conjunctivitis. *Infect Immun.* 1973;8:74.

14. Nurminen M, Leinonen M, Saikku P, Mäkelä PH. The genus-specific antigen of Chlamydia: resemblance to the lipopolysaccharide of enteric bacteria. *Science.* 1983;220:1279.

15. Bavoil PH, Ohlin A, Schachter J. Role of disulfide bonding in outer membrane structure and permeability in *Chlamydia trachomatis. Infect Immun.* 1984;44:479.

16. Schachter J. Biology of *Chlamydia trachomatis.* In: Holmes KK, Sparling PF, Mardh P-A, et al., eds. *Sexually Transmitted Diseases.* New York: McGraw-Hill; 1999:391.

17. Brunham RC, Peeling RW. *Chlamydia trachomatis* antigens: role in immunity and pathogenesis. *Infect Agents Dis.* 1994;3:218.

18. Brunham RC, Plummer F, Stephens RS. Bacterial antigenic variation, host immune response and pathogen-host co-evolution. *Infect Immun.* 1994;61:2273.

19. Brunham R, Yang C, Maclean I, et al. *Chlamydia trachomatis* from individuals in a sexually transmitted disease core group exhibit frequent sequence variation in the major outer membrane protein (omp1) gene. *J Clin Invest.* 1994;94:458.

20. Morrison RP, Manning DS, Caldwell HD. Immunology of *Chlamydia trachomatis* infections: immunoprotective and immunopathologic responses. In: Gallin JI, Fauci AS, Quinn TC, eds. *Advances in Host Defense Mechanisms, Vol. 8: Sexually Transmitted Diseases.* New York: Raven Press; 1992:57.

21. Hayes LJ, Bailey RL, Mabey DC, et al. Genotyping of *Chlamydia trachomatis* from a trachoma-endemic village in the Gambia by a nested polymerase chain reaction: identification of strain variants. *J Infect Dis.* 1992;166:1173.

22. Conway DJ, Holland MJ, Campbell AE, et al. HLA class I and class II polymorphism and trachomatous scarring in a *Chlamydia trachomatis–*endemic population. *J Infect Dis.* 1996;174:643.

23. Kimani J, Maclean IW, Bwayo JJ, et al. Risk factors for *Chlamydia trachomatis* pelvic inflammatory disease among sex workers in Nairobi, Kenya. *J Infect Dis.* 1996;173:1437.

24. Brunham RC, Maclean IW, Binns B, Peeling RW. *Chlamydia trachomatis:* its role in tubal infertility. *J Infect Dis.* 1985;152:1275.

25. Papp JR, Schachter J, Gaydos CA, et al., Centers for Disease Control and Prevention. Recommendations for the laboratory-based detection of *Chlamydia trachomatis* and *Neisseria gonorrhoeae* —2014. *MMWR Morb Mortal Wkly Rep.* 2014;63:02.

26. Centers for Disease Control and Prevention. Sexually transmitted diseases treatment guidelines. *MMWR Morb Mortal Wkly Rep.* 2015;64(RR-03):1-137.

27. Sweet RL, Gibbs R. Sexually transmitted diseases. In: Sweet R, Gibbs R, eds. *Infectious Diseases of the Female Reproductive Tract.* 4th ed. Philadelphia: Lippincott Williams & Wilkins; 2002:118.

28. Hook EW, Handsfield HA. Gonococcal infections in adults. In: Holmes KK, Sparling PF, Mardh P-A, et al., eds. *Sexually Transmitted Diseases.* New York: McGraw-Hill; 1999:451.

29. Sparling PF. Biology of *Neisseria gonorrhoeae.* In: Holmes KK, Sparling PF, Mardh P-A, et al., eds. *Sexually Transmitted Diseases.* New York: McGraw-Hill; 1999:433.

30. Consultation Meeting on Cephalosporin-Resistant Gonorrhea Outbreak Response Plan. *Report of an external consultants' meeting convened by the Division of STD Prevention, National Center for HIV, STD, and TB Prevention, Centers for Disease Control and Prevention (CDC), September 14-15,* 2009:1-12.

31. Centers for Disease Control and Prevention. *Neisseria gonorrhoeae* with reduced susceptibility to azithromycin—San Diego County, California, 2009. *MMWR Morb Mortal Wkly Rep.* 2011;60(579).

32. Centers for Disease Control and Prevention. Summary of notifiable diseases, United States 1992. *MMWR Morb Mortal Wkly Rep.* 1993;41(1).

33. Aral SO, Holmes KK. Social and behavioral determinants of the epidemiology of STDs: industrialized and developing countries. In: Holmes KK, Sparling PF, Mardh P-A, et al., eds. *Sexually Transmitted Diseases.* New York: McGraw-Hill; 1999:39.

34. Pennisi E. Genome reveals wiles and weak points of syphilis. *Science.* 1998;281:324.

35. Radolf JD, Steiner B, Shevchenko D. *Treponema pallidum:* doing a remarkable job with what it's got. *Trends Microbiol.* 1999;7:7.

36. Weinstock GM, Hardham JM, McLeod MP, et al. The genome of *Treponema pallidum:* new light on the agent of syphilis. *FEMS Microbiol Rev.* 1998;22:323.

37. Berman SM. Maternal syphilis: pathophysiology and treatment. *Bull World Health Org.* 2004;82:1.

38. Stokes JH, Beerman H, Ingraham NR. *Modern Clinical Syphilology, Diagnosis and Treatment: Case Study.* 3rd ed. Philadelphia: WB Saunders; 1945.

39. Lukehart SA, Hook EW 3rd, Baker-Zander SA, et al. Invasion of central nervous system by *Treponema pallidum:* implications for diagnosis and treatment. *Ann Intern Med.* 1988;109:855.

40. Tranont EC. Syphilis in adults: from Christopher Columbus to Sir Alexander Flemming to AIDS. *Clin Infect Dis.* 1995;21:1361.

41. Baum EW, Bernhardt M, Sams WM Jr, et al. Secondary syphilis. Still the great imitator. *JAMA.* 1983;249:3069.

42. Larsen SA, Hunter EF, Creighton ET. Syphilis. In: Holmes KK, Mardh P-A, Sparling PF, et al., eds. *Sexually Transmitted Diseases.* New York: McGraw-Hill; 1990:927.

43. Burstain JM, Grimprel E, Lukehart SA, et al. Sensitive detection of *Treponema pallidum* by using the polymerase chain reaction. *J Clin Microbiol.* 1991;29:62.

44. Hicks CB, Benson PM, Lupton GP, Tramont EC. Seronegative secondary syphilis in a patient infected with the human immunodeficiency (HIV) with Kaposi sarcoma: a diagnostic dilemma. *Ann Intern Med.* 1987;107:492.

45. Centers for Disease Control. Current trends: recommendations for diagnosing and treating syphilis in HIV-infected patients. *MMWR Morb Mortal Wkly Rep.* 1988;37:600.

46. Ingraham NR. The value of penicillin alone in the prevention and treatment of congenital syphilis. *Acta Derm Venereol Suppl (Stock).* 1951;31:60.

47. Wendel GD Jr, Stark BJ, Jamison RB, et al. Penicillin allergy and desensitization in serious infections during pregnancy. *New Engl J Med.* 1985;312:1229.

48. World Health Organization. *The Global Elimination of Congenital Syphilis: Rationale and Strategy for Action.* Geneva, Switzerland: WHO Press; 2007:3-6 Available at: <http://www.who.int>.

49. Harter CA, Bernirsche K. Fetal syphilis in the first trimester. *Am J Obstet Gynecol.* 1976;124:705.

50. Nathan L, Bohman VR, Sanchez PJ, et al. In utero infection with *Treponema pallidum* in early pregnancy. *Prenat Diagn.* 1997;17:119.

51. Ingraham NR. The value of penicillin alone in the prevention and treatment of congenital syphilis. *Acta Derm Venereol.* 1951;31:60.

52. Zenker PN, Berman SM. Congenital syphilis: trends and recommendations for evaluation and management. *Pediatr Infect Dis J.* 1991;10:516.

53. Fiumara NJ, Flemming WL, Downing JG, et al. The incidence of prenatal syphilis at the Boston City Hospital. *N Engl J Med.* 1952;247:48.

54. Gomez GB, Kamb ML, Newman LM, et al. Untreated maternal syphilis and adverse outcomes of pregnancy: A systematic review and meta-analysis. *Bull World Health Organ.* 2013;91:217-226.

55. Burton JR, Thorpe EM Jr, Shaver DC, et al. Nonimmune hydrops fetalis associated with maternal infection with syphilis. *Am J Obstet Gynecol.* 1992;167:56.

56. Jacobs A, Rotenberg O. Nonimmune hydrops fetalis due to congenital syphilis associated with negative intrapartum maternal serology screening. *Am J Perinatol.* 1998;15:233.

57. Hollier LM, Harstad TW, Sanchez PJ, et al. Fetal syphilis: clinical and laboratory characteristics. *Obstet Gynecol.* 2001;97:947.

58. Rekart ML, Patrick DM, Chakraborty B, et al. Targeted mass treatment for syphilis with oral azithromycin. *Lancet.* 2003;361:313.

59. Saloojee H, Velaphi S, Goga Y, et al. The prevention and management of congenital syphilis: an overview and recommendations. *Bull World Health Org.* 2004;82:424.

60. Gust DA, Levine WC, St Louis ME, Braxton J, Berman SM. Mortality associated with congenital syphilis in the United States, 1992-1998. *Pediatrics.* 2002;109:E79.

61. Alexander JM, Sheffield JS, Sanchez PJ, et al. Efficacy of treatment for syphilis in pregnancy. *Obstet Gynecol.* 1999;93:5.

62. Sheffield JS, Sanchez PJ, Morris G, et al. Congenital syphilis after maternal treatment for syphilis during pregnancy. *Am J Obstet Gynecol.* 2002;186:569.

63. Wendel GD Jr, Sheffield JS, Hollier LM, et al. Treatment of syphilis in pregnancy and prevention of congenital syphilis. *Clin Infect Dis.* 2002;35: S200.

CHAPTER 53

Maternal and Perinatal Infection in Pregnancy: Viral

HELENE B. BERNSTEIN

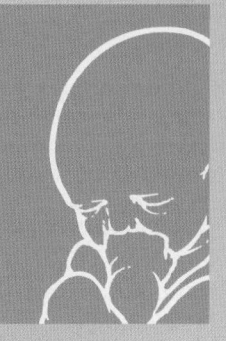

KEY ABBREVIATIONS

Acquired immunodeficiency syndrome	AIDS	Efavirenz	EFV
Antiretroviral	ARV	Enzyme-linked immunosorbent assay	ELISA
American College of Obstetricians and Gynecologists	ACOG	Epstein-Barr virus	EBV
		Erythema infectiosum	EI
Chemokine receptor type 5	CCR5	Fixed-dose combination	FDC
Centers for Disease Control and Prevention	CDC	Glycoprotein	gp
		Hemagglutinin	HA or H
Central nervous system	CNS	Hepatitis A virus	HAV
Combination antiretroviral therapy	cART	Hepatitis B core antigen	HBcAg
Congenital rubella syndrome	CRS	Hepatitis B early antigen	HBeAg
Congenital varicella syndrome	CVS	Hepatitis B immune globulin	HBIG
C-X-C chemokine receptor type 4	CXCR4	Hepatitis B surface antigen	HBsAg
Cytomegalovirus	CMV	Hepatitis B virus	HBV
Deoxyribonucleic acid	DNA	Hepatitis C virus	HCV
Disseminated intravascular coagulopathy	DIC	Hepatitis delta antigen	HDAg
		Hepatitis delta virus	HDV

Herpes simplex virus	HSV	Nucleoside reverse transcriptase inhibitor	NRTI
Human immunodeficiency virus	HIV	Opportunistic infections	OI
Human papillomavirus	HPV	Papanicolaou smear	PAP smear
Immune reconstitution inflammatory syndrome	IRIS	Pediatric AIDS Clinical Trials Group	PACTG
Immunoglobulin	Ig	Pharmacokinetic	PK
Integrase strand transfer inhibitor	INSTI	Polymerase chain reaction	PCR
Intrauterine growth restriction	IUGR	Preexposure prophylaxis	PrEP
Intravenous	IV	Protease inhibitor	PI
Lamivudine	3TC	Rapid influenza diagnostic test	RIDT
Long terminal repeat	LTR	Reverse transcriptase	RT
Measles, mumps, rubella	MMR	Ribonucleic acid	RNA
Mother-to-child transmission	MTCT	Sexually transmitted disease	STD
Mycobacterium avium complex	MAC	Spontaneous rupture of membranes	SROM
Neuraminidase	N or NA	Subacute sclerosing panencephalitis	SSPE
Nevirapine	NVP	Purified protein derivative	PPD
Nonnucleoside reverse transcriptase inhibitor	NNRTI	Tuberculosis	TB
		Varicella zoster immune globulin	VZIG
Nucleic acid test	NAT	Varicella zoster virus	VZV
Nucleic acid sequence-based amplification	NASBA	World Health Organization	WHO
		Zidovudine	ZDV

Viruses have been identified in virtually all organisms. They are among the simplest of living organisms, yet they have significantly influenced history and are an important causative factor for infectious disease. **Viruses are obligate intracellular parasites that utilize the host cell's structural and functional components while exhibiting remarkably diverse strategies for gene expression and replication.** Viral infection ranges from asymptomatic or subclinical to overwhelming and highly lethal, with findings such as meningoencephalitis or hemorrhagic fever with shock. Viral infection is highly variable; many viruses are limited to acute, time-limited infection. However, some viruses establish long-lasting infection. Latent viruses have the capacity to reactivate gene expression many years after acute infection, retroviruses integrate into the host cell genome, and multiple viruses have oncogenic potential.

Virus particles contain nucleic acid and structural proteins, which together are referred to as a *nucleocapsid.* Viral nucleic acid is composed of either DNA or RNA, which may be single or double stranded. Viral genomes can be linear or circular and can exist in multiple segments or as a single segment. Viral genome size ranges from two genes in parvovirus B19 to over 200 genes in cytomegalovirus (CMV). Some viruses have lipid bilayer envelopes external to the nucleocapsid; these envelopes are derived from the host cell and contain viral proteins. Herpes viruses have an additional layer, called a *tegument,* between the nucleocapsid and envelope. Viruses are classified by the International Committee on Taxonomy into orders, families, subfamilies, genera, and species. Classification is based on morphology, nucleic acid type, the presence or absence of an envelope, genome replication strategy, and homology to other viruses.

Infection is typically initiated by the virus binding to a specific host cell receptor. Receptors are normally functional host cell membrane proteins but are also recognized by a viral protein ligand within the viral envelope or nucleocapsid. The viral protein and cellular receptor interaction defines, in part, the host range of the virus, which limits infection to cells that display the appropriate receptor. Virus enters the host cell via translocation of the virion across the plasma membrane; this involves endocytosis or fusion of the viral envelope with the cell membrane. The virus then uncoats its nucleic acid for replication, ultimately leading to viral gene expression and replication. This may occur in either the cytoplasm or nucleus of the cell and may involve integration into the host genome, as in the case of retroviruses. Intracellular assembly of progeny virions occurs followed by release of newly formed virions by cell lysis or by budding from the cell surface, as in the case of most enveloped viruses.

Despite their inability to replicate independently, viruses play a central role in infectious disease, altering the structure and/or the function of the host cell. **For productive infection to occur, viruses must enter cells, replicate their genome, and release infectious virions.** The inability of a virus to complete any of these required steps results in a "nonproductive infection." Viral pathogenesis occurs via several mechanisms and does not require productive infection. These include direct effects on infected host cells, which may result in cell death via lysis or apoptosis. Infected cells can also be killed by antiviral antibody and complement or by cell-mediated immune mechanisms. In addition, some viral genomes encode oncogenes, which can mediate transformation of infected host cells. Viral proteins can also impact the function of uninfected cells, including those of the immune system. Finally, **the host immune response to viral infection encompasses both local and systemic effects via activation of immune cells, the induction of an adaptive immune response, and the release of cytokines, chemokines, and antibodies.** Thus the immune response contributes to or causes the signs and symptoms associated with viral infections, which includes fever, rash, arthralgias, and myalgias. The outcome of viral infection is dependent on host factors such as immune status, age, nutritional status, and genetic background. Genetic factors can alter susceptibility to viral infection, the immune response generated following infection, and the long-term consequences of viral infection.

This chapter discusses many of the viral infections relevant to pregnancy that have significant impact on maternal health and/or pregnancy outcome. The virology, epidemiology, diagnosis, clinical manifestations, management during pregnancy, and impact on the fetus/neonate are reviewed for the viruses listed in Table 53-1.

HUMAN IMMUNODEFICIENCY VIRUS

Virology

Human immunodeficiency virus (HIV) is a member of the Retroviridae family, characterized by spherical, enveloped viruses. The virus envelope surrounds an icosahedral capsid that contains the viral genome and consists of two identical pieces of positive-sense, single-stranded RNA about 9.2 kb long. HIV has a total of nine genes that include three main genes—*gag*, *pol*, and *env*—which are surrounded by long terminal repeat (LTR) regions. The *gag* gene encodes the precursor for the virion capsid proteins, which include the full-length p55 polyprotein precursor and its cleavage products p17 matrix, p24 capsid, p9 nucleocapsid, and p7. The *pol* gene encodes the precursor polyprotein for several viral enzymes including protease, reverse transcriptase, RNase H, and integrase. The *env* gene encodes the envelope glycoprotein (gp160), which is cleaved to the surface unit (gp120) and the transmembrane protein (gp41) necessary for fusion. **Retroviruses are unique because the viral genome is transcribed into DNA via the viral enzyme reverse transcriptase, followed by integration into the host cell genome via the viral enzyme integrase. HIV also has the capacity to become latent within quiescent infected cells, which has made eradication of the virus thus far impossible.**

The HIV envelope glycoprotein (gp120) is a ligand for CD4, the cellular HIV receptor; thus **HIV predominantly infects CD4+ cells, including T cells, monocytes, and macrophages.** Coreceptors required for viral entry and infection have been identified. The two primary HIV coreceptors are the chemokine receptors CXCR4 and CCR5. New infections almost always occur with an HIV strain that utilizes the CCR5 coreceptor, which potentially reflects viral fitness. Individuals homozygous for a 32–base pair deletion within the CCR5 gene are much less likely to become HIV infected, even following significant exposure; moreover, some CCR5 polymorphisms correlate with disease progression of HIV in perinatally infected children and adults.

Epidemiology

The Centers for Disease Control and Prevention (CDC) estimates that over 1.2 million people in the United States are infected with HIV, and 14% of infected individuals are undiagnosed or unaware of their infection.[1] **Most HIV-infected individuals reside outside the United States. Global HIV burden is estimated at 37 million individuals; moreover, women account for more than half of all people living with HIV. In contrast, approximately 50,000 Americans are diagnosed with HIV infection annually; women account for 20% of new HIV infections and 23% of existing infections. Women typically acquire HIV infection by heterosexual contact, and about 65% of new infections occur in black Americans.** White women have the highest percentage of HIV infections attributable to injection drug use (25%), whereas injection drug use accounts for only 14% of HIV infections in Hispanic women and only 11% in black women. Factors associated with an increased prevalence of HIV infection and transmission risk include a high number of sexual contacts, high-risk sexual exposure, receptive anal intercourse, sexual contact with an uncircumcised male, IV drug and/or crack cocaine use, residing in the "inner city," and the presence of other sexually transmitted diseases (STDs), particularly those that cause genital ulcers (herpes, syphilis, chancroid).

HIV infection is limited to humans and chimpanzees, and most infections in the United States are caused by HIV-1, which is divided into three groups: M, N, and O. Over 95% of HIV-1 infections are caused by group M, which is divided into subtypes, or *clades,* A through K. The predominant type of HIV within the United States is clade B, whereas other clades predominate in other regions of the world. HIV-2, a related strain of HIV, is endemic in Africa, Portugal, and France and appears to have a lower vertical transmission rate compared with HIV-1. Much less is known about the treatment of these related viruses given their prevalence in areas of the world where treatment with antiretroviral (ARV) agents is not readily available.

Diagnosis

Historically, HIV infection was diagnosed via virus-specific antibody detection; initial serologic screen was via enzyme-linked immunosorbent assay (ELISA) and either Western blot (WB) or immunofluorescent antibody assay was performed for confirmation. The Western blot identifies antibodies and recognizes specific viral antigens, and it is considered positive when any two of the following three antigens are identified: p24 (capsid), gp41 (envelope), and gp120/160 (envelope). Several salivary and/or rapid blood tests are available with efficacy comparable to ELISA. These tests have a limited ability to diagnose early HIV and HIV-2 infection because they detect HIV-specific immunoglobulin (Ig) G antibodies. **Current recommendations are to screen with an HIV-1/2 antigen/antibody combination immunoassay, or "combo assay," with confirmation of infection with an HIV-1/HIV-2 antibody differentiation immunoassay and HIV-1 nucleic acid test (NAT; Fig. 53-1).**[2] This strategy enables diagnosis of *acute* HIV-1 infection, detection of HIV-2 infection, and faster turnaround time. Enhancements of the combo assay include more accurate HIV-2 diagnosis, p24 antigen assessment (measurable 15 days postinfection), and detection of IgM antibodies (measurable 3 to 5 days after p24 antigen positivity), which enables confirmation of HIV infection days to weeks before the HIV WB becomes positive. Combined with an HIV-1 NAT, this narrows the window between the time of infection and immunoassay reactivity and enables the diagnosis of acute HIV-1 infection, which was not possible using ELISA/WB assessment.[2] Because the risk of HIV transmission from persons with acute and early infection is increased, this strategy may reduce perinatal HIV transmission.

Given the increasing prevalence of HIV infection and studies that demonstrate that identification of HIV-infected pregnant women and early antiretroviral therapy (ART) most effectively prevents perinatal HIV transmission, **both the American College of Obstetricians and Gynecologists (ACOG) and the CDC recommend an "opt out" approach to ensure routine HIV screening for all pregnant women, ideally performed at the first prenatal visit.** The CDC also advocates for repeat testing in the third trimester, citing its cost effectiveness even in areas of low prevalence.[3] A second HIV test in the third trimester

TABLE 53-1   SUMMARY OF ETIOLOGY, DIAGNOSIS, AND MANAGEMENT OF MAJOR PERINATAL VIRAL INFECTIONS

Virus	COMPLICATIONS		DIAGNOSIS		TREATMENT/MANAGEMENT	
	Maternal	Fetal/Neonatal	Maternal	Fetal/Neonatal	Maternal	Fetal/Neonatal
HIV	Opportunistic infection	Perinatal infection	Immunoassay	PCR	cART	cART to reduce perinatal transmission
Influenza	Pneumonia, increased maternal mortality	NA	RT-PCR or immunofluorescence, RIDT for screening	NA	Oseltamivir prophylaxis and treatment, supportive care, vaccinate annually	Maternal vaccination to protect the neonate
Parvovirus B19	Rare	Anemia, hydrops, death	PCR or antibody detection	PCR, ultrasound for anemia	Supportive care	Intrauterine transfusion for severe anemia
Rubeola (measles)	Otitis media, pneumonia, encephalitis	Abortion, preterm delivery	RT-PCR or antibody detection	NA	Supportive care, vaccinate prior to pregnancy	NA
Rubella	Rare	Congenital infection	Antibody detection or RT-PCR	RT-PCR, ultrasound for congenital rubella syndrome	Supportive care, vaccinate prior to pregnancy	Consider pregnancy termination for fetus with CRS
CMV	Chorioretinitis	Congenital infection	PCR	PCR, ultrasound for detection of sequelae	Ganciclovir for severe infection	Consider pregnancy termination for infected fetus with primary maternal infection
HSV	Disseminated infection, primarily in immunocompromised patients	Neonatal infection, intrauterine infection is extremely rare	Examination, PCR, antibody detection	Examination, PCR, antibody detection	Antiviral Tx for infection and prophylaxis to reduce recurrences	Cesarean delivery when mother has active genital lesions
Varicella	Pneumonia, encephalitis, zoster	Congenital or perinatal infection	History, PCR, antibody detection	Ultrasound	VZIG, antivirals for prophylaxis and/or treatment	VZIG, antivirals for prophylaxis and/or treatment
Hepatitis A	Rare	None	RT-PCR or antibody detection	NA	Supportive care, vaccination	IG to neonate if mother acutely infected at delivery
Hepatitis B	Chronic liver disease	Perinatal infection	HBsAg detection, HBV PCR	NA	Supportive care, vaccination; HBIG for exposed, unvaccinated individuals	HBIG and HBV vaccine immediately following delivery. Consider antepartum tenofovir to further reduce transmission
Hepatitis C	Chronic liver disease	Perinatal infection	HCV antibody screen, NAT confirmation	NA	Supportive care, consider antiviral Tx	Maternal treatment may reduce transmission
Hepatitis D	Chronic liver disease	Perinatal infection	Antigen and antibody detection	NA	Supportive care	HBIG and HBV vaccine immediately following delivery
Hepatitis E	Increased mortality	Neonatal infection	RT-PCR, antibody detection	NA	Supportive care	None

cART, combination antiretroviral therapy; *CMV,* cytomegalovirus; *CRS,* congenital rubella syndrome; *HBIG,* HBV immune globulin; *HBsAg,* HBV surface antigen; *HBV,* hepatitis B virus; *HCV,* hepatitis C virus; *HIV,* human immunodeficiency virus; *HSV,* herpes simples virus; *IG,* immune globulin; *NA,* not applicable; *NAT,* nucleic acid test; *PCR,* polymerase chain reaction; *RIDT,* rapid influenza diagnostic test; *RT-PCR,* reverse transcriptase PCR; *VZIG,* varicella zoster immune globulin; *Tx,* treatment.

is recommended for women at increased risk of HIV infection and those living in areas of elevated HIV incidence, which includes residents of Alabama, Connecticut, Delaware, the District of Columbia, Florida, Georgia, Illinois, Louisiana, Maryland, Massachusetts, Mississippi, Nevada, New Jersey, New York, North Carolina, Pennsylvania, Puerto Rico, Rhode Island, South Carolina, Tennessee, Texas, and Virginia as well as women who receive health care in facilities at which prenatal screening identifies at least one HIV-infected pregnant woman per 1000 women screened.

Clinical Manifestations and Staging

The clinical presentation of HIV infection and/or acquired immunodeficiency syndrome (AIDS) depends on when infection

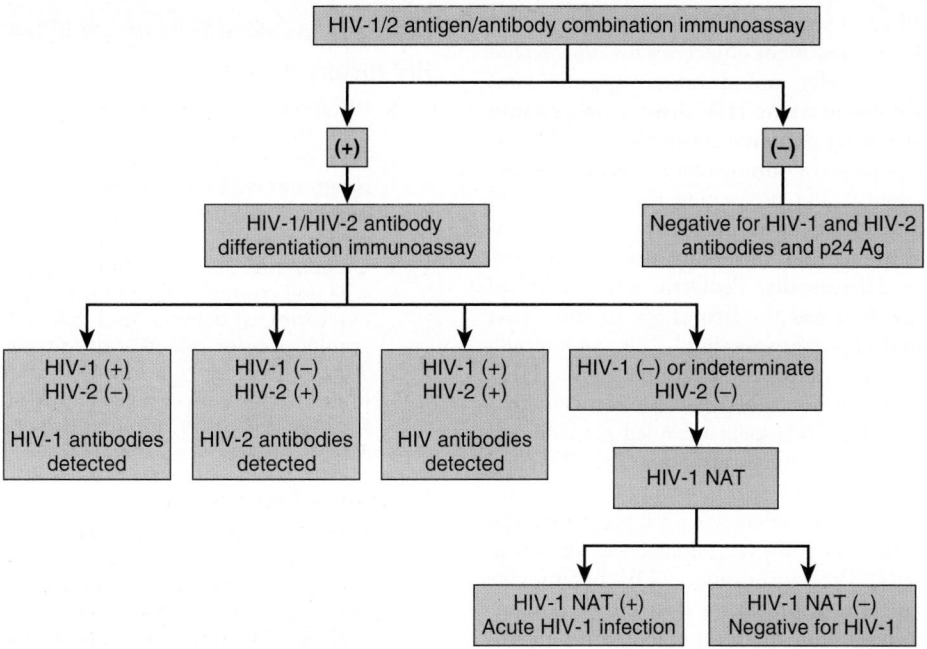

FIG 53-1 Diagnosis of human immunodeficiency virus (HIV) infection. *Ag,* antigen; *HIV,* human immunodeficiency virus; *NAT,* nucleic acid test; *+,* reactive test result; *–,* nonreactive test result.

TABLE 53-2   STAGES OF HIV INFECTION

CDC STAGE	CD4+ T-LYMPHOCYTE COUNT AND PERCENTAGES
Stage 1 (HIV infection)	CD4+ T-lymphocyte count ≥500 cells/μL or ≥ 29%
Stage 2 (HIV infection)	CD4+ T-lymphocyte count 200 to 499 cells/μL or 14% to 29%
Stage 3 (AIDS)	CD4+ T-lymphocyte count <200 cells/μL or <14%

AIDS, acquired immune deficiency syndrome; *CDC,* Centers for Disease Control and Prevention; *HIV,* human immunodeficiency virus.

occurred and whether immunodeficiency resulted. **Following exposure and primary infection, 50% to 70% of individuals infected with HIV develop the acute retroviral syndrome.** At this time patients may have "mononucleosis-like" symptoms that include fever, rigors, pharyngitis, arthralgias, myalgias, maculopapular rash, urticaria, abdominal cramps, diarrhea, headache, and lymphocytic meningitis. The acute phase of infection usually occurs 4 to 6 weeks following HIV exposure and can last several weeks. However, it is uncommon for individuals to be diagnosed during acute infection. Following acute HIV infection, patients enter latent-phase infection, which can last approximately 5 to 10 years in untreated patients and comprises stage 1 and 2 of infection (Table 53-2). During this asymptomatic phase of infection, in the absence of ART, chronic immune activation and progressive destruction of lymphatic tissue ensues.[4] If untreated, most patients will develop stage 3 infection, AIDS, which typically includes one or more of the conditions listed in Box 53-1.

Evolution of Human Immunodeficiency Virus Infection and Treatment

The diagnosis, treatment, and prognosis of HIV infection has improved considerably over the past 30 years. Subsequent to the availability of effective ARVs with fewer adverse effects, HIV

BOX 53-1   AIDS-DEFINING CONDITIONS IN ADULTS

Candidiasis of bronchi, trachea, or lungs
Candidiasis of esophagus*
Cervical cancer, invasive†
Coccidioidomycosis, disseminated or extrapulmonary
Cryptococcosis, extrapulmonary
Cryptosporidiosis, chronic intestinal (>1 month duration)
Cytomegalovirus disease (other than liver, spleen, or nodes), onset at age >1 month
Cytomegalovirus retinitis (with loss of vision)†
Encephalopathy, HIV related
Herpes simplex: Chronic ulcers (>1 month duration) or bronchitis, pneumonitis, or esophagitis (onset at age >1 month)
Histoplasmosis, disseminated or extrapulmonary
Isosporiasis, chronic intestinal (>1 month duration)
Kaposi sarcoma*
Lymphoid interstitial pneumonia or pulmonary lymphoid hyperplasia complex†
Lymphoma, Burkitt (or equivalent term)
Lymphoma, immunoblastic (or equivalent term)
Lymphoma, primary, of brain
Mycobacterium avium complex or *M. kansasii,* disseminated or extrapulmonary*
M. tuberculosis of any site, pulmonary,*† disseminated,* or extrapulmonary*
Mycobacterium, other species or unidentified species, disseminated† or extrapulmonary*
Pneumocystis jiroveci pneumonia*
Pneumonia, recurrent*†
Progressive multifocal leukoencephalopathy
Salmonella septicemia, recurrent
Toxoplasmosis of brain, onset at age >1 month*
Wasting syndrome attributed to HIV

*Condition that might be presumptively diagnosed.
†Only among adults and adolescents aged at least 13 years.
AIDS, acquired immune deficiency syndrome; *HIV,* human immunodeficiency virus.

infection has evolved from a terminal diagnosis to a chronic but treatable life-long disease. **Treatment objectives for *all* infected individuals are to maximally and durably suppress viral load.**[5] **Effective treatment prevents HIV disease progression and transmission, including perinatal transmission.** As treatment has progressed to preserve immunologic function, reducing HIV-related morbidity, and prolonging the duration and quality of life for infected individuals, management recommendations have changed to focus on tolerability, toxicity, and prevention of resistance. **Historically, Pediatric AIDS Clinical Trial Group (PACTG) 076 was the first study to show that ART reduces perinatal HIV transmission.**[6] This randomized, placebo-controlled study comprised treatment-naïve HIV-infected women beyond the fist trimester of pregnancy with a CD4 count above 200/mm³. Treatment included prenatal oral zidovudine (ZDV) and intrapartum intravenous (IV) ZDV, and infants received oral ZDV for 6 weeks following delivery; randomization was ethical because the safety within pregnancy and efficacy of ZDV at the time the study was initiated was unknown. Secondary to reduced HIV transmission, ZDV became the backbone of perinatal HIV treatment for over 20 years. Conversely, updated guidelines limit the recommended use of this drug secondary to toxicity (bone marrow suppression; gastrointestinal [GI] and mitochondrial toxicities such as lipoatrophy, lactic acidosis, and hepatic steatosis; skeletal muscle myopathy; and cardiomyopathy) and the availability of highly effective, well-tolerated therapies with fewer toxic side effects.[5,7] Moreover, combination antiretroviral therapy (cART) has been shown to more effectively limit perinatal HIV transmission.

Ethical Considerations

Pregnant patients should be offered ART based on the same principles used for nonpregnant individuals, taking into account pregnancy-specific maternal or fetal safety issues. **When caring for HIV-infected pregnant women, two separate but related goals emerge: (1) treatment of maternal infection and (2) chemoprophylaxis to reduce the risk of perinatal HIV transmission.** Providers who care for HIV-infected women may encounter patients who decline to start or continue ART. For guidance, the author supports the recommendations of the Panel on Treatment of HIV-Infected Pregnant Women and Prevention of Perinatal Transmission.[5,7] In summary, the provider is responsible for providing information to enable the woman to make an informed choice regarding this and other medical recommendations, including elective cesarean delivery. Coercive and punitive policies undermine trust and the provider-patient relationships. Results can include prenatal care discontinuation or failure to disclose her HIV status to other health care providers, preventing the adoption of behaviors to enhance maternal and fetal well-being. Respecting patient autonomy, we consider it unethical to consider punitive actions against a patient secondary to her decisions regarding her HIV treatment or disclosure of her HIV status. Moreover, disclosure carries risks that range from discrimination to intimate partner violence, making it critical to respect the patient's decision. **Clinicians should be aware of local legal requirements in regard to confidentiality and disclosure of HIV-related health information.**

Management During Pregnancy
Initial Evaluation

Beyond the standard initial antenatal assessment for all pregnant women, including a first-trimester ultrasound to confirm gestational age, evaluation of an HIV-infected pregnant woman

---

BOX 53-2 ASSESSMENT OF HIV DISEASE STATUS

HIV History Review

1. HIV infection duration, transmission route (if known), prior HIV-related illnesses and hospitalizations
2. Prior and ongoing ARV drug use, duration, whether treatment was for maternal benefit and/or to prevent perinatal HIV transmission, adherence and tolerance issues
3. Outcome of HIV-impacted pregnancies
4. CD4 cell counts and HIV viral loads (plasma HIV RNA copies/mL of plasma) and their relationship to ARV, results of prior HIV ARV drug-resistance studies
5. Assess need for opportunistic infection prophylaxis
6. Immunization/infection/serology status with attention to HAV, HBV, HCV, tuberculosis, pneumococcus, and Tdap

Laboratory Assessment

1. CD4 count and HIV viral load
2. ARV drug-resistance studies (genotype preferred) prior to starting or modifying ARV regimens in patients with HIV RNA levels above the threshold for resistance testing (e.g., >500 to 1000 copies/mL)
3. Baseline complete blood cell count with platelets and renal and liver function testing
4. Serologic assessment as required by history and CD4 count (for CD4 <200 cells/mm³, serology for cytomegalovirus and *Toxoplasma gondii* is indicated)
5. HLA-B*5701 testing, if abacavir use is anticipated
6. In PPD-positive patients, chest x-ray to rule out active pulmonary disease
7. If abnormal PAP smear, HPV testing and colposcopy as indicated

---

ARV, antiretroviral; *HAV,* hepatitis A virus; *HBV,* hepatitis B virus; *HCV,* hepatitis C virus; *HIV,* human immunodeficiency virus; *HLA,* human leukocyte antigen; *HPV,* human papillomavirus; *PAP,* Papanicolaou; *PPD,* purified protein derivative; *Tdap,* tetanus, diphtheria, and pertussis (vaccine).

---

should include status assessment as described in Box 53-2. **Plasma HIV RNA (viral load) is determined using reverse transcriptase–polymerase chain reaction (RT-PCR) technology.**[5] If the patient's HIV viral load is undetectable in the absence of treatment, retesting and/or using an alternative assay is recommended (bDNA signal amplification or nucleic acid sequence-based amplification [NASBA] technique).[8] Some patients may have an undetectable viral load; however, the patient could be infected with a non–clade B HIV-1 isolate or HIV-2. None of the above-mentioned assays detect HIV-2 plasma RNA. Consultation with an infectious disease physician with experience in the management of HIV disease can be helpful in these cases or when the woman's genotype and phenotype assay demonstrate significant resistance to ART. Following complete evaluation, recommendations for a plan of HIV-related medical care that includes antepartum, intrapartum, and postpartum care should be provided, taking into account issues described in the following sections.

Antepartum Care

Combination care with at least three drugs from at least two classes of ARVs is standard care for HIV infection in the United States. Patients who enter pregnancy on ART with complete viral suppression should continue their current therapy;

TABLE 53-3   TREATMENT RECOMMENDATIONS FOR ANTIRETROVIRAL-NAIVE PREGNANT WOMEN

PREFERRED BACKBONES AND REGIMENS	FDCs	COMMENT
Two-NRTI Backbones		
TDF/FTC or TDF/3TC	Truvada 200 mg FTC+ 300 mg TDF tablet	The recommended NRTI backbone for nonpregnant adults; can be administered once daily. TDF has potential renal toxicity and should be used with caution in patients with renal insufficiency.
ABC/3TC	Epzicom 300 mg 3TC + 600 mg ABC tablet	Can be administered once daily; ABC is associated with HSRs and should not be used in HLA-B*5701–positive patients; it may be less efficacious than TDF/FTC in patients with HIV RNA level >100,000.
ZDV/3TC	Combivir 150 mg 3TC + 200 mg ZDV tablet	Backbone with the most experience in pregnancy, disadvantages include twice-daily administration and increased toxicity; not a preferred backbone in nonpregnant adults.
PI Regimens		
ATV/r + two-NRTI backbone		Once-daily administration of ATV/r; no longer preferred in nonpregnant adults secondary to increased toxicity-related discontinuation compared with DRV- and RAL-based regimens.
DRV/r + two-NRTI backbone		Twice-daily administration of DRV/r in pregnancy; preferred PI in nonpregnant adults, increasing experience with use in pregnancy.
NNRTI Regimen		
EFV + two-NRTI backbone	Atripla 200 mg FTC + 300 mg TDF + 600 mg EFV tablet	Atripla enables once daily administration of a single tablet regimen; concern due to observed birth defects in primates, although human risk is unconfirmed; postpartum contraception must be ensured; preferred regimen in women who require coadministration of drugs with significant PI interactions.
INSTI Regimen		
RAL + two-NRTI backbone		Twice-daily administration of RAL; preferred NRTI regimen in nonpregnant adults, increasing experience and established PK in pregnancy. Rapid viral load reduction; however, twice daily dosing required.
Alternative Regimens		
RPV/TDF/FTC		Available in coformulated single-pill, once-daily regimen with PK pregnancy data. However, relatively little clinical experience in pregnancy and not recommended for pretreatment HIV RNA >100,000 or CD4 count <200 cells/mm³.
LPV/r + two-NRTI backbone		Twice-daily administration; once-daily LPV/r is not recommended for use in pregnant women; not a preferred PI in adults secondary to higher rates of GI side effects, hyperlipidemia, and insulin resistance.
No Longer Recommended		
SQV/r + two-NRTI backbone		Not recommended based on potential toxicity and dosing disadvantages. Baseline ECG recommended before initiation secondary to potential PR and QT prolongation; contraindicated with preexisting cardiac conduction system disease; large pill burden.
NVP + two-NRTI backbone		No longer recommended secondary to higher adverse event potential, complex lead-in dosing and low resistance barrier. NVP is administered twice daily; caution should be used when initiating ART in women with CD4 count >250 cells/mm³. Use NVP and ABC together with caution; both can cause HSRs within the first few weeks after initiation.

From Panel on Treatment of HIV-Infected Pregnant Women and Prevention of Perinatal Transmission. Recommendations for Use of Antiretroviral Drugs in Pregnant HIV-1-Infected Women for Maternal Health and Interventions to Reduce Perinatal HIV Transmission in the United States. Available at http://aidsinfo.nih.gov/contentfiles/lvguidelines/PerinatalGL.pdf. *3TC*, lamivudine; *ABC*, abacavir; *ART*, antiretroviral therapy; *ATV/r*, atazanavir/ritonavir; *DRV/r*, darunavir/ritonavir; *ECG*, electrocardiogram; *EFV*, efavirenz; *FDC*, fixed-dose combination; *FTC*, emtricitabine; *GI*, gastrointestinal; *HIV*, human immunodeficiency virus; *HLA*, human leukocyte antigen; *HSR*, hypersensitivity reaction; *INSTI*, integrase strand transfer inhibitor; *LPV/r*, lopinavir/ritonavir; *NNRTI*, nonnucleotide reverse transcriptase inhibitor; *NRTI*, nucleotide/nucleoside reverse transcriptase inhibitor; *NVP*, nevirapine; *PI*, protease inhibitor; *PK*, pharmacokinetic; *RAL*, raltegravir; *SQV*, saquinavir; *TDF*, tenofovir disoproxil fumarate; *ZDV*, zidovudine.

if a component of their regimen is contraindicated in pregnancy, the regimen should be altered without therapy interruption. If pregnancy-associated vomiting interferes with ongoing adherence to therapy, antiemetics should be aggressively used prior to discontinuing therapy. Treatment recommendations for ARV-naïve pregnant women are delineated in Table 53-3, and the most commonly used ARTs in pregnancy are described in Table 53-4. **Commonly used drug classes include nucleoside/nucleotide reverse transcriptase inhibitors (NRTIs), nonnucleoside reverse transcriptase inhibitors (NNRTIs), and protease inhibitors (PIs).** Fusion inhibitors (FIs), CCR5 antagonists, and integrase strand transfer inhibitors (INSTIs) have been less commonly used in pregnancy; however, the number of INSTI-treated women who become pregnant will increase because most recommended treatment regimens for nonpregnant adults are INSTI based. Therapeutic considerations include timing of therapy initiation, dosing changes secondary to pregnancy-associated physiologic changes, side effects, drug interactions, teratogenicity, comorbidities, convenience and adherence potential, viral resistance, and the pharmacokinetics and toxicity of transplacentally transferred drugs.

The ideal regimen demonstrates durable virologic suppression with immunologic and clinical improvement, is well tolerated with a simple dosage regimen, and has been shown to be effective in pregnancy in terms of reducing perinatal HIV transmission. ARV drug regimens used today are more convenient and better tolerated than previously utilized regimens, and this has resulted in greater efficacy and improved adherence. At least one NRTI with high placental transfer should be included within the ART regimen if possible; consultation with HIV medicine specialists is advised for women with previous ARV use for maternal indications who demonstrate significant ARV resistance upon testing or when there is a suboptimal response to ART.[7] Up-to-date U.S. treatment recommendations, including a comprehensive review of drug interactions within the adult treatment guidelines, are available online at www.AIDSinfo.nih.gov, and the National Perinatal HIV Hotline (888-448-8765) provides free clinical consultation on all aspects of perinatal HIV care.[7]

Maternal cART should be started as soon as possible and should not be delayed for resistance testing results. Resistance testing should still be performed because it provides important

TABLE 53-4   COMMONLY USED ANTIRETROVIRAL DRUGS IN PREGNANCY

DRUG DOSAGE	FDA PREGNANCY CATEGORY	PHARMACOKINETICS IN PREGNANCY	PREGNANCY CONCERNS AND RECOMMENDATIONS
NRTIs			
Tenofovir disoproxil fumarate (TDF; Viread), 300 mg QD	B	AUC lower in third trimester than postpartum with adequate trough levels in the majority of women. Placental transfer is high.	Twofold increase in birth defects ruled out, 2.2% birth defect prevalence (47 of 2141 births); clinical studies in humans (particularly children) show reversible bone demineralization with chronic use; with HBV coinfection, possible HBV flare when drug is stopped; monitor renal function secondary to potential toxicity.
Lamivudine (3TC; Epivir), 150 mg BID or 300 mg QD	C	PKs are not significantly altered in pregnancy; no change in dose is indicated. Placental transfer is high.	A 1.5-fold increase in birth defects ruled out, with a 3.2% birth defect prevalence (137 of 4418 births). Short-term safety demonstrated for mother and infant; 3TC has antiviral activity against HBV; if coinfected, HBV flare is possible if drug is stopped postpartum.
Emtricitabine (FTC; Emtriva), biologically active form of 3TC, 200 mg QD	B	PK study shows slightly lower levels in third trimester compared with postpartum; no need to increase dose. Placental transfer is high.	Twofold increase in birth defects ruled out, 2.3% birth defect prevalence; antiviral activity against HBV; if coinfected, HBV flare is possible if drug is stopped postpartum.
Abacavir (ABC; Ziagen), 300 mg BID or 600 mg QD	C	PKs are not significantly altered in pregnancy; no change in dose is indicated. Placental transfer is high.	Twofold increase in birth defects ruled out, 3.0% birth defect prevalence (27 of 805 births); hypersensitivity reactions occur in ~5% to 8% of nonpregnant persons; a much smaller percentage are fatal, usually associated with rechallenge. Patients should be educated regarding symptoms, and HLA-B*5701 testing identifies patients at risk.
Zidovudine (ZDV; Retrovir), 300 mg BID	C	PKs are not significantly altered in pregnancy; no dose change is indicated. Placental transfer is high.	1.5-fold increase in birth defects ruled out, 3.2% birth defect prevalence (129 of 4034 births). Short-term safety demonstrated for mother and infant. ZDV is associated with macrocytic anemia.
Didanosine (ddI; Videx), ≥60 kg: 400 mg QD, with TDF 250 mg QD; <60 kg: 250 mg QD, with TDF 200 mg QD	B	PKs are not significantly altered in pregnancy; no change in dose is indicated. Placental transfer is moderate.	Human birth defect rate was 4.8% (20 of 418), compared with 2.7% in the general population; no pattern of defects was discovered. Cases of lactic acidosis, some fatal, have been reported in pregnant women receiving ddI and d4T together; only use if no other alternative is available.
Stavudine (d4T; Zerit), ≥60 kg: 40 mg BID; <60 kg: 30 mg BID	C	PKs are not significantly altered in pregnancy; no change in dose is indicated. Placental transfer is high.	Twofold increase in birth defects ruled out, 2.6% prevalence in birth defects (21 of 809 births); antagonistic with ZDV; cases of fatal lactic acidosis have been reported in pregnant women receiving ddI and d4T together.
NNRTIs			
Efavirenz (EFV; Sustiva), 600 mg QD at or before bedtime	D	AUC decreased during third trimester, compared with postpartum, but nearly all third-trimester subjects exceeded target exposure; no dosage change is indicated. Placental transfer is moderate.	Antiretroviral Pregnancy Registry (prospective) documented birth defects in 20 of 852 live births (2.3%) following first-trimester EFV exposure, including a single NTD with fetal alcohol syndrome and a single case of bilateral facial clefts, anophthalmia, and amniotic band (2.3% birth defect prevalence, twofold increase in overall birth defects ruled out). Retrospective data include six case reports of CNS defects following EFV exposure; however, a meta-analysis of more than 2000 first-trimester EFV-exposed live births showed no increase in overall birth defects (2.0%) and a single NTD (overall incidence 0.07%).[7]
Nevirapine (NVP; Viramune), 200 mg QD for 14 days, then 200 mg BID	C	PKs are not significantly altered in pregnancy; no dose change is indicated. Placental transfer is high.	Twofold increase in birth defects ruled out, 2.9% birth defect prevalence (31 of 1068 births); increased risk of symptomatic, rash-associated, potentially fatal liver toxicity in women with CD4+ counts >250/mm³ when initiating therapy; pregnancy does not increase this risk. Women who become pregnant while taking NVP-containing regimens but are tolerating them well should continue therapy independent of CD4+ count.
Etravirine (ETR; Intelence), 200 mg BID	B	PK data suggest increased exposure in pregnancy of 1.2-1.6 fold. Limited data suggest high placental transfer.	Fewer than 200 first-trimester exposures reported to the Antiretroviral Pregnancy Registry, precluding conclusions regarding birth defect risk.
Rilpivirine (RPV; Edurant), 25 mg QD		Limited PK studies suggest 20% reduced AUC in second trimester and 30% reduction in the third trimester. Placental transfer is unknown.	The limited number of first-trimester exposures reported to the Antiretroviral Pregnancy Registry precludes conclusions regarding birth defect risk.
Protease Inhibitors			
Atazanavir (ATV; Reyataz), PK enhancement required (low-dose RTV), ATV 300 mg + RTV 100 mg QD (increase ATV dose to 400 mg for TDV, EFV, or H2 blocker)	B	PK studies with RTV boosting during pregnancy suggests that standard dosing yields decreased AUC; however, for most pregnant women, no dose adjustment was needed. TDF reduces ATV AUC in all patients by 25%. Placental transfer is low.	Twofold birth defect increase ruled out, 2.2% birth defect prevalence (16 of 922 births). Neurodevelopmental delays have been reported in two studies. ATV-treated adults often have elevated indirect bilirubin levels; increased bilirubin was reported in some infants born to mothers receiving ATV, associated with UGT1A1 genotypes linked to decreased UGT function. Neonatal hypoglycemia has been reported in 3 of 38 ATV-exposed infants.

TABLE 53-4 COMMONLY USED ANTIRETROVIRAL DRUGS IN PREGNANCY—cont'd

DRUG DOSAGE	FDA PREGNANCY CATEGORY	PHARMACOKINETICS IN PREGNANCY	PREGNANCY CONCERNS AND RECOMMENDATIONS
Lopinavir/ritonavir (LPV/r; Kaletra), built in low-dose RTV boosting 400/100 mg BID In second and third trimesters, 600/150 mg BID	C	Once-daily dosing is not recommended in pregnancy. AUC is decreased in second and third trimesters with standard dosing. LPV/r 600 mg/150 mg BID resulted in AUC similar to that of nonpregnant adults receiving LPV/r 400 mg/100 mg. Alternative strategy adds a pediatric LPV/r tablet (100/25 mg) to the standard adult dose. Placental transfer is low.	Twofold increase in birth defect ruled out, 2.2% birth defect prevalence (26 of 1174). Well-tolerated, short-term safety has been demonstrated in Phase I and II studies.
Ritonavir (RTV; Norvir), 100 mg to 400 mg in one or two divided doses as PK enhancer	B	RTV levels are reduced in pregnancy, including low-dose RTV PK enhancement to boost the concentrations of other PIs. Minimal placental transfer to fetus.	Limited experience at full dose in human pregnancy; this agent is currently used as low-dose RTV boosting with other PIs. No evidence of human teratogenicity (twofold increase in birth defects ruled out).
Saquinavir HGC (SQV; Invirase), use with PK enhancement (low-dose RTV), SQV 1000 mg + RTV 100 mg BID	B	PK data suggest that 1000 mg SQV HGC/100 mg RTV twice daily achieves adequate SQV drug levels in pregnant women. Placental transfer to fetus is minimal.	Well-tolerated, short-term safety has been demonstrated for mother and infant for SQV in combination with low-dose RTV boosting. Baseline ECG is recommended before starting because PR and/or QT interval prolongations have been observed.
Indinavir (IDV; Crixivan), prescribe with low-dose RTV boosting (IDV 800 mg + RTV 100 mg) BID	C	Studies using IDV alone showed markedly lower pregnancy levels, compared with postpartum, although HIV RNA suppression was seen. Use only with RTV PK enhancement. Placental transfer to the fetus is minimal.	Twofold increase in birth defect ruled out, 2.4% birth defect prevalence (7/289). Pill burden and renal stone potential are concerns. In rhesus monkeys, neonatal IDV exacerbated transient physiologic hyperbilirubinemia; this was not seen following in utero exposure. Given limited data regarding dosing, trough drug levels should be monitored.
Nelfinavir (NFV; Viracept), 1250 mg BID	B	Using 625-mg tablets, lower AUC and peak levels were seen in the third trimester versus postpartum; however, viral load was suppressed in most women. Placental transfer is minimal.	Twofold increase in overall birth defects ruled out; well-tolerated, short-term safety demonstrated for mother and infant; consider in special circumstances when alternative agents are not tolerated given extensive experience in pregnancy.
Darunavir (DRV; Prezista), PK enhancement required; ARV exp with mutations or pregnancy (DRV 600 mg + RTV 100 mg) BID	C	Used in pregnancy with low-dose RTV boosting; reduced third-trimester plasma concentrations have been observed. Placental transfer is low to moderate.	Experience in human pregnancy is limited with 2.3% (6 of 258 births) birth defect prevalence. Once-daily dosing is not recommended in pregnancy, although 800 mg plus RTV 100 mg twice daily is being investigated.
Fosamprenavir (FPV; Lexiva) Amprenavir prodrug; must use low-dose RTV boosting (FPV 700 mg + RTV 100 mg) BID	C	With RTV boosting, AUC is reduced in the third trimester; however, trough levels appear adequate for patients without PI resistance mutations. Placental transfer is low.	Data are insufficient to assess human teratogenicity. Unboosted FPV and once-daily dosing are not recommended in pregnancy.
Tipranavir (TPV; Aptivus), low-dose RTV PK enhancement required (TPV 500 mg + RTV 200 mg) BID	C	Unknown rate of placental transfer to fetus. Safety and PK data in pregnancy are insufficient to recommend use.	Exposures are insufficient to establish birth defect prevalence.
Integrase Inhibitors			
Raltegravir (RAL; Isentress), 400 mg BID	C	PKs are variable in pregnancy; however, there is no clear relationship between raltegravir concentration and virologic effect in nonpregnant adults. Placental transfer is high.	Severe, potentially life-threatening and fatal skin and hypersensitivity reactions have been reported in nonpregnant adults. One case of markedly elevated liver transaminases was reported with use in late pregnancy. This agent rapidly suppresses viral load, but experience in pregnancy is limited.
Dolutegravir (DTG; Tivicay), 50 mg QD for INSTI-naïve patients	B	No studies of DTG use in pregnancy have been reported; placental transfer occurs in animals.	Exposures are insufficient to establish birth defect prevalence.
Elvitegravir (EVG; Stribild, which includes COBI/ TDF/FTC), 1 tablet daily	B	No studies of EVG use in pregnancy have been reported; breast milk secretion in animals has been reported.	Exposures are insufficient to establish birth defect prevalence.

AUC, area under the curve; *AZT,* azidothymidine; *BID,* twice per day; *CNS,* central nervous system; *COBI,* cobicistat; *ECG,* electrocardiograph; *FTC,* emtricitabine; *H2,* histamine 2; *HBV,* hepatitis B virus; *HGC,* hard gel capsule; *INSTI,* integrase strand transfer inhibitor; *NRTI,* nucleotide/nucleoside reverse transcriptase inhibitor; *NTD,* neural tube defect; *PI,* protease inhibitor; *PK,* pharmacokinetic; *QD,* once per day; *UGT,* uridine diphosphate glucuronosyltransferase; *UGT1A1,* uridine diphosphate glucuronosyltransferase 1.

information for ongoing patient care, and results can be used to modify treatment if needed. Early initiation of therapy is based on the knowledge that comprehensive regimens that comprise antepartum and intrapartum maternal treatment and postpartum infant treatment provide the best protection against perinatal HIV transmission. Additionally, the European National Study of HIV in Pregnancy and Childhood demonstrated that **with longer duration of antenatal ARV prophylaxis, starting prior to 28 weeks' gestation, each additional week of therapy corresponds to a 10% reduced risk of HIV transmission after adjusting for viral load, mode of delivery, and sex of the infant.**[7] Moreover, expanding infant postexposure prophylaxis does not fully substitute for the protective effect of increased maternal ART duration, which also supports early effective maternal treatment. Women with undetectable viral loads should also receive cART because their risk of perinatal transmission is 9.8% if untreated.[9]

Nucleoside/Nucleotide Reverse Transcriptase Inhibitors

Nucleoside/nucleotide reverse transcriptase inhibitors (NRTIs) are used within combination regimens that usually include two NRTIs with either an NNRTI, INSTI, or a PI. Tenofovir (TDF)–emtricitabine (FTC) is the preferred NRTI backbone in treatment-naïve nonpregnant adults, and Table 53-3 shows recommended NRTI backbones for ARV-naïve pregnant women. FTC is the biologically active form of lamivudine (3TC), thus these drugs can be used interchangeably, and there is no benefit to using FTC and 3TC together. Abacavir (ABC) is associated with hypersensitivity reactions. Human leukocyte antigen B (HLA-B) *5701 testing identifies patients at risk; testing should be performed and documented prior to initiating this therapy, and NRTIs are described in Table 53-4. ZDV and 3TC remain a preferred treatment option for treatment-naive pregnant women, despite their toxicity, secondary to extensive experience.[7] **All NRTIs bind to mitochondrial γ-DNA polymerase, potentially causing dysfunction that manifests as clinically significant myopathy, cardiomyopathy, neuropathy, lactic acidosis, or fatty liver—which resembles hemolysis, elevated liver enzymes, low platelets (HELLP) syndrome.** Lactic acidosis and hepatic failure have been noted with long-term combined stavudine and didanosine use, linked to a genetic defect in mitochondrial fatty acid metabolism; therefore this regimen should not be used in pregnancy.[7] Mitochondrial toxicity has been observed in children born to HIV-infected mothers treated with NRTIs, although no increase in mortality was observed.

Nonnucleoside Reverse Transcriptase Inhibitors

Nonnucleoside reverse transcriptase inhibitors (NNRTIs) are typically used with two NRTIs. Efavirenz (EFV) remains the preferred NNRTI in pregnancy; however, tolerability concerns and potential suicidality association led to reclassification to an alternative regimen in nonpregnant adults. EFV is associated with a 2.3% birth defect incidence following first-trimester exposure[9a]; however, EFV remains classified as U.S. Food and Drug Administration (FDA) pregnancy category D based on retrospective studies that have reported central nervous system (CNS) defects. **Current perinatal HIV treatment guidelines support initiation of EFV after the first 8 weeks of pregnancy.**[7] Continuing EFV in virologically suppressed women who present for care in the first trimester is also endorsed because the potential neural tube defect risk is restricted to the first 5 to 6 weeks of pregnancy. This recommendation considers the low likelihood of early pregnancy diagnosis, potential loss of viral control if ARV drugs are changed, and the increased perinatal HIV transmission risk associated with therapy interruption in the first trimester (4.8%).[7] Nevirapine (NVP) is no longer recommended based on its low resistance barrier, high potential for adverse events, and complex lead-in dosing. NVP should not be used for initial treatment in ART-naïve pregnant women with CD4[+] cell counts greater than 250 cells/mm[3]; however, it is safe to continue this drug in women who become pregnant while taking NVP-containing regimens.

Protease Inhibitors

Protease inhibitors (PIs) are characterized by minimal transplacental passage and few adverse side effects, and they are typically paired with two NRTIs. These drugs are ideal for patients who require therapy initiation prior to receiving genotyping results because PI-resistant viruses in ARV-naïve patients are uncommon. And because their short half-life protects against the emergence of resistance with therapy discontinuation, PIs are also a good choice for women who may discontinue therapy postpartum; however, these agents are associated with hyperglycemia in adults, although pregnancy does not seem to increase hyperglycemia.[10] An early glucose challenge test followed by repeat testing after 28 weeks is reasonable in high-risk patients. Conflicting data exist regarding preterm delivery in women who receive PIs. During pregnancy, lower serum concentrations of lopinavir/ritonavir (LPV/r), atazanavir (ATV), and nelfinavir (NFV) have been reported; pregnancy-adjusted dosage regimens are detailed in Table 53-4.[7] Pharmacokinetic (PK) enhancers or boosters—cobicistat (COBI) or low-dose ritonavir, as well as the INSTI elvitegravir (EVG)—improve the PK profiles of several of these drugs via cytochrome (CY) P3A4 inhibition. Although more experience has been reported in pregnancy using ritonavir PK enhancement, multiple fixed-dose combination (FDC) products that incorporate cobicistat are available. Thus providers are likely to encounter women entering pregnancy using cobicistat-containing regimens.

Integrase Strand Transfer Inhibitors

INSTIs are a recently developed class of ARV drugs inhibiting HIV integrase, the enzyme catalyzing insertion of HIV DNA into the human cell genome. Integration is required for replication and stable maintenance of the viral genome, also enabling the establishment of persistent infection. Enzymatic activity consists of two steps: a preparatory step excising two nucleotides from one strand at both ends of the HIV DNA and a final "strand transfer" step inserting viral DNA into an exposed region of cellular DNA. Current integrase inhibitor drugs target the second integration step, strand transfer. Because HIV integrase represents a distinct therapeutic target, integrase inhibitors are expected to maintain activity against HIV that is resistant to other classes of ARV drugs. INSTIs are characterized by their ability to rapidly reduce HIV viral load. Raltegravir (Isentress, RAL) is FDA pregnancy category C and a component of the preferred INSTI regimen in pregnancy.

Hepatitis Coinfection

All HIV-infected women should be screened for hepatitis B virus (HBV) and hepatitis C virus (HCV) unless they are already known to be infected. Recommended screening is via antibody detection, and for HIV-infected women, HBV

TABLE 53-5   PROPHYLACTIC ANTIBIOTIC REGIMENS FOR COMMON OPPORTUNISTIC INFECTIONS

CONDITION	INDICATION FOR PROPHYLAXIS	ANTIBIOTIC REGIMEN
Pneumocystis jiroveci pneumonia	Prior infection or CD4 <200/mm^3	TMP-SMX 1 DS tablet QD indefinitely
Toxoplasma gondii encephalitis	CD4 <100/mm^3, *Toxoplasma* IgG+	TMP-SMX 1 DS tablet QD indefinitely
Mycobacterium tuberculosis infection (i.e., treatment of latent infection)	+PPD >5 mm No active disease on chest radiograph	300 mg INH and 50 mg pyridoxine QD for 9 months
Disseminated *Mycobacterium avium* complex disease	CD4 <50/mm^3	1200 mg azithromycin weekly
Cryptococcosis	CD4 <50/mm^3	Prophylaxis is not recommended in the absence of documented infection; patients treated for acute cryptococcal infection should receive 200 mg fluconazole QD indefinitely.

From Panel on Opportunistic Infections in HIV-Infected Adults and Adolescents. Guidelines for the prevention and treatment of opportunistic infections in HIV-infected adults and adolescents: recommendations from the Centers for Disease Control and Prevention, the National Institutes of Health, and the HIV Medicine Association of the Infectious Diseases Society of America. Available at http://aidsinfo.nih.gov/contentfiles/lvguidelines/adult_oi.pdf.
DS, double strength; *IgG*, immunoglobin G; *INH*, isoniazid; *PPD*, purified protein derivative; *QD*, once per day; *TMP-SMX*, trimethoprim-sulfamethoxazole.

screening should include hepatitis B surface antigen (HBsAg), anti-HBs, and anti-HBc (hepatitis B core). Women with negative screens should receive the HBV vaccine series. Women found to be HBV coinfected should receive ART that uses an NRTI backbone with two drugs active against HIV and HBV; TDF/3TC and TDF/FTC are the preferred NRTI backbones for HIV/HBV coinfected pregnant women. Women with HBV coinfection should have transaminase testing 1 month after initiating ARV and every 3 months thereafter. Differentiating among an HBV flare, immune reconstitution, and drug toxicity can be challenging, and consultation with an expert in HIV and HBV coinfection is recommended.[7] For prophylaxis, the infant should receive HBV immune globulin and the first dose of the HBV vaccine series within 12 hours of birth. HCV therapy is rapidly evolving, and some regimens are safe in pregnancy; therefore HCV coinfected women should be referred to a hepatologist for treatment evaluation. For coinfected patients, delivery planning should be solely based on standard obstetric and HIV-related indications. Coinfected patients should be screened for hepatitis A virus (HAV); and women who are negative for HAV IgG should receive the HAV vaccine series.

Opportunistic Infection Prophylaxis

Patients with a CD4 count below 200 cells/mm^3 should also receive prophylaxis against opportunistic infections (OIs). Transient CD4 count decreases may occur secondary to pregnancy-associated hemodilution; in these cases, the relative percent of CD4+ cells (see Table 53-2) can be used to guide decisions regarding OI prophylaxis. Prophylaxis regimens for *Pneumocystis jiroveci* pneumonia (PJP), toxoplasmosis, tuberculosis (TB), *Mycobacterium avium* complex (MAC), and cryptococcosis are listed in Table 53-5; additional prophylaxis is listed in the Guidelines for the Prevention and Treatment of Opportunistic Infection in HIV-Infected Adults and Adolescents.[4] Prophylactic pyridoxine is increased to 50 mg/day in pregnancy to prevent maternal and fetal neurotoxicity. When untreated HIV patients are diagnosed with a treatable OI—including TB, MAC, PJP, toxoplasmosis, histoplasmosis, HBV, cytomegalovirus (CMV), varicella zoster virus (VZV), or cryptococcal meningitis—providers should be aware of the potential for immune reconstitution inflammatory syndrome (IRIS) when ART is started. In short, IRIS may be observed when the immune system begins to recover and responds to the previously acquired OI with an exaggerated inflammatory response. However, given the goal of reducing perinatal HIV transmission, ART should be started prior to or concurrent with OI treatment.[11]

BOX 53-3   FACTORS THAT INCREASE THE RISK OF PERINATAL HIV TRANSMISSION

History of previous child with HIV infection
Mother with AIDS
Preterm delivery
Decreased maternal CD4 count
High viral load
Firstborn twin
Chorioamnionitis
Modifiable factors (cigarette smoking, illicit drug use, STDs, unprotected sexual intercourse with multiple partners during pregnancy)
Intrapartum blood exposure (e.g., episiotomy, vaginal laceration, forceps delivery)
Delivery following prolonged rupture of membranes
Breastfeeding

AIDS, acquired immune deficiency syndrome; *HIV*, human immunodeficiency virus; *STD*, sexually transmitted disease.

Ongoing Management

In addition to routine prenatal care and evaluation, viral load should be performed monthly when starting a new medication regimen or when a change in viral load is detected. **Patients on stable ART regimens and with suppressed viremia can have viral loads checked each trimester.** CD4 counts can be performed every 3 to 6 months. Vaccinations for pneumococcus and influenza should be given as needed. Coordination of services among prenatal care providers, primary care and HIV specialty care providers, mental health and drug abuse treatment services, and public assistance programs are essential to ensure that infected women remain active participants in their care and that they adhere to their ARV drug regimens.

Factors That Influence Transmission

Perinatal HIV transmission risk is associated with cigarette smoking, illicit drug use, genital tract infections, and unprotected sexual intercourse with multiple partners during pregnancy. Elimination of modifiable risk factors reduces perinatal HIV transmission and improves maternal health. Key factors that influence perinatal HIV transmission are listed in Box 53-3. **Most perinatal HIV transmission occurs within the intrapartum period; thus effective cART or scheduled cesarean delivery in patients without viral suppression substantially reduces transmission.** A minority of infected infants acquire HIV in utero, as characterized by an infant who is positive by polymerase chain reaction (PCR) testing at birth. Most studies were not designed or powered to prevent in utero HIV transmission, however data suggest that early, sustained control of viral replication prevents in utero HIV transmission. The study evaluated perinatal transmission risk factors in women with HIV RNA of fewer than 500 copies/mL at delivery; the overall HIV transmission rate was 0.5% in this population. HIV transmitters were less likely to have received ARV drugs at the time of conception than non-transmitters. Moreover, HIV transmitters were less likely to have HIV RNA of fewer than 500 copies/mL at 14, 28, and 32 weeks of gestation. Among women starting ARV during pregnancy, viral load decreased earlier in nontransmitting women, and both groups initiated therapy at the same time (30 weeks' gestation). **This suggests that early and sustained control of viral replication is associated with decreased HIV transmission, which supports cART initiation as early in pregnancy as possible for all women not treated preconceptionally.**[7,12]

HIV treatment reduces maternal disease progression, and both ART and viral load at delivery are independent risk factors for HIV transmission; **therefore ART is recommended for all women, independent of viral load suppression.** In addition to maternal benefit, this strategy protects neonates born following spontaneous rupture of membranes (SROM) or spontaneous labor that occurs prior to a planned elective cesarean delivery. Mechanisms of protection include using ARVs with good placental transfer and permitting adequate systemic drug levels to be reached in infants at birth. This is likely important when the infant is exposed to virus within the birth canal and is the recipient of a maternal-fetal blood transfusion during uterine contractions. ARVs can also decrease genital tract viral load and can be excreted into genital tract secretions; ZDV and 3TC are present at high concentrations within genital secretions, another potential mechanism of protection against HIV transmission. **Most perinatal HIV transmission in the United States occurs in women who are not known to be HIV infected prior to the birth of their child.** Given this knowledge, it is critical to emphasize the importance of prenatal care, universal HIV testing, and strategies to diagnose acute HIV infection in late pregnancy and prior to delivery and breast feeding.

Invasive Prenatal Testing

If invasive prenatal diagnostic testing is desired, the risks and benefits should be discussed and referral to a genetic counselor made (see Chapter 10). One study assessed vertical HIV transmission following amniocentesis; 1 of 61 infants was infected, which was not significantly different than the transmission rate in women who defer amniocentesis.[13] A second prospective cohort study reported no increase in mother-to-child transmission (MTCT) rates in the 162 women who underwent amniocentesis (of 9302 HIV-infected pregnancies); moreover, no cases of MTCT were identified in 81 women who received ART at the time of amniocentesis.[14] Larger studies are needed to better estimate the risk of HIV transmission following amniocentesis or chorionic villus sampling. However, evidence to date suggests no increased risk of HIV transmission in women with fully suppressed viral loads. Consideration can also be given to noninvasive screening tests such as cell-free fetal DNA (see Chapter 10).

Intrapartum Management of Human Immunodeficiency Virus

Intrapartum IV ZDV is no longer recommended for HIV-infected women who receive a combination ARV with sustained viral suppression (HIV RNA consistently ≤1000 copies/mL during late pregnancy) and no medication adherence concerns.[14] All HIV-infected women should continue ART during the intrapartum period, both for maternal health and to reduce perinatal transmission. Intrapartum ZDV is no longer recommended in virally suppressed women because ZDV therapy to reduce perinatal HIV transmission in cART-treated women has not been evaluated in randomized clinical trials. In addition, multiple studies have shown extremely limited perinatal HIV transmission in women with HIV RNA of fewer than 1000 copies/mL who did not receive intrapartum ZDV. Thus **the newest perinatal HIV treatment guidelines suggest intrapartum ZDV administration consistent with the elective cesarean delivery recommendations.**[7] For virally suppressed patients, neither intervention is expected to further reduce perinatal HIV transmission. Clinicians may also elect to use intrapartum IV ZDV based on clinical judgment.

For intrapartum patients with viral loads greater than 1000, IV ZDV should be given as a loading dose of 2 mg/kg administered over 1 hour, followed by a maintenance dose of 1 mg/kg/hr. Other ART should be taken with a sip of water except stavudine, which is antagonistic to ZDV, therefore it should be withheld. ZDV should be given independent of maternal resistance; it crosses the placenta readily and is metabolized to the active triphosphate form within the placenta, which provides prophylaxis to the infant both before and after exposure. When delivery is indicated for obstetric reasons, delivery must not be delayed for ZDV administration.

During labor, every effort should be made to avoid instrumentation that increases the neonate's exposure to infected maternal blood and secretions. Recommendations include leaving the fetal membranes intact as long as possible, avoiding fetal scalp sampling and fetal scalp electrode placement, and reserving episiotomy and assisted vaginal delivery for select circumstances. If SROM occurs, augmentation and/or induction of labor with pitocin should not be delayed. In cases of uterine atony, methergine should be avoided if possible. PIs are CYP3A4 inhibitors, and concomitant ergotamine use is associated with exaggerated vasoconstrictive responses. NNRTIs are CYP3A4 inducers that have the potential to decrease methergine levels and result in inadequate treatment effect.[7]

Elective Cesarean Delivery

Scheduled cesarean delivery at 38 weeks' gestation, confirmed by early ultrasonography, is recommended for women with HIV RNA levels greater than 1000 copies/mL and for women with unknown HIV RNA levels near the time of delivery. Patients should receive IV ZDV for 3 hours prior to surgery, and prophylactic antibiotics should be administered. These recommendations are based on studies conducted when the majority of HIV-infected women received ZDV monotherapy or no ART, whereas a more recent study of 4864 European women showed that the perinatal HIV transmission rate in women who received at least 14 days of ART was 0.8% regardless of the mode of delivery.[12] CD after onset of labor or SROM does not protect against HIV transmission, so delivery for obstetric indications is recommended in these patients irrespective of viral load.

Scheduled CD is not indicated to prevent HIV transmission in women receiving cART who have plasma HIV RNA levels below 1000 copies/mL. Perinatal HIV transmission in this group of women is 1.0% or less, and no evidence to date suggests any benefit from scheduled CD in patients receiving cART with virologic suppression.[7] Timing and route of delivery influence maternal and neonatal morbidity, and HIV-infected women have increased morbidity and mortality following CD. The risk of complications is related to the degree of immunosuppression and receipt of suppressive cART. Vaginal delivery has the lowest risk of maternal morbidity, scheduled CD is associated with an intermediate risk, and urgent CD has the highest risk of postpartum morbidity.[7,15] Neonatal adverse event risk at 38 weeks' gestation that includes death, respiratory complications, hypoglycemia, sepsis, or neonatal intensive care unit (NICU) admission is 11%, compared with 8% at 39 weeks' gestation; furthermore, infants of HIV-infected mothers have a 4.4% risk of respiratory distress syndrome (RDS) following scheduled CD, compared with 1.6% after vaginal delivery. Given the increased risk of maternal and neonatal adverse events, it is critical to appropriately counsel patients and to respect the patient's autonomy in decision making regarding the route of delivery. In addition, scheduled CD in women with HIV RNA less than 1000 should be performed at 39 weeks or for standard obstetric indications.

Spontaneous Rupture of Membranes

Increasing duration of ruptured membranes is associated with perinatal HIV transmission, but the incremental increased risk of transmission is not clinically significant. Meta-analysis of 4721 deliveries determined that the risk of HIV transmission increases by 2% over the baseline transmission risk (after adjusting for all other factors that influence transmission) for each hour increment following rupture of membranes.[16] Presuming a patient on ART with an undetectable viral load has a baseline perinatal HIV transmission rate of 2%, the risk of transmission after 1 hour of ruptured membranes would be 2.04%, and after 8 hours, the risk of HIV transmission would be 2.32%. Given that prolonged SROM does not appreciably increase HIV transmission risk in term patients, we do not recommend elective CD because it is unlikely to reduce perinatal HIV transmission risk in patients being actively managed using oxytocin for augmentation or induction.

Untreated Women

For HIV-infected women who do not receive ART before labor, IV ZDV should be given during labor. Maternal single-dose NVP is not recommended because there is no added efficacy and a high likelihood of maternal harm, specifically the emergence of a resistant virus. The safest, most effective option to reduce perinatal HIV transmission in this setting is expanded infant prophylaxis.[7] These patients should be referred for HIV care postpartum.

Intrapartum Testing

Rapid HIV testing should be performed for all laboring women without documented HIV status during pregnancy unless the patient declines (opt-out screening) because 40% to 85% of HIV-infected infants in the United States are born to women whose HIV status is unknown prior to delivery. Women with positive rapid HIV testing should be given intrapartum IV ZDV immediately, without awaiting confirmatory testing, and

the pediatrician should be alerted to begin postpartum infant prophylaxis.[7] Following confirmatory HIV antibody testing, these women should receive appropriate assessments to determine their health status, including a CD4 T-lymphocyte count and HIV-1 RNA viral load, and arrangements should be made for establishing HIV care and for providing ongoing psychosocial support after discharge.

Postpartum Care of Women with Human Immunodeficiency Virus

Ideally, women should establish a relationship with an HIV-medicine provider during the latter part of pregnancy to transition into ongoing care after delivery. **Guidelines for managing HIV infection in adults recommend cART for all infected individuals to reduce the risk of disease progression and to prevent HIV transmission, presuming patients are willing and able to commit to therapy and understand the importance of adherence.** This recommendation is based on growing evidence that uncontrolled viremia is associated with the development of non–AIDS-defining diseases that include cardiovascular, renal, and liver diseases; neurologic complications; and malignancies.[5]

Further support is provided by two studies that show delayed disease progression in women who continue cART postpartum. However, the postpartum period poses unique challenges to adherence secondary to the demands of caring for a newborn.[7] Factors to consider regarding postpartum therapy include current treatment guidelines that recommend cART for all HIV-infected individuals to reduce pretreatment CD4 cell counts and trajectory, HIV RNA levels, and adherence issues, and thereby reduce the risk of disease progression and transmission; however, any therapy must consider partner HIV status, future childbearing plans, and patient preference.[5,7]

For patients who continue cART postpartum, standard medication doses can be used immediately following delivery that predominantly affects PIs. If ART is discontinued following delivery, all drugs should be stopped simultaneously unless the patient is on a regimen that contains an NNRTI. Women who receive NNRTI-based regimens should continue the dual-NRTI backbone for at least 7 days after stopping the NNRTI to reduce the development of NNRTI resistance. An alternative, more conservative strategy is to replace the NNRTI with a PI while continuing the NRTIs then to discontinue all the drugs at the same time. The optimal interval between discontinuing an NNRTI and stopping the other ARV drugs is unknown, but at least 7 days is recommended. Drug concentrations may be detectable for more than 3 weeks after EFV discontinuation; therefore some experts recommend continuing other ARV agents or substituting a PI for EFV in addition to the other agents for up to 30 days.[7]

Infant and maternal postpartum ARV prophylaxis significantly lowers, but does not completely eliminate, the risk of postnatal HIV transmission through breast milk. Studies to discern this were performed in areas of the world where formula feeding is not a viable alternative. **Because the benefits of breastfeeding in the United States do not outweigh the risk of HIV transmission, breastfeeding is not recommended for HIV-infected women in the United States.** Contraceptive counseling is a critical aspect of postpartum care. Women should be offered highly effective contraceptives that include long-term reversible methods, implants, injectables, and intrauterine devices (IUDs) to be used in conjunction with condoms to prevent unintended pregnancy.

Infant Screening and Diagnosis

Because the fetus receives maternal IgG by transplacental passage, serologic tests of the HIV-exposed neonate will almost always be positive. In infants, the diagnosis of HIV infection is made by PCR amplification of HIV DNA (more sensitive for the neonatal period) or RNA assays. Virologic tests to diagnose HIV infection should be performed within the first 14 to 21 days of life, at 1 to 2 months, and at 4 to 6 months of age. Two positive tests on different specimens, excluding cord blood, are required to diagnose HIV infection; one positive test is a presumptive diagnosis. HIV is presumptively excluded with two negative tests, one at age 14 days or older and the second at age 1 month or older. Definitive exclusion in a non-breastfed infant is based on two negative tests at age 1 month or older and at age 4 months or older. Further details on case definitions for HIV infection are available from the CDC at www.cdc.gov.[17]

Preconception Counseling for Women With Human Immunodeficiency Virus

Providers should discuss childbearing intentions, including preconception counseling and care, with all patients in a nonjudgmental manner as recommended by the ACOG and the CDC. Issues relevant to HIV-infected women include HIV disease status assessment, hepatitis status assessment, the need for prophylaxis or treatment of opportunistic infections, and evaluating and potentially changing therapy based on the effectiveness and teratogenic potential of drugs in the ARV regimen. Because approximately half of all pregnancies in the United States are unintended, avoiding drugs with teratogenic potential (i.e., EFV) in women of reproductive age should be considered. HIV-infected women are recommended to attain a stable, maximally suppressed viral load prior to conception, because early and sustained control of HIV replication is associated with maximally decreasing perinatal transmission and also reduces sexual transmission.[7] Counseling should review (1) the influence of HIV on pregnancy; (2) appropriate contraceptive options that reduce the likelihood of unintended pregnancy, because ART reduces hormonal contraceptive efficacy (predominantly NNRTIs and PIs); and (3) safe sexual practices that minimize the risk of acquiring sexually transmitted infections or acquiring more virulent or resistant HIV strains.[7] The perinatal treatment guidelines contain detailed, specific information regarding ARV and hormonal contraceptive interactions. Depot medroxyprogesterone acetate (DMPA) can be used without restriction with all ARV, whereas other contraceptives are influenced by ARVs.[7] Women contemplating pregnancy should take a daily multivitamin that includes 400 mg of folic acid to help prevent birth defects.

Human Immunodeficiency Virus Discordant Couples

HIV-uninfected pregnant women with HIV-infected partners may present for consultation. **Recommendations are to review and encourage safe sexual practices, including consistent use of barrier contraception, preexposure prophylaxis (PrEP), and a plan for HIV screening.** As a high-risk patient, first- and third-trimester screening is appropriate. This does not need to include viral load determination, because fourth-generation screening protocols are sufficiently sensitive and have a lower false-positive rate. If women present to labor and delivery without documented negative serology at 36 weeks, rapid intrapartum testing should be performed. Women should also be counseled to recognize the signs and symptoms of acute HIV infection and should be advised to seek immediate care if they experience these symptoms.

Consultation in the preconception period should include screening and treatment of genital tract infections in both partners, because inflammation is associated with viral shedding and increased HIV acquisition for both partners. The HIV-infected partner should be on an ARV regimen with maximal or complete suppression of viral load, which reduces sexual transmission by as much as 96%.[5] Methods of safe conception depend on which partner is HIV infected. For an HIV-infected woman, the safest conception method is artificial insemination. This can be performed in the periovulatory period by the patient at home using a syringe. In discordant couples with an HIV-infected man, the safest reproductive option is using donor sperm from an HIV-uninfected man. If this is not acceptable, semen analysis is recommended (HIV and ARV may reduce sperm count and quality) to prevent unnecessary exposure to infectious genital fluid if the likelihood of getting pregnant is low. Sperm preparation techniques coupled with intrauterine insemination (with or without ovulation induction), in vitro fertilization, or intracytoplasmic sperm injection has been reported to be effective in avoiding seroconversion in uninfected women and offspring. The National Perinatal HIV Hotline (1-888-448-8765) is a resource for a list of institutions that offer reproductive services for HIV-serodiscordant couples. In patients without resources to enable assisted reproductive technology, timed periovulatory unprotected intercourse (condoms should be used at all other times) with a maximally suppressed partner may reduce sexual HIV transmission.

Periconception preexposure prophylaxis (PrEP) may minimize HIV transmission risk within discordant couples. **PrEP is the use of ARV medications by HIV-uninfected individuals to maintain blood and genital drug levels sufficient to prevent HIV acquisition.** Whereas studies have demonstrated that PrEP reduces the risk of HIV acquisition in both men and women, with minimal risk of incident ARV resistance, others have not shown benefit, likely related to adherence issues. One study that investigated PrEP with timed intercourse gave oral TDF at the luteinizing hormone peak with a second oral dose 24 hours later. None of the women became HIV infected, and pregnancy rates were high, plateauing at 75% after 12 attempts. Combination TDF/FTC, currently being evaluated in ongoing trials, is recommended for anyone at ongoing risk of HIV acquisition. Pregnancy is not a contraindication to PrEP.

Counseling and Coordination of Care

Ongoing care of the HIV-infected pregnant woman is enhanced by having a multidisciplinary team, which may include physicians, social workers, a nutritionist, psychologists, and peer counselors. Management should include frequent visits and ongoing discussion regarding adherence to medication regimens to prevent the development of resistance to ARV therapy and to reduce perinatal HIV transmission. Patients should be counseled about the impact of HIV infection on pregnancy, including the risk of perinatal transmission, side effects of medications, potential methods of delivery, and treatment options. **Studies have shown that pregnancy does not affect the progression of HIV disease.** It is unclear whether ART influences preterm delivery, although some reports have shown an increased risk. However, a recent prospective cohort study of over 800 patients who received cART between 2002 and 2008 did not find an increased incidence of preterm birth in women who received PIs.[18] Although a potential increased risk of preterm birth with ART cannot be fully ruled out, the clear maternal health benefits and reduced perinatal HIV transmission support the use of ART during pregnancy. Ascertaining whether the patient has disclosed her HIV serostatus to sex and needle-sharing partners is appropriate. Addressing barriers that prevent disclosure, including recommendations and/or referral for assistance regarding how to safely disclose HIV serostatus, is warranted. Some state and local governments require that clinicians report any known partners of HIV-infected patients to the local health department; thus providers should be aware of regulations that will influence their practice.

For both HIV-infected and exposed women, HIV prevention should be discussed using a straightforward, nonjudgmental approach. Ongoing risk identification should be performed that includes sexual behaviors, IV drug use, sexually transmitted diseases, and untreated psychiatric issues that potentially increase a person's likelihood of engaging in risky behaviors. Behavior interventions, treatment, and avoidance of risk factors should be discussed, emphasizing the importance of consistent condom use and consideration of PrEP even though ART decreases the risk of HIV transmission. Although no reliable data on HIV serodiscordance rates in the United States exist, data on women from sub-Saharan Africa show that women in serodiscordant relationships may be particularly vulnerable to HIV infection.[7]

INFLUENZA
Virology and Epidemiology
Influenza is in the Orthomyxoviridae family, which includes the genera *Influenzavirus A, Influenzavirus B,* and *Influenzavirus C.* Influenza B and C are found almost exclusively in humans, whereas the host range of influenza A includes mammalian and avian species. Influenza virus has a negative-stranded, segmented RNA genome that enables *reassortment,* the rearrangement of viral gene segments in cells infected with two different influenza viruses. This results in the rapid generation of new influenza virus strains (recombinants), which have been responsible for pandemic outbreaks, and is termed *antigenic shift.* Point mutations within the viral genome result in minor, gradual antigenic changes defined as *antigenic drift.* These genetic strategies, combined with a wide host range and our inability to generate a protective immune response against the entire genera, enable influenzavirus to remain an important pathogen that requires annual vaccination. **The World Health Organization (WHO) and U.S. Public Health Service recommend strains to be included in the annual vaccine based on recent prevalence.**

Influenza viruses are enveloped; hemagglutinin (H or HA) and neuraminidase (N or NA) viral glycoproteins are present on the surface, and the virus capsid proteins are M1 and M2. HA binds the cell surface receptor (neuraminic acid), is highly antigenic, and is the target of neutralizing antibodies that protect against infection. NA does not induce neutralizing antibodies; however, antibodies that recognize NA are disease suppressive but permit infection. NA cleaves sialic acid from the infected cell surface, which facilitates virus release (budding) from these cells, and it may remove sialic acid from mucin, enabling cell-free virus to reach epithelial cells. Viral entry begins when HA binds the cell receptor, followed by endocytosis of the viral particle. Within the endocytic compartment, low pH triggers conformational changes in HA, which are required for fusion.

Viral uncoating also requires M2, an ion channel protein that permits influx of H^+ ions into the virus particle, which enables the viral nucleoprotein to enter the cytoplasm.

Influenza strains are named according to their genus (type), the species from which the virus was isolated (omitted if human), and the H and N subtypes. H subtypes confer species specificity, and there is only a single NA subtype for influenza B. **Influenza is spread by respiratory droplets, is highly contagious, and occurs as an epidemic typically during the winter months.** Approximately 50 million cases occur annually in the United States. Children younger than 2 years old and the elderly have the highest hospitalization rates. In 2009, a novel influenza A, H1N1, emerged secondary to complex genetic reassortment. A unique pandemic ensued; 90% of hospitalizations and 87% of deaths occurred in people younger than 65 years. In addition, **788 pregnant women with confirmed or probable H1N1 that resulted in 280 intensive care unit (ICU) admissions and 56 deaths were documented during this pandemic.** The documented case reports potentially underreport infection and overestimate the prevalence of severe illness. The influence of this pandemic can be extrapolated from the mortality rate: **5% of H1N1-related deaths occurred in pregnant women, which represented only 1% of the population; this suggests that pregnant women infected with influenza had an elevated risk of serious illness and death, according to multiple published studies.[19,20]**

Clinical Manifestations
Influenza viruses cause acute upper respiratory tract illness, characterized by the abrupt onset of fever, chills, headache, myalgias, malaise, a dry cough, and nasal discharge. GI manifestations and conjunctivitis can also be present. The incubation period ranges from 1 to 5 days, and most cases of influenza are self-limited. Complications include pneumonia, which occurs in up to 12% of influenza-infected pregnant women,[21] along with Reye syndrome and disseminated intravascular coagulation (DIC). Changes in the immune, cardiac, and respiratory systems likely increase the risk of severe illness in pregnant women infected with influenza.

Diagnosis
Rapid influenza diagnostic tests (RIDTs) are immunoassays that identify influenza A and B viral nucleoproteins in 15 minutes or less. RIDTs are very specific (90% to 95%) but the sensitivity is limited (10% to 70%), with the potential for false-negative results during periods of high influenza incidence. False-positive results occur when influenza is at low prevalence. Some RIDTs distinguish between influenza A and B, but they cannot determine viral subtype. The optimal time of specimen collection is within 48 to 72 hours of illness onset. Confirmation is via RT-PCR, culture, ELISA, or immunofluorescence of respiratory secretions; immunofluorescence and RT-PCR have the most rapid turnaround.

Management of Influenza During Pregnancy
Pregnant women suspected to be infected with influenza should be treated immediately, independent of vaccination status, without waiting for diagnostic confirmation. The recommended treatment for both seasonal and pandemic influenza infection is oseltamivir (Table 53-6); acetaminophen should be used as an antipyretic, and additional recommendations regarding adjunctive therapy are presented in Chapter 38.

TABLE 53-6 ANTIVIRAL MEDICATION DOSING RECOMMENDATIONS FOR INFLUENZA

ANTIVIRAL AGENT	ACTIVITY	ACTION	USE	DOSAGE	DURATION	CONTRAINDICATIONS
Oseltamivir (Tamiflu)	Influenza A and B	NA inhibitor	Treatment	75 mg BID	5 days	None
			Prophylaxis	75 mg QD	7 days	
Zanamivir (Relenza)	Influenza A and B	NA inhibitor	Treatment	10 mg BID inhaled	5 days	Underlying respiratory disease
			Prophylaxis	10 mg QD inhaled	7 days	
Peramivir (Rapivab)	Influenza A and B	NA inhibitor	Treatment	600 mg IV infusion over 15 to 30 min		Category C, limited experience in pregnancy, use only if clearly needed

BID, twice per day; *NA*, neuraminidase; *QD*, once per day.

BOX 53-4 RISK FACTORS FOR SEVERE ILLNESS AND DEATH IN INFLUENZA VIRUS–INFECTED PREGNANT WOMEN

Asthma
Smoking
Obesity
Chronic hypertension
Delayed treatment

The preterm birth rate following pandemic H1N1 infection was 30%. Increased preterm parturition also occurs following seasonal influenza infection, so appropriate monitoring should be undertaken, particularly in women with respiratory compromise.[19,22,23] Early antiviral treatment reduces the duration of the illness, secondary complications, and hospitalizations. Initiating treatment up to 5 days after symptom onset still confers benefit. The risk of severe illness and death is highest in the latter part of pregnancy, compared with the first trimester. Other risk factors are described in Box 53-4.[19,22] The pregnancy-associated risk of illness persists for 2 weeks postpartum.

Chemoprophylaxis should be considered for high-risk, unvaccinated women exposed within 48 hours of presentation (see Table 53-6). Alternative therapy for infection includes amantadine or rimantadine, both of which block M2 channel activity in influenza A. However, significant viral resistance to these drugs limits their effectiveness. **To prevent maternal influenza infection and associated perinatal morbidity and mortality, both the ACOG and the CDC recommend annual vaccination of all pregnant women during influenza season (October to May) using the intramuscular inactivated vaccine.**[24] Maternal vaccination also protects infants up to 6 months of age from influenza infection, has no adverse fetal effects, and is safe in breastfeeding women. **The intranasal vaccine contains live virus and should *not* be used during pregnancy.** The optimal time to vaccinate patients is in October and November to minimize the risk of acquiring influenza. However, vaccination is safe and effective at any time of the year and at any gestational age.

PARVOVIRUS
Virology and Epidemiology
Parvoviruses are small, nonenveloped viruses that contain negative-stranded DNA that encodes two major genes: the REP, or NS, gene encodes functions required for transcription and DNA replication; and the CAP, or S, gene encodes the coat proteins VP1 and VP2. Parvovirus B19 was identified in the 1970s in blood bank specimens and was first linked to sickle cell disease patients with transient aplastic crisis. Parvovirus B19 was then associated with fifth disease, or erythema infectiosum (EI),

and was later linked to hydrops fetalis. Parvoviruses preferentially infect rapidly dividing cells, which explains the observed fetal and neonatal susceptibility. Parvovirus B19 infection is restricted to humans, and the cellular receptor is erythrocyte P antigen, which explains the propensity of this virus to infect red blood cells and their precursors. P antigen is also expressed on megakaryocytes, endothelial cells, placenta, fetal liver, and fetal heart. Parvovirus B19 is spread via respiratory droplets, infected blood products, with hand-to-mouth contact, and perinatally. The incubation period ranges from 4 to 20 days following exposure. Seroprevalence increases with age, and 65% of pregnant women have evidence of prior infection and are immune. Conversely, susceptible women have approximately a 50% risk of seroconversion following exposure to parvovirus B19. Daycare workers, teachers, and parents have all been shown to be at increased risk of seroconversion.

Clinical Manifestations
The most common presentation of B19 parvovirus infection is EI, which is characterized by a facial rash consistent with a slapped-cheek appearance and a reticulated or lacelike rash on the trunk and extremities (Fig. 53-2). The rash is immune-complex mediated and may reappear secondary to temperature changes, sunlight exposure, and stress for several weeks. Infection can also be accompanied by fever, malaise, lymphadenopathy, and symmetric peripheral arthropathy. The hands are most frequently affected followed by the knees and wrists. Symptoms are typically self-limiting but may last for several months. Asymptomatic infection occurs 20% of the time. Persistent parvovirus infection is rare and presents as pure red cell aplasia in patients who fail to mount a neutralizing antibody response.[25] **Fetal infection can be asymptomatic or characterized by aplastic anemia of varying severity. Severe anemia can lead to high-output congestive heart failure and nonimmune hydrops.** Direct infection of the myocardium may also contribute to fetal heart failure.

Diagnosis
Serologic testing via ELISA detects IgG and IgM against B19 parvovirus. However, PCR amplification of viral DNA from maternal or fetal blood is a more sensitive method to confirm acute parvovirus infection because viremia occurs prior to the development of specific antibodies, and viral protein–antibody complexes can result in false-negative serology. Maximum sensitivity is achieved with concurrent serologic and nucleic acid testing.

Management of Parvovirus During Pregnancy
Following exposure to B19 parvovirus in a presumed seronegative woman, serologic and DNA testing should be performed.

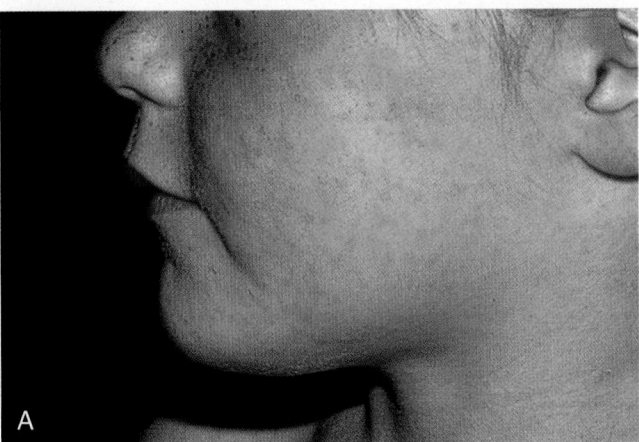

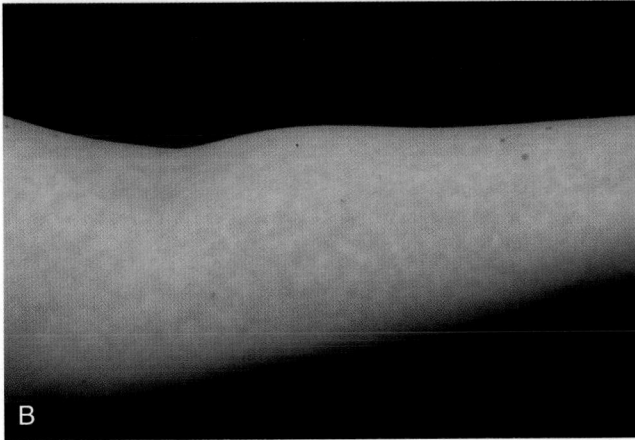

FIG 53-2 A, Characteristic "slapped cheek" rash of erythema infectiosum. **B,** Note lacelike rash on upper extremity. (From Ferri F, et al. *Ferri's Fast Facts in Dermatology.* Philadelphia: Saunders; 2011.)

TABLE 53-7	ASSOCIATION BETWEEN GESTATIONAL AGE AT TIME OF EXPOSURE AND RISK OF FETAL PARVOVIRUS INFECTION

TIME OF EXPOSURE (WEEKS OF GESTATION)	FREQUENCY OF SEVERELY AFFECTED FETUSES
1-12	19%
13-20	15%
>20	6%

The presence of IgG antibody is consistent with prior exposure and/or infection, and no further workup is needed. Susceptible women should have repeat testing performed in about 3 weeks. Pregnant women with confirmed infection should be treated with supportive care because maternal B19 parvovirus infection is usually self-limited. The relationship between the gestational age at the time of exposure to B19 parvovirus and the risk of fetal parvovirus infection that results in a severely affected fetus is shown in Table 53-7. **Serial ultrasounds to evaluate the fetus for hydrops should be performed for 8 to 10 weeks after maternal illness.** If no signs of hydrops are seen during this period, further evaluation is unnecessary. Recent studies have shown that measurement of the fetal middle cerebral artery peak systolic velocity can be useful in documenting fetal anemia prior to the development of hydrops in cases of congenital B19 parvovirus infection.[26]

Fetal infection occurs following approximately 33% of maternal infections.[27] However, the rate of fetal death secondary to intrauterine B19 parvovirus infection is dependent on when maternal infection occurs. Fetal death is rare when maternal infection occurs beyond 20 weeks of gestation, but fetal mortality associated with fetal hydrops is approximately 11% when maternal B19 infection occurs during the first 20 weeks of pregnancy.[28] Although 33% of fetal hydrops will resolve without treatment,[29] there are no reliable predictors for the resolution of hydrops versus fetal death. Thus cordocentesis and intrauterine transfusion are recommended when fetal hydrops is present.[30] Recent studies have documented thrombocytopenia in parvovirus B19–infected fetuses at the time of cordocentesis.[31] However, it is unclear whether any benefit exists to providing platelets at the time of red blood cell transfusion. The majority of fetuses infected with parvovirus B19 demonstrate normal long-term development.[32-34] Rare cases of neurologic morbidity, persistent infection with severe anemia, and other sequelae have been reported following fetal infection.

MEASLES
Virology and Epidemiology
Measles, or rubeola, is an enveloped, negative-stranded RNA virus that is part of the Paramyxoviridae family, which includes respiratory syncytial, canine distemper, mumps, and parainfluenza viruses. Measles' host range is limited to humans, and the envelope of this virus contains fusion and hemagglutinin (HA) proteins; HA binds the cellular receptor, which is a complement regulatory protein, and the fusion protein permits viral entry into the cell. **Rubeola (measles) is one of the most infectious viruses, spread primarily via respiratory droplets; with exposure, 75% to 90% of susceptible contacts become infected.** Although a live, attenuated vaccine is readily available, measles outbreaks in the United States occur among unvaccinated preschoolers, which includes those younger than 15 months; previously vaccinated school-age children; college students; and persons who originated from outside the United States. The incidence of outbreaks in previously vaccinated individuals has been reduced since implementation of a two two-dose vaccination strategy. Until 2014, fewer than 200 cases of measles were diagnosed in the United States annually. However, over 600 measles cases were documented in 2014, which included a large, multistate outbreak linked to an amusement park in California.

Clinical Manifestations
Rubeola has an incubation period of 10 to 14 days. Infected individuals first manifest prodromal symptoms, which may include fever, malaise, myalgias, and headache. This is followed by ocular symptoms that include photophobia and a nonexudative conjunctivitis. Koplik spots, tiny white spots on a red base on the buccal mucosa lateral to the molar teeth, may appear during the prodrome and are pathognomonic for measles infection. If Koplik spots are visualized, they typically appear a day or so prior to the rash and disappear within two days of its appearance. The rash of measles appears between 2 and 7 days following the prodrome and is initially present behind the ears or on the face as a blotchy erythema. The rash then spreads to the trunk, followed by the extremities; the hands and feet may be spared. The rash is initially macular and blanches with pressure but becomes papular and coalescent with a red, nonblanching component (Fig. 53-3). The rash tends to fade after about 5 days, although fever can persist for up to 6 days and may reach

41°C. A productive cough may develop that can persist after defervescence. Lymphadenopathy accompanies the fever and can persist for several weeks.

Complications of rubeola can include laryngitis, bronchiolitis, pneumonia, and otitis media due to secondary bacterial infections. Rare complications include hepatitis, encephalitis, atypical measles, and acute encephalitis. Encephalitis occurs in about 1 in 1000 cases of measles and results from either viral infection of the CNS or a hypersensitivity reaction to systemic viral infection. Symptoms include recurrence of fever and headache, vomiting, and a stiff neck followed by stupor and convulsions. The mortality is 10%, and permanent neurologic sequelae—including mental retardation—develop in 50% of individuals. Atypical measles, which occurs in adults vaccinated with the formalin-inactivated measles vaccine, is characterized by high fever, pneumonia with pleural effusions, obtundation, and a hemorrhagic exanthema. Patients usually have high antibody titers to measles but lack antibodies to the fusion protein. Atypical measles is usually self-limiting, and patients are not contagious to others. A rare complication of measles infection is subacute sclerosing panencephalitis (SSPE), which occurs in 0.5 to 2 per 1000 cases of measles years after the acute infection. SSPE is most common in children who contracted measles prior to 2 years of age and is characterized by progressive neurologic debilitation and a virtually uniformly fatal outcome.

Diagnosis

The diagnosis of measles is usually made based on clinical presentation; as mentioned earlier, Koplik spots are pathognomonic for measles infection. In their absence, diagnosis is based on a history of recent exposure or the presence of a rash. An increase in antibody titer may be detected as early as the first or second day of the rash. Assays for detection of IgM and viral

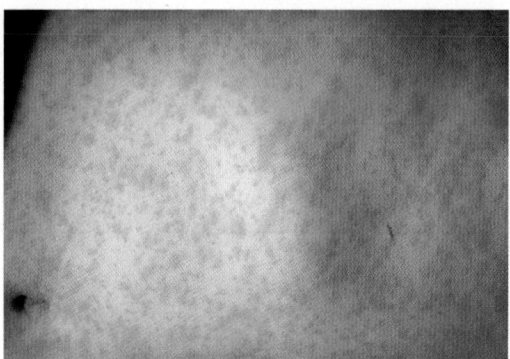

FIG 53-3 Maculopapular rash of measles, or rubeola, showing coalescence of lesions. (Courtesy Centers for Disease Control and Prevention, Dr. Heinz F. Eichenwald.)

RNA are also available. Differential diagnoses include rubella, scarlet fever, infectious mononucleosis, secondary syphilis, toxic shock syndrome, Kawasaki disease, erythema infectiosum, and drug rash. A guide to differentiating some of these illnesses is shown in Table 53-8.[35]

Management of Measles During Pregnancy

Pregnant women with rubeola infection should receive supportive care and should undergo careful observation for evidence of complications. **The largest, most recently reported study of measles in pregnancy revealed that pregnant women were twice as likely to require hospitalization (60%), three times as likely to acquire pneumonia (26%), and six times as likely to die of complications (3%) compared with nonpregnant adults.**[36] Given the higher rate of maternal morbidity and mortality in the setting of measles infection, secondary bacterial infections should be treated promptly with antibiotics. Ribavirin can be considered for cases of viral pneumonia, but it has not been conclusively shown to be of benefit.

The risk of spontaneous abortion and preterm delivery following measles infection during pregnancy is 20% to 60%.[36] If miscarriage does not occur, patients should be counseled that measles does not appear to be associated with an increased risk of congenital malformations and that the risk of congenital measles infection appears to be well below 25%. No congenital measles infections were reported in two recent studies of 98 cases of maternal measles.[36,37] Detailed serial ultrasounds may be performed; evidence of in utero infection includes microcephaly, growth restriction, and oligohydramnios. Reports conflict regarding whether an association exists between measles infection in pregnancy and Crohn disease in offspring, and others have reported an association between measles exposure at the time of birth and the development of Hodgkin disease in children.

The most effective way to prevent measles infection in pregnancy is to ensure vaccination prior to pregnancy using a two-dose series, usually a component of the trivalent measles, mumps, and rubella (MMR) vaccine. This live attenuated vaccine should *not* be given to pregnant women, and patients are recommended to use effective contraception for 3 months after vaccination, although no cases of congenital measles infection have been reported secondary to the measles vaccine.[38] Although most pregnant women will have been previously vaccinated against measles, between 3.2% and 20.5% of pregnant women have either absent or low antibody titers, which would classify them as seronegative.[39] Any pregnant women exposed to measles should have an IgG titer drawn. Seronegative (susceptible) women should be treated with immune globulin intravenously within 6 days of exposure.[38] Neonates delivered

TABLE 53-8	DIFFERENTIAL DIAGNOSIS OF MEASLES					
	CONJUNCTIVITIS	RHINITIS	SORE THROAT	EXANTHEM	LEUKOCYTOSIS	SPECIFIC LABORATORY TESTS
Measles	++	++	−	+	−	+
Rubella	−	±	±	−	−	+
Exanthem subitum	−	±	−	−	−	+
Enterovirus infection	−	±	±	−	−	+
Adenovirus infection	+	+	+	−	−	+
Scarlet fever	±	±	++	−	+	+
Infectious mononucleosis	−	−	++	±	±	+
Drug rash	−	−	−	−	±	−

to a parturient who developed measles within 7 to 10 days of delivery should receive intramuscular (IM) immune globulin. These children should also receive the MMR vaccine at 12 to 15 months of age.[38]

RUBELLA

Virology and Epidemiology

Rubella is a small, spherical, enveloped, single-stranded RNA virus, which is part of the Togaviridae family. Transmission occurs via respiratory droplets and close personal contact. Following infection of respiratory mucosa, virus is found within cervical lymph nodes and disseminates hematogenously. Rubella outbreaks occur in school-age children and in settings where crowded conditions exist such as military bases, religious communities, college campuses, and prisons. As a result of routine vaccination, no recent major outbreaks have occurred in the United States. Elimination of endemic rubella is a national health goal. From 2005 to 2011, a median of 11 rubella cases occurred annually.[38] Most infections occur in foreign-born unvaccinated individuals.

Clinical Manifestations

The incubation period following exposure is 12 to 19 days. However, acute rubella infection is not always diagnosed because 20% to 50% of infections are asymptomatic, and there is no associated prodromal illness. Symptomatic infected patients present with a rash, malaise, fever, conjunctivitis, and generalized lymphadenopathy. The rash is nonpruritic, begins on the face and neck as a faint macular erythema, and spreads rapidly to the trunk and extremities (Fig. 53-4). The rash lasts approximately 3 days and blanches with pressure. Transient polyarthralgias and/or polyarthritis that lasts 5 to 10 days may appear in adolescents and adults following the rash. Rare complications include thrombocytopenic purpura, encephalitis, neuritis, and orchitis.

Diagnosis

Serology is most commonly used to document exposure and/or infection with rubella. IgM specific for rubella is detectable prior to the onset of the rash. Isolation and culture of the virus is possible as is detection of viral RNA by RT-PCR. In cases of suspected congenital rubella infection, RT-PCR can be used to

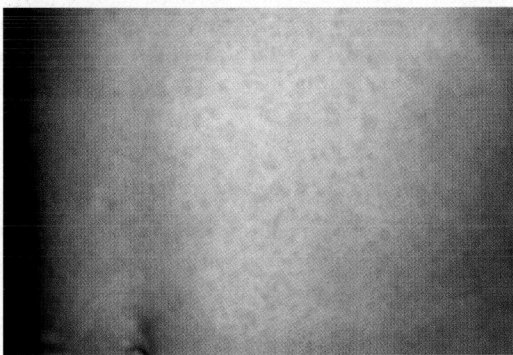

FIG 53-4 This patient presented with a generalized rash on the abdomen caused by German measles (rubella). The rash usually lasts about 3 days and may be accompanied by a low-grade fever. Rubella is caused by a different virus from the one that causes regular measles (rubeola), and immunity to rubella does *not* protect a person from measles, and vice versa. (Courtesy Centers for Disease Control and Prevention.)

detect viral RNA within chorionic villi, fetal blood, and amniotic fluid specimens.

Management of Rubella Infection During Pregnancy

Maternal rubella infection is usually self-limited. However, **congenital rubella infection is associated with miscarriage and stillbirth and can have significant deleterious effects on the fetus.** The primary purpose of the rubella vaccine is to prevent congenital rubella infection, and IVIG administration does not do this. Although this live attenuated vaccine is contraindicated during pregnancy, **no cases of congenital rubella syndrome have been reported in approximately 1000 infants born following inadvertent vaccination during pregnancy.**[38] This indicates that rubella vaccination during pregnancy does not carry a significant risk of birth defects secondary to congenital rubella infection. Therefore therapeutic termination of pregnancy is not recommended in these cases.[38] **Rubella serology is typically performed at the initial prenatal visit to identify women with inadequate levels of antibody.** These women should receive rubella vaccine in the postpartum period. The vaccine is available in monovalent, bivalent (measles-rubella), or trivalent forms (MMR).

Congenital Infection

Only four cases of congenital rubella syndrome (CRS) were documented in the United States from 2005 through 2011.[38] Several retrospective studies have established relationships between the frequency and severity of CRS and the timing of rubella infection in pregnancy. In general, infection in early pregnancy is associated with increased CRS severity. **When maternal infection occurs within the first 12 weeks of pregnancy and is accompanied by a rash, over 80% of fetuses become infected with rubella.**[40] Of these infants, 67% will have findings consistent with CRS.[41] First-trimester infection with rubella is also associated with miscarriage, although some of the women in these studies terminated their pregnancy secondary to exposure. As the pregnancy progresses, the risk of congenital rubella infection decreases: the risk is 54% at 13 to 14 weeks and 25% at the end of the second trimester.[40] The association of congenital rubella infection with CRS also decreases with increasing gestational age, with fetal defects being rare in fetuses infected beyond the 16th week of pregnancy.[40,41] Given that the association of congenital rubella infection and CRS is not absolute at any gestational age, ultrasound may be a useful adjunct in determining whether a fetus is affected, although this technique cannot detect many of the associated abnormalities.

The most common manifestation of congenital rubella infection is growth restriction. Sensorineural hearing loss is the most common single defect associated with CRS and affects up to 90% of congenitally infected infants, and the rate of hearing loss is inversely related to the gestational age of congenital rubella infection.[42] When infection occurs prior to 12 weeks' gestation, other common defects include cardiac lesions (13%), most commonly patent ductus arteriosus, and eye defects (13%) such as cataracts, glaucoma, or retinitis.[41] Other findings consistent with CRS include microphthalmia, microcephaly, cerebral palsy, mental retardation, and intrauterine growth restriction (IUGR). Most of these findings are seen only in fetuses infected within the first 12 weeks of gestation. However, virtually all fetuses infected prior to the 11th week of gestation have CRS.[40] Severe disease can also include thrombocytopenic purpura or hepatosplenomegaly. Fetuses infected between 13 to 16 weeks of gestation have up to a 35% risk of being affected by CRS[40] and typically have hearing loss as their principal manifestation of CRS. Fetuses infected at more advanced gestational ages rarely have sequelae associated with CRS. Following congenital rubella infection, infants may shed virus for up to 1 year after birth. Even in neonates who are asymptomatic at birth, up to one third can manifest long-term complications that include type 1 diabetes mellitus and progressive panencephalitis in the second decade of life.[43,44]

CYTOMEGALOVIRUS INFECTION
Virology and Epidemiology

Cytomegalovirus (CMV) is a large, enveloped, double-stranded DNA virus that is a β-herpesvirus. Herpesviruses have large, complex genomes that replicate in the nucleus of infected cells and enable these viruses to establish acute, persistent, and latent infection. Recurrent CMV infection occurs following reactivation from latently infected cells or by superinfection with a different strain or serotype of virus. CMV is not highly contagious; transmission primarily occurs by contact with infected saliva or urine, and it can also be transmitted via blood or by sexual contact. The incubation period is about 40 days following exposure. Within the United States, primary CMV infection in pregnant women ranges from 0.7% to 4%, and recurrent infection can be as high as 13.5%. Young infants and children with subclinical infection are a major source of infectious CMV; approximately 50% of children who attend daycare actively shed CMV virus in their saliva and/or urine, and fomites within daycare centers are potential sources of CMV infection. Thus **daycare workers are at high risk for infection**. Small children pose an infection risk to family members with annual seroconversion rates of approximately 10% for parents and uninfected siblings.[45] CMV seroprevalence correlates with lower socioeconomic status, birth outside North America, increasing parity and age, abnormal PAP smears, *Trichomonas* infection, and the number of sex partners. CMV infection is also increased in immunocompromised patients. Between 0.2% and 2.2% of infants born in the United States become infected with CMV in utero secondary to maternal infection, and **congenital CMV is the leading cause of hearing loss in children.** Another 6% to 60% of children become infected within the first 6 months of life secondary to intrapartum transmission, environmental exposure, or breastfeeding. However, infants infected peripartum rarely demonstrate serious sequelae of CMV infection.[46]

Clinical Manifestations

Infected patients may be asymptomatic or they may have a mononucleosis-like syndrome with fever, malaise, myalgias, chills, and cervical lymphadenopathy. Infrequent complications include pneumonia, hepatitis, Guillain-Barre syndrome, and aseptic meningitis. Laboratory abnormalities include atypical lymphocytosis, elevated hepatic transaminases, and a negative heterophile antibody response (which distinguishes CMV from Epstein-Barr virus infection).

Diagnosis

Active, maternal CMV infection is best diagnosed by culture, detection of CMV antigens, or DNA PCR of blood, urine, saliva, amniotic fluid, or cervical secretions. Serologic tests are available, but antibody levels may not be detectable for up to 4 weeks after primary infection, and titers can remain elevated; this makes a serologic diagnosis of reinfection difficult. A four-fold increase in IgG titers within multiple specimens suggests active infection. IgM is used to diagnose recent or active infection, but both false-positive and false-negative results can occur. **Routine CMV screening during pregnancy is not recommended secondary to high seroprevalence.** Fetal infection is documented by amniotic fluid culture or PCR, and PCR sensitivity approaches 100% in gestations greater than 21 weeks.[46] Fetal serology and blood culture are much less sensitive. Fetal CMV infection can occur weeks to months following maternal infection; thus repeat testing may be considered at 7-week intervals.[46] **Antepartum CMV detection does not predict the severity of congenital CMV infection, and 80% to 90% of children with congenital CMV infection have no neurologic sequelae.**

Management of Cytomegalovirus During Pregnancy

Pregnant women should be counseled regarding preventive measures: careful handling of potentially infected articles such as diapers, clothing, and toys; avoidance of sharing food and utensils; and frequent hand washing. Antiviral therapy is not indicated in immunocompetent infected individuals, and ganciclovir is not effective for intrauterine treatment of congenital CMV infection. In one trial, passive antepartum maternal immunization of women with primary CMV infection with CMV-specific hyperimmune globulin was associated with decreased congenital CMV infection and fewer infants born with symptomatic CMV disease.[47] However, a follow-up randomized, placebo-controlled trial failed to show reduced infection or reduced sequelae.[48] Thus at this time, **avoiding maternal CMV infection is the only effective prevention for congenital CMV infection.**

Congenital Infection

Congenital CMV infection is diagnosed by the detection of virus or viral nucleic acid within the first 2 weeks of life. **Intrauterine CMV transmission is highest in the third trimester with an overall 30% to 40% risk of fetal transmission.**[49] **However, serious sequelae occur most frequently following first-trimester infection: 24% of infected fetuses have sensorineural hearing loss and 32% have other CNS sequelae.** After the second trimester, 2.5% of infected fetuses demonstrated sensorineural hearing loss and 15% had CNS sequelae.[50] Congenital CMV infection may occur following primary or recurrent CMV infection of pregnant women, but the incidence of serious sequelae is lower following recurrent infection.[51] Most infants with congenital CMV infection exhibit no obvious clinical findings at birth. Nonetheless, **15% of subclinical congenital CMV infection is associated with hearing loss.**[51]

After primary maternal CMV infection, approximately 5% to 18% of infants exhibit serious sequelae, typically following infection during the first half of pregnancy. Clinical findings in these infected infants may include jaundice, petechiae, thrombocytopenia, hepatosplenomegaly, growth restriction, and nonimmune hydrops. Long-term neurologic sequelae include developmental delays, seizure activity, and gross neurologic impairment as well as sensorineural hearing loss.[51] **Ultrasound can be useful in identifying a congenitally infected infant with likely**

impairment. Findings consistent with fetal infection include microcephaly, ventriculomegaly, intracerebral calcifications, ascites, hydrops, echogenic bowel, IUGR, and oligohydramnios. Unusual findings include fetal heart block and meconium peritonitis.[52,53] In the setting of confirmed fetal infection with serial normal ultrasounds, the risk of clinical symptoms of congenital CMV infection following birth is approximately 10%. Thus ultrasound findings, or their absence, are an important factor to consider when counseling.

HERPESVIRUS
Virology and Epidemiology
Herpes simplex virus (HSV) is another large, enveloped, double-stranded DNA virus that replicates in the host cell nucleus. Epithelial cells are the primary targets. However, HSV establishes latency within dorsal root ganglia and can disseminate via hematogenous spread. Latent viral infection can be associated with integration of the viral genome into the host cell DNA. The HSV genome is complex and encodes over 80 polypeptides, including several envelope glycoproteins. Glycoprotein G permits differentiation of two well-defined antigenic and biologic viruses, HSV-1 and HSV-2. HSV-1 is typically associated with nongenital infection, and mouth and lips are the most common sites of viral replication. HSV-1 infection is most prevalent in lower socioeconomic populations, in which 75% to 90% of individuals have antibodies that recognize HSV-1 by 10 years of age. HSV-2 infection is also associated with socioeconomic status and is usually acquired via sexual contact. In the United States, 25% to 65% of individuals have antibodies that recognize HSV-2, and seroprevalence risk correlates with the number of sexual partners. Some individuals have asymptomatic or subclinical primary HSV infections, which account for seropositive patients without a clinical history of infection.

Clinical Manifestations
HSV-1 infection is normally manifested by herpes simplex labialis (cold sores), whereas HSV-2 infection customarily involves the genitals and includes the vulva, vagina, and/or cervix. Painful vesicles appear 2 to 14 days after viral exposure and rupture spontaneously, leaving shallow eroded ulcers (Fig. 53-5). Later in the infection, a dry crust forms, and lesions heal without scarring. Primary infection can be associated with fever, malaise, anorexia, and bilateral inguinal lymphadenopathy, and it is infrequently associated with aseptic meningitis. Women

may have dysuria and urinary retention secondary to urethral involvement. Rates of symptomatic and subclinical HSV shedding from the cervix and vulva during the first 3 months following primary infection are 1% to 3%.

Healing of primary HSV-2 infection may take several weeks and is less severe in individuals with prior HSV-1 infection. Nonprimary first episodes of genital HSV occur when a second HSV strain, either HSV-1 or HSV-2, establishes infection in the presence of preexisting antibodies from a previous infection at a nongenital site. Secondary or recurrent HSV infections usually represent viral reactivation that varies in frequency and intensity. Recurrent infections are typically less severe than primary infections and are associated with fewer lesions and a shorter duration of viral shedding. **One third of HSV-infected individuals have no recurrences, one third have approximately three recurrences per year, and another third have more than three recurrences per year.** Table 53-9 compares clinical findings during primary and recurrent HSV infection. Disseminated HSV infection is rare and arises primarily in immunocompromised individuals, but it can also occur in pregnancy. Disseminated infection is characterized by skin, mucous membrane, and visceral organ involvement, and it may include ocular involvement, meningitis, encephalitis, and ascending myelitis. Prompt treatment with IV acyclovir is indicated for suspected cases of disseminated HSV.

Diagnosis
Definitive diagnosis of active HSV infection is made by viral culture or by nucleic acid detection of HSV, which is faster and more sensitive. Both methods differentiate between HSV-1 and HSV-2. Culture specimens should be collected from fresh vesicles or pustules because viral recovery from crusted lesions is poor; this is not as critical for PCR-based assays. Serology can assess and differentiate primary infection from secondary infection via IgM detection. Cytologic preparations (Tzanck test) show characteristic multinucleated giant cells and intranuclear inclusions. However, this test is rarely performed given the enhanced sensitivity and specificity of culture and nucleic acid detection.

Management of Herpesvirus During Pregnancy
Maternal primary infection with HSV prior to labor does not usually impact the fetus. Intrauterine HSV infection is rare and occurs in approximately 1 in 200,000 deliveries. Sequelae of intrauterine infection include skin vesicles and/or scarring, eye disease, microcephaly, or hydranencephaly. An association between HSV infection in the third trimester of pregnancy and IUGR has also been reported. However, this observation was based on only five patients. Birthweight of infants born to asymptomatic HSV-shedding mothers is lower than those of

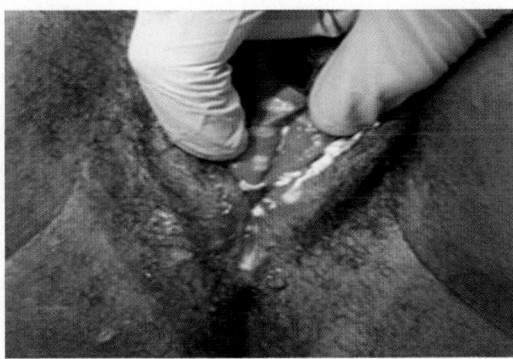

FIG 53-5 Ulcerated lesions characteristic of herpes simplex infection. (From Ferri F, et al. *Ferri's Fast Facts in Dermatology.* Philadelphia: Saunders; 2011.)

TABLE 53-9	COMPARISON OF PRIMARY VERSUS RECURRENT HERPES SIMPLEX VIRUS INFECTION	
STAGE OF ILLNESS	**PRIMARY (DAYS)**	**RECURRENT (DAYS)**
Incubation period and/or prodrome	2-10	1-2
Vesicle, pustule	6	2
Wet ulcer	6	3
Dry crust	8	7
Total	22-30	13-14

TABLE 53-10 HERPES SIMPLEX VIRUS TREATMENT

DRUG	PRIMARY INFECTION	RECURRENT INFECTION	PROPHYLAXIS
Acyclovir	400 mg TID for 7 to 10 days	800 mg BID for 5 days or 800 mg TID for 2 days	400 mg BID
Valacyclovir	1 g BID for 7 to 10 days	500 mg BID for 3 days or 1 g QD for 5 days	500 to 1000 mg QD
Famciclovir	250 mg TID for 7 to 10 days	500 mg followed by 250 mg BID for 2 days or 1 g BID for 1 day	250 mg BID

BID, twice daily; *TID*, three times a day; *QD*, once per day.

nonshedding mothers, but this small observed effect may be due to differences in gestational age at birth.[54] Treatment regimens are described in Table 53-10. **Women with more than two HSV recurrences per year should be offered prophylaxis to decrease the frequency and severity of recurrences.**

Intrapartum HSV exposure is associated with neonatal infection, which complicates approximately 1 in 3500 deliveries in the United States and is associated with significant neonatal morbidity and mortality. Seventy percent of neonatal infection is caused by HSV-2, with a 50% estimated risk of neonatal HSV during primary maternal infection. The incidence of neonatal HSV incidence ranges from 0% to 3% in the setting of recurrent maternal infection.[55] Thus **primary maternal HSV infection, not recurrent infection, accounts for the vast majority of neonatal HSV infections.** ACOG recommends elective cesarean delivery for women with demonstrable genital herpes lesions or prodromal symptoms in labor to reduce the incidence of neonatal HSV infection.[55] However, because 60% to 80% of neonatal HSV infections occur following asymptomatic primary maternal infection, our capacity to prevent neonatal HSV infection by performing cesarean delivery is limited. Cost-benefit analysis of current guidelines for prevention of neonatal HSV infection found that, given the low risk of neonatal HSV transmission with recurrent maternal infection, it requires 1580 elective cesarean deliveries to prevent one neonatal HSV infection.[56]

The duration of ruptured membranes prior to delivery increases the risk of neonatal HSV infection. However, no evidence shows any period of time beyond which cesarean delivery is no longer beneficial. Positive antepartum HSV cultures are not associated with positive cultures at the time of delivery and are not recommended.[57] Prophylactic acyclovir or valacyclovir decreases HSV shedding and outbreaks and reduces the number of cesarean deliveries performed to prevent neonatal HSV infection.[58] This strategy should be considered for women with HSV recurrence during pregnancy. In the case of premature rupture of membranes, acyclovir or other antivirals should be considered in women with active HSV lesions being managed expectantly and taking steroids to enhance fetal lung maturity.[55] In these patients, decisions regarding prophylactic cesarean delivery should be based on the presence of lesions at the time of labor. The risk of neonatal HSV infection in cases of nongenital maternal HSV lesions (i.e., lesions of the thigh, buttocks, or mouth) is low, therefore cesarean delivery is not recommended for these women.

Neonatal Herpes Infection

Factors that predict neonatal HSV transmission include cervical HSV shedding, invasive monitoring, preterm delivery, maternal age younger than 21 years, and HSV viral load.[59] Three patterns of neonatal HSV infections occur with equal frequency. *Local disease* is limited to the skin, eyes, and mouth—so-called SEM disease; this pattern has limited morbidity. *Disseminated*

infection involves multiple visceral organs and includes lungs, liver, adrenal glands, skin, eyes, and brain. Both SEM and disseminated disease are characterized by early presentation (10 to 12 days of life); however, disseminated disease is associated with significant morbidity and mortality. *CNS disease,* which may be associated with skin involvement, occurs later, during the second or third week of life. Following high-dose neonatal acyclovir therapy, 1-year mortality for CNS disease is 29%, and it is 4% for disseminated disease. Despite higher mortality, 83% of disseminated disease survivors have normal neurologic development, whereas only 31% of CNS disease survivors are neurologically intact.[60] Complications of neonatal HSV infection also include DIC and hemorrhagic pneumonitis.

VARICELLA

Virology and Epidemiology

Varicella, or chickenpox, is caused by the varicella zoster virus (VZV), part of the α-herpesvirus subfamily. This enveloped virus contains double-stranded DNA and has at least 69 genes. Viral replication initially occurs within respiratory epithelial cells and is followed by systemic viremia. Long-term latent infection occurs within the nonneuronal cells of the dorsal root ganglia. Humans are the only known host for varicella, a highly contagious disease transmitted by respiratory droplets or close contact. Approximately 95% of susceptible household contacts become infected following exposure, and a 14-day incubation period precedes the emergence of symptoms. Patients are infectious from one day prior to rash appearance until lesions are crusted; immunity following infection is usually life long. Prior to VZV vaccine availability, most natural varicella infections occurred in early childhood, a time when VZV infection is usually self-limited. However, over 50% of varicella-associated mortality occurs in adults, who represent less than 10% of all varicella infections.[61] Most adults (>90%) are VZV immune, even in the absence of a clinical history of chickenpox.

Clinical Manifestations

Infected patients classically present with a centripetal rash characterized by highly pruritic erythematous macules, papules, and vesicles that appear in crops. The rash spreads to the extremities, and evidence of excoriation and scabbed lesions are typically seen. Bacterial superinfection of skin lesions can occur. Fever is common, and infected adults frequently present with malaise, myalgias, arthralgias, and headache. Cough and dyspnea usually occur about 3 days after the appearance of the first skin lesions. Cyanosis, hemoptysis, and pleuritic chest pain are common. **Patients should be carefully observed for the development of varicella pneumonia, which occurs in almost 20% of infections during pregnancy.**[62] Encephalitis is a rare complication of adult VZV infection. Reactivation of latent VZV infection causes herpes zoster or shingles and occurs primarily in the elderly and immunocompromised. Shingles is characterized by a segmentally distributed rash that correlates with specific dermatomes. Pain, itching, and/or paresthesias can occur as a prodrome or with rash appearance. Zoster is usually self-limited, although patients shed infectious virus and can transmit VZV to susceptible individuals.

Diagnosis

Diagnosis is usually made based on exposure history and/or rash. Acute infection can be rapidly diagnosed by PCR amplification of VZV-specific DNA from vesicular fluid and/or throat swabs. Serologic confirmation of exposure via ELISA, which can quantitate VZV-specific IgG and IgM, is most useful for confirming prior exposure. The Tzanck stain identifies multinucleated giant cells within lesions, and varicella can be cultured.

Management of Varicella During Pregnancy

Pregnant women infected with VZV should be offered supportive care that includes calamine lotion, antipyretics, and if necessary, systemic antipruritics. **Oral acyclovir** (800 mg by mouth five times per day) **or valacyclovir** (1 g by mouth three times a day) **are safe in pregnancy and should be given to all infected women because they decrease illness duration if instituted within 24 hours of rash emergence.** Maternal varicella pneumonia is associated with a 5% maternal mortality and presents 3 to 5 days following the rash; patients should be treated with 10 to 15 mg/kg IV acyclovir every 8 hours. **If maternal varicella occurs within 5 days before and 2 days after delivery, varicella zoster immune globulin (VZIG) should be given to the newborn to prevent neonatal varicella.** The infant should be isolated from the mother until all vesicles have crusted over to prevent VZV transmission. If possible, delivery should be delayed 5 to 7 days following the onset of maternal illness to potentially prevent neonatal VZV, which has a 20% to 30% mortality rate.[62]

Prevention includes ascertaining VZV status prior to pregnancy in women without a clinical history of infection and offering live attenuated VZV vaccine (Varivax, Merck) to susceptible women prior to conception. Adults should receive two subcutaneous doses of vaccine 4 to 8 weeks apart. The vaccine is 70% to 80% effective in preventing natural infection, but **this live vaccine is contraindicated during gestation. Pregnancy should be deferred for 3 months following vaccination, although there is no evidence of congenital VZV infection following vaccination during pregnancy.**[63] If a pregnant woman without clinical history of VZV infection or vaccination is exposed to varicella, serology should be performed within 96 hours of exposure. Most patients will be varicella IgG seropositive and not at risk for infection. **With confirmed VZV susceptibility or the inability to obtain serology within 96 hours of exposure, the preferred prophylaxis is high-titer VZIG.**

VariZIG (Emergent Biosolutions) can be obtained 24 hours a day from authorized distributors (1-800-843-7477 in the United States or online at www.fffenterprises.com or at www.asdhealthcare.com/home); the recommended IM dose is 125 U per 10 kg of body weight up to a maximum of 625 U. In the absence of VZIG, IV immune globulin (IVIG) can be substituted at a dose of 400 mg/kg.[64] Prophylactic acyclovir given 800 mg orally five times daily for 5 to 7 days, beginning within 9 days of exposure, is 85% effective at preventing VZV infection in children.[65] Prophylaxis may be combined, which potentially further reduces the risk of maternal varicella infection; a small study that compared postexposure prophylaxis in children found that acyclovir and VZIG together are more efficacious than VZIG alone.[66] Given the time constraints for prophylactic treatment following exposure, consider varicella serologic assessment at the first prenatal visit for women denying a history of VZV infection/vaccination. Results can guide pregnancy management and can identify patient candidates for postpartum vaccination.

Congenital Infection

Congenital varicella infection can lead to spontaneous abortion, intrauterine fetal demise (IUFD), and varicella embryopathy. Congenital varicella syndrome (CVS) is characterized by cutaneous scars, limb hypoplasia and malformed digits, muscle atrophy, microcephaly, cortical atrophy, microphthalmia, cataracts, chorioretinitis, and psychomotor retardation. The frequency of anomalies is low following exposure prior to 13 weeks. Only 0.4% of neonates were born with CVS features in a study of 472 women. The highest risk occurs with maternal infection between 13 and 20 weeks' gestation, with a 2% CVS incidence.[67] No congenital malformations have been observed following maternal infection after 20 weeks' gestation, but neonatal skin lesions and scarring have been noted at birth. Ultrasound examination is preferred for prenatal assessment because serology and VZV DNA do not predict fetal injury.[68] Ultrasound findings suggestive of CVS can include polyhydramnios, hydrops, echogenic foci within abdominal organs, cardiac malformations, limb deformities, microcephaly, and IUGR.[69]

HEPATITIS

Viral hepatitis comprises a spectrum of syndromes that range from subclinical to fulminant disease, and it is caused by several unrelated viruses. Symptoms of acute viral hepatitis may include jaundice, malaise, fatigue, anorexia, nausea, vomiting, and right upper quadrant pain. Hepatic transaminases and bilirubin are moderately to markedly elevated, and liver biopsy shows extensive hepatocellular injury with prominent inflammatory infiltration (Fig. 53-6). Most viral hepatitis infections are self-limited and resolve without treatment, but certain viruses can establish persistent infection, which leads to chronic liver disease (see Chapter 47). The majority of infections in the United States are caused by hepatitis viruses A, B, C, and D, whereas hepatitis E is endemic to Asia, Africa, and Mexico. Other viruses associated

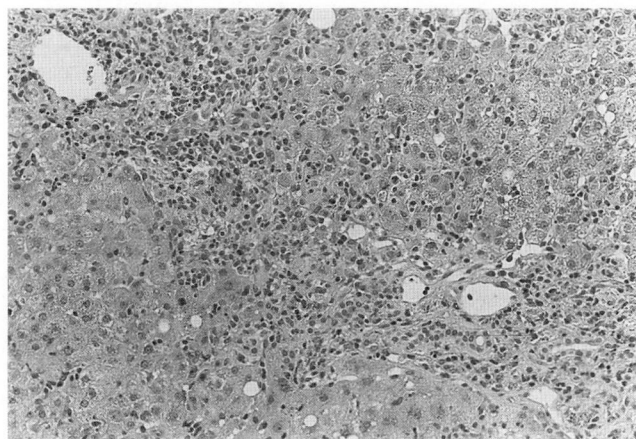

FIG 53-6 Photomicrograph of liver biopsy showing characteristic histologic changes of acute viral hepatitis. Note the intense inflammatory infiltrate.

with liver infection and inflammation (hepatitis) include CMV, HSV, Epstein-Barr virus (EBV), rubella, and yellow fever.[70]

Hepatitis A

Hepatitis A virus (HAV) is a small, single-stranded RNA virus of the Picornaviridae family and is the causative agent for approximately one third of acute hepatitis infections in the United States. HAV transmission primarily occurs via oral-fecal contact. The incidence of HAV in pregnancy is approximately 1 in 1000, and diagnosis is based on HAV IgM and IgG serology or viral nucleic acid detection. The incubation period is approximately 28 to 30 days following exposure. HAV risk factors include contaminated food or water exposure, recent travel outside the United States, illicit drug use, and having a child in daycare. HAV infection is usually self-limited and is restricted to acute infection (not chronic), and fewer than 0.5% of patients require hospitalization. Physical activity should be limited to prevent hepatic trauma, and drugs with potential hepatotoxicity should be avoided. Sexual and household contacts of infected individuals should receive immunoprophylaxis with a single dose of HAV immune globulin and should receive HAV vaccine, an inactive vaccine safe for use in pregnancy.[71] **Perinatal transmission has not been documented; however, infants delivered to an acutely infected mother should receive HAV immune globulin to prevent horizontal transmission following delivery.**[71] HAV infection may be complicated by cholestatic hepatitis, characterized by pruritis, dark urine, direct hyperbilirubinemia, and elevated alkaline phosphatase. This syndrome can last several months. However, long-term prognosis is good, and corticosteroid therapy alleviates symptoms.[70]

Hepatitis B
Virology and Epidemiology

Hepatitis B virus (HBV) is a small, enveloped double-stranded DNA virus in the Hepadnaviridae family. HBV is the etiologic agent of 40% to 45% of hepatitis infections, and it is estimated that 1 million individuals in the United States are chronic viral carriers with 350 million chronically infected individuals worldwide. **In the United States, 5 to 15 per 1000 pregnant women have chronic HBV infection, whereas 1 to 2 per 1000 have acute HBV infection.** The prevalence of HBV is increased in certain populations, which includes Asians, Eskimos, drug addicts, dialysis patients, prisoners, and residents and employees of chronic care facilities.[70] **HBV is transmitted parenterally via sexual transmission and perinatal exposure. Without intervention, infants born to HBsAg-positive mothers have a 90% risk of perinatal HBV infection** (combined prophylaxis to reduce infection is described in the management section). As many as 40% of males and 15% of females with perinatally acquired HBV will die of hepatocellular carcinoma or cirrhosis, which highlights the need for effective prevention.[72]

The postexposure incubation period ranges from 4 weeks to 6 months and is inversely related to viral inoculum. Acute infection is characterized by hepatic inflammation (see Fig. 53-6)[70]; however, less than 1% of acutely infected patients develop fulminant HBV, characterized by massive hepatic necrosis and possible pancreatitis. **Most newly infected adults (85% to 90%) clear their infection, whereas the remaining 10% to 15% become chronically infected. Chronic HBV infection has a 15% to 30% risk of liver cirrhosis and a substantially increased probability of hepatocellular carcinoma.**[70] The three clinically relevant HBV proteins are surface antigen

(HBsAg) or viral envelope glycoprotein; core antigen (HBcAg), associated with viral nucleic acid; and early antigen (HBeAg), a viral protein secreted from infected cells that is not incorporated into virus particles. HBeAg detection normally correlates with HBV DNA greater than 10^6 IU/mL and was used prior to HBV DNA assessment as a marker of viral replication and infectivity. Transition from HBeAg positivity to anti-HBe positivity usually heralds decreased viral replication; however, mutations that induce HBeAg loss with ongoing high-titer HBV replication are documented in long-term infected patients.

Diagnosis

Acute HBV infection is diagnosed by detection of both HBsAg and HBc IgM or HBV DNA detection in HBsAg-negative patients (early acute infection). HBsAg persistence for more than 6 months delineates chronic infection; serologic findings are reviewed in Figure 53-7. Further testing is warranted to assess HBV DNA and hepatic injury, manifested by elevated aminotransferase concentrations. Chronic HBV infection has multiple phases. The immune-tolerant phase is delineated by positive HBsAg and HBeAg and by high HBV DNA in the absence of liver disease. The immune-active phase can be heralded by HBeAg-positive, HBeAg-negative, or anti–HBe-positive serology, with high levels of HBV DNA and fluctuating hepatic inflammation. The inactive phase, or carrier status, is apparent when a person is HBsAg positive and HBeAg negative with an HBV DNA that ranges from 10^1 to 10^5 IU/mL. Patients can transition between phases, which includes reversion from inactive to immune-active infection; therefore ongoing HBV DNA assessment is warranted. Anti-HBs is detected following either infection or vaccination, whereas antibody recognizing HBc or HBe is only detected in HBV-infected patients. Interpretation of HBV serology is reviewed in Table 53-11.

Management of Hepatitis B Virus Infection During Pregnancy

HBV infection is prevented by a recombinant vaccination that is safe in pregnancy and should be offered to patients with significant risk factors, including those with a history of sexually transmitted diseases (STDs), health care workers, and those with infected household or sexual contacts.[73] Several therapies—including lamivudine, tenofovir, and telbivudine—have been used to treat HBV infection during pregnancy. Antepartum treatment for maternal benefit should be coordinated with a hepatologist because optimal treatment duration exceeds that of pregnancy. Amniocentesis is safe in chronically infected women.[74] HBV-infected pregnant women should be vaccinated against HAV to prevent further liver injury. **HBV-infected women can breastfeed because perinatal transmission is not increased in these patients.**[75]

In the United States, all newborns are vaccinated against HBV as part of the CDC's recommendation to decrease HBV prevalence.[76] Infants born to HBsAg-positive mothers should receive the HBV vaccine series *and* HBV immune globulin (HBIG) within 12 hours of birth.[73] Combined active-passive immunization is 85% to 95% effective at preventing perinatal HBV transmission, but this prophylactic regimen is substantially less effective in women with immune-tolerant HBV infection or HBV DNA greater than 200,000 IU/mL (1,000,000 copies/mL). Similar to HIV, perinatal HBV transmission correlates with maternal viral load, but consensus regarding the timing of therapy and HBV DNA concentrations above which antiviral

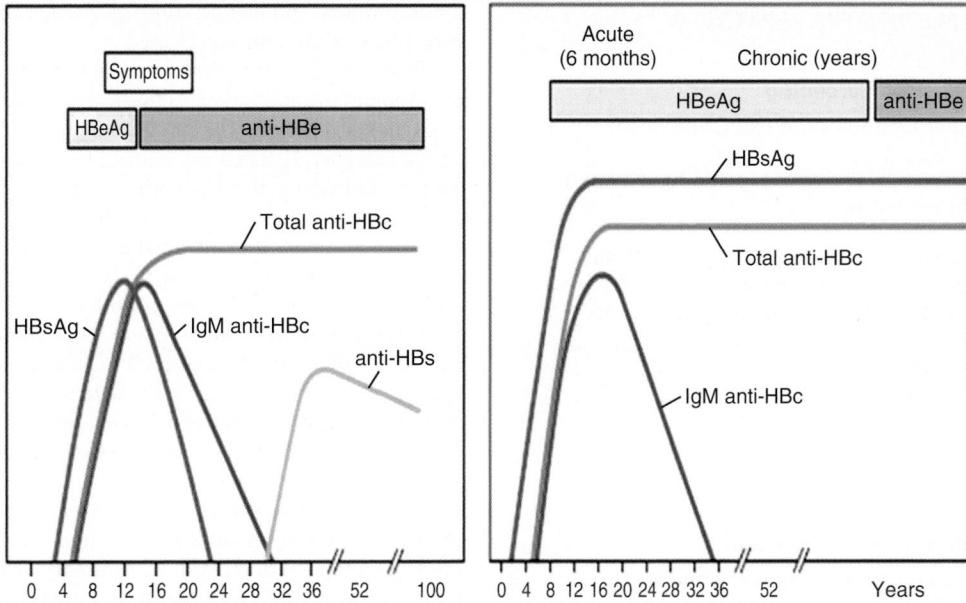

FIG 53-7 Typical course of hepatitis B virus (HBV). *Left,* Typical course of acute HBV. *Right,* Chronic HBV. HBc, hepatitis B core; HBe, early hepatitis B; HBsAg, hepatitis B surface antigen; IgM, immunoglobulin M. (From Koziel MJ, Thio CL. Hepatitis B virus and hepatitis delta virus. In Mandell GL, Bennett JE, Dolin R, eds. *Mandell, Douglas, and Bennett's Principles and Practice of Infectious Disease,* 7th ed., Philadelphia: Elsevier; 2010.)

TABLE 53-11   INTERPRETATION OF HEPATITIS B SEROLOGIC TESTS

TEST	ACUTE INFECTION	IMMUNITY VIA INFECTION	IMMUNITY VIA VACCINATION	CHRONIC INFECTION	INACTIVE PHASE (CARRIER)
HBsAg	+	–	–	+	+
Anti-HBs	–	+	+	–	–
HBeAg	+	–	–	+/–	–
Anti-HBe	–	+/–	–	+/–	+
Anti-HBc*	+	+	–	+	+
IgM anti-HBc	+	–	–	–	–
HBV DNA†	+	–	–	+	+ (Low)
ALT	Elevated	Normal	Normal	Normal-elevated	Normal

From Koziel MJ, Thio CL. Hepatitis B virus and hepatitis delta virus. In Mandell GL, Bennett JE, Dolin R, eds. *Mandell, Douglas, and Bennett's Principles and Practice of Infectious Disease,* 7th ed., Philadelphia: Elsevier; 2010.
*Isolated anti-HBc IgG occurs during acute infection or can indicate remote prior infection (with loss of HBsAg or anti-HBs) or occult infection. HBV DNA assessment and hepatology consult is indicated.
†HBV DNA detection depends on assay sensitivity.
ALT, alanine aminotransferase; *HBc,* hepatitis B core; *HBe,* hepatitis B early antigen; *HBsAg,* hepatitis B surface antigen; *HBV,* hepatitis B virus; *IgM,* immunoglobulin M.

therapy should be considered has yet to be established.[72,77,78] Thus it is reasonable to measure maternal viral load and use the information obtained to educate patients regarding perinatal transmission risk and to consider additional prevention strategies beginning in the third trimester. Antepartum nucleoside/nucleotide analogue therapy combined with HBIG limits intrauterine HBV transmission better than HBIG alone and is recommended in high-risk pregnancies (e.g., in women with prior HBV transmission or high HBV DNA and in those with immune-tolerant infection).[78,79] Oral tenofovir (300 mg once daily) is the first-line HBV treatment secondary to its efficacy, favorable side effect profile, and low rate for the development of drug resistance (compared with lamivudine).[80] Tenofovir has also demonstrated safety in pregnancy secondary to its use as a first-line therapy for HIV infection. Thus preventing drug-resistance development while limiting antepartum/intrapartum HBV transmission risk should be the focus when evaluating patients for adjunctive therapy. Up to 80% to 90% of infants born to women acutely infected with HBV in the third trimester

will be HBsAg positive at birth.[71] However, it is unknown whether antiviral therapy lowers this risk.

Hepatitis C
Virology and Epidemiology

Hepatitis C virus (HCV) is an enveloped, single-stranded RNA virus that consists of six genotypes (1 through 6), and it is part of the Flaviviridae family. HCV is mainly transmitted parenterally and via vertical transmission. The incubation period following exposure is 5 to 10 weeks, and 75% of acute infections are asymptomatic. Sexual HCV transmission risk is substantially lower than with HBV. However, **50% of HCV infections become chronic, which makes it the most common chronic bloodborne pathogen in the United States.** Epidemiologic risk factors include IV drug use, history of blood product transfusion, obesity, and high gravidity. The prevalence of HCV among women of childbearing age in the United States is 1%. However, prevalence in pregnant women using IV drugs may be as high as 70% to 95%.[78] The recent development of highly effective, genotype-specific, HCV-specific protease inhibitors has radically improved disease management. Therapy now has a high likelihood of attaining a sustained virologic response (i.e., cure), reducing morbidity and mortality in infected individuals with a secondary benefit of reducing transmission.

Diagnosis

Recommended screening consists of HCV antibody testing with infection confirmed via a nucleic acid test (NAT) to detect and quantify HCV RNA.[81] **Universal screening is not recommended, but individuals with risk factors should be tested once** (Box 53-5), **and annual testing is recommended for persons injecting drugs or with ongoing HCV exposure risk factors.** Viral load and hepatic transaminase levels vary over time; therefore a single undetectable HCV RNA or normal hepatic transaminase level does not rule out chronic carrier status. HCV RNA also fails to correlate with hepatic inflammation/fibrosis and necessitates ongoing transaminase monitoring.

Hepatitis C Virus in Pregnancy

Perinatal HCV transmission correlates with maternal HCV viral load, and a recent study associated increased transmission with a viral load greater than 600,000 IU/mL. **Perinatal HCV transmission occurs in 3% to 10% of patients with detectable HCV RNA, whereas transmission in the absence of detectable viremia is rare.** Other risk factors for perinatal HCV transmission are maternal IV drug use and HIV coinfection. However, treatment of maternal HIV infection lowers both HIV and HCV transmission.[82] Although HCV transmission risk is increased with invasive fetal monitoring and rupture of membranes more than 6 hours previously, elective cesarean delivery does not reduce perinatal HCV transmission.[83] HCV-infected pregnant women should be immunized against HAV and HBV

if not immune, and breastfeeding by women chronically infected with HCV is not contraindicated.

Until recently, HCV treatment did not offer a high likelihood of virologic cure and was contraindicated in pregnancy secondary to the use of ribavirin. The FDA has designated ribavirin as pregnancy category X based on animal teratogenicity. Preliminary data published by the Ribavirin Pregnancy Registry reported birth defects in 3 of 49 live births (6.1%) and an updated executive summary that included data through February 7, 2014 reported a birth defect rate in liveborn infants following direct exposure of 6.49 (5/77, 95% confidence interval [CI], 2.14 to 14.51).[84] Recent recommendation of a limited duration (12 weeks) of ribavirin-sparing HCV therapy expands treatment options within pregnancy.[78,81] Daily fixed-dose ledipasvir, which inhibits viral phosphoprotein NS5A, and sofosbuvir, an HCV polymerase inhibitor, have been designated as pregnancy category B and are first-line therapy for HCV genotype-1a infection. Sofosbuvir combined with simeprevir, a pregnancy category C protease inhibitor, is another first-line treatment option for HCV genotype-1a infection. In summary, first-line therapeutic regimens compatible with use during pregnancy are available to treat HCV genotypes 1, 4, and 6.[78,81] Recommended regimens for HCV genotypes 2, 3, and 5 contain ribavirin and should be avoided in pregnancy when possible. **Given the potential for curative therapy, patients diagnosed with active HCV infection should be referred to a practitioner prepared to provide comprehensive ongoing management of their HCV disease.** Updated management recommendations are available at www.hcvguidelines.org.[81]

Hepatitis C Virus Preconceptional Counseling

Given the newly developed capacity to effect virologic cure and the ancillary benefit of reducing perinatal transmission, consideration should be given to diagnosing and treating HCV infection prior to conception. No effective HCV vaccine is currently available.

Hepatitis D

Hepatitis delta virus (HDV) is an incomplete RNA virus related to plant viruses. The hepatitis D genome encodes a single nucleocapsid protein, hepatitis delta antigen (HDAg), which is present as two peptides. The short form is required for RNA replication, and the long form is packaged with HDV RNA and the HBsAg envelope glycoprotein. Because HDV utilizes HBV as a helper virus (providing envelope glycoprotein), simultaneous or chronic HBV infection is required for viral replication. HDV is present worldwide with a high prevalence in the Mediterranean basin, Middle East, Central Asia, West Africa, and the Amazon basin. Risk factors include IV drug use and infected blood product exposure. Chronic HDV infection occurs in 1% to 3% of individuals who are simultaneously infected with both HBV and HDV. However, there is a 70% to 80% risk of chronic HDV infection following HDV superinfection of chronic HBV-infected individuals. Patients with chronic HBV and HDV coinfection have a 70% to 80% risk for developing cirrhosis and portal hypertension, and 25% die of hepatic failure. Acute HDV infection is characterized by HDV antigen positivity in the absence of HDV antibody. Chronically infected individuals will have both detectable HDV antigen and HDV antibody. Acute hepatitis D infection is associated with fulminant hepatic failure and a 2% to 20% mortality rate. HDV can be perinatally transmitted.[85] However, **perinatal HBV prophylaxis also effectively**

prevents perinatal HDV transmission given the requirement for HBV coinfection.[71]

Hepatitis E

Hepatitis E virus (HEV) is an enveloped RNA virus that is most closely related to the Togaviridae family, which also includes rubella. Hepatitis E is transmitted by oral-fecal contact and is endemic outside of the United States in regions such as Africa, Asia, and Latin America. Similar to hepatitis A, hepatitis E infection causes only acute disease. Diagnosis can be made by the presence of a specific IgM or of viral nucleic acid (RT-PCR). HEV has four genotypes: genotypes 1 and 2 are nonzoonotic and are present in developing countries, and genotypes 3 and 4 are zoonotic and are present in industrialized countries. The mortality rate following acute hepatitis E infection in the general population is 1%. Significantly higher mortality (up to 20%) has been observed in pregnant women infected with hepatitis E, and genotypes 1 and 2 cause most infections.[86] Maternal morbidity and mortality escalates with increasing gestational age,[71,87] and the preterm delivery rate is estimated to be as high as 66%.[87] **Perinatal hepatitis E transmission is associated with significant perinatal morbidity and mortality.[88]**

COXSACKIE VIRUS

Coxsackie virus is the causative agent of hand, foot, and mouth disease, an enterovirus transmitted through the fecal-oral route. Several serotypes exist, and adult infection typically results in a self-limited febrile illness that requires no treatment.[89] One reported case of coxsackie B virus infection in pregnancy led to acute liver failure, which resolved following expectant management.[90] Coxsackie virus infection during pregnancy has also been associated in several studies with an increased rate of miscarriage[89,91] and an increased rate of insulin-dependent diabetes in offspring,[89,92] although a causative relationship has not been established.

HUMAN PAPILLOMAVIRUS

Human papillomaviruses (HPV) are a group of small DNA viruses. Some types (6 and 11) cause warts, whereas other types (16, 18, 31, 33, 52b, and 58) do not cause warts but are instead highly associated with cervical and oral cancers. Infections are sexually and/or vertically transmitted, and nearly 50% of college-aged women have evidence of infection. Thus prior HPV infection is common in pregnancy; moreover, HPV DNA has been detected in 37% of pregnant women without prior documented infection, which demonstrates an unexpectedly high rate of asymptomatic HPV infection.[93] Anogenital warts, caused by nononcogenic HPV types, are one manifestation of infection and may be managed expectantly. Hormonal effects may cause rapid wart proliferation and growth that necessitates treatment. **Trichloroacetic acid and/or cryotherapy are used to treat anogenital warts in pregnancy because podophyllin is contraindicated.** Little is known regarding the safety of imiquimod cream in pregnancy (category C), and treatment is required for months. Vaginal delivery is not contraindicated, unless the wart burden and position would result in dystocia. Maternal HPV infection with HPV types 6 and 11 is associated with pediatric laryngeal papillomatosis. However, given the high prevalence of maternal HPV infection and the rarity of laryngeal papillomatosis, prophylactic cesarean delivery is not recommended.[93]

Cervical dysplasia is another sequelae of HPV infection. Appropriate workup of abnormal PAP smears should be undertaken independent of pregnancy.

EPSTEIN-BARR VIRUS

The causative agent of infectious mononucleosis is Epstein-Barr Virus (EBV), a member of the Herpesviridae family. Clinical presentation includes malaise, headache, fever, pharyngitis, lymphadenopathy, atypical lymphocytosis, heterophile antibody, and transient mild hepatitis. Infection is typically self-limited. EBV establishes latent, reactivatable infection in B lymphocytes and is also associated with Hodgkin and non-Hodgkin lymphoma. Most adults (>95%) are EBV seropositive, so primary EBV infection in pregnancy is rare. Primary infection and/or reactivation of EBV is not associated with significant adverse pregnancy outcome.[94] An association has been found between EBV reactivation within pregnancy and the development of childhood acute lymphoblastic leukemia in the neonate.[95] In utero EBV transmission has been demonstrated by detection of EBV DNA in neonatal lymphocytes.[96] However, in utero infection has not been directly associated with adverse outcomes. Routine testing is not indicated given the extremely high seroprevalence and the lack of impact on pregnancy.

SMALLPOX

Variola virus is the causative agent of smallpox. Infection is restricted to humans, but it is highly transmissible via airborne droplet inhalation or by direct contact with smallpox lesions.[97] Secondary to widespread vaccination, the last reported smallpox case in the United States was in 1949, and the WHO declared global eradication in 1980. Concerns regarding the potential for variola virus to be used as a bioterrorism agent has led to renewed interest in the presentation and treatment of smallpox disease.

Smallpox infection first presents with a high fever, chills, headache, backache, and vomiting; this differentiates it from chickenpox (varicella), which has a minimal prodrome.[97] Delirium is present in 15%, with some infections progressing to encephalitis. Skin lesions appear 2 to 3 days following the symptom onset and progress from macula to papule to vesicle (Fig. 53-8), vesicle to pustule to scabs, and ultimately form

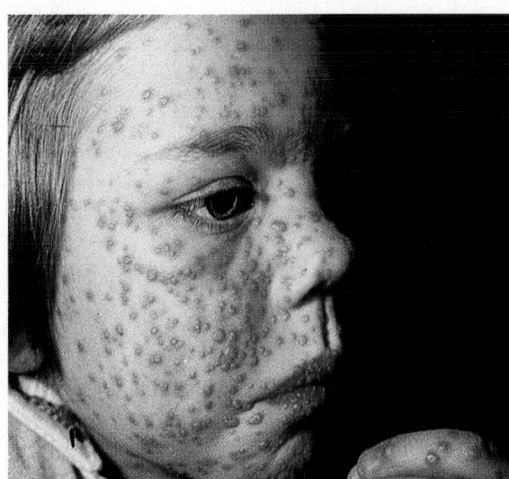

FIG 53-8 Smallpox vesicles, day 3 of clinical infection. (From Tyring S, et al. *Tropical Dermatology*. Edinburgh: Saunders; 2005.)

pitted scars. Smallpox lesions appear in a centrifugal distribution and affect soles and palms, whereas varicella infection exhibits a centripetal lesion distribution that spares the palms and soles. Diagnosis confirmation is via PCR reaction of pustular fluid and/or scabs in a biocontainment facility.

Maternal treatment is supportive; vaccination and containment are critical. Historically, the maternal mortality rate of unvaccinated women was over 60%.[97] Death usually occurs secondary to viral pneumonitis, bacterial pneumonia, or cardiovascular collapse; pregnant women are also at increased risk for hemorrhagic smallpox, a more severe and lethal manifestation of infection. When infection occurs prior to 24 weeks, 75% of pregnancies end in loss or premature delivery. During the latter half of pregnancy, smallpox infection is associated with a 55% preterm delivery rate. Variola virus crosses the placenta, which enables intrauterine infection. During epidemics, the rate of congenital variola infection has ranged from 9% to 60%.

Vaccination within 2 to 3 days of initial exposure affords almost complete protection against disease.[97,98] The currently available vaccine, Dryvax, is composed of live attenuated variola virus. This vaccine has a higher complication risk than other vaccines; sequelae include postvaccinal encephalitis (incidence 12 per million vaccinations, 40% mortality rate), mild generalized vaccinia, and eczema vaccinatum. **Smallpox vaccination is currently restricted to women in military service and researchers who utilize related viruses.** Data on women vaccinated during pregnancy are being compiled in the National Smallpox Vaccine in Pregnancy Registry.[98] Fetal infection following maternal vaccination (fetal vaccinia) is rare and is characterized by skin lesions and internal organ involvement, but it is not associated with fetal malformations. Therefore vaccination is not considered an indication for pregnancy termination. The CDC recommends deferring elective smallpox vaccination during pregnancy; however, immediate vaccination is indicated following smallpox exposure, independent of pregnancy, secondary to the risk of clinical smallpox infection to the mother and fetus.[97]

EBOLA
Virology and Epidemiology
Ebola is an enveloped RNA virus member of the Filoviridae family. The envelope gene encodes two transcription products, GP and sGP, a secreted nonstructural protein. Virus-associated GP binds to target cells and undergoes posttranslational cleavage into GP$_1$ (attachment) and GP$_2$ (fusion) subunits within the endosome, which enables fusion/entry. Ebola is a zoonotic pathogen, and fruit bats are the likely native host and viral reservoir. Transmission occurs via direct contact with body fluids of a person who is sick with or has died of Ebola (blood, vomit, urine, feces, sweat, semen, spit, other fluids) or infected animals (meat). Ebola has been isolated from semen for 3 months following recovery, and **transmission via breastfeeding has been documented.** The incubation period is 2 to 21 days following exposure, and individuals become infectious at symptom onset. Ebola infects macrophages, which leads to massive inflammation, complications, and an outbreak-dependent mortality rate that ranges from 50% to 90%. As of early 2015, only a few cases of Ebola virus disease (EVD) had been reported in the United States (none in pregnancy). The 2015 outbreak involved multiple West African countries: Guinea, Liberia, Nigeria, Senegal, and Sierra Leone. For up-to-date information and recommendations, visit the CDC or WHO sites online.

High-risk exposure includes percutaneous (e.g., needle stick) or mucous membrane contact with blood or body fluids from an EVD patient, exposure to blood or body fluids of a symptomatic EVD patient without appropriate personal protective equipment (PPE), processing blood or body fluids from a symptomatic EVD patient without appropriate PPE or biosafety precautions, or undertaking the following activities without appropriate PPE: direct contact with a dead body (including funeral rites) in Ebola-affected areas, household contact, or providing direct care to a symptomatic EVD patient. Some risk is associated with direct contact with EVD patients with PPE or any direct patient care in EVD-endemic countries and even with a prolonged period within 3 feet of a patient with symptomatic EVD. Low-risk situations include visiting an EVD-endemic country within the past 21 days (with no known exposures), brief proximity to a symptomatic EVD patient, caring for an EVD patient with PPE in a nonendemic country, or air travel with a symptomatic EVD patient.

Clinical Manifestations
Early symptoms include fever, weakness, arthralgias, myalgias, headache, anorexia, and hiccups. Progressive symptoms can include nausea, vomiting, diarrhea, dysphagia, conjunctivitis, abdominal or hepatic tenderness, and unexplained bleeding or bruising. Late symptoms include seizures, chest pain, rash, and miscarriage. Bleeding occurs in approximately 50% of patients and may be solely internal. Otherwise, EVD presents as a nonspecific, severe viral syndrome.

Diagnosis
A *person under investigation* (PUI) is someone who has both an epidemiologic risk factor within the 21 days prior to the onset of symptoms *and* consistent symptoms that include a fever greater than 38.6° C or subjective fever, severe headache, muscle pain, vomiting, diarrhea, abdominal pain, or unexplained hemorrhage. Case confirmation requires laboratory-confirmed diagnostic evidence of Ebola infection. While diagnosis is being considered, the patient should be isolated in a private room with a bathroom. Contact, droplet, and environmental control precautions should be implemented, and appropriate PPE should be consistently used.

All specimens should be collected by staff wearing appropriate PPE and should be handled as category A infectious substances. This includes placing specimens in a leak-proof secondary container, transporting specimens to the laboratory by hand, and avoiding high-traffic areas. Laboratory Response Network laboratories conduct presumptive testing with diagnostic confirmation made by the CDC. Confirmatory testing is via RT-PCR, although virus isolation and serology can also be performed. A negative RT-PCR 72 hours after the onset of symptoms excludes EVD, and a negative RT-PCR more than 48 hours after a positive test fulfills criteria for discontinuing isolation. Given nonspecific symptomatology and the presence of other infectious diseases with similar presentation in EVD endemic areas, differential diagnosis should include malaria, bacterial infection, and Lassa fever, a disease endemic to portions of West Africa with a prevalence of greater than 10,000 cases per year and similar symptoms to early EVD. Diagnostic tests to rule out Lassa fever in patients who test negative for EVD are RT-PCR, antigen detection, and serology.[99]

Management of Ebola in Pregnancy

The critical element of clinical management is prompt patient isolation and implementation of recommended infection-control measures (standard contact and droplet precautions) using appropriate PPE when caring for any PUI and patients with confirmed EVD. CDC guidelines for PPE may be accessed at www.cdc.gov/vhf/ebola/healthcare-us/ppe/guidance.html. Ongoing management consists of supportive care, which includes aggressive IV fluid resuscitation and assessment and correction of electrolyte abnormalities, hypoglycemia, anemia, and coagulopathy. Patients should be assessed for bleeding, secondary infections, and other complications. Empiric broad-spectrum antibiotics should be instituted for suspected infection without awaiting cultures; this is because EVD patients are at risk for sepsis and associated sequelae such as increased vascular permeability, vasodilation, multiple organ failure, and shock. We recommend advanced hemodynamic and fetal monitoring for pregnant women with suspected EVD, maintaining O_2 saturation above 95%, and utilizing vasopressors and ionotropic agents as needed to maintain cardiac output, blood pressure, and tissue perfusion. Symptomatic management of fever, nausea, vomiting, diarrhea, and abdominal pain is warranted.[99]

No evidence suggests that pregnancy increases EVD susceptibility. However, pregnancy is thought to increase disease severity and mortality in the third trimester. Epidemiologic reports suggest a high incidence of miscarriage and fetal loss (greater than 80%). No reports exist of neonatal survival, although intrauterine Ebola transmission was recently reported in two patients: both women recovered, but neither fetus survived.[100] High maternal mortality combined with potentially absent neonatal survival dictates that the primary focus be directed toward optimizing maternal status, recognizing that enhanced monitoring and the capacity for intervention in the United States could be associated with a reduced mortality. Updated guidance can be accessed at www.cdc.gov/vhf/ebola/healthcare-us/hospitals/pregnant-women.html.

KEY POINTS

- Rubella immunization and HBV and HIV infection screening is standard. HIV screening should be performed via an "opt out" approach, and in high prevalence areas, repeat screening in the third trimester should be considered. Varicella screening may be considered in women without a history of infection. Routine CMV screening is not recommended secondary to high seroprevalence.
- The ACOG and the CDC recommend seasonal influenza vaccination (October through May) for all pregnant women with intramuscular inactivated vaccine. HAV and HBV vaccination are also safe in pregnancy and should be offered based on risk and susceptibility. Live attenuated vaccines for rubeola, rubella, and varicella infection should be deferred until after pregnancy.
- Rapid intrapartum HIV testing should be accessible to women without documented HIV status because most perinatally infected infants are born to women unaware of their HIV status.

- The standard of care for HIV infection is cART with at least three drugs from at least two classes of antiretrovirals. Early, sustained control of viral replication is associated with decreased HIV transmission. Fully suppressive preconception therapy is recommended, and cART should be started as early in pregnancy as possible for women entering pregnancy not already on cART.
- Pregnant women suspected to be infected with influenza should receive treatment immediately, without delay for diagnostic confirmation.
- Fetal parvovirus infection may result in fetal anemia and hydrops. Women with documented infection should be screened serially with ultrasound. Middle cerebral artery Doppler studies may also be used.
- Rubeola (measles) is one of the most infectious viruses, and 75% to 90% of exposed, susceptible contacts become infected. Measles infection can cause SSPE, a progressive, uniformly fatal neurologic disease. Infection may originate in individuals born outside the United States, but gaps in vaccination permit the spread of outbreaks in the United States.
- CMV transmission is highest during the third trimester with a 30% to 40% fetal transmission risk. Serious sequelae are most common following first-trimester infection, whereby 24% of infected fetuses have sensorineural hearing loss and 32% have other central nervous system sequelae.
- Susceptible varicella-exposed women should receive VZIG to reduce the risk of infection and transmission. The addition of prophylactic acyclovir may further reduce maternal infection risk.
- Infants born to HBsAg-positive mothers should receive both HBIG and HBV vaccine within 12 hours of birth to reduce perinatal HBV infection. Antepartum tenofovir treatment should also be considered for women at high risk for HBV transmission (HIV coinfection, prior HBV transmission, high HBV loads, or immune-tolerant infection).
- Given the potential to effect virologic cure and the ancillary benefit of reducing perinatal transmission, consideration should be given to diagnosing and treating HCV infection prior to conception. Ribavirin-sparing regimens permit therapy initiation during pregnancy.
- EVD severity and mortality is increased in the third trimester of pregnancy, with almost universal fetal loss. Appropriate infection control combined with hemodynamic monitoring and aggressive maternal care, independent of fetal effects, is recommended.

REFERENCES

1. Centers for Disease Control and Prevention. *Monitoring selected national HIV prevention and care objectives by using HIV surveillance data—United States and 6 dependent areas—2012.* HIV Surveillance Supplemental Report 2014;19(No. 3). Available at <http://www.cdc.gov/hiv/library/reports/surveillance/>.
2. Centers for Disease Control and Prevention and Association of Public Health Laboratories. *Laboratory Testing for the Diagnosis of HIV Infection: Updated Recommendations.* Available at <http://dx.doi.org/10.15620/cdc.23447>.

3. Branson BM, et al. Revised recommendations for HIV testing of adults, adolescents, and pregnant women in health-care settings. *MMWR Recomm Rep.* 2006;55:1-17.

4. Panel on Opportunistic Infections in HIV-Infected Adults and Adolescents. *Guidelines for the prevention and treatment of opportunistic infections in HIV-infected adults and adolescents: recommendations from the Centers for Disease Control and Prevention, the National Institutes of Health, and the HIV Medicine Association of the Infectious Diseases Society of America.* Available at <http://aidsinfo.nih.gov/contentfiles/lvguidelines/adult_oi.pdf>.

5. Panel on Antiretroviral Guidelines for Adults and Adolescents. *Guidelines for the use of antiretroviral agents in HIV-1-infected adults and adolescents.* Department of Health and Human Services. Available at <http://www.aidsinfo.nih.gov/ContentFiles/AdultandAdolescentGL.pdf>.

6. Connor EM, et al. Reduction of maternal-infant transmission of human immunodeficiency virus type 1 with zidovudine treatment. Pediatric AIDS Clinical Trials Group Protocol 076 Study Group. *N Engl J Med.* 1994;331:1173-1180.

7. Panel on Treatment of HIV-Infected Pregnant Women and Prevention of Perinatal Transmission. *Recommendations for Use of Antiretroviral Drugs in Pregnant HIV-1-Infected Women for Maternal Health and Interventions to Reduce Perinatal HIV Transmission in the United States.* Available at: <http://aidsinfo.nih.gov/contentfiles/lvguidelines/PerinatalGL.pdf>.

8. Pas S, et al. Performance Evaluation of the New Roche Cobas AmpliPrep/Cobas TaqMan HIV-1 Test Version 2.0 for Quantification of Human Immunodeficiency Virus Type 1 RNA. *J Clin Microbiol.* 2010;48:1195-1200.

9. Ioannidis JP, et al. Perinatal transmission of human immunodeficiency virus type 1 by pregnant women with RNA virus loads <1000 copies/ml. *J Infect Dis.* 2001;183:539-545.

9a. Antiretroviral Pregnancy Registry Steering Committee. *Antiretroviral Pregnancy Registry international interim report for 1 Jan 1989–31 January 2015.* Wilmington, NC: Registry Coordinating Center; Available at: <http://www.APRegistry.com>.

10. Hitti J, et al. Protease inhibitor-based antiretroviral therapy and glucose tolerance in pregnancy: AIDS Clinical Trials Group A5084. *Am J Obstet Gynecol.* 2007;196:331, e1-7.

11. Kaplan JE, et al. Guidelines for prevention and treatment of opportunistic infections in HIV-infected adults and adolescents: recommendations from CDC, the National Institutes of Health, and the HIV Medicine Association of the Infectious Diseases Society of America. *MMWR Recomm Rep.* 2009;58:1-207.

12. Townsend CL, et al. Low rates of mother-to-child transmission of HIV following effective pregnancy interventions in the United Kingdom and Ireland, 2000-2006. *AIDS.* 2008;22:973-981.

13. Somigliana E, et al. Early invasive diagnostic techniques in pregnant women who are infected with the HIV: a multicenter case series. *Am J Obstet Gynecol.* 2005;193:437-442.

14. Mandelbrot L, et al. Amniocentesis and mother-to-child human immunodeficiency virus transmission in the Agence Nationale de Recherches sur le SIDA et les Hepatites Virales French Perinatal Cohort. *Am J Obstet Gynecol.* 2009;200:160, e1-9.

15. Read JS, Newell MK. Efficacy and safety of cesarean delivery for prevention of mother-to-child transmission of HIV-1. *Cochrane Database Syst Rev.* 2005;(4):CD005479.

16. Duration of ruptured membranes and vertical transmission of HIV-1: a meta-analysis from 15 prospective cohort studies. *AIDS.* 2001;15:357-368.

17. Schneider E, et al. Revised surveillance case definitions for HIV infection among adults, adolescents, and children aged <18 months and for HIV infection and AIDS among children aged 18 months to <13 years–United States, 2008. *MMWR Recomm Rep.* 2008;57:1-12.

18. Patel K, et al. Prenatal protease inhibitor use and risk of preterm birth among HIV-infected women initiating antiretroviral drugs during pregnancy. *J Infect Dis.* 2010;201:1035-1044.

19. Siston AM, et al. Pandemic 2009 influenza A(H1N1) virus illness among pregnant women in the United States. *JAMA.* 2010;303:1517-1525.

20. Louie JK, et al. Pregnancy and severe influenza infection in the 2013-2014 influenza season. *Obstet Gynecol.* 2015;125:184-192.

21. Goodnight WH, Soper DE. Pneumonia in pregnancy. *Crit Care Med.* 2005;33:S390-S397.

22. Varner MW, et al. Influenza-like illness in hospitalized pregnant and post-partum women during the 2009-2010 H1N1 pandemic. *Obstet Gynecol.* 2011;118:593-600.

23. Maternal and Infant Outcomes Among Severely Ill Pregnant and Postpartum Women with 2009 Pandemic Influenza A (H1N1)–United States, April 2009–August 2010. *MMWR Morb Mortal Wkly Rep.* 2011;60:1193-1196.

24. Committee on Obstetric Practice and Immunization Expert Work Group, Centers for Disease Control and Prevention's Advisory Committee on Immunization, United States & American College of Obstetricians and Gynecologists. Committee opinion no. 608: influenza vaccination during pregnancy. *Obstet Gynecol.* 2014;124:648-651.

25. Thurn J. Human parvovirus B19: historical and clinical review. *Rev Infect Dis.* 1988;10:1005-1011.

26. Cosmi E, et al. Noninvasive diagnosis by Doppler ultrasonography of fetal anemia resulting from parvovirus infection. *Am J Obstet Gynecol.* 2002;187:1290-1293.

27. Prospective study of human parvovirus (B19) infection in pregnancy. Public Health Laboratory Service Working Party on Fifth Disease. *BMJ.* 1990;300:1166-1170.

28. Enders M, Weidner A, Zoellner I, Searle K, Enders G. Fetal morbidity and mortality after acute human parvovirus B19 infection in pregnancy: prospective evaluation of 1018 cases. *Prenat Diagn.* 2004;24:513-518.

29. Rodis JF, et al. Management of parvovirus infection in pregnancy and outcomes of hydrops: a survey of members of the Society of Perinatal Obstetricians. *Am J Obstet Gynecol.* 1998;179:985-988.

30. Sahakian V, Weiner CP, Naides SJ, Williamson RA, Scharosch LL. Intra-uterine transfusion treatment of nonimmune hydrops fetalis secondary to human parvovirus B19 infection. *Am J Obstet Gynecol.* 1991;164:1090-1091.

31. De Haan TR, et al. Thrombocytopenia in hydropic fetuses with parvovirus B19 infection: incidence, treatment and correlation with fetal B19 viral load. *BJOG.* 2008;115:76-81.

32. Miller E, Fairley CK, Cohen BJ, Seng C. Immediate and long term outcome of human parvovirus B19 infection in pregnancy. *Br J Obstet Gynaecol.* 1998;105:174-178.

33. Perkin MA, English PM. Immediate and long term outcome of human parvovirus B19 infection in pregnancy. *Br J Obstet Gynaecol.* 1998;105:1337-1338.

34. Rodis JF, et al. Long-term outcome of children following maternal human parvovirus B19 infection. *Obstet Gynecol.* 1998;91:125-128.

35. Brunell PA. Measles. In: Bennett J, Plum F, eds. *Cecil Textbook of Medicine.* Philadelphia: W. B. Saunders Company; 1996:1758-1760.

36. Eberhart-Phillips JE, Frederick PD, Baron RC, Mascola L. Measles in pregnancy: a descriptive study of 58 cases. *Obstet Gynecol.* 1993;82:797-801.

37. Ali ME, Albar HM. Measles in pregnancy: maternal morbidity and perinatal outcome. *Int J Gynaecol Obstet.* 1997;59:109-113.

38. McLean HQ, Fiebelkorn AP, Temte JL, Wallace GS, Centers for Disease Control and Prevention. Prevention of measles, rubella, congenital rubella syndrome, and mumps, 2013: summary recommendations of the Advisory Committee on Immunization Practices (ACIP). *MMWR Recomm Rep.* 2013;62:1-34.

39. Neubert AG, Samuels P, Goodman DB, Rose NC. The seroprevalence of the rubeola antibody in a prenatal screening program. *Obstet Gynecol.* 1997;90:507-510.

40. Miller E, Cradock-Watson JE, Pollock TM. Consequences of confirmed maternal rubella at successive stages of pregnancy. *Lancet.* 1982;2:781-784.

41. Munro ND, Sheppard S, Smithells RW, Holzel H, Jones G. Temporal relations between maternal rubella and congenital defects. *Lancet.* 1987;2:201-204.

42. Control and prevention of rubella: evaluation and management of suspected outbreaks, rubella in pregnant women, and surveillance for congenital rubella syndrome. *MMWR Recomm Rep.* 2001;50:1-23.

43. McIntosh ED, Menser MA. A fifty-year follow-up of congenital rubella. *Lancet.* 1992;340:414-415.

44. Townsend JJ, et al. Progressive rubella panencephalitis. Late onset after congenital rubella. *N Engl J Med.* 1975;292:990-993.

45. Taber LH, Frank AL, Yow MD, Bagley A. Acquisition of cytomegaloviral infections in families with young children: a serological study. *J Infect Dis.* 1985;151:948-952.

46. Stagno S, Britt W. *Cytomegalovirus Infections.* Philadelphia: Elsevier; 2006.

47. Nigro G, Adler SP, La Torre R, Best AM. Passive immunization during pregnancy for congenital cytomegalovirus infection. *N Engl J Med.* 2005;353:1350-1362.

48. Revello MG, et al. A randomized trial of hyperimmune globulin to prevent congenital cytomegalovirus. *N Engl J Med.* 2014;370:1316-1326.

49. Stagno S, et al. Primary cytomegalovirus infection in pregnancy. Incidence, transmission to fetus, and clinical outcome. *JAMA*. 1986;256:1904-1908.

50. Pass RF, Fowler KB, Boppana SB, Britt WJ, Stagno S. Congenital cytomegalovirus infection following first trimester maternal infection: symptoms at birth and outcome. *J Clin Virol*. 2006;35:216-220.

51. Fowler KB, et al. The outcome of congenital cytomegalovirus infection in relation to maternal antibody status. *N Engl J Med*. 1992;326:663-667.

52. Lewis PE, Cefalo RC, Zaritsky AL. Fetal heart block caused by cytomegalovirus. *Am J Obstet Gynecol*. 1980;136:967-968.

53. Pletcher BA, et al. Intrauterine cytomegalovirus infection presenting as fetal meconium peritonitis. *Obstet Gynecol*. 1991;78:903-905.

54. Brown ZA, et al. Asymptomatic maternal shedding of herpes simplex virus at the onset of labor: relationship to preterm labor. *Obstet Gynecol*. 1996;87:483-488.

55. ACOG Practice Bulletin. Clinical management guidelines for obstetrician-gynecologists. No. 82 June 2007. Management of herpes in pregnancy. *Obstet Gynecol*. 2007;109:1489-1498.

56. Randolph AG, Washington AE, Prober CG. Cesarean delivery for women presenting with genital herpes lesions. Efficacy, risks, and costs. *JAMA*. 1993;270:77-82.

57. Arvin AM, et al. Failure of antepartum maternal cultures to predict the infant's risk of exposure to herpes simplex virus at delivery. *N Engl J Med*. 1986;315:796-800.

58. Andrews WW, et al. Valacyclovir therapy to reduce recurrent genital herpes in pregnant women. *Am J Obstet Gynecol*. 2006;194:774-781.

59. Brown ZA, et al. Effect of serologic status and cesarean delivery on transmission rates of herpes simplex virus from mother to infant. *JAMA*. 2003;289:203-209.

60. Thompson C, Whitley R. Neonatal herpes simplex virus infections: where are we now? Hot topics in infection and immunity in children VII. In: Curtis N, Finn A, Pollard AJ, eds. *Advances in Experimental Medicine and Biology*. Vol 697. New York: Springer; 2011:221-230.

61. Varicella-related deaths among adults–United States, 1997. *MMWR Morb Mortal Wkly Rep*. 1997;46:409-412.

62. Chapman S, Duff P. Varicella in pregnancy. *Semin Perinatol*. 1993;17:403-409.

63. Wald ER. Transmission of varicella-vaccine virus: what is the risk? *J Pediatr*. 1998;133:310-311.

64. Smith CK, Arvin AM. Varicella in the fetus and newborn. *Semin Fetal Neonatal Med*. 2009;14:209-217.

65. Asano Y, et al. Postexposure prophylaxis of varicella in family contact by oral acyclovir. *Pediatrics*. 1993;92:219-222.

66. Goldstein SL, Somers MJ, Lande MB, Brewer ED, Jabs KL. Acyclovir prophylaxis of varicella in children with renal disease receiving steroids. *Pediatr Nephrol*. 2000;14:305-308.

67. Enders G, Miller E, Cradock-Watson J, Bolley I, Ridehalgh M. Consequences of varicella and herpes zoster in pregnancy: prospective study of 1739 cases. *Lancet*. 1994;343:1548-1551.

68. Isada NB, et al. In utero diagnosis of congenital varicella zoster virus infection by chorionic villus sampling and polymerase chain reaction. *Am J Obstet Gynecol*. 1991;165:1727-1730.

69. Pretorius DH, Hayward I, Jones KL, Stamm E. Sonographic evaluation of pregnancies with maternal varicella infection. *J Ultrasound Med*. 1992;11:459-463.

70. Wedemeyer H, Pawlotsky JM. Acute viral hepatitis. In: Goldman L, Schafer AI, eds. *Goldman's Cecil Medicine*. Philadelphia: Elsevier; 2012:966-973.

71. ACOG Practice Bulletin No. 86: Viral hepatitis in pregnancy. *Obstet Gynecol*. 2007;110:941-956.

72. Trépo C, Chan HL, Lok A. Hepatitis B virus infection. *Lancet*. 2014;384:2053-2063.

73. Hepatitis B vaccination–United States, 1982-2002. *MMWR Morb Mortal Wkly Rep*. 2002;51:549-552, 563.

74. Davies G, et al. Amniocentesis and women with hepatitis B, hepatitis C, or human immunodeficiency virus. *J Obstet Gynaecol Can*. 2003;25:145-148, 149-152.

75. Hill JB, et al. Risk of hepatitis B transmission in breast-fed infants of chronic hepatitis B carriers. *Obstet Gynecol*. 2002;99:1049-1052.

76. Mast EE, et al. A comprehensive immunization strategy to eliminate transmission of hepatitis B virus infection in the United States: recommendations of the Advisory Committee on Immunization Practices (ACIP) part 1: immunization of infants, children, and adolescents. *MMWR Recomm Rep*. 2005;54:1-31.

77. Wang Z, et al. Quantitative analysis of HBV DNA level and HBeAg titer in hepatitis B surface antigen positive mothers and their babies: HBeAg passage through the placenta and the rate of decay in babies. *J Med Virol*. 2003;71:360-366.

78. Dunkelberg JC, Berkley EM, Thiel KW, Leslie KK. Hepatitis B and C in pregnancy: a review and recommendations for care. *J Perinatol*. 2014;34:882-891.

79. Cholongitas E, Tziomalos K, Pipili C. Management of patients with hepatitis B in special populations. *World J Gastroenterol*. 2015;21:1738-1748.

80. Lok AS, McMahon BJ. Chronic hepatitis B: update 2009. *Hepatology*. 2009;50:661-662.

81. American Association for the Study of Liver Diseases/Infection Disease Society of America/International Antiviral Society–USA. *Recommendations for testing, managing, and treating hepatitis C*. Available at <www.hcvguidelines.org>.

82. Schuval S, et al. Hepatitis C prevalence in children with perinatal human immunodeficiency virus infection enrolled in a long-term follow-up protocol. *Arch Pediatr Adolesc Med*. 2004;158:1007-1013.

83. A Significant Sex–but Not Elective Cesarean Section–Effect on Mother-to-Child Transmission of Hepatitis C Virus Infection. *J Infect Dis*. 2005;192:1872-1879.

84. Roberts SS, et al. The Ribavirin Pregnancy Registry: Findings after 5 years of enrollment, 2003-2009. *Birth Defects Res A Clin Mol Teratol*. 2010;88:551-559.

85. Ramia S, Bahakim H. Perinatal transmission of hepatitis B virus-associated hepatitis D virus. *Ann Inst Pasteur Virol*. 1988;139:285-290.

86. Renou C, Pariente A, Nicand E, Pavio N. Pathogenesis of Hepatitis E in pregnancy. *Liver Int*. 2008;28:1465, author reply 1466.

87. Kumar A, Beniwal M, Kar P, Sharma JB, Murthy NS. Hepatitis E in pregnancy. *Int J Gynaecol Obstet*. 2004;85:240-244.

88. Khuroo MS, Kamili S, Jameel S. Vertical transmission of hepatitis E virus. *Lancet*. 1995;345:1025-1026.

89. Ornoy A, Tenenbaum A. Pregnancy outcome following infections by coxsackie, echo, measles, mumps, hepatitis, polio and encephalitis viruses. *Reprod Toxicol*. 2006;21:446-457.

90. Archer JS. Acute liver failure in pregnancy. A case report. *J Reprod Med*. 2001;46:137-140.

91. Axelsson C, Bondestam K, Frisk G, Bergstrom S, Diderholm H. Coxsackie B virus infections in women with miscarriage. *J Med Virol*. 1993;39:282-285.

92. Dahlquist GG, Ivarsson S, Lindberg B, Forsgren M. Maternal enteroviral infection during pregnancy as a risk factor for childhood IDDM. A population-based case-control study. *Diabetes*. 1995;44:408-413.

93. Worda C, et al. Prevalence of cervical and intrauterine human papillomavirus infection in the third trimester in asymptomatic women. *J Soc Gynecol Investig*. 2005;12:440-444.

94. Eskild A, Bruu AL, Stray-Pedersen B, Jenum P. Epstein-Barr virus infection during pregnancy and the risk of adverse pregnancy outcome. *BJOG*. 2005;112:1620-1624.

95. Lehtinen M, et al. Maternal herpesvirus infections and risk of acute lymphoblastic leukemia in the offspring. *Am J Epidemiol*. 2003;158:207-213.

96. Meyohas MC, et al. Study of mother-to-child Epstein-Barr virus transmission by means of nested PCRs. *J Virol*. 1996;70:6816-6819.

97. Suarez VR, Hankins GD. Smallpox and pregnancy: from eradicated disease to bioterrorist threat. *Obstet Gynecol*. 2002;100:87-93.

98. Women with smallpox vaccine exposure during pregnancy reported to the National Smallpox Vaccine in Pregnancy Registry–United States, 2003. *MMWR Morb Mortal Wkly Rep*. 2003;52:386-388.

99. World Health Organization. *Clinical management of patients with viral haemorrhagic fever: A pocket guide for the front-line health worker*. Available at <www.who.int/csr/resources/publications/clinical-management-patients/en/>.

100. Baggi FM, et al. Management of pregnant women infected with Ebola virus in a treatment centre in Guinea, June 2014. *Euro Surveill*. 2014;19.

Additional references for this chapter are available at ExpertConsult.com.

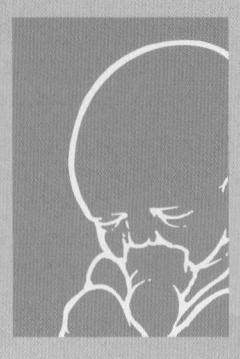

CHAPTER 54

Maternal and Perinatal Infection in Pregnancy: Bacterial

PATRICK DUFF and MEREDITH BIRSNER

KEY ABBREVIATIONS

Acute respiratory distress syndrome	ARDS
Body mass index	BMI
Centers for Disease Control and Prevention	CDC
Central venous pressure	CVP
Computed tomography	CT
Group B *Streptococcus*	GBS
Human immunodeficiency virus	HIV
Listeria monocytogenes	LM
Magnetic resonance imaging	MRI
Methicillin-resistant *Staphylococcus aureus*	MRSA
Nucleic acid amplification test	NAAT
Polymerase chain reaction	PCR
Premature rupture of the membranes	PROM
Systemic immune response syndrome	SIRS

Bacterial infections are the single most common complication encountered by the obstetrician. Some infections, such as puerperal endometritis and lower urinary tract infection, are of principal concern to the mother and pose little or no risk to the fetus or neonate. Others, such as listeriosis and toxoplasmosis, are of greatest threat to the fetus. Still others—such as group B streptococcal infection (GBS), pyelonephritis, and chorioamnionitis—may cause serious morbidity, even life-threatening complications, for both the mother and baby. The purpose of this chapter is to review in detail the major bacterial infections and the key protozoan infection (toxoplasmosis) that the obstetrician confronts in daily clinical practice.

GROUP B STREPTOCOCCAL INFECTION

Epidemiology

Streptococcus agalactiae is a gram-positive encapsulated coccus that produces β-hemolysis when grown on blood agar. **On average, about 20% to 25% of pregnant women in the United States harbor this group B *Streptococcus* (GBS) in their lower genital tract and rectum. GBS is one of the most important causes of early-onset neonatal infection.** The prevalence of neonatal GBS infection now is about 0.5 per 1000 live births, and about 10,000 cases of neonatal streptococcal septicemia occur each year in the United States.[1]

Neonatal GBS infection can be divided into early-onset and late-onset infection, and Table 54-1 summarizes characteristics of both. **About 80% to 85% of cases of neonatal GBS infection are early in onset and result almost exclusively from vertical transmission from a colonized mother.** Early-onset infection presents primarily as a severe pneumonia and overwhelming septicemia. **In preterm infants, the mortality rate from early-onset GBS infection may approach 25%. In term infants, the mortality rate is lower, averaging about 5%.**[2] Late-onset neonatal GBS infection occurs as a result of both vertical and horizontal transmission. It is typically manifested by bacteremia, meningitis, and pneumonia. The mortality rate from late-onset infection is about 5% for both preterm and term infants.[1] Unfortunately, obstetric interventions have proved ineffective in preventing late-onset neonatal infection. Therefore the remainder of this discussion focuses on early-onset infection.

Major risk factors for early-onset infection include preterm labor, especially when complicated by preterm premature rupture of the membranes (PROM); intrapartum maternal fever (chorioamnionitis); prolonged rupture of membranes, defined as greater than 18 hours; previous delivery of an infected infant; young age; and black or Hispanic ethnicity.[1] About 25% of pregnant women have at least one risk factor for GBS infection. The neonatal attack rate in colonized patients is 40% to 50% in the presence of a risk factor and less than 5% in the absence of a risk factor. In infected infants, neonatal

TABLE 54-1 CHARACTERISTICS OF EARLY- AND LATE-ONSET NEONATAL GBS SEPSIS

TYPE OF GBS SEPSIS	TIMING	% OF CASES	RISK FACTORS	INCIDENCE	MORTALITY RATE
Early onset	Within first week	85%	• Gestational age <37 weeks • Preterm premature rupture of membranes • Longer duration of membrane rupture • Intraamniotic infection • Young maternal age • Black or Hispanic race • Prior delivery of an infant with GBS disease	0.34 to 0.37 cases per 1000 live births	2% to 3% (term infants); 20% to 30% (preterm infants)
Late onset	After first week (up to 3 months)	15%	• Gestational age <37 weeks • Black race • Maternal GBS colonization	0.3 to 0.4 cases per 1000 live birth	1% to 2% (term infants); 5% to 6% (preterm infants)

GBS, group B *Streptococcus*.

TABLE 54-2 RELIABILITY OF RAPID DIAGNOSTIC TESTS FOR GROUP B STREPTOCOCCI

TEST	TEST PERFORMANCE			
	SENSITIVITY (%)	SPECIFICITY (%)	PV+ (%)	PV− (%)
Gram stain	34-100	60-70	13-33	86-100
Growth in starch medium	93-98	98-99	65-98	89-99
Antigen detection (coagglutination, latex particle agglutination, enzyme immunoassay)	4-88*	92-100	15-100	76-99
DNA probe[†]	>90	90	61	94

*Sensitivities for identification of heavily colonized women ranged from 29% to 100%.
[†]Specimens were grown in culture for 3.5 hours before the DNA probe was used.

mortality approaches 30% to 35% when a maternal risk factor is present but is less than 5% when a risk factor is absent.[2,3]

Maternal Complications

Several obstetric complications occur with increased frequency in pregnant women who are colonized with GBS. The organism is one of the major causes of **chorioamnionitis** and **postpartum endometritis**. It may cause **postcesarean delivery wound infection**, usually in conjunction with other aerobic and anaerobic bacilli and staphylococci. The organism also is responsible for approximately 2% to 3% of **lower urinary tract infections** in pregnant women.[1] GBS urinary tract infection, in turn, is a risk factor for preterm PROM and preterm labor. For example, Thomsen and colleagues[4] reported a study of 69 women at 27 to 31 weeks' gestation who had streptococcal urinary tract infections. Patients were assigned to treatment with either penicillin or placebo. Treated patients had a significant reduction in the frequency of both preterm PROM and preterm labor.

Other investigations have confirmed the association between GBS colonization and preterm labor and preterm PROM. Women with the latter complication who are colonized with GBS tend to have a shorter latent period and higher frequency of chorioamnionitis and puerperal endometritis compared with noncolonized women.[5]

Diagnosis

The gold standard for the diagnosis of GBS infection is bacteriologic culture. Todd-Hewitt broth or selective blood agar is the preferred medium. **Specimens for culture should be obtained from the lower vagina, perineum, and perianal area using a simple cotton swab.** In recent years, considerable research has been devoted to assessment of rapid diagnostic tests for the identification of colonized women. Table 54-2 summarizes the results of several investigations of rapid diagnostic

tests.[6,7] The information in this table is based on the review by Yancey and associates.[6] These authors noted that, although the rapid diagnostic tests had reasonable sensitivity in identifying heavily colonized patients, they had poor sensitivity in identifying lightly and moderately colonized patients.

Although the first-generation rapid diagnostic tests were not as valuable as originally hoped, Bergeron and colleagues[8] reported exceptionally favorable results with a new polymerase chain reaction (PCR) assay for GBS. In a series of 112 patients, the authors documented a sensitivity of 97%, specificity of 100%, positive predictive value of 100%, and negative predictive value of 99%. This PCR assay now is commercially available and offers clear promise as a rapid test for screening patients at the time of admission for labor. Ahmadzia and colleagues[9] recently reviewed the diagnostic accuracy of intrapartum nucleic acid amplification tests (NAATs) for GBS and reported that the sensitivity ranged from 91% to 94%.

Prevention of Group B Streptococcal Infection

In the past 20 years, several strategies have been proposed for the prevention of neonatal GBS infection.[2,3,10-12] Each strategy has had major imperfections. In 1996, however, the Centers for Disease Control and Prevention (CDC) published a series of recommendations that incorporated the major advantages of previous protocols and minimized some of the more problematic aspects of selected strategies.[12] The initial CDC guidelines recommended either universal culturing of all patients at 35 to 37 weeks' gestation and intrapartum treatment of all colonized women or selective treatment on the basis of identified risk factors. Subsequently, in a large population-based survey, Rosenstein and Schuchat[13] assessed the theoretic impact of the CDC recommendations and showed that a strategy of universal culturing and treatment of all colonized patients would prevent 78% of cases of neonatal infection. In contrast, only 41% of cases

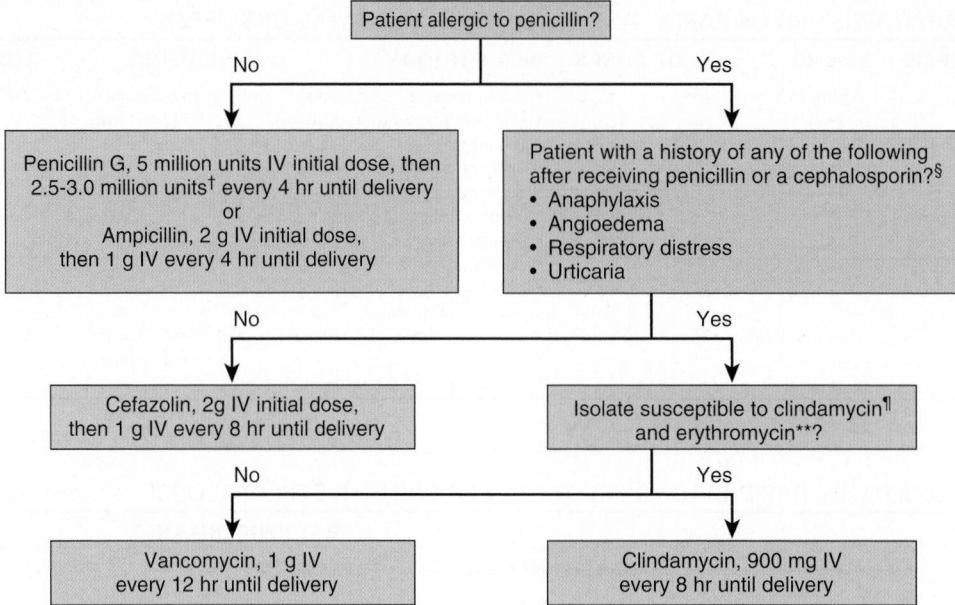

* Broader spectrum agents, including an agent active against GBS, might be necessary for treatment of chorioamnionitis.
† Doses ranging from 2.5 to 3.0 million units are acceptable for the doses administered every 4 hours following the initial dose. The choice of dose within that range should be guided by which formulations of penicillin G are readily available to reduce the need for pharmacies to specially prepare doses.
§ Penicillin-allergic patients with a history of anaphylaxis, angioedema, respiratory distress, or urticaria following administration of penicillin or a cephalosporin are considered to be at high risk for anaphylaxis and should not receive penicillin, ampicillin, or cefazolin for GBS intrapartum prophylaxis. For penicillin-allergic patients who do not have a history of those reactions, cefazolin is the preferred agent because pharmacologic data suggest it achieves effective intraamniotic concentrations. Vancomycin and clindamycin should be reserved for penicillin-allergic women at high risk for anaphylaxis.
¶ If laboratory facilities are adequate, clindamycin and erythromycin susceptibility testing should be performed on prenatal GBS isolates from penicillin-allergic women at high risk for anaphylaxis. If no susceptibility testing is performed, or the results are not available at the time of labor, vancomycin is the preferred agent for GBS intrapartum prophylaxis for penicillin-allergic women at high risk for anaphylaxis.
** Resistance to erythromycin is often but not always associated with clindamycin resistance. If an isolate is resistant to erythromycin, it might have inducible resistance to clindamycin, even if it appears susceptible to clindamycin. If a GBS isolate is susceptible to clindamycin, resistant to erythromycin, and testing for inducible clindamycin resistance has been performed and is negative (no inducible resistance), then clindamycin can be used for GBS intrapartum prophylaxis instead of vancomycin.

FIG 54-1 Recommended regimens for intrapartum antibiotic prophylaxis for prevention of early-onset group B *Streptococcus* (GBS) disease. IV, intravenously.

were prevented when patients were targeted for prophylaxis just on the basis of risk factors. In addition, Locksmith and colleagues[14] confirmed that universal culturing also was of value in decreasing the rate of maternal infection compared with a strategy of only treating on the basis of risk factors.

In 2010, the CDC issued its most recent guidelines for prevention of early-onset GBS infection.[1] **The newest guidelines recommend universal cultures in all patients as the optimal method of prevention. Cultures should be performed at 35 to 37 weeks' gestation. All patients who test positive should receive intrapartum antibiotic prophylaxis with one of the regimens outlined in** Figure 54-1. **Ideally, antibiotics should be administered at least 4 hours before delivery.** DeCueto and coworkers[15] demonstrated that the rate of neonatal GBS infection was reduced significantly when patients were treated for at

least this long. In a subsequent investigation to assess timing of antibiotic prophylaxis, McNanley and associates[16] showed that mean vaginal GBS counts decreased fivefold within 2 hours of antibiotic administration, fiftyfold within 4 hours, and almost a thousandfold within 6 hours.

The new CDC guidelines also addressed issues that previously had been imprecisely defined.[1] **Colonized patients scheduled for a planned cesarean delivery do not require intrapartum prophylaxis. Patients who tested positive for GBS in a previous pregnancy should not be assumed to be colonized and should be retested with each pregnancy.** This recommendation is supported by a later report from Edwards and coworkers.[17] These authors noted that only 59% of patients who were culture positive in a previous pregnancy were positive in the current pregnancy. Conversely, however, **patients who**

TABLE 54-3   INTRAPARTUM ANTIBIOTIC PROPHYLAXIS TO PREVENT EARLY-ONSET GROUP B STREPTOCOCCAL DISEASE

INTRAPARTUM GBS PROPHYLAXIS INDICATED	INTRAPARTUM GBS PROPHYLAXIS NOT INDICATED

• Previous infant with invasive GBS disease
• GBS bacteriuria during any trimester of the current pregnancy
• Positive GBS vaginal-rectal screening culture in late gestation (35 to 37 weeks optimally) during the current pregnancy
• Unknown GBS status at the onset of labor (culture not done, incomplete, or results unknown) and any of the following **intrapartum risk factors**:
  • Delivery at less than 37 weeks
  • Amniotic membrane rupture ≥18 hours
  • Intrapartum temperature ≥100.4° F (≥38.0° C)
  • Intrapartum NAAT positive for GBS
• Presence of one of the above intrapartum risk factors, even if intrapartum NAAT is negative for GBS
• Unknown GBS status at the onset of labor (culture not done, incomplete, or results unknown) and any of the following **intrapartum risk factors**:
  • Delivery at less than 37 weeks
  • Amniotic membrane rupture ≥18 hours
  • Intrapartum temperature ≥100.4° F (≥38.0° C)
  • Intrapartum NAAT positive for GBS
	• Colonization with GBS during a previous pregnancy
	• GBS bacteriuria during a previous pregnancy
	• Negative vaginal and rectal GBS screening culture in late gestation during the current pregnancy regardless of intrapartum risk factors
	• Cesarean delivery performed before onset of labor in a woman with intact amniotic membranes, regardless of GBS colonization status or gestational age

GBS, group B *Streptococcus*; *NAAT*, nucleic acid amplification test.

have GBS bacteriuria in pregnancy, even if treated, should be considered heavily colonized and should be targeted for intrapartum prophylaxis. Moreover, patients who had a previous infant with GBS infection also should be considered colonized and should be treated during labor. Table 54-3 outlines indications and nonindications for intrapartum prophylaxis against GBS.

URINARY TRACT INFECTIONS
Acute Urethritis

Acute urethritis, or acute urethral syndrome, is usually caused by one of three organisms: coliforms (principally *Escherichia coli*), *Neisseria gonorrhoeae,* and *Chlamydia trachomatis.* Coliform organisms are part of the normal vaginal and perineal flora and may be introduced into the urethra during intercourse or when wiping after defecation. *N. gonorrhoeae* and *C. trachomatis* are sexually transmitted pathogens.[18] Patients affected by urethritis typically experience frequency, urgency, and dysuria. Hesitancy, dribbling, and a mucopurulent urethral discharge also may be present. On microscopic examination, the urine usually has white blood cells, but bacteria may not be consistently present. Urine cultures may have low colony counts of coliform organisms, and cultures of the urethral discharge may be positive for gonorrhea and chlamydia. A rapid diagnostic test, such as a NAAT, is now the preferred method for identification of gonorrhea and chlamydia.[18]

Most patients with acute urethritis warrant empiric treatment before the results of laboratory tests are available. Infections caused by coliforms usually respond to the antibiotics described later for treatment of asymptomatic bacteriuria and cystitis. **If gonococcal infection is suspected, the patient should be treated with intramuscular ceftriaxone** (250 mg in a single dose) **plus 1000 mg oral azithromycin.**[19] If the patient is allergic to β-lactam antibiotics, an effective alternative is azithromycin 2000 mg orally in a single dose. This high dose of azithromycin is more likely to be associated with gastrointestinal side effects than more conventional lower doses. An alternative choice in the penicillin-allergic patient is ciprofloxacin 500 mg orally in a single dose. **If chlamydial infection is suspected or**

confirmed, the patient should be treated with azithromycin 1000 mg in a single dose.[1]

Asymptomatic Bacteriuria and Acute Cystitis

The prevalence of asymptomatic bacteriuria in pregnancy is 5% to 10%, and most cases antedate the onset of pregnancy. The frequency of acute cystitis in pregnancy is 1% to 3%. Some cases of cystitis arise de novo, whereas others develop as a result of failure to identify and treat asymptomatic bacteriuria.[20]

E. coli is responsible for at least 80% of cases of initial infections and about 70% of recurrent cases. *Klebsiella pneumoniae* and *Proteus* species also are important pathogens, particularly in patients who have a history of recurrent infection. Up to 10% of infections are caused by gram-positive organisms such as GBS, enterococci, and staphylococci.[18,20]

All pregnant women should have a urine culture at their first prenatal appointment to detect preexisting asymptomatic bacteriuria. If the culture is negative, the likelihood of the patient subsequently developing an asymptomatic infection is less than 5%. **If the culture is positive—defined as greater than 10^5 colonies/mL urine from a midstream, clean-catch specimen—prompt treatment is necessary to prevent ascending infection. In the absence of effective treatment, about one third of pregnant women with asymptomatic bacteriuria will develop acute pyelonephritis.** In a recent report, treatment of asymptomatic bacteriuria was also associated with a reduction in the incidence of low-birthweight babies (relative risk [RR], 0.66; 95% confidence interval [CI], 0.49 to 0.89), but no difference in preterm delivery was seen.[21]

Patients with acute cystitis usually have symptoms of frequency, dysuria, urgency, suprapubic pain, hesitancy, and dribbling. Gross hematuria may be present, but high fever and systemic symptoms are uncommon. In symptomatic patients, the leukocyte esterase and nitrate tests are usually positive. When a urine culture is obtained, a catheterized sample is preferred because it minimizes the probability that urine will be contaminated by vaginal flora. With a catheterized specimen, a colony count greater than 10^2/mL is considered indicative of infection.[22]

TABLE 54-4   ANTIBIOTICS FOR TREATMENT OF ASYMPTOMATIC BACTERIURIA AND ACUTE CYSTITIS

DRUG (TRADE NAME)	STRENGTH OF ACTIVITY	ORAL DOSE	COST
Amoxicillin	Some *Escherichia coli*, most *Proteus* species, GBS, enterococci, some staphylococci	500 mg TID or 875 mg BID	Low
Amoxicillin-clavulanic acid (Augmentin)	Most gram-negative aerobic bacilli and gram-positive cocci	875 mg BID	High
Ampicillin	Some *E. coli*, most *Proteus* species, GBS, enterococci, some staphylococci	250-500 mg 4 times daily	Low
Cephalexin (Keflex)	Most *E. coli*, most *Klebsiella* and *Proteus* species, GBS, staphylococci	250-500 mg 4 times daily	Low
Nitrofurantoin monohydrate macrocrystals—sustained-release preparation (Macrobid)	Most uropathogens except enterococci and *Proteus* species	100 mg BID	Moderate
Double-strength trimethoprim-sulfamethoxazole (Bactrim DS, or Septra DS)	Most uropathogens except some strains of *E. coli*	800 mg/160 mg BID	Low

BID, twice a day; *DS,* double strength; *GBS,* group B streptococci; *TID,* three times a day.

Asymptomatic bacteriuria and acute cystitis characteristically respond well to short courses of oral antibiotics. Single-dose therapy is not as effective in pregnant women as in nonpregnant patients. However, **a 3-day course of treatment appears to be comparable to a 7- to 10-day regimen for an initial infection.**[18] Longer courses of therapy are more appropriate for patients with recurrent infections. Table 54-4 lists several antibiotics of value for treatment of asymptomatic bacteriuria and cystitis.

When sensitivity tests are available—for example, for patients with asymptomatic bacteriuria—they may be used to guide antibiotic selection. When empiric treatment is indicated, the choice of antibiotics should be based on established patterns of susceptibility. **In recent years, 20% to 30% of strains of *E. coli* and more than half the strains of *Klebsiella* have developed resistance to ampicillin.** Thus this drug should not be used when the results of sensitivity tests are unknown unless the suspected pathogen is enterococci, in which case ampicillin or amoxicillin is the drug of choice.[23,24]

When choosing among the drugs listed in Table 54-4, the clinician should consider several factors. First, the sensitivity patterns of ampicillin, amoxicillin, and cephalexin are the most variable. Second, these drugs—along with amoxicillin-clavulanic acid—also have the most pronounced effect on normal bowel and vaginal flora and thus are the most likely to cause diarrhea or monilial vulvovaginitis. In contrast, **nitrofurantoin monohydrate has only minimal effect on vaginal and bowel flora. Moreover, it is more uniformly effective against the common uropathogens, except for *Proteus* species, than trimethoprim-sulfamethoxazole.** Third, **amoxicillin-clavulanic acid and trimethoprim-sulfamethoxazole usually are the best empiric agents for treatment of patients with suspected drug-resistant pathogens.** However, sulfonamides should be avoided in the first trimester of pregnancy because of possible teratogenicity, and they should be avoided immediately prior to delivery because of concern about displacement of bilirubin from protein binding sites, with resultant neonatal jaundice (see Chapter 8).[25]

For patients who have an initial infection and experience a prompt response to treatment, a urine culture for test of cure may not be clinically necessary or cost effective.[18,24] **Cultures during or immediately after treatment are indicated for patients who have a poor response to therapy or who have a history of recurrent infection.** During subsequent clinic appointments, the patient's urine should be screened for nitrites and leukocyte esterase. If either of these tests is positive, repeat urine culture and retreatment are indicated.

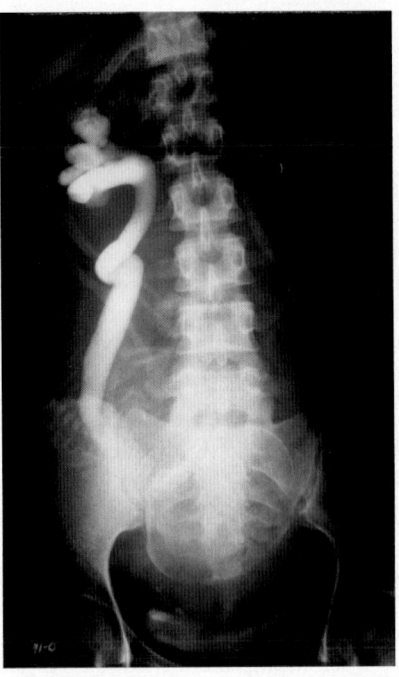

FIG 54-2 Intravenous pyelogram in a pregnant woman shows marked dilation of the right ureter and mild dilation of the renal collecting system.

Acute Pyelonephritis

The incidence of pyelonephritis in pregnancy is 1% to 2%.[20] **Most cases develop as a consequence of undiagnosed or inadequately treated lower urinary tract infection.** Two major physiologic changes occur during pregnancy that predispose to ascending infection of the urinary tract. First, the high concentration of progesterone secreted by the placenta has an inhibitory effect on ureteral peristalsis. Second, the enlarging gravid uterus often compresses the ureters, particularly the right, at the pelvic brim, thus creating additional stasis. Stasis, in turn, facilitates migration of bacteria from the bladder into the ureters and renal parenchyma (Fig. 54-2).

About 75% to 80% of cases of pyelonephritis occur on the right side, 10% to 15% are left sided, and a slightly smaller percentage are bilateral.[20] ***E. coli* is again the principal pathogen.**[20,23] ***K. pneumoniae* and *Proteus* species also are important causes of infection, particularly in women with recurrent episodes of pyelonephritis.** Highly virulent gram-negative bacilli such as *Pseudomonas, Enterobacter,* and *Serratia* are unusual isolates except in immunocompromised patients. Gram-positive cocci do not frequently cause upper tract infection. Anaerobes also are unlikely pathogens unless the patient is chronically obstructed or instrumented.

The usual clinical manifestations of acute pyelonephritis in pregnancy are fever, chills, flank pain and tenderness, urinary frequency or urgency, hematuria, and dysuria. Patients also may have signs of preterm labor, septic shock, and acute respiratory distress syndrome (ARDS). Urinalysis is usually positive for white blood cell casts, red blood cells, and bacteria. Urine colony counts greater than 10^2 colonies/mL in samples collected by catheterization confirm the diagnosis of infection.

Pregnant patients with pyelonephritis may be considered for outpatient therapy if their disease manifestations are mild, they are hemodynamically stable, and they have no evidence of preterm labor.[25] If an outpatient approach is adopted, the patient should be treated with agents that have a high level of activity against the common uropathogens. Acceptable oral agents include amoxicillin-clavulanic acid 875 mg twice daily or double-strength trimethoprim-sulfamethoxazole twice daily for 7 to 10 days. Alternatively, a visiting home nurse may be contracted to administer a parenteral agent such as intravenous (IV) or intramuscular (IM) ceftriaxone 2 g once daily. Although an excellent drug for lower tract infections, nitrofurantoin monohydrate does not consistently achieve the serum and renal parenchymal concentrations necessary for successful treatment of more serious infections.

Patients who appear to be moderately to severely ill or who show any signs of preterm labor should be hospitalized for IV antibiotic therapy. They should receive appropriate supportive treatment and should be monitored closely for complications such as sepsis, ARDS, and preterm labor. One reasonable choice for empiric IV antibiotic therapy is ceftriaxone 2 g every 24 hours. Compared with a first-generation cephalosporin like cefazolin, ceftriaxone has expanded coverage against aerobic gram-negative bacilli and has the advantage of once-daily dosing.[19] If the patient is critically ill or is at high risk for a resistant organism, a second antibiotic, such as gentamicin (7 mg/kg/ideal body weight every 24 hours) or aztreonam (500 mg to 1 g every 8 to 12 hours) should be administered, along with ceftriaxone, until the results of susceptibility tests are available.

Once antibiotic therapy is initiated, about 75% of patients defervesce within 48 hours. By the end of 72 hours, almost 95% of patients are afebrile and asymptomatic.[20] The two most likely causes of treatment failure are a resistant microorganism and obstruction. The latter condition is best diagnosed with computed tomography (CT) scan or renal ultrasonography and typically results from a stone or physical compression of the ureter by the gravid uterus.

Once the patient has begun to defervesce and her clinical condition has improved, she may be discharged from the hospital. Oral antibiotics should be prescribed to complete a total of 7 to 10 days of therapy. Selection of a specific oral agent should be based on considerations of efficacy, toxicity, and expense. A repeat urine culture should be obtained after therapy is completed to ensure that the infection has been adequately treated.

About 20% to 30% of pregnant patients with acute pyelonephritis develop a recurrent urinary tract infection later in pregnancy. The most cost-effective way to reduce the frequency of recurrence is to administer a daily prophylactic dose of an antibiotic such as nitrofurantoin monohydrate 100 mg. Patients receiving prophylaxis should have their urine screened for bacteria at each subsequent clinic appointment. They also should be questioned about recurrence of symptoms. If symptoms recur, or the dipstick test for nitrite or leukocyte esterase is positive, a urine culture should be obtained to determine whether retreatment is necessary.

UPPER GENITAL TRACT INFECTIONS
Chorioamnionitis

Chorioamnionitis—or amnionitis, intraamniotic infection—may present with fever and fetal tachycardia. Because both the mother and infant may experience serious complications when chorioamnionitis is present, prompt diagnosis is imperative.

Epidemiology

Chorioamnionitis occurs in 1% to 5% of term pregnancies.[26] In patients with preterm delivery, the frequency of clinical or subclinical infection may approach 25%.[27] Although chorioamnionitis may result from hematogenous dissemination of microorganisms, it more commonly is an ascending infection caused by organisms that are part of the normal vaginal flora. The principal pathogens are *Bacteroides* and *Prevotella* species, *E. coli*, anaerobic gram-positive cocci, GBS, and genital mycoplasmas.

Several clinical risk factors for chorioamnionitis have been identified. The most important are young age, low socioeconomic status, nulliparity, extended duration of labor and ruptured membranes, multiple vaginal examinations, and preexisting infections of the lower genital tract (e.g., bacterial vaginosis and GBS infection).[26] Antibiotic use in preterm PROM is associated with a statistically significant reduction in chorioamnionitis.[28] In term PROM, consideration should also be given to minimizing use of vaginal digital examinations intrapartum once membrane rupture has occurred, as well as antibiotic prophylaxis, especially when latency greater than 12 hours is expected (see Chapter 30).[29]

Diagnosis

In most situations, the diagnosis of chorioamnionitis can be established on the basis of the clinical findings of maternal fever and maternal and fetal tachycardia in the absence of other localizing signs of infection. In more severely ill patients, uterine tenderness and purulent amniotic fluid may be identified. The disorders that should be considered in the differential diagnosis of intrapartum fever include respiratory tract infection, pyelonephritis, viral syndrome, and appendicitis, but chorioamnionitis should always be the principal consideration.[26]

Laboratory confirmation of the diagnosis of chorioamnionitis is not routinely necessary in term patients who are progressing to delivery. However, in preterm patients who are being evaluated for tocolysis or corticosteroids, laboratory assessment may be of value in establishing the diagnosis of intrauterine infection. In this clinical context, amniotic fluid should be obtained by transabdominal amniocentesis. Table 54-5 summarizes the abnormal laboratory findings that may be present in infected patients.[26,30-33]

Management

Both the mother and infant may experience serious complications when chorioamnionitis is present. Bacteremia occurs in

TABLE 54-5 DIAGNOSTIC TESTS FOR CHORIOAMNIONITIS

TEST	ABNORMAL FINDING	COMMENT
Maternal white blood cell count (WBC)	≥15,000 cells/mm³ with preponderance of leukocytes	Labor and/or corticosteroids may also result in elevation of WBC count.
Amniotic fluid glucose	≤10 to 15 mg	Correlation is excellent with positive amniotic fluid culture and clinical infection.
Amniotic fluid interleukin-6	≥7.9 ng/mL	Correlation is excellent with positive amniotic fluid culture and clinical infection.
Amniotic fluid leukocyte esterase	≥1⁺ reaction	Correlation is good with positive amniotic fluid culture and clinical infection.
Amniotic fluid Gram stain	Any organism in an oil immersion field	Identification of particularly virulent organisms, such as group B streptococci, is possible; however, the test is very sensitive to inoculum effect. In addition, it cannot identify pathogens such as mycoplasmas.
Amniotic fluid culture	Growth of aerobic or anaerobic microorganism	This test is the gold standard, although results are not immediately available for clinical management.
Blood cultures	Growth of aerobic or anaerobic microorganism	Cultures will be positive in 5% to 10% of patients; however, they will usually not be of value in making clinical decisions unless the patient is seriously ill, at increased risk for bacterial endocarditis, immunocompromised, or has a poor response to the initial treatment.

3% to 12% of infected women. When cesarean delivery is required, up to 8% of women develop a wound infection, and about 1% develop a pelvic abscess. Fortunately, maternal death due to infection is exceedingly rare.[26]

Of neonates delivered to mothers with chorioamnionitis, 5% to 10% have pneumonia or bacteremia. The predominant organisms responsible for these infections are GBS and *E. coli*. Meningitis occurs in less than 1% of term infants and in a slightly higher percentage of preterm infants. Mortality due to infection ranges from 1% to 4% in term neonates but may approach 15% in preterm infants because of the confounding effects of other complications such as hyaline membrane disease, intraventricular hemorrhage, and necrotizing enterocolitis.[26]

To prevent maternal and neonatal complications, parenteral antibiotic therapy should be initiated as soon as the diagnosis of chorioamnionitis is made, unless delivery is imminent. Three separate investigations have demonstrated that mother-infant pairs who receive prompt intrapartum treatment have better outcomes than patients treated after delivery.[32-34] The principal benefits of early treatment include decreased frequency of neonatal bacteremia and pneumonia and decreased duration of maternal fever and hospitalization.

The most extensively tested IV antibiotic regimen for treatment of chorioamnionitis is the combination of ampicillin (2 g every 6 hours) **or penicillin** (5 million U every 6 hours) **plus gentamicin** (1.5 mg/kg every 8 hours or 5 to 7 mg/kg/ ideal body weight every 24 hours).[35,36] **The latter regimen of gentamicin is the most cost-effective.**[37,38] **These antibiotics specifically target the two organisms most likely to cause neonatal infection: GBS and *E. coli*.** With rare exceptions, gentamicin is preferred to tobramycin or amikacin because it is available in an inexpensive generic formulation. Amikacin should be reserved for immunocompromised patients who are particularly likely to be infected by highly virulent, drug-resistant aerobic gram-negative bacilli. In patients who are allergic to β-lactam antibiotics, clindamycin (900 mg every 8 hours) should be substituted for ampicillin.[37]

If a patient with chorioamnionitis requires cesarean delivery, a drug with activity against anaerobic organisms should be added to the antibiotic regimen. Either clindamycin (900 mg) or metronidazole (500 mg) is an excellent choice for this purpose. Failure to provide effective coverage of anaerobes may result in treatment failures in 20% to 30% of patients.[37]

Extended-spectrum cephalosporins, penicillins, and carbapenems also provide excellent coverage against the bacteria that

TABLE 54-6 SINGLE AGENTS OF VALUE IN TREATMENT OF CHORIOAMNIONITIS AND PUERPERAL ENDOMETRITIS

DRUG	DOSAGE AND DOSE INTERVAL	RELATIVE COST TO THE PHARMACY*
Extended-Spectrum Cephalosporins		
Cefepime	2 g every 12 hours	Intermediate
Cefotaxime	2 g every 8-12 hours	Intermediate
Cefotetan	2 g every 12 hours	Low
Cefoxitin	2 g every 6 hours	Intermediate
Ceftizoxime	2 g every 12 hours	Intermediate
Extended-Spectrum Penicillins		
Ampicillin-sulbactam	3 g every 6 hours	Low
Mezlocillin	3 to 4 g every 6 hours	Intermediate
Piperacillin	3 to 4 g every 6 hours	Intermediate
Piperacillin-tazobactam	3.375 g every 6 hours	Intermediate
Ticarcillin–clavulanic acid	3.1 g every 6 hours	Low
Carbapenem		
Ertapenem	1 g every 24 hours	High
Imipenem-cilastatin	500 mg every 6 hours	High
Meropenem	1 g every 8 hours	High

*Cost estimates do not include dose preparation fees and administration charges.

cause chorioamnionitis. Dosages and dose intervals for several of these agents are listed in Table 54-6.[19] As a general rule, these drugs are more expensive than the generic combination regimens outlined earlier.

Patients with chorioamnionitis are at increased risk for dysfunctional labor. About 75% require oxytocin for augmentation of labor, and up to 30% to 40% require cesarean delivery, usually for failure to progress in labor. Although chorioamnionitis by itself should not be considered an indication for cesarean delivery, affected patients need close monitoring during labor to ensure that uterine contractility is optimized. In addition, the fetus also needs close surveillance. Fetal heart rate abnormalities such as tachycardia and decreased variability (Fig. 54-3) occur in more than three fourths of the cases, and additional tests such as scalp stimulation may be necessary to evaluate fetal well-being.

Antibiotics usually can be discontinued soon after delivery. Edwards and Duff[39] reported a randomized clinical trial in which patients were treated intrapartum with ampicillin plus gentamicin. In one group of patients, treatment was discontinued after the first postpartum dose of each antibiotic. In the

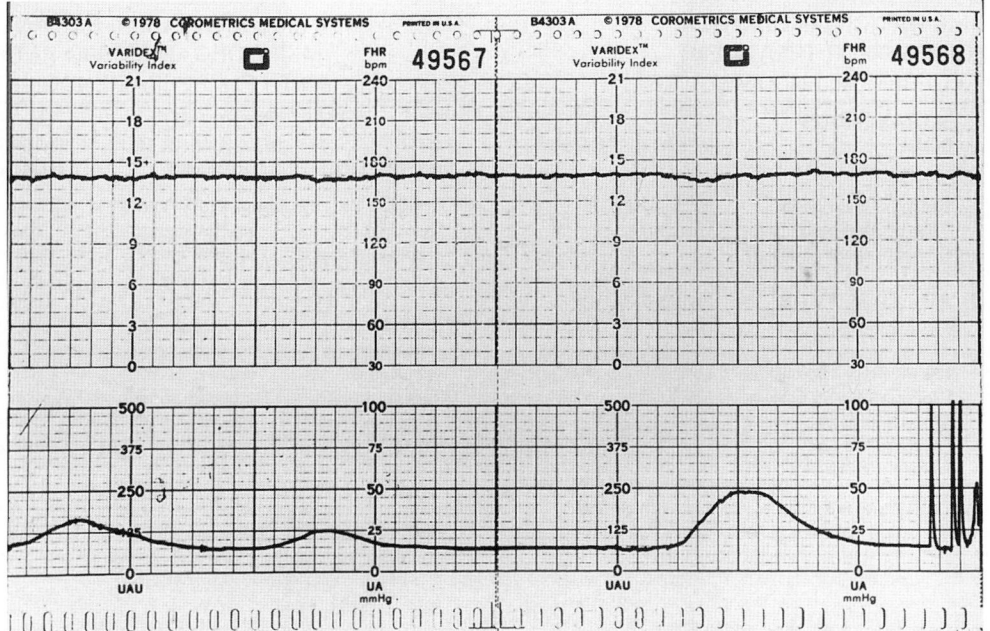

FIG 54-3 Fetal heart tracing from a patient with chorioamnionitis. Note the tachycardia of 170 beats/min and the striking decrease in variability.

second group, patients were treated until they had been afebrile and asymptomatic for 24 hours. Patients in both groups received at least one dose of clindamycin if they delivered by cesarean section. No significant differences in treatment outcome were apparent in the two groups. However, in a follow-up study to the report by Edwards and Duff, Black and colleagues[40] showed that certain patients with chorioamnionitis require more extended treatment. Specifically, those women who are obese—defined as those with a body mass index (BMI) greater than 30—or who have prolonged rupture of membranes (>24 hours) have a significantly increased risk of treatment failure if they receive only a single postpartum dose of antibiotic; they recommended these women be treated postpartum until they have been afebrile and asymptomatic for 24 hours. A recent Cochrane review of antibiotic regimens for chorioamnionitis, however, concluded that limited evidence was available to reveal whether antibiotics should be continued during the postpartum period, which antibiotic regimen should be used, or for what treatment duration.[41] Based on published experience from our institution, we follow the guidelines recommended by Black et al.[40]

Puerperal Endometritis

Epidemiology

The frequency of puerperal endometritis in women who deliver vaginally ranges from 1% to 3%. In women having a scheduled cesarean delivery before the onset of labor and rupture of membranes, the frequency of endometritis ranges from 5% to 10% without antibiotic prophylaxis and is less than 5% with prophylaxis. When cesarean delivery is performed after an extended period of labor and ruptured membranes, the incidence of infection is 30% to 35% without antibiotic prophylaxis and about 60% less with prophylaxis. In indigent patient populations, the frequency of infection may be even higher.[42]

Similarly to chorioamnionitis, endometritis is a polymicrobial infection caused by microorganisms that are part of the normal vaginal flora. These bacteria gain access to the upper genital tract, peritoneal cavity, and occasionally the bloodstream as a result of vaginal examinations during labor and manipulations during surgery. **The most common pathogens are GBS, anaerobic gram-positive cocci, aerobic gram-negative bacilli—predominantly *E. coli, K. pneumoniae,* and *Proteus* species—and anaerobic gram-negative bacilli, principally *Bacteroides* and *Prevotella* species.** *C. trachomatis* is not a common cause of early-onset puerperal endometritis but has been implicated in late-onset infection. The genital mycoplasmas may be pathogens in some patients, but they usually are present in association with more highly virulent bacteria.[42]

The principal risk factors for endometritis are cesarean delivery, young age, low socioeconomic status, extended duration of labor and ruptured membranes, and multiple vaginal examinations. In addition, preexisting infection or colonization of the lower genital tract (gonorrhea, GBS, bacterial vaginosis) also predisposes to ascending infection.

Clinical Presentation and Diagnosis

The diagnosis of postpartum endometritis is based on the presence of fever of 38° C or higher in the absence of any other cause. The presence of either uterine tenderness or purulent or foul-smelling lochia are often used as secondary criteria for the diagnosis of endometritis. Associated findings include malaise, tachycardia, and lower abdominal pain and tenderness. A small number of patients also may have a tender, indurated inflammatory mass in the broad ligament, posterior cul de sac, or retrovesical space.

The initial differential diagnosis of puerperal fever should include endometritis, atelectasis, pneumonia, viral syndrome, pyelonephritis, and appendicitis. Distinction among these disorders usually can be made on the basis of physical examination and a limited number of laboratory tests such as white blood cell count, urinalysis and culture, and in select patients, chest radiograph. Blood cultures should not be done *routinely* because of their expense and their lack of impact on

TABLE 54-7 COMBINATION ANTIBIOTIC REGIMENS FOR TREATMENT OF PUERPERAL ENDOMETRITIS

ANTIBIOTICS	INTRAVENOUS DOSE	RELATIVE COST*
Regimen 1		
Clindamycin *plus*	900 mg every 8 hours	Intermediate
Gentamicin	7 mg/kg ideal body weight every 24 hours[†]	Low
Regimen 2		
Clindamycin *plus*	900 mg every 8 hours	Intermediate
Aztreonam	1 to 2 g every 8 hours	High
Regimen 3		
Metronidazole *plus*	500 mg every 12 hours	Low
Penicillin *or*	5 million U every 6 hours	Low
Ampicillin *plus*	2 g every 6 hours	Low
Gentamicin	7 mg/kg ideal body weight every 24 hours[†]	Low

*Cost estimate does not include dose preparation fees and administration charges.
[†]Single daily dosing of aminoglycoside antibiotics is more effective and less expensive than multidose treatment. In addition, daily dosing is less likely to cause ototoxicity or nephrotoxicity.

TABLE 54-8 TREATMENT OF RESISTANT MICROORGANISMS IN PATIENTS WITH PUERPERAL ENDOMETRITIS

INITIAL ANTIBIOTICS	PRINCIPAL WEAKNESS IN COVERAGE	MODIFICATION OF THERAPY
Extended-spectrum cephalosporins	Some aerobic and anaerobic gram-negative bacilli, enterococci	Change treatment to clindamycin or metronidazole plus penicillin or ampicillin plus gentamicin
Extended-spectrum penicillins	Some aerobic and anaerobic gram-negative bacilli	As above
Clindamycin plus gentamicin or aztreonam	Enterococci, some anaerobic gram-negative bacilli	Add ampicillin or penicillin* Consider substitution of metronidazole for clindamycin

*Ampicillin alone is highly active against enterococci. The combination of penicillin *plus* gentamicin works synergistically to provide excellent coverage against this organism.

clinical decision making. However, they are indicated in patients who have a poor initial response to therapy and in those who seem seriously ill, are immunocompromised, or are at increased risk for bacterial endocarditis.

Management

Patients who have mild to moderately severe infections, particularly after vaginal delivery, can be treated with short IV courses of single agents such as the extended-spectrum cephalosporins and penicillins or carbapenem antibiotics such as imipenem-cilastatin, meropenem, and ertapenem. Table 54-6 lists several antibiotics that have acceptable breadth of coverage against the polymicrobial genital tract flora. Combination antibiotic regimens should be considered for more severely ill patients, particularly those who are indigent and in poor general health. Table 54-7 lists several antibiotic combinations of proven value in treatment of puerperal endometritis. As a general rule, the combination generic drug regimens are less expensive than the single agents whose brand-name patents have yet to expire.

Once antibiotics are begun, approximately 90% of patients defervesce within 48 to 72 hours. When the patient has been afebrile and asymptomatic for 24 hours, parenteral antibiotics should be discontinued and the patient should be discharged. As a general rule, an extended course of oral antibiotics is not necessary after discharge.[37,43] There are at least two notable exceptions to this rule. First, patients who have had a vaginal delivery and who defervesce within 24 hours are candidates for early discharge. In these individuals, a short course of an oral antibiotic such as amoxicillin-clavulanate (875 mg every 12 hours) may be substituted for continued parenteral therapy. Second, patients who have had staphylococcal bacteremia may require a more extended period of administration of parenteral and oral antibiotics with specific antistaphylococcal activity.[44]

Patients who fail to respond to the antibiotic therapy outlined earlier usually have one of two problems. The first is a resistant organism. Table 54-8 lists possible weaknesses in coverage of selected antibiotics and indicates the appropriate change in treatment. **The second major cause of treatment failure is a wound infection,** which may take the form of an incisional abscess or a cellulitis with no actual purulent collection. Incisional abscesses should be opened completely to provide drainage, and a specific antistaphylococcal antibiotic should be added to the treatment regimen. If extensive cellulitis at the margin of the incision is present, an antibiotic with specific coverage against staphylococci should be added, but the wound should not be opened. Vancomycin (1 g IV every 12 hours) is an excellent antistaphylococcal antibiotic, particularly against methicillin-resistant *Staphylococcus aureus* (MRSA).[37] Other possible antistaphylococcal regimens include dalbavancin (1 g in a single dose, repeated in 7 days if necessary), linezolid (600 mg IV every 12 hours), oritavancin (1200-mg single dose), quinupristin/dalfopristin (7.5 mg/kg IV every 8 hours), and telavancin (10 mg/kg IV every 24 hours).[44] Antibiotics may be discontinued once the patient has been afebrile and asymptomatic for a minimum of 24 hours.

When changes in antibiotic therapy do not result in clinical improvement and no evidence of wound infection is present, several unusual disorders should be considered. The differential diagnosis of persistent puerperal fever is summarized in Table 54-9.[42]

Group A *Streptococcus* (GAS) infection is a rare, life-threatening cause of pueperal fever due to *Streptococcus pyogenes*.[45] **Mortality is 30% to 50% when associated with sepsis, known as streptococcal toxic shock syndrome. GAS infections are invasive, and toxin production allows the organism to spread across tissue planes and cause necrosis while evading containment and abscess formation by the maternal immune system. Presentation is atypical and may involve extremes of temperature, unusual and vague pain, and pain in extremities. Endometrial biopsy may be a useful rapid diagnostic tool.** When suspected, invasive GAS infections should be treated emergently with aggressive fluid resuscitation, antibiotic administration (penicillin and clindamycin), and source control that may be extensive and may involve hysterectomy.

Prevention of Puerperal Endometritis

Prophylactic antibiotics clearly are of value in reducing the frequency of postcesarean delivery endometritis, particularly in women having surgery after an extended period of labor and ruptured membranes.[46]

TABLE 54-9 DIFFERENTIAL DIAGNOSIS OF PERSISTENT PUERPERAL FEVER

CONDITION	DIAGNOSTIC TESTS	TREATMENT
Resistant microorganism	Blood culture	Combination antibiotics to cover all possible pelvic pathogens
Wound infection	Physical examination Needle aspiration Ultrasound	Incision and drainage if abscess is present; add antibiotic to cover staphylococci
Pelvic abscess	Physical examination Ultrasound Computed tomography Magnetic resonance imaging	Drainage; combination antibiotics to cover all possible pelvic pathogens
Septic pelvic vein thrombophlebitis	Ultrasound Computed tomography Magnetic resonance imaging	Heparin anticoagulation; combination antibiotics to cover all possible pelvic pathogens
Drug fever	Inspection of temperature graph White blood cell count to identify eosinophilia	Discontinue antibiotics
Mastitis	Physical examination	Add antibiotic to cover staphylococci

Historically, IV prophylactic antibiotics for cesarean delivery were delayed until cord clamping based on several prior studies,[47-50] which showed that the delay decreased the probability that neonates would require evaluations for sepsis without compromising effectiveness. However, a recent Cochrane review of the timing of IV prophylactic antibiotics for cesarean delivery showed that preoperative administration significantly decreases the incidence of composite maternal postpartum infectious morbidity, as compared with administration after cord clamping, with no differences in adverse neonatal outcomes reported.[51] **Women undergoing cesarean delivery should receive antibiotic prophylaxis preoperatively to reduce maternal infectious morbidities.**[52-55]

Tita and associates[56,57] showed that extending the spectrum of antibiotic activity by adding azithromycin (500 mg) to cefazolin (1 g) further reduced the risk for endometritis (RR, 0.41). The use of the broader-spectrum regimen also significantly decreased the rate of wound infection (1.3% vs. 3.1%; $P<.002$). However, a subsequent systematic review revealed that preoperative antibiotic administration *or* the use of extended-spectrum regimens after cord clamping may reduce post–cesarean delivery maternal infection by up to 50%, although the lack of their impact relative to each other has not been studied; therefore a firm recommendation of extended-spectrum antibiotics for all cesarean deliveries is premature.[58] **If preoperative antibiotic prophylaxis is given as it should be, extended-spectrum antibiotics do not seem justified at this point for the vast majority of women.**

Another important step in prevention of endometritis relates to the method of placental delivery. In 1997, Lasley and colleagues[59] conducted a prospective randomized trial (level I evidence) to compare manual removal of the placenta with removal by gentle traction on the umbilical cord. One hundred sixty-five women were randomized to the manual removal arm of the study, and 168 had spontaneous removal of the placenta. All patients in this study received prophylactic antibiotics, usually cefazolin, after the umbilical cord was clamped. In the patients whose placenta was removed by traction on the cord, the rate of endometritis was reduced from 27% to 15% (RR, 0.6; 95% CI, 0.4 to 0.9; $P = .01$).

Subsequently, the Cochrane database[60] evaluated 15 randomized trials ($n = 4694$ patients) to compare different methods of removing the placenta. **A consistent finding in these trials was decreased blood loss, a decreased rate of endometritis, and, subsequently, a shorter duration of hospitalization in women** whose placenta was removed by gentle traction on the umbilical cord.

A previous report by Yancey and associates[61] provides a logical explanation for why manual removal of the placenta is associated with an increased risk for infection. In that study, the authors specifically evaluated the contamination of the surgeon's dominant hand as a result of delivering the infant's head from the lower uterine segment. After this step of the operation, the bacterial contamination of the surgeon's glove was markedly increased. When the surgeon then places this hand behind the placenta to manually extract it, this inevitably introduces many microorganisms into the raw vascular bed beneath the placenta.

Based on the studies outlined earlier, **we recommend that both low- and high-risk patients having cesarean delivery receive antibiotics 30 to 60 minutes before the start of surgery. We recommend use of cefazolin, 1 g if BMI is less than 30 m²/kg (or <80 kg) and 2 g if BMI is greater than 30 m²/kg (or >80 kg), given as a rapid IV infusion.**[62] **We also recommend that, whenever possible, the placenta be removed by traction on the umbilical cord rather than by manual extraction.**

Patients who have an immediate hypersensitivity to β-lactam antibiotics pose a special problem. The best alternative is to administer a single dose of clindamycin (900 mg) plus gentamicin (1.5 mg/kg) before surgery. Although these antibiotics commonly are used for treatment of overt infections, their administration still is warranted in penicillin-allergic patients who are at high risk for postoperative infection.[37]

Serious Sequelae of Puerperal Infection
Wound Infection

Wound infection after cesarean delivery may occur in association with endometritis or as an isolated infection. About 3% to 5% of patients who have a cesarean delivery develop a wound infection (see Chapter 19). The major risk factors for wound infection are listed in Box 54-1. **The principal causative organisms are skin flora** (*S. aureus*, aerobic streptococci) **and the pelvic flora** (aerobic and anaerobic bacilli).[63]

The diagnosis of wound infection should always be considered in patients who have a poor clinical response to antibiotic therapy for endometritis. Clinical examination characteristically shows erythema, induration, and tenderness at the margins of the abdominal incision. When the wound is probed with either a cotton-tipped applicator or fine needle, pus usually exudes. Some patients, however, may have an extensive cellulitis without harboring frank pus in the incision. Clinical examination should be sufficient to establish the correct diagnosis. Nevertheless, culture of the wound exudate is indicated to identify particularly virulent microorganisms such as MRSA.

When pus is present in the incision, the wound must be opened and drained completely. Antibiotic therapy should be modified to provide coverage against staphylococci because some regimens for endometritis may not specifically target this organism. Vancomycin 1 g IV every 12 hours is an excellent choice to cover MRSA.

Once the wound is opened, a careful inspection should be made to be certain that the fascial layer is intact. If it is disrupted, surgical intervention is necessary to reapproximate the fascia. Otherwise, the wound should be irrigated two to three times daily with a solution such as warm saline, a clean dressing should be applied, and the incision should be allowed to heal by secondary intention. In complicated infections, a wound vacuum device may be applied to the wound to facilitate healing. Antibiotics should be continued until the base of the wound is clean and all signs of cellulitis have resolved. Patients usually can be treated at home once the acute signs of infection have subsided.

Necrotizing fasciitis **is an uncommon but extremely serious complication of abdominal wound infection.** It also has been reported in association with infection of the episiotomy site.[64] This condition is most likely to occur in patients with type 1 diabetes mellitus, cancer, or an immunodeficiency disorder. Multiple bacterial pathogens, particularly anaerobes, have been isolated from patients with necrotizing fasciitis.

Necrotizing fasciitis should be suspected when the margins of the wound become discolored, cyanotic, and devoid of sensation. When the wound is opened, the subcutaneous tissue is easily dissected free of the underlying fascia, but muscle tissue is not affected. If the diagnosis is uncertain, a tissue biopsy should be performed and examined by frozen section.

Necrotizing fasciitis is a life-threatening condition that requires aggressive medical and surgical management. Broad-spectrum antibiotics with activity against all potential aerobic and anaerobic pathogens should be administered. Intravascular volume should be maintained with infusions of crystalloid, and electrolyte abnormalities should be corrected. **Finally, and most importantly, the wound must be debrided and all necrotic tissue must be removed.** In many instances, the required dissection is extensive and may best be managed in consultation with an experienced general or plastic surgeon.[65]

Pelvic Abscess

With the advent of modern antibiotics, pelvic abscesses after cesarean or vaginal delivery have become extremely rare. **Less than 1% of patients with puerperal endometritis develop a pelvic abscess.**[42] **When present, abscesses typically are located in the anterior or posterior cul de sac, most commonly the latter, or within the broad ligament.** The usual bacteria isolated from abscess cavities are coliforms and anaerobic gram-negative bacilli, particularly *Bacteroides* and *Prevotella* species.[66]

Patients with an abscess typically experience persistent fever despite initial therapy for endometritis. In addition, they usually have malaise, tachycardia, lower abdominal pain and tenderness, and a palpable pelvic mass anterior, posterior, or lateral to the uterus. The peripheral white blood cell count is usually elevated, and there is a shift toward neutrophils and bands. Ultrasound, CT scan, and magnetic resonance imaging (MRI) may be used to confirm the diagnosis of pelvic abscess.[67] Although CT and MRI may be slightly more sensitive, ultrasound offers the advantages of decreased expense and ready availability.

Patients with a pelvic abscess require surgical intervention to drain the purulent collection. When the abscess is in the posterior cul de sac, colpotomy drainage may be possible, although availability of modern imaging modalities and support from interventional radiologists has made this practice near obsolete. For abscesses located anterior or lateral to the uterus, drainage may be accomplished by CT- or ultrasound-guided placement of a catheter drain.[68] When access is limited or the abscess is extensive, open laparotomy is indicated.

Affected patients should also receive antibiotics with excellent activity against coliform organisms and anaerobes.[37,66] One regimen that has been tested extensively in obstetric patients with serious infections is the combination of penicillin (5 million U IV every 6 hours) or ampicillin (2 g IV every 6 hours) plus gentamicin (7 mg/kg of ideal body weight every 24 hours) plus clindamycin (900 mg IV every 8 hours) or metronidazole (500 mg IV every 12 hours). If a patient is allergic to β-lactam antibiotics, vancomycin (1 g IV every 12 hours) can be substituted for penicillin or ampicillin. Aztreonam (1 g IV every 8 hours) can be used instead of gentamicin when the patient is at risk for nephrotoxicity. Alternatively, the single agents imipenem-cilastatin (500 mg IV every 6 hours), meropenem (1 g every 8 hours), and ertapenem (1 g every 24 hours) provide excellent coverage against the usual pathogens responsible for an abscess. Antibiotics should not be discontinued until the patient has been afebrile and asymptomatic for a minimum of 24 to 48 hours.

Septic Pelvic Thrombophlebitis

Like pelvic abscess, septic pelvic thrombophlebitis is extremely rare; it occurs in 1 in 2000 pregnancies overall and in less than 1% of patients who have puerperal endometritis.[69] Intrauterine infection may cause seeding of pathogenic microorganisms into the venous circulation; in turn, these organisms may damage the vascular endothelium and initiate thrombosis.

Septic pelvic thrombophlebitis occurs in two distinct forms.[69] **The most commonly described disorder is acute thrombosis of one, usually the right, or both ovarian veins** (ovarian vein syndrome).[70] Affected patients typically develop a moderate temperature elevation in association with lower abdominal pain in the first 48 to 96 hours postpartum. Pain usually localizes to the side of the affected vein but may radiate into the groin, upper abdomen, or flank. Nausea, vomiting, and abdominal bloating may be present.

On physical examination, the patient's pulse usually is elevated. Tachypnea, stridor, and dyspnea may be evident if pulmonary embolization has occurred. The abdomen is tender, and bowel sounds are often decreased or absent. Most patients demonstrate voluntary and involuntary guarding, and 50% to 70% have a tender, ropelike mass that originates near one cornua and extends laterally and cephalad toward the upper abdomen. The principal conditions that should be considered in the differential diagnosis of ovarian vein syndrome are pyelonephritis, nephrolithiasis, appendicitis, broad ligament hematoma, adnexal torsion, and pelvic abscess.

The second presentation of septic pelvic vein thrombophlebitis is termed *enigmatic fever*.[71] Initially, affected patients have clinical findings suggestive of endometritis and receive systemic antibiotics. Subsequently, they experience subjective improvement, with the exception of temperature instability. They do not appear to be seriously ill, and positive findings are limited to persistent fever and tachycardia. Disorders that should be considered in the differential diagnosis of enigmatic fever are drug fever, viral syndrome, collagen vascular disease, and pelvic abscess.

The diagnostic tests of greatest value in evaluating a patient with suspected septic pelvic vein thrombophlebitis are CT scan and MRI (Fig. 54-4).[72] These tests are most sensitive in detecting large thrombi in the major pelvic vessels. They are not as useful in identifying thrombi in smaller vessels. In such cases, the ultimate diagnosis may depend on the patient's response to an empirical trial of heparin.[69,73]

Patients with septic pelvic vein thrombophlebitis should be treated with therapeutic doses of either IV unfractionated heparin or low-molecular-weight heparin. Therapy should be continued for 7 to 10 days. Long-term anticoagulation

with oral agents is probably unnecessary unless the patient has massive clotting throughout the pelvic venous plexus or has sustained a pulmonary embolism. Patients should be maintained on broad-spectrum antibiotics throughout the period of heparin administration.

Once medical therapy is initiated, the patient should have objective evidence of a response within 48 to 72 hours. If no improvement is noted, surgical intervention may be necessary.[69,73] The decision to perform surgery should be based on clinical assessment and the relative certainty of the diagnosis. The surgical approach, in turn, should be tailored to the specific intraoperative findings. In most instances, treatment requires only ligation of the affected vessels. Extension of the thrombosis along the vena cava to the point of origin of the renal veins may necessitate embolectomy or placement of an umbrella filter. Excision of the infected vessel and removal of the ipsilateral adnexa and uterus is indicated only in the presence of a well-defined abscess. Whenever any of the previously mentioned procedures are being considered, consultation with an experienced vascular surgeon or interventional radiologist is imperative.

Severe Sepsis

The systemic immune response syndrome (SIRS) is defined by a temperature greater than 38° C, respiratory rate greater than 20/min, heart rate over 90 beats/min, and a peripheral white blood cell count above 12,000/mm³ or below 4000/mm³ or with greater than 10% immature (band) forms. Sepsis is SIRS that results from infection. Severe sepsis is defined by the criteria outlined above plus multiorgan dysfunction. Septic shock is diagnosed when sepsis-induced hypotension is present in association with perfusion abnormalities such as lactic acidosis (serum lactate level of 4.0 mmol/L or more), oliguria, and altered mental status.[74,75]

Septic shock in obstetric patients usually is associated with four specific infections: (1) septic abortion, (2) acute pyelonephritis, (3) chorioamnionitis, or (4) endometritis.[75] Fortunately, fewer than 5% of patients with any of these infections develop septic shock. In the past, **the most common organisms responsible for septic shock were the aerobic gram-negative bacilli, such as** *E. coli and K. pneumoniae and Proteus* along with *Pseudomonas, Enterobacter,* and *Serratia* species.[74] Today, gram-positive organisms have become increasingly important as causative pathogens.[74]

In the early stages of septic shock, patients are usually restless, disoriented, tachycardic, and hypotensive. Although hypothermia is occasionally present, most patients have a relatively high fever (39° to 40° C). Their skin may be warm and flushed owing to an initial phase of vasodilation (warm shock). Subsequently, as extensive vasoconstriction occurs, the skin becomes cool and clammy. Cardiac arrhythmias may be present, and signs of myocardial ischemia may occur. Jaundice, often due to hemolysis, may be evident. Urinary output typically decreases, and frank anuria may develop. Spontaneous bleeding from the genitourinary tract or venipuncture sites may occur as a result of disseminated intramuscular coagulation. Acute respiratory distress syndrome (ARDS) is a common complication of severe sepsis and is associated with manifestations such as dyspnea, stridor, cough, tachypnea, and bilateral rales and wheezing.[74] In addition to these systemic signs and symptoms, affected patients also may have findings related to their primary site of infection such as purulent lochia, uterine tenderness, peritonitis, or flank tenderness.

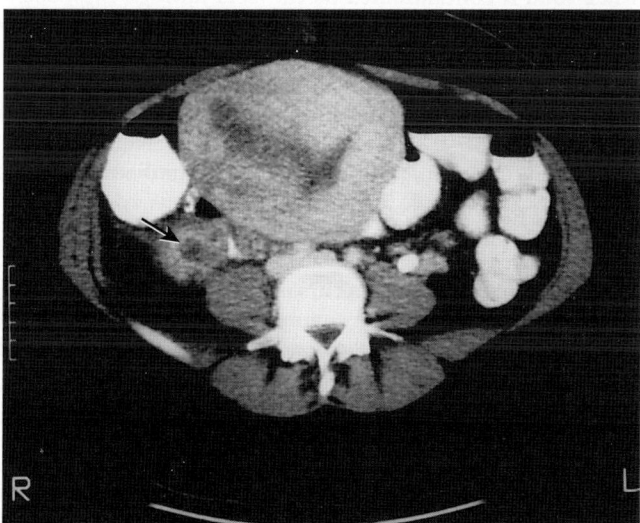

FIG 54-4 Computed tomography scan shows a thrombus (*arrow*) in the right ovarian vein.

The differential diagnosis of septic shock in obstetric patients includes hypovolemic and cardiogenic shock, diabetic ketoacidosis, anaphylactic reaction, anesthetic reaction, and amniotic fluid or venous embolism. Distinction among these disorders usually can be made on the basis of a thorough history and physical examination and a limited number of laboratory studies. The white blood cell count initially may be decreased but, subsequently, it is elevated in most patients. A large percentage of bands is usually evident, and the hematocrit may be decreased if blood loss has occurred. Tests of coagulation such as platelet count, serum fibrinogen concentration, serum concentration of fibrin degradation products, prothrombin time, and activated partial thromboplastin time are frequently abnormal. Serum concentrations of the transaminase enzymes and bilirubin often are increased. Similarly, increased concentrations of blood urea nitrogen and creatinine reflect deterioration of renal function. A chest radiograph is indicated in patients with septic shock to determine whether pneumonia or ARDS is present. In addition, CT scan, MRI, and ultrasound may be of value in localizing an abscess.[68] Affected patients also require electrocardiographic monitoring to detect arrhythmias or signs of ischemic injury.

The first goal of treatment of septic shock is to correct the hemodynamic derangements precipitated by endotoxin. Two large-bore IV catheters and a urinary catheter should be inserted. Isotonic crystalloid such as Ringer's lactate solution or normal saline should be administered, and the infusion should be titrated in accordance with the patient's pulse, blood pressure, and urine output. If the patient is bleeding, packed red cells should be administered; the goal is to maintain a hemoglobin concentration of 7 g/dL. A more restrictive transfusion threshold (7 rather than 9 g/L) has recently been shown to reduce the number of transfusions by approximately 50% without adversely affecting overall mortality.[76]

The goals of fluid resuscitation are to achieve the following:
- Central venous pressure (CVP) of 8 to 12 mm Hg
- Mean arterial pressure of at least 65 mm Hg
- Urine output of at least 0.5 mL/kg per hour
- Central venous oxygen or mixed venous oxygen saturation of 70% or more[76]

If fluid resuscitation is not successful, a vasopressor should be administered. The initial drug of choice is norepinephrine (5 to 15 µg/min), although vasopressin (0.01 to 0.03 U/min) and epinephrine (2 to 10 µg /min) are acceptable alternatives. As a general rule, dopamine should no longer be used as a vasopressor because of its propensity to provoke arrhythmias.[66] Dobutamine (0.5 to 1 µg/kg/min, maximum 40 µg/kg/min) should be used in patients who have a normal CVP but poor cardiac output.[76]

Hydrocortisone (200 to 300 mg/day for 7 days in three or four divided doses or by continuous infusion) should be administered early in the course of septic shock. Although ultimate mortality is not improved, patients who receive corticosteroids have a more rapid reversal of the shock state than those who are not treated.[77,78]

The second objective of treatment is to administer broad-spectrum antibiotics targeted against the most likely pathogens.[19] For genital tract infections, the combination of penicillin (5 million U IV every 6 hours) or ampicillin (2 g IV every 6 hours) plus clindamycin (900 mg IV every 8 hours) or metronidazole (500 mg IV every 8 hours) plus gentamicin (7 mg/kg ideal body weight IV every 24 hours) or aztreonam (1 to 2 g IV every 8 hours) is an appropriate regimen. Alternatively, imipenem-cilastatin (500 mg IV every 6 hours), meropenem (1 g every 8 hours), or ertapenem (1 g IV every 24 hours) can be administered as single agents. Patients also may require surgery; for example, to evacuate infected products of conception, drain a pelvic abscess, or remove badly infected pelvic organs. Indicated surgery never should be delayed because a patient is unstable; operative intervention may be precisely the step necessary to reverse the hemodynamic derangements of septic shock.

Patients with septic shock require meticulous and aggressive supportive care. Core temperature should be maintained as close to normal as possible by use of antipyretics and a cooling blanket. Coagulation abnormalities should be identified promptly and treated by infusion of platelets and coagulation factors, as indicated. Finally, patients should be given oxygen supplementation and should be observed closely for evidence of ARDS, one of the major causes of mortality in cases of severe sepsis.[75] Oxygenation should be monitored by means of a pulse oximeter or radial artery catheter. If evidence of respiratory failure develops, the patient should be intubated and supported with mechanical ventilation.

The prognosis in patients with septic shock clearly depends on the severity of the patient's underlying illness. In previously healthy patients, mortality should not exceed 15%.[79] Fortunately, most obstetric patients are in the latter category; therefore the prognosis for complete recovery is excellent provided that the patient receives competent, timely intervention.

Toxoplasmosis
Epidemiology
Toxoplasma gondii is a protozoan that has three distinct forms: (1) trophozoite, (2) cyst, and (3) oocyst. The life cycle of *T. gondii* is dependent on wild and domestic cats, which are the only host for the oocyst. The oocyst is formed in the cat intestine and is subsequently excreted in the feces. Mammals, such as cows, ingest the oocyst, which is disrupted in the animal's intestine, thus releasing the invasive trophozoite. The trophozoite then is disseminated throughout the body, ultimately forming cysts in brain and muscle.[80]

Human infection occurs when infected meat is ingested or when food is contaminated by cat feces through flies, cockroaches, or fingers. Infection rates are highest in areas of poor sanitation and crowded living conditions. Stray cats and domestic cats that eat raw meat are most likely to carry the parasite. The cyst is destroyed by heat.[80]

About 40% to 50% of adults in the United States have antibody to this organism, and the prevalence of antibody is highest in lower socioeconomic populations. The frequency of seroconversion during pregnancy is 5%, and about 3 in 1000 infants show evidence of congenital infection. Clinically significant congenital toxoplasmosis occurs in about 1 in 8000 pregnancies. Toxoplasmosis is more common in Western Europe, particularly France, most likely because of the practice in that country of eating rare or raw meat. More than 80% of women of childbearing age in Paris have antibody to *T. gondii*, and the incidence of congenital toxoplasmosis is about twice as frequent as that in the United States.[81] Universal screening of pregnant women for toxoplasmosis is not recommended in the United States at this time.[82] Testing is indicated, however, if clinical infection is suspected or if the patient is immunocompromised (e.g., HIV infection). Because the presence of antibodies before pregnancy indicates immunity, the ideal time to test for immunity to toxoplasmosis in women at risk is before conception.[83]

Clinical Manifestations

The ingested organism invades across the intestinal epithelium and spreads hematogenously throughout the body. Intracellular replication leads to cell destruction. Clinical manifestations of infection are the result of direct organ damage and the subsequent immunologic response to parasitemia and cell death. Host immunity is mediated primarily through T lymphocytes.[80]

Most infections in humans are asymptomatic. Even in the absence of symptoms, however, patients may have evidence of multiorgan involvement, and clinical disease can follow a long period of asymptomatic infection. **Symptomatic toxoplasmosis usually presents as an illness similar to mononucleosis.**

In contrast to infection in the immunocompetent host, toxoplasmosis can be a devastating infection in the immunosuppressed patient. Because immunity to *T. gondii* is cell mediated, patients with HIV infection and those treated with chronic immunosuppressive therapy after organ transplantation are particularly susceptible to new or reactivated infection. In these patients, dysfunction of the central nervous system is the most common manifestation of infection. Findings typically include encephalitis, meningoencephalitis, and intracerebral mass lesions (Fig. 54-5). Pneumonitis, myocarditis, and generalized lymphadenopathy also occur commonly.[80]

Diagnosis

The diagnosis of toxoplasmosis in the mother can be confirmed by serologic and histologic methods. Serologic tests that suggest an acute infection include detection of immunoglobulin M (IgM)-specific antibody, demonstration

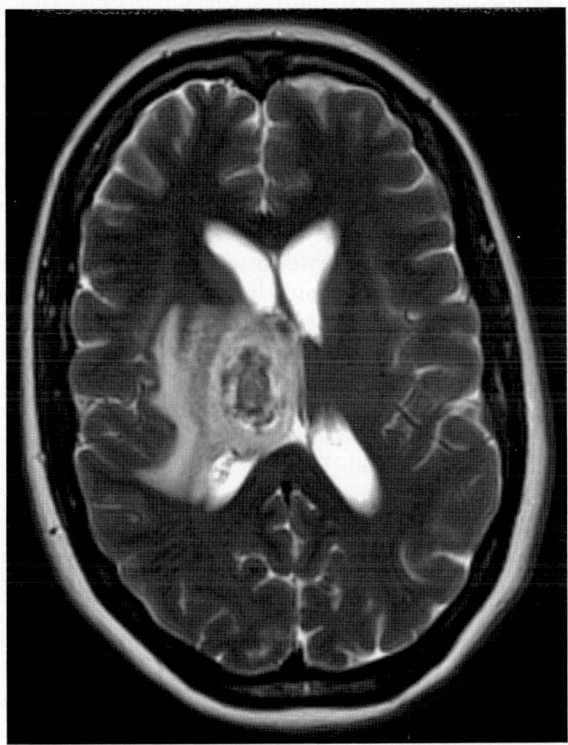

FIG 54-5 Magnetic resonance imaging shows a prominent intracerebral abscess due to toxoplasmosis. (Courtesy Dr. Richard Beegle, Department of Radiology, University of Florida.)

of an extremely high IgG antibody titer (and low IgG avidity), and documentation of IgG seroconversion from negative to positive. Clinicians should be aware that serologic assays for toxoplasmosis are not well standardized. When initial laboratory tests appear to indicate that an acute infection has occurred, repeat serology should be performed in a well-respected reference laboratory (e.g., the Toxoplasma Serology Laboratory of Palo Alto Medical Foundation [www.pamf.org]). In addition, toxoplasmic DNA can be identified in the patient's serum using the PCR test.

T. gondii is most easily identified in lymphatic or brain tissues. Histologic preparations can be examined by light and electron microscopy. For light microscopy, specimens should be stained with either Giemsa or Wright stain.[81,84]

Congenital Toxoplasmosis

Congenital infection can occur if a woman develops acute primary toxoplasmosis during pregnancy. Chronic or latent infection is unlikely to cause fetal injury except perhaps in an immunosuppressed patient. **About 40% of neonates born to mothers with acute toxoplasmosis show evidence of infection. Congenital infection is most likely to occur when maternal infection develops in the third trimester. However, fetal injury is most likely to be severe when maternal infection occurs in the first half of pregnancy.** Less than half of affected infants are symptomatic at birth (Box 54-2).[81,84-85]

The most valuable tests for antenatal diagnosis of congenital toxoplasmosis are ultrasound and amniocentesis.[81,84-85] Ultrasound findings suggestive of infection include ventriculomegaly, intracranial calcifications, microcephaly, ascites, hepatosplenomegaly, and growth restriction. In addition, Hohlfeld and coworkers[86] have now identified a specific gene of *T. gondii* in amniotic fluid using polymerase chain reaction (PCR). In this investigation, 34 of 339 infants had congenital toxoplasmosis confirmed by serologic testing or autopsy. All amniotic fluid specimens from affected pregnancies were positive by PCR, and test results were available within 1 day of specimen collection.

In a subsequent investigation, Romand and colleagues[87] reported that the PCR test had an overall sensitivity of 64% (95% CI, 53% to 75%) for diagnosing congenital toxoplasmosis. No false-positive results were noted, and the positive predictive value was 100%.

Management

Toxoplasmosis in the immunocompetent nonpregnant adult is usually an asymptomatic or self-limited illness and does not require treatment. Immunocompromised patients, however, should be treated, and the regimen of choice is a combination

---

BOX 54-2   CLINICAL MANIFESTATIONS OF CONGENITAL TOXOPLASMOSIS

Rash
Hepatosplenomegaly
Ascites
Fever
Chorioretinitis
Periventricular calcifications
Ventriculomegaly
Seizures
Mental retardation
Uveitis

of oral sulfadiazine (4 g loading dose, then 1 g four times daily) plus pyrimethamine (50 to 100 mg initially, then 25 mg daily). In such patients, extended courses of treatment may be necessary to cure the infection.[84]

Treatment also is indicated when acute toxoplasmosis occurs during pregnancy. Treatment of the mother reduces the risk for congenital infection and decreases the late sequelae of infection.[81,85,88] Pyrimethamine is not recommended for use during the first trimester of pregnancy because of possible teratogenicity, although specific adverse fetal effects have not been documented. Sulfonamides can be used alone, but single-agent therapy appears to be less effective than combination therapy. In Europe, spiramycin has been used extensively in pregnancy with excellent success. It is available for treatment in the United States through the CDC but only after confirmation of maternal infection in a reference laboratory.

Aggressive early treatment of infants with congenital toxoplasmosis is indicated and consists of combination therapy with pyrimethamine, sulfadiazine, and leucovorin for 1 year. Early treatment reduces but does not eliminate the late sequelae of toxoplasmosis, such as chorioretinitis.[89]

In the management of the pregnant patient, prevention of acute toxoplasmosis is of paramount importance. Pregnant women should be advised to avoid contact with cat litter if at all possible, particularly when the cat is allowed to roam outside the home. If they must change the litter, they should do so daily, wear gloves, and wash their hands afterward. They should always wash their hands after preparing meat for cooking and should never eat raw or rare meat. Meat should be cooked thoroughly until the juices are clear. Fruits and vegetables also should be washed carefully to remove possible contamination by oocysts.

Listeriosis

Listeria monocytogenes (LM) is a gram-positive bacillus responsible for severe infections in humans and in a large variety of animal species. It is a facultative intracellular pathogen that invades macrophages and most tissue cells of infected hosts, where it can proliferate. **LM can cause meningitis, encephalitis, bacteremia, and gastroenteritis.** In infected hosts, the bacteria cross the intestinal wall at Peyer patches to invade the mesenteric lymph nodes and blood. The main target organ is the liver, where the bacteria multiply inside hepatocytes. Most disease occurs in patients with impaired cell-mediated immunity; therefore LM is an important cause of severe infections in neonates, pregnant women, elderly people, and transplant recipients. Although dramatic epidemics have received the most publicity, most cases of perinatal listeriosis are isolated.

LM is widespread in nature and can be readily found in soil and vegetation. Seroepidemiologic studies show that the infection is foodborne. Heightened surveillance and quality control by the food industry have been instituted (Box 54-3) and have led to a reduction in the number of cases and deaths from this infection in the past decade. However, most parents are still not aware of the risks of listeriosis and recommended practices for listeriosis prevention, thus they are not taking precautions during their pregnancy to prevent listeriosis.[90] **Because LM can grow and multiply at temperatures as low as 0.5° C (or 32.9° F), refrigerating contaminated foods does not always prevent infection, but cooking contaminated foods at high temperatures consistently destroys the bacteria.** LM can also be contracted through the handling of the products of

> **BOX 54-3** U.S. DEPARTMENT OF AGRICULTURE'S FOOD SAFETY AND INSPECTION SERVICE AND U.S. FOOD AND DRUG ADMINISTRATION'S ADVICE FOR PREGNANT WOMEN TO PREVENT LISTERIOSIS DURING PREGNANCY
>
> - Do not eat hot dogs, luncheon meats, or deli meats unless they are reheated until steaming hot.
> - Do not eat soft cheeses such as feta, Brie, Camembert, blue-veined cheeses, or Mexican-style cheeses such as *queso blanco fresco*. Hard cheeses, semisoft cheeses such as mozzarella, pasteurized processed cheese slices and spreads, cream cheese, and cottage cheese can be safely consumed.
> - Do not eat refrigerated paté or meat spreads. Canned or shelf-stable paté and meat spreads can be eaten.
> - Do not eat refrigerated smoked seafood unless it is an ingredient in a cooked dish such as a casserole. Examples of refrigerated smoked seafood include salmon, trout, whitefish, cod, tuna, and mackerel, which are most often labeled as "nova style," "lox," "kippered," "smoked," or "jerky." This fish is found in the refrigerated section or sold at deli counters of grocery stores and delicatessens. Canned fish such as salmon and tuna or shelf-stable smoked seafood may be safely eaten.
> - Do not drink raw (unpasteurized) milk or eat foods that contain unpasteurized milk.

conception of animals when the miscarriage is due to listeriosis. Therefore it is important for pregnant women who work with animals to avoid hand-to-tissue contact with these materials if possible or to wear gloves if contact cannot be avoided. Owing to the ubiquity of the organism in the environment, outbreaks and sporadic disease continue to occur.[91] A recent outbreak in the United States was attributed to contaminated ice cream.

The incubation period of LM ranges from as little as 1 to 90 days, making identification of the exposure that caused the listeriosis extremely difficult. **Maternal symptoms can vary from flulike or "like food poisoning" to septicemia, meningitis, or pneumonia.** Because no serologic evaluation is reliable, listeriosis is a difficult infection to test for outside the septic peak, when it can be demonstrated in blood cultures. **An exposed pregnant woman with a fever higher than 38.1° C (100.6° F) and signs and symptoms consistent with listeriosis for which no other cause of illness is known should be simultaneously tested and treated for presumptive listeriosis.**[92] **Diagnosis is made primarily by blood culture, and placental cultures should be obtained in the event of delivery.** *Listeria*-specific antibody testing is not routinely available and is neither useful nor recommended in the setting of potential *Listeria* exposure. Amniocentesis may also be considered when clinically appropriate in a symptomatic patient: in such cases, amniotic fluid should be cultured for *Listeria* in addition to other indicated testing. The clinical laboratory should be notified of the clinical concern for *Listeria* specifically because targeted culture techniques are important.[93] **An overall perinatal mortality rate of 50% due to late miscarriage, premature delivery, and stillbirth was recorded before the use of modern therapies.**[94] The clinical characteristics of neonatal listeriosis are similar to neonatal GBS sepsis, with early- and late-onset forms of disease. The mortality rate among liveborn infants is about 10%.[95]

The standard therapy for listeriosis is a combination of ampicillin and gentamicin or, for patients who are intolerant

of β-lactam agents, trimethoprim-sulfamethoxazole. If LM chorioamnionitis is diagnosed preterm, in contrast to other types of chorioamnionitis, in utero therapy with high-dose penicillin or trimethoprim-sulfamethoxazole is possible, and preterm delivery may be avoided.

KEY POINTS

- Overall, without screening and treatment, 85% of neonatal GBS infections are early in onset and result from transmission from a colonized mother.
- All pregnant women should be cultured for cervicovaginal GBS at 35 to 37 weeks' gestation. Culture-positive patients should receive intrapartum antibiotic prophylaxis to prevent early-onset neonatal infection.
- Pregnant patients with GBS bacteriuria should be targeted for intrapartum prophylaxis.
- All pregnant women should have a urine culture at their first prenatal appointment to detect asymptomatic bacteriuria. Infected patients should be treated and then monitored on subsequent prenatal appointments to identify recurrent infection.
- Most cases of pyelonephritis occur as a consequence of undiagnosed or inadequately treated lower urinary tract infections.
- The organisms most likely to cause chorioamnionitis and puerperal endometritis are GBS, E. coli, and gram-positive and gram-negative anaerobes.
- Prophylactic antibiotics are highly effective in preventing post–cesarean delivery endometritis and wound infection. They should be administered before the surgical incision in all cesarean deliveries.
- Resistant organisms and wound infection are the most common causes of persistent fever in patients being treated for puerperal endometritis.
- Septic pelvic thrombophlebitis is another important cause of refractory postoperative fever. This condition is best diagnosed by CT or MRI and is treated with broad-spectrum antibiotics and IV heparin.
- The most common causes of septic shock in obstetric patients are septic abortion, pyelonephritis, chorioamnionitis, and endometritis.
- The two most common methods of transmission of toxoplasmosis are consumption of undercooked beef and contact with cat litter.
- The best diagnostic tests for congenital toxoplasmosis are identification of toxoplasmic DNA in amniotic fluid by polymerase chain reaction and identification of specific fetal injury by ultrasound.
- Pregnant women and immunocompromised patients may reduce their risk for contracting listeriosis by avoiding unpasteurized dairy products.

REFERENCES

1. Prevention of perinatal group B streptococcal disease: revised guidelines from the CDC. *MMWR Morb Mortal Wkly Rep.* 2010;59(RR 10):1.
2. Yancey MK, Duff P. An analysis of the cost-effectiveness of selected protocols for the prevention of neonatal group B streptococcal infection. *Obstet Gynecol.* 1994;83:367.
3. Boyer KM, Gotoff SP. Prevention of early-onset neonatal group B streptococcal disease with selective intrapartum chemoprophylaxis. *N Engl J Med.* 1986;314:1665.
4. Thomsen AC, Morup L, Hansen KB. Antibiotic elimination of group B streptococci in urine in prevention of preterm labor. *Lancet.* 1987;1:591.
5. Newton ER, Clark M. Group B Streptococcus and preterm rupture of membranes. *Obstet Gynecol.* 1988;71:198.
6. Yancey MK, Armer T, Clark P, Duff P. Assessment of rapid identification tests for genital carriage of group B streptococci. *Obstet Gynecol.* 1992;80:1038.
7. Ahmadzia HK, Heine RH. Diagnosis and management of group B Streptococcus in pregnancy. *Obstet Gynecol Clin N Am.* 2014;41:629-647.
8. Bergeron MG, Ke D, Menard C, et al. Rapid detection of group B streptococci in pregnant women at delivery. *N Engl J Med.* 2000;343:175.
9. Ahmadzia HK, Heine P, Brown HL GBS screening: An update on guidelines and methods. *Contemp OBGYN* July 2013.
10. Yow MD, Mason EO, Leeds LJ, et al. Ampicillin prevents intrapartum transmission of group B streptococcus. *JAMA.* 1979;241:1245.
11. Boyer KM, Gadzala CA, Kelly PD, Gotoff SP. Selective intrapartum chemoprophylaxis of neonatal group B streptococcal early-onset disease. III. Interruption of mother-to-infant transmission. *J Infect Dis.* 1983;148:810.
12. Prevention of perinatal group B streptococcal disease: a public health perspective. *MMWR Morb Mortal Wkly Rep.* 1996;45:1.
13. Rosenstein NE, Schuchat A. Opportunities for prevention of perinatal group B streptococcal disease: a multistate surveillance analysis. *Obstet Gynecol.* 1997;90:901.
14. Locksmith GJ, Clark P, Duff P. Maternal and neonatal infection rates with three different protocols for prevention of group B streptococcal disease. *Am J Obstet Gynecol.* 1999;180:416.
15. DeCueto M, Sanchez M-J, Sanpedro A, et al. Timing of intrapartum ampicillin and prevention of vertical transmission of group B streptococcus. *Obstet Gynecol.* 1998;91:112.
16. McNanley AR, Glantz C, Hardy DJ, et al. The effect of intrapartum penicillin on vaginal group B streptococcus colony counts. *Am J Obstet Gynecol.* 2007;197:583e1.
17. Edwards RK, Clark P, Duff P. Intrapartum antibiotic prophylaxis 2: positive predictive value of antenatal group B streptococci cultures and antibiotic susceptibility of clinical isolates. *Obstet Gynecol.* 2002;100:540.
18. Duff P. Urinary tract infections. *Prim Care Update Ob/Gyn.* 1994;1:12.
19. Centers for Disease Control and Prevention—2010 sexually transmitted diseases treatment guidelines. *MMWR.* 2010;59(RR–12):1.
20. Duff P. Pyelonephritis in pregnancy. *Clin Obstet Gynecol.* 1984;27:17.
21. Smaill F, Vazquez JC. Antibiotics for asymptomatic bacteriuria in pregnancy. *Cochrane Database Syst Rev.* 2007;(2):CD000490.
22. Stamm WE, Counts GW, Running KR, et al. Diagnosis of coliform infection in acutely dysuric women. *N Engl J Med.* 1982;307:463.
23. Dunlow S, Duff P. Prevalence of antibiotic-resistant uropathogens in obstetric patients with acute pyelonephritis. *Obstet Gynecol.* 1990;76:241.
24. Stamm WE, Hooton TM. Management of urinary tract infections in adults. *N Engl J Med.* 1993;329:1328.
25. Crider KS, Cleves MA, Reefhuis J, et al. Antibacterial medication use during pregnancy and risk of birth defects. *Arch Pediatr Adolesc Med.* 2009;163:978.
26. Gibbs RS, Duff P. Progress in pathogenesis and management of clinical intraamniotic infection. *Am J Obstet Gynecol.* 1991;164:1317.
27. Armer TL, Duff P. Intraamniotic infection in patients with intact membranes and preterm labor. *Obstet Gynecol Surv.* 1991;46:589.
28. Kenyon S, Boulvain M, Neilson JP. Antibiotics for preterm rupture of membranes. *Cochrane Database Syst Rev.* 2013;(12):CD001058.
29. Saccone G, Berghella V. Antibiotic prophylaxis for term or near-term premature rupture of membranes: metaanalysis of randomized trials. *Am J Obstet Gynecol.* 2015;212:627.e1-627.e9.
30. Romero R, Jimenez C, Lohda AK, et al. Amniotic fluid glucose concentration: a rapid and simple method for the detection of intraamniotic infection in preterm labor. *Am J Obstet Gynecol.* 1990;163:968.
31. Romero R, Yoon BH, Mazor M, et al. The diagnostic and prognostic value of amniotic fluid white blood cell count, glucose, interleukin-6, and Gram stain in patients with preterm labor and intact membranes. *Am J Obstet Gynecol.* 1993;169:805.
32. Sperling RS, Ramamurthy RS, Gibbs RS. A comparison of intrapartum versus immediate postpartum treatment of intra-amniotic infection. *Obstet Gynecol.* 1987;70:861.
33. Gilstrap LC, Leveno KJ, Cox SM, et al. Intrapartum treatment of acute chorioamnionitis: impact on neonatal sepsis. *Am J Obstet Gynecol.* 1988;159:579.
34. Gibbs RS, Dinsmoor MJ, Newton ER, et al. A randomized trial of intrapartum versus immediate postpartum treatment of women with intra-amniotic infection. *Obstet Gynecol.* 1988;72:823.

35. Locksmith GJ, Chin A, Vu T, Shattuck KE, Hankins GD. High compared with standard gentamicin dosing for chorioamnionitis: a comparison of maternal and fetal serum drug levels. *Obstet Gynecol.* 2005;105(3):473-479.

36. Hansen M, Christrup LL, Jarløv JO, Kampmann JP, Bonde J. Gentamicin dosing in critically ill patients. *Acta Anaesthesiol Scand.* 2001;45(6):734-740.

37. Duff P. Antibiotic selection in obstetrics: making cost-effective choices. *Clin Obstet Gynecol.* 2002;45:59.

38. Lyell DJ, Pullen K, Fuh K, et al. Daily compared with 8-hour gentamicin for the treatment of intrapartum chorioamnionitis. A randomized controlled trial. *Obstet Gynecol.* 2010;115:344.

39. Edwards RK, Duff P. Single additional dose postpartum therapy for women with chorioamnionitis. *Obstet Gynecol.* 2003;102:957.

40. Black LP, Hinson L, Duff P. Limited course of antibiotic treatment for chorioamnionitis. *Obstet Gynecol.* 2012;119:1102.

41. Chapman E, Reveiz L, Illanes E, Bonfill Cosp X. Antibiotic regimens for management of intra-amniotic infection. *Cochrane Database Syst Rev.* 2014;(12):CD010976.

42. Duff P. Pathophysiology and management of postcesarean endomyometritis. *Obstet Gynecol.* 1986;67:269.

43. Milligan DA, Brady K, Duff P. Short-term parenteral antibiotic therapy for puerperal endometritis. *J Matern Fetal Med.* 1992;1:60.

44. Drugs for MRSA skin and soft-tissue infections. *Med Lett Drugs Ther.* 2014;56:39.

45. Anderson BL. Puerperal group A streptococcal infection: beyond Semmelweis. *Obstet Gynecol.* 2014;123(4):874-882.

46. Duff P. Prophylactic antibiotics for cesarean delivery: a simple cost-effective strategy for prevention of postoperative morbidity. *Am J Obstet Gynecol.* 1987;157:794.

47. Duff P. A simple checklist for preventing serious complications after cesarean delivery. *Obstet Gynecol.* 2010;116:1393.

48. Howard HR, Phelps D, Blanchard K. Prophylactic cesarean section antibiotics: maternal and neonatal morbidity before or after cord clamping. *Obstet Gynecol.* 1979;53:151.

49. Cunningham FG, Leveno KJ, DePalma RT, et al. Perioperative antimicrobials for cesarean delivery: before or after cord clamping? *Obstet Gynecol.* 1983;62:151.

50. Dinsmoor MJ, Gilbert S, Landon MB, et al. Perioperative antibiotic prophylaxis for non-laboring cesarean delivery. *Obstet Gynecol.* 2008;114:752.

51. Mackeen AD, Packard RE, Ota E, Berghella V, Baxter JK. *Cochrane Database Syst Rev.* 2014;(12):CD009516.

52. Sullivan SA, Smith T, Chang E, et al. Administration of cefazolin prior to skin incision is superior to cefazolin at cord clamping in preventing postcesarean infectious morbidity: a randomized controlled trial. *Am J Obstet Gynecol.* 2007;196:455.e1.

53. Kaimal AJ, Zlatnick MG, Chang YW, et al. Effect of a change in policy regarding the timing of prophylactic antibiotics on the rate of postcesarean delivery surgical-site infections. *Am J Obstet Gynecol.* 2008;199:310.e1.

54. Owens SM, Brozanski BS, Meyn LA, et al. Antimicrobial prophylaxis for cesarean delivery before skin incision. *Obstet Gynecol.* 2009;114:573.

55. Costantine MM, Rahman M, Ghulmiyah L, et al. Timing of perioperative antibiotics for cesarean delivery: a metaanalysis. *Am J Obstet Gynecol.* 2008;199:301.e1.

56. Tita AT, Hauth JC, Grimes A, et al. Decreasing incidence of postcesarean endometritis with extended-spectrum antibiotic prophylaxis. *Obstet Gynecol.* 2008;111:51.

57. Tita AT, Owen J, Stamm AM, et al. Impact of extended-spectrum antibiotic prophylaxis on incidence of postcesarean surgical wound infection. *Am J Obstet Gynecol.* 2008;199:303e1.

58. Tita AT, Rouse DJ, Blackwell S, Saade GR, Spong CY, Andrews WW. Emerging concepts in antibiotic prophylaxis for cesarean delivery: a systematic review. *Obstet Gynecol.* 2009;113(3):675-682.

59. Lasley D, Eblen A, Yancey MK, et al. The effect of placental removal method on the incidence of postcesarean infections. *Am J Obstet Gynecol.* 1997;176:1250.

60. Anorlu RI, Maholwana B, Hofmeyr JG. Methods of delivering the placenta at cesarean section. *Cochran Database Syst Rev.* 2008;(3):CD004737.

61. Yancey MK, Duff P, Clark P. The frequency of glove contamination during cesarean delivery. *Obstet Gynecol.* 1994;83:538.

62. American College of Obstetricians and Gynecologists. Practice Bulletin No. 120: Use of prophylactic antibiotics in labor and delivery. *Obstet Gynecol.* 2011;117(6):1472-1483.

63. Gibbs RS, Blanco JD, St. Clair PJ. A case-control study of wound abscess after cesarean delivery. *Obstet Gynecol.* 1983;62:498.

64. Shy KK, Eschenbach DA. Fatal perineal cellulitis from an episiotomy site. *Obstet Gynecol.* 1979;54:292.

65. Golde S, Ledger WJ. Necrotizing fasciitis in postpartum patients. *Obstet Gynecol.* 1977;50:670.

66. Weinstein WM, Onderdonk AB, Bartlett JG, Gorbach SL. Experimental intra-abdominal abscesses in rats: development of an experimental model. *Infect Immun.* 1974;10:1250.

67. Knochel JQ, Koehler PR, Lee TG, Welch DM. Diagnosis of abdominal abscesses with computed tomography, ultrasound, and ^{111}In leukocyte scans. *Radiology.* 1980;137:425.

68. Gerzof SG, Robbins AH, Johnson WC, et al. Percutaneous catheter drainage of abdominal abscesses: a five-year experience. *N Engl J Med.* 1981;305:653.

69. Duff P, Gibbs RS. Pelvic vein thrombophlebitis: diagnostic dilemma and therapeutic challenge. *Obstet Gynecol Surv.* 1983;38:365.

70. Brown TK, Munsick RA. Puerperal ovarian vein thrombophlebitis: a syndrome. *Am J Obstet Gynecol.* 1971;109:263.

71. Dunn LJ, Van Voorhis LW. Enigmatic fever and pelvic thrombophlebitis. *N Engl J Med.* 1967;276:265.

72. Brown CE, Lowe TW, Cunningham FG, Weinreb JC. Puerperal pelvic vein thrombophlebitis: impact on diagnosis and treatment using x-ray computed tomography and magnetic resonance imaging. *Obstet Gynecol.* 1986;68:789.

73. Duff P. Septic pelvic-vein thrombophlebitis. In: Pastorek JG, ed. *Obstetric and Gynecologic Infectious Disease.* New York: Raven Press; 1994:165.

74. Angus DC, van der Poll T. Severe sepsis and septic shock. *N Engl J Med.* 2013;369:840.

75. Barton JR, Sibai BM. Severe sepsis and septic shock in pregnancy. *Obstet Gynecol.* 2012;120:689.

76. Holst LB, Haase N, Wetterslev J, et al. Lower versus higher hemoglobin threshold for transfusion in septic shock. *N Engl J Med.* 2014;371:1381.

77. DeBacker D, Biston P, Devriendt J, et al. Comparison of dopamine and norepinephrine in the treatment of shock. *N Engl J Med.* 2010;362:779.

78. Sprung CL, Annane D, Keh D, et al. Hydrocortisone therapy for patients with septic shock. *N Engl J Med.* 2008;358:111.

79. Freid MA, Vosti KL. The importance of underlying disease in patients with gram-negative bacteremia. *Arch Intern Med.* 1968;121:418.

80. Krick JA, Remington JS. Toxoplasmosis in the adult: an overview. *N Engl J Med.* 1978;298:550.

81. Daffos F. Prenatal management of 746 pregnancies at risk for congenital toxoplasmosis. *N Engl J Med.* 1988;318:271.

82. Peyron F, Wallon M, Liou C, Garner P. Treatments for toxoplasmosis in pregnancy. *Cochrane Database Syst Rev.* 2000;(2):CD001684.

83. Academy of Pediatrics and the American College of Obstetricians and Gynecologists. *Guidelines for Perinatal Care. 7th edition.* 2012; p433-p434.

84. Egerman RS, Beazley D. Toxoplasmosis. *Semin Perinatol.* 1998;22:332.

85. Desmonts G, Couvreur J. Congenital toxoplasmosis: a prospective study of 378 pregnancies. *N Engl J Med.* 1974;290:1110.

86. Hohlfeld P, Daffos F, Costa JM, et al. Prenatal diagnosis of congenital toxoplasmosis with a polymerase-chain reaction test on amniotic fluid. *N Engl J Med.* 1994;331:695.

87. Romand S, Wallon M, Franck J, et al. Prenatal diagnosis using polymerase chain reaction on amniotic fluid for congenital toxoplasmosis. *Obstet Gynecol.* 2001;97:296.

88. Foulon W, Villena I, Stray-Pedersen B, et al. Treatment of toxoplasmosis during pregnancy: a multicenter study of impact on fetal transmission and children's sequelae at age 1 year. *Am J Obstet Gynecol.* 1999;180:410.

89. Guerina NG, Hsu HW, Meissner HC, et al. Neonatal serologic screening and early treatment for congenital *Toxoplasma gondii* infection. *N Engl J Med.* 1994;330:1858.

90. Cates SC, Carter-Young HL, Conley S, O'Brien B. Pregnant women and listeriosis: preferred educational messages and delivery mechanisms. *J Nutr Educ Behav.* 2004;36:121.

91. MacDonald PD, Whitwam RE, Boggs JD, et al. Outbreak of listeriosis among Mexican immigrants as a result of consumption of illicitly produced Mexican-style cheese. *Clin Infect Dis.* 2005;40:677.

92. Committee on Obstetric Practice, American College of Obstetricians and Gynecologists. Committee Opinion No. 614: Management of pregnant women with presumptive exposure to Listeria monocytogenes. *Obstet Gynecol.* 2014;124(6):1241-1244.

93. SMFM Statement: *Listeria exposure in pregnancy.* August 1, 2014. <https://www.smfm.org/publications/172-smfm-statement-listeria-exposure-in-pregnancy>.

94. McLauchlin J. Human listeriosis in Britain, 1967-85, a summary of 722 cases. 1. Listeriosis during pregnancy and in the newborn. *Epidemiol Infect.* 1990;104:181.

95. Frederiksen B, Samuelsson S. Feto-maternal listeriosis in Denmark 1981-1988. *J Infect.* 1992;24:277.

CHAPTER 55

Mental Health and Behavioral Disorders in Pregnancy

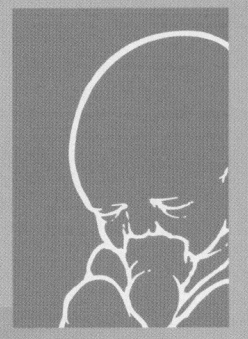

KATHERINE L. WISNER, DOROTHY K.Y. SIT, DEBRA L. BOGEN, MARGARET ALTEMUS, TERI B. PEARLSTEIN, DACE S. SVIKIS, DAWN MISRA, and EMILY S. MILLER

KEY ABBREVIATIONS

American Academy of Neurology	AAN	Intrauterine growth restriction	IUGR
American Academy of Pediatrics	AAP	Low birthweight	LBW
American College of Obstetricians and Gynecologists	ACOG	Lamotrigine	LTG
		Major depressive episode	MDE
Antiepileptic drug	AED	Mood disorders questionnaire	MDQ
Anorexia nervosa	AN	Nortriptyline	NTP
Bipolar disorder	BD	Neonatal abstinence syndrome	NAS
Body mass index	BMI	Nicotine replacement therapy	NRT
Bulimia nervosa	BN	Opioid agonist therapy	OAT
Cognitive behavioral therapy	CBT	Odds ratio	OR
Carbamazepine	CBZ	Postpartum depression	PPD
Concentration/dose (ratio)	C/D	Preterm birth	PTB
Confidence interval	CI	Posttraumatic stress disorder	PTSD
Diagnostic and Statistical Manual of Mental Disorders	DSM	Randomized controlled trial	RCT
		Relative risk	RR
Docosahexaenoic acid	DHA	Small for gestational age	SGA
Edinburgh Postnatal Depression Scale	EPDS	Selective serotonin reuptake inhibitor	SSRI
Electroconvulsive therapy	ECT	Serotonin-norepinephrine reuptake inhibitor	SNRI
Eicosapentaenoic acid	EPA	Substance use disorder	SUD
Fetal alcohol syndrome	FAS	Sudden infant death syndrome	SIDS
Fetal alcohol spectrum disorder	FASD	Thyroid-stimulating hormone	TSH
Food and Drug Administration	FDA	Valproic acid	VPA
Human immunodeficiency virus	HIV		

OVERVIEW

"Mental health is fundamental to health." This statement, made by Surgeon General David Satcher, emphasized the foundation that emotional well-being provides for health. In medical practice, we compartmentalize symptoms and diseases into manageable units; however, the patient comes as an integrated whole. The effect of pathology in any part of the body affects the entire patient. Psychiatric disorders are defined in the *Diagnostic and Statistical Manual of Mental Disorders* (version 5, or *DSM-V*),[1] a classification system that divides mental disorders into types based on criteria sets with defining features. This

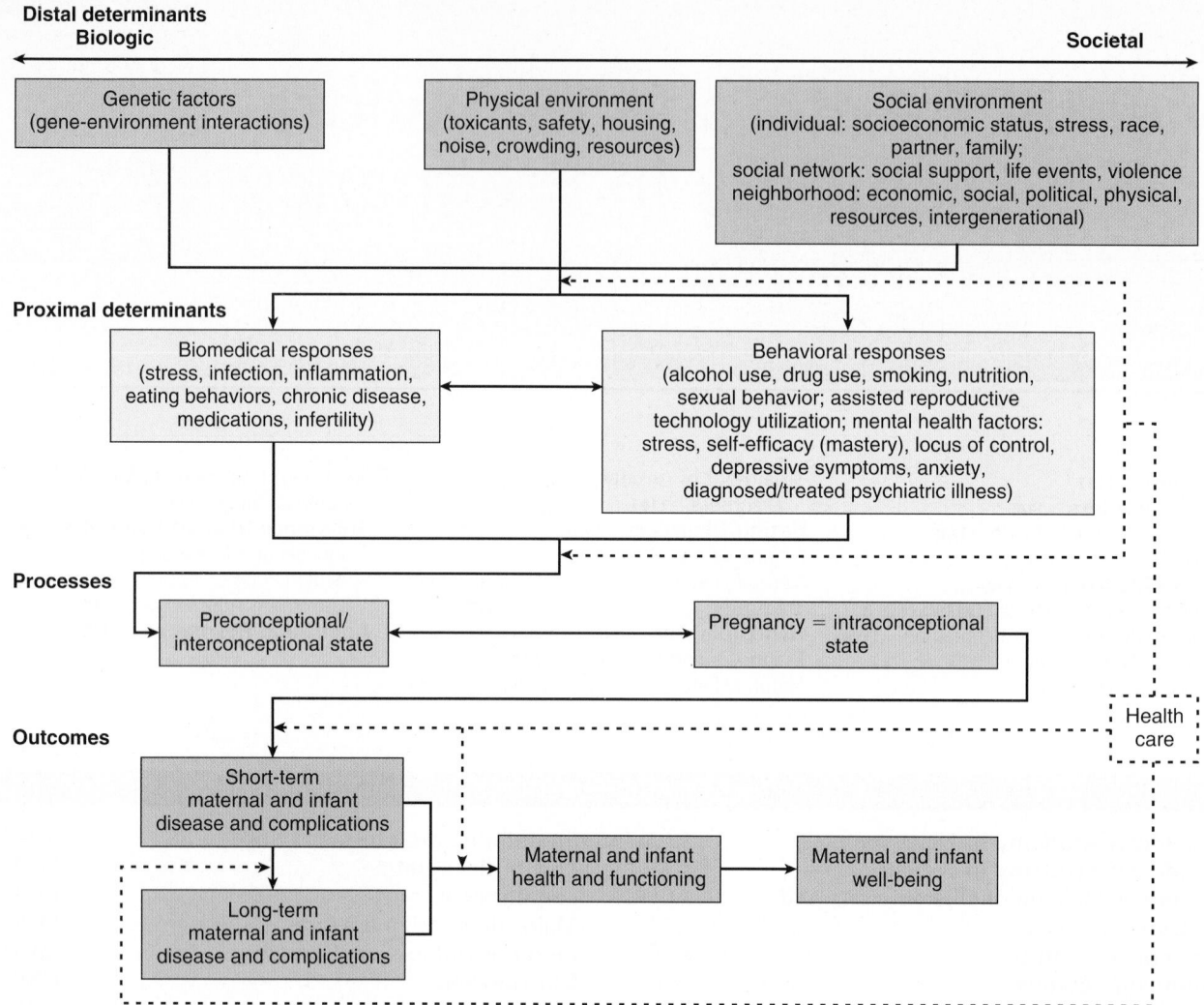

FIG 55-1 Integrated perinatal health framework: a multiple-determinants model with a life-span approach. Illustrative examples are in brackets. (Modified from Misra DP, Guyer B, Allston A. Integrated perinatal health framework. A multiple determinants model with a life span approach. *Am J Prev Med.* 2003;25:65.)

chapter covers the major categories of disorders that affect women of childbearing age. For the pregnant woman and her family, the capacity to function optimally, enjoy relationships, manage the pregnancy, and prepare for birth is critical.

Perinatal health can be conceptualized within a model that integrates the complex social, psychological, behavioral, environmental, and biologic forces that shape pregnancy outcome. Misra and colleagues[2] presented a perinatal framework that integrates a life-span approach with multiple determinants (Fig. 55-1). The model contains four levels that provide a paradigm for the determinants of perinatal health outcomes. The first level in the model is **distal determinants,** which focuses on *distal* (in time) risk factors that place a woman at greater susceptibility to *proximal* (current) risk factors. Distal determinants from biologic, physical, and social domains increase or decrease a woman's likelihood of developing health problems, engaging in high-risk behaviors, or being exposed to potential toxins. Some of the most powerful influences on pregnancy outcome are related to historic women's health factors that occur long before pregnancy, such as maltreatment during childhood.[3] At the next level, **proximal determinants,** risk factors that have a direct impact on a woman's health,

are represented by biomedical and behavioral responses; for example, cigarette smoking. The interaction between *distal* and *proximal* risk factors determines an individual's current overall health status. The relationship between a woman's health status directly before conception and the demands of pregnancy affect perinatal health outcomes. The third level, *processes,* emphasizes the dynamic interaction of preconceptional, interconceptional, and intraconceptional factors on reproductive health. At the fourth level, *outcomes,* the model includes disease, function, and well-being, which provide a comprehensive view of health status.

Each patient comes to pregnancy with sets of malleable risks and assets. To the extent that biopsychosocial exposures with negative impact upon pregnancy outcome can be diminished, eliminated, or replaced with positive factors, pregnancy outcome can be improved. **The role of the physician is to influence the patient's exposures and behaviors to improve the probability of positive reproductive outcomes** (see Fig. 55-1). Childbearing is an ideal time for health interventions because women have contact with professionals and access to health care coverage and are motivated toward positive behaviors to invest in the welfare of their offspring. The role of fathers has recently been identified as a research gap, and opportunity, in perinatal mental health.

The father, partner, or a significant other can be engaged in interventions[4] to reduce maternal stress, encourage prenatal care, and eliminate drug and alcohol use.[5,6]

Our discussion of psychiatric disorders includes five major diagnostic categories that commonly occur in women of childbearing age: (1) mood, (2) anxiety, (3) eating disorders, (4) substance use disorders, and (5) schizophrenia. Our review focuses on the interrelationships among these disorders and their courses during pregnancy and postpartum and during lactation. The impact of childbearing on existing disorders or vulnerabilities in the female patient is reviewed along with episodes that are etiologically related to childbearing.

MOOD DISORDERS

Major Depressive Episode

Diagnosis and Prevalence During Pregnancy and Postpartum

In the DSM-V,[1] a *major depressive episode* (MDE) is defined as at least a 2-week period of either persistent depressed mood or loss of interest or pleasure in daily activities, so-called gatekeeper symptoms, plus four associated symptoms (three if both gatekeeper symptoms are present; see Box 55-1). *Persistent* means the symptom must be present for most of the day nearly every day. The patient also must have impairment of function in interpersonal relationships or work. It is possible to have a *diagnosis* of MDE without the *symptom* of depression. A woman could have persistent loss of interest or pleasure but no sadness and yet have four other symptoms noted in the DSM-V criteria for major depressive disorder. Note that appetite, sleep, and motor activity can be either decreased or increased relative to the woman's norm. A fatigued woman who derives no pleasure from previously enjoyable activities, sleeps 15 hours per day, sits immobile for long periods, and is gaining weight has MDE. A guilt-ridden woman with sadness, 4 hours of sleep nightly, weight loss of 15 pounds, and pacing also has MDE, which may be episodic or chronic.

Nearly twice as many women (12.0%) as men (6.6%) suffer from an MDE each year.[7] Women are at the greatest risk for MDE between 25 and 44 years, the primary age for childbearing. **The period prevalence of MDE is 12.7% during pregnancy** (with 7.5% of women having a new episode), **and 21.9% the year after parturition**[8]; therefore, **MDE is among the most common complications of childbearing.** Mothers at increased risk are disadvantaged,[9] have preterm infants,[10] and are

BOX 55-1   DSM-V CRITERIA FOR MAJOR DEPRESSIVE DISORDER

Over the last 2 weeks, most of the day nearly every day, five of the following (one symptom must be mood or interest) must cause marked distress or impairment in important areas of functioning:
- Depressed mood
- Markedly diminished interest or pleasure
- Significant weight loss or gain unrelated to dieting
- Insomnia or hypersomnia
- Psychomotor agitation/retardation
- Fatigue or loss of energy
- Feelings of worthlessness/guilt
- Diminished ability to concentrate
- Recurrent thoughts of death

in adolescence.[11] Depression persists from months to years after childbirth, with lingering limitations in physical and psychological functioning after recovery.[12] Of women with postpartum MDE, 25% to 50% have episodes that last 7 months or more.[13]

As predicted by the multiple determinants model (see Fig. 55-1), MDE has contributions from several risk factor domains. In women,[14] the strongest predictors were stressful life events, genetic factors, history of an MDE, and high emotional sensitivity. Similarly, stressful life events[15] and a history of MDE in the woman or her family[13] are predictors of postpartum-onset MDE. Women with postpartum MDE are at increased risk (about 25% to 33%) for recurrence after a subsequent birth, and over 40% have nonpostpartum MDE.[16]

The DSM-V[1] allows the designation *with peripartum onset* to specify episodes that begin during pregnancy or within the first 4 weeks postpartum. Epidemiologists have defined the duration of *postpartum* based on data about the break point between elevated risk for psychiatric illness after birth and the baseline risk for episodes in childbearing-aged women.[17] Kendell[18] and Munk-Olsen[19] and their colleagues found a significant peak in the rate of mood disorders in the 90-day period after childbirth. Although the definition of *postpartum* varies, the adverse effects of the disorder for the woman and her family are independent of time of onset.

The most commonly used measure to screen for MDE during childbearing is the Edinburgh Postnatal Depression Scale (EPDS; Fig. 55-2),[20] which has been validated for use both during and after pregnancy. This self-report measure contains 10 items ranked from 0 to 3. Scored by simple addition, the EPDS is free to health care professionals and is available in 23 languages. A cutoff score of greater than or equal to 13 (the sensitivity for identifying MDE is 86%, specificity is 78%, positive predictive value is 73%) was recommended for screening for MDE in clinical settings.[21] For pregnant women the recommended cutoff score is greater than or equal to 15.[22] As with any screening tool, a positive test must be followed by diagnostic evaluation and treatment guidance.[23] The differential diagnosis of MDE in the early postbirth period includes the "baby blues," a transient syndrome that occurs in 80% of mothers that resolves by day 10 postpartum (see Chapter 23).

Natural History Across Childbearing

Periods of hormonal fluctuation—menstrual cycle, pregnancy, postpartum, and perimenopause—are associated with MDE. Investigators have suggested that the rapid change in gonadal steroid concentrations contributes to the etiology of postpartum-onset MDE.[24] The neurobiology of women who develop postpartum depression (PPD) appears especially vulnerable to the mood-destabilizing effects of withdrawal from gonadal steroids.

Postpartum MDE does not differ from MDE at other periods during the childbearing years with respect to clinical presentation and duration of untreated episodes.[23] However, aggressive obsessional thoughts occur more commonly in women who have postpartum-onset MDE compared with those whose depression falls outside the 1-year postbirth period. **Delusions must be differentiated from the far more common obsessional thoughts in the context of depression.**[25,26] *Obsessions are recurrent and persistent thoughts, impulses, or images that are experienced as intrusive and inappropriate and cause marked anxiety or distress.* For example, some mothers have obsessional thoughts about drowning their baby and refuse to

How are you feeling?

As you have recently had a baby, we would like to know how you are feeling now. Please check the answer which comes closest to how you have felt in the past 7 days, not just how you feel today.

1.	I have been able to laugh and see the funny side of things:	Score
	As much as I always could	0
	Not quite so much now	1
	Definitely not so much now	2
	Not at all	3
2.	I have looked forward with enjoyment to things:	
	As much as I ever did	0
	Rather less than I used to	1
	Definitely less than I used to	2
	Hardly at all	3
3.	I have blamed myself unnecessarily when things went wrong:	
	Yes, most of the time	3
	Yes, some of the time	2
	Not very often	1
	No, never	0
4.	I have been anxious or worried for no good reason:	
	No, not at all	0
	Hardly ever	1
	Yes, sometimes	2
	Yes, very often	3
5.	I have felt scared or panicky for no very good reason:	
	Yes, quite a lot	3
	Yes, sometimes	2
	No, not much	1
	No, not at all	0
6.	Things have been getting on top of me:	
	Yes, most of the time I haven't been able to cope at all	3
	Yes, sometimes I haven't been coping as well as usual	2
	No, most of the time I have coped quite well	1
	No, I have been coping as well as ever	0
7.	I have been so unhappy that I have had difficulty sleeping:	
	Yes, most of the time	3
	Yes, sometimes	2
	Not very often	1
	No, not at all	0
8.	I have felt sad or miserable:	
	Yes, most of the time	3
	Yes, quite often	2
	Not very often	1
	No, not at all	0
9.	I have been so unhappy that I have been crying:	
	Yes, most of the time	3
	Yes, quite often	2
	Only occasionally	1
	No, never	0
10.	The thought of harming myself has occurred to me:	
	Yes, quite often	3
	Sometimes	2
	Hardly ever	1
	Never	0

FIG 55-2 Edinburgh Postnatal Depression Scale. (From Cox, JL, Holden JM, Sagovsky R. Detection of postnatal depression. Development of the 10-item Edinburgh Postnatal Depression Scale. *Br J Psych.* 1987;150:782-786.)

bathe the child. Women often have "what if" questions such as, What if I throw the baby over the banister? Obsessions differ from psychotic symptoms because the patient recognizes that the thoughts, impulses, or images are a product of her own mind (not imposed by an external force as might occur in psychosis). Additionally, obsessional visual images may occur but are brief and are perceived as being in the "mind's eye" as opposed to an external hallucination. For example, a woman might have frightening images of her dead baby in a bathtub, but she is aware that the image does not reflect reality. The distinction is important clinically because women with obsessional thoughts are vigilant about preventing any action related to the thought content (e.g., insisting that all kitchen knives be locked away), whereas women with psychosis are at risk for taking action. Although these symptom sets are not mutually exclusive, co-occurrence is very rare.

The physiologic milieu created by MDE adversely impacts maternal function during pregnancy and postpartum.[27] **MDE is associated with poor prenatal care compliance, inadequate nutrition, obesity, smoking, alcohol and drug use, and suicide.** A meta-analysis affirmed that MDE during pregnancy was associated with both low birthweight (LBW) and preterm birth (PTB).[28] Offspring of pregnant women with MDE are at risk for insecure attachment and sleep and eating disorders.[29] Children with in utero exposure to maternal MDE are four times more likely to be depressed at age 16 years.[30]

Psychiatric illness during rapid development of the infant creates a new generation at risk. Maternal depression increases the risk for long-lasting adverse effects such as insecure attachment and poor cognitive performance.[30,31] Other sequelae of maternal mental illness are increased rates of accidental injury, child abuse, neglect, and infanticide.[32] Early identification and intervention for postpartum MDE has the potential to prevent negative sequelae for women and their families. **The relationship between maternal MDE and multiple childhood problems is a continuum that often becomes apparent during pregnancy.**

Treatment of Major Depressive Episode During Pregnancy

The emergence of MDE during childbearing compels a complete medical and family history, review of systems, and physical exam to assess for contributions to depressive symptoms, particularly thyroid abnormalities and anemia. Our experience is that MDE seldom remits with correction of hypothyroidism alone,[33] and treatment for both is required. The use of prescribed and over-the-counter medications, herbal therapies, drugs, and alcohol must be assessed.

Although MDE is a highly prevalent condition, only 1 in 5 Americans receives any guideline-concordant intervention,[34] **and the rate is lower in pregnant women than in nonpregnant women.**[35] In nearly 6500 Medicaid recipients with established MDE treatment, women who became pregnant had a significantly greater drop in both outpatient psychotherapy visits and antidepressant prescription claims compared with matched nonpregnant women, and care did not resume after birth.[36]

Evidence-based treatments for MDE are psychotherapy and antidepressants.[37,38] Studies of interpersonal psychotherapy and pharmacotherapy[39] document both reduced depressive symptoms and improved maternal function following treatment during pregnancy. Psychotherapy is the preferred treatment for most women[34]; however, it is not available in all practice settings,

nor is it feasible for many mothers. Barriers to clinic-based depression care include the physical demands of pregnancy, transportation, childcare for other children, and cost. Adult outpatient settings do not typically offer flexible appointment schedules or allow children on site. If psychotherapy is not feasible, or the woman prefers pharmacotherapy, decision making tends to focus on the potential adverse effects of medication rather than the adverse effects of MDE. The result is often the choice by the woman or her physician to avoid or stop drug treatment to obviate fetal exposure without equal consideration of the risks of MDE to both the mother and fetus.[39] **For most pregnant women, the reality is that accessible and acceptable mental health treatment is very limited.** Low treatment rates are a public health concern given accumulating evidence that MDE increases risk to the pregnant woman and fetus. Federally funded home visitation programs for disadvantaged women are potential adjuncts for collaborative care with obstetricians and mental health professionals to improve rates of depression treatment.[40]

The risk-benefit decision-making process for treatment of MDE during pregnancy was described by representatives from the American Psychiatric Association.[27] **Individually tailored interventions are considered for their capacity to maximize maternal wellness while minimizing adverse effects for the maternal-fetal pair.** The patient and physician both contribute expertise to the process, because the patient's assignment of her own values dictates her choice. For example, some women will not consent to pharmacotherapy during pregnancy regardless of the impairment related to the MDE. Others choose pharmacotherapy because they are not confident that other treatments will be efficacious or because discontinuing medication invariably has been followed by recurrence with psychosocial consequences. The verbal informed consent process promotes the treatment alliance, recognizes the patient's responsibility to make choices for herself and her baby, and provides an opportunity for ongoing assessment of the woman's competence to make decisions.[27]

Although used commonly, the word *safe* is problematic because it implies no possibility of an adverse effect. Confirming any exposure as harmless presents the impossible task of proving no effect on a monumental number of reproductive and developmental outcomes throughout the exposed offspring's lifespan. What can be estimated from available studies is the magnitude of a subset of reproductive risks in antidepressant-treated women.[41] The risks for multiple domains of reproductive toxicity considered in this chapter are miscarriage, intrauterine fetal demise, structural malformations, growth effects, neurobehavioral teratogenicity, and neonatal effects (see Chapter 8). A prominent observation from the literature is the methodologic difficulty of separating the reproductive effects of the drug exposure from the sequelae, both physiologic and psychosocial, of the underlying MDE.

Side Effects of Medical Treatment of Major Depressive Episode During Pregnancy
MISCARRIAGE

In a cohort study[42] of all registered pregnancies in Denmark from 1997 to 2010, the adjusted hazard ratio for miscarriage after exposure to a selective serotonin reuptake inhibitor (SSRI) was 1.27 (95% confidence interval [CI], 1.22 to 1.33) compared with no exposure. However, women who discontinued SSRI treatment 3 to 12 months before pregnancy also had a similar increased hazard ratio of miscarriage (1.24; 95% CI, 1.18 to 1.30). In a population-based Danish cohort study, stillbirth and neonatal mortality were not associated with first-trimester SSRI use.[43]

STRUCTURAL MALFORMATIONS

Studies of first-trimester SSRI exposure do not demonstrate consistent data to support an increased risk for structural malformations. **Two large-scale case control studies[44,45] revealed no increased risk rates overall for malformations, including cardiac anomalies, with SSRI exposure** (combined drugs). Louik and colleagues[45] compared the rates of malformation among 9849 cases and 5860 control infants. Analyses of the associations between individual SSRIs and specific defects showed significant associations between the use of sertraline and omphalocele (odds ratio [OR], 5.7; 95% CI, 1.6 to 20.7) and cardiac septal defects (OR, 2.0; 95% CI, 1.2 to 4.0) and between the use of paroxetine and right ventricular outflow tract obstruction defects (OR, 3.3; 95% CI, 1.3 to 8.8). At the same time, Alwan and colleagues[44] published outcomes from 9622 infants with major birth defects and 4092 control infants born from the National Birth Defects Prevention Study. Maternal SSRI use was associated with anencephaly (OR, 2.4; 95% CI, 1.1 to 5.1); craniosynostosis (OR, 2.5; 95% CI, 1.5 to 4.0), and omphalocele (OR, 2.8; 95% CI, 1.3 to 5.7). In an accompanying editorial, Greene[46] noted that the malformations reported in each study were different and that most had not been previously associated with SSRI exposure.

The relationship between SSRI use in pregnancy and cardiovascular defects has been the focus of recent studies. Bérard and colleagues[47] conducted a population-based cohort study in Quebec of 18,493 depressed or anxious women who were exposed to sertraline ($n = 366$), other SSRIs ($n = 1963$), or a non-SSRI antidepressant ($n = 1296$) and unexposed women in the first trimester. Sertraline use was not significantly associated with the risk of overall major malformations when compared with the no-exposure group. However, sertraline exposure was associated with an increased risk of atrial/ventricular defects (relative risk [RR], 1.34; 95% CI, 1.02 to 1.76) and craniosynostosis (RR, 2.03; 95% CI, 1.09 to 3.75). Exposure to SSRIs other than sertraline during the first trimester of pregnancy was associated with craniosynostosis (RR, 2.43; 95% CI, 1.44 to 4.11) and musculoskeletal defects (RR, 1.28; 95% CI, 1.03 to 1.58). Although analyses were adjusted for potential confounders, data on smoking, folic acid intake, alcohol use, and body mass index (BMI) were missing. Whereas the design included women with a history of depression or anxiety, antidepressant-treated women differ from unmedicated women, which is inherent in observational studies in which randomization is not used.[48,49]

In a Danish study, the rate of congenital heart malformations was similar for pregnancies exposed to continuous SSRI use throughout the first trimester (OR, 2.01; 95% CI, 1.60 to 2.53) and for pregnancies in which SSRI treatment was paused during pregnancy (OR, 1.85; 95% CI, 1.07 to 3.20; $P = .94$).[50] Similar increased risks of specific cardiac malformations were found for individual SSRIs, and no dose-response relationship was observed. Similarly, in a recent American population-based cohort study, Huybrechts and colleagues[51] found no increase in the risk of cardiac malformations attributable to antidepressant use during the first trimester. A total of 64,389 women (6.8%) used antidepressants during the first trimester. Overall, 6403

infants who were not exposed to antidepressants were born with a cardiac defect (72.3/10,000 infants), compared with 580 infants with exposure (90.1/10,000 infants). Associations between antidepressant use and cardiac defects were attenuated with increasing levels of adjustment for confounding. The relative risks of any cardiac defect with the use of SSRIs were 1.25 (95% CI, 1.13 to 1.38) in the unadjusted analysis, and markedly attenuated, 1.12 (95% CI, 1.00 to 1.26), in the analysis restricted to women with depression. Importantly, substantial differences in the characteristics of the patients who were treated, compared with untreated subjects, remained. Stratification according to propensity scoring achieved that comparisons were made between groups with almost identical characteristics. This strategy further attenuated the remaining positive association to 1.06 (95% CI, 0.93 to 1.22). No significant association was observed between the use of paroxetine and right ventricular outflow tract obstruction or between sertraline and ventricular septal defects. A similar pattern of increased risk was reported for cardiac malformations in unadjusted analyses, which became insignificant after adjustment was noted for tricyclic antidepressants (TCAs), serotonin-norepinephrine reuptake inhibitors (SNRIs), bupropion, and other antidepressants.[51]

PRETERM BIRTH AND GROWTH EFFECTS

In a meta-analysis, Grote and colleagues[28] reported that maternal MDE or depressive symptoms during pregnancy increase the risk of PTB and LBW. The associations between antenatal depression and adverse outcome included PTB (RR, 1.13; 95% CI, 1.06 to 1.21) and LBW (RR, 1.18; 95% CI, 1.07 to 1.30) but not intrauterine growth restriction (IUGR). The magnitude of risk for PTB and LBW from gestational depression is comparable to the risk of smoking 10 or more cigarettes a day, but it is modest compared with the higher risks associated with black race and substance abuse.[28] In a prospective study ($n = 238$) of pregnant women with MDE, MDE with SSRI treatment, and controls with neither exposure,[48] women who were either continuously treated with an SSRI (23%) or continuously exposed to MDE (21%) experienced PTB. The rates of late and early PTB were similarly distributed. Postnatal weight, head circumference, and length growth trajectories did not differ across the first year in infants exposed to a selective SNRI or to depression or to neither during pregnancy.[52]

BEHAVIORAL TERATOGENICITY

Behavioral teratogenicity refers to long-term postnatal effects on offspring behavior due to prenatal exposure to agents that affect the central nervous system. Cognitive function, temperament, and overall behavior were similar in children who were exposed prenatally to tricyclics or fluoxetine compared with controls.[53-55] Few data about the postbirth development of individuals exposed in utero to SSRIs have been published; however, all converge on the finding that mental development is similar in exposed compared with unexposed children.[56] Nulman and colleagues[57] conducted intelligence testing on 3- to 7-year-old children who had been exposed in utero to an SSRI ($n = 62$) or venlafaxine ($n = 62$) or depression without medication ($n = 54$) and controls ($n = 62$). Exposure group, drug dose, and duration of drug treatment during pregnancy did not significantly affect cognitive function.

In a longitudinal study,[58] 68 infants with prenatal SNRI ($n = 41$) or major depressive disorder exposure ($n = 27$) and 98 non-exposed controls were evaluated with the Bayley Scales of Infant

Development. Neither prenatal exposure to an SNRI nor an MDD significantly impacted overall scores; however, SNRI exposure was associated with lower psychomotor development scores at 26 and 52 weeks compared with nonexposed infants, although this difference was no longer significant at 78 weeks. Although lower psychomotor scores were observed in the first year, the scores remained well within the normative range and were transient.

NEONATAL EFFECTS

Direct serotonergic effects and/or withdrawal signs can occur in neonates after prenatal exposure to antidepressants. Compared with early gestational SSRI exposure or no exposure, late SSRI exposure incurs an overall risk ratio of 3.0 (95% CI, 2.0 to 4.4) for neonatal behavioral syndrome.[59] Most SSRI-related neonatal case reports involve paroxetine and fluoxetine.[48,59] Neonatal signs include central nervous system, motor, respiratory, and gastrointestinal signs that are usually mild and transient with resolution by 2 weeks of age.[60] A severe syndrome that consists of seizures, dehydration, excessive weight loss, hyperpyrexia, or need for intubation is rare in full-term infants (1/313 cases).[59] Based on the premise that neonatal signs are due to direct pharmacologic effects, tapering and discontinuation of the antidepressant over 10 days to 2 weeks before the delivery date with reintroduction of drug immediately after birth has been suggested[59]; however, data to demonstrate improved outcomes for mothers or newborns have not been published. **If a woman has a history of rapid decompensation during antidepressant taper or discontinuation, this strategy is likely to carry more risk to the maternal-fetal pair than continued treatment.**

Recommendations for Treatment During Pregnancy

The American College of Obstetricians and Gynecologists (ACOG) and the American Psychiatric Association developed a consensus document for antidepressant treatment during pregnancy.[61] For mild cases of MDE in pregnant women, psychotherapy is the treatment of choice as the initial intervention. Depressed pregnant women treated with interpersonal psychotherapy had a significant symptomatic improvement compared with a parenting education control group, and 60% of women achieved remission criteria.[37] Other focused, short-term therapies such as cognitive behavioral therapy (CBT) are also effective options for MDE and may be delivered by nonphysician professionals such as psychologists, psychiatric nurse clinicians, or licensed clinical social workers. The cost and accessibility of depression treatment also impacts treatment selection.

For moderate to severe MDE with marked functional impairment, antidepressant pharmacotherapy or combination therapy (medication and psychotherapy) is appropriate. Established efficacy and tolerability of any antidepressant for the individual woman is a strong consideration in drug choice during the risk-benefit decision-making process. Women with chronic or highly recurrent MDE may be on maintenance antidepressant medication when pregnancy occurs. Maintenance antidepressant treatment is recommended after three or more MDEs due to the near-certain likelihood of recurrence. For pregnant women studied in an academic setting, the risk of relapse for those who discontinued antidepressant usage proximate to conception was significantly greater than women who maintained treatment. Among 82 women who continued their medication, 21 (26%) relapsed compared with 44 (68%) of 65 women who discontinued medication.[62] In contrast,

Yonkers and colleagues[63] found that pregnant women who continued antidepressants experienced the same rate of MDE recurrence as women who stopped in a community sample of obstetric patients. Predictive factors for recurrence in both studies were highly recurrent MDE (four or more episodes prior to pregnancy).

DOSAGE CHANGES ACROSS PREGNANCY

All TCAs and SSRIs are at least partially metabolized by cytochrome P450 (CYP) 2D6,[64] which is induced in pregnancy and results in declining serum concentrations. In a publication about managing tricyclic dosages across pregnancy,[65] a strategy to determine the minimum *effective* dose across gestation was suggested. The women selected a target depressive symptom that was most disturbing, typically insomnia or irritability. Women were asked to contact the physician each time the symptom emerged, and an incremental dose was added. **The dosages increased during the second half of pregnancy and rapidly accelerated in the third trimester. The final dose near term was an average of 1.6 times the nonpregnant dose.**

Similarly, the dose requirements and concentration-dose (C/D) ratios of the SSRIs fluoxetine,[66] citalopram, escitalopram, and sertraline[67] changed during pregnancy and postpartum. In the majority of women, the C/D ratios for the parent compound and primary metabolites decreased between 20 weeks' gestation and delivery, which reflects increased drug metabolism. Pharmacogenetic characterization is not a standard of care for antidepressant therapy; however, Ververs and colleagues[68] showed that CYP 2D6 genotypes predicted plasma paroxetine concentrations during pregnancy. Women who were extensive metabolizers (n = 43) and ultrarapid metabolizers (n = 1) showed steadily *decreasing* plasma paroxetine concentrations across pregnancy. In contrast, plasma paroxetine levels of intermediate metabolizers (n = 25) and poor metabolizers (n = 5) *increased* during pregnancy. Weight gain, maternal age, and smoking did not influence drug concentrations. In extensive and ultrarapid metabolizers, the depressive symptoms increased significantly during the course of pregnancy. Paroxetine is unique among the SSRIs in having 2D6 as the sole metabolic pathway. **For TCAs and most SSRIs, dose requirements often increase during the second half of pregnancy to offset greater drug metabolism. Serial administration of a quantitative depression measure is recommended to identify early symptoms of relapse. The goal is to provide optimal drug dosing across the changing milieu of pregnancy to maximally reduce disease burden.**

INTEGRATIVE TREATMENTS

Known as a treatment for seasonal (winter) MDE, **light therapy** is also efficacious for nonseasonal MDE. Bright light, delivered as an early morning bolus of 10,000 lux illuminance with commercially available boxes, is an efficacious treatment for MDE. The light units conform to stringent standards, with illumination of a broad visual field, lighting from above to avoid glare, and ultraviolet screening. Light therapy for pregnant women with MDE was explored in a small randomized controlled trial (RCT)[69] with bright white versus dim (inactive) arms. The response rates were significantly greater for bright compared with dim light after 5 weeks of 1 hour of early morning light and were comparable to antidepressant treatment. A clinician's guide is available.[70]

Manber and colleagues[71] performed an RCT (n = 150) of **acupuncture treatment** specific to MDE, acupuncture treatment targeted to a condition other than MDE, and a comparison group that received massage. Women who received acupuncture specific for MDE had a significantly greater response rate than those who received the other treatments; again, this response was comparable to that of standard MDE treatments.

Poor nutrition may contribute to the pathogenesis of MDE. Folate and vitamin B_{12} are needed for single-carbon metabolism involved in the synthesis of serotonin and other monoamine neurotransmitters and catecholamines. Folate, B_{12}, iron, zinc, and selenium deficiencies are more common among depressed than nondepressed persons.[72] The depletion of nutrient reserves throughout pregnancy and lactation may increase a woman's risk for MDE. Marginal or low folate status also increases the likelihood of nonresponse to antidepressant medication as well as the probability of relapse. Several RCTs have demonstrated that **folic acid** is an efficacious augmentation strategy for antidepressant medications.[72]

Omega-3 fatty acids are essential long-chain polyunsaturated fatty acids found in nerve cell membranes. Eicosapentaenoic acid (EPA) and docosahexaenoic acid (DHA) are derived primarily from fish. The American diet is relatively deficient in omega-3 compared with omega-6 fatty acids and other fats. Increased requirements during pregnancy raise the risk of deficiency and potentially of MDE. In cross-national studies, an inverse relationship has been shown between per capita fish intake and prevalence rates of MDE, postpartum MDE, and bipolar disorder.[73] Supplementation with 1 gram of EPA and DHA has been recommended for patients with mood disorders.[74] Omega-3 fatty acids have been used to treat perinatal MDE in small RCTs, but efficacy beyond placebo has not been convincingly demonstrated.[73] However, DHA supplementation may attenuate the effects of maternal stress during late pregnancy and can reduce fetal exposure to glucocorticoids in women living in urban low-income environments.[75] Women who received supplementation reported less stress and had lower levels of stress hormones in the third trimester than placebo-treated women. Omega-3 fatty acids have antiinflammatory effects[76] that may contribute to the mechanism of action.

Treatment of Major Depressive Episode in the Postpartum Period

Medications effective for MDE in women outside of childbearing are effective during childbearing.[77] In a randomized comparative efficacy trial, the tricyclic nortriptyline (NTP; $n = 54$) was compared with sertraline ($n = 55$),[78] and the response rates were equal. The dosing started with 10 mg for NTP and 25 mg sertraline for 2 days then 50 mg/day thereafter, and it was increased every 2 weeks to a maximum of 150 and 200 mg/day, respectively. The total side effect burden for both drugs was similar, although the types differed for each drug. A major finding was that the dose of sertraline required for remission in this 8-week, double blind protocol was 100 mg/day or more, with many women requiring 150 to 200 mg/day. **The starting dose of sertraline 50 mg/day was not efficacious in the majority of women, and dose adjustment should be anticipated approximately 2 weeks after treatment initiation.** An RCT of sertraline versus placebo demonstrated efficacy for sertraline[79] with a mean dose of 100 ± 54 mg/day.

In a small novel RCT of the efficacy of estradiol treatment, women with severe postpartum MDE were randomized to placebo or estradiol delivered by transdermal patch (200 μg/day) for 6 months.[80] By 3 months, 80% of the estradiol-treated

and 31% of the placebo-treated group responded. Endometrial changes were found in three participants at the end of the study, despite coadministration of dydrogesterone (10 mg/day, 12 days/month in the final 3 months of the RCT). The changes resolved at follow-up. The inclusion of women who took concurrent antidepressant medications limits the ability to discern an estradiol-specific effect. Little is known about estradiol secretion into breast milk; however, it was not detected in the milk of 18 women who used transdermal estradiol 50 to 100 μg/day for 12 weeks.[81]

Prevention of Postpartum-Onset Major Depressive Episode

To reduce the risk for postpartum MDE, an interpersonal therapy-based group intervention was provided to pregnant women on public assistance. Within 3 months after delivery, 20% of the women in standard care developed postpartum MDE compared with 4% of women who received the intervention.[82] Studies of antidepressants or hormones for the prevention of postpartum MDE are limited to three RCTs,[77] with one small RCT demonstrating the efficacy of sertraline.[83] Women with a history of MDE were treated with sertraline immediately following birth to prevent the onset of MDE. The dosing protocol was, in mg/day, 25 for 4 days, then 40 through week 4, and 75 thereafter. The duration of preventive treatment was a minimum of 6 months. The explanation for sertraline's efficacy is based on its serotonergic impact; therefore, use of another serotonergic drug, particularly one to which the woman had previously responded, is appropriate. Although open studies supported that progesterone prevented recurrence, a placebo-controlled RCT of a synthetic progesterone *increased* the risk of depression after birth.[84]

Treatment During Breastfeeding

The magnitude of antidepressant exposure through breast milk is substantially lower than during pregnancy (Table 55-1). Comprehensive reviews of antidepressant drugs in maternal serum, breast milk, and infant serum have been published.[77] Sertraline or paroxetine (among SSRIs) and nortriptyline (among TCAs) are agents of choice. These drugs are characterized by undetectable or very low breastfed-infant serum concentrations and no reports of adverse events. However, established efficacy of another drug for the woman must be considered strongly in the decision-making process. Although TCAs are reasonable treatments for postpartum MDE, they are second-line drugs due to their toxicity in overdose. More recently released antidepressants are second-line choices for breastfeeding women unless efficacy in prior episodes has been established.

The clinical condition of breastfed infants, particularly those who are sick or LBW, should be monitored to detect adverse effects that may be associated with the maternal drug (behavioral activation or sedation, new-onset feeding or sleeping problems; see Chapter 24). Routine laboratory measurement of serum drug levels in healthy full-term infants is not warranted; however, serum concentrations in preterm and sick infants have not been described and would be a welcome contribution to the literature.

Psychiatric Disorders and Suicidal Ideations

Oates[85] performed an evaluation of the Confidential Enquiry into Maternal Deaths from the United Kingdom. Psychiatric disorder, and suicide specifically, was the leading cause of

TABLE 55-1 SELECTED ANTIDEPRESSANT LEVELS IN BREASTFED INFANTS' SERA

ANTIDEPRESSANT DRUG[†]	SERUM LEVEL RANGE IN BREASTFED INFANTS	TYPICAL MATERNAL DOSE RANGE (mg/day)
Nortriptyline*	Nortriptyline, below limit of quantifiability to 10 ng/mL	50-150; maternal therapeutic serum levels are 50 to 150 ng/mL
Nortriptyline metabolites	E-10-OH–nortriptyline = <4-16 ng/mL Z-10-OH–nortriptyline = <4-17 ng/mL	
Sertraline	Sertraline, below limit of quantifiability to 8 ng/mL	50-200
Sertraline metabolites	Norsertraline, below limit of quantifiability to 26 ng/mL	
Paroxetine	Paroxetine, below limit of quantifiability	10-60
No active metabolites		
Fluoxetine	Fluoxetine, below quantifiability to 340 ng/mL	20-60
Fluoxetine metabolite[‡]	Norfluoxetine, below quantifiability to 265 ng/mL	
Citalopram	Citalopram, below quantifiability to 12.7 ng/mL	20-40
Citalopram metabolite	Desmethylcitalopram, below quantifiability to 3.1 ng/mL	
Venlafaxine	Venlafaxine, below quantifiability to 5 ng/mL	75-300
Venlafaxine metabolite	O-desmethylvenlafaxine, below quantifiability to 38 ng/mL	
Bupropion	Average infant exposure expected to be 2% of the standard maternal dose on a molar basis; infant serum levels not measured in largest series ($n = 10$)[§]	300
Multiple metabolites		

*The most-studied tricyclic antidepressant during breastfeeding, this class of drugs is now used infrequently.
[†]Established efficacy of an antidepressant in a woman is a strong consideration in drug selection.
[‡]As active as fluoxetine, this metabolite has a longer half-life than the parent drug.
[§]Haas JS, et al. Bupropion in breast milk: an exposure assessment for potential treatment to prevent post-partum tobacco use. *Tobacco Control.* 2004;13(1):52-56.

mortality and accounted for 28% of maternal deaths. Women also died of other complications related to psychiatric disorders and substance abuse, and they died violently. In a large scale study[86] of 10,000 women screened with the EPDS, the proportions of response on item 10—"The thought of harming myself has occurred to me"—were for 0, or *never,* 96.81% ($n = 9681$); for 1, or *hardly ever,* 2.46% ($n = 246$); for 2, or *sometimes,* 0.65% ($n = 65$); and for 3, or *yes quite often,* it was .08% ($n = 8$). In this group of 10,000 women screened by phone, 3.2% of women had suicidal ideation.

Suicide assessment requires direct questioning of the patient about her desire to live or die, specific thoughts about killing herself, plans for carrying out the act, and access to and lethality of means.[87] The American Psychiatric Association guidelines for the assessment of suicidal behaviors provide a comprehensive list of questions that help clinicians assess suicidal thoughts, plans, and behaviors.[88] Initial questions address patients' feelings about living (Have you ever thought that life was not worth living? Did you ever wish you could go to sleep and just not wake up?) and are followed by questions that address specific thoughts about death, self-harm, and suicide (Have things ever reached the point that you've thought of harming yourself?). If thoughts of self-harm are endorsed, clinicians should evaluate the details such as the intensity, frequency, timing, persistence, and circumstances. Physicians must also ask whether the patient has made a specific plan for self-harm. Ask about pills, household poisons, and firearms. Has the patient made preparations to enact the plan or for after her death (purchasing the means, writing a will, arranging for child care)? If the safety of the patient is at risk, emergency psychiatric consultation or involuntary commitment is indicated.

The practice guidelines[88] identify situations in which suicide assessment is warranted: emergency department evaluation, an abrupt change in clinical symptoms, lack of improvement or worsening despite treatment, anticipation or experience of an interpersonal loss or stressor (divorce, loss of custody of children, financial loss, legal problems), or a physical illness associated with a threat to life, severe pain, or loss of function. Patients with increased risk are those with previous suicide attempts,

major mood disorders (particularly bipolar disorder), schizophrenia, and substance use.

Bipolar Disorder
Diagnosis and Prevalence
The diagnosis of MDE is limited to the lifetime experience of normal mood with episodes of depression, whereas bipolar disorder (BD) includes normal, depressed, and elevated or irritable mood states (mania or its less intense form, hypomania). Changes in energy and activity levels parallel variations in mood. *Mania* is a persistent, abnormally euphoric, expansive or irritable mood state with inflated self-esteem, agitation, heightened energy, racing thoughts, pressured speech, impulsive behaviors, distractibility, and poor judgment for a minimum of 1 week. Impairment in function must be present. *Hypomania* is defined by a minimum of 4 continuous days of persistent increased creativity, productivity, and sociability or increased irritability that family or coworkers notice. The woman's function may be enhanced by creativity and increased energy. In women, **depression is the predominant mood state and is frequently mistaken for unipolar depression.** Atypical depression—characterized by increased appetite, weight gain, hypersomnia, low energy, heaviness—is more common in women with BD and typically starts in the fall or winter and resolves in spring.

The lifetime prevalence of BD is 1% to 2%.[89,90] BD type I, which affects women and men equally,[91] is characterized by MDE and periods of mania or hypomania.[91] Bipolar variants that are more common in women than men include BD type II (MDE and hypomania), mixed episodes (intermingled manic and depressive symptoms), and rapid cycling (four or more episodes of opposite polarity in one year). Women with BD often have comorbid anxiety disorders, alcohol or substance (especially *Cannabis*) use disorders, bulimia nervosa,[92] childhood or adult physical and/or sexual abuse, and medical problems that include migraines, metabolic syndrome, pain disorders, and hypothyroidism.

The differentiation of MDE from BD is a major challenge, and delays of 7 to 11 years until diagnosis of BD is common.[93]

Prescribing antidepressants without an antimanic drug can complicate treatment by increasing rapid cycling, mania, or mixed episodes. The most commonly used measure is the Mood Disorders Questionnaire (MDQ)[94] shown in Figure 55-3, which assesses lifetime history of mania with 13 yes/no symptoms and two questions: a yes/no query about whether symptoms occurred during the same time period and a designation of the magnitude of the resulting problems (none, minor, moderate, serious). A positive screen requires *more than* seven symptoms during the same period that caused moderate or serious problems. Our team studied use of the MDQ with the EPDS as a combined screening tool in a postpartum population with follow-up diagnosis by a research psychiatric interview.[95] The addition of the MDQ to the EPDS identified BD in 50% of women with traditional scoring, and it reached almost 70% when the MDQ was scored without the impairment criterion. **Based on this study, we recommend the MDQ or a diagnostic assessment for BD be given prior to prescribing antidepressants for a postpartum depressed woman.**

Natural History Across Childbearing

The course of episodes is useful in evaluating recurrence risk during pregnancy. Women with episodes that occur only after delivery are not likely to relapse during pregnancy even without medication.[96] However, women with a chronic course are likely to be symptomatic during pregnancy, and maintenance medication is appropriate. For women with chronic BD, discontinuation of drug treatment proximal to conception incurred a high risk for recurrence (86%) compared with patients who continued treatment (37%).[97] **After delivery, all women with BD are at high risk for recurrent mood episodes.**[98,99]

Postpartum psychosis is typically a manifestation of BD such as mania, mixed state, or depression with psychotic features.[100] It occurs in 1 to 2 per 1000 births in the first month following delivery. Women are more vulnerable to psychosis in the post-birth period than at any other time during their lives. In the first 30 days after birth, a woman is 21.7 times more likely to develop psychosis than in the 2-year period prior to childbirth. If she has not had a child before, she is 35 times more likely to suffer psychosis than women who have children.[101] The magnitude of these relative risks demonstrates that postpartum psychiatric morbidity is a major public health problem.[102,103] The mechanism for the vulnerability of postpartum women with BD for decompensation and psychosis have not been elucidated. Sleep deprivation and marked interference with circadian rhythms related to labor are likely contributors to mood instability.[100] Hormone elevations near the end of gestation and massive postpartum withdrawal also contribute to the risk.[104] **The clinical picture of postpartum psychosis is characterized by rapid onset of hectic mood fluctuations; marked cognitive impairment suggestive of delirium; bizarre behavior; insomnia; visual and auditory hallucinations, including unusual (tactile and olfactory) hallucinations; and impaired judgment and insight.**[105] Specific types of delusional thoughts are related to the risk for infanticide. Delusional altruistic homicide, often associated with maternal suicide, to save both mother and infant "from a fate worse than death" was reported in a review of filicides,[106] that is, killing one's son or daughter. Resnick[106] observed that 40% of the perpetrators of filicide had seen physicians shortly before the tragedy. Sensitive, direct questions about thoughts of harm to the infant are imperative in the examination. Nonjudgmental inquiry can be made as follows: "Some

new mothers have thoughts such as wishing the baby were dead or about harming the baby; has this happened to you?"

The risk for adverse pregnancy outcomes is increased in women with mental illness. A population cohort study demonstrated that women with BD had an increased frequency of placenta previa and antepartum hemorrhage compared with euthymic women.[107]

Treatment of Bipolar Disorder During Childbearing

Medication maintenance is the mainstay of treatment for BD, although psychotherapy and education are also important. Early identification of BD and rapid initiation of treatment results in lower rates of relapse, increased time to recurrence, improved medication adherence, and better function.[108] Because abrupt discontinuation of mood stabilizers increases the risk for recurrence,[109] education about adherence and drug tapering for discontinuation is advisable.

Several classes of drugs are effective for the treatment of mania. Lithium, some antiepileptic drugs (AEDs), and atypical antipsychotic drugs are efficacious; however, these treatments provide response in only 36% to 50% of cases,[1] and patients often receive more than one drug to manage their mood symptoms. **To minimize fetal exposure, strategies include (1) use using the lowest *effective* doses, (2) minimizing the number of drugs taken, and (3) dividing daily doses to avoid high peak serum concentrations, unless compliance will be compromised.**

LITHIUM

Lithium is the standard drug for acute and maintenance therapy for BD. Before initiating lithium treatment, assessment of renal and thyroid function is necessary. The starting dose is 300 mg twice daily. Serum drug concentration and renal function tests should be repeated after 5 to 7 days of treatment. The target serum trough concentration is 0.4 to 1.0 mEq/L at 12 hours. Treatment response is usually achieved at 900 to 1200 mg daily. Due to the physiologic changes of pregnancy, monthly lithium levels are recommended in the first and second trimester with dose adjustment to achieve the prepregnancy concentration that was efficacious. In the final gestational and first postpartum month, weekly lithium levels may need to be measured.[100] Common side effects of lithium include sedation, tremor, renal dysfunction, weight gain, nausea, vomiting, and diarrhea. Toxic effects are associated with somnolence, confusion, severe tremors, renal dysfunction, and intractable vomiting. Women with vomiting are especially vulnerable to toxicity due to fluid loss. Lithium toxicity is managed with drug discontinuation, rehydration therapy, and monitoring of fluid and electrolyte balance and renal function. Diuretics and nonsteroidal antiinflammatory drugs (NSAIDs), which can impair renal clearance, should be avoided in lithium-treated patients.

Lithium exposure during the first trimester was associated with an increased risk for Ebstein anomaly. Subsequent prospective studies demonstrated that the risk was overestimated due to voluntary reporting to a registry, which inflated the number of cases (numerator) and underestimated the magnitude of population exposed (denominator).[100] **The absolute risk of Ebstein anomaly with first-trimester exposure is 1/1000 to 1/2000, 20 to 40 times higher than in the general population.**[100] Lithium-exposed neonates are at risk for being large for gestational age and for hypotonia, feeding difficulties, depressed reflexes, cyanosis, apnea, bradycardia, hypothyroidism,

THE MOOD DISORDER QUESTIONNAIRE

Instructions: Please answer each question to the best of your ability.

	YES	NO
1. Has there ever been a period of time when you were not your usual self and...		
...you felt so good or so hyper that other people thought you were not your normal self or you were so hyper that you got into trouble?	○	○
...you were so irritable that you shouted at people or started fights or arguments?	○	○
...you felt much more self-confident than usual?	○	○
...you got much less sleep than usual and found you didn't really miss it?	○	○
...you were much more talkative or spoke much faster than usual?	○	○
...thoughts raced through your head or you couldn't slow your mind down?	○	○
...you were so easily distracted by things around you that you had trouble concentrating or staying on track?	○	○
...you had much more energy than usual?	○	○
...you were much more active or did many more things than usual?	○	○
...you were much more social or outgoing than usual, for example, you telephoned friends in the middle of the night?	○	○
...you were much more interested in sex than usual?	○	○
...you did things that were unusual for you or that other people might have thought were excessive, foolish, or risky?	○	○
...spending money got you or your family into trouble?	○	○
2. If you checked YES to more than one of the above, have several of these ever happened during the same period of time?	○	○

3. How much of a problem did any of these cause you – like being unable to work; having family, money or legal troubles; getting into arguments or fights? *Please circle one response only.*

No Problem   Minor Problem   Moderate Problem   Serious Problem

	YES	NO
4. Have any of your blood relatives (i.e. children, siblings, parents, grandparents, aunts, uncles) had manic-depressive illness or bipolar disorder?	○	○
5. Has a health professional ever told you that you have manic-depressive illness or bipolar disorder?	○	○

© 2000 by The University of Texas Medical Branch. Reprinted with permission. This instrument is designed for screening purposes only and is not to be used as a diagnostic tool.

FIG 55-3 Mood Disorder Questionnaire. This instrument is designed for screening purposes only and is not to be used as a diagnostic tool. (Courtesy The University of Texas Medical Branch.)

and diabetes insipidus.[100] The neonatal symptoms are temporary and are associated with maternal serum concentrations at delivery of greater than 0.64 mEq/L.[110] The suspension of lithium dosing 24 to 48 hours before a scheduled delivery or at onset of labor reduces the risk for perinatal complications.[110] Developmental milestones are normal in infants exposed in utero to lithium.[100]

VALPROIC ACID

Valproic acid (VPA) was the first AED for mania approved by the Food and Drug Administration (FDA). The starting dose is 500 to 750 mg daily in divided doses, and therapeutic levels range from 50 to 125 µg/mL. Adverse effects include nausea, weight gain, fatigue, tremor, ataxia, diarrhea, abdominal pain, alopecia, hepatitis, thrombocytopenia, and pancreatitis.

Exposure to VPA is associated with increased risk for serious adverse outcomes that include all birth defects (OR, 10.7; 95% CI, 8.2 to 13.3),[111] **developmental delay, and fetal death compared with other AEDs** (see Chapters 8 and 48.)[112] With exposure to multiple AEDs, women have a twofold to fivefold increased risk for major malformations and for having offspring with cognitive impairment compared with monotherapy.[113] Rates of malformations from polytherapy were 6.0% compared with 3.7% for monotherapy.[113,114] VPA is concentrated in the fetal compartment, and provision of the lowest effective dose in divided doses is recommended to avoid high single peak levels.[100] Complications associated with VPA use near delivery include fetal decelerations and infant irritability, jitteriness, feeding difficulties, abnormal tone, hepatic toxicity, hypoglycemia, and reduction in neonatal fibrinogen levels. At birth, cord blood concentrations of VPA can reach twice the maternal levels.[100,113,115]

Meador and colleagues[116] evaluated the intelligence quotient (IQ) in 6-year-old children ($n = 224$) who had been exposed to AEDs in utero, with adjustment for maternal IQ, AED drug type, standardized dose, gestational birth age, and use of periconceptional folate. **The offspring IQs were lower after exposure to VPA** (mean 97; 95% CI, 94 to 101) **than after carbamazepine** (mean 105; 95% CI, 102 to 108; $P = .00015$) **or lamotrigine** (mean 108; 95% CI, 105 to 110; $P = .00003$). A dose-response relationship was observed for VPA, but no other AED, with negative impact on offspring IQ, verbal and nonverbal ability, memory, and executive function. For all AED exposures, the mean IQs were higher in children whose mothers received folate (108; 95% CI, 106 to 111) than in the offspring of non–folate treated mothers (101; 95% CI, 98 to 104; $P = .00009$). Because over half of pregnancies are unplanned and the impact on neural tube development occurs 17 to 30 days postconception, women treated with maintenance VPA are exposed during this critical period, often *before* awareness of pregnancy. **These findings dictate against use of VPA as a first-line drug for childbearing-aged women.**[117]

CARBAMAZEPINE AND OXCARBAZEPINE

Carbamazepine (CBZ) is prescribed at doses between 400 and 1600 mg daily to achieve a target range of 4 to 12 µg/mL. Drug-induced toxicity is usually detectable from clinical symptoms, and the serum level provides objective evidence. During pregnancy, the total AED levels drop, but the amount of unbound bioavailable drug remains constant. Serum concentrations are useful in the assessment of patients with exacerbation of mood symptoms, side effects, and questionable treatment adherence.

Hepatitis, leukopenia, thrombocytopenia, rash, sedation, and ataxia are CBZ side effects. Due to the additive effects on bone marrow suppression, combining CBZ and the antipsychotic clozapine is contraindicated.

The American Academy of Neurology (AAN) committee[113] found no increased risk of major malformations in the offspring of women who received CBZ for epilepsy. However, infants exposed to CBZ had twice the risk for being small for gestational age (SGA) and to have low Apgar scores (<7) at delivery. Exposed children did not have reduced cognitive function on measures of IQ and developmental milestones compared with children who were not exposed to AEDs.[113] Fetal serum levels of CBZ are 50% to 80% of maternal levels.[118] **Because adequate levels of vitamin K are necessary for normal midfacial growth and for the functioning of clotting factors, CBZ exposure in utero could increase the risk of neonatal bleeding.**[100] Some experts recommend treatment with vitamin K 20 mg/day throughout pregnancy[119] and 1 mg intramuscularly to neonates.

Oxcarbazepine has been used to treat mania in divided doses totaling 600 to 1200 mg/day. The parent compound is rapidly metabolized to an active hydroxy metabolite, which undergoes hepatic glucuronidation and renal excretion. Adverse effects are hyponatremia, hypersensitivity reactions, and decreased thyroxine levels (without altered triiodothyronine or thyroid-stimulating hormone [TSH]). Side effects include headaches, dizziness, gait disturbance, fatigue, and concentration changes. In 55 infants exposed in utero to oxcarbazepine (20 combination therapy, 35 monotherapy), one cardiac malformation was reported in an infant also exposed to phenobarbital.[120]

LAMOTRIGINE

Lamotrigine (LTG) is indicated for bipolar depression maintenance therapy.[121] Typical doses range from 50 to 200 mg/day, but doses up to 500 mg/day have been used for long-term treatment of patients with BD. Side effects include headaches, rash, dizziness, diarrhea, abnormal dreams, and pruritus.[117] Aseptic meningitis is a rare but serious potential complication of treatment with LTG. The rash associated with LTG is maculopapular or erythematous in appearance[122] and is associated with rapid dose escalation, combination with VPA, and treatment in adolescents.[123] A retrospective analysis from 12 studies[122] indicated that the rates of benign rash were 8.3% in LTG-treated and 6.4% in placebo-treated patients. In contrast, serious rash occurred in none of the LTG-treated and in only 0.1% of placebo-treated patients. One case of Stevens-Johnson syndrome occurred in an LTG-treated patient. Although this syndrome may be life threatening, the very low risk of serious rash must be weighed against the much more common risks associated with untreated BD.[122]

Continuing LTG reduces the risk of recurrences in pregnant women with BD. Thirty percent of women who continued, versus all who stopped LTG, relapsed during pregnancy (OR, 23.2; 95% CI, 1.5 to 366).[124] Patients who stopped treatment suffered relapses within 2 weeks. Because LTG clearance increases by 65% to 90% in the second and third trimesters compared with preconception, patients usually require higher doses during pregnancy. Guidelines for managing dosing across childbearing have been published.[125] The LTG serum concentration that was efficacious before pregnancy is the target level to be maintained by dose adjustment throughout pregnancy. The metabolism of LTG returns to the prepregnancy state rapidly after birth. To avoid maternal toxicity (dizziness, tremor, and diplopia), the dose should be reduced by 20% to 25% within 3 days of birth and across the first weeks postpartum based on serum concentrations.

The rate of congenital malformations is similar in infants exposed in utero to LTG compared with the general population, but the rate increases when LTG is combined with other AEDs.[113] Recent studies indicate that the risk for orofacial cleft malformations is not increased in LTG-exposed offspring.[126]

ATYPICAL ANTIPSYCHOTICS

Antipsychotic drugs, including the first-generation agents ("typical," such as haloperidol) **and the second-generation agents** ("atypical," such as olanzapine) **are effective treatments for BD** and also for schizophrenia (see the discussion of atypical antipsychotics in the section "Treatment Interventions for Women With Schizophrenia" later in this chapter). Indications include maintenance therapy to prevent recurrence, bipolar depression (quetiapine and combined olanzapine-fluoxetine), and treatment-resistant depression. The usual dose ranges are 5 to 20 mg for olanzapine; 1 to 6 mg for risperidone; 100 to 400 mg, maximum 800 mg, for quetiapine; 80 to 160 mg for ziprasidone; and for aripiprazole, 5 to 30 mg. The initial treatment is started at a lower dose and is titrated against response and tolerance.

The atypical agents are associated with fewer extrapyramidal side effects (tardive dyskinesia, tremor, rigidity, internal restlessness, slowed movements, and dystonia) compared with the older typical antipsychotic agents. Side effects include somnolence, increased hepatic transaminases, and hyperprolactinemia.[127] **In pregnancy, the metabolic side effects of the psychotropic drugs, particularly the atypical agents, are a major concern.**[128] **Patients are at risk for weight gain, metabolic syndrome, elevated triglycerides, and glucose intolerance.**[129] Obesity is associated with complications that include gestational diabetes, preeclampsia, caesarean delivery, and large-for-gestational age (LGA) infants.[130,131]

The reproductive risks of atypical antipsychotics have received minimal research attention. Pregnant women who received either typical or atypical drugs had increased risks for PTB, LBW, and major malformations compared with the general population, but these complications may reflect the effects of the underlying psychiatric disorder. Genetic liability and gene-environment interactions contribute to these outcomes, and maternal risk factors, substance abuse, nutritional status, and the biologic and behavioral concomitants of severe mental illness are likely to be the major determinants of increases in reproductive pathology. Rates of malformations, mainly atrial and ventricular septal defects, are variable; some reports suggest that only infants with exposure to the typical agents were affected,[131] whereas other data demonstrate an increased risk for malformations in women exposed to atypical antipsychotic drugs compared with controls (OR, 2.17; 95% CI, 1.20 to 3.91).[132]

Rates of PTB are increased in patients treated with antipsychotics. However, infants with fetal exposure to the typical drugs weighed less (3158 g ± 440) than the infants exposed to the atypical (3391 g ± 446) or non-antipsychotic drugs (3382 g ± 384).[133] Infants who were significantly LGA were born to mothers who received atypical (20%) compared with typical agents (2%) or non-antipsychotic drugs (3%).[133] In addition, postnatal complications occurred significantly more often in infants prenatally exposed to atypical (15.6%) and typical (21.6%) antipsychotics compared with 4.2% of non–teratogen exposed women. The frequency of stillbirth or

neonatal deaths was not increased compared with the baseline population.

A national pregnancy registry for atypical antipsychotics has been established (http://womensmentalhealth.org/posts/pregnancy-registry). As of April of 2014, 408 women had enrolled with 300 women in the exposed group and 108 women in the comparison group. Rates of major malformations in the two groups were similar: 1.5% (3/200 live births) in the group exposed to atypical antipsychotics and 1.2% (1/84) in the comparison group, a nonsignificant difference but a small sample.

ALTERNATE AND SUPPLEMENTAL TREATMENT OPTIONS

An inverse correlation between omega-3 fatty acid consumption and the prevalence of BD has been demonstrated.[134] An increased duration of remission in patients with BD who were randomized to fish oil versus placebo was reported.[73] Electroconvulsive therapy (ECT) is highly effective for the management of treatment-resistant depression, acute mania, and severe mixed episodes.[100,135] ECT involves delivering an electrical stimulus with a brief pulse device to induce a limited grand mal seizure blocked from peripheral expression by succinylcholine. During ECT, the patient receives short-acting anesthetic agents, which are not likely to cause adverse impact on the mother-infant pair.[100,135]

Prevention of Bipolar Disorder Recurrence Postpartum

The risk for recurrence of mania, depression, or mixed states postpartum is the highest at any point in a woman's life. In women who discontinued lithium therapy,[136] the rates of recurrence in the postpartum period were almost three times that of the nonpregnant women over a similar time (70% vs. 24%). Moreover, among women who had previous postpartum psychosis, more than 40% experienced relapse after declining immediate postpartum lithium prophylaxis, and no woman who began medication immediately postpartum had a recurrence.[96] The postpartum pharmacotherapy plan includes selection of the drugs of past response[100] and educating partners to observe and report early symptoms to prevent episodes.

Breastfeeding for Women with Bipolar Disorder

The mother's desire to breastfeed is an important consideration in the postpartum management (see Chapter 24). Successful lactation may be compromised by not breastfeeding through the night in the early postpartum period; however, sleep deprivation is a major factor in precipitating mania. If a partner or family member can provide support and feed the baby at night, sleep can be preserved.

The American Academy of Pediatrics (AAP)[137] and the AAN[138] concluded that most medications used to treat BD produce breast milk concentrations less than 10% of the mother's weight-adjusted concentrations. A multicenter longitudinal observational study of monotherapy of AEDs examined the impact of breastfeeding on IQ at 3 years age for CBZ, LTG, and VPA.[139] Breastfed children did not differ from formula-fed children. However, the concentrations of LTG in breastfed infants averaged 30% to 35% of that of the mother. The risk for toxicity may be increased in breastfeeding infants of women who receive additional similarly metabolized agents such as lorazepam, aspirin, olanzapine, acetaminophen, and VPA.

Lithium treatment can be managed in breastfeeding women with education and close follow-up.[137,140] In a case series of 10 mother-infant pairs,[140] infant serum lithium concentrations were 25% of maternal levels. In another study of three infants,[141] infant concentrations ranged from 10% to 17% of maternal levels. Caregivers should monitor the infant for signs of toxicity (poor feeding, lethargy, and hypotonia), especially in situations that increase the risk for dehydration (reduced feeding/oral intake, excessive fluid loss or fever).[100] To avoid spuriously high levels of lithium, infant blood samples must be collected in tubes that do not contain lithium heparin as the stabilizing agent.

ANXIETY DISORDERS

Diagnosis and Prevalence

Anxiety disorders comprise panic disorder, generalized anxiety disorder, obsessive-compulsive disorder (OCD), posttraumatic stress disorder (PTSD), and agoraphobia and other phobias. Each of these disorders is distinct and is defined by specific diagnostic criteria according to DSM-V.[1] Many individuals have subclinical anxiety symptoms. **To meet criteria for the diagnosis of an anxiety disorder, the symptoms must cause impairment of functioning.** In women, the lifetime prevalence of anxiety disorders is 5%; panic disorder, 5%; generalized anxiety disorder, 3%; OCD, 6%; social phobia and other specific phobias, 13%; and 10% for and PTSD.[142-144] Multiple anxiety disorders are often present in an individual. Without treatment, anxiety disorders usually have a chronic course. **Although rates of OCD are similar in men and women, all other anxiety disorders are 1.5 to 2 times more common in women. In addition, women with anxiety disorders have an increased risk for development of comorbid MDE.**

Panic attacks are characterized by brief (5- to 15-minute) intense episodes of fear or discomfort that occur in many anxiety disorders and in healthy individuals exposed to acute stress. Symptoms include palpitations, sweating, shortness of breath, choking, nausea, abdominal discomfort, dizziness, unsteadiness, numbness or tingling, chills, hot flashes, or a fear of dying or losing control. Panic disorder is diagnosed when attacks are recurrent or associated with a fear of future attacks. The most disabling consequence of panic disorder is agoraphobia, which occurs in 30% to 40% of women with untreated panic disorder. Patients with agoraphobia restrict activities outside the home or insist on being accompanied by a trusted person due to fear of having a panic attack where help is unavailable.

Generalized anxiety disorder is characterized by excessive worrying about multiple problems. The issues of concern to persons with generalized anxiety disorder are realistic, but the level of worry is much more intense than appropriate. For example, a woman might worry for hours about whether a friend received a thank you note for a gift. Individuals with generalized anxiety disorder have symptoms associated with worry, such as muscle tension, fatigue, headache, nausea, diarrhea, or abdominal pain.

In contrast to generalized anxiety disorder, women with **obsessive-compulsive disorder** focus on more idiosyncratic and often unrealistic concerns. OCD is characterized by disturbing intrusive thoughts and performance of compulsions to temporarily relieve the distress generated by the intrusive thoughts. Obsessional thoughts usually focus on a few key themes: contamination, causing harm, offensive violent or sexual images, religious preoccupations, and urges for symmetry or ordering. Compulsions performed to relieve these intrusive worries include cleaning or washing, checking, repeating, ordering, hoarding, and mental rituals like counting and praying. During pregnancy

and postpartum, contamination concerns and intrusive violent thoughts are particularly common.[145] Differentiating obsessional thoughts and images from delusions and hallucinations can be challenging.[146] **New mothers with OCD may experience disturbing obsessions and mental images of harming their baby. They are highly distressed by these thoughts yet are not at increased risk of harming their infant.**

Exposure to trauma in which a woman experienced or witnessed an event that involved actual or threatened death or serious injury is required for a diagnosis of **posttraumatic stress disorder (PTSD).** The traumatic event is persistently reexperienced in one or more of the following ways: (1) recurrent and intrusive distressing recollections, (2) recurrent distressing dreams, (3) acting or feeling as if the event were occurring in the present (flashbacks), (4) intense distress at cues that remind her of the event, (5) physiologic hyperarousal, and (6) exaggerated startle responses. Symptoms must persist for at least 1 month to meet diagnostic criteria for PTSD. Minimal study has been done of whether birth trauma can result in a new onset or recurrence of PTSD. Preliminary estimates suggest an incidence of 3% for delivery-related PTSD in community samples and as high as 15% in high-risk samples.[147]

Separation anxiety is another type of anxiety focused on potential harm coming to self or others that would disrupt a close relationship. Women with separation anxiety can experience mental distress, nightmares, and physical anxiety symptoms associated with separation or the threat of separation.

Finally, excessive fear of a discrete object or situation constitutes a **phobia.** *Social phobia* refers to disabling fears of speaking or eating in public and fears of humiliation in social interactions. Other common specific phobias are body injury phobia (medical procedures), acrophobia (heights), arachnophobia (spiders), and claustrophobia (enclosed spaces). Individuals with panic disorder often have fear of situations from which they could not escape if they had a panic attack (airplanes). These fears are a feature of panic disorder and agoraphobia and would not warrant a diagnosis of phobia.

Fear of Labor and Delivery

Some women have intense fear of pregnancy and childbirth. About 5% to 10% of pregnant women have extreme fear of delivery, which may be considered a type of phobia. These women often request surgical deliveries to avoid labor. Risk factors for intense fear of delivery and requesting cesarean delivery include preexisting mental illness, history of abuse, poor social support, unemployment, and previous complicated delivery. Focused, short-term psychotherapy may enable these women to accept a vaginal delivery and improve the birth experience.[148]

Natural History Across Childbearing

Pregnancy, delivery, and lactation produce profound changes in physiology, including changes in multiple hormonal and neurotransmitter systems that modulate anxiety symptoms. However, there has been relatively little study of the course of anxiety symptoms or anxiety disorders during pregnancy and postpartum. In one large prospective study, more women scored above threshold on an anxiety scale during weeks 18 and 32 of pregnancy compared with 8 weeks and 8 months postpartum, which suggests that **nonspecific anxiety symptoms worsen during pregnancy. Antenatal anxiety symptoms and anxiety disorders are associated with an increased risk of postpartum** depression, even after controlling for antenatal depression.[149] Anxiety disorders are as common as MDE in the postpartum period.[86] With respect to specific anxiety disorders, preliminary evidence suggests that panic disorder can improve during pregnancy but can recur postpartum. In addition, cessation of breastfeeding may precipitate relapse of panic disorder.[150] Pregnancy and childbirth can trigger the onset of or an exacerbation of preexisting OCD.[145,151] Obsessive-compulsive symptoms are very common in postpartum depression.[152] Intrusive violent thoughts and contamination concerns are quite common in new mothers without psychiatric disorders.[153,154] No information was found on the effects of pregnancy on the course of generalized anxiety disorder, phobias, or PTSD.

Beta-adrenergic agonists such as terbutaline may precipitate panic attacks and other anxiety symptoms during the treatment of premature labor. **Hyperthyroidism is associated with panic attacks, and anxiety and should be considered in the differential diagnosis of postpartum-onset anxiety episodes.**

Effects of Anxiety During Childbearing

Anxiety symptoms and anxiety disorders are associated with an increased risk of preeclampsia and reduced birthweight.[155,156] PTSD, an anxiety disorder associated with marked hyperarousal symptoms including severe insomnia has been associated with increased risk of PTB.[157,158] Less is known about other anxiety disorders and their relationship to delivery complications.[159] Psychosocial stress also has been linked to higher rates of PTB, and several physiologic pathways have been proposed to mediate the association, including autonomic arousal, elevated levels of cortisol and corticotropin-releasing hormone, and systemic inflammation.[160] Lack of sleep, a common symptom of anxiety disorders, can increase inflammatory load and is associated with PTB.[161]

Prenatal anxiety also has been associated with adverse effects on offspring. Fetuses of anxious women show increased heart rate reactivity to maternal stressors, and newborns of highly anxious mothers have reduced heart rate variability and poor autonomic regulation.[162,163] Poor autonomic regulation of heart rate has been linked to impaired emotional regulation in older children and adults. In utero and as newborns, the offspring of anxious women spend more time in deep sleep[162,164] and are more likely to cry excessively.[165]

Maternal anxiety during pregnancy is associated with attention deficits, motor immaturity, and difficult temperament in offspring. In two large prospective longitudinal studies, anxiety during pregnancy increased the risk for hyperactivity, conduct disorder, and anxiety in childhood after controlling for obstetric and sociodemographic risks and for maternal depression.[166-168] Research is needed to understand the contributions of genetic risk factors, parenting behaviors, and the altered uteroplacental milieu to developmental and psychiatric problems in the offspring of anxious mothers.

Treatment of Anxiety Disorders

The boundary between normal and pathologic anxiety cannot be drawn with great precision. **When anxiety substantially impairs work, family, or social adjustment, mental health evaluation is indicated, and treatment is appropriate. Panic disorder responds to most antidepressant medications, which are first-line therapies for this disorder.** Benzodiazepines are also effective but are associated with abuse and physical dependence in a subset of patients. Cognitive behavior therapy (CBT) is a time-limited, structured psychotherapy that is also effective for panic disorder.

In contrast, OCD is effectively treated specifically with the SSRI antidepressants. A behavioral therapy technique, exposure and response prevention, is also effective for OCD. Generalized anxiety disorder responds to a variety of antidepressant medications and to cognitive therapy. PTSD is partially responsive to antidepressants, but psychotherapy or combination treatment is often more effective. The first-line medication treatment for social phobia includes SSRIs and CBT. Specific phobias are treated with focused desensitization therapy rather than medication. An excellent patient educational workbook on anxiety disorders is available (see the resource list at the end of this chapter).

A risk-benefit evaluation for treatments during pregnancy must be individualized for the pregnant woman with anxiety disorder because, like MDE, anxiety can have a negative impact on pregnancy outcome (see Chapter 8). If psychotherapy treatment is refused, not available, or ineffective, pharmacologic treatment should be considered. The use of antidepressants in pregnancy and lactation has been reviewed in the section on major depression. Evidence from the available studies indicates that the teratogenic risk from benzodiazepine exposure, if any, is very small.[169] However, less is known about the effect of benzodiazepines on neurodevelopment. At delivery, neonates exposed to higher doses can have withdrawal seizures or hypotonia.[170]

Benzodiazepines enter breast milk but the concentration in milk varies by drug, dose, and frequency of use. Because alternative treatments are available for anxiety disorders, benzodiazepines often can be avoided or used to treat targeted symptoms for limited periods during pregnancy and lactation. Intermittent use of short half-life benzodiazepines is preferred because chronic use of long-acting benzodiazepines can result in infant sedation, and mothers must be educated to observe for drowsiness and poor feeding. Also, little is known about the degree to which benzodiazepines are absorbed into the circulation of breastfed infants.

EATING DISORDERS

Diagnosis and Prevalence

The classifications of eating disorders have been substantially updated in the "Feeding and Eating Disorders" section of DSM-V.[171] Eating disorders are particularly relevant during pregnancy and lactation, when the increased requirement for food intake can be directly affected by disordered eating. This section will review anorexia nervosa (AN) and bulimia nervosa (BN).

AN is characterized by the restriction of energy intake relative to requirements, which leads to low bodyweight, an intense fear of gaining weight or of becoming fat, or persistent behavior that interferes with weight gain.[171] In addition, women with AN have a disturbance in the way in which their body weight or shape is experienced, they allow an undue influence to be placed on body shape or weight in self-evaluation, and a persistent lack of recognition of the seriousness of the current low body weight is evident. In AN, the body mass index (BMI) is usually less than 18.5 kg/m^2. Although amenorrhea is no longer a required criterion, most women have secondary amenorrhea. The prevalence of AN in adolescents and young adult women is 0.4%. The longitudinal course of AN is variable and includes remission, residual partial symptomatology, or a fluctuating or chronic course. However, the majority of individuals with AN experience remission within 5 years.[171,172] AN is associated with elevated mortality rates (5% per decade) due to both medical complications and increased suicide rates.[171]

Bulimia nervosa (BN) is defined as recurrent episodes of binge eating, a sense of lack of control over eating during the binge episode, and recurrent compensatory methods to prevent weight gain.[171] BN is common and occurs in 1% to 1.5% of young adult women. A *binge* is eating in a discrete period of time (e.g., within 2 hours) an amount of food that is larger than what most people would eat during a similar period of time. Inappropriate compensatory behaviors include self-induced vomiting; laxative, diuretic, or other medication (e.g., ipecac) abuse; fasting; and excessive exercise. **The binge eating and compensatory behaviors must occur at least once a week for 3 months.** Women with BN maintain body weight at or above a normal range. Self-evaluation that is unduly influenced by body shape and weight is also part of the disorder. The longitudinal course of BN can include remission, chronicity, intermittent recurrence, and prolonged disturbed eating behavior. BN has an elevated mortality risk (2% per decade).[171] In women who report lifetime binge eating, both amenorrhea and oligomenorrhea are more common than in women who do not report binge eating.[173] The ratio of women to men with both AN and BN is striking at 10 : 1. **The etiology of eating disorders has contributions from multiple domains: the societal ideal of thinness and encouragement of women to define themselves by the way others perceive them; families that demand conformity and high achievement; genetic susceptibility** (50% to 80% of the variance in liability to AN and BN is accounted for by genetic factors)**; personality traits that include low self-esteem, impulsivity, obsessionality, perfectionism, and emotional instability; and chronic disease, such as diabetes mellitus.**[174,175] Dysregulation of neurotransmitters, neuropeptides, and endocrine factors also likely contribute to etiology. Dieting frequently triggers the onset of an eating disorder in vulnerable individuals.[174]

Women with eating disorders rarely voluntarily disclose their maladaptive eating behaviors, but they may present to their obstetrician-gynecologist with complaints of irregular menses, infertility, sexual dysfunction, unexplained vomiting, fatigue, or palpitations.[174] The obstetrician-gynecologist or primary care clinician can screen for eating disorders with questions about restricted eating, binge eating, purging behavior, and compulsive exercise. Medical examination should include obtaining the patient's weight and evaluation for loss of dental enamel and abrasions on the hands from self-induced vomiting.[174] AN or BN can also present with disruption or cessation of ovulation, and these disorders are included in the differential diagnosis of secondary amenorrhea. Laboratory investigations may disclose abnormalities of electrolytes, blood urea nitrogen, creatinine, amylase, and thyroid indices. The medical consequences of AN and BN are numerous, and the medical complications may be life threatening (Box 55-2). Cardiac rhythm disturbances are common in patients with AN and are usually reversible with improvement in nutritional status. Cardiomyopathy due to chronic ipecac (emetine) abuse in BN may not be reversible.[176] Osteopenia occurs in more than 90% of adult women with AN, and about 40% have osteoporosis at one or more sites.[177] The lumbar spine is most affected. Weight restoration and nutritional replenishment are the ideal treatments for improving bone density. Whereas estrogen supplementation may have a

---

BOX 55-2 PHYSICAL AND LABORATORY FINDINGS IN WOMEN WITH EATING DISORDERS

Common in Women With Eating Disorders

Bradycardia
Hypotension and orthostasis
Hypothermia
Dry skin

More Common in Anorexia Nervosa Due to Severe Calorie Restriction

Emaciated; may wear oversized clothes
Sunken cheeks, sallow skin
Lanugo (fine downy body hair)
Atrophic breasts/atrophic vaginitis
Pitting edema of extremities
Dull, thinning scalp hair
Cold extremities, acrocyanosis
Osteopenia, increased risk of fracture
Constipation
Fluid retention after laxative or diuretic withdrawal
Laboratory: Anemia, ↑ blood urea nitrogen, ↑ cholesterol, ↑ liver function studies, ↑ amylase; ↓ platelets, ↓ magnesium, ↓ zinc, ↓ phosphates, ↓ thyroid. With laxative abuse: metabolic acidosis

More Common in Women Who Purge

Parotitis
Calluses on dorsal hand surface from self-induced emesis
Oral mucosal abrasions
Dental enamel erosion, tooth chipping, extensive cosmetic dental work
Cardiac and skeletal myopathies from ipecac abuse
Laboratory: Metabolic alkalosis, ↓ sodium, ↓ chloride, ↓ potassium, ↑ bicarbonate from purging

---

Data from American Psychiatric Association, *Diagnostic and Statistical Manual*, 5th Edition. Arlington, VA: American Psychiatric Association, 2013; Hay P, et al. Royal Australian and New Zealand College of Psychiatrists clinical practice guidelines for the treatment of eating disorders. *Aust N Z J Psychiatry.* 2014;48(11):977-1008; and Hsu LK. Eating disorders: practical interventions. *J Am Med Womens Assoc.* 2004;59(2): 113-124.

---

promising role, oral contraceptives have not demonstrated consistent benefit.[177] Similarly, data to support bisphosphonate use in AN are conflicting, and the potential teratogenic effects compounded by its long half-life preclude its use for osteoporosis in premenopausal women with AN.[178,179]

Natural History Across Childbearing

Due to anovulation, fertility is often diminished in women with AN or BN due to a reduction in the secretion of gonadotropin-releasing hormone and, in turn, a reduction in both luteinizing hormone and follicle-stimulating hormone. However, if pregnancy is achieved, it can be a stimulus that moves a woman through the continuum from subthreshold symptoms to overt eating disorder.[175] Changing body shape and loss of control of weight gain may reactivate deviant eating patterns and concerns about body shape in women with a history of an eating disorder. Persistence of active eating disorder symptoms and the development of binge eating during pregnancy have been reported. However, several studies have suggested that many pregnant women with BN decrease binge eating and purging. Some women with active eating disorders allow themselves to eat nutritiously and do not purge, with motivation derived from promoting the health of the growing baby.[175] **The optimal treatment of pregnant women with a prior or active eating disorder includes a multidisciplinary team of the obstetrician-gynecologist, nutritionist, and mental health clinician.**[175] Frequent prenatal visits, regular weighing, and enhanced support encourage recommended weight gain and nutrition to ensure fetal well-being. Binge eating during pregnancy may be associated with higher gestational weight gain. BN during pregnancy has been associated with elevated rates of nausea and vomiting, but the risk of hyperemesis gravidarum with BN may not be increased.[180]

A recent systematic review reported that children of mothers with AN have an increased risk of LBW.[181] Inadequate weight gain in pregnancy, elevated risk of miscarriage, IUGR, infants born SGA, microcephaly, PTB, antepartum hemorrhage, and cesarean delivery have also been reported. Some of these adverse pregnancy outcomes may be mitigated in women who gain appropriate weight during pregnancy.[182-184] Eating disorders and food restriction were associated with an increased risk of neural tube defects likely due to decreased folic acid levels.[185] Weight-controlling behaviors that can lead to nutritional deficiencies—including strict dieting, vomiting, and excessive physical exercise—may impact fetal brain development and fetal stress responses.[186] Negative birth outcomes in women with BN have included elevated rates of miscarriage, PTB, and cesarean delivery.[187] Both LBW and macrosomia have been reported in women with BN.

The postpartum period is a time of risk for the onset of MDE and poor maternal adjustment.[174,175] **Women with a history of BN have a threefold increased risk of postpartum MDE compared with women without eating disorders.**[188] Increased stress with a new infant, feelings of lack of control, and a desire to lose pregnancy weight may precipitate recurrence of AN or BN even if the symptoms were under control during pregnancy. The postpartum period is another critical time for a woman with an eating disorder to receive enhanced support and treatment from a multidisciplinary team. Children of mothers with active eating disorders show slower growth in the first year of life[189] and increased psychopathology in childhood and early adolescence.[190]

Treatment of Eating Disorders

Specific treatment goals for patients with eating disorders include establishing healthy eating behaviors; stabilizing nutritional intake and weight; correcting dysfunctional thoughts about weight; and addressing perfectionism, low self-esteem, the pursuit of thinness, mood lability, interpersonal difficulties, and poor coping skills through psychotherapy. Addressing comorbidities such as depression, anxiety, and medical problems are also part of the treatment plan.

Anorexia Nervosa

Women with AN may require hospitalization because of emaciation, severe electrolyte disturbances, depression, suicidality, or failure of outpatient treatment.[191] A structured behavioral inpatient program involves individual and group psychotherapy, meal planning and supervision, nutrition consultation, psychiatric consultation, and medical monitoring.[172,191] Caloric intake that increases too rapidly may lead to *refeeding syndrome,* a serious condition characterized by electrolyte and mineral abnormalities and fluid shifts. Length of inpatient hospitalization and weight achieved at discharge are prognostic predictors,

although 50% of weight-restored women with AN have a relapse in the first year after hospitalization.[192]

Psychotherapies for AN include family therapy, CBT, insight-oriented psychotherapy, supportive clinical management, and interpersonal psychotherapy. No medications are approved by the FDA for the treatment of AN, nor are any recommended by treatment guidelines. Comorbid depression and anxiety often improve with weight gain. Psychotropic medications are usually instituted to treat depression and anxiety or when psychotherapy alone has not been effective. The core symptoms of AN are relatively refractory to psychotropic agents. Studies have included typical antipsychotics, atypical antipsychotics, tricyclics, and SSRIs.[193] Meta-analyses of antipsychotic medications have not demonstrated superiority over placebo for weight gain, decreased anxiety, or improvement in eating disorder cognitions.[194,195]

Relapse prevention is a challenging problem in treating AN, and longitudinal studies demonstrate that AN is a chronic disorder.[172] CBT is helpful in weight-restored women in preventing a relapse of AN. A controlled study showed that fluoxetine was not superior to placebo in weight-restored women also receiving CBT.[192]

Bulimia Nervosa

CBT is the first-line treatment for BN, and both short-term and long-term efficacy has been demonstrated. In CBT, the therapist identifies the stimuli to thought processes and emotions that maintain the binge-purge-starve cycle. The woman develops strategies to manage the disturbed eating, changes the dysfunctional cognitions, and builds alternative ways to manage distress. CBT is a time-limited individual or group psychotherapy. When CBT is not available, self-help manuals and web-based programs utilizing the principles of CBT can be encouraged (see the resource list at the end of this chapter).

Placebo-controlled RCTs with SSRIs, TCAs, and monoamine oxidase inhibitors (MAOIs) have been promising for the reduction of binge eating and purging, although a minority of patients achieve full remission.[193,196] Fluoxetine is FDA approved for BN at a dose of 60 mg/day. Bupropion is contraindicated due to reduced seizure threshold in patients with eating disorders. Many studies of antidepressants also demonstrate reduction of core eating disorder psychopathology such as weight and food preoccupation. The reduction of binge eating and purging frequency with antidepressants is independent of comorbid depression. Adding an antidepressant to CBT is a prudent clinical strategy when depression is comorbid.[172,196] Symptomatic improvement and sustained remission may be maximized with combined CBT and antidepressant medication.

Reduction in binge eating and purging has also been reported with ondansetron and topiramate.[193] Ondansetron is a 5-HT$_3$ antagonist that reduced symptoms compared with placebo, possibly due to regulation of vagal activity. Topiramate has been reported to reduce the number of binge-purge days and to improve self-esteem, eating attitudes, anxiety, and body image. However, topiramate is not recommended as first-line therapy in reproductive-aged women due to increased risk of oral clefts in offspring with first-trimester use.

SCHIZOPHRENIA

Diagnosis and Prevalence

Schizophrenia is a disabling brain disease that affects 1% of the population. The defining feature of schizophrenia is

psychosis, which refers to specific clinical symptoms not to the severity of the episode. Schizophrenia is characterized by delusions (fixed false beliefs), hallucinations, disorganized speech, grossly disorganized behavior or catatonia (displays of bizarre posturing, rigidity, mutism, negativism, purposeless excitement, echolalia), and negative symptoms (lack of emotional expression, apathy) that result in significant social or occupational dysfunction. To have schizophrenia, an individual must exhibit at least two of the specified symptoms, which must have been present for 6 months, and include at least 1 month of active symptoms. The etiology of schizophrenia is unknown, but proposed mechanisms include (1) excessive dopamine transmission; (2) in utero exposure to influenza or other viral agents, which resulted in neurobiologic disruptions[198]; and (3) altered neuroplasticity or neurodevelopmental trajectories.[199] Schizophrenia is distinguished from mood disorders, which may also present with psychosis, by the persistence of hallucinations or delusions when mood symptoms have remitted. The mortality and morbidity of schizophrenia is high, and 10% of patients complete suicide. **Women are more likely to have a later onset, prominent mood symptoms, and a better prognosis than men. The median age of onset is in the late second decade for women. Women have less severe symptoms, fewer hospitalizations, a higher likelihood to return to work, and more social support than men.**[200] **About 67% of women with schizophrenia, compared with 29% of men, are married, and women are twice as likely to have children.**[200]

Natural History Across Childbearing

Women with schizophrenia have lower fertility rates compared with healthy women despite low rates of contraceptive use; irreversible causes of infertility—such as hysterectomy, early menopause, and sterilization—are higher among schizophrenic women.[201] Concurrent maternal smoking, substance use, and socioeconomic problems increase the risk for poor pregnancy outcomes. In a population-based cohort study of over 3000 births from 1980 to1992,[107] **mentally ill women were at increased risk for obstetric complications that included placental abruption** (OR, 2.75; 95% CI, 1.32 to 5.74) **and antepartum hemorrhage** (OR, 1.65; 95% CI, 1.02 to 2.69) **compared with women who did not have psychiatric disorders.** In the first year after delivery, mothers with schizophrenia had high rates of recurrent episodes of psychosis (27%) and depression (38%).[202] Children born to women with schizophrenia are susceptible to subtle neurodevelopmental problems, but the origins (genetic, environment, psychosocial) are complex. Data on the mothers' nutritional status, exposure to psychotropic medications, other prescription or over-the-counter drugs that impact reproductive outcomes, violence, and medical comorbidities are usually lacking from studies.[107]

Extrapolating From Studies on the General Population

Because no specific data for the treatment course in pregnant women with schizophrenia are available, information from the general literature will be reviewed. Stopping antipsychotic treatment results in high relapse rates: 53% of patients who discontinued treatment, compared with 16% who continued treatment for at least 10 months, relapsed during follow-up.[203] Sudden treatment cessation, younger age, early age of illness onset, need for high doses of antipsychotic medication, and recent admission also predicted recurrence. **Because of the high relapse risk without treatment, patients with schizophrenia often** **continue antipsychotic therapy during pregnancy. The preferred drug is the antipsychotic, which provided the greatest symptom reduction and the least side effects for the individual.**[204] If a woman elects to remain monitored without medication, a plan should be developed for reinstituting medication rapidly if prodromal symptoms occur. Services that offer **integrated obstetric and psychiatric management**, pharmacotherapy, parent education groups, and family programs are optimal for promoting positive outcomes.[205]

Treatment Interventions for Women With Schizophrenia

In a large double-blind controlled trial of 1500 patients with schizophrenia, clinical outcomes were similar among groups of patients who received one of four atypical antipsychotics—olanzapine, quetiapine, risperidone, or ziprasidone—or the older antipsychotic perphenazine.[206] The typical antipsychotic perphenazine was as well tolerated as the newer compounds and as effective as three of the four newer agents. Although patients taking olanzapine had lower rates of drug discontinuation and hospitalization, the benefits were offset by higher rates of weight gain and metabolic side effects. Although the study excluded pregnant women, the results have implications for their treatment. The risk-benefit decision may favor the use of typical agents during pregnancy, particularly for women with insulin resistance, obesity, and hypertension. **Control of the psychotic disorder, which usually requires medication continuation, is critical for maternal and fetal health.**[204]

Antipsychotic Drugs During Pregnancy

Clozapine was the first atypical agent to be released; however, burdensome side effects—such as weight gain, tachycardia, dyslipidemia, sedation, and drooling—and mandatory periodic monitoring for agranulocytosis create significant barriers to use (see the earlier section on the use of these drugs to treat bipolar disorder in women of childbearing age). **Clozapine is reserved for patients whose illness is nonresponsive to treatment with less toxic drugs.** Clozapine use in pregnancy has been associated with normal deliveries as well as with gestational diabetes, shoulder dystocia, hypotonia, and neonatal convulsions.[207]

The most available reproductive data among the atypical drugs is for **olanzapine**. Brunner and colleagues[208] reported the outcomes from 610 prospectively identified pregnancies tracked worldwide in Eli Lilly and Company's safety database of voluntary reports. Most women reported olanzapine exposure throughout pregnancy (44.3%) or in the first trimester only (31.5%). The rates of adverse outcomes—such as early pregnancy loss, congenital anomalies, PTB, and stillbirth—did not differ in olanzapine-exposed, compared with nonexposed, women. Olanzapine dosages ranged from 0.6 to 35.0 mg/day, with a mean dosage of 10.3 mg/day.

Risperidone is an atypical agent with diverse receptor-blocking activities. At dosages above 6 mg daily, hyperprolactinemia and motor side effects may emerge. In a postmarketing study of 68 prospectively reported pregnancies with a known outcome, structural malformations occurred in 3.8%, which was consistent with background rates in the general population.[209] Neonatal adaptation difficulties included tremor, jitteriness, irritability, feeding problems, and somnolence.

Quetiapine is an atypical antipsychotic with a wide dose range, with maintenance dosages from 400 to 800 mg/day after initial titration. Side effects include sedation, weight gain, and headache. The few published cases of in utero exposure to quetiapine resulted in normal intrauterine growth, full-term deliveries, and favorable Apgar scores.[204] Yaeger and colleagues[210] presented a sophisticated case discussion of quetiapine treatment of a pregnant woman that provides a clinical review.

Ziprasidone is a suitable choice for managing psychosis, with its neutral effects on weight and lipid and glucose metabolism[211]; however, its use may be associated with prolonged QTc syndrome. Limited information on perinatal exposures with ziprasidone is available. Of 57 cases of known outcomes from gestational exposure, one malformation[212] was observed.

Aripiprazole has novel dopamine antagonist and partial agonist activity. It is indicated for schizophrenia, bipolar mania, mixed episodes, and severe MDE combined with an antidepressant. A recent report from a multicenter cohort study that used prospectively collected data from 2004 to 2011 suggested that exposure to aripiprazole was not associated with increased rates of birth defects, miscarriages, or gestational diabetes compared with nonexposure.[213] However, women treated with aripiprazole may experience declines in the serum concentration of aripiprazole from enhanced hepatic metabolism in pregnancy and could require higher doses.[214] Recent evidence of increased rates of prematurity (11 of 86 [16%] vs. 11 of 172 [7%]) and fetal growth impairment (12 of 86 [19%] vs. 11 of 172 [7%]) in exposed newborns compared with nonexposed newborns could signify concern.[213] However, the findings were difficult to interpret because the majority of women in the exposed group (65%) had received aripiprazole for a brief duration in the first trimester only. In addition, the women receiving aripiprazole also reported high rates of cigarette smoking, a proven risk factor for preterm birth and fetal growth problems.

The longitudinal development of 76 infants exposed throughout pregnancy to atypical antipsychotics was compared with 76 women without mental illness or antipsychotic exposure.[215] At 3 months, the mean scores of cognitive, motor, social-emotional, and adaptive behavior as assessed by the Bayley Scales of Infant Development were significantly lower in exposed infants. However, no significant differences between the two groups were noted at 12 months of age for any of the mean composite scores of the Bayley scales. More infants exposed to atypical antipsychotics had lower birthweight than the controls (13.2% vs. 2.6%, $P = .031$), although no significant differences were reported in mean weight and height at birth between the two groups. In a separate prospective controlled study from 1999 to 2008, investigators examined the outcomes from intrauterine exposure to psychotropic drugs in mother-infant dyads.[215a] Findings suggested 6-month-old infants exposed to antipsychotics ($n = 22$) had significantly lower neuromotor performance on the standardized Infant Neurological International Battery examination compared with infants exposed to antidepressants ($n = 202$) or no psychotropic agents ($n = 85$). Because impaired neuromotor functioning also was associated with maternal disorders, including major depressive disorder or a psychotic disorder, it is still not possible to disentangle the medication effects from the effects of maternal illness.

Optimal maternal and infant outcomes are achieved through individualized treatment planning by a mental health team in collaboration with community programs. The antipsychotic agent associated with the greatest symptom reduction, balanced against its side effects, is the preferred drug for the individual pregnant woman.[204] An additional consideration in risk-benefit discussions is whether that

preferred drug could be replaced by one with a more favorable reproductive risk profile *without* compromising efficacy and tolerability, but no antipsychotic has emerged as definitively more efficacious or having less adverse reproductive effects than any other.[204] Several factors impact the choice of a medication change, including patient and physician concern about the lack of data for the preferred drug—particularly for newer agents—and prior treatment experience with a drug that has less impact on a medical condition that existed before or developed during pregnancy. A factor in every risk-benefit decision is the fact that pregnancy outcome data for drug exposure is inextricably tied to outcomes related to the underlying illness for which the drug is being prescribed.[204]

Antipsychotic Drugs During Breastfeeding

The high concentration of clozapine in breast milk has been attributed to its lipophilicity.[216] The excretion of olanzapine, a highly protein-bound agent, in breast milk has been assessed in small case series. The median estimated dose in infants was 1.6% to 4.0% of the maternal dose.[217] In a woman who took olanzapine (10 mg) daily through childbearing, maternal plasma levels were 33.4 ng/mL at delivery; the infant level was about a third of the maternal level.[218] The breastfed infant's levels were below 2 ng/mL at 2 and 6 weeks. Breastfed infants of mothers taking olanzapine can display somnolence, irritability, tremor, and insomnia.[208]

Three breastfed infants of mothers who were treated with risperidone had nondetectable serum drug metabolite levels and no evidence of adverse reactions.[219] A mother who was treated with risperidone (6 mg/day) provided serial samples of plasma and breast milk every 4 hours over a 24-hour period. The infant drug intake was estimated to be 0.84% of the maternal dose for risperidone, 3.5% for its metabolite, and 4.3% of the weight-adjusted maternal dose.[220]

Six breastfeeding women who received treatment with quetiapine[221] provided breast milk for assay. The total daily infant exposure was less than 0.01 mg/kg/day for five infants and less than 0.10 mg/kg/day for one infant. The estimated dose of ziprasidone received by the breastfed infants was 1.2% of the maternal dose.[222] A woman treated with aripiprazole throughout pregnancy breastfed her full-term infant; at 27 days, no detectable levels of drug or metabolite were found in milk samples.[223]

SUBSTANCE-RELATED DISORDERS
Diagnosis and Prevalence

Children exposed to drugs in utero are more likely to experience a range of physical and neurodevelopmental problems.[224] **In an American national survey,**[225] **5.4% of pregnant women reported illicit drug use in the month prior, and *Cannabis* was the most frequently used substance. Rates were higher in the first (9.0%) and second (4.8%) trimesters than in the third trimester (2.4%). All rates were lower than those found for nonpregnant women from the same age cohort (11.4%).** These data demonstrate that many substance-using women discontinue use when they become pregnant. For women with ongoing substance use disorder (SUD), addiction treatment is the most effective method for improving maternal and infant/child outcomes.[226] **Because addiction often occurs in the context of psychiatric and/or medical comorbidities, poverty, poor nutrition, and violence, comprehensive**

BOX 55-3 DSM-V CRITERIA FOR SUBSTANCE USE DISORDER

1. The substance is often taken in larger amounts or over a longer period than was intended.
2. The desire to cut down or control substance use is persistent, but efforts to do so are unsuccessful.
3. A great deal of time is spent in activities necessary to obtain the substance, use the substance, or recover from its effects.
4. A craving, urge, or a strong desire to use the substance is evident.
5. Recurrent substance use results in a failure to fulfill major role obligations at work, school, or home.
6. Substance use is continued despite having persistent or recurrent social or interpersonal problems caused or exacerbated by the effects.
7. Important social, occupational, or recreational activities are given up or reduced because of substance use.
8. Substance use is recurrent in situations in which it is physically hazardous.
9. Substance use is continued despite knowledge of having a persistent or recurrent physical or psychologic problem that is likely to have been caused or exacerbated by the substance.
10. Tolerance is evident, in either the need for markedly increased amounts of the substance to achieve the desired effect or a markedly diminished effect with continued use of the same amount of the substance.
11. Withdrawal occurs, with either characteristic withdrawal syndrome for the substance or with the substance, or a closely related one, being taken to relieve or avoid withdrawal symptoms.

From American Psychiatric Association (APA). *The Diagnostic and Statistical Manual of Mental Disorders,* Fifth Edition. APA; 2013. Severity ratings range from *mild* (2 to 3 criteria) to *moderate* (4 to 5 criteria) to *severe* (6 to 11 criteria).

TABLE 55-2   SCREENING WITH THE FOUR P'S PLUS

Parents	Did either of your parents ever have a problem with alcohol or drugs?
Partner	Does your partner have a problem with alcohol or drugs?
Past	Have you ever had any beer or wine or liquor?
Pregnancy	In the month before you knew you were pregnant, how many *cigarettes* did you smoke?
	In the month before you knew you were pregnant, how much *beer/wine/liquor* did you drink?

From Chasnoff IJ, Hung WC. *The 4P's Plus.* Chicago: NTI Publishing; 1999.

treatment programs that specialize in the care of pregnant and parenting women play an integral role in improving birth outcomes and increasing the likelihood of recovery from addiction. Criminalization and incarceration of women for prenatal substance use often has deleterious effects and can compromise both maternal and fetal health.[227]

SUDs are diagnosed using the DSM-V,[1] which integrates the two previous categories of substance abuse and dependence from DSM-IV into SUD (Box 55-3). Each class of drugs is evaluated separately and receives its own severity rating based on the number of criteria met for that substance.

Screening, Brief Intervention, and Referral to Treatment

To invest in the health of their baby, pregnant women with SUD are more likely to participate in health care during pregnancy than at other times in their lives.[228] The standard obstetric history includes questions about alcohol, tobacco, and other drug use, and obstetricians can educate women that casual drug use increases risks for adverse maternal and infant outcomes.[229] **Screening, brief intervention, and referral to treatment is an efficient, evidence-based approach to improve perinatal outcomes[230] that is endorsed by ACOG.[226]** Brief interventions range from practitioner advice to reduce or stop drug use to psychoeducational counseling. The practitioner can facilitate access to treatment, and level of care (outpatient, residential) is

determined by severity of addiction and other presenting medical and psychosocial needs.[226]

Screening for substance use and dependence is an integral component of health assessment during obstetric care.[228] Reliable and valid screening tools are useful to identify alcohol, tobacco, and other drug use in pregnant women.[226] For alcohol, the T-ACE mnemonic—which stands for *tolerance-annoyance, cutdown, eye opener*[231]—is a brief, psychometrically sound screening approach to detect drinking in pregnant women (see Chapter 8, Table 8-2). Women with T-ACE scores of 2 and above (range 0 to 5) require follow-up assessment.

Social pressure has increasingly contributed to underreporting of smoking by pregnant women, and multiple-choice questions are recommended to improve disclosure.[232] For drug use, the Drug Abuse Screening Test (DAST-10)[233] focuses on drug use consequences in the prior year. Alternatively, the 4Ps Plus (Table 55-2) was developed specifically to identify pregnant women at risk for prenatal use of alcohol, tobacco, and other drugs. The five-question screen takes less than 1 minute to complete: the first *P* (*Parents*) asks about substance use in family members, the second (*Partner*) asks about partner substance use, and the third (*Past*) asks about *prepregnancy* use of alcohol; questions 4 and 5 (*Pregnancy*) focus on the month prior to pregnancy awareness—one asks about cigarette smoking, the other about alcohol consumption. Targeting the month prior to pregnancy is important because women often use substances at prepregnancy levels until the pregnancy is confirmed, and they stop after early first-trimester exposure has already occurred.

Pregnant women are often reluctant to disclose information about their drug use due to stigma, concern about being judged, or legal consequences. **The practitioner's emotional tone is critical because pregnant women are more likely to divulge substance use when asked by a nonjudgmental care provider.**[228] Alternative to self-report assessments are biologic measures that screen for drug exposure. They include urine, meconium, and hair[234]; however, all have practical limitations.

Specific Drugs of Abuse: Impact and Treatment Approaches

Alcohol

Nearly 1 in 10 pregnant women (9.4%) report alcohol consumption in the past month, 2.3% meet criteria for binge drinking (consuming five or more standard drinks on the same occasion), and 0.4% meet criteria for heavy drinking (binge drinking on each of five or more days in the past month).[225] These rates are lower than those found in nonpregnant women, half of whom report recent alcohol use. Nearly one fourth (24.6%) report recent binge drinking, and 5.3% meet criteria for heavy drinking.

Fetal exposure to alcohol is the most common preventable cause of mental retardation.[227] It also increases the risks for miscarriage, stillbirth, and prematurity. Alcohol is a potent teratogen, and the most severe manifestation of in utero exposure is **fetal alcohol syndrome** (FAS; see Chapter 8). This diagnosis requires maternal alcohol consumption, facial malformations, prenatal or postnatal growth deficits, and lifelong neurodevelopmental disabilities.[235] Affected children have visual, skeletal, and cardiac anomalies. **Recent studies estimate the prevalence of fetal alcohol syndrome to be between 0.2 and 7 per 1000 children**[236] **with an estimated cost of over $4 billion annually.**[237] More broadly, prenatal alcohol consumption can produce a wide range of birth defects and developmental disabilities, known as *fetal alcohol spectrum disorders* (FASDs). With U.S. prevalence between 2% and 5%,[236] FASDs include a broad array of physical defects of the ocular, skeletal, cardiac, and other systems as well as cognitive, behavioral, and adaptive functioning deficits.[238]

Although the negative consequences of heavy drinking during pregnancy—one drink or more per day—are well-known and include FAS and FASD,[239] a meta-analysis also found adverse effects for mild to moderate (one to six drinks per week) and binge drinking (greater than four or five drinks per occasion). Binge drinking during pregnancy was associated with childhood cognitive problems, and moderate drinking was associated with childhood behavior problems.[240] **A question women often ask is whether it is safe to have an occasional glass of wine or a mixed drink while pregnant.** *No amount, gestational time, or type of alcohol use is safe during pregnancy.*[235] If alcohol use in pregnancy is identified, an early ultrasound to establish accurate gestational age dating is recommended. A detailed anatomic survey should be performed, and close monitoring for fetal growth restriction is also warranted.[241]

Research on alcohol intake and breastfeeding is limited. Approximately half of lactating women in Western countries report alcohol use.[242] Alcohol levels in breast milk are similar to maternal blood concentrations; therefore **the AAP recommends abstinence from alcohol during breastfeeding.** If a breastfeeding woman chooses to drink, a practical approach is to counsel her to limit intake to one drink and to wait 2 to 2.5 hours before breastfeeding to allow clearance of the alcoholic beverage from her plasma.[243,244]

MANAGEMENT OF ALCOHOL WITHDRAWAL

Alcohol withdrawal can lead to fetal distress, placental abruption, and preterm delivery.[245] In pregnant women, withdrawal typically begins 6 to 24 hours following cessation of alcohol intake. Early withdrawal signs include anxiety, sleep disturbance, vivid dreams, anorexia, nausea, and headache. Physical signs include tachycardia, elevated blood pressure, hyperactive reflexes, diaphoresis, hyperthermia, and tremor in the hands or tongue. **The peak time for withdrawal seizures is 24 hours after the last drink and is preceded by hyperactive reflexes. Alcohol withdrawal may progress to delirium tremens, which can be fatal to both mother and fetus.**[246]

Medical withdrawal in an inpatient setting is required. Benzodiazepines are common detoxification agents. In a critical review,[247] chlordiazepoxide and diazepam were considered the agents of choice for benzodiazepine treatment during pregnancy. These drugs have differing onset and duration of action and are available in an intravenous formulation. A typical fixed-dose taper starts with chlordiazepoxide (50 mg orally every 6 hours) or lorazepam (2 mg every 6 hours) with dose adjustment until symptoms are controlled. The dose is then tapered by 10% to

25% per day as tolerated. During inpatient care, folic acid and prenatal vitamins should be given daily. Acute management also requires thiamine replacement and maintenance of adequate hydration and electrolyte balance. **Fetal well-being should be monitored.**[246] A patient can be discharged to outpatient treatment when benzodiazepine treatment is no longer required to control symptoms for over 24 hours.[246]

Treatment schedules for medical withdrawal may be fixed dose or symptom based, with severity of withdrawal measured by the revised Clinical Institute Withdrawal Assessment of Alcohol Scale.[248] The withdrawal assessment takes only 2 to 5 minutes to administer and is available online. Symptom-guided withdrawal generally results in more rapid detoxification and lower total doses of benzodiazepine treatment but requires trained staff for implementation. This is particularly relevant for pregnant alcohol-dependent women, in whom lower benzodiazepine doses may suffice due to changes in maternal alcohol metabolism rates.[245,249]

Like alcohol, withdrawal from benzodiazepines is associated with significant morbidity and potential mortality if untreated. Women treated with benzodiazepine drugs that have a short half-life, such as alprazolam, are likely to develop withdrawal more rapidly than with agents with longer half-lives. Acute inpatient withdrawal is often accomplished by a fixed-dose drug taper with substitution of a long-acting benzodiazepine with dosing as needed to treat breakthrough symptoms. Once the patient has achieved a comfortable level of symptom control, the dose is tapered by 10% daily as tolerated. Disulfiram is contraindicated in pregnancy because of the association with birth defects.[250]

Smoking

National survey data[225] **showed that 15.4% of pregnant women reported smoking cigarettes**. Whereas the overall rate of smoking for women in this age group has declined over the past 10 years, rates of prenatal smoking have remained unchanged.[251] Adverse maternal outcomes of prenatal cigarette smoking include thromboembolic disease and respiratory complications. Adverse infant outcomes include spontaneous pregnancy loss, PTB, restricted fetal growth, placenta previa, placental abruption, and premature rupture of membranes.[252] **In the United States, between 23% and 34% of sudden infant death syndrome (SIDS) deaths are attributable to prenatal smoking.**[253] Infants exposed to secondhand smoke are also more likely to have respiratory tract and ear infections and SIDS. An estimated $122 million in health care costs for postpartum infant hospitalization can be ascribed to maternal smoking,[254] and smoking during pregnancy was associated with sleep problems in offspring through age 12.[255]

Women who quit smoking by the first trimester have infants with growth parameters comparable to those born to nonsmokers.[256] **The Five A's—Ask, Advise, Assess, Assist, and Arrange—is an ACOG-endorsed, evidence-based behavioral intervention often provided as part of prenatal care.**[232] **Trained providers spend 5 to 15 minutes at each prenatal visit counseling women who want to quit smoking. To facilitate implementation, computer-delivered Five A's–based brief interventions have been developed.**[257] Smoking "quitlines" (1-800-QUIT-NOW) are effective in assisting pregnant women to stop smoking.[258] Other evidence-based psychosocial strategies to promote prenatal smoking cessation include behavioral incentives, social support, and tailored self-help materials.[226]

Use of nicotine replacement therapy (NRT) in pregnancy remains controversial.[259,260] Nicotine patch use in the second and third trimesters was not associated with maternal or fetal compromise as assessed by using fetal heart rate patterns, amniotic fluid volume, umbilical blood flow, and birthweight.[261] However, a recent RCT of nicotine versus placebo patch in pregnant smokers found no group differences in abstinence rates.[262] Nevertheless, **ACOG supports the use of NRT when nonpharmacologic therapies have proven ineffective.**[263] The antidepressant bupropion is efficacious for smoking cessation, but little research documents use in pregnant women. However, no increase in risk was found for congenital malformations in bupropion–treated pregnant women.[264]

Women who quit smoking in pregnancy tend to relapse within 1 year postpartum.[265] Motivation to breastfeed is an opportunity to support continued cessation or reduction of smoking beyond that achieved during pregnancy. Although the AAP recommends that mothers quit smoking and not smoke around their infants, smoking is not contraindicated during breastfeeding.[137] Nicotine replacement therapy with a patch can also be used with breastfeeding. The 21-mg patch transfers about as much nicotine into breast milk as smoking one pack of cigarettes per day, and the 14 and 7 mg patches transfer even less.[266] To decrease exposure, women can be encouraged to remove the patch at night.

Cannabis

Cannabis is the most commonly used illicit drug in pregnancy, with prevalence rates that range from 2.5% to 5%,[225,267] and women often continue to use throughout their pregnancies.[268] Fewer studies of the impact of *Cannabis* during pregnancy have been conducted than for alcohol, tobacco, cocaine, and opiates. In many reports, prenatal *Cannabis* use is considered a confounding variable when looking at teratogenic effects of other drugs.[269]

Maternal risks of *Cannabis* smoking include carcinogenesis (such as oral cancers) and pulmonary disease. **Although in utero *Cannabis* exposure does not increase the risk for spontaneous abortion or congenital abnormalities,[270,271] it has been associated with IUGR.** *Cannabis*-exposed infants have smaller head circumferences at birth than nonexposed infants, and this difference becomes accentuated in adolescence.[272] Neonatal effects of prenatal *Cannabis* use include exaggerated and prolonged startle reflexes, transient high-pitched cry, and sleep disturbances.[273] In longitudinal studies, in utero *Cannabis* exposure had negative effects on academic achievement,[274] intellectual development,[275] response inhibition,[276] and delinquency.[277] *Cannabis*-exposed children were also more likely to smoke both cigarettes and *Cannabis* than non-*Cannabis* exposed children.[278]

Cannabis and its metabolites pass into breast milk, and concentrations in milk can be substantively higher than those in maternal plasma.[267] There is also some evidence that continued use during lactation can impair first-year neurodevelopment in the infant,[279] and its use by breastfeeding mothers is of concern and is thus contraindicated.[280] As more states legalize medical *Cannabis*, prenatal use for treatment of neurogenic pain or pregnancy-associated hyperemesis will become more common.[281] **No safe threshold limits for *Cannabis* use have been determined, and prenatal use can have long-term negative effects.**[267] Little is known about prenatal exposure to medicinal *Cannabis*.

Data to direct counseling about *Cannabis* use during breastfeeding are limited. **For women who use *Cannabis* daily, the AAP discourages breastfeeding.**[280] Daily use results in high levels of *Cannabis* and its metabolites in breast milk and is associated with neurodevelopmental impairment in the first year of life.[267,279] Women who report infrequent *Cannabis* use should refrain from use during breastfeeding.

Cocaine

Cocaine is a stimulant that can be inhaled, injected, or smoked. It crosses the placenta and the fetal blood-brain barrier. In the mid-1980s, prenatal use of cocaine received considerable media attention. Early studies reported catastrophic effects of prenatal cocaine exposure, and children born to cocaine-abusing mothers were often stigmatized at school and in the community.[282,283] Subsequent studies either failed to replicate previous reports[284] or found that effects were due to co-occurring factors and environmental stressors that form the context in which cocaine addiction often occurs.

Women who use cocaine while pregnant are at increased risk for adrenergic crises that include coronary artery vasospasms and severe hypertension. Notably, β-blockade of these complications is contraindicated because it can lead to unopposed α-adrenergic stimulation. **Fetal consequences of maternal cocaine use include PTB, premature rupture of membranes, placental abruption, and preeclampsia.**[285,286] **Prenatal cocaine exposure is also associated with IUGR,[287] LBW, and SGA.**[288] The relationship between prenatal cocaine exposure and congenital defects is strongly affected by factors associated with cocaine use.[288] In a large prospective blinded study of congenital anomalies in children exposed to cocaine prenatally, no consistent increase or pattern of birth defects was found.[289]

Pregnant cocaine users should be encouraged to stop and be referred for substance-abuse treatment. Acute cocaine intoxication and withdrawal can be treated with supportive measures. Effective psychosocial and behavioral treatments have been developed for pregnant drug-dependent women.[226,290] Communication between prenatal/postpartum care providers and substance-abuse treatment staff is central to the success of such efforts. **The AAP considers cocaine use a contraindication to breastfeeding.**[291]

Methamphetamine

Methamphetamine is a stimulant that results in increased alertness along with hypertension, confusion, decreased appetite, and weight loss.[292] Prenatal methamphetamine use can produce vasoconstriction and restriction of nutrients and oxygen to the fetus.[293] About 5% of American pregnant women have used methamphetamine.[294] Research on methamphetamine-exposed pregnancies remains limited. Gorman and colleagues[295] found that **methamphetamine users were more likely than nonusers to experience gestational hypertension** (OR, 1.8; CI, 1.6 to 2.0), **preeclampsia** (OR, 2.7; CI, 2.4 to 3.0), **intrauterine fetal death** (OR, 5.1; CI, 3.7 to 7.2), **and abruption** (OR, 5.5; CI, 4.9 to 6.3). **They were also more likely to have PTB** (OR, 2.9; 2.7 to 3.1), **neonatal death** (OR, 3.1; CI, 2.3 to 4.2), **and infant death** (OR, 2.5; CI, 1.7 to 3.7). **Children with in utero exposure to methamphetamine displayed greater cognitive problems at age 7.5 years than controls.**[296]

As with other drugs of abuse, prenatal methamphetamine use occurs amid a variety of adverse comorbidities such as psychiatric disorders, other drug use, poor nutrition, lack of health care, and stressful life experiences.[297] Comprehensive harm-reduction models of perinatal care contribute to improved birth outcomes.

For acute methamphetamine intoxication, benzodiazepines and antipsychotic medications calm the agitated, combative, or psychotic patient. No medication is effective for treatment of methamphetamine withdrawal. **The AAP[291] lists amphetamines as contraindicated during breastfeeding.**

Opioids

In the United States, prescription opioid use and misuse has increased dramatically. In a national survey, 4.5 million Americans reported past-month nonmedical use of prescription narcotics, and 1.9 million were diagnosed with opioid use disorder.[255] This escalation is also occurring in pregnant women. In the past decade, prescription opioid use in pregnancy has risen more than fourfold—from 1.2 to 5.6 cases per 1000 live births. Cases of neonatal abstinence syndrome (NAS) also more than doubled during this period, rising from 1.2 to 3.4 per 1000 hospital live births.[298] In a study of pregnant women entering drug abuse treatment over a 20-year time span, **the percentage of opioid-dependent women who reported prescription narcotics as their drug of choice rose from 2% to 28%.**[299]

Opioid-dependent pregnant women who use illicit drugs have a sixfold increase in complications such as PTB, IUGR, fetal distress, meconium aspiration, and LBW.[300,301] Neonatal problems include NAS, neurobehavioral problems, and mortality with a *74-fold increase* in risk for SIDS.[300]

OPIOID AGONIST THERAPY

In a public policy statement, the American Society of Addiction Medicine recommended that pregnant opioid-dependent women be encouraged to initiate opioid agonist therapy (OAT) and continue it through delivery and postpartum. Women who were already receiving OAT prior to becoming pregnant should continue because discontinuation increases the risk for relapse, and detoxification can precipitate fetal distress and comes with higher morbidity and mortality rates. If detoxification is initiated, it should be under medical supervision during the second trimester of pregnancy, when complications are less likely to occur.[227]

Since the 1970s, methadone has been the preferred treatment for opioid-dependent pregnant women (Box 55-4). Methadone is a long acting μ-opioid receptor agonist that provides a steady concentration of opioid in the pregnant woman's bloodstream. Methadone reduces drug craving and prevents negative fetal effects associated with repeated in utero withdrawal from heroin. Methadone maintenance also promotes better adherence to prenatal care and drug abuse counseling because visits can be scheduled to coincide with once-daily methadone dosing. However, **methadone has direct effects on fetal neurobehavioral functions.** The fetuses of women on methadone with uncomplicated pregnancies were evaluated at peak and trough methadone levels.[302] At peak methadone levels, the fetal heart rate was slower, less variable, and displayed fewer accelerations. Fetuses displayed less motor activity, and the integration between heart rate and motor activity was attenuated. Real-time ultrasound recordings at 34 to 37 weeks' gestation were obtained from methadone-treated and untreated women. Both a slower rate and fewer fetal breathing movements were observed for the methadone-treated group regardless of time since the mothers' daily dose.[302]

More recently, **buprenorphine** has been studied as an alternative to methadone. As a partial μ-opioid receptor agonist and κ-receptor antagonist with a half-life of 24 to 60 hours, buprenorphine is effective in the treatment of opioid

---

BOX 55-4   INITIATION OF METHADONE MAINTENANCE TREATMENT IN PREGNANCY

- A medical and substance abuse history should be taken.
- Physical examination is used to evaluate stigmata of intravenous opioid use (needle scars, phlebitis, and skin abscesses).
- Laboratory tests: urine drug testing is used to document opioid and other drug use. Serum infection screening and baseline liver function can be used if hepatitis C infection is known.
- Quantify withdrawal symptoms with a standardized assessment such as the Clinical Opioid Withdrawal Scale (COWS)[320] available online at http://www.csam-asam.org/pdf/misc/COWS_induction_flow_sheet.doc.
- Initial dose of methadone is 10 to 30 mg with additional dosing of 5 to 10 mg every 4 to 6 hours while patient is awake for breakthrough withdrawal symptoms.
- Titrate dose up to relieve withdrawal symptoms for 24 hours with minimal or no craving.
- Methadone has been associated with rate-corrected QTc prolongation and possible consequent cardiac arrhythmia; review personal and family history for risk factors and consider screening electrocardiogram and follow-up evaluation in collaboration with an outpatient methadone clinic.
- When stable, discharge the patient to a methadone clinic to monitor subsequent dosing.
- Evaluate for methadone drug-drug interactions (tricyclic antidepressants, antipsychotic medications, and certain antiemetics and antibiotics are also associated with prolonged QT interval).
- As pregnancy progresses, the same methadone dosage produces lower blood methadone levels, so higher dosing may be required to control symptoms.
- After birth, monitor for signs of overmedication and adjust dosing as needed.

---

dependence. Research with buprenorphine in pregnant women is limited, but it appears to have similar effectiveness to methadone in the treatment of opioid use disorders in pregnancy. Neither methadone nor buprenorphine treatment are associated with increased risk of birth defects. Whereas induction might be easier with methadone than with buprenorphine, a randomized trial of the two **demonstrated a significant reduction in NAS severity for buprenorphine-exposed neonates.**[303] A meta-analysis showed equivalent maternal outcomes for methadone and buprenorphine but improved outcomes for infants.[304,305] If buprenorphine is used in pregnancy, it should be prescribed without naloxone.

PRENATAL CARE

Obstetricians who provide care to pregnant women with opioid use disorder should emphasize several points. First, **maternal and infant outcomes for women who receive OAT during pregnancy are better than those associated with continued prenatal use of illicit opioids.** Both methadone and buprenorphine decrease opioid and other drug abuse, criminal activity, and rates of infection with hepatitis B and C, human immunodeficiency virus (HIV), and sexually transmitted diseases. OAT is associated with lower relapse rates, reduced fetal exposure to illicit drug use, improved adherence to obstetric care, and enhanced neonatal outcomes.[306] Second, **for the majority of pregnant women who receive OAT, standard prenatal care is**

adequate. Providing treatment in an environment where the woman feels safe and supported improves compliance.[307] More intensive care should be reserved for cases where there is a medical indication for closer monitoring. Third, practitioners should inform women that the AAP[280] supports breastfeeding for women receiving OAT regardless of dose. On average, infants receive 2% to 3% of the weight-adjusted maternal methadone dose via breast milk. For mothers treated with OAT, breastfeeding is associated with lower infant treatment rates for NAS and shorter hospital stays.[308-310]

Methadone is metabolized by CYP2B6, CYP2C19, and CYP3A4. Clearance in pregnant women is increased, which results in increased dose requirements across pregnancy, and split dosing may be beneficial.[311] Some women are concerned about increasing their dose and potential harm to the baby. Obstetricians can explain that the higher doses are needed to offset increased clearance related to the physical changes of pregnancy. For mothers compliant with OAT, routine antenatal fetal surveillance is not required.[312] However, if relapse or polysubstance use is suspected, fetal surveillance should be considered in the third trimester.

NEONATAL ABSTINENCE SYNDROME
Whereas 30% to 80% of infants exposed to opioids in utero require treatment for neonatal abstinence syndrome,[313] at this time we cannot predict which infants will require treatment. There is increasing evidence that genetic variability in the opioid receptor may play a role in who develops NAS.[314] NAS is characterized by irritability, tremulousness, sweating, nasal stuffiness, poor suckling, diarrhea, vomiting, and seizures.[315] The incidence of NAS is higher with methadone exposure than with shorter-acting opioids. NAS onset varies across different opioid drugs and can begin as early as 24 hours and as late as 14 days after delivery. Neither the incidence nor severity of NAS correlates with maternal methadone dose at delivery, and NAS can occur in infants born to mothers whose dose is as low as 10 mg per day[316]; therefore **limiting methadone dose to minimize risk of NAS is not warranted.**

ACUTE PAIN MANAGEMENT FOR WOMEN ON OPIOID AGONIST THERAPY
Treatment of acute pain in labor and after delivery is a challenge for women on OAT. After verification of the daily dose, **uninterrupted full-dose maintenance treatment is imperative.** Acute pain should be managed based on clinical evaluation because women who are opioid dependent are likely to need higher doses of narcotics for pain because of tolerance and hyperalgesia.[317] Labor epidural and combined spinal-epidural analgesia are effective,[318] and studies suggest starting analgesia early in labor. Multimodal analgesia—nonsteroidal antiinflammatory drugs (NSAIDs), acetaminophen, and adjuvant drugs that enhance opioid effects, such as TCAs—may be coadministered. For women who require opioids for pain control, dose requirements may be 30% to 100% higher than routine dosing.[319,320] Analgesic dosing should be continuous or scheduled rather than as needed. Mixed agonist and antagonist opioid analgesics—such as pentazocine, nalbuphine, and butorphanol—should be avoided because they may displace the maintenance opioid from receptors and can precipitate acute opioid withdrawal. If methadone or buprenorphine doses were increased antenatally, careful monitoring and consideration of a gradual postpartum dose reduction over 1 to 2 weeks should be considered.[311]

- Mental health is fundamental to health. To the extent that maternal biopsychosocial exposures with negative impact on pregnancy outcomes can be diminished, eliminated, or replaced with positive factors, the risk of poor pregnancy outcome can be reduced.
- Major depression is a treatable illness that is the leading cause of disease burden among girls and women worldwide. The period prevalence of depression is 12.7% during pregnancy, and 7.5% of women have a new (incident) episode.
- A brief and efficient 10-item self-report screening instrument, the Edinburgh Postnatal Depression Scale, is available to screen for perinatal depression. For clinical practice screening, the cutoff scores for probable major depression in postpartum women is 13 or more; for pregnant women, it is 15 or more.
- Women with postpartum depression should be evaluated for bipolar disorder—which is characterized not only by depression but also by episodes of hypomania, mania, or mixed states—before prescribing antidepressant treatment, because antidepressants without a mood stabilizer can result in symptomatic worsening.
- The first-line medications for treatment of a depressed breastfeeding woman are sertraline, paroxetine, and nortriptyline; however, established efficacy of another drug in the individual woman must be considered in the selection of an appropriate medication.
- Abrupt discontinuation of any psychotropic medication creates a higher risk for recurrence than does gradual tapering and discontinuation (over at least 2 weeks).
- Postpartum psychosis is characterized by (1) rapid onset of hectic mood fluctuation, (2) marked cognitive impairment suggestive of delirium, (3) bizarre behavior, (4) insomnia, and (5) visual and auditory, and often unusual (tactile and olfactory), hallucinations. Women with acute-onset postpartum psychosis usually have bipolar disorder.
- The first-line treatment for anorexia nervosa is normalization of eating and weight restoration. Cognitive behavioral therapy is the first-line treatment for bulimia nervosa. Antidepressant medications are the second line treatment for bulimia nervosa, and they can also be useful adjuncts to CBT.
- Antipsychotic drug maintenance treatment and psychosocial support interventions aimed at maximizing function are the mainstays of treatment for schizophrenia.
- Concurrent maternal smoking, substance use, poor nutrition, and socioeconomic problems increase the risk for less optimal pregnancy outcomes.
- The perception of substance use disorders as afflictions solely of poor, minority, and young women is erroneous. Screening measures are available and easy to use, and multidisciplinary treatment intervention results in improved reproductive outcomes.

REFERENCES

1. American Psychiatric Association. *Diagnostic and Statistical Manual of Mental Disorders.* 5th ed. Washington, DC: American Psychiatric Publishing; 2013.
2. Misra DP, Guyer B, Allston A. Integrated perinatal health framework. A multiple determinants model with a life span approach. *Am J Prev Med.* 2003;25(1):65-75.
3. Arnow BA. Relationships between childhood maltreatment, adult health and psychiatric outcomes, and medical utilization. *J Clin Psychiatry.* 2004;65(suppl 12):10-15.
4. Misra DP, et al. Do fathers matter? Paternal contributions to birth outcomes and racial disparities. *Am J Obstet Gynecol.* 2010;202(2):99-100.
5. Teitler J. Father involvement, child health, and maternal health behavior. *Child Youth Serv Rev.* 2001;23:403-425.
6. Oklahoma State Department of Health Maternal and Child Health Service. *Father's Intention of Pregnancy PRAMSGRAM,* 2007. Available at <www.health.ok.gov>; keyword PRAMS.
7. Regier DA, et al. The de facto US mental and addictive disorders service system. Epidemiologic catchment area prospective 1-year prevalence rates of disorders and services. *Arch Gen Psychiatry.* 1993;50(2):85-94.
8. Gaynes BN, et al. Perinatal depression: prevalence, screening accuracy, and screening outcomes. *Evid Rep Technol Assess (Summ).* 2005;119:1-8.
9. Hobfoll SE, et al. Depression prevalence and incidence among inner-city pregnant and postpartum women. *J Consult Clin Psychol.* 1995;63(3):445-453.
10. Logsdon MC, et al. Predictors of depression in mothers of pre-term infants. *J Soc Behav Pers.* 1997;12:73-88.
11. Troutman BR, Cutrona CE. Nonpsychotic postpartum depression among adolescent mothers. *J Abnorm Psychol.* 1990;99(1):69-78.
12. Hays RD, et al. Functioning and well-being outcomes of patients with depression compared with chronic general medical illnesses. *Arch Gen Psychiatry.* 1995;52(1):11-19.
13. O'Hara MW, Neunaber DJ, Zekoski EM. Prospective study of postpartum depression: prevalence, course, and predictive factors. *J Abnorm Psychol.* 1984;93(2):158-171.
14. Kendler KS, et al. The lifetime history of major depression in women. Reliability of diagnosis and heritability. *Arch Gen Psychiatry.* 1993;50(11):863-870.
15. Mazure CM, et al. Adverse life events and cognitive-personality characteristics in the prediction of major depression and antidepressant response. *Am J Psychiatry.* 2000;157(6):896-903.
16. Davidson J, Robertson E. A follow-up study of post partum illness, 1946-1978. *Acta Psychiatr Scand.* 1985;71(5):451-457.
17. Elliott SA, et al. Promoting mental health after childbirth: a controlled trial of primary prevention of postnatal depression. *Br J Clin Psychol.* 2000;39(Pt 3):223-241.
18. Kendell RE, Chalmers JC, Platz C. Epidemiology of puerperal psychoses. *Br J Psychiatry.* 1987;150:662-673.
19. Munk-Olsen T, et al. New parents and mental disorders: a population-based register study. *JAMA.* 2006;296(21):2582-2589.
20. Cox JL, Holden JM, Sagovsky R. Detection of postnatal depression. Development of the 10-item Edinburgh Postnatal Depression Scale. *Br J Psychiatry.* 1987;150:782-786.
21. Cox JL, Holden J. *Perinatal Mental Health: A Guide to the Edinburgh Postnatal Depression Screening Scale.* Bell and Bain Ltd; 2003.
22. Murray L, Cox JL. Screening for depression during pregnancy with the Edinburgh Depression Scale (EPDS). *J Reprod Infant Psychol.* 1990;8:99-107.
23. Wisner KL, Parry BL, Piontek CM. Clinical practice. Postpartum depression. *N Engl J Med.* 2002;347(3):194-199.
24. Bloch M, et al. Effects of gonadal steroids in women with a history of postpartum depression. *Am J Psychiatry.* 2000;157(6):924-930.
25. Wisner KL, Peindl KS, Hanusa BH. Effects of childbearing on the natural history of panic disorder with comorbid mood disorder. *J Affect Disord.* 1996;41(3):173-180.
26. Wisner KL, et al. Obsessions and compulsions in women with postpartum depression. *J Clin Psychiatry.* 1999;60(3):176-180.
27. Wisner KL, et al. Risk-benefit decision making for treatment of depression during pregnancy. *Am J Psychiatry.* 2000;157(12):1933-1940.
28. Grote NK, et al. A meta-analysis of depression during pregnancy and the risk of preterm birth, low birth weight, and intrauterine growth restriction. *Arch Gen Psychiatry.* 2010;67(10):1012-1024.
29. Murray L. The impact of postnatal depression on infant development. *J Child Psychol Psychiatry.* 1992;33(3):543-561.
30. Pawlby S, et al. Antenatal depression predicts depression in adolescent offspring: prospective longitudinal community-based study. *J Affect Disord.* 2009;113(3):236-243.
31. Whiffen VE, Gotlib IH. Infants of postpartum depressed mothers: temperament and cognitive status. *J Abnorm Psychol.* 1989;98(3):274-279.
32. Sanz EJ, et al. Selective serotonin reuptake inhibitors in pregnant women and neonatal withdrawal syndrome: a database analysis. *Lancet.* 2005;365(9458):482-487.
33. Wisner KL, Stowe ZN. Psychobiology of postpartum mood disorders. *Semin Reprod Endocrinol.* 1997;15(1):77-89.
34. Gonzalez HM, et al. Depression care in the United States: too little for too few. *Arch Gen Psychiatry.* 2010;67(1):37-46.
35. Vesga-Lopez O, et al. Psychiatric disorders in pregnant and postpartum women in the United States. *Arch Gen Psychiatry.* 2008;65(7):805-815.
36. Bennett IM, et al. Pregnancy-related discontinuation of antidepressants and depression care visits among Medicaid recipients. *Psychiatr Serv.* 2010;61(4):386-391.
37. Spinelli MG, Endicott J. Controlled clinical trial of interpersonal psychotherapy versus parenting education program for depressed pregnant women. *Am J Psychiatry.* 2003;160(3):555-562.
38. Practice guideline for the assessment and treatment of patients with suicidal behaviors. *Am J Psychiatry.* 2003;160(11 suppl):1-60.
39. Wisner KL, et al. Pharmacotherapy for depressed pregnant women: overcoming obstacles to gathering essential data. *Clin Pharmacol Ther.* 2009;86(4):362-365.
40. Sit DK, et al. Best practices: an emerging best practice model for perinatal depression care. *Psychiatr Serv.* 2009;60(11):1429-1431.
41. Wisner KL. SSRI treatment during pregnancy: are we asking the right questions? *Depress Anxiety.* 2010;27(8):695-698.
42. Andersen JT, et al. Exposure to selective serotonin reuptake inhibitors in early pregnancy and the risk of miscarriage. *Obstet Gynecol.* 2014;124(4):655-661.
43. Jimenez-Solem E, et al. SSRI use during pregnancy and risk of stillbirth and neonatal mortality. *Am J Psychiatry.* 2013;170(3):299-304.
44. Alwan S, et al. Use of selective serotonin-reuptake inhibitors in pregnancy and the risk of birth defects. *N Engl J Med.* 2007;356(26):2684-2692.
45. Louik C, et al. First-trimester use of selective serotonin-reuptake inhibitors and the risk of birth defects. *N Engl J Med.* 2007;356(26):2675-2683.
46. Greene MF. Teratogenicity of SSRIs—serious concern or much ado about little? *N Engl J Med.* 2007;356(26):2732-2733.
47. Bérard A, Zhao JP, Sheehy O. Sertraline use during pregnancy and the risk of major malformations. *Am J Obstet Gynecol.* 2015;212(6):795.e1-795.e12.
48. Wisner KL, et al. Major depression and antidepressant treatment: impact on pregnancy and neonatal outcomes. *Am J Psychiatry.* 2009;166(5):557-566.
49. Palmsten K, Hernandez-Diaz S. Can nonrandomized studies on the safety of antidepressants during pregnancy convincingly beat confounding, chance, and prior beliefs? *Epidemiology.* 2012;23(5):686-688.
50. Jimenez-Solem E, et al. Exposure to selective serotonin reuptake inhibitors and the risk of congenital malformations: a nationwide cohort study. *BMJ Open.* 2012;2(3).
51. Huybrechts KF, et al. Antidepressant use in pregnancy and the risk of cardiac defects. *N Engl J Med.* 2014;370(25):2397-2407.
52. Wisner KL, et al. Does fetal exposure to SSRIs or maternal depression impact infant growth? *Am J Psychiatry.* 2013;170(5):485-493.
53. Nulman I, et al. Neurodevelopment of children exposed in utero to antidepressant drugs. *N Engl J Med.* 1997;336(4):258-262.
54. Nulman I, et al. Child development following exposure to tricyclic antidepressants or fluoxetine throughout fetal life: a prospective, controlled study. *Am J Psychiatry.* 2002;159(11):1889-1895.
55. Casper RC, et al. Length of prenatal exposure to selective serotonin reuptake inhibitor (SSRI) antidepressants: effects on neonatal adaptation and psychomotor development. *Psychopharmacology (Berl).* 2011;217(2):211-219.
56. Suri R, et al. A prospective, naturalistic, blinded study of early neurobehavioral outcomes for infants following prenatal antidepressant exposure. *J Clin Psychiatry.* 2011;72(7):1002-1007.
57. Nulman I, et al. Neurodevelopment of children following prenatal exposure to venlafaxine, selective serotonin reuptake inhibitors, or untreated maternal depression. *Am J Psychiatry.* 2012;169(11):1165-1174.
58. Santucci AK, et al. Impact of prenatal exposure to serotonin reuptake inhibitors or maternal major depressive disorder on infant developmental outcomes. *J Clin Psychiatry.* 2014;75(10):1088-1095.

59. Moses-Kolko EL, et al. Neonatal signs after late in utero exposure to serotonin reuptake inhibitors: literature review and implications for clinical applications. *JAMA*. 2005;293(19):2372-2383.

60. Laine K, et al. Effects of exposure to selective serotonin reuptake inhibitors during pregnancy on serotonergic symptoms in newborns and cord blood monoamine and prolactin concentrations. *Arch Gen Psychiatry*. 2003; 60(7):720-726.

61. Yonkers KA, et al. The management of depression during pregnancy: a report from the American Psychiatric Association and the American College of Obstetricians and Gynecologists. *Gen Hosp Psychiatry*. 2009; 31(5):403-413.

62. Cohen LS, et al. Relapse of major depression during pregnancy in women who maintain or discontinue antidepressant treatment. *JAMA*. 2006;295(5):499-507.

63. Yonkers KA, et al. Does antidepressant use attenuate the risk of a major depressive episode in pregnancy? *Epidemiology*. 2011;22(6):848-854.

64. Samer CF, et al. Applications of CYP450 testing in the clinical setting. *Mol Diagn Ther*. 2013;17(3):165-184.

65. Wisner K, Peindl K, Gigliotti T. Tricyclics vs SSRIs for postpartum depression. *Arch Womens Ment Health*. 1999;1:189.

66. Sit D, et al. Disposition of chiral and racemic fluoxetine and norfluoxetine across childbearing. *J Clin Psychopharmacol*. 2010;30(4):381-386.

67. Sit DK, et al. Changes in antidepressant metabolism and dosing across pregnancy and early postpartum. *J Clin Psychiatry*. 2008;69(4):652-658.

68. Ververs FF, et al. Effect of cytochrome P450 2D6 genotype on maternal paroxetine plasma concentrations during pregnancy. *Clin Pharmacokinet*. 2009;48(10):677-683.

69. Wirz-Justice A, et al. A randomized, double-blind, placebo-controlled study of light therapy for antepartum depression. *J Clin Psychiatry*. 2011;72(7):986-993.

70. Wirz-Justice A, Benedetti F, Terman M. *Chronotherapeutics for affective disorders : a clinician's manual for light and wake therapy*. Vol 12. New York: Karger, Basel; 2009.

71. Manber R, et al. Acupuncture for depression during pregnancy: a randomized controlled trial. *Obstet Gynecol*. 2010;115(3):511-520.

72. Bodnar LM, Wisner KL. Nutrition and depression: implications for improving mental health among childbearing-aged women. *Biol Psychiatry*. 2005;58(9):679-685.

73. Freeman MP, et al. Complementary and alternative medicine in major depressive disorder: the American Psychiatric Association Task Force report. *J Clin Psychiatry*. 2010;71(6):669-681.

74. Freeman MP, et al. Omega-3 fatty acids: evidence basis for treatment and future research in psychiatry. *J Clin Psychiatry*. 2006;67(12):1954-1967.

75. Keenan K, et al. Association between fatty acid supplementation and prenatal stress in African Americans: a randomized controlled trial. *Obstet Gynecol*. 2014;124(6):1080-1087.

76. Wall R, et al. Fatty acids from fish: the anti-inflammatory potential of long-chain omega-3 fatty acids. *Nutr Rev*. 2010;68(5):280-289.

77. Lanza di Scalea T, Wisner KL. Antidepressant medication use during breastfeeding. *Clin Obstet Gynecol*. 2009;52(3):483-497.

78. Wisner KL, et al. Postpartum depression: a randomized trial of sertraline versus nortriptyline. *J Clin Psychopharmacol*. 2006;26(4):353-360.

79. Hantsoo L, et al. A randomized, placebo-controlled, double-blind trial of sertraline for postpartum depression. *Psychopharmacology (Berl)*. 2014;231(5):939-948.

80. Gregoire AJ, et al. Transdermal oestrogen for treatment of severe postnatal depression. *Lancet*. 1996;347(9006):930-933.

81. Perheentupa A, Ruokonen A, Tapanainen JS. Transdermal estradiol treatment suppresses serum gonadotropins during lactation without transfer into breast milk. *Fertil Steril*. 2004;82(4):903-907.

82. Zlotnick C, et al. A preventive intervention for pregnant women on public assistance at risk for postpartum depression. *Am J Psychiatry*. 2006;163(8): 1443-1445.

83. Wisner KL, et al. Prevention of postpartum depression: a pilot randomized clinical trial. *Am J Psychiatry*. 2004;161(7):1290-1292.

84. Lawrie TA, et al. A double-blind randomised placebo controlled trial of postnatal norethisterone enanthate: the effect on postnatal depression and serum hormones. *Br J Obstet Gynaecol*. 1998;105(10):1082-1090.

85. Oates M. Perinatal psychiatric disorders: a leading cause of maternal morbidity and mortality. *Br Med Bull*. 2003;67:219-229.

86. Wisner KL, et al. Onset timing, thoughts of self-harm, and diagnoses in postpartum women with screen-positive depression findings. *JAMA Psychiatry*. 2013;70(5):490-498.

87. Chaudron LH, Caine ED. Suicide among women: a critical review. *J Am Med Womens Assoc*. 2004;59(2):125-134.

88. Practice guideline for the assessment and treatment of patients with suicidal behaviors. *Am J Psychiatry*. 2003;160(11 suppl):1-60.

89. Merikangas KR, et al. Lifetime and 12-month prevalence of bipolar spectrum disorder in the National Comorbidity Survey replication. *Arch Gen Psychiatry*. 2007;64(5):543-552.

90. Merikangas KR, et al. Prevalence and correlates of bipolar spectrum disorder in the world mental health survey initiative. *Arch Gen Psychiatry*. 2011;68(3):241-251.

91. Goodwin FK, Jamison K. *Suicide in Manic-Depressive Disorder*. New York: Oxford University Press; 1990.

92. McElroy SL, et al. Axis I psychiatric comorbidity and its relationship to historical illness variables in 288 patients with bipolar disorder. *Am J Psychiatry*. 2001;158(3):420-426.

93. Baldessarini RJ, Tondo L, Hennen J. Treatment delays in bipolar disorders. *Am J Psychiatry*. 1999;156(5):811-812.

94. Hirschfeld RM, et al. Development and validation of a screening instrument for bipolar spectrum disorder: the Mood Disorder Questionnaire. *Am J Psychiatry*. 2000;157(11):1873-1875.

95. Clark CT, et al. Does screening with the MDQ and EPDS improve identification of bipolar disorder in an obstetrical sample? *Depress Anxiety*. 2015;Under review.

96. Bergink V, et al. Prevention of postpartum psychosis and mania in women at high risk. *Am J Psychiatry*. 2012;169(6):609-615.

97. Viguera AC, et al. Risk of recurrence in women with bipolar disorder during pregnancy: prospective study of mood stabilizer discontinuation. *Am J Psychiatry*. 2007;164(12):1817-1824, quiz 1923.

98. Munk-Olsen T, et al. Risks and predictors of readmission for a mental disorder during the postpartum period. *Arch Gen Psychiatry*. 2009;66(2): 189-195.

99. Harlow BL, et al. Incidence of hospitalization for postpartum psychotic and bipolar episodes in women with and without prior prepregnancy or prenatal psychiatric hospitalizations. *Arch Gen Psychiatry*. 2007;64(1): 42-48.

100. Yonkers KA, et al. Management of bipolar disorder during pregnancy and the postpartum period. *Am J Psychiatry*. 2004;161(4):608-620.

Additional references for this chapter are available at ExpertConsult.com.

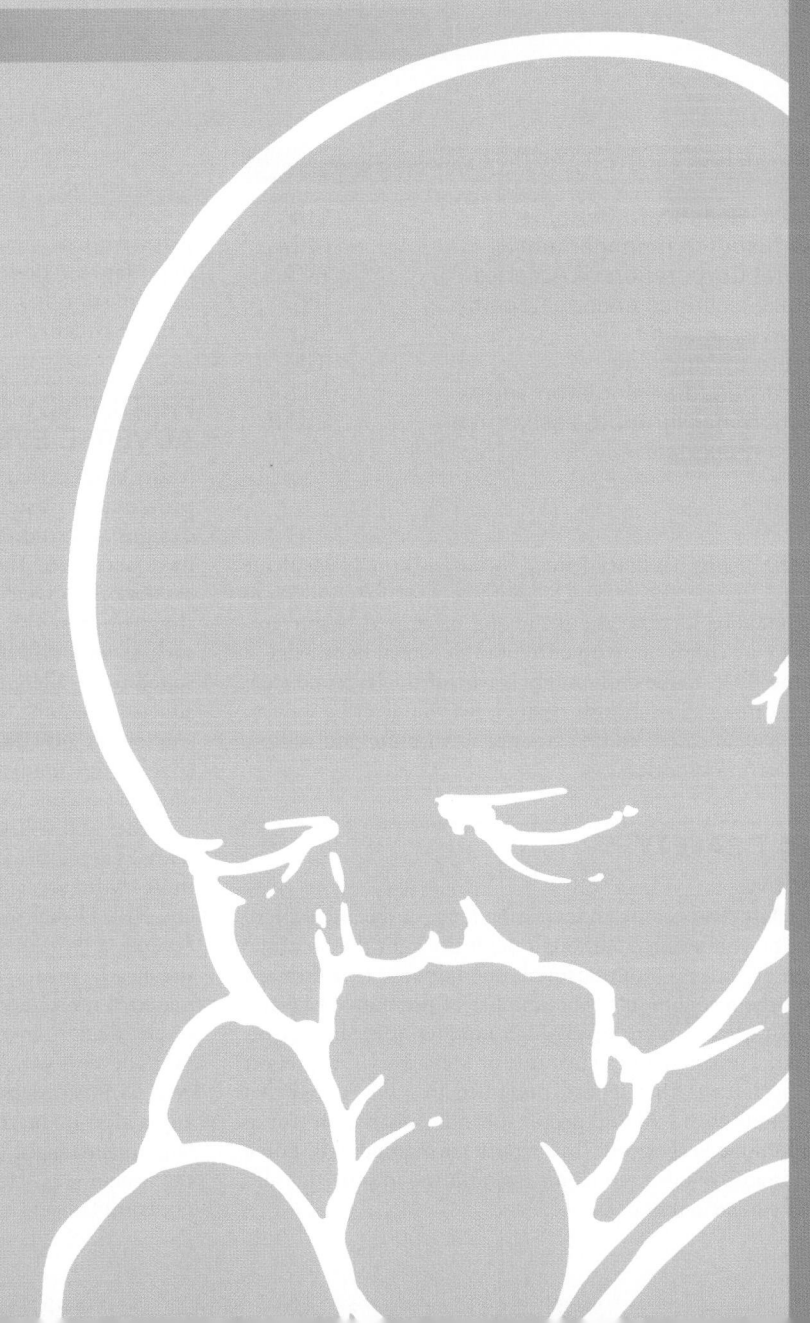

Legal and Ethical Issues in Perinatology

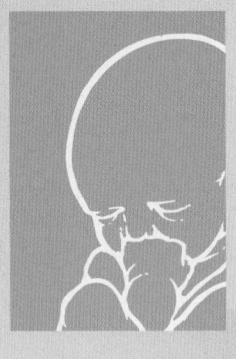

CHAPTER 56

Patient Safety and Quality Measurement in Obstetric Care

WILLIAM A. GROBMAN and JENNIFER L. BAILIT

KEY ABBREVIATIONS

Catholic Healthcare Partners	CHP
Crew resource management	CRM
Hospital Corporation of America	HCA
Hypoxic-ischemic encephalopathy	HIE
Intensive care unit	ICU
Institute of Medicine	IOM
Nulliparous term singleton vertex	NTSV
Situation, background, assessment, recommendation	SBAR

Health care quality has been defined by the Institute of Medicine (IOM) as, "the degree to which health services for individuals and populations increase the likelihood of desired health outcomes and are consistent with current professional knowledge."[1] Under the IOM framework, safety is part of the larger concept of health care quality.[1] In this chapter, we will describe ways to enhance patient safety and to attempt to measure and achieve quality care in obstetrics.

PATIENT SAFETY
Overview

Patient safety has become an increasing focus of the attention of the medical community. Although the reasons for the increased focus are doubtlessly multifactorial, one important contributor has been the recognition of the number of preventable adverse events that occur. The relatively high number of medical errors has been documented in the Institute of Medicine (IOM) report *To Err is Human.* That report, published in 1998, noted that between 44,000 and 98,000 people die in hospitals each year as the result of medical errors.[2] This report, correspondingly, noted the importance of error reduction as a means to improved health care and patient outcomes.

Because obstetric admissions are the leading cause of hospitalization for women in the United States, accounting for over 4 million hospital discharges each year,[3] pregnant women are at particular risk of encountering a medical error. Emphasizing the importance of obstetric safety further is the fact that each obstetric admission has the potential to affect the health not only of a single patient but of both a mother and her infant.

FREQUENCY OF PREVENTABLE OBSTETRIC ADVERSE EVENTS

Many studies that have sought to determine the frequency of preventable obstetric adverse events have used retrospective designs and studied in detail cases in which adverse outcomes have occurred. The overall frequency of preventable adverse events on a given obstetric unit cannot be determined from these studies. This is particularly true given that adverse events, such as administration of a medication to which the patient is stated to be allergic, may occur that do not result in an actual adverse outcome (e.g., anaphylactic shock). However, these studies do give insight into the frequency with which that adverse outcome may have been preventable when such an outcome occurs.

Geller and colleagues[4] analyzed cases of morbidity and mortality that occurred at their institution. These cases included those with severe and "near-miss" morbidity. It should be emphasized that so-called near-miss morbidity is not so named because a woman nearly misses having morbidity but because she nearly misses a mortal event.[5] Thus in their framework, maternal morbidity has a spectrum of severity, and none is more severe than near-miss morbidity. In their study, morbid and mortal events were often found to be preventable, and a *preventable event* was defined as one that could have been avoided by any action or inaction on the part of the health care provider (e.g., mismanagement of patients, failure or delay in diagnosis), the system (e.g., failure in communication), or the patient (e.g., noncompliance). Moreover, women who had the most adverse outcomes were more likely to have had preventable events: 16% of cases with severe morbidity were judged preventable versus 46% of near-miss events and 41% of mortal events.

Berg and colleagues[6] focused exclusively on maternal deaths that occurred in North Carolina. They studied the circumstances that surrounded the pregnancy-related deaths of 108 women between 1995 and 1999. Deaths were considered potentially preventable if (1) preconception care and counseling could have improved outcome; (2) the patient had not adhered to medical advice; (3) the structure and functioning of the health care system was suboptimal; or (4) clinical care was not satisfactory. In their study, 40% of deaths were considered to be preventable, although this frequency significantly differed on the basis of the primary underlying cause of death. For example, 93% of deaths related to hemorrhage, but only 22% of deaths related to cardiomyopathy, were thought to be preventable.

White and associates[7] examined 90 cases that resulted in litigation and in which the claims had been closed. It should be noted that these cases included both gynecology and obstetrics cases, although the majority were related to obstetrics. In their study, 78% of these cases were thought to have a contributing factor that was potentially avoidable. Clark and colleagues[8] also analyzed claims data and focused only on those claims related to perinatal care. Their findings were quite similar to those of White and associates; specifically, they noted that 70% of cases were potentially preventable and related to the care the patient received in the hospital.

Forster and coworkers[9] did attempt to quantify the frequency of adverse events that occur on an obstetric unit through the use of a prospective study. These investigators placed an observer in the labor and delivery unit during the weekday hours of a 6-week period. This observer was trained to ascertain poor patient outcomes, procedural errors, and unsafe working conditions. Cases of concern that were ascertained by the observer were then further evaluated by a multidisciplinary team. The primary outcome of the study was the occurrence of a "quality problem," defined as the occurrence of either an adverse event—that is, an adverse outcome due to health care management, as opposed to progression of natural disease—or a potential adverse event (i.e., "defective processes that have a high likelihood of causing harm"). Of the over 400 patients who were cared for during the study period, 5% experienced a quality problem (i.e., 2% had an adverse event and 3% had a potential adverse event). Sixty-six percent of the adverse events that occurred were judged to be due to errors in health care delivery.

FACTORS THAT CONTRIBUTE TO PREVENTABLE ADVERSE EVENTS

The literature that exists would suggest that multiple contributors are involved in the occurrence of adverse obstetric events. Data from the Joint Commission, for example, illustrate the contributions that multiple factors make in the occurrence of major adverse maternal and perinatal outcomes. For example, their analysis of major maternal adverse events revealed multiple root causes that included lack of adequate communication, training, staffing, and patient assessment.[10] Other investigators similarly have found that preventable adverse events or potential events cannot be traced to one simple and easily remediable cause but are multifactorial and due to a complex interplay of factors. Geller, White, Forster and their colleagues[5,7,9] all have demonstrated the many different factors present at both the

provider and systems level and that have contributed to adverse events.

Despite the many factors that have been implicated in the occurrence of preventable adverse events, it is worth noting that communication and "systems" issues that transcend simple individual error have consistently been found to be predominant etiologies in the occurrence of these events.[5,7,9-11] *Systems issues* is a term that refers to problems that stem not from one individual's actions but from the interconnected relationships of people and institutional policies. **With regard to the sentinel events in maternal care analyzed by the Joint Commission, a communications issue was judged to be a root cause in over 80% of cases.**[10] This frequency far outstripped the next most frequent factors, competency and patient assessment, which were present in fewer than 40% of cases. In their review of closed claims, White and associates[7] noted that inadequate communication among providers was the single most common preventable factor associated with the claim. Similarly, in their prospective study, Forster and colleagues[9] noted that "systems" issues were the most common reason that their trained observer was alerted to further assess for the possibility of a quality problem.

APPROACHES TO IMPROVE OBSTETRIC SAFETY

The previous discussion highlighting the different factors that contribute to patient safety suggests that efforts to improve safety may require multiple different approaches. The potential need for a multifaceted approach is further suggested by the different levels within an organization at which these factors can manifest. **Specifically, key components required for the prevention of adverse events occur at (1) the individual level, such as the level of education or training provided to workers; (2) the group level, as with team effectiveness and communication; and (3) the structural level, like the standardization of processes within an organization.**[11] Correspondingly, attempts to enhance patient safety within obstetrics have utilized, in general, several different types of modalities. The theoretic underpinning to believe that these modalities should be effective—as well as the evidence supporting their use, with a focus on obstetrics—is discussed below.

Checklists and Protocols

Because of the complexity of health care processes and the corresponding potential for errors in communication, one approach to improve patient safety has been the introduction of standardized approaches to patient care. These approaches have taken the form of *protocols,* mandatory items for completion to lead the user to a predetermined outcome, and *checklists,* a list of action items or criteria arranged in a systematic manner that allow the user to record the presence or absence of the individual items listed to ensure that all are considered or completed. Although both are concerned with standardization, checklists provide explicit lists of items, actions thought to act as a cognitive aid due to grouping related items in an organized fashion to improve recall performance.[12]

Pronovost and colleagues[13] demonstrated the potential utility of checklists in their study regarding catheter-related bloodstream infections in the intensive care unit (ICU). In this study, checklists that detailed five key actions required during any central catheter placement were introduced in 108 ICUs throughout the state of Michigan. Of note, these key actions were evidence based; also, the checklists were not merely posted, they were supported by local leaders versed in the supporting evidence, who provided feedback with regard to optimal methods for implementation. Not only did the incidence of catheter-related bloodstream infections significantly decline by 3 months after implementation (incidence rate ratio, 0.62; 95% confidence interval [CI], 0.47 to 0.81), but this incidence continued to decline until 18 months (incidence rate ratio, 0.34; 95% CI, 0.23 to 0.50) after implementation, which was the end point of data collection.

A checklist to guide the administration of oxytocin was developed by Clark and associates,[14] who then implemented this checklist in a private hospital setting. The outcomes of the 100 women prior to checklist implementation were then compared with those of the 100 women who received oxytocin after the implementation. No difference was seen in the duration of labor, duration of oxytocin administration, or operative delivery after implementation, although the maximum dose of oxytocin used was significantly lower, as was the frequency of newborns with one or more complications ($P = .049$).

The potential benefits of a standardized approach to the evaluation and management of preeclampsia has been demonstrated by Menzies and colleagues.[15] After establishing a set of best practices, this group of investigators introduced these practices for preeclampsia management at British Columbia Women's Hospital. Among women with preeclampsia who were managed after the standardized approach was put into place, 0.7% experienced the composite end point of maternal adverse outcomes, which was an 86% reduction compared with the preintervention frequency of 5.1% ($P < .001$). Adverse perinatal outcomes were also reduced, although this finding did not reach statistical significance (odds [OR], 0.65; 95% CI, 0.37 to 1.16).

Nevertheless, a word of caution regarding checklists and protocols is warranted: The mere existence of one of these on a unit cannot be assumed to automatically result in improved care. As demonstrated by Pronovost and associates,[13] the presence of a checklist may enhance care when its components are evidence based and when its use is championed by members of the organization. Moreover, it is ideal to demonstrate—using either traditional scientific or quality improvement study designs—that its introduction is associated with improvement in the care provided or outcomes achieved.[16] Conversely, checklists or protocols can be present but still not translate into any tangible change in health care whatsoever. One set of investigators, for example, observed that the introduction of surgical safety checklists in Ontario, Canada, was not associated with improvements in operative complications or mortality.[17] Bailit and coworkers[18] have demonstrated a similar finding in obstetric care. In their analysis, obstetric units had similar outcomes related to postpartum hemorrhage or shoulder dystocia regardless of whether they had protocols for these events.

Simulation

Simulation refers to the recreation of an actual event that has previously occurred or could potentially occur.[19] **Simulation may be used to enhance patient safety in that an action or procedure can be repeated, thereby improving the execution of that action or procedure without ever exposing providers or patients to harm.** Essentially, simulation of events is an opportunity for health care workers to prepare and train for interventions. Although simulation may have benefits for any type of obstetric procedure (e.g., vaginal delivery), it has often been studied in events such as shoulder dystocia and eclampsia. In these occurrences, simulation may be particularly helpful not only for the novice but even for experienced professionals, who can maintain their skills in managing unpredictable and uncommon events.

Shoulder Dystocia

Data from multiple studies suggest that simulation may enhance several aspects of shoulder dystocia management, which includes communication among the team members, performance of the maneuvers necessary to relieve this problem, and documentation of the event. Moreover, these enhancements have been demonstrated for providers during both their residency training and postresidency experiences.

In a randomized trial, Deering and colleagues[20] demonstrated that those residents who were assigned to train for a shoulder dystocia using an obstetric birth simulator were significantly more likely to utilize maneuvers in a timely and correct fashion in a subsequent simulation than those residents who did not undergo initial simulation training. Furthermore, when judged by a blinded observer, those residents who had undergone simulation training scored higher on measures of overall performance and preparedness.

A study that examined presimulation and postsimulation training outcomes among both residents and attending physicians was performed by Goffman and coworkers.[21] In this study, participants underwent a simulation of a shoulder dystocia event followed by a debriefing that included (1) a brief lecture about shoulder dystocia, (2) a review of the basic maneuvers and a basic algorithm for management of shoulder dystocia, (3) a discussion on optimizing team performance during an obstetric emergency, (4) a review of the key components of documentation, and (5) a review of the digital recording of the simulations and discussion of provider performance. During a second, unanticipated shoulder dystocia simulation, providers demonstrated significant improvements in communication, use of maneuvers, and overall performance.

Similar results were obtained by Crofts and colleagues[22] in their multicenter comparison of presimulation and postsimulation outcomes. This study additionally attempted to ascertain whether high-fidelity simulation using a mannequin with a high degree of biofidelity would enhance performance to a greater extent than low-fidelity simulation using a simple doll-like mannequin by randomizing participants to one of these options. Regardless of randomized group, performance during a simulated shoulder dystocia was improved subsequent to simulation training. Although some measures of performance (e.g., total applied force) were improved to a greater extent in those participants who had undergone high-fidelity training, many other measures (e.g., peak force, use of maneuvers) were no different between the high- and low-fidelity groups. Improvement in performance of simulated shoulder dystocia events has been demonstrated to persist up to 12 months after training.[23]

The previous studies have examined outcomes during simulation events but have not demonstrated improvements in actual clinical outcomes related to simulation training. The few observational studies of clinical outcomes that do exist, however, seem to support the assertion that exposure to simulation may improve outcomes related to shoulder dystocia. In one study at a single institution, investigators examined outcomes both before and after initiation of a shoulder dystocia training program that utilized training in and practice of obstetric maneuvers.[24] After the training program, a significant increase was reported in the frequency with which appropriate maneuvers were used for shoulder dystocia, and a significant reduction was reported in neonatal injury at birth after shoulder dystocia (9.3% to 2.3%; relative risk [RR], 0.25; 95% CI, 0.11 to 0.57). Grobman and associates[25] also used simulation to help train providers to respond to a shoulder dystocia. They did not simulate specific maneuvers but instead emphasized the coordinated response and communication of the team once a shoulder dystocia was diagnosed. After simulation was used in this way, the frequency of brachial plexus palsy at discharge among neonates who had experienced a shoulder dystocia dropped from 7.6% to 1.3% (P = .04).

Eclampsia

Studies that have evaluated simulation training for eclamptic seizure management have demonstrated improvements in response as measured during additional simulations. For example, after having staff in a single tertiary care center participate in simulated eclamptic events with a debriefing session, Thompson and colleagues[26] found that patient resuscitations in posttraining simulation of eclampsia were better managed. Of note, these simulations occurred in the actual delivery unit, as opposed to a separate simulation laboratory, and these researchers used their initial simulations not only for training but also for elucidating site-specific barriers to an optimal response (e.g., an inefficient paging system). This ability of simulation to identify systems-level barriers to best practice has been noted by others as well.[27]

Ellis and colleagues[28] also examined pretraining and posttraining outcomes during eclampsia simulations. In their study, training was associated with an increase in the appropriate and timely completion of desired tasks (e.g., magnesium sulfate administration). Of note, although all participants underwent simulation training, they also were randomized to different training sites (i.e., simulation center vs. hospital unit) and to inclusion of teamwork training in their educational process. Neither site nor supplementary teamwork education was associated with additional improvement.

Other Obstetric Events

Other obstetric events that have been examined in the context of simulation include breech delivery, postpartum hemorrhage, and cord prolapse. In one study focused on breech delivery, after undergoing a simulation of an imminent term vaginal breech, residents took part in a training session with the simulator on the proper techniques for vaginal breech delivery.[29] After this training, residents repeated the standardized simulation. Simulations both before and after training were videotaped and judged by an investigator who was blinded to training status. Scores for skill and safety were significantly greater for residents who participated in the simulated breech delivery after the training. With regard to postpartum hemorrhage, Toledo and colleagues[30] used simulated examples of blood loss volumes to improve care providers' accuracy with regard to blood loss estimation.

Siassakos and colleagues[31] assessed whether clinical outcomes associated with cord prolapse improved after introduction of an obstetric emergency training program that included cord prolapse drills. They found that after these drills, a significant

reduction was reported in diagnosis-to-delivery interval (25 to 14.5 minutes, P < .001), although no significant difference was found in low Apgar scores or rate of admission to the neonatal intensive care unit (NICU).

Draycott and coinvestigators[32] also examined clinical outcomes after introduction of a training session that included fetal heart tracing education and drills in shoulder dystocia, postpartum hemorrhage, eclampsia, twin deliveries, breech deliveries, adult resuscitation (including cardiopulmonary resuscitation), and neonatal resuscitation. After this training, the frequency of hypoxic-ischemic encephalopathy (HIE) decreased by approximately half at their institution (27.3 to 13.6 per 10,000 births, P = .03). This decrease did not seem to be related to other preexisting trends in the frequency of HIE or to changes in the population during the period of study.

Enhancement of Communication

Rather than focus on simulation of specific obstetric events, some investigators have emphasized improvement of communication processes and teamwork in general. **One approach to this is through the establishment of a specific team trained to function and be engaged specifically at the time of obstetric emergencies. One institution, for example, created a "Condition O" team, according to the precepts outlined for rapid-response systems,[33] including (1) case detection that triggers a medical crisis team response, (2) a medical crisis team response available at all times, (3) an evaluation and process improvement system, and (4) an administrative structure to support the system.** After implementation of this system, the investigators reported several quality improvement interventions that were able to be introduced due to case reviews associated with "Condition O" being invoked, although improvements in particular outcomes were not yet demonstrated.

A different approach, in contrast to the one above, is the training for and implementation of standardized communication processes throughout a unit or institution. **One often-cited approach to this type of intervention is *crew resource management* (CRM). This training began—and has continued—in the airline industry, where it was noted that accidents were primarily related to lack of coordination and poor teamwork.[33] CRM seeks to engender effective communication through standardized language, situational awareness, briefing and debriefing, and a leveling of hierarchy that allows all team members to voice concerns over safety.** Some evidence from both observational longitudinal studies and randomized trials suggests that communication training can improve teamwork and communication among providers.[34,35]

In one longitudinal observational study,[36] the introduction of a CRM course at a single institution was noted to be associated with a reduction in high-severity "lawsuits, claims, and observations" (i.e., when the insurance carrier reserves money) by 62%. However, in the one randomized trial that was performed—and in which this CRM course, the MedTeams Labor and Delivery Team Coordination Course, was evaluated—investigators reported that institutions randomized to the intervention were no more likely to reduce the primary measure of obstetric adverse outcomes (mean adverse outcome index) than institutions that received no intervention at all.[37]

Multifaceted Approaches

Some have asserted that the complexity of obstetric care is such that improvements in safety will come not through the

use of one particular intervention but with a multifaceted approach that ultimately results in a fundamental culture change within an institution. Correspondence with principles of high-reliability organizations have helped to guide some of these efforts. Longitudinal observational studies have suggested that the introduction of such programs is associated with outcome improvements. Examples of such programs have been reported by several organizations:

Catholic Healthcare Partners (CHP)[38] instituted a program at 16 sites that included interdisciplinary education, routine medical record reviews to monitor ongoing adherence to appropriate practice, and standardization of forms to encourage adherence with best practices. After introduction of this program, birth trauma rates decreased from 5.0 to 0.17 per 1000 births, and the number of adverse obstetric occurrences (specified birth-related event or injury that might lead to a claim) decreased by 65%, from 7.2 to 2.5 per 1000 births.

Seton Family Hospitals[39] began a program at four sites that included standardization of forms and care processes, introduction of routine communication processes such as situation, background, assessment, recommendation (SBAR); active surveillance of adverse outcomes with temporally proximate feedback; and interdisciplinary obstetric crisis simulation with high-fidelity mannequins. Subsequent to the introduction of this program, birth injury rates declined from a 2-year average of 0.3% to 0.08%, and the average length of stay for infants admitted to the NICU for birth injury declined by 80%.

Yale–New Haven Hospital[40] obstetric department began a program of outside expert review of adverse events, anonymous event reporting, protocol standardization, creation of a patient safety nurse position and patient safety committee, and training in team skills and fetal heart monitoring interpretation. Introduction of this program was associated with a significant reduction ($P = .01$) in their outcome of choice, the mean quarterly adverse outcome index. They have reported that medical liability claims and payments also have been reduced subsequent to the introduction of this program.[41]

Hospital Corporation of America (HCA)[42] instituted a program that included standardized processes, active peer review and feedback, and the empowerment of any member of the health care team to halt care considered possibly dangerous. Subsequent to this program's initiation, a significant reduction was seen ($P < .001$) in the number of professional liability claims per 10,000 deliveries.

Summary

It seems clear that at least some of the adverse outcomes that occur in obstetrics are preventable and that the root causes of these preventable events, although multiple, often involve communication and teamwork. Theory supports various approaches to error reduction, many of which have been used in obstetrics. **Whereas some but not all studies have documented improvements in outcomes related to patient safety initiatives, these studies have been predominantly observational and have used different outcomes—such as provider satisfaction and perception, demonstration of skill acquisition in simulated scenarios, actual care processes, and actual patient outcomes— to assess improvement.** Further work is necessary to understand the best combination of practices and practice methodologies (e.g., simulation on site versus simulation in a laboratory) that most effectively improve care.

MEASUREMENT OF OBSTETRIC QUALITY OF CARE

Measurement is required to understand whether safe care is being provided and whether changes in approaches to patient safety are actually improving the quality of care. Examples of *patient safety measures* are rates of retained surgical sponge or wrong site surgery. A *quality measure* assesses the degree to which maternal and neonatal care is optimized. The following section details different approaches to measurement that have been used in an effort to optimize obstetric care.

Overview

Many types of stakeholders have an interest in quality obstetric care. Patients, doctors, and insurers desire high obstetric quality at an affordable cost. However, each of these groups may perceive quality differently. Patients want to feel that their doctors are caring individuals who produce good outcomes. Doctors want to ensure the best possible outcomes for patients but also, regardless of outcome, they need to be sure they are using best practices. Insurers want to know that the care given is cost effective. Each of these groups wants and needs access to quality measures that reflect their own interests. Thus one of the first steps in measuring quality is to understand who will use the measure and how it will be used.

Quality Measures

The three major categories of quality measures are (1) structural, (2) outcome, and (3) process.[43] *Structural measures* assume that if the hospital contains quality components, the product (medical care) will also be of high quality. Examples of structural measures include board certification, physician licensure, and hospital accreditation. Structural measures are appealing because they are easy to measure and reproduce; however, whereas structural measures may reflect that optimal structures are present, these measures do not guarantee that the different components of the hospital will work well together.

Outcome measures, as indicated by their name, reflect patient outcomes. An example of an outcome measure would be the frequency of maternal mortality or neonatal hypoglycemia. **Because obstetricians generally treat healthy women, adverse outcomes in obstetrics are relatively uncommon. Consequently, the usefulness of many outcome measures, such as maternal mortality, may be limited because most hospitals have few or none of these outcomes to measure.** Furthermore, if outcomes measures are to be maximally useful and reflective of the actual care provided at a given institution, they need to reflect outcomes that the institution can actually affect and should be **risk-adjusted** to account for differences in patients that could materially affect the outcome of interest. For example, although "preterm birth" is an adverse outcome, "frequency of preterm birth" may not be a good measure to reflect patient quality given the lack of useful interventions to prevent this adverse outcome. Also, a comparison of hospitals according to their frequency of peripartum hysterectomies may not reflect comparative quality of care if one hospital is much more likely to care for women with abnormal placentation. One recent investigation has demonstrated that for several adverse obstetric outcomes—severe postpartum hemorrhage, peripartum infection, severe perineal laceration, and a composite adverse neonatal outcome—differences in the characteristics of the patients who are admitted for delivery to different hospitals may materially affect how a hospital is judged to be performing relative to other hospitals with regard to these outcomes.[44] Lastly, outcomes measures may pose distinct challenges in obstetrics, when outcomes of two patients—the mother and the baby—occur. Thus, whereas a hospital may have comparatively good maternal outcomes, it also may have comparatively poor neonatal outcomes, and examination of only one of these sets of outcomes would not fully convey the quality of the care environment.[44]

Process measures reflect practices that physicians or hospitals actually use in their care of patients. An example of a process measure is the frequency with which known group B *Streptococcus* (GBS)–positive women receive appropriate antibiotics. **If a process measure were to conceivably be an adequate reflection of patient safety, there should be evidence that the process is related to improved outcomes.** The most central advantage of a process measure is that it gives direct insight into desired actions within the health care system. Correspondingly, these measures give immediate insight into the processes that need to be attended to in order to enhance patient care. Conversely, one of the disadvantages of process measures is that outcomes are often due to the interplay of many different factors and processes, and improvements in these measures may give false reassurance that improvements in quality of care have been fully realized. Draycott and colleagues[45] have voiced concern that too great a dependence on process measures may obscure the fact that "improvements" in care are not translating to improvement in outcomes. Recent analyses in obstetrics have illustrated this point. Grobman and associates[46] studied care processes and outcomes of over 115,000 women at 25 different hospitals but could not demonstrate that differences in the care provided at the hospitals could account for variation in adverse outcomes that were seen. Similarly, Howell and colleagues[47] studied the frequency of cesarean and elective delivery at less than 39 weeks' gestation among hospitals in New York, but they could find no relationship between how hospitals performed on these measures and the frequency of maternal or neonatal morbidity.

With these considerations in mind, several criteria should be considered in determining whether a measure is a good one. For example, a good measure should (1) balance maternal and neonatal outcomes—that is, it should not reflect improved care for one member of the mother-child dyad while embodying markedly worse care for the other; (2) have the potential to be altered by behaviors within the health care system of interest; (3) be affordable and applicable for use on a larger scale; (4) be acceptable to stakeholders as a meaningful marker of quality; and (5) be reliable and reproducible.[43]

Attempts to Establish Quality Measures

Because measuring the quality of care is a seminal step in both improving patient safety and achieving quality care, many attempts have been made by a multitude of different organizations to determine quality measures in obstetrics. This chapter will not comprehensively review all current quality measures; rather it will present some examples of measures to illustrate the strengths and weaknesses of different choices. The examples will include traditional measures as well as those more recently suggested.

Traditional Measures

The more traditional measures often have been raw frequencies of selected adverse outcomes. One example of this type of measure is maternal mortality. It has been used because it is clearly a profoundly bad outcome, and little potential exists for misascertainment. However, in the modern era within developed countries, maternal mortality is so relatively uncommon that it is difficult to use within a hospital or health care system to reflect quality of health care. Most hospitals will have no maternal mortality even over many years, and few hospitals will have a sufficient number of cases to enable them to use this measure to track their adequacy of care delivery. Furthermore, the absence of this outcome does not mandate that quality care is being provided; lack of quality care may still exist, and short of death, poor outcomes may still be obtained. This does not mean that any maternal mortality should not be fully investigated as a critical part of quality assurance and improvement efforts, only that maternal mortality is unlikely to be useful as a quality marker for intrainstitutional quality tracking and interinstitutional comparisons. Alternatively, in an effort to obtain an outcome measure that still could be used to identify significant adverse maternal events but is more common than maternal mortality, Callaghan and others[48] have advocated that a measure of "severe maternal morbidity" be adopted. This outcome, redefined as the occurrence of an ICU admission or transfusion of at least 4 units of packed red blood cells, occurs nearly 50 times more frequently than maternal mortality.[5,49,50]

Neonatal mortality also has been used as a marker of obstetric quality, although it may be problematic as a marker for obstetric quality for several reasons. First, when a neonate dies, it is unclear to what extent obstetric care, pediatric care, or both may have contributed. Secondly, a large proportion of neonatal mortality is due to prematurity and lethal birth defects, neither of which can be materially affected by obstetric care.[51] Thus the residual fraction of obstetric-related neonatal mortality is relatively small, and once again, it may be so uncommon as to limit its use for evaluation of trends or institutional comparisons.

The cesarean delivery rate has been a common measure used to reflect obstetric quality of care. Whereas debate continues about whether cesarean delivery is a process measure or an outcome measure, it is regardless a flawed measure. First, due to perinatal regionalization, women with greater obstetric complications are concentrated at hospitals best suited to providing specialized care. Thus a comparison of cesarean delivery rates among hospitals without accounting for the differences in patient populations may be misleading. Hospitals with the highest cesarean delivery rates may be giving quality care but have high rates due to their patient population. Conversely, a hospital may be giving poor care and may have an average rate of cesarean delivery, when in fact the cesarean delivery rate should be much lower for their low-risk population.

Newer Approaches to Measures

Although the use of "raw" cesarean delivery rates to measure quality is not ideal, cesarean delivery rates are appealing as a measure because cesarean delivery is an outcome that is easy to ascertain, and it is meaningful to multiple stakeholders. One approach to try and account for population differences among institutions is to calculate and use a "risk-adjusted" cesarean delivery rate as a measure. **Many different techniques for risk-adjustment for cesarean delivery, as well as other obstetric outcomes, have been described.[52-57] Fundamentally, risk adjustment creates a model that predicts what the cesarean delivery rate should be for the particular patient population and allows comparison with the actual rate. By taking** account of differences such as parity, plurality, and comorbidities among populations, risk-adjustment seeks to reflect differences in outcomes related to the health care system rather than the patients who access it.

Risk-adjustment can be used for any outcome but requires formal statistical testing and assessment to demonstrate whether it attains the intended goal of accounting for relevant patient characteristics that contribute to the outcome of interest. For example, a series of risk-adjustment models have been developed and tested for several adverse obstetric outcomes, including severe postpartum hemorrhage, peripartum infection, third- and fourth-degree lacerations, and a composite adverse neonatal outcome.[44]

Another approach to determining an outcome measure that is dependent upon the health care system, rather than the differences in patient populations, is to determine an outcome frequency for a more homogeneous group rather than for all women who receive care. Main and coworkers[58] have suggested, for example, the use of a cesarean delivery rate measure that only assesses women who are nulliparous with a term singleton vertex (NTSV) fetal presentation. Using data from the Sutter Health Care network of 20 birthing units, in which more than 40,000 women deliver each year, these researchers determined age-adjusted NTSV cesarean rates and found that 53% of the variation in these rates was associated with differences in frequency of labor induction and early admission in labor. This finding suggests that some health care practices are associated with the NTSV cesarean rate, and the disadvantage of using this rate is that it excludes women having preterm deliveries or who are multiparous.

One process measure that has recently gained attention is scheduled elective delivery prior to 39 weeks of gestation. This measure has gained popularity as the risks of early-term birth have become better known.[59,60] This process measure has the advantage of being fully under the control of the health care system and does not require risk adjustment. Part of what makes this measure appealing is that it can be calculated from the International Classification of Diseases (edition 9, ICD-9) administrative data, which is already collected and available in hospitals. Nevertheless, one potential difficulty with this measure is the lack of consensus for several indications as to whether they are indeed elective. Also, some have noted that ICD-9 data are not as accurate and complete as data from the medical records and may not provide an accurate assessment. However, a study by Clark and colleagues[61] showed that even when ICD-9 data are used, the majority of cases found to be in violation of a policy against delivery prior to 39 weeks of gestation were true cases of non–medically indicated delivery. Only a minority of cases were due to abstractor error or poor documentation.

The frequency with which antenatal corticosteroids are administered to infants who are delivered at less than 34 weeks is another process measure that has become widely used. This process measure is appealing because of data that show antenatal corticosteroids improve outcomes for premature infants. Nevertheless, this measure does have its disadvantages. Ascertainment of steroid administration can be difficult, especially in a health care setting without electronic medical records (EMRs). Steroids given during the pregnancy, but not during the delivery hospitalization, are time intensive to ascertain because inpatient and outpatient records may need to be reviewed. And whereas 100% administration is the goal, it is not possible to administer corticosteroids to all women prior

to premature delivery due to late patient arrival or emergent circumstances, such as a maternal trauma.

The frequency of neonates who weigh less than 1500 g born outside a tertiary care center is one recently suggested process measure that is appealing because it may reflect adequacy of coordination of an entire health care system. Although data show that very-low-birthweight neonates have worse outcomes when delivered outside a tertiary care center, many incentives may work against delivery at such a location.[62-64] This measure is easy to calculate from birth certificates, and the items from the birth certificate that are needed to calculate the measure are reliable.[42]

The quality measures discussed thus far have represented inpatient care. **Outpatient quality measures do exist, although they are often process measures.** An example of such a measure is the frequency with which pregnant women receive human immunodeficiency virus (HIV) screening early in their antepartum care. One difficulty with these measures has to do with accurate ascertainment, because prenatal care happens in many different settings, and outpatient medical records data are often not in electronic form. Furthermore, whereas hospitals are required to generate administrative data that can be helpful for measuring inpatient quality, outpatient clinics are not required to generate the same kinds of data, and so they do not.

Data Sources

Administrative data, collected primarily for billing or nonmedical purposes, is a rich source of information. Administrative data have the advantages of being complete for the population and relatively cheap to use. **Unfortunately, administrative data often lack the clinical detail needed to make meaningful quality judgments.**[66] Paper-based medical records contain clinical detail but are hard to obtain in a uniform manner for a population and are expensive to collect.

Increasingly, EMRs have been used to provide the basis for quality measures. These data are easy to collect within an institution and have clinical detail. However, because many different types of EMR systems exist, collating medical records information from many sources can be time intensive. **EMRs have the advantage of being able to link outpatient and inpatient information, something that is very difficult to do with administrative data or paper-based medical records.** The types of information that are available from EMRs will increase and improve with time, and there is hope that eventually vital statistics records will be based on actual medical records, rather than on data extraction, thereby making birth certificate data a richer, more accurate source of medical data.

Quality Improvement

The main point of measuring quality of care is to use the measurement tools to improve care. Quality measurement tools allow stakeholders to assess the effects of changes in the system. **There are many ways to accomplish improved quality of care with measurement, but one of the most effective is benchmarking.**[67] *Benchmarking,* also known as *audit and feedback,* is a technique whereby quality is measured, compared with like entities, and then shared back with the participants, often in a blinded manner.** For example, NTSV rates for all the hospitals in a city would be calculated. Each hospital would then receive a graph showing their rate (unblinded) compared with the rates of all the other hospitals (blinded) in the city.

One example of this technique being used was in the Ohio Perinatal Quality Collaborative (OPQC).[68] This group of 20 hospitals in Ohio came together to share data and compare techniques on how to lower the frequency of scheduled deliveries prior to 39 weeks without documentation of a medical indication. Each hospital collected data on scheduled deliveries from $36^{0/7}$ to $38^{6/7}$ weeks in its own institution and submitted the data to a central location for data collation. This data center then created reports that showed each hospital their own rate compared with the rates of all the other hospitals. Each hospital took that information and designed their own program to lower their own frequency. Monthly phone calls allowed hospitals to share their designs and progress. At the initiation of the project, 25% of scheduled deliveries between 36 and $38^{6/7}$ weeks did not have a documented medical indication; this frequency was lowered to less than 5% ($P < .05$) after a year. It was estimated that approximately 1000 births were moved from between $36^{0/7}$ and $38^{6/7}$ to over 39 weeks in the state of Ohio during the 12 months of this effort.

In addition to the collaborative in Ohio, many other quality collaboratives exist across the country.[69] Some are voluntary and others require a fee for participation for the member hospitals. A well-established quality collaborative is the California Maternal Quality Care Collaborative (CMQCC [online at www.cmqcc.org]). In addition to being a resource for members to interact and share data, many quality care collaboratives—including the OPQC and the CMQCC—offer toolkits that allow nonparticipating hospitals to benefit from their quality benchmarks and materials that describe what they have learned by providing data collection tools.

These collaboratives, as well as others, may help to provide insight into the most effective approaches to improving obstetric care. Clark and a group of investigators at Hospital Corporation of America (HCA)[70] compared three methods of implementing change in a labor and delivery unit in an effort to decrease the frequency of elective deliveries prior to 39 weeks. They compared (1) a hard-stop approach, in which physicians were not allowed to schedule deliveries prior to 39 weeks without a medical indication; (2) a soft-stop approach, in which physicians were allowed to schedule deliveries prior to 39 weeks but were told there would be a peer review process to assess whether elective deliveries prior to 39 weeks were occurring; and (3) an education-only approach, in which physicians were educated about relevant issues but no other changes were made. The results of this study showed that both the hard- and soft-stop approaches were associated with changed behavior, whereas the educational approach was not at all effective. Furthermore, the hard-stop strategy was twice as effective as the soft-stop approach.

KEY POINTS

- A proportion of adverse obstetric events have been shown to be preventable; this proportion varies with the clinical circumstances.
- Although multiple factors have been associated with the occurrence of adverse obstetric events, issues with communication have been implicated as a frequent contributor.
- Specific approaches that have been considered to enhance obstetric patient safety include checklists and protocols, simulation, and teamwork training.
- Further investigation is required to understand what approaches and combinations of approaches most improve clinical care and outcomes.
- Quality measures assess the degree to which maternal and neonatal care is optimized.
- Major categories of quality measures include structural, process, and outcome measures.

REFERENCES

1. Lohr KN, Schroeder SA. A strategy for quality assurance in Medicare. *N Engl J Med.* 1990;322:707-712.
2. Institute of Medicine. *To err is human: building a safer health care system.* Washington, DC: National Academy Press; 1999.
3. DeFrances C, Hall M, Podgornik M. *2003 National Hospital Discharge Survey.* Advance data from vital and health statistics. No. 359. Hyattsville, MD: National Center for Health Statistics; 2005.
4. Geller SE, Rosenberg D, Cox SM, et al. The continuum of maternal morbidity and mortality: factors associated with severity. *Am J Obstet Gynecol.* 2004;191:939-944.
5. Geller SE, Rosenberg D, Cox S, Brown M, Simonson L, Kilpatrick S. A scoring system identified near-miss maternal morbidity during pregnancy. *J Clin Epidemiol.* 2004;57:716-720.
6. Berg CJ, Harper MA, Atkinson S, et al. Preventability of pregnancy-related deaths. *Obstet Gynecol.* 2005;106:1228-1234.
7. White AA, Pichert JW, Bledsoe SH, Irwin C, Entman SS. Cause and effect analysis of closed claims in obstetrics and gynecology. *Obstet Gynecol.* 2005;105:1031-1038.
8. Clark SL, Belfort MA, Dildy GA, Meyers JA. Reducing obstetric litigation through alterations in practice patterns. *Am J Obstet.* 2010;112:1279-1283.
9. Forster AJ, Fung I, Caughey S, et al. Adverse events detected by clinical surveillance on an obstetric service. *Obstet Gynecol.* 2006;108:1073-1083.
10. The Joint Commission. *Sentinel Event Alert: Issue 30, Preventing infant death and injury during delivery (Additional Resources).* Available at <http://www.jointcommission.org/sentinel_event_alert__issue_30_preventing_infant_death_and_injury_during_delivery_additional_resources>.
11. Hoff T, Jameson L, Hannan E, Fink E. A Review of the Literature Examining Linkages between Organizational Factors, Medical Errors, and Patient Safety. *Med Care Res Rev.* 2004;61:3-37.
12. Hales BM, Pronovost PJ. The checklist—a tool for error management and performance improvement. *J Crit Care.* 2006;21:231-235.
13. Pronovost P, Needham D, Berenholtz S. An intervention to decrease catheter-related bloodstream infections in the ICU. *N Engl J Med.* 2006;355:2725-2732.
14. Clark S, Belfort M, Saade G, et al. Implementation of a conservative checklist-based protocol for oxytocin administration: maternal and newborn outcomes. *Am J Obstet Gynecol.* 2007;197:480.e1-480.e5.
15. Menzies J, Magee LA, Li J, et al. Instituting surveillance guidelines and adverse outcomes in preeclampsia. *Obstet Gynecol.* 2007;110:121-127.
16. Koetsier A, van der Veer SN, Jager KJ, Peek N, de Keizer NF. Control charts in healthcare quality improvement. A systematic review on adherence to methodological criteria. *Methods Inf Med.* 2012;51:189-198.
17. Urbach DR, Govindrajan A, Saskin R, Wilton AS, Baxter NN. Introduction of surgical safety checklists in Ontario, Canada. *N Engl J Med.* 2014;370:1029-1038.
18. Bailit JL, Grobman WA, McGee P, et al. The association of protocols and perinatal outcomes. *Am J Obstet Gynecol.* 2015;213:86.e1-6.
19. Hunt EA, Shilkofski NA, Atavroudis TA, Nelson KL. Simulation: translation to improved team performance. *Anesthesiol Clin.* 2007;25:301-319.
20. Deering S, Poggi S, Macedonia C, Gherman R, Satin AJ. Improving resident competency in the management of shoulder dystocia with simulation training. *Obstet Gynecol.* 2004;103:1224-1228.
21. Goffman D, Heo H, Pardanani S, Merkatz IR, Bernstein PS. Improving shoulder dystocia management among resident and attending physicians using simulations. *Am J Obstet Gynecol.* 2008;199:294.e1-294.e5.

22. Crofts JF, Bartlett C, Ellis D, Hunt LP, Fox R, Draycott TJ. Training for shoulder dystocia: a trial of simulation using low-fidelity and high-fidelity mannequins. *Obstet Gynecol.* 2006;108:1477-1485.

23. Crofts JF, Bartlett C, Ellis D, Hunt LP, Fox R, Draycott TJ. Management of shoulder dystocia: Skill retention 6 and 12 months after training. *Obstet Gynecol.* 2007;110:1069-1074.

24. Draycott TJ, Crofts JF, Ash JP, et al. Improving neonatal outcome through practical shoulder dystocia training. *Obstet Gynecol.* 2008;112:14-20.

25. Grobman WA, Miller D, Tam K, Hornbogen A, Burke C, Costello R. Outcomes associated with introduction of a shoulder dystocia protocol. *Am J Obstet Gynecol.* 2011;205:513-517.

26. Thompson S, Neal S, Clark V. Clinical risk management in obstetrics: eclampsia drills. *Qual Saf Health Care.* 2004;13:127-129.

27. Osman H, Campbell OM, Nass AH. Using emergency obstetric drills in maternity units as a performance improvement tool. *Birth.* 2009;36:43-50.

28. Ellis D, Crofts JF, Hunt LP, Read M, Fox R, James M. Hospital, simulation center and teamwork training for eclampsia management. *Obstet Gynecol.* 2008;111:723-731.

29. Deering S, Brown J, Hodor J, Satin AJ. Simulation training and resident performance of singleton vaginal breech delivery. *Obstet Gynecol.* 2006;107: 86-89.

30. Toledo P, McCarthy RJ, Burke CA, Goetz K, Wong CA, Grobman WA. The effect of live and web-based education on the accuracy of blood loss estimation in simulated obstetric scenarios. *Am J Obstet Gynecol.* 2010;202: 400.e1-400.e5.

31. Siassakos D, Hasafa Z, Sibanda T, et al. Retrospective cohort study of diagnosis-delivery interval with umbilical cord prolapse: the effect of team training. *BJOG.* 2009;116:1089-1096.

32. Draycott T, Sibanda T, Owen L. Does training in obstetric emergencies improve neonatal outcome? *BJOG.* 2006;113:177-182.

33. Helmreich RL, Merritt AC, Wilhelm JA. The evolution of Crew Resource Management training in commercial aviation. *Int J Aviat Psychol.* 1999;9: 19-32.

34. Alder JR, Christen R, Zemp E, Bitzer J. Communication skills training in obstetrics and gynaecology: whom should we train? A randomized controlled trial. *Arch Gynecol Obstet.* 2007;276:605-612.

35. Haller G, Garnerin P, Morales M, et al. Effect of crew resource management training in a multidisciplinary obstetrical setting. *Int J Qual Health Care.* 2008;20(4):254-263.

36. Pratt SD, Mann S, Salisbury M, et al. John M. Eisenberg Patient Safety and Quality Awards. Impact of CRM-based training on obstetric outcomes and clinicians' patient safety attitudes. *Jt Comm J Qual Patient Saf.* 2007;33: 720-725.

37. Nielsen PE, Goldman MB, Mann S, et al. Effects of teamwork training on adverse outcomes and process of care in labor and delivery: a randomized controlled trial. *Obstet Gynecol.* 2007;109:48-55.

38. Simpson KR, Kort CC, Knox GE. A comprehensive perinatal patient safety program to reduce preventable adverse outcomes and costs of liability claims. *Jt Comm J Qual Patient Saf.* 2009;35:565-574.

39. Mazza F, Kitchens J, Akin M. The road to zero preventable birth injuries. *Jt Comm J Qual Patient Saf.* 2008;34:201-205.

40. Pettker CM, Thung SF, Norwitz ER, et al. Impact of a comprehensive patient safety strategy on obstetric adverse events. *Am J Obstet Gynecol.* 2009;200:492.e1-492.e8.

41. Pettker CM, Thung SF, Lipkind HS, et al. A comprehensive obstetric patient safety program reduces liability claims and payments. *Am J Obstet Gynecol.* 2014;211:319-325.

42. Clark SL, Belfort MA, Byrum SL, Meyers JA, Perlin JB. Improved outcomes, fewer cesarean deliveries, and reduced litigation: results of a new paradigm in patient safety. *Am J Obstet Gynecol.* 2008;199:105.e1-105.e7.

43. Donabedian A. Evaluating the Quality of Medical Care. *Milbank Mem Fund Q.* 1966;44:166-206.

44. Bailit JL, Grobman WA, Rice MM, et al. Risk-adjusted models for adverse obstetric outcomes and variation in risk-adjusted outcomes across hospitals. *Am J Obstet Gynecol.* 2013;209:446.e1-446.e30.

45. Draycott T, Sibanda T, Laxton C, Winter C, Mahmood T, Fox R. Quality improvement demands quality measurement. *BJOG.* 2010;117:1571-1574.

46. Grobman WA, Bailit JL, Rice MM, et al. Can difference in obstetric outcomes be explained by differences in the care provided? The MFMU Network APEX study. *Am J Obstet Gynecol.* 2014;211:147.e1-147.e16.

47. Howell EA, Zeitlin J, Herbert PL, Balbierz A, Egorova N. Association between hospital-level obstetric quality indicators and maternal and neonatal morbidity. *JAMA.* 2014;312(15):1531-1534.

48. Callaghan W, Grobman WA, Main E, Kilpatrick S, D'Alton ME. Facility-based identification of women with severe maternal morbidity: It's time to start. *Obstet Gynecol.* 2014;123:978-981.

49. You WB, Chandrasekaran S, Sullivan J, Grobman WA. Validation of a scoring system to identify women with near-miss maternal morbidity. *Am J Perinatol.* 2012;30:21-24.

50. Grobman WA, Bailit J, Rice MM, et al. Frequency of and factors associated with severe maternal morbidity. *Obstet Gynecol.* 2014;123:804-810.

51. Hein H, Lofgren M. The changing pattern of neonatal mortality in a regionalized system of perinatal care: a current update. *Pediatrics.* 1999;104: 1064-1069.

52. Bailit JL, Love TE, Dawson NV. Quality of obstetric care and risk-adjusted primary cesarean delivery rates. *Am J Obstet Gynecol.* 2006;194:402-407.

53. Keeler E, Park R, Bell R, Gifford DS, Keesey J. Adjusting cesarean delivery rates for case mix. *Health Serv Res.* 1997;32:511-528.

54. Bailit J, Garrett J. Comparison of risk-adjustment methodologies. *Obstet Gynecol.* 2003;102:45-51.

55. Aron D, Harper D, Shepardson L, Rosenthal G. Impact of risk-adjusting cesarean delivery rates when reporting hospital performance. *JAMA.* 1998;279:1968-1972.

56. Glantz JC. Cesarean delivery risk adjustment for regional interhospital comparisons. *Am J Obstet Gynecol.* 1999;181:1425-1431.

57. Gregory KD, Korst LM, Platt LD. Variation in elective primary cesarean delivery by patient and hospital factors. *Am J Obstet Gynecol.* 2001;184: 1521-1532.

58. Main EK, Moore D, Farrell B, et al. Is there a useful cesarean birth measure? Assessment of the nulliparous term singleton vertex cesarean birth rate as a tool for obstetric quality improvement. *Am J Obstet Gynecol.* 2006;194: 1644-1651.

59. Tita AT, Landon MB, Spong CY, et al. Timing of elective repeat cesarean delivery at term and neonatal outcomes. *N Engl J Med.* 2009;360: 111-120.

60. Bailit JL, Gregory KD, Reddy UM, et al. Maternal and neonatal outcomes by labor onset type and gestational age. *Am J Obstet Gynecol.* 2010;202:245.e1-245.e12.

61. Clark SL, Meyers JA, Milton CG, et al. Validation of the joint commission exclusion criteria for elective early-term delivery. *Obstet Gynecol.* 2014;123: 29-33.

62. Warner B, Musial J, Chenier T, Donovan D. The effect of birth hospital type on the outcomes of very low birth weight infants. *Pediatrics.* 2004; 113:35-41.

63. Chien L, Whyte R, Aziz K, Thiessen P, Matthew D, Lee ST. Improved outcome of preterm infants when delivered in tertiary care centers. *Obstet Gynecol.* 2001;98:247-252.

64. Phibbs C, Bronstein J, Buxton E, Phibbs R. The effect of patient volume and level of care at the hospital of birth and neonatal mortality. *JAMA.* 1996;276:1054-1059.

65. Deleted in review.

66. Bailit JL, Ohio Perinatal Quality Collaborative. Rates of labor induction without medical indication are overestimated when derived from birth certificate data. *Am J Obstet Gynecol.* 2010;203:269.e1-269.e3.

67. Jamtvedt G, Young JM, Kristoffersen DT, et al. Audit and feedback: effects on professional practice and health are outcomes. *Cochrane Database Syst Rev.* 2004;2:2.

68. Iams J for the Ohio Perinatal Quality Collaborative. A statewide initiative to reduce inappropriate scheduled births at 36 0/7 to 38 6/7 weeks' gestation. *Am J Obstet Gynecol.* 2010;202:243.e1-243.e8.

69. American College of Obstetricians and Gynecologists. *State Quality Collaboratives Chart.* Available at <http://www.acog.org/About_ACOG/ACOG_Departments/Government_Relations_and_Outreach/-/media/Departments/Government%20Relations%20and%20Outreach/StateQualCollabChart.pdf>.

70. Clark SL, Frye DR, Meyers JA, et al. Reduction in elective delivery at <39 weeks of gestation: comparative effectiveness of 3 approaches to change and the impact on neonatal intensive care admission and stillbirth. *Am J Obstet Gynecol.* 2010;203:449.e1-449.e6.

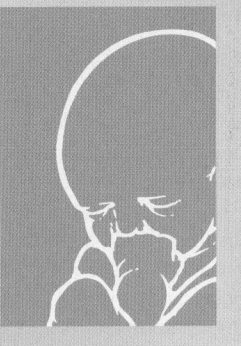

CHAPTER 57

Ethical and Legal Issues in Perinatology

GEORGE J. ANNAS and SHERMAN ELIAS†

KEY ABBREVIATIONS	
American College of Medical Genetics and Genomics	ACMG
American College of Obstetricians and Gynecologists	ACOG
Apolipoprotein E	APOE
Assisted reproductive technology	ART
Cell-free DNA	cfDNA
Chorionic villus sampling	CVS
Chromosomal microarray analysis	CMA
Copy number variant	CNV
Direct to consumer	DTC
Embryonic stem cell	ESC
Food and Drug Administration	FDA
Human immunodeficiency virus	HIV
In vitro fertilization	IVF
Institute of Medicine	IOM
Intrauterine device	IUD
National Institute of Child Health and Human Development	NICHD
National Institutes of Health	NIH
Personal genome service	PGS
Religious Freedom Restoration Act	RFRA
Single nucleotide polymorphism	SNP
Variant of unknown significance	VOUS

Society has great expectations that modern medical technologies will improve longevity and the quality of human life, and nowhere are these expectations higher than in the practice of obstetrics and the desire and expectation of having a healthy child. Along with the rapidly expanding capabilities in diagnosis and treatment, physicians find themselves facing numerous ethical dilemmas while practicing in a legal and social climate in which malpractice suits can threaten even the most competent and conscientious practitioner.

†Deceased.

We cannot address in a single chapter the wide variety of ethical and legal controversies that face contemporary obstetric practice and research. Instead, we focus on selected topics of particular relevance to the practicing obstetrician.

REPRODUCTIVE LIBERTY

Although only about one in four pregnancies ends in elective abortion, abortion has been the most controversial and political medical procedure in the United States for the past four decades. The political debate over abortion has shifted among various dichotomous views of the world: life versus choice, fetus versus woman, fetus versus baby, constitutional rights versus states' rights, government versus physician, and physician and patient versus state legislature. In 2010, the abortion debate came close to derailing the Affordable Care Act, and in 2014, **the U.S. Supreme Court ruled that corporations could have religious beliefs and that these beliefs could permit them not to include some birth control methods** (that the corporation inaccurately thought induced abortion) **in the health insurance plans of their female employees.** Because the 1973 U.S. Supreme Court opinion on *Roe v. Wade* remains so central to the law (and ethics) regarding the physician-patient relationship, as well as federal financing and regulation of clinical medicine and research and of health care insurance itself, **it is essential that obstetricians have a clear understanding of *Roe* and its enduring influence on patient rights—especially reproductive liberty, medical practice, and politics.**[1]

Hundreds of statutes—including relatively new ones that require ultrasound images of the fetus be made available to pregnant women before abortion, suggesting that 20-week-old fetuses feel pain, and requiring that abortion clinics have ready access to hospital emergency departments—and almost two dozen Supreme Court decisions on abortion later, the core legal aspects of *Roe v. Wade*,[2] the most controversial health-related decision ever made by the Court, remain substantially the same as in 1973. Attempts to overturn *Roe* in both the courtroom and the legislature have failed, although they continue. **Pregnant women still have a constitutional right to abortion because the fetus is still not a person under the Constitution.** States still cannot make abortion a crime, either for the woman or the physician, before the fetus becomes viable with the exception of the use of a specific procedure labeled "partial-birth abortion" by Congress. States still can outlaw abortion after the fetus becomes viable, but only if there is an exception that permits abortion to protect the life or health of the pregnant woman. Also, states still can impose restrictions on abortion before fetal viability only if those restrictions do not create an "undue burden" on the pregnant woman, understood as a substantial obstacle that might actually prevent a pregnant woman's obtaining an abortion.

The first case to embrace the concept of reproductive liberty was *Griswold v. Connecticut,* in which the Court ruled in 1965 that a Connecticut statute criminalizing the use of contraceptives violated the constitutional right to privacy that married couples had in sexual relations.[3] Later, in 1972, the Court found that even outside marriage, a person had a "right to privacy … to be free from unwarranted governmental intrusion into matters so fundamentally affecting a person as the decision to bear or beget a child."[4] The following year, in *Roe,* the Court struck down a Texas law that made it a crime for physicians to perform an abortion unless it was necessary to save the life of the patient; there were no exceptions for the woman's health. **The Court held that women have a constitutional right of privacy that is fundamental and "broad enough to encompass a woman's decision … to terminate her pregnancy."**[2] Because the right is fundamental, states that wished to restrict abortion rights were required to demonstrate a compelling interest to restrict the exercise of this right. The Court ruled that the state's interest in the life of the fetus became compelling only at the point of viability, defined as the point at which the fetus can survive independently of its mother. Even after the point of viability, the state cannot favor the life of the fetus over the life or health of the pregnant woman. Under the right of privacy, physicians must be free to use their "medical judgment for the preservation of the life or health of the mother."[2] On the same day that the Court decided *Roe,* it also decided *Doe v. Bolton,*[5] in which the Court defined health very broadly: "The medical judgment may be exercised in the light of all factors—physical, emotional, psychological, familial, and the woman's age—relevant to the well-being of the patient. All these factors may relate to health. This allows the attending physician the room he needs to make his best medical judgment."[5]

Roe and *Doe* together established that both physician and patient were protected by the constitutional right of privacy. In later cases, the Court continued to defer to the medical judgment of the attending physician. For example, in *Planned Parenthood of Central Missouri v. Danforth* in 1976, the Court concluded that state legislatures could not determine when viability occurred; rather this "essentially medical concept … is, and must be, a matter for the judgment of the responsible attending physician."[6] This remains the case today; even as viability in general moves earlier in the pregnancy, it is not up to legislatures or courts to determine when an individual fetus is viable by drawing a line based on the age of the fetus— **the viability of a specific fetus remains a matter of medical judgment to be determined by the attending physicians in a manner consistent with good and accepted obstetric practice.**

By the end of the 1980s, a pattern in Court decisions could be discerned in which abortion regulations that (1) significantly burdened a woman's decision; (2) treated abortion differently from other, similar medical or surgical procedures; (3) interfered with the exercise of professional judgment by the attending physician; or (4) were stricter than accepted medical standards were struck down by the Court.[7] Privacy as a constitutional right became a one-word description of liberty to make decisions regarding marriage, procreation, contraception, sterilization, abortion, family relationships, child rearing, and sexual relationships free of governmental interference.

One strategy to change *Roe* was to change the composition of the Supreme Court by appointing anti-*Roe* justices. Because of new justices on the Court in 1992, in *Planned Parenthood of Southeastern Pennsylvania v. Casey,* the Court had its first real opportunity to overturn *Roe v. Wade.* Many Court observers thought it would. Instead, in an unusual procedure for the Court, three potentially anti-*Roe* justices—Sandra Day O'Connor, David Souter, and Anthony Kennedy—joined together to write a joint opinion confirming the "core holding" of *Roe.* They were joined in most of their opinion by two justices, Harry Blackmun and John Paul Stevens, who would have simply upheld *Roe,* making this a 5-to-4 decision. Most centrally, the authors of the joint opinion believed that although the pressure to overrule *Roe* had grown "more intense," doing so would severely and unnecessarily damage the Court's legitimacy by undermining "the Nation's commitment to the rule of law."[8] Specifically, the three justices wrote that they were reaffirming "*Roe*'s essential holding" that before the point of viability, a woman has a right to choose abortion without undue state interference, and that after the point of viability, the state can restrict abortion "if the law contains exceptions for pregnancies which endanger the woman's life or health," and that "the state has legitimate interests from the outset of the pregnancy in protecting the health of the woman and the life of the fetus that may become a child." The Court applied these principles to uphold laws that mandate much more detailed requirements for abortion, as well as a mandatory 24-hour waiting period, but it struck down a spousal-notification requirement as an "undue burden."

Thus, **after *Casey, Roe* stood for the proposition that pregnant women have a "personal liberty" right—"privacy" went unmentioned—to choose to terminate their pregnancies before the point of viability and that the state cannot "unduly burden" such a right by erecting barriers that effectively prevent the exercise of that choice.**[9] Of course, a major problem was definitional: burdensome regulations were acceptable, "unduly burdensome" ones were not; but it was not clear what qualified as which. Put another way, the state could demonstrate its concern for fetal life by requiring that physicians make women seeking abortions jump through new and burdensome hoops—including offers of detailed and accurate information on abortion, the status of the fetus, adoption, sources of help for childbirth, and a 24-hour waiting period—as long as doing so did not "unduly burden" women by actually preventing them from being able to make a decision to have an abortion.

With the loss of a realistic expectation in 1992 that the Court would overrule *Roe* wholesale without significant changes in the Court's membership, **anti-*Roe* advocates switched strategies dramatically, focusing on criminalizing a specific procedure that they believed would horrify most Americans and that they labeled "partial-birth abortion."** The first such bill passed Congress in 1996 and was vetoed by President Bill Clinton because the prohibition did not contain an exception for the health of the woman, as required by *Roe* and *Casey.* In 1997, this time with the support of the American Medical Association, the bill passed Congress again. President Clinton vetoed it, again for failure to contain a health exception.[10]

Proponents of the ban took their cause to the individual states, most of which enacted substantially identical laws. In 2000, Nebraska's partial-birth abortion law reached the Supreme Court. The Nebraska law carried a penalty of up to 20 years in prison for physicians who performed the procedure. The law reads in relevant part:

No partial-birth abortion shall be performed in this state, unless such a procedure is necessary to save the life of the mother whose life is endangered by a physical disorder, physical illness, or physical injury, including a life-endangering physical condition caused by or arising from the pregnancy itself.

[A "partial-birth abortion" is] an abortion procedure in which the person performing the abortion partially delivers vaginally a living unborn child before killing the unborn child and completing the delivery. ... [The statute further defines the phrase "partially delivers vaginally a living unborn child before killing the unborn child" as] deliberately and intentionally delivering into the vagina a living unborn child, or a substantial portion thereof, for the purpose of performing a procedure that the person performing such procedure knows will kill the unborn child and does kill the unborn child.

This ban applied throughout pregnancy and had no exception to protect the woman's health, only to save her life. In a 5-to-4 opinion in *Stenberg v. Carhart*,[11] the Court found this law unconstitutional for two reasons. First, the description of the banned procedure was too similar to dilation and evacuation (D&E), another procedure that was permitted by the law and widely used for second-trimester abortions. Therefore this law would discourage physicians from using the lawful procedure, which would place an undue burden on their patients. Second, the law failed to provide an exception for instances in which the procedure was deemed necessary by the physician to protect the woman's health, as required by *Roe* and *Casey*. Justice John Paul Stevens, in his concurring opinion, noted that the extreme anti-*Roe* rhetoric as exemplified in the partial-birth abortion debate obscured the fact that during the 27-year period since *Roe* was decided, the core holding of *Roe* "has been endorsed by all but 4 of the 17 Justices who have addressed the issue."

A notable dissenting opinion was written by Justice Kennedy, who had specifically endorsed the core of *Roe* in *Casey*. Kennedy argued that the outlawing of "partial-birth abortion" was consistent with *Casey* because of the interest the state has throughout pregnancy in protecting the life of the fetus that may become a child. In his view, the banned procedure conflates abortion and childbirth in a way that "might cause the medical profession or society as a whole to become insensitive, even disdainful, to life, including life of the human fetus." He also argued that such a ban was not unduly burdensome to women because state legislatures can determine that specific medical procedures, like this one, are not medically necessary.[11]

Justice Stephen Breyer, the author of the *Stenberg* majority opinion, stated that a more precise law, with a health exception, could be constitutional.[11] In 2003, Congress passed a slightly revised law. It did not contain a health exception, but its preface did contain a declaration that the outlawed procedure was *never* medically necessary for the health of the woman. President Bush signed it into law on November 5, 2003. By the time the Court ruled on the constitutionality of this law in April 2007, in *Gonzales v. Carhart*,[12] two important changes had occurred

in the composition of the Court: a new chief justice, John Roberts, replaced the consistently anti-*Roe* Chief Justice William Rehnquist; and Justice Samuel Alito replaced Justice Sandra Day O'Connor, who was consistently pro-*Roe* (as interpreted by the joint opinion in *Casey*). The federal law provides that:

(a) Any physician who, in or affecting interstate or foreign commerce, knowingly performs a partial birth abortion and thereby kills a human fetus shall be fined under this title or imprisoned not more than 2 years, or both. This subsection does not apply to a partial birth abortion that is *necessary to save the life of a mother* whose life is endangered by a physical disorder, physical illness, or physical injury, including a life-endangering physical condition caused by or arising from the pregnancy itself. ...

(b) (1) The term "partial-birth" abortion means an abortion in which the person performing the abortion

(A) *Deliberately and intentionally* vaginally delivers a living fetus until, in the case of a head-first presentation, the *entire fetal head is outside* the body of the mother, *or,* in the case of breech presentation, *any part of the fetal trunk past the navel is outside* the body of the mother, for the purpose of performing an overt act that the person knows will kill the partially delivered living fetus; and

(B) Performs the overt act, other than completion of delivery, that kills the partially delivered living fetus [emphasis added].

The Court decided, 5 to 4, that this new law was constitutional.[12] Justice Kennedy wrote the majority opinion for himself and for Justices Antonin Scalia, Clarence Thomas, and the two new justices. In it he substantially adopts his dissenting opinion in *Stenberg* as the Court's new majority opinion. Although he concludes that his decision is consistent with *Stenberg*, all three U.S. District courts and all three Courts of Appeal that had examined this federal law found it unconstitutional under the principles in *Casey* and *Stenberg*, primarily because of the vagueness of the definition and the lack of a health exception. As to the vagueness argument, Kennedy writes that the new law is no longer vague because it clarifies the distinction between the prohibited procedure, which he calls "intact D&E," and standard D&E abortions because the former requires the delivery of an intact fetus, whereas the latter requires "the removal of fetal parts that are ripped from the fetus as they are pulled through the cervix." In addition, the new federal law specifies fetal landmarks (e.g., the "navel") instead of the vague description of a "substantial portion" of the "unborn child."

Because the law applies to fetuses both before and after the point of viability, Kennedy concedes that under *Casey* the law would be unconstitutional "if its purpose or effect is to place a substantial obstacle in the path of a woman seeking an abortion before the fetus attains viability." Kennedy finds Congress's purpose is twofold: first, lawmakers wanted to "express respect for the dignity of human life" by outlawing "a method of abortion in which a fetus is killed just inches before completion of the birth process," because use of this procedure "will further coarsen society to the humanity of not only newborns, but of all vulnerable and innocent human life. ..." Second, Congress wanted to protect medical ethics, finding that this procedure "confuses the medical, legal, and ethical duties of physicians to preserve and promote life. ..."

The key to Kennedy's legal analysis is his conclusion that these reasons are constitutionally sufficient to justify the ban because under *Casey*: "the State, from the inception of pregnancy, maintains its own regulatory interest in protecting the life of the fetus that may become a child [and this interest] cannot be set at naught by interpreting *Casey's* requirement of a health exception so it becomes tantamount to allowing the doctor to choose the abortion method he or she might prefer." Kennedy then goes on to write that "respect for human life finds an ultimate expression in the bond of love the mother has for her child," and that "while no reliable data" exist on the subject, "it seems unexceptionable to conclude some women come to regret their choice to abort the infant life they once created and sustained. ... Severe depression and loss of esteem can follow." Such regret, Justice Kennedy believes, can be caused or exacerbated if women later learn what the procedure entails, suggesting that physicians fail to describe it to patients because they "may prefer not to disclose precise details of the means [of abortion] that will be used. ..."

The final, critical issue is whether the prohibition would "ever impose significant health risks on women" and whether physicians or Congress should make this determination. Kennedy picks Congress: "The law need not give abortion doctors unfettered choice in the course of their medical practice, nor should it elevate their status above other physicians in the medical community .... Medical uncertainty does not foreclose the exercise of legislative power in the abortion context any more than it does in other contexts." Furthermore, Kennedy argues, the law does not impose an "undue burden" on women for another reason: alternative ways of killing a fetus have not been prohibited. In his words, "If the intact D&E procedure is truly necessary in some circumstances, it appears likely an injection that kills the fetus is an alternative under the Act that allows the doctor to perform the procedure."[12]

Writing for the four justices in the minority, Justice Ruth Bader Ginsburg, the only woman justice on the Court at the time, observes, "Today's decision is alarming. It refuses to take *Casey* and *Stenberg* seriously. It tolerates, indeed applauds, federal intervention to ban nationwide a procedure found necessary and proper in certain cases by the American College of Obstetricians [and Gynecologists] (ACOG). It blurs the line, firmly drawn in *Casey,* between previability and postviability abortions. And, for the first time since *Roe,* the Court blesses a prohibition with no exception safeguarding a woman's health." Ginsburg argues that the majority of the Court has overruled the conclusion in *Stenberg* that a health exception is required when "substantial medical authority supports the proposition that banning a particular abortion procedure could endanger women's health. ..." This conclusion, bolstered by evidence presented by nine professional organizations, including the ACOG, and conclusions by all three U.S. District Courts that heard evidence concerning the Act and its effects, directly contradicted the congressional declaration that "there is no credible medical evidence that partial-birth abortions are safe or are safer than other abortion procedures." Even Justice Kennedy agreed that Congress's finding was untenable.

Justice Ginsburg concludes that this leaves only "flimsy and transparent justifications" for upholding the ban. She rejects those justifications, arguing that the state's interest in "preserving and promoting fetal life" cannot be furthered by a ban that targets only a method of abortion and that cannot save "a single fetus from destruction" by its own terms but may put women's health at risk. Ultimately, she believes that the decision rests entirely on the proposition, never before enshrined in a majority opinion and explicitly repudiated in *Casey,* that "ethical and moral concerns" unrelated to the government's interest in "preserving life" can overcome what had been considered fundamental rights of citizens. The majority seeks to bolster its conclusion

by describing pregnant women as in a fragile emotional state that physicians may take advantage of by withholding information about abortion procedures. Justice Ginsburg concludes that the majority's solution to this hypothetical problem is to "deprive women of the right to make an autonomous choice, even at the expense of their safety." She continues, "This way of thinking [that men must protect women by restricting their choices] reflects ancient notions about women's place in the family and under the Constitution—ideas that have long since been discredited." Ginsburg further notes that the majority simply cannot contain its hostility to reproductive rights as articulated in *Roe* and *Casey,* calling physicians "abortion doctors," describing the fetus as an "unborn child" and as a "baby," labeling second-trimester abortions as "late term," and dismissing "the reasoned medical judgments of highly trained doctors ... as 'preferences' motivated by 'mere convenience.'"[12]

The major change in the law this opinion signals is the new willingness of Congress and the Court to discount the health of pregnant women and the medical judgment of their physicians.[13] This departure from precedent was made possible by categorizing physicians as unprincipled "abortion doctors" and infantilizing pregnant women as incapable of making serious decisions about their lives and health. The majority opinion ignores or marginalizes long-standing principles of constitutional law and substitutes the personal morality of Justice Kennedy and four of his colleagues.

The majority asserts that giving Congress constitutional authority to regulate medical practice is not new but identifies no case in which Congress had ever outlawed a medical procedure. Its reliance on the more than 100-year-old case of *Jacobson v. Massachusetts* is especially inapt.[14] *Jacobson* was about mandatory smallpox vaccination during an epidemic, refusal of which was punishable by a fine. The statute had an exception for "children who present a certificate, signed by a registered physician, that they are unfit subjects for vaccination," and the Court implied that a similar medical exception would be constitutionally required for adults. It is not just abortion regulations that have had a health exception for physicians and their patients—all health regulations have.[15]

On the other hand, **those who expect *Roe* to be overturned by this Court may be disappointed.** Although Justice Alito has replaced Justice O'Connor and is likely to vote in the opposite direction on *Roe*-related issues, Justice Kennedy is the new swing vote on the Court, and he insists that he is upholding the principles of *Roe v. Wade* as reaffirmed in *Casey.* Just as the question of whether a specific abortion regulation was an "undue burden" was once a determination Justice O'Connor could effectively make for the Court, the meaning of *Roe v. Wade* is, at least for now, up to Justice Kennedy. The replacement of two pro-*Roe* justices, Souter and Stevens, with Sonia Sotomayor and Elena Kagan in the Obama administration has made no change in this balance. Nonetheless, there are now three women justices on the Court, and this fact alone will make the Court take women's rights more seriously.

ABORTION POLITICS AND "OBAMACARE"[16,17]

President Barack Obama made it clear during the great debate on health insurance reform that he did not want abortion politics to sabotage his legislation. In his September 10, 2009 speech about health insurance reform to a joint session of Congress, he said, "Under our plan, no federal dollars will be used to fund abortions." **Nonetheless, the centrality of abortion in U.S. politics made it inevitable that abortion funding would play a major role in determining whether there was any health insurance reform law at all.** The debate revolved around the Stupak amendment in the House of Representatives, which provided that "No funds authorized or appropriated by this Act … may be used *to pay for any abortion or to cover any part of the costs of any health plan that includes coverage of abortion,* except in the case where a woman suffers from a physical disorder, physical injury, or physical illness that would, as certified by a physician, place the woman in danger of death unless an abortion is performed, including a life-endangering physical condition caused by or arising from the pregnancy itself, or unless the pregnancy is the result of rape or incest" (italics added). The House passed this amendment by a vote of 240 to 194, with 64 Democrats voting in favor (the House health care bill itself passed 220 to 215). Many thought that the Catholic bishops who lobbied fervently for passage of the Stupak amendment were the most influential in supporting it. More influential, however, was the previously secret fundamentalist Christian political leadership group known alternately as *the Family* or *the Fellowship,* which includes among its members both of the amendment's main sponsors, Bart Stupak (D-MI) and Joe Pitts (R-PA).[16]

The Stupak amendment was defended as merely continuing the practice created by **the Hyde amendment, named after the late Congressman Henry Hyde (R-IL) and attached to every Health and Human Services Appropriations Act passed since 1976;** the Hyde amendment has also been added to appropriations legislation for the Defense Department, the Indian Health Service, and federal employees' health insurance plans. **The Hyde amendment prohibits the use of federal funding for "any abortion" or for any "health benefits coverage that includes abortion" unless the pregnancy is the result of "rape or incest" or "would, as certified by a physician, place the woman in danger of death unless an abortion is performed."** Under the Hyde amendment, states may use their own funds to finance abortion services through their Medicaid programs, and 17 states currently do so.

The U.S. Supreme Court has ruled on the constitutionality of limiting government funding for abortion twice. The first case, in 1977, involved a Connecticut regulation that limited state Medicaid funding to "medically necessary" abortions, thus excluding those not necessary to preserve a woman's life or health. The Court ruled that women have a constitutional right to choose to have an abortion, but the state has no obligation to pay for the exercise of this right and may constitutionally encourage women to continue their pregnancies to term by providing funding for childbirth and not abortion. The state may not constitutionally create obstacles to abortion, but it has no obligation to remove obstacles not of its own making, such as poverty.

Three years after the Connecticut decision, **the Court upheld the Hyde amendment, which prohibited federal funding for medically necessary abortions. Under this ruling, even low-income women who would have devastating health outcomes if they continued a pregnancy could not have an abortion paid for by Medicaid.** In both cases, the Court ruled that the government could make "a value judgment favoring childbirth over abortion and [implement] that judgment by the allocation of public funds." Because the federal government did not make the women poor, and because poverty was their obstacle, no

constitutional requirement exists for the federal government to fund any abortion. Federal funding is a political question to be decided by Congress.

The U.S. Senate bill on health insurance reform, which Majority Leader Harry Reid (D-NV) created by blending bills from two committees, did not contain the Stupak amendment but specifically excluded federal funding for abortions as prohibited by any federal law—including the Hyde amendment—in effect "6 months before the beginning of the plan year involved." States must also ensure that "no federal funds pay or defray the cost" of abortion services in new health plans that cover abortion.

Three major questions were raised about the differences between the House and Senate approaches: Did they fulfill Obama's no-federal-funding promise? Did they follow the Hyde amendment "tradition"? And did they represent good health insurance policy? As for the first question, the Senate version fulfilled the President's promise by requiring abortion funding to come from sources other than federal tax dollars. This aspect of the provision was denigrated as a "bookkeeping trick," but even federal employees who pay for abortions with their government salaries are using funds that came from federal tax dollars. As for the second question, the Stupak amendment goes far beyond the Hyde amendment by prohibiting the use of federal tax dollars not only for abortion itself but also for any health plan available on the proposed exchanges that covers abortion. The goal is to limit access to abortion even when no federal funds are being used for it. The third question relates to public health policy. The Hyde amendment institutionalizes the moral view of some members of Congress that even medically necessary abortions should not be considered health care. After the Democrats lost Ted Kennedy's Senate seat in a special election in Massachusetts—and with it, the 60 votes needed to end a filibuster—the bill previously passed by the Senate became the vehicle for health insurance reform, and a budget "reconciliation" measure (requiring only 51 votes for Senate passage), negotiated by Democratic House and Senate leaders, was used to make modifications to the Senate bill to make it acceptable to the House.

Because the Stupak-Pitts abortion language was not in the Senate bill, it was uncertain whether the 216 House votes needed for passage could be found. **Stupak himself ultimately agreed to vote for the Senate bill as long as President Obama signed an executive order agreeing not to use any aspect of the legislation to fund abortions.** The bill ultimately passed 219 to 212, which suggests that the votes of Stupak and his colleagues were essential. President Barack Obama signed the executive order on March 24 at a private White House event.

Two abortion-related battles followed: the first directly involved the Affordable Care Act (ACA) and its contraception coverage, the second involved research on human embryos. We deal with the ACA controversy first. The ACA's goal is to make comprehensive health insurance available to all Americans. For women, this includes the provision of contraception. Under Health and Human Services (HHS)–promulgated regulations, insurance coverage must include 20 specific contraceptives as recommended by an Institute of Medicine (IOM) panel. Two corporations objected to providing four of these contraceptives, two types of intrauterine devices (IUDs) and the emergency contraceptives Plan B (levonorgestrel) and Ella (ulipristal) to their employees because they believed they could induce abortion.

When it got to the U.S. Supreme Court,[18] the case was based not on the Constitution but on a federal statute, the 1993

Religious Freedom Restoration Act (RFRA), which states that "government shall not substantially burden a person's exercise of religion even if the burden results from a rule of general applicability [unless it] is in furtherance of a compelling governmental interest and is the least restrictive means of furthering that … interest." For RFRA to be relevant, the term "person" must include for-profit corporations. Corporations are legal fictions created entirely by law to protect the interests of real people, including the shareholders and officers of the corporation. Nonetheless, and surprisingly (at least to us), the Court determined that for-profit corporations were persons under the Act and thus could have religious views that the state had to respect.

This left only two remaining legal issues: first, does the state have a compelling interest in covering all 20 contraceptives, and second, is the method of requiring that they be included in employer-provided health insurance policies the "least restrictive means" to do this? The Court quickly answered the first question yes and moved on to the question of least restrictive means, to which it answered no, because the government could accommodate corporations with religious views by granting them an exemption and creating an alternative funding mechanism for the four contraceptives in dispute. This conclusion got five votes but did not satisfy any of the Court's three women justices. For them and Justice Stephen Breyer, Justice Ruth Bader Ginsburg wrote a stinging dissent, noting that the "ability to control their reproductive lives" is central to the ability of women to gain equality in "the economic and social life of the Nation." She also noted that although the majority tried to confine its reasoning to four of the 20 FDA-approved contraceptives, "the Court's reasoning appears to permit commercial enterprises … to exclude from their group health plans all forms of contraceptives." This she added was "a substantial burden on women, especially those earning low wages."

In terms of health care, **the reaction of the ACOG to the opinion seems just about right to us: "This decision inappropriately allows employers to interfere in women's health care decisions … which should be made by a woman and her doctor, based on the patient's needs and her current health."** The ACOG went on to underline that contraceptives and family planning are mainstream medical care and should be treated as such. In their words, **"access to contraception is essential women's health care."**

HUMAN EMBRYONIC STEM CELL RESEARCH FUNDING[19,20]

Embryo research was born political. Expressions of shock and surprise at the 2010 ruling of Federal District Court Judge Royce Lamberth that enjoined federal funding of stem cell research, which was based largely on his reading of an amendment to an appropriations bill, were thus not terribly persuasive. The amendment, known as the *Dickey-Wicker amendment,* provides that no federal funds can be expended by the National Institutes of Health (NIH) for "1) the creation of a human embryo or embryos for research purposes; or 2) research in which a human embryo or embryos are destroyed, discarded, or knowingly subjected to risks of injury or death." The creation and destruction of human embryos for research are deeply tied not only to political and religious debates concerning abortion but also to assisted reproductive technology (ART). In 1979, during the Carter administration, the Ethics Advisory Board of the Department of Health, Education, and Welfare

(forerunner of the Department of Health and Human Services) recommended that the government support research on embryos in order to study and improve ART. Federal research funding was never authorized, and in vitro fertilization (IVF) was introduced into clinical medicine without a research phase. The Reagan administration dissolved the ethics board and ignored its recommendations. The issue was next taken up during the Clinton administration by an NIH Human Embryo Research Panel, which voted on 27 goals of embryo research and recommended seven of these as "acceptable for federal funding" but failed to produce a credible ethical justification for its recommendations, which were widely ignored.[21] Congress, however, responded to the report, and in 1996, President Clinton signed the first appropriations bill containing the Dickey-Wicker amendment, named for its sponsors, Representatives Jay Dickey (R-AR) and Roger Wicker (R-MS). It has been added to NIH appropriations bills every subsequent year, just as the Hyde Amendment restricting abortion funding is added.

The derivation of stem cells from embryos involves destroying the embryo. In 2001, President George W. Bush authorized federal funding for human embryonic stem cell (ESC) research but limited it to cell lines that had been derived before his August 9, 2001 speech—and specifically to cell lines from surplus IVF embryos used with the consent of the couple whose egg and sperm were used to create them. No one challenged this policy as a violation of Dickey-Wicker, perhaps because, as Bush said, the "life and death decision" for these embryos had already been made.

President Barack Obama was well aware that federal funding of ESC research represents a political flash point, but he had promised to rescind the Bush policy, and expanded federal funding of ESC research is widely supported. When Obama announced his new policy to authorize funding for cell lines derived after August 2001, if derived from surplus IVF embryos without the use of federal funds, he knew he could be reawakening the funding debate. He expressed his hope that "Congress will act on a bipartisan basis to provide further support for this research."

Congress did not act. Instead, the debate shifted to the courts, where the core question was whether the new Obama guidelines are consistent with Dickey-Wicker. Lamberth said he believes Dickey-Wicker is "unambiguous" and does not permit the NIH "to separate the derivation of ESCs from research on the ESCs" because "derivation of ESCs from an embryo is an integral step in conducting ESC research." The Obama administration appealed. **The Obama administration's guidelines are based on the political compromise of deriving ESCs only from surplus IVF embryos, and as part of this compromise, the NIH seemed to have conceded that derivation is an integral part of stem cell research, which is why it sets strict limits on the source of the embryos used and the quality of consent obtained.** The political argument for permitting the use of surplus IVF embryos is that these embryos were created for a legitimate reproductive purpose, and when they are no longer wanted for that purpose, their donation for research is ethically preferable to their destruction without any potential societal benefit.[21] Of course, anyone who objects to the creation of embryos for IVF would also object to this compromise. Does Dickey-Wicker permit this political compromise as a matter of law?

President Clinton's National Bioethics Advisory Commission argued in 1999 that it was not ethically reasonable to separate the derivation of stem cells for research from their use in research. The commission believed that the federal government should fund both, for at least as long as the embryos used were those "remaining after infertility treatments." Their reasons were "the close connection in practical and ethical terms between derivation and use of the cells" and the hope that permitting funding for cell derivation could advance science in this area. Lawyers asked by the commission to examine the meaning of Dickey-Wicker concluded that the NIH's distinction between derivation and use of human ESCs was a "reasonable" interpretation of the amendment—but that "there is no indication that either proponents or opponents [of ESC research] contemplated the situation … in which research that destroyed the embryo was separately conducted from research using the cells derived from the embryo."[22]

The Clinton panel's report got less attention than it deserved because at that time the national debate was focused on creating research embryos through cloning (somatic cell nuclear transfer). Bush's Council on Bioethics concentrated on cloning, but it was also the only national ethics panel ever to discuss federal funding as an ethical, rather than political, issue. It concluded that "the decision to fund an activity is … a declaration of official national support and endorsement, a positive assertion that the activity in question is deemed by the nation as a whole … to be good and worthy." Such rhetoric seems disconnected from special-interest legislation[23]; a more honest statement regarding federal funding is that since *Roe v. Wade,* funding for anything remotely related to abortion—and because no one is pregnant, embryo research is indeed only remotely related—has become a potent political liability in Congress. Obama's own ethics panel sensibly stayed out of this political funding debate.

Three paths were open to proponents of federal funding for human ESC research: The first was to mount a vigorous defense in the lawsuit, aiming to persuade the courts that the Obama administration's interpretation of Dickey-Wicker is correct. This strategy ultimately succeeded, and the federal Court of Appeals ruled 2 to 1 in 2011 that Dickey-Wicker permitted the funding of research on human ESCs that had been derived from leftover IVF embryos by nonfederal employees who did not use federal money. We thought this opinion was solid at the time and would prevail, and it has. Nevertheless, we also thought it was reasonable for the Obama administration to seek congressional authorization for its current regulations. However, because this approach would retain Dickey-Wicker and could thus lead to more legal challenges, it would be preferable—and probably more politically feasible—to amend Dickey-Wicker by adding language such as the following: "Nothing in part 2 prohibits the NIH from funding research using embryos created for procreation, including the derivation of stem cells, when the couple no longer wants to use them for procreation and has provided their informed authorization for them to be used in NIH-funded research." Amending the language in this manner would legislatively adopt the ethics position of the Clinton bioethics commission. The third path is continued reliance on private and state funding until sufficient scientific progress is made such that the public demands federal funding for this research.

NIH Director Francis Collins has said that this issue "goes beyond politics … to patients and their families who are counting on us to do everything in our power, ethically and responsibly, to learn how to transform these cells into entirely new therapies." This argument, of course, is itself political; and if Collins is right, **the only place to ultimately resolve the funding issue is in Congress.**

GENETIC COUNSELING, SCREENING, AND PRENATAL DIAGNOSIS[24-26]

In 2013, the American College of Medical Genetics and Genomics (ACMG) opposed legal restrictions on abortion following prenatal diagnosis.[27] The College noted that the entire practice of medical genetics is to provide patients with information to enable the pregnant couple "to choose a safe and personally acceptable management plan" and concluded that "termination of pregnancy for genetic disorders or congenital anomalies that may be diagnosed prenatally is a critically important option …." This statement was prompted by the passage of a North Dakota law outlawing abortion for a "genetic abnormality" defined as "any defect, disease, or disorder that is inherited genetically." The law also has its own nonexclusive list of prohibited indications for abortion: "Any physical disfigurement, scoliosis, dwarfism, Down syndrome, albinism, or any other type of physical or mental disability, abnormality or disease." This law, and proposals like it, are a direct response to the increasing number of genetic tests that can be performed on fetuses and thus the increasing number of conditions for which pregnant women might decide to terminate their pregnancies. North Dakota Governor Jack Dalrymple said he signed this law to challenge the "boundaries of *Roe v. Wade.*" **We have not had to decide what genetic conditions justify abortion before, but the rapid expansion of genetic tests of the fetus makes this a compelling contemporary quandary. Can we simultaneously reject eugenics and discrimination and at the same time provide pregnant women with ever more genomic information about their fetuses?**

Twenty years after *Roe,* a committee of the IOM suggested clinical guidelines for prenatal diagnosis. The committee prophetically anticipated that many more genetic tests would be developed and that "eventually technologies will be available to simultaneously test for hundreds of different disease-causing mutations, either in the same or different genes." **The committee's recommendations, which remain valid today, include the following:**

- Patients must be fully informed about the risks and benefits of testing procedures, their possible outcomes, and alternatives.
- Prenatal diagnosis should only be offered for the diagnosis of genetic disorders and birth defects, not for minor conditions or characteristics or for fetal sex selection.
- Education before and after prenatal screening should be available to patients, and ongoing counseling should be available following pregnancy termination.
- Reproductive genetic services should not be used for the eugenic goal of "improving" the human species.

The recommendations became the foundation upon which professional organizations, most importantly the ACOG and the ACMG, built their own guidelines for prenatal diagnosis. These professional guidelines are used by physicians as the standard of care for their patients. The amount of genetic information that can be obtained from fetuses is so great that it is often difficult for anyone to interpret its meaning or assess the variability and uncertainty of any genetic findings. Sometimes, however, prenatal diagnosis can identify a serious condition, and this information could lead a couple to terminate a pregnancy. The ability to determine the health of the fetus also permits couples who would not otherwise take a chance on having a baby because of the high risk of a serious genetic condition, such as Tay-Sachs disease, to have children without risking birth of an affected child.

Chromosomal microarray analysis (CMA) detects not only entire extra or missing chromosomes but also small losses and gains of segments of DNA throughout the genome, whereas *karyotype analysis* allows detection of extra or missing fragments of chromosomes but only those large enough to be seen under a microscope. These losses and gains of segments of DNA are referred to as *copy number variants* (CNVs), and they can lead to genetic disorders associated with significant disabilities. The National Institute of Child Health and Human Development (NICHD) conducted a large study (*n* = 4406) to compare microarray analysis to karyotype analysis. Samples were split two ways in this study of women undergoing either chorionic villus sampling (CVS) or amniocentesis: standard karyotyping was performed on one portion, and microarray analysis on the other. In 1 in 60 cases in which the karyotype was read as "normal," microarrays revealed a clinically important CNV. When prenatal diagnosis was prompted by a structural abnormality of the fetus seen on an ultrasound and the karyotype was interpreted as "normal," microarray analysis revealed a CNV in almost one in 17 cases.[28] **Clinical dilemmas are sometimes encountered when CMAs show a *variant of unknown (or uncertain) significance* (VOUS),** a change in DNA that has not yet been reliably characterized as benign or pathogenic. Sometimes the answer to the question, "What is the chance of this VOUS leading to a significant problem in my baby?" is that we just do not know. The vast majority of such variants are likely to be just benign variants of no clinical consequences. On the other hand, even if a VOUS is inherited from an apparently "normal" parent, the CNV may cause serious congenital and developmental abnormalities in the child. In such cases, finding a VOUS could lead to questioning whether the parent who transmitted the VOUS is really "normal," or if we need to search for health problems that have not been recognized. In the NICHD study, a VOUS was found in 3.8% of all cases where the karyotype was read as "normal."

The limited time available for decision making makes gathering information quickly imperative, which includes the requirement for testing the parents to determine whether the fetal findings are inherited. Even when a CNV is known to be associated with a well-described genetic syndrome, making a decision about continuing the pregnancy may still be fraught with uncertainty. Genomic information possesses a mythology of precision and determinativeness that it does not deserve. As the medical literature and databases associated with CNVs expand, such diagnostic uncertainties will be less frequent, but they will still occur. While studies continue, **ACOG has recommended that couples who choose chromosomal microarrays should receive both pretest and posttest genetic counseling.** Prenatal counseling is usually described as "nondirective," (i.e., neither for nor against termination of the pregnancy), but this term has no meaning in the context of a genomic VOUS. Physicians must share the uncertainty of diagnosis with their patients and must advise them as best they can without guaranteeing a healthy baby.

For more than three decades, finding a noninvasive way to analyze the genetic makeup of the fetus by identifying fetal cells in the blood of the pregnant woman has been a scientific quest because it could permit prenatal diagnosis without any risk to the fetus. The quest to dependably collect fetal cells from maternal blood has been taken up by private biotech companies. In 1997, it was first reported that fragments of cell-free fetal DNA (cfDNA) circulate in the maternal blood during pregnancy beginning in the early first trimester. About 10% of the DNA in maternal plasma is now known to be of placental origin. This offers the possibility of noninvasive prenatal diagnosis by taking a blood sample from the pregnant woman. The technology currently used for commercial testing is *massively parallel genomic sequencing.*

Within the next few years, noninvasive prenatal detection for the majority of recognized genetic disorders will likely become a reality. The fact that the entire fetal genome is represented in maternal blood opens up the possibility of obtaining fetal DNA fragments that can be assembled into a complete fetal genome readout. A number of substantial hurdles, including the availability of genetic counseling, remain before noninvasive fetal whole-genome sequencing is introduced into clinical practice. First, the cost will have to drop substantially. In this regard, targeting selected genomic regions may prove more efficient and cost effective than deriving the whole genome. On the other hand, isolating and analyzing fetal cells from maternal blood would be more straightforward and presumably less costly. Will noninvasive prenatal testing become "normalized" and routine because of its ease and safety? We think it is inevitable that reasonably priced and accurate genetic and genomic tests based on fetal cells or cfDNA extracted from maternal blood will be offered to all pregnant women. The primary motivation, however, will likely not be medical practice standards but fear of medical malpractice lawsuits. **Obstetricians will likely fear a malpractice lawsuit if a fetus is born with a genetic abnormality, the test for which the couple can credibly explain to a jury that they would have obtained, had they known about it, and that they would have terminated the pregnancy had they known the fetus had the particular genetic condition.** We both believe that physician fear of the extremely unlikely prospect of such a lawsuit is a terrible way to set medical practice standards. Rather **we support professional organizations that set screening standards for their members—and that their members follow them.**

Our current model for prenatal screening and diagnostic testing requires pretest counseling prior to obtaining informed consent, and the obligation to counsel can be seen as inherent in the fiduciary nature of the doctor-patient relationship. For ordinary medical procedures, the physical risks and treatment alternatives—those things that might lead a patient to reject therapy or choose an alternative—are the primary items of information that must be disclosed and should be discussed. Self-determination and rational decision making are the central values protected by informed consent. In the setting of reproductive genetics, what is at stake is the right to decide whether to have genomic testing with emphasis on the right to refuse if the potential harm in terms of stigma or unacceptable choices, including abortion, outweighs the potential benefit for the individual or her family.

New genomic screening and diagnostic tests—including exome and whole-genome sequencing, addressed in Chapter 10—will compete for introduction into routine clinical practice. Some of the critical questions include what information should be provided to which patients, when it should be provided, and how and by whom it should be conveyed. It will soon be impossible to do meaningful counseling about all available genomic testing. Giving too much information (information overload) can amount to misinformation, and it can make the entire counseling process misleading or meaningless. **To prevent disclosure from being pointless or counterproductive, we believe that information-sharing strategies based on general or "generic" consent should be developed for genetic and genomic screening and diagnostic testing**. Their aim would be to provide sufficient information to permit patients to make informed decisions yet avoid the information overload that could lead to "misinformed consent."

Traditionally, the goals of reproductive genetic counseling are to help the person or family to:

Comprehend the medical facts, including the diagnosis, the probable course of the disorder, and the available management choices

Appreciate the way heredity contributes to the disorder and the risk of recurrence in specified relatives

Understand the options for dealing with the risk of recurrence

Choose the course of action most appropriate to them in view of their risk and their family *goals* and act in accordance with that decision

Make the best possible adjustment to the disorder in an affected family member and/or to the risk of recurrence of the disorder

Even knowledgeable couples can become confused, frustrated, and anxious if faced with multiple options for genetic screening and testing. **An approach based on "generic consent,"** which we described in the *New England Journal of Medicine* 20 years ago and still believe in, would not even attempt to describe each of hundreds or thousands of genetic conditions and anomalies to be screened and tested for; instead, **it would emphasize broader concepts and common-denominator issues in genetic and genomic screening.**

We envision a doctor-patient relationship in which patients are told of the availability of a panel of genetic and genomic tests that can be performed on a single blood sample, either for carrier screening or for noninvasive prenatal testing. Couples would be told that these tests would focus on disorders that involve serious physical abnormalities, mental disabilities, or both. Several common examples would be given to indicate the frequency and spectrum of severity of each type or category of genetic condition for which screening or diagnostic testing was being offered. Conditions such as spina bifida and cleft lip, chromosome abnormalities such as Down syndrome and trisomy 18, and single gene disorders such as cystic fibrosis and Tay-Sachs disease might be chosen as representative examples.

In the course of counseling, important factors common to all prenatal screening and diagnostic tests would be highlighted. Among these are their limitations, especially the fact that negative results cannot guarantee a healthy infant. For screening tests, the couple needs to know that additional invasive tests may be needed to establish a diagnosis or clarify confusing or uncertain results. Other considerations that need to be discussed are the costs of testing; options such as adoption, egg or sperm donation, abortion, or acceptance of risks; and issues of confidentiality, including potential disclosure of the results to other family members. If the testing is for carrier status, and a recessive gene is detected in the woman, it must be emphasized that her partner should also be screened.

For prenatal diagnosis, couples should understand that abortion of an abnormal fetus is available, but it is not the only option. For couples who find abortion unacceptable for any indication, prenatal diagnosis may still provide important information. For example, if it becomes known that a baby will be delivered with serious birth defects, choosing to deliver at a tertiary medical center that offers specialized care may optimize the infant's outcome. In some cases, knowing that the fetus has a very serious and incurable disorder may alter the obstetric care for the mother. For example, if the fetus has trisomy 18, the likelihood is high that fetal heart monitoring during labor would show an abnormal tracing. Knowing that the fetus has trisomy 18 could avert performing a cesarean delivery because it would not benefit the infant.

Generic consent to genetic carrier screening and diagnostic testing can be compared with obtaining consent to perform a routine physical examination. Patients know that the purpose of the examination is to locate potential problems likely to require additional follow-up, which could present them with choices they would rather not have to make; essentially, the doctor is looking for trouble, and the patient is hoping no trouble will be found. However, the patient is not generally told about all the possible abnormalities that can be detected by a routine physical examination or routine blood work, only the general purpose of each. On the other hand, **tests that may produce especially sensitive and stigmatizing information, such as screening of blood for the human immunodeficiency virus** (HIV, see Chapter 52), **should not be performed without specific consent.** Similarly, because of its reproductive implications, genetic testing has not traditionally been carried out without specific consent.

What is central in generic consent for genetic and genomic screening and diagnostic testing is not a waiver of the individual patient's right to information. Rather generic consent would reflect **a decision by the medical community that we believe is consistent with the physician's fiduciary obligations to the patient; it is a decision that patients would likely support, that the most reasonable way to conduct genetic and genomic screening and diagnostic testing for multiple diseases simultaneously is to provide basic, general information to obtain consent for the testing and much more detailed information on specific conditions only after they have been detected.** In the vast majority of cases, no such conditions will in fact be found, so this method is also the most efficient and cost effective.

Some patients may require more specific and in-depth information on which to base their decision regarding testing. It is therefore essential to build into the testing program ample opportunity for patients to obtain all the additional information they want or need to help them make decisions. Clinicians, of course, must be open and responsive to the concerns and questions of patients. Counseling could be provided in person by a physician or other health professional. Alternatively, Internet-based audiovisual aids could be used to help ensure consistency in the information provided, improve efficiency, and help respond to the shortage of genetic counselors.

Generic consent for genetic and genomic screening and diagnostic testing should help prevent information overload and wasting time on useless information, especially for carrier screening. It would not, however, solve what is likely to be an even more central question in prenatal genetic testing: **Are there genetic conditions for which testing should *not* be offered to**

prospective parents? Examples might include genes that predispose a person to a particular disease that will not appear until late in life such as Alzheimer disease, Parkinson disease, or breast cancer. From the perspective of the fetus, life with the possibility or even a high probability of developing these diseases in late adulthood is much preferred to no life at all. Thus in this case—unlike that of the fetus with trisomy 18, for example—no reasonable argument could be made that precluding abortion by denying this information could amount to forcing a "wrongful life" on the child.

We should, nonetheless, directly and publicly address the question of whether conditions should exist for which screening of prospective parents or testing of fetuses should *not* be offered as a matter of good medical practice and public policy regardless of the technical ability to do such testing or the wishes of the couple. Offering genetic and genomic screening and diagnostic testing to assist couples in making reproductive decisions is not a neutral activity; rather it implies that some action should be taken on the basis of the results of the test. Simply offering carrier screening for breast cancer or colon cancer genes in the context of preconception care, for example, suggests to couples that artificial insemination, adoption, and even abortion are all reasonable choices if they are found to be carriers of such genes. On the other hand, because of a personal experience with a family member who suffered from one of these adult-onset diseases, a particular couple might see abortion as a reasonable choice under such circumstances, and a practice of keeping such information away from all couples would not be justified. However, **in general we do not believe that pregnancies in women who want to have a child should be terminated for adult-onset diseases. We are all going to die of something, and if we live long enough, that *something* will have a major genetic component; there can be no perfect genome, and the search for it in a fetus will inevitably fail.**

A standard of care for genomic screening and diagnostic testing will inevitably be set, as will a standard for informed consent in the face of hundreds or thousands of available genomic tests. We believe the medical profession should take the lead in setting such standards, and with public input and support, the model of generic consent for genomic screening and diagnostic testing will ultimately be accepted. Other regulators, including the Food and Drug Administration (FDA), will increasingly be involved in setting standards for genomic testing done outside of a physician-patient relationship, usually referred to as *direct-to-consumer* (DTC). In mid-2013, for example, the genetic-testing company 23andMe began running a compelling national television commercial. The ad featured attractive young people saying that for $99, you could learn "hundreds of things about your health," including that you "might have an increased risk of heart disease, arthritis, gallstones, and hemochromatosis." It was the centerpiece of the company's campaign to sign up a million consumers. In November, the FDA sent 23andMe a warning letter, ordering them to "immediately discontinue marketing the PGS [Saliva Collection Kit and Personal Genome Service] until such time as it receives FDA marketing authorization for the [class III] device." One month later, the company announced that it was complying with the FDA's demands and discontinued running its TV commercial.

The 23andMe services rely on single nucleotide polymorphism (SNP) technology to identify genetic markers associated with 254 specific diseases and conditions, although the list has grown over time. The company Web page now boasts "Ongoing reports provided to you as new genetic discoveries are made and as we are able to clear new reports through the FDA." In the past, it said their service could inform people about their health and how to take steps to improve it. In the words of 23andMe's TV commercial, "Change what you can, manage what you can't." The FDA wrote that its main concern was that 23andMe failed to supply any indication that it had "analytically or clinically validated the PGS for its intended uses." The page now states that its service includes "reports that meet FDA standards for being scientifically and clinically valid." The FDA has not yet developed rules for DTC genetic testing, and whether government regulation or private litigation will determine the future contours of DTC genomic sequencing will probably depend on the extent to which consumers and physicians support government regulation.

23andMe had previously framed DTC genetic testing as consumer empowerment that gave people direct access to their genetic information without requiring them to go through a physician or genetic counselor. To oversimplify, the debate has been framed as a struggle between medical (or government) paternalism and an individual's right to their own information. In this sense, it is not so different from the older debate about whether patients should have direct access to their medical records and test results, which was ultimately resolved in favor of direct patient access. We think the day will come when this framing is appropriate, but not until the diagnostic and prognostic capability of genomic information has been clinically validated.

It seems reasonable to predict, for example, that in the next decade or even sooner, a majority of health plans will make it easy for their members to have their entire genome sequenced and linked to their electronic health record, and they will provide software to help their members interrogate their own genomes with or without the help of their physician or a genetic counselor supplied by the health plan. This service will, of course, require a massive data bank of genome reference materials, and the FDA and the National Institute for Standards and Technology are working to establish such a data bank. **Unless genomic tests have been validated, however, genomic information can be misleading or just plain wrong, and this can cause more harm than good in health care settings.** In most cases, family history is likely to be at least as informative about an individual's health risks as SNP-based testing such as that used by 23andMe. In this regard, the FDA's censoring of 23andMe's PGS advertising did not deprive people of useful information; the agency merely asserted its requirement that companies that want to sell their health-related medical devices to the public demonstrate to the FDA that they *work*—in this case, that the tests do what the company asserts that they do. That is traditional consumer protection and what the public expects from the FDA.

Privacy is a closely related issue. How can the extremely private and personal information locked in our DNA be protected from others' using it without our consent for their own purposes or making it available to people or organizations who could use it against us, such as by denying us life or disability insurance? For example, 23andMe has suggested that its longer-range corporate goal is to collect a massive biobank of genetic information that can be used and sold for medical research and could also lead to patentable discoveries. Such uses seem reasonable so long as the consent of the DNA donors is properly obtained and their privacy is protected. Both of these requirements are, however, much more difficult to uphold than 23andMe seems to realize.

Informed consent to genomic testing is currently the subject of a wide-ranging debate, touched off by testing policies published by the ACMG that require that when a physician orders a clinical sequencing test, the testing lab must also test for pathogenic (or probably pathogenic) mutations in 56 genes related to 24 serious disorders. The original report suggested doing away with informed consent, but a later revision included an opt-out provision. People have both a right to know what will be done to diagnose their condition and a right *not* to know information about their genetic predispositions if they do not want to know it. Here, 23andMe had adopted a more rights-respecting mode, telling customers what they will be looking for before they sign up for the genetic testing and giving them a second chance not to find out about the results of specific tests—such as tests for the breast-cancer mutations, Parkinson disease, and Alzheimer disease—after the test is done.

Whether ordered by physicians or by consumers online, whole-genome screening will require more sophisticated informed consent protocols, and we believe that individuals should also retain the right not to have specific genes sequenced at all. Geneticist James Watson set a reasonable standard for nondisclosure when he authorized the publication of his entire genome with one exception: he still refuses to have his apolipo-protein E (*APOE*) status determined because he does not want to know if he is at higher-than-average risk for developing Alzheimer disease. That should be his right and the right of every patient or consumer.

Because of the company's aggressive marketing and refusal to continue negotiations, the FDA shut 23andMe down temporarily. In 2015, the FDA decided it was ready to permit 23andMe to market genetic tests for autosomal recessive disease that could be used by couples to determine whether they both carried such a gene, which would give them a one in four chance of having an affected child. The shutdown provided the opportunity for a serious dialog that could be a basis for setting standards for the entire industry. It could also be a catalyst for creating a regulatory framework for whole-genome–sequencing platforms, which are the future of genomics.[1] It's already a commonplace observation that we will soon have "the $1000 genome with the $1,000,000 interpretation." Put another way, **it is not the cost of the sequencing or the SNP testing that is at the heart of this debate; it is whether the genomic information produced by that sequencing can be used in ways that improve our health.** The goal of both the FDA and 23andMe should be to ensure that genomic information is both accurate and clinically useful. Clinicians will be central to helping consumer-patients use genomic information to make health decisions. Any regulatory regime must recognize this reality by doing more than simply adding the tag line "Ask your physician" on most consumer ads for prescription drugs.

FORCED CESAREAN DELIVERY

Almost 25 years ago, Kolder and colleagues[29] reported a U.S. national survey revealing that court orders had been obtained for cesarean deliveries in 11 states for hospital detentions in two states and for intrauterine transfusions in one state. Among 21 cases in which court orders were sought, the orders were obtained in 86%; in 88% of those cases, the orders were received within 6 hours. Most of the women involved were black, Asian, or Hispanic, and all were poor. Nearly half were unmarried, and one fourth did not speak English as their primary language. In the survey, they also found that 46% of the heads of fellowship programs in maternal-fetal medicine thought that women who refused medical advice and thereby endangered the life of the fetus should be detained, and 47% supported court orders for procedures such as intrauterine transfusions. Until 1990, with the exception of one case in the Georgia State Supreme Court, all cases had been decided by lower courts and therefore had little precedential importance.[30] In most cases, judges were called on an emergency basis and ordered interventions within hours. The judge usually went to the hospital. **Physicians should know what most lawyers and almost all judges know: when a judge arrives at the hospital in response to an emergency call, he or she is acting much more like a lay person than a jurist.** Without time to analyze the issues, without representation for the pregnant woman, without briefing or thoughtful reflection on the situation, in almost total ignorance of the relevant law, and in an unfamiliar setting faced by a relatively calm physician and a woman who can easily be labeled "hysterical," the judge will almost always order whatever the doctor advises.

There is nothing in *Roe v. Wade*,[2] or any other appellate decision, that gives either physicians or judges the right to favor the life or well-being of the fetus over that of the pregnant woman. Nor is there legal precedent for a mother being ordered to undergo surgery (e.g., kidney or partial liver transplantation) to save the life of her dying child. It would be ironic and inconsistent if a woman could be forced to submit to more invasive surgical procedures for the sake of a fetus than for a child. Forcing pregnant women to follow medical advice also places unwarranted faith in that advice. Physicians often disagree about the appropriateness of obstetric interventions, and they can be mistaken.[31] In three of the first five cases in which court-ordered cesarean delivery was sought, the women ultimately delivered vaginally and uneventfully. In the face of such uncertainty—uncertainty compounded by decades of changing and conflicting expert opinion on the management of pregnancy and childbirth—**the moral and legal primacy of the competent, informed pregnant woman in decision making is overwhelming.**[32]

Physicians may feel better after being "blessed" by the judge, but they should not. First, the appearance of legitimacy is deceptive; the judge has acted injudiciously, and no opportunity for meaningful appeal exists. Second, the medical situation has not changed except that more time has been lost that should have been used to continue discussion with the woman directly. Finally, the physician has now helped to transform himself or herself into an agent of the state's authority.[32]

The question of how to deal with a woman who continues to refuse intervention in the face of a court order remains. Do we really want to attempt to restrain and forcibly medicate and operate on a competent refusing adult? Although such a procedure may be legal, it is hardly humane. It is not what one generally associates with modern obstetric care, and it has the potential to cause harm. It also encourages an adversarial relationship between the obstetrician and the patient. Moreover, even from a strictly utilitarian perspective, this marriage of the state and medicine is likely to harm more fetuses than it helps because many women will quite reasonably avoid physicians altogether during pregnancy if failure to follow medical advice can result in forced treatment, involuntary confinement, or criminal charges.

Extending notions of child abuse to "fetal abuse" simply brings government into pregnancy with few if any benefits and with great potential for invasions of privacy and deprivations of liberty. It is not helpful to use the law to convert a woman's and society's moral responsibility to her fetus into the woman's legal responsibility alone.[29] After birth, the fetus becomes a child and can and should thereafter be treated in its own right. Before birth, however, we can obtain access to the fetus only through its mother and, in the absence of her informed consent, can do so only by treating her as a fetal container, a nonperson without rights to bodily integrity.

In 2005, the ACOG revised and updated its 1987 Ethics Committee report on "Patient Choice: Maternal Fetal Conflict," now titled "Maternal Decision Making, Ethics, and the Law,"[33] **which we believe provides thoughtful and useful guidance for the medical practitioner.** The statement highlighted six considerations that we combine into three:

1. Coercive and punitive legal approaches to pregnant women who refuse medical advice fail to recognize that all competent adults are entitled to informed consent and bodily integrity.
2. Court-ordered interventions in cases of informed refusal, as well as punishment of pregnant women for their behavior that may put a fetus at risk, neglect the fact that medical knowledge and predictions of outcomes in obstetrics have limitations ... [and treat medical problems] as if they were moral failings.
3. Coercive and punitive policies are potentially counterproductive in that they are likely to discourage prenatal care and successful treatment, adversely affect infant mortality rates, and undermine the physician-patient relationship ... [and] unjustly single out the most vulnerable women ... and create the potential for criminalization of many types of otherwise legal maternal behavior.

Based on these, the Committee on Ethics made four recommendations, the most central of which are:

1. Pregnant women's autonomous decisions should be respected. ... In the absence of extraordinary circumstances, circumstances that, in fact, the Committee cannot currently imagine, judicial authority should not be used to implement treatment regimens aimed at protecting the fetus, for such actions violate the pregnant woman's autonomy.
2. Pregnant women should not be punished for adverse perinatal outcomes.
3. Policymakers, legislators, and physicians should work together to find constructive and evidence-based ways to address the needs of women with alcohol and other substance abuse problems.

This 2005 statement is even stronger than a 1990 opinion by the District of Columbia Court of Appeals, which ruled that the decision of the pregnant woman must be honored in all but "extremely rare and truly exceptional" cases.[34] ACOG's Ethics Committee "cannot currently imagine" what that "rare and truly exceptional" case might look like.

---

liberty" that is "broad enough to encompass a woman's decision whether or not to terminate a pregnancy" before fetal viability without state interference.

- In *Planned Parenthood of Southeastern Pennsylvania v. Casey* (1992), the U.S. Supreme Court reaffirmed the "core" of *Roe v. Wade* and ruled that before fetal viability, states cannot "unduly burden" a woman's decision to terminate a pregnancy (i.e., although consent and waiting periods may be constitutionally acceptable, states cannot regulate abortion in ways that will actually prevent women from obtaining them).
- *Roe* and *Casey* are critical to understanding the rights of obstetricians, which are derived from the rights of their patients, because they are the major sources of law regarding how far states can go to regulate decisions made in the obstetrician-patient relationship.
- With the exception of a procedure Congress has labeled "partial-birth abortion," unless they contain an exception for the health of the pregnant woman, laws that criminalize abortions are unconstitutional because they are inconsistent with both *Roe* and *Casey*.
- *Roe* has been the source of political controversy since it was decided in 1973. Congress has enacted the Hyde Amendment every year since the mid-1970s, prohibiting the use of federal funds for almost all abortions, and its constitutionality has been upheld by the U.S. Supreme Court. *Roe* motivated the exclusion of abortion funding for Obamacare and ultimately a ruling by the U.S. Supreme Court that for-profit corporations can have religious beliefs, which the government must honor, to not include contraceptive methods the corporation believes induce abortion in the health care insurance made available to their employees.
- The Hyde Amendment was the basis for another similar amendment, the Dickey-Wicker Amendment, which prohibited the use of federal funds for human embryonic stem cell research and was the basis for a temporary injunction that prohibited the NIH from funding such research in 2010 (overturned in 2011) under the Obama administration's human embryonic stem cell research rules.
- To protect patient privacy and autonomy, no information obtained in genetic counseling or screening should be disclosed to any third party without the patient's authorization.
- "Generic" consent for genetic screening that emphasizes broad concepts and common-denominator issues should help maximize rational decision making by preventing information overload and wasting time on useless information.
- Self-determination and rational decision making are the central purposes of informed consent, and information on recommended procedures, risks, benefits, and alternatives should be presented in a way that furthers these purposes.
- Consent of the pregnant woman is a mandatory prerequisite for both investigative procedures and therapy. Her consent must be informed, and she should be told as clearly as possible about the proposed experimental procedures or therapy, its risks to her and her fetus, and

---

KEY POINTS

- In *Roe v. Wade* (1973), the U.S. Supreme Court determined that a fundamental "right to privacy existed in the Fourteenth Amendment's concept of personal

alternatives, success rates, and the likely problems with recuperation.

◆ The fetal-maternal relationship is a unique one that requires physicians to promote a balance of maternal health and fetal welfare while respecting maternal autonomy. Obstetricians should not perform procedures that are refused by pregnant women, although reasonable steps to persuade a woman to change her mind are appropriate.

REFERENCES

1. Annas GJ. The Supreme Court and abortion rights. *N Engl J Med.* 2007;356:2201.
2. *Roe v. Wade,* 410 U.S. 113 (1973).
3. *Griswold v. Connecticut,* 381 U.S. 479 (1965).
4. *Eisenstadt v. Baird,* 405 U.S. 438 (1972).
5. *Doe v. Bolton,* 410 U.S. 179 (1973).
6. *Planned Parenthood of Central Missouri v. Danforth,* 428 U.S. 52 (1976).
7. Elias S, Annas GJ. *Reproductive genetics and the law.* Chicago: Year Book Medical; 1987:145-162.
8. *Planned Parenthood of Southeastern Pennsylvania v. Casey,* 505 U.S. 833 (1992).
9. Annas GJ. The Supreme Court, liberty, and abortion. *N Engl J Med.* 1992;327:651.
10. Annas GJ. Partial-birth abortion, Congress, and the Constitution. *N Engl J Med.* 1998;339:279.
11. *Stenberg v. Carhart,* 530 U.S. 914 (2000).
12. *Gonzales v. Carhart,* 2007 U.S. LEXIS 4338 (2007).
13. Greene MF, Ecker JL. Abortion, health, and the law. *N Engl J Med.* 2004;350:184.
14. *Jacobson v. Massachusetts,* 197 U.S. 11 (1905).
15. Mariner WK, Annas GJ, Glantz LH. *Jacobson v Massachusetts:* it's not your great-great-grandfather's public health law. *Am J Public Health.* 2005;95:581.
16. Annas GJ. Abortion politics and health insurance reform. *N Engl J Med.* 2009;361:2589.
17. Annas GJ, Ruger TW, Ruger JP. Money, sex and religion–the Supreme Court's ACA sequel. *N Engl J Med.* 2014;371:826-866.
18. *Burwell v. Hobby Lobby,* 573 U.S. (2014).
19. Annas GJ. Sudden death for a challenge to federal funding of stem-cell research. *N Engl J Med.* 2011;364:e47.
20. Annas GJ. Resurrection of a stem cell funding barrier: Dickey-Wicker in court. *N Engl J Med.* 2010;362:1259.
21. Annas GJ, Caplan A, Elias S. The politics of human-embryo research: avoiding ethical gridlock. *N Engl J Med.* 1996;334:1329.
22. Ethical Issues in Human Stem Cell Research. *Report and Recommendations of the National Bioethics Advisory Commission.* Vol. 1. Rockville, MD: National Bioethics Advisory Commission; 1999.
23. Annas GJ, Elias S. Politics, moral and embryos: can bioethics in the United States rise above politics? *Nature.* 2004;431:19.
24. Annas GJ, Elias S. *Genomic messages: How the evolving science of genetics affects our health, families, and future.* San Francisco: HarperOne; 2015.
25. Elias S, Annas GJ. Generic consent for genetic screening. *N Engl J Med.* 1994;330:1611.
26. Annas GJ, Elias S. 23andMe and the FDA. *N Engl J Med.* 2014;370:985-988.
27. ACMG statement on access to reproductive options after prenatal diagnosis. *Genet Med.* 2013;15:900.
28. Wapner RJ, Martin CL, Levy B, et al. Chromosomal microarray versus karyotyping for prenatal diagnosis. *N Engl J Med.* 2012;367:2175-2184.
29. Kolder VE, Gallagher J, Parsons MT. Court-ordered obstetrical interventions. *N Engl J Med.* 1987;316:1192.
30. Nelson LJ, Milliken N. Compelled medical treatment of pregnant women. *JAMA.* 1988;259:1060.
31. Notzon FC, Placek PJ, Taffel SM. Comparisons of national cesarean-section rates. *N Engl J Med.* 1987;316:386.
32. Annas GJ. Protecting the liberty of pregnant patients. *N Engl J Med.* 1987;316:1213.
33. ACOG Committee Opinion. *Maternal Decision Making, Ethics, and the Law, No. 321.* Washington DC: American College of Obstetricians and Gynecologist; 1987.
34. *In Re A.C.,* 573 A 2d 1235 (DC App 1990).

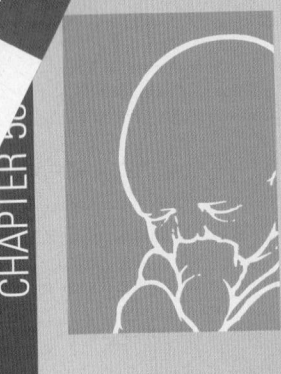

CHAPTER 53

Improving Global Maternal Health: Challenges and Opportunities

GWYNETH LEWIS, LESLEY REGAN, CHELSEA MORRONI, and ERIC R.M. JAUNIAUX

KEY ABBREVIATIONS

Acquired immune deficiency syndrome	AIDS
Cesarean delivery	CD
Contraceptive prevalence rate	CPR
Female genital mutilation/cutting	FGM/C
Global Library of Women's Medicine	GLOWM
Gross national income	GNI
Human immunodeficiency virus	HIV
International Conference on Population and Development	ICPD
International Federation of Obstetricians and Gynecologists	FIGO
Intrauterine device	IUD
Long-acting reversible contraception	LARC
Low-income country	LIC
Millennium development goal	MDG
Middle-income country	MIC
Maternal mortality ratio	MMR
Nongovernmental organization	NGO
Postpartum hemorrhage	PPH
Sexually transmitted infection	STI
Traditional birth attendant	TBA
Tuberculosis	TB
World Health Organization	WHO
United Nations	UN

MATERNAL AND REPRODUCTIVE HEALTH

This chapter can only touch the surface of the complex issues relating to the continuing yet avoidable tragedy of maternal deaths worldwide. However, for those readers for whom it provides the impetus for more in-depth study, many key documents and papers are contained within its references. First, we offer a brief description of the main clinical, health system, and wider social causes and key actions for the prevention of deaths and obstetric complications, particularly in resource-poor countries, and conclude with a summary of the steps that need to be taken at individual, professional, facility, and health system levels and nationally and internationally to help reduce these needless deaths. The section after that provides clinical details on the challenges of preventing, identifying, and managing the main obstetric complications of pregnancy in resource-poor settings, and the final section provides some practical tips for anyone considering working abroad for longer or shorter periods of time.

Maternal Health and the Burden of Death and Disability

"Many Births Mean Many Burials"

—Kenyan Proverb

Every year worldwide, around 290,000 mothers and 3 million babies die at the time of birth, and another 3 million infants are stillborn. Despite recent initiatives, which in some countries have resulted in declines in maternal death rates over the past few years, too little has happened too late. The fact is that the main causes of maternal death and preventive or remediable interventions have been well known for many years, and nearly all of these vulnerable mothers could be saved at little extra cost. Lives would be saved if women had a choice about becoming pregnant, and once pregnant, if they and their babies had access to essential health services that provide evidence-based, technologically appropriate, and affordable interventions even in the poorest countries of the world. This in turn depends on the availability of resources and the recognition and enforcement of the human rights of girls and women. For example, a recent United Nations (UN) report estimated that if all women who actually wanted to avoid pregnancy were able to access and use an effective method of contraception, the number of unintended pregnancies would drop by 70%, and the number of unsafe abortions would drop by 74%. Further, if these women's contraceptive needs were met, and if all pregnant women and their newborn babies received the basic standards of maternity care recommended by the World Health Organization (WHO), the number of maternal deaths would fall by two thirds—from 290,000 down to 96,000—and the number of newborn deaths would fall by more than three quarters, down to 660,000.[1]

Deaths are merely the tip of the iceberg. Globally it is estimated that over 300 million women are living with short- or long-term pregnancy-related complications with around 20 million new cases occurring each year.[2,3] These figures do not reflect other additional yet poorly recognized burdens. In most countries postnatal depression, suicide from puerperal psychosis, and other mental health issues are not even acknowledged as pregnancy-related problems, and the stories of legions of women dying or suffering from these debilitating conditions remain untold.

Babies are affected by their mother's health in pregnancy and birth, and added to the 6 million who die before or just after birth, many more millions are left motherless and less able to thrive. The risk of death for existing children under 5 is doubled if their mother dies in childbirth, which is particularly challenging for girls.[4]

Every maternal death or long-term complication is not only a tragedy for the mother, her partner, and her surviving children, it is also an economic loss to her family, community, and society. Saving mothers lives is also crucial to the wider economy; for example, in Nigeria during 2005, it was estimated that maternal deaths alone led to around $102 million in lost productivity.[5]

A Place Between Life and Death

In developed countries, pregnancy is not generally considered as dangerous, and childbirth is usually regarded as a joyful and positive life-changing event. However, these 11 million births account for only 8% of the annual deliveries worldwide. The same cannot be assumed for the 92% of mothers, some 124,000 million women, living in less developed areas of the world. Of these, approximately 800 will die and 16,000 will suffer severe and long-lasting complications every day.[6,7] Additionally, every day, nearly 8000 babies will die around the time of birth, and another 7000 will be stillborn.[8] **Overall, this burden of maternal and neonatal mortality, including stillbirths, accounts for around 15,800 deaths each day, or 10 lives lost every minute.**

In Chichewa, the national language of Malawi, the word *pakati* refers to pregnancy. Its literal translation means "in the middle between life and death." In other African countries, it is common to hear women in labor using euphemisms such as "I am going to the river to fetch water; I may not come back," or childbirth is described as "slipping on a banana skin at the edge of a cliff with no safety net."

These concerns are all too real for many women, and "a place between life and death" is an accurate description of the 9 months of anxiety and fear that accompany pregnancy and delivery. The World Bank classifies every economy as low, middle, or high income; it uses gross national income (GNI) per capita because GNI is considered to be the single best indicator of economic capacity and progress. Low-income and middle-income economies are collectively referred to as *developing economies.* For the 11 million mothers in high-income countries (HICs), access to quality antenatal, intrapartum, and postnatal care for both mothers and babies is readily available. Another

34 million women will deliver in middle-income countries (MICs), where hospital facilities with variable quality of care or resources such as staff, blood, drugs, or high dependency units may be available. However, for the 90 million mothers in low-income countries (LICs), the situation can be very different, with little or no access to even basic health care, which places the health of both mother and baby at significantly higher risk. The film "Why Did Mrs. X Die: Retold" is available online in several languages (vimeo.com/50848172), and it provides a simple introduction.

Where Mothers Die

Of all the maternal deaths that occur, 99% are in low and middle-income countries, the same as for newborns.[6,9] The WHO defines the *maternal mortality ratio* (MMR) as the number of direct and indirect maternal deaths per 100,000 live births during pregnancy or up to and including 42 days after the end of pregnancy. **The latest UN estimates for 2013 are that the overall global MMR is 210 deaths per 100,000 live births, with an even higher figure (230) for developing regions (LICs and MICs) compared with 12 for developed regions.** The highest regional MMR is 520 for sub-Saharan Africa, followed by 190 for both the Caribbean and Oceania, 170 for Southern Asia (which drops to 140 if India is excluded), 77 for Latin America, 60 for North Africa, and 39 for Central Asia.[6] However, these figures hide wide intercountry and intracountry variations. Overall, Sierra Leone is estimated to have the highest MMR (1100), followed by Chad (980), the Central African Republic (880), and Somalia (850). Ten other African countries have MMRs higher than 500 per 100,000 live births. Due to the sheer weight of its population, the annual deaths of 50,000 mothers in India account for 17% of the global total. This is despite the country having made significant progress in recent years with a concerted effort at national, state, and local levels: the Indian MMR fell from 600 in 1990 to 200 in 2010.[6]

Adolescent Girls and Lifetime Risk of Maternal Death

Ending child marriage is a public health priority. Apart from taking away their childhood, young pregnant girls are more likely to die and are at greater risk of complications. Those under the age of 15 are five times more likely to die of a pregnancy-related cause than women in their twenties.[10] Every year, 3 million undergo unsafe abortions.[9,11] Maternal death is now the leading cause of death for young girls in developing countries, with 15% percent of all deaths worldwide occurring among adolescents.[9,11-13] Compared with mothers aged 20 to 24 years, girls aged between 10 and 19 years have higher risks of obstructed labor, eclampsia, puerperal sepsis, systemic infections, and preterm deliveries and require more cesarean deliveries.[14,15] Their babies also fare worse as a result.

In developing countries, a 15-year-old girl faces a 1:160 risk of dying from a pregnancy-related complication during her lifetime, and this rises to an average risk of 1:38 for those who live in sub-Saharan Africa. The average risk in the most developed countries is 1:3750. In the very worst countries to be born a girl—such as Chad, Niger, and Côte d'Ivoire—the lifetime risk is still between 1:15 and 1:29 despite the fact that these figures have actually been halved over the past 10 years.[6] Even in the developed world, wide variations are seen within a country depending on who the mothers are, where they live, and their social circumstances. In the United Kingdom, for example, vulnerable unemployed women are 10 times more likely to die or suffer complications than women in families where at least one member is employed.[16]

United States

The WHO estimated the overall MMR for the United States to be 28 per 100,000 live births in 2013, which is threefold greater than in Western Europe and Australasia.[6] Indeed, the United States is one of the few countries whose MMR has increased, rather than decreased, in recent years. This may be due to a steady rise in the number of women with advanced maternal age, chronic medical conditions, and obesity coupled with an increasing number of medical interventions, not all of which may be necessary. Recent patient safety research demonstrates that where consistent protocols for diagnosis, management, consultation, or referral of complicated cases are lacking, less optimal maternal outcomes may result.[17]

In the United States, as in many Western countries, the most common obstetric conditions resulting in severe maternal morbidity or mortality are obstetric hemorrhage, severe preeclampsia, and venous thromboembolism.[18] Recent case reviews have highlighted that a significant proportion of the morbidity and mortality from these conditions are due to missed opportunities to improve maternal outcomes. A major challenge is to identify those women who need specialist care at an early stage, without eliminating the category of lower-risk cases. To address this complex problem, a multidisciplinary group of senior health care and birth facility leaders to review and amend current recommendations and plan a national approach to implement improved strategies has recently been convened as the U.S. National Partnership for Maternal Safety.[19]

Mothers Who Survive: Severe Maternal Morbidity

Whereas global maternal deaths may have been neglected until relatively recently, women who suffer from severe maternal morbidity and its long-term sequelae have fared even worse. **It is estimated that 1.1 million of the annual total of 136 million births are complicated by a severe maternal "near-miss" event, after which the mother survived either by chance or following high-quality medical care.** A further 9.5 million women suffer more manageable complications that are still very severe, and 20 million mothers suffer longer-term complications each year.[3] These are conservative estimates.[20]

Whatever the death-to-disability ratio, as with maternal deaths, the numbers will always be too high, and the underlying causes are disturbingly similar. Hence, reducing the risk factors for death will help to decrease the number of significant obstetric complications. Table 58-1 estimates the overall numbers and case fatality rates for the five major global *direct* obstetric complications of pregnancy and the overall numbers of women

affected.[21] **Direct maternal deaths** are those that result from obstetric complications of the pregnancy state (pregnancy, labor, and the puerperium), from interventions, omissions, incorrect treatment, or from a chain of events resulting from any of the above. **Indirect obstetric deaths** are those that result from previous existing disease or disease that developed during pregnancy and which was not due to direct obstetric causes but was aggravated by physiologic effects of pregnancy. **Coincidental maternal deaths** are those from unrelated causes that happen to occur in pregnancy or the puerperium. **Late maternal deaths** include the death of a woman from direct or indirect obstetric causes more than 42 days but less than 1 year after termination of pregnancy.

As stated by Zacharin, "In an unequal world, these women are the most unequal among unequals."[22] Of all the long-term morbidities arising from childbirth, an obstetric fistula is one of the worst. It is estimated that in sub-Saharan Africa and in parts of Asia, between 654,000 to 2 million young women live, usually in isolation and shame, with untreated obstetric fistulae; the annual incidence is 50,000 to 100,000 new cases.[23,24]

Obstetric fistulae are highly stigmatizing, and affected women often become social outcasts. The constant leakage of urine and or fecal matter makes it difficult for them to remain clean, especially in areas with limited access to water, and they most likely will never have children. It is hard to find work; and having failed in their primary objective to have children, they offer little, if any, economic advantage to their families. As a result they are frequently rejected and cast out. The growth in training local surgeons in techniques for simple repair and the ever increasing number of specialist fistula repair centers who also train local staff is slowly helping restore function, fertility, and dignity to these women—but the services available are still few and far between. This is discussed in more depth in the section "Obstructed Labor and Obstetric Fistula."

Babies Who Die

Mothers and their babies are a dyad, inextricably linked, yet all too often the newborn is overlooked when considering policies to reduce the impact of maternal ill health or death. **Around half of the annual 2.6 million stillbirths and 2.9 million deaths in the neonatal period, the first month of life, occur as a result of maternal complications during pregnancy or delivery.**[8] Thus improving maternal care helps more babies survive, and they survive in better condition, which provides a healthier start to life.

Most neonatal deaths (73%) occur during the first week of life with around 36% in the first 24 hours. The major causes are complications that arise from preterm birth (36%), intrapartum asphyxia (23%), and neonatal infections such

TABLE 58-1	ESTIMATED NUMBERS AND INCIDENCE OF THE MAJOR GLOBAL CAUSES OF DIRECT MATERNAL DEATHS AND SEVERE MORBIDITY FOR THE YEAR 2000				
CAUSE	INCIDENCE OF COMPLICATION (% OF LIVE BIRTHS)	NUMBER OF CASES	CASE FATALITY RATE (%)	DEATHS	% OF ALL DIRECT DEATHS
Hemorrhage	10.5	13,795,000	1.0	132,000	28%
Sepsis	4.4	5,768,000	1.3	79,000	16%
Preeclampsia, eclampsia	3.2	4,152,000	1.7	63,000	13%
Obstructed labor	4.6	6,038,000	0.7	42,000	9%
Abortion	14.8	19,340,000	0.3	69,000	15%

Modified from AbouZahr C. Global burden of maternal death. In *British Medical Bulletin. Pregnancy: Reducing Maternal Death and Disability.* British Council. Oxford University Press; 2003, pp. 1-13.

as sepsis, meningitis, and pneumonia, which together contribute 23%.[25] Two thirds of newborn deaths could be prevented if skilled health workers performed effective interventions at birth and during the first week of life.[26]

Labor and the 24 hours surrounding birth are the riskiest times for mother and baby, with 46% of maternal and 40% of neonatal deaths and stillbirths occurring during this period.[27] This fuels the repeated call for more skilled birth attendants to assist at delivery, which should take place in a clean and well-equipped unit with working transport links to more comprehensive facilities capable of managing emergency complications for both mother and baby.

Why Mothers Die
CLINICAL CAUSES

In the most recent WHO analysis of the global causes of maternal death, 73% of the deaths were considered to be due to direct obstetric causes. Of all direct and indirect deaths combined, 27% were due to hemorrhage, 14% to preeclampsia, 11% from puerperal sepsis, 8% from unsafe abortion, 3% from embolism, 3% from obstructed labor, and 7% from other direct causes combined.[28] Virtually all these deaths could be avoided if the maternal and reproductive health services taken for granted in developed countries were available. The other 27% of maternal deaths worldwide are due to indirect causes, most of which result from preexisting underlying medical disorders exacerbated by the mother's pregnant state.

Deaths from illnesses related to human immunodeficiency virus (HIV) and acquired immune deficiency syndrome (AIDS), regarded as indirect deaths, make a major contribution to maternal mortality globally and in some sub-Saharan countries cause more than half of all indirect deaths. In Botswana they account for 56%, and in South Africa and Namibia, the rates are 60%, rising to 67% in Swaziland.[6] In four non-African countries—Ukraine, Bahamas, Thailand, and the Russian Federation—more than 20% of indirect deaths are due to HIV, with the majority being linked to intravenous (IV) drug use.[6] A recent survey predicted that 12% of all deaths during pregnancy and up to 1 year after delivery will result from an HIV-positive pregnancy prevalence rate of 2% and that the MMR will increase to 50% in areas with an HIV-positive pregnancy prevalence rate of 15%.[29]

In developed countries, indirect deaths predominate. The latest U.K. Confidential Enquiry into Maternal Deaths also reported that two thirds of the maternal deaths between the years 2009 and 2012 were due to indirect causes. The risk of a maternal death in the United Kingdom has significantly fallen over the past 10 years from already small numbers. The comparative U.K. MMR, calculated using WHO methods, is now 5.35 deaths per 10,000 live births.[30] The majority of the reported indirect deaths were due to severe medical and mental health problems becoming complicated by pregnancy, such as preexisting cardiac disease, epilepsy, autoimmune disease, and suicide. These causes are now being bolstered by conditions adversely affected by poorer lifestyles such as acquired cardiac disease, hypertension, type 2 diabetes, liver disease, alcohol and drug dependency, and other disorders associated with obesity.[30]

HEALTH SYSTEM FACTORS

A lack of health system planning and resources is one of the largest contributors to the continuing pandemic of maternal ill health and mortality. Many women receive no antenatal care

---

BOX 58-1   BASIC EMERGENCY OBSTETRIC NEWBORN CARE

Basic emergency obstetric and newborn care is critical to reducing maternal and neonatal death. This care, which can be provided with skilled staff in large or small health centers, includes the capabilities for:
- Administering antibiotics, uterotonic drugs (oxytocin), and anticonvulsants (magnesium sulfate)
- Manual removal of the placenta
- Removal of retained products of conception following miscarriage or abortion
- Assisted vaginal delivery, preferably with vacuum extractor
- Basic neonatal resuscitation care

Comprehensive emergency obstetric and newborn care, typically delivered in hospitals, includes all the basic functions above, plus capabilities for:
- Performing cesarean delivery
- Safe blood transfusion
- Provision of care to sick and low-birthweight newborns, including resuscitation

---

at all, and the WHO estimates that only 38% of mothers in low-income countries receive the minimum four antenatal visits they recommend.[31,32] Less than 50% of all women give birth accompanied by a skilled attendant, such as a midwife or doctor,[33] and many lack access to facilities with staff and resources capable of providing basic emergency obstetric or newborn care (Box 58-1) or to higher level services capable of dealing with serious complications or emergencies, such as undertaking life-saving cesarean delivery (CD) for mother or child.[34]

A recent WHO study showed 54 countries that had CD rates lower than 10%, the minimum standard for safe motherhood services, and 69 had rates higher than 15%, all unacceptably high. In 2008, the conservative estimate of the overall rate for Brazil was 45.9%, and it was 30.3% for the United States, compared with 0.7% for Burkina Faso.[35] The study also estimated that in 2008, 3.18 million additional CDs were needed, and 6.20 million unnecessary operations were performed worldwide. The cost of this global "excess" was estimated to amount to approximately $2.32 billion, whereas the cost of the "needed" CDs globally was approximately $432 million.

A critical lack of skilled staff, such as midwives and doctors, is also apparent. It is estimated that the world needs another 350,000 midwives,[36] and doctors are also extremely scarce, especially in the unattractive, remote, and poorer areas of already resource-poor countries. To help address these shortages, task shifting—the transferring of skills and competencies to other trained individuals—is becoming increasingly commonplace. In some countries such as Mozambique, cadres of ancillary staff have been trained as clinical officers—nonphysician clinicians—to perform basic life-saving skills and procedures that include CD, and the results have been impressive.[37]

An emerging issue is that of quality of care. To date, much of the global effort to reduce maternal mortality has focused on increasing access to care; however, the focus is now shifting toward improving and standardizing the variable quality of care that women receive from the health services they have been encouraged to attend. Clinical guidelines and protocols have been developed by the WHO and professional associations, and the use of maternal death reviews to learn lessons to improve care is also having a positive effect.[38]

VULNERABILITY AND UNDERLYING SOCIAL DETERMINANTS

The underlying causes of maternal mortality are complex and multifactorial. For example, although a mother in a resource-poor country may technically be described as dying from a postpartum hemorrhage, the true underlying causes may be very different. She may have died because she had no care, or because she was unable to read the information leaflets about the warning signs and when or where to seek help. Care may have been available but beyond her reach physically or financially. Access to any form of transport in emergency situations is frequently problematic, especially at night. Furthermore, her husband or family members may have prevented her from attending care or lacked the money to pay the necessary bribes to secure her treatment. She may have refused to seek help because she has heard she would be slapped, shouted at, or treated disrespectfully in the health facility. Or she may have overcome all of these obstacles to reach a health care facility only to find poorly trained staff or no staff at all and no medicines, blood products, or equipment and no one capable of performing her life-saving operation. Added to which, she will probably have been in poor physical condition and suffering from anemia and other chronic health disorders. Thus the stated clinical factors surrounding a maternal death provide little or no indication of the underlying causes as to why the woman really died. **Without understanding the wider "causes of the causes," the barriers to safe maternity care cannot be identified and overcome. To help quantify these, it is common for those who work in the field of international women's health to use the "three delays" model as a checklist to help identify the barriers pregnant women face.**[39,40] These barriers may be financial, physical, social, cultural, or medical and may be present in the family, the community, or the health care system. These are inextricably interlinked, and some examples are given in Table 58-2.

"CAUSES OF THE CAUSES"

A recent report into inequalities in health outcomes in England, "Fair Society, Healthy Lives,"[41] states that the "causes of the causes" are the circumstances and societies in which people are born, grow, live, work, and age. Social position, wealth, and education help determine each person's health outcomes and life expectancy. **It estimates that health care services contribute only one third to improvements in life expectancy and that improving life chances and removing inequalities contribute the remaining two thirds.** If this is the case in a developed country, the ratio of inequalities in resource-poor countries must be far higher. Indeed, whether a pregnant woman lives or dies is a lottery that depends almost entirely on where she was born and lives and in what circumstances. Mothers who die are generally the least visible, most vulnerable, and poorest of the poor. Although urban poverty is an increasing problem, most maternal casualties tend to live in rural areas and lack both transport and access to skilled care in health facilities. They are more likely to be illiterate or poorly educated, undertake hard manual work, and find themselves almost permanently pregnant. In societies where social and economic deprivation is rife, so is the absence of laws to protect human rights and promote gender equality in places where those women with the lowest educational achievements are at greatest risk.[42]

The lowly status of girls and women frequently means that they receive the last and least of the family food. General malnourishment, coupled with anemia and micronutrient deficiencies, leads to chronic ill health and multiple comorbidities such

TABLE 58-2	THE THREE DELAYS: EXAMPLES OF BARRIERS TO SAFE, EFFECTIVE MATERNAL CARE
Delay in seeking care	• Traditional beliefs and practices, use of traditional birth attendants • Lack of education and understanding of need for care or warning signs • Mother is not decision maker • Mother has no money and no control over decisions affecting her life • Religious custom and practice
Delay in arriving at a place of care	• No transport • No money • Unofficial bribes • Services patchy or too far away • Concerns about physical abuse by staff in labor • Poor reputation of facilities as "places where women and babies die"
Delay in providing appropriate quality care	• Facilities not equipped to provide basic and/or emergency obstetric care • Lack of suitably trained staff • Poor clinical practice • Little or no use of evidence-based protocols and guidelines • Physical and verbal abuse of women in labor • Lack of blood, medicines, essential equipment, and operating theatres • Frankly harmful care • Intermittent electricity, water, and so on

Modified from Thaddeus S, Maine D. Too far to walk: maternal mortality in context. *Soc Sci Med.* 1994:1091-1110.

as malaria, HIV, or tuberculosis (TB). These women have little or no control over their health, being dependent on male or elder family members to decide whether they should seek care, even in emergencies. Many will become child brides, become pregnant, and be forced to give up any form of education. Female genital mutilation/cutting (FGM/C) is common and is associated with a higher incidence of obstructed labor, emergency cesarean delivery, fetal distress, obstetric fistula, and permanent perineal damage.[43] All of these factors lead to complex pregnancies and higher rates of stillbirth and neonatal death.

WOMEN'S RIGHTS

"Imagine a world where all women enjoy their human rights. Take action to make it happen."
—1998 United Nations Campaign for Human Rights

A further, critically important reason why global efforts to reduce maternal mortality and morbidity have been slow is the low value that society, political, religious, community, and family leaders have placed on women's lives. **As the father of the Safe Motherhood movement, Professor Mahmoud Fathalla, famously said, "Women are not dying of diseases we cannot treat ... they are dying because societies have yet to decide that their lives are worth saving."**[44]

In 1948, the Universal Declaration of Human Rights stated that "all human beings are born free and equal in dignity and rights."[45] The 1995 UN Beijing declaration on women's rights reported that "the full implementation of the human rights of women and of the girl child is an inalienable, integral, and indivisible part of all human rights and fundamental freedoms."[46] By 2009, the UN Human Rights Council had acknowledged that preventable maternal mortality was a human rights violation, and health advocates started using human rights mechanisms to make governments honor their commitment to ensure access to services essential for reproductive health and well-being.

The right to health is a human right, and the health of a nation is determined by the health of its girls and women. Healthy women are more likely to fulfill their potential, nurture healthy families, and contribute to their local and national economies. Ellen Sirleaf Johnson argued that women's socioeconomic empowerment is essential to achieve better health care outcomes, and she ended her 2011 Nobel Prize acceptance speech with a challenge: "Nations thrive when mothers survive, we must strive to keep them alive."[47]

The contribution made by mothers to society is far reaching, and countries that fail to protect and promote women's rights have the worst economic, educational, maternal, and child health outcomes. The application of human rights shifts the understanding of maternal deaths as mere misfortunes that are acts of fate into injustices that the state is obliged to remedy. Using a human rights approach provides valuable tools to hold governments legally accountable to address the preventable causes of maternal mortality and to distribute resources and medicines essential for reproductive health, such as effective contraception and misoprostol to reduce postpartum hemorrhage. For example, when the Sri Lankan government introduced universal education and access to health care, maternal deaths declined significantly for little extra cost.[48] Political will, literacy, and respect for the status and rights of women in society are key components for achieving sustainable health improvements.

Nearly 70 years after the Universal Declaration, many women still struggle to have their basic rights protected. As recently as 2013, objections were raised by certain countries and religious groups to a potential UN statement reaffirming women's rights to education, contraceptive choices, family spacing, and the introduction of declarations against domestic violence, rape, child marriage, and FGM/C. Those who objected considered that upholding these human rights could destroy society by allowing a woman to travel, work, use contraception without her husband's approval, and control her family's spending. These may be extreme views, but there are still far too many countries that turn a blind eye to gender inequalities and violence that includes child marriage, rape, and FGM/C and who do not favor girls receiving primary, let alone secondary, education.

Human rights play an important role in the fight to improve the status of women because they embody a shared set of values that have been enshrined in law. Infringements can be litigated in countries that subscribe to them, but even countries that do not often appear to be sensitive to the charge that they are infringing the human rights of their population. Where the law hinders the use of contraception or does not allow induced abortion, health care professionals invariably find it easier to provide life-saving interventions if they can be reassured that they are protecting the woman's right to life, to benefit from scientific advances, or to avoid discrimination.

Advocacy for women is an obligation for everyone engaged in reproductive health care. This means that all health care professionals need to know how to embed human rights principles into every aspect of their delivery of care. The International Federation of Obstetricians and Gynecologists (FIGO) women's sexual and reproductive rights committee has developed a comprehensive teaching syllabus that can be adapted for use by a wide range of professionals. The clinical knowledge and practical skills required to deliver quality reproductive health care have been built around a core checklist of 10

health-related human rights. The result is a competency-based educational approach that simultaneously advocates for human rights and health by developing standards for performance and tools for training teachers and students in both the classroom and clinical settings. The teaching materials can be freely accessed and downloaded from the Global Library of Women's Medicine (GLOWM).[48b] Experience from the teaching workshops with both laypersons and professional audiences confirms that this approach shifts the teaching of human rights and women's reproductive health from a marginal to a mainstream position in the learning process for all health care professionals.

SEXUAL AND REPRODUCTIVE HEALTH

The lack of universal access to basic sexual and reproductive health services is one of the most significant barriers to reducing maternal morbidity and mortality globally. As stated at the very start of this chapter, but worth repeating here, **a recent report[1] estimated that if all women wanting to avoid pregnancy used an effective method of contraception, the number of unintended pregnancies would drop by 70%, and unsafe abortions would drop by 74%. If these women's contraceptive needs were met, the number of maternal deaths would fall by two thirds, and newborn deaths would decline by more than three quarters,** and the transmission of HIV from mothers to newborns would also be virtually eliminated. Furthermore, it was estimated that contraceptive use averted 272,040 maternal deaths in 2008 and that meeting unmet need for contraception could prevent an additional 104,000 deaths per year, thus preventing a further 29% of maternal mortality.[49] This further reduction by about one third if the unmet need for contraception were met is similar to estimates reported by others,[50] and it underscores the critical role that access to effective contraception plays in preventing maternal mortality and morbidity.

Sexual and reproductive health was formally defined at the 1994 International Conference on Population and Development (ICPD).[51] At its core is the promotion of healthy, voluntary, and safe sexual and reproductive choices for individuals and couples, including decisions about if, when, and with whom to have children. It encompasses highly sensitive and important issues such as sexuality, pregnancy prevention and abortion, gender discrimination, and male/female power relations. Its full attainment depends on the protection of human and reproductive rights. The conference also adopted the goal of ensuring universal access to sexual and reproductive health as part of its framework for a broad set of development objectives and Millennium Development Goals (MDGs) and set very similar objectives in their Target 5:B.[52] Despite these initiatives, an estimated 85 million unintended pregnancies occurred in 2012.[53]

Unintended Pregnancy

An *unintended pregnancy* is one that is mistimed, unplanned, or unwanted at the time of conception,[54,55] and such pregnancies are associated with an array of negative health, economic, social, and psychological outcomes for women and children.[56-60] In 2012, the global unintended pregnancy rate was 53 per 1000 women aged 15 to 44, with the highest rates in Eastern and Middle Africa (108 each) and the lowest in Western Europe (27).[1] Of these 85 million unintended pregnancies, 50% will end in termination,[1] which corresponds to about 1 in 5 of all pregnancies and contributes to the pandemic of unsafe abortion.[61] A further 13% will end in miscarriage, and 38% will result in an unplanned birth.[1] Four out of five pregnancies in the developing world occur among women with no access to modern effective contraception,[59] but even in settings where contraceptive use is comparatively high, unintended pregnancies may still occur when the available contraceptive method fails or because of poor adherence.

Contraception

Voluntary access to family planning—especially modern, effective contraceptive methods for women and men—is crucial to directly improving health outcomes and is positively associated with improvements in educational and economic status.[49,50,62,63] The health benefits include sizable reductions in maternal, newborn, and child morbidity and mortality as well as deaths and complications that arise from unsafe abortion.[60,49,63] At the household level, improved access to family planning services leads to substantial improvements in women's earnings and children's schooling.[62] Nationally, higher levels of uptake correlate with lower fertility rates, which enhance economic growth.[62,64] Conversely, high levels of unwanted fertility correlate with poverty and inequality.[65]

Barriers to contraceptive usage can also be categorized according to the three-delay model described earlier[38] and can occur at the client, health care provider, and health systems level. The most frequently cited reasons for nonuse among women is poor understanding of their risk for pregnancy, concerns about possible side effects, infrequent sexual activity, service fees, or opposition; in the latter, desires of a male partner or religious or cultural reasons are cited. Married women may have little control over contraceptive decision making, which is particularly important when partners differ in their childbearing preferences. Unmarried women frequently have to face strong stigma from judgmental providers if they are sexually active, which in turn reduces these women's ability to obtain needed services. At the provider level, barriers include lack of knowledge or skills, motivation, and bias for or against certain methods, such as intrauterine devices (IUDs). Limiting the provision by certain provider types also blocks uptake: for example, only allowing doctors to insert IUDs or imposing non–evidence-based restrictions on when a method can be started, such as commencing only at the time of menses. Common health system barriers include inadequate human and financial resources and a failure to integrate family planning with other core services such as maternity and child health clinics, delivery, postnatal or postabortion care, and HIV services. Access may also be limited through geographic constraints and lack of equipment and supplies. Shortages of supplies are very common, especially in rural areas. In addition to overcoming provider bias, lack of competency, and health systems issues, most low-resource settings are still in need of educational interventions to increase awareness and understanding for the community as a whole, thereby reducing many of the existing barriers to effective contraceptive use.

Contraceptive prevalence is typically defined as the percentage of women who are currently using, or whose sexual partner is currently using, at least one method of contraception regardless of the method used; usually, it is reported for married or in-union women (women in a stable sexual relationship) aged 15 to 49. **In recent decades, general increases in contraceptive prevalence rates (CPRs) have been seen in most areas of the world, and globally, they increased from 53% in 1990 to 57% to 64% in 2011 through 2012.**[66-71] However, CPRs remain extremely low in parts of Africa with regional estimates of 32%, 19%, and 15% in Eastern, Middle, and Western Africa, respectively,[68] giving a rate of 24% to 30% for Africa overall.[66-71] Wide intercountry variations are also apparent: for example, since 1990, progress in contraceptive use has been made in Rwanda (18% to 50%), Malawi (12% to 45%), and Tanzania (11% to 34%); yet in Sierra Leone and Nigeria, the CPRs for 2010 were 6.7% and 8.6%, respectively.[68] In Southern Africa, rates are now relatively high at 62%, having risen from 47%, and in Southern Asia, rates have risen from 36% to 50% in India and from 34% to 61% in Bangladesh; in addition, substantial gains have been made in Latin America, where the regional CPR is now 73%.[68] Although high and most stable in Europe and North America (72% to 78%), the rates are highest in East Asia, largely attributable to China (83%).[68] Nevertheless, the overall global CPR remains low, and this is a serious obstacle to further improving women's health.

Unmet need for family planning is typically defined as the percentage of women who want to stop or delay childbearing but who are not using any method of contraception to prevent pregnancy. A more useful definition regards both women who use no method or women who use traditional methods as having an unmet need for modern methods, not only because traditional methods have high use-failure rates, but also because, although some women using traditional methods might choose to use these methods, such choices often imply that women perceive other options to be unavailable, or are not fully informed of contraceptive options.[71]

The unmet need for contraception is unacceptably high. Globally, 222 million women who would prefer and are trying to limit or space their pregnancies are not using contraception.[70,71] Around three-quarters of these women live in the world's poorest countries,[72] and the unmet need remains greatest in sub-Saharan Africa (60%) and West and South Asia (50% and 34%, respectively) with disproportionately high levels among illiterate, poor, adolescent, and rural women.[58,50]

The postpartum period is crucially important for contraceptive intervention because rapid repeat pregnancies are associated with poor maternal and infant outcomes. An analysis of data from 27 countries found that 95% of women who were 12 or fewer months postpartum did not want another birth within 2 years, yet 65% of them were not using contraception.[73] Similarly, although most women being treated for complications of induced or spontaneous abortion are in need of effective contraception, data from 17 low-resource countries show that only 1 in 4 of these women were discharged from care with a method in place.[74]

Contraceptive Methods

The type of contraceptive method used is also variable, but choice is critical in relation to efficacy and continued usage, particularly in areas where women find it difficult to attend clinics, or where the service is unavailable or limited by shortages and failure of supplies. Traditional contraceptive techniques such as withdrawal and fertility awareness (natural family planning) are the least effective. The emphasis should be on enabling women and their partners to have access to a wide range of the most effective modern methods. WHO classifies contraceptive methods into effectiveness tiers, which are described in Table 58-3. The effectiveness of the method is critically important for reducing the risk of unintended pregnancy and can be measured either with "perfect use," when the method is used correctly and consistently as directed, or with "typical use," which

TABLE 58-3	EFFECTIVENESS OF CONTRACEPTIVE METHODS BASED ON TYPICAL USE FAILURE RATES

Tier 1 Methods: The Most Effective, Resulting in Less Than 1 Pregnancy per 100 Women in a Year

Permanent contraceptive methods	Male and female sterilization
Long-acting reversible contraceptives (LARCs)	Intrauterine devices (copper bearing or levonorgestrel [LNG] IUDs are effective for 5 to 10 years depending on the IUD)
	Subdermal implant (progestogen only, effective for 3 to 5 years depending on the implant)

Tier 2 Methods: Result in 6 to 12 Pregnancies per 100 Women in a Year

Shorter-acting contraceptive methods	*Injectable contraceptives*
	Progestogen-only injectable contraceptive (requires reinjection every 8 weeks (norethisterone enanthate [NET-EN]) or 12 weeks (depot medroxyprogesterone acetate, [DMPA])
	Oral contraceptives
	Combined oral contraceptive pill (COC; estrogen/progestogen)
	Progestogen-only pill (POP)
	Other methods
	Combined vaginal ring (estrogen/progestogen; the ring is left in the vagina for 3 weeks and then is not used for 1 week)
	Combined patch (estrogen/progestogen; a new patch is applied once a week every week for 3 weeks and then is not used for 1 week)
	Female diaphragms

Tier 3 Methods: Result in 18 or More Pregnancies per 100 Women in a Year

Shorter-acting methods of least contraceptive efficacy	Condoms (male or female)
	Fertility awareness–based methods
	Spermicides

Modified from World Health Organization (WHO). WHO Department of Reproductive Health and Research, Johns Hopkins Bloomsbury School of Public Health/Center for Communications Programs (CCP). Knowledge for health project. Family planning: a global handbook for providers (2011 update). Baltimore/Geneva: CCP and WHO, 2011; and Hatcher RA, Trussell J, Nelson AL, Cates W, Kowal D, Policar M (eds). *Contraceptive Technology.* 20th revised edition. New York: Ardent Media; 2011.

reflects real-world actual use, including inconsistent and incorrect use.[75]

Sterilization, almost exclusively female, is most commonly used in Asia and Latin America. IUDs account for a third of contraceptive use in Asia and are the most commonly used method in some parts.[70] Injectables are the most widely used methods in sub-Saharan Africa and also in Southeast Asia.[70] Oral contraceptives make up nearly half of total contraceptive use in northern Africa, whereas male condoms are the most common method in Central and Western Africa.[72]

The subdermal implant and IUD are the most effective reversible contraceptive methods available and are highly suitable for resource-poor countries because they have failure rates of less than 1% for both perfect and typical use.[75] The failure rates for these methods are very low because they do not require any additional user intervention. Injectable contraceptives, oral contraceptive pills, the hormonal patch, and the vaginal ring all have failure rates of less than 1% with perfect use; however, with typical use, these methods are only 90% to 94% effective.[75] Condoms are 98% effective with perfect use, but the method failure rate increases to 18% to 21% with typical use.[75] *Dual contraception* is defined as the consistent use of a condom, male or female, along with a highly effective nonbarrier method such as hormonal contraception, the copper-bearing IUD, or sterilization. Male and female condoms are the only contraceptive methods available that also protect against sexually transmitted infections (STIs) and HIV; hence using a dual-contraceptive method should be promoted routinely in areas of high STI/HIV prevalence.

Short-acting methods such as condoms and oral and injectable contraceptives are the most commonly used methods in sub-Saharan Africa despite the fact that permanent and LARC methods are much more effective at preventing pregnancy.[76-78] A recent modeling study concluded that if just 20% of the women in sub-Saharan Africa currently using oral contraceptive pills and injectables were to switch to using the more effective subdermal implant, 1.8 million unintended pregnancies, 576,000 abortions (many of them unsafe), and 10,000 maternal deaths would be averted over 5 years.[78] Encouragingly, efforts to achieve the ambitious goal of the 2012 London Summit on Family Planning—to enable an additional 120 million women and girls in the world's poorest countries to access and use lifesaving family planning information, services, and supplies by 2020—appears to be gaining momentum.[79]

Induced Abortion

Even though deaths from unsafe abortion worldwide dropped from 69,000 in 1990 to 47,000 in 2008, the consequences of unsafe abortion remain one of the five leading causes of maternal mortality.[80] However, although the actual numbers may have declined, the proportion of women who die of unsafe abortion has remained stubbornly unchanged at around 9% to 13% of maternal deaths.[28,80] Such deaths can be largely prevented by the provision of safe abortion services offered by trained staff working within an enabling legal framework. Where the in-country laws prevent offering this service, many lives can still be saved by introducing accessible, nonjudgmental, and prompt care for the identification and management of the complications of clandestine unsafe abortions. Only 40% of the world's women have access to safe and legal abortion services within set gestational limits. Elsewhere, access is either absent or is restricted to a lesser or greater degree.[81]

Globally each year, around 44 million abortion procedures take place; about half are unsafe, and the vast majority are due to unintended pregnancies.[82] Unsafe abortions include those undertaken by unskilled providers under unhygienic conditions, those that are self-induced by the woman inserting a foreign object into her uterus or consuming toxic products, and those instigated by physical trauma to a woman's abdomen.[83] Nearly all unsafe abortions (98%), and the deaths that arise as a consequence (99.8%), occur in developing countires.[83] About two thirds of abortion-related deaths occur in sub-Saharan Africa, and one third occur in Asia.[83] **In high-resource regions of the world where safe and legal abortion services are provided, deaths are extremely rare.**[83] The majority of women who seek these procedures in resource-poor countries, where it is usually illegal, will already have had a number of pregnancies. They frequently view their decision to seek an abortion as a last resort—a necessary respite from the exhaustion of incessant childbearing that has left them in very poor health in addition to their family circumstances leaving them with no resources, food, or money to care for another child.

Deaths and disability from unsafe abortion continue to occur, despite major advances in the availability of safe and effective technologies for medically induced abortion, which additionally reduce operative interventions.[84] Complications and causes of death from unsafe abortion include hemorrhage, sepsis, and peritonitis in addition to trauma to the cervix, vagina, uterus, and abdominal organs.[85] Apart from the risk of death, one in four women who undergo an unsafe procedure—an estimated 5 million each year—are likely to develop temporary or life-long disability that requires medical care and includes secondary infertility.[79,83,86]

Induced abortion has existed in all societies since the dawn of time, and evidence shows that wherever they live, and whoever they are, many women will seek an abortion when faced with an unintended pregnancy, irrespective of the legal circumstances.[83,84] For example, the abortion rate of 29 per 1000 women of reproductive age in Africa, where it is mostly illegal, is similar to that of 28 per 1000 women in Europe, where abortion is generally permitted on broad grounds but with limits for gestational age.[81] Where abortion is allowed, very few women resort to unsafe practices, and as a result, morbidity and mortality are extremely low. When made legal, safe and accessible, women's health improves rapidly. In South Africa, for example, the annual number of abortion-related deaths fell by 91% after the liberalization of the abortion law in 1996.[87] When provided in a safe environment by properly trained providers, abortion is one of the safest medical procedures.[83]

Reducing the number of unsafe abortions or promptly identifying and managing their complications are global health priorities. Universal access to legal, safe services for all women is unlikely to be achieved because of the diverse moral, religious, and other contextual issues. It is a highly divisive subject with no easy answers. Nevertheless, whatever stance is taken at a personal, national, or legal level, helping women who are suffering and dying of the complications of unsafe procedures must be part of all programs designed to reduce maternal deaths and disabilities. The first step is to accept that this key health issue should not be swept under the carpet as an inconvenient truth. The second is to develop a program for the management of complications through evidence-based and nonjudgmental national strategies such as the one published in Kenya in 2012 by the Ministry of Medical Services.[88] Bringing the issue of abortion out into the open and acknowledging the problem will go a long way in helping to save lives.

Improving Reproductive Health and Well-Being of All Mothers

Despite intense efforts at many levels, improving the accessibly and quality of care for all of the world's mothers and babies remains a monumental task. Progress has been made, however, in that maternal deaths rates fell 45% between 1990 and 2013 globally. However, in many pockets of the world, rates continue to stagnate or rise, such as in the United States.[6] The international spotlight shone brightly on the problem when Millennium Development Goal 5, agreed to by all UN member states in 1990, challenged low- and middle-income countries to reduce their maternal mortality by 75% by 2015, but now that time has come, and the targets—perhaps in hindsight too ambitious—remain largely unmet.[52,89] The UN has now agreed to new targets, the Sustainable Development Goals, and as currently drafted under Goal 3, *"To ensure healthy lives and promote well-being for all at all ages,"* they propose that by 2030, the overall global MMR should be reduced to less than 70 per 100,000 live births, and preventable neonatal deaths

should be eliminated.[90] These hugely challenging targets will not be met unless action is taken at all levels, and in all sectors, to implement the necessary and fundamental changes that have been described in this chapter. **A recent report estimated that increased coverage and improvement in the quality of maternity services by 2025 could avert 71% of neonatal deaths, 33% of stillbirths, and 54% of maternal deaths at a cost of $1928 for each life saved.**[91] Furthermore, is estimated that contraceptive use averted 272,040 maternal deaths in 2008 and that meeting unmet need for contraception could prevent an additional 104,000 deaths per year.[49]

Making health care welcoming and accessible to all women through improving transport links and eliminating or reducing user fees, scaling up the number of health facilities capable of providing basic emergency and comprehensive emergency obstetric and neonatal care, and increasing the numbers facilities with caring, well-trained midwives, doctors, and other health workers is essential. Developing a culture of quality care must accompany the implementation of appropriate clinical guidelines and protocols, which the WHO and others have already produced, and audits and reviews must be used to assess progress and identify and rectify problems that may be identified. Improving communications and providing a woman with holistic and comprehensive coordinated care during the continuum of her pregnancy—preconception, antenatal, intrapartum, and postnatal care along with postpartum family planning—will also prove crucial. Apart from addressing the clinical quality of care, well-conducted maternal or perinatal death or morbidity reviews also provide in-depth evidence of the underlying reasons why mothers may be dying. Here, their results help not only in the development of accessible maternal and reproductive health services but also with improvements to education and human rights.

Sustained pressure and advocacy for beneficial change, together with leadership and realistic and practical policies, are required from world leaders and influencers, the UN, other international organizations, nongovernmental organizations (NGOs), national governments, and national and local policymakers. Ministers of finance, law, education, transport, and health all need to play their part through enacting human rights legislation, promoting and funding education for girls, and providing better transport links and more medicines, commodities, and other supplies. Essential drugs such as magnesium sulfate are often unavailable or in very short supply, as are blood and fluid replacement, equipment, laboratory reagents, and even generators and clean water. Ministries of health can supply more and better equipped facilities capable of providing care at all levels, and they can create training schools for the extra maternity staff so badly needed in most of the world.

National and local professional associations and individual health care workers can improve the quality of care they provide through the use of evidence-based practice and the development of situationally appropriate clinical guidelines and technologies. They can also ensure continual professional updating and training. Until such time as there are enough midwives and doctors, intermediate-level health care workers trained to undertake tasks traditionally performed by doctors play an invaluable role. A functioning health system also requires an efficient system of communication, referral, and transport. Underpinning and facilitating all of this work should be a supportive national legal and ethical framework that includes policies that strive for equality in women's rights. This is not

BOX 58-2 TWELVE PROPOSITIONS FOR SAFE MOTHERHOOD FOR ALL WOMEN

1. A woman's life is worth saving.
2. Girls should have equal access to food, education, health care, and life opportunities as their brothers.
3. Young girls should not be subject to violence including rape, FGM, and child marriage, and women should not suffer violence in any form.
4. Women should have an equal say in decisions that affect their own and their children's health and well-being.
5. All women must have the basic human right to control their own fertility and reproductive health and plan and space their pregnancies.
6. Pregnancy must be a voluntary choice.
7. Maternity is special and every society has an obligation to make it safe. Safe motherhood is a basic human right enshrined in UN statute.
8. All pregnant women must have access to antenatal/prenatal, birth, and postnatal care as described by WHO and other organizations.
9. All deliveries must be assisted by skilled birth attendants.
10. All women must have access to quality life-saving comprehensive emergency obstetric care if needed.
11. Care must be free or affordable. There should be no bribes or "unofficial" fees.
12. All women should be treated with dignity, respect, and compassion.

Modified from Fathalla M. Ten propositions for safe motherhood for all women. From the Hubert de Watteville Memorial Lecture. Imagine a world where motherhood is safe for all women—you can help make it happen. *Int J Gynaecol Obstet.* 2011;72(3):207-213.

universal. Professor Mahmoud Fathalla once proposed ten steps for safe motherhood, which have been updated and adapted for this chapter.[92] These are listed in Box 58-2, and if accepted by the world's leaders, policymakers, and influencers, the world would be a far safer place for pregnant women and their unborn children.

MAJOR OBSTETRIC COMPLICATIONS: PREVENTION AND MANAGEMENT IN RESOURCE-POOR COUNTRIES

The major complications of pregnancy are similar throughout the world. The outcome for individual women depends upon the care received and the capacity of the local health systems to respond to their needs. Where comprehensive emergency obstetric care is lacking, which includes staff and facilities for cesarean delivery, severe morbidity or death results from prolonged obstructed labor and/or fetal distress and life-threatening hemorrhage.[93]

Postpartum Hemorrhage

The commonest cause of postpartum hemorrhage (PPH) is uterine atony. As discussed in Chapter 18, the risk is highest in mothers with multiple pregnancies, prolonged/obstructed labor, preeclampsia/eclampsia, large uterine fibroids, and grand multiparity (five or more previous deliveries). In resource-poor settings, intrapartum and postpartum hemorrhage continues to be

the leading cause of maternal mortality, accounting for 27% of deaths.[94]

For many pregnant women already suffering from severe chronic anemia due to malnutrition, micronutrient deficiency, sickle cell disease, malaria, or helminthic infections, even a blood loss of 500 mL at delivery can compromise their already challenged hemodynamic state and can result in hypovolemic shock. The prevention or early detection of bleeding and the aggressive use of methods to reduce blood loss are essential. However, blood products and storage facilities are often unavailable,[95] and in an emergency situation, when blood is usually obtained from family members or donors, it is rarely screened for infection and may be diluted with dirty water.

Uterine bimanual massage and uterotonic drugs, if available, should be started at the first sign of atony. Compared with placebo, prophylactic oxytocin decreases PPH greater than 500 mL and reduces the need for therapeutic uterotonics.[96] It is also associated with fewer side effects, specifically nausea and vomiting, and evidence is limited to suggest that prophylactic oxytocin is superior to ergot alkaloids for the routine prevention of PPH. However, once an oxytocic agent has been given, opportunity is limited for further reduction in postpartum blood loss with its use.[97]

Misoprostol, a synthetic prostaglandin E1 analogue, plays a key role in the management of miscarriage.[98] Unlike oxytocin, it is low cost, stable at high temperatures, not degraded by ultraviolet light, and can be used orally or rectally, which makes it particularly useful in areas where skilled health care providers and resources are less available. Recent studies indicate that misoprostol distributed antenatally can be used accurately and reliably by rural Ghanaian and Liberian women after delivery and should be more widely implemented in other countries with high home birth rates.[99,100] Using Misoprostol for PPH prevention appears acceptable to women, but community-based strategies will be needed to increase distribution rates. However, conventional injectable uterotonics are still preferable to either intramuscular prostaglandins or misoprostol for the management of the third stage of labor, especially for low-risk women.[101]

In cases of persistent PPH, aggressive measures to minimize blood loss and secondary infection should be taken, but the availability of facilities and skilled staff to perform balloon tamponade and surgical compression sutures is limited. In facilities unable to provide emergency care, low-technology compression devices can help to stabilize a hemorrhaging mother long enough for her to reach a hospital equipped to provide comprehensive emergency services.[34]

Preeclampsia/Eclampsia

Hypertensive disorders of pregnancy account for 14% of global maternal deaths[28] and are the leading cause of death in some urban areas in low-income countries.[102] They fall into four categories: (1) chronic hypertension, (2) gestational hypertension or pregnancy-induced hypertension (PIH), (3) preeclampsia/eclampsia, and (4) preeclampsia superimposed on chronic hypertension (see Chapter 31).

Preeclampsia and eclampsia are associated with extremes of maternal age (under 17 and over 35 years), nulliparity, multiple pregnancies, preexisting hypertension, preeclampsia in a previous pregnancy, poor socioeconomic circumstances, and illiteracy.[103,104] The increased susceptibility for indigenous African women and blacks living in North America appears to be independent of socioeconomic status and is likely due to biologic or genetic factors.[105,106] However, even in developed countries, identifying women at risk can be difficult.[107] Limited access to antenatal care, little or no screening for high blood pressure and proteinuria, and the wide variations in access to antihypertensive drugs coupled with poor maternal understanding of the signs and symptoms and the need to seek immediate care all help explain the higher mortality from eclampsia in many low- to middle-income countries. Severe morbidity increases eightfold in women with preeclampsia, and it increases sixtyfold after an eclamptic seizure,[103] but the life-threatening neurologic complications and wider organ dysfunctions are reversible if adequate treatment is started in time. **Magnesium sulfate is the drug of choice but is not available in many developing countries. A recent systematic review of the use of magnesium sulfate in low- and middle-income countries found that the majority of women receive less than optimal dosages, usually due to concerns about maternal safety and toxicity, cost, or available resources.**[108]

Training health care and community workers and raising awareness in pregnant women about the signs and symptoms of preeclampsia is essential. Recent evaluation of a clinical model and algorithm in low-income countries has shown a reasonable ability to identify women at increased risk of adverse maternal outcomes associated with hypertensive disorders.[103] Furthermore, a training intervention for health care providers to use an evidence-based protocol for the treatment of preeclampsia and eclampsia has been shown to be effective in reducing the associated case fatality rate.[109]

Sepsis

In the nineteenth and early twentieth century, puerperal sepsis was the major cause of maternal death in industrialized countries; but improvements in hygiene and sanitation, together with the introduction of antibiotics after the Second World War, resulted in its rapid decline.[110] **Nevertheless, perinatal infection still underlies 11% of maternal deaths and 33% of neonatal deaths globally.**[28,111] Poverty contributes significantly to these poor outcomes with clear evidence of an association between poor sanitation, limited access to clean water, and maternal death.[112] Ignorance of both the causes and need to prevent puerperal sepsis is widespread, and in some communities, people still believe illness is due to evil spirits.[113]

For the 50% of women globally who deliver at home attended only by a female relative or untrained traditional birth attendant (TBA), infection is an ever-present danger. Harmful practices are common, such as cutting the cord with broken glass and dressing the stump with cow dung, and despite immunization programs, neonatal tetanus is a frequent problem. Once infected, mothers and babies often lack access to transport, and if they reach a care facility, they frequently find that essential resources such as antibiotics are unavailable. **The WHO guidelines on "the five cleans" needed during delivery**[114] **have led to the introduction of clean birth kits that contain soap, plastic sheeting, gloves, sterile gauze, a razor, and cord ties for use at home births.**[115] These simple kits have achieved a relative reduction in neonatal mortality, particularly in rural areas of developing countries.[116] However, wider interventions that included a skilled birth attendant in the intervention were associated with a greater and more significant reduction in neonatal mortality, omphalitis, and puerperal sepsis.[117] It is therefore considered best practice to provide safe birth kits in the hands of skilled attendants.

Human Immunodeficiency Virus and Malaria

Pregnant women infected with HIV and/or *Plasmodium falciparum* malaria suffer higher complication rates. The MMR for HIV-infected women increases tenfold[118] because their immunodeficiency places them at greater risk of dying of pregnancy-related sepsis. **A recent review estimated the excess mortality attributable to HIV among pregnant and postpartum women to be 994 per 100,000 pregnant women.**[29]

The maternal immune response to malaria is also altered by pregnancy, and the most serious complications—including cerebral malaria, hypoglycemia, pulmonary edema, and severe hemolytic anemia—are more common. Approximately 40% of the world's pregnant women are exposed to malaria infection, and primigravidae are more likely to develop severe maternal anemia and to have low birthweight babies than multigravidae.[119] The fetal and perinatal loss may be as high as 60% to 70% in nonimmune women who contract malaria, and an additional 100,000 infant deaths in Africa result from malaria-induced low birthweight in babies.[120] Malaria infections among pregnant women are less common outside Africa but are more likely to cause severe disease, preterm births, and fetal loss. HIV increases the risk of malaria and its adverse effects, and women with both infections are at particular risk of adverse birth outcomes.[121]

Obstructed Labor and Obstetric Fistula

Worldwide, obstructed labor occurs in an estimated 5% of live births and accounts for 8% of maternal deaths.[122] In sub-Saharan Africa and parts of Asia, as many as 2 million young women are affected and 50,000 to 100,000 new cases occur every year.[123,124] Obstructed labor, or "failure to progress," with or without fetal distress is the main indication for emergency CD worldwide.[125] The problem can be prevented by using a partogram routinely in labor and by resorting to early operative delivery when progress is slow. The partogram is a cheap, graphic record of cervical dilation against time in labor; this simple monitoring tool swiftly identifies when a labor is becoming prolonged, thereby avoiding the development of obstetric fistulae and death from a prolonged obstructed labor or a ruptured uterus.[126] Despite strong advocacy by the WHO and other health care agencies, the global use of partograms is extremely poor, and some senior clinicians wrongly assert that completing the monitoring paperwork is unrealistic for already overworked midwives and doctors.

Obstetric fistulae can occur at any age or parity but are most common in first births, particularly in young girls with a poorly developed pelvis. They are a direct consequence of prolonged obstructed labor where the pressure of the impacted fetus leads to the destruction of the vesicovaginal/rectovaginal septum with subsequent loss of urinary and/or fecal control.[127,128] They can also be due to trauma at the time of pelvic surgery or as a result of rape, and in parts of Africa, some 15% of cases are caused by harmful female genital mutilation/cutting (FGM/C) before or during labor by unskilled birth attendants.[129] The tragedy is that obstructed labor and obstetric fistulae are largely avoidable; a summary of the preventive measures, as described by the WHO, is shown in Table 58-4.

Obstetric fistulae are highly stigmatizing, and affected women who constantly leak urine and fecal matter frequently become social outcasts. Unlikely to have further children or find employment, they are regarded as worthless to their families and are frequently rejected. Specialist fistula repair centers and

TABLE 58-4	PREVENTION OF OBSTETRIC FISTULAE	
TYPE	**WHEN**	**WHAT**
Primary prevention	Before pregnancy	• Eliminate female genital mutilation, early marriage, and early childbearing • Pregnancies are planned
Secondary prevention	During pregnancy	• Skilled antenatal care • During birth, awareness of signs and symptoms of impending fistula such as prolonged labor and the need to seek care • Manage prolonged labor ("Do not let the sun set twice on a laboring woman"*)
		• Easy and early access to facilities equipped to manage essential obstetric care including CD
Tertiary prevention	During and after delivery	• Monitor every labor using partogram to identify women at risk or to monitor those who develop obstructed labor and refer immediately if CD cannot be done in the current facility • Use of indwelling catheters to help enable spontaneous closure of small fistulae in mothers who have survived an obstructed labor • Encourage such women to seek skilled care during next pregnancy and delivery

Modified from Lewis G, de Bernis L. *Obstetric Fistula: Guiding Principles for Clinical Management and Programme Development.* Geneva: World Health Organization; 2006.
*Kenyan proverb.
CD, cesarean delivery.

the training of local surgeons to perform simple repairs helps to restore function, fertility, and dignity to these women, but such services are still beyond the reach of most fistula sufferers.

Cesarean Delivery

Cesarean delivery rates in many resource-poor countries remain much lower than the 10% to 15% cited by the WHO as their target in 1985.[130] In other countries, the rate continues to rise above unacceptably high levels, particularly in private hospitals. **In 2008, the WHO estimated an overall rate of 45.9% for Brazil, 30.3% for the United States, and only 0.7% for Burkina Faso; this equates to 3.18 million CDs that should have been performed, and 6.20 million performed unnecessarily.**[35] The cost of the global "excess" of CD was estimated to be $2.32 billion, whereas the cost of the global unmet need for CD is a mere $432 million.[35] This excess of CD is due to maternal request, increasing maternal age, obesity, poor clinical acumen, risk-averse behaviors, and fear of litigation.[131] However, it is not an operation without sequelae, and the rising incidence of PPH due to placenta increta and/or placenta accreta involving a previous CD scar has risen significantly, as demonstrated by research, in the United Kingdom.[132]

As with all surgical procedures, the benefits and risks must be carefully assessed for both mother and baby. A mother can die of hypovolemic shock after a technically successful CD with average blood loss if she is dehydrated, severely anemic, and unable to cope with an operative insult. If the local health care facility is poorly equipped with no access to emergency resuscitation, blood transfusion, or anesthesia, it may be preferable to delay the CD until transfer to a safer facility can be arranged. However, significant delays in the second stage of labor leads to additional complications that include increased likelihood of hemorrhage, extension of the surgical incision into the vagina or uterine arteries, sepsis, and fistula development.

PRACTICAL ADVICE ON VOLUNTEERING TO WORK OVERSEAS

Many health professionals wish to "give back" to the most vulnerable of the world's citizens; for some, offering their skills in-country is becoming an increasingly popular option. Some choose to work abroad to add experience to their curriculum vitae or when applying for university or higher training, whereas others wish to undertake research or practice their clinical skills.

A growing trend is also to participate in teaching and/or bilateral sustainable support programs in a needy facility organized by their local institutions. Partnering among universities, hospitals, and medical and midwifery schools is also becoming more popular and is a good way to ensure a constant supply of teachers and clinical staff upon which the host institution may have come to rely. Volunteers also play a key role in "training the trainers"—that is, enabling cadres of local staff to act as ongoing trainers in their own country. However, whatever the reasons, volunteering only benefits the local population if the placement is carefully planned, leads to sustainable improvement, and is undertaken with care and understanding.

Well-organized trips conducted sensitively with respect for the mothers, health care workers, and local cultures can be life-enriching experiences for all concerned and yield life-long benefits. However, this is not always the case; at its worst, the arrogant, dismissive, or critical behavior of some volunteers has given so called "volunteerism"[133] a bad reputation locally. Concern exists that such initiatives can lead to exploitation and harm, particularly when projects are only focused on meeting the volunteer's needs or undertaking research that will not benefit the local community. Indeed, in some parts of Africa, what is now referred to as "extraction tourism"—in which only the temporary visitor seems to benefit, often leaving a worse situation and unpleasant feelings behind—is so bad that volunteers are no longer welcome.

For staff working within already well-established exchange schemes, the knowledge of how to prepare and behave should have already been explained, and initial local difficulties have been overcome. However, for others working alone or with small organizations, knowing what to expect and how to plan and conduct the placement is the subject of this section.

In summary, the **key personal qualities** for working abroad include:

1. Compassion and respect
2. Humility and honesty
3. High ethical and moral standards
4. Acceptance of the community and its values and a willingness to behave in a culturally appropriate manner
5. Commitment to promote the welfare of the community you serve first and putting their needs before your own
6. Ability to practice and teach the highest quality evidence-based medicine using sustainable drugs and equipment appropriate for the local circumstances, which will be

available after your departure and, in the case of machinery, will include a source for spare parts so the equipment can be repaired

7. An openness and willingness to learn from local staff, who will have much to teach and share

8. A dedication to ensuring sustainability

9. The ability to resist being openly critical of the lack of resources and poor infrastructure, saying how much better things are at home (staff and patients are all too aware of this)

10. The integrity to follow the same ethical principles you would adhere to in your own institute or country (for research, this is crucial)

Although these principles may seem glaringly obvious, experience has repeatedly shown that failure to follow such simple guidelines can lead to disappointment and frustration on all sides.

Respect

The health staff you will work with and the mothers, babies, and communities you will care for are no different than anywhere else. Even though they may be poor beyond imagination, perhaps have inexplicable customs, and cannot speak your language, each deserves as much respect as you would give all your patients or colleagues at home. They are generally living lives so hard as to be unfathomable, and this deserves recognition, admiration, and compassion. Try to learn a few words of their language, and treat everyone with dignity and respect. Learn about social customs and taboos so you do not inadvertently offend.

Realism

Do not have unrealistic expectations about what can be achieved in the time available to you. In most countries, it takes far longer to organize things, and wheels turn very slowly. Often, a lot of bureaucratic red tape and delay intervenes both before leaving and while in-country. Start organizing your trip months beforehand, and obtain the necessary permissions before you leave. Visas, too, can take time.

Remember that you will not be the first or last volunteer. Volunteering is a growing business, and some popular facilities, like the base camps of Mt. Everest, can become very overcrowded. In some areas, numerous NGOs or other organizations have been seen running the same type of program without joint preplanning or teamwork. This lack of coordination is at best ineffective, and at its worst, disastrous, because it leads to confusion among volunteers and staff, duplication of work, and the waste of very scarce resources. If you wish to work in a particular place, always check who is working there already and contact them. Check with the hosts to see if you would really be welcome, and be sure they are not just being polite to a request from someone they do not know. Rather than just trying to do what you think will help, ask the local staff what would help fill service gaps for them.

Also, be aware that health facilities are generally chronically and completely understaffed with only one or two midwives or doctors to care for numerous patients, at best. As such, they will have little time to teach and nurture inexperienced volunteers because they take up crucial time that could be spent with patients. The paradox is that in wishing to please, they will be polite and may spend too much time with you and not their patients. Such volunteers would probably do better by joining

an already well-established program that can accommodate and acclimatize them. Some larger programs hold predeparture training workshops. In these sessions, be honest about your skills and abilities, and consider how much supervision you would need; then choose your options carefully. You may be welcome, but you will need to be able to step in immediately and pull your own weight rather than becoming an additional burden on an already overstretched staff.

Health Care Staff

The staff you will work with invariably will work longer hours, in far worse conditions, and for far less pay than you. Sometimes they work with no pay at all if money in the health center is limited for a while. In addition, they are rightly proud of what they can achieve with so very little. Although everyone is almost always polite, talking about your own salary or showing large amounts of money is insensitive. However initially surprised or shocked you may be, do not be critical of the facility, lack of resources, or age or type of equipment available. The staff will already be acutely aware of the limitations and will be proud of the innovative local solutions they may have devised to the best of their resources and ability. Although they will have been trained in a variety of institutions, with different knowledge and skills, they will most certainly be more able than you to undertake more complex operations under challenging conditions until you, too, have become expert in their art. Examples of this could include complex fistula repair or even the simple repairs done by the trained former patients of the Addis Ababa Fistula Hospital.

Midwives are the backbone of most maternity services around the world and are widely respected and generally highly competent. Do not underestimate their abilities. They are specialists in "normal" deliveries, and in many places, including the United Kingdom, they teach medical students and junior residents crucial obstetric skills. In European countries, some work as independent autonomous practitioners. In the United Kingdom, midwives are present at every birth, and over 65% of women are delivered with their assistance alone. Either independently or working within a multidisciplinary team for higher risk pregnancies, their skills help improve maternal health care; the latest direct-cause maternal mortality ratio for the United Kingdom, 5.4 per 100,00 live births, is one of the lowest in the world.[30] Other countries with very low death rates are also characterized by the inclusion of their own midwives. They are highly skilled in managing the normal and knowing when to refer for help; the maternal mortality rates in these countries are the lowest in the world. Experienced midwives who work in resource-poor countries will have seen and managed more sick women than most obstetricians in a lifetime. They work without the resources taken for granted elsewhere. A number have a wide variety of other skills, and in certain places—with training, for example—they even undertake cesarean delivery, symphysiotomy, and simple fistulae repair. However, there are far too few midwives, and they are often vastly overworked with intolerably high caseloads and very long shifts. One midwife in a labor ward with 50 or more women is not unusual. Some adopt the babies of mothers who have died, and most are pillars of their community. All will have much to teach you.

In many low-income countries, only a few specialists in obstetrics and gynecology work in the public sector; other health care professionals such as family doctors, medical or clinical officers, or operating theater assistants are trained to perform many routine procedures. In obstetrics, this involves training staff in the competencies to undertake some work traditionally done by maternity health care professionals, doctors, midwives, and nurses—so-called task shifting.[134] **To meet the crisis in human resources all across the developing world, low- and mid-level workers are expanding their skills and taking on new roles according to the competencies in which they have been trained and are able to master.**

Research

Visitors who plan research activities in a foreign country must only undertake these having first obtained national and local ethics committee approval. This can take months, and the process will vary according to local laws. Additionally, the rules in their own institution and country must be followed. If required, consent forms should be obtained from all study participants, having first clearly explained the process in their own language. If a research project is performed in a country with no ethics committee or institutional review board or similar body, researchers should ensure their proposed study adheres to the World Medical Association Declaration of Helsinki.[135]

Research projects should also only focus on interventions that could benefit the women, babies, or communities under consideration. It is not moral or ethical to test drugs, equipment, supplements, vaccines, and so on that will be so expensive as to be unavailable to the women who were the research subjects.

Because of their punishing workload, health care staff in low-income countries have little or no time to prepare papers for publication. However, local researchers should be encouraged and helped to write and author papers, be first author where appropriate, and present their findings at local and international conferences. This not only recognizes their contribution and benefits their careers, it also adds to their knowledge base; such local experience is invaluable when planning appropriate and effective interventions. This support for local doctors is becoming an increasing requirement of those who fund medical and other research programs.

Predeparture Preparation

The following list, although not exhaustive by any means, should help you to start your preparation. Although some general pointers are always helpful, issues specific to the location may apply that you will need to identify and understand. Your hosts can help you in this, but remember: you are ultimately responsible for your health and well-being while in a volunteering program.

Thoroughly research the country and institutions you are planning to visit well in advance of leaving. **Apart from general background, read any WHO, UN, World Bank, and other institutions' in-country fact sheets on the general health of the population as well as in your specific area. Talk with ex-volunteers and find out their practical tips.**

Try to arrange an orientation session about your placement. If it is with a large organization, they may invite you to attend a predeparture meeting to discuss practicalities and your responsibilities. If they are abroad, social media such as Skype are extremely helpful.

Learn about requirements for local medical registration and arrangements for medical indemnity. Ask for their safety briefing packs, and obtain key contact numbers.

Ensure that your passport is valid for at least 6 months beyond the intended length of your entire stay, including any vacation time at the end. Check visa requirements well in advance of your departure by contacting the Embassy or High Commission for the country you are visiting. This may take a long time to complete.

Evaluate your budget. If not provided for you, the cost of subsistence is usually very low, but the cost of accommodation may vary widely. Ask your hosts for their recommendations. Factor in costs for a comprehensive package of personal insurance for health, travel, and loss of possessions.

Consult an established travel center concerning vaccinations and malaria prophylaxis at least 6 months before you travel. Some vaccines, such as against yellow fever, are compulsory to enter many sub-Saharan African countries. The availability of postexposure prophylaxis for HIV is essential in many countries, and you may need to take these supplies with you. Also arrange to take supplies of any essential drugs you personally need because they are unlikely to be widely available elsewhere. You may need to bring these into the country with a letter or confirmatory prescription from your physician.

Contact your licensing body for advice on maintaining your medical licensure and indemnity at home during your placement. Allow yourself maximum time to gain medical registration within the country you are visiting because this can be time consuming.

You will need to protect your pension and take precautions for every eventuality. Research the best options for life insurance.

You will also wish to consider whether you will be taking any drugs or equipment with you and, if so, be sure that you are not at risk of contravening local customs and excise regulations and such. You should check this with your sponsor and on the relevant Web sites.

It is beneficial to arrange for two mentors, one in-country and one at home, to support you. Ask your sponsors to arrange an in-country mentor. Your hospital, professional association, or medical school may be able to put you in touch with colleagues who have experience working in the country and who may be prepared to mentor to you while you are away.

As soon as you arrive, it is essential that you register with the embassy or foreign office of your home country so that they are aware that you are there should there be any emergencies. Many of these organizations use Twitter or other social media to give regular updates of the current political and security climate. Maintain regular contact with your organizing institution and with your mentors.

Keep a diary, take photographs (with permission), and also relax, have fun, make new friends, and enjoy your new environment.

KEY POINTS

♦ Every day, 800 women die as a result of pregnancy or childbirth, and an additional 16,000 develop severe and long-lasting complications.

♦ Every day, 8000 newborn babies die and 7000 are still-born, and more than half of these deaths are from maternal complications.

♦ Adolescent pregnancies account for 11% of all births worldwide, and these young girls and their babies are at far higher risk of death and complications than other mothers.

◆ Of all the maternal and neonatal deaths worldwide, 99% take place in developing countries.

◆ The leading obstetric causes of maternal death in developing countries are hemorrhage, puerperal sepsis, preeclampsia, unsafe abortion, obstructed labor, and embolism. HIV causes a growing number of deaths in countries where it is endemic.

◆ If all pregnant women and their babies could access the maternity care recommended by the WHO, the annual number of maternal deaths would fall by two thirds—from 290,000 to 96,000—and newborn deaths would fall by more than three quarters to 660,000 each year.

◆ If all women had control over their fertility and could access effective contraception, unintended pregnancies would drop by 70%, and unsafe abortions would drop by 74%.

◆ Apart from a lack of skilled health care and other resources, the quality of the care provided also varies widely. The clinical guidelines and protocols set forth by the WHO and professional organizations need to be urgently implemented, and their uptake audited, in developed as well as in developing countries.

◆ Safe motherhood for all women is enshrined as a basic human right by the United Nations, yet many societies have yet to recognize and address this, and they fail to provide the necessary resources to provide adequate reproductive health, maternity, and newborn care or to enact and enforce laws to support equality for women in all aspects of their life, which includes abolition of child marriage and other harmful traditional practices.

◆ A woman's life is always worth saving.

Acknowledgment

The section on the United States was written with assistance by William Callaghan, MD, MPH, chief of Maternal and Infant Health Branch, Division of Reproductive Health, Centers for Disease Control and Prevention, and in collaboration with the American College of Obstetricians and Gynecologists.

REFERENCES

1. Singh S, Darroch JE, Ashford LS. *Adding It Up: Costs and Benefits of Investing in Sexual and Reproductive Health.* New York: Guttmacher Institute and United Nations Population Fund; 2014.
2. World Health Organisation (WHO). *The World Health Report 2005.* Available at: <www.who.int/whr/2005/en>.
3. Hardes K, Gay J, Blanc A. Maternal morbidity: neglected dimension of safe motherhood in the developing world. *Glob Public Health.* 2012; 7(6):603-617.
4. United Nations Children's Fund. *The Progress of the Nations. 2001.* New York: UNICEF; 2001.
5. Islam K, Gurdtham UG. *A systematic review of the estimates of costs-illness associated with maternal and new-born ill-health. Part of the World Health Organisation Maternal-Newborn Health and Poverty series.* Geneva: WHO.; 2005.
6. World Health Organisation. *Trends in maternal mortality: 1990 to 2013. Estimates by WHO, UNICEF, UNFPA, The World Bank and the United Nations Population Division Report 2014.* Geneva: WHO; 2015.
7. Patton GC, Coffey C, Sawyer SM, et al. Global patterns of mortality in young people: a systematic analysis of population health data. *Lancet.* 2009;374:881-892.
8. You D, Bastian P, Wu J, Wardlaw T. *Levels and trends in child mortality. Estimates developed by the UN inter-agency Group for Child Mortality Estimation. Report 2013.* New York: UNICEF, WHO, The World Bank and United Nations; 2013.
9. *World Health Organisation Fact sheet on maternal mortality No 348 updated May 2014.* Available at: <www.who.int/mediacentre/factsheets/fs348/en>.
10. United Nations. *The World's Women. Trends and Statistics 1970-1990.* New York: United Nations; 1991.
11. World Health Organisation media centre. *Adolescent Pregnancy Fact sheet, No 364, Updated September 2014.* Available at: <www.who.int/mediacentre/factsheets/fs364/en>.
12. Patton GC, Coffey C, Sawyer SM, et al. Global patterns of mortality in young people: a systematic analysis of population health data. *Lancet.* 2009;374:881-892.
13. World Health Organisation. *Women and Health: Today's Evidence, Tomorrow's Agenda.* Geneva: WHO; 2009:31.
14. Ganchimeg T, Mori R, Ota E, et al. Maternal and perinatal outcomes among nulliparous adolescents in low- and middle-income countries: a multi-country study. *BJOG.* 2013;120:1622-1630.
15. Ganchimeg T, Ota E, Morisaki N, et al. WHO Multicountry Survey on Maternal Newborn Health Research Network. Pregnancy and childbirth outcomes among adolescent mothers: a World Health Organization multicountry study. *BJOG.* 2014;121(suppl 1):40-48.
16. Lewis G. Saving Mothers' Lives: the continuing benefits for maternal health from the United Kingdom (UK) Confidential Enquires into Maternal Deaths. *Semin Perinatol.* 2012;36:19-26.
17. D'Alton M. *Reducing Maternal Mortality Through Clinical Protocols. Presentation at New York ACOG annual district meeting,* October 2013. Available at: <http://mail.ny.acog.org/website/2013_ADM/Syllabus/5_Fri_DAlton.pdf>.
18. Centers for Disease Control and Prevention (CDC). *Pregnancy Mortality Surveillance System.* Available at: <www.cdc.gov/reproductivehealth/MaternalInfantHealth/PMSS.html>.
19. D'Alton ME, Main EK, Menard MK, Levy BS. The National Partnership for Maternal Safety. *Obstet Gynecol.* 2014;123:973-977.
20. Reichenhiem M, Zylberstajn F, Moraes C, Lobato G. Severe acute obstetric morbidity (near-miss): a review of the relative use of its diagnostic indicators. *Arch Gynecol Obstet.* 2009;280:337-343.
21. AbouZahr C. Global burden of maternal death. In: *British Medical Bulletin. Pregnancy: Reducing maternal death and disability.* British Council: Oxford University Press; 2003:1-13.
22. Zacharin RF. A history of obstetric vesicovaginal fistula. *ANZ J Surg.* 2000;70:851-854.
23. *United Nations Population Fund (UNFPA), FIGO, Columbia University–sponsored Second Meeting of the Working Group for the Prevention and Treatment of Obstetric Fistula.* Addis Ababa: UNFPA; 2002:2002.
24. Stanton C, Holtz S, Ahmed S. Challenges in measuring obstetric fistula. *Int J Gynecol Obstet.* 2007;99:S4-S9.
25. Liu L, Oza S, Hogan D, et al. *Global, regional, and national causes of child mortality in 2000-2013, with projections to inform post-2015 priorities: an updated systematic analysis Lancet, Early Online Publication,* 1 October 2014.
26. World Health Organization (WHO). *Global Health Observatory (GHO) data: Neonatal Mortality.* Available at: <http://www.who.int/gho/child_health/mortality/neonatal_text/en/>.
27. Lawn JE, Blencowe H, Oza S, et al. Every Newborn: progress, priorities, and potential beyond survival. *Lancet.* 2014;384:189-205.
28. Say L, Chou D, Gemill A, et al. Global causes of maternal deaths: a WHO systematic analysis. *Lancet Glob Health.* 2014;2:e323-e333.
29. Calvert C, Ronsmans C. The contribution of HIV to pregnancy-related mortality: a systematic review and meta-analysis. *AIDS.* 2013;27: 1631-1639.
30. Knight M, Kenyon S, Brocklehurst P, Neilson J, Shakespeare J, Kurinczuk JJ, eds. *on behalf of MBRRACE UK. Saving Lives, Improving Mothers' Care - Lessons learned to inform future maternity care from the UK and Ireland. Confidential Enquiries into Maternal Deaths and Morbidity 2009-2012.* Oxford: National Perinatal Epidemiology Unit, University of Oxford; 2014.
31. World Health Organization (WHO). *Global Health Observatory (GHO) data: Antenatal Care.* Available at: <http://www.who.int/gho/maternal_health/reproductive_health/antenatal_care_text/en/>.
32. Villar J, Ba'aqeel H, Piaggio G, et al. WHO antenatal care randomized trial for the evaluation of a new model of routine antenatal care. *Lancet.* 2001;357(9268):1551-1564.
33. World Health Organization (WHO). *World Health Statistics 2014.* Geneva: World Health Organization; 2014.

34. United Nations Population Fund (UNFPA). *Setting standards for emergency obstetric and newborn care*. October 2014. Available at: <http://www.unfpa.org/resources/setting-standards-emergency-obstetric-and-newborn-care>.

35. Gibbons L, Belizá J. *The Global Numbers and Costs of Additionally Needed and Unnecessary Caesarean Sections Performed per Year: Overuse as a Barrier to Universal Coverage*. Geneva: WHO World Health Report; 2010. Background Paper, No 30. Available at: <http://www.who.int/healthsystems/topics/financing/healthreport/30C-sectioncosts.pdf>.

36. International Confederation of Midwives. *The International day of the midwife 2013*. Available at: <http://www.internationalmidwives.org/assets/uploads/documents>.

37. Pereira C, Bugalho A. A comparative study of caesarean deliveries by assistant medical officers and obstetricians in Mozambique. *BJOG*. 1996;103:508-512.

38. van den Broek N, Lewis G, Mathai M. Guest Editors' Choice: Quality of Care supplement. *BJOG*. 2014;121(suppl 4):2-3.

39. Thaddeus S, Maine D. Too far to walk: maternal mortality in context. *Soc Sci Med*. 1994;38:1091-1110.

40. Lewis G. Reviewing maternal deaths to make pregnancy safer. In: Moodley J, ed. *Recent advances in obstetrics*. Vol. 22, No. 3. Elsevier: Best Practice & Research Clinical Obstetrics and Gynaecology; 2008:447-463.

41. UCL Institute of Health Equality. *Fair Society Health Lives (The Marmot Review)*. February 2010. Available at: <http://www.instituteofhealthequity.org/projects/fair-society-healthy-lives-the-marmot-review>.

42. Tunçalp Ö, Souza JP, Hindin MJ, et al. WHO Multicountry Survey on Maternal and Newborn Health Research Network. Education and severe maternal outcomes in developing countries: a multicountry cross-sectional survey. *BJOG*. 2014;121(suppl 1):57-65.

43. Kaplan A, Forbes M, Bonhoure I, et al. Female genital mutilation/cutting in The Gambia: long-term health consequences and complications during delivery and for the newborn. *Int J Womens Health*. 2013;5:323-331.

44. Fathalla M. Human rights aspects of safe motherhood. *Best Pract Res Clin Obstet Gynaecol*. 2006;20(3):409-419.

45. United Nations. *The Universal Declaration of Human Rights*. Available at: <www.un.org/en/documents/udhr>.

46. United Nations Entity for Gender Equality and the Empowerment of Women. *Fourth World Conference on Women: Beijing Declaration*. September 1995. Available at: <http://www.un.org/womenwatch/daw/beijing/beijingdeclaration.html>.

47. Nobel Prize Organization. *A Voice for Freedom! Nobel Lecture by Ellen Johnson Sirleaf, Oslo, Norway*. 10 December 2011. Available at: <www.nobelprize.org/nobel_prizes/peace/laureates/2011/johnson_sirleaf-lecture_en.html>.

48. The World Bank Human Development Network. *Health, Nutrition and Population Series. Investing in maternal health; learning from Sri Lanka and Malaysia*. Washington, DC: 2003.

48b. *Women's Rights, Health, and Empowerment*. Available at: <www.GLOWM.com/womens_health_rights>.

49. Ahmed S, Li Q, Liu L, Tsui AO. Maternal deaths averted by contraceptive use: an analysis of 172 countries. *Lancet*. 2012;380:111-125.

50. Cleland J, Conde-Agudelo A, Peterson H, Ross J, Tsui A. Contraception and health. *Lancet*. 2012;380:149-156.

51. *International Conference on Population and Development Cairo*. Cairo: UNFPA; 1994. Available at: <https://www.unfpa.org/public/icpd>.

52. United Nations Millennium Declaration. *New York, United Nations 2000 (United Nations General Assembly resolution 55/2)*. Available at: <http://www.un.org/millennium/declaration/ares552e.htm>.

53. Sedgh G, Singh S, Hussain R. Intended and unintended pregnancies worldwide in 2012 and recent trends. *Stud Fam Plann*. 2014;45(3):301-314.

54. Centers for Disease Control and Prevention (CDC). *Unintended Pregnancy Prevention*. Available at: <http://www.cdc.gov/reproductivehealth/unintendedpregnancy/>.

55. Santelli J, Rochat R, Hatfield-Timajchy K, et al. Unintended Pregnancy Working Group. The measurement and meaning of unintended pregnancy. *Perspect Sex Reprod Health*. 2003;35(2):94-101.

56. Brown SS, Eisenberg L, eds. *The Best Intentions: Unintended Pregnancy and the Well-Being of Children and Families. Institute of Medicine (US) Committee on Unintended Pregnancies*. Washington D.C.: National Academies Press; 1995.

57. Marston C, Cleland J. Do unintended pregnancies carried to term lead to adverse outcomes for mother and child? An assessment in five developing countries. *Popul Stud (Camb)*. 2003;57(1):77-93.

58. Hardee K, Eggleston E. Unintended pregnancy and women's psychological well-being in Indonesia. *J Biosoc Sci*. 2004;36(5):617-626.

59. Gipson JD, Koenig MA. The effects of unintended pregnancy on infant, child, and parental health: a review of the literature. *Stud Fam Plann*. 2008;39(1):18-38.

60. Tsui AO, McDonald-Mosley R. Family planning and the burden of unintended pregnancies. *Epidemiol Rev*. 2010;32(1):152-174.

61. *Guttmacher Institute, Facts on induced abortion worldwide, In Brief*, 2011. Available at: <http://www.guttmacher.org/pubs/fb_IAW.html>.

62. Canning D, Schultz TP. The economic consequences of reproductive health and family planning. *Lancet*. 2012;380:165-171.

63. Singh S, Darroch JE. *Adding It Up: Costs and Benefits of Contraceptive Services— Estimates for 2012*. New York: Guttmacher Institute and United Nations Population Fund (UNFPA); 2012.

64. Population Reference Bureau. *World Population Data Sheet 2012*. Washington, DC: PRB; 2012.

65. Gillespie D, Ahmed S. Unwanted fertility among the poor: an inequity? *Bull World Health Organ*. 2007;85(2):100-107.

66. World Health Organization (WHO). *Contraceptive prevalence*. Available at: <http://www.who.int/reproductivehealth/topics/family_planning/contraceptive_prevalence/en>.

67. *United Nations Department of Economic and Social Affairs World Contraceptive Use 2011*. Available at: <http://www.un.org/esa/population/publications/contraceptive2011/contraceptive2011.htm>.

68. Alkema L, Kantorova V. National, regional, and global rates and trends in contraceptive prevalence and unmet need for family planning between 1990 and 2015: a systematic and comprehensive analysis. *Lancet*. 2013;381(9878):1642-1652.

69. Alkema L, Kantorova V. National, regional, and global rates and trends in contraceptive prevalence and unmet need for family planning between 1990 and 2015: a systematic and comprehensive analysis. *Lancet*. 2013;381(9878):1642-1652 (Supplement).

70. World Health Organization (WHO). *WHO Department of Reproductive Health and Research, Johns Hopkins Bloomsbury School of Public Health/Center for Communications Programs (CCP). Knowledge for health project. Family planning: a global handbook for providers (2011 update)*. Baltimore, MD/Geneva, Switzerland: CCP and WHO; 2011.

71. World Health Organization (WHO). *WHO Fact Sheet No. 351: Family Planning and Contraception*. May 2015. Available at: <http://www.who.int/mediacentre/factsheets/fs351/en>.

72. Darroch JE, Singh S. Trends in contraceptive need and use in developing countries in 2003, 2008, and 2012: an analysis of national surveys. *Lancet*. 2013;381:1756-1762.

73. Ross J, Winfrey J. Contraception use, intention to use and unmet need during the extended postpartum period. *Int Fam Plan Perspect*. 2001;27:20-27.

74. Kidder E, Sonneveldt E, Hardee K. *Who receives PAC services? Evidence from 14 countries*. Washington, DC: The Futures Group, POLICY Project; 2004.

75. Hatcher RA, Trussell J, Nelson AL, Cates W, Kowal D, Policar M, eds. *Contraceptive Technology*. 20th revised edition. New York, NY: Ardent Media; 2011.

76. Espey E, Ogburn T. Long-acting reversible contraceptives: intrauterine devices and the contraceptive implant. *Obstet Gynecol*. 2011;117:705-719.

77. Trussell J. The essentials of contraception: efficacy, safety, and personal considerations. In: Hatcher RA, Trussell J, Nelson AL, Cates W, Stewart FH, eds. *Contraceptive Technology*. New York: Ardent Media; 2007:221-252.

78. Hubacher D, Mavranezouli I, McGinn E. Unintended pregnancy in sub-Saharan Africa: magnitude of the problem and potential role of contraceptive implants to alleviate it. *Contraception*. 2008;78:73-78.

79. *Family Planning 2020*. Available at: <http://www.familyplanning2020.org>.

80. Åhman E, Shah IH. New estimates and trends regarding unsafe abortion mortality. *Int J Gynecol Obstet*. 2011;115(2):121-126.

81. Center for Reproductive Rights. *A Global View of Abortion Rights*. New York: Center for Reproductive Rights; 2014. Available at: <http://www.reproductiverights.org/document/a-global-view-of-abortion-rights>.

82. Sedgh G, Singh S. Induced abortion: incidence and trends worldwide from 1995 to 2008. *Lancet*. 2012;379(9816):625-632.

83. World Health Organization (WHO). *Unsafe Abortion: Global and Regional Estimates of the Incidence of Unsafe Abortion and Associated Mortality in 2008*. 6th ed. Geneva: World Health Organization; 2011.

84. World Health Organization (WHO). *Safe abortion: technical and policy guidance for health systems*. 2nd ed. Geneva: WHO; 2012.

85. Grimes D, Benson J, Singh S, et al. Unsafe abortion: the preventable pandemic. *Lancet*. 2006;368:1908-1919.

86. Singh S. Hospital admissions resulting from unsafe abortion: estimates from 13 developing countries. *Lancet*. 2006;368(9550):1887-1892.

87. Jewkes R, Rees H. Dramatic decline in abortion mortality due to the Choice on Termination of Pregnancy Act. *S Afr Med J.* 2005;95(4):250.

88. Ministry of Medical Services. *Health Standards and guidelines for reducing morbidity and mortality from unsafe abortion in Kenya.* 2012. Available at: <http://www.safeabortionwomensright.org/>.

89. *Countdown to 2015: Maternal, Newborn, and Child Survival.* Available at: <http://www.countdown2015mnch.org>.

90. United Nations Department of Economic and Social Affairs. *Sustainable Development Knowledge Platform.* Available at: <http://sustainabledevelopment.un.org>.

91. Bhutta ZA, Das JK, Bahl R, et al., for the Lancet Newborn Interventions Review Group; Lancet Every Newborn Study Group. Can available interventions end preventable deaths in mothers, newborn babies, and stillbirths and at what cost? *Lancet.* 2014;384(990):347-370.

92. Fathalla M. Ten propositions for safe motherhood for all women. Adapted and abridged from the Hubert de Watteville Memorial Lecture. Imagine a world where motherhood is safe for all women—you can help make it happen. *Int J Gynaecol Obstet.* 2011;72(3):207-213.

93. World Health Organisation (WHO). *Monitoring emergency obstetric care: a handbook.* Geneva: WHO; 2009.

94. Smith JM, Gubin R, Holston MM, Fullerton J, Prata N. Misoprostol for postpartum hemorrhage prevention at home birth: an integrative review of global implementation experience to date. *BMC Pregnancy Childbirth.* 2013;13:44.

95. Kubio C, Tierney G, Quaye T, et al. Blood transfusion practice in a rural hospital in Northern Ghana, Damongo, West Gonja District. *Transfusion.* 2012;52:2161-2166.

96. Westhoff G, Cotter AM. Prophylactic oxytocin for the third stage of labour to prevent postpartum haemorrhage. *Cochrane Database Syst Rev.* 2013;(10):CD001808.

97. Hofmeyr GJ, Abdel-Aleem H. Uterine massage for preventing postpartum haemorrhage. *Cochrane Database Syst Rev.* 2013;(7):CD006431.

98. World Health Organization (WHO). *Essential Medicines.* Available at: <http://www.who.int/topics/essential_medicines/en/>.

99. Smith JM, Baawo SD, Subah M, et al. Advance distribution of misoprostol for prevention of postpartum hemorrhage (PPH) at home births in two districts of Liberia. *BMC Pregnancy Childbirth.* 2014;14:189.

100. Geller S, Carnahan L, Akosah E, et al. Community-based distribution of misoprostol to prevent postpartum haemorrhage at home births: results from operations research in rural Ghana. *BJOG.* 2014;121:319-325.

101. Tunçalp Ö, Hofmeyr GJ, Gülmezoglu AM. Prostaglandins for preventing postpartum haemorrhage. *Cochrane Database Syst Rev.* 2012;(8):CD000494.

102. Adu-Bonsaffoh K, Samuel OA. Maternal deaths attributable to hypertensive disorders in a tertiary hospital in Ghana. *Int J Gynaecol Obstet.* 2013;123:110-113.

103. Abalos E, Cuesta C, Carroli G, et al. WHO Multicountry Survey on Maternal and Newborn Health Research Network. Pre-eclampsia, eclampsia and adverse maternal and perinatal outcomes: a secondary analysis of the World Health Organization Multicountry Survey. *BJOG.* 2014; 121(suppl 1):14-24.

104. Payne BA, Hutcheon JA, Ansermino JM, et al. A risk prediction model for the assessment and triage of women with hypertensive disorders of pregnancy in low-resourced settings: the miniPIERS (Pre-eclampsia Integrated Estimate of RiSk) multi-country prospective cohort study. *PLoS Med.* 2014;11:e1001589.

105. Urquia ML, Ying I. Serious preeclampsia among different immigrant groups. *J Obstet Gynaecol Can.* 2012;34:348-352.

106. Nakimuli A, Chazara O, Byamugisha J, et al. Pregnancy, parturition and preeclampsia in women of African ancestry. *Am J Obstet Gynecol.* 2014;210:510-520.e1.

107. Giguère Y, Massé J, Thériault S, et al. Screening for pre-eclampsia early in pregnancy: performance of a multivariable model combining clinical characteristics and biochemical markers. *BJOG.* 2015;122(3):402-410.

108. Gordon R, Magee LA, Payne B, et al. Magnesium sulphate for the management of preeclampsia and eclampsia in low and middle-income countries: a systematic review of tested dosing regimens. *J Obstet Gynaecol Can.* 2014;36:154-163.

109. Okonofua FE, Ogu RN, Fabamwo AO, et al. Training health workers for magnesium sulfate use reduces case fatality from eclampsia: results from a multicenter trial. *Acta Obstet Gynecol Scand.* 2013;92:716-720.

110. Loudon I. Maternal mortality in the past and its relevance to developing countries today. *Am J Clin Nutr.* 2000;72:241S-246S.

111. Unicef. *Fact of the week.* Available at: <http://www.unicef.org/factoftheweek/index_51390.html>.

112. Benova L, Cumming O, Campbell OM. Systematic review and meta-analysis: association between water and sanitation environment and maternal mortality. *Trop Med Int Health.* 2014;19:368-387.

113. Yahaya SJ, Bukar M. Knowledge of symptoms and signs of puerperal sepsis in a community in north-eastern Nigeria: a cross-sectional study. *J Obstet Gynaecol.* 2013;33:152-154.

114. World Health Organization (WHO). *Essential newborn care. Report of a technical working group (Trieste, 25–29 April 1994).* Geneva: WHO, Division of Reproductive Health (Technical Support); 1996.

115. Program for Appropriate Technology in Health (PATH). *Basic delivery kit guide (PDF).* Seattle: Program for Appropriate Technology in Health; 2001.

116. Seward N, Osrin D, Li L, et al. Association between clean delivery kit use, clean delivery practices, and neonatal survival: pooled analysis of data from three sites in South Asia. *PLoS Med.* 2012;9:e1001180.

117. Hundley VA, Avan BI. Are birth kits a good idea? A systematic review of the evidence. *Midwifery.* 2012;28:204-215.

118. Moran NF, Moodley J. The effect of HIV infection on maternal health and mortality. *Int J Gynaecol Obstet.* 2012;119:S26-S29.

119. Shulman CE, Dorman EK. Importance and prevention of malaria in pregnancy. *Trans R Soc Trop Med Hyg.* 2003;97:30-35.

120. Desai M, ter Kuile FO, Nosten F, et al. Epidemiology and burden of malaria in pregnancy. *Lancet Infect Dis.* 2007;7:93-104.

121. Ayisi JG, van Eijk AM, ter Kuile FO, et al. The effect of dual infection with HIV and malaria on pregnancy outcome in western Kenya. *AIDS.* 2003;17:585-594.

122. Lewis G, de Bernis L. *Obstetric Fistula: Guiding principles for clinical management and programme development.* Geneva: World Health Organisation; 2006.

123. *UNFPA, FIGO, Columbia University sponsored Second Meeting of the Working Group for the Prevention and Treatment of Obstetric Fistula. Addis Ababa,* 2002.

124. Stanton C, Holtz S, Ahmed S. Challenges in measuring obstetric fistula. *Int J Gynecol Obstet.* 2007;99:S4-S9.

125. Abraham W, Berhan Y. Predictors of labor abnormalities in university hospital: unmatched case control study. *BMC Pregnancy Childbirth.* 2014;14:256.

126. *United States Agency for International Development (USAID) The Partograph: An Essential Tool for Decision-Making during Labor.* Available at: <http://pdf.usaid.gov/pdf_docs/PNACT388.pdf>.

127. Creanga AA, Genadry RR. Obstetric fistulas: a clinical review. *Int J Gynaecol Obstet.* 2007;99:S40-S46.

128. Wall LL. Preventing obstetric fistulas in low-resource countries: insights from a Haddon matrix. *Obstet Gynecol Surv.* 2012;67:111-121.

129. *Faces of dignity: seven stories of girls and women with fistula.* Dar es Salaam, Tanzania: Women's Dignity Project; 2003.

130. World Health Organisation (WHO). Appropriate technology for birth. *Lancet.* 1985;2(8452):436-437.

131. Jauniaux E, Grobman W. Caesarean section: the world's No 1 operation. In: Jauniaux E, Grobman W, eds. *A modern textbook of cesarean section.* Oxford: Oxford University Press; 2015.

132. Fitzpatrick KE, Sellers S, Spark P, Kurinczuk JJ, Brocklehurst P, Knight K. Incidence and risk factors for placenta accreta/increta/percreta in the UK: a national case-control study. *PLoS ONE.* 2012;7(12):e52893.

133. Pezzella AT. Volunteerism and humanitarian efforts in surgery. *Curr Probl Surg.* 2006;43:848-929.

134. Averting Maternal Death and Disability (AMDD). *Task-Shifting: An innovative solution to the human resource crisis.* Available at: <http://www.amddprogram.org/human-resources/task-shifting>.

135. World Medical Association (WMA). *WMA Declaration of Helsinki - Ethical Principles for Medical Research Involving Human Subjects.* Available at: <http://www.wma.net/en/30publications/10policies/b3>.

Appendices

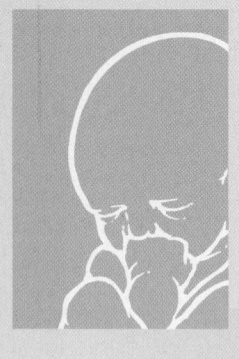

Normal Values in Pregnancy and Ultrasound Measurements

HENRY L. GALAN and LAURA GOETZL

INVASIVE CARDIAC MONITORING

MEASURE	VALUE (36-38 WEEKS)	UNITS
Cardiac output*	6.2 ± 1.0	L/min
Systemic vascular resistance	1210 ± 266	Dyne/cm/sec^{-5}
Heart rate	83 ± 10	Beats/min
Pulmonary vascular resistance	78 ± 22	Dyne/cm/sec^{-5}
Colloid oncotic pressure	18.0 ± 1.5	mm Hg
Mean arterial pressure (MAP)	90.3 ± 5.8	mm Hg
Pulmonary capillary wedge pressure (PCWP)	7.5 ± 1.8	mm Hg
Central venous pressure (CVP)	3.6 ± 2.5	mm Hg
Left ventricular stroke work index	48 ± 6	g/mm^{-2}

Data from Clark SL, Cotton DB, Lee W, et al. Central hemodynamic assessment of normal term pregnancy. *Am J Obstet Gynecol.* 1989;161:1439; Spatling L, Fallenstein F, Huch A, et al. The variability of cardiopulmonary adaptation to pregnancy at rest and during exercise. *Br J Obstet Gynaecol.* 1992;99(Suppl 8):1.
*Cardiac output increases during the first trimester of pregnancy but thereafter is essentially unchanged over the course of pregnancy; heart rate gradually rises 5 to 10 beats/min over the course of pregnancy.

NONINVASIVE CARDIAC MONITORING

MEASURE	10-18 WEEKS	18-26 WEEKS	26-34 WEEKS	34-42 WEEKS
Cardiac output (L/min)	7.26 ± 1.56	7.60 ± 1.63	7.38 ± 1.63	6.37 ± 1.48
Stroke volume (mL)	85 ± 21	85 ± 21	82 ± 21	70 ± 14
Systemic vascular resistance (SVR) (dyne/cm/second^{-5})	966 ± 226	901 ± 224	932 ± 240	1118 ± 325
Heart rate (beats/min)	87 ± 14	90 ± 14	92 ± 14	92 ± 7
Mean arterial pressure (mm Hg)	87 ± 7	84 ± 7	84 ± 7	86 ± 7

Data from Van Oppen CA, Van Der Tweel I, Alsbach JGP, et al. A longitudinal study of maternal hemodynamics during normal pregnancy. *Obstet Gynecol.* 1996;88:40.

ARTERIAL BLOOD GAS VALUES (THIRD TRIMESTER)

	NORMAL ALTITUDE	MODERATE ALTITUDE* (1388 M)
Arterial pH	7.40-7.48	7.44-7.48
Arterial PO_2 (mm Hg)	80-90	78.9-93.5
Arterial PCO_2 (mm Hg)	26.9-32.5	23.9-29.3
Sodium bicarbonate (mEq/L)	19.9-24.1	16.7-20.5

Data from Hankins GD, Clark SL, Harvey CJ, et al. Third trimester arterial blood gas and acid base values in normal pregnancy at moderate altitude. *Obstet Gynecol.* 1996;88:347; and Eng M, Butler J, Bonica JJ. Respiratory function in pregnant obese women. *Am J Obstet Gynecol.* 1975;123:241.
*Provo, Utah.

PULMONARY FUNCTION TESTS

	8-11 WEEKS	20-23 WEEKS	28-31 WEEKS	36-40 WEEKS
Respiratory rate (breaths/min)	15 (14-20)	16 (15-18)	18 (15-20)	17 (16-18)
Tidal volume (mL)	640 (550-710)	650 (625-725)	650 (575-720)	700 (660-755)

Data from Spatling L, Fallenstein F, Huch A, et al. The variability of cardiopulmonary adaptation to pregnancy at rest and during exercise. *Br J Obstet Gynaecol.* 1992;99:1.
Values expressed as median (25th to 75th percentiles).

PULMONARY FUNCTION TESTS, MEAN VALUES

	FIRST TRIMESTER	SECOND TRIMESTER	THIRD TRIMESTER
Mean vital capacity (L)	3.8	3.9	4.1
Mean inspiratory capacity (L)	2.6	2.7	2.9
Mean expiratory reserve volume (L)	1.2	1.2	1.2
Mean residual volume (L)	1.2	1.1	1.0

Data from Gazioglu K, Kaltreider NL, Rosen M, Yu PN. Pulmonary function during pregnancy in normal women and in patients with cardiopulmonary disease. *Thorax.* 1920;25:445; and Puranik BM, Kaore SB, Kurhade GA, et al. A longitudinal study of pulmonary function tests during pregnancy. *Indian J Physiol Pharmacol.* 1994;38:129.

PEAK FLOWS STABLE OVER GESTATION

	PEAK FLOW (L/MIN)
Standing	>320
Sitting	>310
Supine	>300

Data from Harirah HM, Donia SE, Nasrallah FK, et al. Effect of gestational age and position on peak expiratory flow rate: a longitudinal study. *Obstet Gynecol.* 2005;105:372.

LIVER/PANCREATIC FUNCTION TESTS

	FIRST TRIMESTER	SECOND TRIMESTER	THIRD TRIMESTER	TERM
Total alkaline phosphatase (IU/L)	17-88	39-105	46-228	48-249
Gamma glutamyl transferase (IU/L)	2-37	2-43	4-41	5-79
Aspartate transaminase (AST, IU/L)	4-40	10-33	4-32	5-103
Alanine transaminase (ALT, IU/L)	1-32	2-34	2-32	5-115
Total bilirubin (mg/dL)	0.05-1.3	0.1-1.0	0.1-1.2	0.1-1.1
Unconjugated bilirubin (mg/dL)	0.1-0.5	0.1-0.4	0.1-0.5	0.2-0.6
Conjugated bilirubin (mg/dL)	0-0.1	0-0.1	0-0.1	—
Total bile acids (μM/L)	1.7-9.1	1.3-6.7	1.3-8.7	1.8-8.2
Elevated total bile acids (μM/L)	>10	>10	>10	>10
Lactate dehydrogenase (U/L)	78-433	80-447	82-524	—
Amylase (IU/L)	11-97	14-92	14-97	10-82
Lipase (IU/L)	5-109	8-157	21-169	—

Data from Bacq Y, Zarka O, Brechot JF, et al. Liver function tests in normal pregnancy: a prospective study of 103 pregnant women and 103 matched controls. *J Hepatol.* 1996;23:1030; Karensenti D, Bacq Y, Brechot JF, Mariotte N, Vol S, Tichet J. Serum Amylase and lipase activities in normal pregnancy: a prospective case-control study. *Am J Gastroenterol.* 2001;96:697; Larsson A, Palm M, Hansson L-O, Axelsson O. Reference values for clinical chemistry tests during normal pregnancy. *BJOG.* 2008;115:874; Lockitch G. *Handbook of Diagnostic Biochemistry and Hematology in Normal Pregnancy.* Boca Raton, FL: CRC Press; 1993; van Buul EJA, Steegers EAP, Jongsma HW, et al. Haematological and biochemical profile of uncomplicated pregnancy in nulliparous women: a longitudinal study. *Neth J Med.* 1995;46:73; Girling JC, Dow E, Smith JH. Liver function tests in pre-eclampsia: importance of comparison with a reference range derived from normal pregnancy. *BJOG.* 1997;104:246; and Egan N. Reference standard for serum bile acids in pregnancy. *BJOG.* 2012;119;493.

ELECTROLYTES, OSMOLALITY, AND RENAL FUNCTION

	FIRST TRIMESTER	SECOND TRIMESTER	THIRD TRIMESTER	TERM
Total osmolality (mOsm/kg)	267-280	269-289	273-283	271-289
Sodium (mEq/L)	131-139	129-142	127-143	124-141
Potassium (mEq/L)	3.2-4.9	3.3-4.9	3.3-5.2	3.4-5.5
Chloride (mEq/L)	99-108	97-111	97-112	95-111
Bicarbonate (meq/L)	18-26	18-26	17-27	17-25
Urea nitrogen (BUN, mg/dL)	5-14	4-13	3-13	4-15
Creatinine (mg/dL)	0.33-0.80	0.33-0.97	0.3-0.9	0.85-1.1
Serum albumin (g/dL)	3.2-4.7	2.7-4.2	2.3-4.2	2.4-3.9
Uric acid (mg/dL)	1.3-4.2	1.6-5.4	2.0-6.3	2.4-7.2
Urine volume (mL/24 hr)	750-2500	850-2,400	750-2700	550-3900
Creatinine clearance (mL/min)	69-188	55-168	40-192	52-208
Urine protein (mg/24 hr)	19-141	47-186	46-185	—
Urine protein/creatinine ratio (mg/mg); diagnosis of proteinuria	<0.3 Consider 24-hr collection when 0.15 to 0.29	<0.3 Consider 24-hr collection when 0.15 to 0.29	<0.3 Consider 24-hr collection when 0.15 to 0.29	<0.3 Consider 24- hr collection when 0.15 to 0.29

Data from Ezimokhai M, Davison JM, Philips PR, Dunlop W. Non-postural serial changes in renal function during the third trimester of normal human pregnancy. *Br J Obstet Gynaecol.* 1981;88:465; Higby K, Suiter J, Phelps JY, et al. Normal values of urinary albumin and total protein excretion during pregnancy. *Am J Obstet Gynecol.* 1994;171:984; Larsson A, Palm M, Hansson L-O, Axelsson O. Reference values for clinical chemistry tests during normal pregnancy. *BJOG.* 2008;15:874; Lockitch G. *Handbook of Diagnostic Biochemistry and Hematology in Normal Pregnancy.* Boca Raton, FL: CRC Press; 1993; Milman N, Bergholt T, Byg KE, Eriksen L, Hvas AM. Reference intervals for haematologic variables during normal pregnancy and postpartum in 434 healthy Danish women. *Eur J Haematol.* 2007;79:39; van Buul EJ, Steegers EA, Jongsma HW, et al. Haematological and biochemical profile of uncomplicated pregnancy in nulliparous women: a longitudinal study. *Neth J Med.* 1995;46:73; And American College of Obstetricans and Gynecologists. Task Force on Hypertension in Pregnancy, 2013.

CHOLESTEROL AND LIPIDS

	FIRST TRIMESTER	SECOND TRIMESTER	THIRD TRIMESTER	TERM
Total cholesterol (mg/dL)	117-229	136-299	161-349	198-341
HDL (mg/dL)	40-86	48-95	43-92	44-98
LDL (mg/dL)	39-153	41-184	42-224	86-227
VLDL (mg/dL)	10-18	13-23	15-36	25-51
Triglycerides (mg/dL)	11-209	20-293	65-464	103-440

Data from Belo L, Caslake M, Gaffney D, et al. Changes in LDL size and HDL concentration in normal and preeclamptic pregnancies. *Atherosclerois.* 2002;162:425; Desoye G, Schweditsch MO, Pfeiffer KP, Zechner R, Kostner GM. Correlation of hormones with lipid and lipoprotein levels during normal pregnancy and postpartum. *J Clin Endocrinol Metab.* 1987;64:704; Jimenez DM, Pocovi M, Ramon-Cajal J, Romero MA, Martinez H, Grande H. Longitudinal study of plasma lipids and lipoprotein cholesterol in normal pregnancy and puerperium. *Gynecol Obstet Invest.* 1988;25:158; Lain KY, Markovic N, Ness RB, Roberts JM. Effect of smoking on uric acid and other metabolic markers throughout normal pregnancy. *J Clin Endocrinol Metab.* 2005;90:5743; Lockitch G. *Handbook of diagnostic biochemistry and hematology in normal pregnancy.* Boca Raton, FL: CRC Press; 1993.
HDL, high-density lipoprotein; *LDL,* low-density lipoprotein; *TRI,* trimester; *VLDL,* very-low-density lipoprotein.

HEMATOLOGIC INDICES, IRON, AND B$_{12}$

	FIRST TRIMESTER	SECOND TRIMESTER	THIRD TRIMESTER	TERM
White blood cells (10^3/mm^3)	3.9-13.8	4.5-14.8	5.3-16.9	4.2-22.2
Neutrophils (10^3/mm^3)	2.2-8.8	2.9-10.1	3.8-13.1	4.8-12.9
Lymphocytes (10^3/mm^3)	0.4-3.5	0.7-3.9	0.7-3.6	0.9-2.5
Monocytes (10^3/mm^3)	0-1.1	0-1.1	0-1.4	0-0.8
Eosinophils (10^3/mm^3)	0-0.6	0-0.6	0-0.6	—
Basophils (10^3/mm^3)	0-0.1	0-0.1	0-0.1	—
Platelet count (10^9/L)	149-433	135-391	121-429	121-397
Hemoglobin (g/dL)	11.0-14.3	10.5-13.7	11.0-13.8	11.0-14.6
Hematocrit (%)	33-41	32-38	33-40	33-42
Mean cell volume (fL)	81-96	82-97	81-99	82-100
Mean corpuscular hemoglobin (pg)	27-33	—	28-33	28-34
Free erythrocyte protoporphyrin (µg/g)	<3	<3	<3	<3
Ferritin (serum, ng/mL)	10-123	10-101	10-48	10-64
Total iron binding capacity (µg/dL)	246-400	216-400	354-400	317-400
Iron (µg/dL)	40-215	40-220	40-193	40-193
Folate (serum, ng/mL)	2.3-39.3	2.6-15	1.6-40.2	1.7-19.3
Transferrin saturation (%)	>16	>16	>16	>16
B$_{12}$ (pg/mL)	118-438	130-656	99-526	—

Data from American College of Obstetricians and Gynecologists. Anemia in Pregnancy. ACOG Practice Bulletin No. 95. *Obstet Gynecol.* 112:201, 2008; Balloch AJ, Cauchi MN. Reference ranges in haematology parameters in pregnancy derived from patient populations. *Clin Lab Haemetol.* 1993;15:7; Lockitch G. *Handbook of Diagnostic Biochemistry and Hematology in Normal Pregnancy.* Boca Raton, FL: CRC Press; 1993; Malkasian GD, Tauxe WN, Hagedom AB. Total iron binding capacity in normal pregnancy. *J Nuclear Med.* 1964;5:243; Milman N, Agger OA, Nielsen OJ. Iron supplementation during pregnancy. Effect on iron status markers, serum erythropoietin and human placental lactogen. A placebo controlled study in 207 Danish women. *Dan Med Bull.* 1991;38:471; Milman N, Bergholt T, Byg KE, Eriksen L, Hvas AM. Reference intervals for haematologic variables during normal pregnancy and postpartum in 434 healthy Danish women. *Eur J Haematol.* 2007;79:39; Romslo I, Haram K, Sagen N, Augensen K. Iron requirements in normal pregnancy as assessed by serum ferritin, serum transferring saturation and erythrocyte protoporphyrin determinations. *Br J Obstet Gynaecol.* 1983;90:101; Tamura T, Goldenberg RL, Freeberg LE, Cliver SP, Cutter GR, Hoffman HJ. Maternal serum folate and zinc concentrations and their relationship to pregnancy outcome. *Am J Clin Nutr.* 1992;56:365; van Buul EJ, Steegers EA, Jongsma HW, et al. Haematological and biochemical profile of uncomplicated pregnancy in nulliparous women; a longitudinal study. *Neth J Med.* 1995;46:73; Walker MC, Smith GN, Perkins SL, Keely EJ, Garner PR. Changes in homocysteine levels during normal pregnancy. *Am J Obstet Gynecol.* 1999;180:660.

HOMOCYSTEINE, VITAMIN, AND MINERAL LEVELS

	FIRST TRIMESTER	SECOND TRIMESTER	THIRD TRIMESTER	TERM
Homocysteine (µmol/L)	4.1-7.7	3.3-11.0	3.9-11.1	4.7-12.8
Homocysteine (µmol/L), on folate	5.0-7.6	2.9-5.5	3.1-5.8	—
Vitamin D 25(OH)D (ng/mL)	>30	>30	>30	>30
Copper (µg/dL)	69-241	117-253	127-274	163-283
Selenium (µg/L)	98-160	85-164	84-162	84-144
Zinc (µg/dL)	51-101	43-93	41-88	39-71

Data from Izquierdo Alvarez S, Castañón SG, Ruata ML, et al. Updating of normal levels of copper, zinc and selenium in serum of pregnant women. *J Trace Elem Med Biol.* 2007;21:49; Ardawi MS, Nasrat HA, BA'Aqueel HS: Calcium-regulating hormones and parathyroid hormone-related peptide in normal human pregnancy and postpartum: a longitudinal study. *Eur J Endocrinol.* 1997;137:402; Dawson-Hughes B, Heany RP, Holick MF, et al. Estimates of optimal vitamin D status. *Osteopor Int.* 2005;16:713; Lockitch G. *Handbook of Diagnostic Biochemistry and Hematology in Normal Pregnancy.* Boca Raton, FL: CRC Press; 1993; Milman N, Bergholt T, Byg KE, Eriksen L, Hvas AM. Reference intervals for haematologic variables during normal pregnancy and postpartum in 434 healthy Danish women. *Eur J Haematol.* 2007; 79:39; Mimouni F, Tsang RC, Hertzberg VS, Neumann V, Ellis K. Parathyroid hormone and calcitor: changes in normal and insulin dependent diabetic pregnancies. *Obstet Gynecol.* 1989;74:49; Murphy MM, Scott JM, McPartlin JM, Fernandez-Ballart JD: The pregnancy-related decrease in fasting plasma homocysteine is not explained by folic acid supplementation, hemodilution, or a decrease in albumin in a longitudinal study. *Am J Clin Nutr.* 2002;76:614; Qvist I, Abdulla M, Jagerstad M, Svensson S. Iron, zinc and folate status during pregnancy and two months after delivery. *Acta Obstet Gynecol Scand.* 1986;65:15; Walker MC, Smith GN, Perkins SL, Keely EJ, Garner PR. Changes in homocysteine levels during normal pregnancy. *Am J Obstet Gynecol.* 1999;180:660.

CALCIUM METABOLISM

	FIRST TRIMESTER	SECOND TRIMESTER	THIRD TRIMESTER	TERM
Total calcium (mg/dL)	8.5-10.6	7.8-9.4	7.8-9.7	8.1-9.8
Ionized calcium (mg/dL)	4.4-5.3	4.2-5.2	4.4-5.5	4.2-5.4
Parathyroid hormone (pg/mL)	7-15	5-25	5-26	10-17

Data from Ardawi MSM, Nasrat HAN, BA'Aqueel HS. Calcium-regulating hormones and parathyroid hormone-related peptide in normal human pregnancy and postpartum: a longitudinal study. *Eur J Endocrinol.* 1997;137:402; Lockitch G. *Handbook of Diagnostic Biochemistry and Hematology in Normal Pregnancy.* Boca Raton, FL: CRC Press; 1993; Mimouni F, Tsang RC, Hertzberg VS, Neumann V, Ellis K. Parathyroid hormone and calcitrol changes in normal and insulin dependent diabetic pregnancies. *Obstet Gynecol.* 1989;74:49; Pitkin RM, Reynolds WA, Williams GA, Hargis GK. Calcium metabolism in normal pregnancy: a longitudinal study. *Am J Obstet Gynecol.* 1979; 133:781; Seki K, Makimura N, Mitsui C, et al. Calcium-regulating hormones and osteocalcin levels during pregnancy: a longitudinal study. *Am J Obstet Gynecol.* 1991;164:1248.

COAGULATION

	FIRST TRIMESTER	SECOND TRIMESTER	THIRD TRIMESTER	TERM
Prothrombin time (sec)	8.9-12.2	8.6-13.4	8.3-12.9	7.9-12.7
International normalized ratio	0.89-1.05	0.85-0.97	0.81-0.95	0.80-0.94
Partial thromboplastin time (sec)	24.3-38.9	24.2-38.1	23.9-35.0	23.0-34.9
Fibrinogen (mg/dL)	278-676	258-612	276-857	444-670
D-dimer (µg/mL)	0.04-0.50	0.05-2.21	0.16-2.8	—
Antithrombin III (%)	89-112	88-112	81-135	82-138
Antithrombin III deficiency diagnostic criteria	<60%	<60%	<60%	<60%
Protein C, FA (%)	78-121	83-132	73-125	67-120
Protein-C deficiency diagnostic criteria	<60% FA	<60% FA	<60% FA	<60% FA
Protein S, total (%)	39-105	27-101	33-101	—
Protein S, free (%)	34-133	19-113	20-69	37-70
Protein S, FA (%)	57-95	42-68	16-42	—
Protein-S deficiency diagnostic criteria, FA%	NA	<30%	<24%	<24%
Factor II (%)	70-224	73-214	74-179	68-194
Factor V (%)	46-188	66-185	34-195	39-184
Factor VII (%)	60-206	80-280	84-312	87-336
Factor X (%)	62-169	74-177	78-194	72-208
Von Willebrand factor (%)	—	—	121-258	132-260

Data from Cerneca F, Ricci G, Simeone R, et al. Coagulation and fibrinolysis changes in normal pregnancy. Increased levels of procoagulants and reduced levels of inhibitors during pregnancy induce a hypercoagulable state, combined with a reactive fibrinolysis. *Eur J Obstet Gynecol Reprod Biol.* 1997;73:31; Choi JW, Pai SH. Tissue plasminogen activator levels change with plasma fibrinogen concentrations during pregnancy. *Ann Hematol.* 1997;81:611; Faught W, Garner P, Jones G, Ivey B. Changes in protein C and protein S levels in normal pregnancy. *Am J Obstet Gynecol.* 1995;172:147; Francalanci I, Comeglio P, Liotta AA, Cellai AP, Fedi S, Parretti E. D-dimer concentrations during normal pregnancy, as measured by ELISA. *Thromb Res.* 1995;78:399; Lefkowitz JB, Clarke SH, Barbour LA. Comparison of protein S functional and antigenic assays in normal pregnancy. *Am J Obstet Gynecol.* 1996;175:657; Lockitch G. Handbook of diagnostic biochemistry and hematology in normal pregnancy. Boca Raton, FL: CRC Press; 1993; Morse M. Establishing a normal range for d-dimer levels through pregnancy to aid in the diagnosis of pulmonary embolism and deep vein thrombosis. *J Thromb Haemost.* 2004;2:1202; Stirling Y, Woolf L, North WR, Sebhatchian MJ, Meade TW. Haemostasis in normal pregnancy. *Thromb Haemost.* 1984;52:176; Wickstrom K, Edelstam G, Lowbeer CH, Hansson LO, Siegbahn A. Reference intervals for plasma levels of fibroenectin, von Willebrand factor, free protein S and antithrombin during third trimester pregnancy. *Scand J Clin Lab Invest.* 2004;64:31; Inherited thrombophilias in pregnancy. Practice Bulletin No. 138 American College of Obstetricians and Gynecologists. *Obstet Gynecol.* 2013;122:706-717.

FA, functional activity.

INFLAMMATION AND IMMUNE FUNCTION

	FIRST TRIMESTER	SECOND TRIMESTER	THIRD TRIMESTER	TERM
C-reactive protein (mg/L)	0.52-15.5	0.78-16.9	0.44-19.7	—
C3 complement (mg/dL)	44-116	51-119	60-126	64-131
C4 complement (mg/dL)	9-45	10-42	11-43	16-44
Erythrocyte sedimentation rate (mm/h)	4-57	7-83	12-90.5	—
Immunoglobulin A (mg/dL)	21-317	23-343	12-364	14-338
Immunoglobulin G (mg/dL)	838-1410	654-1330	481-1273	554-1162
Immunoglobulin M (mg/dL)	10-309	20-306	0-361	0-320

Data from Saarelainen H, Valtonen P, Punnonen K, et al. Flow mediated vasoldilation and circulating concentrations of high sensitive C-reactive protein, interleukin-6 and tumor necrosis factor-alpha in normal pregnancy—The Cardiovascular Risk in Young Finns Study. *Clin Physiol Funct Imaging.* 2009;29:347; Van den Brock NR, Letsky EA. Pregnancy and the erythrocyte sedimentation rate. *BJOG.* 2001;108:1164; Lockitch G. Handbook of diagnostic biochemistry and hematology in normal pregnancy. Boca Raton, FL: CRC Press; 1993.

ENDOCRINE TESTS

	FIRST TRIMESTER	SECOND TRIMESTER	THIRD TRIMESTER	TERM
Cortisol (µg/dL)	7-23	6-51	12-60	21-64
Aldosterone (ng/dL)	6-104	9-104	15-101	—
Thyroid-stimulating hormone (µIU/mL)	0.1-4.4	0.4-5.0	0.23-4.4	0.0-5.3
Thyroxine, free (ng/dL)	0.7-1.58	0.4-1.4	0.3-1.3	0.3-1.3
Thyroxine, total (µg/dL)	3.6-9.0	4.0-8.9	3.5-8.6	3.9-8.3
Triiodothyronine, free (pg/mL)	2.3-4.4	2.2-4.2	2.1-3.7	2.1-3.5
Triiodothyronine, total (ng/dL)	71-175	84-195	97-182	84-214

Data from Goland R, Jozak S, Conwell I. Placental corticotropin-releasing hormone and the hypercortisolism of pregnancy. *Am J Obstet Gynecol.* 1994;171:1287; Larsson A, Palm M, Hansson L-O, Axelsson O. Reference values for clinical chemistry tests during normal pregnancy. *BJOG.* 2008;15:874; Lockitch G. *Handbook of Diagnostic Biochemistry and Hematology in Normal Pregnancy.* Boca Raton, FL: CRC Press; 1993; Mandel SJ, Spencer CA, Hollowell JG. Are detection and treatment of thyroid insufficiency in pregnancy feasible? *Thyroid.* 2005;15:44; Price A, Obel O, Cresswell J, et al. Comparison of thyroid function in pregnant and non-pregnant Asian and western Caucasian women. *Clin Chim Acta.* 2001;308:91; Bliddal S, Feldt-Rasmussen U, Boas M et al. Gestational-age-specific references ranges from different laboratories misclassifies pregnant women's thyroid status; comparison of two longitudinal prospective cohort studies. *Eur J Endocrinol.* 2013;170;329.

UMBILICAL CORD BLOOD GAS VALUES AND HEMATOLOGIC PARAMETERS*

	ARTERY	VEIN
pH	7.06-7.36	7.14-7.45
PCO_2 (mm Hg)	27.8-68.3	24.0-56.3
PO_2 (mm Hg)	9.8-41.2	12.3-45.0
Base deficit (mmol/L)	0.5-15.3	0.7-12.6
White blood cell count (10^9/L)		11.1-16.2
Red blood cell count (10^{12}/L)		4.13-4.62
Hemoglobin (g/dL)		15.3-17.2
Hematocrit (%)		45.2-50.9
Mean corpuscular volume (fL)		107.4-113.3
Platelet count (10^9/L)		237-321
Reticulocyte count (10^9/L)		145.8-192.6

Data from Eskes TK, Jongsma HW, Houx PC. Percentiles for gas values in human umbilical cord blood. *Eur J Obstet Gynecol Reprod Biol.* 1983;14:341; Mercelina-Roumans P, Breukers R, Ubachs, J, Van Wersch J. Hematological variables in cord blood of neonates of smoking and non-smoking mothers. *J Clin Epidemiol.* 1996;49:449.
*Ranges represent 25th to 75th percentiles.

RELATIONSHIP BETWEEN MEAN AMNIOTIC SAC DIAMETER AND MENSTRUAL AGE

MEAN SAC DIAMETER	PREDICTED AGE (DAYS)	95% CI
2	34.9	34.3-35.5
3	35.8	35.2-36.3
4	36.6	36.1-37.2
5	37.5	37.0-38.0
6	38.4	37.9-38.9
7	39.3	38.9-39.7
8	40.2	39.8-40.6
9	41.1	40.7-41.4
10	41.9	41.6-42.3
11	42.8	42.5-43.2
12	43.7	43.4-44.0
13	44.6	44.3-44.9
14	45.5	45.2-45.8
15	46.3	46.0-46.6
16	47.2	46.9-47.5
17	48.1	47.8-48.4
18	49	48.6-49.4
19	49.9	49.5-50.3
20	50.8	50.3-51.2
21	51.6	51.2-52.1
22	52.5	52.0-53.0
23	53.4	52.9-53.9
24	54.3	53.7-54.8

From Daya S, Wood S, Ward S, et al. Early pregnancy assessment with tranSvaginal ultrasound scanning. *Can Med Assoc J.* 1991;144:444.
CI, confidence interval.

CROWN-RUMP LENGTH (6-18 WEEKS)

CROWN-RUMP LENGTH (MM)	MENSTRUAL AGE (WEEKS)	CROWN-RUMP LENGTH (MM)	MENSTRUAL AGE (WEEKS)	CROWN-RUMP LENGTH (MM)	MENSTRUAL AGE (WEEKS)
1	1	30	10.0	61	12.6
2	2	32	10.1	62	12.6
3	5.9	33	10.2	63	12.7
4	6.1	34	10.3	64	12.8
5	6.2	35	10.4	65	12.8
6	6.4	36	10.5	66	12.9
7	6.6	37	10.6	67	13.0
8	6.7	38	10.7	68	13.1
9	6.9	39	10.8	69	13.1
10	7.1	40	10.9	70	13.2
11	7.2	41	11.0	71	13.3
12	7.4	42	11.1	72	13.4
13	7.5	43	11.2	73	13.4
14	7.7	44	11.2	74	13.5
15	7.9	45	11.3	75	13.6
16	8.0	46	11.4	76	13.7
17	8.1	47	11.5	77	13.7
18	8.3	48	11.6	78	13.8
19	8.4	49	11.7	79	13.9
20	8.6	50	11.7	80	14.0
21	8.7	51	11.8	81	14.1
22	8.9	52	11.9	82	14.2
23	9.0	53	12.0	83	14.2
24	9.1	54	12.0	84	14.3
25	9.2	55	12.1	85	14.4
26	9.4	56	12.2	86	14.5
27	9.5	57	12.3	87	14.6
28	9.6	58	12.3	88	14.7
29	9.7	59	12.4	89	14.8
30	9.9	60	12.5	90	14.9

From Hadlock FP, Shah YP, Kanon DJ, Lindsey JV. Fetal crown-rump length: reevaluation of relation to menstrual age (5-18 weeks) with high-resolution real-time US *Radiology*. 1992;182:501.

HEAD CIRCUMFERENCE

MENSTRUAL AGE (WEEKS)	HEAD CIRCUMFERENCE (CM)				
	3rd	10th	50th	90th	97th
14.0	8.8	9.1	9.7	10.3	10.6
15.0	10.0	10.4	11.0	11.6	12.0
16.0	11.3	11.7	12.4	13.1	13.5
17.0	12.6	13.0	13.8	14.6	15.0
18.0	13.7	14.2	15.1	16.0	16.5
19.0	14.9	15.5	16.4	17.4	17.9
20.0	16.1	16.7	17.7	18.7	19.3
21.0	17.2	17.8	18.9	20.0	20.6
22.0	18.3	18.9	20.12	21.3	21.9
23.0	19.4	20.1	21.3	22.5	23.2
24.0	20.4	21.1	22.4	23.7	24.3
25.0	21.4	22.2	23.5	24.9	25.6
26.0	22.4	23.2	24.6	26.0	26.8
27.0	23.3	24.1	25.6	27.0	27.9
28.0	24.2	25.1	26.6	28.1	29.0
29.0	25.0	25.9	27.5	29.1	30.0
30.0	25.8	26.8	28.4	30.0	31.0
31.0	26.7	27.6	29.3	31.0	31.9
32.0	27.4	28.4	30.1	31.8	32.8
33.0	28.0	29.0	30.8	32.6	33.6
34.0	28.7	29.7	31.5	33.3	34.3
35.0	29.3	30.4	32.2	34.1	35.1
36.0	29.9	30.9	32.8	34.7	35.8
37.0	30.3	31.4	33.3	35.2	36.3
38.0	30.8	31.9	33.8	35.8	36.8
39.0	31.1	32.2	34.2	36.2	37.3
40.0	31.5	32.6	34.6	36.6	37.7

From Hadlock FP, Deter RL, Harrist RB, Park SK. Estimating fetal age: computer-assisted analysis of multiple fetal growth parameters. *Radiology*. 1984;152:497.

ABDOMINAL CIRCUMFERENCE

MENSTRUAL AGE (WEEKS)	ABDOMINAL CIRCUMFERENCE (CM)				
	3rd	10th	50th	90th	97th
14.0	6.4	6.7	7.3	7.9	8.3
15.0	7.5	7.9	8.6	9.3	9.7
16.0	8.6	9.1	9.9	10.7	11.2
17.0	9.7	10.3	11.2	12.1	12.7
18.0	10.9	11.5	12.5	13.5	14.1
19.0	11.9	12.6	13.7	14.8	15.5
20.0	13.1	13.8	15.0	16.3	17.0
21.0	14.1	14.9	16.2	17.6	18.3
22.0	15.1	16.0	17.4	18.8	19.7
23.0	16.1	17.0	18.5	20.0	20.9
24.0	17.1	18.1	19.7	21.3	22.3
25.0	18.1	19.1	20.8	22.5	23.5
26.0	19.1	20.1	21.9	23.87	24.8
27.0	20.0	21.1	23.0	24.9	26.0
28.0	20.9	22.0	24.0	26.0	27.1
29.0	21.8	23.0	25.1	27.2	28.4
30.0	22.7	23.9	26.1	28.3	29.5
31.0	23.6	24.9	27.1	29.4	30.6
32.0	24.5	25.8	28.1	30.4	31.8
33.0	25.3	26.7	29.1	31.5	32.9
34.0	26.1	27.5	30.0	32.5	33.9
35.0	26.9	28.3	30.9	33.5	34.9
36.0	27.7	29.2	31.8	34.4	35.9
37.0	28.5	30.0	32.7	35.4	37.0
38.0	29.2	30.8	33.6	36.4	38.0
39.0	29.9	31.6	34.4	37.3	38.9
40.0	30.7	32.4	35.3	38.2	39.9

From Hadlock FP, Deter RL, Harrist RB, Park SK. Estimating fetal age: computer-assisted analysis of multiple fetal growth parameters. *Radiology*. 1984;152:497.

FEMUR LENGTH

GESTATIONAL AGE (WEEKS)	FEMUR (MM)		
	5th	50th	95th
12	3.9	8.1	12.3
13	6.8	11.0	15.2
14	9.7	13.9	18.1
15	12.6	16.8	21.0
16	15.4	19.7	23.9
17	18.3	22.5	26.8
18	21.1	25.4	29.7
19	23.9	28.2	32.6
20	26.7	31.0	35.4
21	29.4	33.8	38.2
22	32.1	36.5	40.9
23	34.7	39.2	43.6
24	37.4	41.8	46.3
25	39.9	44.4	48.9
26	42.4	46.9	51.4
27	44.9	49.4	53.9
28	47.3	51.8	56.4
29	49.6	54.2	58.7
30	51.8	56.4	61.0
31	54.0	58.6	63.2
32	56.1	60.7	65.4
33	58.1	62.7	67.4
34	60.0	64.7	69.4
35	61.8	66.5	71.2
36	63.5	68.3	73.0
37	65.1	69.9	74.7
38	66.6	71.4	76.2
39	68.0	72.8	77.7
40	69.3	74.2	79.0

From Jeanty P, Cousaert E, Cantaine F, et al. A longitudinal study of fetal limb growth. *Am J Perinatol.* 1984;1:136.

HUMERUS LENGTH

GESTATIONAL AGE (WEEKS)	HUMERUS (MM)		
	5th	50th	95th
12	4.8	8.6	12.3
13	7.6	11.4	15.1
14	10.3	14.1	17.9
15	13.1	16.9	20.7
16	15.8	19.7	23.5
17	21.2	22.4	26.3
18	23.8	25.1	29.0
19	26.3	27.7	31.6
20	28.8	30.3	34.2
21	31.2	32.8	36.7
22	33.5	35.2	39.2
23	33.5	37.5	41.6
24	35.7	39.8	43.8
25	37.9	41.9	46.0
26	39.9	44.0	48.1
27	41.9	46.0	50.1
28	43.7	47.9	52.0
29	45.5	49.7	53.9
30	47.2	51.4	55.6
31	48.9	53.1	57.3
32	50.4	54.7	58.9
33	52.0	56.2	60.5
34	53.4	57.7	62.0
35	54.8	59.2	63.5
36	56.2	60.6	64.9
37	57.6	62.0	66.4
38	59.0	63.4	67.8
39	60.4	64.8	69.3
40	61.9	66.3	70.8

From Jeanty P, Cousaert E, Cantaine F, Hobbins JC, Tack B, et al. A longitudinal study of fetal limb growth. *Am J Perinatol.* 1984;1:136.

TIBIA LENGTH

GESTATIONAL AGE (WEEKS)	TIBIA (MM)		
	5th	50th	95th
12	3.3	8.2	11.2
13	5.6	9.6	13.6
14	8.1	12.0	16.0
15	10.6	14.6	18.6
16	13.1	17.1	21.2
17	15.6	19.7	23.8
18	18.2	22.3	26.4
19	20.8	24.9	29.0
20	23.3	27.5	31.6
21	25.8	30.0	34.2
22	28.3	32.5	36.7
23	30.7	34.9	39.1
24	33.1	37.3	41.6
25	35.4	39.7	43.9
26	37.6	41.9	46.2
27	39.8	44.1	48.4
28	41.9	46.2	50.5
29	43.9	48.2	52.6
30	45.8	50.1	54.5
31	47.6	52.0	56.4
32	49.4	53.8	58.2
33	51.1	55.5	60.0
34	52.7	57.2	61.6
35	54.2	58.7	63.2
36	41.2	60.3	64.8
37	55.8	61.8	66.3
38	58.7	63.2	67.8
39	60.1	64.7	69.3
40	61.5	66.1	70.7

From Jeanty P, Cousaert E, Cantaine F, et al. A longitudinal study of fetal limb growth. *Am J Perinatol.* 1984;1:136.

FIBULA LENGTH

GESTATIONAL AGE (WEEKS)	FIBULA (MM)		
	5th	50th	95th
12	1.7	5.7	9.6
13	4.7	8.7	12.7
14	7.7	11.7	15.6
15	10.6	14.6	18.6
16	13.3	17.4	21.4
17	16.1	20.1	24.2
18	18.7	22.8	26.9
19	21.3	25.4	29.5
20	23.8	27.9	32.0
21	26.2	30.3	34.5
22	28.5	32.7	36.9
23	30.8	35.0	39.2
24	33.0	37.2	41.5
25	35.1	39.4	43.6
26	37.2	41.5	45.7
27	39.2	43.5	47.8
28	41.1	45.4	49.7
29	42.9	47.2	51.6
30	44.7	49.0	53.4
31	46.3	50.7	55.1
32	47.9	52.4	56.8
33	49.5	53.9	58.4
34	50.9	55.4	59.9
35	52.3	56.8	61.3
36	53.6	58.2	62.7
37	54.9	59.4	64.0
38	56.0	60.6	65.2
39	57.1	61.7	66.3
40	58.1	62.8	67.4

From Exacoustos C, Rosati P, Rizzo G, Arduini D. Ultrasound measurements of fetal limb bones. *Ultrasound Obstet Gynecol.* 1991;1:325.

RADIUS LENGTH

GESTATIONAL AGE (WEEKS)	RADIUS (MM)		
	5th	50th	95th
12	3.0	6.9	10.8
13	5.6	9.5	13.4
14	8.1	12.0	16.0
15	10.5	14.5	18.5
16	12.9	16.9	20.9
17	15.2	19.3	23.3
18	17.5	21.5	25.6
19	19.7	23.8	27.9
20	21.8	25.9	30.0
21	23.9	28.0	32.2
22	25.9	30.1	34.2
23	27.9	32.0	36.2
24	29.7	34.0	38.2
25	31.6	35.8	40.0
26	33.3	37.6	41.9
27	35.0	39.3	43.6
28	36.7	41.0	45.3
29	38.3	42.6	46.9
30	39.8	44.1	48.5
31	41.2	45.6	50.0
32	42.6	47.0	51.4
33	44.0	48.4	52.8
34	45.2	49.7	54.1
35	46.4	50.9	55.4
36	47.6	52.1	56.6
37	48.7	53.2	57.7
38	49.7	54.2	58.8
39	50.6	55.2	59.8
40	51.5	56.2	60.8

From Exacoustos C, Rosati P, Rizzo G, Arduini D. Ultrasound measurements of fetal limb bones. *Ultrasound Obstet Gynecol.* 1991;1:325.

ULNA LENGTH

GESTATIONAL AGE (WEEKS)	ULNA (MM)		
	5th	50th	95th
12	2.9	6.8	10.7
13	5.8	9.7	13.7
14	8.6	12.6	16.6
15	11.4	15.4	19.4
16	14.1	18.1	22.1
17	16.7	20.8	24.8
18	19.3	23.3	27.4
19	21.8	25.8	29.9
20	24.2	28.3	32.4
21	26.5	30.6	34.8
22	28.7	32.9	37.1
23	30.9	35.1	39.3
24	33.0	37.2	41.5
25	35.1	39.3	43.5
26	37.0	41.3	45.6
27	38.9	43.2	47.5
28	40.7	45.0	49.3
29	42.5	46.8	51.1
30	44.1	48.5	52.8
31	45.7	50.1	54.5
32	47.2	51.6	56.1
33	48.7	53.1	57.5
34	50.0	54.5	59.0
35	51.3	55.8	60.3
36	52.6	57.1	61.6
37	53.7	58.2	62.8
38	54.8	59.3	63.9
39	55.8	60.4	64.9
40	56.7	61.3	65.9

From Jeanty P, Cousaert E, Cantaine F, et al. A longitudinal study of fetal limb growth. *Am J Perinatol.* 1984;1:136.

FOOT LENGTH

GESTATIONAL AGE (WEEKS)	−2 SD (MM)	MEAN (PREDICTED) (MM)	+2 SD (MM)
12	7	8	9
13	10	11	12
14	13	15	16
15	16	18	20
16	19	21	23
17	22	24	27
18	24	27	30
19	27	30	34
20	30	33	37
21	32	36	40
22	35	39	43
23	37	42	46
24	40	45	50
25	42	47	53
26	45	50	55
27	47	53	58
28	49	55	61
29	51	58	64
30	54	60	67
31	56	62	68
32	58	65	72
33	60	67	74
34	62	69	77
35	64	71	79
36	66	74	82
37	67	76	84
38	69	78	86
39	71	80	88
40	72	81	90

From Mercer BM, Sklar S, Shariatmadar A, Gillieson MS, D'Alton ME. Fetal foot length as a predictor of gestation age. *Am J Obstet Gynecol.* 1987;156:350.
SD, standard deviation.

TRANSCEREBELLAR DIAMETER

AGE (WEEKS)	PERCENTILE VALUES (MM)					MEAN	SD
	5th	10th	50th	90th	95th		
15	14.2	14.5	15.8	17.1	17.4	14.6	1.4
16	14.6	15.0	16.5	17.9	18.3	16.1	1.0
17	15.2	15.6	17.3	18.9	19.3	17.1	1.0
18	15.9	16.4	18.2	19.9	20.5	18.3	1.2
19	16.8	17.3	19.2	21.1	21.7	19.4	1.1
20	17.7	18.3	20.4	22.4	23.0	20.3	1.2
21	18.8	19.4	21.6	23.8	24.5	21.4	1.3
22	19.9	20.5	23.0	25.3	26.0	22.8	1.8
23	21.2	21.8	24.4	26.8	27.6	24.3	1.6
24	22.5	23.2	25.9	28.5	29.3	25.9	1.7
25	23.9	24.6	27.4	30.2	31.0	27.6	1.6
26	25.3	26.0	29.1	31.9	32.8	29.1	1.8
27	26.7	27.6	30.7	33.8	34.7	30.8	1.7
28	28.2	29.1	32.4	35.6	36.6	32.5	1.8
29	29.8	30.7	34.2	35.6	36.6	32.5	1.7
30	31.3	32.2	35.9	39.5	40.6	36.0	2.2
31	32.8	33.8	37.7	41.5	42.6	37.8	2.4
32	34.4	35.4	39.5	43.4	44.7	39.2	2.4
33	35.9	37.0	41.3	45.4	46.7	41.4	2.6
34	37.3	38.5	43.1	47.4	48.8	42.9	2.7
35	38.8	40.0	44.8	49.5	50.9	44.7	3.0
36	40.1	41.4	46.5	51.4	53.0	46.6	3.4
37	41.4	42.8	48.2	53.4	55.0	48.0	3.2
38	42.7	44.1	49.9	55.4	57.1	49.8	3.3

From Chavez MR, Ananth CV, Smulian JC, Lashley S, Kontopoulos EV, Vintzileos AM. Fetal transcerebellar diameter nomogram in singleton gestations with special emphasis in the third trimester: a ccomparison with previously published nomograms. *Am J Obstet Gynecol.* 2003;189:1021.
SD, standard deviation.

AMNIOTIC FLUID INDEX

GESTATIONAL AGE (WEEKS)	2.5TH	5TH	50TH	95TH	97.5TH
16	73	79	121	185	201
17	77	83	128	194	211
18	80	87	133	202	220
19	83	90	138	207	225
20	86	93	141	212	230
21	88	95	144	214	233
22	89	97	146	216	235
23	90	98	147	218	237
24	90	98	148	219	238
25	89	97	148	221	240
26	89	97	148	223	242
27	85	95	148	226	245
28	86	94	148	228	249
29	84	92	147	231	254
30	82	90	147	234	258
31	79	88	146	238	263
32	77	86	146	242	269
33	64	83	145	245	274
34	72	81	144	248	278
35	70	79	142	249	279
36	68	77	140	249	279
37	66	75	138	244	275
38	65	73	134	239	269
39	64	72	130	226	255
40	63	71	125	214	240
41	63	70	119	194	216
42	63	69	112	175	192

From Moore TR, Gayle JE. The amniotic fluid index in normal human pregnancy. *Am J Obstet Gynecol.* 1990;162:1168.

SMALL HEAD CIRCUMFERENCE MEASUREMENTS

AGE (WEEKS)	−2 SD	−3 SD	−4 SD	−5 SD
20	145	131	116	101
21	157	143	128	113
22	169	154	140	125
23	180	166	151	136
24	191	177	162	147
25	202	188	173	158
26	213	198	183	169
27	223	208	194	179
28	233	218	203	189
29	242	227	213	198
30	251	236	222	207
31	260	245	230	216
32	268	253	239	224
33	276	261	246	232
34	283	268	253	239
35	289	275	260	245
36	295	281	266	251
37	301	286	272	257
38	306	291	276	262
39	310	295	281	266
40	314	299	284	270

From Chervenak FA, Jeanty P, Cantraine F, et al. The diagnosis of fetal microcephaly. *Am J Obstet Gynecol.* 1984;149:512.
SD, standard deviation.

UMBILICAL ARTERY RESISTANCE INDEX AND SYSTOLIC/DIASTOLIC RATIO

GA (WEEKS)	5TH PERCENTILE			50TH PERCENTILE			95TH PERCENTILE		
	S/D	PI	RI	S/D	PI	RI	S/D	PI	RI
19	2.93	1.02	0.66	4.28	1.3	0.77	6.73	1.66	0.88
20	2.83	0.99	0.65	4.11	1.27	0.75	6.43	1.62	0.87
21	2.7	0.95	0.64	3.91	1.22	0.74	6.09	1.58	0.85
22	2.6	0.92	0.62	3.77	1.19	0.73	5.85	1.54	0.84
23	2.51	0.89	0.61	3.62	1.15	0.72	5.61	1.5	0.83
24	2.41	0.86	0.6	3.48	1.12	0.71	5.38	1.47	0.82
25	2.33	0.83	0.58	3.35	1.09	0.69	5.18	1.44	0.81
26	2.24	0.8	0.57	3.23	1.06	0.68	5	1.41	0.8
27	2.17	0.77	0.56	3.12	1.03	0.67	4.83	1.38	0.79
28	2.09	0.75	0.55	3.02	1	0.66	4.67	1.35	0.78
29	2.03	0.72	0.53	2.92	0.98	0.65	4.53	1.32	0.77
30	1.96	0.7	0.52	2.83	0.95	0.64	4.4	1.29	0.76
31	1.9	0.68	0.51	2.75	0.93	0.63	4.27	1.27	0.76
32	1.84	0.66	0.5	2.67	0.9	0.61	4.16	1.25	0.75
33	1.79	0.64	0.48	2.6	0.88	0.6	4.06	1.22	0.74
34	1.73	0.62	0.47	2.53	0.86	0.59	3.96	1.2	0.73
35	1.68	0.6	0.46	2.46	0.84	0.58	3.86	1.18	0.72
36	1.64	0.58	0.45	2.4	0.82	0.57	3.78	1.16	0.71
37	1.59	0.56	0.43	2.34	0.8	0.56	3.69	1.14	0.7
38	1.55	0.55	0.42	2.28	0.78	0.55	3.62	1.12	0.7
39	1.51	0.53	0.41	2.23	0.76	0.54	3.54	1.1	0.69
40	1.47	0.51	0.4	2.18	0.75	0.53	3.48	1.09	0.68
41	1.43	0.5	0.39	2.13	0.73	0.52	3.41	1.07	0.67

From Acharya G, Wilsgaard T, Berntsen GK, Maltau JM, Kiserud T. Reference ranges for serial measurements of the umbilical artery Doppler indices in the second half of pregnancy. *Am J Ob Gyn.* 2005;192:937-944.
GA, gestational age; PI, pulsatility index; RI, resistance index; S/D, systolic/diastolic.

MIDDLE CEREBRAL ARTERY PULSATILITY INDEX

AGE (WEEKS)	5TH	10TH	50TH	90TH	95TH
21	1.18	1.26	1.6	2.04	2.19
22	1.25	1.33	1.69	0.15	2.30
23	1.32	1.41	1.78	2.25	2.41
24	1.38	1.47	1.86	2.36	2.52
25	1.44	1.54	1.94	2.45	2.62
26	1.50	1.6	2.01	2.53	2.71
27	1.55	1.65	2.06	2.60	2.78
28	1.58	1.69	2.11	2.66	2.84
29	1.61	1.71	2.15	2.70	2.88
30	1.62	1.73	2.16	2.72	2.90
31	1.62	1.73	2.16	2.71	2.90
32	1.61	1.71	2.14	2.69	2.87
33	1.58	1.68	2.10	2.64	2.82
34	1.53	1.63	2.04	2.57	2.74
35	1.47	1.56	1.96	2.47	2.64
36	1.39	1.48	1.86	2.36	2.52
37	1.30	1.39	1.75	2.22	2.38
38	1.20	1.29	1.63	2.07	2.22
39	1.1	1.18	1.49	1.91	2.05

From Ebbing C, Rasmussen S, Kiserud T. Middle cerebral artery blood flow velocities and pulsatility index and the cerebroplacental pulsatility ratio: longitudinal reference ranges and terms for serial measurements. *Ultrasound Obstet Gynecol.* 2007;30:287.

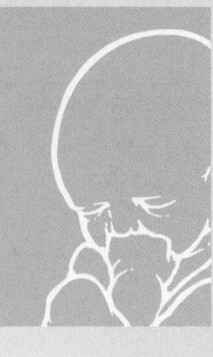

Anatomy of the Pelvis*

STEVEN G. GABBE

KEY POINTS

- To facilitate childbearing, the female pelvis—as opposed to the male pelvis—is characterized by a wider subpubic angle, increased width of the sciatic notch, and greater distance from the symphysis pubis to the anterior edge of the acetabulum.
- The levator ani, the major supporting structure for the pelvic viscera, is a tripartite muscle mass composed of the iliococcygeus, pubococcygeus, and puborectalis; the iliococcygeus is the broadest and most posterior portion.
- Innervation of the levator ani is through the third and fourth sacral nerves.
- The major nerve supply of the perineum is derived from the pudendal nerve. However, the ilioinguinal, genitofemoral, perineal branch of the posterior femoral cutaneous, coccygeal, and last sacral nerve also contribute; thus a pudendal nerve block anesthetizes only a portion of the perineum.
- The internal iliac (hypogastric) artery arises at the level of lumbosacral articulation. It can be distinguished from the external iliac by its smaller size and by its more medial and more posterior position.
- The ureter lies more superficially and is either medial or slightly anterior to the internal iliac artery.
- The cardinal ligaments are located at the base of the broad ligament and are continuous with the connective tissue of the parametrium; they are attached to the pelvic diaphragm through continuity with the superficial superior fascia of the levator ani.
- Because the origin of the uterine artery is variable, its isolation and ligation for control of postpartum bleeding are often fruitless. The uterine artery usually arises as an independent vessel from the internal iliac artery, but it may also arise from the inferior gluteal, internal pudendal, umbilical, or obturator arteries.
- Afferent pain fibers for the uterus, tubes, and ovary enter the cord at T10, T11, and T12; thus spinal or epidural anesthesia must extend to these levels. Fortunately, efferent fibers to the uterus enter above these levels and thus do not interfere with contractions.
- The body of the nonpregnant uterus weighs approximately 70 g, whereas at term it weighs approximately 1100 g.

SUGGESTED READING

1. Moore KL, Dalley AF 2nd. Pelvis and perineum. In: *Clinically Oriented Anatomy*. 6th ed. Baltimore: Lippincott Williams & Wilkins; 2009:326.

*Figures for Appendix II are available at ExpertConsult.com.

Glossary of Key Abbreviations

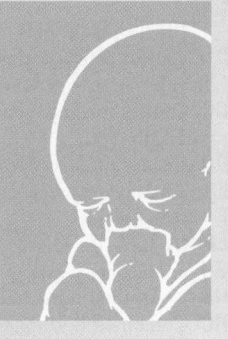

1 Gray 100 cGy or 100 rads
1,25[OH]₂D₃ 1,25-Dihydroxyvitamin D
11β-HSD1 11-β-Hydroxysteroid dehydrogenase type 1
11β-HSD2 11-β-Hydroxysteroid dehydrogenase type 2
17-OH-P 17 α–hydroxyprogesterone caproate
2,3-DPG 2,3-Diphosphoglycerate
3-D Three dimensional
3β-HSD 3β-Hydroxysteroid dehydrogenase (type 1)
3TC Lamivudine
AA Arterioarterial
AABB American Association of Blood Banks
AACE American Association of Clinical Endocrinologists
AAN American Academy of Neurology
AAP American Academy of Pediatrics
aβ2–GP-I Anti-β2–glycoprotein I (antibodies)
AC Abdominal circumference
ACC American College of Cardiology
ACE Angiotensin-converting enzyme
ACEI Angiotensin-converting enzyme inhibitor
AchE Acetylcholinesterase
ACHOIS Australian Carbohydrate Intolerance Study in Pregnant Women Trial Group
ACIP Advisory Committee on Immunization Practices
aCL Anticardiolipin antibodies
ACLS Advanced cardiovascular life support
ACMG American College of Medical Genetics and Genomics
ACNM American College of Nurse Midwives
ACOG American College of Obstetricians and Gynecologists
ACR American College of Rheumatology
ACTG AIDS Clinical Trials Group
ACTH Adrenocorticotropic hormone
AD Abdominal diameter; aortic diameter; atopic dermatitis
ADA American Diabetes Association
ADAMTS-13 von Willebrand cleaving enzyme
ADFLE Autosomal-dominant frontal lobe epilepsy
ADHD Attention-deficit/hyperactivity disorder
ADO Allele dropout
ADP Adenosine diphosphate
ADTLE Autosomal-dominant temporal lobe epilepsy
AED Antiepileptic drug

AEDV Absent end-diastolic velocity
AEP Atopic eruption of pregnancy
AF Amniotic fluid
AFI Amniotic fluid index
AFLP Acute fatty liver of pregnancy
AFP Alpha-fetoprotein
AFV Amniotic fluid volume
AGA Appropriate for gestational age
AHA American Heart Association
AHRQ Agency for Healthcare Quality and Research
AIDS Acquired immunodeficiency syndrome
AII Angiotension II
AIP Acute intermittent porphyria
AIUM American Institute of Ultrasound in Medicine
ALARA As low as reasonably achievable
ALL Acute lymphoblastic leukemia
ALT Alanine aminotransferase
AMA Advanced maternal age
AML Acute myeloid leukemia
AMP Adenosine monophosphate
α-MSH α-Melanocyte–stimulating hormone
AN Anorexia nervosa
ANA Antinuclear antibodies
ANF Atrial natriuretic factor
ANLL Acute nonlymphocytic leukemia
ANP Atrial natriuretic peptide
AP Anteroposterior
APA Antiphospholipid antibody
APC Activated protein C; antigen-presenting cells
APE Acute pulmonary embolus
APGO Association of Professors of Gynecology and Obstetrics
APOE Apolipoprotein E
APR Australian Register of Antiepileptic Drugs in Pregnancy
APS Antiphospholipid syndrome
aPTT Activated partial thromboplastin time
ARDS Acute respiratory distress syndrome; adult respiratory distress syndrome
ARF Acute renal failure
ART Assisted reproductive technology
ARV Antiretroviral
ASA American Society of Anesthesiologists
ASB Asymptomatic bacteriuria
ASD Autism spectrum disorder
AST Aspartate aminotransferase
ATA American Thyroid Association
ATD Antithyroid drugs
ATP Adenosine triphosphate

AV Arteriovenous; atrioventricular
AVM Arteriovenous malformation
AVP Arginine vasopressin
AWHONN Association of Women's Health, Obstetric and Neonatal Nurses
AZA Azathioprine
AZT Azidothymidine
BAFF B-cell activating factor of the tumor necrosis factor family
BCG Bacille Calmette-Guérin
BCR B-cell receptor
BD Bipolar disorder
BDMS Birth defect monitoring system
BFHI Baby-Friendly Hospital Initiative
β-hCG β-human chorionic gonadotropin
BiPAP Bilevel Positive Airway Pressure
BLS Basic life support
BMD Bone mineral density
BMI Body mass index
BN Bulimia nervosa
BNP β-natriuretic peptide; B-type natriuretic peptide; brain natriuretic peptide
BP Blood pressure
BPA Biphenyl A, bisphenol A
BPD Biparietal diameter; bronchopulmonary dysplasia
BPP Biophysical profile
BPS Biophysical profile score
BREG Regulatory B cells
BSA Body surface area
BUN Biochemistry, ultrasound, nuchal translucency; blood urea nitrogen
BV Bacterial vaginosis
C/D Concentration/dose (ratio)
cAMP Cyclic adenosine monophosphate
CA-MRSA Community-acquired methicillin-resistant *Staphylococcus aureus*
CAPS Catastrophic antiphospholipid syndrome
cART Combination antiretroviral therapy
CAT Computed axial tomography
CBAVD Congenital bilateral absence of the vas deferens
CBG Corticosteroid-binding globulin
CBT Cognitive behavioral therapy
CBZ Carbamazepine
ccffDNA Circulating cell-free fetal DNA
CCL2 Monocyte chemotactic protein 1 (MCP-1)
CCL5 Chemokine (C-C motif) ligand 5
CCR CC receptor
CCR5 Chemokine (C-C motif) receptor type 5
cCTG Computerized cardiotocography

CD Cesarean delivery; cluster of differentiation; Crohn disease
CDC Centers for Disease Control and Prevention
CDD Cesarean delivery defect
CEA Carcinoembryonic antigen
CF Cystic fibrosis
CcfDNA Cell-free DNA
CGH Comparative genome hybridization
CHB Congenital heart block
CHC Combined hormonal contraception
CHD Congenital heart disease
CHP Catholic Healthcare Partners
CI Cardiac index; cervical insufficiency; confidence interval
CIITA Class II transactivator
CIN Cervical intraepithelial neoplasia
CL Cervical length
CLD Chronic lung disease
CLIP Corticotropin-like intermediate lobe peptide
CMA Chromosomal microarray analysis
CMACE Centre for Maternal and Child Enquiries
CML Chronic myelocytic leukemia
CMQCC California Maternal Quality Care Collaborative
CMV Cytomegalovirus
CMZ Carbimazole
CNFA Clinically nonfunctioning adenoma
CNS Central nervous system
CNV Copy number variant
CO Cardiac output
CO$_2$ Carbon dioxide
COC Combination oral contraceptive
COP Colloidal oncotic pressure
COX Cyclooxygenase
CP Cerebral palsy
CPAM Congenital pulmonary adenomatoid malformation
CPAP Continuous positive airway pressure
CPD Cephalopelvic disproportion
CPM Confined placental mosaicism
CPR Cerebroplacental Doppler ratio; contraceptive prevalence rate
CPT Current procedural terminology
CrCl Creatinine clearance
CRF Corticotropin-releasing factor
CRH Corticotropin-releasing hormone
CRL Crown-rump length
CRM Crew resource management
CRP C-reactive protein
CRS Congenital rubella syndrome
CS Cesarean section
CSE Combined spinal-epidural
CSF Cerebrospinal fluid
CSII Continuous subcutaneous insulin infusion (pump therapy)
CSL Consortium on Safe Labor
CST Contraction stress test
CT Computed tomography
CTA Computer tomography angiography
CTPA Computed tomography pulmonary angiography
CVP Central venous pressure
CVS Chorionic villus sampling; congenital varicella syndrome
CVT Cerebral vein thrombosis

CXCR C-X-C receptor
CXCR4 C-X-C chemokine receptor type 4
DAT Direct amplification test
DC Dendritic cell; dichorionic
DCC Delayed cord clamping
dDAVP Desmopressin
DES Diethylstilbestrol
DFA Direct fluorescence assays
DHA Dehydroepiandrosterone; docosahexaenoic acid
DHEAS Dehydroepiandrosterone sulfate
DI Diabetes insipidus; disposition index
DIC Disseminated intravascular coagulation
DKA Diabetic ketoacidosis
DMA Disease modifying agent
DMPA Depot medroxyprogesterone acetate
DNA Deoxyribonucleic acid
dNK Decidual natural killer cell
DOC Deoxycorticosterone
DPG Diphosphoglycerate; diphosphatidylglycerol
DPI Dry-powder inhaler
DPPC Dipalmitoylphosphatidylcholine
DRI Daily recommended intake; dietary reference index
DSM *Diagnostic and Statistical Manual of Mental Disorders*
DTC Direct to consumer
DV Ductus venosus
DVP Deepest vertical pocket
DVT Deep venous thrombosis
DZ Dizygotic
EA Early amniocentesis
EASI Extraamniotic saline infusion
EB Elementary bodies
EBV Epstein-Barr virus
EC Emergency contraception
ECC Exocoelomic cavity
ECG Electrocardiogram
ECT Electroconvulsive therapy
ECV External cephalic version
ED Effective dose
EDC Endocrine disrupter chemical; estimated date of confinement
EDD Estimated delivery date
EDSS Expanded disability status scale
EEG Electroencephalogram
EF Ejection fraction
EFM Electronic fetal heart rate monitoring
EFV Efavirenz
EFW Estimated fetal weight
EGD Esophagogastroduodenoscopy
EGF Epidermal growth factor
EGF-R Epidermal growth factor receptor
EGFR Estimated glomerular filtration rate
EI Erythema infectiosum
EIA Enzyme immunoassay
EIAED Enzyme-inducing antiepileptic drug
ELBW Extremely low birthweight
ELISA Enzyme-linked immunosorbent assay
EMA European Medicine Agency
EMG Electromyography
EMR Electronic medical record
EP Ectopic pregnancy
EPA Eicosapentaenoic acid
EPDS Edinburgh Postnatal Depression Scale
EPO Erythropoietin
ER Estrogen receptor

ERCP Endoscopic retrograde cholangiopancreatography
ES Endocrine Society
ESC Embryonic stem cell
ESR Erythrocyte sedimentation rate
ESRD End-stage renal disease
ETG Etonogestrel
EXIT Ex utero intrapartum treatment
FAC Fetal activity count
FAS Fetal alcohol syndrome
FASD Fetal alcohol spectrum disorder
FasL Fas ligand
FAST Focused abdominal sonography for trauma
FASTER First- and Second-Trimester Evaluation of Risk Research Consortium
FBM Fetal breathing movement
FBS Fetal blood sampling
FDA U.S. Food and Drug Administration
FDC Fixed-dose combination
FEV$_1$ Forced expiratory volume in 1 second
FFA Free fatty acid
fFN Fetal fibronectin
FFP Fresh frozen plasma
FGM/C Female genital mutilation/cutting
FGR Fetal growth restriction
FHH Familial hypocalciuric hypercalcemia
FHR Fetal heart rate
FIGO International Federation of Gynecology and Obstetrics
FIHPT Familial isolated primary hyperparathyroidism
FIRS Fetal inflammatory response syndrome
FISH Fluorescence in situ hybridization
FL Femur length
FMC Fetal movement counting
FMH Fetomaternal hemorrhage
FNA Fine-needle aspiration
FNAB Fine-needle aspiration biopsy
FPR False-positive rate
FRC Functional residual capacity
FSH Follicle-stimulating hormone
FT$_3$ Free triiodothyronine
FT$_3$I Free triiodothyronine index
FT$_4$ Free thyroxine
FT$_4$I Free thyroxine index
FVC Forced vital capacity
FVL Factor V Leiden
G6PD Glucose-6-phosphate dehydrogenase
GAG Glycosaminoglycan
GBS Group B *Streptococcus*
G-CSF Granulocyte-colony stimulating factor
g/dL Grams per deciliter
GDM Gestational diabetes mellitus
GDNF Glial cell–derived neurotropic factor
GE Gastroesophageal
GERD Gastroesophageal reflux disease
GFR Glomerular filtration rate
GGTP Gamma glutamyl transpeptidase
GH Gestational hypertension; growth hormone
GLOWM Global Library of Women's Medicine
GLUT1 Glucose transporter 1
GMP Guanosine monophosphate
GNI Gross national income
GP Glycoprotein
GTD Gestational trophoblastic disease

GTT Glucose tolerance test
GU Genitourinary
GVHD Graft-versus-host disease
GWG Gestational weight gain
Gy Gray
H, HA Hemagglutinin
HAART Highly active antiretroviral therapy
HAV Hepatitis A virus
HbA1c Hemoglobin A1c
HBcAg Hepatitis B core antigen
HBIG Hepatitis B immune globulin
HBsAg Hepatitis B surface antigen
HBV Hepatitis B virus
HC Head circumference
HCA Hospital Corporation of America
HCC Hepatocellular cancer
hCG Human chorionic gonadotropin
HCQ Hydroxychloroquine
HCV Hepatitis C virus
HDAC Histone deacetylase
HDAg Hepatitis delta antigen
HDFN Hemolytic disease of the fetus and newborn
HDL High-density lipoprotein
HDN Hemolytic disease of the newborn
HDP Hypertensive disorder of pregnancy
HDV Hepatitis delta virus
HELLP Hemolysis, elevated liver enzymes, low platelet count
HG Hyperemesis gravidarum
HIDA Hepatic iminodiacetic acid scan
HIE Hypoxic-ischemic encephalopathy
HIF Hypoxia inducible factor
HIT Heparin-induced thrombocytopenia
HIV Human immunodeficiency virus
HL Hodgkin lymphoma; humerus length
HLA Human leukocyte antigen
HLA-C Major histocompatibility complex, class I, C antigen
HMD Hyaline membrane disease
HPA Hypothalamic pituitary adrenal
hPL Human placental lactogen
HPV Human papillomavirus
HR Heart rate
HRSA Health Resources and Services Administration
HUS Hemolytic uremic syndrome
Hz Hertz (1 cycle per second)
IA Intermittent auscultation
IAI Intraamniotic infection
IBD Inflammatory bowel disease
IBS Irritable bowel syndrome
ICD Implantable cardioverter-defibrillator
ICH Intracranial hypertension; intracranial hemorrhage
ICP Intrahepatic cholestasis of pregnancy
ICPD International Conference on Population and Development
ICSI Intracytoplasmic sperm injection
ICU Intensive care unit
I-D Induction-to-delivery interval
IDDM Insulin-dependent diabetes mellitus
IDM Infant of a diabetic mother
IDO Indoleamine 2,3 dioxygenase
IFN Interferon
IFN-γ Interferon gamma
IFN–γ-1b Interferon gamma-1b
IFPS Infant Feeding Practices Study

Ig Immunoglobulin
IgA Immunoglobulin A
IGF Insulin-like growth factor
IGF-1 Insulin-like growth factor 1
IGFBP-1 Insulin-like growth factor binding protein 1
IgG Immunoglobulin G
IGRA Interferon-γ release assay
IL Interleukin
IL-1 Interleukin-1
IL-6 Interleukin-6
IM Intramuscular
INH Isoniazid
INHA Inhibin A
iNOS Inducible form of nitric oxide synthase
INR International normalized ratio
INSTI Integrase strand transfer inhibitor
IOM Institute of Medicine
IPT Intraperitoneal transfusion
IPV Internal podalic version
IQ Intelligence quotient
IQR Interquartile range
IRIS Immune reconstitution inflammatory syndrome
ISI Insulin sensitivity index
ITP Idiopathic thrombocytopenic purpura; immune thrombocytopenic purpura
IU International unit
IUD Intrauterine device
IUFD Intrauterine fetal death/demise
IUGR Intrauterine growth restriction
IUPC Intrauterine pressure catheter
IUT Intrauterine transfusion
IV Intravenous
IVC Inferior vena cava
IVF In vitro fertilization
IVH Intraventricular hemorrhage
IVIG Intravenous immunoglobulin
IVP Intravenous pyelogram
IVS Intervillous space
IVT Intravascular transfusion
KB Kleihauer-Betke test
kDa Kilodalton
kHz Kilohertz (1000 cycles per second)
KIR Killer cell immunoglobulin-like receptor
KMC Kangaroo maternal care
KOH Potassium chloride
LABA Long-acting β-agonist
LAC Lupus anticoagulant
LAM Lactational amenorrhea method
LARC Long-acting reversible contraception
LBC Lamellar body count
LBP Lipopolysaccharide binding protein
LBW Low birthweight
LCHAD Long-chain 3-hydroxyacyl coenzyme A dehydrogenase
LCPUFA Long-chain polyunsaturated fatty acid
LDA Low-dose aspirin
LDH Lactate dehydrogenase
LDL Low-density lipoprotein
LEEP Loop electrosurgical excision procedure
LES Lower esophageal sphincter
LGA Large for gestational age
LH Luteinizing hormone
LIC Low-income country

LLETZ Large loop excision of the transformation zone
LM *Listeria monocytogenes*
LMA Laryngeal mask airway
LMNG Liverpool and Manchester Neurodevelopmental Group
LMP Last menstrual period
LMWH Low-molecular-weight heparin
LN Lupus nephritis
LNG Levonorgestrel
LOA Left occiput anterior
LOP Left occiput posterior
LPD Luteal phase defect
LPS Lipopolysaccharide
LRD Limb reduction defect
L/S ratio Lecithin/sphingomyelin ratio
LTBI Latent tuberculosis infection
LTG Lamotrigine
L-thyroxine Levothyroxine
LTR Long terminal repeat
LTRA Leukotriene receptor agonist
LUS Lower uterine segment
LVOT Left ventricular outflow tract
LVP Largest vertical pocket
μg Microgram
MA Microarray
MAC Membrane attack complex; *Mycobacterium avium* complex
MAP Mean arterial pressure
MAS Meconium aspiration syndrome
mBPP Modified biophysical profile
Mc Microchimerism
MC Monochorionic
MCA Middle cerebral artery
MCH Maternal, infant, and child health
MCP-1 Monocyte chemotactic protein 1 (CCL2)
MCV Mean corpuscular volume
MDE Major depressive episode
MDG Millennium development goal
MDI Metered-dose inhaler
MDQ Mood disorders questionnaire
MF Maternal-fetal
MFMU Maternal-Fetal Medicine Units
MHA-TP Microhemagglutination *Treponema pallidum*
MHC Major histocompatibility complex
MHz Megahertz (1 million cycles per second)
MI Mechanical index; myocardial infarction
MIC Middle-income country
MLCK Myosin light-chain kinase
MM Malignant melanoma
MMF Mycophenolate mofetil
mm Hg Millimeters of mercury
MMI Methimazole
MMP Matrix metalloproteinase
MMP-1 Interstitial collagenase
MMP-8 Neutrophil collagenase
MMP-9 Gelatinase B
MMR Maternal mortality ratio; measles, mumps, rubella
MMWR *Morbidity and Mortality Weekly Report*
MODY Maturity-onset diabetes of youth
MoM Multiples of the median
MOMP Major outer membrane protein
MPR Multifetal pregnancy reduction

MPSS Massively parallel DNA shotgun sequencing
MRA Magnetic resonance angiography
MRCP Magnetic resonance cholangiopancreatography
MRI Magnetic resonance imaging
mRNA Messenger RNA
MRSA Methicillin-resistant *Staphylococcus aureus*
MRV Magnetic resonance venogram
MS Multiple sclerosis
MSAFP Maternal serum alpha-fetoprotein
MTCT Mother-to-child transmission
MTX Methotrexate
mV millivolts
MVC Motor vehicle crash
MVP Maximum vertical pocket
MVU Montevideo unit
MZ Monozygotic
N, NA Neuraminidase
NAAPR North American AED Pregnancy Registry
NAAT Nucleic acid amplification test
NAEPP National Asthma Education and Prevention Program
NAFLD Nonalcoholic fatty liver disease
NAFTNet North American Fetal Therapy Network
NAS Neonatal abstinence syndrome
NASBA Nucleic acid sequence-based amplification
NAT Nucleic acid test
NB Nasal bone
NCHS National Center for Health Statistics
NCPP National Collaborative Perinatal Project
ncRNA Noncoding RNA
NDD Neurodevelopmental disorder
NEAD Neurodevelopmental effect of an antiepileptic drug
NEC Necrotizing enterocolitis
NGO Nongovernmental organization
NHANES National Health and Nutrition Examination Survey
NHL Non-Hodgkin lymphoma
NICHD National Institute for Child Health and Human Development
NICU Neonatal intensive care unit
NIH National Institutes of Health
NIPT Noninvasive prenatal testing
NK Natural killer
NLE Neonatal lupus erythematosus
NLR Nod-like receptor
NMDA N-methyl-D-aspartate
NNRTI Nonnucleoside reverse transcriptase inhibitor
NNT Number needed to treat
NO Nitric oxide
NPWT Negative pressure wound therapy
NPY Neuropeptide Y
NRBC Nucleated red blood cell
NRP Neonatal resuscitation program
NRT Nicotine replacement therapy
NRTI Nucleotide/nucleoside reverse transcriptase inhibitor
NS Normal saline
NSAID Nonsteroidal antiinflammatory drug

NSPHPT Neonatal severe primary hyperparathyroidism
NSR Normal sinus rhythm
NST Nonstress test
NT Nuchal translucency
NTD Neural tube defect
NTP Nortriptyline
NTSV Nulliparous term singleton vertex
NVP Nausea and vomiting of pregnancy; nevirapine
NYHA New York Heart Association
O_2 Oxygen
OA Occiput anterior
OAE Otoacoustic emission
OAT Opioid agonist therapy
OC Oral contraceptive
OFD Occipitofrontal diameter
OI Opportunistic infections
OP Occiput posterior
OR Odds ratio
OT Occiput transverse
P450arom P450 cytochrome aromatase
P450scc Cytochrome P450scc
PA Placenta accreta
PABA Para-aminobenzoic acid
PACU Postanesthesia care unit
PAI Plasminogen activator inhibitor
PAI-1 Type 1 plasminogen activator inhibitor
PAMG-1 Placental α-microglobin 1
PAMP Pathogen-associated molecular pattern
Pap smear Papanicolaou smear
PAPP-A Pregnancy-associated plasma protein A
PAWP Pulmonary artery wedge pressure
PAX2 Paired box gene 2
P/C Protein/creatinine (ratio)
PCA Patient-controlled analgesia
PCB Polychlorinated biphenyl
PCEA Patient-controlled epidural analgesia
PCOS Polycystic ovary syndrome
PCR Polymerase chain reaction
PCWP Pulmonary capillary wedge pressure
PD Potential difference
PD-1 Programmed death 1 receptor
PDA Patent ductus arteriosus
PDPH Postdural puncture headache
PDX1 Pancreatic duodenal homeobox 1
PE Preeclampsia; pulmonary embolus
PEEP Positive end-expiratory pressure
PEF Peak expiratory flow
PEFR Peak expiratory flow rate
PEP Polymorphic eruption of pregnancy
PFMT Pelvic floor muscle training
PFP Pruritic folliculitis of pregnancy
PG Pemphigoid gestationis; phosphatidylglycerol
PGC-1α Peroxisome proliferator-activated receptor gamma coactivator
PGD Preimplantation genetic diagnosis
PGE$_1$ Prostaglandin E1 (misoprostol)
PGE$_2$ Prostaglandin E2 (dinoprostone)
PGH Placental growth hormone
PGI$_2$ Prostaglandin I$_2$
PGS Personal genome service; preimplantation genetic screening
PHPT Primary hyperparathyroidism
PICC Peripherally inserted central catheter
PID Pelvic inflammatory disease

PI Protease inhibitor
PJP *Pneumocystis jiroveci* pneumonia
PK Pharmacokinetic
PLGF Placental-like growth factor
PLO Pregnancy and lactation–associated osteoporosis
PMR Perinatal mortality rate
PO Per os (by mouth)
POP Progestin-only oral contraception
PP Prurigo of pregnancy
PPAR Peroxisome proliferator-activated receptor
PPCM Peripartum cardiomyopathy
PPD Postpartum depression; purified protein derivative
PPH Postpartum hemorrhage
PPHN Persistent pulmonary hypertension of the newborn
PPROM Preterm premature rupture of the membranes
PPT Postpartum thyroiditis
PPV Positive predictive value
PR Progesterone receptor
pRBCs Packed red blood cells
PrEP Preexposure prophylaxis
PRES Posterior reversible encephalopathy syndrome
PRIMS Pregnancy and multiple sclerosis
PRL Prolactin
PROM Premature rupture of the membranes
PRR Pattern-recognition receptor
PSV Peak systolic velocity
PTB Preterm birth
PTH Parathyroid hormone
PTHrP Parathyroid hormone–related protein
PTNA Percutaneous needle aspiration
pTREG Peripheral T-regulatory cells
PTSD Posttraumatic stress disorder
PTU Propylthiouracil
PUBS Percutaneous umbilical blood sampling
PUD Peptic ulcer disease
PUFA Polyunsaturated fatty acid
PUVA Psoralen with ultraviolet light A
PVC Premature ventricular contraction
PVH/IVH Periventricular/intraventricular hemorrhage
PVL Periventricular leukomalacia
PVNH Periventricular modular heterotopia
PVR Pulmonary vascular resistance
Qp Pulmonary flow
QPCR Qualitative polymerase chain reaction
Qs Systemic flow
RA Rheumatoid arthritis
RAAS Renin-angiotensin-aldosterone system
RAD Radiation absorbed dose
RANTES (CCL5) Regulated on activation, normal T-cell expressed and secreted
RB Reticulate body
RBC Red blood cell
RCOG Royal College of Obstetricians and Gynaecologists
RCT Randomized controlled trial
RCVS Reversible cerebral vasoconstriction syndrome
RDA Recommended daily allowance
RDS Respiratory distress syndrome
REDV Reversed end-diastolic velocity

REM Rapid eye movement; recurrent early miscarriage
REPL Recurrent early pregnancy loss
RF Rheumatoid factor
RFRA Religious Freedom Restoration Act
Rh(D) Rhesus (D antigen)
RhIG Rhesus immune globulin
RIBA Recombinant immunoblot assay
RIDT Rapid influenza diagnostic test
RIF Rifampin
RLS Restless legs syndrome
RM Recurrent miscarriage
RMR Resting metabolic rate
RNA Ribonucleic acid
ROA Right occiput anterior
ROC Receiver operator characteristic
ROP Retinopathy of prematurity
RPR Rapid plasma reagin
RR Relative risk
RT Reverse transcriptase
RT3U Resin triiodothyronine uptake
RUQ Right upper quadrant
RV Right ventricle
RXR Retinoid X receptor
SAGES Society of American Gastrointestinal and Endoscopic Surgeons
SAH Subarachnoid hemorrhage
SBAR Situation, background, assessment, recommendation
SBO Small bowel obstruction
SCH Subclinical hypothyroidism
SCN1A Sodium channel, voltage-gated, type 1 alpha subunit
SD Standard deviation
S/D Systolic/diastolic (ratio)
SEFW Sonographically estimated fetal weight
sFlt-1 Soluble fms-like tyrosine kinase 1
SGA Small for gestational age
SIDS Sudden infant death syndrome
sIgA Secretory immunoglobulin A
SIRS Systemic immune response syndrome
SIRT1 NAD-dependent deacetylase sirtuin 1
sIUGR Selective intrauterine growth restriction
SLE Systemic lupus erythematosus
SMA Spinal muscular atrophy
SMFM Society for Maternal-Fetal Medicine
SNP Single nucleotide polymorphism
SOAP Society of Obstetric Anesthesia and Perinatology
SP Surfactant protein
SPTA Spatial-peak temporal-average
sPTB Spontaneous preterm birth
SROM Spontaneous rupture of membranes
SS Sjögren syndrome
SSc Systemic sclerosis
SSC Skin-to-skin contact
SSI Surgical site infection
SSKI Saturated solution of potassium iodide
SNRI Serotonin-norepinephrine reuptake inhibitor
SSPE Subacute sclerosing panencephalitis
SSRI Selective serotonin reuptake inhibitor

ST Selective termination
STD Sexually transmitted disease
STI Sexually transmitted infection
SUD Substance use disorder
SUDEP Sudden unexpected death in epilepsy
SV Stroke volume
SVR Systemic vascular resistance
SYS Secondary yolk sac
T$_3$ Triiodothyronine
T$_4$ Thyroxine
T-ACE Tolerance-annoyance, cut down, eye opener
TA-CVS Transabdominal chorionic villus sampling
TAFI Thrombin-activatable fibrinolysis inhibitor
TAPS Twin anemia-polycythemia sequence
TAU Transabdominal ultrasound
TB Tuberculosis
TBA Traditional birth attendant
TBG Thyroxine-binding globulin
TBII Thyroid-binding inhibitor immunoglobulin
TBT Term Breech Trial
TC-CVS Transcervical chorionic villus sampling
TCD Transcerebellar diameter
TCR T-cell receptor
TEE Thermic effect of energy
TEF Thermic effect of food
TF Tissue factor
TFPI Tissue factor pathway inhibitor
TFT Thyroid function test
TGA Transposition of the great arteries
TgAb Antithyroglobulin antibodies
TGC Time gain compensation
TGF-β Transforming growth factor beta
Th Thymus helper
Th1 Helper T-cell type 1
Th2 Helper T-cell type 2
THBR Thyroid hormone–binding ratio
Th cell Helper T cell
TI Thermal index
TIMP Tissue inhibitor of matrix metalloproteinase
TIPS Transjugular intrahepatic portosystemic shunt
TLC Total lung capacity
TLR Toll-like receptor
TLU Translabial ultrasound
TNF-α Tumor necrosis factor alpha
TOLAC Trial of labor after cesarean delivery
TORCH Toxoplasmosis, other infections, rubella, cytomegalovirus, herpes
tPA Tissue plasminogen activator
TPE Total urinary protein excretion
TPN Total parenteral nutrition
TPO Thyroid peroxidase
TPOAb Thyroid peroxidase antibody
TPR Total peripheral resistance
TR-β Thyroid receptor beta
TRAb Thyroid-stimulating hormone receptor antibody

TRAb Thyroid-blocking antibody
TRAIL TNF-related apoptosis-inducing ligand/Apo-2L
TRAP Twin reversed arterial perfusion
TREG Regulatory T cells
TRH Thyroid-releasing hormone; thyrotropin-releasing hormone
TSH Thyroid-stimulating hormone
TSHRAb Thyroid-stimulating hormone receptor antibody
TSI Thyroid-stimulating immunoglobulin
TST Tuberculin skin testing
TT$_3$ Total triiodothyronine
TT$_4$ Total thyroxine
TTP Thrombotic thrombocytopenic purpura
tTREG Thymic T-regulatory cells
TTTS Twin-twin transfusion syndrome
TVCL Transvaginal cervical length
TVU Transvaginal ultrasound
TXA$_2$ Thromboxane A$_2$
UAE Urinary albumin excretion
UC Ulcerative colitis
U-D Uterine incision–delivery interval
UDPGT Uridine diphosphoglucuronosyl transferase
uE$_3$ Unconjugated estriol
UFH Unfractionated heparin
UK United Kingdom
ULvWF Unusually large multimers of von Willebrand factor
UN United Nations
UNICEF United Nations Children's Fund
uPA Urokinase-type plasminogen activator
UPD Uniparental disomy
USDA U.S. Department of Agriculture
USPSTF U.S. Preventive Services Task Force
UTI Urinary tract infection
UVB Ultraviolet light B
V/Q Ventilation-perfusion scan
VAS Vibroacoustic stimulation
VBAC Vaginal birth after cesarean delivery
VDRL Venereal disease research laboratories
VEGF Vascular endothelial growth factor
VKA Vitamin K antagonist
VLBW Very low birthweight
VLDL Very-low-density lipoprotein
VOUS Variants of unknown significance
VPA Valproic acid
VPTD Very preterm delivery
VSD Ventricular septal defect
VTE Venous thromboembolism
VUS Venous ultrasonography
vWD von Willebrand disease
vWF von Willebrand factor
VZIG Varicella zoster immune globulin
VZV Varicella zoster virus
WBC White blood cell
WGA Whole genomic amplification
WHO World Health Organization
ZDV Zidovudine
ZPI Protein Z–dependent protease inhibitor

Index

Page numbers followed by "*f*" indicate figures, "*t*" indicate tables, "*b*" indicate boxes, and "*e*" indicate online-only material.

Cesarean birth/delivery (*Continued*)
  incidence of, 426-427
  indications for, 427-429, 427*f*
  for intrauterine growth restriction,
    764-765
  of large for gestational age (LGA) infants,
    83
  malpresentation
    for abnormal lie, 370
    cesarean delivery, 383
    for compound presentations, 375-376
    deflection attitudes, 371, 371*f*
    shoulder dystocia, 388
    technique of, uterine incision and fetus
      delivery, 370
  maternal complications with trial of labor
    after cesarean birth, 277*t*
  maternal glycemia level and, 880*f*
  on maternal request, 427-429
  in multiple sclerosis, 1046
  pain after, causes of, 344-345
  perimortem, implications of, 574
  in placenta accreta, 457-459, 458*f*-459*f*
  in placenta previa, 403
  in preeclampsia, 686
  with premature rupture of the
    membranes, 650
  in preterm infant, 639
  prior
    multiple, as uterine rupture risk factor,
      416
    as placenta previa risk factor, 401-402
    as uterine rupture risk factor, 416*t*
  rates of, 289-290
  risk and maternal weight gain, 125*f*
  technique of, 429-436
    abdominal closure, 435-436
    abdominal entry, 431-432, 431*f*
    abdominal skin incision, 431-432,
      431*f*
    bladder flap, 432
    delivery, of fetus, 434
    evidence-based recommendations for,
      430*t*
    placental extraction, 434
    postpartum hemorrhage and,
      prevention of, 434
    precesarean antibiotics, 429-430
    precesarean thromboprophylaxis, 430
    prophylactic precesarean interventions,
      430-431
    site preparation, 431
    uterine incision, 432-434, 433*f*
    uterine repair, 434-435, 434*f*-435*f*
  uterine incision
    low transverse (Kerr), 370
    vertical, 370
  vaginal birth after, 444-455
    birthweight, 447
    cervical examinations in, 447
    incision types for, 447
    labor status in, 447
    multiple prior, 447
    planned repeat, risks associated with,
      452
    prior indication for, 447
    prior vaginal delivery, 447
    trends, 444-445, 445*f*

Cesarean birth/delivery (*Continued*)
  trial of labor after
    candidates for, 445
    cost-effectiveness of, 454
    counseling for, 452-454
    induction of labor in, 449-450
    interpregnancy interval in, 449
    labor augmentation, 450
    management of, 452, 453*f*
    maternal complications in, 451*t*
    maternal demographics, 446-447
    number of prior cesarean deliveries
      in, 449
    prior vaginal delivery in, 449
    rates for, 445-446, 446*f*, 446*t*
    risks associated with, 447-454
    success rates for, 447, 447*t*
    uterine closure technique in, 449
    uterine rupture in, 447-448,
      448*t*-450*t*
c-fos, 627
Chemical pneumonitis, 829
Chemicals, pregnancy loss from, 588
Chemokines, 70
  helper T-cells and, 73
  maternal tolerance of fetus through
    regulation of, 77
Chemotherapeutic agents, pregnancy loss
  from, 587
Chemotherapy
  agents, 1058-1059
    alkylating agents, 1059
    antimetabolites, 1058-1059
    antitumor antibiotics, 1059
    platinum agents, 1059
    targeted therapies, 1059
    vinca alkaloids, 1059
  for breast cancer, 1061
  for cervical cancer, 1067
  for colon cancer, 1024
  for colorectal cancer, 1069
  fetal effects of, 145
  for Hodgkin lymphoma, 1062
  for ovarian cancer, 1068
  pharmacology, 1058
  during pregnancy, 1058-1059
Cherney incision, for cesarean delivery, 432
Chest
  bell-shaped, 188.*e*1*f*
  circumference of, changes in, 46
  ultrasound screening for anomalies in,
    186-187
Child marriage, 1197
Chlamydia, 1089-1092
  diagnosis of, 1091
  epidemiology of, 1089-1090
  incidence of, 1089-1090
  pathogenesis of, 1090-1091, 1090*t*
  treatment of, 1091-1092
Chlamydia pneumoniae
  disease spectrum, 1090*t*
  pneumonia and, 830
Chlamydia psittaci, 1090*t*
Chlamydia trachomatis
  abortion and, 586
  acute urethritis, 1133
  premature rupture of the membranes and,
    648

Chlamydia trachomatis (*Continued*)
  recommended treatment regimens for,
    1092*b*
  screening for, 1091*t*
  Th1 and, 73
Chlorambucil, 1059
Chlordiazepoxide
  for alcohol withdrawal, 1167
  fetal effects of, 142
Chlorhexidine, for site preparation, of
  cesarean delivery, 431
Chloride sweat test, for cystic fibrosis, 207
Chloroprocaine
  for paracervical block, 358
  for pudendal nerve block, 358-359
Chloroquine, fetal effects of, 145
Chlorothiazide, in breast milk, 153
Chlorpheniramine
  for atopic dermatitis, 1078-1079
  fetal effects of, 146-147
Cholangiopancreatography, therapeutic
  endoscopic retrograde, 1001
Cholecystitis, 1003
Choledochal cysts, 1003-1004
Choledocholithiasis, 1001, 1003
Cholelithiasis, 1003
  in sickle cell disease, 957
Cholestasis, 53-54
  intrahepatic, of pregnancy, 1008, 1008*t*
  neonatal, 1000
Cholesterol
  increase in pregnancy, 56-57, 57*f*
  normal values in pregnancy, 1216*t*
  placental synthesis of, 20
Choline, supplementation guidelines for,
  131-132
Chorioadenoma destruens, 1072
Chorioamnionitis, 1135-1137
  acute, 77-78
  after premature rupture of the
    membranes, 649-652, 656
  bacterial infection, risk of, 487
  chronic, 77-78
  diagnosis, 1135, 1136*t*
  epidemiology of, 1135
  management of, 1135-1137, 1137*f*
  prolonged second stage of labor and,
    263
  as retained products of conception risk
    factor, 415
  treatment for, 430, 1136*t*
Choriocarcinoma, 1014, 1072-1073, 1072*t*
Chorion, 648
Chorion laeve, 3
Chorionic plate, placental, 3, 3*f*
Chorionic somatotropin, 21
Chorionic villi, 313-314
  surface area of, 314
Chorionic villus sampling (CVS), 211-212,
  211*f*
  for chromosomal abnormalities, 581
  prior to multifetal pregnancy reduction,
    712
  safety of, 211-212
  transabdominal (TA-CVS), 211, 211*f*
  transcervical (TC-CVS), 211, 211*f*
  in twin pregnancies, 212
  in women with bloodborne viruses, 212

Hepatitis C, chorionic villus sampling in women with, 212
Hepatitis coinfection, 1108-1109
Hepatitis E, 1004, 1004t
Hepatocellular carcinoma, 1005-1006
Hepatocellular tumors, 1069
Hepatocyte growth factor, 10-11, 29
Herbal supplements, during pregnancy, 133
Heritable disorders, carrier screening for, 206-208
Heroin, fetal effects of, 151
Herpes (pemphigoid) gestationis, 1081, 1083t
Herpes simplex hepatitis, 1007-1008, 1008t
Herpes simplex virus (HSV), 1119-1120
  clinical manifestations of, 1119, 1119f, 1119t
  diagnosis of, 1119
  epidemiology of, 1119
  management during pregnancy, 1119-1120, 1120t
  neonatal, 1120
  with premature rupture of the membranes, 656
  primary and recurrent compared, 1119, 1119t
  virology of, 1119
Herpes zoster, 1120-1121
Herpesvirus, 1119-1120
Heterochromatic, 85
Heterozygous β-thalassemia, 960
HHS. See Health and Human Services (HHS)
Hidradenitis suppurativa, 1078
High-density lipoprotein (HDL), in diabetes mellitus, 870-871
Higher elevation, residence at, as placenta previa risk factor, 401
Hispanics
  calcium supplementation for, 131
  early-onset group B Streptococcus (GBS) infection, 1130-1131
  obesity in, 122
  preterm birth in, 618f, 621-622
Histology, placental, 9-12
Histone deacetylases (HDACs), 85
Histone modification, 85, 85f
Historic prospective studies, 139
History
  genetic, 194
  obstetric, integrating nutrition into, 122-123
HLA-DRB1 gene, 991
Hodgkin lymphoma, 1062-1063, 1062t, 1063f
Hoffman exercises, 534
Holoprosencephaly
  in diabetes mellitus, 872
  ultrasound screening for, 185, 186.e4f-186.e5f
Homans sign, 966
Homocysteine, 1217t
  in megaloblastic anemia, 956, 956f
Homosexuality, 95-96
Homozygous β-thalassemia, 959-960
Hormonal contraception, of pregnancy prevention, 510-511

Hormones
  fetal
    in cardiovascular system regulation, 32-33
    in growth and metabolism, 28-29
  placental, 20
    estrogens in, 20
    human chorionic gonadotropin in, 20-21
    leptin in, 22
    placental growth hormone in, 22
    placental lactogen in, 21-22
    pregnancy-associated plasma protein A in, 22
    progesterone in, 20
Horner syndrome, 479
Hospital Corporation of America (HCA), 1178
Hospitalization, in multiple gestation pregnancy, 725
Hospitals, maternal transfer to, 630
HOXA10 gene, 84
hPL (human placental lactogen), 21
HPV (human papillomavirus), 1125
H2-receptor blockers, in breast milk, 155
HSV. See Herpes simplex virus (HSV)
Human chorionic gonadotropin (hCG), 20-21, 916
  antiphospholipid syndrome and, 989
  assembly of, 21
  Down syndrome and, 21, 200
  gap junctions, in formation of, 11
  genes for, 20-21
  in hydatidiform mole, 1071f
  isoforms of, 21
  maternal, 54
    thyroid-stimulating hormone (TSH), effect on, 55
  maternal, timing of peak levels in, 21
  physiologic role of, 21
Human embryonic stem cell research funding, 1188-1189
Human endogenous retroviral envelope proteins HERV-W, 11
Human immunodeficiency virus (HIV), 1101-1113
  AIDS-defining conditions in adults, 1103b
  assessment of HIV disease status, 1104b
  as breastfeeding contraindication, 542
  as cause of death, 1199
  chorionic villus sampling in women with, 212
  clinical manifestations and staging of, 1102-1103, 1103t
  counseling and coordination of care and, 1112-1113
  diagnosis of, 1101-1102, 1103f
  discordant couples, 1112
  epidemiology of, 1101
  evolution of, 1103-1104
  genes of, 1101
  infant screening and diagnosis of, 1111
  intrapartum management of, 1110-1111
  management, intrapartum, 1110-1111
    cesarean delivery, elective, 1110-1111
    spontaneous rupture of membranes (SROM), 1111

Human immunodeficiency virus (HIV) (Continued)
    testing, 1111
    untreated women, 1111
  management, ongoing, 1112
  management during pregnancy and, 1104-1110
    ethical considerations and, 1104
    initial evaluation, 1104
    treatment of, 1105t
  National Perinatal HIV Hotline, 1112
  pneumonia and, 829
  postpartum care of women with, 1111
  preconception counseling for women with, 1112
  resource-poor countries and, 1206
  screening for, 112
  treatment
    combination care, 1104-1105
    factors that influence transmission, 1109-1110, 1109b
    invasive prenatal testing, 1110
    non-nucleoside reverse transcriptase inhibitors (NNRTIs), 1104-1105
    of ongoing management of, 1109
    of opportunistic infection prophylaxis, 1109
    protease inhibitors, 1104-1105
  virology, 1101
Human leukocyte antigen (HLA)
  compatible embryos, 214
  cord blood transplantation and, 74
  major histocompatibility complex (MHC) and, 71
  maternal-fetal, disparity in, 79
  maternal tolerance of fetus through, 77
  paternal antigens of fetus and, 78
  T cells and, 72
Human leukocyte C-antigen (HLA-C), extravillous trophoblast cell expression of, 6
Human papillomavirus (HPV), 1125
Human placental lactogen (hPL), 21
Humate-P, for von Willebrand disease, 961-962
Humerus length, normal values in pregnancy, 1220t
Humoral immune responses, 71
Huntington procedure, for uterine inversion, 417-418
HUS. See Hemolytic uremic syndrome (HUS)
Hyaline membrane disease (HMD)
  in diabetes mellitus, 874
  respiratory distress, neonatal, 488
Hyalinization, 500
Hydantoin
  fetal effects of, 140, 140f-141f
  teratogenicity of, 137-138
Hydatidiform mole
  complete mole, 1070-1072
  partial, 1072, 1072f
Hyde amendment, 1187
Hydralazine
  for cardiomyopathy, 820
  fetal effects of, 144
  for hemodynamic management, 825
  for hypertension-eclampsia, 694
  for hypertension-preeclampsia, 684, 686